STERNBERG'S
Diagnostic Surgical Pathology
Fifth Edition

STERNBERG'S
Diagnostic Surgical Pathology

Fifth Edition
Volume 1

Editor
STACEY E. MILLS, M.D.
W. S. Royster Professor of Pathology
Director of Surgical Pathology and Cytopathology
University of Virginia Health System
Charlottesville, Virginia

Associate Editors
DARRYL CARTER, M.D.
Professor Emeritus of Pathology
Yale University School of Medicine
New Haven, Connecticut

JOEL K. GREENSON, M.D.
Professor of Pathology
The University of Michigan Health System
Ann Arbor, Michigan

VICTOR E. REUTER, M.D.
Attending Pathologist, Memorial Hospital;
Professor of Pathology, Weill Medical
College of Cornell University
Memorial Sloan-Kettering Cancer Center
New York, New York

MARK H. STOLER, M.D.
Professor of Pathology & Gynecology
Associate Director of Surgical Pathology and Cytopathology
University of Virginia Health System
Charlottesville, Virginia

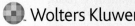 Wolters Kluwer | Lippincott Williams & Wilkins
Health

Philadelphia • Baltimore • New York • London
Buenos Aires • Hong Kong • Sydney • Tokyo

Acquisitions Editor: Jonathan Pine
Managing Editor: Joyce Murphy
Senior Marketing Manager: Angela Panetta
Production Editor: John Larkin
Design Coordinatorr: Stephen Druding
Compositor: ASI/Maryland Composition Co.

Fifth Edition

Fourth Edition by Mills et al: 2004
First, Second, and Third Edition by Sternberg et al: 2000, 1994, 1989

Library of Congress Cataloging-in-Publication Data

Sternberg's diagnostic surgical pathology. — 5th ed. / senior editor, Stacey E. Mills ; editors
Darryl Carter ... [et al.].
    p. ; cm.
  Includes bibliographical references and index.
  ISBN 978-0-7817-7942-5 (alk. paper)
 1. Pathology, Surgical. I. Sternberg, Stephen S. II. Mills, Stacey E. III. Carter, Darryl. IV.
Title: Diagnostic surgical pathology.
  [DNLM: 1. Pathology, Surgical. 2. Diagnostic Techniques and Procedures. WO 142 S839
2010]
  RD57.D53 2010
  617'.075—dc22

                                            2009011562

DISCLAIMER

Care has been taken to confirm the accuracy of the information present and to describe
generally accepted practices. However, the authors, editors, and publisher are not responsible
for errors or omissions or for any consequences from application of the information in this
book and make no warranty, expressed or implied, with respect to the currency, completeness, or accuracy of the contents of the publication. Application of this information in a
particular situation remains the professional responsibility of the practitioner; the clinical
treatments described and recommended may not be considered absolute and universal recommendations.

The authors, editors, and publisher have exerted every effort to ensure that drug selection
and dosage set forth in this text are in accordance with the current recommendations and
practice at the time of publication. However, in view of ongoing research, changes in government regulations, and the constant flow of information relating to drug therapy and drug
reactions, the reader is urged to check the package insert for each drug for any change in
indications and dosage and for added warnings and precautions. This is particularly important when the recommended agent is a new or infrequently employed drug.

Some drugs and medical devices presented in this publication have Food and Drug Administration (FDA) clearance for limited use in restricted research settings. It is the responsibility
of the health care provider to ascertain the FDA status of each drug or device planned for
use in their clinical practice.

To purchase additional copies of this book, call our customer service department at **(800)
638-3030** or fax orders to **(301) 223-2320**. International customers should call **(301) 223-
2300**.

Visit Lippincott Williams & Wilkins on the Internet: **http://www.lww.com**. Lippincott Williams &
Wilkins customer service representatives are available from 8:30 am to 6:00 pm, EST.

Preface to the Fifth Edition

The fifth edition of Sternberg's Diagnostic Surgical Pathology marks two decades of effort by the authors and editors to bring thoughtful diagnostic assistance to surgical pathologists at all levels of training and experience. Our goal has always been to emphasize real life diagnostic problems and pitfalls rather than to simply present "thumbnail sketches" of disease entities. To paraphrase one of our colleagues, "When you already know the diagnosis, almost any pathology textbook will do, but when you really need diagnostic help, this is the textbook you want."

As with prior editions, the fifth brings considerable changes, both welcome and unwelcome, in editorship, authorship and, most importantly, content. Harold Oberman, one of the founding associate editors of this text, died shortly after the publication of the fourth edition. Hal was a superb pathologist and an exemplary human being. We all greatly miss his invariably upbeat and warm persona, as well as his sage advice. We have also lost Andrew Huvos who, along with several colleagues, authored the salivary gland chapter of this text from the beginning. Andy was a world class bone and ENT pathologist with a scholarly and gentlemanly approach to every task that he undertook. He is also greatly missed.

The five years since the publication of the fourth edition have seen major advances throughout surgical pathology. The authors and editors have worked hard to incorporate this new material which continues to fall broadly into the areas of new molecular and immunohistochemical markers for diagnosis and prognosis of neoplasia, improved classification systems for diagnosis and prognosis, the role of pathology in new diagnostic and therapeutic techniques, and the recognition of new entities or variants of entities. Where appropriate updated World Health Organization (WHO) terminology has been employed for tumor diagnosis. A few of the many specific changes include an update on the serrated adenoma and serrated carcinoma pathway; virtually new chapters on salivary gland, larynx, blood vessels, heart, non-melanocytic skin tumors, and placenta; complete updates of the lymph node and bone marrow chapters incorporating the new WHO terminology; and an expanded discussion of the molecular biology of thyroid neoplasia.

For the first time, all illustrations have been color balanced by a single individual to bring uniformity to the color illustrations in the text. Reference lists have been considerably updated and, where possible, older references have been eliminated to save space. The editors wish to especially thank the contributing authors, a veritable "who's who" in surgical pathology, for making the fifth edition of our text the best ever. In addition, we would like to thank Jonathan Pine, Anne Jacobs, Ariel Winter, Teresa Exley, and the staff of Lippincott Williams & Wilkins for their unfaltering, enthusiastic support of our text.

Stacey E. Mills,
Darryl Carter
Joel K. Greenson
Victor E. Reuter
Mark H. Stoler

Preface to the First Edition

We speak of the loneliness of the long-distance runner, but there may be no one lonelier than a surgical pathologist working solo. Those working in large hospitals have the luxury of being able to consult ad lib with one or more pathologists about a given case, and may even have an associate who is a specialist in the area of difficulty. Easy access to consultation is a prerequisite for accurate diagnosis, and, accordingly, for optimal patient care. It is especially critical in those instances when the busy pathologist has a low level of diagnostic doubt, but this is tempered by the need to sign out the case without consultation because of the press of time. Very difficult cases, those readily recognizable as problem cases, are in a sense less troublesome, as the need for a diagnostic consultation is self-evident. Therefore, knowing when and what one doesn't know is of singular importance.

A pathology reference library is the other information source for the working pathologist. Textbook consultation and human consultation go hand-in-hand. In this text we have attempted to emphasize differential diagnosis of the surgical specimen, and to keep to a minimum discussion of the natural history of disease, treatment and autopsy findings. Although no textbook can take the place of a face-to-face discussion of a diagnostic problem (especially over a multi-headed microscope) between two or more pathologists, we have asked our authors to provide the reader with their reasoning in approaching differential evaluation of a biopsy specimen, thereby giving the flavor of a personal consultation. Moreover, the authors for the various chapters have been chosen based not only upon their recognized knowledge of the specific area, but also upon their skill in written communication. Since surgical pathologic diagnosis is a visual exercise, the book is generously illustrated with color and black-and-white photographs. In addition, the chapter authors have been liberal in their use of references, thereby enhancing the value of their presentations for the reader who wishes additional information.

The Section Editors have worked closely with the chapter authors to ensure that the objectives of the text are met; namely, that it is a treatise on the diagnosis of conditions which confront the surgical pathologist. In summary, the goal of the Editors is that this book will be a working companion, and thereby be accorded a place adjacent to the microscope of the reader.

Stephen S. Sternberg
Donald A. Antonioli
Darryl Carter
Joseph C. Eggleston
Stacey E. Mills
Harold A. Oberman

Contributing Authors

N. Volkan Adsay, M.D.
Professor and Vice-Chair, Director of Anatomic Pathology and Laboratory Medicine, Emory University Hospital, Atlanta, Georgia

Geoffrey P. Altshuler, M.B., B.S.
Clinical Professor of Pathology and Pediatrics, Department of Pathology, Children's Hospital, Oklahoma City, Oklahoma

Henry D. Appelman, M.D.
M.R. Abell Professor of Surgical Pathology, University of Michigan, Ann Arbor, Michigan

Pedram Argani, M.D.
Professor of Pathology and Oncology, The Johns Hopkins University, The Johns Hopkins Hospital, Baltimore, Maryland

Kristen A. Atkins, M.D.
Associate Professor of Pathology, University of Virginia Health System, Charlottesville, Virginia

Gustavo Ayala, M.D.
R. Clarence and Irene H. Fulbright Chair in Pathology, Professor Department of Pathology and Scott Department of Urology Director HTAP , Dan L Duncan Cancer Center Baylor College of Medicine, Houston, Texas

Zubair W. Baloch, M.D.
Professor, Pathology and Laboratory Medicine, University of Pennsylvania School of Medicine, Philadelphia, Pennsylvania

Lucia L. Balos, M.D.
Associate Professor, Pathology and Anatomical Sciences, University at Buffalo, Buffalo, New York
Medical Director, Anatomic Pathology, Kaleida Health, Buffalo General Hospital, Buffalo, New York

Jose E. Barreto, M.D.
Professor of Pathology, Universidad Catolica and Instituto de Patologia e Investigacion, Villarrica, Paraguay

Hector Battifora, M.D.
Pathology Consultant, Arcadia, California

J. Bruce Beckwith, M.D.
Adjunct Professor, Pathology and Human Anatomy, Loma Linda University, Loma Linda, California

Daniel M. Berney, M.B., B.Chir., M.A., F.R.C.Path.
Honorary Reader, The Orchid Tissue Laboratory, Center for Molecular Oncology & Imaging, Queen Mary's School of Medicine and Dentistry, London, United Kingdom
Consultant Pathologist, Department of Cellular Pathology, Barts and The London NHS Trust, London, United Kingdom

Gerald J. Berry, M.D.
Professor of Pathology, Stanford University Medical Center, Stanford, California

John S.J. Brooks, M.D.
Professor and Vice Chair, Pathology and Laboratory Medicine, University of Pennsylvania Medical School, Philadelphia, Pennsylvania
Chair and Director of Ayer Laboratories, Pathology, Pennsylvania Hospital of UPHS, Phildelphia, Pennsylvania

Peter G. Bullough, M.D.
Professor of Pathology, Pathology and Laboratory Medicine, Weill-Cornell Medical College, Hospital for Special Surgery, New York, New York

Allen Burke, M.D.
Associate Professor, Pathology, University of Maryland, Baltimore, Maryland
Chairman, Cardiovascular Pathology, Armed Forces Institute of Pathology, Washington, District of Columbia

Jerome S. Burke, M.D.
Adjunct Clinical Professor, Department of Pathology, Stanford University Medical Center, Stanford, California
Senior Pathologist, Department of Pathology, Alta Bates Summit Medical Center, Berkeley, California

Darryl Carter, M.D.
Professor Emeritus, Pathology, Yale University, New Haven, Connecticut

Philip B. Clement, M.D.
Professor Emeritus, Department of Pathology, University of British Columbia, Vancouver, Canada
Consultant Pathologist, Department of Pathology, Vancouver General Hospital, Vancouver, British Columbia, Canada

Harry S. Cooper, M.D.
Senior Member and Vice Chairman, Pathology, Fox Chase Cancer Center, Philadelphia, Pennsylvania

John B. Cousar, M.D.
Professor of Pathology, Department of Pathology, University of Virginia Health System, Charlottesville, Virginia

Christopher P. Crum, M.D.
Professor, Pathology, Harvard Medical School, Boston, Massachusetts
Director, Women's and Perinatal Pathology, Brigham and Women's Hospital, Boston, Massachusetts

Antonio L. Cubilla, M.D.
Professor of Pathology, Universidad Nacional de Asuncion and Instituto de Patologia e Investigacion, Asuncion, Paraguay

Thomas J. Cummings, M.D.
Associate Professor, Department of Pathology, Duke University, Durham, North Carolina

Ronald A. DeLellis, M.D.
Professor and Associate Chair, Department of Pathology and Laboratory Medicine, The Warren Alpert School of Medicine of Brown University, Providence, Rhode Island
Chief, Department of Pathology, Rhode Island Hospital, Providence, Rhode Island

Jonathan I. Epstein, M.D.
The Reinhard Professor of Urologic Pathology, The Johns Hopkins Medical Institutions, Baltimore, Maryland
Director of Surgical Pathology, Department of Pathology, The Johns Hopkins Hospital, Baltimore, Maryland

Lori A. Erickson, M.D.
Associate Professor of Pathology, Laboratory Medicine and Pathology, Mayo Clinic, Rochester, Minnesota

Enid Gilbert-Barness, A.O., M.D., M.B.B.S., F.R.C.P.A., F.R.C.Path., D.Sci.(hc), M.D.(hc)
Professor, Departments of Pathology and Laboratory Medicine, Pediatrics, and Obstetrics and Gynecology, University of South Florida School of Medicine; Director of Pediatric Pathology, Department of Pathology and Laboratory Medicine, Tampa General Hospital, Tampa, Florida

John R. Goldblum, M.D.
Professor of Pathology, Cleveland Clinic Lerner College of Medicine, Anatomic Pathology, Cleveland Clinic, Cleveland, Ohio

Terry L. Gramlich, M.D.
Director of Hepatopathology, AmeriPath Institute of Gastrointestinal Pathology and Digestive Disease, Oakwood Village, Ohio

Joel K. Greenson, M.D.
Professor of Pathology, The University of Michigan Health System, Ann Arbor, Michigan

Elizabeth Harris, M.D.
Gastrointestinal/Liver Pathologist, Associated Pathologists, Brentwood, Tennessee

Clara S. Heffess, M.D.
Chief, Endocrine Division, Department of Endocrine and Otorhinolaryngic-Head and Neck Pathology, Armed Forces Institute of Pathology, Washington, District of Columbia

Reid R. Heffner, Jr., M.D.
Professor and Chair, Pathology and Anatomical Sciences, University at Buffalo School of Medicine and Biomedical Sciences, Buffalo, New York

Michael R. Hendrickson, M.D.
Professor, Pathology, Stanford University School of Medicine, Stanford, California
Professor, Pathology, Stanford Hospital and Clinics, Stanford, California

Michael J. Imber, M.D.
Pathology, Palm Beach Pathology, West Palm Beach, Florida

Carrie Y. Inwards, M.D.
Associate Professor of Pathology, Laboratory Medicine and Pathology, Mayo Clinic, Rochester, Minnesota

Cynthia G. Kaplan, A.B., M.D.
Professor of Pathology, Stony Brook University Medical Center, Stony Brook, New York

Richard L. Kempson, M.D.
Professor, Pathology, Stanford University School of Medicine, Stanford, California
Professor, Pathology, Stanford Hospital and Clinics, Stanford, California

Pawini Khanna, M.D.
Staff Pathologist, Department of Pathology, Bayfront Medical Center, St. Petersburg, Florida

Gordon K. Klintworth, M.D., Ph.D.
Professor of Pathology and Joseph A.C. Wadsworth, Professor of Ophthalmology, Durham, North Carolina

Steven H. Kroft, M.D.
Professor of Pathology, Director of Hematopathology, Medical College of Wisconsin, Milwaukee, Wisconsin

Robert J. Kurman, M.D.
Richard W. TeLinde Distinguished Professor, Departments of Gynecology-Obstetrics and Pathology, Director of Gynecologic Pathology, The Johns Hopkins School of Medicine, Baltimore, Maryland

Ernest E. Lack, M.D.
Director of Anatomic Pathology, Department of Pathology, Washington Hospital Center, Washington, District of Columbia

Howard S. Levin, M.D.
Consultant , Anatomic Pathology, Cleveland Clinic Foundation, Cleveland, Ohio

Virginia A. LiVolsi, M.D.
Professor, Pathology and Laboratory Medicine; Otorhinolaryngology, University of Pennsylvania School of Medicine, Philadelphia, Pennsylvania

Ricardo V. Lloyd, M.D., Ph.D.
Professor of Pathology, Laboratory Medicine and Pathology, Mayo Clinic, Rochester, Minnesota

Teri A. Longacre, M.D.
Professor, Pathology, Stanford University School of Medicine, Stanford, California
Professor, Pathology, Stanford Hospital and Clinics, Stanford, California

William R. Macon, M.D.
Professor of Laboratory Medicine and Pathology, Department of Laboratory Medicine and Pathology, Mayo Clinic, Rochester, Minnesota

Shamlal Mangray, M.B., B.S.
Assistant Professor, Department of Pathology and Laboratory Medicine, The Warren Alpert School of Medicine of Brown University, Providence, Rhode Island
Attending Pathologist, Department of Pathology, Rhode Island Hospital, Providence, Rhode Island

Charles C. Marboe, M.D.
Professor of Clinical Pathology and Vice Chair for Anatomic
Pathology, College of Physicians and Surgeons, Columbia
University, New York, New York

Michael T. Mazur, M.D.
Clinical Professor of Pathology, State University of New York,
Upstate Medical University and Clear Path Diagnostics, Syracuse,
New York

Thomas L. McCurley, M.D.
Associate Professor of Pathology, Director of Immunopathology,
Pathology, Vanderbilt University Medical Center, Nashville,
Tennessee

Paul E. McKeever, M.D., Ph.D.
Professor of Pathology, University of Michigan Medical Center,
Ann Arbor, Michigan

Robert W. McKenna
Professor of Laboratory Medicine and Pathology, University of
Minnesota, Minneapolis, Minnesota

Martin C. Mihm, Jr., M.D.
Professor of Pathology, Massachusetts General Hospital, Harvard
Medical School, Boston, Massachussetts

Rosemary R. Millis, M.D.
Honorary Consultant Pathologist, Hedley Atkins/Cancer Research,
UK Breast Pathology Laboratory, Guy's Hospital, London, United
Kingdom

Stacey E. Mills, M.D.
W. S. Royster Professor of Pathology, Director of Surgical Pathology
and Cytopathology, University of Virginia Health System,
Charlottesville, Virginia

Robert J. Morris, M.D.
Assistant Professor, Dermatology and Pathology, Emory University
School of Medicine, Atlanta, Georgia
Dermatopathologist, Emory University Hospital, Atlanta, Georgia

Tibor Nádasdy, M.D.
Professor, Department of Pathology, Ohio State University,
Columbus, Ohio

George J. Netto, M.D.
Associate Professor, Pathology, The Johns Hopkins Medical
Institutions, Baltimore, Maryland
Associate Professor, Department of Pathology, The Johns Hopkins
Hospital, Baltimore, Maryland

Masayuki Noguchi, M.D.
Professor of Pathology, Institute of Basic Medical Sciences,
University of Tsukuba, Tsukuba, Japan

Marisa R. Nucci, M.D.
Associate Professor, Pathology, Harvard Medical School, Boston,
Massachusetts
Pathologist, Women's and Perinatal Pathology, Brigham and
Women's Hospital, Boston, Massachusetts

David A. Owen, M.B.
Professor of Pathology, University of British Columbia, Pathology
and Laboratory Medicine, Vancouver General Hospital, Vancouver,
British Columbia, Canada

Douglas C. Parker, M.D., D.D.S.
Assistant Professor, Pathology and Dermatology, Emory University
School of Medicine, Atlanta, Georgia
Dermatopathologist, Pathology and Dermatology, Emory University
Hospital, Atlanta, Georgia

Arthur S. Patchefsky, M.D.
Senior Member and Chairman, Pathology, Fox Chase Cancer
Center, Philadelphia, Pennsylvania

James W. Patterson, M.D.
Professor of Pathology and Dermatology, University of Virginia
Health System, Charlottesville, Virginia

Robert E. Petras, M.D.
Associate Clinical Professor of Pathology, Northeastern Ohio
Universities College of Medicine, Rootstown, Ohio
National Director for Gastrointestinal Pathology Services,
AmeriPath Inc., Oakwood Village, Ohio,

Adriano Piris, M.D.
Instructor of Pathology, Massachusetts General Hospital, Harvard
Medical School, Boston, Massachussetts

Nicolas Prieto-Granada, M.D.
Research Fellow, Pathology, Tufts Medical Center, Cambridge,
Massachusetts

Victor E. Reuter, M.D.
Attending Pathologist, Memorial Hospital;
Professor of Pathology, Weill Medical College of Cornell University,
Memorial Sloan-Kettering Cancer Center, New York, New York

Anjali A. Satoskar, M.D.
Assistant Professor, Pathology, Ohio State University, Columbus,
Ohio

Bernd W. Scheithauer, M.D.
Professor of Pathology, Anatomic Pathology, Mayo Clinic,
Rochester, Minnesota

Stuart J. Schnitt, M.D.
Professor of Pathology, Harvard Medical School, Boston,
Massachusets
Director, Division of Anatomic Pathology, Beth Israel Deaconess
Medical Center, Boston, Massachusets

Lynn R. Schoenfield, M.D.
Assistant Professor of Pathology, Cleveland Clinic Lerner College of
Medicine of Case Western Reserve University, Pathology and
Laboratory Medicine Institute, Cleveland Clinic Foundation,
Cleveland, Ohio

Ie-Ming Shih, M.D., Ph.D.
Professor of Pathology, The Johns Hopkins University School of
Medicine, Baltimore, Maryland

Yukio Shimosato, M.D.
Department of Pathology, Keio University School of Medicine,
Tokyo, Japan

Fred G. Silva
Executive Vice President, Secretary and Treasurer, United States
and Canadian Academy of Pathology, Augusta, Georgia

Dale C. Snover, M.D.
Clinical Professor, Laboratory Medicine and Pathology, University of Minnesota Medical School and Fairview Southdale Hospital, Edina, Minnesota

Alvin R. Solomon, M.D.
Professor of Dermatology and Pathology, Oregon Health and Science University, Portland, Oregon

Edward B. Stelow, M.D.
Assistant Professor, Department of Pathology, University of Virginia Health Sciences, Charlottesville, Virginia

Mark H. Stoler, M.D.
Professor of Pathology and Gynecology, Associate Director of Surgical Pathology and Cytopathology, University of Virginia Health System, Charlottesville, Virginia

Steven H. Swerdlow, M.D.
Professor of Pathology, Department of Pathology, Division of Hematopathology, University of Pittsburgh School of Medicine UPMC Presbyterian Hospital, Pittsburgh, Pennsylvania

Lester D.R. Thompson, M.D.
Consultant Pathologist, Department of Pathology, Woodland Hills Medical Center, Woodland Hills, California

Satish K. Tickoo, M.D.
Member, Memorial Hospital, Attending, Department of Pathology, Memorial Sloan-Kettering Cancer Center, New York, New York

Thomas M. Ulbright, M.D.
Lawrence M. Roth Professor of Pathology and Laboratory Medicine, Indiana University School of Medicine, Indianapolis, Indiana

K. Krishnan Unni, M.B., B.S.
Professor Emeritus of Pathology, Department of Laboratory Medicine and Pathology, Mayo Clinic, Rochester, Minnesota

Elsa F. Velazquez, M.D.
Assistant Professor of Pathology, Harvard Medical School, Brigham and Women's Hospital, Boston, Massachusetts

Renu Virmani, M.D.
President and Medical Director, CVPath Institute, Inc., Gaithersburg, Maryland

Kay Washington, M.D., Ph.D.
Professor of Pathology, Vanderbilt University Medical Center, Nashville, Tennessee

Bruce M. Wenig, M.D.
Professor of Pathology, The Albert Einstein College of Medicine, Department of Pathology and Laboratory Medicine, Beth Israel Medical Center, St. Luke's and Roosevelt Hospitals, New York, New York

Mark R. Wick, M.D.
Professor of Pathology, University of Virginia Health System, Charlottesville, Virginia

Jacqueline A. Wieneke, M.D.
Chief, Division of ENT Pathology Pathologist, Department of ENT-Endocrine Pathology, Armed Forces Institute of Pathology, Washington, District of Columbia

Lisa M. Yerian, M.D.
Assistant Professor of Anatomic Pathology, Cleveland Clinic Lerner College of Medicine, Cleveland Clinic, Cleveland, Ohio

Robert H. Young, M.D., F.R.C.Path.
Robert E. Scully Professor of Pathology, Department of Pathology, Harvard Medical School, Boston, Massachusetts
Pathologist, James Homer Wright Pathology Laboratories, Massachusetts General Hospital, Boston, Massachusetts

Richard J. Zarbo, M.D., D.M.D.
Senior Vice-President and Chair, Pathology and Laboratory Medicine, Henry Ford Hospital, Detroit, Michigan

Contents

Douglas C. Parker
Robert J. Morris
Alvin R. Solomon

CHAPTER

1

Nonneoplastic Diseases of the Skin

Nonneoplastic or inflammatory skin diseases encompass a wide array of pathologic processes ranging from autoimmune to infectious to diseases of unknown etiology. In contrast to neoplastic surgical pathology, the histopathology of inflammatory skin diseases frequently does not exhibit a one-to-one correlation with a single diagnosis and requires correlation with the clinical presentation for a definitive diagnosis. In many instances, the dermatologist is neither looking for nor needs a specific histologic diagnosis. For instance, if the clinical differential diagnosis is between atopic dermatitis and psoriasis, the diagnosis of spongiotic dermatitis conveys the essential information to the clinician. Although the diagnosis of many inflammatory skin diseases requires correlation with the clinical features, there are critical diagnoses, such as toxic epidermal necrolysis and staphylococcal scalded skin syndrome, that the surgical pathologist may be asked to differentiate.

The most accurate interpretation of the microscopic pathology of inflammatory skin disease is accomplished if the pathologist is cognizant of the clinical differential diagnosis as well as the histopathologic differential diagnosis. The pathologist must insist that an accurate clinical differential diagnosis or impression be submitted in addition to other data such as the age and sex of the patient and the anatomic site of the biopsy. Although dermatopathology specimens should be interpreted objectively, the final interpretation should always be correlated with the clinical findings.

In this chapter, we have divided nonneoplastic skin diseases into various groups based on histopathologic patterns of inflammation (Tables 1.1 and 1.2). This approach is popular because it furnishes a basis for structured learning of these diseases without a prior knowledge of clinical dermatology. Like all classifications, this approach is not perfect, and it falls short at times because of the incredible complexity of the pathologic processes. Few diseases fit exclusively into only one category. Perhaps the best way to use this morphologic approach is to use the metaphor of a framework and superimposed templates. Think of each pattern as the framework and the specific histologic features of each disease as a template. Mentally superimposing the template then results in a modification of the original pattern. For example, in the diagnosis of lichenoid drug reaction, the pattern of lichenoid interface dermatitis is the framework. Superimposing a template of parakeratosis, eosinophils, and plasma cells over the framework leads to the diagnosis of lichenoid drug eruption. Of course, one must learn to recognize the basic patterns for this system to work effectively.

One final important point concerning the histopathologic interpretation of inflammatory skin diseases is that the lesions are dynamic and change is an intrinsic quality. It must be remembered that a biopsy "captures" the histopathology of the lesion at one point in its evolution. Many inflammatory skin diseases may only be readily diagnosed microscopically at certain points within the spectrum of changes. If a lesion is biopsied early or late in its evolution, the microscopic findings may be nondiagnostic.

SPECIMEN PREPARATION

Careful gross processing of skin biopsies is critical for accurate microscopic interpretation. The shave, punch, and elliptical biopsy techniques are most frequently used to obtain skin specimens for microscopic examination.

The elliptical excision is preferred when the disease process involves the deep dermis or subcutis. Superficial fascia can only be obtained reliably with this technique. In our experience, the "bread-loaf" method (sequential serial sectioning) of cutting skin ellipses is best because it is simple, can be performed rapidly, and ensures adequate sampling of the tissue. The skin ellipse is cut perpendicular to the long axis of the specimen at approximately 3-mm intervals. If the cut surface is marked with ink and each tissue slice is embedded in a separate cassette, it is easy to decide which block to recut if additional sections are needed. Some dermatopathologists prefer to section skin ellipses longitudinally in nonneoplastic lesions. For the most part, the choice is a personal one.

The punch biopsy tool is best used to obtain a cylinder of skin that includes the epidermis, dermis, and a small amount of subcutis. Punch biopsies 4 mm in diameter or greater should be bisected before embedding. Smaller punch biopsy specimens are difficult to bisect and should be embedded intact.

The shave or tangential technique (blade parallel to the skin surface) is of limited value for the study of inflammatory skin diseases because only epidermis and superficial dermis are consistently sampled by this method. Shave biopsy specimens should be bisected or trisected if large enough so that a straight edge is available for microtome sectioning. Applying ink to the cut edge with an applicator stick enables the histotechnologist to identify the cut edge.

Ten percent buffered formalin is an excellent general-purpose fixative for skin specimens. Fixation in B5 solution results in the greater preservation of nuclear detail and is especially useful for evaluating lymphocytic infiltrates clinically suspicious for cutaneous lymphoma.

Hematoxylin and eosin (H&E) is the most commonly used

TABLE 1.1	Definitions of Dermatopathology Terms
Term	Definition
Acantholysis	Disruption of desmosomes that normally join the keratinocytes of the epidermis, resulting in loss of cohesion and rounding up of the affected cells.
Acanthosis	An increase in the thickness of the stratum malpighii.
Bulla	An intraepidermal or subepidermal cavity. Intraepidermal bullae may be secondary to either spongiosis or acantholysis. Subepidermal bullae are formed from extensive papillary dermal edema.
Colloid bodies	Oval to round apoptotic keratinocytes typically found immediately above or below the epidermal basement membrane. These are also referred to as *Civatte bodies.*
Dyskeratosis	Abnormal, premature keratinization of keratinocytes. Dyskeratotic keratinocytes have brightly eosinophilic cytoplasm.
Epidermolysis	A distinctive alteration of the granular layer characterized by perinuclear clear spaces, swollen and irregular keratohyalin granules, and an increase in the thickness of the granular layer. *Acantholysis* and *epidermolysis* are not synonyms; they are different pathologic processes.
Erosion	Partial-thickness loss of the epidermis.
Exocytosis	The presence of inflammatory cells within the epidermis in conjunction with spongiosis.
Hydropic degeneration	See "Vacuolar interface change."
Hyperkeratosis	An increase in the thickness of the stratum corneum. Hyperkeratosis may be either orthokeratotic or parakeratotic in nature. Orthokeratotic hyperkeratosis is an exaggeration of the normal pattern of keratinization (i.e., no nuclei are seen in the stratum corneum). In parakeratotic hyperkeratosis, nuclei are pathologically retained in the stratum corneum.
Leukocytoclasis	Karyorrhexis and destruction of neutrophils. It frequently occurs in the setting of neutrophilic vasculitis (i.e., leukocytoclastic vasculitis).
Lichenoid interface change	Destruction of the basal keratinocytes. Destruction and dyskeratosis result in "remodeling" of the basement membrane zone. A bandlike lymphocytic infiltrate usually accompanies the keratinocyte changes.
Liquefaction degeneration	See "Vacuolar interface change."
Orthokeratosis	See "Hyperkeratosis."
Papillomatosis	Abnormal elongation of the papillary dermis.
Parakeratosis	See "Hyperkeratosis."
Pseudoepitheliomatous hyperplasia	Acanthosis of the epidermis occurring in a pattern that mimics squamous cell carcinoma. *Epithelioma* is an archaic term for carcinoma.
Pustule	An intraepidermal or subepidermal vesicle or bulla filled with neutrophils.
Scale crust	A collection of parakeratotic debris, degenerated inflammatory cells, and tissue exudate on the surface of the epidermis.
Spongiosis	Intercellular intraepidermal edema.
Ulcer	Loss of the entire thickness of the epidermis. The dermis and subcutis may or may not be left intact, depending on the depth of the ulcer.
Vacuolar interface change	Destruction of the basal keratinocytes characterized by the presence of intracytoplasmic vesicles. The vesicles enlarge, and eventually, the basal keratinocytes die; as a result, the integrity of the basal zone of the epidermis is lost.
Vesicle	A small bulla.

TABLE 1.2		
A Few Important Clinical Terms		
Term	Definition	
Bulla	A large, fluid-filled vesicle; may be tense or flaccid.	
Crust	A scab.	
Lichenification	Thickened, rough skin with accentuated skin markings. *Lichenification*, thickening of the skin from chronic rubbing or scratching, is not synonymous with *lichenoid.*	
Macule	A flat change in skin color.	
Nodule	A large, deeply extending papule.	
Papule	A solid elevation of the skin surface.	
Patch	A large macule.	
Plaque	A large, flat-topped papule.	
Scale	Flakes of exfoliated epidermis.	
Vesicle	A small, fluid-filled blister.	

routine stain in dermatopathology, but most special stains used in general surgical pathology are also employed. Specific uses of histochemical stains and immunohistochemistry will be discussed along with the diseases in which their use is of value (1–4).

In dermatopathology, it is important to recreate a three-dimensional mental picture of the two-dimensional microscopic sections. In addition, many inflammatory skin diseases are particularly zonal in their microscopic architecture. Therefore, it is frequently helpful to make either step or serial sections from the paraffin block to maximize the yield of information obtainable from the microscopic sections.

Transverse sectioning of punch biopsies from the scalp is frequently used in the diagnosis of alopecia. A detailed discussion of this technique is beyond the scope of this chapter (5–8).

NORMAL HISTOLOGY

The skin comprises three structures: the epidermis, dermis, and subcutis. The superficial fascia marks the deep boundary between the skin and the underlying soft tissues. Regional anatomic variation of the skin is readily apparent if one compares a specimen from the scalp with one from the palm.

The epidermis is derived from ectoderm and composed of four layers or strata. The stratum corneum is the outermost layer of the epidermis. The fully keratinized cells of this layer are flattened and devoid of nuclei. On acral surfaces (palms and soles), a thin stratum lucidum (clear zone) is present between the stratum corneum and the stratum granulosum. The stratum granulosum is named for the prominent deeply basophilic keratohyalin granules found in flattened keratinocytes. Deep to the stratum granulosum is the stratum spinosum, which is characterized by abundant eosinophilic cytoplasm, ovoid nuclei, and intercellular bridges. The stratum basale (basal cell layer) is the undulating row of cuboidal to columnar cells with minimal cytoplasm and contains proliferating cells for epidermal renewal. The basal cells attach to the basement membrane of the epidermis. The stratum spinosum and the basal cell layer are collectively referred to as the *stratum malpighii.*

Although the majority of cells in the epidermis are keratinocytes, other cell types are present. Melanocytes are neural crest–derived dendritic clear cells situated in the basal zone. The primary function of melanocytes is the production of melanin. Langerhans cells are antigen-processing dendritic cells that are usually interspersed among the keratinocytes of the stratum spinosum but are virtually impossible to see in routine sections. Immunohistochemistry for S-100 protein is positive in both melanocytes and Langerhans cells, but Langerhans cells also express CD1a (9). Merkel cells are sparsely present neuroendocrine cells in the epidermis and function in mechanoreception. Merkel cells are not readily apparent in routine sections (10).

The basement membrane zone that separates the epidermis from the dermis appears to be a homogeneous eosinophilic band with light microscopy but displays a multilayered, complex arrangement at the ultrastructural level. The basement membrane zone is composed of four main layers: the basal cell hemidesmosome, the lamina lucida, the lamina densa, and the sublamina densa.

The most superficial level of the dermis is called the *papillary dermis* because it is located between the downward projections of the epidermis (rete ridges). The dermal papillae have a complex "hand-in-glove" relationship with the epidermal rete ridges. The deep border of the papillary dermis extends to the superficial vascular plexus and reticular dermis. Although it is a small part of the dermis quantitatively, the papillary dermis is important in many inflammatory skin diseases, and it functions as an anatomic buffer zone between the epidermis and reticular dermis.

In addition to its superficial location, the papillary dermis is characterized by a collagen pattern that is distinctively delicate and pale in H&E-stained sections. The adventitial dermis, the fine collagen fibers that invest adnexal structures, blood vessels, and nerves, is continuous with the papillary dermis.

The reticular dermis makes up the bulk of the dermis. Here, the collagen fibers are large, coarse, and brightly eosinophilic. Most of the adnexal structures are found within the reticular dermis. Progressively narrowing projections of the reticular dermis extend in a netlike manner into the subcutis to form the retinacular dermis.

The subcutis is the deepest layer of the skin. It is composed of collagenous septa and lobules of adipocytes. The fibrous septa connect the retinacular dermis with the superficial fascia to which the skin is anchored.

The cutaneous adnexa include hair follicles, sebaceous glands, eccrine glands, and apocrine glands. The hair follicle is a complex structure. The anagen, or growing, hair follicle can be divided into several parts. The deepest part, the hair bulb, is formed from both ectoderm (hair matrix) and mesoderm (dermal papilla). The isthmus extends from the superficial part of the hair bulb to the sebaceous duct. The infundibulum connects the isthmus and sebaceous duct to the epidermis. The intraepidermal portion of the hair follicle is called the *acrotrichium.* The sebaceous lobules empty into the follicle via the short sebaceous duct. An arrector pili muscle attaches to the isthmus below the entrance of the sebaceous duct at an area of the follicle termed the *bulge.*

The telogen, or resting, hair follicle lacks the well-defined components of the anagen, or growing, follicle. Instead, only a small ball of basaloid keratinocytes is located below the level of the sebaceous duct.

Sebaceous glands have a widespread distribution and are typically associated with hair follicles. In the eyelids, they are not associated with hair follicles and are known as the *meibomian glands* and *glands of Zeis.* Sebaceous glands secrete a lipid material known as *sebum.*

The eccrine glands are present at essentially all sites and are composed of a deep dermal or subcutaneous coil, mid dermal coiled and straight ducts, and an intraepidermal acrosyringium. Eccrine ducts are lined by cuboidal epithelial cells surrounded by myoepithelial cells. The eccrine glands' primary function is thermal regulation.

Apocrine glands are much more limited in distribution than eccrine glands and are primarily present in the axillary and anogenital regions. Modified apocrine glands are present in the external ear canal as ceruminous glands and in the eyelid as a gland of Moll. The apocrine epithelium consists of eosinophilic, cuboidal to columnar cells with decapitation secretion. Myoepithelial cells surround the outer portion of the apocrine glands and ducts. Their dermal duct usually ends in the follicular infundibulum, only rarely opening into the surface epidermis. The function of apocrine glands in humans is unknown.

The dermis is rich in blood vessels and lymphatics. The skin vasculature is supplied by perforating arteries of subcutaneous adipose tissue and skeletal muscle. The capillaries, arterioles, and venules of the superficial vascular plexus are located at the junction of the papillary and reticular dermis. Vessels extend from this plexus into the adventitial dermis of the adnexa and also penetrate through the reticular dermis to connect with the deep vascular plexus composed of larger vessels at the level of the deep reticular dermis. From the deep vascular plexus, vessels extend into the fibrous septa of the subcutis.

Aside from specialized end organs such as the Meissner and pacinian corpuscles, the nerves of the dermis are inconspicuous. They progressively decrease in caliber as they become more superficial. In the deep dermis, they usually course adjacent to blood vessels.

INFLAMMATORY SKIN DISEASE

PATTERNS OF EPIDERMAL INFLAMMATION

Spongiotic Dermatitis

Spongiotic dermatitis (11–14) encompasses a wide range of disease processes that is perhaps the most extensive in dermatopathology. Microscopic spongiotic dermatitis loosely correlates with clinical eczematous dermatitis, a spectrum of diseases with equally diverse causes and clinical presentations. The common denominator of spongiotic dermatitis is the presence of intraepidermal edema, which is referred to as *spongiosis* because the clear spaces separating the keratinocytes impart a spongy appearance to the epidermis. Spongiotic dermatitis is subclassified into acute, subacute, and chronic subtypes, depending on the presence or absence of several additional features that are discussed later. These terms relate loosely to the chronologic evolution of the spongiotic lesion. In summary, spongiotic dermatitis comprises a spectrum of histopathologic changes, with the acute and chronic subtypes at the polar ends and the subacute subtype occupying the broad middle.

Epidermal spongiosis, with or without lymphocyte exocytosis, is the main microscopic finding in acute spongiotic dermatitis. Perivascular lymphocytic infiltrates, which are usually localized to the upper dermis, accompany the epidermal spongiosis. In subacute spongiotic dermatitis, parakeratosis, acanthosis, and less commonly papillomatosis are present to varying degrees (Fig. 1.1). The spongiosis ranges from minimal to marked. Eosinophils may be admixed in the inflammatory cell infiltrate, and this finding may be helpful in suggesting an allergic etiology. In contrast to acute and subacute spongiotic dermatitis, chronic spongiotic dermatitis may show little, if any, spongiosis. Acanthosis, parakeratosis, and papillomatosis overshadow spongiosis at this stage in the evolution of the disease. Fibroplasia of the papillary and upper reticular dermis may be present, and the inflammatory cell infiltrates, primarily lymphocytes, range from extensive to scant.

The most important differential diagnosis in this category of diseases is between subacute spongiotic dermatitis and early, patch-stage lesions of the mycosis fungoides type of cutaneous T-cell lymphoma. Dermatologists tend to biopsy long-standing eczematous patches and plaques that do not resolve with topical corticosteroid therapy because the patch stage of cutaneous T-cell lymphoma can clinically mimic eczematous dermatitis. Significant numbers of atypical intraepidermal lymphocytes with convoluted ("cerebriform") nuclei, especially when these are grouped into "Pautrier microabscesses," suggest the diagnosis of mycosis fungoides.

The term *epidermotropism* is used to describe the presence of atypical lymphocytes within the epidermis in cutaneous T-cell lymphoma. Epidermotropism should not be confused with *exocytosis*, the term used to denote the presence of lymphocytes in the epidermis in spongiotic dermatitis. Exocytosis implies the absence of nuclear atypia, but determining whether intraepidermal lymphocytes are atypical can be difficult, especially since the lymphocytes of many spongiotic processes are "activated" and their nuclei are larger with more complex contours than those of small lymphocytes. Associated spongiosis is useful in differentiating between the two because spongiosis is almost always present to some extent in spongiotic dermatitis (exocytosis) but is usually more limited in cutaneous T-cell lymphoma (epidermotropism). A cautious approach to the interpretation of the cytologic features of intraepidermal lymphocytes is essential to avoid confusing spongiotic dermatitis with early, patch-stage lesions of mycosis fungoides. In cases of histopathologic uncertainty, conservative interpretation and clinical correlation are imperative. Additional specimens taken over a period of time may be required before arriving at an accurate diagnosis. Evaluation by molecular techniques for the presence of a T-cell receptor gene rearrangement is an important ancillary study, but correlation with the clinical features is essential.

ACUTE AND SUBACUTE SPONGIOTIC DERMATITIS

Allergic contact dermatitis

CLINICAL FEATURES. Allergic contact dermatitis develops when the skin comes into contact with a substance, such as nickel or the poison ivy plant, to which the patient has been previously sensitized. The dermatitis appears at the site of contact with the offending agent.

HISTOPATHOLOGY. Allergic contact dermatitis begins as acute spongiotic dermatitis, and it may evolve into subacute or chronic spongiotic dermatitis before resolving (11). Typically, the spongiosis is extensive. Spongiotic intraepidermal vesicles may form. Lymphocyte exocytosis is regularly present. Papillary dermal edema may also be present. The dermis typically displays superficial, perivascular, lymphocytic inflammatory infiltrates with varying numbers of admixed eosinophils. The presence of numerous eosinophils helps to differentiate allergic contact dermatitis from other types of spongiotic dermatitis.

Irritant contact dermatitis

CLINICAL FEATURES. Contact with an irritant substance may lead to irritant contact dermatitis (15). Irritants differ from allergens in that no prior sensitization is required for the dermatitis to develop. Soaps and detergents are common irritants.

HISTOPATHOLOGY. The histopathology (15) is similar to that of allergic contact dermatitis except that eosinophils are either not present or rare. Potent irritants may lead to superficial epidermal necrosis associated with intraepidermal neutrophils and a scale crust.

ENDOGENOUS ECZEMA GROUP (ATOPIC DERMATITIS, DYSHIDROSIS, NUMMULAR ECZEMA)

Seborrheic dermatitis

CLINICAL FEATURES. This group of eczematous disorders encompasses many varied clinical presentations ranging from silver dollar–sized patches (nummular eczema) to generalized exfoliative dermatitis (severe atopic dermatitis). These diseases

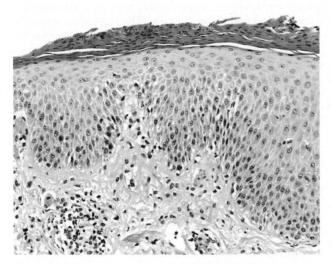

Figure 1.1. Subacute spongiotic dermatitis. Parakeratosis, acanthosis, intraepidermal intercellular edema (spongiosis), lymphocytic exocytosis, and a perivascular lymphocytic infiltrate with occasional eosinophils.

are "endogenous" in the sense that they are not secondary to any known exogenous agents. However, persons with atopic dermatitis are generally more susceptible to irritant contact dermatitis. Therefore, the histologic picture can be a combination of the two processes.

HISTOPATHOLOGY. Generally, these clinically diverse entities are inseparable microscopically, and they encompass the full range from acute to subacute to chronic spongiotic dermatitis. Large spongiotic vesicles may form on the palms or soles in dyshidrosis. A shift from subacute spongiotic dermatitis to a more acute picture may indicate the presence of an irritant dermatitis superimposed on a chronic atopic dermatitis.

PRURIGOFORM ACANTHOSIS (CHRONIC SPONGIOTIC DERMATITIS). Prurigoform acanthosis and chronic spongiotic dermatitis are a class of diseases characterized by irregular acanthosis. Although the two terms may be used as synonyms, *prurigoform acanthosis* implies a position at the extreme end of the spectrum of acanthosis in which epidermal hyperplasia is extensive. This pattern has been separated from acute and subacute spongiotic dermatitis solely for the purpose of pattern recognition. Prurigoform acanthosis and chronic spongiotic dermatitis are the result of sustained irritation of the skin, frequently by rubbing or scratching.

The differential diagnosis of chronic spongiotic dermatitis is similar to that of subacute spongiotic dermatitis, including the mycosis fungoides type of cutaneous T-cell lymphoma. The same histologic criteria used for differentiating acute and subacute spongiotic dermatitis from cutaneous T-cell lymphoma apply to chronic spongiotic dermatitis. Spongiosis is not as prominent, so eliminating cutaneous T-cell lymphoma from the differential diagnosis can be more difficult than in the obvious spongiotic processes. Keratinocytic neoplasms that can be confused with chronic spongiotic dermatitis include hypertrophic actinic keratosis and early squamous cell carcinoma. However, the presence of keratinocyte atypia is useful in differentiating the latter from chronic spongiotic dermatitis.

Lichen simplex chronicus (prurigo nodularis)

CLINICAL FEATURES. The plaques of lichen simplex chronicus (16–18) are scaly, thickened, moderately erythematous, and better demarcated than their more acute counterparts. The term *prurigo nodularis* implies a raised, pruritic nodule. Secondary changes such as excoriation, lichenification, and crusting are common.

HISTOPATHOLOGY. The key finding in this group (16–18) is markedly irregular psoriasiform acanthosis (Fig. 1.2). Both orthokeratosis and parakeratosis are common and sometimes massive. Spongiosis may be absent. When spongiosis is present, it is usually minimal, and it is localized to discrete foci. Fibrosis of the underlying dermis is variable, ranging from linear fibrosis of the papillary dermis to superficial dermal scars. Hyperplasia of small dermal nerve trunks has been observed within the dermal scars.

Pityriasis rosea

CLINICAL FEATURES. Patients presenting with numerous oval patches on the trunk with collarettes of scale in conjunction with a single, larger "herald patch" typify pityriasis rosea (19,20). A link to a viral etiology has been sought and debated in the literature. The clinical differential diagnosis frequently includes secondary syphilis.

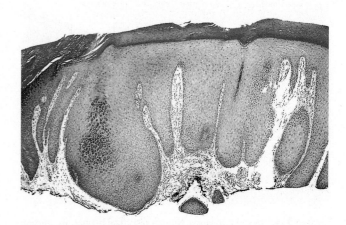

Figure 1.2. Lichen simplex chronicus. Orthokeratosis and hypergranulosis with marked irregular acanthosis with minimal spongiosis. The underlying dermis is fibrotic.

HISTOPATHOLOGY. The histopathology of pityriasis rosea (19,20) is essentially that of subacute spongiotic dermatitis. In most cases, differentiating pityriasis rosea from other forms of subacute spongiotic dermatitis accurately is difficult if not impossible. Papillary dermal microhemorrhage and the presence of discrete mounds of parakeratosis rather than of diffuse parakeratosis are of value in making the diagnosis (Fig. 1.3). The absence of plasma cells from the dermal infiltrate in conjunction with the described epidermal changes aids in separating pityriasis rosea from secondary syphilis, although plasma cells are not always present in the dermal infiltrate of secondary syphilis.

Dermatophytosis

CLINICAL FEATURES. Superficial fungi, or dermatophytes (21), may cause disease of the skin of the scalp (tinea capitis), face (tinea faciale), trunk (tinea corporis), palm (tinea manuum), groin (tinea cruris), or sole (tinea pedis). Scaly, red annular plaques characterize the classic ringworm of tinea corporis, but other presentations frequently pose a diagnostic challenge to

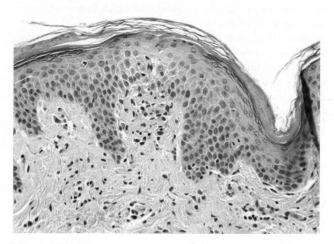

Figure 1.3. Pityriasis rosea. A mound of parakeratosis above minimal focal spongiosis and a perivascular lymphocytic infiltrate in the papillary dermis.

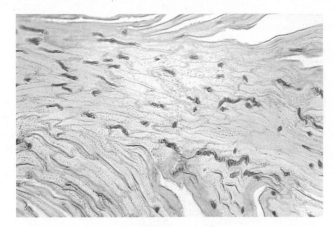

Figure 1.4. Dermatophytosis. Numerous fungal hyphae are present in the stratum corneum in a section stained with periodic acid-Schiff.

clinicians. Fungal infection of the nail (onychomycosis) can also be evaluated by the histologic examination of nail clippings.

HISTOPATHOLOGY. A good clue to the diagnosis of a dermatophyte infection (21) is the finding of neutrophils in the epidermis or stratum corneum in addition to the other changes of spongiotic dermatitis. Frank pustulation may occur. The hyphae are usually limited to the stratum corneum, and they are frequently seen either within or adjacent to a follicular orifice. Hyphae can be seen in sections stained with H&E, but they are much easier to see in sections stained with periodic acid-Schiff (PAS), in which they are diastase resistant (Fig. 1.4). The yeast forms, and the short, thick hyphae of *Pityrosporum* species, as well as the pseudohyphae and budding yeasts of *Candida* species, can be confused morphologically with the true hyphae of dermatophytes. In true dermatophyte fungal infections, slender, septate, or nonseptate hyphae predominate.

ADJUNCTS TO MICROSCOPIC DIAGNOSIS. Fungal cultures from stratum corneum scrapings provide the definitive identification, and these are recommended because they are easy to obtain. *Pityrosporum* yeasts will not grow on routine fungal culture. Dermatophytes can be distinguished from *Candida* species.

Lichen striatus

CLINICAL FEATURES. The linear, small, flesh-colored papules of lichen striatus (22,23) are most commonly found on the extremities of children.

HISTOPATHOLOGY. Despite the inclusion of *lichen* in the name, the major histologic features (22,23) are spongiosis and vacuolar interface change. The spongiotic changes are usually subacute (i.e., accompanied by acanthosis and parakeratosis). The dermal lymphocytic inflammatory infiltrate is present at the dermal-epidermal interface, around the superficial and the deep vascular plexus, and often around eccrine glands.

Stasis Dermatitis

CLINICAL FEATURES. Chronic venous stasis can lead to the development of the scaly erythematous plaques of stasis dermatitis (24) on the lower extremities. Secondary infection and ulcer formation are common.

HISTOPATHOLOGY. In stasis dermatitis (24), subacute spongiotic changes are present over a bandlike zone of dilated capillaries in the papillary dermis. Reticular dermal fibroplasia and

hemosiderin deposits are usually present in older lesions. Hyperplasia of endothelial cells in conjunction with hemosiderin deposition may resemble patch-stage or plaque-stage Kaposi sarcoma.

Psoriasiform Dermatitis

Psoriasiform dermatitis is characterized by regular epidermal acanthosis, parakeratosis, and the absence of a granular layer. The prototype disease of this group is psoriasis vulgaris.

PSORIASIS VULGARIS

CLINICAL FEATURES. Psoriasis (25–29), a common skin disease, is characterized by raised, sharply defined, erythematous plaques with a silvery scale. The typical locations of the plaques include the scalp, elbows, extensor knees, umbilicus, and sacral areas. The degree of involvement ranges from single plaques to generalized exfoliative dermatitis. The pathogenesis of psoriasis is not fully understood.

HISTOPATHOLOGY. Epidermal parakeratosis, absence of the granular layer, regular psoriasiform epidermal acanthosis with suprapapillary plate thinning, increased vascularity of the papillary dermis, and a sparse perivascular lymphocytic infiltrate constitute the more or less constant features of psoriasis (25–29). The elongated and narrowed rete ridges have a "comblike" appearance (Fig. 1.5). Additional diagnostically helpful findings include collections of neutrophils either in the parakeratotic stratum corneum (Munro microabscesses) or at the interface of the stratum malpighii and stratum corneum (spongiform pustules of Kogoj). The latter two changes may be absent in late-stage or partially treated lesions.

PUSTULAR PSORIASIS

CLINICAL FEATURES. This variant of psoriasis (30,31) is characterized by multiple sterile pustules on an erythematous base. It may involve extensive areas, or it can be limited to the palms and soles (*pustulosis palmaris et plantaris*).

HISTOPATHOLOGY. The subcorneal pustules are filled with neutrophils, and they are much larger than the collections of

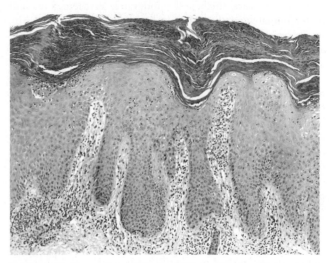

Figure 1.5. Psoriasis vulgaris. Parakeratosis, neutrophils in the stratum corneum, and regular acanthosis with suprapapillary plate thinning. Note the absence of the granular layer. A perivascular lymphocytic infiltrate is present in the papillary dermis.

neutrophils seen in psoriasis vulgaris (30,31). A lymphocytic perivascular infiltrate with a few neutrophils is present in the papillary dermis. The characteristic epidermal features of psoriasis may be absent or well developed in pustular psoriasis lesions.

PITYRIASIS RUBRA PILARIS

CLINICAL FEATURES. Pityriasis rubra pilaris (32,33) frequently presents with erythroderma closely resembling psoriasis. In contrast to psoriasis, pityriasis rubra pilaris is frequently characterized by areas of normal skin (islands of sparring) encompassed by erythematous to salmon-colored scaly plaques (island-sparing) and perifollicular horny spines.

HISTOPATHOLOGY. The microscopic findings in pityriasis rubra pilaris may be nonspecific but can be indistinguishable from those of psoriasis (32,33). Pityriasis rubra pilaris is characterized by both horizontally and vertically alternating tiers of orthokeratosis and parakeratosis in the stratum corneum. Acrotrichial parakeratosis and relatively fewer dermal inflammatory cells may help to differentiate pityriasis rubra pilaris from psoriasis, but clinical correlation is essential.

Lichenoid Interface Dermatitis

Lichenoid interface dermatitis is one of two major inflammatory patterns that primarily involve the epidermal basement membrane zone, hence the use of the term *interface*. The other pattern is vacuolar interface dermatitis (discussed later in this chapter in the section "Vacuolar Interface Dermatitis"). These two patterns can be difficult to separate at times, and both changes may be present in the same lesion.

Lichenoid interface dermatitis is defined by the following two alterations at the basement membrane zone: the destruction of the basal keratinocytes and a bandlike lymphocytic infiltrate of varying density localized to the papillary dermis. The cytoplasm of the altered basal keratinocytes becomes brightly eosinophilic. The nucleus, which is at first pyknotic, is later extruded so that eventually round to oval eosinophilic bodies are found in the lower epidermis and upper papillary dermis. These structures have been termed *colloid bodies or cytoid bodies*. The normally orderly row of cuboidal basal keratinocytes and the sharply defined basement membrane zone are both eventually destroyed. With the regeneration of the keratinocytes, the basement membrane zone takes on a disorderly, irregular appearance. The regular, undulating rete ridge pattern is lost, and the normally cuboidal basal keratinocytes become variable in shape.

A lymphocytic infiltrate is present in the superficial dermis adjacent to the altered keratinocytes. The lymphocytic infiltrate ranges from sparse to dense but is generally moderate to dense. Melanophages may be present in the underlying papillary dermis (pigment incontinence).

The lichenoid interface change frequently overlaps with the vacuolar interface change. Careful examination of the basement membrane zone is essential in distinguishing between the two patterns. Dyskeratosis predominates in the lichenoid pattern, whereas vacuolization of the basal keratinocytes is the hallmark of the vacuolar pattern. A combination of both lichenoid and vacuolar interface changes may be present in certain dermatoses, such as lupus erythematosus.

LICHEN PLANUS

CLINICAL FEATURES. "Purple, pruritic, polygonal papules" accurately sums up the clinical presentation of lichen planus (34–39). The papules tend to occur on the flexor surfaces of the extremities rather than on the dorsal surfaces. In addition, the oral mucosa, nails, and scalp may be affected. When the terminal hairs of the scalp are the primary site of involvement, with resultant alopecia, the term *lichen planopilaris* is used.

HISTOPATHOLOGY. Lichen planus (34–39) is the prototype of lichenoid interface dermatitis (Fig. 1.6). In addition to lichenoid interface change, several other features typify lichen planus histologically. Acanthosis is present, and it may be extreme. However, in a variant of lichen planus that is called *atrophic lichen planus*, the epidermis is atrophic. Hyperkeratosis is a regular feature of lichen planus. The hyperkeratosis is almost always orthokeratotic. The individual keratohyalin granules are larger and more prominent than normal and focally demonstrate a wedge-shaped hypergranulosis. The irregularity of the lichenoid interface change results in the "sawtooth" appearance of the basement membrane zone. Colloid bodies range from abundant to few. Artifactual cleft formation (Max-Joseph space) between the epidermis and papillary dermis is common, and frank hemorrhagic subepidermal bullae may occasionally be seen. The inflammatory cell infiltrate in lichen planus is superficial, typically moderate to dense, predominantly lymphocytic, and displays a bandlike distribution closely approximating the epidermis. Melanophages may be abundant.

In lichen planopilaris, similar changes are seen; however, lichen planopilaris contrasts with ordinary lichen planus in that most of the alteration occurs at the level of the follicular infundibulum. Lichen planopilaris frequently leads to follicular destruction that is characterized by perifollicular lymphocytic infiltrates, remnants of the follicular epithelium, and "naked" hair fibers partly engulfed by mononucleated or multinucleated phagocytes in late-stage lesions.

LICHEN NITIDUS

CLINICAL FEATURES. In lichen nitidus (40), a childhood eruption, groups of pinpoint, round, asymptomatic, flesh-colored papules are located primarily on the trunk, genitalia, abdomen, and forearms.

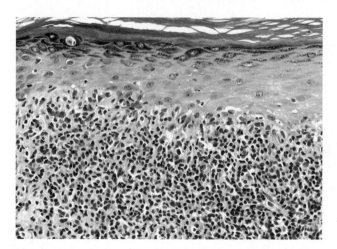

Figure 1.6. Lichen planus. Hypergranulosis, interface alteration with "sawtooth" remodeling of the basement membrane zone, and a superficial, dense bandlike lymphocytic infiltrate.

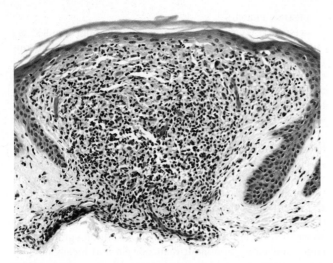

Figure 1.7. Lichen nitidus. The epidermis has a "clawlike" configuration. A lymphohistiocytic infiltrate is present in the papillary dermis.

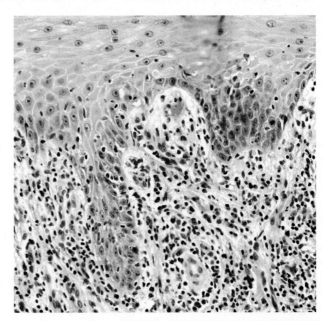

Figure 1.8. Lichenoid drug eruption. The interface alteration with parakeratosis and eosinophils provides a clue to the diagnosis of this type of lichenoid infiltrate.

HISTOPATHOLOGY. Only minimal lichenoid interface change is typically present in lichen nitidus (40). The epidermis has a "clawlike" configuration in which curvilinear fingerlike extensions of the epidermis surround a papillary dermal lymphocytic infiltrate (Fig. 1.7). The dermal infiltrate also contains histiocytes and may be loosely granulomatous. Parakeratosis may be present. Occasional dyskeratotic keratinocytes may be present at the dermal-epidermal junction. As in other lichenoid diseases, the inflammatory cell infiltrate is superficial and closely approximates the epidermis.

LICHENOID DRUG ERUPTION

CLINICAL FEATURES. A lichen planus–like eruption (41,42) may develop after exposure to various drugs and chemicals, such as gold salts, thiazide diuretics, antimalarial drugs, and color film developers.

HISTOPATHOLOGY. Lichenoid drug eruption may closely resemble lichen planus (41,42). Differentiating features of lichenoid drug eruption from lichen planus include epidermal parakeratosis and a more mixed inflammatory infiltrate with eosinophils and plasma cells (Fig. 1.8).

Vacuolar Interface Dermatitis

Vacuolar interface dermatitis is the second of the basement membrane zone "interface" patterns. The term *vacuolar* refers to the finding of intracytoplasmic vacuoles within the cytoplasm of the basal keratinocytes. As in lichenoid interface dermatitis, the end result is an alteration of the normal orderly row of basal cells and the basement membrane. Vacuolar interface change may be present with or without a lymphocytic infiltrate along the basement membrane. Melanophages may be present in the subjacent dermis.

LUPUS ERYTHEMATOSUS

CLINICAL FEATURES. Lupus erythematosus represents a spectrum of disease that can involve virtually any organ and shows a variable serologic profile (43–45). The etiology is unknown but is associated with antibodies and genetic factors. Clinically, lupus erythematosus exhibits a limited cutaneous discoid var-

iant (DLE) and systemic variants including systemic lupus erythematosus (SLE) and subacute cutaneous lupus erythematosus (SCLE). SLE is a systemic disease with protean manifestations. The classic cutaneous presentation is bilateral malar macular erythema. In contrast, discoid lupus erythematosus (DLE) is characterized by the development of sharply circumscribed, erythematous plaques that may be either thick (hypertrophic) or thin (atrophic). Distinctive "carpet tack" follicular keratotic plugs may be present in the plaques. Both SLE and DLE tend to occur on areas exposed to sunlight, such as the face or dorsum of the hand. DLE lesions may precede, develop concomitantly with, or follow the appearance of SLE. Therefore, the histologic diagnosis of DLE does not eliminate the possibility that the patient may also have SLE.

HISTOPATHOLOGY. Histologically, lupus erythematosus (43–45) can be divided into the broad categories of SLE and DLE. Both SLE and DLE (43–45) show a similar range of microscopic features that vary in degree. In DLE, the epidermis ranges from markedly acanthotic to atrophic. The keratinocytes frequently enlarge, becoming pale and angular and imparting a "glazed" appearance to the epidermis. Both acanthosis and atrophy may be present in the same lesion. Hyperkeratosis is frequently marked, and it is usually parakeratotic. Flask-shaped plugs of stratum corneum may fill the follicular orifices. The degree of vacuolar interface change is variable, ranging from focal and relatively inconspicuous to global and extensive (Fig. 1.9A). Colloid bodies and dyskeratotic keratinocytes are usually present, but they are found in smaller numbers than in lichenoid dermatitis. In older lesions, the basement membrane appears thick and irregular. Superficial and deep dermal perivascular lymphocytic infiltrates and peri-infundibular lymphocytic infiltrates are usually present. The lymphocytic infiltrates may also encompass the eccrine glands, and they may extend into the subcutis. Plasma cells are only rarely seen in the inflammatory infiltrates. Increased reticular dermal mucin is present in most cases. This last feature may not be evident in H&S-stained sec-

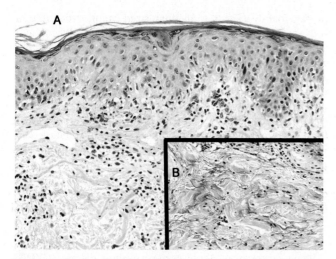

Figure 1.9. Discoid lupus erythematosus. **(A)** Vacuolar interface change is present at the dermal-epidermal junction. Dense lymphocytic infiltrates with admixed melanophages are present in the papillary dermis. **(B)** Increased dermal mucin in the reticular dermis.

tions, so mucin stains, such as the colloidal iron and alcian blue, are particularly helpful (Fig. 1.9B). Basophilic thickening of the adipocyte cell walls may be seen in the subcutis. Adipocyte nuclei are decreased in number, and scattered intralobular lymphocytes are present. When the bulk of the changes are limited to the subcutis, the process is termed *lupus profundus.*

The histopathologic features are usually not as prominent in SLE as in DLE; however, distinction may be very difficult. The epidermis is of normal thickness or is slightly atrophic, and the stratum corneum is usually unaltered. Vacuolar interface change ranges from sparse to extensive. The perivascular dermal lymphocytic infiltrates are usually less dense and more superficial than in DLE. Often, the degree of mucin deposition in the reticular dermis is significantly greater than in DLE.

The differential diagnosis of lupus erythematosus includes diseases characterized by vacuolar interface alteration, such as fixed drug eruption, acute graft-versus-host disease, and dermatomyositis. With the exception of dermatomyositis, the presence of increased dermal mucin and of a deep component of dermal inflammation in lupus erythematosus helps to differentiate it from the other lesions with epidermal interface alteration. In addition to interface diseases, diseases that display superficial and deep perivascular lymphocytic infiltrates, such as polymorphous light eruption (PMLE), can overlap with lupus erythematosus. The distinguishing features include epidermal interface change and increased dermal mucin present in lupus erythematosus and extensive papillary dermal edema in PMLE.

DERMATOMYOSITIS
CLINICAL FEATURES. Poorly demarcated, scaly, erythematous patches are found in dermatomyositis (46,47), a systemic disease that may affect the skin, striated muscles, and other internal organs. A characteristic violaceous "heliotrope" erythema of the upper eyelids and extensor joint surfaces may be seen. Chronic patches can become poikilodermatous (atrophic and telangiectatic with pigmentary change).

HISTOPATHOLOGY. The histologic changes of dermatomyositis (46,47) are frequently indistinguishable from those of SLE. The epidermis is typically atrophic, and vacuolar interface change

is usually prominent and extensive. A sparse, superficial perivascular lymphocytic infiltrate and markedly increased dermal mucin are present in the dermis. The differential diagnosis is similar to lupus erythematosus (discussed earlier in the section "Lupus Erythematosus") and includes both diseases with epidermal interface alteration and those with a superficial and deep lymphocytic infiltrate.

PITYRIASIS LICHENOIDES ET VARIOLIFORMIS ACUTA, PITYRIASIS LICHENOIDES CHRONICA, LYMPHOMATOID PAPULOSIS
CLINICAL FEATURES. Pityriasis lichenoides et varioliformis acuta (PLEVA; also known as Mucha-Habermann disease) and pityriasis lichenoides chronica (PLC) (48–57) overlap clinically and microscopically. PLEVA presents with the sudden onset of crops of small, ulcerated papules, mainly on the trunk, that may heal with superficial scarring—hence, the use of the term *varioliformis* for smallpox (variola) (50). In contrast, PLC presents with red-brown papules that have a characteristic "waferlike" scale. In some patients, lesions of both types coexist.

Lymphomatoid papulosis appears in several different clinical forms, ranging from an eruption virtually identical to PLEVA to large ulcerated plaques and nodules (48–57). Although lymphomatoid papulosis is a self-healing process, the exact relationship between lymphomatoid papulosis and cutaneous lymphoma is not completely clear at this time. In a small but significant percentage of patients, lymphomatoid papulosis, which was originally thought to be a completely benign disease, eventually develops into cutaneous or nodal lymphoma. T-cell receptor gene rearrangements have been documented in lymphomatoid papulosis, but even when present, this finding does not definitely predict an eventual transformation to lymphoma. Clonal gene rearrangements are indicative only of the presence of a clonal population of lymphocytes (54,57). Patients with lymphomatoid papulosis require continued clinical surveillance so that an associated nodal, extranodal, or cutaneous lymphoma can be diagnosed as early as possible.

HISTOPATHOLOGY. Although early lesions may show only marked vacuolar interface change, the histologic counterpart of the ulcerated papules in PLEVA (50) is a broad zone of full-thickness epidermal necrosis. The stratum corneum overlying the zone of necrosis is parakeratotic, and it may contain neutrophils. Florid lymphocyte exocytosis, spongiosis, and erythrocyte extravasation into the epidermis are frequent. The associated lymphocytic infiltrate in the dermis is dense and characteristically "wedge-shaped." The broad base of the wedge extends along the epidermis. The infiltrate becomes less dense and narrower as it descends deeper into the reticular dermis. Large transformed lymphocytes are present in the infiltrates. Penetration of the lymphocytes into vessel walls leads to perivascular hemorrhage.

PLC (49,50) is characterized by similar but less destructive features. A well-developed, sharply demarcated zone of parakeratosis is present. The vacuolar interface change and lymphocyte exocytosis are not usually as extensive as that seen in PLEVA. The wedge-shaped pattern of the dermal inflammatory cells is similar (Fig. 1.10).

In lymphomatoid papulosis (48–57), the epidermal and dermal findings may resemble those of PLEVA or PLC (Fig. 1.11A). However, varying numbers of large, atypical lymphocytes with hyperchromatic, convoluted nuclei are superimposed on the other features (Fig. 1.11B). These cells may closely resemble

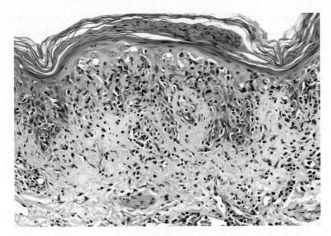

Figure 1.10. Pityriasis lichenoides et varioliformis acuta. Sharply demarcated epidermal parakeratosis, spongiosis, vacuolar interface change with epidermal necrosis, lymphocytic exocytosis, and a dermal lymphocytic inflammatory infiltrate are characteristic.

the atypical lymphocytes of cutaneous T-cell lymphoma, and they have been likened to "lumps of coal." The atypical lymphocytes are most prevalent in the papillary and upper reticular dermis, although some may be epidermotropic. Ki-1 antigen (CD30) is usually detectable in the cytoplasm of the atypical lymphocytes. Classically, three variants of lymphomatoid papulosis are described, but there is often histopathologic overlap between the variants, and correlation with the clinical presentation is essential. The type A variant shows a mixed dermal infiltrate with scattered large, CD30-positive cells, similar to classic type Hodgkin lymphoma. Type B lymphomatoid papulosis is

predominantly a small- to medium-sized lymphocytic infiltrate with absent to rare, large, CD30-positive cells. Type B lymphomatoid papulosis has microscopic overlap with the mycosis fungoides type of cutaneous T-cell lymphoma. Type C lymphomatoid papulosis is characterized by a dense infiltrate with numerous large CD30-positive cells. Type C lymphomatoid papulosis can be virtually indistinguishable from anaplastic large-cell lymphoma, requiring clinical and hematologic correlation for a definitive diagnosis. The clinical history of spontaneously regressing lesions is important in making the diagnosis of lymphomatoid papulosis.

A follicular variant of lymphomatoid papulosis has also been described in which the atypical lymphocytes encompass the follicular infundibula.

ACUTE AND CHRONIC GRAFT-VERSUS-HOST DISEASE

CLINICAL FEATURES. Acute graft-versus-host disease (GVHD) (58,59) is most commonly seen in patients from 10 to 30 days following an allogeneic bone marrow transplant, and it often presents on the acral surfaces and pinnae as an asymptomatic or slightly painful macular eruption. It may progress to a widespread morbilliform or erythrodermic eruption on the trunk and extremities that is difficult to distinguish clinically from a morbilliform drug eruption. Oral mucosal stomatitis and ulcerations may be present.

Chronic GVHD (58,59) typically develops from 100 days after transplant. Two types of chronic GVHD—lichenoid and sclerodermoid—are generally observed.

HISTOPATHOLOGY. The epidermis exhibits vacuolar interface change with associated dyskeratotic keratinocytes and occasional lymphocytes in acute GVHD (Fig. 1.12) (58,59). The degree of epidermal interface alteration ranges from very focal to

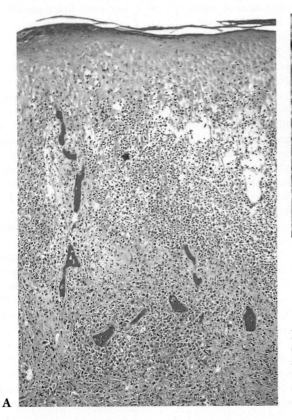

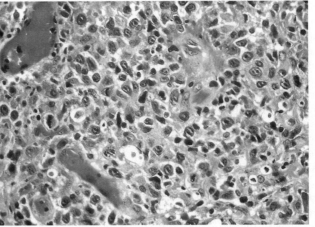

Figure 1.11. Lymphomatoid papulosis. **(A)** The epidermal and dermal alterations resemble pityriasis lichenoides et varioliformis acuta or pityriasis lichenoides chronica. **(B)** Under higher magnification, large atypical lymphocytes with convoluted, bizarrely shaped nuclei are seen. These cells may closely resemble the atypical lymphocytes of mycosis fungoides.

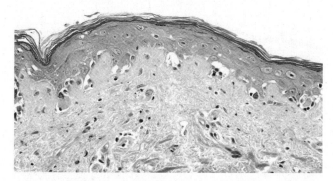

Figure 1.12. Acute graft-versus-host disease. Vacuolar interface alteration with dyskeratotic keratinocytes and a sparse lymphocytic infiltrate.

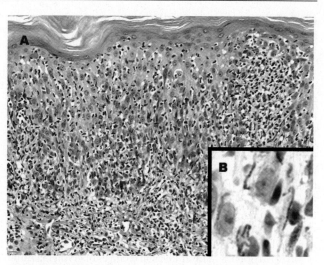

Figure 1.13. Secondary syphilis. **(A)** Psoriasiform epidermal changes and a lichenoid mixed inflammatory infiltrate with plasma cells and focal vacuolar interface change. **(B)** Immunohistochemistry demonstrates spirochete organisms in the epidermis.

extensive with necrosis. The dermis displays a sparse, superficial, perivascular, lymphocytic infiltrate. The presence of at least a small number of intraepidermal lymphocytes is essential because both vacuolar interface change and dyskeratotic keratinocytes may be present in eruptions secondary to cytotoxic chemotherapeutic agents.

The lichenoid form of chronic GVHD (58,59) is identical to lichen planus, and the sclerodermoid variant closely resembles morphea and scleroderma, making clinical correlation essential.

SECONDARY SYPHILIS

CLINICAL FEATURES. Secondary syphilis (60–63) can be a difficult clinical diagnosis because of its ability to mimic many other dermatoses. Asymptomatic, scaly, flesh-colored to erythematous papules or annular plaques are most frequently found on the face and trunk. Characteristic copper-colored macules may occur on the palms and soles. "Moth-eaten" alopecia on the scalp and mucous patches on the tongue are additional clues to the diagnosis.

HISTOPATHOLOGY. The lesions of secondary syphilis (60–63) range from an inconspicuous perivascular lymphocytic infiltrate to a dense, diffuse lymphoplasmacytic infiltrate with extensive vacuolar interface change (Fig. 1.13). In these latter lesions, the epidermis is usually acanthotic. Spongiosis, psoriasiform acanthosis, and lymphocyte exocytosis may be present. The inflammatory cell infiltrate is variable. It may be lichenoid, superficial perivascular, superficial and deep perivascular, or diffuse and granulomatous. This last pattern is most frequently seen in late, resolving lesions. The presence of plasma cells in any cutaneous lymphocytic infiltrate should arouse suspicion of secondary syphilis if the clinical presentation is consistent. Plasma cells may be numerous or sparse, and in some lesions, plasma cells may be absent in secondary syphilis.

Silver impregnation stains, such as the Dieterle, Steiner, and Warthin-Starry stains, are used to stain spirochetes. The organisms are difficult to find in most lesions, so they are best identified in the epidermis or superficial capillary plexus. Recently, immunohistochemistry to demonstrate the infecting organism has been introduced (64).

ADJUNCTS TO MICROSCOPIC DIAGNOSIS. By the time the eruption of secondary syphilis (60–63) is present, the results of serologic studies are usually positive.

FIXED DRUG ERUPTION

CLINICAL FEATURES. The term *fixed drug reaction* (65,66) has its basis on the observation that the repeated administration of certain drugs results in the recurrence of a reddish-brown patch in the same location. Bullae may arise on the patch. Typical sites include the genitalia and face. Tetracycline, barbiturates, and phenolphthalein are among the most common of many offenders.

HISTOPATHOLOGY. Vacuolar epidermal interface alteration with scattered individual and grouped dyskeratotic (necrotic) keratinocytes is characteristic of fixed drug eruptions (65,66) (Fig. 1.14). The affected keratinocytes are found at all levels of the epidermis. Variable numbers of melanophages are typically present in the papillary and upper reticular dermis. In the superficial dermis, there is a perivascular, lymphocytic infiltrate, often admixed with eosinophils. If a bulla is present, it is usually

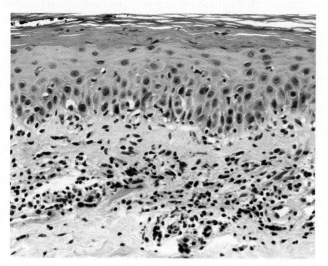

Figure 1.14. Fixed drug eruption. Dyskeratotic keratinocytes, lymphocytic exocytosis, focal vacuolar interface change, and a perivascular lymphocytic infiltrate.

subepidermal, and it occurs in those areas in which the vacuolar interface change is most severe.

ERYTHEMA MULTIFORME

CLINICAL FEATURES. Erythema multiforme (67–71) is a recurrent eruption characterized by a few or many erythematous plaques with an urticarial quality. The diagnostic clinical lesion resembles a target because of the alternating blanched and erythematous rings. Other primary lesions in erythema multiforme include erythematous macules, papules, and bullae, explaining the use of the term *multiforme*. Any part of the integument may be involved, but the distal extremities, especially the palms and soles, and the mucosal surfaces are frequently affected. Although erythema multiforme is often idiopathic, it is commonly secondary to herpes simplex infections, *Mycoplasma* infections, and medications.

HISTOPATHOLOGY. The epidermal changes of erythema multiforme (67–71) are virtually identical to those previously described for fixed drug eruption. Vacuolar interface alteration with associated intraepidermal dyskeratotic keratinocytes is characteristic of erythema multiforme. The degree of vacuolar interface change ranges from focal to marked, and hemorrhagic subepidermal bulla formation may be present (Fig. 1.15). The epidermal changes are essential for the diagnosis; no purely "dermal" form of erythema multiforme exists.

STEVENS-JOHNSON SYNDROME AND TOXIC EPIDERMAL NECROLYSIS

CLINICAL FEATURES. Stevens-Johnson syndrome and toxic epidermal necrolysis (TEN) (72–74) are at the severe, potentially life-threatening end of the erythema multiforme spectrum. Large, flaccid, confluent bullae may involve portions of the skin surface in Stevens-Johnson syndrome and large segments of the skin surface, resulting in total denudation, in TEN. Both disorders include mucosal erosions and ulcers. Frequently associated medications include sulfonamides, anticonvulsants, and nonsteroidal anti-inflammatories, but in some cases, no etiologic association is apparent.

HISTOPATHOLOGY. In fully developed lesions of Stevens-Johnson syndrome and TEN (72–74), the epidermis shows interface alteration with full-thickness necrosis. The epidermis separates from the dermis. Necrotic keratinocytes are present at the edges

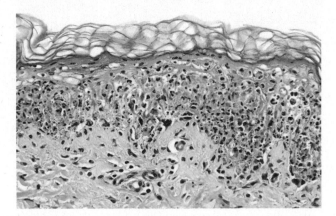

Figure 1.15. Erythema multiforme. Prominent vacuolar interface change and dyskeratotic keratinocytes characterize erythema multiforme.

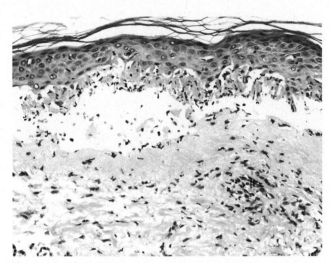

Figure 1.16. Toxic epidermal necrosis. Extensive keratinocyte necrosis below an intact stratum corneum.

of the bullae (Fig. 1.16). The inflammatory cell component is variable.

TEN must be differentiated from the clinically similar staphylococcal scalded skin syndrome. TEN is characterized by epidermal interface alteration with full-thickness epidermal necrosis and subepidermal bulla formation. In contrast, staphylococcal scalded skin syndrome exhibits a superficial plane of cleavage in the granular layer of the epidermis. Superficial epidermal necrosis is also found in necrolytic migratory erythema (glucagonoma syndrome) as well as external chemical and thermal injury. Clinical history is essential in distinction of these three lesions.

Verrucous Acanthosis: Verruca Vulgaris

This category encompasses several hamartomatous and neoplastic entities, such as linear epidermal nevus and seborrheic keratosis, in addition to verruca vulgaris. Verruca vulgaris is discussed in this chapter because it exemplifies the verrucous pattern of acanthosis.

CLINICAL FEATURES. Common warts are typically exophytic verrucous papules that may be single lesions or that may be grouped in a linear configuration. Human papillomavirus is the etiologic agent (75).

HISTOPATHOLOGY. Striking upward displacement of the dermal papillae (papillomatosis) imparts a serrated appearance to the epidermis (75). The stratum corneum is hyperparakeratotic, forming pointed mounds (Fig. 1.17). Extravasated erythrocytes or hemosiderin may be found in the stratum corneum. Large, clumped keratohyalin granules may be present in the thickened granular layer. The dermal papilla show dilated vascular channels. A lymphocytic infiltrate of variable density is usually present in the upper dermis.

Bullous and Pustular Diseases

The category of bullous and pustular diseases encompasses a large number of pathogenetically unrelated entities. The histopathologic classification is usually based on the location of the

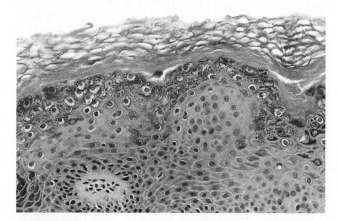

Figure 1.17. Verruca vulgaris. Perinuclear clearing in keratinocytes within the granular layer.

plane of separation—subcorneal, intraepidermal, or subepidermal. The epidermal blistering diseases are subdivided into those with and those without acantholysis. The subepidermal blistering diseases are subdivided into inflammatory and noninflammatory types.

SUBCORNEAL BULLAE WITHOUT ACANTHOLYSIS
Subcorneal pustular dermatosis

CLINICAL FEATURES. In subcorneal pustular dermatosis (also known as Sneddon-Wilkinson disease) (76,77), large flaccid pustules form on the trunk and body folds.

HISTOPATHOLOGY. A large, unilocular subcorneal pustule is present (Fig. 1.18) (76,77). Neutrophils are also found in the subjacent epidermis, which may be psoriasiform. Mixed inflammatory cell infiltrates composed primarily of neutrophils and lymphocytes are located in the superficial dermis.

Scabies

CLINICAL FEATURES. Extremely pruritic erythematous papules and linear "burrows," located especially in the web spaces of the fingers and toes, are characteristic of scabies (78). The causative agent is the human scabies mite.

HISTOPATHOLOGY. The burrow appears microscopically as a cleft in the stratum corneum or upper stratum malpighii con-

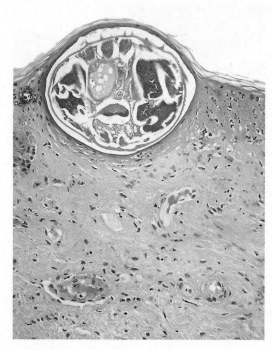

Figure 1.19. Scabies. Mite body parts in a subcorneal burrow.

taining mite body parts (Fig. 1.19) (78). The adjacent epidermis is usually acanthotic, parakeratotic, and spongiotic. Eosinophils are invariably present in the subjacent dermal infiltrates, which are typically dense and extensive.

Acute generalized exanthematous pustulosis

CLINICAL FEATURES. Acute generalized exanthematous pustulosis (AGEP) is characterized by an acute onset of sterile, nonfollicular pustules, usually within hours of beginning a medication (79,80). Common associated agents include beta-lactam and macrolide antibiotics. The eruption resolves after cessation of the suspected medication.

HISTOPATHOLOGY. Lesions of AGEP exhibit intraepidermal and subcorneal pustules with associated spongiosis (79,80). The superficial dermis displays a mixed inflammatory infiltrate with eosinophils. In addition, edema may be present in the papillary dermis. Leukocytoclastic vasculitis may also be seen.

The differential diagnosis of AGEP includes pustular psoriasis, subcorneal pustular dermatosis, bullous impetigo, pustular dermatophyte infection, pemphigus foliaceus, and immunoglobulin A (IgA) pemphigus. Clinical history is crucial in establishing an accurate diagnosis.

SUBCORNEAL BULLAE WITH ACANTHOLYSIS: BULLOUS IMPETIGO

CLINICAL FEATURES. Found primarily in children, bullous impetigo (81) consists of confluent pustules and honey-colored crusts. It usually is a result of a staphylococcal infection.

HISTOPATHOLOGY. The cleavage plane in bullous impetigo (81) either is subcorneal or is within the upper stratum granulosum. The roof of the pustule is parakeratotic stratum corneum, and the floor is formed of keratinocytes, a few or many of which are acantholytic (Fig. 1.20). Neutrophils fill the pustule. Clusters of staphylococci can usually be found with the Brown-Brenn tissue Gram stain.

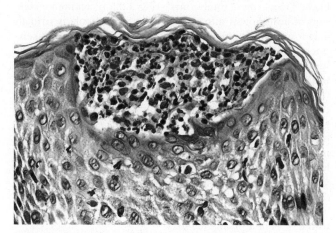

Figure 1.18. Subcorneal pustular dermatosis. The large, unilocular subcorneal pustule is characteristic.

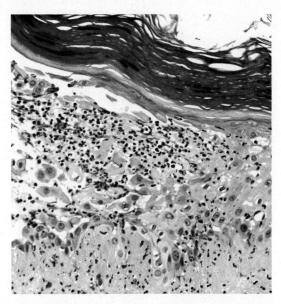

Figure 1.20. Bullous impetigo. The bulla floor is formed from acantholytic keratinocytes. Neutrophils fill the pustule.

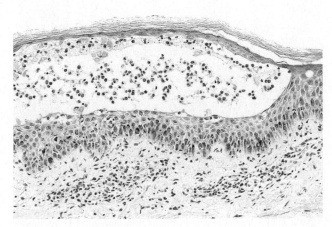

Figure 1.21. Pemphigus foliaceus. A subcorneal bulla with acantholytic keratinocytes and a few inflammatory cells.

The staphylococcal exfoliative toxins A and B target desmoglein 1, a desmosomal cell-cell adhesion molecule that is expressed in the upper levels of the epidermis (81). This correlates with the subcorneal localization of the bullae and epidermal acantholysis.

INTRAEPIDERMAL BULLAE WITHOUT ACANTHOLYSIS: ERYTHEMA TOXICUM NEONATORUM. Spongiotic vesicles and pustules may be present in several of the diseases discussed in the section on acute and subacute spongiotic dermatitis, such as allergic and irritant contact dermatitis. Dermatophyte infections with highly inflammatory species, such as *Trichophyton mentagrophytes*, may result in both spongiotic vesicles and pustules.

CLINICAL FEATURES. This relatively common asymptomatic erythematous pustular eruption (82) is transient, and it is limited to neonates.

HISTOPATHOLOGY. The primary finding in erythema toxicum neonatorum (82) is an intraepidermal pustule filled with eosinophils. The adjacent epidermis is spongiotic.

INTRAEPIDERMAL BULLAE WITH ACANTHOLYSIS
Pemphigus foliaceus and pemphigus erythematosus
CLINICAL FEATURES. Four subtypes of pemphigus (83–85) are commonly recognized. Based on the level of the cleavage plane, pemphigus foliaceus and pemphigus erythematosus are classified as "superficial" types of pemphigus, whereas pemphigus vulgaris and pemphigus vegetans are "deep" forms. Pemphigus foliaceus is frequently not clinically recognized as a "blistering" disease because the bullae may be completely replaced by crusts and erosions by the time the patient seeks care. The trunk tends to be extensively involved. Pemphigus erythematosus presents with similar lesions, but they are located primarily on the face in a malar or seborrheic distribution. Both diseases show antibodies to the cadherin desmosomal protein desmoglein 1 (85).

HISTOPATHOLOGY. The histopathologic features of pemphigus foliaceus and erythematosus are identical (83–85). Acantholysis of the granular layer is the hallmark of the superficial forms of pemphigus. A discrete acantholytic bulla within the granular

layer of the epidermis with few inflammatory cells is characteristic (Fig. 1.21). The acantholytic keratinocytes in the bulla have a rounded appearance. The stratum corneum may be completely denuded, with only the granular layer left on the surface; in older lesions, parakeratosis and acanthosis are found. Eosinophils are frequently present in the adjacent epidermis (eosinophilic spongiosis) and in the subjacent, sparse dermal inflammatory cell infiltrate.

Pemphigus vulgaris, pemphigus vegetans, and paraneoplastic pemphigus
CLINICAL FEATURES. Numerous small, flaccid bullae are present on the scalp and trunk in pemphigus vulgaris (86–92). The oral mucosa is almost invariably involved at some time during the course of the illness. The bullae rupture, leaving erosions that impair swallowing and ultimately lead to starvation and frequently to death. Pemphigus vegetans is much less common than pemphigus vulgaris; it is characterized by intertriginous verrucous plaques. Paraneoplastic pemphigus presents with oral and cutaneous erosions and bullae in patients with an underlying neoplasm, usually lymphoma.

HISTOPATHOLOGY. In pemphigus vulgaris, suprabasal acantholysis (86–92) results in a deep epidermal cleavage plane. The basal keratinocytes remain attached to the basement membrane to form a distinctive single row of cells that have been likened to a "row of tombstones" (Fig. 1.22). Prominent extension of acantholysis into the follicular infundibula is virtually diagnostic of pemphigus vulgaris. Rounded, acantholytic keratinocytes are usually abundant in the blister cavity. Eosinophilic spongiosis is common, and eosinophils are usually present within the blister cavity and within the minimal dermal infiltrate.

Suprabasal acantholysis is more difficult to detect in pemphigus vegetans (86–92). Here, the epidermis is markedly acanthotic, to the point of being verrucous. Large intraepidermal microabscesses filled with eosinophils but only a few acantholytic keratinocytes are characteristic (Fig. 1.23).

In addition to suprabasal acantholysis, dyskeratosis and interface change are present in paraneoplastic pemphigus, resulting in a microscopic appearance resembling that of erythema multiforme or lichen planus (86–92).

ADJUNCTS TO MICROSCOPIC DIAGNOSIS. A direct immunofluorescence examination of specimens from the perilesional skin is essential to confirm the diagnosis of pemphigus (86–92). Immunoglobulin G (IgG) and/or the third component of complement (C3) are present in the intercellular spaces of the epidermis, outlining the keratinocytes. The direct immunofluorescence examination findings are essentially identical in all types of pemphigus, except for paraneoplastic pemphigus, in which, in addition to the intercellular pattern, granular deposits of C3 are present at the dermal-epidermal junction. Antibodies to primarily the cadherin desmosomal protein desmoglein 3 and less commonly desmoglein 1 are present in pemphigus vulgaris (88,89). Antibodies to desmoglein 3 are also present in pemphigus vegetans (86). Paraneoplastic pemphigus exhibits a more numerous antibody profile (91,92). The other acantholytic diseases (benign familial pemphigus, keratosis follicularis, and transient acantholytic dermatosis) are not characterized by intercellular immunoglobulin deposits.

In addition to the direct immunofluorescence procedure, an examination of serum can be performed to detect specific patterns of immunoglobulin deposition on various tissue substrates (indirect immunofluorescence).

Benign familial pemphigus (Hailey-Hailey disease)

CLINICAL FEATURES. Intertriginous vesicles, crusts, and erosions are present in benign familial pemphigus (Hailey-Hailey disease), which is inherited in an autosomal dominant pattern and results from a mutation in an intracellular calcium pump (ATP2C1) (93,94).

HISTOPATHOLOGY. Although suprabasal acantholysis is most prominent, acantholysis is found at all levels of the epidermis in benign familial pemphigus (93). The upper levels of the epidermis appear to be held together loosely by the few remaining intercellular bridges (Fig. 1.24). Few dyskeratotic keratino-

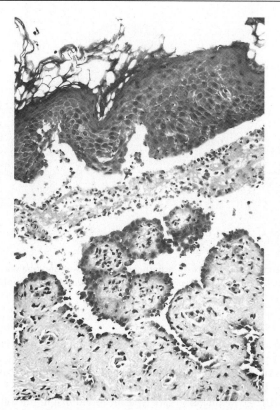

Figure 1.22. Pemphigus vulgaris. Suprabasilar bulla with prominent epidermal acantholysis and a mixed dermal inflammatory infiltrate with eosinophils.

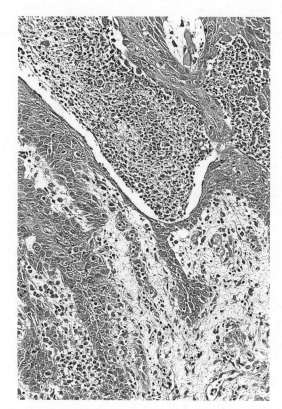

Figure 1.23. Pemphigus vegetans. An intraepidermal microabscess with abundant eosinophils and occasional acantholytic keratinocytes.

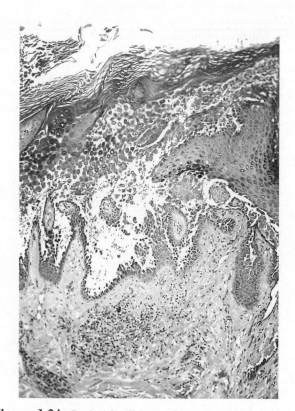

Figure 1.24. Benign familial pemphigus. Prominent epidermal acantholysis with suprabasilar clefting.

cytes are present. Inflammation is minimal, consisting of scattered lymphocytes in the epidermis and papillary dermis.

Keratosis follicularis (Darier disease)

CLINICAL FEATURES. Several different types of skin lesions are found in keratosis follicularis (Darier disease) (95), but crusted, coalescent, scaly papules are most common. They are usually located on the central part of the chest and on the axillae, back, and neck. The disease is inherited in an autosomal dominant pattern and results from a mutation in an intracellular calcium pump (ATP2A2) (96).

HISTOPATHOLOGY. In addition to prominent suprabasal acantholysis, a unique form of dyskeratosis is seen in keratosis follicularis (95,97). The dyskeratotic cells are basophilic, and they have large nuclei. When they are located in the stratum corneum, the dyskeratotic cells are called *grains*. When these cells are located in the granular layer, they are known as *corps ronds* (Fig. 1.25). Other prominent features of keratosis follicularis include marked irregular acanthosis and papillomatosis. Lymphocytic infiltrates may be prominent in the upper dermis.

Transient acantholytic dermatosis (Grover disease)

CLINICAL FEATURES. Scattered, discrete, small, erythematous, pruritic papules on the chest and back constitute the entity known as *transient acantholytic dermatosis*, or Grover disease (98).

HISTOPATHOLOGY. Five different epidermal patterns have been described in transient acantholytic dermatosis (98). The acantholytic patterns resemble pemphigus vulgaris, pemphigus foliaceus, keratosis follicularis, or benign familial pemphigus, but the acantholysis is focal rather than diffuse (Fig. 1.26). In the fifth pattern, acantholytic cells are adjacent to spongiotic foci.

Herpes simplex and herpes zoster infections

CLINICAL FEATURES. After the primary infection (primary herpes simplex or varicella), dormant viral particles reside in sensory ganglia only to erupt at a later date (recurrent herpes simplex or shingles) (99–102). Both eruptions consist of grouped vesicles on an erythematous base. Shingles has a dermatomal distribution. The vesicles eventually turn into pustules and then form crusts before resolving. Many patients experi-

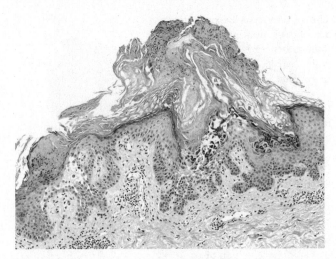

Figure 1.26. Transient acantholytic dermatosis. Suprabasilar epidermal acantholysis. This pattern resembles benign familial pemphigus and pemphigus vulgaris.

ence severe burning pain in the affected region before the eruption appears.

HISTOPATHOLOGY. Distinctive nuclear inclusions in keratinocytes are diagnostic of herpesvirus infection (Fig. 1.27) (99–102). The inclusions are typically found first in the follicular epithelium. Homogenization and peripheral margination of the nuclear chromatin are followed by multiple nucleation of the keratinocytes. The juxtaposed nuclei have molded contours.

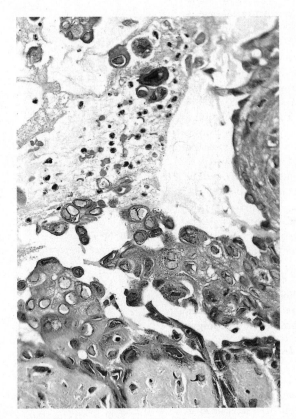

Figure 1.27. Herpesvirus infection. Multinucleated, acantholytic keratinocytes are present on the periphery of the bulla.

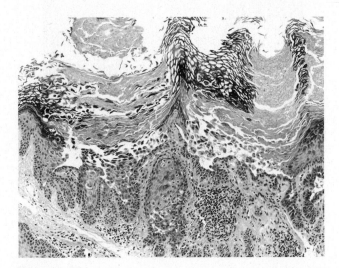

Figure 1.25. Keratosis follicularis. Suprabasal acantholysis and the distinctive large dyskeratotic cells with hyperchromatic nuclei.

The keratinocytes become rounded. Eventually, full-thickness acantholysis and epidermal necrosis develop. The dermal inflammatory cell infiltrate can be extensive. Leukocytoclastic vasculitis may be present. Herpes simplex infection cannot be distinguished from varicella-zoster infection by histology alone; adjunctive studies are required (see next section). Immunohistochemistry for herpes simplex and varicella-zoster can help identify infection in lesions that lack characteristic cytopathic changes.

ADJUNCTS TO MICROSCOPIC DIAGNOSIS. Herpes simplex virus can usually be cultured from vesicles and pustules without difficulty (99–102). Varicella-zoster virus is more difficult to culture, so an examination of exfoliated lesional keratinocytes may be extremely useful. This technique, the Tzanck preparation, consists of opening a vesicle or pustule with a scalpel blade and scraping the lesion base to obtain material for a Giemsa, Wright, or toluidine blue stain of an air-dried smear. The characteristic nuclear changes and multinucleated giant cells are usually readily apparent with this cytologic technique. Other immunologic methods are also available for rapid diagnosis.

SUBEPIDERMAL BULLAE WITH INFLAMMATION

Bullous pemphigoid, cicatricial pemphigoid, and pemphigoid gestationis (herpes gestationis)

CLINICAL FEATURES. Although each of these three diseases is a distinct clinical entity (103–107), all are caused by circulating autoantibodies that are directed against the basement membrane zone proteins. The microscopic appearances of these diseases are similar. Bullous pemphigoid is a blistering eruption characterized by large, tense bullae on the flexor surfaces, trunk, and intertriginous regions. Bullae may arise on an inflammatory urticarial base or on previously normal skin.

The skin lesions of cicatricial pemphigoid are morphologically similar to those of bullous pemphigoid, but they tend to be fewer in number. The mucous membranes of the eyes and oral cavity are the primary sites of involvement. Less commonly, mucosa of the pharynx, esophagus, larynx, and nasal mucosa can be involved. The bullae eventually lead to scarring.

The primary lesion of pemphigoid gestationis is similar to that of bullous pemphigoid as well, but this disease occurs exclusively in pregnant or postpartum women or in women taking oral contraceptives.

HISTOPATHOLOGY. The initial abnormality consists of subepidermal edema (103–107). The subsequent separation of the epidermis from the papillary dermis results in the formation of a subepidermal bulla (Fig. 1.28). Eosinophils, lymphocytes, and neutrophils comprise most of the inflammatory cells in and around the bullae.

ADJUNCTS TO MICROSCOPIC DIAGNOSIS. Linear deposits of IgG and C3 are found along the basement membrane zone in both bullous pemphigoid and cicatricial pemphigoid on direct immunofluorescence examination (103–107). Generally, only C3 is present in pemphigoid gestationis.

Dermatitis herpetiformis

CLINICAL FEATURES. The scalp, extensor surfaces of the extremities, and buttocks are the typical locations on which the grouped, tense, pinhead-sized vesicles of dermatitis herpetiformis are found (108–110). The lesions are extremely pruritic, and patients may present with erosions, rather than intact vesicles, as a consequence of their vigorous scratching. There is a

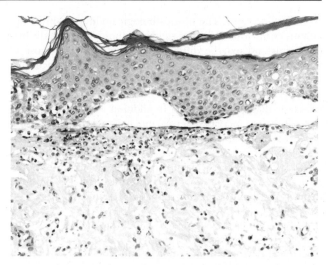

Figure 1.28. Bullous pemphigoid. A subepidermal bulla with a mixed inflammatory infiltrate, including eosinophils.

well-documented association between dermatitis herpetiformis and gluten-sensitive enteropathy (celiac disease).

HISTOPATHOLOGY. Small clusters of neutrophils in the papillary dermis (papillary dermal microabscesses) are pathognomonic of dermatitis herpetiformis (Fig. 1.29) (108–110). Eventually, the epidermis overlying the affected dermal papillae separates to form a row of small subepidermal bullae that may coalesce to form larger bullae. A sparse, predominantly neutrophilic infiltrate is found in the upper reticular dermis.

ADJUNCTS TO MICROSCOPIC DIAGNOSIS. Granular deposits of IgA are invariably present in the papillary dermis of the perilesional skin on direct immunofluorescent examination (108–110).

Linear immunoglobulin A bullous dermatosis

CLINICAL FEATURES. Linear IgA bullous dermatosis (linear IgA disease) (111) presents in childhood or adulthood with bullae in an arcuate configuration on an erythematous base that are distributed primarily over the thighs, buttocks, lower trunk, scalp, face, and genital area.

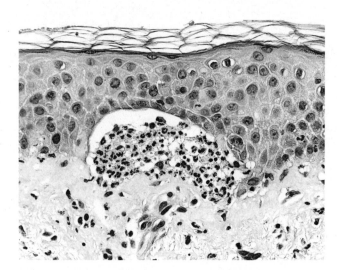

Figure 1.29. Dermatitis herpetiformis. Neutrophilic microabscesses are present in the papillary dermis.

HISTOPATHOLOGY. The histopathologic findings in linear IgA bullous dermatosis (111) are similar to those of dermatitis herpetiformis and may be difficult to distinguish from those of bullous lupus erythematosus. Direct immunofluorescence studies are essential to differentiate linear IgA bullous dermatosis from dermatitis herpetiformis (see following "Adjuncts to microscopic diagnosis" section). In addition to papillary dermal microabscesses, increased dermal mucin is present in the reticular dermis in bullous lupus erythematosus.

ADJUNCTS TO MICROSCOPIC DIAGNOSIS. The linear deposits of IgA at the dermal-epidermal junction on direct immunofluorescent studies in linear IgA disease contrast with the granular deposits of IgA in dermatitis herpetiformis.

SUBEPIDERMAL BULLAE WITHOUT INFLAMMATION
Epidermolysis bullosa

CLINICAL FEATURES. Epidermolysis bullosa (112–114) consists of a group of inherited diseases of structural proteins in the lower epidermis, basement membrane, or upper dermis; they are characterized by blister formation followed by varying degrees of scarring. Bullae tend to form at sites of trauma.

HISTOPATHOLOGY. Although the ultrastructural level of cleavage varies in the different types of epidermolysis bullosa (112–114), all types are characterized by subepidermal bullae on routine histologic sections. The epidermis is intact, and it is separated from the papillary dermis (Fig. 1.30). Minimal inflammation is present in early lesions. The superficial dermis is fibrotic.

Immunofluorescent antigen mapping of the basement membrane zone is used to identify the plane of cleavage and define the type of epidermolysis bullosa.

Porphyria cutanea tarda

CLINICAL FEATURES. Blisters and erosions leading to the formation of small angular scars, changes in pigmentation, and milia are features of porphyria cutanea tarda (115–117). Hypertrichosis may also be seen. The dorsa of the hands and other areas exposed to both sunlight and trauma are commonly involved. Porphyria cutanea tarda is caused by a reduced activity of the uroporphyrinogen decarboxylase enzyme. Urine studies show increased porphyrins in affected patients.

HISTOPATHOLOGY. In addition to the noninflammatory subepidermal bullae, dermal changes usually point to a diagnosis of porphyria cutanea tarda (115–117). The dermal papillae protrude into the blister cavity in a characteristic "festooned" pattern with preservation of their papillary architecture (Fig. 1.31). Another clue to the diagnosis of porphyria cutanea tarda is the presence of "caterpillar bodies," which are eosinophilic, PAS-positive, diastase-resistant linear globules in the epidermis forming the roof of the blister cavity. Both the epidermal basement membrane and the basement membranes of the vessels of the superficial vascular plexus are thickened by PAS-positive, diastase-resistant homogeneous eosinophilic deposits.

Epidermolytic hyperkeratosis

CLINICAL FEATURES. Epidermolytic hyperkeratosis (bullous congenital ichthyosiform erythroderma) (118) is a type of ichthyosis that is inherited in an autosomal dominant manner, resulting from defects in keratins 1 and 10. Rows of confluent, verrucous, scaling papules that are accentuated in the flexural areas arise shortly after birth and persist thereafter.

HISTOPATHOLOGY. The extraordinary histologic finding of epidermolysis is a distinguishing feature of this form of ichthyosis (118). Perinuclear clear spaces, markedly basophilic irregu-

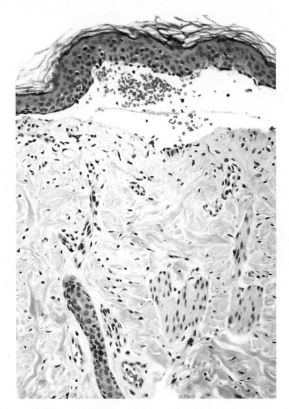

Figure 1.30. Epidermolysis bullosa. A noninflammatory subepidermal cleft overlies a papillary dermal scar.

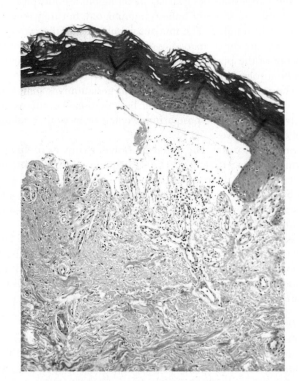

Figure 1.31. Porphyria cutanea tarda. Subepidermal bulla with minimal inflammation. The dermal papillae protrude into the bulla cavity in the characteristic "festooned" pattern.

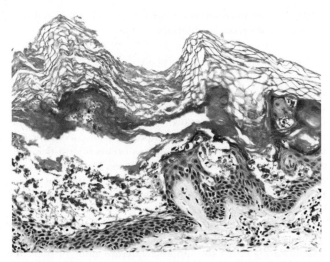

Figure 1.32. Epidermolytic hyperkeratosis. The prominent granular layer is characterized by bizarre, distorted keratohyalin granules (epidermolysis).

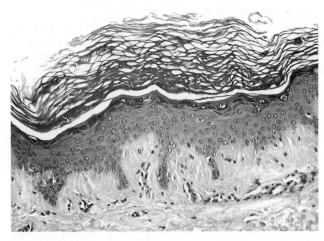

Figure 1.33. Ichthyosis vulgaris. Dense, orthokeratotic hyperkeratosis in an otherwise normal epidermis.

lar keratohyalin granules, and an increase in the thickness of the granular layer constitute epidermolysis (Fig. 1.32). The overlying stratum corneum is hyperkeratotic. A superficial perivascular lymphocytic infiltrate is also present.

"Normal" Epidermis and Dermis

One of the most perplexing situations in dermatopathology occurs when both the epidermis and dermis appear normal. This particular pattern has been termed the *nil lesion*. In addition to the entities described in the next sections, urticaria and telangiectasia macularis eruptiva perstans can present with minimal histologic findings, and these should be considered in the differential diagnosis of microscopically "normal" skin.

VITILIGO
CLINICAL FEATURES. Sharply demarcated depigmented patches that are commonly located on the head and neck, dorsa of the hands, and genitalia characterize vitiligo (119).

HISTOPATHOLOGY. The objective histologic diagnosis of vitiligo (119) is difficult, if not impossible, on routine sections. Melanocytes, which manifest as cells at the dermal-epidermal junction with a clear perinuclear halo, are decreased; this change is best seen by applying the S-100 or melan-A immunoperoxidase stains. However, even when these aids are used, having a control biopsy specimen from adjacent normal skin is helpful for making a semiquantitative estimate of the number of melanocytes present.

ANETODERMA
CLINICAL FEATURES. The lesions of primary anetoderma (120) consist of erythematous macules and urticarial plaques that progress to flaccid, easily reduced, and compressible papules; alternatively, the disease may present as fine, diffuse wrinkling.

HISTOPATHOLOGY. On routine sections, no abnormality is noted in anetoderma (120). However, with elastic tissue stains, a marked reduction or total absence of elastic fibers is revealed in the reticular dermis. The loss of elastic fibers may be limited to the mid reticular dermis. Perivascular mixed inflammatory cell infiltrates may be present in the altered dermis.

ICHTHYOSIS (X-LINKED, LAMELLAR, AND VULGARIS)
CLINICAL FEATURES. Ichthyosis is an inherited skin disease characterized by various patterns of rough scaly patches and plaques (see also "Epidermolytic hyperkeratosis") (121).

HISTOPATHOLOGY. Two types of ichthyosis, X-linked and lamellar, show minimal changes on microscopic examination (121). A third type, ichthyosis vulgaris, is characterized by a decreased or absent granular layer and orthokeratotic hyperkeratosis (Fig. 1.33).

ACANTHOSIS NIGRICANS
CLINICAL FEATURES. Hyperpigmented verrucous plaques are commonly found on the neck, axillae, and groin creases in acanthosis nigricans (122). This disease may be associated with obesity; diabetes mellitus and/or insulin resistance; or malignancy, especially gastrointestinal tumors.

HISTOPATHOLOGY. Orthokeratotic hyperkeratosis and irregular epidermal papillomatosis are present (Fig. 1.34) (122). Contrary to what the term suggests, only slight acanthosis and a minimal increase in melanin are evident.

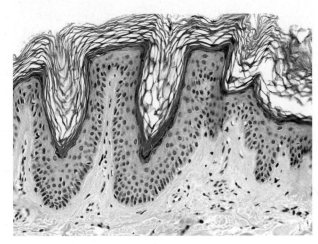

Figure 1.34. Acanthosis nigricans. Orthokeratotic hyperkeratosis and irregular papillomatosis give the epidermis a somewhat verrucous appearance.

TINEA VERSICOLOR

CLINICAL FEATURES. In tinea versicolor (123), *Pityrosporum ovale*, a normal cutaneous flora, can sometimes be pathogenic, leading to the formation of slightly scaly hypopigmented and hyperpigmented macules distributed mainly on the upper trunk and accentuated during the summer.

HISTOPATHOLOGY. Orthokeratotic hyperkeratosis may be the only histologic clue to tinea versicolor (123). A PAS stain will reveal yeast spores and pseudohyphae within the stratum corneum.

POSTINFLAMMATORY PIGMENTARY ALTERATION

CLINICAL FEATURES. Hyperpigmented or variegated macules may occur at the sites of prior inflammatory skin lesions. Determining clinically whether these pigmentary alterations are primary or secondary can be difficult, so a biopsy may be required.

HISTOPATHOLOGY. A sparse, superficial perivascular lymphocytic infiltrate and an increased number of dermal melanophages are present in the upper dermis.

PATTERNS OF DERMAL INFLAMMATION

Although inflammatory diseases of the skin rarely involve either the epidermis or dermis alone, in certain diseases, the diagnostic changes are primarily dermal.

Perivascular Inflammatory Cell Infiltrates

POLYMORPHOUS LIGHT ERUPTION

CLINICAL FEATURES. As the name implies, several different types of clinical lesions may be present in polymorphous light eruption (124). Typically, the patient presents with erythematous papules and vesicles on sun-exposed skin, such as that of the face. Some patients have large plaques, whereas others have only diffuse erythema.

HISTOPATHOLOGY. Superficial and deep perivascular lymphocytic infiltrates are present in polymorphous light eruption (124). The lesions with vesicles may show edema of the papillary dermis (Fig. 1.35), spongiosis, or both, but, in contrast to lupus erythematosus, polymorphous light eruption is associated with minimal or no vacuolar interface change.

GYRATE (FIGURATE) ERYTHEMA

CLINICAL FEATURES. The term *gyrate (figurate) erythema* (125) encompasses several different patterned eruptions, including erythema annulare centrifugum, erythema gyratum repens, and erythema chronicum migrans. The common feature of these eruptions is the presence of multiple waves of curvilinear erythema. Erythema chronicum migrans occurs after a tick bite, and it may be associated with Lyme disease. Erythema gyratum repens is almost invariably associated with an internal malignancy. Erythema annulare centrifugum may be secondary to a variety of infections or other factors.

HISTOPATHOLOGY. The primary histologic finding in gyrate (figurate) erythema is a dense perivascular lymphocytic infiltrate involving either the superficial dermis alone or both the superficial and deep reticular dermis (Fig. 1.36) (125). The lymphocytes are closely adherent to the blood vessel walls and are very well demarcated. In some lesions, a variable amount of epidermal spongiosis may accompany the lymphocytic infiltrates in the dermis.

ARTHROPOD BITE REACTION

CLINICAL FEATURES. A variety of biting insects assault humans. The degree of reaction depends on both the offending agent and the host response (126–129). Insect bites range from small, grouped erythematous papules to large, deep, indurated violaceous nodules that clinically mimic lymphoma.

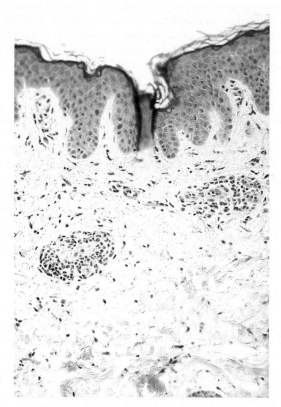

Figure 1.36. Gyrate erythema (erythema annulare centrifugum). Dense superficial perivascular lymphocytic infiltrates closely approximate the dermal blood vessels.

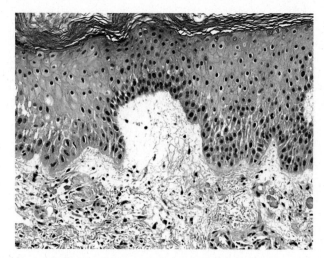

Figure 1.35. Polymorphous light eruption. Perivascular lymphocytic infiltrates are prominent, but both perifollicular inflammation and vacuolar interface change are conspicuously absent.

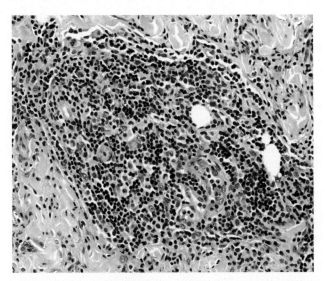

Figure 1.37. Arthropod bite reaction. Lymphocyte hyperplasia consists of a lymphoid follicle with the formation of a germinal center. Eosinophils are usually numerous.

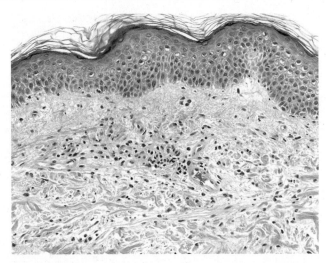

Figure 1.38. Urticaria. A sparse inflammatory infiltrate with scattered eosinophils in the superficial dermis.

HISTOPATHOLOGY. The usual histologic appearance of arthropod bite reaction (126–129) consists of dense, superficial and deep, perivascular lymphocytic infiltrates with numerous admixed eosinophils (Fig. 1.37). Plasma cells are common. Parakeratosis, spongiosis, acanthosis, and epidermal erosions may be present. The extent of lymphocyte proliferation may be so marked that lymphoid follicles with germinal centers are formed. This latter pattern, which is particularly common in tick bite reactions, may closely resemble cutaneous lymphoma. Adnexal structures may be destroyed. In some cases, immunohistochemistry using panels of various monoclonal antibodies to lymphocyte antigens can be helpful in differentiating benign lymphocytic infiltrates from those that are malignant, as can molecular studies and flow cytometric analysis. Clinical correlation is essential in making the diagnosis of cutaneous lymphoma because a significant degree of cytologic atypia may be present in reactive lesions such as insect bites.

URTICARIA

CLINICAL FEATURES. Urticaria, or hives (130,131), can be secondary to ingested substances, including medications; contact with external allergens; systemic infections; malignancies; or physical stimuli, such as heat, cold, pressure, and vibration. The lesions are transient, and they do not remain fixed for longer than approximately 24 hours.

HISTOPATHOLOGY. Sparse perivascular inflammatory cell infiltrates are present in urticaria (Fig. 1.38) (130,131). In some lesions, the inflammatory cells are so inconspicuous that the diagnosis may easily be missed. In early lesions, eosinophils and neutrophils predominate. As the lesions age, the lymphocytes increase in number. Although urticarial lesions appear edematous clinically, detecting edema in the reticular dermis is difficult on routine sections. Edema of the papillary dermis is more easily identified. Vasculitis is generally absent in urticaria. Focal, limited leukocytoclasis and fibrinoid change in vessel walls are indicative of urticarial vasculitis, a clinicopathologic entity that may be associated with lupus erythematosus and hypocomplementemia.

Vasculitis and Vasculopathy

Although perivascular inflammation is present in many cutaneous inflammatory diseases, the term *vasculitis* should be restricted to those processes in which the clinical and histologic manifestations are directly related to the vascular damage. Purpura (nonblanching erythematous macules or papules) is the clinical manifestation of extravasation of red blood cells into the dermis. Microscopically, vasculitis is classified according to the size of the vessel involved (e.g., capillaritis, venulitis) and the type of inflammatory response (leukocytoclastic and/or neutrophilic, lymphocytic, or granulomatous).

Thrombotic occlusion of dermal and subcutaneous blood vessels can occur in various disorders of coagulation, or it can be secondary to cryoprecipitation (cryoglobulinemia or cryofibrinogenemia) leading to cutaneous necrosis without vasculitis (vasculopathy).

CAPILLARITIS (PIGMENTED PURPURAS)

CLINICAL FEATURES. Bilateral nonblanching purpuric and pigmented macules on the ankles and lower legs are collectively called *pigmented purpuras* (132–134). This group includes the progressive pigmentary dermatosis of Schamberg, the purpura annularis telangiectodes of Majocchi, the pigmented purpuric lichenoid dermatitis of Gougerot and Blum, the eczematoid purpura of Doucas and Kapetanakis, and lichen aureus.

HISTOPATHOLOGY. In all of the pigmented purpuras (132–134), pericapillary lymphocytic infiltrates of varying intensity are present in the papillary dermis with the extravasated erythrocytes (Fig. 1.39). Intracellular hemosiderin deposits (iron stain–positive) increase as the lesions progress. The epidermis is either minimally involved, or it is spongiotic. A lichenoid lymphocytic infiltrate with admixed hemosiderin-filled macrophages is present in the Gougerot and Blum type.

LEUKOCYTOCLASTIC VASCULITIS (NECROTIZING VASCULITIS, ALLERGIC VASCULITIS, NEUTROPHILIC VENULITIS)

CLINICAL FEATURES. Palpable purpura, particularly on the lower extremities, is the characteristic clinical lesion of leukocytoclastic vasculitis (135–141). Palpable purpura, fever, arthralgias, abdominal pain, and hematuria comprise the Henoch-

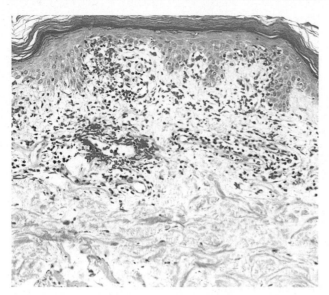

Figure 1.39. Pigmented purpura. Perivascular extravasated erythrocytes in the papillary dermis are characteristic.

Schönlein syndrome. Other diseases that may present with palpable purpura include drug reactions; cryoglobulinemia; connective tissue diseases, such as lupus erythematosus and rheumatoid arthritis; and numerous infections, including viral hepatitis and meningococcemia.

HISTOPATHOLOGY. The histologic hallmark of leukocytoclastic vasculitis is "fibrinoid" (eosinophilic) necrosis of the blood vessel wall, accompanied by fragmented neutrophilic nuclei (leukocytoclasis) (Fig. 1.40) (135–141). Fibrin thrombi may be present in the lumina of involved vessels. Damage to the vessel wall results in the extravasation of erythrocytes. Because the postcapillary venule is the primary target, the changes are usually most marked in the upper dermis, although vessels in the deep dermis and subcutis are also sometimes affected. As the lesion evolves, a mixed inflammatory cell infiltrate replaces the pure neutrophilic one. In the resolving phase, most cells in the infiltrate are lymphocytes, with only a few admixed neu-

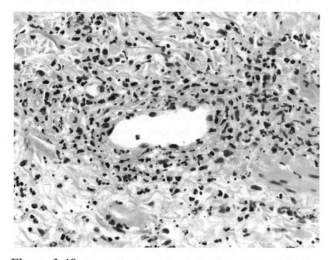

Figure 1.40. Leukocytoclastic vasculitis. Neutrophils with karyorrhexis and fibrinoid necrosis of the vascular wall.

trophils. If the biopsy specimen is taken from a very early or a nearly completely resolved lesion, vessel necrosis may not be found.

ERYTHEMA ELEVATUM DIUTINUM

CLINICAL FEATURES. Erythematous or violaceous nodules and annular plaques are distributed over the joints, especially those of the fingers, wrists, elbows, knees, and toes, in erythema elevatum diutinum (142,143). The older lesions are usually indurated. Erythema elevatum diutinum is frequently associated with human immunodeficiency virus (HIV) disease.

HISTOPATHOLOGY. In addition to a dense, diffuse neutrophilic infiltrate, leukocytoclastic vasculitis is present in early lesions in erythema elevatum diutinum (142,143). Eventually, the number of inflammatory cells decreases as the dermal fibrosis and lamellar "onion skinning" fibroplasia around the vessels increase. In late-stage lesions, the fibrosis predominates, and the neutrophils may be inconspicuous. Extracellular lipid deposits are seen in some late lesions (extracellular cholesterolosis).

GRANULOMA FACIALE

CLINICAL FEATURES. The dusky erythematous papules, plaques, and nodules of granuloma faciale (144) are found primarily on the face, but they may also occur on the trunk.

HISTOPATHOLOGY. Despite its name, granuloma faciale (144) is not a granulomatous dermatitis. The histopathology is similar to that seen in early lesions of erythema elevatum diutinum. A diffuse dermal infiltrate of neutrophils, some of which are karyorrhectic; eosinophils; lymphocytes; and plasma cells is present. Focal vasculitis may be observed. The inflammatory cell infiltrate is eventually replaced by fibroplasia, but this is not as prominent as in erythema elevatum diutinum.

BEHÇET DISEASE

CLINICAL FEATURES. Aphthous ulcers, both oral and genital, may occur in Behçet disease (145). The most characteristic cutaneous lesion is pustular vasculitis, which may be induced by trauma.

HISTOPATHOLOGY. Vasculitis and panniculitis are often combined in the lesions of Behçet disease (145). In addition to leukocytoclastic vasculitis, superficial and deep perivascular and interstitial infiltrates composed of lymphocytes and neutrophils extend through the dermis into the septa and lobules of the subcutis. Some vessels may contain luminal thrombi. Other histologic manifestations of Behçet disease include suppurative folliculitis and intraepidermal or subepidermal vesicles.

POLYARTERITIS NODOSA AND MICROSCOPIC POLYANGIITIS

CLINICAL FEATURES. Polyarteritis nodosa is a systemic vasculitis that involves medium- and small-sized blood vessels (146). A limited cutaneous form occurs in some patients. Cutaneous lesions commonly present as palpable purpura of the lower extremities. Ulceration and infarction may occur. Gastrointestinal lesions can lead to infarction, hemorrhage, and, in some cases, death. Microscopic polyangiitis is a systemic vasculitis that involves small blood vessels and is associated with glomerulonephritis (147,148). Palpable purpura of the lower extremity with occasional ulceration is the typical cutaneous finding.

HISTOPATHOLOGY. The characteristic feature of polyarteritis nodosa is a necrotizing vasculitis involving arteries of the deep dermis and superficial subcutis, especially vessels at the dermal-subcutaneous interface (146). Involvement of these vascular channels may lead to ischemic changes and infarction of the overlying skin. Microscopic polyangiitis shows necrotizing vasculitis of small dermal arteries and can be difficult to differentiate from leukocytoclastic vasculitis (147,148). Distinction from polyarteritis nodosa is based on the size of the arteries involved, clinical presentation, and serologic studies (see following "Adjuncts to microscopic diagnosis" section).

ADJUNCTS TO MICROSCOPIC DIAGNOSIS. Serologic studies are positive for antineutrophil cytoplasmic antibodies (ANCA) in most cases of microscopic polyangiitis (p-ANCA) and are generally negative in polyarteritis nodosa (146–148).

LYMPHOCYTIC VASCULITIS. Lymphocytic vasculitis, which is the destruction of the small blood vessels of the dermis or subcutis by lymphocytes alone, is most commonly seen in pityriasis lichenoides. The presence of perivascular lymphocytes without associated vessel damage is not vasculitis.

GRANULOMATOUS VASCULITIS

CLINICAL FEATURES. Wegener granulomatosis and allergic granulomatosis of Churg and Strauss are types of granulomatous vasculitis (149–154). Both are characterized by the involvement of multiple organs, often including the respiratory tract, kidneys, and heart, in addition to ulcerated cutaneous nodules and plaques.

HISTOPATHOLOGY. Granulomatous vasculitis (149–154) affects the larger arterioles and venules of the deep dermis and subcutis. In addition to a small vessel leukocytoclastic vasculitis, Wegener granulomatosis is characterized by a necrotizing granulomatous infiltrate with large numbers of multinucleated giant cells around medium to large cutaneous vessels. Similar changes are found in allergic granulomatosis, along with abundant eosinophils. Atypical lymphocytes (mainly CD4$^+$ T cells) within a polymorphous, granulomatous infiltrate characterize lymphomatoid granulomatosis (154). These cells are located around the larger blood vessels of the deep dermis, but the granulomatous inflammation may obscure the vasculitis.

ADJUNCTS TO MICROSCOPIC DIAGNOSIS. In most patients, serologic studies are usually positive for ANCAs in Wegener granulomatosis (c-ANCA) and allergic granulomatosis (p-ANCA).

VASCULOPATHY AND ATROPHIE BLANCHE

CLINICAL FEATURES. Cryoprecipitating diseases, including cryoglobulinemia and cryofibrinogenemia, and coagulopathies, such as the antiphospholipid antibody syndromes (caused by lupus anticoagulant or anticardiolipin antibodies), can lead to complete or partial occlusion of the dermal and subcutaneous blood vessels and the formation of necrotic cutaneous plaques or ulcers (155,156).

HISTOPATHOLOGY. Occlusion of the small vessels of the dermis by eosinophilic fibrinoid material leads to the extravasation of erythrocytes (155,156). Inflammation around the affected vessels is minimal or absent. Similar microscopic findings may be found in the lower leg and foot ulcers of atrophie blanche (livedo vasculitis).

Diffuse Dermal Inflammatory Cell Infiltrates

Conditions with diffuse dermal inflammatory cell infiltrates include acute febrile neutrophilic dermatosis, pyoderma gangrenosum, and mastocytosis (157).

ACUTE FEBRILE NEUTROPHILIC DERMATOSIS (SWEET SYNDROME)

CLINICAL FEATURES. Erythematous papules and plaques with superimposed pustules are most commonly found on the upper extremities and face in acute febrile neutrophilic dermatosis (157–160). Fever and leukocytosis may accompany the onset of the skin lesions. Sweet syndrome may precede, may occur simultaneously with, or may follow a diagnosis of hematologic malignancy. It can also occur in association with several other conditions including infections and medications.

HISTOPATHOLOGY. A dense diffuse neutrophilic infiltrate spans the upper and mid reticular dermis (Fig. 1.41) (157–160). Leukocytoclasia is present, but other features of vasculitis are not. Marked papillary dermal edema is often present in early lesions, and subepidermal bullae may be present.

PYODERMA GANGRENOSUM

CLINICAL FEATURES. Pyoderma gangrenosum (161–163) begins as an erythematous papule; this evolves into a pustule that eventually ulcerates. A deep, painful ulcer with undermined violaceous borders is the characteristic clinical lesion. New ulcers develop in areas of trauma (pathergy). Pyoderma gangrenosum is frequently associated with inflammatory bowel disease, multiple myeloma, myeloid leukemia, and hepatitis, although in many cases, other diseases are absent. A bullous form with clinical features that overlap with acute febrile neutrophilic dermatosis has been described, and this variant is highly predictive of an underlying hematologic malignancy.

HISTOPATHOLOGY. The microscopic changes are similar to those of acute febrile neutrophilic dermatosis, but they are more extensive in pyoderma gangrenosum (161–163). A dense dermal neutrophilic infiltrate leads to dermal necrosis and ulceration (Fig. 1.42). Leukocytoclastic vasculitis may be present. Some lesions begin as neutrophilic folliculitis. If the biopsy specimen has been taken from the ulcer edge, the neutrophilic infiltrate may extend beneath intact epidermis, the microscopic equivalent of the undermined borders seen clinically.

MASTOCYTOSIS

CLINICAL FEATURES. Urticaria pigmentosa, the most common form of mastocytosis (164), is characterized by numerous small

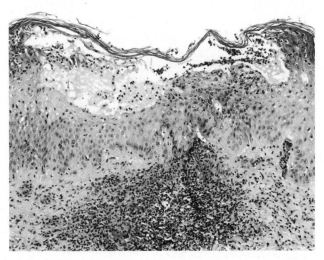

Figure 1.41. Acute febrile neutrophilic dermatosis. A diffuse infiltrate of neutrophils is present in the superficial and mid reticular dermis below an intraepidermal pustule.

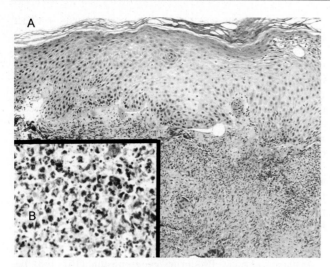

Figure 1.42. Pyoderma gangrenosum. **(A)** A dense neutrophilic infiltrate in the reticular dermis. **(B)** Intact and karyorrhectic neutrophils.

with Leder chloracetate esterase. Immunoperoxidase staining with antibodies directed against the c-Kit antigen is another effective technique for identifying mast cells.

Lipidoses: Xanthelasma and Xanthoma

CLINICAL FEATURES. Xanthelasma (165,166) is characterized by the presence of soft, yellow papules and plaques on the medial eyelids. Xanthomas present as either macules (plane xanthoma), papules (eruptive xanthoma), or nodules (tuberous or tendinous xanthoma). Xanthomas are often distributed over the extensor surfaces of the skin.

HISTOPATHOLOGY. Varying numbers of foamy macrophages infiltrate the dermis in both xanthelasma and xanthomatosis (Fig. 1.44) (165,166). The infiltrate is limited to the upper dermis in xanthelasma, but it occupies the full thickness of the dermis in xanthomatosis. The foam cells have an eccentric nucleus and a large amount of cytoplasm. Multinucleated giant cells may be present. Chronic lesions may become diffusely fibrotic, obscuring the foam cells.

Granulomatous Dermatitis

Granulomas in the dermis and subcutis (167) may be induced by a wide variety of etiologic agents, including many different species of microorganisms and exogenous substances. In addition, endogenous material, most commonly keratinaceous debris forced into the dermis or subcutis from a ruptured epidermoid cyst or dilated hair follicle, will also elicit granulomatous inflammation. The granulomas in granuloma annulare, necro-

yellow-brown papules that urticate when rubbed. Solitary mastocytomas occur most commonly in infants as reddish-tan papules or nodules that also urticate or blister with stroking. Telangiectasia macularis eruptiva perstans is a rare adult form of mastocytosis characterized by telangiectatic red-brown macules. In addition to the skin, mast cell infiltrates may involve the gastrointestinal tract, lymph nodes, liver, spleen, and bone marrow.

HISTOPATHOLOGY. The degree of dermal mast cell infiltration varies greatly between the different clinical types of mastocytosis (Fig. 1.43) (164). Nodular aggregates and diffuse sheets of mast cells are present in the papules and nodules. Variable numbers of eosinophils are present in and around the mast cell infiltrates. Appreciating the subtle increase in perivascular mast cells may be difficult in telangiectasia macularis eruptiva perstans unless special stains are used to highlight the slightly increased number of mast cells around the telangiectatic vessels of the upper dermis. The cytoplasmic mast cell granules show metachromasia (the blue stain colors the granules purple-red) with the toluidine blue and Giemsa stains. The granules also stain

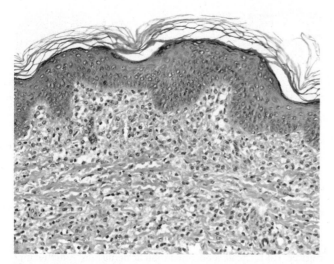

Figure 1.43. Urticaria pigmentosa (mastocytoma). A diffuse infiltrate of mast cells is present in the papillary and upper reticular dermis.

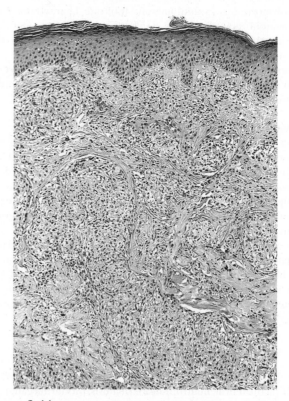

Figure 1.44. Xanthoma. Foamy macrophages fill the upper dermis.

biosis lipoidica, necrobiotic xanthogranuloma, and rheumatoid nodule have been termed *necrobiotic* because the histiocytes cluster around altered collagen fibers. Sarcoidosis and Crohn disease are examples of systemic granulomatous diseases that may present in the skin and subcutis.

SARCOIDOSIS

CLINICAL FEATURES. Cutaneous sarcoidosis (168–171) typically presents as small violaceous to hyperpigmented nodules that may show central clearing. The skin lesions in sarcoidosis are usually asymptomatic. Cutaneous sarcoidosis that occurs on the nose, cheek, and ears is termed *lupus pernio.*

HISTOPATHOLOGY. Well-demarcated granulomas (168–171) are present in any level of the dermis (Fig. 1.45). Epithelioid histiocytes and multinucleated histiocytic giant cells predominate, with a variable lymphocytic infiltrate present at the periphery of the granuloma. The classic sarcoidal granuloma is termed *naked* because of the paucity of lymphocytes in many lesions. The granulomas of sarcoidosis are classified as *nonnecrotizing,* but small areas of necrosis may be present, as may Schaumann or asteroid bodies.

The histologic diagnosis of sarcoidosis in skin is a diagnosis of exclusion. Staining for fungi and acid-fast bacilli should be performed in all cases, in addition to appropriate cultures to rule out infectious causes. Polarization of the specimen should be performed to rule out a foreign body reaction.

INFECTIOUS GRANULOMAS

CLINICAL FEATURES. Many different infectious diseases cause granulomas to form in the skin (172), including leprosy; tuberculosis; atypical acid-fast bacilli infections; deep fungal infections; and protozoal diseases, such as leishmaniasis.

HISTOPATHOLOGY. In microscopic appearance, infectious granulomas (172) range from well-demarcated tuberculoid granulomas to a diffuse inflammatory cell infiltrate with only small, loose granulomas (Fig. 1.46). A central or eccentric focus of neutrophils within a granuloma (necrotizing granuloma) suggests an infectious etiology. Some organisms, such as *Leishmania,* can be found with routine stains, but special stains are usually essential. In skin lesions, the PAS stain is usually preferable to silver stains in searching for fungi because the dermal

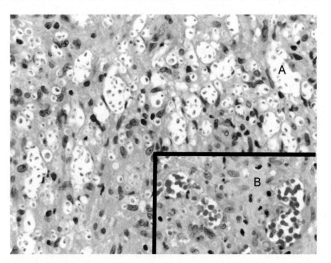

Figure 1.46. Infectious granuloma (cryptococcosis). **(A)** Numerous yeasts are present within epithelioid histiocytes. **(B)** Cryptococcal yeast forms (mucicarmine stain).

reticulum fibers also stain with silver. The Fite modification of the acid-fast stain is superior for staining weakly acid-fast organisms, such as the leprosy bacillus and some atypical mycobacteria.

Perineural granulomas, especially in the mid and deep reticular dermis, require a consideration of leprosy. Granulomas may be only a minor component of the inflammatory cell infiltrate in atypical mycobacterial and *Sporothrix* infections.

GRANULOMAS CAUSED BY EXOGENOUS AND ENDOGENOUS MATERIALS

CLINICAL FEATURES. A wide range of exogenous materials may cause granulomatous inflammation in the skin (173,174). These include beryllium, silica, zirconium, various tattoo pigments, mineral oil, silicone, talc, and starch granules. The keratin proteins in the stratum corneum and the tophaceous urates of gout elicit a marked granulomatous inflammatory response when they come in contact with the dermis.

HISTOPATHOLOGY. Silica granulomas resemble sarcoid, but crystalline material is evident with polarized light. In zirconium and beryllium granulomas, refractile particles cannot usually be detected with polarization (174). Tattoo pigments are irregular, dark intracellular or extracellular granules (Fig. 1.47) (173). Granulomatous dermatitis secondary to the injection of mineral oil or silicone is characterized by large, clear spaces within and between the granulomas and lipid-laden macrophages. Talc is birefringent with polarized light. Starch granules are PAS positive. The inflammatory response to keratinized material consists of poorly formed granulomas with numerous foreign body–type giant cells. Flakes of keratinized material can be found within the inflammation or within the cytoplasm of macrophages.

GRANULOMA ANNULARE

CLINICAL FEATURES. Grouped annular papules, frequently found on the extremities, are characteristic of granuloma annulare (175–177). In rare cases, the papules may be disseminated, and they may be associated with diabetes mellitus. Less common variants of granuloma annulare include perforating granuloma annulare and subcutaneous granuloma annulare.

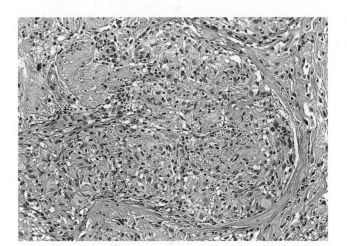

Figure 1.45. Sarcoidosis. A sharply demarcated granuloma composed predominantly of epithelioid histiocytes.

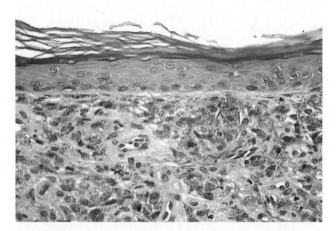

Figure 1.47. Foreign body granuloma (Monsel solution reaction). Intracellular golden brown pigment (ferric subsulfate) is present in the papillary and superficial reticular dermis. The iron pigment stains bright blue with special stains such as Perls Prussian blue.

HISTOPATHOLOGY. Although the concept is somewhat dubious, the primary microscopic finding in granuloma annulare (175–177) has been termed *necrobiosis* (i.e., loose collections of histiocytes that "palisade" around irregular areas of altered dermal collagen). The latter takes on a homogenized appearance, and it is usually associated with an increased quantity of dermal mucin (Fig. 1.48). Lymphocytes may be present at the periphery of the histiocytes. Giant cells are rare. In perforating granuloma annulare, the dermal alteration is superficial, and it is encompassed by epidermis. In the subcutaneous form of granuloma annulare, similar changes are localized to the deep dermis and subcutis.

A clinically significant lesion in the differential diagnosis of granuloma annulare is epithelioid sarcoma. The latter usually has greater cytologic atypia than granuloma annulare, but distinction can be difficult in small biopsies. An immunohistochemical stain for cytokeratin, which is positive in epithelioid sarcoma, is often necessary in this differential diagnosis.

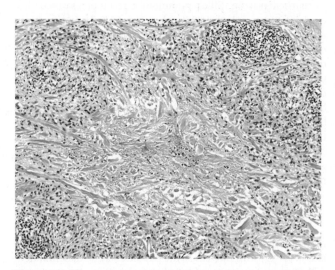

Figure 1.48. Granuloma annulare. Histiocytes and lymphocytes form palisades around altered collagen fibers in the superficial reticular dermis.

NECROBIOSIS LIPOIDICA (NECROBIOSIS LIPOIDICA DIABETICORUM)

CLINICAL FEATURES. The large, yellow atrophic plaques of necrobiosis lipoidica (178,179) are usually located over the shins. When necrobiosis lipoidica is associated with diabetes mellitus, it is termed *necrobiosis lipoidica diabeticorum.*

HISTOPATHOLOGY. The dermal alterations of necrobiosis lipoidica (178,179) are similar to those of granuloma annulare, but they are usually centered deeper in the reticular dermis. In contrast to the more rounded areas of granuloma annulare, the alternating layers of normal and abnormal collagen in necrobiosis lipoidica have a laminated or "sandwiched" appearance. The alteration of dermal collagen is usually more prominent than in granuloma annulare, but a lesser amount of dermal mucin is seen (Fig. 1.49). As the name suggests, lipid deposits may be present in the areas of altered collagen, but this is not typical. The cellular infiltrate around the altered collagen is similar to that of granuloma annulare, except that plasma cells are more common in necrobiosis lipoidica.

NECROBIOTIC XANTHOGRANULOMA

CLINICAL FEATURES. The yellow-red papules, plaques, and nodules of necrobiotic xanthogranuloma (180,181) are usually present around the orbits of older persons, but they may also be found on the neck, trunk, and extremities. The lesions may ulcerate. Necrobiotic xanthogranuloma is frequently associated with a monoclonal IgG paraproteinemia and visceral malignancies.

HISTOPATHOLOGY. Unlike the altered ("necrobiotic") dermal collagen of necrobiosis lipoidica, that of necrobiotic xan-

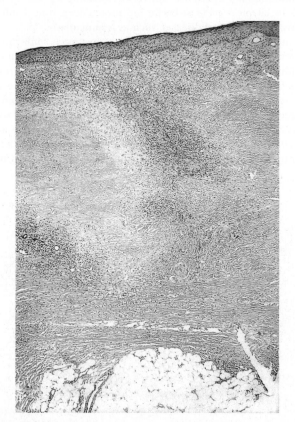

Figure 1.49. Necrobiosis lipoidica. Markedly altered collagen is present between infiltrates of histiocytes, lymphocytes, and plasma cells in a lamellar arrangement ("sandwich" sign).

thogranuloma (180,181) is usually associated with extracellular deposits of lipid, cholesterol clefts, and foam cells. Multinucleated histiocytes, including Touton giant cells, are present. These changes usually extend into the subcutis, resulting in a lobular panniculitis.

RHEUMATOID NODULE

CLINICAL FEATURES. Subcutaneous rheumatoid nodules (182) are found over the extensor aspects of joints such as the elbow. They are usually relatively large nodules, and they may be painful. Rheumatoid nodules occur in adult and juvenile rheumatoid arthritis.

HISTOPATHOLOGY. The histopathology of rheumatoid nodules (182) overlaps with that of deep granuloma annulare and necrobiosis lipoidica. In general, rheumatoid nodules tend to be larger and to be confined to the deep dermis or subcutis (Fig. 1.50). Fibrin may be deposited in the center of the granulomas, as opposed to the mucin deposition of granuloma annulare. Lesions of subcutaneous granuloma annulare can show similar features and require correlation with the clinical and serologic findings for distinction.

Diseases of Hair Follicles and Cartilage

The cutaneous adnexa may be the primary site of dermal inflammation (183,184). The hair follicle with its attached sebaceous gland is the adnexal structure most commonly involved in inflammatory processes.

A discussion of the many different types of hair loss (alopecia) is beyond the scope of this chapter. The reader is referred to the references previously cited for an in-depth discussion of the histopathology of alopecia.

Elastic cartilage is present beneath the dermis in the pinna of the ear and on the nose. Because of this unique anatomic relationship, several diseases specifically involve both the dermis and cartilage.

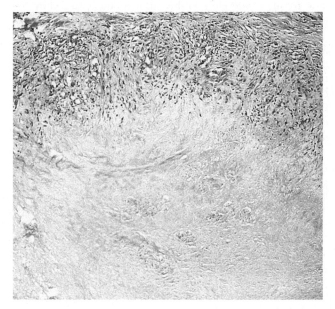

Figure 1.50. Rheumatoid nodule. A large nodule of altered collagen within the deep dermis is surrounded by histiocytes and lymphocytes.

BACTERIAL AND FUNGAL FOLLICULITIS

CLINICAL FEATURES. Bacterial folliculitis (185) is a common skin disorder characterized by tender papulopustules of varying size. Staphylococci are the most common cause of primary bacterial folliculitis.

HISTOPATHOLOGY. Perifollicular neutrophilic infiltrates accompany dilatation of the follicular infundibulum in bacterial folliculitis (185). If the dilatation is extensive, the infundibulum ruptures, with expulsion of the luminal contents into the dermis. The subsequent foreign body–type inflammatory response may destroy the follicle and lead to dermal scar formation.

The inflammatory changes in fungal folliculitis (185), both tinea capitis and tinea corporis, are similar to those of bacterial folliculitis. PAS-positive spores or hyphae are present in or around the hair shafts. In an endothrix infection, the spores are found within the hair shaft. The spores are on the outer surface of the hair shaft in an ectothrix infection. Follicular rupture results in extensive perifollicular granulomatous inflammation (Majocchi granuloma). The follicle is usually destroyed.

ACNE ROSACEA

CLINICAL FEATURES. Erythema of the central part of the face, usually accompanied by acneiform pustules and papules, telangiectasia, and blepharitis, is characteristic of acne rosacea (186,187).

HISTOPATHOLOGY. In contrast to the neutrophilic inflammatory infiltration of bacterial and fungal folliculitis, peri-infundibular lymphocytic or granulomatous inflammation is characteristic of acne rosacea (186,187). The granulomatous inflammation in acne rosacea may be either focally necrotizing or sarcoidal. The latter is indistinguishable from sarcoidosis.

EOSINOPHILIC FOLLICULITIS

CLINICAL FEATURES. Although eosinophilic pustular folliculitis (188–191) is not limited to immunocompromised patients, it frequently occurs in association with HIV disease in the United States. Eosinophilic pustular folliculitis presents with the sudden onset of disseminated follicle-centered pustules, typically on the trunk and less commonly the face.

HISTOPATHOLOGY. Numerous eosinophils infiltrate the hair follicle, particularly the infundibulum, in eosinophilic pustular folliculitis (Fig. 1.51) (188–191). The follicular epithelium is spongiotic. A mixed inflammatory cell infiltrate composed primarily of lymphocytes with a large number of admixed eosinophils is present in the adjacent dermis.

ALOPECIA MUCINOSA (FOLLICULAR MUCINOSIS)

CLINICAL FEATURES. Edematous and erythematous plaques of alopecia with patulous follicular orifices are usually located on the head and neck in alopecia mucinosa (192–197). Alopecia mucinosa in children is a benign, self-limited process, but in adults, follicular mucinosis is frequently a component of cutaneous T-cell lymphoma. *Alopecia mucinosa* is the clinical term, whereas *follicular mucinosis* describes the microscopic findings.

HISTOPATHOLOGY. The keratinocytes of the follicular infundibulum and the outer root sheath are separated by pools of mucin, and they may exhibit a stellate shape in alopecia mucinosa (Fig. 1.52) (192–197). If only a small amount of mucin is present, the condition may mimic follicular spongiosis unless a mucin stain is obtained. A variable number of lymphocytes are within the hair follicle and in the adjacent dermis. The

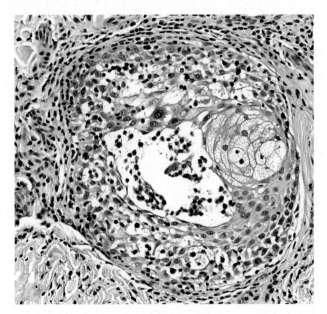

Figure 1.51. Eosinophilic folliculitis. Follicular epithelial spongiosis with an eosinophilic inflammatory infiltrate.

eosinophils are usually admixed. In follicular mucinosis associated with cutaneous T-cell lymphoma, atypical cerebriform lymphocytes are present in the follicle, epidermis, and adjacent dermis.

CHONDRODERMATITIS NODULARIS HELICIS

CLINICAL FEATURES. Chondrodermatitis nodularis (198) presents as an ulcerated painful papule or nodule on the helix of the ear.

HISTOPATHOLOGY. Acanthotic epidermis surrounds the ulcer in chondrodermatitis nodularis (198). Eosinophilic fibrinoid material is present in the ulcer bed. A halo of granulation tissue with prominent small blood vessels is peripheral to the fibrinoid

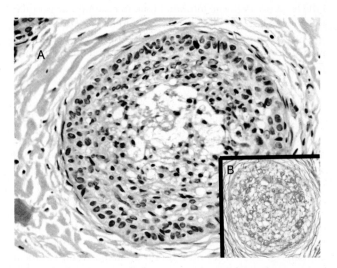

Figure 1.52. Alopecia mucinosa. **(A)** Basophilic mucin deposition within follicular epithelium. **(B)** Colloidal iron stain highlights the increased mucin.

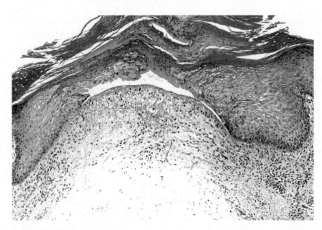

Figure 1.53. Chondrodermatitis nodularis. Marked acanthosis and subjacent fibrinoid changes in the dermis with granulation tissue in the dermis at the periphery of the lesions.

material (Fig. 1.53). The underlying perichondrium is thickened and is infiltrated by inflammatory cells. The cartilage shows degenerative changes, such as a decreased number of chondrocytes, but the dermal and epidermal changes alone are usually sufficient for the diagnosis.

Alterations of Dermal Collagen and Dermal Deposits

The dermal collagen can be altered in many different ways (199). Collagen fibers may be increased or decreased in quantity, or they may be altered in appearance. Deposits of extracellular material may be present.

SCAR, HYPERTROPHIC SCAR, AND KELOID

CLINICAL FEATURES. Scarring is a physiologic response of the dermis to injury (199). When the amount of scar tissue formed is excessive, the term *hypertrophic scar* is used. Keloids (200) are still larger exophytic flesh-colored nodules and plaques that most frequently develop on the earlobes and central chest following trauma or surgery.

HISTOPATHOLOGY. Increased numbers of small blood vessels and granulation tissue are present in young scars (200). The collagen fibers are oriented in a horizontal direction, parallel to the epidermis. As the scar ages, these are replaced by thicker collagen bundles. Excessive, poorly defined nodules of collagen fibers form a hypertrophic scar. Thus, the major morphologic difference between a physiologic scar and a hypertrophic scar is quantitative.

In contrast, large, abnormal, brightly eosinophilic ''glassy'' collagen fibers replace the normal fibrillar collagen in a keloid (Fig. 1.54) (200). Keloids are mostly hypocellular, but cellular islands of fibroblasts are typically interspersed among the abnormal collagen bundles.

SCLERODERMA (SYSTEMIC SCLEROSIS) AND MORPHEA

CLINICAL FEATURES. Although the clinical presentations of morphea and scleroderma (201–207) differ greatly, the two share histologic features that are, for the most part, identical. Scleroderma is a serious systemic disease involving the visceral organs in addition to the skin. In scleroderma, the involved skin first appears edematous and thickened, and it later becomes sclerotic. In contrast, morphea is a purely cutaneous disease

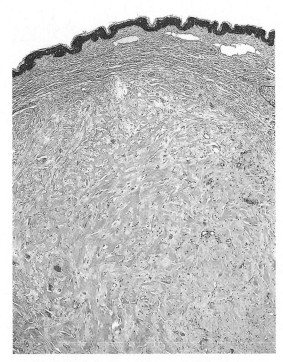

Figure 1.54. Keloid. The entire dermis is expanded by a nodule of thickened, brightly eosinophilic collagen fibers.

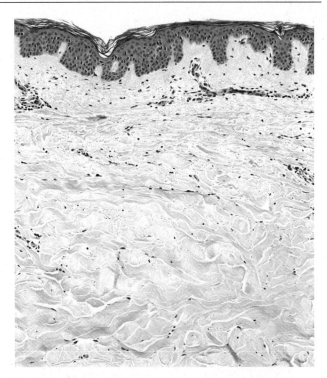

Figure 1.55. Morphea. The dermis is sclerotic, adnexa are decreased, and a lymphocytic infiltrate is present adjacent to an eccrine coil. The reticular dermal-subcutaneous interface is obscured.

that presents with well-defined ivory-white plaques; these may have round, oval, or geographic margins and a violaceous halo.

Although the evidence is controversial, some evidence does exist that indicates that, in some patients, clinical lesions closely resembling or identical to those of morphea are associated with *Borrelia burgdorferi* infection. The sclerodermoid form of chronic GVHD is clinically indistinguishable from scleroderma. Porphyria cutanea tarda may have a sclerodermalike appearance.

HISTOPATHOLOGY. In the early lesions of both morphea and scleroderma (201–207), the change in the collagen may be minimal. Perivascular and periadnexal lymphocytic infiltrates are usually most pronounced in the deep reticular dermis, especially around the eccrine coils. Eventually, the dermis becomes sclerotic; in other words, the normal collagen fiber pattern is replaced by broad, homogeneous eosinophilic fibers. A band of lymphocytes may be found at the junction of the normal and abnormal collagen and may even extend into the subcutis. A characteristic feature of advanced morphea and scleroderma is the blunting of the dermal-subcutaneous interface (Fig. 1.55). The fibrous septa of the subcutis become thickened. The thickened sclerotic dermis imparts a characteristic rectangular shape to the punch biopsy gross specimen. In addition, the lipocytes around the eccrine coils may be decreased in number, or they may be absent. This finding alone is not diagnostic of morphea or scleroderma because lipocytes around the eccrine coils may be lacking in normal skin of the back, a common location for morphea. A "control" biopsy specimen taken from adjacent normal skin for comparison with the abnormally thickened lesional skin is usually helpful.

LICHEN SCLEROSUS

CLINICAL FEATURES. Atrophic, hypopigmented papules coalesce to form patches and plaques in lichen sclerosus et atro-

phicus (208–211). The lesions frequently occur on the trunk and genitalia.

HISTOPATHOLOGY. In lichen sclerosus (208–211), the epidermis is characterized by orthokeratotic hyperkeratosis, atrophy resulting in loss of the rete ridges, and vacuolar interface change. The follicular orifices may be plugged with stratum corneum (Fig. 1.56). The superficial reticular dermis is transformed by homogeneous pale-staining collagen. A bandlike lymphocytic infiltrate is present at the border between the abnormal superficial collagen and the deeper normal fibers.

MYXEDEMA

CLINICAL FEATURES. Myxedema (212) exists in two forms. Generalized myxedema occurs in patients with hypothyroidism. The skin is thickened, dry, and waxy. Hyperthyroid patients have pretibial myxedema, which is characterized by thick, waxy plaques on the shins.

HISTOPATHOLOGY. The microscopic changes of myxedema (212) in both thyroid states are qualitatively identical. Mucin, which is easily demonstrated with mucin stains, separates the collagen bundles of the reticular dermis (Fig. 1.57). Mucin is usually much more abundant in pretibial than in generalized myxedema.

SCLEROMYXEDEMA

CLINICAL FEATURES. Scleromyxedema (212,213) presents with small, dome-shaped, flesh-colored papules on the dorsal hands, axillary folds, and lower extremities; these are accompanied by progressive induration of the skin that may affect mobility. IgG monoclonal paraproteinemia is usually present. The lesions of scleromyxedema are clinically and histologically similar to the fibrosing dermopathy described in renal transplant patients.

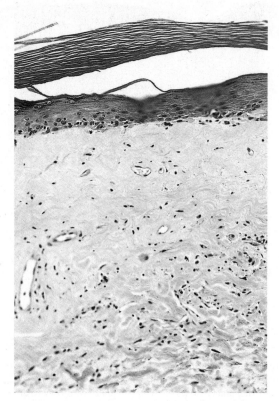

Figure 1.56. Lichen sclerosus et atrophicus. Hyperkeratosis, an atrophic epidermis, and extensive homogenization of the papillary dermal collagen are characteristic. Focal vacuolar interface alteration is often present.

HISTOPATHOLOGY. Increased numbers of fibroblasts, thick collagen bundles, and abundant dermal mucin deposits are present in fully developed lesions of scleromyxedema (Fig. 1.58) (212,213). The mucin stains with colloidal iron or alcian blue at a pH of 2.5, and it is susceptible to hyaluronidase digestion. Older lesions exhibit prominent fibroplasia with less prominent mucin deposition.

NEPHROGENIC SYSTEMIC FIBROSIS (NEPHROGENIC FIBROSING DERMOPATHY)

CLINICAL FEATURES. Nephrogenic systemic fibrosis is a fibrosing condition that develops in patients with renal failure (214). Relatively symmetric erythematous papules and nodules are present in early lesions with coalescence into broad, indurated plaques. The extremities and the trunk are the common sites of involvement, and the face is generally spared. Cutaneous lesions predominate, but lesions have also been demonstrated in internal viscera. Although the exact etiology is not known, studies have shown an association with gadolinium contrast agents (215).

HISTOPATHOLOGY. In early lesions, there is slight dermal fibrosis with increased fibroblast. In well-developed lesions, there is diffuse dermal fibrosis, increased dermal cellularity, and variably increased dermal mucin (214). Inflammation is minimal to mild. Immunohistochemistry for CD34 shows a diffuse pattern of positive cells in the dermis (214).

The histopathology of cutaneous lesions in nephrogenic systemic fibrosis is similar to scleromyxedema. Scleromyxedema

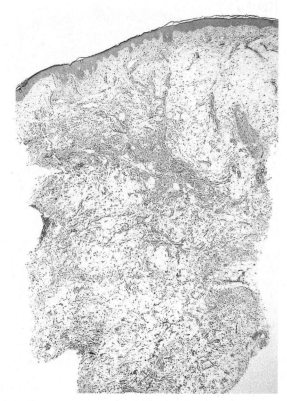

Figure 1.57. Myxedema. The reticular dermal collagen fibers are splayed apart by mucin.

generally shows a greater increase in both dermal mucin and inflammatory cells and lacks the diffuse increase in CD34-positive dermal cells. In addition, the clinical features of the two diseases are distinctly different.

SCLEREDEMA (OF BUSCHKE)

CLINICAL FEATURES. The skin of the upper back is markedly thickened by nonpitting, woody induration. Scleredema (216–218) is usually associated with diabetes mellitus.

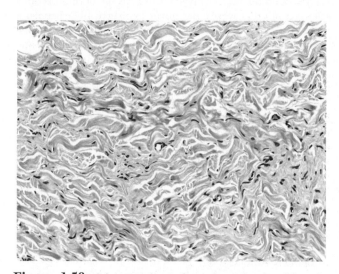

Figure 1.58. Scleromyxedema. Dermal mucin deposition, increased collagen, and fibroblast proliferation are present.

HISTOPATHOLOGY. Despite marked thickening of the dermis in scleredema (216–218), the collagen pattern remains normal. Dermal mucin may not be readily apparent with routine stains, but variably prominent clear spaces are present between the reticular dermal collagen bundles. These spaces are actually filled with mucin. With special stains, the mucin may be abundant, or it may be difficult to demonstrate because it may be removed with aqueous formalin fixation. The use of frozen sections improves the sensitivity of mucin stains. Inflammation, if it is present at all, is minimal.

AMYLOIDOSIS

CLINICAL FEATURES. Primary systemic amyloidosis (219–223) may present with a variety of features, including papules, plaques, tumors, and purpura secondary to minimal trauma. The latter is especially common on the eyelids, and it is referred to as *pinch purpura*. In localized cutaneous amyloidosis, only the skin is involved. This type of amyloidosis occurs in the following three forms: lichenoid, macular, and nodular. Lichen amyloidosis usually presents as pruritic papules and plaques on the pretibial skin. In macular amyloidosis, reticulated hyperpigmentation is present on the upper back. As the name suggests, nodular amyloidosis presents as large nodules, primarily on the lower extremities.

HISTOPATHOLOGY. Primary systemic amyloidosis (219–223) cannot be distinguished from localized cutaneous amyloidosis microscopically. In all types, the amyloid deposition first appears in the basement membranes of the blood vessels and adnexa; this is followed by the replacement of the collagen of the dermal papillae (Fig. 1.59). The deposits have a characteristic pale eosinophilia and a "cracked" appearance. In both lichen and macular amyloidosis, the amyloid deposits are limited to the papillary dermis. In nodular lesions, the amyloid deposits are present throughout the reticular dermis, and they may even extend into the subcutis.

Amyloid deposits stain orange-red with the Congo red stain. Polarization of Congo red–stained sections demonstrates a characteristic apple green dichromism. Thick tissue sections (approximately 10 µm) enhance both the staining and the in-

tensity of the dichromism. Linear, nonbranching amyloid filaments can be demonstrated with electron microscopy.

CALCINOSIS CUTIS AND CALCIPHYLAXIS

CLINICAL FEATURES. Cutaneous calcium deposits appear in several different forms (224–229). These include metastatic calcification, dystrophic calcification, idiopathic calcification, subepidermal calcified nodule, and calciphylaxis. Metastatic calcification occurs most frequently in patients with hyperparathyroidism or chronic renal failure who have abnormal serum calcium and phosphorus values. In dystrophic calcinosis cutis, calcium deposits develop in areas of previously abnormal skin. The serum calcium and phosphorus values are normal. As the name implies, idiopathic calcinosis cutis has no known cause. The following two forms are commonly recognized: tumoral calcinosis, in which large, subcutaneous calcified masses are found; and the more common idiopathic calcinosis of the scrotum, in which small calcified nodules develop in scrotal skin. The subepidermal calcified nodule presents in childhood as a small, flesh-colored, firm papule on the face.

Extensive calcification of the intima and media of the dermal and subcutaneous blood vessels, especially the larger vessels of the subcutis, has been termed *cutaneous vascular calciphylaxis*. Lesions present as painful violaceous nodules and ulcerations typically involving the proximal lower extremities and trunk. This process may result in extensive cutaneous necrosis and may be lethal. Calciphylaxis occurs most frequently in patients with chronic renal failure and abnormal serum calcium and phosphorus metabolism. The specific etiology of this condition is unknown.

HISTOPATHOLOGY. In all of the different types of cutaneous calcification (224–229) except calciphylaxis, the calcium deposits are amorphous, deeply basophilic, extracellular, and dermal. A foreign body reaction consisting of multinucleated giant cells and other inflammatory cells surrounds the calcium deposits (Fig. 1.60). The calcium ranges in quantity from small granules to massive deposits that encompass the entire thickness of the dermis and extend into the subcutis.

The intima and media of large and small blood vessels of the subcutis are extensively calcified in cutaneous calciphylaxis (Fig. 1.61). The calcium deposits are associated with luminal occlusion by thrombi. These changes are most apparent in the vessels adjacent to an ulcer.

Both the von Kossa and alizarin red stains are useful in identifying calcium deposits. The von Kossa stain is not specific for calcium because it reacts with the anion in calcium salts. Alizarin red specifically stains the calcium moiety.

CUTANEOUS GOUT

CLINICAL FEATURES. Gouty deposits in skin (tophi) are uncommon (230,231). They present as firm, deep nodules on the helix of the ear, around the elbows, or on the digits. A chalky material may be extruded from the nodules.

HISTOPATHOLOGY. Tophi are amorphous, pale-staining deposits of monosodium urate crystals in the dermis or subcutis (230,231). The deposits may have a brown tinge, and they are usually surrounded by a foreign body–type granulomatous infiltrate. The deposits frequently calcify, especially when they are large and long-standing. The amorphous deposits are best preserved when the specimen is fixed in anhydrous alcohol rather than in formalin. If any crystals are present in the amorphous aggregates, they can be examined for negative birefringence, a diagnostic characteristic of the monosodium urate crystal.

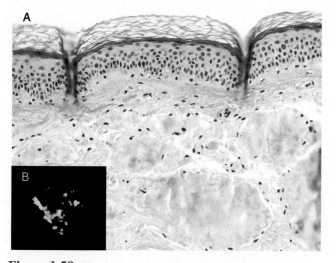

Figure 1.59. Cutaneous amyloidosis. **(A)** Amyloid deposits consisting of amorphous, faintly eosinophilic, acellular material in the superficial dermis. **(B)** The amyloid deposits show apple green dichromism in polarized Congo red–stained sections.

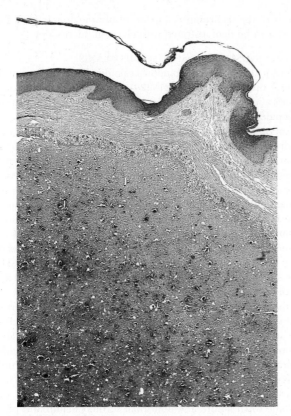

Figure 1.60. Calcinosis cutis. Calcium deposits are deeply basophilic in hematoxylin and eosin–stained sections.

When a primary color compensator lens is positioned between the two polarizing lenses, the crystals appear yellow or blue, depending on the plane of polarization.

Panniculitis

Inflammatory diseases of the subcutis rarely present with diagnostic clinical findings other than a characteristic anatomic lo-

cation or clinical setting (232,233). In addition to the primary diseases of the subcutis discussed in this section, systemic processes such as infectious disease and vasculitis may involve the subcutis. A deep biopsy specimen that includes the full thickness of the subcutis is essential for an adequate microscopic evaluation of panniculitis.

Panniculitis (232,233) can be divided into two anatomic patterns, septal and lobular, depending on whether the major histologic changes are located in the fibrous septa or the adipocyte lobules.

SEPTAL PANNICULITIS. Conditions including septal panniculitis include erythema nodosum and α_1-antitrypsin deficiency panniculitis (234).

Erythema nodosum

CLINICAL FEATURES. Painful tender nodules on the shins are characteristic of erythema nodosum (234–236). Because the inflammation is essentially limited to the subcutis, the nodules are diffuse and poorly demarcated. Erythema nodosum is associated with many diseases, including a variety of infectious diseases, drugs reactions, and sarcoidosis. No clinical association is found in many cases.

HISTOPATHOLOGY. In early lesions of erythema nodosum (234–236), neutrophils and lymphocytes infiltrate the fibrous septa of the subcutis (Fig. 1.62). The inflammatory cells frequently extend for a limited distance into the lobules of the subcutis. As the lesion develops, the lymphocytes and neutrophils decrease while the histiocytes and giant cells increase, imparting a somewhat granulomatous appearance. Eventually, only minimal inflammation remains, and the septa become expanded by fibrosis.

α_1-Antitrypsin deficiency panniculitis

CLINICAL FEATURES. Diffuse indurated erythematous plaques that are frequently mistaken for bacterial cellulitis develop in areas exposed to trauma, such as the extensor surfaces of the arms, legs, and thighs. The plaques eventually break down and drain serosanguineous fluid. The serum levels of α_1-antitrypsin are low. The cutaneous lesions of α_1-antitrypsin deficiency may

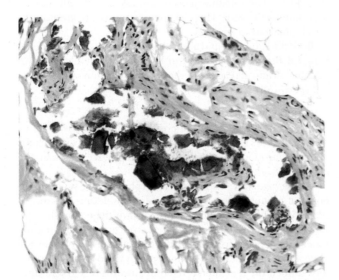

Figure 1.61. Calciphylaxis. The intima and media of large and small blood vessels are extensively calcified. The calcium deposits are often associated with luminal occlusion by thrombi.

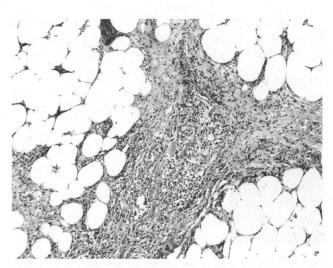

Figure 1.62. Erythema nodosum. A mixed inflammatory cell infiltrate including neutrophils and multinucleated giant cells is present in the septa.

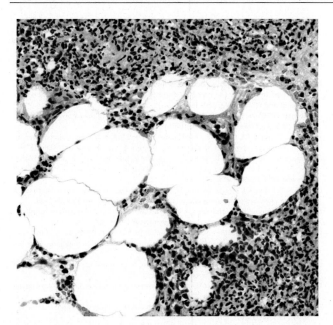

Figure 1.63. α₁-Antitrypsin deficiency panniculitis. A neutrophilic panniculitis that involves both lobules (as shown) and septa. Necrosis is typical.

either precede or follow other visceral manifestations of the disease, such as emphysema and cirrhosis (237–241).

HISTOPATHOLOGY. Initially, diffuse neutrophilic infiltrates extend through the dermis into the septa and lobules of the subcutis (Fig. 1.63) (237–241). As the lesion evolves, the collagen is destroyed (collagenolysis), and the number of inflammatory cells decreases. Eventually, rounded lobules of subcutis are found "floating" in purulent material secondary to lysis of the septal collagen. This change is highly suggestive of α₁-antitrypsin deficiency panniculitis. In draining lesions, channels lined by squamous epithelium extend into and surround the altered dermis, with subsequent transepidermal elimination of the liquefied material. The lesions heal with extensive scarring of the dermis and subcutis.

LOBULAR PANNICULITIS. Nodular vasculitis (erythema induratum), subcutaneous fat necrosis of the newborn, pancreatic fat necrosis, lupus panniculitis, and physical and factitial panniculitis are some of the conditions characterized by lobular panniculitis (242).

Nodular vasculitis (erythema induratum)

CLINICAL FEATURES. This relatively rare form of panniculitis was, in the past, frequently associated with tuberculosis (243–246). The term *nodular vasculitis* is used when no evidence of coexisting tuberculosis is found. The typical location is the posterior calf.

HISTOPATHOLOGY. Nodular vasculitis (243–246) is essentially a granulomatous vasculitis affecting the large vessels of the subcutis, although multiple serial sections may be required to demonstrate the involved vessel. The granulomatous inflammation is present in the lobules of the subcutis. The degree of caseation necrosis is variable.

Subcutaneous fat necrosis of the newborn

CLINICAL FEATURES. Infants with subcutaneous fat necrosis of the newborn (247) are typically in good health. The panniculitis

commonly occurs on the trunk, extremities, buttocks, and cheeks.

HISTOPATHOLOGY. Basophilic fat necrosis and clusters of needlelike clefts are present in the adipocyte lobules, within both lipocytes and histiocytes in subcutaneous fat necrosis of the newborn (247). The clefts may be filled with refractile crystals. Granulomatous inflammation may be present within the altered adipocyte lobules. Small calcium deposits are frequently noted.

Pancreatic fat necrosis

CLINICAL FEATURES. Elevated levels of serum amylase and lipase secondary to pancreatitis or carcinoma of the pancreas can result in panniculitis (248–250). The lesions may be widespread, and they may ulcerate to drain a chalky material.

HISTOPATHOLOGY. In pancreatic fat necrosis (248–250), the affected lipocytes stain deeply basophilic secondary to calcium salt deposition. Loss of the nuclei of the cells results in the formation of characteristic basophilic "rings" (Fig. 1.64). Extracellular granular calcium deposits may be present within the lobules. A granulomatous inflammatory reaction may be present at the periphery of the panniculitis.

Lupus panniculitis

CLINICAL FEATURES. Lupus panniculitis (lupus profundus) (251,252) may develop in a pre-existing lesion of lupus erythematosus or de novo on previously normal skin. In the latter case, it resembles other forms of panniculitis. Lupus panniculitis may develop in patients with either systemic or discoid lupus erythematosus.

HISTOPATHOLOGY. When the lesions exhibit the clinical changes of cutaneous lupus, the typical histologic findings of lupus (i.e., vacuolar interface change and lymphocytic infiltrates) are usually present in the overlying dermis (251,252). If the lesion presents as pure panniculitis clinically, the histologic changes are limited to the subcutis. The adipocyte cell membranes are replaced by basophilic material, and the loss of the nuclei results in the formation of so-called ghost cells. The end result is basophilic sclerosis of the lobule. Dense lymphoplasmacytic infiltrates are present in the lobules and adjacent septa (Fig. 1.65). Mucin deposition may be evident in the overlying dermis and in the septa. Eventually, the altered lobules are replaced by fibrosis.

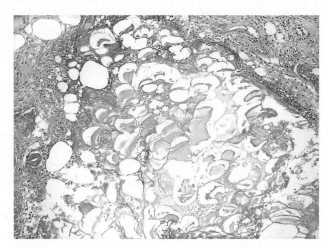

Figure 1.64. Pancreatic fat necrosis. Minimal inflammation, loss of lipocyte basophilia, and small calcium deposits are characteristic.

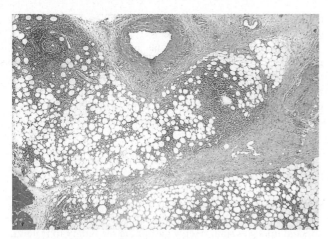

Figure 1.65. Lupus panniculitis. This is an early lesion in which the lymphoplasmacytic lobular infiltrates are extensive and the distinctive basophilia in the lobule is limited.

Physical and factitial panniculitis

CLINICAL FEATURES. Panniculitis (253–255) may result from physical trauma, such as blunt force, pinching, and cold. These and other insults may be inadvertent, or they may be inflicted specifically to cause injury. A variety of foreign substances may be injected into the subcutis to produce an obvious skin lesion for secondary gain.

HISTOPATHOLOGY. Neutrophils are present in the lobules of the subcutis in both mechanically induced panniculitis and panniculitis resulting from the injection of foreign material (253–255). Neutrophils and focal fat necrosis may be the only changes in minimal lesions caused by mechanical trauma, whereas in lesions caused by more violent force, extensive fat necrosis and hemorrhage are seen. Finding identifiable foreign material in lesions induced by injection is surprisingly rare. When factitial panniculitis secondary to injection is suspected, the sections should be examined with polarized light to facilitate the identification of any refractile crystalline material. However, only calcium deposits, mixed neutrophilic and granulomatous infiltrates, and adipocyte necrosis may be present.

The histologic findings in factitial panniculitis overlap with those of α_1-antitrypsin deficiency and infectious panniculitis; therefore, factitial panniculitis is a diagnosis of exclusion that should be made only after appropriate tissue cultures and laboratory studies have yielded negative results, unless confirming clinical evidence is found.

REFERENCES

1. Wallace ML, Smoller BR. Immunohistochemistry in diagnostic dermatopathology. *J Am Acad Dermatol* 1996;34:163–183.
2. White WL. Immunomicroscopy in diagnostic dermatopathology: an update on cutaneous neoplasms. *Adv Dermatol* 1999;14:359–396.
3. Hudson AR, Smoller BR. Immunohistochemistry in diagnostic dermatopathology. *Dermatol Clin* 1999;17:667–689.
4. Schach CP, Smoller BR, Hudson AR, Horn TD. Immunohistochemical stains in dermatopathology. *J Am Acad Dermatol* 2000;43:1094–1100.
5. Headington JT. Transverse microscopic anatomy of the human scalp. A basis for a morphometric approach to disorders of the hair follicle. *Arch Dermatol* 1984;120:449–454.
6. Solomon AR. The transversely sectioned scalp biopsy specimen: the technique and an algorithm for its use in the diagnosis of alopecia. *Adv Dermatol* 1994;9:127–157.
7. Sperling LC, Lupton GP. Histopathology of non-scarring alopecia. *J Cutan Pathol* 1995; 22:97–114.
8. Elston DM, McCollough ML, Angeloni VL. Vertical and transverse sections of alopecia biopsy specimens: combining the two to maximize diagnostic yield. *J Am Acad Dermatol* 1995;32:454–457.
9. McKee PH, Calonje E, Granter SR. The structure and function of skin. In *Pathology of the Skin with Clinical Correlations.* 3rd edition. Philadelphia, PA: Elsevier-Mosby, 2005:16–18.
10. McKee PH, Calonje E, Granter SR. The structure and function of skin. In *Pathology of the Skin with Clinical Correlations.* 3rd edition. Philadelphia, PA: Elsevier-Mosby, 2005:18–20.
11. Ackerman A. Allergic contact dermatitis/nummular dermatitis/dyshidrotic dermatitis/ id reaction. In *Histologic Diagnosis of Inflammatory Skin Disease.* 2nd edition. Baltimore, MD: Williams and Wilkins, 1997:184–186.
12. Kutzner H, Wurzel RM, Wolff HH. Are acrosyringia involved in the pathogenesis of "dyshidrosis"? *Am J Dermatopathol* 1986;8:109–116.
13. Olerud JE, Kulin PA, Chew DE, et al. Cutaneous T-cell lymphoma: evaluation of pretreatment skin biopsy specimens by a panel of pathologists. *Arch Dermatol* 1992;128:501–507.
14. Trautmann A, Altznauer F, Akdis M, et al. The differential fate of cadherins during T-cell–induced keratinocyte apoptosis leads to spongiosis in eczematous dermatitis. *J Invest Dermatol* 2001;117:927–934.
15. Le TK, Schalkwijk J, Van de Kerkhof PC, et al. A histological and immunohistochemical study on chronic irritant contact dermatitis. *Am J Contact Dermatitis* 1998;9:23–28.
16. Doyle JA, Connolly SM, Hunziker N, Winkelmann RK. Prurigo nodularis: a reappraisal of the clinical and histologic features. *J Cutan Pathol* 1979;6:392–403.
17. Harris B, Harris K, Penneys NS. Demonstration by S-100 protein staining of increased numbers of nerves in the papillary dermis of patients with prurigo nodularis. *J Am Acad Dermatol* 1992;26:56–58.
18. Rowland Payne CM, Wilkinson JD, McKee PH, et al. Nodular prurigo—a clinicopathological study of 46 patients. *Br J Dermatol* 1985;113:431–439.
19. El-Shiemy S, Nassar A, Mokhtar M, et al. Light and electron microscopic studies of pityriasis rosea. *Int J Dermatol* 1987;26:237–239.
20. Kempf W, Burg G. Pityriasis rosea—a virus-induced skin disease? An update. *Arch Virol* 2000;145:1509–1520.
21. Gianni C, Morelli V, Cerri A, et al. Usefulness of histological examination for the diagnosis of onychomycosis. *Dermatology* 2001;202:283–288.
22. Taieb A, El Youbi A, Grosshans E, Maleville J. Lichen striatus: a Blaschko linear acquired inflammatory skin eruption. *J Am Acad Dermatol* 1991;25:637–642.
23. Zhang Y, McNutt NS. Lichen striatus. Histological, immunohistochemical, and ultrastructural study of 37 cases. *J Cutan Pathol* 2001;28:65–71.
24. Rao B, Unis M, Poulos E. Acroangiodermatitis: a study of ten cases. *Int J Dermatol* 1994; 33:179–183.
25. Burks JW, Montgomery H. Histopathologic study of psoriasis. *Arch Dermatol* 1943;48: 479–493.
26. Gordon M, Johnson WC. Histopathology and histochemistry of psoriasis. I. The active lesion and clinically normal skin. *Arch Dermatol* 1967;95:402–407.
27. Zip C, Murray S, Walsh NM. The specificity of histopathology in erythroderma. *J Cutan Pathol* 1993;20:393–398.
28. Walsh NM, Prokopetz R, Tron VA, et al. Histopathology in erythroderma: review of a series of cases by multiple observers. *J Cutan Pathol* 1994;21:419–423.
29. Trozak DJ. Histologic grading system for psoriasis vulgaris. *Int J Dermatol* 1994;33:380–381.
30. Prystowsky JH, Cohen PR. Pustular and erythrodermic psoriasis. *Dermatol Clin* 1995;13: 757–771.
31. Altman EM, Kamino H. Diagnosis: psoriasis or not? What are the clues? *Semin Cutan Med Surg* 1999;18:25–35.
32. Magro CM, Crowson AN. The clinical and histomorphological features of pityriasis rubra pilaris. A comparative analysis with psoriasis. *J Cutan Pathol* 1997;24:416–424.
33. Sorensen KB, Thestrup-Pedersen K. Pityriasis rubra pilaris: a retrospective analysis of 43 patients. *Acta Derm Venereol* 1999;79:405–406.
34. Ellis FA. Histopathology of lichen planus based on analysis of one hundred biopsy specimens. *J Invest Dermatol* 1967;48:143–148.
35. Taaffe A. Current concepts in lichen planus. *Int J Dermatol* 1979;18:533–538.
36. Boyd AS, Neldner KH. Lichen planus. *J Am Acad Dermatol* 1991;25:593–619.
37. Bagan-Sebastian JV, Milian-Masanet MA, Penarrocha-Diago M, Jimenez Y. A clinical study of 205 patients with oral lichen planus. *J Oral Maxillofac Surg* 1992;50:116–118.
38. Sanchez-Perez J, De Castro M, Buezo GF, et al. Lichen planus and hepatitis C virus: prevalence and clinical presentation of patients with lichen planus and hepatitis C virus infection. *Br J Dermatol* 1996;134:715–719.
39. Eisen D. The clinical features, malignant potential, and systemic associations of oral lichen planus: a study of 723 patients. *J Am Acad Dermatol* 2002;46:207–214.
40. Mihara M, Nakayama H, Shimao S. Lichen nitidus: a histologic and electron microscopic study. *J Dermatol* 1991;18:475–480.
41. Bleicher PA, Dover JS, Arndt KA. Lichenoid dermatoses and related disorders. I. Lichen planus and lichenoid drug-induced eruptions. *J Am Acad Dermatol* 1990;22:288–292.
42. Halevy S, Shai A. Lichenoid drug eruptions. *J Am Acad Dermatol* 1993;29:249–255.
43. Clark WH, Reed RJ, Mihm MC. Lupus erythematosus. Histopathology of cutaneous lesions. *Hum Pathol* 1973;4:157–163.
44. Ashworth J, Turbitt M, MacKie R. A comparison of the dermal lymphoid infiltrates in discoid lupus erythematosus and Jessner's lymphocytic infiltrate of the skin using the monoclonal antibody Leu 8. *J Cutan Pathol* 1987;14:198–201.
45. Magro CM, Crowson AN, Kovatich AJ, Burns F. Lupus profundus, indeterminate lymphocytic lobular panniculitis and subcutaneous T-cell lymphoma: a spectrum of subcuticular T-cell lymphoid dyscrasia. *J Cutan Pathol* 2001;28:235–247.
46. Hanno R, Callen JP. Histopathology of Gottron's papules. *J Cutan Pathol* 1985;12:389–394.
47. Tsao H, Busam K, Barnhill RL, Haynes HA. Lesions resembling malignant atrophic papulosis in a patient with dermatomyositis. *J Am Acad Dermatol* 1997;36:317–319.
48. Wood GS, Strickler JG, Deneau DG, et al. Lymphomatoid papulosis expresses immunophenotypes associated with T cell lymphoma but not inflammation. *J Am Acad Dermatol* 1986;15:444–448.
49. Wood GS, Strickler JG, Abel EA, et al. Immunohistology of pityriasis lichenoides et varioli-

formis acuta and pityriasis lichenoides chronica. Evidence for their interrelationship with lymphomatoid papulosis. *J Am Acad Dermatol* 1987;16:559–570.
50. Longley J, Demar L, Feinstein RP, et al. Clinical and histologic features of pityriasis lichenoides et varioliformis acuta in children. *Arch Dermatol* 1987;123:1335–1339.
51. Kadin ME. Lymphomatoid papulosis, Ki-1^{+} lymphoma, and primary cutaneous Hodgkin's disease. *Semin Dermatol* 1991;10:164–171.
52. Davis TH, Morton CC, Miller-Cassman R, et al. Hodgkin's disease, lymphomatoid papulosis, and cutaneous T-cell lymphoma derived from a common T-cell clone. *N Engl J Med* 1992;326:1115–1122.
53. Karp DL, Horn TD. Lymphomatoid papulosis. *J Am Acad Dermatol* 1994;30:379–395.
54. El-Azhary RA, Gibson LE, Kurtin PJ, et al. Lymphomatoid papulosis: a clinical and histopathologic review of 53 cases with leukocyte immunophenotyping, DNA flow cytometry, and T-cell receptor gene rearrangement studies. *J Am Acad Dermatol* 1994;30:210–218.
55. Zirbel GM, Gellis SE, Kadin ME, et al. Lymphomatoid papulosis in children. *J Am Acad Dermatol* 1995;33:741–748.
56. Kato N, Matsue K. Follicular lymphomatoid papulosis. *Am J Dermatopathol* 1997;19:189–196.
57. Weinberg JM, Kristal L, Chooback L, et al. The clonal nature of pityriasis lichenoides. *Arch Dermatol* 2002;138:1063–1067.
58. Horn TD, Haskell J. The lymphocytic infiltrate in acute cutaneous allogeneic graft-versus-host reactions lacks evidence for phenotypic restriction in donor-derived cells. *J Cutan Pathol* 1998;25:210–214.
59. Massi D, Franchi A, Pimpinelli N, et al. A reappraisal of the histopathologic criteria for the diagnosis of cutaneous allogeneic acute graft-vs-host disease. *Am J Clin Pathol* 1999;112:791–800.
60. Abell E, Marks R, Jones EW. Secondary syphilis: a clinic-pathological review. *Br J Dermatol* 1975;93:53–61.
61. Noppakun N, Dinehart SM, Solomon AR. Pustular secondary syphilis. *Int J Dermatol* 1987;26:112–114.
62. Lee JY, Hsu ML. Alopecia syphilitica, a simulator of alopecia areata: histopathology and differential diagnosis. *J Cutan Pathol* 1991;18:87–92.
63. Jordaan HF, Louw M. The moth-eaten alopecia of secondary syphilis. A histopathological study of 12 patients. *Am J Dermatopathol* 1995;17:158–162.
64. Phelps RG, Knipsel J, Tu ES, et al. Immunoperoxidase technique for detecting spirochetes in tissue sections. *Int J Dermatol* 2000;39:609–613.
65. Korkij W, Soltani K. Fixed drug eruption. A brief review. *Arch Dermatol* 1984;120:520–524.
66. Fitzpatrick JE. New histopathologic findings in drug eruptions. *Dermatol Clin* 1992;10:19–36.
67. Huff JC, Weston WL, Tonnesen MG. Erythema multiforme: a critical review of characteristics, diagnostic criteria, and causes. *J Am Acad Dermatol* 1983;8:763–775.
68. Cote B, Wechsler J, Bastuji-Garin S, et al. Clinicopathologic correlation in erythema multiforme and Stevens-Johnson syndrome. *Arch Dermatol* 1995;131:1268–1272.
69. Assier H, Bastuji-Garin S, Revuz J, Roujeau JC. Erythema multiforme with mucous membrane involvement and Stevens-Johnson syndrome are clinically different disorders with distinct causes. *Arch Dermatol* 1995;131:539–543.
70. Rzany B, Hering O, Mockenhaupt M, et al. Histopathological and epidemiological characteristics of patients with erythema exudativum multiforme major, Stevens-Johnson syndrome and toxic epidermal necrolysis. *Br J Dermatol* 1996;135:6–11.
71. Roujeau JC. Stevens-Johnson syndrome and toxic epidermal necrolysis are severity variants of the same disease which differs from erythema multiforme. *J Dermatol* 1997;24:726–729.
72. Lyell A. Toxic epidermal necrolysis: an eruption resembling scalding of the skin. *Br J Dermatol* 1956;68:355–361.
73. Roujeau JC, Chosidow O, Saiag P, Guillaume JC. Toxic epidermal necrolysis (Lyell syndrome). *J Am Acad Dermatol* 1990;23:1039–1058.
74. Paquet P, Pierard GE. Erythema multiforme and toxic epidermal necrolysis: a comparative study. *Am J Dermatopathol* 1997;19:127–132.
75. Gross G, Pfister H, Hagedorn M, Gissmann L. Correlation between human papillomavirus (HPV) type and histology of warts. *J Invest Dermatol* 1982;78:160–164.
76. Sanchez NP, Perry HO, Muller SA. On the relationship between subcorneal pustular dermatosis and pustular psoriasis. *Am J Dermatopathol* 1981;3:385–386.
77. Murphy GM, Griffiths WA. Subcorneal pustular dermatosis. *Clin Exp Dermatol* 1989;14:165–167.
78. Hejazi N, Mehregan AH. Scabies: histological study of inflammatory lesions. *Arch Dermatol* 1975;111:37–39.
79. Ronjeau JC, Biolulac-Sage P, Bourseau C, et al. Acute generalized exanthematous pustulosis. Analysis of 63 cases. *Arch Dermatol* 1991;127:1333–1338.
80. Sidoroff A, Halevy S, Bavninck JNB, et al. Acute generalized exanthematous pustulosis (AGEP): a clinical reaction pattern. *J Cutan Pathol* 2001;28:113–119.
81. Amagai M, Matsuyoshi N, Wang ZH, et al. Toxin in bullous impetigo and staphylococcal scalded-skin syndrome targets desmoglein 1. *Nat Med* 2000;6:1275–1277.
82. Freeman RG, Spiller R, Knox JM. Histopathology of erythema toxicum neonatorum. *Arch Dermatol* 1960;82:586–589.
83. Furtado TA. Histopathology of pemphigus foliaceus. *Arch Dermatol* 1959;80:66–71.
84. Landau M, Brenner S. Histopathologic findings in drug-induced pemphigus. *Am J Dermatopathol* 1997;19:411–414.
85. Delmonte S, Kanitakis J, Cozzani E, et al. Diagnosing pemphigus foliaceus: a retrospective analysis of clinical, histological and immunological criteria. *Dermatology* 2001;203:289–293.
86. Becker BA, Gaspari AA. Pemphigus vulgaris and vegetans. *Dermatol Clin* 1993;11:429–452.
87. Woo TY, Solomon AR, Fairley JA. Pemphigus vegetans limited to the lips and oral mucosa. *Arch Dermatol* 1985;121:271–272.
88. Amagai M, Karpati S, Prussick R, et al. Autoantibodies against the amino-terminal cadherin-like binding domain of pemphigus vulgaris are pathogenic. *J Clin Invest* 1992;90:919–926.
89. Emery DJ, Diaz LA, Fairly JA, et al. Pemphigus foliaceus and pemphigus vulgaris autoantibodies react with the extracellular domain of desmogein 1. *J Invest Dermatol* 1995;104:323–328.
90. Virgili A, Trombelli L, Calura G. Sudden vegetation of the mouth. Pemphigus vegetans of the mouth (Hallopeau type). *Arch Dermatol* 1992;128:398–399.
91. Anhalt GJ, Kim SC, Stanley JR, et al. Paraneoplastic pemphigus. An autoimmune mucocutaneous disease associated with neoplasia. *N Engl J Med* 1990;323:1729–1735.
92. Mehregan DR, Oursler JR, Leiferman KM, et al. Paraneoplastic pemphigus: a subset of patients with pemphigus and neoplasia. *J Cutan Pathol* 1993;20:203–210.
93. Galimberti RL, Kowalczuk AM, Bianchi O, et al. Chronic benign familial pemphigus. *Int J Dermatol* 1988;27:495–500.
94. Sudbrak R, Brown J, Dobson-Stone C, et al. Hailey-Hailey disease is caused by mutations in ATP2C1 encoding a novel Ca(2+) pump. *Hum Mol Genet* 2000;9:1131–1140.
95. Gottlieb SK, Lutzner MA. Darier's disease. An electron microscopic study. *Arch Dermatol* 1973;107:225–230.
96. Sakuntabai A, Ruiz-Perez V, Carter S, et al. Mutations in ATP2A2, encoding a Ca2+ pump, cause Darier disease. Nat Genet 1999;21:271–277.
97. Lazaro-Medina A, Robbins TO, Bystryn JC, Ackerman AB. Limitations in the diagnosis of vesiculobullous diseases. *Am J Dermatopathol* 1983;5:7–10.
98. Davis MD, Dinneen AM, Landa N, Gibson LE. Grover's disease: clinicopathologic review of 72 cases. *Mayo Clin Proc* 1999;74:229–234.
99. McSorley J, Shapiro L, Brownstein MH, Hsu KC. Herpes simplex and varicella-zoster: comparative histopathology of 77 cases. *Int J Dermatol* 1974;13:69–75.
100. Stahl RE, Ackerman AB. Ghostly clues to the diagnosis of infections by herpesviruses. *Am J Dermatopathol* 1983;5:33–38.
101. Sangueza OP, Gordon MD, White CR Jr. Subtle clues to the diagnosis of the herpesvirus by light microscopy. Herpetic syringitis. *Am J Dermatopathol* 1995;17:163–168.
102. Barnadas MA, Alegre M, Baselga E, et al. Histopathological changes of primary HIV infection. Description of three cases and review of the literature. *J Cutan Pathol* 1997;24:507–510.
103. Person JR, Rogers RS 3rd. Bullous and cicatricial pemphigoid: clinical, histopathologic, and immunopathologic correlations. *Mayo Clin Proc* 1977;52:54–66.
104. Shornick JK, Bangert JL, Freeman RG, Gilliam JN. Herpes gestationis: clinical and histologic features of twenty-eight cases. *J Am Acad Dermatol* 1983;8:214–224.
105. Ahmed AR, Kurgis BS, Rogers RS 3rd. Cicatricial pemphigoid. *J Am Acad Dermatol* 1991;24:987–1001.
106. Yancey KB, Egan CA. Pemphigoid: clinical, histologic, immunopathologic, and therapeutic considerations. *JAMA* 2000;284:350–356.
107. Liu Z, Diaz LA. Bullous pemphigoid: end of the century overview. *J Dermatol* 2001;28:647–650.
108. Katz SI, Hall RP 3rd, Lawley TJ, Strober W. Dermatitis herpetiformis: the skin and the gut. *Ann Intern Med* 1980;93:857–874.
109. Kaplan RP, Callen JP. Overlapping cutaneous disorders related to dermatitis herpetiformis. *Clin Dermatol* 1991;9:361–380.
110. Warren SJ, Cockerell CJ. Characterization of a subgroup of patients with dermatitis herpetiformis with nonclassical histologic features. *Am J Dermatopathol* 2002;24:305–308.
111. Zhou S, Ferguson DJ, Allen J, Wojnarowska F. The localization of target antigens and autoantibodies in linear IgA disease is variable: correlation of immunogold electron microscopy and immunoblotting. *Br J Dermatol* 1998;139:591–597.
112. Richter BJ, McNutt NS. The spectrum of epidermolysis bullosa acquisita. *Arch Dermatol* 1979;115:1325–1328.
113. Leber K, Shenefelt PD. Congenital erosions. *Arch Dermatol* 2001;137:1521–1526.
114. Fine JD, McGrath J, Eady RA. Inherited epidermolysis bullosa comes into the new millennium: a revised classification system based on current knowledge of pathogenetic mechanisms and the clinical, laboratory, and epidemiologic findings of large, well-defined patient cohorts. *J Am Acad Dermatol* 2000;43:135–137.
115. Cormane RH, Szabo E, Hoo TT. Histopathology of the skin in acquired and hereditary porphyria cutanea tarda. *Br J Dermatol* 1971;85:531–539.
116. Epstein JH, Tuffanelli DL, Epstein WL. Cutaneous changes in the porphyrias. A microscopic study. *Arch Dermatol* 1973;107:689–698.
117. Maynard B, Peters MS. Histologic and immunofluorescence study of cutaneous porphyrias. *J Cutan Pathol* 1992;19:40–47.
118. Mehregan AH. Epidermolytic hyperkeratosis. Incidental findings in the epidermis and in the intraepidermal eccrine sweat duct units. *J Cutan Pathol* 1978;5:76–80.
119. Tobin DJ, Swanson NN, Pittelkow MR, et al. Melanocytes are not absent in lesional skin of long duration vitiligo. *J Pathol* 2000;191:407–416.
120. Carrington PR, Altick JA, Sanusi ID. Atrophoderma elastolytica discreta. *Am J Dermatopathol* 1996;18:212–217.
121. Scheimberg I, Harper JI, Malone M, Lake BD. Inherited ichthyoses: a review of the histology of the skin. *Pediatr Pathol Lab Med* 1996;16:359–378.
122. Curth HO. Classification of acanthosis nigricans. *Int J Dermatol* 1976;15:592–593.
123. Sunenshine PJ, Schwartz RA, Janniger CK. Tinea versicolor: an update. *Cutis* 1998;61:65–68,71–72.
124. Norris PG, Hawk JL. Polymorphic light eruption. *Photodermatol Photoimmunol Photomed* 1990;7:186–191.
125. Kim KJ, Chang SE, Choi JH, et al. Clinicopathologic analysis of 66 cases of erythema annulare centrifugum. *J Dermatol* 2002;29:61–67.
126. Tobias N. Tickbite granuloma. *J Invest Dermatol* 1949;12:255–259.
127. Aberer E, Klade H. Cutaneous manifestations of Lyme borreliosis. *Infection* 1991;19:284–286.
128. Jordaan HF, Schneider JW. Papular urticaria: a histopathologic study of 30 patients. *Am J Dermatopathol* 1997;19:119–126.
129. Hwong H, Jones D, Prieto VG, et al. Persistent atypical lymphocytic hyperplasia following tick bite in a child: report of a case and review of the literature. *Pediatr Dermatol* 2001;18:481–484.
130. Peters MS, Winkelmann RK. Neutrophilic urticaria. *Br J Dermatol* 1985;113:25–30.

131. Stewart GE 2nd. Histopathology of chronic urticaria. *Clin Rev Allergy Immunol* 2002;23: 195–200.
132. Randall SJ, Kierland RR, Montgomery H. Pigmented purpuric eruptions. *Arch Dermatol* 1951;64:177–191.
133. Wong RC, Solomon AR, Field SI, Anderson TF. Pigmented purpuric lichenoid dermatitis of Gougerot-Blum mimicking Kaposi's sarcoma. *Cutis* 1983;31:406–410.
134. Kim HJ, Skidmore RA, Woosley JT. Pigmented purpura over the lower extremities. Purpura annularis telangiectodes of Majocchi. *Arch Dermatol* 1998;134:1477,1480.
135. Braverman IM, Yen A. Demonstration of immune complexes in spontaneous and histamine-induced lesions and in normal skin of patients with leukocytoclastic angitis. *J Invest Dermatol* 1975;64:105–112.
136. Gammon WR, Wheeler CE Jr. Urticarial vasculitis: report of a case and review of the literature. *Arch Dermatol* 1979;115:76–80.
137. Jennette CJ, Milling DM, Falk RJ. Vasculitis affecting the skin. A review. *Arch Dermatol* 1994;130:899–906.
138. Siberry GK, Cohen BA, Johnson B. Cutaneous polyarteritis nodosa. Reports of two cases in children and review of the literature. *Arch Dermatol* 1994;130:884–889.
139. Reinauer S, Megahed M, Goerz G, et al. Schönlein-Henoch purpura associated with gastric *Helicobacter pylori* infection. *J Am Acad Dermatol* 1995;33:876–879.
140. Daoud MS, Hutton KP, Gibson LE. Cutaneous periarteritis nodosa: a clinicopathological study of 79 cases. *Br J Dermatol* 1997;136:706–713.
141. Vidaller A, Sais G. Cutaneous leukocytoclastic vasculitis: the dynamic nature of the infiltrate and the expression of adhesion molecules. *J Cutan Pathol* 2001;28:327–334.
142. McNeely MC, Jorizzo JL, Solomon AR, Peltier FA. Erythema elevatum diutinum. *Clin Rheumatol* 1985;3:17–20.
143. Yiannias JA, El-Azhary RA, Gibson LE. Erythema elevatum diutinum: a clinical and histopathologic study of 13 patients. *J Am Acad Dermatol* 1992;26:38–44.
144. Roustan G, Sanchez Yus E, Salas C, Simon A. Granuloma faciale with extrafacial lesions. *Dermatology* 1999;198:79–82.
145. Magro CM, Crowson AN. Sterile neutrophilic folliculitis with perifollicular vasculopathy: a distinctive cutaneous reaction pattern reflecting systemic disease. *J Cutan Pathol* 1998;25:215–221.
146. Bonsib SM. Polyarteritis nodosa. *Semin Diagn Pathol* 2001;18:14–23.
147. Jeanette JC, Thomas DB, Falk RJ. Microscopic polyangiitis (microscopic polyarteritis). *Semin Diagn Pathol* 2001;18:3–13.
148. Guillevin L, Durand-Gasselin B, Cevallos R, et al. Microscopic polyangiitis: clinical and laboratory findings in eighty-five patients. *Arthritis Rheum* 1999;42:421–430.
149. Churg J, Strauss L. Allergic granulomatosis, allergic angiitis, and periarteritis nodosa. *Am J Pathol* 1951;27:227–231.
150. Daoud MS, Gibson LE, DeRemee RA, et al. Cutaneous Wegener's granulomatosis: clinical, histopathologic, and immunopathologic features of thirty patients. *J Am Acad Dermatol* 1994;31:605–612.
151. Carrington CB, Liebow A. Limited forms of angiitis and granulomatosis of Wegener's type. *Am J Med* 1966;41:497–527.
152. Frances C, Du LT, Piette JC, et al. Wegener's granulomatosis. Dermatological manifestations in 75 cases with clinicopathologic correlation. *Arch Dermatol* 1994;130:861–867.
153. Gibson LE, El-Azhary RA, Smith TF, Reda AM. The spectrum of cutaneous granulomatous vasculitis: histopathologic report of eight cases with clinical correlation. *J Cutan Pathol* 1994;21:437–445.
154. Beaty MW, Toro J, Sorbara L, et al. Cutaneous lymphomatoid granulomatosis: correlation of clinical and biologic features. *Am J Surg Pathol* 2001;25:1111–1120.
155. Gibson GE, Su WP, Pittelkow MR. Antiphospholipid syndrome and the skin. *J Am Acad Dermatol* 1997;36:970–982.
156. Nahass GT. Antiphospholipid antibodies and the antiphospholipid antibody syndrome. *J Am Acad Dermatol* 1997;36:149–168.
157. Jorizzo JL, Solomon AR, Zanolli MD, et al. Neutrophilic vascular reactions. *J Am Acad Dermatol* 1988;19:983–1005.
158. Raimer SS, Duncan WC. Febrile neutrophilic dermatosis in acute myelogenous leukemia. *Arch Dermatol* 1978;114:413–414.
159. Jordaan HF. Acute febrile neutrophilic dermatosis. A histopathological study of 37 patients and a review of the literature. *Am J Dermatopathol* 1989;11:99–111.
160. Von den Driesch P. Sweet's syndrome (acute febrile neutrophilic dermatosis). *J Am Acad Dermatol* 1994;31:535–556.
161. Su WP, Schroeter AL, Perry HO, et al. Histopathologic and immunopathologic study of pyoderma gangrenosum. *J Cutan Pathol* 1986;13:323–330.
162. Davies MG, Hastings A. Sweet's syndrome progressing to pyoderma gangrenosum—a spectrum of neutrophilic skin disease in association with cryptogenic cirrhosis. *Clin Exp Dermatol* 1991;16:279–282.
163. Crowson AN, Mihm MC, Magro C. Pyoderma gangrenosum: a review. *J Cutan Pathol* 2003;30:97–107.
164. Leder LD. Subtle clues to diagnosis by histochemistry. Mast cell disease. *Am J Dermatopathol* 1979;1:261–266.
165. Williford PM, White WL, Jorizzo JL, Greer K. The spectrum of normolipemic plane xanthoma. *Am J Dermatopathol* 1993;15:572–575.
166. Breier F, Zelger B, Reiter H, et al. Papular xanthoma: a clinicopathological study of 10 cases. *J Cutan Pathol* 2002;29:200–206.
167. Rabinowitz LO, Zaim MT. A clinicopathologic approach to granulomatous dermatoses. *J Am Acad Dermatol* 1996;35:588–600.
168. Veien NK, Stahl D, Brodthagen H. Cutaneous sarcoidosis in Caucasians. *J Am Acad Dermatol* 1987;16:534–540.
169. Mana J, Marcoval J, Graells J, et al. Cutaneous involvement in sarcoidosis. Relationship to systemic disease. *Arch Dermatol* 1997;133:882–888.
170. Kim YC, Triffet MK, Gibson LE. Foreign bodies in sarcoidosis. *Am J Dermatopathol* 2000;22:408–412.
171. Gal AA, Koss MN. The pathology of sarcoidosis. *Curr Opin Pulm Med* 2002;8:445–451.
172. Su WP, Kuechle MK, Peters MS, Muller SA. Palisading granulomas caused by infectious diseases. *Am J Dermatopathol* 1992;14:211–215.
173. Dickinson JA. Sarcoidal reactions in tattoos. *Arch Dermatol* 1969;100:315–319.
174. Montemarano AD, Sau P, Johnson FB, et al. Cutaneous granulomas caused by an aluminum-zirconium complex: an ingredient of antiperspirants. *J Am Acad Dermatol* 1997;37:496–498.
175. Umbert P, Winkelmann RK. Histologic, ultrastructural and histochemical studies of granuloma annulare. *Arch Dermatol* 1977;113:1681–1686.
176. Muhlbauer JE. Granuloma annulare. *J Am Acad Dermatol* 1980;3:217–230.
177. McDermott MB, Lind AC, Marley EF, Dehner LP. Deep granuloma annulare (pseudorheumatoid nodule) in children: clinicopathologic study of 35 cases. *Pediatr Dev Pathol* 1998;1:300–308.
178. Gray HR, Grahm JH, Johnson WC. Necrobiosis lipoidica. A histologic and histochemical study. *J Invest Dermatol* 1965;44:369–380.
179. Crosby DL, Woodley DT, Leonard DD. Concomitant granuloma annulare and necrobiosis lipoidica. Report of a case and review of the literature. *Dermatologica* 1991;183:225–229.
180. Finan MC, Winkelmann RK. Histopathology of necrobiotic xanthogranuloma with paraproteinemia. *J Cutan Pathol* 1987;14:92–99.
181. Lebey PB, Determer I, Bazex J, et al. Periorbital papules and nodules. Necrobiotic xanthogranuloma. *Arch Dermatol* 1997;133:99,102.
182. Bennett GA, Zeller JW, Bauer W. Subcutaneous nodules of rheumatoid arthritis and rheumatic fever. *Arch Pathol* 1940;30:70–89.
183. Templeton SF, Solomon AR. Scarring alopecia: a classification based on microscopic criteria. *J Cutan Pathol* 1994;21:97–109.
184. Sperling LC. Scarring alopecia and the dermatopathologist. *J Cutan Pathol* 2001;28:333–342.
185. Elgart ML. Tinea incognito: an update on Majocchi granuloma. *Dermatol Clin* 1996;14:51–55.
186. Marks R. Concepts in the pathogenesis of rosacea. *Br J Dermatol* 1968;80:170–177.
187. Ferrara G, Cannone M, Scalvenzi M, et al. Facial granulomatous diseases: a study of four cases tested for the presence of *Mycobacterium tuberculosis* DNA using nested polymerase chain reaction. *Am J Dermatopathol* 2001;23:8–15.
188. Basarab T, Russell Jones R. HIV-associated eosinophilic folliculitis: case report and review of the literature. *Br J Dermatol* 1996;134:499–503.
189. Blume-Peytavi U, Chen W, Djemadji N, et al. Eosinophilic pustular folliculitis (Ofuji's disease). *J Am Acad Dermatol* 1997;37:259–262.
190. Piantanida EW, Turiansky GW, Kenner JR, et al. HIV-associated eosinophilic folliculitis: diagnosis by transverse histologic sections. *J Am Acad Dermatol* 1998;38:124–126.
191. Ishiguro N, Shishido E, Okamoto R, et al. Ofuji's disease: a report on 20 patients with clinical and histopathological analysis. *J Am Acad Dermatol* 2002;46:827–833.
192. Pinkus H. Alopecia mucinosa. *Arch Dermatol* 1957;76:419–426.
193. Hempstead RW, Ackerman AB. Follicular mucinosis. A reaction pattern in follicular epithelium. *Am J Dermatopathol* 1985;7:245–257.
194. Sentis HJ, Willemze R, Scheffer E. Alopecia mucinosa progressing into mycosis fungoides. A long-term follow-up study of two patients. *Am J Dermatopathol* 1988;10:478–486.
195. Mehregan DA, Gibson LE, Muller SA. Follicular mucinosis: histopathologic review of 33 cases. *Mayo Clin Proc* 1991;66:387–390.
196. Gibson LE, Brown HA, Pittelkow MR, Pujol RM. Follicular mucinosis. *Arch Dermatol* 2002;138:1615.
197. Cerroni L, Fink-Puches R, Back B, Kerl H. Follicular mucinosis: a critical reappraisal of clinicopathologic features and association with mycosis fungoides and Sézary syndrome. *Arch Dermatol* 2002;138:182–189.
198. Santa Cruz DJ. Chondrodermatitis nodularis helicis: a transepidermal perforating disorder. *J Cutan Pathol* 1980;7:70–76.
199. Young EM Jr, Barr RJ. Sclerosing dermatoses. *J Cutan Pathol* 1985;12:426–441.
200. Onwukwe MF. Classification of keloids. *J Dermatol Surg Oncol* 1978;4:534–536.
201. Reed RJ, Clark WH, Mihm MC. The cutaneous collagenoses. *Hum Pathol* 1973;4:165–186.
202. Tremaine R, Adam JE, Orizaga M. Morphea coexisting with lichen sclerosus et atrophicus. *Int J Dermatol* 1990;29:486–489.
203. Buechner SA, Lautenschlager S, Itin P, et al. Lymphoproliferative responses to *Borrelia burgdorferi* in patients with erythema migrans, acrodermatitis chronica atrophicans, lymphadenosis benigna cutis, and morphea. *Arch Dermatol* 1995;131:673–677.
204. Krell JM, Solomon AR, Glavey CM, et al. Nodular scleroderma. *J Am Acad Dermatol* 1995;32:343–345.
205. De Vito JR, Merogi AJ, Vo T, et al. Role of *Borrelia burgdorferi* in the pathogenesis of morphea/scleroderma and lichen sclerosus et atrophicus: a PCR study of thirty-five cases. *J Cutan Pathol* 1996;23:350–358.
206. Fujiwara H, Fujiwara K, Hashimoto K, et al. Detection of *Borrelia burgdorferi* DNA (*B. garinii* or *B. afzelii*) in morphea and lichen sclerosus et atrophicus tissues of German and Japanese but not of US patients. *Arch Dermatol* 1997;133:41–44.
207. Torres JE, Sanchez JL. Histopathologic differentiation between localized and systemic scleroderma. *Am J Dermatopathol* 1998;20:242–245.
208. Uitto J, Santa Cruz DJ, Bauer EA, et al. Morphea and lichen sclerosus et atrophicus. Clinical and histopathologic studies in patients with combined features. *J Am Acad Dermatol* 1980;3:271–279.
209. Meffert JJ, Davis BM, Grimwood RE. Lichen sclerosus. *J Am Acad Dermatol* 1995;32:393–416.
210. Carlson JA, Lamb P, Malfetano J, et al. Clinicopathologic comparison of vulvar and extragenital lichen sclerosus: histologic variants, evolving lesions, and etiology of 141 cases. *Mod Pathol* 1998;11:844–854.
211. Scurry J, Whitehead J, Healey M. Histology of lichen sclerosus varies according to site and proximity to carcinoma. *Am J Dermatopathol* 2001;23:413–418.
212. Stephens CJM, McKee PH, Black MM. The dermal mucinoses. *Advl Dermatol* 1993;8:201–227.
213. Godby A, Bergstresser PR, Chaker B, Pandya AG. Fatal scleromyxedema: report of a case and review of the literature. *J Am Acad Dermatol* 1998;38:289–294.

214. Cowper SE, Su L, Bhawan J, et al. Nephrogenic fibrosing dermopathy. *Am J Dermatopathol* 2001;23:383–393.

215. High WA, Ayers RA, Chandler J, et al. Gadolinium is detectable within the tissue of patients with nephrogenic systemic fibrosis. *J Am Acad Dermatol* 2007;56:21–26.

216. Curtis AC, Shulak BM. Scleredema adultorum. Not always a benign self-limited disease. *Arch Dermatol* 1965;92:526–541.

217. Cole HG, Winkelmann RK. Acid mucopolysaccharide staining in scleredema. *J Cutan Pathol* 1990;17:211–213.

218. Basarab T, Burrows NP, Munn SE, et al. Systemic involvement in scleredema of Buschke associated with IgG-κ paraproteinaemia. *Br J Dermatol* 1997;136:939–942.

219. Black MM. The role of the epidermis in the histopathogenesis of lichen amyloidosus. Histochemical correlations. *Br J Dermatol* 1971;85:524–530.

220. Ratz JL, Bailin PL. Cutaneous amyloidosis. A case report of the tumefactive variant and a review of the spectrum of clinical presentations. *J Am Acad Dermatol* 1981;4:21–26.

221. Libbey CA, Skinner M, Cohen AS. Use of abdominal fat tissue aspirate in the diagnosis of systemic amyloidosis. *Arch Intern Med* 1983;143:1549–1553.

222. Kibbi AG, Rubeiz NG, Zaynoun ST, Kurban AK. Primary localized cutaneous amyloidosis. *Int J Dermatol* 1992;31:95–98.

223. Lee DD, Huang CY, Wong CK. Dermatopathologic findings in 20 cases of systemic amyloidosis. *Am J Dermatopathol* 1998;20:438–442.

224. Woods B, Kellaway TD. Cutaneous calculi. *Br J Dermatol* 1963;75:1–11.

225. Shmunes E, Wood MG. Subepidermal calcified nodules. *Arch Dermatol* 1972;105:593–597.

226. Mehta RL, Scott G, Sloand JA, Francis CW. Skin necrosis associated with acquired protein C deficiency in patients with renal failure and calciphylaxis. *Am J Med* 1990;88:252–257.

227. Dahl PR, Winkelmann RK, Connolly SM. The vascular calcification-cutaneous necrosis syndrome. *J Am Acad Dermatol* 1995;33:53–58.

228. Weenig RH, Sewell LD, Davis MD. Calciphylaxis: natural history, risk factor analysis and outcome. *J Am Acad Dermatol* 2007;56:569–579.

229. Essary LR, Wick MR. Cutaneous calciphylaxis. An underrecognized clinicopathologic entity. *Am J Clin Pathol* 2000;113:280–287.

230. King DF, King LA. The appropriate processing of tophi for microscopy. *Am J Dermatopathol* 1982;4:239.

231. DeCastro P, Jorizzo JL, Solomon AR, et al. Coexistent systemic lupus erythematosus and tophaceous gout. *J Am Acad Dermatol* 1985;13:650–654.

232. Eng A, Aronson IK. Dermatopathology of panniculitis. *Semin Dermatol* 1984;3:1–13.

233. Black MM. Panniculitis. *J Cutan Pathol* 1985;12:366–380.

234. Requena L, Yus ES. Panniculitis. Part I. Mostly septal panniculitis. *J Am Acad Dermatol* 2001;45:163–183.

235. Winkelmann RK, Forstrom L. New observations in the histopathology of erythema nodosum. *J Invest Dermatol* 1975;65:441–446.

236. White WL, Hitchcock MG. Diagnosis: erythema nodosum or not? *Semin Cutan Med Surg* 1999;18:47–55.

237. Rubenstein HM, Jaffer AM, Kudrna JC, et al. α₁-Antitrypsin deficiency with severe panniculitis. Report of two cases. *Ann Intern Med* 1977;86:742–744.

238. Hendrick SJ, Silverman AK, Solomon AR, Headington JT. α₁-Antitrypsin deficiency associated with panniculitis. *J Am Acad Dermatol* 1988;18:684–692.

239. Smith KC, Su WP, Pittelkow MR, Winkelmann RK. Clinical and pathologic correlations in 96 patients with panniculitis, including 15 patients with deficient levels of α₁-antitrypsin. *J Am Acad Dermatol* 1989;21:1192–1196.

240. Edmonds BK, Hodge JA, Rietschel RL. α₁-Antitrypsin deficiency–associated panniculitis: case report and review of the literature. *Pediatr Dermatol* 1991;8:296–299.

241. Geller JD, Su WP. A subtle clue to the histopathologic diagnosis of early α₁-antitrypsin deficiency panniculitis. *J Am Acad Dermatol* 1994;31:241–245.

242. Requena L, Sanchez Yus E. Panniculitis. Part II. Mostly lobular panniculitis. *J Am Acad Dermatol* 2001;45:325–361.

243. Rademaker M, Lowe DG, Munro DD. Erythema induratum (Bazin's disease). *J Am Acad Dermatol* 1989;21:740–745.

244. Chuang YH, Kuo TT, Wang CM, et al. Simultaneous occurrence of papulonecrotic tuberculide and erythema induratum and the identification of *Mycobacterium tuberculosis* DNA by polymerase chain reaction. *Br J Dermatol* 1997;137:276–281.

245. Schneider JW, Jordaan HF. The histopathologic spectrum of erythema induratum of Bazin. *Am J Dermatopathol* 1997;19:323–333.

246. Yus ES, Simon P. About the histopathology of erythema induratum-nodular vasculitis. *Am J Dermatopathol* 1999;21:301–306.

247. Silverman AK, Michels EH, Rasmussen JE. Subcutaneous fat necrosis in an infant, occurring after hypothermic cardiac surgery. Case report and analysis of etiologic factors. *J Am Acad Dermatol* 1986;15:331–336.

248. Szymanski FJ, Bluefarb SM. Nodular fat necrosis and pancreatic disease. *Arch Dermatol* 1961;83:224–229.

249. Dahl PR, Su WP, Cullimore KC, Dicken CH. Pancreatic panniculitis. *J Am Acad Dermatol* 1995;33:413–417.

250. Zellman GL. Pancreatic panniculitis. *J Am Acad Dermatol* 1996;35:282–283.

251. Izumi AK, Takiguchi P. Lupus erythematosus panniculitis. *Arch Dermatol* 1983;119:61–64.

252. Ng PP, Tan SH, Tan T. Lupus erythematosus panniculitis: a clinicopathologic study. *Int J Dermatol* 2002;41:488–490.

253. Forstrom L, Winkelmann RK. Factitial panniculitis. *Arch Dermatol* 1974;110:747–750.

254. Winkelmann RK, Barker SM. Factitial traumatic panniculitis. *J Am Acad Dermatol* 1985;13:988–994.

255. Elston DM, Bergfeld WF, McMahon JT. Aluminum tattoo: a phenomenon that can resemble parasitized histiocytes. *J Cutan Pathol* 1993;20:326–329.

Nonmelanocytic Cutaneous Tumors

The number and variety of cutaneous tumors is truly startling, and for the novice, no doubt intimidating. Virtually every anatomic structure and cell type associated with skin has a nevoid or neoplastic counterpart—in most cases, multiple counterparts—and each of these in turn can present with microscopic variations that create additional diagnostic difficulties.

Although it is beyond the scope of this chapter to cover all of the nonmelanocytic tumors of the skin, I will attempt to discuss some of the most important examples of these tumors and to point the reader to additional resources that will allow exploration of these and other cutaneous neoplasms in greater depth. Tumors will be organized by source, or site of origin, and by microscopic configuration and cytologic features.

The nonmelanocytic tumors can be generally grouped as follows:

1. Epidermal tumors
2. Epithelial cysts
3. Appendageal tumors (i.e., follicular, sebaceous, apocrine, and eccrine)
4. Dermal and/or subcutaneous tumors (including fibrous tissue tumors, vascular tumors, neural tumors, and tumors of fat, muscle, cartilage, and bone)
5. Nonlymphoid infiltrative disorders (composed of "histiocytes" [macrophages] and mast cells)
6. Lymphoid infiltrates (including lymphomas and leukemias)

EPIDERMAL TUMORS

BENIGN EPIDERMAL TUMORS

Lesions with Verruciform Acanthosis

Several benign epithelial proliferations feature a change that can be described as *verruciform acanthosis*, so termed because they mimic the papillomatosis and acanthosis seen in many of the forms of verrucae (warts) produced by human papillomavirus (HPV). Although it might be expected that most verrucae would display typical viropathic changes (e.g., vacuolated granular cells, raisinoid nuclei), it is remarkable how many of those that are biopsied lack these changes. Therefore, verruciform epithelial lesions can create a surprising degree of diagnostic difficulty.

Epidermal nevi are verrucous lesions that are often present at birth or early childhood but occasionally can manifest in adult life. The lesions can be solitary or form linear arrangements, sometimes following the lines of Blaschko. One could consider the *nevus sebaceus* (*organoid nevus*) to represent a variant of epidermal nevus, but because of the latter's association with sebaceous glands, nevoid apocrine structures, and potential development of adnexal neoplasms, it often receives a separate designation. Microscopically, epidermal nevi offer combinations of hyperkeratosis, acanthosis, and papillomatosis that can

be either regular and "church-spired" or quite irregular. Occasionally the papillomatosis is distinctively flat topped (Fig. 2.1). Unusual changes include acantholysis and dyskeratosis of the type seen in the genodermatosis, Darier disease (*acantholytic, dyskeratotic epidermal nevus*) (1,2), or vacuolated keratinocytes with irregularly shaped keratohyalin granules, a change described as *epidermolytic hyperkeratosis* (Fig. 2.2) (3). One variant, called *inflammatory linear verrucous epidermal nevus* (*ILVEN*), features a combination of psoriasiform acanthosis with papillomatosis and alternating ortho- and parakeratosis (Fig. 2.3) (4,5).

Seborrheic keratosis is one of the most common benign epidermal lesions of adult life. It typically presents from the fourth decade and beyond as a rough-surfaced papule, nodule, or plaque on virtually any cutaneous surface other than palms and soles. Sometimes these lesions form large annular plaques or show changes of irritation or inflammation. Pigmented, papillomatous variants arising particularly in the malar regions of African American individuals are termed *dermatosis papulosa nigra*. Seborrheic keratoses are mostly exophytic, showing varying degrees of papillomatosis and acanthosis. They are composed of close-set basaloid cells and often feature "pseudo-horn cysts," which are invaginations of the involved epidermis, filled with keratin, that in cross section appear to be intraepidermal "cysts" (Fig. 2.4). However, there can be considerable microscopic variability among seborrheic keratoses. They can be smooth surfaced and acanthotic, show reticulated downgrowths of interconnecting epidermal cords, or when *irritated*, feature spongiosis and whorled arrangements of keratinocytes (*squamous eddies*) (Fig. 2.5). So-called "clonal" seborrheic keratoses contain discrete clusters of keratinocytes within the epidermis; this may be another manifestation of irritation (Fig. 2.6). Papillomatous variants can closely resemble epidermal nevi. Therefore, when signing out such cases, the age of the patient should be taken into account; lesions resembling seborrheic keratoses in children or young adults are most likely either verrucae or epidermal nevi. It is also likely that lesions resembling seborrheic keratosis that arise in the anogenital region of young adults are actually verrucae (6).

Pseudoepitheliomatous hyperplasia is characterized by extreme acanthosis of the epidermis with extension deep into the dermis. The lesions are often exophytic and verruciform. The microscopic image can raise concerns about squamous cell carcinoma, but there is a lack of cytologic atypia. A variety of conditions can be accompanied by pseudoepitheliomatous hyperplasia, including prurigo nodularis (an exaggerated host response to chronic rubbing and scratching of the skin) (Fig. 2.7), certain deep fungal infections (North American blastomycosis is the prototype), halogenodermas (e.g., bromoderma, iododerma) (Fig. 2.8), and granular cell tumors. The task of the pathologist in these cases is twofold: first, to recognize that the changes are reactive and not neoplastic, and second, to determine the underlying cause if possible. Thus, vertical streaking

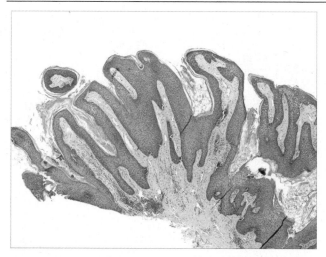

Figure 2.1. Epidermal nevus, showing papillomatosis and acanthosis. Note that the surface papillations are focally flattened.

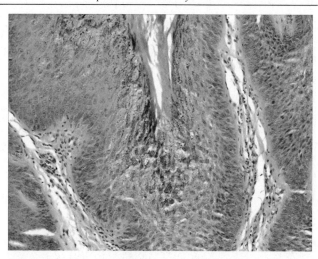

Figure 2.2. Nevoid epidermal lesion showing the changes of epidermolytic hyperkeratosis.

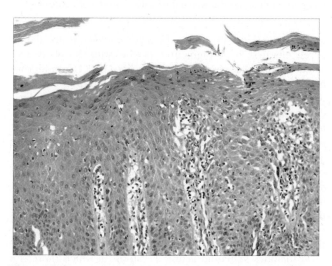

Figure 2.3. Inflammatory linear verrucous epidermal nevus. Note the psoriasiform configuration (complete with neutrophils in the stratum corneum) and alternating hypergranulosis (left) and parakeratosis (right).

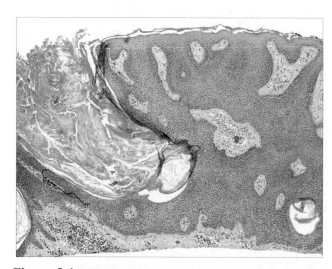

Figure 2.4. Seborrheic keratosis, composed of close-set basaloid cells and pseudo-horn cysts.

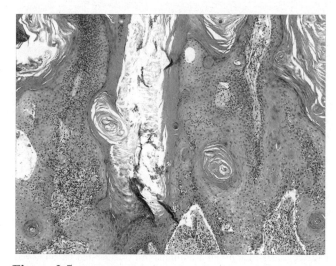

Figure 2.5. Irritated seborrheic keratosis, featuring squamous eddies and spongiotic foci.

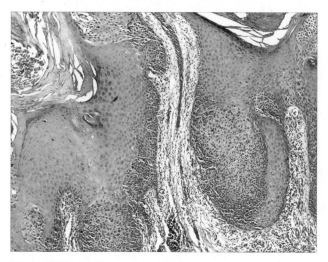

Figure 2.6. ''Clonal'' or nested seborrheic keratosis. The nests do not truly indicate a separate genetic clone of cells and are probably a manifestation of irritation.

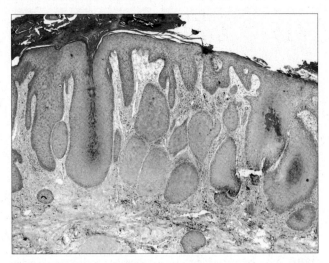

Figure 2.7. Prurigo nodularis, a reactive cutaneous lesion displaying pseudoepitheliomatous hyperplasia.

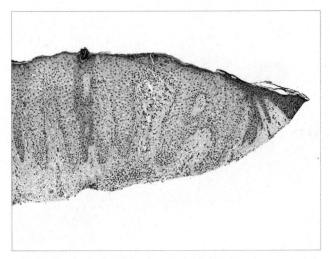

Figure 2.9. Clear cell (pale cell) acanthoma. Note sharp demarcation from adjacent uninvolved epidermis (right) and the intraepidermal portion of an eccrine sweat duct (near left side of figure).

of thick papillary dermal collagen and chronic inflammation tend to accompany prurigo nodules; granulomas and intraepidermal neutrophilic microabscesses are seen in deep fungal infections; neutrophils often accompany halogenodermas; and dermal granular cell elements denote an accompanying granular cell tumor.

Other Benign Epidermal Tumors

Some benign epidermal tumors are smooth surfaced. The *clear cell acanthoma* (*pale cell acanthoma*) is a circumscribed red nodule with peripheral scale that often arises on the leg of middle-aged or older adults (7). Microscopically, these lesions are acanthotic and composed of cells with pale-staining cytoplasm. The surface is smooth and often devoid of stratum corneum or stratum granulosum. A noteworthy finding is that the involved epithelium is sharply demarcated from the adjacent uninvolved epidermis and from adnexal epithelia, a feature of considerable diagnostic

importance (Fig. 2.9) (8,9). *Large-cell acanthomas* are flat to barely elevated, hyperpigmented patches with sharply demarcated borders that also arise in adult life (10). The epidermis may display an exaggeratedly basket-woven stratum corneum, whereas the constituent keratinocytes show cytoplasmic and nuclear enlargement (Fig. 2.10). Basilar hypermelanosis is often identified. These lesions are most often regarded as variants of solar lentigines (11), but because of a degree of keratinocyte atypia and the finding of aneuploidy in one study (12), a case could be made for a low-grade actinic keratosis. *Benign lichenoid keratoses* are characterized by vacuolar alteration of the basilar layer and, at times, a bandlike superficial dermal infiltrate, thereby mimicking the inflammatory dermatosis, lichen planus (Fig. 2.11). These are believed to arise in pre-existing solar lentigines and seborrheic keratoses (13,14). The differential diagnosis includes lichenoid actinic keratosis, in which there is a greater degree of basilar keratinocyte atypia that extends beyond the zone of dermal inflammation. Occasionally, a small

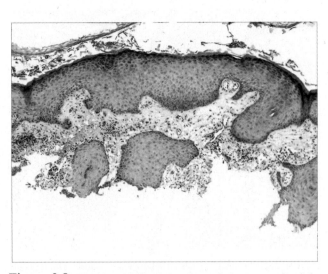

Figure 2.8. Pseudoepitheliomatous hyperplasia as a result of the ingestion of iodides (iododerma).

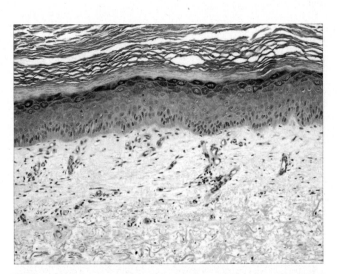

Figure 2.10. Large-cell acanthoma. An exaggerated basket-woven stratum corneum, a prominent granular cell layer, and a spinous layer containing enlarged keratinocytes can be seen.

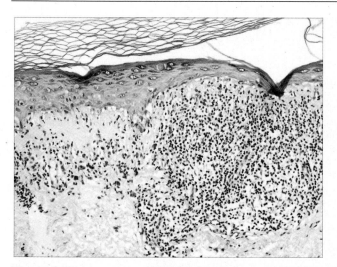

Figure 2.11. Benign lichenoid keratosis. This particular example is a close clinical mimic of lichen planus and would require clinical data for accurate diagnosis.

biopsy of lentigo maligna (or lentiginous melanoma in situ) can show a lichenoid tissue reaction that almost completely obscures the single-cell atypical junctional melanocytic proliferation. If the latter is suspected, additional levels or staining for MART-1 may be useful (15).

EPITHELIAL CYSTS

Classification schemes vary for the cystic epithelial lesions arising in skin. Several of these cystic lesions are conventionally included among the adnexal tumors, but often cysts composed of stratified squamous epithelium (epidermoid cysts, or cysts of follicular origin or differentiation) (16–21) or those containing cilia (an uncommon feature of cutaneous lesions) (22–25) are

classified separately. Tables 2.1 and 2.2 provide a simplified scheme for diagnosing these lesions.

BENIGN ADNEXAL (APPENDAGEAL) TUMORS

There is a startling array of tumors that demonstrate differentiation toward the cutaneous appendages: hair follicle, sebaceous gland, apocrine gland, or eccrine gland. These vary in their degree of differentiation—the degree to which they mimic the normal appendage—and have been classified in descending order of differentiation as hyperplasias or hamartomas, adenomas, and epitheliomas. The theory is that pluripotential stem cells are capable of differentiating toward these epithelial structures.

Several systems have been suggested for classifying the cutaneous adnexal tumors (26–28). Tables of adnexal tumors have been constructed that appear to neatly group these lesions by degree of differentiation and by the appendage to which they appear to be differentiating (29). These schemes have been satisfying in many ways because they at least provide scaffolding upon which to build one's understanding of these tumors. However, problems have arisen with this method, which can be summarized in the following manner:

1. The degrees of differentiation are subject to debate. For example, should syringocystadenoma papilliferum be grouped with the adenomas rather than the epitheliomas? Should poroma be considered an epithelioma rather than an adenoma?
2. The original grouping of sweat gland tumors into either the apocrine or eccrine category was based on a technique called enzyme histochemistry as well as conventional microscopic morphology. In recent years, re-evaluation of these tumors both morphologically and by immunohistochemical methods has resulted in reclassification of many of the sweat gland

TABLE 2.1	Epidermoid Cysts of Follicular Origin/Differentiation	
Cyst Type	*Microscopic Features*	*Comments*
Epidermal (infundibular) cyst (Fig. 2.12)	Stratified squamous epithelium, preserved granular layer, loosely woven lamellated keratin	Milium is a smaller lesion; proliferative variants occur
Human papillomavirus (HPV)–associated cyst	Infundibular type; hypergranulosis, papillomatosis, koilocytic changes	HPV types 57 and 60 have been detected
Pigmented follicular cyst	Infundibular type; multiple pigmented hair shafts in lumen	Hybrid forms occur that also feature trichilemmal keratinization
Cutaneous keratocyst	Festooned configuration; absence of granular layer	Resemble odontogenic keratocysts; seen in nevoid basal cell carcinoma syndrome
Cysts of Gardner syndrome	Infundibular type	Pilomatrixoma-like areas show basaloid cells, shadow cells
Trichilemmal cyst (Fig. 2.13)	Thin wall, lack of granular layer, homogeneous eosinophilic keratin	Alternative terms: pilar cyst, isthmus-catagen cyst; may occur in hybrid forms with infundibular foci; proliferative variants occur
Steatocystoma	Undulating contours, thin-walled, cuticular lining of luminal surface, sebaceous lobules along outer layer of cyst wall	Changes suggest sebaceous ductal differentiation
Dermoid cyst	Infundibular type, with insertion of small follicles; hair shafts in lumen; sebaceous and eccrine elements	Arise along embryonic lines of closure
Eruptive vellus hair cyst	Small cysts arising in association with vellus follicles	May be inherited as autosomal dominant; spontaneous clearing reported

TABLE 2.2	**Ciliated Cysts of the Skin**	
Cyst Type	*Microscopic Features*	*Comments*
Cutaneous endometriosis	Glandular epithelium may contain cilia	Characteristic stroma; poor correlation between histologic features and menstrual cycle; can show decidualized changes
Endosalpingiosis	Columnar epithelial cells with cilia	Arise in periumbilical region after salpingectomy
Mucinous and ciliated vulvar cyst	Cuboidal, tall columnar, or pseudostratified columnar epithelia with mucin and/or cilia	Urogenital sinus origin favored; müllerian or apocrine metaplasia have also been considered
Cutaneous ciliated cyst (Fig. 2.14)	Cuboidal or columnar ciliated epithelium with papillary folds	Solitary lesions, often on lower extremity; possibly müllerian; location resulting from embryonic migration of limb buds
Bronchogenic cyst	Cuboidal or columnar epithelium with cilia and goblet cells	Typical location over suprasternal notch or manubrium
Thyroglossal duct cyst	Occasionally ciliated epithelium with thyroid follicles; lack of smooth muscle or cartilage in cyst wall	Located near hyoid bone; arise from embryonic remnants of the duct
Branchial cleft cyst	Stratified squamous and/or columnar epithelium; surrounding lymphoid tissue	Lateral neck location
Thymic cyst	Resemble bronchogenic cyst but lack goblet cells; thymic tissue and cholesterol granulomas	Located in neck; may arise from embryonic remnants of thymopharyngeal duct

tumors. Thus, many chondroid syringomas (cutaneous mixed tumors) are now regarded as apocrine rather than eccrine in differentiation (30), and acrospiromas can be either apocrine or eccrine (31,32).

3. Although there are certainly many "classic" examples of adnexal tumors, others defy categorization because a given lesion may not only show different lines of differentiation but also different degrees of differentiation. This seems to be a common problem in consultation practice.

4. Adnexal carcinomas do not always fit comfortably into existing classification schemes.

One could argue that the differences among the benign adnexal tumors are largely academic because the precise categorization of tumor rarely seems to make a difference in terms of clinical management. However, some of these tumors have a close relationship to genetically determined syndromes that may have significance in terms of proneness to internal malignancy or other health issues. Examples include multiple trichodiscomas (Birt-Hogg-Dube syndrome) (33), trichilemmomas (Cowden syndrome) (34), or sebaceous tumors (Muir-Torre syndrome) (35). Progression of apparently benign adnexal tumors to malignancy has been reported in several instances (examples include pilomatrixoma, acrospiroma, and poroma). Finally, although knowledge of the precise differentiation pathway may not make a difference in the immediate clinical situation, an understanding of these tumors may lead to discoveries that could have significant impact in other areas of medicine.

Although space considerations limit the ability to consider these lesions in depth, Table 2.3 provides a listing of the most important benign adnexal tumors of skin. Figures 2.15 to 2.18

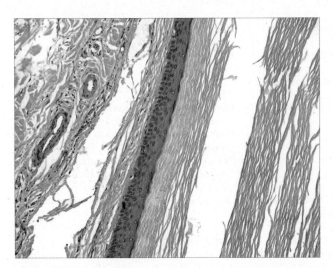

Figure 2.12. Epidermal (infundibular) cyst. The lining is composed of stratified squamous epithelium with a granular cell layer. Keratin contents are identified in the right portion of the figure.

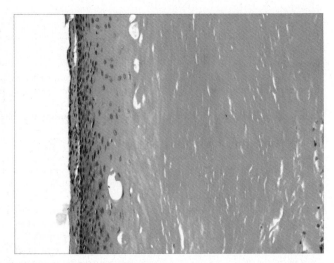

Figure 2.13. Trichilemmal cyst. The lining is composed of stratified squamous epithelium that lacks a granular cell layer and merges imperceptibly with homogeneous, eosinophilic keratin. This is the characteristic mode of keratinization of the follicular isthmus.

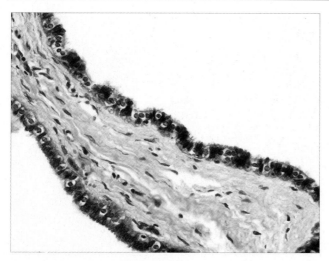

Figure 2.14. Cutaneous ciliated cyst. This one arose in the skin of the lower leg.

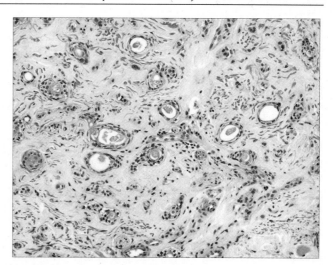

Figure 2.15. Syringoma is a common adnexal tumor of eccrine differentiation often seen in the infraorbital region.

display the microscopic features of four representative tumors: syringoma (Fig. 2.15), trichoepithelioma (Fig. 2.16), syringocystadenoma papilliferum (Fig. 2.17), and eccrine poroma (Fig. 2.18).

ADNEXAL CARCINOMAS

There is a group of malignant epithelial tumors that show some degree of differentiation toward recognizable adnexal struc-

tures, yet display infiltration of connective tissues as well as pleomorphism, cell necrosis, increased mitotic rate, and sometimes atypical mitotic figures. Some of these tumors resemble their counterparts among the benign adnexal tumors, whereas others are microscopically unique. Table 2.4 provides a listing of the important adnexal carcinomas grouped according to their lines of differentiation.

Although some of the adnexal carcinomas are readily iden-

TABLE 2.3	The Benign Adnexal Tumors		
Follicular	*Sebaceous*	*Apocrine*	*Eccrine*
Follicular nevus	Nevus sebaceus (organoid nevus)	Apocrine nevus[c]	Eccrine nevus
Folliculosebaceous cystic hamartoma[a]	Sebaceous hyperplasia	Hidrocystoma, cystadenoma	Hidrocystoma
Dilated pore	Sebaceous adenoma	Hidradenoma papilliferum	Syringoma
Pilar sheath acanthoma	Sebaceoma	Hidradenoma (acrospiroma)[d]	Spiradenoma
Trichofolliculoma[a]		Syringocystadenoma papilliferum	Hidradenoma (poroid)[d]
Trichodiscoma		Tubular apocrine adenoma[e]	Poroma
Fibrofolliculoma		Cylindroma[f]	Papillary eccrine adenoma[e]
Trichilemmoma		Mixed tumor (chondroid syringoma)[g]	Cylindroma[f]
Tumor of the follicular infundibulum			Mucinous syringometaplasia
Trichoadenoma			Mixed tumor (chondroid syringoma)[g]
Trichoepithelioma			
Pilomatrixoma			
Proliferating trichilemmal cyst/tumor			
The trichoblastic tumors[b]			

[a]Some consider trichofolliculoma to represent a later stage in the development of folliculosebaceous cystic hamartoma.
[b]A group of trichoblastic tumors was at first separately categorized because of similarities to the odontogenic tumors. Some authors consider these to be variants of trichoepithelioma.
[c]The apocrine nevus is encountered most often in a nevus sebaceus but may present rarely as an isolated lesion.
[d]The eccrine acrospiroma (clear cell hidradenoma, nodular hidradenoma, solid-cystic hidradenoma) was once considered a single tumor with several different microscopic presentations. There are now believed to be both apocrine (clear and mucinous) and eccrine (poroid and basaloid) types.
[e]There is some disagreement on whether tubular apocrine adenoma and papillary eccrine adenoma are the same or different tumors.
[f]It is not clear whether cylindroma is an apocrine or eccrine tumor.
[g]There are now considered to be both apocrine and eccrine variants of mixed tumor. Apocrine tumors feature cords of epithelial cells and branching ducts, whereas the rare eccrine variant contains small syringoma-like ducts without branching.

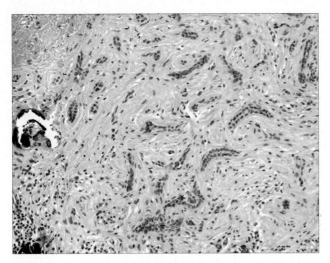

Figure 2.16. Trichoepithelioma, desmoplastic type. Cords of epithelial cells and calcified horn cysts are identified. This is a tumor with follicular differentiation.

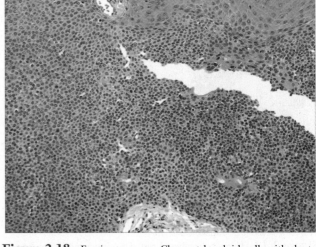

Figure 2.18. Eccrine poroma. Close-set basaloid cells with ductal differentiation are connected to the surface epidermis.

tified as such, through their epidermal relationships or their derivation from/resemblance to benign adnexal tumors, others can closely resemble metastatic tumors from other sites, such as the breast. In these instances, clinical and radiographic data should be considered as important components of the diagnostic process. In addition, immunohistochemical methods have recently been brought to bear on the distinction between primary cutaneous adnexal carcinomas and metastatic carcinomas originating from internal sites; for example, cytokeratin 5/6 and p63 have been recommended because they appear to be preferentially expressed in neoplasms of cutaneous origin (36,37). Two other considerations should be mentioned with regard to the adnexal carcinomas. First, one must be cautious in judging the significance of mitotic activity and nuclear pleomorphism because both of these can be observed in benign adnexal tumors. For example, frequent

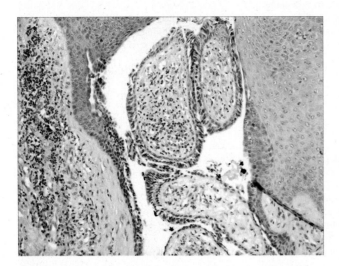

Figure 2.17. Syringocystadenoma papilliferum is generally considered an apocrine tumor. Villi lined by apocrine-type epithelium extend to the epidermal surface.

TABLE 2.4
Adnexal Carcinomas

Follicular Carcinomas
Trichilemmal carcinoma
Pilomatrix carcinoma
Malignant proliferating trichilemmal tumor
Adnexal carcinoma with divergent differentiation
Sebaceous Carcinomas
Basal cell carcinoma with sebaceous differentiation (basosebaceous carcinoma)
Sebaceous carcinoma and variants (basaloid, squamoid, sarcomatoid)
Apocrine Carcinomas
Carcinoma ex dermal cylindroma[a]
Malignant clear cell hidradenoma (acrospiroma)[a]
Ductopapillary apocrine carcinoma
Paget disease, apocrine type
Apocrine signet ring cell adenocarcinoma
Ductal apocrine adenocarcinoma[b]
Eccrine Carcinomas
Porocarcinoma (Fig. 2.19)
Mucinous eccrine carcinoma
Adenoid cystic carcinoma of skin
Papillary digital eccrine adenocarcinoma
Microcystic adnexal carcinoma[c] (Fig. 2.20)
Carcinoma ex eccrine spiradenoma
Malignant mixed tumor of skin[a]
Ductal eccrine adenocarcinoma[b]

[a]The designation of these tumors as either apocrine or eccrine (or both) is subject to debate.
[b]Ductal adenocarcinomas can closely mimic metastatic tumors to the skin, and distinction may depend on clinical data. Recently, immunostains for cytokeratin 5/6 and p63 have been used to address this problem because expression has been found to be more characteristic of cutaneous adnexal carcinomas.
[c]Microcystic adnexal carcinoma combines the features of sclerosing sweat duct carcinoma with microcysts containing trichilemmal-type keratin. It is best known for locally aggressive growth rather than metastasis.

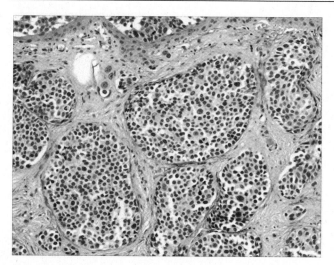

Figure 2.19. Porocarcinoma. Malignant poroid cells involve the epidermis and show dermal invasion.

mitoses can be observed in certain sweat gland tumors, such as acrospiroma, and some proliferating trichilemmal tumors can show both mitoses and foci of nuclear pleomorphisms (38). Therefore, it is important to interpret these features in the overall context of the lesion, keeping in mind both the overall level of differentiation and the presence or absence of infiltration of the surrounding stroma. Second, intermediate levels of malignancy are increasingly being recognized among cutaneous adnexal tumors. An ''intermediate-grade'' lesion shows infiltration of connective tissues at the periphery of the tumor, whereas other histopathologic characteristics of malignancy (e.g., pleomorphism, cell necrosis, mitotic activity) may be inapparent. There is evidence that such tumors are prone to recurrences, sometimes accompanied by greater degrees of cytologic atypia. Examples of such tumors have been seen in association with pilomatrixomas, proliferating trichilemmal tumors, clear cell hidradenomas (acrospiromas), and poromas.

PREMALIGNANT AND MALIGNANT EPIDERMAL TUMORS

Actinic Keratosis

This is a common, sun-induced lesion that most often presents as a rough-surfaced to crusted patch, particularly over the head and neck and extremities. Lesions are variably elevated and can be erythematous, flesh colored, or hyperpigmented. They typically arise in middle-aged to older individuals but can be encountered in young adults as well, and can even be seen in childhood in the rare, recessively inherited disorder xeroderma pigmentosum, which is a condition characterized by abnormal repair of ultraviolet-damaged DNA. Similar keratoses have arisen in individuals exposed to inorganic pentavalent arsenic. Actinic keratoses can progress to invasive squamous cell carcinoma at rates ranging from 0.1% to 10% (39). Metastases from actinic keratosis–related squamous cell carcinomas are uncommon, ranging in incidence from 0.5% to 3.0% (40,41). Microscopically, actinic keratoses often show atypia of the basilar or immediately suprabasilar keratinocytes, with nuclear crowding, pleomorphism, and irregular epithelial budding. Surface maturation of the involved epidermis is often preserved, at least initially, and adnexal epithelium is spared; in fact, it is believed that cells derived from these adnexal structures (e.g., hair follicles, eccrine sweat ducts) are responsible for the preservation of normal-appearing surface epidermis (Fig. 2.21) (42). However, with progression, greater involvement of the adnexa and surface epidermis occurs, so that eventually the entire thickness of epidermis may become atypical. Clinical and microscopic variants include *bowenoid actinic keratosis,* an actinic keratosis that has achieved full-thickness epithelial atypia (i.e., squamous cell carcinoma in situ) and resembles Bowen disease (see next section); *atrophic or hypertrophic actinic keratosis*; the *spreading, pigmented actinic keratosis* (showing overlapping features with solar lentigo) (43,44); and the *acantholytic actinic keratosis,* in which loss of cohesion among atypical basilar keratinocytes creates an image resembling various acantholytic dermatoses (45). The latter lesion can evolve into an invasive, acantholytic (''pseudoglandu-

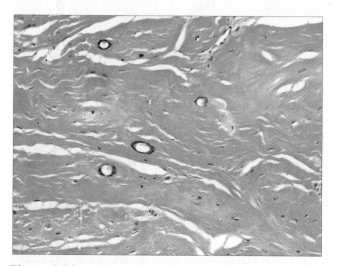

Figure 2.20. Microcystic adnexal carcinoma. Small aggregates of duct-forming epithelial cells extend into the deep dermis.

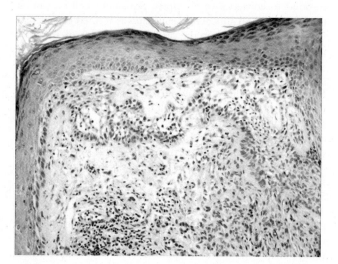

Figure 2.21. Actinic keratosis. Atypical epithelium is identified at the base of the epidermis, separated from it by acantholysis. Atypical keratinocytes also track down a follicular unit (left of figure), but spared follicular epithelium probably accounts for the normal appearance of surface epidermis.

lar'') squamous cell carcinoma. *Lichenoid actinic keratoses* combine the elements of typical actinic keratosis with a bandlike infiltrate that may partly obscure the dermal-epidermal interface (46). Diagnostic challenges may arise when attempting to distinguish actinic keratosis variants from nonmalignant acantholytic dermatoses (e.g., Grover disease, Darier disease), benign lichenoid keratosis, large-cell acanthoma, solar lentigo, or early lentigo maligna. Other malignant or premalignant dermatoses that can microscopically resemble actinic keratosis include superficial basal cell carcinoma and forms of porokeratosis. It is not clear whether there is a difference in prognosis between the bowenoid actinic keratosis and true Bowen disease.

Bowen Disease (Squamous Cell Carcinoma in Situ)

Squamous cell carcinoma in situ of the skin, defined as full-thickness epidermal atypia, can appear in several forms. The best-established type is *Bowen disease*. These lesions appear as erythematous, sometimes pigmented plaques that can develop anywhere on the cutaneous surface, including sun-exposed and non–sun-exposed sites. Plaques can be irregular in shape but tend to be sharply demarcated, and foci of sparing are often identified. Bowen disease can apparently be triggered by several factors. Ultraviolet exposure may be one of these and is at least responsible for the *bowenoid actinic keratosis* referred to earlier. However, the formation of these lesions in sun-protected sites indicates that other carcinogens may be at work; the best established of these are inorganic arsenic exposure and certain types of HPV, particularly HPV-16. Lesions of Bowen disease uncommonly become invasive, but there is evidence that once invasive, these lesions have a high metastatic rate—higher than would be the case for squamous cell carcinomas arising in actinic keratoses. *Bowenoid papulosis* is a condition in which single or multiple papules or plaques develop in the anogenital region (47,48). These are histologically atypical, although they often lack the florid atypia seen in fully developed Bowen disease (47). In this respect, they more closely resemble lesser grades of vulvar intraepithelial neoplasia. Lesions of Bowen disease rarely become invasive, and in fact, they may spontaneously regress or respond to conservative therapies. Squamous cell carcinoma in situ arising on mucocutaneous sites is termed *erythroplasia* (*erythroplasia of Queyrat*, in the case of those arising on the glans penis) (49).

Microscopically, lesions of Bowen disease display full-thickness loss of keratinocyte maturation, with cells showing large, hyperchromatic nuclei, multinucleated keratinocytes, and mitotic figures (some atypical) at all levels of the epidermis (Fig. 2.22). Scattered vacuolated cells can mimic the image of Paget or extramammary Paget disease, or clusters of keratinocytes may produce a ''nested'' configuration. There may be ''skip areas'' of uninvolved epidermis. Typically, there is involvement of follicular epithelium extending to the level of the sebaceous duct. Similar changes are seen in forms of erythroplasia. In bowenoid actinic keratoses, there may be follicular sparing or changes of partial thickness, predominantly basilar atypia at the periphery of the lesions. It is not entirely clear whether the biology of untreated bowenoid actinic keratoses is similar to that of Bowen disease arising in sun-protected sites. In bowenoid papulosis, there are scattered atypical keratinocytes and frequent mitotic figures that are often in the same stage of development, but these tend to occur on a background of more orderly keratinocyte maturation (Fig. 2.23). The differential diagnosis of Bowen

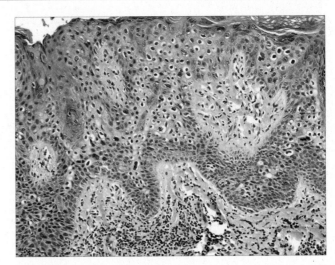

Figure 2.22. Bowen disease (squamous cell carcinoma in situ) showing full-thickness epithelial atypia.

disease, particularly the pagetoid variant, includes Paget disease or extramammary Paget disease, but the latter can usually be recognized by its location, lack of pleomorphism among non-Paget epithelial elements, compression of the basilar layer by Paget cells, and the staining characteristics of Paget cells (e.g., carcinoembryonic antigen, low–molecular-weight cytokeratin positive). Malignant melanoma with pagetoid features also lacks keratinocyte atypia; shows frequent nesting, particularly along the junctional zone, without compression of the basilar layer; and produces a quite different immunoprofile because the neoplastic cells express S-100 protein and other melanocytic antigens. Occasionally, irritated seborrheic keratoses can show some nuclear pleomorphism and mitoses at upper levels of the epidermis, resembling carcinoma in situ and thereby creating considerable diagnostic difficulty. In our experience, this is most common among lesions from elderly individuals and is a particular problem when only partial biopsies are provided (50,51).

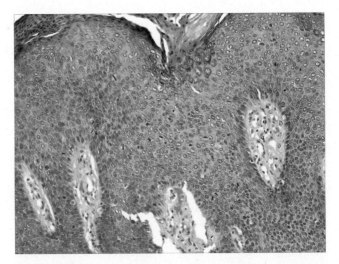

Figure 2.23. Bowenoid papulosis. This lesion shows scattered atypia and mitoses in a background of orderly keratinocyte maturation. Viropathic changes of human papillomavirus can be identified at the epidermal surface.

Keratoacanthoma

In the mid-twentieth century, several authors, notably Rook and Whimster (52) and Musso (53), delineated a proliferative epithelial lesion with resemblances to squamous cell carcinoma that demonstrated spontaneous involution and self-healing. This lesion was termed *keratoacanthoma*. Although widely accepted for years as a pseudomalignancy, many experts currently regard this lesion as a variant form of squamous cell carcinoma (54). This has occurred, in part, because some lesions initially considered keratoacanthomas have metastasized (55) and, in part, because many immunohistochemical, ultrastructural, and genetic investigations have failed to reveal reliable differences from squamous cell carcinoma (56–58).

Keratoacanthomas develop most often in middle-aged to elderly adults, frequently (but not exclusively) on sun-exposed skin. They are rapidly evolving lesions, often developing over a period of 6 to 8 weeks, and present as dome-shaped nodules with central keratin craters. Barring therapeutic intervention, their natural history is to remain stationary for a time and then involute over a 6-month to 1-year period, leaving behind a ragged, crateriform scar. Special varieties include the giant keratoacanthoma *keratoacanthoma centrifugum marginatum*, an expanding, annular lesion; *multiple self-healing epitheliomas of Ferguson-Smith*; and the rare *eruptive keratoacanthomas of Grzybowski*. In cross sections of a fully formed lesion, there is a central keratin crater with a buttresslike arrangement of adjacent, uninvolved epidermis at either site of the crater. Underlying proliferative epithelium extends into the dermis, comprised of cells with glassy-appearing cytoplasm and bland nuclei with low nuclear-to-cytoplasmic ratios. Nuclear pleomorphism and mitotic activity may be observed at the base of the lesion, and perineural infiltration is sometimes identified (59). Intraepidermal neutrophilic microabscesses are commonly found (Fig. 2.24). Although the accompanying dermal infiltrate may contain eosinophils, these can occasionally be found in squamous cell carcinomas and cannot be considered an absolutely reliable diagnostic feature. Findings in involuting keratoacanthomas include apoptotic keratinocytes, a shallow crater with atrophic underlying epithelium, and dermal scar.

Not all pathologists will make a diagnosis of keratoacanthoma, instead preferring a designation such as "squamous cell carcinoma, keratoacanthoma type." I will still render a diagnosis of keratoacanthoma, but the criteria for this diagnosis are fairly strict: (i) the entire lesion must be sampled and displayed in cross section; (ii) the classic microscopic features must be observed, as listed earlier; (iii) there should be a clear clinical description of the lesion, i.e., a rapidly evolving crateriform lesion, with keratoacanthoma as the primary clinical diagnosis, provided by an experienced clinician, preferably a dermatologist; and (iv) there should be no history of immunosuppression.

Squamous Cell Carcinoma

This is the second most common cutaneous malignancy (basal cell carcinoma is most common). It usually presents as an indurated papule or nodule with crusting or ulceration. Squamous cell carcinomas most often arise in actinically damaged skin, particularly in actinic keratoses, but they also develop in mucocutaneous sites, chronic ulcers, burn scars, sinuses, or skin lesions subjected to chronic inflammation or scarring (e.g., discoid lupus erythematosus). They are prone to occur in immunocompromised patients, particularly in renal transplantation patients. The metastatic rate of actinically induced squamous cell carcinomas is low, ranging from 0.5% to 3.0% (41), although from a pathology perspective, the finding of actinic keratosis contiguous to a squamous cell carcinoma is not a useful predictor of metastatic behavior (tumor thickness and depth of invasion are most important in this regard) (60). Metastatic rates are higher among neoplasms arising in other settings, such as mucous membranes or burn scars.

In typical examples, there are masses of epithelial cells within the dermis that display nuclear pleomorphism, atypical mitotic figures, and foci of incomplete keratinization termed *horn pearls* (Fig. 2.25). These epithelial islands extend from the surface epidermis, which usually also displays varying degrees of atypia ranging from actinic keratosis to squamous cell carcinoma in situ. Loss of cohesion of keratinocytes within tumor islands produces an acantholytic, or pseudoglandular, appearance (Fig. 2.26). One variant termed *pseudovascular adenoid squamous cell*

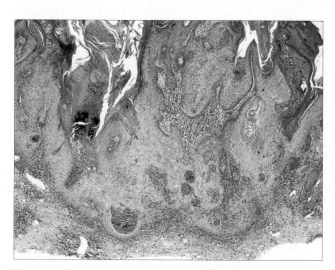

Figure 2.24. Keratoacanthoma showing proliferative epithelium with "glassy" cytoplasm and intraepithelial neutrophilic microabscesses.

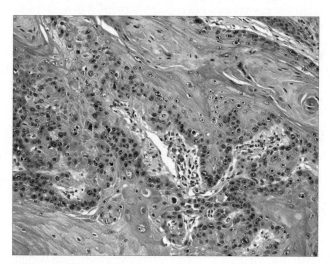

Figure 2.25. Squamous cell carcinoma. Masses of epithelial cells with cytologic atypia and foci of incomplete keratinization are shown.

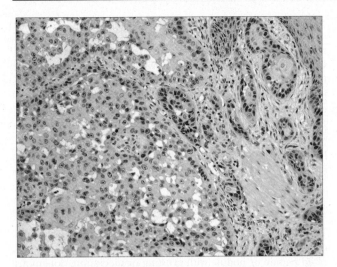

Figure 2.26. Pseudoglandular squamous cell carcinoma. Acantholysis of neoplastic cells produces a glandlike appearance, seen on the right of the figure.

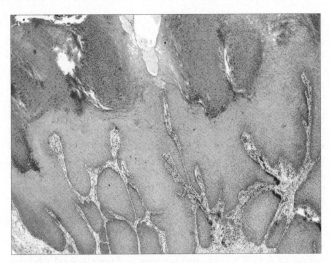

Figure 2.27. Verrucous carcinoma. Marked acanthosis with blunt, "pushing" margins and keratin-filled crypts can be seen.

carcinoma can closely mimic angiosarcoma; it requires careful inspection and sometimes immunohistochemical staining (cytokeratin positive, CD31 negative) for confirmation, although it too may demonstrate biologic aggressiveness (61). *Spindle cell squamous cell carcinoma* raises a differential diagnosis that includes spindle cell malignant melanoma and atypical fibroxanthoma. Epidermal connections are not always demonstrable, and it may be necessary to employ an immunohistochemical panel that includes S-100 protein, CD10, or other markers in addition to cytokeratins. Infiltrative, desmoplastic squamous cell carcinomas may have a higher rate of local recurrence and metastasis compared with neoplasms lacking these features (62). Other variant forms that may be encountered include *signet ring cell squamous cell carcinoma* (63,64) and *carcinosarcoma* (sarcomatoid carcinoma), the latter combining the features of carcinoma and assorted types of sarcomas (65). Invasive squamous cell carcinomas arising from Bowen disease often display basaloid tumor islands with nuclear pleomorphism, resembling the in situ carcinoma of origin or displaying features that more closely resemble an adnexal carcinoma (66,67).

Although the histopathologic diagnosis of cutaneous squamous cell carcinoma is often straightforward, differential diagnostic problems may arise in several circumstances. Issues regarding spindle cell squamous cell carcinoma have already been mentioned. Signet ring cell squamous cell carcinoma can resemble the rare *signet ring cell carcinoma of the eyelids*, a tumor with a high rate of regional or distant metastases (68). Unlike squamous cell carcinoma, the cells of the latter neoplasm may be positive for milk fat globule protein as well as estrogen and progesterone receptors. Furthermore, squamous cell carcinoma can be confused with basal cell carcinoma, or vice versa, in several circumstances (e.g., in instances of bowenoid squamous cell carcinoma or metatypical basal cell carcinoma) (69).

Verrucous Carcinoma

This particularly well-differentiated variant of squamous cell carcinoma develops on the sole of the foot, where it is sometimes called *epithelioma cuniculatum* (a reference to the deep lesional crypts that bear a resemblance to rabbit burrows), but it is also seen in the anogenital region. Lesions on the soles are often clinically thought to represent verrucae, but they are particularly resistant to the usual wart remedies. Although metastases are rare, these lesions can invade and destroy deep structures, and therefore, complete removal is indicated (70,71). Anaplastic transformation can occur spontaneously and, despite earlier teachings, does not always accompany x-ray therapy (72,73).

Microscopic features include hyperkeratosis, parakeratosis, and marked acanthosis that is both exophytic and endophytic. These lesions tend to have blunt, "pushing" margins at the base, although the epithelium often includes keratin-filled crypts containing neutrophils. Cytologic atypia tends to be minimal (Fig. 2.27) but, when found, particularly in the context of dermal invasion, suggests transformation to a biologically more aggressive neoplasm. A relationship with HPV infection is supported by the finding of HPV types 16 and 18, sometimes types 6 and 11, and other HPV types in these lesions (74,75). Resemblances to verrucae, keratoacanthoma, or forms of pseudoepitheliomatous hyperplasia can create diagnostic difficulties, especially when partial or shallow biopsies are submitted for evaluation.

Basal Cell Carcinoma

Basal cell carcinoma is the most common cutaneous malignancy, accounting for approximately 70% of malignant skin tumors (76). With the exception of genetic disorders such as nevoid basal cell carcinoma syndrome (77) or some examples of xeroderma pigmentosum, it typically occurs among adults. Although most often seen in sun-exposed sites, basal cell carcinomas also develop in sun-protected areas. The classical lesion is an ulcerated papule or nodule with a pearly, telangiectatic border, but clinical appearances can vary, and other forms include a sclerotic plaque (*morpheaform basal cell carcinoma*), an erythematous scaly patch (*superficial basal cell carcinoma*), and a pigmented lesion capable of mimicking malignant melanoma (*pigmented basal cell carcinoma*). Basal cell carcinomas are best known for local recurrence or tissue destruction rather than metastasis. However, metastasis has been reported in approximately 0.1% of cases, with involvement of regional lymph nodes, lung, or bone (69). This event is more likely among neglected tumors.

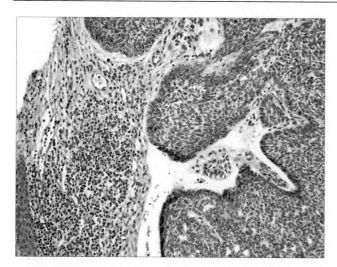

Figure 2.28. Basal cell carcinoma. Macronodular lesion features islands of basaloid cells, peripheral palisading, and cleftlike separations from the adjacent connective tissue.

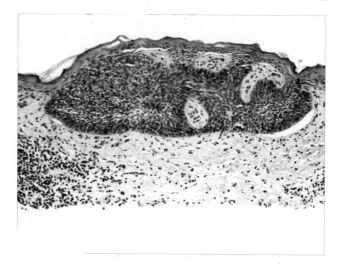

Figure 2.30. Superficial basal cell carcinoma. Islands of basaloid cells are closely associated with the surface epidermis.

The most common histopathologic type of basal cell carcinoma is *nodulocystic*, comprised of rounded lobules of small hyperchromatic cells. There is peripheral palisading of cells, and cleftlike spaces often separate portions of the tumor from the adjacent fibromyxoid stroma (Fig. 2.28). There are several important variant forms. The *infiltrative* basal cell carcinoma features narrow cords of tumor cells within a cellular stroma (Fig. 2.29) (78). When these tumor cells are embedded in a dense, collagenized, hypocellular matrix, the term *morpheaform* basal cell carcinoma is often used (79). The *micronodular* basal cell carcinoma consists of widely scattered small tumor islands, some of which may consist of only a few clustered cells. These may extend deep into the dermis/subcutis and are quite difficult to eradicate (80). *Basosquamous* carcinomas are somewhat controversial; many lesions that receive this designation probably represent keratinizing basal cell carcinomas, but there is another group comprised of neoplastic cells having overlapping features of basal and squamous cell carcinoma that otherwise defy precise categorization (81). Studies indicate that tumors with infiltrative, micronodular, or basosquamous features tend to pursue an aggressive clinical course, and basosquamous carcinomas appear to have a propensity to metastasize.

Other microscopic variants include the *superficial* basal cell carcinoma, in which buds of basaloid cells are identified at the base of the epidermis (Fig. 2.30); the *pigmented* basal cell carcinoma, in which abundant melanocytes and pigment production occur, usually within nodulocystic or superficial tumor types; and reticulated variants, such as the *adenoid* basal cell carcinoma and *fibroepithelioma of Pinkus*. Basal cell carcinomas with sebaceous differentiation (*basosebaceous* basal cell carcinoma) can mimic primary sebaceous neoplasms, and examples of these undoubtedly occur in Muir-Torre syndrome. Unusual forms of basal cell carcinoma feature signet ring, granular, or clear cell changes. Basal cell carcinomas must be distinguished from adnexal tumors such as trichoepithelioma and the basaloid variant of sebaceous carcinoma, basaloid follicular hamartoma, and "cloacogenic" carcinoma. Clear cell variants of basal cell carcinoma can mimic balloon cell melanoma or trichilemmal carcinoma; those with granular cell changes can be distinguished from true granular cell tumors by their distinct fibromyxoid stroma and cytokeratin positivity.

TUMORS OF CONNECTIVE TISSUE

Because several soft tissue tumors also occur in or extend to the skin and are discussed elsewhere, this section will concentrate on those neoplasms that primarily involve the dermis.

CONNECTIVE TISSUE NEVI

These lesions are hamartomas in which collagen is increased in quantity or thickness and may be accompanied by alterations in elastic tissue. They can occur sporadically or as a heritable, autosomal dominant trait. Connective tissue nevi present as indurated papules (82,83) or nodules that may be organized in plaques or appear in disseminated form. The epidermis tends to be uninvolved, although lesions with combined features of

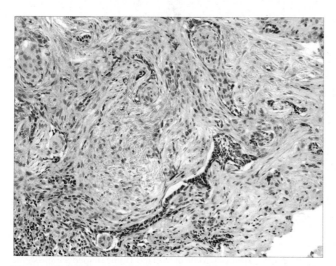

Figure 2.29. Infiltrative basal cell carcinoma showing cords of tumor cells within a cellular stroma.

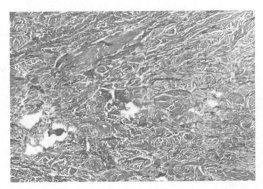

Figure 2.31. Connective tissue nevus. Thickened collagen bundles occupy the dermis.

epidermal nevus or Becker nevus have also been reported (84). In one variant, the *Buschke-Ollendorff syndrome*, connective tissue nevi are associated with osteopoikilosis—sclerotic, stippled densities in long, round, and flat bones. Microscopically, thickened collagen bundles are observed, either in compact or exaggeratedly fenestrated form (Fig. 2.31). Stains such as Verhoeff-van Gieson often show either increased numbers and density of elastic fibers (*nevus elasticus*) or elastic fibers that are fragmented, diminished, or even absent (*nevus anelasticus*) (85,86). Increased quantities of mucin can sometimes be identified (*nevus mucinosus*) (87), and we have observed a few cases in which patchy increases of elastic fibers have been associated with increased quantities of mucin deposition in the same locations (Fig. 2.32). The changes in connective tissue nevi can be subtle, especially in hematoxylin and eosin–stained sections, and diagnosis depends heavily on a high index of suspicion and a good clinical history.

THE ANGIOFIBROMA FAMILY, INCLUDING FIBROUS PAPULE OF THE FACE AND ACQUIRED DIGITAL FIBROKERATOMA

The angiofibroma family is a group of generally acro-located lesions that share as common features dermal fibrosis and vascular proliferation or dilatation. Lesions commonly regarded as belonging to this group include *fibrous papule of the face, pearly penile papules,* the *angiofibromas of tuberous sclerosis, sporadic angiofibromas, digital fibrokeratomas,* and *familial myxovascular fibromas.* I will concentrate on two of these: fibrous papule of the face and acquired digital fibrokeratoma.

Fibrous Papule of the Face

This lesion is typically a firm, dome-shaped lesion arising on the nose or central portions of the face. It is not unusual to encounter several such lesions in an individual patient (88). They are most often flesh colored but may be erythematous or show focal pigmentation. Despite their small size and the small shave biopsies that they usually elicit, these lesions are often recognizable on low-power microscopy. They tend to have gently dome-shaped contours and show both dermal fibrosis and vasodilatation (Fig. 2.33). On occasion, these lesions can show considerable edema. Scattered enlarged, angulated, stellate or multinucleated cells can often be observed in the papillary dermis. These were once suspected to be effete nevus cells, an impression that seemed to be reinforced by the occasional finding of unequivocal nevomelanocytes in these lesions. However, ultrastructural and immunohistochemical studies indicate that these stellate cells are in reality factor XIIIa–positive dermal dendrocytes and that nevus cells, when present, probably represent a coincidental finding (89,90). In recent years, several histologic variants have been reported, including hypercellular, clear cell, pigmented, pleomorphic, inflammatory, granular cell (91), CD34-positive (92), and epithelioid (93) types. These lesions can be mistaken for hemangiomas, telangiectasias, and atypical melanocytic lesions; the latter occurs especially when there is overlying junctional melanocytic hyperplasia, which is a finding that is not unusual in fibrous papules.

Acquired Digital Fibrokeratoma

This lesion presents as a dome-shaped or pedunculated nodule found most commonly in adults on the hands, feet, fingers, and toes (94). The so-called *garlic clove fibromas (Koenen tumors)* that

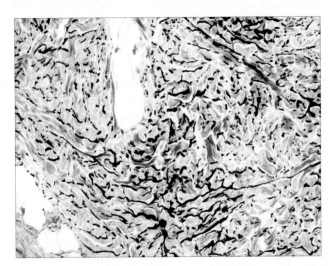

Figure 2.32. Mucinous connective tissue nevus. This Movat pentachrome stain shows aggregates of thickened elastic fibers associated with mucinous deposits.

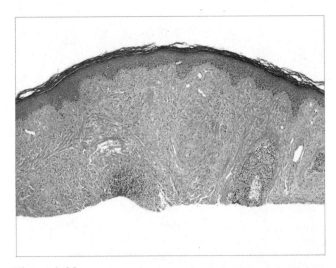

Figure 2.33. Fibrous papule of the face. Dome-shaped papule shows dermal fibrosis and vasodilatation. Scattered spindled to stellate cells are present within the dermis.

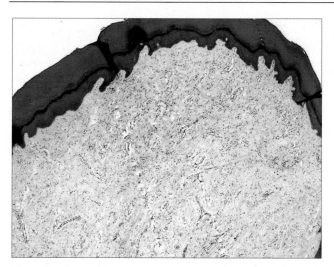

Figure 2.34. Digital fibrokeratoma, featuring hyperkeratosis, acanthosis, thick collagen bundles, and vasodilatation. This example shows increased numbers of fibroblasts.

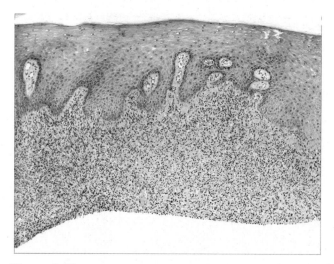

Figure 2.35. Dermatofibroma. Dermal proliferations of small spindled cells with overlying acanthosis are seen.

arise in periungual or subungual tissues of patients with tuberous sclerosis (and sometimes in normal individuals) are also regarded as types of digital fibrokeratomas (95,96). Microscopically, these lesions often appear as elongated or dome-shaped papules, with hyperkeratosis and acanthosis overlying thick collagen bundles that tend to be oriented perpendicularly to the overlying epidermis. Small blood vessels are a prominent feature but may at first glance be inconspicuous because of the density of surrounding collagen. Variant forms may show increased cellularity (fibroblasts) or edema (Fig. 2.34). The differential diagnosis includes particularly supernumerary digits (rudimentary polydactyly), which can closely resemble digital fibrokeratoma clinically and microscopically. However, that lesion is typically present at birth, may be bilateral, and shows prominent nerve bundles in the mid to deep dermis with features of neuroma. In fact, this lesion is believed to occur as the result of autoamputation of a true accessory digit.

DERMATOFIBROMA

Also known by the more generic term *fibrous histiocytoma*, the dermatofibroma is one of the most readily recognizable of the connective tissue tumors, although the variability of its features can create diagnostic difficulties. These lesions present as firm, round papules or small nodules, commonly on the lower legs but also on the arms and trunk. Multiple lesions are not uncommon in otherwise normal individuals, but multiple dermatofibromas have been reported with lupus erythematosus (97), human immunodeficiency virus (HIV) infection (98), and myasthenia gravis (99). Lesions involute even with partial therapy, and recurrences are uncommon, although they are more frequent with certain histologic subtypes, particularly *cellular dermatofibromas*. Recent studies seem to indicate that dermatofibromas are neoplastic (100), although there is a persistent viewpoint that they may represent a kind of reparative process (101).

Microscopically, there is a proliferation of spindled cells between thickened collagen bundles within the dermis, forming a "lens-shaped" zone whose long axis is parallel to the overlying epidermis. The constituent cells apparently consist of dermal

dendrocytes, fibroblasts, and "histiocytes" (macrophages) in varying proportions (Fig. 2.35). At the periphery of the lesion, these spindled cells surround cross-sectional profiles of collagen, a phenomenon sometimes described as "collagen entrapment." With deeper involvement, the proliferations of cells either extend into the subcutis with bulbous, "pushing" margins or infiltrate within connective tissue septa. The epidermis overlying dermatofibromas is typically acanthotic, often with flattening of the bases of rete ridges, although there may also be rete ridge effacement in superficially located tumors. The phenomenon of stromal induction is sometimes seen, in which the involved connective tissue "induces" the formation of basal cell hyperplasia—resembling basal cell carcinoma, or even the formation of follicular units or sebaceous glands. Deeper variants such as the *deep penetrating dermatofibroma* may lack significant epidermal changes (102). Variant forms include the lipidized dermatofibroma, with numerous foamy macrophages, hemorrhage, and Touton-like giant cells, *epithelioid cell histiocytoma* (103–105); *fibrotic* types that can closely resemble sclerotic fibroma (106); *aneurysmal dermatofibroma*, combining features of lipidized dermatofibroma with large blood-filled spaces (Fig. 2.36) (107); and a rare *granular cell dermatofibroma* (108). Occasional dermatofibromas contain cells with large, bizarre, and/or hyperchromatic nuclei (*dermatofibroma with monster cells*) (109), but these lesions nevertheless typically behave in a benign fashion. Occasional mitotic figures can be found in dermatofibromas, but again, they do not appear to denote lesions with more aggressive biologic behavior. Factor XIIIa is commonly expressed in these lesions, although it sometimes appears that expression is confined to dendritic cells accompanying the tumor rather than the major constituent cells (110). On the other hand, the cells of epithelioid cell histiocytoma are often strongly factor XIIIa positive. CD68 and smooth muscle actin may be expressed as well, the latter often in tumors with a myofibroblastic component. The differential diagnosis in a given case can include neurofibroma or spindle cell melanocytic lesions (S-100 positive), leiomyoma (muscle-specific actin and desmin positive), or dermatofibrosarcoma protuberans (CD34 positive).

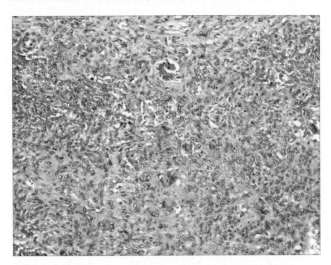

Figure 2.36. Aneurysmal dermatofibroma. This lesion shows considerable hemorrhage, foamy macrophages, and variant forms of Touton giant cells that contain hemosiderin.

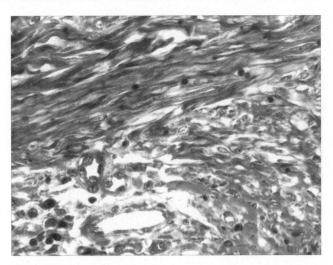

Figure 2.38. Infantile digital fibroma. Phosphotungstic acid-hematoxylin stain shows purple-staining paranuclear inclusion bodies that are about the size of erythrocytes.

FIBROMATOSIS

Forms of fibromatosis can extend into dermis and enter into the differential diagnosis of spindle cell cutaneous lesions, including scar. One unique form of the disease in skin is termed *(recurrent) infantile digital fibroma.* These fibromas manifest as solitary or multiple nodules of the fingers and toes, typically appearing in the first 3 years of life. Although recurrences are common, spontaneous regression may occur (111). On biopsy, there are thick, intersecting collagen bundles and accompanying spindled cells (Fig. 2.37) that contain paranuclear cytoplasmic inclusion bodies roughly the size of erythrocytes. These are eosinophilic with hematoxylin and eosin stain and purple with phosphotungstic acid-hematoxylin (Fig. 2.38). The inclusion bodies are actin positive (112), and ultrastructurally, they consist of bundles of microfilaments with dense bodies. This finding suggests that the constituent cells are actually myofibro-

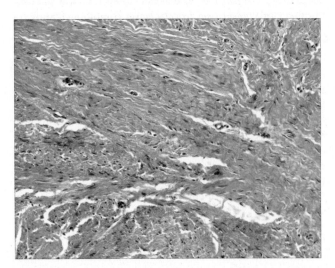

Figure 2.37. Infantile digital fibroma. There are thick, intersecting collagen bundles and accompanying spindled cells, many of which are myofibroblasts.

blasts, and *infantile digital myofibroblastoma* has been proposed as a more accurate name for this tumor (113).

DERMATOFIBROSARCOMA PROTUBERANS

Dermatofibrosarcoma protuberans (DFSP) has been regarded as a fibrous tissue tumor of intermediate malignancy because it is best known for relentless growth and proneness to recurrence rather than metastasis, although the latter definitely occurs and is well documented (114). It is largely a tumor of adults, but there is a closely related pediatric tumor termed *giant cell fibroblastoma.* DFSP most commonly arises on the trunk or proximal extremities, presenting as one or more cutaneous nodules with surrounding induration, indicating subcutaneous growth that is often extensive. This growth pattern sometimes makes complete excision difficult, and recurrences are common. Metastases may develop in about 3% of cases, often with involvement of lymph nodes or the lungs (115).

Microscopically, the tumor is comprised by dense aggregates of spindled cells that form "cartwheel" arrangements (Fig. 2.39) (116). The cells have a monotonous appearance, featuring tapered nuclei and, most often, only sparse mitoses. Subcutaneous involvement is characterized by growth within septa and between adipocytes in horizontal fashion, producing a honeycomb appearance (117). The spindled cells may extend well into the dermis; changes in the overlying epidermis occur (118), but the type of acanthosis seen in dermatofibroma, with flattening of the tips of rete ridges, is rarely observed. Little or no polarizable collagen can be found among neoplastic cells (119). A pigmented variant, known as the Bednar tumor, also features scattered dendritic melanocytes (120). Occasionally, myxoid changes are seen, sometimes, but not invariably, in recurrent lesions (121,122). Fibrosarcoma-like areas occur, and their presence has been associated with local recurrence and metastasis (123,124). CD34 positivity of tumor cells is considered an immunohistochemical hallmark of DFSP (Fig. 2.40) (125).

The differential diagnosis of these tumors includes myofibroma, malignant fibrous histiocytoma (pleomorphic sarcoma), spindle cell melanoma, neurofibroma, and (in the case of myxoid variants) myxoid liposarcoma, in addition to derma-

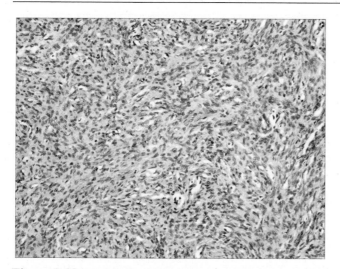

Figure 2.39. Dermatofibrosarcoma protuberans. Dense aggregates of spindled cells forming "cartwheel arrangements." The cells have a monotonous appearance.

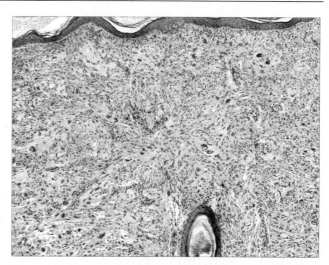

Figure 2.41. Atypical fibroxanthoma. This is an example of the pleomorphic variant of this lesion. It bears a close resemblance to malignant fibrous histiocytoma (pleomorphic sarcoma).

tofibroma. Attention to morphologic details and immunohistochemical analysis usually permit distinction from these other entities.

ATYPICAL FIBROXANTHOMA

Atypical fibroxanthoma (AFX) is a cutaneous mesenchymal tumor that microscopically resembles the soft tissue tumor malignant fibrous histiocytoma/pleomorphic sarcoma (MFH) but has a distinctive clinical presentation and usually a better clinical outcome (126). AFX usually arises in sun-exposed skin of the head and neck region of older adults. It uncommonly develops in younger patients or in other locations; some reports of occurrence in younger individuals may actually have been describing atypical variants of dermatofibroma (e.g., *dermatofibroma with monster cells*). The lesion often presents as an elevated, ulcerated nodule. It responds well to complete surgical excision. Recurrences are uncommon, and metastases are rare. However,

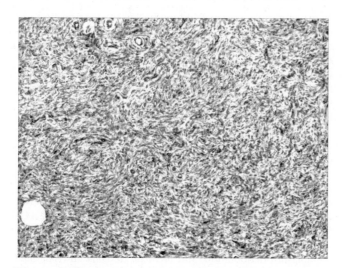

Figure 2.40. Dermatofibrosarcoma protuberans. The constituent cells are CD34 positive, a hallmark of this neoplasm.

metastases have been reported (e.g., to lymph nodes or parotid gland); this usually occurs in deep-seated, recurrent tumors or those that have arisen after radiation therapy (127).

Microscopically, AFX shows a dermal proliferation of polygonal or spindled cells that occasionally contact the overlying or adjacent epidermis, although they lack evidence for *origination* from the epidermis. Some of the cells possess vacuolated, foamy cytoplasm. Pleomorphic variants may feature large, irregularly shaped nuclei with coarse chromatin, prominent nucleoli, and atypical mitotic figures (Fig. 2.41) (128,129). Other variants include *angiomatoid* and *clear cell* types (129) and *AFX with osteoclast-like giant cells* (130–132). A *spindle cell variant* with limited pleomorphism can be difficult to distinguish from a variety of other malignant spindle cell tumors (133). Immunohistochemical study often proves helpful in diagnosis, but usually because negative results help to rule out such potential mimics as spindle cell melanoma (S-100 positive), spindle cell squamous cell carcinoma (cytokeratin positive), or leiomyosarcoma (more uniformly actin positive and desmin positive). A completely reliable positive marker for AFX is highly desirable but has been lacking. However, promising results have been obtained with antibodies to CD10 and CD99 (134).

Microscopic differentiation from MFH has been difficult if not impossible, and clinical features are most often decisive. It is widely believed that AFX is simply a superficial variant of that tumor, but this issue has not been fully resolved by studies of DNA content and proliferative activity (135,136). However, there is a study suggesting that expression of CD74 (LN-2) may help in distinguishing between the two, in that CD74 expression is typical of MFH but most often negative in AFX (137).

NEURAL TUMORS

Although there is considerable variety among the neural tumors that *can* arise in skin, the types of lesions *commonly* found in a cutaneous location are limited, and it is unusual to find neoplasms of ependymal, meningeal, neuronal, or notochordal differentiation. The following represent the most important of the neural tumors from a dermatopathologic perspective.

NEUROFIBROMA

Neurofibromas frequently arise in skin and, in fact, are among the most familiar of cutaneous neoplasms, although variant forms can sometimes create diagnostic difficulties. They most commonly present as isolated soft papules or nodules arising in any cutaneous site (138,139), although in our experience, this presentation is most often encountered in middle-aged to older adults. Occasionally, several such lesions can be seen, in widely scattered or clustered form, in otherwise normal individuals. Multiple neurofibromas, particularly when developing in childhood and presenting together with *café au lait* lesions, strongly suggest a diagnosis of neurofibromatosis of the von Recklinghausen type (140,141). Plexiform neurofibromas can distort the superficial soft tissues and, both on palpation and (as surgical specimens) in cross section, can resemble a "bag of worms." Plexiform neurofibromas have traditionally been regarded as presumptive evidence of neurofibromatosis (142), but recent evidence suggests that this is not invariably the case (143–146).

Microscopically, neurofibromas have a familiar appearance, consisting of scattered spindled cells with "buckled" or "S-shaped" nuclei, within a variably myxoid matrix (147,148). Scattered small vessels and mast cells are common (Fig. 2.42). Although at times the lesions appear to be well demarcated from adjacent dermal connective tissue, they are not encapsulated, and frequently, the lesions merge imperceptibly with dermal collagen. The constituent cells are largely comprised of endoneurial fibroblasts and include Schwann cells and perineurial cells. Myxoid, pigmented, and diffuse types occur, and at times, the small vessel component may be the predominating feature. There is a recently described variant termed *dendritic cell neurofibroma with pseudorosettes* (149). Plexiform neurofibromas show demarcated fascicles of proliferating Schwann cells, separated by a myxofibrous stroma, producing the appearance of miniature nerve trunks (Fig. 2.43) (150).

The most common differential diagnostic consideration is that of melanocytic nevus, sometimes termed *neurotized nevus*. Both are S-100 positive, although neurofibroma would lack other melanocytic markers and would be more likely to be immunoreactive for factor XIIIa (151). Because it makes little difference prognostically whether an isolated, banal lesion is termed neurofibroma or neurotized nevus, we typically do not launch into

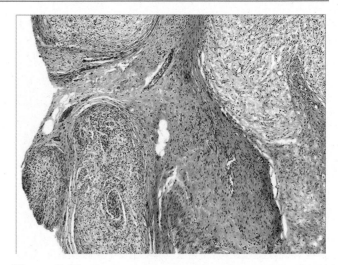

Figure 2.43. Plexiform neurofibroma. Fascicles of cells with the appearance of small nerve trunks, separated by a fibromyxoid stroma, are seen.

an expensive battery of immunohistochemical stains in an attempt to differentiate the two; lesions lacking identifiable nevomelanocytes (usually identifiable as nests or aggregates of cells) and accompanied by small vessels and mast cells are usually termed neurofibroma. A more significant problem is the occasional lesion with hypercellularity, mitotic activity, nuclear atypia, or cell necrosis; such lesions must be distinguished from malignant peripheral nerve sheath tumors. At times, this may be a difficult task, and a given lesion may have to be designated as a "peripheral nerve sheath tumor of indeterminate biologic potential" (150). However, staining for p53 and Ki-67 may help to distinguish malignant peripheral nerve sheath tumors from neurofibroma, which would be expected to be negative for these markers (152,153). Such tumors may also bear a resemblance to desmoplastic malignant melanoma, and therefore, special attention should be paid to any changes at the dermal-epidermal junction, realizing, however, that a proportion of desmoplastic melanomas lack both junctional changes and distinctive melanocytic immunohistochemical markers.

NEURILEMMOMA (SCHWANNOMA)

Neurilemmomas are less common in skin than are neurofibromas. They somewhat resemble solitary neurofibromas clinically, although they are often encapsulated and firmer to palpation, sometimes mimicking epidermal (infundibular) cysts. They are well known to generations of dermatologists as one of the "painful dermal tumors" (154,155). Multiple neurilemmomas can be associated with neurofibromatosis (156) or occur as a noninherited syndrome termed *schwannomatosis* (157).

Microscopically, neurilemmomas are encapsulated and show two major histopathologic patterns: *Antoni A tissue*, consisting of densely aggregated spindle cells whose nuclei form palisaded arrangements, especially around syncytia of cytoplasm (*Verocay bodies*); and *Antoni B tissue*, consisting of sparsely cellular, edematous or myxoid foci (150,158). The latter foci have been considered to represent degenerative change in Antoni A tissue (Fig. 2.44). Mast cells are often numerous in these tumors. Microscopic variants include *glandular* neurilemmoma (probably the result of a metaplastic phenomenon) and *melanotic, plexiform,* and *epithelioid neurilemmomas*. Long-standing and/or traumatized lesions may feature enlarged, hyperchromatic nuclei with occasional mito-

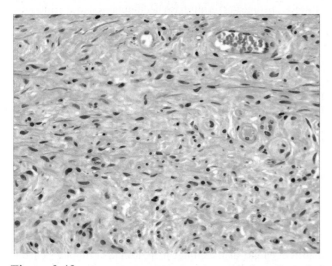

Figure 2.42. Neurofibroma. This view shows typical small spindled cells with "S-shaped" nuclei, mast cells, vessels, and small nerve twigs.

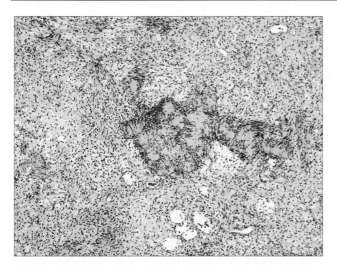

Figure 2.44. Neurilemmoma (Schwannoma). This image shows Antoni A tissue, complete with Verocay bodies, and surrounding Antoni B tissue.

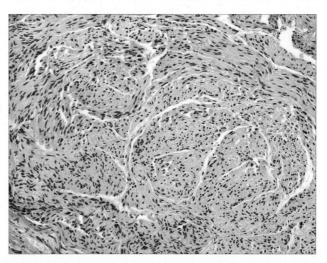

Figure 2.45. Localized, circumscribed neuroma. Fascicles of spindled cells with focal palisading can be identified. Numerous small axons were found in this example.

ses, a change termed *ancient Schwannoma* (159). Malignant change in a cutaneous neurilemmoma is rare (160). The S-100 positivity of neurilemmoma allows distinction from other tumors that exhibit nuclear palisading, such as leiomyoma, and the uncommon neuroid basal cell carcinoma. The localized, circumscribed ("palisaded, encapsulated") neuroma can have overlapping microscopic and immunohistochemical characteristics.

NEUROMAS

There are several types of neuroma that can arise in or involve the skin. Although *traumatic neuroma* has traditionally been considered the most common of these, in our own surgical material, *localized, circumscribed neuroma* (formerly "palisaded, encapsulated" neuroma) is seen most frequently. The latter lesion is generally painless and tends to occur on the central portion of the face (161). The so-called *supernumerary digit* is found at the base of the fifth finger near its ulnar border. The traditional view has been that this lesion represents a kind of "amputation neuroma" (162), the result of autoamputation of a true accessory digit during embryonic life. Although this view has been questioned (163), we recently received a specimen consisting of a true accessory digit, with a polypoid neuroma (supernumerary digit) extending from its surface. Morton neuroma, in reality a fibrosis of the plantar digital nerve, is occasionally encountered in dermatology practice (164,165).

Localized, circumscribed neuromas are considered to be true neoplasms. They are well circumscribed and often possess an attenuated fibrous capsule. Fascicles of bland spindled cells are found, often with demonstrable palisading but without surrounding fibrous sheaths (Fig. 2.45) (166,167). The fascicles often, but not invariably, contain axons (168). S-100 protein staining is regularly demonstrated. Traumatic neuromas are in reality aberrant attempts of reinnervation following disruption of neural axons. Consequently, nerve bundles are surrounded and disrupted by fibrous bands. The supernumerary digit also features small nerves embedded in connective tissue (Fig. 2.46A,B), but small oval structures resembling Meissner bodies are also identified.

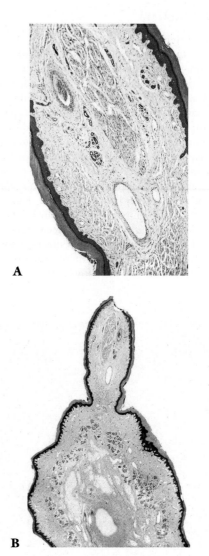

Figure 2.46. Supernumerary digit. **(A)** A typical example, showing polypoid configuration and small nerves embedded in connective tissue. **(B)** This lesion actually arose within a true accessory digit.

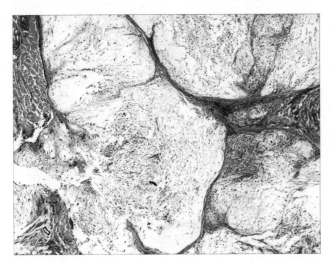

Figure 2.47. Nerve sheath myxoma. Well-demarcated aggregates of spindled cells can be identified within a mucinous matrix.

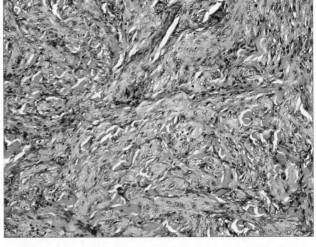

Figure 2.49. Neurothekeoma, cellular type. More solid aggregates of epithelioid cells are present. Nuclear hyperchromasia and mitotic activity are often encountered in these lesions.

NEUROTHEKEOMA

Gallagher and Helwig first introduced this term in 1980 to refer to a group of tumors of presumed nerve sheath origin (169). Since that time, it has become apparent that three somewhat distinctive lesions have become subsumed under this title: the *nerve sheath myxoma*, largely as described by Pulitzer and Reed (170); the *classic neurothekeoma*; and *cellular neurothekeoma* (171). These tumors predominantly affect younger individuals and are most frequently found on the head and neck and upper extremities. They typically present as firm, dome-shaped nodules.

Microscopically, nerve sheath myxomas consist of well-demarcated aggregates of spindled cells that are separated from one another by a markedly mucinous matrix (Fig. 2.47). Classic neurothekeomas are comprised of concentric arrangements of plump spindled to epithelioid cells resembling melanocytic nests. Cytologic atypia ranges from minimal to moderate (Fig. 2.48). In cellular neurothekeoma, there are more solid dermal aggregates of epithelioid cells without formation of discrete

nests as seen in the classic form (Fig. 2.49). Nuclear hyperchromasia and mitotic activity are common in these lesions. On immunohistochemical staining, nerve sheath myxomas are variably positive for S-100 protein, CD57, and epithelial membrane antigen, indicating schwannian and/or perineural differentiation. However, classic and cellular neurothekeomas are negative for these antigens, and in fact, the cellular origin/differentiation of these tumors is problematic. Actin positivity in cellular neurothekeomas has led some to suspect that they are actually variants of epithelioid leiomyoma (172). Local infiltration of deep tissues has been seen in large neurothekeomas, but to date, metastases have not been identified. Tumors with some features of neurothekeoma but showing significant nuclear pleomorphism, necrosis, or atypical mitoses should raise consideration of malignant peripheral nerve sheath tumor or possibly malignant melanoma.

MERKEL CELL CARCINOMA (NEUROENDOCRINE CARCINOMA OF THE SKIN)

Neuroendocrine carcinoma is one of the most biologically aggressive neoplasms of the skin. This primary cutaneous tumor is widely believed to be of Merkel cell origin. The Merkel cell is found in epidermis, oral mucosa, outer follicular sheath, and sweat ducts and is believed to be a specialized neuroepithelial cell that may have a touch receptor function. Merkel cell carcinoma (MCC) typically presents as a violaceous nodule arising in the head and neck region of elderly adults, although exceptions certainly occur (173). Development of MCC in lesions of Bowen disease (squamous cell carcinoma in situ) has been repeatedly described (174–176). Forty percent of these tumors recur locally, and 75% of patients with one or more recurrences develop regional nodal or distant metastases. In most instances, visceral involvement is accompanied by death within 6 months (177,178).

On biopsy, aggregates of small, round tumor cells are found within the dermis. The configurations produced by these cells vary from broad sheets to trabeculae to rounded islands showing organoid growth. Involvement of the overlying epidermis with nestlike arrangements of tumor cells is sometimes noted. Typi-

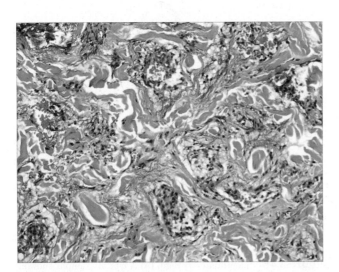

Figure 2.48. Neurothekeoma, classic type. Aggregates of epithelioid cells resemble melanocytic nests.

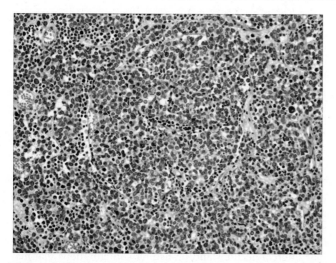

Figure 2.50. Merkel cell carcinoma. Islands of cells showing scant cytoplasm, round to oval nuclei, and evenly distributed chromatin. Nucleoli are inconspicuous.

cally, the cytoplasm is scant, and the nuclei are round to oval with evenly distributed chromatin and inconspicuous nucleoli (Fig. 2.50); mitotic activity is often brisk (173,179). Larger, sometimes giant tumor cells with the same nuclear characteristics are occasionally seen. Divergent squamous and even sweat gland differentiation can be seen in some examples (180,181). Immunohistochemical study shows dotlike paranuclear cytokeratin staining (Fig. 2.51). Cytokeratin 20 is frequently positive, and cells also express neuron-specific enolase, chromogranin, synaptophysin, and a variety of other neural and neuropeptide markers (182).

MCC must be distinguished from neuroendocrine carcinomas metastatic to the skin. The most useful immunohistochemical markers for this purpose are cytokeratin 20 (usually positive in MCC and negative in metastatic neuroendocrine carcinoma) and thyroid transcription factor-1 (TTF-1), which produces the reverse result (183,184). The *Azzopardi phenomenon*—basophilic nucleic acid encrustation of tumoral blood vessels—has been observed in metastatic small-cell pulmonary carcinoma but has only recently been reported in primary MCC of skin (185,186). Other neoplasms that can be confused with MCC (and the immunohistochemical markers that often permit distinction) include non-Hodgkin's lymphoma (CD45 positive) and basal cell carcinoma (Ber-EP4 positive).

VASCULAR TUMORS

Many of the lesions labeled "hemangioma," particularly those arising in childhood, probably represent malformations rather than true neoplasms. However, there is an array of vascular tumors with distinctive microscopic characteristics. Several of these have been linked to infectious agents. Angiosarcoma arises most often in elderly individuals, whereas Kaposi sarcoma can develop in several clinically distinct circumstances.

LOBULAR CAPILLARY HEMANGIOMA

For years, this hemangioma was termed *pyogenic granuloma* because of its resemblance to granulation tissue following infection. The latter name still persists among clinicians but is now a well-established misnomer. Lobular capillary hemangioma (LCH) is a true neoplasm with characteristic microscopic features (187). It typically presents at any age as an erythematous, often polypoid growth on the skin or mucous membranes. It is sometimes, but not always, precipitated by trauma. Development on mucosal surfaces during pregnancy is a recognized phenomenon. *Subcutaneous and intravenous forms of LCH*, as would be expected, have quite different clinical presentations (188,189). The entity known as *acquired tufted hemangioma* is likely another variant of LCH; this presents as enlarging erythematous macules and plaques on the neck and trunk of young individuals (190).

These lesions have in common the proliferation of small vessels that are divided into lobules by fibrous connective tissue (Fig. 2.52) (187). The vessels are lined by plump endothelial cells and surrounded by pericytes. The lobular arrangement of vessels can be obscured by edema and granulation tissue changes that have been superimposed by trauma; this is particularly likely to occur in protuberant lesions. An in-growing collarette of hyperkeratotic epidermis is often seen at the base of polypoid examples of LCH, corresponding to the collarette of

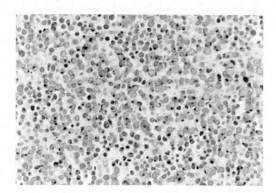

Figure 2.51. Merkel cell carcinoma. This tumor, stained with antibodies to AE1/AE3 cytokeratin, shows dotlike paranuclear staining.

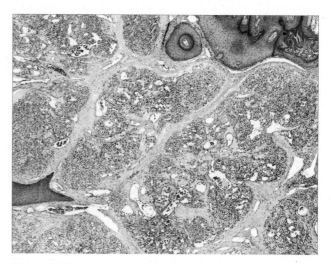

Figure 2.52. Lobular capillary hemangioma. The lobular arrangement of vessels is apparent.

scale noted clinically to surround these lesions. A central vessel with muscular wall resembling a vein may be observed, and fibrosis is observed in the involutional stage. Multiple recurrences (often related to partial removal), regional satellite formation, and disseminated lesions have all been reported, but these are nevertheless benign lesions that ultimately either respond to surgical methods or, in the case of disseminated lesions, may regress spontaneously.

GLOMUS TUMOR

Glomus tumor is one of the most distinctive of the cutaneous vascular tumors. It is composed of elements recapitulating the *Suquet-Hoyer canal*, the arterial segment of the *glomus*, a specialized arteriovenous shunt found primarily in hands, feet, fingers, and toes. This structure is comprised of a narrow lumen lined by a single layer of endothelium, surrounded in turn by four to six layers of glomus cells, which can be regarded as modified smooth muscle cells. Occasionally, these normal structures are found incidentally in biopsies of distal extremities obtained for other reasons and are mistaken for glomus tumors.

The glomus tumor usually presents as a purple nodule, often in a subungual location. These lesions are characteristically painful, a sensation that either arises spontaneously or is elicited by pressure. A variant of this tumor, *glomangioma*, is often solitary but may be multiple and can be inherited as an autosomal dominant trait (191). These lesions occur on the trunk or extremities and are most often painless.

The glomus tumor is well circumscribed or encapsulated and is composed of rather solid aggregates of glomus cells surrounding relatively small vessels (Fig. 2.53) (192), whereas glomangiomas are poorly circumscribed and feature prominent vessels surrounded by only a few layers of glomus cells (193). Immunohistochemistry shows that glomus cells are smooth muscle actin and muscle-specific actin positive and are negative for desmin and markers of endothelial cells (194,195). Multiple nerve fibers can be identified in solitary glomus tumors. Most glomus tumors are benign, but atypical examples exist. The study of atypical glomus tumors by Folpe et al. (196) resulted in a classification scheme that categorizes these lesions as follows: malig-

nant glomus tumor, symplastic glomus tumor, glomus tumor of uncertain malignant potential, and glomangiomatosis. Malignant tumors were considered those with deep location and size greater than 2 cm, or atypical mitotic figures, or moderate to high nuclear grade and five or more mitotic figures per 50 high-power fields. Symplastic glomus tumors featured high nuclear grade but no other malignant features. Metastasis occurred only in the group of tumors fulfilling criteria for malignancy (196).

MICROVENULAR HEMANGIOMA

This lesion arises in sun-damaged skin, especially the arms, of young to middle-aged individuals. Clinically, it has features of a conventional hemangioma, although Kaposi sarcoma is occasionally considered in the differential diagnosis. Microscopic findings include elongated vessels with narrow lumina that display interconnections and branching configurations that may extend into subcutaneous septa (Fig. 2.54). These vessels have venous characteristics. Despite this somewhat unusual configuration, the lesion appears to be relatively confined on low-power inspection, shows minimal if any inflammation, and lacks nuclear atypia or mitotic activity. Significantly, changes expected in Kaposi sarcoma, such as the "promontory sign," hyaline globules, plasma cells, and solid aggregates of spindled cells, are not observed (see Kaposi's sarcoma, pages 60–61) (197–199).

GLOMERULOID HEMANGIOMA

Glomeruloid hemangiomas present as multiple purple or red papules on the trunk and extremities. They may have clinical features resembling a variety of other types of hemangioma, including cherry angioma, cavernous hemangioma, or lobular capillary hemangioma. This type of hemangioma is noteworthy for its association with the *POEMS syndrome* (**p**olyneuropathy, **o**rganomegaly, **e**ndocrinopathies, **s**kin lesions), which in turn is linked to Castleman disease (200,201). Besides the hemangiomas, the skin lesions of POEMS syndrome include sclerodermoid changes, hyperpigmentation, and hypertrichosis.

Glomeruloid hemangiomas are so named because of the dilated vascular spaces containing aggregates of erythrocyte-

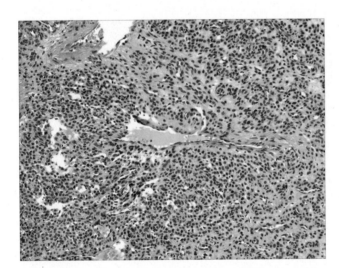

Figure 2.53. Glomus tumor. Dense aggregates of glomus cells surround a dermal vessel.

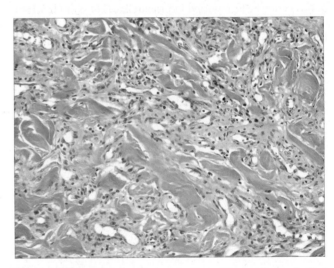

Figure 2.54. Microvenular hemangioma. Elongated vessels show numerous interconnections.

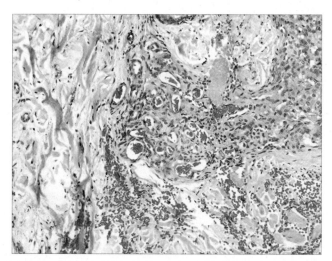

Figure 2.55. Glomeruloid hemangioma. The arrangements of vessels produce a resemblance to renal glomeruli. This lesion occurred in a patient with POEMS syndrome.

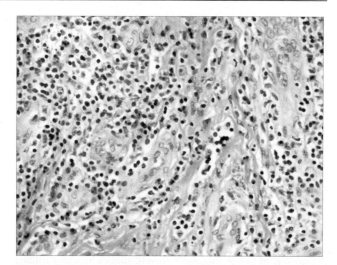

Figure 2.56. Angiolymphoid hyperplasia with eosinophilia. The three components can be identified in this image: vessels with plump endothelial cells, a lymphocytic infiltrate, and numerous eosinophils.

containing capillaries, occasional immature endothelial cells, and eosinophilic globules, producing a resemblance to renal glomeruli (Fig. 2.55) (200,202,203). The globules are PAS positive, diastase resistant, and represent immunoglobulin deposits along with other proteinaceous material. This lesion is widely regarded as a form of reactive cutaneous endothelial hyperplasia, although it is distinct from the lesion termed reactive angioendotheliomatosis (204).

ANGIOLYMPHOID HYPERPLASIA WITH EOSINOPHILIA

Other names for this disorder include *epithelioid* or *histiocytoid hemangioma* (205). Single or multiple reddish-brown papules or nodules occur predominantly in the head and neck region (206). We have observed a patient with chronic lymphocytic leukemia and multiple widespread papular lesions having the microscopic features of angiolymphoid hyperplasia with eosinophilia (ALH). These lesions developed rapidly, superficially resembling a drug eruption. This and other cases raise the question of immune dysregulation as a factor in this condition.

Microscopically, there are three major components: branching vessels with protuberant endothelial cells having the cytologic characteristics of "histiocytes" (macrophages), a lymphocytic infiltrate, and fairly numerous eosinophils (Fig. 2.56) (207–209). The proportions of these three components vary from case to case. In some instances, the vessels predominate, embedded in sclerotic or myxoid connective tissue and associated with a mild lymphocytic infiltrate and few eosinophils; in others, even though all three elements can usually be found, the lymphocytic infiltrate is quite dense, sometimes with germinal center formation. The cutaneous lesions have a benign clinical course.

Kimura disease is often confused or lumped together with ALH, but it should be regarded as a different disease (210). In this disorder, subcutaneous masses occur in the vicinity of the ears and parotid gland, predominantly in young Asian men. Unlike patients with ALH, these patients often have regional lymphadenopathy, hyperglobulinemia (immunoglobulin E), and peripheral eosinophilia (210). Recurrences following sur-

gery are much more common among patients with Kimura disease. Despite some overlapping microscopic changes, lesions of Kimura disease typically have denser lymphoid infiltrates with germinal center formation (205,210), and the endothelial cells of lesional vessels are not always protuberant.

INTRAVASCULAR PAPILLARY ENDOTHELIAL HYPERPLASIA

Also known as *Masson lesion*, this finding follows thrombosis in hemangiomas, hematomas, or dilated vessels, particularly on distal extremities. Trauma is often an initiating factor (211). Lesions appear as tender purpuric nodules. Microscopically, hyalinized papillary fronds lined by plump endothelial cells are identified within a thrombosed vessel (Fig. 2.57), presumably representing organization of the thrombus (211,212). The latter configuration is a key to distinguishing this process from

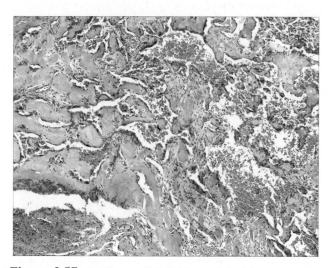

Figure 2.57. Papillary endothelial hyperplasia (Masson). Hyalinized papillary fronds lined by endothelial cells are present within a thrombosed vessel.

angiosarcoma, to which it has a resemblance. However, in addition, the endothelial cells of intravascular papillary endothelial hyperplasia display little atypia or mitotic activity, and necrosis is absent.

BACILLARY ANGIOMATOSIS

The lesions of bacillary angiomatosis are caused by the bacterium *Bartonella henselae* and are particularly observed in patients infected with HIV (213,214). Red to violaceous nodules and plaques develop in virtually any anatomic location. Similar if not identical lesions, called *verruga peruana*, are seen in South America in patients with Carrión disease; in that condition, the causative organism is *Bartonella bacilliformis* (215). On biopsy, the typical protuberant lesion has a collarette at its base and contains vessels with somewhat lobulated arrangements, thus producing an image that more closely mimics lobular capillary hemangioma than Kaposi sarcoma, a significant clinical consideration in HIV-infected patients. The endothelial cells are plump and somewhat "epithelioid" in appearance, and neutrophils are present, even in nonulcerated lesions (Fig. 2.58) (216). Clumps of basophilic bodies, representing the causative organism, can be identified on hematoxylin and eosin staining but are best observed with silver methods such as the Warthin-Starry stain (216,217). The lesions respond to antimicrobial therapy and are becoming less common in view of the improved management of HIV infection and the acquired immunodeficiency syndrome (AIDS).

LYMPHANGIOMAS

Lymphangiomas present predominantly in two forms: as superficial lesions (*lymphangioma circumscriptum*) and as deep-seated lesions with markedly dilated spaces (*deep lymphangioma*), one variety of which is the *cystic hygroma* (218–220). Lymphangioma circumscriptum can develop at any age and has occasionally been seen after radiation therapy. It often presents in the form of grouped papular lesions, occasionally verruciform (221), and

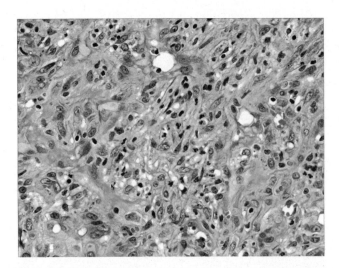

Figure 2.58. Bacillary angiomatosis. Vessels lined by plump, somewhat "epithelioid" endothelial cells are associated with neutrophils in this nonulcerated lesion. Clumps of organisms were identified with a Warthin-Starry stain.

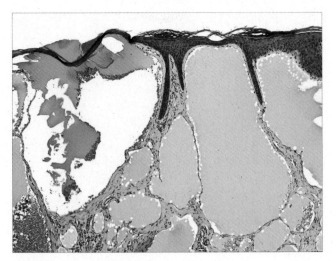

Figure 2.59. Lymphangioma circumscriptum. Thin-walled vessels containing lymph fluid are present within the superficial dermis.

often has the appearance of deep-seated vesicles. Microscopically, there are thin-walled channels, which are sometimes observed to contain lymph fluid, within the superficial dermis, appearing at times to be surrounded by epidermis (Fig. 2.59) (222). Deep lymphangiomas have the appearance of fluctuant nodules and tend to be found in the regions of the head and neck and axillae. Microscopically, there are thin-walled vessels in the dermis and subcutis with flattened endothelium; some are markedly dilated. Scattered mature lymphocytes can be identified in both lesions (218). Lymphangiomas are benign lesions, but recurrences are not uncommon, probably because of the difficulties of defining margins of some of these tumors. D2-40 is a helpful immunohistochemical marker for the endothelial cells of lymphatic vessels (223).

KAPOSI SARCOMA

This well-known tumor has become even better understood in the modern era, as its increasing incidence has accompanied the AIDS pandemic. Kaposi sarcoma arises in four different clinical settings:

1. *Classic Kaposi sarcoma*, in elderly men of Mediterranean origin (224)
2. *African Kaposi sarcoma*, an endemic form occurring among children in certain geographic locations in the African continent (225)
3. *Kaposi sarcoma in immunosuppressed individuals*, including transplantation patients and those who are under therapy for another—usually hematologic—malignancy (226)
4. *AIDS-related Kaposi sarcoma* (227)

Cutaneous lesions may progress through three stages (228). In the macular stage, there are violaceous patches of discoloration that, in some presentations, can be clinically subtle. In the plaque stage, lesions become indurated (therefore palpable) and confluent, and in the tumor stage, solid red-purple nodules are formed. Lesions can develop anywhere, although in the classic form, they are prone to develop on the distal lower extremities. The African form tends to be rapidly progressive, with early development of nodular lesions and involvement of lymph nodes and other organs. Among AIDS patients, Kaposi sarcoma has been most prevalent among homosexual men, although its incidence in this population has been declining.

Regarding pathogenesis, the human leukocyte antigen (HLA)-DR5 allele is overrepresented in Kaposi sarcoma patients compared with the general population (229). Kaposi sarcoma has several characteristics of a true neoplasm, but genomic sequences of human herpesvirus-8 (HHV8) have been detected in Kaposi sarcoma, and immunoreactivity for HHV8 latent nuclear antigen-1 has been found in all of the clinical forms of the disease (230,231). It may be that Kaposi sarcoma results from the effects of this infectious agent in a genetically susceptible host, allowing the virus to express a latent potential for cellular transformation and oncogenesis.

Microscopically, the findings in early macular lesions may be extremely subtle, limited to interconnecting attenuated vessels and scattered spindle cells within the dermis. One helpful finding is the promontory sign, which consists of new vascular channels forming around pre-existing dermal vessels (Fig. 2.60), such that the latter vessels appear to project into the resulting space in the manner of a promontory or cliff (232). Small groupings of vessels may be scattered through the dermis. Apoptosis may be observed among endothelial cells of newly formed blood vessels at this stage (233). In the plaque stage, small vascular channels admix with increased numbers of spindle cells; the latter form small fascicles within the dermis. Branching neovascular spaces appear to dissect between collagen bundles. This is associated with erythrocyte extravasation, hemosiderin deposition, and an inflammatory infiltrate that often includes plasma cells. Distinctive features are the *hyaline globules* found within neoplastic endothelial cells. These are effete erythrocytes that are PAS positive (232,234). Tumor stage lesions show more solid aggregates of spindle cells that contain cytoplasmic vacuoles. Erythrocytes appear to line up between aggregates of spindled cells, producing the "vascular slit" appearance (Fig. 2.61) (232,234). Although the microscopic features of Kaposi sarcoma are characteristic, they can occasionally be mimicked—in early stages by benign vascular proliferations and in later stages by malignant spindle cell tumors of other types, such as spindle cell melanoma, leiomyosarcoma, and spindle cell squamous cell carcinoma. Attention to morphologic

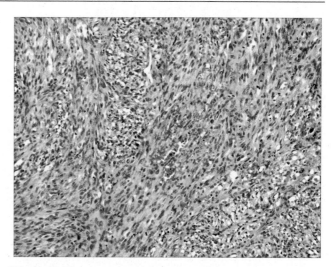

Figure 2.61. Kaposi sarcoma, tumor stage. Solid aggregates of spindled cells with "vascular slit" appearance are seen.

details and use of immunohistochemical panels can usually help to rule out these other entities.

ANGIOSARCOMA

Cutaneous angiosarcoma arises in several different clinical settings: in fields of prior therapeutic irradiation, in areas of chronic lymphedema (so-called *lymphangiosarcoma of Stewart-Treves*), and as idiopathic lesions arising on the scalp or face of elderly individuals (235–238). Lesions consist of macules with bruiselike appearances and violaceous nodules. Metastasis to skin from angiosarcoma arising in the great vessels is also a rare but well-documented cutaneous manifestation of the disease (239). Angiosarcomas are aggressive neoplasms and often lead to death from metastases or unmanageable local disease despite surgery and postoperative irradiation.

Microscopically, there is disordered proliferation of atypical endothelial cells with hyperchromatic nuclei and cytoplasm that can vary from scant to generous in epithelioid variants. Tumor cells line interconnecting, "sieve"-like vascular channels that dissect through dermal and subcutaneous connective tissues, sometimes surrounding adnexal epithelia (Fig. 2.62). Hemorrhage, hemosiderin deposition, and inflammation may accompany the process. Mitotic activity is readily appreciated. Variants include solid spindle cell or epithelioid, granular cell, and pleomorphic types. Some examples of angiosarcoma show only slightly atypical features in the superficial dermis; this can result in erroneous interpretations if only shallow biopsies are performed. Deeper excisional specimens, however, demonstrate the dissecting endothelial profiles that are characteristic of this neoplasm (236,240). Immunohistochemical stains that may be useful in diagnosing angiosarcoma include von Willebrand factor, CD31 (241) and CD34, thrombomodulin, and *Ulex europaeus* lectin. One or more of these stains will ordinarily allow differentiation from tumors that can mimic angiosarcoma, such as other spindle cell sarcomas, epithelioid neoplasms such as melanoma and epithelioid sarcoma, and true squamous cell carcinoma. Unfortunately, certain keratin proteins, particularly keratins 8 and 18, and epithelial tumor-associated glycoproteins, recognized by the B72.3 antibody, can be identified in

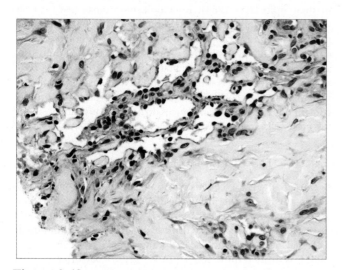

Figure 2.60. Kaposi sarcoma. An example of the "promontory sign" is shown. This biopsy was obtained from a plaque stage lesion.

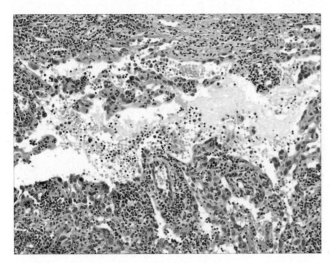

Figure 2.62. Angiosarcoma. Irregular vascular channels are lined by atypical endothelial cells.

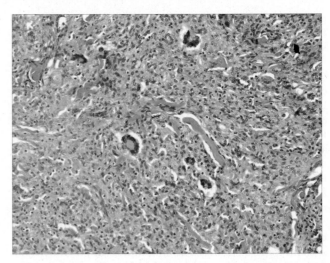

Figure 2.63. Juvenile xanthogranuloma. Touton giant cells are a hallmark of this lesion, although they are not invariably present.

vascular neoplasms, so these should be avoided when evaluating potential tumors of endothelial differentiation (242).

HISTIOCYTIC (MACROPHAGIC) TUMORS

There are several "histiocytic" (macrophagic) proliferations in the skin. Many of these are unusual and quite obscure. For the sake of brevity, I will discuss only two of the most important of these: juvenile xanthogranuloma and Langerhans cell histiocytosis.

JUVENILE XANTHOGRANULOMA

Juvenile xanthogranuloma (JXG) consists of one or more cutaneous or subcutaneous nodules comprised of "histiocytes" (macrophages). Although JXG occurs most commonly in childhood, it can also arise in adult life (243,244). Lesions tend to occur in the head and neck region but can also appear on the trunk or extremities. The typical lesion is a yellow-orange nodule ranging between 0.5 and 1.0 cm in diameter. Although commonly developing in skin, JXG can also arise in deep soft tissue, testis, pericardium, lung, kidney, retroperitoneum, and spleen (244,245). Eye involvement is the best-known extracutaneous complication; anterior chamber hemorrhage and glaucoma are potential complications (246,247). However, cutaneous lesions often involute spontaneously in one to several years (243). Disease associations include neurofibromatosis and juvenile chronic myelogenous leukemia (248), although most often, patients with JXG are otherwise normal. The issue of whether this lesion is reactive or neoplastic has not been completely resolved.

Early lesions show aggregates of macrophages containing small amounts of lipid (249). In fully developed lesions, there are vacuolated or foamy, spindled, or oncocytic cells as well as eosinophils. The classic cell type is the Touton giant cell, featuring a core of eosinophilic cytoplasm, surrounding wreath of

nuclei, and an outer lipid layer (Fig. 2.63) (250). Touton giant cells can be diagnostically useful and are sometimes numerous, but they can also be absent, particularly in deep variants, in late-stage lesions in which fibrosis replaces the cellular elements, and among some juvenile cases (251). Immunohistochemical stains for the cells of JXG include vimentin, the macrophage markers CD68, lysozyme, and HAM56, and factor XIIIa (252).

There are several considerations in the differential diagnosis. Cutaneous lesions of Langerhans cell histiocytosis have cells with reniform nuclei that tend to infiltrate the overlying epidermis, and Touton giant cells are uncommon. S-100 expression is typical in Langerhans cell histiocytosis. Although S-100 positivity has been seen in 25% to 30% of cases of JXG, CD1a, which is a more specific stain for Langerhans cells, has invariably been negative (253). Lipidized dermatofibromas have some features reminiscent of JXG and are factor XIIIa positive, but the morphology of the cellular infiltrate differs, there is overlying epidermal acanthosis, and the occasional Touton-like giant cells tend to be irregular in shape and contain hemosiderin granules in their lipid layer (254). Reticulohistiocytomas feature cells with "ground glass" cytoplasm and nuclei with sharply defined nuclear membranes. Epithelioid melanocytic tumors could be confused with S-100–positive examples of JXG but would usually express other melanocytic markers, such as MART-1 or tyrosinase. Finally, in certain preparations, the rare examples of JXG with small oncocytic cells can mimic mastocytoma, but the constituent cells in those instances do not demonstrate positivity for mast cell markers such as Leder, CD117, or tryptase.

LANGERHANS CELL HISTIOCYTOSIS

Because Langerhans cell histiocytosis is discussed in other chapters in this book, the following discussion will focus on those aspects that are most pertinent to the skin. Langerhans cell histiocytosis is primarily a disease of childhood, although it clearly also occurs in adults, including the elderly (255). Classically, it is divided into three types: (i) *Letterer-Siwe disease*, which is prone to occur early in life and marked by multifocal skin and/or systemic involvement; (ii) *Hand-Schüller-Christian disease,* in which skin lesions can be accompanied by diabetes insipidus, exophthalmos, and bony defects; and (iii) unifocal disease, or *eosinophilic granuloma*, which affects older children and adults and in which skin involvement can accompany lesions of bones and other organs. Variant forms include an eruptive type limited to the skin that occurs in both infants and adults (256), a pulmonary form in young adults related to cigarette smoking (257), a form localized to the genitalia of elderly adults (258), and a rare multifocal type with marked cytologic atypia, termed *Langerhans cell sarcoma* (259). Another form presents at birth or shortly thereafter as single or multiple cutaneous papules and nodules that develop rapidly, ulcerate, and involute spontaneously; this variant is termed *congenital self-healing reticulohistiocytosis* (260). The appearance of lesions can range from crusted hemorrhagic papules in a seborrheic distribution (seen most often in Letterer-Siwe and Hand-Schüller-Christian types) to ulcerated plaques, papules, and nodules. Disease associations can include acute lymphoblastic leukemia, neonatal infection, lymphoma, and virus-associated hemophagocytic syndrome. Prognosis largely depends on the number of organ systems involved, with the poorest survivals being associated with multisystem disease.

Biopsy specimens show aggregates of cells with eosinophilic cytoplasm and nuclei displaying grooves and folds, sometimes producing a reniform appearance (Fig. 2.64) (261). These cells have a distinct tendency to infiltrate the overlying epidermis. In Langerhans cell sarcoma, cells are larger and possess nuclei with abnormal chromatin, prominent nucleoli, and frequent mitotic figures. Extravasated erythrocytes and inflammatory cells, including eosinophils, are frequently identified. The cells have the immunophenotype of Langerhans cells, expressing S-100 protein, CD1a, vimentin, and HLA-DR, and they also stain with peanut agglutinin (262,263). However, unlike normal intraepidermal Langerhans cells, the neoplastic cells express CD4 and placental alkaline phosphatase and show a different adhesion molecule expression profile (264). With electron microscopic analysis, Birbeck granules can be identified in a variable percentage of tumor cells. Morphologically, Langerhans cell histiocytosis can usually be distinguished from potential mimics such as xanthoma disseminatum and cutaneous T-cell lym-

phoma, and the immunohistochemical profile of its constituent cells is decisive.

MAST CELL INFILTRATES

Mast cells are normal constituents of skin, and spindle cell forms can usually be identified in a perivascular distribution. Increased numbers of mast cells can be seen in a variety of inflammatory dermatoses (e.g., arthropod bites, spongiotic [eczematous] dermatitis, some examples of erythema multiforme, and bullous pemphigoid), and they can also be increased in several types of tumors (e.g., neurofibroma and spindle cell lipoma). This fact must be kept in mind when evaluating skin biopsies for a possible mast cell proliferative disorder.

The following discussion is directed toward cutaneous forms of mastocytosis. Regarding the issue of systemic disease, it should be mentioned that clinical involvement in mastocytosis is limited to the skin in approximately 80% of cases. Among those patients who have systemic mastocytosis, approximately half develop skin lesions. The disease in most of these patients tends to follow an indolent clinical course. However, one study did not detect a uniform correlation between the presence or absence of cutaneous involvement and prognosis among patients with systemic mast cell disease.

MASTOCYTOSIS

Cutaneous mastocytosis occurs most commonly in young children but can also occur in adults, particularly those in the third or fourth decades of life (265). An autosomal dominant inheritance pattern has been found in a few instances (266,267), but most often, a family history is not demonstrable. Skin lesions can vary markedly in their appearance, presenting as solitary nodules, widespread maculopapules, nodules, or plaques, or as diffuse erythroderma with thickened skin. Another form, termed *telangiectasia macularis eruptiva perstans* (TMEP), presents with widespread telangiectatic lesions. The erythrodermic form is most common in early infancy, whereas TMEP is characteristic of adults (268,269). Lesions are often hyperpigmented, and the term *urticaria pigmentosa* is sometimes used as a general term for all forms of cutaneous mastocytosis. The pigmentation is believed to result from the effects of mast cell growth factor (a ligand for the product of the C-KIT proto-oncogene), which stimulates both mast cell proliferation *and* melanin production by melanocytes (270).

Lesions of mastocytosis have the property of urticating (producing wheals) when stroked, a phenomenon known as the *Darier sign*. The likelihood of eliciting a positive Darier sign is dependent partly on the mast cell load of a particular lesion (for example, TMEP lesions have relatively few mast cells and are less prone to urticate) and partly on whether or not the mast cells in the tested lesion have recently degranulated. Occasionally, bullae can develop within the lesions, spontaneously or with trauma (271). Other symptoms include pruritus, flushing, dermatographism, and (rarely) diarrhea.

Microscopically, there are increased numbers of mast cells in skin biopsy specimens. In maculopapular lesions and TMEP, the cells are arranged in a perivascular distribution. They are densely aggregated in nodular and erythrodermic types, and in the erythrodermic form, they may create bandlike arrangements in the superficial dermis. Individually, mast cells may be

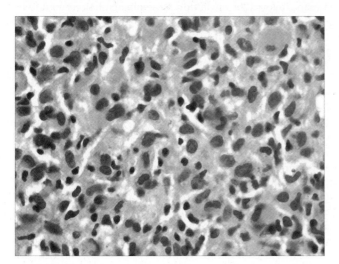
Figure 2.64. Langerhans cell histiocytosis. Note eosinophilic cytoplasm with folded and, in some cases, reniform nuclei. This was one of multiple widespread cutaneous lesions in an adult.

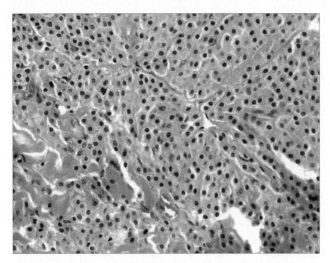

Figure 2.65. Cutaneous mastocytosis. Numerous cells with round to oval nuclei and homogeneous chromatin are present. The cytoplasm of these cells is somewhat granular. Occasional eosinophils can also be identified.

spindled or rounded to oval, the latter being more common in densely cellular variants. They possess granular cytoplasm and round to oval nuclei with homogeneous chromatin (Fig. 2.65). Eosinophils often accompany the lesions, the result of mast cell production of eosinophil chemotactic factor. Mast cells tend not to infiltrate the overlying epidermis. Several different stains are useful for identifying mast cells. Giemsa and toluidine blue stain mast cell granules metachromatically purple, but in some preparations, these stains are difficult to interpret. The Leder (chloroacetate esterase) method stains mast cell cytoplasm intensely red and, in our experience, is a much more satisfying stain. Immunohistochemical stains that are particularly useful include CD117 (c-kit) (272) and tryptase (273).

There are several considerations in the differential diagnosis of cutaneous mastocytosis. First, certain nevi or neoplastic processes can mimic nodular mast cell lesions; these include melanocytic nevi, juvenile xanthogranuloma, and Langerhans cell histiocytosis. Second, as mentioned previously, several inflammatory dermatoses can have increased numbers of mast cells (274). Finally, some mast cell lesions, especially TMEP, have such sparse numbers of mast cells that the diagnosis can be missed entirely. Correct diagnosis requires careful attention to the morphology of the neoplastic cells and evaluation for other cutaneous changes that might suggest an underlying inflammatory dermatosis. In the case of biopsies that show minimal histopathologic changes, an index of suspicion for subtle mast cell disease (such as TMEP) should be maintained. Special stains for mast cells, in the appropriate histopathologic context, can then be decisive.

LYMPHOMA AND LEUKEMIA

There are two particularly significant issues facing pathologists when evaluating cutaneous lymphoid infiltrates. The first is the decision about whether or not an infiltrate is reactive or neoplastic. If it is determined that the infiltrate is neoplastic, then the second decision is to assign the lesion to an appropriate diagnostic category. The first issue typically arises when one is evaluating

a dense dermal lymphoid infiltrate with a few atypical cells and an intermingling of other inflammatory cell types. In these circumstances, morphology can be misleading, and immunophenotyping is not always decisive. The second issue—assigning a lesion to the correct diagnostic category—depends in part on the classification scheme being employed. Several classification systems for lymphomas in general, and cutaneous lymphomas in particular, have been developed over the years, and an unfortunate side effect has been the occasional communication problems among clinicians and pathologists who may be familiar with different systems. However, in recent years, several related systems have become widely adopted; these include the World Health Organization (WHO) classification scheme (275) and the new classification system of cutaneous lymphomas combining the efforts of WHO and the European Organization for Research and Treatment of Cancer (EORTC) (276,277). The latter is founded in part on previous general classifications of lymphomas but takes into account the unique features of cutaneous lymphomas and incorporates the latest immunohistochemical, molecular, and genetic data. Table 2.5 presents the WHO/EORTC classification system (277).

LYMPHOCYTOMA CUTIS

The term *lymphocytoma cutis* (LCC) is used here for localized or disseminated cutaneous proliferations of lymphocytes that are considered benign or reactive in nature. Localized lesions manifest as violaceous tumors that can range up to 4 cm in diameter or as groupings of small pink papules. Disseminated lesions are much less common. Localized lesions preferentially involve the head and neck regions (278).

Although many examples of LCC are idiopathic, lesions can be induced by *Borrelia* infection, sometimes with other cutaneous changes of Lyme disease (279). This may explain older reports of LCC responsive to penicillin. Other causes of LCC include arthropod bites (especially tick bites) not proven to be related to *Borrelia* infection, as a postzoster phenomenon (280); in HIV-infected individuals (281); or after tattoos, exposure to gold and nickel, vaccinations, and taking drugs such as antihistamines and phenytoin (282,283). The natural history of localized lesions is initial enlargement, sometimes over periods of up to 2 years, followed by involution; disseminated lesions tend to be more persistent. Evolution to lymphoma over a period of years has been reported, but some of these cases may have been lymphomas from the beginning that were undetectable with older diagnostic methods.

Microscopic features of LCC can include varying degrees of overlying acanthosis; a patchy, nodular, or diffuse dermal infiltrate composed largely of lymphocytes with a "top-heavy" low-power configuration (i.e., involvement concentrated in the superficial to mid dermis); and a predominance of mature cells with sparse mitoses. Lymphoid follicles with well-formed and sharply delineated germinal centers are sometimes observed (Fig. 2.66). There is often an admixture of other inflammatory cell types, including plasma cells, macrophages (sometimes with granuloma formation), and particularly eosinophils (Fig. 2.67), and tingible body macrophages and proliferative thick-walled vessels are frequently observed (284). However, findings in cutaneous lymphoid infiltrates can vary considerably, and LCC can show a relatively monomorphous cell population, whereas lymphomas can occasionally display any of the morphologic features described earlier. Specific findings to indicate the cause

TABLE 2.5

The WHO/EORTC Classification of Cutaneous Lymphomas

Mature T-Cell and NK-Cell Neoplasms
Mycosis Fungoides (MF)
  Variants of MF
    Pagetoid reticulosis (localized disease)
    Folliculotropic, syringotropic, granulomatous
  Subtype of MF
    Granulomatous slack skin
Sézary Syndrome
CD30$^+$ T-Cell Lymphoproliferative Disorders of the Skin
  Lymphomatoid papulosis
  Primary cutaneous anaplastic large-cell lymphoma
Subcutaneous Panniculitis-Like T-Cell Lymphoma
Primary Cutaneous Peripheral T-Cell Lymphoma (PTL), Unspecified
  Subtypes of PTL
    Primary cutaneous aggressive epidermotropic CD8$^+$ T-cell lymphoma
    Cutaneous gamma/delta-positive T-cell lymphoma
    Primary cutaneous CD4$^+$ small/medium-sized pleomorphic T-cell lymphoma
Extranodal NK/T-Cell Lymphoma, Nasal Type
  Variant of extranodal NK/T-cell lymphoma, nasal type
    Hydroa vacciniforme-like lymphoma
Adult T-Cell Leukemia/Lymphoma
Angioimmunoblastic T-Cell Lymphoma
Mature B-Cell Neoplasms
Cutaneous Marginal Zone B-Cell Lymphoma (MALT Type)
Primary Cutaneous Follicle Center Lymphoma
  Growth patterns
    Follicular
    Follicular and diffuse
    Diffuse
Cutaneous Diffuse Large B-Cell Lymphoma, Leg Type
Cutaneous Diffuse Large B-Cell Lymphoma, Others
Intravascular Large B-Cell Lymphoma
Lymphomatoid Granulomatosis
Chronic Lymphocytic Leukemia
Mantle Cell Lymphoma
Burkitt Lymphoma
Immature Hematopoietic Malignancies
Blastic NK-Cell Lymphoma; CD4$^+$/CD56$^+$ Hematodermic Neoplasm
Precursor Lymphoblastic Leukemia/Lymphoma
  T-lymphoblastic lymphoma
  B-lymphoblastic lymphoma
Myeloid and Monocytic Leukemias
Hodgkin Lymphoma

From Burg G, Kempf W, Cozzio A, et al. WHO/EORTC classification of cutaneous lymphomas 2005: histological and molecular aspects. *J Cutan Pathol* 2005;32:647–674.

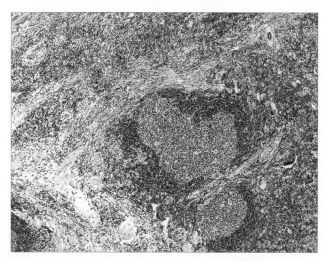

Figure 2.66. Lymphocytoma cutis. Lymphoid follicles with a well-formed germinal center are present in the dermis.

predominantly diploid (286), and molecular studies typically fail to show clonal rearrangements of immunoglobulin heavy-chain or T-cell receptor genes (286,287).

Even immunohistochemistry and molecular analysis can be misleading; for example, proliferation markers can be expressed in benign infiltrates (285), monotypic plasma cells have been found in "benign" cutaneous lymphoid hyperplasia (288), and B-cell clonality has been demonstrated in lesions that appear to be reactive by other methods (289). Nevertheless, a combination of morphologic, immunohistochemical, and molecular techniques leads to a correct diagnosis in most instances. Having said this, there are clearly difficult cases that defy precise classification, at least initially. For those cases, a full description of the findings and the possible interpretations should be provided. The patients should receive close clinical surveillance and possible rebiopsy and should be considered for gene rearrangement studies. I will provide additional clues to the differentiation of LCC from certain lymphomas, particularly marginal

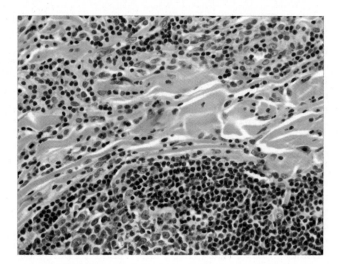

Figure 2.67. Lymphocytoma cutis. Numerous eosinophils can be identified in the dermal infiltrate. A portion of a lymphoid follicle can be seen near the base of this figure.

of a reactive lymphoid process (e.g., tick mouth parts or tattoo pigments) are helpful when present but are lacking in most cases. For this reason, immunohistochemical analysis and molecular genetic studies have assumed increasing importance in diagnosing problematic cutaneous lymphoid proliferations. The lymphocytes of LCC fail to show loss of B-lineage antigens, pan-T-cell antigens, or abnormal coexpression of antigens, and polytypic light chain expression is noted (285). These cells are zone lymphoma and follicular lymphoma, in the discussions that follow.

SELECTED B-CELL LYMPHOMAS

Marginal Zone Lymphoma

Also known as B-cell lymphoma of mucosa-associated lymphoid tissue (*MALT lymphoma*), marginal zone lymphoma (MZL) most often arises in extranodal sites, one of which is the skin. Cutaneous involvement can be primary or secondary to spread from another site. MZL can arise in the setting of chronic inflammation of infectious or autoimmune origin, suggesting a pathogenetic role for chronic antigenic stimulation. In the skin, *Borrelia burgdorferi* infection has been detected by polymerase chain reaction (PCR) methods in some cases (290). Most patients are middle aged and develop red-brown papules or nodules, particularly over the upper half of the body (291). Other symptoms are uncommon, although there have been reports of a hyperviscosity syndrome related to coexistent Waldenström macroglobulinemia (292). Microscopically, there is a dense, diffuse dermal infiltrate composed of small lymphocytes, some of which have features of centrocytes, or marginal zone cells. Both plasma cells and plasmacytoid cells can be identified (293), and some cells display eosinophilic intranuclear inclusions (Dutcher bodies). Reactive germinal centers, sometimes permeated by small neoplastic lymphocytes, and lymphoepithelial lesions may be demonstrated (291). The neoplastic cells have the following immunohistochemical profile: CD20$^+$, CD79a$^+$, CD21$^+$, bcl-2$^+$, bcl-6$^-$, CD5$^-$, CD10$^-$, CD23$^-$, CD35$^-$, and cyclin D1$^-$ (293). Light chain restriction is a regular feature (294). Rearrangements of immunoglobulin heavy- and light-chain genes have been reported (294). Morphologically, there can be a resemblance to reactive lymphoid proliferations (LCC), in that MZL can feature a top-heavy infiltrate, reactive follicles, and occasional eosinophils. However, the findings of diffuse marginal zone cells, sheets of plasma cells (some with Dutcher bodies), and a B-to-T-cell ratio of 3:1 or greater favor the diagnosis of MZL, and immunohistochemical and gene rearrangement studies can be decisive. Primary cutaneous MZL is considered to be a low-grade lymphoma with a good to excellent prognosis.

Follicular Lymphoma

Follicular lymphoma can also arise in the skin or involve it secondarily. It accounts for approximately 40% of all cutaneous B-cell lymphomas (295), and 60% of cutaneous follicular lymphomas are primary lesions. As is true for many lymphomas, follicular lymphoma presents as a violaceous plaque or nodule, quite often in the head and neck region. Microscopically, the dermis is occupied by neoplastic follicles that contain cells with centrocytic, centroblastic, and indeterminate characteristics (Fig. 2.68). Between these follicles are small cells with cleaved nuclear contours. The internal portions of these follicles lack the characteristics of normal, organized germinal centers and their expected tingible body macrophages, apoptosis, and frequent mitotic activity. The neoplastic follicular cells usually have the following immunohistochemical profile: CD20$^+$, CD79$^+$, CD45RA$^+$, CD10$^+$, bcl-2$^+$, bcl-6$^+$, CD5$^-$, CD43$^-$, CD23$^-$, and cyclin D1$^-$ (296). However, bcl-2 and bcl-6 protein expression is not invariably observed in primary cutaneous follicular lymphoma (297). Rearrangement of immunoglobulin heavy- and

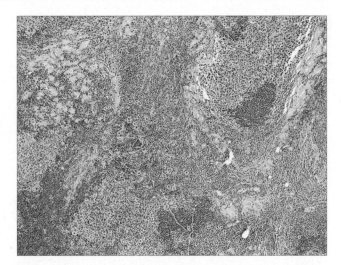

Figure 2.68. Follicular lymphoma. Neoplastic follicles can be identified. The internal portions of these follicles lack the features of normal, organized germinal centers.

light-chain genes is expected. Reactive lymphoid infiltrates (LCC) can bear a morphologic resemblance to follicular lymphoma, but the former feature a greater degree of cellular heterogeneity, more clear-cut polarity of the follicles, and focal germinal centers with tingible body macrophages, apoptosis, and frequent mitotic activity. The immunoprofile also differs considerably, in that LCC fails to show reactivity for CD10, bcl-2, or bcl-6 in the follicular lymphoid aggregates. MZL can also bear a morphologic resemblance to follicular lymphoma, but in this case, immunohistochemistry can be particularly helpful because MZL lacks CD10 and bcl-6 expression. Primary cutaneous follicular lymphomas remain confined to the skin for prolonged periods, and despite recurrences, involvement of extracutaneous sites is unusual (295).

Diffuse Large B-Cell Lymphoma

As the name implies, this group of lymphomas is characterized by diffuse cutaneous infiltration by large neoplastic B cells. Diffuse large B-cell lymphoma (LBCL) can arise de novo or by transformation from either MZL or follicular lymphoma (298). Cutaneous lesions can arise primarily or by secondary spread from another site; they have clinical characteristics similar to those of other B-cell lymphomas and can arise on the head and neck, trunk, and legs. Variant forms include *LBCL, leg type*, a tumor of older adults that tends to have a worse prognosis than those arising in other cutaneous sites (299), and *T-cell–rich B-cell lymphoma*, a variety that can create diagnostic difficulties because of the large numbers of reactive T cells and the relatively small proportion (<10%) of neoplastic B cells (300). Microscopic findings include diffuse dermal growth of medium to large atypical cells that have the characteristics of centroblasts (Fig. 2.69). Nuclei can have several nucleoli and are sometimes multilobated. Anaplastic, spindled, signet ring, immunoblastic, and plasmablastic types can occur, in addition to the previously mentioned T-cell–rich variety (298,301). The usual immunohistochemical profile is as follows: CD20$^+$, CD79a$^+$, CD19$^+$, CD20$^+$, CD22$^+$, bcl-6$^+$, Ki-67$^+$, CD5$^-$, and cyclin D1$^-$ (302). However, approximately 10% of tumors express CD5. Approximately one-half of the tumors can express CD10 and bcl-2, although the

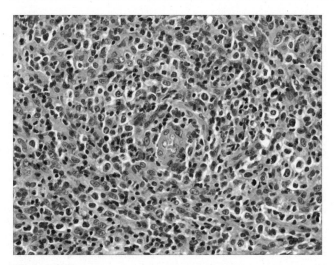

Figure 2.69. Diffuse large B-cell lymphoma. Diffuse dermal growth of medium to large atypical cells.

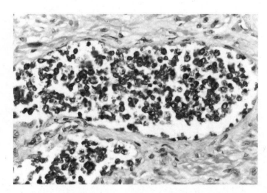

Figure 2.70. Intravascular large B-cell lymphoma. Atypical lymphoid cells are found within dilated cutaneous vessels. These express B-cell lineage antigens.

latter marker is uncommon among primary cutaneous tumors arising in locations other than the legs (303). The T cells are positive for CD3 and CD45RO. CD30 positivity is sometimes seen (regularly in anaplastic types) (304), and the immunoblastic type may express the anaplastic large-cell lymphoma kinase (ALK) protein (298). Light-chain restriction is associated with the ALK-positive and T-cell–rich B-cell variants, and as expected, immunoglobulin heavy- and light-chain gene rearrangements are identified (305). The differential diagnosis of LBCL can be quite broad, in that the neoplastic B cells raise consideration not only of other lymphomas but also other malignancies that feature anaplastic cells, such as poorly differentiated squamous cell carcinoma. Careful attention to morphologic details and immunohistochemical analysis will usually allow distinction. In contrast to T-cell lymphoma, the T cells of T-cell–rich B-cell lymphoma lack significant cytologic atypia, and usually T-cell receptor gene rearrangements are not identified. LBCL is generally regarded as an aggressive tumor, but patients with localized cutaneous disease (with the exception of lesions arising in the legs) generally have an excellent prognosis. Bcl-2 expression or rearrangement of the associated oncogene is considered an adverse prognostic feature in terms of disease-free survival (298).

Angiocentric Lymphomas

There are two important B-cell lymphomas with angiocentric features. The first, *intravascular large B-cell lymphoma*, was once thought to be malignant angioendotheliomatosis until it was determined that the neoplastic cells are lymphoid rather than endothelial in origin (306). This lymphoma occurs in older adults and is characterized by purpuric macules, papules, and nodules together with other signs and symptoms referable to small vessel occlusion, including disseminated intravascular coagulation, hypertension, nephrotic syndrome, and dementia (307). It is a particularly aggressive disease that is only poorly responsive to therapy, although a rare case confined to the skin can have a prolonged course. Microscopically, small cutaneous

vessels contain atypical lymphoid cells (Fig. 2.70) that, in most instances, express B-cell lineage antigens; the typical immunohistochemical profile is CD20+, CD22+, CD79a+, CDCD23−, CD5+/−, CD23−, and cyclin D1−. Negative CD23 and cyclin D1 expression, when combined with CD5 positivity, argue against other B-cell lymphoproliferative lesions that can express CD5 (usually considered a T-cell antigen), such as chronic lymphocytic leukemia and mantle cell lymphoma (308). Light-chain restriction and immunoglobulin heavy-chain gene rearrangements are regularly demonstrated (309). However, a rare T-cell variant of this lymphoma has been reported, and in those cases, the neoplastic cells express CD3 and CD45RO and may show T-cell receptor gene rearrangements (310,311).

The other angiocentric B-cell lymphoma is best known as *lymphomatoid granulomatosis* (LG). In this condition, the lung is the principal site of involvement, but the skin is considered the most common extrapulmonary site (312). LG is a disease of adults and presents with cough, dyspnea, chest pain, and skin lesions that include papules, plaques, and nodules (313,314). Spontaneous regression or response to chemotherapy has been reported, but generally this disorder pursues an aggressive course. LG may result from proliferations of neoplastic B cells that have been transformed by Epstein-Barr virus (EBV) (315). Microscopically, there is an angiocentric dermal infiltrate that can feature vascular occlusion, necrosis, and fibrinoid changes within vessels. The infiltrate is often polymorphous and includes small lymphocytes, macrophages, and plasma cells (312,316). However, variable numbers of large cells (the actual neoplastic cells) are identified (Fig. 2.71). The larger cells can be identified as B cells and express CD20, CD79a, and sometimes CD30 (313,315). EBV RNA can be identified in lesions by in situ hybridization methods, but this has apparently been an easier task in the lung than in skin lesions (317). Rearrangements of the immunoglobulin heavy-chain gene are found, but there are no rearrangements of the T-cell receptor gene. Therefore, it appears that LG is in reality a kind of T-cell–rich B-cell lymphoproliferative disorder (315).

Mantle Cell Lymphoma

Mantle cell lymphoma is thought to be derived from pre–germinal center B cells. It represents approximately 3% to 10% of non-Hodgkin lymphomas and typically presents in middle-aged adults with involvement of lymph nodes, spleen, or bone

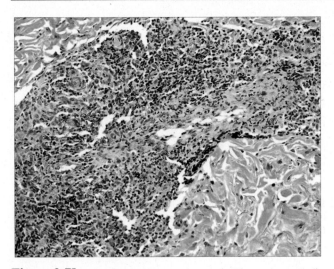

Figure 2.71. Lymphomatoid granulomatosis. The angiocentric infiltrate contains small lymphocytes (T cells) and larger, neoplastic B cells.

marrow. Skin involvement is rare (318,319). This is an aggressive lymphoma, with median survival times of 3 to 5 years (320). Microscopically, there are infiltrates of small- to medium-sized lymphocytes with a resemblance to centrocytes. Scattered macrophages can create a "starry sky" appearance, which is a feature also displayed in Burkitt lymphoma. The typical immunohistochemical profile is CD20$^+$, CD43$^+$, bcl-2$^+$, CD5$^+$, and cyclin D1$^+$ (318,321).

SELECTED T-CELL LYMPHOMAS

Mycosis Fungoides and Related Disorders

Despite the awkward term, first described by Alibert in 1806, *mycosis fungoides* (MF) has been retained because it at least serves to distinguish this unique lymphoma from other cutaneous T-cell lymphomas that have different clinical presentations, clinical courses, and (in some cases) immunohistochemical profiles. It is the most common primary cutaneous T-cell lymphoma and is derived from a mature, postthymic peripheral T cell (322, 323). The incidence and mortality rates appear to be increasing, although it still represents less than 0.5% of all non-Hodgkin lymphomas (324). There is often a history of a preceding eczematous dermatitis, such as contact dermatitis. Early manifestations of the disease are termed *parapsoriasis*, which is a term applied to a group of disorders of which two, *parapsoriasis en plaque* and *retiform (variegate) parapsoriasis*, have a strong association with MF. Although parapsoriasis has been historically considered a precursor of MF, at least by many dermatologists, the prevailing view now seems to be that it represents an early stage of the disease (325,326).

MF typically presents in the form of an erythematous, scaly eruption of long duration, often manifesting as patches or plaques found over the trunk. Eventually these lesions progress to more generalized, infiltrated plaques or tumors that may ulcerate. Generalized erythroderma can be another clinical presentation, sometimes with lymphadenopathy and circulating atypical lymphocytes, which are features of *Sézary syndrome* (see following section on Sézary syndrome). MF can also begin with cutaneous tumors, without progressing through the prolonged

superficial phase. This is known as the *d'emblee* variant, although it is possible that, with modern diagnostic methods, some of these cases may actually represent other varieties of cutaneous T-cell lymphoma (323). Unilesional MF does occur, although by its very nature, it can be difficult to diagnose; it should be distinguished from *pagetoid reticulosis (Woringer-Kolopp disease)*, a limited form of cutaneous T-cell lymphoma that often responds well to local therapy (327,328). Several other conditions are strongly linked with MF; these include *follicular mucinosis (alopecia mucinosa)* and *syringolymphoid hyperplasia*. Both can be associated with or evolve into MF (329,330), although many examples of alopecia mucinosa have a benign clinical course, and idiopathic examples of syringolymphoid hyperplasia have also been described.

The prognosis of MF depends on the extent of disease as reflected in the clinical stage. Those having only plaques and no systemic disease have an overall survival time of greater than 12 years (331), and individuals with limited plaque disease can have survival times approaching age-matched controls. However, patients with advanced cutaneous disease and lymph node and peripheral blood involvement have a median survival time of 5 years, and those with effacement of nodal architecture or visceral disease have a median survival time of 2.5 years (331). *Transformation* to large-cell lymphoma is most often a harbinger of markedly diminished survival (332). The etiology of this lymphoma is still the subject of investigation. Previously, some considered MF to be a disease of "antigen persistence," with eventual breakdown of immune surveillance and evolution of a malignant clone of T cells (333). The current view is that this disease is a malignancy from the very beginning, held in check (at first) by host immunity (322). This concept is supported by the detection of T-cell receptor gene rearrangements early in the course of the disease. The possible role of human T lymphotrophic virus (HTLV-1) or other viruses has also been the subject of investigative studies.

Microscopically, early lesions that were formerly designated parapsoriasis show combinations of parakeratosis, acanthosis, and a mild superficial dermal perivascular or bandlike infiltrate. Some lesions have the configuration of *poikiloderma atrophicans vasculare*: epidermal atrophy, vacuolar degeneration of the epidermal basilar layer, telangiectasia, and pigmentary incontinence (334,335). In *patch stage* lesions, lymphocytes line up along the basilar layer and permeate the epidermis, forming small groups (couplets and triplets) and eventually larger intraepidermal or intrafollicular aggregates termed *Pautrier microabscesses* (Fig. 2.72). This typically occurs in the setting of minimal or absent spongiosis. Although cytologic atypia among lymphocytes is minimal at first, as the disease progresses, there are increasing numbers of small- to medium-sized lymphocytes with hyperchromatic nuclei and irregular, or cerebriform, contours. Papillary dermal collagen becomes thickened and wiry, and atypical lymphocytes appear to permeate this thickened connective tissue (322,336). Admixtures with inflammatory cells, including reactive lymphocytes, plasma cells, eosinophils, or even granulomatous elements, can be seen at first, but as the disease progresses, inflammatory cells are difficult to detect. In *plaque stage* lesions, lymphoid infiltrates become increasingly dense, creating a bandlike configuration in the superficial dermis and a patchy distribution of cells in the deeper dermis. An increasing percentage of intermediate and large lymphocytes can be seen, and often the lymphocytes within the epidermis show greater degrees of atypia than do those in the dermis

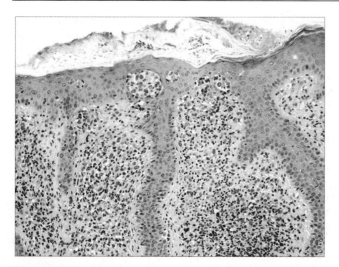

Figure 2.72. Mycosis fungoides. Pautrier microabscesses can be identified within the epidermis.

(337). In *tumor stage* lesions, large atypical cells with numerous mitoses predominate, and often the epidermal involvement diminishes. Transformation to large-cell lymphoma can occur; such lesions contain medium- to large-sized pleomorphic, immunoblastic, large-cell anaplastic, and other unclassified cell types (Fig. 2.73) (332).

The typical immunohistochemical profile is CD2+, CD3+, CD4+, CD5+, and TCRβ+, and CD8− (338). However, reactive CD8+ cells are often identified in the dermal infiltrate. CD7 "dropout" is a helpful feature of MF but is not always easy to discern. Most often, the numbers of CD7-positive cells are diminished rather than absent, particularly when compared with their numbers in benign inflammatory diseases. Loss of CD7 in the epidermal component can be a helpful clue to the diagnosis of MF, and the combination of CD7 deficiency and T-cell receptor γ gene rearrangements is highly specific for the disease (339). A CD8-positive lymphoproliferative disorder with resemblances to MF also occurs; some may refer to this as CD8-

positive MF (340). These tumors may be rapidly progressive and show a poor response to therapy, but indolent examples have also been described.

The diagnosis of MF, particularly in its early stages, can be a major diagnostic challenge. A common problem is the distinction of MF from chronic, reactive inflammatory dermatoses. At present, there is no easy solution to this because the "gold standard" for early diagnosis of MF is still traditional light microscopy (336). Clues to the diagnosis include clustering of lymphocytes within the epidermis, particularly in the absence of spongiosis; lacunae around intraepidermal lymphocytes ("haloed cells"); singly distributed lymphocytes in the basilar epidermis along a broad front; and single lymphocytes permeating wiry papillary dermal collagen. There are several published guidelines to aid in the diagnosis of MF, employing grading systems with major and minor criteria; we have found the one by Guitart et al. (322) to be particularly useful in daily practice. Major criteria are based on the density of the dermal infiltrate, prominence of epidermotropism, and degree of cytologic atypia, and minor criteria include papillary dermal fibroplasia, degree of atypia of intraepidermal lymphocytes, and lack of inflammatory elements. A score of 7 or more is considered diagnostic for MF.

Sézary Syndrome

This form of cutaneous T-cell lymphoma consists of a triad of erythrodermal, lymphadenopathy, and atypical circulating T cells in the peripheral blood. Some consider it the "leukemic" variant of MF (341). It is mainly a disease of adults. Severe pruritus, palmoplantar keratoderma, and nail dystrophy sometimes accompany the process, and on occasion, there can be an eruption of numerous seborrheic keratoses. There are at least 1000 atypical cells (*Sézary cells*) per cubic millimeter of blood (323). Some believe that the diagnosis should require the demonstration of a clonal T-cell population in the peripheral blood (342). This syndrome typically has an aggressive clinical course, and the 5-year survival rates range from 10% to 33%. Treatments have included topical and systemic chemotherapy, monoclonal antibodies, retinoids, cyclosporine, and extracorporeal photopheresis.

On biopsy, lesions of Sézary syndrome often feature significant parakeratosis and acanthosis, sometimes of psoriasiform proportions (343). There may be a bandlike subepidermal lymphocytic infiltrate containing cells with cerebriform nuclei. Epidermotropism and lining up of lymphocytes along the basilar layer can be observed (Fig. 2.74) (344), but these changes may be less pronounced than in patch and plaque stages of typical examples of MF (343). Furthermore, the microscopic changes of nonspecific dermatitis can be seen in up to one-third of cases, making diagnosis a challenging prospect. At times, several biopsies may be necessary before a definitive diagnosis can be rendered. Lymph node infiltration by Sézary cells can also be identified. The immunoprofile is similar to that of MF, so the lymphoid cells usually mark as helper T cells (CD4 positive) (345). There has been a rare case in which CD8-positive, cytotoxic T cells predominated within the epidermis (346). CD7 dropout can occur, but some CD7-positive cases are also encountered. T-cell receptor gene rearrangements are regularly found (342). There appears to be little or no correlation between histopathologic pattern or degree of lymph node involvement and prognosis. However, PAS-positive cytoplasmic

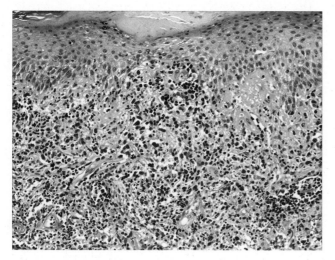

Figure 2.73. Transformed mycosis fungoides. Lymphocytes with large, markedly atypical nuclei can be identified. Many of these are CD30 positive.

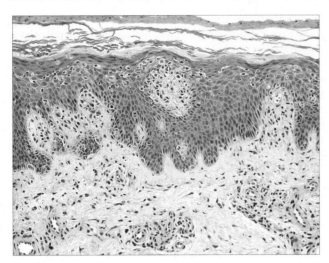

Figure 2.74. Sézary syndrome. Prominent epidermotropism can be observed in this example.

inclusions, large circulating Sézary cells, and large-cell transformation within cutaneous infiltrates are associated with diminished survival (345).

Primary Cutaneous Anaplastic Large-Cell Lymphoma and Lymphomatoid Papulosis

These conditions have as a common thread the cutaneous infiltration of anaplastic CD30-positive cells. Primary cutaneous anaplastic large-cell lymphoma (ALCL) often presents as a single violaceous nodule or multiple grouped nodules confined to one body site (347,348). Microscopically, there is a dense dermal infiltrate of large, pleomorphic or immunoblastic cells that may extend into the subcutis (Fig. 2.75). Many of the cells display abundant, pale to eosinophilic cytoplasm and irregularly shaped or multiple nuclei containing one or more nucleoli (349). Mitoses are frequent. There is a tendency for the neoplastic cells to grow in cohesive aggregates, which can raise the

possibility of malignant melanoma or poorly differentiated squamous cell carcinoma. Accompanying inflammatory cell types can include neutrophils or eosinophils (350). A large proportion of the atypical cells are CD30 positive (348). There is also evidence of T-cell lineage because these cells also express CD2, CD3, CD4, and CD45RO. Loss of certain pan–T-cell antigens is sometimes encountered. Unlike the systemic form of ALCL, primary cutaneous ALCL is negative for anaplastic lymphoma-related tyrosine kinase (ALK-1) in most instances (351). The vast majority of cases show a T-cell receptor gene rearrangement. Unlike systemic ALCL with cutaneous involvement, which responds poorly to chemotherapy and has an adverse prognosis, primary cutaneous ALCL is often an indolent disease; lesions may regress spontaneously, and tumor dissemination occurs only late in the clinical course, if at all (352).

A condition that is probably related to ALCL is *lymphomatoid papulosis*. It was first set apart as a distinct entity by Macaulay, who (along with others) recognized a self-healing eruption of papulonecrotic skin lesions that closely resembled the established cutaneous disease *pityriasis lichenoides et varioliformis acuta* (*Mucha-Habermann disease*) but, on biopsy, featured significant cytologic atypia (353,354). Lymphomatoid papulosis primarily affects adults, with a mean age at diagnosis of 43 years, although children can also have the disorder. Recurrent crops of papulonodules form over the trunk and extremities. These ulcerate and heal with varioliform scars (355). The disease can persist for years without other evidence of malignancy, but a proportion of individuals (10% to 20%) develop malignant lymphoma (356). The lymphomas that occur include MF, Hodgkin disease, and ALCL (348). Lymphomatoid papulosis can be controlled or improved with therapies such as methotrexate and psoralen with ultraviolet-A light (PUVA). Long-term follow-up of these individuals is warranted because of the risk of malignant transformation.

Microscopic changes have been placed into three categories (357,358). *Type A* disease shows large, atypical cells containing large, vesicular nuclei and clumped chromatin (similar to those of ALCL), admixed with small lymphocytes, neutrophils, eosinophils, and macrophages (Fig. 2.76). The image is somewhat reminiscent of Hodgkin disease, and in fact, some of the atypical

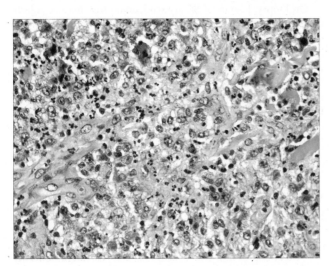

Figure 2.75. Primary cutaneous anaplastic large-cell lymphoma. There is a dense dermal infiltrate of markedly atypical cells, in this case accompanied by numerous neutrophils and eosinophils.

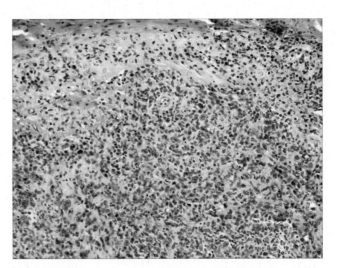

Figure 2.76. Lymphomatoid papulosis. Beneath the epidermis is an infiltrate comprised of markedly atypical cells, many of which are CD30 positive, accompanied by a mixed inflammatory infiltrate.

cells can mimic the Reed-Sternberg cells of the latter condition. *Type B* lesions feature cells with enlarged, hyperchromatic, and convoluted nuclei resembling the cells of MF. Transition between the two forms does occur. The rare *type C* lesion features solid sheets of atypical cells resembling those of ALCL. Immunohistochemically, the atypical cells of lymphomatoid papulosis are often CD4$^+$ and CD8$^-$, although exceptions occur (359). The anaplastic cells that predominate in type A and C lesions are CD30$^+$ (348). The infiltrating cells bear activation and proliferation markers such as CD25 and Ki-67, and cytotoxic granule proteins are also expressed (360). T-cell receptor gene rearrangements can be detected in approximately half of the cases, most often in type B or mixed cases (361). The differential diagnosis includes pityriasis lichenoides et varioliformis acuta, which lacks significant cytologic atypia, and cutaneous Hodgkin disease. With regard to the latter differential, true Reed-Sternberg cells have the immunoprofile of CD30$^+$, CD15$^+$, and CD45R$^-$, whereas the cells of lymphomatoid papulosis are CD30$^+$, CD15$^-$, and CD45R$^+$ (362). Type C lymphomatoid papulosis may be impossible to differentiate from ALCL without clinical data.

LEUKEMIA CUTIS

Skin involvement in patients with leukemia can be categorized as specific leukemic infiltrates and nonspecific manifestations. The latter category will not be discussed here but would include reactive processes such as Sweet syndrome, drug eruptions, or the insect bite–like reactions that have been described in patients with leukemias and lymphomas (363). Specific cutaneous infiltrates have been reported with most leukemias, including acute myeloid leukemia, acute myelomonocytic leukemia, acute erythroleukemia, acute lymphoblastic leukemia, chronic myelogenous leukemia, chronic myelomonocytic leukemia, chronic lymphocytic leukemia, adult T-cell leukemia, T-cell prolymphocytic leukemia, and hairy cell leukemia (364). Cutaneous involvement is particularly common in monocytic and chronic lymphocytic leukemias (364,365). The lesions consist of papules and nodules that are often particularly monomorphous in their appearance; plaques, ulcers, and purpuric lesions also occur. Acute myeloid leukemia is sometimes accompanied by chloroma, a grayish-green tumor that results from the presence of high concentrations of myeloperoxidase in infiltrating myeloblasts (365). The appearance of cutaneous lesions is typically associated with a poor prognosis (366).

Microscopic features include dense dermal infiltrates of atypical cells that permeate collagen bundles and are separated from the epidermis by a grenz zone (Fig. 2.77) (367). A perivascular or periadnexal distribution of the cells is common (364). The specific type of leukemia can often be diagnosed by particular attention to cytologic detail, but this can be aided by histochemistry and immunohistochemistry. Thus, for example, cells of myeloid leukemia express lysozyme, chloroacetate esterase, and myeloperoxidase; monocytic and myelomonocytic leukemias are positive for CD43 and CD68 (368); and acute lymphoblastic leukemia shows the profile of CD19$^+$, CD20$^+$ (sometimes), CD79a$^+$, CD10$^+$, and HLA-DR$^+$. Diagnostic issues arise in cases when there is no other known clinical evidence of leukemia (aleukemia cutis), when there is a question of leukemia versus lymphoma, or when there are only a few leukemic cells obscured by an inflammatory infiltrate (e.g., some examples of Sweet syndrome) (367).

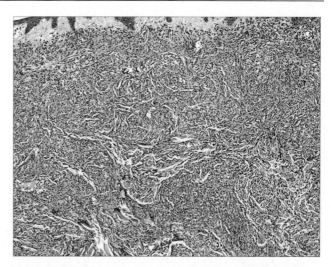

Figure 2.77. Leukemia cutis. There is a dense infiltrate of atypical cells that permeate dermal collagen and are separated from the epidermis by a grenz zone. This biopsy was obtained from a patient with myelomonocytic leukemia.

REFERENCES

1. Starink TM, Woerdeman MJ. Unilateral systematized keratosis follicularis. A variant of Darier's disease or an epidermal naevus (acantholytic dyskeratotic epidermal naevus)? *Br J Dermatol* 1981;105(2):207–214.
2. Demetree JW, Lang PG, St Clair JT. Unilateral, linear, zosteriform epidermal nevus with acantholytic dyskeratosis. *Arch Dermatol* 1979;115(7):875–877.
3. Dudley K, Barr WG, Armin A, Massa MC. Nevus comedonicus in association with widespread, well-differentiated follicular tumors. *J Am Acad Dermatol* 1986;15(5 Pt 2): 1123–1127.
4. Vissers WH, Muys L, Erp PE, de Jong EM, van de Kerkhof PC. Immunohistochemical differentiation between inflammatory linear verrucous epidermal nevus (ILVEN) and psoriasis. *Eur J Dermatol* 2004;14(4):216–220.
5. Ito M, Shimizu N, Fujiwara H, Maruyama T, Tezuka M. Histopathogenesis of inflammatory linear verrucose epidermal naevus: histochemistry, immunohistochemistry and ultrastructure. *Arch Dermatol Res* 1991;283(8):491–499.
6. Zhu WY, Leonardi C, Penneys NS. Detection of human papillomavirus DNA in seborrheic keratosis by polymerase chain reaction. *J Dermatol Sci* 1992;4(3):166–171.
7. Degos R, Civatte J. Clear-cell acanthoma. Experience of 8 years. *Br J Dermatol* 1970;83(2): 248–254.
8. Jones EW, Wells GC. Degos' acanthoma (acanthome a cellules claires). A clinical and histological report of nine cases. *Arch Dermatol* 1966;94(3):286–294.
9. Lupton G, Graham JH. Clear cell acanthoma. *J Cutan Pathol* 1986;13:85.
10. Sanchez Yus E, del Rio E, Requena L. Large-cell acanthoma is a distinctive condition. *Am J Dermatopathol* 1992;14(2):140–147; discussion 148.
11. Roewert HJ, Ackerman AB. Large-cell acanthoma is a solar lentigo. *Am J Dermatopathol* 1992;14(2):122–132.
12. Argenyi ZB, Huston BM, Argenyi EE, Maillet MW, Hurt MA. Large-cell acanthoma of the skin. A study by image analysis cytometry and immunohistochemistry. *Am J Dermatopathol* 1994;16(2):140–144.
13. Panizzon R, Skaria A. Solitary lichenoid benign keratosis: a clinicopathological investigation and comparison to lichen planus. *Dermatologica* 1990;181(4):284–288.
14. Goette DK. Benign lichenoid keratosis. *Arch Dermatol* 1980;116(7):780–782.
15. Wiltz KL, Qureshi H, Patterson JW, Mayes DC, Wick MR. Immunostaining for MART-1 in the interpretation of problematic intra-epidermal pigmented lesions. *J Cutan Pathol* 2007;34(8):601–605.
16. Mieno H, Fujimoto N, Tajima S. Eruptive vellus hair cyst in patients with chronic renal failure. *Dermatology* 2004;208(1):67–69.
17. Mortazavi H, Taheri A, Mansoori P, Kani ZA. Localized forms of steatocystoma multiplex: case report and review of the literature. *Dermatol Online J* 2005;11(1):22.
18. Eiberg H, Hansen L, Hansen C, Mohr J, Teglbjaerg PS, Kjaer KW. Mapping of hereditary trichilemmal cyst (TRICY1) to chromosome 3p24-p21.2 and exclusion of beta-CATENIN and MLH1. *Am J Med Genet A* 2005;133(1):44–47.
19. Cassarino DS, Linden KG, Barr RJ. Cutaneous keratocyst arising independently of the nevoid basal cell carcinoma syndrome. *Am J Dermatopathol* 2005;27(2):177–178.
20. Misago N, Narisawa Y. Verrucous trichilemmal cyst containing human papillomavirus. *Clin Exp Dermatol* 2005;30(1):38–39.
21. Misago N, Abe M, Kohda H. Intradermal dermoid cyst associated with occult spinal dysraphism. *J Dermatol* 1996;23(4):275–278.
22. Chetty R, Reddi A. Rhabdomyomatous multilocular thymic cyst. *Am J Clin Pathol* 2003; 119(6):816–821.
23. Santos LD, Mendelsohn G. Perineal cutaneous ciliated cyst in a male. *Pathology* 2004; 36(4):369–370.

24. Perera GK, Watson KM, Salisbury J, Du Vivier AW. Two cases of cutaneous umbilical endosalpingiosis. *Br J Dermatol* 2004;151(4):924–925.

25. De Giorgi V, Massi D, Mannone F, Stante M, Carli P. Cutaneous endometriosis: non-invasive analysis by epiluminescence microscopy. *Clin Exp Dermatol* 2003;28(3):315–317.

26. McCalmont TH. A call for logic in the classification of adnexal neoplasms. *Am J Dermatopathol* 1996;18(2):103–109.

27. Headington JT. Tumors of the hair follicle. A review. *Am J Pathol* 1976;85(2):479–514.

28. Rosen LB. A review and proposed new classification of benign acquired neoplasms with hair follicle differentiation. *Am J Dermatopathol* 1990;12(5):496–516.

29. Lever WF. *Tumors of the Epidermal Appendages Histopathology of the Skin.* Philadelphia, PA: J. B. Lippincott Company, 1990:579.

30. Hassab-el-Naby HM, Tam S, White WL, Ackerman AB. Mixed tumors of the skin. A histological and immunohistochemical study. *Am J Dermatopathol* 1989;11(5):413–428.

31. Biernat W, Pytel J. Retiform/racemiform neoplasm with features of clear cell hidradenoma. *Am J Dermatopathol* 1999;21(5):479–482.

32. Gianotti R, Alessi E. Clear cell hidradenoma associated with the folliculo-sebaceous-apocrine unit. Histologic study of five cases. *Am J Dermatopathol* 1997;19(4):351–357.

33. Birt AR, Hogg GR, Dube WJ. Hereditary multiple fibrofolliculomas with trichodiscomas and acrochordons. *Arch Dermatol* 1977;113(12):1674–1677.

34. Elston DM, James WD, Rodman OG, Graham GF. Multiple hamartoma syndrome (Cowden's disease) associated with non-Hodgkin's lymphoma. Arch Dermatol 1986;122(5):572–575.

35. Schwartz RA, Torre DP. The Muir-Torre syndrome: a 25-year retrospect. *J Am Acad Dermatol* 1995;33(1):90–104.

36. Ivan D, Hafeez Diwan A, Prieto VG. Expression of p63 in primary cutaneous adnexal neoplasms and adenocarcinoma metastatic to the skin. *Mod Pathol* 2005;18(1):137–142.

37. Qureshi HS, Ormsby AH, Lee MW, Zarbo RJ, Ma CK. The diagnostic utility of p63, CK5/6, CK7, and CK20 in distinguishing primary cutaneous adnexal neoplasms from metastatic carcinomas. *J Cutan Pathol* 2004;31(2):145–152.

38. Cooper PH. Mitotic figures in sweat gland adenomas. *J Cutan Pathol* 1987;14(1):10–14.

39. Salasche SJ. Epidemiology of actinic keratoses and squamous cell carcinoma. *J Am Acad Dermatol* 2000;42(1 Pt 2):4–7.

40. Moller R, Reymann F, Hou-Jensen K. Metastases in dermatological patients with squamous cell carcinoma. *Arch Dermatol* 1979;115(6):703–705.

41. Lund HZ. How often does squamous cell carcinoma of the skin metastasize? *Arch Dermatol* 1965;92:635–637.

42. Mehregan AH. *Pinkus' Guide to Dermatohistopathology.* 4th edition. Norwalk, CT: Appleton-Century-Crofts, 1986.

43. Braun-Falco O, Schmoeckel C, Geyer C. [Pigmented actinic keratoses]. *Hautarzt* 1986;37(12):676–678.

44. James MP, Wells GC, Whimster IW. Spreading pigmented actinic keratoses. *Br J Dermatol* 1978;98(4):373–379.

45. Carapeto FJ, Garcia-Perez A. Acantholytic keratosis. *Dermatologica* 1974;148(4):233–239.

46. Tan CY, Marks R. Lichenoid solar keratosis—prevalence and immunologic findings. *J Invest Dermatol* 1982;79(6):365–367.

47. Patterson JW, Kao GF, Graham JH, Helwig EB. Bowenoid papulosis. A clinicopathologic study with ultrastructural observations. *Cancer* 1986;57(4):823–836.

48. Wade TR, Kopf AW, Ackerman AB. Bowenoid papulosis of the genitalia. *Arch Dermatol* 1979;115(3):306–308.

49. Graham JH, Helwig EB. Erythroplasia of Queyrat. A clinicopathologic and histochemical study. *Cancer* 1973;32(6):1396–1414.

50. Bloch PH. Transformation of seborrheic keratosis into Bowen's disease. *J Cutan Pathol* 1978;5(6):361–367.

51. Marschall SF, Ronan SG, Massa MC. Pigmented Bowen's disease arising from pigmented seborrheic keratoses. *J Am Acad Dermatol* 1990;23(3 Pt 1):440–444.

52. Rook A, Whimster I. Keratoacanthoma—a thirty year retrospect. *Br J Dermatol* 1979;100(1):41–47.

53. Musso L. Spontaneous resolution of a molluscum sebaceum. *Proc R Soc Med* 1950;43(11):838–839.

54. Choonhakarn C, Ackerman AB. Keratoacanthomas: a new classification based on morphologic findings and on anatomic site. *Dermatopathol Pract Concept* 2001;7:7–16.

55. Hodak E, Jones RE, Ackerman AB. Solitary keratoacanthoma is a squamous-cell carcinoma: three examples with metastases. *Am J Dermatopathol* 1993;15(4):332–342; discussion 343–352.

56. Ahmed NU, Ueda M, Ichihashi M. Increased level of c-erbB-2/neu/HER-2 protein in cutaneous squamous cell carcinoma. *Br J Dermatol* 1997;136(6):908–912.

57. Cain CT, Niemann TH, Argenyi ZB. Keratoacanthoma versus squamous cell carcinoma. An immunohistochemical reappraisal of p53 protein and proliferating cell nuclear antigen expression in keratoacanthoma-like tumors. *Am J Dermatopathol* 1995;17(4):324–331.

58. Randall MB, Geisinger KR, Kute TE, Buss DH, Prichard RW. DNA content and proliferative index in cutaneous squamous cell carcinoma and keratoacanthoma. *Am J Clin Pathol* 1990;93(2):259–262.

59. Lapins NA, Helwig EB. Perineural invasion by keratoacanthoma. *Arch Dermatol* 1980;116(7):791–793.

60. Dinehart SM, Nelson-Adesokan P, Cockerell C, Russell S, Brown R. Metastatic cutaneous squamous cell carcinoma derived from actinic keratosis. *Cancer* 1997;79(5):920–923.

61. Nappi O, Wick MR, Pettinato G, Ghiselli RW, Swanson PE. Pseudovascular adenoid squamous cell carcinoma of the skin. A neoplasm that may be mistaken for angiosarcoma. *Am J Surg Pathol* 1992;16(5):429–438.

62. Breuninger H, Schaumburg-Lever G, Holzschuh J, Horny HP. Desmoplastic squamous cell carcinoma of skin and vermilion surface: a highly malignant subtype of skin cancer. *Cancer* 1997;79(5):915–919.

63. Cramer SF, Heggeness LM. Signet-ring squamous cell carcinoma. *Am J Clin Pathol* 1989;91(4):488–491.

64. McKinley E, Valles R, Bang R, Bocklage T. Signet-ring squamous cell carcinoma: a case report. *J Cutan Pathol* 1998;25(3):176–181.

65. Biernat W, Kordek R, Liberski PP, Wozniak L. Carcinosarcoma of the skin. Case report and literature review. *Am J Dermatopathol* 1996;18(6):614–619.

66. Kao GF. Carcinoma arising in Bowen's disease. *Arch Dermatol* 1986;122(10):1124–1126.

67. Escalonilla P, Grilli R, Canamero M, Soriano ML, Farina MC, Manzarbeitia F, et al. Sebaceous carcinoma of the vulva. *Am J Dermatopathol* 1999;21(5):468–472.

68. Wollensak G, Witschel H, Bohm N. Signet ring cell carcinoma of the eccrine sweat glands in the eyelid. *Ophthalmology* 1996;103(11):1788–1793.

69. Farmer ER, Helwig EB. Metastatic basal cell carcinoma: a clinicopathologic study of seventeen cases. *Cancer* 1980;46(4):748–757.

70. McKee PH, Wilkinson JD, Corbett MF, Davey A, Sauven P, Black MM. Carcinoma cuniculatum: a cast metastasizing to skin and lymph nodes. *Clin Exp Dermatol* 1981;6(6):613–618.

71. Schrader M, Laberke HG, Jahnke K. [Lymphatic metastases of verrucous carcinoma (Ackerman tumor)]. *HNO* 1987;35(1):27–30.

72. O'Sullivan B, Warde P, Keane T, Irish J, Cummings B, Payne D. Outcome following radiotherapy in verrucous carcinoma of the larynx. *Int J Radiat Oncol Biol Phys* 1995;32(3):611–617.

73. Youngberg GA, Thornthwaite JT, Inoshita T, Franzus D. Cytologically malignant squamous-cell carcinoma arising in a verrucous carcinoma of the penis. *J Dermatol Surg Oncol* 1983;9(6):474–479.

74. Sasaoka R, Morimura T, Mihara M, Hagari Y, Aki T, Miyamoto T. Detection of human papillomavirus type 16 DNA in two cases of verrucous carcinoma of the foot. *Br J Dermatol* 1996;134(5):983–984.

75. Shroyer KR, Greer RO, Fankhouser CA, McGuirt WF, Marshall R. Detection of human papillomavirus DNA in oral verrucous carcinoma by polymerase chain reaction. *Mod Pathol* 1993;6(6):669–672.

76. Casson P. Basal cell carcinoma. *Clin Plast Surg* 1980;7(3):301–311.

77. Bale AE, Gailani MR, Leffell DJ. Nevoid basal cell carcinoma syndrome. *J Invest Dermatol* 1994;103(5 Suppl):126S–130S.

78. Siegle RJ, MacMillan J, Pollack SV. Infiltrative basal cell carcinoma: a nonsclerosing subtype. *J Dermatol Surg Oncol* 1986;12(8):830–836.

79. Wade TR, Ackerman AB. The many faces of basal-cell carcinoma. *J Dermatol Surg Oncol* 1978;4(1):23–28.

80. Hendrix JD Jr, Parlette HL. Micronodular basal cell carcinoma. A deceptive histologic subtype with frequent clinically undetected tumor extension. *Arch Dermatol* 1996;132(3):295–298.

81. Borel DM. Cutaneous basosquamous carcinoma. Review of the literature and report of 35 cases. *Arch Pathol* 1973;95(5):293–297.

82. Schirren H, Schirren CG, Stolz W, Kind P, Plewig G. Papular elastorrhexis: a variant of dermatofibrosis lenticularis disseminata (Buschke-Ollendorff syndrome)? *Dermatology* 1994;189(4):368–372.

83. Sears JK, Stone MS, Argenyi Z. Papular elastorrhexis: a variant of connective tissue nevus. Case reports and review of the literature. *J Am Acad Dermatol* 1988;19(2 Pt 2):409–414.

84. Fenske NA, Donelan PA. Becker's nevus coexistent with connective-tissue nevus. *Arch Dermatol* 1984;120(10):1347–1350.

85. Wilson BB, Dent CH, Cooper PH. Papular acne scars. A common cutaneous finding. *Arch Dermatol* 1990;126(6):797–800.

86. Kobayasi T, Wolf-Jurgensen P, Danielsen L. Ultrastructure of shagreen patch. *Acta Derm Venereol* 1973;53(4):275–278.

87. Rongioletti F, Rebora A. Mucinous nevus. *Arch Dermatol* 1996;132(12):1522–1523.

88. Graham JH, Sanders JB, Johnson WC, Helwig EB. Fibrous papule of the nose: a clinicopathological study. *J Invest Dermatol* 1965;45(3):194–203.

89. Ragaz A, Berezowsky V. Fibrous papule of the face. A study of five cases by electron microscopy. *Am J Dermatopathol* 1979;1(4):353–356.

90. Nemeth AJ, Penneys NS, Bernstein HB. Fibrous papule: a tumor of fibrohistiocytic cells that contain factor XIIIa. *J Am Acad Dermatol* 1988;19(6):1102–1106.

91. Bansal C, Stewart D, Li A, Cockerell CJ. Histologic variants of fibrous papule. *J Cutan Pathol* 2005;32(6):424–428.

92. Shea CR, Salob S, Reed JA, Lugo J, McNutt NS. CD34-reactive fibrous papule of the nose. *J Am Acad Dermatol* 1996;35(2 Pt 2):342–345.

93. Kucher C, McNiff JM. Epithelioid fibrous papule: a new variant. *J Cutan Pathol* 2007;34(7):571–575.

94. Bart RS, Andrade R, Kopf AW, Leider M. Acquired digital fibrokeratomas. *Arch Dermatol* 1968;97(2):120–129.

95. LoBuono P, Jothikumar T, Kornblee L. Acquired digital fibrokeratoma. *Cutis* 1979;24(1):50–51.

96. Kint A, Baran R. Histopathologic study of Koenen tumors. Are they different from acquired digital fibrokeratoma? *J Am Acad Dermatol* 1988;18(2 Pt 1):369–372.

97. Lin RY, Landsman L, Krey PR, Lambert WC. Multiple dermatofibromas and systemic lupus erythematosus. *Cutis* 1986;37(1):45–47, 49.

98. Murphy SC, Lowitt MH, Kao GF. Multiple eruptive dermatofibromas in an HIV-positive man. *Dermatology* 1995;190(4):309–312.

99. Bargman HB, Fefferman I. Multiple dermatofibromas in a patient with myasthenia gravis treated with prednisone and cyclophosphamide. *J Am Acad Dermatol* 1986;14(2 Pt 2):351–352.

100. Chen TC, Kuo T, Chan HL. Dermatofibroma is a clonal proliferative disease. *J Cutan Pathol* 2000;27(1):36–39.

101. Calonje E. Is cutaneous benign fibrous histiocytoma (dermatofibroma) a reactive inflammatory process or a neoplasm? *Histopathology* 2000;37(3):278–280.

102. Laughlin CL, Carrington PR. Deep penetrating dermatofibroma. *Dermatol Surg* 1998;24(5):592–594.

103. Glusac EJ, McNiff JM. Epithelioid cell histiocytoma: a simulant of vascular and melanocytic neoplasms. *Am J Dermatopathol* 1999;21(1):1–7.

104. Glusac EJ, Barr RJ, Everett MA, Pitha J, Santa Cruz DJ. Epithelioid cell histiocytoma. A report of 10 cases including a new cellular variant. *Am J Surg Pathol* 1994;18(6):583–590.

105. Jones EW, Cerio R, Smith NP. Epithelioid cell histiocytoma: a new entity. *Br J Dermatol* 1989;120(2):185–195.

106. Pujol RM, de Castro F, Schroeter AL, Su WP. Solitary sclerotic fibroma of the skin: a sclerotic dermatofibroma? *Am J Dermatopathol* 1996;18(6):620–624.

107. Santa Cruz DJ, Kyriakos M. Aneurysmal ("angiomatoid") fibrous histiocytoma of the skin. *Cancer* 1981;47(8):2053–2061.

108. Soyer HP, Metze D, Kerl H. Granular cell dermatofibroma. *Am J Dermatopathol* 1997;19(2):168–173.

109. Tamada S, Ackerman AB. Dermatofibroma with monster cells. *Am J Dermatopathol* 1987;9(5):380–387.

110. Calonje E, Fletcher CD. Aneurysmal benign fibrous histiocytoma: clinicopathological analysis of 40 cases of a tumour frequently misdiagnosed as a vascular neoplasm. *Histopathology* 1995;26(4):323–331.

111. Werther K, Seiersen M. [Recurrent infantile digital fibromatosis]. *Ugeskr Laeger* 1997;159(30):4656–4657.

112. Viale G, Doglioni C, Iuzzolino P, Bontempini L, Colombi R, Coggi G, et al. Infantile digital fibromatosis-like tumour (inclusion body fibromatosis) of adulthood: report of two cases with ultrastructural and immunocytochemical findings. *Histopathology* 1988;12(4):415–424.

113. Bhawan J, Bacchetta C, Joris I, Majno G. A myofibroblastic tumor. Infantile digital fibroma (recurrent digital fibrous tumor of childhood). *Am J Pathol* 1979;94(1):19–36.

114. Berbis P, Devant O, Echinard C, Le Treut YP, Dor AM, Privat Y. [Metastatic Darier-Ferrand dermatofibrosarcoma. Review of the literature apropos of a case]. *Ann Dermatol Venereol* 1987;114(10):1217–1227.

115. Kahn LB, Saxe N, Gordon W. Dermatofibrosarcoma protuberans with lymph node and pulmonary metastases. *Arch Dermatol* 1978;114(4):599–601.

116. Taylor HB, Helwig EB. Dermatofibrosarcoma protuberans. *Cancer* 1961;15:717–725.

117. Kamino H, Jacobson M. Dermatofibroma extending into the subcutaneous tissue. Differential diagnosis from dermatofibrosarcoma protuberans. *Am J Surg Pathol* 1990;14(12):1156–1164.

118. Carlson JA, Slominski A, Heasley D, Mihm MC, Toda S. Dermatofibrosarcoma protuberans can induce epidermal hyperplasia that is inversely related to its proximity to the epidermis. *Am J Dermatopathol* 1998;20(4):428–430.

119. Barr RJ, Young EM Jr, King DF. Non-polarizable collagen in dermatofibrosarcoma protuberans: a useful diagnostic aid. *J Cutan Pathol* 1986;13(5):339–346.

120. Dupree WB, Langloss JM, Weiss SW. Pigmented dermatofibrosarcoma protuberans (Bednar tumor). A pathologic, ultrastructural, and immunohistochemical study. *Am J Surg Pathol* 1985;9(9):630–639.

121. Betti R, Inselvini E, Crosti C. Unusual features of primary dermatofibrosarcoma protuberans and its myxoid recurrence. *J Cutan Pathol* 1996;23(3):283–287.

122. Fletcher CD, Evans BJ, MacArtney JC, Smith N, Wilson Jones E, McKee PH. Dermatofibrosarcoma protuberans: a clinicopathological and immunohistochemical study with a review of the literature. *Histopathology* 1985;9(9):921–938.

123. Diaz-Cascajo C, Weyers W, Borrego L, Inarrea JB, Borghi S. Dermatofibrosarcoma protuberans with fibrosarcomatous areas: a clinico-pathologic and immunochemic study in four cases. *Am J Dermatopathol* 1997;19(6):562–567.

124. Hisaoka M, Okamoto S, Morimitsu Y, Tsuji S, Hashimoto H. Dermatofibrosarcoma protuberans with fibrosarcomatous areas. Molecular abnormalities of the p53 pathway in fibrosarcomatous transformation of dermatofibrosarcoma protuberans. *Virchows Arch* 1998;433(4):323–329.

125. Hsi ED, Nickoloff BJ. Dermatofibroma and dermatofibrosarcoma protuberans: an immunohistochemical study reveals distinctive antigenic profiles. *J Dermatol Sci* 1996;11(1):1–9.

126. Bell D. Atypical fibroxanthoma and malignant fibrous histiocytoma. *Am J Dermatopathol* 1979;1(2):185.

127. Helwig EB, May D. Atypical fibroxanthoma of the skin with metastasis. *Cancer* 1986;57(2):368–376.

128. Kroe DJ, Pitcock JA. Atypical fibroxanthoma of the skin. Report of ten cases. *Am J Clin Pathol* 1969;51(4):487–492.

129. Patterson JW, Konerding H, Kramer WM. "Clear cell" atypical fibroxanthoma. *J Dermatol Surg Oncol* 1987;13(10):1109–1114.

130. Khan ZM, Cockerell CJ. Atypical fibroxanthoma with osteoclast-like multinucleated giant cells. *Am J Dermatopathol* 1997;19(2):174–179.

131. Tomaszewski MM, Lupton GP. Atypical fibroxanthoma. An unusual variant with osteoclast-like giant cells. *Am J Surg Pathol* 1997;21(2):213–218.

132. Val-Bernal JF, Corral J, Fernandez F, Gomez-Bellvert C. Atypical fibroxanthoma with osteoclast-like giant cells. *Acta Derm Venereol* 1994;74(6):467–470.

133. Calonje E, Wadden C, Wilson-Jones E, Fletcher CD. Spindle-cell non-pleomorphic atypical fibroxanthoma: analysis of a series and delineation of a distinctive variant. *Histopathology* 1993;22(3):247–254.

134. Mirza B, Weedon D. Atypical fibroxanthoma: a clinicopathological study of 89 cases. *Australas J Dermatol* 2005;46(4):235–238.

135. Michie BA, Reid RP, Fallowfield ME. Aneuploidy in atypical fibroxanthoma: DNA content quantification of 10 cases by image analysis. *J Cutan Pathol* 1994;21(5):404–407.

136. Oshiro Y, Fukuda T, Tsuneyoshi M. Atypical fibroxanthoma versus benign and malignant fibrous histiocytoma. A comparative study of their proliferative activity using MIB-1, DNA flow cytometry, and p53 immunostaining. *Cancer* 1995;75(5):1128–1134.

137. Lazova R, Moynes R, May D, Scott G. LN-2 (CD74). A marker to distinguish atypical fibroxanthoma from malignant fibrous histiocytoma. *Cancer* 1997;79(11):2115–2124.

138. Oshman RG, Phelps RG, Kantor I. A solitary neurofibroma on the finger. *Arch Dermatol* 1988;124(8):1185–1186.

139. Barbagallo JS, Kolodzieh MS, Silverberg NB, Weinberg JM. Neurocutaneous disorders. *Dermatol Clin* 2002;20(3):547–560, viii.

140. Ross DE. Skin manifestations of von Recklinghausen's disease and associated tumors (neurofibromatosis). *Am Surg* 1965;31(11):729–740.

141. Kuo LA, Kuo RS. Plexiform neurofibromatosis: a difficult surgical problem. *Aust N Z J Surg* 1990;60(9):732–735.

142. Wick MR. Malignant peripheral nerve sheath tumors of the skin. *Mayo Clin Proc* 1990;65(2):279–282.

143. Lin V, Daniel S, Forte V. Is a plexiform neurofibroma pathognomonic of neurofibromatosis type I? *Laryngoscope* 2004;114(8):1410–1414.

144. Spinner RJ, Scheithauer BW, Perry A, Amrami KK, Emnett R, Gutmann DH. Colocalized cellular schwannoma and plexiform neurofibroma in the absence of neurofibromatosis. Case report. *J Neurosurg* 2007;107(2):435–439.

145. Marocchio LS, Pereira MC, Soares CT, Oliveira DT. Oral plexiform neurofibroma not associated with neurofibromatosis type I: case report. *J Oral Sci* 2006;48(3):157–160.

146. Fisher DA, Chu P, McCalmont T. Solitary plexiform neurofibroma is not pathognomonic of von Recklinghausen's neurofibromatosis: a report of a case. *Int J Dermatol* 1997;36(6):439–442.

147. Megahed M. Histopathological variants of neurofibroma. A study of 114 lesions. *Am J Dermatopathol* 1994;16(5):486–495.

148. Reed ML, Jacoby RA. Cutaneous neuroanatomy and neuropathology. Normal nerves, neural-crest derivatives, and benign neural neoplasms in the skin. *Am J Dermatopathol* 1983;5(4):335–362.

149. Michal M, Fanburg-Smith JC, Mentzel T, Kutzner H, Requena L, Zamecnik M, et al. Dendritic cell neurofibroma with pseudorosettes: a report of 18 cases of a distinct and hitherto unrecognized neurofibroma variant. *Am J Surg Pathol* 2001;25(5):587–594.

150. Swanson PE, Scheithauer BW, Wick MR. Peripheral nerve sheath neoplasms. Clinicopathologic and immunochemical observations. *Pathol Annu* 1995;30(Pt 2):1–82.

151. Gray MH, Smoller BR, McNutt NS, Hsu A. Immunohistochemical demonstration of factor XIIIa expression in neurofibromas. A practical means of differentiating these tumors from neurotized melanocytic nevi and schwannomas. *Arch Dermatol* 1990;126(4):472–476.

152. Halling KC, Scheithauer BW, Halling AC, Nascimento AG, Ziesmer SC, Roche PC, et al. p53 expression in neurofibroma and malignant peripheral nerve sheath tumor. An immunohistochemical study of sporadic and NF1-associated tumors. *Am J Clin Pathol* 1996;106(3):282–288.

153. McCarron KF, Goldblum JR. Plexiform neurofibroma with and without associated malignant peripheral nerve sheath tumor: a clinicopathologic and immunohistochemical analysis of 54 cases. *Mod Pathol* 1998;11(7):612–617.

154. Whitaker WG, Droulias C. Benign encapsulated neurilemoma: a report of 76 cases. *Am Surg* 1976;42(9):675–678.

155. Buscher CA, Izumi AK. A painful subcutaneous neurilemmoma attached to a peripheral nerve. *J Am Acad Dermatol* 1998;38(1):122–124.

156. Izumi AK, Rosato FE, Wood MG. Von Recklinghausen's disease associated with multiple neurolemomas. *Arch Dermatol* 1971;104(2):172–176.

157. Wolkenstein P, Benchikhi H, Zeller J, Wechsler J, Revuz J. Schwannomatosis: a clinical entity distinct from neurofibromatosis type 2. *Dermatology* 1997;195(3):228–231.

158. Abell MR, Hart WR, Olson JR. Tumors of the peripheral nervous system. *Hum Pathol* 1970;1(4):503–551.

159. Megahed M, Ruzicka T. Cellular schwannoma. *Am J Dermatopathol* 1994;16(4):418–421.

160. McMenamin ME, Fletcher CD. Expanding the spectrum of malignant change in schwannomas: epithelioid malignant change, epithelioid malignant peripheral nerve sheath tumor, and epithelioid angiosarcoma: a study of 17 cases. *Am J Surg Pathol* 2001;25(1):13–25.

161. Dakin MC, Leppard B, Theaker JM. The palisaded, encapsulated neuroma (solitary circumscribed neuroma). *Histopathology* 1992;20(5):405–410.

162. Shapiro L, Juhlin EA, Brownstein MH. "Rudimentary polydactyly": an amputation neuroma. *Arch Dermatol* 1973;108(2):223–225.

163. Brehmer-Andersson EE. Penile neuromas with multiple Meissner's corpuscles. *Histopathology* 1999;34(6):555–556.

164. Reed RJ, Bliss BO. Morton's neuroma. Regressive and productive intermetatarsal elastofibrositis. *Arch Pathol* 1973;95(2):123–129.

165. Young G, Lindsey J. Etiology of symptomatic recurrent interdigital neuromas. *J Am Podiatr Med Assoc* 1993;83(5):255–258.

166. Dover JS, From L, Lewis A. Palisaded encapsulated neuromas. A clinicopathologic study. *Arch Dermatol* 1989;125(3):386–389.

167. Fletcher CD. Solitary circumscribed neuroma of the skin (so-called palisaded, encapsulated neuroma). A clinicopathologic and immunohistochemical study. *Am J Surg Pathol* 1989;13(7):574–580.

168. Kossard S, Kumar A, Wilkinson B. Neural spectrum: palisaded encapsulated neuroma and Verocay body poor dermal schwannoma. *J Cutan Pathol* 1999;26(1):31–36.

169. Gallager RL, Helwig EB. Neurothekeoma—a benign cutaneous tumor of neural origin. *Am J Clin Pathol* 1980;74(6):759–764.

170. Pulitzer DR, Reed RJ. Nerve-sheath myxoma (perineurial myxoma). *Am J Dermatopathol* 1985;7(5):409–421.

171. Rosati LA, Fratamico FC, Eusebi V. Cellular neurothekeoma. *Appl Pathol* 1986;4(3):186–191.

172. Calonje E, Wilson-Jones E, Smith NP, Fletcher CD. Cellular 'neurothekeoma': an epithelioid variant of pilar leiomyoma? Morphological and immunohistochemical analysis of a series. *Histopathology* 1992;20(5):397–404.

173. Smith PD, Patterson JW. Merkel cell carcinoma (neuroendocrine carcinoma of the skin). *Am J Clin Pathol* 2001;115(5 Suppl):S68–S78.

174. Tsuruta D, Hamada T, Mochida K, Nakagawa K, Kobayashi H, Ishii M. Merkel cell carcinoma, Bowen's disease and chronic occupational arsenic poisoning. *Br J Dermatol* 1998;139(2):291–294.

175. Ohnishi Y, Murakami S, Ohtsuka H, Miyauchi S, Shinmori H, Hashimoto K. Merkel cell carcinoma and multiple Bowen's disease: incidental association or possible relationship to inorganic arsenic exposure? *J Dermatol* 1997;24(5):310–316.

176. Schenk P, Konrad K. Merkel cell carcinoma of the head and neck associated with Bowen's disease. *Eur Arch Otorhinolaryngol* 1991;248(8):436–441.
177. Silva EG, Mackay B, Goepfert H, Burgess MA, Fields RS. Endocrine carcinoma of the skin (Merkel cell carcinoma). *Pathol Annu* 1984;19(Pt 2):1–30.
178. Hitchcock CL, Bland KI, Laney RG 3rd, Franzini D, Harris B, Copeland EM 3rd. Neuroendocrine (Merkel cell) carcinoma of the skin. Its natural history, diagnosis, and treatment. *Ann Surg* 1988;207(2):201–207.
179. Hohaus K, Kostler E, Schonlebe J, Klemm E, Wollina U. Merkel cell carcinoma—a retrospective analysis of 17 cases. *J Eur Acad Dermatol Venereol* 2003;17(1):20–24.
180. Walsh NM. Primary neuroendocrine (Merkel cell) carcinoma of the skin: morphologic diversity and implications thereof. *Hum Pathol* 2001;32(7):680–689.
181. Gould E, Albores-Saavedra J, Dubner B, Smith W, Payne CM. Eccrine and squamous differentiation in Merkel cell carcinoma. An immunohistochemical study. *Am J Surg Pathol* 1988;12(10):768–772.
182. Nicholson SA, McDermott MB, Swanson PE, Wick MR. CD99 and cytokeratin-20 in small-cell and basaloid tumors of the skin. *Appl Immunohistochem Mol Morphol* 2000;8(1):37–41.
183. Ordonez NG. Value of thyroid transcription factor-1 immunostaining in distinguishing small cell lung carcinomas from other small cell carcinomas. *Am J Surg Pathol* 2000;24(9): 1217–1223.
184. Lau SK, Luthringer DJ, Eisen RN. Thyroid transcription factor-1: a review. *Appl Immunohistochem Mol Morphol* 2002;10(2):97–102.
185. Vazmitel M, Michal M, Kazakov DV. Merkel cell carcinoma and Azzopardi phenomenon. *Am J Dermatopathol* 2007;29(3):314–315.
186. Wick MR, Patterson JW. Reply to Merkel cell carcinoma and Azzopardi phenomenon. *Am J Dermatopathol* 2007;29(3):315.
187. Mills SE, Cooper PH, Fechner RE. Lobular capillary hemangioma: the underlying lesion of pyogenic granuloma. A study of 73 cases from the oral and nasal mucous membranes. *Am J Surg Pathol* 1980;4(5):470–479.
188. Cooper PH, McAllister HA, Helwig EB. Intravenous pyogenic granuloma. A study of 18 cases. *Am J Surg Pathol* 1979;3(3):221–228.
189. Cooper PH, Mills SE. Subcutaneous granuloma pyogenicum. Lobular capillary hemangioma. *Arch Dermatol* 1982;118(1):30–33.
190. Alessi E, Bertani E, Sala F. Acquired tufted angioma. *Am J Dermatopathol* 1986;8(5): 426–429.
191. Blume-Peytavi U, Adler YD, Geilen CC, Ahmad W, Christiano A, Goerdt S, et al. Multiple familial cutaneous glomangioma: a pedigree of 4 generations and critical analysis of histologic and genetic differences of glomus tumors. *J Am Acad Dermatol* 2000;42(4):633–639.
192. Murad TM, von Haam E, Murthy MS. Ultrastructure of a hemangiopericytoma and a glomus tumor. *Cancer* 1968;22(6):1239–1249.
193. Laymon CW, Peterson WC Jr. Glomangioma (glomus tumor). A clinicopathologic study with special reference to multiple lesions appearing during pregnancy. *Arch Dermatol* 1965; 92(5):509–514.
194. Schurch W, Skalli O, Lagace R, Seemayer TA, Gabbiani G. Intermediate filament proteins and actin isoforms as markers for soft-tissue tumor differentiation and origin. III. Hemangiopericytomas and glomus tumors. *Am J Pathol* 1990;136(4):771–786.
195. Dervan PA, Tobbia IN, Casey M, O'Loughlin J, O'Brien M. Glomus tumours: an immunohistochemical profile of 11 cases. *Histopathology* 1989;14(5):483–491.
196. Folpe AL, Fanburg-Smith JC, Miettinen M, Weiss SW. Atypical and malignant glomus tumors: analysis of 52 cases, with a proposal for the reclassification of glomus tumors. *Am J Surg Pathol* 2001;25(1):1–12.
197. Kim YC, Park HJ, Cinn YW. Microvenular hemangioma. *Dermatology* 2003;206(2):161–164.
198. Black RJ, McCusker GM, Eedy DJ. Microvenular haemangioma. *Clin Exp Dermatol* 1995; 20(3):260–262.
199. Hunt SJ, Santa Cruz DJ, Barr RJ. Microvenular hemangioma. *J Cutan Pathol* 1991;18(4): 235–240.
200. Chan JK, Fletcher CD, Hicklin GA, Rosai J. Glomeruloid hemangioma. A distinctive cutaneous lesion of multicentric Castleman's disease associated with POEMS syndrome. *Am J Surg Pathol* 1990;14(11):1036–1046.
201. Bardwick PA, Zvaifler NJ, Gill GN, Newman D, Greenway GD, Resnick DL. Plasma cell dyscrasia with polyneuropathy, organomegaly, endocrinopathy, M protein, and skin changes: the POEMS syndrome. Report on two cases and a review of the literature. *Medicine (Baltimore)* 1980;59(4):311–322.
202. Kishimoto S, Takenaka H, Shibagaki R, Noda Y, Yamamoto M, Yasuno H. Glomeruloid hemangioma in POEMS syndrome shows two different immunophenotypic endothelial cells. *J Cutan Pathol* 2000;27(2):87–92.
203. Tsai CY, Lai CH, Chan HL, Kuo T. Glomeruloid hemangioma—a specific cutaneous marker of POEMS syndrome. *Int J Dermatol* 2001;40(6):403–406.
204. Rongioletti F, Gambini C, Lerza R. Glomeruloid hemangioma. A cutaneous marker of POEMS syndrome. *Am J Dermatopathol* 1994;16(2):175–178.
205. Rosai J, Gold J, Landy R. The histiocytoid hemangiomas. A unifying concept embracing several previously described entities of skin, soft tissue, large vessels, bone, and heart. *Hum Pathol* 1979;10(6):707–730.
206. Wells GC, Whimster IW. Subcutaneous angiolymphoid hyperplasia with eosinophilia. *Br J Dermatol* 1969;81(1):1–14.
207. Olsen TG, Helwig EB. Angiolymphoid hyperplasia with eosinophilia. A clinicopathologic study of 116 patients. *J Am Acad Dermatol* 1985;12(5 Pt 1):781–796.
208. Mehregan AH, Shapiro L. Angiolymphoid hyperplasia with eosinophilia. *Arch Dermatol* 1971;103(1):50–57.
209. Chan JK, Hui PK, Ng CS, Yuen NW, Kung IT, Gwi E. Epithelioid haemangioma (angiolymphoid hyperplasia with eosinophilia) and Kimura's disease in Chinese. *Histopathology* 1989;15(6):557–574.
210. Urabe A, Tsuneyoshi M, Enjoji M. Epithelioid hemangioma versus Kimura's disease. A comparative clinicopathologic study. *Am J Surg Pathol* 1987;11(10):758–766.
211. Hashimoto H, Daimaru Y, Enjoji M. Intravascular papillary endothelial hyperplasia. A clinicopathologic study of 91 cases. *Am J Dermatopathol* 1983;5(6):539–546.
212. Kuo T, Sayers CP, Rosai J. Masson's "vegetant intravascular hemangioendothelioma": a lesion often mistaken for angiosarcoma—study of seventeen cases located in the skin and soft tissues. *Cancer* 1976;38(3):1227–1236.
213. Cockerell CJ, Whitlow MA, Webster GF, Friedman-Kien AE. Epithelioid angiomatosis: a distinct vascular disorder in patients with the acquired immunodeficiency syndrome or AIDS-related complex. *Lancet* 1987;2(8560):654–656.
214. Plettenberg A, Lorenzen T, Burtsche BT, Rasokat H, Kaliebe T, Albrecht H, et al. Bacillary angiomatosis in HIV-infected patients—an epidemiological and clinical study. *Dermatology* 2000;201(4):326–331.
215. Chian CA, Arrese JE, Pierard GE. Skin manifestations of *Bartonella* infections. *Int J Dermatol* 2002;41(8):461–466.
216. LeBoit PE, Berger TG, Egbert BM, Beckstead JH, Yen TS, Stoler MH. Bacillary angiomatosis. The histopathology and differential diagnosis of a pseudoneoplastic infection in patients with human immunodeficiency virus disease. *Am J Surg Pathol* 1989;13(11): 909–920.
217. LeBoit PE, Berger TG, Egbert BM, Yen TS, Stoler MH, Bonfiglio TA, et al. Epithelioid haemangioma-like vascular proliferation in AIDS: manifestation of cat scratch disease bacillus infection? *Lancet* 1988;1(8592):960–963.
218. Flanagan BP, Helwig EB. Cutaneous lymphangioma. *Arch Dermatol* 1977;113(1):24–30.
219. Palmer LC, Strauch WG, Welton WA. Lymphangioma circumscriptum. A case with deep lymphatic involvement. *Arch Dermatol* 1978;114(3):394–396.
220. Peachey RD, Lim CC, Whimster IW. Lymphangioma of skin. A review of 65 cases. *Br J Dermatol* 1970;83(5):519–527.
221. Mu XC, Tran TA, Dupree M, Carlson JA. Acquired vulvar lymphangioma mimicking genital warts. A case report and review of the literature. *J Cutan Pathol* 1999;26(3):150–154.
222. Whimster IW. The pathology of lymphangioma circumscriptum. *Br J Dermatol* 1976;94(5): 473–486.
223. Fukunaga M. Expression of D2-40 in lymphatic endothelium of normal tissues and in vascular tumours. *Histopathology* 2005;46(4):396–402.
224. Iscovich J, Boffetta P, Franceschi S, Azizi E, Sarid R. Classic Kaposi sarcoma: epidemiology and risk factors. *Cancer* 2000;88(3):500–517.
225. Slavin G, Cameron HM, Forbes C, Mitchell RM. Kaposi's sarcoma in East African children: a report of 51 cases. *J Pathol* 1970;100(3):187–199.
226. Piette WW. The incidence of second malignancies in subsets of Kaposi's sarcoma. *J Am Acad Dermatol* 1987;16(4):855–861.
227. Dezube BJ. AIDS-related Kaposi sarcoma: the role of local therapy for a systemic disease. *Arch Dermatol* 2000;136(12):1554–1556.
228. Cottoni F, Montesu MA. Kaposi's sarcoma classification: a problem not yet defined. *Int J Dermatol* 1996;35(7):480–483.
229. Pollack MS, Safai B, Myskowski PL, Gold JW, Pandey J, Dupont B. Frequencies of HLA and Gm immunogenetic markers in Kaposi's sarcoma. *Tissue Antigens* 1983;21(1):1–8.
230. Warmuth I, Moore PS. Kaposi sarcoma, Kaposi sarcoma-associated herpesvirus, and human T-cell lymphotropic virus type 1. What is the current evidence for causality? *Arch Dermatol* 1997;133(1):83–85.
231. Li N, Anderson WK, Bhawan J. Further confirmation of the association of human herpesvirus 8 with Kaposi's sarcoma. *J Cutan Pathol* 1998;25(8):413–419.
232. Gottlieb GJ, Ackerman AB. Kaposi's sarcoma: an extensively disseminated form in young homosexual men. *Hum Pathol* 1982;13(10):882–892.
233. McNutt NS, Fletcher V, Conant MA. Early lesions of Kaposi's sarcoma in homosexual men. An ultrastructural comparison with other vascular proliferations in skin. *Am J Pathol* 1983;111(1):62–77.
234. Wick MR. Kaposi's sarcoma unrelated to the acquired immunodeficiency syndrome. *Curr Opin Oncol* 1991;3(2):377–383.
235. Alessi E, Sala F, Berti E. Angiosarcomas in lymphedematous limbs. *Am J Dermatopathol* 1986;8(5):371–378.
236. Cooper PH. Angiosarcomas of the skin. *Semin Diagn Pathol* 1987;4(1):2–17.
237. Girard C, Johnson WC, Graham JH. Cutaneous angiosarcoma. *Cancer* 1970;26(4):868–883.
238. Hodgkinson DJ, Soule EH, Woods JE. Cutaneous angiosarcoma of the head and neck. *Cancer* 1979;44(3):1106–1113.
239. Rudd RJ, Fair KP, Patterson JW. Aortic angiosarcoma presenting with cutaneous metastasis: case report and review of the literature. *J Am Acad Dermatol* 2000;43(5 Pt 2):930–933.
240. Rosai J, Sumner HW, Kostianovsky M, Perez-Mesa C. Angiosarcoma of the skin. A clinicopathologic and fine structural study. *Hum Pathol* 1976;7(1):83–109.
241. DeYoung BR, Swanson PE, Argenyi ZB, Ritter JH, Fitzgibbon JF, Stahl DJ, et al. CD31 immunoreactivity in mesenchymal neoplasms of the skin and subcutis: report of 145 cases and review of putative immunohistologic markers of endothelial differentiation. *J Cutan Pathol* 1995;22(3):215–222.
242. Miettinen M, Fetsch JF. Distribution of keratins in normal endothelial cells and a spectrum of vascular tumors: implications in tumor diagnosis. *Hum Pathol* 2000;31(9):1062–1067.
243. Rodriguez J, Ackerman AB. Xanthogranuloma in adults. *Arch Dermatol* 1976;112(1):43–44.
244. Helwig EB, Hackney VC. Juvenile xanthogranuloma (nevoxanthoendothelioma). *Am J Pathol* 1954;30:625–626.
245. Garcia-Pena P, Mariscal A, Abellan C, Zuasnabar A, Lucaya J. Juvenile xanthogranuloma with extracutaneous lesions. *Pediatr Radiol* 1992;22(5):377–378.
246. DeBarge LR, Chan CC, Greenberg SC, McLean IW, Yannuzzi LA, Nussenblatt RB. Chorioretinal, iris, and ciliary body infiltration by juvenile xanthogranuloma masquerading as uveitis. *Surv Ophthalmol* 1994;39(1):65–71.
247. Zimmerman LE. Ocular lesions of juvenile xanthogranuloma. Nevoxanthoendothelioma. *Am J Ophthalmol* 1965;60(6):1011–1035.
248. Zvulunov A, Barak Y, Metzker A. Juvenile xanthogranuloma, neurofibromatosis, and juvenile chronic myelogenous leukemia. World statistical analysis. *Arch Dermatol* 1995;131(8): 904–908.
249. Esterly NB, Sahihi T, Medenica M. Juvenile xanthogranuloma. An atypical case with study of ultrastructure. *Arch Dermatol* 1972;105(1):99–102.

250. Zelger BG, Zelger B, Steiner H, Mikuz G. Solitary giant xanthogranuloma and benign cephalic histiocytosis—variants of juvenile xanthogranuloma. *Br J Dermatol* 1995;133(4):598–604.
251. Sonoda T, Hashimoto H, Enjoji M. Juvenile xanthogranuloma. Clinicopathologic analysis and immunohistochemical study of 57 patients. *Cancer* 1985;56(9):2280–2286.
252. Kraus MD, Haley JC, Ruiz R, Essary L, Moran CA, Fletcher CD. "Juvenile" xanthogranuloma: an immunophenotypic study with a reappraisal of histogenesis. *Am J Dermatopathol* 2001;23(2):104–111.
253. Tomaszewski MM, Lupton GP. Unusual expression of S-100 protein in histiocytic neoplasms. *J Cutan Pathol* 1998;25(3):129–135.
254. Zelger B, Cerio R, Orchard G, Wilson-Jones E. Juvenile and adult xanthogranuloma. A histological and immunohistochemical comparison. *Am J Surg Pathol* 1994;18(2):126–135.
255. Wood C, Wood GS, Deneau DG, Oseroff A, Beckstead JH, Malin J. Malignant histiocytosis X. Report of a rapidly fatal case in an elderly man. *Cancer* 1984;54(2):347–352.
256. Zachariae H. Histiocytosis X in two infants—treated with topical nitrogen mustard. *Br J Dermatol* 1979;100(4):433–438.
257. Vassallo R, Ryu JH, Colby TV, Hartman T, Limper AH. Pulmonary Langerhans'-cell histiocytosis. *N Engl J Med* 2000;342(26):1969–1978.
258. Meehan SA, Smoller BR. Cutaneous Langerhans cell histiocytosis of the genitalia in the elderly: a report of three cases. *J Cutan Pathol* 1998;25(7):370–374.
259. Weiss LM, Grogan TM, Pileri SA, Favara B, Dura T, Paulli M, Feller AC. Langerhans cell sarcoma. In Jaffe ES, Harris NL, Stein H, Vardiman JW, eds. *Tumours of Haematopoietic and Lymphoid Tissues.* Lyon, France: IARC Press, 2001.
260. Hashimoto K, Kagetsu N, Taniguchi Y, Weintraub R, Chapman-Winokur RL, Kasiborski A. Immunohistochemistry and electron microscopy in Langerhans cell histiocytosis confined to the skin. *J Am Acad Dermatol* 1991;25(6 Pt 1):1044–1053.
261. Itoh H, Miyaguni H, Kataoka H, Akiyama Y, Tateyama S, Marutsuka K, et al. Primary cutaneous Langerhans cell histiocytosis showing malignant phenotype in an elderly woman: report of a fatal case. *J Cutan Pathol* 2001;28(7):371–378.
262. Hage C, Willman CL, Favara BE, Isaacson PG. Langerhans' cell histiocytosis (histiocytosis X): immunophenotype and growth fraction. *Hum Pathol* 1993;24(8):840–845.
263. Krenacs L, Tiszalvicz L, Krenacs T, Boumsell L. Immunohistochemical detection of CD1A antigen in formalin-fixed and paraffin-embedded tissue sections with monoclonal antibody 010. *J Pathol* 1993;171(2):99–104.
264. Harrist TJ, Bhan AK, Murphy GF, Sato S, Berman RS, Gellis SE, et al. Histiocytosis-X: in situ characterization of cutaneous infiltrates with monoclonal antibodies. *Am J Clin Pathol* 1983;79(3):294–300.
265. Soter NA. Mastocytosis and the skin. *Hematol Oncol Clin North Am* 2000;14(3):537–555, vi.
266. Shaw JM. Genetic aspects of urticaria pigmentosa. *Arch Dermatol* 1968;97(2):137–138.
267. Oku T, Hashizume H, Yokote R, Sano T, Yamada M. The familial occurrence of bullous mastocytosis (diffuse cutaneous mastocytosis). *Arch Dermatol* 1990;126(11):1478–1484.
268. Hannaford R, Rogers M. Presentation of cutaneous mastocytosis in 173 children. *Australas J Dermatol* 2001;42(1):15–21.
269. Tebbe B, Stavropoulos PG, Krasagakis K, Orfanos CE. Cutaneous mastocytosis in adults. Evaluation of 14 patients with respect to systemic disease manifestations. *Dermatology* 1998; 197(2):101–108.
270. Longley BJ Jr, Morganroth GS, Tyrrell L, Ding TG, Anderson DM, Williams DE, et al. Altered metabolism of mast-cell growth factor (c-kit ligand) in cutaneous mastocytosis. *N Engl J Med* 1993;328(18):1302–1307.
271. Orkin M, Good RA, Clawson CC, Fisher I, Windhorst DB. Bullous mastocytosis. *Arch Dermatol* 1970;101(5):547–564.
272. Hamann K, Haas N, Grabbe J, Czarnetzki BM. Expression of stem cell factor in cutaneous mastocytosis. *Br J Dermatol* 1995;133(2):203–208.
273. Horny HP, Sillaber C, Menke D, Kaiserling E, Wehrmann M, Stehberger B, et al. Diagnostic value of immunostaining for tryptase in patients with mastocytosis. *Am J Surg Pathol* 1998;22(9):1132–1140.
274. Patterson JW, Parsons JM, Blaylock WK, Mills AS. Eosinophils in skin lesions of erythema multiforme. *Arch Pathol Lab Med* 1989;113(1):36–39.
275. Jaffe ES, Harris NL, Stein H, Vardiman JW. Summary of the WHO classification of tumours of haematopooietic and lymphoid tissues. In Jaffe ES, Harris NL, Stein H, Vardiman JW, eds. *Tumours of Haematopoietic and Lymphoid Tissues.* Lyon, France: IARC Press, 2001:10–13.
276. Willemze R, Jaffe ES, Burg G, Cerroni L, Berti E, Swerdlow SH, et al. WHO-EORTC classification for cutaneous lymphomas. *Blood* 2005;105(10):3768–3785.
277. Burg G, Kempf W, Cozzio A, Feit J, Willemze R, et al. WHO/EORTC classification of cutaneous lymphomas 2005: histological and molecular aspects. *J Cutan Pathol* 2005; 32(10):647–674.
278. Bafverstedt B. Lymphadenosis benigna cutis. *Acta Derm Venereol* 1968;48(1):1–6.
279. Hovmark A, Asbrink E, Olsson I. The spirochetal etiology of lymphadenosis benigna cutis solitaria. *Acta Derm Venereol* 1986;66(6):479–484.
280. Roo E, Villegas C, Lopez-Bran E, Jimenez E, Valle P, Sanchez-Yus E. Postzoster cutaneous pseudolymphoma. *Arch Dermatol* 1994;130(5):661–663.
281. Bachelez H, Hadida F, Parizot C, Flageul B, Kemula M, Dubertret L, et al. Oligoclonal expansion of HIV-specific cytotoxic CD8 T lymphocytes in the skin of HIV-1-infected patients with cutaneous pseudolymphoma. *J Clin Invest* 1998;101(11):2506–2516.
282. Lanzafame S, Micali G. [Cutaneous lymphoid hyperplasia (pseudolymphoma) secondary to vaccination]. *Pathologica* 1993;85(1099):555–561.
283. Magro CM, Crowson AN. Drugs with antihistaminic properties as a cause of atypical cutaneous lymphoid hyperplasia. *J Am Acad Dermatol* 1995;32(3):419–428.
284. Patterson JW. Lymphomas. *Dermatol Clin* 1992;10(1):235–251.
285. Medeiros LJ, Picker LJ, Abel EA, Hu CH, Hoppe RT, Warnke RA, et al. Cutaneous lymphoid hyperplasia. Immunologic characteristics and assessment of criteria recently proposed as diagnostic of malignant lymphoma [lymphocytoma]. *J Am Acad Dermatol* 1989; 21(5 Pt 1):929–942.
286. Fan K, Kelly R, Kendrick V. Nonclonal lymphocytic proliferation in cutaneous lymphoid hyperplasia: a flow-cytometric and morphological analysis. *Dermatology* 1992;185(2): 113–119.
287. Braddock SW, Harrington D, Vose J. Generalized nodular cutaneous pseudolymphoma associated with phenytoin therapy. Use of T-cell receptor gene rearrangement in diagnosis and clinical review of cutaneous reactions to phenytoin. *J Am Acad Dermatol* 1992;27(2 Pt 2):337–340.
288. Schmid U, Eckert F, Griesser H, Steinke C, Cogliatti SB, Kaudewitz P, et al. Cutaneous follicular lymphoid hyperplasia with monotypic plasma cells. A clinicopathologic study of 18 patients. *Am J Surg Pathol* 1995;19(1):12–20.
289. Spina D, Miracco C, Santopietro R, Sforza V, Leoncini L, Pacenti L, et al. Distinction between diffuse cutaneous malignant follicular center cell lymphoma and lymphoid hyperplasia by computerized nuclear image analysis. *Am J Dermatopathol* 1993;15(5):415–422.
290. Roggero E, Zucca E, Mainetti C, Bertoni F, Valsangiacomo C, Pedrinis E, et al. Eradication of *Borrelia burgdorferi* infection in primary marginal zone B-cell lymphoma of the skin. *Hum Pathol* 2000;31(2):263–268.
291. Tomaszewski MM, Abbondanzo SL, Lupton GP. Extranodal marginal zone B-cell lymphoma of the skin: a morphologic and immunophenotypic study of 11 cases. *Am J Dermatopathol* 2000;22(3):205–211.
292. Valdez R, Finn WG, Ross CW, Singleton TP, Tworek JA, Schnitzer B. Waldenstrom macroglobulinemia caused by extranodal marginal zone B-cell lymphoma: a report of six cases. *Am J Clin Pathol* 2001;116(5):683–690.
293. Isaacson PG, Muller-Hermelink HK, Piris MA, Berger F, Nathwani BN, Swerdlow SH, Harris NL. Extranodal marginal zone B-cell lymphoma of mucosa-associated lymphoid tissue (MALT lymphoma). In Jaffe ES, Harris NL, Stein H, Vardiman JW, eds. *Tumours of Haematopoietic and Lymphoid Tissues.* Lyon, France: IARC Press, 2001:157–160.
294. Cerroni L, Signoretti S, Hofler G, Annessi G, Putz B, Lackinger E, et al. Primary cutaneous marginal zone B-cell lymphoma: a recently described entity of low-grade malignant cutaneous B-cell lymphoma. *Am J Surg Pathol* 1997;21(11):1307–1315.
295. Aguilera NS, Tomaszewski MM, Moad JC, Bauer FA, Taubenberger JK, Abbondanzo SL. Cutaneous follicle center lymphoma: a clinicopathologic study of 19 cases. *Mod Pathol* 2001;14(9):828–835.
296. de Leval L, Harris NL, Longtine J, Ferry JA, Duncan LM. Cutaneous B-cell lymphomas of follicular and marginal zone types: use of Bcl-6, CD10, Bcl-2, and CD21 in differential diagnosis and classification. *Am J Surg Pathol* 2001;25(6):732–741.
297. Lawnicki LC, Weisenburger DD, Aoun P, Chan WC, Wickert RS, Greiner TC. The t(14; 18) and bcl-2 expression are present in a subset of primary cutaneous follicular lymphoma: association with lower grade. *Am J Clin Pathol* 2002;118(5):765–772.
298. Gatter KC, Warnke RA. Diffuse large B-cell lymphoma. In Jaffe ES, Harris NL, Stein H, Vardiman JW, eds. *Tumours of Haematopoietic and Lymphoid Tissues.* Lyon, France: IARC Press, 2001:171–174.
299. Willemze R, Meijer CJ. EORTC classification for primary cutaneous lymphomas: the best guide to good clinical management. European Organization for Research and Treatment of Cancer. *Am J Dermatopathol* 1999;21(3):265–273.
300. Li S, Griffin CA, Mann RB, Borowitz MJ. Primary cutaneous T-cell-rich B-cell lymphoma: clinically distinct from its nodal counterpart? *Mod Pathol* 2001;14(1):10–13.
301. Cerroni L, El-Shabrawi-Caelen L, Fink-Puches R, LeBoit PE, Kerl H. Cutaneous spindle-cell B-cell lymphoma: a morphologic variant of cutaneous large B-cell lymphoma. *Am J Dermatopathol* 2000;22(4):299–304.
302. Doggett RS, Wood GS, Horning S, Levy R, Dorfman RF, Bindl J, et al. The immunologic characterization of 95 nodal and extranodal diffuse large cell lymphomas in 89 patients. *Am J Pathol* 1984;115(2):245–252.
303. Geelen FA, Vermeer MH, Meijer CJ, Van der Putte SC, Kerkhof E, Kluin PM, et al. bcl-2 protein expression in primary cutaneous large B-cell lymphoma is site-related. *J Clin Oncol* 1998;16(6):2080–2085.
304. Piris M, Brown DC, Gatter KC, Mason DY. CD30 expression in non-Hodgkin's lymphoma. *Histopathology* 1990;17(3):211–218.
305. Sander CA, Kaudewitz P, Kutzner H, Simon M, Schirren CG, Sioutos N, et al. T-cell-rich B-cell lymphoma presenting in skin. A clinicopathologic analysis of six cases. *J Cutan Pathol* 1996;23(2):101–108.
306. Bhawan J, Wolff SM, Ucci AA, Bhan AK. Malignant lymphoma and malignant angioendotheliomatosis: one disease. *Cancer* 1985;55(3):570–576.
307. Gatter KC, Warnke RA. Intravascular large B-cell lymphoma. In Jaffe ES, Harris NL, Stein H, Vardiman JW, eds. *Tumours of Haematopoietic and Lymphoid Tissues.* Lyon, France: IARC Press, 2001:177–178.
308. Khalidi HS, Brynes RK, Browne P, Koo CH, Battifora H, Medeiros LJ. Intravascular large B-cell lymphoma: the CD5 antigen is expressed by a subset of cases. *Mod Pathol* 1998; 11(10):983–988.
309. Chang A, Zic JA, Boyd AS. Intravascular large cell lymphoma: a patient with asymptomatic purpuric patches and a chronic clinical course. *J Am Acad Dermatol* 1998;39(2 Pt 2): 318–321.
310. Lakhani SR, Hulman G, Hall JM, Slack DN, Sloane JP. Intravascular malignant lymphomatosis (angiotropic large-cell lymphoma). A case report with evidence for T-cell lineage with polymerase chain reaction analysis. *Histopathology* 1994;25(3):283–286.
311. Au WY, Shek WH, Nicholls J, Tse KM, Todd D, Kwong YL. T-cell intravascular lymphomatosis (angiotropic large cell lymphoma): association with Epstein-Barr viral infection. *Histopathology* 1997;31(6):563–567.
312. Beaty MW, Toro J, Sorbara L, Stern JB, Pittaluga S, Raffeld M, et al. Cutaneous lymphomatoid granulomatosis: correlation of clinical and biologic features. *Am J Surg Pathol* 2001; 25(9):1111–1120.
313. Jaffe ES, Wilson WH. Lymphomatoid granulomatosis. In Jaffe ES, Harris NL, Stein H, Vardiman JW, eds. *Tumours of Haematopoietic and Lymphoid Tissues.* Lyon, France: IARC Press, 2001:185–187.

314. James WD, Odom RB, Katzenstein AL. Cutaneous manifestations of lymphomatoid granulomatosis. Report of 44 cases and a review of the literature. *Arch Dermatol* 1981;117(4): 196–202.

315. McNiff JM, Cooper D, Howe G, Crotty PL, Tallini G, Crouch J, et al. Lymphomatoid granulomatosis of the skin and lung. An angiocentric T-cell-rich B-cell lymphoproliferative disorder. *Arch Dermatol* 1996;132(12):1464–1470.

316. Kessler S, Lund HZ, Leonard DD. Cutaneous lesions of lymphomatoid granulomatosis. Comparison with lymphomatoid papulosis. *Am J Dermatopathol* 1981;3(2):115–127.

317. Angel CA, Slater DN, Royds JA, Nelson SN, Bleehen SS. Epstein-Barr virus in cutaneous lymphomatoid granulomatosis. *Histopathology* 1994;25(6):545–548.

318. Marti RM, Campo E, Bosch F, Palou J, Estrach T. Cutaneous lymphocyte-associated antigen (CLA) expression in a lymphoblastoid mantle cell lymphoma presenting with skin lesions. Comparison with other clinicopathologic presentations of mantle cell lymphoma. *J Cutan Pathol* 2001;28(5):256–264.

319. Sarikaya I, Patel M, Holder L. Cutaneous mantle cell lymphoma detected with Ga-67 citrate. *Clin Nucl Med* 2000;25(10):849–851.

320. Swerdlow SH, Berger F, Isaacson PI, Muller-Hermelink HK, Nathwani BN, Piris MA, Harris NL. Mantle cell lymphoma. In Jaffe ES, Harris NL, Stein H, Vardiman JW, eds. *Tumours of Haematopoietic and Lymphoid Tissues.* Lyon, France: IARC Press, 2001:168–170.

321. Moody BR, Bartlett NL, George DW, Price CR, Breer WA, Rothschild Y, et al. Cyclin D1 as an aid in the diagnosis of mantle cell lymphoma in skin biopsies: a case report. *Am J Dermatopathol* 2001;23(5):470–476.

322. Guitart J, Kennedy J, Ronan S, Chmiel JS, Hsiegh YC, Variakojis D. Histologic criteria for the diagnosis of mycosis fungoides: proposal for a grading system to standardize pathology reporting. *J Cutan Pathol* 2001;28(4):174–183.

323. Ralfkiaer E, Jaffe ES. Mycosis fungoides and Sezary syndrome. In Jaffe ES, Harris NL, Stein H, Vardiman JW, eds. *Tumours of Haematopoietic and Lymphoid Tissues.* Lyon, France: IARC Press, 2001:216–220.

324. Kim YH, Hoppe RT. Mycosis fungoides and the Sezary syndrome. *Semin Oncol* 1999;26(3): 276–289.

325. Jones REJE. Questions to the editorial board and other authorities. *Am J Dermatopathol* 1986;8:534–545.

326. Simon M, Flaig MJ, Kind P, Sander CA, Kaudewitz P. Large plaque parapsoriasis: clinical and genotypic correlations. *J Cutan Pathol* 2000;27(2):57–60.

327. Mandojana RM, Helwig EB. Localized epidermotropic reticulosis (Woringer-Kolopp disease). *J Am Acad Dermatol* 1983;8(6):813–829.

328. Haghighi B, Smoller BR, LeBoit PE, Warnke RA, Sander CA, Kohler S. Pagetoid reticulosis (Woringer-Kolopp disease): an immunophenotypic, molecular, and clinicopathologic study. *Mod Pathol* 2000;13(5):502–510.

329. Bonta MD, Tannous ZS, Demierre MF, Gonzalez E, Harris NL, Duncan LM. Rapidly progressing mycosis fungoides presenting as follicular mucinosis. *J Am Acad Dermatol* 2000; 43(4):635–640.

330. Zelger B, Sepp N, Weyrer K, Grunewald K. Syringotropic cutaneous T-cell lymphoma: a variant of mycosis fungoides? *Br J Dermatol* 1994;130(6):765–769.

331. Sausville EA, Eddy JL, Makuch RW, Fischmann AB, Schechter GP, Matthews M, et al. Histopathologic staging at initial diagnosis of mycosis fungoides and the Sezary syndrome. Definition of three distinctive prognostic groups. *Ann Intern Med* 1988;109(5):372–382.

332. Cerroni L, Rieger E, Hodl S, Kerl H. Clinicopathologic and immunologic features associated with transformation of mycosis fungoides to large-cell lymphoma. *Am J Surg Pathol* 1992;16(6):543–552.

333. Tan RS, Butterworth CM, McLaughlin H, Malka S, Samman PD. Mycosis fungoides—a disease of antigen persistence. *Br J Dermatol* 1974;91(6):607–616.

334. Altman J. Parapsoriasis: a histopathologic review and classification. *Semin Dermatol* 1984; 3:14–21.

335. McMillan EM, Wasik R, Martin D, Donaldson M, Everett MA. Immuno-electron microscopy of "T" cells in large plaque parapsoriasis. *J Cutan Pathol* 1981;8(5):385–392.

336. Nickoloff BJ. Light-microscopic assessment of 100 patients with patch/plaque-stage mycosis fungoides. *Am J Dermatopathol* 1988;10(6):469–477.

337. Smoller BR, Bishop K, Glusac E, Kim YH, Hendrickson M. Reassessment of histologic parameters in the diagnosis of mycosis fungoides. *Am J Surg Pathol* 1995;19(12):1423–1430.

338. Vonderheid EC, Tan E, Sobel EL, Schwab E, Micaily B, Jegasothy BV. Clinical implications of immunologic phenotyping in cutaneous T cell lymphoma. *J Am Acad Dermatol* 1987; 17(1):40–52.

339. Ormsby A, Bergfeld WF, Tubbs RR, Hsi ED. Evaluation of a new paraffin-reactive CD7 T-cell deletion marker and a polymerase chain reaction-based T-cell receptor gene rearrangement assay: implications for diagnosis of mycosis fungoides in community clinical practice. *J Am Acad Dermatol* 2001;45(3):405–413.

340. Agnarsson BA, Vonderheid EC, Kadin ME. Cutaneous T cell lymphoma with suppressor/cytotoxic (CD8) phenotype: identification of rapidly progressive and chronic subtypes. *J Am Acad Dermatol* 1990;22(4):569–577.

341. Vonderheid EC, Bigler RD, Kotecha A, Boselli CM, Lessin SR, Bernengo MG, et al. Variable CD7 expression on T cells in the leukemic phase of cutaneous T cell lymphoma (Sezary syndrome). *J Invest Dermatol* 2001;117(3):654–662.

342. Russell-Jones R, Whittaker S. T-cell receptor gene analysis in the diagnosis of Sezary syndrome. *J Am Acad Dermatol* 1999;41(2 Pt 1):254–259.

343. Buechner SA, Winkelmann RK. Sezary syndrome. A clinicopathologic study of 39 cases. *Arch Dermatol* 1983;119(12):979–986.

344. Wieselthier JS, Koh HK. Sezary syndrome: diagnosis, prognosis, and critical review of treatment options. *J Am Acad Dermatol* 1990;22(3):381–401.

345. Bernengo MG, Quaglino P, Novelli M, Cappello N, Doveil GC, Lisa F, et al. Prognostic factors in Sezary syndrome: a multivariate analysis of clinical, haematological and immunological features. *Ann Oncol* 1998;9(8):857–863.

346. Piepkorn M, Marty J, Kjeldsberg CR. T cell subset heterogeneity in a series of patients with mycosis fungoides and Sezary syndrome. *J Am Acad Dermatol* 1984;11(3):427–432.

347. Artemi P, Wong DA, Mann S, Regan W. CD30 (Ki-1)-positive primary cutaneous T-cell lymphoma: report of spontaneous resolution. *Australas J Dermatol* 1997;38(4):206–208.

348. Willemze R, Kerl H, Sterry W, Berti E, Cerroni L, Chimenti S, et al. EORTC classification for primary cutaneous lymphomas: a proposal from the Cutaneous Lymphoma Study Group of the European Organization for Research and Treatment of Cancer. *Blood* 1997; 90(1):354–371.

349. Chott A, Kaserer K, Augustin I, Vesely M, Heinz R, Oehlinger W, et al. Ki-1-positive large cell lymphoma. A clinicopathologic study of 41 cases. *Am J Surg Pathol* 1990;14(5):439–448.

350. Simonart T, Kentos A, Renoirte C, Vereecken P, De Dobbeleer G, Dargent JL. Cutaneous involvement by neutrophil-rich, CD30-positive anaplastic large cell lymphoma mimicking deep pustules. *Am J Surg Pathol* 1999;23(2):244–246.

351. Falini B. Anaplastic large cell lymphoma: pathological, molecular and clinical features. *Br J Haematol* 2001;114(4):741–760.

352. Vergier B, Beylot-Barry M, Pulford K, Michel P, Bosq J, de Muret A, et al. Statistical evaluation of diagnostic and prognostic features of CD30 + cutaneous lymphoproliferative disorders: a clinicopathologic study of 65 cases. *Am J Surg Pathol* 1998;22(10):1192–1202.

353. Macaulay WL. Lymphomatoid papulosis. A continuing self-healing eruption, clinically oncocytic differentiation. A report of 3 cases. *J Cutan Pathol* 1996;23(3):254–258

354. Macaulay WL. Lymphomatoid papulosis update. A historical perspective. *Arch Dermatol* 1989;125(10):1387–1389.

355. Sanchez NP, Pittelkow MR, Muller SA, Banks PM, Winkelmann RK. The clinicopathologic spectrum of lymphomatoid papulosis: study of 31 cases. *J Am Acad Dermatol* 1983;8(1): 81–94.

356. Kadin ME. Lymphomatoid papulosis, Ki-1 + lymphoma, and primary cutaneous Hodgkin's disease. *Semin Dermatol* 1991;10(3):164–171.

357. Willemze R, Meyer CJ, Van Vloten WA, Scheffer E. The clinical and histological spectrum of lymphomatoid papulosis. *Br J Dermatol* 1982;107(2):131–144.

358. Willemze R, Scheffer E, Ruiter DJ, van Vloten WA, Meijer CJ. Immunological, cytochemical and ultrastructural studies in lymphomatoid papulosis. *Br J Dermatol* 1983;108(4): 381–394.

359. Davis TH, Morton CC, Miller-Cassman R, Balk SP, Kadin ME. Hodgkin's disease, lymphomatoid papulosis, and cutaneous T-cell lymphoma derived from a common T-cell clone. *N Engl J Med* 1992;326(17):1115–1122.

360. Boulland ML, Wechsler J, Bagot M, Pulford K, Kanavaros P, Gaulard P. Primary CD30-positive cutaneous T-cell lymphomas and lymphomatoid papulosis frequently express cytotoxic proteins. *Histopathology* 2000;36(2):136–144.

361. Whittaker S, Smith N, Jones RR, Luzzatto L. Analysis of beta, gamma, and delta T-cell receptor genes in lymphomatoid papulosis: cellular basis of two distinct histologic subsets. *J Invest Dermatol* 1991;96(5):786–791.

362. Sioutos N, Kerl H, Murphy SB, Kadin ME. Primary cutaneous Hodgkin's disease. Unique clinical, morphologic, and immunophenotypic findings. *Am J Dermatopathol* 1994;16(1): 2–8.

363. Barzilai A, Shpiro D, Goldberg I, Yacob-Hirsch Y, Diaz-Cascajo C, Meytes D, et al. Insect bite-like reaction in patients with hematologic malignant neoplasms. *Arch Dermatol* 1999; 135(12):1503–1507.

364. Ratnam KV, Khor CJ, Su WP. Leukemia cutis. *Dermatol Clin* 1994;12(2):419–431.

365. Braverman IM. *Skin Signs of Systemic Disease.* 2nd edition. Philadelphia, PA: W.B. Saunders, 1981.

366. Su WP, Buechner SA, Li CY. Clinicopathologic correlations in leukemia cutis. *J Am Acad Dermatol* 1984;11(1):121–128.

367. Wong TY, Suster S, Bouffard D, Flynn SD, Johnson RA, Barnhill RL, et al. Histologic spectrum of cutaneous involvement in patients with myelogenous leukemia including the neutrophilic dermatoses. *Int J Dermatol* 1995;34(5):323–329.

368. Canioni D, Fraitag S, Thomas C, Valensi F, Griscelli C, Brousse N. Skin lesions revealing neonatal acute leukemias with monocytic differentiation. A report of 3 cases. *J Cutan Pathol* 1996;23(3):254–258.

CHAPTER

3

Adriano Piris
Nicolas Prieto-Granada
Michael J. Imber
Martin C. Mihm, Jr.

Melanocytic Lesions

The spectrum of benign and malignant melanocytic proliferations is both complex and fascinating. An awareness of the normal developmental biology of the human melanocyte provides diagnostic insight into the morphologic diversity of melanocytic disorders. An understanding of the spectrum of benign proliferative patterns is necessary for recognizing the aberrant histologic and cytologic features of malignant melanoma and precursor lesions.

Melanocytes originate from neural crest precursor cells, which also give rise to peripheral neurons and Schwann cells (1). Cells destined to become epidermal melanocytes migrate to the periderm, where they develop the dendritic morphology and the ultrastructural characteristics of mature melanocytes (2,3). The cytokinetic behavior of melanocytes during embryogenesis and their developmental relationship to other cells of the peripheral nervous system likely are basic factors underlying the morphologic spectrum of benign melanocytic lesions (4–8). The existence of pigmented neurofibromas and melanocytic schwannomas, the association of leptomeningeal melanocytosis with giant congenital melanocytic nevi, and the commonly observed phenomenon of schwannian differentiation or neurotization in acquired melanocytic nevi underscore this point (9). Stromal-epithelial interactions during embryogenesis may influence the development of distinct melanocyte subpopulations that differ in anatomic distribution and the potential to evolve into various types of melanocytic proliferations (10–15).

These properties suggest that the criteria used to distinguish benign from malignant melanocytic proliferations and to identify precursor and borderline lesions must necessarily differ from those applied to epithelial proliferations. The melanocyte is a migratory cell. Its usual location, with dispersion among the epidermal basal keratinocytes, is stable, and evidence of migration and mitotic activity is rare. The melanocytes are held in place with E-cadherin, which is expressed on both keratinocyte and melanocyte surfaces. This appears to be an extremely important molecule for keratinocyte-melanocyte interactions. In the normal homeostatic events of melanocyte migration and proliferation, especially in childhood, the melanocyte downregulates E-cadherin, desmoglein 1, and connexin 43 under the influence of several growth factors. Once the melanocyte divides and repositions itself in the epidermis, then the adhesion molecules reappear (16). The proliferation and migration of melanocytes are also normally seen in regenerating epidermis and in areas of vitiligo undergoing repigmentation (17,18).

The migration of melanocytes across the basement membrane zone of the epidermis and into the papillary dermis is part of the "normal" development of many benign melanocytic lesions, including most of the acquired melanocytic nevi. In addition, upward or lateral migration of melanocytes within the epidermis may be seen in several benign lesions, including the spindle and epithelioid cell nevus and the pigmented spindle cell nevus (19). Therefore, the isolated histologic observation of invasive behavior does not necessarily denote malignancy in a melanocytic lesion because this finding usually suggests an epithelial tumor (20).

BENIGN MELANOCYTIC PROLIFERATIONS

HISTOLOGIC AND CYTOLOGIC CHARACTERISTICS

Most benign lesions that originate from epidermal melanocytes display varying combinations of three proliferative patterns that are readily apparent under low-power examination. *Lentiginous hyperplasia* describes a pattern of crowded single-cell melanocytic growth along the dermal-epidermal junction (Fig. 3.1). This pattern is often seen in compound nevi and lentigines. *Nested proliferation* describes the clonal growth of numerous microanatomically discrete clusters of melanocytes (Fig. 3.2). The distribution of such nests (thèques) of cells within the epidermis or along the junction is often quite characteristic of certain specific types of melanocytic nevi, including the pigmented spindle cell nevus and the spindle and epithelioid cell nevus. Finally, *pagetoid proliferation* describes a pattern of discohesive single-cell growth throughout the entire epidermis (Fig. 3.3). Although pagetoid spread is commonly associated with melanoma, it may be observed in Spitz nevi and in common acquired nevi occurring in acral locations.

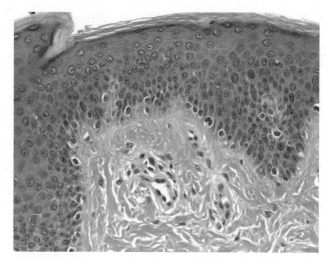

Figure 3.1. Lentiginous melanocytic hyperplasia, benign. The melanocytes are moderately increased in number and lie side by side in the basal layer.

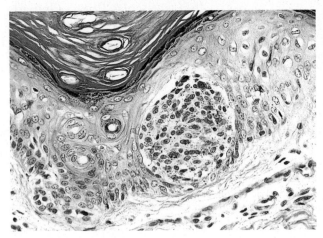

Figure 3.2. Nested melanocytic proliferation, junctional nevus. Cytologically banal-appearing nevomelanocytes proliferate in a well-circumscribed intraepidermal growth center, often referred to as a *thèque* or *nest*.

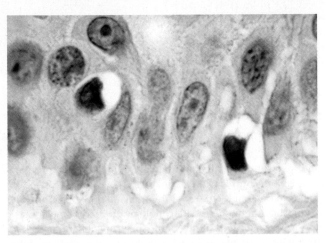

Figure 3.4. Normal melanocyte. The nuclei display characteristic polygonal, hyperchromatic features and appear smaller than the adjacent keratinocyte nuclei. The cytoplasm is collapsed, forming a thin eosinophilic rim about the nucleus. Dendritic processes are evident in one melanocyte as eosinophilic processes extending to the intercellular space of adjacent keratinocytes.

The cytologic characteristics of benign melanocytes or nevus cells are often variable. A comparison of the nuclear features of melanocytes with the features of adjacent normal keratinocyte or endothelial cell nuclei as internal references for nuclear size and detail is often helpful. The nucleus of a normal melanocyte residing within the basal layer of the epidermis typically is somewhat smaller and slightly more hyperchromatic than are the nuclei of nearby keratinocytes (21) (Fig. 3.4). The chromatin pattern is uniform, and no nucleoli are evident. The nuclear contour often appears polygonal or indented, and the cell cytoplasm appears clear as a result of artifactual retraction.

Benign melanocytic lesions do not display anaplastic cytologic characteristics. A wide spectrum of atypical nuclear changes may be seen in such lesions, but these changes generally are reactive, degenerative, or senescent phenomena rather than true anaplastic atypia characteristic of malignant transformation. True hyperchromasia and coarse nuclear membrane

and chromatin clumping are rarely encountered in benign pigment cell lesions. Certain morphologies seem to appear in most benign lesions, whereas other cytologic patterns are typical of specific lesions, such as the Spitz nevus or the pigmented spindle cell nevus.

A symmetric pattern of growth and ultimately of involution is characteristic of benign melanocytic proliferations (22). Histologic symmetry from left to right is readily apparent at low power, and it includes development of the epidermal component that is congruent to that of the dermal component. Simply stated, a junctional melanocytic proliferation synchronously migrates across the dermal-epidermal junction and establishes a dermal component over a lateral dimension that is equal to that of the original epidermal component. The presence of a so-called shoulder of junctional melanocytic hyperplasia lateral to the bulk of an otherwise benign compound lesion reflects aberrant development. Such apparent histologic asymmetry may reflect the asynchronous migration of the junctional melanocyte population into the papillary dermis or the resumption of junctional melanocytic proliferation in what otherwise was a normally evolving lesion.

An apparent vertical gradient of cytologic development that is usually termed *maturation* is present in benign melanocytic proliferations. Cellular pleomorphism and atypical nuclear features are more evident near the epidermal origin of the tumor, with the deeper cells becoming smaller and more cytologically banal. Histologic maturation is likewise evidenced by the progressively smaller size of nevus cell nests or their replacement by discohesively infiltrating single cells at the base of the lesion.

The subsequent involution is symmetric, proceeding from top to bottom, with the replacement of dermal nevomelanocytes by normal dermal connective tissue. A wide spectrum of histologic patterns of senescence may be seen in benign melanocytic lesions. These include schwannian differentiation or neurotization, lipomatous degeneration, and inflammatory regression. A variety of cytologic patterns of senescence may also be observed, including giant cell transformation and balloon cell formation

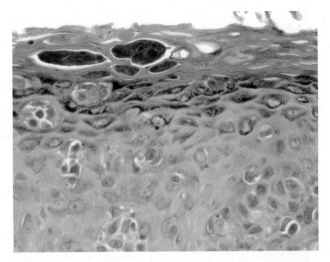

Figure 3.3. Pagetoid spread. Melanocytic cells singly or in nests disposed in an "ascending" array throughout the epidermis are characteristic. This can be observed in both benign and malignant lesions. This example was taken from a superficial spreading melanoma.

(23). In all cases, however, such histologic patterns of senescence appear uniform and symmetric.

ACQUIRED MELANOCYTIC NEVUS

The common acquired melanocytic nevus, or mole, is the most common melanocytic tumor in humans. With increasing age, varying numbers of nevi develop in most persons (24). These usually appear as brown, pigmented lesions that are less than 0.6 cm in diameter, and they may occur anywhere on the skin surface. Common sites include the head and neck, sun-exposed trunk, and extremities. Three major histologic groupings exist that represent stages in the developmental progression of benign nevi, and these often correspond to characteristic gross morphologies (25). The histopathologic alterations observed in these lesions predominantly affect the epidermis and the papillary dermis.

The junctional nevus is the earliest stage of intraepidermal melanocytic proliferation. Nevomelanocytes are dispersed in multiple discrete nests along the dermal-epidermal junction, although lentiginous melanocytic hyperplasia may also be present. Junctional nevi appear clinically as small, slightly raised, and deeply pigmented lesions. The compound melanocytic nevus includes both a junctional component and the infiltration of the dermis by nevus cells distributed singly and in nests. Clinically, such lesions appear elevated or dome shaped, and they are less intensely pigmented than the junctional nevi. The dermal nevus no longer displays a junctional component; nevomelanocytes are confined to the dermis, and they are often associated with varying degrees of senescent histologic change. Clinically, they appear flesh colored or lightly pigmented, and they are dome shaped or pedunculated.

The designations *junctional, dermal,* and *compound* do not refer to the discrete melanocytic entities but rather to the histologically characteristic stages in the natural progression of the common acquired melanocytic nevus. Apparently "intermediate" forms are routinely encountered. The compulsive search for a rare junctional nest of nevus cells for the sake of labeling a predominantly dermal nevus a compound nevus is wasteful, and it overlooks the significance of a developmental spectrum (26).

Certain cytologic features are characteristic of stages in the evolution of melanocytic nevi (Fig. 3.5). The intraepidermal

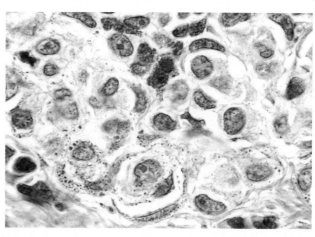

Figure 3.6. Type A nevus cells, compound nevus. Clusters of epithelioid nevus cells with finely granular cytoplasmic melanin pigment deposition, well-demarcated cell boundaries, and eosinophilic nucleoli are characteristically present in the intraepidermal nests and superficial papillary dermal component of the nevus.

nevus cell, referred to as the *epithelioid melanocyte* or *type A nevus cell*, contains a round-to-oval nucleus that is slightly smaller than the nuclei of the adjacent keratinocytes (Fig. 3.6). The nucleus contains finely dispersed chromatin that is similar to that of neuroendocrine cells and occasionally a single, inconspicuous nucleolus. The cytoplasm is prominent, and it often contains moderately coarse melanin granules.

The lymphocyte-like or type B melanocyte is usually part of the dermal component of compound nevi (Fig. 3.7). The nucleus is small and round, and it contains uniformly dispersed chromatin with no apparent nucleoli. Scant, nonpigmented cytoplasm is evident.

The neural or type C nevus cell is often present at the base of melanocytic lesions (Fig. 3.8). This cell is often spindle shaped, and it contains a somewhat smaller oval nucleus with a banal chromatin pattern. These fusiform cells come to rest at, or singly infiltrate, the superficial reticular dermal collagen bundles.

Different patterns of epidermal hyperplasia may be seen in

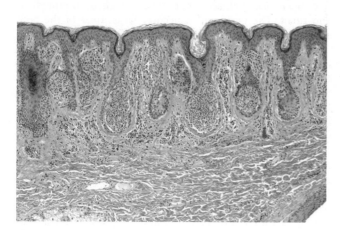

Figure 3.5. Acquired compound nevus. The nevus cells are present in the epidermis and papillary dermis in nests with minimal involvement of the superficial reticular dermis.

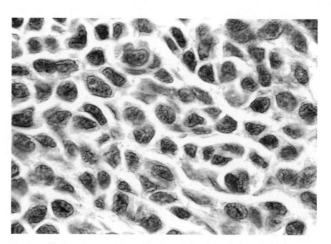

Figure 3.7. Type B nevus cells, compound nevus. Ill-defined aggregates of pleomorphic lymphocyte-like cells infiltrate the mid portion of the lesion. The cells have inapparent nucleoli and scant cytoplasm.

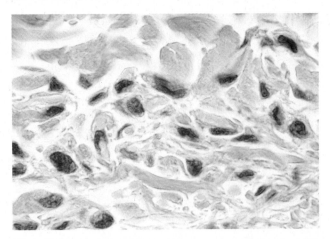

Figure 3.8. Type C nevus cells, compound nevus. Fusiform and spindle nevomelanocytes with scant cytoplasm singly infiltrate the superficial reticular dermis at the base of the lesion.

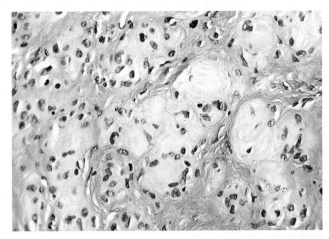

Figure 3.10. Dermal nevus. Extensive neurotization or schwannian differentiation of dermal nevus cells is present. Nests of dermal nevus cells may resemble peripheral neural structures, such as the Wagner-Meissner corpuscle.

association with melanocytic nevi (27,28). Acanthotic epidermal proliferation with pseudo-horn cyst formation may clinically and histologically mimic a seborrheic keratosis. Extensive reticulated epidermal retiform hyperplasia is common in some pedunculated dermal nevi.

A host inflammatory cell response may represent different phenomena. External trauma to a nevus may result from excoriation or plucking hairs. The presence of focal epidermal necrosis, impetiginization, or a foreign body response to keratinous debris suggests such a cause.

Diffuse infiltration of a nevus by lymphocytes and histiocytes with subsequent destruction of pigment-containing cells occurs in the halo nevus (Fig. 3.9) (29,30), a clinical variant in which an enlarging peripheral rim of hypopigmentation surrounds an acquired nevus (31,32). This uncommon form of symmetric inflammatory regression may be genetically determined. It should not be confused with the inflammatory host response seen in dysplastic or malignant melanocytic proliferations.

Long-term clinical observation of benign nevi reveals that most lesions undergo gradual involution (33,34). Residual dermal nevus cells are replaced by fibrous stroma. The subsequent

fibrous papule or fibroepithelial polyp may contain no histologic evidence of a pre-existing pigmented lesion. Melanocytic nevi on occasion display histologic and cytologic variations that reflect senescence. Prominent among the histologic senescent patterns is neurotization, or schwannian differentiation, in which the formation of neuroid structures in loose connective tissue often simulates a neurofibroma (Fig. 3.10). Other less common patterns include lipomatous degeneration, with infiltration of dermal nevi by fat cells, and osseous metaplasia. Cytologic variants include the presence of nevus giant cells or balloon cells (35–37). Such variant histologic and cytologic patterns may also occur in melanoma; therefore, they should never be used as the sole point for discriminating between benign and malignant melanocytic tumors.

CONGENITAL MELANOCYTIC NEVUS

Pigmented lesions occur in approximately 1% of neonates (38). Some of these lesions are lentigines, and other are nevi. Most of the nevi are similar in size to common acquired melanocytic nevi. However, there are distinctive lesions that are quite large. Congenital melanocytic nevi are also more irregular in contour than are acquired nevi, and they are often hair bearing. These have been classified, according to size, as giant, intermediate, and small. The giant nevi can cover large areas of the body and are designated as "bathing trunk nevi" or "garment nevi." These lesions have a somewhat increased risk for malignancy, estimated at between 5% and 10%, depending on the series (39). Histologically, compound and dermal patterns are seen. Some congenital nevi are microscopically indistinguishable from benign acquired nevi. In the most histologically characteristic lesions, the distribution of nevus cells throughout the dermis is more extensive than that seen in acquired nevi, typically involving the lower two-thirds of the reticular dermis and often infiltrating the subcutaneous fat (Fig. 3.11). The presence of nevus cells within cutaneous structures, including sebaceous lobules, multiple arrector pili muscles, and the perineurium of peripheral nerves, is characteristic of congenital nevi and is not seen in acquired nevi (Figs. 3.12 and 3.13) (40,41). The cytologic features of congenital melanocytic nevus cells and their patterns of maturation and senescence differ little from those previously described for acquired nevi (42,43).

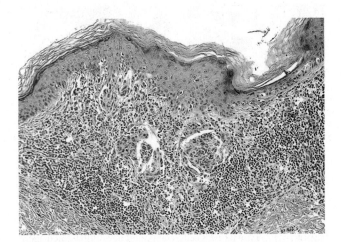

Figure 3.9. Halo nevus. A dense lymphocytic infiltrate obscures residual junctional and dermal nests of nevus cells.

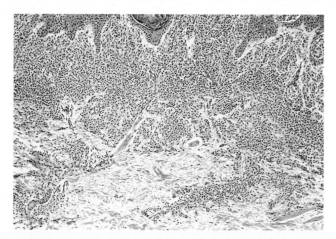

Figure 3.11. Congenital compound nevus. Nevus cells are deep within the reticular dermis and in close association with the appendages.

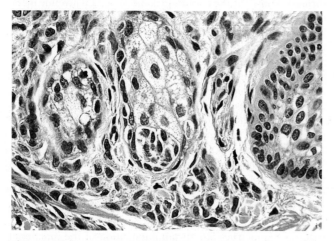

Figure 3.12. Congenital compound nevus. Nevus cells are infiltrating a sebaceous lobule.

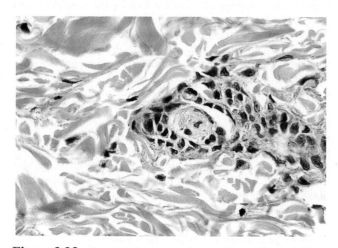

Figure 3.13. Congenital compound nevus. Nevus cells are infiltrating a peripheral nerve twig.

ACRAL MELANOCYTIC NEVI

Melanocytic proliferations occurring in acral skin (hands and feet) consistently exhibit distinct characteristics that can prompt erroneous diagnosis. Dysplastic nevi and Spitz nevi rarely appear in these anatomic sites. Histologically, acral nevi present as lentiginous proliferations. The junctional nested pattern predominates. The melanocytic nests are dyshesive, often irregular in size and shape, and adopt sometimes a crescentic shape and may coalesce (Fig. 3.14). Pagetoid spread is present in up to 61% of all nevi in the palm and soles (44). In the benign lesions, the areas of pagetoid ascent are restricted to the areas of nested proliferation and have benign morphology. In contrast, the pagetoid cells in acral lentiginous melanoma extend well beyond the nests in haphazard array (45–47).

NEVI OF SPECIAL SITES

A percentage of nevi arising in particular anatomic sites have been recently recognized to show unique characteristics. These nevi must be separated from compound congenital nevi, Spitz nevi, and dysplastic nevi arising at these sites. This particular group of lesions exhibits distinct and, at times, worrisome cytologic and architectural features that separate them from the nevi and are the source of possible diagnostic pitfalls. The regions that are known to produce these misleading proliferations are the head and neck, especially the periauricular area; the milk line, extending from the axilla to the groin; and the genital region, especially the vulva. The possible causes that determine these peculiar cytologic and architectural features are unknown. Speculation regarding cause has invoked developmental factors or hormonal changes such as occur in adolescence and pregnancy.

In the head and neck area, these lesions often present diagnostic challenges, especially in the scalp and ear of children and adolescents. These nevi with uncommon characteristics accounted for 10% of scalp nevi in one series (48), whereas in another series of ear and periauricular lesions, they represented

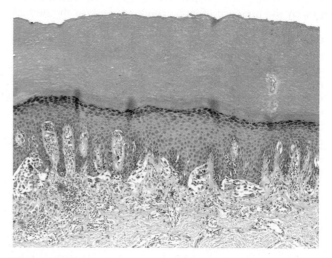

Figure 3.14. Acral nevus. Intraepidermal nests are irregularly disposed at the tips of the rete ridges but also occasionally between the rete ridges. Pagetoid spread is commonly seen, but it is always confined to the areas of nested proliferation. The cells of the dermal nests are characteristically loosely aggregated.

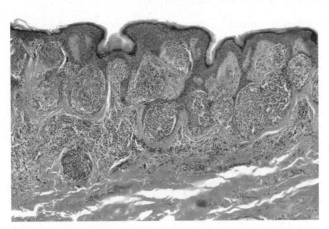

Figure 3.15. Compound nevus with features of nevi of special sites. Large intraepidermal and dermal nevomelanocytic nests are associated with fusion of rete ridges and irregular pigmentation. Dyscohesion of nested nevomelanocytes is frequently observed. These features are commonly seen in lesions in the milk line and genital area.

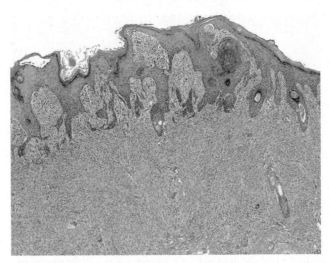

Figure 3.16. Spitz nevus. Large superficial nests become smaller in the reticular dermis and break up into single cells.

42% of the nevi occurring at this site (49). The lesions showed some common features such as poor circumscription with lateral extension of the junctional component and large irregular nests on the tips, on the sides, and in between the rete ridges. However, ear lesions tend to be symmetrical and show stromal fibroplasia, whereas scalp proliferations frequently show a prominent lentiginous component with involvement of follicles and occasional pagetoid spread (48,49). In our experience, scalp lesions have intraepidermal epithelioid cell nests that are finely pigmented and have similar cells in the papillary dermis that are often mistaken for microinvasive melanoma. However, both intraepidermal and dermal cells have atypical but not malignant cytomorphology (50).

Nevi of the milk line, genital nevi, and nevi of flexural sites share several cytologic and architectural features. Nevi of the milk line comprise the axillary folds, the mammary area, the umbilicus, and the inguinal folds. Milk line and genital nevi (Fig. 3.15) share the "nested and dyshesive" pattern, characterized by the presence of large, confluent nests at the dermal-epidermal junction, along with diminished melanocytic cohesion (51). Vulvar nests are often oval and lie along the rete ridges. Other distinctive changes of this group of lesions are stromal fibroplasia, which is usually coarser than in dysplastic nevus, and frequent lentiginous proliferation of the nevomelanocytes. Genital lesions, especially those occurring in the vulva, often show more prominent atypical features, such as moderate to severe cytologic atypia (epithelioid cells with prominent nucleoli) and occasional pagetoid spread. Also, the nests in these genital lesions are large, irregular, and frequently exhibit prominent pigmentation (52).

It is important to keep in mind that all these lesions show invariably benign features such as maturation and absence of dermal mitoses. These represent helpful clues to differentiate these sometimes worrisome looking but benign lesions from dysplastic nevi and malignant melanoma.

SPINDLE AND EPITHELIOID CELL NEVUS (SPITZ NEVUS)

The spindle and epithelioid cell nevus is important because of its histologic similarity to malignant melanoma. This entity was formerly known by the confusing name of benign juvenile melanoma, which nevertheless summarized its clinically benign yet histologically menacing status (53,54). This benign melanocytic lesion often referred to, at present, as the Spitz nevus may occur at all ages, although it is usually observed in children and young adults. Common sites include the head and neck and upper extremities. Clinically, this nevus presents as a small, solitary, dome-shaped dermal nodule. Because of a prominent vascular component in the tumor stroma and a relative lack of melanin pigmentation, it is frequently misdiagnosed clinically as a hemangioma or pyogenic granuloma.

The histologic distribution of nevus cells in the Spitz nevus mirrors that of common acquired nevi, displaying junctional, compound, and dermal forms (Fig. 3.16) (55,56). However, Spitz nevi, like many congenital nevi, usually have a highly prominent dermal component. The overall architecture of the lesion is symmetric, with abrupt attenuation of the junctional nests at the lateral borders. The nevus is composed of varying proportions of spindle and epithelioid melanocytes. Spindle cells are usually present in fascicles arrayed perpendicular to the epidermis, whereas epithelioid cells are dispersed individually throughout the lesion. The overall histologic pattern is often discohesive and infiltrative, in contrast to the confluent and expansile growth pattern of malignant melanoma. The cells taper from a broad base superficially to a narrow "point" in the deep dermis, architecturally resembling an inverted imperfect triangle. Also, the nevus cells mature by becoming smaller from the superficial to the deep part of the tumor (Figs. 3.16 and 3.17).

Because of its atypical cytologic features, the spindle and epithelioid cell nevus is often confused histopathologically with melanoma (57–59). An extreme degree of cellular pleomorphism, particularly of epithelioid melanocytes, may be seen (Fig. 3.18). The nuclei of these cells may be quite large and irregular in contour, and they may contain prominent eosinophilic nucleoli; however, they are otherwise open or vesicular in appearance, and they lack the coarse anaplastic features typical of malignant cells. Often present are eosinophilic cytoplasmic invaginations or "nuclear pseudoinclusions." The presence of mitotic figures and the occasional pagetoid epidermal spread of epithelioid melanocytes may also mimic melanoma.

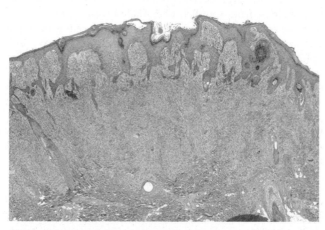

Figure 3.17. Spitz nevus. Benign epidermal hyperplasia overlies a proliferation of spindle cells that form an inverted wedge with the apex in the deep dermis.

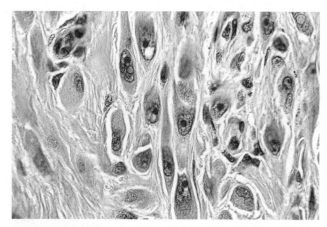

Figure 3.19. Spitz nevus. Fascicles of spindled nevomelanocytes with eosinophilic hyalinized cytoplasm and prominent nucleoli infiltrate the reticular dermis in a "raining down" array perpendicular to the skin surface.

The overwhelming majority of the cells, however, have a benign cytologic appearance that is highlighted by the atypical cells. It is this background of benignity that enables the correct interpretation of the lesion.

Those nevi that contain predominantly spindled melanocytes arranged in fascicles are usually more readily diagnosed than are those lesions consisting largely of pleomorphic epithelioid cells (Fig. 3.19). Several rather unique histologic features are regularly seen in Spitz nevi. These include the deposition of eosinophilic globules of hyalinelike material near the dermalepidermal junction and the artifactual separation of papillary dermal nests from the overlying epidermis (60,61). The tumor stroma may appear quite vascular and edematous. Lymphocytic infiltration is not uncommon, and long-standing lesions may display a densely sclerotic stroma with scattered individual tumor cells trapped amid dermal collagen (62).

Histologic differentiation from melanoma may usually be made based on the overall symmetry of the lesion and the apparent cytologic "maturation" of nevus cells at the base of the lesion. The spindle and epithelioid cell nevus may rarely be a

precursor of melanoma. Careful cytologic study for truly anaplastic nuclear features, bizarre mitoses, and aberrant or asymmetric proliferation should be made in borderline cases (63).

PIGMENTED SPINDLE CELL NEVUS

Regarded as a variant of the Spitz nevus by some authors, the pigmented spindle cell nevus has quite distinctive clinical and histopathologic features that justify its recognition as a separate entity (64,65). This lesion usually occurs as a small (<1 cm), solitary, deeply pigmented yet well-circumscribed maculopapule on the extremities or trunk. Women are more frequently affected than men, and the median age at diagnosis is in the third decade. The intense pigmentation results in a frequent clinical misdiagnosis of superficial spreading melanoma. Unlike the Spitz nevus, the pigmented spindle cell nevus rarely involves the head and neck.

Like other benign nevomelanocytic proliferations, the pigmented spindle cell nevus displays histologic symmetry and cytologic maturation. The histologic appearance is quite characteristic (66). Nests and fascicles of spindle melanocytes arrayed parallel to the long axis of the epidermis are distributed along the dermal-epidermal junction and within the dermal papillae to form a confluent plaque of tumor growth (Fig. 3.20) (67). Junctional and compound varieties are exclusively seen. The base of the lesion usually extends no deeper than the superficial reticular dermis. The overall histologic pattern is one of expansile growth, as opposed to the infiltrative pattern seen at the base of the Spitz nevi.

Unlike Spitz nevus cells, the nevus cells contain abundant melanin pigment, and they are often associated with dense melanophage accumulation. The nuclear characteristics are extremely monomorphous throughout the lesion. A curious cytologic trait of the pigmented spindle cell nevus is the close resemblance of the nevus cell nucleus to the nuclei of nearby epidermal keratinocytes (Fig. 3.21). The nuclei of these nevus cells are generally larger and more open in appearance than are those of the junctional cells of common acquired melanocytic nevi. One or more prominent small nucleoli are typically present. A lymphocytic response may be seen at the base of the lesion. Mitotic figures are uncommon. Although the spectrum

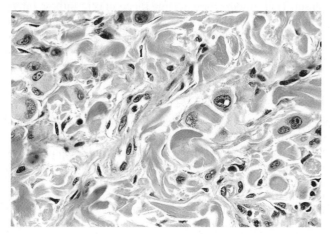

Figure 3.18. Spitz nevus. Cytologically atypical epithelioid nevus cells with prominent nucleoli in the reticular dermis are seen in a background of banal-appearing nevus cells.

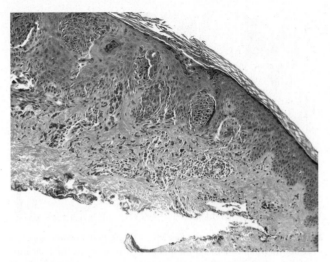

Figure 3.20. Pigmented spindle cell nevus of Reed. Nests of nevus cells are distributed in a plaque along the dermal-epidermal junction and within the dermal papillae. Single-cell infiltration of the epidermis may result in histologic confusion with melanoma.

of senescent patterns has not been fully described in these lesions, the transepidermal elimination of entire junctional nests of nevus cells may be observed (68,69).

DESMOPLASTIC (DERMAL) SPITZ NEVUS

This lesion most often appears in young adulthood, although it can be seen in any age. It usually affects the upper arms or shoulder or the thighs but can be seen anywhere except the palms and soles. It presents as a firm nodule and is most commonly mistaken for a dermatofibroma or even a scar. It may reach 1 cm in diameter. In some cases, the lesion may even resemble a blue nevus.

Histologically, at low-power examination, one appreciates a dense collagenous stroma in which there are scattered promi-

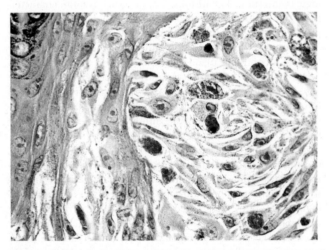

Figure 3.21. Pigmented spindle cell nevus. A nest of heavily pigmented, spindled nevomelanocytes is at the dermal-epidermal junction. Although the individual cells may at first appear atypical, a close inspection reveals size and nuclear morphology similar to those of nearby keratinocytes.

nent cells with large nuclei and often large nucleoli. The cells vary in shape from spindled to epithelioid. On careful inspection, the cells are found to be Spitz nevus–like cells with ample cytoplasm that are hyalinized or foamy but usually are very eosinophilic in appearance. The nuclei show some mild hyperchromasia. Occasionally giant cells are noted. Mitoses are rarely present. There is usually no maturation of the cells, but the cells are all contained in a striking collagenous stroma. One of the principal differential diagnosis problems is the identification of this lesion and the ruling out of desmoplastic malignant melanoma. The presence of the large epithelioid cells is most helpful in identifying the desmoplastic Spitz nevus (70).

ATYPICAL SPITZ NEVI AND SPITZ TUMORS

One of the main problems, microscopically and in the clinical setting, is the issue of atypical spindle and epithelioid proliferations. Clearly some of these atypical proliferations can metastasize and relatively infrequently cause death (71–73). A suggested classification delineates three different groups: the atypical Spitz nevus, the atypical Spitz tumor, and the spitzoid melanomas. The first group exhibits superficial expansile nodules, lack of maturation, or a rare deep mitosis. The spitzoid tumor, on the other hand, is larger than a nevus, often greater than 1 cm in diameter, and extends more deeply into the dermis and subcutaneous fat. Mitoses are much more common and, in some cases, can be as frequent as 2 to 4 per mm^2, depending on the authors. For these lesions, sentinel lymph node biopsy (SLNB) is recommended. The reported range of positivity for SLNB is 26% to 50% (74–76). In our experience (unpublished data), 44% of cases were positive when an SLNB was performed. Although there is limited and short follow-up in for this series, no further progression of these tumors has been reported so far.

Finally, spitzoid melanomas are predominantly dermal-based tumors with severe pleomorphism, frequent atypical mitoses, very striking expansile nodules, and often vascular invasion. Although these lesions have indeterminate prognosis, they are all treated by excision with a 1- to 2-cm margin and an SNLB.

In a recent series of eight children whose first symptoms of melanoma appeared before age 13 years and who all died of the disease, the tumors were all very large and bulky. They exhibited ulceration, necrosis, numerous mitoses, and severe pleomorphism. Their tumors formed large sheets of cells with no intervening stroma and large expansile nodules. Two of the eight patients exhibited tumors that were less than 2 mm in thickness but that were highly pleomorphic and mitotically active (Mihm, unpublished data, 2008).

DERMAL MELANOCYTOSES

Certain acquired and congenital pigmented lesions are associated with proliferative disorders of dermal melanocytes (77). Such dermal melanocytes may be derived from ectopic nests of migratory neural crest cells. These lesions include the common and cellular blue nevus, the Mongolian spot, and the nevi of Ota and Ito. All of these feature delicate spindle cells containing melanin granules dissecting bundles of reticular dermal collagen. The density and distribution of such dermal melanocytes, the degree of melanin pigmentation, and the presence of associated melanophage deposition usually allow the histologic discrimination of these entities (78,79). Clinically, the dermal melanocytoses display a blue or gray color that results from the absorption of the long wavelengths of visible light by dermal melanin and the reflection of the shorter blue wavelengths.

Mongolian Spot

The Mongolian spot is a congenital disorder that possibly results from the aberrant development or migration of epidermal melanocytic precursors. Clinically, the lesion appears as a diffuse area of macular blue-black uniform pigmentation over the lower back or buttocks (80). It is present at birth in most Oriental neonates, and it usually regresses within several years. Ectopic Mongolian spots may occur at other sites.

The biopsy specimens of the involved skin appear normal at low power. High-power study reveals the presence of rare elongated dermal melanocytes containing fine melanin pigment granules. The melanocytes are usually present in the lower two-thirds of the reticular dermis, and they are not associated with melanophage accumulation.

Nevus of Ota and Nevus of Ito

These uncommon pigmented lesions are acquired hamartomas of dermal melanocytes, usually occurring in the first or second decades. They are observed most frequently in Orientals, but they may also occur in Hispanics, blacks, and Native Americans. They appear clinically as macular areas of irregular blue-gray pigmentation (81). The nevus of Ota occurs in periorbital and temporal skin in the distribution of the first and second branches of the trigeminal nerve (82,83). The nevus of Ito occurs over supraclavicular and scapular skin in the distribution of the lateral supraclavicular and brachial nerves (84).

These lesions appear to be histologically distinct from the Mongolian spot. Low-power examination reveals deeply pigmented cells scattered sparsely, usually throughout the entire reticular dermis but sometimes limited only to the upper one-third. Fusiform dermal melanocytes with delicate melanin pigment granules are present with the melanophages, often in a perivascular distribution (Fig. 3.22).

Common Blue Nevus

The common blue nevus is a solitary, small (<1.0 cm), slightly elevated or dome-shaped lesion that often occurs on the dorsa

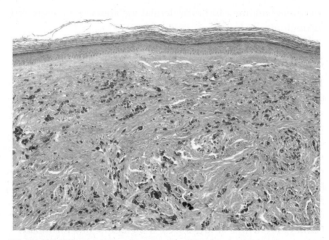

Figure 3.23. Common blue nevus. Dendritic dermal melanocytes are admixed with melanophages in a prominent stroma.

of the hands and feet. It occurs rarely in other organs, including the prostate and uterus (85,86). This is an acquired lesion that is usually seen in adults. A histologic examination at low power reveals a dense, well-circumscribed area of pigment deposition within the dermis (Fig. 3.23) (87). Most of the pigment is within melanophages, often obscuring the background distribution of dermal melanocytes (88). The melanocytic proliferation and pigment deposition may occupy the entire reticular dermis and occasionally the subcutaneous fat. The cells are often distributed in a periadnexal arrangement.

Cellular Blue Nevus

The cellular blue nevus usually occurs on the lower back or buttocks, and it presents as a bluish dermal nodule or plaque measuring more than 1.5 cm in diameter. On microscopic examination, the lesion displays a well-circumscribed cellular mass of interweaving fascicles of unpigmented spindle cells (Fig. 3.24) (89,90). The histologic differential diagnosis may include other cellular spindle cell tumors, such as dermatofibroma and leiomyoma (91). A close examination reveals the presence of

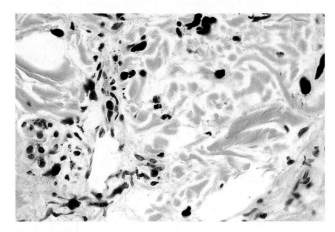

Figure 3.22. Nevus of Ota. The dermal melanocytes exhibit dendrites filled with fine melanin granules.

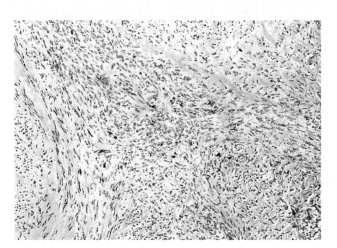

Figure 3.24. Cellular blue nevus. Interweaving fascicles of amelanotic spindle cells contain foci of melanin pigment deposition in both melanophages and dermal melanocytes.

melanin-containing fusiform dermal melanocytes interspersed throughout the lesion.

Pigmented Epithelioid Melanocytoma

The presence of equine melanoma has been recognized for many years. Levene coined the term *equine melanotic disease* (92), which was also likened to a pigmented cellular proliferation in humans by Tuthill et al. (93) and referred to by Clark as "animal-type melanoma." In 1999, Crowson et al. (94) reported six cases of this tumor, one of which metastasized and resulted in death. Carney, in his description of the Carney complex, described a pigmented tumor that he designated as epithelioid blue nevus (95). Zembowicz et al. (96) collected 41 cases of this tumor and reviewed the samples originally described by Carney. From this study, a new designation was formulated, namely, the pigmented epithelioid melanocytoma (96). This terminology was offered to emphasize the apparent indolent course of these lesions, with only one mortality reported. Further support for this unique tumor was found after an extensive comparative microarray analysis of benign nevi, primary melanomas, and equine melanomas. All of these lesions expressed a protein kinase A regulatory subunit type 1 alpha coded by the PRKAR1A gene, whereas 82% of pigmented epithelioid melanocytomas and Carney lesions did not express this product (97).

Clinically the first sign of this lesion is a blue-black plaque or nodule that usually enlarges slowly. The lesions occur commonly on the scalp and extremities and occasionally on the trunk. Although the lesion may first appear as a punctuate discoloration, it can eventually reach the size of 10 to 12 cm. The lesions are usually not associated with other pigmented lesions or history of melanoma.

The low-power picture (Fig. 3.25) is represented by a densely pigmented tumor that affects the entire dermis and even the subcutaneous fat. The tumor in most cases is separated from the epidermis by a grenz zone, but sometimes it involves the epidermis as well. The tumor mass tends to disrupt the normal architecture of the skin. There is sometimes a prominent concentration of cells around the hair follicles. Centrally there is a mass of cells that, toward the periphery, appear to infiltrate

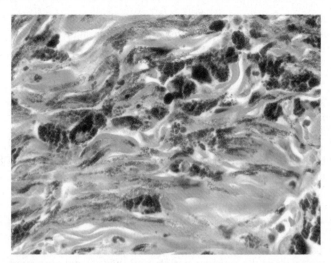

Figure 3.26. Pigmented epithelioid melanocytoma. The densely pigmented dermal melanocytes have characteristic nuclei and display prominent blue nucleoli.

as fascicles. There are areas of epithelioid and spindle cells. On high-power examination, one appreciates that all of the cells have similar nuclei with very large blue nucleoli and, indeed, are all melanocytes (Fig. 3.26). The cytoplasm of the cells is densely pigmented. The spindle cells that first resemble blue nevus cells were found to have thick dendrites containing coarse melanin granules. Only rare melanophages are noted. Mitoses are variable but usually are typical; however, a spectrum of mitotic activity is noted from lesion to lesion. In our experience, this type of lesion, when greater than 2 mm in thickness, will have a positive sentinel lymph node in 44% of cases. To date, these cases are exhibiting indolent behavior with very good prognosis.

MISCELLANEOUS BENIGN MELANOCYTIC LESIONS

Lentigo

The common lentigo or lentigo simplex may be a counterpart to the acquired junctional nevus that differs in the pattern of melanocytic proliferation. Lentigines are acquired lesions, often occurring during childhood; they appear as small, uniformly dark brown macules. They may occur anywhere on the skin, but they show a predilection for acral sites.

Microscopic examination reveals lentiginous melanocytic hyperplasia that is usually distributed along the tips of rete ridges (Fig. 3.27). The adjacent keratinocytes are usually hyperpigmented, and a slight degree of epidermal rete hyperplasia may be present. The histopathologic features are distinguished from those of acquired melanocytic nevi by the absence of nested melanocytic hyperplasia and the infiltration of the papillary dermis by nevomelanocytes (98).

The solar lentigo is a variant that occurs on the sun-exposed skin of older persons. Solar lentigines appear as multiple, often poorly circumscribed areas of macular hyperpigmentation that may exceed 1 cm in diameter (99). Histologically, lentiginous melanocytic hyperplasia is seen in association with marked secondary epidermal rete hyperplasia, sometimes simulating the appearance of a reticulated seborrheic keratosis. At times, how-

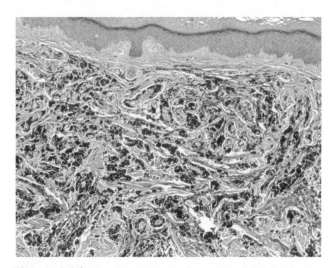

Figure 3.25. Pigmented epithelioid melanocytoma. Numerous melanin-laden cells fill the dermis. Cytologically, all of the cells are heavily pigmented melanocytes with only a rare melanophage admixed.

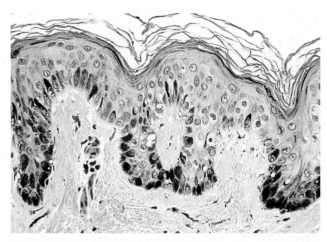

Figure 3.27. Lentigo simplex. Dense melanin deposition in basilar keratinocytes is observed primarily along rete ridges. Lentiginous melanocytic hyperplasia may be obscured by the pigment.

ever, a mixture may be seen in which epidermal atrophy alternates with areas of epidermal hyperplasia.

Combined Nevus

On occasion, elements of two different types of dermal or epidermal melanocytic proliferation may be present in the same pigmented lesion (100). These so-called combined nevi most commonly include components of an acquired melanocytic nevus and the common blue nevus (101). Rarely, Spitz nevus cells may also be present. Combined nevi may display an aberrant histologic pattern of maturation, with pigmented epithelioid type A nevus cells at the base of the lesion instead of at the dermal-epidermal junction. Such variants should be considered in cases that otherwise appear cytologically and architecturally benign. "Inverted" type A cells should be recognized as such, and they should not be mistaken for malignant degeneration simply because they are pigmented and ectopic.

Deep Penetrating Nevus

Clinically, deep penetrating nevi can occur de novo as blue papules or nodules, and often they are mistaken for a blue nevus or nodular melanoma. The more common presentation is in a pre-existing acquired or congenital nevus in which a focal color change raises the possibility of malignant degeneration. This lesion can be mistaken for malignant melanoma reportedly in as many as 40% of cases (102).

Histologically, this relatively uncommon lesion consists of a symmetrical, wedge-shaped proliferation with the base parallel to the long axis of the epidermis and the vertex present in the deep dermis and sometimes in the subcutaneous fat. When it occurs de novo, there is usually an intraepidermal junctional component. When it occurs in a setting of a pre-existing nevus, it usually occurs as a focal transformation in the dermal component of the pre-existing nevus. The types of cells that comprise the deep penetrating nevus are more commonly the inverted type A nevus cells, but sometimes are also spindle cells, type B nevus cells, and blue nevus cells. The inverted type A cells appear pale, epithelioid, and fusiform, occurring in nests often surrounded by melanophages. There is variable but usually

slight melanization of the cytoplasm of the nevus cells. The cellular density in the upper dermis rapidly becomes diminished as the cells follow along the follicles or neurovascular bundles into the deeper tissue. Senescent changes often affect the inverted type A cells with nuclear vacuoles and sometimes hyperchromatic nuclei. Mitoses are very rare and, when present, should lead to multiple sectioning to rule out malignant transformation (103).

Efforts to distinguish this nevus from melanoma by molecular means have resulted in the finding of complete loss of dipeptidyl peptidase IV in malignant melanoma, compared with variable but consistent positivity in the deep penetrating nevi. However, there is a higher expression of MMP-2 and integrin-beta 3 in the advancing front of deep penetrating nevi compared with that of melanoma. This finding can help explain why the pattern of infiltration resembles malignant melanoma in some cases (104).

Intranodal Nevic Nests

The finding of nests of nevic cells in lymph nodes was first reported in 1931 by Stewart and Copeland (105). The incidence of such nevic nests, known as nodal nevi, in lymph nodes draining malignancies ranges from 1% to 22% (106). In the majority of the cases, nodal nevi are intracapsular or intratrabecular, but cases of intraparenchymal nests have been reported (107). The incidence of nodal nevi in sentinel lymph nodes of patients with cutaneous melanomas is 3.9%, which is higher when compared with the incidence in nonsentinel lymph nodes in melanoma patients (1.01%) (108). The origin of these nevus cells is unclear; a possible "benign metastasis-like" mechanism could be involved. One study reports a higher occurrence of nodal nevi with melanomas arising within congenital nevi (109), supporting the "benign metastasis" theory. However, more studies are needed to validate this concept. It is important to emphasize that the pathologist should be aware of the relative high incidence of nodal nevi among sentinel lymph nodes in malignant melanoma to possibly avoid erroneous interpretations. Besides the intracapsular and intraseptal location of the nests, perhaps the more important feature that will help the pathologist make the right call is the benign cytologic and nuclear features of the nevic cells when compared with the pleomorphic epithelioid melanoma cells with nuclear hyperchromasia and pleomorphism.

HISTOPATHOLOGIC CORRELATION WITH ATYPICAL CLINICAL FEATURES

Most common acquired melanocytic nevi and lentigines display symmetry, uniform pigment distribution, and smooth boundaries with adjacent skin. The visual observation of asymmetry, uneven pigment distribution, and irregular or jagged borders within a pigmented lesion is usually a cause for clinical concern. Biopsy or excision is typically performed to rule out the diagnosis of malignant melanoma or a melanoma precursor. In many cases, an atypical-appearing pigmented lesion proves to be microscopically benign.

Histologically benign pigmented lesions may display subtle variations in pigment and melanocyte distribution. These may reflect physiologic or inflammatory characteristics unique to a particular lesion. The observation of such variations is significant if an otherwise histologically benign nevus or lentigo has been removed because of its worrisome clinical appearance. The diagnostic description of such features may provide valuable feedback and reassurance to the clinician.

LENTIGINOUS MELANOCYTIC NEVUS

The most common clinical cause for concern about a pigmented lesion is a reported "changing mole." In an otherwise previously uniform symmetric nevus, such changes typically include an increase in size, the formation of irregular borders with adjacent normal skin, and a peripheral change in color. Although such clinical changes are characteristic of dysplastic nevi, a substantial percentage displays entirely benign cytologic features. Microscopically, the principal correlate is a so-called shoulder area of lentiginous junctional melanocytic proliferation beyond the lateral border of the underlying dermal component. Careful cytologic assessment of the peripheral lentiginous junctional component in addition to that of the more central domain is essential. The absence of significant anaplastic nuclear changes must be confirmed.

The biologic significance of peripheral changes within previously stable nevi is unclear. The idea that most common acquired nevi begin as junctional nevi is widely accepted. Subsequent dermal migration results in the establishment of a dermal component. The lentiginous junctional pattern of melanocytic hyperplasia is typically associated with an active, growing phase. One possibility is that, in many benign changing moles, radial junctional proliferation is reactivated. Because the clinical appearance of reactivated radial proliferation in a benign nevus may be indistinguishable from that of many dysplastic nevi and some superficial spreading melanomas, complete excision and careful histologic study are essential.

RECURRENT MELANOCYTIC NEVUS

For cosmetic reasons, many clinicians prefer to remove acquired melanocytic nevi by a superficial "shave" biopsy and excision technique. Incomplete removal of the nevus may result in the recurrence of a pigmented lesion at the site of prior surgical trauma. Usually, such a recurrence is seen within several months of the procedure (110–115).

Recurrent melanocytic nevi often appear clinically worrisome because of the association of irregular pigmentation with scarring. When the nevus is re-excised, the specimen typically displays a residual dermal nevus component that is separated from the overlying epidermis by a zone of linear cicatricial fibrosis (Figs. 3.28 and 3.29). The overlying epidermis may display lentiginous melanocytic hyperplasia and basilar keratinocytic hyperpigmentation.

REGRESSING MELANOCYTIC NEVUS

The presence of a dense, superficial lymphoid cell infiltrate in an otherwise cytologically benign melanocytic nevus usually reflects inflammatory regression. The best-known example of such regression is the halo nevus, in which inflammatory regression occurs in a symmetric centripetal fashion (Fig. 3.9). Although the clinical appearance of a halo nevus is quite distinct, the microscopic features may be no different from those observed in a changing pigmented lesion in which the progressive change in pigmentation is irregular or asymmetric (116).

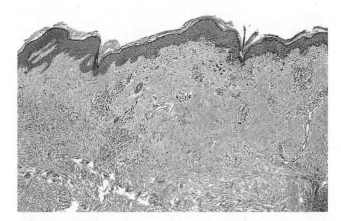

Figure 3.28. Recurrent melanocytic nevus. At low power, a linear fibrotic scar is seen in the superficial dermis between an atrophic epidermis devoid of adnexa and an underlying aggregate of residual dermal nevus cells.

SOLAR LENTIGO

The solar or actinic lentigo is best regarded as a pigmented lesion resulting from chronic sun exposure, as opposed to being a primary neoplasm of epidermal melanocytes or a physiologic variant in cutaneous melanin production and distribution. Thus, tremendous variation in microscopic findings is observed among solar lentigines (Fig. 3.30). Chronic direct ultraviolet damage may selectively affect the dispersal of melanin pigment among basilar keratinocytes. Often, however, melanocytic hyperplasia is simultaneously observed.

The spectrum of changes separating a benign solar lentigo from a pigmented actinic keratosis or lentigo maligna is not always clear. For this reason, caution should be exercised in reporting small biopsy specimens obtained from what otherwise appears to be a large, atypical macular pigmented lesion on chronically sun-damaged skin. The observation of cytologically benign changes within a limited tissue sample from such a lesion does not necessary rule out the presence of adjacent histopathologic atypia.

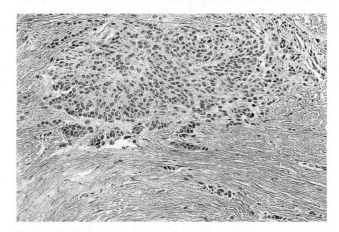

Figure 3.29. Recurrent melanocytic nevus. Lentigo-like basilar hyperpigmentation and melanocytic hyperplasia are in the epidermis overlying the dermal scar. Transepidermal elimination of melanin pigment into the overlying stratum corneum also occurs.

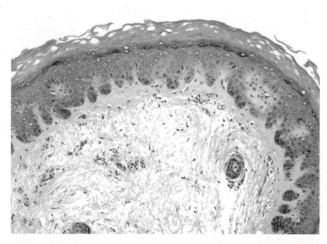

Figure 3.30. Solar lentigo. An irregular pattern of increased melanin pigment within keratinocytes is seen in the epidermis. Solar elastosis, telangiectasia, and slight chronic inflammation are seen in the underlying dermis. Transepidermal elimination of melanin pigment into the overlying stratum corneum also occurs.

CONGENITAL MELANOCYTIC NEVUS

Congenital melanocytic nevi often display an irregular surface contour and pigmentation. This irregularity may reflect the distribution and density of nevomelanocytes within the underlying appendageal epithelium and arrector pili muscles (Figs. 3.11, 3.12, and 3.13). Certain so-called agminate nevi, such as the nevus spilus, are clinically distinguished by an array of discrete, hyperpigmented, slightly raised foci on a hyperpigmented macular background. The microscopic correlate of this visual observation is the nonconfluent distribution of nevomelanocytes in nests or small aggregates within the superficial dermis in association with minimal basilar keratinocytic hyperpigmentation.

Congenital nevi may appear as a localized collection of individual pigmented lesions in a nonrandom, usually linear array. Microscopically, the individual pigmented lesions comprising the array appear indistinguishable from other congenital nevi. The unusual clinical distribution most likely reflects embryologic developmental changes occurring along the Blaschko lines (117). Similar developmental changes are thought to underlie other cutaneous disorders characterized by linear and patterned arrays of discrete lesions, including inflammatory linear verrucous epidermal nevi and incontinentia pigmenti.

In most cases, the history of a pigmented lesion present from birth or the existence of easily recognizable clinical features readily permits a clinical diagnosis. Most congenital nevi are not sampled because they display asymmetric features but because they have changed in appearance. As with most acquired melanocytic nevi in which a change in size or contour is reported, the most common benign microscopic correlate observed is peripheral junctional lentiginous melanocytic hyperplasia.

Atypical pigmented lesions that are reported to be of recent or acquired onset in the nonpediatric population sometimes display features of a benign congenital melanocytic nevus. In view of the stages by which embryonic premelanocytes develop from neural crest cells and migrate to cutaneous epithelium, the microscopic observation of "congenital" features in what is clinically reported to be an "acquired" nevus may reflect a so-called latent congenital nevus. In such a congenital nevus, aberrantly migrating premelanocytes may assume a microanatomic dermal distribution characteristic of congenital nevi, without subsequent gestational proliferation. Only later in life, perhaps secondary to hormonal or developmental signals, may the melanocytic proliferation take place, yielding a clinically acquired but histologically congenital nevus.

MALIGNANT MELANOMA AND PRECURSOR LESIONS

HISTOLOGIC AND CYTOLOGIC CHARACTERISTICS

The diagnosis of malignant melanoma is the most important problem in pigment cell histopathology. The neoplastic transformation of human melanocytes to melanoma may occur directly or via the formation of one or more precursor lesions. Such precursor lesions may include common acquired melanocytic nevi, congenital nevi, and rarely other benign pigmented lesions (118–121). The significance of precursor lesions and the existence of discrete biologic stages of neoplastic melanocytic transformation are supported by both experimental and histopathologic data (122,123). Approximately 60% of melanomas contain histologic remnants of benign pigmented lesions. The accurate recognition of aberrant melanocytic proliferation is therefore necessary to diagnose melanoma consistently and to identify precursor lesions posing a significant clinical risk (124,125).

The spectrum of aberrant melanocytic proliferation may be approached by analyzing the architectural and cytologic features of the lesion, in addition to the host cutaneous response (126). The lateral epidermal margin of melanocytic proliferation is not sharply demarcated, as it is in most benign lesions. Rather, a gradual transition zone usually exists between the lesion and the adjacent normal epidermis. The epidermal features include an extreme degree of hyperplasia of melanocytes in both lentiginous and nested patterns. The dermal-epidermal junction may be obscured by dense accumulations of pigment cells with progressive aberrant growth. Pagetoid spread of melanocytes both individually and in clusters may be observed throughout all levels of the epidermis. Focal epidermal destruction by proliferating cells may result in superficial epidermal erosion or ulceration in fully evolved lesions.

An asymmetric lesional architecture is generally evident in the dermis of both melanomas and precursor lesions (127). Histologic features contributing to this appearance include the focal formation of expansile masses of cells within the dermis and the nonuniform inflammatory regression of the lesion. The dyssynchronous junctional and dermal proliferation results in a histologic "shoulder" of lentiginous hyperplasia along the dermal-epidermal junction lateral to the underlying dermal component. The spread of cells may be seen along dermal eccrine or follicular epithelium in continuity with the adjacent epidermal junctional hyperplasia. This pattern contrasts with the discontinuous appendageal involvement seen in congenital melanocytic nevi.

Anaplastic melanocytic atypia is a feature of malignant melanoma and clinically worrisome precursor lesions, including the dysplastic nevus. Although the cellular pleomorphism and bizarre nuclear features of most melanomas are readily recognized, a spectrum of cytologic changes may be observed. Care must be taken to distinguish the senescent or reactive features commonly seen in benign lesions from the atypia of aberrant proliferations.

Melanocytic atypia may be manifested by varying degrees of nuclear and cytoplasmic change. Atypia in individual cells may be graded as slight, moderate, or severe. Slightly atypical melanocytes display uniformly hyperchromatic nuclei, which are comparable in size to the nuclei of normal keratinocytes or a little larger. Other features include inconspicuous nucleoli, retracted cytoplasm, and inapparent cell boundaries. Moderately atypical cells feature coarse, irregular nuclear membranes with peripheral chromatin condensation. The cytoplasm of these cells contains finely distributed melanin pigment, and cell borders are evident. Severely atypical cells feature extreme nuclear size and hyperchromasia. Atypical mitotic figures, vacuolated nuclei with coarse peripheral chromatin clumping, and irregular eosinophilic nucleoli are characteristic.

Although these patterns of atypia are seen in dysplastic nevi and melanoma, a subtler cytologic finding in aberrant proliferations is the loss of nevomelanocytic maturation at the base of the lesion. Such a loss of normal maturation may reflect a failure to form the so-called type C nevus cells of common acquired nevi or an absence of diminution in cell size at the base of Spitz nevi.

Senescent changes, including the formation of nevus giant cells or balloon cells, are typically seen in benign nevi, but they may also occur in melanoma and premalignant lesions. Therefore, the presence of such findings should not be used to rule out the diagnosis of a worrisome lesion.

Aberrant melanocytic proliferations usually elicit a host inflammatory cell response. The response, which is generally lymphocytic, asymmetrically infiltrates the lesion along its periphery. This pattern is distinct from the diffuse and symmetric infiltrate seen in halo melanocytic nevi. Sequelae of the response include the accumulation of melanophages, dermal fibrosis, and telangiectasia. The presence of extensive regression and dense melanophage activity in the absence of a pigmented lesion is always ominous, and it may indicate the existence of a preceding melanoma or dysplastic nevus.

A variety of immunohistochemical markers are available to assist in discriminating primary or metastatic melanoma from other poorly differentiated or amelanotic malignant tumors (128–130). These include the melanocyte differentiation antigens S-100 protein and melan-A, the melanocyte activation antigen HMB-45, and the tumor proliferation index marker Ki-67 (131–136).

DYSPLASTIC NEVUS

Although Spitz nevi, congenital nevi, and pigmented spindle cell nevi may display cytologic and architectural atypia, dysplastic nevi show consistently distinct abnormalities of cytology and architecture (137). These lesions may arise de novo or in association with a pre-existing nevus. Dysplastic nevi are clinically distinct. They appear as single or multiple slightly raised pigmented lesions that rarely occur before puberty. They are larger than common moles, usually more than 0.6 cm in diameter, and they may occur on any part of the skin surface. The lesion borders are irregular, and variable distribution of pigment is evident on the surface.

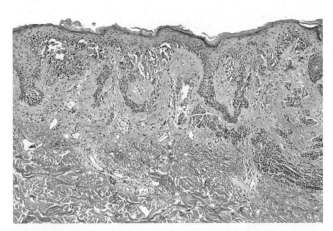

Figure 3.31. Dysplastic nevus. The characteristic cytologic and architectural features are represented by the extension of the intraepidermal atypical nevus cells beyond the dermal component ("shoulder" effect), the fusion of rete ridges, and the stromal changes.

The frequent clinical and histologic observation of dysplastic nevi in persons with sporadic cases of melanoma supports the significance of the dysplastic nevus as a biologic precursor of malignant melanoma but, more importantly, as a marker of increased clinical risk for the development of melanoma (138). Accurate diagnosis and the evaluation of surgical margins for complete excision are therefore important. The presence of multiple dysplastic nevi may identify a person with the dysplastic nevus syndrome (139,140). Persons afflicted with this hereditary autosomal dominant disorder may have hundreds of dysplastic nevi, and one or more primary melanomas are likely to develop eventually (141). Patients are considered to have the syndrome when they have multiple dysplastic nevi and two family members with malignant melanoma.

At first glance, most dysplastic nevi histologically resemble acquired compound melanocytic nevi. However, lentiginous melanocytic hyperplasia extends along the dermal-epidermal junction throughout the lesion and laterally to form a shoulder area beyond the underlying dermal component when it is present (Fig. 3.31). The lesion differs from an acquired nevus, in which symmetry between the epidermal and dermal components is evident. Cytologically, atypical melanocytes are scattered irregularly amid areas of lentiginous and nested melanocytic proliferation (Fig. 3.31). The degree of cytologic atypia may range from mild to severe, but the atypical cells appear against a background of benign nevomelanocytes (142). In contrast, in malignant melanoma, the lesion consists largely of anaplastic cells. Discohesive infiltration of the epidermis by atypical melanocytes is not a feature of dysplastic nevi, and if this is present, melanoma should be considered as a diagnostic possibility. Dysplastic nevi thus exhibit irregular nested and lentiginous proliferation of nevomelanocytes along the dermal-epidermal junction, with individual cells displaying variable atypia.

Characteristic reactive epidermal and dermal changes may be seen in dysplastic nevi. Mild hyperplasia of the epidermal rete is often present, with lamellar condensation of the papillary dermal fibrocytes and eosinophilic concentric fibrosis of the adjacent dermal papillae (Fig. 3.32). Hyperplasia of the dermal papillae may result in the apparent bridging of adjacent tips of

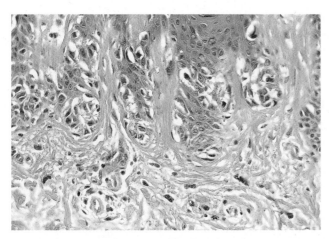

Figure 3.32. Dysplastic nevus. The proliferation of nevomelanocytes exhibits variable and discontiguous atypia and variable distribution of nests. Note the drapelike fibrosis known as lamellar fibroplasia.

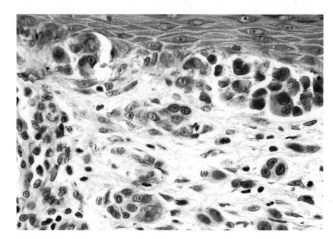

Figure 3.33. Malignant melanoma—radial growth phase. Anaplastic melanocytes are dispersed singly and in small clusters throughout the epidermis and papillary dermis.

rete ridges by melanocytes. A lymphocytic infiltrate is usually in the underlying dermis, and it may contain melanophages. The diagnosis of a dysplastic nevus is established in the presence of the characteristic atypical melanocytic hyperplasia in association with varying degrees of secondary epidermal and dermal changes.

MALIGNANT MELANOMA

Primary malignant melanoma evolves from melanocytic precursors via the formation of intermediate lesions of varying stability (143–146). These precursors, which have already been discussed, include acquired and congenital melanocytic nevi and dysplastic nevi. Histologically distinct forms of primary melanoma also exist, and these may vary in their capacity to metastasize. Recognition of the histologic type of melanoma and a documentation of its features are of prognostic importance.

The major histologic forms of melanoma include superficial spreading melanoma, nodular melanoma, acral lentiginous melanoma, and lentigo maligna melanoma (147–149). Each of these displays characteristic clinical, epidemiologic, and histologic features. Superficial spreading, acral lentiginous, and lentigo maligna melanoma may evolve initially from a slowly growing, plaquelike radial growth phase (RGP) to a rapidly growing, expansile vertical growth phase (VGP). Nodular melanoma displays only an expansile VGP pattern, with no pre-existing RGP.

The histologic recognition of RGP and VGP forms is important because RGP primary melanoma is a clinically benign entity that does not metastasize (150,151). Its removal results in complete cure (152). The transition to VGP melanoma, however, heralds the development of metastatic behavior. In a patient with VGP melanoma, a residual risk for metastasis lingers despite the complete removal of the primary lesion. This risk may be estimated by evaluating other factors, including the depth of penetration of the tumor; its mitotic rate; and the presence or absence of an immune response, epidermal ulceration, and microscopic satellites (153–155).

PRIMARY MELANOMA—RADIAL GROWTH PHASE

RGP melanoma is a slowly developing lesion that may exist for months to years. The tumor appears clinically as a circumferen-

tially enlarging pigmented plaque measuring at least 0.5 to 1 cm in diameter. The border contour is markedly irregular, and areas of intensely black pigmentation are mixed with hypopigmented and erythematous regions that are foci of tumor regression. Pigmented basal cell carcinomas and pigmented seborrheic keratoses may on occasion simulate this appearance.

Microscopically, these tumors display varying degrees of melanocytic hyperplasia that is characterized by severe cytologic atypia and diffuse epidermal infiltration by anaplastic cells (156). The cellular morphology and pattern of infiltration vary with the specific subtype of melanoma—namely, superficial spreading, acral lentiginous, or lentigo maligna. RGP melanoma may be limited to the epidermis; it may be invasive, with superficial infiltration of the papillary dermis; or it may extend to the superficial vascular plexus. Primary melanomas involving the reticular dermis or subcutaneous fat virtually always display VGP characteristics, and thus, they are clinically ominous.

The papillary dermal component of RGP melanomas consists of a mixture of anaplastic single cells and nests infiltrating fibrovascular stroma (Fig. 3.33). The superficially invasive nests of melanoma cells are typically no larger than nests within the epidermis or along the dermal-epidermal junction. The cell population is pleomorphic, the mitotic rate is very low, and a lymphocytic host response is usually present at the base of the lesion. Histologic evidence of a precursor lesion, such as a dysplastic or congenital nevus, is often found.

PRIMARY MELANOMA—VERTICAL GROWTH PHASE

A frequent clinical feature of VGP melanomas is the rapid formation of a discrete pigmented nodule, either within a plaque of RGP melanoma or on otherwise normal skin. The clinical entity of nodular malignant melanoma corresponds to the formation of a VGP melanoma without evident RGP.

VGP melanomas are histologically identified by one or more expansile dermal nodules of anaplastic melanocytes (Fig. 3.34). VGP melanomas usually arise in a pre-existing primary RGP melanoma. The nodule of a VGP melanoma is typically larger than the epidermal or junctional nests comprising the RGP melanoma. The cells tend to be cytologically uniform, and they

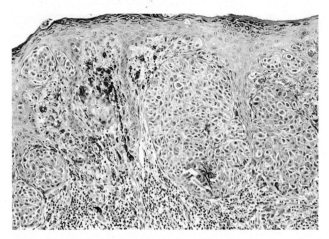

Figure 3.34. Malignant melanoma—vertical growth phase. An expansile nodule of anaplastic cells is infiltrating the papillary dermis. The nodule is clearly larger than the junctional nests of melanoma cells at the left.

are a clone of malignant cells that histologically resemble a tumor metastasis (157). The mitotic rate is higher in VGP melanoma than it is in RGP melanoma, and a host immune response is present less often (158).

The recognition of VGP melanoma is usually straightforward in deep primary lesions of Clark levels IV and V and in most level III lesions. Thin level I or II primary melanomas should be examined carefully for VGP formation because this histologic feature reflects the acquisition of the biologic capacity for metastasis. Approximately 10% of thin primary melanomas displaying VGP features ultimately metastasize, whereas RGP primary melanomas are 100% curable by surgical excision. Extensive stromal fibrosis and melanophage accumulation at the base of a primary lesion that otherwise displays features of radial growth may indicate a regressed primary VGP melanoma, and therefore, it should be reported conservatively.

SUPERFICIAL SPREADING AND NODULAR MELANOMA

This most common form of melanoma occurs in light-skinned persons ranging in age from young adults to the elderly. Risk factors include extensive sun exposure during childhood, a family history of melanoma, large numbers of benign acquired melanocytic nevi, and one or more dysplastic nevi. Superficial spreading melanoma often occurs on the trunk and extremities. The distribution is not limited to areas of direct sun exposure. Although most cases evolve over months to years in a plaquelike growth of primary RGP melanoma before vertical growth develops, the rapid onset of an invasive nodule of primary VGP melanoma may occur without a preceding RGP, which corresponds to the clinical entity of nodular malignant melanoma. The presence and characteristics of the VGP melanoma, not the presence or absence of a pre-existing primary RGP melanoma, determine the prognosis.

The RGP of superficial spreading melanoma displays a pagetoid epidermal infiltration of anaplastic melanocytes against a background of both nested and lentiginous melanocytic hyperplasia. The careful examination of multiple sections through the lesion often reveals a precursor lesion, such as a dysplastic

nevus or congenital nevus. The cytologic features of the VGP component influence the prognosis; patients with VGP lesions containing epithelioid melanoma cells fare worse than those with lesions composed predominantly of spindle cells (159).

LENTIGO MALIGNA

This tumor most often occurs on the sun-exposed skin of elderly persons. Lentigo maligna clinically appears as a slowly growing macular area of irregular hyperpigmentation that may evolve over decades and may measure several centimeters in diameter. Such lesions may resemble solar lentigines or flat pigmented seborrheic or actinic keratoses. Lentigo maligna most often displays only radial growth characteristics, and it is curable by excision or ionizing radiation. Foci of vertical growth may occur in long-standing lesions (160–162).

Histologically, lentigo maligna displays the radial growth of dense lentiginous hyperplasia of predominantly spindle cells along the dermal-epidermal junction against a background of actinic damage, basilar keratinocytic hyperpigmentation, and epidermal atrophy (Fig. 3.35) (163,164). The nested proliferation observed in common superficial spreading lesions is not seen. A common feature is junctional infiltration by anaplastic spindled melanocytes along the follicular and eccrine epithelium. Single-cell infiltration of the papillary dermis may be observed in RGP lesions, and such lesions are referred to as lentigo maligna melanoma, as opposed to simply lentigo maligna. Lesions with VGP formation may appear indistinguishable from the VGP of superficial spreading or nodular melanoma, displaying both epithelioid and spindle cell morphologies (165). Desmoplastic and neurotropic invasive patterns are often associated with VGP formation in lentigo maligna melanoma (166).

ACRAL LENTIGINOUS MELANOMA

Acral lentiginous melanoma is the most common form of melanoma reported in African blacks and Japanese; it accounts for approximately 10% of cases of melanoma in whites (167). Acral

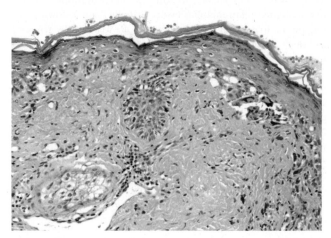

Figure 3.35. Lentigo maligna melanoma. In an atrophic epidermis, there is a predominantly basilar proliferation of single and nested malignant melanocytes with extension to the external root sheath of the follicle. Note multinucleated giant cells and pagetoid spread.

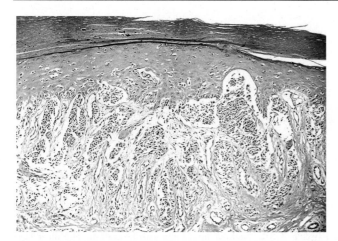

Figure 3.36. Acral lentiginous melanoma. Fascicles of hyperchromatic, spindled pigment cells are superficially infiltrating the dermis of hyperkeratotic acral skin.

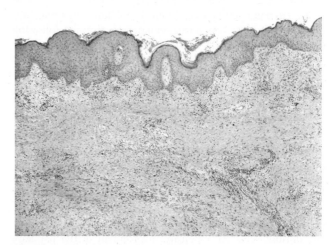

Figure 3.37. Desmoplastic melanoma. Low-power view shows an infiltrative spindle cell component with marked desmoplastic stromal response and foci of chronic inflammation.

lentiginous melanoma occurs most often on the plantar, palmar, subungual, and periungual skin and mucosa, with a peak incidence in the sixth decade (168). The lesions initially appear as densely pigmented macules with irregular borders. Because a thickened, hyperkeratotic epidermis overlies the primary lesion, the clinical appearance may be less ominous than that of other melanomas. The biologic course of acral lentiginous melanoma probably does not differ significantly from the course of the more common superficial spreading type; however, acral melanomas are often relatively advanced at the time of diagnosis (169–171).

The RGP form of acral lentiginous melanoma displays lentiginous hyperplasia of cytologically atypical spindled and dendritic melanocytes, often with accompanying retiform epidermal hyperplasia (Fig. 3.36). Pagetoid infiltration of the epidermis by anaplastic cells is typical, as is the junctional infiltration of the eccrine epithelium, which sometimes extends to involve the eccrine glands of the deep reticular dermis. The VGP form usually consists of spindle cells, and it is often accompanied by epidermal ulceration.

DESMOPLASTIC MELANOMA

Desmoplastic melanoma (DM) represents a unique variant of melanoma. The difference between DM and ordinary melanoma (OM) is supported not only by a different clinical and microscopic appearance, but also by differences in immunohistochemical profile, gene expression profile, and biologic behavior. Clinically, DM is often amelanotic, presenting as a scar, fibroma, or basal cell carcinoma. It has a predilection for sun-exposed areas, especially in the head and neck region, but it can also appear in the acral and mucosal regions. DM presents more often at a later age than OM and with a preference for the male gender. In clinically pigmented lesions, there is usually an accompanying conventional melanocytic component represented by a wide spectrum of lentiginous melanocytic proliferations, from hyperplasia and lentigo maligna to acral and mucosal melanoma (172).

Microscopically, DM is represented by an infiltrating proliferation of pleomorphic and hyperchromatic spindle cells surrounded by a desmoplastic stroma with scattered nidi of chronic

inflammation (Fig. 3.37). The desmoplastic stromal element is composed of abundant collagen and fibroblasts. There is also a variable amount of mucin deposition. The neoplastic spindle cells represent melanocytes with a modified phenotype resembling fibroblasts. Immunohistochemically, they are consistently positive for S-100, focally positive for MART-1, and negative or rarely focally positive for HMB-45. Under the electron microscope, they show granules consistent with premelanosomes. Another frequent finding in these lesions is the presence of extensive perineural and intraneural involvement around the infiltrating edge of the lesion, sometimes discontiguous with the main mass. Therefore, it is important to emphasize the need for careful evaluation of the resected specimen to avoid recurrences.

More recently, DM has been classified in two types by Busam and colleagues. The first type is designated "pure" desmoplastic melanoma, and this designation is used when 90% or more of the lesion is desmoplastic. "Combined" desmoplastic melanoma is the second type, in which less than 90% of the lesion is represented by desmoplasia, with the remaining component having the epithelioid cells of OM. The importance of this classification is that it appears to have prognostic significance, with the pure variant having a better prognosis with less frequency of regional lymph node involvement (173–175).

Busam et al. (176) also showed that desmoplastic melanoma has its own gene expression profile with an upregulation of neurotropic factors and genes involved in the production of extracellular matrix and lower levels of expression of genes related to melanin pigment synthesis.

PROGNOSTIC FACTORS IN MALIGNANT MELANOMA

When reporting malignant melanoma, the general pathologist must document a series of morphologic parameters with the scope of forecasting the course of disease and guiding the clinician toward the appropriate therapeutic approach (177).

Tumor Thickness

Tumor thickness represents the primary determinant of the T classification for staging of melanoma, and the lesions are classified as T1 through T4 depending on the tumor thickness, with breakpoints at less than 1 mm, 1 to 2 mm, 2 to 4 mm, and more than 4 mm. This measurement is performed following the guidelines originally described by Breslow (153), from the granular cell layer to the deepest invasive cell away from adnexal structures. If the lesion is ulcerated, the ulcer bed must be used as the superficial point from which to start the measurement.

Clark Level

Although not a paramount prognostic factor as in previous times, the microanatomic staging of Clark still retains value, especially when considering thin melanomas (<1 mm). The tumors are assigned Clark levels from I to V according to the involvement of the different anatomic subdivisions of the skin: intraepithelial involvement (level I), microinvasive of the papillary dermis (level II), extensive involvement of the papillary dermis sometimes abutting the reticular dermis (level III), significant invasion of the reticular dermis (level IV), and involvement of the subcutaneous fat (level V) (178,179).

Mitotic Rate

As new data continue to emerge from long-term follow-up in some patient cohorts, the presence of dermal mitoses in melanomas is acquiring a more predominant role in prognosis. The Pigmented Lesion/Melanoma Group in Philadelphia has recently validated the concept that the presence of a single mitosis in the vertical growth phase compartment is enough to tilt the balance toward a poorer outcome when compared with melanomas without dermal mitoses (180). Different sets of data pertaining to the number of mitoses are currently under evaluation by the American Joint Committee on Cancer, and the presence of dermal mitoses as well as the mitotic count per square millimeter will take an important place in the new tumor-node-metastasis (TNM) staging.

Tumor-Infiltrating Lymphocytes

It is known that a brisk (diffuse) pattern of lymphocyte infiltration in the tumor results in better outcome than the complete absence of host response, with an intermediate prognosis being reserved for those with a nonbrisk (partial) host response (181). However, this purely morphologic classification fails to fully explain the reasons why patients with diffuse infiltrate fail in the long run to completely control tumor progression. Although several studies have emerged validating the concept of host response in the tumor as a good prognostic indicator, there are still large studies under way to better understand the morphologic and functional heterogeneity of tumor-infiltrating lymphocytes. Only after we have a better understanding of the different functional states and the biochemical pathways leading to inactivation or suppression of their immune function will we be able to better apply different immune therapeutic approaches.

The presence of ulceration is also a strong determinant of prognosis (179). By ulceration we mean not only the focal absence of epithelial surface in a given melanoma, but also the presence of accompanying fibrin and acute inflammation as further proof of a true biologic process (Fig. 3.38). Care must also be exercised when studying a sample that has been previ-

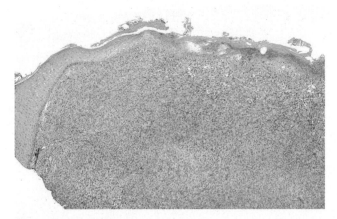

Figure 3.38. Nodular melanoma with ulceration. The ulcer base shows fibrin deposition and neutrophilic debris as evidence of host response and proof of spontaneous ulceration.

ously biopsied, in which case the ulceration with all its attributes would have been the result of the prior procedure and should therefore not be considered.

Other important prognostic indicators include lymphovascular and neural invasion, as well as regression and microscopic satellites. The presence of any of these parameters will increase the likelihood of metastasis and poor outcome.

MOLECULAR PATHOLOGY OF MELANOMA

Over the last several decades, the intricate mechanisms involved in the genesis and maintenance of malignant melanoma have been progressively unraveled. The progression from benign melanocytic lesions, or even benign melanocytes, to a highly malignant tumor involves, as one would expect, dramatic changes in the molecular realm. These alterations affect multiple pathways, such as the tumor suppressor and cell cycle control machinery, and involve the loss of function of the CDKN2A and the PTEN genes. The product of the former, p16/INK4a, inhibits phosphorylation of the Rb protein and prevents transition through the S phase. The alternating reading frame, p14/p19ARF, inhibits the destruction of p53. CDKN2A is the only human gene that affects two major tumor suppressor pathways (Rb and p53). Mutation in PTEN activates the AKT pathway. These events, along with the NRAS and the BRAF (V600E) mutations with subsequent activation of the MAPK pathway, result in perpetuation and proliferation of the malignant cells. The next steps are the invasion of the dermis and the formation of an expansile nodule of vertical growth phase; these involve several alterations of adhesion molecules, such as the switch from the normal E-cadherin to the N-cadherin, the expression of $\alpha V\beta 3$ integrin, and the expression of proteolytic enzymes, such as MMP-2 expression (182,183). A model of this progression of molecular changes is depicted in Figure 3.39.

Melanoma represents a quite heterogeneous group of diseases. This is confirmed at a molecular level with a growing body of evidence that is showing distinct patterns of molecular alterations among tumors that occur in chronically sun-damaged skin, intermittently sun-damaged skin, and skin without sun damage (184–187). This could lead to a possible "molecular classification" of melanoma that would prompt different possible therapeutic measures. Recent studies of the metastatic

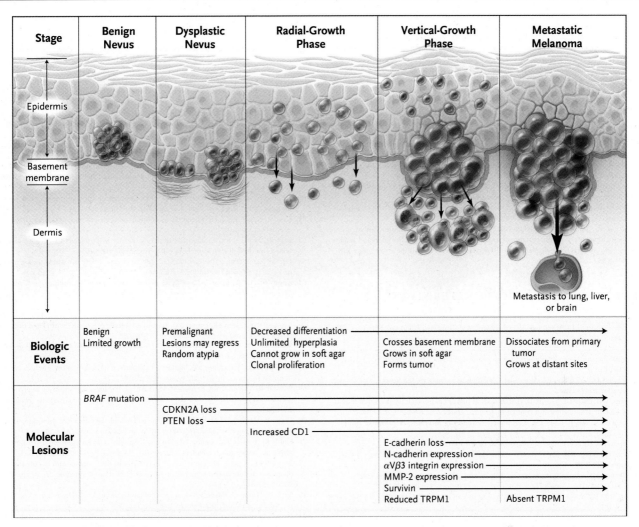

Stage	Benign Nevus	Dysplastic Nevus	Radial-Growth Phase	Vertical-Growth Phase	Metastatic Melanoma

Metastasis to lung, liver, or brain

| **Biologic Events** | Benign Limited growth | Premalignant Lesions may regress Random atypia | Decreased differentiation Unlimited hyperplasia Cannot grow in soft agar Clonal proliferation | Crosses basement membrane Grows in soft agar Forms tumor | Dissociates from primary tumor Grows at distant sites |

| **Molecular Lesions** | *BRAF* mutation | CDKN2A loss PTEN loss | Increased CD1 | E-cadherin loss N-cadherin expression αVβ3 integrin expression MMP-2 expression Survivin Reduced TRPM1 | Absent TRPM1 |

Figure 3.39. Biologic event and molecular changes in the progression of melanoma. At the stage of the benign nevus, BRAF mutation and activation of the mitogen-activated protein kinase (MAPK) pathway occur. The cytologic atypia in dysplastic nevi reflect lesions within the cyclin-dependent kinase inhibitor 2A (CDKN2A) and phosphatase and tensin homologue (PTEN) pathways. Further progression of melanoma is associated with decreased differentiation and decreased expression of melanoma markers regulated by microphthalmia-associated transcription factor (MITF). The vertical growth phase and metastatic melanoma are notable for striking changes in the control of cell adhesion. Changes in the expression of the melanocyte-specific gene melastatin 1 (TRPM1) correlate with metastatic propensity, but the function of this gene remains unknown. Other changes include the loss of E-cadherin and increased expression of N-cadherin, αVβ3 integrin, and matrix metalloproteinase-2 (MMP-2). Reprinted from Miller AJ, Mihm MC Jr. Melanoma. *N Engl J Med* 2006; 355:55.

phenomenon indicate that the primary tumor secretes molecules that prepare a metastatic site for malignant cells. The identification of cancer stem cells suggests a possible role for them in the metastatic phenomenon. Melanoma stem cells have recently been described and may offer further insight into the metastatic melanoma process (188,189). This "molecular dissection" of melanoma gives us invaluable tools to tackle this terrible disease. At the present time, different agents that target several molecular pathways are being tested, bringing a whole new set of treatment options.

REFERENCES

1. Le Douarin NM. Cell line segregation during peripheral nervous system ontogeny. *Science* 1986;231:1515–1522.

2. Yoshida H, Kunisada T, Grimm T, et al. Review: melanocyte migration and survival controlled by SCF/c-kit expression. *J Invest Dermatol Symp Proc* 2001;6:1–5.

3. Christiansen JH, Coles EG, Wilkinson DG. Molecular control of neural crest formation, migration and differentiation. *Curr Opin Cell Biol* 2000;6:719–724.

4. Ito K, Takeuchi T. The differentiation in-vitro of the neural crest cells of the mouse embryo. *J Embryol Exp Morphol* 1984;84:49–62.

5. Quevedo WC, Fleischmann RD. Developmental biology of mammalian melanocytes. *J Invest Dermatol* 1980;75:116–120.

6. Henion PD, Weston JA. Timing and pattern of cell fate restrictions in the neural crest lineage. *Development* 1997;124:4351–4359.

7. Goding CR. Melanocyte development and malignant melanoma. *Forum (Genova)* 2000;3: 176–187.

8. Herlyn M, Berking C, Li G, Styamoorthy K. Lessons from melanocyte development for understanding the biological events in naevus and melanoma formation. *Melanoma Res* 2000;4:303–312.

9. Slaughter JC, Hardman JM, Kempe LG, et al. Neurocutaneous melanosis and leptomeningeal melanomatosis in children. *Arch Pathol* 1969;88:298–304.

10. Medalie DA, Eming SA, Collins ME, et al. Differences in dermal analogs influence subsequent pigmentation, epidermal differentiation, basement membrane, and rete ridge formation of transplanted composite skin grafts. *Transplantation* 1997;64:454–465.

11. Tobin DJ, Bystryn JC. Different populations of melanocytes are present in hair follicles and epidermis. *Pigment Cell Res* 1996;9:304–310.

12. Nakazawa K, Nakazawa H, Collombel C, Damour O. Keratinocyte extracellular matrix-mediated regulation of normal human melanocyte functions. *Pigment Cell Res* 1995;8: 10–18.

13. Suster S. Hyalinizing spindle and epithelioid cell nevus. A study of five cases of a distinctive histologic variant of Spitz's nevus. *Am J Dermatopathol* 1994;16:593–598.

14. Clark WH Jr, Hood AF, Tucker MA, Jampel RM. Atypical melanocytic nevi of the genital type with a discussion of reciprocal parenchymal-stromal interactions in the biology of neoplasia. *Hum Pathol* 1998;29:1S–24S.

15. Smolle J, Hofmann-Wellenhof R, Fink-Puches R. Melanoma and stroma: an interaction of biological and prognostic importance. *Semin Cutan Med Surg* 1996;15:326–335.

16. Haass NK, Herlyn M. Normal human melanocyte homeostasis as a paradigm for understanding melanoma. *J Investig Dermatol Symp Proc* 2005;10:153–163.

17. Breathnach AS. Melanocytes in early regenerated human epidermis. *J Invest Dermatol* 1960; 35:245–251.

18. Staricco RG. Mechanism of migration of the melanocytes from the hair follicle into the epidermis following dermabrasion. *J Invest Dermatol* 1961;36:99–104.

19. Busam KJ, Barnhill RL. Pagetoid Spitz nevus. Intraepidermal Spitz tumor with prominent pagetoid spread. *Am J Surg Pathol* 1995;19:1061–1067.

20. Ainsworth AM, Folberg R, Reed RJ, Clark WH Jr. Melanocytic nevi, melanocytomas, melanocytic dysplasias, and uncommon forms of melanoma. In Clark WH, Goldman LI, Mastrangelo MJ, eds. *Human Malignant Melanoma.* Orlando, FL: Grune & Stratton, 1979: 167–208.

BENIGN MELANOCYTIC PROLIFERATIONS

21. Hu F. Melanocyte cytology in normal skin, melanocytic nevi, and malignant melanomas—a review. In Ackerman AB, ed. *Pathology of Malignant Melanoma.* New York, NY: Masson, 1981:1–21.

22. Urso C, Bondi R. The histological spectrum of acquired nevi. An analysis of the intraepidermal melanocytic proliferation in common and dysplastic nevi. *Pathol Res Pract* 1994;190: 609–614.

23. Bennett DC, Medrano EE. Molecular regulation of melanocyte senescence. *Pigment Cell Res* 2002;4:242–250.

24. Clark WH, Elder DE, Guerry D, et al. A study of tumor progression: the precursor lesions of superficial spreading and nodular melanoma. *Hum Pathol* 1984;15:1147–1165.

25. Eady RA, Gilkes JJ, Jones EW. Eruptive naevi: report of two cases. *Br J Dermatol* 1977;97: 267–278.

26. Masson P. My conception of cellular nevi. *Cancer* 1951;4:9–38.

27. Bentley-Phillips CB, Marks R. The epidermal component of melanocytic nevi. *J Cutan Pathol* 1976;3:190–194.

28. Weedon D. Unusual features of nevocellular nevi. *J Cutan Pathol* 1982;9:284–292.

29. Findlay GH. The histology of Sutton's nevus. *Br J Dermatol* 1957;69:389–394.

30. Swanson JL, Wayte DM, Helwig EB. Ultrastructure of halo nevi. *J Invest Dermatol* 1968;50: 434–437.

31. Wayte DM, Helwig EB. Halo nevi. *Cancer* 1968;22:69–90.

32. Kopf AW, Morrill SD, Silberberg I. Broad spectrum of leukoderma acquisitum centrifugum. *Arch Dermatol* 1965;92:64–68.

33. Stegmaier OC. Natural regression of the melanocytic nevus. *J Invest Dermatol* 1959;32: 413–419.

34. Lund HZ, Stobbe GD. The natural history of the pigmented nevus. Factors of age and anatomic location. *Am J Pathol* 1949;25:1117–1147.

35. Schrader WA, Helwig EB. Balloon cell nevi. *Cancer* 1967;20:1502–1514.

36. Goette DK, Doty RD. Balloon cell nevus. *Arch Dermatol* 1978;114:109–111.

37. Hashimoto K, Bale GF. An electron microscopic study of balloon cell nevi. *Cancer* 1972; 30:530–540.

38. Silvers DN, Helwig EB. Melanocytic nevi in neonates. *J Am Acad Dermatol* 1981;4:166–175.

39. Crowson AN, Magro CM, Mihm MC Jr. The melanocytic proliferations. In *A Comprehensive Textbook of Pigmented Lesions.* Hoboken, NJ: Wiley-Liss, Inc., 2001:209–223.

40. Mark GJ, Mihm MC, Liteplo MG, et al. Congenital melanocytic nevi of the small and garment type—clinical, histologic and ultrastructural studies. *Hum Pathol* 1973;4:395–418.

41. Kuehnl-Petzoldt C, Volk B, Kunze J, et al. Histology of congenital nevi during the first year of life—a study by conventional and electron microscopy. *Am J Dermatopathol* 1984; 6:81–88.

42. Reed RJ. Giant congenital nevi: a conceptualization of patterns. *J Invest Dermatol* 1993; 100:300S–312S.

43. Barnhill RL, Fleischm M. Histologic features of congenital melanocytic nevi in infants 1 year of age or younger. *J Am Acad Dermatol* 1995;33:780–785.

44. Haupt HM, Stern JB. Pagetoid melanocytosis. Histologic features in benign and malignant lesions. *Am J Surg Pathol* 1995;19:792–797.

45. Elder D. Precursors to melanoma and their mimics: nevi of special sites. *Mod Pathol* 2006; 19:S4–S20.

46. Crowson AN, Magro CM, Mihm MC Jr. The melanocytic proliferations. In *A Comprehensive Textbook of Pigmented Lesions.* Hoboken, NJ: Wiley-Liss, Inc., 2001:266–273.

47. LeBoit PE. A diagnosis for maniacs. *Am J Dermatopathol* 2000;22:556–558.

48. Fabrizi G, Pagliarello C, Parente P, et al. Atypical nevi of the scalp in adolescents. *J Cutan Pathol* 2007;34:365–369.

49. Lazova R, Lebster B, Glusac EJ, et al. The characteristic histopathologic features of nevi on and around the ear. *J Cutan Pathol* 2005;32:40–44.

50. Crowson AN, Magro CM, Mihm M C Jr. The melanocytic proliferations. In *A Comprehensive Textbook of Pigmented Lesions.* Hoboken, NJ: Wiley-Liss, Inc., 2001:257–266.

51. Rongioletti F, Ball RA, Marcus R, et al. Histopathological features of flexural melanocytic nevi. A study of 40 cases. *J Cutan Pathol* 2000;27:215–217.

52. Gleason BC, Hirsch MS, Nucci MR, et al. Atypical genital nevi. A clinicopathologic analysis of 56 cases. *Am J Surg Pathol* 2008;32:51–57.

53. Spitz S. Melanomas of childhood. *Am J Pathol* 1948;24:591–609.

54. Allen AC. Juvenile melanomas of children and adults and melanocarcinomas of children. *Arch Dermatol* 1960;82:325–335.

55. Weedon D, Little JH. Spindle and epithelioid cell nevi in children and adults—a review of 211 cases of the Spitz nevus. *Cancer* 1977;40:217–225.

56. Paniago-Pereira C, Maize JC, Ackerman AB. Nevus of large spindle and/or epithelioid cells (Spitz's nevus). *Arch Dermatol* 1978;114:1811–1823.

57. Barnhill RL, Argenyi ZB, From L, et al. Atypical Spitz nevi/tumors: lack of consensus for diagnosis, discrimination from melanoma, and prediction of outcome. *Hum Pathol* 1999; 30:513–520.

58. Zaenglein AL, Heintz P, Kamino H, et al. Congenital Spitz nevus clinically mimicking melanoma. *J Am Acad Dermatol* 2002;47:441–444.

59. Harvell JD, Bastian BC, LeBoit PE. Persistent (recurrent) Spitz nevi: a histopathologic, immunohistochemical, and molecular pathologic study of 22 cases. *Am J Surg Pathol* 2002; 26:654–661.

60. Kamino H, Misheloff E, Ackerman AB, et al. Eosinophilic globules in Spitz's nevi—new findings and a diagnostic sign. *Am J Dermatopathol* 1979;1:319–324.

61. Kamino H, Jagirdar J. Fibronectin in eosinophilic globules of Spitz's nevi. *Am J Dermatopathol* 1984;6:313–316.

62. Barr RJ, Morales RV, Graham JH. Desmoplastic nevus—a distinct histologic variant of mixed spindle cell and epithelioid cell nevus. *Cancer* 1980;46:557–564.

63. Harvell JD, Meehan SA, LeBoit PE. Spitz's nevi with halo reaction: a histopathologic study of 17 cases. *J Cutan Pathol* 1997;24:611–619.

64. Ainsworth AM, Folberg R, Reed RJ, et al. Pigmented spindle cell tumor. In Clark WH, Goldman LI, Mastrangelo MJ, eds. *Human Malignant Melanoma.* Orlando, FL: Grune & Stratton, 1979:179–182.

65. Sau P, Graham JH, Helwig EB. Pigmented spindle cell nevus. *Arch Dermatol* 1984;120:1615.

66. Sagebiel RW, Chinn EK, Egbert BM. Pigmented spindle cell nevus: clinical and histologic review of 90 cases. *Am J Surg Pathol* 1984;8:645–653.

67. Smith NP. The pigmented spindle cell tumor of Reed: an underdiagnosed lesion. *Semin Diagn Pathol* 1987;4:75–87.

68. Sau P, Graham JH, Helwig EB. Pigmented spindle cell nevus: a clinicopathologic analysis of ninety-five cases. *J Am Acad Dermatol* 1993;28:565–571.

69. Barnhill RL, Barnhill MA, Berwick M, Mihm MC Jr. The histologic spectrum of pigmented spindle cell nevus: a review of 120 cases with emphasis on atypical variants. *Hum Pathol* 1991;22:52–58.

70. Crowson AN, Magro CM, Mihm MC Jr. The melanocytic proliferations. In *A Comprehensive Textbook of Pigmented Lesions.* Hoboken, NJ: Wiley-Liss, Inc., 2001:148–155.

71. Smith KJ, Barrett TL, Skelton HG 3rd, et al. Spindle cell and epithelioid cell nevi with atypia and metastasis (malignant Spitz nevus). *Am J Surg Pathol* 1989;13:931–939.

72. Barnhill RL, Argenyi ZB, From L, et al. Atypical Spitz nevi/tumors: lack of consensus for diagnosis, discrimination from melanoma, and prediction of outcome. *Hum Pathol* 1999; 30:513–520.

73. Spatz A, Calonje E, Handfield-Jones S, et al. Spitz tumors in children. A grading system for risk stratification. *Arch Dermatol* 1999;135:282–285.

74. Urso C, Borgognoni L, Saieva C, et al. Sentinel lymph node biopsy in patients with "atypical Spitz tumors." A report on 12 cases. *Hum Pathol* 2006;37:816–823.

75. Su LD, Fullen DR, Sondak VK, Johnson TM, Lowe L. Sentinel lymph node biopsy for patients with problematic spitzoid melanocytic lesions: a report on 18 patients. *Cancer* 2003;97:499–507.

76. Murali R, Sharma RN, Thompson JF. Sentinel lymph node biopsy in histologically ambiguous melanocytic tumors with spitzoid features (so-called atypical spitzoid tumors). *Ann Surg Oncol* 2008;15:302–309.

77. Mevorah B, Frenk E, Delecretaz J. Dermal melanocytosis. *Dermatologica* 1977;154:107–114.

78. Mizoguchi M, Murakami F, Ito M, et al. Clinical, pathological, and etiologic aspects of acquired dermal melanocytosis. *Pigment Cell Res* 1997;10:176–183.

79. Stanford DG, Georgouras KE. Dermal melanocytosis: a clinical spectrum. *Australas J Dermatol* 1996;37:19–25.

80. Kikuchi I, Inoue S. Natural history of the Mongolian spot. *J Dermatol* 1980;7:449–450.

81. Hidano A, Kajima H, Ikeda S, et al. Natural history of nevus of Ota. *Arch Dermatol* 1967; 95:187–195.

82. Ota M, Tanino H. A type of nevus frequently seen in our country: the naevus fusco-caeruleus ophthalmomaxillaris and its relationship to pigmentary changes of the eye. *Tokyo Med J* 1939;63:1243–1245.

83. Kopf AW, Weidman A. Nevus of Ota. *Arch Dermatol* 1962;85:195–208.

84. Mishima Y, Mevorah B. Nevus Ota and nevus Ito in American Negroes. *J Invest Dermatol* 1961;36:133–154.

85. Jao W, Fretzin DF, Christ ML, et al. Blue nevus of the prostate gland. *Arch Pathol* 1971; 91:187–191.

86. Qizilibash AH. Blue nevus of the uterine cervix. *Am J Clin Pathol* 1973;59:803–806.

87. Dorsey CS, Montgomery H. Blue nevus and its distinction from mongolian spot and the nevus of Ota. *J Invest Dermatol* 1954;22:225–236.

88. Carr S, See J, Wilkinson B, et al. Hypopigmented common blue nevus. *J Cutan Pathol* 1997;24:494–498.

89. Rodriquez HA, Ackerman LV. Cellular blue nevus—clinicopathologic study of forty-five cases. *Cancer* 1968;21:393–405.

90. Lambert WC, Brodkin RH. Nodal and subcutaneous cellular blue nevi—a pseudometastasizing pseudomelanoma. *Arch Dermatol* 1984;120:367–370.

91. Michael M, Kerekes Z, Kinkor Z, et al. Desmoplastic cellular blue nevi. *Am J Dermatopathol* 1995;17:230–235.

92. Levene A. Equine melanotic disease. *Tumori* 1971;57:133–168.

93. Tuthill RJ, Clark WH Jr, Levene A. Pilar neurocristic hamartoma: its relationship to blue nevus and equine melanotic disease. *Arch Dermatol* 1982;118:592–596.

94. Crowson AN, Magro CM, Mihm MC Jr. Malignant melanoma with prominent pigment synthesis: "animal type" melanoma—a clinical and histological study of six cases with a consideration of other melanocytic neoplasms with prominent pigment synthesis. *Hum Pathol* 1999;30:543–550

95. Carney JA, Ferreiro JA. The epithelioid blue nevus. A multicentric familial tumor with important associations, including cardiac myxoma and psammomatous melanotic schwannoma. *Am J Surg Pathol* 1996;20:259–272.

96. Zembowicz A, Carney JA, Mihm MC. Pigmented epithelioid melanocytoma: a low-grade melanocytic tumor with metastatic potential indistinguishable from animal-type melanoma and epithelioid blue nevus. *Am J Surg Pathol* 2004;28:31–40.

97. Zembowicz A, Knoepp SM, Bei T, Stergiopoulos S, Eng C, Mihm MC, Stratakis CA. Loss of expression of protein kinase a regulatory subunit 1 alpha in pigmented epithelioid melanocytoma but not in melanoma or other melanocytic lesions. *Am J Surg Pathol* 2007; 31:1764–1775.

MISCELLANEOUS BENIGN MELANOCYTIC LESIONS

98. Hirone T, Eryu Y. Ultrastructure of giant pigment granules in lentigo simplex. *Acta Derm Venereol Suppl (Stockh)* 1978;58:223–229.

99. Mehregan AH. Lentigo senilis and its evolution. *J Invest Dermatol* 1975;65:429–433.

100. Fletcher V, Sagebiel RW. The combined nevus. In Ackerman AB, ed. *Pathology of Malignant Melanoma.* New York, NY: Masson, 1981:273–283.

101. Leopold JG, Richards DB. The interrelationship of blue and common nevi. *J Pathol* 1968; 95:37–43.

102. Robson A, Morley-Quante M, Hempel H, et al. Deep penetrating nevus: clinicopathological study of 31 cases with further delineation of histological features allowing distinction from other pigmented benign melanocytic lesions and melanoma. *Histopathology* 2003;43: 529–537.

103. Crowson AN, Magro CM, Mihm MC Jr. The melanocytic proliferations. In *A Comprehensive Textbook of Pigmented Lesions.* Hoboken, NJ: Wiley-Liss, Inc., 2001:186–192.

104. Roesch A, Wittschier S, Becker B, Landthaler M, Vogt T. Loss of dipeptidyl peptidase IV immunostaining discriminates malignant melanomas from deep penetrating nevi. *Mod Pathol* 2006;19:1378–1385.

105. Stewart FW, Copeland MM. Neurogenic sarcoma. *Am J Cancer* 1931;15:1235–1320.

106. Holt JB, Sangueza OP, Levine EA, et al. Nodal melanocytic nevi in sentinel lymph nodes. Correlation with melanoma-associated cutaneous nevi. *Am J Clin Pathol* 2004;121:58–63.

107. Biddle DA, Evans HL, Kemp BL, et al. Intraparenchymal nevus cell aggregates in lymph nodes: a possible diagnostic pitfall with malignant melanoma and carcinoma. *Am J Surg Pathol* 2003;27:673–681.

108. Carson KF, Wen DR, Li PX, et al. Nodal nevi and cutaneous melanomas. *Am J Surg Pathol* 1996;20:834–840.

109. Fontaine D, Parkhill W, Greer W, et al. Nevus cells in lymph nodes: an association with congenital cutaneous nevi. *Am J Dermatopathol* 2002;24:1–5.

110. Schoenfeld RJ, Pinkus H. The recurrence of nevi after incomplete removal. *Arch Dermatol* 1958;78:30–35.

111. Cox AJ, Walton RG. The induction of junctional changes in pigmented nevi. *Arch Pathol* 1965;79:428–434.

112. Imagawa I, Endo M, Morishima T. Mechanism of recurrence of pigmented nevi following dermabrasion. *Acta Derm Venereol Suppl (Stockh)* 1976;56:353–359.

113. Park HK, Leonard DD, Arrington JH, et al. Recurrent melanocytic nevi: clinical and histologic review of 175 cases. *J Am Acad Dermatol* 1987;17:285–292.

114. Sexton M, Sexton CW. Recurrent pigmented melanocytic nevus: a benign lesion, not to be mistaken for malignant melanoma. *Arch Pathol Lab Med* 1991;115:122–126.

115. Curley RK, Fallowfield ME, Cook MG, Marsden RA. Effect of incisional biopsy on subsequent histology of melanocytic naevi. *Br J Dermatol* 1990;123:504–506.

116. Mooney MA, Barr RJ, Buxton MG. Halo nevus or halo phenomenon? A study of 142 cases. *J Cutan Pathol* 1995;22:342–348.

117. Happle R. Lyonization and the lines of Blaschko. *Hum Genet* 1985;70:200–206.

MALIGNANT MELANOMA AND PRECURSOR LESIONS

118. Richardson SK, Tannous ZS, Mihm MC Jr. Congenital and infantile melanoma: review of the literature and report of an uncommon variant, pigment-synthesizing melanoma. *J Am Acad Dermatol* 2002;47:77–90.

119. Fishman C, Mihm MC Jr, Sober AJ. Diagnosis and management of nevi and cutaneous melanoma in infants and children. *Clin Dermatol* 2002;20:44–50.

120. Granter SR, McKee PH, Calonje E, et al. Melanoma associated with blue nevus and melanoma mimicking cellular blue nevus: a clinicopathologic study of 10 cases on the spectrum of so-called 'malignant blue nevus.' *Am J Surg Pathol* 2001;25:316–323.

121. Scalzo DA, Hida CA, Toth G, et al. Childhood melanoma: a clinicopathological study of 22 cases. *Melanoma Res* 1997;7:63–68.

122. Clark WH Jr, Ainsworth AM, Bernardino EM, et al. The developmental biology of primary human malignant melanomas. *Semin Oncol* 1975;2:83–103.

123. Hussein MR, Wood GS. Molecular aspects of melanocytic dysplastic nevi. *J Mol Diagn* 2002; 4:71–80.

124. Reed RJ, Ichinose H, Clark WH, Mihm MC. Common and uncommon melanocytic nevi and borderline melanomas. *Semin Oncol* 1975;2:119–147.

125. Reed RJ, Clark WH Jr, Mihm MC. Premalignant melanocytic dysplasias. In Ackerman AB, ed. *Pathology of Malignant Melanoma.* New York, NY: Masson, 1981:159–183.

126. Reed RJ. A classification of melanocytic dysplasias and malignant melanomas. *Am J Dermatopathol* 1984;6:195–206.

127. Barnhill RL, Mihm MC Jr. The histopathology of cutaneous malignant melanoma. *Semin Diagn Pathol* 1993;10:47–75.

128. Smoller BR. Immunohistochemistry in the diagnosis of melanocytic neoplasms. *Pathology (Phila)* 1994;2:371–383.

129. Shea CR, Prieto VG. Recent developments in the pathology of melanocytic neoplasia. *Dermatol Clin* 1999;17:615–630, ix.

130. Smoller BR. Immunohistochemistry in the diagnosis of malignant melanoma. *Clin Dermatol* 1991;9:235–241.

131. Busam KJ, Jungbluth AA. Melan-A, a new melanocytic differentiation marker. *Adv Anat Pathol* 1999;6:12–18.

132. Smoller BR, McNutt NS, Hsu A. HMB-45 recognizes stimulated melanocytes. *J Cutan Pathol* 1989;16:49–53.

133. Orchard GE. Comparison of immunohistochemical labelling of melanocyte differentiation antibodies melan-A, tyrosinase and HMB 45 with NKIC3 and S100 protein in the evaluation of benign naevi and malignant melanoma. *Histochem J* 2000;32:475–481.

134. Orosz Z. Melan-A/Mart-1 expression in various melanocytic lesions and in non-melanocytic soft tissue tumours. *Histopathology* 1999;34:517–525.

135. Lohmann CM, Iversen K, Jungbluth AA, et al. Expression of melanocyte differentiation antigens and Ki-67 in nodal nevi and comparison of Ki-67 expression with metastatic melanoma. *Am J Surg Pathol* 2002;26:1351–1357.

136. Busam KJ, Chen Y-T, Old LJ, et al. Expression of melan-A (MART1) in benign melanocytic nevi and primary cutaneous malignant melanoma. *Am J Surg Pathol* 1998;22:976–982.

137. Murphy GF, Mihm MC Jr. Recognition and evaluation of cytological dysplasia in acquired melanocytic nevi. *Hum Pathol* 1999;30:506–512.

138. Rhodes AR, Harrist TJ, Day CL, et al. Dysplastic melanocytic nevi in histologic association with 234 primary cutaneous melanomas. *J Am Acad Dermatol* 1983;9:563–574.

139. Elder DE, Goldman LI, Goldman SC, et al. Dysplastic nevus syndrome: a phenotypic association of sporadic cutaneous melanoma. *Cancer* 1980;46:1787–1794.

140. Clark WH, Reimer RR, Greene M, et al. Origin of familial malignant melanomas from heritable melanocytic lesions—the B-K mole syndrome. *Arch Dermatol* 1978;114:732–738.

141. Greene MH, Goldin LR, Clark WH Jr, et al. Familial cutaneous malignant melanoma: autosomal dominant trait possibly linked to the Rh locus. *Proc Natl Acad Sci U S A* 1983; 80:6071–6075.

142. Rhodes AR, Melski JW, Sober AJ, et al. Increased intraepidermal melanocyte frequency and size in dysplastic melanocytic nevi and cutaneous melanoma. A comparative quantitative study of dysplastic melanocytic nevi, superficial spreading melanoma, nevocellular nevi, and solar lentigines. *J Invest Dermatol* 1983;80:452–459.

143. Halpern AC, Schuchter LM. Prognostic models in melanoma. *Semin Oncol* 1997;24:S2–S7.

144. Elder DE, Van Belle P, Elenitsas R, et al. Neoplastic progression and prognosis in melanoma. *Semin Cutan Med Surg* 1996;15:336–348.

145. Slominski A, Wortsman J, Carlson AJ, et al. Malignant melanoma. *Arch Pathol Lab Med* 2001;125:1295–1306.

146. Crowson AN, Magro CM, Sanchez-Carpintero I, Mihm MC Jr. The precursors of malignant melanoma. *Recent Results Cancer Res* 2002;160:75–84.

147. Elder DE, Jucovy PM, Tuthill RJ, Clark WH. The classification of malignant melanoma. *Am J Dermatopathol* 1980;2:315–320.

148. McGovern VJ, Mihm MC, Bailly C, et al. The classification of malignant melanoma and its histologic reporting. *Cancer* 1973;32:1446–1457.

149. Mihm MC, Lopansri S. A review of the classification of malignant melanoma. *J Dermatol* 1979;6:131–142.

150. Guerry D 4th, Synnestvedt M, Elder DE, Schultz D. Lessons from tumor progression: the invasive radial growth phase of melanoma is common, incapable of metastasis, and indolent. *J Invest Dermatol* 1993;100:342S–345S.

151. King R, Googe PB, Mihm MC Jr. Thin melanomas. *Clin Lab Med* 2000;20:713–729.

152. Elder DE, Guerry D 4th, Epstein MN, et al. Invasive malignant melanomas lacking competence for metastasis. *Am J Dermatopathol* 1984;6:55–61.

153. Breslow A. Thickness, cross-sectional areas and depth of invasion in the prognosis of cutaneous melanoma. *Ann Surg* 1970;172:902–906.

154. Balch CM, Wilkerson JA, Murad TQ, et al. The prognostic significance of ulceration of cutaneous melanoma. *Cancer* 1980;45:3012–3017.

155. Day CL, Harrist TJ, Gorstein F, et al. Malignant melanoma. Prognostic significance of "microscopic satellites" in the reticular dermis and subcutaneous fat. *Ann Surg* 1981;194: 108–112.

156. Reed RJ, Clark WH Jr, Mihm MC. Premalignant melanocytic dysplasias. In Ackerman AB, ed. *Pathology of Malignant Melanoma.* New York, NY: Masson, 1981:159–183.

157. Herlyn M, Balaban G, Bennicelli J, et al. Primary melanoma cells of the vertical growth phase: similarities to metastatic cells. *J Natl Cancer Inst* 1985;74:283–289.

158. Pierard GE, Pierard-Franchimont C. The proliferative activity of cells of malignant melanomas. *Am J Dermatopathol* 1984;6:317–323.

159. Day CL, Harrist TJ, Mihm CM. Classification of malignant melanomas according to the histologic morphology of melanoma nodules. *J Dermatol Surg Oncol* 1982;8:874–876.

160. Tannous ZS, Lerner LH, Duncan LM, et al. Progression to invasive melanoma from malignant melanoma in situ, lentigo maligna type. *Hum Pathol* 2000;31:705–708.

161. Flotte TJ, Mihm MC Jr. Lentigo maligna and malignant melanoma in situ, lentigo maligna type. *Hum Pathol* 1999;30:533–536.

162. Auslender S, Barzilai A, Goldberg I, et al. Lentigo maligna and superficial spreading melanoma are different in their in situ phase: an immunohistochemical study. *Hum Pathol* 2002;33:1001–1005.

163. Clark WH, Mihm MC. Lentigo maligna and lentigo-maligna melanoma. *Am J Pathol* 1969; 55:39–67.

164. Kaufmann R, Nikelski K, Weber L, Sterry W. Amelanotic lentigo maligna melanoma. *J Am Acad Dermatol* 1995;32:339–342.

165. Skelton HG, Smith KJ, Laskin WB, et al. Desmoplastic malignant melanoma. *J Am Acad Dermatol* 1995;32:717–725.

166. Wharton JM, Carlson JA, Mihm MC Jr. Desmoplastic malignant melanoma: diagnosis of early clinical lesions. *Hum Pathol* 1999;30:537–542.

167. Kerl H, Hodl S, Stettner H. Acral lentiginous melanoma. In Ackerman AB, ed. *Pathology of Malignant Melanoma*. New York, NY: Masson, 1981:217–242.

168. Arrington JH, Reed RJ, Ichinose H, Krementz ET. Plantar lentiginous melanoma. A distinct variant of human cutaneous malignant melanoma. *Am J Surg Pathol* 1977;1:131–143.

169. Jimbow K, Ikeda S, Takahashi H, et al. Biological behavior and natural course of acral malignant melanoma. Clinical and histologic features and prognosis of palmoplantar, subungual, and other acral malignant melanomas. *Am J Dermatopathol* 1984;6:43–53.

170. Clark WH, Bernardino EA, Reed RJ, Kopf AW. Acral lentiginous melanomas including melanomas of mucous membranes. In Clark WH, Goldman LI, Mastrangelo MJ, eds. *Human Malignant Melanoma*. New York, NY: Grune & Stratton, 1979:109–124.

171. Cascinelli N, Zurrida S, Galimerti V, et al. Acral lentiginous melanoma: a histological type without prognostic significance. *J Dermatol Surg Oncol* 1994;20:817–822.

DESMOPLASTIC MELANOMA

172. Crowson N, Magro CM, Mihm MC Jr. Desmoplastic melanoma. In *A Comprehensive Textbook of Pigmented Lesions*. Hoboken, NJ: Wiley-Liss, Inc., 2001:332–336.

173. Busam KJ. Cutaneous desmoplastic melanoma. *Adv Anat Pathol* 2005;12:92–102.

174. Busam KJ, Mujumbar U, Hummer AJ, et al. Cutaneous desmoplastic melanoma. Reappraisal of morphologic heterogeneity and prognostic factors. *Am J Surg Pathol* 2004;28:1518–1525.

175. Hawkins WG, Busam KJ, Ben-Porat L, et al. Desmoplastic melanoma: a pathologically and clinically distinct form of cutaneous melanoma. *Ann Surg Oncol* 2005;12:207–213.

176. Busam KJ, Zhao H, Coit DG, et al. Distinction of desmoplastic melanoma from non-desmoplastic melanoma by gene expression profiling. *J Invest Dermatol* 2005;124:412–419.

PROGNOSTIC FACTORS IN MALIGNANT MELANOMA

177. Clark WH Jr, From L, Bernardino EA, et al. The histogenesis and biologic behavior of primary human malignant melanoma of the skin. *Cancer Res* 1969;29:705–727.

178. Clark WH Jr, Elder DE, Guerry D 4th, et al. Model predicting survival in stage I melanoma based on tumor progression. *J Natl Cancer Inst* 1989;81:1893–1904.

179. Balch CM, Buzaid AC, Soong SJ, et al. Final version of the American Joint Committee on Cancer staging system for cutaneous melanoma. *J Clin Oncol* 2001;19:3635–3648.

180. Gimotty PA, Guerry D, Ming ME, et al. Thin primary cutaneous malignant melanoma: a prognostic tree for 10-year metastasis is more accurate than American Joint Committee on Cancer staging. *J Clin Oncol* 2004;18:3668–3676.

181. Clemente CG, Mihm MC Jr, Bufalino R, et al. Prognostic value of tumor infiltrating lymphocytes in the vertical growth phase of primary cutaneous melanoma. *Cancer* 1996;77:1303–1310.

MOLECULAR PATHOLOGY OF MELANOMA

182. Miller AJ, Mihm MC Jr. Melanoma. *N Engl J Med* 2006;355:51–65.

183. Fecher LA, Cummings SD, Keefe MJ, et al. Toward a molecular classification of melanoma. *J Clin Oncol* 2007;25:1606–1620.

184. Bastian BC, Kashani-Sabet M, Hamm H, et al. Gene amplifications characterize acral melanoma and permit the detection of occult tumor cells in the surrounding skin. *Cancer Res* 2000;60:1968–1973.

185. Bastian BC, Olshen AB, LeBoit PE, et al. Classifying melanocytic tumors based on DNA copy number changes. *Am J Pathol* 2003;163:1765–1770.

186. Curtin JA, Fridlyand J, Kageshita T, et al. Distinct sets of genetic alterations in melanoma. *N Engl J Med* 2005;353:2135–2147.

187. Curtin JA, Busam K, Pinkel D, et al. Somatic activation of KIT in distinct subtypes of melanoma. *J Clin Oncol* 2006;24:4340–4346.

188. Li F, Tiede B, Massague J, et al. Beyond tumorigenesis: cancer stem cells in metastasis. *Cell Res* 2006;17:3–14.

189. Schatton T, Murphy GF, Frank NY, et al. Identification of cells initiating human melanomas. *Nature* 2008;451:345–349.

CHAPTER

4

Reid R. Heffner, Jr.
Lucia L. Balos

Muscle Biopsy in Neuromuscular Diseases

This chapter is designed to provide the surgical pathologist a concise discussion of commonly biopsied nonneoplastic neuromuscular diseases. In this pragmatic approach, the focus is on morphology and on those disorders amenable to diagnosis by morphologic techniques. Readers who wish to acquire a more detailed understanding of the field are referred elsewhere (1–11).

PLANNING AND PROCEDURES

CLINICAL INFORMATION

At our institution, to encourage the clinician to provide clinical data that may be essential to biopsy interpretation, the requesting physician is asked to complete and return a form to the pathology laboratory with the tissue specimen. This form requests only essential data, and it is not so lengthy that compliance is discouraged. The biopsy specimen is reviewed by the pathologist. In more complicated cases, the clinician may be given a preliminary diagnosis, while additional information is requested. In this regard, the telephone is almost as useful as the microscope in interpreting muscle biopsy specimens.

COLLECTION AND PREPARATION OF THE MUSCLE BIOPSY SPECIMEN

Ideally, muscle biopsies should be performed by persons skilled in biopsy technique and with knowledge of specimen submission procedures. The requesting physician, who is familiar with the patient, is obligated to ensure that an appropriate muscle is sampled. The biopsy specimen should be representative of the disease process. For example, if the symptoms involve the legs rather than the arms, a specimen from the upper extremity cannot be expected to reflect the disease process accurately. Moreover, the specimen should be obtained from a muscle in which the disease process is active and evolving. A specimen from a severely affected muscle, in which marked weakness or atrophy is present, is generally characterized by end-stage disease that is difficult to interpret, much like end-stage renal disease.

An accurate pathologic diagnosis depends on the proper preparation of the muscle sample. Because of the unique requirements for handling the muscle specimen, it must be received at times when experienced technical assistance is available. Two separate specimens are routinely requested (Fig. 4.1).

Before excision, the first specimen is maintained in an isometric state by introducing it into a muscle clamp, which prevents the contraction artifact caused by cutting the muscle and immersing it in fixative. Because the muscle is placed in the instrument lengthwise, the specimen is already oriented for processing. Inasmuch as the biopsy specimen must extend entirely across the clamp, an acceptable sample size of at least 0.5 cm in diameter and 1 cm in length must be provided. The specimen should be of sufficient size to permit the adequate observation of the pathologic process. The fixed sample can be used for paraffin sections, 1-μm to 2-μm resin-embedded sections, and electron microscopic studies. Practically speaking, the pathologist with some experience can see sufficient detail in resin sections, making ultrastructural examination unnecessary in many cases.

A second fresh specimen measuring about $1.0 \times 0.5 \times 0.5$ cm is used for the preparation of frozen sections. A variety of flash-freezing techniques have been described (12,13). Whatever technique is selected, the freezing process must proceed with extreme rapidity. In our laboratory, serial frozen sections are routinely stained with hematoxylin and eosin (H&E), rapid Gomori trichrome (RTC), adenosine triphosphatase (ATPase) at pH 9.4, and nicotinamide adenine dinucleotide, reduced (NADH-TR). When other stains, such as periodic acid-Schiff (PAS) for glycogen, fat stains, phosphorylase, and additional histochemical stains, are warranted, they are performed. Frozen tissue also may be used for immunofluorescence microscopy or biochemical analysis.

INTERPRETATION OF THE MUSCLE BIOPSY SPECIMEN

NORMAL MUSCLE

In the evaluation of the muscle biopsy specimen, familiarity with the normal structure is the basis for understanding the diversity of pathologic reactions that occur in neuromuscular disease. The reader is referred elsewhere for a more detailed discussion of the light microscopy, histochemistry, and electron microscopy of normal muscle (1–11). The myocyte is a multinucleated, syncytium-like cell with a shape resembling an elongated cylinder, although the normal adult fiber is not truly round but,

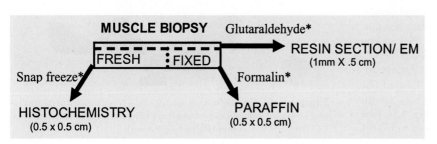

Figure 4.1. Suggested division of a routine skeletal muscle biopsy specimen, fixation (*asterisk*), and method of processing.

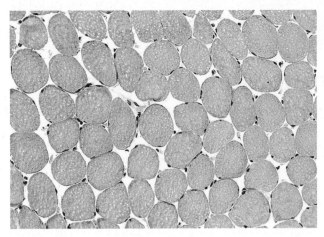

Figure 4.2. Normal muscle (transverse section). The fibers are typically polygonal, and the sarcolemmal nuclei are located peripherally.

TABLE 4.1		

Fiber Typing in Skeletal Muscle

	Type 1	Type 2
Color	Red	White
Adenosine triphosphatase activity (pH 9.4)	Low	High
Oxidative enzyme content	High	Low
Glycogen	Low	High
Phosphorylase	Low	High
Lipid content	High	Low

instead, is polygonal or multifaceted in cross section (Fig. 4.2). The sarcolemmal nuclei are ordinarily located peripherally, with four to six per fiber in transverse sections. The diameter of the fibers depends on several factors. In general, powerful proximal muscles are made up of fibers with a mean diameter (85 to 90 µm) greater than that (20 µm) of smaller, distal, or ocular muscles, which are devoted to finely coordinated activity. Fiber size is greater in males than in females, probably because of hormonal influences and the general propensity of males to engage in more strenuous physical activity. That exercise encourages fiber hypertrophy in both sexes is well established. Muscle fibers in children and the elderly are smaller than those in young, healthy adults.

In vertebrates, notably certain species of birds, one can distinguish between red (e.g., soleus) and white (e.g., pectoralis) muscles, with the color of red muscles being a consequence of their greater myoglobin content. Red muscle, with its larger mitochondrial population and higher capillary density, is adapted to aerobic respiration and is designed for postural or sustained activity. White muscle, which contains fewer mitochondria and abundant glycogen, is capable of anaerobic respiration; it is more suited to sudden and intermittent action. Although an entire muscle in lower animals may be composed of either red or white fibers, human muscle is constructed of both fiber types, which are arranged in a mixed mosaic pattern resembling a checkerboard. The location of the muscle in the body and its function determine the proportion of type 1 and type 2 fibers, but the average muscle has about twice as many type 2 fibers (60% to 65%) as type 1 fibers (35% to 40%).

Fiber typing, the demonstration of the histochemical properties of muscle fibers within a biopsy specimen, is accomplished by carrying out histoenzymatic reactions in frozen sections (Table 4.1). Fiber types are not evident in slides stained with H&E. Most laboratories use two complementary histochemical reactions for this purpose. The myofibrillar ATPase reaction is considered to be the most reliable method for distinguishing fiber types. A spectrum of staining patterns can be achieved by manipulating the pH during the procedure. In the standard or alkaline ATPase reaction conducted at a pH of 9.4, type 1 fibers appear light, and they can be seen better in sections counterstained with eosin. Type 2 fibers appear dark (Fig. 4.3). Fibers with intermediate staining properties are not seen in the alka-

line reaction. When the pH of the incubating solution is reduced to the acidic range in the so-called reverse ATPase reaction, type 1 fibers are very dark, type 2A fibers are very light, and the staining intensity of type 2B fibers is intermediate. Commercial antibodies to slow (type 1) and fast (type 2) myosin are now available. By means of immunostaining, fiber typing with results similar to those obtained with ATPase reactions can be achieved in paraffin sections (14).

The oxidative enzyme reactions, such as the NADH-TR reaction, reflect the concentration of mitochondria within the myofibers. The fiber staining is essentially the opposite of that seen in the alkaline ATPase reaction. Thus, intensely stained fibers are designated as type 1 (oxidative), and lighter fibers are designated as type 2. Typically, oxidative enzyme reactions further divide type 2 fibers into two subpopulations. Type 2B fibers are very lightly stained, whereas the staining intensity of type 2A fibers is intermediate between that of type 1 and that of 2B. The myofibrillary network is stained such that the sarcoplasm has a somewhat granular appearance.

All muscle fibers contain phosphorylase, as well as glycogen; these are more abundant in type 2 (glycolytic) fibers. Some laboratories take advantage of the histochemical reaction for phosphorylase, or the PAS stain, as a means of fiber typing, but our experience dictates that such staining is unpredictable. We restrict use of the phosphorylase reaction to cases of possible enzyme deficiency (McArdle disease). Lipid vacuoles are more numerous in the sarcoplasm of type 1 fibers, yet fat stains seldom

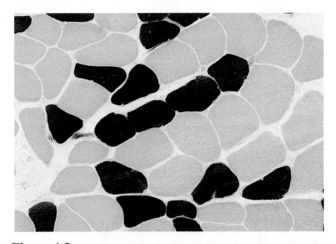

Figure 4.3. Normal muscle. In the alkaline adenosine triphosphatase (ATPase) reaction, type 1 fibers are light, and type 2 fibers are dark (ATPase, pH 9.4, counterstained with eosin).

demonstrate an unequivocal difference between fiber types. Fat stains are valuable when the diagnosis of lipid storage disease is suspected.

ARTIFACTS

Among the most unavoidable and disturbing artifacts is the vacuolation produced by improper freezing of the muscle biopsy specimen (Fig. 4.4). It may also occur after improper transport or storage that allows thawing of the sample. This type of artifact may simulate pathologic change, such as vacuolar myopathy, or it may distort pathologically altered fibers, thereby precluding proper interpretation. In contrast to pathologic vacuoles, the vacuoles associated with the artifact are in the more slowly frozen or earliest thawing portion of the specimen, which is generally in the center or at the periphery of the tissue block, respectively. Vacuoles tend to affect every fiber in the region of artifact and may be arranged in a gradient according to size. Where the artifact is minimal, small vacuoles are numerous in each fiber and are uniform in size, and they are located between the myofibrils. In poorly frozen regions, larger clear vacuoles are found within the sarcoplasm. These ice crystals typically assume linear, triangular, rectangular, trapezoidal, and other noncircular geometric forms.

With severe contraction artifact in longitudinal sections, dark contraction bands alternate with lucent, disrupted zones within the fiber (Fig. 4.5). The latter appear as jagged cracks in the sarcoplasm in transversely oriented sections. Contraction artifact is most noticeable at the edges of the specimen. This artifact is commonly seen in unclamped specimens, when plastic disposable clamps that only partially prevent contraction are used or when the muscle is injected with local anesthetic. Contraction artifact renders muscle particularly unfit for electron microscopy. The orderly structural landmarks are obliterated by myofibrillar fragmentation and disorientation.

A frequent artifact occurs in frozen sections when the section lifts off the slide. The staining intensity of the fibers varies, and a variety of striped or ring structures result from curling or wrinkling of the fibers (Fig. 4.6).

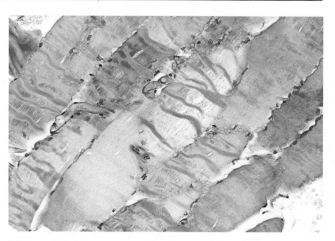

Figure 4.5. Contraction artifact. Darker contraction bands and disrupted lucent zones are seen in several longitudinally oriented fibers (periodic acid-Schiff stain).

PATHOLOGIC REACTIONS OF MUSCLE IN A REVIEW OF THE BIOPSY

When evaluating muscle biopsies, the surgical pathologist is likely to come across one or more of the reactions described in the following pages. None of the pathologic changes that may be observed in the muscle biopsy specimen is totally specific for a single disease, although each has diagnostic significance because it is restricted to one disease or a limited number of diseases. The presence of each pathologic change described in the following sections should engender a differential diagnosis in the mind of the observer. Arrival at a precise diagnosis involves correlation not only with the clinical information and laboratory test results, but also with the sum of the pathologic findings, often producing a pathologic pattern or signature of the disease process. The pathologic changes described here are arbitrarily divided into two categories—those seen in fixed tissue by routine light microscopy and those seen in frozen sections, usually in histochemical preparations. This division obviously is artificial because many changes are visible in both

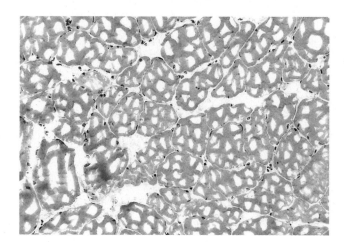

Figure 4.4. Freezing artifact. Extensive vacuolar change is caused by improper freezing. Many of the vacuoles have linear, noncircular geometric shapes.

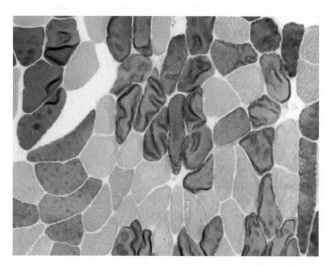

Figure 4.6. Frozen section has partially lifted off the slide. Tissue twists create artifact seen as fiber curling with striped and ring structures in the fibers (ATPase, pH 9.4, counterstained with eosin).

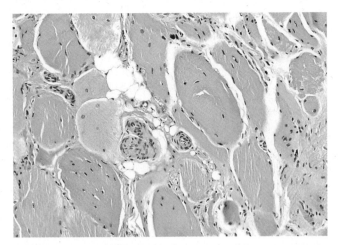

Figure 4.7. Nuclear internalization. Many fibers contain one or more internal, often pyknotic nuclei.

permanent and frozen sections, but it denotes which of the two techniques tends to be superior in demonstrating a particular abnormality. All of the pathologic changes discussed here can be appreciated under the light microscope and are visible only in greater detail ultrastructurally. Therefore, a description of the fine structure of each change accompanies the description of the light microscopic features.

OBSERVATIONS IN ROUTINE PARAFFIN SECTIONS

Nuclear Changes

The most frequent abnormality involving the nucleus is internalization. According to quantitative studies, the nuclei in cross sections of normal muscle are peripheral or subsarcolemmal in 97% to 99% of fibers. In specimens from patients with neuromuscular disease, the counts of internal nuclei typically are commonly elevated in 5% to 10% of fibers. Although the sarcoplasmic integrity appears undisturbed, such fibers usually are mildly or moderately altered in size (Fig. 4.7). This inconstancy of nuclear position is of no specific diagnostic import, and it is a reaction to a variety of diverse injuries. However, if most of the fibers contain randomly distributed internal nuclei, the diagnosis of myotonic dystrophy should be strongly considered (Table 4.2). The virtually pathognomonic criterion of centronuclear myopathy is the presence of a single central or paracentral nucleus within nearly every fiber. As opposed to nuclear internalization in the absence of injury to the sarcoplasm, after sarcoplasmic necrosis, the nuclei may no longer be fixed in a peripheral location. They commonly migrate internally in degenerating

TABLE 4.2
Conditions in Which Internal Nuclei Have Diagnostic Significance
Myotendinous insertion
Centronuclear myopathy
Myotonic dystrophy
Fiber regeneration
Fiber atrophy

and regenerating fibers, no matter what the cause. Severely atrophic fibers also contain multiple pyknotic nuclei that seem to remain intact, forming clusters as the sarcoplasm is progressively diminished in volume.

Ring Fibers

The ring is formed by a peripheral bundle of myofibrils that is directed circumferentially, encircling the inner portion of the myofiber, which otherwise appears normal in disposition and structure. In cross sections of muscle, the striated annulation is oriented in the transverse plane rather than in the longitudinal axis of the fiber (Fig. 4.8). The striations are easily visible in PAS-stained sections, resin sections, and ultrastructurally; under the electron microscope, the abnormally oriented myofibrils usually exhibit a normal architecture except for the hypercontraction of the sarcomeres (15). Although ring fibers have been reported in a variety of diseases, they are most consistently observed in limb-girdle dystrophy and myotonic dystrophy. Large numbers of ring fibers especially favor the latter diagnosis.

Hyaline Fibers

Hyaline fibers are pathologically rounded and enlarged. They are more deeply stained than normal fibers, whether in paraffin or frozen sections stained with H&E, trichrome, PAS, or histochemical methods (Fig. 4.9). The sarcoplasm is smudged and homogeneous. The hyaline fiber is a bona fide pathologic change in tissue unaffected by contraction artifact, and in many instances, it represents an early stage of cell necrosis (16). Serial sections through the same fiber may reveal zones of unequivocal necrosis and phagocytosis adjacent to hyalinization. Hyaline fibers are most commonly encountered in Duchenne muscular dystrophy, and they are most numerous in this condition.

Fiber Necrosis

The initial sign of necrosis in light microscopic sections is an alteration in the tinctorial properties of the muscle fiber that is perhaps best appreciated in H&E stains. The acutely necrotic fiber first stains more intensely eosinophilic and then pales to

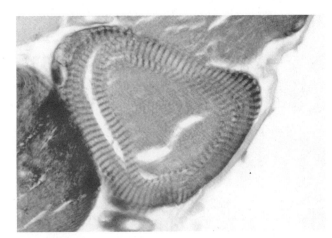

Figure 4.8. Ring fiber. Circumferential orientation of the peripheral myofibrils produces a striated ring that encircles a transversely sectioned fiber in the center of the field (periodic acid-Schiff stain).

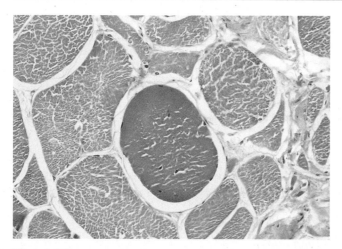

Figure 4.9. Hyaline fiber. The fiber in the center of the photograph is rounded, and it has dark, opaque sarcoplasm.

TABLE 4.3

Fiber Necrosis Seen in the Biopsy Specimen

Pathologic Features	Disease
Small groups of necrotic fibers	Duchenne dystrophy
Perifascicular necrosis	Dermatomyositis
Random fiber necrosis	PM, IBM
Infarcts with large areas of necrosis	PAN
Extensive, diffuse	Rhabdomyolysis in patients with CPT deficiency, alcoholics, military recruits

CPT, carnitine palmitoyltransferase; IBM, inclusion body myositis; PAN, polyarteritis nodosa; PM, polymyositis.

a wan shade of pink. Simultaneously, the appearance of the sarcoplasm is transformed from striated to coarsely granular. The nuclei become pyknotic, fragmented, and finally no longer visible. As the necrotic process culminates, the sarcoplasm assumes a vacuolated or fragmented texture, and phagocytosis of the necrotic cell begins (Fig. 4.10). With the intensification of the phagocytic process, the sarcoplasm is evacuated by macrophages that occupy the residual spaces. Often, even before the total removal of the necrotic sarcoplasmic debris, the phase of regeneration has supervened; therefore, both regenerative and phagocytic activity may be seen in the same fiber. Necrosis may be a part of the pathologic response in many muscle diseases, but it is prevalent in Duchenne muscular dystrophy and the inflammatory myopathies (Table 4.3).

Fiber Regeneration

Fiber necrosis generally acts as a stimulus for subsequent regeneration. Hence, the presence of regenerating fibers in a biopsy specimen, even in the absence of necrotic fibers, is a likely indicator of previous necrosis or of fiber necrosis in adjacent muscle

that has escaped sampling. The regeneration of fibers is believed to arise by two independent routes. When the necrosis of a myofiber is segmental, the regenerative activity originates from sprouts of sarcoplasm at the viable segments adjacent to the damaged sarcoplasm. The satellite cells are a second source of regeneration following injury to the muscle cell as these cells are transformed into myoblasts (17). Current evidence indicates that the satellite cells with the restorative capacity to form new muscle play a more important role than sarcoplasmic sprouting. Regenerating fibers are most readily visualized in H&E sections by the basophilia of their sarcoplasm. The nuclei, which are often eccentric in location and which may be focally increased in number, are larger than normal, with vesicular chromatin and prominent nucleoli (Fig. 4.11). Ultrastructurally, the regenerating fibers are replete with ribosomes, which explains the sarcoplasmic basophilia at the light microscopic level (18).

Inclusions

Inclusions may be located within the sarcolemmal nuclei or within the sarcoplasm. Nuclear inclusions suggest the diagnosis of oculopharyngeal dystrophy or inclusion body myositis. Sarco-

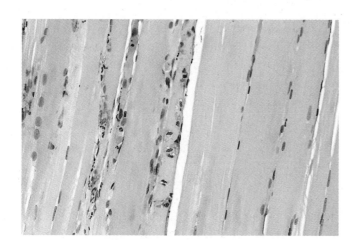

Figure 4.10. Fiber necrosis. The necrotic process in the fiber at the center of this longitudinal section is recognized by a loss of cross striations and early phagocytosis.

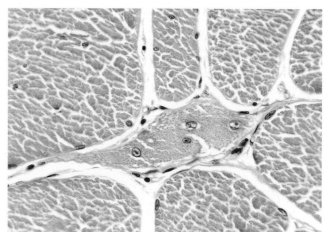

Figure 4.11. Regenerating fibers. Sarcolemmal nuclei are large and vesicular, and they contain prominent nucleoli. The sarcoplasm is basophilic.

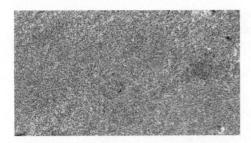

Figure 4.12. Oculopharyngeal muscular dystrophy. High-power electron micrograph showing intranuclear inclusion composed of 8.5-nm tubulofilamentous material.

TABLE 4.4	
Inflammation Seen in the Biopsy Specimen	
Pathologic Features	*Disease*
Perivascular, angiocentric	DM, connective tissue disease, FSHD
Endomysial, around fibers	PM, IBM, viral
Nodular	Rheumatoid arthritis, granulomas
Polymorphous with eosinophils	PAN, drug reactions, trichinosis, eosinophilic fasciitis

DM, dermatomyositis; FSHD, facioscapulohumeral dystrophy; IBM, inclusion body myositis; PAN, polyarteritis nodosa; PM, polymyositis.

plasmic inclusions suggest the diagnosis of myofibrillar myopathy or inclusion body myositis. In oculopharyngeal dystrophy, nuclear inclusions are difficult to detect by light microscopy. Electron microscopic examination of the muscle tissue is likely to reveal nuclear inclusions composed of 8.5-nm unbranched tubular structures (Fig. 4.12). These inclusions contain the protein PABP2, which accumulates in the sarcolemmal nuclei as a result of short expansions of GCG repeats in the poly(A) binding protein gene on chromosome 14q11–13.

Nuclear inclusions in inclusion body myositis are faintly pink to wine colored in H&E stains, and they often fill the nucleus, leaving a rim of peripheral chromatin (Fig. 4.13). Pink or red inclusions may also be seen in the sarcoplasmic rimmed vacuoles. Under the electron microscope, these inclusions, which consist of membranous whorls and bundles of filaments measuring 15 to 18 nm in diameter, may be present in few fibers, and they are extremely difficult to identify. The filaments were once thought to be of viral origin, perhaps from the mumps virus. They are now considered β-amyloid fibrils (see "Inclusion Body Myositis" section). Because the filaments are sparse, Congo red stains tend to be negative despite contrary claims in the literature. In the myofibrillar myopathies, the inclusions represent focal collections of intermediate filaments such as desmin, which form poorly defined, smudged areas within the fibers. In hyaline body myopathy, the inclusions, which contain myosin filaments, are subsarcolemmal, well-defined, and slightly different in texture from the surrounding sarcoplasm.

Inflammation

Interstitial inflammatory infiltrates are most frequently encountered in immunologically mediated or idiopathic inflammatory myopathies (Table 4.4). Most important among these are polymyositis (PM), dermatomyositis (DM), and inclusion body myositis, which make up 29% of all cases in our files. The inflammatory cells in PM invade the endomysium, sometimes enveloping necrotic fibers. Sheets of inflammatory cells expand the endomysial spaces in acute, more severe disease (Fig. 4.14). In DM, they surround intramuscular blood vessels with minimal infiltration of the vascular walls. The inflammatory cells are mononuclear in type, chiefly consisting of mature lymphocytes. Plasma cells are a minor part of the inflammatory response. Rare eosinophils are seen, and neutrophils are absent. A similar pattern of inflammation is seen in facioscapulohumeral dystrophy, a disorder distinguished from PM and DM by its clinical features.

An inflammatory myopathy histologically identical to PM and DM may accompany any of the systemic connective tissue diseases. However, crucial differences among several of these collagen vascular disorders are diagnostically reliable. Nodular infiltrates composed largely of plasma cells are highly suggestive of rheumatoid arthritis. Polyarteritis nodosa and systemic lupus erythematosus, on the other hand, are typically associated with a vasculitis. Polyarteritis nodosa shows an affinity for larger vessels, especially arteries, within the epimysium and perimysium. The entire wall of the vessel may be infiltrated by inflammatory

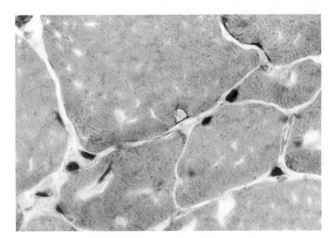

Figure 4.13. Inclusion body myositis. An intranuclear inclusion is shown at the center of the picture. The inclusion is eosinophilic and smudged; it is located within a sarcolemmal nucleus.

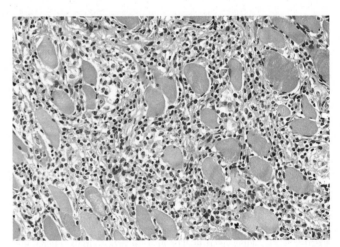

Figure 4.14. Inflammatory myopathy. Sheets of lymphocytes expand the endomysial spaces and surround the fibers.

cells, which usually include conspicuous eosinophils. In systemic lupus erythematosus, the affected vessels are smaller in caliber, and they exhibit fibrinoid necrosis. Areas of vascular injury attract neutrophils, and the remnant of their breakdown, nuclear dust, is also seen. With the use of immunohistochemical techniques, deposits of immunoglobulin and complement can be demonstrated at sites of vascular injury in both conditions.

Granulomatous inflammation may be indicative of sarcoidosis or idiopathic granulomatous myositis, a chronic progressive myopathy of middle-aged women without systemic manifestations (19,20). The granulomas in both are sharply circumscribed and nonnecrotizing. They invade and expand the interstitium, and they are composed of lymphocytes, epithelioid histiocytes, and multinucleated giant cells. *Trichinella* infestation may elicit a granulomatous response in muscle that usually contains numerous eosinophils. Other microbial agents, including bacteria, fungi, and viruses, may cause inflammatory myopathy, but a muscle biopsy is not routinely a part of the diagnostic investigation of these infections.

Fibrosis and Fatty Infiltration

The factors that provoke interstitial fibrosis and fatty replacement of muscle have not been adequately investigated, but they are the bequest of chronic neuromuscular disease of both myopathic and neurogenic origin. Even the most seasoned pathologist experiences difficulty in interpreting the biopsy specimen with marked fibrosis or fatty infiltration because, at this juncture in the natural history of the disease, the active pathologic process has probably subsided and the opportunity of discovering specific pathologic changes is irretrievably lost. Because end-stage muscle is unlikely to provide information relevant to the patient's diagnosis, the biopsy of a severely involved muscle should be discouraged whenever possible.

OBSERVATIONS IN FROZEN SECTIONS

Atrophy and Hypertrophy

One of the most demanding challenges the surgical pathologist must face is the muscle biopsy specimen in which atrophy or hypertrophy is the major finding. The usefulness of histochemistry can be considerable in this situation. Because the muscle fiber depends on neural and other influences for survival, the disruption of these influences results in the atrophy of the fiber. The most common form of atrophy in neuromuscular disease is that caused by denervation. In addition, the maintenance of muscle fiber integrity requires regular activity. Disuse, as may occur with prolonged bed rest, can lead to muscle atrophy. Finally, a reduction in fiber volume may be a complication of aging, ischemia, or poor nutrition.

Hypertrophy, by comparison, is principally a consequence of an increase in muscular work, either during exercise or as a compensatory reaction of normal, intact fibers to the atrophy of others in their midst. In an evaluation of fiber size, the measurement of cell diameters may be fruitful. Morphometric analysis of the muscle specimen is indicated in the event that changes in fiber diameters are minimal and subtle. Morphometry can be performed manually with an eyepiece micrometer or electronically with a computer-assisted image analyzer (21). To obtain statistically significant morphometric data, the lesser diameter of each muscle fiber should be measured, and the minimum number of fibers in the sample should be 200.

TABLE 4.5
Diseases with Prominent Type 1 Fiber Atrophy
Myotonic dystrophy
Nemaline myopathy
Centronuclear myopathy
Congenital fiber–type disproportion

The atrophic or hypertrophic process may be selective, involving only one fiber type, or nonselective (22). Selective atrophy of type 1 fibers is seen most commonly in myotonic dystrophy, but is also seen in distal myopathy, nemaline myopathy, centronuclear myopathy, and congenital fiber–type disproportion (Table 4.5). Type 2 fiber atrophy (Fig. 4.15) is observed in myasthenia gravis, acute denervation, disuse, and systemic malignancy (23). In our experience, more than half of such cases are attributable to corticosteroid therapy (Table 4.6). Hypertrophy restricted to type 1 fibers is relatively specific for infantile spinal muscular atrophy (ISMA), although such hypertrophy may develop in normal athletes who undergo endurance training. Type 2 fiber hypertrophy has been reported in runners, notably sprinters, and in congenital fiber–type disproportion. Nonselective alterations in fiber size are somewhat uninformative from a diagnostic standpoint. Denervation accounts for a large proportion of cases of nonselective atrophy but certainly not all of them. Hypertrophy involving both major fiber types is frequently noted in limb-girdle dystrophy, inclusion body myositis, myotonia congenita, and acromegaly.

The pattern of atrophy may be diagnostic in some atrophic diseases. Grouped atrophy, which is recognized as a clustering of five or more small angular fibers, is essentially pathognomonic for chronic neurogenic disorders (Fig. 4.16). Panfascicular atrophy, an extreme version of grouped atrophy wherein the vast majority of fibers in each fascicle are severely atrophic, is a distinctive feature of ISMA. Perifascicular atrophy typifies DM, in which fiber atrophy is limited mainly to the periphery of the fascicles. Unfortunately, in many muscle biopsy specimens, atrophic fibers are randomly situated in the section. This pattern of atrophy is totally nonspecific.

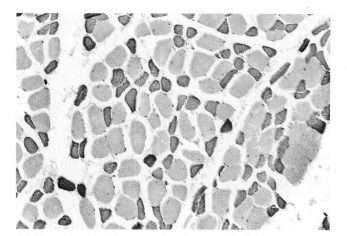

Figure 4.15. Type 2 atrophy in a patient with malignancy and cachexia (immunostain for fast myosin).

TABLE 4.6

Diseases with Prominent Type 2 Fiber Atrophy

Corticosteroid therapy and hypercorticoidism
Myasthenia gravis
Disuse atrophy
Acute denervation
Paraneoplastic myopathy

Fiber Shape

Assessing fiber shape may be more advantageous in frozen sections than in paraffin sections because the fiber arrangement is more compact in the latter. In contrast to the normal polygonal contour of the myofiber viewed in the transverse plane, rounded fibers favor a myopathic process, particularly muscular dystrophy or congenital myopathy. In denervating diseases, excluding ISMA, which is characterized by rounded atrophic fibers, the atrophic fibers are angular or ensiform (Fig. 4.17). These fibers appear flattened and narrow with tapered or pointed ends. Angulated fibers are also found in myasthenia gravis, disuse, myotonic dystrophy, and steroid myopathy.

CHANGES IN THE HISTOCHEMICAL PROFILE

The normal checkerboard staining paradigm that is so familiar in histoenzymatic reactions may fall victim to certain pathologic conditions. Predominance of one fiber population is emblematic of the congenital myopathies. Type 1 fiber predominance is found in central core disease, nemaline myopathy, centronuclear myopathy, and some cases of congenital fiber–type disproportion (Table 4.7). In chronic denervation, the normal checkerboard pattern is replaced by large groups of fibers with identical histochemical properties. So-called type grouping (Fig. 4.18) is a result of reinnervation of the denervated muscle (24). Normal anatomic and physiologic principles help to explain type grouping. The muscle fibers in each motor unit are of a single histochemical type. The neuron, through its axon and intramuscular branches (nerve twigs), which innervate the individual fibers, governs the fiber type in the motor unit. Reinnervation of a type 1 fiber by a type 2 nerve twig has been shown experimentally to convert the fiber from type 1 to type 2. The

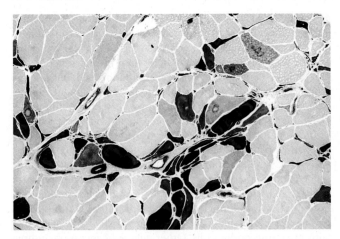

Figure 4.17. Neurogenic atrophy. Many atrophic fibers are angular (adenosine triphosphatase, pH 9.4).

opposite occurs with a type 2 fiber and a type 1 twig. Thus, when neighboring denervated fibers of differing histochemical types undergo reinnervation by collateral sprouts from a single axon that has remained viable, all of the fibers are converted to one histochemical type, and type grouping results.

Fiber Splitting

Muscle fibers that have become hypertrophic are most likely to split into smaller subunits of two or more smaller fibers that appear to be mature myocytes with intact sarcoplasm. Before splitting is concluded, the fiber assumes a segmented appearance as slitlike spaces form invaginations between individual segments (Fig. 4.19). Within each space, the extensions of the plasma membrane remain continuous around the dividing portions of the cell. Fiber splitting is conspicuous in limb-girdle dystrophy and in some cases of denervation and inclusion body myositis (25).

Mottled Fibers

The peculiar, uneven staining reaction of mottled or moth-eaten fibers is satisfactorily demonstrated only in oxidative enzyme preparations. Multiple minute zones of weak enzyme activity with irregular and poorly delimited borders are randomly dispersed in the sarcoplasm (Fig. 4.20). Ultrastructurally, mottled areas reveal a lack of mitochondria and the destruction of the myofilaments. The fact that the ultrastructural integrity of much of the cell sarcoplasm between the zones of mottling is preserved upholds the notion that the mottled fiber has the capacity for recovery and that it represents a form of reversible injury. Moth-eaten fibers are numerous in facioscapulohumeral

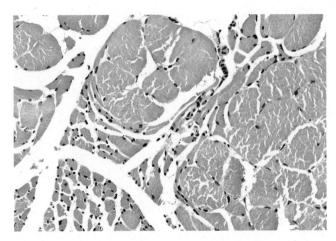

Figure 4.16. Chronic neurogenic atrophy. Grouping of many small angular fibers is evident.

TABLE 4.7

Diseases with Fiber Type Predominance

Central core disease (type 1)
Multicore disease (type 1)
Nemaline myopathy (type 1)
Centronuclear myopathy (type 1)
Denervation with type grouping (type 1, type 2, or both)

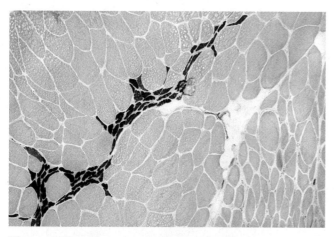

Figure 4.18. Chronic denervation with reinnervation. Type grouping replaces the normal checkerboard staining pattern (adenosine triphosphatase, pH 9.4).

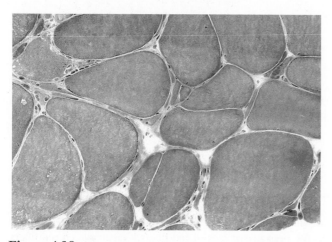

Figure 4.19. Fiber splitting. Several hypertrophic fibers are seen. The fiber at the bottom and center is divided into two smaller subunits (frozen section, rapid Gomori trichrome).

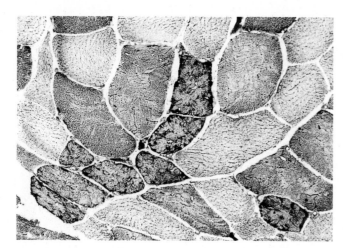

Figure 4.20. Mottled fibers. The sarcoplasm appears moth eaten as a result of the presence of patchy areas of poor staining (nicotinamide adenine dinucleotide, reduced).

and limb-girdle dystrophy and, in a review of our experience, denervation.

Cores and Targets

Oxidative enzyme reactions are the ideal technique for identifying cores that appear as regions of depleted or absent enzyme activity (Fig. 4.21). Ultrastructurally and in resin sections, distinguishing between structured and unstructured cores is possible (26). The cross-banding pattern is evident in the structured core, whereas cross striations are absent from the unstructured core, which perhaps represents a later stage in core development. Cores cannot be regarded as a specific pathologic finding because they occur in a variety of diseases. In our experience, they are most prevalent in neurogenic atrophy, being encountered more frequently than target fibers. As a nonspecific change, cores are present in less than 10% of fibers, whereas they are numerous and are located more often in type 1 fibers in central core disease. Although cores are single and centrally placed within the fiber in classic central core disease, they may be multiple and eccentric in other conditions.

For diagnostic purposes, target fibers are considered pathognomonic for neurogenic atrophy (27), but unfortunately, they are identified in less than 25% of cases. Despite certain similarities, targets and cores differ in several ways. The target has a greater diameter than the core, and it virtually always occurs singularly within the fiber. As opposed to the core, which extends the entire length of the fiber, the target typically spans only a few sarcomeres. Of greatest significance is the three-zone structure of the target fiber. The central zone, which resembles the unstructured core, is surrounded by an intermediate zone, which is darkly stained in oxidative enzyme reactions (Fig. 4.22). This rim, which is not part of a core lesion, sharply contrasts with the third zone, the outer normal portion of the fiber. The term *targetoid* refers to corelike lesions that lack the intermediate zone or rim of increased oxidative enzyme activity. *Targetoids* and *cores* essentially are identical, and the terms are often used interchangeably.

Nemaline Rods

Rods were first recognized in nemaline myopathy, a congenital and nonprogressive muscle disease of childhood (28). The

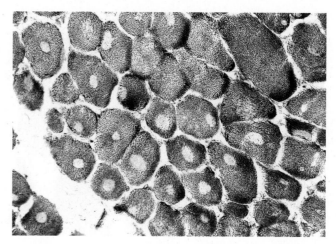

Figure 4.21. Central core disease. The focal areas of reduced enzyme activity are single, and they are centrally positioned within many fibers (nicotinamide adenine dinucleotide, reduced).

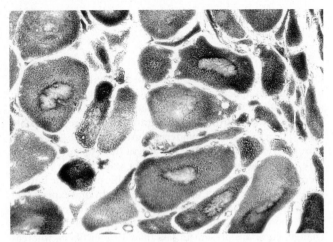

Figure 4.22. Neurogenic atrophy. In target fibers, an inner, un-stained zone is surrounded by a rim of increased enzyme activity (nico-tinamide adenine dinucleotide, reduced).

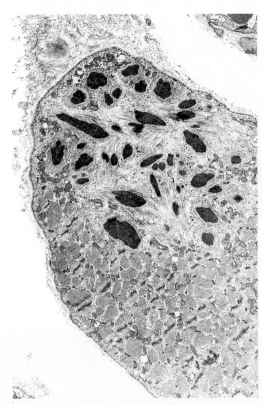

Figure 4.24. Nemaline myopathy. Ultrastructurally, rods are osmio-philic and elongated or rectangular, resembling Z-bands.

name *nemaline* is derived from the Greek root *nema* ("thread" or "threadlike") to emphasize the pathologic marker of this disorder. The threads or rods tend to cluster beneath the sarco-lemma. Rods easily escape detection in H&E sections, and they are suitably visualized in RTC stains on frozen sections (Fig. 4.23) or in resin sections. Ultrastructurally, the rods are osmio-philic oblong or rectangular structures with a greatest dimen-sion of 6 to 7 μm (Fig. 4.24). Their latticelike appearance resem-bles that of the normal Z-band (29), lending credence to the concept that they originate from, and perhaps are proliferations of, Z-bands. Since the original description of nemaline myopa-thy, it has become increasingly evident that rods are not unique to a single disease entity. Occasional rods in a small number of fibers have been reported in muscle specimens of muscular dystrophy and PM, for example. One cannot be comfortable with the diagnosis of nemaline myopathy unless, in the appro-priate clinical setting, many fibers in the specimen contain rods and they are numerous within each fiber.

Mitochondrial Abnormalities

Abnormalities of mitochondria occur in a wide variety of dis-eases (30–32). They may be generalized disorders, or they may be limited to skeletal muscle. The mitochondrial abnormalities are similar in all of these diseases, and they are often recognized by the presence of ragged red fibers. Classic ragged red fibers are readily identified by the RTC method, in which intensely red, subsarcolemmal protrusions from the cell surface give the margins of involved fibers an irregular, ragged appearance (Fig. 4.25). Such fibers are surrounded by prominent, sometimes

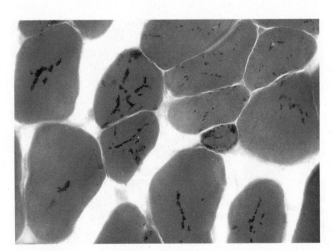

Figure 4.23. Nemaline myopathy. Collections of dark, rod-shaped structures are evident in many of the fibers (frozen section, rapid Go-mori trichrome).

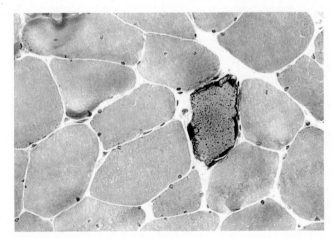

Figure 4.25. Ragged red fiber. Collections of mitochondria appear as red-stained, irregular, subsarcolemmal areas within the involved fiber (frozen section, rapid Gomori trichrome).

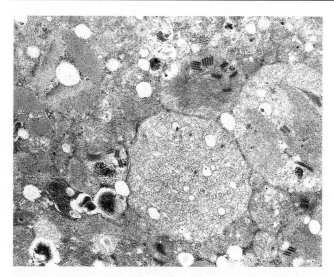

Figure 4.26. Mitochondrial myopathy. Ragged red fiber is seen with abnormally large mitochondria, several of which contain paracrystalline inclusions.

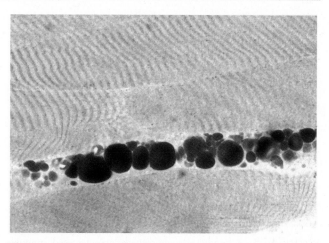

Figure 4.27. Lipid storage myopathy. Numerous osmiophilic, lipid-containing vacuoles are evident in the sarcoplasm of the fiber at the center (resin section, toluidine blue).

dilated capillaries that appear to indent them and to be increased in number. Ragged red fibers are equally impressive in oxidative enzyme reactions, especially succinate dehydrogenase reactions, in which large collections of mitochondria are seen as dark, coarsely granular deposits that not only may be subsarcolemmal but may also diffuse throughout the fiber.

Electron microscopy shows that ragged red fibers contain accumulations of mitochondria that are enlarged and deformed. Their cristae are excessively numerous and disorganized, or they may be concentrically arranged. Among the commonly encountered matrix inclusions are glycogen aggregates, clear vacuoles, floccular densities, myelin figures, and paracrystalline structures having a square or rectangular conformation and resembling a parking lot or grid (Fig. 4.26). Paracrystalline inclusions appear to arise from neighboring cristae and to consist of parallel, intersecting membranes separated by lucent spaces. These inclusions contain mitochondrial creatine kinase and perhaps other proteins.

Vacuolar Change

Vacuoles may contain abnormal quantities of glycogen or lipid (Table 4.8). Hence, routine microscopic sections with vacuolar change of an unexplained nature should be stained with PAS and oil red O or other suitable fat stains. We prefer to use resin sections, in which the osmiophilic fat deposits are more clearly demonstrated than they are in routine fat stains (Fig. 4.27). An abundance of lipid within myofibers is a relatively specific finding that is usually indicative of a lipid storage disease or mitochondrial myopathy, with the latter frequently being recognized by the presence of ragged red fibers. Although deposits of glycogen raise the specter of carbohydrate storage disease or other disorders affecting glycogen metabolism, such as hypothyroidism (33), they can be an incidental, fortuitous finding in virtually any disorder. Especially when only one or two fibers in the specimen are involved and the vacuoles are crescentlike, subsarcolemmal, and visible primarily in PAS stains, they are probably of no clinical significance.

The so-called rimmed vacuole has received attention as a diagnostic criterion of oculopharyngeal dystrophy (34), distal myopathy (35), and inclusion body myositis (36). The vacuole is sharply demarcated and is filled with granular material (Fig. 4.28) that may form a surrounding red rim in RTC stains performed on frozen sections. Ultrastructurally, this type of vacuole is not always enclosed by a membrane, and it contains whorling membranous profiles in addition to tubular filaments. The rimmed vacuole is believed to be derived from the autophagic vacuole, which classically is membrane bound and is a repository for the debris of autodigestion.

NEUROMUSCULAR DISEASES

The muscle biopsy is only one facet of the overall diagnostic evaluation of the patient. It must not be interpreted in a vacuum

TABLE 4.8	Sarcoplasmic Vacuoles Seen in the Biopsy Specimen
Pathologic Features	*Disease*
In center of specimen, often arranged in size gradient	Freezing artifact
Often subsarcolemmal, PAS positive	Glycogen storage
In scattered fibers; small, round, osmiophilic; ORO positive	Lipid storage, mitochondrial myopathies
Rimmed, ubiquitin-positive	IBM, distal myopathy, OPMD
IBM, inclusion body myositis; OPMD, oculopharyngeal dystrophy; ORO, oil red O; PAS, periodic acid-Schiff.	

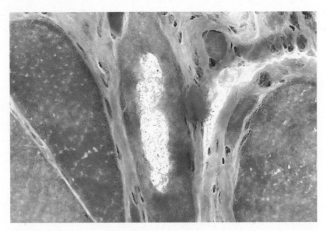

Figure 4.28. A rimmed vacuole contains abundant red, granular material (frozen section, rapid Gomori trichrome).

without a consideration of the clinical history, physical examination findings, and the results of all pertinent laboratory tests. This section provides the background needed to interpret the biopsy findings in the context of the clinical setting. Those neuromuscular diseases that are most often encountered and in which the muscle biopsy significantly contributes to the diagnosis are emphasized. An abbreviated classification of neuromuscular disease, which is based on more than 25 years of experience and 5000 consecutive, unselected muscle biopsies performed at our institution, is provided in Table 4.9. The percentage of cases in each major category offers a relative idea of the incidence of disease in the general population and certainly of the diseases likely to come to biopsy. From a statistical standpoint, the most important neuromuscular diseases are either inflammatory (28% of cases) or neurogenic (27% of cases), more than 80% of which are associated with peripheral neuropathy. Despite our best efforts, we were unable to render a diagnosis in approximately 5% of biopsies, so the diagnosis in these pathologic reports must be descriptive without a definitive interpretation.

MUSCULAR DYSTROPHIES

The rather meaningless term *dystrophy*, which literally means "deficient nutrition," was popularized toward the close of the

TABLE 4.9

Incidence of Neuromuscular Diseases Based on 5000 Muscle Biopsies Performed at the State University of New York, Buffalo

Disease	Percentage (%)
Inflammatory myopathies	28
Neurogenic diseases	27
Metabolic diseases	20
Miscellaneous	11
Dystrophies	6
Congenital myopathies	3
No definitive diagnosis	5

nineteenth century, when the pathogenesis of the muscular dystrophies was totally mysterious. The muscular dystrophies, which share certain clinical and pathologic attributes, have long been considered part of a common rubric. In general, the initial symptoms are manifested during childhood or young adulthood. The cardinal symptom is muscular weakness that is steadily and unremittingly progressive. Most forms of dystrophy are genetic (Table 4.10); hence, a family history of similar symptoms can be elicited in many cases. However, each dystrophy is in fact a unique entity with its own special features. The pathologic criteria of fiber necrosis, regeneration, and reactive fibrosis that once unified this group of myopathies are obsolete. Except for the Duchenne and Becker forms of dystrophy, these findings occur in the latest stages of disease but not in biopsy specimens.

Duchenne Muscular Dystrophy

Duchenne muscular dystrophy (DMD) is not only the most common member of this family of diseases, but it is also the most malignant and relentless. According to genetic mapping studies, the DMD gene is located in band Xp21 of the short arm of the X chromosome (37,38). The gene has been identified as a 14-kb coding sequence within 2.5 to 3.0 Mb of DNA, and it is the largest known human gene. Presumably, the extraordinary size of the gene is responsible for the high rate of mutations, accounting for approximately two-thirds of DMD cases. With the use of complementary DNA probes, exonic or multiple exonic deletions have been demonstrated in 65% of patients with DMD (39). The identification of such deletions permits an accurate diagnosis, including carrier and prenatal detection (40). Patients with DMD lack the gene product dystrophin, a 427-kd, rod-shaped protein that is found predominantly in skeletal muscle and also in smooth and cardiac muscle (41). Dystrophin is localized to the sarcolemmal membrane and is presumed to promote membrane stability, particularly during muscle contraction (42,43). Dystrophin has been shown to be attached to the sarcolemma by a transmembrane glycoprotein complex (see "Limb-Girdle Dystrophy" section), with the N-terminal being bound to F-actin within the sarcoplasm and the C-terminal being bound to β-dystroglycan (44), in addition to dystrobrevin and syntrophin (Fig. 4.29).

As an X-linked recessively inherited disorder, DMD almost exclusively affects boys who are neurologically intact at birth. However, by the time the child attempts to stand or walk, the first signs of overt disease are noticeable. A subtle awkwardness gradually gives way to pelvifemoral and scapulohumeral weakness, sparing the muscles of facial expression and swallowing. A paradoxical enlargement of selected muscles that also are weak and flabby is characteristic of DMD. This pseudohypertrophy, which is associated with fatty infiltration and reactive fibrosis, is especially apparent in the calves and buttocks. Mild mental stolidity that cannot be explained on the basis of physical incapacitation is considered intrinsic to the disease. Death is often hastened by an insidious cardiomyopathy leading to sinus tachycardia, cardiac arrhythmias, and congestive heart failure. An extremely high level of serum creatine kinase is an early indicator of this form of dystrophy, and it may actually precede the pathologic alterations in muscle.

In the muscle biopsy specimen, fiber necrosis and regeneration are much more striking and more widespread than in other dystrophies, as are the large number of hyaline fibers. Necrotic and regenerating fibers are frequently seen in clusters. Patchy

TABLE 4.10	Genetics of Neuromuscular Disease	
Disease	*Gene (Protein)*	*Chromosome*
Dystrophinopathies		
Duchenne	Dystrophin	Xp21
Becker	Dystrophin	Xp21
Facioscapulohumeral dystrophy	FRGI?	4q35
Limb-girdle muscular dystrophies		
LGMD 1A	Myotilin	5q31
LGMD 1B	LMNA (laminA/C)	1q21
LGMD 1C	CAV3 (caveolin3)	3p25
LGMD 2A	CAPN3 (calpain3)	15q15
LGMD 2B	DYSF (dysferlin)	2p12–24
LGMD 2C	γ-Sarcoglycan	13q12
LGMD 2D	α-Sarcoglycan	17q21
LGMD 2E	β-Sarcoglycan	4q12
LGMD 2F	δ-Sarcoglycan	5q33–34
LGMD 2G	Telethonin	17q11–12
LGMD 2H	TRIM32	9q31–34
LGMD 2I	Fukutin-related protein	19q13.3
LGMD 2J	Titin	2q31
LGMD 2K	POMT1	9q34
Oculopharyngeal muscular dystrophy	PABP2	14q11–13
Congenital muscular dystrophy		
Fukuyama type	FCMD (fukutin)	9q31–33
Merosin deficiency	LAMA2 (laminin α2)	6q2
Myotonic muscular dystrophy	DMPK (myotonin kinase)	19q13.2–13.3
Congenital myopathies		
Central core disease	RYR1	19q12–13.1
Nemaline myopathy	TPM3 (α-tropomyosin)	1q22
	NEB (nebulin)	2q13–33
Centronuclear myopathy (X-linked)	MTM1 (myotubularin)	Xq27–28
Myofibrillar myopathy	Desmin	2q35
	CRYAB (αβ-crystalline)	11q21–33

?, possibly.

endomysial fibrosis, a predictable nonspecific reaction to injury in chronic muscle disease, is conspicuous during the early phases of DMD, and it is disproportionately greater than the destruction of muscle cells. Immunostains are now available for detecting membrane-associated dystrophin (45,46). Whereas normal muscle specimens contain fibers that virtually all stain positively (Fig. 4.30), in DMD, very few, if any, fibers show sarcolemmal staining. The absence of immunoreactivity is essentially diagnostic of the disease.

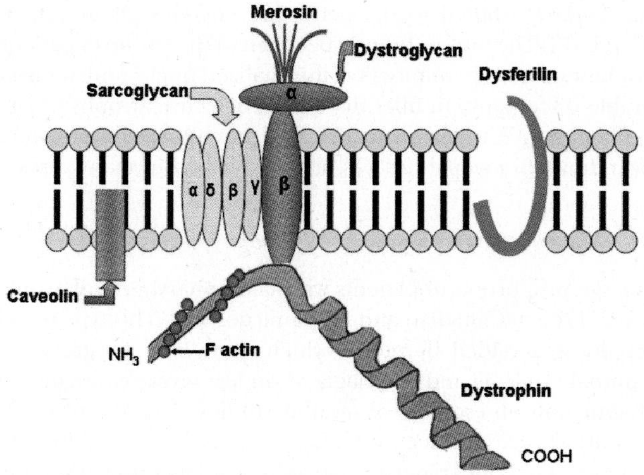

BECKER MUSCULAR DYSTROPHY

DMD is allelic with Becker dystrophy, a mild form of X-linked dystrophy. The symptoms in Becker dystrophy are less severe than in DMD, and the rate of progression is slower. Although patients with DMD lack dystrophin, the muscle of patients with Becker dystrophy typically contains dystrophin, which may be sufficient in quantity but is abnormal in molecular size or structure (47,48). The pathologic changes are similar to, but less severe than, those of DMD.

Facioscapulohumeral Dystrophy

Facioscapulohumeral dystrophy is a comparatively mild myopathy that principally involves the voluntary musculature of the face, shoulders, and upper extremities. This disease exhibits an autosomal dominant inheritance pattern in most families, with an onset in the second and third decades. The gene locus is believed to be in the q35 subtelomeric region of chromosome 4 (49). The normal gene locus, near or within the FRG1 gene,

Figure 4.29. Sarcoplasmic membrane demonstrating the relationship of dystrophin to dystrophin-associated glycoproteins.

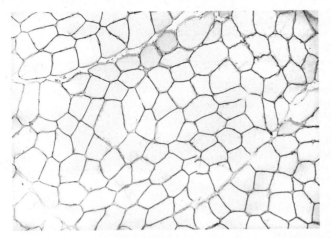

Figure 4.30. Normal immunostaining pattern for dystrophin. The sarcolemmal regions of the fibers are outlined.

is comprised of 11 to 100 D_4Z_4 repeats (50,51). By a deletion process within the 3.3-kb portion of the gene, the number of repeats in facioscapulohumeral dystrophy is reduced to fewer than nine. Muscle pseudohypertrophy is not an expected part of the clinical picture, as it is in DMD, nor is a loss of mental agility or cardiac dysfunction. The biopsy specimen reveals many atrophic muscle fibers, often clustered or grouped together, in the absence of significant fiber necrosis or regeneration. Moth-eaten fibers tend to be numerous in oxidative enzyme reactions. The presence of inflammatory cells, which are visualized as small foci of perivascular mature lymphocytes, separates facioscapulohumeral dystrophy from the other dystrophies in which this pattern of inflammation is absent. The inflammation is associated with the early stages of disease, and it becomes less remarkable with the passage of time.

Limb-Girdle Dystrophy

Limb-girdle dystrophy is not a single disease entity, but rather a collection of myopathies tenuously bound together by a common thread—the involvement of proximal axial muscles (52). Most cases are characterized by an onset in late adolescence or young adulthood, the gradual deterioration of muscle function over a long time span, and autosomal recessive inheritance (types 2A to 2K), although dominant inheritance is also known (types 1A to 1D). Pseudohypertrophy is noted in approximately one-third of patients. Some cases have been associated with a sarcoglycan deficiency, most commonly a lack of adhalin or α-sarcoglycan, for which the abnormal gene locus is at 17q12 (53). To date, four sarcoglycans (α to δ) have been described. Cases of recessively inherited limb-girdle dystrophy have been reported in association with an absence of each of these sarcoglycans (54). The sarcoglycans are a transmembrane complex adjacent to the dystroglycan couplet to which dystrophin is connected. In summary, the types 2C, 2D, 2E, and 2F sarcoglycanopathies have been related to genetic defects on chromosome loci 13q12, 17q12–21, 4q12, and 5q33, respectively. Type 2A is caused by a mutation in the gene coding for calpain 3, a calcium-activated protease.

Type 2B has emerged as perhaps the most common of the limb-girdle dystrophies and deserves more attention. Type 2B shares the same gene locus as Miyoshi-type distal myopathy but

is phenotypically quite distinct. The dysferlin gene, DYSF, is a large 150-kb coding region on chromosome 2p13 that codes for a membrane-associated protein (55). Dysferlinopathy has an onset in young adults with proximal weakness more pronounced in the legs and a very high serum creatine kinase. A more recently described limb-girdle dystrophy involves the Z-band–associated protein telethonin, the gene locus for which is chromosome 17q11–12 (56). These patients present at age 2 to 15 years with proximal and distal muscle involvement. Mutations in the gene for titin were first described in patients from Finland (57). Some authors classify titinopathy, a dominantly inherited late-onset myopathy, as a distal myopathy because there is predominant lower leg involvement. The salient histologic abnormalities in the limb-girdle dystrophies as a whole are marked nuclear internalization and a variability in fiber diameters that is accentuated by dramatic fiber hypertrophy. The hypertrophic process induces fiber splitting, which may be widespread. Dysferlinopathy is distinguished by mild chronic inflammation. Immunostains may show upregulation of major histocompatibility complex (MHC) class I antigen on muscle fiber membranes. Rimmed vacuoles are found in cases of telethonin and titin deficiency.

Distal Myopathy

Distal myopathy, which has a debatable lineage as a true dystrophy because of its rather atypical clinical features, is a rare illness that has been regarded by some as a variant of inclusion body myositis. At least four forms of this heterogeneous disease have been described in addition to the hereditary variant of inclusion body myositis. The largest experience with this disorder comes from the Scandinavian countries, where the Welander form of distal myopathy is dominantly inherited; this form occurs more frequently in males and progresses in indolent fashion. The initial expressions of disease are not detected until the ages of 50 to 70 years, and distal, not proximal, muscles are primarily affected. Welander myopathy is linked to chromosome 2p13, suggesting that it is allelic with Miyoshi myopathy, an early-onset distal myopathy with recessive inheritance. Miyoshi myopathy, which has been described in Japan and other parts of Asia, has been mapped to 2p12–14, which is the locus of the dysferlin gene. Several non-Scandinavian forms of late-onset, dominantly inherited, distal myopathies remain poorly understood. One of these, which is also classified as limb-girdle dystrophy type 2G, has been attributed to the gene that encodes telethonin on 17q11–12. The muscle biopsy specimen in this group of patients contains abnormal numbers of internalized nuclei and a considerable discrepancy in fiber diameters. Selective atrophy of type 1 fibers in Welander myopathy and rimmed vacuoles in non-Scandinavian myopathies has been described in many cases.

Oculopharyngeal Muscular Dystrophy

A large proportion of patients with oculopharyngeal dystrophy are of French-Canadian and Hispanic descent. This type of dystrophy is heralded by ptosis, which sometimes progresses to ophthalmoplegia and dysphagia or, in less severe cases, muscle dysfunction on esophageal motility studies. A cardiomyopathy causing cardiac conduction defects has been reported in some patients. Oculopharyngeal dystrophy is a late-onset myopathy that begins in middle life and has a benign outcome. The musculature reveals mild dystrophic change with nuclear internalization, fiber atrophy, and interstitial fibrosis. In many cases, a distinctive aspect of the pathologic picture is the presence of rimmed vacuoles. Electron microscopic examination of the muscle tissue may reveal nuclear inclusions composed of unbranched tubulofilamentous structures with an outer diameter of 8.5 nm (Fig. 4.12). These inclusions contain the protein PABP2, which accumulates in the sarcolemmal nuclei as a result of short expansions of GCG repeats in the poly(A) binding protein gene on chromosome 14q11–13. The normal coding region has six triplet repeats, whereas in this dominantly inherited disorder, small $(GCG)_{8-13}$ expanded segments are found in the affected PABP2 gene (58).

Myotonic Muscular Dystrophy

Myotonic muscular dystrophy (MyD) is a common multiple-organ disorder. Its prevalence exceeds that of DMD in some geographic regions of the United States. Although MyD is dominantly inherited, the penetrance is quite unpredictable, so the age at onset ranges from infancy to later adulthood, typically during the third or fourth decade, and the combinations of clinical symptoms are variable. Muscle weakness is first expressed in the facial muscles and the acral muscles of the extremities. Among the classic presenting signs are ptosis, an expressionless visage, and dysphagia. Myotonia, an inability of the muscle to relax once it has contracted, is a sine qua non of MyD, and this generally is one of the first signals of impending myopathy. This curious manifestation of membrane instability may be elicited by vigorous voluntary muscle contraction or by percussion with a reflex hammer. Using electromyography (EMG) to substantiate myotonia may be necessary when it is clinically silent. Common systemic manifestations include cataracts in 90% of patients, testicular atrophy, diabetes mellitus and other endocrine disturbances, cardiomyopathy, and mild dementia. Special radiologic and physiologic techniques are able to demonstrate smooth muscle dysfunction in the gut, urinary bladder, and uterus. The MyD gene, which is 200 kb in length, is located in the q13.2–13.3 region of chromosome 19. A mutation in the gene is associated with an insertion of CTG repeats (59). The normal gene has up to 40 repeats, whereas the MyD gene may contain from 50 to several hundred repeats (60). The MyD gene codes for myotonin protein kinase, the function of which is unclear.

When the muscle tissue is studied at an early stage of the disease, a multitude of pyknotic internal nuclei, selective atrophy of type 1 fibers, and ring fibers are encountered. In material obtained from patients with chronic, long-standing MyD, finding dystrophic changes—fiber destruction, regeneration, and reactive fibrosis—is not surprising.

CONGENITAL MYOPATHIES

Although the designation *congenital myopathy* has become thoroughly entrenched in the medical lexicon and is unlikely to be replaced by an alternate term in the near future, it is imprecise and misleading. For example, data indicate that certain myopathies that are congenital in a true sense, such as some lipid and glycogen storage diseases, are arbitrarily excluded from this designation. Furthermore, despite the name, the symptoms are not invariably present at birth.

Nonetheless, these conditions share several features. The patient frequently is afflicted at an early age, exhibiting signs of the floppy infant syndrome (61). Such a child suffers from weakness that is more extreme proximally, hypotonia, and listlessness. As inherited diseases, cases of congenital myopathy are often familial. In contrast to the dystrophies, the congenital myopathies follow a clinical course that is quite benign and that, at times, remits. Because the congenital myopathies are not easily distinguished on clinical grounds, muscle biopsy is an indispensable diagnostic tool. The application of techniques such as enzyme histochemistry and electron microscopy beginning in the late 1950s fostered the discovery of several previously unrecognized neuromuscular diseases, some of which had formally been relegated to the realm of the muscular dystrophies, and launched a new era in diagnostic pathology. As a result, many of the congenital myopathies are named for a characteristic, if not a unique, morphologic attribute.

Central Core Disease

Central core disease was the first in a long succession of congenital myopathies to be delineated (62). In most cases, a lack of muscular vitality is noted in infancy, and this condition is the legacy of its dominant inheritance. The gene locus has been discovered in the q13.1 band of chromosome 19 (63). More than 17 missense mutations have been reported in the RYR1 gene, the majority of which involve the N terminus or the rod domains of the ryanodine receptor protein that is a portion of the calcium release channel of the sarcoplasmic reticulum. Mutations of the RYR1 gene predispose the individual to malignant hyperthermia. Muscle involvement is likely to be mild, proximal, and nonprogressive. In the biopsy specimen, a multiplicity of muscle fibers harbor a single, centrally located defect or core. More than one core per fiber may be encountered, and the proportion of core-containing fibers is inconsistent from case to case. A predominance of type 1 fibers is frequently evident in this condition.

Multicore Disease

Multicore (minicore) disease is characterized by type 1 fiber predominance and minute corelike structures in the majority of muscle fibers. Multicores, which tend to be numerous within each fiber, are often globular or sometimes disklike in longitudinal sections (Fig. 4.31). Such cores are pale in most stains, including PAS, trichrome, and NADH-TR. Ultrastructurally, the cores exhibit disorganization of the myofibrils and the loss of organelles, such as mitochondria. At least some cases of multicore disease may actually be a form of central core disease, inasmuch as their gene locus is also on 19q13 and the RYR1 gene is involved (64,65). Clinically, multicore disease is a congenital, usually nonprogressive myopathy in which generalized weakness and hypotonia are seen (66,67). In some patients, the facial or extraocular muscles are involved.

Nemaline (Rod) Myopathy

Nemaline myopathy, which is more prevalent in females, may be transmitted as a dominant or recessive trait. Mutations have been detected in five thin filament genes, including slow α-tropomyosin (TPM3) and nebulin (NEB) (68). The ebbing of strength is often more pronounced in the facial and proximal limb muscles. Facial dysmorphism in which the face is elongated, the jaw is prognathic, and the palate is highly vaulted

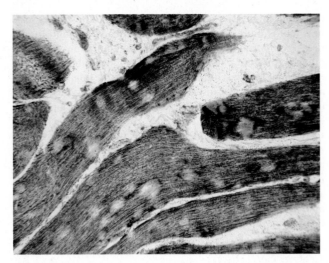

Figure 4.31. Multicore disease. Numerous small globular-shaped cores are seen in the fibers. Cores appear unstained with oxidative enzyme reactions (nicotinamide adenine dinucleotide, reduced).

may alert the clinician to the diagnosis. Histochemical reactions reveal a selective atrophy of oxidative fibers in some cases. The rods tend to be located in the majority of fibers, and they are very numerous.

Centronuclear Myopathy

In centronuclear myopathy, the genetic determinants and the age at onset are not at all uniform. The pattern of inheritance may be dominant, recessive, or X-linked. In X-linked disease, the abnormal gene MTM1 is located on chromosome Xq27–28. More than 140 mutations have been reported in MTM1, which encodes myotubularin with an active site of tyrosine phosphatase (69). The disease may be fully expressed in infancy, or it may emerge from apparent dormancy at any time from childhood to the seventh decade. Some progression of weakness is typical, but the degree of disability is variable. Extraocular palsies and facial asthenia occur simultaneously with the involvement of the appendicular muscles. Pathologically, a central or paracentral nucleus that is identified within most muscle fibers resembles those indigenous to the fetal myotube stage of development—hence, the application of the term *myotubular myopathy* to this disorder (70). The theory that this entity may represent an arrest in muscle maturation in utero has not met with enthusiastic acceptance. These nuclei exceed the normal size, and they have a vesicular chromatin network (Fig. 4.32). The sarcoplasm surrounding the central nucleus is disrupted ultrastructurally, and it may appear clear or vacuolated in frozen sections. The fibers, as if they are mimicking myotubes, contain few, if any, nuclei in a sarcolemmal or peripheral location.

Congenital Fiber–Type Disproportion

Name chosen for this myopathy is somewhat unsatisfactory because it fails to specify the essential pathologic findings—the atrophy of type 1 fibers and the hypertrophy of type 2 fibers (Fig. 4.33). Glycolytic fibers may be rare as a result of the type 1 predominance. When congenital fiber–type disproportion occurs in families, it is assumed to be an inherited affliction, but the mechanism of inheritance has not been firmly established.

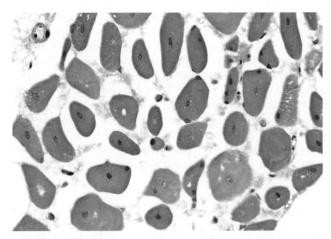

Figure 4.32. Centronuclear myopathy. Most fibers contain a central or paracentral nucleus.

The harbingers of this illness, which are frequently detectable at birth, are a paucity of motor activity and diminished muscle tone. The deterioration of muscle function tends to continue throughout the first decade and then to cease or even to undergo reversal. Skeletal deformities, which are exemplified by hip dislocation, kyphoscoliosis, and joint contractures, occur in more than half of all patients (71).

Myofibrillar Myopathies

This heterogeneous group of diseases, also known as the protein surplus myopathies (72,73), is characterized by the accumulation of intermediate filaments including desmin, actin, myosin, αβ-crystalline, and myotilin within the fibers, only one of which is generally overabundant in a given patient. These accumulations typically form some sort of sarcoplasmic inclusions or foci of myofibrillar material that can best be seen in frozen sections. These are often adult-onset, autosomal dominantly inherited, slowly progressive conditions that feature myopathy with wasting. Affected patients have distal weakness, dysphagia, and cardiac muscle involvement. The best known type is desmin myopa-

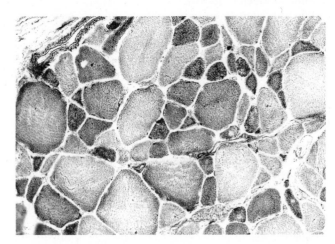

Figure 4.33. Congenital fiber–type disproportion with hypertrophy of some type 2 fibers and atrophy of type 1 fibers (nicotinamide adenine dinucleotide, reduced).

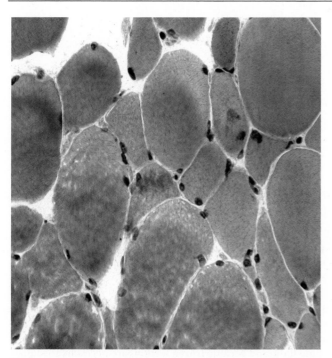

Figure 4.34. Desmin myopathy. Two fibers contain slightly basophilic smudged regions within the sarcoplasm, which represent collections of myofibrillar material (frozen section, rapid Gomori trichrome).

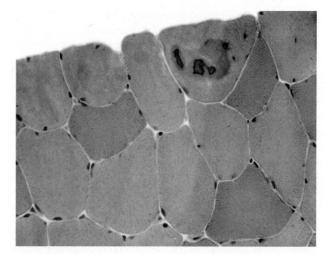

Figure 4.35. Cytoplasmic body. Circumscribed inclusion with three dense, red central foci surrounded by green filamentous material (paraffin, Gomori trichrome stain).

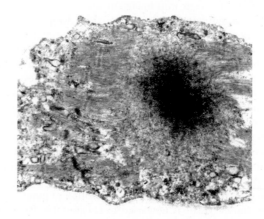

Figure 4.36. Under the electron microscope, the cytoplasmic body is composed of a dense osmiophilic filamentous core surrounded by a more lucent array of filaments radiating outward.

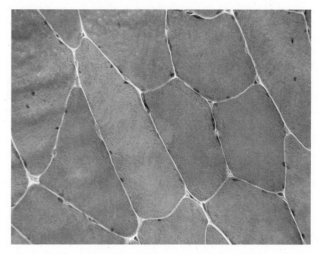

Figure 4.37. Hyaline body has distinct margins and a subsarcolemmal location. The finely red granular appearance of the mitochondria in the normal sarcoplasm is absent from the more dense, homogeneous look of the hyaline body (frozen section, rapid Gomori trichrome).

thy, a disease with an onset usually in childhood or early adulthood (74). In some cases, a missense mutation or deletion involves the desmin gene located on 2q35 (75). In a similar phenotype, mutations in the CRYAB gene on chromosome 11q21–23 that encodes αβ-crystalline, a cytoplasmic heat shock protein, have been reported. In frozen sections stained with RTC, smudged, basophilic, or purple filamentous areas are seen in the sarcoplasm of some fibers (Fig. 4.34). These are unstained in NADH-TR reactions but are highlighted in immunostains for desmin. Under the electron microscope, such regions contain electron-dense accumulations that are both granular and filamentous. They often are arranged in register with the Z-bands. A second feature of desmin myopathy is the presence of cytoplasmic bodies. These are best seen in RTC stains that allow identification of one or two dense, red-staining centers surrounded by lighter, green-staining regions with a circumscribed border (Fig. 4.35). Under the electron microscope, cytoplasmic bodies are filamentous and feature a dark center surrounded by loosely arranged radiating fibrils (Fig. 4.36). Hyaline bodies are the mark of hyaline body myopathy, which may present as the scapuloperoneal syndrome. Hyaline bodies contain myosin, and in some cases, mutations of the MYH7 myosin gene located on chromosome 14q have been described. Hyaline bodies tend to be round, well circumscribed, and subsarcolemmal (Fig. 4.37). They have an opaque quality when compared with the surrounding normal sarcoplasm. They are composed of filamentous material when studied by electron microscopy.

INFLAMMATORY AND IMMUNE-MEDIATED MYOPATHIES

Polymyositis and Dermatomyositis

Polymyositis (PM) and dermatomyositis (DM) are common myopathies in adults. They are more prevalent in women between the ages of 20 and 40 years. The muscular weakness is proximal, somewhat abrupt in onset, and rapidly progressive over a period of several weeks. Thereafter, remissions and exacerbations punctuate the course, such that the benefits of corticosteroids, which are the treatment of choice for this disorder, are difficult to evaluate in an individual patient. Myalgias, dysphagia, and malaise are frequent concomitant symptoms. DM is diagnosed in the presence of a violaceous rash on the eyelids, face, and extensor surfaces of the limbs, especially the digits. Corroborative laboratory studies include an elevation of the erythrocyte sedimentation rate and serum creatine kinase level in both diseases. Several autoantibodies can be demonstrated in the serum of patients with PM. Many of these detect overlap syndromes. Anti–Jo-1, an antisynthetase antibody, is a marker for coexistent interstitial lung disease. Anti–PM-1 (anti–PM-scl) antibody is associated with PM and scleroderma. Small, brief, and polyphasic motor units are noted in EMG recordings in PM and DM. In approximately 20% of cases, DM is said to be associated with neoplasia, especially carcinoma of the lung, colon, or breast, and this paraneoplastic syndrome may precede the discovery of the tumor by several months. PM is much less commonly found to occur with malignancies.

PM is an autoimmune disease in which lymphocytes (predominantly T cells) have become sensitized to muscle antigens. A cell-mediated response leads to the necrosis of muscle fibers and subsequent regeneration (76). Approximately 75% of cells in the endomysium are CD8+ cytotoxic lymphocytes. As one might predict, muscle fibers that do not normally express major histocompatibility antigens have MHC class I antigen on the sarcolemmal surface when they are examined by immunoperoxidase techniques (77). This immunostaining pattern is also observed in DM. Immunoglobulin and complement deposits have been reported in some patients with PM (78), but neither we nor several other investigators have been able to confirm this observation. In our laboratory, the deposition of immune reactants in muscle tissue is now used to exclude the diagnosis of PM (79). In long-standing disease, fiber necrosis and the inflammatory reaction are generally absent. Instead, the biopsy is likely to reveal fiber atrophy and endoperimysial fibrosis. DM is essentially an angiopathy involving muscle and skin (80). Subcutaneous tissues, the intestine, and the peripheral nerves may also be involved in children. In a typical case, perivascular lymphocytic infiltrates are present without a true vasculitis. The inflammatory response in muscle is minimal or absent in some cases. Perifascicular atrophy is considered a hallmark of the disease (Fig. 4.38). Deposits of immunoglobulins and complement can be demonstrated within the intramuscular blood vessel walls, and they are presumably related to immunologically mediated capillary damage that results in a reduction in the size of the vascular bed (81,82). Perifascicular atrophy is also thought to be caused by this ischemic process. Undulating tubular arrays of unknown significance have been identified in endothelial cells by electron microscopy (83). However, these are difficult to find in a biopsy specimen, and they are not specific for DM.

Inclusion Body Myositis

Inclusion body myositis, an inflammatory myopathy, causes a withering of acral muscles, especially those in the extensor compartment of the arm. The disease seems to affect persons between the ages of 50 and 70 years and men more than women, in whom the pace of deterioration is slow (84). In contrast to

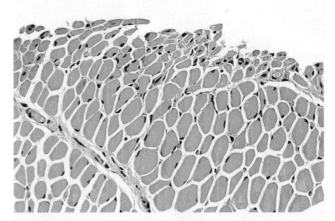

Figure 4.38. Dermatomyositis. The fibers at the edge of the fascicle at the top are atrophic.

PM and DM, inclusion body myositis does not respond to steroid therapy. Because the microscopic picture simulates that of several other diseases, all of which may sometimes be seen in the same slide, and because frozen sections are necessary for a diagnosis, the muscle biopsy specimen in inclusion body myositis may be misinterpreted. The first clue to the diagnosis is a specimen with many small, angular, often grouped fibers, which suggests denervation, with inflammation. Fiber hypertrophy and fiber splitting, which are rare findings in other inflammatory myopathies, are typical features. In addition to lymphocytic inflammation, which is minimal or absent in almost half of the cases, there is variable fiber necrosis and regeneration. Detection of MHC class I antigen expression on the sarcolemma of the fibers is accomplished with immunostaining. The upregulation of expression may be even more robust than in PM and DM (85). The biopsy may show rimmed vacuoles, inclusion bodies, and ragged red fibers. The vacuoles can be immunostained for ubiquitin, and they contain amyloid, which is difficult to visualize with Congo red stains (86,87). Inclusions located in the sarcolemmal nuclei and sarcoplasm are almost invariably overlooked in paraffin sections. Nuclear inclusions are faintly pink in H&E stains, and they often fill the nucleus, leaving a rim of peripheral chromatin (Fig. 4.13). Pink or red inclusions may also be seen in the sarcoplasmic rimmed vacuoles. Under the electron microscope, these inclusions, which consist of membranous whorls and bundles of filaments measuring 15 to 18 nm in diameter, may be present in few fibers. The filaments are at times difficult to identify (Fig. 4.39). The filaments were once thought to be of viral origin, perhaps from the mumps virus (88). They are now considered to be β-amyloid fibrils (89) and other proteins such as tau. Finally, the frequent presence of ragged red fibers implies an abnormality of mitochondria, which reportedly is related to multiple deletions in the mitochondrial DNA (90).

Viral Myositis

Several viral diseases are associated with myalgia and weakness of varying severity. The influenza virus and coxsackievirus are especially known for causing myositis as part of a generalized viral illness. Other viruses that have been implicated in the pathogenesis of myositis are the parainfluenza, hepatitis B, and en-

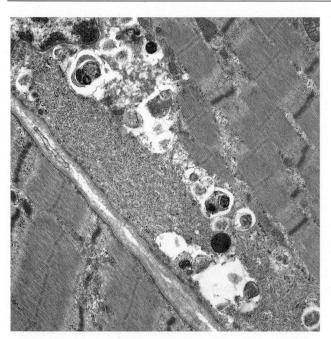

Figure 4.39. A portion of two fibers can be seen. In the upper fiber, the ultrastructural appearance of a rimmed vacuole filled with membranous profiles is illustrated. Note the collection of filaments in the lower left part of the upper fiber.

terocytopathogenic human orphan (ECHO) viruses. In severe cases, myoglobinuria and marked weakness, which may be progressive, are reported. However, viral myositis is self-limited in most instances, and biopsies are not performed. In acquired immunodeficiency syndrome (AIDS), neuromuscular complications are common, but these are usually caused by peripheral nerve disease (91). Cases of human immunodeficiency virus (HIV) myositis closely resemble PM pathologically, with cell necrosis and inflammation mainly composed of lymphocytes (92,93). The noteworthy finding of nemaline rods in some patients with HIV myopathy is of uncertain pathogenesis. The presence of multinucleated giant cells similar to that described in the brains of AIDS patients has also been reported in muscle.

METABOLIC DISEASES

Carbohydrate Storage Diseases

ACID MALTASE DEFICIENCY. Type 2 glycogenosis, which is transmitted as a recessive trait, is classically a fatal systemic disease of infants, who exhibit progressive weakness, hypotonia, macroglossia, cardiomyopathy, and organomegaly. The neuromuscular symptoms overshadow those referable to other organs, and they may be reminiscent of limb-girdle dystrophy or a congenital myopathy when the onset is delayed to late childhood or adulthood (94). The prognosis is considerably brighter in the adult form of the deficiency. Muscle biopsy reveals PAS-positive, diastase-labile vacuoles of varying sizes that replace much of the sarcoplasm of the fibers. At the electron microscopic level, membrane-bound, glycogen-filled vacuoles constitute presumptive evidence of acid maltase deficiency. Because enzyme activity cannot be demonstrated histochemically, biochemical analysis of muscle tissue is required for a definitive diagnosis. The gene for this disease is located on chromosome

17 at q21–23. Numerous mutations have been reported, the most common of which is found at exon 18.

MCARDLE DISEASE. Myophosphorylase deficiency (type 5 glycogenosis) is a recessively inherited disorder with onset in childhood or adolescence. It is characterized by muscle weakness, pain, and stiffness that is exacerbated by exercise. The inability of patients to generate lactate during ischemic exercise because they are unable to break down α-1,4-glucoside linkages properly is the basis for the tourniquet test, at the end of which venous blood analysis fails to show a normal elevation of lactic acid. Histologically, many crescentic, PAS-positive vacuoles are observed in a subsarcolemmal location (Fig. 4.40). Ultrastructurally, collections of glycogen granules are visualized within the vacuoles. One can arrive at the correct diagnosis by using histochemical reactions that disclose an absence of phosphorylase activity. The lack of the enzyme is associated with several different point mutations in the coding region located on chromosome 11 at q13 (95).

PHOSPHOFRUCTOKINASE DEFICIENCY. Phosphofructokinase (PFK) deficiency (type 7 glycogenosis, Tarui disease) is a recessively inherited disease resembling McArdle disease. The gene for myopathy resides on chromosome 12q13. More than 15 mutations in the PFK-M gene are known. With an onset that typically occurs in childhood, the clinical manifestations include muscular pain and stiffness induced by exercise. Prolonged exercise may be associated with nausea, vomiting, severe weakness, prostration, and myoglobinuria. In some patients, progressive muscle weakness develops that seems unrelated to exercise or activity. Hemolytic anemia has been described in a few patients, and it presumably is related to erythrocyte PFK deficiency. As in McArdle disease, the anticipated rise in the blood lactate does not occur in the ischemic forearm test. In frozen sections, PAS-positive crescents are seen adjacent to the sarcolemma of the muscle fibers. Under the electron microscope, an abundance of β-glycogen particles is found within the crescents and between the myofibrils. PFK deficiency can be demonstrated histochemically. However, histochemical stains are somewhat unreliable, so the results should be confirmed by biochemical analysis.

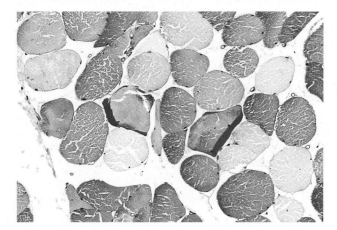

Figure 4.40. McArdle disease. Dark, subsarcolemmal crescents in two fibers contain abundant period acid-Schiff (PAS)–positive material (frozen section, PAS).

Lipid Storage Diseases

CARNITINE DEFICIENCY. Carnitine is necessary for the entry of long-chain fatty acids into the mitochondria for oxidative metabolism (96). Carnitine deficiency can be systemic, or it may be confined to skeletal muscle. In either case, slowly progressive and mild muscular weakness may date from infancy to middle age. Systemic disease that usually is secondary to acyl-coenzyme A dehydrogenase deficiency or one of the organic acidurias is recognized by acute encephalopathy, heart failure, hepatic dysfunction, hypoglycemia, and abnormally low plasma carnitine levels. The major pathologic change is the diffuse vacuolization of muscle fibers. Vacuoles of variable size are conveniently identified in fat stains and resin sections and by electron microscopy. The latter may reveal dysmorphic, enlarged mitochondria filled with paracrystalline inclusions.

CARNITINE PALMITOYLTRANSFERASE DEFICIENCY. Patients with this condition experience weakness, myalgias, and recurrent myoglobinuria precipitated by exercise or fasting. The lipid vacuoles within the muscle fibers may be normal or excessive. The mitochondria are morphologically unremarkable. A deficiency of carnitine palmitoyltransferase (CPT), which is most often a recessively inherited trait, can be detected only by biochemical methods. CPT is an enzyme system that promotes the transport of long-chain fatty acids across the mitochondrial membrane. Unlike shorter chain fatty acids, long-chain fatty acids, which are a major energy source for striated muscle, cannot enter the mitochondria directly. This problem is overcome by a series of steps beginning within the cytoplasm at the outer mitochondrial membrane, where long-chain fatty acids are esterified to acyl-coenzyme A (acyl-CoA). The inner mitochondrial membrane does not permit the passage of acyl-CoA, so the acyl group is transferred to the carrier carnitine by the enzyme CPT I. Once the acyl group is across the inner membrane of the mitochondrion, a second acyltransferase, CPT II, catalyzes the re-formation of acyl-CoA, making it available for β-oxidation. The free carnitine is released into the cytosol for reuse. CPT deficiency in the muscle usually involves CPT II, the gene for which is situated on chromosome 1p32. More than 15 mutations have been described that often result from a missense Ser113Leu mutation (97).

ACYL-COENZYME A DEHYDROGENASE DEFICIENCIES. This group of recessively inherited myopathies is a well-recognized cause of lipid storage myopathy, which may be a result of a deficiency of short-, medium-, long-, or very long–chain acyl-CoA dehydrogenase enzyme. Two main forms of dehydrogenase deficiency exist. The infantile form is associated with cardiomyopathy, liver involvement, hypoglycemia, and neurologic findings such as hypotonia and seizures. The later onset form begins in older children and may manifest mainly as a myopathy. These patients, who most often have very long–chain acyl-CoA dehydrogenase deficiency, suffer weakness, myalgias, and recurrent myoglobinuria like CPT deficiency.

Mitochondrial Myopathies

The morphologic abnormalities involving mitochondria are similar in all of the mitochondrial myopathies, for the most part differing only in severity. Obviously, therefore, rendering a definitive diagnosis based on morphologic criteria alone is not possible because the mitochondrial myopathies constitute a heterogeneous and complex group from the clinical, biochemical, and genetic points of view (98,99).

These myopathies may be primary or secondary. In the primary disorders, the initial and predominant pathologic events involve the mitochondria. Typically, a genetic defect and a biochemical derangement that may be related to a defect in mitochondrial metabolism are present. Several mitochondrial myopathies, including those seen in aging, are generalized disorders involving many organs in addition to the skeletal muscle (100,101). Progressive ptosis and ophthalmoplegia are striking in the Kearns-Sayre syndrome (102) and in oculocraniosomatic neuromuscular disease with ragged red fibers (103). In the secondary disorders, an underlying clinical condition, such as lipid storage disease or hypothyroidism, is present, and the mitochondrial changes are only one aspect of the total pathologic process.

KEARNS-SAYRE SYNDROME. The onset of this sporadic disease usually occurs before the age of 20 years, beginning with ptosis, progressive external ophthalmoplegia, and pigmentary retinal degeneration. Other common features are heart block, cerebellar ataxia, and very short stature. Most cases are reported with a defect in the cytochrome oxidase system that results from a variety of deletions in the mitochondrial DNA (104,105). The deletions are large (up to 5 kb), and they affect several genes at once. A frequent mutation is a deletion of 4977 base pairs that has been called the *common deletion*.

MYOPATHY, ENCEPHALOPATHY, LACTIC ACIDOSIS, STROKE SYNDROME. Myopathy, encephalopathy, lactic acidosis, stroke (MELAS) syndrome is caused by a point mutation in the tRNA$^{Leu(UUR)}$ mitochondrial gene, often with an A→G mutation in base pair 3243. The genetic defect may be associated with an abnormality in complex I of the respiratory chain. MELAS occurs in children, resulting in muscle weakness, seizures, stroke, dementia, and lactic acidosis. Computed tomography (CT) may show calcifications in the basal ganglia. Abnormal mitochondria are seen in the smooth muscle elements of blood vessels during the ultrastructural examination (106). Ragged red fibers stain positively for cytochrome oxidase and succinate dehydrogenase in histochemical preparations.

MYOCLONUS EPILEPSY WITH RAGGED RED FIBERS SYNDROME. A point mutation (A8344G) in the mitochondrial tRNA^{Lys} gene is responsible for myoclonus epilepsy with ragged red fibers (MERRF) syndrome (107). This maternally inherited syndrome is associated with a defect in complex IV of the respiratory chain. The clinical manifestations, which begin in childhood, include myoclonus, ataxia, and dementia. In muscle biopsy specimens stained histochemically, ragged fibers are positive for succinate dehydrogenase but negative for cytochrome oxidase.

Myoadenylate Deaminase Deficiency

Adenylate deaminase, or adenosine monophosphate deaminase (AMPD), is an enzyme found in skeletal muscle; a deficiency may lead to exercise intolerance in some patients, who experience aches and muscular cramps without significant muscle weakness on neurologic examination (108,109). AMPD deficiency is also reported in asymptomatic patients, in whom it appears to be a clinically incidental finding. Myoadenylate deaminase, which converts AMP to ammonia and inosine monophosphate, can be detected with histochemical or biochemical techniques. The gene coding for deaminase in muscle (AMPD1) is situated on chromosome 1p21. Patients with clinical disease have a truncated deaminase peptide that often is the consequence of a nonsense mutation (C→T transition) at nucleotide 34 of the AMPD1 gene.

Critical Care Myopathy

This entity occurs in acutely ill patients, who are usually admitted to the intensive care unit. Profound generalized weakness, often affecting the respiratory muscles, is rapidly progressive, although it is reversible if it is recognized early and is properly treated. The condition is potentiated by treatment with steroids and muscle relaxants, such as vecuronium and pancuronium (110). Many patients with this disease are reported to have a selective loss of myosin filaments that can be detected by electron microscopic examination of the biopsy specimen (111). In frozen sections, the affected fibers, which tend to be numerous, are angular and unstained in ATPase reactions at any pH, reflecting the deficiency of myosin.

Neuromuscular Junction Disorders

Both immune-mediated and congenital disorders have been described. The congenital myasthenic syndromes are rare and are reviewed elsewhere (112). The weakness tends to fluctuate, and it generally affects the extraocular muscles, with ptosis being a common symptom. The course is generally slowly progressive. EMG, rather than muscle biopsy, is important in establishing the diagnosis. In most biopsies, an investigation of the endplates is not practical because these structures are localized at the innervation zone, which can be properly identified only by electric stimulation during the biopsy procedure.

MYASTHENIA GRAVIS. Myasthenia gravis, which is more frequent in young adult women, is characterized by the insidious onset of easy fatigability in the extraocular and facial muscles. The clinical diagnosis depends on a positive response to anticholinesterase agents and a decrement in motor action potentials during repetitive stimulation. In our experience, the muscle biopsy specimen is often normal, or it may be characterized by a nonspecific pattern of atrophy. The typical finding of moderate to severe type 2 fiber atrophy is encountered in a minority of cases. Research has shown that patients with myasthenia gravis synthesize antibodies to the postsynaptic membrane of the motor endplate; these block neuromuscular transmission and damage the endplate region (113,114). Ultrastructurally, the junctional folds of the endplates are simplified, and the synaptic clefts are widened (115).

EATON-LAMBERT SYNDROME. This immune-mediated disorder is usually associated with malignancy. Approximately 60% of patients are found to have small-cell lung carcinoma. The myasthenic syndrome is related to an antibody to the calcium channel in the presynaptic membrane of the motor endplate that results in a reduced quantal release of acetylcholine from the nerve terminal (116). Freeze fracture electron microscopic studies have demonstrated a loss of active zone particles on the

P-face of the synaptic membrane. These particles correspond to the site of the calcium channels.

Denervating Diseases

OVERVIEW. Neurogenic atrophy of muscle results from injury to the peripheral nervous system, either the anterior horn cell or its axon. The pathogenesis of the denervating condition cannot be determined by examining a muscle biopsy specimen because the histologic changes affecting the muscle are the same in all denervating diseases, except in infants. In early denervation, the selective atrophy of type 2 fibers is frequently the only abnormality, so the diagnosis of denervation depends on confirmatory clinical information. With continuing denervation, the proportions of atrophic type 1 and type 2 fibers become relatively equal. At first, denervated fibers are randomly scattered rather than being grouped together. Chronic denervation is characterized by grouped fiber atrophy in addition to type grouping and target fiber formation (117). Immunohistochemistry may be useful in confirming or discovering the process of denervation (118). In normal fibers, neural cell adhesion molecule (N-CAM) staining can only be seen at the neuromuscular junctions, but denervated fibers demonstrate N-CAM staining of the entire sarcolemma. Neuronal nitric acid synthase (nNOS) is absent from denervated fibers. When fibers are then reinnervated, nNOS expression reappears in the sarcolemmal membrane.

DENERVATION IN INFANTS. ISMA is the most common neurogenic disease in young children. The condition is familial, and it most often is inherited as an autosomal recessive trait. Several genes probably play a role in this disease, but the most important is the telomeric SMN1 gene located on chromosome 5q11.2–13.3 (119). The most severe cases are associated with large deletions of SMN1. The age at onset, which ranges from birth to early childhood, dictates the natural history. In general, the earlier the onset is, the more unfavorable the prognosis. The average life expectancy in this disease is approximately 12 months. Infants typically exhibit the floppy infant syndrome, with severe weakness, a weak cry, poor suck, and respiratory difficulties, although cognitive function is normal. Fasciculations are difficult to appreciate except in the tongue. The pathologic picture differs from that of other neurogenic atrophies in that the atrophic process, which is caused by lower motor neuron disease, is widespread, involving virtually every fascicle. Most fibers in each fascicle are small and rounded (Fig. 4.41). Among the denervated fibers are counterparts that are normal in diameter or hypertrophic. The enlarged fibers are predominantly type 1 in many cases, although in our experience, the hypertrophy of both major fiber types does occur. Splitting of hypertrophic fibers, on the other hand, does not.

PITFALLS

The submission of a specimen with insufficient clinical data may lead to a delay in the diagnosis or to an incorrect diagnosis. The clinical information guides the investigation of the biopsy specimen beyond the routine workup. Several special techniques are available, but from a practical and economic standpoint, not all of them can be used in every case. As an example,

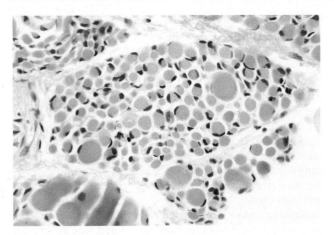

Figure 4.41. Infantile spinal muscular atrophy. Most of the fibers in the fascicle are atrophic and rounded.

myopathy in thyroid disease or during statin therapy is characterized by nonspecific features, which in the absence of a proper history may leave the pathologist with the sense that the workup is incomplete. The clinician sending the biopsy in this situation may simply want to know if the patient has myopathy and what its features are. More troublesome is biopsy accompanied by an incorrect clinical diagnosis, which may trap the pathologist into a lengthy pointless workup or an error in diagnosis. Whenever the diagnosis and the pathologic findings do not match, communication with the contributor is a wise decision.

Expecting the muscle biopsy specimen to show any significant change when the patient is free of muscle weakness on physical examination is generally unreasonable. The pathologist should proceed with caution in a biopsy from a patient without weakness. Some patients experience only intermittent weakness and are not weak at the time of the exam. Many of these patients complain of pain or cramps, suggesting a metabolic myopathy.

In several diseases (Table 4.11), the muscle biopsy is a low-yield diagnostic procedure in all but the most sophisticated laboratories because either nonspecific changes or an absence of pathologic changes is encountered. In others, the weakness is of physiologic origin without a morphologic correlate, and a biopsy is contraindicated.

An inadequate specimen is one of the most important reasons why a muscle biopsy is a noncontributory procedure. As discussed in the "Planning and Procedures" section, the biopsy should represent the disease. If symptoms are limited to the leg muscles, a biopsy of the arm is likely to be normal. A muscle in which there is an active disease process is more apt to contain diagnostic features. Severely involved muscle in which the disease process has been long standing and chronic often results in a biopsy with end-stage disease and nonspecific findings. Another type of inadequate specimen is the one with only a few fibers. Such biopsies, which are often obtained by inexperienced clinicians, should be interpreted with a comment on the limited size.

Muscles subjected to prior trauma or affected by an unrelated disease process should not be sampled. Needle tracts produced during EMG studies or intramuscular injections of therapeutic medications are a common type of traumatic injury. The changes in such muscles—fiber necrosis, regeneration, inflammation, and endomysial fibrosis—mimic those of certain neuromuscular diseases, and they can mislead the pathologist. The biopsy specimen should be taken from the belly of the muscle, away from tendinous insertions, the normal histologic features of which may be misinterpreted as pathologic. At the tendinous interface, muscle fibers typically vary more in size; the internal nuclei are numerous; and the fibers are separated by trabeculae of dense collagen as they attach to the tendon (Fig. 4.42). Similar but less pronounced features are found at the interface of muscles and fascia. The interfaces should not be confused with fibrosis.

Certain muscles are commonly biopsied, and the pathologist becomes familiar with their appearance. Not all muscles look alike. The pathologist should be careful when receiving an unfamiliar muscle. For example, the paraspinal muscles normally contain increased numbers of internal nuclei, and groups of fascicles are separated by abundant connective tissue that resembles fibrosis. In more distal leg muscles such as the gastrocnemius, subclinical disc disease can cause the picture of denervation, which is unrelated to the disease for which the biopsy was obtained.

Vacuolization of the fibers is a frequent consequence of improper freezing, transport, or storage of the specimen. These ice crystals must be distinguished from pathologic vacuoles seen in storage diseases. Ice crystals tend to be linear or assume non-

TABLE 4.11

Diseases and Other Conditions Associated with Neuromuscular Symptoms, Most Commonly Weakness, in Which the Muscle Biopsy Is a Low-Yield or Contraindicated Procedure

Electrolyte disturbances
Most endocrine diseases
Malignant hyperthermia
Myasthenic syndromes
Myotonic disorders
Old age
Periodic paralysis
Poor nutrition

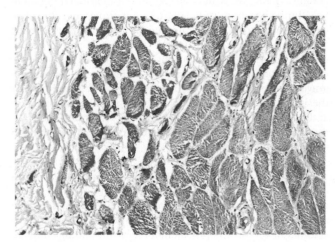

Figure 4.42. Tendinous insertion. In this location, the muscle fibers normally vary in size, and they are often surrounded by fibrous tissue (Gomori trichrome).

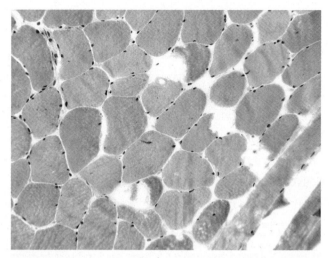

Figure 4.43. Muscle specimen submitted in saline. Fluid between fibers mimics edema. Several fibers are damaged and disrupted and appear blown out.

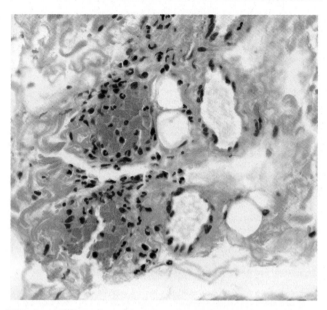

Figure 4.44. During the biopsy procedure, the muscle has been roughly handled, leading to a pseudovasculitis in the perimysium. Neutrophils are marginating in the vessel lumina and beginning to traverse the vessel walls.

circular shapes in contrast to pathologic vacuoles, which tend to be round. PAS and fat stains should be used to rule out lipid and glycogen storage whenever there is a question about the origin of the vacuoles.

Specimens submitted in saline or kept too moist show fluid accumulation between the fibers that resembles edema. The fibers are also often vacuolated, disrupted, or "blown out" as though they exploded (Fig. 4.43). These changes, which may be mistaken for an acute myopathy with edema and fiber necrosis, occur in the absence of inflammation or phagocytosis that would be expected in a pathologic reaction. Such mishandling may result in a loss of enzyme staining and the false impression of an enzyme deficiency.

A common problem encountered in reviewing muscle biopsies is the significance of small fibers. The portion of the biopsy crushed by the teeth at the ends of the clamp should not be submitted for processing because of crush artifact, which can leave all the fibers intact but appearing atrophic. Some biopsies come from the elderly. It is important to remember that, with aging, there is fiber atrophy. The fiber diameters in a 75-year-old patient are one-half the diameters of a 25-year-old patient. A final caveat regarding atrophy is related to steroid myopathy. Some patients undergoing a biopsy, especially those in whom inflammatory myopathy is suspected, have already been treated with corticosteroids, which causes fiber atrophy, mainly of type 2 fibers. The lack of a proper history may lead to a misinterpretation in these cases.

Fatty infiltration can be a sign of chronic muscle disease, which must be distinguished from the fatty infiltration occurring in obese people. In chronic disease, there are usually other pathologic findings such as variation in fiber size and fibrosis.

We receive many biopsies with the diagnosis of inflammatory myopathy. The presence of neutrophils is a very unusual finding in true disease and represents a red flag. Almost always when neutrophils are seen, especially when they penetrate the vessel walls and when they collect within the vascular lumina (margination), they represent a pseudovasculitis, an acute inflammatory reaction to the trauma of the biopsy itself (Fig. 4.44). In our experience, this finding occurs when the biopsy procedure was done by an inexperienced individual whose surgery took an excessive amount of time and likely involved rough handling of the tissue.

REFERENCES

GENERAL REFERENCES

1. Carpenter S, Karpati G. *Pathology of Skeletal Muscle.* New York, NY: Oxford University Press, 2001.
2. DeGirolami U, Smith TW. Pathology of skeletal muscle diseases. *Am J Pathol* 1982;107:235–276.
3. Dubowitz V, Sewry CA. *Muscle Biopsy. A Practical Approach.* Philadelphia, PA: Saunders, 2007.
4. Engel AG, Franzini-Armstrong C, eds. *Myology.* New York, NY: McGraw-Hill, 1994.
5. Heffner RR, ed. *Muscle Pathology.* New York, NY: Churchill Livingstone, 1984.
6. Heffner RR. Diseases of skeletal muscle. In Nelson JS, Parisi JE, Mena H, Schochet SS, eds. *Principles and Practice of Neuropathology.* New York, NY: Oxford, 2003:525–577.
7. Heffner RR. Muscle pathology for the general pathologist. *Adv Pathol Lab Med* 1995;8:169–200.
8. Heffner RR, Schochet SS. Skeletal muscle. In Damjanov I, Linder J, eds. *Anderson's Pathology.* St. Louis, MO: Mosby, 1996:2653–2690.
9. Karpati G, ed. *Structural and Molecular Basis of Skeletal Muscle Diseases.* Basel, Switzerland: ISN Neuropath Press, 2002.
10. Mastaglia FL, Walton JN, eds. *Skeletal Muscle Pathology.* Edinburgh, United Kingdom: Churchill Livingstone, 1992.
11. Walton JN, Karpati G, Hilton-Jones D, eds. *Disorders of Voluntary Muscle.* 6th edition. Edinburgh, United Kingdom: Churchill Livingstone, 1994.

TECHNIQUES

12. Bossen EH. Collection and preparation of the muscle biopsy. In Heffner RR, ed. *Muscle Pathology.* New York, NY: Churchill Livingstone, 1984:11–14.
13. Pamphlett R. Muscle biopsy. In Mastaglia FL, Walton JN, eds. *Skeletal Muscle Pathology.* Edinburgh, United Kingdom: Churchill Livingstone, 1992:95–121.
14. Jay V, Becker LE. Fiber-type differentiation by myosin immunohistochemistry on paraffin-embedded skeletal muscle. *Arch Pathol Lab Med* 1994;118:917–918.

GENERAL REACTIONS

15. Heffner RR. Electron microscopy of disorders of skeletal muscle. *Ann Clin Lab Sci* 1975;5:338–347.
16. Cullen MJ, Fulthrope JJ. Stages in fiber breakdown in Duchenne muscular dystrophy. *J Neurol Sci* 1975;24:179–200.

17. Chou SM, Nonaka I. Satellite cells and muscle regeneration in diseased human skeletal muscles. *J Neurol Sci* 1977;34:131–145.
18. Mastaglia FL, Dawkins RL, Papadimitriou JM. Morphological changes in skeletal muscle after transplantation: a light and electron-microscopic study of the initial phases of degeneration and regeneration. *J Neurol Sci* 1975;25:227–247.
19. Hewlett RH, Brownell B. Granulomatous myopathy: its relationship to sarcoidosis and polymyositis. *J Neurol Neurosurg Psychiatry* 1975;38:1090–1099.
20. Lynch PG, Bansal DV. Granulomatous polymyositis. *J Neurol Sci* 1973;18:1–9.
21. Bennington JL, Krupp M. Morphometric analysis of muscle. In Heffner RR, ed. *Muscle Pathology.* New York, NY: Churchill Livingstone, 1984:43–71.
22. Engel WK. Selective and nonselective susceptibility of muscle fiber types. A new approach to human neuromuscular diseases. *Arch Neurol* 1970;22:97–117.
23. Barron SA, Heffner RR. Weakness in malignancy: evidence for a remote effect of tumor on distal axons. *Ann Neurol* 1978;4:268–274.
24. Karpati G, Engel WK. "Type grouping" in skeletal muscles after experimental reinnervation. *Neurology* 1968;18:447–455.
25. Swash M, Schwartz MS, Sargeant MK. Pathogenesis of longitudinal splitting of muscle fibres in neurogenic disorders and in polymyositis. *Neuropathol Appl Neurobiol* 1977;4:99–115.
26. Neville HE, Brooke MH. Central core fibers: structured and unstructured. In Kakulas BA, ed. *Basic Research in Myology. Proceedings of the Second International Congress on Muscle Diseases, Perth, Australia.* Amsterdam, The Netherlands: Excerpta Medica, 1973:497–511.
27. Engel WK. Muscle target fibers, a newly recognized sign of denervation. *Nature* 1961;191:389–390.
28. Shy GM, Engel WK, Sommers JE, Wanko T. Nemaline myopathy: a new congenital myopathy. *Brain* 1963;86:793–810.
29. Price HM, Gordon GB, Pearson CM, et al. New evidence for excessive accumulation of Z-band material in nemaline myopathy. *Proc Natl Acad Sci U S A* 1965;54:1398–1406.
30. Zeviani M, Lamantea E. Genetic disorders of the mitochondrial OXPHOS system. *Science Med* 2007;10:154–167.
31. Bauserman SC, Heffner RR. Mitochondrial myopathies. In Heffner RR, ed. *Muscle Pathology.* New York, NY: Churchill Livingstone, 1984:109–123.
32. Tassin S, Brucher JM. The mitochondrial disorders: pathogenesis and aetiological classification. *Neuropathol Appl Neurobiol* 1982;8:251–263.
33. Norris FH, Panner BJ. Hypothyroid myopathy. *Arch Neurol* 1966;14:574–589.
34. Neville HE, Brooke MH. Muscle biopsy in the diagnosis of oculopharyngeal myopathy. *J Neuropathol Exp Neurol* 1974;33(Abstr):193.
35. Markesbery WR, Griggs RC, Herr B. Distal myopathy: electron microscopic and histochemical studies. *Neurology* 1977;27:727–735.
36. Carpenter S, Karpati G, Heller I, Eisen A. Inclusion body myositis: a distinct variety of idiopathic inflammatory myopathy. *Neurology* 1978;28:8–17.

MUSCULAR DYSTROPHIES

37. Hejtmancik JF, Harris SG, Tsao CC, et al. Carrier diagnosis of Duchenne muscular dystrophy using restriction fragment length polymorphisms. *Neurology* 1986;36:1553–1562.
38. Lindenbaum RH, Clarke G, Patel C, et al. Muscular dystrophy in an X;1 translocation female suggests that Duchenne locus is on X chromosome short arm. *J Med Genet* 1979;16:389–392.
39. Koenig M, Hoffman EP, Bertelson CJ, et al. Complete cloning of the Duchenne muscular dystrophy (DMD) cDNA and preliminary genomic organization of the DMD gene in normal and affected individuals. *Cell* 1987;50:509–517.
40. Prior TW. Genetic analysis of the Duchenne muscular dystrophy gene. *Arch Pathol Lab Med* 1991;115:984–990.
41. Hoffman EP, Fischbeck K, Brown RH, et al. Characterization of dystrophin in muscle biopsy specimens from Duchenne and Becker muscular dystrophy patients. *N Engl J Med* 1988;318:1363–1368.
42. Fong P, Turner PR, Denetclaw WF, et al. Increased activity of calcium leak channels in myotubes of Duchenne human and mdx mouse origin. *Science* 1990;250:673–676.
43. Hoffman EP, Brown RH, Kunkel LM. Dystrophin: the protein product of the Duchenne muscular dystrophy locus. *Cell* 1987;51:919–928.
44. Worton R. Muscular dystrophies: diseases of the dystrophin-glycoprotein complex. *Science* 1995;270:755–756.
45. Uchino M, Araki S, Miike T, et al. Localization and characterization of dystrophin in muscle biopsy specimens from Duchenne muscular dystrophy and various neuromuscular disorders. *Muscle Nerve* 1989;12:1009–1016.
46. Ohlendieck K, Matsumura K, Ionasescu VV, et al. Duchenne muscular dystrophy: deficiency of dystrophin-associated proteins in the sarcolemma. *Neurology* 1993;43:795–800.
47. Koenig M, Beggs AH, Moyer M, et al. The molecular basis for Duchenne versus Becker muscular dystrophy: correlation of severity with type of deletion. *Am J Hum Genet* 1989;45:498–506.
48. Liechti-Gallati S, Koenig M, Kunkel LM, et al. Molecular deletion patterns in Duchenne- and Becker-type muscular dystrophy. *Hum Genet* 1989;81:343–348.
49. Sarfarzi M, Wijmenga C, Upadhyaya M, et al. Regional mapping of facioscapulohumeral muscular dystrophy gene on 4q35. *Am J Hum Genet* 1992;51:396–403.
50. Lemmers RJ, deKievit P, Sandkuijl L, et al. Facioscapulohumeral muscular dystrophy is uniquely associated with one of the two variants of the 4q subtelomere. *Nat Genet* 2002;32:235–236.
51. Lemmers RJ, Osborn M, Haaf T, et al. D4F104S1 deletion in facioscapulohumeral muscular dystrophy. *Neurology* 2003;61:178–183.
52. Chutkow JG, Heffner RR Jr, Kramer AA, Edwards JA. Adult-onset autosomal dominant limb-girdle muscular dystrophy. *Ann Neurol* 1986;20:240–248.
53. Duggan DJ, Gorospe JF, Fanin M, et al. Mutations in the sarcoglycan genes in patients with myopathy. *N Engl J Med* 1997;336:618–624.

54. Dubowitz V. The muscular dystrophies—clarity or chaos? *N Engl J Med* 1997;336:650–651.
55. Matsuda C, Hayashi YK, Ogawa M, et al. The sarcolemmal proteins dysferlin and caveolin 3 interact in skeletal muscle. *Hum Mol Genet* 2001;10:1761–1766.
56. Moreira ES, Wiltshire TJ, Gaulkner G, et al. Limb girdle muscular dystrophy type 2G is caused by mutations in the gene encoding the sarcomere protein telethonin. *Nat Genet* 2002;24:163–166.
57. Udd B, Vihola A, Sarparanta J, et al. Titinopathies and extension of the M-line mutation phenotype beyond distal myopathy and LGMD2J. *Neurology* 2005;64:636–642.
58. Becher MW, Morrison L, Davis LE, et al. Oculopharyngeal muscular dystrophy in Hispanic New Mexicans. *JAMA* 2001;286:2437–2440.
59. Caskey CT, Pizzuti A, Fu YH, et al. Triplet repeat mutations in human disease. *Science* 1992;256:785–788.
60. Abruzzese C, Porrini SC, Mariani B, et al. Instability of a permutation allele in homozygous patients with myotonic dystrophy type 1. *Ann Neurol* 2002;52:435–441.

CONGENITAL MYOPATHIES

61. Greenfield JG, Cornman T, Shy GM. The prognostic value of the muscle biopsy in the "floppy infant." *Brain* 1958;81:461–484.
62. Shy GM, Magee KR. A new congenital non-progressive myopathy. *Brain* 1957;79:610–621.
63. Haan EA, Freemantle CJ, McCure JA, et al. Assignment of the gene for central core disease to chromosome 19. *Hum Genet* 1990;86:187–190.
64. Ferreiro A, Monnier N, Romero NB, et al. A recessive form of central core disease, transiently presenting as multi-minicore disease, is associated with a homozygous mutation in the ryanodine receptor type 1 gene. *Ann Neurol* 2002;51:750–759.
65. Jungbluth H, Davis MR, Muller C, et al. MRI of muscle in congenital myopathies associated with RYR1 mutations. *Neuromuscul Disord* 2004;14:785–790.
66. Heffner RR, Cohen M, Duffner P, Daigler G. Multicore disease in twins. *J Neurol Neurosurg Psychiatry* 1976;39:602–606.
67. Shuaib A, Martin JM, Mitchell LB, Brownell AK. Multicore myopathy. *Can J Neurol Sci* 1988;15:10–14.
68. Ryan MM, Schnell C, Strickland CD, et al. Nemaline myopathy: a clinical study of 143 cases. *Ann Neurol* 2001;50:312–320.
69. Laporte J, Biancalana V, Tanner SM, et al. MTM1 mutations in X-linked myotubular myopathy. *Hum Mutat* 2000;15:393–409.
70. Spiro AJ, Shy GM, Gonatas NK. Myotubular myopathy. Persistence of fetal muscle in an adolescent boy. *Arch Neurol* 1966;14:1–14.
71. Clancy RR, Kelts KA, Oehlert JW. Clinical variability in congenital fiber-type disproportion. *J Neurol Sci* 1980;46:257–266.
72. deBleecker JL, Engel AG, Ertl BB. Myofibrillar myopathy with abnormal foci of desmin positivity. *J Neuropathol Exp Neurol* 1996;55:563–577.
73. Goebel HH, Borchet A. Protein surplus myopathies and other rare congenital myopathies. *Semin Paediatr Neurol* 2002;9:160–170.
74. Pellissier JF, Pouget J, Charpin C, Figarella D. Myopathy associated with desmin intermediate filaments. *J Neurol Sci* 1989;89:49–61.
75. Dalakas MC, Park KY, Semino-Mora C, et al. Desmin myopathy, a skeletal myopathy with cardiomyopathy caused by mutations in the desmin gene. *N Engl J Med* 2000;342:770–780.

INFLAMMATORY AND IMMUNE-MEDIATED MYOPATHIES

76. Heffner RR. Inflammatory myopathies. A review. *J Neuropathol Exp Neurol* 1993;52:339–350.
77. Emslie-Smith AM, Arahata K, Engel AG. Major histocompatibility complex class I antigen expression, immunolocalization of interferon subtypes, and T cell-mediated cytotoxicity in myopathies. *Hum Pathol* 1989;20:224–231.
78. Oxenhandler R, Adelstein EH, Hart MN. Immunopathology of skeletal muscle. The value of direct immunofluorescence in the diagnosis of connective tissue disease. *Hum Pathol* 1977;8:321–328.
79. Heffner RR, Barron SA, Jenis EH, Valeski JE. Skeletal muscle in polymyositis. Immunohistochemical study. *Arch Pathol Lab Med* 1979;103:310–313.
80. Carpenter S, Karpati G. The pathological diagnosis of specific inflammatory myopathies. *Brain Pathol* 1992;2:13–19.
81. Kissel TJ, Mendell JR, Rammohan K, et al. Microvascular deposition of complement membrane attack complex in dermatomyositis. *N Engl J Med* 1986;314:329–334.
82. Carpenter S, Karpati G, Rothman S, et al. The childhood type of dermatomyositis. *Neurology* 1976;26:952–962.
83. Banker BQ. Dermatomyositis of childhood. Ultrastructural alterations of muscle and intramuscular blood vessels. *J Neuropathol Exp Neurol* 1975;34:46–75.
84. Carpenter S, Karpati G, Heller I, et al. Inclusion body myositis: a distinct variety of idiopathic inflammatory myopathy. *Neurology* 1978;28:8–17.
85. Jain A, Sharma MC, Sarkar C, et al. Major histocompatibility complex class I and II detection as a diagnostic tool in idiopathic inflammatory myopathies. *Arch Pathol Lab Med* 2007;131:1070–1076.
86. Askanas V, Serdaroglu P, Engel WK, Alvarez RB. Immunocytochemical localization of ubiquitin in inclusion body myositis allows its light-microscopic distinction from polymyositis. *Neurology* 1992;42:460–461.
87. Askanas V, Engel WK, Alvarez RB. Enhanced detection of Congo red–positive amyloid deposits in muscle fibers of inclusion body myositis and brain of Alzheimer's disease using fluorescence technique. *Neurology* 1993;43:1265–1267.
88. Chou SM. Inclusion body myositis: a chronic persistent mumps myositis? *Hum Pathol* 1986;17:765–777.
89. Askanas V, Alvarez RB, Engel WK, et al. Beta-amyloid precursor epitopes in muscle fibers of inclusion body myositis. *Ann Neurol* 1993;34:551–560.

90. Santorelli FM, Sciacco M, Tanji K, et al. Multiple mitochondrial DNA deletions in sporadic inclusion body myositis: a study of 56 patients. *Ann Neurol* 1996;39:789–795.

91. Lange DJ, Britton CB, Younger DS, Hays AP. The neuromuscular manifestations of HIV infections. *Arch Neurol* 1988;45:1084–1088.

92. Bailey RO, Turok DI, Jaufmann BP, Singh JK. Myositis and AIDS. *Hum Pathol* 1987;18: 749–751.

93. Simpson DM, Bender AN. HIV-associated myopathy: analysis of 11 patients. *Ann Neurol* 1988;24:79–84.

METABOLIC DISEASES

94. Engel AG, Gomez MR, Seybold ME, Lambert EH. The spectrum and diagnosis of acid maltase deficiency. *Neurology* 1973;23:95–106.

95. Tsujino S, Shanske S, DiMauro S. Molecular genetic heterogeneity of myophosphorylase deficiency (McArdle's disease). *N Engl J Med* 1993;329:241–245.

96. DiMauro S, Trevisan C, Hays A. Disorders of lipid metabolism in muscle. *Muscle Nerve* 1980;3:369–388.

97. Haap M, Thamer C, Machann J, et al. Metabolic characterization of a woman homozygous for the Ser113Leu missense mutation in carnitine palmitoyl transferase II. *J Clin Endocrinol Metab* 2002;87:2139–2143.

98. DiMauro S, Bonilla E, Zeviani M, et al. Mitochondrial myopathies. *Ann Neurol* 1985;17: 521–538.

99. Johns DR. Mitochondrial DNA and disease. *N Engl J Med* 1995;333:638–644.

100. Mendell JR. Mitochondrial myopathy in the elderly: exaggerated aging in the pathogenesis of disease. *Ann Neurol* 1995;37:3–4.

101. Johnson W, Karpati G, Carpenter S, et al. Late-onset mitochondrial myopathy. *Ann Neurol* 1995;37:16–23.

102. Berenberg RA, Pollock JN, DiMauro S, et al. Lumping or splitting: "ophthalmoplegia-plus" or Kearns-Sayre syndrome? *Ann Neurol* 1977;1:37–54.

103. Olson W, Engel WK, Walsh GO, Einaugler R. Oculocraniosomatic neuromuscular disease with "ragged-red" fibers. *Arch Neurol* 1972;26:193–211.

104. Sparaco M, Bonilla E, DiMauro S, Powers JM. Neuropathology of mitochondrial encephalomyopathies due to mitochondrial DNA defects. *J Neuropathol Exp Neurol* 1993;52:1–10.

105. Moraes CT, DiMauro S, Zeviani M, et al. Mitochondrial DNA deletions in progressive external ophthalmoplegia and Kearns-Sayre syndrome. *N Engl J Med* 1989;320:1293–1299.

106. Clark JM, Marks MP, Adalsteinsson E, et al. MELAS: clinical and pathologic correlations with MRI, xenon/CT, and MR spectroscopy. *Neurology* 1996;46:223–227.

107. Silvestri G, Ciafaloni E, Santorelli FM, et al. Clinical features associated with the A→G transition at nucleotide 8344 of mtDNA ("MERRF mutation"). *Neurology* 1993;43: 1200–1206.

108. Fishbein WN, Armbrustmacher VW, Griffin JL. Myoadenylate deaminase deficiency: a new disease of muscle. *Science* 1978;200:545–548.

109. Keleman J, Rice DR, Bradley WG, et al. Familial myoadenylate deaminase deficiency and exertional myalgia. *Neurology* 1982;32:857–863.

110. DeJonghe B, Sharshar T, Lefaucheur JP, et al. Paresis acquired in the intensive care unit *JAMA* 2002;288:2859–2867.

111. Al-Lozi MT, Pestronk A, Yee WC, et al. Rapidly evolving myopathy with myosin-deficient muscle fibers. *Ann Neurol* 1994;35:273–279.

NEUROMUSCULAR JUNCTION DISORDERS

112. Hanti D, Richard P, Koenig J. Congenital myasthenic syndromes. *Curr Opin Neurol* 2004; 17:539–551.

113. DeBaets MH, Oosterhuis HJGH, eds. *Myasthenia Gravis.* Ann Arbor, MI: CRC Press, 1993.

114. Engel AG, Lambert EH, Howard FM. Immune complexes (IgG and C3) at the motor endplate in myasthenia gravis. Ultrastructural and light microscopic localization and electrophysiologic correlations. *Mayo Clin Proc* 1977;52:267–280.

115. Santa T, Engel AG, Lambert EH. Histometric study of neuromuscular junction ultrastructure. I. Myasthenia gravis. *Neurology* 1972;22:71–82.

116. Nagel A, Engel Ag, Lang B, et al. Lambert-Eaton myasthenic syndrome IgG depletes presynaptic membrane active zone particles by antigenic modulation. *Ann Neurol* 1988; 24:552–558.

DENERVATION

117. Armbrustmacher VW. Skeletal muscle in denervation. *Pathol Annu* 1978;13:1–33.

118. Gosztonyi G, Naschold U, Grozdanoviv Z, et al. Expression of Leu-19 (CD56, N-CAM) and nitric oxide synthase (NOS) 1 in denervated and reinnervated human skeletal muscle. *Microsc Res Tech* 2001;55:187–197.

119. Feldkotter M, Schwarzer V, Wirth R, et al. Quantitative analyses of SMN 1 and SMN 2 based on real-time light cycler PCR: fast and highly reliable carrier testing and prediction of severity of spinal muscular atrophy. *Am J Hum Genet* 2002;70:358–368.

Disorders of Soft Tissue

Soft tissue tumors (STTs) are said to be uncommon, but are they really? Certainly, one could never judge from the voluminous literature on the subject; reports pertaining to STTs rival those on lymphomas in frequency, and articles on the subject appear in virtually every issue of each pathology journal. This body of work gives testament to the variety of lesions encountered and the diagnostic difficulties they cause. A conservative estimate of the incidence of STTs would include the number of sarcomas expected per year (9,220 in 2007) (1) and an appraisal of the ratio of benign mesenchymal neoplasms relative to sarcomas (possibly 10 to 1 or higher). Reactive lesions such as fasciitis would be added to the total to give a fairly large figure. Such a calculation still does not truly indicate how often the pathologist is faced with a diagnostic problem related to this field. The first issue is definitional—only entities encountered within the soft tissues are quantified, but pathologists see identical tumors within other body sites (e.g., skin, organs), and the real scope of the matter is better thought of in terms of total mesenchymal lesions. Counting organ-based mesenchymal tumors is virtually impossible. Second, pathologists consider a "soft tissue" tumor whenever they are faced with a potential mimic, and many melanomas, carcinomas, and lymphomas can arouse such thoughts. Third, even the malignancies are underestimated because tumors from the skin and uncoded locations are not counted as "connective tissue" sarcomas. Clearly, pathologists deal with questions pertaining to this field much more often than is generally stated if these other elements are entered in the equation.

This chapter provides a problem-oriented approach that emphasizes diagnosis from the routinely stained section. When data are available, they are summarized in tabular form that highlights the clinical presentation and provides a guide to the natural history of these tumors. The text concentrates on histologic features, and diagnostic criteria are discussed in a practical way. The supplemental information includes an account of the differential diagnostic possibilities and ancillary diagnostic techniques. The tables are meant to help the pathologist act as an information resource to the clinician. However, the survival data in the tables, although for the most part gleaned from major series, are based on cases that have accumulated over several decades. Survival data found in clinical oncology group studies are usually far superior for most sarcomas, with overall 5-year survival rates of 60% to 70% or higher.

Literature references highlight only classic descriptions and key molecular and marker findings. In this era of electronic online databases, readers are encouraged to search for much more detailed information on the numerous entities discussed in this chapter.

PHILOSOPHIC APPROACH TO THE DIAGNOSIS OF SOFT TISSUE TUMORS—AN OVERVIEW

The topic of STTs can be confusing to the novice, and before diagnostic competence can be achieved, a general understanding of the field is necessary. To this end, one should first become familiar with benign lesions that mimic sarcomas to prevent the possibility of overdiagnosis. Malignant lesions can then be reviewed and can be placed in context.

Can some method of examination be applied to this vast field to minimize errors? A step-by-step process is perhaps the easiest way to approach each case; this might be called the "skeptical approach" to STT diagnosis. A series of crucial questions should be answered in a defined order. First, regardless of the histology of the lesion, one must ask, "*Is the lesion really a neoplasm?*" (In other words, from the start, all lesions should be considered reactive until proven otherwise.) After all, several pseudosarcomas may have a brisk mitotic rate, yet these are not only benign but often nonneoplastic. Therefore, the mitotic rate alone cannot be relied on as a criterion for either neoplasm or malignancy; instead, the type of differentiation in the lesion must first be decided in many instances. Some lesions require only a quick glance before malignancy is diagnosed. These tumors generally exhibit a high degree of cellularity, necrosis, and an enormous number of mitotic figures per high-power field (hpf). In contrast, reactive lesions often follow certain histopathologic rules and exhibit architectural organization.

The second question is, "*Is the lesion malignant?*" (That is, the lesion should be considered benign until certain criteria are met.) The only presumptive sign of malignancy is necrosis; without necrosis, nuclear pleomorphism and cellularity must be evaluated in context.

The third question is, "*Is the lesion necessarily a sarcoma?*" Could it be a carcinoma or melanoma mimicking sarcoma? (That is, the lesion should be considered a nonsarcomatous malignancy before it is accepted as a sarcoma.) Organ-based "sarcomas," particularly those in the breast, esophagus, and respiratory tract, should be considered pseudosarcomatous carcinomas until further evidence to the contrary accumulates. Ancillary techniques, such as immunohistochemistry and ultrastructural examination, are often required to make this distinction with certainty. Melanoma is one of the great histologic mimickers; it may simulate undifferentiated pleomorphic sarcoma (UPS; previously called malignant fibrous histiocytoma [MFH]), myxofibrosarcoma, leiomyosarcoma, epithelioid sarcoma, malignant peripheral nerve sheath tumors (MPNSTs), and, if it is vacuolated, even liposarcoma. Any lesion with both an epithelioid and spindle cell pattern should be approached with the idea of excluding melanoma before a sarcoma is considered. Although the presence of intranuclear cytoplasmic inclusions within a melanoma is not entirely specific, it may be a helpful morphologic feature hinting at that possibility.

After the first three questions have been answered, one may then proceed to the fourth and final question, "*What is the type of differentiation displayed by the putative sarcoma?*" Depending on the answer to this question, one must determine whether criteria for that phenotypic malignancy are satisfied. The all-important mitotic rate determines malignancy in certain tumor types

TABLE 5.1

Phenotypes of Soft Tissue Tumors for Which Mitotic Rate Determines Malignancy

Fibroblastic tumors
Solitary fibrous tumors
Smooth muscle tumors
Nerve sheath tumors
Granular cell tumors

(Table 5.1). For some phenotypes such as smooth muscle tumors, both the site and mitotic rate are crucial in this determination. The use of this approach aids greatly in (a) the elimination of certain bizarre, but benign, mesenchymal lesions from the malignant roster; (b) the recognition of pleomorphic, but clearly benign, tumors; and (c) the correct classification of nonsarcomas (pseudosarcomatous carcinomas and melanomas), which require a different therapeutic approach.

RECOGNITION OF PSEUDOSARCOMAS

Table 5.2 lists the lesions that mimic sarcomas. Knowledge of the histologic appearance of these lesions is critical to prevent incorrect diagnoses of sarcoma. The following discussion provides some insight into this group of lesions.

Some of the most rapidly growing but relatively small mesenchymal lesions are benign. Any tumor with a tissue culture–like character, as is found in fasciitis and myositis, should be considered benign until it is proven otherwise. Circumscribed and encapsulated fatty lesions with either spindle cells or highly

TABLE 5.2

Pseudosarcomas

Nodular fasciitis
Proliferative fasciitis
Proliferative myositis
Proliferative peribursitis
Postoperative spindle cell nodule
Spindle cell and/or pleomorphic lipoma
Lipoblastoma
Cellular angiolipoma
Bizarre leiomyoma
Fetal rhabdomyoma
Pyogenic granuloma
Papillary endothelial hyperplasia
Atypical fibrous polyps
Myxoma
Myositis ossificans
Others
Nonmesenchymal lesions
  Sarcomatoid renal cell carcinoma
  Pseudosarcomatous carcinoma
  Giant cell carcinoma
  Carcinoma with osteoclast-like giant cells
  Melanoma
  Lymphoma (anaplastic, interdigitating types)
  Follicular dendritic cell tumor

pleomorphic "floret" cells but *without* increased vasculature should also be considered benign. Bizarre nuclear features may be encountered in a host of benign soft tissue lesions, both reactive and neoplastic; for example, leiomyomas and neurofibromas may contain these features. Any circumscribed vascular lesion or a vascular lesion with a lobular architecture, such as that seen in pyogenic granuloma, should be considered benign. Last, a great majority of sarcomas are highly vascular, even if this fact is less than completely appreciated at the light microscopic level. For that reason, relatively avascular lesions can be considered benign, as the intramuscular myxoma exemplifies.

RECOGNITION OF OTHER TUMORS MIMICKING SARCOMAS

Tumors occurring primarily in organs should be considered carcinomas until they are proven otherwise. After all, a variety of carcinomas may mimic fibrosarcoma or UPS/MFH with osteoclast-like giant cells; these may occur in the breast, pancreas, bladder, and other sites (2–4). Tumors resembling the collagenized or storiform type of UPS/MFH often turn out to be pseudosarcomatous carcinomas, as frequently occurs in the larynx (5). Renal cell carcinoma may have a sarcomatoid appearance, a possibility that is well known; therefore, a clear cell component in a possible sarcoma should alert one to this possibility. Stains for epithelial markers should be initiated.

Lymphoma may not only mimic the small round cell tumors, but may also simulate the pleomorphic and inflammatory types of UPS/MFH. Only careful attention to nuclear detail (the majority of lymphomas contain irregular indentations in nuclear outline) alerts one to this possibility. Also, newly recognized lymphoma variants, such as follicular dendritic cell tumor (6,7), the interdigitating reticulum cell tumor (8), and anaplastic large-cell lymphoma (9), may also be mistaken for sarcomas.

SPINDLE CELL CARCINOMA

Spindle cell carcinoma is deceptive, and because routine cytokeratin (CK) markers are frequently absent, it continues to be misdiagnosed as sarcoma. The transformation of a squamous cell carcinoma into a spindle cell carcinoma is a recognized phenomenon in a variety of mucosal sites, such as the larynx, the oral and nasal cavities, and the skin. In fact, it is a form of metaplasia into a fibroblast-like appearance. Several studies note that this change may be accompanied by a gain of vimentin and smooth muscle actin (SMA) along with the complete or nearly complete loss of CK reactivity (10–13). The histologic appearance of a brightly eosinophilic tumor at low power is typical. Furthermore, most cases are not highly pleomorphic but, instead, uniform. The spindle cells are elongated, with open oval nuclei and prominent nucleoli, and they have "plump" cytoplasm, meaning they are wide with some cytoplasm on the sides of the nuclei (Fig. 5.1). These features are not seen in smooth muscle and many "fibrohistiocytic" tumors. Usually, only a focal storiform pattern is seen. A reticulin stain may demonstrate elongated groups of cells surrounded by reticulin. These features should raise the suspicion of a possible spindle cell carcinoma. Studies continue to find a frequent absence of standard CKs AE1/3 and CAM5.2, but if a series of CK subsets is used, approximately 70% of cases are positive (14). Wide-spectrum screening of CK has been shown to be more

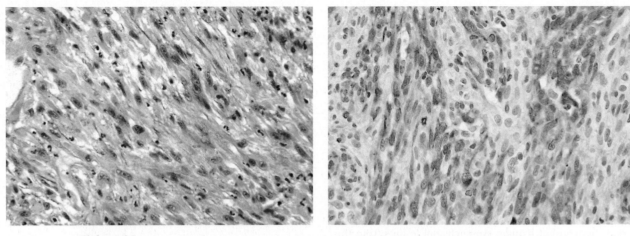

Figure 5.1. Spindle cell squamous carcinoma. Most cases have streaming eosinophilic spindle cells with plump cytoplasm and enlarged nuclei with nucleoli **(A)**; all cells look roughly similar, in contrast to atypical fibroxanthoma. Whereas high–molecular-weight cytokeratin (34bE12) **(B)** often stains the tumor, some cases may show only focal staining, and 30% are negative with cytokeratin subset antibodies.

useful in some situations (15). In skin and mucosal sites, this diagnosis should be considered before that of mesenchymal tumors, such as atypical fibroxanthoma.

SPINDLE CELL MELANOMA

When a melanoma mimics a sarcoma (16–19), its recognition may be based on the presence of separated cords (streaks of spindled tumor cells separated by fibrous tissue on either side—a kind of incomplete nest), a nesting pattern, or the failure to exhibit a completely idealized pattern (e.g., failure to exhibit a well-defined alternating fascicle pattern for leiomyosarcoma, failure to exhibit an excellent storiform pattern or extensive sclerosis for UPS/MFH). Only a high index of suspicion helps one eliminate melanomas from the ranks of sarcomas. In particular, spindle cell or desmoplastic melanoma, whether in a skin primary tumor or a metastasis, may truly simulate a nerve sheath or schwannian tumor because it has a neurosarcomatous ultrastructure and melanosomes may be difficult to find. A key helpful feature is the common diffuse S-100 positivity that is present, in contrast to MPNST. Even in the skin, an intraepidermal melanocytic component may be absent, signifying the lack of this important clue (20). Furthermore, HMB-45, which is present so frequently in ordinary melanoma, is also lacking in up to 75% of cases of desmoplastic melanoma (19,21). Thus, as in spindle cell carcinoma, caution must be used in the interpretation of negative results. Newer markers, such as melan-A, tyrosinase, and microphthalmia transcription factor (22,23), may assist in difficult cases.

RECOGNITION OF THREE MAJOR CATEGORIES

The statement that the two major sarcoma categories are the round cell sarcomas and the spindle cell sarcomas has been made. However, such a formulation is too simplified. The categories are not necessarily pure; for example, rhabdomyosarcoma (RMS), a "round" cell tumor, may have a spindled histology, and it may be included in the differential diagnosis of

spindle cell sarcomas, such as leiomyosarcoma. Dividing sarcomas into three categories, with the third category labeled "other" or "odd," is better. A variety of unusual sarcoma types, each with its own natural history and behavior, are encountered. For example, angiosarcoma, Kaposi sarcoma, paraganglioma, epithelioid sarcoma, clear-cell sarcoma, rhabdoid sarcoma, and alveolar soft part sarcoma would all belong to the third group. Clearly, these do not fit neatly into the round cell and spindle cell categories, and just as clearly, the biologic behavior of each differs; furthermore, each requires an individualized therapeutic approach. On the contrary, the therapy for particular adult spindle cell sarcomas (those of "fibrohistiocytic," nerve sheath, and smooth muscle origin) remains similar, although newer chemotherapy agents are beginning to target specific types such as leiomyosarcoma. Such histology-specific therapies will be increasingly important in the future. Critically important in dealing with this group of tumors is the enumeration of the pathologic characteristics of prognostic significance. Round cell sarcomas often have a rapid course, but as a group, they are also chemosensitive; a large fraction of these sarcomas is potentially curable.

IMPORTANCE OF LINE OF DIFFERENTIATION ("HISTOGENESIS")

The line of differentiation is not particularly important, as yet, for the treatment of many adult spindle cell sarcomas, including most high-grade pleomorphic tumors, and it may not be discernible. Referring to the line of differentiation a tumor exhibits, rather than its histogenesis, is best because of lineage infidelity in tumor progression. However, a pathologist who correctly identifies the *tumor phenotype* (the line of differentiation rather than the cell of origin) of a sarcoma and who renders a specific diagnosis performs a valuable service to the clinician. The treating physician may then refer to the literature on a specific sarcoma for guidance. Classifying RMS tumors correctly, for example, is particularly important because these are treated very differently from other tumors. A correct diagnosis of an unusual sarcoma (e.g., epithelioid sarcoma) likewise alerts the clinician to the likely natural history and potential prognostic factors. Thus, tumor phenotype or line of differentiation remains important, and it will become more so once effective targeted therapy is identified for each tumor.

ORIGIN AND ETIOLOGY OF SARCOMAS

SCOPE OF DIAGNOSTIC ISSUES

To give some perspective on sarcoma diagnosis, there are at least nine tumor phenotypes (smooth and skeletal muscle, lipocytic, vascular, etc.), each of which is complicated by multiple distinctive sarcoma subtypes, resulting in more than 100 sarcoma subtypes.

OVERVIEW

Although the speculation has been that most sarcomas arise from a primitive uncommitted mesenchymal cell, this idea seems less than completely tenable when one considers that the vast majority of sarcomas are indeed of a *single* phenotype and that they remain true to that phenotype throughout their natural history. Occasional sarcomas do "dedifferentiate," or transform, a phenomenon that is discussed later. True malignant mesenchymomas, with their multiple phenotypes, are exceedingly rare. Thus, sarcomas quite likely arise from an abnormal event occurring in a cell of an already committed mesenchymal phenotype, even though such a cell may seem primitive and without visible differentiation.

Do sarcomas arise from benign STTs? The visualization of this phenomenon is rare (24–28). Most sarcomas appear to arise de novo. However, one may occasionally conjecture about the possibility of an associated low-grade or benign lesion; in some gastrointestinal stromal tumors, an adjacent nodule has absolutely bland histology. Similarly, a nerve sheath lesion with a long clinical duration (even if those occurring in neurofibromatosis are excluded) may give rise to this suspicion, and bland nerve sheath regions can be identified in several nerve sheath sarcomas. Thus, a two-step carcinogenic process is suspected in a few sarcomatous tumors, but the vast majority appears to provide no such clue.

SARCOMA NOT OTHERWISE SPECIFIED

Even with technologic advances such as the electron microscope and monoclonal antibodies, occasional sarcomas (roughly 5%) may not be definitively characterized. Therefore, using the term *sarcoma not otherwise specified (NOS)* for these lesions is appropriate. However, some qualifier should be used as a clinical guide (e.g., spindle cell sarcoma NOS or round cell sarcoma NOS). If such a lesion is encountered, a listing of all the attempts to assign the lesion to a particular diagnostic category should be included within the pathology report.

The etiology of sarcomas remains elusive, except in postradiation tumors. Some sarcomas occur in the setting of familial genetic syndromes, such as Li-Fraumeni syndrome (p53 germline mutation) (29) and RB (retinoblastoma) gene mutations (30). Weak associations have been made with polychlorinated biphenyls and polyaromatic hydrocarbons and with dioxin (31–36). However, the latter association is very weak, and it may not be borne out by future work. Diet has been investigated

only rarely (37). In some cases, these tumors may develop in a prior injection site, a phenomenon supported by animal studies (38,39). A viral etiology of Kaposi sarcoma is now accepted, with the agent being the human herpesvirus-8 (HHV8) or Kaposi sarcoma herpesvirus (KSHV) (see "Kaposi Sarcoma"), and some leiomyosarcomas in patients with acquired immunodeficiency syndrome (AIDS) have been associated with the Epstein-Barr virus (40,41).

TISSUE SECTIONS

As a general rule, a minimum of *one block per centimeter of greatest tumor dimension* should be processed; more material may be submitted, depending on the variable nature of the sectioned surface. This general rule must be tempered by the size of the tumor. In small tumors, some sections could include both the marginal and peripheral areas, whereas the remaining sections are obtained from the center of the lesion; thus, in a small lesion of approximately 3 cm, four to five sections might be obtained. In large lesions (5 to 10 cm), 8 to 10 sections may be required. In very large lesions (10 to 20 cm), 10 to 15 sections may be obtained if the lesion is relatively uniform. When sections are obtained, documenting (a) necrosis (by including it in a section with viable tissue), (b) any unusual appearance seen at gross examination, (c) the margins, and (d) the relationships to surrounding structures is important. When preoperative chemotherapy has been administered, a cross-sectional area of the tumor should be submitted to evaluate the percentage of necrosis and fibrosis.

COMMENT ON MARGINS

A thin, stretched *fascial* lateral margin (even when it is 1 to 2 mm) is a complete surgical margin, and such areas do *not* generally give rise to recurrences. These may be described as "close," but the tumor is really contained in that direction, and that area should be described as a fascial margin. In contrast, the cut surgical margins, if they are "close," are a major concern, and in such situations, the margin should be described in a note or comment. Multiple ink colors are now commonly used, and reports should include distances to various margins in a properly oriented specimen.

EVALUATION OF PROGNOSTIC FACTORS

The gross and microscopic evaluation of a neoplasm is of critical importance to the clinician in determining the prognosis. In a sense, this information is even more vital than the exact histogenetic origin of the neoplasm. The evaluation must begin with a gross assessment of the lesion. The entire lesion should be inked, the exterior should be dabbed with fixative to ensure that the ink adheres, and the margins should be adequately sampled. The presence and degree of necrosis should be recorded because this affects tumor grade. Communication with the surgeons is vital for an understanding of their impression of the closest margin. Furthermore, *a diagnosis is incomplete without an assigned grade and a comment on the status of margins.*

The grade of a sarcoma (see "Grade" under later "Evaluation of Prognostic Factors" section) is absolutely key to the subsequent clinical management, and its absence from a report will result in a call from clinicians. As with other tumor sites, use of a tumor template is recommended.

RECOMMENDATIONS FOR THE FINAL PATHOLOGY REPORT

The final pathology report should contain all relevant gross and microscopic descriptive information, and it should be able to stand alone if all of the blocks and slides from a case are lost. In this day of frequent second opinions and detailed therapeutic protocols, standardizing reports of sarcomas is even more important. To that end, the ideal pathology report contains a detailed gross description, particularly of the following: (a) size—in three dimensions—of the lesion, (b) the overall color and texture of the lesion, (c) the variable areas in the lesion, and (d) the extent of visible necrosis. How closely the lesion approaches any of the margins should be specified with precise measurements. Within the gross description, a guide or diagram of labeled sections is often helpful in reconstructing the lesion later. The value of a microscopic description (or comment) is enhanced when it includes information concerning the shape and size of cells, the characteristic patterns that were noted, and any ancillary studies that were performed. The actual wording of the diagnosis should include tumor size, grade, and modifiers such as "superficial," "deep," and "intramuscular." When preoperative chemotherapy has been administered, the percent necrosis/fibrosis should be recorded, supplying the clinician with valuable data on the effectiveness of therapy. A comment on the margins should be incorporated into the report, and a tumor template is recommended.

CONSULTATION

Because of the overall rarity of STTs and the tremendous variation in histologic patterns, even within a given sarcoma phenotype, the suggestion is that consultation be sought in difficult cases, particularly when the original pathologist receives only a handful of cases per year. Sending a case for consultation is also important when immunohistochemistry or electron microscopy may provide important information regarding the patient's treatment and management. To save time, recut sections should be accompanied by at least one representative block or 5 to 10 unstained slides.

LIMITATIONS OF PROCEDURES

FROZEN SECTION

One should not try to make a specific diagnosis (unless it is obvious) from intraoperative frozen sections, but instead, one should attempt to decide whether the lesion is malignant. If this determination cannot be made with confidence, one can resort to terms such as "spindle cell tumor of unknown malignant potential"; even this noncommittal diagnosis guides the surgeon, who may then elect complete excision or await the final report.

ASPIRATION BIOPSY CYTOLOGY

The use of aspiration biopsy cytology in the diagnosis of sarcomas has been successful in the hands of expert cytopathologists, particularly when ancillary techniques, such as electron microscopy and immunohistochemistry, are applied. Indeed, both the overall sensitivity and specificity have been estimated to be 95% (42). However, this high diagnostic yield is undoubtedly related to experience, and those who see only an occasional cytologic aspirate of a sarcoma are unlikely to match this rate. Also, unless small chunks of tissue are available, the pathologist does not have the added benefit of visualizing the morphologic pattern of the lesion. Therefore, a certain amount of interpretive caution is mandated, particularly when a distinction must be made between benign and malignant lesions.

NEEDLE AND INCISIONAL BIOPSY

Because of the presence of variable patterns within any given STT, particularly malignant lesions, the application of a needle biopsy technique can give rise to difficulties. Once again, those who have a great deal of experience with the technique clearly report excellent results in predicting the ultimate diagnosis. Kissin et al. (43), for example, report an overall diagnostic yield of 84% and an accuracy of 90%, and they highly recommend the use of this technique in planning a definitive primary surgical procedure. On the other hand, both they and other pathologists stress the possibility of a sampling error with incisional biopsy or needle biopsy. Underestimation of tumor grade is a recurring problem with needle biopsies as a result of sampling error. Therefore, samples obtained with this approach may be unrepresentative of a neoplasm, and this possible shortcoming should be recognized and communicated to the clinicians planning further therapy.

EXCISIONAL BIOPSY

Material may also be received from an "excisional biopsy." In this form, a rim of normal or marginal tissue may or may not be present, and occasionally, the surgeon may mention that the lesion was "shelled out." Some sarcomas are sufficiently circumscribed to be shelled out, yet they are malignant lesions. Even so, the excisional biopsy should be treated as if it is the definitive surgical procedure, and all margins should be inked and well sampled. Experience with the excisional biopsy has shown that *it is an inadequate approach* to sarcomas because of the presence of tumor at or near marginal areas.

CURRENT SARCOMA THERAPY

Wide local excision (a minimum of 1- to 2-cm margins of normal tissue) has been the most common current approach to sarcomas, and a compartmentectomy is often performed whenever this is possible. In the hands of an experienced sarcoma surgeon, a biopsy is performed in such a manner that it can be incorporated by this complete resection procedure. Increasingly, resections are being performed with smaller margins (2 mm to 1 cm) in an attempt to spare function. The addition of postoperative irradiation has been effective in drastically reducing local recurrence, allowing the wide local excision to replace amputation in many instances. Chemotherapy of advanced or metastatic disease continues to have a low response rate of about

15% to 20%, and complete responses are rare. Commonly, preoperative chemotherapy is administered after a diagnostic biopsy of high-grade sarcoma, and the percent necrosis/fibrosis is recorded. Adjuvant chemotherapy is occasionally used, but it is of unproven value for most sarcomas. Adjuvant chemotherapy is often administered now for some rare but aggressive tumors, such as angiosarcoma and synovial sarcoma, through the use of histology-specific protocols. Furthermore, future protocols ought to exclude tumors smaller than 5 cm.

METHODS OF DETERMINING LINE OF DIFFERENTIATION

Major advances have been made in the diagnosis of STTs as a result of the application of ancillary techniques (e.g., immunohistochemistry, electron microscopy, cytogenetics) within recent years. A brief discussion of each of these methods is presented with the intent of increasing awareness of their usefulness and limitations.

CYTOGENETICS IN SARCOMAS

The analysis of chromosomal patterns in sarcomas over two decades has demonstrated that several STTs with recognizable nonrandom chromosomal aberrations occur (Table 5.3) (44–46). The chromosomal translocations are specific for various neoplastic phenotypes and may have diagnostic value. Processing tissue for cytogenetic analysis is encouraged for those pathologists who have access to this technology in their region.

Newer fluorescence in situ hybridization (FISH) techniques are being applied in some diagnostic laboratories. With further developments in the molecular analysis of sarcomas, molecular assays will likely complement or replace cytogenetic karyotyping (47).

MOLECULAR DIAGNOSIS OF SOFT TISSUE TUMORS

The molecular diagnosis of STTs is a rapidly advancing field, and selected information is supplied in Table 5.4. The findings are clearly useful diagnostically. Specific tumor growth is apparently related to the activation of transcription factors through the formation of new fusion proteins. Some tumors have more than one genetic change, and some genes are involved in multiple tumor types. In the future, molecular microchips testing any given tumor for a panel of genetic changes will become available, making assays simpler and the diagnosis easier. The usefulness of molecular analysis in sarcoma prognosis has been documented, particularly in Ewing sarcoma and primitive neuroectodermal tumors (PNETs) (48), alveolar RMS (49), and synovial sarcoma (50).

OVERVIEW OF IMMUNOHISTOCHEMISTRY

The application of immunohistochemical techniques has had a major impact on the diagnosis of soft tissue lesions. Most laboratories use the avidin-biotin or streptavidin techniques because of their increased sensitivity, and frequently, automated equipment is used along with a panel of markers. The usefulness of

TABLE 5.3	Nonrandom Chromosomal Abnormalities in Soft Tissue Tumors
Tumor Type	*Abnormality*
Synovial sarcoma	t(X;18)(p11.2;q11.2)
Liposarcoma, myxoid	t(12;16)
Rhabdomyosarcoma, alveolar	t(2;13)(q37;q14); del(13)(q14)
Rhabdomyosarcoma, embryonal	t(8;11)(q12;q21); +11 (trisomy); del(11)
Ewings/PNET family	t(11;22)(q24;q12), and i(11)
Desmoplastic small cell tumor	t(11;22)(p13;q12)
Clear cell sarcoma	t(12;22)(q13;q12)
Epithelioid sarcoma	t(8;22)(q22;q11); +2
Chondrosarcoma, myxoid	t(9;22)(q31;q12.2)
Fibrosarcoma, infantile	+8, +11, +17 (trisomies)
MPNST in neurofibromatosis	t(17;22)(q21;q13.1;?)
Undifferentiated pleomorphic sarcoma (MFH)	del(1;q11); others, complex
Leiomyosarcoma	t(12;14); others
Alveolar soft part sarcoma	der17 t(X;17)
Pigmented villonodular synovitis	+7 (trisomy)
Fibromatosis (desmoid)	del(5)(q13–q31); +8; +20 (trisomies)
Neurofibroma	t(1;22)
Atypical lipoma	r(?3)(ring)
Lipoma	t(3;12)(q28;q14); 3 groups
Leiomyoma, uterus	del(7)(q21); t(12;14)(q14–15;q23–24)
Plexiform fibrohistiocytic tumor	−6, −8; deletions
Dermatofibrosarcoma	t(17;22)(q22;q13)
Low-grade fibromyxoid sarcoma	t(7,16) (q32–34;p11); t(11,16) (p11;p11)

MFH, malignant fibrous histiocytoma; MPNST, malignant peripheral nerve sheath tumor; PNET, primitive neuroectodermal tumor; ?, unknown.

TABLE 5.4	Molecular Biology of Soft Tissue Tumors	
Tumor	*Affected Genes*	*Prognosis*
Dermatofibrosarcoma	COL1A1-PDGFB	
Ewing sarcoma/PNET	EWS-FLI1	Favorable if type 1
	EWS-ETV1	
	EWS-ERG	
Alveolar rhabdomyosarcoma	PAX3-FKHR	
	PAX7-FKHR	Favorable over PAX3
Myxoid liposarcoma	EWSR1/FUS-DDIT3	
Clear cell sarcoma	EWS-ATF1	
Synovial sarcoma	SYT-SSX1	
	SYT-SSX2	Favorable over SSX1
Myxoid chondrosarcoma	EWS-CHN	
Desmoplastic small-cell tumor	EWS-WT1	
Giant cell tumor of tendon sheath	COL6A3-CSF1	
Low-grade fibromyxoid sarcoma	FUS-CREB3L2 or FUS-CREB3L1	
Alveolar soft part sarcoma	ASPL-TFE3	

PNET, primitive neuroectodermal tumor.

immunohistochemistry stems from several facts, including the following: (a) some soft tissue phenotypes are associated with an identifiable marker protein; (b) marker proteins are often preserved in paraffin-embedded tissue blocks; (c) the sensitivity and specificity of markers have been reasonably good (although major exceptions do exist, creating problems that are discussed later); and (d) new markers are forthcoming. With the increased sensitivity resulting from antigen unmasking through microwave pretreatment and the like, a high percentage of tumors do stain. However, widespread use has led to the identification of nonspecific reactions; therefore, the results of this procedure must be subjected to strict interpretive caution with a foreknowledge of possible aberrant reactions. Furthermore, a panel approach using multiple markers is generally employed. With this technology, approximately 50% to 75% of all STTs contain relatively specific immunoreactivity, enabling the confirmation of a given phenotype or line of differentiation. Emphasis should always be placed on interpretation within the context of the standard histologic features. Typical marker profiles for STTs are listed in Table 5.5.

Problems with Immunohistochemistry

Serious interpretative difficulties have arisen within the past several years as numerous immunohistochemical markers have been applied to the vast array of mesenchymal lesions. The work of many authors has highlighted problems relating to nonspecificity on the one hand and aberrant immunoreactivity on the other.

MARKER NEGATIVITY. One crucial fact seems to have been forgotten whenever stains are assessed for diagnosis or a contribution to the literature—any given marker does not react with 100% of its proper tumor type. In fact, most studies show that only 50% to 90% of given tumor types contain reactivity for the specific marker tested. Even with antigen retrieval, not all cases react. Therefore, the significant lesson that must be relearned is that one may make a correct diagnosis in the face of marker negativity. For example, not all RMS tumors are desmin positive, not all malignant nerve sheath tumors are S-100 positive, and

not all monophasic synovial sarcomas are CK positive. In such instances, substantial other support is required, but in certain cases, some blocks are useless. Therefore, perfection in an immunohistochemical marker should not be expected.

NONSPECIFICITY. The initial rush of enthusiasm accompanying the appearance of a new ''specific'' marker is often replaced with harsh realism once the marker is subjected to a series of scientific studies. The results frequently show that the marker is useful but less than completely specific. For example, as a group, the muscle markers were originally thought to be specific for the smooth and skeletal muscle cell types, but actins react with myofibroblastic and fibrohistiocytic lesions, with SMA expected in myofibroblasts. Hence, marker reactivity alone does not lead to a correct diagnosis; the cell and nuclear size and shape, growth pattern, tumor location, and patient information must be integrated with the results of marker staining.

ABERRANT IMMUNOREACTIVITY. The phenomenon of marker staining occurring when it is theoretically unexpected is referred to as *aberrant immunoreactivity*. This began with a report of the epithelial marker CK in nonepithelial neoplasms, such as leiomyosarcoma (51), and since then, CK has been identified in nearly every mesenchymal phenotype and tumor. This reactivity is real, it has reflected actual protein expression whenever it has been studied, and it represents the neoplastic expression of markers seen in either the fetal state or in the process of proliferation itself (52,53). The problem also involves the other intermediate filaments—neurofilaments can be found in RMS (54), and desmin can be found in endothelial tumors and rare carcinomas (J.S.J.B., personal observation, 1993). Several leukocytic antibodies stain mesenchymal cell types, and skeletal muscle actin antibodies rarely can stain smooth muscle tumors. Pathologists must take this phenomenon into account in the interpretation of immunohistochemistry. Luckily, most instances of aberrant reactivity show only patchy rather than diffuse staining.

Such aberrant immunoreactivity likely is the result of the direct visualization of the generation of neoplastic heterogeneity resulting from gene de-repression during tumor progression. In fact, a closer examination of aberrant immunoreactivity may

TABLE 5.5	Immunohistochemical Marker Profiles of Soft Tissue Tumors[a]												
	DES	*CMA*	*SMA*	*CD34*	*S-100*	*NSE*	*SYN*	*CK*	*EMA*	*F13a*	*CD68*	*F8*	*CD31*
Rhabdomyosarcoma	++	+	−*	−	+/−	+/−	+/−	−*	−	−	−	−	−
Neuroblastoma	−	−	−	−	+/−	+	+	−	−	−	−	−	−
Extraskeletal Ewing	−	−	−	−	−	+/−	+/−	−	−	−	−	−	−
Rhabdoid sarcoma	+/−	+/−	−	−	−	−	−	+	+	−	−	−	−
Desmoplastic SRCT	++	−	−	−	+/−	++	−*	++	++	−	−	−	−
Liposarcoma	−*	−	−	+/−	+	−	−	−	−	−	−	−	−
Leiomyosarcoma	+	++	++	+	+/−	−	−	+/−	+/−	+	+	−	−
MPNST	+/−	−	−*	−	++	+	−	−*	+	+/−	+/−	−	−
Synovial sarcoma	−	−	−	−*	−*	+/−	−	++	++	−	−	−	−
Fibromatosis	+/−	+	++	−	−	−	−	−	−	−	−	−	−
Solitary fibrous tumor	−	−	−	++	−	−	−	−	−	−	−	−	−
Fibrosarcoma	−	−	−	−	−	−	−	−	−	+	+	−	−
Nodular fasciitis	−	+/−	++	−	−	−	−	−	−	−	+/−	−	−
BFH	−	−	−*	−	−	−	−	−	−	++	−	−	−
DFSP	−	−	−	++	−	−	−	−	−	−	+/−	−	−
UPS/MFH	−*	−*	+/−	+/−	−	+/−	−	−*	+/−	+	+	−	−
Dedifferentiated areas[b]	+/−	+/−	+/−	+	+/−	−	−	−*	−	+	+	−	−
Epithelioid sarcoma	−	−	−	++	−	+/−	−	++	++	−	−	−	−
Angiosarcoma	+/−	−	−*	++	−	−	−	+/−	−	−	−	++	+
Epithelioid hemangioendothelioma	+/−	−	−	++	−	−	−	+/−	−	−	−	++	+
Kaposi sarcoma	+/−	−	+/−	++	−	−	−	−	−	−	−	+/−	+
Paraganglioma	−	−	−	−	+	+	+	−	−	−	−	−	−
Chondrosarcoma	−	−	−	−	++	−	−	+/−	+/−	−	−	−	−
Chordoma	−	−	−	−	++	−	−	++	++	−	−	−	−
Clear cell sarcoma	−	−	−	−	++	−	−	−	+/−	−	−	−	−
Alveolar soft part sarcoma	+	+	−	−	−	−	−	−	−	−	−	−	−

[a]Interpretive caution and correlation with histology are vital; no stain is diagnostic in and of itself.
[b]Dedifferentiated regions of tumors such as leiomyosarcoma, liposarcoma, and chondrosarcoma most frequently lose, but may retain, antigen expression.
BFH, benign fibrous histiocytoma; CD68, factor VIII–related antigen; CK, cytokeratin; CMA, common muscle actin (HHF35); DES, desmin; DFSP, dermatofibrosarcoma protuberans; EMA, epithelial membrane antigen; F13a, factor XIIIa; MPNST, malignant peripheral nerve sheath tumor; NSE, anti–neuron-specific enolase; S-100, S-100 antigen; SMA, smooth muscle actin; SRCT, small round cell tumor; SYN, synaptophysin; UPS/MFH, undifferentiated pleomorphic sarcoma/malignant fibrous histiocytoma; ++, strongly reactive in most cases; +, positive reaction; −, pertinent negatives in a panel approach; +/−, occasional, usually focal, reactions; *, typically negative, but rare positive results reported (see text).

explain why spindle cell carcinomas and carcinosarcomas exist; one hypothesis that has been proposed is that the successive loss of one marker (CK) through the clonal expansion of an epithelial neoplasm is followed by the gain of another marker (e.g., vimentin, desmin), with a consequent shift in morphologic appearance. The fundamental significance of this hypothesis lies in its denial of the need for stem cells or primitive precursors in the development of multiple-lineage neoplasms.

GENERAL MARKERS

Vimentin has been hailed as the intermediate filament for mesenchymal tissues because it is found within essentially all normal mesenchymal tissue elements and most sarcomas. However, vimentin immunoreactivity is not that informative from a diagnostic viewpoint because many tumors, including carcinomas and melanoma, contain vimentin. In mesenchymal tumors, vimentin can best be used in three situations. First, as Battifora (55) demonstrated, vimentin staining highlights those areas on a slide that are likely to contain other forms of reactivity; it acts as a test of a block for marker reactivity in general, and it localizes regions for proper interpretation. Second, vimentin positivity helps confirm a diagnosis in those few tumors, such as epithelioid sarcoma, known to coexpress CK and vimentin. Third, vimentin reactivity provides a better visualization of the cell shape, which may aid in tumor identification.

Several STTs may express specific collagen types, but the collagen typing of sarcomas appears to be a complex affair, and some time may elapse before specific patterns of collagen immunoreactivity become helpful diagnostically. Immunoreactive laminin is commonly seen in neoplasms demonstrating a basal lamina ultrastructurally (schwannian and smooth muscle lesions) (56). Although laminin was not identified in fibroblastic tumors (56), fibroblastic and/or fibrohistiocytic processes appear to be capable of laminin production (57).

CD34, AN ANCILLARY MARKER

CD34 is a 110-kd transmembrane glycoprotein found on human hematopoietic progenitor cells and vascular endothelial cells; it may play a role in cell adhesion and signal transduction. The first reported antibody to CD34 was MY10, raised against a human myeloid leukemia cell line; this differs somewhat from a more common CD34 antibody, QBEND/10. In 1990, Ramani et al. (58) first used CD34 as a vascular marker. Other studies of vascular lesions soon followed, and they showed its sensitivity for endothelial neoplasms; CD34 decorates 70% to 80% of angiosarcomas, 90% of Kaposi sarcomas, and 100% of epithelioid hemangioendotheliomas.

Clearly, CD34 has a much broader reactivity (Table 5.6) (59,60). Three important CD34-positive lesions are solitary fibrous tumors, gastrointestinal stromal tumors, and dermatofibrosarcoma protuberans (DFSP) (61). Some lipomatous tumors, such as spindle cell lipoma and the fibrous areas of atypical lipomatous tumor, are also positive for CD34.

In normal skin, a select group of fibroblastic cells and dermal dendrocytes display CD34. Cohen et al. (62) demonstrated the usefulness of CD34 in distinguishing DFSP from benign fibrous histiocytoma/dermatofibroma (BFH/DF); 88% of DFSPs are CD34 positive, whereas BFH/DF is characteristically CD34 negative. Occasional BFH cases contain CD34, particularly at the periphery; this finding should not deter one from the diagnosis. Therefore, CD34 can be used with factor XIIIa (F13a) to sort out particular differential diagnoses, such as (a) Kaposi sarcoma (CD34$^+$/F13a$^+$) versus BFH/DF (CD34$^-$/F13a$^+$) and (b) DFSP (CD34$^+$/F13a$^-$) versus BFH/DF (CD34$^-$/F13a$^+$).

Finally, CD34 is absent in practically all carcinomas, but it is present in up to 50% of epithelioid sarcomas. Thus, only the following three tumors appear to be simultaneously positive for CK and CD34: epithelioid sarcoma, epithelioid angiosarcoma, and glandular schwannoma.

BCL-2, AN ANCILLARY MARKER

BCL-2 is actually a family of proteins involved in the apoptosis pathway in cell growth and death. BCL-2 is present in selected STTs (e.g., solitary fibrous tumor, synovial sarcoma, DFSP), and if it is used as an ancillary or confirmatory marker, it does have a role in the diagnosis of STTs (63).

ENDOTHELIAL MARKERS

CD31, AN ENDOTHELIAL MARKER

CD31 is a 130-kd membrane glycoprotein (gp IIa) of the immunoglobulin supergene family expressed in some hematopoietic cells and endothelial cells (64). Originally called *PECAM-1* (*platelet endothelial cell adhesion molecule*), CD31 was first reported to have 100% sensitivity and specificity for endothelial lesions; other studies reported reactivity in 78% of 27 angiosarcomas stained (65), in epithelioid angiosarcomas, and in all Kaposi sarcomas (66). CD31 appeared more sensitive than factor VIII–related antigen in detecting tumors of endothelial derivation when these two markers were compared head to head. Work on angiosarcomas has confirmed the excellent sensitivity of CD31 in these malignancies.

Despite the high specificity reported for CD31, weak immunostaining has been noted in carcinoma and mesothelioma (67), and it has been detected by immunoblotting and by polymerase chain reaction in a group of solid tumor cell lines (68). Furthermore, membrane staining is present on histiocytes and macrophages, a possible source of confusion. Thus, there is a lack of absolute specificity of CD31 for endothelial cells, and interpretation should take this into account.

FACTOR VIII–RELATED ANTIGEN

One of the most specific markers for a soft tissue phenotype is factor VIII–related antigen. Produced by endothelial cells, this large protein has been identified in numerous benign and malignant endothelial lesions. For optimal results, trypsinization is commonly performed to detect it. Factor VIII–related antigen can be useful in detecting poorly differentiated angiosarcomas and in clarifying the nature of other lesions. This antigen may be found to some degree in lymphatic endothelium and lymphangiomas (69) but only focally in Kaposi sarcoma (70). When compared with CD31, factor VIII–related antigen is not as sensitive.

Ulex lectin may be observed in endothelial cells, but it is not specific; both epithelial tumors and epithelioid sarcoma (71) also may be decorated by the stain. Thus, few pathologists use ulex now. Blood group antigens also appear on endothelial cells

TABLE 5.6	CD34 in Soft Tissue Lesions: Juxtaposition of Positive and Negative Tumors
CD34-Positive Lesions	*CD34-Negative Lesions*
Solitary fibrous tumor (90%)	Fibrosarcomatous mesothelioma, fibromatosis
DFSP (>90%)	Benign fibrous histiocytoma/dermatofibroma (5%+)
Kaposi sarcoma	Spindle cell hemangioma
	Synovial sarcoma
Smooth muscle tumors, nongastrointestinal (33%–50%)	Atypical fibroxanthoma
Gastrointestinal stromal tumors, epithelioid (80%–90%)	Undifferentiated pleomorphic sarcoma/MFH (5%–10%)
Angiosarcoma, including epithelioid (66%)	Melanoma
Epithelioid hemangioendothelioma	Carcinoma (1%+)
Neuroma/neurofibroma (60%–90%)	Fibrosarcoma (and carcinoma)
Epithelioid sarcoma (60%)	Rhabdomyosarcoma
	Nodular fasciitis

DFSP, dermatofibrosarcoma protuberans; MFH, malignant fibrous histiocytoma.

and tumors of endothelial origin, including poorly differentiated angiosarcomas; however, whether the loss of these antigens is related to biologic potential is uncertain.

FIBROHISTIOCYTIC MARKERS

No specific markers for the "fibrohistiocytic" phenotype are known. Because of the poor specificity of α_1-antichymotrypsin, α_1-antitrypsin, lysozyme, and ferritin, these markers are no longer used. Muscle markers stain a percentage of fibrohistiocytic lesions (see "Muscle Markers"), so these can be used to advantage in limited situations.

CD68, A "HISTIOCYTIC" MARKER

CD68 is a 110-kd glycoprotein found in the lysosomes of monocytes and macrophages and in the primary granules of neutrophils. KP1 is a commercially available CD68 monoclonal antibody raised against a lysosomal fraction of human lung macrophages; other CD68 antibodies include Y2/131, Y1/82A, Ki-M6, Ki-M7, and PG-M1 (72). The histiocyte-like lineage of the stromal cells in nodular tenosynovitis and pigmented villonodular synovitis has been documented with CD68. A similar diffuse reaction is observed in giant cell tumor of soft parts. When one is faced with the differential diagnosis of epithelioid sarcoma versus a reactive granulomatous process, CD68 is useful as a counterpoint to CK. The many tumor-infiltrating histiocytes within a variety of neoplasms—carcinomas, sarcomas, and melanomas—are highlighted with CD68 antibody and should not be confused with tumor reactivity.

Initial reports of prominent CD68 reactivity in UPS/MFH raised questions concerning a possible histiocytic histogenesis. However, a high percentage of positive cells clearly is consistent with reactive histiocytes. Nonetheless, UPS/MFH tumor cells do exhibit variable CD68 (KP1) reactivity (73,74), possibly in approximately 90% of cases. In my experience, the percentage of CD68-positive MFH cases is closer to 40% to 50% after instances with floridly positive benign histiocytes but negative tumor cells have been subtracted. The significance of this finding has been modified by the realization that any tumor with lysosomal granules may be positive for CD68 (Table 5.7). Granular cell tumors are typically CD68 positive (75), along with some

TABLE 5.7

CD68 in Soft Tissue Tumors

Positive Lesions	Cases (%)
Dermatofibrosarcoma	33
Fibrosarcoma	50
Leiomyosarcoma	22–85
Undifferentiated pleomorphic sarcoma/MFH	30–90
Angiomatoid fibrous histiocytoma	45
Neurofibroma	100
Schwannoma	87
Granular cell tumor	100
Malignant peripheral nerve sheath tumor	36–67
Melanoma	97

MFH, malignant fibrous histiocytoma.

TABLE 5.8

Factor XIIIa in Soft Tissue Lesions: Juxtaposition of Positive and Negative Lesions

Positive Tumors	Percentage (%)	Negative Tumors
BFH/DF	90	Dermatofibrosarcoma
Myxofibrosarcoma	80	Myxoid liposarcoma
Angiomatoid FH	10	PFHT
Fibrosarcoma	25	Fibromatosis
JXG		Histiocytosis X
RH/MR		Angiohistiocytoma
SHML		Granular cell tumor
Leiomyosarcoma	50	Leiomyoma
Neurofibroma	100	Schwannoma
MPNST	16	Synovial sarcoma
		Nodular fasciitis

BFH/DF, benign fibrous histiocytoma/dermatofibroma; FH, fibrous histiocytoma; JXG, juvenile xanthogranuloma; MPNST, malignant peripheral nerve sheath tumor; PFHT, plexiform fibrohistiocytic tumor; RH/MR, reticulohistiocytoma, multicentric reticulohistiocytosis; SHML, sinus histiocytosis with massive lymphadenopathy (Rosai-Dorfman disease).

nerve sheath tumors and many other tumors, including carcinomas and melanomas (76). CD68 can be expected in cells that exhibit phagolysosomes or lysosome-like granules, indicating phagocytosis or autophagy. Large studies of CD68 have affirmed its wide spectrum of reactivity and nonspecificity (76). Because of this lack of fidelity to the histiocytic lineage and its reactivity in diverse tumors, CD68 cannot be used as a diagnostic criterion for UPS/MFH.

FACTOR XIIIA, A HISTIOCYTIC MARKER

An intracellular form of the fibrin-stabilizing factor, F13a, is the last enzyme generated in the fibrin coagulation cascade. Normally present in the serum, it may be subject to uptake by tumor cells. F13a is routinely expressed by histiocytes, such as the so-called dermal dendrocytes in the skin and similar cells in other sites (77). Table 5.8 lists the common reactions with the F13a marker. F13a can be of use in the differential diagnosis of BFH/DF versus DFSP (78) and in that of juvenile xanthogranuloma (79) versus histiocytosis X. Most BFHs show prominent reactivity. Hyperplasia of the dermal dendrocytes accounts for the reactivity in Kaposi sarcoma (80). With regard to the F13a reactivity commonly found in UPS/MFH (81), most of the positive cells appear to be infiltrating histiocyte-like cells rather than true tumor cells. Although F13a is said to be of some help in distinguishing UPS/MFH from other spindle cell sarcomas, reactivity can be significant in leiomyosarcomas and MPNSTs. It seems doubtful that it is lineage restricted. F13a should be used with extreme caution, and one should realize that it is only an "ancillary" marker.

MUSCLE MARKERS

DESMIN

The intermediate filament desmin is a sensitive marker for muscle lesions found in tumors of both smooth and skeletal muscle origin. In skeletal muscle, it links Z-bands of adjacent myofibrils. More than 90% of RMS cases are positive, including those that are very poorly differentiated. In several comparative studies, desmin has been proven to be superior to other muscle markers for the identification of RMS (82,83). In smooth muscle tumors, the immunoreactivity for desmin is variable, depending particularly on tumor site. Esophageal and uterine tumors essentially always appear positive for desmin, whereas a proportion in the soft tissue (84–86) and skin appear to be less immunoreactive. This problem is in part a consequence of fixation; desmin is affected adversely by formalin fixation. However, certain normal smooth muscle phenotypes, particularly those around vessels, are known to be negative for desmin. Desmin staining has been favorably affected by antigen retrieval methods.

Desmin can be found in 17% of nonmyogenic STTs (87,88). Therefore, desmin positivity indicates a *myoid* phenotype, not necessarily a muscle phenotype. Myofibroblastic tumors, such as fibromatosis, may contain at least focal desmin reactivity, and sometimes, the reactivity is diffuse. This might cause an erroneous diagnosis of leiomyosarcoma if one depends on the immunoprofile alone. The fact that some cases of UPS/MFH also contain spotty desmin (87,89) may be explained by the presence of myofibroblasts ultrastructurally. Thus, if one is faced with a possible desmin-positive pleomorphic sarcoma, UPS/MFH should be considered together with pleomorphic rhabdomyosarcoma and leiomyosarcoma, and the growth pattern and histologic features should be taken into account.

MYOGLOBIN

Myoglobin is found exclusively in skeletal muscle lesions. Although it is specific for RMS, its sensitivity is far less than that of desmin (90,91). It tends to stain cells with relatively abundant cytoplasm. More specific skeletal muscle markers have largely replaced it.

MUSCLE-SPECIFIC ACTIN

In the 1980s, monoclonal antibodies to muscle-specific actin (HHF35, or MSA) and myosin were described. MSA decorates most leiomyomatous tumors and cases of RMS. Like desmin, MSA is not specific for muscle phenotypes because lesions of myofibroblastic and fibrohistiocytic origin may be positive for MSA (92). Unlike desmin, MSA stains myoepithelial lesions, which may be mistaken for smooth muscle tumors in several organs. Although actins are produced by pericytes, the typical hemangiopericytoma (HPC) is negative for MSA, although myopericytoma is positive.

SMOOTH MUSCLE ACTIN

SMA is restricted in its recognition of actin isoforms; it does not detect other α-actins (skeletal and cardiac) or γ-SMA. SMA is readily identified in smooth muscle neoplasms (93), but it is also found in nonmuscle lesions with a so-called myoid phenotype. With regard to this, understanding that myofibroblastic lesions, such as nodular fasciitis (NF) and fibromatosis, are SMA positive is crucial (94,95); the recognition of this helps prevent their overdiagnosis as leiomyosarcoma, and it can be used to significant advantage in certain differential diagnoses (e.g., fasciitis vs. fibrosarcoma). In reality, SMA expression is the hallmark of the myofibroblastic phenotype (SMA$^+$/MSA$^+$/DES$^-$)

(96). Other tumors showing some SMA-positive myoid reactivity are fibrohistiocytic tumors (97,98), ossifying fibromyxoid tumor (99), some gastrointestinal stromal tumors, endometrial stromal tumors (100), and the dedifferentiated areas of liposarcoma (101).

Despite its name, SMA reactivity can be seen in the following: rhabdomyoma (102); some cases of RMS (103), particularly the botryoid type (J.S.J.B., personal observation, 1998); spindle cell carcinomas (11); myoepitheliomas (104); mesothelioma (105); and melanoma (106). Finally, although angiosarcomas are generally SMA negative, reactivity in rare cases (107) has apparently signified the presence or induction of a pericytic cell type.

MYOD1, MYOGENIN, CALPONIN, AND CALDESMON

MyoD1 is a myogenic regulatory gene on the short arm of chromosome 11 that encodes a 45-kd nuclear phosphoprotein expressed only in skeletal muscle (nuclear reactivity). It transactivates other myogenic genes (myogenin and myf5) in the process of development before the other myogenic proteins, such as desmin. In diagnostic pathology, it clearly is a useful marker for RMS (101,108). MyoD1 had been used to support the myogenic origin of alveolar soft part sarcoma (109), but reactivity was not nuclear, and other studies have refuted this finding (110).

Myogenin immunoreactivity appears to be specific for the skeletal muscle phenotype. The majority of cases of RMS are positive with nuclear staining (108,111).

Calponin is another marker present in smooth muscle; it is found in leiomyosarcoma, myoepithelioma, and myofibroblastic tumors. However, it is not specific, and reactivity can be seen in epithelium and other mesenchymal tumors (112–114). It can complement SMA in putative leiomyosarcomas negative for other myoid markers.

Caldesmon, specifically h-caldesmon, the high–molecular-weight form, is more specific for smooth muscle than is calponin, and it is not found in myofibroblastic lesions, such as fibromatosis or in fibrohistiocytic tumors (114).

Other muscle markers (e.g., titin, Z-band protein, isoenzymes of creatine kinase) are not used diagnostically.

NEURAL MARKERS

For neural tumors, markers can be roughly divided into those that mark lesions of neuronal origin (e.g., neurofilament) and those that react with nonneuronal elements, including Schwann cell lesions (e.g., S-100 protein). Neurofilament, the intermediate filament of neurons, is of value in identifying peripheral tumors, such as neuroblastoma and ganglioneuroblastoma (115–117). Importantly, it does not react with nonneuronal nerve sheath lesions. PNETs, or neuroepitheliomas, also contain neurofilament. Originally, neuron-specific enolase was considered fairly specific for neuronal lesions, as well as selected other tumors. However, this has turned out not to be the case, and a vast array of human tumors contain immunoreactive neuron-specific enolase (118). Thus, the usefulness of this protein as a marker is limited, and the meaning of its immunoreactivity is unclear, despite the availability of monoclonal antibodies to the supposedly more specific γ-isoenzyme. Neuron-specific enolase must never be used alone, the results must be interpreted with extreme caution, and it must be used only when necessary.

Synaptophysin and, to a lesser extent, chromogranin are additional proteins to mark neuroblastoma, PNET, and paraganglioma (119,120).

S-100 PROTEIN

Despite all that has been written about it, S-100 antigen is nonetheless quite useful in diagnostic immunohistochemistry, even though it is found in a wide variety of tissues and cell types. In mesenchymal cells, S-100 immunoreactivity is found within chondrocytes, adipocytes, and lesions of schwannian origin. Because the differential diagnosis of a problematic soft tissue lesion rarely involves more than one of these three phenotypes at the same time, S-100 immunoreactivity has real meaning. Between 50% and 75% of MPNSTs are positive for S-100 (121–123). Indeed, a positive result of an S-100 test, particularly if it is floridly positive, can be taken as supportive evidence for a tumor of schwannian derivation in the presence of the appropriate histology. Occasional cases of leiomyosarcoma exhibit some S-100 immunoreactivity, usually weak staining that likely is caused by the less specific α-subunit of S-100. Perineural cells and tumors thereof are S-100 negative but epithelial membrane antigen (EMA) positive (124). Clear cell sarcoma is another S-100–positive tumor, and the cartilaginous areas in chondromatous tumors are immunoreactive. Although S-100 should theoretically stain most myxoid liposarcomas, many are negative or show only focal positivity. Therefore, a negative S-100 result should be considered inconclusive. Interestingly, the dedifferentiated areas of liposarcoma are S-100 negative, as are cases of myxofibrosarcoma. Hashimoto et al. (125) emphasized its usefulness in distinguishing pleomorphic liposarcoma from myxofibrosarcoma. Other S-100–positive tumors include ossifying fibromyxoid tumor (126) and some cases of synovial sarcoma (127).

CD57, OR LEU-7

CD57 has also been reported in lesions of nerve sheath origin; although this may be a nonspecific reaction (128), it does have limited usefulness. Likewise, the specificity of myelin basic protein within selected lesions, particularly those of schwannian origin, is doubtful. Desmin has been detected in rare nerve sheath lesions (129).

NESTIN

This is relatively common in MPNST, but strong reactivity may also be identified in RMS, leiomyosarcoma, melanoma, and some UPS/MFH (130).

CD99, or MIC2

MIC2 is a 30- to 32-kd cell surface glycoprotein marker encoded by a pseudoautosomal gene on chromosomes X and Y. With the monoclonal antibodies that are used (O13, 12E7, and HBA71), CD99 is uniformly expressed as membrane staining in Ewing sarcoma and PNET, but it is absent in neuroblastoma (131). However, like other surface markers, CD99 is not specific, and it can occasionally be seen in RMS, lymphoma, mesothelioma, UPS/MFH, synovial sarcoma, solitary fibrous tumor, nuchal fibroma, and desmoplastic small round cell tumor, among others (131,132).

EPITHELIAL MARKERS

The two sarcomas that characteristically display epithelial markers are synovial sarcoma and epithelioid sarcoma. Biphasic synovial sarcomas are essentially always positive for CK (133) and EMA (134), whereas monophasic tumors exhibit CK and EMA immunoreactivity in approximately 75% to 90% of cases. However, these two markers may not always be present in the same tumor; therefore, performing tests for both increases the diagnostic yield. Epithelioid sarcoma is also frequently positive for CK and EMA (135). Other tumors, such as rhabdoid sarcoma of soft tissue and chordoma, frequently exhibit CK immunoreactivity.

Aberrant CK immunoreactivity can be found in many other sarcomas and in virtually every mesenchymal phenotype. CK has been reported in a significant percentage of smooth muscle tumors (136), UPS/MFH (137), and vascular tumors, including angiosarcoma (138,139). Other tumors, such as nerve sheath lesions, occasionally exhibit this phenomenon. This has complicated the interpretation of epithelial markers in mesenchymal tumors and spindle cell lesions in general. When frozen tissues are tested, more tumors and a greater percentage of cells are found positive than in the tests of paraffin samples. Luckily, aberrant CK in paraffin sections is rarely diffuse; instead, it marks only individual cells widely scattered throughout a given tumor (i.e., a pattern that is different from that of carcinomas and the epithelium-like sarcomas). Nonetheless, the problem of distinguishing the latter from other sarcomas and sarcomas from spindle cell carcinomas is more complicated. To confuse matters further, nearly half of all spindle cell carcinomas fail to exhibit standard epithelial markers, as my personal experience also supports. Old-fashioned histochemistry in the form of a reticulin stain is a helpful adjunct in the differential diagnosis of such carcinomas and various sarcomas. Thus, islands of cells surrounded by reticulin provide additional support for a diagnosis of monophasic synovial sarcoma in a CK-positive spindly and cellular lesion with fibrosarcomatous or hemangiopericytomatous areas.

EMA does not exhibit complete specificity either. EMA immunoreactivity has been detected in MPNSTs and leiomyosarcomas. Usually, however, the immunoreactivity is focal, and the diagnosis is relatively evident. EMA reactivity in nerve sheath tumors may reflect a perineural cell element (124). When a large series of mesenchymal tumors was tested, promiscuous EMA reactivity was the rule (140), so again, positivity is not definitive for any tumor type.

OTHER MARKERS

MDM2 and CDK4

These two markers have substantial specificity for liposarcoma including both well-differentiated and dedifferentiated forms (141). Reactivity reflects corresponding molecular changes in liposarcoma. Indeed, use of these markers has demonstrated that many retroperitoneal UPSs/MFHs are in fact dedifferentiated liposarcomas.

WT1

Although this marker was originally identified as present in most desmoplastic small round cell tumors, immunoreactivity and mRNA expression have since been observed in many sarcoma types, where it may have prognostic import (142).

PROGNOSTIC IMMUNOHISTOCHEMISTRY

Relatively few studies have focused on the usefulness of oncoprotein and proliferation markers in assessing patient prognosis in soft tissue sarcomas. Therefore, no conclusive prognostic markers are available, although the following proteins have been studied in selected tumors: p53 (143), Rb protein (144), Ki-67 (145), MDM2 (146), vascular endothelial growth factor (VEGF) (147), and adhesion molecules (148). The nm23 gene has also been evaluated (149). WT1 and p16 may have prognostic value.

ELECTRON MICROSCOPY

Electron microscopy is a well-studied technology, so it is discussed only briefly here. Review articles on STT ultrastructure are fairly common (150,151), and further references are provided under the relevant individual headings. Table 5.9, a partial summary of electron microscopy findings, is meant to be a starting point for the ultrastructure of STT. Electron microscopy, which is more expensive than immunohistochemistry and is occasionally subject to artifact and sampling error, is nonetheless an extremely valuable diagnostic adjunct, particularly in the significant minority of marker-negative cases. In the hands of experts, ultrastructural analysis is at least at good as, if not better than, immunohistochemistry. Most institutions lack expertise in the soft tissue field, and interpretation can be difficult for the novice.

EVALUATION OF PROGNOSTIC FACTORS

GRADE

The grading of sarcomas (152–157) has always been complex, variable, and somewhat subjective because agreed-on standards are lacking. The area is made all the more confusing when certain lesions are excluded from the grading process and are assigned automatic grades. The rationale for automatic grading is based on the knowledge of the natural history; nonmetastatic lesions, such as DFSP and well-differentiated liposarcoma, have been assigned to grade 1, whereas highly metastatic aggressive tumors, such as RMS, synovial sarcoma, and angiosarcoma, have been assigned to grade 3. Still other lesions are denied the appropriateness of grade 1 type (e.g., epithelioid and clear cell sarcomas).

The following four types of grading systems are in use: (a) the original three-tiered system proposed by the American Joint Committee on Cancer (152); (b) another three-tiered system based on necrosis (National Institutes of Health system) (153); (c) a combination of differentiation, mitotic rate, and necrosis (French Federation of Cancer Centers Sarcoma Group system) (154,158,159); and (d) the ''low/high'' two-tiered system used by surgeons (surgical staging system) (160). In the older, widely used American Joint Committee on Cancer system, the automatic grading already discussed was used, and only the category of spindle cell sarcomas permitted assignment to all three grades. However, the exact histologic distinction between grades was not clarified. Traditionally, the degree of cellularity, pleomorphism, and mitotic activity determined the grade of spindle cell sarcoma. Costa et al. (153) defined the key importance of necrosis in determining the prognosis. Therefore, they assigned cases with no necrosis to grade 1, cases with 15% necrosis to grade 2, and cases with more than 15% necrosis to grade 3. This system had definite predictive value, but they studied very few cases of RMS, and they did not address the question

TABLE 5.9	**Electron Microscopy in Selected Soft Tissue Tumors**
Type	*Characteristics*
Rhabdomyosarcoma	Glycogen, Z-bands or thick/thin filaments, or filaments with dilated endoplastic reticulum
Ewing sarcoma	No key feature, few organelles, glycogen
Synovial sarcoma	Spaces with microvilli-like processes, cell junctions, external lamina
Malignant peripheral nerve sheath tumor	Interdigitating cell processes, complete or partial external lamina, mesaxon formation, junctions, pinocytosis
Leiomyosarcoma	Filaments with dense bodies (actin/myosin), pinocytosis, external lamina
Undifferentiated pleomorphic sarcoma-MFH	Histiocyte-like cells: prominent lysosomes, Golgi, no lamina, surface ruffles
	Fibroblastic cells: abundant dilated rough endoplastic reticulum, filaments (vimentin), no lamina, surface ruffles
Liposarcoma	Lipid and partial external lamina in immature cells
Epithelioid sarcoma	Prominent masses of filaments, cell processes, intercellular junctions
Clear cell sarcoma	Schwannian features with interdigitating cell processes, melanosomes in 60%–70%

MFH, malignant fibrous histiocytoma.

of whether certain histologic types have a poor prognosis in the absence of necrosis. Multivariate analyses have documented the prognostic importance of necrosis, tumor size, mitotic rate, depth, and status of margins (161,162).

The issue is confounded by the fact that no one system has been universally accepted. Some authors have proposed a two-tiered system—a low and a high grade—that is helpful for planning surgery. However, because most sarcomas are not low grade, this produces an inordinate number of high-grade lesions, and thus, it is not a true prognostication scheme. Furthermore, histologic features may affect some automatically graded tumors, such as synovial sarcoma and angiosarcoma, such that automatic grading is made unduly deceptive. A generally acceptable grading system must be simple, and it should be able to be applied without exception. The French system is based on key factors like necrosis and mitotic rate proven to affect prognosis; it is being used increasingly in this country. However, until agreement is reached on a grading system, pathologists may continue to use any one of several systems, while alerting clinicians about which grading system is being used. Using multiple systems is also appropriate—for example, "sarcoma, high-grade, grade 2 of 3 with French system."

STAGING SYSTEM

The current staging system for sarcomas is critically dependent on the grade assignment, further emphasizing the need for a uniform grading system. In the American Joint Committee on Cancer staging system, the first three stages are essentially defined as equivalent to the three histologic grades. If lymph node involvement is present, the tumor is assigned to stage IIIC. Stage IV is any tumor, regardless of grade, with either distant metastasis or local involvement of the bone or nerve. When this system is used, the respective 5-year and 10-year survival rates are as follows: for stage I, 75% and 63%; stage II, 55% and 40%; stage III, 29% and 19%; and stage IV, 7% and 3%.

FUTURE PROGNOSTICATION

At some point, a different system may be identified to provide patients and clinicians with a true assessment of an individual patient's prognosis, such as a prognostic score based on proven factors.

OTHER PROGNOSTIC FEATURES, INCLUDING DNA PLOIDY

Factors such as tumor size, depth, and location are accepted prognostic indicators. In general, the prognosis is more favorable if a tumor is small, if it is superficial rather than deep, and if it is distal rather than proximal. The degree of cellular differentiation, a feature that is frequently difficult to quantify, nonetheless appears to have some impact on the prognosis. DNA flow cytometric analysis has shown a rough correlation between ploidy and grade, but the lack of aneuploidy does not imply a low grade; several highly aggressive grade 3 tumors (e.g., angiosarcoma, RMS) are frequently diploid. Several studies have documented the effect of DNA ploidy on sarcoma prognosis. In childhood tumors such as neuroblastoma, aneuploidy is a favorable finding; in RMS, the data are complex, but aneuploidy may again be favorable in some instances. In adult sarcomas, the opposite is true; aneuploidy has been shown, in general, to be unfavorable for sarcomas and specifically for certain histologies, such as uterine leiomyosarcoma, gastrointestinal stromal tumors, synovial sarcoma, epithelioid sarcoma, clear cell sarcoma, and possibly MFH. The S-phase percentage may be important, as two studies have shown (163,164).

OTHER STUDIES AND FUTURE PROSPECTS

Surprisingly, certain STTs contain hormonal receptors of one kind or another, and they occasionally respond to antihormonal therapy (165–167). In the future, cell proliferation markers and oncogene proteins or messages may assist in the assignment of patients to favorable or unfavorable prognostic categories. With immunotherapeutic approaches gaining promise, the local interaction between immune effector cells and sarcoma cells (168,169) merits further investigation. With UPS/MFH as an example, a favorable prognostic significance has been demonstrated for human leukocyte antigen (HLA)-DR–positive tumor cells (170) and for HSP-27 (heat shock protein) positivity (171). Interestingly, molecular findings that were previously documented to be important diagnostically are also turning out to have prognostic significance in Ewing sarcoma, RMS, and synovial sarcoma (48–50). Finally, mutation analysis with targeted molecule-based therapy, which has already been used in gastrointestinal stromal tumors, will be important in the future.

SARCOMA SYNDROMES

Many genetic and clinical syndromes are associated with mesenchymal tumors, in addition to that which usually comes to mind—namely, neurofibromatosis (172). The clinical group can be subdivided into those with a constellation of findings, such as Carney myxoma syndrome (173–175), and those related to laboratory information, such as hypercalcemia (176) and hypoglycemia (177). The Carney triad is the association between gastric leiomyosarcoma, pulmonary chondroma, and paraganglioma (178); pathologists should consider it when any one of these tumors is encountered. Kasabach-Merritt syndrome is defined as disseminated intravascular coagulation resulting from benign (179) or malignant (180) vascular tumors. Tryptophan ingestion and eosinophilic fasciitis and/or myalgia syndrome (181,182) is another such association. Genetic sarcoma syndromes include the spectrum of cancer families with sarcomas, as well as the following: breast, lung, endometrial, and adrenal carcinomas (183,184); Gardner syndrome (lipomas, mesenteric fibromatosis) (185); tuberous sclerosis (hamartomas, renal angiomyolipomas) (186); and Bannayan syndrome (lipomas, hemangiomas, macrocephaly) (187), to mention only a few.

SOFT TISSUE LESIONS: LESIONS MIMICKING SARCOMAS (PSEUDOSARCOMAS)

NODULAR FASCIITIS

Nodular fasciitis (NF), which is commonly mistaken for a sarcoma, is a reactive proliferation (188–193) characterized by extremely rapid growth (more so than the usual sarcoma); it achieves its small size of 2 to 3 cm in a matter of weeks. Lesions are only rarely larger or of longer duration (3 months to 1 year).

A few patients report pain and a history of trauma to the area. Most cases occur in persons between the ages of 20 and 50 years, with men and women being equally affected. NF is commonly found on the forearm, arm, face, and shoulder, although it may occur in any exterior location. NF, which is usually well circumscribed, is tan to gray-white with a myxoid appearance, and it is not very distinctive from other tumors grossly.

In NF, several histologic findings are key, the most important

of which is apparent at low power; nearly all cases have a characteristic architecture in the form of a *zonation effect* (Fig. 5.2). The center is hypocellular, and it may have an eosinophilic fibrinous area; alternatively, some cases show central light hyalinization. At the periphery, the appearance is more hypercellular, with small vessels in a lobular array abutting a collagenized zone. In between, spindly cells populate a loose myxoid area. The lesion typically is located just above the muscle layer, with

Figure 5.2. Nodular fasciitis. Note the deep tumor above the muscle along the fascial plane (**A**). Organization is apparent from the periphery to the center (**B**): fibrous tissue with lobules of capillaries (*bottom, zone 1*), radiating vessels and myxoid tissue (*zone 2*), and a hypocellular fibrin-like region centrally (*top, zone 3*). Foamy histiocytes and lymphocytes accompany a loose array of spindly cells with a tissue culture quality (**C**). These cells are diffusely positive for smooth muscle actin (**D**).   *(continues)*

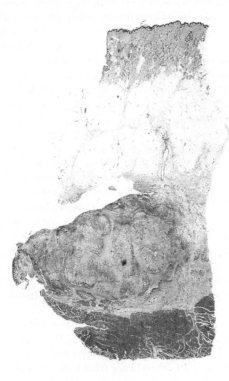

A

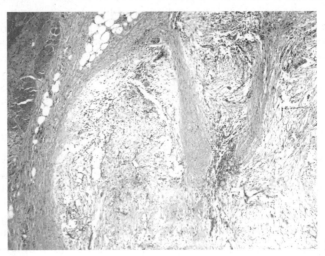

B

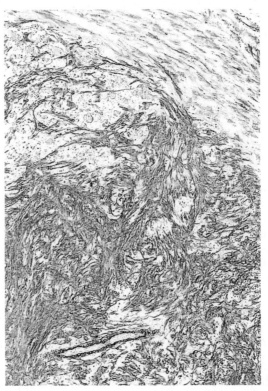

C

D

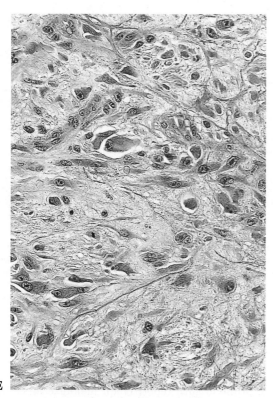

E

Figure 5.2. *(Continued)* In the proliferative variant, individual cells have copious cytoplasm and oval nuclei, like ganglion cells (**E**).

the lateral thick bands of collagen representing the fascial layer. The predominant cell is a variably sized bipolar spindle cell with long cytoplasmic processes. Scattered cells have the characteristic tripolar or stellate shape of the myofibroblast, the cell type identified ultrastructurally. Immunohistochemically, many of these cells exhibit strong and diffuse staining with SMA (Fig. 5.2D) (94,95), which can be used to diagnostic advantage. Some cells may react with MSA, but desmin is often absent. Although the cells may appear worrisome with their active enlarged vesicular nuclei and nucleoli, they are uniform with no pleomorphism. The hallmark is the loose arrangement of the cells in a "tissue culture"–like manner. Although most cases have a random pattern, some "cellular" variants contain storiform areas, interconnecting bundles, or cystic areas focally, even in the same lesion; in these tumors, small microcysts with mucin should be searched for at low power. An inflammatory component of lymphocytes and macrophages is practically always present to some degree; scattered mast cells and histiocytic giant cells can also be seen. Thus, CD68 shows many histiocytes and giant cells, unlike fibromatosis and fibrosarcoma. Plasma cells and neutrophils are rare; large numbers of these should cause alarm (192) because they are a common component of tumors such as the inflammatory fibrous histiocytoma. Scattered red blood cells are often seen, and they may be superficially reminiscent of Kaposi sarcoma; however, the pattern is different, the lesion is too deep, and hemosiderin is hardly ever found. Lastly, *mitotic activity* may be prominent. Most cases contain 1 to 5 mitotic figures per 5 hpf; lesions with a higher mitotic rate should be viewed with caution because they may be a malignant process. Nonetheless, NF is the classic example of an important dictum—nonmalignant reactive lesions may be quite mitotically active.

Perhaps the simplest and most useful subclassification of NF is that of Bernstein and Lattes (192). They divide NF into the following five subtypes: (a) the usual type already described; (b) the reactive type, with its radially oriented vessels around a central loose area, which corresponds to the "repair" variant of Allen (189); (c) the cellular type, with microcysts and little or no zonation effect and imperfect storiform regions resembling fibrous histiocytoma; (d) a metaplastic type, with focal osteoid or chondroid metaplasia; and (e) the proliferative type, which is the same as "proliferative fasciitis" described by others and which Bernstein and Lattes and others believe is part of the spectrum of NF. Shimizu et al. (193) analyzed 250 cases and noted that the three subtypes they described were related to the duration of the lesion; the myxoid type had a short history, the cellular type was of intermediate duration, and the fibrous type had the longest duration. DNA ploidy results are diploid in this and in related reactive proliferations (194).

The most common diagnostic difficulty arises with other fibrous tumors, including fibromatosis, fibrosarcoma, BFH, and MFH. However, unlike NF, each of these has a uniform pattern, and none has the microcysts often seen in the cellular NF variant. Neither fibromatosis nor fibrosarcoma has the loose texture of NF; a uniformly collagenized matrix distinguishes the former, whereas the tight "herringbone" pattern separates the latter. The inflammatory MFH subtype may offer the most significant problem, but nuclear atypia, foam cells, plasma cells, and neutrophils are not found in NF. Differentiation between cellular NF and a deep BFH is occasionally extremely difficult; the factors that favor fibrous histiocytoma include a more superficial location, a closely knit pattern of cells, wide storiform areas, a lack of microcysts, and an infiltrating border. Nuclear pleomorphism favors a fibrohistiocytic lesion. Problematic is distinction from the rare low-grade myofibroblastic sarcoma that mimics fasciitis and is often superficial; however, it lacks microcysts and CD68-positive histiocytes and giant cells and has an infiltrative border.

The points to remember in the diagnosis of this lesion are that (a) the nuclei of NF are never hyperchromatic or pleomorphic, (b) NF is never seen extending to skin except on the face, (c) the average mitotic rate in NF is 1 per hpf, (d) plasma cells and neutrophils are unusual in NF, and (e) NF manifests rapid growth. The diagnosis of NF by aspiration biopsy cytology, although possible, is probably hazardous. Bernstein and Lattes (192) have elegantly demonstrated that NF is clearly a reactive and, generally, a nonrecurrent lesion. Of their 134 cases, all of the recurrent cases were rediagnosed as something else on review, and even partially excised NF did not recur. If all of the reports are surveyed, well-documented NFs are found to recur rarely (1% of cases) (193).

PROLIFERATIVE FASCIITIS

Proliferative fasciitis (195) resembles NF in the following respects: the location within deep tissues, the small size, the presence of a zonation pattern, and the loose quality of cell growth. Strikingly different are the cells themselves. More polygonal in shape, they have abundant eosinophilic cytoplasm surrounding very large, but oval to round, vesicular nuclei with prominent nucleoli that highly resemble ganglion cells (Fig. 5.2). They are dispersed singly within a slightly myxoid or collagenized stroma, and they are more common around the central fibrinous area than at the periphery. To those familiar with it, the lesion is unique, and it is not easily mistaken for anything else. Unlike NF, it occurs in an older age group (older than 50 years), but otherwise, it has a similar presentation and a nonrecurrent natural history.

PROLIFERATIVE MYOSITIS

Proliferative myositis (196) is a related reactive lesion in which ganglion-like cells proliferate between muscle fibers and then separate each of them so that, at low power, a distinctive "checkerboard" appearance is visible. These cells resemble fibroblasts ultrastructurally and immunohistochemically, and they are clearly nonmuscular. Although the checkerboard pattern is occasionally mimicked by an infiltrating lymphoma or infantile fibromatosis, in neither of these lesions are the cells as unusual looking or as dispersed.

PROLIFERATIVE PERIBURSITIS

Proliferative peribursitis (197) is an angiomyxoid tumorlike mass occurring near joints and ligaments. Although this lesion does not have a classic zonation pattern, it does exhibit organization into vascular and nonvascular regions. Clusters of vessels, sometimes with a nodular configuration, occupy the myxoid substance (Fig. 5.3), along with actin-positive spindle cells that have bipolar and stellate shapes. As in other reactive lesions, small numbers of lymphocytes and histiocytes are found, and the spindled cells are dispersed evenly throughout. Sometimes, small rounded histiocytes contain vacuoles, and they can mimic lipoblasts. Many lesions contain cysts, some of which resemble ganglion cysts, whereas others have a definite synovial lining. Dense scarring may also be present.

This highly vascular lesion is different from the hypovascular juxta-articular myxoma, and it can be mistaken for myxoid liposarcoma; it is distinguished from liposarcoma by its variability from area to area, the lack of lipoblasts, and the stellate nature of the putative myofibroblasts causing it. Although it can be seen in any age group, proliferative peribursitis typically presents as a complication of previous joint disease (e.g., degenerative joint disease, ruptured ganglion cyst), and multiple dislocations or external trauma have been noted in these patients.

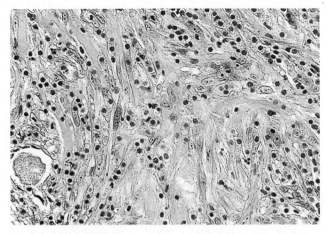

Figure 5.4. Postoperative spindle cell nodule. In this bladder tumor, plump fibroblasts that have large nuclei with nucleoli are disturbing. However, they occur singly, and they are accompanied by an inflammatory cell infiltrate.

POSTOPERATIVE SPINDLE CELL NODULE

Although postoperative spindle cell nodule does not occur in the soft tissues, it does raise the differential diagnosis of sarcoma. In the original report (198), tumorlike masses of the vagina, prostatic urethra, or bladder developed within 5 weeks to 3 months after a prior surgical procedure. An edematous ulcerating lesion with infiltrating borders emerged. Plump spindle cells with abundant amphophilic cytoplasm are found, accompanied by a prominent chronic inflammatory infiltrate and even extravasated red blood cells (Fig. 5.4). The mitotic rate may vary between 1 and 25 per 10 hpf. Although the postoperative spindle cell nodule simulates sarcoma, the cells are not hyperchromatic, and atypical mitotic figures are not seen; the myxoid quality with cell separation and inflammation, when combined with the history, are characteristic. Immunohistochemically, the proliferating cells have the staining pattern of myofibroblasts (positive for desmin and muscle actin), but they may display CK reactivity, which causes spindle cell carcinoma

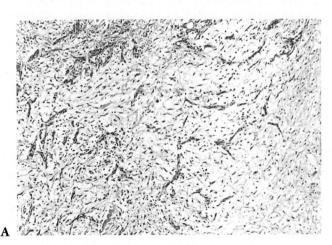 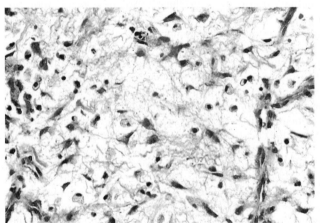

A   B

Figure 5.3. Proliferative peribursitis. At low power, an angiomyxoid lesion mimics myxoid liposarcoma, but the vessels are thicker than capillaries (**A**). At high power, the vessels have a cuff of pericytes, and stellate or tripolar myofibroblasts proliferate in a single-cell fashion (**B**). As in fasciitis, scattered lymphocytes and histiocytes are present.

to be considered in the differential diagnosis. The postoperative spindle cell nodule is not limited to the genitourinary tract, but it may rarely be seen in the endometrium. Similar reactive lesions known as *pseudosarcomatous fibromyxoid tumors* also occur in the genitourinary tract, but they are not associated with antecedent surgery or trauma (199,200).

LESSONS FROM REACTIVE LESIONS: COMMON FEATURES

Every one of the aforementioned reactive conditions shares several of the following features: a myofibroblastic cell type, a loose to myxoid pattern, and a sprinkling of lymphocytes and small round histiocytes of both eosinophilic monocytoid and foam cell types. The repair mechanism of mesenchymal tissue seems to follow this programmatic format regardless of location in the body.

SPINDLE CELL LIPOMA

The name *spindle cell lipoma* is highly descriptive of the pathology—an ordinary lipoma with a quite variable content of bland spindle cells (Fig. 5.5). The following two variations are found: the more common myxoid lesion and a nonmyxoid fibrous type. Notably absent from either type are the lipoblasts and the capillary network of liposarcoma. The spindle cells morphologically remind one of those seen in neurofibroma. The nuclei may be wavy, and they seem to stream along in the same direction. In actuality, distinguishing between a neurofibroma and a fibrous histiocytoma deep within fat can be difficult in those cases in which spindle cells predominate. The spindle cell lipoma (201,202), however, fails to exhibit a storiform pattern; it is frequently more cellular than the usual neurofibroma; and it is S-100 negative and CD34 positive. Its clinical presentation is characteristic, with a vast majority of lesions occurring on the back of the neck or on the shoulder in elderly men; however, odd locations have been reported. In the fibrous variant, thin bands of collagen accompany the proliferation in a manner that is similar to that seen in solitary fibrous tumor. For the tumor to recur is unusual.

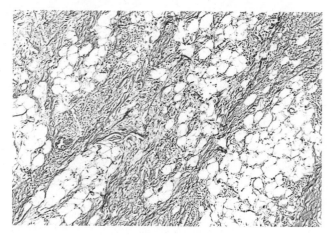

Figure 5.5. Spindle cell lipoma. A proliferation of adipocytes is transected by disorganized bands of collagen containing spindle cells. In some cases, the spindle cells may be predominant.

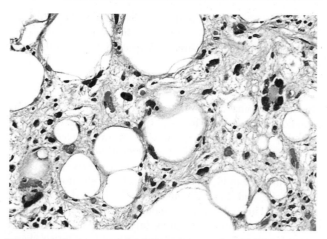

Figure 5.6. Pleomorphic lipoma. The characteristic floret cells are large pleomorphic cells with nuclei around the cell periphery. Adjacent fat cells are variably sized, and additional smaller spindle cells are present.

PLEOMORPHIC LIPOMA

As the name implies, this unusual but benign tumor (203,204) is characterized by very large cells against a background of fibroadipose tissue; practically all cases are superficial—in the subcutaneous tissue. The following four histologic features should be noticed: (a) circumscription with encapsulation (unlike liposarcoma), (b) a wreathlike arrangement of the nuclear lobes in the characteristic "floret" cells (Fig. 5.6), (c) a lack of prominent vascularity, and (d) a rarity of lipoblasts. Smaller spindly cells with elongated nuclei in a lightly collagenized background are also seen, and these are reminiscent of spindle cell lipoma. The clinical setting of this CD34-positive tumor is similar to that of spindle cell lipoma; it is a superficial tumor found almost exclusively on the back of the neck in older men. Cases in women or unusual locations are infrequent. At one time, the floret cells were considered pathognomonic for this tumor, but they can occasionally be identified in liposarcoma. Extremely rare mitotic figures and a large size do not detract from the diagnosis. No aggressive behavior has been reported; however, one or two instances of local recurrence have been documented. Pleomorphic lipoma is rare, being only one-tenth as common as the spindle cell lipoma, which in turn accounts for only 1.5% of all adipocyte tumors. The cytogenetic findings show a relationship to spindle cell lipoma and clearly differ from those of atypical lipoma (205).

LIPOBLASTOMA

Vellios et al. (206) initially described the benign fatty tumor called *lipoblastoma*. It characteristically occurs on the extremities of young children, particularly boys, before the age of 3 years (206), but rare cases can occur in adulthood. In this lesion, prominent fibrous septa divide the adipose tissue into lobules, and a light myxoid quality is visible at low power. A range of differentiation, from unvacuolated spindle cells within the myxoid matrix to increasingly larger and more vacuolated cells to the mature adipocyte, can be noted at high power. Despite the presence of these scattered developing lipoblasts, the lesion lacks the capillary network of liposarcoma. If these lesions are followed for some time, they gradually mature, with the disappearance of the spindle and myxoid elements. The clinician should have a natural reluctance to diagnose liposarcoma in children because such lesions are exceedingly rare at that age.

CELLULAR ANGIOLIPOMA

Most angiolipomas are easily recognized as the mainly fatty subcutaneous tumors that they are. Unusual cases may manifest; examples include an overgrowth of the vascular component mimicking Kaposi sarcoma (207) or even other solid lesions, such as smooth muscle tumors. Because the vessels are probably small venules, spindle cells representing pericytes dominate the appearance, and these are intermingled with endothelial cells (Fig. 5.7). The cellular angiolipoma is set apart from Kaposi sarcoma by the following features: (a) it is deeper because it is a subcutaneous tumor; (b) it is circumscribed; (c) it nearly always contains small vessel thrombi; and (d) it incorporates mature fat (however little) within its confines. Some of the atypical vascular lesions of the breast bear a resemblance to these tumors.

BIZARRE LEIOMYOMA

That pleomorphism is not a sine qua non for sarcoma is best exemplified by this highly pleomorphic but benign smooth muscle tumor, which is most frequently found in the uterus. Under various designations (e.g., atypical, symplastic, apoplectic), these tumors are characterized by quite large, atypical-appearing nuclei in an otherwise classic smooth muscle tumor (Fig. 5.8). They tend to be small and to have either very few or no mitotic figures. Whenever nuclear atypia is encountered in a putative soft tissue or retroperitoneal leiomyoma, mitoses should be sought very carefully, and a malignant diagnosis should be seriously considered.

FETAL AND GENITAL RHABDOMYOMA

The fetal rhabdomyoma, which is occasionally confused with the better differentiated myotubular forms of RMS, occurs mainly in the head and neck of toddlers (208). A similar lesion

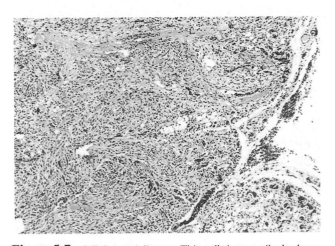

Figure 5.7. Cellular angiolipoma. This well-circumscribed subcutaneous tumor is composed nearly entirely of a vascular proliferation; on closer inspection, scattered fat cells are noted. Some of the blood-filled spaces contain thrombi.

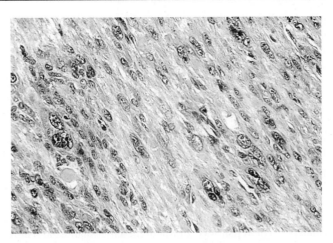

Figure 5.8. Bizarre leiomyoma. Enlarged pleomorphic nuclei were found in this uterine tumor; however, a careful search proved the well-sampled lesion to be completely nonmitotic.

is found in the adult female genital tract (209). Small parallel bundles of easily recognized rhabdomyocytes are separated by thin strands of collagen and vascular tissue or by less differentiated cells. The rhabdomyocyte groups intersect in a random fashion, although the entire lesion retains an architectural structure of separated bundles of streaming tumor cells (Fig. 5.9). The nuclei are bland in appearance, and only occasional

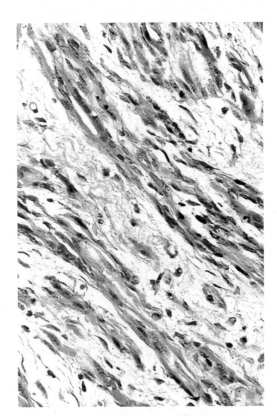

Figure 5.9. Rhabdomyoma, genital type. In the "separated bundle" pattern, fibrous tissue is seen on either side of spindling groups of cells; this pattern may be a finding in superficial epithelioid malignant schwannoma or, as seen here, in genital rhabdomyoma; note the long cytoplasmic extensions with parallel sides, peculiar to skeletal muscle tumors.

nucleoli can be seen. Notably, the tumor lacks mitotic activity, a cambium layer, and the jaggedly infiltrating pattern of RMS at its periphery. Thus, whereas the rhabdomyoma is not really circumscribed, most tumor cells tend to stop at roughly the same location in the lateral and deep aspects of the tumor. When the fetal type is highly cellular and compact, it becomes more difficult to distinguish from RMS (210). In the female genital tract, the genital type occurs at a rather advanced mean age (36 years) in comparison with genital RMS, and it is much less cellular than the fetal type already described.

PAPILLARY ENDOTHELIAL HYPERPLASIA

Although papillary endothelial hyperplasia (211–213) may commonly be mistaken for an angiosarcoma, these can be easily differentiated. First, most of these reactive lesions occur within a vessel or a vessel-like structure, and therefore, unlike the malignant tumor, they are circumscribed. Second, the nuclei are quite bland. Third, rather than ramifying the vascular channels, the papillary formations tend to occupy a contiguous large space that can be traced around much of the proliferation (Fig. 5.10). In foci, a fibrin-like matrix probably representing a stage of an organizing thrombus is observed in this lesion. Although the lesion may occur almost anywhere, it is frequently found on the fingers as a painful nodule. Pathologists should be aware that it can proliferate in a hematoma or blood-filled space within another tumor, causing further confusion, or that it can result from procedures such as fine-needle aspiration of organs, where it is noncircumscribed, simulating angiosarcoma even further.

ATYPICAL FIBROUS POLYPS

Atypical fibrous polyps are unusual but benign lesions (211–213) that occur most often around orifices such as the nose, vagina, and anus, although they also form elsewhere. Within what otherwise is bland fibrous tissue, highly atypical cells are seen superficially resembling those in a sarcoma. However, unlike the latter, atypical fibrous polyps exhibit multiple but uni-

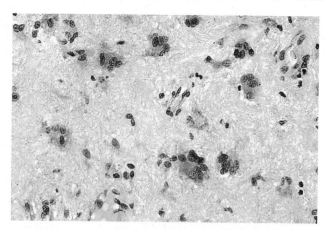

Figure 5.11. Atypical fibrous polyp. Protruding nodules in various sites are composed of collagen punctuated by individually scattered fibroblasts, some of which have "pleomorphic" nuclei; the latter are actually multiple lobes of the same size rather than true bizarre nuclei.

form oval nuclear lobes that all are the same size (Fig. 5.11). These lobes are often clustered, and they overlap (similar to the "floret" cell). Another characteristic is that the atypical cells are scattered singly throughout the lesions, never appearing to group. Therefore, another rule of STT pathology is that neoplasms tend to exhibit crowding and adjacent cell growth, in contrast to the single-cell growth of reactive fibroblastic lesions. Furthermore, cells with multiple nuclear lobes are not truly atypical or pleomorphic and should be ignored when considering malignancy.

GIANT CELL FIBROBLASTOMA

Giant cell fibroblastomas are discussed in "Dermatofibrosarcoma Protuberans."

MYXOMA

Myxoma is an extremely gelatinous lesion that commonly appears as a circumscribed mass deep within the muscle, usually in an extremity (214,215). Strangely enough for a nearly avascular lesion (Table 5.10, Fig. 5.12), an occasional myxoma may reach a considerable size (10 to 13 cm). The bulk of the lesion consists of a slightly basophilic proteoglycan matrix, and at high power, only a few stellate or bipolar cells with oval nuclei are seen (Fig. 5.12). Unlike myxoid liposarcoma, the lesion is circumscribed and very hypocellular, and it lacks any significant vascularity. An inapparent architecture is present; toward the periphery, an increased number of spindle cells abut on a lightly collagenized capsule. Centrally, a mucinous cyst or focal eosinophilic fibrinous quality can often be appreciated. These attributes suggest a reactive lesion; indeed, the myxoma rarely, if ever, recurs. The differential diagnosis includes nerve sheath myxoma, in which attention to the periphery shows parallel layers of spindly cells with wavy nuclei representing the nerve. The cardiac myxoma (216,217) is different because it contains endothelial cells in a fibrinous or myxoid matrix; although some consider this a peculiar reorganizing thrombus, chromosomal aberrations (449) and aneuploidy in some may signal a neoplastic nature. The cardiac myxoma is a frequent component of the Carney syndrome (173).

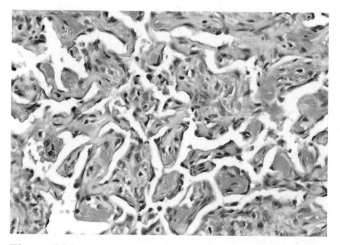

Figure 5.10. Papillary endothelial hyperplasia. Papillary structures project into a large continuous space, unlike the less ramifying channels of angiosarcoma; cores of either cellular collagen or fibrin are lined by bland cells without the tufting noted in angiosarcoma.

TABLE 5.10		Differential Diagnosis of Myxoid Lesions: Histology and Histochemistry					
Tumor	Nodules	Vessels[a]	Cellularity	Pleomorphism	Mitoses	IHC	
Myxoma	S	+/−	+/−	−	− (+/−)	Myoid$^{+/-}$	
Angiomyxoma, superficial	M	+	+	−	+/−	—	
Angiomyxoma, aggressive	S	+	+	−	+/−	Des$^+$, MSA$^-$	
Angiomyofibroblastoma	S	+	+	−	+/−	Des$^+$, MSA$^-$	
Myxofibrosarcoma	S or M	+ +	+ + +	+/+ +	+ +	Myoid$^{+/-}$	
Myxoid liposarcoma	S or M	+ +	+ +	−	+	S-100	
Myxoid chondrosarcoma	M	+	+	−	+/−	S-100; CK$^-$	
Myoepithelioma	M	+	+	−	+	CK, p63	

[a]See text and schematic (Fig. 5.33) for vessel description.
CK, cytokeratin; Des, desmin; IHC, immunohistochemistry; M, multiple; MSA, muscle-specific actin; S, single; +, present; + + +, strongly present; −, not present; +/−, rare or focal.

MYOSITIS OSSIFICANS

Massive calcification and other events occur quickly in myositis ossificans (218). Within the span of 4 to 6 weeks after the commonly associated traumatic injury, pain and tenderness develop, followed by a mass lesion within the extremity musculature, typically in a young male patient (Fig. 5.13). The massive calcification of the lesion is apparent on radiographic study, and histologically, it has the configuration of lamellar bone. It is a solitary and well-circumscribed lesion with organization into the following three zones: a periphery of well-formed lamellar bone gradually maturing from poorly formed trabeculae of osteoid in the middle zone and, in the center, a fibroblastic proliferation with remarkable similarity to NF. Older, mature lesions resemble soft tissue osteomas. Before the lesion is well developed, it may resemble osteosarcoma, but, in extraosseous osteosarcomas, the osteoid is located more centrally, which is the reverse of myositis. Rarely, malignant transformation has occurred within myositis ossificans (24); although this term is a misnomer, it has nonetheless been retained. Like other reactive lesions, myositis ossificans shows zonation at low power.

OTHERS

Many other pseudosarcomatous lesions (198,219–230) have been recognized, and considering them in the differential diagnosis and keeping the possibility of a sarcoma mimic in mind at all times are important. To reiterate, the possibility of spindle cell carcinoma should always be entertained whenever a lesion is in or near an organ or the skin; likewise, melanoma is always part of the differential diagnosis.

FIBROUS LESIONS

NF, proliferative myositis, and atypical fibrous polyps have already been described in "Soft Tissue Lesions: Lesions Mimicking Sarcomas (Pseudosarcomas)."

EOSINOPHILIC FASCIITIS AND EOSINOPHILIA-MYALGIA SYNDROME

In 1975, Shulman described a diffuse fasciitis with eosinophilia, a fibrosing inflammatory condition of skin, subcutaneous tissue, and fascia that has come to be known as *eosinophilic fasciitis* (231). Patients had painful symmetric thickenings, particularly on the thighs. The infiltrates of eosinophils were typically accompanied by clusters of lymphocytes, mast cells, and histio-

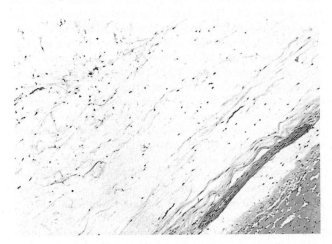

Figure 5.12. Intramuscular myxoma. This markedly hypocellular lesion is well circumscribed and nearly avascular. No pleomorphism is present.

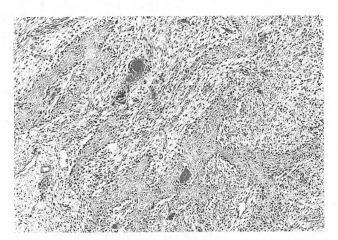

Figure 5.13. Myositis ossificans. Parallel arrays of immature osteoid arise from a fasciitis-like background to form bony trabeculae; the nuclei are disturbing because of prominent nucleoli. Such osteoid is found at the periphery of myositis and panniculitis ossificans, lesions that form swiftly.

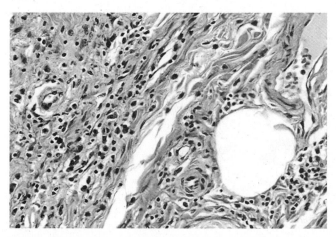

Figure 5.14. Eosinophilic fasciitis. A woody, firm subcutaneous lump in the thigh consists of fibrosis with prominent eosinophils, mast cells, lymphocytes, and plasma cells. Often, perivascular lymphoid cuffs are present, and focal myositis is rarely seen.

cytes, and the resultant lesions were either fibrotic or fibromyxoid (Fig. 5.14). Myopathy was observed only occasionally. In 1990, the ingestion of L-tryptophan became associated with a similar disease, the eosinophilia-myalgia syndrome, which is characterized by myositis and neuritis. After a flurry of articles and investigations, a toxin contaminating the drug during manufacturing was identified as a likely cause of eosinophilia-myalgia syndrome (232–234). The pathologic findings of eosinophilia-myalgia syndrome overlap with those of eosinophilic fasciitis, and only a history of L-tryptophan can distinguish between the two.

TUMEFACTIVE FIBROINFLAMMATORY LESIONS

Cases in which the surgeon observes a tumor but the biopsy specimen shows only fibrosis and mild inflammation are referred to as *tumefactive fibroinflammatory lesions*. Many such cases present as head and neck tumors, although they can also be seen on the extremity (235). The fibrosis is characteristically dense, and occasionally, obliterated vascular structures are identified on elastic stain. The etiology is unknown.

Focal myositis is another histologically bland entity with a mass-forming presentation (236)

RETROPERITONEAL FIBROSIS

Although true fibromatosis of the retroperitoneum may occur in Gardner syndrome, most cases of retroperitoneal fibrosis do not appear to be a proliferation of fibroblasts as much as they do a scarring process (237). Fibrosis with clusters of lymphocytes and plasma cells is found. Occasionally, large presacral masses can be seen (238). The pathogenesis may be related to autoimmunity or to certain drugs, such as methysergide.

KELOID

The keloid, which is easily recognized as a hypertrophic scar, is typified by the presence of very thick, highly eosinophilic collagen bands. The reason for mentioning this entity is that

the presence of such "keloidal collagen" in another lesion, such as fibromatosis, may provide a clue to its fibroblastic nature.

FIBROMA

A true circumscribed fibroma is rare in the soft tissues. Hypocellularity accompanied by dense collagen is the main feature in the sclerotic fibroma (239), but pleomorphic skin tumors have been described (240). If a pleomorphic fibroma is a consideration, excluding the desmoplastic melanoma with an S-100 stain is wise.

Better known are the examples of *fibroma of tendon sheath* (241). In the usual clinical setting, a male patient between 30 and 50 years of age presents with a nodule on the fingers, hands, or wrist. These well-circumscribed, generally small tumors may be lobulated. The dense collagen is variably stained, and small vascular slits in the tumor separate the widely scattered spindled fibroblasts. Focally, the lesions may be cellular, particularly at the periphery, but mitotic figures are scarce. This lesion is probably reactive, and it may represent a burned-out "giant cell tumor of tendon sheath"; however, giant cells are rarely seen, and this assertion has been criticized. A subtype with pleomorphism in which giant nuclei are dispersed singly, as in atypical fibrous polyps, has been described (242).

The *nuchal fibroma* often occurs on the back of the neck and presents as fibrofatty tissue with very dense collagen and occasional cartilaginous metaplasia (243).

Associated with the polyposis syndrome, the Gardner fibroma is a highly collagenized and hypocellular tumor similar to nuchal fibroma occurring predominately in the back, chest wall, and flank (244).

COLLAGENOUS FIBROMA

Collagenous fibroma, which was originally called *desmoplastic fibroblastoma* (245), is a subcutaneous lesion without primitive elements (246). It most closely resembles a very hypocellular fibromatosis with scattered stellate spindle cells, some of which show SMA positivity. Although some lesions are infiltrative, most have a capsule. No recurrences have been reported.

ANGIOFIBROMA AND GIANT CELL ANGIOFIBROMA

Angiofibroma is a tumor that occurs in young male patients, particularly in the nasopharynx (247) (see Chapter 21). It consists of fibroblastic cells proliferating among large open blood vessels. Because the vessels are indigenous to the area, an angiofibroma actually resembles fibromatosis with vessels. *Giant cell angiofibroma* is an entity occurring in the orbital region. A fibrous lesion, it resembles a large, atypical fibrous polyp (248). *Cellular angiofibroma* is another lesion with fibrous tissue, bland cells, and occasionally fat (248). The tumor cells are CD34 positive, so distinguishing these angiofibromas from a spindle cell lipoma with many spindle cells is difficult. These lesions may belong to the solitary fibrous group.

ELASTOFIBROMA

Nearly every example of elastofibroma has occurred in the mid back and scapular region (249,250). On low power, it appears

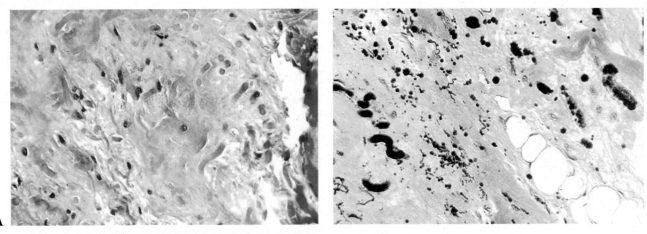

Figure 5.15. Elastofibroma. Unusual thick, wormlike fibers are embedded in this lesion, a fibrofatty mass (**A**). On elastic stain (**B**), the abnormal quantity and shapes of elastic fibers can be readily identified.

to be a fibroblastic or fibrofatty proliferation that is densely collagenized, but with higher power, circular and snakelike eosinophilic bands of elastic tissue are noted (Fig. 5.15). Usually, these elastic fibers have a beaded appearance and constitute most of the stroma. The underlying cause of this pseudotumor produced by abnormal elastogenesis is unknown, but the surgically excised lesion has no tendency to recur.

FIBROUS PROLIFERATIONS OF CHILDHOOD

A delineation of every fibrous proliferation that may occur in children would be voluminous (251). Practically all such lesions are associated with a characteristic age and location, and they may be solitary or multiple; recurrence or regression may or may not occur. When such lesions are encountered, some of which may simulate fibrosarcoma or other sarcomas, consulting soft tissue or pediatric pathology texts or review articles is best. Only selected features of certain lesions are discussed here. The *fibrous hamartoma of infancy* is a solitary, poorly circumscribed proliferation in which loosely shaped spindle cells are found in organoid nodules within fatty tissue (252). In *infantile digital fibromatosis*, the pathognomonic feature is the presence of small, round intracytoplasmic inclusions approximately the size of a lymphocyte nucleus; they are periodic acid-Schiff (PAS) negative, and they apparently consist of actin filaments (253). In *infantile myofibromatosis*, small bundles of spindle-shaped cells resemble smooth muscle (254). Cutaneous nodules, gingival hypertrophy, and flexure contractures characterize the mesenchymal dysplasia known as *juvenile hyaline fibromatosis*, which is probably inherited as an autosomal-recessive trait (255). The amorphous hyaline substance found within it has areas resembling keloidal collagen. *Fibromatosis colli* presents as a rapidly growing mass in the second to fourth week of life, and microscopically, it appears as a diffuse scar within skeletal muscle. In *calcifying aponeurotic fibroma* (256), ill-defined and painless masses appear on the hands and feet of children between the ages of 10 to 15 years; in the classic lesion, primitive mesenchy-

mal cells resembling fibromatosis or fibrosarcoma occur in nodules surrounding central calcification.

ANGIOMYXOID LESIONS, INCLUDING ANGIOMYOFIBROBLASTOMA

ANGIOMYOFIBROBLASTOMA

Angiomyofibroblastoma is comprised of small spindle cells accompanied by small but widely arced vessels (257–259). Pleomorphism is absent, and the tumor is circumscribed (Fig. 5.16; see Table 5.10 for the differential diagnosis). Unlike aggressive angiomyxoma, with which angiomyofibroblastoma may be confused, it is more vascular and does not have vessels that are open and round. It can also be mistaken for liposarcoma, but no true lipoblasts are found. The immunoprofile, which was originally reported to be distinct, is the same as that of aggressive angiomyxoma—it is positive for desmin but negative for MSA and SMA; thus, the distinction between the two entities must

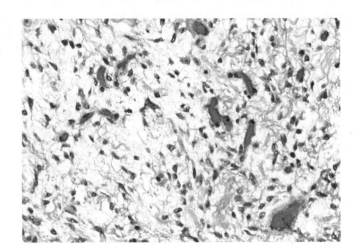

Figure 5.16. Angiomyofibroblastoma. Small cells, some stellate in appearance, proliferate in a loose myxoid matrix accompanied by short capillary vessels. No lipoblasts are seen, and the cells are positive for desmin (see text).

be based on the hematoxylin and eosin appearance (260). Rare sarcomatous transformation has been noted (261).

SUPERFICIAL ANGIOMYXOMA

Described in detail by Allen et al. (262), the superficial angiomyxoma is a cutaneous and subcutaneous multinodular hypocellular myxoma-like tumor that may contain epithelial elements in the form of squamous inclusions. The recurrence rate is higher for lesions with epithelial elements (60%) than for those that do not have them (20%). Some cases are related to Carney syndrome (see Table 5.10 and Fig. 5.33 for the differential diagnosis).

AGGRESSIVE ANGIOMYXOMA

Aggressive angiomyxoma (see Chapter 51) also occurs in male patients, and it is found on nongenital regions of the body (263,264); it can be distinguished from angiomyofibroblastoma by its large size, infiltrating border, and thick rounded vessels (see Table 5.10 and Fig. 5.33 for the differential diagnosis). With only a 30% recurrence rate, it is not as aggressive as originally thought.

INFLAMMATORY MYOFIBROBLASTIC TUMOR ("PSEUDOTUMOR")

This myofibroblastic proliferation (227,265–268) may be seen in a wide variety of locations in both children and adults. Typically, inflammatory myofibroblastic tumor is a circumscribed but nonencapsulated lesion; it contains spindle cells proliferating in a background of fibrosis with lymphocytes; plasma cells; histiocytes; foamy macrophages; and, occasionally, eosinophils and neutrophils. In some cases, the stroma is sclerotic and hypocellular, whereas in other cases, numerous SMA-positive spindle cells with pale eosinophilic cytoplasm are noted (Fig. 5.17). Nuclear pleomorphism and atypical mitoses are absent. The inflammatory myofibroblastic tumor, which was thought to be reactive in nature at one time, is a true neoplasm with the potential for recurrence (35%) and multifocality; clonal cytogenetic findings support this view. The cases originally described as inflammatory fibrosarcoma are generally considered to belong to this group of lesions (269). Molecular findings show that the inflammatory myofibroblastic tumor demonstrates a fusion of the TPM3 or TPM4 (tropomyosin) gene to the ALK (anaplastic lymphoma kinase) gene, and 40% to 60% of cases are immunoreactive with the ALK antibodies ALK1 or p80 (270).

FIBROMATOSIS

Several fibromatoses occur in adults (271–274), mainly in two distinctly different forms. First, lesions occurring on the hands and feet (palmar and plantar, respectively) appear as contractures with small nodules; cellular fibrotic lesions with variable amounts of collagen are seen among the tendinous tissue. Although they are frequently multinodular, a single dominant nodule may be present. The lesions are rarely misdiagnosed. Unlike the proliferation in scars, proliferation in fibromatosis is uniform and relatively hypovascular, and it lacks hemosiderin. Although the palmar and plantar fibromatoses may recur locally after excision, they are localized problems without the same potential for growth and infiltration that is seen in the desmoid tumors.

The second, or desmoid, type of fibromatosis is noted clinically as a large mass, often on the abdomen or trunk. Here, a uniformly cellular appearance is typical (Fig. 5.18). The fibroblasts in one plane are bipolar with attenuated to invisible cytoplasm and a thin, oval, pointed nucleus. In another plane, the cells are polygonal or stellate, and the periphery of the cytoplasm appears to merge imperceptibly with the surrounding collagen, indicating an intimate relationship with it. This feature is a general aid in identifying cells as myofibroblastic. Infiltration of the surrounding tissues is typical. As a rule, the cells in the fibromatoses are quite evenly scattered, and the overall cellularity is low to intermediate. In other words, cellularity is never marked, and the cells rarely touch one another. Mitoses are usually not identified, or they are rare. The immunoprofile with its SMA-positive myoid reaction can be used to advantage

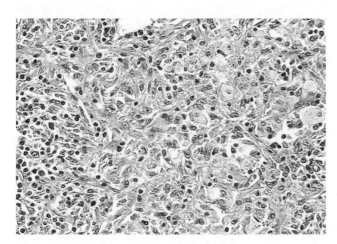

Figure 5.17. Inflammatory myofibroblastic tumor. In a tumor sprinkled with lymphocytes, plasma cells, and foamy histiocytes, eosinophilic spindle cells are seen in the background. Pleomorphism and necrosis are notably absent, and mitotic activity is virtually lacking.

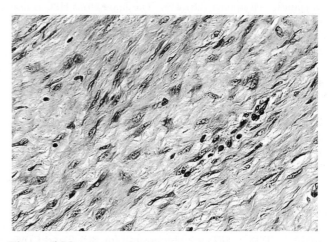

Figure 5.18. Fibromatosis. Fibroblasts proliferate on a continuous bed of collagen, with each cell separated from the others. In most cells, the cytoplasm is inapparent. When a cell is cut en face (*center*), the cytoplasm is visible, but it merges imperceptibly with the collagen bed, a telltale sign indicating the close relationship between the fibroblast and its product.

in the differential diagnosis. Beta-catenin nuclear positivity can be supportive of the diagnosis, but it is neither absolutely necessary nor specific (275). This lesion has been demonstrated to be clonal (276), and therefore, it is probably neoplastic. The abdominal and pelvic fibromatoses occur almost exclusively in female patients, and they can be more myxoid; some of these are hormonally responsive. In Gardner syndrome (277), the fibromatoses commonly are mesenteric and postoperative, and the rate of recurrence is higher (185).

Fibromatosis often recurs, but if it is left alone, it may solidify and stop growing. Cytogenetic findings may predict recurrence (278). Disagreement exists about the ultimate treatment; some recommend only an initial wide excision, followed by observation in the hope that growth may cease, whereas others recommend radiotherapy, which may have long-term untoward consequences. Because of the excellent results in radiotherapy series, postoperative radiation is frequently recommended. In adults, the distinction between an aggressive fibromatosis and a low-grade fibrosarcoma is based on the mitotic rate; any significant and consistent mitotic rate higher than 5 per 10 hpf in a fibroblastic tumor warrants its designation as a low-grade, well-differentiated fibrosarcoma, which should be treated in a similar manner. Congenital and infantile forms of fibromatosis are highly cellular and mitotically active, and these mimic fibrosarcoma (279).

SOLITARY FIBROUS TUMOR

Tumors described originally as localized fibrous mesothelioma have come to be known as *solitary fibrous tumors* (*SFTs*) because they clearly are not of mesothelial origin (280–283). SFTs develop not only from the pleura, but also near other serosal surfaces, such as the pericardium, peritoneum, and the surface of the liver. Significantly, they may develop without an association to a serosal surface, such as in the mediastinum, orbit, thyroid, or nasal cavity; and now, they are also commonly reported in the soft tissues.

SFTs belong to the category of fibroblastic tumors because some authors note a histologic identity similar to that of previously reported breast tumors and perhaps the fibrous variant of spindle cell lipoma (284,285). The lipomatous HPC is now regarded to belong to the SFT group of tumors as well (286), and indeed, essentially all HPCs are now considered SFTs (287). SFTs rarely express actin (and desmin), and they have (myo)fibroblastic ultrastructural features. Regardless of location, they are histologically identical to those in the pleura, which are composed of nondescript bland and uniform spindle cells dispersed among elongated, thin, parallel collagen bands in a "patternless" pattern (Fig. 5.19). The nuclei are small, and mitoses are difficult to find in the average case. Foci of storiform or hemangiopericytomatous growth are typical. Actually, the parallel arrangement of the collagen bundles is a characteristic design that is not seen in fibromatosis; the consistent CD34 positivity is another feature distinguishing SFT from fibromatosis (288). Therefore, two markers distinguish between these two collagenized tumors—fibromatosis (SMA$^+$/CD34$^-$) and SFT (SMA$^-$/CD34$^+$). SFTs are also positive for BCL-2 and CD99. Most benign-appearing SFTs behave in a benign fashion (289). Sarcoma is part of the differential diagnosis, and needle biopsy specimens may be misinterpreted as fibrosarcoma. If an uncommon cellular tumor is encountered, the following criteria developed for malignancy in pleural tumors (283) are applicable in

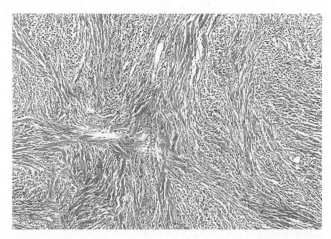

Figure 5.19. Solitary fibrous tumor. The thin parallel strands of collagen set this lesion apart. The spindle cells are bland and nondescript, but they may exist in storiform or pericytomatous patterns.

soft tissue (290,291): increased cellularity, necrosis, pleomorphism, and an increased mitotic rate (>4 per 10 hpf). In rare cases, malignant SFTs appear to occur as fibrosarcomatous progression next to benign-appearing SFTs.

MYOFIBROBLASTOMA FAMILY

PALISADED MYOFIBROBLASTOMA

Also known as *intranodal hemorrhagic spindle tumor with amianthoid fibers*, this tumor was simultaneously described by two groups as a lesion that is found exclusively in inguinal lymph nodes (292,293). It is composed of a spindle cell proliferation replacing the substance of a lymph node and is accompanied by hemorrhage and irregular knots of collagen bundles (the amianthoid fibers with a crystalline appearance). The spindle cells have elongated nuclei that often show nuclear palisading similar to that of a nerve sheath tumor (Fig. 5.20). Their cytoplasm is

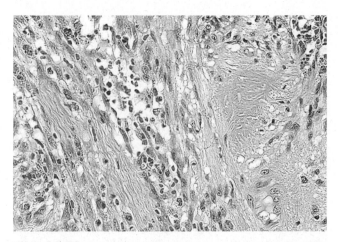

Figure 5.20. Palisaded myofibroblastoma. This intranodal tumor resembles a hemorrhagic neurilemoma with nuclear palisading (present elsewhere); here, extravasated red blood cells are found among elongated spindled cells, and the eosinophilic material constitutes the crystal-like amianthoid fibers, which are virtually pathognomonic.

eosinophilic and tapered, giving a myoid quality and raising the possibility of smooth muscle origin. With actin immunoreactivity, the cell type is likely either a myofibroblast or a specialized smooth muscle cell. The lesion mimics Kaposi sarcoma and a node-based hemorrhagic schwannoma, but neither of these has the characteristic fibers, and the tumor is negative for S-100. This unusual lesion has been reported in other locations (294–296). No evidence of aggressive behavior or even local recurrence has been found.

OTHER MYOFIBROBLASTOMAS

Myofibroblastomas have been seen in sites other than lymph nodes, including the paratesticular region (297), breast (284), meninges, soft tissues (294,296), and tongue.

OSSIFYING FIBROMYXOID TUMOR

An ossifying fibromyxoid tumor (OFMT) is a distinctly unusual tumor (126,298). The presence of both calcification and ossification in irregular trabecula-like formations throughout the tumor or concentrated at the periphery raises the clinical diagnosis of a calcified soft tissue mass, such as a synovial sarcoma or osteosarcoma. Usually, a well-circumscribed mass approximately 4 cm in size is found in the subcutaneous tissue or muscle of the upper and lower extremities. More than 80% of cases have had an incomplete shell of mature bone in the capsular region. Small rounded cells may exist either as sheets of poorly differentiated cells or as unusual cords and strings suspended in a loose stroma (Fig. 5.21). Two-thirds of the cases show S-100 positivity; approximately one-third have desmin. Local recurrence has been noted in 25% of cases, and metastatic disease has been reported in 1 of 41 initial patients. The origin of this tumor is unresolved, although it may be related to S-100–positive chondroid or schwannian SFTs. Evidence for a Schwann cell origin includes the presence of a basal lamina and an absence of type II collagen. Atypical and malignant variants have been reported (126), but there is a nearly negligible rate of metastasis in OFMT.

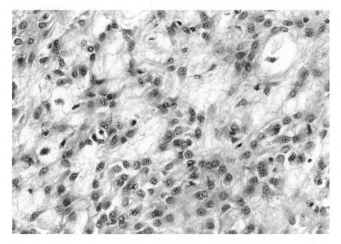

Figure 5.21. Ossifying fibromyxoid tumor. Strings, cords, and clusters of cells with modest eosinophilic cytoplasm are found in a fibromyxoid matrix. Not shown is the calcification typically seen in the capsule.

FIBROSARCOMAS

WELL-DIFFERENTIATED FIBROSARCOMA

In adults, the distinction between an aggressive fibromatosis and a well-differentiated fibrosarcoma is based on the mitotic rate; any significant and consistent mitotic rate of more than 5 per 10 hpf in a fibroblastic tumor warrants designation as a low-grade fibrosarcoma.

INFLAMMATORY FIBROSARCOMA

Inflammatory fibrosarcoma is considered a variant of inflammatory pseudotumor and/or myofibroblastic tumor with multicentricity (see "Inflammatory Myofibroblastic Tumor").

MYOFIBROSARCOMA

Rare tumors of malignant myofibroblasts have been reported (299,300). Most of these are low-grade tumors, also known as low-grade myofibroblastic sarcoma according to the new World Health Organization classification (287). Composed of SMA-positive myofibroblasts, the tumors mimic both NF (although they are infiltrative, have a deeper intramuscular location, and lack histiocytic giant cells) and leiomyosarcoma (although they lack the alternating fascicular pattern of a smooth muscle proliferation). Desmin positivity may be seen alone or in combination with SMA. High-grade pleomorphic myofibrosarcomas resemble UPS/MFH, but they exhibit prominent rather than spotty SMA reactivity (301).

MYXOINFLAMMATORY FIBROBLASTIC SARCOMA

Two series of unusual tumors occurring mainly on the hands and feet have been reported (302,303). The tumors were found in both men and women of all ages, and the morphology was most reminiscent of either inflammatory pseudotumor or myxofibrosarcoma with extensive chronic inflammation. No other tumor has the following constellation of morphologic findings: (a) an infiltrative subcutaneous tumor with a multinodular appearance; (b) areas of dense fibrosis with prominent chronic inflammation; (c) myxoid areas with both spindled and epithelioid cells; (d) scattered pleomorphic cells resembling Reed-Sternberg cells with prominent eosinophilic nucleoli ("virocytes"); and (e) mucin-filled cells in the myxoid areas with a basophilic wispy cytoplasm similar to the extracellular matrix. Positive markers included vimentin, focal weak CK in some, and focal CD68. Recurrences were noted in 25% to 67% of patients, and metastatic disease was rare.

MYXOFIBROSARCOMA

The term *myxofibrosarcoma* was originally applied to very low-grade lesions similar to myxoid MFH (304,305), but it has come to encompass all cases previously termed myxoid MFH (287) (see Table 5.10 and Fig. 5.29D); therefore, it is discussed here rather than in the section on UPS/MFH.

The tumor previously known as the *myxoid variant of MFH* is more common but less aggressive than the storiform-pleomorphic type, although it is more recurrent locally (306). Unlike myxoid liposarcoma, it is often found in the subcutaneous location and exhibits several distinctive histologic features. First, pleomorphism is prominent, in contrast to the remarkably uniform nature of the much smaller nuclei in most myxoid liposarcomas; furthermore, it is characteristically an S-100–negative tumor, unlike some liposarcomas. Second, the cells have a stellate or tripolar shape, like myofibroblasts (see Fig. 5.29D). Third, the vessels are recognizably different, being thick walled and often curved with a wide arc. They are not isolated fine capillaries; instead, they are associated with an eosinophilic substance, and the adherent tumor cells add to their thick appearance at low power (see Fig. 5.33 for comparison with other myxoid tumors). Fourth, another differentiating feature is the presence of nonmyxoid UPS/MFH-like elements in many cases. Originally, the definition required more than 50% myxoid histology (306), which conferred a better prognosis, but the requirement for the myxoid component has been decreased to 10% (287,307). Regardless, because this tumor is related to the higher grade tumor previously known as MFH, a further study of myxofibrosarcoma may provide clues to the origin of UPS/MFH.

Recently, an epithelioid variant of myxofibrosarcoma has been described with epithelioid cells surrounded by varying amounts of myxoid matrix, growing in sheets, with pleomorphic cells; this variant recalls a differential diagnosis of melanoma, carcinoma, and other epithelioid tumors (308).

FIBROSARCOMA

The following two highly cellular variations of fibrosarcoma exist: infantile fibrosarcoma and adult fibrosarcoma. In infants and children (309,310), fibrosarcoma is a mitotically active, locally aggressive tumor with a specific gene fusion (TEL-TRKC) and a relationship to congenital mesoblastic nephroma. In the past, tumors in adults labeled as fibrosarcomas constituted a high percentage of soft issue sarcomas. More recently, the total number of cases with this designation has decreased precipitously for several reasons. First, pleomorphic fibroblastic tumors in adults are now conventionally called undifferentiated pleomorphic sarcoma (UPS/MFH). Second, with the use of immunohistochemical techniques, it has become apparent that several lesions may mimic fibrosarcoma in adults, particularly nerve sheath sarcomas and synovial sarcoma. Clear examples of fibrosarcoma exist in adults, but this designation should be limited to lesions with the following characteristics: (a) an overall highly cellular spindle cell pattern; (b) a herringbone pattern in which sheets of cells intersect at acute angles (Fig. 5.22); (c) an absence of pleomorphism; and (d) an absence of immunohistochemical staining for S-100 or CK. Furthermore, marker-negative cases should be subjected to ultrastructural examination to allow more specific diagnoses in several instances. When this designation is used, high-grade fibrosarcoma in adults is exceedingly rare.

LOW-GRADE FIBROMYXOID SARCOMA

This deceptively bland sclerosing lesion, which is similar in appearance to both fibromatosis and a nerve sheath tumor, does metastasize (311–313). Many of the cases reported thus far have been in female patients, and most of these sarcomas have been identified after the metastases appeared. The metastases develop years after the removal of a primary tumor. A slight whirling, partially storiform appearance is noted, and the areas may be extremely hypocellular with myxoid nodules. The cells are

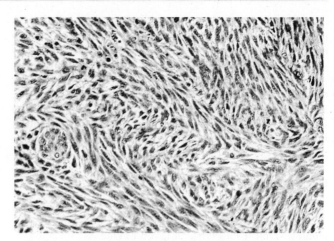

Figure 5.22. Fibrosarcoma. Highly cellular streams of nuclei intersect at acute angles, giving rise to the nonspecific "herringbone" pattern. Lack of specific features and negative marker studies force a default to this diagnosis of exclusion. Synovial sarcoma and malignant peripheral nerve sheath tumor should be considered when this is seen.

small, thin, and spindly, and occasionally, the nuclei are bent and wavy. However, the lesion is negative for S-100, and mitotic activity in the primary lesion can be extremely low.

Some cases may clearly have giant rosettes, and the tumor originally described as *hyalinizing spindle cell tumor with giant rosettes* (314) undoubtedly is really one end of the fibromyxoid sarcoma spectrum (315). At low power, the tumor resembles a nerve sheath tumor because the hyalinizing rosettes are reminiscent of palisading Verocay bodies. However, these rosettes are large, and they have a collagenized core, and the remainder of the lesion is composed of small spindle cells in a storiform or random distribution (Fig. 5.23). Rare S-100–positive cells are visible in the rosettes, with the rest of the tumor being S-100 negative and CD34 negative. The rate of metastases is less than 10% for all variants. Low-grade fibromyxoid sarcoma has a translocation of t(7,16)(q32-34;p11) or t(11,16)(p11;p11), resulting in FUS-CREB3L2 or FUS-CREB3L1 gene fusions.

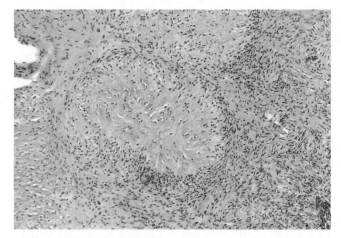

Figure 5.23. Low-grade fibromyxoid sarcoma. At medium power, a giant rosette is surrounded by proliferating cells with small nuclei. Adjacent spindle cells lack pleomorphism and exhibit a vague storiform pattern.

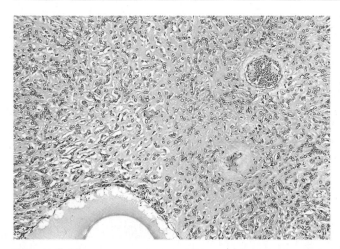

Figure 5.24. Sclerosing epithelioid fibrosarcoma. Within a highly collagenized matrix, groups of cells grow in cords and nests; the vesicular nature of the nuclei can barely be appreciated in this medium-power view.

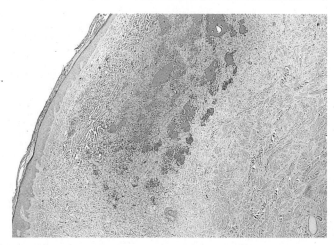

Figure 5.25. Aneurysmal variant of benign fibrous histiocytoma. Below a hyperplastic epidermis, a dermal spindle cell lesion contains lakes of blood; no endothelial lining of the lakes will be found.

SCLEROSING EPITHELIOID FIBROSARCOMA

In the first series of 25 cases of this unusual tumor, young persons from 20 to 50 years of age had deep tumors on the lower extremity (316,317). Uniform cellular proliferation was found in distinct nests or cords of epithelioid cells with abundant cytoplasm. Prominent hyaline sclerosis, which was noted in all cases, surrounded the nests (Fig. 5.24), and foci of conventional fibrosarcoma were occasionally seen. The mitotic rate averaged 4 per 10 hpf, and a few cases showed chondro-osseous differentiation. The tumors were positive for vimentin, and they occasionally stained with EMA, S-100, and CK. The frequent recurrence in 53% of cases and metastases in 43% of cases attest to its aggressiveness, but the course may be long (5 to 15 years), thus suggesting a new form of low-grade fibrosarcoma. Ultrastructural examination may be necessary to classify the tumor correctly and to exclude the pure epithelioid variant of synovial sarcoma, with which it can be confused.

FIBROHISTIOCYTIC ("FIBROCYTIC") LESIONS

It is now accepted that tumors in this category are not related to true histiocytic lineage (monocyte/macrophage bone marrow–derived cell), but rather are probably derived from a peculiar type of fibroblastic mesenchymal cell. Therefore, the term *fibrocytic* is gaining acceptance for this group of lesions.

BENIGN FIBROUS HISTIOCYTOMA

BFH usually presents as a small dermal nodule at almost any age (318). When the tumor is highly sclerotic and hypocellular, it may be termed *DF*. When lesions are larger and more cellular, the hallmark of fibrohistiocytic lesions, the storiform pattern, is seen. In these lesions, the small spindly cells are tightly arranged, and they have very thin, elongated nuclei with scanty cytoplasm. The nuclei have pointed ends, and they practically touch one another, unlike those seen in most smooth muscle lesions. The storiform arrangement is best envisioned as a cart-

wheel configuration of cells emanating from a common point. Within each portion of the cartwheel, the cells line up in a parallel array, although they lack the nuclear palisading of a schwannoma. An infiltrating border is typical, and recurrence is more likely if the lesion is incompletely excised or it extends into the subcutaneous fat (319). BFHs of deeper soft tissue are rarely encountered (320), and they raise the possibility of the malignant counterpart; the benign tumor lacks pleomorphism, and mitoses are uncommon. If a lesion is round rather than flat and it is less than 2 or 3 cm in size, fibrous histiocytoma is a more likely diagnosis than DF.

Related lesions include DF with monster cells, cutaneous histiocytoma, and the epithelioid variant (321–323). Occasional aneurysmal or "angiomatoid" variants also occur (Fig. 5.25).

ATYPICAL FIBROUS HISTIOCYTOMA

In reality, a spectrum of lesions, ranging from the completely bland BFH to the lesion with marked nuclear pleomorphism called *atypical fibrous histiocytoma* (*AFH*), exists (324). In contrast to an *atypical fibroxanthoma* (*AFX*) (see "Atypical Fibroxanthoma"), the AFH commonly presents on the extremities of young to middle-aged adults, rather than on sun-exposed areas, including the head and neck, of older patients.

PLEXIFORM FIBROHISTIOCYTIC TUMOR

In this tumor of children and young adults (325,326), separated nodules surrounded by a rim of fibrous tissue proliferate in the deep dermis and subcutaneous fat. Fibrohistiocytic cells and multinucleated giant cells populate the nodules, accompanied by a chronic inflammatory infiltrate. The combination of giant cells and stromal cells is reminiscent of the giant cell tumor of tendon sheath to some degree, but the superficial location is incorrect. As a rule, mitotic figures are rare (0 to 2 per 10 hpf), but exceptions do occur. Some nodules appear predominantly fibroblastic. Most of these patients are female. In one study, local recurrence developed in more than one-third of the patients, and 2 of 32 tumors metastasized to the local lymph nodes; distant metastases were not observed (325). The differential diagnosis includes ordinary fibrous histiocytoma, plexiform

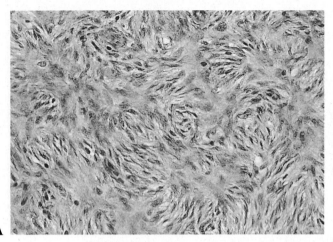

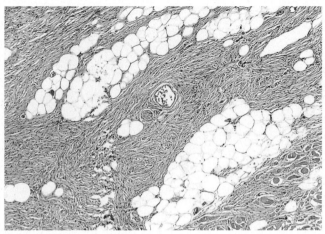

A   **B**

Figure 5.26. Dermatofibrosarcoma protuberans. The cartwheel or storiform pattern without pleomorphism is typical of dermatofibrosarcoma. Note the thin nuclei, lack of perceptible cell borders, and overall tight quality of the pattern **(A)**. Similar cells occur in small fibrous histiocytomas, which, however, lack the plaquelike growth in the dermis or the prominent layered invasion of the subcutaneous fat **(B)**.

tumors (e.g., neurofibroma), fibromatosis, giant cell tumor of soft tissue, and epithelioid sarcoma. The results of studies including SMA positivity suggest that this may be another myofibroblastic proliferation. Atypical and widely metastatic variants have been described (327,328).

DERMATOFIBROSARCOMA PROTUBERANS

DFSP is discussed elsewhere in this text (see Chapter 2). It is the storiform tumor par excellence, with each and every field showing this characteristic pattern (Fig. 5.26). Other tumors may also show this pattern (Table 5.11). Although the tumor is highly cellular, the nuclei are once again quite thin, with an innocuous appearance. Mitoses are difficult to find, and the lesion is concerning only because of its propensity for local recurrence. In larger, bosselated tumors bulging from the skin surface, the diagnosis is evident (329); however, in smaller lesions, in which DFSP appears to merge with its "relative," the fibrous histiocytoma, the immunoprofile is distinctly different because DFSP (CD34$^+$/F13a$^-$) stain reactions differ from those in BFH (CD34$^-$/F13a$^+$). A plaquelike growth of significant size (larger than 2 to 3 cm) should probably be clinically required.

The myxoid variant may be confused with liposarcoma, but it differs in its very superficial location either directly under the epidermis or in the subcutaneous tissues (330). DFSP may also be pigmented (331), it may acquire a granular cell cytoplasm (332), and it may "dedifferentiate" with fibrosarcoma-like or MFH-like areas.

Some primary DFSPs or recurrences exhibit fibrosarcomatous transformation (DFSP-FS) (333–335). The fibrosarcomatous component is highly cellular, may lose the storiform pattern, frequently retains its CD34 positivity, and exhibits a much higher mitotic rate (>7 per 10 hpf). When such transformation occurs, it is often visible as a dominant gross nodule, and the rate of recurrence and metastases is much higher. Because of its gene fusion COL1A1-PDGFB, patients with recurrences and metastases of DFSP may be treated with imatinib mesylate (Gleevec).

GIANT CELL FIBROBLASTOMA

Giant cell fibroblastoma, which is frequently mistaken for a sarcoma, is rare fibroblastic tumor that occurs mainly in boys younger than 10 years of age (336,337). The tumors are superficial, and they are found in a variety of locations. The lesions may be highly sclerotic and hypocellular, with widely scattered

TABLE 5.11	Differential Diagnosis of Tumors with a Partial Storiform or Hemangiopericytoma-Like Pattern
Storiform Pattern	*Hemangiopericytoma-Like Pattern*
Dermatofibrosarcoma	Cellular hemangioma (infantile hemangioendothelioma)
Undifferentiated pleomorphic sarcoma (MFH and dedifferentiated tumors)	Glomus tumor
Leiomyosarcoma (focal)	Mesenchymal chondrosarcoma
Nerve sheath tumors	Leiomyosarcoma (focal)
Liposarcoma (focal)	Undifferentiated pleomorphic sarcoma/MFH (focal)
Fibromatosis (focal)	Synovial sarcoma
Nodular fasciitis	Nerve sheath tumors
Thymoma (focal)	Solitary fibrous tumor
	Thymoma (rare)
MFH, malignant fibrous histiocytoma.	

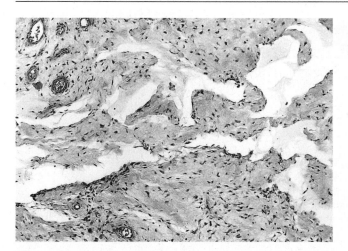

Figure 5.27. Giant cell fibroblastoma. Wide vessel-like spaces with basophilic ground substance are typical of this tumor, which also contains a collagenous background with scattered and occasional atypical cells.

atypical cells; alternatively, the regions may be quite cellular with prominent thick-walled vessels. Adipose tissue is often seen. One telltale characteristic is the formation of wide, vessel-like spaces (Fig. 5.27) that are incompletely lined by fibroblastic cells (negative for factor VIII and nonendothelial). The lesion may resemble (a) a neurofibroma with ancient change, (b) a liposarcoma lacking capillary vascularity, or (c) a peculiar angiosarcoma in which the huge spaces are unusual and only incompletely lined. Approximately half of patients experience local recurrence, but no metastases have occurred. This odd lesion has acquired the designation *childhood DFSP* because occasional cases show zones consistent with the storiform adult tumor (338), and adult DFSPs may contain giant cell fibroblastoma–like areas (339).

UNDIFFERENTIATED PLEOMORPHIC SARCOMA (PREVIOUSLY CALLED MALIGNANT FIBROUS HISTIOCYTOMA)

Undoubtedly, this tumor will be renamed in the future; some have suggested that it does not exist (340) or that it should be called *pleomorphic fibrosarcoma* (341). As mentioned earlier, lesions in this group of tumors bear no relationship to the true histiocyte, and therefore, MFH is a misnomer.

As seen in Table 5.12A, the term MFH was used to encompass a group of tumor subtypes, and now most of them have been renamed or indeed expanded into a spectrum of lesions. Aside from myxofibrosarcoma (discussed above), each of these will be described here. Only the common storiform/pleomorphic type still carries the "MFH" designation preceded by undifferentiated pleomorphic sarcoma (UPS/MFH-SP), as included in the new World Health Organization classification (342). Here it is considered a true entity, however misnamed, in this text.

In most modern tallies, the UPS/MFH complex had clearly been the most common soft tissue sarcoma (343–346), accounting for approximately 20% to 25% of cases. Some now suggest that the specific storiform/pleomorphic UPS/MFH accounts for as little as 5% of adult sarcomas, with myxofibrosarcoma constituting much of the remainder. It may occur in virtually any site of the body, including within the visceral organs. The lower extremity is the most frequent site, and UPS/MFH is likely the most common tumor of the thigh, with liposarcoma being a close second. Morphologically, the different varieties of the complex (Table 5.12A) resemble a wide variety of other tumors and makes the differential diagnosis lengthy. When all of the forms are considered, several generalizations emerge. First, the prognosis varies considerably by specific subtype, with the superficial types (cutaneous UPS/MFH and angiomatoid) having the most favorable prognosis, and the deeper lesions (UPS/MFH-SP and malignant giant cell types) having the worst prognosis (Table 5.12B). Second, many deep extremity cases may be cured by wide local excision. Third, the latter two tumors are generally considered high grade (grade 2 or 3). Fourth, the prognosis varies with size (small), depth (superficial), location (distal is better than proximal), presence of a lymphocytic host response, and grade. In presentation, they are similar to most sarcomas, producing mass lesions.

The essence of UPS/MFH is pleomorphism. In daily practice, pathologists have a tendency to misuse the words *pleomorphism* and *pleomorphic* to characterize peculiar-looking cells. A strict definition of the terms is a mean variation in cytoplasmic and nuclear size throughout a tumor. To be a useful classifier

TABLE 5.12A	Terminology Relating to UPS/MFH Subtypes
Old Term	*New Term*
MFH, storiform-pleomorphic	UPS
MFH, myxoid	Myxofibrosarcoma
MFH, histiocytoid (rare variant)	Myxofibrosarcoma, epithelioid
MFH, angiomatoid	Angiomatoid FH
MFH, giant cell	Giant cell tumor of soft tissue
	Giant cell tumor of low malignant potential
	UPS, giant cell type
MFH, inflammatory	Other tumors: dedifferentiated liposarcoma, inflammatory myofibroblastic tumor
	UPS, inflammatory
AFX	Atypical fibrous histiocytoma (AFH), younger patients
	Atypical fibroxanthoma (AFX), older patients, sun-exposed skin
	UPS/MFH superficial, large tumors

AFH, atypical fibrous histiocytoma; AFX, atypical fibroxanthoma; FH, fibrous histiocytoma; LPS, liposarcoma; MFH, malignant fibrous histiocytoma; UPS, undifferentiated pleomorphic sarcoma.

TABLE 5.12B	Undifferentiated Pleomorphic Sarcoma (MFH): Natural History of Tumors Previously Characterized as MFH Subtypes[a]					
	AFX/SMFH	*UPS-SP*	*MyxoFS*	*UPS/Giant*	*Inflammatory*	*Angiomatoid*
Relative percentage	—	20%	60%	3%–10%	3%–5%	Rare
Average age (yr)	39 (A)[b], 69 (B)[b]	~60	65	56	50–55	~15
Sex (M/F)	2.0	~1.5	1.8	1.3	~1.5	1.6
Sites	A, trunk, limbs; B, head/neck	Leg (thigh); arm; trunk; retroperitoneum	Leg (thigh); arm; trunk; head/neck	Leg (thigh); trunk	Retroperitoneum; trunk; thigh	Arm (elbow); thigh
Other	From sun exposure; small, ulcerated	66% >5 cm deep and large do worse	>50%, myxoid; 70%, subcutaneous	Short duration; occasional osteoid	Fever; high WBC count; large	Subcutaneous; 88% <30 yr; 2.5 cm
Recurrence	9%	38%–51%	52%–61%	53%	High	63%
Metastases	~1%	38%–42%	23%–35%	53%–60%	High	<1%
Survival						
Percentage	NA	46%	—	63%	~100%	1%
DOD						
2 yr	NA	68%	—	—	—	—
5 yr	NA	30%–42%[c]	65%–100%	31%–33%	0–44%	—
10 yr	NA	—	52%	—	11%	—

[a]See text for information on each entity.
[b]Two age peaks are defined by location in older literature; tumors in younger patients are now referred to as atypical fibrous histiocytoma (AFH).
[c]Literature data on MFH series; current survival of all sarcomas is 60% to 70% at 5 years, and storiform/pleomorphic UPS/MFH and myxofibrosarcoma are representative.
AFX/SMFH, atypical fibroxanthoma/superficial malignant fibrous histiocytoma; DOD, dead of disease; F, female; M, male; MFH, malignant fibrous histiocytoma; MyxoFS, myxofibrosarcoma; NA, not applicable; SP, storiform/pleomorphic; UPS, undifferentiated pleomorphic sarcoma; WBC, white blood cell.

in daily practice, evaluation of this characteristic should occur at low to medium power, thus dividing soft tissue tumors into "uniform" or "pleomorphic" categories. At that power, pleomorphism is an outstanding feature in UPS/MFH. Whereas other tumors, such as liposarcoma and RMS, do exhibit pleomorphism, they tend to do so within the constraints of their phenotype (i.e., they still look like the cell of origin). In contrast, the bizarre UPS/MFH cell has certain characteristics. In its largest form, it has voluminous cytoplasm that may be pale to highly eosinophilic and that occasionally is vacuolated. The cell may range in size from very large to huge; indeed, it may be the most expansive tumor cell in existence. Notably, the cytoplasm does not have the granular or fibrillar appearance of rhabdomyoblasts; however, it may be multivacuolated, simulating a lipoblast. The vacuoles in myxofibrosarcoma are composed of proteoglycan material (Table 5.13). Unlike the cells in leiomyosarcoma, which have elongated, tapering cytoplasm, the UPS/MFH cells may be oval or spindled, but they are shorter and do not show long stretches of streaming cells or fascicular growth. Unlike smooth muscle cells, the spindled cells often lack defined cell borders. The nuclear characteristics are also quite typical, with highly bizarre shapes and multiple nuclear lobes of differing sizes. The nucleoli may be not only prominent but also quite large. The nucleus tends to have a thick membrane and, more often than not, exhibits a jagged outline that may be termed "irregularly irregular." Occasionally, the nuclei contain eosinophilic inclusions similar to those of melanoma

or display clear nuclear vacuoles, such as those that may be seen in liposarcoma.

With strict adherence to the histologic features mentioned earlier, coupled with the skeptical approach and a search for more specific morphologic patterns (e.g., alternating fascicles in leiomyosarcoma), many of the mimics of UPS/MFH can and should be eliminated.

The UPS/MFH cell appears to be a peculiar form of mesenchymal cell—possibly fibroblastic—with a propensity to develop such unusual features. Although it may exhibit immunoreactivity with markers such as CD68, surface marker analysis by several investigators has shown that it does not resemble cells of the bone marrow–derived monocyte, macrophage, and histiocyte series (347). As a mesenchymal cell, it retains the ability to produce laminin, and through chromosomal progression, "histiocyte-like" cells emerge from fibroblast-like cells (348). Compared with most other soft tissue phenotypes, this cell is probably more primitive developmentally.

UPS/MFH tends to be overdiagnosed, a point that Fletcher (340) properly emphasizes. Nonetheless, cytogenetic studies appear to support the idea that this tumor is different from other pleomorphic tumors (349). Hopefully, careful attention to a strict definition of a storiform pattern, when combined with the realization that UPS/MFH-like areas may accompany phenotypically different sarcomas (350) or carcinomas, will alleviate the stress on the use of this term.

Prognostic markers of significance in UPS/MFH include p53 and MIB1 (351).

TABLE 5.13	Cytoplasmic Vacuolation in Soft Tissue Tumors	
Tumor	*Substance*	*Differential Features*
Liposarcoma	Lipid	Vacuole indents nucleus with scalloped appearance; positive fat stain; S-100 positive
Vascular tumors (endothelial)	None (a lumen)	Vacuole may be septate; no effect on nucleus; reticulin outlines groups of cells; rare red blood cells in vacuoles; factor VIII antigen positive
Smooth muscle tumors	None (artifact)	Vacuole not present in nonformalin fixatives; perinuclear with occasional indentation of nucleus; nonvacuolated spindle areas usually present
Rhabdomyosarcoma	Glycogen	Juxtanuclear and PAS positive in larger tumor cells; desmin and muscle actin positive
Myxofibrosarcoma	Proteoglycans	Nucleus not usually indented; seen mainly in pleomorphic cells; alcian blue–positive; fat stain, $+/-$; S-100-negative
Chordoma	Proteoglycans	No effect on nucleus; PAS positive; cytokeratin positive
(Paraganglioma)	?	Indents nucleus; positive argyrophilic stains
(Melanoma)	?	Rare cases are highly vacuolated; may be septate; S-100 positive
(Lymphoma)	Immunoglobin	Clear or eosinophilic PAS-positive inclusion; light chain positive in small-cell ("signet ring") lymphoma; LCA positive

Small intranuclear vacuoles are characteristic of myxoma, lipomatous, and nerve sheath tumors; they may occasionally be seen in other tumors, such as MFH. Cytoplasmic vacuoles are frequently mimicked by extracellular vacuolization, which is common in any myxoid lesion. The differential should include other tumors (in parentheses).
LCA, leukocyte common antibody; MFH, malignant fibrous histiocytoma; PAS, periodic acid-Schiff; ?, unidentified.

ATYPICAL FIBROXANTHOMA (AND SUPERFICIAL UPS/MFH)

AFX entity is covered in detail in Chapter 2. If a tumor occurs in older patients (>50 years) and occurs on sun-exposed skin, the AFX designation is appropriate. Similar tumors in other settings are better termed AFH, as discussed earlier. Both AFX and AFH bear histologic similarity to the deeper forms of UPS/MFH, and as such, it is the most superficial type of this neoplasm, although it is small and generally innocuous (352). Tumors that are large (>3 cm) and involve the subcutaneous tissues may be called (superficial) UPS/MFH. As in deep UPS/MFH, pleomorphic cells are apparent at low power, but a great variability in the accompanying smaller cells is also noted. Cells with angulated and curved nuclei are present, as well as an inflammatory component (Fig. 5.28). The immunoprofile is similar to that of UPS/MFH. The variants include a nonpleomorphic type and cases with benign giant cells. Unlike AFH,

AFX lacks a grenz zone or space below the epidermis and the classic features of BFH (324).

AFX and AFH must be included in the frequent differential diagnosis of spindle cell superficial skin lesions, namely, spindle cell squamous carcinoma and melanoma, both of which occasionally harbor cellular pleomorphism. Spindle cell squamous carcinoma tends to have cells that are plumper, wider, and more eosinophilic, with some grouping focally (Fig. 5.1). A storiform pattern is only rarely found; in such instances, immunohistochemical techniques are required to make the diagnosis. CK may be absent in a substantial proportion of spindle cell squamous tumors. With melanoma, attention to the epidermal surface, the more smoothly contoured nucleus, and the presence of separated bundles of cells and sprinkling of lymphocytes permit distinction. AFX and AFH are S-100 negative, although S-100–positive Langerhans histiocytes can be identified. The rare older reports of metastatic AFX implied its malignant potential (353), but those cases probably represented the larger superficial UPS/MFH. The smaller lesions of AFH and AFX are now considered not to have metastatic potential, although problems may arise with repeated local recurrences.

UNDIFFERENTIATED PLEOMORPHIC SARCOMA (STORIFORM-PLEOMORPHIC)

Storiform-pleomorphic UPS/MFH remains a common adult sarcoma. Although it usually appears as a white to pale yellow tumor, occasional examples presenting as hemorrhagic cysts can be deceptive, and they can simulate hematomas (a type of "clinging" sarcoma); only the scattered tumor cells clinging to the edge reveal the correct diagnosis. Infrequently, a purely storiform variant without pleomorphism occurs, giving rise to a so-called DFSP-like variant, which must be distinguished from the deep BFH. Its deep location and increased mitotic rate attest to its malignant nature; this is the exception to the rule that cellular uniformity is seldom seen in UPS/MFH. The previously designated "histiocytoid" form is now subsumed into the epithelioid myxofibrosarcoma, in which very rounded or epithelioid cells predominate. Here, many cells generally are of the

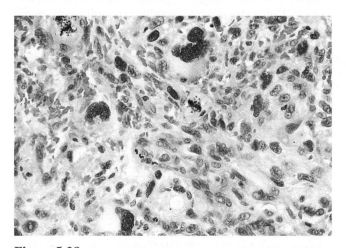

Figure 5.28. Atypical fibroxanthoma (AFX). In contrast to spindle cell carcinoma (Fig. 5.1), the cell shape and size vary markedly in this lesion. The smaller cells of AFX lack prominent cell borders and have oval or angulated and bent nuclei, unlike those of carcinoma.

same size with moderate amounts of dense eosinophilic cytoplasm, but scattered bizarre cells are positioned throughout. The distinction from a carcinoma is related to its discohesive quality, and tightly grouped nesting tumor cells are not found.

The vast majority of such lesions show the combination of a storiform pattern and the pleomorphic cells previously described (Fig. 5.29A,B). Many tumors are highly sclerotic, with broad areas of hyaline collagen and only sparsely scattered cells. Necrosis is the rule rather than the exception. In more cellular areas, the tumor giant cells are accompanied by smaller spindled to rounded cells with either round or quite irregular nuclei. The storiform pattern is not necessarily present in every field or every slide. Nonetheless, it consists of cells emanating from a common focus, a pattern that is often repetitive in the areas in which it is found. It should be identified more than just focally because several tumors have a focal storiform pattern (Table 5.11). Realizing that lengthy streams of spindle cells ("directional streaming") are only occasionally found is important; if they are identified with any frequency, a pleomorphic or dedifferentiated leiomyosarcoma should be considered. Several cases may be accompanied by a variable host response in the form of lymphocytes and plasma cells. This host response should not be confused with the inflammatory UPS/MFH, in which neutrophils predominate. As in all types of UPS/MFH, the male patients outnumber the female patients, and most tumors are quite large and deeply situated. UPS/MFH is the most common postradiation sarcoma (354).

Pleomorphic hyalinizing angiectatic tumor of soft parts (355) may enter into consideration because of the bizarre cells; however, this tumor is much more sclerotic and nonmitotic, it has CD34-positive fibroblasts, and it contains unusual dilated vessels with a fibrinous quality.

MYXOID MALIGNANT FIBROUS HISTIOCYTOMA

See "Myxofibrosarcoma" and Tables 5.10 and 5.12A,B for a discussion of tumors previously called myxoid malignant fibrous histiocytoma.

GIANT CELL TUMORS INCLUDING UNDIFFERENTIATED PLEOMORPHIC SARCOMA/ MALIGNANT FIBROUS HISTIOCYTOMA WITH GIANT CELLS

In recent years, studies have demonstrated that giant cell–rich tumors constitute a family of neoplasms ranging from benign to borderline malignant to fully malignant (see Table 5.12A) (356,357). Common to all three tumor types are osteoclast-like true histiocytic giant cells and oval to spindled histiocyte-like stromal cells that exhibit at least focal CD68 positivity. The giant cells have anywhere from 20 to 100 nuclei, with all of the nuclei or nuclear lobes being small and round to oval. The nuclei of the smaller stromal cells resemble those of the giant cells, as is the case in giant cell tumor of bone. Cases lacking atypia are designated giant cell tumor of soft tissue (GCT-ST) and typically occur as multinodular masses in the subcutis; mitoses are present, angiolymphatic invasion may be seen, but necrosis is absent and metastases rarely occur. When mild to moderate atypia is present, the term giant cell tumor of low malignant potential (GCT-LMP) has been suggested.

The fully malignant form is a recognizable subtype (358,359). In the past, this was called *malignant giant cell tumor*

of soft parts; the current designation is undifferentiated pleomorphic sarcoma with giant cells (UPS/MFH-GC). Again, the evenly dispersed osteoclast-like giant cells are clearly visible, as are the stromal cells. However, the hallmark of fully malignant UPS/ MFH-GC is that it contains *two* types of giant cells—namely, the osteoclast-like type and the more characteristic pleomorphic UPS/MFH cells previously described (Fig. 5.29C). Although these hyperchromatic bizarre cells may be outnumbered, they are always present. Similar tumors may arise from tendon sheaths (360).

Pseudosarcomatous carcinomas of various organs mimic this pattern, so care must be taken to eliminate that possibility. Because occasional cases may have small foci of osteoid, the differential diagnosis also includes extraskeletal osteosarcoma. Even melanoma may simulate this tumor. When this morphology occurs as a second pattern in another tumor, such as leiomyosarcoma (361), it may be considered a type of dedifferentiation. Although the prognosis of this type of UPS/MFH is said to be similar to that of the storiform pleomorphic type (Table 5.12B), highly aggressive and rapidly spreading forms have been seen.

INFLAMMATORY MALIGNANT FIBROUS HISTIOCYTOMA

The original description of inflammatory UPS/MFH was a highly aggressive lesion initially misdiagnosed as reactive (362,363), and importantly, the inflammatory cells consisted predominantly of neutrophils, giving the tumor an abscess-like appearance. However, many cases previously diagnosed as this entity have been shown to be variants of other specific entities such as dedifferentiated liposarcoma in the retroperitoneum or inflammatory myofibroblastic tumor (342,364). Most such cases have a marked infiltrate of lymphocytes and plasma cells. Instead of highly pleomorphic cells, scattered atypical cells with enlarged vesicular nuclei with prominent nucleoli have been seen (Fig. 5.29D). Scattered lymphocytes and foamy histiocytes are also present, and atypical mitoses can be found. The differential diagnosis includes the following: (a) reactive abscess–like lesions; (b) xanthogranulomatous pyelonephritis with extension to the retroperitoneal area; and (c) other lesions with prominent inflammation (Table 5.12A). A diagnosis of this type is incorrect if only lymphocytes, plasma cells, or eosinophils are present. The variant with neutrophils is extraordinarily rare and extremely aggressive. Patients may have fever and a leukocytosis mimicking an infectious process. Immunohistochemical studies (363) have effectively excluded the possibility that inflammatory UPS/MFH represents a form of Hodgkin or non-Hodgkin lymphoma, both of which are in the differential diagnosis.

Cases dominated by chronic inflammation, such as variants of well-differentiated or dedifferentiated retroperitoneal liposarcoma, should be excluded before the diagnosis is made (364).

ANGIOMATOID FIBROUS HISTIOCYTOMA

In the light of more recent follow-up data, this tumor has been downgraded to a "fibrohistiocytic" tumor of so-called intermediate malignancy, and it should not be considered a fully sarcomatous member of the UPS/MFH group (365,366). Its placement in the fibrohistiocytic category is also questioned, with the World Health Organization classification delegating the angiomatoid fibrous histiocytoma to the uncertain histogenesis

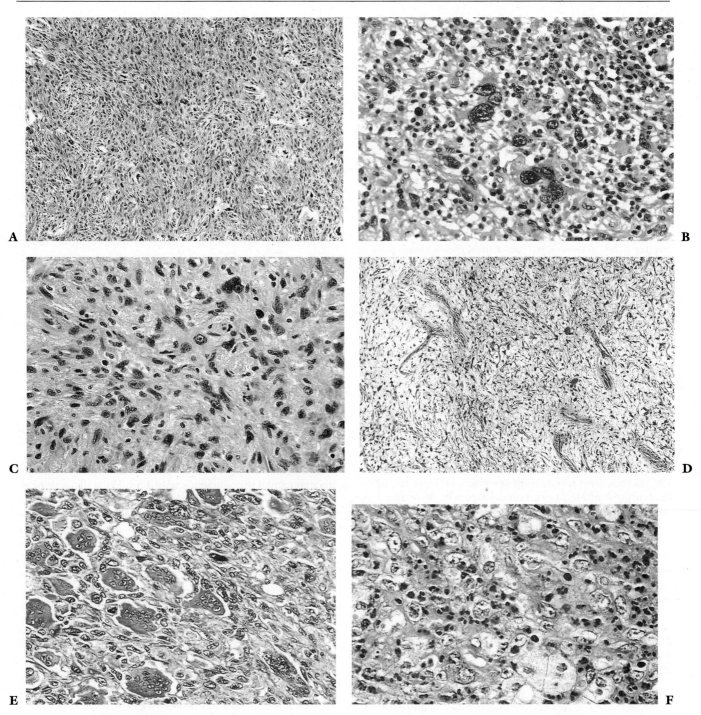

Figure 5.29. **(A)** Undifferentiated pleomorphic sarcoma (malignant fibrous histiocytoma [UPS/MFH]), storiform/pleomorphic. At medium power, pleomorphic nuclei are scattered among smaller cells growing in a vague storiform pattern. At high power, truly bizarre nuclei in huge cells are often found, and they may be accompanied by an inflammatory infiltrate **(B)**. In many cases, the smaller spindle cells exhibit irregular nuclear shapes that differ from one another; note also the lack of well-defined cell borders **(C)**. **(D)** Myxofibrosarcoma. At medium power, one notices the following three features: the pleomorphic nuclei, the cell strands indicating a stellate cell shape, and the scattered vessels with long arcs. In contrast to the thin and smaller arced vessels of myxoid liposarcoma, these vessels are thicker and less frequent (Fig. 5.33). **(E)** Giant cell tumor of soft tissue. The following two types of large cells are often, but not always, found: the osteoclast-like giant cells, which are true nontumoral histiocytes, and the malignant tumor giant cells with their enlarged nuclei. **(F)** UPS/MFH, inflammatory type. In contrast to a cluster of benign foamy histiocytes, the malignant nuclei of this tumor are larger and vesicular but not bizarre. They are immersed in a sea of neutrophils and other inflammatory cells. *(continued)*

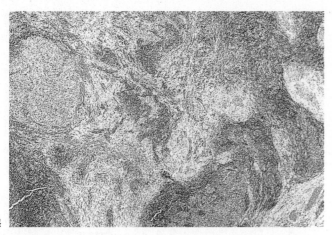

G

Figure 5.29. *(Continues)* **(G)** Angiomatoid fibrous histiocytoma. At low power, a key feature is the common dark cuff of lymphoid cells complete with the germinal center seen at the bottom; lighter tumor nodules proliferate in the center and at the top left.

group (287). This often cystic and hemorrhagic tumor is unlike the common type of UPS/MFH in the following ways: (a) it occurs at a very young age; (b) it is practically always a superficial subcutaneous nodule with a lymphoid cuff (Fig. 5.29E); (c) it frequently lacks pleomorphism as a dominant feature; (d) it often exhibits immunoreactive CD68, EMA, and desmin; (e) it is diploid in DNA content; and (f) only 2% of patients with this tumor die of metastatic disease (367). Histologically, sheets of fibroblast-like or histiocyte-like cells with oval nuclei and nucleoli occur within a circumscribed nodule that is often surrounded by a lymphocytic cuff. Hemosiderin is commonly present, and the proliferation tends to grow without an overt storiform pattern. Molecular analysis has demonstrated the presence of the FUS-ATF1 fusion gene (368). The more bland-appearing cutaneous benign aneurysmal fibrous histiocytoma is unrelated and is part of the differential diagnosis (369). Because this is clearly the most benign of all fibrohistiocytic malignancies, pathologists and clinicians must recognize the marked difference between these and modify treatment accordingly.

UNDIFFERENTIATED PLEOMORPHIC SARCOMA/MALIGNANT FIBROUS HISTIOCYTOMA AS A FINAL COMMON PATHWAY

Occasional sarcomas exhibit two patterns. The first is usually easily recognizable (e.g., liposarcoma, leiomyosarcoma, or chondrosarcoma), and the second pattern is very similar, if not identical, to UPS/MFH. These tumors are referred to as *dedifferentiated*, but this historical term is meant to convey a transformation resulting from tumor progression. Specific markers of the more recognizable phenotype are present, but they are commonly lost in the dedifferentiated UPS/MFH portion (370,371). Because of the frequent occurrence of the phenomenon, it has been proposed that UPS/MFH is a type of final common pathway (370); this hypothesis appears to be supported by further studies (372,373). The implications of this are as follows: (a) a putative primary UPS/MFH may be a dedifferentiated tumor in disguise, and the periphery of all UPS/MFH-like tumors should be well sampled to search for other phenotypic patterns; (b) an UPS/MFH-like metastasis may have arisen from another sarcoma type; and (c)

the UPS/MFH cell is placed in a primitive position in mesenchymal differentiation. Approximately 2.5% of all sarcomas exhibit this phenomenon (373).

Although *retrodifferentiation*—the direct change of a differentiated cell to an undifferentiated one—is generally said not to occur, such a change can be envisioned as the result of tumor progression and clonal evolution whereby the differentiated cells gradually lose the functional genetic messages that produce differentiation in the first place. By this mechanism, the process could be explained without resorting to the reasoning that all mesenchymal tumors derive from completely undifferentiated cells. Furthermore, the direct metaplasia of one differentiated cell to another without an undifferentiated intermediary has been established in the laboratory. Experimental evidence confirms the unstable nature of UPS/MFH cells and the potential for phenotypic and immunophenotypic alteration (374).

LESIONS OF ADIPOSE TISSUE

Lipoblastoma, spindle cell lipoma, and *pleomorphic lipoma* were discussed earlier in this chapter (see Figs. 5.5 and 5.6).

LIPOMA VARIATIONS

Lipomas are quite easily recognized as encapsulated proliferations of mature adipocytes. Unlike the adipocytes in the atypical variant (well-differentiated liposarcoma), the adipocytes in the usual lipoma have lipid vacuoles that are uniform in size. Some lipomas exhibit prominent vascularity, usually at the periphery. These have been called *angiolipomas*, and they are one of the few painful STTs (see Table 5.19) that are distinctly different clinically from ordinary lipomas. The angiolipoma is seen in young persons, often appearing on the arm as a small, firm subcutaneous nodule. In occasional cases, the vascular proliferation, which consists not of pure endothelial capillaries but rather of thick-walled vessels with pericytes, may be exceedingly prominent (see Fig. 5.7), mimicking either a highly cellular angioma or even Kaposi sarcoma. However, the circumscription of the lesion, as well as the scattered adipocytes, helps to define this unusual form. Occasionally, deep vascular tumors are incorrectly called *angiolipomas*; these are better termed *intramuscular hemangiomas*, and they consist of venous, arterial, and capillary vascular malformations with associated fat (375). *Intramuscular angioma* is a term that has been introduced to include similar lesions that may have lymphatic elements. Angiomyolipomas have islands of smooth muscle in addition to the adipose tissue and vascular elements. The smooth muscle element can be quite striking and even granular in nature; the long granular processes may cause confusion with rhabdomyomatous elements. The tumor is positive for HMB-45, and it contains unusual crystalloids. Although it characteristically occurs in the kidney as part of the tuberous sclerosis complex, occasional cases have been reported elsewhere. As highly pleomorphic tumors, angiomyolipomas mimic sarcomas and carcinomas, but they are basically benign with only rare exceptions (376). Deep intramuscular forms of lipoma also occur (377), particularly in the paraspinal region. Here, the tumors are rarely encapsulated, and they frequently recur.

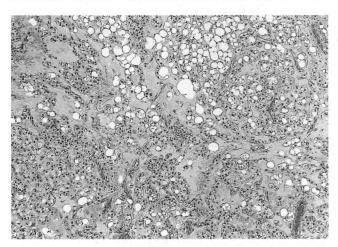

Figure 5.30. Chondroid lipoma. The combination of mature adipocytes (visible at the top of this field) with clusters of less differentiated cells in a loose chondroid matrix is typical.

Some cases of *hibernoma*, a tumor of brown fat with multivacuolated cytoplasm, may contain large areas of white fat elements, making the diagnosis more difficult and causing liposarcoma to be included in the differential diagnosis (378).

CHONDROID LIPOMA

As the name *chondroid lipoma* suggests, this unusual tumor has two components—mature adipose tissue and islands and nests of eosinophilic vacuolated cells resembling both lipoblasts and chondroblasts (379,380). The tumor is well circumscribed, and it has a myxoid matrix (Fig. 5.30). Stains show that the lesion is positive for S-100 and CD68, and some cases are CK positive. Its appearance is similar to that of both liposarcoma and myxoid chondrosarcoma, which are entities that must be excluded.

LIPOSARCOMA

Forms of liposarcoma (381–387) fall into the following three groups conceptually: (a) atypical lipomatous tumor, or well-differentiated liposarcoma, with or without dedifferentiation (DD-LPS); (b) the myxoid and round cell and/or cellular myxoid spectrum; and (c) pleomorphic liposarcoma.

ATYPICAL LIPOMATOUS TUMOR

The atypical lipomatous tumor (ALT) encompasses the previously designated well-differentiated liposarcoma (WD-LPS) when it occurs in the periphery; retroperitoneal tumors may still, however, be called WD-LPS. This common form of liposarcoma never metastasizes (Table 5.14), and it frequently is only a local problem that, nonetheless, may require wide local excision. Clinicians should be alerted to the well-known problem of local recurrence and encouraged to excise such tumors fully, especially because peripheral tumors may still exhibit dedifferentiation (388). With this designation, the distinction between pleomorphic lipoma and ALT or WD-LPS becomes less important because both are only local problems. However, floret cells and lipoblasts may be found in both, but the circumscription of the former is distinctive, and the different cytogenetic findings underscore distinctly separate entities (389).

Microscopically, the ATL or WD-LPS is an easily recognized fatty lesion dissected by fibrous tissue septa. Characteristically, the septa are cellular, and they contain small spindle cells, a feature that may be noted at low power. Occasionally, highly pleomorphic cells also hug the septa adjacent to the fibrous tissue. Clear-cut, large, bizarre lipoblasts (Fig. 5.31) can be identified by the vacuoles indenting the nucleus (the definition of a lipoblast). Interestingly, many of these tumors show a high degree of variability in the size of the lipocytes, another feature that is noticeable at low power. The random distribution of the pleomorphic nuclei is again visible at low power. As is common in all types of liposarcoma, encapsulation is often mimicked; however, the capsule is never thick, and small islands of tumor cells may be present in the adjacent soft tissue. Therefore, all such lesions must be excised widely regardless of the terminology used.

Dedifferentiation in ATL or WD-LPS is characterized by solid tumor foci without adipocytes and may be low or high grade based on cellularity and the mitotic rate, not on the mere pres-

TABLE 5.14	Liposarcoma: Natural History and Subtypes				
	All Types	ATL/WD-LPS	Myxoid	Cellular Myxoid Round Cell	Pleomorphic
Relative percentage	16%–18%	~45%	~25%	~15%	~10%
Average age (yr)	53	56	46	43	57
Sites	Leg (thigh); retroper; trunk; arm	Retroper; extremities; inguinal region	Extremities (thigh)	Extremities; trunk; retroper	Retroper; extremities
Other	Retroper cases do worse	Wide local excision needed	Multiple local recurrences	Short course seen with myxoid and pleomorphic	Seen with all other types
Local	>50%	15%–53%	43%–53%	85%	30%–73%
Recurrence	10%	10%	11%	10%	9%
Metastases	40%	0	~33%	High rate	High rate
Survival					
5 yr	57%–70%	70%–85% (83%)	47%–77% (80%)	18%–40% (25%)	21%–33% (43%)
10 yr	50%–53%	50%	45%–50%	8%–15%	20%

ATL/WD-LPS, atypical lipoma/well-differentiated liposarcoma; retroper, retroperitoneum.

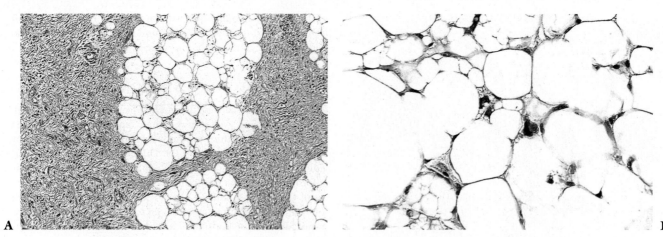

Figure 5.31. Liposarcoma, well-differentiated atypical lipoma. Fibrous septa with more cells than ordinary fibrous tissue (cellular septa) are often found in this tumor **(A)**. At high power, pleomorphic nuclei are widely scattered among fat cells of variable size **(B)**. A well-differentiated adipocyte tumor on the exterior of the body is referred to as an *atypical lipoma*, for which complete excision should be sought.

ence of pleomorphism (390). Occasionally, the surgeon resects only the firm dedifferentiated area, creating the possibility of misdiagnosis as UPS/MFH; thus, any potential UPS/MFH should be considered a possible WD-LPS and the fatty tissue at the edge of the tumor should be examined carefully for the presence of lipoblasts or cellular septa.

MYXOID LIPOSARCOMA

The one type of sarcoma that can be most easily diagnosed on frozen section is the myxoid liposarcoma. This is because of its absolutely classic appearance—a hypocellular myxoid lesion composed of uniform and small cells with variable cellularity and a diagnostic rich capillary network that creates a "chicken wire" appearance (Fig. 5.32). Sometimes, the identification of lipoblasts in this myxoid subtype is difficult, but its low-power vascular pattern is distinctive in comparison with that of other

myxoid tumors (Fig. 5.33). The nucleus is small and oval with finely dispersed chromatin, and nucleoli are frequently lacking. Mitoses are uncommon, except in the more cellular examples. The uniformity of this tumor directly contrasts with the pleomorphism of myxofibrosarcoma. A guide to the differential diagnosis of myxoid lesions is provided in Table 5.10. One nearly pathognomonic pattern, the presence of lymphangioma-like or lacelike pools secondary to degeneration within the tumor, may occur.

Although pathologists tend to lump all myxoid liposarcomas together, clearly low-grade hypocellular examples and more cellular grade 2 tumors are encountered. The myxoid subtype may be accompanied by focal cellular or round cell (and grade 3) morphology. A significant percentage of liposarcomas have varied histology, with myxoid, cellular/round cell, and even pleomorphic regions. When this is the case, the lesion should be graded according to the least differentiated region. There is a

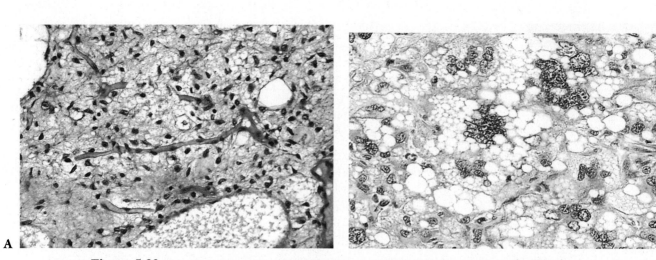

Figure 5.32. Liposarcoma, myxoid and pleomorphic. A delicate, branching capillary network courses through the uniform and bland small cells of the myxoid liposarcoma **(A)**; lipoblasts can be difficult to locate, and the lymphangioma-like cystic degeneration (*bottom*) is nearly unique. One type of pleomorphic liposarcoma **(B)** has cells with multiple grapelike vacuoles. A cellular or round cell component may accompany either form.

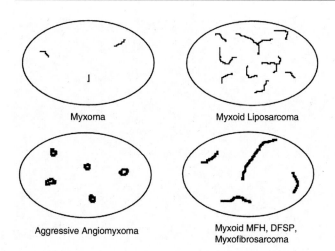

Figure 5.33. Schematic of vessels in myxoid tumors. Circular vessels with thick rims set aggressive angiomyxoma apart from other angiomyxoid lesions. The myxoma is nearly always hypovascular. The very frequent small capillaries seen in myxoid liposarcoma form a network, and they have a small arc—in other words, they would form small circles if the arc were complete. In contrast, the vessels of myxoid malignant fibrous histiocytoma are less frequent and thicker because pericytes or tumor cells are attached, and they have wider arcs.

spectrum between myxoid and round cell liposarcoma proven by cytogenetic and molecular studies (391), and the term "cellular myxoid" type is gradually replacing the historical "round cell" nomenclature. The natural history of the myxoid subtype is one of either complete cure or multiple local recurrences, followed by eventual metastases after several years. Of all liposarcomas, the myxoid type is the second most common (Table 5.13).

CELLULAR MYXOID, OR ROUND CELL, LIPOSARCOMA

Sheets of cells with a variable degree of eosinophilic cytoplasm constitute *round cell liposarcoma*, the older term for this lesion, which, with its densely placed cells, is basically at the end of a spectrum of the myxoid type. Vascularity in the form of a capillary network is present, although this is sometimes partly or completely obscured. The nuclei are mostly uniform, but they are somewhat larger than those seen in the myxoid type, and nucleoli are displayed. A high mitotic rate usually accompanies this subtype. The eosinophilic cytoplasm may appear somewhat granular; however, in most tumors, small cytoplasmic vacuoles can be seen. This lipocytic differentiation often clusters, and characteristic lipoblasts are present. In discussions of the dividing lines between regular and cellular tumors, studies have agreed that the percentage of cellular areas serves as a guide for distinguishing grade 2 tumors (<25%) from grade 3 tumors (>25%) (392,393). The natural history of round cell liposarcoma is extremely aggressive, as Table 5.13 indicates.

PLEOMORPHIC LIPOSARCOMA

Pleomorphic liposarcoma occurs in two forms. In the less common form, multivacuolated giant cells (Fig. 5.32) are present in a lesion that otherwise closely resembles round cell liposarcoma

(394,395). The vacuoles are characteristically small and numerous within the tumor giant cells. Occasionally the smaller cells have plump cytoplasm diffusely throughout a tumor, giving rise to the epithelioid subtype (396). In the second and more common form, tumors resembling UPS/MFH contain definite lipoblastic differentiation in the form of pleomorphic lipoblasts scattered about. This is to be distinguished from tumors that have prominent well-differentiated liposarcoma and a second component of pleomorphic sarcoma; although these tumors have been mistaken for *pleomorphic liposarcoma*, calling these *dedifferentiated liposarcomas*, as is conventional for other tumors, is more appropriate. Whereas the usual liposarcoma manifests S-100 immunoreactivity to a variable degree, these dedifferentiated or UPS/MFH-like areas are S-100 negative. The realization that dedifferentiation commonly occurs in the larger retroperitoneal liposarcomas, at which point metastatic disease may become apparent, is important (Table 5.13). The diagnosis of such dedifferentiation requires a highly cellular tumor with a mitotic rate of at least 5 per 10 hpf (385); this criterion avoids the overidentification of the common fibrous areas in well-differentiated liposarcomas of the retroperitoneum as fibrous areas, which are hypocellular, having only scattered pleomorphic cells.

DIFFERENTIAL DIAGNOSIS

The differential diagnosis of vacuolated soft tissue lesions is presented in Table 5.14. Liposarcoma tends to occur in the deep soft tissues, as opposed to the more superficial, subcutaneous benign lipocytic tumors. Some liposarcomas may contain focal HPC-like areas, but this rarely is a problem in the differential diagnosis. In occasional cases, sclerosis may occur, and the cells may take on a neural appearance, but the rich capillary network is diagnostic. The distinction between a myxoid liposarcoma and the myxoid variant of DFSP can be histologically difficult; however, the latter is usually a highly superficial lesion adjacent to the skin. In myxofibrosarcoma (myxoid UPS/MFH), the pleomorphic cells may be vacuolated, but they lack lipid. In addition, there are fewer vessels made thicker as a result of the adherence of pleomorphic cells. The thin vessels of myxoid liposarcoma have a curving radius that is smaller than that of the thicker, widely arcing vessels of myxofibrosarcoma (myxoid UPS/MFH) (Fig. 5.33).

Finally, recurrent liposarcomas may lack any lipocytic differentiation, and they may exhibit a variety of histologic patterns (386). Most liposarcomas occur in the extremities, particularly the thigh (Table 5.13). However, trunk and retroperitoneal tumors together account for more than 40% of cases. Patients with retroperitoneal tumors have a poorer 5-year survival rate (41%) than patients with extremity tumors (71%). Although the tumor may occur in childhood, most patients are between 40 and 60 years of age. For all liposarcomas, patients younger than 50 years of age fare better. As with other sarcomas, a tumor size of less than 5 cm is a favorable sign. This is also one of the STTs that may be multicentric.

SMOOTH MUSCLE LESIONS

Bizarre leiomyoma is discussed earlier in this chapter.

LEIOMYOMA

Most benign smooth muscle tumors are easily recognized because of the convergence of the following attributes: (a) a spin-

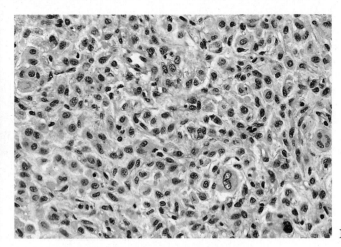

Figure 5.34. Leiomyoma. In the center, the blunt-ended elongated nuclei typical of a smooth muscle proliferation are seen along with cells coursing perpendicular to the plane of section above and below (**A**). Epithelioid variants are rare in soft tissue; here, a gastric gastrointestinal stromal tumor (GIST) contains round cells with smaller oval nuclei (**B**).

dle cell lesion, with cells that have elongated, tapering eosinophilic cytoplasm; and (b) an elongated but blunt-ended nucleus. In benign lesions, the nucleus tends to be finely stippled, whereas in malignant lesions, the cells often have vesicular nuclei with nucleoli and an increased mitotic rate. The pattern of growth is also characteristic; the cells grow in long directional streams or sweeps that are grouped together as a bundle or fascicle. In any given section, these bundles tend to intersect at right angles, producing circular silhouettes when they are viewed against the plane of section (Fig. 5.34). This is referred to as the *alternating fascicle (bundle) pattern*. Rare cases may have a granular cytoplasm (397).

Some benign lesions exhibit a great deal of vasculature in the form of thick-walled veins or arteries; these have been termed *angiomyomas* or *vascular leiomyomas*. Still others have a rounded cell morphology throughout the lesion (Fig. 5.34), which gave rise to the term *epithelioid leiomyoma*. The differential diagnosis of the latter tumor is provided in Table 5.15. Although occasional epithelioid examples are highly vacuolated and although they were at one time referred to as *leiomyoblastomas*, particularly when they were located in the gastrointestinal tract, this vacuolization is largely an artifact of fixation (Table 5.14), and they are now referred to as gastrointestinal stromal tumors (GIST). Therefore, the term *leiomyoblastoma* has been abandoned. In

the female genital tract, unusual benign growths occur either throughout a region of the uterine muscle (intravenous leiomyomatosis) or throughout the peritoneal cavity (leiomyomatosis peritonealis disseminata).

Although leiomyomas of deep soft tissue and retroperitoneum may exist (398–400), they are extremely rare, and extreme caution should be exercised when such a diagnosis is made; any mitotic activity or necrosis in a deep leiomyomatous tumor is cause for alarm.

LEIOMYOSARCOMA

The cellular characteristics of the benign smooth muscle tumors that were previously described are retained in most leiomyosarcomas (LMSs). Significantly, the definition of a malignant smooth muscle tumor varies according to the site, with the criteria between uterine and nonuterine lesions differing drastically (Table 5.16). In counting mitoses, the clinician should realize that the size of a high-power field varies considerably, depending on the characteristics of the microscope (401,402). Many LMSs occur in the uterus, and these are discussed in detail in the relevant chapter.

In the soft tissues, LMSs may arise from medium or large veins (403), such as the inferior vena cava (404); such cases show a marked female predominance, and their presentation includes ascites and leg edema. Retroperitoneal cases also show a female predominance (405), and as a rule, the tumors are highly aggressive, easily recognized smooth muscle lesions. These patients historically have had a 5-year survival rate of 29%.

Skin and subcutaneous tissue tumors are quite different (397,406,407). Male patients greatly outnumber female patients, and the overall survival rates are far superior because of the superficial location. These tumors characteristically occur in the hair-bearing regions of the extremities, and pain and ulceration are commonly noted. The mitotic rates may be quite low (Table 5.16). Epithelioid (407) and granular cell (397) morphology may be observed in skin and subcutaneous tumors, as well as in deep tumors (408). Location is again important; the often low-grade dermal tumors lack metastatic potential,

TABLE 5.15

Sarcomas with Epithelioid Morphology

Epithelioid sarcoma
Rhabdoid sarcoma
Synovial sarcoma, epithelioid variant
Leiomyosarcoma, epithelioid variant
Myxofibrosarcoma, epithelioid variant
Malignant peripheral nerve sheath tumor, epithelioid variant
Angiosarcoma, epithelioid variant
Epithelioid hemangioendothelioma
Liposarcoma, round cell/epithelioid variant
Alveolar soft part sarcoma

TABLE 5.16	Mitotic Count and Malignancy in Smooth Muscle Tumors				
Site	*Benign*	*UMP[a]*	*Malignant*		*Malignant Features*
Skin/subcutaneous	0 per 10 hpf	–	1 per 10 hpf, if consistent 2 per 10 hpf = definite		Nuclear pleomorphism
Retroperitoneum	0 per 10 hpf	+	1–4 per 10 hpf 5 per 10 hpf = definite		Size >7.5 cm; necrosis
Vascular	0 per 10 hpf	+	1–4 per 10 hpf		Large size, necrosis
Soft tissue	0 per 10 hpf	+	1–2 per 10 hpf		Depth important

[a]The term *smooth muscle tumor of uncertain malignant potential (UMP)* may be used when mitotic counts are few and not present throughout. Leiomyomas of deep soft tissue should have very few mitoses and otherwise completely benign morphology. hpf, high-power field.

whereas subcutaneous tumors metastasize in approximately 30% to 40% of cases.

Deep intramuscular LMSs are also reported, some with dedifferentiation (84), myxoid morphology (409), rhabdomyoblastic differentiation (410), or osteoclast-like giant cells (411). The myxoid subtype can be deceptive, with a highly aggressive course in the absence of significant mitotic activity. Children may rarely harbor LMSs (412).

Aside from the usual spindle cell type with the alternating bundle pattern previously described (Fig. 5.35) and the epithelioid type, LMS can be pleomorphic (413). However, it must be stressed that pleomorphism is neither a requirement nor a criterion for a malignant diagnosis, as was noted earlier in this chapter. A distinction must also be made between (a) pleomorphic LMS, in which the pleomorphism occurs within the bounds of recognizable smooth muscle features ("pleomorphism within a phenotype"), and (b) the dedifferentiated LMS, in which two patterns are present, with the second pattern being UPS/MFH-like or containing giant cells.

LEIOMYOSARCOMA AND EPSTEIN-BARR VIRUS

Several reports have documented an association between Epstein-Barr virus and smooth muscle tumors in a variety of sites, including the adrenal gland and soft tissue (414–416). Many of these cases have occurred in patients with AIDS or human immunodeficiency virus (HIV) infection, and some

have been seen after transplantation. LMSs in immunocompetent patients are not associated with Epstein-Barr virus infection.

LESIONS OF STRIATED MUSCLE

Fetal rhabdomyoma was described earlier in this chapter (see Fig. 5.9).

ADULT RHABDOMYOMA

In addition to fetal rhabdomyoma, which has already been discussed, an adult form occurs that consists of highly differentiated cells growing in sheets (102). The cytoplasm is abundant, and it is distinctly granular and fibrillar. It is easily recognized despite the presence of cytoplasmic vacuolization and the formation of so-called spider cells. The intracytoplasmic glycogen and rodlike crystals (jackstraws) are usually identifiable. Typically, this form of rhabdomyoma develops in the head and neck region, particularly in the pharynx and larynx. The cardiac rhabdomyoma is a small lesion encountered in association with tuberous sclerosis, and it is probably a result of a hamartomatous process (417).

RHABDOMYOSARCOMA

Oddly enough, the vast majority of RMS tumors (418–420) do not occur in the extremities, where the bulk of the skeletal muscle resides. Rather, a host of classic locations have been described, each with its own typical histology and natural history (Table 5.17). Although most cases occur in the first decade of life (Tables 5.17 and 5.18), this is not true of paratesticular and extremity cases, both of which are found in adolescence. Rarely, cases occur congenitally or in adults older than 40 years (90,421,422). Most cases of adult pleomorphic RMS diagnosed in the past likely were examples of UPS/MFH. The natural history of RMS is that of a highly aggressive tumor that either kills the patient or is cured by modern chemotherapy. Although the prognosis does depend on factors such as the site (Table 5.17) and histology, it depends mostly on the group (a type of staging). In general, patients in groups I or II, who have either completely resected disease or microscopic disease remaining, respectively, are frequently cured. In contrast, patients in groups III or IV, who have locally unresectable or metastatic disease, respectively, frequently die despite chemotherapeutic measures.

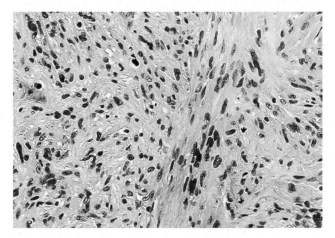

Figure 5.35. Leiomyosarcoma. The alternating fascicle pattern (parallel and perpendicular to the plane of section) and blunt-ended nuclei are recognizable in this cutaneous tumor, which had a prominent mitotic rate (4 per 10 hpf); only minor pleomorphism is present.

TABLE 5.17	Characteristics of Rhabdomyosarcoma by Site							
	All Cases	*Head/Neck (Non-Orbit)*	*Orbit*	*Paratesticular*	*Other GU*	*Extremities*	*Retroperitoneal*	*Trunk*
Incidence	—	24%–29%	7%–19%	20%	4%	14%–23%	8%	8%
Average age (yr)	5–7	5–7	5–7	15	5–7	14	6	—
Sex (M/F)	3/2	—	—	—	—	1/1	3/2	—
Histology	—	80%–90% E	70% E	90% E	75% B	40% A	85% E	50% A
LN mets	10%–20%	—	—	40%	High rate	High rate	—	—
2-yr DFS	—	51%	77%	80%	68%	42%	42%	50%

Head and neck tumors in parameningeal locations (middle ear, nasopharynx, sinus) have a worse prognosis than other head tumors. The cure rate for orbital tumors is high (as with paratesticular cases). Paratesticular rhabdomyosarcoma is one of the most favorable types, but it is subject to late relapse; lymphadenectomy is the usual procedure, but this need not be done for cases without pelvic lymphadenopathy. Note that the extremity is the least frequent major site (behind head/neck, orbit, and paratesticular cases); extremity cases have the highest relapse rate and the lowest survival rate. The data are from many intergroup reports. Data are based on Intergroup Rhabdomyosarcoma Study literature from the 1980s to 1990s giving comparative information; current survival may be superior.
A, alveolar types; B, botryoid; DFS, disease-free survival; E, embryonal; F, female; GU, genitourinary; LN mets, lymph node metastases; M, male.

Rhabdomyosarcoma Classification

The Intergroup Rhabdomyosarcoma Study grew dissatisfied with the predictive value of the conventional classification, so it has designated tumors as either favorable (botryoid, well-differentiated or spindle cell, and most embryonal RMS tumors) or unfavorable (423,424). The unfavorable tumors are those that have anaplastic features or alveolar histology or those that are very poorly differentiated with monomorphous round cell morphology, such as the solid variant of alveolar RMS. With this designation, the unfavorable category comprises approximately 20% of cases, and its 2-year, disease-free survival rate is 72%, versus 89% for favorable cases. If a tumor has any alveolar morphology, it should be classified thus.

Embryonal Rhabdomyosarcoma

Most RMS tumors are classified as embryonal; these tumors consist of sheets of poorly to moderately differentiated cells with a rounded morphology. In contrast to the nucleus in Ewing sarcoma, the nucleus in RMS is eccentric (Fig. 5.36A), and the rest of the cytoplasm appears more granular and eosinophilic. Such cells are present, at least focally, in most cases. As the cells

TABLE 5.18
Sarcomas by Peak Age Group
Younger than 10 years
Rhabdomyosarcoma
Neuroblastoma
Fibrosarcoma
Between 11 and 40 years
Synovial sarcoma
Epithelioid sarcoma
Clear cell sarcoma
Nerve sheath sarcoma
Epithelioid hemangioendothelioma
Mesenchymal chondrosarcoma
Extraskeletal Ewing sarcoma
Alveolar soft part sarcoma
Older than 40 years—all other types

become larger, the cytoplasm may appear fibrillar, and it may encircle the nucleus. Cross-striations are uncommon; they are present in approximately half of embryonal RMS cases (20% of alveolar RMS). Thus, these striations cannot be used as the sole criterion for the diagnosis, and they may actually be found in other tumors disguised in the form of trapped skeletal muscle fibers. Again, in contrast to Ewing sarcoma, RMS exhibits occasional spindling, and in such fields, the characteristic "strap" cells may be identified. The cytoplasmic borders run in parallel for a certain length *without tapering*. When such cells are present throughout RMS, the tumor mimics the myotubular stage of normal muscle development, and the lesion is considered well differentiated. This occurrence has been called *spindle cell RMS* or *leiomyomatous RMS* to call attention to the confusion it may cause (425). Whereas childhood cases of spindle cell RMS have an excellent prognosis, the rare cases in adults do not (426). The embryonal pattern is the most common type of RMS in practically all sites.

Botryoid Rhabdomyosarcoma

RMS cases that occur near a lumen or a space (e.g., genitourinary tract, female reproductive tract, conjunctiva) are most often of the botryoid type. This much more myxoid tumor is a variant of the embryonal type, and it has a very typical low-power appearance in which the density of cells is greatest just below the adjacent epithelium (Fig. 5.36B,C). This area is known as the *cambium layer*. Usually, the characteristic small strap cells are located at the junction of this layer with the more myxoid underlying regions. In all, this type accounts for approximately 25% of all RMS cases; roughly 75% of all botryoid tumors occur in the genitourinary tract.

Alveolar Rhabdomyosarcoma

Alveolar RMS affects patients at an older mean age than do the other types of RMS, and it is frequently observed in adolescents with lesions on the extremities and trunk. This histologic type has the worst prognosis when all other variables are held constant. The tumor is divided by small fibrous septa between which tumor cells float discohesively in oval or elongated spaces (Fig.

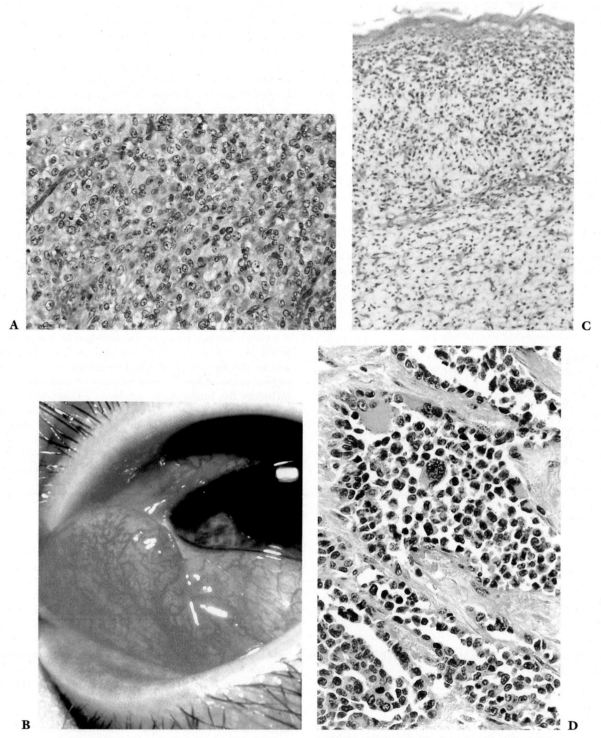

Figure 5.36. Rhabdomyosarcoma. In the embryonal type **(A)**, round cells with small oval nuclei and scanty eosinophilic cytoplasm are seen. The eccentric placement of the nucleus in the cytoplasm is a helpful diagnostic characteristic. Such cells grow in sheets without other features. The botryoid type bulges into a space, which, in this case, is the orbital conjunctiva **(B)** (courtesy of Dr. Ralph Eagle, Temple University, Philadelphia, PA); the dense aggregation of cells below the epithelium **(C)** is its hallmark (known as the *cambium layer*). Underneath, the loose texture is pronounced, and differentiating strap cells can be found. In most examples of the alveolar type, the alveolar morphology is obvious when they are well formed and striking **(D)**. The tumor cells either grip fibrous septa around the alveoli or lie discohesively in the space; large pleomorphic cells with abundant cytoplasm are infrequent but diagnostic, especially in the solid variant or when alveoli are less conspicuous.

5.36D). Cells at the periphery of the alveoli hug these septa. Although the differentiation may vary from case to case, most of the tumors are largely noncytoplasmic, and only scattered eosinophilic cells can be seen. Multinucleated giant cells with a wreath of nuclei are a frequent finding in alveolar rhabdomyosarcoma but not in the other types. Little in the way of spindle-shaped cells is identified. Muscle markers are often reactive. The solid variant fails to form the nearly pathognomonic alveolar spaces, except in very small foci. This form can be recognized by the presence of the aforementioned tumor giant cells. Alveolar RMS may present with bone marrow metastases or tumor cell leukemia (427). Molecular analysis of this type may be important prognostically (see "Molecular Diagnosis of Soft Tissue Tumors").

Molecular Prognosis

The molecular analysis, which is becoming so helpful in classifying small round cell tumors, may also be important prognostically because PAX7-FKHR alveolar RMS tumors have a more favorable clinical course than do PAX3-FKHR tumors (49,428).

Pleomorphic Rhabdomyosarcoma

Pleomorphic RMS is rare; the examples designated as such in the past were more likely UPS/MFH. RMS tumors in children with some pleomorphism are, by current convention, subsumed into the embryonal group. However, unusual childhood and rare adult cases can be found (101,350). The cells are reminiscent of those seen in rhabdomyoma, with abundant eosinophilic and granular cytoplasm. The cell shape may be elongated and boxcarlike or round to polygonal. Unlike the nuclei of UPS/MFH, the nuclei in pleomorphic RMS are usually regular, single, and round; if multiple nucleation is seen, the nuclear lobes are nearly the same size. Such cases may possibly be considered variants of the embryonal type with more prominent cytoplasmic differentiation.

VASCULAR LESIONS

Papillary endothelial hyperplasia was described earlier in this chapter (see Fig. 5.10).

LOBULAR CAPILLARY HEMANGIOMA (PYOGENIC GRANULOMA)

This relatively common, reddish-blue, small cutaneous lesion may appear in almost any site, but it tends to occur on the lips and face of pregnant women (429,430). The frequent mitoses and enlarged endothelial nuclei may initially be disturbing at high power, but a low-power view discloses an organized architecture for this lesion (Fig. 5.37). Particularly at the lateral edges, a lobular arrangement wherein groups of capillaries proliferate but abruptly stop is noted. A thin collagen layer surrounds each lobule. This arrangement is disrupted at the base, where irregularly shaped larger vascular channels reside and presumably communicate with the proliferation. At this location, some anastomosing channels resembling angiosarcoma can occasionally be identified, but they are focal, not an integral part of the lesion. At a higher power, another discriminating feature of benign vascular lesions is apparent; the small capillary

endothelium-lined spaces are also surrounded by a perithelial or pericytic layer of cells. This double layer of cells, which is also seen in intramuscular angiomatosis, is not seen in the clonal angiosarcoma. Frequently, the pyogenic granuloma, which is more properly called *lobular capillary hemangioma*, contains a superficial region of ulceration in which neutrophils abound in the more superficial lobules. The lobular capillary hemangioma may be reactive or neoplastic, but despite its relationship to pregnancy and the oral contraceptive pill, it lacks steroid hormone receptors.

HEMANGIOMA

A tremendous variety is seen in hemangiomas, which range from (a) the cavernous type, in which very large spaces are separated by fibrous tissue, to (b) the capillary type, which lacks fibrous septa and may be quite cellular. The venous hemangioma is another form containing smooth muscle encircling the vascular spaces. Occasional hemangiomas develop within muscle (intramuscular type). These are noncircumscribed tumors that particularly form in the muscles of the thigh in young adults; pain is a frequent symptom. The intramuscular type is often accompanied by adipose tissue, and it may recur; however, it is clearly benign. It can be distinguished from angiosarcoma by the presence of a two-cell layer (endothelial and perithelial) and by the formation of round to elongated vascular spaces without anastomoses. Special subtypes of hemangioma exist, including the multicentric cutaneous glomeruloid hemangioma; this has a characteristic appearance within dilated vascular channels, and it is associated with Castleman disease and POEMS (polyneuropathy, organomegaly, endocrinopathy, M-protein, skin changes) syndrome (431). An excellent review of all congenital vascular lesions and malformations and their associated syndromes appears in Silverman (432).

Cellular (Juvenile) Hemangioma

Previously called *juvenile hemangioendothelioma*, cellular hemangioma is an immature form of capillary hemangioma, with practically all cases occurring in children younger than 1 year of age. It may be found in a variety of sites, but it is common in the cheek or periparotid region (433,434). The histologic appearance is characteristic, with plump polygonal cells that grow in sheets and areas that resemble hemangiopericytoma (HPC). Unlike the cells of HPC, those of cellular hemangioma have more cytoplasm and contain vacuoles, and a reticulin stain outlines groups of cells surrounding a space, as opposed to outlining the individual cells in HPC. Also, unlike the cells of HPC, the cells lining the luminal spaces appear exactly like those between the luminal structures (i.e., they are all endothelial). Numerous mitotic figures may be noted, but the lesions are clearly benign, and they may even regress. In some cases, the areas have easily recognizable hemangioma, and this type of maturation is often seen at the periphery.

Epithelioid Hemangioma

In some endothelial tumors, the cells are quite plump, and they may be rounded, giving an "epithelioid" or "histiocytoid" appearance (Table 5.15). The concept of a "histiocytoid hemangioma" is important (435) because it enables the recognition of a group of peculiar lesions. However, lesions that form distinct clinicopathologic entities with different biologic potentials

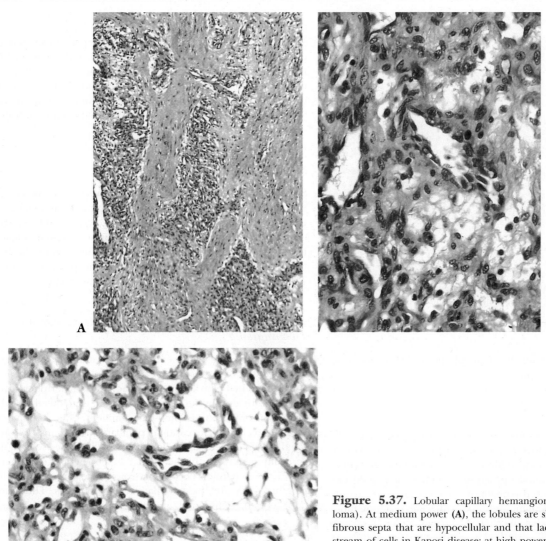

Figure 5.37. Lobular capillary hemangioma (pyogenic granuloma). At medium power (**A**), the lobules are sharply demarcated by fibrous septa that are hypocellular and that lack the denser spindly stream of cells in Kaposi disease; at high power (**B**), dilated capillary vessels have an eosinophilic outline resulting from a pericyte layer. In an inflamed case, the double lining of endothelial and perithelial cells typical of many nonclonal vascular lesions is more easily seen (**C**).

still retain their own designation. *Epithelioid hemangioma* is the accepted term for the lesion formerly known as *angiolymphoid hyperplasia with eosinophilia* (436). Eosinophilic plump and vacuolated endothelial cells (Fig. 5.38) proliferate in small groups and occasional sheets within a fibrous background, and they are typically accompanied by lymphoid aggregates and eosinophils. Often found as a subcutaneous lump in the head and neck, epithelioid hemangioma, with its prominent lymphocytic component and blood vessels, bears a superficial resemblance to Kimura disease. Unlike epithelioid hemangioma, however, Kimura disease lacks epithelioid morphology, and it is essentially geographically restricted to Japan (437). Epithelioid hemangioma may recur, and it may be seen with HIV infection. Epithelioid endothelial cells may also be identified in other hemangiomas, epithelioid hemangioendothelioma (see "Epithelioid Hemangioendothelioma"), and some angiosarcomas.

Spindle Cell Hemangioma

Spindle cell hemangioma (438), which was originally called *spindle cell hemangioendothelioma*, resembles some cases of Kaposi

sarcoma, and separating the two may be difficult. Clinically, spindle cell hemangioma resembles Kaposi sarcoma, with multiple nodules on the extremities of young male patients, but no association has been found with HIV or HHV8. Histologically, bland spindle cells flourish between vascular lumina, and extravasated red blood cells are present, as is seen in Kaposi sarcoma (Fig. 5.39). Several features help to separate spindle cell hemangioma from Kaposi sarcoma. First, spindle cell hemangioma is a nodular or multinodular lesion in which large cavernous spaces are filled with blood, some of which contain partially organized thrombi. Calcified nodules or phleboliths may be noticed at low power, and some nodules are intravascular. Second, scattered vacuolated cells may be discerned either lining the channels or surrounding the blood-filled spaces; these resemble signet ring cells to some degree, and they are not identified in Kaposi sarcoma. Third, spindle cell hemangioma lacks a prominent lymphoplasmacytic response. Scattered hemosiderin granules may be detected. The low-power architectural features of spindle cell hemangioma with central hemorrhagic spaces and phleboliths are the important clues for the differential diagnosis with Kaposi sarcoma. The proposed notion is that

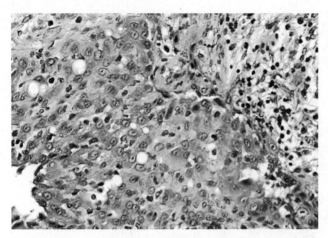

Figure 5.38. Epithelioid hemangioma (angiolymphoid hyperplasia with eosinophilia). In a subcutaneous nodule with a lymphoid cuff, sheets of epithelioid endothelial cells are appreciated; these have intracytoplasmic vacuoles, and they are often present within the larger vessels found centrally in the lesion. Lymphocytes and eosinophils are easily visible.

spindle cell hemangioma is not neoplastic, and this appears to be an accepted concept.

Tufted Angioma

Tufted angioma, also known as *angioblastoma of Nakagawa*, is an acquired benign cutaneous vascular neoplasm that is most often seen in infants or young children (439). The lesions present as indolent, but occasionally progressive, tender, ill-defined erythematous macules and papules on the neck or upper trunk. Despite their enlargement over time, with some reaching more than 10 cm in diameter, the clinical course is benign. A characteristic "cannonball" distribution of the vascular nodules is seen, with a pattern similar to that of lobular capillary hemangioma. A crescent-shaped or dilated vascular channel is at the edge of each nodule. Two cell types are described, and occasionally, crystalline material can be identified in the cytoplasm.

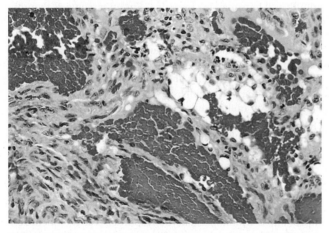

Figure 5.39. Spindle cell hemangioma. Although the spindle cells can mimic Kaposi sarcoma, the vacuolated endothelial cells are unique to spindle cell hemangioma. Here, they are found lining blood-filled channels.

Microvenular Hemangioma

Microvenular hemangioma is an acquired cutaneous hemangioma that presents as an asymptomatic, small, well-circumscribed red papule on the limbs and trunk of young adults, and it may clinically mimic Kaposi sarcoma (440). Irregular, narrow branching vessels are lined by flat or slightly plump endothelial cells without atypia. They dissect a sclerotic stroma in an infiltrative manner.

Sinusoidal Hemangioma

Sinusoidal hemangioma is a variant of cavernous hemangioma that occurs in middle-aged adults, predominantly women (441). It has a characteristic appearance and grows as a nodule in the dermis or subcutaneous tissue. This circumscribed hemorrhagic lesion has a lobular growth pattern and intercommunicating thin-walled blood vessels containing pseudopapillary structures. Thrombosis with dystrophic calcification can occur.

Hobnail Hemangioma, or Targetoid Hemosiderotic Hemangioma

Occurring on the trunk or extremities of young to middle-aged adults, this lesion presents as a small, solitary purple papule surrounded by a pale halo and occasionally by a peripheral ring (442). In the dermis, an irregular, dilated, thin-walled vascular channel proliferation is lined by prominent, often hobnail endothelial cells with occasional papillary projections. Extravasated red blood cells and inflammatory cells may be seen in the surrounding stroma. In the deeper subcutaneous component, the vascular channels become narrowed, they dissect the collagen, and they are lined by flat endothelial cells. The lesion appears to be self-limited, and excision is curative.

ANGIOMATOSIS

The involvement of a large portion of the body (skin to deep muscle or multiple muscle compartments) with a benign but diffuse vascular proliferation is termed *angiomatosis* (443). Small, meandering capillaries or small venules may be seen, or the lesion may be composed of a mixture of larger venous channels and capillaries. Some cutaneous forms of angiomatosis appear reactive (444).

BACILLARY ANGIOMATOSIS

Unusual cutaneous lesions resembling histiocytoid hemangioma were originally described in patients with AIDS and were called *epithelioid angiomatosis*. Subsequently, similar lesions associated with the cat-scratch bacillus were termed *epithelioid hemangioma-like vascular proliferation*, but the entity has come to be known as *bacillary angiomatosis* (445). Clinically, bacillary angiomatosis most commonly presents as a cutaneous disease characterized by multiple friable angiomatous papules or erythematous papules with and without crusts; it is visibly similar to pyogenic granuloma and Kaposi sarcoma. Systemic symptoms, such as fever, chills, night sweats, and weight loss, are common. Other organs and systems may be involved, including the liver, spleen, lymph nodes, and mucosal surfaces of the conjunctivae and respiratory tract. Presentation as a primary STT has been reported (446), as has bone involvement as osteomyelitis and coexistence with Kaposi sarcoma elsewhere.

Histologically, bacillary angiomatosis resembles lobular capillary hemangioma. Indeed, the early cases were also termed *disseminated pyogenic granuloma*. The lesions are often polypoid with epithelial collarettes. Granulation tissue–like clusters of small rounded vessels are present, separated by bands of fibrosis; plump endothelial cells and neutrophils also abound. Perithelial cells surround the small vessels. As in granulation tissue, myofibroblasts may be seen, but the tight streaming bundles of spindle cells of Kaposi sarcoma are absent. Granular eosinophilic or, less often, basophilic material representing the bacilli may be observed, but this can be mistaken for fibrin; the Warthin-Starry stain can be used to detect and to confirm the bacterial nature. Immunohistochemically, the vessels show strong factor VIII reactivity, whereas Kaposi sarcoma does not. The lesion is caused by several agents, including *Bartonella henselae* and *claridgeiae*. Because some cases have been associated with Epstein-Barr virus in AIDS, this lesion may also represent a nonspecific response to infection by various agents.

VASCULAR TRANSFORMATION OF SINUSES

Vascular transformation of sinuses is a morphologic spectrum of vascular proliferation that was originally described as being limited to the nodal sinuses without involvement of the actual capsule (Fig. 5.40). At low power, most cases are recognizable because of the prominence of red blood cell–filled spaces limited to the nodal sinuses. At high power, in most cases, the spaces are dilated and circular with very few, if any, spindled cells among them. No evidence of intraparenchymal or intracapsular involvement has been found. However, the morphologic spectrum has been expanded to include those cases with spindle cells, which may display an almost identical appearance to Kaposi sarcoma with parenchymal involvement (447). Eosinophilic globules and extravasation of red cells may be seen, thus adding to the confusion. However, fibrosis between spindle cells is usually present in vascular transformation of sinuses but not in nodal Kaposi sarcoma; in addition, the well-formed spindle cell fascicles of Kaposi sarcoma are not seen in vascular transfor-

mation of sinuses. Vascular transformation of sinuses may infiltrate the nodal capsule, another difference from Kaposi sarcoma. The cellular form is the subtype that most resembles Kaposi sarcoma, but this form does have delicate sclerosis and a fibrohistiocyte-like delicate storiform pattern. This means that fibrosis and/or sclerosis should be sought when any nodal tumor resembling Kaposi sarcoma is encountered.

ENDOTHELIAL TUMORS OF INTERMEDIATE MALIGNANCY

KAPOSIFORM HEMANGIOENDOTHELIOMA

Kaposiform hemangioendothelioma, a distinctive, locally aggressive vascular tumor often occurring in the retroperitoneum of young children, may cause thrombocytopenia (i.e., Kasabach-Merritt syndrome with disseminated intravascular coagulation) (448). Large, invasive tumors contain solid nodules of spindle cells with slitlike spaces similar to those of Kaposi sarcoma; however, the nodules are surrounded by fibrous bands, unlike those seen in Kaposi sarcoma. The skin is another common site for this tumor, where it presents as ill-defined plaques. Infiltration may cause intra-abdominal masses, or it may surround the internal organs, such as the kidneys, pancreas, adrenal glands, and gut. The large size of these lesions, their position in the body, and a lack of PAS-positive hyalin globules distinguish them from Kaposi sarcoma. Rare adult tumors have been described (449).

RETIFORM HEMANGIOENDOTHELIOMA

This unusual dermal and subcutaneous tumor forms vascular channels, but they ramify through the tissue in a dispersed fashion; small cells with small, naked nuclei appear as knots or tufts in the lumina (450) (Fig. 5.41). No vacuoles or growth in cords, such as occurs in epithelioid hemangioendothelioma, are seen. This entity is considered a tumor of intermediate malignancy, but it only rarely metastasizes. Retiform hemangioendothelioma should be considered in the differential diagnosis of angio-

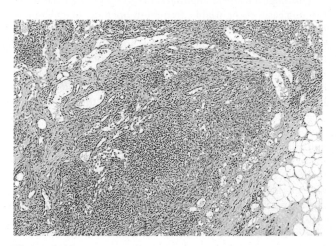

Figure 5.40. Vascular transformation of sinuses. In this lymph node, open vascular channels occupy the sinuses beneath the uninvolved capsule. In addition, spindle cells proliferate along the sinuses and in the parenchyma. Note the small foci of fibrosis.

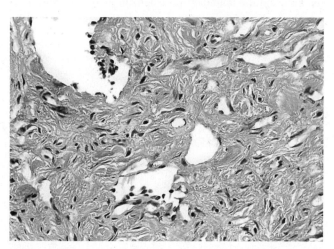

Figure 5.41. Retiform hemangioendothelioma. The vascular structures in this lesion may be open or closed. In open vessels, the small, bland hobnail nuclei are often seen protruding into the lumen; no mitoses or atypia is seen. Closed vessels resemble ramifying cords of cells within the fibrous tissue.

sarcoma. The newly described papillary intralymphatic angioendothelioma is a related entity with larger dilated lymphatic channels (451).

MALIGNANT ENDOTHELIAL TUMORS

EPITHELIOID HEMANGIOENDOTHELIOMA

Because epithelioid hemangioendothelioma is endothelial in origin and it is capable of metastasis, this tumor is a low-grade form of angiosarcoma expressing unusual histology (452,453). Soft tissue cases commonly occur on an upper or lower extremity and display striking angiocentricity, with growth within and around large veins or arteries. However, it may also occur within organs, such as the liver (hepatic hemangioendothelioma, which is often mistaken for sclerosing cholangiocarcinoma) and lungs (intravascular bronchoalveolar tumor).

Regardless of the site, the histology is similar. Although any tumor may contain highly cellular areas, the much more typical pattern is sclerotic, with tumor cells growing in single-cell strands (Fig. 5.42). Its vascular nature is betrayed by the formation of large vacuoles, which are frequently septate (Fig. 5.42, Table 5.13). Single red blood cells may be found within the vacuoles, identifying the vacuoles as being vascular in origin. An elastic stain is often helpful for delineating the occasionally obliterated and inapparent host vessel. When sheets of tumor cells are found, a reticulin stain will outline small groups with a nesting pattern mimicking that of carcinoma. Although the nuclei may vary from small and pyknotic to large and oval with nucleoli, occasional cases have prominent nuclear pleomorphism.

Most of these tumors have an extremely low mitotic rate, with an average of 1 to 2 mitotic figures per 10 hpf. In the soft tissue, the recurrence rate is 10%, and more than 20% of cases metastasize to the lymph nodes, lungs, or liver. The differential diagnosis includes other epithelioid or histiocytoid endothelial lesions, but the sclerotic pattern with strings of tumor cells is nearly diagnostic. Myxoid chondrosarcoma, another tumor with a stringlike pattern, may be excluded by its lack of vascular markers and the abundant proteoglycan matrix. Finally, a related tumor has a polymorphic appearance, including angiosarcoma-like areas (454).

ANGIOSARCOMA

Somewhere between a one-third and one-half of all angiosarcomas occur in the skin (455,456), particularly on the head and neck of elderly patients. Men are affected more commonly than women, and the tumor appears as either reddish-blue nodules or, more commonly, flat spreading bruises. They may expand to quite a large size, and their full extent is frequently underestimated by the clinician. Because of this ''iceberg'' effect, the local excision is often inadequate, and recurrence is common. In this form, early metastatic disease develops in a high percentage of patients, and the overall prognosis is poor. Less common are those cases that develop in the deep soft tissue in association with the major vessels (453,457). Most studies have failed to identify HHV8 as a causative agent (458).

Two other presenting forms of angiosarcoma are common. In patients with long-standing lymphedema, the risk for the development of angiosarcoma in the affected extremity is increased (459). In the days of radical breast surgery for cancer, postmastectomy angiosarcoma developed in the arm after a latent period of about 10 years in several cases. These patients were frequently in the seventh decade of life, and they had a mean survival time of 19 months. The other common site is within the breast (460,461); this form affects patients in the third and fourth decades of life. Although the tumors may be small, they frequently produce diffuse enlargement of the breast with overlying skin discoloration. The histology can be deceptively bland, and realizing that a full spectrum of benign vascular lesions of the breast must also be considered is important. The location within the breast may provide some clue because many superficial cutaneous or subcutaneous vascular lesions are commonly benign; in contrast, mammary angiosarcoma involves the actual breast parenchyma. An increasing number of mammary angiosarcomas have been reported after radiation therapy for localized breast cancer (462); in the same postradiation setting, so-called atypical vascular lesions of the mammary skin have been recently reported and form irregular spaces without nuclear atypia (463).

Histologically, most angiosarcomas disclose their nature by forming easily recognizable, frequently open vascular channels. Unlike those of benign tumors, these channels freely anastomose and branch. They are lined by ''too many cells'' to cover the space, and these cells are plump, with prominent, hyperchromatic nuclei. In addition, tufts of endothelial cells protrude into the vascular channels. In the skin, the existing collagen bundles frequently serve as a ''scaffold'' for the proliferation (Fig. 5.43A), and these small circular, separated pillars are a clue to the diagnosis. Occasionally, the cutaneous forms are epithelioid in appearance, with round to polygonal cells growing in diffuse sheets. This cutaneous and highly aggressive epithelioid variant (Fig. 5.43B) should be distinguished from the epithelioid hemangioendothelioma, a tumor of much lower malignant potential. In this more poorly differentiated form, the cells commonly have enlarged nuclei with nucleoli, and the only hint of the vascular structure is found either at the edge with vessel formation or centrally with the septate vacuole (Fig. 5.43B). Deep soft tissue variants of epithelioid angiosarcoma may arise from the arterial endothelium (457,464). A granular variant has also been described. Still other forms may resemble

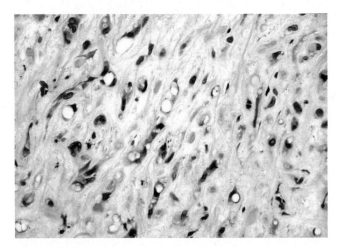

Figure 5.42. Epithelioid hemangioendothelioma. This is a sclerosing tumor in which thin strands of tumor cells proliferate. Some of the cells have septate vacuoles, typical of endothelial cells.

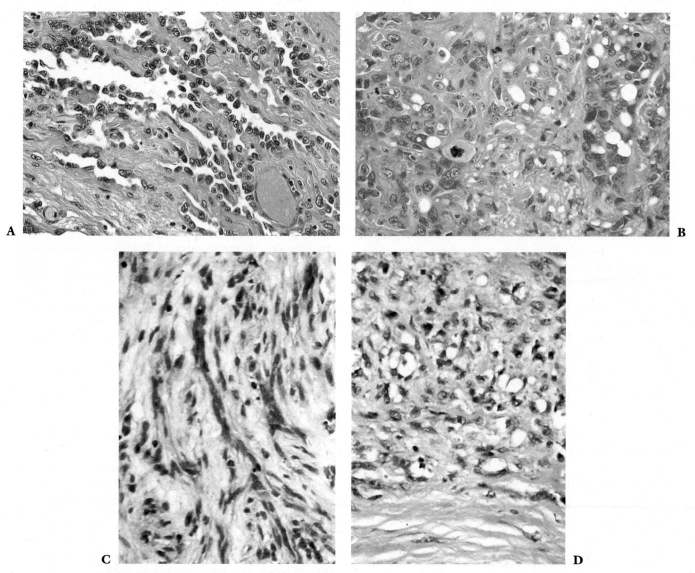

Figure 5.43. Angiosarcoma. The existing collagen serves as a "scaffold" for the hyperchromatic and tufting endothelial cells in angiosarcoma (**A**). Too many cells line the anastomosing spaces, and atypia is present. In poorly differentiated epithelioid cases (**B**), vacuoles are often seen, and when two vacuoles abut each other, a septate vacuole is produced. This is a clue to the endothelial nature of the lesion, especially if a red blood cell is found in a vacuole. A sclerosing angiosarcoma (**C, D**) may be mistaken for fibromatosis, but it has a double row of nuclei in a branching pattern (**C**); open channels and septate vacuoles are found focally (**D**).

Kaposi sarcoma, or they may be extremely bloody, with great similarity to choriocarcinoma, particularly in the lung. Highly cellular cases may spindle, resembling fibrosarcoma, but open vascular channels are usually visible in foci. Lastly, a peculiar sclerosing form resembles fibromatosis (Fig. 5.43C,D). However, the use of high power demonstrates that the cells grow in thin strands that frequently branch and that there is often have a double row of cells. Occasionally, the cells split apart, forming vascular channels, or they have septate vacuoles with red cells.

The differential diagnosis includes pseudoangiomatous carcinoma when the skin is involved (465) and mesothelioma when the serous membranes are involved (466). Although hemangioendothelioma-like sheets of epithelioid cells are seen in the pleura ("pseudomesothelioma"), the channels are formed focally, so these cases should be regarded as angiosarcomas (466). Regardless of the site, angiosarcoma is a highly aggressive lesion,

and in most instances, the degree of differentiation or grade does not affect the overall survival, except in the breast, where a relationship between histologic grade and survival does appear to exist.

KAPOSI SARCOMA

Three points should be made about Kaposi sarcoma. First, it may or may not be a fully malignant neoplasm (467,468), and it may be cytogenetically polyclonal (469). Second, its clinical forms are misunderstood. In the classic elderly patients formerly documented, more internal visceral involvement was found than is currently appreciated (470); in cases associated with homotransplantation, regression is common if the immunosuppression is halted (468). Furthermore, in the AIDS population, regression and long survival may occur (471), and survival is related more to immunologic status than to the bulk or distribution of the lesions. Third, although many cases are histologically straightforward (a uniform and bland proliferation of eosinophilic spindly cells showing directional streaming), it is not generally realized that Kaposi sarcoma may be mistaken for the following in the skin: (a) inflammatory dermatosis (472); (b) pyogenic granuloma, which lacks a spindle cell element (473); (c) angiodermatitis or pseudo-Kaposi sarcoma, which is a *lobular* proliferation of capillaries separated by fibrous tissue rather than spindle cells below hyperplastic or ulcerated epithelium and that contains prominent hemosiderin; (d) bacillary angiomatosis, an epithelioid, vascular tumor–like lesion that lacks spindle cells and that is the result of a bacterial infection; and (e) angiosarcoma, in which a spindly component accompanies the formation of anastomosing channels in rare cases of Kaposi sarcoma. In the lymph node, the vascular transformation of sinuses should be considered; in contrast to Kaposi sarcoma, this is a hemangioma-like lesion with blood-filled spaces and mild fibrosis.

Kaposi sarcoma has been shown to be caused by a virus, HHV8 (474,475). The findings include HHV8 identified by in situ hybridization in the spindle cells (476), seroconversion to HHV8 before the development of Kaposi sarcoma, and the resolution of Kaposi sarcoma after protease-induced seronegativity. However, the virus can be found in the blood of people who do not have Kaposi sarcoma (477) and in body cavity lymphomas as well.

PERICYTIC (PERIVASCULAR) TUMORS

GLOMUS TUMOR

The glomus tumor, which is derived from a specialized pericyte, frequently occurs in the subungual portion of the finger and less frequently on other parts of the extremity and trunk (478). The histology is variable, with prominent vasculature being noted in all cases. Sometimes, these vessels are surrounded by a sharply demarcated cuff of cells with prominent eosinophilic cytoplasm (Fig. 5.44). Well-defined cell borders, which give an "epithelioid" appearance, are often seen, but the cell borders

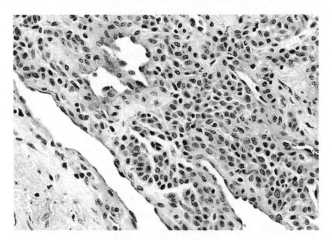

Figure 5.44. Glomus tumor. Small rounded cells with eosinophilic cytoplasm cluster around and between gaping vascular spaces. The nucleus is generally round to slightly oval.

TABLE 5.19
Frequently Painful Soft Tissue Lesions
Glomus tumor
Angiolipoma
Neuroma
Vascular leiomyoma (angiomyoma)
Cutaneous leiomyosarcoma
Clear cell sarcoma
Calcified synovial sarcoma

may be indistinct. In some cases, the sheets of cells appear to be punctuated by vascular spaces. In still others, the vascular spaces are indeed huge (glomangioma), and they may have muscular walls (glomangiomyoma). The nucleus is usually small and round with finely dispersed chromatin. Desmin reactivity can be an aid to diagnosis (479,480), as well as reactivity with SMA. Most patients are young adults, either male or female, who present with pain, particularly on exposure to cold. Rare glomus tumors that are cellular with mitoses and nuclear atypia are called *atypical glomus tumors* or *glomangiosarcoma* (481); metastases occur in nearly 40% of these patients. The differential diagnosis of painful STTs is listed in Table 5.19.

LYMPHANGIOMYOMA, OR LYMPHANGIOMYOMATOSIS

Lymphangiomyoma is often associated with the tuberous sclerosis complex (186,482); its molecular biology suggests causation through TSC2 mutations (483). The tumor, which was originally described long ago in isolated case reports, has been incorporated into a family of neoplasms with perivascular epithelioid cell differentiation that are known as *PEComas* (see "Perivascular Epithelioid Cell Tumors"). Lymphangiomyomatosis is a well-recognized clinical entity characterized by a chylous pleural effusion or ascites that appears almost exclusively in female patients. Tumors in the mediastinum and lung are common, but they occasionally occur in the retroperitoneum. In the lung, they typically are multiple, and they appear as stellate lesions containing slips of smooth muscle around spaces filled with the proteinaceous lymph fluid. Cells other than smooth muscle may be present. Such tumors may be found diffusely throughout the lungs, and they frequently replace the local lymph nodes. Pericytomatous histology is the rule in the larger, bulky masses. The clinical course is variable, with resectable cases doing well; those patients with diffuse pulmonary involvement usually have a progressive course and die after long periods. Antihormonal therapy has had a major impact on the management of this disease because the tumors may exhibit steroid hormone receptors (482). Single lung transplants have also been performed.

HEMANGIOPERICYTOMA

HPC is rapidly becoming nonexistent. Although a description is included, it is becoming clear that HPC is related, if not identical, to SFT (342), and the historical criteria for malignant HPC are similar to those for SFT.

What is HPC? At this point, it is mainly a pattern. First, it is clearly *not* a wide variety of lesions that histologically manifest

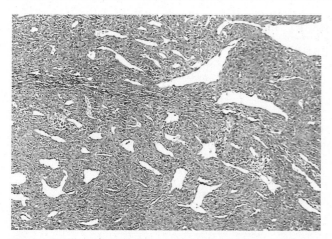

Figure 5.45. Pericytomatous pattern. The pattern seen here, with dilated vascular spaces (some having a staghorn or bifid shape) evenly dispersed among tumor cells, is nonspecific; the workup of such a lesion includes an assessment of other patterns and immunohistochemistry.

the nonspecific branching and staghorn open vascular pattern (Table 5.11 and Fig. 5.45) (484–486). Although Stout originally described HPC, he himself rejected most diagnosed cases. Therefore, HPC is a *diagnosis of exclusion* that is most frequently mimicked by synovial sarcoma, which may occasionally present as a pure HPC lesion; many blocks or additional tissue are required from the synovial sarcoma to demonstrate the epithelial differentiation. Thus, any CK immunoreactivity is quite important, and its presence excludes HPC as a diagnosis. If focal cartilage is present in the form of small islands, the diagnosis becomes mesenchymal chondrosarcoma. MPNSTs also exhibit this growth pattern, so these should be excluded.

Any tumor with a focal HPC pattern should be diagnosed as another specific entity; if the pattern is consistent throughout (Fig. 5.45) and negative for muscle, nerve sheath, and epithelial markers but positive for CD34 and CD99, then SFT should be the diagnosis in most instances (342). Thus, current practice dictates not only eliminating many other lesions but also searching for the thin bands of collagen that characterize SFT, and malignancy can be evaluated on that basis.

Lesions reported as HPCs may be associated, like SFT, with hypoglycemia and Castleman disease (487), and they may exhibit lipomatous differentiation (488).

MYOPERICYTOMA

Tumors of true pericytic origin have been described (489,490); these do, in contrast to HPC, contain myoid markers. These tumors have spindle cells with eosinophilic cytoplasm, like smooth muscle cells, and they have been called *myopericytomas.* A special form of HPC in the nasal sinuses may belong to this category because muscle markers are expressed (491). Myopericytomas have a characteristic concentric ring–like perivascular growth pattern that is seen best in the less cellular areas of the tumor or at its periphery. Immunohistochemically, SMA is often reactive, and desmin may be found in some tumors. Tumors such as angioleiomyoma and vascular leiomyoma may be considered to be within the family of myopericytic lesions.

PERIVASCULAR EPITHELIOID CELL TUMOR (PECOMA)

For a discussion of PEComas, see the relevant section at the end of this chapter.

LESIONS OF SUPPOSEDLY SYNOVIAL ORIGIN

GIANT CELL TUMOR OF TENDON SHEATH

This lesion occurs in the following two clinically different forms: a localized form, which is also called *nodular tenosynovitis* and has been shown to be polyclonal, and a diffuse form known as *pigmented villonodular synovitis* (*PVNS*) (492,493). The nodular type is usually a small, circumscribed, lobulated mass affecting mainly the hands, although nonarticular arm and leg lesions have been recognized. Most of the tumors are cellular, with numerous multinucleated benign giant cells evenly dispersed throughout the lesion. Accompanying these are variable numbers of inflammatory cells, such as lymphocytes and histiocytes, and rounded stromal cells. Hemosiderin is typically present, and it occasionally is prominent. The lesion has cleftlike spaces, and a scattered mitotic figure may be found. The lesion is CD68 positive, and desmin-positive, dendrite-like cells can be seen (494). Although the lesion is clearly benign, local recurrence develops in approximately 20% of cases.

In the diffuse form, which is less common, the knee and ankle joints are generally affected by a florid papillary synovitis, and the histology is similar to that of the nodular type. The lesion is not encapsulated, but instead, it grows around the joint cavity, with extension into the soft tissue. These lesions are much more locally aggressive, eroding joints and recurring in nearly half the cases.

Both tumor types contain the COL6A3-CSF1 gene fusion (495).

MALIGNANT GIANT CELL TUMOR OF TENDON SHEATH

Although the malignant giant cell tumor of tendon sheath is similar in histology to tenosynovitis, these very rare tumors appear more aggressive at the time of recurrence, and they may metastasize (360). Such recurrences resemble the aggressive bone tumor, but they (and so-called malignant PVNS) have areas without multinucleated giant cells, more tightly compact mononuclear cells arranged in sheets, necrosis, and a high mitotic rate (>10 mitotic figures per 20 hpf). The distinction from giant cell UPS/MFH, which may be moot, relates to location near a joint and lack of bizarre pleomorphic cells.

SYNOVIAL SARCOMA

Synovial sarcoma is a misnomer because this malignancy is only rarely found within joints and it has no immunocytochemical relationship to the CK-negative normal synovium (496–501). Nonetheless, the vast body of the existing literature favors the retention of this phraseology rather than the adoption of a new term. In the distant past, only the biphasic variant was recognized. A monophasic variant was gradually accepted, and with the advent of immunohistochemistry, this variant has come to

TABLE 5.20	Synovial Sarcoma: Clinical Characteristics	

| | Synovial Sarcoma[a] | |
	Regular	Calcified
Average age (yr)	~30	26
Sex (M/F)	~1.2	~1.9
Sites	Extremities (knee region, thigh, foot, hand)	Extremely (94%)
Other	Pain in ~25%; long duration; late metastases; death	Pain in 40%; long duration
Recurrence[b]	32%–55%	32%
Metastases	52%–74%	25%
Survival		
Percentage DOD	High	23%
5 yr	36%–69% (50%)	83%
10 yr	30%–38%	66%

[a]Approximate recent averages are given in parentheses.
[b]Recurrence means local recurrence.
DOD, dead of disease; F, female; M, male.

outnumber the biphasic type by a ratio of 2 to 1 in relatively recent series. Although synovial sarcoma is commonly referred to as a highly aggressive tumor, an analysis of various series (Table 5.20) and a comparison with other sarcomas have failed to demonstrate much of a survival difference between synovial sarcoma and other sarcomas at 5 years. Some patients die of the disease quite early, but in a fair proportion, the clinical course is prolonged, with late recurrences, metastases, and death even beyond 10 years. Some studies point to a high degree of chemosensitivity, with even metastatic disease showing regression (501). This is particularly true in childhood synovial sarcoma. The newer survival data are superior to those of the past, and the traditional approach to these tumors must change accordingly. For example, synovial sarcoma was commonly assigned to grade 3 morphology, which was a practice based on scanty evidence and a lack of careful examination of the histologic features. In the study of Cagle et al. (499), the noticeable survival difference depended on the overall percentage of glandular elements and the mitotic rate. For low-risk patients whose tumors contained more than 50% glandular elements and less than 15 mitoses per 10 hpf, the survival rate at 3 years and probably at 5 years was 100%, whereas for high-risk patients whose tumors were monophasic and less glandular with a higher mitotic rate, the 3-year survival rate was 43%, decreasing to approximately 20% at 5 years. Some studies have noted that patients with biphasic or more glandular tumors have a more favorable prognosis, but most agree there is no survival advantage. The recommendation is that this tumor be treated more scientifically and that the system developed by Cagle and colleagues be applied to accumulate more data for future analysis.

The prognosis in synovial sarcoma is related to the size and the margin status (498,502). An analysis of DNA ploidy results has shown a survival advantage for those patients with diploid tumors. The molecular analysis of synovial sarcoma is diagnostic (the SYT-SSX1 or SYT-SSX2 fusion gene is specific) (503), and it is also prognostic because the course is more favorable for patients who have tumors with translocation of the SSX2 gene (Table 5.4) (50).

Histologically, no other tumor in the body resembles the biphasic synovial sarcoma variant. The glandular element (Fig.

5.46A), which is clearly epithelial both immunohistochemically and ultrastructurally, is found in variable amounts, and the glands are usually quite elongated. In some cases, the glandular element outlines very large cystic spaces into which thick fronds protrude. The epithelium secretes a mucicarmine-positive and PAS-positive substance, and it is limited by a basement membrane. The cells have abundant pink cytoplasm and oval nuclei. The other component is a variably cellular, but usually highly dense, population of spindled cells, which are often erroneously referred to as *stromal cells*. The oval nuclei have a "blastic" appearance resulting from the finely dispersed chromatin, and they frequently abut each other, often overlapping. The spindle cells have very scanty cytoplasm that is inapparent, except in the more hypocellular areas. As in nerve sheath lesions, alternating hypocellular and hypercellular regions can be seen. At low power, most of these tumors have a nodular pattern, and they infiltrate the surrounding tissues. Even in biphasic tumors, a hemangiopericytomatous pattern is not uncommon. If the tumor is on the chest wall, the density of the spindle cell component and the lack of papillary structures in the epithelial component can usually distinguish it from mesothelioma, the other biphasic tumor.

The monophasic variant may easily simulate fibrosarcoma, MPNST, SFT/HPC, and mesenchymal chondrosarcoma. In other words, because of the high degree of cellularity, a herringbone pattern or an HPC pattern (Fig. 5.46B) may predominate. However, clues to the real nature of the tumor include the presence of small, oval, overlapping nuclei (Fig. 5.46A), the identification of rare clusters of more plump and eosinophilic cells (Fig. 5.46C), the lack of the nervelike wavy nucleus, the lack of any cartilaginous differentiation, and the location. The imperceptible clusters of epithelioid cells (Fig. 5.46C) can be identified on reticulin stain (Fig. 5.46D), which can be used to support the diagnosis even if markers such as CK (Fig. 5.46E) are negative. Essentially, any highly cellular tumor with the aforementioned differential diagnosis occurring on the extremity of a young adult ought to be considered a monophasic synovial sarcoma until it is proven otherwise. The use of immunohistochemistry has been extremely valuable in this regard because nearly 90% of all monophasic tumors contain at least focal,

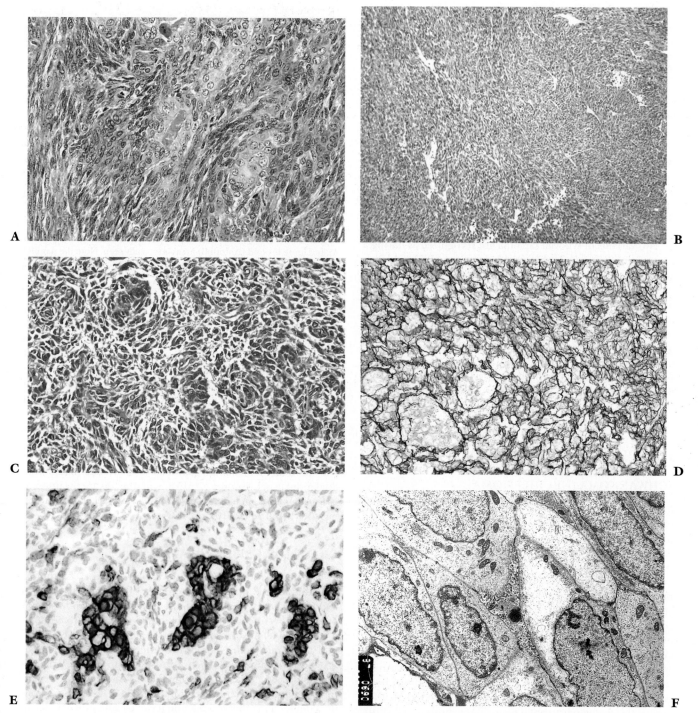

Figure 5.46. Synovial sarcoma. The biphasic type frequently has an obvious glandular component, which here is noted by its lighter cytoplasm and intraluminal material. Note the small, oval but overlapping nuclei in the spindle component (**A**). Many monophasic cases contain the pericytomatous pattern (**B**), but solid areas are also present; a careful search revealed focal cell clusters (**C**), indicating epithelial differentiation. A reticulin stain is useful to locate them and to document their epithelial nesting pattern (**D**). Cytokeratin decorates both the glands and the scattered spindle cells (**E**). Ultrastructurally, thin spaces with microvilli are found in these fibrosarcoma-like tumors, confirming the diagnosis (**F**).

but definite, CK or EMA expression. Indeed, synovial sarcomas contain specific CKs—CK7 and CK19—in comparison with tumors that have aberrant expression (133,504). Other epithelial markers, such as EMA, are helpful if they can be identified, but they are less specific (298). Synovial sarcomas are also positive for BCL-2 and CD99 (60%) and occasionally for S-100 (30%) (127); they are negative for CD34. Many cases are calponin positive, and focal SMA staining may be seen as well. Ultrastructurally, even the fibrosarcoma-like areas of monophasic synovial sarcoma contain a morphologic marker—the slitlike glandular spaces with microvilli (Fig. 5.46F). To reiterate, a high degree of suspicion should be aroused by a finding of the aforementioned clusters, which on reticulin stain, are outlined like nests in an epithelial tumor (Fig. 5.46D). Given the proper clinical setting, this is sufficient evidence for the diagnosis (Tables 5.18 and 5.20).

Two variants of synovial sarcoma are recognized as having a prognostic impact. A highly calcified variant (505), which is commonly biphasic, with a much less aggressive natural history has been described (Table 5.20). Poorly differentiated monophasic cases are more mitotically active, with vesicular nuclei that are slightly larger than those of the typical case (506,507); this variant has an unfavorable course. A rare example is the myxoid synovial sarcoma (508), and a purely epithelial monophasic synovial sarcoma is exceptional; both of these have been described. The latter exhibit the pericytomatous pattern, but they have circular nests that are noted only on reticulin stain (509).

PERIPHERAL NERVE SHEATH LESIONS

SCHWANNOMA (NEURILEMOMA)

Encapsulation combined with a dimorphic histology (cellular or Antoni A regions with loose myxoid Antoni B areas) defines this benign tumor, which is also known as *neurilemoma*. The schwannoma can be found at almost any site, but it is more common on the head and neck and extremities, where the tumors arise from small- to medium-sized nerves. Despite the neural origin, most lesions are painless, and only those that are larger or are undergoing cystic degeneration cause pain. Uncommonly, large tumors are found in the posterior mediastinum or the retroperitoneum. The typical tumor is solitary, occurring in a middle-aged adult. A rare example has been associated with von Recklinghausen neurofibromatosis. An occasional cutaneous schwannoma may exhibit a plexiform growth pattern, which should not cause confusion with neurofibroma; this type can be seen in neurofibromatosis type 2 (510), as can schwannomatosis (511).

Microscopically, the tip to the diagnosis is the dimorphic growth pattern (Fig. 5.47). The Antoni A regions are cellular, but they lack the mitotic figures of a malignant nerve sheath tumor. Even when very rare mitotic figures are present, the identification of an encapsulated schwannian tumor implies benignity; hypercellular tumors with scattered mitoses have been termed *cellular schwannomas* (see "Cellular Schwannoma"). The nuclei are elongated, they are occasionally pointed, and they frequently are wavy and undulating. In the classic example, rows of nuclei line up in a "nuclear palisade." Still other frequent formations include whorls of nervelike structures and the Verocay body (eosinophilic cell bodies nearly encircled by rows of

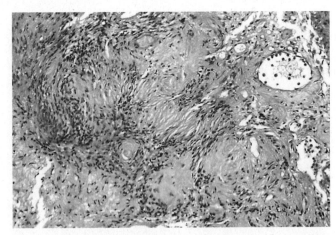

Figure 5.47. Schwannoma. A dimorphic pattern of cellular (Antoni A) and loose myxoid (Antoni B) areas is typically seen. Note the parallel rows of nuclei (nuclear palisading).

nuclei). The Antoni B areas are hypocellular, and the cells lack orientation. They are loosely arranged in a myxoid matrix accompanied by thin strands of collagen. Occasional mast cells may be identified in the Antoni B area. In addition, thick-walled vessels are unusually prominent. Degeneration with cyst formation should not be mistaken for necrosis, and rare atypical nuclei (so-called ancient change) should not be taken as a sign of malignancy. At the periphery and toward either end, the remnants of the originating nerve can sometimes be detected. S-100 reactivity is constant. Rare variants include pigmented (melanotic) schwannoma (512); neuroblastoma-like schwannoma (513); benign glandular schwannoma (514); pseudoglandular schwannoma (515); and the distinctly unusual psammomatous melanotic schwannoma, a marker for Carney myxoma syndrome (516).

GRANULAR CELL SCHWANNOMA

The lesion previously known as *granular cell tumor* is a tumor with abundant cytoplasm, pyknotic nuclei, and growth in cords and trabeculae. Cytoplasmic granularity may be seen in several other tumors, including ameloblastoma (517), DF (335), leiomyoma and leiomyosarcoma (397), angiosarcoma (518), UPS/MFH, and melanoma; however, in the schwannoma type, the PAS-positive granules, which correspond to the autophagosomes ultrastructurally, show significant variation in size, ranging from minute to large and globular (Fig. 5.40). This variability is not seen in other lesions, and it can be a helpful diagnostic clue. CD68 reactivity is nearly always present. In light of its S-100 reactivity and its occasional appearance as part of neurofibromatosis, the designation *granular cell schwannoma* has gained acceptance. A malignant counterpart has similar morphology but with rare mitoses or necrosis (Fig. 5.40; see "Malignant Granular Cell Tumor").

CELLULAR SCHWANNOMA

Occasional highly cellular nerve sheath tumors may be mistaken for malignancy, of which the cellular schwannoma is a prime example (519,520). This lesion, which was originally described by Woodruff and colleagues in 1981, may be quite large, and it may show nuclear pleomorphism and several mitotic figures (up to 4 per 10 hpf, on average). Sheets of eosinophilic cells with bullet-shaped nuclei are characteristic, and they are often the hallmarks of a schwannoma; hyalinized thick vessels and foamy histiocytes are also seen. The key feature is a thick capsule, often with prominent lymphoid aggregates. Cellular schwannoma is found mainly in the paravertebral region of the retroperitoneum, mediastinum, and pelvis. Unlike MPNST, it exhibits strong, diffuse S-100 reactivity, a diagnostic feature.

NEUROFIBROMA

Unlike schwannoma, the neurofibroma is an unencapsulated nerve sheath lesion that may occur in the following forms: (a) a solitary localized nodule; (b) a diffuse thickening of the skin and subcutaneous tissues; or (c) a "plexiform" tumor, a worm-like, multinodular growth within major or minor nerves. Although only the last form is characteristic of neurofibromatosis, that autosomal-dominant disease may also produce solitary or diffuse lesions. The neurofibroma may be found virtually anywhere in the skin or subcutaneous tissues, and it is usually seen in young adults.

The neurofibroma differs from the schwannoma in that a single uniform pattern is noted at low power (Fig. 5.48A). The borders infiltrate the adjacent dermis and adipose tissue, even in the apparently circumscribed nodular type. In both the nodular and diffuse forms, the skin appendages are frequently surrounded by the proliferation. Although deeper tumors may be either quite myxoid or extensively collagenized, the more superficial cutaneous types are moderately cellular. The cells have scanty but extensively elongated cytoplasm, appearing as extremely thin, lightly eosinophilic fibrillar structures. The nucleus may be oval, but it often is wavy or comma shaped (Fig. 5.48B). Randomly dispersed, highly pleomorphic nuclei should be ignored; they represent a type of degenerative phenomenon called *ancient change* (Fig. 5.48C). Thin axonal processes usually can be demonstrated with silver stains or neurofilament immunoreactivity. The overall cellularity of a neurofibroma, unlike that of many other tumors, is quite uniform throughout, and

the typical benign tumor is never highly cellular. Very rarely, these tumors may be pigmented, granular, epithelioid, or even cellular in appearance (521); however, any epithelioid morphology should be viewed with caution, and it should be accompanied by search for mitotic figures.

In the plexiform type (Fig. 5.48A), the cellular proliferation expands contiguous nerves, which, at low power, appear as small nodules with a dense eosinophilic rim representing the remnant of the original nerve (522). Circular structures of fibrillar eosinophilic material outlined by nuclei are reminiscent of Wagner-Meissner corpuscles (523). Approximately 10% of patients with the diffuse form have neurofibromatosis. This diffuse form may be confused with spindle cell lipoma when it occurs predominantly within the fatty tissue; however, it is much less spindly and more evenly cellular, and it is not circumscribed. Tumors with hybrid morphology (combined schwannoma and neurofibroma) can also be identified (524).

PERINEURIAL CELL TUMOR

This rare tumor, which is similar in all respects to neurofibroma but which lacks both Schwann cells and S-100 immunoreactivity, has been termed *perineurial cell tumor*, or perineurioma (525–527). The perineurial cell of normal nerves and the corresponding tumor are positive for EMA. Sclerosing variants with dense fibrosis and long, thin streaks of linear cytoplasm have been reported. Thus, if the pathologist encounters a neurofibroma-like, S-100–negative nerve sheath tumor, it may still be of nerve sheath origin, and EMA reactivity should be checked.

NEUROFIBROMATOSIS

Neurofibromatosis, a single-gene disorder, is a relatively common autosomal-dominant condition affecting 1 in 3000 liveborn children (528). Although its penetrance is nearly 100%, the expression of the gene varies greatly. The disease takes two forms. In the better recognized form, which is referred to as *von Recklinghausen disease* (neurofibromatosis type 1), patients have multiple café-au-lait spots and dermal neurofibromas. In

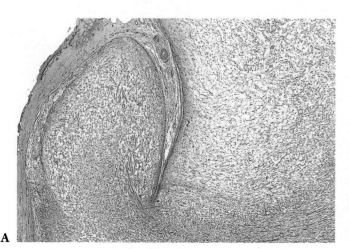

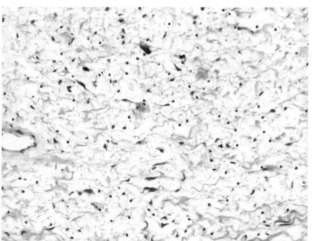

A   **B**

Figure 5.48. Neurofibroma. One of several expanded nerves is seen in plexiform neurofibroma (**A**). Neurofibromas are usually uniformly hypocellular and slightly myxoid, with an undulating fibrillar background (**B**); they may show nuclear atypia ("ancient change"), which should not be misconstrued as a sign of malignancy.

the more unusual neurofibromatosis type 2, patients have predominantly bilateral acoustic neuromas (schwannomas) that are associated with other brain and spinal cord tumors. The gene for neurofibromatosis type 1 has been mapped to chromosome 17, and its large protein product has been analyzed. It is diagnosed based on the presence of any *two* of the following:

1. At least five café-au-lait spots larger than 5 mm (six larger than 15 mm if the patient is prepubertal)
2. Two or more neurofibromas of any type or one plexiform type
3. Multiple large freckles in the axillary or inguinal regions
4. Sphenoid wing dysplasia
5. Bilateral optic nerve gliomas
6. Multiple iris nodules (Lisch spots)
7. A first-degree relative with the preceding criteria

In addition to cutaneous tumors, patients may exhibit solitary deep tumors; diffuse gastrointestinal ganglioneuromatosis; brain and spinal cord tumors, including meningiomas and ependymomas; and occasionally, malignant progression within a neurofibroma. Estimates of the rate of malignancy in neurofibromatosis type 1 are quite variable, but the more recent figures put it at 3.6% to 4.6%. Interestingly, the phenomenon of divergent differentiation is far more common in the malignant tumors of patients with neurofibromatosis type 1. A significant percentage of patients with neurofibromatosis type 1 die early, but a much higher percentage has a favorable long-term survival.

MALIGNANT PERIPHERAL NERVE SHEATH TUMOR

Because not all of the tumors in this group are clearly schwannian in origin, *MPNST* is the preferred terminology. Must an association with a small or large nerve be present for the diagnosis to be made? A high percentage of MPNSTs do come practically labeled as such by the surgeon who has noted this relationship (529–531). Several series have documented tumors in the absence of such a nerve but with identical histology and an identical course. Therefore, the diagnosis can be made on morphologic grounds alone if attention is paid to nuclear features, and the focal expression of S-100 protein fur-

ther supports this diagnosis in a spindle cell sarcoma. With many MPNSTs, the first impression is that of a highly cellular, fibrosarcoma-like tumor, such as the one depicted in Figure 5.22. A search for more specific features should ensue. The morphologic features that, if they are present in combination, help confirm the diagnosis of MPNST include the following: (a) alternating hypocellular and hypercellular regions; (b) the appearance of the thin, wavy, comma-shaped or bullet-shaped nuclei (Fig. 5.49A), particularly in hypocellular areas; (c) nuclear palisading, which may, however, also be prominent in a leiomyosarcoma; (d) nervelike whorls (Fig. 5.49B) or tactoid bodies resembling Wagner-Meissner corpuscles; (e) a prominent, thick-walled vasculature; and (f) heterologous elements. For example, isolated RMS elements in a spindle cell sarcoma (''Triton'' tumor; see ''Divergent Differentiation'') practically identify the spindle cell element as being of nerve sheath origin. Such muscle differentiation is often found at the junction between the hypercellular and hypocellular regions.

With regard to distribution, MPNSTs occur almost anywhere in the body, including the skin, head and neck, and retroperitoneum, but a peripheral location on the extremities is more common in the solitary (non–neurofibromatosis type 1) form, whereas central lesions on the trunk or head and neck predominate in neurofibromatosis (Table 5.21). The limb-girdle regions are commonly affected in either type. Tumors in patients with neurofibromatosis type 1 tend to occur at an earlier age, and a male predominance is noted. When MPNSTs are associated with neurofibromatosis type 1, they can develop from long-standing benign neurofibromas. Otherwise, documentation of an MPNST arising from a precursor lesion is exceedingly rare. Occasional MPNSTs are associated with pain and paresthesias, although most are without other symptoms.

Several histologic types of MPNST exist. Some cases resemble fibrosarcoma, having a very dense population of spindle cells with fascicles intersecting at acute angles (the herringbone pattern). This is perhaps the most common pattern, but hypocellular areas can generally be found with the characteristic wavy (but also bullet-shaped) nuclei. The presence of these alternating hypercellular and hypocellular areas is suggestive of nerve sheath origin, and it is reminiscent of benign schwannian tumors. Other tumors resemble neurofibromas. In this subtype,

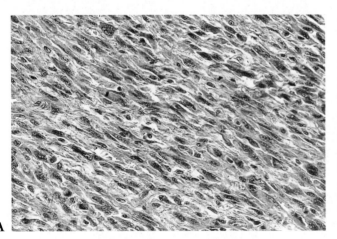
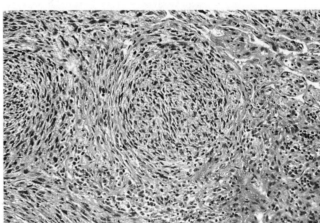

A   B

Figure 5.49. Malignant peripheral nerve sheath tumor. In this mitotically active and cellular tumor, occasional nuclei have a bullet shape—blunt at one end and pointed at the other **(A).** In a spindle cell sarcoma, nervelike whorls **(B)** are another clue to a nerve sheath origin.

TABLE 5.21	Characteristics of Malignant Peripheral Nerve Sheath Tumors				
	Spindled[a]			*Divergent Differentiation*[a]	
	Solitary	VRN	Epithelioid[b]	Triton	Glandular
Relative percentage	~50%	~40%	~5%	~5%	<1%
Average age (yr)	40	29	3–35	30	29
Percentage VRN	—	—	?	66	87
M/F	—	—	1.5	1.0	0.66
Common sites	Peripheral: retroperitoneum extremities; trunk; girdles; head and neck	Central: trunk; girdles; extremities; head and neck	Major nerves of legs (sciatic); arm	Thigh; neck; back; buttock	Neck; back
Other	May occur after radiation	5% VRN develop MPNST; risk = 4,600×	Mixed cases with spindle cells more common	20% had other elements	
LR	38%–80%	45%–75%	~50%	60%	75%
Metastases	16%–42%	39%–63%	~60%	48%	33%
Survival					
Percentage DOD	—	—	50%	72%	77%
5 yr	23%–75%	15%–37%	—	For all divergent cases	
10 yr	34%	9%	—	Crude 2 yr = 27% Crude 5 yr = 13%	

[a]Based on literature summary of 67 Triton tumors + 16 pure glandular MPNSTs. Twelve cases with other types of differentiation (cartilage, bone), as well as rare benign glandular cases, are not included.
[b]Pure cases only.
DOD, dead of disease; F, female; LR, local recurrence; M, male; MPNST, malignant peripheral nerve sheath tumor; VRN, von Recklinghausen disease.

the pathologist must ignore the bizarre nuclear changes in assessing malignancy and instead search for mitotic figures. Mitoses are important (Table 5.1); they are not identified in benign lesions, and any significant mitotic rate (>1 mitotic figure per 20 hpf) can be construed as evidence of potentially malignant behavior in a neurofibromatous lesion. Although definitive criteria have not been systematically studied, such a low rate should act as an overall guide because these tumors can be lethal (530). In this regard, erring on the side of calling a lesion a low-grade MPNST to effect a wider local excision and possibly to prevent further biologic aggression is perhaps more important. One hint of malignancy in a neurofibroma-like tumor is the presence of focal densely cellular regions or necrosis.

Occasional cases display extreme nuclear pleomorphism with a UPS/MFH-like appearance, a type found in cases of neurofibromatosis type 1. Perhaps the most difficult variant to diagnose is the purely epithelioid type (Table 5.21) (532), which accounts for approximately 5% of all MPNSTs. Epithelioid tumors (Table 5.15) may easily cause confusion with carcinoma or melanoma. The epithelioid type grows in a nodular pattern and practically always exhibits necrosis. The epithelioid cells are closely packed, and they grow in sheets. However, small foci of spindling with more classic nerve sheath morphology are virtually always found in the areas of hypocellularity, exemplifying the rule that a focal part is often the key to the whole. The cytoplasm of the epithelioid cells is pale, and the nuclei are usually rounded with either evenly dispersed chromatin or prominent nucleoli. The intranuclear cytoplasmic inclusions of melanoma are lacking, and a reticulin stain fails to demonstrate the nesting pattern of the carcinoma. Incidentally, this epithelioid type should not be confused with the much more primitive-appearing neuroepithelioma (PNET) of neuronal, as opposed to nerve sheath, origin. Additional assistance can be gained by

staining such a tumor for CK and S-100 antigen; only the latter should be present, and it is seen in 50% to 75% of all MPNSTs. Significantly, S-100 in MPNSTs is never diffuse, and its positivity is strong, as in the cellular schwannoma; caution should be taken in diagnosing such a case. Finally, some MPNSTs show perineurial differentiation, which is recognized by their significant EMA immunoreactivity (533).

DIVERGENT DIFFERENTIATION

The capacity of nerve sheath tumors to exhibit so-called heterotopic elements is derived from their origin in the neural crest (534–537), where the mesenchymal tissue is pluripotent, forming the entire soft tissue of the head. Thus, in addition to RMS elements (malignant Triton tumor) (535,538), one may find cartilage or chondrosarcoma, osteoid or osteosarcoma, and angiosarcoma. A peculiar finding is the occasional case with glandular differentiation, which was described by Woodruff and Christensen (537). The glandular component, which has intestinal characteristics, can occur by itself; it can appear benign or malignant (539); and it can contain evidence of neuroendocrine differentiation. These tumors with divergent differentiation have the worst prognosis of all the MPNSTs (Table 5.21), and they occur more frequently in neurofibromatosis type 1.

PRIMITIVE NEUROECTODERMAL TUMOR

See "Soft Tissue Ewing Sarcoma and/or Primitive Neuroectodermal Tumor Family" in "Unusual Lesions" for a discussion of these tumors.

OSTEOCARTILAGINOUS LESIONS

Myositis ossificans is discussed in "Soft Tissue Lesions: Lesions Mimicking Sarcomas (Pseudosarcomas)."

EXTRASKELETAL CHONDROMAS AND OSTEOMAS

Easily recognizable benign cartilaginous and osseous tumors may occur within the soft tissues. Chondromas tend to be more common on the hands and in the head and neck region, and because of the lack of pleomorphism or mitotic figures, they are easily identified as benign lesions. Chondroid tissue along with giant cells and spindle cells in a pericytomatous pattern may occur in the very unusual tumor associated with hypophosphatemia.

EXTRASKELETAL CHONDROSARCOMA

Aside from the rare well-differentiated chondrosarcoma of the soft tissues (540), two main groups of soft tissue chondrosarcomatous tumors exist. So-called extraskeletal myxoid chondrosarcoma has a highly recognizable morphologic appearance, but it is now considered to be a tumor of uncertain origin (287); nevertheless, it is discussed here (541–543). The extraskeletal myxoid chondrosarcoma has a lobular or nodular growth pattern, and in contrast to other myxoid lesions (Table 5.10), it has cells that often display a characteristic arrangement with the eosinophilic and granular cells with circular nuclei growing in "strings" or in single file, like the spokes of a wheel, from the periphery to the center of the lobules (Fig. 5.50). In areas of marked cellularity, this pattern is absent. Like the mucous substance of other chondrocytic lesions, that of extraskeletal myxoid chondrosarcoma is not sensitive to hyaluronidase. S-100 immunoreactivity is seen in only a minority of cases, as is synaptophysin. Molecular analysis (Table 5.4) shows the presence of an EWS-NR4A3(TEC) fusion (544). Its clinical course is often indolent. The majority of cases are low grade (Table

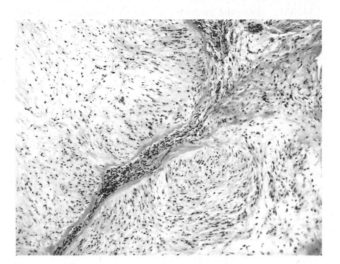

Figure 5.50. Myxoid chondrosarcoma. In this lobule at medium power, the myxoid substance is occupied by thin cords or strands of cells radiating toward the periphery, like spokes of a wheel.

5.22), with late recurrences developing 10 to 15 years after the diagnosis; however, a more rapid course is possible, particularly with the high-grade cellular variants.

Extraskeletal myxoid chondrosarcoma may be confused with *soft tissue myoepitheliomas* (see "Myoepithelioma and Mixed Tumors"). Mesenchymal chondrosarcoma is usually a lesion of bone; however, it does rarely occur in soft tissue as well (545–547). One form is easy to recognize because large areas of well-differentiated cartilaginous or chondrosarcomatous tissue are present and these are accompanied by a population of tightly packed small, round, primitive-appearing cells. The tumor is more difficult to recognize when the cartilaginous foci are extremely small and widely scattered. In these cases, the small primitive cell component frequently grows in a hemangiopericytomatous pattern; the diagnosis rests on recognition of the sometimes minute areas of cartilaginous differentiation. Indeed, this *bimorphic* pattern, even when it is nearly concealed, is pathognomonic. The tumor may be thought of as an HPC with cartilaginous differentiation. Immunohistochemistry may be helpful because the chondroid element can be confirmed with S-100 staining, and the cytogenetic findings differ from those of the myxoid type. This is another tumor that may show CD99 staining. Patients with mesenchymal chondrosarcoma experience late local recurrence and metastasis relatively often and die after 5 to 15 years (Table 5.22).

MYOEPITHELIOMA AND MIXED TUMORS

Myxoid tumors with epithelial or myoepithelial differentiation are termed *soft tissue myoepitheliomas and mixed tumors* (104,548); a tumor is mixed if it resembles the pleomorphic adenoma of the salivary gland. The myxoid tumors simulate extraskeletal myxoid chondrosarcoma but contain CK-positive, SMA-positive, calponin-positive, and S-100–positive spindle cells. These stains should be performed when extraskeletal myxoid chondrosarcoma is being considered. Some consider *parachordoma* to belong to this group, but others believe that it is a separate entity (549).

EXTRAOSSEOUS OSTEOSARCOMA

In the soft tissue, osteosarcoma may exhibit all the various histologic features found in the corresponding bone tumor. In contrast to primary bone tumors, most STTs occur in middle-aged and elderly patients (550–554). They may present with pain of long duration in the affected region. Rare examples have been known to arise from myositis ossificans, at injection sites, from heterotopic ossification in dermatomyositis, or in the skin (553). Other characteristics, including the highly aggressive nature of this tumor, are listed in Table 5.22. The zonation pattern of myositis ossificans is not found; instead, the advancing edge of this tumor is highly cellular, without osteoid formation. As with osseous and cartilaginous tumors arising in bone, the pathologist should be reluctant to diagnose extraskeletal osteosarcoma in the digits; in such locations, benign fibro-osseous pseudotumor (555) or reactive periostitis is more common, and it may be difficult to diagnose because it lacks the typical zoning of myositis ossificans. Extraskeletal osteosarcoma can arise in the postradiation setting, and on rare occasions, it can exhibit a markedly well-differentiated morphology or small-cell features.

TABLE 5.22		Characteristics of Extraskeletal Sarcomas		
			Chondrosarcoma	
	Ewing/PNET	*Mesenchymal*	*Myxoid*	*Osteosarcoma*[a]
Average age (yr)	~20	~30	44–49	>50
Age range (yr)	1–63	19–61	13–89	6–80
Common sites	Paravertebral; leg; chest wall	Head and neck (orbit, meninges); extremity (thigh)	Extremities (thigh, knee)	Extremities (thigh); girdles
Other	Deep; periosteal	Some long duration; x-ray shows stippled diffuse calcifications	Pain in 30%; some long duration	Pain in 10%–33%; radiograph shows spotty calcifications
Local recurrence	27%	44% (66%)[b]	41%–57%	42%[c]–76%
Metastases	65%	50% (60%)[b]	14%–28%	63%–80%
Time to failure	Short	Short	Variable	7–14 mo
Survival				
Percentage DOD	63% (65% DF on chemotherapy)	30% (74%)[b]	28%–53%	High
5 yr	Low	55%[b]	High	~25%
10 yr	—	27%[b]		

[a]Taken from the four largest series.
[b]Combined bone and soft tissue data.
[c]Most recent data.
DF, disease free; DOD, dead of disease; PNET, peripheral neuroectodermal tumor.

UNUSUAL LESIONS

MESENCHYMOMA

This term is falling out of favor because it is not a well-defined category, and many tumors may contain a focus of another type of differentiation (e.g., chondrolipoma). In addition, malignant tumors such as myxoid liposarcoma may have foci of cartilage and bone; dedifferentiated liposarcoma may show smooth muscle or chondro-osseous elements; and MPNSTs exhibit divergent differentiation. Thus many so-called malignant mesenchymomas (556,557) are now considered variants of other sarcoma types. This term may be avoided, and the tumor may instead be described as having various elements, as one would do for a germ cell tumor, for example.

Likewise, benign mesenchymomas (558,559) are often admixtures of fat and fibrous tissue, along with selected other elements; reference to the dominant line of differentiation is now preferred. Some of these unusual proliferations may be hamartomatous rather than neoplastic in nature.

ALVEOLAR SOFT PART SARCOMA

No other sarcoma has quite the same appearance as alveolar soft part sarcoma (560–562). Most lesions contain large areas with an alveolar pattern, which is well illustrated by a reticulin stain that shows surrounding nests rather than individual cells. The cells themselves are *uniform*, and they have large, round nuclei with a single prominent nucleus, together with granular eosinophilic or clear cytoplasm (Fig. 5.51). PAS-positive, diastase-resistant crystalline material (apparently containing monocarboxylate transporter 1 and its chaperone CD147) can be found in most cases, but its quantity is quite variable. A common feature is vascular invasion. As a rule, mitoses are scarce. Unu-

sual variants without much alveolar formation and scattered pleomorphic cells have been reported. Unlike the cells of paragangliomas, those of alveolar soft part sarcoma are frequently discohesive, and they lack nuclear pleomorphism. Unlike the alveoli of alveolar RMS, these alveoli are not elongated and are not separated by fibrous tissue, and the cells are much larger than primitive myocytes. The tumor may closely resemble areas in renal cell carcinoma, which must be included in the differential diagnosis, along with melanoma, metastatic adrenal carcinoma (often pleomorphic), and clear cell sarcoma. The natural history can be quite prolonged (Table 5.23).

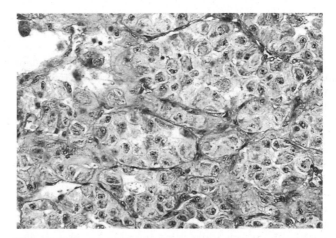

Figure 5.51. Alveolar soft part sarcoma. A thin microvasculature surrounds the nests of large polygonal cells, giving the impression of solid alveoli or an organoid appearance; the cells have uniform round nuclei with prominent nuclei and abundant cytoplasm, which shows noticeable granular clumping. The clumps correspond to crystalline material and stain with periodic acid-Schiff.

TABLE 5.23	Characteristics of Some Unusual Sarcomas			
	Rhabdoid	*Epithelioid*	*Clear Cell*	*Alveolar Soft Part*
Average age (yr)	<1	28	32	<30
Age range (yr)	14–36	4–90	7–83	0–74
Major sites	Pelvis; girdles; neck; central nervous system; heart	Hand; distal arm; leg	Foot; ankle; lower extremity (arm)	Extremity (thigh); buttock; orbit
Other	Rapid growth; most die <1 yr	Long duration; pain in 22%; multiple recurrences; late deaths	Long duration; pain; tenderness in 50%; multiple recurrences; late deaths	Vascular bruit present; late recurrennces
Local recurrence	NA	77%	45%	20%–33%
Metastases	~100%	45%	46%	~66%
Survival				
Percentage DOD	82%	31%	44%	Eventually most
5 yr	—	60%–70%	High	59%–67%
10 yr	—	25%–50%	—	47%

DOD, dead of disease.

The histogenesis of this tumor has been argued ever since its description in 1952. Interest has centered on a myogenic origin as a result of the finding of desmin, actin, and other muscle markers (562). In contrast to my previous results, I have seen several examples with both desmin and MSA; this staining is never extensive. A skeletal muscle origin is not supported by the detection of cytoplasmic MyoD1 protein because more specific MyoD1 nuclear staining is absent (562). Whether this unusual lesion derives from a specialized muscle cell or another cell type is still an open question. No one has yet reported the presence of myoglobin.

A molecular analysis of this neoplasm has demonstrated the presence of an unbalanced translocation der(17)t(X;17), with a corresponding ASPL-TFE3 fusion gene specific for the lesion (563). Interestingly, a subset of distinctive renal tumors in childhood possesses the same gene fusion, although the translocation in these cases is balanced (564). TFE3 immunoreactivity may be useful in the diagnosis of alveolar soft part sarcoma.

MALIGNANT GRANULAR CELL TUMOR

Although clear-cut examples of malignant granular cell tumor exist in the literature, some reports are not accurate (565). The tumor closely resembles the benign granular cell tumor (granular schwannoma) and grows in sheets (Fig. 5.52) without the organoid pattern of alveolar soft part sarcoma. Instead, nests and cords of PAS-positive granular cells are found in the dermis and subcutaneous fat, exactly the same as in the benign variant. Some authors state that certain metastasizing granular cell tumors are virtually indistinguishable from the benign type, and only the presence of metastasis may ultimately prove a tumor to be malignant. However, the following microscopic features favor a diagnosis of malignancy: (a) necrosis; (b) large vesicular nuclei with nucleoli, which is in contrast to the pyknotic type of the benign variant; (c) wide cellular sheets; (d) any tendency to a spindle cell morphology; and (e) any appreciable mitotic rate (566,567). The tumor size is not a distinguishing feature because more than half of the accepted cases are smaller than 5 cm. A tumor with any of the preceding features might be

labeled as a *tumor of uncertain malignant potential* before the appearance of metastatic disease to ensure a close follow-up. Although a mitotic rate of greater than 2 per 10 hpf has been mentioned as being a distinguishing feature, many of the reports in the literature describe tumors with fewer mitoses. Considering any tumor with any mitoses worrisome and those with a consistent mitotic rate of 1 per 10 hpf as malignant seems wise; wide local excision is advised in such cases. Importantly, the tipoff to look for mitoses is the presence of many cells with enlarged vesicular nuclei.

Concerning the cell of origin, most malignant granular cell tumors are positive for S-100 and CD68 (567,568), and therefore, they morphologically, ultrastructurally, and immunohistochemically resemble the benign granular cell tumor, a tumor of altered Schwann cells. Although the lesion is fairly characteristic, granular variants of squamous cell carcinoma, melanoma, smooth muscle tumors, or even angiosarcoma should be considered in the differential diagnosis, similar to that discussed for

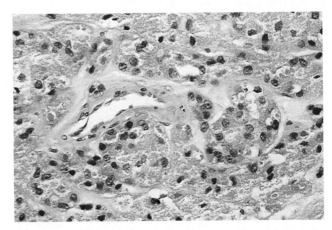

Figure 5.52. Malignant granular cell tumor. Unlike its benign counterpart, this tumor has vesicular nuclei with nucleoli; rare mitoses were found elsewhere. These features alone are worrisome; spindling areas and necrosis clinch the diagnosis. Note the intracytoplasmic globules of various sizes.

benign granular cell schwannoma; immunohistochemistry should be used to exclude them from consideration. When the literature up to 1992 was summarized, malignant granular cell tumors had a high rate of local recurrence (70%); they were much more common in female patients; they occurred in any site of the body; and they were quite lethal, with 65% of patients dying of disease within 4 to 5 years. In newer series with cases diagnosed prospectively, a significant proportion of patients are living disease free.

RHABDOID TUMORS

Although rhabdoid sarcoma (extrarenal rhabdoid tumor) exhibits one of the most characteristic cell types in soft tissue pathology, it is a controversial entity (569–574), and its very existence as a separate tumor has been called into question. The issues are highlighted in review articles (573,574). The peculiar and "pathognomonic" feature of the tumor is the presence of intracytoplasmic inclusions (Fig. 5.53), which ultrastructurally prove to be whorls of intermediate filaments. They appear either as pale circular regions outlined by a more eosinophilic rim of cytoplasm or as densely eosinophilic inclusions. However, similar cells have been documented in a wide variety of sarcomas and indeed in carcinomas and melanoma. Its distinction from epithelioid sarcoma may at times be difficult, if not impossible. In addition to the rhabdoid cells, the tumor shows a sheetlike growth pattern of rounded cells that may initially be confused with an embryonal RMS because of the presence of eccentric eosinophilic cytoplasm. Most tumors contain no evidence of tumor cell spindling. Therefore, the question arises of whether all rhabdoid tumors are really other neoplasms with a dominance of these cells or whether at least some tumors remain a separate entity. For now, the following path is recommended: if only rare to scattered "rhabdoid" cells are seen in a tumor, the clinician should search for a more specific finding, such as striations; if a tumor is completely populated by these cells, then the term *rhabdoid sarcoma* or *extrarenal rhabdoid tumor* may be applied, with reservations about its exact origin being noted. Extrarenal rhabdoid tumor is the counterpart of the tumor described in the kidneys of young children that is called

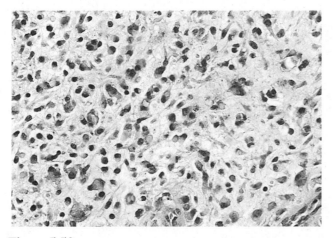

Figure 5.53. Rhabdoid tumor. Intracytoplasmic pale inclusions (intermediate filament whorls ultrastructurally) are seen in this case. These may be encountered in a wide variety of tumors, but they must predominate in any "rhabdoid" sarcoma.

inclusion body sarcoma. Like the renal tumor, the extrarenal rhabdoid tumor is highly aggressive and lethal, occurring in a wide variety of locations in patients mostly younger than 20 years (Table 5.23).

Immunohistochemically, rhabdoid tumors resemble epithelioid sarcoma (positive for vimentin, CK, and EMA), although they do not display either the combined epithelioid-spindly pattern or the cohesive nature of the latter. Desmin and other muscle markers are not expressed, but CD99 and synaptophysin have been found focally in some cases. These neoplasms typically exhibit monosomy 22 or the partial deletion of 22q11.2 where the INI1/SMARCB1 gene resides (575).

EPITHELIOID SARCOMA

Often, the clinical appearance alone allows epithelioid sarcoma to be recognized (576–581). Several cases have a subcutaneous or deep dermal location, and after a time, these cases appear as prominent nodules raised above the skin surface with central ulceration. Multiple nodules of this type may occur in a line from the wrist progressing toward the elbow. Still other cases have a more deep-seated location, and their presentation is less obvious. Microscopically, the tumor is a mixture of spindled and rounded or polygonal eosinophilic cells with small nuclei, only some of which have nucleoli. These spindled and epithelioid cells appear to merge imperceptibly (Fig. 5.54). Significantly, the growth pattern is nodular with central necrosis, and frequently, an inflammatory cell infiltrate in the form of lymphocytes and plasma cells occupies the periphery. For this reason, the differential diagnosis includes inflammatory processes, such as a rheumatoid nodule. However, the cells of epithelioid sarcoma are more densely eosinophilic, the nuclei are more vesicular than those of palisading histiocytes, and the immunohistochemical profile is completely different. Broad areas of fibrosis and hyalinization may occur in some cases, wherein the cells appear to radiate from a central scarred area. Some fibrosing cases are bland, resembling a fibroma. Rhabdoid cells may be apparent, and a pseudoangiomatous pattern may be noted. The so-called *proximal* type contains sheets of cells with prominent nucleoli resembling a poorly differentiated carcinoma (579). Synovial sarcoma, angiosarcoma, melanoma, and other epithelioid lesions (Table 5.15), including poorly differentiated carcinoma, are part of the differential diagnosis. Immunohistochemically, the tumor is clearly epithelium-like, with CK and EMA commonly being present, which has led to the use of the term *carcinoma of soft tissue*. CD34 reactivity, which is found in more than 50% of cases (580), helps distinguish epithelial sarcomas from carcinomas, which are negative for CD34. Oddly, endothelial differentiation has also been reported. A new marker, INI1, can be helpful diagnostically because epithelioid sarcomas lose nuclear INI1 immunoreactivity (581).

The clinical characteristics of this slowly growing tumor are listed in Table 5.23. Local recurrence is highly likely, with the subsequent appearance of metastases in a high percentage of cases. The indolent yet doggedly persistent nature of this tumor should be a factor in determining therapy. Amputation, although not part of the management of most other sarcomas, is definitely a consideration, but attempts to avoid it are increasingly successful. Favorable prognostic factors include the following: small size (<2 cm); female sex; low mitotic rate (1 per 10

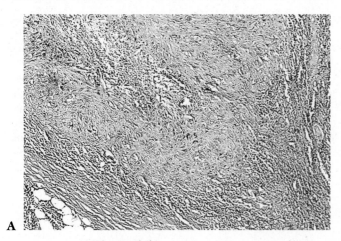
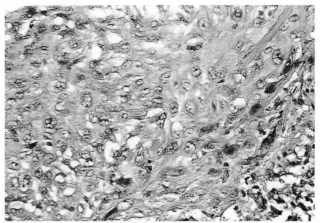

Figure 5.54. Epithelioid sarcoma. At low power, a tumor nodule is enveloped by a fibroinflammatory cuff (**A**). Note the central necrosis. At high power (**B**), round to spindly cells with eosinophilic cytoplasm form a sheet at the periphery of the nodule. Prominent nucleoli can be seen.

hpf); absence of necrosis, vascular invasion, or nodal metastasis; and DNA diploidy.

CLEAR CELL SARCOMA

The most recognizable feature of clear cell carcinoma is its growth pattern (582–585). Although the tumor often grows in sheets, nests of tumor cells are seen divided by fine fibrous tissue septa (Fig. 5.55A); this feature can best be illustrated with a reticulin stain, in which nests rather than cells are outlined (this is one of the few sarcomas with this reticulin pattern). The cells characteristically have a round to oval nucleus with a central prominent nucleolus. The nuclei are markedly uniform, and essentially no pleomorphism is present. Although the name implies a cell with clear cytoplasm, occasional cases have a more eosinophilic cytoplasm resembling that of melanomas. Indeed, one designation for this tumor is *melanoma of soft parts*. Like melanomas, the tumors frequently contain melanin, which can be identified on Fontana or argyrophilic stains. Also similar to melanomas, the lesions are commonly S-100 positive (Fig. 5.55B), they often stain with HMB-45 and other melanoma markers, and they may rarely contain aberrant CK. Glycogen is also present in the tumor, which characteristically develops on a lower extremity of young patients, commonly causing pain. This is a slowly growing lesion of long duration. The prognosis is better if the lesion is small (<5 cm) and superficial and if the DNA content is diploid. Importantly, this is one of the sarcoma types—along with RMS, synovial sarcoma, and UPS/MFH—that commonly metastasize to regional lymph nodes; therefore, the nodes should be critically examined by clinicians. Cytogenetic abnormalities have been described (Table 5.3). Like epithelioid sarcoma, clear cell sarcoma is an aggressive tumor, but it has a variable course (Table 5.23). Molecular analysis (Table 5.4) has revealed an EWS-ATF1 fusion (585).

SOFT TISSUE EWING SARCOMA AND/OR PRIMITIVE NEUROECTODERMAL TUMOR FAMILY

Because both display similar cytogenetic features, proto-oncogene expression, cell culture, and immunohistochemical abnormalities, Ewing sarcoma (EWS) and PNET are currently viewed as the ends of a spectrum of a family of tumors (586–589),

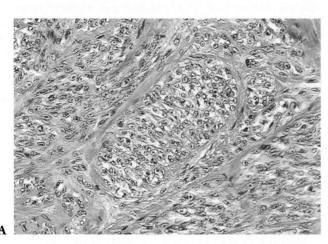
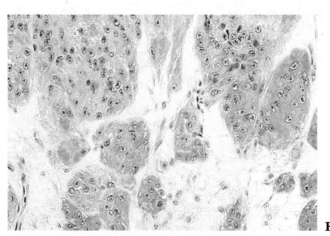

Figure 5.55. Clear cell sarcoma. Unlike other sarcomas, this tumor forms nests that are surrounded by fine pink collagen bands (a reticulin stain would trace the same outline around nests). The cells are uniform, with clear to eosinophilic cytoplasm and central nucleoli (**A**). Most cases are strongly positive for S-100 (**B**).

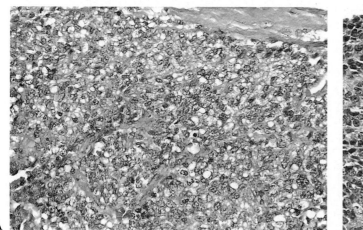
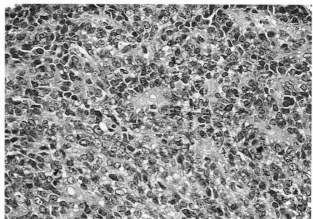

A   B

Figure 5.56. Spectrum of Ewing sarcoma and peripheral primitive neuroectodermal tumor (PNET). At the Ewing sarcoma end of the spectrum **(A)**, sheets of small cells have uniform nuclei and a bubbly appearance caused by abundant glycogen; no spindling or rosettes or any markers of neural differentiation are found. In contrast, many but not all PNETs **(B)** contain rosettes, the morphologic hallmark of this small round cell tumor. The nuclei have dispersed chromatin and a finely granular quality.

with Ewing sarcoma generally lacking the neural features and markers of PNET.

Ewing sarcoma and/or PNET commonly occur in persons younger than 30 years of age. Histologically, Ewing sarcoma of soft tissue resembles the primary bone neoplasm. It is a small round cell sarcoma wherein the nuclei are incredibly uniform, round to oval, vesicular or finely stippled, and approximately the size of those seen in large-cell lymphoma (Fig. 5.56). However, the cells lack the thick nuclear rims and nucleoli that are so prominent in large-cell lymphoma. In addition, unlike in lymphoma, the tumor occurs in broad sheets and lobules that are frequently separated by thick fibrous septa; however, this distinction can be difficult in some cases. Most lesions are PAS positive and diastase sensitive, indicating the presence of glycogen. Apart from lymphoma, the tumor must be distinguished from RMS; EWS lacks any significant eosinophilic cytoplasm and evidence of spindling. The PNET end of the spectrum displays rosettes or neural markers, but it is otherwise similar. In some cases of PNET, the nucleoli are prominent, and the cells lack the vacuolated or clear cytoplasm seen in typical EWS. Although a variety of names have been applied, terms such as *peripheral* cannot be used to encompass all PNETs because several of them occur on the trunk and chest wall (e.g., so-called Askin tumor). Notably, the karyotype of PNET differs from that of neuroblastoma (Table 5.3), and the karyotype of olfactory neuroblastoma is also different (590).

CD99 occurs very frequently in the EWS/PNET family of tumors, and it is an aid in the diagnosis; however, it is not specific, and no diagnosis should rely on this marker alone. Chloroma, another tumor in the differential diagnosis, is frequently CD99 positive; a myeloperoxidase stain aids in this distinction. For PNET, the immunohistochemical demonstration of neural markers (neurofilament, synaptophysin, chromogranin, and S-100) documents neuronal differentiation, in addition to the less sensitive neuron-specific enolase. An antibody to FLI-1 may aid in the diagnosis of small round cell tumors (591). The unusual nature of this tumor family is further highlighted by the identification of a variety of intermediate filaments within the tumors, indicating that they may be the ultimate pluripotential

mesenchymal tumors. Dual-phenotype tumors (ectomesenchymomas) with PNET and RMS have been reported.

The exact fusion type of the molecular diagnostic finding EWS–FLI-1 (Table 5.4) has been shown to be of prognostic value (48), and peripheral blood testing may identify patients at high risk for recurrence (592). The reader is referred to reviews of the molecular biology of EWS and/or PNET (593–595).

In the past, a rapid clinical course was the rule, but data from the Intergroup Rhabdomyosarcoma Study and European studies have indicated a high rate of complete clinical response and an overall 65% disease-free survival rate (Table 5.22) (596). The prognosis of patients with tumors of this family was said to depend on the presence or absence of neural markers; those who had tumors with neural markers (i.e., PNETs) were initially reported to have a more unfavorable course. However, at present, the survival between the two ends of this spectrum does not appear to differ (589).

DESMOPLASTIC SMALL ROUND CELL TUMOR

Desmoplastic small round cell tumor has a unique morphology and immunoprofile (597–600). It affects young adult patients, predominantly men, and the patients typically present with abdominal pain, distention, and occasionally ascites. Large tumor masses involve the mesentery and pelvis with multiple peritoneal implants. Cases have presented in the testis, pleura, and other sites. Cytogenetically, a translocation, t(11;22), that is similar, but not identical, to that of EWS and/or PNET has been described (601), and molecular studies show an EWS-WT1 gene fusion (599,602).

On section, the desmoplastic small round cell tumor is gray-white with myxoid areas and necrotic foci. Histologically, the low-power appearance has a characteristic pattern in which nests of tumor are surrounded and dominated by a desmoplastic stroma (Fig. 5.57), similar to that seen in metastatic carcinoid tumor. Within variably sized nests, the small tumor cells have a scanty cytoplasm, indistinct cell borders, and a round to slightly spindled shape. The nuclei are small, oval, and uniform with

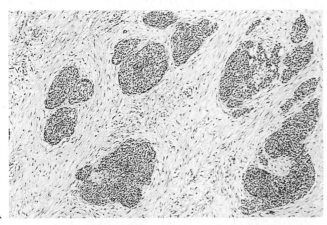
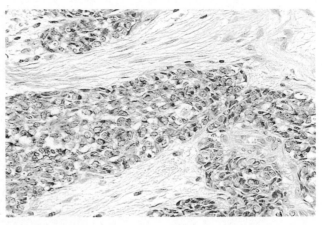

Figure 5.57. Desmoplastic small round cell tumor. Islands of small tumor cells are trapped within a desmoplastic stroma (**A**). Perinuclear, dotlike desmin immunoreactivity (**B**) is typical of this neoplasm, which is also cytokeratin positive.

hyperchromatic nuclei and inconspicuous nucleoli; pleomorphism is not generally seen. Numerous mitoses and occasional rhabdoid-type cells are present. Some nests contain central necrosis and peripheral palisading; gland formation may rarely be identified. The impression is that of a small round cell tumor of childhood with epithelial or neuroendocrine features.

Immunohistochemically, the unique pattern is a combination of epithelial, neural, and muscle markers. CK, EMA, neuron-specific enolase, desmin, and vimentin are identified in most cases (598). An antibody to WT1 is reactive and is useful in the diagnosis (603). Interestingly, the desmin positivity is often perinuclear and dotlike. The combination of CK and desmin immunoreactivity has allowed the diagnosis to be made cytologically (604). Because fetal mesothelium is positive for both CK and desmin, the current theory is that desmoplastic small round cell tumor may be a ''mesothelioblastoma.'' Ultrastructurally, little differentiation is visible, with scanty organelles, including ribosomes, mitochondria, and intracytoplasmic glycogen. Intermediate filaments are prominent, and they sometimes form perinuclear clusters. Rarely, dense-core, neurosecretory-type granules have been seen.

The natural history of the tumor is that of an extremely aggressive lesion that is only partially responsive to chemotherapy. Most patients die of disease 6 months to 4 years after diagnosis.

PERIVASCULAR EPITHELIOID CELL TUMORS (PECOMAS)

Studies have now linked a group of tumors to an origin from the perivascular epithelioid cell, including angiomyolipoma; clear cell ''sugar'' tumor of the lung; clear cell myomelanocytic tumor of the falciform ligament (605); lymphangioleiomyomatosis (see ''Lymphangiomyoma, or Lymphangiomyomatosis''); and unusual clear cell ''PEComas'' of the uterus, pancreas, thigh, heart, and other sites (606). Several of these tumors are commonly associated with tuberous sclerosis. As a group, they are positive for melanoma markers (HMB-45, melan-A, tyrosinase, and microphthalmia transcription factor) and muscle markers (SMA, MSA, and calponin), and almost

70% are negative for S-100. They may mimic clear cell sarcoma and cutaneous melanoma.

POSTRADIATION SOFT TISSUE SARCOMAS

Virtually any histologic type can occur in the postradiation therapy setting (107,354,607). The most common histology reported in the soft tissue is UPS/MFH, but leiomyosarcoma, liposarcoma, MPNST, synovial sarcoma, angiosarcoma, extraskeletal osteosarcoma, and others have all been observed. One of the biggest misconceptions is that the time interval needs to be 10 years or more after radiation; in fact, these postradiation sarcomas can occur as early as 2 years after radiation.

REFERENCES

1. Jemal A, Murray T, Siegel R, et al. Cancer statistics, 2007. *CA Cancer J Clin* 2007;57:43–66.
2. Factor S, Biempica L, Ratner I, et al. Carcinoma of the breast with multinucleated reactive stromal giant cells. *Virchows Arch A Pathol Anat Histopathol* 1977;374:1–12.
3. Rosai J. Carcinoma of pancreas simulating giant cell tumor of bone. Electron-microscopic evidence of its acinar cell origin. *Cancer* 1968;22:333–344.
4. Zukerberg LR, Armin AR, Pisharodi L, Young RH. Transitional cell carcinoma of the urinary bladder with osteoclast-type giant cells: a report of two cases and review of the literature. *Histopathology* 1990;17:407–411.
5. Alguacil Garcia A, Alonso A, Pettigrew NM. Sarcomatoid carcinoma (so-called pseudosarcoma) of the larynx simulating malignant giant cell tumor of soft parts. A case report. *Am J Clin Pathol* 1984;82:340–343.
6. Perez-Ordonez B, Erlandson RA, Rosai J. Follicular dendritic cell tumor—report of 13 additional cases of a distinctive entity. *Am J Surg Pathol* 1996;20:944–955.
7. Chan JK, Fletcher CD, Nayler SJ, Cooper K. Follicular dendritic cell sarcoma—clinicopathologic analysis of 17 cases suggesting a malignant potential higher than currently recognized. *Cancer* 1997;79:294–313.
8. Monda L, Warnke R, Rosai J. A primary lymph node malignancy with features suggestive of dendritic reticulum cell differentiation. A report of 4 cases. *Am J Pathol* 1986;122: 562–572.
9. Chan JK, Buchanan R, Fletcher CD. Sarcomatoid variant of anaplastic large cell Ki-1 lymphoma. *Am J Surg Pathol* 1990;14:983–988.

SPINDLE CELL CARCINOMA

10. Ellis GL, Langloss JM, Heffner DK, Hyams VJ. Spindle cell carcinoma of the aerodigestive tract. An immunohistochemical analysis of 21 cases. *Am J Surg Pathol* 1987;11:335–342.
11. Nakhleh RE, Zarbo RJ, Ewing S, et al. Myogenic differentiation in spindle cell (sarcomatoid) carcinomas of the upper aerodigestive tract. *Appl Immunohistochem* 1993;1:58–68.
12. Zarbo RJ, Crissman JD, Venkat H, Weiss MA. Spindle cell carcinoma of the upper aerodi-

gestive tract mucosa. An immunohistologic and ultrastructural study of 18 biphasic tumors and comparison with seven monophasic spindle cell tumors. *Am J Surg Pathol* 1986;10: 741–753.

13. Smith KJ, Skelton HG, Morgan AM, et al. Spindle cell neoplasms coexpressing cytokeratin and vimentin (metaplastic squamous cell carcinoma). *J Cutan Pathol* 1992;19:286–293.

14. Cheney RT, Kim J, Brooks JS. Cytokeratin profile of spindle cell squamous carcinoma. *Mod Pathol* 1997;10:42A.

15. Adem C, Reynolds C, Adlakha H, et al. Wide spectrum screening keratin as a marker of metaplastic spindle cell carcinoma of the breast: an immunohistochemical study of 24 patients. *Histopathology* 2002;40:556–562.

16. Bhutta S, Mirra JM, Cochran AJ. Myxoid malignant melanoma: a previously undescribed histologic pattern noted in metastatic lesions and a report of four cases. *Am J Surg Pathol* 1986;10:203–211.

17. Dabbs D, Bolen J. Superficial spreading malignant melanoma with neurosarcomatous metastasis. *Am J Clin Pathol* 1984;82:109–114.

18. Weidner N, Flanders DJ, Jochimsen PR, Stamler FW. Neurosarcomatous malignant melanoma arising in a neuroid giant congenital melanocytic nevus. *Arch Dermatol* 1985;121: 1302–1306.

19. Carlson JA, Dickersin GR, Sober AJ, Barnhill RL. Desmoplastic neurotropic melanoma: a clinicopathologic analysis of 28 cases. *Cancer* 1995;75:478–494.

20. Jain S, Allen PW. Desmoplastic malignant melanoma and its variants. A study of 45 cases. *Am J Surg Pathol* 1989;13:358–373.

21. Blessing K, Sanders DS, Grant JJ. Comparison of immunohistochemical staining of the novel antibody melan-A with S100 protein and HMB-45 in malignant melanoma and melanoma variants. *Histopathology* 1998;32:139–146.

22. Koch MB, Shih IP, Weiss SW, Folpe AL. Microphthalmia transcription factor and melanoma cell adhesion molecule expression distinguish desmoplastic/spindle cell melanoma from morphologic mimics. *Am J Surg Pathol* 2001;25:58–64.

23. Busam KJ, Iversen K, Coplan KC, Jungbluth AA. Analysis of microphthalmia transcription factor expression in normal tissues and tumors, and comparison of its expression with S-100 protein, gp100, and tyrosinase in desmoplastic malignant melanoma. *Am J Surg Pathol* 2001;25:197–204.

CLASSIFICATION AND ETIOLOGY

24. Huvos A. The spontaneous transformation of benign into malignant soft tissue tumors. *Am J Surg Pathol* 1985;9:7–14.

25. Carstens PH, Schrodt GR. Malignant transformation of a benign encapsulated neurilemoma. *Am J Clin Pathol* 1969;51:144–149.

26. Eckardt J, Ivins J, Perry H, Unni K. Osteosarcoma arising in heterotopic ossification of dermatomyositis: case report and review of the literature. *Cancer* 1981;48:1256–1261.

27. Lee JM, Baumgartner FJ, Shellans S, et al. Degeneration and sarcomatous transformation of a retroperitoneal leiomyoma. *Eur J Surg* 1996;162:337–340.

28. Rossi S, Fletcher CD. Angiosarcoma arising in hemangioma/vascular malformation—report of four cases and review of the literature. *Am J Surg Pathol* 2002;26:1319–1329.

29. Varley JM, Evans DG, Birch JM. Li-Fraumeni syndrome—a molecular and clinical review. *Br J Cancer* 1997;76:1–14.

30. Weichselbaum RR, Beckett M, Diamond A. Some retinoblastomas, osteosarcomas, and soft tissue sarcomas may share a common etiology. *Proc Natl Acad Sci U S A* 1988;85: 2106–2109.

31. Johnson ES. Association between soft tissue sarcomas, malignant lymphomas, and phenoxy herbicides/chlorophenols: evidence from occupational cohort studies. *Fundam Appl Toxicol* 1990;14:219–234.

32. Eriksson M, Hardell L, Adami HO. Exposure to dioxins as a risk factor for soft tissue sarcoma: a population-based case-control study. *J Natl Cancer Inst* 1990;82:486–490.

33. Wingren G, Fredrikson M, Brage HN, et al. Soft tissue sarcoma and occupational exposures. *Cancer* 1990;66:806–811.

34. Hajdu SI. The health effects of agrichemicals: herbicides and soft tissue sarcomas. *Hum Pathol* 1993;24:1383–1384.

35. Grimalt JO, Sunyer J, Moreno V, et al. Risk excess of soft-tissue sarcoma and thyroid cancer in a community exposed to airborne organochlorinated compound mixtures with a high hexachlorobenzene content. *Int J Cancer* 1994;56:200–203.

36. Kogevinas M, Kauppinen T, Winkelmann R, et al. Soft tissue sarcoma and non-Hodgkin's lymphoma in workers exposed to phenoxy herbicides, chlorophenols, and dioxins: two nested case-control studies. *Epidemiology* 1995;6:396–402.

37. Tavani A, Pregnolato A, Negri E, et al. Diet and risk of lymphoid neoplasms and soft tissue sarcomas. *Nutr Cancer* 1997;27:256–260.

38. Gemmill LT. The issue of injection site sarcomas. *J Am Vet Med Assoc* 1997;210:889–890.

39. Hendrick MJ, Brooks JJ. Postvaccinal sarcomas in the cat: histology and immunohistochemistry. *Vet Pathol* 1994;31:126–129.

40. McClain KL, Leach CT, Jenson HB, et al. Association of Epstein-Barr virus with leiomyosarcomas in young people with AIDS. *N Engl J Med* 1995;332:12–18.

41. Rogatsch H, Bonatti H, Menet A, et al. Epstein-Barr virus–associated multicentric leiomyosarcoma in an adult patient after heart transplantation—case report and review of the literature. *Am J Surg Pathol* 2000;24:614–621.

BIOPSY PROCEDURES

42. Kilpatrick SE, Cappellari JO, Bos GD, et al. Is fine-needle aspiration biopsy a practical alternative to open biopsy for the primary diagnosis of sarcoma? Experience with 140 patients. *Am J Clin Pathol* 2001;115:59–68.

43. Kissin M, Fisher C, Carter R, et al. Value of tru-cut biopsy in the diagnosis of soft tissue tumors. *Br J Surg* 1986;73:742–744.

CYTOGENETICS AND MOLECULAR BIOLOGY

44. Sreekantaiah C. The cytogenetic and molecular characterization of benign and malignant soft tissue tumors. *Cytogenet Cell Genet* 1998;82:13–29.

45. Fletcher CD, Dal Cin P, De Wever I, et al. Correlation between clinicopathological features and karyotype in spindle cell sarcomas—a report of 130 cases from the CHAMP Study Group. *Am J Pathol* 1999;154:1841–1847.

46. Mertens F, Strömberg U, Mandahl N, et al. Prognostically important chromosomal aberrations in soft tissue sarcomas: a report of the Chromosomes and Morphology (CHAMP) Study Group. *Cancer Res* 2002;62:3980–3984.

47. Barr FG, Chatten J, D'Cruz CM, et al. Molecular assays for chromosomal translocations in the diagnosis of pediatric soft tissue sarcomas. *JAMA* 1995;273:553–557.

48. De Alava E, Kawai A, Healey JH, et al. EWS-FL11 fusion transcript structure is an independent determinant of prognosis in Ewing's sarcoma. *J Clin Oncol* 1998;16:1248–1255.

49. Kelly KM, Womer RB, Sorensen PH, et al. Common and variant gene fusions predict distinct clinical phenotypes in rhabdomyosarcoma. *J Clin Oncol* 1997;15:1831–1836.

50. Ladanyi M, Antonescu CR, Leung DH, et al. Impact of SYT-SSX fusion type on the clinical behavior of synovial sarcoma: a multi-institutional retrospective study of 243 patients. *Cancer Res* 2002;62:135–140.

IMMUNOHISTOCHEMISTRY

51. Brown D, Theaker J, Banks P, et al. Cytokeratin expression in smooth muscle and smooth muscle tumours. *Histopathology* 1987;11:477–486.

52. Franke WW, Jahn L, Knapp AC. Cytokeratins and desmosomal proteins in certain epithelioid and non-epithelial cells. In Osborn M, Weber K, eds. *Cytoskeletal Proteins in Tumor Diagnosis.* Boston, MA: Current Communications in Molecular Biology, Cold Spring Harbor Laboratory, 1989:151–172.

53. Von Koskull H, Virtanen I. Induction of cytokeratin expression in human mesenchymal cells. *J Cell Physiol* 1987;133:321–329.

54. Miettinen M, Rapola J. Immunohistochemical spectrum of rhabdomyosarcoma and rhabdomyosarcoma-like tumors. Expression of cytokeratin and the 68-kD neurofilament protein. *Am J Surg Pathol* 1989;13:120–132.

55. Battifora H. Assessment of antigen damage in immunohistochemistry. The vimentin internal control. *Am J Clin Pathol* 1991;96:669–671.

56. Miettinen M, Foidart JM, Ekblom P. Immunohistochemical demonstration of laminin, the major glycoprotein of basement membranes, as an aid in the diagnosis of soft tissue tumors. *Am J Clin Pathol* 1983;79:306–311.

57. Soini Y, Autio-Harmainen H. Tumor cells of malignant fibrous histiocytomas express mRNA for laminin. *Am J Pathol* 1991;139:1061–1068.

CD34

58. Ramani P, Bradley NJ, Fletcher CD. QBEND/10, a new monoclonal antibody to endothelium: assessment of its diagnostic utility in paraffin sections. *Histopathology* 1990;17: 237–242.

59. Aiba S, Tabata N, Ishii H, et al. Dermatofibrosarcoma protuberans is a unique fibrohistiocytic tumour expressing CD34. *Br J Dermatol* 1992;127:79–84.

60. Sirgi KE, Wick MR, Swanson PE. B72.3 and CD34 immunoreactivity in malignant epithelioid soft tissue tumors: adjuncts in the recognition of endothelial neoplasms. *Am J Surg Pathol* 1993;17:179–185.

61. Van de Rijn M, Rouse RV. CD34: a review. *Appl Immunohistochem* 1994;2:71–80.

62. Cohen PR, Rapin RP, Farhood AI. Dermatofibroma and dermatofibrosarcoma protuberans: differential expression of CD34 and factor XIIIa [review]. *Am J Dermatopathol* 1994; 16:573–574.

63. Miettinen M, Sarlomo-Rikala M, Kovatich AJ. Cell-type- and tumour-type-related patterns of bcl-2 reactivity in mesenchymal cells and soft tissue tumours. *Virchows Arch Int J Pathol* 1998;433:255–260.

CD31

64. Newman PJ, Berndt MC, Gorski J, et al. PECAM-1 (CD31) cloning and relation to adhesion molecules of the immunoglobulin gene superfamily. *Science* 1990;247:1219–1222.

65. Miettinen M, Lindenmayer AE, Chaubal A. Endothelial cell markers CD31, CD34, and BNH9 antibody to H- and Y-antigens—evaluation of their specificity and sensitivity in the diagnosis of vascular tumors and comparison with von Willebrand factor. *Mod Pathol* 1994; 7:82–90.

66. Uccini S, Ruco LP, Monardo F, et al. Co-expression of endothelial cell and macrophage antigens in Kaposi's sarcoma cells. *J Pathol* 1994;173:23–31.

67. De Young BR, Frierson HF Jr, Ly MN, et al. CD31 immunoreactivity in carcinomas and mesotheliomas. *Am J Clin Pathol* 1998;110:374–377.

68. Tang DG, Chen YQ, Newman PJ, et al. Identification of PECAM-1 in solid tumor cells and its potential involvement in tumor cell adhesion to endothelium. *J Biol Chem* 1993; 268:22883–22894.

FACTOR VIII–RELATED ANTIGEN

69. Schneiderman H, Gruhn J. Metachronous axillary and splenic lymphangiomatosis: demonstration of immunoreactive factor VIII–related antigen. *Am J Clin Pathol* 1983;79: 625–627.

70. Auerbach H, Brooks JJ. Kaposi's sarcoma: observations and a hypothesis. *Lab Invest* 1985; 52:4A.

71. Wick MR, Manivel JC. Epithelioid sarcoma and epithelioid hemangioendothelioma: an immunocytochemical and lectin-histochemical comparison. *Virchows Arch A Pathol Anat Histopathol* 1987;410:309–316.

CD68

72. Weiss LM, Arber DA, Chang KL. CD68: a review. *Appl Immunohistochem* 1994;2:2–8.

73. McHugh M, Miettinen M. KP1 (CD68): its limited specificity for histiocytic tumors. *Appl Immunohistochem* 1994;2:186–190.

74. Smith ME, Costa MJ, Weiss SW. Evaluation of CD68 and other histiocytic antigens in angiomatoid malignant fibrous histiocytoma. *Am J Surg Pathol* 1991;15:757–763.

75. Dei Tos AP, Doglioni C, Laurino L, Fletcher CD. KP1 (CD68) expression in benign neural tumours. Further evidence of its low specificity as a histiocytic/myeloid marker. *Histopathology* 1993;23:185–187.

76. Gloghini A, Rizzo A, Zanette I, et al. KP1/CD68 expression in malignant neoplasms including lymphomas, sarcomas, and carcinomas. *Am J Clin Pathol* 1995;103:425–431.

77. Sueki H, Whitaker D, Buchsbaum M, Murphy GF. Novel interactions between dermal dendrocytes and mast cells in human skin. Implications for hemostasis and matrix repair. *Lab Invest* 1993;69:160–172.

FACTOR XIIIa

78. Zelger B, Sidoroff A, Stanzl U, et al. Deep penetrating dermatofibroma versus dermatofibrosarcoma protuberans. A clinicopathologic comparison. *Am J Surg Pathol* 1994;18: 677–686.

79. Misery L, Boucheron S, Claudy AL. Factor XIIIa expression in juvenile xanthogranuloma. *Acta Derm Venereol* 1994;74:43–44.

80. Kanitakis J, Roca-Miralles M. Factor-XIIIa–expressing dermal dendrocytes in Kaposi's sarcoma. A comparison between classical and immunosuppression-associated types. *Virchows Arch A Pathol Anat Histopathol* 1992;420:227–231.

81. Cerio R, Spaull J, Oliver GF, Jones WE. A study of factor XIIIa and MAC 387 immunolabeling in normal and pathological skin. *Am J Dermatopathol* 1990;12:221–233.

MUSCLE MARKERS

82. Dickman PS, Triche TJ. Extraosseous Ewing's sarcoma versus primitive rhabdomyosarcoma: diagnostic criteria and clinical correlation. *Hum Pathol* 1986;17:881–893.

83. Eusebi V, Rilke F, Ceccarelli C, et al. Fetal heavy chain skeletal myosin. An oncofetal antigen expressed by rhabdomyosarcoma. *Am J Surg Pathol* 1986;10:680–686.

84. Hashimoto H, Daimaru Y, Tsuneyoshi M, Enjoji M. Leiomyosarcoma of the external soft tissues. A clinicopathologic, immunohistochemical, and electron microscopic study. *Cancer* 1986;57:2077–2088.

85. Gabbiani G, Kapanci Y, Barazzone P, Franke W. Immunochemical identification of intermediate-sized filaments in human neoplastic cells. A diagnostic aide for the surgical pathologist. *Am J Pathol* 1981;104:206–216.

86. Miettinen M, Lehto VP, Badley RA, Virtanen I. Expression of intermediate filaments in soft-tissue sarcomas. *Int J Cancer* 1982;30:541–546.

87. Rangdaeng S, Truong LD. Comparative immunohistochemical staining for desmin and muscle-specific actin: a study of 576 cases. *Am J Clin Pathol* 1991;96:32–45.

88. Truong LD, Rangdaeng S, Cagle P, et al. The diagnostic utility of desmin: a study of 584 cases and review of the literature. *Am J Clin Pathol* 1990;93:305–314.

89. Lawson C, Fisher C, Gatter K. An immunohistochemical study of differentiation in malignant fibrous histiocytoma. *Histopathology* 1987;11:375–384.

90. Brooks JJ. Immunohistochemistry of soft tissue tumors. Myoglobin as a tumor marker for rhabdomyosarcoma. *Cancer* 1982;50:1757–1763.

91. Eusebi V, Ceccarelli C, Gorza L, et al. Immunocytochemistry of rhabdomyosarcoma. The use of four different markers. *Am J Surg Pathol* 1986;10:293–299.

92. Roholl PJ, Elbers HR, Prinsen I, et al. Distribution of actin isoforms in sarcomas: an immunohistochemical study. *Hum Pathol* 1990;21:1269–1274.

93. Schurch W, Skalli O, Seemayer TA, Gabbiani G. Intermediate filament proteins and actin isoforms as markers for soft tissue tumor differentiation and origin. I. Smooth muscle tumors. *Am J Pathol* 1987;128:91–103.

94. Montgomery EA, Meis JM. Nodular fasciitis: its morphologic spectrum and immunohistochemical profile. *Am J Surg Pathol* 1991;15:942–948.

95. Tomasek J, Rayan GM. Correlation of alpha-smooth muscle actin expression and contraction in Dupuytren's disease fibroblasts. *J Hand Surg [Am]* 1995;20:450–455.

96. Estes JM, Vande Berg JS, Adzick NS, et al. Phenotypic and functional features of myofibroblasts in sheep fetal wounds. *Differentiation* 1994;56:173–182.

97. Calonje E, Wadden C, Wilson-Jones E, Fletcher CD. Spindle cell non-pleomorphic atypical fibroxanthoma: analysis of a series and delineation of a distinctive variant. *Histopathology* 1993;22:247–254.

98. Calonje E, Mentzel T, Fletcher CD. Cellular benign fibrous histiocytoma. Clinicopathologic analysis of 74 cases of a distinctive variant of cutaneous fibrous histiocytoma with frequent recurrence. *Am J Surg Pathol* 1994;18:668–676.

99. Schofield JB, Krausz T, Stamp GW, et al. Ossifying fibromyoid tumour of soft parts: immunohistochemical and ultrastructural analysis. *Histopathology* 1993;22:101–112.

100. Franquemont DW, Frierson HF Jr, Mills SE. An immunohistochemical study of normal endometrial stroma and endometrial stromal neoplasms: evidence for smooth muscle differentiation. *Am J Surg Pathol* 1991;15:861–870.

101. Wesche WA, Fletcher CD, Dias P, et al. Immunohistochemistry of MyoD1 in adult pleomorphic soft tissue sarcomas. *Am J Surg Pathol* 1995;19:261–269.

102. Kapadia SB, Meis JM, Frisman DM, et al. Adult rhabdomyoma of the head and neck: a clinicopathologic and immunophenotypic study. *Hum Pathol* 1993;24:608–617.

103. Tallini G, Parham DM, Dias P, et al. Myogenic regulatory protein expression in adult soft tissue sarcomas: a sensitive and specific marker of skeletal muscle differentiation. *Am J Pathol* 1994;144:693–701.

104. Kilpatrick SE, Hitchcock MG, Kraus MD, et al. Mixed tumors and myoepitheliomas of soft tissue—a clinicopathologic study of 19 cases with a unifying concept. *Am J Surg Pathol* 1997;21:13–22.

105. Kung IT, Thallas V, Spencer EJ, Wilson SM. Expression of muscle actins in diffuse mesotheliomas. *Hum Pathol* 1995;26:565–570.

106. Banerjee SS, Bishop PW, Nicholson CM, Eyden BP. Malignant melanoma showing smooth muscle differentiation. *J Clin Pathol* 1996;49:950–951.

107. Parham DM, Fisher C. Angiosarcomas of the breast developing post radiotherapy. *Histopathology* 1997;31:189–195.

108. Cessna MH, Zhou H, Perkins SL, et al. Are myogenin and MyoD1 expression specific for rhabdomyosarcoma? A study of 150 cases, with emphasis on spindle cell mimics. *Am J Surg Pathol* 2001;25:1150–1157.

109. Rosai J, Dias P, Parham DM, et al. MyoD1 protein expression in alveolar soft part sarcoma as confirmatory evidence of its skeletal muscle nature. *Am J Surg Pathol* 1991;15:974–981.

110. Wang NP, Bacchi CE, Jiang JJ, et al. Does alveolar soft-part sarcoma exhibit skeletal muscle differentiation? An immunocytochemical and biochemical study of myogenic regulatory protein expression. *Mod Pathol* 1996;9:496–506.

111. Dias P, Chen B, Dilday B, et al. Strong immunostaining for myogenin in rhabdomyosarcoma is significantly associated with tumors of the alveolar subclass. *Am J Pathol* 2000;156: 399–408.

112. Yamamura H, Yoshikawa H, Tatsuta M, et al. Expression of the smooth muscle calponin gene in human osteosarcoma and its possible association with prognosis. *Int J Cancer* 1998; 79:245–250.

113. Nagao T, Sugano I, Ishida Y, et al. Salivary gland malignant myoepithelioma—a clinicopathologic and immunohistochemical study of ten cases. *Cancer* 1998;83:1292–1299.

114. Sakamoto A, Oda Y, Yamamoto H, et al. Calponin and h-caldesmon expression in atypical fibroxanthoma and superficial leiomyosarcoma. *Virchows Arch Int J Pathol* 2002;440: 404–409.

NEURAL MARKERS

115. Trojanowski J, Lee V, Schlaepfer W. An immunohistochemical study of human central and peripheral nervous tumors using monoclonal antibodies against neurofilaments and glial filaments. *Hum Pathol* 1984;15:248–257.

116. Sasaki A, Ogawa A, Nakazato Y, Ishida Y. Distribution of neurofilament protein and neuron-specific enolase in peripheral neuronal tumors. *Virchows Arch A Pathol Anat Histopathol* 1985;407:33–34.

117. Mukai M, Torikata C, Iri H, et al. Expression of neurofilament triplet proteins in human neural tumors. An immunohistochemical study of paraganglioma, ganglioneuroma, ganglioneuroblastoma, and neuroblastoma. *Am J Pathol* 1986;122:28–35.

118. Dranoff G, Bigner D. A word of caution in the use of neuron-specific enolase expression in tumor diagnosis. *Arch Pathol Lab Med* 1984;108:535.

119. Hachitanda Y, Tsuneyoshi M, Enjoji M. Expression of pan-neuroendocrine proteins in 53 neuroblastic tumors: an immunohistochemical study with neuron-specific enolase, chromogranin, and synaptophysin. *Arch Pathol Lab Med* 1989;113:381–384.

120. Gould V, Lee I, Wiedenmann B, et al. Synaptophysin: a novel marker for neurons, certain neuroendocrine cells, and their neoplasms. *Hum Pathol* 1986;17:979–983.

121. Nakajima T, Watanabe S, Sato Y, et al. An immunoperoxidase study of S100 protein distribution in normal and neoplastic tissues. *Am J Surg Pathol* 1982;6:715–727.

122. Weiss SW, Langloss JM, Enzinger FM. Value of S-100 protein in the diagnosis of soft tissue tumors with particular reference to benign and malignant Schwann cell tumors. *Lab Invest* 1983;49:299–308.

123. Daimaru Y, Hashimoto H, Enjoji M. Malignant peripheral nerve-sheath tumors (malignant schwannomas). An immunohistochemical study of 29 cases. *Am J Surg Pathol* 1985;9: 434–444.

124. Theaker JM, Fletcher CD. Epithelial membrane antigen expression by the perineurial cell: further studies of peripheral nerve lesions. *Histopathology* 1989;14:581–592.

125. Hashimoto H, Daimaru Y, Enjoji M. S-100 protein distribution in liposarcoma. An immunoperoxidase study with special reference to the distinction of liposarcoma from myxoid malignant fibrous histiocytoma. *Virchows Arch A Pathol Anat Histopathol* 1984;405:1–10.

126. Kilpatrick SE, Ward WG, Mozes M, et al. Atypical and malignant variants of ossifying fibromyxoid tumor—clinicopathologic analysis of six cases. *Am J Surg Pathol* 1995;19: 1039–1046.

127. Guillou L, Wadden C, Kraus MD, et al. S100 protein reactivity in synovial sarcomas—a potentially frequent diagnostic pitfall: immunohistochemical analysis of 100 cases. *Appl Immunohistochem* 1996;4:167–175.

128. Swanson PE, Manivel JC, Wick MR. Immunoreactivity for Leu-7 in neurofibrosarcoma and other spindle cell sarcomas of soft tissue. *Am J Pathol* 1987;126:546–560.

129. Wick MR, Swanson PE, Scheithauer BW, Manivel JC. Malignant peripheral nerve sheath tumor. An immunohistochemical study of 62 cases. *Am J Clin Pathol* 1987;87:425–433.

130. Shimada S, Tsuzuki T, Kuroda M, et al. Nestin expression as a new marker in malignant peripheral nerve sheath tumors. *Pathol Int* 2007;57:60–67.

131. Stevenson AJ, Chatten J, Bertoni F, et al. CD99 (p30/32 MIC2) neuroectodermal/Ewing's sarcoma antigen as an immunohistochemical marker: review of more than 600 tumors and the literature experience. *Appl Immunohistochem* 1994;2:231–240.

132. Zamecnik M, Michal M. Nuchal-type fibroma is positive for CD34 and CD99. *Am J Surg Pathol* 2001;25:970.

EPITHELIAL MARKERS

133. Miettinen M, Limon J, Niezabitowski A, Lasota J. Patterns of keratin polypeptides in 110 biphasic, monophasic, and poorly differentiated synovial sarcomas. *Virchows Arch Int J Pathol* 2000;437:275–283.

134. Fisher C. Synovial sarcoma: ultrastructural and immunohistochemical features of epithelial differentiation in monophasic and biphasic tumors. *Hum Pathol* 1986;17:996–1008.

135. Chase DR, Enzinger FM. Epithelioid sarcoma. Diagnosis, prognostic indicators, and treatment. *Am J Surg Pathol* 1985;9:241–263.

136. Gown AM, Boyd HC, Chang Y, et al. Smooth muscle cells can express cytokeratins of "simple" epithelium: immunocytochemical and biochemical studies in vitro and in vivo. *Am J Pathol* 1988;132:223–232.

137. Litzky LA, Brooks JJ. Aberrant expression of cytokeratin in malignant fibrous histiocytoma and spindle cell tumors. *Mod Pathol* 1992;5:30–34.

138. Gray MH, Rosenberg AE, Dickersin GR, Bhan AK. Cytokeratin expression in epithelioid vascular neoplasms. *Hum Pathol* 1990;21:212–217.

139. Palman C, Brooks JJ, LiVolsi VA. Aberrant expression of cytokeratin in vascular tissues and tumors. *Mod Pathol* 1990;3:77A.

140. Swanson PE, Scheithauer BW, Manivel JC, Wick MR. Epithelial membrane antigen reactivity in mesenchymal neoplasms: an immunohistochemical study of 306 soft tissue sarcomas. *Surg Pathol* 1992;2:313–322.

141. Sirvent N, Coindre JM, Maire G, et al. Detection of MDM2-CDK4 amplification by fluorescence in situ hybridization in 200 paraffin-embedded tumor samples: utility in diagnosing adipocytic lesions and comparison with immunohistochemistry and real-time PCR. *Am J Surg Pathol* 2007;31:1476–1479.

142. Coosemans A, Nik SA, Caluwaerts S, et al. Upregulation of Wilms' tumour gene 1 (WT1) in uterine sarcomas. *Eur J Cancer.* 2007;43:1630–1637.

PROGNOSTIC MARKERS

143. Golouh R, Bracko M, Novak J. Predictive value of proliferation-related markers, p53, and DNA ploidy for survival in patients with soft tissue spindle cell sarcomas. *Mod Pathol* 1996;9:919–924.

144. Würl P, Meye A, Lautenschläger C, et al. Clinical relevance of pRb and p53 co-overexpression in soft tissue sarcomas. *Cancer Lett* 1999;139:159–165.

145. Huuhtanen RL, Blomqvist CP, Wiklund TA, et al. Comparison of the Ki-67 score and S-phase fraction as prognostic variables in soft tissue sarcoma. *Br J Cancer* 1999;79:945–951.

146. Würl P, Lautenschläger C, Meye A, et al. A multifactorial prognostic model for adult soft tissue sarcoma considering clinical, histopathological and molecular data. *Anticancer Res* 2000;20:2065–2072.

147. Würl P, Taubert H, Meye A, et al. Expression of vascular endothelial growth factor and its receptor flk-1 in soft tissue sarcomas: correlation to cathepsin expression and prognosis. *Acta Histochem Cytochem* 1998;31:55–63.

148. Maula S, Huuhtanen RL, Blomqvist CP, et al. The adhesion molecule CD44v6 is associated with a high risk for local recurrence in adult soft tissue sarcomas. *Br J Cancer* 2001;84:244–252.

149. Royds JA, Robinson MH, Stephenson T, et al. The association between *nm23* gene expression and survival in patients with sarcomas. *Br J Cancer* 1997;75:1195–1200.

ELECTRON MICROSCOPY

150. Harris M. Differential diagnosis of spindle cell tumors by electron microscopy—personal experience and a review. *Histopathology* 1981;5:81–105.

151. Nakanishi I, Katsuda S, Ooi A, et al. Diagnostic aspect of spindle cell sarcomas by electron microscopy. *Acta Pathol Jpn* 1983;33:425–437.

GRADE AND STAGE

152. Russell WO, Cohen J, Enzinger F, et al. A clinical and pathological staging system for soft tissue sarcomas. *Cancer* 1977;40:1562–1570.

153. Costa J, Wesley RA, Glatstein E, Rosenberg SA. The grading of soft tissue sarcomas. Results of a clinicohistopathologic correlation in a series of 163 cases. *Cancer* 1984;53:530–541.

154. Trojani M, Contesso G, Coindre J, et al. Soft-tissue sarcomas of adults: study of pathological prognostic variables and definition of a histopathological grading system. *Int J Cancer* 1984;33:37–42.

155. Bodaert A, DeMascarel I, DeMascarel A, Goussot J. Reproducibility of a histopathologic grading system for adult soft tissue sarcoma. *Cancer* 1986;58:306–309.

156. Myhre-Jensen O, Kaae S, Madsen E, Sneppen O. Histopathological grading in soft-tissue tumours: relation to survival in 261 surgically treated patients. *Acta Pathol Microbiol Immunol Scand A* 1983;91:145–150.

157. Suit H, Mankin H, Schiller A, et al. Staging systems for sarcoma of soft tissue and sarcoma of bone. *Cancer Treat Symp* 1985;3:29–36.

158. Coindre JM, Terrier P, Bui NB, et al. Prognostic factors in adult patients with locally controlled soft tissue sarcoma: a study of 546 patients from the French Federation of Cancer Centers Sarcoma Group. *J Clin Oncol* 1996;14:869–877.

159. Guillou L, Coindre JM, Bonichon F, et al. Comparative study of the National Cancer Institute and French Federation of Cancer Centers Sarcoma Group grading systems in a population of 410 adult patients with soft tissue sarcoma. *J Clin Oncol* 1997;15:350–362.

160. Enneking WF, Spanier SS, Goodman MA. A system for the surgical staging of musculoskeletal sarcoma. *Clin Orthop* 1980;1:106–120.

161. Lewis JJ, Leung D, Casper ES, et al. Multifactorial analysis of long-term follow-up (more than 5 years) of primary extremity sarcoma. *Arch Surg* 1999;134:190–194.

162. Coindre JM, Terrier P, Guillou L, et al. Predictive value of grade for metastasis development in the main histologic types of adult soft tissue sarcomas—a study of 1,240 patients from the French Federation of Cancer Centers Sarcoma Group. *Cancer* 2001;91:1914–1926.

DNA PLOIDY AND PROGNOSIS

163. Huuhtanen RL, Blomqvist CP, Wiklund TA, et al. S-phase fraction of 155 soft tissue sarcomas—correlation with clinical outcome. *Cancer* 1996;77:1815–1822.

164. Gustafson P, Fernö M, Åkerman M, et al. Flow cytometric S-phase fraction in soft-tissue sarcoma: prognostic importance analysed in 160 patients. *Br J Cancer* 1997;75:94–100.

165. Kinzbrunner B, Ritter S, Domingo J, Rosenthal C. Remission of rapidly growing desmoid tumors after tamoxifen therapy. *Cancer* 1983;52:2201–2204.

166. Brentani M, Pacheco M, Oshima C, et al. Steroid receptors in breast angiosarcoma. *Cancer* 1983;51:2105–2111.

167. Weiss SW, Langloss JM, Shmookler BM, et al. Estrogen receptor protein in bone and soft tissue tumors. *Lab Invest* 1986;54:689–694.

168. Walter S, Govoni D, Bottazzi B, Mantovani A. The role of macrophages in the regulation of primary tumor growth. *Pathobiology* 1991;59:239–242.

169. Restifo NP, Esquivel F, Asher AL, et al. Defective presentation of endogenous antigens by a murine sarcoma: implications for the failure of an anti-tumor immune response. *J Immunol* 1991;147:1453–1459.

170. Brooks JJ, Hergan R, Ryan L. Malignant fibrous histiocytoma (MFH): prognostic value of HLA-Dr paraffin immunoreactivity. *Mod Pathol* 1992;5:4A.

171. Têtu B, Lacasse B, Bouchard HL, et al. Prognostic influence of HSP-27 expression in malignant fibrous histiocytoma: a clinicopathological and immunohistochemical study. *Cancer Res* 1992;52:2325–2328.

SARCOMA SYNDROMES

172. Riccardi VM. Neurofibromatosis: past, present, and future. *N Engl J Med* 1991;324:1283–1285.

173. Carney JA, Hruska LS, Beauchamp GD, Gordon H. Dominant inheritance of the complex of myxomas, spotty pigmentation, and endocrine overactivity. *Mayo Clin Proc* 1986;61:165–172.

174. Carney JA. The complex of myxomas, spotty pigmentation, and endocrine overactivity. *Arch Intern Med* 1987;147:418–419.

175. Koopman RJ, Happle R. Autosomal dominant transmission of the NAME syndrome (nevi, atrial myxoma, mucinosis of the skin and endocrine overactivity). *Hum Genet* 1991;86:300–304.

176. Choi YS, Lundy RO. Rhabdomyosarcoma and hypercalcemia. *Arch Intern Med* 1989;149:1189.

177. Cole FH Jr, Ellis RA, Goodman RC, et al. Benign fibrous pleural tumor with elevation of insulin-like growth factor and hypoglycemia. *South Med J* 1990;83:690–694.

178. Carney JA. The triad of gastric epithelioid leiomyosarcoma, pulmonary chondroma, and functioning extra-adrenal paraganglioma: a five-year review. *Medicine (Baltimore)* 1983;62:159–169.

179. Gengenbach S, Ridker PM. Left ventricular hemangioma in Kasabach-Merritt syndrome. *Am Heart J* 1991;121:202–203.

180. Arcomano MA, Shulkin BL, Petry NA, Wahl RL. Metastatic angiosarcoma with thrombocytopenia and intratumoral indium-111–platelet deposition. *J Nucl Med* 1991;32:2278–2280.

181. Varga J, Griffin R, Newman JH, Jimenez SA. Eosinophilic fasciitis is clinically distinguishable from the eosinophilia-myalgia syndrome and is not associated with L-tryptophan use. *J Rheumatol* 1991;18:259–263.

182. Winkelmann RK, Connolly SM, Quimby SR, et al. Histopathologic features of the L-tryptophan–related eosinophilia-myalgia (fasciitis) syndrome. *Mayo Clin Proc* 1991;66:457–463.

183. Garber JE, Goldstein AM, Kantor AF, et al. Follow-up study of twenty-four families with Li-Fraumeni syndrome. *Cancer Res* 1991;51:6094–6097.

184. Lynch H, Katz D, Bogard P, Lynch J. The sarcoma, breast cancer, lung cancer, and adrenocortical carcinoma syndrome revisited: childhood cancer. *Am J Dis Child* 1985;139:134–136.

185. Burke AP, Sobin LH, Shekitka KM, et al. Intra-abdominal fibromatosis: a pathologic analysis of 130 tumors with comparison of clinical subgroups. *Am J Surg Pathol* 1990;14:335–341.

186. Shepherd CW, Gomez MR, Lie JT, Crowson CS. Causes of death in patients with tuberous sclerosis. *Mayo Clin Proc* 1991;66:792–796.

187. Moretti-Ferreira D, Koiffmann CP, Souza DH, et al. Macroencephaly, multiple lipomas, and hemangiomata (Bannayan-Zonana syndrome): genetic heterogeneity or autosomal dominant locus with at least two different allelic forms? *Am J Med Genet* 1989;34:548–551.

FASCIITIS, REACTIVE

188. Konwaler B, Keasbey L, Kaplan L. Subcutaneous pseudosarcomatous fibromatosis (fasciitis). *Am J Clin Pathol* 1955;25:241–252.

189. Allen PW. Nodular fasciitis. *Pathology* 1972;4:9–26.
190. Wirman J. Nodular fasciitis. A lesion of myofibroblasts. *Cancer* 1976;38:2378–2389.
191. Meister P, Buckmann FW, Konrad E. Extent and level of fascial involvement in 100 cases with nodular fasciitis. *Virchows Arch A Pathol Anat Histopathol* 1978;380:177–185.
192. Bernstein KE, Lattes R. Nodular (pseudosarcomatous) fasciitis, a nonrecurrent lesion: clinicopathologic study of 134 cases. *Cancer* 1982;49:1668–1678.
193. Shimizu S, Hashimoto H, Enjoji M. Nodular fasciitis: an analysis of 250 patients. *Pathology* 1984;16:161–166.
194. El-Jabbour JN, Wilson GD, Bennett MH, et al. Flow cytometric study of nodular fasciitis, proliferative fasciitis, and proliferative myositis. *Hum Pathol* 1991;22:1146–1149.
195. Chung EB, Enzinger FM. Proliferative fasciitis. *Cancer* 1975;36:1450–1458.
196. Enzinger FM, Dulcey F. Proliferative myositis. Report of thirty-three cases. *Cancer* 1967;20:2213–2223.
197. Brooks JJ. Proliferative periburitis: a pseudosarcoma with angiomyxoid features occurring near joints and ligaments. (In preparation)
198. Proppe KH, Scully RE, Rosai J. Postoperative spindle cell nodules of genitourinary tract resembling sarcomas. A report of eight cases. *Am J Surg Pathol* 1984;8:101–108.
199. Ro JY, Ayala AG, Ordonez NG, et al. Pseudosarcomatous fibromyxoid tumor of the urinary bladder. *Am J Clin Pathol* 1986;86:583–590.
200. Sahin AA, Ro JY, El-Naggar AK, et al. Pseudosarcomatous fibromyxoid tumor of the prostate: a case report with immunohistochemical, electron microscopic, and DNA flow cytometric analysis. *Am J Clin Pathol* 1991;96:253–258.

SPINDLE AND PLEOMORPHIC LIPOMA

201. Enzinger FM, Harvey DA. Spindle cell lipoma. *Cancer* 1975;36:1852–1859.
202. Fletcher CD, Martin Bates E. Spindle cell lipoma: a clinicopathological study with some original observations. *Histopathology* 1987;11:803–817.
203. Shmookler BM, Enzinger FM. Pleomorphic lipoma: a benign tumor simulating liposarcoma. A clinicopathologic analysis of 48 cases. *Cancer* 1981;47:126–133.
204. Azzopardi JG, Iocco J, Salm R. Pleomorphic lipoma: a tumour simulating liposarcoma. *Histopathology* 1983;7:511–523.
205. Fletcher CD, Akerman M, Dal Cin P, et al. Correlation between clinicopathological features and karyotype in lipomatous tumors—a report of 178 cases from the Chromosomes and Morphology (CHAMP) Collaborative Study Group. *Am J Pathol* 1996;148:623–630.
206. Vellios F, Baez J, Schumacker H. Lipoblastomatosis: a tumor of fetal fat different from hibernoma. *Am J Pathol* 1958;34:1149–1158.

LEIOMYOMA AND RHABDOMYOMA

207. Hunt SJ, Santa Cruz DJ, Barr RJ. Cellular angiolipoma. *Am J Surg Pathol* 1990;14:75–81.
208. Dehner LP, Enzinger FM, Font RL. Fetal rhabdomyoma. An analysis of nine cases. *Cancer* 1972;30:160–166.
209. Gold J, Bossen E. Benign vaginal rhabdomyoma: a light and electron microscopic study. *Cancer* 1976;32:2283–2294.
210. Kodet R, Fajstavr J, Kabelka Z, et al. Is fetal cellular rhabdomyoma an entity or a differentiated rhabdomyosarcoma? A study of patients with rhabdomyoma of the tongue and sarcoma of the tongue enrolled in the intergroup rhabdomyosarcoma studies I, II, and III. *Cancer* 1991;67:2907–2913.

PAPILLARY ENDOTHELIAL HYPERPLASIA

211. Eusebi V, Fanti P, Fedeli F, Mancini A. Masson's intravascular vegetant hemangioendothelioma. *Tumori* 1980;66:489–498.
212. Salyer W, Salyer D. Intravascular angiomatosis: development and distinction from angiosarcoma. *Cancer* 1975;36:995–1001.
213. Amerigo J, Berry C. Intravascular papillary endothelial hyperplasia in the skin and subcutaneous tissue. *Virchows Arch A Pathol Anat Histopathol* 1980;387:81–90.

MYXOMA

214. Hashimoto H, Tsuneyoshi M, Daimaru Y, et al. Intramuscular myxoma. A clinicopathologic, immunohistochemical, and electron microscopic study. *Cancer* 1986;58:740–747.
215. Miettinen M, Hockerstedt K, Reitamo J, Totterman S. Intramuscular myxoma—a clinicopathological study of twenty-three cases. *Am J Clin Pathol* 1985;84:265–272.
216. Boxer M: Cardiac myxoma: an immunoperoxidase study of histogenesis. *Histopathology* 1984;8:861–872.
217. Dewald GW, Dahl RJ, Spurbeck JL, et al. Chromosomally abnormal clones and nonrandom telomeric translocations in cardiac myxomas. *Mayo Clin Proc* 1987;62:558–567.

MYOSITIS OSSIFICANS, OTHER

218. Sumiyoshi K, Tsuneyoshi M, Enjoji M. Myositis ossificans. A clinicopathologic study of 21 cases. *Acta Pathol Jpn* 1985;35:1109–1122.
219. Thompson J, Van der Walt J. Nodular fibrous proliferation (nodular pseudotumor) of the tunica vaginalis testis. *Histopathology* 1986;10:741–748.
220. Hutter R, Foote F, Francis K, Higinbotham N. Parosteal fasciitis. *Am J Surg* 1962;104:800–807.

221. Kwittken J, Branche M. Fasciitis ossificans. *Am J Clin Pathol* 1969;51:251–255.
222. Patchefsky AS, Enzinger FM. Intravascular fasciitis: a report of 17 cases. *Am J Surg Pathol* 1981;5:29–36.
223. Weiss SW, Enzinger FM, Johnson FB. Silica reaction simulating fibrous histiocytoma. *Cancer* 1978;42:2738–2743.
224. Hizawa K, Inaba H, Nakanishi S, et al. Subcutaneous pseudosarcomatous polyvinylpyrrolidone granuloma. *J Surg Pathol* 1984;8:393–398.
225. Weidner N, Askin F, Berthrong M, et al. Bizarre (pseudomalignant) granulation-tissue reactions following ionizing radiation exposure: a microscopic, immunohistochemical, and flow cytometric study. *Cancer* 1987;59:1509–1514.
226. Umlas J, Federman M, Crawford C, et al. Spindle cell pseudotumor due to *Mycobacterium avium-intracellulare* in patients with acquired immunodeficiency syndrome (AIDS): positive staining of mycobacteria for cytoskeleton filaments. *Am J Surg Pathol* 1991;15:1181–1187.
227. Hurt MA, Santa Cruz DJ. Cutaneous inflammatory pseudotumor: lesions resembling "inflammatory pseudotumors" or "plasma cell granulomas" of extracutaneous sites. *Am J Surg Pathol* 1990;14:764–773.
228. Albores-Saavedra J, Manivel JC, Essenfeld H, et al. Pseudosarcomatous myofibroblastic proliferations in the urinary bladder of children. *Cancer* 1990;66:1234–1241.
229. Allenby PA, Boesel CP, Marsh WL Jr. Diffuse angiomatosis of the extremities presenting as a sarcoma. *Arch Pathol Lab Med* 1991;115:425–426.
230. Suster S, Rosai J. Hamartoma of the scalp with ectopic meningothelial elements: a distinctive benign soft tissue lesion that may simulate angiosarcoma. *Am J Surg Pathol* 1990;14:1–11.

EOSINOPHILIC FASCIITIS, FIBROSIS

231. Michet C, Doyle J, Ginsburg W. Eosinophilic fasciitis. Report of 15 cases. *Mayo Clin Proc* 1981;56:27–34.
232. Jaffe I, Kopelman R, Baird R, et al. Eosinophilic fasciitis associated with the eosinophilia-myalgia syndrome. *Am J Med* 1990;88:542–546.
233. Varga J, Uitto J, Jimenez SA. The cause and pathogenesis of the eosinophilia-myalgia syndrome. *Ann Intern Med* 1992;116:140–147.
234. Herrick MK, Chang Y, Horoupian DS, et al. L-Tryptophan and the eosinophilia-myalgia syndrome: pathologic findings in eight patients. *Hum Pathol* 1991;22:12–21.
235. Savage PD, Wick MR, Thompson RC, Skubitz KM. Tumefactive fibroinflammatory lesion of the extremity: report of a case and review of the literature. *Arch Pathol Lab Med* 1991;115:230–232.
236. Moskovic E, Fisher C, Westbury G, Parsons C. Focal myositis, a benign inflammatory pseudotumour: CT appearances. *Br J Radiol* 1991;64:489–493.
237. Jones J, Ross E, Matz L, et al. Retroperitoneal fibrosis. *Am J Med* 1970;48:203–208.
238. Amis ES Jr. Retroperitoneal fibrosis. *AJR Am J Roentgenol* 1991;157:321–329.

FIBROMAS

239. Donati P, Amantea A, Carducci M, Balus L. Sclerotic (hypocellular) fibromas of the skin. *Br J Dermatol* 1991;124:395–396.
240. Layfield LJ, Fain JS. Pleomorphic fibroma of skin: a case report and immunohistochemical study. *Arch Pathol Lab Med* 1991;115:1046–1049.
241. Chung EB, Enzinger FM. Fibroma of tendon sheath. *Cancer* 1979;44:1945–1954.
242. Lamovec J, Bracko M, Voncina D. Pleomorphic fibroma of tendon sheath. *Am J Surg Pathol* 1991;15:1202–1205.
243. Balachandran K, Allen PW, MacCormac LB. Nuchal fibroma: a clinicopathological study of nine cases. *Am J Surg Pathol* 1995;19:313–317.
244. Coffin CM, Hornick JL, Zhou H, Fletcher CD. Gardner fibroma: a clinicopathologic and immunohistochemical analysis of 45 patients with 57 fibromas. *Am J Surg Pathol* 2007;31:410–416.
245. Evans HL. Desmoplastic fibroblastoma—a report of seven cases. *Am J Surg Pathol* 1995;19:1077–1081.
246. Nielsen GP, O'Connell JX, Dickersin GR, Rosenberg AE. Collagenous fibroma (desmoplastic fibroblastoma): a report of seven cases. *Mod Pathol* 1996;9:781–785.
247. Beham A, Fletcher CD, Kainz J, et al. Nasopharyngeal angiofibroma: an immunohistochemical study of 32 cases. *Virchows Arch A Pathol Anat Histopathol* 1993;423:281–285.
248. Tos AP, Seregard S, Calonje E, et al. Giant cell angiofibroma—a distinctive orbital tumor in adults. *Am J Surg Pathol* 1995;19:1286–1293.
249. Nagamine N, Nohara Y, Ito E. Elastofibroma in Okinawa. A clinicopathologic study of 170 cases. *Cancer* 1982;50:1794–1805.
250. Fukuda Y, Miyake H, Masuda A, Masugi Y. Histogenesis of unique elastophilic fibers of elastofibroma: ultrastructural and immunohistochemical studies. *Hum Pathol* 1987;18:424–429.

FIBROUS PROLIFERATIONS

251. Dehner L, Askin F. Tumors of fibrous tissue origin in childhood: a clinicopathologic study of cutaneous and soft tissue neoplasms in 66 children. *Cancer* 1976;38:888–900.
252. Enzinger F. Fibrous hamartoma of infancy. *Cancer* 1965;18:241–248.
253. Iwasaki H, Kikuchi M, Ohtsuki I, et al. Infantile digital fibromatosis: identification of actin filaments in cytoplasmic inclusions by heavy meromysin binding. *Cancer* 1983;52:1653–1661.
254. Chung EB, Enzinger FM. Infantile myofibromatosis. *Cancer* 1981;48:1807–1818.

255. Remberger K, Krieg T, Kunze D, et al. Fibromatosis hyalinica multiplex (juvenile hyaline fibromatosis): light microscopic, electron microscopic, immunohistochemical and biochemical findings. *Cancer* 1985;56:614–624.
256. Allen PW, Enzinger FM. Juvenile aponeurotic fibroma. *Cancer* 1970;26:857–867.

ANGIOMYOFIBROBLASTOMA, ANGIOMYXOMA

257. Fletcher CD, Tsang WY, Fisher C, et al. Angiomyofibroblastoma of the vulva: a benign neoplasm distinct from aggressive angiomyxoma. *Am J Surg Pathol* 1992;16:373–382.
258. Ockner DM, Sayadi H, Swanson PE, et al. Genital angiomyofibroblastoma—comparison with aggressive angiomyxoma and other myxoid neoplasms of skin and soft tissue. *Am J Clin Pathol* 1997;107:36–44.
259. Laskin WB, Fetsch JF, Mostofi FK. Angiomyofibroblastoma-like tumor of the male genital tract—analysis of 11 cases with comparison to female angiomyofibroblastoma and spindle cell lipoma. *Am J Surg Pathol* 1998;22:6–16.
260. Granter SR, Nucci MR, Fletcher CD. Aggressive angiomyxoma: reappraisal of its relationship to angiomyofibroblastoma in a series of 16 cases. *Histopathology* 1997;30:3–10.
261. Nielsen GP, Young RH, Dickersin GR, Rosenberg AE. Angiomyofibroblastoma of the vulva with sarcomatous transformation ("angiomyofibrosarcoma"). *Am J Surg Pathol* 1997;21:1104–1108.
262. Allen PW, Dymock RB, MacCormac LB. Superficial angiomyxomas with and without epithelial components. Report of 30 tumors in 28 patients. *Am J Surg Pathol* 1988;12:519–530.
263. Steeper TA, Rosai J. Aggressive angiomyxoma of the female pelvis and perineum. Report of nine cases of a distinctive type of gynecologic soft-tissue neoplasm. *Am J Surg Pathol* 1983;7:463–475.
264. Iezzoni JC, Fechner RE, Wong LS, Rosai J. Aggressive angiomyxoma in males—a report of four cases. *Am J Clin Pathol* 1995;104:391–396.

INFLAMMATORY MYOFIBROBLASTIC TUMOR

265. Facchetti F, De Wolf Peeters C, De Weber I, Frizzera G. Inflammatory pseudotumor of lymph nodes: immunohistochemical evidence for its fibrohistiocytic nature. *Am J Pathol* 1990;137:281–289.
266. Coyne JD, Wilson G, Sandhu D, Young RH. Inflammatory pseudotumour of the urinary bladder. *Histopathology* 1991;18:261–264.
267. Tang TT, Segura AD, Oechler HW, et al. Inflammatory myofibrohistiocytic proliferation simulating sarcoma in children. *Cancer* 1990;65:1626–1634.
268. Ramachandra S, Hollowood K, Bisceglia M, Fletcher CD. Inflammatory pseudotumour of soft tissues: a clinicopathological and immunohistochemical analysis of 18 cases. *Histopathology* 1995;27:313–323.
269. Meis JM, Enzinger FM. Inflammatory fibrosarcoma of the mesentery and retroperitoneum: a tumor closely simulating inflammatory pseudotumor. *Am J Surg Pathol* 1991;15:1146–1156.
270. Cook JR, Dehner LP, Collins MH, et al. Anaplastic lymphoma kinase (ALK) expression in the inflammatory myofibroblastic tumor—a comparative immunohistochemical study. *Am J Surg Pathol* 2001;25:1364–1371.

FIBROMATOSIS

271. Allen PW. The fibromatoses: a clinicopathologic classification based on 140 cases. *Am J Surg Pathol* 1977;1:255–270.
272. Reitamo JJ, Hayry P, Nykyri E, Saxen E. The desmoid tumor. I. Incidence, sex-, age- and anatomical distribution in the Finnish population. *Am J Clin Pathol* 1982;77:665–673.
273. Hayry P, Reitamo JJ, Totterman S, et al. The desmoid tumor. II. Analysis of factors possibly contributing to the etiology and growth behavior. *Am J Clin Pathol* 1982;77:674–680.
274. Weiss SW. Proliferative fibroblastic lesions. From hyperplasia to neoplasia. *Am J Surg Pathol* 1986;10:14–25.
275. Carlson JW, Fletcher CD. Immunohistochemistry for beta-catenin in the differential diagnosis of spindle cell lesions: analysis of a series and review of the literature. *Histopathology* 2007;51:509–514.
276. Li MM, Cordon-Cardo C, Gerald WL, Rosai J. Desmoid fibromatosis is a clonal process. *Hum Pathol* 1996;27:939–943.
277. Richards R, Rogers S, Gardner E. Spontaneous mesenteric fibromatosis in Gardner's syndrome. *Cancer* 1981;47:597–601.
278. Fletcher JA, Naeem R, Xiao S, Corson JM. Chromosome aberrations in desmoid tumors: trisomy 8 may be a predictor of recurrence. *Cancer Genet Cytogenet* 1995;79:139–143.
279. Schmidt D, Klinge P, Leuschner I, Harms D. Infantile desmoid-type fibromatosis. Morphological features correlate with biological behaviour. *J Pathol* 1991;164:315–319.

SOLITARY FIBROUS TUMOR

280. Witkin GB, Rosai J. Solitary fibrous tumor of the upper respiratory tract: a report of six cases. *Am J Surg Pathol* 1991;15:842–848.
281. Goodlad JR, Fletcher CD. Solitary fibrous tumour arising at unusual sites: analysis of a series. *Histopathology* 1991;19:515–522.
282. Masson EA, MacFarlane IA, Graham D, Foy P. Spontaneous hypoglycaemia due to a pleural fibroma: role of insulin-like growth factors. *Thorax* 1991;46:930–931.
283. England DM, Hochholzer L, McCarthy MJ. Localized benign and malignant fibrous tumors of the pleura: a clinicopathologic review of 223 cases. *Am J Surg Pathol* 1989;13:640–658.

284. Wargotz ES, Weiss SW, Norris HJ. Myofibroblastoma of the breast. Sixteen cases of a distinctive benign mesenchymal tumor. *Am J Surg Pathol* 1987;11:493–502.
285. Magro G, Bisceglia M, Michal M, Eusebi V. Spindle cell lipoma-like tumor, solitary fibrous tumor and myofibroblastoma of the breast: a clinico-pathological analysis of 13 cases in favor of a unifying histogenetic concept. *Virchows Arch Int J Pathol* 2002;440:249–260.
286. Guillou L, Gebhard S, Coindre JM. Lipomatous hemangiopericytoma: a fat-containing variant of solitary fibrous tumor? Clinicopathologic, immunohistochemical, and ultrastructural analysis of a series in favor of a unifying concept. *Hum Pathol* 2000;31:1108–1115.
287. Fletcher CD, Unni KK, Mertens F. Pathology and genetics of tumours of soft tissue and bone. In Kleihues P, Sobin LH, eds. *World Health Organization Classification of Tumours.* Lyons, France: IARC Press, 2002:86–89.
288. Suster S, Nascimento AG, Miettinen M, et al. Solitary fibrous tumors of soft tissue—a clinicopathologic and immunohistochemical study of 12 cases. *Am J Surg Pathol* 1995;19:1257–1266.
289. Brunnemann RB, Ro JY, Ordonez NG, et al. Extrapleural solitary fibrous tumor: a clinicopathologic study of 24 cases. *Mod Pathol* 1999;12:1034–1042.
290. Hanau CA, Miettinen M. Solitary fibrous tumor: histological and immunohistochemical spectrum of benign and malignant variants presenting at different sites. *Hum Pathol* 1995;26:440–449.
291. Nielsen GP, O'Connell JX, Dickersin GR, Rosenberg AE. Solitary fibrous tumor of soft tissue: a report of 15 cases, including 5 malignant examples with light microscopic, immunohistochemical, and ultrastructural data. *Mod Pathol* 1997;10:1028–1037.

MYOFIBROBLASTOMAS

292. Suster S, Rosai J. Intranodal hemorrhagic spindle cell tumor with "amianthoid" fibers: report of six cases of a distinctive mesenchymal neoplasm of the inguinal region that simulates Kaposi's sarcoma. *Am J Surg Pathol* 1989;13:347–357.
293. Weiss SW, Gnepp DR, Bratthauer GL. Palisaded myofibroblastoma: a benign mesenchymal tumor of lymph node. *Am J Surg Pathol* 1989;13:341–346.
294. Harkin JC, Webb SV. Soft-tissue tumor with abnormal amianthoid collagen fibers. *Arch Pathol Lab Med* 1990;114:1281–1282.
295. Fletcher CD, Stirling RW. Intranodal myofibroblastoma presenting in the submandibular region: evidence of a broader clinical and histologic spectrum. *Histopathology* 1990;16:287–294.
296. Herrera GA, Johnson WW, Lockard VG, Walker BL. Soft tissue myofibroblastomas. *Mod Pathol* 1991;4:571–577.
297. Bégin LR, Frail D, Brzezinski A. Myofibroblastoma of the tunica testis: evolving phase of so-called fibrous pseudotumor? *Hum Pathol* 1990;21:866–868.

OSSIFYING FIBROMYXOID TUMOR

298. Enzinger FM, Weiss SW, Liang CY. Ossifying fibromyxoid tumor of soft parts: a clinicopathological analysis of 59 cases. *Am J Surg Pathol* 1989;13:817–827.

MYOFIBROSARCOMA, FIBROBLASTIC SARCOMA

299. Eyden BP, Christensen L, Tagore V, Harris M. Myofibrosarcoma of subcutaneous soft tissue of the cheek. *J Submicrosc Cytol Pathol* 1992;24:307–313.
300. Montgomery E, Goldblum JR, Fisher C. Myofibrosarcoma—a clinicopathologic study. *Am J Surg Pathol* 2001;25:219–228.
301. Montgomery E, Fisher C. Myofibroblastic differentiation in malignant fibrous histiocytoma (pleomorphic myofibrosarcoma): a clinicopathological study. *Histopathology* 2001;38:499–509.
302. Montgomery EA, Devaney KO, Giordano TJ, Weiss SW. Inflammatory myxohyaline tumor of distal extremities with virocyte or Reed-Sternberg–like cells: a distinctive lesion with features simulating inflammatory conditions, Hodgkin's disease, and various sarcomas. *Mod Pathol* 1998;11:384–391.
303. Meis-Kindblom JM, Kindblom LG. Acral myxoinflammatory fibroblastic sarcoma—a low-grade tumor of the hands and feet. *Am J Surg Pathol* 1998;22:911–924.

MYXOFIBROSARCOMA

304. Merck C, Angervall L, Kindblom LG, Oden A. Myxofibrosarcoma. A malignant soft tissue tumor of fibroblastic-histiocytic origin. A clinicopathologic and prognostic study of 110 cases using multivariate analysis. *Acta Pathol Microbiol Immunol Scand Suppl* 1983;282:1–40.
305. Angervall L, Kindblom LG, Merck C. Myxofibrosarcoma. A study of 30 cases. *Acta Pathol Microbiol Scand [A]* 1977;85A:127–140.
306. Weiss SW, Enzinger FM. Myxoid variant of malignant fibrous histiocytoma. *Cancer* 1977;39:1672–1685.
307. Mentzel T, Calonge E, Wadden C, et al. Myxofibrosarcoma—clinicopathologic analysis of 75 cases with emphasis on the low-grade variant. *Am J Surg Pathol* 1996;20:391–405.
308. Nascimento AF, Bertoni F, Fletcher CD. Epithelioid variant of myxofibrosarcoma: expanding the clinicomorphologic spectrum of myxofibrosarcoma in a series of 17 cases. *Am J Surg Pathol* 2007;31:99–105.

OTHER FIBROSARCOMAS

309. Chung EB, Enzinger FM. Infantile fibrosarcoma. *Cancer* 1976;38:729–739.
310. Soule EH, Pritchard DJ. Fibrosarcoma in infants and children: a review of 110 cases. *Cancer* 1977;40:1711–1721.

311. Evans HL. Low-grade fibromyxoid sarcoma. A report of two metastasizing neoplasms having a deceptively benign appearance. *Am J Clin Pathol* 1987;88:615–619.

312. Goodlad JR, Mentzel T, Fletcher CD. Low-grade fibromyxoid sarcoma: clinicopathological analysis of eleven new cases in support of a distinct entity. *Histopathology* 1995;26:229–237.

313. Dvornik G, Barbareschi M, Gallotta P, Palma PD. Low-grade fibromyxoid sarcoma. *Histopathology* 1997;30:274–276.

314. Lane KL, Shannon RJ, Weiss SW. Hyalinizing spindle cell tumor with giant rosettes—a distinctive tumor closely resembling low-grade fibromyxoid sarcoma. *Am J Surg Pathol* 1997;21:1481–1488.

315. Folpe AL, Lane KL, Paull G, Weiss SW. Low-grade fibromyxoid sarcoma and hyalinizing spindle cell tumor with giant rosettes—a clinicopathologic study of 73 cases supporting their identity and assessing the impact of high-grade areas. *Am J Surg Pathol* 2000;24:1353–1360.

316. Meis-Kindblom JM, Kindblom LG, Enzinger FM. Sclerosing epithelioid fibrosarcoma—a variant of fibrosarcoma simulating carcinoma. *Am J Surg Pathol* 1995;19:979–993.

317. Reid R, Barrett A, Hamblen DL. Sclerosing epithelioid fibrosarcoma. *Histopathology* 1996;28:451–455.

FIBROUS HISTIOCYTOMA

318. Gonzalez B. Benign fibrous histiocytoma of the skin. An immunohistochemical analysis of 30 cases. *Pathol Res Pract* 1985;180:486–489.

319. Franquemont DW, Cooper PH, Shmookler BM, Wick MR. Benign fibrous histiocytoma of the skin with potential for local recurrence: a tumor to be distinguished from dermatofibroma. *Mod Pathol* 1990;3:158–163.

320. Fletcher CD. Benign fibrous histiocytoma of subcutaneous and deep soft tissue: a clinicopathologic analysis of 21 cases. *Am J Surg Pathol* 1990;14:801–809.

321. Beham A, Fletcher CD: Atypical 'pseudosarcomatous' variant of cutaneous benign fibrous histiocytoma: report of eight cases. *Histopathology* 1990;17:167–169.

322. Cerio R, Spaull J, Jones EW. Histiocytoma cutis: a tumour of dermal dendrocytes (dermal dendrocytoma). *Br J Dermatol* 1989;120:197–206.

323. Singh Gomez C, Calonje E, Fletcher CD. Epithelioid benign fibrous histiocytoma of skin: clinico-pathological analysis of 20 cases of a poorly known variant. *Histopathology* 1994;24:123–129.

324. Kaddu S, McMenamin ME, Fletcher CD. Atypical fibrous histiocytoma of the skin—clinicopathologic analysis of 59 cases with evidence of infrequent metastasis. *Am J Surg Pathol* 2002;26:35–46.

PLEXIFORM FIBROHISTIOCYTIC TUMOR

325. Enzinger FM, Zhang RY. Plexiform fibrohistiocytic tumor presenting in children and young adults. An analysis of 65 cases. *Am J Surg Pathol* 1988;12:818–826.

326. Zelger B, Weinlich G, Steiner H, et al. Dermal and subcutaneous variants of plexiform fibrohistiocytic tumor. *Am J Surg Pathol* 1997;21:235–241.

327. Fisher C. Atypical plexiform fibrohistiocytic tumour. *Histopathology* 1997;30:271–273.

328. Salomao DR, Nascimento AG. Plexiform fibrohistiocytic tumor with systemic metastases—a case report. *Am J Surg Pathol* 1997;21:469–476.

DERMATOFIBROSARCOMA PROTUBERANS

329. Fletcher CD, Evans BJ, MacArtney JC, et al. Dermatofibrosarcoma protuberans: a clinicopathological and immunohistochemical study with a review of the literature. *Histopathology* 1985;9:921–938.

330. Frierson HF, Cooper PH. Myxoid variant of dermatofibrosarcoma protuberans. *Am J Surg Pathol* 1983;7:445–450.

331. Ding JA, Hashimoto H, Sugimoto T, et al. Bednar tumor (pigmented dermatofibrosarcoma protuberans). An analysis of six cases. *Acta Pathol Jpn* 1990;40:744–754.

332. Banerjee SS, Harris M, Eyden BP, Hamid BN. Granular cell variant of dermatofibrosarcoma protuberans. *Histopathology* 1990;17:375–378.

333. Brenner W, Schaefler K, Chhabra H, Posteo A. Dermatofibrosarcoma protuberans metastatic to a regional lymph node. *Cancer* 1975;36:1897–1902.

334. O'Connell JX, Trotter MJ. Fibrosarcomatous dermatofibrosarcoma protuberans: a variant. *Mod Pathol* 1996;9:273–278.

335. Goldblum JR, Reith JD, Weiss SW. Sarcomas arising in dermatofibrosarcoma protuberans—a reappraisal of biologic behavior in eighteen cases treated by wide local excision with extended clinical follow-up. *Am J Surg Pathol* 2000;24:1125–1130.

336. Shmookler BM, Enzinger FM, Weiss SW. Giant cell fibroblastoma: a juvenile form of dermatofibrosarcoma protuberans. *Cancer* 1989;64:2154–2161.

337. Goldblum JR. Giant cell fibroblastoma—a report of three cases with histologic and immunohistochemical evidence of a relationship to dermatofibrosarcoma protuberans. *Arch Pathol Lab Med* 1996;120:1052–1055.

338. Alguacil-Garcia A. Giant cell fibroblastoma recurring as dermatofibrosarcoma protuberans. *Am J Surg Pathol* 1991;15:798–801.

339. Beham A, Fletcher CD. Dermatofibrosarcoma protuberans with areas resembling giant cell fibroblastoma: report of two cases. *Histopathology* 1990;17:165–167.

UNDIFFERENTIATED PLEOMORPHIC SARCOMA (MALIGNANT FIBROUS HISTIOCYTOMA)

340. Fletcher CD. Pleomorphic malignant fibrous histiocytoma: fact or fiction? A critical reappraisal based on 159 tumors diagnosed as pleomorphic sarcoma. *Am J Surg Pathol* 1992;16:213–228.

341. Brooks JJ. Fact or fiction: malignant fibrous histiocytoma. *Am J Surg Pathol* 1992;16:1023–1024.

342. Fletcher CD, Unni KK, Mertens F, eds. *Pathology and Genetics of Tumours of Soft Tissue and Bone.* Lyon, France: World Health Organization Classification of Tumours, IARC Press, 2002:110–126.

343. Weiss SW, Enzinger FM. Malignant fibrous histiocytoma: an analysis of 200 cases. *Cancer* 1978;41:2250–2266.

344. Bertoni F, Capanna R, Biagini R, et al. Malignant fibrous histiocytoma of soft tissue. An analysis of 78 cases located and deeply seated in the extremities. *Cancer* 1985;56:356–367.

345. Enjoji M, Hashimoto H, Tsuneyoshi M, Iwasaki H. Malignant fibrous histiocytoma. A clinicopathologic study of 130 cases. *Acta Pathol Jpn* 1980;30:727–741.

346. Reddick R, Michelitch H, Triche T. Malignant soft tissue tumors (malignant fibrous histiocytoma, pleomorphic liposarcoma, and pleomorphic rhabdomyosarcoma): an electron microscopic study. *Hum Pathol* 1979;10:327–343.

347. Soini Y, Miettinen M. Immunohistochemistry of markers of histiomonocytic cells in malignant fibrous histiocytomas. *Pathol Res Pract* 1990;186:759–767.

348. Genberg M, Mark J, Hakelius L, et al. Origin and relationship between different cell types in malignant fibrous histiocytoma. *Am J Pathol* 1989;135:1185–1196.

349. Schmidt H, Körber S, Hinze R, et al. Cytogenetic characterization of ten malignant fibrous histiocytomas. *Cancer Genet Cytogenet* 1998;100:134–142.

350. Schürch W, Bégin LR, Seemayer TA, et al. Pleomorphic soft tissue myogenic sarcomas of adulthood—a reappraisal in the mid-1990s. *Am J Surg Pathol* 1996;20:131–147.

351. Jensen V, Sorensen FB, Bentzen SM, et al. Proliferative activity (MIB-1 index) is an independent prognostic parameter in patients with high-grade soft tissue sarcomas of subtypes other than malignant fibrous histiocytomas: a retrospective immunohistological study including 216 soft tissue sarcomas. *Histopathology* 1998;32:536–546.

ATYPICAL FIBROXANTHOMA

352. Jacobs D, Edwards W, Ye R. Metastatic atypical fibroxanthoma of skin. *Cancer* 1975;35:457–463.

353. Sankar NM, Pang KS, Thiruchelvam T, Meldrum-Hanna WG. Metastasis from atypical fibroxanthoma of skin. *Med J Aust* 1998;168:418–419.

354. Laskin WB, Silverman TA, Enzinger FM. Postradiation soft tissue sarcomas: an analysis of 53 cases. *Cancer* 1988;62:2330–2340.

PLEOMORPHIC HYALINIZING ANGIECTATIC TUMOR

355. Smith ME, Fisher C, Weiss SW. Pleomorphic hyalinizing angiectatic tumor of soft parts—a low-grade neoplasm resembling neurilemoma. *Am J Surg Pathol* 1996;20:21–29.

GIANT CELL TUMORS OF SOFT TISSUE

356. Oliveira AM, Dei Tos AP, Fletcher CD, Nascimento AG. Primary giant cell tumor of soft tissues—a study of 22 cases. *Am J Surg Pathol* 2000;24:248–256.

357. O'Connell JX, Wehrli BM, Nielsen GP, Rosenberg AE. Giant cell tumors of soft tissue—a clinicopathologic study of 18 benign and malignant tumors. *Am J Surg Pathol* 2000;24:386–395.

358. Guccion JG, Enzinger FM. Malignant giant cell tumor of soft parts. An analysis of 32 cases. *Cancer* 1972;29:1518–1529.

359. Salm R, Sissons H. Giant cell tumors of soft tissues. *J Pathol* 1972;107:27–39.

360. Bertoni F, Unni KK, Beabout JW, Sim FH. Malignant giant cell tumor of the tendon sheaths and joints (malignant pigmented villonodular synovitis). *Am J Surg Pathol* 1997;21:153–163.

361. Mentzel T, Calonje E, Fletcher CD. Leiomyosarcoma with prominent osteoclast-like giant cells: analysis of eight cases closely mimicking the so-called giant cell variant of malignant fibrous histiocytoma. *Am J Surg Pathol* 1994;18:258–265.

INFLAMMATORY TUMORS OF SOFT TISSUE

362. Kyriakos M, Kempson RL. Inflammatory fibrous histiocytoma. An aggressive and lethal lesion. *Cancer* 1976;37:1584–1606.

363. Khalidi HS, Singleton TP, Weiss SW. Inflammatory malignant fibrous histiocytoma: distinction from Hodgkin's disease and non-Hodgkin's lymphoma by a panel of leukocyte markers. *Mod Pathol* 1997;10:438–442.

364. Coindre JM, Hostein I, Maire G, et al. Inflammatory malignant fibrous histiocytomas and dedifferentiated liposarcomas: histological review, genomic profile, and MDM2 and CDK4 status favour a single entity. *J Pathol* 2004;203:822–830.

365. Costa MJ, Weiss SW. Angiomatoid malignant fibrous histiocytoma: a follow-up study of 108 cases with evaluation of possible histologic predictors of outcome. *Am J Surg Pathol* 1990;14:1126–1132.

366. Enzinger FM. Angiomatoid malignant fibrous histiocytoma: a distinct fibrohistiocytic tumor of children and young adults simulating a vascular neoplasm. *Cancer* 1979;44:2147–2157.

367. Pettinato G, Manivel JC, DeRosa G, et al. Angiomatoid malignant fibrous histiocytoma: cytologic, immunohistochemical, ultrastructural, and flow cytometric study of 20 cases. *Mod Pathol* 1990;3:479–487.

368. Waters BL, Panagopoulos I, Allen EF. Genetic characterization of angiomatoid fibrous histiocytoma identifies fusion of the FUS and ATF-1 genes induced by a chromosomal translocation involving bands 12q13 and 16p11. *Cancer Genet Cytogenet* 2000;121:109–116.

369. Santa Cruz DJ, Kyriakos M. Aneurysmal ("angiomatoid") fibrous histiocytoma of the skin. *Cancer* 1981;47:2053–2061.

370. Brooks JJ. The significance of double phenotypic patterns and markers in human sarcomas. A new model of mesenchymal differentiation. *Am J Pathol* 1986;125:113–123.

371. Wick MR, Siegal GP, Mills SE, et al. Dedifferentiated chondrosarcoma of bone. An immunohistochemical and lectin-histochemical study. *Virchows Arch A Pathol Anat Histopathol* 1987;411:23–32.

372. Roholl PJ, Rutgers DH, Rademakers LH, et al. Characterization of human soft tissue sarcomas in nude mice. Evidence for histogenic properties of malignant fibrous histiocytomas. *Am J Pathol* 1988;131:559–568.

373. Hashimoto H, Daimaru Y, Tsuneyoshi M, Enjoji M. Soft tissue sarcoma with additional anaplastic components: a clinicopathologic and immunohistochemical study of 27 cases. *Cancer* 1990;66:1578–1589.

374. Roholl PJ, Prinsen I, Rademakers LP, et al. Two cell lines with epithelial cell-like characteristics established from malignant fibrous histiocytomas. *Cancer* 1991;68:1963–1972.

LIPOMA AND VARIANTS

375. Beham A, Fletcher CD. Intramuscular angioma: a clinicopathological analysis of 74 cases. *Histopathology* 1991;18:53–59.

376. Ferry JA, Malt RA, Young RH. Renal angiomyolipoma with sarcomatous transformation and pulmonary metastases. *Am J Surg Pathol* 1991;15:1083–1088.

377. Kindblom LG, Angervall L, Stener B, Wickbom I. Intermuscular and intramuscular lipomas and hibernomas. A clinical, roentgenologic, histologic, and prognostic study of 46 cases. *Cancer* 1974;33:754–762.

378. Furlong MA, Fanburg-Smith JC, Miettinen M. The morphologic spectrum of hibernoma—a clinicopathologic study of 170 cases. *Am J Surg Pathol* 2001;25:809–814.

379. Meis JM, Enzinger FM. Chondroid lipoma: a unique tumor simulating liposarcoma and myxoid chondrosarcoma. *Am J Surg Pathol* 1993;17:1103–1112.

380. Gisselsson D, Domanski HA, Höglund M, et al. Unique cytological features and chromosome aberrations in chondroid lipoma—a case report based on fine-needle aspiration cytology, histopathology, electron microscopy, chromosome banding, and molecular cytogenetics. *Am J Surg Pathol* 1999;23:1300–1304.

LIPOSARCOMA

381. Evans HL, Soule EH, Winkelmann RK. Atypical lipoma, atypical intramuscular lipoma, and well-differentiated retroperitoneal liposarcoma: a reappraisal of 30 cases formerly classified as well-differentiated liposarcoma. *Cancer* 1979;43:574–584.

382. Azumi N, Curtis J, Kempson RL, Hendrickson MR. Atypical and malignant neoplasms showing lipomatous differentiation: a study of 111 cases. *Am J Surg Pathol* 1987;11:161–183.

383. Enterline HT, Culberson J, Rochlin D, Brady L. Liposarcoma—a clinical and pathologic study of 53 cases. *Cancer* 1960;13:932–950.

384. Enzinger F, Winslow D. Liposarcoma: a study of 103 cases. *Virchows Arch A Pathol Anat Histopathol* 1962;335:367–388.

385. Evans HL. Liposarcoma: a study of 55 cases with a reassessment of its classification. *Am J Surg Pathol* 1979;3:507–523.

386. Snover D, Sumner H, Dehner L. Variability of histologic pattern in recurrent soft tissue sarcomas originally diagnosed as liposarcoma. *Cancer* 1982;49:1005–1015.

387. Orson G, Sim F, Reiman H, Taylor W. Liposarcoma of the musculoskeletal system. *Cancer* 1987;60:1362–1370.

388. Brooks JJ, Connor AM. Atypical lipoma of the extremities with dedifferentiation: implications for management. *Surg Pathol* 1990;3:169–178.

389. Rosai J, Akerman M, Cin PD, Weiss SW. Combined morphologic and karyotypic study of 59 atypical lipomatous tumors—evaluation of their relationship and differential diagnosis with other adipose tissue tumors. *Am J Surg Pathol* 1996;20:1182–1189.

390. Henricks WH, Chu YC, Goldblum JR, et al. Dedifferentiated liposarcoma—a clinicopathological analysis of 155 cases with a proposal for an expanded definition of dedifferentiation. *Am J Surg Pathol* 1997;21:271–281.

391. Knight JC, Renwick PJ, Dal Cin P, et al. Translocation t(12;16)(q13;p11) in myxoid liposarcoma and round cell liposarcoma: molecular and cytogenetic analysis. *Cancer Res* 1995;55:24–27.

392. Smith TA, Easley KA, Goldblum JR. Myxoid/round cell liposarcoma of the extremities—a clinicopathologic study of 29 cases with particular attention to extent of round cell liposarcoma. *Am J Surg Pathol* 1996;20:171–180.

393. Kilpatrick SE, Doyon J, Choong PF, et al. The clinicopathologic spectrum of myxoid and round cell liposarcoma—a study of 95 cases. *Cancer* 1996;77:1450–1458.

394. Miettinen M, Enzinger FM. Epithelioid variant of pleomorphic liposarcoma: a study of 12 cases of a distinctive variant of high-grade liposarcoma. *Mod Pathol* 1999;12:722–728.

395. Gebhard S, Coindre JM, Michels JJ, et al. Pleomorphic liposarcoma: clinicopathologic, immunohistochemical, and follow-up analysis of 63 cases—a study from the French Federation of Cancer Centers Sarcoma Group. *Am J Surg Pathol* 2002;26:601–616.

396. Miettinen M, Enzinger FM. Epithelioid variant of pleomorphic liposarcoma: a study of 12 cases of a distinctive variant of high-grade liposarcoma. *Mod Pathol* 1999;12:722–728.

LEIOMYOMA AND LEIOMYOSARCOMA

397. Mentzel T, Wadden C, Fletcher CD. Granular cell change in smooth muscle tumours of skin and soft tissue. *Histopathology* 1994;24:223–231.

398. McWilliam LJ, Pitt M. Intraneural leiomyoma. *Histopathology* 1995;26:195–197.

399. Billings SD, Folpe AL, Weiss SW. Do leiomyomas of deep soft tissue exist? An analysis of highly differentiated smooth muscle tumors of deep soft tissue supporting two distinct subtypes. *Am J Surg Pathol* 2001;25:1134–1142.

400. Paal E, Miettinen M. Retroperitoneal leiomyomas—a clinicopathologic and immunohistochemical study of 56 cases with a comparison to retroperitoneal leiomyosarcomas. *Am J Surg Pathol* 2001;25:1355–1363.

401. Donhuijsen K. Mitosis counts: reproducibility and significance in grading of malignancy. *Hum Pathol* 1986;17:1122–1125.

402. Baak JP. Mitosis counting in tumors. *Hum Pathol* 1990;21:683–685.

403. Farshid G, Pradhan M, Goldblum J, Weiss SW. Leiomyosarcoma of somatic soft tissues—a tumor of vascular origin with multivariate analysis of outcome in 42 cases. *Am J Surg Pathol* 2002;26:14–24.

404. Mingoli A, Feldhaus RJ, Cavallaro A, Stipa S. Leiomyosarcoma of the inferior vena cava: analysis and search of world literature on 141 patients and report of three new cases. *J Vasc Surg* 1991;14:688–699.

405. Shmookler BM, Lauer DH. Retroperitoneal leiomyosarcoma. A clinicopathologic analysis of 36 cases. *Am J Surg Pathol* 1983;7:269–280.

406. Kaddu S, Beham A, Cerroni L, et al. Cutaneous leiomyosarcoma. *Am J Surg Pathol* 1997;21:979–987.

407. Suster S. Epithelioid leiomyosarcoma of the skin and subcutaneous tissue: clinicopathologic, immunohistochemical, and ultrastructural study of five cases. *Am J Surg Pathol* 1994;18:232–240.

408. Piana S, Roncaroli F. Epithelioid leiomyosarcoma of retroperitoneum with granular cell change. *Histopathology* 1994;25:90–93.

409. Rubin BP, Fletcher CD. Myxoid leiomyosarcoma of soft tissue, an underrecognized variant. *Am J Surg Pathol* 2000;24:927–936.

410. Roncaroli F, Eusebi V. Rhabdomyoblastic differentiation in a leiomyosarcoma of the retroperitoneum. *Hum Pathol* 1996;27:310–313.

411. Matthews TJ, Fisher C. Leiomyosarcoma of soft tissue and pulmonary metastasis, both with osteoclast-like giant cells. *J Clin Pathol* 1994;47:370–371.

412. Somerhausen NDA, Fletcher CD. Leiomyosarcoma of soft tissue in children—clinicopathologic analysis of 20 cases. *Am J Surg Pathol* 1999;23:755–763.

413. Oda Y, Miyajima K, Kawaguchi K, et al. Pleomorphic leiomyosarcoma—clinicopathologic and immunohistochemical study with special emphasis on its distinction from ordinary leiomyosarcoma and malignant fibrous histiocytoma. *Am J Surg Pathol* 2001;25:1030–1038.

414. Jenson HB, Leach CT, McClain KL, et al. Benign and malignant smooth muscle tumors containing Epstein-Barr virus in children with AIDS. *Leuk Lymphoma* 1997;27:303–314.

415. Kingma DW, Shad A, Tsokos M, et al. Epstein-Barr virus (EBV)–associated smooth-muscle tumor arising in a post-transplant patient treated successfully for two PT-EBV–associated large cell lymphomas—case report. *Am J Surg Pathol* 1996;20:1511–1519.

416. Hill MA, Araya JC, Eckert MW, et al. Tumor specific Epstein-Barr virus infection is not associated with leiomyosarcoma in human immunodeficiency virus–negative individuals. *Cancer* 1997;80:204–210.

RHABDOMYOSARCOMA

417. Burke AP, Virmani R. Cardiac rhabdomyoma: a clinicopathologic study. *Mod Pathol* 1991;4:70–74.

418. Enzinger FM, Shiraki M. Alveolar rhabdomyosarcoma. An analysis of 110 cases. *Cancer* 1969;24:18–31.

419. Soule EH, Geitz M, Henderson ED. Embryonal rhabdomyosarcoma of the limbs and limb-girdles. A clinicopathologic study of 61 cases. *Cancer* 1969;23:1336–1346.

420. Seidal T, Kindblom LG. The ultrastructure of alveolar and embryonal rhabdomyosarcoma. A correlative light and electron microscopic study of 17 cases. *Acta Pathol Microbiol Immunol Scand [A]* 1984;92:231–248.

421. Miettinen M. Rhabdomyosarcoma in patients older than 40 years of age. *Cancer* 1988;62:2060–2065.

422. Seidal T, Kindblom LG, Angervall L. Rhabdomyosarcoma in middle-aged and elderly individuals. *APMIS* 1989;97:236–248.

423. Ruymann F, Heyn R, Ragab A, et al. Completely resected rhabdomyosarcoma: the effect of unfavorable histology on survival. *Proc Am Soc Clin Oncol Abst C* 1984;334(Abstr):86.

424. Newton WA Jr, Gehan EA, Webber BL, et al. Classification of rhabdomyosarcomas and related sarcomas—pathologic aspects and proposal for a new classification. Intergroup Rhabdomyosarcoma Study. *Cancer* 1995;76:1073–1085.

425. Cavazzana AO, Schmidt D, Ninfo V, et al. Spindle cell rhabdomyosarcoma: a prognostically favorable variant of rhabdomyosarcoma. *Am J Surg Pathol* 1992;16:229–235.

426. Rubin BP, Hasserjian RP, Singer S, et al. Spindle cell rhabdomyosarcoma (so-called) in adults—report of two cases with emphasis on differential diagnosis. *Am J Surg Pathol* 1998;22:459–464.

427. Fitzmaurice RJ, Johnson PR, Liu Yin JA, Freemont AJ. Rhabdomyosarcoma presenting as "acute leukaemia." *Histopathology* 1991;18:173–175.

428. Sorensen PH, Lynch JC, Qualman SJ, et al. PAX3-FKHR and PAX7-FKHR gene fusions are prognostic indicators in alveolar rhabdomyosarcoma: a report from the Children's Oncology Group. *J Clin Oncol* 2002;20:2672–2679.

HEMANGIOMAS

429. Mills SE, Cooper PH, Fechner RE. Lobular capillary hemangioma: the underlying lesion of pyogenic granuloma. A study of 73 cases from the oral and nasal mucous membranes. *Am J Surg Pathol* 1980;4:470–479.

430. Nichols GE, Gaffey MJ, Mills SE, Weiss LM. Lobular capillary hemangioma: an immunohistochemical study including steroid hormone receptor status. *Am J Clin Pathol* 1992;97:770–775.

431. Chan JK, Fletcher CD, Hicklin GA, Rosai J. Glomeruloid hemangioma: a distinctive cutaneous lesion of multicentric Castleman's disease associated with POEMS syndrome. *Am J Surg Pathol* 1990;14:1036–1046.

432. Silverman RA. Hemangiomas and vascular malformations. *Pediatr Clin North Am* 1991;38:811–834.

433. Goldman R, Perzik S. Infantile hemangioma of the parotid gland: a clinicopathological study of 15 cases. *Arch Otolaryngol* 1969;90:605–608.

434. Nagao K, Matsuzaki O, Shigematsu H, et al. Histopathologic studies of benign infantile hemangioendothelioma of the parotid gland. *Cancer* 1980;46:2250–2256.

435. Rosai J, Gold J, Landy R. The histiocytoid hemangiomas: a unifying concept embracing several previously described entities of skin, soft tissue, large vessels, bone, and heart. *Hum Pathol* 1979;10:707–730.

436. Fetsch JF, Weiss SW. Observations concerning the pathogenesis of epithelioid hemangioma (angiolymphoid hyperplasia). *Mod Pathol* 1991;4:449–455.

437. Urabe A, Tsuneyoshi M, Enjoji M. Epithelioid hemangioma versus Kimura's disease. A comparative clinicopathologic study. *Am J Surg Pathol* 1987;11:758–766.

438. Perkins P, Weiss SW. Spindle cell hemangioendothelioma—an analysis of 78 cases with reassessment of its pathogenesis and biologic behavior. *Am J Surg Pathol* 1996;20:1196–1204.

439. Padilla RS, Orkin M, Rosai J. Acquired "tufted" angioma (progressive capillary hemangioma). A distinctive clinicopathologic entity related to lobular capillary hemangioma. *Am J Dermatopathol* 1987;9:292–300.

440. Hunt SJ, Santa Cruz DJ, Barr RJ. Microvenular hemangioma. *J Cutan Pathol* 1991;18:235–240.

441. Calonje E, Fletcher CD. Sinusoidal hemangioma: a distinctive benign vascular neoplasm within the group of cavernous hemangiomas. *Am J Surg Pathol* 1991;15:1130–1135.

442. Guillou L, Calonje E, Speight P, et al. Hobnail hemangioma—a pseudomalignant vascular lesion with a reappraisal of targetoid hemosiderotic hemangioma. *Am J Surg Pathol* 1999;23:97–105.

443. Rao VK, Weiss SW. Angiomatosis of soft tissue: an analysis of the histologic features and clinical outcome in 51 cases. *Am J Surg Pathol* 1992;16:764–771.

444. McMenamin ME, Fletcher CD. Reactive angioendotheliomatosis—a study of 15 cases demonstrating a wide clinicopathologic spectrum. *Am J Surg Pathol* 2002;26:685–697.

445. Koehler JE, Sanchez MA, Garrido CS, et al. Molecular epidemiology of *Bartonella* infections in patients with bacillary angiomatosis-peliosis. *N Engl J Med* 1997;337:1876–1883.

446. Schinella RA, Greco MA. Bacillary angiomatosis presenting as a soft-tissue tumor without skin involvement. *Hum Pathol* 1990;21:567–569.

447. Chan JK, Warnke RA, Dorfman R. Vascular transformation of sinuses in lymph nodes: a study of its morphological spectrum and distinction from Kaposi's sarcoma. *Am J Surg Pathol* 1991;15:732–743.

HEMANGIOENDOTHELIOMAS

448. Zukerberg LR, Nickoloff BJ, Weiss SW. Kaposiform hemangioendothelioma of infancy and childhood: an aggressive neoplasm associated with Kasabach-Merritt syndrome and lymphangiomatosis. *Am J Surg Pathol* 1993;17:321–328.

449. Mentzel T, Mazzoleni G, Dei Tos AP, Fletcher CD. Kaposiform hemangioendothelioma in adults—clinicopathologic and immunohistochemical analysis of three cases. *Am J Clin Pathol* 1997;108:450–455.

450. Calonje E, Fletcher CD, Wilson-Jones E, Rosai J. Retiform hemangioendothelioma: a distinctive form of low-grade angiosarcoma delineated in a series of 15 cases. *Am J Surg Pathol* 1994;18:115–125.

451. Fanburg-Smith JC, Michal M, Partanen TA, et al. Papillary intralymphatic angioendothelioma (PILA)—a report of twelve cases of a distinctive vascular tumor with phenotypic features of lymphatic vessels. *Am J Surg Pathol* 1999;23:1004–1010.

452. Weiss SW, Enzinger FM. Epithelioid hemangioendothelioma: a vascular tumor often mistaken for a carcinoma. *Cancer* 1982;50:970–981.

453. Mentzel T, Beham A, Calonje E, et al. Epithelioid hemangioendothelioma of skin and soft tissues: clinicopathologic and immunohistochemical study of 30 cases. *Am J Surg Pathol* 1997;21:363–374.

454. Nascimento AG, Keeney GL, Sciot R, Fletcher CD. Polymorphous hemangioendothelioma—a report of two cases, one affecting extranodal soft tissues, and review of the literature. *Am J Surg Pathol* 1997;21:1083–1089.

ANGIOSARCOMA

455. Rosai J, Sumner H, Kostianovsky M, Perez-Mesa C. Angiosarcoma of the skin: a clinicopathologic and fine structural study. *Hum Pathol* 1976;7:83–109.

456. Mark RJ, Poen JC, Tran LM, et al. Angiosarcoma: a report of 67 patients and a review of the literature. *Cancer* 1996;77:2400–2406.

457. Meis-Kindblom JM, Kindblom LG. Angiosarcoma of soft tissue—a study of 80 cases. *Am J Surg Pathol* 1998;22:683–697.

458. Martinez-Escribano JA, Gil-Mateo MD, Miquel J, et al. Human herpesvirus 8 is not detectable by polymerase chain reaction in angiosarcoma. *Br J Dermatol* 1998;138:546–547.

459. Maddox JC, Evans HL. Angiosarcoma of skin and soft tissue: a study of forty-four cases. *Cancer* 1981;48:1907–1921.

460. Rosen PP, Kimmel M, Ernsberger D. Mammary angiosarcoma: the prognostic significance of tumor differentiation. *Cancer* 1988;62:2145–2151.

461. Merino M, Berman M, Carter D. Angiosarcoma of the breast. *Am J Surg Pathol* 1983;7:53–60.

462. Moskaluk CA, Merino MJ, Danforth DN, Medeiros LJ. Low-grade angiosarcoma of the skin of the breast: a complication of lumpectomy and radiation therapy for breast carcinoma. *Hum Pathol* 1992;23:710–714.

463. Brenn T, Fletcher CD. Radiation-associated cutaneous atypical vascular lesions and angiosarcoma: clinicopathologic analysis of 42 cases. *Am J Surg Pathol* 2005;29:983–996.

464. Fletcher CD, Beham A, Bekir S, et al. Epithelioid angiosarcoma of deep soft tissue: a distinctive tumor readily mistaken for an epithelial neoplasm. *Am J Surg Pathol* 1991;15:915–924.

465. Banerjee SS, Eyden BP, Wells S, et al. Pseudoangiosarcomatous carcinoma: a clinicopathological study of seven cases. *Histopathology* 1992;21:13–23.

466. Zhang PJ, LiVolsi VA, Brooks JJ. Malignant epithelioid vascular tumors of the pleura: report of a series and literature review. *Hum Pathol* 2000;31:29–34.

KAPOSI SARCOMA

467. Costa J, Rabson AS. Generalised Kaposi's sarcoma is not a neoplasm. *Lancet* 1983;1:58.

468. Brooks JJ. Kaposi's sarcoma: a reversible hyperplasia. *Lancet* 1986;2:1309–1311.

469. Delli-Bovi PD, Donti E, Knowles DM, et al. Presence of chromosomal abnormalities and lack of AIDS retrovirus DNA sequences in AIDS-associated Kaposi's sarcoma. *Cancer Res* 1986;46:6333–6338.

470. Cox FH, Helwig EB. Kaposi's sarcoma. *Cancer* 1959;12:289–298.

471. Real FX, Krown SE. Spontaneous regression of Kaposi's sarcoma in patients with AIDS. *N Engl J Med* 1985;313:1659.

472. Blumenfeld W, Egbert BM, Sagebiel RW. Differential diagnosis of Kaposi's sarcoma. *Arch Pathol Lab Med* 1985;109:123–127.

473. Templeton AC. Kaposi's sarcoma. *Pathol Annu* 1981;16:315–336.

474. Chang Y, Cesarman E, Pessin MS, et al. Identification of herpesvirus-like DNA sequences in AIDS-associated Kaposi's sarcoma. *Science* 1994;266:1865–1869.

475. Chang Y. Kaposi's sarcoma and Kaposi's sarcoma-associated herpesvirus (human herpesvirus 8): where are we now? *J Natl Cancer Inst* 1997;89:1829–1831.

476. Li JJ, Huang YQ, Cockerell CJ, Friedman-Kien AE. Localization of human herpes-like virus type 8 in vascular endothelial cells and perivascular spindle-shaped cells of Kaposi's sarcoma lesions by in situ hybridization. *Am J Pathol* 1996;148:1741–1748.

477. Kikuta H, Itakura O, Ariga T, Kobayashi K. Detection of human herpesvirus 8 DNA sequences in peripheral blood mononuclear cells of children. *J Med Virol* 1997;53:81–84.

GLOMUS TUMOR

478. Tsuneyoshi M, Enjoji M. Glomus tumor: a clinicopathologic and electron microscopic study. *Cancer* 1982;50:1601–1607.

479. Brooks JJ, Miettinen M, Virtanen I. Desmin immunoreactivity in glomus tumors. *Am J Clin Pathol* 1987;87:292.

480. Porter PL, Bigler SA, McNutt M, Gown AM. The immunophenotype of hemangiopericytomas and glomus tumors, with special reference to muscle protein expression: an immunohistochemical study and review of the literature. *Mod Pathol* 1991;4:46–52.

481. Folpe AL, Fanburg-Smith JC, Miettinen M, Weiss SW. Atypical and malignant glomus tumors—analysis of 52 cases, with a proposal for the reclassification of glomus tumors. *Am J Surg Pathol* 2001;25:1–12.

LYMPHANGIOMYOMATOSIS

482. Taylor JR, Ryu J, Colby TV, Raffin TA. Lymphangioleiomyomatosis—clinical course in 32 patients. *N Engl J Med* 1990;323:1254–1260.

483. Smolarek TA, Wessner LL, McCormack FX, et al. Evidence that lymphangiomyomatosis is caused by TSC2 mutations: chromosome 16p13 loss of heterozygosity in angiomyolipomas and lymph nodes from women with lymphangiomyomatosis. *Am J Hum Genet* 1998;62:810–815.

HEMANGIOPERICYTOMA

484. Nappi O, Ritter JH, Pettinato G, Wick MR. Hemangiopericytoma: histopathological pattern or clinicopathologic entity? *Semin Diagn Pathol* 1995;12:221–232.

485. Enzinger FM, Smith BH. Hemangiopericytoma. An analysis of 106 cases. *Hum Pathol* 1976;7:61–82.

486. McMaster MJ, Soule EH, Ivins JC. Hemangiopericytoma. A clinicopathologic study and long-term follow-up of 60 patients. *Cancer* 1975;36:2232–2244.

487. Gerald W, Kostianovsky M, Rosai J. Development of vascular neoplasia in Castleman's disease: report of seven cases. *Am J Surg Pathol* 1990;14:603–614.

488. Nielsen GP, Dickersin GR, Provenzal JM, Rosenberg AE. Lipomatous hemangiopericytoma: a histologic, ultrastructural and immunohistochemical study of a unique variant of hemangiopericytoma. *Am J Surg Pathol* 1995;19:748–756.

489. Granter SR, Badizadegan K, Fletcher CD. Myofibromatosis in adults, glomangiopericytoma, and myopericytoma—a spectrum of tumors showing perivascular myoid differentiation. *Am J Surg Pathol* 1998;22:513–525.

490. McMenamin ME, Fletcher CD. Malignant myopericytoma: expanding the spectrum of tumours with myopericytic differentiation. *Histopathology* 2002;41:450–460.

491. Eichhorn JH, Dickersin GR, Bhan AK, Goodman ML. Sinonasal hemangiopericytoma: a reassessment with electron microscopy, immunohistochemistry, and long-term follow-up. *Am J Surg Pathol* 1990;14:856–866.

GIANT CELL TUMOR OF TENDON SHEATH

492. Ushijima M, Hashimoto H, Tsuneyoshi M, Enjoji M. Giant cell tumor of the tendon sheath (nodular tenosynovitis). A study of 207 cases to compare the large joint group with the common digit group. *Cancer* 1986;57:875–884.
493. Ushijima M, Hashimoto H, Tsuneyoshi M, Enjoji M. Pigmented villonodular synovitis. A clinicopathologic study of 52 cases. *Acta Pathol Jpn* 1986;36:317–326.
494. Folpe AL, Weiss SW, Fletcher CD, Gown AM. Tenosynovial giant cell tumors: evidence for a desmin-positive dendritic cell subpopulation. *Mod Pathol* 1998;11:939–944.
495. West RB, Rubin BP, Miller MA, et al. A landscape effect in tenosynovial giant-cell tumor from activation of CSF1 expression by a translocation in a minority of tumor cells. *Proc Natl Acad Sci USA.* 2006;103:690–695.

SYNOVIAL SARCOMA

496. Machen SK, Easley KA, Goldblum JR. Synovial sarcoma of the extremities—a clinicopathologic study of 34 cases, including semi-quantitative analysis of spindled, epithelial, and poorly differentiated areas. *Am J Surg Pathol* 1999;23:268–275.
497. Bergh P, Meis-Kindblom JM, Gherlinzoni F, et al. Synovial sarcoma—identification of low- and high-risk groups. *Cancer* 1999;85:2596–2607.
498. Singer S, Baldini EH, Demetri GD, et al. Synovial sarcoma: prognostic significance of tumor size, margin of resection, and mitotic activity for survival. *J Clin Oncol* 1996;14: 1201–1208.
499. Cagle LA, Mirra JM, Storm FK, et al. Histologic features relating to prognosis in synovial sarcoma. *Cancer* 1987;59:1810–1814.
500. Evans HL. Synovial sarcoma: a study of 23 biphasic and 17 probable monophasic examples. *Pathol Annu* 1980;15(Pt 2):309–332.
501. Rosen G, Forscher C, Lowenbraun S, et al. Synovial sarcoma: uniform response of metastases to high-dose ifosfamide. *Cancer* 1994;73:2506–2511.
502. Lewis JJ, Antonescu CR, Leung DH, et al. Synovial sarcoma: a multivariate analysis of prognostic factors in 112 patients with primary localized tumors of the extremity. *J Clin Oncol* 2000;18:2087–2094.
503. Urschel JD, Anderson TM, Whooley BP. Finger clubbing and a lung mass—solitary fibrous tumor of the pleura. *Chest* 1999;115:1735–1737.
504. Smith TA, Machen SK, Fisher C, Goldblum JR. Usefulness of cytokeratin subsets for distinguishing monophasic synovial sarcoma from malignant peripheral nerve sheath tumor. *Am J Clin Pathol* 1999;112:641–648.
505. Varela Duran J, Enzinger FM. Calcifying synovial sarcoma. *Cancer* 1982;50:345–352.
506. Folpe AL, Schmidt RA, Chapman D, Gown AM. Poorly differentiated synovial sarcoma—immunohistochemical distinction from primitive neuroectodermal tumors and high-grade malignant peripheral nerve sheath tumors. *Am J Surg Pathol* 1998;22:673–682.
507. Van de Rijn M, Barr FG, Xiong QB, et al. Poorly differentiated synovial sarcoma—an analysis of clinical, pathologic, and molecular genetic features. *Am J Surg Pathol* 1999;23: 106–112.
508. Krane JF, Bertoni F, Fletcher CD. Myxoid synovial sarcoma: an underappreciated morphologic subset. *Mod Pathol* 1999;12:456–462.
509. Weidner N, Goldman R, Johnston J. Epithelioid monophasic synovial sarcoma. *Ultrastruct Pathol* 1993;17:287–294.

SCHWANNOMA, GRANULAR, CELLULAR

510. Ishida T, Kuroda M, Motoi T, et al. Phenotypic diversity of neurofibromatosis 2: association with plexiform schwannoma. *Histopathology* 1998;32:264–270.
511. Evans DG, Mason S, Huson SM, et al. Spinal and cutaneous schwannomatosis is a variant form of type 2 neurofibromatosis: a clinical and molecular study. *J Neurol Neurosurg Psychiatry* 1997;62:361–366.
512. Lowman R, LiVolsi VA. Pigmented (melanotic) schwannomas of the spinal canal. *Cancer* 1980;46:391–397.
513. Fisher C, Chappell ME, Weiss SW. Neuroblastoma-like epithelioid schwannoma. *Histopathology* 1995;26:193–194.
514. Brooks JJ, Draffen RM. Benign glandular schwannoma. *Arch Pathol Lab Med* 1992;116: 192–195.
515. Ferry JA, Dickersin GR. Pseudoglandular schwannoma. *Am J Clin Pathol* 1988;89:546–552.
516. Thornton CM, Handley J, Bingham EA, et al. Psammomatous melanotic schwannoma arising in the dermis in a patient with Carney's complex. *Histopathology* 1992;20:71–73.
517. Hoke HF, Harrelson AB. Granular cell ameloblastoma with metastasis to the cervical vertebrae. Observations on the origin of the granular cells. *Cancer* 1967;20:991–999.
518. McWilliams LJ, Harris M. Granular cell angiosarcoma of the skin: histology, electron microscopy and immunohistochemistry of a newly recognized tumor. *Histopathology* 1985; 9:1205–1216.
519. White W, Shiu MH, Rosenblum MK, et al. Cellular schwannoma: a clinicopathologic study of 57 patients and 58 tumors. *Cancer* 1990;66:1266–1275.
520. Casadei GP, Scheithauer BW, Hirose T, et al. Cellular schwannoma: a clinicopathologic, DNA flow cytometric, and proliferation marker study of 70 patients. *Cancer* 1995;75: 1109–1119.

NEUROFIBROMA

521. Liapis H, Dehner LP, Gutmann DH. Neurofibroma and cellular neurofibroma with atypia: a report of 14 tumors. *Am J Surg Pathol* 1999;23:1156–1157.

522. McCarron KF, Goldblum JR. Plexiform neurofibroma with and without associated malignant peripheral nerve sheath tumor: a clinicopathologic and immunohistochemical analysis of 54 cases. *Mod Pathol* 1998;11:612–617.
523. Watabe K, Kumanishi T, Ikuta F, Olyake Y. Tactile-like corpuscles in neurofibromas: immunohistochemical demonstration of S-100 protein. *Acta Neuropathol (Berl)* 1983;61:173–177.
524. Feany MB, Anthony DC, Fletcher CD. Nerve sheath tumours with hybrid features of neurofibroma and schwannoma: a conceptual challenge. *Histopathology* 1998;32:405–410.
525. Ushigome S, Takakuwa T, Hyuga M, et al. Perineurial cell tumor and the significance of the perineurial cells in neurofibroma. *Acta Pathol Jpn* 1986;36:973–987.
526. Robson AM, Calonje E. Cutaneous perineurioma: a poorly recognized tumour often misdiagnosed as epithelioid histiocytoma. *Histopathology* 2000;37:332–339.
527. Mentzel T, Dei Tos AP, Fletcher CD. Perineurioma (storiform perineurial fibroma): clinicopathological analysis of four cases. *Histopathology* 1994;25:261–267.
528. Friedman JM, Birch PH. Type 1 neurofibromatosis: a descriptive analysis of the disorder in 1,728 patients. *Am J Med Genet* 1997;70:138–143.

MALIGNANT PERIPHERAL NERVE SHEATH TUMOR

529. Ducatman BS, Scheithauer BW, Piepgras DG, et al. Malignant peripheral nerve sheath tumors. A clinicopathologic study of 120 cases. *Cancer* 1986;57:2006–2021.
530. Trojanowski J, Kliman G, Proppe K. Malignant tumors of neurosheath origin. *Cancer* 1980; 46:1202–1212.
531. Hruban RH, Shiu MH, Senie RT, Woodruff JM. Malignant peripheral nerve sheath tumors of the buttock and lower extremity: a study of 43 cases. *Cancer* 1990;66:1253–1265.
532. Laskin WB, Weiss SW, Bratthauer GL. Epithelioid variant of malignant peripheral nerve sheath tumor (malignant epithelioid schwannoma). *Am J Surg Pathol* 1991;15:1136–1145.
533. Hirose T, Scheithauer BW, Sano T. Perineurial malignant peripheral nerve sheath tumor (MPNST)—a clinicopathologic, immunohistochemical, and ultrastructural study of seven cases. *Am J Surg Pathol* 1998;22:1368–1378.
534. Ducatman BS, Scheithauer BW. Malignant peripheral nerve sheath tumors with divergent differentiation. *Cancer* 1984;54:1049–1057.
535. Brooks JS, Freeman M, Enterline HT. Malignant "Triton" tumors. Natural history and immunohistochemistry of nine new cases with literature review. *Cancer* 1985;55: 2543–2549.
536. Brooks JJ. Malignant schwannomas with divergent differentiation including "Triton" tumor. In Williams CJ, Krikorian JG, Green MR, et al., eds. *Textbook of Uncommon Cancer.* Chichester, United Kingdom: John Wiley & Sons, 1988:653–668.
537. Woodruff JM, Christensen WN. Glandular peripheral nerve sheath tumors. *Cancer* 1993; 72:3618–3628.
538. Woodruff JM, Chernik NL, Smith MC, et al. Peripheral nerve tumors with rhabdomyosarcomatous differentiation (malignant "Triton" tumors). *Cancer* 1973;32:426–439.
539. Allegranza A, Ferraresi S, Luccarelli G. Malignant glandular schwannoma: a case with favourable prognosis. *Histopathology* 1988;12:549–552.

CHONDROSARCOMA

540. Mackenzie DH. The unsuspected soft tissue chondrosarcoma. *Histopathology* 1983;7: 759–766.
541. Enzinger FM, Shiraki M. Extraskeletal myxoid chondrosarcoma. An analysis of 34 cases. *Hum Pathol* 1972;3:421–435.
542. Antonescu CR, Argani P, Erlandson RA, et al. Skeletal and extraskeletal myxoid chondrosarcoma—a comparative clinicopathologic, ultrastructural, and molecular study. *Cancer* 1998;83:1504–1521.
543. Meis-Kindblom JM, Bergh P, Gunterberg B, Kindblom LG. Extraskeletal myxoid chondrosarcoma—a reappraisal of its morphologic spectrum and prognostic factors based on 117 cases. *Am J Surg Pathol* 1999;23:636–650.
544. Labelle Y, Bussières J, Courjal F, Goldring MB. The EWS TEC fusion protein encoded by the t(9;22) chromosomal translocation in human chondrosarcomas is a highly potent transcriptional activator. *Oncogene* 1999;18:3303–3308.
545. Nakashima Y, Unni KK, Shives TC, et al. Mesenchymal chondrosarcoma of bone and soft tissue. A review of 111 cases. *Cancer* 1986;57:2444–2453.
546. Swanson PE, Lillemoe TJ, Manivel JC, Wick MR. Mesenchymal chondrosarcoma: an immunohistochemical study. *Arch Pathol Lab Med* 1990;114:943–948.
547. Granter SR, Renshaw AA, Fletcher CD, et al. CD99 reactivity in mesenchymal chondrosarcoma. *Hum Pathol* 1996;27:1273–1276.

MYOEPITHELIOMA

548. Michal M, Miettinen M. Myoepitheliomas of the skin and soft tissues—report of 12 cases. *Virchows Arch Int J Pathol* 1999;434:393–400.
549. Folpe AL, Agoff SN, Willis J, Weiss SW. Parachordoma is immunohistochemically and cytogenetically distinct from axial chordoma and extraskeletal myxoid chondrosarcoma. *Am J Surg Pathol* 1999;23:1059–1067.

OSTEOSARCOMA

550. Bane BL, Evans HL, Ro JY, et al. Extraskeletal osteosarcoma: a clinicopathologic review of 26 cases. *Cancer* 1990;65:2762–2770.

551. Lee JS, Fetsch JF, Wasdhal DA, et al. A review of 40 patients with extraskeletal osteosarcoma. *Cancer* 1995;76:2253–2259.
552. Jensen ML, Schumacher B, Jensen OM, et al. Extraskeletal osteosarcomas—a clinicopathologic study of 25 cases. *Am J Surg Pathol* 1998;22:588–594.
553. Kobos JW, Yu GH, Varadarajan S, Brooks JS. Primary cutaneous osteosarcoma. *Am J Dermatopathol* 1995;17:53–57.
554. Ahmad SA, Patel SR, Ballo MT, et al. Extraosseous osteosarcoma: response to treatment and long-term outcome. *J Clin Oncol* 2002;20:521–527.
555. Dupree W, Enzinger F. Fibro-osseous pseudotumor of the digits. *Cancer* 1986;58:2103–2109.

MESENCHYMOMA

556. Klima M, Smith M, Spjut H, Root E. Malignant mesenchymoma: case report with electron microscopy. *Cancer* 1975;36:1086–1094.
557. Brady MS, Perino G, Tallini G, et al. Malignant mesenchymoma. *Cancer* 1996;77:467–473.
558. Wolthers O, Stellfeld M. Benign mesenchymoma in the trachea of a patient with the nevoid basal cell carcinoma syndrome. *Laryngol Otol* 1987;101:522–526.
559. Mann S, Russell P, Wills EJ, et al. Benign vaginal mesenchymoma showing mature skeletal muscle, smooth muscle, and fatty differentiation: report of a case. *Int J Surg Pathol* 1996;4:49–54.

ALVEOLAR SOFT PART SARCOMA

560. Lieberman PH, Brennan MF, Kimmel M, et al. Alveolar soft-part sarcoma. A clinicopathologic study of half a century. *Cancer* 1989;63:1–13.
561. Auerbach HE, Brooks JJ. Alveolar soft part sarcoma. A clinicopathologic and immunohistochemical study. *Cancer* 1987;60:66–73.
562. Wang NP, Bacchi CE, Jiang JJ, et al. Does alveolar soft part sarcoma exhibit skeletal muscle differentiation? An immunocytochemical and biochemical study of myogenic regulatory protein expression. *Mod Pathol* 1996;9:496–501.
563. Ladanyi M, Lui MY, Antonescu CR, et al. The der(17)t(X;17)(p11;q25) of human alveolar soft part sarcoma fuses the *TFE3* transcription factor gene to *ASPL*, a novel gene at 17q25. *Oncogene* 2001;20:48–57.
564. Argani P, Antonescu CR, Illei PB, et al. Primary renal neoplasms with the *ASPL-TFE3* gene fusion of alveolar soft part sarcoma—a distinctive tumor entity previously included among renal cell carcinomas of children and adolescents. *Am J Pathol* 2001;159:179–192.

MALIGNANT GRANULAR CELL TUMOR

565. Brooks JJ. Malignant granular cell tumors ("myoblastomas"). In Williams CJ, Krikorian JG, Green MR, et al., eds. *Textbook of Uncommon Cancer*. Chichester, United Kingdom: John Wiley & Sons, 1988:669–682.
566. Casorzo L, Fessia L, Sapino A, et al. Extraskeletal Ewing's tumor with translocation t(11;22) in a patient with Down syndrome. *Cancer Genet Cytogenet* 1989;37:79–84.
567. Fanburg-Smith JC, Meis-Kindblom JM, Fante R, Kindblom LG. Malignant granular cell tumor of soft tissue—diagnostic criteria and clinicopathologic correlation. *Am J Surg Pathol* 1998;22:779–794.
568. Troncoso P, Ordonez NG, Raymond AK, Mackay B. Malignant granular cell tumor: immunocytochemical and ultrastructural observations. *Ultrastruct Pathol* 1988;12:137–144.

RHABDOID TUMOR

569. Weeks DA, Beckwith JB, Mierau GW. Rhabdoid tumor: an entity or a phenotype. *Arch Pathol Lab Med* 1989;113:113–114.
570. Tsokos M, Kouraklis G, Chandra RS, et al. Malignant rhabdoid tumor of the kidney and soft tissues: evidence for a diverse morphological and immunocytochemical phenotype. *Arch Pathol Lab Med* 1989;113:115–120.
571. Molenaar WM, DeJong B, Dam-Meiring A, et al. Epithelioid sarcoma or malignant rhabdoid tumor of soft tissue? Epithelioid immunophenotype and rhabdoid karyotype. *Hum Pathol* 1989;20:347–351.
572. Kodet R, Newton WA Jr, Sachs N, et al. Rhabdoid tumors of soft tissues: a clinicopathologic study of 26 cases enrolled on the Intergroup Rhabdomyosarcoma Study. *Hum Pathol* 1991;22:674–684.
573. Parham DM, Weeks DA, Beckwith JB. The clinicopathologic spectrum of putative extrarenal rhabdoid tumors. *Am J Surg Pathol* 1994;18:1010–1029.
574. Wick MR, Ritter JH, Dehner LP. Malignant rhabdoid tumors: a clinicopathologic review and conceptual discussion. *Semin Diagn Pathol* 1995;12:233–248.
575. Biegel JA, Zhou JY, Rorke LB, et al. Germ-line and acquired mutations of *INI1* in atypical teratoid and rhabdoid tumors. *Cancer Res* 1999;59:74–79.

EPITHELIOID SARCOMA

576. Enzinger FM. Epithelioid sarcoma. A sarcoma simulating a granuloma or a carcinoma. *Cancer* 1970;26:1029–1041.
577. Prat J, Woodruff JM, Marcove RC. Epithelioid sarcoma: an analysis of 22 cases indicating the prognostic significance of vascular invasion and regional lymph node metastasis. *Cancer* 1978;41:1472–1487.

578. Chase DR, Enzinger FM. Epithelioid sarcoma. Diagnosis, prognostic indicators, and treatment. *Am J Surg Pathol* 1985;9:241–263.
579. Guillou L, Wadden C, Coindre JM, et al. "Proximal-type" epithelioid sarcoma, a distinctive aggressive neoplasm showing rhabdoid features—clinicopathologic, immunohistochemical, and ultrastructural study of a series. *Am J Surg Pathol* 1997;21:130–146.
580. Miettinen M, Fanburg-Smith JC, Virolainen M, et al. Epithelioid sarcoma: an immunohistochemical analysis of 112 classical and variant cases and a discussion of the differential diagnosis. *Hum Pathol* 1999;30:934–942.
581. Modena P, Lualdi E, Facchinetti F, et al. SMARCB1/INI1 tumor suppressor gene is frequently inactivated in epithelioid sarcomas. *Cancer Res* 2005;65:4012–4019.

CLEAR CELL SARCOMA

582. Enzinger FM. Clear cell sarcoma of tendons and aponeuroses: an analysis of 21 cases. *Cancer* 1965;18:1163–1173.
583. Lucas DR, Nascimento AG, Sim FH. Clear cell sarcoma of soft tissues: Mayo Clinic experience with 35 cases. *Am J Surg Pathol* 1992;16:1197–1204.
584. Montgomery EA, Meis JM, Ramos AG, et al. Clear cell sarcoma of tendons and aponeuroses: a clinicopathologic study of 58 cases with analysis of prognostic factors. *Int J Surg Pathol* 1993;1:89–100.
585. Sandberg AA, Bridge JA. Updates on the cytogenetics and molecular genetics of bone and soft tissue tumors: clear cell sarcoma (malignant melanoma of soft parts). *Cancer Genet Cytogenet* 2001;130:1–7.

EWING SARCOMA/PRIMITIVE NEUROECTODERMAL TUMOR

586. Angervall L, Enzinger FM. Extraskeletal neoplasm resembling Ewing's sarcoma. *Cancer* 1975;36:240–251.
587. Lawlor ER, Mathers JA, Bainbridge T, et al. Peripheral primitive neuroectodermal tumors in adults: documentation by molecular analysis. *J Clin Oncol* 1998;16:1150–1157.
588. Dehner LP. The evolution of the diagnosis and understanding of primitive and embryonic neoplasms in children: living through an epoch [Review]. *Mod Pathol* 1998;11:669–685.
589. Parham DM, Hijazi Y, Steinberg SM, et al. Neuroectodermal differentiation in Ewing's sarcoma family of tumors does not predict tumor behavior. *Hum Pathol* 1999;30:911–918.
590. Argani P, Perez-Ordoñez B, Xiao H, et al. Olfactory neuroblastoma is not related to the Ewing family of tumors—absence of *EWS/FLI1* gene fusion and MIC2 expression. *Am J Surg Pathol* 1998;22:391–398.
591. Folpe AL, Hill CE, Parham DM, et al. Immunohistochemical detection of FLI-1 protein expression—a study of 132 round cell tumors with emphasis on CD99-positive mimics of Ewing's sarcoma/primitive neuroectodermal tumor. *Am J Surg Pathol* 2000;24:1657–1662.
592. West DC, Grier HE, Swallow MM, et al. Detection of circulating tumor cells in patients with Ewing's sarcoma and peripheral primitive neuroectodermal tumor. *J Clin Oncol* 1997;15:583–588.
593. Ladanyi M. Diagnosis and classification of small round cell tumors of childhood. *Am J Pathol* 1999;155:2181–2182.
594. De Alava E, Gerald WL. Molecular biology of the Ewing's sarcoma/primitive neuroectodermal tumor family. *J Clin Oncol* 2000;18:204–213.
595. Sandberg AA, Bridge JA. Updates on cytogenetics and molecular genetics of bone and soft tissue tumors: Ewing sarcoma and peripheral primitive neuroectodermal tumors. *Cancer Genet Cytogenet* 2000;123:1–26.
596. Oberlin O, Le Deley MC, Bui BN, et al. Prognostic factors in localized Ewing's tumours and peripheral neuroectodermal tumours: the third study of the French Society of Paediatric Oncology (EW88 study). *Br J Cancer* 2001;85:1646–1654.

DESMOPLASTIC SMALL ROUND CELL TUMOR

597. Gerald WL, Miller HK, Battifora H, et al. Intra-abdominal desmoplastic small round cell tumor: report of 19 cases of a distinctive type of high-grade polyphenotypic malignancy affecting young individuals. *Am J Surg Pathol* 1991;15:499–513.
598. Gerald WL, Ladanyi M, De Alava E, et al. Clinical, pathologic, and molecular spectrum of tumors associated with t(11;22)(p13;q12): desmoplastic small round cell tumor and its variants. *J Clin Oncol* 1998;16:3028–3036.
599. Wolf AN, Ladanyi M, Paull G, et al. The expanding clinical spectrum of desmoplastic small round cell tumor: a report of two cases with molecular confirmation. *Hum Pathol* 1999;30:430–435.
600. Lae ME, Roche PC, Jin L, et al. Desmoplastic small round cell tumor—a clinicopathologic, immunohistochemical, and molecular study of 32 tumors. *Am J Surg Pathol* 2002;26:823–835.
601. Biegel JA, Conard K, Brooks JJ. Translocation (11;22)(p13;q12): primary change in intra-abdominal desmoplastic small round cell tumor. *Genes Chromosomes Cancer* 1993;7:119–121.
602. De Alava E, Ladanyi M, Rosai J, Gerald WL. Detection of chimeric transcripts in desmoplastic small round cell tumor and related developmental tumors by reverse transcriptase polymerase chain reaction—a specific diagnostic assay. *Am J Pathol* 1995;147:1584–1591.
603. Hill DA, Pfeifer JD, Marley EF, et al. WT1 staining reliably differentiates desmoplastic small round cell tumor from Ewing sarcoma/primitive neuroectodermal tumor—an immunohistochemical and molecular diagnostic study. *Am J Clin Pathol* 2000;114:345–353.
604. Setrakian S, Gupta PK, Heald J, Brooks JJ. Intra-abdominal desmoplastic small round cell

tumor: report of a case diagnosed by fine needle aspiration cytology. *Acta Cytol* 1992;36: 373–376.

PERIVASCULAR EPITHELIOID CELL TUMOR

605. Folpe AL, Goodman ZD, Ishak KG, et al. Clear cell myomelanocytic tumor of the falciform ligament/ligamentum teres—a novel member of the perivascular epithelioid clear cell family of tumors with a predilection for children and young adults. *Am J Surg Pathol* 2000; 24:1239–1246.

606. Vang R, Kempson RL. Perivascular epithelioid cell tumor ('PEComa') of the uterus—a subset of HMB-45–positive epithelioid mesenchymal neoplasms with an uncertain relationship to pure smooth muscle tumors. *Am J Surg Pathol* 2002;26:1–13.

607. Wiklund TA, Blomqvist CP, Räty J, et al. Postirradiation sarcoma: analysis of a nationwide cancer registry material. *Cancer* 1991;68:524–531.

Joint Diseases

ARTHRITIS

The normal joint is painless, provides the required range of motion, and in use remains stable. Failure of joint function is characterized by pain, limitation of motion, and instability and is generally referred to as *arthritis*. To understand the nature of this large group of common diseases, it is first necessary to consider how the morphology of the joint provides for normal function.

Three anatomic features are important: (a) the shape of the articulating surfaces, (b) the integrity of the ligaments and musculotendinous structures around the joint as well as their nerve supply, and (c) the mechanical properties of the extracellular matrices of the ligaments, cartilage, and bone. Dysfunction may begin in any one of the structures that make up the joint; however, at the time of the initial clinical assessment, most of the structures of the joint may be involved, and therefore, it is difficult for the physician to determine the primary cause (1).

GENERAL FEATURES OF THE ARTHRITIC JOINT

The alterations observed in the tissues of an arthritic joint may be divided into two categories: those that are evidence of injury and those that can be regarded as reparative or reactive (2). An obvious sign of injury in the cellular component of the cartilage is the death of a significant number of chondrocytes (Fig. 6.1). On occasion, even complete necrosis of the chondrocytes may be observed. Perhaps more obvious injury is seen in the extracellular matrix. Depletion of proteoglycan in the cartilage matrix is seen in a section, stained by hematoxylin and eosin, as a diminution in basophilic staining; this may be highlighted by the use of specific stains for proteoglycans such as safranin O or Alcian blue (Fig. 6.2). Collagen injury is recognized by vertical and horizontal clefts within the cartilage matrix (Fig. 6.3) (3). A significant feature of damaged articular cartilage is an irregular, thickened, granular tidemark indicating disturbed calcification, which is frequently associated with duplication of the tidemark.

Cartilage regeneration or repair usually presents either as a proliferation of chondrocytes within the damaged cartilage or as a proliferation of new cartilage cells from the underlying bone and from the periphery of the joint (Fig. 6.4). The proliferative cartilage is likely to be more cellular than normal cartilage and demonstrates increased proteoglycan synthesis and, on polarized light microscopy, a different organization of the collagenous component of the extracellular matrix (Fig. 6.5).

In the adjacent subchondral bone, injury is evidenced by superficial bone necrosis, microfractures within the superficial bone trabeculae, and the development of localized areas of bone lysis, microscopically characterized by replacement of bone tissue by fibromyxomatous tissue, which may on occasion be cystic.

Reparative changes in the bone are seen as an increase in osteoblastic activity in the subarticular region with new bone formation and thickening of the subchondral trabeculae. A reparative process that is commonly present in arthritic joints is remodeling of the articular surface. This takes place particularly at the periphery of the joint, where, through the process of endochondral ossification, proliferating cartilage is transformed into bony spurs covered by cartilage or osteophytes, which serve to redistribute the load over the articulating surfaces (4).

The synovium lining of an arthritic joint usually shows hyperplasia or hypertrophy of the synovial lining cells, as well as varying degrees of inflammation (Fig. 6.6). Because the hyperplastic synovium of an arthritic joint becomes traumatized in the course of use, some degree of hemosiderin deposition is common. In those diseases in which rapid breakdown of the joint surface occurs (e.g., Charcot joint and rapidly destructive osteoarthritis), pieces of bone and cartilage may be found within the synovial membrane, surrounded by histiocytes and chronic inflammatory cells.

Large pieces of detached cartilage or cartilage and bone within the joint space (*loose bodies*) may increase in size because of cellular proliferation at their surface, and as they steadily enlarge, the center of these loose bodies becomes necrotic and calcified (Fig. 6.7). In a resected loose body, it may be possible to see concentric rings of calcification, indicating the history of its growth (Fig. 6.8). Sometimes the loose bodies secondarily become attached to the synovium and are invaded by blood vessels. Through the process of endochondral ossification, these attached and revascularized loose bodies may become converted to nodules of viable bone within the synovium. It is important to distinguish these secondary posttraumatic osteochondral loose bodies from primary synovial chondromatosis, as discussed later in this chapter.

OSTEOARTHRITIS

In most cases, osteoarthritis arises as a result of mechanical dysfunction after trauma. However, in general, the onset of clinical disease in *osteoarthritis* does not occur until late middle age. Clinically, the most common presenting joints are the first metatarsophalangeal, lumbar spine, knee, and hip. Although more than one joint may be affected, the disease usually is limited to either one joint or the same joint bilaterally.

An x-ray image generally shows deformity, loss of the joint space, osteophyte formation, sclerosis of the subchondral bone, and often migration of the joint (Fig. 6.9). Frequently, lytic "cystic" lesions can be seen in the subchondral bone, particularly in the case of arthritis of the hip.

The most significant macroscopic features of an osteoarthritic joint are damage to the articular cartilage, bone loss, and an alteration in the shape of the articulating surface. In large portions of the joint, presumably weight bearing, the cartilage may be entirely absent. The exposed underlying bone may have

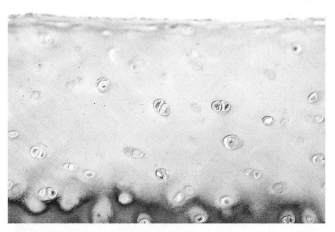

Figure 6.1. Articular cartilage taken from an osteoarthritic metatarsal phalangeal joint. Although the surface of the cartilage appears flat and intact, there are many ghost chondrocytes as well as marked irregularity of the tidemark.

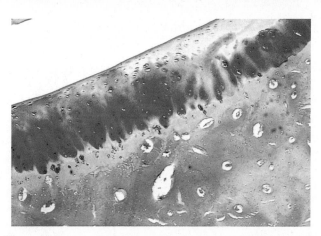

Figure 6.2. A photomicrograph of an articular surface stained with safranin O, a quantitative stain for sulfated proteoglycans. A lack of staining in the upper part of the articular cartilage (right) is indicative of diminished proteoglycans, which would result in a loss of the normal turgor of the cartilage in this region.

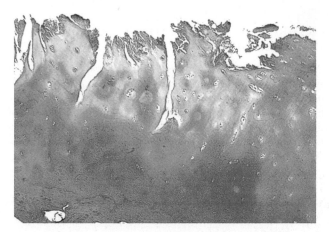

Figure 6.3. Cartilage removed from an osteoarthritic hip joint to demonstrate matrix damage at the surface. The normally smooth surface is disrupted, and both small and large clefts can be seen extending into the substance of the hyaline cartilage.

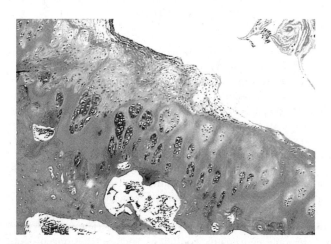

Figure 6.4. Cartilage removed from an osteoarthritic femoral head, demonstrating both intrinsic and extrinsic cartilage regeneration. The intrinsic cartilage regeneration is seen in the form of clones of chondrocytes within the cartilage matrix. Many of these clones contain as many as 20 chondrocytes. On the surface of the cartilage is extrinsic repair in the form of fibrocartilage extending over the surface from the periphery of the joint.

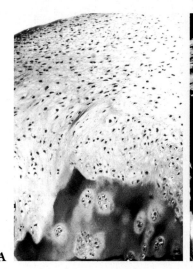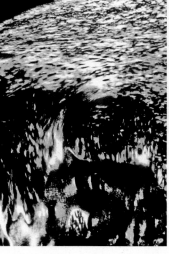

Figure 6.5. **(A)** The articular surface of an arthritic joint demonstrating extrinsic reparative fibrocartilage, which has extended over the remnants of the original articular hyaline cartilage. **(B)** The same field photographed with polarized light shows the coarse and more disorganized collagen fibers in the reparative cartilage.

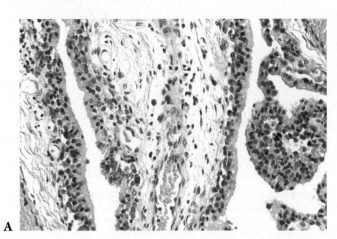
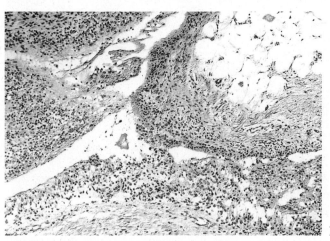

A   **B**

Figure 6.6. **(A)** Synovial tissue obtained from a patient with osteoarthritis. The cellular synovial lining is both hypertrophied and hyperplastic. **(B)** Although osteoarthritis is a noninflammatory form of arthritis, there may be marked chronic inflammation resulting from the breakdown products of the destroyed cartilage, as seen in this photograph.

a polished, smooth appearance generally described as *eburnation*. The cartilage that remains is often somewhat discolored and, instead of its usual smooth and shiny appearance, is rough and velvety. When the joint is sectioned, the bone underneath the eroded articular surface is sclerotic. In addition, fibrous walled cysts filled with mucoid fluid may be seen immediately below the surface. At the periphery of the joint, bony outgrowths, or osteophytes, are frequently present (Fig. 6.10).

In most cases of osteoarthritis, microscopic evidence of both injury and repair are present in the cartilage and bone without any significant inflammatory component, although occasionally scattered perivascular lymphocytes and even lymphoid follicles may be seen within the synovial membrane (Fig. 6.11) (5).

In some neuropathic conditions, such as tabes dorsalis and the peripheral neuropathies of diabetes or pernicious anemia, one may observe rapidly destructive osteoarthritis complicated by multiple loose bodies, severe subluxation, and even dislocation. This type of joint is usually referred to as a *Charcot joint* (6) and is characterized histologically by extreme deformity and bone and cartilage detritus seen within the synovial membrane (Figs. 6.12 and 6.13).

ARTHRITIS SECONDARY TO SUBCHONDRAL INSUFFICIENCY FRACTURE

Primary subchondral fractures in the femoral head occur in stress osteopathy in young military trainees; *insufficiency fractures* occur in renal transplantation recipients and, most commonly in my experience, in elderly osteoporotic women. Reports of this fracture type have stressed the importance of its differentiation from osteonecrosis, especially when one uses magnetic res-

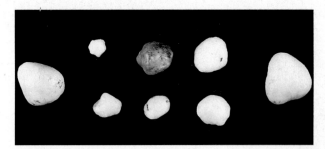

Figure 6.7. A group of osteocartilaginous loose bodies removed from an osteoarthritic knee joint. Note the irregular, but smooth, contours as well as the variation in size. Loose bodies such as these may become secondarily attached to the synovial membrane, where they may be revascularized, so on histologic examination, there is viable bone within that center as well as active endochondral ossification. When free in the joint, loose bodies may grow by cartilage replication on the surface of the loose body.

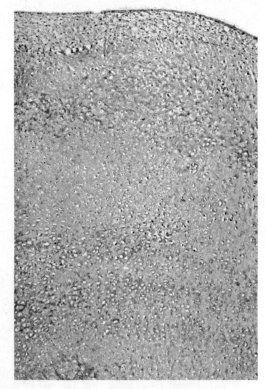

Figure 6.8. A photomicrograph of a portion of one of the loose bodies shown in Figure 6.7 that demonstrates irregular, but concentric, rings of calcification and cartilage replication on its surface.

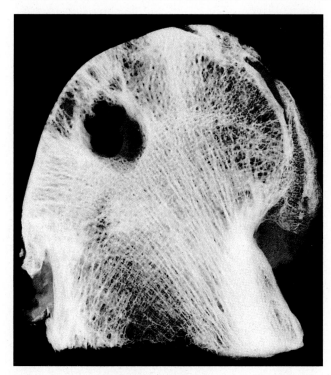

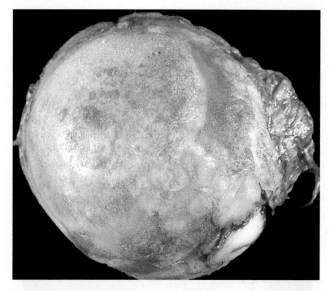

Figure 6.10. A femoral head removed from a patient with osteoarthritis of the hip joint. There is extensive loss of the articular cartilage with exposure of polished, eburnated bone and remnants of degenerated cartilage around the periphery of eburnated areas. The small nodules of cartilage in the center of the eburnated zone are tufts of regenerative cartilage growing up from the underlying subchondral bone. In favorable circumstances, this regenerative cartilage may eventually cover the entire articular surface.

Figure 6.9. A radiograph of a 4-mm slice taken through the center of an osteoarthritic femoral head to demonstrate the gross anatomic features of osteoarthritis. There has been loss of bone substance superiorly and laterally with a loss of the normal sphericity of the femoral head. Along this surface, the articular cartilage has been lost. The subchondral bone is sclerotic as a result of the thickening of the trabeculae in reaction to the loss of cartilage. Beneath the articular surface is a large lytic defect, a subchondral bone cyst, which is a characteristic finding in osteoarthritis where the cartilage has been lost. New bone formation extends over much of the medial surface and over the periphery of the joint. These osteophytes should be regarded as reparative phenomena that are restoring the joint contour.

granulomatous tissue are usually observed in the narrow spaces, in which small fragments of bone and articular cartilage embedded in amorphous eosinophilic debris are found surrounded by aggregated epithelioid histiocytes and giant cells (9–11). We now believe that in most cases, rapidly destructive arthrosis of the hip and other joints is the result of insufficiency fracture.

RHEUMATOID ARTHRITIS

Rheumatoid arthritis is a relatively common inflammatory disease affecting men and women of all ages, with a peak incidence in

onance imaging, because the initial diagnosis will affect management of the patient. Many clinically reported cases have resolved after conservative therapy without progressing to collapse or requiring surgery. However, in my own experience, histologic evidence of subchondral fracture as the cause of acute onset of hip pain in elderly women has become increasingly commonplace. In the published cases of insufficiency fracture, shortly after the onset of the hip pain, radiographic changes were reported as unremarkable (which would seem to be inconsistent with the severity of the reported pain in these patients); however, magnetic resonance imaging has shown a pattern of bone marrow edema. Histopathologically, the most characteristic finding in the cases reported was the presence of fracture callus and granulation tissue along both edges of a fracture line paralleling the articular surface (Fig. 6.14) (7).

First reported in the literature by Postel and Kerboull in 1970 (8), *rapidly destructive arthrosis* of the hip joint is a relatively uncommon form of arthritis that is seen mostly in elderly women. Rapidly destructive arthrosis is characterized by rapid joint destruction within 6 to 12 months, and disappearance of the joint space is the typical initial finding on radiographs, followed by rapid disappearance of the femoral head.

Some patients with subchondral insufficiency fracture go on to show rapid disappearance of the hip joint space and the superficial portion of the marrow space. Round to oval foci of

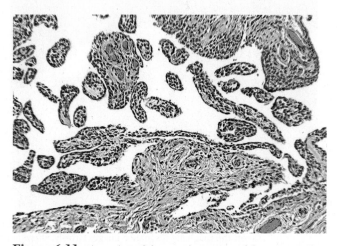

Figure 6.11. A portion of the synovium removed from an osteoarthritic joint. The synovium can be seen in papillary folds, and the synovial lining can be observed in places that are hypertrophied and hyperplastic. There is fibrosis, with focal myxoid change, of the underlying fibroadipose tissue and occasional focal collections of chronic inflammatory cells.

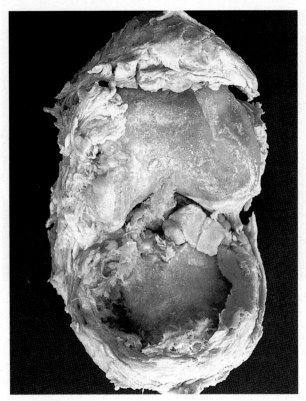

Figure 6.12. The knee joint of a patient with Charcot arthropathy. The patella and femoral condyles are in the upper part of the figure; the lower part of the figure shows the grossly distorted articular surface of the tibia. Note the complete loss of cartilage over the articulating surfaces. The cruciate ligaments are not in evidence. The menisci are grossly degenerated, and the synovium is very proliferative and stained by hemosiderin. Obvious osteocartilaginous loose bodies are present in the posterior aspect of the joint.

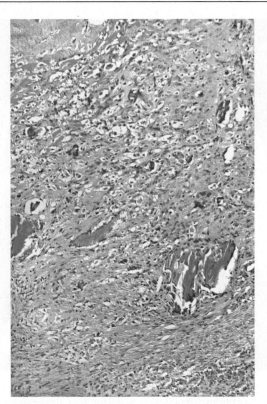

Figure 6.13. Synovium from the joint demonstrated in Figure 6.12. There is histiocytic infiltration of the synovial tissue with collections of both fibrin and hemosiderin. Small fragments of bone (detritus) are present throughout the field. The largest pieces of bone are phagocytosed by histiocytes and giant cells at the periphery.

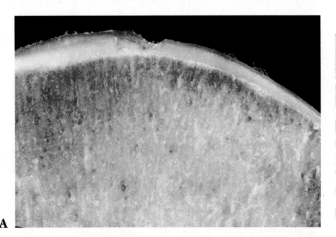
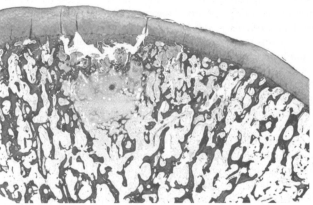

A   B

Figure 6.14. **(A)** A section through a femoral head removed with a clinical diagnosis of osteonecrosis based on the magnetic resonance image. Grossly, there is no evidence of osteonecrosis, and the only abnormality noted was a narrow band of hyperemia in the subchondral region. **(B)** Microscopic examination revealed a subchondral fracture with reparative tissue.

young adults and menopausal women. There is often a genetic predisposition, and the disease is characterized by immune-driven chronic inflammation. Rheumatoid factors are detectable in the serum in most cases. Although rheumatoid arthritis is a multiorgan disease, the main target organs are the synovial lining of joints, bursae, and tendon sheaths. Marked by a variable course, including exacerbations and remissions of disease activity, many cases are chronic and progressive and result in severe disability and sometimes death.

In the acute stage of rheumatoid arthritis, aspiration of the joint may reveal an inflammatory exudate with many polymorphonuclear leukocytes, even suggesting the possibility of septic arthritis. In general, the cell counts in rheumatoid arthritis are lower (<75,000) than those seen in septic arthritis (>100,000).

The principal morphologic feature of rheumatoid arthritis is joint destruction and, unlike osteoarthritis, there is little evidence of reparative tissue, proliferative cartilage, bone sclerosis, or osteophytes (8). The most characteristic microscopic feature is a chronic exudative inflamed synovium characterized by hypertrophy and hyperplasia of the synovial lining cells with focal fibrinous exudation at the surface and an infiltration of the superficial synovium by lymphocytes and plasma cells (Fig. 6.15). Many of the plasma cells contain a smooth eosinophilic cytoplasmic inclusion or Russell body. Lymphoid follicles are not uncommon. The inflamed synovium eventually extends over the articular surface from the joint periphery to form a covering or *pannus* that destroys the underlying cartilage both by interfering with chondrocyte nutrition and by enzymatically degrading the matrix (Fig. 6.16). The end result of this inflammatory destruction of the articular surfaces may be fusion of the joint either by fibrous granulation tissue or, rarely, by bone (12–14).

In addition to the destruction of the articular surface by the inflamed synovium, there also is extension of the inflamed synovium into the capsular tissue and periarticular supportive tissues. Destruction of these tissues results in instability of the joint, leading to joint subluxation and the severe deformity so characteristic of rheumatoid arthritis. Another microscopic feature of rheumatoid arthritis that is not always appreciated is

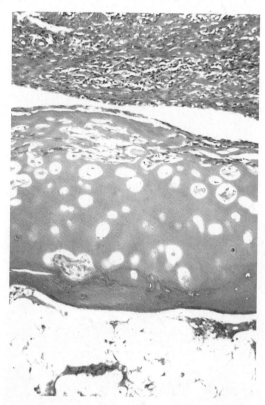

Figure 6.16. Articular cartilage with overlying pannus taken from a patient with rheumatoid arthritis that demonstrates the chronic inflammation and large areas of lysis around the chondrocytes within the articular cartilage. These enlarged chondrocyte lacunae are often referred to as *Weichselbaum lacunae* and are typically found in rheumatoid arthritis.

that chronic inflammatory tissue is also typically present in the subchondral bone. On occasion, the articular cartilage is destroyed not only from above by the inflamed synovium, but also from below by chronically inflamed tissue in the subchondral bone (Fig. 6.17).

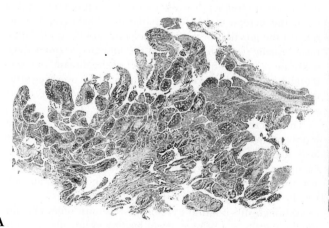

A

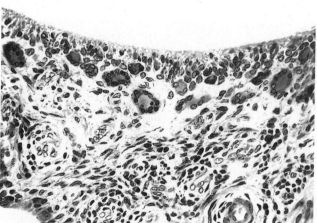

B

Figure 6.15. **(A)** A low-power view of the synovial membrane removed from a patient with rheumatoid arthritis that demonstrates the papillary appearance of the synovium and intense inflammatory infiltration, with many lymphoid follicles. The surface of the synovium may have large collections of fibrin. **(B)** A higher power view of the proliferative synovial lining, which often has giant cell forms.

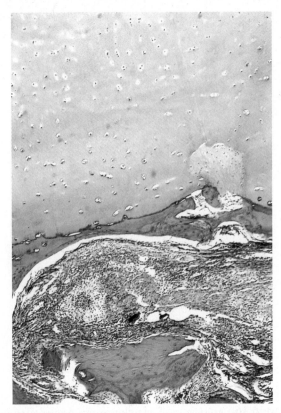

Figure 6.17. Articular cartilage and underlying subchondral bone from a patient with rheumatoid arthritis. Note the extensive chronic inflammation in subchondral bone, a finding typical of rheumatoid arthritis.

Approximately 25% of patients with rheumatoid arthritis develop rheumatoid nodules. These nodules are found in subcutaneous sites, especially along the extensor surfaces of the forearm and the elbow, as well as the shin. Less often they may occur in visceral organs, especially the heart, lung, and gastrointestinal tract, and even in the synovial membrane itself. Histologically, the rheumatoid nodule is characterized by an irregular central zone of fibrinoid necrosis surrounded by palisaded histiocytes, giant cells, and a cuff of chronic inflammatory cells (Fig. 6.18).

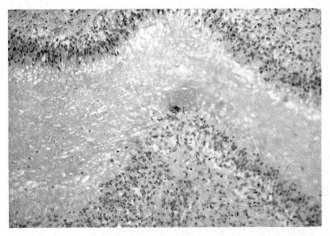

Figure 6.18. A portion of a rheumatoid nodule demonstrating the central irregular area of fibrinoid necrosis surrounded by palisaded histiocytes and chronic inflammatory cells.

With the destruction of the articular cartilage, the inflammatory component tends to regress, and in patients who have had total joint surface replacements, even without synovectomy, the synovitis in that joint tends to become much less severe. Conversely, in a rheumatoid joint that has been treated by synovectomy without resection of the articular bone, the inflammatory synovium may reappear, and the progression of the disease is only temporarily halted by synovial excision.

Involvement of the spine occurs in more than 50% of patients with rheumatoid arthritis. Most commonly, the cervical spine is involved. Bony erosion and apophyseal joint space narrowing are common and may result in ankylosis. Erosions of the odontoid process occur in approximately one-third of patients as a result of weakening of the transverse and apical ligaments by the inflamed synovium. Therefore, minor trauma may result in atlantoaxial subluxation or basilar invagination and sudden death.

OSTEONECROSIS

Osteonecrosis is a common late complication of fractured neck of the femur and, together with idiopathic segmental subchondral infarction, is a significant cause of hip arthritis. In idiopathic disease, not only the hip but also the knee and other major joints may be affected (15). The clinical symptoms result from fractures through the articular surfaces and follow collapse of the underlying necrotic infarcted bone segment. Also probably contributing to collapse is the reparative granulation tissue that forms around the margin of the infarct and destroys the bone at this site (16–18).

Some of the risk groups are patients who have been treated with corticosteroids, alcoholics, and persons affected by sickle cell disease or Gaucher disease. More than 50% of cases exhibit bilateral or other joint involvement, a finding indicating the systemic nature of the disease.

Gross examination of the articular surface of a joint resected from a patient with early clinical osteonecrosis is likely to reveal a fairly intact articular cartilage, although the cartilage is often folded and cracked at the edge of the necrotic area as a result of fracture (Fig. 6.19). Section through the infarcted zone has a characteristic yellow, opaque, chalky appearance in the affected subchondral bone and, at the periphery of the infarct, a rim of hyperemic fibrous tissue. Beyond the infarcted zone, the bone trabeculae are frequently thickened by reparative bone, giving rise to the increase in density seen on clinical radiographs. Fractures at the junction of the necrotic bone and the granulation tissue usually result in collapse of the infarcted segment (Fig. 6.20); moreover, with the progression of the disease, one sees flattening of the joint surface, detachment of the overlying articular cartilage, and loss of bony tissue leading to secondary osteoarthritis (Fig. 6.21).

The microscopic recognition of necrotic bone depends mostly on the identification of necrosis of the marrow fat and associated hematopoietic tissue. In the bone itself, the osteocytic lacunae may be enlarged and empty, or they may be of normal size with pyknotic nuclei, depending on the time span over which the necrosis occurred (Fig. 6.22).

Although subchondral osteonecrosis is most often encountered clinically as a primary event leading eventually to severe arthritis, osteonecrosis may also secondarily complicate existing cases of arthritis (19).

Some cases that would have been diagnosed, until quite recently, as osteonecrosis on the basis of magnetic resonance im-

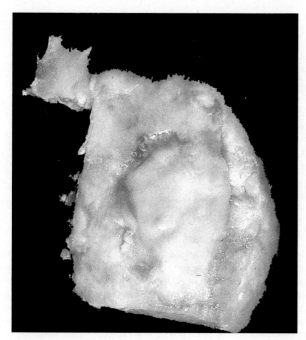

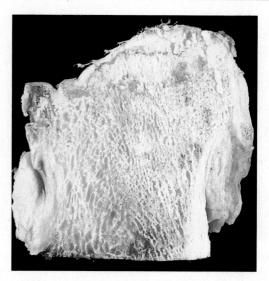

Figure 6.21. The cut surface of the femoral head from a patient with long-standing osteonecrosis in which the necrotic segment has collapsed, with subsequent deformity of the articulating surface and secondary clinical osteoarthritis.

Figure 6.19. The articular surface of the medial femoral condyle of the knee in a case of avascular necrosis. The depression around the necrotic fragment is the result of the underlying fracture (see also Figs. 6.20 and 6.21).

aging and even histopathologic features are now recognized to have resulted from subchondral insufficiency fractures as previously discussed.

GOUT

Clinical *gout* is the result of an inflammatory response to monosodium urate monohydrate crystals that may form as a result of

hyperuricemia. Hyperuricemia may result from diet, increased cell breakdown associated with malignancy, or genetic factors. Contributing factors are hypertension, renal impairment, and the use of diuretics.

In both the primary and the secondary forms of gout, hyperuricemia results in the deposition of monosodium urate crystals in joints and visceral organs (20,21). The kidney is frequently affected, and uric acid stones are present in nearly all patients with gout.

Acute gouty arthritis is generally monoarticular and seems to have a predilection for the lower extremity, particularly the first metatarsophalangeal joint. In the early stages of the disease, the patient's symptoms may be attributed to sepsis. However, examination of the aspirated fluid by polarized light microscopy

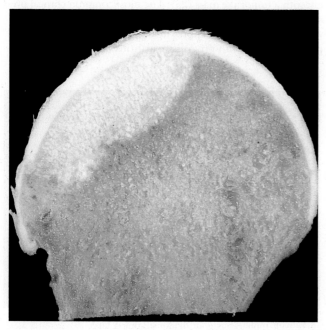

Figure 6.20. The femoral head demonstrating a large area of subchondral necrosis (avascular necrosis, osteonecrosis).

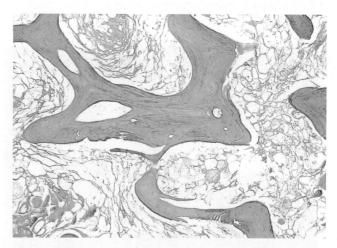

Figure 6.22. Portion of the necrotic bone, illustrated grossly in Figure 6.21, showing complete saponification of the marrow fat together with the absence of viable osteocytes within the bone tissue itself. (Microscopically, the marrow is a much more sensitive indicator of necrosis than is the bone.)

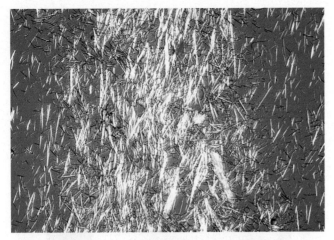

Figure 6.23. Sodium biurate crystals precipitated from the synovial fluid of a patient with gout. The sodium biurate crystals are strongly negatively birefringent (polarized light).

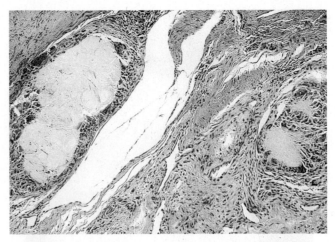

Figure 6.25. Part of the periphery of the tophaceous deposits illustrated in Figure 6.24 that demonstrates the appearance of the crystalline deposits under transmitted light microscopy with surrounding histiocytes, giant cells, and chronic inflammatory cells. Polarization of properly preserved tissue in such a case may demonstrate the refractile urate crystals in these amorphous deposits. (Frequently, the crystals can be demonstrated only by polarized light microscopy of an unstained section.)

will, in all cases, demonstrate the presence of strongly negatively birefringent needle-shaped crystals (Fig. 6.23) (22).

Continued deposition of monosodium urate crystals eventually results in chronic tophaceous gout. Tophaceous (chalky) deposits around joints eventually erode into the bone and articular cartilage and cause large periarticular defects that may be seen on radiologic examination (Fig. 6.24). Histologically, the resected tophi consist of large crystalline deposits rimmed by histiocytes and giant cells and surrounded by fibrous tissue (Fig. 6.25). During the course of the routine staining of histologic sections, the crystals, which are water soluble, are usually removed; however, examination of unstained sections by polarized light generally clearly demonstrates the crystalline nature of the deposits.

CALCIUM PYROPHOSPHATE CRYSTAL DEPOSITION DISEASE

Small deposits within the articular tissues of a chalky white material is a common finding in arthritic joints and more usually is the result of *calcium pyrophosphate deposition disease* (CPPD). The disease may be familial or may be associated with other metabolic disease such as hyperparathyroidism, hemochromatosis, hypothyroidism, or even gout itself. However, most cases lack such associations.

The nomenclature of this disease has been confusing. The term *chondrocalcinosis* has been used by radiologists to describe calcium deposits in the knee menisci of elderly patients. The term *pseudogout* has been used by rheumatologists to describe those patients with CPPD who present with an acute swollen joint mimicking gout. Very rarely, a patient with CPPD will present with a tumorlike mass (23). The most common clinical presentation of a patient with CPPD is similar to that of a patient with osteoarthritis, and approximately 50% of clinically affected patients present with progressive arthritis that often affects sev-

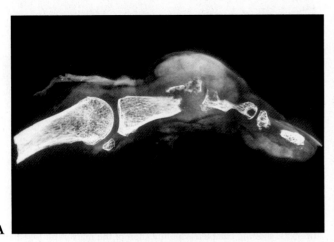

A

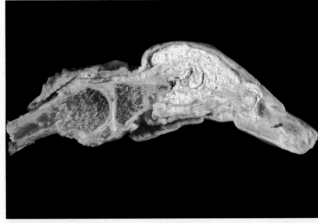

B

Figure 6.24. **(A)** Radiograph of a little finger of a patient with tophaceous gout demonstrating a large periarticular deposit around the proximal interphalangeal joint with extensive bone erosion and joint destruction. **(B)** Cut surface of the specimen illustrated in **A**. Note the chalky white appearance of the gouty deposits.

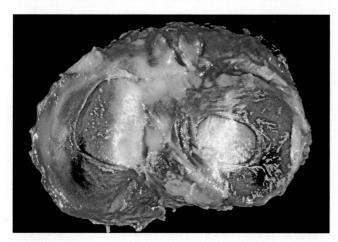

Figure 6.26. The articular surface of the tibia from a patient with hemochromatosis and calcium pyrophosphate deposition disease. Note the discoloration of the cartilage and the menisci and the linear deposits of chalky white material within the menisci as well as in the articular cartilage.

eral joints. The onset of the disease is usually in the fourth decade of life (24–28).

Gross examination of the affected tissues reveals small chalky white deposits (Fig. 6.26), which on microscopic examination, in contrast to uric acid deposits, show small rhomboidal crystals that are weakly positively birefringent (Fig. 6.27). (Because on occasion there may be some histiocytic and giant cell reaction around these crystalline deposits, it is important that they be distinguished from uric acid crystals.)

HYDROXYAPATITE DEPOSITION AND RELATED CONDITIONS

Deposition of calcium hydroxyapatite in soft tissues, which must be distinguished from gout and CPPD, may be associated with trauma, scleroderma, renal failure, hyperparathyroidism, sarcoidosis, metastatic disease, myeloma, or hypermetabolic states (29–31).

Metastatic calcification is a problem particularly in patients with disturbed calcium homeostasis and hypermetabolic states (e.g., hyperparathyroidism, Paget disease) who may have undergone prolonged bed rest. The calcification, which may be both intracellular and extracellular, is likely to occur in the kidneys, alveolar walls of the lungs, cornea, conjunctiva, and gastric mucosa (i.e., those areas subject to large pH changes), as well as in the media and intima of the blood vessels.

In foci of coagulation necrosis, caseous necrosis, and fat necrosis, the dead tissue that does not undergo rapid absorption frequently becomes calcified. This type of calcification, which is not related to any disturbance in calcium homeostasis, is called *dystrophic calcification.* Of particular interest to orthopaedic surgeons is the calcification that is common in tendons, ligaments, and bursae, presumably after mechanical trauma. A common clinical presentation is a painful shoulder that corresponds anatomically to the insertion of the supraspinatus muscle onto the humerus. Gross examination reveals amorphous chalky white deposits, and microscopic studies reveal that the calcium is isolated in fibrous or fatty tissue or may be present with chronic inflammatory cells including, at times, multinucleated giant cells (Fig. 6.28).

Tumoral calcinosis is a rare condition that mostly affects blacks in otherwise good health. Characteristically, blood phosphate levels are elevated. The disease usually presents in the second decade of life and is characterized by deposition of painless calcific masses around the hips, elbows, shoulders, and gluteal area (i.e., areas subject to movement or pressure). Rarely, intraosseous deposits also may occur (Fig. 6.29) (32).

SEPTIC ARTHRITIS

Joint infection may be caused by hematogenous infection of the synovium, decompression of contiguous osteomyelitis, or direct inoculation of a joint after trauma or surgery. With total joint replacement and arthroscopy now such common procedures, postsurgical infection is one of the most common causes of the septic joint.

Septic arthritis is relatively common in neonates and infants, in whom it affects the hip, knee, or ankle, and severe residual growth disturbances may result from damage to the growth car-

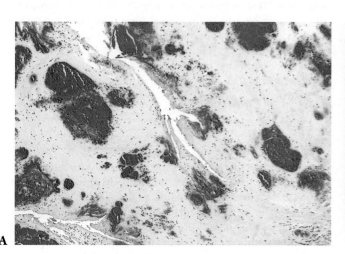

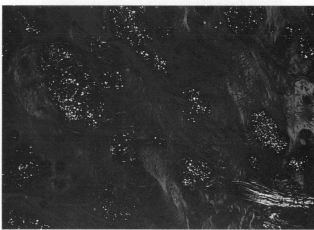

A   B

Figure 6.27. **(A)** A portion of the meniscus demonstrated in Figure 6.26 showing the calcified deposits of crystalline material within the fibrocartilage of the meniscus. **(B)** A polarized light image of the same field to show the refractile crystals within these calcified deposits.

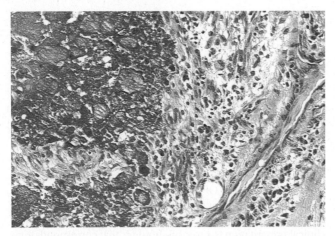

Figure 6.28. A photomicrograph to demonstrate calcium hydroxyapatite deposit with histiocyte, giant cell, and chronic inflammatory response.

tilage (Fig. 6.30) (33,34). Other groups of patients particularly susceptible to septic arthritis are debilitated older adults with rheumatoid arthritis or other chronic inflammatory joint diseases and immunocompromised patients. The diagnosis is established by joint aspiration. To increase the likelihood of bacterial growth, the aspirate should be inoculated into the culture medium as soon as possible after collection.

Suppurative arthritis as a complication of gonorrhea is now rare. However, it is an important diagnostic alternative to bear in mind because the true nature of the disease is likely to be missed unless a careful history is taken. As with other forms of

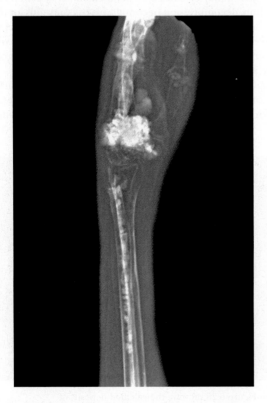

Figure 6.29. Calcium deposits in the soft tissues and in the radius of a patient with tumoral calcinosis.

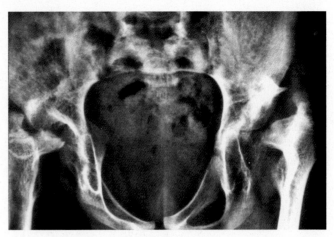

Figure 6.30. Radiograph of the pelvis of a 7-year-old boy with a history of multiple joint infections. Destruction of the articular cartilage and subchondral bone has led to total disappearance of both femoral heads and acetabula with disintegration of the hip joints, which is characteristic of late septic arthritis.

bacterial arthritis, the knee joints are usually the first to be affected, but multiple joint involvement is much more common in patients with gonorrhea than in those with other types of infection. Patients with syphilis may also develop arthritis, either as a result of the extension of gummatous osteitis into a joint or as a complication of congenital syphilis.

Pyogenic osteomyelitis of the vertebral column is less common than infections of the appendicular skeleton. The disease may be seen at any age but is most common after the sixth decade. It should always be considered in the differential diagnosis of back pain in elderly patients. The predisposing factors include systemic urinary tract infection, diabetes, and, in younger patients, immunodeficiency disease and intravenous drug addiction (35). The lumbar spine is involved twice as frequently as the thoracic spine, whereas the cervical spine is only rarely affected.

Retropharyngeal abscesses may arise from cervical infections, and abscess in the paraspinal muscle may follow thoracic infections. Abscess in the psoas muscle sheath may spread to the groin or even to the popliteal fossa. The central nervous system can become contaminated by spread of the infection into the neural canal, resulting in meningitis. The adjacent vertebra is often infected by spread along the vertebral ligaments; the intervertebral disc may become sequestrated and eventually be destroyed.

TUBERCULOSIS

Tuberculosis affecting the bones and joints results from hematogenous spread from elsewhere in the body, usually from the lungs. In most patients, foci of infection within the bone coexist with involvement of the adjacent joint, most commonly the spine, hips, and knees. Tuberculosis of the spine and hip is most commonly seen in children, in contrast to tuberculosis of the knee, which is most commonly seen in adults.

In roentgenograms of the hip and knee joints, tuberculosis is generally associated with marginal erosions of the bone and

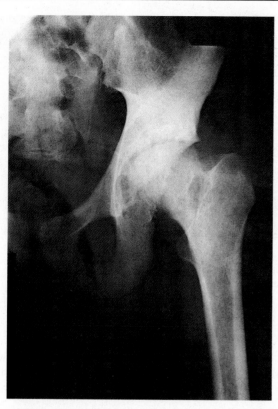

Figure 6.31. Tuberculosis of the hip joint. Note the concentric narrowing of the joint together with erosive changes that are present on both sides of the joint.

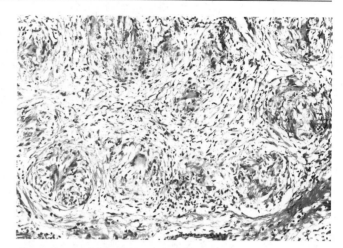

Figure 6.32. Synovium contains multiple close-packed nodules of pale histiocytes and giant cells with minimal lymphocytic cuffing typical of sarcoidosis.

necrosis, the very prominent epithelioid cells, and the paucity of lymphocytes around the granulomas should alert the pathologist to the correct diagnosis (Fig. 6.32).

TISSUE RESPONSE TO ARTIFICIAL JOINT IMPLANTS

Today, *total joint replacement* for the treatment of arthritis has become commonplace. Implants sometimes fail because of infection or mechanical failure; as a result, the surgical pathologist often must examine tissue from around failed joint implants. In the case of infection, there will be signs of both acute and chronic inflammation in the joint tissues and around the prosthesis. In the case of mechanical failure, debris generated by the various components of the artificial joint may produce a granulomatous reaction (37–39).

Wear debris is most often from one of three sources: the metallic component of the joint, the high-density polyethylene, or the methyl methacrylate that is frequently used as grout to hold the prosthetic parts in place. The metallic debris sometimes results in a gray-black discoloration of the synovial tissues as well as the reactive tissue surrounding the prosthesis. This discoloration is particularly prominent with the use of prostheses manufactured from titanium (40). Microscopic examination of such tissue shows irregular metal fragments, measuring between 1 and 3 μm, usually within histiocytes (Fig. 6.33).

High-density polyethylene results in threadlike fragments that may measure up to 10 to 20 μm in length and are present within histiocytes and giant cells. However, the polyethylene fragments become apparent only when the tissue is examined by polarized light (Fig. 6.34). Occasionally, the reaction is so severe that a giant cell pseudotumor results, often with erosion of the periarticular bone.

In routine histologic preparations, methyl methacrylate is dissolved from the tissue during normal tissue processing, and microscopic examination reveals only the spaces where the cement had previously been (Fig. 6.35). The cement fragments vary considerably in size; the smallest fragments are less than 1 μm in diameter, whereas the largest fragments are 100 μm or

destruction of the subchondral bone on both sides of the joint with subsequent loss of the joint space (Fig. 6.31). Histologic examination of the affected tissue reveals the typical granulomatous lesions. Mycobacterial infections in patients with acquired immunodeficiency syndrome (AIDS) may lack a granulomatous reaction and may have only a diffuse infiltration of histiocytes that usually contain numerous acid-fast organisms (36).

In bone and joint lesions, it is often difficult to demonstrate the acid-fast bacilli, and definitive diagnosis depends on culture. Unfortunately, the disease may not have been suspected preoperatively, and in some cases of total joint replacement for arthritis, the diagnosis of tuberculosis is made only after gross and microscopic examination of the resected joint.

When granulomatous infection is suspected, it is important to make direct smears and cultures for both acid-fast organisms and fungi. The common fungal conditions found in bone that give rise to granulomatous infection are blastomycosis, coccidioidomycosis, and cryptococcosis. Sporotrichosis may result from direct contamination of a joint by a puncture wound from a rose thorn.

SARCOIDOSIS

Approximately 10% of patients with *sarcoidosis* have joint involvement. Most of these patients have polyarticular migratory arthritis that rapidly resolves. However, a few patients may develop chronic granulomatous arthritis that may be difficult to differentiate from tuberculosis, although the lack of caseation

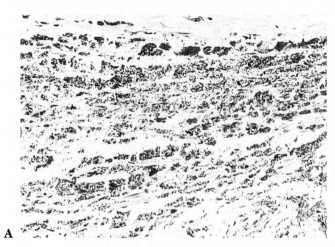
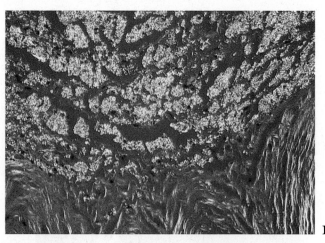

A   B

Figure 6.33. **(A)** Extensive intracytoplasmic metallic particles from a patient with a failed hip prosthesis. Such deposits may be found in the synovial and capsular tissue around the joint and sometimes may be observed in the tissue around the stem of the prosthesis within the bone. **(B)** Another field of metallic debris within capsular tissue from a patient with a failed prosthesis that shows refraction around the edges of the opaque metal fragments.

greater. In addition to the large pieces of cement that are generally associated with giant cells, one also may see masses of foamy histiocytes, which presumably are secondary to very finely powdered cement. These fragments cannot be demonstrated in the tissue section because of preparative techniques.

Silicone rubber has also been used for the manufacture of prosthetic implants, particularly to replace the small joints of the hands and wrists. Fragmentation of the silicone leads to a severe histiocytic and giant cell reaction, and the included silicone particles have a characteristic bosselated and faintly yellow appearance, which is refractile, although not birefringent (Fig. 6.36) (41,42).

In all the removed prostheses examined in our department, wear debris has been found on microscopic examination, either in the synovium, bone marrow spaces, or surrounding soft tissue. There appears to be a good correlation among the amount of wear debris, the duration of the implant, and the patient's level of activity. The more active the patient is, as determined by distance walked and other physical activities, the more wear debris and tissue reaction are generally present in the tissue.

HOFFA DISEASE (SYNOVIAL LIPOMATOSIS)

Hoffa disease, or synovial lipomatosis, is a rare condition most often presenting clinically as enlargement of the infrapatellar fat pad, with resulting pain or deep aching in the anterior compartment of the knee. However, the condition may occur rarely in any joint (43).

Macroscopically, the affected synovium has a marked papillary, yellow, and fatty appearance. Microscopically, there is mild hyperplasia of the synovial lining cells with abundant unremarkable fat extending to the synovial lining. Occasionally, a mild to moderate chronic inflammatory infiltrate may be present (Fig. 6.37).

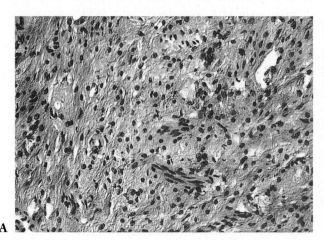
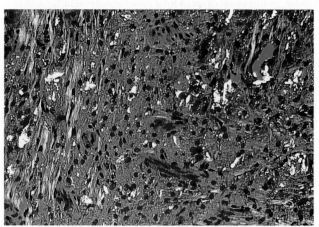

A   B

Figure 6.34. **(A)** The synovial reaction around a failed knee prosthesis that demonstrates many foamy histiocytes with occasional giant cells. **(B)** Innumerable refractile fragments of polyethylene within the histiocytes and giant cells from the same lesion.

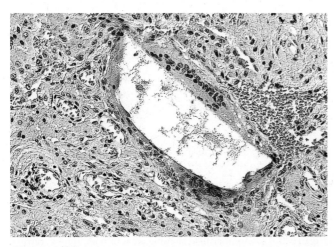

Figure 6.35. The reactive tissue around a failed hip prosthesis shows a large defect surrounded by multinucleated giant cells that contained a particle of methyl methacrylate cement. The cement has been dissolved by the processing technique, and only particles of barium sulfate, which are mixed with the cement to make it radiographically opaque, can be seen within the defect at this time.

PIGMENTED VILLONODULAR SYNOVITIS

Pigmented villonodular synovitis is a locally aggressive benign tumor of the synovium of joints and tendon sheaths. It is commonly seen in the synovial lining of the flexor tendons of the hand and in the synovium of the knee, as well as less commonly in other joints. The lesion is either asymptomatic or only mildly painful; in tendon sheaths, the lesion, often referred to as a giant cell tumor of the tendon sheath, usually presents as a swelling, whereas in the knee, villous and multinodular lesions clinically present with effusions. In general, the condition is confined to one joint or tendon sheath; multiple sites are only rarely involved (44–47).

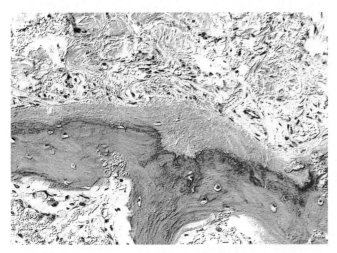

Figure 6.36. Portion of bone and periosteal tissue removed from a patient with a failed Silastic implant. Throughout the tissue and even within the substance of the bone, collections of a bosselated yellowish material, which is the disintegrated Silastic, can be seen. On occasion, this material may cause a histiocyte and giant cell reaction sufficient to mimic an intraosseous tumor radiographically.

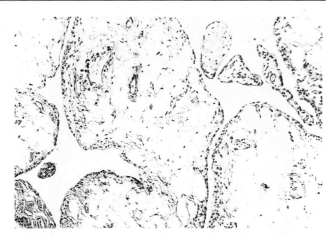

Figure 6.37. Synovium of a patient with Hoffa disease that shows fatty infiltration of the subsynovial tissue.

In most cases, the lesion is a solitary nodule. In large joints, nodules are generally asymptomatic. Large joint cases presenting clinically usually consist of multiple nodules, often with associated hyperplastic villous changes in the synovium and extensive hemosiderin deposition (Figs. 6.38 and 6.39). All lesions grossly appear cream colored or tan and have a firm, nodular consistency.

Microscopically, the characteristic findings are nodules of proliferating, collagen-producing polyhedral epithelioid cells, often with scattered, multinucleated giant cells. Iron deposits and aggregates of foam cells may be present, but these are usually seen in the periphery of the lesion and are most consistent with secondary changes after hemorrhage into the lesion (Fig. 6.40). Abundant collagen may be evident in patients with long-standing disease (Fig. 6.41). In general, the lesion is noninflammatory or has only sparse lymphocytes and plasma cells. Very rare cases of malignant degeneration have been described (48). Pigmented villonodular synovitis must be distinguished from hemosiderotic synovitis, which is seen in patients with chronic intra-articular bleeding (e.g., hemophilia). Although hemosiderotic synovitis contains a significant amount of pigment, mainly

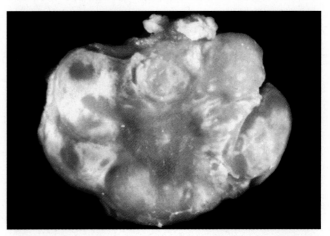

Figure 6.38. The cut surface of a lesion of pigmented villonodular tenosynovitis removed from the finger of a patient. Note the variegated appearance with nodules of fibrosis and lipid deposits with focal hemosiderin pigmentation, particularly around the periphery of the lesion.

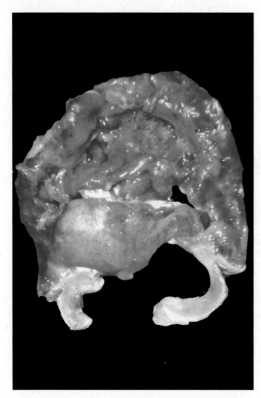

Figure 6.39. A portion of the synovium removed from a patient with pigmented villonodular synovitis of the knee joint. There is a marked papillary proliferation of the synovial tissue, which grossly is mahogany brown. The extent of involvement can be gauged from the attached menisci.

within the synovial lining cells, it lacks the distinct submembranous mononuclear and giant cell proliferation that characterizes pigmented villonodular synovitis (Fig. 6.42) (49,50).

PRIMARY SYNOVIAL CHONDROMATOSIS

Primary synovial chondromatosis is characterized by the proliferation of irregular islands of cellular cartilaginous metaplasia

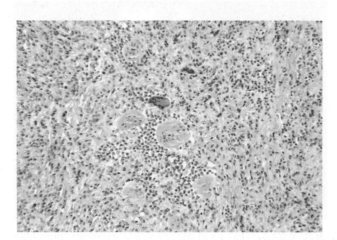

Figure 6.40. Pigmented villonodular synovitis showing the plump histiocytic cells with occasional giant cells and focal hemosiderin deposits.

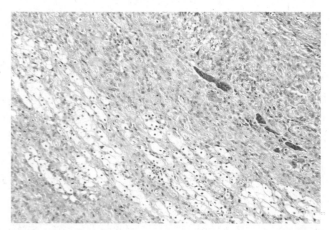

Figure 6.41. Another field showing areas of both fibrous scarring and lipid-laden histiocytes. The scar tissue has a trabeculated, almost "bony" appearance.

within the synovium of a joint (or tendon sheath), generally without any underlying arthritis (51,52). This finding distinguishes it from the much more commonly observed cartilaginous loose bodies in the joints and synovial tissues of patients with various types of arthritis.

Grossly, the affected joint cavity may contain hundreds of cartilaginous loose bodies, although the articular surfaces of the joint are likely to be intact. The synovial membrane contains many cartilaginous nodules ranging in size from 1 to 2 mm to several centimeters (Fig. 6.43).

Microscopically, nodular foci of chondrometaplasia occur in the synovium, characterized by markedly disorganized clumps of cartilage cells with some cytologic atypia (Fig. 6.44). This disordered appearance helps to differentiate primary synovial chondromatosis from the much more common secondary chondromatosis, which occurs in association with osteoarthritis and traumatic loose bodies.

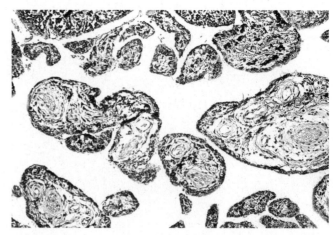

Figure 6.42. Synovium obtained from a patient with hemophilia with severe hemosiderotic synovitis. The hemosiderin is confined mainly to the synovial lining cells, and within the synovium, there is no histiocytic or giant cell proliferation, as would occur in pigmented villonodular synovitis. Grossly, both lesions appear mahogany brown. However, hemosiderotic synovitis generally has a much finer villous appearance, in contrast to the plump papillary pattern seen in pigmented villonodular synovitis.

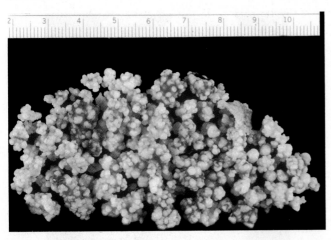

Figure 6.43. Tissue obtained from the knee joint of a patient with synovial chondromatosis. In this condition, the synovium is filled with minute cartilaginous bodies, many of which may be free within the synovial cavity. These synovial cartilaginous bodies may undergo secondary endochondral ossification and thus may appear radiodense on clinical radiographs.

Primary synovial chondromatosis frequently recurs after excision. Very rarely, malignant degeneration has been reported. In a few cases, pressure erosion of adjacent bone may lead to difficulty in differentiation from an intraosseous chondrosarcoma.

OSTEOCHONDRITIS DISSECANS

Osteochondritis dissecans is a benign noninflammatory condition of diarthrodial joints that affects young adults. The disorder is characterized by a well-demarcated fragment of bone and overlying articular cartilage, which may or may not be separated from the articular surface at the time of presentation. The condition usually involves the lateral aspect of the medial femoral

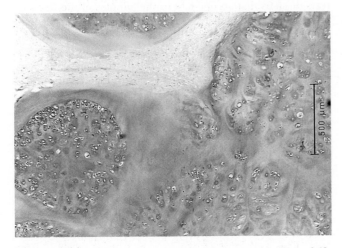

Figure 6.44. Portion of the synovium demonstrated in Figure 6.42. The cartilaginous nodules are extremely cellular, and the deposition of the chondrocytes is in the form of irregular clones lacking the regularity of the chondrocytes seen in the more commonly encountered loose bodies associated with osteoarthritis. (Compare with Fig. 6.8.)

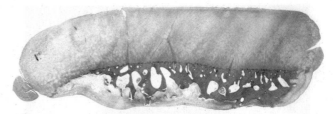

Figure 6.45. A loose body originating from the articular surface of a patient with osteochondritis dissecans. (The bone may or may not be necrotic, depending on whether the loose body is still attached to the affected epiphysis.)

condyle of the knee and, less often, the posteromedial aspect of the talus or anterolateral aspect of the capitellum. Patients complain of joint pain, often with joint effusions and occasional locking of the joint.

Although osteochondritis dissecans usually is unilateral, it may be bilateral and symmetric. Familial cases have been reported. The underlying defect in osteochondritis dissecans may be an accessory center of ossification, although trauma must play an important role in the initiation of clinical disease.

Radiographs reveal a well-demarcated defect in the articular surface of the affected joint. The gross resected specimen usually is a flat, smooth nodule formed of avascular bone, with overlying viable articular cartilage. A layer of dense fibrous connective tissue, or fibrocartilage, usually forms on the bony surface of the osteochondral fragment (Fig. 6.45). Treatment consists of reattachment of the loose body (when feasible) or excision.

MENISCAL TEARS

The menisci are composed mainly of collagen, and the principal orientation of their collagen fibers is circumferential to withstand the circumferential tension within the meniscus during normal loading. Some radially disposed fibers probably act as ties to resist longitudinal splitting of the menisci, which could result from undue compression (53). The menisci of young persons are usually white, translucent, and supple on palpation. In older persons, the menisci lose their translucency and become more opaque, yellow, and less supple.

Lacerations of the meniscus cause symptoms that require surgical treatment in two groups of patients: the young, in whom injury is frequently related to athletic activity; and older persons, in whom degeneration leads to laceration. Most lacerations take place in the posterior horn of the meniscus and, more commonly, in the medial meniscus. They usually occur as clefts that run along the circumferentially directed collagen fibers. Over time, such a cleft may extend to the medial margin of the meniscus and may create a tag (Fig. 6.46). Extension of the tear may lead to the bucket-handle deformity. Sometimes the meniscus is detached, usually posteriorly. A horizontal cleavage in the posterior horn of the meniscus is found at autopsy in more than 50% of older persons.

The advent of arthrography and arthroscopy assisted in the clinical diagnosis of tears in the menisci. These techniques help to localize tears and facilitate partial meniscectomy.

Torn menisci may have evidence of both injury and repair. However, it is often difficult to determine whether degenerative

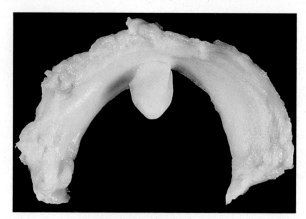

Figure 6.46. A medial meniscus removed from the knee of a patient with long-standing symptoms. A smooth tag that has developed from a linear tear of the posterior horn is seen extending into the joint space. The margins of the tag have become smooth over time.

changes result from, or contribute to, the tear. When present, repair is likely to be confined to the outer third of the meniscus, where there is normally a blood supply (54).

DISC HERNIATION

The intervertebral disc comprises a nucleus pulposus, consisting mainly of water and proteoglycan within an annulus of obliquely oriented collagen fibers and confined superiorly and inferiorly by the cartilaginous endplate. Because the water in the nucleus is incompressible, loads are transmitted hydrodynamically from one vertebra to the next through the cartilage and bony endplates, whereas radial forces are absorbed through the tension in the fibers of the annulus (55).

The disc of the young adult, with its bulging mucoid nucleus pulposus, dense collagenous annulus fibrosus, and well-defined cartilaginous endplates, can be clearly differentiated from that of the elderly person, with its shrunken, yellowed, and dehydrated nucleus pulposus. In general, acute displacement of the disc tissue is a disease of people in their third and fourth decades. It is less likely to occur or to cause significant compromise of the neural canal or foramen in an older person in whom disc tissue, especially the nucleus pulposus, is shrunken and dehydrated.

Displacement of disc tissue (usually the nucleus pulposus) from the intervertebral disc space may occur anteriorly, posterolaterally, superiorly, or inferiorly. Displacement of disc tissue anteriorly usually produces asymptomatic spondylosis deformans, whereas displacement posterolaterally produces pressure on the nerve roots or encroachment on the contents of the spinal canal. Displacement superiorly or inferiorly into the adjacent vertebral bodies leads to the development of Schmorl nodes.

Displacement of the nuclear tissue requires prior traumatic laceration of the annular fibers where the collagen bundles attach to the vertebral bodies by Sharpey fibers. Such tears are usually associated with torsion and compression injuries and result from the sudden application of load.

Spondylosis deformans, as a result of anterior protrusion, is one of the most common forms of spinal disease seen radiographi-

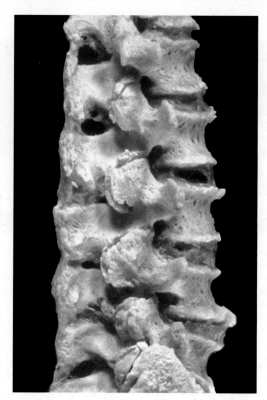

Figure 6.47. A postero-oblique view of the lumbar spine of an elderly man. There is severe arthritis of the facet joints together with exuberant marginal osteophytes, particularly anteriorly. The intervertebral foramina are narrowed, and the osteophytic extension into them may cause nerve root compression.

cally and at autopsy. By the age of 50 years, it is present in more than half the population. It occurs more frequently in people engaged in occupations that require heavy physical labor. The lumbar spine is the site most commonly affected (Fig. 6.47).

Posterolateral displacement is found at autopsy in approximately 50% of older persons, mostly in the lumbar region of the spine. The basis for posterior disc displacement is the small tears or clefts that accumulate in the annulus of the disc as a result of the stress of daily activities. Clinical symptoms depend on the amount of disc tissue displaced and its proximity to neural structures. Surgically removed material usually displays evidence of matrix degeneration and cell death along with regenerative clones of chondrocytes (Fig. 6.48). Late recurrence of pain may result from further displacement of disc tissue or from scarring, which is sometimes accompanied by calcification and ossification. The relative infrequency of osteophyte formation in the posterior aspect of the vertebral body results from the firm attachment of the disc to the posterior longitudinal ligament. Disc degeneration and consequent narrowing of the intervertebral space will lead to facet joint arthritis and often to instability. Further injury to the subchondral bone plate will result in severe osteoarthritis of the intervertebral joint.

GANGLION

A *ganglion* is a fibrous-walled cyst filled with clear mucinous fluid, usually without a recognizable lining of differentiated

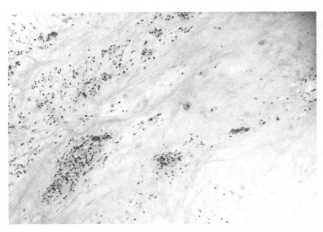

Figure 6.48. Tissue removed from a herniated intervertebral disc. There are fragments of irregular fibrillar matrix, some of which appear necrotic but within which are small foci of proliferating cartilage cells and focal perivascular inflammatory tissue.

cells. These cysts occur in the soft tissues, usually dissecting between tissue planes, and are often seen around the hands and feet, particularly on the extensor surfaces near joints. The most common location is around the wrist joint. Similar cystic lesions may be seen in the parameniscal tissue of the knee joint, usually in the lateral meniscus (Fig. 6.49), as well as in the lumbar spine.

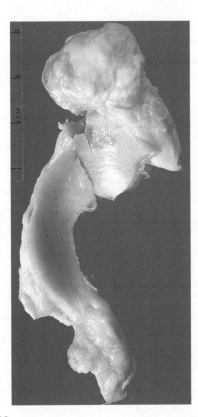

Figure 6.49. A lateral meniscus removed from a patient with symptoms of internal derangement of the knee. Attached to the perimeter of the posterior horn of the meniscus is a fibrous-walled cyst, which was filled with clear mucoid fluid.

Ganglia may arise as herniations of the synovium; alternatively, they may arise from mucinous degeneration within dense fibrous connective tissue, possibly secondary to repeated trauma, especially on the extensor surfaces of the hands and feet. Rarely, a communication with the joint cavity is demonstrable. On occasion, ganglia may erode the adjacent bone and may become totally intraosseous. The most common site for an intraosseous ganglion is the medial malleolus of the tibia (56). On microscopic examination, the wall of the cyst is generally fibrous and lined by flattened cells; inflammation may be observed if the cyst previously has been ruptured.

BURSITIS

Bursitis is characterized by pain, redness, and swelling in and around one of the many bursae that lie between the muscles, tendons, and bony prominences, especially around the joints. It commonly results from chronic trauma and is frequently seen in the shoulders of professional athletes and in the prepatellar and infrapatellar bursae of those who kneel. Bursitis is sometimes seen as a complication of rheumatoid arthritis, particularly in the popliteal area (Baker cyst). Bursitis may also result from infection, as in tuberculous infection of the trochanteric bursae. Sometimes extensive calcification may complicate a chronically inflamed bursa.

On gross examination of an inflamed bursa, the wall of the bursal sac is usually markedly thickened, and the lining is often erythematous and shaggy as a result of fibrinous exudation into the cavity. Microscopic examination generally shows chronic inflammation and scarring.

MORTON NEUROMA

Morton neuroma is a distinct clinicopathologic entity characterized by thickening and degeneration of one of the interdigital nerves of the foot, most commonly that between the third and fourth metatarsal heads (57). The patient, usually a woman, experiences sharp shooting pains that are worse when standing. These pains characteristically begin in the sole of the foot and radiate to the exterior surface. At surgery, a fusiform swelling proximal to the bifurcation of the plantar interdigital nerve is usually seen. When dissected, the resected specimen usually includes the neurovascular bundle (Fig. 6.50).

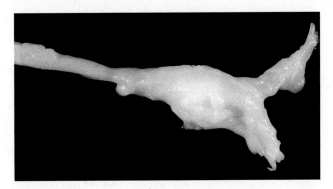

Figure 6.50. A segment of the plantar interdigital nerve resected from the space between the third and fourth metatarsal heads in a patient with Morton neuroma. There is fusiform swelling of the neurovascular bundle just proximal to the bifurcation.

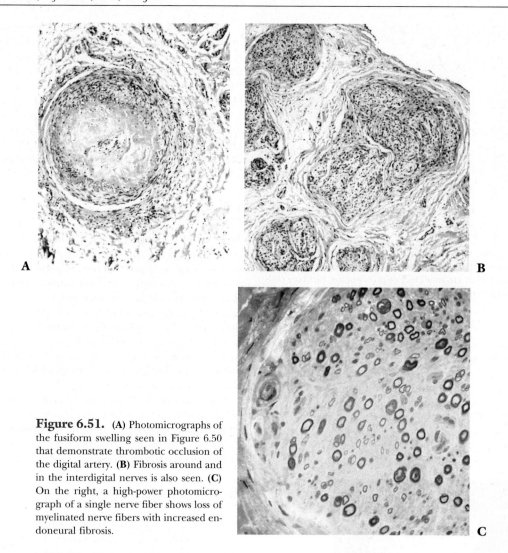

Figure 6.51. **(A)** Photomicrographs of the fusiform swelling seen in Figure 6.50 that demonstrate thrombotic occlusion of the digital artery. **(B)** Fibrosis around and in the interdigital nerves is also seen. **(C)** On the right, a high-power photomicrograph of a single nerve fiber shows loss of myelinated nerve fibers with increased endoneural fibrosis.

Characteristic microscopic features include the following: endarterial thickening of the digital artery, often with thrombosis and occlusion of the lumen; extensive fibrosis both around and within the nerve, giving rise to demyelinization and a marked depletion of axons within the digital nerve; and evidence of Schwann cell and fibroblast proliferation (Fig. 6.51). These findings are most consistent with recurrent nerve trauma, probably caused by wearing poorly fitting shoes. Morton neuroma should be differentiated from amputation (traumatic) neuroma, which may also occur in the interdigital nerves of the feet, although much more rarely.

REFERENCES

1. Bullough PG. Pathology. In Klippel JH, Dieppe P, eds. *Rheumatology.* London, United Kingdom: Mosby, 1998:8.1–8.8.
2. Nakata K, Bullough PG. The injury and repair of human articular cartilage: a morphological study of 192 cases of coxarthrosis. *Nippon Seikeigeka Gakkai Zasshi* 1986;60:763–775.
3. Hunter DJ, Li J, Lavalley M, Bauer DC, Nevitt M, Degroot J, et al. Cartilage markers and their association with cartilage loss on MRI in knee osteoarthritis: the Boston Osteoarthritis Knee Study. *Arthritis Res Ther* 2007;9:R108.
4. Macys JR, Bullough PG, Wilson PD Jr. Coxarthrosis: a study of the natural history based on a correlation of clinical, radiographic, and pathologic findings. *Semin Arthritis Rheum* 1980;10:66–80.
5. Benjamin M, McGonagle D. Histopathologic changes at "synovio-entheseal complexes" suggesting a novel mechanism for synovitis in osteoarthritis and spondyloarthritis. *Arthritis Rheum* 2007;56:3601–3609.
6. Eichenholtz SN. *Charcot Joints.* Springfield, IL: Charles C. Thomas, 1966.
7. Yamamoto T, Schneider R, Bullough PG. Insufficiency subchondral fracture of the femoral head. *Am J Surg Pathol* 2000;24:464–468.
8. Postel M, Kerboull M. Total prosthetic replacement in rapidly destructive arthrosis of the hip joint. *Clin Orthop Relat Res* 1970;72:138–144.
9. Yamamoto T, Bullough PG. The role of subchondral insufficiency fracture in rapid destruction of the hip joint: a preliminary report. *Arthritis Rheum* 2000;43:2423–2427.
10. Yamamoto T, Schneider R, Bullough PG. Subchondral insufficiency fracture of the femoral head: histopathologic correlation with MRI. *Skeletal Radiol* 2001;30:247–254.
11. Yamamoto T, Schneider R, Iwamoto Y, Bullough P. Histopathologic prevalence of subchondral insufficiency fracture of the femoral head. *Ann Rheum Dis* 2008;67:150–153.
12. Ainola MM, Mandelin JA, Liljestrom MP, Li TF, Hukkanen MV, Konttinen YT. Pannus invasion and cartilage degradation in rheumatoid arthritis: involvement of MMP-3 and interleukin-1beta. *Clin Exp Rheumatol* 2005;23:644–650.
13. Rhodes LA, Conaghan PG, Radjenovic A, Grainger AJ, Emery P, McGonagle D. Further evidence that a cartilage-pannus junction synovitis predilection is not a specific feature of rheumatoid arthritis. *Ann Rheum Dis* 2005;64:1347–1349.
14. Firestein GS. Rheumatoid synovitis and pannus. In Klippel JH, Dieppe P, eds. *Rheumatology.* London, United Kingdom: Mosby, 1998:13.1–13.24.
15. Bullough PG, DiCarlo EF. Subchondral avascular necrosis: a common cause of arthritis. *Ann Rheum Dis* 1990;49:412–420.
16. Glimcher MJ, Kenzora JE. The biology of osteonecrosis of the human femoral head and its clinical implications: II. The pathological changes in the femoral head as an organ and in the hip joint. *Clin Orthop Relat Res* 1979;139:283–312.
17. Bullough PG, Kambolis CP, Marcove RC. Bone infarctions not associated with caisson disease. *J Bone Joint Surg Am* 1965;47A:477–491.
18. Catto M. A histological study of avascular necrosis of the femoral head after transcervical fracture. *J Bone Joint Surg Am* 1965;47:749–776.
19. Franchi A, Bullough PG. Secondary avascular necrosis in coxarthrosis: a morphologic study. *J Rheumatol* 1992;19:1263–1268.
20. Pillinger MH, Rosenthal P, Abeles AM. Hyperuricemia and gout: new insights into pathogenesis and treatment. *Bull NYU Hosp Jt Dis* 2007;65:215–221.
21. Boss GR, Seegmiller JE. Hyperuricemia and gout. Classification, complications and management. *N Engl J Med* 1979;300:1459–1468.

22. Gatter RA. The compensated polarized light microscope in clinical rheumatology. *Arthritis Rheum* 1974;17:253–255.

23. Sissons HA, Steiner GC, Bonar F, May M, Rosenberg ZS, Samuels H, et al. Tumoral calcium pyrophosphate deposition disease. *Skeletal Radiol* 1989;18:79–87.

24. McCarty DJ. Crystals and arthritis. *Dis Mon* 1994;40:255–299.

25. Markel SF, Hart WR. Arthropathy in calcium pyrophosphate dihydrate crystal deposition disease. Pathologic study of 12 cases. *Arch Pathol Lab Med* 1982;106:529–533.

26. Reginato AJ, Schumacher HR, Martinez VA. The articular cartilage in familial chondrocalcinosis. Light and electron microscopic study. *Arthritis Rheum* 1974;17:977–992.

27. Cheung HS. Role of calcium-containing crystals in osteoarthritis. *Front Biosci* 2005;10:1336–1340.

28. Resnick D, Niwayama G, Goergen TG, Utsinger PD, Shapiro RF, Haselwood DH, et al. Clinical, radiographic and pathologic abnormalities in calcium pyrophosphate dihydrate deposition disease (CPPD): pseudogout. *Radiology* 1977;122:1–15.

29. Rosenthal AK. Calcium crystal deposition and osteoarthritis. *Rheum Dis Clin North Am* 2006;32:401–412.

30. Rosenthal AK. Update in calcium deposition diseases. *Curr Opin Rheumatol* 2007;19:158–162.

31. Russell RG, Kanis JA. Ectopic calcification and ossification. In Nordin BEC, ed. *Metabolic Bone and Stone Disease.* Edinburgh, United Kingdom: Churchill Livingstone, 1993.

32. Slavin RE, Wen J, Kumar D, Evans EB. Familial tumoral calcinosis. A clinical, histopathologic, and ultrastructural study with an analysis of its calcifying process and pathogenesis. *Am J Surg Pathol* 1993;17:788–802.

33. Lipsky BA, Weigelt JA, Gupta V, Killian A, Peng MM. Skin, soft tissue, bone, and joint infections in hospitalized patients: epidemiology and microbiological, clinical, and economic outcomes. *Infect Control Hosp Epidemiol* 2007;28:1290–1298.

34. Green NE, Edwards K. Bone and joint infections in children. *Orthop Clin North Am* 1987;18:555–576.

35. Gifford DB, Patzakis M, Ivler D, Swezey RL. Septic arthritis due to pseudomonas in heroin addicts. *J Bone Joint Surg Am* 1975;57:631–635.

36. Bender BL, Yunis EJ. Disseminated nongranulomatous *Mycobacterium avium* osteomyelitis. *Hum Pathol* 1980;11:476–478.

37. Moran E, Masters S, Berendt AR, McLardy-Smith P, Byren I, Atkins BL. Guiding empirical antibiotic therapy in orthopaedics: the microbiology of prosthetic joint infection managed by debridement, irrigation and prosthesis retention. *J Infect* 2007;55:1–7.

38. Berendt AR, McLardy-Smith P. Prosthetic joint infection. *Curr Infect Dis Rep* 1999;1:267–272.

39. Mendes DG, Figarola F, Bullough PG, Loudis P. High density polyethylene prosthetic femoral head replacement in the dog. *Clin Orthop Relat Res* 1975;274–283.

40. Black J, Sherk H, Bonini J, Rostoker WR, Schajowicz F, Galante JO. Metallosis associated with a stable titanium-alloy femoral component in total hip replacement. A case report. *J Bone Joint Surg Am* 1990;72:126–130.

41. Kircher T. Silicone lymphadenopathy: a complication of silicone elastomer finger joint prostheses. *Hum Pathol* 1980;11:240–244.

42. Gordon M, Bullough PG. Synovial and osseous inflammation in failed silicone-rubber prostheses. *J Bone Joint Surg Am* 1982;64:574–580.

43. Hallel T, Lew S, Bansal M. Villous lipomatous proliferation of the synovial membrane (lipoma arborescens). *J Bone Joint Surg Am* 1988;70:264–270.

44. Mendenhall WM, Mendenhall CM, Reith JD, Scarborough MT, Gibbs CP, Mendenhall NP. Pigmented villonodular synovitis. *Am J Clin Oncol* 2006;29:548–550.

45. Adem C, Sebo TJ, Riehle DL, Lohse CM, Nascimento AG. Recurrent and non-recurrent pigmented villonodular synovitis 1. *Ann Pathol* 2002;22:448–452.

46. Docken WP. Pigmented villonodular synovitis. *Ann Rheum Dis* 1997;56:336.

47. Docken WP. Pigmented villonodular synovitis: a review with illustrative case reports. *Semin Arthritis Rheum* 1979;9:1–22.

48. Layfield LJ, Meloni-Ehrig A, Liu K, Shepard R, Harrelson JM. Malignant giant cell tumor of synovium (malignant pigmented villonodular synovitis). *Arch Pathol Lab Med* 2000;124:1636–1641.

49. Arnold WD, Hilgartner MW. Hemophilic arthropathy. Current concepts of pathogenesis and management. *J Bone Joint Surg Am* 1977;59:287–305.

50. Rodriguez-Merchan EC. Pathogenesis, early diagnosis, and prophylaxis for chronic hemophilic synovitis. *Clin Orthop Relat Res* 1997;343:6–11.

51. Villacin AB, Brigham LN, Bullough PG. Primary and secondary synovial chondrometaplasia: histopathologic and clinicoradiologic differences. *Hum Pathol* 1979;10:439–451.

52. Murphey MD, Vidal JA, Fanburg-Smith JC, Gajewski DA. Imaging of synovial chondromatosis with radiologic-pathologic correlation. *Radiographics* 2007;27:1465–1488.

53. Bullough PG, Munuera L, Murphy J, Weinstein AM. The strength of the menisci of the knee as it relates to their fine structure. *J Bone Joint Surg Br* 1970;52:564–567.

54. Arnoczky SP, Warren RF. The microvasculature of the meniscus and its response to injury. An experimental study in the dog. *Am J Sports Med* 1983;11:131–141.

55. Bullough PG, Boachie-Adjei O. *Atlas of Spinal Diseases.* New York, NY: Gower Medical Publishing, 1988.

56. Kambolis C, Bullough PG, Jaffe HI. Ganglionic cystic defects of bone. *J Bone Joint Surg Am* 1973;55:496–505.

57. Morscher E, Ulrich J, Dick W. Morton's intermetatarsal neuroma: morphology and histological substrate. *Foot Ankle Int* 2000;21:558–562.

Nonneoplastic Diseases of Bones

This chapter discusses the three main classes of bone disease, other than neoplasms, of concern to the surgical pathologist: metabolic disease, traumatic lesions, and infections. The chapter begins with a brief discussion of bone structure and tissue preparation.

TISSUE STRUCTURE

Most of the organ systems that present to the surgical pathologist consist of cellular tissues. The connective tissues are made up principally of an extracellular matrix, which serves a mechanical function (1). In general, most of the symptoms of connective tissue disease are a result of structural failure of the extracellular matrix (e.g., fracture).

Connective tissues (e.g., ligaments, tendons, bone, cartilage) are subjected principally to three types of applied stress: compression, tension, and shear. The constituents of the extracellular matrix are ideally suited to resisting one or another of these types of stress. Whereas collagen resists tension, hydroxyapatite in the bone and the large globular proteoglycan aggregates in the cartilage are particularly well suited to resisting compression. Thus, the combination of matrix constituents in each type of tissue reflects the types of stresses that are applied to it.

The extracellular matrix is synthesized and, to a greater or lesser extent, broken down by its intrinsic cells (i.e., fibroblasts, osteoblasts, and chondroblasts) (2). The matrix has a very definite microarchitecture designed to resist the forces that act on the anatomic structure (3,4). For example, collagen fibers run more or less parallel to the length of the ligaments and tendons. Similarly, within the cancellous bone, the trabeculae are arranged along the principal lines of stress. The cortex is thicker in the middle of the shaft of a long bone to resist bending forces, whereas the cancellous bone is concentrated at the ends of the long bones to resist the mainly compressive forces that are common at that site. It is important for the surgical pathologist to understand these physiologic and anatomic principles because without them it is not easy to interpret the histologic findings in diseased connective tissues.

METHODS OF EXAMINATION

Specimens received by the surgical pathologist from orthopaedic operations often consist of fragments of bone and soft tissue without obvious anatomic landmarks. However, when a large piece of bone is submitted, anatomic landmarks should be carefully sought (5). The bony specimens should be cut into thin slices of 3 or 4 mm with a band saw. The cut surfaces of the bone should be gently washed and brushed with a nail brush to remove the bone dust, which otherwise may cause histologic artifacts. The color of the bone should be noted; necrotic or dead bone is likely to have an opaque and yellow appearance, whereas living bone appears translucent and pink. An obvious increase or decrease in bone density should be sought, as should localized lesions. Obviously, some experience is required to perform the examination, and we have found that a dissecting microscope, such as is used in the operating room, is useful for this purpose. Another useful adjunct to the gross examination is the preparation of radiographs of the sliced bone specimens. These can be very helpful in defining both the texture and margins of a lesion, which may not be immediately apparent on gross examination; we have found this technique to be particularly useful in looking for the nidus of an osteoid osteoma (Fig. 7.1).

The routine sectioning of bone after embedding requires that calcium be removed from the bone before histologic sections are prepared. Calcium can be removed successfully and relatively quickly if some simple guidelines are followed. First, before decalcification, the tissue must be well fixed. Second, slices, not whole specimens, should be decalcified. Third, it must be realized that as the calcium is removed by acid, the acid is neutralized. Therefore, it is necessary that an adequate amount of acid be used, the acid be changed frequently, and a shaker be used to ensure that the acid thoroughly infiltrates the specimen. Following decalcification, all the acid must be washed out of the specimen; otherwise, poor staining may result. Washing for at least 12 hours in running water usually ensures good differentiation of the hematoxylin and eosin stain.

Scanning electron microscopy has proved useful for studying bone texture (6). Transmission electron microscopy may be useful in the differential diagnosis of certain tumors (7).

Histomorphometry, which is the quantification of morphologic features at the tissue and cellular levels, can further define the metabolic diseases of bone (8). The parameters indicative of bone formation include the percentages of active osteoblastic surface, osteoid surface, and mineralizing surface. Those indicative of bone mineralization include osteoid volume and mineral apposition rate. Those indicative of bone resorption include total eroded surface and active osteoclastic surface. Table 7.1 summarizes these parameters in the various metabolic bone diseases. Pathologists often say, "I don't need a number to make the diagnosis of osteoporosis." This is true, but morphometry helps clarify the dynamics of the disease and subtle alterations in the balance between osteoblast formative activity and osteoclast resorption. Morphometry enhances the assessment of metabolic bone disease by supplementing the information gained from qualitative visual examination with quantitative information. Furthermore, the discipline required to make objective measurements can only improve visual diagnostic acumen.

METABOLIC DISEASES

The quality and quantity of the extracellular matrix of the bone reflect cellular activity (9–11). Osteoblasts synthesize the collag-

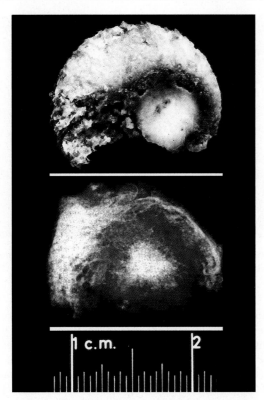

Figure 7.1. Photograph (*above*) of a section through a gross specimen of an osteoid osteoma with a specimen radiograph (*below*). The lucent area around the nidus represents fibrovascular tissue. (See text for technique.)

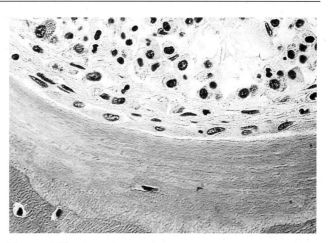

Figure 7.2. Bone trabeculae showing a layer of plump osteoblasts at the surface.

is often referred to as *cell coupling* or *linkage*. The rate of matrix production is reflected in the cytologic appearance of the osteoblasts, which range from flat (inactive) to plump (active) (Fig. 7.2). As bone formation proceeds, some of the osteoblasts are buried within the matrix and become osteocytes. The osteocytes maintain contact with each other and with the surface osteoblasts through cellular processes that run through a network of canaliculi within the bone matrix to form a functional syncytium, which is thought to play a major role in both mineral and structural homeostasis (Fig. 7.3). Osteoblastic activity is probably positively influenced by increased physical activity, parathyroid hormone, and certain growth factors. Activity of the osteoblasts is suppressed by inactivity and steroid hormones (12–14).

When the osteoblasts synthesize collagen, it is deposited in parallel layers to produce the lamellar pattern that characterizes normal adult bone (Fig. 7.4). Time is required to achieve this high degree of organization, and when bone is formed and deposited rapidly, as in the fetus, a fracture callus, or certain

enous matrix of the bone and regulate its mineralization. Osteoclasts, which may be multinucleated, are fewer in number than osteoblasts and are responsible for removing bone. For the amount of bone in the skeleton to stay the same, the rate of production must equal the rate of resorption; this equilibrium

TABLE 7.1	Parameters Indicative of Bone Formation					
	Disease					
Parameter	*Secondary Active Osteoporosis*	*Senile Active Osteoporosis*	*Vitamin D Deficiency Osteomalacia*	*Paget Disease*	*Hyperparathyroidism*	*Aluminum Toxicity*
Cancellous bone volume	D	D	N or I	I	I	N or I
Mineralized cancellous bone volume	D	D	N or D	I	I	N or I
Osteoid volume	N or I	N or I	I	I	I	I
Osteoid surface	N or I	N or I	I	I	I	I
Osteoid thickness	N or I	N or I	I	I	I	I
Osteoblast surface	N or I	N or D	I	I	I	D or 0
Mineralizing surface	N	N or D	N or D	N or I	I	D or 0
Mineral apposition rate	N or I	D	D	N or I	I	D or 0
Osteoid maturation rate	N or I	I	I	N	N	I
Eroded surface	I	N or I	I	I	I	N or I
Osteoclast surface	I	N or D	I	I	I	N or D
Osteoclast number	I	N or D	I	I	I	N or D

D, decrease; I, increased; N, normal.

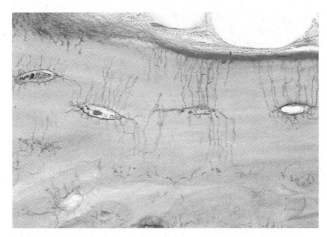

Figure 7.3. Photomicrograph demonstrating osteocytes and osteocytic canaliculi.

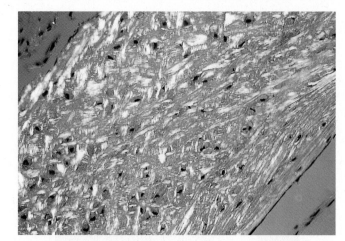

Figure 7.5. Disordered arrangement of the collagen in immature woven bone. Polarized light.

neoplastic and hypermetabolic states, it is less obviously organized, and the collagen has a basketlike weave. This type of bone is referred to as *woven* or *immature bone* (Fig. 7.5). It is never a normal microscopic finding and should alert the pathologist to look for underlying pathology. (The microscopic examination of collagen is greatly aided by the use of polarized light, which demonstrates not only the collagen fibers but also their organization.)

The distribution of calcium in bone cannot be studied by examining decalcified sections. However, it is possible to study the mineralization of the matrix if undecalcified sections are prepared. For the study of those diseases in which disturbed mineralization is suspected, this examination is essential (15). When the organic matrix is first deposited by the osteoblast, it is not mineralized; therefore, a layer of unmineralized matrix, termed *osteoid*, is always present at the formative surface of bone (Fig. 7.6). Normally, this layer is very thin because the time between matrix deposition and subsequent mineralization is short; however, when the rates of deposition and mineralization are unbalanced, the amount and extent of the osteoid increase, and hyperosteoidosis may develop. Hyperosteoidosis occurs basically for three reasons. First, in any condition in which bone

formation is increased, the osteoid surfaces are both more extensive and thicker (e.g., fracture callus, Paget disease, hyperparathyroidism). Second, the mineralization of bone depends on the presence of many substances, including calcium, phosphorus, vitamin D, and alkaline phosphatase. If the amount of any of these substances is inadequate, mineralization is delayed, perhaps markedly. Third, the presence in bone of certain inhibitory or toxic substances, such as aluminum, iron, and fluoride, may block mineralization, even though the amounts of calcium, alkaline phosphatase, and vitamin D in the tissues are adequate.

Tetracycline binds to actively mineralizing surfaces and exhibits fluorescence in ultraviolet light on microscopic examination, and these features have made it a valuable aid in the study of bone and bone diseases (16). Pulsed doses of tetracycline can be administered to a patient before biopsy to determine the extent of mineralization and the amount of bone formed over a given time (Fig. 7.7). Additionally, the morphology of the tetracycline labels reflects the cause of the disease process. When mineralization is blocked, especially in an aluminum-associated disease, the label is not taken up. On the other hand, in patients with vitamin D deficiency, the labels are often exten-

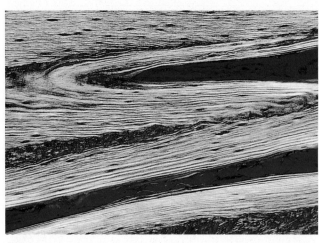

Figure 7.4. Lamellar arrangement of normal adult bone. Polarized light.

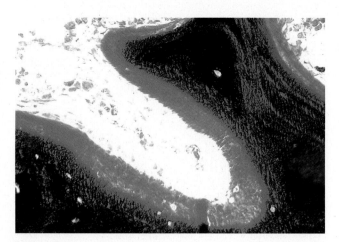

Figure 7.6. A section of undecalcified bone demonstrating a layer of unmineralized bone (osteoid) at the surface. The osteoid in this section is stained red, and the mineralized bone is black.

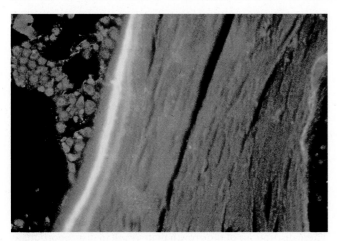

Figure 7.7. Photomicrograph taken with ultraviolet illumination to show two tetracycline labels at the bone formative surfaces. Oxytetracycline gives a green fluorescence, and the demeclocycline (Declomycin) gives a yellow fluorescence.

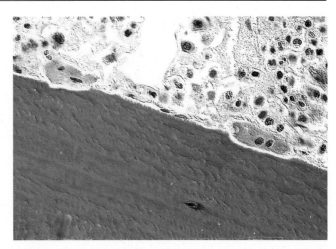

Figure 7.9. The irregular eroded surface associated with osteoclastic activity. Two osteoclasts are seen at the surface lying in shallow depressions, or Howship lacunae.

sive and smudged, whereas they are sharp in persons with normal bone formation (Fig. 7.8). (It should be noted that tetracycline may be passively absorbed onto a recently resorbed surface and thus confuse interpretation.)

The resorption of bone by osteoclasts, rather than reflecting physiologic calcium homeostasis, is primarily associated with maintenance of the structural integrity of the skeleton. Morphologically, osteoclasts, which are large cells containing approximately two to four nuclei, adhere to the bone surface and are seen in depressions referred to as *Howship lacunae* or *resorption bays* (Fig. 7.9). In cancellous bone, resorption is generally limited to the bone surface, and the portions of the surface that have been resorbed can be recognized by an irregular, scalloped appearance, which contrasts with the smooth surface of formative or resting bone. Eventually, the resorptive surfaces are again covered by osteoblasts, and new bone forms on them. The junction between the original resorbed surface and the new bone is marked on sections stained with hematoxylin and eosin by a sharp basophilic line referred to as a *reversal front* or *cement line* (Fig. 7.10) (17).

In diseases characterized by increased modeling, such as Paget disease and osteoporosis, the osteoclastic activity, although often markedly increased, is generally confined to the surface. However, in hyperparathyroidism, whether primary or secondary, the osteoclasts characteristically tunnel into the mineralized bone matrix, creating a "wormhole" appearance referred to as *dissecting resorption*. However, regardless of the cause or patterns of resorption, the architecture of the bone is distorted in all pathologic resorptive states.

Cortical bone in adults is composed of closely applied, densely compact cylindric units called *osteons* (Fig. 7.11). Primary osteons are formed in juveniles by the ingrowth of periosteal blood vessels that follow a "cutting cone" of osteoclasts, which tunnel through the existing cortex deposited by the periosteum. The tunnel, or haversian canal, formed by the osteoclasts and containing the vessels is subsequently partially filled in by osteoblasts, which deposit concentric layers of bone matrix. Secondary and subsequent osteons are formed during the process of remodeling by the outgrowth from existing haversian

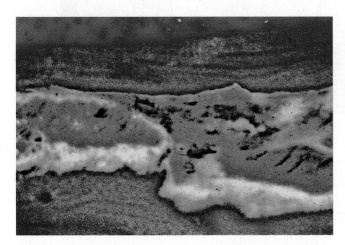

Figure 7.8. Photomicrograph demonstrating a smudged tetracycline label at the mineralization front in a patient with osteomalacia.

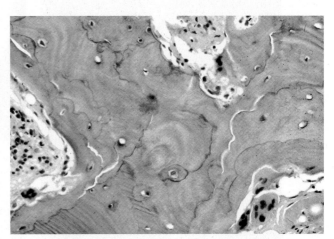

Figure 7.10. Photomicrograph demonstrating cement line in bone from a patient with advanced Paget disease. Numerous wavy blue cement lines seen throughout the specimen create a mosaic pattern in the bone.

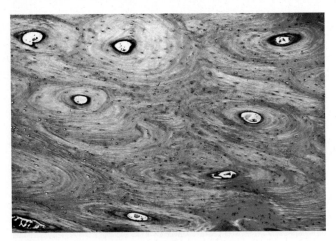

Figure 7.11. Haversian systems in cortical bone.

systems of new vessels; these are also preceded by a cluster of osteoclasts.

ABNORMAL FORMATION OF THE ORGANIC MATRIX

The synthesis of collagen by the cells may be abnormal because of either genetic or acquired conditions. Examples of the former are osteogenesis imperfecta and Ehlers-Danlos syndrome, whereas examples of the latter are scurvy and lathyrism. Today, the condition most likely to be seen by the surgical pathologist is osteogenesis imperfecta.

Osteogenesis Imperfecta

Osteogenesis imperfecta, one of the most common of the congenital connective tissue matrix diseases, comprises several distinct syndromes, some inherited as an autosomal dominant trait and others as a recessive trait; still others occur as spontaneous mutations. Persons with these various syndromes have in common a short stature and a propensity for fracture. Many of the patients also have poorly formed dentin, hearing loss, and frequently blue sclerae. Most of their clinical problems are caused by fractures, and those more severely affected, during the course of their childhood, sustain hundreds of major and minor fractures. The fractures occur more often in the lower limbs and, in a significant number of cases, involve the growth plates around the knee joints, giving rise eventually to growth plate fragmentation. Subsequent independent growth of the cartilage fragments causes swelling of the epiphyseal end of the bone. The deformed bone end filled with nodules of cartilage has been likened, on x-ray films, to a bag of popcorn (Fig. 7.12). These disruptions of the growth plate result in disproportionate shortening of the lower limbs in affected persons (18).

Bone samples from patients with the severe congenital form of osteogenesis imperfecta characteristically lack an organized trabecular pattern. The osteocytes are crowded within the bone, reflecting diminished collagen synthesis by the crowded osteoblasts at the surface. Frequently, large areas of woven bone are seen. In less severely affected persons, the bone is generally lamellar in pattern, although even in this bone, the osteocytes are crowded and the lamellae may be thinner than those in age-matched controls (Fig. 7.13). The lack of collagen synthesis by osteoblasts results in severely osteoporotic bone, which in turn leads to the numerous fractures characteristic of this condition.

ABNORMAL MINERALIZATION

The mineralization of bone depends on several factors, including vitamin D, calcium, phosphate, and alkaline phosphatase,

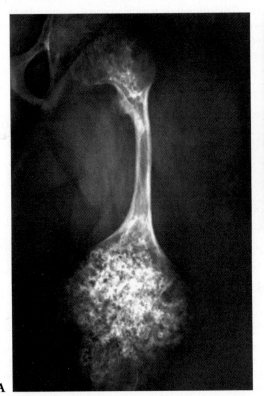

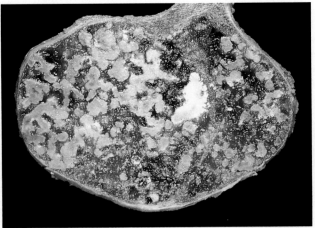

Figure 7.12. (A) Pelvis and femur of a patient with osteogenesis imperfecta. Marked swelling of the distal end of the femur with numerous dense, circular calcified inclusions creates an appearance that has been likened to a bag of popcorn. **(B)** The sectioned lower end of the femur shown in **A** demonstrates that the calcified lesions seen on the x-ray film are in fact cartilaginous nodules. These nodules arise from fragmentation of the epiphyseal growth plate.

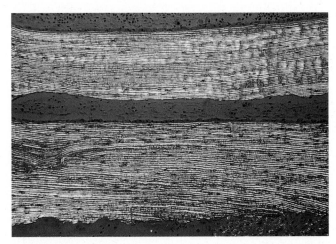

Figure 7.13. Polarized light photomicrograph demonstrating the fine lamellar pattern seen in patients with osteogenesis imperfecta. This photograph should be contrasted with Figure 7.4.

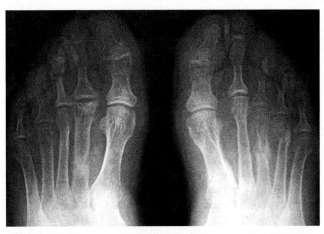

Figure 7.14. Clinical radiograph of both feet to demonstrate bilateral stress fractures of the metatarsal bones. The fracture lines are transverse, which is characteristic of insufficiency fractures in osteomalacia.

and it may be disturbed by the presence of certain metals, such as lead, strontium, iron, and aluminum.

Because the routine microscopic examination of bone requires decalcification of the tissue before embedding and sectioning, disease resulting from abnormal mineralization is likely to be overlooked by pathologists unless the clinician has alerted them to the possibility. Plastic embedding can be used to prepare undecalcified sections. If small pieces of only cancellous bone are used, even paraffin-embedded undecalcified tissue may provide adequate sections for diagnosis.

Osteomalacia and Rickets

In general, the terms *osteomalacia* (in adults) and *rickets* (in children) are used to describe those diseases that result from a deficiency in vitamin D, an abnormality in the metabolism of vitamin D, or a deficiency of calcium in the diet. The most common symptom of osteomalacia is bone pain, which is usually generalized and often vague. In addition, the low calcium level may cause muscle weakness, which is often profound (19). Radiographic examination reveals generalized osteopenia with the classic finding of multiple bilateral and symmetric partial linear fractures of the bone, commonly referred to as *insufficiency fractures* (Fig. 7.14).

On microscopic examination, the most striking abnormalities are a massive increase in the amount of unmineralized bone (up to 40% or 50% of the total bone volume) and disorganization of the trabecular architecture. The mineralization front, which is the junction between the osteoid and mineralized bone, is very irregular, granular, and fuzzy. In addition to an increase in osteoid volume, bone volume is often increased overall as a consequence of increased osteoblastic activity (Fig. 7.15).

Rickets is the childhood manifestation of osteomalacia. In childhood, the anatomic changes are found most characteristically around the metaphyses of the most rapidly growing bones—that is, around the knee and wrist joints. On x-ray films, the epiphyseal growth plates are irregular and broadened and have a characteristic cup shape. Microscopically, the growth plate is thickened and poorly defined, especially on its metaphyseal side, where tongues of uncalcified cartilage can be seen

extending into the metaphysis. As in adults, the bone shows extensive, wide osteoid seams.

In addition to the classic forms of osteomalacia and rickets secondary to calcium and vitamin D deficiencies, severe osteomalacia may occasionally be secondary to hypophosphatemia. Usually, the hypophosphatemia is the result of increased urinary phosphate loss, which may be the consequence of a primary renal tubular defect, diuretic therapy, or hyperparathyroidism. Very rarely, hypophosphatemia is associated with hormone-producing soft tissue tumors, particularly benign fibrovascular tumors, resulting in oncogenic osteomalacia. In this instance, resection of the tumor generally results in complete resolution of the osteomalacia. Therefore, it is important to look for an occult tumor in cases of osteomalacia without a clear cause (20,21).

Hypophosphatasia

Hypophosphatasia (not to be confused with hypophosphatemia) is a rare genetic disease characterized by a disturb-

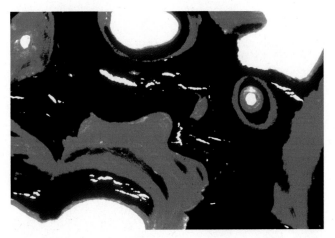

Figure 7.15. Photomicrograph of a section of undecalcified bone shows the extent of bone that is unmineralized. The portion stained red is unmineralized osteoid, and the portion stained black contains hydroxyapatite.

ance in the synthesis of the enzyme alkaline phosphatase (22). It takes two forms. The first is inherited as an autosomal recessive trait that manifests as severe disease in infants. In general, when hypophosphatasia is diagnosed in infants younger than 6 months of age, it follows a rapidly progressive fatal course. The second form is an autosomal dominant condition that may not become evident until adulthood. In these cases, the disease is less severe and often asymptomatic.

The disorder is characterized clinically by decreased levels of alkaline phosphatase in the blood, bone, intestines, liver, and kidneys. The serum phosphorus and calcium levels are usually normal. In less severe cases, hypophosphatasia may not present clinically until the fourth, fifth, or sixth decade of life. Patients often have a childhood history of a rickets-like disorder, short stature, and deformed extremities.

Microscopic examination of the tissue from affected infants reveals increased osteoid and irregular epiphyseal cartilage with lengthened chondrocyte columns. Histopathologic examination of bone from adult patients reveals an osteomalacic picture, with increased quantities of unmineralized bone. Unlike the osteomalacia of vitamin D deficiency, that of hypophosphatasia is characterized by a paucity of osteoblasts.

Metal Toxicity

After the introduction of renal dialysis, many patients undergoing this procedure were treated with large doses of antacids to bind dietary phosphate and thereby prevent hyperphosphatemia. Eventually, it became apparent that the aluminum in the antacid had been incorporated into the bone and other body tissues of these patients. Several disease states resulted, most importantly aluminum-induced encephalopathy and aluminum-induced bone disease (23). In aluminum-induced bone disease, the amount of osteoid in the skeletal tissues may be considerably elevated; however, in this form of hyperosteoidosis, unlike that of vitamin D deficiency, the mineralization front is well demarcated, and the osteoblastic activity is minimal. Aurintricarboxylic acid stain can be used to demonstrate aluminum along the mineralization front (Fig. 7.16).

To a much lesser extent, both iron (24) and fluoride interfere with the deposition of calcium within bone. In conditions

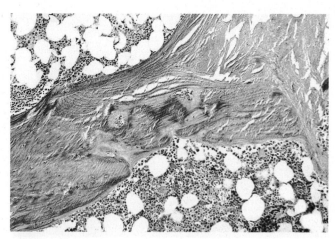

Figure 7.17. Undecalcified bone obtained from a patient treated with sodium fluoride shows a patchy basophilia, typically seen in the thickened bone of patients treated with fluoride.

characterized by high levels of iron (e.g., thalassemia) or fluoride (e.g., fluorosis), osteoid on the surface of the bone is increased (Fig. 7.17).

ABNORMAL RESORPTION

Several conditions are characterized by increased resorption of bone, including hyperparathyroidism, Paget disease, and osteoporosis. Osteopetrosis is also thought to be a disease related to abnormal resorption; although osteoclasts are frequently abundant, they appear not to resorb the calcified cartilage in bone formed by endochondral ossification.

Hyperparathyroidism

The overproduction of parathyroid hormone may be either a primary or a secondary phenomenon. The most common cause of primary hyperparathyroidism is an adenoma of one of the parathyroid glands; more rarely, it is a carcinoma or hyperplasia of obscure origin. Hyperparathyroidism is characterized biochemically by marked hypercalcemia and hypophosphatemia. The patients are usually young to middle-aged adults who present with a history of recurrent kidney stones, peptic ulcer, or less specific complaints, such as nausea, vomiting, weakness, and headaches (25). Although kidney disease is the most common clinical presentation, bone disease is present in approximately one-fourth of patients in the form of bone pain or, rarely, pathologic fracture.

Secondary hyperparathyroidism is generally the result of chronic renal failure in which, in association with phosphate retention, hypocalcemia develops. This process initiates compensatory or secondary hyperparathyroidism (26).

Whether the disease is primary or secondary, the radiologic and pathologic features found in the bone are similar (27). Roentgenographic examination may reveal diffuse osteopenia, but the most characteristic findings are seen on roentgenograms of the hand, where erosion of the tufts of the phalanges and subperiosteal cortical resorption, especially on the radial

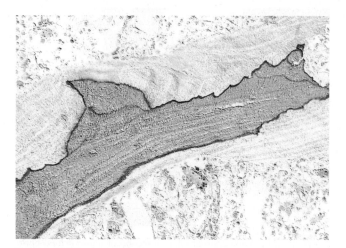

Figure 7.16. A biopsy specimen obtained from a patient with aluminum toxicity has been stained to show localization of aluminum at the mineralization front.

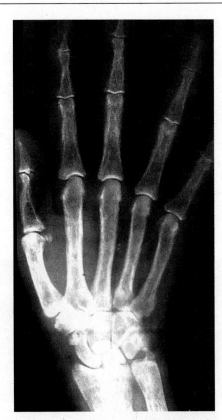

Figure 7.18. Clinical radiograph of the hand of a patient with hyperparathyroidism shows resorption of the tufts of the terminal phalanges and characteristic subperiosteal resorption of the radial side of the middle and proximal phalanges.

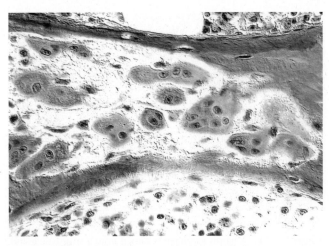

Figure 7.19. Photomicrograph of a biopsy specimen from a patient with hyperparathyroidism demonstrates osteoclastic dissecting resorption. At the surface, a layer of unmineralized bone appears as red seams on the bone surface.

side of the phalanges, are apparent (Fig. 7.18). Very rarely, large lytic lesions mimicking bone tumors may develop within the skeleton. These lesions, known as *brown tumors* because of their color, may be solitary or multiple, and when multiple, they give rise to the classic presentation described by von Recklinghausen—osteitis fibrosa cystica. When solitary, they may be mistaken for an aneurysmal bone cyst or a giant cell tumor.

On microscopic examination, the characteristic finding in hyperparathyroidism is increased osteoclastic activity; burrowing of the osteoclasts into the bone matrix creates a tunneled appearance (Fig. 7.19). In addition to increased resorption, bone formation is markedly increased, and this is often associated with peritrabecular fibrosis (Fig. 7.20). On occasion, the peritrabecular fibrosis must be distinguished from the changes associated with myelofibrosis. Whereas in myelofibrosis the increased fibrous tissue is generally distributed diffusely throughout the bone marrow, in hyperparathyroidism, the fibrosis hugs the trabecular surface. Another differential diagnostic consideration is the acute phase of Paget disease. In Paget disease, the osteoclasts are generally at the surface of the bone trabeculae, and they do not form tunnels. Furthermore, the osteoclasts of Paget disease frequently contain many more nuclei than the osteoclasts of hyperparathyroidism. Nevertheless, because it is not always possible to distinguish the two conditions microscopically, the clinical presentation and the biochemical findings are essential for making the correct diagnosis.

A brown tumor consists of numerous giant cells, generally associated with interstitial hemorrhage marked by hemosiderin

deposition (Fig. 7.21). Between the giant cells are plump proliferating fibroblasts, and often the lesion is quite vascular. On occasion, it may be difficult to differentiate this lesion from a giant cell tumor, although the giant cells in the latter are generally uniformly distributed throughout the lesion, interstitial hemorrhage is absent, and the stromal cells are not fibroblastic in type. A more difficult differential diagnosis may be between a brown tumor of hyperparathyroidism and a giant cell reparative granuloma; again, the clinical history and biochemical findings should help.

Once hyperparathyroidism is controlled, by either resection of the parathyroid tumor or medical control of the hyperphosphatemia, the radiographic and histologic changes rapidly regress.

Paget Disease

Paget disease, which is very common in northern Europeans but rare in blacks and Asians, is in most instances monostotic,

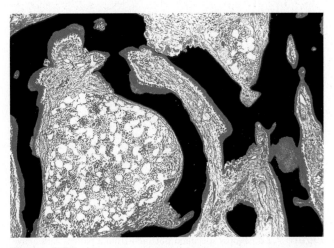

Figure 7.20. Photomicrograph of a patient with secondary hyperparathyroidism shows typical peritrabecular fibrosis in addition to osteoid seams and evidence of resorption. Peritrabecular fibrosis is associated with a marked increase in bone turnover and should be distinguished from diffuse marrow fibrosis in myeloid metaplasia.

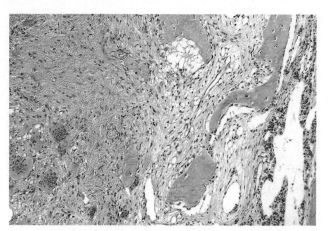

Figure 7.21. A biopsy specimen obtained from a large lytic lesion in the bone of a patient with hyperparathyroidism. Numerous giant cells and a brownish staining of the stroma are evident, together with reactive bone and cyst formation. This appearance is characteristic of a brown tumor but can be confused with a giant cell tumor.

asymptomatic, and discovered only incidentally during the course of a roentgenographic examination. Although any bone can be affected, the disease most commonly develops in the axial skeleton (spine, pelvis, and skull). In a small number of affected persons, the lesions are widespread and polyostotic, and it is these patients who are likely to come to the attention of a physician. The usual complaints are bone pain or symptoms of one of the complications of the disease, which include fracture, arthritis, and, most seriously but very rarely, a malignant tumor (28,29).

It has been suggested that Paget disease results from a viral infection of the osteoclasts that leads to a localized massive increase in osteoclastic activity (30). Associated with this active osteoclastic resorption is a reactive osteoblastic deposition of new bone, and in the acute phase of the disease, most of the new bone formed is of the woven type (Fig.

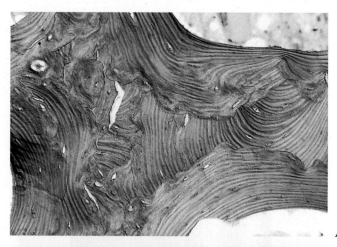

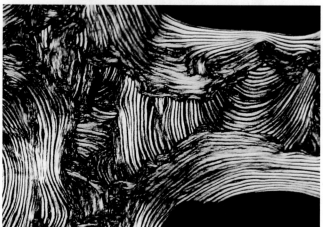

Figure 7.23. **(A)** Thickened trabecular bone obtained from a patient with burned-out Paget disease. An increase in the number of cement lines and marked irregularity of the microarchitecture of the bone tissue are apparent in this partially polarized hematoxylin and eosin section. **(B)** A fully polarized image showing the disordered arrangement of the lamellar bone fragments, which are more obvious.

7.22). The consequence is that the bone rapidly becomes completely disorganized. Additionally, because of the rapidity of bone turnover, the number of reversal fronts, or cement lines, also increases, so that not only the overall architecture of the bone but also the microarchitecture is markedly disturbed (Fig. 7.23). The radiologic appearance reflects the underlying morphologic changes. In the early stages of Paget disease, radiolucency may be striking, but in the later stages, the bone density increases, the trabecular architecture becomes more disturbed, and the normally clear distinction between cortical and cancellous bone is lost (Fig. 7.24). In some cases, the radiographic changes may be confused with those of a primary or metastatic tumor. In most instances, a biopsy should make the diagnosis clear.

The marked increase in bone formation is generally associated with very high levels of alkaline phosphatase, although the blood levels of calcium and phosphorus are generally normal. However, hypercalcemia is an occasional complication following prolonged bed rest in a patient with extensive involvement, and renal calculi may develop in such cases.

Progressive bone deformity in patients with Paget disease results from the rapid rate of bone modeling and repeated mi-

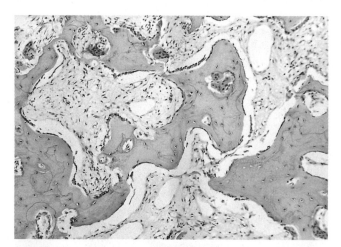

Figure 7.22. Biopsy specimen obtained from a patient with active Paget disease shows irregular and disorganized trabeculae lined by plump osteoblasts and numerous multinucleated osteoclasts. The bone trabeculae are hypercellular and have a woven pattern. The giant cell osteoclasts with many nuclei, such as are seen here, are typical of Paget disease.

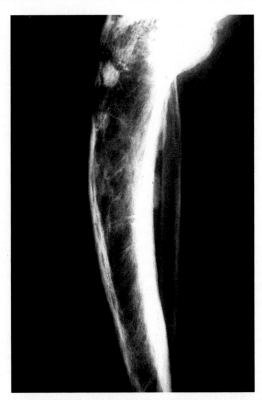

Figure 7.24. Clinical radiograph of the leg of a patient with Paget disease. The tibia is anteriorly bowed with thickening of the cortex and a coarsening of the trabecular architecture. Note the adjacent unaffected fibula for comparison.

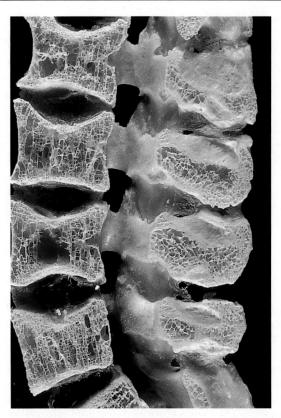

Figure 7.25. A portion of the lumbar spine of a patient with severe osteoporosis. Crush fractures with subsequent deformity of the vertebrae are seen. The loss of cancellous bone is obvious. The accentuation of the vertical trabeculae should be noted.

crofracture of the bone. Rarely, incomplete cortical fractures progress to complete fractures. (Despite the increase in bone density in Paget disease, the disturbed microarchitecture leads to bone weakness with an increased tendency to fracture.)

Sarcoma has been said to develop in 1% to 2% of patients with widespread Paget disease, but if one considers the asymptomatic cases that are discovered only incidentally, either by roentgenographic survey or at autopsy, the overall incidence of sarcoma in Paget disease must be much lower. (Note that sarcoma is associated not just with widespread disease; it also may occur in a monostotic focus.)

Arthritis is a common presenting symptom of Paget disease. It results from rapid remodeling of the bone end, which disturbs the proportions of the articular surfaces of the affected joint (31). This disturbance in turn leads to a functional failure of the joint, with erosion of the articular cartilage and the development of osteoarthritis.

Osteoporosis

A decrease in the density of the skeleton (osteopenia) may result from any number of factors, including disturbances in collagen formation, hematologic or endocrine abnormalities, neoplastic disorders, and immobilization. However, the term *osteoporosis* is generally applied to either a generalized senile or postmenopausal loss of bone that has become severe enough to result in

fractures, usually in the spine, wrist, or hip (32,33). The most common type of fracture is the vertebral compression fracture (Fig. 7.25), which causes a loss of height and the dowager's hump seen in elderly persons. On x-ray examination, flattening of the vertebral bodies is associated with widening and swelling of the intervertebral disc and gives rise to the so-called fish mouth appearance. The thoracic spine and upper lumbar spine are most frequently affected by fracture (34).

On histologic examination, osteoporotic bone generally shows no abnormal mineralization but rather a considerable porosity of cancellous bone, the trabeculae of which have become thin and strikingly disconnected from one another (Fig. 7.26). Close examination of the bone surfaces generally reveals an increase in resorptive activity, manifested as either an increased number of osteoclasts or an increased percentage of the surface with resorptive pitting (35). In our experience, resorptive activity in osteoporotic patients is approximately twice that in age-matched controls (Fig. 7.27). In patients with osteoporosis, biopsies are frequently performed to evaluate the effects of treatment, and it is important to point out that the heterogeneity of the structure of bone is such that changes in bone volume should be evaluated with great care. On the other hand, the bone biopsy can be very useful for assessing cellular activity and can indicate whether or not a decrease in resorptive activity has been coupled with an increase in the rate of bone formation (36). (Treatment with fluoride leads to recognizable alterations in trabecular architecture and changes in mineralization and, consequently, is no longer used. The treatment most

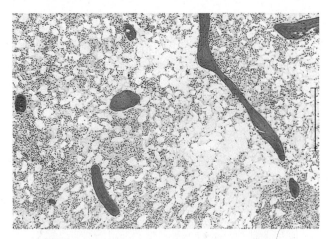

Figure 7.26. A biopsy specimen from a patient with osteoporosis has scant, disconnected, and thin bone trabeculae.

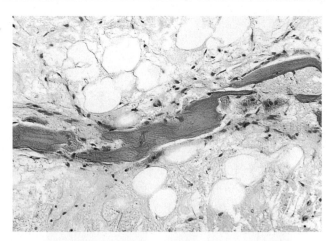

Figure 7.28. Marked osteoclastic resorption of bone trabeculae in transient osteoporosis with edema and mild fibrotic changes in the bone marrow. Further examination of this section might reveal hypervascularity of the marrow in other areas.

frequently used at present is the administration of one of the bisphosphonates. Parathyroid hormone [PTH] is also occasionally used.)

TRANSIENT OSTEOPOROSIS. Occasionally, a younger patient may experience bone pain, usually in a lower extremity, that is associated roentgenographically with localized patchy osteopenia. The lesions of transient localized osteoporosis are generally juxta-articular in location and may spontaneously remit with reossification. In some cases, they are migratory, giving rise to the term *transient migratory osteoporosis* (37,38). Histologic examination of such bone reveals only disconnected bone trabeculae, often with evidence of fat necrosis, hyperemia of the bone marrow space, and increased resorptive activity (Fig. 7.28).

Osteopetrosis

Osteopetrosis is a rare congenital disorder in which the density of all bones is markedly increased (39). The long bones are usually shortened and frequently exhibit a modeling defect (the Erlenmeyer flask deformity) characterized by loss of the normal

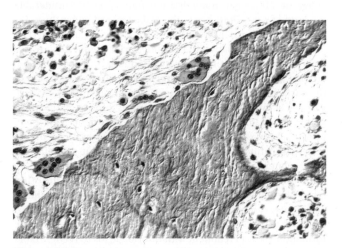

Figure 7.27. A portion of a biopsy specimen obtained from a patient with severe osteoporosis shows increased surface osteoclast activity.

metaphyseal flare. Despite the increase in bone density, the disease is often complicated by multiple fractures resulting from a disturbed microarchitecture. Anemia is caused by a marked reduction in the marrow space.

Two clinical presentations have been recognized. A severe form usually causes death in utero or in early childhood and appears to be inherited as an autosomal recessive trait. In a less severe form, patients reach adult life; this form is inherited as an autosomal dominant condition.

The clinical diagnosis may be delayed until adulthood, and the condition is usually detected because of a pathologic fracture or as an incidental radiologic finding. In such cases, the osteopetrosis must be differentiated from widespread osteoblastic metastases, myelosclerosis, and Paget disease.

Radiologic examination may reveal a uniform opacity of the skeletal tissue or, particularly in the pelvic and peripheral bones, alternating areas of affected and apparently normal bone that result in a peculiar striped appearance of the tissue. Occasionally, spinal involvement may give rise to spondylolisthesis as a consequence of fractures through the pars interarticularis in the lumbar region.

On gross examination, the density of the affected bones is increased, and they may weigh two to three times more than normal despite usually being somewhat smaller than normal. On sectioning, the bone tissue is very compact, showing a complete loss of the normal architecture.

Microscopic examination reveals extremely dense and irregular bone trabeculae, nearly all of which have a central core of cartilage (Fig. 7.29). Although a paucity of osteoclasts has been reported in osteopetrosis, microscopic examination shows that the osteoclasts are often abundant (Fig. 7.30). However, electron microscopic studies have demonstrated that these osteoclasts lack ruffled borders, and although they are close to the bone, they do not show the normal cytologic features of actively resorbing osteoclasts.

In osteopetrotic mice, normal bone and cartilage resorption has been restored after the transplantation of normal bone marrow or splenic cells. This procedure has also been tried in humans (40).

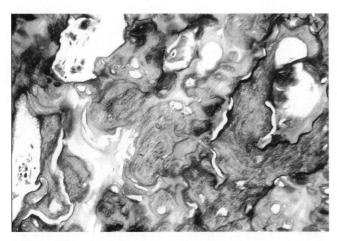

Figure 7.29. Photomicrograph of a biopsy specimen from a patient with osteopetrosis. Extremely irregular and thickened bone trabeculae and cores of blue calcified cartilage are evident throughout the section.

POSTTRAUMATIC LESIONS

FRACTURE OF THE BONE

A fracture is related to both mechanical injury and the strength of the bone. With the obvious exception of severe trauma, such as that sustained in motorcycle accidents and other forms of violence, many of the fractures seen in clinical practice are pathologic fractures caused by either weakened bone, osteoporosis in the elderly, or local bone disease, including tumor and infection (41). Another important contributing factor to fracture is a lack of coordination in both elderly persons and young children (42).

Most fractures through cortical bone have a spiral configuration that results from the combination of the direction of the force applied to the bone and the microstructure of the bone itself. When the structure of the bone is very disturbed, as, for example, in Paget disease or osteopetrosis, the fracture may be transverse, so that it simulates a break in a piece of chalk. Repeated stress to a bone, as, for example, in long-distance running, marching, or ballet dancing, may result in the develop-

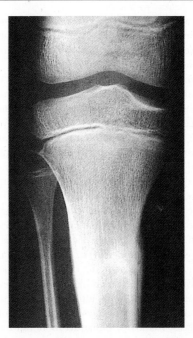

Figure 7.31. Clinical radiograph taken from a teenage runner demonstrates a sclerotic lesion in the upper third of the diaphysis of the tibia. There is an overlying periosteal reaction, and a slight lytic defect is seen at the surface. This lesion is a stress fracture, but in the absence of any history of trauma, it could be mistaken for a malignant lesion.

ment of incomplete stress or fatigue fractures through its cortex (Fig. 7.31). Such lesions may occur without an obvious history of significant mechanical trauma, and the nature of the lesion may therefore be misinterpreted by the clinician, radiologist, and pathologist as a neoplasm. Similarly, repeated trauma at ligamentous and tendinous insertions may lead to pseudosarcomatous avulsion fractures at these sites (Fig. 7.32). Avulsion fractures are most commonly seen around the pelvis, particularly at the origin of the adductor muscles along the inferior

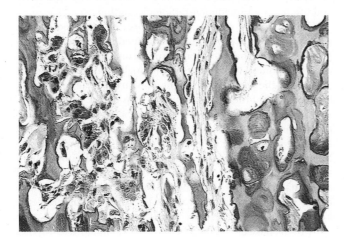

Figure 7.30. Numerous osteoclast-like cells in osteopetrosis. Note the abundant calcified cartilage within this section in addition to some areas of bone.

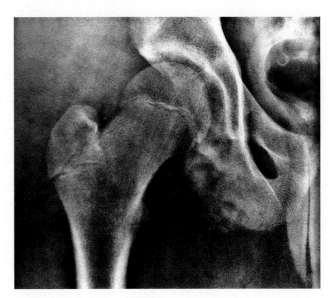

Figure 7.32. Clinical radiograph demonstrates an avulsion injury of the ischial tuberosity. Because of its fragmented appearance, the lesion could easily be mistaken for a neoplasm.

pubic ramus and at the lower end of the thigh, where the adductor muscles insert. In young children, avulsion fractures of the tibial tubercle cause fragmentation of that structure, which results in a lesion known as *Osgood-Schlatter disease.*

When a fracture occurs, the degree of injury to the tissue depends on the direction and magnitude of the force applied. The bone fragments may be displaced, the fragments may be numerous (comminuted fracture), the skin overlying the fracture may be perforated (compound fracture), and in some cases, soft tissue may be interposed between the fractured ends of the bone. For these and other reasons, the histologic appearance of the reparative tissue surrounding a fracture may vary greatly. Generally, tissue that has been obtained within a few days after the injury shows evidence of acute damage and hemorrhage. The bone immediately adjacent to the fracture site is necrotic, and in certain anatomic locations, such as the femoral neck, carpal scaphoid, and patella, the bone necrosis may be extensive because of the anatomy of the local vascular supply (Fig. 7.33). Extensive necrosis is likely to delay healing.

Tissue obtained 1 to 2 weeks after a fracture is usually markedly cellular and frequently hypervascular. Within the proliferating fibroblasts, islands of immature bone and cartilage are being formed. The hypercellularity, disordered organization, and matrix production may give rise to a pseudosarcomatous appearance (Fig. 7.34). Because a biopsy is not likely to have been performed unless the clinician has failed to recognize the traumatic nature of the patient's problem, the pseudosarcomatous appearance of the callus may lead to serious errors in interpretation by the pathologist.

The amount of callus produced around a fracture depends on several factors, including the degree of instability and the vascularity of the injured bone. The amount of callus is usually increased in unstable fractures. In poorly vascularized areas of the skeleton (e.g., the mid shaft of the tibia), callus formation may be scant; consequently, healing may be delayed, sometimes indefinitely. This delay gives rise to chronic nonunion of the fracture site and rarely the development of a pseudoarthrosis, or false joint.

Once the callus is sufficient to immobilize the fracture site, repair takes place between the fractured cortical and medullary

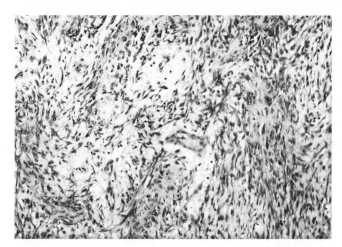

Figure 7.34. Hypercellular callus at the early stage of fracture healing. The immature matrix formation and irregular arrangement of the proliferating fibroblastic cells, often with many mitotic figures, may cause a mistaken diagnosis of malignancy.

bones. When union has been achieved, the callus is remodeled and eventually disappears. Very little callus is produced when a fracture is treated with rigid internal or external surgical fixation, after which primary healing of the bone proceeds without the abundant external callus generally associated with unstable fractures.

BONE INFARCTION

Death of bone tissue following an interruption of its blood supply is a feature of almost all fractures. Localized bone infarcts also occur relatively frequently in patients with sickle cell anemia and Gaucher disease (43). They also used to be common in caisson workers with decompression sickness. Infarcts may also develop in patients with connective tissue diseases, such as rheumatoid arthritis and lupus erythematosus, who have been treated with corticosteroids.

In many cases, infarction involves the femoral head or other convex articular surfaces (see Chapter 6). However, on rare occasions, infarction may affect the metaphysis of a long bone or even a flat bone. The lesions may be multiple and symmetric and often are an incidental radiologic finding.

The early stage of a bone infarct can be observed only at autopsy; it appears grossly as an elongated pale area with a hyperemic border that is rather sharply demarcated from the surrounding bones. At this stage, not enough time has elapsed for changes in the architecture of the bone trabeculae to develop, and therefore, little if any change is seen on the radiograph.

Microscopically, irregular cystic spaces are seen in the marrow that result from the breakdown of the walls of fat cells, and extensive calcification may be noted focally. The bone trabeculae are nonviable, as evidenced by lacunae that do not contain stainable osteocytes. However, the most obvious evidence of early infarction is found in bone that contains hematopoietic tissue, where, because such tissue is extremely vulnerable to ischemia, only ghost cells are seen (Fig. 7.35).

With the passage of time, ingrowth of granulation tissue takes place at the periphery of the lesion, and "creeping substitution" of the nonviable cancellous bone with new, viable bone layered on the trabecular surfaces is seen at the periphery of the infarct.

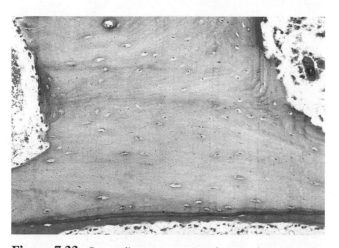

Figure 7.33. Bone adjacent to a recent fracture shows extensive necrosis with empty lacunae and poorly staining matrix. Necrosis of the tissue adjacent to the fracture site is to be expected, and extensive fragmentation of the bone can delay healing of the fracture.

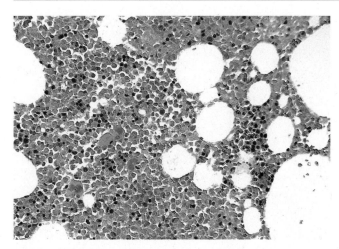

Figure 7.35. Infarcted hematopoietic bone marrow. The pyknotic basophilic nucleated red cells stand out in a background of ghost cells. Note also the variation in the fat globules.

In most cases, the healing process is aborted, and a rim of highly collagenized connective tissue forms about the periphery of the lesion. This connective tissue wall becomes infiltrated with calcium salts (Fig. 7.36).

Radiographs of the lesion in the later stages of development have a typical appearance. A moderately thick radiopaque serpentine border can be observed that often outlines an elongated area of central radiolucency (Fig. 7.37). This appearance has been likened to a coil of smoke. In some cases, particularly

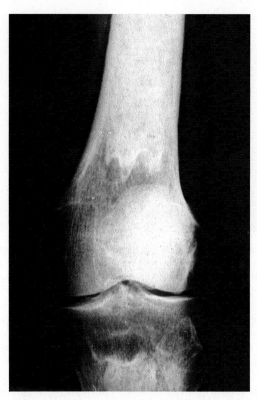

Figure 7.37. Multiple bone infarcts in caisson disease. Marked increased central density in the lower diaphysis and metaphysis of the femur is sharply demarcated from the surrounding tissue. Such a lesion could be mistaken for a calcified enchondroma.

in solitary lesions, radiographs may suggest a calcified enchondroma. Usually, however, the foci of calcified matrix in enchondroma or chondrosarcoma are discrete and scattered diffusely throughout the lesion, and the margin of the lesion is not so clearly outlined as in an infarct.

The occasional development in a bone infarct of a malignant spindle cell tumor, usually a malignant fibrous histiocytoma, is a well-recognized complication (44).

MYOSITIS OSSIFICANS CIRCUMSCRIPTA

Myositis ossificans circumscripta is a solitary, nonprogressive, benign ossifying lesion of soft tissues that often develops close to a bone (see Chapter 5) (45). The patient usually presents with a lump in a muscle that has been evident for some weeks and may be somewhat painful. A history of trauma can usually be elicited, but the traumatic incidents are more often than not trivial in nature. A radiograph taken soon after the onset of symptoms may not reveal any calcification, but within 1 to 2 weeks, a poorly defined area of opacification appears. During succeeding weeks, the periphery of this shadow becomes increasingly well delineated from the surrounding soft tissue (Fig. 7.38). Magnetic resonance imaging allows a much earlier diagnosis but may cause confusion because of the pseudosarcomatous appearance microscopically.

Gross examination of a focus of myositis ossificans circumscripta that has been present for 1 or 2 months reveals a circumscribed shell of bony tissue with a soft, reddish-brown central area. The lesion is usually 2 to 5 cm in diameter and adheres to the surrounding muscle (Fig. 7.39).

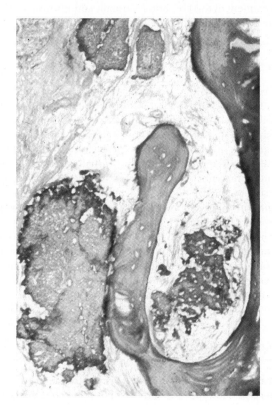

Figure 7.36. Calcium deposition in necrotic marrow in a bone infarct. Heavy deposition of calcium may lead to increased radiodensity on clinical radiographs.

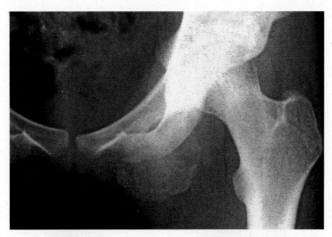

Figure 7.38. Clinical radiograph of a young woman 1 month postpartum in whom pubic pain developed shortly after childbirth. A well-defined ossifying mass is seen in the soft tissue adjacent to the pubis.

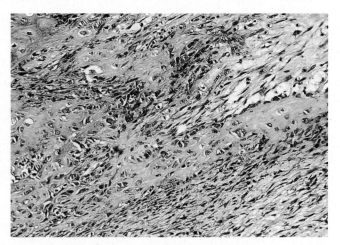

Figure 7.40. The center of the tissue shown in Figure 7.39 demonstrates immature bone formation with cellular fibrous tissue. The irregularity and cellularity demonstrated here could cause concern and lead to an erroneous diagnosis of sarcoma.

The microscopic examination of myositis ossificans circumscripta reveals an irregular mass of active, immature fibroblasts in the center of the lesion, with foci of interstitial hemorrhage that are rarely extensive. At some distance from the center of the lesion, depending on the age of the entity, small foci of osteoid production can be seen. The resulting tissue may be disorganized and hypercellular (Fig. 7.40). Near the periphery, more and more clearly defined trabeculae are evident. The bone is usually of the immature woven type, with large, round,

and crowded osteocytes. However, in long-standing lesions, the bone may be mature and have a lamellar pattern.

It may be difficult on the basis of histologic evidence alone to differentiate a focus of myositis, especially in its acute stage, from a sarcoma. Careful correlation of the clinical and radiologic findings is thus essential. An important distinction to be emphasized is that whereas myositis ossificans is most mature at the periphery and least mature at the center, the opposite is true of osteosarcoma.

Treatment of this condition is usually conservative, with excision of the mass an option.

REACTIVE PERIOSTITIS

Reactive periostitis is a rare calcifying and ossifying soft tissue lesion that occurs most often in the hands and less often in the feet (46). The lesion is likely to originate along the margin of a phalanx, and although no mineralization may be seen on radiographic studies obtained in the early stages at the time of clinical presentation, calcification is usually present. A history of trauma may not be given, but it is generally believed that the lesion of reactive periostitis, like those of myositis ossificans circumscripta and subungual exostosis (to which reactive periostitis is closely related), is posttraumatic. Microscopically, especially in the early phases, the disordered fibroblastic proliferation, mitotic activity, and immature bone formation may suggest osteosarcoma. However, as in myositis ossificans, maturation of the tissue is seen toward the periphery of the lesion, and the edge of the lesion is usually encased in a shell of bone.

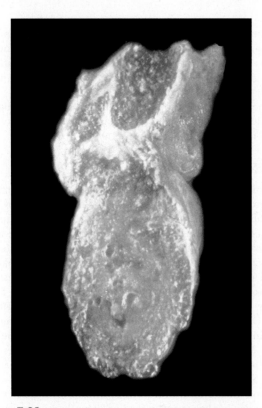

Figure 7.39. Gross photograph of the specimen removed from the patient shown in Figure 7.38. A segment of normal bone is seen in the upper part of the photograph, and immediately beneath this segment is a well-circumscribed mass with peripheral ossification.

BONE INFECTION

Clinically significant inflammation is most frequently the result of infection. However, it is important to remember that inflammation also occurs in response to other pathologic processes, including trauma, some metabolic diseases (e.g., gout), and even neoplasia.

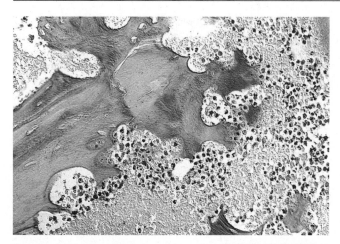

Figure 7.41. Biopsy specimen of osteomyelitis demonstrating polymorphonuclear leukocyte infiltration with necrosis and focal erosion of the bone tissue secondary to enzymatic digestion.

Infection of the bones and joints is caused by microbial organisms that are either blood-borne (hematogenous infection) or implanted directly into the bone through an open wound.

In general, most bone infections are pyogenic (Fig. 7.41), whereas joint infections are granulomatous (see Chapter 6) (47). In the developed world, the incidence of infection in the skeletal tissues has markedly declined since the advent of antibiotics (48). Today, most cases of bone infection are seen in elderly debilitated persons, in young immunocompromised persons, or often as complications of surgery or compound fractures (49,50).

Occasionally, the differential diagnosis is problematic, especially when osteomyelitis must be differentiated from round cell tumors and eosinophilic granuloma. Diagnostic problems are encountered not only radiologically and clinically (Ewing tumor may present with fever and an increased sedimentation rate), but also microscopically, especially with small crushed specimens, in which tumor cells and inflammatory cells may be difficult to distinguish. In such cases, the diagnosis of osteomyelitis may depend on the results of intraoperative cultures in combination with the patient's subsequent postoperative course. The importance of obtaining an adequate amount of culture material and prompt inoculation of the material into a transport medium cannot be overemphasized.

HEMATOGENOUS OSTEOMYELITIS

Most patients with acute hematogenous osteomyelitis are children. *Staphylococcus aureus*, *Streptococcus pyogenes*, and *Haemophilus influenzae* are the most commonly isolated microbes. The most frequent sites of pediatric osteomyelitis are areas of rapid growth and areas at increased risk for trauma: the distal femur, proximal femur, proximal tibia, proximal humerus, and distal radius. The large caliber of the metaphyseal veins in children results in a marked slowing of blood flow, so that traumatized tissue is predisposed to thrombosis and subsequent colonization by blood-borne bacteria.

Hematogenous osteomyelitis is uncommon in healthy adults. However, as the number of debilitated persons has increased (e.g., patients with chronic immunodeficiency disease or drug addiction), so has the number of adults with osteomyelitis. *S. aureus* is the most commonly isolated pathogen, although infec-

tions with Gram-negative rods and yeasts are also seen in intravenous drug users. Infecting bacteria are carried into the blood from the skin or injected from unclean hypodermic needles. Additionally, injected drugs are often "cut," contaminating needles with particulate matter. The occluded microvasculature then provides a ready site for bacterial colonization. Local pain may be the sole clinical finding, so that the diagnosis of osteomyelitis is delayed. The focus is usually the spine or pelvis.

In elderly persons, especially those with genitourinary infections, opportunistic bacteria selected out by repeated antibiotic use, usually *Pseudomonas aeruginosa*, gain access to the spine, possibly via the Batson venous plexus.

Another group of elderly patients in whom osteomyelitis may be a problem are those with peripheral vascular insufficiency, which in many cases is associated with diabetes. In these patients, the infection usually involves the small bones of the feet. The etiology is frequently polymicrobial.

Adults with bone infections often present only with pain; thus, a diagnosis of osteomyelitis may not at first be obvious. The accompanying radiographic bone changes may easily be misinterpreted by the radiologist as a malignant tumor. The clinical diagnosis may be further confused by negative cultures resulting from the inappropriate empiric use of antibiotics.

It can be affirmed that there is no single test that can serve as definitive for the diagnosis of musculoskeletal infection. The most useful tests have been shown to be (a) an erythrocyte sedimentation rate greater than 30 mm/hr; (b) C-reactive protein greater than 10 mg/L; and (c) a positive culture on aspiration.

OSTEOMYELITIS RESULTING FROM THE DIRECT INOCULATION OF BACTERIA

Now that acute hematogenous osteomyelitis of childhood occurs much less frequently, posttraumatic osteomyelitis has become the more common clinical problem, usually following puncture wounds, traffic accidents, or surgery.

Iatrogenic infections may be associated with the fixation of a simple or compound fracture or with prosthetic joint replacement. (More than 500,000 prosthetic joint replacements are performed each year in the United States alone.) After a total joint replacement procedure, infection may occur as an acute complication of the operation or present insidiously many months or even years later.

Late infection of total joint replacement occurs in 1% to 2% of cases. The differential clinical diagnosis from aseptic loosening of the arthroplasty may be difficult; however, an erythrocyte sedimentation rate greater than 30 mm/hr is helpful. At reoperation, frozen section has been widely used as an adjunct to diagnosis. It is important to analyze at least two or three samples, avoiding obvious fibrin and preferably using granulation tissue. At least 10 polymorphonuclear cells per high-power field are generally accepted as being predictive of infection (51–54).

CHRONIC OSTEOMYELITIS

With the mortality rate reduced to almost zero, few people die of hematogenous osteomyelitis. However, chronic disease develops in from 15% to 30% of patients (Fig. 7.42). In children, and less rarely in adults, chronic osteomyelitis may present as a solitary radiolucent lesion with a sclerotic margin in the metaphyseal region of a long bone; this is usually referred to as

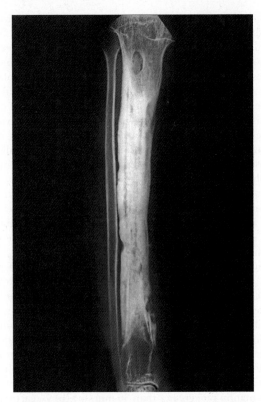

Figure 7.42. Clinical radiograph of the leg of a patient with long-standing osteomyelitis shows a central sequestrum of necrotic bone surrounded by thickened exuberant periosteal new bone, which constitutes the involucrum.

Brodie abscess. Chronic osteomyelitis is frequently the result of either inadequate antibiotic treatment or the incomplete surgical debridement of necrotic bone. Necrotic bone within the affected areas (the sequestrum) protects bacteria from even high levels of appropriate antibiotics. Furthermore, the formation of bacterial biofilms—sessile microbial communities with inherent resistance to antimicrobial agents—contributes to the genesis of chronic osteomyelitis. The biofilm acts as a "nidus" of infection, and acute disease results when host defenses cannot eliminate the released bacteria. Biofilms associated with osteomyelitis are usually comprised of a mixture of various bacterial and fungal species, and the disease does not resolve until the sessile population is surgically removed.

Squamous cell carcinoma in association with a chronic fistula has been reported to be a late sequela of chronic osteomyelitis in approximately 1% of patients, occurring up to 30 to 40 years after the original infection (55). Systemic amyloidosis may also be a complication of chronic osteomyelitis.

CHRONIC MULTIFOCAL OSTEOMYELITIS

Chronic recurrent multifocal osteomyelitis, now a recognized variant of osteomyelitis in children and young adults, is characterized by low-grade fever, local swelling and pain, and radiologic findings suggesting osteomyelitis or a round cell neoplasm (56,57). Bone-seeking isotopes may reveal multiple asymptomatic sites of involvement. The lesions occur mainly in the metaphyses of tubular bones and in the clavicles and are sometimes symmetric.

Cultures are negative for bacterial, fungal, and viral organisms. The clinical course is characterized by intermittent periods of exacerbation and improvement during several years. In some patients, the recurrence of associated skin lesions (pustulosis palmoplantaris) closely parallels exacerbation of the bone lesions.

On microscopic examination, acute inflammation with polymorphonuclear leukocyte predominance occurs in the early phases of the disease, and fibrosis of the marrow with chronic inflammation occurs in the later phases. The most common finding is subacute or chronic osteomyelitis with a predominance of plasma cells. Fragments of necrotic bone with associated multinucleated giant cells are a common finding.

REFERENCES

1. Carando S, Portigliatti Barbos M, Ascenzi A, Boyde A. Orientation of collagen in human tibial and fibular shaft and possible correlation with mechanical properties. *Bone* 1989;10: 139–142.
2. Marks SC Jr, Popoff SN. Bone cell biology: the regulation of development, structure, and function in the skeleton. *Am J Anat* 1988;183:1–44.
3. Frank CB, Woo SL, Andriacchi T. Normal ligament: structure, function and composition. In Woo SL-Y, Buckwalter JA, eds. *Injury and Repair of the Musculoskeletal Soft Tissues.* Park Ridge, IL: American Academy of Orthopaedic Surgeons, 1988:45–101.
4. Buckwalter JA, Einhorn TA, Simon SR. *Orthopaedic Basic Science: Biology and Biomechanics of the Musculoskeletal System.* Rosemont, IL: American Academy of Orthopaedic Surgeons, 2000.
5. Dickson G. *Methods of Calcified Tissue Preparation.* New York, NY: Elsevier, 1984.
6. Boyde A, Maconnachie E, Reid SA, Delling G, Mundy GR. Scanning electron microscopy in bone pathology: review of methods, potential and applications. *Scan Electron Microsc* 1986;Pt 4:1537–1554.
7. Steiner GC. Tumors and tumor like conditions of bone and joints. In Johannessen JV, ed. *Electron Microscopy in Human Medicine.* New York, NY: McGraw-Hill, 1981:54–140.
8. Bullough PG, Bansal M, DiCarlo EF. The tissue diagnosis of metabolic bone disease. Role of histomorphometry. *Orthop Clin North Am* 1990;21:65–79.
9. Bilezikian JP, Raisz LG, Rodan GA. *Principles of Bone Biology.* San Diego, CA: Academic Press, 2002.
10. Parfitt AM. Renal bone disease: a new conceptual framework for the interpretation of bone histomorphometry. *Curr Opin Nephrol Hypertens* 2003;12:387–403.
11. Porter GA, Gurley M, Roth SI. Bone. In Sternberg S, ed. *Histology for Pathologists.* Philadelphia, PA: Lippincott-Raven, 1997:85–106.
12. Parfitt AM, Qiu S, Rao DS. The mineralization index—a new approach to the histomorphometric appraisal of osteomalacia. *Bone* 2004;35:320–325.
13. Als OS, Gotfredsen A, Christiansen C. The effect of glucocorticoids on bone mass in rheumatoid arthritis patients. Influence of menopausal state. *Arthritis Rheum* 1985;28:369–375.
14. Dalle Carbonare L, Chavassieux PM, Arlot ME, Meunier PJ. Bone histomorphometry in untreated and treated glucocorticoid-induced osteoporosis. *Front Horm Res* 2002;30:37–48.
15. Anderson C. *Manual for the Examination of Bone.* Boca Raton, FL: CRC Press, 1982.
16. Milch R, Rall D, Tobie J. Fluorescence of tetracycline antibiotics in bone. *J Bone Joint Surg Am* 1958;40:897–910.
17. Sokoloff L. Note on histology of cement lines. In Kenedi RM, ed. *Perspectives in Biomedical Engineering; Proceedings of a Symposium Organized in Association with the Biological Engineering Society.* Baltimore, MD: University Park Press, 1973:314.
18. Bullough PG, Davidson DD, Lorenzo JC. The morbid anatomy of the skeleton in osteogenesis imperfecta. *Clin Orthop Relat Res* 1981;159:42–57.
19. Doppelt SH. Vitamin D, rickets, and osteomalacia. *Orthop Clin North Am* 1984;15:671–686.
20. Kaul M, Silverberg M, Dicarlo EF, Schneider R, Bass AR, Erkan D. Tumor-induced osteomalacia. *Clin Rheumatol* 2007;26:1575–1579.
21. Nuovo MA, Dorfman HD, Sun CC, Chalew SA. Tumor-induced osteomalacia and rickets. *Am J Surg Pathol* 1989;13:588–599.
22. Whyte MP. Hypophosphatasia. In Scriver CR, ed. *The Metabolic and Molecular Bases of Inherited Disease.* New York, NY: McGraw-Hill, 1995:4605.
23. Sherrard DJ, Andress DL. Aluminum-related osteodystrophy. *Adv Intern Med* 1989;34: 307–323.
24. Gratwick GM, Bullough PG, Bohne WH, Markenson AL, Peterson CM. Thalassemic osteoarthropathy. *Ann Intern Med* 1978;88:494–501.
25. Khan A, Bilezikian J. Primary hyperparathyroidism: pathophysiology and impact on bone. *CMAJ* 2000;163:184–187.
26. Freemont AJ. The pathology of dialysis. *Semin Dial* 2002;15:227–231.
27. Elder G. Pathophysiology and recent advances in the management of renal osteodystrophy. *J Bone Miner Res* 2002;17:2094–2105.
28. Paget J. On a form of chronic inflammation of bones (Osteitis deformans). *Clin Orthop Relat Res* 1966;49:3–16.
29. Smith J, Botet JF, Yeh SD. Bone sarcomas in Paget disease: a study of 85 patients. *Radiology* 1984;152:583–590.
30. Basle MF, Mazaud P, Malkani K, Chretien MF, Moreau MF, Rebel A. Isolation of osteoclasts from Pagetic bone tissue: morphometry and cytochemistry on isolated cells. *Bone* 1988;9: 1–6.

31. Goldman AB, Bullough P, Kammerman S, Ambos M. Osteitis deformans of the hip joint. *AJR Am J Roentgenol* 1977;128:601–606.

32. Raisz LG. Pathogenesis of postmenopausal osteoporosis. *Clin Orthop Relat Res* 2001;2:5–12.

33. Becker C. Pathophysiology and clinical manifestations of osteoporosis. *Clin Cornerstone* 2006; 8:19–27.

34. Avioli L. *The Osteoporotic Syndrome: Detection, Prevention, and Treatment*. San Diego, CA: Academic Press, 2000.

35. Anonymous. *Proceeding of the NIH Consensus Development Conference on Osteoporosis Prevention, Diagnosis, and Therapy*. Bethesda, MD: National Institutes of Health, 2000:86.

36. Chavassieux P, Meunier PJ. Histomorphometric approach of bone loss in men. *Calcif Tissue Int* 2001;69:209–213.

37. Lakhanpal S, Ginsburg WW, Luthra HS, Hunder GG. Transient regional osteoporosis. A study of 56 cases and review of the literature. *Ann Intern Med* 1987;106:444–450.

38. Miyanishi K, Yamamoto T, Nakashima Y, et al. Subchondral changes in transient osteoporosis of the hip. *Skeletal Radiol* 2001;30:255–261.

39. Shapiro F, Glimcher MJ, Holtrop ME, Tashjian AH Jr, Brickley-Parsons D, Kenzora JE. Human osteopetrosis: a histological, ultrastructural, and biochemical study. *J Bone Joint Surg Am* 1980;62:384–399.

40. Marks SC Jr. Osteopetrosis—multiple pathways for the interception of osteoclast function. *Appl Pathol* 1987;5:172–183.

41. Heppenstall R. *Fracture Treatment and Healing*. Philadelphia, PA: Saunders, 1980.

42. Ogden JA. *Skeletal Injury in the Child*. New York, NY: Springer, 2000.

43. Bullough PG, Kambolis CP, Marcove RC, et al. Bone infarctions not associated with caisson disease. *J Bone Joint Surg Am* 1965;47A:477–491.

44. Mirra JM, Bullough PG, Marcove RC, Jacobs B, Huvos AG. Malignant fibrous histiocytoma and osteosarcoma in association with bone infarcts; report of four cases, two in caisson workers. *J Bone Joint Surg Am* 1974;56:932–940.

45. Norman A, Dorfman HD. Juxtacortical circumscribed myositis ossificans: evolution and radiographic features. *Radiology* 1970;96:301–306.

46. Spjut HJ, Dorfman HD. Florid reactive periostitis of the tubular bones of the hands and feet. A benign lesion which may simulate osteosarcoma. *Am J Surg Pathol* 1981;5:423–433.

47. Green NE, Edwards K. Bone and joint infections in children. *Orthop Clin North Am* 1987; 18:555–576.

48. Waldvogel FA, Papageorgiou PS. Osteomyelitis: the past decade. *N Engl J Med* 1980;303: 360–370.

49. Gifford DB, Patzakis M, Ivler D, Swezey RL. Septic arthritis due to pseudomonas in heroin addicts. *J Bone Joint Surg Am* 1975;57:631–635.

50. Nade S. Infection after joint replacement—what would Lister think? *Med J Aust* 1990;152: 394–397.

51. Della Valle CJ, Sporer SM, Jacobs JJ, Berger RA, Rosenberg AG, Paprosky WG. Preoperative testing for sepsis before revision total knee arthroplasty. *J Arthroplasty* 2007;22:90–93.

52. Bori G, Soriano A, Garcia S, Mallofre C, Riba J, Mensa J. Usefulness of histological analysis for predicting the presence of microorganisms at the time of reimplantation after hip resection arthroplasty for the treatment of infection. *J Bone Joint Surg Am* 2007;89: 1232–1237.

53. Wong YC, Lee QJ, Wai YL, Ng WF. Intraoperative frozen section for detecting active infection in failed hip and knee arthroplasties. *J Arthroplasty* 2005;20:1015–1020.

54. Lonner JH, Desai P, Dicesare PE, Steiner G, Zuckerman JD. The reliability of analysis of intraoperative frozen sections for identifying active infection during revision hip or knee arthroplasty. *J Bone Joint Surg Am* 1996;78:1553–1558.

55. Greenspan A, Norman A, Steiner G. Case report 146. Squamous cell carcinoma arising in chronic, draining sinus tract secondary to osteomyelitis of right tibia. *Skeletal Radiol* 1981; 6:149–151.

56. El-Shanti HI, Ferguson PJ. Chronic recurrent multifocal osteomyelitis: a concise review and genetic update. *Clin Orthop Relat Res* 2007;462:11–19.

57. Solheim LF, Paus B, Liverud K, Stoen E. Chronic recurrent multifocal osteomyelitis. A new clinical-radiological syndrome. *Acta Orthop Scand* 1980;51:37–41.

Carrie Y. Inwards
K. Krishnan Unni

Bone Tumors

Neoplasms and tumorlike conditions of bone are rare. Thus, orthopedic surgeons, radiologists, and pathologists generally have little experience with these lesions. Bone tumors also tend to affect young children and adolescents. These factors are a cause of concern for the surgical pathologist dealing with a bone tumor because a diagnosis of sarcoma will result in extensive surgery and, in most cases, chemotherapy with or without radiotherapy. Historically, the diagnosis of a sarcoma often mandated amputation surgery and carried a poor prognosis. However, in recent years, significant advances in diagnosis and treatment have improved the outlook for these patients, most of whom are candidates for limb-sparing surgery and many of whom survive their sarcoma. Advances in pathologic diagnosis include immunohistochemical, cytogenetic, and molecular techniques. These are part of the continued search for prognostic factors related to the host and the tumor that are important in predicting behavior and guiding treatment.

Medicine in general is becoming a multidisciplinary science. A prime example of a multidisciplinary approach to patient care is orthopedic oncology. To arrive at a correct diagnosis for a bone tumor, orthopedic surgeons, radiologists, and pathologists must cooperate. The team caring for patients with bone tumors also includes medical oncologists, radiation oncologists, and physiatrists. In the initial stages of diagnosis and evaluation, however, the first three members of the team—orthopedic surgeon, radiologist, and pathologist—play the key role. Good communication among these specialists ensures that mistakes are kept to a minimum. A surgical pathologist attempting to diagnose a bone lesion without the aid of clinical information and roentgenographic appearance is at a great disadvantage.

The clinical features are of relatively little significance in most bone lesions. Most patients experience pain, swelling, or both. Clinical information actually may be misleading. For example, a patient with Ewing sarcoma may present with fever and an increased erythrocyte sedimentation rate, features that suggest a diagnosis of osteomyelitis. Furthermore, the roentgenographic appearance of Ewing tumor can simulate that of osteomyelitis. This similarity can lead to a tragic delay in the diagnosis of Ewing sarcoma. However, the age of the patient and the location of the lesion in a given bone are key pieces of information.

Its appearance on the roentgenogram can be considered the gross manifestation of a bone lesion. Roentgenograms help in defining the exact location of a lesion and its aggressiveness. Plain roentgenograms are generally helpful in differentiating benign lesions from malignant ones. The interphase between the lesion and the bone involved is of paramount importance. A lesion that is well marginated is likely to be benign, whereas one with poorly defined margins is more likely to be aggressive. The pattern of periosteal new bone formation is also important. Thick, continuous, organized periosteal new bone is usually indicative of a benign lesion, whereas a discontinuous, poorly organized reaction with an onionskin or spiculated appearance suggests a rapidly growing lesion.

There are, of course, limitations in the interpretation of roentgenograms. A certain amount of bone has to be destroyed in the medullary cavity before the lesion becomes apparent. Some permeative lesions, such as Ewing sarcoma, may be present despite a normal-appearing plain film. Some benign lesions, such as aneurysmal bone cysts or even osteoblastomas, may look very aggressive on roentgenograms. We do not believe that the surgical pathologist should refuse to diagnose a bone tumor if roentgenograms are not available. If the histologic evaluation reveals an osteosarcoma, the diagnosis is osteosarcoma—irrespective of what the roentgenographic appearance may be. In contrast, in other cases, such as low-grade cartilage tumors, a diagnosis should not be made without roentgenographic correlation.

Several additional imaging modalities, such as computed tomography (CT) and magnetic resonance imaging (MRI), are very useful in defining the extent of a bone or soft tissue lesion. These modalities, however, do not supplant plain roentgenograms for diagnostic purposes.

CLASSIFICATION

The classification that is used more or less universally is the one first proposed by Lichtenstein (1). This is based either on the cytologic characteristics of the neoplastic cells or the matrix produced by the neoplasm. The different entities are divided into benign and malignant counterparts. This division does not mean that benign neoplasms undergo malignant change. Such a transformation is unusual, in our experience. However, classification into benign and malignant counterparts is a convenient way to remember the different entities (2).

The classification scheme has some inconsistencies. We do not consider it to be a histogenetic classification because we do not believe that we know the cell of origin of most of these neoplasms. The classification is based more on the appearance of the tumor cells. However, we do use terms such as *tumors of unknown origin* that suggest that we do know the cell of origin of the other neoplasms.

METHODS OF BIOPSY

Material can be obtained from a bone neoplasm for diagnosis by several different methods. The classic method is an open biopsy carried out with the patient under general anesthesia. It is important that the surgeon, pathologist, and radiologist communicate so that the best method of biopsy and the best site for the biopsy can be determined.

We routinely perform frozen sections on bone biopsy specimens. Frozen sections offer several advantages. First, we can determine the adequacy of the biopsy specimen. Some bone neoplasms, such as Ewing sarcoma, tend to be very necrotic. If all the biopsy material shows only necrotic tissue, the final diagnosis cannot be made. We think all pathologists should be able to determine the adequacy of a biopsy specimen on frozen section. The frozen section diagnosis may also allow for immediate treatment. This advantage is becoming less important in high-grade malignant tumors, such as osteosarcomas, which are treated with chemotherapy before the definitive surgical procedure is undertaken. However, we still make frozen section diagnoses in many conditions, such as giant cell tumors and chondrosarcomas, for which definitive treatment can be carried out at the time of the biopsy. We also use frozen sections to check margins. In resections and amputations, the surgeon usually sends in a marrow sample from the margin in situ. It is nearly impossible to check margins adequately on large soft tissue extensions of bone tumors or large soft tissue sarcomas. Another advantage of frozen section diagnosis is the recognition of an infectious cause of the lesion. Obtaining material for culture at the time of surgery is obviously important.

Needle biopsy is another method of diagnosing bone tumors. The amount of diagnostic material varies depending on the size of the needle used for the procedure, which can range from 18 to 11 or 12 gauge.

A needle biopsy is frequently performed by a radiologist under CT or ultrasonographic guidance. The specimen typically consists of a smear and biopsy tissue obtained most often with a 14- to 18-gauge needle. We believe that the needle biopsy is a good diagnostic procedure if adequate material is obtained. This technique is especially useful in documenting metastatic malignant disease or a recurrent tumor. However, it has some limitations when used in diagnosing primary bone neoplasms. Needle biopsies are not well suited for diagnosing cartilage tumors and cystic lesions, such as aneurysmal bone cysts. We think that some lesions, such as osteoblastomas, may be overdiagnosed as osteosarcoma with such limited amounts of tissue. A positive diagnosis on the needle biopsy may have the advantage of reducing cost in cases of high-grade malignant lesions, especially because many of these tumors are treated with preoperative chemotherapy, radiotherapy, or both. We see no special advantage in performing needle biopsies in obviously benign lesions, such as chondromyxoid fibroma and fibrous dysplasia, that require only surgical management.

HANDLING OF SPECIMENS

No special laboratory equipment is required for handling bone biopsy specimens obtained from patients with neoplastic conditions. Most bone neoplasms have soft areas that can be processed without decalcification. Hence, with rare exception, permanent slides should be prepared within 24 hours for many bone biopsy specimens. Only occasionally have we seen an osteoid osteoma or a parosteal osteosarcoma mineralized to the extent that no section could be obtained without prior decalcification. If the biopsy specimen received contains both soft and hard fragments, it is important to separate the hard material from the soft tissue, especially in the case of small-cell neoplasms, such as malignant lymphomas, which may be extensively permeative and may even invoke a sclerotic reaction in medullary bone. We use the point of a scalpel blade to tease out small fragments of fleshy tissue from between bone trabeculae. This

tissue can be used for permanent sections and, if necessary, special studies. Decalcified sections are useful for studying low-power morphologic features.

For decalcification, we fix the specimen in 10% formaldehyde for at least 1 hour. Then the tissue is placed in a rapid decalcifying agent until soft enough for processing. It is important to take very thin slices of bone to minimize the time required for decalcification. Most specimens should be decalcified within 24 hours. Occasionally, with extremely sclerotic bone, it may be necessary to decalcify for a longer period. Some small specimens require only hours of decalcification. It is important to check the specimen periodically to ensure that excessive decalcification, which results in a lack of cytologic detail, does not occur.

Most malignant specimens consist of resection samples. We usually dissect away all the soft material, leaving only the involved bone and soft tissue extension of the neoplasm, if any. Margins of soft tissue extensions are examined on frozen section, if necessary. Using a band saw, we bivalve the bone with the tumor. The band saw is kept in a room that can be closed so that laboratory personnel are not exposed to the bone dust. Even thin slices of bone can be prepared for decalcification with the band saw. However, a hand-held saw may be preferable to take thin sections for decalcification. The gross specimen is washed with running water, and a brush is used to remove bone dust. This step minimizes the artifacts that may otherwise be present in sections. Amputation specimens are handled in the same way as resection specimens.

Most osteosarcoma specimens are resected tissue obtained after preoperative chemotherapy. Good evidence shows that the prognosis of these patients is related to the amount of necrosis present at the time of the resection. Hence, it is important that pathologists study the specimen to calculate the amount of necrosis. We routinely decalcify one thin macrosection of the entire specimen, including the bone and the tumor, cut parallel to the initial plane of sectioning. The entire slice is then submitted for sectioning. The effect of chemotherapy may appear as areas of fibrosis, granulation tissue, frank necrosis, or, most commonly, dense bone formation within the marrow spaces.

We believe it is impossible to be precise about the percentage of necrosis in these specimens. However, we can be fairly accurate in calculating the area of viable tumor in relation to the area of necrotic tumor. The identification of viable tumor may also be difficult. One frequently observes enlarged hyperchromatic nuclei embedded in sclerotic bone. It is difficult to determine whether this represents viable tumor and, if so, the percentage of the lesion that is viable. Despite these drawbacks, this calculation has prognostic significance.

GRADING AND STAGING OF BONE TUMORS

Formerly, a good system for staging bone and soft tissue neoplasms was not available. Largely through the efforts of Enneking et al. (3), orthopedic oncologists from Florida, a staging system has become universally accepted that is based on two criteria: the histologic grade and the anatomic location of the tumor.

The first criterion for the staging system is the grade of the neoplasm. Several different systems are used for grading sarcomas. In one system proposed by the National Cancer Institute, necrosis is a very important factor in grading neoplasms (4). The authors believed that the more necrotic the tumor is, the worse the prognosis. We agree that high-grade tumors tend to be more necrotic. However, we do not use necrosis as one of the criteria for grading. We suspect that necrosis may be an independent prognostic criterion. The grading system we use is based predominantly on the cytologic characteristics of the tumor cells (5). It follows the criteria laid down by Broders (6) more than 80 years ago. If the tumor cells closely resemble the cells from which they are supposed to arise, the tumor is well differentiated. If a tumor is so undifferentiated that one can hardly recognize the normal counterpart, the tumor is poorly differentiated. We grade most bone tumors from 1 to 4, depending on the nuclear changes and, to a lesser extent, the cellularity of the lesion. In the staging system of Enneking and colleagues, tumors are classified as low grade or high grade. The low-grade tumors in the Enneking system are grades 1 and 2 in the Broders system, and the high-grade tumors in the Enneking system are grades 3 and 4 in the Broders system.

The anatomic location of the tumor depends on whether the lesion is confined to one compartment or involves more than one compartment. For bone tumors, lesions confined within the bone are considered to be in one compartment, and lesions that have broken through the bone into soft tissues are considered to involve two compartments.

Low-grade tumors are considered stage I. High-grade tumors are considered stage II. A neoplasm of any grade that has metastasized is considered stage III. Each stage comprises subdivisions A and B, depending on whether the tumor involves one compartment or more than one compartment. The staging system appears in Table 8.1.

This staging system is not perfect. For instance, it does not take into consideration the small-cell malignant lesions of bone. However, it is a simple, reproducible system that can be used by orthopedic oncologists around the world. We believe that a simple but imperfect system that will be used is better than a perfect but complicated system that will seldom be used.

The staging system is also related to concepts about surgical margins (7). A pseudocapsule is formed by the compression of surrounding normal tissues when a tumor invades soft tissue. A zone of increased vascularity is present between the pseudocapsule and surrounding normal tissues. This is considered the reactive zone. The terms surgeons use to describe margins are defined as follows:

1. *Intralesional margin.* After a curettage or debulking procedure, microscopic evidence of the lesion is found at the margin.
2. *Marginal margin.* The lesion is shelled out, usually with the pseudocapsule; no normal tissue is removed.
3. *Wide margin.* The entire tumor is removed with the pseudocapsule, the reactive zone, and a cuff of normal tissue surrounding it.
4. *Radical margin.* The entire compartment bearing the tumor is removed completely. For instance, a radical margin for an osteosarcoma of the distal femur involves disarticulation of the hip.

In the surgical staging system, the term *radical* does not refer to radical surgery; even a hemipelvectomy may be a marginal excision, depending on the extent and anatomic location of the tumor. The surgical staging system is very important because it provides a common language for all physicians interested in bone and soft tissue tumors.

NEOPLASMS OF BONE

SMALL-CELL NEOPLASMS

The classification scheme generally used for bone tumors, which includes Ewing tumor with tumors of unknown origin, has been modified slightly to include Ewing sarcoma with small-cell malignant lesions. This seems more reasonable because the differential diagnosis of Ewing tumor involves other small-cell malignant lesions. Although metastatic small-cell malignant tumors, such as small-cell carcinoma of the lung and neuroblastoma metastatic to bone, are in the differential diagnosis, they are discussed with metastatic carcinoma in general. In this section, they are discussed only insofar as they are involved in the differential diagnosis.

Myeloma

Myeloma is the most common primary bone neoplasm. It accounts for approximately 1% of all types of malignancies and slightly more than 10% of hematologic malignancies.

Bone pain is the most frequent symptom of myeloma. Many patients present with pathologic fracture, and a biopsy is performed during surgery for the fracture. Patients with involvement of the spine commonly present with spinal cord compression. Myeloma is more commonly seen in middle-aged and elderly persons. Of 1027 patients in a Mayo Clinic study of multiple myeloma, 2% were younger than 40 years, and 38% were 70 years of age or older (8). Myeloma usually involves adult bones that contain hematopoietic marrow. Patients with myeloma are usually anemic. Their peripheral blood smears typically show features of a normochromic, normocytic anemia with rouleaux. Electrophoresis and immunoelectrophoresis performed with both serum and urine can detect a monoclonal protein in almost all cases of multiple myeloma (99%) at the time of diagnosis.

Conventional radiographs show a skeletal abnormality in approximately 80% of patients at the time of diagnosis. Roentgenograms generally show multiple, punched-out, purely lytic

TABLE 8.1			
Staging of Bone Neoplasms			
Stage	*Grade[a]*	*Site[b]*	*Metastasis[c]*
IA	1	T1	M0
IB	1	T2	M0
IIA	2	T1	M0
IIB	2	T2	M0
IIIA	1, 2	T1	M1
IIIB	1, 2	T2	M1

[a]1, low grade; 2, high grade.
[b]T1, involves one compartment; T2, involves more than one compartment.
[c]M0, no metastatic tumor; M1, metastatic lesions present.

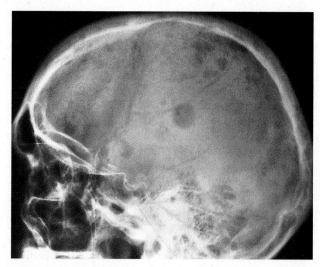

Figure 8.1. Roentgenogram of myeloma shows multiple purely lytic defects involving the skull.

holes in the bone (Fig. 8.1). Typically, myeloma is not associated with any sclerosis. A small percentage of patients with myeloma present with diffuse osteopenia.

The gross appearance is typically described as that of "currant jelly." The lesion is soft and red. However, many myelomas have a "fish flesh" appearance, similar to that of lymphomas.

Histologically, myeloma consists of neoplastic cells that cytologically resemble normal plasma cells. Features that aid in the recognition of these as abnormal plasma cells are an eccentric nucleus with coarsely clumped nuclear chromatin, variability in cell shape, more prominent nucleoli, and multiple nucleation (Fig. 8.2). The cytologic appearance in myeloma can range from cells closely simulating plasma cells to cells with an anaplastic appearance devoid of easily recognizable plasmacytic features. Myelomas frequently exhibit a sinusoidal vascular pattern similar to that of endocrine neoplasms. From 10% to 15% of myelomas contain deposits of amyloid. The amyloid may be in the wall of vessels or appear as masses within the neoplasm. Rarely, the amyloid is so massive in association with a giant cell reaction

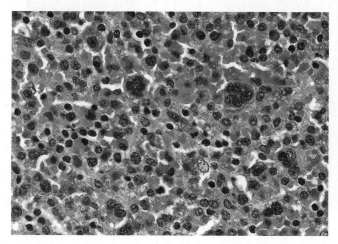

Figure 8.2. Myeloma with sheets of plasma cells, some of which are multinucleated. The cytoplasm is abundant, and the nuclei are situated eccentrically.

that it may mask an underlying myeloma. In our experience, any amyloid deposit in the bone is evidence of an underlying systemic plasma cell dyscrasia rather than an "amyloidoma," except in the rare instance of amyloid deposits in patients undergoing long-term hemodialysis (9). This has also been the experience of others (10).

Although most myelomas are multiple, a small percentage of patients have a solitary plasmacytoma (11–13). Solitary plasmacytomas of bone most commonly involve the spine. The patients are somewhat younger than those with multiple myeloma. Although in most cases this type of bone lesion progresses to multiple myeloma, the overall survival of patients with a solitary plasmacytoma is better than that of patients who present with multiple myeloma.

The term *osteosclerotic myeloma* refers to the plasma cell dyscrasias seen in patients with polyneuropathy, organomegaly, endocrinopathy, serum M-protein, and skin changes: the POEMS (Crow-Fukase) syndrome (14,15). The osteosclerotic bone lesions may be single or multiple. Bone tissue from these sites consists of a plasmacytoma surrounded by sclerotic bone. Oftentimes, the sclerotic bone predominates, and only small clusters or nests of tumor are present. Immunohistochemical stains for kappa (κ) and lambda (λ) light chains aid in confirming clonality. The patients tend to be younger, and the clinical course may be protracted. However, even patients with multiple myeloma may experience long-term survival (8).

The differential diagnosis of myeloma includes chronic osteomyelitis with a predominance of plasma cells. Almost without exception, chronic osteomyelitis shows capillary proliferation in the background, simulating that seen in granulation tissue, and at least a sprinkling of other inflammatory cells, such as lymphocytes, eosinophils, and neutrophils.

Immunohistochemistry can be helpful in the differential diagnosis. A monoclonal cytoplasmic staining pattern for κ or λ light chain establishes a diagnosis of malignant disease. If carcinoma is a consideration, keratin stains can be helpful. Myeloma cells should be negative with keratin markers. Epithelial membrane antigen is not useful, however, because some myelomas stain with antibodies to this antigen. Myelomas stain positive for CD138. However, because some carcinomas can also show positive immunoreactivity with CD138, it is important to correlate a positive stain with other clinicopathologic findings.

The histologic distinction between myeloma and lymphoma can occasionally be difficult. In the vast majority of cases, careful attention to clinical and laboratory information solves the problem. In addition, myeloma and lymphoma can usually be distinguished through the use of immunoperoxidase stains. Myeloma cells show strong cytoplasmic immunoglobulin light chain stain restriction and are weakly positive or negative for CD45 and CD20, the B-cell–lineage marker. In contrast, most B-cell lymphomas show the converse staining pattern, with strong positivity for CD45 and CD20 and little reactivity for CD138 and immunoglobulin light chains.

Lymphoma

Lymphoma of bone can be either a primary tumor or a manifestation of more generalized disease (16,17). Primary lymphomas of bone have been reported as comprising approximately 7% of malignant bone tumors and 5% of extranodal lymphomas (18). A modest male predominance is noted, and most often, it is a disease of young and older adults. However, lymphoma of bone can occur in children, although it is only about one-tenth as common as Ewing sarcoma (19,20). Any portion of the skeleton may be involved, but the most frequently affected sites are the femur and pelvic bones. Patients with lymphoma generally have bone pain at presentation and may have systemic symptoms. Patients with involvement of the spine may present with symptoms referable to spinal cord compression.

Roentgenograms generally show extensive involvement of the bone with a permeative destructive process (Fig. 8.3). A mixture of lysis and sclerosis is characteristic in lymphoma. Periosteal new bone formation is rarely seen. Results of bone scans are characteristically positive in lymphoma. A negative bone roentgenogram with a positive bone scan should arouse suspicion of lymphoma. MRI may also show extensive permeation of marrow that may not be obvious on plain roentgenograms.

The gross appearance of lymphoma is that of the usual fish flesh. Occasionally, however, lymphoma is associated with extreme bone sclerosis, and the tumor may not be obvious. Such specimens may require extensive decalcification that may result in loss of detail of the tumor cells. Hence, it is important to try to separate even small fragments of soft material from within the interstices of the bone for separate processing.

The microscopic appearance of malignant lymphoma of bone is variable (21). Under low power, the lesion is permeative, leaving behind normal structures such as bony trabeculae (Fig. 8.4A) and marrow fat. The bony trabeculae may be thickened. It is not uncommon for lymphoma of bone to be associated with significant crush artifact. Although it may be difficult at times to assess the cytologic features, most lymphomas have a polymorphic appearance with scattered small lymphocytes in the background (Fig. 8.4B). These features are helpful in the differential diagnosis, especially when used in distinguishing lymphoma from the monomorphic appearance of Ewing sarcoma. Most lymphomas of bone are classified as diffuse large B-cell lymphomas. It is extremely unusual for a low-grade or follicular lymphoma to create a mass lesion in bone. Occasionally, lymphomas contain dense sclerosis. Under these circumstances, the cells may be elongated and even have a storiform pattern. This can lead to a mistaken diagnosis of sarcoma (Fig. 8.4C) (22). Immunohistochemical studies are an essential part of the diagnostic workup for lymphoma. The panel should include markers against B cells (CD20 and CD79a), T cells (CD3), and leukocyte common antigen (CD45). CD30 is helpful when anaplastic large-cell lymphoma and classic Hodgkin lymphoma are the differential diagnosis.

The differential diagnosis includes chronic osteomyelitis, myeloid sarcoma (granulocytic sarcoma), and carcinoma. The mixed cell infiltrate of lymphoma may lead to a mistaken diagnosis of chronic osteomyelitis. The clinical and roentgenographic appearances also may be similar. However, lymphoma lacks the granulation tissue appearance of osteomyelitis. In rare instances, immunohistochemical studies may be necessary to establish the diagnosis. Myeloid sarcoma may present as a mass lesion in bone (23–25). It can occur de novo or concurrently with acute myeloid leukemia or a myeloproliferative disorder.

It is not possible to definitively diagnose myeloid sarcoma on sections stained only with hematoxylin and eosin. Eosinophilic metamyelocytes are helpful if present, but they are absent in 50% to 70% of cases. One should suspect myeloid sarcoma in the differential diagnosis with lymphoma when the tumor cells express CD45 without CD20 or CD45RO (26). In addition, the vast majority of cases are positive for CD43 (27). Additional markers that are quite specific for myeloid processes include myeloperoxidase, lysozyme, and CD33. Myeloid sarcoma can also show monocytic differentiation that is reflected in positive reactivity with CD68. Metastatic large-cell undifferentiated carcinoma may be difficult to differentiate from lymphoma. Immunohistochemical stains for keratin and hematopoietic markers are helpful in resolving this problem.

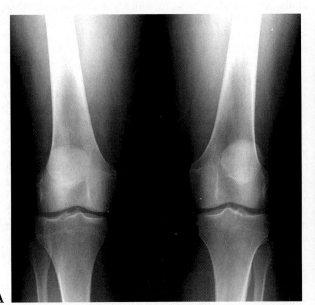
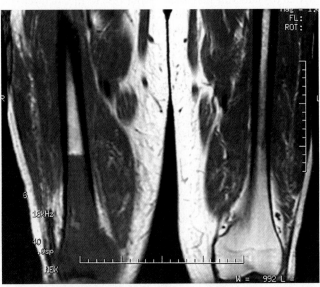

A   **B**

Figure 8.3. Malignant lymphoma of bone. **(A)** Anteroposterior radiograph of the knees shows a subtle region of increased density in the right medial femoral condyle. **(B)** The coronal T1-weighted magnetic resonance image (MRI) shows a large infiltrative tumor in the distal right femur that extends from the distal diaphysis to the end of the bone. The MRI findings are out of proportion to what is predicted on the radiograph, and this imaging feature is highly suggestive of a diagnosis of lymphoma.

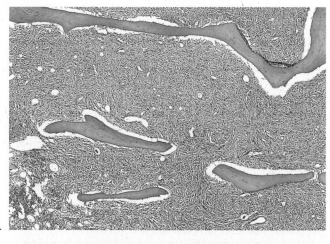

A

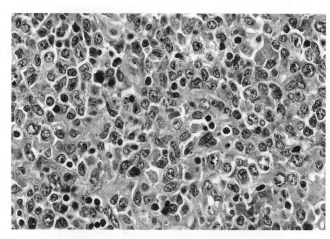

B

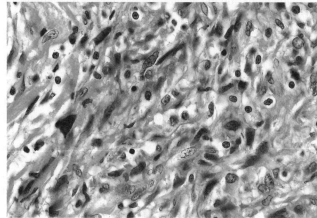

C

Figure 8.4. Malignant lymphoma of bone. **(A)** Tumor diffusely permeates the marrow. The pre-existing trabecular bone is intact. **(B)** Polymorphic appearance with a lack of uniformity in nuclear size and shape. **(C)** Fibrosis and spindling suggest a diagnosis of sarcoma.

Hodgkin lymphoma may appear as a mass lesion in bone. Most commonly, involvement of bone is a late manifestation of classical Hodgkin lymphoma. Rarely, bone involvement is the presenting sign of Hodgkin lymphoma (28–30). Hodgkin lymphoma that involves the skeleton usually affects the spine. Almost without exception, lymph nodes are involved, especially para-aortic lymph nodes. A diagnosis of Hodgkin lymphoma should be considered when the biopsy specimen shows a mixed cell infiltrate with inflammatory cells, particularly eosinophils, and rare pleomorphic cells. The Reed-Sternberg cells stain with CD30, PAX5, and oftentimes with CD15, and are negative with CD45.

Ewing Sarcoma

In the past, Ewing sarcoma was considered the most lethal of all bone neoplasms. Modern therapeutic approaches with radiation and chemotherapy have improved the prognosis considerably. Ewing sarcoma is rare, making up approximately 8.6% of all malignant bone tumors in the Mayo Clinic series. A distinct predilection for males is noted. Most patients are young; however, it is unusual to see Ewing sarcoma in patients younger than 5 years, an age group in which metastatic neuroblastoma is more common. Any portion of the skeleton may be involved, but the long bones are the most typical sites. The lesion usually involves the shaft of the bone. Patients with Ewing sarcoma usually have localized pain or swelling at presentation. However, some have systemic manifestations, such as fever, weight loss,

and an increased erythrocyte sedimentation rate, suggesting the possibility of osteomyelitis.

Askin et al. (31) described a small-cell tumor of the thoracopulmonary region in children and suggested that it was neurally derived. Since then, the term *peripheral neuroectodermal tumor* (*PNET*) has become an accepted diagnostic designation. The histologic appearance is marked by a small round cell tumor with tumor cells arranged in a lobular pattern and with rosettes. Studies have shown that Ewing sarcoma is of neuroectodermal origin, but with limited neural differentiation, whereas PNET demonstrates more definite neural features (32). They have similar immunohistochemical, cytogenetic, and molecular features, and therefore, both belong within the Ewing sarcoma family of tumors (33–38).

On roentgenograms, Ewing tumors tend to be extensive, sometimes involving an entire bone. The lesion is usually a permeative, destructive process, with multiple tiny areas of destruction involving the bone. Nevertheless, large geographic areas of destruction may be seen. Typically, Ewing tumor produces a pronounced reactive new bone formation of the periosteum, giving rise to an onionskin appearance (Fig. 8.5). CT and MRI studies are very useful in defining the extent of the tumor.

The gross appearance of Ewing sarcoma is that of a white, fleshy neoplasm (Fig. 8.6). The tumor may appear liquid and resemble pus. Large areas of necrosis are common.

Ewing sarcoma is composed of small, round, uniform nuclei with clear cytoplasm and indistinct cytoplasmic bodies (Fig. 8.7A). Any clear-cut spindling of the nucleus should rule out a

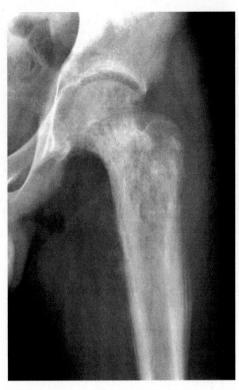

Figure 8.5. Roentgenogram of Ewing tumor shows a destructive lesion with periosteal new bone formation giving rise to an onionskin appearance.

diagnosis of Ewing sarcoma. Special stains usually show glycogen within tumor cells. Mitotic figures may be present, but usually they are not numerous. Large areas of necrosis may be found, and residual tumor may be present only around vascular spaces. The tumor cells may be arranged around small spaces, giving rise to a pseudorosette formation. Occasionally, Ewing tumors

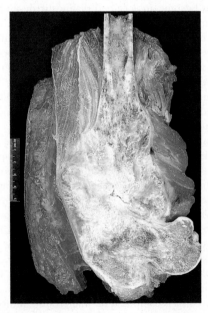

Figure 8.6. Gross appearance of a large Ewing tumor of the femur with pathologic fracture. The tumor is soft and fleshy.

contain cells that are larger and more irregular than those seen in typical Ewing sarcoma. These have been referred to as examples of large-cell or atypical Ewing sarcoma.

Immunohistochemical studies may be helpful in diagnosing Ewing sarcoma. CD99, a p30/32^{MIC2} gene product, is a cell surface glycoprotein expressed in Ewing sarcomas and PNETs. Strong membrane staining for CD99 is consistently seen in Ewing sarcoma. However, CD99 expression can be seen in other malignant neoplasms, including sarcomas and carcinomas, and hematopoietic lesions, such as lymphoblastic lymphomas and acute lymphocytic leukemias (39–43). FLI-1 is another sensitive, but not specific, marker for Ewing sarcoma that may be helpful in an immunohistochemical panel (44). Ewing sarcoma also occasionally stains for cytokeratin (45). Therefore, careful clinical, radiographic, and histologic correlation is necessary when immunohistochemical results are interpreted.

Cytogenetic and molecular genetic studies can be useful adjunctive tools in diagnosing Ewing sarcoma (46). The t(11;22) (q24;q12) chromosomal translocation or variants thereof are detectable in more than 95% of Ewing sarcomas and PNETs. The breakpoints of these translocations have indicated the involvement of the EWS gene on chromosome 22, the FL1-1 gene on chromosome 11, and the ERG gene on chromosome 21. This results in the production of the fusion genes EWS-FL1-1 for t(11;22) and EWS-ERG for t(21;22), which can be detected by reverse transcriptase polymerase chain reaction (RT-PCR) and fluorescence in situ hybridization (FISH) techniques (47–49). The EWS-FLI-1 fusion gene is present in up to 95% of Ewing sarcomas, whereas EWS-ERG is identified in approximately 5% of tumors. Other translocations are seen in less than 1% of tumors (33).

Several attempts have been made to correlate histologic features with prognosis in Ewing sarcoma. It has been suggested that growth with a filigree pattern, atypical histologic features (Fig. 8.7B), and necrosis are all associated with a poorer prognosis (50–52).

The differential diagnosis includes metastatic neuroblastoma and malignant lymphoma. Other small-cell malignant lesions, such as small-cell osteosarcoma and mesenchymal chondrosarcoma, are ruled out by matrix within the neoplasm. Metastatic neuroblastoma usually is not a problem because most often it is already known that the patient has a neuroblastoma. Rarely, the diagnosis can be very difficult. If the lesion shows a clear-cut rosette formation and a neurofibrillary background, the diagnosis of neuroblastoma is obvious. However, some neuroblastomas do not show such differentiation. We think the clinical features must be of paramount importance in this differentiation. When we see a bone biopsy specimen from a patient of approximately 2 years of age or younger, we always consider the possibility of metastatic neuroblastoma. Malignant lymphomas usually develop in older patients, and the infiltrate is polymorphic. In a small percentage of cases, it can be impossible to histologically distinguish lymphoma from Ewing sarcoma. Immunohistochemical stains and, at times, RT-PCR and FISH are critical in this situation. B-cell lymphoblastic lymphomas are often positive with CD99. Therefore, the addition of CD79a, CD10, CD34, and TdT to the immunohistochemical panel can be helpful in distinguishing lymphoblastic lymphoma from Ewing sarcoma, which should be negative with these markers.

Treatment of patients with Ewing sarcoma is based on multiagent systemic chemotherapy (neoadjuvant treatment), combined with delayed surgical removal of the tumor (when feasi-

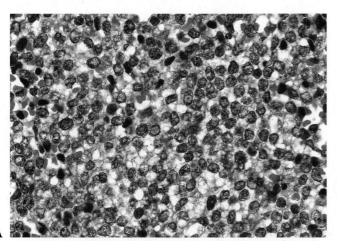

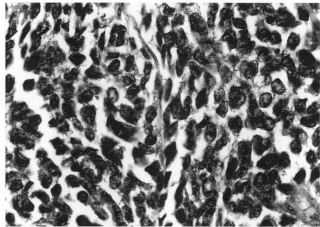

A   B

Figure 8.7. Ewing tumor. **(A)** High-power appearance of uniform round nuclei and indistinct cytoplasmic borders. **(B)** High-power view of "large-cell" tumor. The nuclei are more pleomorphic than in classic Ewing tumor.

ble) and/or radiation therapy. The prognosis of patients with Ewing sarcoma has improved considerably over the years since the introduction of modern intensive chemotherapy combined with an increased use and improved techniques of surgery. Five-year and 10-year survival rates of 57% and 49%, respectively (53), 5-year overall survival rates of 65% (54), and overall survival rates of 61% to 72% (55) have been reported. Pathologists play an important role in determining prognosis because the histologic percentage of chemotherapy-induced necrosis in the resected tumor is strongly related to prognosis (56–58).

CHONDROID TUMORS

Chondroid lesions comprise the second largest single group of neoplasms of bone.

Benign Chondroid Tumors

OSTEOCHONDROMA. Osteochondroma is the most common benign bone tumor. Historically, there has been debate regarding whether osteochondromas represent a developmental aberration or a benign neoplasm. More recently, the discovery of clonal chromosomal abnormalities in osteochondromas has provided evidence that they represent a true neoplasm (59,60). Moreover, clonal karyotypic abnormalities leading to the loss or rearrangement of 8q24.1 or 11p11-12, the chromosomal loci of the EXT1 and EXT2 genes, have been detected as somatic aberrations in both sporadic and hereditary osteochondromas (61,62).

The size of osteochondromas is quite variable. If they are small, they do not cause symptoms, so their true incidence is unknown. Symptoms may develop as a consequence of size, impingement on adjacent structures such as nerves, or fracture through the stalk, causing pain. Most osteochondromas seen in a surgical practice are in young patients, and a distinct male predominance is noted. The most common site is the metaphysis of long bones, although rarely, flat bones are also affected. Roentgenograms show a mushroomlike growth that extends away from the nearest joint. The cortex of the underlying bone is continuous with the cortex of the stalk of the osteochondroma. Similarly, the medullary cavity is continuous with the

medullary cavity of the stalk (Fig. 8.8). Grossly, one sees a cartilage cap that matures into bone and becomes the stalk (Fig. 8.9). The cap is usually regular and thin. A thick cartilage cap with a bosselated surface suggests the development of secondary chondrosarcoma.

Microscopically, the surface of an osteochondroma shows a pink fibrous capsule that is the periosteum of the underlying bone. The chondrocytes are within lacunae and tend to have a columnar arrangement toward the base, where they undergo

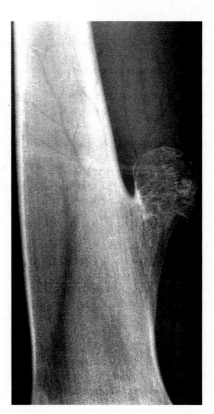

Figure 8.8. Roentgenogram of osteochondroma of the femur. Note that the medullary cavity of the lesion is continuous with the medullary cavity of the bone. The cortices are similarly continuous.

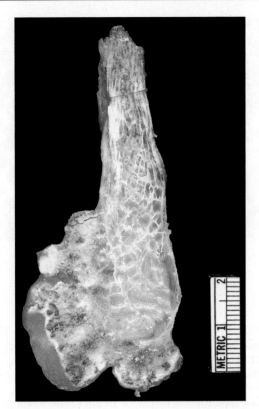

Figure 8.9. Gross specimen of osteochondroma. Sessile osteochondroma of the distal femur is shown. The smooth, pale blue cartilage cap has a thickness of less than 1 cm.

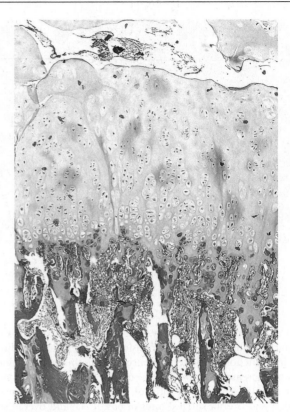

Figure 8.10. Osteochondroma. The cartilage cap matures into underlying cancellous bone. Note the orderly arrangement of the cartilage cells at the base of the cartilage cap.

endochondral ossification (Fig. 8.10). Between the bony trabeculae of the stalk, one sees fatty or hematopoietic marrow. The proliferation of spindle cells between the bony trabeculae should arouse suspicion of a parosteal osteosarcoma. A minority of patients have hereditary multiple exostoses. The transmission is autosomal dominant. Genetic linkage studies have implicated the EXT1 and EXT2 genes in the majority of cases (63,64). These patients frequently have other skeletal abnormalities. The roentgenographic, gross, and microscopic features of such osteochondromas are identical to those in patients with solitary exostosis.

Rarely, a bursa overlies the osteosarcoma. This leads to rapid growth and a mass effect that may arouse suspicion of chondrosarcoma (65).

The most important differential diagnosis is secondary chondrosarcoma. Because most secondary chondrosarcomas that arise in osteochondromas are low grade, the diagnosis cannot be based purely on the histologic findings. Roentgenographically, a thick or irregular cartilage cap and areas of lucency within the cartilage are worrisome features. Grossly, a bosselated, thick cartilage cap with cystic change within the cartilage is a troubling feature. Microscopically, secondary chondrosarcomas are extremely well differentiated, but invasion of surrounding tissues is evidence of sarcomatous change (66). Rare examples of dedifferentiated chondrosarcoma arising in pre-existing osteochondroma have also been reported (67).

CHONDROMA. The term *chondroma* can be used for a benign neoplasm composed of cartilage. These cartilage tumors can occur within the bone (enchondroma), on the surface of

the bone (periosteal chondroma), or in the soft tissues (soft tissue chondroma).

Enchondromas usually do not cause symptoms, so their true incidence is unknown. No sex predilection is noted, and any age group can be involved. Most enchondromas in surgical series involve the small bones of the hands and feet. Roentgenographically, enchondromas affecting the larger bones appear as circumscribed lesions in the metaphysis or diaphysis of long bones (Fig. 8.11). The lesion does not show aggressive invasion into or through the cortex. However, occasionally there is minimal erosion of the cortical bone. Usually flecks of calcification are seen within the neoplasm. Grossly, the lesion is well circumscribed and has the pale blue appearance typical of cartilage. The lesion is solid and does not show any myxoid change. Microscopically, enchondromas are hypocellular with few, if any, doubly nucleated cells. The lesion may have a multifocal appearance within the bone. However, there is no destructive permeation of pre-existing medullary or cortical bone (Fig. 8.12). The matrix does not show significant myxoid change (Fig. 8.13), but areas of degenerative necrosis may be focally present.

Enchondromas of the small bones of the hands and feet are somewhat different. Roentgenograms show thinning of the overlying cortex but no penetration into soft tissues. This feature frequently results in pathologic fracture, so that pain may be the presenting symptom. Microscopically, enchondromas involving the small bones of the hands and feet are hypercellular, with frequent doubly nucleated cells and myxoid change in the matrix (Fig. 8.14). In other words, the histologic appearance is generally that of a grade 1 chondrosarcoma. However, if the

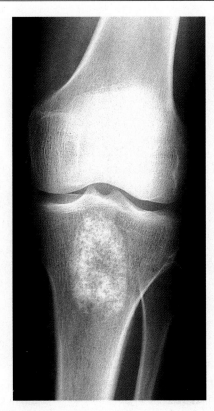

Figure 8.11. Enchondroma of the proximal tibia with uniform mineralization. The lesion is circumscribed and does not invade the cortex.

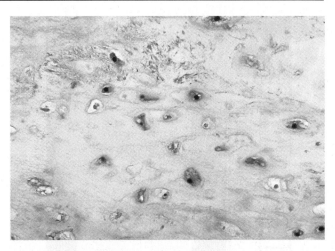

Figure 8.13. High-power appearance of an enchondroma of the femur. The tumor is hypocellular, and the nuclei are small.

roentgenographic appearance is that of a benign lesion, such histologic changes can be ignored.

The differential diagnosis of enchondroma is chondrosarcoma. A painful chondroid neoplasm in a large bone in an adult patient should be viewed with suspicion. The roentgenograms generally show expansion of the bone, cortical thickening, and destructive erosion or permeation of the cortex. Any marked myxoid change in the matrix is a worrisome sign in a large bone cartilage tumor. Permeation, manifested as marrow spaces filled with the neoplasm and entrapment of pre-existing bony trabeculae, is the most important sign of malignancy. In small bone

cartilage tumors, the chondroid neoplasm must permeate the cortex into soft tissue before a histologic diagnosis of chondrosarcoma can be made.

Rarely, a cartilage tumor occurs on the surface of a bone (periosteal chondroma) (Fig. 8.15) (68). This lesion tends to be smaller than 3 cm and appears on roentgenograms as a saucerized, well-demarcated lucency on the cortex. Histologically, at low power, the lesion shows no tendency to permeate surrounding tissue. However, the lesion is hypercellular, may be myxoid, and has doubly nucleated cells that may be quite hyperchromatic (Fig. 8.16). These changes do not denote malignancy if the lesion is small and the roentgenograms support a benign process.

Neoplasms composed of hyaline cartilage are unusual in the soft tissues except in the hands and feet (69–73). Histologically, they resemble synovial chondromatosis and may indeed represent this entity. The lesion is lobulated, and the chondrocytes often occur in clusters. The cells may be quite hyperchromatic, and doubly nucleated cells may be common. Despite all of these worrisome histologic features, the clinical behavior is always that of a benign lesion. The tumor may recur locally, but malignant transformation is extremely rare.

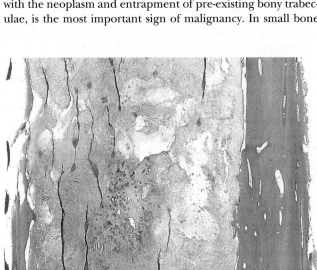

Figure 8.12. Low-power appearance of an enchondroma involving the fibula: a sharp cortical boundary without evidence of permeation.

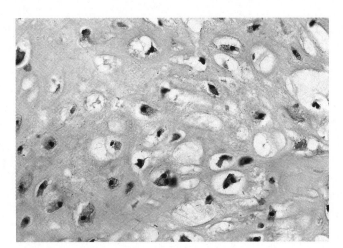

Figure 8.14. Enchondroma of the phalanx. The tumor is hypercellular and contains enlarged nuclei.

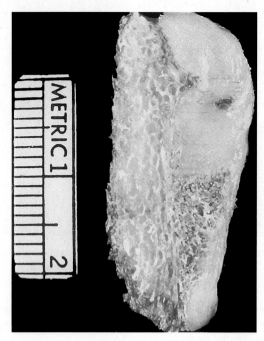

Figure 8.15. Periosteal chondroma. The lesion is on the surface of the bone, well circumscribed, and small.

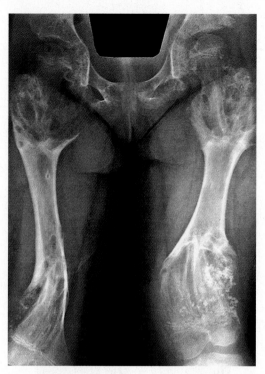

Figure 8.17. Roentgenogram of the legs in a patient with Ollier disease. In each femur, cartilaginous masses involve both ends of the bone.

A small number of patients have multiple cartilaginous lesions at presentation. This condition, generally considered a congenital nonhereditary disorder, has been termed *Ollier disease*. In Ollier disease, multiple masses of cartilage tend to involve the ends of long bones and the flat bones (Fig. 8.17). These patients also have skeletal deformities secondary to the cartilaginous masses. There may be a tendency to involve half the skeleton. The biopsy specimen from such a lesion usually shows hypercellularity, doubly nucleated cells, and hyperchromasia of the nuclei, suggesting a diagnosis of low-grade chondrosarcoma. However, if the roentgenographic features are those of Ollier disease, such changes should be ignored. Most lesions tend to regress when the skeleton matures, although rare instances of chondrosarcoma have occurred in patients with Ollier disease (74). An even smaller minority of patients

have multiple chondroid lesions in the bones and associated soft tissue hemangiomas. This disorder has been termed *Maffucci syndrome*. It has been suggested that Maffucci syndrome is associated with a high incidence of malignancy, either in the skeleton or in visceral organs (75).

CHONDROBLASTOMA. Chondroblastoma is a benign chondroid neoplasm that occurs predominantly in the second decade of life. A slight male predominance is noted, and any bone in the skeleton may be involved, although most lesions occur at the ends of long bones. Patients with chondroblastoma involving the skull bones tend to be older (76). Most reports of chondroblastoma emphasize the epiphyseal location of the lesion (77–80). Patients generally experience bone pain.

The roentgenographic appearance is quite characteristic. The lesion is extremely well circumscribed, and the epicenter is almost always in the epiphysis (Fig. 8.18) (81). More than 50% involve the epiphysis and extend to the metaphysis. A well-circumscribed lesion involving the epiphysis and metaphysis of a patient with an open epiphyseal plate is characteristic of chondroblastoma. Approximately 15% of the lesions involve the apophysis, especially the greater trochanter of the femur. Approximately one-third of chondroblastomas show mineral on roentgenograms.

Grossly, chondroblastomas tend to be white and firm. Rarely, the lesion is cystic. Microscopically, chondroblastoma is composed of a mixture of mononuclear cells and giant cells. The mononuclear cells tend to have oval nuclei with a longitudinal groove similar to that seen in Langerhans cell histiocytosis. The cells tend to have either clear or pink cytoplasm and distinct cytoplasmic outlines. Although the cytologic features of chondroblastoma are usually quite characteristic, we do not believe

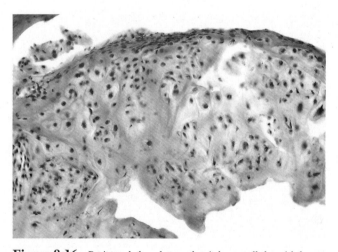

Figure 8.16. Periosteal chondroma that is hypercellular with large, atypical chondrocytes.

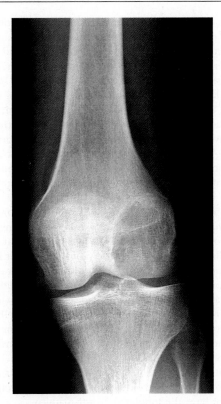

Figure 8.18. Chondroblastoma of the distal femur. The lesion extends to the articular cartilage, is extremely well circumscribed, and has a sclerotic rim.

that a firm diagnosis of chondroblastoma can be made without identification of either chondroid differentiation in the matrix (Fig. 8.19) or the characteristic "chicken wire" calcification (Fig. 8.20). In a study of a large number of chondroblastomas, chondroid differentiation was identified in 95% of the cases, and calcific deposits were identified in 35% of cases (76). The chondroid areas tend to have a pink matrix rather than the blue matrix typical of cartilage tumors. More than one-third of chondroblastomas are associated with secondary aneurysmal bone cysts. The aneurysmal bone cyst may be a predominant feature, and a chondroblastoma may be present only as a small

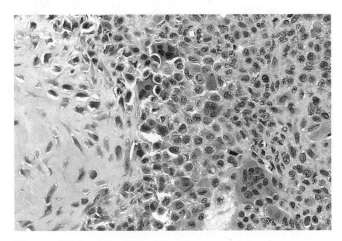

Figure 8.19. Chondroblastoma with eosinophilic chondroid matrix, giant cells, and mononuclear cells.

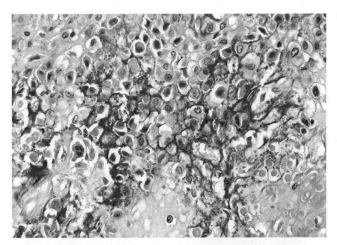

Figure 8.20. Chondroblastoma with mononuclear cells, distinct cytoplasmic borders, and characteristic deposits of calcification between the cells.

mural nodule. This has no clinical significance. Mitotic figures are commonly found within the mononuclear cells. In approximately one-fourth of chondroblastomas, pigment is within the mononuclear cells, particularly when the skull bones are involved. Vascular invasion is distinctly uncommon.

Chondroblastomas are benign lesions but may recur locally and even be somewhat aggressive locally. A small percentage of chondroblastomas metastasize to the lungs (82–85). Generally, the metastasis tends to be localized, and the patients survive after removal of the metastatic lesion. However, multiple metastatic neoplasms, which develop in some patients, may prove fatal (86). No histologic features predict a propensity for pulmonary metastasis.

The differential diagnosis usually involves giant cell tumor and chondromyxoid fibroma. Giant cell tumors and chondroblastomas both occur in the epiphysis, but giant cell tumors almost always develop after the epiphyseal plate has closed. Chondroid differentiation and calcific deposits should separate chondroblastoma from giant cell tumor. Chondroblastomas and chondromyxoid fibromas share several histologic features. Chondromyxoid fibromas tend to be metaphyseal, whereas chondroblastomas are typically epiphyseal.

CHONDROMYXOID FIBROMA. Chondromyxoid fibroma is an extremely rare benign cartilaginous neoplasm of bone. There were only 52 examples in the Mayo Clinic files before 2007, and a review from the Rizzoli Institute revealed only 27 cases (87). The patients are generally in the second and third decades of life, and the lesion typically involves the metaphysis of long bones (88). Occasionally it presents as a juxtacortical tumor (89). Chondromyxoid fibroma tends to develop in the small bones of the feet. Roentgenograms show an extremely well-circumscribed, purely lytic defect in the metaphysis of long bones (Fig. 8.21). The lesion generally has a sclerotic margin that may be scalloped, similar to that in metaphyseal fibrous defects.

Grossly, chondromyxoid fibromas tend to be small and may resemble hyaline cartilage. They usually do not show gross myxoid change.

Microscopically, chondromyxoid fibroma is always well circumscribed. Any permeation of surrounding tissue should be

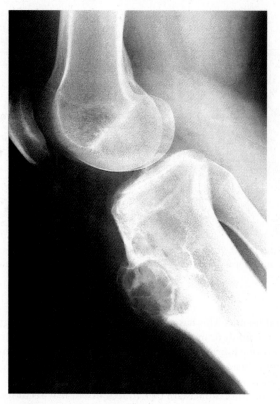

Figure 8.21. Chondromyxoid fibroma seen as a well-circumscribed lytic defect of the proximal tibia.

viewed with suspicion. Another characteristic low-power feature is the lobulated appearance of the neoplasm (Fig. 8.22A). The lobules may be large or small. Characteristically, the center of the lesion is hypocellular, and the periphery is hypercellular. Benign giant cells are usually found at the periphery of lobules. The cells are oval or stellate (Fig. 8.22B). They may be enlarged and hyperchromatic, suggesting malignancy. Clear-cut hyaline cartilage differentiation is seen in only a small percentage of cases. The matrix appears blue or myxoid. The peripheral cellu-

lar areas may have nuclei simulating those in chondroblastoma. Secondary changes, such as aneurysmal bone cyst, may be seen.

Chondromyxoid fibroma is a benign process, and a simple curettage is usually curative. However, recurrences may appear, and even soft tissue implants have been described (90). In a study of a large series of chondromyxoid fibroma of bone, no malignant transformation was found (91). However, another study included two examples of malignant transformation of chondromyxoid fibroma, one with and one without prior radiation (88). Although few in number, the majority of chondromyxoid fibromas that have been studied on a cytogenetic level have shown complex abnormalities involving chromosome 6 (92).

The differential diagnosis includes chondrosarcoma, chondroblastoma, and fibrous dysplasia with myxoid change. A very myxoid chondrosarcoma can have a lobulated appearance and stellate cells, simulating chondromyxoid fibroma. It is important to remember that chondromyxoid fibromas always have a benign appearance, whereas chondrosarcomas should show an aggressive appearance on roentgenograms. Usually, a lobulated chondrosarcoma does not have the distinctly hypocellular center and hypercellular periphery seen in chondromyxoid fibroma. Chondrosarcomas also tend to permeate surrounding bone. Chondroblastomas do not generally have a lobulated growth pattern. An extremely myxoid fibrous dysplasia may be mistaken for chondromyxoid fibroma. However, fibrous dysplasia does not have the lobulated growth pattern.

Malignant Chondroid Tumors

CONVENTIONAL CHONDROSARCOMA. Chondrosarcomas are the third most common malignant bone neoplasm (less common than only myeloma and osteosarcoma). It has been recognized for some time that chondrosarcoma is not a stereotypical disease but has variants (93). The term *conventional chondrosarcoma* is used for the most common variety, which is composed of hyaline cartilage and tends to involve the larger bones of adult patients. Although any portion of the skeleton may be affected, a distinct predilection for bones close to the axial skeleton, such as the pelvic and shoulder girdles, is noted. Chon-

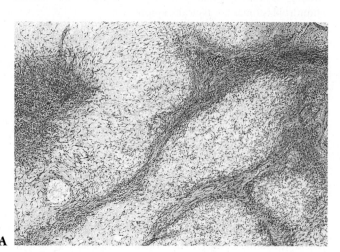

A

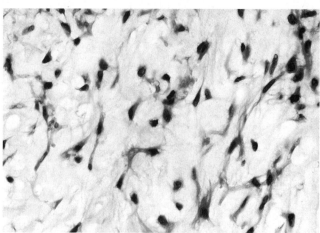

B

Figure 8.22. Chondromyxoid fibroma. **(A)** An irregularly shaped hypocellular center is surrounded by a cellular spindle cell stroma. **(B)** The lobules contain tumor cells with small nuclei and eosinophilic cytoplasmic extensions within a myxoid background.

drosarcoma involving the small bones of the hands and feet, the jawbones, and the skull is decidedly unusual (94). However, chondrosarcomas may occur in the nose and larynx (95). There is a definite male predilection, and chondrosarcoma generally occurs in adult patients. Chondrosarcoma is unusual in patients younger than 16 years of age (96). Patients present with swelling or pain. Rarely, the presenting symptom is a pathologic fracture.

Roentgenograms may suggest a specific diagnosis in chondrosarcoma. The lesions typically involve the diaphysis or metaphysis of long bones. In the ilium, the periacetabular region is preferred. Fluffy calcification is usually present, but the distribution is not uniform. The margins are poorly defined. The cortex may show thickening or destructive erosion, often associated with permeation into surrounding soft tissue. The combination of expansion of bone with thickening of the cortex, although present in only approximately one-fourth of cases, is practically diagnostic of chondrosarcoma (Fig. 8.23A). Periosteal new bone formation is unusual.

The gross appearance of chondrosarcoma is characteristic (Fig. 8.23B). The tumor has the pearly white or light blue appearance of cartilage. Foci of calcification may be seen grossly. Any myxoid change in a cartilage tumor of a large bone that may result in the formation of small cysts is suspect for chondrosarcoma (Fig. 8.24).

Well-differentiated chondrosarcomas are difficult to diagnose based purely on the histologic findings. Chondrosarcomas are not well-circumscribed lesions but tend to permeate marrow spaces, entrapping trabecular bone (Fig. 8.25). A myxoid change in the matrix suggests malignancy. The nuclei tend to crowd together and to be doubly nucleated and hyperchromatic (Figs. 8.26 and 8.27). The chondrocytes are within lacunae and

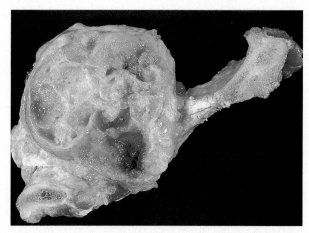

Figure 8.24. Chondrosarcoma involving the acetabulum. The myxoid quality of the matrix has led to focal cystic change.

do not spindle as a rule. Large areas of spindling in a cartilage tumor should be reason enough to diagnose either chondroblastic osteosarcoma or dedifferentiated chondrosarcoma.

Several studies have shown the usefulness of grading in determining the prognosis of a patient with chondrosarcoma (97–101). We grade chondrosarcomas primarily on the basis of the cellularity of the tumor and the nuclear changes of the chondrocytes. Low-grade chondrosarcomas tend to be less cellular than higher grade chondrosarcomas, and the nuclear changes are much more pronounced in higher grade chondrosarcomas; chondrosarcomas are graded only as 1, 2, or 3. The

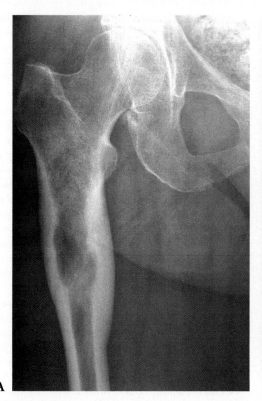

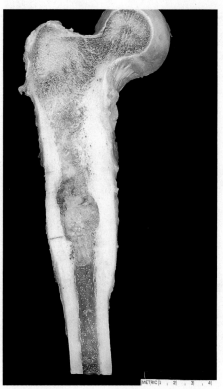

A   **B**

Figure 8.23. Grade 1 chondrosarcoma of the femoral shaft. **(A)** Roentgenogram shows erosion of markedly thickened cortices. **(B)** Corresponding gross specimen.

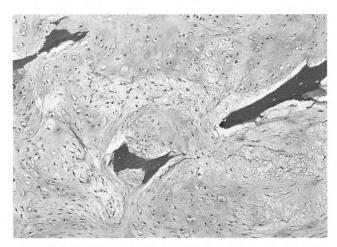

Figure 8.25. Grade 1 chondrosarcoma permeating pre-existing trabecular bone and filling the marrow spaces.

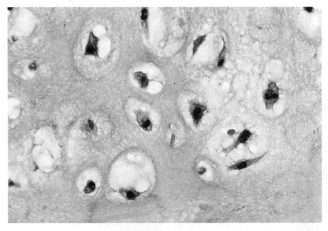

Figure 8.26. High-power appearance of grade 1 chondrosarcoma. A few doubly nucleated cells and moderate atypia are present.

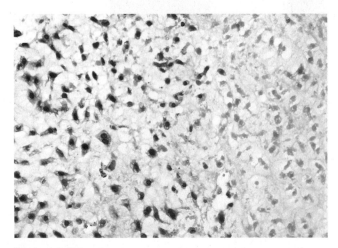

Figure 8.27. High-power appearance of grade 2 chondrosarcoma with necrosis (*right*). The nuclei are crowded and hyperchromatic.

malignant tumor that has areas of spindling and thus is grade 4 should be called either *chondroblastic osteosarcoma* or *dedifferentiated chondrosarcoma.* Mitotic figures are rare in chondrosarcomas and thus are not useful for grading, as suggested by others (98).

The most effective treatment for chondrosarcoma is surgical removal with a wide margin. Adjunctive chemotherapy and radiation do not alter outcome. Five-year survival does not mean cure for patients with chondrosarcomas. In a study of chondrosarcoma involving the long bones and limb girdle from the Mayo Clinic, the 5-year survival rate was 77%, although patients continued to have local recurrence or even distant metastasis up to 20 years later. The risk for distant metastasis was 4% for grade 1 tumors but 30% for higher grade tumors (102). Another study of chondrosarcoma from the Massachusetts General Hospital found a longer duration of survival in patients with low-grade tumors who had a resection with wide margins (103).

It is well recognized that differentiation between a low-grade chondrosarcoma and an enchondroma can be difficult (104). One has to use the cytologic changes, myxoid quality of the stroma, and permeative characteristics in an attempt to make this distinction. However, we rely heavily on the roentgenographic appearance to distinguish between enchondroma and chondrosarcoma. The term *aggressive enchondroma* is sometimes used for tumors with histologic and radiographic features that are not diagnostic of chondrosarcoma but more worrisome than those typically seen in enchondroma. Large, painful lesions situated toward the axial skeleton are likely to be chondrosarcomas, whereas painless, small lesions and especially lesions in the small bones are likely to be benign.

The rules for diagnosing chondrosarcoma in a small bone of the hand or foot are different from those for the diagnosis in larger bones. Enchondromas of the small bones look quite worrisome cytologically, and taken out of context, they may be mistaken for chondrosarcoma. However, one has to see permeation of the tumor through the cortex into soft tissues before a diagnosis of chondrosarcoma can be made in a small bone; chondrosarcomas do occur in small bones, and several reports have confirmed deaths from pulmonary metastasis (105–107).

SECONDARY CHONDROSARCOMA. Most chondrosarcomas apparently arise de novo. In the Mayo Clinic files, however, approximately 14% of chondrosarcomas were secondary to a pre-existing condition. Chondrosarcomas may arise in an exostosis (Fig. 8.28), either as a solitary lesion or multiple lesions, or in a patient with chondrodysplasia. The diagnosis of a secondary chondrosarcoma is usually quite difficult because the tumor is low grade. However, any change in the size or symptom pattern of a pre-existing lesion should arouse suspicion of a secondary chondrosarcoma. Because most secondary chondrosarcomas are low grade, the prognosis should be excellent (66,108). We believe that solitary enchondromas rarely, if ever, become malignant.

Patients with secondary chondrosarcomas are generally younger than those with conventional chondrosarcomas. However, conventional chondrosarcoma can occur in young patients. Some studies have suggested that the prognosis in children with chondrosarcoma is worse than the prognosis in adults (109), but this has not been our experience (96). One must be careful to exclude chondroblastic osteosarcoma from any series of chondrosarcomas in children. Chondroblastic osteosarcomas are much more common than chondrosarcomas in children.

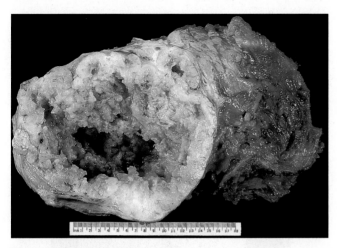

Figure 8.28. Chondrosarcoma arising in an osteochondroma. The lesion shows central necrosis and cystic change.

PERIOSTEAL CHONDROSARCOMA. Most chondroid lesions on the surface of bone are benign. Even those that show cytologic atypia tend to behave in a benign fashion and should be considered periosteal chondromas. Rarely, however, one sees a purely hyaline cartilage malignant tumor on the surface of bone. It tends to be larger than a periosteal chondroma, usually more than 5 cm in greatest dimension. The roentgenograms tend to show poor circumscription, and microscopically, the tumor nodules permeate surrounding soft tissue. The truly malignant quality of the lesion is emphasized by the rare occurrence of metastasis (68).

CLEAR CELL CHONDROSARCOMA. This is an unusual variant of chondrosarcoma that tends to occur at the ends of long bones. Clear cell chondrosarcoma typically presents radiographically as a geographic lytic lesion located in the epimetaphyseal region of long bones (Fig. 8.29). Lesions in the axial skeleton are usually expansile and destructive (110). Microscopically, clear cell chondrosarcomas are composed of cells with well-defined cytoplasmic membranes, a clear cytoplasm, and a centrally placed round nucleus with an occasional prominent nucleolus (Fig. 8.30). The cells tend to be arranged in lobules. Benign giant cells are usually found at the edge of the lobules. Characteristically, trabeculae of woven bone are present in the center of the lobules (Fig. 8.31). In approximately 50% of the cases, one sees areas of conventional low-grade chondrosarcoma (111). Secondary aneurysmal bone cyst–like changes may also be seen in clear cell chondrosarcoma. Clear cell chondrosarcoma exhibits the clinical behavior of a low-grade chondrosarcoma and has a tendency to metastasize relatively late. In the last report from the Mayo Clinic, the 10-year overall survival rate was 89%, and the disease-free survival rate was 69% (112). Only a few rare examples of dedifferentiated clear cell chondrosarcoma have been described (113).

DEDIFFERENTIATED CHONDROSARCOMA. Dedifferentiated chondrosarcoma was delineated as a distinct entity in 1971 (114). Since then, the lesion has been well accepted as an entity, although the term *dedifferentiated chondrosarcoma* has been questioned (115). Dedifferentiated chondrosarcoma is diagnosed when a low-grade chondrosarcoma is juxtaposed with a high-

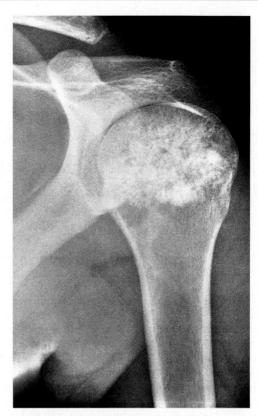

Figure 8.29. Clear cell chondrosarcoma of the proximal humerus. The lesion is heavily mineralized, extends to the end of the bone, and appears well circumscribed.

grade spindle cell sarcoma. The spindle cell sarcoma most commonly shows features of a fibrosarcoma, a malignant fibrous histiocytoma, or an osteosarcoma. Patients with dedifferentiated chondrosarcoma are older than patients with other spindle cell sarcomas of bone. These lesions occur in the same location as chondrosarcomas, such as the pelvic and shoulder girdles. Roentgenograms may have the appearance of chondrosarcoma, or more commonly, they may show areas of chondrosarcoma next to malignant neoplasms that appear to be highly aggressive

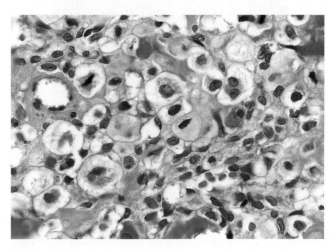

Figure 8.30. Clear cell chondrosarcoma with round nuclei, clear cytoplasm, and well-defined boundaries.

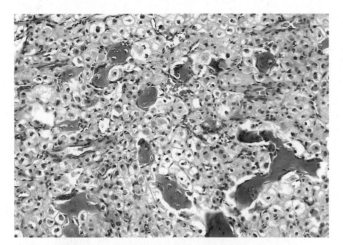

Figure 8.31. Clear cell chondrosarcoma with faint lobulation, woven bone, and clear cells.

(Fig. 8.32) (116). Grossly, one recognizes clear-cut cartilage tumor and, in close proximity, the fish flesh appearance of a sarcoma (Fig. 8.33). Microscopically, one finds a well-differentiated chondrosarcoma next to a high-grade spindle cell sarcoma (Fig. 8.34), which may show osteoid production.

All reports have confirmed the original impression that patients with dedifferentiated chondrosarcoma have a very poor prognosis (117–120). Even patients with the rare dedifferentiated chondrosarcoma arising in osteochondroma have a poor survival (67,121).

The differential diagnosis includes chondroblastic osteosar-

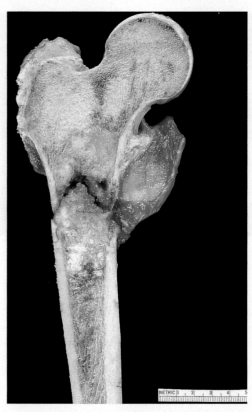

Figure 8.33. Dedifferentiated chondrosarcoma of the proximal femur associated with pathologic fracture. The medullary portion has the gross appearance of chondrosarcoma, but the soft tissue mass medially has the fleshy appearance of a high-grade sarcoma.

coma. Chondroblastic osteosarcoma is characterized by the gradual transition from a high-grade cartilaginous neoplasm to a spindle cell malignant lesion. However, in dedifferentiated chondrosarcoma, the change from a low-grade chondrosarcoma to a high-grade spindle cell malignant neoplasm is abrupt. Chondroblastic osteosarcomas generally occur in young patients, whereas dedifferentiated chondrosarcoma is a disease of

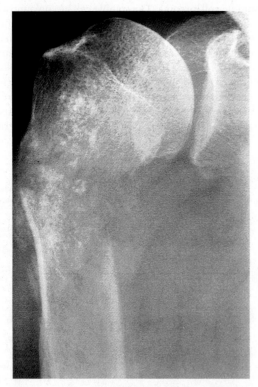

Figure 8.32. Roentgenogram shows dedifferentiated chondrosarcoma of the proximal humerus. The mineralization is consistent with cartilage, and a very aggressive-looking area is located medially.

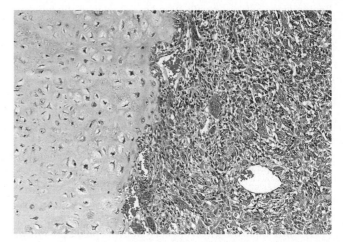

Figure 8.34. Dedifferentiated chondrosarcoma. Chondrosarcoma (*right*) is juxtaposed with high-grade malignant fibrous histiocytoma (*left*).

older persons. This distinction is important because the prognosis is considerably worse in dedifferentiated chondrosarcoma than in chondroblastic osteosarcoma.

MESENCHYMAL CHONDROSARCOMA. Mesenchymal chondrosarcoma is an unusual tumor first described as a distinct entity in 1959 (122). Approximately one-third of all mesenchymal chondrosarcomas appear to arise in the soft tissues. Their histologic features and clinical behavior are similar to those of the skeletal counterpart. A slight female predominance is noted, and the tumor is generally found in young adults. Any portion of the skeleton may be involved, but there is a definite tendency for involvement of the jawbones and ribs (123). The roentgenographic features are somewhat nonspecific. The appearance is usually that of a malignant tumor with or without calcification. Grossly, the lesion is usually pink and fleshy, mimicking other sarcomas. However, foci of calcification are usually present.

The microscopic appearance of mesenchymal chondrosarcoma is characteristic. Islands of well-differentiated cartilage are juxtaposed with a small, round to oval cell malignant lesion (Figs. 8.35 and 8.36). The small malignant cells may be arranged around vascular spaces, giving rise to a hemangiopericytomatous pattern. When the tumor was originally described, it was thought that the cartilaginous nodules had to appear completely benign. With experience, however, came the realization that the chondroid islands may have the appearance of a low-grade chondrosarcoma. The chondroid islands may undergo calcification or even ossification. Although the small malignant cells are usually round to oval, simulating Ewing sarcoma, foci of frank spindling may be found. Benign giant cells are very unusual.

The prognosis of mesenchymal chondrosarcoma is unpredictable. Some patients have metastases at presentation and die very soon afterward. Others survive for a long time, sometimes even after metastasis. Some authors have subdivided mesenchymal chondrosarcomas into those with and those without a hemangiopericytomatous pattern (124), suggesting that this feature is of prognostic significance. This has not been our experience (125).

The differential diagnosis includes all small-cell malignant lesions, such as Ewing sarcoma, lymphoma, and small-cell osteo-

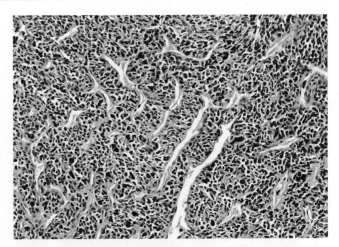

Figure 8.36. Small oval cells arranged around vascular spaces produce a hemangiopericytomatous pattern.

sarcoma. However, any chondroid lobules should separate lymphoma and Ewing sarcoma. Well-differentiated cartilage is unusual in small-cell osteosarcoma.

OSTEOGENIC TUMORS

Osteogenic tumors are considered as one group because their common characteristic is the production of an osteoid, or bony, matrix by the tumor cell. They are also divided into benign and malignant counterparts, although the transformation of benign lesions into malignant ones almost never occurs.

Benign Osteogenic Tumors

OSTEOID OSTEOMA. Osteoid osteomas are rare neoplasms with very characteristic symptoms. Patients present with pain that is usually worse at night and almost immediately relieved by aspirin. The lesion may be associated with synovitis, which causes pain if it is close to a joint. The origin of the exquisite pain of osteoid osteoma is unknown, but several theories have been suggested, including the production of prostaglandins by the lesion (126).

Osteoid osteoma occurs predominantly in the second decade of life, and a pronounced male preference is noted. The lesion involves the metaphysis or shaft of long bones, and the cortex tends to be affected. The roentgenographic appearance is typical, consisting of a radiolucent nidus that is usually surrounded by an extensive sclerotic zone (Fig. 8.37) (127). The sclerosis may be so extensive that the nidus is difficult to localize (128). This difficulty may lead to multiple surgical procedures to remove the osteoid osteoma (129). The best imaging study to demonstrate osteoid osteoma is CT, preferably with the use of bone windows.

The gross appearance of osteoid osteoma is typical. It is important that the surgical pathologist examine the gross specimen for a nidus and not submit the entire tissue mass removed by the surgeon for decalcification. The nidus is small, red, and granular. It is softer than the surrounding sclerotic tissue and usually stands out from the surrounding sclerotic bone (Fig. 8.38). If several fragments of sclerotic bone are received, it may be necessary to obtain a roentgenogram of the specimen to

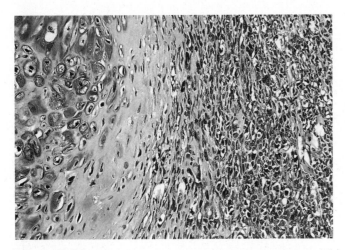

Figure 8.35. Mesenchymal chondrosarcoma with cartilage and small blue cells.

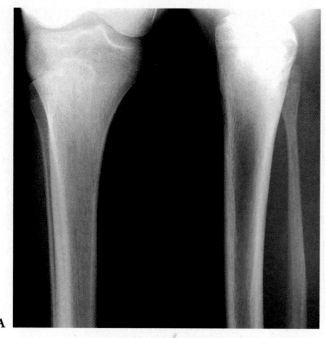

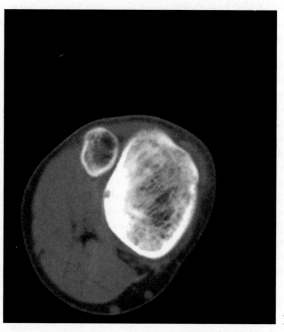

A   **B**

Figure 8.37. Osteoid osteoma of the proximal tibia. **(A)** Anteroposterior and lateral radiographs of the proximal tibia show an ill-defined region of sclerosis in the proximal tibia posteriorly. **(B)** The axial computed tomogram shows a tiny lytic intracortical lesion in the proximal tibial metaphysis posteriorly with associated medullary sclerosis. The imaging features are characteristic of osteoid osteoma.

help identify the nidus. The surgeon usually requests a roentgenogram of the involved bone to ensure that the area of involvement has been removed.

The histologic appearance of osteoid osteoma is also typical. One sees an extremely well-circumscribed lesion composed of anastomosing bony trabeculae (Fig. 8.39). Mineralization of the bone is variable. The bony trabeculae are rimmed by osteoblasts. The spaces between the trabeculae show capillary proliferation and few cells. Benign giant cells are almost always found.

The treatment of osteoid osteoma is either surgical removal or CT-guided radiofrequency ablation (130,131). The relief of symptoms is so dramatic that the patient usually realizes on

recovery from anesthesia that the lesion has been removed. Recurrences are unusual, although they have been reported (132).

The differential diagnosis includes osteomyelitis and osteoblastoma. A localized area of osteomyelitis, termed *Brodie abscess*, can simulate osteoid osteoma clinically and roentgenographically. Histologically, however, a Brodie abscess does not resemble an osteoid osteoma.

Osteoblastomas and osteoid osteomas are related conditions, and they may be histologically indistinguishable (133). Arbitrarily, a lesion smaller than 1.5 cm in diameter is considered an osteoid osteoma, and a lesion larger than 1.5 cm is considered an osteoblastoma.

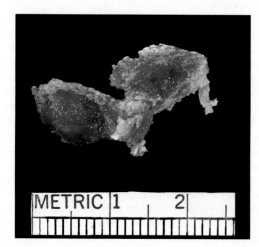

Figure 8.38. Gross appearance of osteoid osteoma. The round red nidus (left) is easily pulled away from the surrounding cortical bone (right).

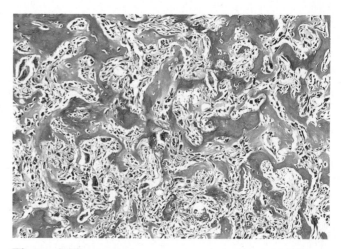

Figure 8.39. Osteoid osteoma with anastomosing trabeculae of woven bone.

OSTEOBLASTOMA. Benign osteoblastoma is an unusual neoplasm, approximately one-fourth as common as osteoid osteoma. Similar to osteoid osteoma, the lesion shows a marked male predominance and usually affects young patients. Unlike osteoid osteoma, the lesion tends to involve the spine, especially the posterior elements. In the long bones, it generally affects the diaphysis. Rarely, it occurs as a periosteal-based tumor (134). In approximately one-fourth of cases, the lesion appears aggressive and simulates malignancy (135). In some cases, however, a nidus seen on roentgenograms suggests a large osteoid osteoma.

The gross appearance is also variable. The lesion is by definition larger than 1.5 cm in dimension, and it appears red, granular, and well circumscribed. An area of surrounding sclerosis may or may not be present.

Microscopically, an osteoblastoma resembles an osteoid osteoma. The nidus is composed of anastomosing bony trabeculae rimmed by osteoblasts (Fig. 8.40). The spaces between the trabeculae are loose and quite vascular. No sheets of spindle cells are seen. It is important to examine the edges of an osteoblastoma because the tumor should not show any permeation. The term *epithelioid multinodular osteoblastoma* refers to osteoblastomas characterized by clusters of epithelioid osteoblasts, often without matrix, arranged in multiple nodules (136).

The diagnostic problems with osteoblastoma have been summarized by Dorfman and Weiss (137). Some osteoblastomas have bizarre hyperchromatic nuclei, and these tumors have been termed *pseudomalignant osteoblastomas* (138). Schajowicz and Lemos (139) introduced the term *malignant osteoblastoma* to refer to a lesion that resembles an osteoblastoma but is locally aggressive. Dorfman and Weiss (137) introduced the term *aggressive osteoblastoma* for the same entity. The main histologic finding for this diagnosis appears to be epithelioid osteoblasts. We find the concept of aggressive osteoblastoma to be somewhat nebulous. In studies of a large number of cases, aggressive osteoblastoma could not be separated out as a distinct entity (140,141). Several examples of transformation of an osteoblastoma to an osteosarcoma have been reported (142,143). However, it is difficult to be sure that these lesions were not osteosarcomas to begin with. Distinguishing between osteoblastoma and osteosarcoma can be extremely difficult; the term *osteosarcoma resembling osteoblastoma* has been used for these diffi-

cult lesions (144). The most important single criterion to separate an osteosarcoma from an osteoblastoma is lack of permeation in the latter. All the proposed criteria are fallible.

Toxic osteoblastoma is a rare variant of osteoblastoma associated with systemic manifestations, including weight loss, fever, and generalized periostitis (145–147).

The differential diagnosis includes osteosarcoma and osteoid osteoma. As previously stated, osteoid osteoma is defined by the size of the nidus. We have already referred to the difficulty in distinguishing osteoblastoma from osteosarcoma.

OSTEOMA. Osteomas are rare benign overgrowths of bone. Most involve the mandible and maxilla and may manifest as a mass in the sinus. They may be associated with Gardner syndrome (148). An osteoma of the skull may be a response to an invading meningioma. Rarely, an osteoma is seen on the surface of a long bone.

Malignant Osteogenic Tumors

The definition of osteosarcoma requires that the malignant tumor produce osteoid matrix. By this definition, osteosarcoma can be divided into several subtypes, depending on the clinical, roentgenographic, and microscopic features. Some of these subtypes have prognostic significance, whereas others do not (149).

CONVENTIONAL OSTEOSARCOMA. Conventional osteosarcoma is a high-grade malignant neoplasm that occurs predominantly in the metaphysis of the long bones of adolescents and young adults. A definite male predominance is noted, and it is very unusual to see osteosarcoma in patients younger than 5 years. The distal femur and proximal tibia are the most common sites, and the metaphysis is preferentially involved. Approximately 10% of osteosarcomas occur in the diaphysis, but they tend to be unusual types of osteosarcoma. Patients usually present with pain or swelling. Pathologic fracture is uncommon.

The roentgenographic features of osteosarcoma are quite variable. Almost always, the lesion appears as an area of geographic destruction with extension into soft tissues (Fig. 8.41). Reactive new bone formation is present at the junction of the cortex and where the periosteum has been lifted off by the tumor. This area has been referred to as the *Codman triangle*. The lesion generally contains mineralization but may be purely lytic.

Grossly, osteosarcoma typically forms a large mass extending into the soft tissue. The epiphyseal plate usually acts as a barrier, and both the proximal and distal margins are generally well defined (Fig. 8.42). The lesion may be soft and fleshy or gritty, depending on the amount of osteoid produced. Approximately one-fourth of lesions contain large amounts of cartilage and may simulate chondrosarcoma in appearance.

By definition, conventional osteosarcoma is a spindle cell neoplasm that is high grade and produces osteoid matrix. Conventional osteosarcoma can be further subdivided into osteoblastic, fibroblastic, and chondroblastic types, depending on the predominant matrix.

Approximately 50% of all conventional osteosarcomas are osteoblastic. The osteoid is usually a fine, lacelike pink matrix (Figs. 8.43 and 8.44). The amount of mineralization in the matrix is quite variable. Less commonly, the osteoid is organized in a trabecular fashion. Approximately 25% of osteosarcomas

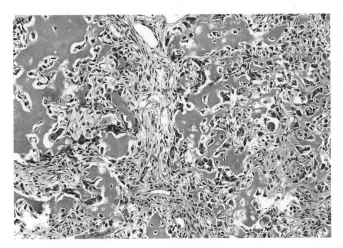

Figure 8.40. Osteoblastoma. The histologic appearance is identical to that of osteoid osteoma.

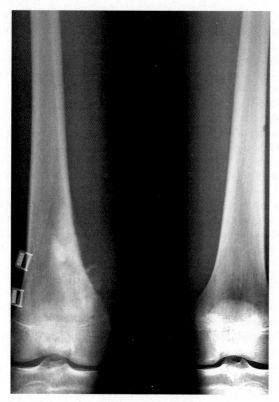

Figure 8.41. Conventional osteosarcoma involving the distal femoral metaphysis. The lesion is very dense, and new bone formation in the soft tissues results in a sunburst pattern.

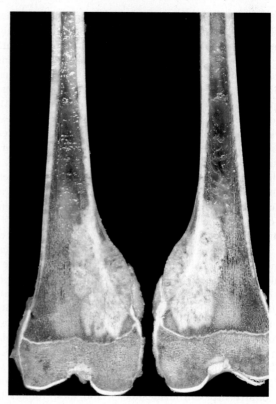

Figure 8.42. Gross specimen of conventional osteosarcoma corresponding to the lesion shown in Figure 8.41. Note that the epiphyseal plate acts as a relative barrier.

show purely spindle cell growth with only small foci of matrix. This variation is referred to as *fibroblastic osteosarcoma.*

Approximately 25% of osteosarcomas show a predominantly chondroid differentiation. The cartilage usually appears malignant, with hyperchromasia and hypercellularity. Spindling occurs at the periphery of the lobules of cartilage, and one sees osteoid production either between the spindle cells or in the center of the chondroid lobules (Fig. 8.45). Even if clear-cut osteoid production is absent, a high-grade chondroid neoplasm with sheets of spindle cells in a young patient should be considered a chondroblastic osteosarcoma. Some osteosarcomas have plump cells with pink cytoplasm resembling epithelial cells (150). In approximately one-fourth of all osteosarcomas, benign giant cells are scattered throughout. Rarely, the giant cells are so predominant that the lesion is mistaken for a giant cell tumor. The finding of an apparent giant cell tumor in the metaphysis of a young patient should arouse suspicion of an osteosarcoma.

Osteosarcoma tends to metastasize to the lungs. CT has improved our ability to detect micrometastatic spots. Together, advances in imaging, diagnosis, surgical technique, and instrumentation; adjuvant therapy; and the basic knowledge of tumor biology have resulted in quantum improvements in the control of local and systemic disease. During the past 3 decades, the 5-year survival rate of patients with localized high-grade osteosarcoma has risen from less than 20% to 50% to 75% (151–156).

Most osteosarcomas are resected after preoperative chemotherapy. The incidence of amputation for osteosarcoma has diminished dramatically. Most authors now believe that the amount of necrosis observed after chemotherapy correlates with

prognosis. Hence, it is important for surgical pathologists to evaluate the extent of necrosis in resected osteosarcoma (157,158).

The method used for evaluating the extent of necrosis varies. We simply take one slice of the entire tumor, including the involved bone, decalcify it, and embed the whole slice. One generally sees areas of fibrosis, frank necrosis, loose fibrovascular connective tissue simulating granulation tissue, or, most commonly, large amounts of thick sclerotic bone replacing the marrow cavity. Sometimes, it is difficult to decide whether some

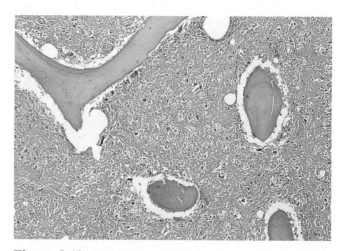

Figure 8.43. Osteoblastic osteosarcoma permeating pre-existing trabeculae of bone.

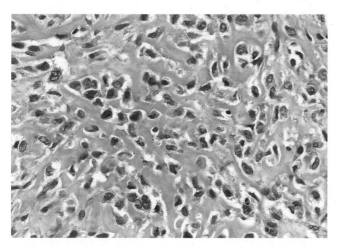

Figure 8.44. Osteoblastic osteosarcoma with finely ramifying matrix between tumor cells.

cells are viable. It is generally agreed that if doubt exists, the cells should be considered viable.

POSTRADIATION SARCOMA. It has long been recognized that osteosarcoma may develop in bones in the field of radiation (159). The exact incidence is unknown. There is a latent period, usually averaging 17 years. The amount of radiation involved varies, ranging from 12 to 240 Gy. Most commonly, the dose is between 40 and 60 Gy (160). The bone with sarcomas may have been irradiated during treatment for a nonosseous neoplasm or may have been included in the field of radiation during treatment for a bone neoplasm, such as a giant cell tumor. The sarcoma may be fibrosarcoma, osteosarcoma, or malignant fibrous histiocytoma. In our experience, almost all of these sarcomas are high-grade malignant tumors and histologically indistinguishable from conventional osteosarcoma. The reported survival rates of patients with postirradiation sarcoma have been poor (161–163). However, the prognosis of patients with peripheral resectable sarcomas is good if a wide surgical margin can be achieved (161).

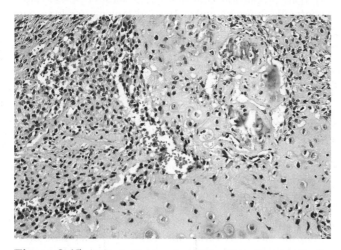

Figure 8.45. Chondroblastic osteosarcoma from the scapula of a 16-year-old boy. Lobules of malignant-appearing cartilage are surrounded by atypical spindle cells associated with osteoid production.

PAGET SARCOMA. Paget disease is a well-known predisposing condition for the development of osteosarcoma. The exact incidence of sarcoma arising in Paget disease is unknown but is generally considered to be less than 1%. A patient with Paget disease who experiences increasing localized pain may have a sarcoma. Patients with Paget sarcoma are much older than those with conventional osteosarcoma. The roentgenograms show classic features of Paget disease and an area of destruction. The histologic appearance is that of high-grade sarcoma, which may be osteosarcoma, fibrosarcoma, or malignant fibrous histiocytoma. Several studies have confirmed the extremely poor prognosis associated with Paget sarcoma (164–166).

TELANGIECTATIC OSTEOSARCOMA. The criteria we use to diagnose telangiectatic osteosarcoma are as follows:

1. The roentgenogram shows a purely lytic destructive lesion simulating the appearance of an aneurysmal bone cyst (Fig. 8.46).
2. The gross appearance is that of spaces separated by septa or a large cavity containing blood (Fig. 8.47).
3. Histologically, the lesion consists of spaces separated by septa (Fig. 8.48). The septa contain highly malignant cells (Fig. 8.49).

On the basis of these criteria, telangiectatic osteosarcoma is an extremely uncommon tumor. When Matsuno et al. (167) reviewed the Mayo Clinic files for osteosarcoma in 1976, they found 25 cases. At that time, the prognosis for telangiectatic osteosarcoma appeared to be worse than that for conventional osteosarcoma, but other authors disputed this point (168). In a

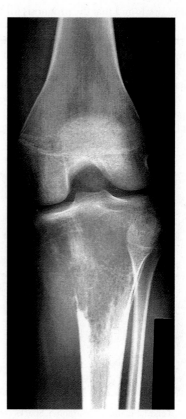

Figure 8.46. Roentgenogram of telangiectatic osteosarcoma of the proximal tibia. The destructive process is purely lytic.

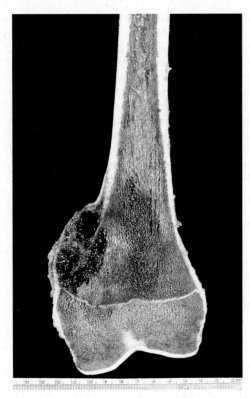

Figure 8.47. Gross specimen of telangiectatic osteosarcoma with tumor in the distal femur. The neoplasm has the appearance of a bag of blood.

later study (169), we found that the prognosis for telangiectatic osteosarcoma had improved considerably; it now seems to be the same as that for conventional osteosarcoma. In the later study, the prognosis did not appear to be related to the use of chemotherapy.

Even if telangiectatic osteosarcoma does not differ prognostically from conventional osteosarcoma, we believe that it should be separated as an entity because it is still mistaken for an aneurysmal bone cyst. The roentgenographic, gross, and mi-

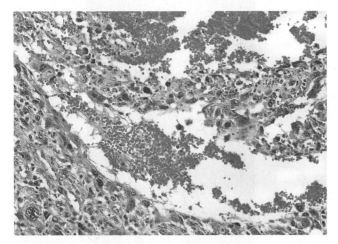

Figure 8.48. Telangiectatic osteosarcoma. Spaces containing blood are separated by septa. The cells appear malignant even at this level of magnification.

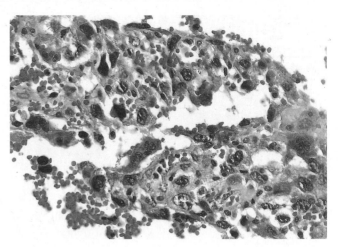

Figure 8.49. Marked nuclear pleomorphism in a telangiectatic osteosarcoma.

croscopic features may all be similar. The distinction has to be made purely on the basis of whether cytologically malignant cells are within the septa in telangiectatic osteosarcoma.

LOW-GRADE CENTRAL OSTEOSARCOMA. An osteosarcoma so well differentiated that it simulated fibrous dysplasia was first described in 1977 (170). The appearance of only a few reports of this entity since then attests to its rarity. We have only 22 examples in the Mayo Clinic files. Patients with low-grade osteosarcoma are generally older than patients with conventional osteosarcoma. The symptoms tend to be prolonged. The distal end of the femur is the most common site. Roentgenographically, the lesions are usually large, with frequent extraosseous extension (Fig. 8.50). Typically, much of the lesion is well circumscribed, and only focal areas suggest an aggressive growth pattern. Grossly, the lesion is firm and fibrous, lacking the fish flesh appearance of a high-grade osteosarcoma.

Histologically, the lesion is a spindle cell neoplasm that is hypocellular with much collagen production. The nuclei show only subtle signs of atypia, and mitotic figures are uncommon (Fig. 8.51). The amount of bone produced varies, and occasionally, bone production simulates that in fibrous dysplasia. Most importantly, however, low-grade osteosarcoma tends to permeate the surrounding bone and soft tissues, whereas fibrous dysplasia is well circumscribed (Fig. 8.52). The prognosis in low-grade osteosarcoma is excellent, but high-grade osteosarcoma eventually develops in up to 15% of patients in whom the tumor recurs (171).

SMALL-CELL OSTEOSARCOMA. Occasionally, an osteosarcoma has very small malignant cells simulating those in Ewing sarcoma, but the tumor clearly produces a matrix material. We diagnose small-cell osteosarcoma only if the tumor cells have produced mineralizing matrix material. Small-cell osteosarcoma is an extremely uncommon neoplasm, and the prognosis seems to be poor (172,173).

All of the previously described tumors occur predominantly within the medullary cavity, although rarely, some have been reported to develop in the cortex (174).

In addition to the clinicopathologic features in the different entities, the site of the tumor may be important in prognosis.

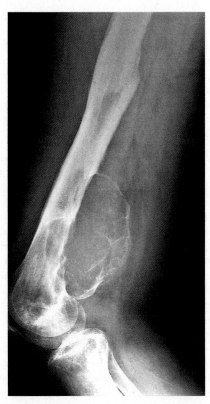

Figure 8.50. Roentgenogram of central low-grade osteosarcoma showing extension into soft tissue posteriorly.

For instance, patients with osteosarcomas of the jaw have traditionally fared better than patients with conventional osteosarcoma (175). However, patients with osteosarcoma of the skull tend to do very poorly (176).

SURFACE OSTEOSARCOMAS
Parosteal osteosarcoma. Parosteal osteosarcoma was first described in 1951 (177). It shows a definite female predilection, unlike most other osteosarcomas. The patients tend to be older than those with conventional osteosarcoma; most of them are

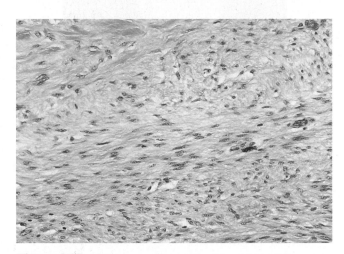

Figure 8.51. High-power appearance of low-grade osteosarcoma. The stroma is hypocellular with only slight atypia of the spindle cells.

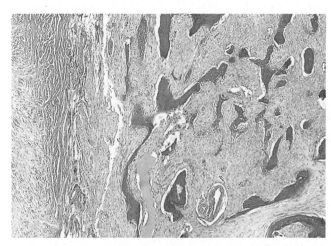

Figure 8.52. Low-grade osteosarcoma invading surrounding skeletal muscle.

in the third and fourth decades of life (178). The tendency to involve the posterior aspect of the distal femur is very striking; approximately 70% of the tumors are at this site. Patients generally describe a painless swelling, and the usual dysfunction is inability to flex the knee. Roentgenographically, parosteal osteosarcoma is seen as a heavily ossified mass on the surface of the bone. Usually, continuity is lacking between the lesion and the underlying marrow (Fig. 8.53). Grossly, parosteal osteosarcoma is a mass that is firm to hard. Areas of cartilage may be recognized, and the cartilage may be in the form of a cartilage

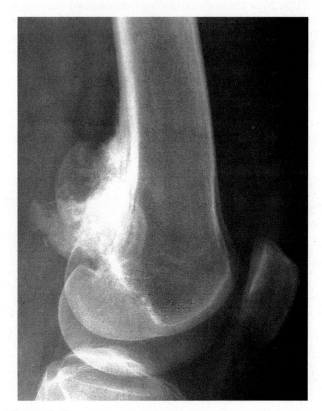

Figure 8.53. Parosteal osteosarcoma in the form of a heavily mineralized mass attached to the posterior aspect of the distal femoral metaphysis.

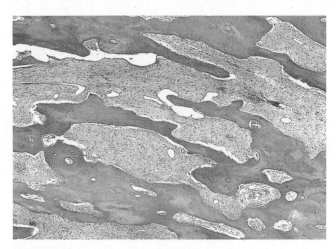

Figure 8.54. Parosteal osteosarcoma. Note the hypocellular spindle cell stroma and long seams of trabecular bone.

plate. Any soft areas should be sampled to exclude high-grade osteosarcoma.

Microscopically, parosteal osteosarcoma is a low-grade neoplasm. The tumor is composed of a hypocellular growth of spindle cells with subtle cytologic atypia (Figs. 8.54 and 8.55). Mitotic figures are rare. Bone production consists of well-formed bone trabeculae or woven bone. Various amounts of cartilage may be seen. The cartilage may be arranged at the periphery and have the appearance of a cap. Most parosteal osteosarcomas are grade 1. A small percentage with slightly increased cellularity and cytologic atypia are grade 2. In a study by Okada et al. (178), 37 of 226 parosteal osteosarcomas showed foci of high-grade osteosarcoma, either initially or at the time of recurrence. This process has been termed *dedifferentiation* (179–181). Medullary involvement may occur in parosteal osteosarcoma. In one study, it was found in approximately 25% of tumors (178).

With adequate treatment, the prognosis for patients who have parosteal osteosarcoma is excellent. Local recurrence is the rule with inadequate excision. However, metastatic spread of parosteal osteosarcoma is extremely rare unless the tumor is dedifferentiated. The differential diagnosis includes osteochon-

droma and myositis ossificans. In osteochondroma, the roentgenograms show clear-cut continuity between the involved bone and the osteochondroma. No such continuity is seen in parosteal osteosarcoma. In osteochondroma, fatty or hematopoietic marrow is present between the bony trabeculae. In parosteal osteosarcoma, spindle cell proliferation occurs. Myositis ossificans does not show attachment to the underlying bone on roentgenograms and appears much more active histologically than parosteal osteosarcoma.

Periosteal osteosarcoma. Periosteal osteosarcoma was first described as a distinct entity in 1976 (182). The tumor is predominantly chondroblastic and therefore was first considered to be chondrosarcoma (183). Patients with periosteal osteosarcoma tend to be in the same age group as those with conventional osteosarcoma. A slight female predominance is noted. Any portion of the skeleton may be affected, but most tumors involve the diaphysis of the femur or tibia. Roentgenograms show a lucent defect on the surface of the cortex, with spicules of bone extending into the soft tissues (Fig. 8.56). By definition, medullary involvement should be absent (Fig. 8.57). Histologically, periosteal osteosarcoma is moderately differentiated, taking the form of a predominantly chondroblastic grade 2 or 3 osteosarcoma. The cartilage appears to be arranged in lobules with peripheral spindling (Fig. 8.58). Typically, the center of the lobule of the cartilage shows bone formation, giving rise to a feathery appearance (Fig. 8.59). The prognosis of patients with periosteal osteosarcoma is better than for those with conventional medullary osteosarcoma. One study found an 83% survival rate for patients with periosteal osteosarcoma (184).

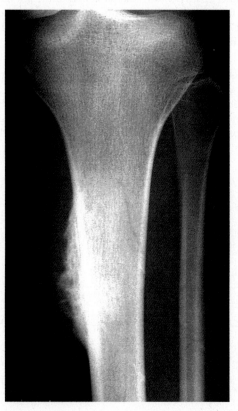

Figure 8.56. Periosteal osteosarcoma of the proximal tibia. The lesion is lightly mineralized and on the surface of the bone.

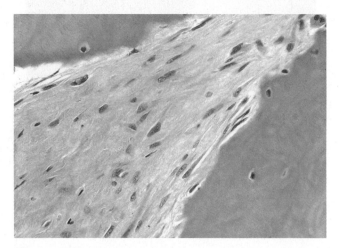

Figure 8.55. High-power appearance of parosteal osteosarcoma. The spindle cells demonstrate minimal atypia, and the bone appears to arise directly from the spindle cells.

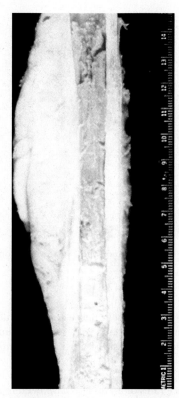

Figure 8.57. Periosteal osteosarcoma on the surface of the femoral diaphysis. The marrow is not involved.

High-grade surface osteosarcoma. This very rare neoplasm occurs predominantly on the surface of bone (185,186). The roentgenograms show a lesion on the surface of bone with variable mineralization. Grossly, the tumor has the fish flesh appearance of a high-grade sarcoma. Microscopically, high-grade surface osteosarcoma has the appearance of conventional osteosarcoma, with markedly pleomorphic tumor cells. The prognosis seems to be similar to that for conventional osteosarcoma (187).

This subclassification of types of osteosarcoma may appear excessively detailed and cumbersome. However, it is important

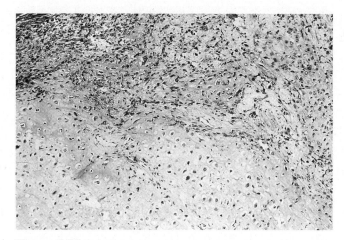

Figure 8.58. Periosteal osteosarcoma composed of lobules of cartilage with peripheral spindling.

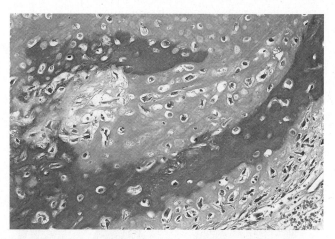

Figure 8.59. Bone formation in the center of a cartilaginous lobule in periosteal osteosarcoma.

to remember the different types so that they can be recognized when seen; some of them also are of prognostic significance.

TUMORS OF UNKNOWN ORIGIN

Benign Tumors of Unknown Origin: Giant Cell Tumor

Giant cell tumor of bone is one of the few neoplasms of bone with a distinct predilection for skeletally mature women. Most patients are in the third and fourth decades of life. Any patient with a giant cell tumor who is younger than 20 years is likely to be female and have a mature skeleton.

Any portion of the skeleton may be involved, but a definite predilection for the ends of long bones is noted. The distal femur, proximal tibia, distal radius, and sacrum are the four most common locations, in that order. Although the sacrum is one of the more frequent locations for a giant cell tumor, the spine above the level of the sacrum is rarely involved. Most giant cell–containing lesions of the small bones are giant cell lesions, such as aneurysmal bone cysts or giant cell reparative granulomas, rather than true giant cell tumors. However, true giant cell tumors do occur in the small bones of the hands and feet, and they tend to be more aggressive in their local behavior (188,189). Approximately 1% of giant cell tumors present as multiple synchronous or metachronous tumors (190).

Roentgenograms show a purely lytic destructive lesion involving the end of the bone and extending up to the articular cartilage. Mineralization within the lesion is distinctly unusual in giant cell tumors. The lesion is usually poorly defined and may simulate a malignant tumor (Fig. 8.60). A giant cell tumor recurring in the soft tissues characteristically produces an eggshell type of ossification around the lesion (191). The roentgenographic appearance has been graded according to the degree of destruction of bone, but this scale has not been related to clinical behavior (192).

The gross appearance of a giant cell tumor is usually quite characteristic. The lesion is soft and dark brown (Fig. 8.61). Many giant cell tumors, however, appear fleshy white or pink. Collections of foam cells may be seen as areas of yellow discoloration. Many giant cell tumors show partial or predominant cyst formation.

Microscopically, giant cell tumors consist of multinucleated

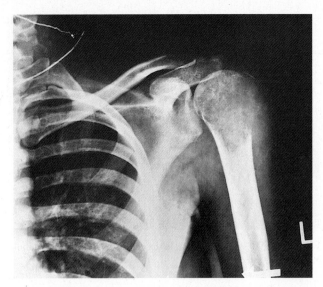

Figure 8.60. Roentgenogram of giant cell tumor of the proximal humerus. The lesion is lytic and appears to be very aggressive.

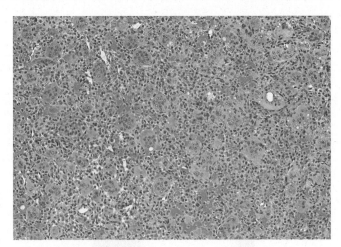

Figure 8.62. Giant cell tumor with a mixture of mononuclear cells and giant cells.

giant cells and mononuclear cells. The giant cells are usually distributed uniformly throughout the lesion (Fig. 8.62). The giant cells may contain as few as 10 or as many as 50 nuclei. The mononuclear cells are round to oval, and the nuclei resemble those in the giant cells (Fig. 8.63). Although mitotic activity may be brisk in the mononuclear cells, the nuclei lack atypia. Atypical mitotic figures should not be seen in a classic giant cell tumor.

Although most giant cell tumors have the classic appearance previously described, variations occur. It is not uncommon to see areas of secondary aneurysmal bone cyst in giant cell tumors. They may be focal or dominant. Collections of foam cells are quite common in giant cell tumors. The mononuclear cells tend to spindle out in these foam cell areas and may even have a storiform pattern. Occasionally, the spindling cells with the storiform pattern dominate the appearance of the giant cell tumor itself. In the areas where the lesion extends to the soft tissue,

bone tends to form as a shell. Rarely, one finds abundant new bone formation in the substance of a giant cell tumor. This may lead to a mistaken diagnosis of an osteoblastoma or even an osteosarcoma.

The histologic grading of giant cell tumors is not useful. Local recurrence rates of up to 30% have been reported (193). The recurrence rate varies depending on the location of the tumor and type of treatment. Rarely, a benign giant cell tumor metastasizes to the lung or even lymph nodes (194–196). The metastatic lesion is usually solitary, and patients have a good prognosis if the lesion is removed. In some cases, however, diffuse metastasis develops from a giant cell tumor that histologically appears benign. Some of these patients have died of the tumor, although spontaneous regression of the metastasis has been reported (195). Flow cytometric determination of the DNA content of the tumor cells has not been useful in predicting which benign giant cell tumors will metastasize (197).

The differential diagnosis of giant cell tumors includes a variety of conditions associated with giant cells, including aneurysmal bone cysts, osteosarcomas, hyperparathyroidism, and chondroblastomas. Calcification or chondroid differentiation

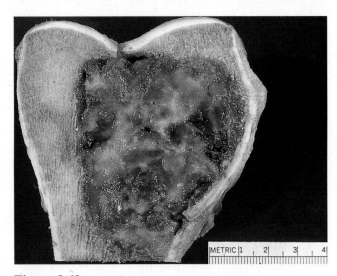

Figure 8.61. Giant cell tumor in the distal femur. The lesion extends to the end of the bone.

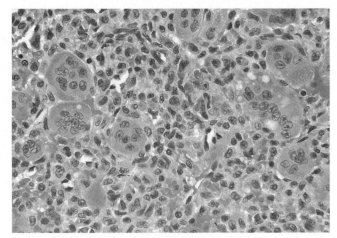

Figure 8.63. High-power appearance of giant cell tumor. The nuclei of the giant cells are similar to those of the mononuclear cells.

should separate chondroblastoma from a giant cell tumor. Most other giant cell–containing lesions are metaphyseal or diaphyseal, whereas giant cell tumors tend to be epiphyseal. Giant cell tumors have been shown to express p63, suggesting that this may be a useful biomarker to differentiate giant cell tumor from other giant cell–rich tumors (198).

Malignant Tumors of Unknown Origin

MALIGNANCY IN GIANT CELL TUMORS. Malignancy in giant cell tumors is extremely uncommon (199,200). Establishing the diagnosis of malignancy in giant cell tumors requires previous documentation of a benign giant cell tumor in the same location or clear-cut areas of benign giant cell tumor juxtaposed with spindle cell sarcoma at the time of biopsy. The former is much more common than the latter, for which the term *primary malignant giant cell tumor* has been used. A spindle cell sarcoma with abundant giant cells is insufficient for a diagnosis of malignancy in giant cell tumors. In the Mayo Clinic files, 31 of the 36 malignant giant cell tumors were judged to have developed after the treatment of a benign giant cell tumor. Twenty-five of these 31 tumors had previously been irradiated. Only five patients were shown to have malignancy in a giant cell tumor at the time of diagnosis.

The skeletal distribution of malignant giant cell tumors is the same as that for giant cell tumors. The patients are somewhat older, with most tumors occurring in the fourth and fifth decades of life. The roentgenographic appearance may be that of a typical giant cell tumor or of malignancy. Histologically, secondary malignant giant cell tumors do not show any evidence of a benign giant cell tumor. They have the appearance of osteosarcoma, fibrosarcoma, or malignant fibrous histiocytoma. In primary malignant giant cell tumors, one sees distinct areas of a classic benign giant cell tumor juxtaposed with a spindle cell sarcoma. The prognosis in cases of malignant giant cell tumor is the same as in cases of spindle cell sarcoma.

ADAMANTINOMA. Classic adamantinoma is a rare low-grade malignant bone tumor that has a pronounced tendency to involve the tibia (80% to 85% of cases) (201). In 10% to 15% of cases, the lesion is also found in the ipsilateral fibula. Some of the remaining most frequent sites include the humerus, ulna, and femur. Most patients are young adults; men and women are affected almost equally. The patients usually present with pain or swelling. The duration of the symptoms can be remarkably long, and approximately one-fourth of all patients have symptoms for more than 5 years (202).

Roentgenograms show large lesions involving the shaft of the bone. Usually, both the cortex and the medullary cavity are involved (Fig. 8.64), but some lesions are purely cortical. The lesion is composed of large areas of sclerosis interspersed with areas of lucency. Generally, one area of destruction dominates, usually in the mid portion of the lesion. Rarely, an adamantinoma occurs in the metaphysis or in the end of the bone and may be purely lytic.

Grossly, adamantinomas tend to be firm and fibrous. Occasionally, areas of cystic change are seen.

Typically, adamantinomas have epithelial islands in a fibrous stroma. The relative amounts of epithelium and fibrous stroma vary. The epithelial cells are usually arranged in clusters with a central loose area and peripheral palisading (203–207). The epithelial component stains positive with keratin markers. Sev-

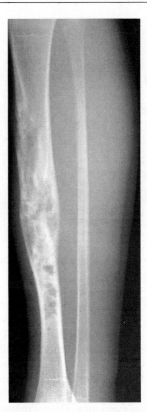

Figure 8.64. Adamantinoma extensively involving the shaft of the tibia with a mixture of lysis and sclerosis. The cortices and medullary cavity are both involved.

eral patterns of growth, including tubular, basaloid, spindle cell, and squamous, can be seen in adamantinoma. Distinct squamous differentiation is uncommon, and keratin production is even less common (Fig. 8.65). The epithelial cells show little mitotic activity and only mild to moderate cytologic atypia. A small percentage of adamantinomas have a purely spindling pattern (Fig. 8.66). Even these spindle cells tend to cluster and merge into a less cellular stroma.

It has long been recognized that fibrous dysplasia-like or osteofibrous dysplasia–like areas may be seen in adamantinoma,

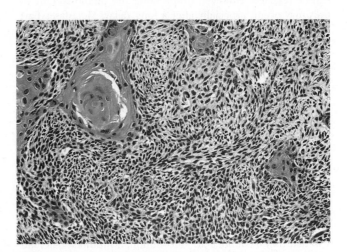

Figure 8.65. Adamantinoma. Spindle cells are shown with focal squamous differentiation.

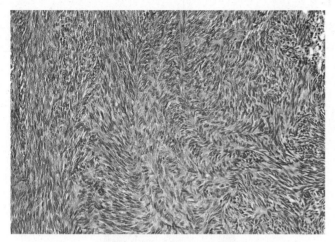

Figure 8.66. A cellular spindling pattern in adamantinoma.

particularly at the periphery of the lesion (208–210). Tumors characterized by a predominance of osteofibrous tissue containing small groups of inconspicuous epithelial cells have been termed osteofibrous-like adamantinoma or differentiated adamantinoma. These small groups or nests of inconspicuous epithelial cells should be visible on routine hematoxylin and eosin sections; however, keratin stains may be helpful in confirming the hematoxylin and eosin impression. Prominent osteofibrous dysplasia–like change has been used as evidence that osteofibrous dysplasia may be a regressive form of adamantinoma (211). Others believe that these osteofibrous dysplasia–like adamantinomas are precursors of classic adamantinoma (203,212,213). While this debate continues, there have not been any widely accepted convincing cases of osteofibrous dysplasia evolving to adamantinoma or vice versa. There are two cases reported in the literature of progression from differentiated to classic adamantinoma (203). More recently, trisomies 7, 8, 12, and/or 21 have been reported in a few examples of osteofibrous dysplasia, adamantinoma, and osteofibrous dysplasia–like adamantinoma, which suggests a common pathogenesis of osteofibrous dysplasia and adamantinoma (212).

Classic adamantinomas are usually treated surgically with an en bloc resection. The prognosis is very favorable if the lesion can be resected. However, lymph node and pulmonary metastasis may occur, especially after a long delay. Metastases have been reported in approximately 15% to 30% of cases. More conservative treatment with lesser surgical margins is usually considered for osteofibrous dysplasia–like adamantinomas because nearly all of these tumors behave in a benign fashion.

The differential diagnosis primarily includes metastatic carcinoma. It is unusual to see metastatic carcinoma below the level of the knee. Patients with adamantinoma are usually younger than those with metastatic carcinoma. The epithelial cells of adamantinoma appear distinctly less malignant than those of carcinoma.

VASCULAR TUMORS

Benign Vascular Tumors

Vascular tumors of bone are uncommon. Symptomatic hemangiomas are extremely uncommon. Many of the vascular neoplasms of the spine described at the time of autopsy may not

be true neoplasms. Most hemangiomas are asymptomatic and found incidentally on roentgenograms obtained for some other reason, especially roentgenograms of the skull taken to investigate headaches. An occasional hemangioma of a vertebral body may present with compression fracture, extension into the spinal canal, and therefore spinal cord compression. A distinct female predilection is noted, and patients in any age group may be affected. Although any portion of the skeleton may be involved, in a surgical series, most lesions are in the spine, skull, and jaws.

The roentgenographic appearance of a hemangioma can be diagnostic, especially in the spine or skull. In the skull, hemangiomas tend to have a sunburst appearance because of the presence of trabecular bone. In the spine, the appearance on CT has been likened to a polka dot (because of the bony trabecula) (Fig. 8.67). In long bones, vascular tumors tend to appear as areas of lucency and, hence, to be nonspecific.

The gross appearance is that of a hemorrhagic mass. If an entire portion of the skull is excised, one may find that trabeculae of bone are responsible for the sunburst appearance on the roentgenogram.

Microscopically, hemangiomas tend to be either capillary or cavernous. Reactive new bone formation is frequently present and may lead to a mistaken diagnosis of osteoblastoma. The endothelial cells are small, and the nuclei do not show atypia. Epithelioid hemangioma is a histologic variant of hemangioma characterized by a lobular growth pattern and epithelioid endothelial cells lining well-formed capillary-like vessels (214).

The clinical behavior of a hemangioma is that of a benign process. Some patients may have serious sequelae of a hemangioma of a vertebra.

The differential diagnosis includes a low-grade angiosarcoma/hemangioendothelioma. The distinction between a hemangioma and a low-grade angiosarcoma can be difficult and must be based on the cytologic changes of the endothelial cells.

An uncommon condition called *Gorham disease* may be related to hemangiomas. In this condition, dissolution of large segments of bone is seen in one geographic area of the body

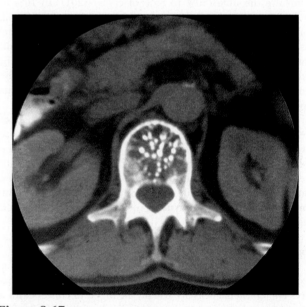

Figure 8.67. Computed tomogram of hemangioma involving the vertebral body. Note the polka dot appearance.

(215). The biopsy findings may be completely nonspecific in examples of disappearing bone disease (massive osteolysis or Gorham disease). Occasionally, one finds vascular proliferation (216). The cause of Gorham disease is unknown.

Malignant Vascular Tumors

ANGIOSARCOMA (HEMANGIOENDOTHELIOMA). We consider the terms *angiosarcoma*, *hemangioendothelial sarcoma*, and *hemangioendothelioma* to be synonymous. Any portion of the skeleton may be involved, with only one-third of the lesions affecting the long tubular bones. Approximately one-third of patients with angiosarcoma have multicentric disease. Typically, the multiple lesions tend to congregate in one geographic area, such as an entire leg. However, the lesions may be widely separated; for example, both hands or both feet may be involved. Localized pain is the usual symptom.

The radiographic features of angiosarcoma of bone are nonspecific and therefore usually insufficient to suggest a precise diagnosis (217). The roentgenograms of high-grade tumors show purely lytic areas of destruction, with little or no reactive new bone formation. Multiple osteolytic areas in one extremity strongly suggest the diagnosis of angiosarcoma (Fig. 8.68).

Grossly, the lesions tend to be red and hemorrhagic. Microscopically, angiosarcomas are characterized by anastomosing channels lined by atypical-appearing endothelial cells (Figs. 8.69 and 8.70). Papillary tufting within the endothelial spaces is distinctly unusual. Benign giant cells may be present and may mask the underlying neoplasm. Inflammatory infiltrates, especially eosinophils, are not uncommon. Reactive new bone formation is also found in a small number of cases.

A small minority of tumors have an epithelioid appearance (218–221). This histologically distinct subgroup has been termed *epithelioid hemangioendothelioma*. The tumor tends to be slightly lobulated and may have a myxoid or chondroid background. The endothelial cells appear epithelial, with prominent pink cytoplasm. Cytoplasmic vacuoles are also prominent.

Angiosarcomas are graded predominantly according to the cytologic atypia of the endothelial cells. Patients with low-grade angiosarcoma have an excellent prognosis, whereas those with high-grade tumors have a poor prognosis (222,223). However, some studies have suggested that the prognosis in angiosarcoma

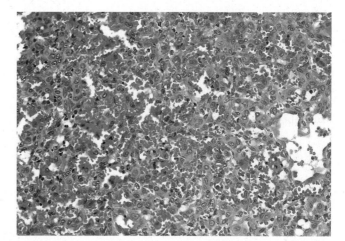

Figure 8.69. Grade 2 hemangioendothelioma. A vessel-forming growth pattern with blood-filled spaces is evident.

of bone is unpredictable (224). Patients with epithelioid hemangioendothelioma have an excellent prognosis unless the visceral organs are involved (221).

Treatment involves surgical ablation. Some patients have responded favorably to radiation therapy. When angiosarcoma of bone is diagnosed, multicentricity should be sought.

The differential diagnosis of a low-grade angiosarcoma includes hemangioma. This distinction is based on assessment of cytologic atypia and the extent of a vasoformative growth and invasion of pre-existing bone. A high-grade angiosarcoma may have large areas of spindling and simulate a high-grade spindle cell sarcoma. Immunostains can be helpful in the differential diagnosis of malignant vascular tumors since the majority is positive with factor VIII and CD31. Tumors with an epithelioid appearance may be mistaken for metastatic carcinoma. Keratin and epithelial membrane antigen immunostains may not be helpful in making the distinction between carcinoma and angiosarcoma or epithelioid hemangioendothelioma because all of these tumors may be positive with these markers. The differential is further complicated because vascular tumors and metastatic carcinoma can present with radiographic evidence of multicentric disease.

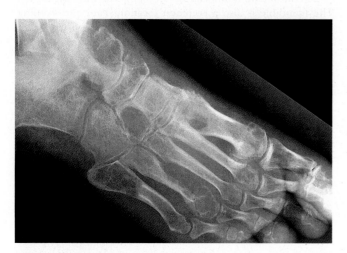

Figure 8.68. Multicentric hemangioendothelioma involving multiple bones of the foot.

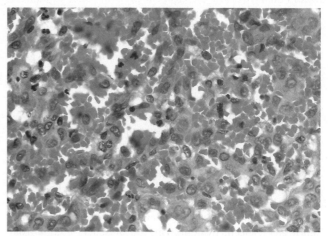

Figure 8.70. Grade 2 hemangioendothelioma. Malignant endothelial cells line the vascular spaces.

HEMANGIOPERICYTOMA. It is extremely uncommon to find hemangiopericytoma as a primary bone tumor (see Chapter 5). If it is found in bone, the possibility of metastasis from a hemangiopericytoma of the meninges should be considered. The histologic features are the same as those in soft tissue hemangiopericytomas—that is, a consistent pattern of round to oval cells arranged around deformed vascular spaces. Most hemangiopericytomas of bone are malignant (225,226).

FIBROHISTIOCYTIC TUMORS

Benign Fibrous Histiocytoma

In this extremely uncommon neoplasm of bone, the tumor cells are spindle shaped and arranged in a storiform pattern. Foam cells are frequently found. Benign giant cells are distributed unevenly in the lesion. The histologic description fits that of a metaphyseal fibrous defect or nonossifying fibroma. Indeed, the term *benign fibrous histiocytoma of bone* is applied when the lesion has the histologic characteristics of a nonossifying fibroma but the clinical or roentgenographic findings do not support the diagnosis. Patients with metaphyseal fibrous defects are usually younger than 20 years of age. Those with benign fibrous histiocytoma are usually adults. Metaphyseal fibrous defects, of course, occur in the metaphysis of long bones. Benign fibrous histiocytomas tend to develop in unusual locations, such as the pelvic bones. Pain may indicate that the lesion is a true neoplasm and not a fibrous defect. In all reported series, the clinical behavior has been that of a benign tumor (227,228).

Malignant Fibrous Histiocytoma

The term *malignant fibrous histiocytoma (MFH)* is synonymous with *pleomorphic malignant histiocytoma* and *undifferentiated high-grade pleomorphic sarcoma*. The criteria for diagnosis of MFH arising in bone and soft tissue are identical. MFH comprises a group of pleomorphic sarcomas that show no definable line of differentiation. MFH of bone is a very uncommon diagnosis. One reason is that the histologic features of MFH tend to merge into those of fibrosarcoma and fibroblastic osteosarcoma. For the same histologic grade of tumors, this distinction has no prognostic significance (229).

Malignant fibrous histiocytoma tends to affect males and females equally. It lacks the clear-cut predominance in patients in the second decade of life and instead is distributed rather evenly in different age groups. Any portion of the skeleton may be affected, but the metaphysis of long bones is preferred. Many high-grade sarcomas secondary to other conditions, such as infarct (230) and prior irradiation (231), show histologic features of MFH. The symptoms are nonspecific, usually consisting of pain or swelling. Roentgenograms nearly always show a purely lytic process and destruction of the cortex (232).

Grossly, MFH has the fish flesh appearance of most high-grade sarcomas. Areas of yellow discoloration caused by foam cells may be grossly evident.

Malignant fibrous histiocytoma is composed of a spindle cell proliferation arranged in a storiform pattern or has highly malignant cells with a histiocytic quality, including abundant pink cytoplasm. Benign giant cells and even malignant giant cells are almost always seen. By definition, the presence of chondroid or osteoid matrix rules out a diagnosis of MFH. Some authors have subdivided MFH of bone into fibroblastic, histiocytic, and

malignant giant cell tumor types (233). Whether this subclassification is of clinical significance is not clear.

The evidence so far suggests that the clinical behavior of MFH of bone is no different from that of a high-grade fibrosarcoma or osteosarcoma (234–238).

The differential diagnosis of primary MFH of bone encompasses other high-grade sarcomas, including fibrosarcoma, leiomyosarcoma, osteosarcoma, and dedifferentiated chondrosarcoma. Immunohistochemical smooth muscle markers are helpful in separating MFH from leiomyosarcoma. Any neoplastic osteoid matrix rules out a diagnosis of MFH. The high-grade sarcomatous component of dedifferentiated chondrosarcoma may be composed of MFH. Therefore, misdiagnosis may result from sampling error if this is the only component seen in biopsy tissue. Fibrosarcomas tend not to be as pleomorphic as MFHs and generally do not have giant cells. The most important differential diagnostic considerations are malignant lymphoma and metastatic sarcomatoid carcinoma. Malignant lymphomas, as previously described, may have spindling qualities and even a storiform pattern. If one finds extensive lymphocytic infiltrates and a predominantly permeative lesion without a large area of destruction, one should consider the possibility of malignant lymphoma. A multicentric MFH usually means malignant lymphoma. Metastatic sarcomatoid carcinoma, especially from a renal or pulmonary primary, can show features that overlap with MFH. The possibility of a sarcomatoid carcinoma should be considered with any spindle cell neoplasm in a patient around the age of 60 years. A thorough clinical and radiographic examination is the best way to avoid mistaking a sarcomatoid carcinoma as MFH. Immunostains for keratin markers may or may not be helpful.

FIBROUS TUMORS

Desmoplastic Fibroma

The term *borderline* is meant to describe an entity that may be locally aggressive but lacks the potential for distant spread. Jaffe (239) first delineated desmoplastic fibroma but discussed it with fibrosarcoma, pointing out the similarity with the latter. Only 14 examples of desmoplastic fibroma are recorded in the Mayo Clinic files.

The most common locations are the pelvis and long bones. The mandible is also a common location. Pain and swelling are the usual symptoms. Roentgenograms show purely lucent metaphyseal lesions associated with moderate expansion of the bone.

Grossly, the lesion is white and fibrous. Microscopically, desmoplastic fibromas are the intraosseous counterpart of desmoid tumors. The lesion is a hypocellular spindle cell lesion with abundant collagen production (Fig. 8.71). The cells lack cytologic atypia, and mitotic figures are rare. The lesion also contains thin-walled, dilated vascular channels similar to those in desmoid tumors.

Lesional curettage leads to recurrence. Resections, however, are almost always followed by cure (240).

Fibrosarcoma

Fibrosarcoma is the only malignant fibrous tumor of bone. Fibrosarcoma can be defined as a malignant spindle cell tumor

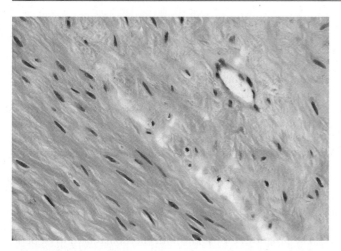

Figure 8.71. Desmoplastic fibroma. Hypocellular spindle cell proliferation is associated with abundant collagen production.

in which no matrix production is identified. Males and females are equally affected with fibrosarcoma. As with MFH, no marked predilection for the second decade of life is noted. Any portion of the skeleton may be involved, although 50% of the tumors are in the metaphysis of long bones. Pain or swelling is the usual symptom.

The roentgenographic features of fibrosarcoma are quite nonspecific. A low-grade fibrosarcoma may appear benign on roentgenograms. Usually, however, a purely lucent destructive lesion involves the metaphysis. Periosteal new bone formation may be seen.

The gross pathologic features are also nonspecific. Fibrosarcomas have the fish flesh appearance usually associated with spindle cell sarcomas.

Microscopically, fibrosarcomas have spindle cells with various degrees of anaplasia (Fig. 8.72). Low-grade fibrosarcomas are hypocellular, with spindle cells that are arranged in a herringbone pattern and produce large amounts of collagen. As the degree of malignancy increases, the lesion becomes hypercellular, and the cells tend to become more hyperchromatic. Mitotic figures are more abundant in high-grade tumors. The

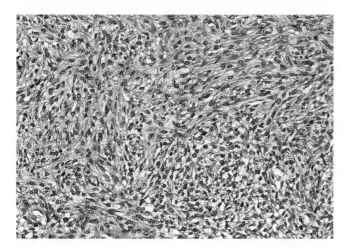

Figure 8.72. Fibrosarcoma with fascicles of spindle cells. The lesion is quite cellular.

prognosis seems to correlate well with the histologic grade of the neoplasm (241). Two unusual histologic features of fibrosarcoma must be remembered. Some fibrosarcomas have very small cells simulating those of Ewing tumor. However, the spindling nature of the neoplasm should rule out the diagnosis of Ewing sarcoma. Some fibrosarcomas produce an abundant myxoid matrix that may make the tumor cells appear deceptively bland.

Approximately one-fourth of all fibrosarcomas listed in the Mayo Clinic files appear to be secondary tumors—that is, tumors secondary to a pre-existing condition such as an infarct, Paget disease, or prior irradiation.

The differential diagnosis includes desmoplastic fibroma at the less severe end of the spectrum of malignancy and metastatic sarcomatoid carcinoma at the more severe end.

Several reports on primary leiomyosarcoma of bone have been published (242,243). The prognosis seems to be the same as that for fibrosarcoma. If a spindle cell neoplasm of bone, especially in a woman, has a myogenic quality, the possibility of a metastatic leiomyosarcoma (especially from the uterus) should be considered.

NOTOCHORDAL TUMORS

Chordoma

Chordoma is a malignant tumor that arises from remnants of the notochord. The vast majority occur in the axial skeleton. However, a small number of tumors have been reported as representing primary extra-axial chordomas in bone and soft tissue (244). Small masses of apparently ectopic notochordal rests, called *ecchordosis physaliphora*, have been described (245). These are not clinically significant, however, and are incidental findings at the time of autopsy.

Chordomas affect men much more often than women and are distinctly uncommon in patients younger than 20 years of age. However, chordomas have been reported rarely in children and young adults (246–250). The tumors in this age group tend to occur in the base of the skull and the cervical spine, and some have been reported to show an aggressive clinical behavior. In the Mayo Clinic files, more than half of all chordomas involved the sacrum, and 37% involved the clivus. The remaining tumors affected the cervical spine, lumbar spine, and thoracic spine, in that order. Patients usually present with pain. Lesions of the sacrum may be difficult to identify roentgenographically, so treatment may be delayed.

Roentgenograms show irregular areas of destruction involving the midline of the sacrum, the body of the vertebra, and the clivus. Residual osseous trabeculae and amorphous masses of calcific material may be seen. When chordoma involves the sacrum, the extension is almost always into the presacral space.

Grossly, chordoma is a soft, lobulated, gray-brown tumor that appears somewhat mucoid (Fig. 8.73).

Histologically, one of the most characteristic features of a chordoma is its lobulated appearance. If enough tissue is examined, chordomas always show lobules of tumor separated by fibrous septa (Fig. 8.74). Lobulation may not be apparent if only a small amount of biopsy tissue is available for review. Within the lobule, small round cells without significant cytologic pleomorphism are arranged in a cordlike fashion in a myxoid stroma. The cells may appear extremely epithelial or may be spindled. In many of the tumor cells, vacuolization of the cytoplasm gives

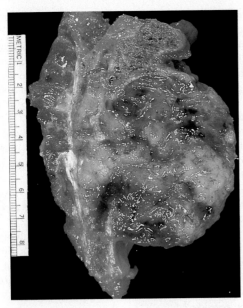

Figure 8.73. Resected specimen of chordoma of the sacrum. The tumor extends anteriorly and appears myxoid.

rise to a bubbly appearance termed *physaliphorous*. However, we find the lobulated growth pattern and the cord arrangement of the cells much more useful than the physaliphorous cells in diagnosing chordoma. The presence of foci containing pleomorphic cells does not seem to affect the prognosis adversely. Cellular and poorly differentiated histologic variants of chordoma have been described in skull base tumors occurring in children and adolescents (246). The poorly differentiated variant is associated with a poorer prognosis when compared to the other variants. Brachyury appears to be a very sensitive and specific immunohistochemical marker for chordoma (251). Chordomas also express keratin markers and epithelial membrane antigen. They show variable staining with S-100 protein.

In 1973, Heffelfinger et al. (252) described chordomas at the base of the skull with a predominant chondroid differentia-

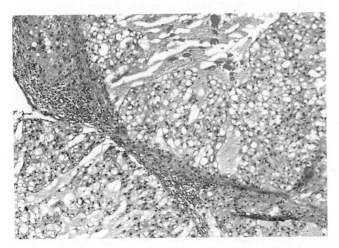

Figure 8.74. Chordoma with the diagnostic features of lobulation, myxoid matrix, and vacuolated cells in a cord arrangement.

tion and termed them *chondroid chordomas* (Fig. 8.75). These were associated with a much better prognosis than conventional chordomas in the same location. Chondroid chordomas contain variable amounts of chondroid tissue admixed with typical chordoma; thus, sampling can be a problem. Both components are positive for keratin (253–255). The main consideration in the histologic differential in this setting is chondrosarcoma, which should be positive for S-100 and negative for keratin. It is important to make this distinction because chondrosarcomas at the base of the skull have a better prognosis than chordoma at the same site (256).

Transformation of a chordoma into a high-grade spindle cell sarcoma (dedifferentiation) has been noted to occur with (257,258) and without (259) irradiation. The prognosis in these cases seems to be worse.

The prognosis for patients with chordomas used to be poor because of the location of the tumors. Although some series have reported high rates and early occurrence of metastasis (260,261), most patients survive for a long time, although with neurologic deficits. The prognosis improved remarkably after the advent of resective surgery for the sacrum and spine (262–264).

The differential diagnosis includes chondrosarcoma, metastatic carcinoma, and myxopapillary ependymoma. Because both metastatic carcinomas and chordomas are positive for keratin markers, brachyury can be helpful in making the distinction. In addition, chordomas often show some immunoreactivity for S-100 protein, whereas carcinomas are negative. Chondrosarcomas may grow in a lobulated fashion but lack the fibrous septa. Immunohistochemical stains are helpful in distinguishing chondrosarcoma from chordoma because chordomas are positive for keratin markers and chondrosarcomas are negative. Myxopapillary ependymomas do not stain for epithelial markers (265).

Giant Notochordal Rest

Giant notochordal rest (GNR) is a recently described entity that has also been termed *giant notochordal hamartoma* and *intraosseous benign notochord cell tumor* (266–268). Although it is a lesion of notochordal origin, its histologic features are bland when compared with conventional chordoma. It is composed of a uniform, sheetlike proliferation of cells resembling fat at low magnification (Fig. 8.76). The cells contain small, round nuclei that contain fine nuclear chromatin surrounded by clear to faintly eosinophilic cytoplasm with varying amounts of vacuolization. Unlike chordoma, the lesion lacks lobulation, syncytial cords and stands of tumor cells, prominent mucinous extracellular matrix, and a destructive growth pattern. GNR typically shows strong and diffuse immunoreactivity with keratin.

GNR and chordoma show differing radiographic features. Imaging studies of chordomas show a large, lytic, and destructive tumor, often associated with a soft tissue mass. In contrast, the roentgenograms and CT scans of a GNR are normal or show minimal sclerosis. However, MRI studies show a lesion with low T1- and high T2-weighted signal intensities and no soft tissue mass.

So far, it appears that the biologic behavior of GNR is that of a benign or indolent lesion. Therefore, patients with a GNR do not need the aggressive treatment required to treat a conventional chordoma.

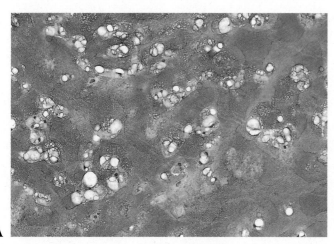

A

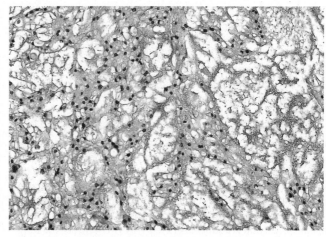

B

Figure 8.75. Chondroid chordoma with cartilage (**A**) and cords (**B**).

NEURAL TUMORS: NEURILEMOMA

Neurogenic tumors of bone are extremely rare. We have not seen a neurofibroma within bone, even in patients with neurofibromatosis.

Neurilemoma is an extremely uncommon benign lesion of bone. Many large neurilemomas that develop around the sacrum involve bone. However, it is difficult to know whether they are primary in the sacrum or affect it secondarily. We have found only 14 examples of neurilemoma in the Mayo Clinic files. The lesions tend to involve the mandible. Other portions of the skeleton also have been reported to be involved (269–271). One of the most important features of neurilemoma is that the roentgenograms always show an extremely well-circumscribed lesion. A diagnosis of neurilemoma is not tenable if the roentgenographic appearance suggests malignant disease. Microscopically, neurilemomas have the classic appearance of neurilemomas elsewhere; that is, they are spindle cell lesions with a palisading growth pattern. Treatment is conservative removal, and the prognosis is good.

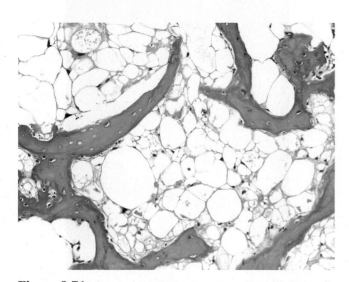

Figure 8.76. Giant notochordal rest composed of clear cells with minimal cytologic nuclear atypia filling the intertrabecular marrow.

LIPOGENIC TUMORS

Benign Lipogenic Tumors: Lipoma

Lipogenic tumors are extremely uncommon in bone (272). We have identified only eight examples of intraosseous lipoma in the Mayo Clinic files. Although the tumor has been described to involve any portion of the skeleton, a predilection for the calcaneus has been noted (273). Roentgenograms typically show rarefaction of the bone, with a central area of calcification similar to that in infarcts. Histologically, fat replaces bone, with a central focus of calcification. We have not seen malignant transformation of a lipoma, although this has been described (274).

Malignant Lipogenic Tumors: Liposarcoma

Liposarcomas are extremely uncommon in bone. Most liposarcomas in bone are either metastatic or a direct extension of soft tissue liposarcoma. We have seen only one example of a myxoid liposarcoma with round cell features that was apparently primary in bone.

CONDITIONS SIMULATING NEOPLASMS OF BONE

Conditions that simulate primary neoplasms of bone may cause considerable diagnostic problems. A variety of conditions must be considered in the differential diagnosis of a primary bone neoplasm. Some of these are quite common, whereas others are very rare.

METASTATIC CARCINOMA

Metastatic carcinoma is by far the most common malignant neoplasm involving bone. It tends to develop in older adults and is localized in the axial skeleton or the pelvic or shoulder girdle. It is extremely uncommon to see metastatic carcinoma below the level of the knee and elbow joints. In most instances, the primary site is identifiable, and a biopsy may be performed only to establish the diagnosis of metastatic carcinoma in the skeleton. Needle biopsies are ideal for confirming the diagnosis of metastatic carcinoma.

A small percentage of metastatic carcinomas have no apparent primary site (275). Even in this circumstance, the histologic diagnosis of metastatic carcinoma is usually not difficult.

When an adult patient presents with multiple bone lesions, the differential diagnosis usually centers on metastatic carcinoma, multiple myeloma, and lymphoma. Results of isotope bone scans are almost always positive in metastatic carcinoma, whereas they are generally negative in myeloma. Hence, negative findings on an isotope bone scan strongly favor a diagnosis of multiple myeloma. Detection of a monoclonal protein in the serum or urine also supports a diagnosis of myeloma. A physical examination with radiographic and laboratory studies usually discloses the site of a primary carcinoma. The most common primary sites that are sources of metastases to bone are the lung, breast, prostate, and kidney. It is unusual, in our experience, for follicular carcinoma of the thyroid to present as a metastatic bone tumor, especially with an occult primary lesion.

When metastatic carcinoma is diagnosed, the surgical pathologist may or may not be able to predict the primary site. Some unusual primary malignant lesions, such as hepatocellular carcinoma and cylindroma of the salivary gland, are so characteristic that one can predict the primary site. However, when the lesion is an undifferentiated adenocarcinoma or squamous cell carcinoma, one can only suggest possible primary sites. A variety of immunostains such as prostate markers, keratin stains, CDX2, and thyroid transcription factor-1 can be helpful in suggesting primary sites.

One of the more difficult diagnostic problems is sarcomatoid carcinoma metastatic to bone (Fig. 8.77). We try to avoid mistaking this for a primary neoplasm by considering the possibility of a sarcomatoid carcinoma in any adult patient with a spindling malignant tumor of bone. Generally speaking, the cells of metastatic spindling carcinomas are much plumper than those of primary sarcomas of bone. Sampling may also reveal obvious areas of carcinoma. However, these criteria are not infallible. Immunohistochemical studies may be of great help in separating a true sarcoma from a sarcomatoid carcinoma (276), although these tests do not always make the separation. In our experience, a sarcomatoid renal cell carcinoma (277) is the most common mimic of a primary sarcoma of bone. We have seen metastatic renal cell carcinomas simulate fibrosarcoma, MFH, and even osteosarcoma. A good clinical examination, including intravenous pyelography and CT of the chest and abdomen, is indicated when the possibility of a metastatic sarcomatoid carcinoma arises. Despite all precautions, however, an occasional erroneous diagnosis of sarcoma, when the lesion is a sarcomatoid carcinoma, is inevitable.

The identification of a possible primary site in a patient with a metastatic carcinoma from an unknown primary tumor is of more than academic interest. Patients with tumors such as breast carcinoma and prostate carcinoma may survive a long time with skeletal metastasis, whereas those with lung cancer typically succumb quickly.

ANEURYSMAL BONE AND OTHER CYSTS

Several cystic conditions of bone may simulate primary neoplasms.

Aneurysmal Bone Cyst

Aneurysmal bone cyst (ABC) is an uncommon bone tumor that may grow rapidly and recur locally. Until recently, the cause of ABCs was unknown, but recent findings have confirmed its clonal neoplastic nature (278). ABC-like areas may also occur in association with other neoplasms, especially giant cell tumor of bone, chondroblastoma, and fibrous dysplasia (279,280). Secondary ABC is rarely associated with malignant disease.

ABC occurs predominantly in the first two decades of life. Most lesions arise in the long bones, where they involve the metaphysis. When an ABC affects the vertebral column, the dorsal elements are usually involved.

Roentgenograms show a lytic destructive lesion in the metaphysis of long bones involving the bone eccentrically and producing a "blowout" appearance (Fig. 8.78). The soft tissue ex-

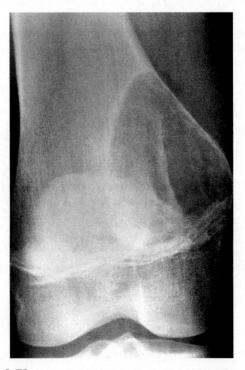

Figure 8.78. Aneurysmal bone cyst in the distal femoral metaphysis. The lesion is eccentric and expands the bone.

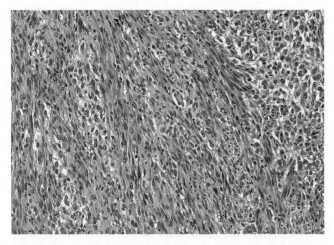

Figure 8.77. Metastatic sarcomatoid carcinoma with features resembling those of a spindle cell sarcoma. The primary tumor was in the lung.

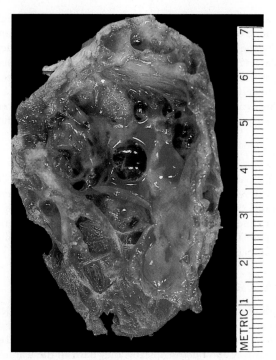

Figure 8.79. Gross specimen of an aneurysmal bone cyst. The lesion consists of blood-filled spaces separated by delicate septa.

tension usually is surrounded by a rim of reactive new bone formation that produces an eggshell appearance. The margins may be indistinct, and the lesion may simulate a malignant tumor. CT scans show fluid levels in ABCs, which are considered to be a helpful feature (281). This finding, however, does not rule out a diagnosis of telangiectatic osteosarcoma. MRI shows a honeycomb appearance with fluid levels.

The surgeon usually describes the lesion as a cavity, in which bleeding may be brisk (Fig. 8.79). Characteristically, the surgical pathologist receives a very small amount of tissue from what appears to be a large lesion on the roentgenogram. Microscopically, ABCs are composed of spaces separated by septa (Fig. 8.80). The spaces contain either serum or blood. The septum is composed of a loose arrangement of spindle cells interposed

with benign giant cells. Typically, one finds a very fine line of osteoid, termed *fibro-osteoid*, just beneath the lining of the septum. It has been shown that the lining cells of the septum are not endothelial (282). Almost all ABCs have areas in which the lesion is more or less solid. Here, one finds a loose arrangement of spindle cells with brisk mitotic activity but no cytologic atypia. Fine lacelike osteoid or trabecular osteoid is usually seen. Also, a peculiar calcified matrix is quite characteristic of ABCs (283,284).

Occasionally, an ABC appears firm and fleshy grossly and completely solid microscopically, with no cystic cavities (285). This lesion has been called a *solid aneurysmal bone cyst.* The solid areas show spindle cell proliferation with giant cells and osteoid production similar to that seen in the more solid areas of conventional ABC (Fig. 8.81). The resemblance has led to the concept that these solid lesions are a form of ABC, which was posteriorly confirmed by molecular analysis.

Cytogenetic and molecular genetic studies have shown that approximately 70% of ABCs contain USP6 fusion genes (286). The most common is CDH11-USP6, but several others have been described (287). Interestingly, most of the USP6 fusion partners are genes highly expressed during the process of osteoblastic development and differentiation, which suggests that ABC is a primitive bone tumor with incipient osteoblastic differentiation. USP6 fusion genes have also been found in the so-called giant cell reparative granuloma (solid variant of ABC). In addition, USP6 fusion genes have not been found in secondary ABC, cherubism, and brown tumor, which supports the idea that these are distinct morphologic or biologic entities (288).

ABCs are benign, and simple curettage is the treatment of choice. However, they recur locally in approximately 20% of cases, especially in those with centrally located tumors (286). It seems that the status of the molecular abnormalities is not associated with the clinical outcome. Even the recurrences should be treated conservatively.

The differential diagnosis includes giant cell tumor and osteosarcoma. Some ABCs have large numbers of benign giant cells, and this may lead to a mistaken diagnosis of giant cell tumor. However, the background cells in ABCs are more fibrogenic, and they occur in the metaphysis of long bones in young people. Telangiectatic osteosarcoma resembles an ABC at low power. Under high power, however, the cells in the stroma of

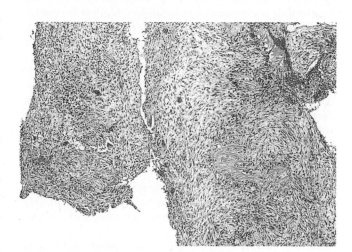

Figure 8.80. Aneurysmal bone cyst. Spaces are separated by septa that contain fibroblasts and benign giant cells.

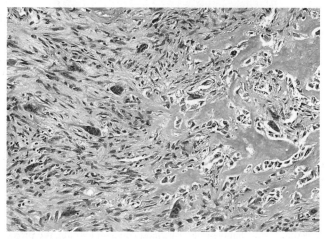

Figure 8.81. "Solid" aneurysmal bone cyst with loosely arranged spindle cells, benign giant cells, and reactive bone.

telangiectatic osteosarcoma are highly pleomorphic, whereas ABCs have no cytologic atypia. Solid ABCs may be mistaken for low-grade osteosarcomas. However, low-grade osteosarcomas are hypocellular, whereas ABCs are cellular and mitotically active.

Simple Cyst

Simple cysts of bone occur predominantly in the proximal humerus and proximal femur in patients in the first and second decades of life (289). Boys are affected much more often than girls, and the patients usually have pathologic fractures at presentation. The roentgenograms show trabeculated lesions involving the metaphysis and extending up to the epiphyseal plate (Fig. 8.82). The lesion does not expand the bone.

Grossly, the lesion is a cyst containing straw-colored or blood-tinged fluid and a thin lining. Microscopically, the lining is composed of spindle cells and a few giant cells. Some simple cysts contain a peculiar calcified matrix that probably represents mineralized fibrin.

Simple cysts may be found in unusual locations, such as the ilium and calcaneus. The patients tend to be older. Treatment consists of injection of methylprednisolone acetate (290) or the creation of simple burr holes (291). It is unusual to receive material from simple cysts in surgical pathology. Curettage and bone grafting are performed only if other methods of treatment fail or the radiographic features are questionable.

Ganglion Cyst

Cysts containing mucoid material similar to that found in the common ganglia around the wrist are seen uncommonly within

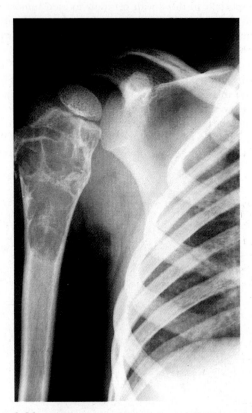

Figure 8.82. Simple cyst in the most common location, the proximal humerus. The lesion extends up to the epiphyseal plate, is centrally located, and does not expand the bone.

bone. They may be either an extension of a soft tissue ganglion into bone or a primary lesion in the bone (292). They tend to involve the ends of long bones, extending up to the articular cartilage (293). Histologically, the cyst is usually composed of fibrous tissue without an epithelial lining, and it contains mucoid material (294).

The treatment of these lesions is simple curettage. Awareness of this type of lesion should preclude any mistaken diagnosis.

Cysts of Degenerative Joint Disease

In some patients with severe degenerative joint disease, a cystic lesion develops in subchondral bone. The cyst may even be expansile (295). The roentgenographic diagnosis is usually easy because the lesion is always associated with severe degenerative disease of the nearest joint. Grossly, the cyst usually contains mucoid material. Microscopically, it has no lining.

Epidermoid Cyst

Islands of squamous cell epithelium may become embedded in bone and produce an expansile lesion. Most of these lesions develop in the skull, but they may also occur in the distal phalanx. Grossly and microscopically, they have all the features of an epidermoid cyst of the skin. Another condition related to epidermoid cyst is subungual keratoacanthoma. As the name indicates, this type of cyst occurs in the nail bed and produces well-defined lytic defects of the underlying bone. The lesion is composed of proliferating squamous cells with abundant pink cytoplasm similar to that in the cells in classic keratoacanthoma of the skin. The well-circumscribed nature of the lesion on roentgenograms should prevent a mistaken diagnosis of squamous cell carcinoma.

FIBROUS DYSPLASIA AND OSTEOFIBROUS DYSPLASIA

Fibrous dysplasia is a benign osteofibrous lesion that may occur as a single focus in bone or be multifocal. Multifocal occurrence associated with skin pigmentation, endocrine hyperactivity, and precocious puberty (especially in girls) is called *Albright syndrome* (296). Fibrous dysplasia (usually polyostotic) associated with intramuscular myxomas is known as *Mazabraud syndrome* (297). An activating point mutation of the alpha subunit of the stimulatory G-protein gene (GNAS) at the Arg codon has been identified in fibrous dysplasia (monostotic and polyostotic) and in lesional tissue of patients with Albright syndrome (298,299).

Most patients with fibrous dysplasia are younger than 30 years. The most common locations are the jawbones, skull, ribs, and proximal femur. Patients may present with a pathologic fracture, especially if the proximal femur is involved. Those with involvement of the skull and jaws may present with deformities. Those with involvement of the ribs are usually older, possibly because the lesions are asymptomatic and detected incidentally on chest roentgenograms.

Roentgenographically, fibrous dysplasia appears as a well-defined area of rarefaction that usually has a sclerotic rim (Fig. 8.83). The lucent area may be somewhat hazy, and the term *ground glass* has been applied.

Grossly, fibrous dysplasia is firm and fibrous and may be gritty. Microscopically, fibrous dysplasia shows a hypocellular proliferation of plump spindle cells with collagen production.

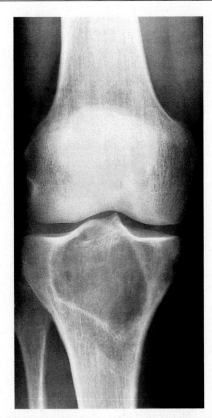

Figure 8.83. Fibrous dysplasia involving the proximal tibia. The lesion is well demarcated and has a sclerotic rim.

sia have many islands of benign-appearing cartilage (300). This appearance is especially common in the region of the femoral neck. Occasionally, fibrous dysplasia contains marked myxoid change, and this may lead to a mistaken diagnosis of fibromyxoma or chondromyxoid fibroma. Fibrous dysplasias with secondary ABCs may be associated with rapid growth and be worrisome for malignant change (301,302). Some examples of fibrous dysplasia, especially in the skull and jawbones, contain bone in the form of spherules resembling the psammomatous calcifications of meningiomas. However, this appearance is not unique to these locations.

Malignant transformation is uncommon in fibrous dysplasia. In many reports, malignant transformation in fibrous dysplasia probably represents dedifferentiation of low-grade osteosarcoma. However, several reports of malignant change in fibrous dysplasia have been published (303,304). In a Mayo Clinic study of 28 examples of sarcoma arising in fibrous dysplasia, 13 arose after radiation, and the others were not associated with radiotherapy (305). Nineteen patients had monostotic fibrous dysplasia, and nine had polyostotic disease.

Osteofibrous dysplasia is a fibro-osseous lesion that occurs exclusively in the tibia or fibula (or both), usually in children in the first decade of life (306–308). Patients frequently have a pathologic fracture at presentation. Roentgenographically, the lesion tends to affect the cortex of the tibia (Fig. 8.85), whereas fibrous dysplasia affects the medullary cavity. Histologically, it shows features that are similar to those seen in fibrous dysplasia. Both lesions are composed of a spindle cell proliferation with the production of immature woven bone. However, the bone trabeculae in osteofibrous dysplasia are more prominently

The spindle cells usually are not arranged in any meaningful fashion, but occasionally, a storiform arrangement is seen. The cells lack cytologic atypia, and mitotic figures are rare. The diagnostic feature of fibrous dysplasia is the production of woven bone (Fig. 8.84), which arises directly from the spindle cells. Osteoblastic rimming is usually not seen. However, bone with osteoblastic rimming does not rule out the diagnosis of fibrous dysplasia.

Fibrous dysplasia may display several unusual histologic changes that hinder the diagnosis. Some cases of fibrous dyspla-

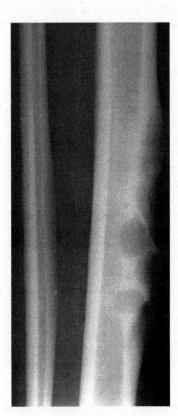

Figure 8.85. Osteofibrous dysplasia involving the cortex of the tibia.

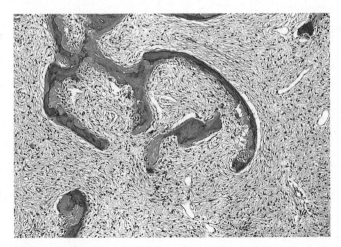

Figure 8.84. Fibrous dysplasia with spindle cell proliferation and characteristic metaplastic bone formation.

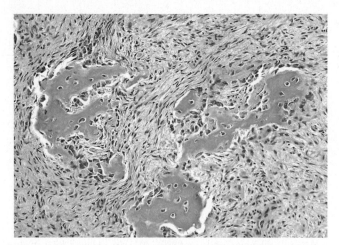

Figure 8.86. Osteofibrous dysplasia. The lesion appears more "active" than fibrous dysplasia. The bony trabeculae are rimmed with osteoblasts.

rimmed with osteoblasts (Fig. 8.86) than in classic fibrous dysplasia. Another distinguishing feature is the presence of keratin-positive spindle cells, which are seen in the majority of osteofibrous dysplasias and not in fibrous dysplasia (309). The prognosis in osteofibrous dysplasia is excellent, and the lesion tends to regress as the patient matures.

Osteofibrous dysplasia and adamantinoma have similar roentgenographic features, and adamantinomas frequently contain areas histologically identical to osteofibrous dysplasia. In particular, it can be difficult to make the distinction between osteofibrous dysplasia and osteofibrous dysplasia–like adamantinoma because of somewhat subtle differences (see "Adamantinoma" section).

METAPHYSEAL FIBROUS DEFECTS

Metaphyseal fibrous defects have been known by other names, such as *fibroma, nonossifying fibroma,* and *fibrous cortical defect.* We prefer the term *metaphyseal fibrous defect* because it describes the location of the lesion and the probability that this is not a true neoplasm. Metaphyseal fibrous defects are not uncommon but are usually incidental findings. Some patients are younger than 20 years, and a slight male predominance is noted. The defect occurs in the metaphysis of long bones, especially the distal femur, distal tibia, and proximal tibia. The roentgenograms may be diagnostic and show a lucent, elongated defect involving both the cortex and the medulla or just the cortex, and a sclerotic undulating margin produces a scalloped appearance (Fig. 8.87).

Grossly, the lesion is well circumscribed, red, and granular. Microscopically, metaphyseal fibrous defects show a spindle cell proliferation with a very characteristic storiform arrangement (Fig. 8.88). Mitotic figures are common in the spindle cells, but cytologic atypia is absent. Benign giant cells are usually found but are not prominent. Hemosiderin pigment, foam cells, and even cholesterol crystals are common.

Metaphyseal fibrous defects do not need to be treated unless pathologic fracture is a concern because of the size of the lesion (310). Simple curettage is sufficient. Rarely, patients present

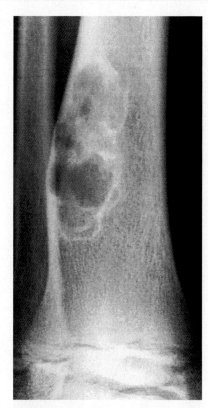

Figure 8.87. Metaphyseal fibrous defect involving the distal tibia. A sclerotic margin gives rise to a scalloped appearance.

with multiple metaphyseal fibrous defects, together with skin pigmentation, mental retardation, and endocrine abnormalities (311,312). These lesions tend to regress when the patient matures, just as the solitary lesions do.

A related condition has been called *periosteal desmoid* (313). These are small irregularities in the distal cortex of the femur, usually discovered incidentally. Histologically, only bland fibrous tissue is found. The name is unfortunate because it suggests an aggressive neoplasm. In fact, periosteal desmoid is an incidental finding of no clinical significance, and the term *cortical irregularities of the femur* has been used (314).

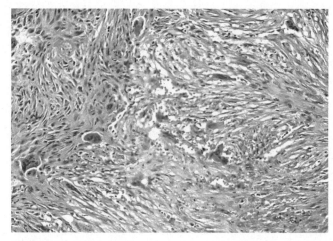

Figure 8.88. Metaphyseal fibrous defect composed of spindle cells in a storiform pattern and scattered benign giant cells.

FRACTURE CALLUS

Fracture callus usually is not a diagnostic problem because the diagnosis is clinically obvious. Histologically, spindle cell proliferation occurs with cartilage and bone. The cartilage may be quite hypercellular and worrisome for a chondrosarcoma. However, the orderly maturation to trabecular-appearing bone is typical of a reactive process and does not suggest a neoplasm. It is important when a fracture callus is diagnosed to make sure that the lesion is not a pathologic fracture and that the real lesion has not been overlooked.

In some situations, the clinical diagnosis is not so obvious. Stress fractures can appear as tumors, and the fracture lines may be overlooked. This occurrence may be associated with extensive periosteal new bone formation that can simulate the appearance of a small-cell neoplasm on the roentgenogram. Another common problem has been referred to as *insufficiency fractures* (315). These tend to occur in the pelvic region of postmenopausal women. The bone scan findings are usually positive in the sacrum and pubis, so metastatic carcinoma is suspected. The biopsy specimen shows only reactive new bone formation. Recognition of this entity avoids unnecessary biopsies.

MYOSITIS OSSIFICANS

Myositis ossificans, or heterotopic ossification, may occur in muscle or soft tissue (see Chapter 5). The patient may or may not have an associated history of trauma. The lesion grows rather rapidly and may be mistaken for a neoplasm. However, heterotopic ossification develops much faster than most neoplasms. The roentgenographic findings are usually negative for the first 2 to 3 weeks. After approximately the third week, mineralization usually occurs at the periphery with a central lucency. This appearance is also present on CT scans and helps the radiologist make an accurate diagnosis.

Grossly, the lesion is well circumscribed. If the surgeon has trouble removing the lesion, it probably is not heterotopic ossification. Microscopically, heterotopic ossification shows a zonation phenomenon first described by Ackerman (316). The central portion of heterotopic ossification is composed of a proliferation of loosely arranged spindle cells. Mitotic activity is usually brisk, but cytologic atypia is absent (Fig. 8.89). The lesion tends to mature toward the periphery, producing osteoid

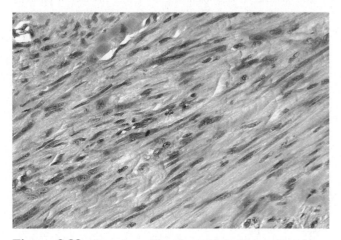

Figure 8.89. Central portion of myositis ossificans. Loosely arranged spindle cells with mitotic activity and no cytologic atypia.

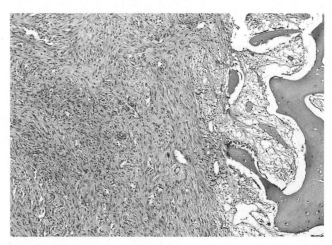

Figure 8.90. Myositis ossificans with zonation. The central cellular portion (*left*) matures into bone (*right*).

rimmed with osteoblasts, and this in turn matures into trabecular bone (Fig. 8.90). The edge of the lesion usually has mineral in the form of an eggshell. Heterotopic ossification can occur in different parts of the body and may have unusual histologic features (317,318).

An unusual form of myositis ossificans tends to be generalized and may lead to immobilization and even death. These patients usually have associated skeletal anomalies that frequently involve the small bones of the hands and feet (319–321). In rare instances, malignancy has arisen in heterotopic ossification (322).

OSTEOMYELITIS AND CARCINOMA IN OSTEOMYELITIS

Osteomyelitis is not usually difficult to identify because the clinical and roentgenographic features are characteristic. However, osteomyelitis can resemble neoplasms, especially after antibiotic treatment (323). Acute osteomyelitis can simulate neoplasms such as Ewing tumor and malignant lymphoma on roentgenograms. Osteomyelitis appears as a permeative, destructive lesion with periosteal new bone formation. Chronic osteomyelitis can produce geographic areas of destruction simulating a neoplasm such as a giant cell tumor, or it may take the form of a focal abscess simulating osteoid osteoma. Grossly, the appearance of acute osteomyelitis is well known. However, some neoplasms, such as Ewing sarcoma, may have the same gross appearance. The microscopic appearance of osteomyelitis depends on the stage. In the acute phase, capillary proliferation and reactive new bone formation are associated with an acute inflammatory infiltrate. In the chronic stages, the lesion is composed predominantly of plasma cells and lymphocytes. The plasma cellular infiltrate may be so heavy that it simulates a neoplasm.

Osteomyelitis is usually solitary, but rare examples of multifocal osteomyelitis that may be viral have been reported (324,325).

Many biopsy samples of osteomyelitis are pyogenic. However, occasionally a granulomatous appearance caused by infectious agents, such as tuberculosis or blastomycosis, is seen. Small, nonspecific granulomas are not unusual in pyogenic osteomyelitis. They can simulate the granulomatous appearance of sarcoidosis, which occasionally involves bone. Special stains and cultures are necessary to make a definitive diagnosis of infection.

The development of malignant disease in osteomyelitis of long duration, especially with a draining sinus, is a rare but well-known complication. Most patients have an extremely well-differentiated squamous cell carcinoma. Patients usually state that their sinuses have been draining for several years and that the lesion has become more painful and more foul smelling. The histologic appearance is that of an extremely well-differentiated squamous cell carcinoma. If squamous epithelium is present within the bone, the lesion has to be considered a squamous cell carcinoma. Because most patients have low-grade squamous cell carcinoma, the prognosis is excellent (326,327). Rarely, other malignant neoplasms, such as fibrosarcoma, have been reported in chronic osteomyelitis (328).

LANGERHANS CELL HISTIOCYTOSIS

Langerhans cell histiocytosis is a disease of unknown cause and diverse manifestations. In 1953, Lichtenstein (329) proposed that the disease entities known as *eosinophilic granuloma, Hand-Schüller-Christian disease*, and *Letterer-Siwe disease* all share a common pathologic appearance. This view was challenged by Lieberman et al. (330). They suggested that Letterer-Siwe disease is not a specific entity but may involve several pathologic processes. Good evidence, however, suggests that at least some examples of disseminated disease with features of Letterer-Siwe syndrome are actually Langerhans cell histiocytosis (331,332). It was once thought that Langerhans cell histiocytosis most likely was a reactive disorder rather than a neoplastic process. However, studies have demonstrated clonality in Langerhans cell histiocytosis, supporting a neoplastic origin (333).

The clinical features of Langerhans cell histiocytosis depend on the extent of involvement. Patients with solitary disease often have localized pain. Patients with disseminated disease may have lymphadenopathy, skin lesions, or diabetes insipidus, and the roentgenographic features are usually quite characteristic. In the skull, Langerhans cell histiocytosis manifests as an area of lucency that has a hole-in-hole appearance because of the different rates of destruction of the two tables of the bone. In long bones, lucent areas are frequent, with pronounced, benign-appearing, reactive new bone formation.

Histologically, Langerhans cell histiocytosis is notable for the characteristic histiocytic cells known as *Langerhans cells*. These have an oval nucleus with a longitudinal groove, resulting in a coffee-bean appearance (Fig. 8.91). The histiocytes tend to be in clusters and associated with eosinophils. Areas of necrosis and giant cell reaction are common in Langerhans cell histiocytosis of bones. Other inflammatory cells, such as plasma cells and lymphocytes, are also frequently found. Mitotic figures, including occasional atypical mitotic figures, are not uncommon.

The differential diagnosis includes osteomyelitis on the one hand and malignant lymphoma on the other. In a rare instance, only special stains separate an unusual form of osteomyelitis from Langerhans cell histiocytosis. Langerhans cells are usually positive for S-100 protein; however, CD1a and Langerin (CD207) are more specific markers of Langerhans cells (334, 335). In malignant lymphoma, the characteristic nuclear features of Langerhans cells are absent. Lymphoid immunohistochemical markers can also be helpful in separating lymphoma from Langerhans cell histiocytosis.

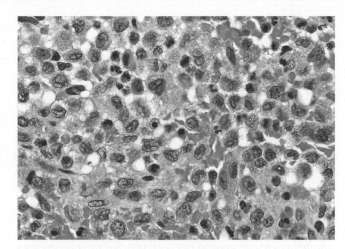

Figure 8.91. Langerhans cell histiocytosis. The loosely arranged histiocytes have oval nuclei with longitudinal grooves. A sprinkling of eosinophils and a giant cell are present.

Some authors have suggested that the histologic features are correlated with prognosis in Langerhans cell histiocytosis (336). However, several other studies suggest that the stage of the disease is a much more important prognostic indicator than the histologic appearance in Langerhans cell histiocytosis (337, 338). Kilpatrick et al. (339), in a large series on Langerhans cell histiocytosis of bone, found hepatosplenomegaly, thrombocytopenia, young age at diagnosis, and polyostotic occurrence (three bones or more) to be associated with a poor prognosis.

PAGET DISEASE

Paget disease is a disorder of unclear etiology. It is characterized by an abnormal osteoclastic-osteoblastic remodeling of bone that leads to deformity, pathologic fractures, and enlargement of single or multiple bones. Genetic factors are known to play a role in the development of Paget disease, with mutations affecting different components of the RANK-NF-κB signaling pathway (340,341). It is unclear whether exposure to environmental factors, such as viruses, is also related to manifestation of the disease. It is unusual to see Paget disease in patients younger than 40 years. The lesion is generally asymptomatic or may produce pain. The disease may also be severe, with resulting deformities (342). Although any portion of the skeleton may be involved, the pelvis is most commonly affected (343).

The roentgenographic appearance of Paget disease correlates to the phase of the disease and therefore includes a spectrum of lytic, mixed lytic and sclerotic, and sclerotic findings. Paget disease always extends to the end of a bone. Both the cortical and the medullary bone are thickened and irregular. The demarcation between normal bone and afflicted bone is quite sharp and pointed, resembling a flame or a blade of grass. Rarely, extension of the lesion into soft tissues in examples of florid Paget disease suggests a malignant change (344). Occasionally, Paget disease appears as a pure area of lysis that may suggest a neoplasm (345).

The histologic appearance is quite typical, although not diagnostic. Thickening of the bone is irregular. Characteristically, irregular blue lines in the bone produce a mosaic appearance. Other features are increased osteoclastic and osteoblastic activity and a fine fibrosis in the marrow. Although the mosaic appearance draws attention to the possibility of Paget disease, we find that the increased osteoclastic and osteoblastic activity is more helpful in diagnosing Paget disease. However, we believe that Paget disease cannot be diagnosed unless the roentgenograms support the diagnosis. Pagetoid bone is associated with a variety of conditions, including metastatic carcinoma and fibrous dysplasia.

HYPERPARATHYROIDISM

It is unusual for the effects of primary hyperparathyroidism to become a skeletal problem. Whenever a lesion containing giant cells occurs in an unusual location, the possibility of hyperparathyroidism should be considered. A surgical pathologist is more likely to see a biopsy specimen from a patient with secondary hyperparathyroidism (346,347).

MASTOCYTOSIS

Mastocytosis, an uncommon disorder, may appear as skin lesions (urticaria pigmentosa) or as a systemic disorder with or without skin involvement. The prognosis is generally good for patients with skin involvement but unpredictable for those with systemic mast cell disease. Patients with systemic mast cell disease have associated malignant disease that may lead to death (348). Very rare instances of mast cell leukemia with an extremely poor prognosis have also been described (349).

Patients with systemic mast cell disease may present with vague symptoms or symptoms associated with the gastrointestinal tract or skeleton. Approximately one-fourth of patients with systemic mast cell disease have symptoms related to the skeleton, such as fractures or osteoporosis (350). Almost 60% of patients with systemic mast cell disease have roentgenographic evidence of skeletal involvement, either diffuse osteoporosis or focal lesions that show a mixture of osteolysis and osteosclerosis (351).

Histologically, mast cell disease is characterized by the diffuse involvement of bone or, more commonly, focal lesions. These lesions tend to be paratrabecular aggregates with the appearance of microgranulomas (Fig. 8.92). Mast cells are oval to spindle shaped and contain relatively clear cytoplasm. They are frequently associated with eosinophils. A tryptase immunoperoxidase stain can be helpful in identifying mast cells.

The prognosis in mast cell disease is unpredictable, but mastocytosis is rarely the cause of death.

CHEST WALL HAMARTOMA

Chest wall hamartoma is an extremely rare tumor. It was first described in 1972 as intrathoracic mesenchymoma (352). Although the authors had at least one patient who survived with no treatment, the lesion has been mistaken for a malignant tumor. Several articles since then have confirmed the benignity of this lesion (353,354).

The lesion, usually consisting of multilobular masses, involves the chest wall of newborns and infants. It may be large enough to interfere with normal delivery. Roentgenograms show a large lesion of one or more ribs that deforms the involved ribs. Grossly, the lesions tend to have islands of cartilage and cysts. Microscopically, chest wall hamartoma has nodules of cartilage that may be hypercellular and mistaken for chondrosarcoma. Typically, the cartilage matures into trabecular bone and resembles an epiphyseal plate. Areas of spindle cell proliferation with giant cells and clear-cut areas of ABC formation are seen.

The prognosis in chest wall hamartoma is excellent, and the patients may or may not require treatment.

SYNOVIAL CHONDROMATOSIS

Synovial chondromatosis is an uncommon disease that is always monoarticular and tends to involve the large joints, especially the knees and the hips (see Chapter 6). However, smaller joints, such as the temporomandibular joint, also have been reported to be affected.

The patients are usually adults, but the lesion has also been reported in children (355). Pain, swelling, or limited motion is usual at presentation. The roentgenograms may be negative, reveal diffuse swelling of the joint, or, most characteristically, show calcific densities within the joint (356).

Grossly, the synovium appears thickened, with scattered chondroid nodules. To make a diagnosis of synovial chondromatosis microscopically, one must identify nodules of cartilage within the synovium. Clusters of chondrocytes tend to be arranged in lobules (Fig. 8.93). The chondrocytes may be doubly nucleated with atypia that is moderate to marked. The atypia may be so pronounced that, out of context, the diagnosis of chondrosarcoma is entertained. However, if the lesion is within the joint and the chondrocytes have a characteristic clustering pattern, the atypia can be ignored. In rare instances, chondrosarcoma has arisen in association with synovial chondromatosis. Marked myxoid change of the matrix, loss of the clustering arrangement, and spindling of the nuclei are associated with chondrosarcoma of the synovium (357).

Synovial chondromatosis is a primary condition of the synovium and tends to recur locally. True synovial chondromatosis must be differentiated from secondary osteocartilaginous loose bodies associated with other primary conditions of the joint, such as degenerative disease. These bodies simply represent the growth of fragments of articular cartilage. They do not show the lobulation, clustering, and cytologic atypia of synovial chondromatosis.

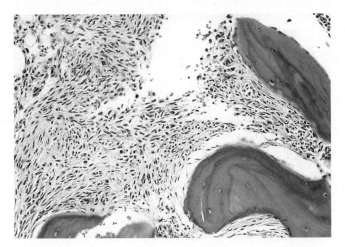

Figure 8.92. Mast cells forming paratrabecular aggregates. The cells are oval and have distinct outlines. The bone is thickened.

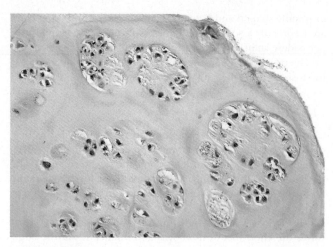

Figure 8.93. Synovial chondromatosis. Although quite cellular, the clustering arrangement is typical.

BONE INFARCT

Aseptic necrosis of the femoral head is the best known example of an infarct of bone. However, infarcts may occur in other locations, especially in the metaphyseal region of long bones. Patients with bone infarcts may have pain, or the lesions may be incidental findings on roentgenograms, which show an area of lucency surrounded by calcification. This finding may lead to a mistaken diagnosis of cartilaginous neoplasm. However, in chondroid neoplasms, calcification is more diffuse, whereas it tends to be peripheral in infarcts. Histologically, bone infarcts have bony trabeculae with loss of osteocytes. This sign may not be reliable because osteocytes can be lost even in normal bone with decalcification. Infarcts also show fat necrosis in the marrow, which is eventually replaced by calcification. The combination of empty bone lacunae and amorphous calcification in the marrow is diagnostic of infarcts. Rarely, sarcomas arise in association with an infarct.

MYOFIBROMATOSIS (CONGENITAL FIBROMATOSIS)

Myofibromatosis is a rare disease that usually occurs in newborn infants. It may appear as a single nodule in the soft tissue, multiple nodules involving the skeleton and soft tissues, or a diffuse form with involvement of visceral organs. Only the last condition is associated with a poor prognosis. The other lesions tend to resolve spontaneously. The solitary form of myofibromatosis can occur in bone (358). In a series of patients with myofibromatosis of bone, their ages ranged from 6 months to 16 years (median age, 15.5 months) (359). The roentgenograms generally show a well-circumscribed lucency of bone.

Microscopically, spindle cell proliferation with pink cytoplasm yields a myoid appearance. The cells are loosely arranged, and the background appears myxoid or chondroid. The cells tend to be arranged in nodules and have either areas of prominent slitlike vascular spaces or spindle cell proliferation with a hemangiopericytomatous pattern. The importance of recognizing congenital fibromatosis is that it is frequently mistaken for sarcoma and the patient is overtreated.

NEUROPATHIC JOINT

Neuropathic joint is also known as *Charcot joint*. Whenever radiographic evidence of rapid dissolution of bone is found at a joint, neuropathic joint should be suspected. Microscopically, neuropathic joints are marked by fibroblastic proliferation, reactive new bone formation, and very characteristic shards of bone and cartilage embedded in the fibroblastic proliferation. The cause of neuropathic joints may be peripheral neurologic disease associated with diabetes mellitus or spinal cord problems, such as syringomyelia. The rapid dissolution of the bone may lead to a mistaken diagnosis of a malignant lesion.

SUBUNGUAL EXOSTOSIS AND SUBUNGUAL KERATOACANTHOMA

In subungual (Dupuytren) exostosis, a rare condition, an osteocartilaginous lesion forms under the nail bed, predominantly that of the great toe (360,361). Although traditionally regarded as a reactive proliferative process, recent identification of a recurrent t(X;6) translocation in subungual exostoses suggest that they are neoplastic lesions (362,363). Subungual exostosis tends to occur mainly in males and affects persons in the second and third decades of life. The patient has a mass lesion that sometimes causes ulceration of the nail. The roentgenograms show a calcifying lesion projecting from the distal portion of the phalanx. Microscopically, spindle cell proliferation on the surface of the cartilage has the appearance of a cap. Mature trabecular bone formation under the cartilage cap produces the appearance of an osteochondroma. However, the location and the spindle cell proliferation separate subungual exostosis from an osteochondroma. The lesion may appear quite cellular with mitotic activity and be mistaken for a sarcoma. The treatment is simple excision, and recurrences are not uncommon.

Subungual keratoacanthoma is a rare lesion that occurs under the nail bed and produces a characteristic well-circumscribed defect of the underlying phalanx. Histologically, the lesion shows a proliferation of squamous cells with large amounts of cytoplasm and marked keratinization. The lesion is benign, and only conservative treatment is required (364). Squamous cell carcinomas also occur under the nail bed. However, they tend to be a chronic problem, whereas keratoacanthomas are usually rapidly progressive. Keratoacanthomas generally form a well-defined defect in the bone, whereas squamous cell carcinomas tend to permeate bone.

BIZARRE PAROSTEAL OSTEOCHONDROMATOUS PROLIFERATION

Bizarre parosteal osteochondromatous proliferation (BPOP) was first described by Nora et al. (365) in 1983. Similar to subungual exostosis, BPOP has been thought to most likely represent a reactive lesion. However, recent cytogenetic studies have indicated that t(1;17)(q32;q21) and variant translocations involving 1q32 are unique and common to the lesion (366,367). Unlike subungual exostosis, BPOPs involve the small bones of the hands more often than the small bones of the feet. They also occur away from the nail bed. Approximately 25% affect large bones (368). Roentgenographically, the lesion appears as a mineralizing mass attached to the underlying cortex, but not continuous with it as in an osteochondroma.

Histologically, BPOP has similarities to both subungual exos-

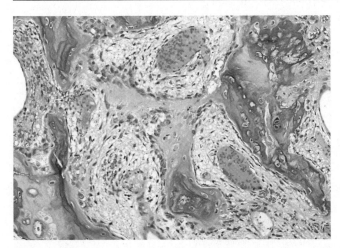

Figure 8.94. Bizarre parosteal osteochondromatous proliferation with blue cartilage maturing into bone.

tosis and osteochondroma. A prominent cartilaginous component is seen with maturation into bone. Unlike osteochondroma, this disorder shows spindle cell proliferation between bony trabeculae. Very characteristic irregular maturation of the cartilage in the bone produces a zone of chondro-osteoid with a blue tinctorial quality (Fig. 8.94). This quality is so characteristic that the diagnosis usually can be made without knowledge of the clinical circumstances.

BPOP is benign but has some propensity for local recurrence.

SINUS HISTIOCYTOSIS WITH MASSIVE LYMPHADENOPATHY

First described by Rosai and Dorfman (369), this condition of unknown cause has long been known to affect extranodal sites, including bone. In a large review of sinus histiocytosis with massive lymphadenopathy (370), the skeleton was the fifth most common site of extranodal involvement with sinus histiocytosis. Bone involvement occurs in less than 5% to 10% of cases, and skeletal lesions are usually multifocal (371). Most of these patients also have lymphadenopathy and diseases in other organs. However, occasionally patients present with a solitary lesion of bone without additional clinical manifestations.

The diagnosis of sinus histiocytosis with massive lymphadenopathy rests on the histologic appearance. In bone, areas of fibrosis, a polyclonal plasma cell proliferation, lymphocytes, and numerous histiocytes are generally seen. Most characteristic are the histiocytes that possess abundant pale eosinophilic or foamy cytoplasm surrounding enlarged, round, or oval vesicular nuclei. One of the hallmarks of the histiocytes is lymphophagocytosis or emperipolesis, a phenomenon in which lymphocytes are found within the cytoplasm of the histiocytes. Lymphocyte phagocytosis by the histiocytes is also very characteristic and therefore extremely helpful in making the diagnosis of sinus histiocytosis with massive lymphadenopathy. The most useful immunohistochemical marker for sinus histiocytosis with massive lymphadenopathy is the histiocytic expression of S-100 protein. The histiocytes also express additional macrophage markers such as CD68 and HAM56. This is a rare condition involving bone, but it is important to remember the entity to avoid the mistaken diagnosis of malignant disease.

REFERENCES

GENERAL REFERENCES

1. Lichtenstein L. Classification of primary tumors of bone. *Cancer* 1951;4:335–341.
2. Unni KK. *Dahlin's Bone Tumors: General Aspects and Data on 11,087 Cases.* 5th edition. Philadelphia, PA: Lippincott-Raven Publishers, 1996.
3. Enneking WF, Spanier SS, Goodman MA. Current concepts review. The surgical staging of musculoskeletal sarcoma. *J Bone Joint Surg Am* 1980;62:1027–1030.
4. Costa J, Wesley RA, Glatstein E, et al. The grading of soft tissue sarcomas. Results of a clinicohistopathologic correlation in a series of 163 cases. *Cancer* 1984;53:530–541.
5. Unni KK, Dahlin DC. Grading of bone tumors. *Semin Diagn Pathol* 1984;1:165–172.
6. Broders AC. Squamous-cell epithelioma of the lip: a study of five hundred and thirty-seven cases. *JAMA* 1920;74:656–664.
7. Bertoni F, Present DA, Enneking WF. Staging of bone tumors. *Contemp Issues Surg Pathol* 1988;11:47–83.

MYELOMA

8. Kyle RA, Gertz MA, Witzig TE, et al. Review of 1027 patients with newly diagnosed multiple myeloma. *Mayo Clin Proc* 2003;78:21–33.
9. Casey TT, Stone WJ, DiRaimondo CR, et al. Tumoral amyloidosis of bone of beta 2-microglobulin origin in association with long-term hemodialysis: a new type of amyloid disease. *Hum Pathol* 1986;17:731–738.
10. Pambuccian SE, Horyd ID, Cawte T, et al. Amyloidoma of bone, a plasma cell/plasmacytoid neoplasm. Report of three cases and review of the literature. *Am J Surg Pathol* 1997;21:179–186.
11. Woodruff RK, Malpas JS, White FE. Solitary plasmacytoma. II: Solitary plasmacytoma of bone. *Cancer* 1979;43:2344–2347.
12. Bataille R, Sany J. Solitary myeloma: clinical and prognostic features of a review of 114 cases. *Cancer* 1981;48:845–851.
13. Frassica DA, Frassica FJ, Schray MF, et al. Solitary plasmacytoma of bone: Mayo Clinic experience. *Int J Radiat Oncol Biol Phys* 1989;16:43–48.
14. Resnick D, Greenway GD, Bardwick PA, et al. Plasma-cell dyscrasia with polyneuropathy, organomegaly, endocrinopathy, M-protein, and skin changes: the POEMS syndrome. Distinctive radiographic abnormalities. *Radiology* 1981;140:17–22.
15. Kelly JJ Jr, Kyle RA, Miles JM, et al. Osteosclerotic myeloma and peripheral neuropathy. *Neurology* 1983;33:202–210.

MALIGNANT LYMPHOMA

16. Jones D, Kraus MD, Dorfman DM. Lymphoma presenting as a solitary bone lesion. *Am J Clin Pathol* 1999;111:171–178.
17. Howat AJ, Thomas H, Waters KD, et al. Malignant lymphoma of bone in children. *Cancer* 1987;59:335–339.
18. Kitsoulis P, Vlychou M, Papoudou-Bai A, et al. Primary lymphomas of bone. *Anticancer Res* 2006;26(1A):325–337.
19. Pettit CK, Zukerberg LR, Gray MH, et al. Primary lymphoma of bone. A B-cell neoplasm with a high frequency of multilobated cells. *Am J Surg Pathol* 1990;14:329–334.
20. Glotzbecker MP, Kersun LS, Choi, JK, et al. Primary non-Hodgkin's lymphoma of bone in children. *J Bone Joint Surg* 2006;88-A(3):583–594.
21. Ostrowski ML, Unni KK, Banks PM, et al. Malignant lymphoma of bone. *Cancer* 1986;58:2646–2655.
22. Kluin PM, Slootweg PJ, Schuurman HJ, et al. Primary B-cell malignant lymphoma of the maxilla with a sarcomatous pattern and multilobated nuclei. *Cancer* 1984;54:1598–1605.
23. Meis JM, Butler JJ, Osborne BM, et al. Granulocytic sarcoma in nonleukemic patients. *Cancer* 1986;58:2697–2709.
24. Welch P, Grossi C, Carroll A, et al. Granulocytic sarcoma with an indolent course and destructive skeletal disease. Tumor characterization with immunologic markers, electron microscopy, cytochemistry, and cytogenetic studies. *Cancer* 1986;57:1005–1010.
25. Neiman RS, Barcos M, Berard C, et al. Granulocytic sarcoma: a clinicopathologic study of 61 biopsied cases. *Cancer* 1981;48:1426–1437.
26. Goldstein NS, Ritter JH, Argenyi ZB, et al. Granulocytic sarcoma: potential diagnostic clues from immunostaining patterns seen with anti-lymphoid antibodies. *Int J Surg Pathol* 1995;2:177–186.
27. Traweek ST, Arber DA, Rappaport H, et al. Extramedullary myeloid cell tumors. An immunohistochemical and morphologic study of 28 cases. *Am J Surg Pathol* 1993;17:1011–1019.
28. Newcomer LN, Silverstein MB, Cadman EC, et al. Bone involvement in Hodgkin's disease. *Cancer* 1982;49:338–342.
29. Klein MJ, Rudin BJ, Greenspan A, et al. Hodgkin disease presenting as a lesion in the wrist. A case report. *J Bone Joint Surg Am* 1987;69:1246–1249.
30. Ostrowski ML, Inwards CY, Strickler JG, et al. Osseous Hodgkin disease. *Cancer* 1999;85:1166–1178.

EWING TUMOR

31. Askin FB, Rosai J, Sibley RK, et al. Malignant small cell tumor of the thoracopulmonary region in childhood: a distinctive clinicopathologic entity of uncertain histogenesis. *Cancer* 1979;43:2438–2451.

32. Noguera R, Triche TJ, Navarro S, et al. Dynamic model of differentiation in Ewing's sarcoma cells. Comparative analysis of morphologic, immunocytochemical and oncogene expression parameters. *Lab Invest* 1992;62:143–151.

33. Sandberg AA, Bridge JA. Updates on cytogenetics and molecular genetics of bone and soft tissue tumors: Ewing sarcoma and peripheral primitive neuroectodermal tumors. *Cancer Genet Cytogenet* 2000;123:1–26.

34. Yunis EJ. Ewing's sarcoma and related small round cell neoplasms in children. *Am J Surg Pathol* 1986;1(10 Suppl):54–62.

35. Ushigome S, Shimoda T, Takaki K, et al. Immunocytochemical and ultrastructural studies of the histogenesis of Ewing's sarcoma and putatively related tumors. *Cancer* 1989;64: 52–62.

36. Tsuneyoshi M, Yokoyama R, Hashimoto H, et al. Comparative study of neuroectodermal tumor and Ewing's sarcoma of the bone. Histopathologic, immunohistochemical and ultrastructural features. *Acta Pathol Jpn* 1989;39:573–581.

37. Ladanyi M, Heinemann FS, Huvos AG, et al. Neural differentiation in small round cell tumors of bone and soft tissue with the translocation t(11;22)(q24;q12): an immunohistochemical study of 11 cases. *Hum Pathol* 1990;21:1245–1251.

38. Navarro S, Cavazzana AO, Llombart-Bosch A, et al. Comparison of Ewing's sarcoma of bone and peripheral neuroepithelioma. An immunocytochemical and ultrastructural analysis of two primitive neuroectodermal neoplasms. *Arch Pathol Lab Med* 1994;118: 608–615.

39. Stevenson AJ, Chatten J, Bertoni F, et al. CD99 (p30/32^{MIC2}) neuroectodermal/Ewing's sarcoma antigen as an immunohistochemical marker: review of more than 600 tumors and the literature experience. *Appl Immunohistochem* 1994;2:231–240.

40. Hess E, Cohen C, DeRose PB, et al. Nonspecificity of p30/32^{MIC2} immunolocalization with the O13 monoclonal antibody in the diagnosis of Ewing's sarcoma: application of an algorithmic immunohistochemical analysis. *Appl Immunohistochem* 1997;5:94–103.

41. Riopel M, Dickman PS, Link MP, et al. MIC2 analysis in pediatric lymphomas and leukemias. *Hum Pathol* 1994;25:396–399.

42. Vartanian RK, Sudilovsky D, Weidner N. Immunostaining of monoclonal antibody O13 (anti-MIC2 gene product [CD99]) in lymphomas: impact of heat-induced epitope retrieval. *Appl Immunohistochem* 1996;4:43–55.

43. Lucas DR, Bentley G, Dan ME, et al. Ewing sarcoma versus lymphoblastic lymphoma. A comparative immunohistochemical study. *Am J Clin Pathol* 2001;115:11–17.

44. Folpe AL, Hill CE, Parham DM, et al. Immunohistochemical detection of FLI1 protein expression: a study of 132 round cell tumors with emphasis on CD99-positive mimics of Ewing's sarcoma/primitive neuroectodermal tumor. *Am J Surg Pathol* 2000;24:1657–1662.

45. Gu M, Antonescu CR, Guiter G, et al. Cytokeratin immunoreactivity in Ewing's sarcoma. Prevalence in 50 cases confirmed by molecular diagnostic studies. *Am J Surg Pathol* 2000; 24:410–416.

46. Folpe AL, Goldblum JR, Rubin BP, et al. Morphologic and immunophenotypic diversity in Ewing family tumors. A study of 66 genetically confirmed cases. *Am J Surg Pathol* 2005; 29:1025–1033.

47. Delattre O, Zucman J, Melot T, et al. The Ewing family of tumors—a subgroup of small-round-cell tumors defined by specific chimeric transcripts. *N Engl J Med* 1994;331:294–299.

48. Scotlandi K, Serra M, Manara MC, et al. Immunostaining of the p30/32^{MIC2} antigen and molecular detection of EWS rearrangements for the diagnosis of Ewing's sarcoma and peripheral neuroectodermal tumor. *Hum Pathol* 1996;27:408–416.

49. Bridge JA, Sandberg AA. Cytogenetic and molecular genetic techniques as adjunctive approaches in the diagnosis of bone and soft tissue tumors. *Skeletal Radiol* 2000;29: 249–258.

50. Kissane JM, Askin FB, Foulkes M, et al. Ewing's sarcoma of bone: clinicopathologic aspects of 303 cases from the Intergroup Ewing's Sarcoma Study. *Hum Pathol* 1983;14:773–779.

51. Hartman KR, Triche TJ, Kinsella TJ, et al. Prognostic value of histopathology in Ewing's sarcoma. Long-term follow-up of distal extremity primary tumors. *Cancer* 1991;67:163–171.

52. Llombart-Bosch A, Contesso G, Henry-Amar M, et al. Histopathological predictive factors in Ewing's sarcoma of bone and clinicopathological correlations. A retrospective study of 261 cases. *Virchows Arch A Pathol Anat Histopathol* 1986;409:627–640.

53. Bacci G, Longhi Al, Ferrari S, et al. Prognostic factors in non-metastatic Ewing's sarcoma tumor of bone: an analysis of 579 patients treated at a single institution with adjuvant or neoadjuvant chemotherapy between 1972 and 1998. *Acta Oncol* 2006;45:469–475.

54. Rodriguez-Galindo C, Liu T, Krasin MJ, et al. Analysis of prognostic factors in Ewing sarcoma family of tumors: review of St. Jude Children's Research Hospital studies. *Cancer* 2007;110:375–384.

55. Grier HE, Krailo MD, Tarbell NJ, et al. Addition of ifosfamide and etoposide to standard chemotherapy for Ewing's sarcoma and primitive neuroectodermal tumor of bone. *N Engl J Med* 2003;348:694–701.

56. Aparicio J, Munarriz B, Pastor M, et al. Long-term follow-up and prognostic factors in Ewing's sarcoma. A multivariate analysis of 116 patients from a single institution. *Oncology* 1998;55:20–26.

57. Bacci G, Ferrari S, Bertoni F, et al. Prognostic factors in nonmetastatic Ewing's sarcoma of bone treated with adjuvant chemotherapy: analysis of 359 patients at the Istituto Ortopedico Rizzoli. *J Clin Oncol* 2000;18:4–11.

58. Wunder JS, Paulian G, Huvos AG, et al. The histological response to chemotherapy as a predictor of the oncological outcome of operative treatment of Ewing's sarcoma. *J Bone Joint Surg Am* 1998;80:1020–1033.

59. Bridge JA, Bhatia PS, Anderson JR, et al. Biologic and clinical significance of cytogenetic and molecular cytogenetic abnormalities in benign and malignant cartilaginous lesions. *Cancer Genet Cytogenet* 1993;69:79–90.

60. Mertens F, Rydholm A, Kreicbergs A, et al. Loss of chromosome band 8a24 in sporadic osteocartilaginous exostoses. *Genes Chromosomes Cancer* 1994;9:8–12.

61. Bridge JA, Nelson M. Orndal C, et al. Clonal karyotypic abnormalities of the hereditary multiple exostoses chromosomal loci 8q24.1 (EXT1) and 11p11-12 (EXT2) in patients with sporadic and hereditary osteochondromas. *Cancer* 1998;92:1657–1663.

62. Hameetman L, Szuhai K, Yavas A, et al. The role of EXT1 in nonhereditary osteochondroma: identification of homozygous deletions. *Natl Cancer Inst* 2007;99:396–406.

CHONDROID TUMORS

63. Legeai-Mallet L, Margaritte-Jeannin P, Lemdani M, et al. An extension of the admixture test for the study of genetic heterogeneity in hereditary multiple extoses. *Hum Genet* 1997; 99:298–302.

64. Raskind WH, Conrad EU III, Matsushita M, et al. Evaluation of locus heterogeneity and EXT1 mutations in 34 families with hereditary multiple exostoses. *Hum Mutat* 1998;11: 231–239.

65. Borges AM, Huvos AG, Smith J. Bursa formation and synovial chondrometaplasia associated with osteochondromas. *Am J Clin Pathol* 1981;75:648–653.

66. Ahmed AR, Tan TS, Unni KK, et al. Secondary chondrosarcoma in osteochondroma; report of 107 patients. *Clin Orthop Relat Res* 2003;411:193–206.

67. Staals, EL, Bacchini P, Bertoni F. Dedifferentiated chondrosarcomas arising in preexisting osteochondromas. *J Bone Joint Surg Am* 2007;89:987–993.

68. Nojima T, Unni KK, McLeod RA, et al. Periosteal chondroma and periosteal chondrosarcoma. *Am J Surg Pathol* 1985;9:666–677.

69. Boriani S, Bacchini P, Bertoni F, et al. Periosteal chondroma. A review of twenty cases. *J Bone Joint Surg Am* 1983;65:205–212.

70. Bauer TW, Dorfman HD, Latham JT Jr. Periosteal chondroma. A clinicopathologic study of 23 cases. *Am J Surg Pathol* 1982;6:631–637.

71. Lichtenstein L, Goldman RL. Cartilage tumors in soft tissues, particularly in the hand and foot. *Cancer* 1964;17:1203–1208.

72. Dahlin DC, Salvador AH. Cartilaginous tumors of the soft tissues of the hands and feet. *Mayo Clin Proc* 1974;49:721–726.

73. Chung EB, Enzinger FM. Chondroma of soft parts. *Cancer* 1978;41:1414–1424.

74. Liu J, Hudkins PG, Swee RG, et al. Bone sarcomas associated with Ollier's disease. *Cancer* 1987;59:1376–1385.

75. Lewis RJ, Ketcham AS. Maffucci's syndrome: functional and neoplastic significance. Case report and review of the literature. *J Bone Joint Surg Am* 1973;55:1465–1479.

76. Kurt AM, Unni KK, Sim FH, et al. Chondroblastoma of bone. *Hum Pathol* 1989;20:965–976.

77. Schajowicz F, Gallardo H. Epiphysial chondroblastoma of bone. A clinico-pathological study of sixty-nine cases. *J Bone Joint Surg Br* 1970;52:205–226.

78. Springfield DS, Capanna R, Gherlinzoni F, et al. Chondroblastoma. A review of seventy cases. *J Bone Joint Surg Am* 1985;67:748–755.

79. Huvos AG, Marcove RC. Chondroblastoma of bone. A critical review. *Clin Orthop* 1973; 95:300–312.

80. Dahlin DC, Ivins JC. Benign chondroblastoma. A study of 125 cases. *Cancer* 1972;30: 401–413.

81. McLeod RA, Beabout JW. The roentgenographic features of chondroblastoma. *Am J Roentgenol Radium Ther Nucl Med* 1973;118:464–471.

82. Kahn LB, Wood FM, Ackerman LV. Malignant chondroblastoma. Report of two cases and review of the literature. *Arch Pathol* 1969;88:371–376.

83. Green P, Whittaker RP. Benign chondroblastoma. Case report with pulmonary metastasis. *J Bone Joint Surg Am* 1975;57:418–420.

84. Riddell RJ, Louis CJ, Bromberger NA. Pulmonary metastases from chondroblastoma of the tibia. Report of a case. *J Bone Joint Surg Br* 1973;55:848–853.

85. Wirman JA, Crissman JD, Aron BF. Metastatic chondroblastoma: report of an unusual case treated with radiotherapy. *Cancer* 1979;44:87–93.

86. Kyriakos M, Land VJ, Penning HL, et al. Metastatic chondroblastoma. Report of a fatal case with a review of the literature on atypical, aggressive, and malignant chondroblastoma. *Cancer* 1985;55:1770–1789.

87. Gherlinzoni F, Rock M, Picci P. Chondromyxoid fibroma. The experience at the Istituto Ortopedico Rizzoli. *J Bone Joint Surg Am* 1983;65:198–204.

88. Wu CT, Inwards CY, O'Laughlin S, et al. Chondromyxoid fibroma of bone: a clinicopathologic review of 278 cases. *Hum Pathol* 1998;29:438–446.

89. Baker AC, Rezeanu L, O'Laughlin S, et al. Juxtacortical chondromyxoid fibroma of bone: a unique variant—a case study of 20 patients. *Am J Surg Pathol* 2007;31:1662–1668.

90. Kyriakos M. Soft tissue implantation of chondromyxoid fibroma. *Am J Surg Pathol* 1979; 3:363–372.

91. Zillmer DA, Dorfman HD. Chondromyxoid fibroma of bone: thirty-six cases with clinicopathologic correlation. *Hum Pathol* 1989;20:952–964.

92. Smith CA, Magenis RE, Himoe E, et al. Chondromyxoid fibroma of the nasal cavity with an interstitial insertion between chromosomes 6 and 19. *Cancer Genet Cytogenet* 2006;171: 97–100.

93. Dahlin DC. Chondrosarcoma and its "variants." *Monogr Pathol* 1976;17:300–311.

94. Saito K, Unni KK, Wollan PC, et al. Chondrosarcoma of the jaw and facial bones. *Cancer* 1995;76:1550–1558.

95. Lewis JE, Olsen KD, Inwards CY. Cartilaginous tumors of the larynx: clinicopathologic review of 47 cases. *Ann Otol Rhinol Laryngol* 1997;106:94–100.

96. Young CL, Sim FH, Unni KK, et al. Chondrosarcoma of bone in children. *Cancer* 1990; 66:1641–1648.

97. Meachim G. Histological grading of chondrosarcomata. *J Bone Joint Surg Br* 1979;61: 393–394.

98. Evans HL, Ayala AG, Romsdahl MM. Prognostic factors in chondrosarcoma of bone: a clinicopathologic analysis with emphasis on histologic grading. *Cancer* 1977;40:818–831.

99. Gitelis S, Bertoni F, Picci P, et al. Chondrosarcoma of bone. The experience at the Istituto Ortopedico Rizzoli. *J Bone Joint Surg Am* 1981;63:1248–1257.

100. Pritchard DJ, Lunke RJ, Taylor WF, et al. Chondrosarcoma: a clinicopathologic and statistical analysis. *Cancer* 1980;45:149–157.

101. Henderson ED, Dahlin DC. Chondrosarcoma of bone—a study of two hundred and eighty-eight cases. *J Bone Joint Surg Am* 1963;45:1450–1458.

102. Bjornsson J, McLeod RA, Unni KK, et al. Primary chondrosarcoma of long bones and limb girdles. *Cancer* 1998;83:2105–2119.
103. Lee FY, Mankin HJ, Fondren G, et al. Chondrosarcoma of bone: an assessment of outcome. *J Bone Joint Surg Am* 1999;81:326–338.
104. Mirra JM, Gold R, Downs J, et al. A new histologic approach to the differentiation of enchondroma and chondrosarcoma of the bones. A clinicopathologic analysis of 51 cases. *Clin Orthop* 1985;201:214–237.
105. Dahlin DC, Salvador AH. Chondrosarcomas of bones of the hands and feet—a study of 30 cases. *Cancer* 1974;34:755–760.
106. Karabela-Bouropoulou V, Patra-Malli F, Agnantis N. Chondrosarcoma of the thumb: an unusual case with lung and cutaneous metastases and death of the patient 6 years after treatment. *J Cancer Res Clin Oncol* 1986;112:71–74.
107. Ogose A, Unni KK, Swee RG, et al. Chondrosarcoma of small bones of the hands and feet. *Cancer* 1997;80:50–59.
108. Garrison RC, Unni KK, McLeod RA, et al. Chondrosarcoma arising in osteochondroma. *Cancer* 1982;49:1890–1897.
109. Huvos AG, Marcove RC. Chondrosarcoma in the young. A clinicopathologic analysis of 79 patients younger than 21 years of age. *Am J Surg Pathol* 1987;11:930–942.
110. Collins MS, Koyama T, Swee RG, et al. Clear cell chondrosarcoma: radiographic, computed tomographic, and magnetic resonance findings in 34 patients with pathologic correlation. *Skeletal Radiol* 2003;32:12:687–694.
111. Bjornsson J, Unni KK, Dahlin DC, et al. Clear cell chondrosarcoma of bone. Observations in 47 cases. *Am J Surg Pathol* 1984;8:223–230.
112. Itala A, Leerapun T, Inwards C, et al. An institutional review of clear cell chondrosarcoma. *Clin Orthop Relat Res* 2005;440:209–212.
113. Kalil RK, Inwards CY, Unni KK, et al. Dedifferentiated clear cell chondrosarcoma. *Am J Surg Pathol* 2000;24:1079–1086.
114. Dahlin DC, Beabout TW. Dedifferentiation of low-grade chondrosarcomas. *Cancer* 1971; 28:461–466.
115. Johnson S, Tetu B, Ayala AG, et al. Chondrosarcoma with additional mesenchymal component (dedifferentiated chondrosarcoma). I. A clinicopathologic study of 26 cases. *Cancer* 1986;58:278–286.
116. Littrell LA, Wenger DE, Wold LE, et al. Radiographic, CT, and MR imaging features of dedifferentiated chondrosarcomas: a retrospective review of 174 de novo cases. *Radiographics* 2004;24:1397–1409.
117. Capanna R, Bertoni F, Bettelli G, et al. Dedifferentiated chondrosarcoma. *J Bone Joint Surg Am* 1988;70:60–69.
118. Frassica FJ, Unni KK, Beabout JW, et al. Dedifferentiated chondrosarcoma. A report of the clinicopathological features and treatment of seventy-eight cases. *J Bone Joint Surg Am* 1986;68:1197–1205.
119. Dickey ID, Rose PS, Fuchs B, et al. Dedifferentiated chondrosarcoma: the role of chemotherapy with updated outcomes. *J Bone Joint Surg Am* 2004;86-A:2412–2418.
120. Staals EL, Bacchini P, Bertoni F. Dedifferentiated central chondrosarcoma. *Cancer* 2006; 106:2682–2691.
121. Matsuno T, Ichioka Y, Yagi T, et al. Spindle-cell sarcoma in patients who have osteochondromatosis. A report of two cases. *J Bone Joint Surg Am* 1988;70:137–141.
122. Lichtenstein L, Bernstein D. Unusual benign and malignant chondroid tumors of bone: a survey of some mesenchymal cartilage tumors and malignant chondroblastic tumors, including a few multicentric ones, as well as many atypical benign chondroblastomas and chondromyxoid fibromas. *Cancer* 1959;12:1142–1157.
123. Vencio EF, Reeve CM, Unni KK, et al. Mesenchymal chondrosarcoma of the jaw bones. Clinicopathologic study of 19 cases. *Cancer* 1998;82:2350–2355.
124. Huvos AG, Rosen G, Dabska M, et al. Mesenchymal chondrosarcoma. A clinicopathologic analysis of 35 patients with emphasis on treatment. *Cancer* 1983;51:1230–1237.
125. Nakashima Y, Unni KK, Shives TC, et al. Mesenchymal chondrosarcoma of bone and soft tissue: a review of 111 cases. *Cancer* 1987;57:2444–2453.

OSTEOGENIC TUMORS

126. Makley JT, Dunn MJ. Prostaglandin synthesis by osteoid osteoma (Letter). *Lancet* 1982;2: 42.
127. Swee RG, McLeod RA, Beabout JW. Osteoid osteoma: detection, diagnosis, and localization. *Radiology* 1979;130:117–123.
128. Marcove RC, Heelan RT, Huvos AG, et al. Osteoid osteoma. Diagnosis, localization, and treatment. *Clin Orthop* 1991;267:197–201.
129. Sim FH, Dahlin DC, Beabout JW. Osteoid osteoma: diagnostic problems. *J Bone Joint Surg Am* 1975;57:154–159.
130. Rosenthal DL, Hornicek FJ, Wolfe MW, et al. Percutaneous radiofrequency coagulation of osteoid osteoma compared with operative treatment. *J Bone Joint Surg Am* 1998;80: 815–821.
131. Muscolo DL, Velan O, Pineda Acero G, et al. Osteoid osteoma of the hip. Percutaneous resection guided by computed tomography. *Clin Orthop* 1995;310:170–175.
132. Regan MW, Galey JP, Oakeshott RD. Recurrent osteoid osteoma. Case report with a ten-year asymptomatic interval. *Clin Orthop* 1990;253:221–224.
133. De Souza Diaz L, Frost HM. Osteoid osteoma–osteoblastoma. *Cancer* 1974;33:1075–1081.
134. Mortazavi SM, Wenger D, Asadollahi S, et al. Periosteal osteoblastoma: report of a case with a rare histopathologic presentation and review of the literature. *Skeletal Radiol* 2007; 36:259–264.
135. McLeod RA, Dahlin DC, Beabout JW. The spectrum of osteoblastoma. *Am J Roentgenol* 1976;126:321–325.
136. Filippi RZ, Swee RG, Unni KK. Epithelioid multinodular osteoblastoma: a clinicopathologic analysis of 26 cases. *Am J Surg Pathol* 2007;31:1265–1268.
137. Dorfman HD, Weiss SW. Borderline osteoblastic tumors: problems in the differential diagnosis of aggressive osteoblastoma and low-grade osteosarcoma. *Semin Diagn Pathol* 1984;1:215–234.
138. Mirra JM, Kendrick RA, Kendrick RE. Pseudomalignant osteoblastoma versus arrested osteosarcoma: a case report. *Cancer* 1976;37:2005–2014.
139. Schajowicz F, Lemos C. Malignant osteoblastoma. *J Bone Joint Surg Br* 1976;58:202–211.
140. Lucas DR, Unni KK, McLeod RA, et al. Osteoblastoma: clinicopathologic study of 306 cases. *Hum Pathol* 1994;25:117–134.
141. Della Rocca C, Huvos AG. Osteoblastoma: varied histological presentations with a benign clinical course. An analysis of 55 cases. *Am J Surg Pathol* 1996;20:841–850.
142. Merryweather R, Middlemiss JH, Sanerkin NG. Malignant transformation of osteoblastoma. *J Bone Joint Surg Br* 1980;62:381–384.
143. Seki T, Fukuda H, Ishii Y, et al. Malignant transformation of benign osteoblastoma. A case report. *J Bone Joint Surg Am* 1975;57:424–426.
144. Bertoni F, Unni KK, McLeod RA, et al. Osteosarcoma resembling osteoblastoma. *Cancer* 1985;55:416–426.
145. Mirra JM, Cove K, Theros E, et al. A case of osteoblastoma associated with severe systemic toxicity. *Am J Surg Pathol* 1979;3:436–471.
146. Yoshikawa S, Nakamura T, Takagi M, et al. Benign osteoblastoma as a cause of osteomalacia. A report of two cases. *J Bone Joint Surg Br* 1977;59:279–286.
147. Dale S, Breidahl WH, Baker D, et al. Severe toxic osteoblastoma of the humerus associated with diffuse periostitis of multiple bones. *Skeletal Radiol* 2001;30:464–468.
148. Haggitt RC, Reid BJ. Hereditary gastrointestinal polyposis syndromes. *Am J Surg Pathol* 1986;10:871–887.
149. Dahlin DC, Unni KK. Osteosarcoma of bone and its important recognizable varieties. *Am J Surg Pathol* 1977;1:61–72.
150. Deyrup AT, Montag AG. Epithelioid and epithelial neoplasms of bone. *Arch Pathol Lab Med* 2007;131:205–216.
151. Dahlin DC, Coventry MB. Osteogenic sarcoma. A study of six hundred cases. *J Bone Joint Surg Am* 1967;49:101–110.
152. Rosen G, Marcove RC, Caparros B, et al. Primary osteogenic sarcoma: the rationale for preoperative chemotherapy and delayed surgery. *Cancer* 1979;43:2163–2177.
153. Edmonson JH, Green SJ, Ivins JC, et al. A controlled pilot study of high-dose methotrexate as postsurgical adjuvant treatment for primary osteosarcoma. *J Clin Oncol* 1984;2:152–156.
154. Taylor WF, Ivins JC, Unni KK, et al. Prognostic variables in osteosarcoma: a multi-institutional study. *J Natl Cancer Inst* 1989;81:21–30.
155. Bielack SS, Kempf-Bielack B, Delling G, et al. Prognostic factors in high-grade osteosarcoma of the extremities or trunk: an analysis of 1,702 patients treated on neoadjuvant cooperative osteosarcoma study group protocols. *J Clin Oncol* 2002;2:776–790.
156. Meyers PA, Schwartz, CL, Krailo MD, et al. Osteosarcoma: the addition of muramyl tripeptide to chemotherapy improves overall survival—a report from the Children's Oncology Group. *J Clin Oncol* 2008;26:633–638.
157. Raymond AK, Ayala AG. Specimen management after osteosarcoma chemotherapy. *Contemp Issues Surg Pathol* 1988;11:157–181.
158. Bacci G, Ferrari S, Bertoni F, et al. Histologic response of high-grade nonmetastatic osteosarcoma of the extremity to chemotherapy. *Clin Orthop Relat Res* 2001;386:186–196.
159. Cahan WG, Woodard HQ, Higinbotham NL, et al. Sarcoma arising in irradiated bone: report of eleven cases. *Cancer* 1948;1:3–29.
160. Arlen M, Higinbotham NL, Huvos AG, et al. Radiation-induced sarcoma of bone. *Cancer* 1971;28:1087–1099.
161. Inoue YZ, Frassica FJ, Sim FH, et al. Clinicopathologic features and treatment of postirradiation sarcoma of bone and soft tissue. *J Surg Oncol* 2000;75:42–50.
162. Weatherby RP, Dahlin DC, Ivins JC. Postradiation sarcoma of bone: review of 78 Mayo Clinic cases. *Mayo Clin Proc* 1981;56:294–306.
163. Huvos AG, Woodard HQ, Cahan WG, et al. Postradiation osteogenic sarcoma of bone and soft tissues. A clinicopathologic study of 66 patients. *Cancer* 1985;55:1244–1255.
164. Wick MR, Siegal GP, Unni KK, et al. Sarcomas of bone complicating osteitis deformans (Paget's disease): fifty years' experience. *Am J Surg Pathol* 1981;5:47–59.
165. Huvos AG, Butler A, Bretsky SS. Osteogenic sarcoma associated with Paget's disease of bone. A clinicopathologic study of 65 patients. *Cancer* 1983;52:1489–1495.
166. Deyrup AT, Montag AG, Inwards, CY, et al. Sarcomas arising in Paget disease of bone: a clinicopathologic analysis of 70 cases. *Arch Pathol Lab Med* 2007;131:942–946.
167. Matsuno T, Unni KK, McLeod RA, et al. Telangiectatic osteogenic sarcoma. *Cancer* 1976; 38:2538–2547.
168. Huvos AG, Rosen G, Bretsky SS, et al. Telangiectatic osteogenic sarcoma: a clinicopathologic study of 124 patients. *Cancer* 1982;49:1679–1689.
169. Mervak TR, Unni KK, Pritchard DJ, et al. Telangiectatic osteosarcoma. *Clin Orthop* 1991; 270:135–139.
170. Unni KK, Dahlin DC, McLeod RA, et al. Intraosseous well-differentiated osteosarcoma. *Cancer* 1977;40:1337–1347.
171. Kurt AM, Unni KK, McLeod RA, et al. Low-grade intraosseous osteosarcoma. *Cancer* 1990; 65:1418–1428.
172. Sim FH, Unni KK, Beabout JW, et al. Osteosarcoma with small cells simulating Ewing's tumor. *J Bone Joint Surg Am* 1979;61:207–215.
173. Nakajima H, Sim FH, Bond JR, et al. Small cell osteosarcoma of bone. Review of 72 cases. *Cancer* 1997;79:2095–2106.
174. Kyriakos M. Intracortical osteosarcoma. *Cancer* 1980;46:2525–2533.
175. Clark JL, Unni M, Dahlin DC, et al. Osteosarcoma of the jaw. *Cancer* 1983;51:2311–2316.
176. Nora FE, Unni KK, Pritchard DJ, et al. Osteosarcoma of extragnathic craniofacial bones. *Mayo Clin Proc* 1983;58:268–272.
177. Geschickter CF, Copeland MM. Parosteal osteosarcoma of bone: a new entity. *Ann Surg* 1951;133:790–806.
178. Okada K, Frassica FJ, Sim FH, et al. Parosteal osteosarcoma. A clinicopathological study. *J Bone Joint Surg Am* 1994;76:366–378.
179. Sheth DS, Yasko AW, Raymond AK, et al. Conventional and dedifferentiated parosteal osteosarcoma. Diagnosis, treatments and outcome. *Cancer* 1996;78:2136–2145.
180. Wold LE, Unni KK, Beabout JW, et al. Dedifferentiated parosteal osteosarcoma. *J Bone Joint Surg Am* 1984;66:53–59.

181. Bertoni F, Bacchini P, Staals, et al. Dedifferentiated parosteal osteosarcoma: the experience of the Rizzoli Institute. *Cancer* 2005;103:2373–2382.
182. Unni KK, Dahlin DC, Beabout JW. Periosteal osteogenic sarcoma. *Cancer* 1976;37: 2476–2485.
183. Schajowicz F. Juxtacortical chondrosarcoma. *J Bone Joint Surg Br* 1977;59:473–480.
184. Rose PS, Dickey ID, Wenger, DE, et al. Periosteal osteosarcoma: long-term outcome and risk of late recurrence. *Clin Orthop Relat Res* 2006;451:50–54.
185. Wold LE, Unni KK, Beabout W, et al. High-grade surface osteosarcomas. *Am J Surg* 1984; 8:181–186.
186. Okada K, Unni KK, Swee RG, et al. High-grade surface osteosarcoma. A clinicopathologic study of 46 cases. *Cancer* 1999;85:1044–1054.
187. Staals EL, Bacchini P, Bertoni F. High-grade surface osteosarcoma. A review of 25 cases from the Rizzoli Institute. *Cancer* 2008;112:1592–1599.

GIANT CELL TUMOR

188. Biscaglia R, Bacchini P, Bertoni F. Giant cell tumor of the bones of the hand and foot. *Cancer* 2000;88:2022–2032.
189. Wold LE, Swee RG. Giant cell tumor of the small bones of the hands and feet. *Semin Diagn Pathol* 1994;1:173–184.
190. Hoch B, Inwards C, Sundaram M, et al. Multicentric giant cell tumor of bone. Clinicopathologic analysis of thirty cases. *J Bone Joint Surg Am* 2006;88:1998–2008.
191. Cooper KL, Beabout JW, Dahlin DC. Giant cell tumor: ossification in soft-tissue implants. *Radiology* 1984;153:597–602.
192. Campanacci M, Baldini N, Boriani S, et al. Giant-cell tumor of bone. *J Bone Joint Surg Am* 1987;69:106–114.
193. Balke M, Schremper L, Gebert C, et al. Giant cell tumor of bone: treatment and outcome of 214 cases. *J Cancer Res Clin Oncol* 2008;134:969–978.
194. Bertoni F, Present D, Sudanese A, et al. Giant-cell tumor of bone with pulmonary metastases. Six case reports and a review of the literature. *Clin Orthop* 1988;237:275–285.
195. Bertoni F, Present D, Enneking WF. Giant-cell tumor of bone with pulmonary metastases. *J Bone Joint Surg Am* 1985;67:890–900.
196. Siebenrock KA, Unni KK, Rock MG. Giant-cell tumour of bone metastasising to the lungs. A long-term follow-up. *J Bone Joint Surg Br* 1998;80:43–47.
197. Ladanyi M, Traganos F, Huvos AG. Benign metastasizing giant cell tumors of bone. A DNA flow cytometric study. *Cancer* 1989;64:1521–1526.
198. Dickson BC, Shu-Qiu L, Wunder JS, et al. Giant cell tumors of bone express p63. *Mod Pathol* 2008;21:369–375.
199. Marui T, Yamamoto T, Yoshihara H, et al. De novo malignant transformation of giant cell tumor of bone. *Skeletal Radiol* 2001;30:104–108.
200. Bertoni F, Bacchini P, Staals EL. Malignancy in giant cell tumor of bone. *Cancer* 2003;97: 2520–2529.

ADAMANTINOMA

201. Jain D, Jain VK, Vasishta RK, et al. Adamantinoma: a clinicopathological review and update. *Diagn Pathol* 2008;3:8.
202. Keeney GL, Unni M, Beabout JW, et al. Adamantinoma of long bones. A clinicopathologic study of 85 cases. *Cancer* 1989;64:730–737.
203. Hazelbag HM, Taminiau AH, Fleuren GH, et al. Adamantinoma of the long bones: a clinicopathological study of thirty-two patients with emphasis on histological subtype, precursor lesion, and biological behavior. *J Bone Joint Surg Am* 1994;76:1482–1499.
204. Rosai J. Adamantinoma of the tibia. Electron microscopic evidence of its epithelial origin. *Am J Clin Pathol* 1969;51:786–792.
205. Rosai J, Pinkus GS. Immunohistochemical demonstration of epithelial differentiation in adamantinoma of the tibia. *Am J Surg Pathol* 1982;6:427–434.
206. Mori H, Yamamoto S, Hiramatsu K, et al. Adamantinoma of the tibia. Ultrastructural and immunohistochemical study with reference to histogenesis. *Clin Orthop* 1984;190:299–310.
207. Benassi MS, Campanacci L, Gamberi G, et al. Cytokeratin expression and distribution in adamantinoma of the long bones and osteofibrous dysplasia of tibia and fibula: an immunohistochemical study correlated to histogenesis. *Histopathology* 1994;25:71–76.
208. Dockerty MB, Meyerding HW. Adamantinoma of the tibia: report of two new cases. *JAMA* 1942;119:932–937.
209. Cohen DM, Dahlin DC, Pugh DG. Fibrous dysplasia associated with adamantinoma of the long bones. *Cancer* 1962;15:515–521.
210. Weiss SW, Dorfman HD. Adamantinoma of long bone. An analysis of nine new cases with emphasis on metastasizing lesions and fibrous dysplasia-like changes. *Hum Pathol* 1977;8: 141–153.
211. Czerniak B, Rojas-Corona RR, Dorfman HD. Morphologic diversity of long bone adamantinoma: the concept of differentiated (regressing) adamantinoma and its relationship to osteofibrous dysplasia. *Cancer* 1989;64:2319–2334.
212. Gleason BC, Leigl-Atzwanger B, Kozakewich HP, et al. Osteofibrous dysplasia and adamantinoma in children and adolescents: a clinicopathologic reappraisal. *Am J Surg Pathol* 2008;32:363–376.
213. Gleason BC, Leigl-Atzwanger B, Kozakewich HP, et al. Osteofibrous dysplasia and adamantinoma in children and adolescents: a clinicopathologic reappraisal. *Am J Surg Pathol* 2008;32:363–376.

VASCULAR TUMORS

214. O'Connell JX, Kattapuram SV, Mankin HJ, et al. Epithelioid hemangioma of bone. A tumor often mistaken for low-grade angiosarcoma or malignant hemangioendothelioma. *Am J Surg Pathol* 1993;17:610–617.
215. Gorham LW, Stout AP. Massive osteolysis (acute spontaneous absorption of bone, phantom bone, disappearing bone): its relation to hemangiomatosis. *J Bone Joint Surg Am* 1955; 37:985–1004.
216. Halliday DR, Dahlin DC, Pugh DG, et al. Massive osteolysis and angiomatosis. *Radiology* 1964;82:637–644.
217. Wenger DE, Wold LE. Malignant vascular lesions of bone: radiologic and pathologic features. *Skeletal Radiol* 2000;29:619–631.
218. Weiss SW, Enzinger FM. Epithelioid hemangioendothelioma: a vascular tumor often mistaken for a carcinoma. *Cancer* 1982;50:970–981.
219. Maruyama N, Kumagai Y, Ishida Y, et al. Epithelioid haemangioendothelioma of the bone tissue. *Virchows Arch A Pathol Anat Histopathol* 1985;407:159–165.
220. Tsuneyoshi M, Dorfman HD, Bauer TW. Epithelioid hemangioendothelioma of bone. A clinicopathologic, ultrastructural, and immunohistochemical study. *Am J Surg Pathol* 1986; 10:754–764.
221. Kleer CG, Unni M, McLeod RA. Epithelioid hemangioendothelioma of bone. *Am J Surg Pathol* 1996;20:1301–1311.
222. Wold LE, Unni KK, Beabout JW, et al. Hemangioendothelial sarcoma. *Am J Surg Pathol* 1982;6:59–70.
223. Campanacci M, Boriani S, Giunti A. Hemangioendothelioma of bone: a study of 29 cases. *Cancer* 1980;46:804–814.
224. Volpe R, Mazabraud A. Hemangioendothelioma (angiosarcoma) of bone: a distinct pathologic entity with an unpredictable course? *Cancer* 1982;49:727–736.
225. Wold LE, Unni KK, Cooper KL, et al. Hemangiopericytoma of bone. *Am J Surg Pathol* 1982;6:53–58.
226. Tang JS, Gold RH, Mirra JM, et al. Hemangiopericytoma of bone. *Cancer* 1988;62:848–859.

FIBROHISTIOCYTIC TUMORS

227. Bertoni F, Calderoni P, Bacchini P, et al. Benign fibrous histiocytoma of bone. *J Bone Joint Surg Am* 1986;68:1225–1230.
228. Clarke BE, Xipell JM, Thomas DP. Benign fibrous histiocytoma of bone. *Am J Surg Pathol* 1985;9:806–815.
229. Nishida J, Sim FH, Wenger DE, et al. Malignant fibrous histiocytoma of bone. A clinicopathologic study of 81 patients. *Cancer* 1997;79:482–493.
230. Mirra JM, Gold RH, Marafiote R. Malignant (fibrous) histiocytoma arising in association with a bone infarct in sickle-cell disease: coincidence or cause-and-effect? *Cancer* 1977;39: 186–194.
231. Huvos AG, Woodard HQ, Heilweil M. Postradiation malignant fibrous histiocytoma of bone. A clinicopathologic study of 20 patients. *Am J Surg Pathol* 1986;10:9–18.
232. Feldman F, Lattes R. Primary malignant fibrous histiocytoma (fibrous xanthoma) of bone. *Skeletal Radiol* 1977;1:145–160.
233. Huvos AG, Heilweil M, Bretsky SS. The pathology of malignant fibrous histiocytoma of bone. A study of 130 patients. *Am J Surg Pathol* 1985;9:853–871.
234. Taconis WK, van Rijssel TG. Fibrosarcoma of long bones. A study of the significance of areas of malignant fibrous histiocytoma. *J Bone Joint Surg Br* 1985;67:111–116.
235. Nakashima Y, Morishita S, Kotoura Y, et al. Malignant fibrous histiocytoma of bone. A review of 13 cases and an ultrastructural study. *Cancer* 1985;55:2804–2811.
236. Ghandur-Mnaymneh L, Zych G, Mnaymneh W. Primary malignant fibrous histiocytoma of bone: report of six cases with ultrastructural study and analysis of the literature. *Cancer* 1982;49:698–707.
237. Capanna R, Bertoni F, Bacchini P, et al. Malignant fibrous histiocytoma of bone. The experience at the Rizzoli Institute: report of 90 cases. *Cancer* 1984;54:177–187.
238. McCarthy EF, Matsuno T, Dorfman HD. Malignant fibrous histiocytoma of bone: a study of 35 cases. *Hum Pathol* 1979;10:57–70.

FIBROUS TUMORS

239. Jaffe HL. *Tumors and Tumorous Conditions of the Bones and Joints*. Philadelphia, PA: Lea & Febiger, 1958:298–313.
240. Inwards CY, Unni KK, Beabout JW, et al. Desmoplastic fibroma of bone. *Cancer* 1991;68: 1978–1983.
241. Jeffree GM, Price CH. Metastatic spread of fibrosarcoma of bone. A report on forty-nine cases, and a comparison with osteosarcoma. *J Bone Joint Surg Br* 1976;58:418–425.
242. Myers JL, Arocho J, Bernreuter W, et al. Leiomyosarcoma of bone. A clinicopathologic, immunohistochemical, and ultrastructural study of five cases. *Cancer* 1991;67:1051–1056.
243. Angervall L, Berlin O, Kindblom LG, et al. Primary leiomyosarcoma of bone: a study of five cases. *Cancer* 1980;46:1270–1279.

NOTOCHORDAL TUMORS

244. Tirabosco RT, Mangham DC, Rosenberg, AE, et al. Brachyury expression in extra-axial skeletal and soft tissue chordomas: a marker that distinguishes chordoma from mixed tumor/myoepithelioma/parachordoma in soft tissue. *Am J Surg Pathol* 2008;32:572–580.
245. Ulich TR, Mirra JM. Ecchordosis physaliphora vertebralis. *Clin Orthop* 1982;163:282–289.
246. Hoch BL, Nielsen GP, Liebsh NG, et al. Base of skull chordomas in children and adolescents: a clinicopathologic study of 73 cases. *Am J Surg Pathol* 2006;30:811–818.
247. Wold LE, Laws ER Jr. Cranial chordomas in children and young adults. *J Neurosurg* 1983; 59:1043–1047.
248. Coffin CM, Swanson PE, Wick MR, et al. Chordoma in childhood and adolescence: a clinicopathologic analysis of 12 cases. *Arch Pathol Lab Med* 1993;117:927–933.
249. Borba LAB, Al-Mefty O, Mrak RE, et al. Cranial chordomas in children and adolescents. *J Neurosurg* 1996;84:584–591.

250. Sibley RK, Day DL, Dehner LP, et al. Metastasizing chordoma in early childhood: a pathological and immunohistochemical study with review of the literature. *Pediatr Pathol* 1987;7:287–301.

251. Vujovic S, Henderson SR, Presneau N, et al. Brachyury, a crucial regulator of notochordal development, is a novel biomarker for chordomas. *J Pathol* 2006;209:157–165.

252. Heffelfinger MJ, Dahlin DC, MacCarty CS, et al. Chordomas and cartilaginous tumors at the skull base. *Cancer* 1973;32:410–420.

253. Rosenberg AE, Brown GA, Bhan AK, et al. Chondroid chordoma—a variant of chordoma. A morphologic and immunohistochemical study. *Am J Clin Pathol* 1994;101:36–41.

254. Salisbury JR. Demonstration of cytokeratins and an epithelial membrane antigen in chondroid chordoma. *J Pathol* 1987;153:37–40.

255. Mitchell A, Scheithauer BW, Unni KK, et al. Chordoma and chondroid neoplasms of the spheno-occiput. *Cancer* 1993;72:2943–2949.

256. Rosenberg AE, Nielsen GP, Keel SB, et al. Chondrosarcoma of the base of the skull. A clinicopathological study of 200 cases with emphasis on its distinction from chordoma. *Am J Surg Pathol* 1999;23:1370–1378.

257. Belza MG, Urich H. Chordoma and malignant fibrous histiocytoma. Evidence for transformation. *Cancer* 1986;58:1082–1087.

258. Miettinen M, Lehto VP, Virtanen I. Malignant fibrous histiocytoma within a recurrent chordoma. A light microscopic, electron microscopic, and immunohistochemical study. *Am J Clin Pathol* 1984;82:738–743.

259. Makek M, Leu HJ. Malignant fibrous histiocytoma arising in a recurrent chordoma. Case report and electron microscopic findings. *Virchows Arch A Pathol Anat Histopathol* 1982;397:241–250.

260. Chambers PW, Schwinn CP. Chordoma. A clinicopathologic study of metastasis. *Am J Clin Pathol* 1979;72:765–776.

261. Volpe R, Mazabraud A. A clinicopathologic review of 25 cases of chordoma (a pleomorphic and metastasizing neoplasm). *Am J Surg Pathol* 1983;7:161–170.

262. Kaiser TE, Pritchard DJ, Unni KK. Clinicopathologic study of sacrococcygeal chordoma. *Cancer* 1984;53:2574–2578.

263. Bergh P, Kindblom L, Gunterberg B, et al. Prognostic factors in chordoma of the sacrum and mobile spine: a study of 39 patients. *Cancer* 2000;88:2122–2134.

264. Fuchs B, Dickey ID, Yaszemski MJ, et al. Operative management of sacral chordoma. *J Bone Joint Surg Am* 2005;87:2211–2216.

265. Miettinen M. Chordoma. Antibodies to epithelial membrane antigen and carcinoembryonic antigen in differential diagnosis. *Arch Pathol Lab Med* 1984;108:891–892.

266. Mirra JM, Brien EW. Giant notochordal hamartoma of intraosseous origin: a newly reported benign entity to be distinguished from chordoma. Report of two cases. *Skeletal Radiol* 2001;30:698–709.

267. Kyriakos M, Totty WG, Lenke LG. Giant vertebral notochordal rest: a lesion distinct from chordoma: discussion of an evolving concept. *Am J Surg Pathol* 2003;27:396–406.

268. Yamaguchi T, Suzuki S, Ishiiwa H, et al. Benign notochordal cell tumors: a comparative histological study of benign notochordal cell tumors, classic chordomas, and notochordal vestiges of fetal intervertebral discs. *Am J Surg Pathol* 2004;28:756–761.

NEURAL TUMORS

269. Divertie MB, Dahlin DC. Neurilemmoma of rib: report of a case. *Dis Chest* 1963;44:635–637.

270. Gordon EJ. Solitary intraosseous neurilemmoma of the tibia: review of intraosseous neurilemmoma and neurofibroma. *Clin Orthop* 1976;117:271–282.

271. Dalinka MK, Cannino C, Patchefsky AS, et al. Case report 12. *Skeletal Radiol* 1976;1:123–124.

LIPOGENIC TUMORS

272. Milgram JW. Intraosseous lipomas. A clinicopathologic study of 66 cases. *Clin Orthop* 1988;231:277–302.

273. Gunterberg B, Kindblom LG. Intraosseous lipoma. A report of two cases. *Acta Orthop Scand* 1978;49:95–97.

274. Milgram JW. Malignant transformation in bone lipomas. *Skeletal Radiol* 1990;19:347–352.

METASTASES TO BONE

275. Simon MA, Karluk MB. Skeletal metastases of unknown origin. Diagnostic strategy for orthopedic surgeons. *Clin Orthop* 1982;166:96–103.

276. Ogawa K, Kim YC, Nakashima Y, et al. Expression of epithelial markers in sarcomatoid carcinoma: an immunohistochemical study. *Histopathology* 1987;11:511–522.

277. Tomera KM, Farrow GM, Lieber MM. Sarcomatoid renal carcinoma. *J Urol* 1983;130:657–659.

ANEURYSMAL BONE CYST

278. Oliveira AM, Hsi BL, Weremowicz S, et al. USP6 (Tre2) fusion oncogenes in aneurysmal bone cyst. *Cancer Res* 2004;64:1920–1923.

279. Levy WM, Miller AS, Bonakdarpour A, et al. Aneurysmal bone cyst secondary to other osseous lesions. Report of 57 cases. *Am J Clin Pathol* 1975;63:1–8.

280. Martinez V, Sissons HA. Aneurysmal bone cyst. A review of 123 cases including primary lesions and those secondary to other bone pathology. *Cancer* 1988;61:2291–2304.

281. Hudson TM. Fluid levels in aneurysmal bone cysts: a CT feature. *AJR Am J Roentgenol* 1984;142:1001–1004.

282. Alles JU, Schulz A. Immunocytochemical markers (endothelial and histiocytic) and ultrastructure of primary aneurysmal bone cysts. *Hum Pathol* 1986;17:39–45.

283. Gold RH, Mirra JM. Case report 234. Aneurysmal bone cyst of left scapula with intramural calcified chondroid. *Skeletal Radiol* 1983;10:57–60.

284. Vergel De Dios AM, Bond JR, Shives TC, et al. Aneurysmal bone cyst. A clinicopathologic study of 238 cases. *Cancer* 1992;69:2921–2931.

285. Sanerkin NG, Mott MG, Roylance J. An unusual intraosseous lesion with fibroblastic, osteoclastic, osteoblastic, aneurysmal and fibromyxoid elements. "Solid" variant of aneurysmal bone cyst. *Cancer* 1983;51:2278–2286.

286. Oliveira AM, Perez-Atayde AR, Inwards CY, et al. USP6 and CDH11 oncogenes identify the neoplastic cell in primary aneurysmal bone cysts and are absent in so-called secondary aneurysmal bone cysts. *Am J Pathol* 2004;165:1773–1780.

287. Oliveira AM, Perez-Atayde AR, Dal Cin P, et al. Aneurysmal bone cyst variant translocations upregulate USP6 transcription by promoter swapping with the ZNF9, COL1A1, TRAP150, and OMD genes. *Oncogene* 2005;24:3419–3426.

288. Sukov WR, Franco MF, Erickson-Johnson M, et al. Frequency of USP6 rearrangements in myositis ossificans, brown tumor, and cherubism: molecular cytogenetic evidence that a subset of "myositis ossificans-like lesions" are the early phases in the formation of soft-tissue aneurysmal bone cyst. *Skeletal Radiol* 2008;37:321–327.

BENIGN BONE CYSTS

289. Boseker EH, Bickel WH, Dahlin DC. A clinicopathologic study of simple unicameral bone cysts. *Surg Gynecol Obstet* 1968;127:550–560.

290. Scaglietti O, Marchetti PG, Bartolozzi P. The effects of methylprednisolone acetate in the treatment of bone cysts. Results of three years' follow-up. *J Bone Joint Surg Br* 1979;61:200–204.

291. Chigira M, Maehara S, Arita S, et al. The aetiology and treatment of simple bone cysts. *J Bone Joint Surg Br* 1983;65:633–637.

292. Schajowicz F, Clavel Sainz M, Slullitel JA. Juxta-articular bone cysts (intra-osseous ganglia): a clinicopathological study of eighty-eight cases. *J Bone Joint Surg Br* 1979;61:107–116.

293. Sim FH, Dahlin DC. Ganglion cysts of bone. *Mayo Clin Proc* 1971;46:484–488.

294. Bauer TW, Dorfman HD. Intraosseous ganglion: a clinicopathologic study of 11 cases. *Am J Surg Pathol* 1982;6:207–213.

295. Glass TA, Dyer R, Fisher L, et al. Expansile subchondral bone cyst. *AJR Am J Roentgenol* 1982;139:1210–1211.

FIBROUS DYSPLASIA, FIBROUS DEFECTS

296. Dockerty MB, Ghormley RK, Kennedy RLJ, et al. Albright's syndrome (polyostotic fibrous dysplasia with cutaneous pigmentation in both sexes and gonadal dysfunction in females). *Arch Intern Med* 1945;75:357–375.

297. Lassance Cabral CE, Guedes P, Fonseca T, et al. Polyostotic fibrous dysplasia associated with intramuscular myxomas: Mazabraud's syndrome. *Skeletal Radiol* 1998;27:278–282.

298. Weinstein LS, Shenker A, Gejman PV, et al. Activating mutations of the stimulatory G protein in the McCune-Albright syndrome. *N Engl J Med* 1991;325:1688–1695.

299. Bianco P, Riminucc M, Majolagbe A, et al. Mutations of the GNAS1 gene, stromal cell dysfunction, and osteomalacic changes in non-McCune-Albright fibrous dysplasia of bone. *J Bone Miner Res* 2000;15:120–128.

300. Ishida T, Dorfman HD. Massive chondroid differentiation in fibrous dysplasia of bone (fibrocartilaginous dysplasia). *Am J Surg Pathol* 1993;17:924–930.

301. Simpson AH, Creasy TS, Williamson DM, et al. Cystic degeneration of fibrous dysplasia masquerading as sarcoma. *J Bone Joint Surg Br* 1989;71:434–436.

302. Diercks RL, Sauter AJ, Mallens WM. Aneurysmal bone cyst in association with fibrous dysplasia. A case report. *J Bone Joint Surg Br* 1986;68:144–146.

303. Feintuch TA. Chondrosarcoma arising in a cartilaginous area of previously irradiated fibrous dysplasia. *Cancer* 1973;31:877–881.

304. Huvos AG, Higinbotham NL, Miller TR. Bone sarcomas arising in fibrous dysplasia. *J Bone Joint Surg Am* 1972;54:1047–1056.

305. Ruggieri P, Sim FH, Bond JR, et al. Malignancies in fibrous dysplasia. *Cancer* 1994;73:1411–1424.

306. Campanacci M, Laus M. Osteofibrous dysplasia of the tibia and fibula. *J Bone Joint Surg Am* 1981;63:367–375.

307. Nakashima Y, Yamamuro T, Fujiwara Y, et al. Osteofibrous dysplasia (ossifying fibroma of long bones). A study of 12 cases. *Cancer* 1983;52:909–914.

308. Blackwell JB, McCarthy SW, Xipell JM, et al. Osteofibrous dysplasia of the tibia and fibula. *Pathology* 1988;20:227–233.

309. Sweet DE, Vinh TN, Devaney K. Cortical osteofibrous dysplasia of long bone and its relationship to adamantinoma. A clinicopathological study of 30 cases. *Am J Surg Pathol* 1992;16:282–290.

310. Arata MA, Peterson HA, Dahlin DC. Pathological fractures through non-ossifying fibromas. Review of the Mayo Clinic experience. *J Bone Joint Surg Am* 1981;63:980–988.

311. Campanacci M, Laus M, Boriani S. Multiple non-ossifying fibromata with extraskeletal anomalies: a new syndrome? *J Bone Joint Surg Br* 1983;65:627–632.

312. Mirra JM, Gold RH, Rand F. Disseminated nonossifying fibromas in association with café-au-lait spots (Jaffe-Campanacci syndrome). *Clin Orthop* 1982;168:192–205.

313. Kimmelstiel P, Rapp IH. Cortical defect due to periosteal desmoids. *Bull Hosp Joint Dis* 1951;12:286–297.

314. Barnes GR Jr, Gwinn JL. Distal irregularities of the femur simulating malignancy. *Am J Roentgenol Radium Ther Nucl Med* 1974;122:180–185.

TRAUMATIC LESIONS

315. Cooper KL, Beabout JW, Swee RG. Insufficiency fractures of the sacrum. *Radiology* 1985; 156:15–20.
316. Ackerman LV. Extra-osseous localized non-neoplastic bone and cartilage formation (so-called myositis ossificans): clinical and pathological confusion with malignant neoplasms. *J Bone Joint Surg Am* 1958;40:279–298.
317. Dupree WB, Enzinger FM. Fibro-osseous pseudotumor of the digits. *Cancer* 1986;58: 2103–2109.
318. Spjut HJ, Dorfman HD. Florid reactive periostitis of the tubular bones of the hands and feet. A benign lesion which may simulate osteosarcoma. *Am J Surg Pathol* 1981;5:423–433.
319. Smith R. Myositis ossificans progressiva: a review of current problems. *Semin Arthritis Rheum* 1975;4:369–380.
320. Smith R, Russell RG, Woods CG. Myositis ossificans progressiva. Clinical features of eight patients and their response to treatment. *J Bone Joint Surg Br* 1976;58:48–57.
321. Cramer SF, Ruehl A, Mandel MA. Fibrodysplasia ossificans progressiva: a distinctive bone-forming lesion of the soft tissue. *Cancer* 1981;48:1016–1021.
322. Eckardt JJ, Ivins JC, Perry HO, et al. Osteosarcoma arising in heterotopic ossification of dermatomyositis: case report and review of the literature. *Cancer* 1981;48:1256–1261.

OSTEOMYELITIS AND CARCINOMA

323. Cabanela ME, Sim FH, Beabout JW, et al. Osteomyelitis appearing as neoplasms. A diagnostic problem. *Arch Surg* 1974;109:68–72.
324. Björkstén B, Boquist L. Histopathological aspects of chronic recurrent multifocal osteomyelitis. *J Bone Joint Surg Br* 1980;62:376–380.
325. Jurik AG, Helmig O, Ternowitz T, et al. Chronic recurrent multifocal osteomyelitis: a follow-up study. *J Pediatr Orthop* 1988;8:49–58.
326. Fitzgerald RH Jr, Brewer NS, Dahlin DC. Squamous-cell carcinoma complicating chronic osteomyelitis. *J Bone Joint Surg Am* 1976;58:1146–1148.
327. McGrory JE, Pritchard DJ, Unni KK, et al. Malignant lesions arising in chronic osteomyelitis. *Clin Orthop* 1999;362:181–189.
328. Akbarnia BA, Wirth CR, Colman N. Fibrosarcoma arising from chronic osteomyelitis. Case report and review of the literature. *J Bone Joint Surg Am* 1976;58:123–125.

LANGERHANS HISTIOCYTOSIS

329. Lichtenstein L. Histiocytosis X: integration of eosinophilic granuloma of bone, "Letterer-Siwe disease," and "Schüller-Christian disease" as related manifestations of single nosologic entity. *Arch Pathol* 1953;56:84–102.
330. Lieberman PH, Jones CR, Dargeon HW, et al. A reappraisal of eosinophilic granuloma of bone, Hand-Schüller-Christian syndrome and Letterer-Siwe syndrome. *Medicine (Baltimore)* 1969;48:375–400.
331. Novice FM, Collison DW, Kleinsmith DM, et al. Letterer-Siwe disease in adults. *Cancer* 1989;63:166–174.
332. Simmons PS, Wold LE, Elveback LR, et al. Prognostic factors and management of histiocytosis X. *J Pediatr* 1981;98(Abstr):1023.
333. Willman CL, Busque L, Griffith BB, et al. Langerhans'-cell histiocytosis (histiocytosis X)—a clonal proliferative disease. *N Engl J Med* 1994;331:154–160.
334. Emile JF, Wechsler J, Brousse N, et al. Langerhans' cell histiocytosis. Definitive diagnosis with the use of monoclonal antibody O10 on routinely paraffin-embedded samples. *Am J Surg Pathol* 1995;19:636–641.
335. Lau SK, Chu PG, Weiss LM. Immunohistochemical expression of Langerin in Langerhans cell histiocytosis and non-Langerhans cell histiocytic disorders. *Am J Surg Pathol* 2008;32: 615–619.
336. Newton WA Jr, Hamoudi AB. Histiocytosis: a histologic classification with clinical correlation. *Perspect Pediatr Pathol* 1973;1:251–283.
337. Nezelof C, Frileux-Herbet F, Cronier-Sachot J. Disseminated histiocytosis X: analysis of prognostic factors based on a retrospective study of 50 cases. *Cancer* 1979;44:1824–1838.
338. Risdall RJ, Dehner LP, Duray P, et al. Histiocytosis X (Langerhans' cell histiocytosis). Prognostic role of histopathology. *Arch Pathol Lab Med* 1983;107:59–63.
339. Kilpatrick SE, Wenger DE, Gilchrist GS, et al. Langerhans' cell histiocytosis (histiocytosis X) of bone. A clinicopathologic analysis of 263 pediatric and adult cases. *Cancer* 1995;76: 2471–2484.

PAGET DISEASE

340. Layfield R. The molecular pathogenesis of Paget disease of bone. *Expert Rev Mol Med* 2007; 9:1–13.
341. Reddy SV. Etiologic factors in Paget's disease of bone. *Cell Mol Life Sci* 2006;63:391–398.
342. Frame B, Marel GM. Paget disease: a review of current knowledge. *Radiology* 1981;141: 21–24.
343. Guyer PB, Chamberlain AT, Ackery DM, et al. The anatomic distribution of osteitis deformans. *Clin Orthop* 1981;156:141–144.
344. Bowerman JW, Altman J, Hughes JL, et al. Pseudo-malignant lesions in Paget's disease of bone. *Am J Roentgenol Radium Ther Nucl Med* 1975;124:57–61.
345. Eisman JA, Martin TJ. Osteolytic Paget's disease. Recognition and risks of biopsy. *J Bone Joint Surg Am* 1986;68:112–117.

HYPERPARATHYROIDISM

346. Vigorita VJ, Einhorn TA, Phelps KR. Microscopic bone pathology in two cases of surgically treated secondary hyperparathyroidism. Report of a distinct skeletal lesion. *Am J Surg Pathol* 1987;11:205–209.
347. Present D, Calderoni P, Bacchini P, et al. Brown tumor of the tibia as an early manifestation of renal osteodystrophy. A case report. *Clin Orthop* 1988;231:303–306.

MAST CELL DISEASE

348. Travis WD, Li CY, Bergstralh EJ. Solid and hematologic malignancies in 60 patients with systemic mast cell disease. *Arch Pathol Lab Med* 1989;113:365–368.
349. Travis WD, Li CY, Hoagland HC, et al. Mast cell leukemia: report of a case and review of the literature. *Mayo Clin Proc* 1986;61:957–966.
350. Travis WD, Li CY, Bergstralh EJ, et al. Systemic mast cell disease. Analysis of 58 cases and literature review. *Medicine (Baltimore)* 1988;67:345–368.
351. Barer M, Peterson LF, Dahlin DC, et al. Mastocytosis with osseous lesions resembling metastatic malignant lesions in bone. *J Bone Joint Surg Am* 1968;50:142–152.

MESENCHYMOMA

352. Blumenthal BI, Capitanio MA, Queloz JM, et al. Intrathoracic mesenchymoma. Observations in two infants. *Radiology* 1972;104:107–109.
353. McLeod RA, Dahlin DC. Hamartoma (mesenchymoma) of the chest wall in infancy. *Radiology* 1979;131:657–661.
354. Odell JM, Benjamin DR. Mesenchymal hamartoma of chest wall in infancy: natural history of two cases. *Pediatr Pathol* 1986;5:135–146.

SYNOVIAL CHONDROMATOSIS

355. Carey RP. Synovial chondromatosis of the knee in childhood. A report of two cases. *J Bone Joint Surg Br* 1983;65:444–447.
356. Murphey MD, Vidal JA, Fanburg-Smith JC, et al. Imaging of synovial chondromatosis with radiologic-pathologic correlation. *Radiographics* 2007;27:1465–1488.
357. Bertoni F, Unni KK, Beabout JW, et al. Chondrosarcomas of the synovium. *Cancer* 1991; 67:155–162.

CONGENITAL FIBROMATOSIS

358. Kindblom LG, Angervall L. Congenital solitary fibromatosis of the skeleton: case report of a variant of congenital generalized fibromatosis. *Cancer* 1978;41:636–640.
359. Inwards CY, Unni KK, Beabout JW, et al. Solitary congenital fibromatosis (infantile myofibromatosis) of bone. *Am J Surg Pathol* 1991;15:935–941.

SUBUNGUAL AND PAROSTEAL TUMORS

360. Miller-Breslow A, Dorfman HD. Dupuytren's (subungual) exostosis. *Am J Surg Pathol* 1988; 12:368–378.
361. Landon GC, Johnson KA, Dahlin DC. Subungual exostoses. *J Bone Joint Surg Am* 1979;61: 256–259.
362. Zambrano E, Nose V, Perez-Atayde AR, et al. Distinct chromosomal rearrangements in subungual (Dupuytren) exostosis and bizarre parosteal osteochondromatous proliferation (Nora lesion). *Am J Surg Pathol* 2004;28:1033–1039.
363. Storlazzi CT, Wozniak A, Panagopouls I, et al. Rearrangement of the COL12A1 and COL4A5 genes in subungual exostosis: molecular cytogenetic delineation of the tumor-specific translocationt(X;6)(q13–14;q22). *Int J Cancer* 2005;118:1972–1976.
364. Keeney GL, Banks PM, Linscheid RL. Subungual keratoacanthoma. Report of a case and review of the literature. *Arch Dermatol* 1988;124:1074–1076.
365. Nora FE, Dahlin DC, Beabout JW. Bizarre parosteal osteochondromatous proliferations of the hands and feet. *Am J Surg Pathol* 1983;7:245–250.
366. Nilsson M, Domanski HA, Mertens F, et al. Molecular cytogenetic characterization of recurrent translocation breakpoints in bizarre parosteal osteochondromatous proliferation (Nora's lesion). *Hum Pathol* 2004;35:1063–1069.
367. Zambrano E, Nose V, Perez-Atayde AR, et al. Distinct chromosomal rearrangements in subungual (Dupuytren) exostosis and bizarre parosteal osteochondromatous proliferation (Nora lesion). *Am J Surg Pathol* 2004;28:1033–1039.
368. Meneses MF, Unni KK, Swee RG. Bizarre parosteal osteochondromatous proliferation of bone (Nora's lesion). *Am J Surg Pathol* 1993;17:691–697.

SINUS HISTIOCYTOSIS WITH MASSIVE LYMPHADENOPATHY

369. Rosai J, Dorfman RF. Sinus histiocytosis with massive lymphadenopathy. A newly recognized benign clinicopathological entity. *Arch Pathol* 1969;87:63–70.
370. Foucar E, Rosai J, Dorfman R. Sinus histiocytosis with massive lymphadenopathy (Rosai-Dorfman disease): review of the entity. *Semin Diagn Pathol* 1990;7:19–73.
371. Gaitonde S. Multifocal extranodal sinus histiocytosis with massive lymphadenopathy: an overview. *Arch Pathol Lab Med* 2007;131:1117–1121.

CHAPTER

9

Darryl Carter
Stuart J. Schnitt
Rosemary R. Millis

The Breast

Breast cancer is the most common malignancy in women, affecting one in eight in the Western world. Advances in imaging techniques and the increased use of needle biopsy have greatly assisted the preoperative evaluation of breast lesions but, in a large proportion of cases, differentiation between benign and malignant lesions still rests on histologic examination. As a result, breast biopsies form a major part of the workload of most surgical pathology laboratories, and their number has increased along with the use of breast cancer screening programs throughout the world. In the management of patients with breast disease, close cooperation between surgeon, medical oncologist, radiation oncologist, radiologist, and pathologist is always of the utmost importance. The pathologist should be well acquainted with the clinical and mammographic findings and must ensure that they do not conflict with the histologic diagnosis. Most diagnostic errors can be avoided if the pathologist (a) correlates the gross and microscopic appearances and specimen x-ray images, when relevant; (b) is familiar with the architecture and cellular relationships of the normal breast; and (c) is aware of particular patterns of benign breast disease that can mimic carcinoma.

BREAST SPECIMENS

The gross examination of mammary tissue includes both inspection and palpation and may be aided in many instances by x-ray examination. It is always advantageous to obtain tissue in the fresh state, even if frozen section is not to be performed. This not only facilitates the assessment of abnormalities but also allows tissue to be set aside for special studies, as necessary. The gross examination should include an assessment of the features listed in Table 9.1. In most cases, a preliminary diagnosis can be made at this stage. The contrasting macroscopic features of carcinoma and fibroadenoma (the most common benign mammary tumor) are listed in Table 9.2 and illustrated in Figures 9.1 and 9.2. In certain instances, however, the gross appearance can be misleading; some types of carcinoma, particularly mucinous and medullary carcinoma, have a smooth, rounded outline and a soft consistency. Infiltrating lobular carcinoma may be extremely diffuse and difficult to see on gross examination, and palpation may be more helpful than visual inspection. Conversely, a number of benign lesions can mimic carcinoma on gross examination (Table 9.3).

It is difficult to lay down rigid guidelines regarding the number of blocks that should be obtained from specimens because the circumstances differ from case to case. It is important, however, that tumors be sampled thoroughly because their microscopic appearance may vary from area to area. Both the center and periphery of tumors should be sampled, as well as the surrounding tissue. Malignant change may be far more extensive than is suspected on gross examination. When possible, a section including the largest full-cut face of a tumor should be submitted in one block. Because noninvasive carcinoma may be an incidental finding, it is always important to sample apparently normal tissue, including that around an obviously benign lesion. Sampling should concentrate on the nonfatty component of specimens and, as is discussed later, areas of mammographic abnormality. The likelihood of detecting significant pathologic changes in fatty tissue that are not also present in the nonfatty component of the specimen is extremely low (1).

CATEGORIES OF SPECIMEN

FROZEN SECTION

In recent years, because of changes in clinical practice, the use of the frozen section to diagnose mammary carcinoma has de-

---

TABLE 9.1

Features to be Recorded on Gross Examination of a Breast Biopsy Specimen

General features
State of specimen (fresh/fixed)
Type of specimen (e.g., excision biopsy, microdochectomy)
Side (left/right)
Size (three dimensions)
Consistency
Other features (e.g., presence of cysts)
Dominant lesion (when present)
Site
Size (maximum diameter most important); in the case of small carcinomas, this should be confirmed on microscopic examination
Outline: irregular or smooth, clearly or poorly defined
Relationship to surrounding tissue (e.g., protrudes from or contracts into)
Texture/consistency
Color
Proximity to specimen margins
X-ray appearance (when relevant)

TABLE 9.2	Contrasting Gross Features of Typical Infiltrating Carcinoma and Fibroadenoma	
	Infiltrating Carcinoma	*Fibroadenoma*
Outline	Irregular[a]	Smooth; may be rounded or lobulated
Relationship to surrounding tissue	Fixed; concave cut face	Mobile; protruding, convex cut face
Texture/consistency	Hard, gritty ("unripe pear")	Rubbery, uniform; may have a clefted cut face
Color	Variable; often streaked with yellow (elastic tissue)	Variable but uniform in any one lesion; often glistening

[a]Certain special types of invasive carcinoma (mucinous and medullary) have a rounded outline.

clined. Malignancy is usually diagnosed by either core needle biopsy or open excisional biopsy of ambulatory patients. The need to consider treatment alternatives precludes the use of frozen section diagnosis immediately before definitive treatment (2). Frozen sections may be appropriate for the confirmation of a cytologic diagnosis of carcinoma or the evaluation of surgical margins. If frozen section is undertaken and any doubt arises about the diagnosis, a final decision should be deferred until processed tissue is available. Difficulties with frozen sections are usually attributable to sampling errors, technical problems, or, occasionally, histologic misinterpretation. Errors in interpretation arise particularly with sclerosing lesions (sclerosing adenosis, radial scar, ductal adenoma), epithelial hyperplasia, papillary lesions, and fat necrosis. The diagnosis of in situ

carcinoma can also cause problems, not only because it may be difficult to distinguish from benign epithelial hyperplasia but also because stromal invasion cannot always be excluded in the small sample usually examined.

NEEDLE BIOPSY

The use of needle biopsy, both fine-needle aspiration (aspiration cytology) and tissue core, in the assessment of breast disease has dramatically increased. Tissue core biopsy has the advantage of allowing histologic rather than cytologic assessment; the proportion of indeterminate and inadequate specimens is far less; and distinction between in situ and invasive carcinoma may be

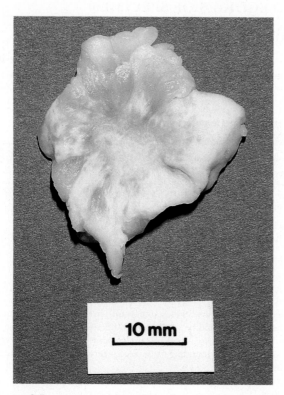

Figure 9.1. Cut surface of a biopsy specimen containing a typical infiltrating carcinoma. The irregular outline of the tumor and contraction from the surrounding tissue produce a slightly concave cut surface.

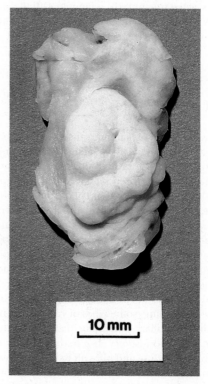

Figure 9.2. Cut surface of a biopsy specimen containing a typical fibroadenoma. The lesion has a smooth, rounded outline with a suggestion of a lobulated structure, and it protrudes from the surrounding breast tissue.

TABLE 9.3

Benign Lesions That Most Frequently Mimic Carcinoma on Gross Examination

Radial scar
Ductal adenoma
Duct ectasia
Reactive fibrosis around cysts

more readily accomplished. In addition, prognostic indicators (ER, PR, HER2/*neu*, etc.) can be evaluated in many core needle biopsies. However, it may be possible to process and report aspirated samples more quickly, allowing assessment of the adequacy of the sample and, in some situations, diagnosis at the time of the initial outpatient visit. In the evaluation of tissue core biopsy samples, problems are encountered because of the limited size of the specimen and, not infrequently, the presence of crush artifact. Other problems include destruction of the lesional tissue by hemorrhage or infarction and displacement of benign epithelium to simulate invasive carcinoma (3), although displacement of malignant epithelium from in situ carcinoma has also been reported following localization by guide-wire for excision of a mammographic abnormality (4). Needle biopsy of nonpalpable lesions requires radiographic guidance by either ultrasonography or stereotactic mammography. In the case of needle core biopsies performed to evaluate microcalcification, it is important that calcifications be identified on radiographs of the core biopsy samples (5) and confirmed in the histologic sections. However, calcifications imaged on radiographs are often larger than those seen microscopically. Calcification may rarely be seen in aspirated material. Uncertainty in the interpretation of a needle biopsy specimen should lead to open biopsy. In patients receiving neoadjuvant therapy, core needle biopsy specimens may be the only histologic material available if the tumor regresses completely as a consequence of therapy.

OPEN BIOPSY

Open biopsy may take the form of either (a) an incisional biopsy in which only part of the lesion is sampled, or (b) an excisional biopsy intended to remove the lesion in its entirety. The latter may also be referred to as a *lumpectomy*, *partial mastectomy*, or *tylectomy*. The amount of tissue removed varies considerably and may be an entire quadrant of the breast. In centers practicing conservation treatment, excision of the carcinoma usually forms part of the definitive therapy, and histologic assessment of the surgical margins is particularly important. During the operation, some surgeons rely on the gross appearance alone, whereas others ask for a frozen section evaluation of the margins. However, full evaluation of margins on frozen section may be too time-consuming to be useful. Assessment of specimen x-ray images has been used to note the proximity of a neoplasm to the surgical margins, but is not reliable (6). Touch preps have been advocated to evaluate margins rapidly. Although the exact techniques used to assess neoplastic involvement of tumor margins vary, it is always important to ink the surface of the specimen before dissection. This may be facilitated, particularly in the case of fresh specimens, if the surface is thoroughly blotted dry, or dipped briefly into alcohol or acetone, both before and after application of the dye. This procedure helps fix the

dye onto the surface of the specimen and limit its spread into the planes of the underlying tissue. The use of several different colored dyes to mark the margins helps in the recognition of orientation of sections. This is possible only if the specimen is oriented by the surgeon with the use of clips, sutures of different lengths, or some other means at the time of excision. Identification of the location of the nipple allows orientation of the specimen in the direction of the ducts, which may be important when the extent of ductal carcinoma in situ (DCIS) is defined.

Localization biopsies of clinically occult lesions, detected by mammography, present special problems. When carcinoma involves the margin, it should be noted whether the involvement is focal or diffuse and whether the involvement is by in situ or invasive carcinoma. When the margin is not involved, its distance from the carcinoma should be reported in millimeters. Each excision margin should be included on at least one section and, ideally, there should be two or three sections from the margin closest to the grossly identified neoplasm. If resection is found to be incomplete and the specimen has been oriented to allow a determination of which margin is involved, re-excision of only the appropriate area may sometimes be carried out. Some surgeons prefer to perform shave biopsies of the wall of the cavity that is left after the excision biopsy has been performed. Alternatively, the outer wall of the excision biopsy specimen can be shaved. The use of the shaved margin method may result in overestimation of the extent of tumor and the use of perpendicular margins may result in underestimation (6).

MICRODOCHECTOMY

Microdochectomy, a procedure used to investigate patients with discharge from a nipple, aims to remove the diseased duct system. It is helpful if the surgeon marks the apex of the specimen with a suture and leaves a probe in the affected duct. The specimen may be dissected either by opening the duct with fine scissors or by making serial slices across the duct lumen. We favor the latter method. The former technique may dislodge very small lesions. When such specimens are reported, it is always important to state whether a cause of the discharge has been demonstrated; if not, continued clinical follow-up may be required because the lesional tissue may not have been removed.

MASTECTOMY

Although the increased use of conservation therapy in the treatment of breast cancer has resulted in more limited specimens, mastectomy, when carried out, always necessitates a thorough gross description (7). Again, correct orientation of the specimen is facilitated if markers are inserted at the time of operation. These should be placed at the 12 o'clock position on the skin ellipse and in the axilla. The axillary portion can be divided into three levels (Fig. 9.3) on radical mastectomy specimens, which are uncommon in current clinical practice. In the absence of muscle resection, levels must be marked intraoperatively. As part of the gross examination, the size and appearance of the skin ellipse and nipple should be noted, and the site and size of any biopsy incision should be recorded. After ink has been applied to the deep specimen margin, the breast is usually sliced serially in the sagittal plane from its posterior aspect. If the skin is left intact, the specimen can later be reconstructed if examination of more tissue is necessary. Any abnormalities

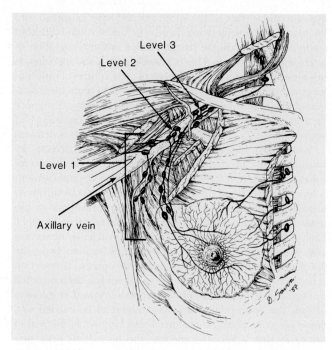

Figure 9.3. Diagram of the anatomy of the breast and axilla, with particular reference to lymphatic drainage. The axillary lymph nodes can be divided into three groups according to their relationship to the pectoralis minor muscle (in the diagram, the central portion of this muscle has been removed for clarity): level 1 (low) nodes lie below and lateral to the pectoralis minor, level 2 (middle) nodes lie beneath the muscle, and level 3 (high) nodes lie above and medial to the muscle.

found within the breast tissue should be carefully described and localized, with particular attention paid to the features listed in Table 9.1. The general appearance of the remaining breast tissue should also be noted. Blocks should be obtained from any abnormal area, including any previous biopsy site if present, and from the deep margin closest to the tumor or biopsy site. At least one block should be obtained from each quadrant, and another block should be obtained parallel to the skin in the subareolar region to sample the major ducts.

Careful manual palpation of the tissue is the generally accepted practice for locating axillary lymph nodes. The number found per axilla varies, depending on the extent of the axillary dissection. Special techniques, including radiographic imaging and clearing methods, may increase the yield of lymph nodes. Examination of multiple levels of each block of lymph nodes and immunohistochemical study with the use of epithelial markers may help detect small metastases, but the significance of the additional information gained by these laborious techniques remains to be determined (8,9). Conservation treatment of mammary carcinoma often includes axillary dissection. The tissue containing the nodes may be removed in continuity with that containing the carcinoma; more often, it is separate. Careful orientation of the specimen, as previously described, may be important.

SENTINEL LYMPH NODE BIOPSY

Excision of the sentinel lymph node(s) is being used increasingly as an alternative to traditional axillary dissection (10). The sentinel lymph node(s) is identified by the surgeon following injection of the affected breast with dye and/or radioactive-labeled tracer and then submitted to the pathologist. At some institutions, the sentinel node is examined intraoperatively by frozen section or cytologic (touch preparation) examination. Sentinel lymph nodes require more extensive pathologic evaluation than do nodes procured via standard axillary dissection. Paraffin blocks of sentinel nodes should be sectioned at three levels (10). Although immunohistochemical stains for cytokeratin and molecular techniques have been used to detect occult metastases in sentinel and nonsentinel lymph nodes, the clinical value of these adjunctive procedures has not been established (10).

SPECIAL TECHNIQUES

SPECIMEN RADIOGRAPHY AND LOCALIZATION BIOPSY

The mammographic appearance of carcinoma and benign breast lesions is described briefly in Table 9.4. The handling of mammographically detected lesions is time-consuming but, for an accurate assessment, consistent methods must be used (11). Radiologic signs of malignancy may or may not be accompanied by a palpable abnormality. In the absence of any clinical sign, a mammographically suspect lesion must be localized preoperatively. The technique most frequently used is the insertion of a fine hooked wire, which serves to guide the surgeon. After excision, the specimen should be radiographically examined and the findings compared with the preoperative mammogram (Fig. 9.4) to ensure that the lesional tissue and the wire have been removed. Specimen radiography should be performed while the patient is still in the operating room so that further tissue can be removed if necessary. An x-ray image of the specimen must be sent along with the specimen to the pathologist, with the area in question clearly indicated.

TABLE 9.4	**Contrasting Mammographic Appearances of Carcinoma and Benign Lesions**
Carcinoma	*Benign Lesions*
Opacity with irregular, spiculated margins	Opacity with smooth margins
Trabecular distortion	
Fine calcifications grouped closely together; may be rodlike or branched	Coarser calcifications widely dispersed; often have rounded, smooth outline
Asymmetric changes	Symmetric changes
Secondary signs (e.g., nipple retraction, skin thickening)	

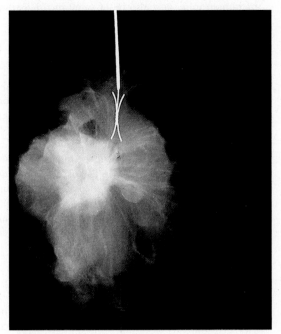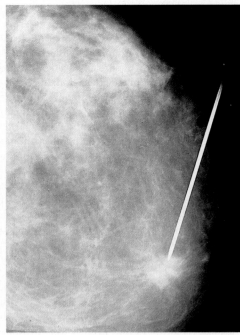

Figure 9.4. Comparison of the x-ray image of the excised specimen with the preoperative mammogram allows confirmation that the suspect density has been removed. The guide-wire introducer is seen in the mammogram, whereas the guide-wire is observed in situ in the specimen radiograph. Histologic study showed an infiltrating ductal carcinoma.

Microcalcification is the most frequent mammographic sign of a clinically occult tumor (Figs. 9.5 and 9.6), but it is usually confined to the DCIS of a carcinoma. Confirmation of the presence of calcium is not usually a problem, but it may require additional slides and even x-ray examination of the blocks. When extensive study is carried out, it should be remembered that calcifications seen on slides are significantly smaller than those visualized by the radiologist on x-ray film. Other mammographic signs of malignancy, however, such as architectural dis-

tortion, may be more difficult to match with those on the original mammogram. Compression of the excised specimen during the x-ray examination may help detect the abnormality. Occasionally, when the tissue has been excised, a palpable abnormality becomes apparent. Otherwise, frozen section is not recommended in this situation because (a) many mammographically detected abnormalities are small, and (b) histologic interpreta-

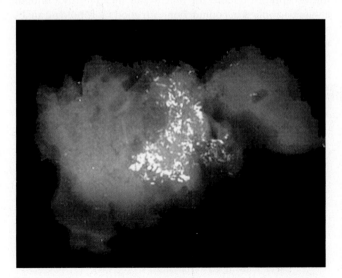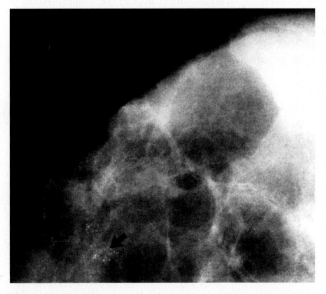

Figure 9.5. Specimen radiograph. This excised mass shows an extensive rodlike or casting pattern of calcification, which is typical and virtually diagnostic of poorly differentiated, high-grade ductal carcinoma in situ with comedo necrosis.

Figure 9.6. Mammogram showing a localized focus of clusters of fine, granular, sandlike particles of calcification (*arrow*). This pattern of calcification is typical of well-differentiated, low-grade ductal carcinoma in situ, but a similar appearance may be seen in benign lesions.

tion is often difficult (2). The entire specimen should be sliced at 2- to 3-mm intervals. In the absence of an obvious gross lesion, all the slices should, if possible, be processed. If this is not feasible, blocks should include both the mammographic abnormality and the immediately surrounding tissue. All areas containing microcalcification should be examined. Selection of the involved areas is facilitated by further x-ray examination after the tissue has been finely sliced. If the specimen proves to contain carcinoma, additional sampling may be necessary. This is particularly important in cases of DCIS because it helps the examiner to assess the extent of disease, determine whether foci of infiltration exist, and demonstrate the relationships to the margins. If each slice is processed separately, the extent of the lesion can be deduced by counting the number of slices involved (11). If microscopic examination fails to confirm the presence of calcification, x-ray examination of the paraffin blocks may help to locate the exact site of the calcium within the tissue. Calcium oxalate crystals (weddellite), in contrast to the more common calcium phosphate, do not stain with hematoxylin and so are not easily seen in slides stained with hematoxylin and eosin, nor do they stain with von Kossa stain (12,13). The crystals, however, are readily seen by polarized light microscopy. Although either form of calcification may present as a mammographic abnormality, calcium oxalate crystals are usually associated with benign mammary lesions—in particular, cystic change and apocrine metaplasia. The histology report of all specimens removed as a result of a mammographic abnormality should include a comparison of the mammographic and gross findings, in addition to a comparison of the mammographic and histologic findings.

OTHER IMAGING TECHNIQUES

Both ultrasonography and magnetic resonance imaging may also provide useful information in the evaluation of patients with breast symptoms. The former is particularly helpful in distinguishing cystic from solid lesions, whereas the latter, in conjunction with mammography, may aid in the detection, diagnosis, and staging of breast cancer and in the differentiation of postsurgical scarring from tumor recurrence in patients whose breast carcinoma was previously treated with conservation therapy (14). Other imaging techniques, including scintimammography, positron emission tomography, and particularly digital mammography, may also be of value in the assessment of patients with breast disorders.

SUBGROSS EXAMINATION

Subgross examination, which is best suited to research laboratories, has greatly enhanced the knowledge and understanding of mammary tissue and its abnormalities, particularly by defining the site of origin of many pathologic entities. Samples are fixed, sliced, stained, dehydrated with alcohol, and then cleared with methyl salicylate (15). A dissecting or stereoscopic microscope can be used to examine the tissue slices, and abnormal areas may be selected for further histologic examination. Similar techniques for the stereoscopic examination of paraffin-embedded tissue blocks have also been reported and are used to evaluate the distribution of pathologic lesions in the mammary tree (16,17).

ANCILLARY STUDIES

A knowledge of estrogen and progesterone receptor status is important, primarily as a guide to the choice of systemic treatment in patients with breast carcinoma, but also as a prognostic indicator, albeit a weak one. Immunohistochemical analysis of hormone receptor status has largely replaced hormone receptor cytosol assays (18). Among several advantages, this has facilitated the evaluation of small specimens, from which it would not be possible to obtain sufficient fresh tissue for cytosol assays. Evaluation of other prognostic factors and factors predictive of response to therapy is discussed below.

Electron microscopy is usually not required in the routine diagnosis of breast disease. It may occasionally be helpful in a problem case to distinguish among carcinoma, sarcoma, and lymphoma. However, in most situations, immunohistochemistry has largely supplanted the use of electron microscopy (19). A general outline of the use of histochemical and immunohistochemical techniques appears in Tables 9.5 and 9.6. Immunohistochemistry has largely supplanted histochemical stains, with the exception of stains for mucin and melanin; they should always be applied in conjunction with good morphologic analysis. It should be used as an adjunct to a histologic diagnosis and never to make a diagnosis in isolation.

TABLE 9.5	Use of Histochemistry in Breast Pathology
Type of Pathology	*Stain*
Histologic typing	
Mucinous (colloid) carcinoma	Mucin stains (e.g., PAS + alcian blue)
Adenoid cystic carcinoma	Mucin stains (e.g., PAS + alcian blue)
Carcinoma with neuroendocrine features	Argyrophil stains (e.g., Grimelius)
Differential diagnosis	
Carcinoma versus sarcoma or lymphoma	Mucin stains
	Reticulin
Primary versus secondary carcinoma	Mucin stains
	Elastic stains
	Other stains (e.g., for melanin)
Paget disease versus Bowen disease or malignant melanoma	Mucin melanin stains (for further details, see Table 9.19)
PAS, periodic acid-Schiff.	

TABLE 9.6	Most Common Uses of Immunohistochemistry in Breast Pathology

- Assessment of estrogen and progesterone receptor status by using specific antibodies to the receptor proteins.
- Assessment of HER2/*neu* protein overexpression by using specific antibodies to the HER2/*neu* protein. Usually supported by FISH evaluation for amplification.
- Distinguishing in situ from invasive carcinomas by using antibodies to myoepithelial cell markers (e.g., actins, calponin, smooth muscle myosin heavy chain, p63) and basement membrane proteins (e.g., type IV collagen, laminin).
- Assessment of metastatic lesions for possible breast origin by using antibodies to estrogen receptor, gross cystic disease fluid protein-15, cytokeratins, and other markers, depending on the clinical circumstances, anatomic location, and histologic differential diagnosis.
- Evaluation of spindle cell lesions (metaplastic carcinoma vs. mesenchymal lesion) by using antibodies to cytokeratins and mesenchymal markers (e.g., CD34).
- Evaluation of vascular and pseudovascular lesions (e.g., PASH).
- Distinguishing ductal from lobular in situ carcinomas by using antibodies to E-cadherin.
- Distinguishing high-grade sarcomas, for example, angiosarcoma with CD31, factor VIII-related antigen.

THE PATHOLOGY REPORT

This vital component of the diagnostic process not only records whether a lesion is benign or malignant, but also conveys data related to extent and prognosis, and thus treatment planning (7). In addition, it may be used for academic review in research and teaching. The report should therefore state whether a lesion is benign or malignant; if it is the latter, the features listed in Table 9.7 should all be recorded. The use of a synoptic or checklist-type format has been recommended to ensure a uniform system of reporting and increase the likelihood that all clinically important information is provided (20).

THE NORMAL BREAST

Even though the normal mammary epithelium comprises only a minor component of the total breast tissue mass, most of the diseases affecting the breast arise from it. The epithelium is arranged in the form of 10 to 15 segments, each consisting of a branching structure that has been likened to a flowering tree (21). The lobules represent the flowers, which drain into duct-ules and ducts (twigs and branches) (Fig. 9.7); these in turn drain into the collecting ducts (trunk) that open onto the surface of the nipple. Just below the nipple, the ducts are expanded to lactiferous sinuses. The epithelium throughout the duct system is bilayered, consisting of an inner epithelial layer and an outer myoepithelial layer. The importance of this double cell layer cannot be overemphasized because it is one of the main guides to the distinction between benign and malignant lesions.

The lobule, together with its terminal duct, has been called the *terminal duct lobular unit* (TDLU). The normal lobule consists of a variable number of blind-ended terminal ductules, alternatively called *acini*, each of which has a typical double epithelial cell layer. The acini are surrounded by loose fibrovascular intralobular stroma, which contrasts with the denser and less cellular interlobular stroma (Fig. 9.8). Elastic tissue, normally present in variable amounts around ducts, is absent from the lobules. The luminal epithelium of the resting breast is cuboidal or columnar. The outer basal or myoepithelial layer, although always present, is variably distinctive. In fresh tissue, myoepithelial cells can be demonstrated by staining for alkaline phosphatase activity, whereas in fixed tissue they can be demonstrated by immunohistochemical methods with antibodies to myoepithelial cell markers, such as actins, calponin, smooth

TABLE 9.7	Features to Be Recorded on Histologic Examination of Invasive Breast Carcinoma

Histologic type
Histologic grade
Presence and type of any associated in situ carcinoma
Presence or absence of vascular (angiolymphatic) invasion
Maximum diameter of invasive component
Size and extent (proportion) of in situ component
Margin status
Presence of calcification (if noted on mammogram) and location
Correlation with mammogram when relevant
Steroid hormone receptor and HER2/*neu* status when relevant
Other prognostic and predictive markers, when relevant
Other significant features (e.g., Paget disease of the nipple)
Lymph node status when relevant (total number of nodes, number of deposits >2 cm, presence of extracapsular invasion)
Pathologic stage (T and N status)

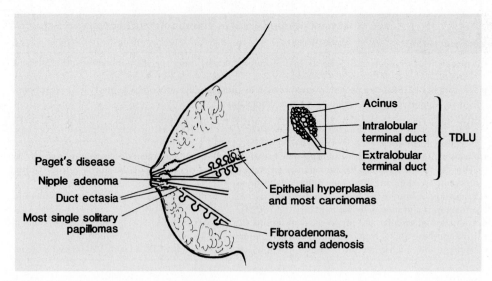

Figure 9.7. A schematic representation of the breast indicating the sites of origin of pathologic lesions.

muscle myosin heavy chain, high–molecular-weight cytokeratins, and p63. Epithelial cells are differentiated by their keratin profile and staining for GCDFP-15. The TDLU is the physiologically active area of the breast and the site of origin of most pathologic lesions. Familiarity with the cyclic changes in the normal lobule is basic to the interpretation of breast histology.

The size of the mammary lobules and the number of acini are extremely variable. This may be partly related to the pa-

tient's age, but also to the plane of the section. Changes in the mammary lobules occur in association with the menstrual cycle (22), with variation in the epithelial and stromal components. In the early follicular phase, the stroma is dense and collagenized and the epithelium is columnar with only one type of cell apparent. The later follicular phase is characterized by distinct epithelial and myoepithelial cell types and a dense and fibrous lobular stroma (see Fig. 9.9). In the luteal phase, the lobular stroma is looser and more myxoid; both epithelial and myoepithelial cell layers are evident; and the acinar lumens are progressively distended with eosinophilic secretion. These changes may not be observed synchronously in all lobules.

During pregnancy and lactation, the number of lobules and acini within each lobule increase at the expense of the interlobular and intralobular stroma. Luminal epithelial cells have cytoplasmic vacuoles, which often protrude into the lumen (Fig. 9.10). The florid changes in both nuclei and cytoplasm seen in pregnancy and lactation can be alarming to the inexperienced observer; areas of infarction, which occasionally develop in the

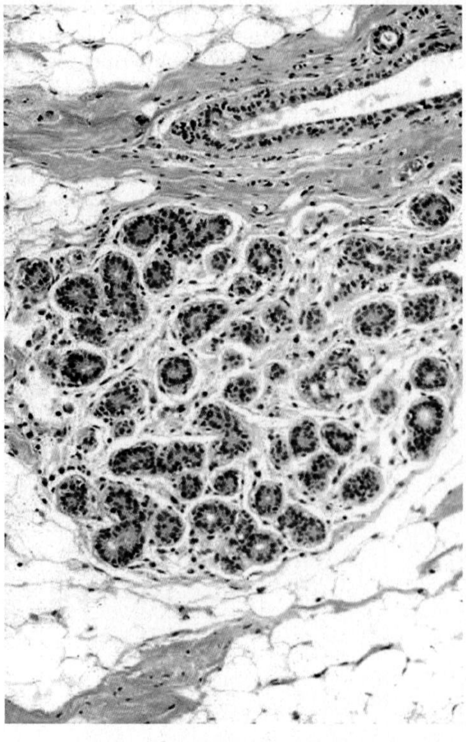

Figure 9.8. Lobule and duct in early proliferative phase. The lobular stroma and epithelium are distinct from the interlobular stroma. The stroma is loose and moderately cellular. Acini are evident as rounded structures with little secretion. Myoepithelial layer is not prominent.

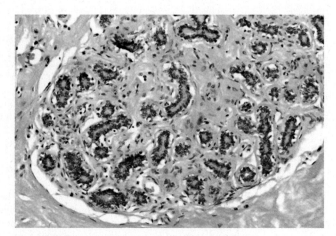

Figure 9.9. Lobule in late proliferative phase. Lobular stroma is denser and more fibrous. Epithelial/myoepithelial layers are clearly evident.

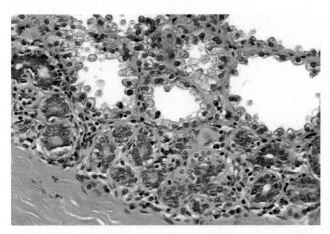

Figure 9.10. Partially lactating lobule. The stroma in the lactating zone is not evident, nor are the myoepithelial cells. Epithelial cells are cuboidal with vacuolated cytoplasm and prominent, hyperchromatic nuclei.

breast during pregnancy, may compound the problem (23). When lactation ceases, the lobules involute and return to normal resting appearance, but involution usually proceeds unevenly and takes several months. Involuting lobules are irregular in contour and frequently infiltrated by lymphocytes and plasma cells. With increasing age, particularly after the menopause, gradual atrophy of the lobular acini occurs, together with a loss of specialized intralobular stroma. The postmenopausal breast normally consists largely of adipose tissue containing a few residual ducts and vessels in interlobular stroma.

Occasionally, an isolated lobule showing secretory changes may be seen in the nonpregnant breast. Although this is often called a *residual lactating lobule*, it may occur in a nulliparous woman.

Most pathologic changes in the breast have been termed either *lobular* or *ductal*, in that lesions so designated were thought to arise from either the lobular acini or the larger ducts. In more recent years, however, this assumption has been questioned. Subgross studies (15,21) have shown that most lesions originally termed *ductal* (e.g., cysts, ductal epithelial hyperplasia, and DCIS) actually arise from the TDLU, which "unfolds" with coalescence of the acini to produce larger structures resembling ducts. Indeed, the only common benign lesion thought to arise from the large or medium-sized duct rather than from the TDLU is the solitary intraductal papilloma. Also found in breast tissue are intramammary lymph nodes, which are more frequent than previously recognized and may be identified on routine mammograms (24).

Sections of the breast and overlying skin from the nipple and subareolar region have a characteristic appearance. The epidermis contains occasional clear cells that must not be confused with Paget cells and that are cytologically benign. Some of these cells are clear keratinocytes, whereas others are thought to be derived from epidermally located mammary acinar epithelium. Although the areola lacks pilosebaceous units, sebaceous glands are present, related to the lactiferous ducts. Sometimes, these glands drain via the lactiferous duct lumina and thus terminate in a common ostium, or they may terminate directly in the epidermis adjacent to the lactiferous ducts. During pregnancy, the glands become increasingly prominent, resulting in the formation of small elevations called *Montgomery tubercles*. Nu-

merous bundles of smooth muscle are a distinctive feature of the subareolar region. Apocrine glands are also frequently present.

NIPPLE LESIONS

Lesions of the nipple present special diagnostic problems due in part to their location, but also because of the special features they present.

PAGET DISEASE OF THE NIPPLE

Paget disease of the nipple is seen clinically as a red, weeping, often crusted lesion of the nipple and may be indistinguishable from eczema. On microscopic examination, the epidermis is seen to be permeated by malignant cells arranged either singly, in groups, or, more rarely, in tubules (Fig. 9.11). The cells may be sparse, or they may be so numerous that they completely efface and destroy the epidermis. Paget cells have large nuclei, prominent nucleoli, and abundant pale-staining cytoplasm that often contains mucin. Because of shrinkage artifact, the cells sometimes appear to lie within a space. The underlying dermis shows variable degrees of telangiectasia and chronic inflammation. In almost every case of mammary Paget disease, an underlying carcinoma is found. This is nearly always of ductal type and may be either pure in situ carcinoma (nearly always of high grade, poorly differentiated type) or a combination of in situ and infiltrating carcinoma.

Paget disease occurs in 1% to 2% of all patients with mammary carcinoma. Although occasionally the in situ carcinoma is restricted to a single duct beneath the nipple, generally it is widespread throughout the breast (25). The occurrence of a solitary focus of in situ carcinoma in a large duct beneath the nipple appears to be one instance in which carcinoma truly originates in a large duct rather than in the TDLU. The histogenesis of Paget cells has been a matter of controversy, but immunohistochemical studies have confirmed their glandular epithelial immunophenotype, thereby supporting the theory of cell migration from an origin in the duct system of the breast (or possibly from epidermally located mammary ductal epithelial cells) (26). The microscopic appearance of Paget disease of the nipple can sometimes be confused with that of either superficial

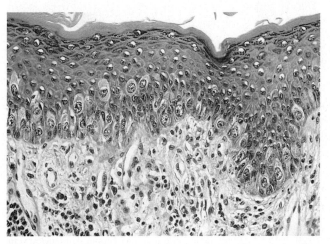

Figure 9.11. Paget disease of the nipple. The epidermis is infiltrated by large Paget cells with abundant pale cytoplasm, large vesicular nuclei, and prominent nucleoli.

TABLE 9.8	Histochemical and Immunohistochemical Stains Helpful in the Differential Diagnosis of Paget Disease of the Nipple, Bowen Disease, and Superficial Spreading Malignant Melanoma		
	Paget Disease	*Bowen Disease*	*Malignant Melanoma*
Glycogen	+ / −	+	−
Mucin	+[a]	−	−
Melanin	−[a]	−	+
Simple epithelial cytokeratins	+	−	−
Keratinocyte cytokeratins	−	+	−
Neuroectodermal and melanoma markers (e.g., S100, NKl-C3, HMB-45)	+ / −	−	+
Epithelial membrane antibodies (e.g., EMA, HMFG)	+	−	−
HER2/*neu*	+	−	−

[a]Mucin is not always present in Paget cells and melanin occasionally is.
+, Usually present; + / −, variably present; −, usually absent; EMA, epithelial membrane antigen.

spreading melanoma or Bowen disease, both of which may rarely occur in the region of the nipple. Features helpful in the differential diagnosis include the presence of multinucleated giant cells and individual cell keratinization in Bowen disease. In malignant melanoma, tumor cells come into direct contact with and invade the underlying dermis, whereas Paget cells remain within the epidermis. It should be noted that in some cases, Paget cells may contain melanin pigment; therefore, the presence of such pigment within pagetoid cells in the epidermis does not necessarily define the cells as those of malignant melanoma. A distinction should also be made from direct invasion of the epidermis by an underlying carcinoma.

Histochemical and immunohistochemical stains that may be helpful in the differential diagnosis of Paget disease are listed in Table 9.8. The cells of Paget disease of the nipple, together with the underlying carcinoma, nearly always express the HER2/*neu* oncoprotein (Fig. 9.12). Antibodies to this protein, together with antibodies to low–molecular-weight cytokeratins,

can sometimes help to make the diagnosis in difficult cases and when the Paget cells are few and far between (26). As discussed previously, clear cells occasionally occur in the epidermis of the normal nipple (Toker clear cells) and should not be mistaken for the cells of Paget disease.

NIPPLE ADENOMA (FLORID PAPILLOMATOSIS OF THE NIPPLE)

Nipple adenoma is a relatively uncommon entity that the unwary may easily mistake for carcinoma. The condition has also been called *florid papillomatosis of the nipple, florid adenomatosis, subareolar duct papillomatosis,* or *erosive adenomatosis*. It is most common in the fourth decade but may be seen in women of any age, and also occurs in men. The soreness, ulceration, and swelling of the nipple, sometimes with discharge, may simulate Paget disease of the nipple (27).

The gross appearance is usually that of an ill-defined nodule (Fig. 9.13). At low power, the lesion has a rounded outline and

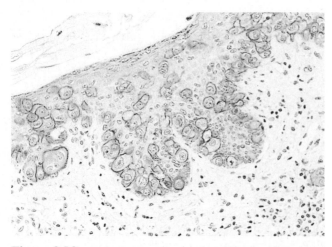

Figure 9.12. Paget disease of the nipple. Nipple skin labeled with an antibody to HER2/*neu* shows striking membrane staining of Paget cells, a reaction typical of Paget disease. Coexistent underlying poorly differentiated, high-grade ductal carcinoma in situ stained similarly.

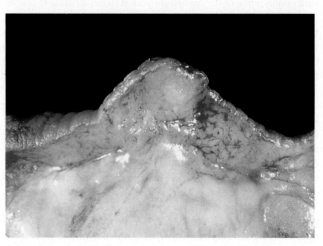

Figure 9.13. Nipple adenoma. In this photograph of a nipple specimen, a rounded gray-white nodule is seen immediately below the nipple skin.

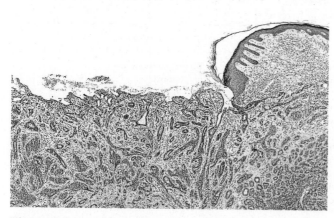

Figure 9.14. Nipple adenoma. This low-power photograph shows the interface of the lesion with the nipple surface. The glandular epithelium produces the clinical appearance of an "erosion." Note the abrupt transition to squamous epithelium. The haphazardly arranged bilayered tubules exhibit varying degrees of dilation and epithelial hyperplasia.

is composed of haphazardly arranged, proliferating, tubular structures surrounded by a varying amount of fibrous stroma (Fig. 9.14). The epithelial tubules, with their columnar cells, may extend to the surface of the nipple, in which case an abrupt transition to the stratified squamous epithelium is seen (Fig. 9.14). They are of various sizes and shapes, simulating infiltrating carcinoma. Lobular architecture is lacking, probably because the lesion arises from the larger ducts rather than from the lobules.

At high power, two cell types lining most of the tubules can usually be discerned (see Fig. 9.91). Different degrees of epithelial hyperplasia may be seen, sometimes distending and occluding the glandular lumina (Fig. 9.15). The epithelial cells are usually cuboidal or columnar, but apocrine and squamous metaplasia both occur. As in many other lesions of the breast, stromal sclerosis sometimes distorts the glandular structures. Apparent involvement of muscle bundles may be seen, usually without reaction, and mitotic figures may be present, although not in

abundance. Necrosis is rare. Rosen and Caicco (28) described three distinct growth patterns of nipple adenoma, but these do not appear to have any prognostic significance. The lesion is generally considered entirely benign, but occasional cases of coexistent or subsequent carcinoma have been reported (28,29). The lesion may recur if it is incompletely excised. Nipple adenomas should be differentiated from syringomatous adenoma of the nipple (Table 9.9) and from an unusual subareolar papillary intraductal proliferative lesion called *subareolar sclerosing duct hyperplasia* (30). The latter abnormality is located beneath the areola without involvement of the surface of the nipple, but it may be associated with a nipple discharge. Although small ducts manifesting intraluminal papillary proliferation are present at the periphery of subareolar sclerosing duct hyperplasia, the lesion is distinctive because of the central sclerosis that results in entrapped and distorted ducts, analogous to the findings in a radial scar.

SYRINGOMATOUS ADENOMA OF THE NIPPLE

These rare tumors are composed of poorly circumscribed collections of small, bilayered epithelial tubular structures, solid islands of cells, and squamous cysts set within a fibrous stroma that can show myxoid or hyaline change. The tubular structures often have a comma-shaped extension similar to that seen in other syringomatous tumors (Fig. 9.16). Calcification may be present within the epithelial structures. Infiltration between glandular structures and muscular and perineural invasion are common (31,32). This lesion has features similar to those of the low-grade adenosquamous carcinoma that occasionally arises within the parenchyma of the breast (see section "Metaplastic Carcinoma" below). In the nipple region, syringomatous adenoma appears to behave in a benign fashion, but complete excision with a clear margin is advisable because recurrence has been recorded (31,32). Syringomatous adenoma may be histologically confused with tubular carcinoma, which rarely occurs in the nipple. Features helpful in the differential diagnosis of nipple adenoma, syringomatous adenoma, and tubular carcinoma are listed in Table 9.9.

GENERAL GUIDELINES FOR THE HISTOPATHOLOGIC INTERPRETATION OF BREAST TISSUE

A thorough understanding of the appearance of the normal breast is essential to the assessment of pathologic lesions. As discussed previously, most lesions arise within the TDLU. In most benign lesions, some lobular architecture is retained, although this may be severely distorted, and frequently the specialized stroma is no longer discernible. With the exception of microglandular adenosis, in all benign lesions, however florid, the two cell layers (epithelium and myoepithelium) comprising the glandular elements are retained.

Nonneoplastic benign epithelial changes affecting the TDLU can be divided broadly into four categories:

1. Metaplastic change within the epithelium (e.g., apocrine metaplasia)
2. Distortion of pre-existing glandular components (e.g., cystic change)

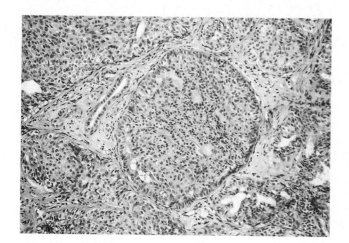

Figure 9.15. Nipple adenoma. This high-power view shows the marked degree of epithelial hyperplasia that may be seen in these lesions.

TABLE 9.9	Contrasting Features of Nipple Adenoma (Florid Papillomatosis), Syringomatous Adenoma, and Tubular Carcinoma		
	Nipple Adenoma	*Syringomatous Adenoma*	*Tubular Carcinoma*
Site	Areolar and subareolar	Subareolar	Breast parenchyma
Glandular distribution and overall outline	Circumscribed	Haphazard	Haphazard
Glandular shape	Variable	Comma-shaped	Rounded and angulated
Lining epithelium	Two cell types	Two cell types	One cell type
Cytologic atypia and mitoses	Uncommon	Absent	Present
Luminal bridging	Absent	Absent	Often present
Basement membrane	Present	Present	Absent
Squamous metaplasia	Sometimes present	Present	Absent
Changes in adjacent ducts	Papillary proliferation	Nil	Ductal carcinoma in situ may be present
Surrounding stroma	Normal	Normal	Reactive and cellular

3. An increased number of glandular components, termed *adenosis*
4. An increased number of epithelial cells within pre-existing glandular components, variously called *epithelial hyperplasia*, *epitheliosis*, and *papillomatosis.*

These changes are frequently accompanied by alterations in the stroma, usually in the form of an increase in fibrous tissue and sometimes in elastic tissue.

In many benign lesions, a combination of these changes is seen, such as (a) cystic change with apocrine metaplasia, or (b) the coexistence of adenosis, sclerosis, elastosis, cyst formation, and epithelial hyperplasia in a radial scar. When breast tissue is examined, an initial low-power assessment is necessary to establish the presence or absence of an overall lobular architecture, and a high-power view is needed to confirm the presence or absence of the two cell types characteristic of benign lesions. Most benign lesions retain these two characteristics.

In contrast to the benign changes previously described, infiltrating carcinoma lacks retention of a lobular pattern. The proliferating epithelial components are randomly arranged and variable in size, and they consist of only one cell type (except in a few rare malignancies, most notably adenoid cystic carcinoma). Although tubule formation is seen in well-differentiated

carcinomas, the tubules are lined by a single type of cell without a myoepithelial component.

In many instances, one can avoid an overdiagnosis of malignancy by acquiring familiarity with the benign lesions that may mimic carcinoma. Lesions that commonly cause problems are the following:

1. Sclerosing lesions (sclerosing adenosis, radial scar, ductal adenoma), which may be mistaken for infiltrating carcinoma. The presence of apocrine metaplasia or coexisting cancerization by DCIS can cause particular problems (see sections "Sclerosing Adenosis," "Radial Scar and Complex Sclerosing Lesion," and "Ductal Carcinoma in Situ").
2. Benign epithelial hyperplasia of ductal type, which may be mistaken for carcinoma in situ (see section "Epithelial Hyperplasia").
3. Benign intraductal papilloma. Differentiation between benign and malignant papillary lesions is frequently difficult. Sclerosis within an intraductal papilloma further compounds the problem and may mimic infiltrating carcinoma. Similar problems can also occur with ductal adenomas (see sections "Papillary Lesions" and "Ductal Adenoma").
4. Physiologic hyperplasia. Florid hyperplastic changes seen in the secretory breast (during pregnancy and lactation) can be alarming to the uninitiated (see section "The Normal Breast").
5. Reactive changes. Occasionally, chronic inflammation around a cyst or in an area of fat necrosis, when viewed at low power, resembles infiltrating carcinoma (see section "Cysts").
6. Treatment-induced changes. Epithelial atypia may be striking. Radiation and chemotherapy can both induce these changes (see section "Changes Induced by Therapy").

Before making a diagnosis of malignancy, particularly on frozen section or when dealing with a small tissue sample (e.g., needle core), the practitioner should always ask the question, Could these changes be caused by a benign lesion?

BENIGN BREAST DISEASE

As stated in the discussion of the normal breast, a wide variety of physiologic changes affect the mammary epithelium. They do not usually occur uniformly throughout the tissue and, as a

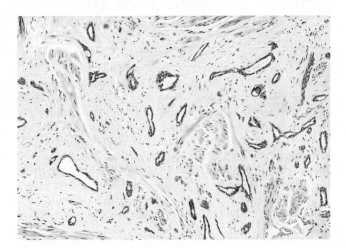

Figure 9.16. Syringomatous adenoma of the nipple. This view shows the many typical bilayered tubules. Some are comma-shaped and others infiltrate muscle bundles.

TABLE 9.10	Definitions of Terms Used in Benign Breast Disease
Term	*Definition*
Adenosis	An increased number, or enlargement, of glandular components
Epithelial hyperplasia (papillomatosis/epitheliosis)	An increased number of epithelial cells within preexisting glandular components
Cysts	Pathologically dilated sacs lined by epithelium and containing fluid
Epithelial metaplasia	Change from one fully differentiated type of epithelium to another not normally found at that site
Papilloma	A structure composed of fibrovascular cores covered by epithelium

result, such changes may produce clinical abnormalities. Not every breast biopsy sample contains pathologic changes; provided that care has been taken in sampling the specimen, the pathologist should not be afraid of recording the presence of normal breast tissue.

The term *benign breast disease* encompasses a wide range of lesions. Some are well-defined entities (e.g., fibroadenoma and duct papilloma), but a large number of biopsy specimens exhibit a mixture of changes affecting the TDLU. Through the years, a number of terms have been used to describe these changes, many of which may represent extremes of physiologic change rather than true pathologic lesions. Several all-embracing terms denote a wide spectrum of different appearances. The term *fibrocystic change* is the most frequently used, but it should always be accompanied by a full description of the individual components within the biopsy specimen. This has important prognostic significance in that, as is discussed later, only certain specific lesions are considered to carry an increased risk for subsequent carcinoma. It is also important that the terms used to describe benign breast disease be clearly defined. Definitions of the most frequently used terms appear in Table 9.10.

METAPLASTIC EPITHELIAL CHANGE

Metaplastic change is common within breast epithelium and is nearly always of apocrine type, in which the luminal epithelial cells resemble those of apocrine glands. The cells are larger than normal, with abundant granular eosinophilic cytoplasm, and show apical luminal bleb formation (Fig. 9.17). Ill-defined supranuclear vacuoles are often present. The nuclei are of variable size and may be either hyperchromatic or vesicular, but they generally have prominent nucleoli. Sometimes, the cytologic features of apocrine epithelium can be worrisome. This is especially true in the setting of other florid, benign epithelial changes, particularly sclerosing adenosis and intraductal epithelial hyperplasia. Once the apocrine nature of the cells has been recognized, however, care should be exercised in the interpretation of such cytologic features. This problem is discussed further in subsequent sections.

The presence of apocrine metaplasia within a background of adenosis has been termed *apocrine adenosis* (33). This term has also been used in other contexts—namely, apocrine metaplasia specifically within sclerosing adenosis (34) and a distinctive form of adenosis associated with adenomyoepithelioma (35).

Another change sometimes encountered in the breast epithelium is so-called columnar cell change, in which acini are variably dilated and lined by columnar epithelial cells with oval to elongated nuclei. Apical cytoplasmic snouts are often present at the luminal surface of these cells (Fig. 9.18). The term *colum-*

nar alteration with apocrine snouts and secretions (CAPSS) has been used for this appearance (36). Atypical hyperplasia in this setting has been described as *flat epithelial atypia* (FEA) (37) (see Fig. 9.19). Sometimes the luminal epithelial cells exhibit abundant clear cytoplasm, and it has been postulated that such clear cell metaplasia is a form of eccrine differentiation rather than a response to hormonal stimulation, as was previously suggested (38,39) (Fig. 9.20). This change has been noted in benign lesions and otherwise normal breast epithelium. Squamous metaplasia occasionally occurs in benign lesions, most often in duct papillomas and adenomas and in benign phyllodes tumors; more rarely, it occurs in radial sclerosing lesions and fibroadenomas, and it is also seen infrequently in otherwise normal structures. In at least some instances, the squamous cells appear to arise from myoepithelium rather than luminal epithelium (40). Except that their nature should be recognized, apocrine,

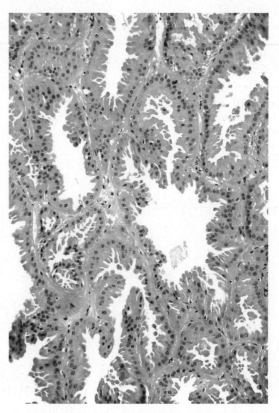

Figure 9.17. Apocrine metaplasia of the luminal epithelium lining cysts. The cells have abundant granular eosinophilic cytoplasm and show apical bleb formation.

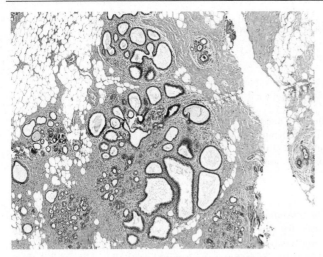

Figure 9.18. Columnar cell change (also known as *blunt duct adenosis*). The acini are dilated with columnar luminal cells and myoepithelium. The lobular architecture and specialized intralobular stroma are retained.

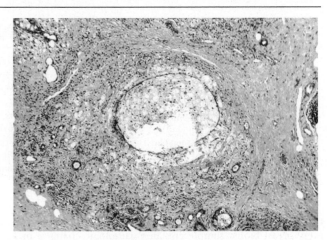

Figure 9.21. Cystic change. The duct is virtually obliterated by foamy histiocytes around and in the lumen.

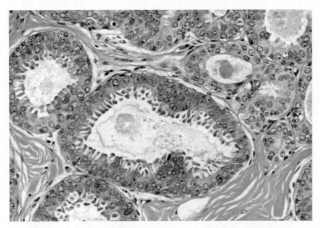

Figure 9.19. Flat epithelial atypia. Columnar cell change with prominent apocrine snouts and secretions. There is a hyperplasia of the epithelial cells with more than one layer of cells evident. In some of the ducts, the nuclei are atypical.

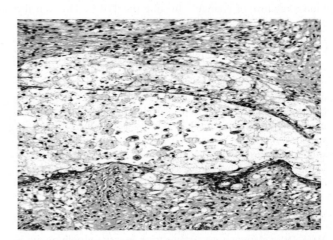

Figure 9.22. Cystic change. At higher magnification, the epithelial cells of the duct are almost all destroyed by the inflammatory reaction, and fibrosis is beginning around the duct.

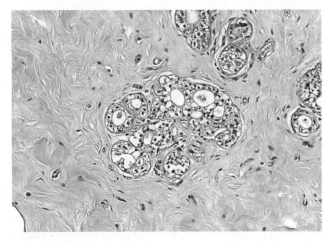

Figure 9.20. Clear cell metaplasia. The luminal epithelial cells have abundant clear cytoplasm.

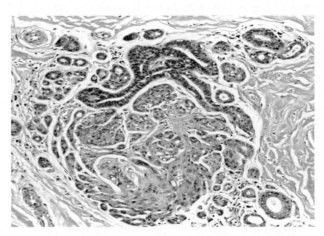

Figure 9.23. Sclerosing adenosis. At low power, the lobular architecture remains intact, but sclerosis distorts the epithelial structures. The nodular area in the center can be shown to be mostly myoepithelium.

columnar, clear cell, and squamous cell changes are of no known clinical significance.

CYSTS

Cyst formation is one of the most common changes seen in breast tissue and is frequently seen in combination with other benign lesions. As described in the section "The Normal Breast," it is generally accepted that cysts arise from lobular acini that coalesce (Figs. 9.21 and 9.22). The cysts are lined by a double cell layer, and the luminal epithelium frequently shows apocrine metaplasia. Cystic change does not usually cause major diagnostic problems; however, minor problems in interpretation may be encountered in the following situations:

1. In large cysts, the epithelial lining may be partially, if not entirely, lost.
2. An inflammatory reaction around a cyst, particularly when accompanied by fibrosis, can be mistaken for infiltrating carcinoma on low-power examination.
3. An intense inflammatory reaction consisting mainly of foamy macrophages may be all that remains at the site of a cyst and may be mistaken for fat necrosis.
4. Elastic tissue can be demonstrated around ectatic ducts.
5. The differentiation of benign cysts from the rare condition of cystic hypersecretory DCIS is discussed later (see section "Cystic Hypersecretory Ductal Carcinoma in Situ").

ADENOSIS

The term *adenosis*, defined in Table 9.8, indicates an increase in the number of glandular elements. Although this is usually taken to imply pathologic change, the term *simple adenosis* has been used to describe an increase in the size and number of lobules that can occur under the influence of hormonal stimulation. Strictly speaking, the lobular proliferation seen in pregnancy is a "physiologic" form of adenosis.

Sclerosing Adenosis

The best recognized pathologic form of adenosis is sclerosing adenosis, in which a numeric increase in the glandular elements is accompanied by stromal proliferation, producing glandular compression and distortion within an expanded lobular unit. It is especially important to be familiar with this form of adenosis because it can mimic carcinoma mammographically and histologically. Particular difficulty can occur with frozen sections and small tissue samples, but problems will be reduced if attention is paid to the aforementioned general guidelines. In cases of sclerosing adenosis, low-power examination reveals multiple nodular areas with retention of the overall lobular architecture (Fig. 9.23). These nodules are usually rounded and well defined. The numerous tubules, although frequently compressed and distorted, retain their two cell layers, but this feature may not be evident in each individual tubule (Fig. 9.24). The compression of the glandular components is more marked at the center of the lesion, whereas the caliber of those at the periphery is greater. Myoepithelial proliferation is often a major component of the lesion, and sometimes sheets of these cells are present. Confirmation of the myoepithelial phenotype by immunohistochemistry may be helpful. Microcalcification is frequently seen within the glandular lumina (Fig. 9.24). The fi-

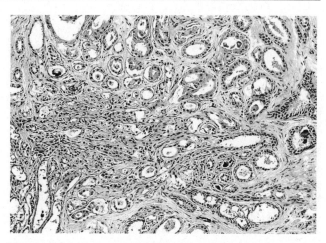

Figure 9.24. Sclerosing adenosis. At high power, compression and distortion of the epithelial components are evident, particularly in the central part of the lesion, where the double cell layer is less obvious. Note the foci of microcalcification.

brous stroma is usually dense and often hyalinized, and elastic tissue may be prominent. Compression of the tubules occludes their lumina in many areas, resulting in an infiltrative growth pattern. Actual invasion of nerves (Fig. 9.25) and vessels, although uncommon, is a well-recognized phenomenon associated with sclerosing adenosis and should not be taken as an indication of malignancy. The proliferating epithelial cells lack atypical features, but a particularly worrisome picture may be seen when apocrine metaplasia is also present (33,34). Recognition of the metaplastic nature of the epithelial cells is therefore especially important in the context of sclerosing adenosis. As discussed previously, the term *apocrine adenosis* has been used to describe this phenomenon (34). The term *atypical apocrine adenosis* (Fig. 9.26) has been used when these metaplastic cells are considered to show atypia (41,42). The difficulty of distinguishing the latter, which may show alarming cytology, from simple apocrine epithelium on the one hand and from apocrine carcinoma in situ on the other makes the study of so-called apocrine adenosis in relation to the incidence of subsequent carcinoma a somewhat controversial subject. When sclerosing

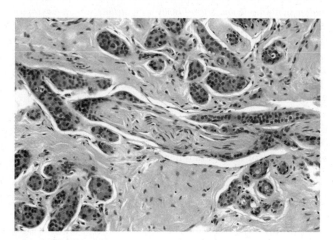

Figure 9.25. Sclerosing adenosis with perineural invasion. The perineural space is distended by bland epithelium in association with sclerosing adenosis.

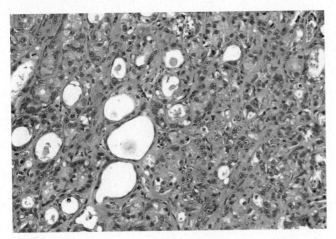

Figure 9.26. Atypical apocrine sclerosing lesion. The presence of apocrine cells in the setting of sclerosing adenosis can be confused with invasive cancer.

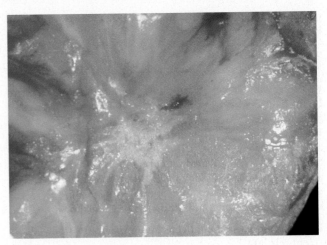

Figure 9.27. Radial scar. On gross examination, this stellate lesion closely resembles an infiltrating carcinoma.

adenosis occurs in an area of in situ carcinoma, the differential diagnosis from infiltrating carcinoma may be difficult. This problem is discussed later.

The diagnosis of sclerosing adenosis should not present a problem if attention is paid to the features previously mentioned. On initial low-power examination, sclerosing adenosis may be mistaken for infiltrating lobular carcinoma; however, on high-power examination, confusion with tubular carcinoma is more likely to occur. Features that distinguish sclerosing adenosis from tubular carcinoma are listed in Table 9.9. In difficult cases, immunohistochemistry may be helpful in the identification of both myoepithelial cells and basement membranes (Table 9.6). Sclerosing adenosis is most often a minor microscopic change, but in some instances it may be more extensive, producing a mammographic or palpable abnormality. The term *nodular adenosis*, or *adenosis tumor*, has been applied to florid examples of sclerosing adenosis that result in palpable lesions, sometimes seen as rounded, pink, granular areas on gross examination.

Radial Scar and Complex Sclerosing Lesion

A variety of terms, including *radial scar, complex sclerosing lesion, radial sclerosing lesion, scleroelastotic scar, stellate scar, nonencapsulated sclerosing lesion, indurative mastopathy, benign sclerosing ductal proliferation,* and *sclerosing papillary proliferation,* have been used for this histologically complex lesion, which typically contains adenosis, epithelial hyperplasia, and, frequently, cyst formation. The term *radial scar* has been reserved by some for individual lesions of less than 1 cm; larger, more complex lesions, frequently with more pronounced architectural disturbance (possibly resulting from the convergence of several adjacent radial scars), have been termed *complex sclerosing lesions.* The number of synonyms for this lesion reflects the controversy surrounding its genesis and its variable microscopic appearance.

Radial scar can mimic carcinoma both mammographically and on gross examination because it has a stellate appearance with central sclerosis and elastosis (Fig. 9.27). The distinction from infiltrating carcinoma can also be difficult on histologic examination. For a summary of those features helpful in the differential diagnosis of benign sclerosing lesions and infiltrating carcinoma, see Table 9.11. Radial scars are generally nonpal-

pable, often multiple, and frequently bilateral. They are often discovered as an incidental finding in breast specimens, but may be detected mammographically. They appear grossly as firm, chalky white lesions with an irregular outline. The stellate appearance is caused by bands of dense, fibrous connective tissue extending outward from the central core. The overall low-power appearance has been likened to the head of a flower (Fig. 9.28). The characteristic feature is a central elastotic scar containing relatively few glandular structures. Surrounding the central scar there may be lobules, sometimes distorted by sclerosis, and/or ducts with epithelial hyperplasia, which may be atypical or, rarely, contain intraductal carcinoma. It is the small, entrapped epithelial structures in the central scar that may simulate carcinoma. High-power examination of the central area shows a haphazard arrangement of irregular, small tubules with a double cell layer discernible in at least some of the structures (Figs. 9.29 and 9.30). These are surrounded by dense collagen and elastic tissue, which is characteristic of the lesion and may be a dominant finding. In the outer epithelial components, apocrine metaplasia and calcification may be present. Radial scars are often associated with other benign lesions, particularly sclerosing adenosis. Although the clinical significance of radial scars remains controversial (43,44), most authorities consider them to be benign mimics of cancer (45). However, an increased incidence of carcinoma and *atypical ductal hyperplasia* (ADH) appears to be associated with large radial scars, particularly in women older than 50 years (46). In addition, a clinical follow-up study has suggested that radial scars are associated with an increased risk for subsequent breast cancer, particularly when found in breasts that exhibit other benign proliferative lesions (47). The size and histologic features of radial scar should be reported with that diagnosis.

Radial scars are being seen with increasing frequency because they produce mammographic abnormalities that may be impossible to distinguish from those of infiltrating carcinoma; therefore, they are commonly detected during breast cancer screening programs. The possible confusion of these lesions with carcinoma is accentuated in core needle biopsy specimens because appreciation of its overall architecture may not be possible in a small sample, and the central scar may mimic cancer unless the characteristic features are noticed.

TABLE 9.11	Contrasting Features of Sclerosing Adenosis, Radial Scar, Tubular Carcinoma, and Microglandular Adenosis			
	Sclerosing Adenosis	*Radial Scar*	*Tubular Carcinoma[a]*	*Microglandular Adenosis*
Glandular distribution and overall pattern	Lobular outline, rounded	"Flower head"	Haphazard, stellate	Haphazard, usually no lobular outline
Glandular shape	Variable, with small, compressed lumina	Centrally small, with variably shaped lumina; peripherally dilated	Angulated with open lumina	Rounded with open lumina
Intraluminal secretion	Rare	Centrally rare	Uncommon	Striking, colloid-like
Lining epithelium	Two cell types (luminal epithelium and myoepithelium)	Two cell types (myoepithelium variably distinct centrally, luminal epithelium frequently hyperplastic peripherally)	One cell type	One cell type
Cytologic atypia	Nil	Nil	Usually mild	Nil
Cytoplasmic protrusions (apical snouts)	Uncommon	Centrally uncommon	Present	Absent
Luminal bridging	Absent	Centrally absent	Frequently present	Absent
Basement membrane	Present	Present	Absent	See text
Stroma	Fibrous or hyaline	Centrally hyaline with elastosis	Desmoplastic (reactive and cellular)	Collagenous or fatty; hypocellular

[a]Very occasionally, a coincidental carcinoma is seen in association with one of the benign lesions described.

Tubular Adenosis

Tubular adenosis is an unusual, benign lesion that may be misinterpreted as carcinoma (48). Microscopic examination reveals a haphazard proliferation of uniform, elongated, sinuous tubules with a bilayered structure of both luminal epithelium and myoepithelium. This lesion lacks the circumscription characteristic of most other types of adenosis. Luminal secretions are usually present and microcalcification is frequent. The rare occurrence of cancerization of this lesion by DCIS adds to the difficulties of differential diagnosis (38).

Microglandular Adenosis

Microglandular adenosis, another uncommon form of adenosis, is the one benign lesion in which the rule of "two cell types"

is broken (39–41). The proliferating tubules are lined by a single epithelial layer and lack an outer myoepithelial mantle. The arrangement of the tubules is haphazard; they are small, regular, and rounded without angulation (Fig. 9.31). Eosinophilic, periodic acid-Schiff (PAS)–positive, diastase-resistant material is frequently seen within the lumina, as are calcium deposits. The epithelial cells are cuboidal or flattened without apical snouts and are cytologically benign. The cells are occasionally vacuolated and contain cytoplasmic PAS-positive material. Staining for basement membrane by the PAS method is usually negative, but complete reticulin rings can be demonstrated around the tubules by silver impregnation techniques.

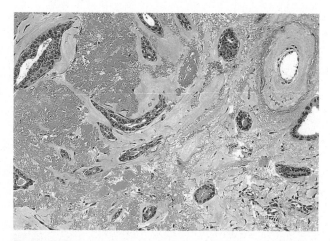

Figure 9.29. The center of a radial scar. The features are similar to those of sclerosing adenosis, with distorted, often compressed, tubular structures lined by a double cell layer. In this example, myoepithelial cells are obvious. Note the dark pink stroma, representing elastosis, a characteristic feature of many such lesions. In some preparations, the elastosis stain is paler.

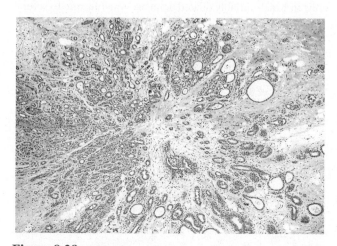

Figure 9.28. Radial scar. At low power, it resembles the head of a flower, with a fibroelastotic, relatively acellular center surrounded by dilated glandular structures showing various degrees of epithelial hyperplasia.

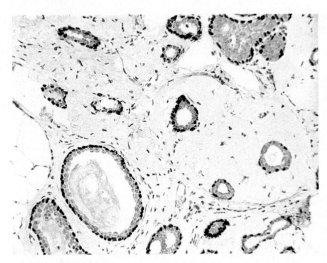

Figure 9.30. Radial scar. The entrapped benign glands are sur-rounded by myoepithelial cells, which show strong nuclear staining for p63.

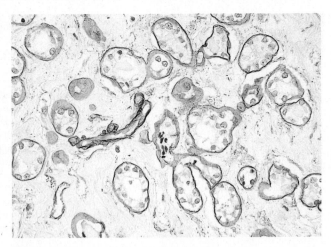

Figure 9.32. Microglandular adenosis. Immunohistochemistry for collagen IV demonstrates a complete ring of basement membrane around individual tubules.

Immunohistochemistry with basement membrane markers such as laminin and collagen IV (Fig. 9.32), in addition to electron microscopy, confirms the presence of an intact basement membrane around the epithelial structures and the absence of myoepithelial cells. Most reports on microglandu-lar adenosis indicate that it is entirely benign (49–51). How-ever, atypical forms of this lesion have been described (Fig. 9.33) (atypical microglandular adenosis) (52). In addition, carcinoma can rarely arise in or in conjunction with micro-glandular adenosis (52–53), and some of these carcinomas have distinctive features.

The term *secretory adenosis* has been used to describe a lesion architecturally similar to microglandular adenosis but in which myoepithelial cells are evident around the tubular structures (54). Whether or not tubular adenosis and secretory adenosis are separate entities is not apparent.

Blunt Duct Adenosis (Columnar Cell Change and Columnar Cell Hyperplasia)

The term *blunt duct adenosis* has been used by different authors to describe different lesions. Most often, this term has been used to describe a lesion such as that illustrated in Figure 9.18. The lobular architecture is well maintained, usually with reten-tion of the specialized stroma. The acini, which may be in-creased in number, are distorted and variably dilated. Indeed, it is debated whether acinar formation occurs at all or whether, as the name implies, the process results from the proliferation of terminal ducts without the development of true acini. The luminal cells lining these spaces are typically columnar and often show apical snouts. It has been proposed that lesions with this constellation of histologic features be termed *columnar cell change* when only one or two layers of epithelial cells are present and *columnar cell hyperplasia* when more than two epithelial cell layers are seen (55). Included within this category are lesions designated as *columnar alteration with prominent apical snouts and secretions* (CAPSS). *Flat epithelial atypia* (FEA) is a descriptive term that encompasses changes in the breast terminal duct lobular units in which variably dilated acini are lined by one to several

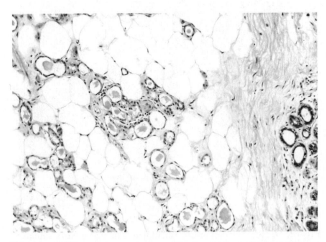

Figure 9.31. Microglandular adenosis (MGA). Haphazardly ar-ranged tubules, containing eosinophilic periodic acid-Schiff (PAS)–positive secretions, are lined by a single layer of cytologically benign luminal epithelium. The myoepithelial mantle is absent, whereas in the adjacent ducts and acini a myoepithelial layer is apparent.

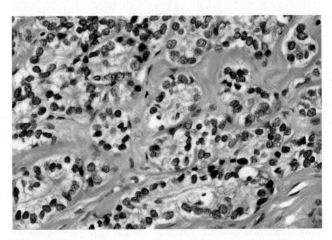

Figure 9.33. Atypia in microglandular adenosis. Atypical hyperpla-sia of the epithelium in MGA can be mistaken for invasive cancer.

layers of epithelial cells, which are usually columnar in shape and which display low-grade cytologic atypia (Fig. 9.19). Observational studies have suggested that at least some FEAs may represent either a precursor of ductal carcinoma in situ (DCIS) or early DCIS. However, the few follow-up studies of these lesions suggest that the risk of local recurrence or progression to invasive carcinoma is extremely low (37).

EPITHELIAL HYPERPLASIA

The term *epithelial hyperplasia* indicates a proliferation of epithelial cells within pre-existing glandular structures. *Ductal epithelial hyperplasia* is synonymous with *intraductal hyperplasia, epitheliosis, hyperplasia of usual type,* and *usual ductal hyperplasia* (UDH). The latter is the term used in the most recent World Health Organization classification (46). No universally recognized entity is termed *lobular hyperplasia.* The distinction between benign ductal epithelial hyperplasia and other intraductal epithelial proliferative lesions (ADH, DCIS) is sometimes problematic, and the diagnosis of ductal epithelial hyperplasia can raise some of the most difficult problems in the study of breast pathology (Table 9.12). It must be accepted, however, that a gray area exists about which even the most experienced pathologists do not always agree. This has been emphasized by a study showing considerable disagreement in the evaluation of a small group of such lesions by pathologists with a particular interest and experience in breast pathology (56). However, agreement can be improved if carefully defined histologic criteria are used (57). Although ancillary techniques, including assessment of proliferative activity, morphometry, and immunohistochemistry with various antibodies (particularly antibodies to high–molecular-weight cytokeratins, such as cytokeratins 5 and 6), have shown some overall differences between the groups, they do not allow clear separation in individual cases.

Usual Ductal Hyperplasia

UDH varies in extent from a few foci to widespread involvement of large areas of glandular tissue. The degree of hyperplasia within each glandular structure also varies. Several systems for grading the degree of hyperplasia have been described on the assumption that a spectrum of changes exists, ranging from normal to hyperplasia to atypia to carcinoma in situ (58). However, the concept that progression through these stages, both histologically and biologically, occurs is not accepted by all (59). Certain architectural and cytologic features are characteristic of DCIS, and these hallmarks must be present before a diagnosis of carcinoma in situ can be made. It is probable that even though some hyperplastic lesions are committed to developing into an invasive carcinoma, others are merely markers of an increased risk for the subsequent development of invasive malignancy and never actually progress themselves.

The changes seen in UDH range from mild hyperplasia, in which the proliferating epithelium is more than two cells but no more than four cells thick, to moderate hyperplasia, marked by considerable encroachment and bridging of the lumen (Fig. 9.34), to florid hyperplasia, with distention and obliteration of the lumen (Fig. 9.35). The differentiation of UDH from carcinoma in situ rests on a variety of features, listed in Table 9.10.

Low-power features characteristic of benign hyperplasia include the following:

1. The spaces between the proliferating cells are irregular and often slitlike, and they appear "compressible" (Fig. 9.34). They are frequently concentrated around the periphery of the glandlike space. Micropapillary projections, if present, are elongated (often tapering) or tuftlike, and they can resemble the pattern of hyperplasia seen in gynecomastia (60). The occasional presence of stromal cores results in true papillary structures. Islands of stroma may be seen within a solid

TABLE 9.12	**Contrasting Features of Epithelial Hyperplasia (Epitheliosis) and Ductal Carcinoma in Situ**	
	Epithelial Hyperplasia	*Well-Differentiated/Low-Grade Ductal Carcinoma in Situ*
Pattern	Varied	Recognized patterns of ductal carcinoma in situ
Spaces	Irregular, slitlike, mainly peripheral	Regular, rounded, rigid throughout space
Bridges	Long axis of nuclei parallel to bridge	Long axis of nuclei haphazard or at right angles ("Roman arches")
Streaming pattern	Yes (sometimes subtle)	No
Cells	Polymorphic; myoepithelial,[a] Lymphocytes Peripheral myoepithelial layer often obvious, sometimes hyperplastic	Monotonous; epithelial cells are the proliferating layer (except peripheral myoepithelium, which may be stretched, attenuated, incomplete, and inconspicuous. Non-proliferative)
Apocrine metaplasia	May be focally present	Absent[b]
Cell margins	Often indistinct	Usually more defined
Nuclear morphology	No malignant features	Malignant features present but may be subtle
Nuclear spacing	Irregular, often overlapping	Evenly spread
Necrosis/hemorrhage	Rare	May be present, sometimes marked
Periductal fibrosis and inflammation	Uncommon	May be present, sometimes marked
Adjacent changes	May merge with other benign lesions	May be adjacent to benign lesions but does not merge (except for multiple papillomas; see text)

[a]The spindle-shaped cells, although termed *myoepithelial*, do *not* show positive staining with α-actin.
[b]In situ carcinoma with apocrine features does occur but usually involves the whole lesion, and the cells have obvious malignant features.

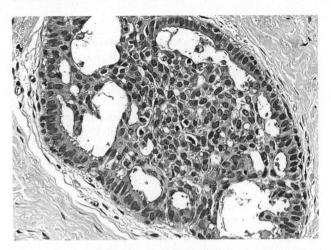

Figure 9.34. Usual ductal hyperplasia. The proliferating epithelial cells are polymorphic, and the nuclei seem to touch and mold in some areas. The intercellular spaces are irregular in both size and shape.

proliferation of epithelium. Stromal cores, or islands, are always lined by a myoepithelial layer.
2. The cells are unevenly arranged. In some areas, the nuclei are densely crowded; in others, they are more widely separated.
3. Necrosis and hemorrhage are rare.
4. Periductal stromal changes, such as fibrosis, elastosis, and chronic inflammation, are uncommon.

High-power features characteristic of benign hyperplasia include the following:

1. Cell and nuclear size, shape, and placement vary. A polymorphic cell population consists of epithelium, spindle-shaped "myoepithelial" cells, and varying numbers of lymphocytes and histiocytes.
2. Apocrine metaplasia is often present. This is usually focal, but hyperplastic lesions composed entirely of apocrine cells also occur. As discussed previously, the cytologic appearance

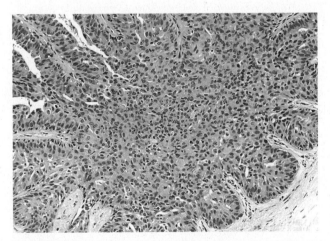

Figure 9.35. Usual ductal hyperplasia. A duct is virtually occluded by a solid sheet of cells. Occasional irregular spaces are present, particularly in the upper half of the field. The polymorphic nature of the cells is evident, with a mixture of round and spindle-shaped nuclei. The latter are aligned to give an impression of "streaming" in some areas.

of apocrine cells can be worrisome, but carcinoma should not be diagnosed without unequivocal evidence of malignancy.
3. The nuclei of proliferating cells are often parallel to one another; this arrangement creates the impression of "streaming" (Fig. 9.35).
4. When epithelial bridges form, the nuclei of the proliferating cells lie parallel to the line of the bridge, and the bridges often taper in the center.
5. Cytologic features of malignancy are absent. In particular, nucleoli are inconspicuous and mitoses are infrequent. Abnormal mitotic figures are not seen.

Some features, such as microcalcification and foam cells, are seen in both benign and malignant lesions; in our experience, they are of no help in distinguishing between the two.

In the differential diagnosis of UDH and carcinoma in situ, all the features listed must be taken into account because no single feature is conclusive.

Atypical Ductal Hyperplasia

The term *atypical ductal hyperplasia* has been poorly defined in the past, with the result that its significance, particularly in terms of risk for subsequent carcinoma, has been unclear. Careful studies have attempted to resolve the problem by more clearly defining the histologic appearance of *atypical hyperplasia* (61,62). As originally described, it is an unusual entity, but it is probably currently overdiagnosed. The diagnosis should be made only when lesions have some of the features of DCIS but fall short of the fully developed picture. Both architectural and cytologic features should be taken into account. However, the diagnostic criteria for atypical hyperplasia of ductal type are not yet precisely defined. This is partly because neither DCIS nor ADH is a single histologic entity; rather, each encompasses a variety of patterns so that strict histologic criteria are difficult to define. It also remains to be established whether ADH is a step in a progression between hyperplasia and carcinoma in situ, or whether it merely comprises a variety of patterns in which benignity and malignancy cannot be distinguished with certainty. This may be because the features of in situ carcinoma are not fully developed within individual glandular components. Follow-up studies indicate that some patients with ADH will progress to develop lesions recognizable as DCIS or invasive cancer. The use of the ADH term to describe DCIS lesions of limited extent remains controversial as well. Page and Rodgers (62) stated that when diagnostic features of DCIS are present, they must be seen in at least two glandular spaces; otherwise, they are classified as ADH lesions. On the other hand, Tavassoli and Norris (63) considered that when diagnostic features of DCIS exist, the area involved should be at least 2 mm in extent, regardless of the number of ducts involved, before the diagnosis of DCIS is applied; if less than 2 mm in extent, the term ADH was used. Follow-up data are consistent with the notion that minimal areas of DCIS, however defined, have the same prognosis as larger DCIS lesions.

The risk for subsequent invasive carcinoma is discussed later; the fact that this risk applies to both breasts is compelling evidence that ADH is indeed different from DCIS, in which the subsequent risk is highest in the contiguous area (64).

To summarize, the term *atypical ductal hyperplasia* should be applied only to lesions in which the diagnosis of carcinoma

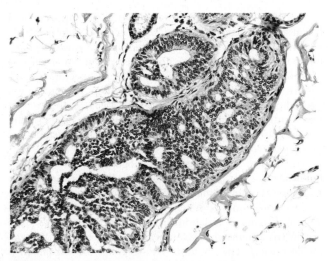

Figure 9.36. Atypical ductal hyperplasia. The periphery of the proliferating epithelium has a cribriform pattern, and the cells are relatively uniform. However, in central areas the cells are more irregularly arranged, with areas of nuclear crowding and overlapping, and the cell margins are indistinct.

in situ is seriously considered, but in which the features are insufficiently developed for a definite diagnosis of DCIS to be made (Figs. 9.36 and 9.37). Much work remains to be done in this area.

IN SITU CARCINOMA

The term *in situ carcinoma* is used to describe a proliferation of presumably malignant epithelial cells that remain confined by a basement membrane. The significance of this arrangement lies in the fact that no lymphatics or blood vessels are present in the epithelial layer, so metastatic spread cannot occur until malignant cells cross the basement membrane. This classic view

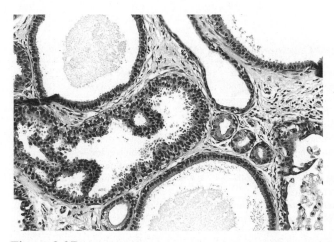

Figure 9.37. Atypical ductal hyperplasia. In this example, the duct in the center of the field shows epithelial proliferation protruding as arches. Even though the cells are uniform, they are irregularly arranged, with crowding and overlapping. These latter features, together with involvement of just this one duct, in a lobule, leads to a diagnosis of atypical hyperplasia.

has been modified in the light of electron microscopic and immunohistochemical findings, which have shown both a discontinuous basement membrane and the occasional extension of cells across the membrane (65,66). Nevertheless, the division into in situ and infiltrating carcinoma on the basis of light microscopy studies continues to be of significant clinical value. When the diagnosis of carcinoma in situ is made, it is always important to exclude the presence of small foci of invasive carcinoma by examining multiple blocks of tissue and, if any suspect areas are found, multiple levels. Most in situ carcinomas are detected either by mammography or as an incidental finding in tissue adjacent to a palpable benign lesion. Sometimes, however, DCIS may produce a mass or present as Paget disease of the nipple or a nipple discharge. In situ carcinoma is divided into ductal and lobular types, based on the architectural and cytologic features of the proliferation rather than on its anatomic location within the ductal–lobular system because it is thought that both types arise from the TDLU.

DUCTAL CARCINOMA IN SITU

Recognition is growing of the heterogeneous nature of DCIS in terms of clinical features, histology, biology, and, most importantly, clinical behavior. Traditionally, DCIS has been subclassified on the basis of architectural pattern rather than cytologic features. However, such classification has proven unsatisfactory for several reasons. Although small lesions may show only one pattern, larger lesions frequently show considerable variation from slide to slide, within one slide, and even sometimes within a single involved TDLU or individual glandular component. Furthermore, the criteria are subjective and poorly defined, and interobserver variation is considerable. These facts are reflected in the varying incidence rates for the different subtypes in reported series of DCIS, and they may account for the differences in the incidence rates of subsequent invasive carcinoma reported for the various subtypes of DCIS in patients undergoing treatment with less than mastectomy. Because DCIS is being diagnosed more frequently, largely as a consequence of the increased use of mammography in breast cancer screening programs, it is becoming urgent that the biologic implications of such a diagnosis are understood (67,68). The increased use of conservation therapy for invasive carcinoma has led to a call for similar treatment for in situ carcinoma. Numerous trials are currently under way to evaluate the best treatment for DCIS but, to gain the most benefit from these studies, it is imperative that more attention be paid to the different histologic features of DCIS, both to understand its biology and to devise a more reproducible classification.

Although several studies suggest that recurrence following DCIS treated by conservation therapy is more frequent in patients with high-grade, poorly differentiated lesions (69–72), some reports indicate that recurrence in patients with low-grade, well-differentiated DCIS increases with a longer follow-up (73,74).

Although any new classification should attempt to reflect the biology of in situ carcinoma, it is also essential that the classification adopted be not only clinically relevant but also readily reproducible among different groups of pathologists.

Within the existing classification, clear differences are found between the major patterns. The most notable of these are nuclear grade, the presence or absence of necrosis, and the presence or absence of architectural differentiation (cell polarization). In addition, the evaluation of several biologic markers, such as proliferative activity, estrogen and progesterone receptor status, and oncoprotein production, suggests that biologic differences correlate with the histologic features (75).

Initial attempts to improve the classification divided DCIS into two broad groups, termed variously *comedo* and *noncomedo*, *high-grade* and *low-grade*, and *large cell* and *small cell*. However, evidence is increasing that division into two categories is an oversimplification, and several proposed systems divide DCIS into three categories (Table 9.13). Most of these are based on cytonuclear grade and the presence or absence of necrosis, but in one classification the secondary feature is the presence or absence of architectural differentiation, as manifested by the polarization of cells. Thus, general agreement has been reached in regard to the category that includes lesions with the least differentiated nuclei. The debate centers around whether division of the better differentiated lesions should be based on the presence or absence of necrosis or cell polarization or only on cytonuclear features. Lagios (76) was the first to emphasize the value of nuclear grade in the classification of DCIS, and he used a combination of nuclear grade, architectural growth pattern, and necrosis to define four categories, later contracted to three (76). In a selected group of patients, the risk for local recurrence following lumpectomy was significantly greater after the excision of high-grade lesions than after the excision of low-grade lesions. In Nottingham, DCIS was divided into pure comedo DCIS, DCIS with necrosis (non–pure comedo), and DCIS without necrosis (71). These two systems were used in the development of the Van Nuys classification, which includes all cases with poorly differentiated nuclei in a high-grade group; the remaining cases of non–high-grade DCIS are divided according to the presence or absence of necrosis (69). A group of European pathologists proposed classifying DCIS into poorly, intermediately, and well-differentiated groups (77). Division is based primarily on cytonuclear differentiation and secondarily on architectural differentiation—which refers to the polarization of cells around intercellular spaces within the ductal lumen and over the surface of papillae. It has yet to be ascertained which of the aforementioned classifications will be the most widely accepted.

At a 1997 consensus conference (78), it was suggested that because all the major classifications reflect nuclear grade, DCIS should be categorized primarily according to nuclear grade, but that other features (particularly the presence or absence of necrosis and cellular polarization and the architectural growth pattern) should also be recorded. In addition, margins, lesion size, microcalcification associated with DCIS, correlation of DCIS with specimen x-ray and mammographic findings, and the presence of any microinvasion should all be documented in the pathology report.

The nuclear grade is usually homogeneous within a lesion but, when it is not, the proportion of each grade and the size and amount of the highest grade or percentage relevant to the entire lesion should be stated. High-grade nuclei are pleomorphic, with marked variation in size and shape, and they are usually large (more than 2.5 times the size of normal duct epithelial nuclei). The contours are irregular; the chromatin is coarse and irregularly distributed or vesicular; and the nucleoli are prominent and often multiple. Mitoses are usually present and often numerous. Low-grade nuclei are rounded and uniform in size and shape, and they are monotonous and monomorphic in appearance. Even though they are larger than those of the normal breast (1.5 to 2 times the size of normal duct epithelial nuclei), they are usually smaller than high-grade nuclei. The nuclear contour is smooth and rounded or oval; the chromatin is diffuse and fine; and the nucleoli are inconspicuous or absent. These features, together with the uniform spacing of the cells, give the lesions a strikingly monotonous appearance. Mitoses are few or absent. Intermediate-grade nuclei are the most difficult to define. Although they are pleomorphic, they do not show such marked variation in shape, size, and outline as high-grade nuclei. The size is usually intermediate; the chromatin is fine to coarse; nucleoli, although evident, are not prominent; and mitoses, although often present, are not frequent.

Necrosis should be carefully assessed and not confused with secretion or apoptosis. By definition, ghost cells and karyorrhectic debris should be present. Comedo-type necrosis consists of a central zone of necrosis within a duct. Punctate necrosis is not zonal.

TABLE 9.13	**Proposed Classifications for Ductal Carcinoma in Situ (DCIS)**		
Lagios (70)	**High-grade DCIS**	**Intermediate-grade DCIS**	**Low-grade DCIS**
	High nuclear grade	Intermediate nuclear grade	Low nuclear grade
	Comedo necrosis	Punctate necrosis	Necrosis absent
Nottingham (72)	**Pure comedo DCIS**	**DCIS with necrosis**	**DCIS without necrosis**
	Central comedo necrosis surrounding sheets of large pleomorphic cells	Central necrosis Noncomedo surrounding pattern	Necrosis absent
Van Nuys (69)	**High-grade DCIS**	**Non–high-grade DCIS with necrosis**	**Non–high-grade DCIS without necrosis**
	High nuclear grade	Non–high nuclear grade	Non–high nuclear grade
		Necrosis present	Necrosis absent
Holland and Hendricks (European Working Group) (79)	**Poorly differentiated DCIS**	**Intermediately differentiated DCIS**	**Well-differentiated DCIS**
	Poorly differentiated nuclei	Intermediately differentiated nuclei	Well-differentiated nuclei
	Cellular polarization minimal or absent	Cellular polarization present, not prominent	Cellular polarization prominent
NHSBSP/EEC (77)	**High-grade DCIS**	**Intermediate-grade DCIS**	**Low-grade DCIS**
	High nuclear grade	Intermediate nuclear grade	Low nuclear grade

DCIS, ductal carcinoma in situ; EEC, European Economic Community; NHSBSP, National Health Service Breast Screening Programme.

Architectural differentiation (cell polarization) is the feature used in the DCIS classification described by Holland et al. (77). It is defined as polarization or radial orientation of the apices of the tumor cells toward intercellular spaces. A series of such formations results in a true cribriform pattern. Sometimes the intercellular spaces, or lumina, are very small, or cellular orientation is present without the formation of a true lumen, so that a rosette-like appearance results that may be seen in the solid pattern of DCIS. Polarization over cellular protuberances and bridges and over micropapillae is seen in the true micropapillary and clinging patterns of DCIS. Although the apices of the cells covering the cellular protrusions are oriented toward the duct lumen, polarization is not always as easy to see in these latter patterns as it is in the cribriform and solid patterns. Architectural differentiation usually parallels nuclear differentiation; it is minimal or absent in DCIS composed of cells of high nuclear grade but marked in DCIS composed of cells of low nuclear grade.

The architectural growth pattern should be described as comedo, solid, cribriform, papillary, micropapillary, or clinging. According to the criteria of Holland et al. (77), a true cribriform or micropapillary pattern is seen only when cell polarization is present. The appearance resembling a cribriform or micropapillary pattern, sometimes seen in DCIS of high nuclear grade, is usually a pseudopattern because cell polarization is absent.

The assessment of surgical margins and extent of disease is also of extreme importance.

High-Grade Ductal Carcinoma in Situ, Poorly Differentiated Ductal Carcinoma in Situ, Comedo Ductal Carcinoma in Situ

The distinction between DCIS with cells of high nuclear grade and benign disease does not usually present a problem because the component cells of DCIS have overt malignant features. Architectural differentiation (cell polarization), as described by Holland et al. (77), is usually absent or minimal, although it may be present around a few intercellular spaces. Central comedo-type necrosis is generally associated with high-grade nuclei and is a defining feature in some classifications, but not others (Table 9.13, Fig. 9.38). Necrosis is occasionally so extensive that

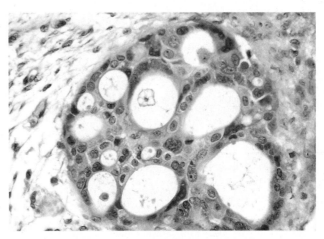

Figure 9.39. Ductal carcinoma in situ, poorly differentiated, high-grade type. This example shows pseudocribriform architecture and no necrosis. However, the malignant cells are large and pleomorphic, with coarse, clumped nuclear chromatin.

only a few cells are seen at the periphery of the glandular lumen. Such lesions form part of the spectrum of DCIS with a clinging pattern. Some classifications accept that the malignant cells occasionally produce a solid sheet filling the duct lumen without central necrosis. Alternatively, the cells may grow in a pseudocribriform or pseudomicropapillary pattern (without cell polarization) (Fig. 9.39). Autophagocytosis is frequently seen within sheets of malignant cells. The calcification, so often found within the central necrotic material, is amorphous and generally produces a typical branching, linear, or casting pattern on mammograms that is usually diagnostic of malignancy (79) (Fig. 9.5). The involved ducts may be very distended, and this type of DCIS is often quite large and may result in a palpable abnormality in the breast. This is partly a consequence of the surrounding stromal reaction, which is usually more evident in this pattern of DCIS than in others. Cancerization of the lobules is frequent. When present, Paget disease of the nipple is almost invariably associated with DCIS composed of cells with high-grade nuclei.

Low-Grade Ductal Carcinoma in Situ, Well-Differentiated Ductal Carcinoma in Situ

This type of DCIS is at the other end of the spectrum of classifications based primarily on nuclear grade. Most cases of the Van Nuys non–high-grade DCIS without necrosis and the Nottingham DCIS without necrosis probably fall into this category. DCIS composed of cells of low nuclear grade is sometimes difficult to differentiate from ductal epithelial hyperplasia. The most striking feature is the monotonous appearance of the cells. The growth pattern of most lesions of this group is true cribriform (Fig. 9.40), micropapillary (Fig. 9.41), or, less frequently, solid (Fig. 9.42). Prominent, uniform cell polarization (architectural differentiation) is seen. In the cribriform pattern, lumina between the proliferating cells are geometric, punched out, rigid, and rounded (Fig. 9.40), and they are usually evenly distributed within the cell masses. The cells within the center of the proliferating strands forming the bridges and arcades are arranged regularly or lie at a right angle to the plane of the cellular strands. In the micropapillary pattern, proliferating cells extend into the lumen of the glandular structure, but with-

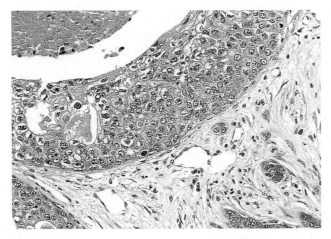

Figure 9.38. Ductal carcinoma in situ, poorly differentiated, high-grade type with a comedo pattern. The proliferating malignant cells are large and pleomorphic, and a central area of necrosis can be seen at the top of the figure.

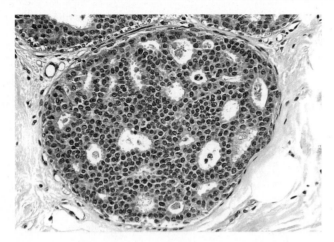

Figure 9.40. Ductal carcinoma in situ, well-differentiated, low-grade type with a cribriform pattern. The malignant cells are polarized around sharply defined spaces. The cells are relatively small and monomorphic. The overall appearance is monotonous.

out a fibrovascular stalk. The papillae frequently have a clublike appearance, and cells are evenly distributed within them (Fig. 9.41), but the micropapillae may join to form lumens, which are less regular in size and shape and more slitlike than in a true cribriform pattern. Occasionally, true papillae with fibrovascular cores are associated with the micropapillae. Small rosettes of cells with surface polarization, apparently separated from the papillae, are often seen floating free within the duct lumen. When the growth pattern is solid, a pattern of small, incompletely formed intercellular spaces with polarization of

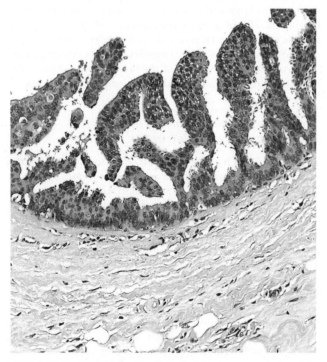

Figure 9.41. Ductal carcinoma in situ, well-differentiated, low-grade type with a micropapillary pattern. The proliferating cells protrude as fronds into the duct lumen, some producing a clublike appearance that lacks a fibrovascular core.

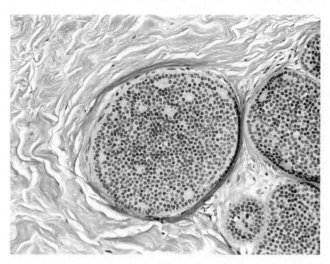

Figure 9.42. Ductal carcinoma in situ, well-differentiated, low-grade type with a solid pattern. The duct is completely obliterated by relatively small neoplastic cells that have a uniform, monotonous appearance. In some areas, polarization of cells is evident, producing a microacinar or rosette-like appearance.

the surrounding cells usually results in a rosette-like appearance (Fig. 9.42). Necrosis is rarely associated with cells of low nuclear grade, and its absence is one of the defining features of some classifications, but the presence of small, focal areas of necrosis is allowed in others (Table 9.13). However, secretions are frequently seen within the duct lumen and should not be mistaken for necrosis. Calcification is not as frequent as in poorly differentiated DCIS and, when present, it is usually rounded and laminated or psammomatous and deposited within the secretions. Such calcification produces clusters of granular, sandlike particles on mammograms (Fig. 9.6), but this pattern is not as distinctive as that of the calcification seen in poorly differentiated, high-grade DCIS, in that similar patterns may also occur in benign lesions (70). Some patterns of well-differentiated DCIS are difficult to distinguish from lobular carcinoma in situ (LCIS). Furthermore, some in situ carcinomas may show mixed ductal and lobular features.

Intermediate-Grade Ductal Carcinoma in Situ, Intermediately Differentiated Ductal Carcinoma in Situ

The third type of DCIS in classifications based primarily on a three-tier nuclear grade system is composed of cells with intermediate-grade nuclei. Its features are intermediate between those of high-grade, poorly differentiated types and low-grade, well-differentiated types. In the classification of Holland et al. (77), the presence of cell polarization is important, although this is not as prominent and uniform as in the well-differentiated type (Fig. 9.43). The growth pattern varies and may be solid, cribriform (Fig. 9.43), micropapillary, or clinging. Necrosis may or may not be present. Calcification, when present, may be laminated or amorphous (77).

In the Van Nuys and Nottingham classifications, the presence or absence of necrosis is the defining feature that divides the non–high-grade types of DCIS.

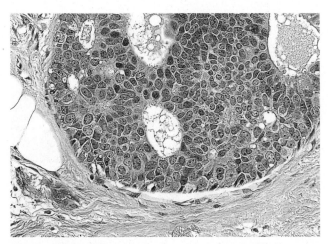

Figure 9.43. Ductal carcinoma in situ, intermediately differentiated, intermediate grade with a cribriform pattern. Although evident, the polarization of cells around spaces is not as marked, and the nuclear pleomorphism is greater than that in low-grade, well-differentiated cases.

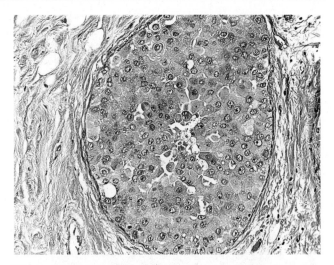

Figure 9.44. Ductal carcinoma in situ, apocrine type. The cells in this example of ductal carcinoma in situ possess abundant eosinophilic cytoplasm.

Clinging Ductal Carcinoma in Situ

The terms *clinging DCIS* and *clinging carcinoma* have been applied to two histologically distinct lesions, both characterized by one or two cell layers confined to the periphery of the involved spaces. In the first lesion, the cells lining the involved spaces have high-grade nuclei. In these cases, central necrosis may be evident, and such lesions are examples of poorly differentiated DCIS (80,81). Other lesions included in the category of clinging DCIS by some authorities (80,81) are composed of smaller, more uniform cells with low-grade nuclei, characteristic of well-differentiated DCIS. In many such lesions, the cells are columnar. Although lesions of this type are sometimes seen in conjunction with low-grade DCIS that has a cribriform or micropapillary pattern, they are being encountered with increasing frequency as isolated lesions in breast biopsy specimens obtained to assess mammographic microcalcifications. This pattern is not universally recognized as representing fully developed DCIS, and some consider it to be part of the spectrum of ADH (61,62) or columnar cell hyperplasia with atypia (45). Such lesions do not appear to be associated with as high a risk for breast cancer as fully developed forms of low-grade DCIS (81,82).

Apocrine Ductal Carcinoma in Situ

Apocrine change within DCIS is not unusual and is probably underrecognized in lesions diagnosed as DCIS. The same criteria applied in the diagnosis of nonapocrine DCIS should be used, and in most cases this does not present a problem (Fig. 9.44). Occasionally, however, benign apocrine hyperplasia may have a worrisome appearance, and the differential diagnosis with DCIS is difficult. In our view, DCIS should be diagnosed only when the characteristic cytologic and architectural features are present.

An intermediate category of intraductal apocrine lesions has been suggested. O'Malley et al. (83) use nuclear features and lesion extent to define a borderline category between usual apocrine lesions and well-differentiated, low-grade apocrine DCIS. Tavassoli and Norris (84) also use quantitative criteria to measure nuclear size, degree of hyperplasia, and lesion extent to define four groups of lesions: atypical apocrine metaplasia; atypical apocrine hyperplasia; poorly differentiated, high-grade (necrotic) DCIS; and well-differentiated, low-grade (nonnecrotic) DCIS.

Neuroendocrine (Argyrophilic) Ductal Carcinoma in Situ

A solid pattern of DCIS with neuroendocrine histologic features has been recognized (85,86). Such lesions are usually seen in elderly patients, who often present with a blood-stained nipple discharge. The involved glandular elements are often markedly distended. The proliferating cells have a polygonal, oval, or spindle morphologic appearance and granular eosinophilic cytoplasm with intervening fibrovascular cores and septa. Rosettes and ribbons may be evident, as may mucin production and microglandular spaces (87). In some examples, the component cells are a mixture of spindle cells and argyrophilic signet ring cells (87) (Fig. 9.45). Because of the frequent lack of overt cytologic atypia, this type of DCIS can easily be misdiagnosed as benign. Small foci of invasive carcinoma are present in a significant number of cases, and in one series, invasion was associated with endocrine DCIS in 20 of 34 cases. In another 18 cases, nearby papillomas were colonized by endocrine DCIS (78). "Solid papillary carcinoma" of the breast would appear to be related to, if not identical with, neuroendocrine DCIS (88).

Signet Ring Cell Ductal Carcinoma in Situ

In situ ductal carcinomas consisting predominantly of signet ring cells have been described (89). However, signet ring cell formation is probably more commonly seen in in situ lobular carcinomas.

Cystic Hypersecretory Ductal Carcinoma in Situ

This is an uncommon pattern of DCIS (90). The gross appearance is characteristic, consisting of cysts filled with viscid mate-

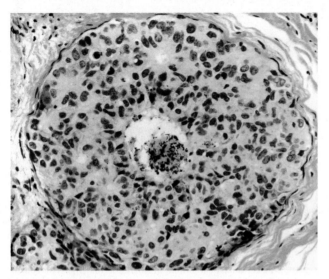

Figure 9.45. Ductal carcinoma in situ, endocrine type. The cells are pleomorphic and there is central necrosis. Pseudorosettes are formed by the proliferating cells. Immunostain for synaptophysin was positive.

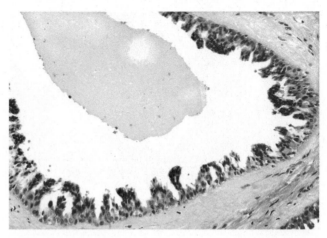

Figure 9.47. Ductal carcinoma in situ, cystic hypersecretory type. In this high-power view, the distinctive micropapillary pattern of the neoplastic epithelium is evident surrounding the central secretions.

rial. Microscopic examination reveals multiple cyst-like structures containing homogeneous eosinophilic material that resembles thyroid colloid. Some are lined by histologically benign, flat, or columnar epithelium. Others, unlike simple cysts, have a lining epithelium that shows various degrees of hyperplasia, with foci of DCIS that have a micropapillary or cribriform pattern. The lining cells may exhibit secretory activity, with features reminiscent of the lactating breast (Figs. 9.46 and 9.47). Stains for mucin show focal positivity within the epithelial cells; most of the cyst contents are negative. This lesion can easily be overlooked and should be borne in mind when apparently

benign cysts are examined. Occasionally, hyperplasia is seen without fully developed carcinoma in situ. Such lesions are termed *cystic hypersecretory hyperplasia* (91).

DCIS WITH BASAL-LIKE PHENOTYPE

Bryan, Schnitt, and Collins (92) identified a group of DCIS cases that were negative for estrogen receptor, progesterone receptor, and HER2/*neu* (triple-negative) and expressed basal cytokeratins, epidermal growth factor receptor (EGFR), or both, and suggested that they might represent precursors to invasive basal-like carcinomas. Livasy et al. (93) studied 245 cases of pure DCIS and found 61% to be Luminal A type (ER+, HER2−), 9% Luminal B (ER+, HER2+), 16% HER2 (HER2+, ER−) and 8% to be basal-like (ER−, HER2−, EGFR+, and/or cytokeratin 5/6+). The basal-like lesions were associated with unfavorable prognostic markers, including high-grade nuclei, p53 overexpression, and elevated Ki-67 index.

DUCTAL CARCINOMA IN SITU INVOLVING LOBULES (CANCERIZATION OF LOBULES)

When DCIS is extensive, it is frequently seen within obviously lobular structures (Fig. 9.48). The term *cancerization of lobules* has been used to describe this finding. It is nearly always associated with one of the typical patterns of DCIS previously described, but very occasionally it occurs alone. The appearance should not be misinterpreted as invasive carcinoma, a possibility that is enhanced when the process is further complicated by the presence of sclerosing adenosis (94,95). The differentiation from invasive carcinoma and the differentiation of lobular cancerization by DCIS from LCIS are discussed later.

EXCLUDING INVASIVE CARCINOMA

In all cases of in situ carcinoma, it is important that the lesional tissue be examined thoroughly to exclude small foci of invasion, but invasion should not be diagnosed unless the evidence is unequivocal. Some authorities report invasion only when the interlobular stroma is involved and not when the only apparent invasion is basement membrane disruption within lobular

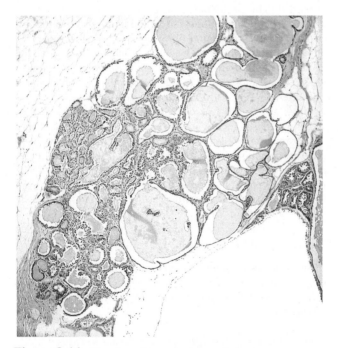

Figure 9.46. Ductal carcinoma in situ, cystic hypersecretory type. Multiple glandular structures show varying degrees of dilation and contain homogeneous material resembling thyroid colloid.

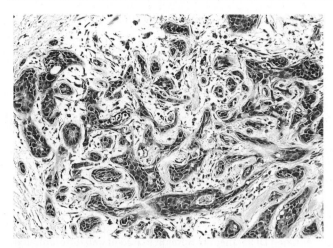

Figure 9.48. Lobular cancerization by ductal carcinoma in situ in an area of sclerosing adenosis. The overall lobular architecture is retained. The acinar pattern is disturbed by the sclerosing process and further distorted and distended by cohesive sheets of moderately large, pleomorphic malignant cells. This pattern of cancerization is particularly prone to misinterpretation as invasion. Elsewhere, typical high-grade, poorly differentiated ductal carcinoma in situ with a comedo pattern was present.

stroma (85). The immunohistochemical demonstration of myoepithelial cells or basement membrane components may be of help in evaluating possible foci of invasion. Small foci of invasion have been found more frequently in extensive DCIS lesions and in those of high nuclear grade (70,76). The presence of microinvasion—invasive foci less than 1 mm in diameter—has little effect on prognosis.

OTHER IMPORTANT FEATURES OF DUCTAL CARCINOMA IN SITU

Following excision, DCIS most often recurs at the site of the previous lesion. This observation indicates that recurrence represents residual disease left behind at the time of initial surgery, and underscores the importance of excision margins in the treatment of DCIS. What comprises a clear margin, however, has not been well defined. The elegant three-dimensional studies of the distribution of DCIS in the mammary tree carried out by Faverly et al. (16) have a significant bearing on the surgical approach to DCIS. These studies have shown that poorly differentiated DCIS nearly always (90% of cases) exhibits a continuous growth pattern, with no gaps between the foci of DCIS. In well-differentiated DCIS, on the other hand, gaps are frequent, with normal epithelium seen between foci of DCIS. The growth pattern is defined as multifocal when the gaps are smaller than

40 mm and multicentric when they are larger than 40 mm. In only one case of DCIS, among 80 studied, were the gaps larger than 40 mm. In most (92%) of the cases of well-differentiated DCIS, the gaps were smaller than 10 mm. This means that a 10-mm surgical margin will theoretically guarantee clearance in most cases. These and other studies (96,97) negate the previously held view that DCIS is a multicentric process in most cases. When cases of DCIS are examined, the width of the nearest surgical margin should be recorded by the pathologist.

In addition to type of DCIS and the clearance margins, the size of a lesion may play a major role in dictating the most appropriate therapy for DCIS. These features are interrelated to some extent, in that low-grade, well-differentiated DCIS is more likely to be small and circumscribed, so that excision is easier, whereas high-grade, poorly differentiated DCIS is more often extensive and, in practice, more often incompletely excised. One exception to this general rule is DCIS with a micropapillary architectural pattern; studies have found that lesions with this pattern, regardless of nuclear grade, are frequently large (72,98). Furthermore, well-differentiated, low-grade DCIS is more likely to lack calcification, so the extent of the lesion on a mammogram is more difficult to define. Also, as mentioned, three-dimensional studies have shown that the growth pattern is usually discontinuous, so the assessment of excision is more difficult. When calcification is present within DCIS, mammographic assessment of the extent of the lesion can be helpful in planning surgery. In earlier studies, Holland et al. (86) found that the mammographic extent and histologic extent were more consistent in poorly differentiated than in well-differentiated lesions. With "state-of-the-art" mammography, however, such discrepancies have become less apparent (79). Evaluation of the extent of DCIS can be difficult because several adjacent sections may be involved. Careful correlation of the histologic with the gross examination findings and, when available, the results of specimen radiology is essential. Advocates of large, whole-mount sections claim that this is an area in which the technique can be of particular value. The evaluation of margins can also raise major problems in that no definition of a negative, close, or involved margin has been accepted. From a practical point of view, it is best to consider a margin positive when DCIS touches the surgical margin. In other situations, the distance between the edge of the DCIS and the margins should be recorded in millimeters or fractions thereof.

Silverstein et al. (99) proposed a prognostic index for DCIS based on histologic type, excision margin, and tumor size (Van Nuys prognostic index) (Table 9.14). They found that all three features were related independently to recurrence, but when the scores for each feature were combined, a stronger prognostic indicator was obtained. Each feature is scored from 1 through 3, and the scores are added together to give a combined

TABLE 9.14	Van Nuys Prognostic Index for Ductal Carcinoma in Situ		
	Score		
Feature	*1*	*2*	*3*
Lesion size	≤15 mm	16–40 mm	>40 mm
Margin	≥10 mm	1–9 mm	<1 mm
Histology	Non–high grade without necrosis	Non–high grade with necrosis	High grade

score from 3 through 9. However, in a more recent study from this group, neither lesion size nor histology provided additional prognostic information in patients with a margin width of more than 10 mm, suggesting that margin status is the most important of these three factors (100).

Through the years, many studies of biologic marker expression in DCIS have been carried out. The most recent studies have used immunohistochemical methods to demonstrate marker expression. Although the application of histologic classification, antibodies, and scoring methods has not been consistent, the results have shown general agreement (75). Poorly differentiated, high-grade DCIS usually has a high proliferation index; frequently expresses the c-*erb*-B2 oncoprotein; and more often expresses p53 protein than other types, but it is more likely to be negative for estrogen and progesterone receptors. Low-grade, well-differentiated DCIS usually has a low proliferative index; rarely expresses either c-*erb*-B2 oncoprotein or p53 protein; and is nearly always positive for estrogen and progesterone receptors. Intermediate types of DCIS show intermediate patterns of marker expression.

Angiogenesis is another feature that has been studied in DCIS. An increase in stromal microvessels has been reported, particularly in high-grade DCIS (101,102). The aforementioned associations underscore the biologic heterogeneity of DCIS. Moreover, the results of one study have indicated that, when used in conjunction with local excision and radiation therapy, tamoxifen significantly reduces the risk for local recurrence only among patients with estrogen receptor–positive DCIS (103). Therefore, determination of the estrogen receptor status of DCIS by immunohistochemistry is now being used with increasing frequency to guide patient management. At the present time, none of the other biologic markers has a clinical role.

Research on genetic alterations in DCIS has also provided new insights into these lesions. Studies have indicated that the number and type of chromosomal alterations differ according to DCIS pattern and grade (104,105). For example, comparative genomic hybridization analysis has been used to show that high-grade DCIS lesions exhibit more numerous chromosomal losses and gains than do low-grade lesions (106). Furthermore, the particular chromosomal loci that are altered appear to vary according to the grade of DCIS, with losses of material on chromosomes 17p and 16q particularly common in low-grade DCIS, gains of 1q and losses of 11q common in intermediate-grade DCIS, and gains of 17q and 11q common in high-grade DCIS (107). It is hoped that further understanding of the genetic and molecular alterations in these lesions will lead to a biologically based classification system of DCIS.

DISTINGUISHING DUCTAL CARCINOMA IN SITU FROM EPITHELIAL HYPERPLASIA

In many cases of DCIS, no diagnostic problem arises; however, on occasion, differentiation from benign intraductal epithelial hyperplasia can be extremely difficult. The distinguishing features have been discussed and are listed in Table 9.10.

To summarize, low-power features suggestive of DCIS are the following:

1. Intercellular spaces and luminal bridges appear "rigid."
2. Necrosis is present.
3. The cells are evenly distributed.

High-power features suggestive of DCIS are the following:

1. Only one cell type is seen (i.e., the population is monomorphic).
2. Foci of apocrine metaplasia are not seen.
3. The nuclei do not show streaming. The nuclei of cells forming bridges or lining spaces are either randomly arranged or are oriented perpendicular to the bridges or radially around the spaces.
4. Cytologic features suggestive of malignancy are usually discernible. Although in well-differentiated, low-grade DCIS nuclear pleomorphism may be minimal, the cells are usually hyperchromatic with at least one prominent nucleolus, and the nuclear-to-cytoplasmic ratio is increased. Mitotic figures are variable. They are frequent in high-grade, poorly differentiated DCIS; they are difficult to find in well-differentiated, low-grade DCIS.

Use of the term *atypical ductal hyperplasia* should be reserved for cases showing some of the aforementioned features but not the full picture of DCIS.

PAPILLARY LESIONS

There are several lesions of the breast with a papillary structure—a fibrovascular core covered by epithelium. Papillomatosis is a diffuse, intraductal lesion with papillary or micropapillary (papillary configuration without the fibrovascular core). Localized intraductal lesions present as grossly evident tumorous masses and include solitary papillomas, multiple papillomas, juvenile papillomatosis and intracystic papillary carcinoma (IPC).

Four categories of papillary carcinoma of the breast have been distinguished: (a) the previously described variants of DCIS—a noninvasive carcinoma extending into the medium and smaller ducts throughout the breast tissue, which is not evident grossly as a single tumor and may be papillary or, more frequently, micropapillary; (b) intracystic papillary carcinoma (IPC), a larger (greater than 5 mm in diameter), grossly evident tumor found mostly in a cystically dilated duct; (c) invasive papillary carcinoma, a rare form of invasive carcinoma characterized by a papillary structure and frequently associated with one of the noninvasive forms. IPC may also infiltrate with a papillary pattern into the duct wall; (d) a fourth type of carcinoma with papillary features is the micropapillary form of invasive carcinoma, often with extensive angiolymphatic invasion, which is discussed below.

INTRADUCTAL PAPILLOMAS

The differential diagnosis of papillomas from IPCs is confounded by the relative rarity and the relatively benign clinical course of the IPC. Papillomas occur in all age groups, in all areas of the breast, and present as lumps, with or without bloody nipple discharge. They can best be found by dissection of the ductal system, as discussed above under "Microdochectomy." Grossly, they may be associated with large- or medium-size ducts to which they are confined (Fig. 9.49). Microscopically, they usually have prominent fibrovascular cores, but they may be

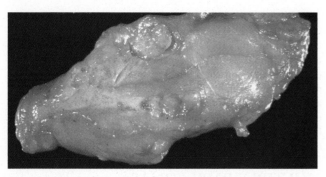

Figure 9.49. A benign intraductal papilloma removed by microdochectomy (see above). The duct has been opened longitudinally and the papilloma appears as a circumscribed nodule.

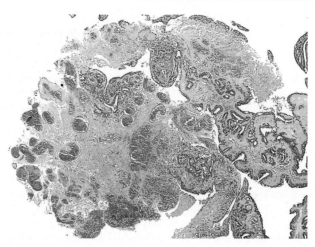

Figure 9.51. A partly infarcted benign intraductal papilloma.

quite cellular and irregular (Fig. 9.50), and they may have all the patterns shown as ductal hyperplasia.

The following are the features most helpful in distinguishing between benign and malignant lesions:

1. Benign papillomas have well-developed fibrovascular cores. In the classic form, these consist of arborescent fronds (Fig. 9.50), but often the papillae are broad and clublike, containing numerous glandular components that result in an adenomatous pattern.
2. The cardinal feature of a benign papillary lesion is the presence of two types of epithelial cell, both covering the fibrovascular core and lining the glandular components within the broader papillae. The myoepithelial layer is variably distinctive but always present. In problematic cases, myoepithelial cells can be highlighted by immunostaining.
3. The luminal epithelium of a benign papilloma may show a variety of changes; epithelial hyperplasia is often present, apocrine metaplasia is frequent, and, rarely, squamous metaplasia occurs.

Infarction of benign papillomas is not uncommon (Fig. 9.51) and may account for the blood-stained nipple discharge (108).

The presence of infarction and hemorrhage is, however, not helpful in distinguishing between benign and malignant lesions.

Some of the most alarming appearances in benign papillomas are produced by intense peripheral fibrosis with subsequent trapping of epithelial elements (Fig. 9.52). This results in a pattern similar to that previously described in other sclerosing lesions and may raise a suspicion of infiltrating carcinoma. The presence of the two cell types (myoepithelium and luminal epithelium) in at least some of the trapped components indicates the benign nature of the lesion. Lesions in which sclerosis is extreme, especially with obliteration of the ductal lumen, have been termed *ductal adenomas*. These are discussed later.

In the differentiation of benign from malignant papillary lesions, careful attention to low- and high-power views is essential. The low-power view indicates (a) the papillary nature of the lesion, and (b) the size of the fibrovascular cores. Usually,

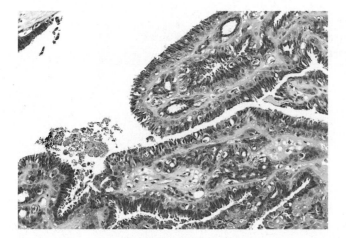

Figure 9.50. A benign intraductal papilloma with arborescent papillary fronds and well-developed fibrovascular cores. These are covered by two cell types—a basal or myoepithelial layer and a luminal epithelial layer, which are readily seen in this example.

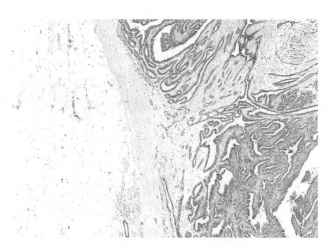

Figure 9.52. Periphery of a benign intraductal papilloma showing fibrosis with trapping of glandular components. Even at this magnification, the papilloma is obviously benign, an important feature in correctly interpreting the sclerotic area at the periphery as entrapment, similar to what is seen in a benign colon polyp. The immunohistochemical demonstration of two cell types (epithelium and myoepithelium) will confirm the benign nature of the lesion.

the outline of an encompassing duct wall can be discerned, even in cases with sclerosis and entrapment of epithelial structures. High-power examination permits an assessment of the other epithelial changes previously described, the most important of which is the presence of two cell types covering the fronds and lining the contained epithelial elements. Finally, the generally benign appearance of the lesion precludes the diagnosis of carcinoma.

Three other points related to the diagnosis of benign papillomas merit mention. First, in the presence of a heavy, blood-stained discharge, organization can occasionally lead to the formation of a so-called granulation tissue polyp. This should not be mistaken for a true papilloma. Second, in sections from the region of the lactiferous sinus, tangential cuts of the tortuous ducts with a pleated contour may give the false impression of a papilloma. Third, partial involvement of a benign papilloma by DCIS does sometimes occur.

In addition to the difficulties and controversy over the diagnosis of intraductal papilloma, and perhaps in part because of these difficulties, uncertainty persists over the precancerous significance of intraductal papillomas. Most authors believe that intraductal papillomas of the breast are rarely associated with invasive carcinoma during the follow-up period. Kraus and Neubecker (109), Hendrick (110), Haagensen et al. (111), Hart (112), and Lewison and Lyons (113) reported a total of 427 cases of intraductal papillomas of the breast in which carcinoma developed during the follow-up period in only two patients (0.4%) during a follow-up that ranged from 5 to 22 years. Three other series of papillomas—by Buhl-Jorgensen et al. (114), Moore et al. (115) and Kilgore et al. (116)—showed the development of cancer in 19 of 235 cases during a follow-up period of 4 months to 16 years. Carter (117) reported on 64 cases of intraductal papillomas of the breast followed for a period of 5 to 17 years. Six recurred as papillomas, and six patients went on to develop breast cancer. Two of the patients who developed carcinoma of the breast were among six with multiple papillomas. In 14 patients, there was distinct hyperplasia or papillomatosis of the associated ducts. Two of these patients developed breast cancer. Among 44 patients in whom there were only nonproliferative cystic changes or fibroadenomas, only 5% developed carcinoma. Rosen (118) reviewed the literature of 612 solitary papillomas treated by excision and found 11 ipsilateral carcinomas (2%), 10 contralateral carcinomas (2%), and 3 bilateral carcinomas (0.3%) in follow-up. He concluded that solitary papillomas were not precancerous. Page et al. (119) conducted a case control study of women with papillomas that contained areas of atypical hyperplasia and found them to have a fourfold increase in risk of cancer compared to women with excision of papillomas that lacked atypia. Table 9.15 lists the features that distinguish papilloma from intracystic papillary carcinoma.

MULTIPLE PAPILLOMAS

Although relatively few cases of multiple papillomas have been reported, there is a strong suggestion from this limited literature that they are significantly precancerous lesions. To distinguish multiple papillomas from papillomatosis, a size cutoff at least 3 mm in diameter has been suggested. Histologically, each of the papillomas has the appearance of solitary papilloma as described above. A fibrovascular core and epithelial/myoepithelial configuration can be discerned. They tend to be cellular and florid but, even in cases with associated invasive carcinoma, atypia may be absent. Associated carcinomas are of any type (mostly invasive ductal) and are not often papillary. Haagensen (111) considered multiple intraductal papillomas to be precancerous. Murad, Contesso and Mourisse (120) reported a high rate of recurrence and malignant transformation in women with multiple papillomas compared to no cancer and only one recurrence among 73 women with solitary papilloma. Ohuchi, Abe, and Kasai (121) reported three-dimensional serial reconstructions of breasts with papillomas in which they found solitary papillomas originating in large ducts, whereas multiple papillomas arose in association with terminal duct/lobular units. Six of 16 (37.5%) of the peripheral or multiple papilloma cases were associated with carcinomas, but none of the nine solitary papillomas that originated centrally was associated with carcinoma. Papotti et al. (122) found similar results.

JUVENILE PAPILLOMATOSIS

In 1980, Rosen et al. (123) described 37 cases of juvenile papillomatosis of the breast in which the average age was 19, with a

TABLE 9.15	Contrasting Features of Benign Papilloma and Intra-cystic Papillary Carcinoma	
	Benign Papilloma	*Papillary Carcinoma*
Fibrovascular cores	Well developed	Usually delicate or absent
Luminal epithelium	May show features of benign hyperplasia with oval nuclei perpendicular to central core	Variable in thickness; sometimes tall
Myoepithelium	Present, usually prominent	Generally absent; occasionally focally present, but no continuous layer
Nuclei	Benign	Malignant features present, but may be subtle; sometimes open and clear
Apocrine metaplasia	Frequent	Rare
Surrounding tissue	Often benign lesions	Ductal carcinoma in situ, or even invasive carcinoma may be present
Clinical presentation	Nipple discharge frequent	Nipple discharge less common; usually presents as a mass

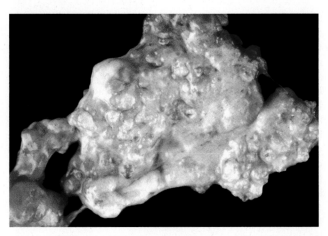

Figure 9.53. Juvenile papillomatosis. This gross photograph shows the nodularity of juvenile papillomatosis. The lesion is made up of multiple papillary structures as well as dilated cysts filled with cheesy material.

range from 10 to 44. The patients presented with a localized multinodular mass (Fig. 9.53) that, microscopically, was characterized by the presence of numerous papillomas, some with cytologic atypia, and numerous dilated cysts that were so impressive that the lesion was referred to as "Swiss cheese disease" of the breast. Sclerosing adenosis often accompanied the papillomas. In 1982, Rosen et al. (124) described 41 patients with juvenile papillomatosis, followed for a median of 14 years. Age of diagnosis ranged between 15 and 35 years, with a median of 19 years. Fifty-eight percent of the patients had a positive family history for breast carcinoma, and six had bilateral juvenile papillomatosis. Of the four patients (10%) who subsequently developed breast cancer, all had bilateral disease originally, a recurrence of the juvenile papillomatosis after primary excision, and a family history of breast cancer. None of the patients with non-recurrent unilateral unicentric juvenile papillomatosis was found to have subsequently developed carcinoma of the breast. Bazzocchi et al. (125) reported 13 cases of juvenile papillomatosis with an average age of 25 years. A family history of breast cancer was reported in 33% of the cases. Coexistent carcinoma was found in 15% of the cases.

Another lesion occurring in adolescent and young women in which the predominant feature is epithelial hyperplasia, often with a papillary pattern and without the prominent cyst formation described previously, has been termed *papillary duct hyperplasia* (126).

PAPILLOMAS WITH ATYPIA (ATYPICAL PAPILLOMAS)

Some intraductal papillomas may exhibit areas of epithelial proliferation that fulfill the criteria for the diagnosis of ADH or DCIS (most often of the low-grade variety). However, the classification of such lesions, particularly when the proliferation fulfills the qualitative criteria for the diagnosis of DCIS, varies among authors. In general, the classification has been based largely on the extent of the atypical proliferation within the papillary lesion. For example, Tavassoli (127) uses the designation "atypical papilloma" if the atypical changes involve less than one-third of the papilloma and "carcinoma arising in a papilloma" when the atypical population of cells involves at least one-third

but less than 90% of the lesion. Page et al. (128) have stated that "any area of uniform histology and cytology consistent with non-comedo DCIS" within a papilloma larger than 3 mm should be considered DCIS within a papilloma, whereas foci with the same qualitative features but 3 mm or smaller in size are classified as ADH within a papilloma. Of note, using these definitions, the investigators found that the risk for subsequent breast cancer associated with ADH within a papilloma was similar to the risk associated with atypical hyperplasia in the breast parenchyma (relative risk [RR], 4 to 5). However, in contrast to the patients with ADH within parenchyma, the patients with ADH in the papillomas were at risk for cancer largely confined to the ipsilateral breast, in the area of the original papilloma.

Intracystic Papillary Carcinoma

Intracystic papillary carcinomas (IPCs) are rare, accounting for 0.5% to 1% of breast cancers. They are usually found in older women, may be bulky lesions, and are usually located away from the nipple. Grossly, they are circumscribed, cystic, and often necrotic. Microscopically, they have a papillary configuration with fibrovascular cores covered by a single or multiple layers of cells, but other DCIS patterns, such as cribriform or micropapillary, may also be present. Kraus and Neubecker (109) described 21 patients with papillary carcinoma, and the criteria they used are classic (see Table 9.13). Their differentiation from benign intraductal papillomas has already been considered. The most important features in carcinoma are (a) the absence of a regular myoepithelial layer, which may be focal but not continuous (129), and (b) the usually delicate nature of the fibrovascular papillary cores, which may consist of little more than capillaries supported by a small amount of fibrous stroma (Fig. 9.54). As a result, the capillary endothelium may be seen adjacent to epithelial cells and can be mistaken for a myoepithelial layer. Occasional micropapillae (papillary projections of epithelial cells without a fibrovascular core) may be present. The malignant epithelial cells usually have a strikingly monomorphic appearance that may first alert one to the malignant nature of the lesion. The cells are generally well differentiated, often with minimal characteristics of malignancy. They sometimes

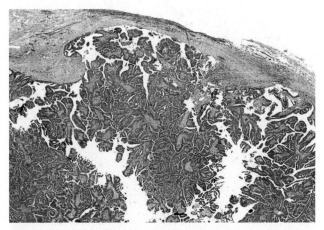

Figure 9.54. Intracystic papillary carcinoma (IPC). The intraductal localization of this expansive tumor is readily appreciated at low power. The tumor consists of papillary components. Some of the papillae have fibrovascular cores; others are slender. All are covered by a single type of epithelium.

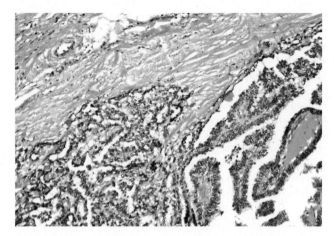

Figure 9.55. Intracystic papillary carcinoma. Fibrovascular cores covered by a single layer of epithelium without an intervening myoepithelial layer are evident. Invasion of the cyst wall has occurred.

have tall, oval nuclei that lie perpendicular to the core. The degree of epithelial proliferation varies from one lesion to another; sometimes the papillae are covered by only one or two layers of epithelial cells, whereas in other cases solid sheets of cells are interspersed with only small islands of stroma. As in benign papilloma, fibrosis around a malignant papilloma may entrap epithelium. This appearance should not be mistaken for invasion. However, invasion into the duct wall and periductal stroma may occur (Fig. 9.55). Collins et al. (129,130) used the term *encapsulated papillary carcinoma* when the myoepithelial layer was not identifiable. Metastases from this invasion are rare, but have been observed (Fig. 9.56).

Stewart (131) used the term *noninfiltrating papillary carcinoma* to refer to a lesion "limited to the mammary duct system and affecting the large, medium, or small radicals" and separately described intracystic carcinoma. A number of authors have dis-

tinguished diffuse intraductal carcinoma or DCIS from the localized, so-called intracystic papillary carcinomas. Carter et al. (132) reported a group of 41 cases of intracystic papillary carcinomas, and subcategorized them as IPC alone, IPC with DCIS, and IPC with invasive carcinoma and distinguished from the DCIS and/or invasive carcinoma that often accompanies them. Patients with invasive carcinoma and DCIS behaved as expected from these associated lesions. Those with IPC alone had a very benign follow-up, even with excisional therapy. Lefkowitz et al. (132) described 77 cases of intracystic papillary carcinoma of the breast and also distinguished the cases into three categories: IPC alone, IPC associated with DCIS, or IPC associated with invasive carcinoma. The follow-up data were similar. Leal et al. (133) reported 29 additional cases of IPC, divided as IPC alone, IPC with DCIS, and IPC with invasive carcinoma, and had similar follow-up data.

LOBULAR NEOPLASIA (ATYPICAL LOBULAR HYPERPLASIA AND LOBULAR CARCINOMA IN SITU)

Lobular epithelial proliferations do not show the variation of change evident in ductal proliferations. Atypical lobular hyperplasia (ALH) is, however, a well-recognized entity and better defined than its ductal counterpart (Fig. 9.57). The features distinguishing ALH from LCIS are detailed in Table 9.16. The diagnostic criteria parallel those for ADH, in that some of the features of in situ carcinoma are seen. In LCIS, the incidence of multifocality is high (90% in some series), and bilateral disease is frequent (134).

On low-power examination, the overall lobular architecture is retained, although individual acini are enlarged and distended, in contrast to those of surrounding normal lobules; the lumina are obliterated (Fig. 9.58). High-power examination shows a monomorphic population of cells completely filling the lumina. The proliferating cells are smaller than those in DCIS but larger than normal mammary epithelial cells, and the nuclear-to-cytoplasmic ratio is increased. Nuclear pleomorphism is less pronounced than in DCIS, and mitotic figures are infrequent. In many cases, a notable feature is the lack of cellular

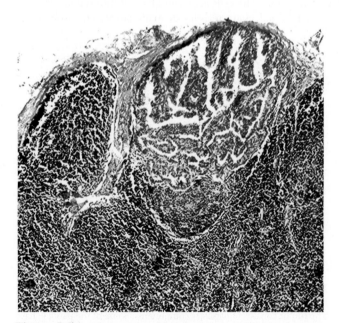

Figure 9.56. Metastatic papillary carcinoma. Axillary node metastasis from the IPC shown in Figure 9.54.

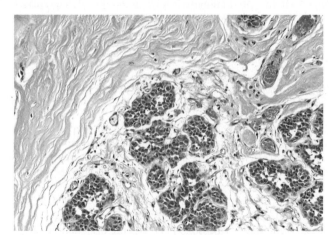

Figure 9.57. Atypical lobular hyperplasia. The incomplete obliteration of acinar lumina is apparent. A relatively monomorphic proliferation of cells has partially effaced normal architecture.

TABLE 9.16	Contrasting Features of Atypical Lobular Hyperplasia and Lobular Carcinoma in Situ	
	Atypical Lobular Hyperplasia	*Lobular Carcinoma in Situ*
Distention of acini	Less distended and distorted	Distended and distorted
Degree of involvement	Often only part of lobular unit units	Major part of one or more lobular units
Luminal obliteration	Incomplete. If complete, no distention	Complete, except if Pagetoid
Cellular composition	Less monotonous; may be variable cell types; less regularly spaced	Round, regular, monotonous; one cell type; evenly spaced
Cellular cohesion	More cohesive	Noncohesive
Spread to ducts	Pagetoid spread may occur, but less well developed	Pagetoid spread and other forms (see text)

cohesion. Good fixation is essential when this feature is assessed. Although cell size varies somewhat from lesion to lesion, the variation is not as marked as in DCIS. Calcification is much less frequent, and the stromal changes sometimes seen in DCIS are not usually present.

Another feature associated with LCIS is pagetoid spread of the malignant cells into ductlike structures. In this pattern, malignant cells spread between an intact epithelium on the luminal surface and the underlying myoepithelial cells (Fig. 9.59). On occasion, this occurs in a nodular fashion, producing what has been described as a cloverleaf pattern. A pagetoid pattern of spread may occasionally be seen in DCIS, but is infrequent.

Rarely, in situ carcinomas composed of cells that have the cytologic features of LCIS may exhibit comedo necrosis. In addition, a variant of LCIS composed of cells with more nuclear atypia and pleomorphism than are seen in the classic form of LCIS has been described (134).

LCIS must be distinguished from cancerization of lobules by DCIS (135). The distinguishing features are listed in Table 9.17. The most important of these is the cytologic appearance of the malignant cells, presence or absence of a pattern, and the associated changes in the breast. DCIS is usually found in ducts when cancerization of the lobules occurs. However, LCIS and DCIS can occur side-by-side and sometimes even within the same TDLU (136.) E-cadherin staining is of questionable value in borderline cases.

As mentioned in the case of DCIS, it is always important to exclude the presence of associated invasive carcinoma. This problem may be compounded by sclerosing adenosis occurring within an area of LCIS (137). The problem of microinvasion from LCIS rarely occurs, however.

RELATIONSHIP OF BENIGN BREAST DISEASE TO RISK FOR SUBSEQUENT CARCINOMA, AND THE CLINICAL SIGNIFICANCE OF IN SITU CARCINOMA

For many years, the relationship of benign breast disease to the risk for subsequent carcinoma was controversial. Of the several reasons for the controversy, the most important was past inconsistencies in defining benign breast disease, not only in the field of pathology but also in radiologic and clinical practice.

Cohort studies performed during the past two decades, which have included a careful pathologic classification of benign breast disease, are beginning to resolve this problem (58,62,63,64,138,139). The most important message is that most women with benign breast disease are not at increased risk for subsequent carcinoma, which is confined to those whose biopsy specimens show proliferative epithelial changes. Although a small risk is associated with intraductal papilloma, sclerosing adenosis, and UDH (RR, 1.5 to 2.0), it is only in cases with evidence of atypical hyperplasia that the risk is substantially increased (RR, 4.0 to 5.0). The risk is related to both breasts.

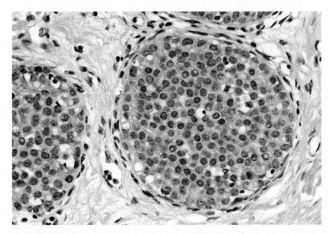

Figure 9.58. Lobular carcinoma in situ. The lobular architecture is retained. The acini are distended by a monomorphic population of cells, and the lumina are completely obliterated. The cells are smaller and less pleomorphic than those seen in lobular cancerization by ductal carcinoma in situ (Fig. 9.48). Intracellular lumens, especially seen near the basement membrane, may be a prominent feature.

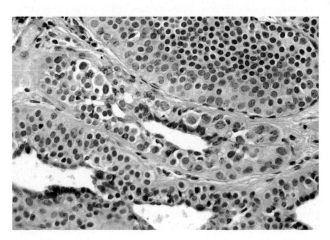

Figure 9.59. Lobular carcinoma in situ showing pagetoid spread within a duct. The neoplastic cells are insinuated between the intact luminal epithelium and the underlying myoepithelium and basement membrane.

TABLE 9.17	Contrasting Features of Cancerization of Lobules by Ductal Carcinoma in Situ and Lobular Carcinoma In Situ	
	Cancerization of Lobules	*Lobular Carcinoma in Situ*
Lobular architecture	Retained	Retained
Pattern within spaces	Recognized patterns of DCIS, but may be solid sheets of cells	Solid sheets of cells
Necrosis	May be present	Usually absent
Cellular features	Usually large, often pleomorphic	Smaller, more uniform; intracytoplasmic lumina often present
Cellular cohesion	Cohesive	Noncohesive
Mitoses	Variable, may be frequent	Infrequent
Changes in surrounding ducts	Recognized patterns of DCIS	Recognized patterns of LCIS
Inflammatory response in surrounding stroma	May be marked	Usually absent
Fibroplasia in surrounding stroma	May be marked	Usually absent
Immunohistochemistry	Cells positive for E-cadherin and negative for high–molecular-weight cytokeratin	Cells negative for E-cadherin and positive for high–molecular-weight cytokeratin

DCIS, ductal carcinoma in situ; LCIS, lobular carcinoma in situ.

A strong interaction with family history has also been noted. Studies have found the risk to be markedly increased in women who have atypical hyperplasia and a first-degree relative with breast cancer (58,62,138,139), but this association may be largely limited to premenopausal women. Atypical hyperplasia is seen in only about 4% of all otherwise benign breast biopsy specimens in symptomatic women, but the incidence is increased in specimens obtained to evaluate mammographic abnormalities (62,138).

It should be noted, however, that debate continues about the significance of cystic change without epithelial hyperplasia. Although studies by Dupont and Page (58) and by London et al. (59) indicate that cystic change is not a risk factor on its own, many authorities consider that cysts, particularly of apocrine type, are a marker for subsequent malignancy (140). Furthermore, Dupont et al. (58,138) have found that cysts elevate breast cancer risk if they are associated with epithelial hyperplasia, or occur in women with a family history.

Follow-up studies of patients with LCIS treated by biopsy alone indicate that subsequent invasive carcinoma will develop in approximately 20% to 35% of cases (134). One study shows that this risk does not decrease with time (141). The subsequent carcinomas may occur in either breast, and one-third do not become apparent for as long as 20 years (142). The invasive carcinomas in these patients may be of ductal or lobular type, although the proportion of invasive lobular carcinomas is higher in this group than in breast cancer patients generally (134).

There are fewer studies with long-term follow-up of patients with DCIS treated by biopsy alone, and the data are more controversial, with quoted incidence rates of subsequent invasive carcinoma ranging from 25% to 75% (142,143). Subsequent tumors usually occur in the same breast and the same quadrant as the previous biopsy specimen, and are always of ductal type. In one series, the average time to diagnosis was 10 years (114). Despite the apparent discrepancy in the follow-up data, it is probable that the incidence of subsequent carcinoma is low following the removal of small, inconspicuous lesions, usually of low-grade, well-differentiated type, many of which may have previously been diagnosed as benign (142,143). A much higher

incidence has been reported in association with palpable lesions with a comedo pattern (142,143). In a study of small, mammographically detected foci of DCIS less than 25 mm in diameter treated by excision alone, the overall recurrence rate was only 10% (79). Half of the recurrent lesions were invasive, and nearly all occurred in cases with a high-grade comedo pattern. More recent studies have also noted a higher incidence of recurrence after the removal of lesions with a high nuclear grade and necrosis (69,72). As previously indicated, however, the evidence for behavioral differences in subtypes of DCIS is very preliminary, and continued evaluation is needed. More studies to ascertain the significance of histologic features, based on more reproducible criteria, as have been outlined, are needed to understand the clinical significance of DCIS and plan appropriate treatment. The margin status and possibly the size of the lesion must also be considered, along with the mode of presentation and the biologic features, such as oncoprotein expression and estrogen receptor status (67,68).

The presence of extensive DCIS comprising more than 25% of the whole tumor, together with in situ carcinoma in the tissue around infiltrating tumors, has been found to be associated with a high rate of local recurrence following conservation therapy for invasive mammary carcinoma (144). This is probably related to considerable residual DCIS in the treated breast around the biopsy site (145). Extensive in situ carcinoma in association with invasive breast carcinomas is regarded as a strong risk factor for recurrence following conservation therapy for mammary carcinoma, particularly when the resection margins are involved. At some centers this is an indicator for re-excision before radiotherapy (145).

INFILTRATING (INVASIVE) CARCINOMA

Infiltrating breast cancers constitute a heterogeneous group of lesions that differ in clinical presentation, radiographic characteristics, pathologic features, and biologic potential. The most widely used classification of invasive breast cancers is that of the World Health Organization (second edition) (146). This classification scheme is based on the growth pattern and cytologic features of the invasive tumor cells, and does not imply histogenesis or site of origin within the mammary duct system. For example, although the classification system recognizes invasive carcinomas designated as *ductal* or *lobular*, this is not meant to indicate that the former originate in extralobular ducts and the latter in lobules. Subgross whole-organ sectioning has demonstrated that most invasive breast cancers arise in the TDLU, regardless of histologic type (15).

The most common histologic type of invasive breast cancer by far is invasive (infiltrating) ductal carcinoma (147–149). In fact, invasive ductal carcinoma is diagnosed by default because this tumor type is defined as a type of cancer "not classified into any of the other categories of invasive mammary carcinoma" (15). To emphasize this point further, and to distinguish these tumors from invasive breast cancers with specific or special histologic features (e.g., invasive lobular, tubular, mucinous, medullary, and other rare types), some authorities prefer the term *infiltrating ductal carcinoma, not otherwise specified* (NOS) (147) or *infiltrating carcinoma of no special type* (NST) (149).

The distribution of histologic types of invasive breast cancer has varied among published series (Table 9.18). These differences may be related to a number of factors, including the nature of the patient population and variability in the confines of definition for the different histologic types. In general, special-type cancers comprise approximately 20% to 30% of invasive carcinomas, and at least 90% of a tumor should demonstrate the defining histologic characteristics of a special-type cancer before it is designated as being of that histologic type (149,150).

A classification is of value only if it is of both clinical and pathologic significance. As previously discussed, DCIS and LCIS appear to differ in biologic behavior. When infiltrating carcinoma is considered, however, the difference between ductal and lobular carcinomas is less clear. The morphologic appearances of the two tumors are distinct, and they do also show some differences in clinical behavior. Lobular carcinoma is more often multifocal and bilateral than is ductal carcinoma, and differences have been found in the pattern of metastases from the two tumor types (151–153). Because certain variants of infiltrating lobular carcinoma have been described relatively recently, further studies are needed before the full significance of these patterns is understood. In addition to this broad subdivision, a number of special types of mammary carcinomas are recognized, most of which are probably variants of the ductal type. Although these comprise only a small proportion of infiltrating tumors, they are important because some of them are associated with a more favorable prognosis. Others, seen extremely rarely, are worthy of distinction so that the significance of their morphologic appearance may become better understood. The grading of infiltrating carcinoma is also an important form of classification from the point of view of prognosis.

The incidence rates of the different types of carcinoma given in Table 9.18 are based on those seen in a general hospital practice. Although minor geographic variations are seen, more significant differences are noted in carcinomas detected in screening centers. In particular, many screening centers detect a higher proportion of tumors of special type, particularly tubular carcinomas.

The incidence of microinvasive carcinoma is also high in screen-detected lesions. *Microinvasion* is defined as the presence of one or more foci of invasion, none larger than 1 mm in maximum diameter, and is typically identified in a lesion that is predominantly DCIS, most often of high grade. Immunohistochemistry (Table 9.6) can sometimes be helpful in the evaluation when the presence of invasion is doubtful.

The gross features of a typical infiltrating carcinoma are contrasted with those of a fibroadenoma in Table 9.2 and illustrated in Figure 9.1. In most cases, the diagnosis of carcinoma is strongly suspected based on the gross examination. Some benign lesions, however, mimic carcinoma; these are listed in Table 9.3. Attention has been drawn to the importance of correlating the gross and microscopic appearances. Caution should always be exercised in making a diagnosis of malignancy in the absence of confirmatory gross evidence.

INFILTRATING DUCTAL CARCINOMA (INFILTRATING CARCINOMA, NOT OTHERWISE SPECIFIED; INFILTRATING CARCINOMA OF NO SPECIAL TYPE)

Infiltrating ductal carcinoma (infiltrating carcinoma NOS; infiltrating carcinoma NST) is ductal carcinoma without any special feature that would allow it to be classified as one of the distinctive subtypes. It is the most common type of infiltrating mammary carcinoma. The gross appearance is usually typical (Table 9.2), with an irregular stellate outline. Some tumors have a more circumscribed or nodular outline, but the cut face of the tumor always blends into the surrounding tissue and is not elevated.

Microscopically, at low power, randomly arranged epithelial elements are seen. Myoepithelial cells are absent. Tubule forma-

| TABLE 9.18 | Histologic Types of Invasive Breast Cancer in Four Large Series Before the Widespread Use of Mammographic Screening |

Histologic Type

Study	No. of Cancers	Ductal[a] (%)	Lobular (%)	Medullary (%)	Mucinous (%)	Tubular (%)	Tubular Mixed (%)	Mixed (%)	Other (%)
Fisher et al. (147)	1000	53	5	6	2	1	—	32	—
Rosen (148)	857	75	10	9	2	2	—	—	—
Ellis et al. (150)	1547	49	16	3	1	2	14	14	2
Page and Anderson (149)	Not stated	70	10	5	2	3	2	—	8

[a]In some series, designated *not otherwise specified* (NOS) or *no special type* (NST).

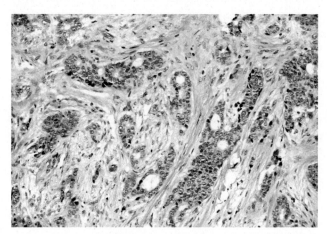

Figure 9.60. Infiltrating ductal carcinoma NOS. The carcinoma grows in tubules and solid trabeculae. The nuclei show relatively little pleomorphism, and the rate of mitotic activity is low. Desmoplastic reaction of the stroma is a dominant feature.

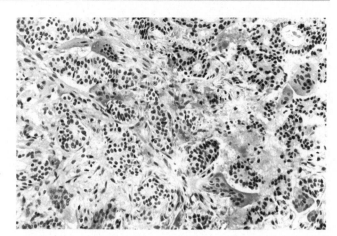

Figure 9.62. Infiltrating ductal carcinoma grade 1. The presence of numerous osteoclast-like giant cells within the stroma is a notable and unusual feature.

tion may be pronounced, focally present, or totally absent (Figs. 9.60 and 9.61). Other arrangements include trabeculae or large groups of malignant cells. When large sheets of cells are present, necrosis may be seen. Occasionally, this may be so marked that pseudocysts form. The malignant cells vary in appearance. In some tumors, cellular or nuclear pleomorphism is minimal (Fig. 9.60), whereas in others it is marked (Fig. 9.61), sometimes with multinucleated giant forms. The degree of mitotic activity also varies. Mucin can usually be demonstrated within the tubular lumina as well as intracellularly. A number of changes may be seen in the epithelium, including apocrine and squamous metaplasia. These are usually focal, but occasionally they predominate.

As in carcinomas from many other sites, the amount of stroma varies. Its composition also ranges from fibroblastic to densely hyaline, and the stroma contains varying amounts of collagen, extracellular mucin, and elastic tissue. Often, the fibroblastic, or desmoplastic, reaction to the growth of malignant cells is the predominant feature of the tumor mass. Tumors with a large amount

of dense hyaline stroma were previously termed *scirrhous.* In some carcinomas, the stroma is uniformly distributed, but in others the center of the tumor is fibrotic and relatively acellular, with the malignant epithelial components seen mainly at the periphery. The degree of lymphoplasmacytic reaction varies considerably and may be minimal, moderate, or marked. Calcification is relatively frequent, usually within the epithelial components but occasionally within the stroma. Other rare features are stromal, osteoclast-like giant cells (154,155) (Fig. 9.62) and giant cell granulomas within the stroma.

With adequate sampling, in situ carcinoma can usually be demonstrated in association with most infiltrating carcinomas of this type. It is nearly always ductal but occasionally lobular, or both forms may be seen simultaneously.

Invasion of small vascular spaces should be sought in all infiltrating carcinomas because it is of prognostic significance (Fig. 9.63). True vascular space invasion should not be confused with the artifactual retraction of groups of malignant cells from surrounding stroma. It is usually most easily identified at the periphery of tumors. Detection may be facilitated by immunohisto-

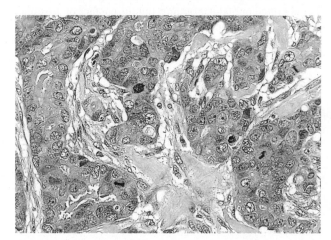

Figure 9.61. Infiltrating ductal carcinoma NOS. This carcinoma is less well-differentiated than the one in Figure 9.47. Nuclear pleomorphism is marked, and a high mitotic rate is evident. A suggestion of lumen formation is seen on the left side of the figure, an unusual feature for such a high-grade tumor.

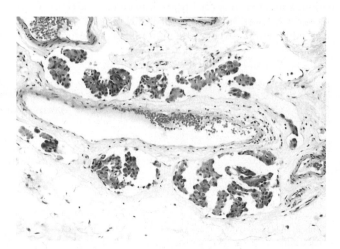

Figure 9.63. Lymphatic permeation by infiltrating ductal carcinoma. The endothelial lining cells of the lymphatic vessel are clearly seen, as is an adjacent venule.

chemistry (Table 9.6). Although such small vessel involvement is most often termed *lymphatic vessel invasion*, it is not usually possible to distinguish between small capillaries and lymphatics on routinely stained sections. Tumor emboli within large blood vessels are only uncommonly encountered. Perineural invasion may also be seen.

GRADING

Nuclear grading is based on nuclear pleomorphism and mitotic activity (156), but in clinical practice it has largely been replaced by histologic grading.

Several systems of histologic grading have been described. The system most widely used, based on that of Bloom and Richardson (157) as modified by Elston and Ellis (158), is described in Table 9.19. This system includes an assessment of tubule formation, nuclear pleomorphism, and mitotic activity. The mitotic activity score should take into account the size of the high-power field used. Although some tumor types are partly defined by their histologic grade (e.g., tubular carcinomas are by definition grade 1 and medullary carcinomas are by definition grade 3), Elston and Ellis (158) advocate the histologic grading of all invasive breast cancers.

With all grading systems, wide sampling is important because some tumors vary markedly in appearance from area to area. Although considerable interobserver variation may be seen in grading systems, if strict criteria are applied, more consistent results giving good prognostic information can be obtained.

PROGNOSTIC AND PREDICTIVE FACTORS

Prognostic factors provide information useful in assessing the outcome at the time of diagnosis, whereas *predictive factors*

TABLE 9.19

Histologic Grading

Feature	Score
Tubule formation (extent within tumor)	
>75%	1
10%–75%	2
<10%	3
Nuclear pleomorphism	
Small, regular, uniform	1
Moderate variation in shape and size	2
Marked variation in shape and size	3
Mitotic count per 10 hpf (dependent on microscopic field area)	
Field diameter 0.59 mm diameter/0.274-mm² area	
0–9	1
10–19	2
>20	3
Field diameter 0.44-mm diameter/0.152-mm² area	
0–5	1
6–10	2
>11	3

Total score: 3–5, grade 1, well differentiated; 6–7, grade 2, moderately differentiated; 8–9, grade 3, poorly differentiated.
hpf, high-power field.

provide information about the likelihood of response to a given therapy. Traditional prognostic factors in patients with invasive breast cancer include lymph node status (the single most important prognostic factor), tumor size, histologic type, and histologic grade. Lymphatic vessel invasion is also considered by many to be an important prognostic factor. Numerous other biologic markers have been proposed as aids to assess the prognosis in mammary carcinoma. These include the following: markers of proliferation (e.g., S-phase fraction, thymidine labeling index, and immunostaining with antibodies to Ki-67); oncoproteins (in particular HER2/*neu* or c-*erb*-B2); tumor suppressor genes (e.g., p53); angiogenesis, as indicated by stromal microvessel density; and bone marrow micrometastases, among others. These should all be included in the pathology report; a synoptic report is useful as a prompt to make sure that all prognostic factors have been addressed and reported.

Estrogen and progesterone receptor status are weak prognostic factors, but they are powerful predictive factors used in assessing the likelihood of response to hormonal therapy (159). The assessment of estrogen and progesterone receptors has been greatly facilitated by the development of antibodies that work consistently well in fixed tissue, so that such assessment has become a part of routine practice. The measurement of HER2/*neu* protein overexpression by immunohistochemistry or HER2/*neu* gene amplification by fluorescence in situ hybridization currently has an established role in decision making regarding patient management, particularly in the selection of patients for treatment with trastuzumab (Herceptin), a monoclonal antibody that targets the HER2/*neu* protein (160), and for other chemotherapy as well. Recently, the American Society of Clinical Oncology (ASCO) and the College of American Pathologists (161) have issued guidelines for performance and evaluation of HER2/*neu* testing. They found that neither immunohistochemistry (IHC) nor fluorescent in situ hybridization (FISH) techniques had superiority when they were performed under optimal conditions. HER2 positivity was considered when there was IHC positivity of 30% or more, 3+ uniform intense membrane staining, or a FISH result demonstrating more than six copies of HER2 genes per nucleus or a FISH ratio (HER2 gene signals to chromosome 17 centromere signals) of more than 2.2. A negative result was IHC staining of 0 or 1+, a FISH result with less than four HER2 gene copies per nucleus, or a FISH ratio of less than 1.8. Equivocal results require additional action for final determination. EGFR status is also under consideration as a predictive factor, and it may be evaluated by IHC, FISH, or by determination of specific mutation. Its predictive value is not as well established as that of the steroid hormone receptors and HER2/*neu*, at this time. The ASCO guidelines for breast markers currently include estrogen and progesterone receptors, HER2/*neu*, several serum markers, and certain multiparameter gene expression arrays (162).

With additional therapies targeted at specific tumor molecules on the horizon, it is probable that the immunohistochemical detection of such targets will become increasingly valuable. At present, the lymph node status, tumor size, histologic type, histologic grade, and presence or absence of lymphatic vessel invasion remain the best independent prognostic indicators (160).

SPECIAL TYPES OF MAMMARY CARCINOMA

INFILTRATING LOBULAR CARCINOMA

The reported incidence of infiltrating lobular carcinoma varies considerably, in part because this entity has been better recognized in recent years (163,164).

The gross features may be typical, as described in Table 9.2, but infiltrating lobular carcinoma is often poorly defined and difficult to see, radiographically and grossly, because it insinuates itself into normal stroma without distorting it. Palpation of the specimen may be a better guide to the presence of the tumor than inspection. The modified grading system of Bloom and Richardson (157,158) can be applied to lobular carcinomas and can separate these tumors into different prognostic groups.

Classic Infiltrating Lobular Carcinoma

The histologic appearance of classic infiltrating lobular carcinoma is illustrated in Figure 9.64. The malignant cells lack cohesion and are arranged individually or linearly in single files, or as narrow trabeculae within the stroma. The lack of cohesion in these tumors is particularly distinctive; in one article, 56% of a series of lobular carcinomas showed truncation mutations in the E-cadherin adhesion molecule gene (165). In addition, almost all infiltrating lobular carcinomas lack E-cadherin protein expression by immunohistochemistry. The wide separation of the malignant cells may lead to underdiagnosis of these tumors, particularly in frozen sections or in lymph nodes. A "targetoid" arrangement is often present around residual normal mammary structures, which are more often seen within lobular carcinomas than in ductal tumors. "Skip areas"—that is, foci of infiltrating carcinoma separated by areas of uninvolved mammary tissue—are a common feature of lobular carcinomas, giving the appearance of multifocality.

The malignant cells are usually smaller and less pleomorphic than those of ductal carcinoma, and they have fewer mitotic figures. Necrosis is rarely, if ever, present. Intracellular mucin is frequent. Although the classic "bull's-eye" appearance of in-

tracytoplasmic lumina seen with the combined alcian blue/PAS stain is said to be typical of lobular carcinoma, both in situ and invasive (166), in our experience it is also seen in ductal carcinoma. Antibodies to epithelial membrane antigen can also be used to demonstrate intracytoplasmic lumina, which are found in adenocarcinomas from various sites but are almost always present within mammary carcinomas of lobular type (167). Foci of signet ring cells occur.

As in ductal carcinomas, the amount and nature of the stroma vary considerably, and although the stroma may be dense and hyaline with abundant elastic tissue, some invasive lobular carcinomas elicit little or no desmoplastic reaction. Probably for this reason, lobular carcinomas can be difficult to detect mammographically. Vascular permeation is more difficult to identify in these tumors. LCIS is associated with most, but not all, infiltrating lobular carcinomas.

Variants of Infiltrating Lobular Carcinoma

In addition to the classic pattern of infiltrating lobular carcinoma, other patterns have been categorized as variants of this type of tumor (163,164,168). Most show similar cytologic features and exhibit the cellular discohesion characteristic of lobular carcinoma. Sometimes, the malignant cells grow in *solid* sheets that engulf normal structures and infiltrate the fat in a growth pattern similar to that seen in lymphoma (solid variant) (Fig. 9.65). When the sheets of cells are smaller and arranged in rounded aggregates, the pattern has been termed *alveolar* (Fig. 9.66), and it may be difficult to distinguish this variant of invasive lobular carcinoma from LCIS (169). Occasionally, the cells form tubules, but these are usually small and poorly developed (Fig. 9.67). Tumors with this feature have been referred to as *tubulolobular* (170). Other variants differ in cellular morphology. Signet ring cells may be found in lobular carcinomas (168). LiVolsi and Merino (171) described a *signet ring* variant of invasive lobular carcinoma, in which signet ring cells were the predominant feature (Fig. 9.68), and reported that it had a propensity to metastasize to the gastrointestinal and urinary tract.

A *pleomorphic variant of invasive lobular carcinoma* is well de-

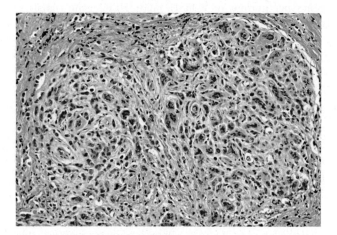

Figure 9.64. Infiltrating lobular carcinoma, classic pattern. The cells invade singly and as single files of cells and lack cohesion. The "targetoid" arrangement of the files of cells invading around normal structures is characteristic. The desmoplastic reaction seen in the ductal carcinoma is lacking.

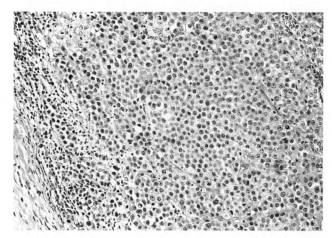

Figure 9.65. Infiltrating lobular carcinoma, solid variant. The cells show features similar to those seen in classic infiltrating lobular carcinoma, but little, if any, intervening stroma is present. Such tumors may be mistaken for malignant lymphoma.

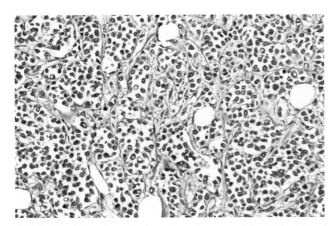

Figure 9.66. Infiltrating carcinoma, alveolar variant. The cytologic appearance is similar to that seen in classic lobular carcinoma, but the cells are arranged in small, solid nests separated by thin, fibrovascular septa. The appearance mimics the pattern of lobular carcinoma in situ.

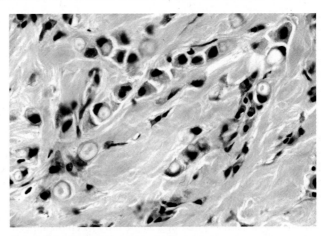

Figure 9.68. Invasive lobular carcinoma, signet ring variant. The cells contain vacuole-like spaces, which stain for mucus. However, the spaces are intracellular lumina.

scribed. The histologic appearance is that of classic lobular carcinoma, but the nuclei are more anaplastic, pleomorphic, and mitotically active (Fig. 9.69), sometimes with apocrine or histiocytoid features of cytoplasmic differentiation (172–174). However, the typical pattern of infiltration and lack of cellular cohesion indicate that these lesions are of lobular type.

It is unusual for any of these variants to be seen in pure form; areas of classic infiltrating lobular carcinoma are nearly always seen. Skip areas are common in all patterns. Associated in situ carcinoma, when present, is most often of lobular type. It has been reported that the various histologic patterns of lobular carcinoma are of prognostic significance; tumors with the classic pattern are associated with the most favorable outcome, and those with the pleomorphic pattern the least favorable (172–175). The classic pattern is most often associated with the multifocality and bilaterality that is the hallmark of lobular carcinoma (175).

Classic invasive lobular carcinomas typically express estrogen and progesterone receptors and rarely show overexpression of the HER2/*neu* protein (176) or accumulation of the p53 gene product (177). Gross cystic disease fluid protein is seen in about one-third of all invasive lobular carcinomas, but is present in the vast majority of lesions with prominent signet ring cell features (178). Although pleomorphic lobular carcinomas are also often positive for estrogen and progesterone receptors, they also frequently show HER2/*neu* protein overexpression and p53 protein accumulation (179,180).

Although typical infiltrating ductal carcinoma and typical infiltrating lobular carcinoma can easily be distinguished, some tumors show features of both types or indeterminate features. This should not be surprising in view of reports suggesting that some invasive ductal carcinomas exhibit cytogenetic alterations similar to those seen in invasive lobular carcinomas (181,182). Some authorities categorize such lesions histologically as invasive carcinomas with ductal and lobular features, whereas others classify them as ductal carcinoma NOS. Immunohistochemical

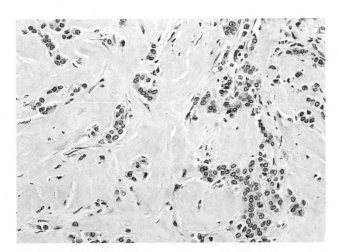

Figure 9.67. Infiltrating lobular carcinoma, tubulolobular variant. In this example, much of the tumor shows microtubule formation. These tubules are small and often poorly formed, with indistinct lumina. Such tumors have been called *tubulolobular carcinomas.* A mixture of tubular and lobular carcinoma, on the other hand, should be reported as a mixed tumor.

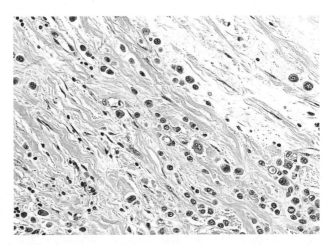

Figure 9.69. Infiltrating lobular carcinoma, pleomorphic variant. Despite the growth pattern and lack of cohesion typical of lobular carcinoma, a high degree of nuclear pleomorphism is present. The eosinophilic cytoplasm is suggestive of apocrine differentiation. Signet ring cells are present.

staining for E-cadherin and cytokeratin 8 has been proposed as a useful adjunct in making the distinction between ductal and lobular carcinomas (183). Occasionally, carcinomas are a genuine mixture of these two histologic types.

TUBULAR CARCINOMA

Tubular carcinoma has been recognized to be associated with a particularly favorable prognosis (184,185). Although its overall incidence is low (Table 9.18), it is higher in tumors detected by mammography. The gross features do not differ from those of a typical infiltrating carcinoma (Table 9.2), but the tumors are usually smaller than 2 cm. Microscopically, this tumor is an extremely well-differentiated carcinoma consisting of irregularly arranged tubules lined by a single layer of epithelial cells with little pleomorphism and a low mitotic rate. Cytoplasmic apical snouts are frequently seen. The glandular lumina are open and the tubules are characteristically angulated (Fig. 9.70). Occasionally, trabecular bars are present, although branching and anastomosis of tubules are not features. The stroma is abundant and usually cellular. Elastosis may be prominent. DCIS is frequently an associated finding and, when present, it is usually of well-differentiated, low-grade type with a cribriform or micropapillary pattern. The well-differentiated appearance of tubular carcinoma may lead to underdiagnosis. The lesions with which it is most frequently confused are sclerosing adenosis, radial scar, and microglandular adenosis. Features helpful in the differential diagnosis are listed in Table 9.11.

In some carcinomas, the pattern is entirely tubular. In others, the tubular component is mixed with different types of carcinomas, usually ductal carcinoma NOS (carcinoma NST), but sometimes other types, including invasive lobular carcinoma. The terms *tubular NOS* and *tubular mixed* have been applied on occasion to tumors with these mixed patterns. Although the question of what proportion of a tumor must have a tubular pattern for it to be classified as a true tubular carcinoma has caused some disagreement, the term *tubular carcinoma* is best reserved for carcinomas in which the pattern is at least 90% tubular. Such tumors are associated with a particularly favorable prognosis (185,186). However, tumors in which the pat-

tern is more than 75% tubular are also associated with a more favorable prognosis than other ductal carcinomas NOS (carcinomas NST) (185).

The expression of various biologic markers in tubular carcinomas generally reflects the well-differentiated nature of these lesions and their good prognosis. The tumors are typically positive for estrogen and progesterone receptors (185–192) and are almost always diploid, have a low proliferative rate, and rarely show HER2 overexpression or p53 protein accumulation (185,193–195). In comparison with invasive carcinomas of NST, tubular carcinomas exhibit fewer overall chromosomal changes; more often show losses of 16q; and less often show losses of 17p (196).

INFILTRATING CRIBRIFORM CARCINOMA

This relatively uncommon pattern of carcinoma has been described as a specific entity (197). The infiltrating component of the tumor has a cribriform pattern reminiscent of DCIS of cribriform type, with which it is frequently associated (Fig. 9.71). The tumor is rare but worthy of distinction because it carries a favorable prognosis, similar to that of tubular carcinoma (198). Tumors with a mixed cribriform and tubular pattern are often found. Areas of invasive cribriform carcinoma may also be associated with typical infiltrating ductal carcinoma NOS (carcinoma NST), but such tumors do not carry the very favorable prognosis associated with either the pure cribriform pattern or mixed cribriform and tubular pattern.

MUCINOUS CARCINOMA

Mammary mucinous carcinomas are also known as *colloid, mucoid,* or *gelatinous carcinomas.* Like medullary carcinomas, they have a rounded outline and a soft texture, and they may be large. The cut surface has a characteristic glistening, gelatinous appearance. Mucinous carcinoma is usually seen in elderly patients and is generally considered to carry a favorable prognosis (184,185), although occasional articles have suggested that on long-term follow-up, the prognosis may not be so good (199).

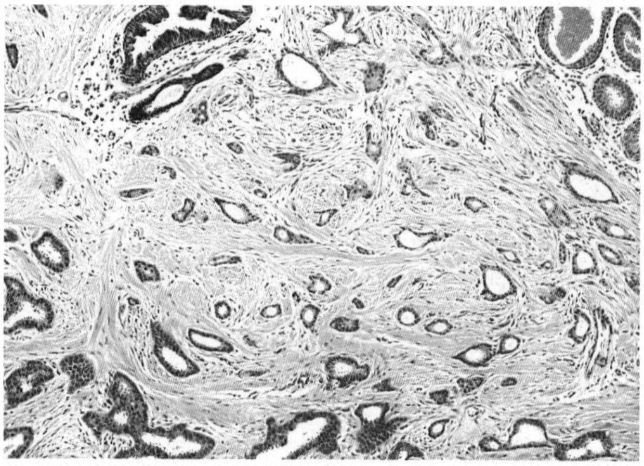

Figure 9.70. Tubular carcinoma composed of open tubules with angulated outlines. These are lined by a single layer of well-differentiated cells having luminal protrusions (apical snouts). The intervening stroma is fibroblastic.

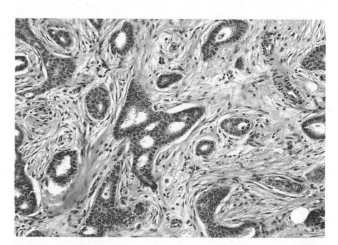

Figure 9.71. Infiltrating cribriform carcinoma. This pattern may be mixed with tubular carcinoma (Fig. 9.70). The relatively well-differentiated malignant cells are arranged in a cribriform pattern, similar to that seen in ductal carcinoma in situ. In this example, luminal cytoplasmic bleb formation is seen.

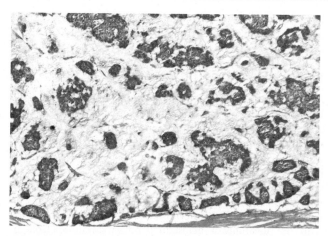

Figure 9.72. Mucinous carcinoma. Clumps of tumor cells lie within pools of mucin, without apparent fibrous reaction.

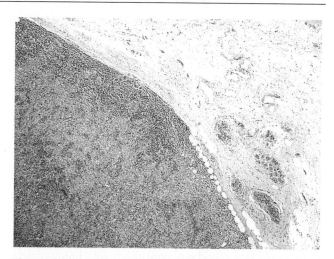

Figure 9.73. Medullary carcinoma. At low power, the tumor has a sharply defined, rounded outline. A dense chronic inflammatory stromal reaction can be appreciated. No ductal carcinoma in situ is seen.

In our experience, if strict diagnostic criteria are applied, the prognosis for patients with pure mucinous carcinoma is excellent (200). Microscopically, the tumor is composed of groups of malignant cells showing little pleomorphism and a low mitotic rate; the cells are set within pools of extracellular mucin surrounded by bands of fibrous connective tissue (Fig. 9.72). The mucin may be difficult to see in conventional hematoxylin and eosin sections, but it is clearly demonstrated by alcian blue or PAS techniques. A small amount of intracellular mucin may also be present. Calcification is rare. Argyrophilia can be demonstrated in the malignant cells of some mucinous carcinomas. This feature, together with certain morphologic characteristics, has been used to subdivide mucinous carcinomas into two types (201–203). Type A tumors, characterized by trabeculae and by ribbons and rings of malignant cells with minimal intracytoplasmic mucin, are not argyrophilic. Type B tumors, characterized by sheets and clumps of tumor cells with little pleomorphism and often with abundant intracytoplasmic mucin, are usually argyrophilic. However, no one has reliably shown a prognostic difference between these two groups. An in situ ductal component may be present and may also show marked mucin production.

The expression of various biologic markers in mucinous carcinomas generally reflects the good prognosis associated with these lesions, which are typically positive for estrogen and progesterone receptors (203,204) and usually do not overexpress the HER2/*neu* protein or show p53 protein accumulation (192–194). In addition, mucinous carcinomas exhibit substantially fewer and simpler chromosomal abnormalities than invasive carcinomas of NST (205–207).

Although the term *mucinous carcinoma* should be applied only to tumors showing the aforementioned features throughout, areas with a mucinous appearance are not infrequently seen in combination with other infiltrating carcinomas, most commonly infiltrating ductal carcinoma NOS. It is usually considered that if 90% of a carcinoma is of a certain type, it should be so designated, but mucinous carcinomas are an exception because the favorable prognostic implication applies only to tumors consisting entirely of the mucinous pattern (150,170,173). The differential diagnosis of mucinous carcinoma is from the pseudotumorous mucocele-like lesion, which is discussed at the end of the chapter.

MEDULLARY CARCINOMA

Interobserver agreement in making this diagnosis is notably lacking (208,209). If strict criteria are applied, this type of carcinoma is uncommon, accounting for fewer than 1% of all infiltrating mammary carcinomas, in our experience and that of some others (210). If strict criteria are applied, this type of carcinoma is uncommon, accounting for fewer than 1% of all infiltrating mammary carcinomas. However, some authorities report an incidence between 2% and 5%, illustrating the variation in the application of diagnostic criteria (158).

Medullary carcinomas have a characteristic gross and mammographic appearance, being soft and circumscribed and often of considerable size. On microscopic examination, the well-demarcated outline is confirmed (Fig. 9.73). The predominant growth pattern is syncytial, with broad anastomosing bands or sheets of malignant cells set within sparse stroma (Fig. 9.74). This pattern should constitute more than 75% of the tumor. The stromal lymphoplasmacytic response is marked, sometimes with germinal center formation. Necrosis is frequent, although of limited extent. The malignant cells are large, with marked

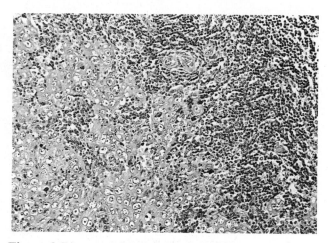

Figure 9.74. Medullary carcinoma. At higher power, poorly differentiated tumor cells show a syncytial growth pattern in which individual cell borders are not readily observed.

nuclear pleomorphism, prominent nucleoli, and frequent mitotic figures. Tumor giant cells are not uncommon. The cells sometimes have a squamoid appearance and may manifest true squamous metaplasia. Mucin is rarely present, and calcification has not been described. Typical medullary carcinoma is not associated with DCIS. The syncytial growth pattern, circumscription, and lymphoplasmacytic response are the most important of the diagnostic criteria (211). The lymphoplasmocytic response is mandatory for better prognosis.

Tumors that do not conform precisely to these criteria have been classified as *atypical medullary carcinomas* (212). Such tumors have the same growth pattern as typical medullary carcinomas but lack no more than two of the classic microscopic features. The criteria for the diagnosis of typical and atypical medullary carcinoma are listed in Table 9.20.

Although some studies have found medullary carcinoma to be associated with a good prognosis, this is not a universal finding. The inconsistency may be related to interobserver variability in making the diagnosis (158,211).

The prognosis of lesions designated atypical medullary carcinoma was originally reported to be between that of typical medullary carcinoma and that of infiltrating ductal carcinoma without special features (182). However, in more recent studies, no survival advantage was noted for patients with atypical tumors (158,210,213), whereas in another report, tumors with only one atypical feature were found to have the same favorable prognosis as that associated with typical medullary tumors (214). Therefore, the usefulness of this designation must be considered questionable.

The expression of biologic markers in medullary carcinomas is more reflective of the aggressive histologic features of these tumors than of the favorable prognosis reported by some investigators. Estrogen and progesterone receptor positivity has only uncommonly been reported (190–192,209), and HER2/*neu* overexpression has been reported only infrequently (193,194). The triple-negative profile suggests consideration of the basal-like carcinoma category; the histology and BRCA-1 association are also consistent. A number of studies have indicated that medullary carcinomas and invasive carcinomas with medullary features are particularly common in women with mutations in the breast cancer susceptibility gene BRCA-1 (215). Complex chromosomal alterations are seen much more often in medullary than in tubular and mucinous carcinomas (206). Most medullary carcinomas are aneuploid and are associated with p53 protein accumulation (195).

INFILTRATING PAPILLARY CARCINOMA

Although infiltrating carcinomas with a predominantly papillary pattern have been described (216) and are said to be associated with a relatively favorable prognosis, in our experience invasive cancers with a papillary pattern are rare. Some tumors with extensive necrosis have a pseudopapillary pattern. Because both the diagnosis and prognosis of papillary carcinoma are controversial, the term *infiltrating papillary carcinoma* should be used with caution and applied only to tumors containing true papillary structures. Furthermore, when this tumor pattern is seen, the possibility of metastatic papillary carcinoma from another site, such as ovary, should be considered. Calcification is often present in such lesions, which are frequently accompanied by foci of DCIS, also with a micropapillary or true papillary architectural pattern.

INVASIVE MICROPAPILLARY CARCINOMA

Invasive micropapillary carcinoma appears to be associated with a poor prognosis (217–222). These lesions are characterized by clusters of cells in a micropapillary or tubular–alveolar arrangement that appear to be suspended in a clear space, or in some cases a mucinous or aqueous-type fluid. The micropapillary clusters lack fibrovascular cores. The cell clusters appear to have an "inside-out" arrangement, with the apical surface polarized to the outside. The appearance may mimic that of serous papillary carcinoma of the ovary or may simulate lymphatic and vascular space invasion (217) (Fig. 9.75). True lymphatic and vascular space invasion has been reported in 33% to 67% of cases and may be extensive (217,218,221). Cytologically, the cells comprising the invasive micropapillary carcinoma usually have low- to intermediate-grade nuclei. In most reported cases, invasive micropapillary carcinomas have been admixed to a variable degree with invasive carcinoma NOS or, in a minority of cases, with mucinous carcinoma. However, the prognosis appears to be adversely affected when the micropapillary pattern is present focally or diffusely within the tumor (218,222). In immunohistochemical studies of invasive micropapillary carcinoma, 72% to

TABLE 9.20	Histologic Criteria for the Diagnosis of Medullary Carcinoma with Lymphoid Stroma and Atypical Medullary Carcinoma
Typical Medullary (All the following features)	*Atypical Medullary (Features of typical medullary but no more than two atypical features)*
Predominant syncytial growth pattern (>75%)	Predominant syncytial growth (>75%) must be present
Other typical features	Atypical features
Circumscribed margin both macroscopically and microscopically	Focal areas of infiltration at tumor margins
Marked or moderate lymphoplasmacytic stromal reaction	Absent or mild lymphoplasmacytic reaction, or at margin only
Pleomorphic nuclei with high mitotic rate	Uniform nuclei with infrequent mitoses
Absence of tubule formation	Focal tubule formation
No in situ component (but not a disqualifying feature)	In situ carcinoma present (not always considered an atypical feature)

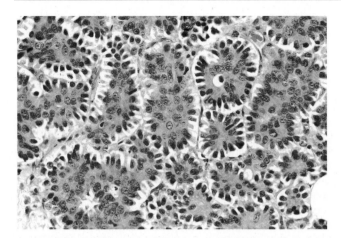

Figure 9.75. Invasive micropapillary carcinoma. Clusters of neoplastic cells are present within clear spaces separated by fibrovascular tissue.

75% were positive for estrogen receptor and 45% were positive for progesterone receptor. HER2/*neu* overexpression was observed in 36% of cases, and p53 protein accumulation was seen in 12% of cases, with 66% positive for Bcl-2 (223).

ADENOID CYSTIC CARCINOMA

This tumor, uncommon in the breast, is histologically identical to its counterpart in the salivary gland (Fig. 9.76). However, in the breast it is associated with a very favorable prognosis (224,225). On microscopic examination, the tumor may be confused with cribriform carcinoma (either in situ or invasive), but the two can be distinguished by the presence or absence of the two cell types (luminal epithelial and myoepithelial) that comprise adenoid cystic carcinoma. Mucin stains are also of value; the large cystic spaces contain hyaluronidase-sensitive, alcian blue positive mucin that does not stain with PAS, whereas the small, indistinct, true glandular spaces contain PAS-positive, diastase-resistant mucin. These two patterns of mucin secretion are particularly well demonstrated by the combined alcian blue

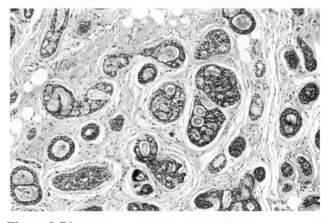

Figure 9.76. Adenoid cystic carcinoma. The tumor is composed of basaloid cells with scanty cytoplasm. A cribriform pattern is seen, but the large spaces are pseudocysts lined by basement membrane material and contain alcian blue–positive mucin, whereas the smaller true glandular lumina contain periodic acid-Schiff (PAS)–positive, diastase-resistant material.

and PAS stain. Immunohistochemically, antibodies to basement membrane components outline the pseudocystic spaces, and antibodies specific for luminal and myoepithelial cells highlight the dual cell population (226,227). A peculiar intraductal proliferation called collagenous spherulosis can mimic the appearance of adenoid cystic carcinoma closely. C-kit has been reported as a relatively constant finding in adenoid cystic carcinomas and a useful tool for distinguishing adenoid cystic carcinoma from collagenous spherulosis (228).

However, collagenous spherulosis is found in ducts and is usually quite limited in extent; it is discussed and illustrated at the end of this chapter. A solid variant of adenoid cystic carcinoma composed primarily of basaloid cells has been described (226). Most reports indicate that adenoid cystic carcinomas are usually negative for estrogen and progesterone receptors. However, estrogen receptor positivity rates of 26% and 46% were reported in two series (224,225).

Other types of carcinoma, more often seen in the salivary gland or skin but rarely reported in the breast, include mucoepidermoid tumor (229,230), clear cell hidradenoma (231), and eccrine spiradenoma (232). Pleomorphic adenoma and syringomatous tumor, the latter occasionally occurring in the region of the nipple, are discussed elsewhere.

CARCINOMAS WITH NEUROENDOCRINE DIFFERENTIATION (CARCINOID TUMOR, ARGYROPHIL CARCINOMA)

Carcinomas with histologic and histochemical and immunohistochemical features of carcinoid tumors have been described in the breast. Several studies have also shown that argyrophilia can be demonstrated in infiltrating ductal carcinomas NOS without carcinoid features (233). A high proportion of mucinous carcinomas, some in situ carcinomas, and a few infiltrating lobular carcinomas are also argyrophilic (85–87, 200–204,234). However, tumors with the histologic appearance of carcinoid tumors and immunohistochemical documentation of chromogranin A, synaptophysin, and neuron-specific enolase positivity have been described (235). Upalakalin et al. (236) reviewed 59 carcinoid tumors in the breast and found 21% were metastatic to the breast from other locations, including the intestine and lung. Composite tumors—part neuroendocrine carcinoma and part invasive ductal carcinoma—have also been described.

Tsang and Chan (86) described 34 cases of endocrine carcinoma of the breast—14 purely DCIS and 20 with invasion. The majority of cells were immunohistochemically marked with chromogranin A, synaptophysin, and neuron-specific enolase. Papillomas in the vicinity invariably showed pagetoid involvement by the DCIS cells. Festoons and pseudorosettes were prominent. All cases were also immunoreactive for estrogen and progesterone receptor.

SECRETORY OR JUVENILE CARCINOMA

Carcinoma of the breast in children is rare. When it does occur, it is usually of secretory type (237). Although such tumors in children and adults younger than 30 years are associated with a very favorable prognosis, they occasionally occur in older women, in whom the prognosis may not be quite so good; late recurrence and even metastases have been recorded (238–240). On gross examination, secretory carcinomas are usually small

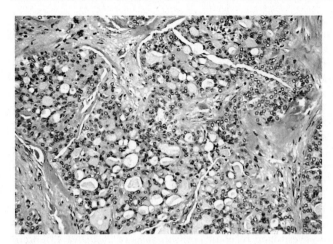

Figure 9.77. Secretory carcinoma. The tumor consists of several merging epithelial islands. The malignant epithelial cells show little pleomorphism and have abundant cytoplasm. They are arranged around irregular spaces. Secretions are within the spaces and, at higher power, can also be seen within the cytoplasm of some of the surrounding cells.

and well circumscribed. On microscopic examination, islands of irregular tubular and papillary structures are seen that contain eosinophilic, PAS-positive, diastase-resistant material (Fig. 9.77). The malignant cells show minimal pleomorphism and few, if any, mitoses. The cytoplasm is pale-staining and usually plentiful. On sections stained with hematoxylin and eosin it may be difficult to decide how much of the tumor is invasive and how much is in situ.

APOCRINE CARCINOMA

The presence of focal areas of cells with abundant granular eosinophilic cytoplasm resembling apocrine metaplasia is not uncommon in invasive mammary carcinomas. However, tumors composed predominantly or entirely of apocrine cells are less frequent and probably account for fewer than 0.5% of all mammary carcinomas (241,242) (Fig. 9.78). The prognosis of such carcinomas has not been demonstrated to differ from that of

infiltrating ductal carcinomas NOS of similar grade. Although most apocrine carcinomas appear to be variants of ductal carcinoma, apocrine features are occasionally seen in tumors that otherwise have the characteristics of infiltrating lobular carcinoma (171,173). Pure DCIS with apocrine features occurs somewhat more frequently.

METAPLASTIC CARCINOMA

Carcinomas showing extensive "metaplastic" changes to spindle cells, squamous cells, and heterologous mesenchymal elements are well recognized in the breast. In most such tumors, areas of infiltrating ductal carcinoma (even though sometimes very small and focal) can be demonstrated, frequently with transition to the metaplastic element. Various terms have been applied to these tumors, and in recent years several methods of subclassification have been recommended (243–250). Debate regarding the prognosis of the tumors is considerable; some series show a generally poor outcome with little variation between microscopic subgroups (244,250), and others claim that subclassification can delineate tumors with different prognoses (245–249). The most frequent metaplastic element is that of pleomorphic spindle cells producing the appearance of a fibrosarcomatous or high-grade sarcoma NOS (sarcoma NST). Other tumors contain osteosarcomatous (Fig. 9.79) and chondrosarcomatous growth patterns or, more rarely, leiomyosarcomatous and rhabdomyosarcomatous components (246–251). More than one sarcomatous element may be present within a tumor.

The term *spindle cell carcinoma* has been reserved by some to describe tumors composed predominantly of bipolar spindle cells of relatively bland appearance, with only mild to moderate atypia, arranged in interweaving bundles (246–251). Such tumors frequently also contain areas of squamous differentiation. In some spindle cell tumors, the malignant cells are so bland that distinction from benign spindle cell proliferations, such as fibromatosis, can be difficult (252).

The term *matrix-producing carcinoma* has been used to describe metaplastic carcinomas in which an apparently abrupt

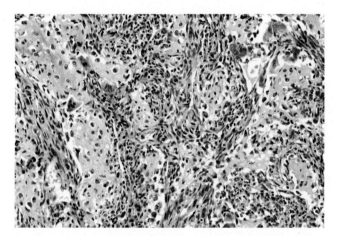

Figure 9.79. Metaplastic carcinoma (sarcomatoid type). This tumor is composed of interlacing bundles of spindle-shaped cells having the pattern of a spindle cell sarcoma NOS. Elsewhere, areas of conventional adenocarcinoma merged with this pattern. The malignant spindle cell population reacted with cytokeratin antibodies. It is also producing an osteoid-like matrix. Rare osteoclast-like giant cells are present.

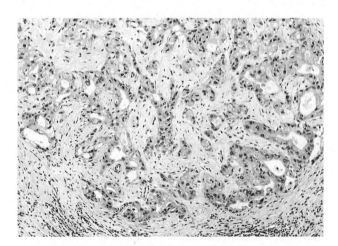

Figure 9.78. Apocrine carcinoma. In this tumor, the malignant cells have typical eosinophilic, and relatively abundant, cytoplasm.

transition occurs from carcinoma to an osseous (Fig. 9.79) or cartilaginous matrix without an intervening transitional phase (245). A more favorable prognosis has been claimed for this latter group of tumors, and for the spindle cell carcinomas described previously, than for other metaplastic carcinomas (245,246). Extensive sampling of metaplastic tumors may be needed to identify typical carcinomatous foci and distinguish them from true sarcomas because of differences in biologic behavior and response to therapy. Immunohistochemistry is of particular value in evaluating tumors that lack evident carcinoma. Although pseudosarcomatous elements may stain with vimentin and sometimes other mesenchymal markers, it is nearly always possible to demonstrate epithelial markers (cytokeratin positivity) in at least occasional cells (243,245–250). In some tumors, only high–molecular-weight cytokeratin reactivity is seen. Other special stains are of limited value; mucin is not usually present and elastosis is rare, but reticulin stains can sometimes be helpful in showing the characteristic mazelike pattern of carcinoma. Electron microscopy may also identify the true epithelial nature of the cells (244,246). Lymph node metastases may appear as carcinomatous or pseudosarcomatous elements. The incidence of lymph node metastases from metaplastic carcinomas is lower than might be anticipated, and spread via the bloodstream may occur. The results of estrogen and progesterone receptor studies in metaplastic carcinomas are typically negative, regardless of the histologic subtype examined.

Pure squamous cell carcinoma of the breast is rare (248,253), although squamoid or even true squamous differentiation is not uncommon in infiltrating ductal carcinoma NOS. As already mentioned, this is particularly true in medullary carcinoma and spindle cell tumors. The pure squamous cell carcinoma of the breast is usually large, with a central cystic cavity lined by malignant squamous epithelium. The prognosis of these tumors is controversial, but a particularly poor outcome has been reported in squamous cell carcinomas showing acantholysis (254). This feature may produce a pattern easily mistaken for angiosarcoma, but adequate sampling, aided by immunohistochemistry, usually reveals the carcinomatous nature of the tumor.

One uncommon variant of metaplastic carcinoma is *low-grade adenosquamous carcinoma* (255,256). It has features similar to those of the syringomatous tumor that occurs in minor salivary glands, the microcystic adnexal carcinoma of the skin seen characteristically in the region of the lip, and the syringomatous adenoma of the nipple, described later. As in these latter lesions, an infiltration of tubules, some with a "tadpole" or "comma" morphologic appearance, is seen. In places, squamous differentiation is evident (Fig. 9.80). A suggestion of two cell layers may also be observed. Some reports, however, have disputed the presence of a second so-called myoepithelial layer around any of the malignant tubules, and have interpreted such structures as entrapped benign glands incorporated into the margins of the lesion (256). An association has been observed between low-grade adenosquamous carcinoma and sclerosing adenosis, radial scar, ductal adenoma, papilloma, and adenomyoepithelioma, which suggests that these entities may form part of a broad spectrum of adenomyoepithelial lesions, a proposal that may reconcile some of the conflicting views in the literature (256–258).

BASAL-LIKE CARCINOMAS

Microarray profiling has identified subtypes of invasive carcinomas based upon their immunohistochemical profiles: luminal

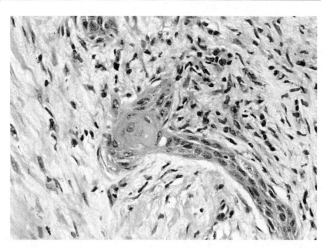

Figure 9.80. Low-grade adenosquamous carcinoma. In this photograph, one of the distinctive tadpole-shaped epithelial structures seen in these lesions shows obvious squamous differentiation.

A, (ER+, HER2−) luminal B (ER+, HER2+), HER2 overexpressing (ER−, HER2+) and basal-like (ER−, HER2−, EGFR+, and/or CK5/6+). The basal-like subtype is associated with poorer clinical outcomes and is the type associated with BRCA-1–related breast cancer. Histologically, most basal-like carcinomas are grade 3 ductal carcinomas or metaplastic carcinomas with geographic necrosis, pushing borders and a stromal lymphocytic response (259). Rakha et al. (260) found 16% of cases were triple-negative (ER−, PR−, HER2−). The majority of these cases were grade 3, ductal/NST carcinomas with larger size, pushing margins, poorer Nottingham prognostic index, development of recurrence and distant metastases, and poorer outcome. They were also associated with loss of androgen receptor and E-cadherin, and expression of basal cytokeratins (CK5/6 and 14) and p53. Kim et al. (261) compared carcinomas with basal-like phenotype to those overexpressing HER2/*neu* and found the latter to be more aggressive.

MYOEPITHELIAL-TYPE CARCINOMA

Rakha et al. (262) described carcinomas expressing myoepithelial-like proteins (SMA and/or p63) making up about 13% of a large group of invasive carcinomas. Histologically, they were ductal/NST, tubular-mixed and medullary-like carcinomas with loss of tubule formation, marked cellular pleomorphism, poorer Nottingham prognostic index, and development of distal metastases. They also showed loss of steroid hormone receptors, FHIT proteins, and expression of p53 and EGFR. They were found more frequently in younger patients. Histologically, they had central acellular zones and expressed E-cadherin.

OTHER CARCINOMAS WITH PARTICULAR HISTOLOGIC FEATURES

The cells in some carcinomas show other particular cytologic features, such as abundant cytoplasmic lipid (263,264) or glycogen (265,266). Some carcinomas have histiocytoid features that may represent a variant of apocrine change occurring in either lobular or dual carcinoma (172). The term *myoblastoid carcinoma* has been used for the latter tumors (267). Although focal changes are relatively common, it is rare for tumors to consist predominantly or exclusively of cells with any one of the afore-mentioned features. When this does happen, they should be classified accordingly. However, little evidence is available to show any prognostic significance of these features. Histologic changes that may affect the stroma, such as osteoclast-like giant cells and granulomatous reactions, have already been mentioned.

CARCINOMAS WITH UNIQUE CLINICAL MANIFESTATIONS

INFLAMMATORY CARCINOMA

The diagnosis of inflammatory carcinoma is based on clinical criteria and it is treated differently with multimodality therapy. It is a clinical description of the red, warm, edematous appearance of the breast. Outcome is often poor, despite the marked improvement achieved with current management. However, evaluation of clinical criteria may be equivocal and skin biopsy may be carried out to identify carcinomatous dermal lymphatic permeation, which is usually present. Charafe-Jauffret et al. (268) found most inflammatory carcinomas were E-cadherin–positive, ER-negative, and positive for MIB1, MUC1, and HER2/*neu*.

CARCINOMA OF THE MALE BREAST

Carcinoma of the breast is uncommon in men, accounting for fewer than 1% of all breast cancers. It tends to occur in a somewhat older age group in men than in women, with the peak in the seventh decade. Clinical gynecomastia has not been shown to be a risk for carcinoma. However, an increased incidence of breast cancer in men with Klinefelter syndrome has long been recognized (269). Male breast cancer has also been linked extensively to mutations of BRCA2 and also to a lesser extent to mutations in BRCA1. Tchou et al. studied 41 men with breast cancer and found point mutations in BRCA1 in 4 and in BRCA2 in 11 of them (270). The prognosis, when related to the tumor size, malignancy grade, and number of positive axillary lymph nodes, is equivalent in male and female patients (271,272).

Special types of mammary carcinoma, such as mucinous, medullary, tubular, and apocrine carcinoma, may be seen in men (272), but most are of the ductal type. Because of the absence of lobules in the normal male breast, reports of unequivocal lobular carcinoma, either invasive or in situ, are rare. However, invasive papillary carcinomas are seen with increased frequency. Paget disease is comparatively more common in men, and half of these patients have a palpable breast mass with axillary lymph node metastases (273).

CHANGES INDUCED BY THERAPY

CHEMOTHERAPY

Recent years have seen a trend toward the treatment of breast cancer with primary chemotherapy, particularly in premenopausal patients whose tumors are inoperable at the time of presentation; the rationale is that such treatment may facilitate subsequent breast conservation. A number of histologic

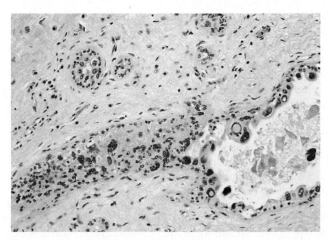

Figure 9.81. Changes after chemotherapy. Residual ductal carcinoma in situ from a patient treated with neoadjuvant chemotherapy. The malignant cells show degenerative nuclear changes. The surrounding tissue is fibrotic with a scattered lymphocytic infiltrate. This appearance is but one of many that may be seen after chemotherapy.

changes are seen following neoadjuvant chemotherapy (Fig. 9.81). These include necrosis, cellular fibrosis, sclerosis, lymphocytic infiltration, and the presence of hemosiderin-laden macrophages. Nuclear enlargement and vacuolization of both the nuclei and the cytoplasm of malignant cells is a frequent but not universal finding. The nuclear changes may confound grading of the tumor (274,275).

RADIATION CHANGES

With the widespread use of conservation therapy (often including radiotherapy) for mammary carcinoma, histologic changes induced by radiation are frequently seen. In addition to the vascular and stromal changes already well known at other sites, marked epithelial atrophy, intralobular fibrosis, and epithelial atypia (particularly in the TDLUs) may develop (276). The latter produces a striking appearance (Fig. 9.82) that may cause

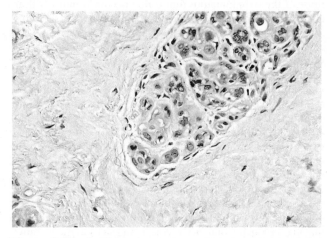

Figure 9.82. Radiation change. Breast tissue from a patient previously treated by tumorectomy and radiotherapy for primary breast carcinoma. The acini show epithelial atrophy with associated intralobular fibrosis, but the most striking feature is the marked epithelial atypia. This should not be misinterpreted as malignant change. Mitotic activity is absent.

malignancy to be suspected, particularly in needle biopsy samples. As discussed later in this chapter, fat necrosis is often seen at the site of a boost radiation dose, which sometimes constitutes part of conservation therapy (277).

METASTATIC CARCINOMA WITHIN THE BREAST

Most malignancies seen in the breast are primary carcinomas. Occasionally, however, the breast is the site of metastasis from a primary tumor elsewhere in the body. Such a tumor can easily be misdiagnosed unless one is aware of the possibility. A full knowledge of the clinical history is therefore important, and tumors showing none of the typical patterns of mammary carcinoma should arouse suspicion. The differential diagnosis is particularly difficult in a needle biopsy specimen. The presence of in situ carcinoma is indicative of a mammary primary, but its absence does not exclude it. A wide variety of tumors have been reported to metastasize to the breast, but the most frequent are lung carcinoma and malignant melanoma (278,279). Metastasis from the contralateral breast can also occur, and this may be difficult to distinguish from a new primary.

Generally, metastatic lesions consist of single or multiple rounded nodules. When the histologic appearance of the metastatic lesion resembles that of the primary tumor, the diagnosis should not be a problem. In many cases, however, the metastatic tumor is anaplastic, and differentiation from a primary mammary carcinoma is difficult. A rounded outline and the absence of in situ change are both suggestive of a metastasis. Often, multiple satellite nodules with widespread lymphatic emboli are present (275). The use of special stains, including immunohistochemistry, may also be helpful; in particular, elastosis has not been demonstrated in secondary tumors. Immunohistochemical evaluation for TTF-1 may be of some value in detecting metastasis from pulmonary adenocarcinoma.

METASTATIC CARCINOMA FROM THE BREAST

Metastases from mammary carcinoma may be seen at virtually any site, but the most common are lymph nodes, bone, lung, and liver. Differences have been reported in the distribution of metastases from ductal and lobular carcinoma (151–153), the latter having a propensity to spread to viscera, particularly the gastrointestinal tract. The retroperitoneum, endometrium, and meninges are also more commonly involved by lobular carcinoma. Occasionally, breast cancer may present as a metastasis, most frequently in an axillary lymph node. In most such cases, a primary carcinoma can eventually be detected pathologically within the breast that has a histologic appearance similar to that of the lymph node metastasis. Some of the primary tumors are extremely small, and a few, apparently, purely in situ. In approximately two-thirds of the cases, the carcinoma has an apocrine appearance (280).

AXILLARY LYMPH NODES

Axillary lymph node metastases are usually easy to identify on histologic examination, but sometimes unusual patterns are

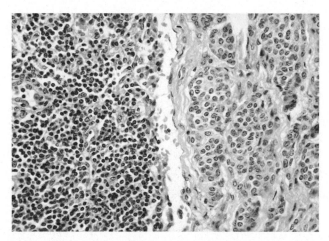

Figure 9.83. Nevus cell nests within the capsule of an axillary lymph node. The cells have a "packeted" appearance. Immunohistochemistry showed positive staining with S-100 antibody and negative staining with epithelial markers.

seen. Occasionally, the metastasis mimics the appearance of in situ carcinoma (Fig. 9.75). Lobular carcinoma may completely obliterate the nodal structure and resemble malignant lymphoma. Metastatic carcinoma confined to the sinuses must be distinguished from sinus histiocytosis; conversely, sinus histiocytosis can mimic metastatic carcinoma.

The term *micrometastases* is used to describe deposits smaller than 2 mm in maximum diameter. The clinical significance of micrometastases detected on sections routinely stained with hematoxylin and eosin, and of "occult" micrometastases detected by immunohistochemistry, is as yet unknown (10). Nevertheless, immunohistochemistry may be of value in cases in which foci suspected of being metastases are encountered. Benign lesions within lymph nodes can be mistaken for metastatic carcinoma. Giant cell and epithelioid granulomas are well recognized occurrences in regional lymph nodes draining carcinomas at various sites and are occasionally seen in the axilla. Foreign body reaction to silicone gel has also been reported in the axillary lymph nodes of patients with breast prostheses (281). Nevus cell nests within the capsule are rare but are particularly likely to occur within the axillary nodes (Fig. 9.83). They are always confined to the capsule or fibrous trabeculae of the node (282,283). Immunohistochemical markers help to distinguish them from metastatic carcinoma.

Another uncommon but well-recognized phenomenon is the presence of benign ectopic epithelium within lymph nodes (Fig. 9.84). These foci may resemble normal mammary epithelium or show benign pathologic changes (284,285). A carcinoma apparently arising in ectopic breast tissue in an axillary lymph node has been reported (286).

TUMORS WITH MIXED EPITHELIAL AND STROMAL COMPONENTS

FIBROADENOMA AND VARIANTS

Fibroadenoma

Fibroadenoma is the most common benign breast lesion and occurs usually in young women. It is considered to arise in the

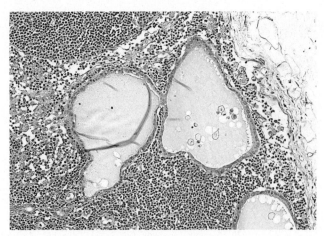

Figure 9.84. Benign epithelial inclusion within an axillary lymph node. These are possibly of mammary epithelial or adnexal origin. This lesion shows benign architectural and cytologic features and must not be misinterpreted as metastatic carcinoma.

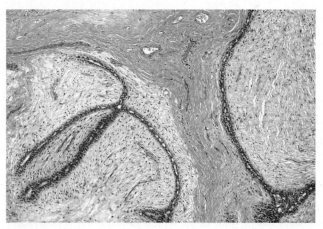

Figure 9.86. Fibroadenoma. In this higher-power view of a fibroadenoma with an intracanalicular pattern, the epithelial components are compressed and elongated. It is also possible to discern that the epithelium is composed of two cell types. Demarcation between lobular and interlobular stroma is evident.

lobule, but whether it represents a true neoplasm or merely a distortion of lobular architecture is debated. The gross features have been described and illustrated (Fig. 9.2) and contrasted with those of carcinoma in Table 9.2. Fibroadenomas are multiple in about 20% of cases.

The microscopic appearance confirms the rounded outline and shows a lesion with proliferation of both stromal and epithelial elements. Classically, two patterns have been described: (a) a pericanalicular pattern, in which the stroma surrounds rounded epithelial elements (Fig. 9.85), and (b) an intracanalicular pattern, in which the epithelial elements are distorted, stretched, and compressed by the proliferating stroma (Fig. 9.86). The patterns frequently occur together but are not thought to have any special clinical significance. On high-power examination, the epithelial components are seen to be lined by the usual two cell types. Several changes may occur within the epithelial elements, including apocrine metaplasia and varying degrees

of epithelial hyperplasia. The latter, when severe, may give cause for concern. Another change that can appear alarming is sclerosing adenosis (23) (Fig. 9.87). A tissue core sample of such a lesion may be difficult to interpret, particularly if apocrine metaplasia is also present. Cystic change is not uncommon. Squamous metaplasia is rarely seen. Secretory changes during pregnancy and lactation may affect the epithelium, whereas in fibroadenomas from elderly patients the epithelium is frequently atrophic. Fibroadenomas that contain cysts larger than 3 mm, sclerosing adenosis, epithelial calcifications, or papillary apocrine change have been called *complex fibroadenomas* (287). In one clinical follow-up study, complex fibroadenomas were reported to be associated with a greater risk for subsequent breast cancer than fibroadenomas lacking such changes (287).

Although, as mentioned, epithelial hyperplasia may be severe, carcinoma in situ within a fibroadenoma is rare, and the diagnosis should not be made unless the classic features listed in Table 9.10 are clearly seen. When carcinoma in situ does

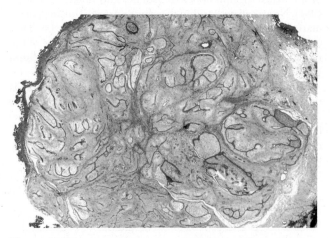

Figure 9.85. Fibroadenoma showing demarcation from the surrounding compressed breast tissue. Although the growth pattern is mixed, it is predominantly pericanalicular. The glandular components are mainly small and rounded, but some are dilated. The pattern is lobular with separation of the pinker interlobular stroma from the bluer lobular stroma.

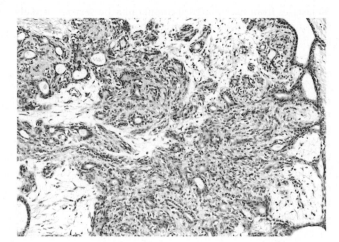

Figure 9.87. Fibroadenoma in which an area of sclerosing adenosis is present. A needle core biopsy specimen of such a lesion could be difficult to interpret. Despite considerable distortion of the glandular elements, two cell types are clearly apparent in many areas.

occur, it is more frequently found to be lobular than ductal (288). In one study, the in situ lesion was found to be confined to the fibroadenoma in 80% of cases (289). Infiltrating carcinoma may also involve a fibroadenoma, sometimes accompanying an in situ lesion, and may occasionally be confined within the fibroadenoma.

The stromal element in fibroadenomas varies in consistency. Myxoid change is relatively common. Hyaline stromal change is seen usually in older patients, in whom it accompanies epithelial atrophy and, not infrequently, contains deposits of calcification.

Heterologous stromal elements are rarely present. When they do occur, adipose tissue is most common, although cartilage, bone, and smooth muscle have all been reported. In the syndrome described by Carney and Toorkey (290)—consisting of a familial complex of myxomas occurring in the breast, heart, or skin; endocrine overactivity; spotty pigmentation; and schwannomas—the myxoid component in the breast may take the form of a fibroadenoma-like lesion. Another uncommon feature is the presence of multinucleated stromal giant cells (291). These can produce a striking low-power picture, but the cytologic features, although bizarre, are benign, and mitotic figures are not seen.

Infarction in a fibroadenoma is unusual but occurs most frequently during pregnancy and lactation, when its appearance may give rise to diagnostic difficulties.

Fibroadenomatoid Hyperplasia

The term *fibroadenomatoid hyperplasia* is used to describe changes resembling those seen in a fibroadenoma but affecting individual or sometimes multiple adjacent lobules without the formation of a discrete mass.

Juvenile Fibroadenoma

Fibroadenoma in adolescence usually has the same appearance as that already described, although sometimes the pattern is more obviously lobular. The term *juvenile fibroadenoma* generally applies to a variant lesion that often grows rapidly and may produce marked distortion of the breast (291,292). Although called *juvenile*, it also occurs in older women. Microscopic examination reveals hyperplasia of both the stromal and epithelial components (Fig. 9.88), with the former manifesting increased

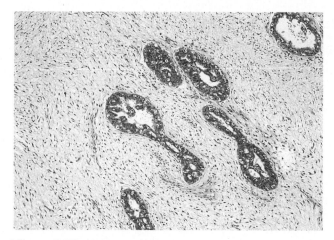

Figure 9.88. Juvenile fibroadenoma. A higher-power view of the lesion in Figure 9.81 shows the typical so-called gynecomastoid pattern of epithelial hyperplasia. Distinctive tufts of cells protrude into the lumen.

cellularity and the latter hyperplasia, often with the tufted pattern characteristic of gynecomastia or virginal hypertrophy (60).

Juvenile fibroadenomas should be distinguished from benign phyllodes tumors. In contrast to benign phyllodes tumors, juvenile fibroadenomas usually have a pericanalicular growth pattern, and the epithelial hyperplasia is a more prominent feature. Stromal cellularity is less and the cells show no periductal concentration, no atypia, and few mitoses, if any. Although some degree of stromal overgrowth with separation of the glandular elements may be present, this again is less prominent than in benign phyllodes tumors, and large areas of stroma devoid of epithelium are not seen. Distinction between the two is important because juvenile fibroadenomas should be treated by excision with preservation of as much of the surrounding normal tissue as possible, whereas in the case of benign phyllodes tumors, a rim of normal tissue should be included in the excision. The degree of epithelial hyperplasia can occasionally be severe and worrisome. In one study, it was recommended that the term *juvenile fibroadenoma* be reserved for lesions with severe atypical hyperplasia (258). Even so, no relationship has been shown with subsequent carcinoma, and simple excision is adequate treatment.

Occasionally, juvenile fibroadenomas are multiple or bilateral, or both, and they may recur repeatedly. The breast can sometimes contain innumerable lesions of various sizes and has been likened to a sack of marbles. This condition is more common in black than in white women and typically presents in the early teens. The fibroadenomas may recur rapidly after excision, and the histologic appearance in this situation may be that of a conventional or juvenile fibroadenoma; moreover, these patterns may coexist. The rapidity and frequency of recurrence usually wane after the third decade (292,293,294).

Giant Fibroadenoma

The term *giant fibroadenoma* is best avoided because its exact meaning is a source of confusion.

Tubular Adenoma

Tubular adenomas are well-demarcated lesions that have features in common with fibroadenomas; on occasion, areas with the typical appearance of both are seen within the same tumor (295). It is debatable whether tubular adenoma should be considered a separate entity or merely a variant of fibroadenoma in which the epithelial element has outgrown the stroma. The hyperplasia of the stroma seen in fibroadenomas is lacking in tubular adenomas. These relatively rare lesions usually occur in young women. Although, like fibroadenomas, they are well defined on gross examination, they are softer in texture and characteristically tan-brown. Histologic examination shows proliferating tubules closely packed together, with little or no surrounding fibrous stroma (Fig. 9.89). Although variable in amount, the stroma does no more than provide a supporting framework. A stromal lymphocytic infiltrate may be present. Lesions with more stroma resemble closely packed hyperplastic lobules. Adenomas in which the tubules are closely arranged in a back-to-back fashion can have a particularly worrisome appearance. The tubules are lined by a double cell layer, but the myoepithelial cells, although often remarkably inconspicuous, can always be demonstrated immunohistochemically with anti-

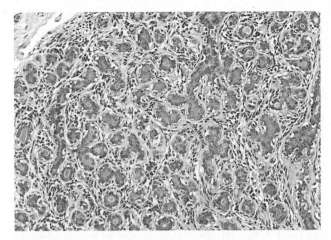

Figure 9.89. Tubular adenoma. In contrast to a fibroadenoma, the lesion is composed predominantly of proliferating epithelial components with only supporting stroma. The myoepithelium is variably conspicuous, and lymphocytes are scattered in the stroma. The lesion has a rounded outline, clearly demarcated from the surrounding tissue.

bodies to myoepithelial cell elements. However, tubular adenoma should also be distinguished from carcinoma based on the marked uniformity of the tubules, lack of cytologic atypia, absence of desmoplastic stromal reaction, and overall circumscription of the lesion.

Lactating Adenoma

This lesion is similar to the tubular adenoma but shows prominent lactational change (295). It is seen only in pregnancy and more likely is a coalescence of hyperplastic lobules rather than a true adenoma. Focal infarction of such lesions is not uncommon.

PHYLLODES TUMOR

The term *phyllodes tumor* is recommended in the World Health Organization classification for the tumor previously called *cystosarcoma phyllodes*. The latter term indicated a large, fleshy tumor with a leaflike appearance on the cut surface, and was not originally intended to denote malignancy. Although phyllodes tumors share many features with fibroadenomas, they are more likely to recur; some are locally aggressive and can even metastasize. It should be emphasized, however, that most of these lesions, although they have a tendency to recur locally, are entirely benign. The reported incidence of malignancy varies considerably. This is partly because it may be difficult to distinguish between benign and malignant lesions histologically (295,296); many lesions have a borderline appearance, and some with an apparently benign appearance have been reported to behave aggressively, and vice versa.

Phyllodes tumors generally occur in an older age group than fibroadenomas; most patients are middle-aged or elderly. They are rare in children, and malignant phyllodes tumors in persons younger than 20 years of age are exceptional (297). Patients with phyllodes tumors often have a history of a rapidly enlarging tumor, sometimes at the site of a pre-existing, long-standing mass. The pathologic assessment of these lesions requires not only that they be differentiated from fibroadenomas but also that benign and malignant phyllodes tumors be separated.

Phyllodes tumors are usually larger than fibroadenomas and often have surface projections. The latter is an important feature because incomplete removal of the projections is thought to be the cause of local recurrence. The cut surface of the tumor often has a cleft, sometimes cauliflower-like appearance resulting from the frequent presence of an exaggerated intracanalicular growth pattern. Although usually firm and rubbery, phyllodes tumors may be soft, with gelatinous areas. They may also contain foci of necrosis and hemorrhage, which are suggestive of malignancy.

On microscopic examination, phyllodes tumors have the basic architecture of a fibroadenoma, but usually with a prominent intracanalicular pattern (Fig. 9.90). The most important distinguishing feature, however, is the stromal hypercellularity. Even so, the distinction between a cellular fibroadenoma and a benign phyllodes tumor is difficult in some cases. No one histologic feature will always provide an absolute and universally accepted distinction between the two, and the stromal cellularity of these lesions sometimes overlaps (298). Stromal cellularity is the most important feature, but in some tumors with a relatively low level of stromal cellularity, other features (such as stromal nuclear pleomorphism or the mitotic rate, architecture, and stromal overgrowth) indicate a diagnosis of phyllodes tumor rather than fibroadenoma. The increased stromal cellularity seen in phyllodes tumors is usually most pronounced immediately adjacent to the epithelial components. Metaplasia within the stroma occurs more frequently than in fibroadenomas; fat, bone, cartilage, and skeletal muscle have all been recorded. The epithelial component also shows a variety of appearances; hyperplasia is common, and squamous metaplasia is seen more often than in fibroadenomas, although apocrine metaplasia is less frequent. The malignant element of phyllodes tumors, when present, is the stroma. Very rarely, carcinoma in situ arises within the epithelial component of a phyllodes tumor.

Because the microscopic appearance of phyllodes tumors may vary considerably from area to area, thorough sampling is important to assess the malignant potential of the stromal component. Features suggestive of malignancy are the following:

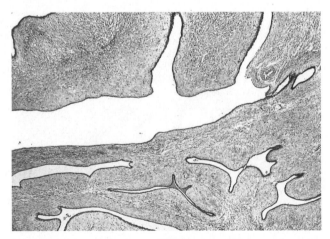

Figure 9.90. Phyllodes tumor. This low-power view demonstrates the exaggerated intracanalicular growth pattern and increased stromal cellularity that is usually most marked adjacent to the epithelial elements.

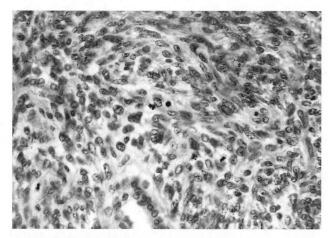

Figure 9.91. Malignant phyllodes tumor. The stromal cells show nuclear hyperchromasia, pleomorphism, and numerous mitotic figures. The overtly malignant pattern is that of an undifferentiated sarcoma.

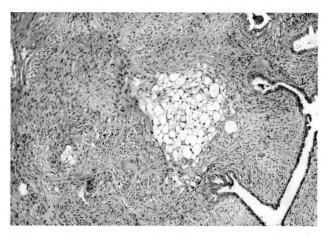

Figure 9.92. Malignant phyllodes tumor with liposarcomatous element.

1. Increased mitotic activity (Fig. 9.91) is frequently quoted as the most important feature in the differentiation between benign and malignant phyllodes tumors; however, it is also the most difficult to define. The question of what constitutes increased activity and so indicates malignancy is a source of considerable disagreement. In our experience, mitotic activity is common adjacent to the epithelial component of all phyllodes tumors; therefore, increased activity away from the ducts is most significant. Most accounts refer to the number of mitoses per 10 high-power fields, but make no attempt to define the size of the high-power field. Many articles suggest that a mitotic rate of more than 5 per 10 high-power fields indicates malignancy. However, in the absence of any other worrying feature, a mitotic rate of 10 per average (0.44-mm field diameter) 10 high-power fields is probably more significant.
2. Marked atypia of the stromal cells.
3. Comparative overgrowth of the stromal component with areas devoid of epithelial elements (''stromal overgrowth''). When this is present, fields examined with a low-power objective consist only of stroma.
4. An infiltrating (not a pushing) margin.
5. Necrosis and hemorrhage.

A ''borderline'' category has been used on occasion for tumors wherein the microscopic distinction between benign and malignant characteristics is especially problematic.

Distinction of fibroadenoma from phyllodes tumor on needle biopsy may be especially difficult because of limited material and heterogeneity in phyllodes tumors. Lee et al. (299) found the presence of cellular stroma and stromal overgrowth (defined as a 10× field without epithelium) predictive of phyllodes tumor. Jacobs et al. (300) found the mitotic index most useful.

All phyllodes tumors, whether benign or malignant, tend to recur locally, particularly when the lesion has been inadequately excised by enucleation without a surrounding rim of normal tissue. A margin of at least 1 cm of normal breast surrounding all aspects of the tumor is preferred. Most tumors can safely be treated by wide local excision, but simple mastectomy should be considered for patients who have a lesion with microscopic features suggesting a particularly aggressive behavior or a very large lesion. Mastectomy should also be considered when the size of the breast does not permit adequate margins by wide excision. Recurrence is best related to inadequacy of excision rather than to the histologic features of the tumor (301,302). However, large tumors and those with an irregular margin or marked stromal overgrowth are particularly likely to recur.

Recurrent phyllodes tumors may contain both stromal and epithelial components, although the predominance of the stromal portion is often increased. Furthermore, the recurrence may exhibit more malignant characteristics than the original neoplasm.

Despite the difficulties reported in the literature in distinguishing between benign and malignant phyllodes tumors, most of those that behave in a truly aggressive fashion and metastasize have an obviously sarcomatous stroma and do not present a diagnostic problem.

Typically, the malignant stroma resembles a high-grade sarcoma NOS but, on occasion, specific lines of differentiation may be observed taking the form of liposarcoma (Fig. 9.92), osteosarcoma, or, rarely, chondrosarcoma. The presence of malignant heterologous elements is a sign of a particularly poor prognosis (301,302). Tumor size is a poor predictor of prognosis. Although large tumors have a higher rate of recurrence, this may well be related to inadequate excision rather than malignant potential. It has been suggested that flow cytometric analysis of ploidy and S-phase fraction may provide additional prognostic information in phyllodes tumors (303,304). Immunoreactivity for the p53 protein is associated with high-grade histology but does not appear to be of prognostic value independently (305).

Metastases usually present after chest wall recurrence and most often involve the lungs. They generally consist only of the stromal component of the tumor and are usually bloodborne. Axillary dissection is therefore not indicated. On occasion, careful examination may be required to distinguish a metastasis from a primary neoplasm at the metastatic site.

PURE MESENCHYMAL TUMORS

As already emphasized, most pathologic lesions in the breast arise from the epithelium. However, the stroma may also give rise to neoplasms; in general, these are similar in appearance to mesenchymal lesions seen at other sites. Most benign and malignant mesenchymal lesions occurring in the body have been described in the breast. From the viewpoint of differential diagnosis, only the more frequent and important are described in the following paragraphs.

BENIGN TUMORS

Lipoma

Lipoma is the most common benign mesenchymal tumor to occur in the breast, where it shows a range of appearances similar to those seen elsewhere in the body. Occasionally, normal glandular structures are incorporated within the substance of a lipoma; such lesions have been called *adenolipomas*.

Vascular Lesions

Benign vascular lesions of the breast parenchyma are most often incidental microscopic findings and may be divided into four categories: *perilobular hemangiomas, angiomatoses, venous hemangiomas,* and *hemangiomas involving the mammary subcutaneous tissue* (306–309). Of these, the perilobular hemangioma is the most common (Fig. 9.93). Subcutaneous angiomas may arise within the region of the breast, but any vascular lesion within the substance of the breast that produces a palpable mass should raise the suspicion of angiosarcoma. However, benign palpable angiomas do sometimes occur, and the differential diagnosis of angiomatous lesions is outlined in Table 9.21.

Other Benign Mesenchymal Neoplasms

Leiomyoma is uncommon in the breast but can occur in the region of the nipple (310) and even more rarely in the substance of the breast (311). Neurilemoma and neurofibroma are occasionally encountered. Chondrolipomatous, chondro-osseous, and osseous tumors are very rare (312). These latter tumors are composed entirely of mature mesenchymal tissue, although normal mammary epithelium may occasionally be incorporated within them.

Certain benign tumors, although rarely seen in the breast,

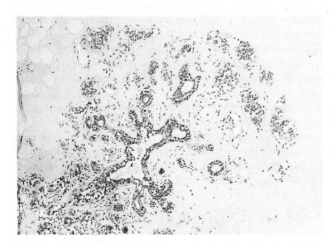

Figure 9.93. Perilobular hemangioma. This benign, typically incidental lesion manifests as a cluster of thin-walled capillaries around a terminal duct lobular unit.

TABLE 9.21	
Contrasting Features of Hemangioma and Low-Grade Angiosarcoma	
Hemangioma	*Angiosarcoma*
May not be in breast; rarely >2 cm	In breast; usually >2 cm
Circumscribed outline	Irregular outline
Divided into lobules by fibrous septa	No fibrous septa
Mostly isolated, unconnected vascular spaces; anastomosing channels, when present, are simple	Complex, serpiginous; anastomosing vascular channels
Atypia and mitoses absent	Atypia and mitoses present in some areas
Adjacent to or surround lobules	Invade and expand lobules
Feeder vessels may be present	Feeder vessels not apparent

are important in that they may be mistaken for carcinoma on gross, mammographic, and microscopic examination. These include infiltrative fibromatosis and granular cell tumors (313,314). The appearance of these lesions does not differ from those described elsewhere in the body.

MALIGNANT TUMORS

Angiosarcoma

Although the terms *angioma* and *angiosarcoma* strictly refer to tumors of both lymphatic and vascular channels, in the breast they are usually applied to tumors arising from blood vessels. Angiosarcoma is rare, accounting for fewer than 1% of all malignant mammary lesions, but it is important because in the past it was frequently misdiagnosed as a benign lesion. Although benign angiomas can occur in the breast, they rarely present as a palpable abnormality. The salient points that differentiate benign mammary angiomas from angiosarcomas are listed in Table 9.21. Previously, all angiosarcomas were considered to be highly aggressive malignancies but histologic stratification reveals quite different prognostic groups (315,316). Low-grade angiosarcomas have a survival of more than 75%, whereas high-grade angiosarcomas have a survival of less than 15%. On gross examination, angiosarcomas are usually poorly defined, consisting of spongy hemorrhagic tissue. Microscopically, numerous anastomosing vascular channels are seen; in low-grade lesions, these may have a deceptively benign appearance (Fig. 9.94). Extensive sampling, however, should reveal areas in which the endothelial cells display malignant features, with pleomorphism, hyperchromasia, and rare mitotic figures. Intermediate-grade lesions exhibit marked endothelial proliferation with papillary projections into the vascular lumina and readily apparent mitoses. High-grade tumors have a more solid appearance, with only slitlike remnants of vascular channels (Fig. 9.95), marked pleomorphism, and mitotic activity. Areas of hemorrhage and necrosis are often present in these more aggressive lesions. Well-formed vascular channels are frequently seen around the periphery of an otherwise poorly differentiated lesion. Immunohistochemical staining for factor VIII–related antigen, CD31, and CD34 is usually seen in well-differentiated parts of angiosarcomas, but may be weak or negative in poorly differentiated areas (316).

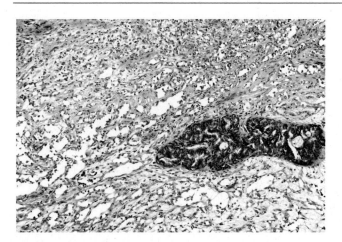

Figure 9.94. Angiosarcoma, low grade. The breast tissue is infiltrated by numerous well-formed, anastomosing vascular channels. The appearance is deceptively benign.

Following excision of an angiosarcoma, local recurrence is common. As with other sarcomas, metastasis occurs via the bloodstream.

Postmastectomy Lymphangiosarcoma (Stewart-Treves Syndrome)

These rare tumors, originally reported in the arms of patients who had undergone mastectomy many years before, arise in sites of chronic lymphedema (317). It is more common when the axilla has been radiated as well as surgically altered. Histologically, areas of dilated vessels are often found in association with poorly differentiated areas of malignant tumor. Although the specific vascular nature of the lesion has been questioned, immunohistochemical studies have confirmed its endothelial origin (318). The outcome is poor.

Radiation-Induced Sarcoma

Sarcoma arising at the site of radiotherapy for carcinoma of the breast is rare but may occur in either bone or soft tissue. Such

tumors are now much less common than previously reported, despite the large number of patients treated with this modality. The interval between radiation therapy and the occurrence of sarcoma is extremely variable; it usually exceeds a decade but, on rare occasions, tumors arise within half that time (319).

The range of tumor types is wide and includes fibrosarcoma, pleomorphic sarcoma NOS, angiosarcoma, and osteochondroid tumors. Most postirradiation angiosarcomas are high-grade neoplasms, akin to those occurring in chronic lymphedema (Stewart-Treves syndrome); however, low-grade angiosarcomas may also occur. The growth pattern of an epithelioid angiosarcoma may closely resemble that of carcinoma exhibiting radiation changes (319).

The occurrence of angiosarcoma, in either the residual breast or overlying skin of patients receiving conservation therapy for mammary carcinoma that has included radiation, has become well recognized (320). Because most patients described have also had lymphedema of the breast and skin, the relative roles of radiotherapy and lymphatic stasis in the etiology of these tumors remains unclear. Most cases have arisen within a relatively short period after therapy (286).

In addition to angiosarcoma, Fineberg and Rosen (321) have described atypical vascular lesions following radiotherapy. Although these lesions appear to be benign, their true biologic significance has yet to be determined.

Other Sarcomas of the Breast

Pure sarcomas, without an associated epithelial component, occasionally occur in the breast (297,322–324). Although rare, they should be distinguished on the one hand from metaplastic carcinoma, and on the other from a malignant phyllodes tumor that has outgrown its epithelial component. Wide sampling of such lesions is important (261). The most common pattern is that of a fibroblastic neoplasm with the pattern of a fibrosarcoma or high-grade sarcoma NOS. Sarcomas with the pattern of osteosarcoma, liposarcoma, and even leiomyosarcoma and rhabdomyosarcoma have also been described (322,323). Several malignant mesenchymal elements may coexist. When such lesions are reported, all the sarcomatous elements present should all be listed (324).

TUMORS OF LYMPHOID AND HEMATOPOIETIC CELLS

LYMPHOMA

The breast is a recognized site of disseminated extranodal lymphoma. However, primary lymphoma of the breast also occurs, although it is an uncommon tumor and accounts for fewer than 1% of all malignant mammary neoplasms. Primary lymphoma is almost always of non-Hodgkin type, and the most commonly observed type is a diffuse, large B-cell lymphoma (325). Follicular and mantle zone lymphomas are also seen. Most such lymphomas presented in stage IE or IIE. In one study, 11% were bilateral upon presentation. Five-year overall survival was 82%. Patients with more indolent lymphomas had 92% overall survival and 76% progression-free survival (325). One type that affects young women and is often associated with pregnancy is a Burkitt-type lymphoma that is frequently bilateral. Most such lesions have been described in Africa (326). The diffuse, large

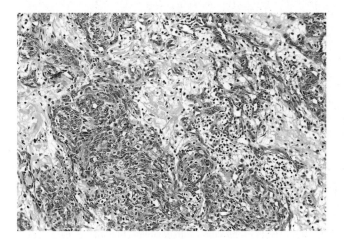

Figure 9.95. Angiosarcoma, high grade. This tumor consists of a solid mass composed of epithelioid endothelial cells. The cells are pleomorphic and hyperchromatic with increased mitotic activity.

B-cell type type affects older women and presents with clinical features identical to those of carcinoma of the breast. A more rounded outline, however, may suggest the possibility of a lymphoma. This latter type is usually a B-cell lymphoma. Some studies have suggested that a significant proportion are lymphomas arising from the mucosa-associated lymphoid system ("maltomas") (327,328), although this view is disputed (329–331). Microscopically, the appearance is the same as that of malignant lymphoma at other sites. Differentiation must be made from anaplastic carcinomas and the solid variant of lobular carcinoma (329), and immunohistochemistry is of value in this situation.

OTHER HEMATOPOIETIC TUMORS

Infrequently, the breast is involved by leukemia of either lymphatic or myeloid type. Extramedullary plasmacytoma also occurs at this site, although most of these cases represent extension from a lesion in an underlying rib.

Rarely, a florid, reactive, inflammatory cell infiltrate characterized by a polymorphic lymphoid cell population with germinal center formation may occur in the breast and raise the question of a lymphoproliferative lesion. Immunohistochemistry may be helpful in demonstrating the polyclonal nature of the cells, thereby distinguishing this process from a lymphoma. Although the term *pseudolymphoma* has been used in the past to describe such lesions, it has fallen out of favor. Some lesions previously diagnosed as such have subsequently evolved into B-cell lymphomas. Moreover, the seemingly polyclonal nature of the lesion may mask a monoclonal population of cells that can be revealed by genotypic analysis (332).

ROSAI-DORFMAN DISEASE

The rare occurrence of this lesion within the breast has been well documented (333).

OTHER BENIGN TUMORS

DUCTAL ADENOMA

The lesions termed *ductal adenomas* are thought to arise in medium-sized ducts rather than from the large ducts immediately below the nipple, and therefore they usually present as a palpable lump rather than as a nipple discharge. They may also present as a mammographic abnormality. Clinically and radiologically, the lesions can mimic carcinoma; on gross examination, although they usually consist of single or multiple rounded lesions, their gritty texture and elastic streaks may be strongly suggestive of malignancy. As with all sclerosing lesions, histologic diagnosis may be particularly difficult on frozen section and tissue core biopsy.

On low-power examination, the lesions are rounded and frequently bounded by the dense, fibrous wall of the distended duct within which they arise (Figs. 9.96 and 9.97). Within the nodule, proliferating epithelial structures are seen without a papillary growth pattern. Although tubule formation is recognized in some areas, many of these are compressed and distorted by sclerosis of the stroma, resulting in a pseudoinfiltrative pattern. Focal areas of tubular dilation, epithelial hyperplasia, and cyst formation may also be seen. In some lesions, the sur-

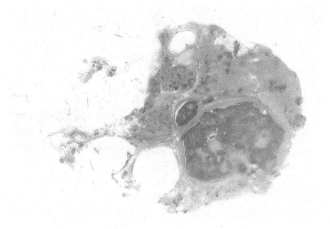

Figure 9.96. Benign ductal adenoma. In this very low-power view, dense, fibrous tissue can be seen around most of the lesion. Within the center, proliferating epithelial components are juxtaposed with areas of dense fibrosis.

rounding fibrous wall is less apparent, and direct growth into the adjacent tissues appears to occur. The margin, however, remains well demarcated, and the outline is rounded and pushing. Tumors with marked central fibrosis and elastosis are strikingly similar to radial sclerosing lesions. The stroma may also show myxoid change and, rarely, cartilaginous metaplasia.

High-power examination confirms the presence of two cell types lining the epithelial components. The myoepithelial cells are sometimes difficult to see but are often markedly hyperplastic. The luminal cells frequently show apocrine metaplasia and, sometimes, squamous metaplasia (Fig. 9.98). Calcification may be present.

It is difficult to know how best to classify this lesion, and although the term *ductal adenoma* has gained wide acceptance, it is a misnomer in the strict sense of the word *adenoma*. Some of the lesions described by Azzopardi and Salm (334) almost certainly evolve from severe fibrosis within a benign ductal pap-

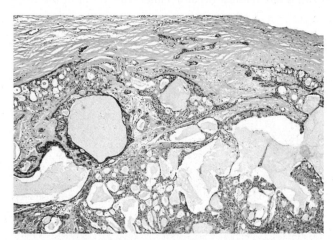

Figure 9.97. Ductal adenoma. These lesions vary considerably in appearance, with proliferation and metaplasia of both luminal and myoepithelial components. This example exhibits epithelial hyperplasia, apocrine metaplasia, and cystic dilation of some of the glandular components.

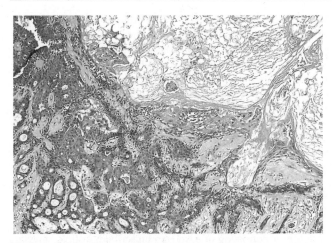

Figure 9.98. Ductal adenoma. This example exhibits squamous metaplasia with keratinization.

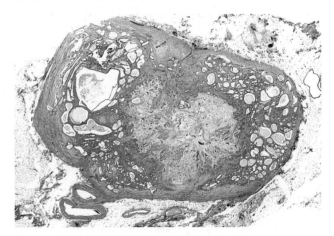

Figure 9.99. Pleomorphic adenoma. The circumscribed tumor nodule has a central cartilaginous pattern and a periphery of epithelial elements.

illoma (335); some resemble pleomorphic adenomas of salivary glands; some have been included in the category of adenomyoepitheliomas; and others are placed under the heading of complex sclerosing lesions. Ductal adenomas may also occur as part of the inheritable complex of myxomas, spotty pigmentation, endocrine overactivity, and schwannomas described by Carney and Toorkey (336). Some ductal adenomas, particularly those with a myxoid stroma, are more reminiscent of pleomorphic adenomas of the salivary gland (302). Reports of adenomyoepitheliomas have also included lesions that could be classified as ductal adenomas, albeit with evidence of myoepithelial hyperplasia (337). Ductal adenomas are frequently accompanied by other benign changes, including cysts, sclerosing adenosis, and ductal epithelial hyperplasia (Fig. 9.94).

PLEOMORPHIC ADENOMA

Although this benign tumor occurs only rarely in the breast, its recognition is important because it can easily be mistaken for carcinoma (338–340). Histologically, the neoplasm is identical to pleomorphic adenoma (benign mixed tumor) occurring in salivary glands and is characterized by a dual population of luminal epithelial and myoepithelial cells with a mucinous and myxoid stroma in which pseudocartilage, true chondroid and osteoid change may occur (Fig. 9.99). The myoepithelial cells may take on a clear or spindled appearance (Fig. 9.100) and are demonstrable with immunostains for p63, calponin, smooth muscle actin, and S-100 protein. The differential diagnosis ranges from benign lesions such as ductal adenoma on the one hand to carcinoma with mucoid, myxoid, cartilaginous, or osteoid change on the other. Some examples of ductal adenoma show a marked resemblance to pleomorphic adenoma, and occasional lesions have features of both (334). Pleomorphic adenomas have also been described arising in close association with benign papillomas and sclerosing adenosis (338). Differentiation from carcinoma, especially mucinous carcinoma, is sometimes difficult and depends on the benign nature of the epithelial cells and demonstration of the two-cell types characteristic of pleomorphic adenoma. Immunohistochemistry may be of help (338).

ADENOMYOEPITHELIOMA

The proliferation of myoepithelial cells is a frequent finding in a wide range of well-defined mammary lesions. Through the years, several articles have described adenomyoepithelioma and myoepithelioma as specific entities. However, the same term has been used to describe several different entities with varying contributions of epithelial and myoepithelial components (27,337,341–343). Some of these appear to be similar, if not identical, to lesions that are already well recognized but in which myoepithelial proliferation is sometimes a significant component. These include ductal adenoma and sclerosing adenosis. It is evident, therefore, that the term *adenomyoepithelioma*, which represents a spectrum of lesions, needs better definition. Some distinctive tumors do appear to be composed of epithelial and myoepithelial cells, with the latter component forming a significant part of the neoplasm (Fig. 9.101). The behavior of such lesions is uncertain, but some appear to have low-grade malignant potential with a tendency for local recurrence and rarely metastasis (344).

A distinctive pattern of adenosis has been described in association with neoplasms considered to be adenomyoepitheliomas.

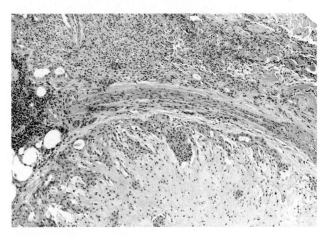

Figure 9.100. Pleomorphic adenoma. At higher magnification, the cartilaginous differentiation and the epithelial elements of the tumor are evident. Myoepithelial cells appear as clear cells.

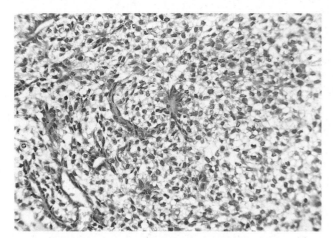

Figure 9.101. Adenomyoepithelioma. In a high-power view, the two cell types of this lesion are clearly seen. Proliferating fusiform and cuboidal clear myoepithelial cells, reactive immunohistochemically with α-actin, surround compressed tubules lined by luminal-type epithelium.

The lesion has been termed *adenomyoepithelioma with a distinctive type of apocrine adenosis* by Eusebi et al. (27), and *adenomyoepithelial adenosis* and *low-grade malignant adenomyoepithelioma* by Kiaer et al. (342). It is characterized by two components: (a) glandular elements lined by epithelial cells, frequently having features suggestive of apocrine differentiation, with an outer myoepithelial layer, and (b) solid nests of cells, composed mainly of proliferating myoepithelial cells with clear cytoplasm but containing occasional lumina lined by epithelium similar to that lining the glandular elements (Fig. 9.102). The myoepithelial component of the lesion distinguishes it from microglandular adenosis. The behavior of this lesion is unpredictable, and local recurrence has been reported (27,342).

Occasionally, unusual but obviously malignant lesions with evidence of both myoepithelial and epithelial components are encountered. In malignant adenomyoepitheliomas, the histo-

logically malignant areas are focal within an otherwise apparently benign neoplasm (258,344). Either or both of these components may be malignant. It has further been suggested that some metaplastic carcinomas, including the low-grade adenosquamous carcinoma, may be myoepithelial in origin (255–257). Adenocarcinoma arising within or following an adenomyoepithelioma has been reported rarely (258,337). Tumors with wholly myoepithelial characteristics have also been described (337–343).

MYOFIBROBLASTOMA

This distinctive stromal tumor, described by Wargotz et al. (345), is probably the same as the spindle cell tumor of the breast previously identified by Toker et al. (346). It is a very rare tumor consisting of a well-circumscribed, nodular mass of haphazardly arranged bundles of spindle cells interspersed with bands of collagen. Myofibroblastomas must be distinguished on the one hand from reactive processes and benign spindle cell lesions, such as fasciitis, fibromatosis, leiomyomas, and nerve sheath tumors, and on the other hand from sarcomas and metaplastic carcinomas (347).

INFLAMMATORY LESIONS

Inflammatory lesions of the breast are usually a clinical problem and are generally treated without resort to biopsy. Acute inflammation with abscess formation is most frequent during lactation. Tuberculosis involving the breast is rare but well documented (348); it may be mistaken clinically for carcinoma (349). Various mycotic and parasitic infestations have also been reported (350).

The differential diagnosis of granulomatous lesions in the breast, apart from infectious agents, should include sarcoidosis, foreign body reaction, fat necrosis, and granulomatous mastitis. Other systemic diseases, such as the vasculitides, may also occur in the breast.

LACTIFEROUS DUCT FISTULA

In this condition, which occurs typically in premenopausal parous women, a fistulous tract forms between a lactiferous duct and the surface of the areola. The tract is lined by stratified squamous epithelium or granulation tissue. The lesion is related to recurrent episodes of subareolar abscess formation (351).

FOREIGN BODY REACTION

Foreign body reaction occurs after foreign material has been introduced into the breast, most often during biopsy or surgery, or accidentally. Silicone results in granuloma formation when introduced into the breast either by direct injection or leakage through a silicone-filled mammary prosthesis. Many mammary prostheses are now saline-filled because of difficulties encountered in the use of silicone (352).

Silicone implants may result in complications necessitating surgical intervention (353). The most common of these is capsular contraction, which produces distortion or excessive firmness of the breast. Capsular contraction is an exaggerated normal response to foreign material, which microscopically is seen as an increase in dense collagen around the implant. Synovium-

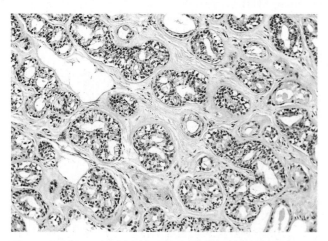

Figure 9.102. Adenomyoepithelioma with adenomyoepithelial adenosis. The two components of this lesion are clearly seen. A small number of simple tubules lined by two cell layers—luminal cells with apocrine features and an outer myoepithelial layer—are present. These are intermingled with more complex islands of cells, composed of proliferating myoepithelium around residual lumina lined by epithelium similar to that seen in the smaller tubules.

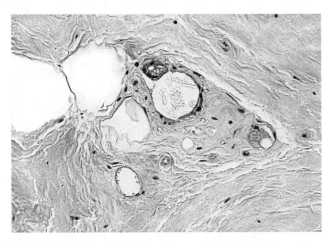

Figure 9.103. Reaction to a silicone implant. Spaces containing strands of colorless material, consistent with the elastomer shell, are within an area of dense fibrosis. Occasional foreign-body giant cells are also seen.

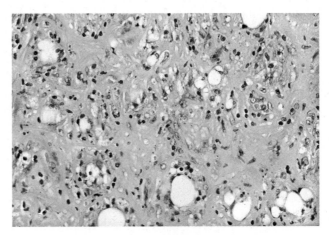

Figure 9.104. Fat necrosis. Fat necrosis results from injury, most often following a biopsy. The reacting histiocytes may be impressive and misleading. Identification of the setting in which they occur and the vacuoles containing fat are helpful in correct identification of the process.

like metaplasia of the wall of the surrounding capsule has also been described (354). Rupture of a gel implant with diffusion of silicone into the breast, hematoma, and wound infection are other complications of silicone implants.

Foreign body reaction can develop around the various components of implants. Fragments of polyurethane foam, which was used to coat some implants, produce angular and curvilinear birefringent, crystal-like structures. Crumpled strands and sheets of colorless material represent the silicone elastomer shell of the implant (Fig. 9.103). Silicone gel leakage characteristically produces oval, cystic spaces that appear empty or contain amorphous, smoothly round, or oval material that is not birefringent with polarized light (321). Silicone can diffuse to a variety of sites in the body, and silicone lymphadenopathy has been reported in axillary lymph nodes; hematogenous dispersion can also occur (353).

FAT NECROSIS

Necrosis of fat also elicits a granulomatous, foreign body–type reaction. Patients with this condition usually have a history of trauma, usually surgical. Fat necrosis is also seen at the site of radiation implants, which are sometimes used in conservation therapy. On clinical and mammographic examination, fat necrosis may be indistinguishable from carcinoma (277). Grossly, the necrotic fat has a characteristically opaque, bright yellow appearance. Microscopically, areas of necrotic fat are surrounded by chronic inflammatory cells, such as lymphocytes, foamy histiocytes, and often multinucleated giant cells. Deposits of hemosiderin are common. Sometimes, inflammatory cells appear to surround a cavity, and, in long-standing lesions, fibrosis and even calcification may be seen within the cavity wall (Fig. 9.104). The term *membranous fat necrosis* has been used to describe these cyst-like lesions (355).

CHRONIC GRANULOMATOUS MASTITIS (PERILOBULAR MASTITIS)

The cause of this uncommon lesion is obscure. It usually presents as a mass, nearly always in young, parous women, and

is often related to recent pregnancy. Clinically, the lesion can simulate carcinoma. Sinus formation is a common complication. Bilateral disease sometimes occurs. On histologic examination, necrotizing granulomas often accompanied by suppuration are seen confined to the lobules (356). These are composed of histiocytes, giant cells of Langhans type, and neutrophils, in addition to variable numbers of lymphocytes and plasma cells. Microabscesses may form (Fig. 9.105). The condition must be distinguished from other causes of granulomatous reaction within the breast, such as sarcoidosis, tuberculosis, and fungal infections. Microorganisms should always be sought.

DUCT ECTASIA (PERIDUCTAL MASTITIS)

Duct ectasia is another inflammatory condition of unknown cause that has been variously called *plasma cell mastitis*, *mastitis obliterans*, and *comedo mastitis*. Nipple retraction and discharge

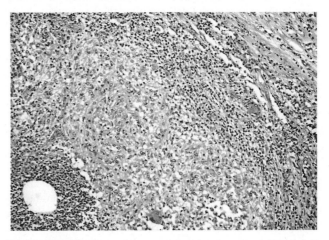

Figure 9.105. Granulomatous mastitis. The granulomatous nature of the inflammation is evident. Histiocytes, plasma cells, lymphocytes, and giant cells of Langhans type predominate, but large numbers of neutrophils are seen in the top left corner of the field. The clear round spaces are thought to represent lipid.

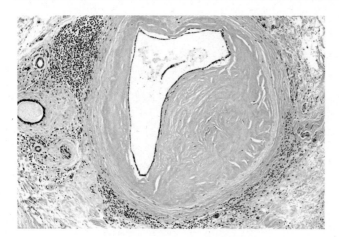

Figure 9.106. Duct ectasia. A dilated ducts with extensive periductal fibrosis and associated patchy chronic inflammatory cell reaction.

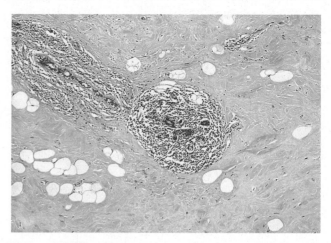

Figure 9.107. Lymphocytic mastopathy. The atrophic terminal duct lobular unit, surrounded by a well-defined, dense lymphocytic infiltrate, is set within a markedly fibrotic stroma.

may be present, mimicking carcinoma clinically. On radiologic examination, calcification may be seen and the lesion mimics duct ectasia or, rarely, DCIS. In the intermediate stages of the disease, dilated ducts containing soft, yellowish-green material sometimes grossly simulate DCIS with a comedo pattern.

In contrast to the inflammation seen in granulomatous mastitis, in duct ectasia the inflammation is entirely periductal and, in the early stages of the disease, confined to the large subareolar ducts (357). Later, an entire mammary segment may be involved. Initially, lymphocytes and plasma cells surround dilated ducts containing amorphous debris and foamy histiocytes. The lining epithelium may be hyperplastic but is more commonly attenuated and may be replaced entirely by granulation tissue, often containing foreign-body giant cells and foamy macrophages. As the disease advances, progressive periductal fibrosis develops (Fig. 9.106), with eventual obliteration of the duct lumen. In the late stages, the lesion may be difficult to recognize, but elastic stains outline the site of the original duct (357). This may consist of an obliterated lumen often surrounded by a ring of small, epithelium-lined tubular structures, sometimes referred to as the *garland pattern*, or one or two epithelium-lined spaces may be seen to one side of an obliterated duct. In the early stages of the condition, the presence of elastic tissue enables duct ectasia to be distinguished from cysts because the latter are derived from lobules and therefore lack elastic tissue in their walls. Changes similar to those of classic duct ectasia are sometimes seen in association with intraductal papillary lesions, presumably secondary to obstruction.

DIABETIC MASTOPATHY AND LYMPHOCYTIC MASTOPATHY (LYMPHOCYTIC LOBULITIS)

Whether these are distinct, separate entities or part of the same spectrum is a matter of debate. The condition affects young to middle-aged women and often is associated with Type 1 diabetes or other manifestations of, and associations with, autoimmunity (358–362). The lesion usually presents as either a lump or a nodularity in the breast and is typically painful. Presentation as a nonpalpable, mammographic abnormality has also been described. One or more lesions may develop, and they may be bilateral. Dense fibrosis, lobular atrophy, and aggregates of lymphocytes are seen in a perivascular and perilobular distribution (Fig. 9.107). The lesions appear to progress through a stage

of initial inflammation that is followed by increasing lobular atrophy and sclerosis with resolution of the inflammatory components. The latter consist mainly of B lymphocytes and only a few T cells. Prominent epithelioid stromal cells were initially noted in patients with diabetes (360). Such cells, however, have also been found in the absence of diabetes. They are usually oval- or spindle-shaped and may have granular cytoplasm. A positive immunohistochemical reaction with anti–smooth muscle actin and a negative reaction for cytokeratin has raised the possibility that they are of myofibroblastic origin. The morphologic features of these cells can be alarming, and they should not be mistaken for infiltrating carcinoma (360). Changes similar to those already described may be an incidental finding in breast tissue from diabetic patients without symptoms (329).

The frequent presence of circulating autoantibodies associated with HLA-DR3, -DR4, or -DR5 in patients with lymphocytic lobulitis supports the concept of an autoimmune origin (358,359).

MISCELLANEOUS BENIGN LESIONS AND CHANGES

GYNECOMASTIA

Enlargement of the male breast (gynecomastia) often occurs briefly at puberty, but usually recedes promptly. It may also occur in response to hormonal stimulation. The process may be localized or generalized and can affect one or both breasts (363,364), although clinical unilateral involvement is most common. The histologic appearance varies with the duration of the condition. In all stages, the number of ducts is increased, and they may be dilated. In the early stages, there is epithelial hyperplasia with a characteristic pattern of tapering tufts of epithelium protruding into the lumen, similar to that sometimes seen in benign epithelial hyperplasia in women (51) and in the epithelial component of many juvenile fibroadenomas. The epithelial hyperplasia seen in the early stages can be florid and produce a worrisome appearance, but distinction from carcinoma in situ can be made by applying the criteria previously described. The periductal stroma is loose, vascular, and cellular and may contain lymphocytes and plasma cells (Figs. 9.108 and 9.109). In later stages, there is progressive fibrosis and hyalinization of the stroma and atrophy of

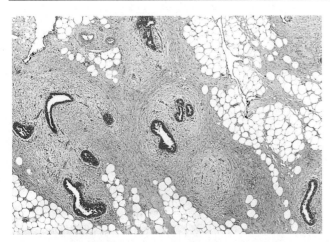

Figure 9.108. Gynecomastia at an early stage showing proliferation of ducts without lobules. The periductal stroma is loose and vascular and contains lymphocytes and plasma cells.

the epithelium. Although true lobule formation is not usually present, lobules are sometimes seen, but agreement has not been reached regarding whether this feature is limited to cases with a known endocrine cause (364). However, lobular development may occur with hormonal stimulation.

EFFECTS OF ANDROGEN THERAPY

Long-term androgen therapy may be administered in female-to-male transsexuals before surgical removal of the breasts. No distinctive histology has yet been reported in such patients (365).

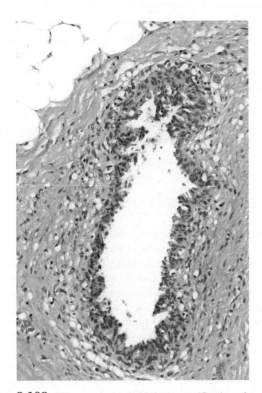

Figure 9.109. Gynecomastia. At higher magnification, the myxoid stroma and the markedly active epithelium are evident.

JUVENILE, VIRGINAL, OR PHYSIOLOGIC HYPERTROPHY

Rapid and distressing enlargement of one or, more frequently, both breasts, which are often asymmetric, occasionally occurs in adolescence. Histologic examination shows features strikingly similar to those of gynecomastia: abundant connective tissue and duct proliferation, frequently with epithelial hyperplasia but little or no lobule formation (293).

MACROMASTIA IN PREGNANCY

Massive enlargement of the breast associated with pregnancy is less common than juvenile hypertrophy (366). This condition commences early in pregnancy, with rapid and massive bilateral breast enlargement. The breasts are erythematous, edematous, and painful, and ulceration of the overlying skin may develop. Regression after parturition is typical, but involution may not be complete, and recurrence in subsequent pregnancies is usual.

HAMARTOMA (FIBROADENOLIPOMA)

In the strict sense, *mammary hamartoma* is a misnomer, but this term has been used to describe a lesion with the characteristic mammographic appearance of a clearly demarcated density (367,368). Clinically, it may simulate a fibroadenoma, but it is often impalpable. It is usually readily enucleated and grossly consists of a smooth, well-circumscribed, usually ovoid or lenticular mass of tissue with no distinguishing feature (369–371). Histologic examination shows mammary tissue that may be normal or exhibit a variety of benign changes (Fig. 9.110). The stroma contains varying amounts of adipose tissue. The fibrous component may predominate and result in lobular attenuation. The changes of pseudoangiomatous hyperplasia, described in the next section, also may be present (370). This is an underrecognized condition, largely because good clinicopathologic correlation is required to make the diagnosis (368,370,372). The lesion has been called by various names, including *adenolipoma*,

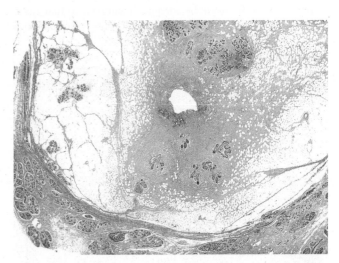

Figure 9.110. Mammary hamartoma. This rounded, well-defined lesion is distinct from the surrounding breast tissue. Histologic examination shows glandular breast tissue with no distinctive features. The overall gross and microscopic appearances, taken together, are in keeping with a diagnosis of mammary hamartoma.

fibroadenolipoma, mastoma, and *postlactational breast tumor.* The myoid or muscular hamartoma is closely related but has the additional feature of a smooth muscle stromal element, and rare examples of chondroid islands in the fat have been reported (369,372).

PSEUDOANGIOMATOUS STROMAL HYPERPLASIA

Pseudoangiomatous stromal hyperplasia (PASH) is a proliferation of myofibroblasts, which may be mistaken for well-differentiated angiosarcoma (373). It is found in premenopausal women and postmenopausal women on hormone replacement therapy, and varies in size from microscopic fields to localized, palpable masses, to (rarely) bilateral breast enlargement. It is often found in other benign proliferative lesions, especially fibroepithelial lesions, and is often seen in gynecomastia (370,373–376). In the most common form, apparently anastomosing, slitlike spaces, lined by flattened spindle cells, intersect hyalinized mammary stroma (Fig. 9.111). Their spindled nuclei are usually attenuated and amitotic. Immunostaining is positive with antibodies to CD34, vimentin, and actin, but staining for factor VIII–related antigen and keratin is negative. In unusual examples, the myofibroblasts proliferate to become *fascicular,* which gives the appearance of a spindle-cell neoplasm. Rarely, nuclear atypia and mitotic figures have been observed. It can present as a rapidly enlarging mass lesion (377).

MUCOCELE-LIKE LESIONS

The differential diagnosis of mucinous carcinomas is primarily from mucocele-like lesions, which is a term used by Rosen (378) to describe mucus-filled cysts lined by flattened epithelium with focal areas of hyperplasia often producing a papillary pattern. Extrusion of mucin into the surrounding stroma is a frequent feature (Fig. 9.112), and it is important to distinguish those extrusions from mucinous carcinoma. Subsequent studies have highlighted the association of some mucocele-like tumors with ADH, carcinoma in situ, and mucinous carcinoma (379,380). Therefore, when mucocele-like lesions are encountered, it is important that the tissue be adequately sampled so that carcinoma can be excluded. Because calcification is present in a

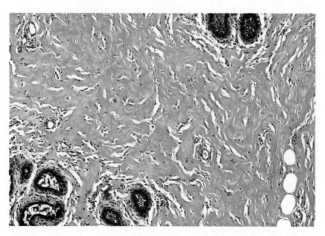

Figure 9.111. Pseudoangiomatous stromal hyperplasia. Slitlike spaces lined by flattened, fusiform cells intersect the stroma of this mammary hamartoma. These should not be mistaken for blood vessels.

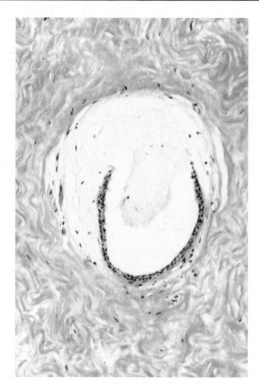

Figure 9.112. Mucocele-like lesion. Mucus-filled, cystlike spaces are lined by cuboidal to low-columnar epithelial cells. Extensive extravasation of mucus is evident at the side of the duct.

high proportion of cases, many of these lesions are detected by mammography (379).

Galactocele

This uncommon lesion occurs following the abrupt suppression of lactation. Beneath the areola, a milk-filled cavity forms; on histologic examination, this consists of dilated, anastomosing, epithelium-lined channels. The luminal epithelium may show secretory activity. Leakage of the cyst contents into the surrounding tissue may lead to a lipo-granulomatous reaction (381), and sometimes a focal collection of foamy macrophages containing milk may be seen, even in the absence of a classic galactocele (382).

COLLAGENOUS SPHERULOSIS

Collagenous spherulosis is found in mammary lobules and small ducts, generally as a coincidental finding (383–385). It is usually quite limited in extent, but its appearance closely mimics adenoid cystic carcinoma. Rounded, acellular, eosinophilic, fibrillar material, or hyaline, amorphous material surrounded by epithelium is seen, in lobular acini and small ducts (Fig. 9.109). The surrounding cells are elongated and spindle-shaped (Fig. 9.113). The central material is immunoreactive with antibodies to collagen type IV (Fig. 9.114). Immunohistochemistry and electron microscopy have demonstrated basement membrane components within the deposits and evidence of myoepithelial differentiation in the surrounding cells, suggesting that this material is a product of myoepithelial cells (384). The lesion is

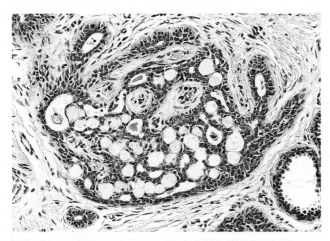

Figure 9.113. Collagenous spherulosis. Rounded deposits of fibrillar and hyaline material are surrounded by proliferating epithelial cells. The cells immediately adjacent to the deposits are sometimes spindle-shaped.

frequently associated with other entities, including radial sclerosing lesions and adenosis. Its occurrence within areas of ductal epithelial hyperplasia has led to the suggestion that the change represents marked myoepithelial differentiation within epithelial hyperplasia. The main importance of recognizing this entity is to appreciate its benign nature and distinguish it from carcinoma because the features can be confused with those of adenoid cystic or signet ring cell carcinoma. C-kit has been shown to be expressed in adenoid cystic carcinomas and not in collagenous spherulosis (228). The differential expression can be exploited to differentiate the two entities. Rarely, LCIS may involve a focus of collagenous spherulosis. In this situation, the appearance may mimic that of DCIS (386).

STROMAL GIANT CELLS

Bizarre stromal giant cells have already been mentioned in the section on fibroadenoma, but they may also be seen in other benign breast lesions and in otherwise normal breast tissue (387) (Fig. 9.111). They are of no known significance.

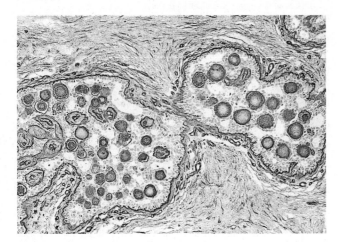

Figure 9.114. Collagenous spherulosis, stained with an antibody to collagen IV. Note the striking positive immunostaining of the "collagen balls."

REFERENCES

1. Schnitt SJ, Wang HH. Histologic sampling of grossly benign breast biopsies. How much is enough? *Am J Surg Pathol* 1989;13:505–512.
2. Oberman HA. A modest proposal. *Am J Surg Pathol* 1992;16:69–70.
3. Lee KC, Chan JKC, Ho LC. Histologic changes in the breast after fine-needle aspiration. *Am J Surg Pathol* 1994;18:1039–1047.
4. Youngston BJ, Cranor M, Rosen PP. Epithelial displacement in surgical pathology specimens after needling procedures. *Am J Surg Pathol* 1994;18:896–903.
5. Liberman L, Evans WP 3rd, Dershaw DD, et al. Radiography of microcalcifications in stereotaxic mammary core biopsy specimens. *Radiology* 1994;190:223–225.
6. Lee CH, Carter D. Detecting residual tumor after excisional biopsy of impalpable breast carcinoma: efficacy of comparing preoperative mammograms with radiographs of the biopsy specimen. *Am J Roentgenol* 1995;164: 81–86.
7. Recommendations for the reporting of breast carcinoma. *Hum Pathol* 1996; 27:220–224.
8. Kingsley WB, Peters GN, Cheek JH. What constitutes adequate study of axillary lymph nodes in breast cancer? *Ann Surg* 1984;201:311–314.
9. Hartveit F, Samsonen G, Tangen M, et al. Routine histological investigation of the axillary nodes in breast cancer. *Clin Oncol* 1982;8:121–126.
10. Schwartz GF, Giuliano AE, Veronesi U. Proceedings of the consensus conference on the role of sentinel lymph node biopsy in carcinoma of the breast, April 19–22, 2001, Philadelphia, Pennsylvania. *Cancer* 2002;94:2542–2551.
11. Zafrani B, Contesso G, Eusebi V, et al. Guidelines for the pathological management of mammographically detected breast lesions. *Breast* 1995;4:52–56.
12. Tornos C, Silva E, El-Naggar A, et al. Calcium oxalate crystals in breast biopsies. The missing microcalcifications. *Am J Surg Pathol* 1990;14:961–968.
13. Going JJ, Anderson TJ, Crocker PR, et al. Weddellite calcification in the breast: eighteen cases with implications for breast cancer screening. *Histopathology* 1990;16:119–124.
14. Orel SG, Schnall MD. MR imaging of the breast for the detection, diagnosis, and staging of breast cancer. *Radiology* 2001;220:13–30.
15. Wellings SR, Jensen HM, Marcum RG. Atlas of subgross pathology of the human breast with special reference to possible cancerous lesions. *J Natl Cancer Inst* 1975;55:231–273.
16. Faverly D, Holland R, Burgers L. An original stereomicroscopic analysis of the mammary gland tree. *Virchows Arch A Pathol Anat Histopathol* 1992;421:115–119.
17. Going JJ, Moffat DF. Escaping from flatland: clinical and biological aspects of human mammary duct anatomy in 3 dimensions. *J Pathol* 2004; 203:538–544.
18. Barnes DM, Millis RR. Oestrogen receptors: the history, the relevance and the methods of evaluation. In Kirkham N, Lemoine NR, eds. *Progress in Pathology.* Vol 2. New York: Churchill Livingstone, 1995:89–114.
19. Dabbs DJ. Diagnostic immunohistochemistry of the breast. In Dabbs DJ, ed. *Diagnostic Immunohistochemistry.* New York: Churchill Livingstone, 2002:536–558.
20. Henson DE, Oberman HA, Hutter RV. Practice protocol for the examination of specimens removed from patients with cancer of the breast; a publication of the Cancer Committee, College of American Pathologists, and the Task Force for Protocols on the Examination of Specimens from Patients with Breast Cancer. *Arch Pathol Lab Med* 1997;121:27–33.
21. Jensen HM. Breast pathology, emphasizing precancerous and cancer-associated lesions. In Bulbrook RO, Taylor DJ, eds. *Commentaries on Research in Breast Disease.* Vol 2. New York: Alan R. Liss, 1981:41–86.
22. Longacre TA, Bartow SA. A correlative morphologic study of human breast and endometrium in the menstrual cycle. *Am J Surg Pathol* 1986;10:382–393.
23. Oberman HA. Benign breast lesions confused with carcinoma. In McDivitt R, Oberman H, Ozzello L, et al., eds. *The Breast.* Baltimore: Williams & Wilkins, 1984:1–33.
24. Egan RL, McSweeney MB. Intramammary lymph nodes. *Cancer* 1983;51:1838–1842.
25. Chaudary MA, Millis RR, Lane EB, et al. Paget disease of the nipple: a ten-year review including clinical, pathological and immunohistochemical findings. *Breast Cancer Res Treat* 1986;8:139–146.
26. Kohler S, Rouse RV, Smoller BR. The differential diagnosis of pagetoid cells in the epidermis. *Mod Pathol* 1998;11:79–92.
27. Perzin KH, Lattes R. Papillary adenoma of the nipple (florid papillomatosis, adenoma, adenomatosis). A clinicopathologic study. *Cancer* 1972;29:996–1009.
28. Rosen PP, Caicco JA. Florid papillomatosis of the nipple. A study of 51 patients, including nine with mammary carcinoma. *Am J Surg Pathol* 1986;10:87–101.
29. Jones MW, Tavassoli FA. Coexistence of nipple duct adenoma and breast carcinoma: a clinicopathological study of 5 cases and review of literature. *Mod Pathol* 1995;8:633–636.
30. Rosen PP. Subareolar sclerosing duct hyperplasia of the breast. *Cancer* 1987;59:1927–1930.
31. Rosen PP. Syringomatous adenoma of the nipple. *Am J Surg Pathol* 1983;7:739–745.
32. Jones MW, Norris HJ, Snyder RC. Infiltrating syringomatous adenoma of the nipple. A clinical and pathological study of 11 cases. *Am J Surg Pathol* 1989;13:197–201.
33. Rosen PP, Oberman HA. Tumors of the mammary gland. In Rosai J, Sobin LH, eds. *Atlas of Tumor Pathology,* Fascicle 7. Washington, DC: Armed Forces Institute of Pathology, 1993: 50–58.
34. Simpson JF, Page DL, Dupont WD. Apocrine adenosis—a mimic of mammary carcinoma. *Surg Pathol* 1990;3:289–299.
35. Eusebi V, Casadei GP, Bussolati G, et al. Adenomyoepithelioma of the breast with a distinctive type of apocrine adenosis. *Histopathology* 1987;11:305–315.
36. Abdel-Fatah TM, Powe DG, Hodi Z, Reis-Filho JS, Ellis IO. High frequency of co-existence of columnar cell lesions, lobular neoplasia and low grade ductal carcinoma-in-situ with invasive tubular carcinoma and invasive lobular carcinoma. *Am J Surg Pathol* 2007;31: 417–426.
37. Schnitt SJ. The diagnosis and management of pre-invasive breast disease: flat epithelial atypia classification, pathologic features and clinical significance. *Breast Cancer Res* 2003; 5:263–268.
38. Vina M, Wells CA. Clear cell metaplasia of the breast: a lesion showing eccrine differentiation. *Histopathology* 1989;15:85–92.

39. Tavassoli FA, Yeh IT. Lactational and clear cell changes of the breast in nonlactating, nonpregnant women. *Am J Clin Pathol* 1987;87:23–29.
40. Raju GC. The histological and immunohistochemical evidence of squamous metaplasia from the myoepithelial cells in the breast. *Histopathology* 1990;17:272–275.
41. Carter DJ, Rosen PP. Atypical apocrine metaplasia in sclerosing lesions of the breast: a study of 51 patients. *Mod Pathol* 1991;4:1–5.
42. Seidman JD, Ashton M, Lefkowitz M. Atypical apocrine adenosis of the breast—a clinicopathological study of 37 patients with an 8.7-year follow-up. *Cancer* 1996;77:2529–2537.
43. Linell F, Ljungberg O, Andersson I. Breast carcinoma: aspects of early stages, progression and related problems. *Acta Pathol Microbiol Scand [A]* 1980;272[Suppl]:14–62.
44. Fisher ER, Palekar AS, Sass R, et al. Scar cancers: pathologic findings from the National Surgical Adjuvant Breast Project (protocol No. 4) IX. *Breast Cancer Res Treat* 1983;3:39–59.
45. Andersen JA, Gram JB. Radial scar in the female breast. A long-term follow-up study of 32 cases. *Cancer* 1984;53:2557–2560.
46. Sloane JP, Mayers MM. Carcinoma and atypical hyperplasia in radial scars and complex sclerosing lesions: importance of lesion size and patient age. *Histopathology* 1993;23: 225–231.
47. Jacobs TW, Byrne C, Colditz G, et al. Radial scars in benign breast-biopsy specimens and the risk of breast cancer. *N Engl J Med* 1999;340:430–436.
48. Lee K-C, Chan JKC, Gwi E. Tubular adenosis of the breast: a distinctive benign lesion mimicking invasive carcinoma. *Am J Surg Pathol* 1996;20:46–54.
49. Millis RR, Eusebi V. Microglandular adenosis of the breast. *Adv Anat Pathol* 1995;2:10–18.
50. Clement PB, Azzopardi JG. Microglandular adenosis of the breast: a lesion simulating tubular carcinoma. *Histopathology* 1983;7:169–180.
51. Tavassoli FA, Norris HJ. Microglandular adenosis of the breast. A clinicopathologic study of 11 cases with ultrastructural observations. *Am J Surg Pathol* 1983;7:731–737.
52. James BA, Cranor ML, Rosen PP. Carcinoma of the breast arising in microglandular adenosis. *Am J Clin Pathol* 1993;100:507–513.
53. Koenig C, Dadmanesh F, Bratthauer GL, et al. Carcinoma arising in microglandular adenosis: an immunohistochemical analysis of 20 intraepithelial and invasive neoplasms. *Int J Surg Pathol* 2000;8:303–315.
54. Tavassoli FA. Benign lesions. In Tavassoli FA. *Pathology of the breast.* Stamford, CT: Appleton & Lang, 1999:145.
55. Schnitt SJ, Vincent-Salomon A. Columnar cell lesions of the breast. *Adv Anat Pathol* 2003; 110:113–124.
56. Rosai J. Borderline epithelial lesions of the breast. *Am J Surg Pathol* 1991;15:209–221.
57. Schnitt SJ, Connoly JL, Tavassoli FA, et al. Interobserver reproducibility in the diagnosis of ductal proliferative breast lesions using standardized criteria. *Am J Surg Pathol* 1992;16: 1133–1143.
58. Dupont WD, Page DL. Risk factors for breast cancer in women with proliferative breast disease. *N Engl J Med* 1985;312:146–151.
59. Azzopardi JG. Benign and malignant proliferative epithelial lesions of the breast: a review. *Eur J Cancer Clin Oncol* 1983;19:1717–1720.
60. Tham K-T, Dupont WD, Page DL, et al. Micro-papillary hyperplasia with atypical features in female breasts, resembling gynecomastia. *Prog Surg Pathol* 1989;10:101–109.
61. Page DL, Dupont WD. Anatomic markers of human premalignancy and risk of breast cancer. *Cancer* 1990;66:1326–1335.
62. Page DL, Rodgers LW. Combined histologic and cytologic criteria for the diagnosis of mammary atypical ductal hyperplasia. *Hum Pathol* 1992;23:1095–1097.
63. Tavassoli FA, Norris HJ. A comparison of the results of long-term follow-up for atypical intraductal hyperplasia and intraductal hyperplasia of the breast. *Cancer* 1990;65:518–529.
64. London SJ, Connolly JL, Schnitt SJ, et al. A prospective study of benign breast disease and the risk of breast cancer. *JAMA* 1992;267:941–944.
65. Ozzello L. Ultrastructure of intra-epithelial carcinomas of the breast. *Cancer* 1971;28: 1508–1515.
66. Gusterson BA, Warburton MJ, Mitchell D, et al. Distribution of myoepithelial cells and basement membrane proteins in the normal breast and in benign malignant breast diseases. *Cancer Res* 1982;42:4763–4770.
67. Feig SA. Clinical significance of ductal carcinoma in situ of the breast. *Semin Breast Dis* 2000;3:8–13.
68. Shoker BS, Sloane JP. DCIS grading schemes and clinical implications. *Histopathology* 1999; 35:393–400.
69. Silverstein MJ, Poller DN, Waisman JR, et al. Prognostic classification of breast ductal carcinoma in situ. *Lancet* 1995;345:1154–1157.
70. Lagios MD, Margolin FR, Westdahl PR, et al. Mammographically detected duct carcinoma in situ. Frequency of local recurrence following tylectomy and prognostic effect of nuclear grade on local recurrence. *Cancer* 1989;63:618–624.
71. Poller D, Silverstein M, Galea M. Ductal carcinoma in situ of the breast: a proposal for a new simplified histological classification, association between cellular proliferation and c-*erb*B-2 protein expression. *Mod Pathol* 1994;7:257–262.
72. Bellamy COC, McDonald C, Salter DM, et al. Noninvasive ductal carcinoma of the breast: the relevance of histologic categorization. *Hum Pathol* 1993;24:16–23.
73. Solin LJ, Kurtz J, Forquet A, et al. Fifteen-year results of the treatment of breast-conserving surgery and definitive breast irradiation for the treatment of ductal carcinoma in situ of the breast. *J Clin Oncol* 1995;14:754–763.
74. Page DL, Dupont WD, Rogers LW, et al. Continued local recurrence of carcinoma 15–25 years after a diagnosis of low-grade ductal carcinoma in situ of the breast treated only by biopsy. *Cancer* 1995;76:1197–1199.
75. Millis RR, Bobrow LG, Barnes DM. Immunohistochemical evaluation of biological markers in mammary carcinoma in situ: correlation with morphological features and recently proposed schemes for histological classification. *Breast* 1996;5:113–122.
76. Lagios MD. Duct carcinoma in situ. Pathology and treatment. *Surg Clin North Am* 1990; 70:853–871.
77. Holland F, Peterse JL, Millis RR, et al. Ductal carcinoma in situ: a proposal for a new classification. *Semin Diagn Pathol* 1994;11:167–180.
78. Schwartz GF. Consensus conference on the classification of ductal carcinoma in situ. *Cancer* 1997;80:1798–1802.
79. Holland R, Hendricks J. Microcalcifications associated with ductal carcinoma in situ: mammographic-pathologic correlations. *Semin Diagn Pathol* 1994;11:181–192.
80. Azzopardi JG. Underdiagnosis of malignancy. In Bennington J, ed. *Problems in Breast Pathology.* Philadelphia: WB Saunders, 1979:192–239.
81. Eusebi V, Feudale E, Foschini MP, et al. Long-term follow-up of in situ carcinoma of the breast. *Semin Diagn Pathol* 1994;11:223–235.
82. Bijker N, Peterse JL, Duchateau L, et al. Risk factors for recurrence and metastasis after breast-conserving therapy for ductal carcinoma-in-situ: analysis of European Organization for Research and Treatment of Cancer Trial 10853. *J Clin Oncol* 2001;19:2263–2271.
83. O'Malley FP, Page DL, Nelson EH, et al. Ductal carcinoma in situ of the breast with apocrine cytology: definition of a borderline category. *Hum Pathol* 1994;25:164–168.
84. Tavassoli FA, Norris HJ. Intraductal apocrine carcinoma: a clinicopathologic study of 37 cases. *Mod Pathol* 1994;7:813–818.
85. Cross AS, Azzopardi JG, Krausz T, et al. A morphological and immunocytochemical study of a distinctive variant of ductal carcinoma in situ of the breast. *Histopathology* 1985;9: 21–37.
86. Tsang WYW, Chan JKC. Endocrine ductal carcinoma in situ (E-DCIS) of the breast. *Am J Surg Pathol* 1996;20:921–943.
87. Maluf HM, Zukerberg LR, Dickerson GR, et al. Spindle cell argyrophilic mucin-producing carcinoma of the breast. Histological, ultrastructural and immunohistochemical studies of two cases. *Am J Surg Pathol* 1991;15:677–686.
88. Maluf HM, Koerner FC. Solid papillary carcinoma of the breast. *Am J Surg Pathol* 1995; 19:1237–1244.
89. Fisher ER, Brown R. Intraductal signet ring carcinoma. A hitherto undescribed form of intraductal carcinoma of the breast. *Cancer* 1985;55:2533–2537.
90. Rosen PP, Scott M. Cystic hypersecretory duct carcinoma of the breast. *Am J Surg Pathol* 1984;8:31–41.
91. Guerry P, Erlandson RA, Rosen PP. Cystic hypersecretory hyperplasia and cystic hypersecretory duct carcinoma of the breast. Pathology, therapy and follow-up of 39 patients. *Cancer* 1988;61:1611–1620.
92. Bryan BB, Schnitt SJ, Collins LC. Ductal carcinoma-in-situ with basal-like phenotype: a possible precursor to invasive basal-like breast cancer. *Mod Pathol* 2006;19:617–621.
93. Livasy CA, Perou CM, Karaca G, et al. Identification of a basal-like subtype of breast ductal carcinoma-in-situ. *Hum Pathol* 2007;38:197–204.
94. Eusebi V, Collina G, Bussolati G. Carcinoma in situ in sclerosing adenosis of the breast: an immunocytochemical study. *Semin Diagn Pathol* 1989;6:146–152.
95. Oberman HA, Markey BA. Non-invasive carcinoma of the breast presenting in adenosis. *Mod Pathol* 1991;4:31–35.
96. Page DL, Anderson TJ, Connolly JL, et al. Extent of invasive disease. In Page D, Anderson T, eds. *Diagnostic Histopathology of the Breast.* New York: Churchill Livingstone, 1987: 278–281.
97. Holland R, Hendricks JHCL, Verbeek ALM, et al. Extent, distribution, and mammographic/histological correlations of breast ductal carcinoma in situ. *Lancet* 1990; 335:519–522.
98. Patchefsky AS, Schwartz GF, Finkelstein SD, et al. Heterogeneity of intraductal carcinoma of the breast. *Cancer* 1989;63:731–741.
99. Silverstein MJ, Lagios MD, Craig PH, et al. A prognostic index for ductal carcinoma in situ of the breast. *Cancer* 1996;77:2267–2274.
100. Silverstein MJ, Lagios MD, Groshen S, et al. The influence of margin width on local control of ductal carcinoma in situ of the breast. *N Engl J Med* 1999;340:1455–1461.
101. Guidi AJ, Fischer L, Harris JR, et al. Microvessel density and distribution in ductal carcinoma in situ of the breast. *J Natl Cancer Inst* 1994;86:614–619.
102. Engels K, Fox SB, Whitehouse RM, et al. Distinct angiogenic patterns are associated with high-grade in situ ductal carcinomas of the breast. *J Pathol* 1997;181:207–212.
103. Allred DC, Bryant J, Land S, et al. Estrogen receptor expression as a predictive marker of the effectiveness of tamoxifen in the treatment of DCIS: findings from NSABP protocol B-24. *Breast Cancer Res Treat* 2002;76[Suppl 1]:S36.
104. Tsuda H, Fukutomi T, Hirohashi S. Pattern of gene alterations in intraductal breast neoplasms associated with histological type and grade. *Clin Cancer Res* 1995;1:261–267.
105. Buerger H, Otterbach F, Simon R, et al. Comparative genomic hybridization of ductal carcinoma in situ of the breast—evidence of multiple genetic pathways. *J Pathol* 1999;187: 396–402.
106. Lakhani SR. The transition from hyperplasia to invasive carcinoma of the breast. *J Pathol* 1999;187:272–278.
107. Van Diest PJ. Ductal carcinoma in situ in breast carcinogenesis. *J Pathol* 1999;187:383–384.
108. Flint A, Oberman HA. Infarction and squamous metaplasia of intraductal papilloma. A benign breast lesion that may simulate carcinoma. *Hum Pathol* 1984;15:764–767.
109. Kraus FT, Neubecker RD. The differential diagnosis of papillary tumors of the breast. *Cancer* 1962;15:444–455.
110. Hendrick JW. Intraductal papilloma of the breast. *Surg Gynecol Obstet* 1957;105:215–223.
111. Haagensen CC, Stout AP, Phillips JS. The papillary neoplasms of the breast. I. Benign intraductal papilloma. *Ann Surg* 1951;133:18–36.
112. Hart D. Intracystic papillomatous tumors of the breast. *Arch Surg* 1927;14:793–835.
113. Lewison EF, Lyons JG Jr. Relationship between benign breast disease and cancer. *Arch Surg* 1953;66:94–114.
114. Buhl-Jorgensen SE, Fischerman K, Johansen H, et al. Cancer in intraductal papilloma and papillomatosis. *Surg Gynecol Obstet* 1968;127:1307–1316.
115. Moore SW, Pearce J, Ring E. Intraductal papilloma of the breast. *Surg Gynecol Obstet* 1961; 112:153–158.
116. Kilgore QR, Fleming R, Ramos N. The incidence of cancer with nipple discharge and the risk of cancer in the presence of papillary disease of the breast. *Surg Gynecol Obstet* 1953; 96:649–660.

117. Carter D. Intraductal papillomas of the breast: a study of 78 cases. *Cancer* 1977;39: 1689–1692.
118. Rosen PP. Arthur Purdy Stout and papilloma of the breast. Comments on the occasion of his 100th birthday. *Am J Surg Pathol* 1986;10:100–107.
119. Page DL, Salhany, Jenson RA. Subsequent breast cancer risk after biopsy with atypia in a breast papilloma. *Cancer* 1996;78:258–266.
120. Murad TM, Contesso G, Mourisse H. Papillary tumors of large lactiferous ducts. *Cancer* 1981;48:122–133.
121. Ohuchi N, Abe R, Kasai M. Possible cancerous change of intraductal papillomas of the breast. A 3-D reconstruction of 25 cases. *Cancer* 1984;54:605–611.
122. Papotti M, Gugliotta P, Ghiringhello B, et al. Association of breast carcinoma and multiple intraductal papillomas: an histological and immunohistochemical investigation. *Histopathology* 1984; 8:963–975.
123. Rosen PP, Cantrell B, Mullen DL, et al. Juvenile papillomatosis (Swiss cheese disease) of the breast. *Am J Surg Pathol* 1980;4:3–12.
124. Taffurelli M, Santini D, Martinelli G, et al. Juvenile papillomatosis of the breast. A multidisciplinary study. *Pathol Annu* 1991;26:25–35.
125. Bazzochi F, Santini D, Matinelli G, et al. Juvenile papillomatosis (epitheliosis) of the breast. A clinical and pathological study of 13 cases. *Am J Clin Pathol* 1986;86:745–748.
126. Wilson M, Cranor ML, Rosen PP. Papillary duct hyperplasia of the breast in children and young women. *Mod Pathol* 1993;5:570–574.
127. Tavassoli FA. *Pathology of the Breast.* 2nd edition Stamford, CT: Appleton & Lange, 1999: 343–354.
128. Page DL, Salhany KE, Jensen RA, et al. Subsequent breast carcinoma risk after biopsy with atypia in a breast papilloma. *Cancer* 1996;78:258–266.
129. Raju UB, Lee MW, Zarbo RJ, et al. Papillary neoplasia of the breast: immunohistochemically defined myoepithelial cells in the diagnosis of benign and malignant papillary breast lesions. *Mod Pathol* 1989;2:569–576.
130. Collins LC, Carlo VP, Hwang H, Barry TS, Gown AM, Schnitt SJ. Intracystic papillary carcinoma of the breast: a re-evaluation using a panel of myoepithelial markers. *Am J Surg Pathol* 2006;30:1002–1007.
131. Stewart FW. *Atlas of Tumor Pathology*, Fasc 34. Tumors of the Breast. Washington, DC: Armed Forces Institute of Pathology, 1950:18, 53.
132. Carter D, Orr SL, Merino MJ. Intracystic papillary carcinoma of the breast after mastectomy, radiotherapy or excisional biopsy alone. *Cancer* 1983;52:14–19.
133. LefkowitzM, Lefkowitz W, Wargotz ES. Intraductal (intracystic) papillary carcinoma of the breast and its variants: a clinicopathologic study of 77 cases. *Hum Pathol* 1994;25: 802–809.
134. Leal C, Costa I, Fonseca D, et al. Intracystic (encysted) papillary carcinoma of the breast: a clinical, pathological and immunohistochemical study. *Hum Pathol* 1998;29:1097–1104.
134. Schnitt SJ, Morrow M. Lobular carcinoma in situ: current concepts and controversies. *Semin Diagn Pathol* 1999;16:209–223.
135. Kerner H, Lichtig C. Lobular cancerization: incidence and differential diagnosis with lobular carcinoma in situ of breast. *Histopathology* 1986;10:621–629.
136. Rosen PP. Co-existent lobular carcinoma in situ and intraductal carcinoma in a single lobular-duct unit. *Am J Surg Pathol* 1980;4:241–246.
137. Fechner RE. Lobular carcinoma in situ in sclerosing adenosis. A potential source of confusion with invasive carcinoma. *Am J Surg Pathol* 1981;5:233–239.
138. Dupont WD, Parl FF, Hartmaan WH, et al. Breast cancer risk associated with proliferative breast disease and atypical hyperplasia. *Cancer* 1993;71:1258–1265.
139. Carter CL, Corle DK, Micozzi MS, et al. A prospective study of the development of breast cancer in 16,692 women with benign breast disease. *Am J Epidemiol* 1988;128:467–477.
140. Dixon JM, Lumsden AM, Miller WR. The relationship of cyst type to risk factors for breast cancer and the subsequent development of breast cancer in patients with breast cystic disease. *Eur J Cancer Clin Oncol* 1985;21:1047–1050.
141. Bodian CA, Perzin KH, Lattes R. Lobular neoplasia—long-term risk of breast cancer and relation to other factors. *Cancer* 1996;78:1024–1034.
142. Rosen PP, Braun DW Jr, Kinne DE. The clinical significance of preinvasive breast carcinoma. *Cancer* 1980;46:919–925.
143. Page DL, Dupont WD, Rogers LW, et al. Intraductal carcinoma of the breast: follow-up after biopsy only. *Cancer* 1982;49:751–758.
144. Schnitt SJ, Connolly JL. Pathologic risk factors for local recurrence in patients with invasive breast cancer treated with conservative surgery and radiation therapy. *Semin Breast Dis* 1999;2:230–239.
145. Holland R, Connolly JR, Gelman R, et al. The presence of an extensive intraductal component following a limited excision correlates with prominent residual disease in the remainder of the breast. *J Clin Oncol* 1990;8:113–118.
146. World Health Organization. Histological typing of breast tumours. *Tumori* 1982;68: 181–198.
147. Fisher ER, Gregorio RM, Fisher B, et al. The pathology of invasive breast cancer. A syllabus derived from findings of the National Surgical Adjuvant Breast Project (protocol No. 4). *Cancer* 1975;36:1–85.
148. Rosen PP. The pathological classification of human mammary carcinoma: past, present and future. *Ann Clin Lab Sci* 1979;9:144–156.
149. Page DL, Anderson TJ. *Diagnostic histopathology of the breast.* Edinburgh: Churchill Livingstone, 1987.
150. Ellis IO, Galea M, Broughton N, et al. Pathological prognostic factors in breast cancer. II. Histological type. Relationship with survival in a large study with long-term follow-up. *Histopathology* 1992;20:479–489.
151. Harris M, Howell A, Chrissohou M, et al. A comparison of the metastatic pattern of infiltrating lobular and infiltrating ductal carcinoma of the breast. *Br J Cancer* 1984;50: 23–30.
152. Du Toit R, Locker AP, Ellis IO, et al. An evaluation of differences in prognosis, recurrence patterns and receptor status between invasive lobular and other invasive carcinomas of the breast. *Eur J Surg Oncol* 1991;17:251–257.
153. Dixon AR, Ellis IO, Elston CW, et al. A comparison of the clinical metastatic patterns of invasive lobular and ductal carcinomas of the breast. *Br J Cancer* 1991;63:634–635.
154. Holland R, van Haelst U. Mammary carcinoma with osteoclast-like giant cells. Additional observations on six cases. *Cancer* 1984;53:1963–1973.
155. Tavassoli FA, Norris HJ. Breast carcinoma with osteoclast-like giant cells. *Arch Pathol Lab Med* 1986;110:636–639.
156. Black MM, Speer FD. Nuclear structure in cancer tissues. *Surg Gynecol Obstet* 1957;105: 97–102.
157. Bloom HJG, Richardson WW. Histological grading and prognosis in breast cancer. A study of 1,409 cases of which 359 have been followed for 15 years. *Br J Cancer* 1957;11:359–377.
158. Elston CW, Ellis IO. Pathological prognostic factors in breast cancer. I. The value of histological grade in breast cancer: experience from a large study with long-term follow-up. *Histopathology* 1991;19:403–410.
159. Schnitt SJ. Traditional and newer pathologic factors. *J Natl Cancer Inst Monogr* 2001;30: 22–26.
160. Schnitt SJ, Jacobs TW. Current status of HER2 testing: caught between a rock and a hard place. *Am J Clin Pathol* 2001;116:806–810.
161. Wolff AC, Hammond ME, Schwartz JN, et al. American Society of Oncology/College of American Pathologists guideline recommendations for human epidermal growth factor receptor 2 testing in breast cancer. *J Clin Oncol* 2007;25:118–145.
162. Harris L, Fritsche H, Mennel R, et al. American Society of Clinical Oncology 2007 update of recommendations for the use of tumor markers in breast cancer. *J Clin Oncol* 2007; 25(33):5287–5312.
163. Martinez V, Azzopardi JG. Invasive lobular carcinoma of the breast: incidence and variants. *Histopathology* 1979;3:467–488.
164. Van Bogaert L-J, Maldague P. Infiltrating lobular carcinoma of the female breast. Deviations from the usual histopathologic appearance. *Cancer* 1980;45:979–984.
165. Berx G, Cleton-Jansen AM, Strumane K, et al. E-cadherin is inactivated in a majority of invasive human lobular breast cancers by truncation mutations throughout its extracellular domain. *Oncogene* 1996;13:1919–1925.
166. Gad A, Azzopardi JG. Lobular carcinoma of the breast: a special variant of mucin-secreting carcinoma. *J Clin Pathol* 1975;28:711–716.
167. Quincey C, Raitt N, Bell J, et al. Intracytoplasmic lumina—a useful diagnostic feature of adenocarcinomas. *Histopathology* 1991;19:83–87.
168. Raju U, Ma CK, Shaw A. Signet ring variant of lobular carcinoma of the breast: a clinicopathological and immunohistochemical study. *Mod Pathol* 1993;6:516–520.
169. Nesland JM, Grude TH, Ottestad L, et al. Invasive lobular carcinoma of the breast. The importance of an alveolar growth pattern. *Pathol Annu* 1992;23:233–247.
170. Fisher ER, Gregorio RM, Redmond C, et al. Tubulolobular invasive breast cancer: a variant of lobular invasive cancer. *Hum Pathol* 1977;8:679–683.
171. Merino MJ, Livolsi VA. Signet ring carcinoma of the female breast: a clinicopathologic analysis of 24 cases. *Cancer* 1981;48:1830–1837.
172. Dixon JM, Anderson TJ, Page DL, et al. Infiltrating lobular carcinoma of the breast. *Histopathology* 1982;6:149–161.
173. Walford N, Ten Velden J. Histiocytoid breast carcinoma: an apocrine variant of lobular carcinoma. *Histopathology* 1989;14:515–522.
174. Eusebi V, Magalhaes F, Azzopardi JG. Pleomorphic lobular carcinoma of the breast: an aggressive tumor showing apocrine differentiation. *Hum Pathol* 1992;23:655–662.
175. Di Costanzo D, Rosen PP, Gareen I, et al. Prognosis in infiltrating lobular carcinoma. An analysis of "classical" and variant tumors. *Am J Surg Pathol* 1990;14:12–23.
176. Porter PL, Garcia R, Moe R, et al. C-erbB-2 oncogene protein in in situ and invasive lobular breast neoplasia. *Cancer* 1991;68:331–334.
177. Domagala W, Markiewski M, Kubiak R, et al. Immunohistochemical profile of invasive lobular carcinoma of the breast: predominantly vimentin and p53 protein negative, cathepsin D and oestrogen receptor positive. *Virchows Arch A Pathol Anat Histopathol* 1993; 423:497–502.
178. Mazoujian G, Bodian C, Haagensen DE Jr, et al. Expression of GCDFP-15 in breast carcinomas. Relationship to pathologic and clinical factors. *Cancer* 1989;63:2156–2161.
179. Radhi JM. Immunohistochemical analysis of pleomorphic lobular carcinoma: higher expression of p53 and chromogranin and lower expression of ER and PgR. *Histopathology* 2000;36:156–160.
180. Middleton LP, Palacios DM, Bryant BR, et al. Pleomorphic lobular carcinoma: morphology, immunohistochemistry, and molecular analysis. *Am J Surg Pathol* 2000;24:1650–1656.
181. Nishizaki T, Chew K, Chu L, et al. Genomic alterations in lobular breast cancer by comparative genomic hybridization. *Int J Cancer* 1997;74:513–517.
182. Roylance R, Gorman P, Harris W, et al. Comparative genomic hybridization of breast tumours stratified by histological grade reveals new insights into the biological progression of breast cancer. *Cancer Res* 1999;59:1433–1436.
183. Lehr HA, Folpe A, Yaziji H, et al. Cytokeratin 8 immunostaining pattern and E-cadherin expression distinguish lobular from ductal breast carcinoma. *Am J Clin Pathol* 2000;114: 190–196.
184. Rosen PP, Groshen S, Kinne DW, et al. Factors influencing prognosis in node-negative breast carcinoma: analysis of 767 T1 N0 M0/T2 N0 M0 patients with long-term follow-up. *J Clin Oncol* 1993;11:2090–2100.
185. Diab SG, Clark GM, Osborne CK, et al. Tumor characteristics and clinical outcome of tubular and mucinous breast carcinomas. *J Clin Oncol* 1999;17:1442–1448.
186. Deos PH, Norris HJ. Well-differentiated (tubular) carcinoma of the breast. A clinicopathologic study of 145 pure and mixed cases. *Am J Clin Pathol* 1982;78:1–7.
187. McBoyle MF, Razek HA, Carter JL, et al. Tubular carcinoma of the breast: an institutional review. *Am Surg* 1997;63:639–644; discussion 644–645.
188. Winchester DJ, Sahin AA, Tucker SL, et al. Tubular carcinoma of the breast. Predicting axillary nodal metastases and recurrence. *Ann Surg* 1996;223:342–347.
189. Berger AC, Miller SM, Harris MN, et al. Axillary dissection for tubular carcinoma of the breast. *Breast J* 1996;2:204.
190. Reiner A, Reiner G, Spona J, et al. Histopathologic characterization of human breast

cancer in correlation with estrogen receptor status. A comparison of immunocytochemical and biochemical analysis. *Cancer* 1988;61:1149–1154.

191. Helin HJ, Helle MJ, Kallioniemi OP, et al. Immunohistochemical determination of estrogen and progesterone receptors in human breast carcinoma. Correlation with histopathology and DNA flow cytometry. *Cancer* 1989;63:1761–1767.

192. Stierer M, Rosen H, Weber R, et al. Immunohistochemical and biochemical measurement of estrogen and progesterone receptors in primary breast cancer. Correlation of histopathology and prognostic factors. *Ann Surg* 1993;218:13–21.

193. Soomro S, Shousha S, Taylor P, et al. c-erbB-2 expression in different histological types of invasive breast carcinoma. *J Clin Pathol* 1991;44:211–214.

194. Somerville JE, Clarke LA, Biggart JD. c-erbB-2 overexpression and histological type of in situ and invasive breast carcinoma. *J Clin Pathol* 1992;45:16–20.

195. Rosen PP, Lesser ML, Arroyo CD, et al. p53 in node-negative breast carcinoma: an immunohistochemical study of epidemiologic risk factors, histologic features, and prognosis. *J Clin Oncol* 1995;13:821–830.

196. Waldman FM, Hwang ES, Etzell J, et al. Genomic alterations in tubular breast carcinomas. *Hum Pathol* 2001;32:222–226.

197. Page DL, Dixon JM, Anderson TJ, et al. Invasive cribriform carcinoma of the breast. *Histopathology* 1983;7:525–536.

198. Venable JG, Schwartz AM, Silverberg SG. Infiltrating cribriform carcinoma of the breast: a distinctive clinicopathologic entity. *Hum Pathol* 1990;21:333–338.

199. Clayton F. Pure mucinous carcinomas of the breast: morphologic features and prognostic correlates. *Hum Pathol* 1986;17:34–38.

200. Fentiman IS, Millis RR, Smith P, et al. Mucoid breast carcinomas: histology and prognosis. *Br J Cancer* 1997;75:1061–1065.

201. Capella C, Eusebi V, Mann B, et al. Endocrine differentiation in mucoid carcinoma of the breast. *Histopathology* 1980;4:613–630.

202. Coady AT, Shousha S, Dawson PM, et al. Mucinous carcinoma of the breast: further characterization of its three subtypes. *Histopathology* 1989;15:617–626.

203. Rasmussen BB, Rose C, Christensen I. Prognostic factors in primary mucinous breast carcinoma. *Am J Clin Pathol* 1987;87:155–160.

204. Avisar E, Khan MA, Axelrod D, et al. Pure mucinous carcinoma of the breast: a clinicopathologic correlation study. *Ann Surg Oncol* 1998;5:447–451.

205. Toikkanen S, Eerola E, Ekfors TO. Pure and mixed mucinous breast carcinomas: DNA stemline and prognosis. *J Clin Pathol* 1988;41:300–303.

206. Adeyinka A, Mertens F, Idvall I, et al. Cytogenetic findings in invasive breast carcinomas with prognostically favourable histology: a less complex karyotypic pattern? *Int J Cancer* 1998;79:361–364.

207. Fujii H, Anbazhagan R, Bornman DM, et al. Mucinous cancers have fewer genomic alterations than more common classes of breast cancer. *Breast Cancer Res Treat* 2002;76:255–260.

208. Gaffey MJ, Mills SE, Frierson HF, et al. Medullary carcinoma of the breast: interobserver variability in histopathologic diagnosis. *Mod Pathol* 1995;8:31–38.

209. Pedersen L, Holck S, Schiodt T, et al. Inter- and intraobserver variability in the histopathological diagnosis of medullary carcinoma of the breast, and its prognostic implications. *Breast Cancer Res Treat* 1989;14:91–99.

210. Rapin V, Contesso G, Mouriesse H, et al. Medullary breast carcinoma. A re-evaluation of 95 cases of breast cancer with inflammatory stroma. *Cancer* 1988;61:2503–2510.

211. Pedersen L, Zedeler K, Holck S, et al. Medullary carcinoma of the breast—prevalence and prognostic importance of classical risk factors in breast cancer. *Eur J Cancer* 1995;31A:2289–2295.

212. Ridolfi RL, Rosen PP, Port A, et al. Medullary carcinoma of the breast. A clinicopathologic study with 10-year follow-up. *Cancer* 1977;40:1365–1385.

213. Fisher ER, Kenny JP, Sass R, et al. Medullary cancer of the breast revisited. *Breast Cancer Res Treat* 1990;16:215–229.

214. Wargotz ES, Silverberg SG. Medullary carcinoma of the breast: clinicopathologic study with appraisal of current diagnostic criteria. *Hum Pathol* 1988;19:1340–1346.

215. Lakhani SR, Jacquemier J, Sloane JP, et al. Multifactorial analysis of differences between sporadic breast cancers and cancers involving BRCA1 and BRCA2 mutations. *J Natl Cancer Inst* 1998;90:1138–1145.

216. Fisher ER, Palekar AS, Redmond C, et al. Pathologic findings from the National Surgical Adjuvant Breast Project (protocol No. 4). VI. Invasive papillary cancer. *Am J Clin Pathol* 1980;73:313–322.

217. Siriaunkgul S, Tavassoli FA. Invasive micropapillary carcinoma of the breast. *Mod Pathol* 1993;6:660–662.

218. Luna-More S, Gonzalez B, Acedo C, et al. Invasive micropapillary carcinoma of the breast. A new special type of invasive mammary carcinoma. *Pathol Res Pract* 1994;190:668–674.

219. Middleton LP, Tressera F, Sobel ME, et al. Infiltrating micropapillary carcinoma of the breast. *Mod Pathol* 1999;12:499–504.

220. Paterakos M, Watkin WG, Edgerton SM, et al. Invasive micropapillary carcinoma of the breast: a prognostic study. *Hum Pathol* 1999;30:1459–1463.

221. Walsh MM, Bleiweiss IJ. Invasive micropapillary carcinoma of the breast: eighty cases of an underrecognized entity. *Hum Pathol* 2001;32:583–589.

222. Nassar H, Wallis T, Andea A, et al. Clinicopathologic analysis of invasive micropapillary differentiation in breast carcinoma. *Mod Pathol* 2001;14:836–841.

223. Luna-More S, de los Santos F, Breton JJ, et al. Estrogen and progesterone receptors, c-erbB-2, p53, and Bcl-2 in thirty-three invasive micropapillary breast carcinomas. *Pathol Res Pract* 1996;192:27–32.

224. Kleer CG, Oberman HA. Adenoid cystic carcinoma of the breast. Value of histologic grading and proliferative activity. *Am J Surg Pathol* 1998;22:569–575.

225. Arpino G, Clark GM, Mohsin S, et al. Adenoid cystic carcinoma of the breast. Molecular markers, treatment, and clinical outcome. *Cancer* 2002;94:2119–2227.

226. Shin SJ, Rosen PP. Solid variant of mammary adenoid cystic carcinoma with basaloid features: a study of nine cases. *Am J Surg Pathol* 2002;26:413–420.

227. Rosen PP. Adenoid cystic carcinoma of the breast. A morphologically heterogeneous neoplasm. *Pathol Annu* 1989;24:237–254.

228. Rabban JT, Swain RS, Zaloudek CJ, Chase DR, Chen YY. Immunophenotype overlap between adenoid cystic carcinoma and collagenous spherulosis of the breast: potential diagnostic pitfalls using myoepithelial markers. *Mod Pathol* 2006;19:1351–1357.

229. Patchefsky AS, Frauenhoffer CM, Krall RA, et al. Low-grade mucoepidermoid carcinoma of the breast. *Arch Pathol Lab Med* 1979;103:196–198.

230. Hastrup N, Sehested M. High-grade mucoepidermoid carcinoma of the breast. *Histopathology* 1985;9:887–892.

231. Finck FM, Schwinn CP, Keasbey LE. Clear cell hidradenoma of the breast. *Cancer* 1968;22:125–135.

232. Draheim JH, Neubecker RD, Sprinz H. An unusual tumor of the breast resembling eccrine spiradenoma. *Am J Clin Pathol* 1959;31:511–516.

233. Miremadi A, Pinder S, Lee AHS, et al. Neuroendocrine differentiation and prognosis in breast adenocarcinoma. *Histopathology* 2002;40:215–222.

234. Papotti M, Macri L, Finzi G, et al. Neuroendocrine differentiation in carcinomas of the breast: a study of 51 cases. *Semin Diagn Pathol* 1989;6:174–188.

235. Zekioglu O, Erhan Y, Ciris M, Bayramoglu H. Neuroendocrine differentiated carcinomas of the breast: a distinct entity. *Breast* 2003;12:251–257.

236. Upalakalin JN, Collins LC, Tawa N, Parangi S. Carcinoid tumors of the breast. *Am J Surg* 2006;191:799–805.

237. McDivitt RW, Stewart FW. Breast carcinoma in children. *JAMA* 1966;195:388–390.

238. Krausz T, Jenkins D, Grontoft O, et al. Secretory carcinoma of the breast in adults: emphasis on late recurrence and metastasis. *Histopathology* 1989;14:25–36.

239. Rosen PP, Cranor ML. Secretory carcinoma of the breast. *Arch Pathol Lab Med* 1991;115:141–144.

240. Tavassoli FA, Norris HJ. Secretory carcinoma of the breast. *Cancer* 1980;45:2404–2413.

241. Eusebi V, Millis RR, Cattani MG, et al. Apocrine carcinoma of the breast. A morphologic and immunocytochemical study. *Am J Pathol* 1986;123:532–541.

242. Abati AD, Kimmel M, Rosen PP. Apocrine mammary carcinoma. A clinicopathologic study of 72 cases. *Am J Clin Pathol* 1990;94:371–377.

243. Eusebi V, Cattani MG, Ceccarelli C, et al. Sarcomatoid carcinomas of the breast: an immunocytochemical study of 14 cases. *Prog Surg Pathol* 1989;10:83–99.

244. Oberman HA. Metaplastic carcinoma of the breast. *Am J Surg Pathol* 1987;11:918–929.

245. Wargotz ES, Norris HJ. Metaplastic carcinomas of the breast. I. Matrix-producing carcinoma. *Hum Pathol* 1989;20:628–635.

246. Wargotz ES, Deos PH, Norris HJ. Metaplastic carcinomas of the breast. II. Spindle cell carcinoma. *Hum Pathol* 1989;20:732–740.

247. Wargotz ES, Norris HJ. Metaplastic carcinomas of the breast. III. Carcinosarcoma. *Cancer* 1989;64:1490–1499.

248. Wargotz ES, Norris HJ. Metaplastic carcinomas of the breast. IV. Squamous cell carcinoma of ductal origin. *Cancer* 1990;65:272–276.

249. Wargotz ES, Norris HJ. Metaplastic carcinomas of the breast. V. Metaplastic carcinoma with osteoclastic giant cells. *Hum Pathol* 1990;21:1142–1150.

250. Pitts WC, Rojas VA, Gaffey MJ, et al. Carcinomas with metaplasia and sarcomas of the breast. *Am J Clin Pathol* 1991;95:623–632.

251. Gersell DJ, Katzenstein A-L. Spindle cell carcinoma of the breast. A clinicopathologic and ultrastructural study. *Hum Pathol* 1981;12:550–561.

252. Gobbi H, Simpson JF, Borowsky A, et al. Metaplastic breast tumors with a dominant fibromatosis-like phenotype have a high risk of local recurrence. *Cancer* 1999;85:2170–2182.

253. Eggers JW, Chesney TM. Squamous cell carcinoma of the breast: a clinicopathologic analysis of eight cases and review of the literature. *Hum Pathol* 1984;15:526–531.

254. Eusebi V, Lamovec J, Cattani MG, et al. Acantholytic variant of squamous-cell carcinoma of the breast. *Am J Surg Pathol* 1986;10:855–861.

255. Rosen PP, Ernsberger D. Low-grade adenosquamous carcinoma. A variant of metaplastic mammary carcinoma. *Am J Surg Pathol* 1987;11:351–358.

256. Van Hoeven K, Drudis T, Cranor ML, et al. Low-grade adenosquamous carcinoma of the breast. *Am J Surg Pathol* 1993;17:248–258.

257. Foschini MP, Pizzicannella G, Peterse JL, et al. Adenomyoepithelioma of the breast associated with low-grade adenosquamous and sarcomatoid carcinomas. *Virchows Arch* 1995;427:243–250.

258. Rasbridge SA, Millis RR. Adenomyoepithelioma of the breast with malignant features. *Virchows Arch* 1998;432:123–130.

259. Livasy CA, Karaca G, Nanda R, et al. Phenotypic evaluation of the basal-like subtype of invasive breast carcinoma. *Mod Pathol* 2006;19:264–271.

260. Rakha EA, El-Sayed ME, Green AR, Lee AH, Robertson JF, Ellis IO. Prognostic markers in triple negative breast cancer. *Cancer* 2007;109:25–32.

261. Kim MJ, RO JY, Ahn SH, Kim HH, Kim SB, Gong G. Clinicopathologic significance of the basal-like subtype of breast cancer: a comparison with hormone receptor and HER2/neu-overexpressing phenotypes. *Hum Pathol* 2006;37:1217–1226.

262. Rakha EA, Putti TC, Abd El-Rehim DM, et al. Morphological and immunophenotypic analysis of breast carcinomas with basal and myoepithelial differentiation. *J Pathol* 2006;208:495–506.

263. Fisher ER, Gregorio R, Kim WS, et al. Lipid in invasive cancer of the breast. *Am J Clin Pathol* 1977;68:558–561.

264. Van Bogaert L-J, Maldague P. Histologic variants of lipid-secreting carcinoma of the breast. *Virchows Arch A Pathol Anat Histopathol* 1977;375:345–353.

265. Fisher ER, Tavares J, Bulatao IS, et al. Glycogen-rich, clear cell breast cancer: with comments concerning other clear cell variants. *Hum Pathol* 1985;16:1085–1090.

266. Hull MT, Warfel KA. Glycogen-rich clear cell carcinomas of the breast. A clinicopathologic and ultrastructural study. *Am J Surg Pathol* 1986;10:553–559.

267. Eusebi V, Foschini MP, Bussolati G, et al. Myoblastomatoid (histiocytoid) carcinoma of the breast: a type of apocrine carcinoma. *Am J Surg Pathol* 1995;19:553–562.

268. Charafe-Jauffret E, Tarpin C, Bardou VJ, et al. Immunophenotypic analysis of inflammatory breast cancers: identification of an "inflammatory signature." *J Pathol* 2004;202:265–273.

269. Jackson AW, Muldal S, Ockey CH, et al. Carcinoma of the male breast in association with the Klinefelter syndrome. *Br Med J* 1965;1:223–225.

270. Tchou J, Ward MR, Volpe P, et al. Large genomic rearrangement in BRCA1 and BRCA2 and clinical characteristics of men with breast cancer in the United States. *Clin Breast Cancer* 2007;7:627–633.

271. Goss PE, Reid C, Pintilie M, et al. Male breast carcinoma. A review of 229 patients who presented to the Princess Margaret Hospital during 40 years: 1955–1996. *Cancer* 1999;85:629–639.

272. Burga AM, Fadare O, Lininger RA, Tavassoli FA. Invasive carcinomas of the male breast: a morphologic study of the distribution of histologic types and metastatic patterns in 778 cases. *Virchows Arch* 2006;449:507–512.

273. Serour F, Birkenfeld S, Amsterdam E, et al. Paget disease of the male breast. *Cancer* 1988; 62:601–605.

274. Frierson HF, Fechner RE. Histologic grade of locally advanced infiltrating ductal carcinoma after treatment with induction of chemotherapy. *Am J Clin Pathol* 1994;102:154–157.

275. Honkop AH, Pinedo HM, Dejong JS, et al. Effects of chemotherapy on pathological characteristics of locally advanced breast cancer. *Am J Clin Pathol* 1997;107:211–218.

276. Schnitt SJ, Connolly JL, Harris J, et al. Radiation-induced changes in the breast. *Hum Pathol* 1984;15:545–550.

277. Chaudary MA, Girling A, Girling S, et al. New lumps in the breast following conservation treatment for early breast cancer. *Breast Cancer Res Treat* 1988;11:51–58.

278. McIntosh IH, Hooper AA, Millis RR, et al. Metastatic carcinoma within the breast. *Clin Oncol* 1976;2:393–401.

279. Vergier B, Trojani M, de Mascarel I, et al. Metastases to the breast: differential diagnosis from primary breast carcinoma. *J Surg Oncol* 1991;48:112–116.

280. Rosen PP, Kimmel M. Occult breast carcinoma presenting with axillary lymph node metastases: a follow-up study of 48 patients. *Hum Pathol* 1990;21:518–523.

281. Truong LD, Cartwright J, Goodman MD, et al. Silicone lymphadenopathy associated with augmentation mammoplasty. Morphological features of nine cases. *Am J Surg Pathol* 1988; 12:484–491.

282. Johnson WT, Helwig EB. Benign nevus cells in the capsule of lymph nodes. *Cancer* 1969; 23:747–753.

283. Ridolfi RL, Rosen PP, Thaler H. Nevus cell aggregates associated with lymph nodes: estimated frequency and clinical significance. *Cancer* 1977;39:164–171.

284. Edlow D, Carter D. Heterotopic epithelium in axillary lymph nodes: report of a case and review of the literature. *Am J Clin Pathol* 1973;59(5):666–673.

285. Turner DR, Millis RR. Breast tissue inclusions in axillary lymph nodes. *Histopathology* 1980; 4:631–636.

286. Walker AN, Fechner RE. Papillary carcinoma arising from ectopic breast tissue in an axillary lymph node. *Diagn Gynecol Obstet* 1982;4:141–145.

287. Dupont WD, Page DL, Parl FF, et al. Long-term risk of breast cancer in women with fibroadenoma. *N Engl J Med* 1994;331:10–15.

288. Yoshida Y, Takaoka M, Fukumoto M. Carcinoma arising in fibroadenoma: case report and review of the world literature. *J Surg Oncol* 1985;29:132–140.

289. Diaz NM, Palmer JO, McDivitt RW. Carcinoma arising within fibroadenomas of the breast. A clinicopathologic study of 105 patients. *Am J Clin Pathol* 1991;95:614–622.

290. Carney JA, Toorkey BC. Myxoid fibroadenoma and allied conditions (myxomatosis) of the breast. A heritable disorder with special associations including cardiac and cutaneous myxomas. *Am J Surg Pathol* 1991;15:713–721.

291. Berean K, Tron VA, Churg A, et al. Mammary fibroadenoma with multinucleated stromal giant cells. *Am J Surg Pathol* 1986;10:823–827.

292. Pike AM, Oberman HA. Juvenile (cellular) adenofibromas. A clinicopathologic study. *Am J Surg Pathol* 1985;9:730–736.

293. Oberman HA. Breast lesions in the adolescent female. *Pathol Annu* 1979;14:175–201.

294. Mies C, Rosen PP. Juvenile fibroadenoma with atypical epithelial hyperplasia. *Am J Surg Pathol* 1987;11:184–190.

295. Hertel BF, Zaloudek C, Kempson RL. Breast adenomas. *Cancer* 1976;37:2891–2905.

296. Lindquist KD, van Heerden JA, Welland LH, et al. Recurrent and metastatic cystosarcoma phyllodes. *Am J Surg* 1982;144:341–343.

297. Azzopardi JG. *Problems in Breast Pathology.* Philadelphia: WB Saunders, 1979:346–378.

298. Moffat CJC, Pinder SE, Dixon AR, et al. Phyllodes tumours of the breast: a clinicopathological review of 32 cases. *Histopathology* 1995; 27:205–218.

299. Lee AH, Hodi Z, Ellis IO, Elston CW. Histological features useful in the distinction of phyllodes tumor and fibroadenoma on needle core biopsy of the breast. *Histopathology* 2007;51:336–344.

300. Jacobs TW, Chen YY, Guinee DG, Jr., et al. Fibroepithelial lesions with cellular stroma on breast core needle biopsy: are there predictors of outcome on surgical excision. *Am J Clin Pathol* 2005;124:342–354.

301. Murad TM, Hines JR, Beal J, et al. Histopathological and clinical correlations of cystosarcoma phyllodes. *Arch Pathol Lab Med* 1988;112:752–756.

302. Cohn-Cedermark G, Rutqvist LE, Rosendahl I, et al. Prognostic factors in cystosarcoma phyllodes. A clinicopathologic study of 77 patients. *Cancer* 1991;68:2017–2022.

303. El-Naggar AK, Ro JY, McLemore D, et al. DNA content and proliferative activity of cystosarcoma phyllodes of the breast. Potential prognostic significance. *Am J Clin Pathol* 1990;93:480–485.

304. Palko MJ, Wang SE, Shackney SE, et al. Flow cytometric S-fraction as a predictor of clinical outcome in cystosarcoma phyllodes. *Arch Pathol Lab Med* 1990;114:949–952.

305. Tse, GMJ, Putti TC, Kung FYL, et al. Increased p53 protein expression in malignant mammary phyllodes tumors. *Mod Pathol* 2002;15:734–740.

306. Jozefczyk MA, Rosen PP. Vascular tumors of the breast. II. Perilobular hemangiomas and hemangiomas. *Am J Surg Pathol* 1985;9:491–503.

307. Rosen PP. Vascular tumors of the breast. III. Angiomatosis. *Am J Surg Pathol* 1985;9:652–658.

308. Rosen PP, Jozefczyk MA, Boram LH. Vascular tumors of the breast. IV. The venous hemangioma. *Am J Surg Pathol* 1985;9:659–665.

309. Rosen PP. Vascular tumors of the breast. V. Nonparenchymal hemangiomas of mammary subcutaneous tissues. *Am J Surg Pathol* 1985;9:723–729.

310. Nascimento AG, Karas M, Rosen PP, et al. Leiomyoma of the nipple. *Am J Surg Pathol* 1979;3:151–154.

311. Bascain A, Ferrara G, Orabona P, et al. Smooth muscle tumours of the breast: clinicopathologic features of two cases. *Tumori* 1994;80:241–245.

312. Lugo M, Reyes JM, Puton PB. Benign chondrolipomatous tumours of the breast. *Arch Pathol Lab Med* 1982;106:691–692.

313. Wargotz ES, Norris HJ, Austin RM, et al. Fibromatosis of the breast. A clinical and pathological study of 28 cases. *Am J Surg Pathol* 1987;11:38–45.

314. DeMay RM, Kay S. Granular cell tumor of the breast. *Pathol Annu* 1984;19 Pt 2:121–148.

315. Donnell RM, Rosen PP, Lieberman PH, et al. Angiosarcoma and other vascular tumors of the breast. Pathologic analysis as a guide to prognosis. *Am J Surg Pathol* 1981;5:629–642.

316. Merino MJ, Carter D, Berman M. Angiosarcoma of the breast. *Am J Surg Pathol* 1983;7:53–60.

317. Woodward AH, Ivins JC, Soule EH. Lymphangiosarcoma arising in chronic lymphedematous extremities. *Cancer* 1972;30:562–572.

318. Miettinen M, Lehto V-P, Virtanen I. Postmastectomy angiosarcoma (Stewart-Treves syndrome). Light-microscopic, immunohistological and ultrastructural characteristics of two cases. *Am J Surg Pathol* 1983;7:329–339.

319. Kuten A, Sapir D, Cohen Y, et al. Postirradiation soft tissue sarcoma occurring in breast cancer patients: report of seven cases and results of combination chemotherapy. *J Surg Oncol* 1985;28:168–171.

320. Badwe RA, Hanby AM, Fentiman IS, et al. Angiosarcoma of the skin overlying an irradiated breast. *Breast Cancer Res Treat* 1991;19:69–72.

321. Fineberg S, Rosen PP. Cutaneous angiosarcoma and atypical vascular lesions of the skin and breast after radiation therapy for breast carcinoma. *Am J Clin Pathol* 1994;102:757–763.

322. Going JJ, Lumsden AM, Anderson TJ. A classical osteogenic sarcoma of the breast: histology, immunohistochemistry and ultrastructure. *Histopathology* 1986;10:631–641.

323. Austin RM, Dupree WB. Liposarcoma of the breast: a clinicopathologic study of 20 cases. *Hum Pathol* 1986;17:906–913.

324. Callery CD, Rosen PP, Kinne DW. Sarcoma of the breast. A study of 32 patients with reappraisal of classification and therapy. *Ann Surg* 1985;201:527–532.

325. Ganjoo K, Advani R, Mariappan MR, McMillan A, Horning S. Non-Hodgkin's lymphoma of the breast. *Cancer* 2007;110:25–30.

326. Hugh JC, Jackson FI, Hanson J, et al. Primary breast lymphoma. An immunohistologic study of 20 new cases. *Cancer* 1990;66:2602–2611.

327. Lamovec J, Jancar J. Primary malignant lymphoma of the breast. Lymphoma of the mucosa-associated lymphoid tissue. *Cancer* 1987;60:3033–3041.

328. Cohen PL, Brooks JJ. Lymphomas of the breast. A clinicopathological and immunohistological study of primary and secondary cases. *Cancer* 1991;67:1359–1369.

329. Bobrow LG, Richards MA, Happerfield LC, et al. Breast lymphomas: a clinicopathologic review. *Hum Pathol* 1993;24:57–64.

330. Arber DA, Simpson JF, Weiss LM, et al. Non-Hodgkin's lymphoma involving the breast. *Am J Surg Pathol* 1994;18:288–295.

331. Abbondanzo SL, Seidman JD, Lefkowitz M, et al. Primary diffuse large B-cell lymphoma of the breast: a clinicopathologic study of 31 cases. *Pathol Res Pract* 1996;192:37–43.

332. Rosen PP, Oberman HA. Tumors of the mammary gland. In Rosai J, Sobin LH, eds. *Atlas of Tumor Pathology*, Fascicle 7. Washington, DC: Armed Forces Institute of Pathology, 1993:337–339.

333. Green I, Dorfman RF, Rosai J. Breast involvement by extranodal Rosai-Dorfman disease: report of seven cases. *Am J Surg Pathol* 1997;21:664–668.

334. Azzopardi JG, Salm R. Ductal adenoma of the breast: a lesion which can mimic carcinoma. *J Pathol* 1984;144:15–23.

335. Lammie GA, Millis RR. Ductal adenoma of the breast—a review of fifteen cases. *Hum Pathol* 1989;20:903–908.

336. Carney JA, Toorkey BC. Ductal adenoma of the breast with tubular features. A probable component of the complex of myxomas, spotty pigmentation, endocrine overactivity and schwannomas. *Am J Surg Pathol* 1991;15:722–731.

337. Tavassoli FA. Myoepithelial lesions of the breast. Myoepitheliosis, adenomyoepithelioma and myoepithelial carcinoma. *Am J Surg Pathol* 1991;15:554–568.

338. Moran CA, Suster S, Carter D. Benign mixed tumors (pleomorphic adenomas) of the breast. *Am J Surg Pathol* 1990;14:913–921.

339. Chen KTK. Pleomorphic adenoma of the breast. *Am J Clin Pathol* 1990;93:792–794.

340. Diaz NM, McDivitt RW, Wick MR. Pleomorphic adenoma of the breast: a clinicopathologic and immunohistochemical study of 10 cases. *Hum Pathol* 1991;22:1206–1214.

341. Zarbo RJ, Oberman HA. Cellular adenomyoepithelioma of the breast. *Am J Surg Pathol* 1983;7:863–870.

342. Kiaer H, Nielsen B, Paulsen S, et al. Adenomyoepithelial adenosis and low-grade malignant adenomyoepithelioma of the breast. *Virchows Arch A Pathol Anat Histopathol* 1984;405:55–67.

343. Erlandson RA, Rosen PP. Infiltrating myoepithelioma of the breast. *Am J Surg Pathol* 1982; 6:785–793.

344. Loose JH, Patchefsky AS, Hollander IJ, et al. Adenomyoepithelioma of the breast. *Am J Surg Pathol* 1992;16:868–876.

345. Wargotz ES, Weiss SW, Norris HJ. Myofibroblastoma of the breast. Sixteen cases of a distinctive benign mesenchymal tumor. *Am J Surg Pathol* 1987;11:493–502.

346. Toker C, Tang C-K, Whitely JF, et al. Benign spindle cell breast tumor. *Cancer* 1981;48:1615–1622.

347. McMenamin ME, DeSchryver K, Fletcher CDM. Fibrous lesions of the breast. A review. *Int J Surg Pathol* 2000;8:99–108

348. Hale JA, Peters GN, Cheek JH. Tuberculosis of the breast: rare but still extant. Review of the literature and report of an additional case. *Am J Surg* 1985;150:620–624.

349. Shinde SR, Chandawarkar RY, Deshmukh SP. Tuberculosis of the breast masquerading as carcinoma: a study of 100 patients. *World J Surg* 1995;19:379–381.

350. Azzopardi JG. Miscellaneous entities. In Bennington JL, ed. *Problems in Breast Pathology.* Philadelphia: WB Saunders, 1979:400.

351. Anonymous. Mammillary fistula. *Lancet* 1986;2:438–439.

352. Angell M. Evaluating the health risks of breast implants: the interplay of medical science, the law and public opinion. *N Engl J Med* 1996; 334:1513–1518.

353. Kossovsky N, Freiman CJ. Silicone breast implant pathology: clinical data and immunological consequences. *Arch Pathol Lab Med* 1994;118:686–693.

354. Hameed MR, Erlandson R, Rosen PP. Capsular synovial-like hyperplasia around mammary implants similar to detritic synovitis. *Am J Surg Pathol* 1995;19:433–438.

355. Coyne JD, Parkinson D, Baildam AD. Membranous fat necrosis of the breast. *Histopathology* 1996;28:61–64.

356. Going JJ, Anderson TJ, Wilkinson S, et al. Granulomatous lobular mastitis. *J Clin Pathol* 1987;40:535–540.

357. Azzopardi JG. Cystic disease: duct ectasia: fat necrosis; "fibrous disease of the breast." In Bennington JL, ed. *Problems in Breast Pathology.* Philadelphia: WB Saunders, 1979:57–89.

358. Schwartz IS, Strauchen JA. Lymphocytic mastopathy. An autoimmune disease of the breast? *Am J Clin Pathol* 1990;93:725–730.

359. Lammie GA, Bobrow LG, Staunton MDM, et al. Sclerosing lymphocytic lobulitis of the breast—evidence for an autoimmune pathogenesis. *Histopathology* 1991;19:13–20.

360. Ashton AM, Lefkkowitz M, Tavassoli A. Epithelioid stromal cells in lymphocytic mastitis—a source of confusion with invasive carcinoma. *Mod Pathol* 1994;7:49–54.

361. Morgan MC, Weaver MG, Crowe JP, et al. Diabetic mastopathy: a clinicopathologic study in palpable and nonpalpable breast lesions. *Mod Pathol* 1995;8:349–354.

362. Ely KA, Tse G, Simpson JF, et al. Diabetic mastopathy. A clinicopathologic review. *Am J Clin Pathol* 2000;113:541–545.

363. Bannayan GA, Hadju SI. Gynecomastia: clinicopathologic study of 351 cases. *Am J Clin Pathol* 1972;57:431–437.

364. Anderson JA, Gram JB. Gynaecomasty. Histological aspects in a surgical material. *Acta Pathol Microbiol Immunol Scand [A]* 1982;90:185–190.

365. Burgess HE, Shousha S. An immunohistochemical study of the long-term effects of androgen administration on female-to-male transsexual breast: a comparison with normal female breast and male breast showing gynaecomastia. *J Pathol* 1993;170:37–43.

366. Beischner NA, Hueston JH, Pepperell RJ. Massive hypertrophy of the breasts in pregnancy: report of 3 cases and review of the literature, "never think you've seen everything." *Obstet Gynecol* 1989;44:234–243.

367. Linell F, Ostberg G, Soderstrom J, et al. Breast hamartomas. An important entity in mammary pathology. *Virchows Arch A Pathol Anat Histopathol* 1979;383:253–264.

368. Daya D, Trus T, Dsouza TJ, et al. Hamartoma of the breast, an underrecognized breast lesion—a clinicopathological and radiographic study of 25 cases. *Am J Clin Pathol* 1995; 108:685–689.

369. Oberman HA. Hamartomas and hamartoma variants of the breast. *Semin Diagn Pathol* 1989;6:135–145.

370. Fisher CJ, Hanby AM, Robinson L, et al. Mammary hamartoma—a review of 35 cases. *Histopathology* 1992;20:99–106.

371. Charpin C, Mathoulin MP, Andrac L, et al. Reappraisal of breast hamartomas: a morphological study of 41 cases. *Pathol Res Pract* 1994;190:362–371.

372. Daroca PJ Jr, Reed RJ, Love GL, et al. Myoid hamartomas of the breast. *Hum Pathol* 1985; 16:212–219.

373. Vuitch MF, Rosen PP, Erlandson RA. Pseudoangiomatous hyperplasia of mammary stroma. *Hum Pathol* 1986;17:185–191.

374. Anderson C, Ricci A, Pedersen CA, et al. Immunocytochemical analysis of estrogen and progesterone receptors in benign stromal lesions of the breast. *Am J Surg Pathol* 1991;15: 145–149.

375. Powell CM, Cranor ML, Rosen PP. Pseudoangiomatous stromal hyperplasia (PASH): a mammary stromal tumor with myofibroblastic differentiation. *Am J Surg Pathol* 1995;19: 270–277.

376. Ibrahim RE, Sciotto CG, Weidner N. Pseudoangiomatous hyperplasia of mammary stroma. Some observations regarding its clinicopathological spectrum. *Cancer* 1989;63:1154–1167.

377. Taira N, Ohsumi S, Aogi K, et al. Nodular pseudoangiomatous stromal hyperplasia of mammary stroma in a case showing rapid tumor growth. *Breast Cancer* 2005;12:331–336

378. Rosen PP. Mucocele-like tumors of the breast. *Am J Surg Pathol* 1986;10:464–469.

379. Chinyama CN, Davies JD. Mammary mucinous lesions: congeners, prevalence and important pathological associations. *Histopathology* 1996;29:533–539.

380. Hamele-Bena D, Cranor ML, Rosen PP. Mammary mucocele-like lesions: benign and malignant. *Am J Surg Pathol* 1996;20:1081–1085.

381. Ironside JW, Guthrie W. The galactocoele: a light- and electron-microscopic study. *Histopathology* 1985;9:457–467.

382. Rytina ERC, Coady AT, Millis RR. Milk granuloma: an unusual appearance in lactational breast tissue. *Histopathology* 1990;17:466–468.

383. Clement PB, Young RH, Azzopardi JG. Collagenous spherulosis of the breast. *Am J Surg Pathol* 1987;11:411–417.

384. Wells CA, Wells CW, Yeomans P, et al. Spherical connective tissue inclusions in epithelial hyperplasia of the breast ("collagenous spherulosis"). *J Clin Pathol* 1990;43:905–908.

385. Mooney EE, Kayani N, Tavassoli FA. Spherulosis of the breast. A spectrum of mucinous and collagenous lesions. *Arch Pathol Lab Med* 1999;123:626–630.

386. Sgroi D, Koerner FC. Involvement of collagenous spherulosis by lobular carcinoma in situ. *Am J Surg Pathol* 1995;19:1366–1370.

387. Rosen PP. Multinucleated mammary stromal giant cells. A benign lesion that simulates invasive carcinoma. *Cancer* 1979;44:1305–1308.

CHAPTER

10

Paul E. McKeever

The Brain, Spinal Cord, and Meninges

TERMS AND ABBREVIATIONS USED IN THIS CHAPTER

α-ACT: α-antichymotrypsin macrophage marker; AFP: α-feto-protein; CADASIL: cerebral autosomal dominant arteriopathy with subcortical infarcts and leukoencephalopathy; CD45rb: LCA: leukocyte common antigen; CD3: T-cell–specific marker; CD20: L26, B-cell–specific marker; CD68: KP-1, macrophage marker; CISH: chromogenic in situ hybridization; CK: cytokeratin; EBV, Epstein-Barr virus; EMA: epithelial membrane antigen; epithelioid: cells with distinct cytoplasm and nonfibrillar cellular margins that resemble epithelial cells; ECM: extracellular matrix; fibrillar: cells that extend cytoplasmic processes bound by plasma membranes (unipolar, bipolar, or multipolar); FISH: fluorescent in situ hybridization; GFAP: glial fibrillary acidic protein constituent of glial fibrils (intermediate filament); gliosis: brain reaction to injury remotely similar to systemic fibrosis; HV: herpes virus; HSV: herpes simplex virus; HCG: human chorionic gonadotropin; Ig: immunoglobulin; IHC: immunohistochemistry; κ and λ: kappa and lambda light-chain subclasses of immunoglobulin molecules; NF: neurofilament; PCR: polymerase chain reaction; PLAP: placental alkaline phosphatase; PNET: primitive neuroectodermal tumor; PML: progressive multifocal leukoencephalopathy; S-100: highly acidic small protein soluble in 100% ammonium sulfate; syncytial: cells that have no cytoplasmic borders by light microscopy; TTF-1: thyroid transcription factor 1, a protein present in thyroid and large-cell lung neoplasms.

This chapter focuses on the diagnosis of neurosurgical biopsy and resection specimens from the central nervous system and within the cranial-spinal vault. It is organized by major etiologic categories of disease processes: infectious/inflammatory, cerebrovascular, neoplastic, degenerative, developmental, toxic/metabolic, and traumatic diseases. The focus is on those diseases seen by the surgical pathologist. Extensive recent comprehensive reviews of different fields of neuropathology are also available (1–8). The evaluation of lesions of the pituitary gland and sellar region are reviewed in Chapter 12.

The approach to diagnosis employed in this chapter relies principally on histologic evaluation of hematoxylin and eosin (H&E)-stained sections, with incorporation of smear preparations, histochemical stains, electron microscopy, and immunohistochemical preparations as supplemental aids in diagnosis.

Tables 10.1 through 10.21 provide information about pathologic entities to assist in reading the text and diagnosing cases. Suspected specific disease can be checked directly on the individual table where its key structural, chemical, and topographic features are listed. The text and figures elaborate upon the information in the tables. Features of unknown cases may be found in the tables, which should be helpful to the diagnostician. For example, if the lesion is a mass, specific tables summarize differential features depending on whether the mass is composed of fibrillar cells (Table 10.10, see Fig. 10.39); epithelioid cells (Table 10.11, see Fig. 10.125); more than one type of cell (Table 10.12, see Fig. 10.110); small anaplastic cells (Table 10.13, see Fig. 10.81); or syncytial cells (Table 10.14, see Fig. 10.88).

ALGORITHMIC APPROACH TO DIAGNOSIS EMPLOYING TABLES AND TEXT

An example of a case interpreted from start to finish employing an algorithmic approach and the tables and text is presented in Figure 10.1. As in any other organ system, an algorithmic approach to specimens, at the time of frozen section and subsequently, is valuable. It prevents overlooking key etiologic considerations including secondary pathologic processes.

1. *Neoplasm or Not Neoplasm:* This hypercellular lesion is composed of pleomorphic cells with atypical nuclei, which indicate neoplasm. If the lesion were not neoplastic, other etiologic categories, including infectious, inflammatory, toxic-metabolic, traumatic, vascular, developmental, and degenerative, would be considered.

2. *Primary or Metastatic:* These cells are fibrillar. They are plump and large, but not spindled or vacuolated. The neoplastic cell nuclei are moderately pleomorphic; the cells have small

---

TABLE 10.1

Indications for Intraoperative Consultation at Biopsy

Lesion requires proper surgical sampling of tissue for diagnosis and grading
Lesion may require special tissue processing
Culture for microorganisms
Fixation for electron microscopy
Fixation for immunohistochemistry
Touch preparation
Other special processing
Diagnosis affects immediate surgical procedure

TABLE 10.2	**Surgery Directed Toward a Neurologic Symptom or Specific Disease**

CONFIRMATORY FEATURES OF SUSPECTED DISEASE

Symptom/Suspected Disease	Structures	Reactant	Locations[a]
Herpes simplex encephalitis	Encephalitis (Table 10.3), Cowdry A amphophilic nuclear inclusions of 90-nm to 100-nm "target" capsids	HSV antigen	Temporal or basilar frontal lobe, CNS; frequently bilateral
Toxoplasmosis	Necrosis containing 3-nm to 5-nm tachyzoites; (cysts); (inflammation)[b]	Toxoplasma antigen	CNS, frequent multiple lesions
Progressive multifocal leukoencephalopathy	Demyelination, bizarre, glial, amphophilic nuclear inclusions of 15-nm to 25-nm or 30-nm to 40-nm diameter	JC/SV40 antigen, myelin, neurofilament	Cerebral white matter, CNS
Dementia/Creutzfeldt-Jakob disease	Cytoplasmic vacuoles indenting nuclei, gliosis (Table 10.3)	GFAP, prion (DANGER)	Bilateral cerebral cortex, gray matter
Small-vessel disease	Vasculitis or arterial sclerosis or congophilic angiopathy	Amyloid, iron	Cerebrum, CNS; frequent multiple lesions
Dementia/Alzheimer disease	Argyrophilic plaques; neurofibrillary tangles of bihelical filaments	Neurofilament, tau	Bilateral cerebral cortex
Demyelination	Loss of myelin, gitter cells, with or without axonal preservation	Myelin, neurofilament	Cerebral white matter, CNS
Epilepsy	Low-grade glioma or ganglioglioma (Table 10.10), or gliosis (Tables 10.3 and 10.18), or vascular malformation	GFAP, neurofilament, synaptophysin, iron	Temporal lobe, cerebral cortex

[a]Most common or most specific location is listed first.
[b]Parentheses around a differential feature indicate an uncommon feature very useful in differential diagnosis when found.
CNS, central nervous system; GFAP, glial fibrillary acidic protein; HSV, herpes simplex virus; JC, JC virus; SV, simian virus.

TABLE 10.3	**Differential Features of Cells Infiltrating Central Nervous Parenchyma**

DIFFERENTIAL FEATURES

Diagnosis	Structures	Reactant	Locations[a]
Gliosis[b]	Cells are fibrillar, uncrowded; round or oval nuclei	GFAP in glial filament	CNS
Macrophages	Cells and nuclei are round to elongated; cell content reflects injury	KP-1; α-ACT	CNS, meninges
Encephalitis and/or cerebritis	Perivascular mixture of inflammatory cells	CD3, CD20, LCA, κ and λ Ig, α-ACT; KP-1, microorganism	CNS gray matter, CNS
Hemorrhage	Red blood cells or macrophages with hemosiderin	Fibrin, iron	Deep cerebrum, cerebellum, CNS
Margin of gliomas[c]	Cells are fibrillar; angular nuclei indent each other; (mitoses)[c,d]	GFAP	CNS
Lymphoma	Perivascular, noncohesive small, round cells	CD3, CD20, LCA, κ and λ Ig	Deep cerebrum, CNS; meninges

[a]Most common or most specific location is listed first.
[b]Nonspecific reaction to injury.
[c]Suspicion of margin of glioma on frozen section should be followed by a request for another, more central biopsy. Mitoses suggest margin of a high-grade glioma.
[d]Parentheses around a differential feature indicate an uncommon feature that is very useful in differential diagnosis when it is found.
α-ACT, α-antichymotrypsin macrophage marker; CNS, central nervous system; GFAP, glial fibrillary acidic protein; Ig, immunoglobulin; LCA, leukocyte common antigen (CD45/45R).

TABLE 10.4

Viral Inclusions in the Central Nervous System

	Nucleus	Cytoplasm
Neurons		
Herpes simplex and zoster	+	−
Rabies	−	+
SSPE (measles)	+	−
Oligodendrocytes		
PML (JC virus)	+	−
SSPE (measles)	+	−
Various cells (endothelial, ependymal, glial)		
Cytomegalovirus	+	+

PML, progressive multifocal leukoencephalopathy; SSPE, subacute sclerosing panencephalitis.

processes emanating from them. The lesion lacks rosettes. There is a vessel cuffed by many small, reactive-appearing mononuclear cells. There is no evidence of microvascular proliferation and neither necrosis nor mitotic activity is identified. No epithelial elements are recognized. The findings are those of a primary CNS neoplasm rather than a metastatic lesion (Tables 10.10 and 10.11).

3. *Glial, Neuronal, and Other Primary Considerations:* Possible primary CNS neoplasm diagnoses in Table 10.10 include giant-cell astrocytoma, gemistocytic astrocytoma, ganglion-cell tumor, or histiocytosis (Fig. 10.1). Although nuclei of the lesional cells have a slight resemblance to neuronal nuclei, their chromatin is more condensed. Their cytoplasm is pink without purple Nissl substance of neurons. Bielschowsky stain reveals passing axons of parenchyma

TABLE 10.5

Causes to Consider in Intracranial Hematoma

Traumatic
 Cerebral contusion
 Epidural or subdural hematoma
Infectious and inflammatory
 Vasculitis
 Fungus (mycotic aneurysm)
Developmental vascular
 Vascular malformation (arteriovenous, malformation, cavernous angioma)
 Aneurysm
Hematologic
 Thrombocytopenia
 Sickle cell anemia
Neoplastic
 Primary (high-grade glioma)
 Metastatic (e.g., melanoma, renal cell carcinoma)
 Leukemia (chloroma in acute myelogenous leukemia)
Vascular
 Amyloid angiopathy
 Hypertension
 Conversion of ischemic infarct
Toxic-metabolic: Anticoagulation-related

infiltrated by this neoplasm, but no silver staining of neoplastic cells (Fig. 10.1); neoplastic cells were also negative for synaptophysin, a neuronal marker (not shown). Aggregate features do not support a ganglion-cell tumor. The neoplastic cells are positive for the intermediate filament glial fibrillary acidic protein (GFAP), a marker that accentuates their fibrillarity and confirms their astrocytic nature (Fig. 10.1). The related text in this chapter describes differences between gemistocytic astrocytoma and giant-cell astrocytoma. Gemistocytic astrocytomas resemble reactive astrocytes and have abundant, plump, hyaline cytoplasm and peripheralized nuclei. Macrophages (histiocytes) are GFAP-negative and lack the fibrillary structure highlighted by GFAP, arguing against the diagnosis histiocytosis. Neoplastic cells are negative for the T-lymphocyte marker CD45RO (Fig. 10.1D) and the B-lymphocyte marker CD20 (Fig. 10.1E), whereas polyclonal perivascular lymphocytes are positive. Therefore, the aggregate histologic, histochemical, and IHC findings support the diagnosis of gemistocytic astrocytoma. Most gemistocytic astrocytomas are grade II, although they tend to progress to a higher grade. Grading is further discussed in the "Gemistocytic Astrocytoma," "Diffuse Astrocytoma," and "Anaplastic Astrocytoma" sections. Other algorithmic approaches to the brain biopsy are available (9,10).

CLINICAL AND RADIOGRAPHIC PERSPECTIVE OF LESIONS

Biopsies should be examined with knowledge of the clinical history. If a specific diagnosis or differential is not suspected preoperatively, at the least a major neurologic symptom (e.g., weakness or visual loss) or category of neurologic disease (e.g., refractory epilepsy) is usually available to focus the search for a diagnosis (Table 10.2). The pathologist should always know, at a minimum, the age and sex of the patient, the precise location of the targeted lesion, and imaging characteristics. Knowledge about past medical history (e.g., previous CNS or primary neoplasms, connective tissue disease, immunosuppressive disease) is critical to interpretation. Likewise, knowledge about preoperative therapy (e.g., corticosteroids, chemotherapy, radiation therapy, radiosurgery) is also critical to interpretation of findings (e.g., necrosis, vascular fibrosis).

Certain pathologic entities predominate in pediatric, adult, or geriatric age categories as described in the text. A communication system between the operating rooms and the pathology diagnostic rooms is especially important to share relevant clinical and pathologic observations on individual cases examined by frozen section (Table 10.1).

Radiology provides extremely valuable gross pathologic information—most importantly, computed axial tomography (CT scan) and magnetic resonance imaging (MRI); use of contrast and special imaging techniques (e.g., diffusion- and perfusion-weighted imaging) add additional data in characterizing normal and abnormal structures. Emerging imaging techniques including MR spectroscopy (evaluation of chemical components in a lesion) offer additional information about specific lesions (6,11).

TABLE 10.6   Vascular Malformations

Malformation[a]	Vessels	Neuropile	Gliosis and Hemosiderin-Laden Macrophages
Arteriovenous malformation	Arteries, veins, arterialized veins	Absent, except around feeding vessels	Present[b]
Cavernous angioma	Compact cluster thin-walled to thick-walled vessels, mineralization	Absent usually	Present[b]
Capillary telangiectasia	Capillaries, thin-walled	Admixed	Absent
Venous malformation	Veins, often dilated	Admixed	Absent
Varix	Vein, dilated (vein of Galen)	Absent	Absent unless ruptured

[a]Location: Each can be found anywhere in the central nervous system; capillary telangiectasias often in brainstem and venous malformations in the spinal leptomeninges.

[b]Gliosis and hemosiderin-laden macrophages are consistent with leakage; they serve as a seizure focus, and they signal a tendency for spontaneous hemorrhage.

TABLE 10.7   Relative Frequency of Most Common Pediatric and Adult Brain Neoplasms

CHILDREN			ADULTS		
Location	Diagnosis and Frequency		Location	Diagnosis and Frequency	
Anterior fossa	Miscellaneous	33%	Anterior fossa	Gliomas (cerebrum)[a]	33%
				Meningiomas (dura)	13%
				Metastases (cerebrum)	12%
				Pituitary adenomas (sella)	5%
				Miscellaneous	4%
			Total		67%
Posterior fossa	Astrocytomas (cerebellum)[a]	26%			
	Medulloblastomas (cerebellum)	24%			
	Ependymomas (fourth ventricle)	14%	Posterior fossa	Schwannomas (8th cranial nerve)	8%
	Miscellaneous	3%		Miscellaneous	25%
Total		67%	Total		33%

[a]Most common site in parentheses. See entry in text for other locations.

TABLE 10.8

World Health Organization Criteria for Grading of Astrocytomas

Grade	Nomenclature	Histologic Features
1	Pilocytic	Circumscribed; biphasic: bipolar piloid cells and multipolar cells; microcysts, Rosenthal fibers, and granular bodies; may or may not have rare mitotic figures, vascular proliferation, or focal necrosis
2	Diffuse	Moderate hypercellularity of monotonous cells; mild nuclear atypia; no or minimal mitotic activity
3	Anaplastic	Increased cellularity and diffuse infiltration; increased nuclear atypia; increased mitotic activity
4	Glioblastoma	Vascular proliferation or necrosis; crowded anaplastic cells; marked nuclear atypia; brisk mitotic activity

From Louis DN, Ohgaki H, Wiestler OD, Cavenee WK. *World Health Organization Classification of Tumours: Pathology and Genetics of Tumors of the Nervous System.* Geneva: IARC Press, 2007, with permission.

TABLE 10.9

World Health Organization Criteria for Grading of Oligodendrogliomas

Grade	Nomenclature	Histologic Features
2	Oligodendroglioma	Moderate cellularity; homogeneously round nuclei, "fried egg" halo (paraffin); fine capillary network; mineralization (microcalcifications)
3	Anaplastic oligodendroglioma	Increased cellularity; high mitotic rate; marked cytologic atypia; microvascular proliferation; necrosis

From Louis DN, Ohgaki H, Wiestler OD, Cavenee WK. *World Health Organization Classification of Tumours: Pathology and Genetics of Tumors of the Nervous System.* Geneva: IARC Press, 2007, with permission.

| TABLE 10.10 | Differential Diagnosis of a Mass of Fibrillar Cells | | |

DIFFERENTIAL FEATURES

Diagnosis[a]	Structures	Reactant	Locations[b]
Fibrosis	Spindle cells of meningeal or perivascular origin	Collagen; reticulin	Meninges, CNS
Granuloma	Like fibrosis with "whorls" and inflammation	Microorganisms	Basal meninges, CNS
Pilocytic astrocytoma	Hypercellularity; hairlike fibrillarity; Rosenthal fibers; microcysts	GFAP	Cerebellum, thalamus/hypothalamus, optic nerve, CNS
Astrocytoma	Hypercellularity; angular nuclei cluster and indent each other; infiltrates CNS	GFAP	Cerebrum, brainstem, spinal cord, CNS
Anaplastic astrocytoma	Increase in above features; mitoses	GFAP	Cerebrum, brainstem, CNS
Gemistocytic astrocytoma	Hypercellularity; cells swollen with hyaline pink cytoplasm and eccentric pleomorphic nuclei; infiltrates CNS	GFAP	Cerebrum
Giant-cell astrocytoma	Giant astrocytes with thick fibrils; large round or oval nuclei	GFAP	Lateral ventricle, subependymal
Astroblastoma	Perivascular rosettes with expanded glial cell processes	Nonfibrillar GFAP	Cerebrum, CNS
Pleomorphic xanthoastrocytoma	Pleomorphic cells are often vacuolated	GFAP, reticulin, lipid	Leptomeninges, cerebral cortex
Ependymoma	Hypercellularity; ependymal and/or perivascular rosettes; round or oval nuclei, cilia, and basal bodies	GFAP, EMA	Cerebrum, cerebellum, spinal cord, CNS
Tanycytic ependymoma or subependymoma	Combination of astrocytoma and ependymoma; round or oval nuclei cluster among fibrillar mats; ependymal cytology	GFAP	Spinal cord, fourth ventricle, subependymal, CNS
Anaplastic ependymoma	Above features with mitoses; necrosis	GFAP, S-100	Cerebrum, cerebellum
Giloblastoma multiforme	Regions of coagulation necrosis; mitoses; pleomorphism; endothelial proliferation	GFAP, S-100	Cerebrum, CNS
Gilosarcoma	Glioblastoma plus fibrosarcoma intermixed	GFAP, reticulin, collagen	Cerebrum
Ganglion-cell tumors	Binucleated and pleomorphic neurons; diagnosis dependent on gliomatous and neuroblastic elements	GFAP, synaptophysin, PGP 9.5; neurofilament, Nissl	Cerebrum, CNS
Central neurocytoma	Round cells and nuclei; thin fibrils near vessels	Synaptophysin, neurofilament	Septum pellucidum, lateral ventricles, CNS
Pineocytoma	Normal pineal structures	Synaptophysin, neurofilament	Pineal
Fibroblastic meningioma	Spindle cells; interdigitating cell processes and desmosomes; (thick collagen); (whorls)[c]	Vimentin, EMA, reticulin, progesterone receptor	Falx, tentorium, meninges; choroid plexus
Fibrosarcoma/malignant fibrous histiocytoma	Hypercellular; pleomorphic spindle cells and nuclei; mitoses; necrosis	Reticulin, collagen	Meninges, CNS
Schwannoma	Verocay bodies; Antoni A and B; thin pericellular basement membrane	Reticulin, S-100, collagen	8th cranial nerve, spinal roots, PNS
Neurofibroma	Multiple cell types spread axons	Neurofilament, myelin, S-100, Leu-7	Spinal root, PNS; cranial nerve
Histiocytosis	Sheetlike pattern of macrophages, fibroblasts, and leukocytes	α-ACT, S-100	Parasellar, CNS, systemic
Hemangioblastoma	Multivacuolated stromal cells between many capillaries; hypervascularity; (fibrillarity is frozen section artifact)	Cytoplasmic lipid, reticulin, factor VIII	Cerebellum, spinal cord, CNS
Melanoma	Anaplasia, mitoses, necrosis	Melanin, HMB45 antigen; S-100	CNS or meninges, frequent, multiple metastases; systemic

[a]The order of tabulated lesions follows their order in text.
[b]Most common or most specific location is listed first.
[c]Parentheses around a differential feature indicate an uncommon feature that is very useful in differential diagnosis when it is found.
α-ACT, α-antichymotrypsin macrophage marker; CNS, central nervous system; EMA, epithelial membrane antigen; GFAP, glial fibrillary acitic protein; PNS, peripheral nervous system; PTAH, phosphotungstic acid hematoxylin.

TABLE 10.11	Differential Diagnosis of a Mass of Epithelioid Cells			

	DIFFERENTIAL FEATURES			
Diagnosis[a]	Structures	Reactant	Locations[b]	
Gitter cells or xanthogranuloma	Crowded macrophages engorged with lipid vacuoles; eccentric nucleus; noncohesive cells	α-ACT; KP-1; muramidase	CNS	
Oligodendroglioma	Round cells and nuclei with prominent peri-nuclear halos; nests of cells between delicate vessels	Leu-7, S-100; del 1p 19q	Cerebrum, CNS	
Anaplastic oligodendroglioma	Above features with mitoses and pleomorphism	Above markers	Cerebrum, CNS	
Choroid plexus papilloma	Large mass with structure of choroid plexus	Laminin, cytokeratin, transthyretin, mucin[c]	Fourth ventricle, lateral ventricle, cerebellopontine angle, choroid plexus	
Choroid plexus carcinoma	Above features with anaplasia and mitoses; (necrosis)	Cytokeratin, (transthyretin, mucin)	Above lesions	
Medulloepithelioma	Columnar epithelium with "basement membrane" on both surfaces; fibrovascular base for papillae and tubules	Nestin	Deep cerebrum, cauda equina, CNS	
Meningioma	Whorls, psammoma bodies, interdigitating cell processes and desmosomes; (thick collagen)	Vimentin, EMA, progesterone receptors	Falx, tentorium; meninges; choroid plexus; (extracranial)	
Chordoma	Masses or cords of physaliphorous cells	Cytokeratin, EMA; (mucin)	Sacrococcygeal tissues, cauda equina, clivus, spinal canal	
Paraganglioma	Nests of clear or granular cells surrounded by many capillaries	Chromogranin	Petrous ridge, spinal cord, epidural	
Pituitary adenoma	Secondary granules	Pituitary peptides; chromogranin	Sellar, suprasellar	
Endodermal sinus tumor	Schiller-Duvall bodies	AFP	Pineal, parasellar	
Embryonal carcinoma	Anaplasia, mitoses	AFP, (PLAP)	Pineal, parasellar	
Hemangioblastoma	Multivacuolated stromal cells between many capillaries; hypervascularity	Cytoplasmic lipid, reticulin, factor VIII	Cerebellum, spinal cord, CNS	
Craniopharyngioma	Squamous, adamantinomatous	Cholesterol cytokeratin	Suprasellar, sellar	
Carcinoma	Distinct margin with CNS; anaplasia, mitoses, necrosis	Cytokeratin, EMA, (mucin)	Cerebrum, cerebellum, meninges, CNS; frequent multiples masses; systemic	
Melanoma	Anaplasia, mitoses, necrosis	Melanin, HMB45, tyrosinase	Above locations	

[a]The order of tabulated lesions follows their order in text.
[b]Most common or most specific location is listed first.
[c]Parentheses around a differential feature indicate an uncommon feature that is very useful in differential diagnosis when it is found.
α-ACT, α-antichymotrypsin macrophage marker; AFP, α-fetoprotein; CNS, central nervous system; EMA, epithelial membrane antigen; PLAP, placental alkaline phosphatase.

Major categories of lesions of the brain, spinal cord, and meninges, such as solitary or multiple masses, cysts, vascular malformations, or abscesses, are likely to be recognized by imaging or upon viewing a gross specimen. The neurosurgical lesions summarized in Tables 10.6 through 10.19 are usually focal, whereas the lesions in the biopsies directed toward a neurologic disease tend to be more diffuse (Table 10.2). One particularly problematic diagnosis is vasculitis that can be focal, multifocal, or diffuse. If you are lucky enough to be consulted on any multifocal case, advise the surgeon to target a new or subacute radiographic lesion.

Multiple lesions can be produced by neoplasms or by inflammatory, vascular, and infectious diseases. If inflammation or infection is suspected prior to or seen at biopsy, cultures for appropriate microorganisms should be sent in sterile containers directly from the Operating Room to Microbiology. The "M-rule" for common multiple CNS neoplasms includes metastases, malignant lymphoma, melanoma, and (late stages only) medulloblastoma.

In some settings (e.g., in a patient with neurologic deficits), a biopsy is performed in a desperate attempt to find a diagnosis. In such a setting, to optimize the probability of a pathologic diagnosis, the biopsy should be directed at a region of recent radiologic abnormality such as contrast enhancement, and optimally should include (a) dura, (b) arachnoid, (c) gray matter, and (d) white matter. In the setting of radiologic lesions, biopsy of a normal radiologic region or a so-called unguided or undirected ("blind") biopsy is, in our experience, a useless waste of everyone's time. It is a ritual that helps the clinician say that everything was tried on a moribund patient.

The tomographic density of hemorrhage is sufficiently unique at certain stages of organization to preoperatively iden-

	TABLE 10.12	**Differential Diagnosis of a Mass of Conspicuously Different Cells**		

		DIFFERENTIAL FEATURES		
Diagnosis[a]	*Structures*	*Reactant*	*Locations[b]*	
Oligoastrocytoma	Mixture of astrocytoma (Table 10.10) and oligodendroglioma (Table 10.11)	GFAP, Leu-7, S-100	Cerebrum, CNS	
Anaplastic oligoastrocytoma	Above features with mitoses and pleomorphism, necrosis, MVP	GFAP, Leu-7, S-100	Cerebrum, CNS	
Glioblastoma or gliosarcoma with epithelial metaplasia	Structures of glioblastoma or gliosarcoma (Table 10.10) plus epithelial regions	GFAP, S-100, cytokeratin, EMA	Cerebrum, CNS	
Ependymoma/ malignant ependymoma	Structures of ependymoma or malignant ependymoma (Table 10.10) plus epithelioid cells	GFAP	Cerebellum, cerebrum, spinal cord, CNS	
Myxopapillary ependymoma	Cuboidal and/or columnar epithelium on hyaline fibrovascular papillae; variable fibrillarity	Mucin, GFAP	Regions of the filum terminale	
Ganglion cell tumors	Binucleated and pleomorphic neurons plus glioma (Table 10.10) plus fibrosis plus inflammation	GFAP, synaptophysin, PGP 9.5, neurofilament, Nissl, collagen, reticulin	Cerebrum, CNS	
Desmoplastic medulloblastoma	Regions of medulloblastoma (Table 10.13) and desmoplasia (Table 10.10)	Synaptophysin, S-100, reticulin, (neurofilament); (GFAP)[c]	Lateral cerebellum, CNS, meninges; (extra-axial)	
Transitional meningioma	Regions of fibrous (Table 10.10) and syncytial (Table 10.14) meningioma	Vimentin, EMA, reticulin, PR	Falx, tentorium; meninges; choroid plexus	
Germinoma	Regions of large epithelioid cells and small lymphocytes	PLAP, CD117	Pineal, parasellar, CNS	
Teratoma	Well-differentiated tissues from more than one germinal layer; may contain another germ cell tumor component (Table 10.11)	Mucin, collagen, GFAP; others	Pineal, suprasellar, sacrococcygeal	
Choriocarcinoma	Syncytial and cytotrophoblast	Human chorionic gonadotropin	Pineal, parasellar, CNS[d]	
Desmoplastic carcinoma	Regions of carcinoma (Table 10.11) and fibrosis (Table 10.10) plus inflammation	Cytokeratin, EMA; (mucin); (TTF-1)	Cerebrum, cerebellum, meninges, CNS, frequent multiple masses, systemic	
Melanoma	Regions of fibrillar and epithelioid melanoma (Tables 10.10 and 10.11) GFAP, Leu-7, S-100	Melanin, HMB45 antigen, S-100, tyrosinase	Cerebrum, cerebellum, meninges, CNS; frequently multiple masses, systemic	

[a]The order of tabulated lesions follows their order in text.
[b]Most common or most specific location is listed first.
[c]Parentheses around a differential feature indicate an uncommon feature that is very useful in differential diagnosis when it is found.
[d]As a primary midline tumor or metastasis to the CNS from a pelvic or gonadal primary tumor.
CNS, central nervous system; EMA, epithelial membrane antigen; GFAP, glial fibrillary acidic protein; PLAP, placental alkaline phosphatase; MVP, microvascular proliferation; PR, progesterone receptors; TTF-1, thyroid transcription factor 1.

tify hemorrhage as a major component of a lesion. In general, calcifications and relationships with the skull are resolved well by CT. Gray and white matter, edema, and melanin are resolved well by MRI. Vascular abnormalities are frequently appreciated clinically and angiographically. CT or MRI angiography of flow voids is sometimes sufficient and is less invasive than classic angiography.

INTRAOPERATIVE CONSULTATION

Certain entities that may be either suspected clinically or suggested on cytologic preparation and frozen section can affect the immediate surgical procedure (see "Primary Open Biopsy"

section and Table 10.1). Most significantly, attempts at total resection are often made for these neoplasms: meningiomas, schwannomas, solitary metastases, cysts, ependymomas, hemangioblastomas, cerebellar pilocytic astrocytomas, and craniopharyngiomas. Therefore, assessment of such specimens requires careful clinicopathologic correlation at the time of the primary operation, and intraoperative consultation guides the procedure.

Any undefined lesion should be biopsied and inspected by both cytologic preparation and frozen sections. Cytologic preparations add fine nuclear detail and the presence or absence of (a) glial-type processes, (b) discohesiveness in pituitary adenomas, oligodendrogliomas, medulloblastomas, and lymphomas, and (c) "epithelioid" features, with cellular cohesion (suggesting junctions) in carcinomas. The value of such preparations

TABLE 10.13	Differential Diagnosis of a Mass of Small, Crowded, Anaplastic Cells		
	DIFFERENTIAL FEATURES		
Diagnosis	*Structures*	*Reactant*	*Locations[a]*
Ependymoblastoma	Like PNET; ribbons or cords of cells; true ependymal rosettes	GFAP, S-100	Cerebrum, cerebellum
Medulloblastoma, pineoblastoma, neuroblastoma, or PNET	Slight fibrillarity; (Homer Wright rosettes); (palisades); "carrot" nuclei; (neural or glial foci)[b]	Synaptophysin; PGP 9.5; (S-100); (neurofilament); (GFAP)	Cerebellum, brainstem, pineal, CNS; (extra-axial)
Rhabdomyosarcoma or medullomyoblastoma	Muscle striations	Desmin, muscle specific actin, SMA	Pineal, cerebellum, CNS
Hemangiopericytoma	Hypercellularity; thick pericellular matrix, mitoses	Reticulin	Falx, tentorium; meninges; (extracranial)
Lymphoma	Noncohesive, round cells; vascular wall invasion	Reticulin, collagen, L26, UCHL1, LCA, monoclonal κ and λ Ig	Deep cerebrum, CNS, meninges; may be multiple
Small-cell carcinoma	Cohesive cells; (epithelioid); (desmosomes)	Cytokeratin, EMA	CNS, meninges; frequent multiple masses, systemic

[a]Most common or most specific location is listed first.
[b]Parentheses around a differential feature indicate an uncommon feature that is very useful in differential diagnosis when it is found.
CNS, central nervous system; EMA, epithelial membrane antigen; GFAP, glial fibrillary acidic protein; Ig, immunoglobulin; LCA, leukocyte common antigen; PGP, protein gene product; PNET, primitive neuroectodermal tumor; UCHL1, T-lymphocyte marker CD45RO; SMA, smooth muscle actin.

has been demonstrated (12,13) and, in some centers, intraoperative diagnosis is based only on evaluation of cytologic preparations. Although smear and crush preparations may be done, touch preparations minimize effort and artifact. Touch a glass slide to the wet tissue and then immediately fix it in ethanol before it dries. Stain with H&E or with a cytologic stain.

Difficult access to, and fragility of, central nervous tissue places a high premium on obtaining tissue suitable for diagnosis during the first surgical procedure and avoiding secondary biopsy after a primary nondiagnostic biopsy (4). The goal of the pathologist in the intraoperative setting is not to definitively diagnose and grade every case but, rather, to (a) ensure that a lesional tissue has been obtained for subsequent diagnosis and grading; (b) to ensure the lesional tissue has been appropriately sampled (e.g., that high grade features are noted on a suspected glioblastoma based on imaging features); (c) to provide sufficient preliminary diagnostic information to optimize surgery;

and (d) to perform appropriate special tissue processing (Table 10.1). Optimizing surgery depends upon the individual case and upon whether open biopsy or stereotactic needle biopsy is being done (see sections below).

Given the constraints of intraoperative evaluation of tissue, including sampling limitations and freezing artifact, precise diagnosis is often neither possible nor necessary for a successful intraoperative consultation. The surgical pathologist need only go as far as necessary with her/his diagnosis (e.g., high-grade glioma, metastatic neoplasm, atypical lymphoid infiltrate suspicious for lymphoma, abundant neutrophils suggestive of abscess, granulomatous inflammation) to guide the surgery without attempting to make complex diagnoses that optimally employ paraffin sections. The pathologist's microscopic impression, even if rendered as a differential, guides the surgical procedure.

In the setting of a glial neoplasm, it is not wise to offer a

TABLE 10.14	Differential Diagnosis of a Mass That Includes Syncytial Cells		
	DIFFERENTIAL FEATURES		
Diagnosis	*Structures*	*Reactant*	*Locations[a]*
Meningiomas	Whorls, psammoma bodies; interdigitating cell processes and desmosomes; (thick collagen)[b]	Vimentin, epithelial membrane antigen, PR	Falx, tentorium meninges; choroid plexus; (extracranial)
Anaplastic meningioma	Decrease in above features; mitoses, necrosis; central nervous system invasion	Above chemicals	Above locations
Choriocarcinoma	Syncytium usually mixed with cytotrophoblast (Table 10.12)	Human chorionic gonadotropin	Pineal, suprasellar

[a]Most common or most specific location is listed first.
[b]Parentheses around a differential feature indicate an uncommon feature very useful in differential diagnosis when it is found.
PR, progesterone receptors.

TABLE 10.15	World Health Organization Criteria for Grading of Meningiomas[a]

Meningioma (grade I)
  Fails to meet diagnostic criteria below
  <4 mitotic figures per 10 hpf (0.16 mm^2)
Atypical meningioma (grade II)
  Increased mitotic activity: 4–19 per 10 hpf (0.16 mm^2)
    OR three or more of the following:
  Increased cellularity
  Small cells with high nuclear:cytoplasmic ratio
  Prominent nucleoli
  Sheetlike and/or patternless growth pattern
  Foci of "spontaneous" or "geographic" necrosis
Anaplastic meningioma (grade III)
  Increased mitotic activity >19 per 10 hpf (0.16 mm^2)
    OR
  "Malignant" and/or anaplastic cytologic appearance (e.g., resembling sarcoma, carcinoma, melanoma)

[a]Brain invasion not a criterion for increased grade; WHO grade II also assigned to intracranial clear-cell and chordoid meningiomas; WHO grade III assigned to rhabdoid and papillary meningiomas.
Modified from Louis DN, Ohgaki H, Wiestler OD, Cavenee WK. *World Health Organization Classification of Tumours of the Central Nervous System.* Geneva: IARC Press, 2007.

TABLE 10.16	Histiocytoses Affecting the Central Nervous System Compared with Macrophages

Disease	Characteristic Histology	CD68 (KP-1)	S-100	CD1a	Birbeck Granules (EM)
Macrophage	Foamy, epithelioid, multinucleated giant cells	+	−	−	−
Erdheim-Chester	Touton giant cells	+	+/−[a]	−	−
Rosai-Dorfman	Emperipolesis	+	+	−	−
Langerhans histiocytosis	Reniform nuclei, eosinophilic cytoplasm	+	+	+	+

[a]S-100 has been positive in some, but not all, cases of Erdheim-Chester disease.
EM, electron microscopy.

TABLE 10.17	Carcinomas and Melanoma Metastatic to Brain

Primary Tumor	Frequency with Which the Primary Tumor Metastasizes to the Brain	Frequency of a Brain Metastasis Originating from the Primary Tumor
Lung	26%–42%	35%
Breast	15%–25%	20%
Skin (melanoma)	39%–92%	10%
Kidney	10%–25%	10%
Gastrointestinal tract	5%–7%	5%
Choriocarcinoma	High	Low
All others	Variable	<20%

TABLE 10.18	Differential Diagnosis of Cyst with Wall of Fibrillar Cells		
	DIFFERENTIAL FEATURES		
Diagnosis	*Structures*	*Reactant*	*Locations[a]*
Cavitary gliosis	Wall of gliosis (Table 10.3)	GFAP in glial filaments	Cerebrum, CNS
Abscess	Wall of granulation tissue; fibrosis (Table 10.10); inflammation and gliosis; purulent contents	Collagen, reticulin, L26, UCHL1, LCA, κ and λ Ig, α-ACT, microorganisms	Basal frontal and temporal lobes, CNS
Cystic astrocytoma	Wall of pilocytic astrocytoma (Table 10.10)	GFAP	Cerebellum, CNS
Hemangioblastoma	Wall of gliosis; mural nodule of hemagioblastoma (Table 10.3)	Cytoplasmic lipid, reticulin, factor VIII	Cerebellum, CNS
Glial cyst, simple cyst, or wall of syrinx	Wall of gliosis (Table 10.10); Rosenthal fibers	GFAP in glial filaments	Pineal, cerebellum, and spinal cord; brainstem
Pineal cyst	Wall of fibrillary cells, rarely ependymal		Pineal
Meningeal cyst	Wall of dura, arachnoid; syncytial cells	Collagen, PR	Spinal epidural surface

[a]Most common or most specific location is listed first.
α-ACT, α-antichymotrypsin macrophage marker; CNS, central nervous system; GFAP, glial fibrillary acidic protein; Ig, immunoglobulin; LCA, leukocyte common antigen; UHCL1, T-lymphocyte marker CD45RO; PR, progesterone receptors.

grade during intraoperative frozen section or touch preparation interpretation. Because gliomas are quite heterogeneous, diagnostic features that affect the classification and grade may be revealed only in the "permanent" specimens, and not on frozen section. For instance, oligodendroglial elements in a mixed glioma may not be well represented or recognized on the frozen material; the characteristic halo is a paraffin-embedding artifact. A diagnosis of "primary glial neoplasm with abundant mitotic activity, at least WHO grade III," or "high-grade glioma," effectively characterizes a biopsy when malignant glial cells are unequivocally identified on cytologic and frozen section preparations, and allows for the later identification of oligodendroglial and other elements not evident on the fresh sample.

The intraoperative consultation provides the opportunity to obtain tissue for microbiologic culture, special fixation (e.g., lymphoma), and special processing (e.g., flow cytometry, cytogenetics, molecular evaluation, and electron microscopy) when preliminary assessment deems it necessary or pragmatic (see "Tissue Processing" below).

SUMMARY POINTS ABOUT INTRAOPERATIVE CONSULTATION

I. *Be Prepared:*
   A. *History:* Patient age, duration of symptoms, and surgical location are minimum.
   B. *Radiography:* View images and/or read reports. On reports, objective findings trump interpretation. Are there one or more masses? Infiltrative? Enhancing?

TABLE 10.19	Differential Diagnosis of a Cyst with Wall Lined by Epithelium		
	DIFFERENTIAL FEATURES		
Diagnosis	*Structures*	*Reactant*	*Locations[a]*
Cystic craniopharyngioma	Wall of adamantinomatous or incompletely keratinized squamous epithelium; cyst contains "motor oil"	Cytokeratin, cholesterol	Suprasellar, sella
Ependymal cyst	Columnar epithelium usually ciliated	GFAP	Spinal cord, brain
Colloid cyst	Fibrous wall lined by inner ciliated and/or nonciliated simple columnar epithelium; cyst contains colloid and cell ghosts	Mucin	Third ventricle
Dermoid cyst	Epidermoid cyst features plus adnexa of skin; cyst contains sebum, squames, and hair	Keratin, cholesterol	Midline cerebellum, fourth ventricle, skull, spinal dura, cauda equina
Epidermoid cyst	Fibrous wall lined by inner keratinizing stratified squamous epithelium; cyst contains waxy squames	Keratin, cholesterol	Cerebellar pontine angle, temporal lobe, spinal dura, pineal, sella, brainstem, central nervous system
Enterogenous cyst	Columnar epithelium cyst contains mucin; rests on collagen	Mucin	Spinal cord

[a]Most common or most specific location is listed first.
GFAP, glial fibrillary acidic protein.

TABLE 10.20	Inclusion Immunophenotype			
Inclusion	*Ubiquitin (HAR)[a]*	*Tau (HAR)[a]*	*α-Synuclein (Formic Acid)[a]*	*β-Amyloid (Formic Acid)[a]*
AD tangles and neurites	+	+	−	−
AD neuritic plaque	+ Neurites	+ Neurites	+/− Plaque	+ Plaque
Lewy bodies and neurites	+	−	+	−
Pick bodies and neurites	+	+	−[b]	−
Frontotemporal dementia or motor neuron disease	+	−	−	−
Mutiple system atrophy	+ GCIs	+/− GCIs	+ GCIs	−

[a]Preferred antigen retrieval technique.
[b]Labeling of Pick bodies and neurites has reported with proteinase K antigen retrieval.
AD, Alzheimer disease; GCIs, glial cytoplasmic inclusions; HAR, heat antigen retrieval, microwave in citrate buffer.

C. *Check for prior specimens:* Slides and reports.

II. **New Specimen:** Both cytologic and frozen sections preferred.

III. **Observations:**

A. *Cell type:* Fibrillar, epithelioid, mixed, small and crowded, or syncytial (e.g., fibrillar*)

B. *Major features:* Such as mass; marked cellular and nuclear pleomorphism*

TABLE 10.21

Findings in Surgically Resected Temporal Lobes in Setting of Seizure Disorder

Minimal or nonspecific changes
  Minimal or no histologic abnormality (25%)[a]
  Gliosis (34%)
  Subpial gliosis, enhanced
  CA1 and dentate gyrus neuron loss
  Perivascular hemosiderin-laden macrophages
Neoplastic
  Glioma (12%)
  Dysembryoplastic neuroepithelial tumor
  Ganglioglioma
Infectious and inflammatory (3%)
  Encephalitis and meningoencephalitis
  Rasmussen encephalitis
Traumatic remote traumatic contusion (5%)
Developmental migrational
  Cortical dysplasia/hamartoma (4%)
  Microdysgenesis
  Tuber
  Cyst
Developmental vascular
  Vascular malformation (arteriovenous malformation or cavernous angioma) (2%)
  Sturge-Weber syndrome
Vascular: remote infarct (4%)
Reaction to monitoring
  Arachnoid fibrosis; chronic inflammation, including hemosiderin-laden macrophages
  Needle monitoring tract damage: macrophages, hemosiderin-laden macrophages, gliosis

[a]Percentages are estimated frequencies of the more common findings.

C. *Differential (Dif):* Such as glioblastoma (GbM), giant-cell astrocytoma (GCA), pleomorphic xanthoastrocytoma (PXA), sarcoma (Src), or melanoma (Mel)*

IV. **Narrow the Differential:** Check excluding and corroborating features (e.g., for above Dif*).

A. *Location:* Entirely extramedullary (e.g., outside of CNS [excludes GbM, GCA]); skull invasion (favors Src, Mel); subependymal (favors GCA)

B. *Radiography:* Diffuse margin with CNS (favors GbM)

C. *Duration of symptoms:* For a new mass, <3 mo favors GbM, Src, Mel

D. *Microscopic features:*
1. No mitoses (favors GCA, PXA)
2. Granular bodies (favors PXA)
3. Necrosis (favors GbM, Src, Mel)
4. Microvascular proliferation (favors GbM)
5. Intercellular collagen (favors PXA, Src)

*The differential (set in parentheses) of a mass with fibrillar cells of marked cellular and nuclear pleomorphism is a single algorithmic example of how to use the summary points.

CATEGORIES OF SURGICAL SPECIMENS

Optimal management of a specimen requires knowledge of the aim of the procedure. Three major types of neurosurgical procedures routinely yield tissue: (a) primary biopsies, (b) secondary biopsies, and (c) therapeutic resections. A primary biopsy seeks a diagnosis. Secondary biopsies may try again to establish a diagnosis, or monitor consequences of therapy. Biopsies can be performed using CT- or MRI-guided stereotactic needle biopsy or using an open technique. Therapeutic resections attempt gross total excision of lesional tissue. Individual cases may combine more than one procedure at a single operation. For example, open biopsy for diagnosis of an intramedullary spinal cord tumor may proceed directly to a therapeutic resection if the intraoperative evaluation suggests ependymoma.

PRIMARY OPEN BIOPSY

The primary biopsy for diagnosis is critical. The craniotomy and open biopsy, where the neurosurgeon "turns a flap" by sawing

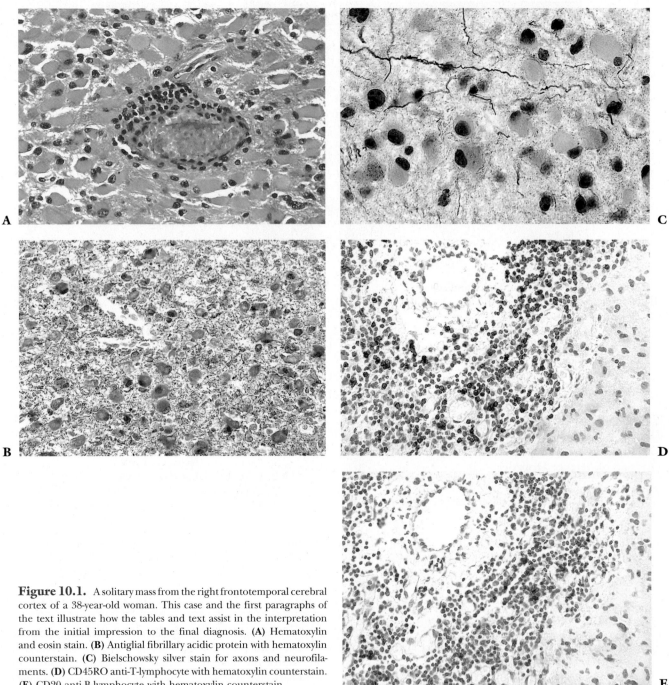

Figure 10.1. A solitary mass from the right frontotemporal cerebral cortex of a 38-year-old woman. This case and the first paragraphs of the text illustrate how the tables and text assist in the interpretation from the initial impression to the final diagnosis. **(A)** Hematoxylin and eosin stain. **(B)** Antiglial fibrillary acidic protein with hematoxylin counterstain. **(C)** Bielschowsky silver stain for axons and neurofilaments. **(D)** CD45RO anti-T-lymphocyte with hematoxylin counterstain. **(E)** CD20 anti-B-lymphocyte with hematoxylin counterstain.

through, and temporarily opening, a portion of the calvarium, affords a macroscopic view of the lesion. In some centers, localization of the lesion is aided by intraoperative imaging, including MRI. The pathologist's database should include the preoperative radiologic data as well as macroscopic findings in situ, either by direct observation or by conversation with the neurosurgeon. Descriptive observations of the margin, color, consistency, precise point of attachment, and immediate surroundings of a lesion are frequently helpful. Because an open biopsy provides surgical latitude from biopsy to total resection, it is important to recognize resectable tumors whenever possible during surgery. Resectable tumors include meningiomas, carcinomas, adeno-

mas, schwannomas, pilocytic astrocytomas, and many ependymomas.

STEREOTACTIC NEEDLE BIOPSY

Radiographically guided stereotactic needle biopsies of vital and sensitive locations through a small hole in the skull are increasing in frequency (14). Needle biopsy specimens have requirements for tissue handling similar to open biopsy specimens, with the following exceptions.

Radiographs substitute for direct visual inspection of the lesion in situ. This and the small size of the specimen confound even the most careful attempts at proper sampling of the lesion. Movement of a centimeter or less may result in totally necrotic or gliotic nondiagnostic tissue. This so-called black box effect requires that sampling of needle biopsies for diagnosis be monitored with frozen sections. However, the intraoperative interpretation does not affect the immediate surgical procedure with regard to therapy because excision of the lesion is not intended.

Better results come from examining both whole-cell cytology and frozen section histology than from either alone, but special care is needed to avoid harming tiny stereotactic biopsies by touching and drying. One approach is to freeze the entire tissue and touch only the gauze pad it came on to a slide for cytology. When the pathologist indicates that a diagnostic region has been sampled, the neurosurgeon should take a second sample for permanent section from the same region, extruding it directly into fixative. Those who excessively ponder the macroscopic appearance of this tiny tissue fragment under powerful lights risk a dried, nondiagnostic sample.

The most important task for the pathologist during stereotactic surgery is to advise the surgeon of the likelihood that he or she is sampling the lesion itself, rather than normal, gliotic, or otherwise nondiagnostic tissue (Fig. 10.2). Frequently, initial biopsies yield minimally abnormal tissue and lesional tissue is identified on subsequent biopsies, or an initial biopsy may yield low-grade features when high-grade features are suspected radiologically. The features to look for are addressed in the "Tumor and Tumor Margin" section below.

The most frequent lesions to be approached by stereotactic biopsy are suspected gliomas in critically sensitive regions of the brain, including speech and motor cortex, thalamus, basal ganglia, and brainstem. Lesions in less sensitive regions should be approached by open biopsy to provide a better tissue sample than needle biopsy. Lesions firmer than gliomas, particularly common in the pineal region, tend to resist the needle. The relative difficulty of capture of the stereotactic specimen is an important clue to its diagnosis because gliomas and lymphomas tend to be easily obtained, whereas others are difficult. The presence of a large vessel in a needle biopsy specimen is a matter of concern that should be reported to the neurosurgeon.

Stereotactic biopsies of cystic lesions yield a lower percentage of positive diagnoses than do those of solid tumors because of the difficulty of obtaining diagnostic tissue from a mural nodule or the wall of a lesion. Stereotactic biopsies of tumors with architectural and cytologic appearance similar to normal tissue (e.g., choroid plexus and choroid plexus papilloma, pineal and pineocytoma) can be reported as the appropriate type of tissue, with a comment about the need for neuroanatomical and clinical correlation to rule out the possibility of normal structure. Stereotactic biopsies of pineal tumors present problems analogous to the problems the fabled elephant presented to the six blind men (Fig. 10.2).

SECONDARY BIOPSY

Secondary biopsies are repeat biopsies of the lesion or its immediate vicinity. The need for a secondary biopsy following a nondiagnostic primary biopsy can usually be avoided by adequate sampling of the tissue at the primary biopsy. Most helpful in

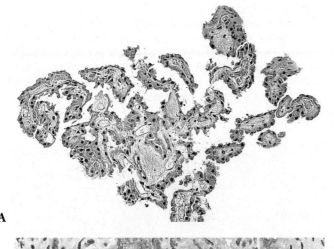

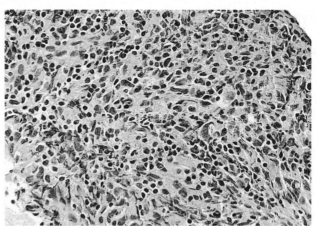

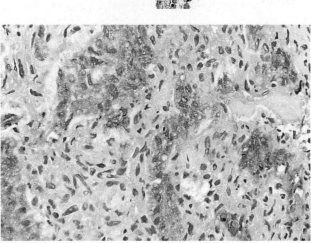

Figure 10.2. Stereotactic biopsy of pineal tumor. The first biopsy from this patient revealed epithelium on a fibrous base resembling choroid plexus epithelium (**A**). Another biopsy revealed germinoma (**B**). Still another specimen from this second biopsy was α-fetoprotein–positive (**C**), and it contained Schiller-Duvall bodies (not shown) in a focus of yolk sac tumor.

this regard is monitoring the primary biopsy procedure with frozen sections (Table 10.1). The proper time to render the judgment that a specimen is nondiagnostic is during the biopsy procedure, allowing the surgeon the opportunity to obtain another specimen.

BIOPSY AFTER THERAPY

Accurate diagnosis is enhanced when the patient's clinical status and the type of neurosurgical procedure are understood. Moreover, ancillary microscopic findings may be helpful. One of many examples is the significance of necrosis in a cerebral astrocytoma. Spontaneous coagulation necrosis in a diffuse cerebral astrocytoma is a feature of a glioblastoma multiforme. On the other hand, if necrosis is found in an astrocytoma biopsied after cytotoxic or radiotherapy, it may simply represent a good therapeutic response (Fig. 10.3).

Exceptionally problematic are biopsies after radiotherapy, chemotherapy, or vascular embolization of tumors. Even the previous surgical procedure can radically alter the appearance of a neoplasm (Fig. 10.4). Previous treatment information should be obtained prior to rendering an opinion. Primary biopsies for diagnosis after the initiation of such therapy should be discouraged.

Other biopsies intentionally monitor the effects of therapy. Months or years following tissue diagnosis and radiotherapy of a glioma, a radiologic abnormality or declining clinical status may prompt another biopsy to distinguish between recurrence of tumor and radiation necrosis.

THERAPEUTIC RESECTION

If the initial operation for diagnosis was incomplete, a second operation may be done to achieve a therapeutic effect. Other operations are primary resections of brain, often the temporal lobe, to treat medically refractory seizure foci. Categories of therapeutic resection include gross total (100% removal of visible mass), radi-cal subtotal (95% to 99% removal), subtotal (75% to 95% removal), and partial (10% to 75% removal) resection.

If the lesion was removed with a Cavitron ultrasonic aspirator (CUSA), tissue obtained from the suction collection device retains diagnostic features and immunoreactivity. However, tissue artifact is common and easy to confuse with necrosis in aspirated specimens. Blue-tinged necrosis and linear streaks of nuclear material suggest artifact.

The pathologist should compare prior diagnostic findings to the remaining lesion. Familiarity with the histologic appearance of a lesion on previous biopsy is critical to accurate interpretation (Fig. 10.4). If the resection is performed months or years following the primary biopsy, the pathologist may be expected to render an opinion about the effect of therapy. Evidence of treatment response, such as necrosis and vascular fibrosis, should be noted (Fig. 10.3).

Alternatively, the second procedure is performed with therapeutic intent, such as to place a wafer impregnated with a chemotherapeutic agent. In such cases, specific histologic features (e.g., definitive features of glioblastoma) may be necessary to qualify for specific treatment protocols for placement of the wafer.

MACROSCOPIC SPECIMEN INTERPRETATION AND PROCESSING

All specimens should be examined for arachnoid, gray matter, and white matter. To optimize evaluation, sectioning of specimens with identifiable architecture should be performed perpendicular to the meninges, from arachnoid through gray matter to white matter.

Many lesions are macroscopically evident in biopsy specimens. Yellow or firm gray or white matter typically corresponds to gliosis. Solid tissue that is not discernible as either gray matter or white matter typically represents an abnormal mass. Some tumors are often semiliquid and gelatinous in nature (oligodendrogliomas, lymphomas, pituitary adenomas). See Tables 10.11

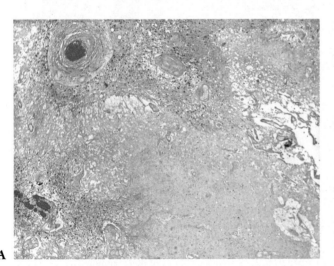

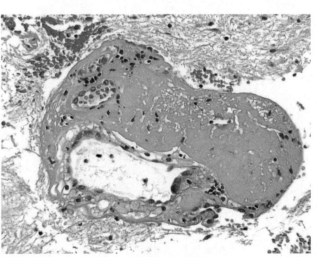

A   B

Figure 10.3. Treatment effects. Largely necrotic lesion in a young man a year after radiation therapy to a total dose of 81 Gy along with concurrent Temodar chemotherapy for his glioblastoma shows **(A)** radiation effects, including fibrinoid necrosis of vascular walls and extensive tissue coagulation necrosis with beginning cavitation; **(B)** vessel has cavitation, macrophages, and fibrinoid material (FM) in its wall. Small vessels within the FM resemble revascularization in a thrombus.

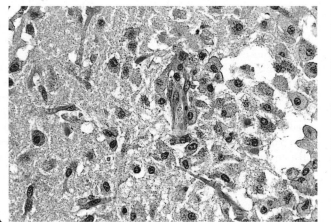
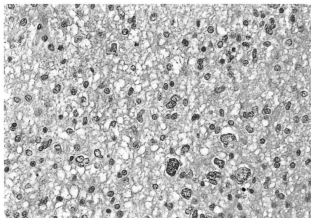

A **B**

Figure 10.4. This frontal lobe specimen resected 24 days after an initial biopsy simulates an organizing infarct (**A**). The original biopsy revealed an obvious glioma (**B**).

through 10.13 for diagnosis by distinguishing features. Multiplicity of masses is usually impossible to establish from the neurosurgical specimen alone; it requires radiographic correlation.

Flat tissue no thicker than 3 mm that is neither dura nor arachnoid may represent the wall of a cyst (see Tables 10.18 and 10.19). This can be compared and verified with the in situ or radiographic impressions of the lesion. Intracranial and intraspinal cysts are often fragmented in the course of their removal.

A vascular conglomerate larger than the usual aggregates of arachnoidal vessels may represent a vascular malformation (Table 10.6). Vascular malformations involve meninges and/or parenchyma and are often associated with recent or chronic hemorrhage.

Necrosis of the CNS parenchyma or of tumors is initially very soft and friable. It cavitates with age more rapidly in CNS parenchyma than in tumors. It can be clear, white, or yellow depending on the state of microcavitation and macrophage reaction. The arachnoid is typically preserved despite underlying parenchymal necrosis.

Although clinical diagnosis is variable, radiographic and macroscopic examination often do not distinguish inflammatory from other lesions. This must be done microscopically, as described in Tables 10.2 through 10.19 and the accompanying text and figures.

Some lesions have many of the features described above. A mass may contain regions of necrosis or hemorrhage. Arteriovenous malformations and cavernous angiomas are commonly linked with hemorrhage. Macroscopic cysts may occur within a mass, especially within cystic astrocytomas, oligodendrogliomas, craniopharyngiomas, and teratomas. Therefore, all tissue regions should be adequately sampled, particularly any interface between lesion and recognizable brain.

MARGINS

Assessment of margins in the resection of many CNS lesions, particularly diffuse gliomas, is an unrealistic goal. Due to limitations of access, CNS lesions are frequently resected piecemeal and with the use of combined ultrasound and suction. Although a gross total resection is attempted in some cases, guided by imaging studies, most adult primary gliomas manifest a diffusely

infiltrative growth pattern that defies even radical resections attempted in the past, and are considered nonresectable. Some exceptions exist, with, for example, a pilocytic astrocytoma from the cerebellum of a child or a dysembryoplastic neuroepithelial tumor from the cerebrum. See further considerations below in the "Glioma" section. In rare cases, an en bloc excision of an entire neoplasm (e.g., a meningioma) is obtained. It is best to mark the margin of tissue around such an intact specimen with ink, unless the surgeon requests otherwise.

TISSUE PROCESSING

General Considerations

1. Squash/smear/touch preparations
2. Unfrozen routine permanent paraffin sections
3. Frozen sections
4. Electron microscopy (EM) (retain a small portion in a fixative for EM, if necessary)
5. Frozen tissue, for possible future molecular diagnostic studies (freeze fresh tissue as soon as possible and store)
6. Other (microbiology, flow cytometry, cytogenetics, molecular diagnostics)

Routine Fixation

In most cases, with the critical exception of suspected hematopoietic neoplasms, fixation of biopsy and resection specimens in formalin and routine processing is sufficient to meet diagnostic needs.

Electron Microscopic Fixation

Glutaraldehyde fixation of a small portion of a lesion can be done any time after formalin fixation, making it easy to save tiny pieces of wet tissue in formalin in case EM is needed. It may be needed for (a) poorly differentiated or unusual tumors; (b) differential that includes a lesion best confirmed by EM-like ependymoma; (c) toxic-metabolic disease; and (d) infection. Saving a bit of tissue for possible future EM evaluation until completion of a challenging case is smart. Keeping it in formalin in its original jar is easy.

Hematopoietic Specimens

When a hematopoietic lesion is identified intraoperatively or suspected clinically, the specimen should be treated like a lymph node biopsy. Nuclear morphology is a key element of hematopoietic diagnoses. As such, a portion of the specimen should be fixed in a mercuric chloride-formalin fixative (e.g., B5) or, alternatively, zinc-containing fixative. The cassette must be marked to indicate that removal of the metallic fixative is required after the appropriate fixation interval. If enough tissue is available, a suspected hematopoietic lesion can also be placed in cell culture medium and sent for flow cytometric evaluation for phenotypic characterization. Touch preparations are often useful, especially intraoperatively. A portion can also be flash-frozen to accommodate molecular evaluation and labile antigen evaluation by IHC; retaining a frozen section specimen in the frozen state can accomplish this goal simply and effectively.

Microbiological Workup Recommendations

Cultures usually are more sensitive than other methods (including molecular methods) to detect organisms that grow in vitro. If an infectious etiology is suspected intraoperatively, it is critical that the surgeon be notified of the possibility immediately so that optimal samples for bacterial (aerobic and anaerobic), mycobacterial, fungal, and viral cultures can be obtained by the surgeon from the sterile operating field and sent directly to the microbiology laboratory. Saving a small, fixed portion of the lesion for possible EM evaluation and freezing another small piece is wise.

Molecular Diagnosis

Incorporation of genetic data into the assessment of a CNS neoplasm is now well established for glial neoplasms and is emerging for other lesions including infections. Formalin-fixed, paraffin-embedded tissue sections can be used for most of the techniques, including IHC, fluorescent in situ hybridization (FISH), in situ hybridization (ISH), and polymerase chain reaction (PCR) techniques. Other techniques require unfixed tissue for evaluation. When abundant lesional tissue is present, the pathologist is wise to snap-freeze a portion and store it at -80 °C. Retaining the frozen specimen in a frozen state can accomplish this, assuming adequate tissue is available for permanent sections.

Toxic-Metabolic Processes

When a biopsy from a patient with suspected toxic-metabolic disorder is performed (e.g., for a suspected lysosomal storage disease, mitochondrial cytopathy, or cerebral autosomal dominant arteriopathy with subcortical infarcts and leukoencephalopathy [CADASIL]), representative gray and white matter should be fixed in formalin for routine processing; retained in formalin or glutaraldehyde for possible electron microscopic evaluation; and frozen for possible biochemical studies if enough tissue is available to meet histologic needs.

HIGH-RISK INFECTIOUS DISEASE CASE CONSIDERATIONS

Universal precautions prevent transmission of most infectious diseases from central nervous specimens to pathologists and assistants. However, biopsies obtained from (a) patients with known HIV infection/AIDS, and (b) patients with a clinical differential diagnosis that includes Creutzfeldt-Jakob disease (CJD) require special consideration and handling (4,15).

Minimization of risk to laboratory personnel includes (a) advance warning by neurosurgeons when operations are performed on high-risk patients; (b) cytologic preparations instead of frozen sections on specimens from these patients, and only if needed to confirm lesional tissue; (c) declining frozen sections from patients with a clinical differential diagnosis that includes CJD; and (d) proper handling of specimens once received in the laboratory.

Human Immunodeficiency Virus (HIV)

Brain biopsies obtained from patients with known HIV infection or acquired immunodeficiency syndrome (AIDS) are usually tested for infectious processes (e.g., toxoplasmosis) and neoplasm (e.g., lymphoma or other neoplasms). HIV is inactivated by formalin, so, after fixation, there is minimal risk of handling specimens from such patients. Cytologic preparations often provide assurance of lesional tissue. However, if a frozen section is necessary from such a specimen, decontamination of the cryostat should be carried out by using and replacing a disposable blade, removing all freezing medium debris, and wiping surfaces that came into contact with the specimen with a solution of 10% bleach in water. Use of a separate cryostat for such specimens, when available, can minimize downtime in a busy frozen section laboratory.

Prion Diseases, Including Creutzfeldt-Jakob Disease

Biopsy for possible CJD requires a compelling clinical reason, such as a treatable disease being in the clinical differential. A neurologist with expertise in prion diseases should certify all biopsies for dementia: (a) Is there a possibility of prion disease or not? (b) Could the patient have another treatable cause of the dementia? Without an affirmative answer to both questions, biopsy is not appropriate because of the concern of contamination of surgical and pathology personnel.

If biopsy is undertaken, frozen sections should not be done. Specimens must include (a) tissue for formalin fixation, and (b) snap-frozen tissue for Western blot and gene sequencing evaluation. It is also desirable to collect blood for germline comparison. Prior to biopsy, the neurosurgeon should confer with the neurologist to sample an appropriate portion of brain, depending on symptoms. In addition to gray matter, white matter and meninges should be sampled.

The National Prion Disease Pathology Surveillance Center (NPDPSC) at Case Western University is funded and equipped for molecular diagnosis of prion diseases. For Western blot, the NPDPSC requests at least 10 mg of tissue (pea-sized or 0.5 cm diameter) for biopsies. Put tissue into a small plastic vial and screw on the cap. Put the vial into a biohazard bag and close bag. Store initially in a -70 °C freezer until it can be sent by overnight mail to the NPDPSC on a Monday or Tuesday at this address: Diane Kofskey for Dr. Gambetti; National Prion Disease Pathology Surveillance Center; Division of Neuropathology, Rm. 418; Case Western Reserve University; 2085 Adelbert Road; Cleveland, OH 44106; Phone: 216-368-0819; Fax: 216-368-2546.

In the rare biopsied case in which CJD is in the differential, decontamination of tissue for histologic processing, sectioning, and examination can be obtained as follows. Specimens should be sectioned to fit into cassettes (see special notes below); if desired, a small portion of cortex can be placed into glutaraldehyde for possible electron microscopic evaluation. The cassettes are (a) placed into 10% buffered formalin for fixation for at least 24 hours; (b) transferred to undiluted, 95% to 100% formic acid for 1 hour; (c) then returned to fresh 10% formalin for another 48 hours or more before routine processing. Although of very low risk, embedded tissue should be handled as if infectious—sectioned by an experienced technologist using disposable blades, with incineration of all section waste and wiping of microtome and cutting station with bleach or 2N NaOH. Histologic and many IHC evaluations are minimally impeded by the formic acid processing. Disposable towels, gloves, and equipment should be used in initial processing and subsequently incinerated. Contaminated surfaces can be cleaned using 5% bleach (corrosive for steel instruments) or 2N NaOH (incompatible with aluminum) with prolonged exposure (15 minutes up to 2 hours) for equipment (4,15). More information is available online at http://www.pathology.med.umich.edu/Safety%20Manual/CJD%20Final.pdf.

Special Notes

1. Cassettes should be labeled with pencil as formic acid will dissolve away even the ink specially formulated for histologic processing.
2. Normal plastic cassettes are resistant to formic acid, but the thin plastic netting of cassettes designed for small biopsies will dissolve in formic acid, so a small biopsy should be wrapped in lens paper to keep it in the cassette. Metal tops should not be used.

HISTOCHEMICAL AND IMMUNOHISTOCHEMICAL EVALUATION

Special stains (16), IHC stains, and cytologic techniques that aid the diagnosis of specific entities at biopsy are described in Tables 10.2 and 10.10 through 10.20. Routinely use a standard tissue control that contains regions both positive and negative for the IHC marker under evaluation. If possible, choose a block with the lesion of interest that also contains tissue with known positive and negative regions to use as an internal standard tissue control (i.e., the edge of a tumor with gliotic brain and vessels for GFAP IHC).

Polarization microscopy quickly reveals mature collagen fibers and hair shafts (see Fig. 10.133 in the "Dermoid Cyst" section below). On the Congo red stain, polarization distinguishes light yellow-green amyloid from whiter collagen (17).

Individual neoplasms may lack a marker generally representative of its category. Others may lose expression of markers as they progress to higher grades of malignancy. Because these factors or technical reasons may cause individual neoplasms to fail to label for a marker, a positive immunostaining result is more meaningful than a negative result.

Based on initial histologic findings, one can construct a differential diagnosis for which a group of appropriate special stains can be assembled from information in the text and tables

here. To minimize redundancy, positive rather than negative features are emphasized below, under each entity. Depending on difficulty, the differential can be solved on H&E or IHC (18).

There are many web sites for locating IHC expertise, reagents, and suppliers. www.biocompare.com searches for very specific reagents and their suppliers. www.histonet.org provides numerous comments, recipes, and images from histology and histochemistry professionals. Our UM IHC laboratory professionals often use the antibody name in Google searches to find new antibodies.

ELECTRON MICROSCOPY

The importance of electron microscopy (EM) in cranial and spinal diagnostic neuropathology has been diminished by faster IHC. However, EM is valuable in defined settings in which IHC cannot distinguish among specific subtypes of tumor (19). Unlike largely confirmatory IHC, EM shows many latent structures that may point to a new direction in interpretation. At times, it is the only path to a definitive answer. For example, among various clear-cell tumors, basal bodies, cilia, elongated junctions, and microvillous lumens distinguish clear-cell ependymoma from oligodendroglioma. EM can be a valuable adjunct to diagnosis in specific settings; see the "Tissue Processing section" above.

EM is needed to confirm certain metabolic diseases. Specimens from sites other than brain are frequently biopsied for evaluation of various metabolic diseases that affect the CNS, such as neuronal ceroid-lipofuscinosis, the various lysosomal storage diseases, leukodystrophies, mitochondrial encephalopathies, and vascular diseases including CADASIL (19).

REACTIVE CHANGES

GLIOSIS

Gliosis is a reaction of the CNS to injury of the brain or spinal cord (see Fig. 10.5A). It identifies abnormal CNS tissue. Gliosis is defined as either (a) increased number of astrocytes, or (b) increased number and length of process or increased cytoplasmic synthesis of GFAP representing a gemistocytic astrocyte. Although subtle changes such as astrocyte swelling with fluid occur earlier, gliosis is usually appreciated on H&E-stained slides within 2 weeks after an injury. Because nearly any injury of the CNS can cause gliosis, it is not diagnostic of a specific pathologic entity.

Anti-GFAP IHC differentiates subtle forms of gliosis (Table 10.3). When this differentiation is critical, an age-matched control slide from the same region of normal CNS should be stained concurrently. Compared to control, look for a greater number of astrocytes, a greater number and density of cell processes, and the presence of a GFAP-positive gemistocytic appearance.

The problem of distinguishing gliosis from low-grade glioma is challenging and is described below (see "Gliomas"). Gliosis does not expand, although gliotic parenchyma may surround an expanding tumor. "Pure" gliosis, which lacks noticeable CNS parenchyma, is associated with long-standing cysts (Table 10.18). In contrast to microcysts of gliomas (see Fig. 10.32 in the "Gliomas" section), these cysts are macroscopic, confluent, and often have numerous residual macrophages. However, in the absence of evidence of another origin, the possibility of neoplastic origin of such cysts must still be considered. In gliosis, astrocytes respect each other's space and show more uniform spacing between individual glial cells than in the margin of a glioma (see Fig. 10.5A; also see Figs. 10.23, 10.24, and 10.35 below). The nuclear:cytoplasmic ratio of gliosis is less than that of a glioma. Excessive fibrillarity and Rosenthal fibers do not distinguish gliosis from glioma (see Figs. 10.35 and 10.40 in the "Gliomas" section).

MACROPHAGES, MICROGLIAL CELLS

Macrophages present as (a) granular or foamy macrophages, (b) microglial cells with rod-shaped nuclei, or (c) epithelioid macrophages with or without multinucleated giant cells. They may be seen, in variable and sometimes striking abundance, in any condition that involves tissue disruption, including infectious, inflammatory, necrotic, traumatic, degenerative, and neoplastic processes (20–22). The origin of these cells is variable among lesions, and consists of some combination of (a) "native" parenchymal microglial cells, which can proliferate along with (b) blood-derived macrophages entering the brain parenchyma in response to damage (21). The fate of the latter cells may be to remain at the site of injury or migrate to the perivascular space (22). Because distinction among these origins is not useful diagnostically, the inclusive term *macrophages* can be employed.

In the brain, a useful diagnostic for macrophages is CD68 (KP-1) IHC (see Fig. 10.25 in the "Demyelination" section below), and it frequently identifies considerably more macrophages than are anticipated by H&E evaluation. A special stain for myelin (e.g., Luxol fast blue-hematoxylin and eosin [LFB-H&E]) (see Fig. 10.19 in the "Progressive Multifocal Leukoencephalopathy" section below), identifies engulfed myelin debris and a stain for axons (see Fig. 10.26 in the "Demyelination" section below) helps to distinguish between necrotic CNS tissue (axons disintegrate and leave axonal debris in macrophages) and demyelination (foamy macrophages contain myelin but not axonal debris). GFAP IHC is helpful to discern

gemistocytic reactive astrocytes from macrophages. Reactive macrophages must be distinguished from the histiocytoses; see the "Histiocytosis" section below.

Foamy macrophages are common in infarct and demyelination; their lysosomes are loaded with cellular debris and may contain yeast forms and other organisms. Macrophages swollen plump by phagocytosis within the CNS are called *granular* or *gitter cells* (Figs. 10.4A and 10.5B). Hemosiderin-laden macrophages can be noted around organizing hemorrhages, traumatic lesions, and some vascular malformations. Large, rounded cells with foamy cytoplasm and eccentric nuclei, having the appearance of macrophages, present occasionally as a part of such rare lesions as xanthogranulomas of choroid plexus. They are occasionally evident in various brain tumors, along with lymphocytes. Lipid-laden macrophages can be distinguished from amebae in the rare amebic brain abscess by their larger and more distinct nuclei and less chromatin clumping than amebae, and by their CD68 positivity (see the "Infectious Disease, Parasites" section below).

Epithelioid macrophages are activated but nonfoamy macrophages identified in granulomatous inflammation in infectious (e.g., fungus, AFB) and inflammatory (e.g., sarcoid) diseases of the CNS.

Microglial cells are macrophages that closely resemble antigen-presenting dendritic cells seen elsewhere in the body, and play a key role in response to a variety of etiologic insults (21,22). They have a spindle-shaped nucleus and no discernible cytoplasm, and must be distinguished from the so-called naked nuclei of infiltrating glioma and endothelial cell nuclei. They are CD68-positive (see Fig. 10.25). They are notably seen diffusely in brain tissue or as small aggregates, so-called microglial nodules, in viral and rickettsial diseases, and around dying neurons (neuronophagocytosis; see Fig. 10.7). When a microglial nodule is accompanied by multinucleated giant cells, HIV encephalitis is a strong possibility.

GRANULOMATOUS INFLAMMATION

Granulomatous inflammation is defined by both cell types and architecture. Cells include infiltrates of (a) activated, epitheli-

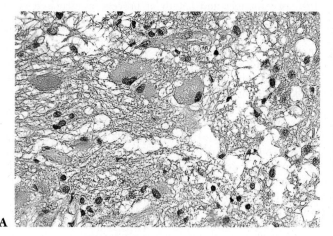
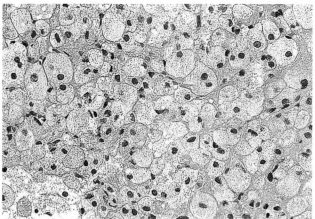

Figure 10.5. Reactive changes. Common reactions to injury in the central nervous system include gliosis (**A**) and "gitter cell" reaction of macrophages filled with neutral fat (**B**). The gliosis occurred in edematous brain near a metastatic carcinoma. The macrophages are in a subacute infarct clinically suspected to be a glioma.

oid macrophages with or without multinucleated giant cells, and (b) lymphoid cells. Foamy macrophages may or may not be seen. Architecturally, the infiltrate may form nodules, or granulomas, with or without central necrosis. Identification of granulomatous inflammation raises the differential of infectious or autoimmune inflammatory conditions. Granulomatous inflammation is common in the setting of bacterial (tuberculosis, syphilis, Whipple disease), fungal, and parasitic infections. These entities must be distinguished from rare, noninfectious granulomatous processes that can affect the CNS, including systemic lupus erythematosus (SLE), Wegener granulomatosis, sarcoidosis, rheumatoid meningitis, and Crohn disease. If a histiocytic process is in the differential diagnosis, IHC for S-100 and CD1a can be performed (see the "Histiocytosis" section below).

PERIVASCULAR INFLAMMATION

Virtually any irritation of the CNS can stimulate accumulation of cells around blood vessels (Fig. 10.6), including surgical wounds and implants (23). Macrophages ingest the irritant or injured cellular constituents and move them to the perivascular space (22). In the absence of classic lymph nodes in the brain, this perivascular region is where cells that respond to antigens intermingle. Depending on severity and duration of illness, the perivascular inflammation varies substantially. Old hemorrhage is characterized mainly by perivascular macrophages laden with hemosiderin. Viral or autoimmune encephalitis produces a maximal response, with abundant perivascular macrophages and lymphocytes along with parenchymal infiltrates of microglial cells and microglial nodules.

MENINGEAL FIBROSIS

Meningeal fibrosis develops following traumatic injuries, meningitis, vasculitis involving meningeal vessels, radiation therapy, or as a desmoplastic response to a tumor, especially if the tumor triggers massive vascular proliferation. Multifocal fibrosclerosis with hypertrophic intracranial pachymeningitis is a firm, fibrous lesion with dural thickening, frequently found in conjunction with an intracranial pseudotumor (24). Arachnoiditis ossificans deposits bone within the chronic inflammatory response.

INFECTIOUS DISEASES

In a symptomatic patient with imaging findings suggesting an infectious or inflammatory disease, when evaluation of cerebrospinal fluid (CSF) is unrevealing, biopsy is undertaken to attempt establish a definitive diagnosis and rule out other processes (see Fig. 10.9). Optimal sampling by biopsy that (a) includes dura, arachnoid, and gray and white matter, and (b) is performed in the site of a radiologically enhancing lesion markedly improves the chance of reaching a diagnosis.

When biopsy is performed, the principal goal of the surgical pathologist in this setting is to evaluate features of infectious and inflammatory processes, and rule out ischemic damage and neoplasm. Check the history; the immunocompromised patient is particularly susceptible to CNS infection. Specific susceptibilities are found below.

MICROBIAL CULTURE

If an infectious etiology is suggested at the time of biopsy, the surgeon must be notified to send cultures (see "Tissue Processing").

SPECIAL STAINS

A combination of histochemical microbial stains is employed in the setting of inflammation to evaluate for organisms and assess for specific cell types. IHC or in situ hybridization may help to identify organisms, particularly toxoplasma, viruses (including herpes, cytomegalovirus [CMV], and JC virus), fungi, and *Rickettsia* (25). Available molecular biologic approaches for identification of microorganisms vary among institutions. Some require frozen section, but PCR usually can be performed on

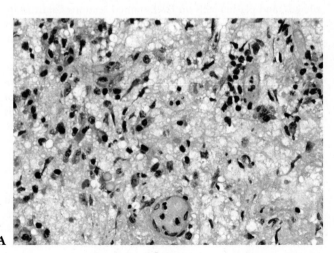

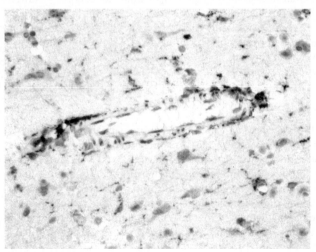

A **B**

Figure 10.6. **(A)** Perivascular mixed inflammatory infiltrate is composed of lymphocytes, plasma cells, and macrophages around but not within vessel walls. **(B)** Chronic encephalitis stained with CD68 shows elongated microglial macrophages within brain tissue and around vessels, but not within the vascular wall. Note the normal thin endothelial lining (compare with vasculitis, Fig. 10.25C,D).

DNA extracted from paraffin-embedded sections of tissue following deparaffinization steps. Most useful is the ability to detect mycobacteria, in the setting of necrotizing granulomatous inflammation, and assess tuberculosis (TB) or not TB. Cultures for TB are more sensitive but they take much longer.

Electron microscopy has a role in the identification of microorganisms that do not grow in culture and are hard to stain, including viruses, Whipple bacillus, amebae, and spirochetes.

MENINGITIS, CEREBRITIS (FOCAL ENCEPHALITIS), MYELITIS

The terms *meningitis*, *cerebritis*, and *myelitis* literally mean inflammation of the meninges (dura or leptomeninges), cerebral parenchyma, or spinal cord parenchyma, respectively (26). Acute (neutrophils), chronic (lymphocytes and macrophages), and granulomatous (round, fibrous clusters of lymphocytes and epithelioid macrophages) inflammation can be identified. These forms of inflammation can be seen in infectious processes and in autoimmune inflammatory processes. In general, inflammation is not a prominent feature in neoplastic processes, and caution must be exercised in a hypercellular lesion with a large number of macrophages and other inflammatory cells. However, inflammatory infiltrates can be seen in neoplastic processes, especially perivascular lymphocytic infiltrates (particularly common in lymphomas, gangliogliomas, gemistocytic astrocytomas, and oligodendrogliomas) and macrophages mixed with neoplastic cells, but they are a secondary feature.

The term *cerebritis* has been used to describe a focal cerebral encephalitis of bacterial origin that is not sufficiently encapsulated to be an abcess (26,27). Unfortunately, cerebritis is confusing since it excludes CNS structures posterior to the cerebrum, leaving cumbersome alternatives like *cerebellitis*, *mesencephalitis*, or *brainstemitis*. I prefer the term *focal encephalitis* to cerebritis. Focal encephalitis (FE) precedes frank abscess formation but requires early biopsy to be seen. FE may be sterile or may contain an infectious agent. Its inflammatory infiltrate is composed of neutrophils, macrophages, lymphocytes, and plasma cells, with or without parenchymal necrosis (Figs. 10.6 and 10.7). FE is found around septic thromboemboli, neoplasms, ruptured vascular malformations, infarcts, or traumatic lesions. Meningitis may precede FE. The above features also apply to focal myelitis. Septic FE is usually caused by bacterial agents, most often streptococci or staphylococci, and less frequently by Gram-negative organisms such as *Escherichia coli*, *Pseudomonas*, or *Haemophilus influenzae*.

ENCEPHALITIS

The term *encephalitis* literally means brain inflammation. Viruses and *Rickettsia* usually cause inflammation of brain tissue that is more diffuse than that caused by bacteria, and may involve more than the cerebrum. By convention, this brain inflammation is usually called encephalitis (26). Most viral infections are self-limited and cause inflammation that resolves without permanent brain damage. Other infections, emphasized in the section "Viruses," below, can result in a serious necrotizing process.

MYELITIS AND TRANSVERSE MYELITIS

Myelitis and so-called transverse myelitis (specifically inflammation of the spinal cord parenchyma) present clinically with

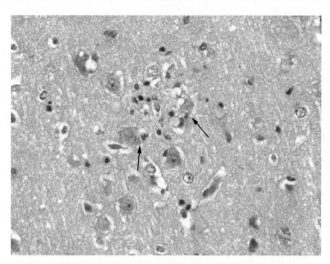

Figure 10.7. Chronic encephalitis. The hallmark of chronic encephalitis is neuronophagia, the "eating of neurons." Lymphocytes recognize infected neurons, even ones such as these that show no inclusions, and direct microglial macrophages to eat them (*arrows*). Notice that these infected neurons are not hypoxic, they have not lost their purple cytoplasmic Nissl substance, nor have they turned orange. When there is no encephalitis, the most common cause of neuronophagia is hypoxic damage to neurons.

symptoms that can involve sensory, motor, and autonomic modalities of variable severity. The etiology is often illusive, but etiologies include infectious (HSV, CMV, etc.), inflammatory (multiple sclerosis [MS], connective tissue disease, etc.), vascular (infarct due to thrombosis), developmental (vascular malformation), traumatic, and iatrogenic processes (28,29). Workup is based on imaging and CSF and serum evaluation; biopsy is occasionally performed to search for etiology.

ABSCESS

An abscess, typically preceded by focal encephalitis or cerebritis, combines features of inflammation, gliosis, and fibrosis. A mixture of polymorphonuclear leukocytes, lymphocytes, macrophages, and plasma cells on H&E-stained sections confirms inflammation (Fig. 10.8). Polymorphism of inflammatory components can be verified by finding mixed B- and T-cell lymphocytes admixed with CD68-positive macrophages.

The wall of a brain abscess consists of collagen and reactive gliosis. The collagen layer is formed by fibroblasts that migrate out from the surrounding blood vessels. Thus, the thickness of this layer varies depending upon the number of viable vessels and their distance from the abscess as well as on the age of the abscess. Because collagen is rare within the CNS, its presence is an important diagnostic feature of an abscess (Table 10.18). Collagen may be difficult to distinguish from fibrillary gliosis on a slide stained with H&E. Points to remember are the extracellular and often wavy appearance of collagen compared with the intracellular fibrillar character of gliosis. Collagen will polarize yellow-white on H&E- or Congo red–stained sections, whereas gliosis will not. If there is any doubt, it is best to stain histochemically for collagen or reticulin, or stain immunohistochemically for collagen type IV.

Other entities that produce collagen within the CNS may be confused with the wall of an abscess (Tables 10.10 through

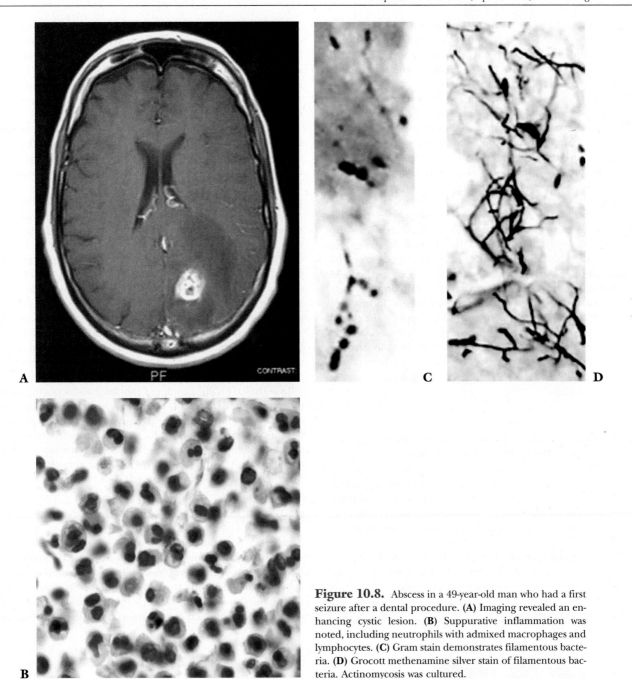

Figure 10.8. Abscess in a 49-year-old man who had a first seizure after a dental procedure. **(A)** Imaging revealed an enhancing cystic lesion. **(B)** Suppurative inflammation was noted, including neutrophils with admixed macrophages and lymphocytes. **(C)** Gram stain demonstrates filamentous bacteria. **(D)** Grocott methenamine silver stain of filamentous bacteria. Actinomycosis was cultured.

10.12, 10.18, 10.19). Sarcomatous and desmoplastic neoplasms, and various cysts with collagenous walls, generally lack an inflammatory component. Notable exceptions are cysts that have ruptured and exuded material foreign to the CNS, such as colloid or squamous epithelial cells (see Fig. 10.132 in the "Common Metastatic Tumors" section below, and Table 10.19). If this material is not detectable within the inflammatory reaction to the cyst, clinical and pathologic correlation assists the interpretation. These other lesions that combine collagen and inflammation are sterile in situ and do not contain microorganisms.

Nocardial abscesses of the cerebrum and the spinal cord are rising in frequency in drug addicts. Multiple microabscesses should be considered in the differential diagnosis of encepha-

lopathy in hospitalized patients with chronic disease, immunosuppression, and sepsis (26).

MYCOBACTERIA, SPIROCHETES, AND WHIPPLE DISEASE

Suppurative bacterial infections have been discussed above under cerebritis, meningitis, and abscess. Here consideration will be given to several special diseases, including tuberculosis, syphilis, and Whipple disease (30,31).

Tuberculosis and atypical mycobacteria can involve any region of the CNS, principally manifesting as meningitis and meningoencephalitis (31). AFB stains are useful, but slower cultures are more sensitive. A role for PCR in identifying and speciating mycobacteria has been established (32). In human immunodeficiency virus (HIV)-infected patients, newly acquired tuberculosis can spread readily and progress rapidly to active disease. Tuberculosis can be the first clinical manifestation of immunodeficiency in these patients.

The frequency of neurosyphilis continues to increase in AIDS patients (30). Microscopic examination reveals focal lymphoplasmacytic inflammatory infiltrates in a predominantly perivascular arrangement. Syphilis contributes to the list of the differential diagnoses of granulomatous inflammations. Silver stains for spirochetes do not work well in brain due to background staining. Special identification procedures are available at the Centers for Disease Control and Prevention (CDC).

Whipple disease rarely presents as a primary brain disease, and even then usually with concomitant gastrointestinal symptoms. The diagnosis can be made by brain biopsy. Histologic features include PAS-positive, diastase-resistant macrophages, microgranulomas, giant multinucleated cells, perivascular lymphocytes, and reactive microglia (Fig. 10.9). Supplemental data come from immunohistochemical evaluation for group B streptococci and electron microscopy (33). Biopsy of the central cingulate gyrus, mediobasal temporal region, and insular cortex yields the most diagnostic tissue. Electron microscopy can confirm the presence of a characteristic bacillus that has been named *Tropheryma whippelii*.

FUNGI

Fungal organisms that involve the CNS include those presenting as (a) *yeast forms* (Fig. 10.10), including *Cryptococcus neoformans*, coccidioides, histoplasmosis, candida, and blastomycosis; and (b) *hyphal forms* (Fig. 10.11), including the zygomycetes (mucor and rhizopus, rhizomucor), *Aspergillus*, and pseudoallescheria. Involvement of the CNS can be via a hematogenous route (e.g., from a primary pulmonary source) or via direct extension from an infected sinus.

Fungal organisms tend to involve the meninges, in some cases presumably passing from subarachnoid space along perivascular spaces to involve parenchyma. Vascular wall invasion is common in hyphal forms, which may lead to catastrophic rupture and hemorrhage.

Variable inflammatory infiltrates are elicited by fungi, most often chronic and granulomatous. When fungi are suspected, use of both GMS and PAS is recommended because some forms stain better with one than the other stain (Fig. 10.11). Mucicarmine is of value in evaluating the capsule of *Cryptococcus*. This relatively nonantigenic capsule delays the inflammatory response to *Cryptococcus*.

Cryptococcal meningitis is the most common form of fungal meningitis, with a variable inflammatory response, often minimal in acute infections and in the setting of AIDS (Fig. 10.10). Chronic infections can produce granulomatous inflammation. Histoplasmosis, blastomycosis, and coccidioidomycosis can present as CNS parenchymal lesions, after presumed dissemination from lung, with variable suppurative to granulomatous inflammatory reactions; characteristic yeast forms can be identified by H&E, GMS, and PAS (Fig. 10.10). Candida can also involve the CNS as intraparenchymal masses; inflammation is typically acute (27). Zygomycetes organisms tend to be angiocentric and angioinvasive (Fig. 10.11). Zygomycetes may involve brain by direct extension from a nasal sinus infection; diabetic patients appear to be at particular risk of such infections (34).

Assessment includes the identification of hyphal or yeast forms and an attempt at identification of the organism. Ideally, a portion of the specimen is sent for culture and specific identification. The report of hyphal organisms as suspicious for aspergillosis (based on dichotomous branching and septa formation) or zygomycetes (based on ribbonlike hypha of varying width, absence of definite septa, and right-angle branching) should be confirmed by culture, IHC, or ISH. Pseudallescheria can appear histologically as hyphae with acute branches and septa, and treatment is different (35). Histologic consultation with a microbiologist prior to reporting is wise.

PARASITES

A variety of parasitic organisms can involve the CNS, including endemic organisms or exotic organisms most frequently seen in immigrants or travelers (36–39). Important parasites include (a) protozoa, including toxoplasma and amebae; (b) the pork tapeworm *Taenia solium*; and (c) schistosoma, a trematode. The organisms can be seen at various stages of their development

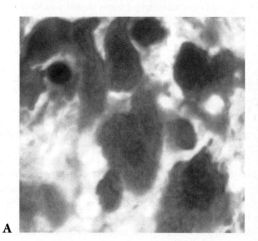
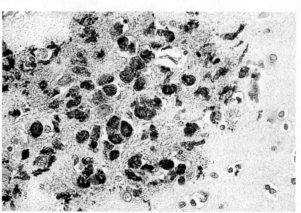

A   **B**

Figure 10.9. Whipple disease of the central nervous system. Typical cluster of reactive cells stained with periodic acid-Schiff stain (**A**) and by immunoperoxidase for anti-group B *Streptococcus* (**B**). (**B**, Courtesy of Dr. M.E. Velasco, Medical College of Ohio, Toledo, Ohio.)

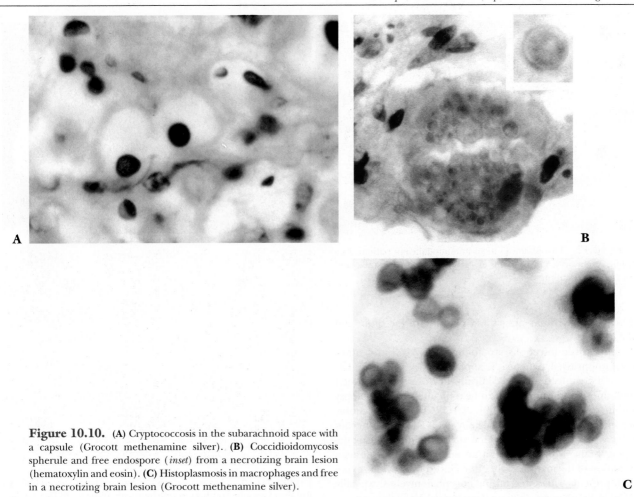

Figure 10.10. **(A)** Cryptococcosis in the subarachnoid space with a capsule (Grocott methenamine silver). **(B)** Coccidioidomycosis spherule and free endospore (*inset*) from a necrotizing brain lesion (hematoxylin and eosin). **(C)** Histoplasmosis in macrophages and free in a necrotizing brain lesion (Grocott methenamine silver).

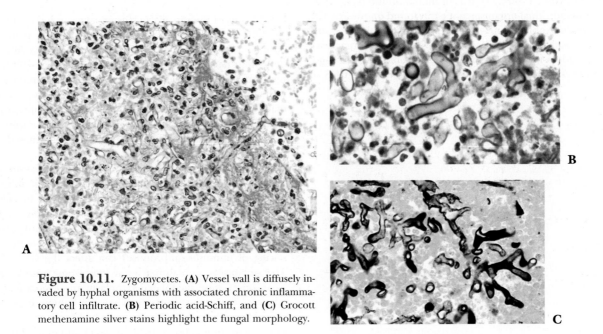

Figure 10.11. Zygomycetes. **(A)** Vessel wall is diffusely invaded by hyphal organisms with associated chronic inflammatory cell infiltrate. **(B)** Periodic acid-Schiff, and **(C)** Grocott methenamine silver stains highlight the fungal morphology.

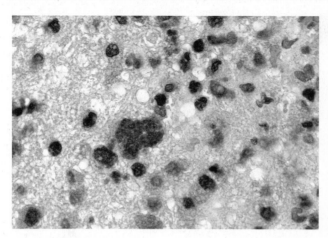

Figure 10.12. Toxoplasmosis in an immunodeficient patient. Amphophilic pseudocyst full of a cluster of bradyzoites is irregular and larger than surrounding cells.

and involve the leptomeninges and neuropil of the brain and spinal cord.

Opportunistic infections are common in AIDS and other immunosuppressed patients. Toxoplasmosis is the most frequent of these infections, and clinically the differential between toxoplasmosis and lymphoma can be difficult, requiring biopsy if antimicrobial therapy fails (39). A TORCH (toxoplasmosis, other infections, rubella, cytomegalovirus [CMV], and herpes simplex virus [HSV]) organism that affects the intrauterine developing brain, toxoplasmosis in an adult likely represents a reactivation of dormant parasites introduced by previous exposure. It presents with a necrotizing encephalomyelitis, typically multifocal by imaging, that is characterized by ill-defined necrotic lesions containing thin-walled cysts filled with bradyzoites ("slow [growing] animal"; dark-staining dot-like structures representing nuclei, and individual tachyzoites "fast [growing] animal" (Figs. 10.12 and 10.13). IHC or immunofluorescence pinpoints the individual organism, not easily found on routine H& E sections. Toxoplasma may coexist with candida in the same patient as well as with *Cryptococcus*, CMV, and other organisms. Rarely, toxoplasmosis is complicated by cerebral hemorrhage.

Neurocysticercosis, the result of migration to the CNS of

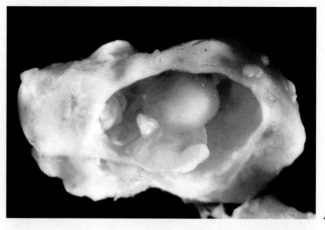

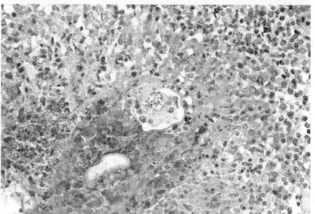

Figure 10.14. (A) Cysticercosis cyst resected from the cerebral hemisphere of a young South American man with seizures. (B) Degenerating schistosome egg in the center surrounded by heavy mixed inflammatory infiltrate. *(A, Courtesy of Dr. D. Burns, University of Texas Southwestern, Dallas, Texas.)*

larval forms of the tapeworm *Taenia solium*, is a common parasitic infection of the CNS found occasionally in people who have been in developing countries. About 50% to 70% of patients with neurocysticercosis present with seizures (36). Some resected specimens are tan, firm nodules containing a cavity with either a cystic region (Fig. 10.14A) or grumous, gray-yellow material. Microscopically, pale eosinophilic membranes separate the cavity from gliotic brain parenchyma with chronic perivascular inflammation. The characteristic invaginated scolex may be seen.

Schistosomiasis in the CNS is the result of migration of eggs of the organisms. The eggs characteristically elicit an intense, granulomatous inflammatory response and can be misinterpreted radiologically as a high-grade neoplasm (Fig. 10.14B).

Amebae, including *Naegleria* and, less commonly, *Acanthamoeba, Sappinia diploidea,* and *Balamuthia* (seen mostly in the setting of immunocompromise) can affect the CNS (37,38). The organisms, containing a nucleus (some with a distinct karyosome), have vacuolated cytoplasm and can easily be mistaken for foamy macrophages. They may contain ingested red cells. Macrophages can be distinguished from amebae in the rare amebic brain abscess by their larger and more distinct nuclei and less chromatin clumping than amebae; the organisms are negative for CD68.

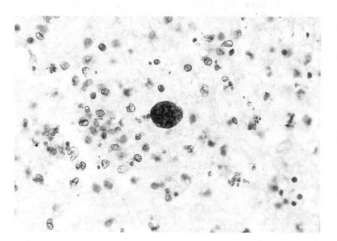

Figure 10.13. Cyst and free tachyzoites immunostained for *Toxoplasma* antigen (immunoperoxidase with hematoxylin counterstain).

Exotic CNS infections often occur in AIDS patients. They include trypanosomiasis and strongyloidiasis.

VIRUSES

A large number of viruses affect the CNS, with or without systemic (especially respiratory system) involvement; with variability among seasons and geographical regions (e.g., presence of specific vectors); and with considerable variation in clinical presentation (40,41). It is highly likely that viral infections have been significantly underreported as the result of difficulty in identifying the etiologic agent.

Most diagnostic tools are clinical and include serologic (serum or CSF, usually with a rise between acute and convalescent specimens); PCR (serum, CSF, or brain); culture on mosquito or mammalian cell line or by intracranial inoculation into suckling mice (blood, CSF, brain tissue); or immunocytochemical (brain and other organ tissues) evaluations. CSF or postmortem brain specimens can be evaluated at reference laboratories or the CDC.

Histologically, most viral encephalitides induce perivascular lymphocytic cuffing. This (an increased number of parenchymal microglial cells) and neuronophagia ("neuron eating"; Fig. 10.7) raise suspicion of a viral infection. Some viruses produce recognizable inclusions (Table 10.4), many of which can be identified with IHC or ISH. Neuronal inclusion bodies are (a) in nuclei with herpesviruses and measles virus of subacute sclerosing panencephalitis (SSPE); and (b) in cytoplasm in rabies. Oligodendrocyte nuclear inclusions are seen in progressive multifocal leukoencephalopathy (PML) and SSPE. CMV induces inclusions in the nucleus and cytoplasm of endothelial cells, ependymal cells, and glial cells. Many viruses do not manifest inclusions, including HIV, poliovirus, and arboviruses including West Nile virus.

Enteroviruses and Arboviruses

In acute viral meningitis and meningoencephalitis, it is estimated that enterovirus infections (e.g., coxsackievirus, echovirus) cause between 60% and 90% of cases, and that arbovirus infections (e.g., Eastern equine, St. Louis, West Nile, etc.) comprise many of the remaining cases (41). Pathologic findings in cases described to date are nonspecific, without characteristic inclusions.

West Nile Virus

This arbovirus, a member of the *Flaviviridae* family, has recently emerged in the United States and Canada, with mosquito and bird vectors and hosts, and involvement of humans (40). Transmission by blood transfusion and organ transplantation has been documented recently. Symptoms are variable, multisystemic, and nonspecific, and include fever, myalgia, lymphadenopathy, rash, and headache. Neurologic symptoms include headache, encephalopathy, and diffuse weakness, including acute flaccid paralysis (40,42,44). A proportion of cases are fatal, and fatalities occur principally in the elderly—most with underlying systemic diseases.

The findings are nonspecific. They include a patchy meningitis, encephalitis, and polio-like myelitis with variable but, in some cases, severe involvement of the substantia nigra, brainstem (particularly the medulla), and cerebellum. Perivascular

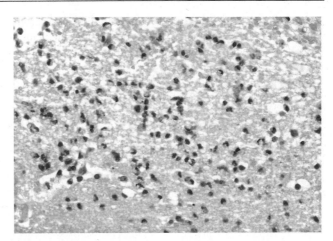

Figure 10.15. Inflammatory infiltrate in herpes simplex virus encephalitis. *(Courtesy of Dr. F. Stephen Vogel, Duke University Medical Center, Durham, North Carolina.)*

inflammation with evidence of meningoencephalitis and, in some cases, microglial nodules and neuronophagia can be seen (42,44). Anterior horn cells appear to be targeted in some patients, providing a substrate for the weakness (42). Of the involved regions, only the cerebrum and cerebellum are reasonable biopsy candidates. Laboratory diagnosis is based predominantly on serology (45). Additional information on this and other arboviruses is available from the Arbovirus Diagnostic Laboratory in Fort Collins, Colorado.

Herpes Simplex Virus (HSV)

The most common cause of nonepidemic encephalitis is herpes simplex virus (HSV) (Tables 10.2 and 10.3). The process is usually localized to the temporal and frontal lobes. When suspected by clinical and imaging findings, the diagnosis of HSV can be made by CSF culture, serology, and PCR evaluation rather than biopsy. Biopsy of the medial portion of a temporal lobe is still carried out in some cases. In the acute and subacute phase, perivascular inflammation, composed predominantly of lymphocytes mixed with macrophages, is accompanied by varying degrees of necrosis and hemorrhage (Fig. 10.15). Inclusion bodies are not easy to find in small brain biopsies (Fig. 10.16).

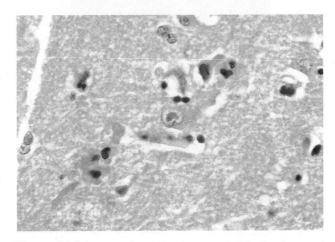

Figure 10.16. Herpes simplex virus encephalitis. Cowdry type A inclusion body in the center. *(Courtesy of Dr. F. Stephen Vogel, Duke University Medical Center, Durham, North Carolina.)*

Sensitive and specific methods of identification include in situ hybridization and IHC. Electron microscopy also may demonstrate viral particles but is less sensitive and less specific.

Cytomegalovirus (CMV)

CMV infection in an adult likely represents reactivation of dormant disease (27,43). Histologic findings vary from cells with typical CMV inclusions with virtually no associated inflammation, to severe necrotizing ependymitis and meningoencephalitis. Other lesions may be complicated by CMV infection. IHC, in situ hybridization, and PCR are useful techniques for detecting the virus in paraffin-embedded tissue.

Progressive Multifocal Leukoencephalopathy (PML)

PML is the result of activation of the DNA papovavirus, predominantly JC virus (rarely, SV-40 virus), in the brain. The disease is typically seen in the setting of severe immunodeficiency (e.g., AIDS) and lymphoproliferative disorder and associated treatment; occasional cases occur in the setting of immunosuppression after solid organ transplant and in connective tissue diseases (e.g., lupus) treated with immunosuppression (46).

PML manifests as multiple discrete foci of demyelination. Radiographically, it may simulate multiple sclerosis or a mass (Fig. 10.17). Brain biopsy frequently shows an active to subacute process, (a) typically with abundant foamy macrophages, many of which, on LFB-H&E stain, contain myelin; (b) marked reactive gliosis with many astrocytes manifesting bizarre, anaplastic nuclei that can be confused with glioma; and (c) glassy nuclear inclusions in oligodendrocytes that enlarge the nucleus and marginate the chromatin (Figs. 10.18 and 10.19). Perivascular infiltrates of mature lymphocytes are prominent in some cases. The histologic findings of PML are similar in patients with and without AIDS, although bizarre astrocytes are less frequent, and perivascular inflammatory cells more frequent, in AIDS patients. Diagnosis of PML can be confirmed by IHC, in situ hybridization (Fig. 10.19), or electron microscopy (1,27,47).

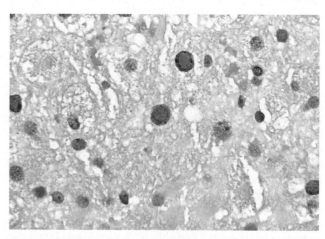

Figure 10.18. Progressive multifocal leukoencephalopathy. An infected oligodendroglial nucleus is enlarged by a pink-purple (amphophilic) accumulation of virions and peripheralization of chromatin.

Subacute Sclerosing Panencephalitis (SSPE)/Measles

Subacute sclerosing panencephalitis (SSPE) is a rare disease, with a relatively high incidence in Asia and the Middle East. This slowly progressive disease is caused by a persistant infection of immune-resistant measles virus, usually in unvaccinated or late-vaccinated children. Optimal testing involves identification of antimeasles antibodies, both IgG and IgM in both the CSF and serum. Brain biopsy is rarely performed. When undertaken, viral encephalitis-type changes predominate and there is loss of myelin in subcortical white matter (27). Nuclear inclusions may be detected in neurons and oligodendroglial cells by H&E. IHC or in situ hybridization evaluation detects measles virus antigen.

HIV/AIDS

The CNS is significantly affected by HIV- and AIDS-related diseases. Such diseases can be classified as primary (due directly to HIV) and secondary, with opportunistic diseases resulting

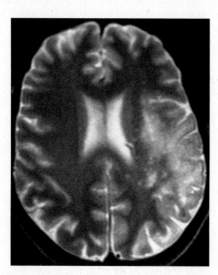

Figure 10.17. Progressive multifocal leukoencephalopathy simulates an edematous mass in this T2-weighted magnetic resonance image from a patient with severe immunodeficiency. (*Courtesy of Dr. Herbert Ichinose and Dr. Joseph Epps, Jr., Pendleton Memorial Methodist Hospital, New Orleans, Louisiana.*)

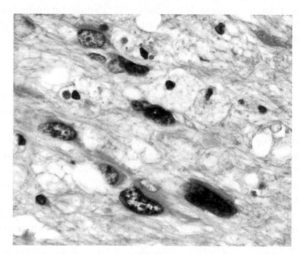

Figure 10.19. Deep white-matter lesion from a 54-year-old woman treated with immunosuppressives for lupus. Astrocytes manifest strikingly atypical nuclei. Abundant foamy macrophages contain blue balls of myelin, which is consistent with demyelination.

from the immunodeficiency. Primary and secondary CNS disease were very common in the early era of AIDS, with neurologic symptoms at clinical presentation and CNS abnormalities noted in more than half of patients (3,48). Highly active antiretroviral therapy (HAART) has markedly altered the disease course, but not eliminated CNS diseases (49,50).

The primary and secondary disease processes in HIV infection and AIDS produce a spectrum of neuropathology, beginning with cerebritis, meningitis, encephalitis, and vascular pathology, and ending with degenerative-metabolic changes and neoplasia.

PRIMARY MANIFESTATIONS OF HUMAN IMMUNODEFI-CIENCY VIRUS (HIV). HIV causes several primary CNS diseases, including (a) HIV encephalitis, (b) leukoencephalopathy and vacuolar myelopathy, and (c) lymphocytic meningitis (50). These changes can be seen in biopsies of secondary lesions (e.g., toxoplasmosis or lymphoma) or in cerebral biopsies carried out to assess the etiology of unanticipated cognitive decline and detect a treatable cause of disease (see previous section, "High-Risk Infectious Disease Case Considerations" for tissue handling).

The hallmarks of HIV encephalitis, considered pathognomonic of the disease, are multinucleated giant cells in the setting of microglial nodules, which form multiple foci of various sizes within white and gray matter (Fig. 10.20). Nonspecific viral encephalitis changes are also noted, including microglial nodules without giant cells. By IHC, the giant cells can contain abundant HIV markers, including p23.

HIV leukoencephalopathy is characterized by diffuse damage to the white matter with loss of myelin, reactive astrogliosis, multinucleated cells, and macrophage infiltrates with scant lymphocytic infiltrates.

Lymphocytic meningitis is still another primary manifestation of HIV infection and is remarkable for heavy lymphocytic infiltrates within the leptomeninges and perivascular spaces. HIV cerebral vasculitis and granulomatous angiitis may occur with lymphocytic or lymphoplasmohistiocytic-multinucleated giant-cell infiltration of cerebral vessel walls, occasionally accompanied by necrosis.

Since the onset of HAART, the severity and incidence of

primary HIV encephalitis and leukoencephalopathy has decreased (49,50). However, a new form of HIV encephalitis, with severe leukoencephalopathy and intense perivascular macrophage and lymphocyte infiltrates, has been described—postulated to be a response of the revived immune system (49).

SECONDARY MANIFESTATIONS OF AIDS AND OTHER IMMUNOSUPPRESSION: INFECTIONS AND NEOPLASTIC PROCESSES. A wide range of opportunistic diseases occur secondary to the immunosuppression caused by AIDS as well as in the context of therapy-related immunosuppression (3). The organisms of note include (a) fungi, including *Cryptococcus neoformans* (Fig. 10.10) and candida; (b) viruses, including the JC virus (Figs. 10.17 through 10.21) and CMV; (c) parasites, including toxoplasmosis (Figs. 10.12 and 10.13); and (d) bacteria, including *Listeria monocytogenes, H. influenzae, Streptococcus pneumonia, Staphylococcus epidermidis,* and *Pseudomonas* (27). Many viral and parasitic diseases likely represent reactivation of the infectious agent, which had been encountered in the past and held in check by the normal immune system.

Primary CNS lymphoma is a well-recognized neoplasm in AIDS (see "Lymphoma," below). Other neoplasms can (rarely) involve the CNS in the setting of immunosuppression, including Kaposi sarcoma and leiomyosarcoma.

HAART allows recovery of the immune system in many patients with AIDS and prevents the immunodeficiency with early treatment. This has markedly decreased the incidence of some secondary, opportunistic disease processes. However, the incidence of PML and lymphoma has not been clearly reduced, and it is possible that PML may shift toward a more chronic disease in treated patients (49).

PRION DISEASES

"PRION" was coined from PROteinaceous INfectious particle with the vowels transposed (4). The counterpart of the pathogenic prion protein is a normal constituent of neurons, white blood cells, and other cell membranes with a still-undefined function (4). When an abnormal tertiary structure is acquired,

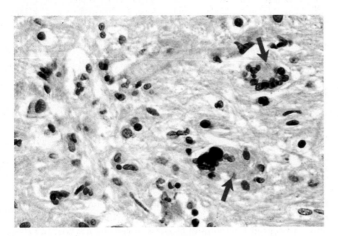

Figure 10.20. Human immunodeficiency virus encephalitis. Multinucleated giant cells (*arrows*) in the setting of a loosely formed microglial nodule accompanied by gliosis. (*Courtesy of Dr. Javad Towfighi, Penn State University, Hershey, Pennsylvania.*)

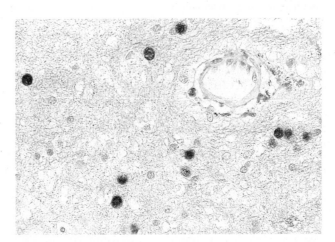

Figure 10.21. Progressive multifocal leukoencephalopathy. Cytochemical detection of JC viral sequences by in situ hybridization in larger nuclei stained blue by alkaline phosphatase reaction product. Negative nuclei counterstain pink, and perivascular macrophages contain light brown cytoplasmic granules. (*Courtesy of Dr. Ricardo Lloyd, Mayo Clinic, Rochester, Minnesota.*)

the protein both (a) becomes resistant to normal protein degradation, and (b) has the autocatalytic capacity to convert the tertiary structure of other prion proteins to the pathogenic conformation. As this cycle continues, an increasing percentage of normal protein is converted into the pathogenic prion configuration.

Several forms of prion disease affect man, including (a) the most common sporadic form, Creutzfeldt-Jacob disease (CJD), in which no germline mutation is present; (b) familial forms, with germline mutations, including Gerstmann-Sträussler-Scheinker, familial CJD, and fatal familial insomnia (FFI); and (c) acquired forms, including Kuru (passed from person to person by the eating of the human brain of dead relatives) variant CJD (see below), and iatrogenic CJD (patients receiving growth hormone derived from pooled cadaver pituitaries, contaminated neurosurgical and ophthalmologic surgical equipment, depth electrodes, or contaminated transplanted tissue [dura, cornea]) (27). Sporadic CJD is the most common of these. Prion diseases, known as "transmissible spongiform encephalopathies," occur sporadically in humans, cows, sheep (scrapie), goats, mink, cats, deer, and elk. Variant CJD appears to have arisen in cows in the setting of use of sheep tissue, including scrapie-containing brain as cattle feed, and was perpetuated by inclusion of affected cow nervous tissue in feed. In man and animals, these diseases are uniformly fatal.

Clinical diagnosis of CJD is difficult and imprecise, especially at early stages. Detection of the 14-3-3 protein in CSF is a valuable but imperfect tool (51). Because many CNS diseases can increase 14-3-3, its utility for CJD may tilt toward a negative 14-3-3 ruling out CJD, rather than a positive 14-3-3 confirming CJD. Ultimately, histopathologic and molecular evaluations of brain tissue are the gold standard for diagnosis (52).

Key considerations for biopsy of a "possible CJD" case include a reasonable chance to find a treatable cause of the cognitive deficits and safety of operating room and pathology staff. Biopsy for the identification of a prion-related disease is not warranted if the clinical suspicion is very high, based on clinical features (rapid progression of the disease), brain imaging studies, electrodiagnostic studies (EEG), and confirmatory serologic and CSF studies that exclude other explanations (e.g., stroke, vasculitis, meningoencephalitis).

Histologic Appearance

Several histologic changes are evidence of prion disease, including a combination of neuropil vacuolation and gliosis (53). Histologic changes in CJD include (a) vacuolation of the neuropil, with involvement of all six cortical layers in cerebrum, or with diffuse involvement of the cerebellar molecular layer (Figs. 10.22 and 10.23); (b) reactive gliosis that is particularly prominent in late stages of the disease (Fig. 10.24); and (c) occasional plaques of amyloid-like material in the neocortex in new-variant CJD. By H&E, a few vacuoles in the neuropil are glassy or lightly eosinophilic rather than clear. Microglial cells are increased in number, but perivascular inflammatory infiltrates are negligible.

Lack of identification of diagnostic histologic changes from a single biopsy site does not rule out CJD because (a) different subtypes of the disease exist, variable with the mutation in the prion protein, with variably cortical predominant, basal ganglia predominant, thalamus predominant, and hippocampal predominant disease; and (b) considerable variation can be seen from gyrus to gyrus in CJD and at different stages of the disease

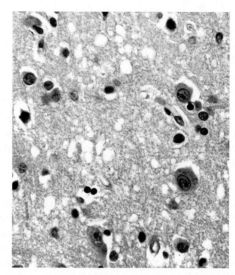

Figure 10.22. Creutzfeldt-Jakob disease. Biopsy of the cerebral frontal lobe from a 57-year-old man with suspected Alzheimer disease. Coalescing round vacuoles and gliosis are present in the neuropil. Some of the vacuoles have a glassy appearance, rather than a punched-out look. These involved all six cortical layers (cresyl violet with eosin).

(54,55). A diagnostic pitfall—diffuse cortical vacuolization—is a common finding in advanced Alzheimer disease. Superficial cortical vacuolization occurs in ischemia and in frontotemporal dementia; the vacuoles in these cases are clear, punched-out, and different from those in CJD. Processing artifacts can produce vacuoles that encircle neurons, vessels, and glia; these are larger than CJD vacuoles. Nonetheless, because many vacuoles are not related to prions, molecular diagnosis of prions is needed to confirm suspicions based on vacuoles.

Immunohistochemistry

IHC after protease predigestion of normal prion proteins helps identify protease-resistant prion protein. However there is a

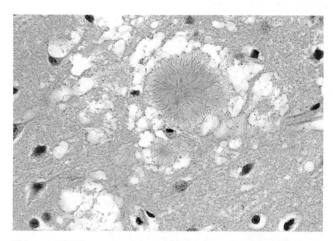

Figure 10.23. Variant Creutzfeldt-Jakob disease. This variant is from the cerebral cortex of a 29-year-old woman in the United Kingdom who experienced 17 months of progressive dementia, ataxia, and chorea. Fibrillary plaques composed of prion protein resemble skyrocket bursts, and they are surrounded by very coarse spongiform changes in the neuropil. (*Courtesy of Dr. Jeanne E. Bell, National CJD Surveillance Unit, Western General Hospital, Edinburgh, United Kingdom.*)

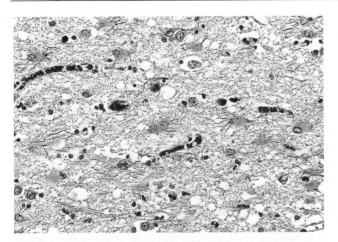

Figure 10.24. Familial Creutzfeldt-Jakob disease. Most of the neurons have been lost and replaced by gliosis in this case. Phosphotungstic acid hematoxylin stain highlights gliotic fibrils and vacuolated neuropils.

fairly high background labeling among the IHC techniques, challenging their sensitivity and specificity (53,54). Specifically, most available antibodies manifest some degree of background labeling of neurons in control cases, and they can stain neuritic plaques. These should be interpreted only by an experienced observer.

Molecular Diagnosis

The gold standard of identification of the prion protein is molecular evaluation for the protease-digestion–resistant protein by Western blot, performed in specialized medical centers and at the National Prion Disease Pathology Surveillance Center in Cleveland, Ohio (52; see "High-Risk Infectious Disease Case Considerations" section above). Sporadic CJD lacks a germline mutation, which can be confirmed by sequencing of the prion protein gene to rule out known familial CJD variants.

Variant CJD/"Mad Cow Disease"

In the mid-1990s "new-variant" CJD (vCJD) emerged in Great Britain and France, originally called "mad cow disease." It has been linked by molecular analysis to the eating of meat from cows with bovine spongiform encephalopathy (BSE), in most cases through contamination of the meat with brain and other highly infected tissue during slaughter and butchering. The previously postulated "species barrier" to transmission was broached (53). By early 2003, approximately 135 cases of new-variant CJD had been reported, most cases diagnosed in the United Kingdom.

In the United Kingdom and Europe, the BSE epidemic is now ending and the number of cases is decreasing, thanks to the strict control of animal foodstuff that was the main source of prion contamination (56). BSE in North America (two cases to date) may be at its beginning. Significant measures have been adopted to reduce the risk from recycling of infection via feed, but it remains to be seen whether they are watertight (57).

Despite vCJD being a small fraction of prion diseases, it is a major public health and economic concern. After halting all imports of U.S. beef in 2003, the Japanese government decided in December 2005 to allow importation of beef from the United

States derived from young cattle from which specified risk materials are removed (58). Rapid tests for misfolded PrP in central nervous tissue of slaughter cattle now allows hope for better monitoring (57), provided our hands are on our wallets and our heads out of the sand.

The histologic appearance of vCJD differs from sporadic CJD. In the cerebral and cerebellar cortex, (a) striking stellate, "florid" plaques composed of prion protein, easily seen by H& E, labeled by PAS and anti-prion protein antibodies; (b) coarse vacuolization, rather than the fine vacuolation of CJD; and (c) marked gliosis are the most and consistent neuropathologic features (Fig. 10.23) (53). These cerebral cortical plaques and coarse spongiform features have not been seen among typical sporadic CJD cases. Similar plaques can be noted in the cerebellum of sporadic CJD (4,55).

Hereditary Prion Diseases

The vacuolization, neuron loss, and gliosis in hereditary prion disorders such as Gerstmann-Sträussler-Scheinker syndrome (GSS), fatal familial insomnia (FFI), and familial CJD (Fig. 10.24) are similar to sporadic CJD and kuru (27). These diseases are rarely biopsied.

INFLAMMATORY DISEASES

Causes of inflammatory diseases of the CNS are elusive because there is considerable overlap in their clinical and histologic findings. A range of inflammatory diseases affects the brain, including connective tissue diseases, sarcoid, and rheumatoid disease. They variably affect leptomeninges, blood vessels, and brain tissue. Altered mental status and meningeal changes invite biopsy to evaluate etiology and to rule out infections. Optimal sampling that includes dura, arachnoid, and gray matter in the area of a radiological enhancement improves the chance of reaching a lesion.

GRANULOMATOUS INFLAMMATION

Inflammatory diseases can present a granulomatous appearance, with or without distinct granuloma formation, with or without regions of necrosis. See "Granulomatous Inflammation" in the "Reactive Changes" and "Infectious Diseases" sections above.

Granulomatous inflammation can also be seen in the setting of dural, leptomeningeal, or parenchymal involvement of the CNS by Wegner granulomatosis and rheumatoid arthritis. Granulomatous meningitis has a predilection for the base of the brain. Neurosarcoidosis is always a diagnosis of exclusion in cases of granulomatous inflammation. Infection must be ruled out first. Sarcoid typically affects the leptomeninges and blood vessels of the brain or spinal cord. Lesions contain lymphocytic leptomeningeal infiltration, slight lymphocytic cuffing of intraparenchymal vessels, scattered small leptomeningeal and parenchymal noncaseating granulomas, and mild reactive astrocytosis, especially in the white matter, with only moderate loss of myelin.

SMALL-VESSEL DISEASE AND VASCULITIS

Brain biopsies performed in search of small-vessel disease, particularly vasculitis, frequently do not provide a satisfactory correlation between the pathologic specimen and the radiographic data, although step-sectioning through the entire block of tissue may occasionally yield diagnostic material. Small vessels are primarily affected in isolated angiitis of the CNS, and both angiography and leptomeningeal plus parenchymal biopsy of a radiographic lesion are essential to the diagnosis (59–61).

Criteria for diagnosis of vasculitis include both (a) vessel wall inflammation, and (b) vessel wall damage and destruction. Chronic, healed, or resolving vasculitis manifests irregular vessel wall fibrosis, often with partial damage of elastica. H&E, trichrome, type IV collagen, and elastic stains are keys to confirming vasculitis.

Temporal arteritis is a common disorder that affects small- to medium-sized arteries of elderly women. It is often biopsied bilaterally (60). The disease particularly affects the intima, with giant cells a prominent part of the infiltrate. Although uncommon, systemic lupus erythematosus (SLE) affects the CNS more frequently than other collagen diseases (61). Rarely, SLE produces microinfarcts and necrotizing vasculitis with thrombosis. Isolated angiitis and arteritis associated with collagen vascular disease, infection, toxins, and granulomatous disease can cause strokes in young people (62).

A multitude of diseases are responsible for individual cases of vasculitis. Cerebral angiitis can be a part of systemic vasculitis in mixed cryoglobulinemia and Wegener disease. Isolated, primary CNS angiitis may include inflammation of very small vessels (59). Angiitis also occurs in association with herpes varicella-zoster virus (63), relapsing polychondritis, and Behçet disease (66). Lymphomatoid granulomatosis is a process that spans inflammatory and neoplastic entities. It is discussed under "Neoplastic Diseases, Lymphoma."

Intrathecal methotrexate therapy can cause mineralizing microangiopathy (64). Meningovascular syphilis and associated vasculitis is rising in frequency associated with AIDS. Illicit drugs, such as cocaine, heroin, and amphetamines, affect not only the cardiac vessels but also cerebral vessels, and can cause cerebral vasculitis associated with intraparenchymal or subarachnoid hemorrhage (65).

DEMYELINATION

Demyelination results principally from (a) presumed autoimmune etiologies such as multiple sclerosis (MS) or acute disseminated encephalomyelitis (ADEM, perivenous demyelination) (67); (b) infectious etiologies, most notably PML (see "Infectious Disease" section above); and (c) toxic metabolic etiologies, including the leukodystrophies (e.g., Gaucher disease, adrenoleukodystrophy). Survivors of carbon monoxide poisoning and patients with long-standing hypertension and atherosclerosis can have diffuse cerebral hemisphere white matter demyelinating lesions that can histologically mimic the demyelination of MS in surgical specimens. The absence of a margin with less affected brain may help distinguish this from MS plaques, which typically have a sharp margin.

Demyelinating diseases are usually investigated clinically without biopsy (Table 10.2). Exceptions occur with unusual clinical presentations where the clinical diagnosis is unknown or unclear. For instance, active MS lesions can be mistaken radiologically for neoplasm (68). Demyelination due to a primary viral process (PML, HIV leukoencephalitis, CMV, varicella-zoster) is also occasionally seen at biopsy; these entities are considered in the "Viruses" section above. The leukodystrophies are very rarely seen by the surgical pathologist.

Histology

Primary, acute demyelinating lesions histologically show destruction of myelin and abundant foamy macrophages containing myelin debris and lipid droplets (Fig. 10.25). There is relative sparing of axons in demyelinating disease, although a fraction of axons are lost in chronic MS. In contrast, axonal loss precedes myelin loss in an infarct (Fig. 10.26). The amount of gliosis increases with the chronicity of the lesion.

Histochemically, special stains for myelin (Luxol fast blue-hematoxylin and eosin [LFB-H&E]) and axons (Bodian or Bielschowsky silver stain, or neurofilament IHC) help to distinguish between (a) demyelination (foamy macrophages containing LFB-positive myelin debris present with axons mostly retained intact in brain tissue); and (b) necrosis, including infarct (axons lost), and Wallerian degeneration (myelin loss is secondary to axonal loss). GFAP stain helps discern gemistocytic reactive astrocytes from macrophages; CD68 and CD45/45RB identify macrophages and lymphocytes. If the lesion was induced by a virus, neuronal or oligodendroglial intranuclear inclusions may be found, particularly at the periphery of the lesion.

Multiple Sclerosis

The major demyelinating disorder of adults is MS. MS is likely an autoimmune disease (69). Despite an immense amount of sophisticated research spanning the past three decades, much remains unknown about this disease. It remains uncertain why some areas of myelin are attacked and others remain spared.

MS manifests acute (or "active"), subacute, and chronic lesions. The former are those that are typically seen at biopsy from a patient suspected of having something other than MS (Fig. 10.25). Due to loss of integrity of the blood–brain barrier, they can have imaging characteristics that mimic a malignant neoplasm (68). MS should be differentiated from other disorders that have similar lesions, including Behçet disease and late-onset forms of leukodystrophies.

Acute Disseminated Encephalomyelitis (ADEM)

Perivenous demyelination is a prominent pathologic finding in postinfectious and postvaccination encephalomyelitis, which is thought to be an autoimmune phenomenon initiated by a viral pathogen, most commonly varicella-zoster and influenza (67,70–72). ADEM is in some cases associated with hemorrhage. It is rarely biopsied. If biopsied, identification of its perivascular pattern of demyelination is important. The demyelination of MS extends beyond vessels to a confluent patch or plaque.

Differential Diagnosis

A demyelinating lesion may be confused with neoplastic disease. Gliosis in the subacute demyelinating lesion can be robust, with large astrocytes with chromosomes spread apart in their cytoplasm (so-called Creutzfeldt cells), mimicking glioma cells (68). In addition, macrophages can accumulate in large numbers in an active region of demyelination to the extent that they mimic glioma, especially oligodendroglioma; or they may mimic hemangioblastoma. Leu-7– and S-100–positive oligodendroglio-

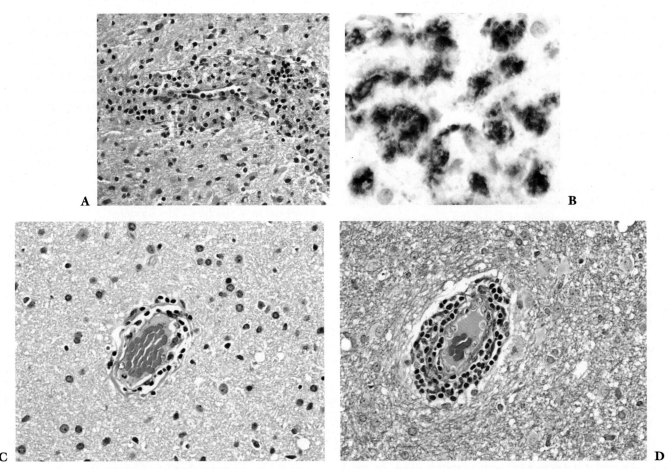

Figure 10.25. Vascular involvement in multiple sclerosis (MS) (**A, B**) compared with vasculitis (**C, D**). Active MS lesion presented on MRI as ring enhancing lesion in a 24-year-old woman. (**A**) Abundant plump cells and scant lymphocytes around blood vessel, but not in its wall. Initial impression could mistake this lesion for vasculitis or glioma. (**B**) CD68 immunostain identifies the plump cells as macrophages. Active vasculitis presented on MRI as severe white-matter disease with patchy enhancement in a 32-year-old woman. (**C**) Lymphocytes and macrophages penetrate the pink necrotic wall of the vessel and insinuate between collagen fibers. Endothelium is swollen. (**D**) Trichrome stain reveals vascular wall penetration and plump endothelium.

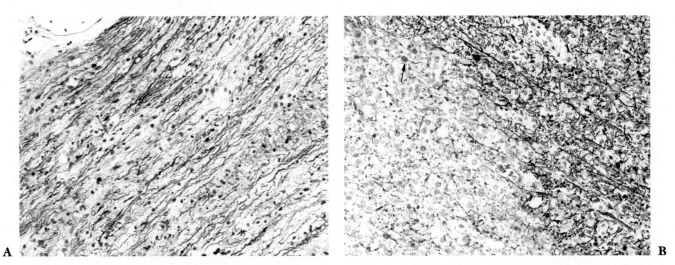

Figure 10.26. Two different white-matter lesions are each stained for neurofilaments, with hematoxylin counterstain for nuclei. (**A**) Demyelination is hard to see except for some pale, lipid-filled macrophages (*arrow*) between straight brown axons. Axons are spared in demyelination. (**B**) Focal white-matter necrosis produced the pale side of this image in this small infarct. Necrotic axons become very pale and finally disintegrate into small beads that are eaten by macrophages. Some damaged axons swell (*arrow*).

mas have fewer cytoplasmic vacuoles and more central nuclei than lipid-laden CD68-positive macrophages. Hemangioblastomas are more vascular than oligodendrogliomas (see Fig. 10.5B; and Figs. 10.54 and 10.120 in the "Tumors" section below). LFB-H&E stain will reveal phagocytosis of myelin in a demyelinating lesion.

CEREBROVASCULAR DISEASES

INFARCT

Infarction of CNS parenchyma is a common pathologic process often associated with clinical stroke. Thrombosis of an atherosclerotic artery or emboli of blood clot or of atherosclerotic plaque commonly causes infarcts. Other etiologies include coagulopathy, amyloid angiopathy, local vasospasm, major changes in blood pressure, CADASIL, mitochondrial encephalopathy with lactic acidosis and strokes (MELAS), and infectious and inflammatory processes. Infarcts can occur in young adults with normal arteries as a result of a severe episode of hypotension, or in association with coagulopathy or cerebral vasospasm (73).

Representative portions of the specimens should be submitted for histologic evaluation to optimize evaluation of blood vessels by sectioning perpendicular to the surface of the brain, and by including arachnoid, gray matter, and white matter. Vessels are carefully examined for evidence of embolism, arteriosclerosis, atherosclerosis, amyloid angiopathy (see "Amyloid Angiopathy" section below), and an infectious-inflammatory process (see "Small-Vessel Diseases" below). If mitochondrial disease and CADASIL have not been ruled out, then portions of gray matter and gray–white matter junction should be saved for possible EM examination.

In CNS tissue, the age of the infarct is evaluated for active changes and evidence of organization, and classified as acute, subacute, or remote. Special stains for axons (Bodian or Bielschowsky silver stain, neurofilament IHC) help to distinguish between necrotic tissue (axons missing or disintegrated) and demyelination (axons retained).

INTRACRANIAL HEMORRHAGE

Clotted blood or hematoma removed from an intracranial location represents a common surgical neuropathology specimen. Such a specimen can be removed from the epidural, subdural, subarachnoid, or intraparenchymal regions. Possible causes of intracranial hemorrhage are summarized in Table 10.5 (74).

The contribution of the surgical pathologist to such specimens lies in careful macroscopic and microscopic inspection of the material and clinicopathologic correlation with (a) evaluation of potential etiologies for intracranial hemorrhage, including clinically unsuspected causes, such as a cryptic vascular malformation, vascular disease, or neoplasm; and (b) approximate dating of the hematoma as acute, subacute, or chronic.

Close macroscopic examination of aspiration collection device contents and resected specimens should be done, submitting for histologic evaluation representative brain parenchyma and other solid regions when present. At least one cassette of hematoma, or more as indicated by gross findings, should be submitted for processing. Bone fragments may represent bone dust generated during the surgery or may be secondary to traumatic injury.

Microscopic examination of the hematoma can roughly distinguish among (a) *acute hemorrhage* (minutes to hours old, in which white-cell nuclei are intact and no evidence of organization is noted); (b) *subacute hemorrhage* (days old, in which white-cell nuclei are karyorrhectic and macrophages ingesting red cells are noted); and (c) *remote or chronic hemorrhage* (weeks to years old, with hemosiderin containing macrophages and ingrowth of blood vessels and fibroblasts in the meninges), and reactive astrocytes surrounding the lesion (in parenchymal lesions). Hemosiderin is evident 4 days after hemorrhage and reactive astrocytes 2 weeks after hemorrhage. Both persist indefinitely.

Epidural and Subdural Hemorrhage

Epidural hemorrhage typically results from trauma, most frequently with temporal bone fracture and rupture of the middle meningeal artery. Most such evacuated specimens contain acute hematoma.

Subdural hemorrhages may or may not follow known trauma (75). They are most common in elderly patients with some degree of cerebral atrophy (and bridging vein susceptibility to tear), as well as in patients with systemic cancer (76) and CNS tumors in postoperative settings (75). Acute subdural hematoma is, as a rule, removed by aspiration; contents may come for evaluation in a suction collection device. Subacute or chronic subdural hematomas require excision and histologic evaluation of the subdural membranes to rule out a neoplasm.

Left in situ, subdural hematoma organization continues for weeks. Fibrotic membranes are formed on both sides of a hematoma. The membrane on the dural (outer) side forms first and is usually about 2 to 5 cells thick in a 5-day-old subdural hematoma, and approximately 12 cells thick after a week; it eventually may become as thick as normal dura. Movat pentachrome stain distinguishes new membrane collagen, which stains green from dura (which stains yellow). The membrane on the arachnoid (inner) side of the clot organizes more slowly than the dural membrane and is often not evident in a surgical specimen. Hematomas may re-bleed and contain admixed acute, subacute, and chronic changes, confusing the picture. As organization proceeds, abundant hemosiderin-containing macrophages are present. In chronic membranes, eosinophils can be very numerous. Long-standing hematomas may calcify.

Subarachnoid Hemorrhage

Rupture of a saccular aneurysm of the circle of Willis causes subarachnoid hemorrhage, the contents of which may or may not be evacuated (73). Occasionally, these aneurysms also rupture into brain tissue. Any systemic disease with a bleeding tendency can elicit meningeal hemorrhage, but nonaneurysmal bleeds rarely require surgical intervention. Subarachnoid extension from an intraparenchymal hemorrhage that ruptures into the ventricular space is also common.

Hemorrhage into Brain Parenchyma

Intraparenchymal hemorrhage has many potential causes, including iatrogenic hemorrhage, and often accompanies other lesions within the CNS (Table 10.5) (73). A hemorrhage may remain relatively circumscribed within the brain or may present as a rapidly expanding mass that requires rapid removal, resulting in a specimen containing acute hemorrhage. Massive hemorrhage displaces and compresses the surrounding brain tissue. Smaller hemorrhages may be subacute or chronic. With time, rarefaction of the brain parenchyma eventually forms a slit or a cystic cavity lined by gliosis mixed with macrophages, blood pigment deposits, and occasionally partially lysed red blood cells.

The hemorrhages in hypertensive individuals occur most commonly in the putamen, thalamus, cerebrum, pons, and cerebellum. A surgical specimen from a massive hypertensive hemorrhage consists of a large amount of acute hemorrhage, although subacute changes may be seen as well, suggesting previous limited hemorrhage. Portions of edematous brain tissue with petechial hemorrhages and characteristic arterioles with sclerosis as a result of replacement of smooth muscle by collagen are occasionally evident on examination. A clue to hypertensive origin of a hemorrhage is atherosclerotic damage to intact arterioles and small arteries in any brain tissue resected with the hematoma, often with fragmentation and reduplication of elastic tissue or intramural lipidized macrophages (3).

Arteriovenous malformations (AVMs) and cavernous angiomas are vascular malformations with risk of hemorrhage. See the "Vascular Malformation" section below.

Subarachnoid aneurysms occasionally rupture into the brain, but radiography reveals their nature. Other causes of intracerebral hemorrhage include exposure to cold, medications (e.g., anticoagulation therapy), and surgery, particularly cardiac surgery and carotid endarterectomy (74,75).

VASCULAR MALFORMATION

Most vascular malformations are developmental in origin, likely dating to embryonic maldevelopment, with some familial cases identified (75,77). Vascular malformations can occur anywhere in the brain, spinal cord, and associated leptomeninges (Fig. 10.27).

Four types of vascular malformations are generally recognized: capillary telangiectasia, cavernous angioma, arteriovenous malformation (AVM), and venous malformation (Table 10.6) (77,78). A dilation of a venous structure, or varix, is one type of venous malformation; the most common example is the great vein of Galen malformation. Sturge-Weber disease (cerebrofacial or cerebrotrigeminal angiomatosis) typically manifests a "port wine" type hemangioma of the face and an underlying complex vascular malformation that involves the leptomeninges and cortex. The vessels are often mineralized, and cortical mineralization by CT scan is a useful marker of the lesion. Resection is carried out in the setting of intractable seizures.

Histologic distinction among these malformations takes into account (a) the size of and nature of the vessels involved, including the presence or absence of large arterialized vessels; (b) the presence or absence of nervous tissue interposed among the vessels; (c) the presence or absence of hemosiderin-laden macrophages suggesting leakage of vessels; and (d) reactive gliosis surrounding and intermixed with the vessels (Table 10.6).

Arteriovenous malformations (AVMs) and cavernous angiomas are the two vascular malformations most relevant to the surgical pathologist. Because their vessels tend to leak and induce gliosis, cavernous angiomas and AVMs can present with seizure disorder. Both lesions can also cause spontaneous hemorrhage. Best seen by trichrome or elastic stains, AVMs manifest artery–vein connections with associated arterialization of veins. *Arterialization* is thickening of a venous wall to the point where it resembles an artery, possibly due to fibrotic reaction to shunted arterial blood. Arteries show irregular duplication or loss of elastin (Fig. 10.28). Thrombi are common. In AVMs discovered without hemorrhage, the risk of hemorrhage has been estimated to be 1.3% to 4.0% yearly, with morbidity following hemorrhage of 53% to 81% and mortality of 10.0% to 17.6%. Surgical treatment offers good prognosis and seizure and hemorrhage control (77,78).

In a small biopsy sample with abundant hemosiderin within a highly cellular matrix, an AVM or cavernous angioma may be confused with the edge of a hemorrhage, infarct, inflammatory focus, or neoplasm. Demonstrate the abnormal vessels with Movat or other elastic and collagen stains, plus the reactive macrophages and glia with CD68 and GFAP, to avoid the confusion. Inflamed vessels are common in vascular malformations.

SUPERIOR SAGITTAL SINUS THROMBOSIS

Thrombosis of the superior sagittal sinus is occasionally encountered. Sinus thrombosis followed by venous infarction may

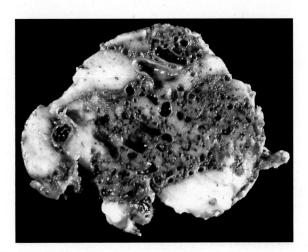

Figure 10.27. This arteriovenous malformation demonstrates the classic feature of brain parenchyma between abnormal vessels. The vascular walls vary in thickness, even around the circumference of the individual vessels.

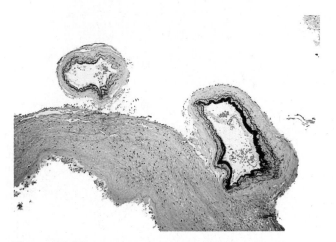

Figure 10.28. Incomplete and focally reduplicated elastic lamina in vessels from an arteriovenous malformation. Elastic stain.

occur, usually as a complication of a pre-existing infectious disease, connective tissue disease, or in the setting of hypercoagulability. Occasionally surgical decompression is done. The specimen of clotted blood is treated identical to any hematoma, with histologic evaluation and evaluation for tumor, infectious agents, and other possible etiologic entities.

AMYLOID ANGIOPATHY

Amyloid deposition restricted to the CNS is a frequent form of localized amyloidosis. It is due to deposition of a CNS type of beta-amyloid rather than the proteins seen in systemic amyloidosis. Cerebral amyloid (congophilic) angiopathy is seen in elderly patients with or without dementia and in cases of familial (hereditary) amyloidosis (79). Leukoencephalopathy is a feature of amyloid angiopathy. Microinfarcts or small foci of early ischemic damage with hemosiderin deposits may be associated findings in cases of amyloid angiopathy of leptomeningeal and superficial cortical arteries.

Cerebral amyloid angiopathy (CAA) results from deposition of beta-amyloid in the cerebral vessels and associated vessel wall injury. Although CAA may be suspected by H&E stain, based on a smudgy appearance of vessel walls and loss of smooth muscle nuclei, confirmation is required. Amyloid fibrils can be identified by (a) histochemical stains, including Congo red stain (salmon orange) with confirmation by polarization ("Granny Smith apple green") or thioflavin T stain (requires fluorescence microscopy), or (b) immunostaining for beta-amyloid (Fig. 10.29). CAA can be graded using the Vonsattel criteria as absent, mild (focal deposition of amyloid in vessel walls), moderate (circumferential deposition of amyloid, loss of smooth muscle cell nuclei, and vessel-in-vessel appearance), and severe (vessel wall damage, aneurysm formation). Only severe CAA and fibrinoid necrosis of vessel walls appear to be associated with "lobar" hemorrhage (79). A granulomatous reaction to the amyloid is seen in some cases.

Cerebral parenchyma from hematoma specimens from adult patients must be submitted for careful histologic evaluation for

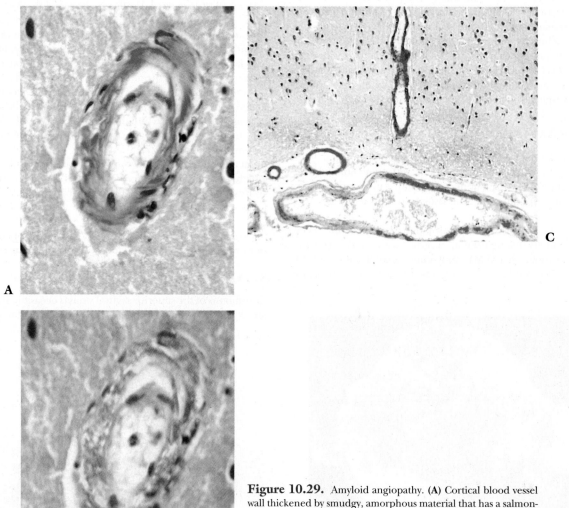

Figure 10.29. Amyloid angiopathy. **(A)** Cortical blood vessel wall thickened by smudgy, amorphous material that has a salmon-orange tincture with Congo red stain; the deposition is circumferential and smooth muscle nuclei are lost focally. **(B)** Polarization microscopy reveals a Granny Smith apple green color, in contrast to collagen, which would have polarized yellow-white. **(C)** β-amyloid immunoperoxidase labels multiple blood vessels with the red chromogen aminoethyl carbazole (AEC). *(A and B, Courtesy of Dr. Dennis Burns, University of Texas Southwestern, Dallas, Texas.)*

amyloid deposition in blood vessels because amyloid angiopathy may provide an unanticipated etiology for the hemorrhage, and this is an important finding for patient management.

SMALL-VESSEL DISEASES

Most of the small-vessel disease entities have inflammatory etiologies (vasculitis), and are discussed in the ''Inflammatory Disease'' section. CADASIL and arteriosclerosis are vasculopathies but are not inflammatory.

Cerebral Autosomal Dominant Angiopathy with Subcortical Infarcts and Leukoencephalopathy (CADASIL)

Presenting with migraine headaches, strokes, and generalized, progressive neurologic deficits including dementia, CADASIL is a rare disorder due to Notch3 gene (chromosome 19) mutations (80). Mutation evaluation can be performed at commercial laboratories on DNA extracted from white blood cells. Imaging identifies infarct-like lesions and white-matter disease (leukoencephalopathy). Although biopsy of the brain can be undertaken for diagnosis, the characteristic vascular changes can also be identified in biopsies of more accessible skin and muscle (81). By light microscopy, the affected vessels have a thickened appearance with a basophilic, granular material seen by H&E stain. This granular material is PAS-positive and it displaces smooth muscle cells, seen best when stained for smooth muscle actin. Electron microscopy reveals dark, granular osmophilic deposits (GRODs) immediately adjacent to smooth muscle cells. IHC evaluation for Notch3 protein deposition has been described.

Arteriosclerosis

Causes of CNS arteriosclerosis are hypertension, diabetes, and aging. Walls of small arteries are thickened with hyalinized collagen. Perivascular macrophages may be present. They may contain light brown, iron-negative phagolysosomes or dark brown, iron-positive hemosiderin.

VASCULAR DEMENTIA, MULTI-INFARCT VASCULAR DEMENTIA

The concept of so-called vascular dementia is controversial, and detailed discussion is beyond the scope of this chapter (2,4). A review of the topic from the neuropathology perspective concludes that vascular dementia has perhaps 7% to 10% prevalence (82). Vascular dementia is a diagnosis that should not be rendered on a surgical specimen.

TUMORS

The neoplasms of the brain that predominate in adults differ from those seen in children (Table 10.7). More pediatric neoplasms occur in the posterior fossa than in the anterior fossa, whereas the opposite is true of adult neoplasms.

GRADING MALIGNANT POTENTIAL OF TUMORS

The World Health Organization (WHO) sponsors a uniform terminology and grading system of brain tumors (8). Histologic criteria of malignancy are applied by WHO to gliomas and some other tumors. Starting with the most benign as grade I, numerical grades II, III, and IV represent increasing malignancy (Tables 10.8 and 10.9). Some prefer using grades 1, 2, 3, and 4 because these are not affected by double vision. Numerical grades assigned by WHO are used in this chapter.

ASSAYS OF PROLIFERATIVE CAPACITY

Proliferation antigens such as MIB-1 (Fig. 10.30) and proliferating cell nuclear antigen (PCNA), are nuclear antigens that appear during one or more proliferative phases of the cell cycle. Positive nuclei stain brown, and percentage of positive nuclei divided by total nuclei can be counted and calculated. This is called a labeling index (LI) or proliferation index (PI). This PI is usually sampled in regions of highest proliferation called ''hot spots.'' A simple way to do this is to dot ''hot spots'' with a pen under a $10\times$ objective, and count these regions under a $40\times$ objective (83). Ki-67 predicts survival among fibrillary astrocytic neoplasms (84,85). These PIs augment prognostication by standard histopathologic criteria.

The MIB-1 antibody detects Ki-67 epitopes in paraffin sections of formalin-fixed tissue. Studies have revealed the prognostic value of MIB-1 labeling indices. In one analysis, MIB-1 PI was the only independent predictor of survival (86). Among only grade II astrocytoma patients, MIB-1 distinguishes tumors with good prognosis by their low labeling indices (84). Lower MIB-1 PIs are found in younger patients with glioblastomas, and they have a significantly better prognosis than do older patients (83).

As valuable as it is to assessment of proliferative capacity, the MIB-1 PI is a semiquantitative assay based upon a qualitative staining method. Thus, MIB-1 staining methods and counting criteria vary among laboratories. A published value of PIs may not be relevant to a different laboratory. This means that individual laboratories should set their own standards for PIs based upon their previous cases. Organizations that standardize assays worldwide might contribute to standardization of MIB-1 staining methods and counting criteria.

Basic points of information about MIB-1 include the ability of reactive and inflammatory changes to produce conspicuous

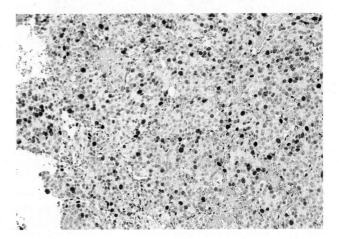

Figure 10.30. MIB-1, as an indicator of proliferative index of a neoplasm, reveals many positive brown nuclei, reflecting a high proliferation index in this anaplastic oligodendroglioma.

PIs, easily as high as most gliomas of low or intermediate grade (in our laboratory, up to 20%). Thus, a good pathologist and H&E stain is essential to setting the context for interpretation of the MIB-1 PI. A check on nuclear features of MIB-1–positive cells can reveal very important data: rounded nuclei of reactive cells or leukocytes; elongated nuclei in astrocytoma cells mixed with other glioma cells; more mitoses than seen on other stains (they look like dark granola). Always consider structure and context when interpreting this and other stains.

MOLECULAR EVALUATION

Molecular data regarding tumors can have diagnostic, prognostic, and therapeutic implications (87). For example, combined 1p and 19q deletions in oligodendrogliomas are associated with enhanced chemoresponsiveness and improved prognosis (88). In addition, several other molecular markers are providing useful diagnostic and prognostic information. For example, EGFR amplification may be useful in distinguishing high-grade astrocytoma from anaplastic oligodendroglioma; n-Myc amplification has prognostic significance in medulloblastomas; and INI1 studies are useful in the diagnosis of the atypical teratoid-rhabdoid tumor (AT/RT).

GLIOMAS

Glioma is a term that embraces astrocytoma, glioblastoma, ependymoma, and oligodendroglioma, and their various subtypes and combinations. An important general rule is that gliomas tend to contain GFAP and lack collagen, reticulin, and fibronectin in their parenchyma, distinguishing them from nonglial neoplasms (Fig. 10.31) (89,90). However, oligodendroglioma cells are more variable in their GFAP expression; like other gliomas, they contain less specific glial proteins such as Leu-7 and S-100 protein (89–92). Uncommon variants like xanthoastrocytomas may have parenchymal reticulin. The term *glioma* is too vague for a final diagnosis of properly sampled permanent histologic

sections. However, the term is useful when frozen sectioning obscures the subtype of a glioma or when the central tumor is missing.

Clinical needs are expanding the pathologist's role in the interpretation of gliomas. The particular effectiveness of combined procarbazine, chloroethylcyclohexylnitrosourea, and vincristine (PCV) chemotherapy for gliomas with an oligodendroglial component has increased the value of recognizing this component (91). Moreover, molecular methods of defining oligodendrogliomas have been proposed (93).

Postoperative systemic thromboses are a major complication of brain tumor surgery. The pathologist may be able to predict patients likely to encounter this difficulty by noting in the report tumors (usually malignant gliomas) that contain thrombosed vessels (94).

This chapter emphasizes grading consistent with the WHO international classification of tumors (8). There are other grading systems, each with its own merit (95). To avoid confusion, the grade number should state the grading system used. Because it is felt that tumors get worse (progress) via second, third, or multiple focal changes, the highest grade identified in the specimen is the one reported, even if this grade does not predominate. The histologic term *low-grade* applied to astrocytomas and other gliomas does not necessarily imply a benign neoplasm or even a favorable prognosis. Grade II is generally a slow-growing but diffuse glioma that cannot be totally removed and will eventually kill the patient, assuming no other major health issues. The designation *benign*, implying that, once removed, the neoplasm will not recur, is frequently used only for pilocytic astrocytomas and for certain neuronal tumors and ependymomas. Most of these are considered grade I. Even these tumors need to be in favorable locations and have distinct margins to have a good chance for cure.

Tumor and Tumor Margin

It is important to recognize two types of specimens from a potential glioma (96–100). The first type is the tumor epicenter (Tables 10.10 through 10.12), which has cellular density exceeding that of surrounding brain (Figs. 10.4B and 10.32). To obtain optimal tissue, it is best to monitor each glioma biopsy with

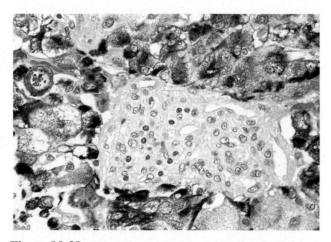

Figure 10.31. Keys to interpreting the glial fibrillary acidic protein (GFAP) stain. The endothelial cells that comprise the prominent central microvascular proliferation lack brown GFAP immunolabeling, and they serve as a critical internal negative control of the stain. Cytologically neoplastic cells with pleomorphic nuclei of this glioblastoma are identified as neoplastic glia because their cytoplasm is positive by GFAP immunolabeling. Note the single mitotic figure in a GFAP-positive cell.

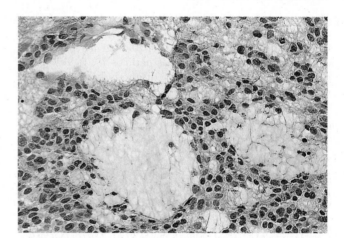

Figure 10.32. The microcysts in this glioma contain cells and eosinophilic proteinaceous material. The long, empty cavity in the corner of this frozen section is the result of cryostat artifact.

cytologic and frozen sections, and to indicate clearly specimens which are not satisfactory (Table 10.1; see also the "Intraoperative Consultation" section). Unless the glioma is an unequivocal glioblastoma, grading of malignancy is best saved for permanent sections after optimal evaluation of the entire sample (Tables 10.10 through 10.12). Some gliomas are highly vascular (97). The most confusing gliomas are multicentric, raising the question of metastatic disease (see "Lymphoma" and "Carcinoma" below) (99).

The second type of specimen is CNS parenchyma infiltrated by the margin of the glioma, and is a product of the infiltrative nature of many gliomas (8). It is often impossible to determine the histologic grade and type of glioma giving rise to an infiltrative margin of neoplastic glia when only the margin is available for examination. This should be explained to the surgeon during the operation, affording the surgeon the opportunity to obtain a better specimen.

Farther from the glioma itself, neoplastic glia in CNS parenchyma are difficult to distinguish from gliosis. Features that distinguish glioma cells from gliosis and normal parenchyma include pleomorphism, nuclear hyperchromasia, nuclear cluster formation (Fig. 10.33), nuclear molding, mitoses, and calcifications. Mitoses are rare in low-grade gliomas and are exceptionally rare in gliosis, even when associated with demyelination (68). Mitoses suggest not only that the tumor is a glioma, but also that it is a high-grade malignancy. Abnormal variations in size and shape of glial nuclei are more frequent than mitoses in margins of gliomas.

Gliomas expand whereas gliosis contracts. This important feature is difficult to confirm without serial radiographs and in situ observation of confluence of the actual mass and its margin to exclude the possibility of gliosis around a tumor or a cyst.

Granular calcifications scattered among hypercellular glia favor glioma over gliosis or normal white matter. Caution is required not to overinterpret calcifications associated with neurons and neuropil within 0.5 cm of a large mass. Lack of calcification is not useful in this context because microscopic calcifications are evident in only one-fourth of ependymomas and one-eighth of astrocytomas (98). Although microcysts, calcifications, and mitoses are important diagnostic features of gliomas, they are not seen in every case and are infrequent within the margins

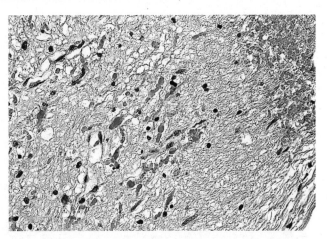

Figure 10.34. Gliosis. Cellular density increases slightly from one side of the field to the other. The elongated and beaded Rosenthal fibers in the center vary more in size and shape than the erythrocytes at the side, and they are not as orange. A nearby epidermoid cyst (not shown) produced this area of gliosis.

of gliomas invading CNS parenchyma (Tables 10.8 through 10.10).

Another important feature distinguishing the margin of a glioma from gliosis is cellular density. Cellular density is relatively constant in white matter, whereas cellular density in gray matter varies in a predictable laminar pattern reflecting the neuroanatomical arrangement of neurons and accompanying glia. Gliosis may show an even distribution of cellular density (Fig. 10.24) or a subtly increasing gradient of density from one side of the section to the other (Fig. 10.34). Certain gliomas exhibit uneven distribution of cellular density (Fig. 10.35). Others obscure the junction between gray and white matter. Still others spawn secondary structures of Scherer, the most distinctive being subpial and perineuronal gliomatosis (Fig. 10.36). These are collections of neoplastic glia beneath the pia or around neurons (100).

A helpful feature to consider is nuclear spacing. Glial nuclei in normal or gliotic parenchyma do not touch each other (Figs. 10.24 and 10.34). Glioma nuclei frequently touch and even indent one another (Figs. 10.35 through 10.37B). Strangely, this nuclear affinity often persists among scattered clusters of cells in the diffuse margins of gliomas.

Nuclear pleomorphism and hyperchromasia is valuable in distinguishing margins of gliomas (Fig. 10.33). Because the nuclei of gliomas are more pleomorphic than normal or gliotic CNS parenchyma, this helps to identify a glioma (4). Difficulties arise in judging the amount of pleomorphism and hyperchromasia because it requires a quantitative judgment, which is more difficult to perceive than a qualitative distinction. It is facilitated by close quality control of tissue processing.

Away from the tumor epicenter, diffuse astrocytomas may show only rare cells with atypical nuclei, no definitive, recognizable tumor. Rare gliomas produce diffuse and extensive involvement of the CNS called *gliomatosis cerebri*. The surgical diagnosis of gliomatosis cerebri requires correlation of MRI and biopsy (96).

Astrocytomas

Astrocytomas are among the most fibrillar of CNS neoplasms (Table 10.10). They present a number of difficult problems of

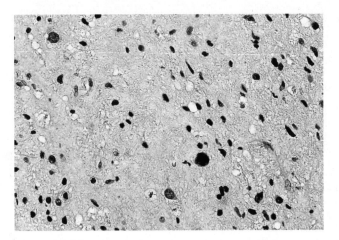

Figure 10.33. Margin of glioma. Pleomorphic and hyperchromatic nuclei cluster and touch one another among the axons of cerebral white matter. A few normochromatic nuclei provide a normal baseline.

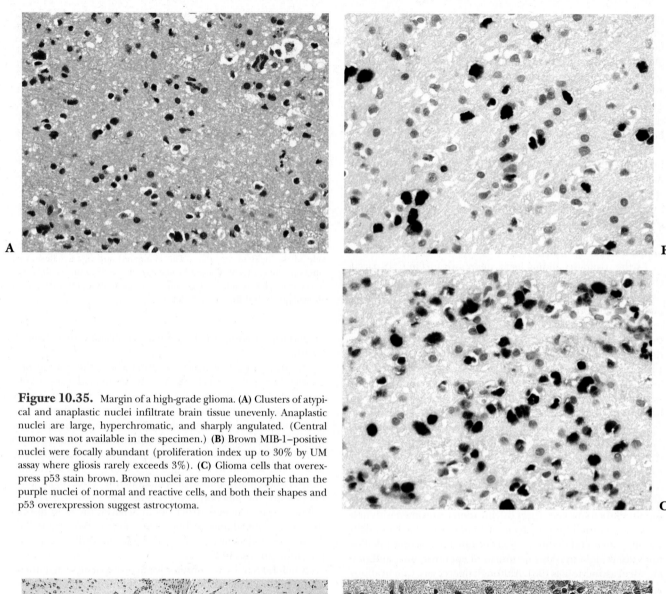

Figure 10.35. Margin of a high-grade glioma. **(A)** Clusters of atypical and anaplastic nuclei infiltrate brain tissue unevenly. Anaplastic nuclei are large, hyperchromatic, and sharply angulated. (Central tumor was not available in the specimen.) **(B)** Brown MIB-1–positive nuclei were focally abundant (proliferation index up to 30% by UM assay where gliosis rarely exceeds 3%). **(C)** Glioma cells that overexpress p53 stain brown. Brown nuclei are more pleomorphic than the purple nuclei of normal and reactive cells, and both their shapes and p53 overexpression suggest astrocytoma.

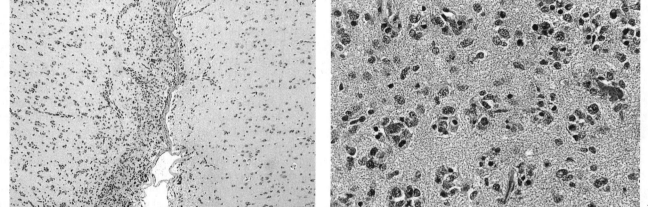

Figure 10.36. Secondary structures of Scherer. **(A)** Adjacent gyri are minimally and maximally infiltrated with glioma cells. Perivascular, perineuronal, and subpial gliomatoses are prominent in the maximally infiltrated gyrus. The pink arachnoid membrane in the center between gyri is not infiltrated. **(B)** Perineuronal gliomatosis. Neoplastic glia surround normal cerebral neurons at the margin of a glioma like ants around honey drops. This sample does not indicate the grade of glioma in the tumor itself.

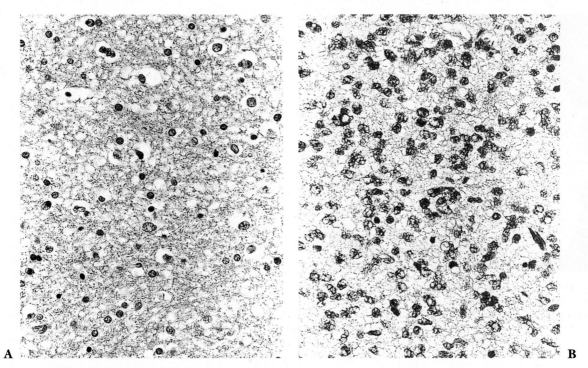

Figure 10.37. This partial resection of temporal lobe was diagnosed as "gliosis" **(A)**. A diffusely infiltrating World Health Organization grade 2 astrocytoma presented 10 years later near the site of the previous resection **(B)**.

recognition. Among the most treacherous is distinguishing low-grade astrocytoma from gliosis (Fig. 10.37; Tables 10.3 and 10.8 through 10.10). Features that distinguish astrocytoma from gliosis or normal parenchyma are described above (see "Gliomas"). One of these features, microcystic degeneration, is more typical of astrocytoma than other gliomas and is simplest to recognize on unfrozen tissue sections. On frozen sections, microcysts differ from ice artifact by their protein content (Fig. 10.32).

Astrocytomas as a group tend to be more fibrillar than other gliomas except tanycytic ependymomas and subependymomas (Table 10.10). Astrocytomas contain GFAP, although the amount is variable. GFAP is the single most important IHC marker distinguishing astrocytomas from nearly all nonglial neoplasms (89,90).

Astrocytomas are a heterogeneous group of neoplasms with numerous subtypes (101,102). Because some designations of subtypes emphasize grading (low-grade, anaplastic, and glioblastoma), whereas others emphasize structural differences (pilocytic, gemistocytic, and cystic), overlap in nomenclature is unavoidable. The most significant structural differences are ones that indicate a different prognosis. These include the pilocytic astrocytoma, which can frequently be cured by surgical removal in a clinically resectable region like cerebellum; and the gemistocytic astrocytoma, which has a poorer prognosis than is suggested by standard histologic criteria. Because of their importance to prognosis, these are described individually.

CYSTIC ASTROCYTOMA. Cystic astrocytomas are not a specific type or grade of tumor, but are a group of entities easily confused. They require a similar approach to avoid confusion. Macroscopically, cystic astrocytomas are usually low-grade astrocytomas, unless the cysts contain necrosis. Although macroscopic cysts can occur in almost any astrocytoma, they are most

frequent in low-grade pilocytic astrocytomas of the cerebellum (see "Pilocytic Astrocytoma" below). They must be distinguished from hemangioblastoma (Table 10.10) (see "Hemangioblastoma" below). There is some question whether the simple cyst of the cerebellum is derived from a cystic astrocytoma of extremely low grade. The first approach to both of these questions is to encourage the neurosurgeon to search diligently for a nodule on the inner wall of the cyst (mural nodule). This can be facilitated by radiography and by intraoperative microscopic consultation. If the entire cyst is removed, then the pathologist submits all thick and translucent gray material, vascular material, and enigmatic material for paraffin sections.

PILOCYTIC ASTROCYTOMA—GRADE I. The pilocytic astrocytoma is about the only good news in the astrocytoma series because it has a better prognosis than its diffuse counterparts, especially when it occurs in a resectable location like the cerebellum (103–105). Even this is tempered by the facts that adequate surgical removal of a pilocytic astrocytoma depends on its location, and that some pilocytic astrocytomas develop multicentric disease (106). The 10-year survival of supratentorial cases is 100% after gross total resection and 74% after subtotal resection or biopsy (104). Some pilocytic astrocytomas have surprisingly discrete margins, but others show local microscopic infiltration despite a well-demarcated MR image (1).

Most, but not all, pilocytic astrocytomas occur in children or young adults. They are most abundant in the posterior fossa, where they represent the majority of childhood astrocytomas (Table 10.7). They are also found around the third ventricle, thalamus, hypothalamus, and neurohypophysis, where they can be difficult to control due to their location near clinically sensitive brain structures (Fig. 10.38) (107). Cerebral hemispheric

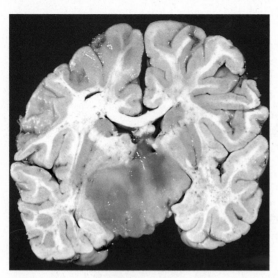

Figure 10.38. This peri–third-ventricular pilocytic astrocytoma in a 13-month-old patient escaped therapy. Nonetheless, its margin with the brain is typically discrete. The tumor parenchyma is light gray. Darker regions are mucinous cysts and clusters of microcysts. *(Courtesy of Dr. Patricia Uherova, University of Michigan, Ann Arbor, Michigan.)*

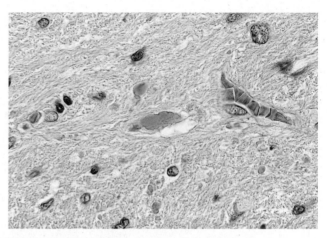

Figure 10.40. Pilocytic astrocytoma, cerebellar, from a mural nodule in a cystic lesion. Rosenthal fibers in the central field mingle with protein droplets. Both are pinker and less uniform in diameter than the erythrocytes lateral to them.

pilocytic astrocytomas are less common but important to recognize to ensure appropriate treatment (103).

Because of its usual benign nature, it is important to distinguish the pilocytic astrocytoma from other astrocytomas (Tables 10.8, 10.10, and 10.18). *Pilocytic* means "hair cell," one of the major features of this astrocytoma. Parallel bundles of elongated, fibrillar cytoplasmic processes resemble mats of hair (Fig. 10.39A). These hairlike processes contain large amounts of glial fibrils that stain well with either PTAH or IHC evaluation for GFAP (Fig. 10.39B).

Rosenthal fibers are highly eosinophilic, hyaline structures (Fig. 10.34 and 10.40). They are round, oval, or beaded, with slightly irregular margins, resembling cracked glass, resulting from their formation within glial processes. In contrast to erythrocytes, they are pink rather than orange and have greater variation in size and shape. They contain ubiquinated alpha B-crystallin, which can be identified by IHC. Although Rosenthal

fibers assist in distinguishing the pilocytic astrocytoma from other variants, they are of no value in differentiating astrocytomas from gliosis, since they occur in both. They indicate chronicity of a process—reactive (e.g., gliosis adjacent to an abscess wall) or neoplastic (e.g., gangliogliomas).

Eosinophilic granular bodies consist of droplets of protein sometimes found in association with Rosenthal fibers. These protein droplets are usually intracellular, but occasionally are extracellular and up to 40 μm in diameter. Their bright pink color, similar to Rosenthal fibers, distinguishes them from mucoid degeneration in oligodendrogliomas. They are PAS-positive and can be IHC stained with alpha 1-antichymotrypsin. They should not be confused with lipid-laden macrophages that have multiple clear vacuoles (Fig. 10.5) or with hemosiderin-laden macrophages. These eosinophilic changes in cytoplasm and fibrils cannot be used in isolation to grade astrocytomas because they are occasionally found in higher-grade neoplasms.

Pilocytic astrocytomas are often microcystic, and they may be macrocystic. In the cerebellum, the cysts can be quite large, necessitating a search by the neurosurgeon for a mural nodule.

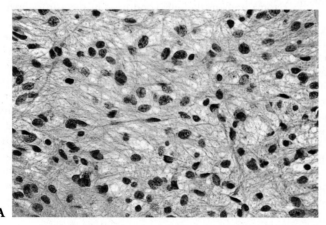 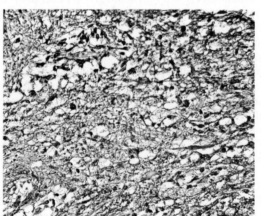

Figure 10.39. Pilocytic astrocytoma. **(A)** This low-grade glioma manifests both bipolar neoplastic cells with elongated, hairlike processes projecting from either end and other neoplastic cells with multiple processes. **(B)** Glial fibrillary acidic protein immunoperoxidase is strongly positive in the processes of the neoplastic cells.

This mural nodule and its solid counterpart are often very vascular and resemble a hemangioblastoma, particularly on frozen section when the hemangioblastoma cells appear fibrillar (102). Unlike hemangioblastoma, the mural nodule of a pilocytic astrocytoma contains GFAP-positive neoplastic astrocytes negative for lipids on staining. Calcifications favor an astrocytoma.

The *pilomyxoid astrocytoma* (PMA) is a relative of the pilocytic astrocytoma typically found in very young children (months to 2 years). It tapers to rare in older patients, but the exact incidence is unknown due to its scarcity. It has bipolar cells that cluster around vessels, but its parenchyma is more pilocytic than ependymomatous. This angiocentricity and its mucinous matrix characterize the PMA (108). Perhaps partly because its most common location is near hypothalamus and optic chiasm (where it is hard to remove) and near meninges, local recurrence and CSF spread are more common with PMAs than pilocytic astrocytomas. PMA is considered a grade II rather than a grade I.

Pilocytic astrocytomas rarely manifest malignant degeneration to grade III, indicated by hypercellularity, mitoses, and necrosis. Endothelial proliferation or invasion of the subarachnoid space does not alone signal a bad prognosis.

DIFFUSE ASTROCYTOMA—GRADE II. The term *diffuse* has been generally accepted to distinguish grade II astrocytomas from the more circumscribed grade I astrocytomas like the pilocytic astrocytoma. Common sense argues for this definitive terminology that emphasizes resectability, and simplifies grading of low-grade astrocytomas.

The term *diffuse* appropriately describes these neoplasms because their margin gradually diminishes in cellularity. Within the extensive margin, neoplastic cells intermingle with CNS parenchyma (Fig. 10.33) (4). These astrocytomas can be particularly difficult to distinguish from gliosis in small samples. Look for atypical nuclei (hyperchromatic and pleomorphic nuclei) with regional crowding in astrocytomas. Some low-grade astrocytomas produce no tumor that can be distinguished from brain parenchyma, but, rather, only a diffuse infiltration of the parenchyma that resembles the margin of a glioma (see "Tumor and Tumor Margin," above). Diffuse invasion of CNS parenchyma may also be evident by formation of secondary structures of Scherer (see "Gliomas," above).

The diffuse nature of growth and infiltration of low-grade astrocytomas demonstrates why they are so seldom cured despite their relatively benign histology. Postoperative survival averages 7 years, but the range of individual survival is large. In adequate specimens, MIB-1 aids estimation of survival (84). Astrocytomas have a worse prognosis when located in the brainstem.

Protoplasmic, fibrillary, and gemistocytic astrocytomas are all diffuse astrocytomas. Special features of gemistocytic astrocytomas are described separately below because they can be confused with reactive astrocytes and with oligodendroglial minigemistocytes.

Protoplasmic astrocytoma. The historical diagnosis of protoplasmic astrocytoma is rare, and has diminished by encroachment of new diagnoses (e.g., pilomyxoid astrocytoma) and broadening of others (e.g., oligoastrocytoma). They are presently an endangered species, which unfortunately does not help the patient with one. Protoplasmic astrocytomas are thought to have small-cell bodies, round to oval nuclei, few cellular pro-

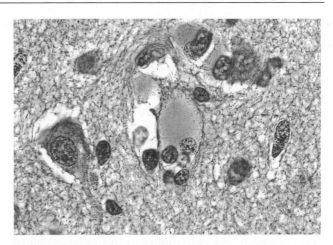

Figure 10.41. Gemistocytic astrocytoma. Plump gemistocyte in the center contains hyaline pink cytoplasm and lacks purple Nissl substance, in contrast to the more angular neuron nearby. Although the nuclear: cytoplasmic ratio of the neuron appears greater than that of the gemistocyte, the neuron, in contrast to the gemistocyte, may be a few feet long.

cesses, and numerous microcysts filled with faintly purple mucoid material.

Fibrillary astrocytoma. Fibrillary astrocytomas are common. They are a mixture of (fibrillary) cellular processes and nuclei of greater angularity and density than CNS parenchyma (Fig. 10.4B). They contain more cytoplasm and their cellular processes are longer and with more glial fibrillary acidic protein (GFAP) than protoplasmic astrocytomas. Both subtypes produce microcysts; however, microcysts are particularly prominent in protoplasmic astrocytomas in which case they tend to degenerate into macrocysts (1). Prognostic implications of these two categories of low-grade astrocytoma are unclear. On the other hand, gemistocytic astrocytomas tend to progress to higher grades quite easily (see "Gemistocytic Astrocytoma," below).

Gemistocytic astrocytoma. Gemistocytes are conspicuous within this variant of diffuse astrocytoma (Table 10.10). They are astrocytes with a distended, hyaline, pink cytoplasm packed with GFAP fibrils (Figs. 10.1, 10.41, and 10.42). Their nuclei are

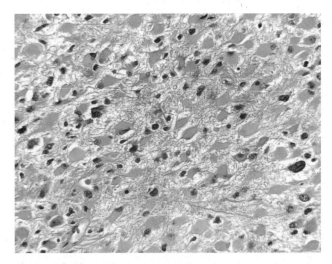

Figure 10.42. Gemistocytic astrocytoma has long cytoplasmic processes and nuclei of various shapes, including long, bowtie, boomerang, and teardrop nuclei. Compare this with minigemistocytes (also known as microgemistocytes) in some oligodendrogliomas (Fig. 10.56).

pleomorphic and often are at the rim of the cell, producing a bizarre caricature of a reactive astrocyte (Fig. 10.42). In practice, distinction from reactive gemistocytes is best done using the greater nuclear hyperchromasia and elongation (e.g., "boomerang" nuclei) of neoplastic gemistocytes. Perivascular cuffs of polyclonal lymphocytes are common in gemistocytic astrocytoma. Neoplastic gemistocytes should comprise approximately 20% or more of the neoplasm to merit the name gemistocytic astrocytoma. Gemistocytic astrocytomas frequently are clinically aggressive, can progress quickly to anaplastic astrocytoma, and generally produce a poorer prognosis than suggested by their histologic grade.

Differential diagnosis. The differential diagnosis of astrocytomas includes an oligodendroglioma, so care must be taken to rule out an admixed or separate oligodendroglioma component. Look for at least some oddly shaped or elongated nuclei in astrocytomas. In contrast, an oligodendroglioma is distinguished by abundant to ubiquitous round nuclei, often surrounded by clear, perinuclear halos. Thin, branching capillaries favor oligodendroglioma. At biopsy, cytologic preparations (12) are often more informative than frozen sections in distinguishing these two gliomas. The classic or pure oligodendroglioma cell often has a 1p and/or 19q chromosomal deletion, and has little or no GFAP. Look for long GFAP-positive cellular processes and/or p53 overexpression in astrocytoma cells (109).

Gemistocytic astrocytoma cells must be distinguished from the now-called minigemistocytes of oligodendroglioma. Look for monotonous small, round nuclei in minigemistocytes. Gemistocytic cells in an astrocytoma must be distinguished from reactive astrocytes. Reactive astrocytes are well spaced and do not crowd each other, like the trees in an orchard; their nuclei are generally round or oval, uniform in size, and, although enlarged with an open chromatin pattern, are not atypical (hyperchromatic, pleomorphic). Gemistocytic astrocytomas can be distinguished from gangliogliomas by their lack of dysplastic and/or neoplastic neurons (Fig. 10.1) and from subependymal giant-cell tumors by their smaller nuclei and greater tendency to infiltrate CNS.

Summary Points About Diffuse Astrocytoma

- Key microscopic findings: Infiltrating glial cells with atypical nuclei and some elongated nuclei; fibrillary cellular processes; at least focally hypercellular. Absent or extremely rare mitotic figures (Table 10.8); necrosis or microvascular proliferation are absent.
- IHC and molecular findings: Astrocytomas express GFAP and S-100 in the cell body and long cellular processes. High MIB-1 suggests short survival (84). p53 overexpression, found in about half of diffuse astrocytomas, is helpful in distinguishing gliosis from glioma.

GLIOMATOSIS CEREBRI. The ultimate manifestation of diffuse growth (or of widespread neoplastic transformation) is gliomatosis cerebri, where neoplastic glia spread widely throughout the brain, sometimes manifesting a peculiar, almost neuroanatomical distribution in gray or white matter. It involves more than two cerebral lobes and is frequently bilateral (8,100). Involvement of thalamus and basal ganglia is common. Gliomatosis cerebri was considered a high-grade malignant glioma, but long survivors are known (110). Survival (96) and molecular

(111) studies confirm that gliomatosis cerebri is a subtype of astrocytoma that can be graded like astrocytoma. The grade is usually III, sometimes II or IV.

ANAPLASTIC ASTROCYTOMA—GRADE III. The designation *anaplastic* emphasizes the grade of malignancy. Mitoses are considered a feature of anaplastic astrocytomas because the percentage of mitoses in low-grade diffuse astrocytomas is so low that the standard microscopic section of biopsy material usually does not yield conspicuous mitoses (Tables 10.8, 10.10 through 10.12). Phosphohistone H3 (PHH3) is a specific IHC marker of cells undergoing mitosis. PHH3 staining helps to identify and quantify mitoses, which helps to distinguish anaplastic astrocytomas from grade II astrocytomas (112).

Quantitative features shared by high-grade gliomas are increased cellular density, increased nuclear pleomorphism, and increased nuclear hyperchromatism (Fig. 10.43). It is difficult to objectify such quantitative criteria without morphometry. Our rule of thumb for evaluating cellular density is that the average distance between a nucleus and its nearest neighbor (not actually touching) should be less than the average nuclear diameter before the density is considered conclusive evidence of anaplasia. Forty percent of anaplastic astrocytomas show loss of DNA from the long arm of chromosome 19 (113,114).

The lack of foci of coagulation necrosis and lack of microvascular proliferation in an astrocytic glioma distinguishes anaplastic astrocytomas from glioblastomas (Table 10.10), but individual cells with pyknotic nuclei may be interspersed in anaplastic astrocytomas. Care must be taken to discern any oligodendroglioma component of a glial neoplasm; foci of necrosis are acceptable for the diagnosis of an anaplastic oligoastrocytoma. Likewise, the possibility of an ependymoma must be ruled out. Check for perivascular pseudorosettes and true ependymal rosettes.

Average survival of patients with anaplastic astrocytoma is slightly more than 2 years. Rare anaplastic astrocytomas are associated with hereditary colonic polyposis or neurofibromatosis (4,113).

OTHER VARIANTS OF ASTROCYTOMA. **Subependymal giant-cell astrocytoma (SEGA).** The SEGA has a distinctive loca-

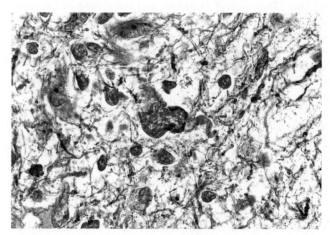

Figure 10.43. Anaplastic astrocytoma. Pleomorphism of nuclei in glial fibrillary acidic protein (GFAP)-positive cells is conspicuous (immunoperoxidase anti-GFAP with hematoxylin).

tion, histology, and association with tuberous sclerosis (115). Tuberous sclerosis is an autosomal dominant syndrome that causes hamartomas and benign neoplasms. It is associated with mutations in the TSC1 gene on chromosome 9q34 and the TSC2 gene on chromosome 16p13.3. These tumor suppressor genes produce proteins hamartin and tuberin (116). The tumor arises from the medial portion of the floor of the lateral ventricle in the region where subependymal nodules of giant astrocytes, called "candle gutterings," are frequently found. The tumor grows into the lateral ventricle and may obstruct the foramen of Monro. It is composed of giant astrocytes with large nuclei and prominent nucleoli (Fig. 10.44). Although pleomorphic, their nuclei lack sharp angulations. These cells may contain stainable glial filaments (Fig. 10.44B), but lack Nissl substance. Some have neurofilaments. These giant astrocytes and their characteristically thick cytoplasmic processes have a tendency to form disoriented fascicles. Their pleomorphism is at variance with their relatively benign behavior. It is very important to recognize this histologic entity because necrosis, endothelial proliferation, and mitoses are neither as common nor as ominous as in diffuse cerebral astrocytomas.

Astroblastoma. The existence of astroblastoma as a pure pathologic entity is debated. Its grade has not been established (8). Astroblastic "rosettes" resemble perivascular pseudorosettes of ependymomas except that the astroblastic processes remain thick throughout the entire distance from cell body to adventitia of the vessel (115). Foot processes may even thicken near the adventitia (Fig. 10.45). Because other gliomas may have foci like this, the pattern must predominate in a well-circumscribed tumor to be an astroblastoma. Although astroblastomas express focal GFAP, they do not stain with PTAH. This dichotomy may be due to expression of a nonfibrillar form of the GFAP molecule.

Pleomorphic xanthoastrocytoma (PXA). The PXA is a bizarre, supratentorial astrocytoma of young people that often involves both the leptomeninges and cerebral cortex (117). It occasionally hemorrhages (118). Its fibrillarity and its pleomorphic, hyaline, lipid-laden, giant cells, and multinucleated cells are clues to its diagnosis. Protein granular degeneration may be

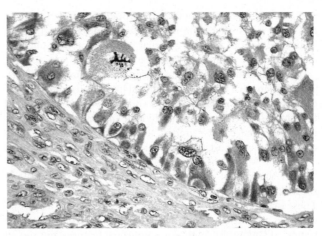

Figure 10.45. Astroblastic processes highlighted with glial fibrillary acidic protein stain are thick near the vascular adventitia, and they may even expand into foot processes.

prominent, similar to pilocytic astrocytoma. Intracellular lipid content is an important feature, and the empty round vacuoles are seen well in paraffin sections after GFAP staining. Astrocytes are confirmed by demonstrating strongly GFAP-positive cells, often with histiocytic features. These cells are often surrounded by reticulin fibers, which break a general rule that glioma cells lack reticulin. Neuronal elements in some tumors suggest that some pleomorphic xanthoastrocytomas may be the glial portion of a ganglioglioma (119).

Granular cell tumors. Location, location, location. This problem with granular cell tumors reaches beyond semantics to prognosis. In the infundulum, they are circumscribed and benign, but in the cerebrum they are usually infiltrative and malignant (101,120; compare with Chapter 12, The Pituitary and Sella Region). Their histologic features are the same: plump, round cells filled with cytoplasmic granules. These cells are PAS– and S-100–positive but often GFAP-negative.

Cerebral granular cell tumors are variants of astrocytomas

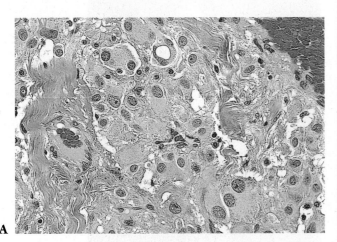

A

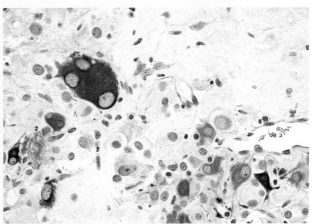

B

Figure 10.44. Subependymal giant-cell astrocytoma. **(A)** Huge cells with large nuclei and abundant, finely granular cytoplasm mingle with bright pink cellular processes. Despite their size, most nuclei are round to oval with delicately stippled chromatin and no mitoses. This tumor grew into the third ventricle of a 21-year-old man with tuberous sclerosis. **(B)** Typical mixture of glial fibrillary acidic protein (GFAP)-positive and -negative cells in a subependymal giant-cell astrocytoma. This tumor was negative with neuronal markers (immunoperoxidase anti-GFAP with hematoxylin).

and glioblastomas. They need to be properly identified to avoid confusion with other tumors (including neuroendocrine and histiocytic tumors and the granular cells common in pilocytic astrocytomas) and macrophage reactions.

Glioneuronal tumor with neuropil-like islands (GNTNI). The glioneuronal tumor with neuropil-like islands is a rare, infiltrating astrocytoma that contains rounded islands of neuropil that stains for synaptophysin within the tumor. It is an infiltrating tumor that can be graded II or III by criteria for more common forms of astrocytoma (8).

There is work to be done classifying the tumors listed in the "Other Variants of Astrocytoma" section. For example, neuropil-like islands are a defining characteristic of the GNTNI. These islands within this tumor raise questions about its classification as an astrocytoma rather than as a mixed glial-neuronal tumor. SEGA and PXA also show neuronal features, but not all tumors show them. SEGA and PXA could be split into pure and mixed varieties, like the split of desmoplastic infantile astrocytoma and desmoplastic infantile ganglioglioma. Such splits are reasonable if they demonstrate prognostic or therapeutic value.

GLIOBLASTOMA MULTIFORME (GLIOBLASTOMA)—GRADE IV. Glioblastoma is now considered the most malignant astrocytoma. In fact, it is a glioma that may be uniformly undifferentiated, but often also contains focal astrocytoma, less often oligodendroglioma, and, rarely, ependymoma. Most commonly, a lower-grade glioma may progress to glioblastoma over time, and many of these progressions are associated with specific genetic alterations, including loss of genetic material in chromosome 10 (121). A de novo glioblastoma appears to exist as well and manifests EGFR amplification, a separate molecular alteration from the glioblastoma arising from a low-grade astrocytoma that is often associated with a p53 mutation rather than epidermal growth factor receptor (EGFR) amplification (122).

Although most glioblastomas are supratentorial (Figs. 10.46 and 47), they also occur in the brainstem, uncommonly in the cerebellum, and rarely in the spinal cord. They are even more devastating in these locations than in the cerebrum, due to smaller spaces for their expansion.

A malignant astrocytoma with the additional feature of either necrosis or microvascular proliferation is now considered a glioblastoma (101) (Table 10.8) (Figs. 10.48 through 10.50). Other malignant features of glioblastomas include hypercellularity, bizarre nuclei, multinucleated cells, mitoses (Fig. 10.49), and abnormal mitotic spindles (Fig. 10.50). Unfortunately, the heterogeneity of glioblastomas for these histologic features compromises diagnoses obtained on small biopsies (such as stereotactic needle biopsies) and jeopardizes accurate grading (123).

Microvascular proliferation (increased density of cells in vascular walls) is an important characteristic of grade IV diffuse astrocytomas. Formerly called endothelial proliferation, microvascular proliferation is a criterion of glioblastoma in diffuse astrocytomas that also have cytologic anaplasia (Fig. 10.50). Endothelial proliferation is a qualitative feature that is relatively simple to recognize in either of its two forms. One form is simply an increase in the number of nuclei within the vascular wall, and the other form is the formation of multiple lumina within the vascular structure so that it resembles a renal glomerulus.

Most confusion arises in distinguishing glioblastoma from malignant meningioma and from carcinoma. Unlike many metastases, the glioblastoma is nearly always solitary upon first encounter, although it may have already invaded across the midline via the corpus callosum, massa intermedia, or anterior

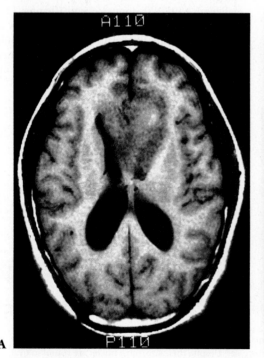 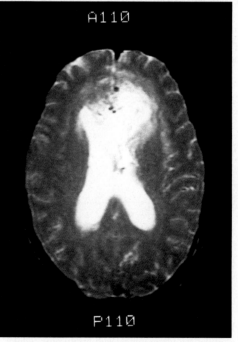

Figure 10.46. Frontal glioblastoma multiforme. This glioma in this 40-year-old man has crossed the midline, and it involves both frontal lobes on magnetic resonance images. **(A)** Heterogeneous signal on a T1-weighted image. **(B)** Bright signal on a T2-weighted image. *(Courtesy of Dr. James Brunberg, University of Michigan, Ann Arbor, Michigan.)*

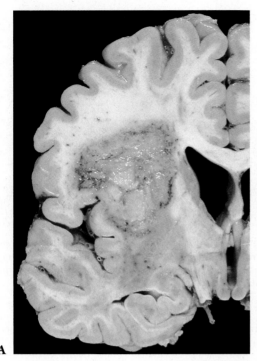
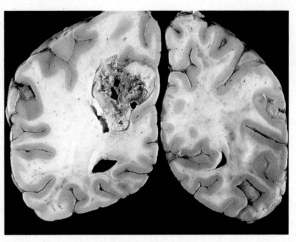

Figure 10.47. Glioblastoma. **(A)** This untreated glioblastoma was observed in an 84-year-old man. Considerable spontaneous necrosis is noted grossly. **(B)** Left parietal glioblastoma in this 44-year-old woman contains multiform regions of light tan neoplasm, shaggy white necrotic neoplasm, blue-gray semitranslucent fibrovascular tissue, brown hemorrhage, and dark cavities. Its margin with the brain appears distinct despite microscopic invasion. This is common in fast-growing glioblastoma, and it has been called a *pseudocapsule* (*B, Courtesy of Dr. Leslie Bruch, Washington University, St. Louis, Missouri.*)

commissure to produce a so-called butterfly lesion. Unlike carcinoma and meningioma, glioblastomas are fibrillar rather than epithelioid or syncytial (Tables 10.10, 10.11, 10.12, and 10.14). Although the rapid growth of a glioblastoma may produce a "pseudocapsule," neoplastic glia are evident beyond this margin within the parenchyma, often forming secondary structures of Scherer (see "Gliomas," above). Glioblastoma contains

GFAP (Fig. 10.31) lacking in carcinoma and malignant meningioma, although either nonglial neoplasm may trap islands of CNS parenchyma and stimulate gliosis (121).

Molecular oncology provides insights into the variable responses of glioblastomas to chemotherapy. O6 methylguanine DNA methyltransferase (MGMT) is a DNA-repair enzyme. It removes methyl groups from O6 methylguanine, an abnormal

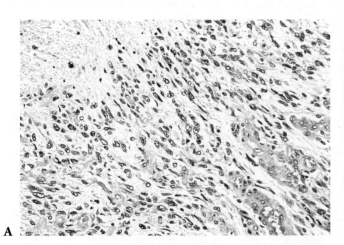
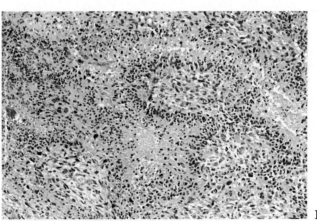

Figure 10.48. Glioblastoma. **(A)** Coagulation necrosis in the pale corner is key to the diagnosis of glioblastoma. Microvascular proliferation (formerly "endothelial proliferation") thickens vascular walls in the opposite corner of this field. This is the contemporary term for hypertrophy and hyperplasia of various cells in the vessel wall. **(B)** Focally, neoplastic cells surround the necrotic tumor, a feature of glioblastoma called *perinecrotic pseudopalisades.*

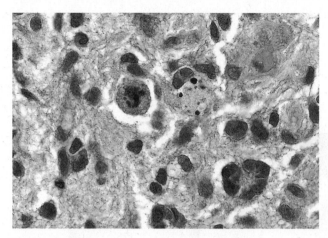

Figure 10.49. Glioblastoma. Anaplastic astrocytes should be evident in addition to coagulation necrosis and/or endothelial proliferation to confirm a glioblastoma. Mitoses, multinucleated tumor cells, and karyorrhectic cells occur.

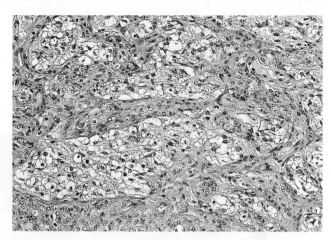

Figure 10.51. Gliosarcoma. Interwoven bands of dark pink fibrovascular and light pink glial tissue are seen in this right temporal lobe gliosarcoma. The neoplasm is hypercellular and pleomorphic, and it contains mitoses in both tissues.

guanine harmful to DNA, good when protecting normal cells. But MGMT also removes methyl groups from O6 methylguanine glioblastoma cells produced by alkylating chemotherapy agents like temozolomide, hindering the effect of these important drugs. But nearly half of glioblastoma cannot produce MGMT, rendering these tumors sensitive to alkylating agents. This can be detected by PCR, thus predicting which patients have glioblastomas sensitive to temozolomide (96). This test is not generally available now, but it may be available in the next few years (124).

GLIOSARCOMA—GRADE IV. A gliosarcoma is a mixture of glioblastoma and sarcoma. Regions of collagen-positive and GFAP-negative sarcoma cells bridge the glioblastoma in a marbled configuration (Tables 10.10 and 10.12; Figs. 10.51 and 10.52). It is critical for the pathologist to be aware of this entity because of the tendency for radiologists and neurosurgeons to interpret superficial, well-circumscribed gliosarcomas as meningioma. Tumor progression from gliosarcomas to pure sarcoma lacking GFAP-positive cells can occur (125). Aberrant expres-

sion of epithelial markers and lipid production is occasionally seen in gliosarcoma and in glioblastoma (126).

Oligodendrogliomas

Oligodendrogliomas must be distinguished from astrocytomas because their prognoses and treatments differ. On average, an oligodendroglioma of the same grade as an astrocytoma has a better prognosis than the astrocytoma and is more susceptible to combined chemotherapy than the astrocytoma. The most useful markers of oligodendrogliomas are structural features seen on H&E: cells with uniformly round nuclei that all look alike. These cells often show perinuclear halos on paraffin sections (127).

Every year or two a new immunohistochemical marker of oligodendroglioma emerges, but none has lasted. Arguably the best positive marker right now seems to be deletions on the short arm of chromosome 1 (1p) and the long arm of chromosome 19 (19q) (128–130). GFAP is useful combined with structural features, the most important of which is round nuclei.

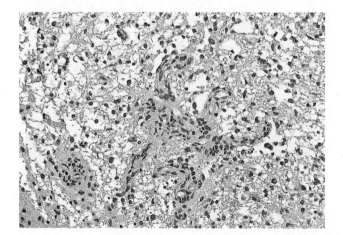

Figure 10.50. Glioblastoma. Branching microvascular proliferation is prominent. This finding and cytologic features of anaplastic astrocytes are sufficient criteria for glioblastoma.

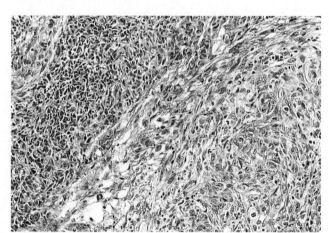

Figure 10.52. Gliosarcoma. Sarcomatous regions of gliosarcoma produce collagen stained blue, whereas red regions of glioma lack collagen (trichrome stain).

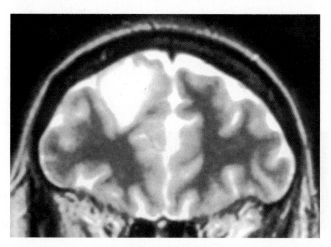

Figure 10.53. Oligodendroglioma. Imaging of a frontal lobe lesion in a young woman with new-onset seizures reveals a relatively circumscribed lesion.

Classic oligodendroglioma have little or no GFAP; less classic oligodendroglioma have some cells with GFAP only in their cell bodies or in short processes.

OLIGODENDROGLIOMA—GRADE II. The oligodendroglioma, found frequently in the temporal and frontal lobes of young adults (Fig. 10.53), and its anaplastic counterparts have been found to respond to combined PCV chemotherapy [procarbazine, chloroethylcyclohexylnitrosourea (CCNU), and vincristine (PCV)] (129). This chemotherapy responsiveness has put a premium on its recognition. Those anaplastic oligodendrogliomas that manifest losses in the short arm of chromosome 1 (1p) are particularly sensitive to PCV chemotherapy; thus, molecular characterization of tumors with oligodendroglioma components is being used as a guide to therapy (128).

Oligodendrogliomas can be found in pure forms or, commonly, found mixed with astrocytoma. The pure oligodendroglioma differs from other gliomas, except for a few ependymomas, in having an epithelioid rather than a fibrillar appearance (Table 10.11) (Fig. 10.54). This appearance is most evident within the central portion of the neoplasm, which is most crowded with neoplastic cells. Well-differentiated oligodendrogliomas ("classic" oligodendrogliomas) are characterized by remarkably round and regular nuclei centrally placed within cells, which on paraffin-embedded tissue manifest a perinuclear halo and thereby resemble a fried egg (Table 10.9). These can diffusely infiltrate brain tissue (Fig. 10.55). They have a fine capillary network, described as "chicken wire," which can segregate the parenchyma into small lobules, and they often have admixed multifocal regions of mineralization (Fig. 10.54). Because it is an artifact of fixation, the absence of perinuclear halos, as in frozen section preparations, does not rule out oligodendroglioma; it may merely reflect prompt fixation. Deletions in chromosomes 1p and19q have been shown to be markers of classic oligodendroglial histology (131–133). Assuming the continued absence of at least one sensitive and specific IHC marker for oligodendroglioma cells, the combined 1p/19q chromosomal marker will eventually be incorporated into diagnostic criteria for oligodendrogliomas (Fig. 10.55B).

Pure oligodendrogliomas are easily diagnosed histologically. However, identifying the oligodendroglioma component in the mixed glioma, oligoastrocytoma, is difficult. This difficulty in the past has been complicated by the lack of a specific marker for oligodendroglioma that withstands paraffin embedding limits the usefulness of immunostaining. Oligodendrogliomas are highly variable in their GFAP expression and, in fact, many oligodendrogliomas are negative (Fig. 10.56). The marker MAP-2 strongly labels many oligodendroglial cells, and this may be a much needed marker (134). The broad specificity of Leu-7 and S-100 limits their use. However, an oligodendroglioma invading the meninges can be differentiated from a meningioma by its positivity with the Leu-7 monoclonal antibody, since meningiomas are typically negative.

The category of oligodendroglioma has been broadened to include some tumors formerly considered astrocytic or mixed gliomas. "Minigemistocytes" or "microgemistocytes" are now considered oligodendroglial (92). Nuclei of minigemistocytes have clumped and marginated chromatin and are slightly larger than those of nonneoplastic oligodendroglia. Their nuclei are

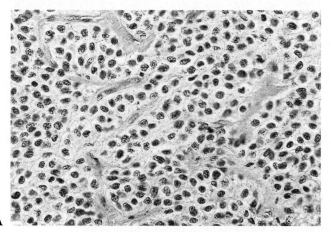

A

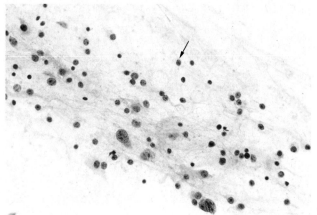

B

Figure 10.54. Oligodendrogliomas. **(A)** A delicate fibrovascular stroma divides groups of cells with perinuclear halos into nests. **(B)** Intraoperative cytologic preparation of another grade II oligodendroglioma shows cells with round nuclei of various sizes larger than nonneoplastic glia (*arrow*). Cytologic preparations lightly touched to a slide and immediately fixed show oligodendroglial nuclear features better than do frozen sections.

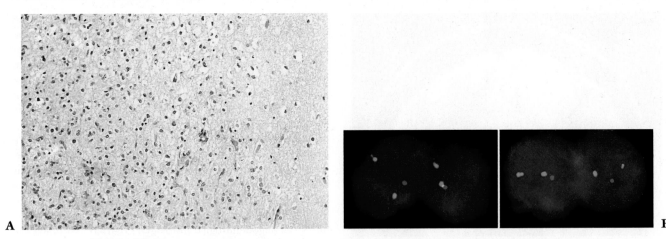

A   B

Figure 10.55. Oligodendrogliomas. **(A)** Neoplastic cells with perinuclear halos infiltrate the brain paren-chyma. This diffuse margin of infiltration distinguishes oligodendroglioma from neoplasms with cells of similar appearance, such as meningiomas, pituitary adenomas, and most carcinomas. **(B)** In each of two blue-stained nuclei on the left, the red probe shows a 1p deletion. On the right, a different red probe shows a 19q deletion in both nuclei. Green control probes show the expected two copies per diploid nucleus. *(Fluorescence in situ hybridization images contributed by Dr. Philip J. Boyer, Department of Pathology, University of Colorado Health Science Center, Denver, Colorado.)*

smaller and rounder than gemistocytes in gemistocytic astrocy-tomas. Minigemistocytes classically have only a ball of GFAP immunoreactivity near their nucleus, but many are not classic and have GFAP in their short processes (Fig. 10.56).

The epithelioid appearance of pure oligodendrogliomas imi-tates true epithelial neoplasms and other gliomas with epitheli-oid features (Tables 10.11 and 10.12) (135). Suprasellar oligo-dendrogliomas may be mistaken for pituitary adenomas. Oligodendrogliomas near sites frequented by meningiomas may be confused with meningotheliomatous meningiomas or with lipoid metaplasia in meningiomas. Anaplastic oligodendro-gliomas simulate metastatic carcinoma, particularly renal cell carcinoma. More than two-thirds of oligodendrogliomas con-tain microscopic calcifications that distinguish them from he-

mangioblastoma and most metastatic carcinomas. A pure oligo-dendroglioma is actually less fibrillar than the neuroectodermal tumors it imitates, including central neurocytoma and clear-cell ependymoma.

If the margin of the neoplasm is sampled in addition to the central region, even macroscopically discrete oligodendroglio-mas have a more diffuse margin with CNS parenchyma than do adenomas, carcinomas, and meningiomas (Fig. 10.55). Second-ary structures are frequent, especially perineuronal gliomatosis (see ''Astrocytomas'' and ''Gliomas,'' above). Precise localiza-tion of the biopsy specimen is helpful because oligodendroglio-mas do not originate from the adenohypophysis or dura and rarely invade them. A panel of immunostains for chromogranin and pituitary hormones identifies adenomas, and epithelial

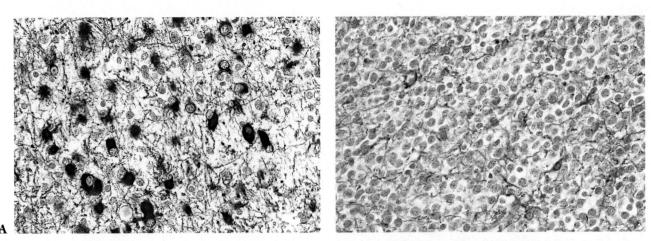

A   B

Figure 10.56. Both these right temporal lobe tumors are called *oligodendrogliomas*, primarily based on the roundness of their nuclei. **(A)** This tumor from a 44-year-old woman contains numerous glial fibrillary acidic protein (GFAP)-positive minigemistocytes with round nuclei and relatively short processes. **(B)** This tumor from a 29-year-old woman has classic GFAP-negative neoplastic cells. Both tumors have intermingled GFAP-positive processes from trapped reactive astrocytes with smaller nuclei.

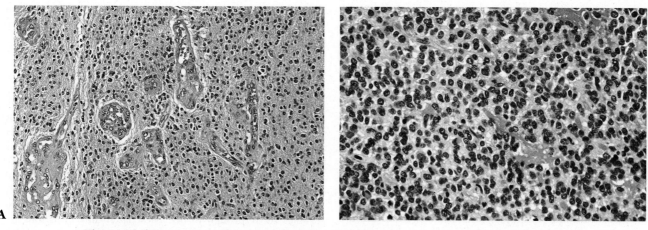

Figure 10.57. Anaplastic oligodendroglioma from the left frontal lobe of a 35-year-old woman. **(A)** Microvascular proliferation (*arrow*). **(B)** Another region of this tumor is crowded with cells. Conspicuously atypical nuclei are predominantly round and hyperchromatic. Mitoses are common.

membrane antigen (EMA) distinguishes meningiomas from oligodendrogliomas.

ANAPLASTIC OLIGODENDROGLIOMA (MALIGNANT OLIGODENDROGLIOMA)—GRADE III. The features of anaplastic transformation in oligodendroglioma (Fig. 10.57) include increased cellularity, nuclear atypia, necrosis, and increased mitotic activity (Tables 10.9 and 10.11). Limited amounts of microvascular proliferation are frequently present in oligodendrogliomas, and in isolation cannot be considered evidence of malignant transformation. Better prognosis and sensitivity to PCV or Temodar chemotherapy is particularly well defined in the subset of these tumors with losses in chromosome 1p. Because of their link to better prognosis and sensitivity to chemotherapy, testing for deletions in chromosomes 1p and 19q is fast becoming the standard of care for gliomas. PCR, FISH, and CGH tests are available (136). Tests are available at various laboratories, including the Mayo Clinic in Rochester, Minnesota, and Massachusetts General Hospital in Boston.

Oligoastrocytomas

Oligoastrocytomas are mixed gliomas composed of both astrocytoma and oligodendroglioma, as described in their respective sections. Depending on its degree of malignancy, an individual tumor can be either low grade (grade II) or high grade (grade III).

OLIGOASTROCYTOMA (MIXED OLIGODENDROGLIOMA-ASTROCYTOMA)—GRADE II. This is a mixed glioma composed of both diffuse astrocytoma and oligodendroglioma, grade II. The potential utility of PCV chemotherapy in a mixed tumor in which an oligodendroglioma element is present is not as well defined in this group as in pure oligodendroglioma.

Difficulties are encountered in determining whether individual tumors contain a mixture of both oligodendroglial and astrocytic elements and whether both are neoplastic. Each element must be conspicuous on histologic grounds for this diagnosis. The elements may be intermixed or clustered in separate regions. Neoplastic cells can be assessed for astrocytic phenotype with GFAP immunostaining. Definitive phenotypic iden-

tification of oligodendroglial elements is problematic, but MAP-2 IHC has shown promise (134).

The true oligodendroglial cells must be distinguished from infiltrating macrophages swollen with lipid (Fig. 10.5). The former have neoplastic nuclei more centrally placed within the cells than within swollen macrophages and a single large perinuclear halo (Fig. 10.54) instead of multiple small phagocytic vacuoles (Fig. 10.4A). Oligoastrocytomas can undergo anaplastic transformation to grade III neoplasms. One study has shown that deletions on 1p identify two subgroups of oligoastrocytomas. Those without deletions behave like grade II or III diffuse astrocytomas, including shorter survival. Oligoastrocytoms with deletions on 1p behave like grade II or III oligodendrogliomas that have 1p loss, including longer survival (130).

ANAPLASTIC OLIGOASTROCYTOMA (MIXED OLIGODENDROGLIOMA-ASTROCYTOMA)—GRADE III. Features of anaplastic transformation in either the oligodendroglioma component, astrocytoma component, or both components of an oligoastrocytoma (which connote a higher grade) include a combination of increased cellularity, nuclear atypia, cellular pleomorphism, and a high mitotic rate. Microvascular proliferation and necrosis may be identified but need not be present. Distinction of anaplastic oligoastrocytoma from glioblastoma can be difficult. If we see either microvascular proliferation or necrosis in the astrocytic component, we interpret the tumor to be glioblastoma.

Gliomas Associated with Radiation

Malignant astrocytic gliomas are the most frequent types of gliomas to arise subsequent to radiotherapy. Most of these are either anaplastic astrocytomas or glioblastomas. Many arise 5 to 25 years following treatment of a pituitary adenoma or craniopharyngioma. No radiation-specific histologic features occur in malignant gliomas that arise years after radiotherapy.

The incidence of astrocytomas and glioblastomas during this postradiotherapy time interval is conspicuously higher than their incidence in the general population (137). They fulfill standard criteria of correlation with radiation by being different from patients' first tumors and occurring in the field of prior

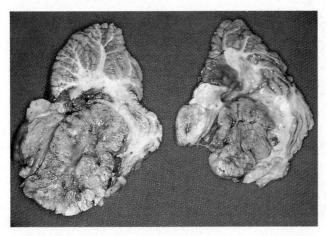

Figure 10.58. Ependymoma. In contrast to medulloblastoma, this red and brown nodular ependymoma has a distinct margin with cerebellar parenchyma. *(Courtesy of Dr. Samuel Hicks, University of Michigan, Ann Arbor, Michigan.)*

radiation. In addition, the interval between first and second tumor presentation precludes the presence of the second (malignant) tumor during radiation.

Ependymomas

Ependymomas are glial neoplasms that occur almost exclusively adjacent to a ventricle in the cerebral hemispheres, in the brainstem, and in spinal cord. Many ependymomas have a relatively discrete margin with brain (Fig. 10.58) compared with fibrillary gliomas, which manifest an infiltrative margin. Thus, total removal is possible for some, but not all, ependymomas. The cellular conformations of ependymomas vary between fibrillar and epithelial, posing special problems of differentiation not only from other gliomas, but also from carcinomas and meningiomas (Tables 10.10 through 10.14). These latter differentiations are facilitated by recalling that even epithelioid ependymomas frequently stain with anti-GFAP, have distinctive ultrastructure, and contain at least a few cells with fibrillar processes. A good place to look for these few fibrillar processes is around vessels. In contrast to nonglial neoplasms, aggregated ependymoma cells lack a basement membrane. Reticulin and type IV collagen

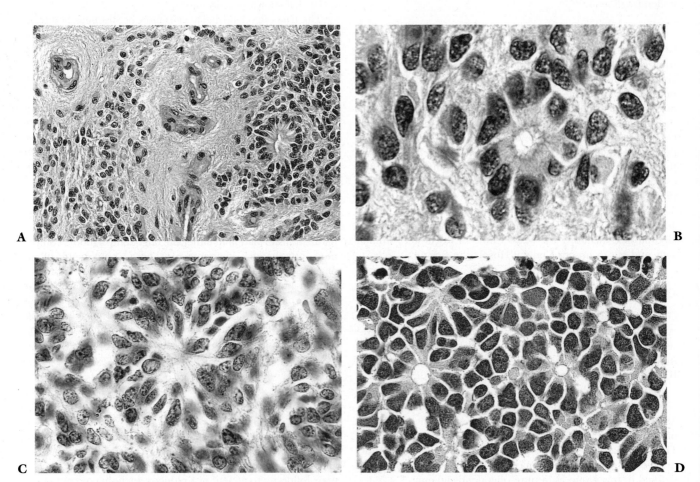

Figure 10.59. Rosette stone. Rosettes are useful in identifying brain tumors. The perivascular rosettes in the center of this illustration are more numerous than the nearby true rosette in this and in most ependymomas (**A**). True ependymal rosettes always have a lumen lined with ependymal cells, whether it is elongated (**A**) or round (**B**). Cilia may protrude into this lumen. Fibrillary rosettes (Homer Wright rosettes) contain cellular processes in their centers (**C**), and they occur in primitive neuroectodermal tumors, medulloblastomas, pineoblastomas, and neuroblastomas. Flexner rosettes, which are found in retinoblastoma and less commonly in pineoblastomas, have a lumen with a hypereosinophilic border (**D**). The border is a mixture of cytoplasmic processes resembling photoreceptors and acid mucosubstances.

stains show no fibrils in these aggregates, and this distinguishes them from vascular adventitia.

Look for rosettes as phenotypic evidence to confirm suspicion of an ependymoma (Tables 10.10 through 10.12). The true ependymal rosette, or luminal rosette, consists of ependymal cells evenly spaced perpendicular to and forming a central lumen (Fig. 10.59). Close light microscopic examination of the lumen may reveal microvilli or cilia. True rosettes may be found in individual cases of any of the ependymoma variants, but some samples of ependymoma lack true rosettes. At the outer portion of the rosettes, cells blend into parenchyma. Some tumors show expanded ependymal rosettes and others have long ependymal linings that do not close into rosettes.

Perivascular pseudorosettes of ependymomas (Fig. 10.60A) have a fibrillar zone ("spokes of the wheels") that is at least two nuclear or three erythrocyte diameters wide around central vessels ("hubs of the wheels"). With the majority of tumor vessels involved, a characteristic pattern of halos around vessels resembling atolls with light, sandy beaches is evident at low magnification. This phenomenon is due to thin tapering of the neoplastic cell processes as they extend around a blood vessel.

The thin processes are in distinction to the thick processes of astroblastic formations. Perivascular rosettes resemble other gliovascular structures (GVSs) in astrocytomas and glioblastomas, but GVSs have more narrow and uneven fibrillar zones. Perivascular rosettes are more common than true ependymal rosettes in ependymomas.

Ependymomas express GFAP (Fig. 10.60B). Both astrocytomas and ependymomas show GFAP, but GFAP highlights perivascular rosettes in ependymomas, making it useful in some cases. Ultrastructural findings in ependymomas include perivascular rosettes, cilia, basal bodies, and microvillous inclusions (Fig. 10.60C). Electron microscopy is critical in diagnosis of some variants. Ependymomas uncommonly and only focally express cytokeratin or EMA, but these markers contribute to identification when positive (Fig. 10.60D).

The described general features of ependymoma are useful in identifying the variants of ependymoma described below, except where specifically excluded.

SUBEPENDYMOMA—GRADE I. The subependymoma occurs in the wall of a ventricle, protruding into the ventricular

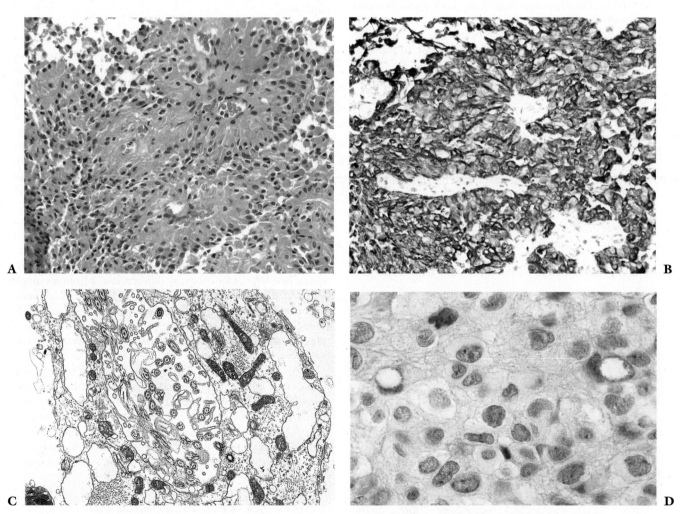

Figure 10.60. Ependymoma. **(A)** Prominent perivascular rosettes (also known as pseudorosettes) are noted in this ependymoma. **(B)** Glial fibrillary acidic protein labels the neoplastic cell processes; blood vessel–related cells are negative. **(C)** Ultrastructural evaluation is needed when rosettes are not evident. It reveals microvillous cytoplasmic structures, cilia, and basal bodies. **(D)** EMA stains rosettes and microvillous inclusions in this ependymoma.

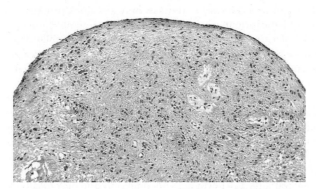

Figure 10.61. Subependymoma. This neoplasm protrudes into the fourth ventricle of a 60-year-old man. It forms zones with many nuclei near other zones with many cellular processes.

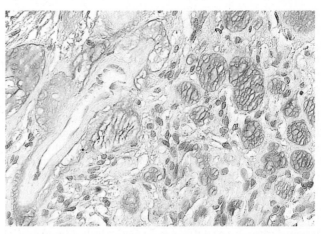

Figure 10.63. Perivascular and parenchymal blue mucin in a myxopapillary ependymoma from the cauda equina.

space (Fig. 10.61). Its histologic features closely resemble those of tanycytic ependymoma, but the tanycytic ependymoma is most common in the spinal cord rather than in a ventricle. Adding to this trap for the unwary, the namesake of the tanycytic ependymoma, the tanycyte, is an elongated cell normally found just beneath the ependymal lining of a ventricle, particularly the third ventricle. The tanycyte has been also suggested to be the cell of origin of the chordoid glioma of the third ventricle (138).

The subependymoma is lobular. It has clusters of nuclei surrounded by fibrillar cellular processes. These processes resemble those of astrocytomas. Key to recognition of a subependymoma are its ventricular location, and its nuclei with smooth, rounded borders and with distinctly light and dark regions of chromatin ("salt and pepper" chromatin). These round to oval ependymal nuclei are rarely elongated or spindled. Mitoses are rare to absent. A subependymoma that is completely resected usually does not recur.

MYXOPAPILLARY EPENDYMOMA—GRADE I. This type of ependymoma that appears the least glial is almost totally confined to the region of the filum terminale, cauda equina, sacrum, and adjacent extravertebral soft tissues (Figs. 10.62 and

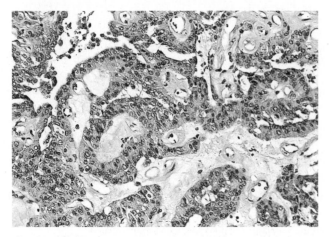

Figure 10.62. Myxopapillary ependymoma. It originated in the filum terminale of a 40-year-old woman. It has papillae of epithelioid cells and blue-tinged mucin.

10.63). This location distinguishes the myxopapillary ependymoma from various other tumors, including choroid plexus papilloma.

Although the differential features of ependymomas described above can be useful, the peculiar morphology and growth of myxopapillary ependymoma pose unique problems. They are tabulated as tumors containing two different cell types because careful search usually reveals both epithelial and fibrillar cells (Table 10.12). However, individual samples of tumor vary from this general pattern. The most difficult variants of myxopapillary ependymoma to recognize are those that are nearly all myxoid or epithelial. The highly myxoid variety may produce cords of cells in a mucoid matrix resembling chordoma, a neoplasm found in the same location. Lack of physaliphorous cells and presence of GFAP are features that distinguish the myxopapillary ependymoma from chordoma.

Fibrillary myxopapillary ependymomas may be confused with fibrous meningioma and schwannoma. The epithelial and the papillary variants may resemble carcinoma or meningioma (see Fig. 10.62). Stainable mucin in the myxopapillary ependymoma (see Fig. 10.63) helps to differentiate it from meningioma, which rarely produces mucin (4), and from schwannoma. Mucin in vascular walls (mucoid degeneration) is particularly characteristic of myxopapillary ependymomas. The GFAP stain differentiates the positive myxopapillary ependymoma from carcinoma and meningioma.

In contrast to metastatic carcinoma, myxopapillary ependymomas lack malignant cytology and are focally fibrillar. Paragangliomas may mimic myxopapillary ependymomas (see Fig. 10.108 in the "Neuroendocrine Tumors" section below), although presence of mucin and absence of secretory granules distinguishes the latter tumor (see Fig. 10.63). Cilia and basal bodies are harder to find in this tumor than in other ependymomas.

Although given a grade I by WHO, some myxopapillary ependymomas behave aggressively and become unresectable (139).

EPENDYMOMA (LOW-GRADE EPENDYMOMA)—GRADE II. The designation *low-grade* is often dropped and this group is referred to simply as ependymoma. The rosettes described above and the nuclear features of well-differentiated ependymomas distinguish them from astrocytomas. Nuclei of ependymomas are typically round or oval with prominent light and dark regions stained with hematoxylin (see Fig. 10.59). In the parenchyma away from rosettes, nuclei tend to be more uniformly crowded than astrocytoma nuclei and less crowded than in medulloblastomas and primitive neuroectodermal tumors (see Fig. 10.59A).

Epithelioid ependymomas occasionally have a remarkably distinct margin with CNS parenchyma imitating margins of nonglial neoplasms. Anti-GFAP stain for glial filaments is extremely helpful in differentiating these ependymomas (Fig. 10.60B) from carcinomas, pituitary adenomas, craniopharyngiomas, and meningiomas (Tables 10.11 through 10.14). The stain accentuates fibrillar cellular processes that distinguish the ependymoma.

Papillary ependymomas closely resemble choroid plexus papillomas. Solid regions of ependymoma parenchyma where neoplastic cells grow on one another rather than on fibrovascular stroma are accentuated by reticulin stains (Fig. 10.64).

Histologic grade is less predictive of survival in ependymoma than in astrocytoma (139,142). Radiographic evidence of residual disease after surgery predicts markedly reduced survival, placing a premium on correct intraoperative diagnosis and gross total removal.

Interesting but unchallenging variants of ependymoma were described above. Variants of ependymoma that are likely to be confused with other tumors are specifically highlighted directly below.

Clear cell ependymoma. These uncommon gliomas, usually supratentorial, closely resemble oligodendrogliomas (Fig. 10.65). They must be distinguished from oligodendroglioma and central neurocytoma. The latter tumor can be identified by its synaptophysin positivity. Some but not all specimens of clear-cell ependymoma show a focal rosette or two. I have not found EMA reliable in distinguishing this variant. The ultrastructural features of clear-cell ependymomas are ependymal, and electron microscopy is recommended to identify these neoplasms (140,141). Individual clear-cell ependymomas can be either grade II or grade III.

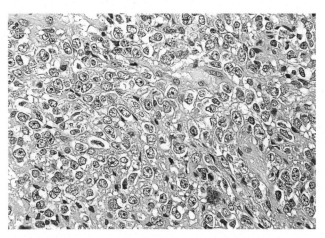

Figure 10.65. Clear-cell ependymoma. The neoplastic cells mimic oligodendroglia or small neurons. The ultrastructure of this tumor resembled that in Figure 10.60C, with numerous cilia and basal bodies.

Tanycytic ependymoma. Tanycytic ependymomas are usually found within the spinal cord parenchyma (Fig. 10.66). They have both ependymal and astrocytic features. Their high degree of fibrillar cellular processes resembles astrocytomas. Key to their recognition are nuclei with smooth, rounded borders and with distinctly light and dark regions of chromatin ("salt and pepper" chromatin). Even when elongated, these nuclei resemble those of other ependymomas. Architecture is a key diagnostic feature: They typically form zones replete with nuclei and other zones where fibrillar cellular processes predominate (Figs. 10.61 and 10.66). These zones are larger and less linear than rhythmic palisades or Verocay bodies (Figs. 10.35 and 10.61; and see Fig. 10.105 in the "Peripheral Nerve Sheath Tumors" section below). They are not limited to alignment along vessels like perivascular rosettes of other ependymomas (Fig. 10.60).

Like the low-grade ependymoma, their margins with surrounding parenchyma tend to be discrete and potentially resectable, which is the surgical reason to distinguish them from diffuse astrocytomas. It is frequently important to inquire about the tumor margin and inform the surgeon of this variant during

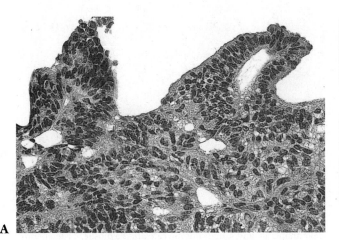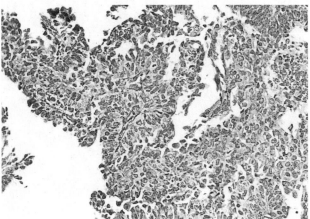

A **B**

Figure 10.64. Papillary ependymoma. The epithelioid cells line lumina and form solid regions of parenchyma (**A**). Reticulin stain shows that many of these epithelial cells do not rest directly on vessels (**B**).

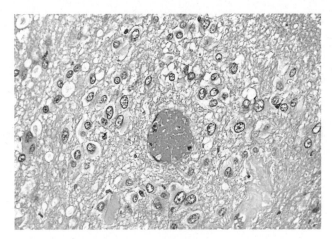

Figure 10.66.   Tanycytic ependymoma. Solitary intramedullary neoplasm in the spinal cord of a 44-year-old man.

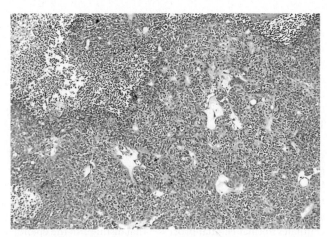

Figure 10.68.   Ependymoblastoma. Vague ribbons packed with cells alternate with necrotic regions. Numerous true ependymal rosettes are present.

the operation to ensure appropriate consideration of resection. These neoplasms are ependymomas rather than astrocytomas. When the diagnosis of tanycytic ependymoma is in doubt, ultrastructural confirmation of its typical ependymal features is recommended.

ANAPLASTIC EPENDYMOMA (MALIGNANT EPENDYMOMA)—GRADE III. Anaplastic ependymomas are uncommon. Although often found in the cerebrum or cerebellum of children and young adults, they are not limited to these ages or locations. Key diagnostic criteria for anaplasia include (a) increased cellularity, (b) nuclear anaplasia, and (c) brisk mitotic activity (Fig. 10.67A) (101). Vascular proliferation—intramural or glomeruloid (Fig. 10.67B)—and necrosis (including pseudopalisading necrosis) may be seen; however, necrosis in an otherwise low-grade ependymoma does not confer the diagnosis of anaplasia or of glioblastoma. These tumors can be discrete or have an

infiltrative margin. Architectural features, including perivascular rosettes, are reduced in number but aid the distinction of this tumor from high-grade astrocytoma. Although anaplastic ependymoma is listed in Table 10.10 among fibrillary neoplasms, ependymomas with many epithelioid cells can also be anaplastic (Table 10.12). Histopathologic features of malignancy do not accurately predict poor survival (142).

EPENDYMOBLASTOMA—GRADE IV. This is a rare tumor characterized by conspicuous hypercellularity and ependymal rosettes (Table 10.13) (Fig. 10.68). It is featured as an embryonal tumor in some classifications. It is included here because of its structural features, which most closely resemble ependymoma. Distinguishing ependymomas from ependymoblastoma is difficult and important to clinical management.

Most cases occur in infants and children. The tumor is highly

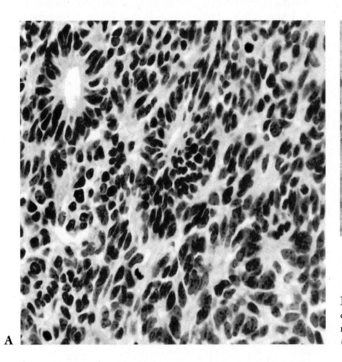

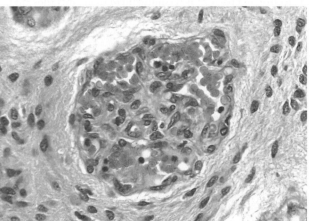

Figure 10.67.   Anaplastic ependymoma. **(A)** High cellularity, nuclear anaplasia, and a high mitotic rate are diagnostic. True ependymal rosettes are noted. Other regions contained perivascular rosettes (not shown). **(B)** Glomeruloid microvascular proliferation.

cellular, with mitoses and necrosis. It lacks multinucleation and giant cells and has little or no endothelial proliferation (143). The ependymoblastoma is biologically malignant and infiltrates the leptomeninges, eventually spreading along CSF pathways like a medulloblastoma.

NEURONAL TUMORS

Within this group of tumors that contain an abnormal proliferation of neurons is a spectrum of neoplastic growth potential ranging from the most benign gangliocytoma to the rare ganglioglioma with glioblastoma in its glial component (Tables 10.10 and 10.12) (4). Most ganglion cell neoplasms have a better prognosis than gliomas that superficially resemble them, and therefore their proper identification is important (144).

Gangliocytoma—Grade I and Ganglioglioma—Grade I (Rarely up to Grade III)

These tumors may arise anywhere (145,146) but are most common in the cerebrum, particularly the temporal lobe. Distinction of a ganglion cell tumor from developmental lesions cortical dysplasia and tubers can be difficult; see the "Cortical Malformation" section below.

The identification and evaluation of ganglion cell neoplasms has four important stages. The first is recognition of neurons (Fig. 10.69). Many neoplastic cells, particularly cells of glioblastomas, melanomas, and astrocytomas, resemble neurons by their large size or prominent nucleoli. These cells lack Nissl substance, which characterizes true neurons. Although Nissl substance can often be appreciated by cytoplasmic basophilia on H&E-stained slides, use of neuronal immunolabels (including synaptophysin, Neu-N, and neurofilament along with GFAP) can help discern the phenotype of atypical cells (145).

If neurons have been identified, the next step in recognition of a ganglion cell tumor is confirmation that the neurons are neoplastic. Neuronal tumors typically manifest both (a) histologic abnormalities, including abnormal neuronal clustering and loss of orderly distribution; and (b) cytologic abnormalities,

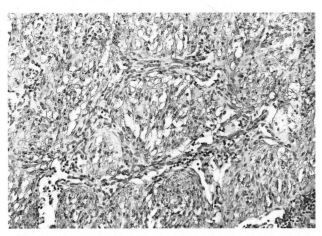

Figure 10.70. Ganglioglioma. This tumor from the right temporal lobe of a 16-year-old girl exhibits S-100 protein–positive parenchyma and bands of S-100–negative fibrovascular tissue with mononuclear cells.

including binucleation, cytologic atypia (e.g., large and bizarre nuclei, hyperchromatism), and neurons of various stages of development (Fig. 10.69) (27). Mitotic activity may also be apparent but MIB-1 reactivity in neurons is more common.

A common error is to interpret a field of entrapped normal neurons infiltrated by glioma cells as a ganglioglioma. Frequently, clustered adjacent to ganglion cells are either other ganglion cells or smaller neurons. Ganglion cell tumors may provide clues of their true nature by displaying heavy bands of fibrous tissue or perivascular round cells (Fig. 10.70), but these are not invariably present.

Once a ganglion cell neoplasm has been identified, the glial element must be evaluated. A section lightly stained for GFAP with IHC (less than half the usual time in DAB substrate) and fully counterstained with hematoxylin facilitates this determination by providing a better view of glial nuclei. If the light brown cells appear reactive, cluster near the margin of the neoplasm, and do not meet the criteria of neoplasia described for low-

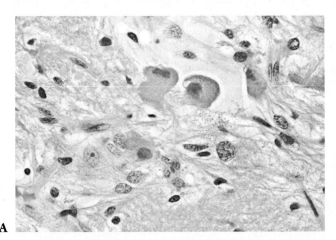

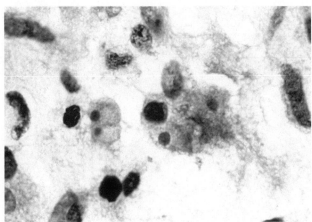

A **B**

Figure 10.69. Ganglioglioma. **(A)** Abnormally clustered and cytologically atypical neurons with large nuclei and large nucleoli; a central neuron has discernible basophilic Nissl substance peripherally. Astrocytes with spindle-shaped nuclei manifesting mild nuclear atypia. **(B)** Both large and small binucleated neurons in the stereotactic biopsy of a solitary right thalamic ganglioglioma in a 13-year-old girl contain large round nucleoli and Nissl substance.

grade astrocytoma, the tumor is a gangliocytoma or central neurocytoma (see below). If the GFAP-positive cells are neoplastic but not anaplastic, the neoplasm is a ganglioglioma. If these glial elements are anaplastic (see "Anaplastic Astrocytoma" and "Glioblastoma" sections), the neoplasm is an anaplastic ganglioglioma. Grading of gangliogliomas relies on grading of the glial component corresponding to the criteria of astrocytomas. Rarely, the glial component is a glioblastoma.

Rosenthal fibers and granular bodies are commonly seen in ganglion cell tumors and signify chronicity. Perivascular cuffs of lymphocytes are common in gangliogliomas.

Dysplastic Gangliocytoma of the Cerebellum (DGC)

The DGC is an unusual variant of a gangliocytoma, also known as Lhermitte-Duclos disease. Hyperplastic and disordered granular cell neurons enlarge a part of the cerebellum (Fig. 10.71). The neoplastic potential of this tumor, which looks dysplastic, is indicated by some tumors that have recurred following surgery. Some DGCs are familial, associated with Cowden syndrome, or with multiple hamartoma-neoplasia syndrome (147).

Dysembryoplastic Neuroepithelial Tumor (DNT)—Grade I

The dysembryoplastic neuroepithelial tumor may be the small, almost hamartomatous counterpart of a ganglioglioma or glioma. It is, on macroscopic or low-power microscopic evaluation, multinodular within the cerebral cortex, most often cortex of the temporal lobe. Some are cystic (Fig. 10.72). Some are incidental findings, and some are associated with long-standing partial complex seizure disorders in adolescents and young adults. The nodules are composed (a) principally of cells that resemble oligodendroglioma, and (b) neurons that often appear to float within pools of Alcian blue positive acid mucopolysaccharide (Fig. 10.73) (148). In practice, identification of neurons is often difficult; immunolabeling for synaptophysin, neurofilaments, and Neu-N can help discern the neuronal component. Its low MIB-1 proliferation index, mature histotopographic appearance, and association with cortical dysplasia suggest a maldevelopmental origin (149).

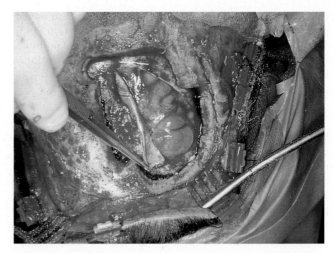

Figure 10.72. Dysembryoplastic neuroepithelial tumor. Forceps retract the dura to reveal one of multiple brown cortical nodules next to a lighter, translucent, bulging cyst. *(Courtesy of Dr. Donald Ross, University of Michigan, Ann Arbor, Michigan.)*

Oligodendrogliomas mimic DNTs; both tumors are frequently microcystic. Retrospective assessment of resected tumors diagnosed as "oligodendroglioma" and then "cured" has revealed some cases of DNT. A multinodular architecture and identification of neurons floating in "pools of mucin" near bundles of axons flanked by oligodendroglia are key histologic features in diagnosing DNTs.

Central Neurocytoma—Grade II

This tumor has stimulated much interest because of its structural beauty, hidden identity, and relatively benign prognosis. Initially it was considered grade I by WHO, but now is labeled grade II. It most commonly grows into the lateral or third ventricle from the septum pellucidum or foramen of Monro, although cases not associated with the ventricle have been reported (Fig. 10.74) (150,151). It is the most common neoplasm involving the septum pellucidum in young adults.

Careful application of diagnostic tools facilitates proper

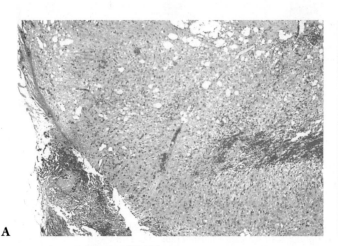
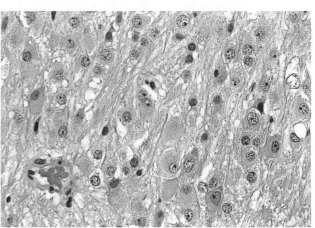

A   B

Figure 10.71. Dysplastic gangliocytoma of the cerebellum. The molecular and granular cell layers of this enlarged folium are obscured by hyperplastic neurons **(A)**. The neurons are large with prominent nucleoli and occasional binucleated cells **(B)**. *(Courtesy of Dr. Qazi Azher, Hurley Medical Center, Flint, Michigan.)*

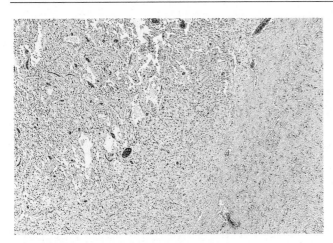

Figure 10.73. Dysembryoplastic neuroepithelial tumor. This small cortical tumor nodule has a relatively discrete margin and a regular distribution of benign cells. *(Courtesy of Dr. Jonathan Fratkin, University of Mississippi Medical Center, Jackson, Mississippi.)*

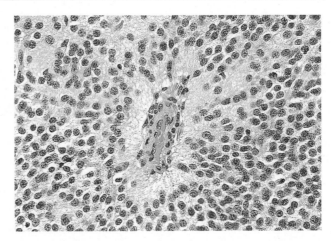

Figure 10.75. Central neurocytoma. Its fibrillar perivascular zone and round cells with halos around the round nuclei imitate ependymoma and oligodendroglioma.

identification of the central neurocytoma, which for years has been mistaken for a glioma (Fig. 10.75). The tumor consists of a homogeneous population of cells with a neuroendocrine nucleus and modest cytoplasm. The neoplastic cells of central neurocytomas express synaptophysin and Neu-N and are usually negative for GFAP, although reactive astrocytes commonly mix with tumor cells. Homer Wright rosettes and ganglionic cells are uncommon features that are useful in individual cases (151). Although radiotherapy has been used, a good prognosis usually follows total surgical excision (150). However, rare anaplastic variants have been reported.

Electron microscopy first defined the central neurocytoma by revealing microtubules, 100- to 200-nm dense-core vesicles, and clear vesicles to confirm this "Cinderella tumor" to be of true neuronal lineage. Today, IHC suffices to confirm most central neurocytomas.

Desmoplastic Infantile Ganglioglioma (DIG)—Grade I

Desmoplastic infantile gangliogliomas often attain considerable size and resemble very fibrous gangliogliomas (Fig. 10.76). These neoplasms are found in patients less than 18 months of age, are frequently cystic, and often involve the meninges (152).

Cerebellar Liponeurocytoma (Grade I to II)

Although first described years ago, and often called a lipomatous medulloblastoma, there has been excitement about categorizing this tumor as a distinct pathologic entity. This cerebellar neoplasm grows in adults of mean age of 50 years. Some of its cells contain lipid (153). These and the other cells are variably immunoreactive for neuronal (synaptophysin and MAP-2) and glial (GFAP) markers. It partly resembles a medulloblastoma but has better cytologic differentiation, low mitotic activity, and a better prognosis. Because it usually expresses neuronal and glial markers, it would make sense to consider the cerebellar liponeurocytoma to be a mixed neuronal-glial tumor.

PINEAL PARENCHYMAL TUMORS

Intraoperative diagnostic surgical pathology of these tumors is among the most challenging areas of the clinical neuropathology practices. One must have a firm grasp of the normal histology of the gland obtained from examination of the normal pineal gland and its variations. All of the submitted specimen should be examined.

Pineal tumors include tumors of the native pineal parenchymal neurons, but also astrocytomas, germ cell tumors, meningiomas, and metastases. These latter tumors are described in their respective sections. Pineal cysts are common; see "Cyst" section, below.

Pineal parenchymal tumors arise from pineocytes, manifest-

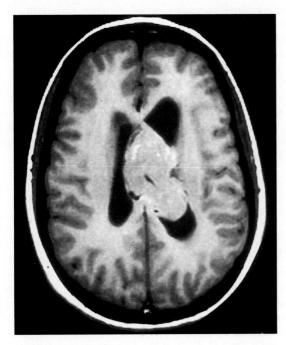

Figure 10.74. Central neurocytoma. A typical midline intraventricular location of this large central neurocytoma in a 27-year-old woman is shown on T1-weighted magnetic resonance image. *(Courtesy of Dr. James Brunberg, University of Michigan, Ann Arbor, Michigan.)*

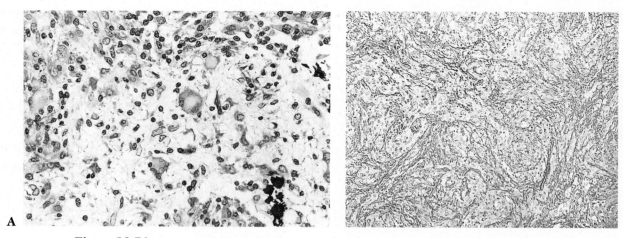

Figure 10.76. Desmoplastic infantile ganglioglioma. This massive tumor of the left cerebral hemisphere of a 7-month-old boy contains abnormal binucleated neurons and glia **(A)**, mixed with a complex network of desmoplasia stained with reticulin stain **(B)**.

ing mixed photoreceptor and neuroendocrine features (154,155). IHC for synaptophysin identifies their neuronal phenotype. Other markers like chromogranin, Tau, neurofilament, and neuron-specific enolase (NSE) are sometimes used, but are less reliable than synaptophysin. Retinal S-antigen reactivity reflects their photosensory differentiation (18).

Pineocytoma—Grade II

This neoplasm simulates the histologic appearance of normal pineal gland (Table 10.10), but has hypercellularity beyond that of the normal pineal gland. Neoplastic cells with uniformly round nuclei are divided by fibrovascular stroma into expanded lobules. They manifest pineocytomatous rosettes, a cluster of neurons with processes directed centrally (Fig. 10.77). These are often larger than other fibrillar rosettes. Nuclear atypia is minimal and mitotic figures are scant (154).

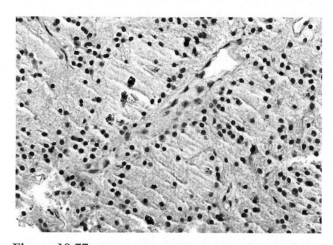

Figure 10.77. Pineocytoma. Neoplastic cells with round nuclei form nests and surround fibrillary zones that resemble huge, loose Homer Wright rosettes. These large, fibrillar rosettes are typical of well-differentiated pineal cell tumors, but they are not always evident in small samples. *(Courtesy of Dr. Uma P. Kalyan-Raman, University of Illinois College of Medicine, Peoria, Illinois.)*

Pineal Parenchymal Tumor of Intermediate Differentiation

Pineal parenchymal tumors of intermediate differentiation and malignancy sit at the interface between pineocytoma and pineoblastoma. There is a marked increase in cellularity from that seen in pineocytoma, and pineocytomatous rosettes are rare (Fig. 10.78A). Nuclei manifest only mild atypia and are generally homogeneous in appearance. Mitotic figures are identified in greater numbers than in pineocytoma.

Pineoblastoma—Grade IV

Pineoblastoma consists of sheets of crowded, highly anaplastic, undifferentiated-appearing neoplastic cells, manifesting focal nuclear moulding, with a high mitotic rate resembling medulloblastoma/PNET and retinoblastoma (Fig. 10.78B). Flexner-Wintersteiner rosettes similar to those in retinoblastoma can be identified in a few cases (Fig. 10.59). Necrosis can be present and extensive.

In some tumors, intermixed regions ranging from pineocytoma, pineal parenchymal tumor of intermediate malignancy, and pineoblastoma can be identified. The presence of pineoblastoma connotes increased malignancy and the higher grade is given.

UNDIFFERENTIATED AND MULTIPOTENTIAL TUMORS

Medulloblastoma—Grade IV

The medulloblastoma is a common primitive neuroectodermal tumor that arises in the cerebellum or in the roof of the fourth ventricle (Figs. 10.79 through 10.81) (Table 10.13). It is most common in children, but also occurs in young adults; it is rare in patients over age 35 (156,157). It is often associated with isochromosome 17q (one chromosome composed of two long arms of chromosome 17) (156). Because it spreads along CSF pathways, treatment should be directed at the entire neuraxis. About 5% of medulloblastomas metastasize to a systemic location, particularly to bone. The younger age of most patients with

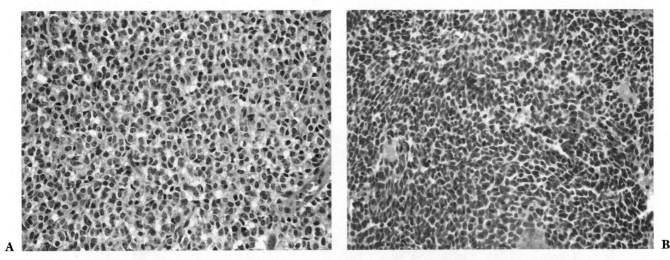

A B

Figure 10.78. Pineal tumors. **(A)** This pineal parenchymal tumor of intermediate differentiation has high cellularity but relatively monomorphous appearance and scant mitotic activity. **(B)** This pineoblastoma demonstrates high cellularity, marked nuclear pleomorphism, and a high mitotic rate.

this medulloblastoma and its cerebellar location are helpful, but not diagnostic.

Medulloblastoma is a small, round, blue cell tumor with marked hypercellularity, anaplastic nuclei, and a high nuclear cytoplasmic ratio (Fig. 10.81), similar to that seen in pineoblastoma (Fig. 10.78B). Its neuronal phenotype is demonstrated by positivity of a proportion of neoplastic cells for synaptophysin (Fig. 10.81C). Regardless of its other lines of differentiation, neuronal differentiation has come to be one defining characteristic of medulloblastoma, albeit minimal and focal at times. Hence, the questionable use of the glial, neuronal, and endo-

crine marker, neuron-specific enolase (NSE) to "show" neuronal differentiation. Until discovery of a truly neuron-specific subtype of NSE, it should be used only with caution and backup in this context. Synaptophysin is better.

Regions of glial differentiation can be noted histologically and confirmed by GFAP IHC. Electron microscopy can adjunctively confirm the neural nature of neoplastic cells. Occasional nonglial differentiation, particularly soft tissue cells, reflects its multipotential nature. Its appearance must be distinguished from small-cell undifferentiated carcinoma and lymphoma (see Fig. 10.113 in the "Hematopoietic and Lymphoid Neoplasms" section, and Figs. 10.126 and 10.127 in the "Common Metastatic Tumors" section) (Table 10.13).

Fibrillarity is extremely important to the diagnosis of medulloblastoma, and must be carefully assessed. Although neither small-cell carcinoma nor lymphoma is fibrillar, primary CNS lymphoma diffusely infiltrates CNS parenchyma to the point where it becomes mixed with normal and reactive fibrillar cells

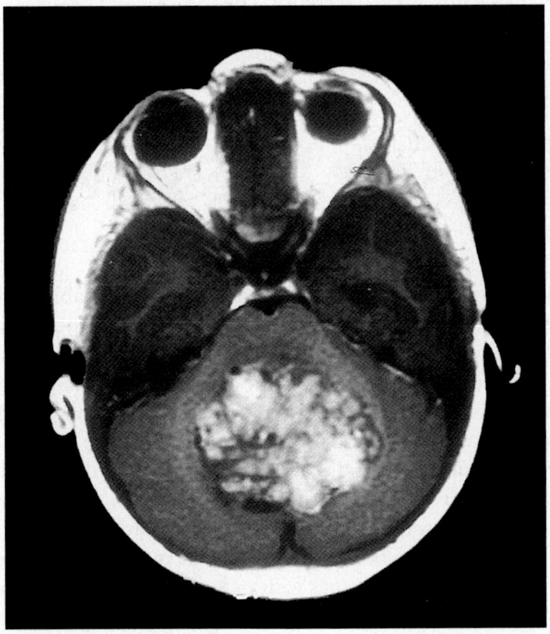

Figure 10.79. Medulloblastoma. This brain magnetic resonance image is from a 2.5-year-old girl with a large midline cerebellar medulloblastoma. The T1-weighted image enhances heterogeneously after contrast is administered. *(Courtesy of Dr. James Brunberg, University of Michigan, Ann Arbor, Michigan.)*

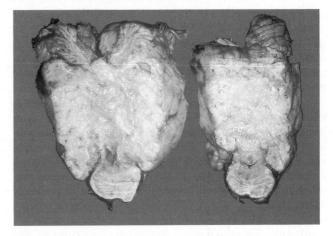

Figure 10.80. Medulloblastoma. The solid, light gray, semitranslucent medulloblastoma infiltrates the cerebellum and effaces the cerebellar folia. *(Courtesy of Dr. Samuel Hicks, University of Michigan, Ann Arbor, Michigan.)*

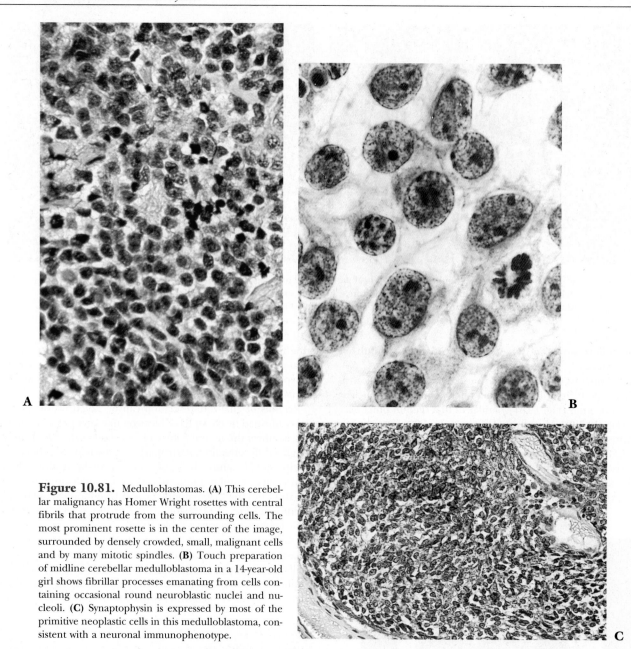

Figure 10.81. Medulloblastomas. **(A)** This cerebellar malignancy has Homer Wright rosettes with central fibrils that protrude from the surrounding cells. The most prominent rosette is in the center of the image, surrounded by densely crowded, small, malignant cells and by many mitotic spindles. **(B)** Touch preparation of midline cerebellar medulloblastoma in a 14-year-old girl shows fibrillar processes emanating from cells containing occasional round neuroblastic nuclei and nucleoli. **(C)** Synaptophysin is expressed by most of the primitive neoplastic cells in this medulloblastoma, consistent with a neuronal immunophenotype.

(see Fig. 10.113D). Thus, the fibrillar cellular processes must come directly from the neoplastic cells to indicate medulloblastoma (Fig. 10.81). Rosettes with cores filled with fibrils (Homer Wright rosettes) in CNS are characteristic of medulloblastomas (see Fig. 10.59C); however, many biopsy samples of medulloblastoma consist of sheets of neoplastic cells with only vague to nonexistent rosettes. Some biopsies contain rhythmic palisades of tumor cells with fibrils resembling those seen in gliomas. Elongated nuclei resembling carrots are seen more often in medulloblastomas (Fig. 10.81A) than in lymphomas, provided all tissue has been properly handled and immediately fixed.

DESMOPLASTIC MEDULLOBLASTOMA—GRADE IV. Regions of this medulloblastoma variant are called desmoplastic: They have both abundant reticulin and crowded, proliferating cells. Segregated by the desmoplasia are pale islands of tissue that lack reticulin and are less crowded with cells (Table 10.12). These islands show neuronal markers like synaptophysin and relatively low proliferation (158). These islands are called reticulin-free zones, and they give the desmoplastic medulloblastoma a nodular appearance, even on H&E stains (Fig. 10.82).

Desmoplastic medulloblastomas were once more broadly defined to include non-nodular desmoplastic medulloblastomas (158). However, the nodularity is associated with a better prognosis than that seen in other medulloblastomas. In fact, the more nodularity the better the prognosis, in general. Some infants have medulloblastomas with extensive nodularity of large reticulin-free zones, and seem to be particularly responsive to treatment (159).

ANAPLASTIC AND LARGE-CELL MEDULLOBLASTOMAS. Medulloblastoma children whose tumors show large cells, nuclei, and nucleoli have particularly poor survival compared to

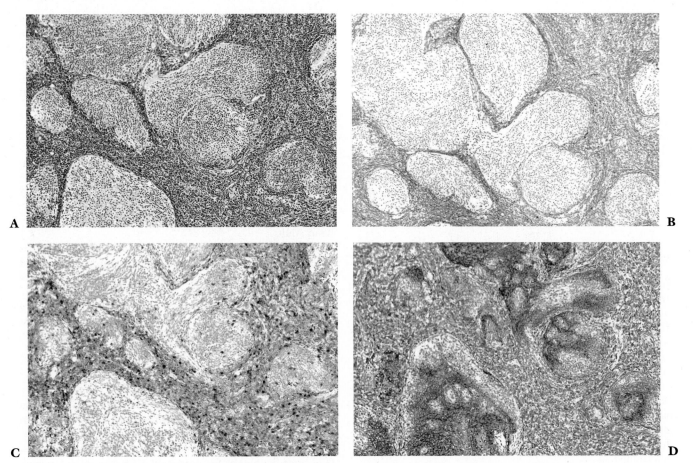

Figure 10.82. Four nearby sections of a desmoplastic medulloblastoma. **(A)** Pale islands of less cell density are surrounded by a densely cellular sea. **(B)** The sea contains reticulin and the islands do not. **(C)** The sea contains most of the proliferating cells, stained brown with MIB-1. **(D)** The islands express synaptophysin, reflecting their neuronal differentiation.

children afflicted by other types of medulloblastomas (160). These prognostic features legitimize the large-cell medulloblastoma (LCM) variant. The LCM variant also has many mitoses and apoptotic nuclei. Other more variable features of LCM are conspicuous cytoplasm, cells that wrap around each other, and round or vesicular nuclei. One or more markers induced by hepatocyte growth factor, including c-Myc, eventually may help distinguish LCM from other medulloblastomas (161).

Anaplastic medulloblastomas have the same features described for LCM. The term *anaplastic medulloblastoma* implies that other medulloblastomas are not anaplastic. The nomenclature would be simplified and clarified by replacing the term anaplastic medulloblastoma with large-cell medulloblastoma.

MEDULLOMYOBLASTOMA—GRADE IV. This rare neoplasm occurs in the midline posterior fossa of children and contains smooth or striated muscle fibers. In this regard, mesenchymal expression by medulloblastomas is not limited to muscle cell lineage (162). For reasons unknown to this old neuropathologist, muscle differentiation has historically been retained as defining a subcategory of medulloblastoma. PTAH stain, electron microscopy for sarcomeres and myofibrils, or IHC for desmin and muscle-specific actin markers (Table 10.13) confirm muscular differentiation.

Medullomyoblastomas are mixtures of stainable muscle cells

and small neuroectodermal cells resembling medulloblastoma, in contrast to pure primary intracranial rhabdomyosarcomas that do not include cells derived from neuroectoderm. Synaptophysin facilitates detection of these neuroectodermal cells.

Primitive Neuroectodermal Tumors (PNETs)—Grade IV

PNETs are composed of very crowded, small blue cells with high nuclear:cytoplasmic ratios; pleomorphic and hyperchromatic nuclei; and often mitoses and apoptosis. Markers of neuronal differentiation, such as synaptophysin and protein gene product (PGP 9.5), aid identification of PNET that resemble a medulloblastoma (Fig. 10.82) (163,164).

CENTRAL PRIMITIVE NEUROECTODERMAL TUMOR (cPNET)—GRADE IV. The cPNET is also known as a central nervous system primitive neuroectodermal tumor. Classic cPNET resembles the cerebellar medulloblastoma. Recent nomenclature identifies cPNET within any region of the CNS other than cerebellum, and broadens its definition to include a variety of other rare CNS tumors, including neuroblastoma, ganglioneuroblastoma, medulloepithelioma, and ependymoblastoma (8).

Although cPNETs express NSE, so do most gliomas. I prefer

more specific markers of neuronal differentiation, such as synaptophysin, to confirm a cPNET. cPNETs have occurred in patients with renal tumors and neural tube defects (163,164). Expression of a variety of other neuroectodermal antigens reflects the embryonal nature of these neoplasms (18).

PERIPHERAL PRIMITIVE NEUROECTODERMAL TUMOR (PPNET)—GRADE IV. pPNET also occurs in peripheral locations (see also the "Ewing Tumor" section, pages 241–243 in Chapter 8, Bone Tumors). pPNETs are associated with the t(11,22)(q24;q12) chromosomal translocation, and stain with MIC-2. Sites include those that arise from neural crest derivatives, gonads, chest wall, and bone. Rare pPNETs arise in the craniospinal vault (165). pPNET is highly aggressive; it recurs locally and metastasizes.

Medulloepithelioma—Grade IV

Keys to the recognition of this rare neoplasm are its occurrence in children under 6 years and its distinctive tubular and papillary epithelial growth pattern (Fig. 10.83) (Table 10.11) (8). Although the medulloepithelioma resembles metastatic carcinoma, the patient's age and lack of a primary neoplasm militates against the latter diagnosis. Choroid plexus carcinoma is more difficult to distinguish from medulloepithelioma, unless origin from a more differentiated papilloma can be determined. Dense pink material on the apical surface of medulloepithelioma cells and foci of neuroblastic differentiation help to distinguish it. The basal portion of its epithelium stains strongly for nestin. How this might help with the differential remains to be determined.

Atypical Teratoid/Rhabdoid Tumor—Grade IV

Infants and young children suffer from this rare and highly malignant tumor (166). It frequents the posterior fossa and metastasizes early through the CSF.

Malignant cells have more pink cytoplasm, and are more epithelial than medulloblastoma. Vacuolated cells and cells with rhabdoid features may be found. The tumor contains multiple different antigens and many intermediate filament types—almost always vimentin and EMA, and often focal GFAP, cytokeratin, neurofilaments, or muscle actin. Synaptophysin and chromogranin may be present. Atypical teratoid/rhabdoid tumors have abnormalities of chromosome 22, which helps to distinguish them from other primitive neuroectodermal tumors, including medulloblastoma, a tumor with which they are often confused (166). AT/RT lack the INI1 gene product.

CHOROID PLEXUS EPITHELIAL TUMORS

Choroid plexus neoplasms are uncommon. Most appear in childhood. Location is particularly important for the diagnosis of primary tumors of the choroid plexus (Table 10.11). They can occur in any portion of choroid plexus, but are more frequent in the lateral ventricles of children and the fourth ventricle of adults.

Focal GFAP reactivity in certain choroid plexus papillomas (CPPs) suggests focal ependymal differentiation. This has led to some to classify CPP among gliomas. A rare event in neuropathology, "Lumpers" may prevail over "Splitters." The separate classification of CPP is retained here because CPPs are predominantly epithelioid, and epithelioid tumors are the most likely to enter the differential diagnosis of CPP, atypical CPP, and choroid plexus carcinoma (CPC).

Choroid Plexus Papilloma—Grade I

Clinical and radiographic features often include hydrocephalus. The tumor must be larger than normal choroid plexus to occasion the diagnosis of choroid plexus papilloma, because its microscopic features are very similar to normal choroid plexus. Thus, needle biopsy for suspected CCP cannot be recommended (Fig. 10.2). Like the normal choroid plexus, CCPs have a well-defined fibrovascular core lined by epithelial cells. However, the epithelial lining of papillomas is more distinctly crowded and piled-up–appearing (Fig. 10.84) rather than the

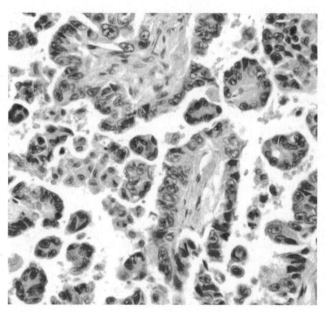

Figure 10.84. Choroid plexus papilloma. This solitary tumor in the cerebellopontine angle is composed of columnar epithelial cells manifesting mild cytologic pleomorphism and piling up on each other; the tumor cells surround a fibrovascular stroma.

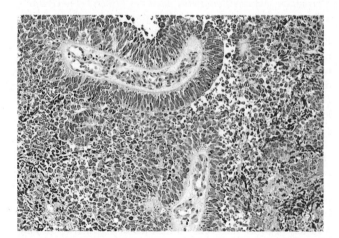

Figure 10.83. Medulloepithelioma. The anaplastic cells of this papillary neoplasm form a pseudostratified epithelium with dense material on its surface.

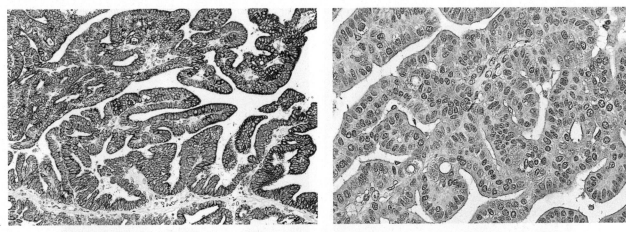

Figure 10.85. Choroid plexus papilloma. This typical choroid plexus papilloma from the lateral ventricle of a child expresses CAM5.2 cytokeratin **(A)** and transthyretin (prealbumin) **(B)**.

simple cuboidal epithelium of normal choroid plexus (Fig. 10.2A). Pigmented, oncocytic, osteogenic, and adenomatous variants of papillomas are uncommon variants (167–169). Cytologically, mild but minimal nuclear pleomorphism, atypia, and hyperchromicity can be noted, in contrast to the homogeneous population of uniformly sized, round nuclei in normal choroid plexus (Fig. 10.2A). Immunoreactivity for cytokeratin (Fig. 10.85A) and transthyretin (Fig. 10.85B) is present in choroid plexus epithelial cells (167). Some papillomas express GFAP, and some express synaptophysin.

The differential diagnosis includes primary tumors, including papillary variant of ependymoma and metastatic tumors, including papillary variants of thyroid, breast, renal, and ovarian carcinomas. In contrast to papillary ependymoma, the choroid plexus papilloma contains a single layer of columnar to cuboidal epithelial cells over a basement membrane, and fibrovascular stroma positive for type IV collagen, reticulin, and laminin (Tables 10.10 through 10.12) (see "Ependymoma," above). The choroid plexus papilloma lacks the necrosis and anaplasia seen in metastatic papillary carcinoma. The papilloma coexpresses CAM5.2, vimentin, and S-100 protein, a usual triad in carcinoma.

A potentially confusing neoplasm, the papillary variant of myxopapillary ependymoma, occurs in a different location than the choroid plexus papilloma. Mucin production in the choroid plexus papilloma, lack of whorls, and lack of solid, syncytial foci distinguish it from papillary meningioma.

Atypical Choroid Plexus Papilloma—Grade II

The concept of an "atypical" choroid plexus papilloma, at the interface between papilloma and carcinoma, has been raised. Criteria have been suggested for this entity: 2 or more mitoses per 10 randomly selected high-power fields (170).

Choroid Plexus Carcinoma—Grade III

The choroid plexus carcinoma (anaplastic choroid plexus papilloma) is a very rare neoplasm that is difficult to distinguish from metastatic carcinoma. The neoplasm architecturally consists of sheets of anaplastic cells, often with regions of necrosis; papillary features may be difficult to distinguish. In some cases, a transitional zone between papilloma and carcinoma of the choroid plexus is identified. Primary carcinoma of the choroid plexus so closely resembles metastatic carcinoma that the latter must be carefully excluded before making the diagnosis of primary choroid plexus carcinoma. The paucity of appropriate primary systemic carcinomas in children facilitates diagnosis of choroid plexus carcinoma in them (171).

MENINGEAL AND RELATED TUMORS

Meningiomas—Grade I

Meningeal location is a major discriminator of meningioma from other primary intracranial neoplasms (Tables 10.10 through 10.12 and 10.14). Most meningiomas are attached to dura, facilitating their recognition. Frequent locations are parasagittal, falx cerebri (Fig. 10.86), over the cerebral convexities, olfactory groove, sphenoid ridge, near the sella (107), foramen magnum, tentorium cerebelli, cerebellopontine angle, and spinal canal (172,173). Less commonly, meningiomas arise from the choroid plexus and, very rarely, within the CNS parenchyma itself (174). Choroid plexus, intraparenchymal, central pontine angle, and spinal meningiomas are the most diagnostically challenging because certain variants of meningioma mimic other tumors found in these locations, and meningioma may be forgotten in the differential. Macroscopically, meningiomas are firm with tiny nodules (Fig. 10.87).

The incidence of multiple meningiomas is between 1% and 6%. Only a fraction of them are associated with von Recklinghausen neurofibromatosis (NF-1) (8). Although the NF-1 gene is on chromosome 17, the classic genetic abnormality in meningioma is loss in chromosome 22.

Because the various histologic patterns of meningioma are highly diversified, few generalizations are applicable to every individual tumor. Nonetheless, the most common patterns of growth are (a) meningothelial, with syncytial and epithelioid cells and indistinct cell borders, (Fig. 10.88); (b) fibroblastic, consisting of spindle-shaped cells with indistinct cell boundaries (Fig. 10.91); and (c) transitional, including both meningothelial and fibroblastic, and classic whorls (Fig. 10.92). Psammoma bodies are common but highly variable in number from case to case.

Certain features should be recognized as evidence of menin-

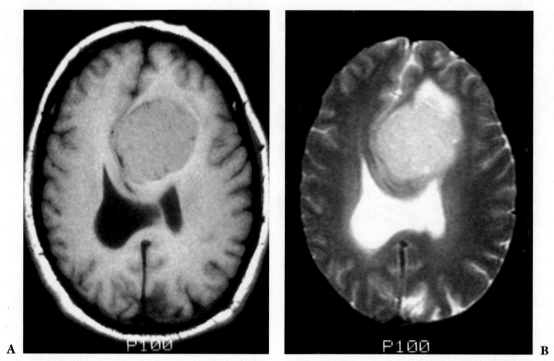

Figure 10.86. Large, falcine meningioma. This neoplasm in this 48-year-old man distorts the frontal lobes and lateral ventricles on magnetic resonance images. **(A)** The T1-weighted signal is well demarcated and is darker than white matter. **(B)** T2-weighted signal shows focal edema rostral to the tumor. *(Courtesy of Dr. James Brunberg, University of Michigan, Ann Arbor, Michigan.)*

gioma in any tumor from the craniospinal vault (173). A syncytial appearance (Fig. 10.88) is a distinctive feature of meningothelial meningiomas and a focal feature of other subtypes of meningioma (Table 10.14). The structural bases of this syncytial appearance are numerous tightly interdigitating cellular processes held together by desmosomes, not a true syncytium (Fig. 10.89). These structures confirm meningioma by electron microscopy in rare cases that cannot be confirmed by epithelial membrane antigen (EMA) IHC.

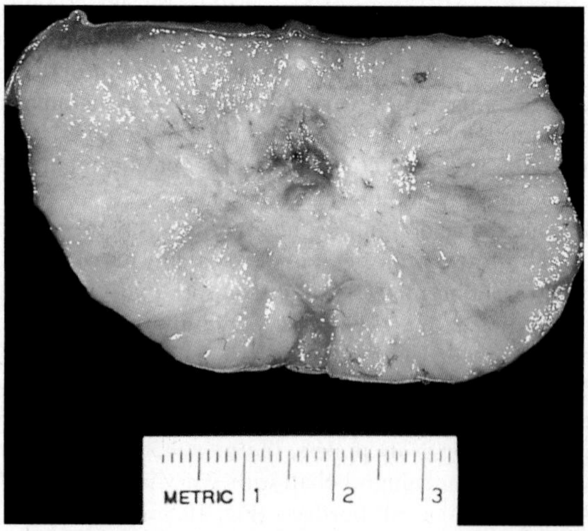

Whorls and psammoma bodies typify meningiomas (Figs. 10.92 and 10.93). Psammoma bodies are concentrically laminated calcifications. Most meningiomas contain EMA, which distinguishes them from gliomas (Fig. 10.90 and 10.91B) (172,173). Vimentin and S-100 protein expression should be used only in combination with other markers because many tumors other than meningioma express these markers (18).

In contrast to gliomas, cells with large or hyperchromatic nuclei are not evidence of aggressive growth. Instead, specific subtypes identified by their structural and histochemical features, cytology, mitotic activity, and brain invasion are guides to aggressive growth.

MENINGOTHELIAL MENINGIOMA (SYNCYTIAL MENINGIOMA)—GRADE I. This is the classic syncytial meningioma (Fig. 10.88), which resembles the small clusters of meningeal cells found normally in the meninges and choroid plexus. Its features are described above, but whorls and psammoma bodies are often sparse (Table 10.14).

Its syncytial appearance, whorls, psammoma bodies, and its usual dural attachment distinguish this meningioma from neoplasms other than meningioma. Meningothelial meningioma occasionally appears epithelioid and simulates ependymoma, but the meningioma lacks GFAP.

These meningiomas can be confused with oligodendrogliomas. Epithelial membrane antigen reactivity identifies the meningiomas. The margin of a meningioma with CNS parenchyma is more discrete than that of a glioma. Equivocal cases require electron microscopy as described above (Fig. 10.89).

Figure 10.87. Fibroblastic meningioma. Taken from the right parietal dura of a 65-year-old woman, this meningioma has a bosselated surface of multiple tan nodules separated by fibrous tissue. It contains regions of red surgical hemorrhage, white collagen, and yellow lipoid metaplasia. *(Courtesy of Dr. Walter Henricks, University of Michigan, Ann Arbor, Michigan.)*

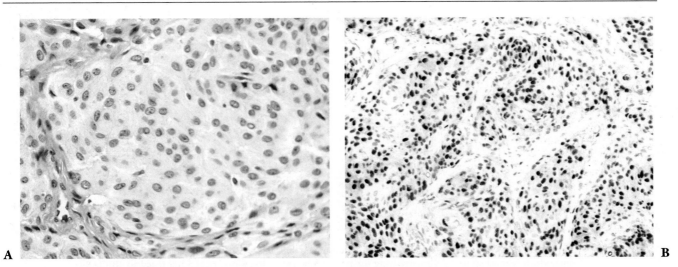

A   B

Figure 10.88. Meningothelial meningioma. This was a left frontal meningeal tumor in a 59-year-old man.
(A) Its indistinct cellular boundaries and syncytial appearance reflect tightly interdigitating cellular processes
too small to see without electron microscopy (see next Fig. 10.89). Its nuclei are round to oval with smooth
membranes, finely stippled chromatin, and small nucleoli. A few nuclei have light pink cytoplasmic inclusions.
At the edge of the image, vascular tissue surrounds this nest of cells. **(B)** Nests of meningioma cells are highlighted by their brown nuclei stained for progesterone receptors (PR). Vascular septae that segregate these
nests are negative for PR.

**FIBROBLASTIC MENINGIOMA (FIBROUSMENINGIOMA)—
GRADE I.** Fibroblastic meningiomas are firm tumors composed
of spindle cells (Table 10.10). They resemble schwannomas,
fibrillary astrocytomas, and pilocytic astrocytomas. This resemblance produces confusion in regions where more than one of
these tumors is found, specifically the cerebellopontine angle,
spinal nerve routes, cauda equina, and CNS parenchyma (Fig.
10.91). Fibrous meningiomas express at least focal EMA, which
distinguish them from schwannomas and astrocytomas (18).

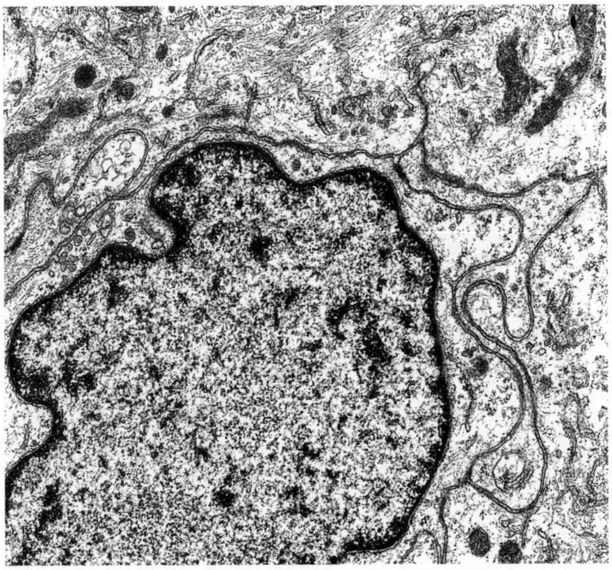

Fibrous meningiomas often have very thick bundles of collagen within tumor parenchyma. This excludes schwannoma and
astrocytoma from the differential diagnosis.

**TRANSITIONAL MENINGIOMA (MIXED MENINGIOMA)—
GRADE I.** Transitional meningiomas are composed of syncytial
and fibroblastic components as described above. The presence
of cells intermediate between syncytial and fibroblastic justi-
fies their designation as transitional (4). Prominent whorls,
psammoma bodies, and clusters of syncytial cells make these
very common meningiomas among the easiest to identify with
H&E (Fig. 10.92).

PSAMMOMATOUS MENINGIOMA—GRADE I. Psammomatous meningiomas are often found in the spinal region. They
are crowded with psammoma bodies. This benign variant is recognized as meningioma by finding syncytial cells between the
conspicuous, concentrically laminated psammoma bodies (Fig.
10.93).

**HEMANGIOBLASTIC, ANGIOBLASTIC, AND ANGIOMATOUS
MENINGIOMAS—GRADE I.** Angiomatous meningioma has features typical of a benign meningioma but in addition contains
many small or large vascular channels (4). These may predominate over its meningothelial elements (Fig. 10.94). An angiomatous meningioma can closely resemble hemangioblastoma or
become sclerotic.

It has become popular to call all of these vascular subtypes
of meningioma "angiomatous" meningioma. The rationale for
keeping separate subtypes is to recall that meningiomas mimic
other tumors (i.e., some meningiomas can mimic hemangioblastomas). Unlike hemangioblastoma, most of these meningiomas contain meningothelial cells concentrically wrapped
around small blood vessels and capillaries. In the face of such
mimicry, confirmation of meningioma is positive staining for

Figure 10.89. Recurrent meningothelial meningioma. It spread
along the dura at the base of the skull in a 40-year-old man. Ultrastructurally, it contains tightly interdigitating cellular processes and desmosomes.

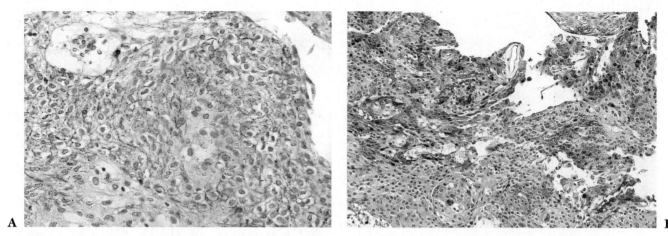

A   B

Figure 10.90. Meningioma. Epithelial membrane antigen lines the cell surfaces of regions of this meningioma, which is attached to the dura overlying the frontal lobe (**A**). It has widespread S-100 reactivity (**B**).

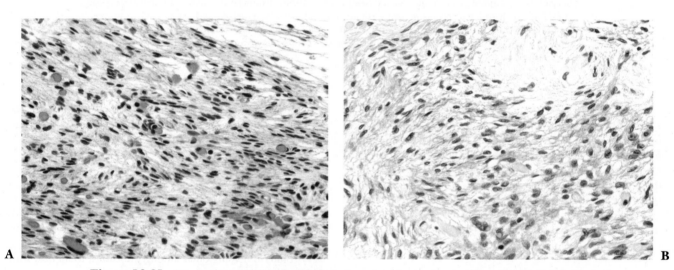

A   B

Figure 10.91. Fibroblastic meningioma. Right frontal meningeal tumor in a younger than usual patient, an adolescent boy. (**A**) The tumor has elongated cells and nuclei that resemble a schwannoma. (**B**) Epithelial membrane antigen expression confirms meningioma.

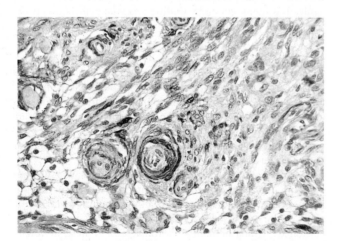

Figure 10.92. Transitional meningioma. S-100 protein is only focally present in this cerebellopontine angle transitional meningioma with lipoid metaplasia and whorls.

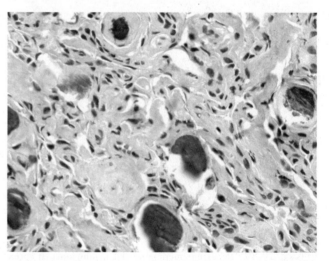

Figure 10.93. Psammomatous meningioma. This cervical intradural, extramedullary tumor shows abundant psammoma bodies, many of which have calcified.

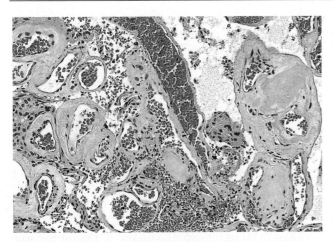

Figure 10.94. Angiomatous meningioma. This tumor resembles a vascular malformation, except for its clusters of meningothelial cells between the vessels.

PR and/or EMA, and confirmation of hemangioblastoma is positive staining for NSE and/or EGFR.

OTHER MENINGIOMAS OF GRADE I. Dual epithelial and mesenchymal components of meningiomas have spawned a plethora of proposed variant types of meningiomas. Recognizing these other variants helps to avoid mistaking them for other entities, including ones requiring different treatments (175–182). Variants include lipoblastic (181), arachnoid trabecular (177), microcystic (180), lymphoplasmacytic-rich (4), osteogenic (178), cartilaginous (178), secretory (182) (Fig. 10.95), and mucoid (176) meningiomas. Keys to distinguishing these variants of meningioma from carcinoma and sarcoma are finely granular chromatin, few mitoses, and meningothelial features. Adequate sampling and inspection usually reveal foci with a syncytial pattern, whorls, or at least a tendency of meningeal cells to flatten and encircle vessels; but ultrastructural confirmation is the key to difficult cases.

Aggressive or Malignant Meningiomas

BRAIN INVASION. Invasion of adjacent cerebral parenchyma or invasion of small blood vessels within the tumor is considered to connote a *higher risk of recurrence* of a meningioma. At this time, evidence of brain invasion is not one of the factors that is invoked in grading and does not constitute a criterion for increased grade (8). Brain invasion is considered more ominous than dural invasion, the latter a common finding in low- and high-grade meningiomas.

MENINGIOMA—GRADE II. Certain histologic features of meningioma, such as chordoid or clear-cell features, are associated with aggressive behavior and a tendency to recur. They and atypical meningioma are given an intermediate grade of II.

CHORDOID MENINGIOMA—GRADE II. The chordoid meningioma variant is particularly vexing due to its similarity to chordoma. It is found in childhood more often than most meningiomas (179). It is distinguished by its meningothelial features and lack of cytokeratin (Fig. 10.96). Its diagnosis carries a WHO grade of II because of its tendency to recur.

ATYPICAL MENINGIOMA—GRADE II. This subtype of meningioma need not show any chordoid or clear-cell features (183). Theoretically, any lower-grade subtype could be an atypical meningioma, but most atypical meningiomas would otherwise be considered meningothelial if they had fewer of the features in the criteria described below.

Specific criteria for the distinction between benign meningioma and atypical meningioma are summarized in Table 10.15. Using these criteria, the diagnosis of atypical meningioma can be made in a meningioma that manifests between 4 and 19 mitotic figures in 10 high-power fields (hpfs) (Fig. 10.97A). As described by Dr. Arie Perry of the Dept. of Pathology and Immunology, Washington University School of Medicine, St. Louis, Missouri, these 10 hpfs are chosen to find the "hot spots" of highest mitotic activity before starting to count. By comparing fields at intermediate to high magnification, these hot spots

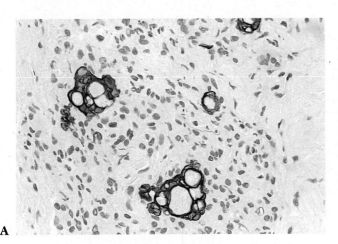
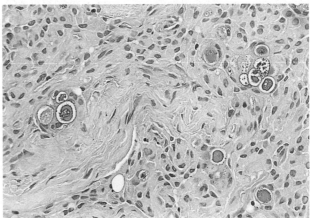

A **B**

Figure 10.95. Secretory meningioma. Although most meningioma cells are negative, these strikingly CAM5.2 cytokeratin-positive (**A**) structures resemble acini. Unlike carcinoma, its cytologic features are benign and meningothelial. Typically, focal clusters of immunoreactive cells surround "secretory" globules that are periodic acid-Schiff–positive (**B**).

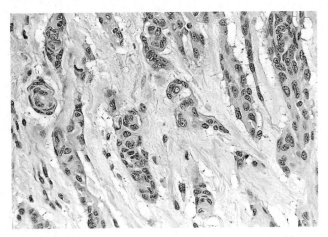

Figure 10.96. Chordoid meningioma. Cords of cells between myxoid collagen resemble chordoma except for their meningothelial nuclei and whorl formation.

correlate to some extent with the histologic features described below (184).

An alternative route to the diagnosis of atypical meningioma is to find three or more specific histologic features from among increased cellularity; small cells with a high N:C ratio; prominent nucleoli; patternless, sheetlike growth; and foci of spontaneous or "geographic" necrosis. These may be spotted at low magnification. They are recognized to correspond to a neoplasm that is likely to be more aggressive than grade I meningiomas, and to recur locally (184). Seemingly subjective criteria have been quantified. For example, increased cellularity was defined as ≥53 nuclei/hpf diameter (184).

Although not currently a component of the WHO criteria, chromosomal abnormalities (in addition to the standard loss of chromosome 22) or MIB-1 may forecast increased aggressiveness (8,183).

In a tumor in which atypical findings are noted, but findings fall short of criteria for diagnosis of atypical meningioma, I use a diagnosis of "Meningioma, grade I, with (either 1 or 2) atypical features." Although the WHO grade in this case would still be I, the clinicians are alerted to watch that meningioma.

Intervention prior to surgery has the potential to introduce pitfalls in surgical neuropathology. Vascular embolization even a day or two prior to surgery (in an attempt to limit bleeding, a significant intraoperative complication) may produce iatrogenic necrosis (Fig. 10.98). Care is needed to determine whether necrosis is spontaneous or the tumors were embolized prior to surgery. Although these emboli are often visible in the specimen, the surgeon will know whether they were used. If necrosis is the only feature in an otherwise benign, embolized meningioma, it should not be interpreted as pathologic.

CLEAR CELL MENINGIOMA—GRADE II. One of the many reasons to subclassify meningiomas is to identify more aggressive variants. This subtype is an example. Although it looks benign, many clear-cell meningiomas are biologically aggressive. At present, its location in the cranial vault influences its higher grade, compared with spinal clear-cell meningiomas (8). A mixture of clear cells and meningothelial features are keys to its diagnosis (185). Cytoplasmic glycogen helps to confirm the diagnosis (Fig. 10.99). This variant is particularly common in the lumbar and cerebellopontine angle regions.

MENINGIOMAS OF GRADE III. Certain histologic features of meningioma, such as chordoid or clear-cell features, are associated with very aggressive behavior and are given the highest grade recognized as a meningioma, grade III.

RHABDOID MENINGIOMA—GRADE III. This uncommon morphologic variant of meningioma is a highly aggressive tumor. Barely cohesive cells depart from the usual syncytial appearance of meningioma. They are filled with abundant eosinophilic cytoplasm (186). Hyaline perinuclear inclusions contain whorls of intermediate filaments seen by electron microscopy,

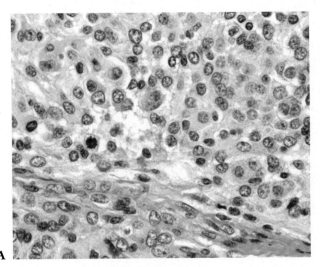

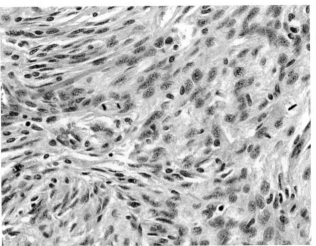

A   B

Figure 10.97. Atypical and anaplastic meningiomas. **(A)** This atypical meningioma had five mitotic figures in 10 high-power fields. **(B)** This anaplastic meningioma was rapidly increasing in size in the left parietal region of a 67-year-old man. It has both meningothelial and sarcomatoid cells. Some of its 27 mitotic figures in 10 high-power fields are shown here. One shows its mitotic spindle organizers.

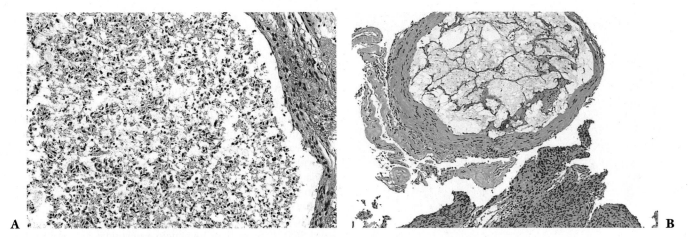

Figure 10.98. Early necrosis in meningioma. This meningioma (**A**) was embolized with 45-μm to 150-μm contour emboli, Avitene powder, and gelatin foam (**B**) by interventional angiography 1 day before surgery. Discohesive cells contain pyknotic or eosinophilic nuclei.

with IHC reactivity for vimentin. These push the meningothelial nuclei to the side of the cell.

When this variant occurs within a classic meningioma or as a recurrence, it is easy to recognize. Rare tumors are entirely rhabdoid, making them more difficult to identify and distinguish from epithelioid and gemistocytic gliomas. In such cases, location, pattern of brain invasion, vimentin predominance and EMA reactivity, and ultrastructure reveal their true identity.

Within the cranial vault, the rhabdoid phenotype is an ominous feature. It usually signals a poor prognosis.

PAPILLARY MENINGIOMA—GRADE III. Papillary configurations in meningiomas are rare, but they are prognostically associated with high rates of local recurrence and metastases. The papillae have a vascular core (Fig. 10.100), and may form by edematous or necrotic loosening of the surrounding tumor cells (4).

The recognition of a papillary meningioma in other than dural locations characteristic for meningioma is difficult. Papillary meningiomas resemble papillary ependymomas, choroid plexus papillomas, and carcinomas. Look for other histologic

regions of the tumor to detect features more characteristic of meningioma. Use EMA and, if necessary, electron microscopy.

ANAPLASTIC MENINGIOMA (MALIGNANT MENINGIOMA)—GRADE III. Anaplastic meningiomas (Fig. 10.97B) tend to be lobulated and circumscribed neoplasms that usually retain enough histologic features in their more differentiated regions to be recognized as meningiomas. Histologic criteria that confer the designation anaplastic meningioma include either (a) 20 or more mitotic figures per 10 hpfs, or (b) regions with malignant, anaplastic cytology, resembling a sarcoma, carcinoma, or melanoma (187) (Table 10.15). MIB-1 labeling indices, although not a criterion for advancing the grade of the tumor, are high in most anaplastic meningiomas (188). The median survival of patients is 2 years (187).

Anaplastic meningiomas may be confused with anaplastic gliomas and glioblastomas, particularly when the high-grade glioma stains equivocally for GFAP and invades the meninges; or, alternatively, when an anaplastic meningioma stains poorly for EMA. Even when invading brain, a meningioma has a more discrete margin than do most gliomas, and does not form sec-

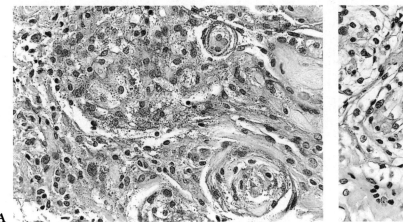

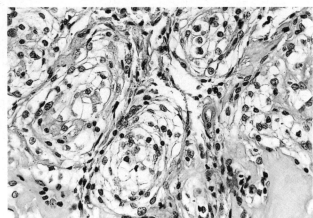

Figure 10.99. Clear-cell meningioma. This tumor has recurred several times in the lumbar spinal dura of this 43-year-old man. Its cells contain glycogen seen with the periodic acid-Schiff stain (**A**) and confirmed by digestion with diastase (**B**).

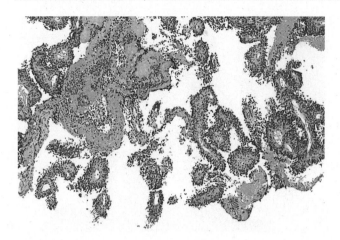

Figure 10.100. Papillary meningioma. The papillae are composed of syncytial cells making rosettes around the vessels.

ondary structures of Scherer. Often the invasive front of a meningioma is discrete or proceeds along vessels, trapping islands of gliotic CNS parenchyma along the way. This pattern is distinct from the individual neoplastic glial cells, which wander many centimeters throughout the CNS parenchyma surrounding gliomas. If none of the above is conclusive, use electron microscopy.

Hemangiopericytoma—Grade II or III

This highly cellular and mitotically active neoplasm, rich in pericellular reticulin, has features similar to hemangiopericytomas (HPCs) elsewhere in the body. This lesion was previously considered an "angioblastic" variant of meningioma. Correct diagnosis is critical because HPCs are biologically aggressive; approximately 60% to 80% of HPCs recur and 23% to 64% metastasize (bone, liver, lung, CNS) (4,189).

Histologically, HPCs are distinguished from meningiomas by their uniform hypercellularity, relatively homogeneous appearance of cells, uniform and higher mitotic index, "staghorn" vascular pattern, and microscopic tendency to bulge into vascular lumina without bursting through the endothelium (Fig. 10.101) (Tables 10.13 and 10.14) (189). HPC nuclei are less pleomorphic and less spindled than fibrosarcoma. Histochemically, the hemangiopericytoma can also be distinguished from such malignant neoplasms as malignant gliomas and metastatic carcinomas by foci of extensive basement membrane or reticulin around every cell, highlighted by a silver or type IV collagen stain (Fig. 10.101). HPCs lack the "ropey" collagenous connective tissue of the solitary fibrous tumor (SFT) (Fig. 10.102) (172).

IHC distinguishes many meningeal HPCs from meningioma and SFT. A majority of hemangiopericytomas are positive for factor 13a and Leu-7 and also positive for CD34. Unfortunately, staining of meningioma, SFT, and meningeal HPC overlap (190,191), so caution is necessary in interpretation; see comparison with SFT below (192,193).

Solitary Fibrous Tumor

The meningeal solitary fibrous tumor (SFT) is found in many locations, including mediastinum and pleura. Unfortunately, when in the dura, it is often not recognized (172). The SFT typically presents as a dural-based lesion in the cranium and spinal canal with occasional intra-axial (lateral ventricle, spinal cord) presentation, but can recur and metastasize (Fig. 10.102) (192–194). SFT and can be confused histologically with a fibrous meningioma and HPC. It consists of a relatively monomorphic population of spindle cells with the characteristic presence of abundant, "ropey" collagen intimately admixed with the neoplastic cells. Characteristically, the neoplastic cells are diffusely and strongly immunoreactive for CD34 and also label with CD99 and BCL2, although they are negative for EMA. In

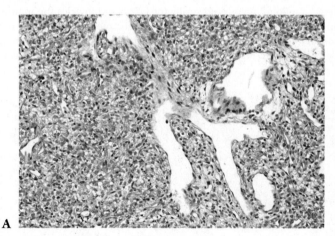

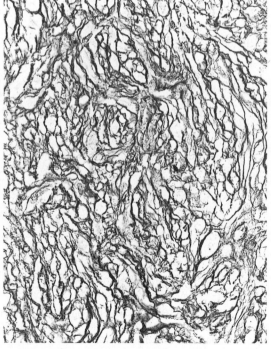

Figure 10.101. Hemangiopericytoma. Multiple recurrent tumor in the left parietal meninges of a 64-year-old woman. Neoplastic cells distort vascular lumina **(A)**. Reticulin surrounds each individual cell **(B)**.

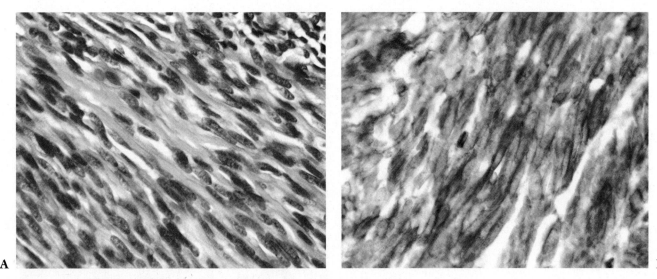

Figure 10.102. Solitary fibrous tumor. This dura-based tumor is from a 43-year-old woman. **(A)** The spindle cell tumor has prominent admixed collagen bundles. **(B)** CD34 immunostain labels the neoplastic cells. The cells were negative for epithelial membrane antigen (not shown).

contrast and important in differential diagnosis, CD34 labeling is diffuse but weaker in HPC and patchy and weak in fibrous meningiomas (193,194). Some HPC are also SFT.

Chordoma

Location is central to the diagnosis of chordoma (Table 10.11). The embryonic notochord is a midline structure prescribing the sites of chordomas. Most chordomas occur at either end of the primitive notochord, approximately 40% in the clivus and 45% in the sacrum; the rest occur from notochord vestiges along the spinal column, 10% along cervical, 2% along thoracic, and 2% along lumbar portions of the spine. Because of their propensity to slowly invade surrounding tissues, including bone, the precise anatomic origin of individual chordomas is often difficult to establish.

''Physaliphorous cells'' of chordomas contain large, characteristic intracytoplasmic vacuoles (Fig. 10.103). Because the cells frequently grow in cords, these vacuoles occasionally line up like beads on a string, differing from the principal differential diagnostic entities—chondrosarcoma and other chondroid neoplasms, which have individual or paired cells embedded in a myxoid matrix (195–198). IHC clearly differentiates these entities: chordomas express S-100, cytokeratin, EMA, and 5'-nucleotidase; whereas chondrosarcomas express S-100 but lack the other antigens (18). The ''chordoid meningioma'' lacks cytokeratin expression.

The vacuoles of physaliphorous cells contain mucin and glycogen (Fig. 10.103), unlike watery perinuclear oligodendroglial vacuoles and the multiplicity of smaller lipid vacuoles of hemangioblastomas (Fig. 10.54, and see Fig. 10.119 in the ''Neuroendocrine Tumors'' section below). By electron microscopy, chordomas have desmosomes and distinctive mitochondrial-rough endoplasmic reticulum complexes, both of which chondrosarcomas lack (195).

Malignant histologic transformation of chordoma is uncommon. Despite this, relentless local invasion of clinically sensitive regions results in a poor long-term prognosis.

Chordomas can contain chondroid elements. The resulting chondroid chordomas may have slightly longer patient survival than do regular chordoma. They contain regions of classical chordoma that are positive for EMA, cytokeratin, and S-100; and chondroid regions that are S-100–positive and lack EMA and cytokeratin (195). Some pathologists prefer to interpret such tumors as either chordomas or low-grade chondrosarcomas.

Chondroma and Chondrosarcoma

Chondroid neoplasms with conspicuous cartilage formation have distinct features that are readily identified. They occur infrequently in the meninges, and rarely within the choroid plexus or CNS parenchyma. Midline chondroid lesions, particularly those arising in the base of the skull, clivus, or the region of the cauda equina, should prompt consideration of chordoma.

The mesenchymal chondrosarcoma is rare. It originates in the intracranial and spinal meninges and cauda equina in childhood and young adulthood (199). It resembles hemangiopericytoma except for islands of atypical cartilage or chondrosarcoma.

Poorly differentiated chondrosarcomas are rare, and usually involve the meninges. They can be difficult to distinguish from other sarcomas and from meningeal gliomatosis and carcinomatosis. A key feature is evidence of cartilage production, which is often sparse (199). Presence of S-100 protein as evidence of chondroid differentiation must be interpreted cautiously in meningeal and CNS neoplasms because most gliomas, chordomas, melanomas, nerve sheath tumors, and some meningiomas contain S-100 protein (4,173) (see Figs. 10.70 and 10.90).

Other Sarcomas—Grade III to IV

Sarcomas are discussed in more detail in Chapter 5, Disorders of Soft Tissue. Only specifics related to the CNS and meninges are mentioned here. Sarcomas and melanomas are unusual among brain tumors in that they may arise as a primary meningeal tumor, a primary CNS parenchymal tumor, or as a metas-

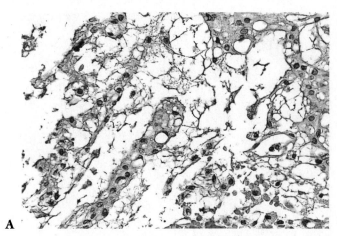

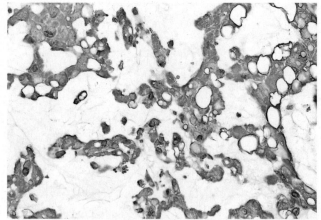

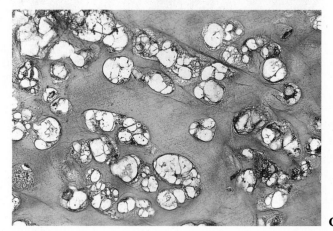

Figure 10.103. Chordoma. Cords of physaliphorous cells sit in mucin (**A**). The cells are positive for CAM 5.2 cytokeratin (**B**) and for mucin (**C**). The tumor also was positive for vimentin and S-100 protein (not shown).

tasis from other parts of the body (197–200). The latter two entities are very rare. A few sarcomas grow out from mixed tumors (200), and the rare mesenchymal chondrosarcoma resembles a mixed tumor (199). Reported incidences of primary intracranial sarcomas vary from 0.08% to 4.3%, the former percentage being more contemporary (197). This lower incidence partly reflects application of ultrastructure and IHC to identify the lymphoid or neuroectodermal nature of entities previously thought to be sarcoma, such as the primary brain lymphoma and the giant-cell glioblastoma (92). Malignant fibrous histiocytoma (MFH) and myogenic sarcoma were more common than fibrosarcoma in one group of cases (197). Liposarcomas are rare within the craniospinal vault.

The key to differentiating sarcoma from other malignant meningeal neoplasms is its lack of features of glial and meningeal cells (4). Lack of GFAP-positive neoplastic glia distinguishes sarcoma from glioblastoma invading the meninges and from gliosarcoma (125). Total lack of meningeal histology distinguishes sarcoma from anaplastic meningioma (Tables 10.10 and 10.14).

Prior radiation correlates with a significant percentage of intracranial sarcomas, particularly in the sellar region after radiotherapy for craniopharyngioma or adenoma (198). Patients with sarcomas that follow sellar radiation succumb within months due to local tumor invasion.

PERIPHERAL NERVE SHEATH TUMORS—GRADE I–IV

Peripheral nerve sheath tumors are discussed in more detail in Chapter 5, Disorders of Soft Tissue. Within the craniospinal

vault, benign nerve sheath tumors (grade I) can be subclassified as either schwannoma or neurofibroma as described under these headings (Table 10.10). Malignant peripheral nerve sheath tumors (MPNSTs, grade IIs to IV) arise either in the setting of neurofibroma or de novo; only very rare example of MPNSTs arising in the setting of schwannoma have been identified. There is an increased incidence of MPNST in neurofibromatosis type 1 (NF-1).

Immunohistochemically, schwannomas and neurofibromas are robustly positive for S-100 protein and Leu-7; both can be positive for GFAP; both are negative for epithelial membrane antigen (EMA) and keratin. MPNSTs tend to have markedly reduced expression of S-100.

Schwannoma (Neurilemoma, Neurinoma)—Grade I

Schwannomas tend to arise on peripheral aspects of, and compress, nerves and can be encapsulated (Table 10.10). They consist of a relatively pure population of Schwann cells and characteristically manifest Antoni A (cellular) and Antoni B (vacuolated) regions, although less commonly in the cerebellopontine angle (CPA) than at other sites. They often have collagenized vessel walls and perivascular hemosiderin deposition. They lack admixed axons.

Within the cranial vault, nearly all schwannomas are attached to the 8th cranial nerve (Fig. 10.104), from which the confusing clinical term *acoustic neuroma* is derived. Few schwannomas are attached to the 5th or 7th, and even fewer to other cranial nerves. Within the spinal canal, schwannomas are usually at-

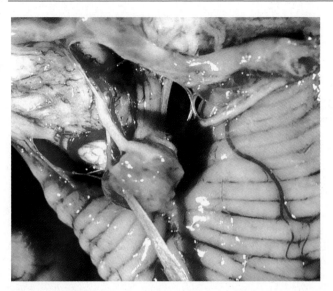

Figure 10.104. Schwannoma. A peripheral nerve sheath tumor exophytically arises in the cerebellopontine angle between the white brainstem and red-streaked cerebellum. It lies directly adjacent to the white 8th cranial nerve.

tached to a sensory (dorsal) spinal nerve root. They may secondarily extend into the cord itself, or very rarely originate within the spinal cord.

Bilateral 8th nerve schwannomas indicate neurofibromatosis type 2 (NF-2). Unusual locations and associations with gliomas, meningiomas, and meningeal proliferation are also seen with NF-2 (201,202). The NF-2 gene is a complex gene on chromosome 22q12. It encodes information for a protein called merlin or schwannomin (8).

The differential diagnosis of schwannoma and neurofibroma includes fibroblastic meningioma (Fig. 10.91), solitary fibrous tumor (Fig. 10.102), tanycytic ependymoma, subependymoma (Fig. 10.61), and astrocytoma (Fig. 10.39). Schwannoma can be

distinguished from astrocytoma and ependymoma by its abundant parenchymal basement membranes that stain well with type IV collagen (Fig. 10.105B). Focal reactivity of some schwannomas with anti-GFAP requires care in the use of these antisera to dissect a differential.

Fibroblastic meningiomas are difficult to distinguish histologically from schwannomas when the specimen lacks characteristic features of meningioma, such as meningeal whorls and psammoma bodies. Antoni A and B growth patterns resemble fibroblastic meningiomas (Fig. 10.91). Verocay bodies (Fig. 10.105) are more distinctive of schwannomas than the Antoni patterns, but are not seen in all schwannomas. An IHC panel including EMA and type IV collagen resolves most cases. Schwannomas have more continuous basement membranes all along the exterior surface of their cells than do the meningiomas or gliomas in the differential. The basement membranes are seen with the aid of type IV collagen stain or electron microscopy on the most difficult cases (Table 10.10). They lack EMA found in meningiomas.

Neurofibroma—Grade I

Neurofibromas arise and infiltrate within nerves and, thus, neoplastic cells are intimately admixed with axons. Schwann cells, perineurial cells, fibroblasts, and mast cells are admixed. They generally lack Antoni A and B regions; their vessels are typically thin-walled and lack perivascular hemosiderin deposition. They often have a myxoid extracellular matrix.

Plexiform neurofibromas are associated with neurofibromatosis type 1 (NF-1), caused by a mutation in chromosome 17q12, and are associated with the "neurofibromin" gene product. The vast majority of neurofibromas, including those in NF-1, occur outside of the craniospinal vault.

Perineurioma—Grades I–III

Perineurial cells are specialized epithelioid myofibroblasts with tight junctions that normally compose the perineurium, a spe-

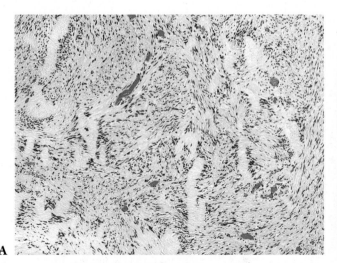

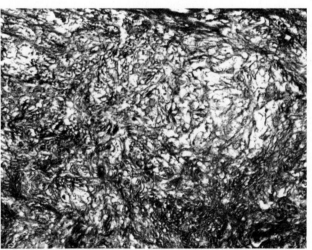

A   B

Figure 10.105. Schwannoma. **(A)** Antoni A pattern with palisades of nuclei and fibrils called Verocay bodies in a schwannoma of the right 8th cranial nerve in a 33-year-old man. Verocay bodies should be viewed at a low power like this to be appreciated. (Compare with palisades of nuclei and fibrils of a subependymoma in Figure 10.61.) **(B)** Schwannomas have basement membranes surrounding each cell, turning them dark brown with a type IV collagen stain. This is from the right brachial plexus of a 72-year-old man.

cialized nerve sheath that forms a protective barrier of 6 to 10 concentric cell layers around nerve fascicles. Perineuriomas are their neoplastic counterparts. Intraneural perineuriomas are benign grade I tumors that enlarge nerve diameters—enlargement that can involve a considerable length of the nerve. Soft tissue perineuriomas can be benign or malignant.

Intraneural perineuriomas swell the nerve from within. They form concentric layers of spindled cells and collagen around axons that resemble whorls or onion bulbs. Because classic onion bulbs are formed by Schwann cells in the context of chronic demyelination, the perineurioma must form pseudo-onion bulbs. Because perineurioma cells are EMA-positive and S-100-protein–negative, these pseudo-onion bulbs are easily distinguished from onion bulbs of Schwann cells with the opposite staining pattern. Perineurioma cells are also positive for vimentin, and surrounded by type IV collagen. Being located within the endoneurium of a peripheral nerve distinguishes the perineurioma from a fibrous meningioma.

Malignant Peripheral Nerve Sheath Tumor (MPNST)—Grades II–IV

Malignant nerve sheath tumors are very rare within the cranial cavity (Table 10.10). They arise in peripheral nerves, frequently in the context of NF-1 (202). They usually arise in the context of a neurofibroma, with a transition demonstrable histologically, but also can arise de novo. They only rarely originate from schwannoma or ganglioneuroblastoma.

Histologic features in MPNST are variable among tumors. In resections, identification of infiltration within a nerve is a critical architectural feature. The tumor shows (a) marked hypercellularity, either diffuse or variable from region to region, of cells with spindle-shaped nuclei manifesting tapered ends, less often epithelioid; (b) nuclear pleomorphism; and (c) often but not always brisk mitotic activity, which may include abnormal mitoses (Fig. 10.106). Necrosis distinguishes grade IV MPNST, which is the most common grade on adequate samples of tumor. Grade II tumors mimic neurofibromas (NFs), but their nuclei are darker than and three times the size of NF

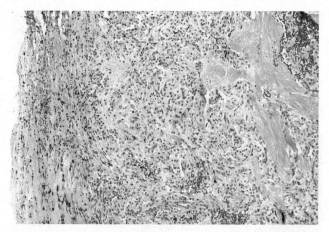

Figure 10.107. Paraganglioma. This tumor has clusters of cells separated by fibrovascular stroma (Zellballen).

nuclei (8). Immunohistochemically, in most MPNSTs, expression of S-100 protein is markedly reduced, with identification in only scattered cells or absent expression. In MPNST, p53 is high and S-100 low, whereas these stains are just the oposite in NF. Epithelial differentiation, regions of rhabdomyosarcoma ("Triton tumor") and chondrosarcoma, are identified in some tumors and should be reported in the diagnosis. Full examination of resections and evaluation of prior biopsies are critical to correct diagnosis.

NEUROENDOCRINE TUMORS (SEE ALSO SECTION IV, "ENDOCRINE SYSTEM")

Paraganglioma—Grade I

Paragangliomas can be identified within the spinal canal (Fig. 10.107) and can grow into the posterior fossa from the temporal bone (115). As in other sites, neuroendocrine cells have a cytoplasmic granularity, and often form nests (Zellballen) between numerous thin-walled vessels (203). Regions of ganglion cell

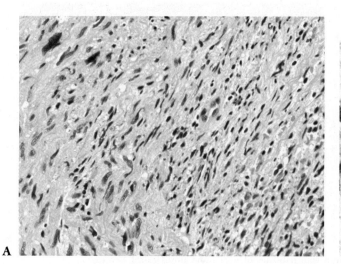

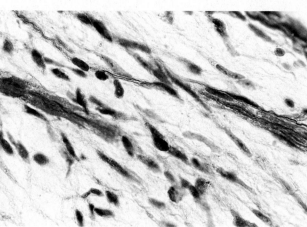

Figure 10.106. Malignant peripheral nerve sheath tumors (MPNSTs). **(A)** This MPNST invaded nerves in the left brachial plexus of a 15-year-old boy. It has a fascicular pattern of pleomorphic cells that are predominantly spindled with hyperchromatic nuclei. **(B)** This MPNST in the cauda equina of a 45-year-old man grew within the nerve fascicles spreading apart black axons surrounded by blue myelin.

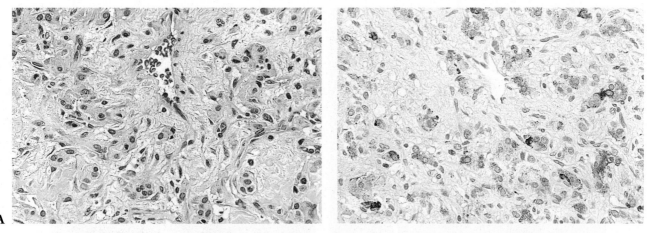

Figure 10.108. Paraganglioma. This tumor from the cauda equina of a 55-year-old man imitates a myxopapillary ependymoma (**A**). However, immunoperoxidase stains revealed that its cells contain chromogranin (**B**) and that they were glial fibrillary acidic protein negative (not shown).

differentiation can be seen in some tumors. By location and structure, the differential of paragangliomas includes angiomatous meningiomas, myxopapillary ependymomas (Fig. 10.108), hemangioblastomas, and renal cell carcinomas. Abundant secretory granules are demonstrated by immunostaining for chromogranin only in the paraganglioma, and these neurosecretory granules are also visible ultrastructurally. For paragangliomas near the nervous system, chromogranin discriminates paragangliomas from other tumors better than synaptophysin. Paragangliomas with well-formed Zellballen are distinct from the more intimate mixture of capillary and stromal cells in hemangioblastoma; the latter have vacuolated cells, which are not noted in the paraganglioma (Fig. 10.107, and see Figs. 10.119 through 10.121 in the "Hemangioblastoma (Capillary Hemangioblastoma)—Grade I" section below).

Pituitary Adenoma—Grade I

Pituitary adenomas are covered in Chapter 12, The Pituitary and Sellar Region. Pituitary adenomas occasionally grow dorsally into the base of the brain and imitate oligodendroglioma, ependymoma, or meningioma (Table 10.11). Adenomas are distinguished from these other entities by immunopositivity for chromogranin. Expression of specific pituitary peptide hormones is present in all but null-cell adenomas, and usually restricted to less than three hormones. EM also identifies neurosecretory granules.

Neuroendocrine Carcinoma

Pituitary carcinoma is defined by metastasis to a location remote from the sella, including the CNS parenchyma, remote subarachnoid space, or extracranial metastasis (e.g., lymph nodes, lung, bone, liver). Other neuroendocrine carcinomas found in the brain typically come from systemic primaries, such as small-cell carcinoma of the lung. These are discussed with metastatic carcinomas. See also Chapter 11.

GERM CELL TUMORS

Germ cell tumors are discussed in Chapter 55, Sex Cord—Stromal, Steroid Cell, and Germ Cell Tumors of the Ovary, and

Chapter 47, Testicular and Paratesticular Tumors. They are mentioned here in relation to specific associations with the CNS, and their differential diagnosis. Within the cranial vault, 95% of primary germ cell tumors are found along the midline in the pineal and suprasellar regions, especially the former. About one-tenth involve both regions and one-fourth arise in the suprasellar cistern (204,205). A review of parasellar germ cell tumors is available (107). The sacrococcygeal teratoma occurs at the base of the spine.

Problems with appropriately classifying a pineal tumor can be encountered with stereotactic needle biopsies and even open biopsies resulting from an incomplete sample of tissue and mechanical problems in removal (Fig. 10.2). All such biopsies should be monitored with frozen sections and touch preparations.

In assessing the differential diagnosis, it is important to appreciate the proximity of the pineal gland to deep cerebrum, cerebellum, ventricles, and brainstem, and the proximity of the suprasellar region to deep cerebrum, ventricles, and the sella (204). Brain tumors in these regions, which must be considered in the differential diagnosis, vary with the histologic type of germ cell tumor, as noted below.

Germinoma

Germinomas are the most common intracranial germ cell neoplasm (204–210). Their predominance in adolescence and puberty aids recognition of many intracranial germinomas (Figs. 10.109 and 10.110). They can be admixed with other germ cell tumors (Fig. 10.2). Rare germinomas occur in various dysgenetic syndromes (207,210). Pineal and parasellar germinomas resemble their gonadal counterparts in having two distinct cell types: (a) large, neoplastic, epithelioid cells contain large, round, vesicular nuclei with irregular and pleomorphic nucleoli and abundant PAS-positive cytoplasm; and (b) nests of polyclonal lymphocytes (Fig. 10.110) (211), occasionally complicated by granulomatous inflammation. This inflammation can confound interpretation (208). The nuclei of the small lymphocytic component crush and smear easily in stereotactic biopsies, leaving streaks of hematoxylin. The lymphocytes may be so numerous that they obscure the large-cell component.

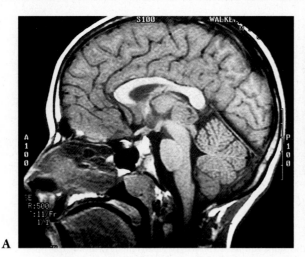
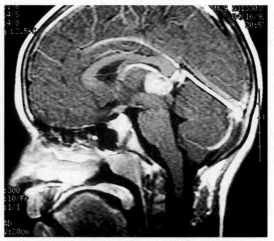

Figure 10.109. Pineal germinoma. These sagittal T1-weighted magnetic resonance images are from a pineal germinoma in a 15-year-old boy. **(A)** The midline tumor density resembles gray matter. **(B)** The tumor enhances brightly with contrast medium. *(Courtesy of Dr. James Brunberg, University of Michigan, Ann Arbor, Michigan.)*

The large nuclei of the germinoma cells are more uniform than the striking nuclear anaplasia seen in embryonal carcinoma. Mitotic figures are easy to find, nucleoli are irregular, and necrosis is common in germinomas.

In contrast to pineal parenchymal tumors and gliomas, germinomas have no cells intermediate between small (lymphocytes) and large (germinoma) cells. This pattern is diagnostic if sufficient tissue is available (Table 10.12).

CD117 (c-kit) stains 100% of intracranial germinomas in one study, and it often outperforms other markers (212). Placental alkaline phosphatase (PLAP) can be localized by IHC in 93% of germinomas and 25% of embryonal carcinomas (107). Although this marker distinguishes germinomas from gliomas, about 13% of systemic carcinomas express PLAP (213). In addition to this, similarities in lymphocytes and in cytokeratin (CK) and EMA reactivity of large cells obscure distinctions between germinoma and some carcinomas. In such instances, solitary midline location in the absence of systemic neoplasia suggests germinoma, because carcinomas similar to germinoma are met-astatic and usually lateral. CK and EMA may be more useful in differentiating carcinomas from suprasellar germinomas than from pineal germinomas, because suprasellar germinomas often lack these carcinoma markers (209).

The lymphocytic component of germinoma stains with CD45RB, CD3, and CD20, distinguishing these cells from neuroectodermal and glial cells (211). Their small size and regular nuclear features also distinguish them from the anaplastic cells in malignant small-cell neoplasms (Table 10.13).

Germinomas are very radiosensitive, leading to better outcomes than their features suggest. Metastases are uncommon, and are often associated with surgical procedures (206).

Teratoma

Teratomas contain a variety of tissues derived from all three germinal layers (Table 10.12). Most CNS teratomas are well differentiated and are histologic grade I. Mature teratomas have well-differentiated representatives of all three embryonic tissue

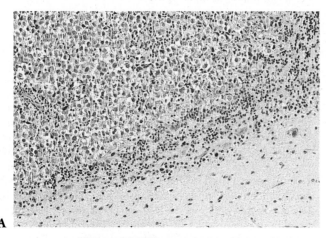
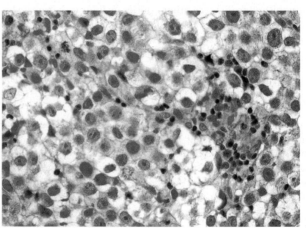

Figure 10.110. Germinoma. **(A)** This tumor recurred in the cerebellum (*bottom*) 13 years after surgery and radiation therapy completed in adolescence. Cerebellar granular neurons in a diagonal band across the field slightly resemble the tumor lymphocytes, but the neoplastic large cells are distinctive. **(B)** The high-power view demonstrates the biphasic appearance with neoplastic cells and reactive lymphocytes.

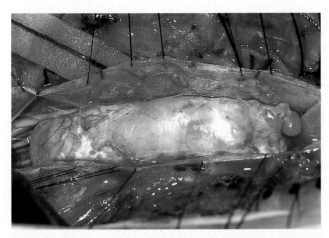

Figure 10.111. Teratoma. Partially cystic solitary intradural tumor near the sacral spinal cord. Angiomatous regions (*blue-brown*), squamous epithelium (*pearly white*), gray glial tissue, yellow adipose tissue, and translucent columnar epithelial-lined cysts are present in the tumor.

layers, including neuroectodermal (107,214,215). Solid or cystic foci of epithelium are mixed with glandular or tubular structures. These are separated by mesenchymal proliferation. Glial and neuronal tissue is common and cartilage is occasionally present. The immunohistochemical profile varies and reflects the tissues present.

Immature teratomas have less differentiated elements from all or any of the three germinal layers. Histologically immature elements that are prognostically important include embryonal neuroepithelial structures that resemble medulloepithelioma, neuroblastoma, retinoblastoma, or ependymoblastoma. Half of the patients with intracranial immature teratomas die within 1 year, but maturation of the teratoma is occasionally observed (216).

Pineal teratomas are more common in males. Sacrococcygeal teratomas are more common in females (214).

The most common diagnostic problem results from incomplete sampling (Fig. 10.111). A region of a teratoma with neuroglial differentiation may resemble various types of glioma. This can be rectified by appraisal of the entire tumor. Finally, teratomas from any CNS location may contain elements of another, less benign, germ cell tumor (107). The prognosis is that of the most malignant germ cell element found.

Other Germ Cell Tumors and Mixed Germ Cell Tumors

Choriocarcinoma contains huge syncytial and smaller trophoblastic cells (syncytiotrophoblasts and cytotrophoblasts). Schiller-Duval bodies identify yolk sac (endodermal sinus) tumors (107). Most yolk sac tumors and embryonal carcinomas express alpha-fetoprotein (AFP) (215). The majority of choriocarcinomas contain human chorionic gonadotropin (HCG) (217). These markers in tissue aid diagnosis, and in serum and CSF they aid monitoring for possible recurrence. Unlike germinoma, lymphocytes are not prominent in pure choriocarcinoma, embryonal carcinoma, or endodermal sinus tumors. However, mixtures of these other germ cell tumors and germinoma occur (Fig. 10.2). The prognosis of these tumors is worse

than that of germinoma, giving special import to correct classification of intracranial germ cell and mixed tumor types (107).

An unusual new mixed tumor has been described by Valdez (218). It is a germinoma in which the lymphocyte population is a lymphoma. The therapeutic susceptibility and prognosis of this "gerlymphoma" is as yet unknown.

In the brain, embryonal carcinomas and endodermal sinus tumors may resemble malignant meningioma, metastatic carcinoma, and choroid plexus carcinoma. Choriocarcinoma also resembles metastatic carcinoma, as well as glioblastoma. Presence of AFP or HCG distinguishes some of these germ cell tumors but is most useful in a panel of stains (204) (Tables 10.11 and 10.12).

HEMATOPOIETIC AND LYMPHOID NEOPLASMS

Lymphoma

Lymphomas involving the CNS can be either "primary," appearing first in the CNS; and "secondary," coming from peripheral lymphoma with involvement of CNS parenchyma, dura, and nerve roots (219–226).

PRIMARY CNS LYMPHOMA. *Primary CNS lymphoma* is defined as presentation of lymphoma in the CNS without evidence of systemic lymphoma. This neoplasm involves the cerebral hemispheres most commonly, but also may arise in the cerebellum, brainstem, or spinal cord. Leptomeninges may be involved, usually by secondary spreading. Patients with primary CNS lymphoma may develop subsequent systemic lymphoma, including unusual places such as testes.

After an apparent sharp increase in the rate of primary CNS lymphoma (222,226), a more recently observed reduction in rate was noted (224). The increased incidence is likely due to its occurrence among immunosuppressed patients and in patients with AIDS (219,222). Primary CNS lymphomas that arise in immunocompromised patients produce a distinctly poorer prognosis than those in the immunocompetent (226). Survival in AIDS patients with CNS lymphomas depends on the extent of immunosuppression, clinical condition prior to therapy, and spread of tumor (219).

SECONDARY CNS LYMPHOMA. In patients with peripheral lymphoma, secondary involvement of the nervous system can occur, with a frequency estimated at 5% to 29% of patients, with data principally from the pre-AIDS era (220–222). Secondary involvement can be in the dura, leptomeninges, cranial nerves, peripheral nerves, intravascular region, or CNS parenchyma.

POSTTRANSPLANTATION LYMPHOPROLIFERATIVE DISEASE (PTLD). In the setting of organ transplantation and associated immunosuppression, similar to that seen elsewhere in the body, a range of "posttransplantation lymphoproliferative disorders" can develop (227). Diagnosis is challenging (228). Aggregate histologic, IHC, and molecular workup is necessary to distinguish between (a) lymphoid/plasmacytic hyperplasia (polyclonal, no immunoglobulin ([Ig] gene rearrangement); (b) atypical hyperplasia/B-cell hyperplasia and lymphoma (monoclonal, Ig rearrangement present); and (c) diffuse, large-B-cell immunoblastic lymphoma (monoclonal). The Epstein-Barr virus (EBV) can be identified in most PTLD lymphoma cases (223).

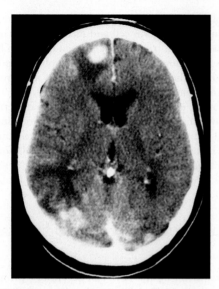

Figure 10.112. Primary CNS diffuse, large-B-cell lymphoma. This neoplasm in a 64-year-old woman manifests multiple masses that enhance after contrast on this computed tomography image. *(Courtesy of Dr. Stephen Gebarski, University of Michigan, Ann Arbor, Michigan.)*

DIAGNOSIS. Diagnosis of primary CNS lymphoma requires procurement of adequate specimens at biopsy (see "Tissue Processing" section above) for identification and subclassification of the lymphoma subtype. The radiographic appearance, particularly of the multicentric variety, is helpful (Fig. 10.112). Toxoplasmosis is the common differential challenge and classically has more radiographically identified lesions than does lymphoma.

The vast majority of CNS lymphomas are diffuse, large B-cell lymphomas (Fig. 10.113). Involvement of the CNS and meninges by T-cell lymphomas, other non-Hodgkin lymphomas, or Hodgkin lymphoma is rare (221). Steroid treatment before biopsy should be avoided if clinically feasible, since it destroys diagnostic cells. Although necrotic cells retain their CD20 positivity, it is not wise to make diagnoses on necrotic cells.

CNS lymphoma is frequently centered on blood vessels with invasion of both brain parenchyma and blood vessel walls. This is best appreciated with a stain that both differentiates the vascular wall from parenchyma and consistently demonstrates fine nuclear morphology, such as Masson trichrome, anti-type IV collagen, or anti-GFAP with hematoxylin counterstain. In this way, monomorphic lymphoma cells in both vessels and brain can be distinguished from dimorphic cellular patterns such as desmoplasia and microvascular proliferation of undifferentiated carcinoma, medulloblastoma, and glioma (Table 10.12). Lymphoma is more prone to crush artifact (Fig. 10.114) than the other tumors.

The vast majority of primary and secondary CNS lymphomas are classified using WHO criteria as diffuse, large-B-cell lymphomas (223). H&E and IHC-stained paraffin sections are sufficient for diagnosis and B-cell marker immunophenotyping in more than 70% of cases with a panel including CD20, CD3, and CD45RB. Some pathologists employ the B-cell marker CD79a as well. Lymphomas often contain polyclonal reactive lymphoid elements, including CD3-positive T cells, which may be recognized by their smaller size and benign nuclei. Identification of monotypic expression of kappa- and lambda-light chain, evalu-

ated by IHC or in situ hybridization, is a helpful feature. Ancillary studies, such as immunoglobulin gene rearrangement, can be performed on paraffin-embedded or frozen tissue.

Extreme care in interpreting fibrillarity and glioma markers is required because, although typically vasculocentric, lymphoid cells can individually infiltrate the CNS parenchyma and mix with gliosis, giving the superficial appearance of a glioma (Fig. 10.113D). Carefully inspect the nuclei of CD20+ versus GFAP+ cells to find which are neoplastic. The accurate identification of a suspected primary CNS lymphoma requires careful attention to other neoplasms that closely resemble it, including primitive neuroectodermal tumors and undifferentiated small-cell carcinoma (Table 10.13). If hematopoietic markers are negative, synaptophysin, S-100, or cytokeratin may mark PNET, glioma, or carcinoma. If the reniform nuclear morphology and abundant cytoplasm of a histiocytic lesion is noted, inclusion of S-100 and CD1a may provide useful data.

EBV-RELATED PROCESSES. In addition to that seen in PTLD, EBV is identified and may be the driver in lymphomatoid granulomatosis and the lymphoma seen in AIDS and other cases of immunosuppression. Identification of EBV is not a diagnostic criterion for these processes but is helpful in the diagnosis of lymphomatoid granulomatosis.

Lymphomatoid Granulomatosis

Lymphomatoid granulomatosis (LG) is a lymphoproliferative disease that spans the boundaries of inflammatory disease, vasculitis, and neoplasm. It histologically manifests (a) angiocentric inflammation, including lymphocytes with atypical nuclear features; and (b) angiodisruptive vessel wall injury. Well-formed granulomas are typically absent (223). LG is an EBV-related process, and identification of EBV by in situ hybridization of IHC is very helpful in the diagnosis. LG can progress to lymphoma, and is seen associated with AIDS (229). CNS involvement is almost always seen in the setting of concomitant pulmonary disease.

Dural, Subarachnoid, and Nerve Lymphoma (Neurolymphomatosis)

Lymphoma can also target the (a) dura, (b) leptomeningeal space, and (c) cranial and peripheral nerve roots and nerves (Fig. 10.115). Lymphoma in these locations is usually diagnosed by identification of neoplastic lymphocytes in CSF cytology specimens rather than by biopsy (230).

Intravascular Lymphoma

Although rare, the CNS is one of the sites of predilection for intravascular lymphoma, a variant of large-B-cell lymphoma. Rather than extensively invading blood vessel walls, the neoplastic cells fill blood vessel lumens. The clinical presentation mimics vasculitis. The cells have an atypical cytologic appearance, arousing suspicion for neoplasm. Most are positive for CD20, facilitating their diagnosis.

Leukemia

Leukemia can involve the arachnoid, cranial, and peripheral nerve roots and brain parenchyma. The diagnosis of leukemia

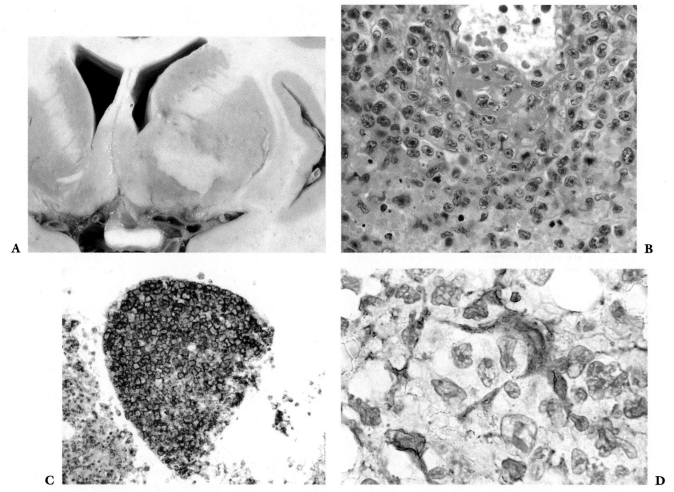

Figure 10.113. Primary CNS diffuse, large-B-cell lymphoma. **(A)** A plaquelike lesion consisting of a largely necrotic tumor involves the right putamen and globus pallidus. **(B)** Vasculocentric infiltration of lymphoma into the blood vessel wall; vessel lumen at the middle top, necrosis at the bottom. **(C)** Neoplastic cells are strongly CD20-positive; scant admixed CD3 cells were present (not shown). **(D)** As a potential pitfall of interpretation, intermixed glial fibrillary acidic protein-positive astrocytes with light, small nuclei are reactive; the fibrillar processes belong to the astrocyte.

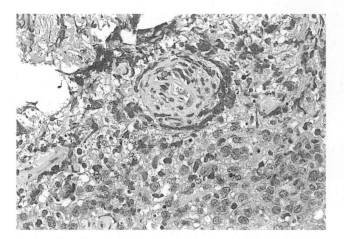

Figure 10.114. Primary CNS lymphoma. Needle biopsy shows nuclear smearing artifacts. Malignant cells with prominent nucleoli invade the brain parenchyma and vessel wall.

within the craniospinal vault is usually established by examination of CSF cytology. Intraparenchymal and meningeal mass lesions and hemorrhages can occur in the setting of a blast crisis of more than 300,000 leukocytes per cubic millimeter, resulting in intravascular leukostasis. These are most common in acute myelogenous leukemia, and they require surgical removal.

Histiocytoses

Histiocytoses predominate in children and young adults. CNS involvement can be primary in the dura, leptomeninges, or parenchyma or secondary to skull, vertebral, or systemic involvement. The parasellar and cavernous sinus regions are particularly susceptible and, as a result, diabetes insipidus and optic symptoms are common.

The key histologic and immunohistochemical components of these diseases are summarized in Figures 10.116 through 10.118 and in Table 10.16 (231–234). Variably dense, polarizable collagen is typically admixed with all of them, making bi-

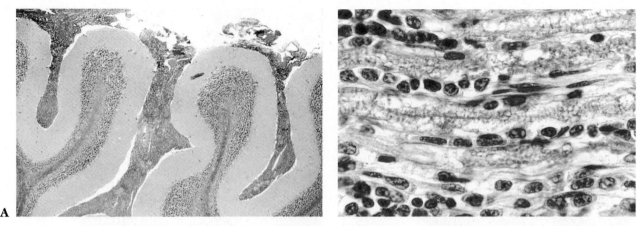

Figure 10.115. Large-B-cell lymphoma. It diffusely involves **(A)** the subarachnoid space and **(B)** nerve root (neurolymphomatosis) with neoplastic cells diffusely infiltrating among myelinated axons (Luxol-fast blue; hematoxylin and eosin).

opsy and resection difficult. All have a mixed inflammatory infiltrate rich in macrophages. *Erdheim-Chester disease* of the CNS, typically seen in the context of long bone and organ system disease, has characteristic Touton giant cells that are CD68 positive and CD1a-negative (231) (Fig. 10.116). *Rosai-Dorfman disease* ("sinus histocytosis with massive lymphadenopathy") can be seen with or without systemic disease. It is characterized by *emperipolesis*, the engulfment by macrophages of intact lymphocytes (234). The macrophages are CD68-and S-100–positive, and CD1a-negative (Fig. 10.117). *Langerhans cell histiocytosis* can be seen as a lytic skull lesion or parasellar mass. The diagnostic Langerhans cells have abundant eosinophilic cytoplasm and reniform nuclei. These cells are S-100– and CD1a-positive (Fig. 10.118) and contain Birbeck granules by electron microscopy. Xanthoma disseminatum (juvenile xanthogranulomatosis) has

also been described in the CNS; concomitant skin involvement is characteristic (232).

As with all macrophage-rich lesions, histochemical stains to evaluate for microorganisms are necessary. Microbiologic cultures are recommended, when possible.

MISCELLANEOUS INTRACRANIAL OR SPINAL MASSES

Lipoma

Lipomas are rare and are rarely excised. Possibly reflecting their heterotopic origin during embryogenesis, lipomas frequent midline locations, near the corpus callosum, quadrigeminal plate, hypothalamus, spinal canal, or cauda equina. They are composed of mature adipose tissue, but they also may contain

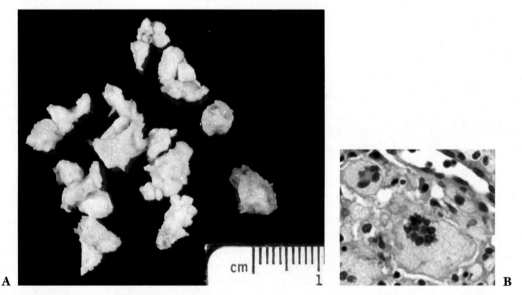

Figure 10.116. Erdheim-Chester disease. **(A)** Fragments of an orange-yellow, markedly fibrous, dura-based mass. **(B)** The mixed inflammatory infiltrate includes lymphocytes and foamy histocytes, some with a central ring of nuclei surrounding an eosinophilic core, and Touton giant cells. The histocytes were S-100–positive and CD1a-negative (not shown).

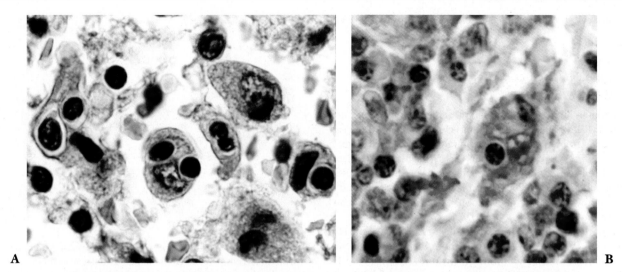

Figure 10.117. Rosai-Dorfman disease. **(A)** Emperipolesis of intact lymphocytes by macrophages is shown. **(B)** The macrophages are strongly S-100–positive. They were also CD1a-negative (not shown).

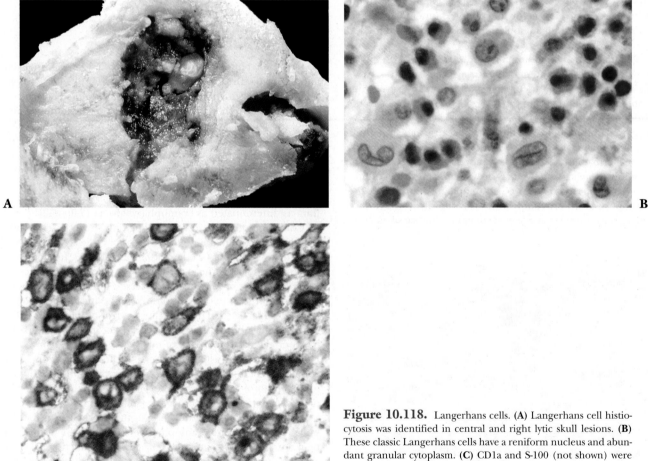

Figure 10.118. Langerhans cells. **(A)** Langerhans cell histiocytosis was identified in central and right lytic skull lesions. **(B)** These classic Langerhans cells have a reniform nucleus and abundant granular cytoplasm. **(C)** CD1a and S-100 (not shown) were strongly positive in the Langerhans cells.

Schwann cells, bone, cartilage, or hamartomatous blood vessels (4).

Hemangioblastoma (Capillary Hemangioblastoma)—Grade I

The capillary hemangioblastoma resembles an endocrine neoplasm (Fig. 10.119) (235–237). It has close juxtaposition of capillary and stromal cells, and occasionally shows secretory granules or expresses erythropoietin (238). Its pink, vacuolated stromal cells contain neuron-specific enolase (NSE), present in neuroendocrine cells (235), but it lacks an endocrine gland of origin in any of its principal locations (cerebellum, spinal cord, and meninges).

Some hemangioblastomas are associated with the von Hippel-Lindau (VHL) complex, having more than one lesion or a hemangioblastoma in an unusual location (237). The VHL tumor suppressor gene is located on chromosome 3p25-26 and is also associated with endolymphatic sac tumors (239). The VHL protein is angiogenic.

Because the hemangioblastoma is nonfibrillar, it should not masquerade as an astrocytoma. However, this may occur. Cerebellar hemangioblastomas often manifest as neoplastic mural nodules within a cystic cavity. Biopsies of the cyst wall will show gliosis and Rosenthal fibers, and mimic a pilocytic astrocytoma—a relatively common cerebellar neoplasm. If in doubt, ask the surgeon to inspect for, and sample, mural nodules. Even within this tumor, hemangioblastomas occasionally show GFAP staining (236).

When a hemangioblastoma is sectioned on a cryostat at biopsy, the high lipid content of the stromal cells ruptures, resulting in an artifactual resemblance to a fibrillar astrocytoma (Table 10.10). A lipid stain can be applied to the frozen section to identify fat droplets in hemangioblastoma (Fig. 10.120). Cytologic preparations help with the biopsy because they show nonfibrillar stromal cells with large nuclei and vacuoles.

On permanent sections, the epithelioid nature of the hemangioblastoma is usually intact, leaving one more feat of mimicry—its similarity to renal cell carcinoma. Although most of the important differential features are described under carcinoma, more uniform nuclear chromatin, absence of necrosis,

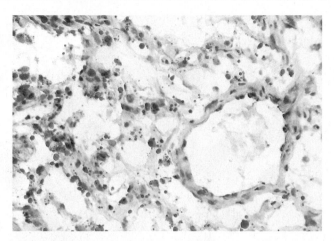

Figure 10.120. Hemangioblastoma. After frozen sectioning ruptures stroma cells, a hemangioblastoma resembles an astrocytoma. However, the hemangioblastoma contains red-orange lipid (oil red-O).

small nucleoli, fewer mitoses, and intimate arrangement of capillaries and stromal cells suggest hemangioblastoma (Fig. 10.119). Vascularity in both tumors can be highlighted by reticulin and CD34. In contrast to renal cell carcinoma, hemangioblastoma stromal cells tend to stain for NSE and not EMA (Fig. 10.121) (235,237).

Craniopharyngioma—Grade I

The epithelial appearance of craniopharyngioma is discussed and illustrated in Chapter 12, The Pituitary and Sellar Region. However, its distinction from other brain tumors is discussed here. A properly sampled craniopharyngioma, including a sample of the solid mass associated with cystic craniopharyngiomas, is difficult to confuse with other brain tumors because of its distinctive adamantinomatous and/or keratinizing epithelium (Tables 10.11 and 10.19). Three of four craniopharyngiomas calcify, helping to distinguish them from metastatic carcinoma, which in brain rarely calcifies and rarely has squamous epithelium as differentiated as craniopharyngioma (240–242).

Confusion can arise from sampling only the intensely gliotic margin of craniopharyngioma, which may closely resemble a pilocytic astrocytoma (see Figs. 10.34 and 10.40). Juvenile predominance, location near the third ventricle, and presence of Rosenthal fibers occur in both processes. Communication with the neurosurgeon to obtain solid tissue is critical. After biopsy, the highly reactive and fibrillar gliosis surrounding a craniopharyngioma may be distinguished from pilocytic astrocytoma by its lower cellularity and lack of microcysts (107). In contrast to lighter contents of astrocytoma cysts, craniopharyngioma cyst contents possess the color and consistency of motor oil, containing cholesterol crystals, cholesterol clefts, reactive giant cells, or a focal deposit of keratin-laden epithelial cells.

The occurrence of transitional tumors between Rathke pouch derivatives and craniopharyngioma blurs the distinction between them (242). On small biopsies, the distinction between a cystic craniopharyngioma, Rathke cyst with epithelial metaplasia, and epidermoid cyst can be difficult (Table 10.19) (115). Xin and collaborators addressed these small biopsies with cytokeratin subtype analyses. They found that Rathke cysts express cytokeratin 8 and 20, and the others do not (241).

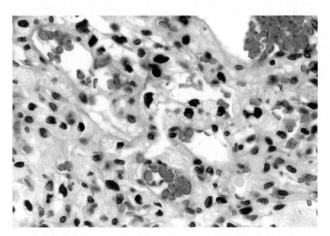

Figure 10.119. Hemangioblastoma. This mural nodule is from a cerebellar cyst in a 23-year-old man. The lesion consists of numerous thin-walled capillaries with admixed vacuolated stromal cells.

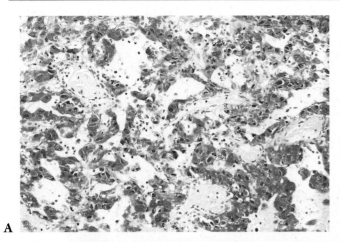

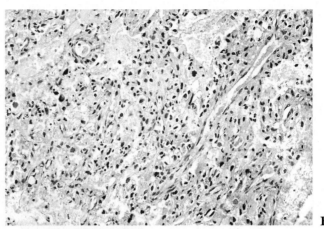

A

B

Figure 10.121. Cerebellar hemangioblastoma. This patient had both von Hippel-Lindau complex and primary renal cell carcinoma. His cerebellar hemangioblastoma was positive for neuron-specific enolase **(A)** and negative for epithelial membrane antigen **(B)**.

Desmoplastic Small-Cell Tumor—Grade IV

One of these tumors has been reported exclusively within the cranium (243). It usually occurs in the abdomen of children and young adults. It is composed of well-defined nests of small, round, primitive cells separated by abundant desmoplastic stroma. Its t(11;22)(p13;q12) chromosomal translocation is similar to the translocation of peripheral PNET (see "Primitive Neuroectodermal Tumors" section above).

COMMON METASTATIC TUMORS

When a lesion appears neoplastic, the pathologist must consider and distinguish between primary CNS neoplasms and metastatic neoplasm. Many neoplasms metastasize to the CNS from known primary sites. However, even in this advanced age of imaging, pathologic identification of unexpected carcinoma in the brain of an adult presenting with seizures or ataxia is a common and regular occurrence. The overwhelming predominance of metastatic neoplasms to the brain is from carcinomas or melanoma, with occasional germ cell neoplasms identified.

Carcinoma

Nearly all intracranial carcinomas are metastases from extracranial primaries. This section emphasizes these carcinomas.

Rare primary brain carcinomas occur in the choroid plexus, from germ cell tumors of the pineal and suprasellar regions, and from cysts. These are described with their less malignant counterparts.

The hallmark of carcinoma as it relates to the CNS and meninges is its distinctively epithelial structure (Figs. 10.122 through 10.127) (Table 10.11). Table 10.17 summarizes the chances that a primary malignant neoplasm will metastasize to the brain. It also shows the likelihood that a brain metastasis came from various primaries (244–248). To understand this table, look at the rows for skin and breast. The most common neoplasm that metastasizes to CNS from skin is melanoma (Figs. 10.128 and 10.129). However, although melanomas commonly metastasize to the CNS, only about 10% of brain metastases come from melanoma because melanoma is a relatively rare

neoplasm. Breast carcinomas (Fig. 10.124) have a lower tendency to metastasize to the brain (15% to 25%) than melanomas; however, approximately 20% of metastases found in the brain come from breast carcinomas because breast carcinomas are more common than melanomas.

The primary site of tumors metastatic to the vertebral column that cause secondary impingement on the spinal canal is often known at the time of biopsy or resection, and most commonly includes prostate, breast, or hematopoietic origin neoplasms.

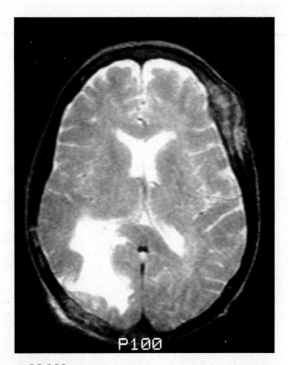

Figure 10.122. Cerebral metastasis of breast carcinoma. This carcinoma metastasized both to the meninges and to the posterior cerebrum of this 70-year-old woman. The cerebral metastasis gives a T2-weighted signal that is brighter than metastasis to the meninges because of the surrounding cerebral edema. *(Courtesy of Dr. James Brunberg, University of Michigan, Ann Arbor, Michigan.)*

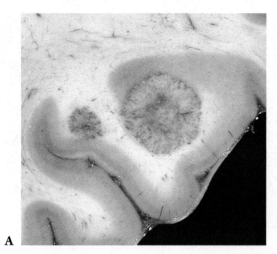

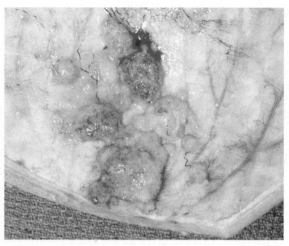

A   **B**

Figure 10.123. Metastatic carcinoma. **(A)** This metastatic lung carcinoma caused the two centrally necrotic lesions at the gray–white matter junction. **(B)** This prostate carcinoma is extensively metastatic to the dura.

Metastatic carcinoma uncommonly produces carcinomatous meningitis, seen on biopsy or CSF cytology. Carcinomatous meningitis is a poor prognostic sign.

The site of metastasis within the craniospinal vault is of little help in identifying metastatic carcinoma from other lesions such as glioma or abscess unless there are multiple locations ("M-rule") (Figs. 10.122 and 10.123). Clinical uncertainty about diagnosis results in a relatively high number of resections of solitary rather than multiple CNS metastases. Metastatic carcinoma metastasizes to regions of the brain approximately in proportion to volume of CNS tissue, leading to its prominence in cerebrum. But metastases also occur in the cerebellum, brainstem, spinal cord, pituitary, and pineal. Some neoplasms metastasize to dura, including breast and prostate carcinoma (Fig. 10.123B). Certain regions are particularly hazardous to interpret (e.g., the pineal and hypophyseal regions, which are the sites of primary germ cell tumors that resemble carcinoma).

The histologic hallmarks of carcinoma metastatic to the CNS are an epithelial appearance, with discrete cell boundaries like cobblestones in an old road; and a distinct, pushing rather than infiltrative tumor margin with CNS parenchyma (Figs. 10.124 through 10.126). Small-cell carcinoma is one exception: It can also focally but insidiously infiltrate the brain (Fig. 10.127).

Immunohistochemistry in the Differential of Site of Origin of a Metastatic Carcinoma

Although general surgical pathology acumen is important in generating a differential of possible primary sites of metastasis, IHC plays important roles in confirmation of metastasis from a known primary, or suggesting potential sites for a tumor of unknown primary. The panel of immunostains employed varies among pathologists (18,246,247,249). Thyroid transcription factor 1 (TTF-1), positive in most lung and thyroid adenocarcinomas and negative in other adenocarcinomas, is an important new marker in the diagnostic arsenal (250). A reasonable panel of immunostains would include cytokeratin CAM 5.2 along with

Figure 10.124. Metastatic papillary carcinoma. This papillary carcinoma metastatic to the cerebrum from the breast imitates papillary meningioma and choroid plexus carcinoma. Note gliosis in the adjacent brain.

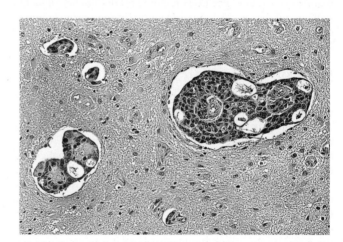

Figure 10.125. Metastatic lung adenocarcinoma. The biopsy of a left parietal mass revealed clusters of epithelioid, cohesive cells manifesting lumen formation and producing mucin. Characteristic of metastatic neoplasms, the neoplastic cells grew along the perivascular space of Virchow-Robin, surrounding and compressing central vessels, but did not invade adjacent brain parenchyma. Note the reactive gliosis of the adjacent parenchyma.

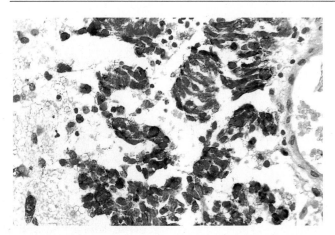

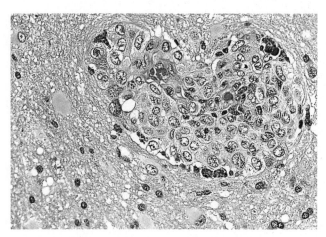

Figure 10.126. Metastatic small-cell carcinoma. This small-cell neoplasm was resected from the cerebellum of an elderly woman. Histologically, a small-cell neoplasm was present; it consisted of tightly clustered cells with a high nuclear:cytoplasmic ratio and focal nuclear molding. A lung lesion was subsequently identified. Neoplastic cells are cytokeratin cell adhesion molecule 5.2-positive. The neoplastic cells were negative for CD45RB (leukocyte common antigen) and S-100 protein (not shown).

Figure 10.128. Metastatic melanoma. This dark invader of the right frontal lobe of a 52-year-old woman presents little diagnostic challenge as one of three pigmented metastases from a cutaneous primary tumor overlying the scapula. The pleomorphic epithelioid cells cluster around a vessel rather than infiltrating the gliotic brain parenchyma.

cytokeratin CK7 and CK20, TTF-1, and, in the right clinical setting, prostate-specific antigen (PSA) (251). Interpretation must be made in the light of histologic features. Most breast and lung adenocarcinomas are pancytokeratin-, CAM 5.2-, and CK7-positive and CK20-negative; most lung adenocarcinomas are TTF-1–positive, and positivity markedly reduces the likelihood of nonpulmonary primaries. Colon carcinoma is typically CK20-positive and CK7-and TTF-1–negative. Diagnosis of gastric and pancreaticobiliary carcinoma is more challenging, with variable CK7 and CK20 expression. Essentially all prostate carcinomas are positive for CAM 5.2 and PSA.

Renal cell carcinomas are challenging immunodiagnostically. Most are positive for CAM 5.2 and negative for CK20; a few are positive for CK7; TTF-1 is negative. Its large, clear cells aid its identification.

DIFFERENTIAL DIAGNOSIS FROM PRIMARY CNS TUMORS. Within CNS parenchyma, few neoplasms other than glioblastoma or anaplastic glioma show the intensity of nuclear pleomorphism, profuse mitotic abnormalities, or spontaneous tumor necrosis present in metastatic carcinomas. Distinct epithelial borders and lack of fibrillar cytoplasmic processes contrast with the pattern of glioblastoma.

The distinct cell borders in carcinomas are not identified in meningiomas where a syncytial appearance is often noted, with indistinct cell boundaries. Only rare secretory meningiomas contain cytokeratin, but can be distinguished from carcinoma metastatic to the meninges by their pattern of multifocal clusters of cytokeratin-positive meningothelial cells around a negative "secretion." Most cells of secretory meningioma are cytokeratin-negative (Fig. 10.95). Low-grade meningiomas lack the abundant mitoses and regions of necrosis often found in metastatic carcinomas.

Although primary choriocarcinoma occurs in the pineal and suprasellar regions, often in association with other germ cell tumors, metastatic choriocarcinoma from an extracranial primary lacks predilection for these specific sites. Choriocarcinoma metastatic to the brain frequently is hemorrhagic. Rare choriocarcinomas have been found within spontaneous intracranial hemorrhages. Beta-HCG is a useful marker in distinguishing choriocarcinoma from beta-HCG–negative carcinomas, other germ cell tumors, and glioblastomas (107) (Tables 10.10 through 10.12).

Metastatic renal cell carcinoma must be distinguished from hemangioblastoma (Fig. 10.119), angiomatous meningioma (Fig. 10.94), oligodendroglioma (Fig. 10.57), and chordoma (Fig. 10.103). These neoplasms all contain distinct epithelial cell borders. Presence of EMA and CK help distinguish renal cell carcinoma from cerebellar hemangioblastoma and oligodendroglioma (244). Angiomatous meningioma lacks CK, and chordoma has specific location and ultrastructure.

Metastatic small-cell carcinoma (Fig. 10.26) can be very difficult to distinguish from medulloblastoma/PNET and lymphoma (Figs. 10.83, 10.115, and 10.126) and can invade the brain (Fig. 10.127). Small-cell carcinoma typically manifests a

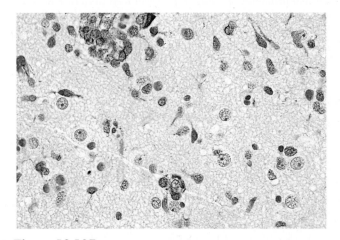

Figure 10.127. Metastatic small cell carcinoma. Cytokeratin cell adhesion molecule 5.2 reactivity of these infiltrative atypical malignant cells with unipolar processes is a clue to their origin. This pulmonary oat cell carcinoma metastasized to brain.

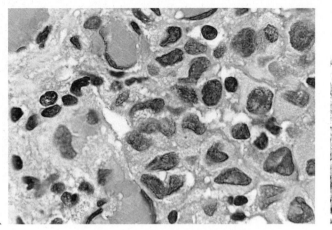

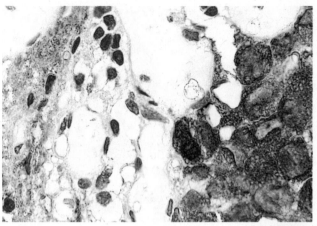

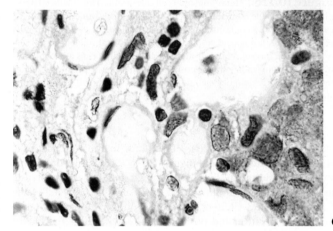

Figure 10.129. Metastatic melanoma. This light-colored melanoma metastatic to the left temporal lobe of a 32-year-old man **(A)** has more S-100 protein reactivity than does the adjacent CNS parenchyma on the left **(B)**, and it is uniquely HMB45-positive **(C)**.

rim of epithelial cytoplasm and cohesive nonfibrillar cells, lacking in lymphoma and medulloblastoma/PNET. Cytokeratin CAM 5.2 and EMA are expressed by small-cell carcinoma (Fig. 10.126). Carcinoma cells lack CD3 and CD20. Electron microscopy can demonstrate epithelial borders of such cells and may reveal desmosomes or neuroendocrine features.

Melanocytosis, Melanocytoma, and Melanoma

Nearly all intracranial melanomas are metastases from extracranial primaries. This section emphasizes these melanomas first. Less common primary brain melanomas are described after metastatic melanomas, along with melanocytomas and other primary melanocytic entities.

METASTATIC MELANOMA. Metastatic melanoma can be either the simplest or most difficult neoplasm to recognize in the CNS, depending on its pigmentation and growth pattern (Tables 10.10 to 10.12). Melanomas with radiographic evidence of a multiplicity of lesions (''M-rule''), an epithelial appearance, features of malignancy, and presence of melanin are easy to recognize (Fig. 10.128). Solitary tumors with fibrillar or spindle cells, and without pigment, are more difficult. Considering melanoma as a possible diagnosis is critical.

Melanomas are often strongly S-100–positive (Fig. 10.129), a marker of low specificity in brain because it stains many CNS tumors (18). HMB-45 and MART-1/MelanA IHC procedures identify most melanomas metastatic to CNS (Fig. 10.129). Al-

though the spectrum of HMB-45 and MART-1/MelanA reactivity on other CNS neoplasms remains to be confirmed, other pigmented tumors may be positive. I have found tyrosinase to be the most specific marker of melanocytic tumors in brain.

PRIMARY MELANOCYTOSIS, MELANOCYTOMA, AND MELANOMA. The number of benign arachnoid melanocytes varies among individuals, and can be appreciated by MRI (252). Abnormal proliferation of these cells can lead to diffuse melanocytosis that shows no mass, to melanocytoma that is a relatively benign mass, or to malignant melanoma (253,254). In addition, primary melanomas can occasionally develop, sometimes in association with melanocytoma, and can disseminate in the leptomeninges (253).

Rare meningioma, schwannoma, ependymoma, neuroblastoma, and PNET contain melanin (115). They must be distinguished by their individually described features.

Hematopoietic Malignancies

Lymphomas and leukemias can penetrate normal tissue barriers and traffic through the bloodstream, obscuring the definition of metastatic (e.g., angiocentric lymphomas and leukemic hemorrhages). These entities are described above in the section ''Hematopoietic and Lymphoid Neoplasms.'' In general, lymphomas that secondarily involve the CNS enter via its coverings (skull, vertebra, or meninges) or via the blood. Plasmacytomas and myelomas rarely involve CNS directly, but they do involve its bony coverings. As a site relatively resistant to penetration of some chemotherapy agents, aggressively treated hematopoietic malignancies may be found in the CNS or CSF after systemic remission.

CYSTS

Cysts differ from cystic tumors by their lack of a solid nodule of tissue. This simple fact is critical to distinguish glial cysts from cystic gliomas with mural nodules, and epithelial cysts from cystic craniopharyngiomas.

A group of slow-growing CNS neoplasms often present as a cystic lesion, including pilocytic astrocytoma of the posterior fossa, hemangioblastoma, and ganglioglioma. In an adult, metastatic carcinoma is occasionally cystic. In some cases, the mural nodule is difficult to discern. The mural nodule is typically the principal region of tumor growth and biopsy. Resection of this region is critical to accurate diagnosis.

Often the cyst wall is lined by astrocytes, frequently admixed with numerous glial fibrils and Rosenthal fibers. Careful determination whether the gliosis constitutes or surrounds the wall, and whether this wall is part of a pilocytic astrocytoma should be made (Figs. 10.34 and 10.40).

Glial Cyst, Simple Cyst, and Wall of Syrinx

The common denominator of these cysts of various locations and obscure etiologies is that their wall is lined only by gliosis (Table 10.18). Their location influences their names. Appropriately lined cysts are often called glial cysts and, in the cerebellum, simple cysts. A syrinx is a dissection of white matter of the brainstem or spinal cord that is not in continuity with the ventricle or spinal canal and is not lined by ependymal cells. Surgical specimens from the wall of a syrinx usually come from the spinal cord.

Histologic characteristics of these cysts are described above (see "Gliosis"). It is sometimes only with the passage of time that these cysts are proven not to be associated with low-grade astrocytomas. As much tissue as possible should be sampled from specimens of these cysts.

Pineal Cyst

Cysts that resemble the glial cyst described above are common in the pineal gland (Fig. 10.130) (255,256). They are biopsied when mistaken for a cystic neoplasm radiologically. The dense gliosis that lines these cysts, often replete with Rosenthal fibers, has been mistaken for a pilocytic astrocytoma. Also, the cyst compresses adjacent pineal parenchyma, imparting the appearance of increased cellularity, making distinction from a pineal parenchymal tumor difficult. Pineal cysts lack epithelial and mesenchymal features of germ cell neoplasm, teratoma, enterogenous cyst, epidermoid cyst, and dermoid cyst (see Figs. 10.133 through 10.136). Radiography reveals a solid, often enhancing, tumor associated with glioma, germ cell neoplasm, and teratoma, but not with a pineal cyst (255,256).

Neuroepithelial Cyst and Ependymal Cyst

These cysts have an epithelioid surface resting on either a fibrillary glial or a fibrous collagen base (Fig. 10.131). They occur

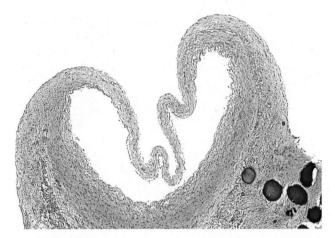

Figure 10.130. Pineal cyst. This cyst is intact and partly collapsed. Its fibrillar, reactive glial lining is pinker than the surrounding pineal gland, which contains dark, round, purple calcifications.

in brain and spinal cord (Table 10.19). They rarely rupture to cause sterile meningitis (257).

Colloid Cyst

Location is a key feature of colloid cyst, more precisely called colloid cyst of the third ventricle (Table 10.19). Its location in the third ventricle, usually near the choroid plexus and foramen of Monro, helps distinguish the colloid cyst from other cysts that superficially resemble it (enterogenous cysts, ependymal cysts, and Rathke cleft cysts) but occur in different locations. The simple columnar and cuboidal epithelium, which may be flattened to simple squamous epithelium, often contains a mixture of ciliated and nonciliated cells. The topographic distribution of the epithelial cells suggests respiratory origin (258), and the cilia taper distally to resemble sensory cilia, suggesting an olfactory origin. The cyst contents are predominantly carboxymucins, rendering them PAS- and Alcian blue-positive (259).

Colloid cysts present little diagnostic challenge provided their location is remembered. An exception is a previously ruptured and inflamed colloid cyst that may mimic an abscess or

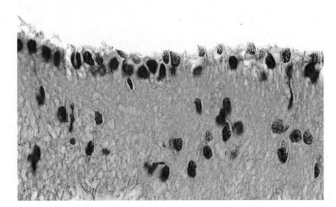

Figure 10.131. Neuroepithelial cyst. Ciliated columnar cells, without evidence of mucin production, which is consistent with ependymal cells, rest on a glial base.

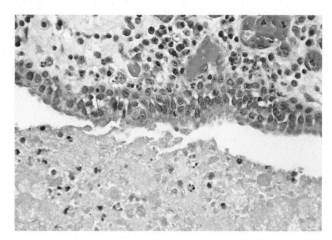

Figure 10.132. Colloid cyst. The ruptured cyst presented as a third ventricular mass. Note the columnar epithelial layer of cells.

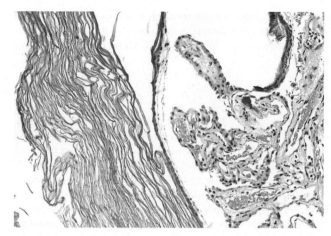

Figure 10.134. Epidermoid cyst. The thin, squamous epithelial lining in the center of the field produced the squames nearby. No adnexal structures are present, ruling out a dermoid cyst. The choroid plexus lies on the right side of this field.

ventriculitis unless the colloid material or epithelium can be identified (Fig. 10.132). Use of a keratin immunostain facilitates identification of the epithelial elements.

Dermoid Cyst

Dermoid cysts are most frequently midline cysts, possibly from the embryonic inclusions of skin at the time of closure of the neural groove. They occur between the cerebellar hemispheres, in the fourth ventricle, in the lumbosacral region of the cord, and in the skull. They may involve CNS parenchyma and/or meninges (4).

The neurosurgeon can frequently alert the pathologist to the possibility of a dermoid cyst from its gross characteristics (Table 10.19). After hair and squamous epithelium are identified in a cyst (Fig. 10.133) within the cranial vault or spinal canal, few alternative lesions are possible other than teratoma. Although meticulous sampling and failure to find tissue elements other than fibrous tissue, skin, and adnexa suggest dermoid cyst, some suspect these cysts may be mature teratomas, especially if minute evidence of other germinal layers is found.

Ruptured dermoid cysts can cause sterile, chemical meningitis and inflammation resembling an abscess. Squamous epithelial cells or cholesterol clefts identified within the inflammation are clues to its cause, but such elements can be seen in a ruptured or operated craniopharyngioma as well.

Epidermoid Cyst

Epidermoid cysts contrast with the previously described dermoid cyst by their lack of adnexal structures, including hair. They contain only keratinized squamous epithelium and its byproducts, making the cyst contents soft, waxy, white, and pearly (Table 10.19).

Although they are more common in lateral than midline sites, location is not as helpful as gross and microscopic appearance in identifying epidermoid cysts because they have been found in many different locations. Frequent locations are the cerebellopontine angle (Fig. 10.134), around the pons, near the sella, within the temporal lobe, in the diploë, and in the spinal canal. The cautions about sampling a teratoma and about

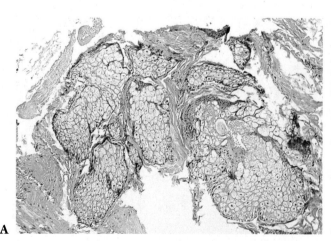

A

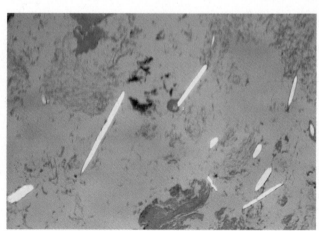

B

Figure 10.133. Dermoid cyst. **(A)** Adnexal structures abound in the collagenous wall of this cyst. A round hair shaft is speckled brown and pink. In one corner, the lumen contains squamous epithelial debris (squames). **(B)** The hair shafts are highlighted with polarized light.

rupture of cyst contents described for dermoid cysts also pertain to epidermoid cysts.

In the suprasellar and sellar regions, distinction from cystic craniopharyngioma requires careful sampling of all tissue, thick or thin. Observation of a solid tumor with typical morphology (e.g., adamantinomatous) is diagnostic of craniopharyngioma, and its absence upon complete sampling suggests an epidermoid cyst. Because craniopharyngiomas have recently been found negative for cytokeratin subtypes CK8 and CK20, this may provide support for the diagnosis of cyst on an incomplete biopsy specimen (when the specimen is positive for these subtypes) (241).

Rarely, carcinoma arises within an epidermoid cyst (4). Solid tumor harboring malignant squamous cells indicates the diagnosis.

Enterogenous Cyst

Enterogenous cysts are recognized as intradural cysts, usually attached to the spinal cord (Fig. 10.135), in children and adults, but similar cysts within the spinal cord have been described in infants (115). The cyst is lined by columnar epithelium that secretes mucus (Fig. 10.136; Table 10.19). The epithelium is usually nonciliated and resembles intestinal epithelium or, more rarely, bronchial epithelium (260).

MENINGEAL CYST

A cyst in the posterior or lateral epidural space in the spinal canal, or overlying the hemispheres, lined only by fibrous tissue

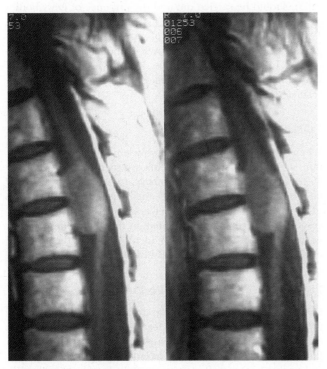

Figure 10.135. Enterogenous cyst in this 60-year-old woman compresses the spinal cord at the midthoracic vertebral level, and it does not enhance after contrast medium (*right*) on T1-weighted magnetic resonance images. (*Courtesy of Dr. James Brunberg, University of Michigan, Ann Arbor, Michigan.*)

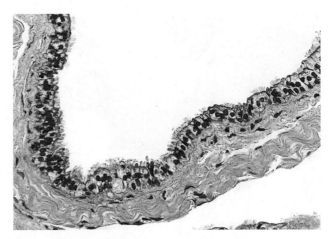

Figure 10.136. Enterogenous cyst. Ciliated, mucus-secreting epithelium rests on a fibrous base.

resembling dura and lacking arachnoid membrane, is a meningeal cyst or diverticulum (Table 10.18). A subdural or subarachnoid cyst with a thinner wall than the epidural cyst, protruding toward or into brain or spinal cord, is an arachnoid cyst. Other cysts have variable thickness more difficult to categorize. Progesterone receptors distinguish this group of cysts from other cysts (Fig. 10.137) (261).

DEGENERATIVE DISEASES—SURGICAL FOCUS ON DEMENTIA

The neurodegenerative diseases of adults are traditionally subdivided into (a) memory disorders: Alzheimer disease (AD), Lewy body disease (LBD) including Parkinson disease (PD), and frontotemporal dementia (FTD); (b) disorders of movement: Huntington disease, Parkinson disease (PD), progressive supranuclear palsy (PSP); and (c) motor neuron diseases (spinal muscular atrophy, amyotrophic lateral sclerosis) (2,3).

Most patients with suspected degenerative diseases are not biopsied. This section will concentrate on dementing diseases that can be found on a brain biopsy.

Dementia, a progressive and persistent alteration and decline of the normal cognitive state, can be a symptom of various etiologic processes, including degenerative, infectious (viral meningoencephalitis), inflammatory, demyelinating, cerebrovascular, neoplastic, and toxic-metabolic (Lafora body disease) diseases. This section deals principally with the most common degenerative diseases (see also "Viruses," including "HIV," "Prion Diseases," "Demyelination," and "Cerebrovascular Diseases" sections).

The principal goal of a cortical biopsy in the setting of a dementing disease lacking a clinical diagnosis is evaluation for treatable versus untreatable disease. See (a) CJD provisos, and (b) "Tissue Processing—High Risk" sections above. Identification of the classic hallmark lesions of the degenerative diseases can be valuable in explaining a patient's cognitive decline (Table 10.20; Fig. 10.138) and ruling out other etiologies of significance.

ALZHEIMER DISEASE—A TAUOPATHY

Alzheimer disease (AD) is the most common neurodegenerative disease that causes dementia. Diagnostic and staging criteria

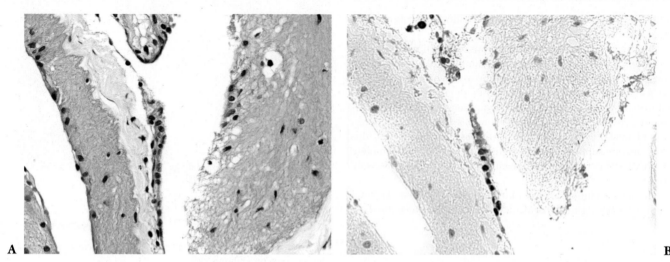

Figure 10.137. Arachnoid cyst. From the posterior fossa of a 2-year-old boy, this cyst has a thin, collagenous membrane covered with meningothelial cells. The membrane itself lies on brain tissue. In similar fields of nearby sections, the collagenous membrane is best appreciated in **A**, and the progesterone-receptor–positive meningothelial cells in **B**. Distinguishing between pinker and tighter brain tissue and wavy strands of collagen is tricky. Take every occasion to compare them side-by-side.

have been established (262–264). Hallmark and diagnostic histologic features include the presence of (a) *neurofibrillary tangles* in the cytoplasm of intact neurons, a major constituent of which is abnormally phosphorylated tau, composed ultrastructurally of paired helical filaments; (b) *neuritic plaques* present in the neuropile composed of aggregates of amyloid with admixed abnormal axons and dendrites; and (c) *dystrophic neurites*, containing deposits of tau (Fig. 10.138). In contrast, diffuse amyloid plaques lacking associated neurites, common in the aging brain, are of unknown significance but do not correlate with dementia. Tau immunostain optimally identifies neurites and tangles (Table 10.20). Silver stains such as Bielschowsky and Gallyas identify neuritic plaques and neurofibrillary tangles but have high background. Evaluation for tangles and amyloid by use of thioflavin S and thioflavin T is inexpensive but requires use of a fluorescence microscope.

In the setting of a biopsy, the presence of neuritic plaques and neurofibrillary tangles can be reported as "Alzheimer disease–type changes," and semiquantification (sparse, moderate, numerous) using CERAD charts can be carried out (263). Identification in the neocortex of a moderate number of neuritic plaques and/or neurofibrillary tangles, although not definitive, likely connotes some component of AD. Absence of AD changes does not rule out AD. For instance, intermediate Braak and Braak stage AD (262), which may be clinically symptomatic, may show minimal pathology in a cortical biopsy.

LEWY BODY DISEASE (LBD)/PARKINSON DISEASE (PD)—A SYNUCLEINOPATHY

Lewy body disease (also known as dementia with Lewy bodies [DLB] and diffuse Lewy body disease [DLBD]) is the second most common disease associated with dementia in autopsy series, but notoriously difficult to diagnose clinically. Consensus criteria have been developed and validated for the clinical and autopsy diagnosis of LBD and a staging system has been proposed (265,266). LBD occurs in "pure" cases, but concomitant AD and PD is most common.

The hallmark lesion, the "Lewy body," is accompanied by the presence of dystrophic "Lewy neurites," neuronal loss, and gliosis. In comparison to the Lewy bodies of the brainstem substantia nigra, "cortical" Lewy bodies, which develop in neurons of the limbic lobe and the neocortex, are difficult to recognize in H&E-stained sections (Fig. 10.138).

In the setting of a biopsy, IHC for ubiquitin or, better, alpha-synuclein, a specific and sensitive marker for LBD changes (265), should be carried out and the presence of Lewy bodies and Lewy neurites diagnosed as LBD-type changes (Table 10.20). Although identification of several Lewy bodies in a single sulcal region likely is diagnostic of the neocortical component of LBD, without an autopsy, definitive diagnosis should not be made, and a report should state "Lewy body disease–related changes."

COMBINED AD/LBD

When ubiquitin or, optimally, α-synuclein immunostain evaluation is employed, features of LBD are seen in approximately 30% of patients with AD; conversely, most patients with LBD have some element of AD change identifiable. Features of both of these diseases can be identified at biopsy (3). These two processes likely have an additive effect in the dementing process. At the time of biopsy, descriptive identification of the presence or absence of changes of AD and LBD is a pragmatic approach.

FRONTOTEMPORAL DEMENTIA

Following evaluation of a biopsy specimen for histologic features of AD and LBD, look for features of the frontotemporal dementia (FTD) group of diseases. Subclassification includes Pick disease, corticobasal degeneration, progressive supranuclear palsy, FTD with Parkinsonism linked to chromosome 17, and frontotemporal lobar degeneration with or without motor neuron disease (267–270).

Most forms of frontotemporal dementia manifest vacuolation of the superficial cortical layers, ballooned neurons, and

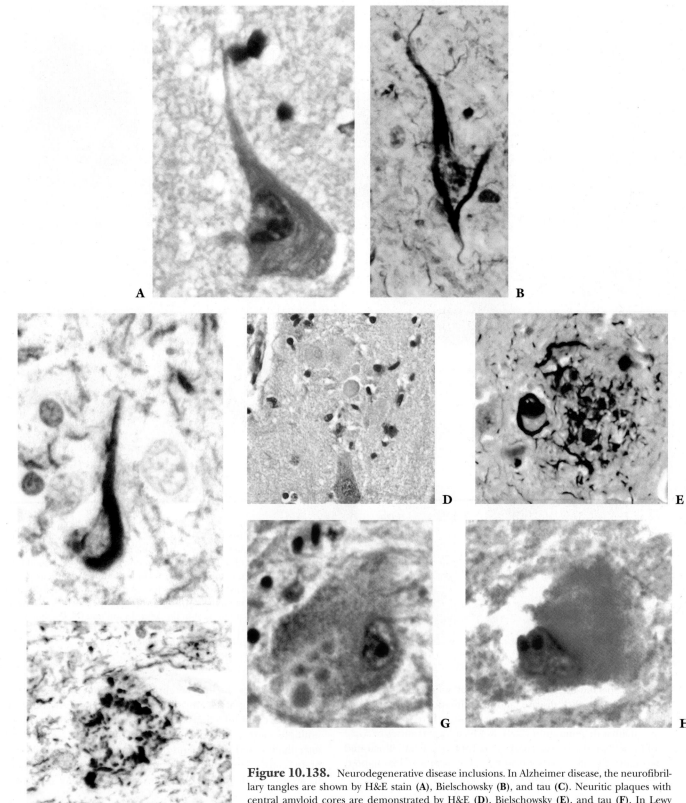

Figure 10.138. Neurodegenerative disease inclusions. In Alzheimer disease, the neurofibrillary tangles are shown by H&E stain **(A)**, Bielschowsky **(B)**, and tau **(C)**. Neuritic plaques with central amyloid cores are demonstrated by H&E **(D)**, Bielschowsky **(E)**, and tau **(F)**. In Lewy body disease, Lewy bodies are demonstrated in substantia nigra neurons **(G)** and cortical neurons by H&E **(H)** *(continues)*

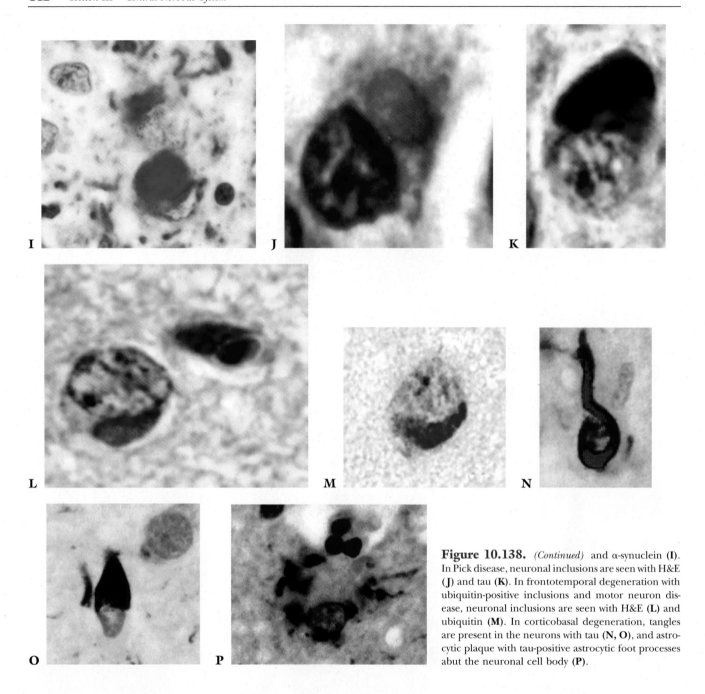

Figure 10.138. *(Continued)* and α-synuclein **(I)**. In Pick disease, neuronal inclusions are seen with H&E **(J)** and tau **(K)**. In frontotemporal degeneration with ubiquitin-positive inclusions and motor neuron disease, neuronal inclusions are seen with H&E **(L)** and ubiquitin **(M)**. In corticobasal degeneration, tangles are present in the neurons with tau **(N, O)**, and astrocytic plaque with tau-positive astrocytic foot processes abut the neuronal cell body **(P)**.

gliosis. Specific inclusions include silver stain and tau-positive Pick bodies in Pick disease, and ubiquitin-positive cytoplasmic inclusions that are tau-and α-synuclein–negative in frontotemporal lobar degeneration (269). Key histologic features of some of these diseases are summarized in Table 10.20 and illustrated in Figure 10.138. Others are outside of the scope of this chapter, and are covered by definitive texts (2,3).

OTHER DEMENTIAS

Additional causes of dementia include Lafora disease (Fig. 10.139), neuronal ceroid lipofuscinosis, adrenoleukodystrophy, and others reviewed elsewhere (27,271,272). Some of these can be diagnosed on brain biopsy or biopsy of other sites. Nondegenerative causes of dementia are addressed in their appropri-

ate section. These include cerebrovascular dementias associated with multiple infarcts, amyloid angiopathy, and CADASIL; inflammatory and infectious dementias associated with vasculitis, multiple sclerosis, TB, cryptococcosis, syphilis, PML, AIDS, viral encephalitis, and prions; and dementia associated with diffuse brain tumors. Toxic, metabolic, and traumatic causes of dementia are usually diagnosed clinically or at autopsy, not surgically.

DEVELOPMENTAL DISEASES AND SEIZURE SURGERY

A variety of developmental disorders affecting the CNS are examined in the setting of surgical pathology (1,3,4).

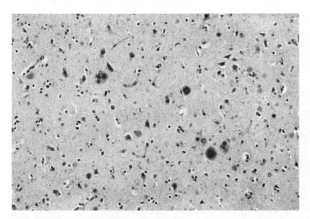

Figure 10.139. Multiple Lafora bodies of various size and structure. Brain biopsy.

MENINGOCELES, MENINGOMYELOCELES, MENINGOENCEPHALOCELES

In the setting of a vertebral and/or cranial bone developmental defect, portions of meninges and, in some cases, either spinal cord (meningomyelocele) or brain (meningoencephalocele) can herniate and lead to discernible lesions in the neonatal period (3). The correct diagnosis of these lesions is assisted by correlation of macroscopic and microscopic findings with operative and radiographic findings. The role of the diagnostic pathologist is to (a) identify and name the various components of the resected lesion, albeit often resected piecemeal; and (b) rule out the presence of other lesions such as an epidermoid or dermoid cyst, teratoma (mature or immature), and other neoplasms. The neural tissues can be chaotically admixed with reactive gliosis, fibrous connective tissue, vessels, and inflammation, and are difficult to discern. Immunostains for synaptophysin and GFAP can help identify neural elements. Choroid plexus can be identified in some meningomyeloceles and meningoencephaloceles. When the herniated tissue has become infected due to compromise in the overlying skin, considerable inflammation can be present, and a search for bacterial and fungal elements is necessary.

NASAL ENCEPHALOCELES, NASAL GLIAL HETEROTOPIAS ("NASAL GLIOMAS")

Nasal encephaloceles and nasal glial heterotopias are members of a spectrum of lesions that can be seen in the nasal region, most commonly in childhood. If not identified at birth, they can present with a CSF leak or recurrent meningitis. Nomenclature remains controversial. Nasal encephaloceles typically are identified in association with a discernible cranial bone defect (273), whereas nasal glial heterotopias may or may not have an associated cranial bone defect (1). Both are generally considered to represent anteriorly displaced heterotopic CNS tissue. They have negligible malignant potential (274). The name *nasal glioma* in the clinical, surgical, and radiologic literature is misleading. Because the term *glioma* has specific neoplastic connotations, it is best avoided. Although characteristically located in the nasal region, similar heterotopic lesions can rarely be identified in other skull and scalp locations (1).

Resection specimens of these displaced tissues, often received in fragments and associated with respiratory mucosa,

contain glial cells, most commonly in interlacing fascicles and admixed fibrovascular connective tissue. Immunostain evaluation reveals that the constituent glial cells are positive for GFAP, which labels delicate astrocytic processes, confirming the impression of astrocyte phenotype. Neurons and axons can be encountered, as identified by cytologic characteristics, silver stain, and neurofilament protein or synaptophysin immunostain. The principal differential diagnosis is well-differentiated teratoma. Radiologic and in situ correlation is critical to the appropriate diagnosis.

CORTICAL MALFORMATIONS

Most commonly seen by the surgical pathologist in resection specimens from patients manifesting seizures, a variety of malformations of the cortical architecture can be identified (275). Resected cortical regions should be sectioned perpendicular to the arachnoid surface to include arachnoid, gray matter, and white matter.

Use of neuronal markers, including Neu-N, synaptophysin, and neurofilament along with GFAP, facilitates the identification of abnormal regions of cortex, in contrast to normal surrounding regions, and helps with phenotypic identification of abnormal cells.

Microdysgenesis is a term used to describe a group of lesions noted only microscopically and not radiologically, including (a) focal oligodendroglial clusters, often interspersed with ganglion cells, in gray or white matter; (b) oligodendroglial hyperplasia with findings of hypercellularity of oligodendrocytes, but findings that fall short of oligodendroglioma; and (c) isolated neurons in the white matter, greater than normal for site (275). *Cortical dysplasia* (focal cortical dysplasia) can be noted radiologically and often grossly by a blurring of the gray–white matter junction and consists histologically of disrupted cortical architecture with unusual enlarged cells, some with cytologic features of neurons, some with features of astrocytes, and some with features of both (1). *Cortical tubers*, usually in tuberous sclerosis patients, manifest cortical dysplasia and, in addition, manifest a prominent number of the enlarged, ballooned cells, most notable at the gray–white matter junction, which can express both GFAP and neuronal antigens.

The histologic distinction between cortical dysplasia and cortical tubers on one hand and gangliocytic neoplasms on the other can be difficult. Neuronal neoplasms typically manifest both (a) architectural abnormalities, including abnormal neuronal clustering and loss of orderly distribution; and (b) cytologic abnormalities, including binucleation, cytologic atypia (e.g., large and bizarre nuclei, hyperchromatism), neurons of various stages of development; and (c) increased cellular density and proliferation (27).

EPILEPSY SURGERY

About 80% of complex partial seizures originate in the temporal lobe, but can occur in any lobe or in a full hemisphere (e.g., in Rasmussen encephalitis). Intractable seizures, resistant to pharmacologic therapies, are debilitating and markedly limit the patient's quality of life. Radical neurosurgical procedures such as temporal lobectomy (hippocampus, temporal neocortex, and often amygdala) and hemispherectomies are performed after extensive imaging studies and, often, mapping of regions to localize the seizure focus. In a carefully selected popu-

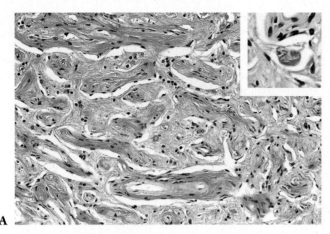
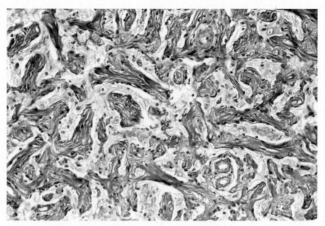

A   B

Figure 10.140. Meningioangiomatosis, sporadic, from cortex in a 16-year-old boy with seizures. **(A)** Prominent perivascular fibrosis is noted in the cortex (H&E stain). **(B)** Trichrome stain highlights fibrosis and entrapped neuropil. Inset: Tangle in neuron. Perivascular cells are characteristically negative for epithelial membrane antigen and glial fibrillary acidic protein (not shown).

lation of patients with defined epileptogenic foci and regions of electrophysiology and/or imaging abnormality, results range between freedom from seizures and marked reduction in seizures (276,277). Risks in such surgery include introduction of a new seizure focus resulting from the brain tissue reaction to the surgery along with typical surgical risks (hemorrhage, infection, etc.).

Correct positioning of the specimen by the neurosurgeon and cross sections that optimally section through the hippocampus are critical. GFAP identifies gliosis. Synaptophysin, Neu-N, or neurofilament helps evaluate for disordered neuronal architecture. Incorporation of findings on imaging studies and knowledge about use of depth or surface electrode monitoring is important to microscopic interpretation.

As summarized in Table 10.21, a variety of changes can be identified in the resected specimens, some known preoperatively, some unsuspected (3,278,279). The critical role of the pathologist is in ruling out neoplasm, either anticipated by imaging studies or occult. Primary intracerebral tumors presenting with medically refractory epilepsy are usually low-grade dysembryoplastic neuroepithelial tumors (DNTs), oligodendrogliomas, astrocytomas, and gangliogliomas. Meningioangiomatosis, a hamartomatous lesion, is usually unsuspected. It is seen sporadically and in NF-2, often dural-based and variably mineralized, and often misinterpreted clinically as meningioma (Fig. 10.140) (1).

The clinical term *mesial temporal sclerosis* (MTS) corresponds histologically to the common, striking reduction in the number of hippocampal pyramidal and, in some cases, dentate gyrus neurons accompanied by gliosis. The most common MTS shows severe neuronal loss in the Sommer sector (H1) and the end folium (H3-5) of the large pyramidal neurons in the Ammon horn, with sparing of neurons between these regions (H2) and sparing of the tiny neurons in the dentate (276). Whether such a change is a result of seizure activity (and hypothesized transient ischemia) or is the cause of the seizures is debatable. Subpial gliosis is a common finding in resected temporal lobes, and is of uncertain significance.

Iatrogenic changes due to electrode monitoring are common and include arachnoid changes (fibrosis and mononuclear-cell infiltrate, including hemosiderin-laden macro-

phages). With depth electrodes, cortical lesions include a track of encephalomalacia with associated lymphocytes, macrophages, hemorrhage, and early gliosis in the surgical specimen.

Various infectious and inflammatory processes can lead to seizures. For instance, about 50% to 70% of patients with neurocysticercosis present with seizures (36) (Fig. 10.14A). Rasmussen encephalitis is an uncommon but notable disease, with loss of cognitive skills, intractable seizures, and atrophy of one hemisphere, associated with antibodies against the GluR3 glutamate receptor. Biopsy or hemispherectomy is carried out in some cases. Findings are nonspecific inflammation with microglial cells without evidence of virions (279).

ACKNOWLEDGMENTS

The following colleagues at the University of Michigan, Penn State University, University of Texas Southwestern Medical Center, and University of Colorado Health Science Center provided particularly valuable assistance. Dr. Philip Boyer provided tables, figures, and references, and updated some material. Dr. Mila Blaivas provided figures and commentary. Dr. Joseph Parisi provided some tables. Drs. Javad Towfighi and Dennis Burns provided figures. Drs. Mila Blaivas, Jeanne Bell, Larry Junck, and Ricardo Lloyd provided key citations. I thank Dianna Banka, Nicole Cheesman, Melissa Mills, and Peggy Otto for their skill and patience in preparing this chapter. Joseph Mailloux provided electron micrographs of high quality. Mark Deming and Elizabeth Walker carefully prepared the illustrations. Immunohistologists and histopathologists in the University of Michigan Medical Center Pathology Laboratories prepared fine microscopic slides.

REFERENCES

1. Burger PC, Scheithauer BW, Vogel FS. *Surgical Pathology of the Nervous System and its Coverings.* 4th edition New York: Churchill Livingstone, 2002.
2. Dickson DW. *Neurodegeneration: The Molecular Pathology of Dementia and Movement Disorders.* Basel: ISN Neuropath Press, 2003.
3. Ellison D, Love S., Chimelli L, et al., eds. *Neuropathology.* 2nd Philadelphia: Mosby, 2004.
4. Garcia JH, Budka H, McKeever PE, et al., eds. *Neuropathology: The Diagnostic Approach.* Philadelphia: Mosby, 1997.

5. Prayson R. *Neuropathology*. Philadelphia: Elsevier Churchill Livingstone, 2005.
6. Gujar SK, Maheshwari S, Bjorkman-Burtscher I, et al. Magnetic resonance spectroscopy. *J Neuro-Ophthalmol* 2005; 25(3):217–226.
7. Love S, Louis DN, Ellison DW. *Greenfield's Neuropathology*. 8th edition New York: Hodder Arnold, 2008.
8. Louis DN, Ohgaki H, Wiestler OD, et al. The 2007 WHO classification of tumours of the central nervous system. *Acta Neuropathol* 2007;114:97–109.
9. Kleinschmidt-DeMasters BK, Prayson RA. An algorithmic approach to the brain biopsy—part I. *Arch Pathol Lab Med* 2006;130(11):1630–1638.
10. Prayson RA, Kleinschmidt-DeMasters BK. An algorithmic approach to the brain biopsy—part II. *Arch Pathol Lab Med* 2006;130(11):1639–1648.
11. Sundgren PC, Fan X, Weybright P, et al. Differentiation of recurrent brain tumor versus radiation injury using diffusion tensor imaging in patients with new contrast-enhancing lesions. *Magc Reson Imag* 2006;24:1131–1142.
12. Inagawa H, Ishizawa K, Hirose T. Qualitative and quantitative analysis of cytologic assessment of astrocytoma, oligodendroglioma and oligoastrocytoma. *Acta Cytologica* 2007;51: 900–906.
13. Firlik KS, Martinez AJ, Lunsford LD. Use of cytological preparations for the intraoperative diagnosis of stereotactically obtained brain biopsies: a 19-year experience and survey of neuropathologists. *J Neurosurg* 1999;91:454–458.
14. Rajshekhar V. Current status of stereotactic biopsy. *Stereotact Funct Neurosurg* 2001;76: 137–139.
15. Rutala WA, Weber DJ. Creutzfeldt-Jakob disease: recommendations for disinfection and sterilization. *Clin Infect Dis* 2001;32:1348–1356.
16. McKeever PE, Balentine JD. Histochemistry of the nervous system. In Spicer SS, ed. *Histochemistry in Pathologic Diagnosis*. New York: Marcel-Dekker; 1987:871–957.
17. Prophet EB, Mills B, Arrington JB, Sobin LH. *Laboratory Methods in Histotechnology*. Washington, DC: AFIP, 1992.
18. McKeever PE: Immunohistochemistry of the nervous system. In Dabbs DJ, ed. *Diagnostic Immunohistochemistry*. 2nd edition Philadelphia: Churchill Livingstone, 2006:746–816.
19. Mrak RE. The big eye in the 21st century: the role of electron microscopy in modern diagnostic neuropathology. *J Neuropathol Exp Neurol* 2002;61:1027–1039
20. Danton GH, Dietrich WD. Inflammatory mechanisms after ischemia and stroke. *J Neuropathol Exp Neurol* 2003;62:127–136.
21. Kreutzberg GW. Microglia: a sensor for pathological events in the CNS. *Trends Neurosci* 1996;19:312–318.
22. McKeever PE, Balentine JD. Macrophage migration through the brain parenchyma to the perivascular space following particle ingestion. *Am J Pathol* 1978;93:153–164.
23. Del Bigio MR. Biologic reactions to cerebrospinal fluid shunt devices: a review of the cellular pathology. *Neurosurgery* 1998;42:319–325.
24. Berger JR, Snodgrass S, Glaser J, et al. Multifocal fibrosclerosis with hypertrophic intracranial pachymeningitis. *Neurology* 1989;39:1345–1349.
25. Thomson RB Jr., Bertram H. Laboratory diagnosis of central nervous system infections. *Infect Dis Clin North Am* 2001;15:1047–1071.
26. Falcone S, Post MJ. Encephalitis, cerebritis, and brain abscess: pathophysiology and imaging findings. *Neuroimaging Clin N Am* 2000;10:333–353.
27. Graham DI, Lantos PL. *Greenfield's Neuropathology*. 7th edition New York: Hodder, 2002.
28. Jacob A, Weinshenker BG. An approach to the diagnosis of acute transverse myelitis. *Sem Neurol* 2008;28:105–120.
29. Wingerchuk DM, Lucchinetti CF. Comparative immunopathogenesis of acute disseminated encephalomyelitis, neuromyelitis optica, and multiple sclerosis. *Current Opinion Neurol* 2007;20:343–350.
30. Johnson PC, Farnie MA. Testing for syphilis. *Dermatol Clin* 1994;12:9–17.
31. Morrison A, Gyure KA, Stone J, et al. Mycobacterial spindle cell pseudotumor of the brain: a case report and review of the literature. *Amer J Surg Path* 1999;23:1294–1299.
32. Park do Y, Kim JY, Choi KU, et al. Comparison of polymerase chain reaction with histopathologic features for diagnosis of tuberculosis in formalin-fixed, paraffin-embedded histologic specimens. *Arch Pathol Lab Med* 2000;127:326–330.
33. Schwartz MA, Selhorts JB, Ochs AL, et al. Oculomasticatory myorhythmia: a unique movement disorder occurring in Whipple's disease. *Ann Neurol* 1986;20:677–683.
34. Frater JL, Hall GS, Procop GW. Histologic features of zygomycosis: emphasis on perineural invasion and fungal morphology. *Arch Pathol Lab Med* 2001;125:375–378.
35. Nesky MA, McDougal EC, Peacock Jr JE. *Pseudallescheria boydii* brain abscess successfully treated with voriconazole and surgical drainage: case report and literature review of central nervous system pseudallescheriasis. *Clin Infect Dis* 2000;31:673–677.
36. Carpio A, Escobar A, Hauser WA. Cysticercosis and epilepsy: a critical review. *Epilepsia* 1998;39:1025–1040.
37. Martinez AJ, Visvesvara GS. Free-living, aquatic and opportunistic amebas. *Brain Pathol* 1997;7:583–598.
38. Gelman BB, Popov V, Chaljub G, et al. Neuropathological and ultrastructural features of amebic encephalitis caused by Sappinia diploidea. *J Neuropathol Exper Neurol* 2003;62: 990–998.
39. Nath A, Sinai AP. Cerebral toxoplasmosis. *Curr Treat Options Neurol* 2003;5:3–12.
40. Campbell GL, Marfin AA, Lanciotti RS, Gubler DJ. West Nile virus. *Lancet Infect Dis* 2002; 2:519–529.
41. Cassady KA, Whitley RJ. Pathogenesis and pathophysiology of viral infections of the central nervous system. In Scheld WM, Whitley RJ, Durack DT, eds. *Infections of the Central Nervous System*. 2nd edition Philadelphia: Lippincott-Raven, 1997:7–22.
42. Leis AA, Fratkin J, Stokic DS. West Nile poliomyelitis. *Lancet Infect Dis* 2003;3:9–10.
43. Maschke M, Kastrup O, Diener HC. CNS manifestations of cytomegalovirus infections: diagnosis and treatment. *CNS Drugs* 2002;16:303–315.
44. Sampson BA, Ambrosi C, Charlot A, et al. The pathology of human West Nile virus infection. *Hum Pathol* 2000;31:527–531.
45. Batalis NI, Galup L, Zaki SR, et al. West Nile virus encephalitis. *Am J Forensic Med Pathol* 2005;26:192–196.
46. Ahmed F, Aziz T, Kaufman LD. Progressive multifocal leukoencephalopathy in a patient with systemic lupus erythematosus. *J Rheumatol* 1999;26:1609–1612.
47. Ironside JW, Lewis FA, Blythe D, et al. The identification of cells containing JC papovavirus DNA in progressive multifocal leukoencephalopathy by combined in situ hybridization and immunocytochemistry. *J Pathol* 1989;157:291–297.
48. Budka H. Neuropathology of myelitis, myelopathy, and spinal infections in AIDS. *Neuroimag Clin North Am* 1997;7:639–650.
49. Gray F, Chretien F, Vallat-DeCouvelaere AV, et al. The changing pattern of HIV neuropathology in the HAART era. *J Neuropathol Exp Neurol* 2003; 62:429–440.
50. Vago L, Bonetto S, Nebuloni M, et al. Pathological findings in the central nervous system of AIDS patients on assumed antiretroviral therapeutic regimens: retrospective study of 1597 autopsies. *AIDS* 2002;16:1925–1928.
51. Burkhard PR, Sanchez JC, Landis T, et al. CSF detection of the 14-3-3 protein in unselected patients with dementia. *Neurol* 2001;56:1528–1533.
52. Castellani RJ, Parchi P, Madoff L, et al. Biopsy diagnosis of Creutzfeldt-Jakob disease by western blot: a case report. *Hum Pathol* 1997;28:623–641.
53. Ironside JW, Head MW, Bell JE, et al. Laboratory diagnosis of variant Creutzfeldt-Jakob disease. *Histopathology* 2000;37:1–9.
54. Kovacs GG, Head MW, Hegyi I, et al. Immunohistochemistry for the prion protein: comparison of different monoclonal antibodies in human prion disease subtypes. *Brain Pathol* 2002;12:1–11.
55. Parchi P, Giese A, Capellari S, et al. Classification of sporadic Creutzfeldt-Jakob disease based on molecular and phenotypic analysis of 300 subjects. *Ann Neurol* 1999;46:224–233.
56. Crozet C, Lehmann S. Prions: where do we stand 20 years after the appearance of bovine spongiform encephalopathy? *Med Sci (Paris)* 2007;23:1148–1157.
57. Bradley R, Liberski PP. Bovine spongiform encephalopathy (BSE): the end of the beginning or the beginning of the end? *Folia Neuropathologica* 2004;42(Suppl A):55–68.
58. Sugiura K, Smith GC. A comparison of the risk of bovine spongiform encephalopathy infectivity in beef from cattle younger than 21 months in Japan with that in beef from the United States assessed by the carcass maturity score. *J Food Protection* 2008;71:802–806.
59. Block F, Reith W. Isolated vasculitis of the central nervous system. *Radiologe* 2000;40: 1090–1097.
60. Boyev LR, Miller NR, Green WR. Efficacy of unilateral versus bilateral temporal artery biopsies for the diagnosis of giant cell arteritis. *Am J Ophthalmol* 1999;128:211–215.
61. Jennekens FG, Kater L. The central nervous system in systemic lupus erythematosus. Parts 1 and 2. *Rheumatology* 2002;41:605–630.
62. Lanthier S, Lortie A, Michaud J, et al. Isolated angiitis of the CNS in children. *Neurology* 2001;56:837–842.
63. McKelvie PA, Collins S, Thyagarajan D, et al. Meningoencephalomyelitis with vasculitis due to varicella zoster virus: a case report and review of the literature. *Pathology* 2002;34: 88–93.
64. Phanthumchinda K, Intragumtornchai T, Kasantikul V. Stroke-like syndrome, mineralizing microangiopathy, and neuroaxonal dystrophy following intrathecal methotrexate therapy. *Neurology* 1991;41:1847–1848.
65. Sloan MA, Kittner SJ, Rigamonti D, et al. Occurrence of stroke associated with use/abuse of drugs. *Neurology* 1991;41:1358–1364.
66. Wechsler B, Vidaihet M, Piette JC, et al. Cerebral venous thrombosis in Behcet's disease: clinical study and long-term follow-up of 25 cases. *Neurology* 1992;42:614–618.
67. Dangond F, Lacomis D, Schwartz RB, et al. Acute disseminated encephalomyelitis progressing to hemorrhagic encephalitis. *Neurology* 1991;41:1697–1698.
68. Zagzag D, Miller DC, Kleinman GM,. et al. Demyelinating disease versus tumor in surgical neuropathology. Clues to a correct pathologic diagnosis. *Am J Surg Pathol* 1993;17:537–545.
69. Barnett MH, Sutton I. The pathology of multiple sclerosis: a paradigm shift. *Curr Opin Neurol* 2006;19(3):242–247.
70. Tenembaum S, Chitnis T, Ness J, et al. International Pediatric MS Study Group. Acute disseminated encephalomyelitis. *Neurology* 2007;68(16 Suppl 2):S23–S36.
71. Menge T, Hemmer B, Nessler S, et al. Acute disseminated encephalomyelitis: an update. *Arch Neurol* 2005;62(11):1673–1680.
72. Menge T, Kieseier BC, Nessler S, et al. Acute disseminated encephalomyelitis: an acute hit against the brain. *Curr Opin Neurol* 2007;20(3):247–254.
73. Bernardini GL, DeShaies EM. Critical care of intracerebral and subarachnoid hemorrhage. *Curr Neurol Neurosci Rep* 2001;1:568–576.
74. Abrahams NA, Prayson RA. The role of histopathologic examination of intracranial blood clots removed for hemorrhage of unknown etiology: a clinical pathologic analysis of 31 cases. *Ann Diagn Pathol* 2000;4:361–366.
75. Favre J, Taha JM, Burchiel KJ. An analysis of the respective risks of hematoma formation in 361 consecutive morphological and functional stereotactic procedures. *Neurosurgery* 2002;50:48–57.
76. Minette SE, Kimmel DW. Subdural hematoma in patients with systemic cancer. *Mayo Clin Proc* 1989;64:637–642.
77. Challa VR, Moody DM, Brown WR. Vascular malformations of the central nervous system. *J Neuropathol Exp Neurol* 1995;54:609–621.
78. Fleetwood IG, Steinberg GK. Arteriovenous malformations. *Lancet* 2002;359:863–873.
79. Vonsattel JP, Myers RH, Hedley-Whyte ET, et al. Cerebral amyloid angiopathy without and with cerebral hemorrhages: a comparative histologic study. *Ann Neurol* 1991;30:637–649.
80. Markus HS, Martin RJ, Simpson MA, et al. Diagnostic strategies in CADASIL. *Neurology* 2002;59:1134–1138.
81. Mayer M, Straube A, Bruening R, et al. Muscle and skin biopsies are a sensitive diagnostic tool in the diagnosis of CADASIL. *J Neurol* 1999;246:526–532.
82. Jellinger KA. Vascular-ischemic dementia: an update. *J Neural Transm Suppl* 2002;62:1–623.
83. McKeever PE, Junck L, Strawderman MS, et al. Proliferation index is related to patient age in glioblastoma. *Neurology* 2001;56:1216–1218.
84. McKeever PE, Strawderman MS, Yamini B, et al. MIB-1 proliferation index predicts survival among patients with grade II astrocytoma. *J Neuropathol Exp Neurol* 1998;57:931–936.

85. Montine TJ, Vandersteenhoven JJ, Aguzzi A, et al. Prognostic significance of Ki-67 proliferation index in supratentorial fibrillary astrocytic neoplasms. *Neurosurgery* 1994;34:674–678.

86. Sallinen PK, Haapasalo HK, Visakorpi T, et al. Prognostication of astrocytoma patient survival by Ki67 (MIB-1), PCNA, and S-phase fraction using archival paraffin-embedded samples. *J Pathol* 1994;174:275–282.

87. Fuller CE, Perry A. Molecular diagnostics in central nervous system tumors. *Adv Anat Pathol* 2005 Jul;12(4):180–194.

88. Cairncross G, Berkey B, Shaw E, et al. Phase III trial of chemotherapy plus radiotherapy compared with radiotherapy alone for pure and mixed anaplastic oligodendroglioma: Intergroup RTOG 9402. *J Clin Oncol* 2006; 24:2707–2714.

89. Cáccamo DV, Rubinstein LJ. Tumors: applications of immunocytochemical methods. In Garcia JH, Budka H, McKeever PE, Sarnat HB, Sima AAF, eds. Neuropathology: The Diagnostic Approach. Philadelphia: Mosby. 1997:193–218.

90. Chronwall BM, McKeever PE, Kornblith PL. Glial and nonglial neoplasms evaluated on frozen section by double immunofluorescence for fibronectin and glial fibrillary acidic protein. *Acta Neuropathol (Berl)* 1983;59:283–287.

91. Ino Y, Betensky RA, Zlatescu MC, et al. Molecular subtypes of anaplastic oligodendroglioma: implications for patient management at diagnosis. *Clin Cancer Res* 2001;7:839–845.

92. McKeever PE. Insights about brain tumors gained through immunohistochemistry and in situ hybridization of nuclear and phenotypic markers. *J Histochem Cytochem* 1998;46: 585–594.

93. Reifenberger G, Louis DN. Oligodendroglioma: toward molecular definitions in diagnostic neuro-oncology. *J Neuropathol Exp Neurol* 2003;62:111–126.

94. Rodas RA, Fenstermaker RA, McKeever PE, et al. Intraluminal thrombosis in brain tumor vessels correlates with postoperative thrombotic complications. *J Neurosurg* 1998;89: 200–205.

95. Nataf F, Koziak M, Ricci AC, et al. Results of the Sainte-Anne–Lyons series of 318 oligodendroglioma in adults. *Neuro-Chirurgie* 2005;51(Pt 2):329–351.

96. Vates GE, Chang S, Lamborn KR, et al. Gliomatosis cerebri: a review of 22 cases. *Neurosurg* 2003;53:261–271.

97. Lombardi D, Scheithauer BW, Piepgras D, et al. Angioglioma and the arteriovenous malformation-glioma association. *J Neurosurg* 1991;75:589–599.

98. Martin F Jr, Lemmen LJ. Calcification in intracranial neoplasms. *Am J Pathol* 1952;28: 1107–1129.

99. Pell MF, Revesz T, Thomas DG. Multicentric malignant glioma. *Br J Neurosurg* 1991;5: 631–634.

100. Yamada SM, Hayashi Y, Takahashi H, et al. Histological and genetic diagnosis of gliomatosis cerebri. *J Neuro-Oncol* 2001;52:237–240.

101. Burger PC, Scheithauer BW. *Atlas of Tumor Pathology, Series 4, Fascicle 7. Tumors of the Central Nervous System.* Washington, DC: Armed Forces Institute of Pathology, 2007.

102. Burger PC, Vogel FS. Frozen section interpretation in surgical neuropathology. I. Intracranial lesions. II. Intraspinal lesions. *Am J Surg Pathol* 1977–8;1:323–347;2:81–95.

103. Clark GB, Henry JM, McKeever PE. Cerebral pilocytic astrocytoma. *Cancer* 1985;56: 1128–1133.

104. Forsyth PA, Shaw EG, Scheithauer BW, et al. 51 cases of supratentorial pilocytic astrocytomas: a clinicopathologic, prognostic, and flow cytometric study. *Cancer* 1993;72: 1335–1342.

105. Hayostek C, Shaw EG, Scheithauer BW, et al. Astrocytomas of the cerebellum. A comparative clinicopathologic study of pilocytic and diffuse astrocytomas. *Cancer* 1993;72:856–869.

106. Mamelak AN, Prados MD, Obana WG, et al. Treatment options and prognosis for multicentric juvenile pilocytic astrocytoma. *J Neurosurg* 1994; 81:24–30.

107. McKeever PE, Blaivas M, Gebarski SS. Sellar tumors other than adenomas. In Thapar K, Kovacs K, Scheithauer BW, Lloyd RV, eds. *Diagnosis and Management of Pituitary Tumors.* Totowa, NJ: The Humana Press, Inc., 2000.

108. Komotar RJ, Burger PC, Carson BS, et al. Pilocytic and pilomyxoid astrocytomas. *Neurosurg* 2004;54:72–79.

109. Rasheed BK, McLendon RE, Herndon JE, et al. Alterations of the TP53 gene in human gliomas. *Cancer Res* 1994;54:1324–1330.

110. Blumbergs PC, Chin DK, Hallpike JF. Diffuse infiltrating astrocytoma (gliomatosis cerebri) with twenty-two-year history. *Clin Experimental Neurol* 1983;19:94–101.

111. Braeuninger S, Schneider-Stock R, Kirches E, et al. Evaluation of molecular genetic alterations associated with tumor progression in a case of gliomatosis cerebri. *J Neuro-Oncology* 2007;82(1):23–27.

112. Colman H, Giannini C, Huang L, et al. Assessment and prognostic significance of mitotic index using the mitosis marker phospho-histone H3 in low and intermediate-grade infiltrating astrocytomas. *Am J Surg Pathol* 2006;30:657–664.

113. Newton HB, Rosenblum MK, Malkin MG. Turcot's syndrome. Flow cytometric analysis. *Cancer* 1991;68:1633–1639.

114. Von Deimling A, Bender B, Jahnke R, et al. Loci associated with malignant progression in astrocytomas: a candidate on chromosome 19q. *Cancer Res* 1994;54:1397–1401.

115. Russell DS, Rubinstein LJ. *Pathology of Tumours of the Nervous System.* Baltimore: Williams & Wilkins, 1989.

116. Plank TL, Yeung RS, Henske EP. Hamartin, the product of the tuberous sclerosis 1 (TSC1) gene, interacts with tuberin and appears to be localized to cytoplasmic vesicles. *Cancer Res* 1998;58:4766–4770.

117. Giannini C, Scheithauer BW, Burger PC, et al. Pleomorphic xanthoastrocytoma: what do we really know about it? *Cancer* 1999;85:2033–2045.

118. Levy RA, Allen R, McKeever PE. Pleomorphic xanthoastrocytoma presenting with massive intracranial hemorrhage. *AJNR* 1996;17:154–156.

119. Powell SZ, Yachnis AT, Rorke LB, et al. Divergent differentiation in pleomorphic xanthoastrocytoma. Evidence for a neuronal element and possible relationship to ganglion cell tumors. *Am J Surg Pathol* 1996;20:80–85.

120. Dickson DW, Suzuki KI, Kanner R, et al. Cerebral granular cell tumor: immunohistochemical and electron microscopy study. *J Neuropathol Exp Neurol* 1996;45:304–314.

121. McKeever PE. Laboratory methods of brain tumor analysis. In Nelson JS, Mena H, Parisi

JE, Schochet Jr SS, eds. *Principles and Practice of Neuropathology.* 2nd edition New York: Oxford, 2003.

122. Kleihues P, Ohgaki H. Primary and secondary glioblastoma: from concept to clinical diagnosis. *Neuro-Oncol* 1999;1:44–51.

123. Paulus W, Peiffer J. Intratumoral histologic heterogeneity of gliomas. A quantitative study. *Cancer* 1989;64:442–447.

124. Hegi ME, Diserens AC, Gorlia T, et al. MGMT gene silencing and benefit from temozolomide in glioblastoma. *New Eng J Med* 2005;352:997–1003.

125. McKeever PE, Wichman A, Chronwall BM, Thomas C, Howard R. Sarcoma arising from a gliosarcoma. *South Med J* 1984;77:1027–1032.

126. Rosenblum MK, Erlandson RA, Budzilovich GN. The lipid-rich epithelioid glioblastoma. *Am J Surg Pathol* 1991;15:925–934.

127. Giannini C, Scheithauer BW, Weaver AL, et al. Oligodendrogliomas: reproducibility and prognostic value of histologic diagnosis and grading. *J Neuropathol Exp Neurol* 2001;60: 248–262.

128. Reifenberger G, Louis DN. Oligodendroglioma: toward molecular definitions in diagnostic neuro-oncology. *J Neuropathol Exp Neurol* 2003;62:111–126.

129. Smith JS, Perry A, Borell TJ, et al. Alterations of chromosome arms 1p and 19q as predictors of survival in oligodendrogliomas, astrocytomas, and mixed oligoastrocytomas. *J Clin Oncol* 2000;18:636–645.

130. Eoli M, Bissola L, Bruzzone MG, Pollo B, et al. Reclassification of oligoastrocytomas by loss of heterozygosity studies. *Int J Cancer* 2006;119:84–90.

131. Aldape K, Burger PC, Perry A. Clinicopathologic aspects of 1p/19q loss and the diagnosis of oligodendroglioma. *Arch Pathol Lab Med* 2007;131:242–251.

132. Mokhtari K, Paris S, Aguirre-Cruz L, et al. Olig2 expression, GFAP, p53 and 1p loss analysis contribute to glioma subclassification. *Neuropathol Appl Neurobiol* 2005;31:62–69.

133. Mokhtari K, Paris S, Aguirre-Cruz L, et al. Clinicopathologic aspects of 1p/19q loss and the diagnosis of oligodendroglioma. *Arch Pathol Lab Med* 2007;131(2):242–251.

134. Suzuki SO, Kitai R, Llena J, et al. MAP-2e, a novel MAP-2 isoform, is expressed in gliomas and delineates tumor architecture and patterns of infiltration. *J Neuropathol Exp Neurol* 2002;61:403–412.

135. Koperek O, Gelpi E, Birner P, et al. Value and limits of immunohistochemistry in differential diagnosis of clear cell primary brain tumors. *Acta Neuropathol* 2004;108:24–30.

136. Mohapatra G, Betensky RA, Miller ER, et al. Glioma test array for use with formalin-fixed, paraffin-embedded tissue: array comparative genomic hybridization correlates with loss of heterozygosity and fluorescence in situ hybridization. *J Mol Diagn* 2006; 8:268–276.

137. Kitanaka C, Shitara N, Nakagomi T, et al. Postradiation astrocytoma: report of two cases. *J Neurosurg* 1989;70:469–474.

138. Sato K, Kubota T, Ishida M, et al. Immunohistochemical and ultrastructural study of chordoid glioma of the third ventricle: its tanycytic differentiation. *Acta Neuropathologica* 2003;106:176–180.

139. Ross DA, McKeever PE, Sandler HM, et al. Myxopapillary ependymoma. *Cancer* 1993;71: 3114–3118.

140. Min KW, Scheithauer BW. Clear cell ependymoma: a mimic of oligodendroglioma: clinicopathologic and ultrastructural considerations. *Am J Surg Pathol* 1997;21(7):820–826.

141. Kawano N, Yada K, Aihara M, et al. Oligodendroglioma-like cells (clear cells) in ependymoma. *Acat Neuropathol (Berl)* 1984;3:122–127.

142. Ross GW, Rubinstein LJ. Lack of histopathological correlation of malignant ependymomas with postoperative survival. *J Neurosurg* 1989;70:31–36.

143. Mork SJ, Rubinstein LJ. Ependymoblastoma: a reappraisal of a rare embryonal tumor. *Cancer* 1985;55:1536–1542.

144. Oberc-Greenwood MA, McKeever PE, Kornblith PL, et al. A human ganglioglioma containing paired helical filaments. *Hum Pathol* 1984;15:834–838.

145. Wirnsberg GH, Becker H, Ziervogel K, Hofler H. Diagnostic immunohistochemistry of neuroblastic tumors. *Am J Surg Pathol* 1992;15:49–57.

146. Karamitopoulou E, Perentes E, Probst A, et al. Ganglioglioma of the brain stem: neurological dysfunction of 16-year duration. *Clin Neuropathol* 1995;14:162–168.

147. Lindboe CF, Helseth E, Myhr G. Lhermitte-Duclos disease and giant meningioma as manifestations of Cowden's disease. *Clin Neuropathol* 1995;14:327–330.

148. Daumas-Duport C. Dysembryoplastic neuroepithelial tumors. *Brain Pathol* 1993;3: 283–295.

149. Prayson RA, Morris HH, Estes ML, et al. Dysembryoplastic neuroepithelial tumor: a clinicopathologic and immunohistochemical study of 11 tumors including MIB1 immunoreactivity. *Clin Neuropathol* 1996;15:47–53.

150. Figarella-Branger D, Pellissier JF, Daumas-Duport C, et al. Central neurocytomas. Critical evaluation of a small-cell neuronal tumor. *Am J Surg Pathol* 1992;16:97–109.

151. Yasargil MG, von Ammon K, von Deimling A, et al. Central neurocytoma: histopathological variants and therapeutic approaches. *J Neurosurg* 1992;76:32–37.

152. Vandenberg SR, May EE, Rubinstein LJ, et al. Desmoplastic supratentorial neuroepithelial tumors of infancy with divergent differentiation potential ("desmoplastic infantile gangliogliomas"). Report on 11 cases of a distinctive embryonal tumor with favorable prognosis. *J Neurosurg* 1987;66:58–71.

153. Gonzalez-Campora R, Weller RO. Lipidized mature neuroectodermal tumour of the cerebellum with myoid differentiation. *Neuropathol Appl Neurobiol* 1998;397–402.

154. Lutterbach J, Fauchon F, Schild SE, et al. Malignant pineal parenchymal tumors in adult patients: patterns of care and prognostic factors. *Neurosurg* 2002;51:44–55.

155. McKeever, PE. Immunohistochemistry of the nervous system. In Dabbs DJ, ed. *Diagnostic Immunohistochemistry.* New York: Churchill Livingstone, 2002.

156. Giordana MT, Migheli A, Pavanelli E. Interphase cytogenetics of medulloblastoma: isochromosome 17q is a constant finding. *J Neuropathol Exp Neurol* 1997;56:609.

157. Roberts RO, Lynch CF, Jones MP, Hart MN. Medulloblastoma: a population-based study of 532 cases. *J Neuropathol Exp Neurol* 1991;50:134–144.

158. Katsetos CD, Herman MM, Frankfurter A, et al. Cerebellar desmoplastic medulloblastomas. A further immunohistochemical characterization of the reticulin-free pale islands. *Arch Pathol Lab Med* 1989;113:1019–1029.

159. Rutkowski S, Bode U, Deinlein F, et al. Treatment of early childhood medulloblastoma by positive chemotherapy alone. *N Eng J Med* 2005;352:978–986.
160. McManamy CS, Lamont JM, Taylor RE, et al. Morphophenotypic variation predicts clinical behavior in childhood non-desmoplastic medulloblastomas. *J Neuropathol Exp Neurol* 2003; 62:627–632.
161. Li Y, Guessous F, Johnson EB, et al. Functional and molecular interactions between the HGF/c-Met pathway and c-Myc in large-cell medulloblastoma. *Lab Invest* 2008;88(2): 98–111.
162. Kleihues UE, Smith TW, DeGirolami U, et al. Medulloblastoma with cartilaginous differentiation. *Arch Pathol Lab Med* 1989;113:84–88.
163. Bonnin JM, Rubinstein LJ, Palmer NF, et al. The association of embryonal tumors originating in the kidney and in the brain; a report of seven cases. *Cancer* 1984;54:2137–2146.
164. Freyer DR, Hutchinson RJ, McKeever PE. Primary primitive neuroectodermal tumor of the spinal cord associated with neural tube defect. *Pediatr Neurosci* 1989;15:181–187.
165. Mobley BC, Roulston D, Shah, GV, et al. Peripheral PNET/Ewing sarcoma in the craniospinal vault: case reports and review. *Human Pathol* 2005;37:845–853.
166. Rorke LB, Packer R, Biegel J. Central nervous system atypical teratoid/rhabdoid tumors of infancy and childhood. *J Neuro-Oncol* 1995;24:21–28.
167. Albrecht S, Rouah E, Becker LE, et al. Transthyretin immunoreactivity in choroid plexus neoplasms and brain metastases. *Mod Pathol* 1991;4:610–614.
168. Andreini L, Doglioni C, Giangaspero F. Tubular adenoma of choroid plexus: a case report. *Clin Neuropathol* 1991;10:137–140.
169. Watanabe K, Ando Y, Iwanaga H, et al. Choroid plexus papilloma containing melanin pigment. *Clin Neuropathol* 1995;14:159–161.
170. Jeibmann A, Hasselblatt M, Gerss J, et al. Prognostic implications of atypical histologic features in choroid plexus papilloma. *J Neuropathol Exp Neurol* 2006;65:1069–1073.
171. Imaya H, Kudo M. Malignant choroid plexus papilloma of the IV ventricle. *Childs Nerv Syst* 1991;7:109–111.
172. Johnson MD, Powell SZ, Boyer PJ, et al. Dural lesions mimicking meningiomas. *Hum Pathol* 2002;33:1211–1226.
173. Meis JM, Ordonez NG, Bruner JM. Meningiomas: an immunohistochemical study of 50 cases. *Arch Pathol Lab Med* 1986;110:934–937.
174. Salvati M, Artico M, Lunardi P, et al. Intramedullary meningioma: case report and review of the literature. *Surg Neurol* 1992;37:42–45.
175. Riemenschneider MJ, Perry A, Reifenberger G. Histological classification and molecular genetics of meningiomas. *Lancet Neurol* 2006;5(12):1045–1054.
176. Chen WYK, Kepes JJ. Extensive intracellular mucoid changes in meningiomas: a manifestation of polyvinylpyrrolidone (PVP) effect on tissues with mesenchymal characteristics. *J Neuropathol Exp Neurol* 1985;44:360.
177. Ito H, Kawano N, Yada K, et al. Meningiomas differentiating to arachnoid trabecular cells: a proposal for histological subtype "arachnoid trabecular cell meningioma." *Acta Neuropathol (Berl)* 1991;82:327–330.
178. Kepes JJ. Presidential address: the histopathology of meningiomas. A reflection of origins and expected behavior. *J Neuropathol Exp Neurol* 1986;45:95–107.
179. Kobata H, Kondo A, Iwasaki K, et al. Chordoid meningioma in a child. *J Neurosurg* 1998; 88:319–323.
180. Kulah A, Ilcayto R, Fiskeci C. Cystic meningiomas. *Acta Neurochir (Wien)* 1991;111:108–113.
181. Lattes R, Bigotti G. Lipoblastic meningioma: "vacuolated meningioma." *Hum Pathol* 1991; 22:164–171.
182. Louis DN, Hamilton AJ, Sobel RA, et al. Pseudopsammomatous meningioma with elevated serum carcinoembryonic antigen: a true secretory meningioma. Case report. *J Neurosurg* 1991;74:129–132.
183. Cerdá-Nicolás M, Lopez-Ginés C, Peydr-Olaya A, et al. Histologic and cytogenetic patterns in benign, atypical, and malignant meningiomas. Does correlation with recurrence exist? *Int J Surg Pathol* 1995;2:301–310.
184. Perry A, Stafford, SL, Scheithauer BW, et al. Meningioma grading: an analysis of histologic parameters. *Am J Surg Pathol* 1997;21:1455–1465.
185. Gokden M, Roth KA, Carroll SL, et al. Clear cell neoplasms and pseudoneoplastic lesions of the central nervous system. *Sem Diagnostic Pathol* 1997;14:252–269.
186. Kepes JJ, Moral LA, Wilkinson SB, et al. Rhabdoid transformation of tumor cells in meningiomas. *Am J Surg Pathol* 1998;22: 231–238.
187. Perry A, Scheithauer BW, Stafford SL, et al. "Malignancy" in meningiomas: a clinicopathologic study of 116 patients, with grading implications. *Cancer* 1999;85:2046–2056.
188. Prayson RA. Malignant meningioma: a clinicopathologic study of 23 patients including MIB-1 and p53 immunohistochemistry. *Am J Clin Pathol* 1996;105:719–726.
189. Mena H, Ribas JL, Pezeshkpour GH, et al. Hemangiopericytoma of the central nervous system: a review of 94 cases. *Hum Pathol* 1991;22:84–91.
190. Perry A, Scheithauer BW, Nascimento AG. The immunophenotypic spectrum of meningeal hemangiopericytoma: a comparison with fibrous meningioma and solitary fibrous tumor of meninges. *Am J Surg Pathol* 1997;21:1354–1360.
191. Rajaram V, Brat DJ, Perry A. Anaplastic meningioma versus meningeal hemangiopericytoma: immunohistochemical and genetic markers. *Hum Pathol* 2004;35:1413–1418.
192. Martin AJ, Fisher C, Igbaseimokumo U, et al. Solitary fibrous tumours of the meninges: case series and literature review. *J Neurooncol* 2001;54:57–69.
193. Tihan T, Viglione M, Rosenblum MK, et al. Solitary fibrous tumors in the central nervous system. A clinicopathologic review of 18 cases and comparison to meningeal hemangiopericytomas. *Arch Pathol Lab Med* 2003;127:432–439.
194. Vorster SJ, Prayson RA, Lee JH. Solitary fibrous tumor of the thoracic spine. Case report and review of the literature. *J Neurosurg* 2000;92(Suppl 2):217–220.
195. Persson S, Kindblom LG, Angervall L. Classical and chondroid chordoma. A light-microscopic, histochemical, ultrastructural and immunohistochemical analysis of the various cell types. *Pathol Res Pract* 1991;187:828–838.
196. Fletcher CDM, Mertens F, eds. *World Health Organization Classification of Tumors Pathology and Genetics of Tumors of Soft Tissue and Bone.* Lyon, France: IARC Press, 2002.
197. Paulus W, Slowik F, Jellinger K. Primary intracranial sarcomas: histopathological features of 19 cases. *Histopath* 1991;18:395–402.
198. Powell HC, Marshall LF, Igneizi RJ. Post-irradiation pituitary sarcoma. *Acta Neuropathol (Berl)* 1977;39:165–167.
199. Rushing EJ, Mena H, Smirniotopoulos JG. Mesenchymal chondrosarcoma of the cauda equina. *Clin Neuropathol* 1995;14:150–153.
200. Skullerud K, Stenwig AE, Brandtzaeg P, et al. Intracranial primary leiomyosarcoma arising in a teratoma of the pineal area. *Clin Neuropathol* 1995;14:245–248.
201. Geddes JF, Sutcliffe JC, King TT. Mixed cranial nerve tumors in neurofibromatosis type 2. *Clin Neuropathol* 1995;14:310–313.
202. Scheithauer BW, Woodruff JM, Erlandson RA. *Tumors of the Peripheral Nervous System.* Washington, DC: American Registry of Pathology, 1999.
203. Silverstein AM, Quint DJ, McKeever PE. Intradural paraganglioma of the thoracic spine. *Am J Neuroradiol* 1990;11:614–616.
204. Bjornsson J, Scheithauer BW, Okazaki H, et al. Intracranial germ cell tumors: pathobiological and immunohistochemical aspects of 70 cases. *J Neuropathol Exp Neurol* 1985;44:32–46.
205. Jennings MT, Gelman R, Hochberg F. Intracranial germ-cell tumors: natural history and pathogenesis. *J Neurosurg* 1985;63:155–167.
206. Haw C, Steinbok P, Ventriculoscope tract recurrence after endoscopic biopsy of pineal germinoma. *Pediatr Neurosurg* 2001;34:215–217.
207. Konig R, Schonberger W, Grimm W. Mediastinal teratocarcinoma and hypophyseal stalk germinoma in a patient with Klinefelter syndrome. *Klin Padiatr* 1990;202:53–56.
208. Kraichoke S, Cosgrove M, Chandrasoma PT. Granulomatous inflammation in pineal germinoma. A cause of diagnostic failure of stereotaxic brain biopsy. *Am J Surg Pathol* 1988; 12:655–660.
209. Nakagawa Y, Perentes E, Ross GW, et al. Immunohistochemical differences between intracranial germinomas and their gonadal equivalents. An immunoperoxidase study of germ cell tumours with epithelial membrane antigen, cytokeratin, and vimentin. *J Pathol* 1988; 156:67–72.
210. Sugita K, Izumi T, Yamaguchi K, et al. Cornelia de Lange syndrome associated with a suprasellar germinoma. *Brain Dev* 1986;8:541–546.
211. Vaquero J, Coca S, Magallon R, et al. Immunohistochemical study of natural killer cells in tumor-infiltrating lymphocytes of primary intracranial germinomas. *J Neurosurg* 1990; 72:616–618.
212. Nakamura H, Takeshima H, Makino K, Kuratsu J. C-kit expression in germinoma: an immunohistochemistry-based study. *J Neuro-Oncol* 2005;75:163–167.
213. Wick MR, Swanson PE, Manivel JC. Placental-like alkaline phosphatase reactivity in human tumors: an immunohistochemical study of 520 cases. *Hum Pathol* 1987;18:946–954.
214. Gonzalez-Crussi F, Winkler RF, Mirkin DL. Sacrococcygeal teratomas in infants and children: relationship of histology and prognosis in 40 cases. *Arch Pathol Lab Med* 1978;102: 420–425.
215. Norgaard-Pedersen B, Lindholm J, Albrechtsen R, et al. Alpha-fetoprotein and human chorionic gonadotropin in a patient with a primary intracranial germ cell tumor. *Cancer* 1978; 41: 2315–2320.
216. Shaffrey ME, Lanzino,. Lopes MB, et al. Maturation of intracranial immature teratomas. *J Neurosurg* 1996;85:672–676.
217. Kohyama S, Uematsu M, Ishihara S, et al. An experience of stereotactic radiation therapy for primary intracranial choriocarcinoma. *Tumori* 2001;87:162–165.
218. Valdez R, McKeever P, Finn WG, et al. Composite germ cell tumor and B-cell non-Hodgkin's lymphoma arising in the sella turcica. *Hum Pathol* 2002;33:1044–1047.
219. Carbone A. AIDS-related non-Hodgkin's lymphomas: from pathology and molecular pathogenesis to treatment. *Hum Pathol* 2002;33:392–404.
220. Davenport RD, O'Donnell LJ, Schnitzer B, et al. Non-Hodgkin's lymphoma of the brain following Hodgkin's disease: an immunohistochemical study. *Cancer* 1991;67:440–443.
221. Ferracini R, Bergmann M, Pileri S, et al. Primary T-cell lymphoma of the central nervous system. *Clin Neuropathol* 1995;14:125–129.
222. Fine H, Mayer R. Primary central nervous system lymphoma. *Ann Intern Med* 1993;119: 1093–1104.
223. Jaffee ES, Harris NL, Stein H, et al. *World Health Organization Classification of Tumors, Pathology, and Genetics of Tumors of Haematopoietic and Lymphoid Tissues.* Lyon, France: IARC Press, 2001.
224. Kadan-Lottick NS, Skluzacek MC, Gurney JG. Decreasing incidence rates of primary central nervous system lymphoma. *Cancer* 2002;95:193–202.
225. Lai R, Rosenblum MK, DeAngelis LM. Primary CNS lymphoma: a whole-brain disease? *Neurology* 2002;59:1557–1562.
226. Miller D, Hochberg F, Harris N, et al. Pathology with clinical correlations of primary central nervous system non-Hodgkin's lymphoma. *Cancer* 1994;74:1383–1397.
227. Dean AF, Diss TC, Wotherspoon AC, et al. Histologic, molecular, and radiologic characterization of resolving cerebral posttransplant lymphoproliferative disorder. *Pediatr Res* 1997; 41:651–656.
228. Niaudet P. Postransplant lymphoproliferative disease following renal transplantation: a multicenter retrospective study of 41 cases observed between 1992 and 1996. *Transplant Proc* 1998;30:2816–2817.
229. Anders KH, Latta H, Chang BS, Tomiyasu U, Quddusi AS, Vinters HV. Lymphomatoid granulomatosis and malignant lymphoma of the central nervous system in the acquired immunodeficiency syndrome. *Hum Pathol* 1989;20:326–334.
230. Diaz-Arrastia R, Younger DS, Hair L, et al. Neurolymphomatosis: a clinicopathologic syndrome re-emerges. *Neurology* 1992;42:1136–1141.
231. Adle-Biassette H, Chetritt J, Bergemer-Fouquet AM, et al. Pathology of the central nervous system in Chester-Erdheim disease: report of three cases. *J Neuropathol Exp Neurol* 1997; 56:1207–1216.
232. Chepuri NB, Challa VR. Xanthoma disseminatum: a rare intracranial mass. *Am J Neuroradiol* 2003;24:105–108.
233. Eriksen B, Janinis J, Variakojis D, et al. Primary histiocytosis X of the parieto-occipital lobe. *Hum Pathol* 1988;19:611–614.

234. Kim M, Provias J, Bernstein M. . Rosai-Dorfman disease mimicking multiple meningioma: case report. *Neurosurg* 1995;36:1185–1187.

235. Feldenzer JA, McKeever PE. Selective localization of gamma-enolase in stromal cells of cerebellar hemangioblastomas. *Acta Neuropathol (Berl)* 1987;72:281–285.

236. McComb RD, Eastman PJ, Hahn FJ, et al. Cerebellar hemangioblastoma with prominent stromal astrocytosis: diagnostic and histogenetic considerations. *Clin Neuropathol* 1987;6: 149–154.

237. Rubio A, Meyers SP, Powers JM, et al. Hemangioblastoma of the optic nerve. *Hum Pathol* 1994;25:1249–1251.

238. Tachibana O, Yamashima T, Yamashita J. Immunohistochemical study of erythropoietin in cerebellar hemangioblastomas associated with secondary polycythemia. *Neurosurgery* 1991;28:24–26.

239. Vortmeyer AO, Huang SC, Koch CA, et al. Somatic von Hippel-Lindau gene mutations detected in sporadic endolymphatic sac tumors. *Cancer Res* 2000;60:5963–5965.

240. Kahn EA, Gosch HH, Seeger JF, et al. Forty-five years experience with craniopharyngiomas. *Surg Neurol* 1973;1:5–12.

241. Xin W, Rubin MA, McKeever PE. Differential expression of cytokeratins 8 and 20 distinguishes craniopharyngioma from Rathke cleft cyst. *Arch Pathol Lab Med* 2002;126: 1174–1178.

242. Yamada H, Haratake J, Narasaki T, et al. Embryonal craniopharyngioma. Case report of the morphogenesis of a craniopharyngioma. *Cancer* 1995;75:2971–2977.

243. Tison V, Cerasoli S, Morigi F, et al. Intracranial desmoplastic small-cell tumor. Report of a case. *Am J Surg Pathol* 1996;20:112–117.

244. Andrew SM, Gradwell E. Immunoperoxidase labeled antibody staining in differential diagnosis of central nervous system haemangioblastomas and central nervous system metastases of renal carcinomas. *J Clin Pathol* 1986;39:917–919.

245. Aronson SM, Garcia JH, Aronson BE. Metastatic neoplasms of the brain: their frequency in relation to age. *Cancer* 1964;17:558–565.

246. Chu P, Wu E, Weiss LM. Cytokeratin 7 and cytokeratin 20 expression in epithelial neoplasms: a survey of 435 cases. *Mod Pathol* 2000;13:962–972.

247. DeYoung BR, Wick MR. Immunohistologic evaluation of metastatic carcinomas of unknown origin: an algorithmic approach. *Semin Diagn Pathol* 2000;17:184–193.

248. Le Chevalier T, Smith FP, Caille P, et al. Sites of primary malignancies in patients presenting with cerebral metastases: a review of 120 cases. *Cancer* 1985;56:880–882.

249. Becher MW, Abel TW, Thompson RC, et al. J Immunohistochemical analysis of metastatic neoplasms of the central nervous system. *Neuropathol Exp Neurol* 2006;65(10):935–944.

250. Srodon M, Westra WH. Immunohistochemical staining for thyroid transcription factor-1: a helpful aid in discerning primary site of tumor origin in patients with brain metastases. *Hum Pathol* 2002;33:642–645.

251. McKeever PE. *New Methods of Brain Tumor Analysis.* Washington, DC: American Registry of Pathology, 2006:1–51, and illus. pp. 1–29.

252. Gebarski SS, Blaivas MA. Imaging of normal leptomeningeal melanin. *Am J Neuroradiol* 1996;17:55–60.

253. Lopez-Castilla J, Diaz-Fernandez F, Soult JA, et al. Primary leptomeningeal melanoma in a child. *Pediatr Neurol* 2001;24:390–392.

254. Painter TJ, Chaljub G, Sethi R, et al. Intracranial and intraspinal meningeal melanocytosis. *AJNR Am J Neuroradiol* 2000; 21:1349–1353.

255. Fetell MR, Bruce JN, Burke AM, et al. Non-neoplastic pineal cysts. *Neurology* 1991;41: 1034–1040.

256. Rushing EJ, Mena J, Ribas JL. Primary pineal parenchymal lesions: a review of 53 cases. *J Neuropathol Exp Neurol* 1991;50:364.

257. Kuroda Y, Abe M, Nagumo F, et al. Neuroepithelial cyst presenting as recurrent aseptic meningitis. *Neurology* 1991;41:1834–1835.

258. Ho KL, Garcia JH. Colloid cysts of the third ventricle: ultrastructural features are compatible with endodermal derivation. *Acta Neuropathol* 1992;83:605–612.

259. McKeever PE, Hall BJ, Spicer SS. The origin of colloid cysts of the third ventricle. *J Neuropathol Exp Neurol* 1978;37:658.

260. Whiting DM, Chou SM, Lanzieri CF, et al. Cervical neurenteric cyst associated with Klippel-Feil syndrome: a case report and review of the literature. *Clin Neuropathol* 1991;10:285–290.

261. Go KG, Blankenstein MA, Vroom TM, et al. Progesterone receptors in arachnoid cysts. *Acta Neurochirurgica* 1997;139(4):349–354.

262. Braak H, Braak E. Neuropathological staging of Alzheimer-related changes. *Acta Neuropathologica* 1991;82:239–259.

263. Mirra SS, Heyman A, McKeel D, et al. The consortium to establish a registry for Alzheimer's disease (CERAD). Part II. Standardization of the neuropathologic assessment of Alzheimer's disease. *Neurology* 1991;41:479–486.

264. Anonymous. Consensus recommendations for the postmortem diagnosis of Alzheimer's disease. National Institute on Aging and Reagan Institute Working Group on diagnostic criteria of the neuropathological assessment of Alzheimer's disease. *Neurobiol Aging* 1997; 18:S1–S2.

265. Braak H, Del Tredici K, Rub U, et al. Staging of brain pathology related to sporadic Parkinson's disease. *Neurobiol Aging* 2003;24:197–211.

266. McKeith IG, Ballard CG, Perry RH, et al. Prospective validation of consensus criteria for the diagnosis of dementia with Lewy bodies. *Neurology* 2000;54:1050–1058.

267. Dickson DW, Bergeron C, Chin SS, et al. Office of Rare Diseases of the National Institutes of Health. Office of Rare Diseases neuropathologic criteria for corticobasal degeneration. *J Neuropathol Exp Neurol* 2002; 61:935–946.

268. Foster NL, Wilhelmsen K, Sima AA, et al. Frontotemporal dementia and parkinsonism linked to chromosome 17: a consensus conference. *Ann Neurol* 1997;41:706–715.

269. Kertesz A, Kawarai T, Rogaeva E, et al. Familial frontotemporal dementia with ubiquitin-positive, tau-negative inclusions. *Neurology* 2000;54: 818–827.

270. McKhann GM, Albert MS, Grossman M, et al. Work Group on Frontotemporal Dementia and Pick's Disease. Clinical and pathological diagnosis of frontotemporal dementia: report of the Work Group on Frontotemporal Dementia and Pick's Disease. *Arch Neurol* 2001; 58:1803–1809.

271. Coker SB. The diagnosis of childhood neurodegenerative disorders presenting as dementia in adults. *Neurology* 1991;41:794–798.

272. Drury I, Blaivas M, Abou-Khalil BW, et al. Biopsy results in a kindred with Lafora disease. *Arch Neurol* 1993;50:102–105.

273. Hoving EW. Nasal encephaloceles. *Childs Nerv Syst* 2000; 16:702–706.

274. Patterson K, Kapur S, Chandra RS. ''Nasal gliomas'' and related brain heterotopias: a pathologist's perspective. *Pediatr Pathol* 1986;5:353–362.

275. Hardiman O, Burke T, Phillips J, et al. Microdysgenesis in resected temporal neocortex: incidence and clinical significance in focal epilepsy. *Neurology* 1988;38:1041–1047.

276. Bruton, CJ. The neuropathology of temporal lobe epilepsy. In Russel G, Marley E, Williams P, eds. *Maudsley Monographs Number Thirty-One.* New York: Oxford University Press, 1988: 1–94.

277. Devlin AM, Cross JH, Harkness W, et al. Clinical outcomes of hemispherectomy for epilepsy in childhood and adolescence. *Brain* 2003;126:556–566.

278. Frater JL, Prayson RA, Morris III HH, et al. Surgical pathologic findings of extratemporal-based intractable epilepsy: a study of 133 consecutive resections. *Arch Pathol Lab Med* 2000; 124:545–549.

279. Prayson RA, Frater JL. Rasmussen encephalitis: a clinicopathologic and immunohistochemical study of seven patients. *Am J Clin Pathol* 2002;117:776–782.

CHAPTER

11

Ricardo V. Lloyd
Lori A. Erickson

The Neuroendocrine and Paracrine Systems

This chapter is divided into two parts. The first part outlines the neuroendocrine system and presents an overview of the diffuse or dispersed neuroendocrine system (DNS), to help the general surgical pathologist gain a panoramic view of this complex system. Methods of analysis of tumors of the DNS are also presented because some of these techniques are indispensable for the diagnosis of many neuroendocrine neoplasms. The second part of the chapter discusses examples of specific lesions of the DNS. Some of the less common DNS tumors are presented, along with differential diagnoses, because the more common lesions are covered in detail in other areas of the text.

The DNS consists of a wide variety of cells that are present in the central and peripheral nervous system and in many classic endocrine organs (Table 11.1). The cells of the DNS have also been referred to historically as *paraneurons* (1). These cells share the ability to produce many biologically active amines, peptides, and other substances. These substances may act as neurotransmitters, as true hormones, or as paracrine regulators. *Paracrine regulation* refers to the production of amines and hormones by cells that exert a local effect on the target cells by diffusion through the extracellular space. The production of somatostatin by the pancreatic islets, which regulate insulin and glucagon production in neighboring islet cells, is an example of paracrine regulation. The cells and neoplasm of the neuroendocrine and paracrine systems make up the DNS.

DEVELOPMENT OF THE DISPERSED NEUROENDOCRINE SYSTEM CONCEPT

Feyrter (2) considered the clear cells of the gastrointestinal tract to be peripheral endocrine or paracrine cells. The detailed study of neuroendocrine cells by Pearse (3,4) led to the development of the concept of amine precursor uptake and decarboxylation (APUD). Although the APUD concept provided a unifying theory for explaining some endocrine diseases and ectopic hormone productions, the hypothesis that the cells were all of neural crest origin, as postulated by Pearse, was later disproved by the experiments of LeDouarin (5) and others. The current neuroendocrine classification of cells and tumors uses immunohistochemical (IHC), ultrastructural, and molecular biological features to define members of the DNS (6–8).

CELLS AND NEOPLASMS OF THE DISPERSED NEUROENDOCRINE SYSTEM

The principal cells and neoplasms that form the DNS are listed in Table 11.1. The steroid-producing endocrine cells of the adrenal cortex, ovary, and testis, as well as the thyroid hormone-producing follicular cells in the thyroid gland, do not form part of the DNS. Cells and neoplasms of the DNS may be divided into the following two principal groups: (a) those of neural type, which include neuroblastomas, pheochromocytomas, and paragangliomas; and (b) those of epithelial type, which include carcinoids and neuroendocrine neoplasms from many sites. Many of these neoplasms have distinct clinicopathologic features, so precise classification by the pathologist is necessary for optimal clinical management. Although the term *carcinoid tumor* has been broadly used to refer to many neoplasms derived from the DNS (9), this term should be restricted to the traditional tumors of the gastrointestinal tract and lungs. The most recent World Health Organization recommendation for the general endocrine tumor classification includes (10):

1. Well-differentiated endocrine tumors
2. Well-differentiated endocrine carcinomas
3. Poorly differentiated endocrine (small-cell) carcinomas
4. Mixed exocrine-endocrine tumors

Many broad-spectrum IHC markers are available to aid in the diagnosis of neuroendocrine neoplasms. The principal markers include chromogranins and synaptophysin. Other markers that can be helpful but are of more limited use include neuron-specific enolase (NSE); proconvertases PC1/PC3 and PC2; bombesin and/or gastrin-releasing peptide (GRP); CD57 (Leu-7/HNK-1); synaptic vesicle protein 2; PGP9.5; and others (11). Although silver stains, such as Grimelius (12) and Churukian-Schenk (13) argyrophilic stains (a histochemical reaction in which the endocrine cells take up silver ions, but a reducing agent is needed to produce a positive reaction) and the Masson-Fontana argentaffin stain (a histochemical reaction in which the endocrine cells take up and reduce silver ions without a reducing agent), are helpful in characterizing some neuroendocrine neoplasms, the great variability in silver stains leads to less consistent results than those yielded by IHC stains. However, IHC stains are not without problems. Interlaboratory variability resulting from use of different antibodies and different techniques remains a serious problem. Despite this variability, the predictability and reproducibility of standardized IHC reagents, such as monoclonal antibodies, has made the use of these reagents to characterize neuroendocrine neoplasms widely accepted.

GENERAL NEUROENDOCRINE MARKERS

CHROMOGRANIN/SECRETOGRANIN

The chromogranin/secretogranin (Cg/Sg) family is composed of several acidic proteins that are present in the secretory gran-

TABLE 11.1	Cells and Neoplasms of the Dispersed Neuroendocrine System[a]	
Cell	*Neoplasms*	*Hormones/Amines*
Adrenal medulla	Pheochromocytoma, neuroblastoma, and ganglioneuroma	Enkephalins, catecholamines, VIP, and SRIF
Biliary tract and liver	Benign and malignant tumors	Serotonin, catecholamines, and miscellaneous peptides
Bronchopulmonary tree	Neuroendocrine tumors (including "carcinoids")	GRP, ACTH, endorphin, calcitonin, catecholamines, and serotonin
Gastrointestinal tract	Benign and malignant tumors (including "carcinoids")	Gastrin, SRIF, GRP, VIP, secretin, enteroglucagon, PP, serotonin, catecholamines, cholecystokinin, insulin, and glucagon
Hypophysis	Adenomas and carcinomas	ACTH, GH, FSH, LH, PRL, TSH, β-endorphin, calcitonin, catecholamines, and MSH
Merkel cells of skin	Neuroendocrine (Merkel cell) carcinoma	Calcitonin, catecholamines, PP, and VIP
Pancreatic islet	Benign and malignant tumors	Insulin, PP, glucagon, SRIF, VIP, gastrin, catecholamines, and serotonin
Paraganglion	Paragangliomas	Enkephalin, catecholamines, and VIP
Parathyroid	Adenomas and carcinomas	Parathyroid hormone catecholamines
Thyroid C-cell	Medullary thyroid carcinoma	Calcitonin, somatostatin, ACTH, CGRP, and catecholamines
Miscellaneous neuroendocrine cells in breast, cervix, kidney, larynx, ovary, paranasal sinus, prostate, testis, and other sites	Benign and malignant tumors and mixed tumors	Miscellaneous peptides, serotonin, and catecholamines

[a]The hypothalamus and pineal gland are also members of the dispersed neuroendocrine system.
ACTH, adrenocorticotropic hormone; CGRP, calcitonin gene-related peptide; FSH, follicle-stimulating hormone; GH, growth hormone; GRP, gastrin-releasing peptide; LH, luteinizing hormone; MSH, melanocyte-stimulating hormone; PP, pancreatic polypeptide; PRL, prolactin; SRIF, somatostatin; TSH, thyroid-stimulating hormone; VIP, vasoactive intestinal polypeptide.

ules of neuroendocrine cells. The three major Cg/Sg proteins are currently designated as chromogranin A, B, and secretogranin II (Sg II). The distribution of chromogranin A has been studied extensively in human tumors (14). It is present in most neuroendocrine cells and neoplasms. However, most neoplasms with only a few endocrine secretory granules, such as small-cell carcinomas of the lung, do not react strongly with chromogranin A antibodies (14). Because of their widespread distribution and high degree of specificity, chromogranins A and B and Sg II are excellent markers for neuroendocrine cells and neoplasms (15,16).

SYNAPTOPHYSIN

This 38-kd molecule is a component of the membrane of presynaptic vesicles. It is widely distributed in neurons and neuroendocrine cells and their neoplasms, and it is another broad-spectrum neuroendocrine marker that is localized in cytoplasmic vesicles rather than in secretory granules (15,17). Some endocrine tumors that are not members of DNS, such as adrenal cortical adenomas and carcinomas, may express synaptophysin; thus, this marker should be used with other neuroendocrine markers, such as chromogranin. Many other related vesicle proteins, such as synaptobrevin, syntaxin, synaptogranin, SNAP-25B, and rabphilin 3A, have been found to be associated with cytoplasmic vesicles (18). However, their clinical use and specificity as broad-spectrum neuroendocrine markers has not been demonstrated.

NEURON-SPECIFIC ENOLASE

The neuron-specific enolase (NSE) enzyme, which is also known as γ-enolase, is a highly sensitive (albeit not too specific) marker for neuroendocrine cells and tumors. It is commonly found in neurons, peripheral nerves, and neuroendocrine cells (19). Some nonneuroendocrine cells and neoplasm also react with antisera against NSE. In the diagnosis of neuroendocrine tumors, NSE should be used only with other broad-spectrum markers of neuroendocrine cells.

PROCONVERTASES

The proconvertases (PCs) are recently described enzymes that process propeptides into active peptides within cells. Some of these, including PC1/PC3 and PC2, are highly specific for neuroendocrine cells and tumors (20), and they can be used as specific neuroendocrine markers.

BOMBESIN/GASTRIN-RELEASING PEPTIDE AND CD57 (LEU-7/HNK-1)

Bombesin is a tetradecapeptide originally isolated from amphibian skin. It is present in many endocrine cells as well as in central and peripheral neurons (21). GRP, the proposed mammalian analogue of bombesin, has been found in many lung and gastrointestinal endocrine tumors (22) and can be used as a broad-spectrum marker for many endocrine neoplasms.

CD57 (Leu-7/HNK-1), a monoclonal antibody that was produced against a T-cell leukemia cell line, recognizes natural killer cells in blood and lymphoid tissues. It also reacts with small-cell carcinomas of the lung, as well as with pheochromocytomas and other neuroendocrine neoplasms (23,24).

OTHER IMMUNOHISTOCHEMICAL MARKERS

With advances in proteomics, newer neuroendocrine markers are being discovered. A promising new marker is synaptic vesicle protein 2, which is associated with secretory granules and which should serve as a good complement to chromogranin and synaptophysin (25). Many other IHC markers, such as PGP9.5, antibodies against enzymes in the synthetic pathways for peptide hormones, and CD56 (neural cell adhesion molecules), have been used to characterize some neuroendocrine cells and tumors (13). However, these are generally used as second or adjunctive markers in problematic cases.

REGULATORY PEPTIDES AND AMINES

A broad spectrum of peptides and amines is present in cells and tumors of the DNS (see Table 11.1). Although the biologic function of many of these is known, some of these substances are without known activity. The localization of peptides may be of some help in characterizing certain neuroendocrine neoplasms. However, ectopic production of peptides is a common phenomenon, so the presence of a specific peptide may not be helpful in characterizing unusual neuroendocrine neoplasms. Although most neuroendocrine tumors express broad-spectrum markers such as chromogranin and synaptophysin, specific peptides are not commonly found in specific tumor types. For example, calcitonin is frequently expressed by medullary thyroid carcinomas and atypical laryngeal carcinoids, but may also be expressed ectopically in other tumors (Table 11.2).

ULTRASTRUCTURAL CHARACTERISTICS OF NEUROENDOCRINE CELLS AND NEOPLASMS

When the differential diagnosis of an anaplastic neoplasm includes a neuroendocrine carcinoma, the presence of secretory granules on ultrastructural examination can be helpful in establishing the diagnosis of a malignant neuroendocrine neoplasm. Cytoplasmic secretory granules usually have a central or eccentric core of variable density and limiting membrane. The size of the secretory granules ranges from 50 to 400 nm (Fig. 11.1). Although the morphology of secretory granules in many normal neuroendocrine cells can be used as an aid in recognizing spe-

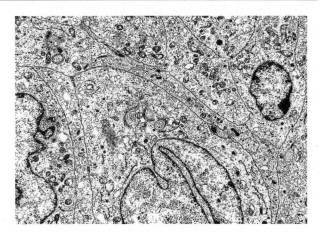

Figure 11.1. Neuroendocrine carcinoma of lung from a patient with Cushing syndrome. The carcinoma was positive for adrenocorticotropic hormone and corticotropin-releasing hormone by immunostaining. Neurosecretory granules ranging in size from 100 to 300 nm in diameter are present in the cytoplasm (8600×).

cific cell types, these distinct morphologic granule features are not often seen in neuroendocrine neoplasms. Recent studies have shown that several hormones and amines, such as calcitonin and somatostatin, may be stored in the same secretory granules in medullary thyroid carcinomas (26) and that Cg/Sg proteins form a major constituent of the secretory granule (14,15).

IN SITU HYBRIDIZATION AND POLYMERASE CHAIN REACTION

Localization of the mRNA for specific peptides and other neuroendocrine markers by in situ hybridization (ISH) is another useful technique for characterizing neuroendocrine cells and neoplasms (8,27). Some neuroendocrine neoplasms may contain mainly the mRNA but not the translated product for specific hormones, so detection of the mRNA within the cells can help to establish the diagnosis (27) (Fig. 11.2). However, most neuroendocrine tumors contain enough peptides, hormones, or broad-spectrum markers to be detected by IHC techniques. A notable exception is the production of ectopic hormones by neuroendocrine tumors, in which ISH offers some advantages because of the retention of intracytoplasmic mRNA. The use of the polymerase chain reaction (PCR) to amplify small

TABLE 11.2	Sites of Eutopic and Ectopic Hormone Production of Common Neuroendocrine Hormones	
Hormone	*Produced by Cells/Tumors*	*Other Relatively Frequent Sites of Production*
Calcitonin	C-cell/medullary thyroid carcinoma	Laryngeal NE tumors; pancreatic NE tumors
ACTH	Pituitary/pituitary adenomas	Pancreatic NE tumors; lung NE tumors; pheochromocytomas
CRH	Hypothalamic neuromas	Pancreatic NE tumors
GH	Pituitary/pituitary adenomas	Pancreatic NE tumors
GHRH	Hypothalamic neuromas	Pancreatic NE tumors
Pancreatic polypeptide	Pancreatic islet/pancreatic NE tumors	Intestinal NE tumors (hindgut carcinoids)
Somatostatin	Pancreatic islet/pancreatic NE tumors, duodenum, stomach	Intestinal NE tumors (hindgut carcinoids)

ACTH, adrenocorticotropic hormone; CRH, corticotropin-releasing hormones; GH, growth hormone; GHRH, growth hormone–releasing hormone; NE, neuroendocrine.

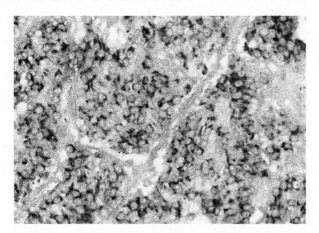

Figure 11.2. In situ hybridization localizing chromogranin A RNA diffusely in a retroperitoneal neuroendocrine tumor (in situ hybridization with a digoxigenin-labeled probe cocktail of chromogranin A and B with streptavidin nitroblue tetrazolium-5-bromo-4-chloro-3-indolyl phosphate [NBT-BCIP] detection).

amounts of DNA and of reverse transcriptase-PCR to amplify specific products starting with RNA is becoming more common in diagnostic pathology (28,29). A combination of PCR and ISH has helped to amplify and to visualize specific RNA and DNA targets that are expressed in low abundance in tissue sections (30).

MULTIPLE ENDOCRINE NEOPLASIA SYNDROMES

The development of hyperplasia and neoplasias involving multiple organs of the DNS is usually a familial condition. The term *multiple endocrine neoplasia* (MEN) is applied to this syndrome. Several distinct patterns of familial MEN are observed; these are inherited as autosomal dominant traits with a high degree of penetrance. In type I, the principal organs affected include the pituitary, pancreas, and parathyroid (31). Some patients may also have the Zollinger-Ellison syndrome with peptic ulceration. Type 2a usually involves the thyroid C cells and the adrenal medulla, as well as the parathyroids (32). Type 2b also involves the thyroid C cells and adrenal medulla, and it is associated with mucosal neuromas (33). The studies of DeLellis and Wolfe (26) have shown that hyperplasias usually precede neoplasias in MEN syndromes involving the C cells of the thyroid and the adrenal medulla. The genes for MEN1 (MENIN) and MEN2a and 2b (rearranged during transfection [RET] proto-oncogenes) have been characterized extensively (32,34). The availability of these genetic markers has facilitated screening and early diagnosis of MEN2a and 2b in affected families (35), although no general screening tests for MEN1 are available to date (36).

ECTOPIC HORMONE PRODUCTION

Ectopic or inappropriate hormone secretion is characterized by the production of hormones by a tumor in which the parent tissue from which the tumor was derived does not produce the hormone. The DNS provides a general unifying concept explaining ectopic hormone production by many endocrine tumors. Some nonneuroendocrine tumors, such as squamous cell

carcinomas of the lungs, hepatocellular carcinomas, and some sarcomas, may be associated with ectopic hormone production (37). Ectopic hormone production by some neoplasms, such as the production of adrenocorticotropin (ACTH) by pancreatic endocrine neoplasms, may be associated with a more biologically aggressive tumor (38) (Table 11.2). One of the most commonly produced ectopic hormones associated with hypercalcemia is parathyroid hormone–related protein (39). This protein is produced by parathyroid neoplasms as well as by many neuroendocrine and other tumors, and it is a major cause of hypercalcemia associated with malignancy (39).

Many of the common neuroendocrine neoplasms are discussed elsewhere in this book, so they are mentioned in this chapter only in discussions or differential diagnoses. These include pheochromocytomas, paragangliomas, medullary thyroid carcinomas, melanomas, pancreatic and gastrointestinal neuroendocrine neoplasms, and neuroendocrine neoplasms of the lungs. The terminology used in this chapter is from the most recent World Health Organization recommendation for general endocrine tumor classification (10).

NEUROENDOCRINE NEOPLASMS

THYMUS

Thymic neuroendocrine neoplasms have features of cells and tumors of the DNS, including dense-core secretory granules. These tumors should not be considered to be thymomas because they are not made up of thymic epithelial cells or lymphocytes (40). Some thymic neuroendocrine tumors are associated with Cushing syndrome (41).

Thymic neuroendocrine tumors can range from completely encapsulated to large, invasive tumors. They are usually lobulated and the cut surface is solid and tan or gray. Focal necrosis and hemorrhage are common; however, cystic changes, which are often seen in thymomas, are not present.

Microscopic examination shows fibrous trabeculae with lobules of tumor cells, anastomosing bands of tumor cells (Fig. 11.3), or radial arrangement of tumor cells around a central lumen. Lymphocytes are usually sparse or absent. The ultrastructural examination usually shows small, secretory granules

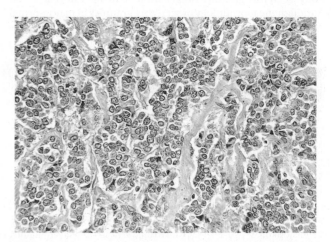

Figure 11.3. Thymic neuroendocrine tumor with a trabecular pattern of growth. The neoplasm was positive for chromogranin A and serotonin by immunostaining.

of 100 to 450 nm in diameter. IHC studies reveal NSE, as well as chromogranin, immunoreactivity in most tumors. ACTH, somatostatin, calcitonin, and other peptides have also been found (41,42). Because thymic neuroendocrine tumors have a broad range of histologic appearances, the differential diagnosis includes many lesions. Epithelial thymomas, germ cell tumors, and lymphomas are nonneuroendocrine tumors that should be considered in the differential diagnosis. IHC staining for broad-spectrum neuroendocrine markers, such as chromogranins and synaptophysin, can usually exclude these other tumors. Parathyroid and thyroid neoplasms; paragangliomas; and other metastatic neuroendocrine carcinomas, including poorly differentiated (small-cell) neuroendocrine carcinomas, medullary thyroid carcinomas, pulmonary neuroendocrine tumors, and pancreatic neuroendocrine tumors, should all be part of the differential diagnosis. IHC staining does not differentiate between thymic neuroendocrine tumors and other neuroendocrine neoplasms.

SKIN

The Merkel cells and the neuroendocrine carcinoma of the skin have features of neuroendocrine differentiation, including the presence of dense-core secretory granules and the production of various peptides and amines (43-46). Merkel cell carcinomas commonly arise in the dermis and subcutaneous tissues in older adult patients, although they are occasionally seen in younger patients (46). The most frequent sites are the head and neck, but they are also commonly found on the extremities. The histologic features of these neoplasms include round cells with scanty amounts of cytoplasm. The vesicular nuclei often contain one or more nucleoli. The ultrastructural examination reveals small, dense-core secretory granules between 70 and 150 nm in diameter. Collections of perinuclear intermediate filaments and cytoplasmic spinous processes are often seen on ultrastructural examination as well. The IHC characterization reveals NSE, chromogranin A, vasoactive intestinal peptide, calcitonin, pancreatic polypeptide, and other peptides (44–46).

The differential diagnosis of primary neuroendocrine carcinomas of the skin includes lymphomas, metastatic carcinomas, and poorly differentiated adnexal skin neoplasms. Neuroendocrine markers and electron microscopy can readily establish the neuroendocrine nature of the neoplasm, but they cannot exclude a metastatic small-cell neuroendocrine carcinoma from almost any organ. The use of antibodies to cytokeratin 20 (Fig. 11.4) is useful for separating pulmonary and other metastatic small cell carcinomas from neuroendocrine carcinoma of the skin (47).

LARYNX

Neuroendocrine carcinomas of the larynx are uncommon tumors (48–51). These tumors can range from small polypoid to large, bulging masses with gray-white or tan cut surfaces. The microscopic features of the small-cell neuroendocrine carcinoma are similar to the tumors of the lung, consisting of cells with small amounts of cytoplasm, small nuclei, and coarse chromation. The laryngeal neuroendocrine carcinomas (atypical carcinoids) have moderate to abundant cytoplasm, and they can be arranged in nests, cords, ribbons, or acini (Fig. 11.5). Ultrastructural study usually reveals small secretory granules ranging from 70 to 250 nm in diameter. The IHC characteriza-

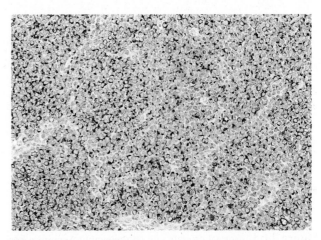

Figure 11.4. Neuroendocrine (Merkel cell) carcinoma showing strong staining for cytokeratin 20. Some tumor cells have a distinct juxtanuclear pattern of staining. This marker is useful in distinguishing between a Merkel cell carcinoma and metastatic small-cell carcinoma from the lung (immunoperoxidase stain).

tion usually shows chromogranin A and NSE. Chromogranin A is present focally in the small-cell variant of neuroendocrine carcinoma. Calcitonin, somatostatin, and serotonin are also commonly found. Woodruff et al. (50) found calcitonin in 67% of the atypical laryngeal carcinoids.

The differential diagnosis includes conventional laryngeal epidermoid carcinoma, medullary thyroid carcinoma, paraganglioma, metastatic neuroendocrine carcinoma, and lymphoma. The presence of immunoreactive calcitonin in these tumors, especially in a metastatic site in the neck, may lead to an erroneous diagnosis of metastatic medullary thyroid carcinoma (MTC). In the author's experience, MTC is positive for thyroid transcription factor 1 whereas laryngeal neuroendocrine carcinomas are negative for this marker.

PROSTATE

Prostatic neuroendocrine cells and carcinomas, including poorly differentiated endocrine (small-cell) carcinomas, have

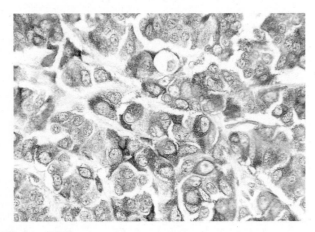

Figure 11.5. Laryngeal well-differentiated neuroendocrine carcinoma (atypical carcinoid) staining positively for chromogranin A. The carcinoma was also diffusely positive for calcitonin (immunoperoxidase stain).

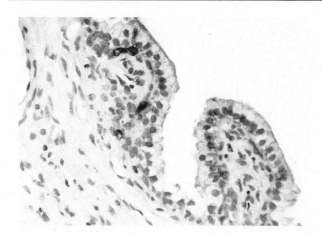

Figure 11.6. Normal prostate with chromogranin A–positive neuroendocrine cells. (Immunoperoxidase stain.)

been described by various authors (52–57). Some prostatic neuroendocrine carcinomas may produce adrenocorticotropic hormone (ACTH), causing Cushing syndrome (57). Several peptide hormones, including calcitonin, bombesin, and somatostatin, have been identified in the normal human prostate (Fig. 11.6) (53). The histologic features of prostatic neuroendocrine tumors range from adenocarcinomas with mixed neuroendocrine carcinoma (Fig. 11.7) to poorly differentiated endocrine (small-cell) carcinomas (52). The secretory granules vary greatly in morphology and size. IHC studies of prostate neuroendocrine carcinomas have shown that the tumors express peptides, as well as prostatic markers, such as prostate-specific antigen (54).

BREAST

Neuroendocrine neoplasms (carcinoids) of the breast have remained controversial since the early description by Cubilla and Woodruff and others (58–60). Argyrophilia and dense-core secretory granules have been observed in breast carcinomas (51,53). Chromogranin A immunoreactivity has been reported in up to 40% of breast carcinomas (58,60). In addition, chromogranin A and B mRNA have been detected in argyrophilic

breast carcinomas, indicating that this endocrine marker is synthesized by the tumor cells (60). Positive immunoreactivity for chromogranin and/or synaptophysin in at least 50% of the tumor cells has been designated as neuroendocrine breast carcinoma by some investigators (61). Ectopic production of ACTH, causing Cushing syndrome, has been observed in a patient with infiltrating ductal carcinomas (62). Neuroendocrine neoplasms of the breast usually represent multidirectional or divergent differentiation of adenocarcinomas with some endocrine features. A recent report by Sapino et al. (61) studied neuroendocrine breast carcinomas, which were defined as having at least 50% immunoreactivity for chromogranin or synaptophysin. An analysis of the clinical outcomes showed that mucinous differentiation was associated with low-grade tumors, and, more importantly, that histologic grade was more important than the immunophenotype in determining prognosis (61). Occasionally, a midgut carcinoid tumor metastatic to the breast may present as a primary breast carcinoma (Fig. 11.8). Positive staining with the Masson-Fontana argentaffin stain, which is present in midgut carcinoids, helps to separate carcinoids of the breast from metastatic midgut carcinoids.

OVARY AND TESTES

Neuroendocrine neoplasms (carcinoids) of the ovary and testes have been well documented. These neoplasms often arise as an

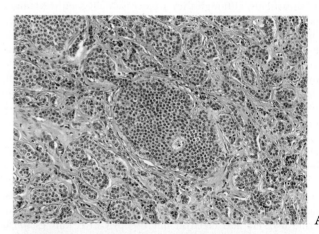

A

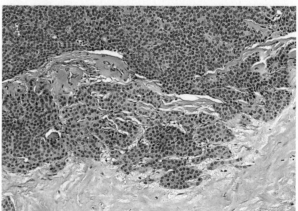

B

Figure 11.8. **(A)** Well-differentiated neuroendocrine carcinoma (carcinoid) of the jejunum with mixed insular and trabecular patterns. **(B)** Metastatic jejunal carcinoid to the breast. The tumor cells were positive with the Masson-Fontana silver stain, confirming that it was a metastasis from the jejunum.

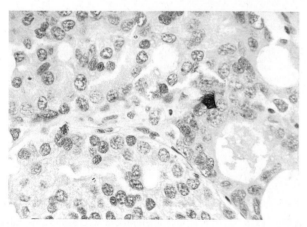

Figure 11.7. Prostatic adenocarcinomas with scattered cytologically malignant neuroendocrine cells revealed by chromogranin A immunostaining. (Immunoperoxidase stain.)

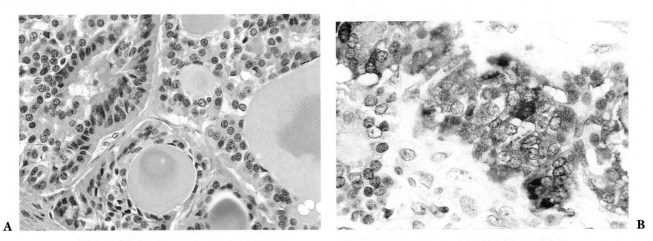

Figure 11.9. Ovarian well-differentiated neuroendocrine tumor (stromal carcinoid). **(A)** A mixture of colloid-filled thyroid follicles and neuroendocrine cells is present. **(B)** Positive immunostaining for calcitonin is present in the ovarian stromal carcinoid. (Immunoperoxidase stain.)

element within a teratoma in the ovary, but they can also occur in pure form in both ovary and testes. The patterns include insular, trabecular, and stromal carcinoids in the ovary (Fig. 11.9). Ultrastructural examination often shows secretory granules of variable sizes. Recent IHC studies have shown a broad spectrum of peptides. Chromogranin, thyroglobulin, calcitonin, serotonin, somatostatin, glucagon, insulin, and gastrin have been found in these neoplasms (Figs. 11.9 and 11.10) (63–65). The differential diagnosis of ovarian carcinoid tumors includes granulosa cell tumor, Sertoli-Leydig cell tumor, and metastatic carcinoid tumors.

Low-grade testicular neuroendocrine neoplasms (carcinoids) occur predominantly as pure carcinoid tumors, unlike their ovarian counterparts (66). They often show an insular pattern similar to midgut carcinoids, and they are usually argentaffin-positive. The carcinoid syndrome is rarely produced by these tumors, although rare cases associated with the carcinoid syndrome have been reported (67). Ultrastructural studies show variable numbers of dense-core secretory granules. IHC studies of testicular carcinoids have found vasoactive intestinal polypeptide serotonin and substance P immunoreactivity (67).

The differential diagnosis includes lymphomas, Leydig cell tumors, small-cell carcinomas, neuroblastomas, and metastatic carcinoid tumors. Metastatic carcinoid tumors must be excluded before a diagnosis of a primary testicular carcinoid neoplasm can be established (68).

UTERINE CERVIX

Primary neuroendocrine carcinomas of the uterine cervix are uncommon neoplasms (69–72). They have been divided into well-differentiated neuroendocrine carcinomas and poorly differentiated (small-cell) neuroendocrine carcinoma types, with the latter tumors having a much worse prognosis (70). The light-microscopic appearance varies from solid tumor nests to insular, trabecular, spindle cell, or glandular patterns of round polygonal cells with large nuclei and small nucleoli (Figs. 11.11 and 11.12). The carcinomas are commonly argyrophilic. Electron-microscopic studies show dense-core granules ranging from 150 to 300 nm in diameter. Neurosecretory granules may be a variable; in the series of Barrett et al. (69), only 7 of 20 cases had neurosecretory granules. IHC studies have shown that

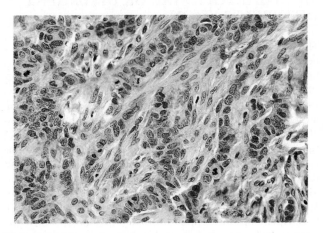

Figure 11.10. Well-differentiated neuroendocrine carcinoma (atypical carcinoid) of the cervix. This neoplasm has a prominent trabecular pattern.

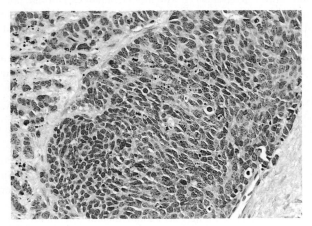

Figure 11.11. Poorly differentiated neuroendocrine carcinoma of the cervix with histologic features similar to small-cell carcinoma of the lung.

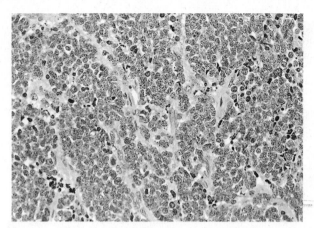

Figure 11.12. Neuroendocrine carcinoma of the urinary bladder. The tumor cells have large nuclei and scanty amounts of cytoplasm. Immunostaining was diffusely positive for neuron-specific enolase and focally for chromogranin A.

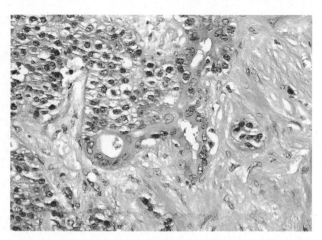

Figure 11.13. Ductuloinsular tumor of the pancreas showing multidirectional differentiation. The duct cells were positive for carcinoembryonic antigen, whereas the endocrine cells expressed chromogranin A.

most neoplasms contain serotonin. Vasoactive intestinal polypeptide, somatostatin, pancreatic polypeptide, and ACTH may also be present (70). Silva et al. (69) described an intermediate cell type of endocrine carcinoma of the cervix that was associated with a poor prognosis when compared to that of adenocarcinoma of the cervix. Studies using ISH have shown that poorly differentiated (small-cell) neuroendocrine carcinoma of the cervix is frequently associated with human papillomavirus type 18 (71). In a study of 23 poorly differentiated (small-cell) neuroendocrine carcinomas of the cervix, Conner et al. (73) concluded that early diagnosis and combined therapeutic modalities could lead to longer survival in some patients. These tumors frequently express chromogranin, synaptophysin, and neural cell adhesion molecule (72). The differential diagnosis of neuroendocrine carcinomas of the uterine cervix includes lymphoma, poorly differentiated carcinomas, and metastatic neuroendocrine carcinomas.

URINARY BLADDER

Poorly differentiated neuroendocrine (small-cell) carcinoma of the urinary bladder (Fig. 11.13) has been observed in association with transitional-cell carcinoma, adenocarcinoma, and squamous-cell carcinomas, or as a homogeneous neoplasm in about half the cases (74–76). In many cases, in situ transitional-cell carcinoma is present. The histologic patterns range from sheets or irregular nests of tumor cells to a trabecular growth pattern. Necrosis and a high mitotic rate are common. The Azzopardi phenomenon with hematoxylin deposits around blood vessels may be seen in some cases. Ultrastructural studies show sparse, dense-core secretory granules in some cases, whereas slender cytoplasmic processes are frequently seen (76). IHC stains are positive for NSE and serotonin diffusely, whereas focal staining for chromogranin A may be present. Cytokeratin immunoreactivity is common, whereas rare tumors may contain immunoreactive vasoactive intestinal polypeptide and other neuropeptides.

The differential diagnosis should include metastatic neuroendocrine carcinoma from the prostate, cervix, and colon and lymphomas. The presence of a transitional-cell carcinoma component or carcinoma in situ helps to establish the bladder

as the primary site. Small-cell carcinoma of the urinary bladder, like other small carcinomas, is a highly lethal neoplasm.

MISCELLANEOUS NEUROENDOCRINE TUMORS

Neuroendocrine tumors have been found in many unusual primary sites. Some of these include esophagus (77), kidney (78), paranasal sinus (79), liver (80), gallbladder (81), middle ear (82), eye, orbit (83), and mesentery (84). The neuroendocrine carcinomas of the colon and rectum (85) and ampullary region (86) are highly aggressive neoplasms. Primary hepatic carcinoid tumors are very rare (87), so a small primary site outside of the liver must be exhaustively excluded before this diagnosis is made. Not only have some of these neoplasms been immunoreactive for broad-spectrum markers, such as chromogranin A and NSE, but they also have been found to have insulin and gastrin in a few cases (86). These tumors may occasionally be associated with clinical syndromes.

NEOPLASMS WITH MULTIDIRECTIONAL OR DIVERGENT DIFFERENTIATION

The presence of endocrine cells in nonendocrine tumors has been well documented in many organs, including prostate (52), breast (60), skin (46), endometrium (88), pancreas (89), lungs (90), adrenal glands (91), thyroid (92), and many others (93,94). Divergent or multidirectional differentiation of tumors, which is seen in some neoplasms, includes the production of mucin by endocrine tumors, such as goblet cell carcinoid tumors of the appendix (95); mixed follicular-medullary thyroid carcinoma of the thyroid, producing both calcitonin and thyroglobulin (96); and ductuloinsular tumors of the pancreas with endocrine and glandular differentiation (97) (Fig. 11.13). Multidirectional differentiation is observed in some hepatocellular carcinoma with endocrine differentiation in which the tumor cells express albumin and endocrine markers (87) (Fig. 11.14). The percentage of neuroendocrine cells in neoplasms with divergent differentiation may be important for determin-

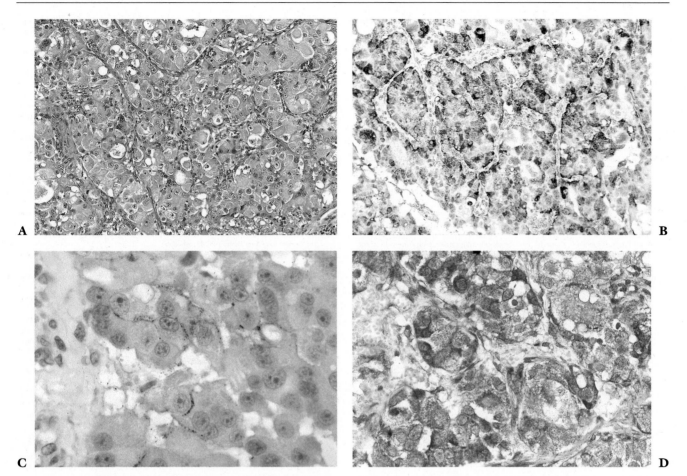

Figure 11.14. Hepatocellular carcinoma with neuroendocrine differentiation. **(A)** Hematoxylin-stained and eosin-stained sections show pleomorphic cells with abundant cytoplasm. **(B)** The tumor cells are positive for chromogranin A. **(C)** A canalicular pattern of staining with a polyclonal carcinoembryonic antigen antibody is observed. **(D)** The tumor cells are also positive for albumin mRNA by in situ hybridization. (Immunoperoxidase and in situ hybridization stains.)

ing prognosis such as is seen in carcinomas of the colon and rectum (98), whereas, in breast carcinomas with divergent differentiation, the tumor grade is much more important than the endocrine differentiation in determining the prognosis (61).

Evidence from experimental models indicates that one cell can give rise to both endocrine and exocrine patterns of differentiation (99,100). Molecular studies have shown that poorly differentiated neuroendocrine carcinomas and associated adenocarcinomas of the colon appear to be derived from the same cell of origin (101). In these mixed endocrine-exocrine carcinomas, it is usually the most aggressive cell population that drives the clinical behavior of the tumor (100). Knowledge about the pathogenesis of these tumors will come from further studies in stem cell (102,103) and molecular biology (104,105). An example of the merging of such studies is the recent discovery that neurogenin 3, a transcription factor required for endocrine cell differentiation in the developing pancreas, is also needed for the development of endocrine cells in the intestine and gastric epithelium (106). The practical implication of these observations for the surgical pathologist is that a combination of various diagnostic modalities, including conventional special stains, electron microscopy, IHC, and molecular studies may be necessary, in addition to clinical–pathologic correlations, to arrive at the most precise diagnosis and classification of neu-

roendocrine neoplasms. These approaches are even more important as specific targeted therapies are being developed for specific neoplasms (100).

REFERENCES

1. Fujita T. Present status of paraneuron concept. *Arch Histol Cytol* 1989;52 Suppl:1–8.
2. Feyrter F. [The problem of the peripheral endocrine (paracrine) glands of man]. *Wien Klin Wochenschr* 1954;66:572–575.
3. Pearse AG. The APUD cell concept and its implications in pathology. *Pathol Annu* 1974; 9:27–41.
4. Pearse AG, Takor T. Embryology of the diffuse neuroendocrine system and its relationship to the common peptides. *Fed Proc* 1979;38:2288–2294.
5. Le Douarin NM. *The Neural Crest.* Cambridge, England: Cambridge University Press, 1982.
6. Lloyd RV. Overview of neuroendocrine cells and tumors. *Endocr Pathol* 1996;7:323–328.
7. Lloyd RV. Use of molecular probes in the study of endocrine diseases. *Hum Pathol* 1987; 18:1199–1211.
8. DeLellis RA, Wolfe HJ. New techniques in gene product analysis. *Arch Pathol Lab Med* 1987;111:620–627.
9. DeLellis RA, Dayal Y, Wolfe HJ. Carcinoid tumors. Changing concepts and new perspectives. *Am J Surg Pathol* 1984;8:295–300.
10. DeLellis RA, Lloyd RV, Heitz PV, Eng C, eds. *Pathology and Genetics—Tumours of Endocrine Organs.* Lyon, France: IARC Press, 2004.
11. DeLellis RA, Shin SJ. Diagnostic immunohistochemistry of endocrine tumors. In DJ Dabbs, ed. *Diagnostic Immunohistochemistry.* New York: Churchill Livingstone, 2002, 209–240.
12. Grimelius L. A silver nitrate stain for alpha-2 cells in human pancreatic islets. *Acta Soc Med Ups* 1968;73:243–270.
13. Smith DM, Jr., Haggitt RC. A comparative study of generic stains for carcinoid secretory granules. *Am J Surg Pathol* 1983;7:61–68.

14. Wilson BS, Lloyd RV. Detection of chromogranin in neuroendocrine cells with a monoclonal antibody. *Am J Pathol* 1984;115:458–468.

15. Wiedenmann B, Huttner WB. Synaptophysin and chromogranins/secretogranins—widespread constituents of distinct types of neuroendocrine vesicles and new tools in tumor diagnosis. *Virchows Arch B Cell Pathol Incl Mol Pathol* 1989;58:95–121.

16. Schmid KW, Kroll M, Hittmair A, et al. Chromogranin A and B in adenomas of the pituitary. An immunohistochemical study of 42 cases. *Am J Surg Pathol* 1991;15:1072–1077.

17. Gould VE, Lee I, Wiedenmann B, et al. Synaptophysin: a novel marker for neurons, certain neuroendocrine cells, and their neoplasms. *Hum Pathol* 1986;17:979–983.

18. Ybe JA, Wakeham DE, Brodsky FM, Hwang PK. Molecular structures of proteins involved in vesicle fusion. *Traffic* 2000;1:474–479.

19. Lloyd RV, Warner TF. Immunohistochemistry of neuron-specific enolase. In RA DeLellis, ed. *Advances in Immunochemistry.* New York: Masson, 1984, 27–140.

20. Scopsi L, Gullo M, Rilke F, et al. Proprotein convertases (PC1/PC3 and PC2) in normal and neoplastic human tissues: their use as markers of neuroendocrine differentiation. *J Clin Endocrinol Metab* 1995;80:294–301.

21. Wharton J, Polak JM, Bloom SR, et al. Bombesin-like immunoreactivity in the lung. *Nature* 1978;273:769–770.

22. Bostwick DG, Roth KA, Evans CJ, et al. Gastrin-releasing peptide, a mammalian analog of bombesin, is present in human neuroendocrine lung tumors. *Am J Pathol* 1984;117:195–200.

23. Bunn PA, Jr., Linnoila I, Minna JD, et al. Small-cell lung cancer, endocrine cells of the fetal bronchus, and other neuroendocrine cells express the Leu-7 antigenic determinant present on natural killer cells. *Blood* 1985;65:764–768.

24. Tischler AS, Mobtaker H, Mann K, et al. Anti-lymphocyte antibody Leu-7 (HNK-1) recognizes a constituent of neuroendocrine granule matrix. *J Histochem Cytochem* 1986;34:1213–1216.

25. Portela-Gomes GM, Lukinius A, Grimelius L. Synaptic vesicle protein 2, a new neuroendocrine cell marker. *Am J Pathol* 2000;157:1299–1309.

26. DeLellis RA, Wolfe HJ. The pathobiology of the human calcitonin (C)-cell: a review. *Pathol Annu* 1981;16:25–52.

27. Hamid Q, Corrin B, Sheppard MN, et al. Expression of chromogranin A mRNA in small-cell carcinoma of the lung. *J Pathol* 1991;163:293–297.

28. Shibata D, Martin WJ, Arnheim N. Analysis of DNA sequences in forty-year-old paraffin-embedded thin-tissue sections: a bridge between molecular biology and classical histology. *Cancer Res* 1988;48:4564–4566.

29. Qian X, Lloyd RV. Recent developments in signal amplification methods for in situ hybridization. *Diagn Mol Pathol* 2003;12:1–13.

30. Long AA, Komminoth P, Lee E, Wolfe HJ. Comparison of indirect and direct in-situ polymerase chain reaction in cell preparations and tissue sections. Detection of viral DNA, gene rearrangements and chromosomal translocations. *Histochemistry* 1993;99:151–162.

31. Wermer P. Genetic aspects of adenomatosis of endocrine glands. *Am J Med* 1954;16:363–371.

32. Chandrasekharappa SC, Guru SC, Manickam P, et al. Positional cloning of the gene for multiple endocrine neoplasia-type 1. *Science* 1997;276:404–407.

33. Sipple JH. The association of pheochromocytoma with carcinoma of the thyroid gland. *Am J Med* 1961;31:163–166.

34. Komminoth P, Muletta-Feurer S, Saremaslani P, et al. Molecular diagnosis of multiple endocrine neoplasia (MEN) in paraffin-embedded specimens. *Endocr Pathol* 1995;6:267–278.

35. Eng C. Multiple endocrine neoplasia type 2 and the practice of molecular medicine. *Rev Endocr Metab Disord* 2000;1:283–290.

36. Marx SJ, Agarwal SK, Kester MB, et al. Multiple endocrine neoplasia type 1: clinical and genetic features of the hereditary endocrine neoplasias. *Recent Prog Horm Res* 1999;54:397–438;discussion 438–399.

37. DeLellis RA, Xia L. Paraneoplastic endocrine syndromes: a review. *Endocr Pathol* 2003;14:303–317.

38. Clark ES, Carney JA. Pancreatic islet cell tumor associated with Cushing's syndrome. *Am J Surg Pathol* 1984;8:917–924.

39. Matsushita H, Usui M, Hara M, et al. Co-secretion of parathyroid hormone and parathyroid-hormone-related protein via a regulated pathway in human parathyroid adenoma cells. *Am J Pathol* 1997;150:861–871.

40. Rosai J, Higa E. Mediastinal endocrine neoplasm, of probable thymic origin, related to carcinoid tumor. Clinicopathologic study of 8 cases. *Cancer* 1972;29:1061–1074.

41. Wick MR, Rosai J. Neuroendocrine neoplasms of the mediastinum. *Semin Diagn Pathol* 1991;8:35–51.

42. Huntrakoon M, Lin F, Heitz PU, Tomita T. Thymic carcinoid tumor with Cushing's syndrome. Report of a case with electron microscopic and immunoperoxidase studies for neuron-specific enolase and corticotropin. *Arch Pathol Lab Med* 1984;108:551–554.

43. Frigerio B, Capella C, Eusebi V, et al. Merkel cell carcinoma of the skin: the structure and origin of normal Merkel cells. *Histopathology* 1983;7:229–249.

44. Gould VE, Moll R, Moll I, et al. Neuroendocrine (Merkel) cells of the skin: hyperplasias, dysplasias, and neoplasms. *Lab Invest* 1985;52:334–353.

45. Sibley RK, Dahl D. Primary neuroendocrine (Merkel cell?) carcinoma of the skin. II. An immunocytochemical study of 21 cases. *Am J Surg Pathol* 1985;9:109–116.

46. Dinh V, Feun L, Elgart G, Savaraj N. Merkel cell carcinomas. *Hematol Oncol Clin North Am* 2007;21:527–544.

47. Chan JK, Suster S, Wenig BM, Tsang WY, et al. Cytokeratin 20 immunoreactivity distinguishes Merkel cell (primary cutaneous neuroendocrine) carcinomas and salivary gland small-cell carcinomas from small-cell carcinomas of various sites. *Am J Surg Pathol* 1997;21:226–234.

48. Blok PH, Manni JJ, van den Broek P, van Haelst UJ, Slooff JL. Carcinoid of the larynx: a report of three cases and a review of the literature. *Laryngoscope* 1985;95:715–719.

49. Wenig BM, Gnepp DR. The spectrum of neuroendocrine carcinomas of the larynx. *Semin Diagn Pathol* 1989;6:329–350.

50. Woodruff JM, Huvos AG, Erlandson RA, Shah JP, Gerold FP. Neuroendocrine carcinomas of the larynx. A study of two types, one of which mimics thyroid medullary carcinoma. *Am J Surg Pathol* 1985;9:771–790.

51. Woodruff JM, Senie RT. Atypical carcinoid tumor of the larynx. A critical review of the literature. *ORL J Otorhinolaryngol Relat Spec* 1991;53:194–209.

52. di Sant'Agnese PA. Divergent neuroendocrine differentiation in prostatic carcinoma. *Semin Diagn Pathol* 2000;17:149–161.

53. di Sant'Agnese PA, de Mesy Jensen KL, Churukian CJ, Agarwal MM. Human prostatic endocrine-paracrine (APUD) cells. Distributional analysis with a comparison of serotonin and neuron-specific enolase immunoreactivity and silver stains. *Arch Pathol Lab Med* 1985;109:607–612.

54. Huang J, Yao JL, di Sant'Agnese PA, Yang Q, et al. Immunohistochemical characterization of neuroendocrine cells in prostate cancer. *Prostate* 2006;66:1399–1406.

55. Ro JY, Tetu B, Ayala AG, Ordonez NG. Small-cell carcinoma of the prostate. II. Immunohistochemical and electron microscopic studies of 18 cases. *Cancer* 1987;59:977–982.

56. Vuitch MF, Mendelsohn G. Relationship of ectopic ACTH production to tumor differentiation: a morphologic and immunohistochemical study of prostatic carcinoma with Cushing's syndrome. *Cancer* 1981;47:296–299.

57. Wenk RE, Bhagavan BS, Levy R, et al. Ectopic ACTH, prostatic oat cell carcinoma, and marked hypernatremia. *Cancer* 1977;40:773–778.

58. Bussolati G, Papotti M, Sapino A, et al. Endocrine markers in argyrophilic carcinomas of the breast. *Am J Surg Pathol* 1987;11:248–256.

59. Cubilla AL, Woodruff JM. Primary carcinoid tumor of the breast. A report of eight patients. *Am J Surg Pathol* 1977;1:283–292.

60. Sapino A, Righi L, Cassoni P, et al. Expression of the neuroendocrine phenotype in carcinomas of the breast. *Semin Diagn Pathol* 2000;17:127–137.

61. Sapino A, Papotti M, Righi L, et al. Clinical significance of neuroendocrine carcinoma of the breast. *Ann Oncol* 2001;12(Suppl 2):S115–S117.

62. Woodard BH, Eisenbarth G, Wallace NR, et al. Adrenocorticotropin production by a mammary carcinoma. *Cancer* 1981;47:1823–1827.

63. Sporrong B, Falkmer S, Robboy SJ, et al. Neurohormonal peptides in ovarian carcinoids: an immunohistochemical study of 81 primary carcinoids and of intraovarian metastases from six mid-gut carcinoids. *Cancer* 1982;49:68–74.

64. Stagno PA, Petras RE, Hart WR. Strumal carcinoids of the ovary. An immunohistologic and ultrastructural study. *Arch Pathol Lab Med* 1987;111:440–446.

65. Ueda G, Sato Y, Yamasaki M, et al. Strumal carcinoid of the ovary: histological, ultrastructural, and immunohistological studies with anti-human thyroglobulin. *Gynecol Oncol* 1978;6:411–419.

66. Berdjis CC, Mostofi FK. Carcinoid tumors of the testis. *J Urol* 1977;118:777–782.

67. Leake J, Levitt G, Ramani P. Primary carcinoid of the testis in a 10-year-old boy. *Histopathology* 1991;19:373–375.

68. Ordonez NG, Ayala AG, Sneige N, Mackay B. Immunohistochemical demonstration of multiple neurohormonal polypeptides in a case of pure testicular carcinoid. *Am J Clin Pathol* 1982;78:860–864.

69. Silva EG, Kott MM, Ordonez NG. Endocrine carcinoma intermediate cell type of the uterine cervix. *Cancer* 1984;54:1705–1713.

70. Tsunoda S, Jobo T, Arai M, et al. Small-cell carcinoma of the uterine cervix: a clinicopathologic study of 11 cases. *Int J Gynecol Cancer* 2005;15:295–300.

71. Barrett RJ, 2nd, Davos I, Leuchter RS, Lagasse LD. Neuroendocrine features in poorly differentiated and undifferentiated carcinomas of the cervix. *Cancer* 1987;60:2325–2330.

72. Stoler MH, Mills SE, Gersell DJ, Walker AN. Small-cell neuroendocrine carcinoma of the cervix. A human papillomavirus type 18-associated cancer. *Am J Surg Pathol* 1991;15:28–32.

73. Conner MG, Richter H, Moran CA, et al. Small-cell carcinoma of the cervix: a clinicopathologic and immunohistochemical study of 23 cases. *Ann Diagn Pathol* 2002;6:345–348.

74. Mills SE, Wolfe JT, 3rd, Weiss MA, et al. Small-cell undifferentiated carcinoma of the urinary bladder. A light-microscopic, immunocytochemical, and ultrastructural study of 12 cases. *Am J Surg Pathol* 1987;11:606–617.

75. Blomjous CE, Vos W, De Voogt HJ, et al. Small-cell carcinoma of the urinary bladder. A clinicopathologic, morphometric, immunohistochemical, and ultrastructural study of 18 cases. *Cancer* 1989;64:1347–1357.

76. Grignon DJ, Ro JY, Ayala AG, et al. Small-cell carcinoma of the urinary bladder. A clinicopathologic analysis of 22 cases. *Cancer* 1992;69:527–536.

77. Reyes CV, Chejfec G, Jao W, Gould VE. Neuroendocrine carcinomas of the esophagus. *Ultrastruct Pathol* 1980;1:367–376.

78. Stahl RE, Sidhu GS. Primary carcinoid of the kidney: light and electron microscopic study. *Cancer* 1979;44:1345–1349.

79. Kameya T, Shimosato Y, Adachi I, et al. I. Neuroendocrine carcinoma of the paranasal sinus: a morphological and endocrinological study. *Cancer* 1980;45:330–339.

80. Gould VE, Banner BF, Baerwaldt M. Neuroendocrine neoplasms in unusual primary sites. *Diagn Histopathol* 1981;4:263–277.

81. Wada A, Ishiguro S, Tateishi R, et al. Carcinoid tumor of the gallbladder associated with adenocarcinoma. *Cancer* 1983;51:1911–1917.

82. Murphy GF, Pilch BZ, Dickersin GR, et al. Carcinoid tumor of the middle ear. *Am J Clin Pathol* 1980;73:816–823.

83. Riddle PJ, Font RL, Zimmerman LE. Carcinoid tumors of the eye and orbit: a clinicopathologic study of 15 cases, with histochemical and electron microscopic observations. *Hum Pathol* 1982;13:459–469.

84. Barnardo DE, Stavrou M, Bourne R, Bogomoletz WV. Primary carcinoid tumor of the mesentery. *Hum Pathol* 1984;15:796–798.

85. Gaffey MJ, Mills SE, Lack EE. Neuroendocrine carcinoma of the colon and rectum. A clinicopathologic, ultrastructural, and immunohistochemical study of 24 cases. *Am J Surg Pathol* 1990;14:1010–1023.

86. Zamboni G, Franzin G, Bonetti F, et al. Small-cell neuroendocrine carcinoma of the ampullary region. A clinicopathologic, immunohistochemical, and ultrastructural study of three cases. *Am J Surg Pathol* 1990;14:703–713.

87. Andreola S, Lombardi L, Audisio RA, et al. A clinicopathologic study of primary hepatic carcinoid tumors. *Cancer* 1990;65:1211–1218.

88. Inoue M, Ueda G, Yamasaki M, et al. Immunohistochemical demonstration of peptide hormones in endometrial carcinomas. *Cancer* 1984;54:2127–2131.

89. Kloppel G. Mixed exocrine-endocrine tumors of the pancreas. *Semin Diagn Pathol* 2000; 17:104–108.

90. Brambilla E, Lantuejoul S, Sturm N. Divergent differentiation in neuroendocrine lung tumors. *Semin Diagn Pathol* 2000;17:138–148.

91. Tischler AS. Divergent differentiation in neuroendocrine tumors of the adrenal gland. *Semin Diagn Pathol* 2000;17:120–126.

92. Papotti M, Volante M, Komminoth P, et al. Thyroid carcinomas with mixed follicular and C-cell differentiation patterns. *Semin Diagn Pathol* 2000;17:109–119.

93. Chejfec G, Capella C, Solcia E, et al. Amphicrine cells, dysplasias, and neoplasias. *Cancer* 1985;56:2683–2690.

94. DeLellis RA, Tischler AS, Wolfe HJ. Multidirectional differentiation in neuroendocrine neoplasms. *J Histochem Cytochem* 1984;32:899–904.

95. Rodriguez FH, Jr., Sarma DP, Lunseth JH. Goblet cell carcinoid of the appendix. *Hum Pathol* 1982;13:286–288.

96. Papotti M, Negro F, Carney JA, et al. Mixed medullary-follicular carcinoma of the thyroid. A morphological, immunohistochemical and in situ hybridization analysis of 11 cases. *Virchows Arch* 1997;430:397–405.

97. Reid JD, Yuh SL, Petrelli M, Jaffe R. Ductuloinsular tumors of the pancreas: a light, electron microscopic and immunohistochemical study. *Cancer* 1982;49:908–915.

98. Grabowski P, Schonfelder J, Ahnert-Hilger G, et al. Expression of neuroendocrine markers: a signature of human undifferentiated carcinoma of the colon and rectum. *Virchows Arch* 2002;441:256–263.

99. Bjerknes M, Cheng H. The stem-cell zone of the small intestinal epithelium. III. Evidence from columnar, enteroendocrine, and mucous cells in the adult mouse. *Am J Anat* 1981; 160:77–91.

100. Volante M, Rindi G, Papotti M. The grey zone between pure (neuro)endocrine and non-(neuro)endocrine tumours: a comment on concepts and classification of mixed exocrine-endocrine neoplasms. *Virchows Arch* 2006;449:499–506.

101. Vortmeyer AO, Lubensky IA, Merino MJ, et al. Concordance of genetic alterations in poorly differentiated colorectal neuroendocrine carcinomas and associated adenocarcinomas. *J Natl Cancer Inst* 1997;89:1448–1453.

102. Odorico JS, Kaufman DS, Thomson JA. Multilineage differentiation from human embryonic stem cell lines. *Stem Cells* 2001;19:193–204.

103. Jiang Y, Jahagirdar BN, Reinhardt RL, et al. Pluripotency of mesenchymal stem cells derived from adult marrow. *Nature* 2002;418:41–49.

104. Onuki N, Wistuba, II, Travis WD, et al. Genetic changes in the spectrum of neuroendocrine lung tumors. *Cancer* 1999;85:600–607.

105. Agarwal SK, Guru SC, Heppner C, et al. Menin interacts with the AP1 transcription factor JunD and represses JunD-activated transcription. *Cell* 1999;96:143–152.

106. Jenny M, Uhl C, Roche C, et al. Neurogenin3 is differentially required for endocrine cell fate specification in the intestinal and gastric epithelium. *Embo J* 2002;21:6338–6347.

The Pituitary and Sellar Region

Of the wide variety of lesions that affect the sellar region, pituitary adenomas are by far the most common. With the development of immunocytology, the pathologist can now engage in clinical correlation with endocrinologists and neurosurgeons and plays an integral role in the management of patients with sellar lesions. In this chapter, these processes are put into perspective for the surgical pathologist. The complex anatomy of the sellar region brings a wide variety of lesions into the clinicopathologic differential diagnosis. Only those unique or common to this location are discussed.

THE NORMAL PITUITARY

ANTERIOR LOBE

The anterior pituitary is roughly divided into a central *mucoid wedge* and lateral components termed *acidophilic wings* (Fig. 12.1). The term mucoid refers to the abundance of basophilic, periodic acid-Schiff (PAS)–positive cells concentrated and often clustered in this mid portion of the gland. These cells are engaged in the production of adrenocorticotropic hormone (ACTH) and related molecules. Thyrotropic hormone (TSH)–producing cells are far smaller in number and more anteriorly situated. Follicle-stimulating hormone (FSH)– and luteinizing hormone (LH)–producing cells are widely and individually distributed throughout the gland. The lateral wings contain the majority of growth hormone (GH) and prolactin (PRL) cells, both of which are variably granulated and eosinophilic. The morphologic features of anterior pituitary cells, as well as the biochemical characteristics of their hormone products, are summarized in Table 12.1. The region of the intermediate lobe, a well-developed structure in lower animals, is vestigial in humans and consists primarily of a distinctive form of corticotropic cell and glandular spaces. The latter are remnants of the Rathke cleft and are lined by cuboidal to columnar, ciliated, or mucin-producing cells and only occasionally by granulated adenohypophyseal cells. A sleeve of anterior pituitary tissue extends upward along the anterior aspect of the pituitary stalk and consists mainly of LH/FSH and ACTH cells, all of which are prone to squamous metaplasia with age (1). Salivary gland rests, serous in type, are encountered at the base of the pituitary stalk.

On hematoxylin and eosin (H&E) stain, anterior pituitary cells vary greatly in appearance (Fig. 12.2). Arranged in cords surrounded by a rich network of capillaries (Fig. 12.3), they were once grouped on the basis of tinctorial characteristics as acidophilic, basophilic, or chromophobic. The current classification is based on hormone content as visualized by immunohistochemistry and ultrastructure (Figs. 12.4 and 12.5 and Table 12.1). The same is true of pituitary adenomas (Tables 12.2 and 12.3) (2). Electron microscopy has played a pivotal role in classifying pituitary cells and their tumors. Classification based solely on histochemical stains is no longer recommended because it provides little insight into functional differentiation, which can only be obtained by correlative immunohistochemical and, where needed, ultrastructural studies. These methods have shown GH and PRL cells to be histogenetically related, as are cells engaged in glycoprotein hormone (LH, FSH, and TSH) production. The cells of the anterior pituitary are not limited to the production of these hormones; they have been shown to contain various other peptides (3), as well as growth factors (4).

Ultrastructurally, anterior pituitary cells are epithelial in nature and possess the full complement of organelles required for hormone production and export. Identification of normal and neoplastic pituitary cell types requires attention to such features as cell shape; the content and disposition of organelles; the presence or absence and arrangement of filaments; and of course, the number, size, electron density, and shape of secretory granules (Table 12.3). The mechanisms of hormone secretion vary from transmembrane diffusion to the actual expulsion of secretory granules, a characteristic of PRL cells (5). Folliculostellate cells akin to sustentacular cells in the paraganglia are also encountered in the anterior pituitary (3,6). Small in number, their immunoreactivity for S-100 protein, glial fibrillary acidic protein, galectin 3, and annexin 1 and their lack of synaptophysin staining distinguish them from the hormone-producing cells. The function of folliculostellate cells is controversial, but it appears to be diverse. Their products include growth and inhibitory factors, cytokines, and others. It has even been suggested that they represent stem cells.

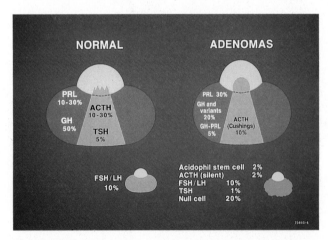

Figure 12.1. Schematic of the normal pituitary in horizontal section. Note the proportions and distribution of normal cells and of adenomas. To a significant extent, the locations of growth hormone (GH), prolactin (PRL), and adrenocorticotropic hormone (ACTH) adenomas correspond to the locations of their normal cellular counterparts. Clinically "silent" tumors without endocrine function are usually macroadenomas without specific localization (lower right).

TABLE 12.1	Cells and Hormones of the Normal Pituitary					
Cell	Product	Percentage of Cells	Location	Characteristics	Histochemical Staining[a]	Immunoperoxidase Staining
Somatotroph	Growth hormone (GH)	50%	Lateral wings	Polypeptide; 191 amino acids; molecular weight (MW), 22,000	A–C (densely to sparsely granulated); eosin, phloxine; orange G	GH[b]
Lactotroph	Prolactin (PRL)	10%–30% (pregnancy, 50%)	Lateral wings	Polypeptide; 198 amino acids; MW, 23,500	A–C (densely to sparsely granulated): eosin, phloxine; Brookes' carmoisine; Herlant's erythrosine	PRL[b]
Corticotroph	Adrenocorticotropic hormone (ACTH) and related hormones	10%–20%	Concentrated in mucoid wedge; often clustered	Polypeptide; 39 amino acids; MW, 4507	B; periodic acid-Schiff (PAS); lead hematoxylin	ACTH, β-lipotropin (LPH), endorphins, melanocyte-stimulating hormones
Gonadotroph	Luteinizing hormone (LH) and follicle-stimulating hormone (FSH)[c]	10%	Generalized	LH[c]: glycoprotein; 115 amino acids; MW, 28,260	B; PAS; aldehyde fuchsin; aldehyde thionin	LH, FSH, ± α-subunit
Thyrotroph	Thyrotropic hormone (TSH)[c]	5%	Concentrated in anterior mucoid wedge	Glycoprotein; 201 amino acids; MW, 28,000. The β-subunit consists of 110 amino acids with one carbohydrate moiety.	B; PAS; aldehyde fuchsin; aldehyde thionin	TSH ± α-subunit

[a]A, acidophilic; B, basophilic; C, chromophobic.
[b]Rare acidophilic stem cells, presumed to be precursor cells producing both GH and PRL, are present in the normal pituitary.
[c]FSH, LH, and TSH have a common 92–amino acid, 14,000–molecular weight glycoprotein α-subunit, and they are produced in the same cell.

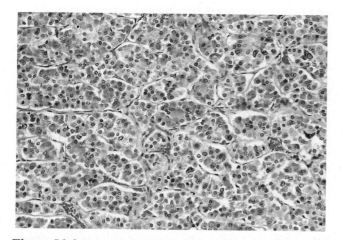

Figure 12.2. Normal anterior pituitary. Note the variation in cellular granularity. The staining ranges from acidophilic to chromophobic; several dark-staining basophils are also present.

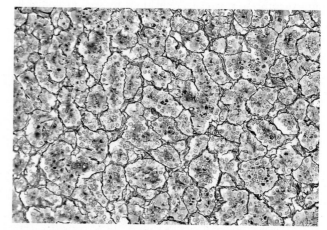

Figure 12.3. Normal anterior pituitary. Acini and cords of cells are demonstrated (reticulin stain).

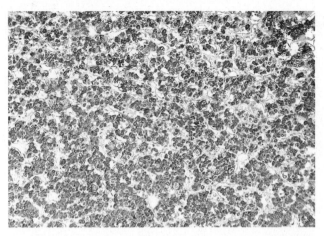

Figure 12.4. Normal growth hormone (GH) cells. The high density of these cells in the lateral wing of the anterior lobe, which here are seen immunostained for GH, is sufficient to mimic adenomas, particularly on frozen section.

POSTERIOR LOBE

The pituitary stalk and the posterior or "neural" lobe represent part of a neurosecretory unit that begins in the magnocellular neurons of the supraoptic and paraventricular nuclei. Coursing via the stalk to the posterior lobe, their unmyelinated axons and terminations carry and store the hormones vasopressin and oxytocin. In their course, the 1-nm diameter axons often show the formation of swellings (Herring bodies) in which neurosecretory materials accumulate. The two hormones, each associated with its respective carrier protein (neurophysin), are aldehyde fuchsin and aldehyde thionin positive and chromalum hematoxylin positive. Pituicytes, modified glial cells of primarily astrocytic type, are found throughout the posterior lobe (Fig. 12.6). At the ultrastructural level, axons and their swellings (Herring bodies) and terminations contain secretory granules of varying electron density, as well as multilamellar bodies and electron lucent vesicles (7). In intimate association with the pituicyte processes, axonal terminations are seen to abut or lie

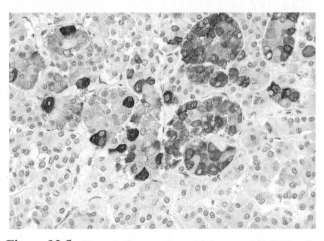

Figure 12.5. Normal adrenocorticotropic hormone (ACTH) cells. The nodularity normally exhibited by some ACTH cells may be mistaken for pituitary hyperplasia, particularly in the setting of Cushing disease when no adenoma is identified.

within perivascular spaces. Lastly, scattered corticotropic cells are a normal feature of the posterior lobe (Fig. 12.7). Derived from the intermediate lobe, they appear to be physiologically distinct from anterior lobe corticotrophs (ACTH-secreting cells). Their accumulation with age, a process termed *basophil invasion* of the posterior lobe, is of unknown clinical significance. Such cells are thought to give rise to so-called silent corticotroph cell adenomas (3,8).

PITUITARY ADENOMAS

In neurosurgical series, pituitary adenomas represent 10% to 20% of intracranial neoplasms. This high frequency is attributable to the introduction of radioimmunoassay for the detection of hormone elevations, as well as to the ready demonstration of even very small microadenomas by modern neuroimaging techniques. A higher proportion of functioning adenomas (65%) occurs in surgical series, whereas clinically nonfunctioning tumors predominate in autopsy series (9). Incidental or subclinical adenomas are encountered in nearly 25% of autopsies (Figs. 12.8 and 12.9) (10). No correlation is observed between their immunophenotype and endocrine findings (11). The majority are either null cell adenomas (50%) or prolactinomas (45%). Approximately 3% of all adenomas are associated with multiple endocrine neoplasia type 1 (MEN1) (12–14). Occasional tumors, usually GH-producing adenomas, arise in Carney complex (15). For an in-depth discussion of the endocrinologic aspects of pituitary tumors, the reader is referred to authoritative texts (16–18).

Multiple adenomas, although common in autopsy series (10,11,19,20), are encountered in less than 1% of surgical specimens (Fig. 12.9) (21). Coexistence of ACTH and PRL cell adenomas is most common, which is not surprising given the high incidence of incidental PRL cell adenomas in autopsy series (11). The distinction of two tumors in a single biopsy specimen is often difficult and may require both immunocytochemical and ultrastructural confirmation (21).

CLASSIFICATION OF PITUITARY ADENOMAS

In broad terms, the World Health Organization (WHO) and Systematized Nomenclature of Medicine (SNOMED) classify adenohypophyseal tumors as typical and atypical adenomas (WHO 8272/0 and 8272/1), as well as carcinomas (WHO 8272/3) (22).

Until recent years, advances in the medical and surgical management of adenomas exceeded progress in surgical pathology. As was previously stated, the complex histochemical stains that were once used are of little value in the characterization of normal or adenomatous pituitary tissue. For example, the eosinophilic adenomas once considered solely GH producing may manufacture GH, PRL, or both. Alternatively, they may lack hormone immunoreactivity altogether, with eosinophilia being a result of oncocytic change. Although basophilic adenomas are PAS positive and are usually associated with Cushing disease, weakly PAS-reactive tumors may also produce FSH/LH and/or TSH, with or without α-subunit. Lastly, chromophobic adenomas may either lack hormone staining or may contain any of the full range of pituitary hormones. The classification of adenomas and their clinicopathologic and immunocytochemical features are summarized in Table 12.2. Note that all adenomas are synap-

TABLE 12.2   Pituitary Adenomas: Clinical and Pathologic Characteristics

Adenoma Type	Incidence	Clinical	Staining	Hormone	Blood	Immunoreaction	Gross Features Size	Invasion
Lactotropic adenomas								
Sparsely granulated	25%	Amenorrhea and/or galactorrhea; impotence	C	PRL	+	+	33% micro/ 67% macro	52% overall
Densely granulated	1%	Amenorrhea and/or galactorrhea; impotence	A	PRL	+	+		
Somatotropic adenomas								
Sparsely granulated	5%	Acromegaly or gigantism	C-A	GH	+	+	14% micro/ 86% macro	50% overall
Densely granulated	5%	Acromegaly or gigantism	A	GH	+	+		
Adenomas with combined lactotropic and somatotropic features								
Mixed GH cell/PRL cell	5%	Acromegaly or gigantism ± hyperprolactinemia	A/C	GH/PRL	+/+	+/+	26% micro/ 74% macro	31% overall
Mammosomatotroph	3%	Acromegaly or gigantism ± hyperprolactinemia	A	GH/PRL	+/+	+/+	50% micro/ 50% macro	
Acidophil stem cell	1%	Hyperprolactinemia or "nonfunctional"; only occasional acromegaly	C	GH/PRL	±/+	+/+	Usually invasive macroadenomas	
Corticotropic adenomas								
Cushing	10%	Hypercortisolism	B	ACTH, β-LPH, endorphins, and POMC	+	+	87% micro/ 13% macro	8%/ 62%
Nelson	2%	Pigmentation; mass symptoms	B-C	ACTH, β-LPH, endorphins, and POMC	+	+	100% macro	82%
Crooke cell	<1%	Hypercortisolism	B-C	ACTH, β-LPH, endorphins, and POMC	+	+	25% micro/ 75% macro	85%
Silent corticotropic	3%	Mass symptoms; hypopituitarism	B-C	ACTH, β-LPH, endorphins, and POMC	−	+	100% macro	82%
Glycoprotein adenomas								
Gonadotropic	7%–15%	Setting of hypogonadism; functionally silent; mass effects	C-B	FSH and LH	15%	+ (± α-subunit)	5% micro/ 95% macro	21%
Thyrotropic	1%	Setting of hypothyroidism or hyperthyroidism	C-B	TSH	+	+ (± α-subunit)	Usually invasive macroadenomas	75%
Plurihormonal adenomas	10%	Usually acromegaly ± hyperprolactinemia; glycoprotein hormone production rarely expressed	C-A	Usually GH, PRL, and TSH, α-subunit; includes other unusual combinations	+/±/−	Usually +/+/+	25% micro/ 75% macro	52%
Silent subtype 3	3%	Mass effects; hyperprolactinemia or GH effects	C to mild A	No specific hormone	−	Scant to variable GH (10%), PRL (10%), or TSH; rare ACTH	Usually macro	Frequent
Null cell adenomas	20%							
Nononcocytic	14%	Visual symptoms; hypopituitarism; headaches	C	None ± mild hyperprolactinemia as a result of pituitary stalk compression	−	−	5% micro/ 95% macro	42%
Oncocytic	6%	Visual symptoms; hypopituitarism; headaches	A	None ± mild hyperprolactinemia as a result of pituitary stalk compression	−	−	5% micro/ 95% macro	

ACTH, adrenocorticotropic hormone; FSH, follicle-stimulating hormone; GH, growth hormone; LH, luteinizing hormone; LPH, lipotropin; POMC, pro-opiomelanocortin; PRL, prolactin; TSH, thyrotrophic hormone. C, chromophobic; A, acidophilic; B, basophilic.

TABLE 12.3 Pituitary Adenomas: Ultrastructural Features

Ultrastructural Type	Cell	Nucleus	Rough Endoplasmic Reticulum	Golgi	Granule Morphology	Miscellaneous
Prolactin cell adenoma						
Densely granulated adenoma	Round to oval	Eccentric, oval to irregular	Peripheral parallel stacks	Prominent, ring shaped	400–1200 nm (600 nm average), electron dense, round to irregular	
Sparsely granulated adenoma	Polyhedral	Oval to irregular	"Nebenkern" (concentric whorl) formation	Abundant, ring shaped or convoluted	150–500 nm (250 nm average), electron dense, round to irregular	Misplaced exocytosis
Growth hormone cell adenoma						
Densely granulated adenoma	Round to oval	Central, round to oval, prominent nucleolus	Moderate, peripheral parallel arrays	Prominent, spherical, numerous vesicles	300–600 nm, electron dense, spherical, apposed limiting membrane	
Sparsely granulated adenoma	Pleomorphic	Single to multiple, eccentric, irregular	Prominent, peripheral parallel rows or scattered	Abundant, ring shaped	400–450 nm, electron dense, occasionally 100–250 nm	Paranuclear fibrous bodies, multiple centrioles, smooth endoplasmic reticulum, tubular aggregates in endothelial cells
Adenoma with combined prolactin and growth hormone cell features						
Mixed growth hormone cell–prolactin cell adenoma	Variable proportions of sparsely and densely granulated growth hormones and prolactin cells with morphologic features noted above					
Mammosomatotroph cell adenoma	Polyhedral	Oval to irregular	Well developed	Prominent, numerous immature secretory vesicles	Two populations: 150–450 nm, electron dense, round to oval, apposed limiting membrane; 350–2000 nm, variably electron dense, elongated, loose limiting membrane (intracellular and extracellular); abundant	
Acidophil stem cell adenoma	Elongated	Irregular	Poorly to moderately developed	Moderate; few associated secretory granules	50–300 nm, electron dense; sparse	Paranuclear fibrous bodies, smooth endoplasmic reticulum, multiple centrioles, misplaced exocytosis, frequent abnormal or giant mitochondria, variable oncocytic transformation

(continues)

Ultrastructural Type	Cell	Nucleus	Rough Endoplasmic Reticulum	Golgi	Granule Morphology	Miscellaneous
Corticotroph cell adenoma						
Densely or sparsely granulated adenoma	Round, angular, or elongate	Round to oval	Abundant, short profiles	Prominent	250–700 nm, round to heart or tear-drop shaped, slightly irregular, variably electron dense, often peripheral location	Perinuclear and cytoplasmic 70-Å microfilaments; enigmatic body (large paranuclear lysosome)
Nelson syndrome	As above but with little or no microfilaments					
Crooke cell adenoma	As above but with marked to massive accumulation of macrofilaments					
Silent corticotroph cell adenoma	Resembles densely or sparsely granulated Cushing adenoma					
Silent subtype 1						
Silent subtype 2	Small polyhedral	Centrally placed	Numerous	Prominent	150–300 nm, irregular drop-shaped; sparse	No perinuclear and cytoplasmic microfilaments
Glycoprotein adenoma						
Gonadotroph cell adenoma	Small to medium, angular to elongated	Oval	Sparse	Moderate, occasionally dilated Vacuolar ("honeycomb") transformation in females	Less than 150 nm, electron dense ± lucent halo, often peripheral location or in processes abutting capillaries; sparse	Scattered cytoplasmic microtubules
Thyrotroph cell adenoma	Small; angular cells with elongated processes	Irregular to oval	Poorly developed profiles	Moderate	50–250 nm, electron dense with lucent halo, often peripheral location or in processes abutting capillaries; sparse	Scattered cytoplasmic microtubules, occasional large lysosomes
Plurihormonal adenomas	This heterogeneous group of adenomas varies greatly in ultrastructural appearance; some tumors are monomorphous, whereas others consist of two or three distinct cell types					
Silent subtype 3	Irregular polar	Pleomorphic with spheridia	Moderate	Prominent, multifocal	200 nm, cytoplasm and particularly in processes	Abundant smooth endoplasmic reticulum
Null cell adenoma						
Nononcocytic adenoma	Small polyhedral	Irregular, indented	Sparse stacks, some ribosomal clusters	Moderate	100–250 nm, electron dense ± lucent halo; sparse	Microtubules, annulate lamellae
Oncocytic adenoma ("pituitary oncocytoma")	Large polyhedral	Irregular, indented	Sparse stacks, some ribosomal clusters	Moderate	100–250 nm, electron dense ± lucent halo; sparse	Abundant light and dark mitochondria, microtubules

See references 2, 3, 24, 29, 30, 31, and 268

465

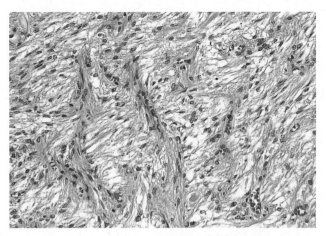

Figure 12.6. Posterior pituitary. The posterior lobe consists of the axonal processes and terminations of the vasopressin and oxytocin-producing supraoptic and paraventricular nuclei. In addition, endothelial cells and pituicytes, modified astrocytes, contribute to its cellularity.

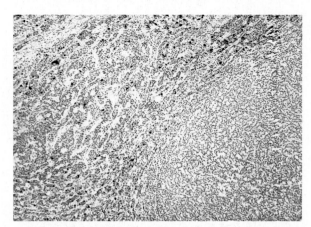

Figure 12.9. Multiple microadenomas. One is a large and fully developed null cell tumor (right), whereas the other is a minute prolactinoma (upper left) still showing residual acinar architecture. Note the presence of occasional normal gonadotropic cells entrapped in the early lesion, whereas the larger tumor is monomorphous (immunoperoxidase preparation and antiluteinizing hormone).

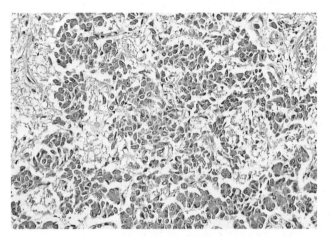

Figure 12.7. Basophil invasion. A normal feature of the posterior lobe is the presence of adrenocorticotropic hormone cells at its interface with the anterior lobe (periodic acid-Schiff).

tophysin immunoreactive but not all stain for chromogranin; the same is true of keratins and epithelial membrane antigen (23).

Electron microscopy has revealed much about the nature of normal pituitary cells (24) and their respective tumors. At present, its value is underrated (25), but it provided the underpinnings of a logical classification of pituitary adenomas and continues to play a valuable role in the diagnosis of unusual adenoma types and the expanding spectrum of rare sellar region tumors (Table 12.3) (26,27). The reader is referred to several comprehensive reviews of pituitary adenomas (18,28–31). The major adenoma subgroups are discussed in turn in the following sections.

METHODS IN PITUITARY PATHOLOGY

Cell biology studies have provided abundant data regarding the nature and behavior of pituitary adenomas. Etiologic and genetic factors underlying their genesis are discussed elsewhere (31). Whether pituitary adenomas are monoclonal or multiclonal in nature has been a subject of debate (32), but X chromosome inactivation studies have shown that they are clonal lesions (33,34). However, cell proliferation studies using flow cytometry (S-phase analysis) (35,36), as well as Ki-67 (36–38) and bromodeoxyuridine (BrDU) labeling (39), do show a correlation between elevated indices and the capacity of a tumor to invade and/or metastasize. The same is true of mitotic indices (40) and p53 protein immunoreactivity (41). Topoisomerase (42) and cyclo-oxygenase (43) immunoreactivity are also indicators of proliferative activity. Metalloproteinase expression has been shown to be invasion associated (44). Despite reports to the contrary (45), DNA ploidy analysis is of limited use in identifying invasive and aggressive lesions (35,46). The same is true of the silver-staining nucleolar organizing region (AgNOR) analysis (47,48).

In situ hybridization permits the identification of hormone mRNA expression, a modality useful in the study of so-called silent adenomas (see below). The degree of secretory activity exhibited by pituitary adenomas shows little correlation with

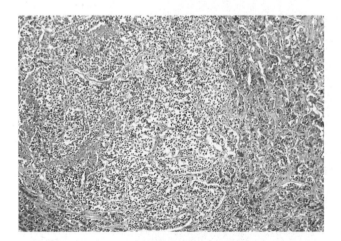

Figure 12.8. Microadenoma. Relative circumscription and early compression of surrounding parenchyma are seen. The acinar architecture is effaced.

cell proliferation. Although immunostains permit the crude quantification of hormones within cells, they yield no information regarding rates of secretion. The latter can be estimated in vitro by the reverse hemolytic plaque assay (49). This method and more conventional tissue culture methods remain experimental modalities. The same is true of immunoelectron microscopy, which permits the identification of one or more hormones or other substances within single cells, specific organelles, or even secretory granules.

BASIC PATHOLOGY OF PITUITARY ADENOMAS

Pituitary adenomas show somewhat of a predilection for women in the third to sixth decades of life. No age group is exempt, including childhood, a period wherein 2% of all adenomas occur (50–52). ACTH-producing tumors are those most often encountered in pediatric patients (51). Such adenomas are thought to be more aggressive in children (52). The vast majority of pituitary adenomas are sporadic, but MEN1, Carney complex, and McCune-Albright syndrome predispose to their development (53). Those that are associated with MEN1 tend to be plurihormonal, macroadenomas, and invasive (54).

As a rule, endocrinologically functional tumors are often small, whereas silent or nonfunctioning tumors are large, coming to attention only as a result of mass effects. A convenient distinction of *microadenomas*, which are radiographically defined as tumors 1 cm in size or smaller, from *macroadenomas*, which are tumors exceeding 1 cm, has long been in use (55). *Diffuse adenomas* are ones that fill and expand the sella, often compressing the residual gland into a thin membrane. Larger or *massive* adenomas often efface the sellar floor, displace surrounding structures, and undergo suprasellar extension. *Giant adenomas*, which are presently defined as adenomas greater than 4 cm in maximal dimension, are very uncommon (56). It is of note that pituitary adenomas, regardless of size, are rarely associated with diabetes insipidus. Gross, operatively or radiographically apparent invasion is not limited to macroadenomas. In any case, it predisposes patients to tumor recurrence (57). Surgical specimens only infrequently include dura or bone. Nonetheless, the frequency of microscopic dural invasion, when systematically sought, is common, ranging from 65% to 95%, depending on tumor size (58). Thus, documenting the presence of invasion by microscopy is of little use unless bone involvement is seen.

The development of at least some adenomas is thought to proceed through an early stage of hyperplasia (Fig. 12.9). An intermediate-phase lesion, wherein acinar expansion is marked and cellular monomorphism is nearly complete, is the *tumorlet* (59,60). As dissolution of acinar architecture ensues and compression of surrounding pituitary parenchyma becomes apparent, the microadenoma stage is reached (Figs. 12.8 and 12.10). Although condensation of pituitary stroma does take place around these enlarging lesions, pituitary adenomas do not possess a true capsule. With continued enlargement, they expand the sella, often asymmetrically, and demineralize its floor. Elevation of the sellar diaphragm is common, as is the extension of tumor through its frequently incompetent diaphragmatic opening. The result of significant suprasellar extension is chiasmal compression (Fig. 12.11) with visual disturbance, typically bitemporal hemianopsia. Massive suprasellar extension may result in the deep indentation of the brain in the region of the third ventricle. Extension into the middle,

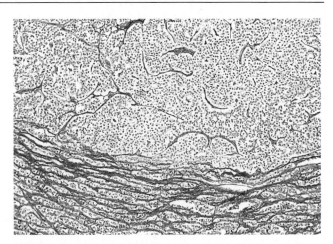

Figure 12.10. Pituitary adenoma. The lack of reticulin content and the compression of surrounding parenchyma are demonstrated (reticulin stain).

anterior, or, less often, posterior fossa may also be seen. Lateral growth into the cavernous sinus may occur through infrequent naturally occurring discontinuities in the fibrous membrane separating the sella from the sinus (61) or by way of invasion. Invasive and malignant pituitary tumors are discussed later.

Rare adenomas are ectopic, actually arising outside the sella (62). Origin in a teratoma is a novel presentation (63). Abscess formation within the substance of an adenoma has been described (64,65), but in most instances, it is a postoperative complication. Another, albeit late, complication of adenoma irradiation is the induction of sarcoma formation, which is more often a fibrosarcoma than an osteosarcoma (66). Postirradiation gliomas are far less common (67).

Pituitary apoplexy, which is defined as rapid enlargement of an adenoma by intratumoral hemorrhage and variable infarction, may be a surgical emergency (Fig. 12.12). Alternatively, the process may undergo subclinical evolution. Seen in approximately 10% of operated adenomas, it takes the form of hemorrhagic, necrotic, or cystic foci (68–72). Apoplexy affects all types of adenoma, but large, nonfunctioning tumors are particularly prone. The specimens usually consist of blood and necrotic tumor. Identification of the underlying tumor is aided by reti-

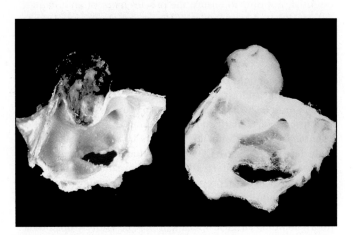

Figure 12.11. Pituitary macroadenoma. Thinning and demineralization of the sellar floor, as well as suprasellar extension, are seen.

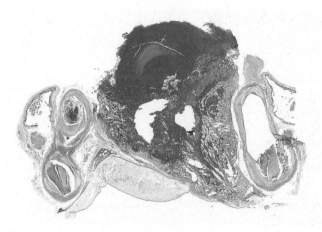

Figure 12.12. Pituitary apoplexy. The sellar region in coronal sections shows a massive hemorrhage within a macroadenoma. (Courtesy of Dr. K. Kovacs, St. Michael's Hospital, Toronto, Ontario, Canada.)

culin stains, which highlight the abnormal stromal pattern of the adenoma (Fig. 12.13). As a rule, such tissue is unsuitable for immunohistochemical characterization.

THE ROLE OF THE PATHOLOGIST

The assessment of pituitary adenomas begins at the time of surgery. Although smears or frozen sections may be performed to identify the tumor, systematic assessment of resection margins is an unrealistic endeavor. Total excision is complicated by factors such as irregular tumor shape, lack of cleavage planes and of a capsule, and grossly inapparent foci of dural invasion (Fig. 12.14). Furthermore, because of lack of stroma, the soft consistency of adenomas obscures landmarks and may even promote contamination of the operative field.

Pituitary adenomas exhibit various growth patterns (Fig. 12.15). Their recognition, although of no prognostic significance, is worthwhile because a spectrum of lesions enters into the differential diagnosis. The number of diagnostic possibilities is markedly reduced by attention to such factors as the presence or absence of sellar enlargement and clinical and biochemical data regarding hormone secretion and hyperfunction. A working relationship between the pathologist and surgeon is essential, not only to ensure the procurement of an adequate specimen but also to maximize clinicopathologic correlation.

SPECIMEN HANDLING

Fresh tissues should be promptly transported from the operating room on a moist Telfa pad; delayed fixation and drying artifact must be avoided. Smears are preferable to touch preparations and particularly to frozen sections in the assessment of adenomas. Stained with H&E, smears best demonstrate cytologic detail (Fig. 12.16). Cytologic methods obviate the mechanical and freezing artifacts that affect permanent sections and immunocytochemical preparations. Once the tissues are frozen, they often show nonspecific or reduced immunoreactivity. Furthermore, they are useless for ultrastructural study. Minute, poorly handled surgical specimens may be entirely unsuitable for diagnosis.

Following intraoperative study, the specimen should be for-

malin fixed only after a minute portion, at minimum a single 1-mm fragment, has been placed in glutaraldehyde for possible ultrastructural study. In a pinch, formalin-fixed tissue does nicely. Accurate sampling for electron microscopy is essential; unlike more rubbery, normal adenohypophyseal tissue, adenoma is readily identified by its soft, almost creamy texture. With an adequate sample, consideration can be given to freezing a portion for biochemical or genetic studies. When diagnostic tissue is scant or no lesion is identified on cytologic or frozen section assessment, the entire specimen should be step sectioned to obtain H&E and unstained slides.

In addition to the preparation of an H&E-stained slide, consecutive microsections should be cut for both PAS and reticulin stains, as well as immunostains for pituitary hormones. Performance of a full hormone battery, including GH, PRL, ACTH, LH, FSH, TSH, and α-subunit, requires at least eight unstained microsections. Recutting blocks after having prepared only a single H&E section wastes tissue and may compromise the diagnosis. Although a battery approach is preferable, immunostains can be selectively applied, depending on the clinical setting. As noted later, hyperprolactinemia at levels less than 150 ng/mL does not indicate tumoral PRL production. Instead, it may be a result of *stalk section effect* (pituitary stalk compression), which interferes with PRL-inhibiting factor (dopamine) delivery to the anterior lobe (73,74). If lack of PRL staining is not demonstrated, valuable time may be lost in useless endocrine therapy directed at a presumed PRL cell adenoma. In the setting of Cushing disease, immunostains for ACTH are particularly useful in confirming the presence of a small, often fragmented pituitary adenoma. In large institutions with advanced endocrine and neurosurgical departments, the full spectrum of antibodies for pituitary hormones is usually applied to all but the adenomas of Cushing disease, the tumors of which are monotypic. As stated earlier, electron microscopy plays an important, albeit defined, role in the assessment of adenomas.

PROLACTIN CELL ADENOMA

Nearly half of functional pituitary adenomas are, at least in part, PRL-producing tumors. So-called prolactinomas or lactotropic tumors are composed entirely of PRL cells. Prolactinomas are the most frequently occurring adenoma in MEN1 (14). On the other hand, isolated familial prolactinomas are rare (75). Whereas estrogens cause prolactinomas in experimental animals and pregnancy may be associated with enlargement of some, these agents alone are generally incapable of inducing prolactinomas in humans (76–78). Microadenomas generally occur in reproductive-age women who exhibit exquisite sensitivity to PRL excess by manifesting with amenorrhea, galactorrhea, or both. In men and postmenopausal women, prolactinomas often appear to be clinically nonfunctional, growing to macroadenoma dimensions and exhibiting invasion (79). One study suggests that the basis for this relative aggressiveness lies in differences in proliferative activity (80). Approximately 50% of prolactinomas are grossly or radiographically invasive at initial surgery. Not surprisingly, the frequency of invasion increases with tumor size. Serum PRL levels are uniformly elevated in patients with prolactinomas, although the levels range from little more than normal (approximately 20 ng/mL) to extremely high (≥2000 ng/mL). As a rule, PRL levels correlate with the tumor size (81,82). As noted earlier, mild increases of PRL

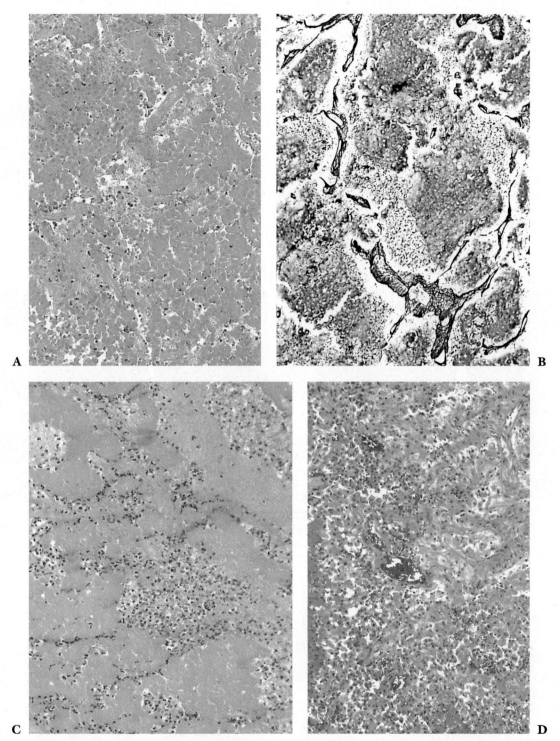

Figure 12.13. Pituitary apoplexy. **(A)** Hematoxylin and eosin–stained sections of such specimens often show only hemorrhage and extensive necrosis. **(B)** The underlying pattern of adenoma is highlighted by reticulin stain. **(C)** In the subacute phase, aggregates of polymorphonuclear leukocytes should not be mistaken for infection. **(D)** In chronic phases, ingrowth of granulation tissue may be conspicuous.

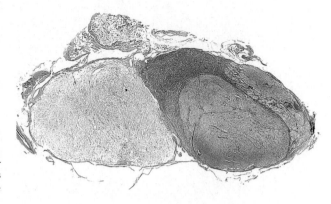

Figure 12.14. Microinvasive adenoma. This whole-mount sagittal section of the pituitary demonstrates the adenoma. Note the irregular outlines of the tumor, as well as the early invasion of the dural capsule, on the anterior aspect of the gland.

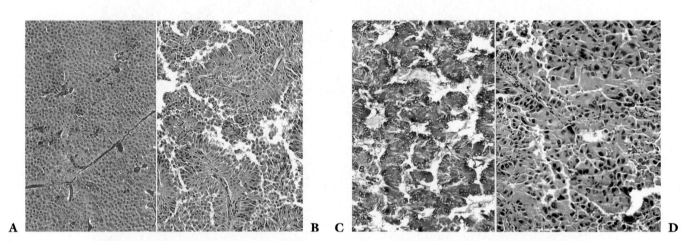

A   B   C   D

Figure 12.15. Pituitary adenomas. The hematoxylin and eosin–stained appearance of these adenomas, which include diffuse (**A**), papillary (**B**), ribbon (**C**), and pleomorphic (**D**) patterns, illustrates their broad morphologic spectrum and highlights the diagnostic use of immunohistochemistry.

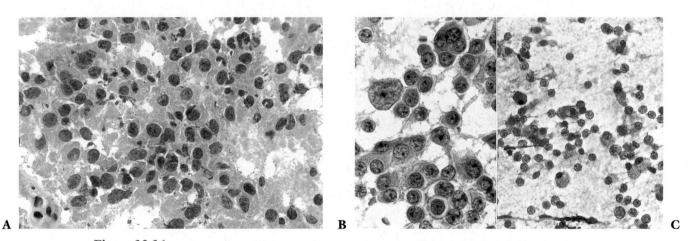

A   B   C

Figure 12.16. Pituitary adenoma. This is a comparison of a hematoxylin and eosin–stained frozen section (**A**) and a touch preparation (**B**). The latter shows excellent cytologic detail, including prominence of nucleoli, binucleation, nuclear atypia, the presence of a mitosis, and cytoplasmic uniformity. A touch preparation from normal pituitary tissue is far less cellular; it shows variation in cytoplasmic staining; and it lacks both nuclear abnormalities, as well as mitoses (**C**).

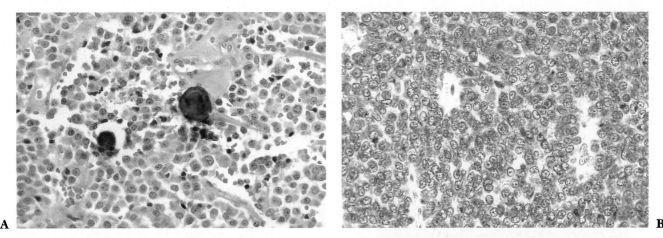

Figure 12.17. Prolactin cell adenomas. These are nearly all chromophobic, and they often contain spherical microcalcifications **(A)**. Immunoreactivity for prolactin shows a characteristic globular reaction in the paranuclear Golgi zone **(B)**.

(<150 ng/mL) may be a result of "stalk section effect" and are not diagnostic of adenoma (73,74).

Nearly all prolactinomas are sparsely granulated and thus chromophobic (Fig. 12.17). Densely granulated (eosinophilic) examples are rare. Approximately 10% to 20% of prolactinomas feature psammomatous microcalcification (83). The latter is usually scant but may be so abundant that it forms a "pituitary stone." The presence of microcalcifications in an adenoma strongly suggests the diagnosis of prolactinoma, as does the rare finding of spherical amyloid bodies (Fig. 12.18) (84). Immunoreactivity for PRL is typically strong but is paranuclear in location (Fig. 12.17). The ultrastructural features of PRL cell ade-

noma are distinctive (Table 12.3) and include abundant rough endoplasmic reticulum, as well as "misplaced exocytosis" or granule extrusion between neoplastic cells (85,86).

Given the efficacy of dopamine agonist therapy, the frequency of prolactinomas in surgical series has dramatically decreased from 30% to 10%. These agents produce atrophy of tumoral cells with resultant tumor shrinkage or arrest; the effect is reversible with cessation of therapy and thus not curative. The morphologic effects of such dopamine agonists as bromocriptine have been well characterized (87–89). They include diminution of cell size, condensation of nuclei, reduction in synthetic and secretory organelles, cessation of granule extrusion,

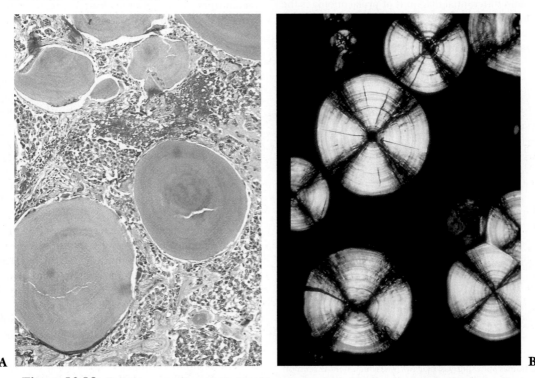

Figure 12.18. Prolactinoma with amyloid deposition. Such spherical bodies are virtually diagnostic of a prolactin cell adenoma (B, polarization).

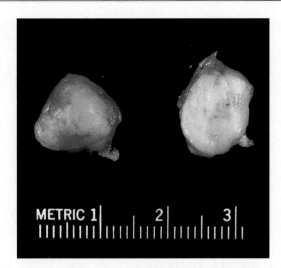

Figure 12.19. Bromocriptine effect. This dopamine agonist and prolactin inhibitor produces not only involution and shrinkage of prolactin cell adenomas, but also marked interstitial fibrosis. Such adenomas may be grossly firm and rubbery.

and interstitial collagen deposition. Necrosis plays no significant part. Perhaps because of uneven D2 receptor loss, these changes may not affect all tumor cells. When administered long term, they may induce dense tumoral fibrosis (Figs. 12.19 and 12.20). Whether the latter complicates eventual resection is unclear.

Small tumor size and normalization of PRL levels after surgical or medical therapy of prolactinoma are favorable prognostic features. Macroadenomas in postreproductive females and particularly in males are prone to recur (90,91). Surgery is the principal therapy, but medical treatment, including a GH receptor antagonist (92), plays a major role and has met with real success. The main differential diagnosis of prolactinoma is the acidophil stem cell adenoma (93) (see "Acidophil Stem Cell Adenoma" section). Key distinguishing features include its often large size in the presence of low PRL levels, minor immu-

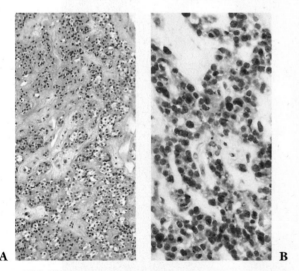

Figure 12.20. Treated prolactin (PRL) cell adenoma. Microscopically, these adenomas show perivascular fibrosis, which here is seen on hematoxylin and eosin stain **(A)** and on immunostain for PRL **(B)**, the reactivity of which persists.

noreactivity for both PRL and GH, and distinctive ultrastructure features.

GROWTH HORMONE–PRODUCING ADENOMAS

GROWTH HORMONE CELL ADENOMA

Two disorders are associated with GH-producing adenomas. These include gigantism, which begins in childhood or adolescence, and acromegaly, a far more common disease affecting adults. Their pathologic basis differs.

Although 25% of adenomas are associated with clinical or immunocytologic evidence of GH production, only a minority makes GH alone (94,95). The vast majority of adenomas produce both GH and PRL or are plurihormonal, also expressing TSH and/or α-subunit. Precursor lesions of GH cell adenomas include somatotroph hyperplasia caused by ectopic production of growth hormone–releasing hormone (GHRH) by a variety of endocrine tumors and in the McCune-Albright syndrome (53,96). GH adenomas also occur in Carney complex (53,97). The pathology of GH-producing or somatotropic tumors has been extensively studied (18,95,98–100). Nearly all are solitary, but GH-producing adenomas account for the majority of multiple adenomas in surgical series (21).

Eosinophilic and chromophobic forms of GH cell adenoma occur with equal frequency. Both result in acromegaly or enlargement of acral parts of the body. Facial changes are conspicuous. These effects are largely mediated by insulin-like growth factor-1 (IGF-1), a substance produced by the liver and more reliably elevated than GH levels. The histologic patterns of GH cell adenomas are often nonspecific and diffuse, but nuclear pleomorphism and multinucleation are most often seen in sparsely granulated (chromophobic) tumors. The latter often show only scant GH immunoreactivity (Fig. 12.21). In contrast, densely granulated eosinophilic tumors stain strongly (Fig. 12.22). A characteristic of chromophobic lesions is the presence of paranuclear, eosinophilic, low–molecular-weight keratin-containing "fibrous bodies." At the ultrastructural level, these consist of intermediate filament whorls, often enmeshing organelles (Table 12.3). Similar structures are seen in a variety of neuroendocrine neoplasms, but their presence in a pituitary adenoma indicates somatotropic differentiation. Sparsely granulated GH cells do not occur in the normal pituitary. In contrast, the cells of densely granulated tumors resemble normal GH cells, their eosinophilia being a result of abundant larger secretory granules. Such tumors lack fibrous bodies. Although the endocrinologic features and secretory activity of eosinophilic and chromophobic variants of GH cell adenoma are similar, chromophobic tumors are more aggressive. In at least one large study (101), no microadenomas were found among the chromophobic lesions, which were three times more invasive than eosinophilic tumors. Some GH adenomas may even produce GHRH, with the presumed result being autostimulation. Such adenomas are more aggressive than those not producing this hypothalamic releasing hormone (102). On rare occasion, GH adenomas show neuronal metaplasia (see below) (103). Clinically nonfunctional or "silent GH cell adenomas" are rare (104).

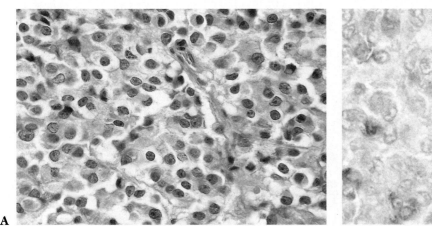
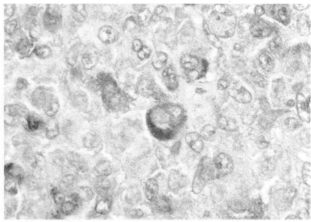

Figure 12.21. **(A)** Growth hormone cell adenoma, sparsely granulated (chromophobic) type. Note the presence of paranuclear hyaline bodies. **(B)** Immunoreactivity for growth hormone may be weak and present in only a portion of cells.

Medical treatment of GH-producing adenomas involves the use of long-acting somatostatin analogs, such as octreotide. Morphologically, their effect varies but includes mild to moderate interstitial fibrosis (105). As a rule, tumor shrinkage is minor despite reduction in GH levels (105).

PLURIHORMONAL GROWTH HORMONE–PRODUCING ADENOMAS

The majority of acromegaly-associated adenomas produce not only GH, but also PRL and one or more glycoprotein hormones, usually TSH and/or α-subunit (94,95). Immunoreactivity for LH or FSH is exceptional (106). Hypersecretion of PRL may be clinically or biochemically apparent, but TSH secretion is rarely expressed, even at the biochemical level. Most plurihormonal tumors are macroadenomas. A majority show radiographic or gross operative invasion. This group of tumors is of particular pathologic interest because they may consist of one, two, or three ultrastructurally distinct cell types, including GH, PRL, and/or TSH cells (Table 12.3).

MIXED GROWTH HORMONE CELL–PROLACTIN CELL ADENOMA

As has already been noted, most GH-producing adenomas also secrete PRL. Indeed, nearly 40% of acromegalic patients have hyperprolactinemia. Because any number of lesions in the sellar region may be associated with hyperprolactinemia as a result of stalk section effect, a diagnosis of GH adenoma with a PRL-producing component cannot be made without immunocytologic confirmation.

The predominant clinical feature of the mixed GH cell–PRL cell adenoma is acromegaly. The effects of concomitant GH and PRL elevation are not always apparent. Such tumors, which are variably acidophilic, are of interest because they are composed of two distinct, albeit related, cell types—somatotrophs and lactotrophs (Fig. 12.23) (107). They represent approximately 5% of pituitary adenomas and are relatively indolent in behavior. Both GH and PRL immunoreactivity are strong. Distinguishing them ultrastructurally from the acidophil stem cell adenoma is important but generally easy. The latter, an aggressive form of GH- and PRL-producing adenoma, shows

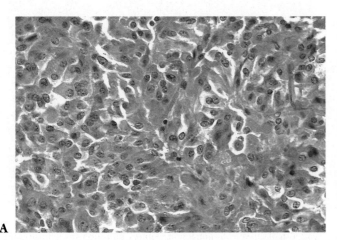
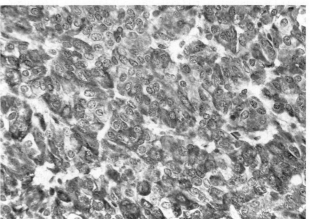

Figure 12.22. **(A)** Growth hormone (GH) cell adenoma, densely granulated (eosinophilic) type. Note the prominent acidophilia and the lack of fibrous bodies. **(B)** GH immunoreactivity is strong.

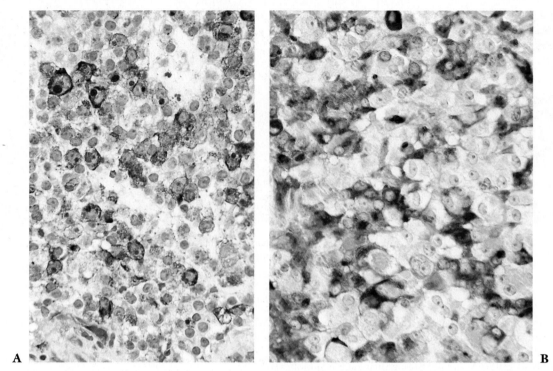

Figure 12.23. Mixed growth hormone (GH) cell–prolactin (PRL) cell adenomas. Such tumors consist of two distinct cell populations, one of which is reactive for GH (**A**) and one of which is reactive for PRL (**B**).

much less hormone reactivity and masquerades as a prolactinoma, with GH elevation and acromegaly being infrequent (Table 12.3) (93).

MAMMOSOMATOTROPH CELL ADENOMA

This unusual GH- and PRL-producing tumor represents only 1% of pituitary adenomas and is the most common tumor underlying gigantism or unrestrained somatic growth. It is of interest because this well-differentiated, eosinophilic tumor is composed of a single cell type sharing ultrastructural features of both GH and PRL cells. Key features include densely granulated cells resembling somatotrophs but exhibiting both large (up to 1500 nm) granules and misplaced exocytosis, a feature of lactotrophs (108,109). Immunoreactivity for both hormones is strong. Like the mixed GH cell–PRL cell adenoma, it results in acromegaly, and it is also relatively indolent in behavior. Again, making a distinction from acidophil stem cell adenoma is essential (Table 12.3).

ACIDOPHIL STEM CELL ADENOMA

This unique form of pituitary adenoma is uncommon and comprises less than 1% of all adenomas and 5% of GH-producing tumors. It is composed of immature cells, perhaps stem cells, of the acidophil (GH and PRL cell) line. Small numbers of acidophil stem cells are found in the normal pituitary. On light microscopy, acidophil stem cell adenomas are either chromophobic or somewhat oncocytic in appearance (Fig. 12.24). As a rule, acidophil stem cell adenoma shows greater immunoreactivity for PRL than for GH, which may be lacking. Ultrastructurally, the tumor consists of a single, rather poorly differentiated cell type showing features intermediate between GH cells

(fibrous bodies) and PRL cells (misplaced exocytoses) (Table 12.3) (93). Secretory granules are sparse and small. An often conspicuous feature is the presence of giant mitochondria, which may be apparent on light microscopy as cytoplasmic vacuoles, some approaching the size of the nucleus. Electron microscopy is required to establish a firm diagnosis of acidophil stem cell adenoma (Table 12.3).

Acidophil stem cell adenomas are either clinically nonfunctioning or produce mild hyperprolactinemia. GH levels are often normal, and acromegaly is an uncommon finding. The majority are obviously growing, invasive macroadenomas (26).

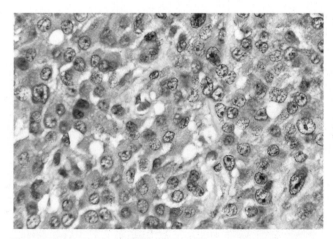

Figure 12.24. Acidophil stem cell adenoma. Although definitive diagnosis of this uncommon lesion requires immunohistochemistry and electron microscopy, hematoxylin and eosin stains may show paranuclear vacuolization, a feature corresponding to giant mitochondria.

The diagnosis is of clinical importance because acidophil stem cell adenomas may be clinically mistaken for prolactinoma. Unlike the latter, they fail to respond to dopamine agonist therapy; only normal PRL cells are suppressed by the treatment.

EXTRAPITUITARY DISEASE AND GROWTH HORMONE EXCESS

This topic was briefly alluded to earlier. Although the older literature states that up to 50% of lung and gastric carcinomas contain GH (110), few, if any, examples have been adequately documented (111). Acromegaly in association with an extrasellar neoplasm is usually a result of ectopic secretion of GHRH by a neuroendocrine neoplasm, such as bronchial carcinoid tumor, pancreatic islet cell tumor, or pheochromocytoma (112–116). In such cases, the pituitary is enlarged and shows GH cell hyperplasia, a reversible alteration.

CORTICOTROPH CELL ADENOMAS

Adenomas that produce ACTH fall into three major groups: endocrinologically active tumors associated with either Cushing disease or Nelson syndrome (117–120) and clinically nonfunctioning or *silent corticotropic adenomas*.

CUSHING DISEASE

Although Cushing disease is rarely caused by corticotroph cell hyperplasia, the vast majority of cases are caused by an ACTH-producing adenoma. The incidence of the disease is 1 to 10 cases per million per year. Up to 3.5% of cases occur in the setting of MEN1 (121). However, isolated familial Cushing disease is very rare (122).

ACTH-producing tumors represent nearly 15% of all adenomas. Affected patients vary greatly in age (peak incidence is 30 to 40 years), and the female-to-male ratio is 8:1. Blood ACTH levels may be high but are generally less than 200 pg/mL. To document the pituitary source of ACTH at petrosal sinus sampling, a pituitary-peripheral gradient greater than 2 establishes the diagnosis of Cushing disease. A low value, especially after corticotropin-releasing hormone (CRH) stimulation, indicates

an extrapituitary source. Although adrenal insufficiency is associated with nodular ACTH cell hyperplasia, "tumorlets," and even small adenomas, adrenal failure (Addison disease) plays no clinically significant role in the genesis of ACTH cell adenomas (59).

Most ACTH cell tumors (87%) are microadenomas (mean size, 5 mm), but some measure no more than 1 to 2 mm. At surgery, only approximately 15% to 20% of all ACTH cell adenomas are found to be invasive (123), a factor clearly underlying persistent disease and recurrence. Invasion is directly linked to tumor size because it is much less common in microadenomas (8%) than in macroadenomas (62%). Postoperative remission is achieved in 90% of microadenomas but only 65% of macroadenomas. Thus, tumor size and invasiveness determine surgical success (124). Patients with Cushing disease die not as a result of endocrine imbalance, but of cardiac complications.

Most functional ACTH adenomas arise in the midline of the pituitary, the so-called mucoid wedge. Occasional examples are posteriorly situated and must be distinguished from clinically insignificant foci of basophil invasion. The latter cells lie enmeshed in posterior lobe axons. Of double adenomas in surgical specimens, the combination of an ACTH cell adenoma and a prolactinoma is best known (125,126). ACTH adenomas are associated with two transcription factors, neuD1 (127) and Tpit (128).

On light microscopy, ACTH adenomas are amphophilic or basophilic and often strongly PAS positive (Fig. 12.25). Immunohistochemistry shows not only the presence of ACTH, but also the presence of other hormones derived from the pro-opiomelanocortin (POMC) precursor molecule. Among these are β-lipotropin, endorphin, enkephalins, and melanocyte-stimulating hormone (MSH). The ultrastructural features of ACTH adenomas are distinctive and include an abundance of secretory granules ranging in configuration from round to heart or teardrop shaped and with varying electron density, as well as perinuclear cytoplasmic intermediate filament bundles composed of keratin (Table 12.3). Their presence explains the variable cytokeratin immunoreactivity of corticotropic adenomas. Neuronal metaplasia is rarely seen (129).

In Cushing disease, the extratumoral pituitary typically shows Crooke hyaline change, which is the result of massive perinu-

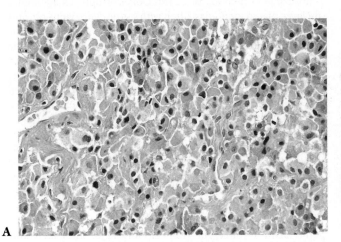 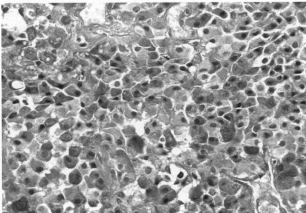

A   **B**

Figure 12.25. Corticotropic adenomas. These are amphophilic and granule rich (**A**), as well as periodic acid-Schiff positive (**B**).

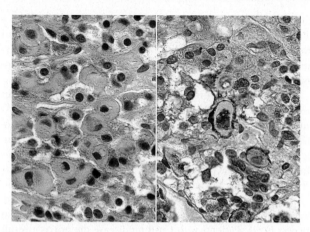

Figure 12.26. Adrenocorticotropic hormone (ACTH)–producing adenoma. Crooke hyaline change in the corticotropic cells of the nontumorous pituitary is a regular accompaniment of ACTH-producing adenomas, but it may be found in association with hypercortisolemia of any cause. The peripherally situated hyaline band (*left*) is composed of cytokeratin, and thus, it is not ACTH immunoreactive (*right*).

clear accumulation of cytokeratin filaments (Fig. 12.26). The change results from glucocorticoid feedback on the pituitary and presumably acts as a physical barrier to granule secretion. On occasion, ACTH cell adenomas per se show extensive Crooke change (130,131). Although unconfirmed, this may reflect the presence of functioning glucocorticoid receptors on adenoma cells. Crooke cell adenomas are aggressive tumors with high rates of invasion (132). Crooke cell carcinoma is rare.

NELSON SYNDROME

The lesion underlying this disorder, now decreasing in frequency, has long been said to involve a small ACTH cell adenoma, one undetectable by radiographic means and thus prompting an adrenalectomy. Continued tumor growth is then furthered by lack of inhibitory feedback effects of glucocorticoids (Nelson syndrome). An additional mechanism involves adrenalectomy after incomplete resection of an invasive macroadenoma. In any case, the tumors of Nelson syndrome are often aggressive (117). Most become or are invasive macroadenomas (123). Unlike Cushing adenomas, the adenomas of Nelson syndrome are variably PAS positive. Ultrastructurally, perinuclear cytoplasmic microfilament bundles are sparse or absent. Crooke hyaline change is lacking in extratumoral ACTH cells. At least 20% of patients with Nelson syndrome reportedly die of their tumor; a similar number are cured by surgery (117). Malignant transformation of Nelson adenomas accounts for a significant proportion of pituitary carcinomas (see "Pituitary Carcinoma" section later in this chapter) (133).

SILENT CORTICOTROPH CELL ADENOMAS

Some patients with ACTH immunoreactive tumors present without evidence of hormone excess. These uncommon "silent" variants of corticotropic adenomas occur in two forms: either basophilic (densely granulated; subtype 1) or chromophobic (sparsely granulated; subtype 2) (134). Their PAS positivity and ACTH immunoreactivity differ, being stronger in subtype 1 tumors. Both tumors are unassociated with serum ACTH elevation

or clinical signs of glucocorticoid excess. Some have suggested that silent corticotroph adenomas are incapable of hormone secretion, whereas others have found that they elaborate abnormal forms of high–molecular-weight ACTH, ACTH-related peptides (135), or endorphins (136). Silent corticotroph cell adenomas may arise from intermediate lobe corticotrophs, a cell population physiologically distinct from ACTH cells of the anterior lobe (8). The ultrastructure of these two adenoma subtypes differs (Table 12.3). Type 1 tumors resemble ordinary Cushing adenomas, whereas type 2 tumors possess far fewer and smaller granules and lack intermediate filaments. Because silent corticotroph adenomas are endocrinologically inactive and only rarely become functional (137), most grow to macroadenoma proportions and are invasive. Occasionally, in approximately 35% of cases, these tumors, particularly subtype 1 tumors, undergo spontaneous infarction (pituitary apoplexy). Silent adenomas are more aggressive and recur more often than those of Cushing disease.

EXTRAPITUITARY DISEASE AND ADRENOCORTICOTROPIN HORMONE EXCESS

In 10% to 25% of cases, Cushing syndrome is the result of ectopic ACTH production by a neoplasm, most often a neuroendocrine tumor of the lung, such as a bronchial carcinoid tumor or a small-cell carcinoma. In such instances, ACTH levels are markedly elevated, and the adrenal glands undergo massive cortical hyperplasia. The pituitary, which is normal in size, shows only Crooke hyaline change. Ectopic production of CRH by neuroendocrine tumors has also been reported. In such instances, the pituitary shows marked ACTH cell hyperplasia (138).

GONADOTROPH CELL ADENOMA

Tumors producing LH and FSH are relatively common and represent the majority of nonfunctioning adenomas. Gonadotroph derived, they are well characterized in both morphologic (139) and clinical (140,141) terms. Few are associated with MEN1 (142). Most occur in older adults, with men being preferentially affected. Elevation of serum LH and FSH levels is best seen in males because physiologic elevation of gonadotropins is normal after menopause (143). Gonadotroph cell adenomas are large macroadenomas, often with suprasellar extension, and they cause pressure-related neurologic and visual symptoms (72%), as well as hypopituitarism (67%) (141). Radiographic or gross apparent invasiveness is noted in only 20% to 30% of cases (123,141). Only approximately 5% of gonadotropic adenomas require reoperation (140). Pituitary apoplexy is a recognized complication. Not surprisingly, occasional examples are incidental findings.

Unlike normal gonadotrophs, the adenoma cells are polygonal to elongated. Some are diffuse in pattern, but others show perivascular pseudorosettes or even papillae. Chromophobic or oncocytic, they contain only scant, peripherally situated, PAS-positive granules. Immunostains show reactivity for FSH and/or LH and often for the α-subunit as well. Chromogranin staining is strong. MIB-1 labeling is typically low (<3%). Steroidogenic factor 1 (SF1), the transcription factor associated with gonadotrophs, is also demonstrable (144). Ultrastructurally, gonadotroph cell adenomas feature polar cells with process formation and small numbers of minute secretory granules disposed beneath the plasmalemma. Inexplicably, gonadotroph cell adenomas in men differ from those in women. The latter exhibits the characteristic "honeycomb transformation" of Golgi complexes (Table 12.3) (139). Because gonadotroph cell adenomas share many features of null cell adenoma, including frequent oncocytic change and scant LH/FSH immunoreactivity (145), their distinction may not be possible on immunostains alone.

THYROTROPH CELL ADENOMA

Thyrotropic tumors are the least common of the pituitary adenomas. The majority of these adenomas occur in adults and affect females (146). TSH-producing adenomas are seen in the setting of MEN1 and Carney complex, some as plurihormonal lesions (147,148). Most arise in the setting of hyper- or hypothyroidism (149–151). For example, one autopsy study showed that both TSH cell hyperplasia and an increase in TSH-containing adenomas accompany hypothyroidism (60). A significant number cause elevated serum TSH levels in association with normal triiodothyronine and thyroxine levels, a condition termed "inappropriate TSH elevation" (152). Administration of thyrotropin-releasing hormone does not further increase TSH levels, thus distinguishing TSH adenoma from pituitary resistance to thyroid hormone. In the setting of hypothyroidism, combined TSH and PRL cell hyperplasia causes pituitary enlargement that may mimic an adenoma (see below) (153). Most TSH adenomas are invasive (75%) and aggressive (146). Thus, medical therapy and/or radiotherapy are often required.

Most TSH adenomas are invasive macroadenomas, and some are sclerotic in texture. The majority of these adenomas are chromophobic tumors showing only mild PAS positivity. In addition to containing TSH (Fig. 12.27), most are also immunoreactive for α-subunit. Ultrastructurally, their cells resemble normal thyrotrophs, featuring processes containing microtubules, prominence of lysosomes, and sparse, minute secretory granules (Table 12.3).

NULL CELL ADENOMA

Approximately 20% of all pituitary adenomas show no clinical and only scant or no immunocytochemical evidence of hormone production (154). Despite synaptophysin and chromogranin staining and the presence of secretory granules, such tumors are relatively devoid of organelles and lack specific differentiation—hence the term *null cell adenoma*. The synonym *undifferentiated cell adenoma* that was once applied should be avoided because it wrongly implies anaplasia and aggressive behavior. Whether null cell adenomas represent a distinct clinicopathologic entity is unsettled. Increasingly sensitive immunohistochemical methods suggest a relationship to gonadotropic adenomas (145,155–157). Interestingly, no transcription factor staining has been demonstrated (158).

Most null cell adenomas occur after age 40 and come to clinical attention as a result of mass effects. Thus, the majority of patients show laboratory evidence of hypopituitarism. Virtually all null cell adenomas are macroadenomas, but only a minority (40%) are radiographically or grossly invasive (123,141). Thus, their prognosis is favorable, with a recurrence rate of approximately 10% (141,159). No association with MEN1 or Carney complex has been found.

At the light microscopic level, null cell adenomas are PAS negative and, depending on mitochondrial content, either chromophobic or acidophilic (oncocytic) (Fig. 12.28) (24,160). The latter distinction is of no clinical significance; thus, the designation "pituitary oncocytoma" is of no utility. Furthermore, other adenomas, such as acidophil stem cell and gonadotroph adenomas, may also be oncocytic. Immunoreactivity for pituitary hormones, if present, takes the form of α-subunit or scant LH/FSH staining. MIB-1 labeling indices are low (161). Ultrastructurally, null cell adenomas contain only sparse, small, subplasmalemmal secretory granules in association with poorly developed organelles (Table 12.3).

SILENT ADENOMA, SUBTYPE 3

Truly unclassifiable pituitary adenomas are rare. Most are plurihormonal and exhibit unusual hormone combinations (95). At

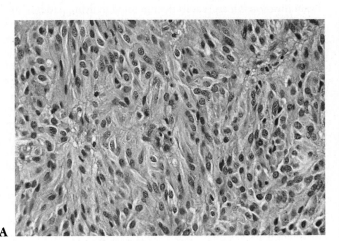
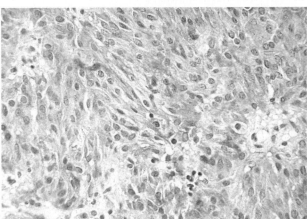

A   **B**

Figure 12.27. Thyrotropic adenoma. Glycoprotein adenomas often contain spindle-shaped cells (**A**), and they show little or no periodic acid-Schiff reactivity. In this example, the immunoreaction for thyroid-stimulating hormone varies in intensity (**B**).

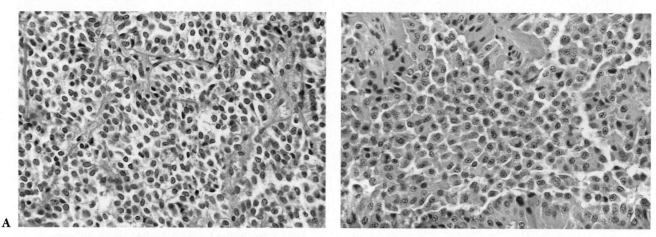

Figure 12.28. Null cell adenoma. These are typically chromophobic (**A**), but they may also be oncocytic as a result of mitochondrial accumulation (**B**), which is a finding of no clinical importance. Null cell tumors show little or no immunoreactivity.

least one other characterized adenoma of unknown cytogenesis occurs with some regularity. This adenoma, termed *silent adenoma, subtype 3* (162), was once included among variants of silent corticotroph cell adenoma. The tumor shows no sex predilection but differs in presentation by gender. In female patients, it usually occurs between 20 and 35 years of age and often mimics prolactinoma. In men, most present as nonfunctioning macroadenomas, but a minority are associated with acromegaly. Histologically, most subtype 3 adenomas are chromophobic, with their sizable cells showing some degree of nuclear pleomorphism and nucleolar prominence. PAS stains are usually negative. Minor positivity for any pituitary hormone may be seen, particularly PRL, GH, and/or TSH, but some are immunonegative. ACTH staining is rare. Electron microscopy shows polar cells, which is suggestive of glycoprotein differentiation (Table 12.3), in addition to pleomorphic nuclei containing multiple spheridia. Both rough and smooth endoplasmic reticula are abundant, whereas secretory granules are sparse and small.

The behavior of silent adenoma, subtype 3, is aggressive, with a rather high frequency of invasion and of recurrence (162,163). Despite frequent PRL immunoexpression, dopamine agonist treatment is ineffective.

INVASIVE AND ATYPICAL ADENOMAS

As previously noted, radiographic or grossly evident invasion of the dura or of sellar bone is commonly observed in pituitary adenomas. Although its overall incidence is 35%, the frequency of invasion varies from 20% to 80%, depending on tumor type (Table 12.2) (123). Because microscopic dural invasion (Fig. 12.14) is of little clinical significance, being seen in 80% to 95% of sampled paratumoral dura, and is related to tumor size (58), only radiographic or grossly apparent invasion is considered relevant with regard to tumor recurrence and treatment planning.

The term *atypical adenoma* was coined to denote tumors that, based on mitotic activity, MIB-1 labeling, and p53 immunoexpression, were likely to be invasive (38,41) and, presumably, recur. The relationship of such atypia to actual recurrence re-

mains to be confirmed (36). The molecular genetic basis of aggressive and/or invasive behavior is becoming better understood.

PITUITARY CARCINOMA

Pituitary carcinomas are rare; only approximately 100 cases have been reported (164–168). Like adenomas, they are derived from secretory cells of the pituitary. Most occur in gradual transition from typical or atypical, often invasive macroadenomas. The latency period is generally 5 to 10 years. Few arise de novo. Only adults have been affected. Most pituitary carcinomas and their metastases are endocrinologically functional, with PRL or ACTH being the principal products (133,169); TSH carcinoma is very uncommon (170). Nonfunctioning tumors, such as silent corticotropic, gonadotropic, and null cell adenomas, comprise approximately 20% of pituitary carcinomas (167,168,171). The designation "pituitary carcinoma" is predicated on the finding of one or more of the following: (a) discontinuous spread within the cerebrospinal space; (b) extracranial metastases, typically to liver, bone, lymph node, or lung, by way of the bloodstream or lymphatics; or (c) gross brain invasion. Of these parameters, brain invasion is least readily documented in living patients and therefore contestable as a criterion. Whether a diagnosis of pituitary carcinoma can be made in the absence of these features remains to be seen (30,167). Light microscopic or cytologic features alone are of little use in establishing the diagnosis of carcinoma. Although cytologic atypia and a brisk mitotic index are predictive of aggressive behavior, some show neither. Nonetheless, significant differences between adenoma, invasive adenoma, and pituitary carcinoma have been documented in terms of presence of mitotic activity, percentage of cells in mitosis (40), MIB-1 labeling (38), and p53 expression (41). Ultrastructural studies of pituitary carcinomas often show some loss of differentiation (172). Neuronal metaplasia is rarely seen (173). Even an example of ectopic pituitary carcinoma has been described (174).

To some extent, the prognosis of pituitary carcinoma varies in relation to histologic grade. One sizable study found that 66% of patients died within 1 year of the first metastasis (167). Another study found that 80% of all patients died within 8 years (167). The diagnosis most appropriate for tumors with cytological malignant features but without metastatic disease remains to be determined (175).

PITUITARY ADENOMA WITH NEURONAL METAPLASIA (GANGLIOCYTOMA)

As noted earlier, neurons are occasionally found within the substance of pituitary adenomas (103). Most are sparsely granulated GH-producing adenomas associated with acromegaly. The neurons in such tumors often produce GHRH (103). Similarly, CRH-producing neurons have been observed with Cushing disease (129). The light microscopic, ultrastructural, and immunocytologic features of the neurons vary in terms of cell size, nuclear number, and content of Nissl substance (Fig. 12.29). Such lesions were once termed *adenohypophyseal neuronal choristoma* because the neurons were thought to be heterotopic and implicated in the genesis of the adenoma (176). More recent studies indicate that the neurons arise by metaplasia from adenoma cells (103) because they contain not only neurofilament protein, synaptophysin, and chromogranin, but also hypothalamic-releasing hormones and the same pituitary hormones as the associated adenoma. Occasional keratin staining of the neurons also supports the metaplasia concept. In addition, ultrastructure demonstrates the presence of cells with features intermediate between those of adenoma cells and neurons (103). The behavior of such lesions is that of the underlying adenoma. Neuronal metaplasia is rarely seen in pituitary carcinoma (173). Lastly, not all sellar gangliocytic lesions are associated with adenoma.

SPINDLE CELL ONCOCYTOMA

This rare, only recently described (177) tumor of adulthood simulates a nonfunctioning pituitary macroadenoma, often with conspicuous suprasellar extension. It consists of mitochondria-rich, spindle and epithelioid cells with variable atypia, but only rarely mitotic activity, increased MIB-1 labeling, or necrosis (Fig. 12.30). The immunotype includes staining for vimentin, epithelial membrane antigen (EMA), S-100 protein, galectin 3, and annexin 1. Synaptophysin stains are negative, and granules are absent or nearly so at the ultrastructural level. Spindle cell oncocytomas may be derived from the folliculostellate cells of the anterior pituitary. Most behave in a benign manner, but recurrences can be seen. Only exceptional examples undergo invasive, destructive growth (178,179).

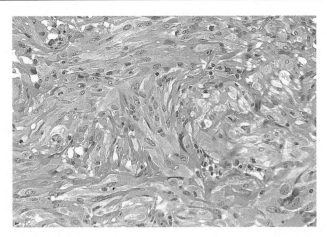

Figure 12.30. Spindle cell oncocytoma. This rare spindle and epithelioid neoplasm of the sella may be derived from folliculostellate cells.

PITUITARY HYPERPLASIA

The most common cause of pituitary hyperplasia is pregnancy, during which PRL cells undergo reversible hypertrophy and proliferation in association with transdifferentiation of GH to PRL cells (180,181).

Clinically significant hyperplasia of adenohypophyseal cells is very uncommon (Table 12.4) (18). With regard to GH excess, it is seen most often in the setting of GHRH-induced acromegaly (112–116) and is the mechanism underlying gigantism (182). Pituitary hyperplasia is seen in several inherited conditions, including the McCune-Albright syndrome (183) and Carney complex (15,184). It is also the basis of Cushing syndrome because of ectopic CRH production (120) and is seen in Addison disease (59). Pituitary enlargement caused by TSH and PRL cell hyperplasia occurs in hypothyroidism (60,153). Rare causes of pituitary hyperplasia include idiopathic hypothalamic dysfunction (185) and hypothalamic neuronal hamartoma (186).

Given the regional variation in cell distribution within the normal adenohypophysis, a diagnosis of diffuse hyperplasia is

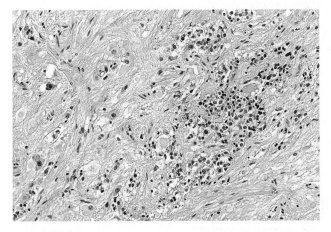

Figure 12.29. Gangliocytoma of the pituitary. This was composed of hypothalamic-type neurons situated within the substance of a growth hormone cell adenoma. Immunostains show that the neurons contain growth hormone–releasing hormone.

TABLE 12.4

Pituitary Hyperplasia

Prolactin cell
   Pregnancy and lactation
   Estrogen treatment
   Hypothyroidism (thyrotropin-releasing hormone effect)
   Cushing disease (uncommon)
Growth hormone cell
   Hypothalamic neuronal hamartoma (growth hormone–releasing hormone)
   Neuroendocrine neoplasm (ectopic growth hormone-releasing hormone)
Corticotroph cell
   Neuroendocrine neoplasm (corticotropin-releasing hormone)
   Addison's disease (corticotrophin-releasing hormone effect)
Gonadotroph cell
   Klinefelter and Turner syndrome
   Hypothalamic neuronal hamartoma (luteinizing hormone-releasing hormone)
Thyrotroph cell
   Hypothyroidism (thyrotropin-releasing hormone effect)

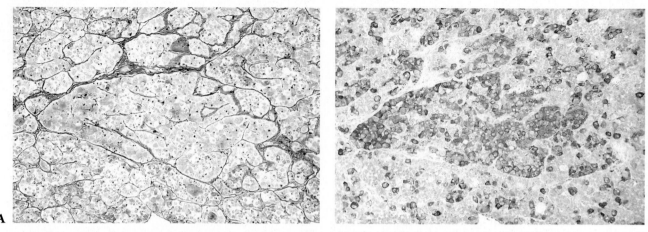

A   **B**

Figure 12.31. Adrenocorticotropic hormone (ACTH) cell hyperplasia. This case of idiopathic ACTH cell hyperplasia, which is presumably caused by hypothalamic dysfunction, illustrates the expansion of the acinar pattern on reticulin stain **(A)** and a corresponding marked increase of ACTH immunoreactive cells **(B)**. Such hyperplastic nodules were present throughout the serially sectioned gland.

impossible to make on a limited biopsy. It requires cell counts on hypophysectomy or autopsy specimens. Even nodular hyperplasia, particularly of the ACTH cells, poses a diagnostic challenge because such cells are normally disposed in small nodules. Microscopically, nodular pituitary hyperplasia consists of an increase in a specific cell type with associated expansion of acini, a feature best appreciated on reticulin stain (Fig. 12.31). When the causes are successfully treated, resolution of the hyperplasia and shrinkage of the sella ensue.

MISCELLANEOUS SELLAR TUMORS AND CYSTS

The histopathologic spectrum of nonadenomatous sellar lesions is highly varied. Only the most common are specifically discussed. Unusual processes are summarized and referenced in Table 12.5. The immunohistochemical differential diagnosis of frequently occurring sellar tumors that mimic pituitary adenoma is presented in Table 12.6.

TABLE 12.5	Miscellaneous Lesions of the Pituitary and Sellar Region
Benign neoplasms	**Vascular lesions**
Pituitary adenoma (2,3,5,24,30,268)	Pituitary infarction (234,283)
Meningioma (269)	Pituitary apoplexy (69,70)
Postirradiation meningioma (270)	Aneurysm (284)
Craniopharyngioma, adamantinomatous (187,190,193)	**Cysts**
Craniopharyngioma, papillary (193,197)	Rathke cleft cyst (199–204)
Granular cell tumor (207,209,210)	Epidermoid cyst (285,286)
Pituicytoma (215–217)	Dermoid cyst (287)
Glomangioma (273)	**Malignant neoplasms**
Gangliocytoma of pituitary (129)	Chordoma (288,289)
Hypothalamic neuronal hamartoma (186)	Germ cell tumors (290)
Schwannoma (271)	Hemangiopericytoma (291)
Paraganglioma (272)	Postirradiation neoplasms (66,67)
Glomangioma (273)	Metastatic carcinoma (223)
Spindle cell oncocytoma (177)	Metastatic carcinoma to pituitary adenoma (230)
Histiocytosis X (218)	Metastatic lymphoma and/or leukemia (228,229)
Hemangioma (274)	Plasmacytoma (292,293)
Hemangioblastoma (275)	**Infectious diseases**
Myxoma (276)	Bacterial abscess (64,192,205)
Fibrous dysplasia of bone	Tuberculosis
Giant cell tumor of bone (277)	Fungal abscess (294)
Inflammatory disorders	Cysticercosis (295)
Mucocele (278)	Hydatid cyst (296)
Lymphocytic hypophysitis (236,239,279)	**Medical diseases**
Sarcoidosis (280)	Hemosiderosis and/or hemochromatosis (297)
Giant cell granuloma (281,282)	Mucopolysaccharidoses (298)
Erdheim-Chester disease (218)	**Physical injury**
Rosai-Dorfman disease (260,261)	Trauma (299)
	Radionecrosis (300)

TABLE 12.6 Immunohistochemistry of Sellar Region Tumors

Tumor	Periodic Acid-Schiff/ Diastase	Pituitary Hormones	Epithelial Membrane Antigen	Cytokeratin (CK)	S-100 Protein	Synaptophysin (SYN)	Chromogranin	Carcinoembryonic Antigen (CEA)	Placental Alkaline Phosphatase	Leukocyte Common Antigen	Vimentin	Other Markers
Pituitary adenoma	+/+; (ACTH > LH, FSH, TSH)	+ (Null cell – except α-subunit)	+ (ACTH)	+ (ACTH & GH)	–	+	+ (Null cell, LH/FSH, TSH)	–	–	–	–	–
Metastatic carcinoma	±	–	+	+	±	±	±	±	±	–	±	–
Lymphoma	–	–	–	–	–	–	–	–	–	+	–	CD20, CD3, CD30
Plasmacytoma or myeloma	± (30%)	–	±	±	–	–	–	–	–	±	–	CD138 MUM1, kappa & lambda
Germinoma	+/–	–	–	± (10%–20%)	–	–	–	–	+	–	± (15%)	CD117, Oct 4
Pituicytoma	–	–	±	–	+	–	–	–	–	–	+	GFAP, TTF1
Spindle cell oncocytoma	–	–	+	–	+	–	–	–	–	–	+	Galectin 3, annexin 1
Granular cell tumor	+/+	–	–	–	+	–	–	±[a]	–	–	+	CD68
Langerhans cell histiocytosis	–	–	–	–	+	–	–	–	–	–	–	CD1a, langerin
Chordoma	+/–	–	+	+[b]	+	–	–	± (10%)	–	–	+	Brachyury
Meningioma	±[b]	–	+	±[b]	±	–	–	±[b]	–	–	+	Progesterone receptor
Hemangiopericytoma	–	–	–	–	–	–	–	–	–	–	+	CD34, BCL2, CD99

[a] Nonspecific reaction with lysosomes.

[b] Secretory variant of meningioma contains PAS positive pseudopsammoma bodies; surrounding cells are CEA reactive and CK reactive.

ACTH, adrenocorticotropic hormone-producing adenoma; FSH, follicle-stimulating hormone-producing adenoma; GH, growth hormone-producing adenoma; LH, luteinizing hormone-producing adenoma; TSH, thyrotrophic hormone-producing adenoma.

ADAMANTINOMATOUS CRANIOPHARYNGIOMA

Craniopharyngiomas represent 1% to 2% of all intracranial neoplasms and are the most common tumor of childhood and adolescence. More than 50% of patients are less than 20 years old. Only rare congenital examples are seen in neonates. Craniopharyngiomas are histologically related to Rathke cleft cysts because both are derived from the pituitary anlage. Most adamantinomatous craniopharyngiomas are suprasellar. Although 25% have an intrasellar component, purely intrasellar examples are uncommon (187). Rare examples are situated entirely within the nasopharynx, sphenoid bone, a sinus, or even the optic chiasm.

Averaging 3 to 4 cm in diameter, craniopharyngiomas produce compressive effects, including visual disturbance, hydrocephalus, endocrine abnormalities such as growth retardation, diabetes insipidus, and hyperprolactinemia caused by stalk effect. Sites of extension include the third ventricle; less often the anterior, middle, or posterior fossae; and rarely the nasopharynx. Most are adherent to adjacent brain tissue. Approximately 85% feature cysts containing cholesterol-rich fluid likened to machine oil. Calcifications are often radiographically evident, but bone formation is uncommon. Tooth formation, a pathologic curiosity (188), underscores the similarity of craniopharyngioma to adamantinoma.

The histologic appearance of adamantinomatous craniopharyngiomas is diagnostic (Fig. 12.32). They consist of complex epithelium-producing "wet keratin," calcific debris, cholesterol crystals, and fibrous stroma. Whereas the diagnosis can be made based on finding the characteristic epithelium or wet keratin, a presumptive diagnosis can be made based on cholesterol-rich, xanthogranulomatous tissue alone. The notion that xanthogranuloma of the sellar region (189) is a distinct entity is questionable. It may be simply a manifestation of tissue degeneration, generally in a cystic tumor, such as craniopharyngioma or Rathke cleft cyst. Unlike epidermoid cysts, which feature orderly maturation of a thin layer of squamous epithelium with resultant wafer-thin squamous cells, craniopharyngiomas demonstrate a complex, epithelial growth in cords and islands. A layer of tall, basaloid epithelium surrounds the islands of obviously squamoid cells, which in turn undergo transition to loose tissue termed *stellate reticulum* and wet keratin (Fig. 12.32). The pro-

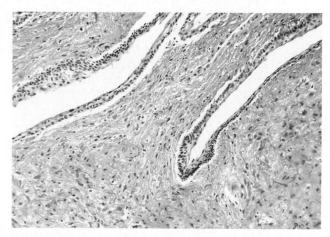

Figure 12.33. Craniopharyngioma. These typically incite marked gliosis in the adjacent brain parenchyma, and the gliosis should not be mistaken for glioma. The irregular tumor configuration results in the pseudoinvasion of their surroundings.

cess of keratinization differs from that of epidermoid cysts because it is not associated with a granular layer. Craniopharyngiomas directly abut brain parenchyma, producing an irregular interface that resembles parenchymal invasion and is associated with gliosis that may be so pronounced that it mimics pilocytic astrocytoma (Fig. 12.33).

Occasional craniopharyngiomas show a mixed pattern of adamantinomatous and, to a lesser extent, ordinary stratified squamous epithelium (Fig. 12.34) (190). This explains the occasional difficulty in distinguishing a limited biopsy of craniopharyngioma from epidermoid cyst. Squamous metaplasia in a Rathke cleft cyst may pose a similar problem. Melanin formation is a curiosity (191). Superimposed abscess formation is a rare complication of craniopharyngioma (192).

Although craniopharyngiomas are benign, their often incomplete excision results in frequent recurrence (193). Factors associated with recurrence include cytologic atypia and mitotic activity, tumor size exceeding 3 cm, and abnormalities of cerebrospinal fluid (CSF). Intracranial spread by way of CSF is rare (194), but surgical implantation may be seen (195). Although

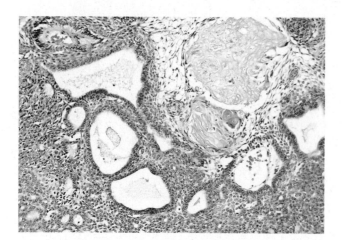

Figure 12.32. Craniopharyngioma. This example shows the typical complex pattern of squamous epithelial growth ranging from dense to loose with peripheral palisading, microcyst formation, and keratinization.

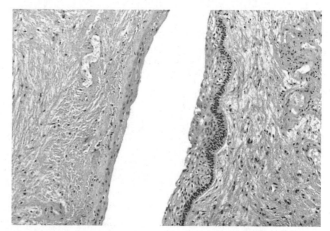

Figure 12.34. Craniopharyngioma. This neoplasm had a biphasic growth pattern consisting of typical adamantinoma-like, as well as ordinary, stratified squamous epithelium. A small biopsy from such a lesion may be mistaken for an epidermoid cyst.

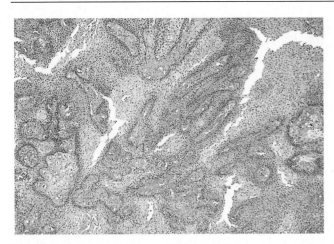

Figure 12.35. Craniopharyngioma, papillary type. Note the prominent stratified squamous component, the lack of cholesterol-rich debris, and the formation of papillae.

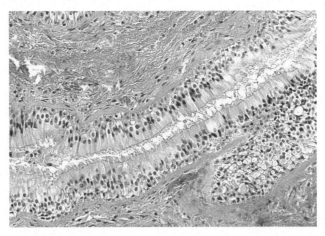

Figure 12.36. Rathke cleft cyst. The unilocular structure is lined by columnar, ciliated, and mucin-producing epithelium. Secretory adenohypophyseal cells are occasionally identified.

the treatment of craniopharyngiomas is primarily surgical, radiation therapy does play a role. Malignant transformation to squamous cell carcinoma is rare (196).

PAPILLARY CRANIOPHARYNGIOMA

Comprising 10% of craniopharyngiomas, the papillary variant of craniopharyngioma is distinctive. It affects adults and often involves or lies within the third ventricle. Furthermore, it contains clear fluid and lacks calcifications (197). Microscopically, the sheets of mature squamous epithelium dehisce, forming perivascular pseudopapillae. Little or no keratin production is seen (Fig. 12.35). Unlike the irregular interface of adamantinomatous craniopharyngiomas with the adjacent brain, papillary tumors are smoothly contoured and separate more readily. As a result, less than 10% of papillary tumors recur (193,197). Rare examples of intracranial metastasis by way of the CSF or surgical implantation have been documented (198).

RATHKE CLEFT CYST

These distinctive cysts originate in remnants of the Rathke pouch, which is a normal microscopic finding at the interface of the anterior and posterior lobes (199). Symptomatic Rathke cleft cysts are uncommon. Most measure 1 cm or more (200–204). With continued growth, they produce visual disturbance, hypopituitarism, or diabetes insipidus. Stalk section effect often results in hyperprolactinemia.

Histologically, Rathke cleft cysts are thin walled, contain mucoid fluid, and are lined by a variety of epithelia, including cuboidal to columnar, ciliated or goblet cells, as well as occasional adenohypophyseal cells (Fig. 12.36). Given the high frequency of subclinical pituitary adenomas (10), the finding of an occasional Rathke cleft cyst in association with an adenoma is not surprising. Squamous metaplasia may supervene. The same is true of xanthogranulomatous change, which may totally obscure the cyst lining. Abscess formation is a rare complication of Rathke cleft cyst (205,206). The prognosis of surgically treated cysts is excellent; even subtotal resection is curative (204).

NEURONAL AND GLIAL LESIONS OF THE SELLAR REGION

HYPOTHALAMIC NEURONAL HAMARTOMA

On rare occasions, hamartomas composed of hypothalamic neurons form clinically symptomatic suprasellar masses (Fig. 12.37). Many are associated with endocrine dysfunction, most often precocious puberty caused by the production of luteinizing hormone–releasing hormone (LHRH) (185). Others may elaborate GHRH and become associated with acromegaly (115). The pituitary may show either hyperplasia or an adenoma of the LH/FSH or GH cells (176). Hypothalamic neuronal hamartoma are benign. Resection, when possible, is curative. These are readily distinguished from ganglioglioma by their resemblance to normal hypothalamic tissue (Fig. 12.37) and lack of an astrocytic component.

GRANULAR CELL TUMOR

Most granular cell tumors affecting the pituitary are asymptomatic and arise in the stalk or posterior lobe. Such incidental,

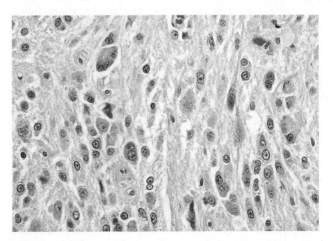

Figure 12.37. Hypothalamic neuronal hamartoma. The ganglion cells of this large lesion, which was present for more than 40 years, were engaged in the production of growth hormone–releasing hormone. An associated growth hormone cell adenoma was found, presumably the result of long-term stimulation.

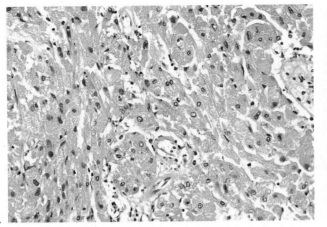
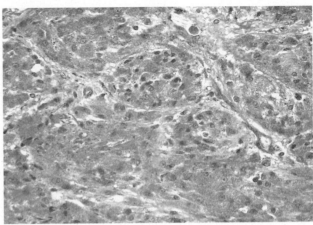

A

B

Figure 12.38. Granular cell tumor of the pituitary stalk **(A)**. This nodular mass, lying largely in the suprasellar area, was associated with hyperprolactinemia as a result of "stalk effect." Such tumor cells are filled with periodic acid-Schiff–positive lysosomes **(B)**.

microscopic "tumorlettes" are seen in 10% to 17% of autopsies (207,208). Multifocality is common. Their cellular origin is from pituicytes, which are functionally specialized, osmosensitive astrocytes of the neurohypophysis. In contrast, symptomatic granular cell tumors of the neurohypophysis are rare, with less than 100 having been reported to date. They exhibit no diagnostic clinical or radiographic features and are hormonally inactive (209–213). Their peak incidence is in the fifth decade, and the female-to-male ratio is 2:1. Symptoms include mass effects, such as visual field defects, hypopituitarism, and diabetes insipidus resulting from stalk effect. Hyperprolactinemia is also common. On magnetic resonance imaging (MRI), granular cell tumors are solid, markedly enhancing, noncalcified, intra- or suprasellar masses simulating pituitary adenomas. At surgery, they are firm, gray-tan, and prone to bleed. Although granular cell tumors are generally benign, they may slowly recur and are occasionally aggressive, exhibiting increased MIB-1 labeling and p53 immunoreactivity (213). Aggressive surgery and adjuvant irradiation improve survival (212).

Granular cell tumors of the pituitary consist of large, polygonal cells that form sheets or ill-defined lobules and that possess round, peripherally situated nuclei with delicate chromatin and uniform nucleoli (Fig. 12.38). Cytoplasmic granularity is prominent as a result of an abundance of PAS-positive, diastase-resistant lysosomes (Fig. 12.38). Mitoses are absent. Lymphocytic infiltrates may be focally evident. The principal differential diagnosis is a pituitary adenoma with oncocytic features. Pituitary adenomas lack significant PAS positivity and are filled with phosphotungstic acid hematoxylin (PTAH)–positive mitochondria. Conversely, granular cell tumors lack synaptophysin staining and show cytoplasmic NSE and CD68 immunoreactivity (214). GFAP and S-100 protein reactivity may be weak or negative. Electron microscopy shows the organelle-poor cells to contain abundant lysosomes, some of which are engaged in autophagocytosis. Secretory granules are absent.

PITUICYTOMA

This well-differentiated glial neoplasm of the sellar or suprasellar area arises from pituicytes, which are functionally specialized glia of the posterior pituitary. Clinically, it affects mainly adults; presents with headaches, visual disturbance, and hypopituitarism; and mimics the radiographic and operative appearance of pituitary adenoma. Only rarely has it occurred in association

with MEN1 (215). Radiographically, pituicytomas are well circumscribed, solid, and contrast enhancing. Microscopically, they are noninfiltrative and composed of vague lobules and sheets of spindled cells with relatively abundant cytoplasm and round-to-oval nuclei. They are somewhat fascicular or swirling in architecture (Fig. 12.39) and appear astrocytic. Atypia is minimal, and mitoses are exceptional. Immunostains show strong reactivity for S-100 protein, vimentin, and TTF1 but generally less or little staining for GFAP. Ultrastructurally, the cells possess processes and contain intermediate filaments but lack surface specialization such as microvilli or cilia. The differential diagnosis includes normal neurohypophysis, which can be mimicked by hypocellular pituicytomas and pilocytic astrocytomas. Also in the differential diagnosis is spindle cell oncocytoma, a tumor composed of spindle and epithelioid cells lacking immunoreactivity for GFAP and instead showing staining for S-100 protein and EMA. The distinction from normal adenohypophysis rests on finding abundant axons, some with swellings (Herring bodies). The distinction from pilocytic astrocytoma usually depends on finding biphasic (compact and microcystic) architecture in association with Rosenthal fibers and granular bodies, all of which are alien to pituicytoma. The biologic behavior of pituicy-

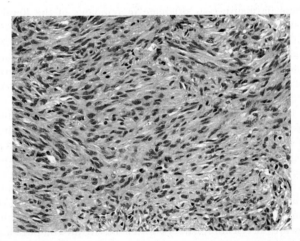

Figure 12.39. Pituicytoma. This distinctive glial neoplasm consists of spindle cells often disposed in a tufted pattern (hematoxylin and eosin, 250× magnification).

Chapter 12 • The Pituitary and Sellar Region 485

tomas suggests that they are benign but capable of slow recurrence after subtotal resection (216,217).

MISCELLANEOUS TUMORS

LANGERHANS CELL HISTIOCYTOSIS

Although variants of Langerhans histiocytosis include eosinophilic granuloma, Hand-Schüller-Christian disease, and Letterer-Siwe disease, only approximately 50% are readily classifiable according to this scheme (218). Involvement of the nervous system is seen in approximately 25% of cases and is almost always associated with bony lesions. Because the disorder involves mainly the hypothalamus, pituitary stalk, and posterior lobe, diabetes insipidus is a constant. Hypothalamic dysfunction that is permanent in nature is also frequent; this is particularly true of GH deficiency (219). Isolated infundibular involvement is rare (220). Anatomically, the anterior lobe is spared.

Making a histologic diagnosis may be difficult because the disease passes through stages. In active lesions, the histiocytes are associated with giant cells, lymphocytes, plasma cells, eosinophils in greatly varying numbers, and reactive astrocytes (Fig. 12.40). The Langerhans histiocytes, which are characterized by their large, folded nuclei, are immunoreactive for the nonspecific markers of S-100 protein and CD1A, as well as Langerin (CD207), a relatively specific marker associated with the formation of Birbeck granules (221). Reactivity for S-100 protein is not always seen. The same is true of the ultrastructurally diagnostic Birbeck granules.

SALIVARY GLAND–LIKE TUMORS OF THE SELLAR REGION

A spectrum of salivary gland–like neoplasms rarely occurs in the sellar region (222). These neoplasms are no doubt linked to salivary gland rests normally occurring at this location. Such glands typically reside on the superior aspect of the gland overlying the posterior lobe. Secondary involvement of the sella and perisellar structures by locally invasive or malignant salivary gland tumors is very uncommon.

METASTATIC NEOPLASMS

Pituitary/sellar metastases, particularly of mammary, lung, or gastrointestinal carcinoma, are often encountered at autopsy (223,224). In contrast, symptomatic deposits are very uncommon in the absence of a known primary (225). In one series, metastases masquerading as primary tumors prompted less than 1% of surgeries for pituitary adenoma (225). Patients are typically middle age or older and are often female. Symptoms include visual disturbance, hypopituitarism, and diabetes insipidus. The posterior lobe is more often affected given its direct arterial supply. Involvement of the anterior lobe is secondary from surrounding affected bone and/or dura or from posterior lobe deposits (Fig. 12.41). Microscopically, anterior lobe involvement consists of permeation of sinusoidal vessels and/or filling of acini. Because symptomatic pituitary/sellar metastases are a manifestation of late-stage disease, the prognosis is poor, even after surgical decompression and radiotherapy (225).

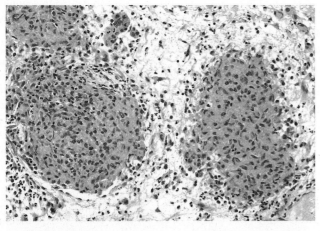

A

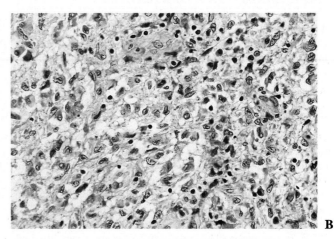

B

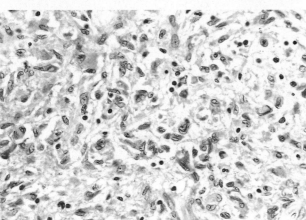

C

Figure 12.40. Langerhans cell histiocytosis. The infiltrate, which affects the hypothalamus, pituitary stalk, and posterior lobe, consists of Langerhans histiocytes forming either epithelioid clusters (**A**) or diffuse infiltrates (**B**). Such cells are S-100 protein immunoreactive (**C**).

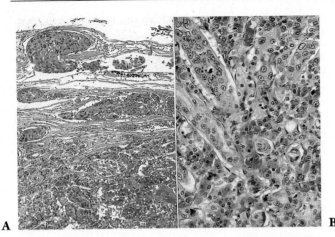

A   **B**

Figure 12.41. Metastatic carcinoma. The involvement of sellar bone and dura **(A)** usually precedes involvement of the anterior lobe, wherein sinuses are often filled by tumor **(B)**.

Lymphoma is rarely primary in the pituitary and/or sellar region (226). One such lesion reportedly arose in a pituitary adenoma (227). Secondary involvement of the pituitary in acute and chronic leukemia is more often an autopsy finding (228,229). On rare occasion, metastases are found within the substance of a suddenly enlarging pituitary adenoma (230–232).

INFLAMMATORY DISORDERS

A variety of inflammatory processes affect the pituitary gland. Chief among these are lymphocytic hypophysitis, granulomatous (giant-cell hypophysitis), and xanthomatous hypophysitis (233). Each is discussed in turn in the following sections.

LYMPHOCYTIC HYPOPHYSITIS

Pituitary insufficiency of pregnancy and of the postpartum period is most often a result of hypovolemic shock with resultant capillary thrombosis and ischemic necrosis (Sheehan syndrome) (234). In recent years, however, a large number of well-documented cases of autoimmune adenohypophysitis have been reported, particularly in association with pregnancy. This was the subject of a recent comprehensive literature review (235). In one series (236), nearly 20% of women were affected during the postpartum period; of these, nearly 25% exhibited some degree of pituitary hypofunction. Combinations of PRL, ACTH, LH/FSH, and TSH deficiency may be seen. Hyperprolactinemia may also be seen in early phase disease. Humoral and cellular immune mechanisms mediate the disorder. Antipituitary antibodies are demonstrable (237). The lymphocytic infiltrate resides in the anterior pituitary and consists of B and T cells of both CD4$^+$ and CD8$^+$ type (238). In conjunction, inflammation may also occur in other endocrine organs, such as the thyroid and/or ovaries. On occasion, isolated pituitary hormone deficiency results, such as deficiency of ACTH, PRL, or TSH (239–241).

Patients typically present with postpartum pituitary failure and occasionally signs of mass effect, including headache and visual field defects (242). Males and aged females are only infre-

quently affected (243). Neuroimaging often mimics pituitary adenoma. Because pregnancy is known to cause PRL cell hyperplasia and accelerated growth of PRL cell adenomas and because hyperprolactinemia is common in lymphocytic hypophysitis, establishing the correct diagnosis requires a biopsy. Treatment consists of biopsy or decompression, as well as hormone replacement. Although surgery results in relief of headaches and improved vision, no reversal of endocrine deficits is seen; long-term hormone replacement is required (242).

Unlike the soft, creamy texture of a pituitary adenoma, the lymphocytic hypophysitis specimens are typically firm and yellow. Microsections show lymphoplasmacytic cells in the interstitium and within the acini, with necrosis lacking (Fig. 12.42). Germinal centers are occasionally seen. Although scant clusters of epithelioid histiocytes may be encountered, well-formed granulomas are not. Thus, distinguishing lymphocytic hypophysitis from sarcoidosis, giant-cell granuloma, or infection of the pituitary generally poses no problem (see following section). The same is true of the focal, clinically insignificant lymphocytic infiltrates that are occasionally observed in the normal pituitary. Lastly, T-cell–rich inflammation, possibly an antitumor immune response, has been described in a rare PRL cell adenoma (244).

GRANULOMATOUS HYPOPHYSITIS (GIANT-CELL GRANULOMA) OF THE PITUITARY

This rare, idiopathic inflammatory disorder (245–248) affects the anterior pituitary of adults but, unlike lymphocytic hypophysitis, shows no sex predilection or association with pregnancy. Hypopituitarism occurs in the majority, but diabetes insipidus does not. On occasion, the process is accompanied by a similar giant-cell reaction in other endocrine organs, including the thyroid and/or ovaries.

Unlike sarcoidosis, a systemic disease that, when involving the CNS, primarily affects the hypothalamus and posterior pituitary, granulomatous hypophysitis is limited to the sellar region, usually involving the adenohypophysis alone. Microscopically, it is characterized by well-formed, noncaseating granulomas without an appreciable lymphocytic infiltrate (Fig. 12.43). Lack of necrosis distinguishes it from tuberculosis. Organisms are not seen on special stains. Parenchymal destruction with fibrosis

Figure 12.42. Lymphocytic hypophysitis. Note the architectural disarray and the destruction of the pituitary cords as a result of lymphoplasmacytic inflammation and fibrosis.

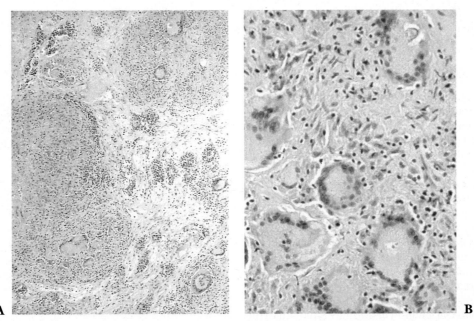

Figure 12.43. Granulomatous hypophysitis (Giant cell granuloma) of the pituitary. This noncaseating process was limited to the anterior pituitary, it contained no stainable microorganisms, and it resolved after biopsy (**A**). Resultant hypopituitarism was noted. The multinucleate giant cells show occasional Schaumann bodies (**B**).

is the end result. Nonspecific granulomatous hypophysitis may accompany rupture of a Rathke cleft cyst (249).

XANTHOMATOUS HYPOPHYSITIS

This poorly understood lesion was only recently described (250), and few reports have followed (233,251). All patients have been females with variable anterior lobe dysfunction and occasional diabetes insipidus. Often partially cystic and fluid containing, the biopsy shows infiltration by xanthic histiocytes negative for organisms. The cells are immunoreactive for CD68 but are S-100 protein and CD1A negative. No Birbeck granules are identified.

SARCOIDOSIS

This idiopathic, multisystem granulomatous disorder affects the CNS in 5% to 10% of cases. Adults are usually affected, particularly black women. Termed "neurosarcoidosis," it most often involves the basal meninges and brain parenchyma (ventricular region, optic nerves, and posterior fossa structures); hypothalamic/pituitary involvement is seen in 10% of cases. Isolated pituitary disease has been reported in only two instances (252). Lastly, one case of pituitary adenoma containing sarcoidal infiltrates has been reported (253). Neurosarcoidosis only rarely occurs in isolation; concurrent systemic disease is the rule. Hypothalamic pituitary involvement results in anterior pituitary hypofunction, diabetes insipidus, and hyperprolactinemia (254). The sella is generally not enlarged. Grossly, the specimen appears firm and yellow. Sections show noncaseating granulomatous inflammation primarily involving the leptomeninges and neural tissue. The discrete granulomas are often sur-

rounded by lymphocytic cuffs (Fig. 12.44). Although necrosis is not evident, focal fibrinoid change may be seen. Multinucleate giant cells are common, but the presence of Schaumann bodies varies greatly. By definition, special stains for microorganisms are negative. Burned-out foci appear as fibrous scars containing only occasional chronic inflammatory or histiocytic giant cells. Despite medical therapy, improvement in hormone deficiency is uncommon (254). In contrast to sarcoidosis, giant-cell granuloma of the pituitary involves the anterior lobe and is unassociated with significant systemic disease. Granulomatous hypophysitis may also follow interferon and ribavirin treatment

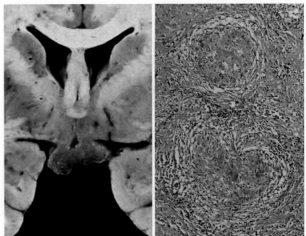

Figure 12.44. Sarcoidosis involving hypothalamus, pituitary stalk and posterior lobe. Note typical yellow discoloration of the hypothalamus (**A**) Numerous discrete noncaseating granulomas are surrounded by cuffs of lymphocytes (**B**).

(255). Lastly, a pituitary adenoma with noncaseating granulomatous inflammation has also been reported (256).

ERDHEIM-CHESTER DISEASE

This multisystem histiocytosis is characterized pathologically by xanthogranulomatous infiltrates, and it is defined clinically and radiologically by bone involvement. Symmetric sclerosis of long bones with increased uptake on bone scan is a constant and pathognomonic finding. Visceral involvement varies, but it is seen in more than half of the cases; sites commonly affected include the retroperitoneum, kidneys, orbits, skin, pericardium, and lungs. Central nervous system involvement may take the form of dural and parenchymal infiltrates affecting mainly the cerebellum and brainstem. These are diffuse or localized and are often grossly yellow. Involvement of the hypothalamus and pituitary gland is very uncommon (257,258). Posterior lobe involvement is the rule and often results in diabetes insipidus. Histopathologic verification of the diagnosis of Erdheim-Chester disease usually involves the biopsy of bone, skin, and orbital or retroperitoneal lesions. These feature S-100 and CD1a immunonegative histiocytes and Touton giant cells (Fig. 12.45). Birbeck granules are absent.

ROSAI-DORFMAN DISEASE

This uncommon disorder, first described as affecting lymph nodes, rarely also involves the pituitary and sellar region with resultant diabetes insipidus and pituitary dysfunction (259–261). Microscopy reveals S-100 protein immunopositive histiocytes showing lymphocyte emperipolesis.

EMPTY SELLA SYNDROME

Empty sella syndrome may be of the primary or secondary type. Both feature reduction in volume of sellar contents. The primary form results from chronic compression of the gland as a result of the downward herniation of the arachnoid membrane

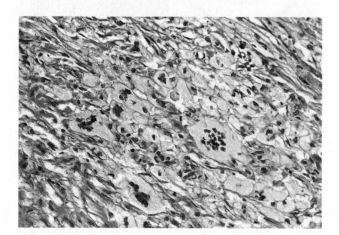

Figure 12.45. Erdheim-Chester disease. Note the macrophages and Touton-type giant cells. Such tumors lack S-100 protein and CD1a staining, as well as Birbeck granules.

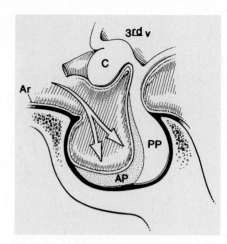

Figure 12.46. Primary empty sella syndrome. An arachnoidal diverticulum extends into the sella through an incompetent sellar diaphragm to compress the pituitary gland. Chiasmal prolapse or traction on the pituitary stalk may produce visual symptoms or hyperprolactinemia, respectively.

through an incompetent sellar diaphragm (Figs. 12.46). An association with intracranial hypertension is seen in approximately 75% of cases (262). Based on autopsy studies, nearly 50% of adults have a diaphragmatic defect measuring 5 mm or greater, with a fully developed primary empty sella being present in approximately 5% (263). The lesion is essentially an intrasellar arachnoidocele, and although sometimes not associated with pituitary dysfunction, it is mainly caused by glucocorticoid or isolated GH deficiency (264,265). Shunt placement for reduction of CSF pressure may be beneficial (262). Secondary empty sella syndrome differs. Its causes include spontaneous infarction of the gland, as occurs in postpartum pituitary necrosis (Sheehan syndrome characterized by panhypopituitarism but not diabetes insipidus) (266); surgical extirpation of a sellar tumor; hemorrhagic infarction of an adenoma (pituitary apoplexy) (267); and pituitary atrophy after irradiation of the sellar region.

Whatever the cause, empty sella syndrome may result in (a) visual field defects, some of which are caused by chiasmal prolapse, or (b) impaired pituitary function. Hyperprolactinemia may be seen a result of traction on the pituitary stalk (257). Diabetes insipidus is encountered. With the advent of modern imaging techniques, patients infrequently come to surgery. When they do, the disappointing specimen consists of little more than a fragment of arachnoid membrane. Given the relatively high frequency of subclinical pituitary adenomas in normal individuals (10), it is not surprising that empty sella syndrome is occasionally associated with a microadenoma.

ACKNOWLEDGMENT

The authors are indebted to Dr. Queenie Lau of Brisbane, Australia for her invaluable assistance and detailed editing in updating this chapter.

REFERENCES

1. Asa SL, Kovacs K, Bilbao JM. The pars tuberalis of the human pituitary. A histologic, immunohistochemical, ultrastructural and immunoelectron microscopic analysis. *Virchows Arch A Pathol Anat Histopathol* 1983;399:49–59.

2. Horvath E, Kovacs K. Ultrastructural classification of pituitary adenomas. *Can J Neurol Sci* 1976;3:9–21.
3. Horvath E, Kovacs K. The adenohypophysis. In *Functional Endocrine Pathology*. Cambridge, MA: Blackwell Scientific, 1998:247–281.
4. Ren P, Scheithauer BW, Halper J. The immunohistochemical localization of TGFa, EGF, IGF-1, and TGFb in the human pituitary gland. *Endocr Pathol* 1994;5:40–48.
5. Ryder DR, Horvath E, Kovacs K. Fine structural features of secretion in adenomas of human pituitary gland. *Arch Pathol Lab Med* 1980;104:518–522.
6. Horvath E, Kovacs K. Folliculo-stellate cells of the human pituitary: a type of adult stem cell? *Ultrastruct Pathol* 2002;26:219–228.
7. Scheithauer BW, Horvath E, Kovacs K. Ultrastructure of the neurohypophysis. *Microsc Res Tech* 1992;20:177–186.
8. Horvath E, Kovacs K, Lloyd RV. Pars intermedia of the human pituitary revisited: Morphologic aspects and frequency of hyperplasia of POMC-peptide immunoreactive cells. *Endocr Pathol* 1999;10:55–64.
9. Earle KM, Dillard SH Jr. Pathology of adenomas of the pituitary gland. In Kohler PO, Ross GT, eds. *Diagnosis and Treatment of Pituitary Tumors: Proceedings of a Conference (International Congress Series #303)*. New York, NY: Excerpta Medica, Elsevier Publishers, 1973.
10. Costello RT. Subclinical adenoma of the pituitary gland. *Am J Pathol* 1936;12:205–214.
11. McComb DJ, Ryan N, Horvath E, et al. Subclinical adenomas of the human pituitary. New light on old problems. *Arch Pathol Lab Med* 1983;107:488–491.
12. Bahn RS, Scheithauer BW, van Heerden JA, et al. Nonidentical expressions of multiple endocrine neoplasia, type I, in identical twins. *Mayo Clin Proc* 1986;61:689–696.
13. Scheithauer BW, Laws ER Jr, Kovacs K, et al. Pituitary adenomas of the multiple endocrine neoplasia type I syndrome. *Semin Diagn Pathol* 1987;4:205–211.
14. Verges B, Boureille F, Goudet P, et al. Pituitary disease in MEN type 1 (MEN1): data from the France-Belgium MEN1 multicenter study. *J Clin Endocrinol Metab* 2002;87:457–465.
15. Kurtkaya-Yapicier O, Scheithauer BW, Carney JA, et al. Pituitary adenoma in Carney complex: an immunohistochemical, ultrastructural, and immunoelectron microscopic study. *Ultrastruct Pathol* 2002;26:345–353.
16. Melmed S. *The Pituitary*. Cambridge, MA: Blackwell Scientific, 1995.
17. Thomer MO, Vance ML, Laws ER Jr. The anterior pituitary. In Wilson JD, Foster DW, Kronenberg HN, eds. *Williams Textbook of Endocrinology*. Philadelphia, PA: WB Saunders, 1998:249–340.
18. Horvath E, Scheithauer BW, Kovacs K, et al. Hypothalamus and pituitary. In Graham DI, Lantos PL, eds. *Greenfield's Neuropathology*. 7th edition. London, United Kingdom: Arnold Publishers, 2002:983–1062.
19. Kontogeorgos G, Kovacs K, Horvath E, et al. Multiple adenomas of the human pituitary. A retrospective autopsy study with clinical implications. *J Neurosurg* 1991;74:243–247.
20. Buurman H, Saeger W. Subclinical adenomas in postmortem pituitaries: classification and correlations to clinical data. *Eur J Endocrinol* 2006;154:753–758.
21. Kontogeorgos G, Scheithauer BW, Horvath E, et al. Double adenomas of the pituitary: a clinicopathological study of 11 tumors. *Neurosurgery* 1992;31:840–849; discussion 849.
22. Lloyd RV, Kovacs K, Young WF Jr, et al. Pituitary tumors: introduction. In DeLellis RA, Lloyd RV, Heitz PU, Eng C, eds. *World Health Organization Classification of Tumours: Pathology and Genetics of Tumours of Endocrine Organs*. Lyon, France: IARC Press, 2004:9–13.
23. Lloyd RV, Scheithauer BW, Kovacs K, et al. The immunophenotype of pituitary adenomas. *Endocr Pathol* 1996;7:145–150.
24. Kovacs K, Horvath E. Tumors of the pituitary gland. In *Atlas of Tumor Pathology. 2nd series. Fascicle 21*. Washington, DC: Armed Forces Institute of Pathology, 1986:16–50.
25. Asa SL. *Tumors of the Pituitary Gland*. 3rd edition. Washington, DC: Armed Forces Institute of Pathology, 1998.
26. Horvath E, Kovacs K, Singer W, et al. Acidophil stem cell adenoma of the human pituitary: clinicopathologic analysis of 15 cases. *Cancer* 1981;47:761–771.
27. Coire CI, Horvath E, Kovacs K, et al. A composite silent corticotroph pituitary adenoma with interspersed adrenocortical cells: case report. *Neurosurgery* 1998;42:650–654.
28. Scheithauer BW, Kovacs K, Horvath E. The adenohypophysis. In Lechago J, Gould VE, eds. *Bloodworth's Endocrine Pathology*. 3rd edition. Baltimore, MD: Williams & Wilkins, 1997: 85–152.
29. Horvath E, Scheithauer BW, Kovacs K. Hypothalamus and pituitary. In Graham DI, Lantos PL, eds. *Greenfield's Neuropathology*. 7th edition. London, United Kingdom: Arnold, 2002: 983–1062.
30. Kovacs K, Scheithauer BW, Horvath E, et al. The World Health Organization classification of adenohypophysial neoplasms. A proposed five-tier scheme. *Cancer* 1996;78:502–510.
31. DeLellis RA, Lloyd RV, Heitz PU, et al., eds. Tumours of the pituitary. In *World Health Organization Classification of Tumours – Pathology and Genetics of Tumours of Endocrine Organs*. Lyon, France: IARC Press, 2004:9–48.
32. Clayton RN, Farrell WE. Clonality of pituitary tumours: more complicated than initially envisaged? *Brain Pathol* 2001;11:313–327.
33. Jacoby LB, Hedley-Whyte ET, Pulaski K, et al. Clonal origin of pituitary adenomas. *J Neurosurg*.1990;73:731–735.
34. Alexander JM, Biller BM, Bikkal H, et al. Clinically nonfunctioning pituitary tumors are monoclonal in origin. *J Clin Invest* 1990;86:336–340.
35. Anniko M, Tribukait B, Wersall J. DNA ploidy and cell phase in human pituitary tumors. *Cancer* 1984;53:1708–1713.
36. Scheithauer BW, Gaffey TA, Lloyd RV, et al. Pathobiology of pituitary adenomas and carcinomas. *Neurosurgery* 2006;59:341–353; discussion 341–353.
37. Knosp E, Kitz K, Perneczky A. Proliferation activity in pituitary adenomas: measurement by monoclonal antibody Ki-67. *Neurosurgery* 1989;25:927–930.
38. Thapar K, Kovacs K, Scheithauer BW, et al. Proliferative activity and invasiveness among pituitary adenomas and carcinomas: an analysis using the MIB-1 antibody. *Neurosurgery* 1996;38:99–106; discussion 106–107.
39. Nagashima T, Murovic JA, Hoshino T, et al. The proliferative potential of human pituitary tumors in situ. *J Neurosurg* 1986;64:588–593.
40. Thapar K, Yamada Y, Scheithauer B, et al. Assessment of mitotic activity in pituitary adenomas and carcinomas. *Endocr Pathol* 1996;7:215–221.
41. Thapar K, Scheithauer BW, Kovacs K, et al. p53 expression in pituitary adenomas and carcinomas: correlation with invasiveness and tumor growth fractions. *Neurosurgery* 1996; 38:765–770; discussion 770–771.
42. Vidal S, Kovacs K, Horvath E, et al. Topoisomerase II alpha expression in pituitary adenomas and carcinomas: relationship to tumor behavior. *Mod Pathol* 2002;15:1205–1212.
43. Onguru O, Scheithauer BW, Kovacs K, et al. Analysis of Cox-2 and thromboxane synthase expression in pituitary adenomas and carcinomas. *Endocr Pathol* 2004;15:17–27.
44. Gong J, Zhao Y, Abdel-Fattah R, et al. Matrix metalloproteinase-9, a potential biological marker in invasive pituitary adenomas. *Pituitary* 2008;11:37–48.
45. Hulting AL, Askensten U, Tribukait B, et al. DNA evaluation in growth hormone producing pituitary adenomas: flow cytometry versus single cell analysis. *Acta Endocrinol (Copenh)* 1989;121:317–321.
46. Ahyai A, Hori A, Bockermann V, et al. Impulse cytophotometric DNA analysis in pituitary adenomas. *Neurosurg Rev* 1988;11:77–86.
47. Stefaneanu L, Horvath E, Kovacs K. Argyrophil organizer region proteins (AgNORs) in adenohypophysial cells and adenomas of the human pituitary. *Mod Pathol* 1989;2:192–199.
48. Hucumenoglu S, Kaya H, Kotiloglu E, et al. AgNOR values are not helpful in the differential diagnosis of pituitary adenomas. *Clin Neurol Neurosurg* 2002;104:293–299.
49. Neill JD, Frawley LS. Detection of hormone release from individual cells in mixed populations using a reverse hemolytic plaque assay. *Endocrinology* 1983;112:1135–1137.
50. Kanter SL, Mickle JP, Hunter SB, et al. Pituitary adenomas in pediatric patients: are they more invasive? *Pediatr Neurosci* 1985;12:202–204.
51. Kane LA, Leinung MC, Scheithauer BW, et al. Pituitary adenomas in childhood and adolescence. *J Clin Endocrinol Metab* 1994;79:1135–1140.
52. Leinung MC, Kane LA, Scheithauer BW, et al. Long term follow-up of transsphenoidal surgery for the treatment of Cushing's disease in childhood. *J Clin Endocrinol Metab* 1995; 80:2475–2479.
53. Horvath A, Stratakis CA. Clinical and molecular genetics of acromegaly: MEN1, Carney complex, McCune-Albright syndrome, familial acromegaly and genetic defects in sporadic tumors. *Rev Endocr Metab Disord* 2008;9:1–11.
54. Trouillas J, Labat-Moleur F, Sturm N, et al. Pituitary tumors and hyperplasia in multiple endocrine neoplasia type 1 syndrome (MEN1): a case-control study in a series of 77 patients versus 2509 non-MEN1 patients. *Am J Surg Pathol* 2008;32:534–543.
55. Hardy J, Vezina JL. Transsphenoidal neurosurgery of intracranial neoplasm. *Adv Neurol* 1976;15:261–273.
56. Mortini P, Barzaghi R, Losa M, et al. Surgical treatment of giant pituitary adenomas: strategies and results in a series of 95 consecutive patients. *Neurosurgery* 2007;60:993–1002; discussion 1003–1004.
57. Rauhut F, Clar HE, Bamberg M, et al. Diagnostic criteria in pituitary tumour recurrence: combined modality of surgery and radiotherapy. *Acta Neurochir (Wien)* 1986;80:73–78.
58. Selman WR, Laws ER Jr, Scheithauer BW, et al. The occurrence of dural invasion in pituitary adenomas. *J Neurosurg* 1986;64:402–407.
59. Scheithauer BW, Kovacs K, Randall RV. The pituitary gland in untreated Addison's disease. A histologic and immunocytologic study of 18 adenohypophyses. *Arch Pathol Lab Med* 1983;107:484–487.
60. Scheithauer BW, Kovacs K, Randall RV, et al. Pituitary gland in hypothyroidism. Histologic and immunocytologic study. *Arch Pathol Lab Med* 1985;109:499–504.
61. Yokoyama S, Hirano H, Moroki K, et al. Are nonfunctioning pituitary adenomas extending into the cavernous sinus aggressive and/or invasive? *Neurosurgery* 2001;49:857–862; discussion 862–863.
62. Lloyd RV, Chandler WF, Kovacs K, et al. Ectopic pituitary adenomas with normal anterior pituitary glands. *Am J Surg Pathol* 1986;10:546–552.
63. Axiotis CA, Lippes HA, Merino MJ, et al. Corticotroph cell pituitary adenoma within an ovarian teratoma. A new cause of Cushing's syndrome. *Am J Surg Pathol* 1987;11:218–224.
64. Nelson PB, Haverkos H, Martinez AJ, et al. Abscess formation within pituitary tumors. *Neurosurgery* 1983;12:331–333.
65. Robinson B. Intrasellar abscess after transsphenoidal pituitary adenomectomy. *Neurosurgery* 1983;12:684–686.
66. Waltz TA, Brownell B. Sarcoma: a possible late result of effective radiation therapy for pituitary adenoma. Report of two cases. *J Neurosurg* 1966;24:901–907.
67. Menon G, Nair S, Rajesh BJ, et al. Malignant astrocytoma following radiotherapy for craniopharyngioma. *J Cancer Res Ther* 2007;3:50–52.
68. Wakai S, Fukushima T, Teramoto A, et al. Pituitary apoplexy: its incidence and clinical significance. *J Neurosurg* 1981;55:187–193.
69. Mohr G, Hardy J. Hemorrhage, necrosis, and apoplexy in pituitary adenomas. *Surg Neurol* 1982;18:181–189.
70. Ebersold MJ, Laws ER Jr, Scheithauer BW, et al. Pituitary apoplexy treated by transsphenoidal surgery. A clinicopathological and immunocytochemical study. *J Neurosurg* 1983;58: 315–320.
71. Cardoso ER, Peterson EW. Pituitary apoplexy: a review. *Neurosurgery* 1984;14:363–373.
72. Ahmed M, Rifai A, Al-Jurf M, et al. Classical pituitary apoplexy presentation and a follow-up of 13 patients. *Horm Res* 1989;31:125–132.
73. Randall RV, Scheithauer BW, Laws ER Jr, et al. Pseudoprolactinomas. *Trans Am Clin Climatol Assoc* 1983;94:114–121.
74. Lees PD, Pickard JD. Hyperprolactinemia, intrasellar pituitary tissue pressure, and the pituitary stalk compression syndrome. *J Neurosurg* 1987;67:192–196.
75. Berezin M, Karasik A. Familial prolactinoma. *Clin Endocrinol (Oxf)* 1995;42:483–486.
76. Corenblum B, Donovan L. The safety of physiological estrogen plus progestin replacement therapy and with oral contraceptive therapy in women with pathological hyperprolactinemia. *Fertil Steril* 1993;59:671–673.
77. Kovacs K, Stefaneanu L, Ezzat S, et al. Prolactin-producing pituitary adenoma in a male-to-female transsexual patient with protracted estrogen administration. A morphologic study. *Arch Pathol Lab Med* 1994;118:562–565.

78. Wingrave SJ, Kay CR, Vessey MP. Oral contraceptives and pituitary adenomas. *Br Med J* 1980;280:685–686.
79. Randall RV, Scheithauer BW, Laws ER Jr, et al. Pituitary adenomas associated with hyperprolactinemia: a clinical and immunohistochemical study of 97 patients operated on transsphenoidally. *Mayo Clin Proc* 1985;60:753–762.
80. Calle-Rodrigue RD, Giannini C, Scheithauer BW, et al. Prolactinomas in male and female patients: a comparative clinicopathologic study. *Mayo Clin Proc* 1998;73:1046–1052.
81. Ma W, Ikeda H, Yoshimoto T. Clinicopathologic study of 123 cases of prolactin-secreting pituitary adenomas with special reference to multihormone production and clonality of the adenomas. *Cancer* 2002;95:258–266.
82. Nishioka H, Haraoka J, Akada K, et al. Gender-related differences in prolactin secretion in pituitary prolactinomas. *Neuroradiology* 2002;44:407–410.
83. Lipper S, Isenberg HD, Kahn LB. Calcospherites in pituitary prolactinomas. A hypothesis for their formation. *Arch Pathol Lab Med* 1984;108:31–34.
84. Landolt AM, Kleihues P, Heitz PU. Amyloid deposits in pituitary adenomas. Differentiation of two types. *Arch Pathol Lab Med* 1987;111:453–458.
85. Robert F, Hardy J. Prolactin-secreting adenomas. A light and electron microscopical study. *Arch Pathol* 1975;99:625–633.
86. Horvath E, Kovacs K. Pathology of prolactin cell adenomas of the human pituitary. *Semin Diagn Pathol* 1986;3:4–17.
87. Tindall GT, Kovacs K, Horvath E, et al. Human prolactin-producing adenomas and bromocriptine: a histological, immunocytochemical, ultrastructural, and morphometric study. *J Clin Endocrinol Metab* 1982;55:1178–1183.
88. Barrow DL, Tindall GT, Kovacs K, et al. Clinical and pathological effects of bromocriptine on prolactin-secreting and other pituitary tumors. *J Neurosurg* 1984;60:1–7.
89. Mori H, Mori S, Saitoh Y, et al. Effects of bromocriptine on prolactin-secreting pituitary adenomas. Mechanism of reduction in tumor size evaluated by light and electron microscopic, immunohistochemical, and morphometric analysis. *Cancer* 1985;56:230–238.
90. Delgrange E, Trouillas J, Maiter D, et al. Sex-related difference in the growth of prolactinomas: a clinical and proliferation marker study. *J Clin Endocrinol Metab* 1997;82:2102–2107.
91. Webster J, Page MD, Bevan JS, et al. Low recurrence rate after partial hypophysectomy for prolactinoma: the predictive value of dynamic prolactin function tests. *Clin Endocrinol (Oxf)* 1992;36:35–44.
92. van der Lely AJ, Hutson RK, Trainer PJ, et al. Long-term treatment of acromegaly with pegvisomant, a growth hormone receptor antagonist. *Lancet* 2001;358:1754–1759.
93. Horvath E, Kovacs K, Singer W, et al. Acidophil stem cell adenoma of the human pituitary. *Arch Pathol Lab Med* 1977;101:594–599.
94. Horvath E, Kovacs K, Scheithauer BW, et al. Pituitary adenomas producing growth hormone, prolactin, and one or more glycoprotein hormones: a histologic, immunohistochemical, and ultrastructural study of four surgically removed tumors. *Ultrastruct Pathol* 1983;5:171–183.
95. Scheithauer BW, Horvath E, Kovacs K, et al. Plurihormonal pituitary adenomas. *Semin Diagn Pathol* 1986;3:69–82.
96. Scheithauer BW, Horvath E, Kovacs K, et al. Pathology of pituitary adenomas and pituitary hyperplasia (Chapter 7). In Thapar K, Kovacs K, Scheithauer BW, et al., eds. *The Pituitary: Diagnosis and Management of Pituitary Tumors.* Boca Raton, FL: Humana Press, 2001:91–154.
97. Carney JA, Hruska LS, Beauchamp GD, et al. Dominant inheritance of the complex of myxomas, spotty pigmentation, and endocrine overactivity. *Mayo Clin Proc* 1986;61:165–172.
98. Horvath E, Scheithauer BW, Kovacs K. Morphologic aspects of growth hormone-producing pituitary adenomas with emphasis on novel concepts. In Ludecke DK, Tolis G, eds. *Growth Hormone, Growth Factors, and Acromegaly.* Volume 3. New York, NY: Raven Press, 1987:107–114.
99. Laws ER Jr, Scheithauer BW, Carpenter S, et al. The pathogenesis of acromegaly. Clinical and immunocytochemical analysis in 75 patients. *J Neurosurg* 1985;63:35–38.
100. Kovacs K, Horvath E. Pathology of growth hormone-producing tumors of the human pituitary. *Semin Diagn Pathol* 1986;3:18–33.
101. Robert F. Electron microscopy of human pituitary tumors. In Tindall GT, Collins WF, eds. *Clinical Management of Pituitary Disorders.* New York, NY: Raven Press, 1979:113–131.
102. Thapar K, Kovacs K, Stefaneanu L, et al. Overexpression of the growth-hormone-releasing hormone gene in acromegaly-associated pituitary tumors. An event associated with neoplastic progression and aggressive behavior. *Am J Pathol* 1997;151:769–784.
103. Horvath E, Kovacs K, Scheithauer BW, et al. Pituitary adenoma with neuronal choristoma (PANCH): composite lesion or lineage infidelity? *Ultrastruct Pathol* 1994;18:565–574.
104. Klibanski A, Zervas NT, Kovacs K, et al. Clinically silent hypersecretion of growth hormone in patients with pituitary tumors. *J Neurosurg* 1987;66:806–811.
105. Ezzat S, Horvath E, Harris AG, et al. Morphological effects of octreotide on growth hormone-producing pituitary adenomas. *J Clin Endocrinol Metab* 1994;79:113–118.
106. Kontogeorgos G, Kovacs K, Scheithauer BW, et al. Alpha-subunit immunoreactivity in plurihormonal pituitary adenomas of patients with acromegaly. *Mod Pathol* 1991;4:191–195.
107. Corenblum B, Sirek AM, Horvath E, et al. Human mixed somatotrophic and lactotrophic pituitary adenomas. *J Clin Endocrinol Metab* 1976;42:857–863.
108. Horvath E, Kovacs K, Killinger DW. Mammosomatotroph cell adenoma of the human pituitary. *Proc Electron Microsc Soc Am* 1980;38:726.
109. Felix IA, Horvath E, Kovacs K, et al. Mammosomatotroph adenoma of the pituitary associated with gigantism and hyperprolactinemia. A morphological study including immunoelectron microscopy. *Acta Neuropathol* 1986;71:76–82.
110. Beck C, Burger HG. Evidence for the presence of immunoreactive growth hormone in cancers of the lung and stomach. *Cancer* 1972;30:75–79.
111. Melmed S, Ezrin C, Kovacs K, et al. Acromegaly due to secretion of growth hormone by an ectopic pancreatic islet-cell tumor. *N Engl J Med* 1985;312:9–17.
112. Thorner MO, Perryman RL, Cronin MJ, et al. Somatotroph hyperplasia. Successful treatment of acromegaly by removal of a pancreatic islet tumor secreting a growth hormone-releasing factor. *J Clin Invest* 1982;70:965–977.
113. Scheithauer BW, Carpenter PC, Bloch B, et al. Ectopic secretion of a growth hormone-releasing factor. Report of a case of acromegaly with bronchial carcinoid tumor. *Am J Med* 1984;76:605–616.
114. Asa SL, Kovacs K, Thorner MO, et al. Immunohistological localization of growth hormone-releasing hormone in human tumors. *J Clin Endocrinol Metab* 1985;60:423–427.
115. Sano T, Asa SL, Kovacs K. Growth hormone-releasing hormone-producing tumors: clinical, biochemical, and morphological manifestations. *Endocr Rev* 1988;9:357–373.
116. Garcia-Luna PP, Leal-Cerro A, Montero C, et al. A rare cause of acromegaly: ectopic production of growth hormone-releasing factor by a bronchial carcinoid tumor. *Surg Neurol* 1987;27:563–568.
117. Wilson CB, Tyrrell JB, Fitzgerald PA, et al. Neurosurgical aspects of Cushing's disease and Nelson's syndrome. In Tindall GT, Collins WF, eds. *Clinical Management of Pituitary Disorders.* New York, NY: Raven Press, 1979:229–238.
118. Robert F, Pelletier G, Hardy J. Pituitary adenomas in Cushing's disease. A histologic, ultrastructural, and immunocytochemical study. *Arch Pathol Lab Med* 1978;102:448–455.
119. Robert F, Hardy J. Human corticotroph cell adenomas. *Semin Diagn Pathol* 1986;3:34–41.
120. Lloyd RV, Chandler WF, McKeever PE, et al. The spectrum of ACTH-producing pituitary lesions. *Am J Surg Pathol* 1986;10:618–626.
121. Ballard HS, Frame B, Hartsock RJ. Familial multiple endocrine adenoma-peptic ulcer complex. 1964. *Medicine (Baltimore)* 1991;70:281–283; discussion 283–285.
122. Gardner DF, Barlascini CO Jr, Downs RW Jr, et al. Cushing's disease in two sisters. *Am J Med Sci* 1989;297:387–389.
123. Scheithauer BW, Kovacs KT, Laws ER Jr, et al. Pathology of invasive pituitary tumors with special reference to functional classification. *J Neurosurg* 1986;65:733–744.
124. Stevenaert A, Perrin G, Martin D, et al. [Cushing's disease and corticotrophic adenoma: results of pituitary microsurgery]. *Neurochirurgie* 2002;48:234–265.
125. Lecomte P, Jan M, Combe H, et al. Les adenomes hypophysaires multiples. *Rev Fr Endocrinol Clin* 2000:41–56.
126. Wynne AG, Scheithauer BW, Young WF Jr, et al. Coexisting corticotroph and lactotroph adenomas: case report with reference to the relationship of corticotropin and prolactin excess. *Neurosurgery* 1992;30:919–923.
127. Oyama K, Sanno N, Teramoto A, et al. Expression of neuro D1 in human normal pituitaries and pituitary adenomas. *Mod Pathol* 2001;14:892–899.
128. Legius E, Marchuk DA, Collins FS, et al. Somatic deletion of the neurofibromatosis type 1 gene in a neurofibrosarcoma supports a tumour suppressor gene hypothesis. *Nat Genet* 1993;3:122–126.
129. Asa SL, Kovacs K, Tindall GT, et al. Cushing's disease associated with an intrasellar gangliocytoma producing corticotrophin-releasing factor. *Ann Intern Med* 1984;101:789–793.
130. Horvath E, Kovacs K, Josse R. Pituitary corticotroph cell adenoma with marked abundance of microfilaments. *Ultrastruct Pathol* 1983;5:249–255.
131. Felix IA, Horvath E, Kovacs K. Massive Crooke's hyalinization in corticotroph cell adenomas of the human pituitary. A histological, immunocytological, and electron microscopic study of three cases. *Acta Neurochir (Wien)* 1981;58:235–243.
132. George DH, Scheithauer BW, Kovacs K, et al. Crooke's cell adenoma of the pituitary: an aggressive variant of corticotroph adenoma. *Am J Surg Pathol* 2003;27:1330–1336.
133. Gaffey TA, Scheithauer BW, Lloyd RV, et al. Corticotroph carcinoma of the pituitary: a clinicopathological study. Report of four cases. *J Neurosurg* 2002;96:352–360.
134. Horvath E, Kovacs K, Killinger DW, et al. Silent corticotropic adenomas of the human pituitary gland: a histologic, immunocytologic, and ultrastructural study. *Am J Pathol* 1980;98:617–638.
135. Reincke M, Allolio B, Saeger W, et al. A pituitary adenoma secreting high molecular weight adrenocorticotropin without evidence of Cushing's disease. *J Clin Endocrinol Metab* 1987;65:1296–1300.
136. Trouillas J, Girod C, Sassolas G, et al. A human beta-endorphin pituitary adenoma. *J Clin Endocrinol Metab* 1984;58:242–249.
137. Tan EU, Ho MS, Rajasoorya CR. Metamorphosis of a non-functioning pituitary adenoma to Cushing's disease. *Pituitary* 2000;3:117–122.
138. Raux Demay MC, Proeschel MF, de Keyzer Y, et al. Characterization of human corticotrophin-releasing hormone and pro-opiomelanocortin-related peptides in a thymic carcinoid tumour responsible for Cushing's syndrome. *Clin Endocrinol (Oxf)* 1988;29:649–657.
139. Horvath E, Kovacs K. Gonadotroph adenomas of the human pituitary: sex-related fine-structural dichotomy. A histologic, immunocytochemical, and electron-microscopic study of 30 tumors. *Am J Pathol* 1984;117:429–440.
140. Young WF Jr, Scheithauer BW, Kovacs KT, et al. Gonadotroph adenoma of the pituitary gland: a clinicopathologic analysis of 100 cases. *Mayo Clin Proc* 1996;71:649–656.
141. Ebersold MJ, Quast LM, Laws ER Jr, et al. Long-term results in transsphenoidal removal of nonfunctioning pituitary adenomas. *J Neurosurg* 1986;64:713–719.
142. Kannuki S, Matsumoto K, Sano T, et al. Double pituitary adenoma—two case reports. *Neurol Med Chir (Tokyo)* 1996;36:818–821.
143. Daneshdoost L, Gennarelli TA, Bashey HM, et al. Recognition of gonadotroph adenomas in women. *N Engl J Med* 1991;324:589–594.
144. Asa SL, Bamberger AM, Cao B, et al. The transcription activator steroidogenic factor-1 is preferentially expressed in the human pituitary gonadotroph. *J Clin Endocrinol Metab* 1996;81:2165–2170.
145. Kontogeorgos G, Kovacs KT, Horvath E, et al. Null cell adenomas, oncocytomas, and gonadotroph adenomas of the human pituitary: an immunocytochemical and ultrastructural analysis of 300 cases. *Endocr Pathol* 1993;4:20–27.
146. Sanno N, Teramoto A, Osamura RY. Long-term surgical outcome in 16 patients with thyrotropin pituitary adenoma. *J Neurosurg* 2000;93:194–200.
147. Burgess JR, Shepherd JJ, Greenaway TM. Thyrotropinomas in multiple endocrine neoplasia type 1 (MEN-1). *Aust N Z J Med* 1994;24:740–741.
148. Kirschner LS, Carney JA, Pack SD, et al. Mutations of the gene encoding the protein kinase A type I-alpha regulatory subunit in patients with the Carney complex. *Nat Genet* 2000;26:89–92.
149. Katz MS, Gregerman RI, Horvath E, et al. Thyrotroph cell adenoma of the human pituitary

gland associated with primary hypothyroidism: clinical and morphological features. *Acta Endocrinol (Copenh)* 1980;95:41–48.

150. Fatourechi V, Gharib H, Scheithauer BW, et al. Pituitary thyrotropic adenoma associated with congenital hypothyroidism. Report of two cases. *Am J Med* 1984;76:725–728.

151. Girod C, Trouillas J, Claustrat B. The human thyrotropic adenoma: pathologic diagnosis in five cases and critical review of the literature. *Semin Diagn Pathol* 1986;3:58–68.

152. Gharib H, Carpenter PC, Scheithauer BW, et al. The spectrum of inappropriate pituitary thyrotropin secretion associated with hyperthyroidism. *Mayo Clin Proc* 1982;57:556–563.

153. Pioro EP, Scheithauer BW, Laws ER Jr, et al. Combined thyrotroph and lactotroph cell hyperplasia simulating prolactin-secreting pituitary adenoma in long-standing primary hypothyroidism. *Surg Neurol* 1988;29:218–226.

154. Martinez AJ. The pathology of nonfunctional pituitary adenomas. *Semin Diagn Pathol* 1986; 3:83–94.

155. Asa SL, Gerrie BM, Singer W, et al. Gonadotropin secretion in vitro by human pituitary null cell adenomas and oncocytomas. *J Clin Endocrinol Metab* 1986;62:1011–1019.

156. Black PM, Hsu DW, Klibanski A, et al. Hormone production in clinically nonfunctioning pituitary adenomas. *J Neurosurg* 1987;66:244–250.

157. Kovacs K, Asa SL, Horvath E. Null cell adenomas of the pituitary: attempts to resolve their cytogenesis. In Lechago J, Kameya T, eds. *Endocrine Pathology Update*. Philadelphia, PA: Field and Wood, 1992.

158. Kovacs K, Horvath E, Ryan N, et al. Null cell adenoma of the human pituitary. *Virchows Arch A Pathol Anat Histol* 1980;387:165–174.

159. Lillehei KO, Kirschman DL, Kleinschmidt-DeMasters BK, et al. Reassessment of the role of radiation therapy in the treatment of endocrine-inactive pituitary macroadenomas. *Neurosurgery* 1998;43:432–438; discussion 438–439.

160. Kovacs K, Horvath E. Pituitary "chromophobe" adenoma composed of oncocytes. A light and electron microscopic study. *Arch Pathol* 1973;95:235–239.

161. Schmid M, Munscher A, Saeger W, et al. Pituitary hormone mRNA in null cell adenomas and oncocytomas by in situ hybridization comparison with immunohistochemical and clinical data. *Pathol Res Pract* 2001;197:663–669.

162. Horvath E, Kovacs K, Smyth HS, et al. A novel type of pituitary adenoma: morphological features and clinical correlations. *J Clin Endocrinol Metab* 1988;66:1111–1118.

163. Horvath E, Kovacs K, Smyth HS, et al. Silent adenoma subtype 3 of the pituitary—immuno-histochemical and ultrastructural classification: a review of 29 cases. *Ultrastruct Pathol* 2005; 29:511–524.

164. U HS, Johnson C. Metastatic prolactin-secreting pituitary adenoma. *Hum Pathol* 1984;15: 94–96.

165. Plangger CA, Twerdy K, Grunert V, et al. Subarachnoid metastases from a prolactinoma. *Neurochirurgia (Stuttg)* 1985;28:235–237.

166. Nudleman KL, Choi B, Kusske JA. Primary pituitary carcinoma: a clinical pathological study. *Neurosurgery* 1985;16:90–95.

167. Pernicone PJ, Scheithauer BW, Sebo TJ, et al. Pituitary carcinoma: a clinicopathologic study of 15 cases. *Cancer* 1997;79:804–812.

168. McCutcheon IE, Pieper DR, Fuller GN, et al. Pituitary carcinoma containing gonadotropins: treatment by radical excision and cytotoxic chemotherapy: case report. *Neurosurgery* 2000;46:1233–1239; discussion 1239–1240.

169. Holthouse DJ, Robbins PD, Kahler R, et al. Corticotroph pituitary carcinoma: case report and literature review. *Endocr Pathol* 2001;12:329–341.

170. Mixson AJ, Friedman TC, Katz DA, et al. Thyrotropin-secreting pituitary carcinoma. *J Clin Endocrinol Metab* 1993;76:529–533.

171. Roncaroli F, Nose V, Scheithauer BW, et al. Gonadotropic pituitary carcinoma: HER-2/neu expression and gene amplification. Report of two cases. *J Neurosurg* 2003;99:402–408.

172. Scheithauer BW, Fereidooni F, Horvath E, et al. Pituitary carcinoma: an ultrastructural study of eleven cases. *Ultrastruct Pathol* 2001;25:227–242.

173. Scheithauer BW, Horvath E, Kovacs K, et al. Prolactin-producing pituitary adenoma and carcinoma with neuronal components—a metaplastic lesion. *Pituitary* 1999;1:197–205.

174. Hosaka N, Kitajiri S, Hiraumi H, et al. Ectopic pituitary adenoma with malignant transformation. *Am J Surg Pathol* 2002;26:1078–1082.

175. Mamelak AN, Carmichael JP, Park P, et al. Atypical pituitary adenoma with malignant features. *Pituitary* 2008;Oct 24 (Epub).

176. Asa SL, Scheithauer BW, Bilbao JM, et al. A case for hypothalamic acromegaly: a clinicopathological study of six patients with hypothalamic gangliocytomas producing growth hormone-releasing factor. *J Clin Endocrinol Metab* 1984;58:796–803.

177. Roncaroli F, Scheithauer BW, Cenacchi G, et al. "Spindle cell oncocytoma" of the adenohypophysis: a tumor of folliculostellate cells? *Am J Surg Pathol* 2002;26:1048–1055.

178. Kloub O, Perry A, Tu PH, et al. Spindle cell oncocytoma of the adenohypophysis: report of two recurrent cases. *Am J Surg Pathol* 2005;29:247–253.

179. Dahiya S, Sarkar C, Hedley-Whyte ET, et al. Spindle cell oncocytoma of the adenohypophysis: report of two cases. *Acta Neuropathol* 2005;110:97–99.

180. Scheithauer BW, Sano T, Kovacs KT, et al. The pituitary gland in pregnancy: a clinicopathologic and immunohistochemical study of 69 cases. *Mayo Clin Proc* 1990;65:461–474.

181. Stefaneanu L, Kovacs K, Lloyd RV, et al. Pituitary lactotrophs and somatotrophs in pregnancy: a correlative in situ hybridization and immunocytochemical study. *Virchows Arch B Cell Pathol Incl Mol Pathol*. 1992;62:291–296.

182. Zimmerman D, Young WF Jr, Ebersold MJ, et al. Congenital gigantism due to growth hormone-releasing hormone excess and pituitary hyperplasia with adenomatous transformation. *J Clin Endocrinol Metab* 1993;76:216–222.

183. Kovacs K, Horvath E, Thorner MO, et al. Mammosomatotroph hyperplasia associated with acromegaly and hyperprolactinemia in a patient with the McCune-Albright syndrome. A histologic, immunocytologic and ultrastructural study of the surgically-removed adenohypophysis. *Virchows Arch A Pathol Anat Histopathol* 1984;403:77–86.

184. Pack SD, Kirschner LS, Pak E, et al. Genetic and histologic studies of somatomammotropic pituitary tumors in patients with the "complex of spotty skin pigmentation, myxomas, endocrine overactivity and schwannomas" (Carney complex). *J Clin Endocrinol Metab* 2000; 85:3860–3865.

185. Young WF Jr, Scheithauer BW, Gharib H, et al. Cushing's syndrome due to primary multinodular corticotrope hyperplasia. *Mayo Clin Proc* 1988;63:256–262.

186. Judge DM, Kulin HE, Page R, et al. Hypothalamic hamartoma: a source of luteinizing-hormone-releasing factor in precocious puberty. *N Engl J Med* 1977;296:7–10.

187. Laws ER Jr. Transsphenoidal microsurgery in the management of craniopharyngioma. *J Neurosurg* 1980;52:661–666.

188. Seemayer TA, Blundell JS, Wiglesworth FW. Pituitary craniopharyngioma with tooth formation. *Cancer* 1972;29:423–430.

189. Paulus W, Honegger J, Keyvani K, et al. Xanthogranuloma of the sellar region: a clinico-pathological entity different from adamantinomatous craniopharyngioma. *Acta Neuropathol* 1999;97:377–382.

190. Petito CK, DeGirolami U, Earle KM. Craniopharyngiomas: a clinical and pathological review. *Cancer* 1976;37:1944–1952.

191. Harris BT, Horoupian DS, Tse V, et al. Melanotic craniopharyngioma: a report of two cases. *Acta Neuropathol* 1999;98:433–436.

192. Obrador S, Blazquez MG. Pituitary abscess in a craniopharyngioma. Case report. *J Neurosurg* 1972;36:785–789.

193. Duff JM, Meyer FB, Illstrup DM, et al. Long-term outcomes for surgically resected craniopharyngiomas. *Neurosurgery* 2000;46:291–302; discussion 302–305.

194. Gupta K, Kuhn MJ, Shevlin DW, et al. Metastatic craniopharyngioma. *AJNR Am J Neuroradiol* 1999;20:1059–1060.

195. Ishii K, Sugita K, Kobayashi H, et al. Intracranial ectopic recurrence of craniopharyngioma after Ommaya reservoir implantation. *Pediatr Neurosurg* 2004;40:230–233.

196. Kristopaitis T, Thomas C, Petruzzelli GJ, et al. Malignant craniopharyngioma. *Arch Pathol Lab Med* 2000;124:1356–1360.

197. Crotty TB, Scheithauer BW, Young WF Jr, et al. Papillary craniopharyngioma: a clinicopathological study of 48 cases. *J Neurosurg* 1995;83:206–214.

198. Elmaci L, Kurtkaya-Yapicier O, Ekinci G, et al. Metastatic papillary craniopharyngioma: case study and study of tumor angiogenesis. *Neuro Oncol* 2002;4:123–128.

199. McGrath P. Cysts of sellar and pharyngeal hypophyses. *Pathology* 1971;3:123–131.

200. Weber EL, Vogel FS, Odom GL. Cysts of the sella turcica. *J Neurosurg* 1970;33:48–53.

201. Yoshida J, Kobayashi T, Kageyama N, et al. Symptomatic Rathke's cleft cyst. Morphological study with light and electron microscopy and tissue culture. *J Neurosurg* 1977;47:451–458.

202. Steinberg GK, Koenig GH, Golden JB. Symptomatic Rathke's cleft cysts. Report of two cases. *J Neurosurg* 1982;56:290–295.

203. Barrow DL, Spector RH, Takei Y, et al. Symptomatic Rathke's cleft cysts located entirely in the suprasellar region: review of diagnosis, management, and pathogenesis. *Neurosurgery* 1985;16:766–772.

204. Tomlinson FH, Scheithauer BW, Young WF, et al. Rathke's cleft cyst—a clinicopathologic study of 31 cases. *Brain Pathol* 1994;4:453.

205. Obenchain TG, Becker DP. Abscess formation in a Rathke's cleft cyst. Case report. *J Neurosurg* 1972;36:359–362.

206. Israel ZH, Yacoub M, Gomori JM, et al. Rathke's cleft cyst abscess. *Pediatr Neurosurg* 2000; 33:159–161.

207. Luse SA, Kernohan JW. Granular-cell tumors of the stalk and posterior lobe of the pituitary gland. *Cancer* 1955;8:616–622.

208. Boecher-Schwarz HG, Fries G, Bornemann A, et al. Suprasellar granular cell tumor. *Neurosurgery* 1992;31:751–754; discussion 754.

209. Liwnicz BH, Liwnicz RG, Huff JS, et al. Giant granular cell tumor of the suprasellar area: immunocytochemical and electron microscopic studies. *Neurosurgery* 1984;15:246–251.

210. Schlachter LB, Tindall GT, Pearl GS. Granular cell tumor of the pituitary gland associated with diabetes insipidus. *Neurosurgery* 1980;6:418–421.

211. Cohen-Gadol AA, Pichelmann MA, Link MJ, et al. Granular cell tumor of the sellar and suprasellar region: clinicopathologic study of 11 cases and literature review. *Mayo Clin Proc* 2003;78:567–573.

212. Schaller B, Kirsch E, Tolnay M, et al. Symptomatic granular cell tumor of the pituitary gland: case report and review of the literature. *Neurosurgery* 1998;42:166–170; discussion 170–171.

213. Vogelgesang S, Junge MH, Pahnke J, et al. August 2001: sellar/suprasellar mass in a 59-year-old woman. *Brain Pathol* 2002;12:135–136, 139.

214. Kurtin PJ, Bonin DM. Immunohistochemical demonstration of the lysosome-associated glycoprotein CD68 (KP-1) in granular cell tumors and schwannomas. *Hum Pathol* 1994; 25:1172–1178.

215. Brat DJ, Scheithauer BW, Staugaitis SM, et al. Pituicytoma: a distinctive low-grade glioma of the neurohypophysis. *Am J Surg Pathol* 2000;24:362–368.

216. Figarella-Branger D, Dufour H, Fernandez C, et al. Pituicytomas, a mis-diagnosed benign tumor of the neurohypophysis: report of three cases. *Acta Neuropathol* 2002;104:313–319.

217. Schultz AB, Brat DJ, Oyesiku NM, et al. Intrasellar pituicytoma in a patient with other endocrine neoplasms. *Arch Pathol Lab Med* 2001;125:527–530.

218. Kepes JJ, Kepes M. Predominantly cerebral forms of histiocytosis-X. A reappraisal of "Gagel's hypothalamic granuloma," "granuloma infiltrans of the hypothalamus" and "Ayala's disease" with a report of four cases. *Acta Neuropathol* 1969;14:77–98.

219. Donadieu J, Rolon MA, Pion I, et al. Incidence of growth hormone deficiency in pediatric-onset Langerhans cell histiocytosis: efficacy and safety of growth hormone treatment. *J Clin Endocrinol Metab* 2004;89:604–609.

220. Horn EM, Coons SW, Spetzler RF, et al. Isolated Langerhans cell histiocytosis of the infundibulum presenting with fulminant diabetes insipidus. *Childs Nerv Syst* 2006;22: 542–544.

221. Lau SK, Chu PG, Weiss LM. Immunohistochemical expression of langerin in Langerhans cell histiocytosis and non-Langerhans cell histiocytic disorders. *Am J Surg Pathol* 2008;23: 615–619.

222. Hampton TA, Scheithauer BW, Rojiani AM, et al. Salivary gland-like tumors of the sellar region. *Am J Surg Pathol* 1997;21:424–434.

223. Teears RJ, Silverman EM. Clinicopathologic review of 88 cases of carcinoma metastatic to the pituitary gland. *Cancer* 1975;36:216–220.

224. Heshmati HM, Scheithauer BW, Young WF Jr. Metastases to the pituitary gland. *Endocrinologist* 2002;12:45–49.

225. Branch CL Jr, Laws ER Jr. Metastatic tumors of the sella turcica masquerading as primary pituitary tumors. *J Clin Endocrinol Metab* 1987;65:469–474.

226. Kaufmann TJ, Lopes MB, Laws ER Jr, et al. Primary sellar lymphoma: radiologic and pathologic findings in two patients. *AJNR Am J Neuroradiol* 2002;23:364–367.

227. Kuhn D, Buchfelder M, Brabletz T, et al. Intrasellar malignant lymphoma developing within pituitary adenoma. *Acta Neuropathol* 1999;97:311–316.

228. Masse SR, Wolk RW, Conklin RH. Peripituitary gland involvement in acute leukemia in adults. *Arch Pathol* 1973;96:141–142.

229. Nemoto K, Ohnishi Y, Tsukada T. Chronic lymphocytic leukemia showing pituitary tumor with massive leukemic cell infiltration, and special reference to clinicopathological findings of CLL. *Acta Pathol Jpn* 1978;28:797–805.

230. Molinatti PA, Scheithauer BW, Randall RV, et al. Metastasis to pituitary adenoma. *Arch Pathol Lab Med* 1985;109:287–289.

231. James RL Jr, Arsenis G, Stoler M, et al. Hypophyseal metastatic renal cell carcinoma and pituitary adenoma. Case report and review of the literature. *Am J Med* 1984;76:337–340.

232. Zager EL, Hedley-Whyte ET. Metastasis within a pituitary adenoma presenting with bilateral abducens palsies: case report and review of the literature. *Neurosurgery* 1987;21: 383–386.

233. Tashiro T, Sano T, Xu B, et al. Spectrum of different types of hypophysitis: a clinicopathologic study of hypophysitis in 31 cases. *Endocr Pathol* 2002;13:183–195.

234. Sheehan HL, Stanfield JP. The pathogenesis of postpartum necrosis of the anterior lobe of the pituitary gland. *Acta Endocrinol (Copenh)* 1961;37:479.

235. Caturegli P, Newschaffer C, Olivi A, et al. Autoimmune hypophysitis. *Endocr Rev* 2005;26: 599–614.

236. Asa SL, Bilbao JM, Kovacs K, et al. Lymphocytic hypophysitis of pregnancy resulting in hypopituitarism: a distinct clinicopathologic entity. *Ann Intern Med* 1981;95:166–171.

237. Takao T, Nanamiya W, Matsumoto R, et al. Antipituitary antibodies in patients with lymphocytic hypophysitis. *Horm Res* 2001;55:288–292.

238. Gutenberg A, Buslei R, Fahlbusch R, et al. Immunopathology of primary hypophysitis: implications for pathogenesis. *Am J Surg Pathol* 2005;29:329–338.

239. Jensen MD, Handwerger BS, Scheithauer BW, et al. Lymphocytic hypophysitis with isolated corticotropin deficiency. *Ann Intern Med* 1986;105:200–203.

240. Horvath E, Vidal S, Syro LV, et al. Severe lymphocytic adenohypophysitis with selective disappearance of prolactin cells: a histologic, ultrastructural and immunoelectron microscopic study. *Acta Neuropathol* 2001;101:631–637.

241. Hashimoto K, Yamakita N, Ikeda T, et al. Longitudinal study of patients with idiopathic isolated TSH deficiency: possible progression of pituitary dysfunction in lymphocytic adenohypophysitis. *Endocr J* 2006;53:593–601.

242. Leung GK, Lopes MB, Thorner MO, et al. Primary hypophysitis: a single-center experience in 16 cases. *J Neurosurg* 2004;101:262–271.

243. Bensing S, Hulting AL, Hoog A, et al. Lymphocytic hypophysitis: report of two biopsy-proven cases and one suspected case with pituitary autoantibodies. *J Endocrinol Invest* 2007; 30:153–162.

244. Vajtai I, Sahli R, Kappeler A. Pituitary prolactinoma with T cell rich inflammatory infiltrate: a possible example of antitumoral immune response to be differentiated from lymphocytic hypophysitis. *Acta Neuropathol* 2006;111:397–399.

245. Cooper R, Belilos E, Drexler S, et al. Idiopathic giant-cell granulomatous hypophysitis mimicking acute meningitis. *Am J Med Sci* 1999;318:339–342.

246. Fujiwara T, Ota K, Kakudo N, et al. Idiopathic giant cell granulomatous hypophysitis with hypopituitarism, right abducens nerve paresis and masked diabetes insipidus. *Intern Med* 2001;40:915–919.

247. Bhansali A, Velayutham P, Radotra BD, et al. Idiopathic granulomatous hypophysitis presenting as non-functioning pituitary adenoma: description of six cases and review of literature. *Br J Neurosurg* 2004;18:489–494.

248. Scanarini M, d'Avella D, Rotilio A, et al. Giant-cell granulomatous hypophysitis: a distinct clinicopathological entity. *J Neurosurg* 1989;71:681–686.

249. Roncaroli F, Bacci A, Frank G, et al. Granulomatous hypophysitis caused by a ruptured intrasellar Rathke's cleft cyst: report of a case and review of the literature. *Neurosurgery* 1998;43:146–149.

250. Folkerth RD, Price DL Jr, Schwartz M, et al. Xanthomatous hypophysitis. *Am J Surg Pathol* 1998;22:736–741.

251. Deodhare SS, Bilbao JM, Kovacs K, et al. Xanthomatous hypophysitis: a novel entity of obscure etiology. *Endocr Pathol* 1999;10:237–241.

252. Pillai P, Ray-Chaudhury A, Ammirati M, et al. Solitary pituitary sarcoidosis with normal endocrine function. *J Neurosurg* 2008;108:591–594.

253. Rubin MR, Bruce JN, Khandji AG, et al. Sarcoidosis within a pituitary adenoma. *Pituitary* 2001;4:195–202.

254. Bihan H, Christozova V, Dumas JL, et al. Sarcoidosis: clinical, hormonal, and magnetic resonance imaging (MRI) manifestations of hypothalamic-pituitary disease in 9 patients and review of the literature. *Medicine (Baltimore)* 2007;86:259–268.

255. Tebben PJ, Atkinson JL, Scheithauer BW, et al. Granulomatous adenohypophysitis after interferon and ribavirin therapy. *Endocr Pract* 2007;13:169–175.

256. Scheithauer BW, Silva AI, Atkinson JL, et al. Pituitary adenoma with tumoral granulomatous reaction. *Endocr Pathol* 2007;18:86–90.

257. Gharib H, Frey HM, Laws ER Jr, et al. Coexistent primary empty sella syndrome and hyperprolactinemia. Report of 11 cases. *Arch Intern Med* 1983;143:1383–1386.

258. Kovacs K, Bilbao JM, Fornasier VL, et al. Pituitary pathology in Erdheim-Chester disease. *Endocr Pathol* 2004;15:159–166.

259. Ng HK, Poon WS. Sinus histiocytosis with massive lymphadenopathy localized to the sella. *Br J Neurosurg* 1995;9:551–555.

260. Kelly WF, Bradey N, Scoones D. Rosai-Dorfman disease presenting as a pituitary tumour. *Clin Endocrinol (Oxf)* 1999;50:133–137.

261. Woodcock RJ Jr, Mandell JW, Lipper MH. Sinus histiocytosis (Rosai-Dorfman disease) of the suprasellar region: MR imaging findings—a case report. *Radiology* 1999;213:808–810.

262. Maira G, Anile C, Mangiola A. Primary empty sella syndrome in a series of 142 patients. *J Neurosurg* 2005;103:831–836.

263. Bergland RM, Ray BS, Torack RM. Anatomical variations in the pituitary gland and adjacent structures in 225 human autopsy cases. *J Neurosurg* 1968;28:93–99.

264. Del Monte P, Foppiani L, Cafferata C, et al. Primary "empty sella" in adults: endocrine findings. *Endocr J* 2006;53:803–809.

265. Durodoye OM, Mendlovic DB, Brenner RS, et al. Endocrine disturbances in empty sella syndrome: case reports and review of literature. *Endocr Pract* 2005;11:120–124.

266. Ozkan Y, Colak R. Sheehan syndrome: clinical and laboratory evaluation of 20 cases. *Neuro Endocrinol Lett* 2005;26:257–260.

267. Weiss RE. Empty sella following spontaneous resolution of a pituitary macroadenoma. *Horm Res* 2003;60:49–52.

268. Girod C, Mazzuca M, Trouillas J. Light microscopy, fine structure and immunohistochemistry studies of 278 pituitary adenomas. In Derome PJ, Gedynak CP, Peillon F, eds. *Pituitary Adenomas.* Esciepios, Paris; 1980.

269. Solero CL, Giombini S, Morello G. Suprasellar and olfactory meningiomas. Report on a series of 153 personal cases. *Acta Neurochir (Wien)* 1983;67:181–194.

270. Spallone A. Meningioma as a sequel of radiotherapy for pituitary adenoma. *Neurochirurgia (Stuttg)* 1982;25:68–72.

271. Goebel HH, Shimokawa K, Schaake T, et al. Schwannoma of the sellar region. *Acta Neurochir (Wien)* 1979;48:191–197.

272. Bilbao JM, Horvath E, Kovacs K, et al. Intrasellar paraganglioma associated with hypopituitarism. *Arch Pathol Lab Med* 1978;102:95–98.

273. Asa SL, Kovacs K, Horvath E, et al. Sellar glomangioma. *Ultrastruct Pathol* 1984;7:49–54.

274. Sansone ME, Liwnicz BH, Mandybur TI. Giant pituitary cavernous hemangioma: case report. *J Neurosurg* 1980;53:124–126.

275. Dan NG, Smith DE. Pituitary hemangioblastoma in a patient with von Hippel-Lindau disease. Case report. *J Neurosurg* 1975;42:232–235.

276. Nagatani M, Mori S, Takimoto N, et al. Primary myxoma in the pituitary fossa: case report. *Neurosurgery* 1987;20:329–331.

277. Wolfe JT 3rd, Scheithauer BW, Dahlin DC. Giant-cell tumor of the sphenoid bone. Review of 10 cases. *J Neurosurg* 1983;59:322–327.

278. Gerlings PG. Sphenoid sinus mucocoele presenting as hypophyseal tumour. *Acta Neurochir (Wien)* 1982;61:167–171.

279. Portocarrero CJ, Robinson AG, Taylor AL, et al. Lymphoid hypophysitis. An unusual cause of hyperprolactinemia and enlarged sella turcica. *JAMA* 1981;246:1811–1812.

280. Vesely DL, Maldonado A, Levey GS. Partial hypopituitarism and possible hypothalamic involvement in sarcoidosis: report of a case and review of the literature. *Am J Med* 1977; 62:425–431.

281. del Pozo JM, Roda JE, Montoya JG, et al. Intrasellar granuloma. Case report. *J Neurosurg* 1980;53:717–719.

282. Taylon C, Duff TA. Giant cell granuloma involving the pituitary gland. Case report. *J Neurosurg* 1980;52:584–587.

283. Wolman L. Pituitary necrosis in raised intracranial pressure. *J Pathol Bacteriol* 1956;72:575.

284. White JC, Ballantine HT Jr. Intrasellar aneurysms simulating hypophyseal tumours. *J Neurosurg* 1961;18:34–50.

285. Boggan JE, Davis RL, Zorman G, et al. Intrasellar epidermoid cyst. Case report. *J Neurosurg* 1983;58:411–415.

286. Salyer D, Carter D. Squamous carcinoma arising in the pituitary gland. *Cancer* 1973;31: 713–718.

287. Gluszcz A. A cancer arising in a dermoid of the brain. A case report. *J Neuropathol Exp Neurol* 1962;21:383–387.

288. Belza J. Double midline intracranial tumors of vestigial origin: contiguous intrasellar chordoma and suprasellar craniopharyngioma. Case report. *J Neurosurg* 1966;25:199–204.

289. Mathews W, Wilson CB. Ectopic intrasellar chordoma. Case report. *J Neurosurg* 1974;40: 260–263.

290. Bjornsson J, Scheithauer BW, Okazaki H, et al. Intracranial germ cell tumors: pathobiological and immunohistochemical aspects of 70 cases. *J Neuropathol Exp Neurol* 1985;44:32–46.

291. Mangiardi JR, Flamm ES, Cravioto H, et al. Hemangiopericytoma of the pituitary fossa: case report. *Neurosurgery* 1983;13:58–62.

292. Sanchez JA, Rahman S, Strauss RA, et al. Multiple myeloma masquerading as a pituitary tumor. *Arch Pathol Lab Med* 1977;101:55–56.

293. Urbanski SJ, Bilbao JM, Horvath E, et al. Intrasellar solitary plasmacytoma terminating in multiple myeloma: a report of a case including electron microscopical study. *Surg Neurol* 1980;14:233–236.

294. Goldhammer Y, Smith JL, Yates BM. Mycotic intrasellar abscess. *Am J Ophthalmol* 1974;78: 478–484.

295. Rafael H, Gomez-Llata S. Intrasellar cysticercosis. Case report. *J Neurosurg* 1985;63: 975–976.

296. Ozgen T, Bertan V, Kansu T, et al. Intrasellar hydatid cyst. Case report. *J Neurosurg* 1984; 60:647–648.

297. Bergeron C, Kovacs K. Pituitary siderosis. A histologic, immunocytologic, and ultrastructural study. *Am J Pathol* 1978;93:295–309.

298. Schochet SS Jr, McCormick WF, Halmi NS. Pituitary gland in patients with Hurler syndrome. Light and electron microscopic study. *Arch Pathol* 1974;97:96–99.

299. Ceballos R. Pituitary changes in head trauma (analysis of 102 consecutive cases of head injury). *Ala J Med Sci* 1966;3:185–198.

300. Fajardo LF. Endocrine organs. In *Pathology of Radiation Injury.* New York, NY: Masson, 1982.

Zubair W. Baloch
Virginia A. Livolsi

Pathology of Thyroid and Parathyroid Disease

This chapter will review the pathology of lesions of the thyroid and parathyroid that are of importance to the practicing surgical pathologist and cytopathologist.

The thyroid gland is affected by several pathologic lesions that are manifested by varied morphologies. Despite the large number of lesions, it is convenient to consider them as divided into two major types: those that show a diffuse pattern and those that produce nodules. Diffuse thyroid lesions are those that are associated with conditions affecting the entire gland, such as hyperplasias and thyroiditis. Nodular lesions comprise those disorders that produce a clinical nodule and consist of nonneoplastic hyperplasias as well as benign and malignant tumors. This chapter will review the pathology of the thyroid including both neoplastic and nonneoplastic conditions. A major emphasis will be the recognition of thyroid neoplasms and, in particular, thyroid malignancies. To appreciate some of the pathologic variations that may affect the thyroid, an understanding of normal thyroid development and anatomy is useful.

THYROID DEVELOPMENT

The thyroid begins to develop between weeks 2 and 3 of gestation, and development is completed by week 11 (1). The gland develops from three structures: one median anlage and two lateral anlagen. The median anlage develops from the base of the tongue in the foramen cecum. The median anlage descends from the tongue to its final position in the anterior neck along the thyroglossal duct. Following the median anlage descent and expansion to its final position, the thyroglossal duct then atrophies, although the duct may persist, become cystic in nature, and possibly even develop papillary thyroid carcinoma in thyroid tissue present in its wall. The lateral anlage develops from what has been termed the ''fourth-fifth'' branchial pouch, which contains the ultimobranchial body. The ultimobranchial body is associated with calcitonin-secreting cells (C cells). Fusion of the median and both lateral anlagen occurs in the upper lateral aspect of the gland; C cells predominate in this area. Solid cell nests composed of collections of stratified epithelial cells with focal mucin production and cyst formation are believed to be remnants of the ultimobranchial body and may be seen in up to 30% of adult thyroids (Fig. 13.1) (2–4).

DEVELOPMENTAL ANOMALIES

The most common anomalies encountered with the thyroid gland include abnormalities in gland development. Thyroid maldescent can result in the presence of lingual thyroid located in the back of the tongue; as this tissue grows, it could become a surgical emergency in young children (Fig. 13.2) (5). It is critical to be aware that in patients with lingual thyroid, this may be the only thyroid that is present. Therefore, its removal could result in profound acute hypothyroidism. Thyroid tissue

can be found in any location along the thyroglossal duct. In fact, more than 60% of thyroglossal duct cysts will contain thyroid tissue in the wall. Because of its close association with the development of other tissues, thyroid tissue may be seen in association with the esophagus, larynx, trachea, jugular carotid lymph nodes, soft tissues of the neck, and even heart and great vessels (6,7).

Because of the intimate developmental relationships, derivatives of the branchial or pharyngeal pouches (parathyroid tissue, salivary gland remnants, and thymus) can sometimes be found in the thyroid (Fig. 13.3). Developmental considerations also explain the finding of normal thyroid tissue in the cervical fat or muscle (8). Fat, cartilage, or muscle may occasionally be found within the thyroid capsule (9,10). These minor abnormalities of development must be remembered lest they be confused with infiltrative neoplastic growth.

Benign-appearing thyroid tissue in lymph node tissue should be evaluated with extreme caution. It is believed by some, but not all, that lymph nodes medial to the jugular vein may contain benign thyroid tissue within the capsule (11). These thyroid inclusions must be contained within the capsule and must be composed of normal-appearing thyroid without atypical nuclei, psammoma bodies, or papillary group formation (12,13). Although normal thyroid tissue may be present in soft tissues of the lateral neck, thyroid tissue in a lymph node lateral to the jugular vein, no matter how benign appearing, represents metastatic papillary carcinoma (14).

Occasionally, the thyroid gland may not develop or only partially develop. Thyroid hemiaplasia is much more common than complete aplasia, although hemiaplasia is quite rare. Thyroid hemiagenesis has been associated with Graves disease, although the exact nature of this association is not known (15).

ANATOMY OF THE THYROID

The normal adult thyroid consists of two lobes connected by an isthmus. The normal gland weight ranges from 14 to 18 g and depends on sex, size, and nutritional status of the individual, as well as appropriate iodine intake (4,16). The parathyroids and recurrent laryngeal nerves lie behind the gland (17). The superior and inferior thyroidal arteries supply the gland. The intraglandular and subcapsular lymphatics drain into the internal jugular lymph nodes (4,18).

Thyroid tissue is light brown in color and firm in consistency. Nodules are not uncommon in the euthyroid adult population (19). Microscopically, the thyroid is composed of follicles lined by epithelial cells that surround the central colloid; 20 to 40 follicles make up a lobule (Fig. 13.4) (19). Birefringent crystalline material (shown by chemical analysis and x-ray diffraction analysis to be calcium oxalate) is commonly found in the colloid of normal or diseased thyroids (20). Small collections of C cells are situated within the confines of the basement membrane of

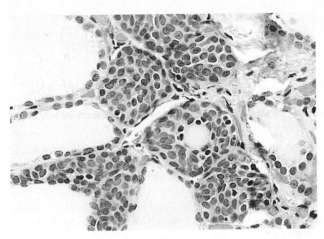

Figure 13.1. Ultimobranchial body rest in thyroid showing solid cell nests with focal cyst formation. The ultimobranchial body is believed to give rise to the thyroid C cells.

the thyroid follicles. Difficult to identify by ordinary histologic stains, the normal C cells can be identified by immunostaining for calcitonin (21).

Ultrastructural studies of normal thyroid show that the follicular cells are arranged in a single layer around the central colloid (22). The cells contain liposomes and a complement of endoplasmic reticulum and small mitochondria. The nuclei are round with homogeneous chromatin. Well-developed desmosomes and terminal bars separate cells. In the interstitium, numerous fenestrated capillaries are noted (22). The C cells are found within the confines of the basement membranes of the follicles. In the cytoplasm of these C cells, numerous double membrane-bound neurosecretory granules containing calcitonin are found (21,23).

DIFFUSE THYROID ENLARGEMENTS

THE THYROIDITIDES

Although occasionally presenting as nodules or asymmetric enlargement of the gland, thyroiditis commonly involves the thyroid diffusely.

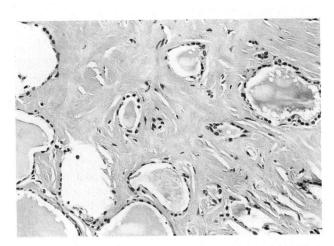

Figure 13.2. High-power view of lingual thyroid showing thyroid follicle surrounded by dense fibrous tissue. This was an incidental finding at surgery in a patient with head and neck squamous cell carcinoma.

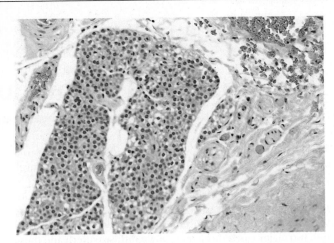

Figure 13.3. Parathyroid tissue involving capsule of the thyroid. Most parathyroid tissue associated with the thyroid is present within the thyroid capsule. Occasionally intrathyroidal parathyroid tissue may be seen.

Acute Thyroiditis

Acute thyroiditis is rare and is almost always a result of infection, although acute thyroiditis may be encountered in the thyroid shortly after radiation exposure (24–26). The disease is most commonly encountered in malnourished children, elderly debilitated adults, immunocompromised individuals, or in otherwise healthy patients following trauma to the neck. Most patients present with painful enlargement of the gland. Grossly, the gland often appears normal but may be focally or diffusely softened with areas of purulence. Microscopically, acute inflammation with microabscess formation is present. Microorganisms may be seen. A variety of organisms cause thyroiditis including bacteria, fungi, and viruses (26,27). In individuals with human immunodeficiency virus infection, the occurrence of *Pneumocystis carinii* infection has been reported.

Granulomatous Thyroiditis

Granulomatous subacute thyroiditis, also referred to as nonsuppurative thyroiditis or de Quervain disease, is a rare entity that

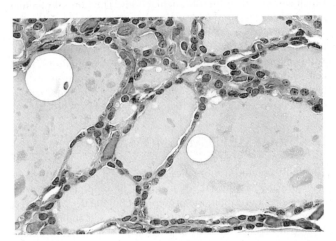

Figure 13.4. Normal thyroid follicles lined by a single layer of flat cuboidal follicular epithelial cells. A rich vascular network is observed between the follicles.

usually presents in women and has been associated with HLA-Bw35 (26,28). The changes seen in the gland are most likely a result of the response of the thyroid to systemic viral infection; some authors suggest that it represents actual viral infection of the gland. A viral cause for this disorder can be supported by both clinical and epidemiologic studies. "Epidemics" of subacute thyroiditis have been reported (29). Most patients with subacute thyroiditis recover without any permanent damage to the thyroid. However, some studies have reported end-stage hypothyroidism in 5% to 9% of patients (28).

Grossly the thyroid is asymmetrically enlarged and firm. Irregular white-tan lesions or several small poorly demarcated nodules may simulate carcinoma (26,30). Microscopically, early in the disease, there is loss of the follicular epithelium and colloid depletion. Leakage of stored hormone occurs, and clinical hyperthyroidism may result. The inflammatory response, which is composed initially of polymorphonuclear leukocytes and even microabscesses, progresses until lymphocytes, plasma cells, and histiocytes become the major inflammatory cells. A rim of histiocytes and giant cells replaces the follicular epithelium, giving rise to a granulomatous appearance. A central fibrotic reaction occurs. Recovery is associated with regeneration of follicles from the viable edges of the involved areas (26,31).

Palpation Thyroiditis

Palpation thyroiditis (multifocal granulomatous folliculitis) is found in 85% to 95% of surgically resected thyroids and probably represents the thyroid's response to minor trauma. The histologic features of this lesion include multiple isolated follicles or small groups of follicles that show partial or circumferential loss of epithelium and replacement of the lost epithelium by inflammatory cells, predominantly macrophages (Fig. 13.5). The lesions most likely regress and sometimes need to be differentiated from C-cell hyperplasia and ultimobranchial body remnants (32).

AUTOIMMUNE THYROID DISEASE

Autoimmune thyroid disease (AITD) encompasses a spectrum of clinical and morphologic entities in which interrelationships

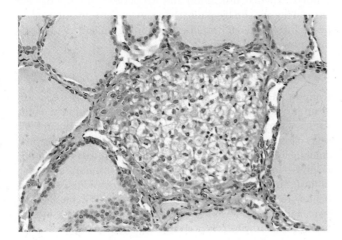

Figure 13.5. "Palpation thyroiditis" in a thyroid removed for papillary thyroid carcinoma. This form of thyroiditis is characterized by the presence of histiocytes and lymphocytes, is usually focal, and is associated with minor trauma to the gland.

are speculative but that share certain features suggesting their autoimmune etiology. The spectrum includes diffuse toxic goiter (Graves disease) associated with hyperthyroidism on the one hand and lymphocytic thyroiditis (Hashimoto disease) associated with hypothyroidism on the other. However, in between, various lesions associated with hyperthyroidism, hypothyroidism, or euthyroidism can be found. This section briefly summarizes the current thinking on autoimmunity as related to thyroid disease and discusses the pathologic aspects of the autoimmune entities most commonly seen in surgical practice.

The early work of Volpe and colleagues suggested that AITD involves an inherited defect in immune surveillance (33). The current understanding is that AITD is a polygenetic disease in which susceptibility genes and environmental initiators act together to initiate both cellular and humoral immune responses against the thyroid gland (34,35). Genome-wide screening and linkage analyses have identified several chromosomal foci that are linked to AITD. These are *HT-1* (chromosome 13q33) and *HT-2* (chromosome 12q22) for Hashimoto thyroiditis and *GD-1* (chromosome 14q31), *GD-2* (chromosome 20q11.2), and *GD-3* (chromosome Xq21) for Graves disease. In addition, several other genes have been proposed as susceptibility or immunoregulatory genes. These include major histocompatibility complex (chromosome 6), cytotoxic T-lymphocyte–associated antigen-4 (*CTLA-4*) gene (chromosome 2), *CD40* (chromosome 20), thyroglobulin gene (chromosome 8), and the autoimmune regulator gene (chromosome 21) (35–38). The exact mechanism of involvement of environmental factors in AITD is still not clearly understood; however, it is theorized to include dietary iodide, medication, and infection (38).

PATHOLOGY OF AUTOIMMUNE THYROID DISEASE

The presence of lymphoid cells in the substance of the thyroid parenchyma probably reflects an abnormal immunologic state. However, the interrelationships among classic chronic thyroiditis, its variants, and "nonspecific" thyroiditis are problematic.

The morphologic and immunopathologic overlap between nonspecific lymphocytic thyroiditis and Hashimoto disease suggests that they represent a spectrum of autoimmune injury (37,39–41).

In Hashimoto thyroiditis (42,43), the gland is firm and symmetrically enlarged, weighing from 25 to 250 g (43). Normal thyroid lobulation is accentuated by interlobular fibrosis. The thyroid has a tan-yellow appearance attributed to the abundant lymphoid tissue. The thyroid follicles are small and atrophic. Colloid appears dense or may be absent. Follicular cells are metaplastic and include oncocytic (Hürthle cell), clear cell, and squamous types (Fig. 13.6) (25,26,43). In the stroma and in atrophic follicles, a lymphoplasmacytic infiltration with well-developed germinal centers is found. Variable degrees of interlobular fibrosis are seen. The nuclei of the follicular epithelial cells often show nuclear clearing, enlargement, and overlapping; this reactive nuclear change can be mistaken for foci of papillary thyroid carcinoma (Fig. 13.6) (26,44). Apoptosis is believed to be the mechanism for thyroid follicular cell destruction in Hashimoto disease (45).

The lymphocytic infiltrate is composed of both T and B cells in an almost 1:1 ratio, differing from the peripheral blood, which shows T-cell predominance (46). T lymphocytes within

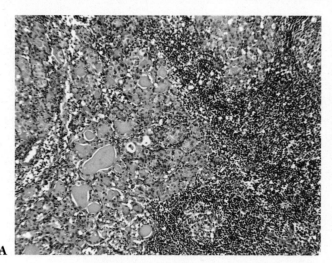 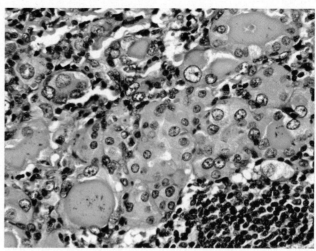

A   B

Figure 13.6.   **(A)** The thyroid in Hashimoto disease shows a dense lymphoplasmacytic infiltrate with germinal
center formation. The follicular epithelium often shows Hürthle cell change. **(B)** Often, the follicular epithelium
adjacent to the inflammatory cell infiltrate of autoimmune thyroiditis shows "clear" chromatin similar to the
nuclear changes seen in papillary thyroid carcinoma. These changes are often seen scattered throughout the
inflamed gland and should not be misinterpreted as papillary carcinoma.

the thyroid are predominantly suppressor type, whereas the peripheral blood of these patients contains mostly helper T cells (47). The B cells are usually of the immunoglobulin (Ig) G-κ subclass.

Patients with Hashimoto thyroiditis are at increased risk of neoplasia with the most common malignancy being malignant lymphoma, B-cell type (48,49). In addition, patients with Hashimoto disease may be prone to the development of plasmacytomas within the gland (50). A peculiar variant of mucoepidermoid carcinoma, known as sclerosing mucoepidermoid carcinoma with eosinophilia, has been recognized in patients with Hashimoto disease (51).

CHRONIC LYMPHOCYTIC THYROIDITIS CLASSIFICATION

Mizukami et al. (52) established a new classification of chronic lymphocytic thyroiditis. This classification is useful because it allows one to see that the mere presence of lymphocytes in the thyroid does not indicate autoimmune disease. They divided their patients into four groups:

1. Chronic thyroiditis, oxyphilic: This group contains patients with classic Hashimoto disease histology.
2. Chronic thyroiditis, mixed: This group shows less of an infiltrate than group 1 with minimal fibrosis. Patients demonstrate normal thyroid, hyperthyroidism, or hypothyroidism.
3. Chronic thyroiditis, hyperplastic: This group shows glandular hyperplasia associated with only a small lymphocytic reaction. Most patients are hyperthyroid.
4. Chronic thyroiditis, focal: This group shows only a focal lymphocytic reaction, and most patients are euthyroid.

FIBROSING VARIANT OF HASHIMOTO THYROIDITIS

The fibrous or fibrosing variant of Hashimoto thyroiditis comprises approximately 10% to 13% of all cases of Hashimoto

disease. Pathologically, the thyroid architecture is destroyed with severe follicular atrophy, dense keloid-like fibrosis, and prominent squamous or epidermoid metaplasia of the follicular epithelium.

Several other fibrosing entities, such as Riedel disease, tumefactive fibrosis of the head and neck, and fibrous atrophy (idiopathic myxedema), need to be differentiated from the fibrosing variant of Hashimoto disease. In fibrosing thyroiditis, the sclerosis is confined to the thyroid, and the lobular architecture of the gland is maintained (52,53).

PAINLESS/SILENT THYROIDITIS

Painless thyroiditis is an autoimmune disease that causes painless enlargement of thyroid gland along with brief hyperthyroidism followed by hypothyroidism. It can occur in the postpartum period and is called postpartum thyroiditis. Mizukami et al. (54) analyzed 26 biopsies from patients with painless thyroiditis. All showed follicular disruption and lymphocytic infiltration, but stromal fibrous and oxyphilic changes were rare. Subset analysis of the intrathyroidal lymphocytes showed similarities to Hashimoto thyroiditis (54,55).

FOCAL NONSPECIFIC THYROIDITIS

Lymphocytic infiltration of the thyroid is found more frequently at autopsy and in surgical specimens since the addition of iodide to the water supplies of the United States approximately 60 years ago (56). It has been suggested that iodide (iodine) may combine with a protein, act as an antigen, and evoke an immune response localized to the thyroid gland. Postmortem studies indicate an incidence of focal lymphocytic thyroiditis of approximately 15% to 20% in women; it is found rarely in men. Kurashima and Hirokawa (39) believe that focal lymphocytic infiltration of the thyroid represents an immunologic disorder associated with aging.

Focal aggregates of lymphocytes and, occasionally, germinal center formation are noted, but oncocytes are rarely present. Follicular atrophy is also rare (39).

OTHER ENTITIES WITH LYMPHOCYTES IN THE THYROID

Diffuse Toxic Goiter/Graves Disease

Autoimmune hyperthyroidism occurs predominantly in women (female-to-male ratio of approximately 9:1) (40). Patients with Graves disease show a genetic predisposition to the disease, and their relatives have an unusually high incidence of other autoimmune disorders; the gland is infiltrated by lymphocytes (41,57). Similarities to Hashimoto thyroiditis include an apparently genetically determined defect in suppressor T cells with consequent proliferation of thyroid-directed B cells, which produce antithyroid autoantibodies. These antibodies (thyroid receptor antibodies [TRAbs]) are directed against the thyrotropin receptor complex of the follicular epithelial cell, which they stimulate to grow and function (34,58). Hence, the gland enlarges and secretes increased amounts of thyroid hormones, resulting in clinical hyperthyroidism.

Grossly, the thyroid in Graves disease is diffusely and usually symmetrically enlarged, with weights of 50 to 150 g. Vascularity is marked. Histologic examination shows retention of lobular architecture, prominent vascular congestion, and follicular hyperplasia. The follicular cells are columnar with enlarged nuclei. Colloid is virtually absent. Papillary infoldings of the follicular epithelium are also seen. The follicular cells in Graves disease can demonstrate marked nuclear chromatin clearing, which in combination with papillary hyperplasia can be mistaken for papillary carcinoma (59). However, at low-power magnification, the diffuse nature of the process can be a clue that one is dealing with a nonneoplastic process. Lymphocytes are often found in the stroma. Within the follicular centers, B cells predominate; T lymphocytes, especially helper subsets, are seen in a perifollicular location (60). In a diffuse goiter removed from a hyperthyroid patient, the absence of stromal lymphocytes should raise the possibility of a secondary form of hyperthyroidism, such as a pituitary lesion (measurements of thyroid-stimulating hormone will resolve this issue).

Therapy-induced changes in histology include decreased vascularity and involution of the follicular epithelium with repletion of colloid after iodide therapy. Beta-blocking drugs and thiouracil do not alter the morphology (61,62); however, radioactive iodine treatment can show follicular atrophy and fibrosis (63). Lymphoid infiltration, which is sometimes associated with follicular center formation, is often seen in patients with classic hyperthyroid Graves disease. The lymphoid cells are usually found only in the interfollicular stroma and do not encroach upon the follicles themselves. The follicles show marked epithelial hyperplasia, and unless presurgical iodide treatment has been administered, fibrosis is unusual (62).

Toxic Nodular Goiter

In glands with hyperfunctioning follicular nodules, lymphocytic collections can be seen; in unusual cases, this occurs outside the capsule of the nodule (64).

Drug-Associated Thyroiditis

Some medications may result in pathologic changes in the thyroid. It is often not possible to determine whether the drug has induced thyroiditis or has uncovered pre-existing subclinical thyroid disease. Certain drugs are associated with morphologic changes. Goiter commonly develops in patients treated with lithium for prolonged periods. Hypothyroidism occurs in 3% to 12% of such cases (65,66).

Lymphocytic thyroiditis is also believed to be associated with the addition of iodine to diets. In a study of 10,000 Japanese children between the ages of 6 and 18 years, the incidence of biopsy-proven lymphocytic thyroiditis was 5.3 per 1000 in a high-iodine area compared with an incidence of a 1.4 per 1000 in a low-iodine zone (67).

Thyroid functional abnormalities have been recognized in patients taking amiodarone, an iodine-containing cardiotropic drug (68). Alves et al. (68) reported that in 104 patients on chronic amiodarone treatment, 32% developed hypothyroidism, and 23% developed hyperthyroidism. The histologic changes described by Smyrk et al. (69) included follicular damage and disruption, epithelial cell vacuolization, and macrophagic and lymphocytic reaction to degenerating follicles. By electron microscopy, a lamellar configuration was seen in a few lysosomes.

Atkins et al. (70) described hypothyroidism occurring in several patients receiving interleukin-2 (IL-2) and lymphokine-activated killer cell therapy for advanced cancers and postulated that the therapy unmasked a subclinical autoimmune thyroiditis; the hypothyroidism appeared to be associated with a favorable tumor response in these patients.

Papillary Cancer

Scattered lymphocytic infiltrates are often seen at the periphery of thyroid neoplasms, particularly in the vicinity of the infiltrative edges of papillary cancer (71,72). Volpe (73) suggests that the lymphoid infiltrate results from a "local antigenic perturbation" to altered antigen on the tumor cells.

FIBROSING THYROID LESIONS

Several entities can result in significant fibrosis in the thyroid. Fibrosing thyroid lesions include the fibrosing variant of Hashimoto thyroiditis and fibrous atrophy, which were discussed earlier.

RIEDEL THYROIDITIS

Riedel thyroiditis (also known as Riedel disease, invasive fibrous thyroiditis, or Riedel struma) has been incorrectly included among the thyroiditides (74). It is not really a disorder of the thyroid but one that involves the thyroid as well as other structures in the neck or even systemic structures. Riedel disease is an extremely rare entity with an incidence of 0.05% of surgical thyroid diseases and a female predominance. Most patients are euthyroid, although hypothyroidism and hyperthyroidism have been reported (75).

Descriptions of the thyroid range from stony hard or woody fixed; the term *ligneous thyroiditis* has been used (75). When the lesion is confined to the neck, no systemic abnormalities are found; however, in some patients, the neck lesion represents part of a systemic disease; retroperitoneal, mediastinal, or retroorbital fibrosis as well as sclerosing cholangitis may occur (76–78). In the review by Schwaegerle et al. (75), 34% of patients with Riedel disease reported after 1960 had other fibrosing lesions. Familial cases with multifocal involvement have been described (79). No etiologic relationship to drug intake has been suggested for isolated Riedel disease.

Grossly, the fibrosis involves all or part of the thyroid and is described as woody and very hard. Extension of the fibrosis beyond the thyroid is characteristic. Clinically and grossly, the lesion may be confused with carcinoma. Histologically, the involved portions of the gland are destroyed and replaced by keloid-like fibrous tissue associated with lymphocytes and plasma cells. The fibrous tissue extends into muscle, nerves, and fat and entraps blood vessels. In approximately 25% of cases, the parathyroid glands are also encased (75,78). There is an associated vasculitis (predominantly a phlebitis) with frequent thrombosis (74,78). In 25% of cases of Riedel disease, an adenoma is identified centrally in the fibrotic mass (74). Although the relationship between the adenoma and the fibrous reaction is unknown, the fibrous tissue proliferation may be a reaction to the adenoma or its products.

Quantitative studies of the Ig-containing cells in fibrous Hashimoto thyroiditis show that cells containing κ-light chains outnumber λ-containing cells (64% vs. 36%), whereas in Riedel disease, λ-containing cells comprise more than 70% of the immunocyte population (80). In Hashimoto thyroiditis, IgA cells make up approximately 15% of the lymphocytes, whereas in Riedel disease, IgA-containing plasma cells comprise approximately 45% of the immunocyte population. The immunologic evaluation supports the separation of the distinctive Riedel lesion from other thyroiditides.

COMBINED RIEDEL DISEASE AND HASHIMOTO THYROIDITIS

In rare instances, the thyroid gland can show features of both Riedel disease and Hashimoto thyroiditis. The histologic picture resembles Riedel disease, whereas the serology shows thyroglobulin and microsomal antibodies seen in Hashimoto thyroiditis (81,82).

RADIATION FIBROSIS

Reaction of the thyroid to radiation can result in a variety of complications that are related to dose in cases of external radiation to the gland. When radioiodine is administered, hypothyroidism is common, and the incidence increases with time (83).

Pathologic changes occur in the thyroid after external radiation in approximately 75% of cases and include foci of follicular hyperplasia (88%), lymphocytic infiltration (67%), oncocytic metaplasia (42%), fibrosis (25%), and adenomatous nodule formation (51%) (Fig. 13.7) (84).

Months or years after radioiodine, a grossly shrunken and fibrotic gland results that histologically shows fibrosis, follicular atrophy, oncocytic and squamous metaplasia, lymphocytic infiltration, and nuclear abnormalities. Vascular change (intimal thickening and sclerosis of arterial walls often with inflammatory cell cuffing) is characteristic of radiation damage (84).

AMYLOIDOSIS

Amyloid is found in the thyroid in three different settings. The most common of these is the amyloid in the stroma of medullary thyroid carcinoma (85). Amyloid goiter is a tumefactive mass of amyloid associated with a foreign body giant-cell response and with adipose tissue. It is associated with systemic amyloid-

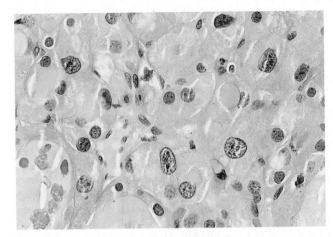

Figure 13.7. This nodule from a patient with nodular goiter shows random nuclear atypia. This change is often seen in the thyroid after radiation exposure.

osis. Another complication of systemic amyloidosis is amyloid deposition in the thyroid stroma and in glandular and periglandular blood vessels. Hypothyroidism may result (86,87).

FIBROSIS CAUSED BY COLLAGEN VASCULAR DISEASE

Approximately 14% to 24% of patients with scleroderma experience thyroid dysfunction as a result of interfollicular fibrosis, and 5% show evidence of chronic lymphocytic thyroiditis. The fibrosis may be caused by vascular sclerosis, which is common in scleroderma (88,89).

PIGMENTS IN THE THYROID

Pigmentation of the thyroid may be caused by iron (hemosiderin) deposition in sites of bleeding or may be found in disorders of iron metabolism such as hemochromatosis. In the former, the pigment is found in macrophages, whereas in the latter, it is present in the follicular epithelium (Fig. 13.8) (90).

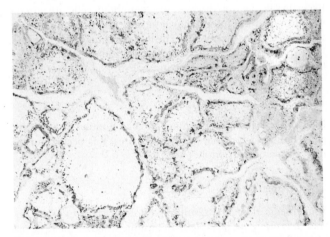

Figure 13.8. A Prussian blue stain for iron in a patient with hemochromatosis shows extensive iron deposition in follicular epithelial cells.

In patients on chronic minocycline therapy (or occasionally other tetracycline antibiotics), deposition of minocycline-associated pigment produces coal-black coloration of the thyroid. These effects appear to be related to interactions of minocycline with thyroid peroxidase, the key enzyme in thyroid hormone synthesis (91). Histologically, a granular, dustlike precipitate of black-brown pigment is noted in the apical portions of the follicular epithelial cells (90,92). Only rarely are abnormalities of thyroid function noted in these cases.

NODULAR THYROID ENLARGEMENTS

This category consists of thyroid lesions that present as solitary or multiple nodules: benign nodular goiter, toxic nodules, and benign and malignant neoplasms. The nodular thyroid lesions are of most interest to surgeons and patients because the major differential diagnostic possibility is cancer. This section describes the gross and microscopic morphology of the various thyroid nodular lesions.

LESIONS CHARACTERIZED BY A PAPILLARY PATTERN

Papillary thyroid lesions include papillary carcinoma, papillary hyperplasia (often associated with hyperfunction), and papillary change in an adenoma or adenomatous follicular nodule.

PAPILLARY CARCINOMA OF THE THYROID

In the United States, thyroid carcinoma comprises approximately 1% of all cancers and accounts for 0.2% of cancer deaths. Most of these cancers are of the papillary type. This is the most common malignant tumor of the gland in countries having iodine-sufficient or iodine-excess diets and comprises approximately 80% of thyroid malignancies in the United States (93). These common tumors tend to be biologically indolent and have an excellent prognosis (>90% survival at 20 years) (93,94). The tumors invade lymphatics, leading to multifocal lesions and to regional node metastases. Venous invasion rarely occurs, and metastases outside the neck are unusual (5% to 7% of cases) (71,95,96).

Papillary carcinoma can occur at any age and rarely has been diagnosed as a congenital tumor (97). Most tumors are diagnosed in patients in the third and fifth decades (98,99). Women are affected more than men in ratios of 2:1 to 4:1 (99).

Etiologic Factors

Etiologic factors for papillary carcinoma are not well established; various cellular and genetic mechanisms/targets have been studied in the development of papillary carcinoma.

Iodine

The addition of iodine to the diet in endemic goiter areas in Europe and South America has been associated with a decreased incidence of follicular cancer and an increase in papillary carcinoma (100,101).

External Radiation

External radiation probably plays a role in the development of papillary cancer (102). The average time from radiation expo-

sure to tumor development has classically been reported as 20 years; however, development time is variable, particularly following major nuclear facility accidents such as that seen in Chernobyl. A great increase in the incidence of papillary carcinoma in Belarus and Ukraine has been apparent since the Chernobyl nuclear accident (103). The increased incidence was seen predominantly in young children from that area who had been exposed to the radiation. Most reported tumors following this nuclear disaster have been papillary carcinomas, many of which show aggressive histologic features including extracapsular extension and vascular invasion (103,104).

Autoimmune Disease

Some authors believe that patients with Graves disease have a higher than expected incidence of papillary cancer (105); other studies disagree (106). Many studies indicate that up to one-third of papillary cancers arise in the setting of chronic thyroiditis. However, these studies tend to lack serologic proof of preexisting thyroiditis (107). Follow-up studies of patients with documented thyroiditis indicate that the tumor that arises much more frequently in these glands is malignant lymphoma, not papillary cancer (discussed subsequently) (108). Because papillary cancer and thyroiditis are both common conditions, the possibility of coincidental coexistence is more likely than an etiologic relationship (109). However, recent molecular data have shown that foci of atypical follicular epithelium in chronic thyroiditis do show loss of heterozygosity for various tumor suppressor genes and RET/PTC rearrangements (110).

Hormonal and Reproductive Factors

Papillary carcinoma is more common in women than men. Some studies have suggested the role of various hormonal factors in the development of papillary carcinoma; these include increased parity, late age at the onset of first pregnancy, fertility problems, and oral contraceptive use (111). Lee et al. (112) have shown that estradiol promotes cell proliferation via enhancement of antiapoptotic signaling pathway in a human papillary thyroid carcinoma cell line; interestingly, this growth-promoting effect of estradiol was attenuated by tamoxifen.

Genetic Syndromes

Papillary carcinomas have been described in patients with familial adenomatous polyposis coli (FAP), Cowden syndrome, hereditary nonpolyposis colon cancer syndrome (HNPCC), Peutz-Jeghers syndrome, and ataxia telangiectasia (113,114).

FAP is caused by germline mutations of the adenomatous polyposis coli (*APC*) gene. Thyroid carcinoma, mostly papillary carcinoma (>95% of cases), occurs in 1% to 2% of patients with FAP; all of these patients show germline mutations of the *APC* gene; however, somatic mutations of or loss of heterozygosity (LOH) for the *APC* gene are not found in thyroid tumors. Interestingly, a majority of these tumors do show activation of RET/PTC1 in thyroid tumors, suggesting a possible association between *APC* and RET/PTC in the development of this particular subset of familial papillary carcinoma (115,116).

Cowden syndrome is characterized by formation of hamartomas in several organs and a high risk of developing breast and thyroid cancer. The genetic locus for Cowden syndrome has been mapped to chromosome 10q23.3 and is also known as

PTEN, which is a protein tyrosine phosphatase and exerts its tumor suppressor effects by antagonizing protein tyrosine kinase activity. Interestingly, *PTEN* mutation or gene deletion is noted in 26% of benign tumors but only in 6.1% of malignant tumors of the thyroid (117,118).

Thyroid and Parathyroid Adenomas

Occasionally, papillary cancers arise in benign nodules or adenomas (119,120). This may result merely from a malignant tumor arising in a nodular area of the gland instead of in a nonnodular zone (i.e., it is likely to be a random event of location and not indicate a casual relationship). Several authors have described the association of papillary carcinoma and parathyroid adenoma or hyperplasia. Both types of lesions are associated with a history of low-dose external radiation to the neck (119).

Pathology

The gross appearance of papillary thyroid cancer is quite variable (71,121). The lesions may appear anywhere within the gland. By definition, typical papillary carcinomas are greater than 1.0 to 1.5 cm, often averaging 2 to 3 cm, although lesions may be quite large (Fig. 13.9). The lesions are firm and usually white in color with an invasive appearance. Lesional calcification is a common feature. Because of extensive sclerosis, the lesion may grossly resemble a scar. In addition, cyst formation may be observed. In fact, some lesions may rarely be completely cystic, making diagnosis difficult (122,123). Necrosis (in the absence of a prior needle biopsy) is not a feature of typical papillary carcinoma and suggests a higher grade lesion (124).

Microscopically, papillary carcinomas share certain features. The neoplastic papillae contain a central core of fibrovascular (occasionally just fibrous) tissue lined by one layer or, occasionally, several layers of cells with crowded oval nuclei (Fig. 13.10). In contrast, hyperplasia of thyroid follicles may sometimes exaggerate into papillary change; there is infolding of the lining epithelium composed of columnar cells with basal round and uniform nuclei. There is either no central core or a core of edematous or myxomatous paucicellular stroma often including small follicles (subfollicle formation) (106,121–123).

Psammoma bodies that represent the "ghosts" of dead papillae are differentiated from dystrophic calcifications by lamellations (Fig. 13.10) (125). True psammoma bodies are formed by focal areas of infarction of the tips of papillae attracting calcium that is deposited on the dying cells. Progressive infarction of the papillae and ensuing calcium deposition lead to lamellation (126). Psammoma bodies are usually present within the cores of papillae or in the tumor stroma, but not within the neoplastic follicles. Only rarely are psammoma bodies found in benign conditions in the thyroid (127).

The nuclei of papillary cancer have been described as clear, ground-glass, empty, or Orphan Annie–eyed (Fig. 13.10). These nuclei are larger and more oval than normal follicular nuclei and contain hypodense chromatin (122,128). In papillary cancer, these nuclei often overlap one another. Although cleared nuclei are characteristic of papillary carcinoma, autoimmune thyroiditis, particularly Hashimoto disease, often shows similar nuclear changes (41). Intranuclear inclusions of cytoplasm are often found. Another characteristic of the papillary cancer nucleus is the nuclear groove (123,128). Nuclear grooves may be seen in other thyroid lesions including Hashimoto disease, adenomatous hyperplasia, and diffuse hyperplasia, as well as in follicular adenomas (particularly hyalinizing trabecular neoplasm) (129,130). For the most part, nuclear grooves are more commonly seen in papillary carcinoma than in other thyroid lesions; however, the mere presence of nuclear grooves is not diagnostic for papillary carcinoma.

Most of these tumors will be composed predominantly or focally of papillary areas. A large number will contain follicular areas as well (131). The tumor cells are usually columnar. Clear nuclei are found in more than 80% of such lesions, intranuclear inclusions are found in approximately 80% to 85%, and nuclear grooves are seen in almost all cases. Mitoses are exceptional in usual papillary carcinoma. Psammoma bodies are found in approximately 40% to 50% of cases (123), but their presence in thyroid tissue indicates that a papillary carcinoma is most

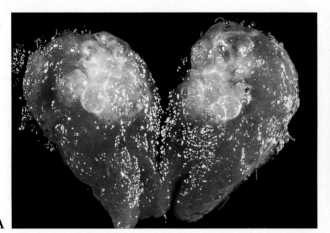
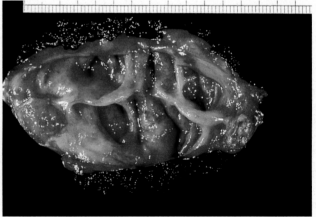

A   **B**

Figure 13.9. **(A)** Gross picture of a papillary thyroid carcinoma showing a yellow-white infiltrative mass with evidence of fibrous strands. **(B)** Gross picture of a papillary thyroid carcinoma with extensive cyst formation. Note the smooth lining to the cyst wall. This lesion was also associated with cystic lymph node metastases, which were the first presenting sign of tumor. These lesions can be difficult to diagnose, particularly on fine-needle aspiration, because the papillary carcinoma cells may be only focally present in the cyst wall.

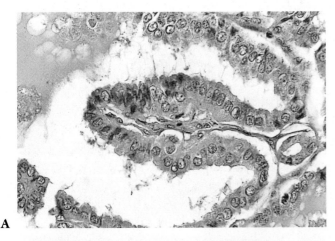

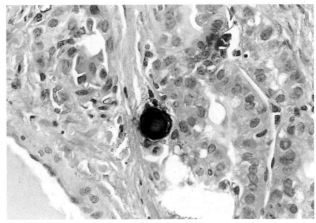

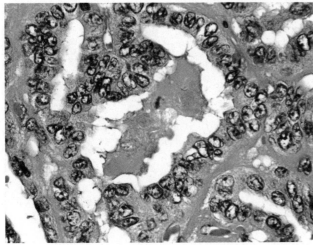

Figure 13.10. **(A)** Microscopic examination of a papilla in papillary carcinoma. Even at this power, nuclear clearing, elongation, and overlapping are identified. The papillary group shows a nonedematous vascular core (200×). **(B)** Psammoma body formation is common in papillary thyroid carcinoma. **(C)** High-power view of papillary carcinoma nuclei showing nuclear clearing, enlargement, overlapping, and intranuclear grooves (400×).

likely present somewhere in the gland. The finding of psammoma bodies in a cervical lymph node is strong evidence of a papillary cancer in the thyroid (14).

Many papillary carcinomas (approximately 15% to 45%) contain foci of squamous differentiation (132). Almost all papillary carcinomas show areas of desmoplasia either in the central portions of the tumor or at the peripheral zones of the lesions. Even in encapsulated lesions, sclerosis is seen in areas of capsular penetration (133).

Scattered lymphocytes are common at the invasive edges of the tumor (121,134). Rarely, an intense lymphocytic infiltrate is seen, but it is localized to the invasive tumor foci and does not indicate a pre-existing underlying chronic thyroiditis (121). Cyst formation may occur and, in fact, may be so striking that the diagnosis of papillary carcinoma is difficult to make, particularly if the lesion has metastasized to neck lymph nodes, making the distinction (particularly on a clinical basis) from a branchial cleft cyst difficult (135).

Papillary carcinoma invades the glandular lymphatics, which accounts for the high incidence of regional node metastases (93,122,123). Papillary carcinoma can also present as multifocal tumors within the same gland. It has been shown that papillary carcinomas are clonal proliferations. The monoclonal nature of papillary carcinoma has been proven by molecular biology techniques. In view of these studies, it is believed that multifocality of papillary carcinoma must be a result of intrathyroidal lymphatic spread rather than multifocal primary tumors. Re-

cent RET/PTC and LOH studies have shown that multifocal papillary microcarcinomas can be separate primaries instead of intraglandular spreading from one tumor source (136,137).

What does this multifocality mean with regard to therapy and prognosis? Some argue that because of multifocal microscopic lesions, the entire gland should be excised; others indicate that more conservative surgery (lobectomy or lobectomy and isthmusectomy) followed by thyroid suppression is adequate because the tumors are often hormonally controllable (138,139). The low frequency of local recurrence in the opposite thyroid lobe and the long-term follow-up studies of conservatively treated patients showing excellent results suggest that the second viewpoint is the wiser one. Of course, treatment of extrathyroidal or massive papillary cancer requires more radical procedures (140).

Venous invasion can be identified in up to 7% of papillary cancers (122). It has been suggested that cases with histologic vascular invasion may be considered as a sign of an increased tendency toward hematogenic invasion and consequent increase in the relative percentage of metastases (141).

Regional lymph node metastases are extremely common (≥50%) at initial presentation of usual papillary cancer (Fig. 13.11). This feature does not adversely affect long-term prognosis (142,143). Hence, attempts at staging papillary carcinoma may have minimal clinical significance. Some patients will present with cervical node enlargement and will have no obvious thyroid tumor. Frequently the nodal metastasis will involve one

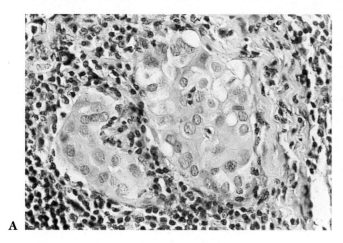

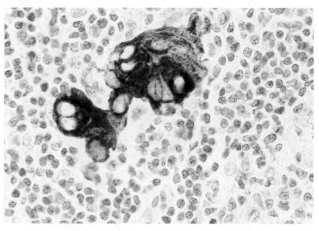

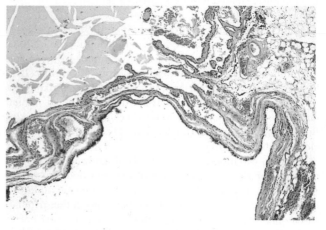

Figure 13.11. **(A)** Small focus of epithelial cells identified in a neck dissection for head and neck squamous carcinoma. **(B)** Immunostaining for cytokeratin reveals that these cells are epithelial in nature. **(C)** Immunostaining for thyroglobulin confirms that the epithelial cells are consistent with metastatic thyroid carcinoma. A subsequent thyroidectomy confirmed the presence of papillary carcinoma.

node that may be cystic (Fig. 13.12) (144). The histology of the nodal metastases in papillary cancer may appear papillary, mixed, or follicular (Fig. 13.13) (122).

Histologic grading is of no use in papillary carcinoma because more than 95% of these lesions are grade 1. In some tumors, either in the primary site or in recurrences, areas of poorly differentiated cancer characterized by solid growth of

tumor, necrosis, mitotic activity, and cytologic atypia can be found. Such lesions have a much more guarded prognosis (124). Anaplastic change in a papillary cancer can occur, although it is uncommon (145).

Distant metastases of papillary carcinoma to lungs and bones occur in 5% to 7% of cases (93,95). Despite the presence of multiple metastases, however, survival may still be prolonged,

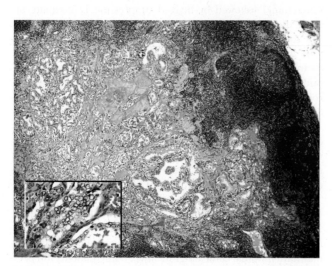

Figure 13.12. Metastatic papillary carcinoma in a neck lymph node. The inset shows the diagnostic nuclear features.

Figure 13.13. Metastatic papillary carcinoma with extensive cyst formation in a neck lymph node. These lesions may be confused clinically with branchial cleft cysts, particularly in patients with no known history of thyroid carcinoma.

especially if the metastases can be treated with radioiodine (146). In ordinary papillary carcinoma, death is uncommon (93).

Ultrastructure

The electron microscopic appearance of papillary carcinoma includes a nucleus with dispersed chromatin and highly infolded nuclear membrane, cytoplasmic intranuclear inclusions, and a cytoplasm that contains many mitochondria and numerous cytoplasmic filaments (22,147). Keratohyaline granules have been found in tumors with squamous foci (22).

Immunohistochemistry

Immunostaining shows that most papillary cancers contain thyroglobulin and TTF-1. Several reports have been published regarding the use of various immunohistochemical markers that can differentiate papillary carcinoma from other follicular-derived lesions of the thyroid. From an extensive list of these markers, the ones that have shown some promise include cytokeratin-19, HBME-1, and galectin-3 (148–150). However, none of these have proven to be specific because all can be expressed in some benign lesions of thyroid. Therefore, some authors have proposed that diagnosis of papillary cancer should be carried out by using an immunopanel consisting of the markers previously mentioned (150).

The other markers that have been explored in the diagnosis of papillary carcinoma include S-100 protein, blood group antigens, estrogen receptors, CD15, and CD57 (151–153).

Flow Cytometry

Although the great majority of papillary thyroid cancers are diploid, the literature suggests that up to 20% may show aneuploid or at least nondiploid subpopulations (154). It has been shown that aneuploid tumors often are associated with a more aggressive clinical course (154,155); however, multivariate analysis has not shown that ploidy is an independent prognostic factor.

Molecular Pathology of Papillary Carcinoma

In the past decade, the literature on thyroid has been focused mainly on the role of various biologic events and genetic determinants in the pathogenesis of various thyroid tumors.

Rearrangements of the *RET* gene, known as *RET/PTC*, have been identified in papillary carcinoma of thyroid (156–159). The *RET* proto-oncogene is normally expressed in cells of neural crest origin and plays a role in kidney and gastrointestinal neuronal development. It is located on chromosome 10q11.2 and cell membrane receptor tyrosine kinase. In normal thyroid, wild-type *RET* is only expressed in C cells and not follicular cells. *RET/PTC* seen in papillary carcinomas occurs as a result of fusion of the tyrosine kinase domain of RET to the 5′ portion of the various genes (156). To date, 11 novel types of rearrangements have been described in papillary carcinoma. *RET/PTC1* and *RET/PTC3* are the most common forms that occur in sporadic papillary carcinoma. *RET/PTC1* is formed by fusion of *RET* to *H4*, and *RET/PTC3* occurs as a result of fusion of *RET* to the *ELE1* gene (160).

RET/PTC expression in thyroid follicular cells of transgenic mice leads to development of thyroid tumors with histologic features of papillary thyroid carcinoma (161). Similarly, transfection of follicular cells in tissue culture by *RET/PTC* causes the cells to demonstrate nuclear features of papillary carcinoma (162). The prevalence of *RET/PTC* in papillary carcinoma varies significantly among various geographic regions (163,164); in the United States, it ranges from 11% to 43% (165). In sporadic tumors, *RET/PTC1* is the most common form of rearrangement (60% to 70%), followed by *RET/PTC3* (20% to 30%) (165). The other rare forms of *RET/PTC* rearrangements have been mainly found in radiation-induced papillary carcinomas (166). Several studies have shown a strong association between radiation-induced papillary carcinoma and expression of *RET/PTC*; in papillary carcinoma, among children affected by the Chernobyl nuclear accident, *RET/PTC3* was found to be the most common form of rearrangement, followed by *RET/PTC1* (166,167).

Recently, it has been shown that *RET/PTC* expression can also occur in some benign lesions. These include hyalinizing trabecular adenoma, Hashimoto thyroiditis, and hyperplastic nodules and follicular adenoma (168–170).

Several authors have suggested an association between Hashimoto thyroiditis and papillary carcinoma (168,169); however, others have suggested that this association is most likely incidental because both are common (109). Recently, two independent studies have shown high prevalence of *RET/PTC* in histologically benign thyroid tissue affected by Hashimoto thyroiditis; these studies concluded that thyroiditic glands harbor multiple foci of papillary carcinoma that are not identified by histologic examination only (168,171). However, a study by Nikiforova et al. (109) has disputed these findings and failed to reproduce these results.

RET/PTC has been identified in benign thyroid nodules, especially the ones that are seen in patients with a history of external radiation. However, the significance of this still remains controversial and needs to be further elucidated by examination of a large cohort of cases (170). Activation of the *RAS* oncogene is considered to be an important mechanism by which human cancer develops. *RAS* has been shown to regulate several pathways that contribute to cellular transformation, including the Raf/MEK/ERK pathway. Numerous studies confirm that the Raf/MEK/ERK pathway is a significant contributor to the malignant phenotype associated with deregulated *RAS* signaling.

An activating mutation in *BRAF* has been described in 29% to 69% of human papillary thyroid cancers. *BRAF* activating mutations in thyroid cancer are almost exclusively the *BRAF V600E* mutation and have been found in 29% to 69% of papillary thyroid cancers, 13% of poorly differentiated cancers, and 10% of anaplastic cancers (172–174). The role of *BRAF* as an oncogenic-initiating event in thyroid follicular cells has been confirmed in mice models (174).

There is practically no concordance between papillary carcinoma with *RET/PTC*, *BRAF*, or *RAS* mutations. The lack of this overlap provides strong evidence of this signaling pathway for thyroid follicular cells to develop into papillary carcinoma (175).

Prognostic Factors

Poor prognostic factors in papillary carcinoma include older age at diagnosis, male sex, large tumor size, and extrathyroidal growth. Pathologic variables associated with a more guarded prognosis include less differentiated or solid areas, vascular invasion, and aneuploid cell population (176,177).

The most widely accepted system of staging solid organ malignancies is the postoperative tumor-node-metastasis (pTNM) system, which is endorsed by both the International Union against Cancer (UICC) and the American Joint Commission on Cancer (AJCC). Generally, this system stages malignant lesions according to the tumor size and invasiveness, nodal spread, and distant metastases. On the basis of this AJCC staging system, all patients younger than 45 years of age with papillary thyroid cancer or follicular thyroid cancer have stage I disease unless they have distant metastases, in which circumstance the disease is classified as stage II. Older patients (≥45 years of age) with node-negative papillary or follicular microcarcinoma (T1N0M0) have stage I disease. Intrathyroidal tumors 1.1 cm or larger are stage II, and either nodal involvement or extrathyroid invasion in older patients with papillary or follicular thyroid carcinoma leads to a classification of stage III (178,179).

Some studies have shown that *RET/PTC* expression in papillary carcinoma can be associated with aggressive biologic behavior (180), whereas others have reported just the opposite (i.e., that *RET/PTC* expression is more commonly seen in slow-growing and clinically indolent tumors) (181). It is also suggested that different rearrangements of *RET/PTC* are associated with different biologic behavior (182). Nikiforov (165) found a significant difference in local recurrence and distant metastases between tumors with *RET/PTC1* and *RET/PTC3* expression. Cetta et al. (183) reported similar findings.

It has been shown that papillary carcinoma with *BRAF* mutations follows an aggressive clinical course (i.e., extrathyroidal extension and more advanced clinical stage). In addition, aggressive phenotype of papillary carcinoma, such as tall-cell variant, is associated with high prevalence of *BRAF* mutations (184).

Several other biologic markers have been suggested as prognostic predictors in papillary carcinoma; these include p53, Ki-67, cell cycle proteins, proliferating cell nuclear antigen (PCNA), bcl-2, cathepsin D, and topoisomerase II (185–187).

SUBTYPES OF PAPILLARY CARCINOMA

Papillary Microcarcinoma (Occult Papillary Carcinoma)

According to the World Health Organization (WHO), papillary microcarcinoma is defined as a tumor measuring 1 cm or less; however, some experts have also defined tumors measuring up to 1.5 cm as microcarcinomas (188,189). Other terms for these lesions have included occult papillary carcinoma, occult sclerosing carcinoma, small papillary carcinoma, and nonencapsulated sclerosing tumor. These lesions are quite common as incidental findings at autopsy or in thyroidectomy for benign disease or in completion thyroidectomies in patients with a history of carcinoma involving the opposite thyroid lobe. The incidence of these lesions has varied significantly with the study, but papillary microcarcinoma has been reported in up to 36% of carefully sectioned thyroid specimens (189–191). Harach et al. (192) suggested that tumors measuring less than 5 mm (minute papillary carcinomas) should be considered a normal finding and should be left untreated (192). However, lymph node metastases from lesions less than 0.5 cm are known (193,194). Distant metastases, although very rare, are also documented (194). The

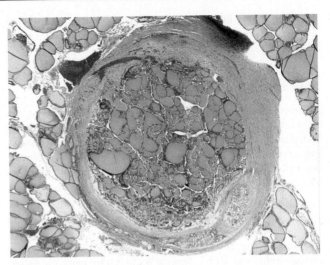

Figure 13.14. Papillary microcarcinoma in a patient with a benign follicular nodule. This lesion was an incidental finding in the thyroid lobectomy specimen.

small papillary carcinoma is a nonencapsulated, sclerotic, white to tan nodule often located subcapsularly. Histologically, the tumors may be totally follicular or show papillary areas as well (Fig. 13.14). Sclerosis may be prominent; the lesions infiltrate the surrounding thyroid (195).

A familial form of papillary microcarcinoma has been recognized; these tumors are characterized by multifocality with increased tendency toward vascular and lymphatic invasion, distant metastasis, and even death (196).

It is important to recognize that the incidentally found microcarcinoma confined within the thyroid is probably of no clinical importance and should not be overtreated. Therefore, some authors have suggested the term *papillary microtumor* to prevent aggressive management (197).

Follicular Variant of Papillary Cancer

The follicular variant of papillary carcinoma is a distinctive papillary carcinoma variant. The incidence of this variant is difficult to determine because, in the past, some of these lesions have been classified as follicular carcinomas or adenomas. Grossly and histologically, the tumor may appear encapsulated (Fig. 13.15) (198,199). Despite the almost total follicular pattern in the primary site, features that suggest that a tumor is a follicular variant of papillary cancer include clear nuclei, psammoma bodies, and desmoplastic response at invasive areas (198). Immunohistochemical staining shows the presence of low– and high–molecular-weight cytokeratins and HBME-1, which may aid in differentiating this lesion from follicular adenomas and carcinomas (190,191). The prognosis of the follicular variant is apparently similar to usual papillary cancer, although there may be a greater risk for this variant to metastasize outside the neck and for vascular invasion; regional nodal metastases are less common than in classic papillary cancer (198,199).

Two distinct types of follicular variants include the diffuse follicular variant and the encapsulated follicular variant (198,200). In the diffuse follicular variant, the gland is diffusely replaced by tumor. Lymph node and distant metastases are common in these patients. The prognosis appears to be poor in

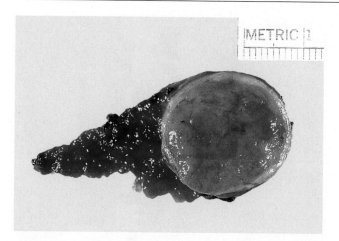

Figure 13.15. The follicular variant of papillary carcinoma may grossly appear as a circumscribed nodule resembling a follicular adenoma. Microscopic examination shows a follicular architecture with nuclear features of typical papillary thyroid carcinoma.

these patients, although only a handful of cases have been described (200).

The encapsulated follicular variant refers to the follicular variant, that is characterized by the presence of a capsule around the lesion. These lesions are associated with an excellent prognosis. In some cases, the diagnosis of this particular variant of papillary carcinoma can be difficult because of the presence of multifocal rather than diffuse distribution of nuclear features of papillary thyroid carcinoma (201,202). Because of this peculiar morphologic presentation, these tumors can be misdiagnosed as adenomatoid nodule or follicular adenoma (201). Some authors have suggested that these tumors be classified as "tumors of undetermined malignant potential" as a result of the excellent prognosis (203); however, others have shown that some cases belonging in this category can lead to distant metastasis (204).

Tall-Cell Variant

Hawk and Hazard (205) found that the tall-cell variant made up approximately 10% of the papillary cancers they studied (205). The tumor is large (>6 cm) (Fig. 13.16), extends extra-

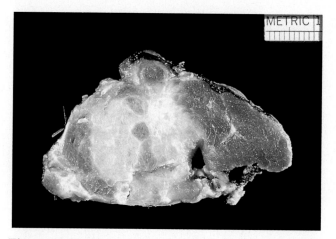

Figure 13.16. Gross photo of a tall-cell variant of papillary carcinoma showing a large, infiltrative, white-tan lesion.

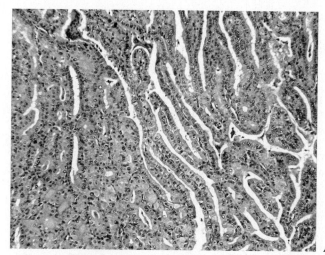

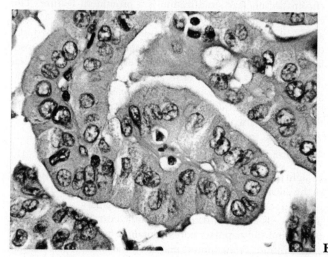

Figure 13.17. Tall-cell variant of papillary carcinoma. Low-power view shows a papillary architecture (**A**), and high-power view shows large elongated tumor cells (cell height three times the width), abundant eosinophilic cytoplasm, and nuclear changes of papillary carcinoma (**B**).

thyroidally, and shows mitotic activity and vascular invasion more often than usual papillary cancer. The tumor tends to occur in older adult patients (205–207).

The tall-cell variant is three times as tall as it is wide, and its cytoplasm is often eosinophilic (Fig. 13.17) (188). In fact, these tumors may be referred to as "pink-cell" variant of papillary carcinoma. Tall cells should represent 50% or more of the papillary carcinoma cells to make the diagnosis of tall-cell variant (208). The tumors show an extensive papillary pattern, often with a heavy lymphocytic infiltration present in or around the papillae. Some tall-cell tumors arise in glands with extensive histologic evidence of chronic thyroiditis. Dedifferentiation to squamous cell carcinoma has been described. Local recurrences with invasion of the trachea can be seen, and this complication may be fatal (209). Flow cytometry studies, although limited in number, have failed to reveal differences between typical papillary carcinoma and the tall-cell variant (210). The prognosis for this variant is less favorable than for usual papillary cancer, although it is believed that the poor outcome in these tumors may be secondary to the fact that these tumors are often associated with poor prognostic variables such as older age, extrathyroidal spread, necrosis, high mitotic rate, and distant metastases (207,211).

Columnar Cell Variant

The columnar cell variant is a rare form of papillary carcinoma. (Some authors believe that it is so unusual a tumor that it deserves its own category and should not be placed in the papillary group [212,213]). The tumor needs to be distinguished from other papillary carcinomas because this lesion is associated with an extremely poor outcome, with most deaths occurring within 5 years of diagnosis (212,214). Grossly, the tumors often measure more than 6 cm. The tumor is characterized microscopically by papillary growth. Tall columnar cells line the papillae. The nuclear features are usually not those of typical papillary carcinomas. The nuclei are hyperchromatic with a punctate chromatin; nuclear stratification is a prominent feature. The cells usually have scant cytoplasm, which can be clear. Mitoses are frequently seen. Psammoma bodies are rare. Extrathyroidal extension is common, as are distant metastases (214). Encapsulated variants, which may have a better prognosis, have been described (215). Because of its aggressive behavior, the actual classification of this lesion as a variant of papillary carcinoma has been controversial, although most authors include this lesion in the papillary carcinoma classification (214).

Warthin-Like Variant

By light microscopy, these tumors resemble a "Warthin tumor" of the salivary gland. These tumors usually arise in a background of lymphocytic thyroiditis and show papillary architecture. Tumor cells with abundant eosinophilic cytoplasm line the papillae, and the papillary cores contain a brisk lymphoplasmacytic infiltrate. Some tumors may show transition to tall-cell variant, which usually occurs at the invasive edge of tumor. Limited follow-up has shown that these tumors in their pure form follow a clinical course similar to conventional papillary carcinoma (216,217).

Diffuse Sclerosis Variant

The diffuse sclerosis variant of papillary carcinoma is rare, representing only approximately 3% of all papillary carcinomas (218). The tumor, which most often affects children and young adults, may present as bilateral goiter. The tumor permeates the gland outlining the intraglandular lymphatics. Tumor papillae have associated areas of squamous metaplasia. Numerous psammoma bodies are found (Fig. 13.18). Lymphocytic infiltrates are found around the tumor foci. The lesions tend to recur in the neck and have a somewhat more serious prognosis than usual childhood papillary cancer. These lesions appear to represent 10% of the papillary carcinomas seen in children exposed to the radioactive iodine released after the Chernobyl accident (218–220). Although the tumors often show extracapsular extension, distant and nodal metastases, and a decreased disease-free survival when compared with the usual type of papillary carcinoma, mortality is low.

Solid Variant

A solid growth pattern is noted in many papillary carcinomas. When the solid growth represents greater than 50% of the

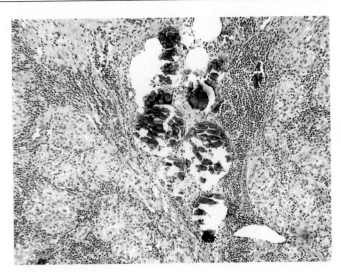

Figure 13.18. Diffuse sclerosis variant showing solid tumor nests and numerous psammoma bodies. Notice the lymphocytic infiltrates around the tumor foci.

tumor mass, a diagnosis of solid variant of papillary carcinoma may be made (Fig. 13.19) (221). The solid variant is most commonly seen in children and has been reported in more than 30% of patients with papillary carcinoma after the Chernobyl nuclear accident (104). The nuclear features are those of papillary carcinoma. It is important to recognize these lesions as papillary carcinomas and not to overdiagnose them as more aggressive tumors such as insular carcinoma (discussed later in the chapter). The prognosis is controversial, with some studies showing outcomes similar to typical papillary carcinoma and other studies showing more aggressive behavior (222). A study in adults has shown that solid papillary carcinoma has a similar and only slightly less favorable prognosis than the usual type. This differs from poorly differentiated thyroid cancer defined predominantly by the presence of necrosis (124).

Harach and Williams (223) designated papillary cancers with solid growth pattern in children as "childhood thyroid carcinoma." These tumors are widely invasive throughout the thyroid. Almost half of these cases are associated with history of external radiation to the head and neck region (223).

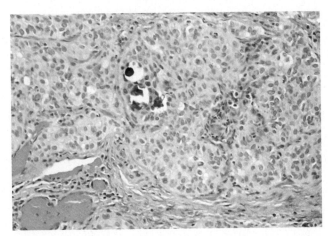

Figure 13.19. Solid variant of papillary carcinoma with focal calcifications and psammoma bodies.

Encapsulated Variant

The encapsulated variant presents grossly as an adenoma and comprises from 8% to 13% of papillary cancers (215,224). Microscopically, such lesions usually show total encapsulation; however, there are cytologic features of papillary cancer, including nuclear changes and psammoma bodies. Some of these lesions will show focal invasion into the capsule. The prognosis is excellent.

Other Variants

Rare variants of papillary cancer for which prognostic data are not well established include the spindle cell variant, the clear-cell variant, the oxyphilic (Hürthle cell) variant (225), papillary carcinoma with lipomatous stroma (226), papillary carcinoma with fasciitis-like stroma (227), myxoid variant (228), and cribriform variant (113) seen in patients with familial adenomatous polyposis.

PAPILLARY HYPERPLASIA

Papillary hyperplasia, which is seen in untreated autoimmune hyperthyroidism (Graves disease), congenital errors of thyroid metabolism, and hyperfunctioning foci in goitrous glands, shows overgrowth of the follicular epithelium. The cell growth involves both hypertrophy and hyperplasia; infoldings (i.e., papillations) form. Diffuse papillary hyperplasia is distinguished from papillary carcinoma by the preservation of the gland architecture, the diffuse character of the lesion, and the normal nuclei. In toxic nodular goiter, the changes are similar but the lesion tends to be focal. Nuclear characteristics differentiate the lesion from cancer (131,229).

Papillary Hyperplasia in Follicular Nodule

Well-circumscribed solitary thyroid nodules may show a microscopic appearance of papillary growth. However, the papillae contain extremely edematous stalks with follicles in them (Fig. 13.20). The nuclei are round and not clear; there are no psammoma bodies. Some of these nodules produce a warm or hot

appearance on scan (14,230). At times, areas in nodular goiters will show a focally similar papillary appearance; these areas are often associated with hemorrhage and edema. Although papillary adenoma has been used as a diagnostic term for these lesions, it should not be used because it has been applied to several lesions from hyperplastic ones to encapsulated papillary carcinomas. It has been shown by immunohistochemistry that papillary hyperplastic nodules are negative for HBME-1 and focally positive for CK-19. This can be helpful to differentiate these nodules from papillary carcinoma in diagnostically challenging cases (231).

LESIONS WITH FOLLICULAR ARCHITECTURE

The majority of thyroid lesions (physiologic hyperplasia, benign nodular lesions, and neoplasms) display a macrofollicular or microfollicular pattern. The thyroid lesions in this histologic category include those found in patients with congenital disorders of thyroid metabolism (inborn errors of thyroid metabolism and dyshormonogenetic goiter) and disorders of the thyroid in diffuse toxic goiter (autoimmune hyperthyroidism [Graves disease] and Basedow disease). In some of these conditions, hypothyroidism is found; in others, hyperfunction is present; and in still others, euthyroidism is present.

When the thyroid cannot produce normal amounts of thyroid hormone, the pituitary secretes increased amounts of thyrotropin (thyroid-stimulating hormone [TSH]), which, in turn, directs the thyroid follicular cells to produce more thyroid hormones—thyroxine and triiodothyronine (T_4 and T_3). The cells undergo hyperplasia and hypertrophy. The thyroid gland enlarges and, in some cases, nodules form. Causes of this type of hyperplasia include dyshormonogenetic goiter, TSH-producing pituitary adenomas, trophoblastic disease, inadequate dietary iodine, and goitrogenic drugs.

In autoimmune hyperthyroidism (diffuse toxic goiter or Graves disease), hyperplasia and hypertrophy result from TSH-mimicking Igs (thyrotropin receptor antibodies) that attach to the receptor on the follicular cell membrane and trigger the intracellular sequence of events that enables increased thyroid hormone production.

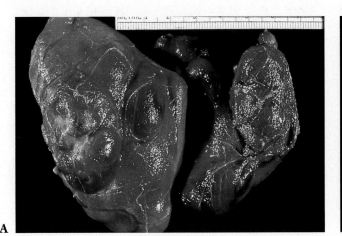
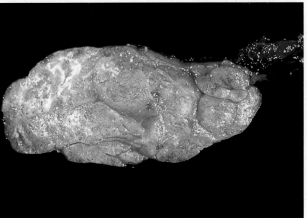

A   B

Figure 13.20. **(A)** Papillary hyperplastic nodule showing papillae lined by small round follicular cells and subfollicle formation. **(B)** Low-power microscopic view of multinodular goiter showing multiple nodules of thyroid follicles of varying size.

INBORN ERRORS OF THYROID METABOLISM—GENETIC DISORDERS

Inborn errors of thyroid metabolism consist of a spectrum of inherited biochemical abnormalities that can affect any step in the pathway of thyroid hormone synthesis, secretion, or action. Differences in the clinical symptoms and presentations depend on whether the defect is complete or incomplete, whether the change is qualitative or quantitative, which enzyme or protein is involved, and the degree of compensation of the individual. If the defect is severe, neonatal hypothyroidism (cretinism) occurs (232–234).

The morphology of the thyroid in patients with dyshormonogenesis is similar despite the different biochemical abnormalities (235). The gland is usually enlarged and nodular. Secondary changes including hemorrhage and fibrosis can be found. Microscopically, the changes consist of extreme follicular hyperplasia. Most nodules show microfollicular or trabecular patterns (236). Clear-cell change may be seen. Cytologic atypia is very common and may be so severe as to suggest a malignancy (237). However, true invasive growth is extremely rare, so care must be taken to not overdiagnose malignancy.

NODULAR THYROID DISEASE AND HYPERTHYROIDISM

Descriptions of clinical hyperthyroidism in patients with nodular glands have been attributed to Plummer and Goetsch. The gland may be multinodular, or only a solitary mass may be present (238).

Toxic Nodular Goiter

In toxic nodular goiter, the clinical symptoms complex of hyperthyroidism is associated with a nodular gland. This cause of hyperthyroidism is more commonly seen in older individuals. This histology is similar to diffuse toxic goiter with the changes occurring within nodules (239).

Toxic Nodule (Adenoma, Carcinoma)

Rarely, a solitary nodule will function autonomously and produce clinical hyperfunction. Most of these are benign nodules;

only rare examples of documented follicular carcinomas producing hyperthyroidism are known (240).

Central Hyperthyroidism

The pituitary and, more rarely, hypothalamic causes of hyperthyroidism have been documented in some patients (241). The thyroid in these cases is enlarged but often only slightly. Histologically, the appearance mimics the hyperplasia seen in autoimmune hyperthyroidism, except that lymphocytic infiltration is absent or minimal.

Other Causes of Hyperthyroidism

Other causes of clinical hyperthyroidism include gestational trophoblastic disease (242), struma ovarii (243), subacute thyroiditis (discussed previously), painless thyroiditis (discussed previously), rapidly growing tumors in the gland with thyroid destruction, excess exogenous thyroid hormone ingestion (244), ectopic production of TSH and thyrotropin-releasing hormone (TRH), and peripheral and generalized resistance to thyroid hormone (245). In some of these conditions, the histologic changes are well described (i.e., subacute thyroiditis and rapidly growing tumor in the gland produce destruction of the thyroid with release of stored hormone into the circulation); in others, the histology is poorly documented.

FOLLICULAR THYROID NODULES

NODULAR GOITER

The incidence of nodular goiter depends on the criteria used to define it. Approximately 2% to 4% of the population has a clinical mass. Approximately 10% of thyroids removed at autopsy will contain nodules, usually multiple, but up to 40% to 50% of thyroids will harbor microscopic nodules (246,247). Although multinodular goiter can be associated with hyperfunction (248), the patient is usually euthyroid.

Grossly, nodular goiters range from slightly to massively enlarged glands (weights of 50 to >800 g can be found) with intact capsules and a bumpy external surface (Fig. 13.21). Sectioning

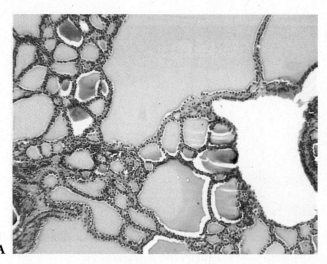

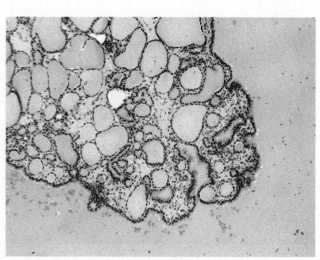

A   B

Figure 13.21. **(A)** Multinodular goiter showing asymmetric enlargement of thyroid lobes. **(B)** Cut section of multinodular goiter showing multiple tan nodules with focal fibrosis.

will show multiple nodules of varying consistency separated by variable amounts of normal-appearing thyroid (Fig. 13.21). The nodules are composed chiefly of brown thyroid tissue; fibrous bands and calcification are often noted. Microscopically, colloid lakes alternating with normal to hyperplastic-appearing foci of thyroid, hemorrhage, siderosis, fibrosis, calcification, and even bone are found (Fig. 13.20). Variable amounts of lymphocytic infiltrate will also be found, possibly reflecting an immunologic abnormality (247).

Why do nodules occur? The work of Struder and colleagues (249,250) suggests that certain follicular cells or groups of cells are intrinsically more rapidly growing than their neighbors. The initial proliferation is polyclonal, involving one follicle or, more likely, a group of follicles. Adjacent follicles remain quiescent. In the process, vascular compression in the stroma leads to focal ischemia, necrosis, and inflammatory changes. Later, the same process may affect another group of follicles until large zones of the thyroid are affected. As the process continues, the secondary phenomena—hemorrhage, fibrosis, and calcification—take place. While these changes occur, the hormonal stimuli to the gland continue. Distortion of the vascular supply and the presence of dilated follicles filled with colloid interfere with the distribution of iodide and thyrotropin. Some parts of the gland will be exposed to excess thyrotropin, and focal hyperplasia may occur; other areas will have relative iodide or thyrotropin deficiency leading to zones of atrophy (249,250).

What can be said about solitary follicular nodules that histologically, at least, appear identical to the multiple nodules seen in nodular goiter? Are these then regenerative, proliferative nodules, but not neoplasms; or alternatively, do these represent true benign follicular adenomas? Many pathologists prefer the less definitive term "adenomatous or adenomatoid follicular nodule" for such lesions, avoiding the issue of histogenesis.

Hicks et al. (251) and Namba and Fagin (252), using genetic analysis technology that had previously proved clonal origin of colonic adenomas and parathyroid adenomas, found that solitary thyroid follicular nodules were clonal; hence, they are follicular adenomas.

FOLLICULAR ADENOMA

A follicular adenoma or solitary adenomatous or adenomatoid nodule is defined as a benign encapsulated mass of follicles, usually showing a uniform pattern throughout the confined nodule (Fig. 13.22) (208,253). Adenomas are solitary; indeed, if there are multiple nodules in a lobe or a thyroid gland, it is probably more appropriate to diagnose multinodular goiter with adenomatous change (adenomatous hyperplasia). The features Meissner used to distinguish histologically between adenoma and adenomatous nodules included encapsulation, uniformity of pattern within the adenoma, and compression of the surrounding gland by the adenoma and its capsule.

Descriptive terms that have been used to delineate the patterns seen in follicular adenomas include macrofollicular, simple, microfollicular, fetal, embryonal, and trabecular. However, because these patterns have no clinical import, it is not necessary to subdivide thyroid adenomas. Relatively common changes found in adenomas include hemorrhage, edema, and fibrosis, especially in the central portions of the tumor. Calcification may be seen. Lesions that have undergone fine-needle aspiration (FNA) biopsy may show necrosis, increased mitotic activity, and cellular atypia in the area of the needle tract. Rare adenomas with fat, cartilage, or signet ring cells may be seen (14,208).

Whether or not some solitary follicular nodules have the biologic potential to become carcinoma is unknown; the findings of aneuploid cell populations in 27% of such lesions suggest that some of these may represent carcinoma in situ (154). The solitary follicular lesion removed by lobectomy, when it is adequately studied, shows no evidence of invasion and will neither recur nor metastasize. (Enucleation of follicular adenomas

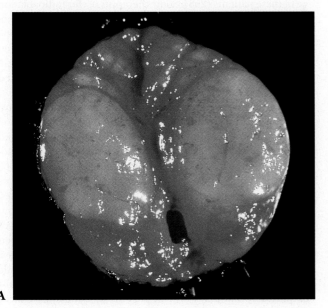

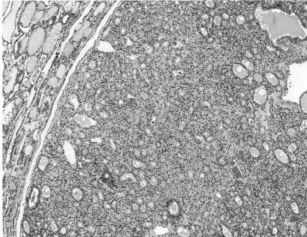

A   **B**

Figure 13.22. **(A)** Gross follicular adenoma showing a tan-brown circumscribed nodule. **(B)** A low-power view of follicular adenoma showing a thinly encapsulated, microfollicular pattern tumor with no capsular or vascular invasion.

should be mentioned here only to be condemned as a surgical procedure. The pathologic evaluation of these lesions requires analysis of the tumor-capsule-thyroid interface.)

Occasionally, a follicular adenoma will contain bizarre cells (i.e., will show random, often marked cytologically atypical cells with huge hyperchromatic nuclei); sometimes multinucleated cells may be seen. These lesions are benign.

HYALINIZING TRABECULAR ADENOMA/ NEOPLASM OF THE THYROID

The hyalinizing trabecular adenoma is a follicular-derived lesion that has a distinctive histology (254). Microscopically, these adenomas grow in nests that are surrounded by dense hyaline stroma. The histology is reminiscent of that seen in paragangliomas; however, the tumor is derived from the follicular epithelium (Fig. 13.23). The nuclear features of the follicular cells are similar to those seen in papillary carcinoma (254). By immunohistochemistry, the cells of hyalinizing trabecular adenoma stain positive for thyroglobulin and cytokeratin 19 and negative for calcitonin, although the presence of other neuroendocrine markers has been described (255,256).

Some authors have recently proposed that these adenomas actually represent a variant of papillary carcinoma. This is because of similar nuclear cytology, immunoprofile, and *RET* oncogene rearrangements in both tumors (257,258). However, to date, no *BRAF* mutations have been seen in these tumors, and a benign behavior has thus far been described in all cases of hyalinizing trabecular adenoma (259). Therefore, until metastatic behavior is described in a case of hyalinizing trabecular adenoma, these tumors can be designated as hyalinizing trabecular neoplasm.

ATYPICAL FOLLICULAR ADENOMA

Atypical follicular adenoma, a term proposed by Hazard and Kenyon (260), includes those follicular tumors that show pathologically disturbing features (spontaneous necrosis, infarction, numerous mitoses, or unusual cellularity) but do not show invasive characteristics on careful examination. The overwhelming majority of the atypical adenomas behave clinically in a benign fashion.

FOLLICULAR CARCINOMA OF THE THYROID

Follicular carcinoma comprises approximately 5% of thyroid cancers; however, in iodide-deficient areas, this tumor is more prevalent, making up 25% to 40% of thyroid cancers (261,262). When iodide is added to the diet, papillary cancer increases, and follicular tumors decrease (101). The true incidence of follicular carcinoma is difficult to determine because the follicular variant of papillary carcinoma may still be placed into this category (263). Risk factors include iodine deficiency, older age, female gender, and radiation exposure. Clinically, follicular carcinoma usually presents as a solitary mass in the thyroid (262).

Follicular carcinoma has a marked propensity for vascular invasion (not lymphatics). It is possible that follicular cancers produce certain factors that alter the venous endothelium, allowing the tumor easy access (261,262,264). In any event, follicular carcinoma avoids lymphatics; hence, true embolic lymph node metastases are exceedingly rare (265).

Follicular carcinoma disseminates hematogenously and metastasizes to bone, lungs, brain, and liver (Fig. 13.24A) (266). Follicular cancer metastases will usually be treatable by radioiodine if there is no normal thyroid tissue present in the neck. For this reason, many surgeons consider total thyroidectomy appropriate therapy for encapsulated follicular cancers (267). Because it is very difficult, if not impossible, to render a definitive cancer diagnosis on an FNA sample or frozen section of such a tumor, delayed completion thyroidectomy may be necessary (267).

Alternatively, because the disease-free interval after lobectomy or cure of these encapsulated lesions is so great, completion thyroidectomy may represent "overkill" in a large percentage of these patients (268). Some therapists prefer radioablation of the residual thyroid either when the definite diagnosis of cancer is made or if and when metastases first appear (269). Total thyroidectomy appears warranted in those individuals who present with metastatic disease and in whom the primary is still untreated (270). Certainly, lymph node dissection is not warranted because these tumors do not spread to nodes (270).

Patients who have follicular carcinoma that is widely invasive fare poorly (261). However, those individuals with encapsulated follicular tumors confined to the thyroid enjoy a prolonged survival (>80% at 10 years) (262). Several studies have addressed those factors (clinical and pathologic) that are associated with a worse outcome (271,272). Poor prognostic factors include the presence of metastases, multiple sites of metastases, age over 50 years, large tumor size, extensive vascular invasion, extracapsular extension, and poorly differentiated areas of tumor (273). Studies using multivariate analysis have identified age over 45 years, extrathyroidal extension, distant metastases, and tumor size greater than 4 cm as independent prognostic factors in follicular carcinoma (274). An extremely significant complication that may occur in patients with follicular cancer is transformation into anaplastic cancer (275); this may occur de novo in an untreated follicular lesion or in metastatic foci (276).

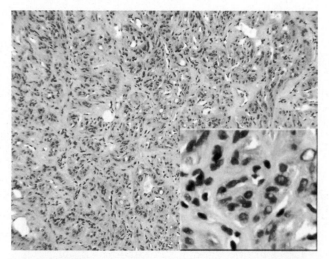

Figure 13.23. Histologic examination of a hyalinizing trabecular adenoma shows multiple nests of thyroid follicular epithelium surrounded by a vascular network. The appearances are similar to those seen in a paraganglioma; however, the epithelial cells are derived from follicular epithelium. Note that the nuclei appear similar to those of papillary carcinoma (*inset*).

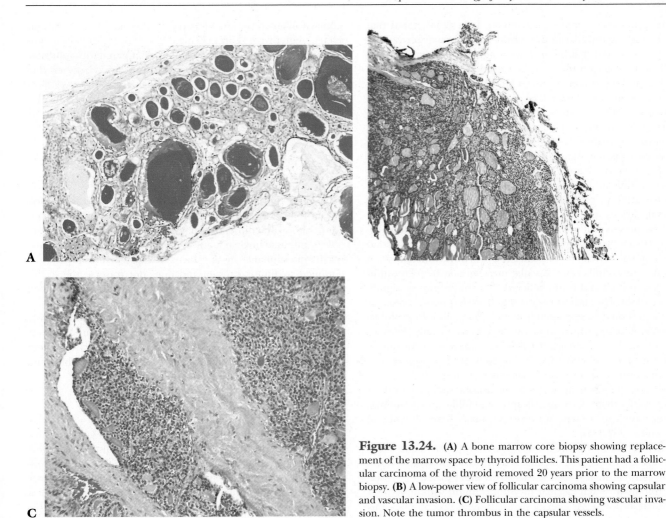

Figure 13.24. (A) A bone marrow core biopsy showing replacement of the marrow space by thyroid follicles. This patient had a follicular carcinoma of the thyroid removed 20 years prior to the marrow biopsy. (B) A low-power view of follicular carcinoma showing capsular and vascular invasion. (C) Follicular carcinoma showing vascular invasion. Note the tumor thrombus in the capsular vessels.

Pathology

The widely invasive follicular carcinoma is a tumor that is clinically and surgically recognized as a cancer; the role of the pathologist in its diagnosis is to confirm that it is of thyroid origin and is a follicular neoplasm (14). Lang et al. (271) noted that 80% of the patients with widely invasive cancers developed metastases and approximately 20% died of tumor. Woolner (277) found a 50% fatality rate for widely invasive tumors compared with a rate of only 3% in those with minimal invasion (277). Many of these tumors contain poorly differentiated areas and should be diagnosed as "poorly differentiated follicular carcinomas."

Only the pathologist, upon examining well-fixed histologic sections, can diagnose the minimally invasive follicular carcinoma. These lesions are not diagnosable by FNA cytology because the diagnosis requires the demonstration of invasion at the edges of the lesion; therefore, sampling of the center, as in obtaining a cytologic sample, cannot be diagnostic (278).

Similar problems exist in evaluating such lesions by frozen section. Some authors recommend that intraoperative assessment of such lesions should involve the examination of frozen sections from three or four separate areas of the nodule (279). This wastes resources and rarely gives useful diagnostic information. The surgeon should have removed the lobe involved by the nodule, and if it is a follicular carcinoma that is only minimally invasive, the appropriate therapy has probably already been accomplished. Because only a small number of these lesions will show evidence of invasion at the time of permanent section (i.e., the majority of them are benign) and because overdiagnosis is more dangerous for the patient than is the delay in making a definitive diagnosis, we discourage frozen section evaluation of these nodules (280).

Grossly, the minimally invasive follicular carcinoma resembles a follicular adenoma; the lesion is well encapsulated. The thickness of the capsule is prominent and is often thicker than that seen in follicular adenoma. Microscopically, the tumor demonstrates a microfollicular or trabecular pattern with regular, small round follicles (208,262,281). Hemorrhage, necrosis, or even tumor infarction may be noted, and significant mitotic activity is often found (264).

What are the minimum criteria for making this diagnosis? Invasion of the capsule, invasion through the capsule, and invasion into veins in or beyond the capsule represent the diagnostic criteria for carcinoma in a follicular thyroid neoplasm (Fig. 13.24B,C). The criterion for vascular invasion applies *solely and strictly to veins in or beyond the capsule* because tumor plugs within capillaries in the substance tumor have no apparent diagnostic and prognostic importance (201,262). The definition of capsular invasion is controversial (201). Lang and Georgii (282) and Franssila et al. (283) require penetration of the capsule to diagnose a follicular tumor as carcinoma. Lida (284) noted that distinguishing capsular invasion from trapping may prove difficult; he required that the invasive tongues of tumor sever and deflect the collagen fibers in the capsule (284).

Is capsular invasion insufficient for the diagnosis of follicular cancer? Kahn and Perzin (281) found that only one in seven patients (14%) with capsular invasion demonstrated metastases. Evans (285) noted that capsular invasion was only present in three of seven patients (43%) with metastases. However, in these three patients, metastases were already present at initial diagnosis. However, those authors who diagnose tumors with capsular invasion only as atypical adenomas indicate a benign clinical course after thyroid lobectomy. Periods of follow-up differ among various series.

The presence of vascular invasion is also indicative of malignancy in a follicular tumor. Invasion of vessels within or beyond the lesional capsule is necessary for a definitive diagnosis of vascular invasion because vascular invasion may be seen within the lesion itself and is not believed to be of prognostic significance (286). The authors believe that those lesions with vascular invasion should be separated from the minimally invasive follicular carcinomas, which show capsular invasion only. Perhaps use of the term *angioinvasive follicular carcinoma* is warranted because it is believed that the angioinvasive lesions have a greater probability of recurrence and metastasis (201).

Although most recurrences or metastases will appear within 5 years after thyroidectomy, encapsulated follicular carcinomas notoriously can present as metastases many years after initial resection (262,285).

In our practice, we use the terms *minimally invasive* and *angioinvasive carcinoma*. The former is applied to those cases that show only capsular or transcapsular invasion; the latter is used for tumors in which vascular invasion is found with or without capsular invasion. As previously mentioned, we propose this distinction based on the belief that angioinvasive tumors have greater propensity toward distant metastasis (201).

None of the ancillary techniques assist in differentiating benign from malignant follicular tumors. Ultrastructural, morphometric, and flow cytometric analyses have not helped in distinguishing these lesions (287,288). Approximately 60% of follicular carcinomas will show aneuploid cell populations. Backdahl (289) analyzed 65 follicular thyroid tumors (26 benign tumors and 39 carcinomas). He noted that of the 20 patients with cancer who survived, 19 had diploid tumors; whereas 17 of 19 patients who died of carcinoma had tumors with aneuploid DNA patterns.

All follicular carcinomas express thyroglobulin and show a similar cytokeratin profile to normal thyroid parenchyma. Some authors have shown that HBME-1 is exclusively expressed in 90% to 100% of follicular carcinomas and not adenomas. However, others have reported HBME-1 expression in adenomatoid nodules and follicular adenomas (152,255,290).

Molecular Biology of Follicular Carcinoma

A specific translocation t(2;3) leads to the expression of PAX8-peroxisome proliferator–activated receptor-γ (PPAR-γ) chimeric protein; initial studies by Kroll and colleagues have demonstrated that this translocation is specific to follicular carcinoma (291,292). However, follow-up studies employing immunohistochemistry and molecular biology have shown that PPAR-γ expression can occur in some cases of follicular ade-

noma, follicular variant of papillary thyroid carcinoma, and even benign thyroid parenchyma (293–295). *RAS* mutations are more frequent in follicular carcinoma compared with follicular adenoma; some authors have found an association between *RAS* mutations and clinically aggressive follicular carcinomas (296). LOH on chromosomes 10q and 3p can be seen in follicular carcinoma, suggesting a role of tumor suppressor genes in its pathogenesis (297,298).

WELL-DIFFERENTIATED FOLLICULAR "TUMORS OF UNDETERMINED MALIGNANT POTENTIAL"

This designation has been recently proposed in thyroid pathology for follicular-patterned encapsulated tumors that have been controversial and difficult to diagnose as a result of (a) questionable or minimal nuclear features of papillary thyroid carcinoma, or (b) questionable or one focus of capsular invasion that is confined to tumor capsule and does not traverse the entire thickness of capsule and lacks any nuclear features of papillary thyroid carcinoma (203).

This terminology may be extremely helpful to pathologists in the diagnoses of certain follicular-patterned lesions; however, these terms are proposed on the basis of data that lack complete clinical follow-up. Therefore, clinicians may find it problematic to establish treatment strategies.

HÜRTHLE CELL LESIONS

Hürthle cells are derived from follicular epithelium and are characterized morphologically by large size, distinct cell borders, voluminous granular cytoplasm, large nucleus, and prominent nucleolus (299). Ultrastructural studies have shown that the cytoplasmic granularity is produced by huge mitochondria filling the cell (300). Studies by Harcourt-Webster and Stott (301) and Tremblay and Pearse (302) have shown that these cells contain high levels of oxidative enzymes.

Hürthle cells can be found in several conditions in the thyroid (nodular goiter, nonspecific chronic thyroiditis, long-standing hyperthyroidism, chronic lymphocytic thyroiditis [Hashimoto disease], and nodules and neoplasms); they cannot be considered specific for any disease entity (303,304).

Nodules of Hürthle cells are not all neoplastic. In fact, the majority represents Hürthle cell change of pre-existing follicular adenomatous nodules in goiters or thyroiditis (303).

The clinical behavior in Hürthle cell neoplasms has elicited debate in the literature. Some authors cite 80% or more of these lesions as benign, whereas others consider all such lesions malignant (305–307). Because most Hürthle cell neoplasms are follicular in pattern, the criterion for distinguishing benign from malignant is the same as for follicular neoplasms (i.e., the identification of capsular or vascular invasion) (299,308). However, the pathologic criterion for malignancy is met more frequently for tumors composed of Hürthle cells than for their non-Hürthle counterparts (299,308). Thus, whereas 2% to 3% of solitary encapsulated follicular tumors of the thyroid show invasive characteristics, 30% to 40% of such lesions with Hürthle cell cytology will have such features. In addition, whereas true follicular carcinomas of the thyroid rarely, if ever, metastasize embolically to lymph nodes, approximately 30% of Hürthle cell carcinomas do metastasize to lymph nodes (299,306,308).

Most Hürthle cell neoplasms of the thyroid are solitary mass lesions that show complete or partial encapsulation. They are

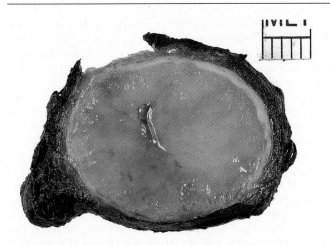

Figure 13.25. Gross Hürthle cell adenoma showing a circumscribed orange-brown lesion. Diagnosis relies on histologic examination with thorough examination of the capsule.

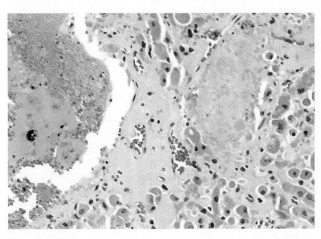

Figure 13.27. Extensive necrosis in a Hürthle cell nodule following fine-needle aspiration. It is often difficult to evaluate these lesions because of extensive artifact.

distinguished from the surrounding thyroid by their distinctive brown to mahogany color (Figs. 13.25 and 13.26). Rarely, a Hürthle cell neoplasm may undergo spontaneous infarction. Extensive infarction may also be seen following FNA biopsy (Fig. 13.27) (308,309).

The claim that all Hürthle cell neoplasms should be considered malignant or potentially malignant, especially if 2 cm or greater in size, is no longer considered valid. Many studies from the United States and Europe (310,311) indicate that benign Hürthle cell neoplasms exist. Size, nuclear atypia, multinucleation, cellular pleomorphism, mitoses, and histologic pattern of the lesion are not predictive of behavior (299,308). Both benign and malignant tumors can show calcifications, which may be confused with psammoma bodies, but these calcifications are present within the colloid (304).

Pathologic criteria for malignancy—vascular invasion, transcapsular penetration, and destructive capsular invasion—can predict the clinical behavior of these tumors. The distinction between benign and malignant Hürthle cell tumors is made by the pathologic evaluation of the mass, applying strict criteria as previously noted for the non-Hürthle follicular tumors. In the

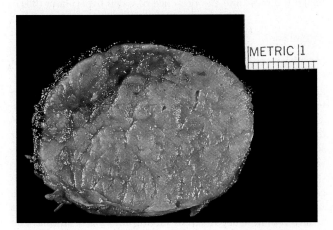

Figure 13.26. Gross Hürthle cell carcinoma showing a mahogany brown multilobated mass with gross evidence of hemorrhage and necrosis. This lesion showed capsular and vascular invasion.

absence of invasion, a Hürthle cell thyroid tumor should be considered benign (304,308,312). Total thyroidectomy is not needed for all Hürthle cell neoplasms (313,314).

By immunohistochemistry, Hürthle cell lesions are positive for thyroglobulin and TTF-1. Carcinoembryonic antigen (CEA) expression has been described in some but not all series. Hürthle cell lesions are positive for S-100 protein (315,316). In addition, galectin 3 may potentially serve as a marker in difficult differential diagnosis cases involving Hürthle cell adenomas and Hürthle cell carcinomas (317).

In the histologically defined carcinomas, flow cytometric data may provide prognostic aid. Carcinomas that show an aneuploid pattern may behave more aggressively than those that are diploid. Biologically and histologically benign oxyphilic tumors of the thyroid can show aneuploid DNA patterns. However, such a finding does not indicate malignant behavior. Approximately 20% to 50% of Hürthle cell tumors that are histologically malignant and aneuploid are more aggressive biologically and clinically than diploid Hürthle cell cancers (318,319).

Molecular Biology of Hürthle Cell Tumors

Hürthle cell tumors are biologically different from other follicular-derived tumors (320,321). *H-ras* mutations are more frequent in Hürthle cell carcinoma than follicular carcinoma (296,322). Segev et al. (323) have shown that Hürthle cell tumors show a high percentage of allelic alterations compared with other follicular-derived tumors. Maximo et al. (324) studied the relationship between mitochondrial DNA alterations and thyroid tumorigenesis. This study showed that Hürthle cell tumors display a relatively higher percentage of common deletions of mitochondrial DNA compared with other follicular-derived tumors. In addition, Hürthle cell tumors also showed germline polymorphisms of the *ATPase 6* gene, which is required for the maintenance of mitochondrial DNA (324). It is postulated that Hürthle cell tumors may develop in thyroid gland via two different mechanisms. The presence of abundant and abnormal mitochondria in the cytoplasm of the neoplastic Hürthle cells may be seen either throughout the tumor, suggesting that the neoplastic transformation occurred in cells with abnormal mitochondrial DNA (i.e., de novo transformation), or limited to some portions of tumor, indicating that abnormalities in mitochondrial DNA occurred after the tumor originated from the follicular cells (324,325).

C-CELL LESIONS

The hormone calcitonin was discovered and characterized in the early 1960s; the thyroid C cell had been described in many animal species by the end of the 19th and early 20th centuries. In the early 1960s, pathologists were defining the morphology of the tumor now known as medullary carcinoma (326,327). In 1966, Williams (328) proposed that medullary carcinoma might be derived from the C cell and predicted that if the C cell was the source of calcitonin, then the tumors might also produce this hormone.

The C cells are derived embryologically from the neural crest and migrate into the thyroid along with the ultimobranchial body. Hence, these two elements may be closely associated in the adult thyroid; however, the ultimobranchial body itself does not show calcitonin immunoreactivity and should not be considered as hyperplastic C cells (329,330). In humans, C cells are found along the lateral aspects of the thyroid lobes in the upper two-thirds of the gland. The C cells comprise less than 0.1% of the thyroid mass in humans (331,332). Wolfe et al. (331,332) showed C-cell distribution in the thyroid by immunohistochemistry. The number of C cells in the thyroid differs according to age. They identified larger numbers of these cells in infants and children under the age of 6 years than in adults. In children, groups of up to 6 cells can be seen, with as many as 100 cells noted in a low-power microscopic field. In adult glands, no more than 10 cells should be found in a low-power field.

Clusters of C cells in adults have been described in endocrinologically normal adults. O'Toole et al. (333) examined thyroid glands from forensic autopsies and recognized a trend toward increased numbers of these cells in older individuals (>60 years old); however, they noted large standard deviations. This remains a problem area for pathologists.

MEDULLARY THYROID CARCINOMA

Medullary thyroid carcinoma is rare and comprises less than 10% of all thyroid malignancies (334,335). This tumor is of great diagnostic importance because of its aggressiveness, its close association with multiple endocrine neoplasia (MEN) syndromes (MEN2A and MEN2B), and a relationship to a C-cell hyperplasia as the probable precursor lesion (336). Although the majority of medullary carcinomas are sporadic, approximately 10% to 20% are familial. Because these familial cases have been identified, a gene associated with medullary carcinoma has been identified on chromosome 10 and involves mutations in the *RET* oncogene (336,337). The clinical features are similar in both sporadic and familial cases that are symptomatic (334). Medullary carcinoma can affect patients of any age; however, most affected individuals are adults with an average age of approximately 50 years (334,335). In familial cases, though, children can be affected; also in these instances, the age of diagnosis tends to be younger (mean age of approximately 20 years). Although sporadic medullary carcinomas are seen more commonly in women, familial cases have an equal sex ratio because an autosomal dominant mode of inheritance is present (338,339).

Most patients with medullary carcinoma will present with a thyroid nodule that is painless but firm. In up to 50% of cases, obvious nodal metastases will be present at the time of diagnosis. Distant metastases to lung, bone, or liver may also be noted initially in approximately 15% to 25% of cases (340). When the tumor produces excess hormone other than calcitonin, the presenting symptoms may be related to that hormone hypersecretion (e.g., adrenocorticotropic hormone [ACTH], prostaglandin) (341,342).

In the familial forms, there are associated endocrine or neuroendocrine lesions. Sipple syndrome (MEN2 or MEN2A) is familial and consists of medullary thyroid cancer and C-cell hyperplasia, adrenal pheochromocytoma and adrenal medullary hyperplasia, and parathyroid hyperplasia (343,344). Although most affected patients will have the complete syndrome, not every patient will manifest each of these lesions. Studies have shown that the gene responsible for familial medullary carcinoma is *RET* (337); mutations in *RET* (different from the *RET* translocation in papillary carcinoma) are found in the tumors and germline of patients with familial medullary carcinomas and the MEN2 syndromes (345). Mutations in specific codons have been correlated with clinical behavior and symptomatology in some families (345–347). MEN2B consists of medullary thyroid carcinoma and C-cell hyperplasia, pheochromocytoma and adrenal medullary hyperplasia, mucosal neuromas, gastrointestinal ganglioneuromas, and musculoskeletal abnormalities (348–352). These patients may have familial disease (present in >50%); some cases arise apparently as spontaneous mutations. These patients have biologically aggressive medullary carcinoma and may succumb to metastases at an early age. MEN2B shows similarity to von Recklinghausen disease because, in neurofibromatosis, similar lesions are found in the gastrointestinal tract and pheochromocytomas are common. Nerve growth factor has been identified in some medullary carcinomas of these patients; it has been postulated that this product of the tumor may be responsible for the neural lesions seen in patients with MEN2B (353). However, the neural lesions often precede the development of medullary cancer by many years. In MEN2B, the tumor and germline mutations in *RET* are found on codon 918, which is an intracellular focus of the *RET* oncogene (354).

The pathologist may contribute to the determination of familial rather than sporadic disease if, upon examining a medullary carcinoma of the thyroid, he or she notes multifocal or bilateral tumors and the presence of C-cell hyperplasia (334).

Pathology

Medullary carcinoma is usually located in the area of highest C-cell concentration (i.e., the lateral upper two-thirds of the gland). In familial cases, multiple small nodules may be detected grossly, and rarely, lesions may be found in the isthmus. The tumors range in size from barely visible to several centimeters. Many medullary carcinomas are grossly circumscribed, but some will show infiltrative borders (Fig. 13.28). Some tumors will show gross necrosis and hemorrhage (208,334).

The typical medullary carcinoma may be microscopically circumscribed or, more likely, may be freely infiltrating into the surrounding thyroid. The pattern of growth is of tumor cells arranged in nests separated by varying amounts of stroma. The tumor nests are composed of round, oval, or spindle-shaped cells; there often is isolated cellular pleomorphism or even multinucleated cells (Fig. 13.29). The nuclei are uniform; the nu-

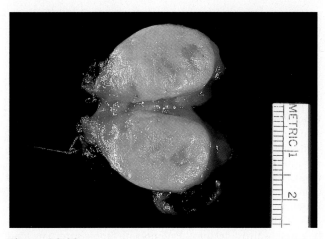

Figure 13.28. Gross medullary carcinoma showing a relatively circumscribed tan-brown mass with focal hemorrhage.

clear-to-cytoplasmic ratio is low. Intranuclear cytoplasmic inclusions are commonly noted. Mitoses can be seen. The tumor stroma characteristically contains amyloid, although this is not necessary for the diagnosis; approximately 25% of medullary carcinomas do not contain amyloid (Fig. 13.29). The amyloid is most likely derived from precalcitonin, and indeed, immuno-

histochemical stains for calcitonin often stain the amyloid. Calcifications in areas of amyloid deposition are characteristically present. The tumors commonly invade lymphatics and veins (208,334,355).

Several medullary carcinoma variants have been described. In the papillary variant, a papillary or pseudopapillary growth pattern is identified. The pseudopapillary variant is more common and probably results from fixation artifact (356). The true papillary variant is extremely rare and needs to be differentiated from typical papillary thyroid carcinoma; nuclear morphology is the most important distinguishing feature. The follicular variant is characterized by the presence of follicles, glands, or tubules. Care must be rendered to determine that the follicular structures are not just entrapped normal thyroid within the lesion (356,357). Some medullary carcinomas are grossly and microscopically encapsulated (358,359). Mendelsohn and Oertel (360) reported a series of encapsulated thyroid lesions classified as atypical adenomas and showed that many of these were medullary cancers containing immunoreactive calcitonin. The follow-up in encapsulated medullary carcinomas indicates that they have a more benign prognosis than usual medullary tumors. The histologic differential diagnosis for the encapsulated variant includes hyalinizing trabecular adenoma. Immunohistochemistry for calcitonin will be positive in the medullary carcinoma but not within the hyalinizing trabecular adenoma. In

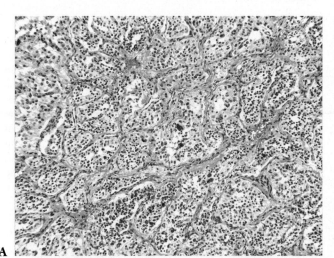

A

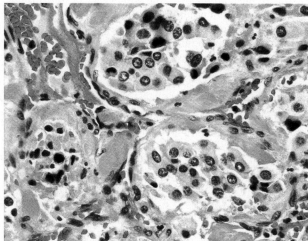

B

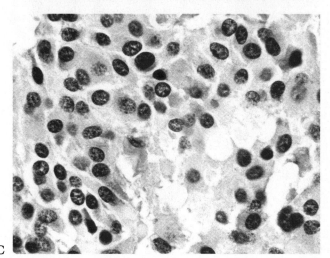

C

Figure 13.29. **(A)** Low-power view of medullary carcinoma showing nests of cells surrounded by dense pink stroma containing amyloid. **(B)** Medullary carcinoma showing sheets of neoplastic C cells surrounded by amyloid. **(C)** Higher-power view of medullary carcinoma showing round uniform cells with a punctate chromatin pattern and mild variation in nuclear size.

the past, some authors have used the term *C-cell adenoma* to describe encapsulated variants of medullary carcinoma; however, this terminology is not favored (361). The small-cell variant of medullary carcinoma has also been described (362). These tumors look like pulmonary small-cell carcinoma, from which they need to be distinguished, if possible. The prognosis is worse than for typical medullary carcinoma. Although calcitonin expression may not always be seen, the small-cell variant of medullary carcinoma often expresses CEA and calcitonin gene–related peptide, just as other types of medullary carcinoma do (362). The giant-cell variant is rare and is characterized by large atypical cells admixed with areas of typical medullary carcinoma (363). Because of the presence of large atypical cells, this variant needs to be differentiated from anaplastic thyroid carcinoma, a tumor with a worse prognosis when compared with medullary carcinoma. The clear-cell variant is a rare form of medullary carcinoma and is characterized by cells with abundant clear cytoplasm (364). Immunohistochemical stains reveal the presence of calcitonin in the lesional cells. Differential diagnostic consideration for this variant includes follicular-derived neoplasms with clear-cell cytoplasm as well as metastatic renal cell carcinoma. Other variants of medullary carcinoma include oncocytic and squamous variants (365). Immunohistochemical stains are often needed to establish the correct diagnosis.

Up to 40% of medullary carcinomas contain mucin, most of which is extracellular; intracytoplasmic mucin can be seen in approximately 15% of medullary carcinomas (366). Rare tumor may contain melanin pigment, the significance of which is not known (367). By immunohistochemistry, the majority of medullary carcinomas express low–molecular-weight cytokeratin, calcitonin, and calcitonin gene–related peptide (Fig. 13.30) (368). In addition, many tumors express CEA, which may also be elevated in the serum (Fig. 13.30) (369). A variety of other peptides may be found in tumor cells including somatostatin, vasoactive intestinal peptide, and synaptophysin (370,371). Some studies have also identified polysialic acid (neural cell adhesion molecule) in medullary carcinomas but not in other thyroid tumors (372).

Occasional lesions (and often these are small-cell type) do not contain immunoreactive calcitonin. To accept a calcitonin-free tumor of the thyroid as a medullary carcinoma, it should arise in a familial setting or occur in a thyroid with unequivocal C-cell hyperplasia. Immunoreactivity for calcitonin gene–related peptide would add proof to the histogenetic nature of such a lesion.

Prognostic Factors

From the clinical standpoint, stage is the most important variable for prognosis (373–375). A tumor confined to the thyroid without nodal or distant metastases is associated with prolonged survival (375). Several researchers have found that younger patients (<40 years old), especially women, fare somewhat better than the whole group of medullary cancer patients (374,376). Patients who are discovered by screening because they are members of affected families often have very small tumors and can be cured by thyroidectomy. Patients with Sipple syndrome tend to have less aggressive tumors than the sporadic group, whereas patients with MEN2B have aggressive lesions (375,377). Pathologic features that have been related to prognosis include tumor pattern, amyloid content, pleomorphism, necrosis, and mitotic activity (375,378). Small-cell medullary carcinomas and those tumors with extensive areas of necrosis, marked cellular pleomorphism, and high mitotic activity are associated with poor prognosis (378). Encapsulated tumors and tumors with uniform cytology and abundant amyloid tend to be indolent tumors. Schroder et al. (378) found that aneuploidy was associated with a poor outcome.

MIXED FOLLICULAR AND MEDULLARY CARCINOMA

These controversial tumors show thyroglobulin and calcitonin immunoreactivity and ultrastructural evidence of differentiation along two cell lines (379,380). Some of the series of these tumors may have been confusing, with trapping of follicles at the invading edge of the medullary carcinoma and diffusion of thyroglobulin into the medullary carcinoma; this may result in diagnosis of mixed tumors showing immunostaining for both hormones (380). Caution should be taken when making the diagnosis of mixed medullary and follicular-derived carcinomas.

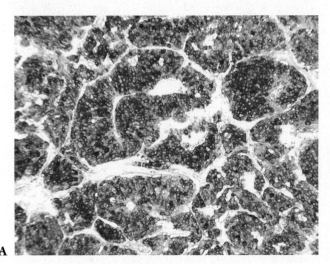

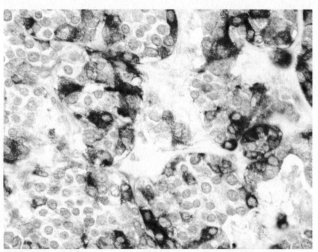

A   **B**

Figure 13.30. **(A)** Calcitonin immunostaining in medullary carcinoma shows strong reactivity in neoplastic cells. **(B)** Immunostaining for carcinoembryonic antigen is often positive as well.

C-CELL HYPERPLASIA

The definition of C-cell hyperplasia is difficult. The lower limit of C-cell hyperplasia and the upper limit of normal C-cell mass are not clear. Various studies show C-cell clusters in adults that, taken alone, could fit into the category of C-cell hyperplasia. Yet O'Toole et al. (333) and Gibson et al. (381) noted these clusters of C cells at autopsy in apparently endocrinologically normal individuals. Conversely, the lower limit of medullary carcinoma and upper limit of C-cell hyperplasia is difficult to define. DeLellis and Wolfe (382) state that C-cell hyperplasia ranges from diffuse increase in the cells to nodules of C-cell–replacing follicles, and once the basement membrane of the follicle is breached, medullary carcinoma should be diagnosed. However, Carney et al. (383) point out that it is not always obvious that the basement membrane has been crossed.

In the classic case of C-cell hyperplasia, the lesion appears as multifocal areas of increased numbers of amphophilic large cells replacing follicular epithelium and also replacing follicles completely forming nodules (Fig. 13.31). More specific definitions of C-cell hyperplasia include more than 50 C cells per low-power field and more than 40 C cells/cm^2 to more than 50 C cells per three low-power fields (384,385). With these definitions, C-cell hyperplasia is seen not only in patients with MEN syndromes or familial medullary carcinoma (386), but also in patients with hyperparathyroidism, chronic hypercalcemia of other causes, Hashimoto disease, residual thyroid tissue following removal of medullary cancer (sporadic type), and even thyroid tissue adjacent to nonmedullary carcinomas (385,387). Because C-cell hyperplasia may be associated with so many lesions, the exact significance using these various definitions cannot be determined. One of the best ways to distinguish C-cell hyperplasia is by routine histologic examination. C-cell hyperplasia associated with familial medullary carcinoma and MEN syndromes is readily observed on routine hematoxylin and eosin (H&E) stains (388,389). The cells are often large and show significant nuclear atypia as well as occasional features of medullary carcinoma. On the other hand, secondary C-cell hyperplasia is often only observed by immunohistochemical staining for calcitonin and quantitative analysis. Therefore, the actual diagnosis of

C-cell hyperplasia may be made by routine histologic examination for the presence of C cells by H&E stains. Micromedullary carcinoma can be found in glands removed prophylactically because of positive genetic testing for RET mutations (390). These carcinomas are similar to micropapillary carcinomas; that is, they measure ≤1 cm. In the familial setting, there is usually associated C-cell hyperplasia (195).

Micromedullary carcinomas are also being recognized as sporadic tumors in thyroid lobes or glands removed for benign nodules or for nonmedullary cancer. These lesions show a rounded or focally infiltrative pattern of growth, may contain amyloid, and are not necessarily associated with C-cell hyperplasia. The glands frequently show chronic lymphocytic thyroiditis. In the absence of symptomatic hypercalcitoninemia, or lymph node metastases, these lesions are cured by their simple removal (195,391).

POORLY DIFFERENTIATED CARCINOMA ("INSULAR" CARCINOMA)

Poorly differentiated thyroid carcinoma is a follicular-derived carcinoma with a prognosis between well-differentiated thyroid carcinomas (papillary or follicular) and anaplastic thyroid carcinoma (124,392,393). The term *insular* has been used to describe the lesion's histologic growth pattern, which is somewhat "carcinoid-like"; however, solid and trabecular growth patterns do occur (394). The incidence of this tumor appears to vary with differing geographic locations, with incidence as high as 5% described in Italy but a much lower incidence in the United States (394–396). In some classifications, insular carcinoma is classified under follicular carcinoma.

The lesions are often large, gray-white in color, and infiltrative and show extensive necrosis (Fig. 13.32). Microscopically, the tumor is composed of round cells with evenly distributed nuclear chromatin and inconspicuous nucleoli. The tumor cell can be arranged in nests enveloped by a well-developed capillary framework (i.e., insular pattern, solid sheets, or trabeculae) (Fig. 13.33). Necrosis, vascular invasion, and mitoses are prominent features (124,393). The tumor cells should stain positive for thyroglobulin and negative for calcitonin. Poorly differen-

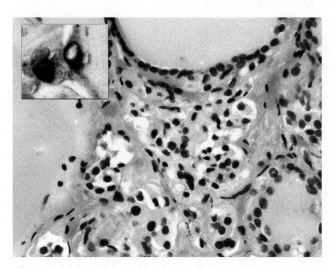

Figure 13.31. Example of a C-cell nodular proliferation in a patient with a history of multiple endocrine neoplasia type 2A. The inset shows the confirmatory immunostains for calcitonin.

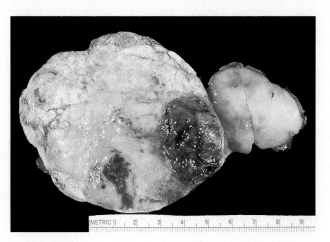

Figure 13.32. Gross poorly differentiated (insular) carcinoma showing a large yellow-white tumor mass with gross evidence of hemorrhage and necrosis.

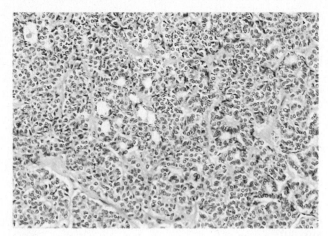

Figure 13.33. Histologic examination of poorly differentiated (insular pattern) carcinoma often shows a neuroendocrine growth pattern similar to that seen in carcinoid. The tumor cells show mitotic activity and necrosis are often present, but they are thyroglobulin positive.

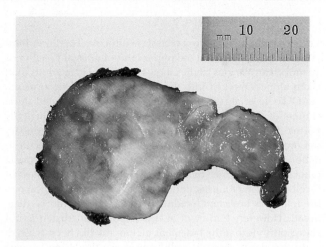

Figure 13.34. Gross anaplastic thyroid carcinoma showing a large yellow, tan, white mass with areas of hemorrhage.

tiated carcinoma is associated with a worse prognosis than well-differentiated thyroid carcinomas but a significantly better prognosis than anaplastic thyroid carcinoma. Insular, solid, and trabecular growth patterns have been described as focal features in otherwise well-differentiated thyroid carcinomas by some authors (393); the better differentiated tumors include papillary carcinoma, including the follicular variant, and follicular carcinoma (124,321,393).

It has been shown that the extent of poorly differentiated components in a well-differentiated thyroid tumor can affect the prognosis; tumors with more than 10% of the poorly differentiated component are associated with frequent regional recurrences, distant metastases, and poor prognosis (397).

ANAPLASTIC THYROID TUMORS

Anaplastic carcinomas are a group of high-grade thyroid carcinomas that are usually undifferentiated histologically and have an extremely poor prognosis, with many patients surviving less than 6 months following diagnosis (145,398). Synonyms for anaplastic carcinoma include undifferentiated, dedifferentiated, and sarcomatoid carcinoma. These tumors represent approximately 5% of thyroid malignancies. The tumor is more commonly seen in older adult women who present with a rapidly enlarging mass, which often results in dyspnea. Risk factors are largely unknown but may include a history of radiation and iodine deficiency (399). A precursor well-differentiated thyroid carcinoma (papillary, follicular, or Hürthle cell) may be observed (400,401).

Grossly, the tumors are large with extensive intrathyroidal and extrathyroidal invasion (Figs. 13.34 and 13.35). Surgical resection is often not performed because the lesion's extent and diagnosis are commonly made on biopsy. The tumor invades extensively in the thyroid tissue, resulting in parenchymal destruction, which may be associated with transient hyperthyroidism. Necrosis, vascular invasion, and mitoses are quite prominent (401). Histologically, a variety of patterns have been described (261,402–405). The tumors are usually made up of a variety of cell types. Most tumors are composed of giant cells

and spindle cells, although "squamoid" differentiation is seen in about one-third of cases (401,406). Osteoclast-like giant cells are a common feature (407). A "paucicellular" variant of anaplastic carcinoma has been described; it is characterized by dense fibrosis, calcification, and a poor patient outcome (408). Spindle cell squamous anaplastic carcinoma may be the result of transformation of tall-cell papillary carcinoma (409).

Electron microscopic and immunohistologic studies have indicated that almost all anaplastic thyroid tumors are indeed epithelial in nature (410,411). The cells contain many cytoplasmic organelles and dense bodies similar to those found in follicular epithelium. By immunohistochemistry, anaplastic thyroid carcinomas should be positive for cytokeratin (411). Thyroglobulin immunostaining is often negative (412).

Small-cell carcinoma of the thyroid is extremely rare. Numerous studies have shown conclusively that many tumors that would have been classified as small-cell carcinoma represent either medullary carcinoma, small-cell malignant lymphoma, poorly differentiated carcinoma of follicular derivation (insular variant), or a metastasis to the thyroid (usually but not always from a lung primary) (413).

THYROID SARCOMA

Sarcomas of the thyroid are rare; fibrosarcomas, leiomyosarcomas, and angiosarcomas have been described (414–416). Angiosarcoma of thyroid has been most commonly described from the Alpine regions of Europe. Clinically, the affected patients resemble those with anaplastic carcinoma. By gross and histologic examination, these tumors resemble angiosarcomas of soft tissue (416,417).

LYMPHOCYTIC LESIONS AFFECTING THE THYROID

Malignant Lymphoma

Malignant lymphoma may involve the thyroid as part of systemic lymphoma (secondary lymphoma) or may arise primarily in the thyroid (108). Approximately 20% of patients dying of generalized malignant lymphoma will show thyroid involvement at au-

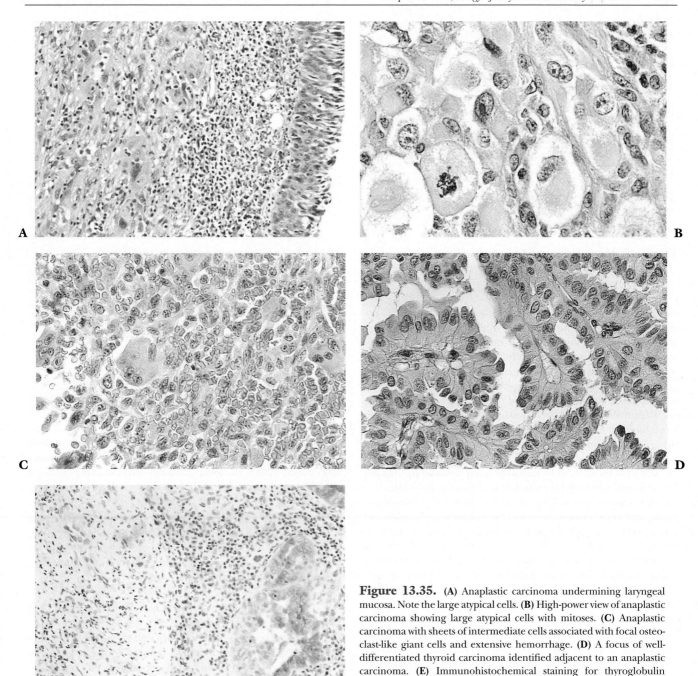

Figure 13.35. **(A)** Anaplastic carcinoma undermining laryngeal mucosa. Note the large atypical cells. **(B)** High-power view of anaplastic carcinoma showing large atypical cells with mitoses. **(C)** Anaplastic carcinoma with sheets of intermediate cells associated with focal osteoclast-like giant cells and extensive hemorrhage. **(D)** A focus of well-differentiated thyroid carcinoma identified adjacent to an anaplastic carcinoma. **(E)** Immunohistochemical staining for thyroglobulin shows focal positivity in a well-differentiated area of the tumor (*right*) and negative reactivity in the anaplastic component (*left*).

topsy. Thyroid replacement is rarely extensive enough to produce clinical hypothyroidism (108,418).

Of all thyroid malignancies, 1% to 3.5% are malignant lymphomas. Primary malignant lymphoma of the thyroid usually arises in an immunologically abnormal gland, usually one affected by chronic lymphocytic thyroiditis (48,419). Clinically, thyroid lymphoma affects women more frequently than men (ratio of 2.5 to 8.4:1). Most patients are older (age 50 to 80 years). The mass, often arising in patients with Hashimoto disease, is rapidly growing and may extend outside the gland (420,421). An immunologically abnormal tissue produces the background for lymphoma development. However, rarely, lymphomas may arise in normal glands. It is important not to view

autoimmune thyroiditis as a premalignant condition because thyroid lymphoma is so rare. The lymphoid tissue present in the thyroid has been considered part of the mucosal-associated lymphoid tissue (MALT) system; lesions of similar MALT might be expected to occur in patients with primary thyroid lymphoma. Gastrointestinal and thyroid lymphomas occur too frequently in the same patient to be considered coincidental (considering the relative rarity of extranodal lymphoma) (420).

Grossly, most thyroid lymphomas appear as large fleshy tan or gray masses often extending outside the thyroid capsule. Infiltration of the residual thyroid tissue may be seen. The nontumoral thyroid may show the gross appearance of lymphocytic thyroiditis, although the findings often depend on the amount

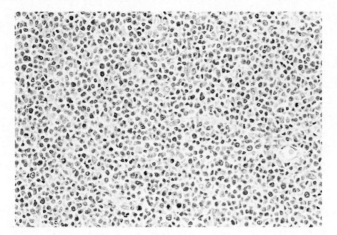

Figure 13.36. Diffuse large-cell lymphoma arising in a patient with Hashimoto thyroiditis.

of thyroid tissue uninvolved by the tumor. The microscopic appearance of thyroid lymphomas resembles lymphoma occurring in other sites. The gamut of small-, intermediate-, and large-cell lesions are found; sometimes nodular areas are noted, although a diffuse pattern is more common. The most common histologic subtype is large-cell diffuse lymphoma (Fig. 13.36). Some tumors demonstrate a plasmacytoid appearance, whereas others show features of immunoblastic sarcoma. Immunophenotyping studies indicate that most thyroid lymphomas are of B-cell lineage (48,108). Epstein-Barr virus has been identified in some cases (422,423).

The tumors often disclose areas of zonal necrosis. Infiltration of surrounding thyroid is seen. It is common to see infiltration of lymphocytes into residual thyroid follicles; sometimes the malignant cells replace the follicular epithelium. Invasion beyond the thyroid itself, into surrounding strap muscles and soft tissue, is seen in 50% to 60% of cases. Approximately 25% of cases will show vascular invasion. A common histologic finding is the so-called "lymphoepithelial lesion"; in the thyroid, this consists of thyroid follicles stuffed with neoplastic lymphoid cells that sometimes partially or totally replace the follicular epithelium (108,423).

When a diagnosis of thyroid lymphoma is made, careful clinical staging of the disease is warranted. Treatment for thyroid lymphoma depends on the staging results. If the disease is widespread, chemotherapy is the choice; however, if the tumor is localized to the gland only or the regional lymph nodes, radiation therapy with or without adjuvant chemotherapy appears warranted. The prognosis for localized thyroid lymphoma is excellent. More than 50% to 80% of affected patients survive 10 years (108,423).

Other Hematopoietic Lesions in the Thyroid

Infiltration of the thyroid gland is rare in patients with systemic myeloma; from 0% to 2.6% of patients in large series of cases of multiple myeloma will show thyroid involvement. Extramedullary plasma cell tumors have been reported in the thyroid. Microscopically, the lesion consists of sheets of mature plasma cells replacing thyroid. Capsular extension or penetration can be seen. Differentiation to large-cell lymphoma may be evident (50,424).

Other lesions that may rarely involve the thyroid include chronic leukemias (425), signet cell lymphoma (426), Hodgkin disease (427,428), mycosis fungoides, chloroma, histiocytosis (429), and Rosai-Dorfman disease (430).

UNUSUAL THYROID TUMORS

Squamous Cell Lesions

Squamous cells can be identified in the thyroid in a variety of conditions including developmental rests, inflammatory processes, and neoplasms. Thymic remnants, remnants of the thyroglossal duct, and ultimobranchial body rest (solid cell nests) can be identified in some carefully sectioned thyroids (132,431).

Metaplastic Squamous Lesions of the Thyroid

Inflammatory or destructive processes associated with reparative phenomena can give rise to squamous cells in the thyroid. It is believed that most of these represent metaplasia of follicular epithelium (132).

Squamous Cells in Thyroid Neoplasms

ADENOMAS: ADENOMATOID NODULES. Squamous metaplasia is rare in benign adenomatous nodules but may be seen in those that have been aspirated or biopsied (432).

PAPILLARY CARCINOMA. Squamous or squamoid areas can be found focally in approximately 16% to 40% of ordinary papillary cancers (208). Franssila (433) did not note any prognostic significance to this focal finding.

DIFFUSE SCLEROSIS VARIANT OF PAPILLARY CARCINOMA. As noted earlier, this unusual variant of papillary carcinoma is characterized by diffuse, often bilateral, involvement of the thyroid by a papillary tumor with many psammoma bodies and prominent squamous metaplasia (434).

MUCOEPIDERMOID CARCINOMA AND SCLEROSING MUCOEPIDERMOID CARCINOMA WITH EOSINOPHILIA. These are rare but distinctive variants of thyroid carcinoma. Mucoepidermoid carcinoma of thyroid origin is composed of solid masses of squamoid cells and mucin-producing cells, sometimes forming glands (51,435). The nuclei may on occasion show a ground-glass appearance, and psammoma bodies may be found. Some authors consider that this lesion is a variant of papillary carcinoma; all cases show thyroglobulin and TTF-1 expression (436,437). The prognosis of thyroid mucoepidermoid carcinoma is quite good. Lesions may metastasize to regional nodes and rarely distantly. Death from disease is rare (51,438).

Sclerosing mucoepidermoid carcinoma with eosinophilia is usually seen in a background of lymphocytic thyroiditis and is characterized by tumor cells arranged in small sheets, anastamosing trabeculae, and narrow strands associated with dense fibrosis and numerous eosinophils (Fig. 13.37). Although these lesions may metastasize to lymph nodes and show extracapsular spread, vascular invasion, and perineural invasion, death as a result of disease is uncommon. The tumor cells stain negative for thyroglobulin and calcitonin and positive for cytokeratin (51,436,439).

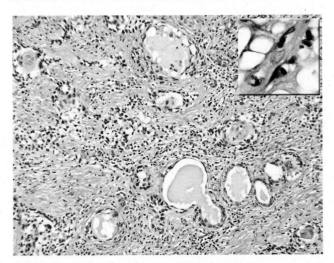

Figure 13.37. Sclerosing mucoepidermoid carcinoma with eosinophilia showing tumor cells arranged in cords, tubules, and glands with background sclerosis and eosinophilic infiltration (inset).

At present, there is no consensus regarding the origin of these tumors. Initial studies postulated origin from intrathyroidal ectopic salivary gland rests. Franssila et al. (440) and Harach (438) suggested origin from vestiges of ultimobranchial body (solid cell nests), and others have suggested follicular origin. Recent studies have suggested that based on the immunoprofile, both of these tumors have different origins; mucoepidermoid carcinoma shows follicular derivation, and sclerosing mucoepidermoid carcinoma is derived from ultimobranchial body rests/solid cell nests (51,441).

SQUAMOUS CELL CARCINOMA OF THE THYROID. Primary squamous cell carcinoma of the thyroid is very rare. Thyroid squamous cancer occurs in older adult patients who present with histories of goiter (442). The tumors resemble squamous carcinomas of other organs and range from well-differentiated to poorly differentiated lesions, with or without keratinization. Origin in abnormal thyroids is common, and as such, these tumors clinically and pathologically share features with anaplastic thyroid cancers. The prognosis is also similar; these tumors are radioresistant and often rapidly fatal (442,443).

METASTATIC SQUAMOUS CARCINOMA IN THE THYROID. Far more common than the primary tumors, metastatic squamous cell carcinoma can involve the thyroid (132). Direct extensions from laryngeal or esophageal primaries are probably encountered most often. Hematogenous metastases from lung or other primary sites also occur (the latter are often noted at autopsy; thyroid dysfunction is rare). Metastatic squamous cell carcinomas usually present grossly and microscopically as multiple nodules (132,443).

CLEAR-CELL TUMORS. Thyroid tumors with clear cells fall into the following four groups: primary follicular-derived lesions with clear cells, medullary cancer, parathyroid tumors, and metastatic kidney cancer (364,444,445).

Follicular cells in the thyroid may undergo a variety of metaplastic changes: squamous, oncocytic, and occasionally clear cell. Thyroid nodules and neoplasms can take on clear-cell cytol-

ogy. Clear cells may be caused by formation of intracytoplasmic vesicles, glycogen accumulation, fat accumulation, or deposition of intracellular thyroglobulin. Clear-cell neoplasms of thyroid follicular cell origin form a spectrum of tumors—some papillary, some follicular, and some anaplastic. Often, oncocytic cells are found in close association with the clear cells. Some clear-cell follicular tumors are benign, and some of these are distinctive lesions showing signet ring cells, called signet ring adenomas (444,446).

Rarely, tumors of follicular origin will show clear cells because of intracytoplasmic fat accumulation. In some examples, fat admixed with thyroid follicles is found; these lesions have been termed *adenolipomas, thyrolipomas,* or *hamartomas,* and they are benign. In a few instances, fat and amyloid have been admixed and formed a thyroid mass (447,448).

Various authors have estimated the incidence of true intrathyroidal parathyroid tissue (as distinguished from parathyroid tissue abutting the thyroid capsule) to be 0.2%. On rare occasions, such glands may be affected by hyperplasia or neoplasia; hyperparathyroidism may result. If the tumor is solid, it may exhibit clear-cell cytology and be confused with a primary thyroid neoplasm (449–451).

The frequency of solitary renal cancer metastases to the thyroid seems disproportionate to the frequency of kidney carcinoma. It is unclear why this tumor often spreads to the thyroid. The thyroid metastasis may be the initial manifestation of the kidney neoplasm, or the thyroid metastasis may be solitary and represent the only spread of the disease. In patients with a history of kidney cancer, the time interval between the initial renal neoplasm resection and the thyroid metastasis may be many years (452). In our experience and that reported in the literature, the usual renal carcinoma that spreads to the thyroid is clear-cell carcinoma. Often it presents as a solitary nodule. The histopathologic distinction between a clear-cell thyroid tumor and renal cancer metastasis in the thyroid may be quite difficult. Stains for immunoreactive thyroglobulin, if positive, are very helpful, but metastatic tumors may take up thyroglobulin from the surrounding gland (diffusion artifact) (452,453).

METASTATIC TUMORS TO THE THYROID. Metastases may reach the thyroid by direct extension from tumors in adjacent structures, by retrograde lymphatic spread, or hematogenously. Carcinomas of the larynx, pharynx, trachea, and esophagus may invade the thyroid directly. Often, multiple areas of the gland are involved; distinction from thyroid primary is usually not difficult. Retrograde extension through lymphatic routes into the thyroid is unusual. In theory, at least, any tumor involving cervical lymph nodes could extend into the thyroid by this mechanism. Hematogenous metastases to the thyroid vary according to tumor type (452,454). Virtually any malignant tumor may metastasize to the thyroid; some of these may resemble primary lesions. A metastasis should always be considered when the histology is unusual for a thyroid primary. Some patients may have a history of cancer elsewhere, but this is not always the case. In surgical series, carcinomas of the kidney and colon and melanoma are most commonly found (454,455); the incidence of these tumor types in thyroid metastases is disproportionate to the frequency of occurrence of these tumors. Grossly, such lesions are often solitary, circumscribed masses; they may appear quite compatible with a primary tumor. Histologically, the neoplasm may also be a single nodule. Resemblance to colonic adenocarcinoma, breast cancer, or pigmented melanoma reassures the pathologist that this is a metastasis. However, clear-cell carcinoma of the kidney, as has been noted, may present a problem (452).

TUMORS WITH THYMIC OR RELATED BRANCHIAL POUCH DIFFERENTIATION. On rare occasions, thymic tissue may be located intrathyroidally. Rarely, thymomas may arise in these thymic rests (456,457). *Spindle epithelial tumor with thymus-like differentiation (SETTLE)* occurs in children and young adults. By light microscopy, the tumor shows an admixture of spindle and epithelioid cells. Squamous differentiation resembling Hassall corpuscles can occur. Tumor cells usually stain positive for cytokeratins, smooth muscle actin, and muscle-specific actin and are negative for thyroglobulin and calcitonin (457–459). *Carcinoma showing thymus-like differentiation (CASTLE)* resembles thymic carcinoma by morphology. Some cases may appear similar to lymphoepithelioma-like carcinoma of thymus (460). By immunohistochemistry, these tumors are positive for cytokeratin, CD5, and bcl-2 and negative for thyroglobulin and calcitonin (460,461).

TERATOMAS. Clinically, teratomas present in neonates or infants under the age of 1 year as huge midline neck masses. Often these tumors measure 10 cm or more (462,463). Approximately 35% of women who deliver babies with teratomas experience polyhydramnios in pregnancy. A significant number of cases reported in series and reviews have been identified in stillborns. Grossly, most of these tumors are predominantly or partially cystic. Histologically, the teratomas in newborns and young infants have contained elements of all three germ layers and have been benign. There does not appear to be an increased association of congenital abnormalities in these children. Teratomas of the thyroid in adults differ from those in newborns because they are more frequently malignant (464,465). It seems likely that these lesions conform to immature teratomas or malignant germ cell neoplasms arising in the gonads.

OTHER MESENCHYMAL LESIONS. Primary mesenchymal lesions of thyroid are rare; hemangioma (466), neurilemoma, leiomyoma, leiomyosarcoma (414,467), and solitary fibrous tumor can occur in thyroid (415,468).

Thyroid Tumors in Unusual Locations

LINGUAL THYROID. Although clinically significant, lingual thyroid is an unusual disorder; microscopic remnants of thyroid tissue have been described in 9.8% of tongues examined at autopsy. Grossly, lingual thyroid appears as a mass at the base of the tongue. Histologic examination discloses normal-appearing thyroid follicles interdigitated with skeletal muscle fibers. Rare cases of thyroid carcinoma arising in lingual thyroid are recorded (469,470).

CARCINOMA ARISING IN ASSOCIATION WITH THYROGLOSSAL DUCT. Neoplasms arising in association with the thyroglossal duct might be expected to be squamous carcinomas, but these are extremely rare (471,472); indeed, most tumors occurring in this setting have been thyroid carcinomas, and most are described as papillary (472). Nussbaum et al. (473) described one case of anaplastic carcinoma apparently arising in thyroglossal duct remnants. Medullary carcinoma has not

been described; because the parafollicular cells are not found in the median thyroid, this is not unexpected.

Thyroglossal duct–associated carcinoma is rare and comprises less than 1% of all thyroid cancers. The sex ratio favors females (1.5:1); this is interesting because benign thyroglossal cysts are more common in males. Most patients are adults, although a few have been diagnosed in children under the age of 10 years. The symptoms consist of a midline neck swelling, which has been noted by the patient for a period of days to "many years." Most of the tumors measure between 2 and 3 cm, although lesions as large as 12 cm have been reported (471,474,475).

The clinical presentation of thyroglossal duct carcinoma is identical to that of benign thyroglossal duct cysts (i.e., a swelling in the anterior neck). Grossly, the lesions are usually cystic, but portions of the cyst may be occupied by solid or even obviously papillary tissue. Microscopically, the most common tumor type is papillary carcinoma, which makes up approximately 95% of thyroglossal duct carcinomas (475). Rare cases of squamous or epidermoid carcinoma have been reported (476); these probably are the only tumors that arise from the duct itself (i.e., the lining epithelium). Therapy is similar to that for benign thyroglossal duct cyst (i.e., the Sistrunk procedure), which involves removal en bloc of the cyst and the hyoid bone (477).

When the diagnosis of thyroglossal cyst–associated thyroid cancer is made, the question of its origin arises. Does this tumor represent a metastasis from a primary lesion in the gland, or is the primary site in the region of the gland or in the region of the cyst? In rare cases in which the thyroid was examined pathologically, areas of papillary carcinoma were found in the gland (402,475). Most authors studying this problem conclude that the thyroglossal carcinoma is a primary tumor arising in remnants of thyroid associated with the duct; in those few cases where intrathyroidal tumor has been found, this was considered a separate primary (402,471).

The behavior of thyroglossal duct–associated papillary carcinoma resembles that of thyroid papillary cancer in general. Metastases to lymph nodes have been documented. Death as a result of tumor has rarely been reported (402,471).

INTRATRACHEAL AND INTRALARYNGEAL THYROID CARCINOMA. Malignant tumors arising in thyroid tissue located within the trachea or larynx are very rare but have been reported (478).

FROZEN SECTION DIAGNOSIS AND THE THYROID

Before the advent of fine-needle and large-bore needle biopsy, the method most used in diagnosis of thyroid nodules was intraoperative frozen section. The nodule, or preferably the thyroid lobe, was excised, and a representative portion (preferably encompassing nodule-capsule-thyroid interface) was prepared for frozen section and intraoperative interpretation by a pathologist. In those cases in which the diagnosis of papillary, medullary, or anaplastic cancer was given, appropriate surgery was immediately undertaken.

Even with frozen section, however, despite recommendations of sampling two or even four different areas, the diagnosis of follicular carcinomas is notoriously difficult. In many cases, the diagnosis rendered is "follicular lesion—diagnosis deferred to permanent sections" (280).

Several studies have evaluated frozen section and FNA diagnostic results for thyroid nodules (403,479,480). Although frozen section diagnosis may be specific (90% to 97%), it is not sensitive (60%) (280,404). In addition, deferred diagnoses at frozen section do nothing to alter the operative procedure or guide the surgeon. Frozen section results influenced the surgical approach in only a small percentage of cases. Also, in the era of cost containment, it does not seem justified to perform frozen sections for the intraoperative diagnosis of thyroid nodules; this is even truer if a preoperative FNA has been performed with malignant or suspicious results (404).

GROSS EXAMINATION AND HISTOPATHOLOGIC REPORTING OF THYROID RESECTION SPECIMENS

The pertinent clinical history of the patient should be part of the gross examination of thyroid specimens. This includes age and sex of the patient, relevant history (history of head and neck radiation, family history of thyroid disease or tumors, previous treatment, and history of FNA and cytologic diagnosis), and type of surgical procedure (partial, near total, or total thyroidectomy). The laboratory data (e.g., thyroid function tests, thyroid antibodies, serum calcitonin) and radiologic studies (e.g., ultrasound, thyroid scan) should be included.

The surgeon should orient the specimen. Gross examination should include weight and measurement (in three dimensions) of the specimen and description of external and cut surface (color and consistency). If there are nodules present, each should be described (size, location, and characteristics such as encapsulation, solid, cystic, calcification, and FNA track[s]). If the specimen contains regional nodes, levels and characteristics of any grossly involved nodes should be described. Presence of any parathyroid glands should also be mentioned.

The number of sections submitted for histopathologic examination is determined by the gross findings. For inflammatory lesions such as Graves disease and Hashimoto thyroiditis, which cause diffuse enlargement of thyroid, we recommend one block for every 5 g of tissue. In case of encapsulated solitary or dominant nodule, we recommend submitting the entire circumference of nodule. All sections should include tumor capsule with main tumor mass, along with a margin of normal-appearing thyroid parenchyma. For nonencapsulated or partially encapsulated nodules, one section per 0.5 cm should be submitted.

The final pathology report for thyroid tumors should include histologic type of the tumor, number of foci or multicentricity, encapsulation, presence of tumor capsule and vascular invasion (both at the periphery and beyond the tumor), extrathyroidal extension, and extent of the disease in the contralateral lobe. If lymph node dissection has been performed, the presence of metastases by number and size should be recorded. It is important to document extranodal extension. The number of parathyroids along with their location, if possible, should be documented. Additional findings in the thyroid such as goiter, thyroiditis, and benign tumors should be documented.

A majority of thyroid nodules undergo preoperative FNA; therefore, it is important that FNA diagnosis be correlated with the histologic findings, and this can be documented in the final pathology report.

FINE-NEEDLE ASPIRATION OF THE THYROID

In recent years, FNA has emerged as the first step in the diagnostic management of thyroid nodules. It has proven to be a cost-

effective tool in the selection of patients requiring surgical intervention, halving the number of patients undergoing thyroid surgery and doubling the incidence of malignancy in the resected specimens. To the patient's advantage, the technique is rapid and well tolerated and can be therapeutic for cystic lesions. However, specimen collection, preparation, and interpretation must be optimized for the full benefits of thyroid FNA to be realized (405,481–484).

TECHNIQUE

In general, a 25-gauge needle attached to a 10-cc syringe is used for thyroid aspiration to minimize bleeding, and the angle of approach is medial to lateral, placing the needle below the strap muscles and in front of the trachea, making short, rapid strokes with only slight changes in direction. Larger needles (23-gauge) may be used to drain cysts, followed by reaspiration of any remaining solid areas with a 25-gauge needle (405,485).

SPECIMEN ADEQUACY AND REPORTING

On-site microscopic assessment, with reaspiration when necessary, can minimize the number of inadequate specimens. Although it is generally agreed that the presence of follicular cells is a minimum requirement for thyroid FNA adequacy, the absolute number of cells is subject to debate (486). Adequacy criteria of five to six groups of well-preserved follicular cells, with each group containing 10 or more cells, are proposed by some authors (487). Others require 8 to 10 fragments of well-preserved follicular cells on at least two smears (405). Yet cases with abundant colloid and macrophages and only rare follicular cells may be reported descriptively as "suggestive of" or "consistent with" nodular goiter, with a caveat that the epithelial component is scant. Studies have shown average insufficiency rates in the 15% to 20% range. The nondiagnostic thyroid aspirate can pose a dilemma in clinical management, with cancer rates as high as 25% among nondiagnostic thyroid FNAs (488). These figures serve to emphasize the importance of incorporating clinicoradiographic factors such as patient age, sex, history of prior irradiation, and lesion characteristics (>3 cm, solid/cystic) along with the FNA results when selecting patients for thyroid surgery (278,489).

BENIGN NONNEOPLASTIC LESIONS

Chronic Lymphocytic Thyroiditis

FNAs from autoimmune (Hashimoto) thyroiditis are generally moderately cellular, characterized by a mixed population of mature and transformed lymphocytes, plasma cells, histiocytes, and occasional tingible-body macrophages. This inflammatory component is accompanied by aggregates of follicular cells, Hürthle cells, and scant colloid (Fig. 13.38). In the proper clinical setting, FNA is highly effective in confirming the diagnosis of chronic lymphocytic thyroiditis; however, difficulties can be encountered in distinguishing between lymphocytic thyroiditis and Hürthle cell neoplasm (490). Thorough sampling is critical to maximize detection of associated neoplasms, in particular papillary carcinoma and lymphoma. Lymphomas arising in the setting of Hashimoto thyroiditis are most often large-cell type (491) and may be recognized in aspirate material by a monotonous population of large atypical lymphoid cells. The FNA find-

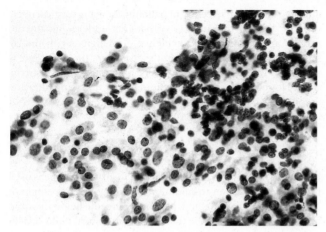

Figure 13.38. Aspiration biopsy specimen from chronic lymphocytic (Hashimoto) thyroiditis showing Hürthle cells intermixed with chronic inflammatory cells (note abundant, ill-defined cytoplasm of Hürthle cells).

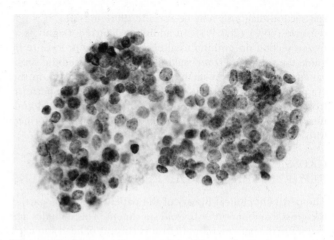

Figure 13.40. Follicular adenoma aspirate showing prominent nuclear crowding and syncytial three-dimensional arrangement.

ing of a predominant or atypical lymphoid population in the setting of Hashimoto thyroiditis should prompt immunophenotyping evaluation either by immunocytochemistry or flow cytometry (491).

Nodular Goiter

FNAs from nodular goiter yield abundant colloid; scant to moderate amounts of follicular epithelium, appearing predominantly as flat sheets, occasionally accompanied by Hürthle cell change; and a variable reactive component consisting of macrophages, fibroconnective tissue, and inflammatory cells. Aspirates of hyperplastic nodules exhibit a more abundant epithelial component that retains bland, uniform morphology and a background of abundant colloid (405,492). The reactive component predominates in aspirates of hemorrhagic cysts, yielding numerous hemosiderin-laden macrophages along with abundant colloid. However, it should be noted that up to 15% of cystic lesions might represent cystic degeneration of a neoplasm, most commonly papillary carcinoma (493,494). This highlights the im-

portance of repeat sampling of any solid areas remaining after cyst drainage and provides a rationale for surgical removal of large, persistent cysts.

NEOPLASTIC LESIONS

Follicular Lesions/Neoplasms

FNA specimens from follicular neoplasms are cellular with scant to absent colloid. The follicular epithelium appears in syncytial fragments with microfollicular or trabecular patterns. Both morphologic and morphometric studies have emphasized the features of increased nuclear size, nuclear pleomorphism, and crowding as helpful in the specific cytologic diagnosis of follicular carcinoma (278,495). However, in routine practice, most follicular carcinomas and follicular adenomas have a similar cytologic pattern (Figs. 13.39 to 13.41). This pattern may be indistinguishable, in 15% to 25% of cases, from hyperplastic nodule in goiter (278,496). Similarly, overlapping cytologic criteria occur between follicular neoplasms and follicular variant of papillary carcinoma, particularly when the characteristic nuclear changes are focal and not adequately sampled or are

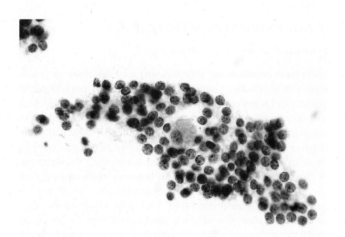

Figure 13.39. Follicular epithelial cells from benign thyroid (nodular goiter; follicular cells appearing as a flat sheet, accompanied by macrophage).

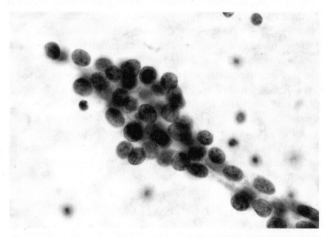

Figure 13.41. Aspirate from follicular carcinoma. Note relative nuclear enlargement of follicular cell nuclei with nuclear overlapping and crowding in the follicular neoplasms compared with the goiter aspirate.

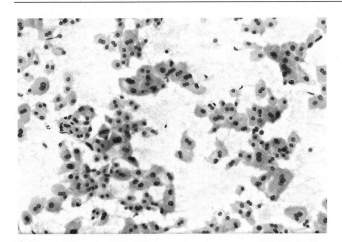

Figure 13.42. Aspirate smear of Hürthle cell adenoma showing cell discohesion, numerous cells with abundant, well-defined cytoplasm, binucleation, and multinucleation.

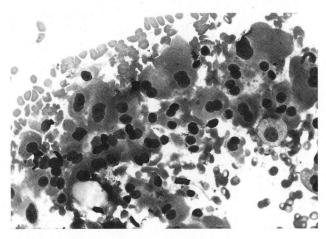

Figure 13.44. Hürthle cell adenoma aspirate showing only slight variation in nuclear size and shape.

poorly visualized in the aspirated material. Generous sampling and optimal specimen preparation minimize these limitations of FNA in distinguishing among follicular lesions. Overall, the incidence of malignancy in nodules with a cytologic diagnosis of follicular neoplasm ranges from 15% to 30% (497).

Hürthle Cell Neoplasms

Hürthle cell neoplasm aspirates are cellular, with scant colloid, and contain cells with abundant, granular cytoplasm and central round nuclei that often have prominent nucleoli. The cells are loosely cohesive, appearing in aggregates, singly, in monolayers, or in follicular patterns (Fig. 13.42) (498). It has been suggested that nonmacrofollicular architecture, absence of colloid, absence of inflammation, and presence of transgressing blood vessels in thyroid FNA specimens is highly predictive of Hürthle cell neoplasm (499,500). Marked nuclear atypia and binucleation may be common in both Hürthle cell adenomas and carcinomas and cannot be used as indicators of malignancy (Figs. 13.43 and 13.44) (500). Ordinary follicular cells are scarce (<10%), and a lymphocytic infiltrate is absent. The differential

diagnosis includes chronic lymphocytic thyroiditis, medullary carcinoma, and, rarely, papillary carcinoma (particularly tall-cell, Hürthle cell, or Warthin tumor–like variants) (217,501).

Papillary Carcinoma

FNA specimens from papillary carcinomas show a wide range of cytologic patterns. High cellularity is a common feature, and colloid is usually scant. The epithelium may appear as true papillary fragments (Fig. 13.45) but more commonly is arranged in multilayered syncytial fragments or branched sheets (Fig. 13.46). A predominant follicular pattern can be seen, particularly in the follicular variant of papillary carcinoma (Fig. 13.47). Nuclear enlargement and pleomorphism are present, along with nuclear crowding, fine powdery chromatin, nuclear grooves, and sharply defined intranuclear cytoplasmic inclusions (Fig. 13.48). The cytoplasm is usually dense and cyanophilic. Strict attention must be paid to finding a set of diagnostic criteria, rather than single isolated features, to arrive at the proper diagnosis (502–504). True papillary fragments with fibrovascular cores are seen in benign processes; nuclear grooves

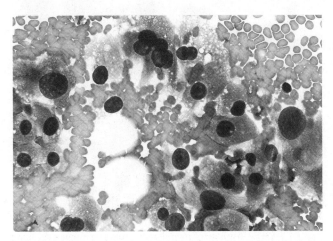

Figure 13.43. Aspirate from mild chronic thyroiditis demonstrating marked nuclear enlargement and pleomorphism. (Compare with the blander nuclei of the Hürthle cell adenoma depicted in Fig. 13.44.)

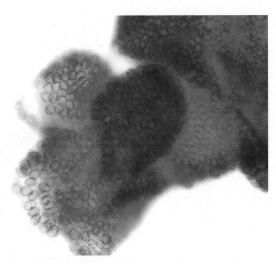

Figure 13.45. A papillary fragment from a papillary carcinoma aspirate showing nuclear features of papillary thyroid carcinoma.

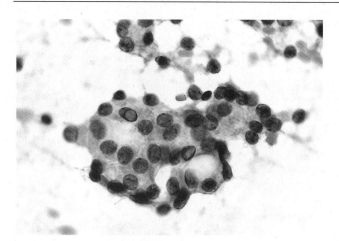

Figure 13.46. Prominent follicular pattern in an aspirate from papillary carcinoma, follicular variant. Note intranuclear inclusion and groove.

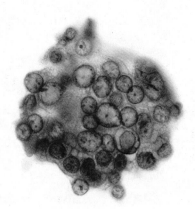

Figure 13.48. Nuclear features of enlargement and crowding. Fine, powdery chromatin and grooves are demonstrated in this aspirate of papillary carcinoma.

have been found in 40% of nonpapillary lesion tissue sections (129,130), and intranuclear inclusions may rarely be seen in follicular and Hürthle cell neoplasms and medullary carcinomas (405). Nuclear grooves and inclusions can appear together in aspirates of hyalinizing trabecular neoplasm of thyroid (505). The features of multinucleated giant cells, seen in 55% to 100% of cases, and psammoma bodies, although not specific for papillary carcinoma, are helpful associated findings. There is much evidence now that the various subtypes of papillary carcinomas can be reliably distinguished in cytologic specimens (502,506,507).

Medullary Carcinoma

FNAs from medullary carcinoma are generally highly cellular, composed of loosely cohesive sheets and nests of cells. Occasionally, paucicellular specimens obscured by blood are encountered. The tumor cells have abundant, granular cytoplasm that appears ill-defined and contains small eosinophilic granules on Romanowsky-stained preparations in 5% to 20% of cells (Fig.

13.49) (508–510). Eccentrically placed, round nuclei impart a plasmacytoid look to the cells in some medullary tumors (Fig. 13.49), whereas in others, a more spindled or pleomorphic morphology predominates. The nuclear chromatin is coarsely or finely stippled, and intranuclear cytoplasmic inclusions may be seen. In the minority of aspirates, the epithelial component is accompanied by amyloid appearing as amorphous globules or irregularly shaped fragments, resembling colloid. Positive immunohistochemical staining for calcitonin is highly specific for medullary carcinoma; however, sensitivity may be as low as 55% to 60% in cytologic material (508,510,511).

Anaplastic Carcinoma

The clinical presentation of a rapidly growing, infiltrative thyroid mass in an older adult patient is an important clue to the

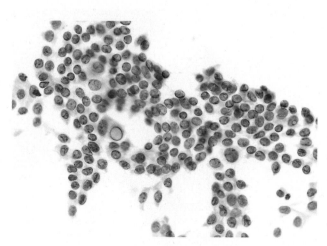

Figure 13.47. Papillary thyroid carcinoma aspirate exhibiting branched sheets, nuclear pleomorphism, and intranuclear pseudoinclusions.

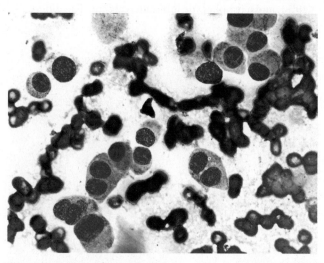

Figure 13.49. Aspirate of medullary thyroid carcinoma exhibiting uninucleated and binucleated cells with eccentrically placed nuclei (plasmacytoid appearance) and cytoplasm containing prominent granules.

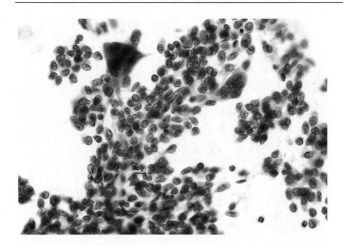

Figure 13.50. Anaplastic carcinoma aspirate demonstrating pleomorphic spindle cells appearing singly and as multinucleated osteoclast-like giant cells.

diagnosis of anaplastic carcinoma. By histology, anaplastic carcinoma of thyroid may exhibit predominantly epithelial or "sarcomatous" patterns, including fibrosarcoma-like, malignant fibrous histiocytoma–like, and osteoclastoma-like appearances, among others (Fig. 13.50). The cytologic pattern of these tumors is equally varied, but marked cellular pleomorphism and anaplasia, accompanied by a necrotic, inflammatory background, are the hallmarks (512,513).

Other Malignancies

The thyroid gland may be a primary site of lymphoma or secondarily involved by systemic disease. Most thyroid gland lymphomas are of the large-cell type and appear cytologically as a monotonous population of round cells with scant cytoplasm, finely granular chromatin, and prominent nucleoli. Background features of cytoplasmic fragmentation (lymphoglandular bodies) and karyorrhexis suggest that the abnormal cells are of lymphoid origin, but special immunophenotyping studies are used to confirm monoclonality (514,515).

Metastatic tumors to the thyroid gland make up a small proportion of thyroid malignancies (453). Over a 25-year period at the Mayo Clinic, 2.6% of thyroid malignancies were metastatic tumors from other sites (453). Kini (405) reports 22 cases out of 593 thyroid cancers (3.7%) over 9 years. In a series by Michelow and Leiman (516), a rate as high as 7.5% (21 metastatic tumors of 280 neoplastic thyroid lesions) was reported (516). Lung, kidney, breast, and malignant melanoma are reported to be the most common primary sites to metastasize to thyroid, followed by isolated cases from a wide variety of sites. Yet the majority of thyroid nodules (71%) that develop in patients with known prior malignancy are benign; thus, FNA can play a particularly important role in these patients.

Ancillary Studies

Effective criteria for the cytologic diagnosis of thyroid lesions are well established, yet areas of diagnostic uncertainty remain. This has led to a search for useful markers of thyroid malignancy that can be applied to cytologic specimens. Studies of vimentin, lectins, and different molecular-weight cytokeratins as indica-

tors of thyroid malignancy have met with only limited success, particularly in cytologic material. More promising results have been reported in studies describing the immunodetection of thyroperoxidase (TPO) (517), CD44 (518), HBME-1 (519), galectin 3, *RET* proto-oncogene (520), and *BRAF* oncogene mutations (521,522) in malignant follicular-derived lesions of thyroid. However, all these markers, except *BRAF* oncogene mutations, can also be detected in some FNA specimens from benign lesions.

Other ancillary techniques including flow cytometric measurement of ploidy and proliferation and enumeration of argyrophilic nucleolar organizing region-associated proteins have not proven to be of value in distinguishing between benign and malignant thyroid disease (523).

Sequelae of Thyroid Fine-Needle Aspiration

Ranges of tissue effects have been described in thyroid resections following FNA. In a comprehensive review of 3000 thyroidectomies, LiVolsi and Merino (524) observed post–FNA biopsy changes in 300 cases (524). Similar rates of tissue damage have been reported by others (525,526). The observed tissue alterations are grouped into acute (within 3 weeks of FNA) and chronic categories. The acute changes include hemorrhage, granulation tissue, giant cells, hemosiderin-laden macrophages, necrosis, and, rarely, infarction (Fig. 13.51). Among the chronic changes are various types of metaplasias (oncocytic, spindle cell, and squamous), linear fibrosis, infarction, pseudoinvasion of the capsule, random nuclear atypia, and papillary degeneration. Case reports have appeared in the literature of infarction or even complete disappearance of Hürthle cell nodules (375,527) following FNA. Kini's review (525) of post–FNA biopsy infarction of thyroid neoplasms reports 27 cases with partial to total infarction of the resected lesion (nine of the cases had undergone large-needle biopsies in addition to FNA). In several of these cases, careful examination was required to identify the thin rim of neoplastic tissue at the periphery of these infarcted nodules to reconcile the apparent cytohistologic discrepancies (525). These reports highlight the critical importance of providing information on prior FNA procedure and the cytologic diagnosis to the pathologist handling subsequent tissue samples of a thyroid nodule.

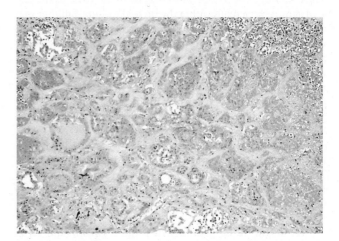

Figure 13.51. Histologic section of a resected thyroid nodule showing an area of infarction following fine-needle aspiration.

PARATHYROID PATHOLOGY

EMBRYOLOGY

The parathyroids develop from the third and fourth branchial pouches with cellular proliferation beginning in the 8- to 10-mm embryo. The thymus and parathyroid complex are derived from the third branchial pouch. These tissues migrate downward, and the parathyroids cease to migrate, remaining at the lower poles of the thyroid. The fourth branchial pouch, or the fourth and fifth pharyngeal complex, gives rise to the superior parathyroid glands and through the ultimobranchial body to the parafollicular or C cells in the lateral thyroid. The superior parathyroids in the usual state remain adjacent to the upper poles of the thyroid. Hence, although from the numbers designated for the pouches it would be expected that the superior parathyroid gland would arise from branchial pouch 3 and the lower ones from pouch 4, the reverse is true. Thus, the inferior parathyroids migrating with thymus come to rest below the parathyroids derived from branchial pouch 4 (528).

However, the migratory patterns in this area of embryology are quite variable, with numerous anatomic variations occurring in normal adults. These variations can produce difficulties in surgical explorations of the neck.

ANATOMY AND HISTOLOGY

The variation in location of the glands can present problems in exploration of the neck. Thus, in searching for abnormal parathyroid tissue in patients with hypercalcemia, there may be difficulty in locating the diseased gland(s); conversely, the surgeon who is operating in the neck for other reasons such as thyroid or laryngeal disease may inadvertently traumatize or remove parathyroid glands because of the problems with anatomic position, which can be considered normal variants (529,530).

Eighty percent or more of normal adults have four parathyroid glands. However, careful autopsy dissection studies have indicated that anywhere from 1 to 12 parathyroid glands can occur. The most common variations are three glands found in approximately 1% to 7% of studied individuals and five glands found in 3% to 6% of studied individuals (531).

The exact location of the four parathyroid glands varies. Thus, the superior parathyroids may be found close to the thyroid capsule or actually within the thyroid capsule, but they may also be located behind the pharynx or the esophagus, lateral to the larynx, or behind any part of the thyroid (greater variability is seen in the lower parathyroids). The lower glands lie usually near the lower pole of the thyroid, although they may be found in other locations in the lower neck behind the thyroid, paratracheally, or close to or within the thymus in the superior mediastinum. The glands tend to be bilaterally symmetric in location (530,531).

The parathyroid glands measure between 2 and 7 mm in length, 2 and 4 mm in width, and 0.5 and 2 mm in thickness. They are kidney bean–shaped, soft, and brown to rust in color. However, color varies with extracellular fat content, the degree of vascular congestion, and the number of oxyphils that are present (528).

The weight of the parathyroids is quite variable and varies with sex, race, and overall nutritional status of the individual. The combined weight of all parathyroid tissues is approximately

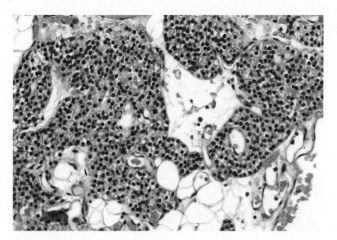

Figure 13.52. Normal parathyroid gland in a middle-aged man. Note admixture of parenchymal cells and fat.

120 mg in a normal adult male and approximately 145 mg in an adult female. Weights of individual glands range from 30 to 70 mg, with averages of approximately 35 to 55 mg (528,529,532).

Microscopic examination shows that each parathyroid gland is surrounded by a thin fibrous capsule that extends into the parenchyma as fibrous septa dividing the gland into lobules (Fig. 13.52). The parenchymal cells of the parathyroids are arranged in cords and nests around capillaries. Small clusters of cells are interspersed with foci of adipose tissue. However, there is variability in the location and interrelationships between the fat and parenchymal cells in the parathyroid gland so that biopsies from specific areas of the parathyroid may be predominantly fat, predominantly parenchyma, or a mix of these two (Figs. 13.53 and 13.54). In both normal and hyperfunctioning glands, follicles surrounding colloid-like material can be found (533). Whether this colloid-like substance is or is not related to amyloid remains controversial (533).

In the adult, the parathyroid is composed of chief and oxyphil cells; fibrous stroma, which is usually thin and delicate; and variable amounts of fat. Historically, the cell-to-fat ratio of 50:50 has been accepted as normal for adults. However, numerous

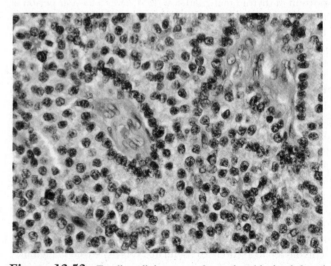

Figure 13.53. Totally cellular area of parathyroid gland found within thymus.

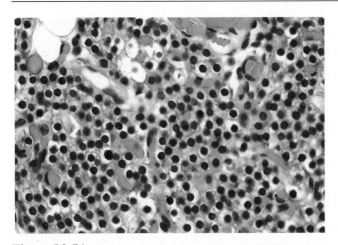

Figure 13.54. Parathyroid parenchyma; note vascularity.

studies have indicated that individuals dying without hormonal dysfunction show parathyroids in which the stromal fat is significantly less than 50% (534). It may be as little as 10%. In fact, numerous studies, including those of Dufour and colleagues and Decker and colleagues (534–536), show that a figure of approximately 17% fat is normal in an adult parathyroid gland. Cell-to-fat ratios in terms of stromal fat serve little purpose in microscopic interpretation of functional status. Densitometry measurements show that the parenchymal cell mass accounts for 74% of parathyroid weight (533).

Normal parathyroid epithelial cells include chief cells, oxyphils, and clear cells, which reflect different morphologic expressions of the same parenchymal cell. The chief cell is polyhedral in shape and poorly outlined, measures 6 to 8 nm in diameter, and contains amphophilic to slightly eosinophilic cytoplasm and a sharp, nuclear membrane. Intracellular fat is found in normal chief cells. Clear cells represent chief cells in which there is an excessive amount of glycogen in the cytoplasm (531,533).

Oxyphils that are initially found around the time of puberty and rarely in childhood apparently increase with age and may form small microscopic nodules. The oxyphil cell in the parathyroid, as in other organs, is large, measuring approximately 10 nm in diameter, and has a well-demarcated cell membrane, eosinophilic granular cytoplasm, and a pyknotic nucleus (531).

Intracellular fat content may be helpful in defining functional status. Thus, in chief cells, which make up the predominant cells in the parathyroid, intracellular fat (i.e., intracytoplasmic fat) is found in the overwhelming majority of cells in the euparathyroid state (approximately 80% of cells) (534).

Ultrastructurally, the chief cells undergo a cyclic process during synthesis and secretion of parathyroid hormones, with the hormone being synthesized on Golgi apparatus–associated membrane-bound secretory granules. These cells eventually secrete these particles of hormone into the surrounding milieu. Little lipid is present in the active parathyroid cell, which in the euparathyroid state is approximately 20% of the parenchymal cell population (533).

DISEASES OF THE PARATHYROID

Surgical pathologists dealing with the parathyroid virtually always evaluate parathyroid tissue in patients who have hypercalcemia.

Primary hyperparathyroidism is defined as the disease in which, in the absence of a known stimulus, one or more parathyroid glands secrete excess parathyroid hormone and produce hypercalcemia. Serum calcium ranges from 11 to 18 mg/dL, with most asymptomatic patients found in the lower end of the spectrum.

The prevalence of primary hyperparathyroidism is estimated as 1 to 5 cases per 1000 adults (0.1% to 0.5%). Women are affected more commonly than men. Most of these patients are asymptomatic and are diagnosed through routine screening tests for serum calcium (537,538).

The etiology of primary hyperparathyroidism is unknown; although in some families, genetics play a role (MEN syndromes) (discussed later in the chapter).

Irradiation to the head and neck has been postulated as a cause of hyperparathyroidism. Thyroid abnormalities have been seen in such cases (539,540). In a certain number of individuals with hyperparathyroidism, predominantly adenomas, a history of irradiation to the head and neck may be elicited, although the magnitude of this association is not clear. Prinz et al. (539) found that 67% of individuals in their series with combined thyroid and parathyroid tumors reported a history of irradiation.

PATHOLOGY OF THE PARATHYROID GLANDS IN PRIMARY HYPERPARATHYROIDISM

Three subgroups of pathologic lesions are found in patients with primary hyperparathyroidism: adenoma, multigland hyperplasia, double adenoma, atypical adenoma, and, rarely, carcinoma.

Parathyroid Adenoma

Parathyroid adenoma is responsible for hyperparathyroidism in 30% to 90% of cases. The wide range of variation indicates both pathologic interpretation and surgical interpretation of the disease. In fact, for practical purposes, the estimate that 75% to 80% of primary hyperparathyroidism is caused by a solitary adenoma seems correct (Fig. 13.55) (537,541).

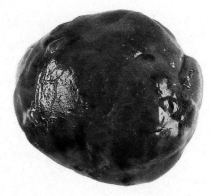

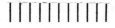

Figure 13.55. Gross parathyroid adenoma; note yellow tissue (right), which is the rim of the normal gland.

Evidence supports a clonal origin for parathyroid adenomas (542). Arnold et al. (540), using restriction fragment length polymorphism techniques, showed that nonfamilial solitary parathyroid lesions were monoclonal neoplasms.

Grossly, parathyroid adenomas tend to be located more commonly in the lower glands than in the upper glands, although one study found the reverse to be true (541). Typically, the adenoma is an oval red-brown nodule that is smooth, circumscribed, or encapsulated. The lesion, which often replaces one parathyroid gland, may show areas of hemorrhage and, if large, cystic degeneration (543–545). Occasionally in small adenomas, a grossly visible rim of normal yellow-brown parathyroid tissue may be seen (546). Weights of adenomas vary from 300 mg to several grams. The size ranges from less than 1 cm to more than 3 cm (537).

Microscopically, adenomas are usually encapsulated lesions composed of parathyroid chief cells arranged within a delicate capillary network recapitulating endocrine tumors in general (Figs. 13.54 and 13.56). Rarely, lobules and sometimes nodules may be formed. Stromal fat is usually absent. Unless very large, approximately 50% of adenomas disclose a normal rim or even atrophic parathyroid tissue outside the adenoma capsule. The cells in the rim tend to be smaller and more uniform, with stromal and cytoplasmic fat abundant in the rim but absent in the adenoma. However, the absence of a rim does not preclude the diagnosis of adenoma because large tumors may have overgrown the pre-existing normal gland or the rim may have been lost during sectioning (532,548).

In large tumors, zones of fibrosis may be found in addition to hemorrhage, cholesterol clefts, and hemosiderin, as well as occasional areas of calcification. Rarely, lymphocytes are noted within an adenoma. Thymic tissue may be found in association with an adenoma, or an adenoma may be found within the thymus (Fig. 13.53) (548,549). Follicles may be found in adenomas, causing diagnostic confusion with thyroid tissue (Figs. 13.57 and 13.58). The cells in adenoma range from bland to severely atypical (550). Most cells composing the lesion have relatively small, uniform, dark nuclei. Usually focally, bizarre multinucleated cells with dark, crinkled nuclei can be seen. These nuclei probably represent degenerative changes rather than malignant or premalignant potential (550). It has been stated that mitotic activity is never found in a parathyroid ade-

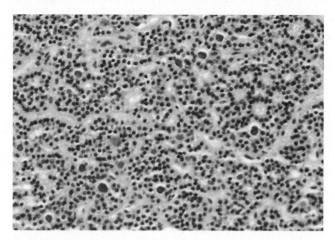

Figure 13.57. Parathyroid adenoma with formation of microfollicles; confusion with hyperplastic thyroid can occur at intraoperative evaluation.

noma and that its presence should lead one to suspect the possibility of a malignant neoplasm (551–553). This particular area, however, is fraught with difficulty and debate.

The nonadenomatous glands harbored in a patient with a parathyroid adenoma may show normal to increased cytoplasmic fat content and normal weight (554).

In approximately 10% of cases, microscopic examination of biopsies from "normal" glands shows areas of hypercellularity, so-called microscopic hyperplasia. Although this may represent a true parenchymal cell increase, the difficulty in defining normal (as noted previously) or, more likely, sampling errors probably account for this (62,555).

Oxyphilic or oncocytic adenomas do occur and can function. These tumors tend to be larger than chief cell adenomas, and the serum calcium levels tend to be minimally elevated (556,557).

Parathyroid adenomas in ectopic locations should not be unexpected in light of the embryologic development of the parathyroid glands (548,558). Thus, when hyperparathyroidism occurs in such an individual and no adenoma or abnormal glands are identified in the neck, ectopic locations that should be considered include the mediastinum with or without associated thymic tissue, behind the esophagus, or even intrathyroi-

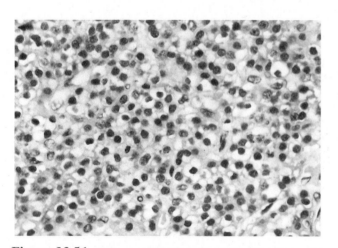

Figure 13.56. Diffuse proliferation of parathyroid cells in adenoma; note total absence of stromal fat.

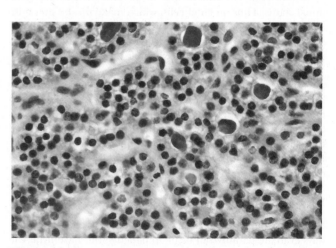

Figure 13.58. Higher-power magnification view of Figure 13.57.

dal. Sophisticated imaging techniques and scans, venous sampling, or arteriography may be helpful in locating abnormal parathyroid tissue (548,559–561). However, despite many attempts to determine the best imaging technique for localizing abnormal parathyroid tissue, the best "technique" for successful identification of abnormal parathyroid glands is an experienced surgeon (562,563).

The concept of double adenomas has lost favor in the literature (564). Many patients who have so-called double adenomas will, over a period of time, return with recurrent hyperparathyroidism and, in fact, have four-gland hyperplasia. To confirm the diagnosis of double adenoma, one must find two glands that are enlarged and histologically abnormal; the remaining glands must be normal, there should be a negative family history of parathyroid disease, and permanent cure on long-term follow-up by excision of the enlarged glands alone should be noted. Very few cases of double adenomas fulfilling these criteria are found in the literature. With the advent of intraoperative parathyroid hormone assay, cases of double adenoma can be detected at initial neck exploration (565–568). We have seen eight cases of such patients over a 10-year period at our institution.

Primary Parathyroid Hyperplasia

Primary parathyroid hyperplasia is divided into two main groups: the common group, which is chief cell hyperplasia, and the less common group, which is water clear-cell hyperplasia.

Chief cell hyperplasia accounts for 15% of hyperparathyroidism in most series, although some reports indicate that approximately half of primary hyperparathyroidism is produced by hyperplasia (531,569–572). The reasons for this probably lie in discrepancies in pathologic interpretation (531). Approximately 30% of patients with chief cell hyperplasia have familial hyperparathyroidism or one of the syndromes of MEN (573,574).

Grossly, all four glands are enlarged equally or nonequally. If unequal in size, the lower glands are usually larger. Occasionally, one gland is much larger than the others and conveys the surgical impression of an adenoma. The weight of all four glands ranges from 150 mg to more than 20 g, but usually it is in the range of 1 to 3 g (575,576).

Microscopically, one can see diffuse chief cells or nodules increase in hyperplasia, with solid masses of cells with minimal to no fat. Usually they are all chief cells with rare oxyphils. Nodular or pseudoadenomatous hyperplasia consists of circumscribed nodules of chief, transitional, or oxyphil cells; each nodule is devoid of fat, and there is little fat in the intervening stroma. Usually in hyperplasia, there is no rim of normal tissue. Bizarre nuclei are rarely found in primary hyperplasia. Mitoses, however, may occasionally be identified (531,572,577). Therapy in this disease is directed at removing all parathyroid tissue with or without autotransplantation (572,576).

Clear-cell or water clear-cell hyperplasia is very rare and is the only condition of the parathyroid in which the superior glands are larger than the lower glands (578,579). Total weights of such parathyroids always exceed 1 g and usually weigh from 5 to 10 g. The glands are irregular and show pseudopods and cysts; a distinct mahogany color is seen grossly. Histologically, the glands are composed of diffuse sheets of clear cells without any mixture of other type. No rim is present. A Swedish study

indicated that water clear-cell hyperplasia is strongly associated with blood group O (578).

Atypical Parathyroid Adenoma

Some solitary parathyroid tumors demonstrate features of carcinoma but lack infiltrative growth, vascular invasion, or metastasis at presentation. Such neoplasms have been called "atypical adenoma," indicating potential but not overt characteristics for malignant behavior. The features of concern include desmoplastic reaction, mitoses, nuclear atypia, and necrosis. Long-term follow-up studies of large series of such cases are needed to determine the risk of malignant (metastatic) potential of such tumors (580–583).

Parathyroid Carcinoma

Parathyroid carcinoma is responsible for approximately 1% to 2% of primary hyperparathyroidism. There is clinically an unusual scenario with an almost equal gender ratio, which is uncommon in parathyroid adenomas and usual hyperplasias, in which women predominate. The incidence of benign hyperparathyroidism appears to increase with age; however, patients with parathyroid carcinoma tend to be somewhat younger and are almost always symptomatic with very high levels of serum calcium. Very rarely, parathyroid carcinoma can occur in the setting of familial endocrine disease (584–592).

Clinically, patients with parathyroid carcinoma show high calcium levels of approximately 15 mg/dL. Many have polyuria, polydysplasia, nausea, vomiting, weight loss, and constipation (589). They may also have bone pain, renal stones, and other symptoms related to hypercalcemia. An important clinical clue is the presence of a palpable mass in the neck on physical examination. The mass may be clinically thought to be a thyroid nodule (553).

Parathyroid carcinomas tend to be large (average weight, 12 g) and characteristically show a histology with trabecular arrangement of tumor cells divided by thick fibrous bands and capsular and blood vessel invasion in the presence of mitotic figures (553,591,593). Because mitotic figures are virtually never found in a benign parathyroid adenoma, their presence in tumor cells should raise the suspicion of malignancy (Figs. 13.59 and 13.60). However, this has been called into question,

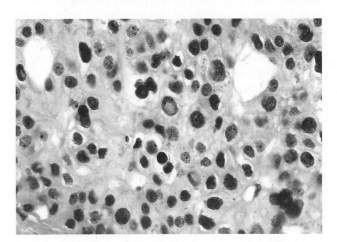

Figure 13.59. Parathyroid carcinoma. Note nuclear pleomorphism and intranuclear inclusion.

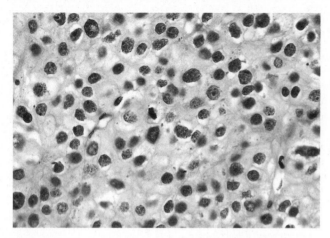

Figure 13.60. Parathyroid carcinoma; mitosis is shown in the center of the photograph.

and parathyroid tumors with mitotic activity may, in fact, be benign (594). However, long-term follow-up in the reported series is quite brief, and there is a long natural history to parathyroid carcinoma, so all of the answers are not yet available (594). Mitotic activity in secondary hyperparathyroidism is not to be equated with malignancy, and mitotic activity may occasionally be found in primary hyperparathyroidism as well (594–596).

The presence of capsular invasion is not equated with malignancy because large parathyroid adenomas may have undergone prior hemorrhage with consequent fibrosis and trapping of tumor cells within the capsule. Vascular invasion is difficult to define except if seen outside the vicinity of the neoplasm (597). An important clue to the diagnosis of parathyroid carcinoma is the surgical finding of adherence or invasion into local structures, which should raise the suspicion of a carcinoma. Metastases at the time of presentation are unusual but may be found in the regional lymph nodes. There may be local invasion into nerves, soft tissue, and the esophagus as well. Rarely, nonfunctioning parathyroid carcinomas have been described. These lesions tend to be large and composed of clear cells (598). The prognosis of parathyroid carcinoma is usually one of an indolent malignancy. Metastases may occur in up to one-third of cases and are found in regional lymph nodes, bone, lung, and liver. Many patients, however, survive for long periods of time. Multiple recurrences are known over a 15- and 20-year period. The severity of the symptoms caused by metastatic disease is directly related to tumor burden, which is related to the parathyroid hormone produced (586,587,591,597,599,600).

The development of carcinoma in the setting of four-gland hyperplasia is rare but has been reported. Similarly, rare cases of parathyroid carcinoma arising in secondary hyperparathyroidism have been reported. The hyperparathyroidism–jaw tumor (HPT-JT) syndrome is an autosomal dominant disorder characterized by the occurrence of parathyroid tumors, which may be carcinomas in approximately 15% of patients, and ossifying fibromas that usually affect the mandible and/or the maxilla (601–603). The gene causing HPT-JT, referred to as *HRPT2*, is located on chromosome 1q31.2 and consists of 17 exons that encode a 531–amino acid protein named parafibromin (604). Although the role of parafibromin in the etiology of parathyroid carcinoma is still unknown, immunohistochemical analyses have shown reduced parafibromin expression in para-

thyroid carcinomas compared with parathyroid adenomas (553,605,606). Cetani et al. (604) have shown that negative parafibromin staining is almost invariably associated with *HRPT2* mutations and confirm that loss of parafibromin staining strongly predicts parathyroid malignancy.

Multiple Endocrine Neoplasia Syndromes

The syndromes of MEN1 (Wermer syndrome) and MEN2 (Sipple syndrome) are associated with pathologic changes in parathyroids. In MEN1, pathologic changes similar to adenomatous or pseudoadenomatous chief cell hyperplasia (previously described) are found. In MEN2, the parathyroids tend to show a diffuse hyperplasia, but occasionally, one gland is involved, suggesting an "adenoma." In this syndrome, the hyperparathyroidism is found more commonly in patients with mutations in specific codons of ret oncogene and less often in families with less common ret mutations. Parathyroid abnormalities are much less common in other variants of MEN2 syndrome (573,607–612).

Familial hyperparathyroidism shows the pathologic alterations of chief cell hyperplasia similar to Wermer syndrome (613).

Unusual Lesions of the Parathyroid

PARATHYROID CYSTS. Cysts of the parathyroid glands are unusual and may present and be clinically misinterpreted as thyroid nodules. They occur more frequently in women than in men; usually are large, ranging from 1 to 6 cm; and may be located in many parathyroids, although most are found in the lower glands. Occasionally they may be found in the mediastinum, mimicking superior/anterior mediastinal masses (614).

Grossly, these cysts are almost always unilocular and smooth walled and contain water fluid with high parathyroid hormone content (615–617). Histologically, one layer of clear epithelium containing glycogen lines them. The cyst wall is fibrous with fragments of smooth muscle and nests of normal parathyroid tissue. It is unclear how these cysts arise. Microcysts are found in approximately half of normal parathyroids and might possibly enlarge by accumulation of secretion, or they fuse and produce grossly visible cysts. The cysts may arise from embryologic remnants of pharyngeal pouches in the neck undergoing cystic degeneration and entrapping portions of parathyroid tissue. Many people believe, however, that parathyroid cysts represent degenerated parathyroid adenomas, and in some cases, in fact, the cysts have been associated with hyperparathyroidism (544,618,619). However, this is uncommon, and only a few functional cysts have been reported. It may be that different parathyroid cysts have different origins, although they pathologically resemble one another.

LIPOADENOMA-HAMARTOMA OF THE PARATHYROID. These tumors present as masses that histologically are composed of parathyroid cells arranged in nests similar to normal parathyroid but are intimately associated with large areas of adipose tissue (620). The lesion may be functional or nonfunctional and usually is circumscribed but rarely encapsulated. In unusual examples, a rim of normal parathyroid tissue is present at the periphery (527,621,622). In some instances, at least one other histologically normal parathyroid was recognized. In some, there is an unusual myxomatous stroma, and other mesenchymal elements including metaplastic bone may be found. Of 17 cases so described, more than three-fourths functioned, although with relatively low levels of hypercalcemia (527, 621,622).

PARATHYROMATOSIS. Rare instances of hyperparathyroidism caused by primary hyperplasia can show nests of hyperplastic parathyroid cells in the neck outside of hyperplastic glands (623–625). In the individuals reported, these were discovered at the first neck exploration, so that spillage during prior surgery could be excluded. In each of these patients, there was no evidence of malignancy (625,626). Reddick et al. (627) postulated that during embryologic development, nests of pharyngeal tissue containing parathyroid cells might be scattered throughout the adipose tissue of the neck and mediastinum. Normally, these nests are inconspicuous. However, in the process of diffuse hyperplasia of the parathyroids, all functioning tissue may become hyperplastic and appear as separate fragments on histologic evaluation (627).

In patients who undergo neck surgery and in whom an abnormal parathyroid is disrupted, spillage of the abnormal parathyroid tissue can result in "take" in the vascular wound and lead to "secondary parathyromatosis." This condition has been most commonly reported in patients with secondary hyperparathyroidism caused by renal disease. The scattered hyperplastic hyperfunctioning parathyroid tissue can continue to produce parathyroid hormone and may clinically simulate the metabolic consequences of a parathyroid carcinoma (624).

THE INTRAOPERATIVE ASSESSMENT OF PARATHYROID

In the intraoperative assessment of parathyroid pathology, it cannot be stated strongly enough that there must be close communication between the surgeon and pathologist during surgery. The pathologist needs to be apprised of the gross findings and cannot work in a vacuum. What is recommended is as follows. The largest parathyroid gland found is resected in toto; the pathologist weighs it, measures it, and examines it histologically. If the gland shows diffuse growth of chief cells, maybe a normal-appearing rim, a lack of fat, and bizarre nuclei, a diagnosis of presumed adenoma can be rendered (628–633).

If the histology is that of hypercellularity but criteria for adenoma are not seen, biopsy of at least one more gland is needed, and in fact, in many centers, pathologists prefer to have the largest abnormal gland and at least a biopsy of one more gland. Weight ratio of parenchymal cells to fat and normal or abundant intracytoplasmic fat content in the second gland strongly support that the first one is an adenoma (632,634).

In normal parathyroid glands, 80% of the cells are in the nonsecretory phase and contain intracytoplasmic fat. The following question may be asked: Is the fat stain useful in distinguishing hyperplasia from adenoma, since all hyperfunctioning glands should be fat depleted? The advocacy of fat stains (Sudan IV, oil red O, or toluidine blue) on parathyroid tissue removed at surgery has come into vogue. The scenario is as follows. A sample of an enlarged parathyroid gland is sent for frozen section, and by H&E stain, it is hypercellular with little or no stromal fat. Thus, it represents either an adenoma or a hyperplastic gland and is not normal. A biopsy of a second parathyroid is frozen and is normocellular or minimally hypercellular. Fat

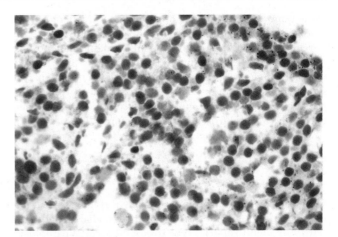

Figure 13.61. Oil red O stain on frozen section of normal parathyroid gland. Note intracellular fat.

stain shows abundant cytoplasmic fat in the latter biopsy; hence, this is a normal gland. The enlarged gland, which shows minimal to no fat, represents an adenoma. Some authors have proposed the use of rapid (30 seconds) toluidine blue stain on parathyroid frozen sections to highlight the intracellular fat. This method is faster to perform and interpret than oil red O stain (534,635–637).

Many authors have cautioned, however, that the fat stain cannot be the sole procedure on which to base a diagnosis because, although the fat stain is helpful, it is only helpful in approximately 80% of cases and must be considered as an adjunctive technique in light of gross findings, gland weight, and size; it cannot be relied upon by itself (Figs. 13.61 and 13.62) (536,635,637).

Rapid parathyroid hormone assay along with frozen section can be helpful in indicating the successful excision of abnormal parathyroid gland(s). The samples for parathyroid hormone assay are taken preoperatively from thyroid veins. The samples are procured again after the removal of the suspected abnormal parathyroid gland(s); a successful removal of the abnormal gland is accompanied by a rapid decrease in parathyroid hormone (638,639).

From our own experience, it should be stressed that the

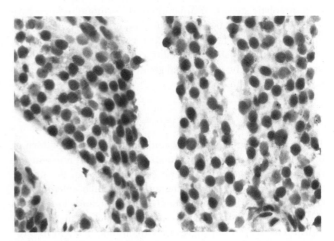

Figure 13.62. Oil red O stain of parathyroid adenoma. Note total absence of fat.

tissue removed should always be examined intraoperatively by frozen section to confirm that it is indeed a parathyroid gland. Rarely, removal of a thyroid nodule will result in a false-positive result with the rapid parathyroid hormone assay (632).

Some surgeons prefer a "biochemical frozen section"; by sending a biopsy for intraoperative parathyroid hormone assay if that is increased, they confirm that tissue is parathyroid, and excise it. No actual frozen section is required (639).

OTHER TYPES OF HYPERPARATHYROIDISM

Secondary Hyperparathyroidism

Secondary hyperparathyroidism, usually a result of renal disease, is relatively common in the age of hemodialysis and renal transplantation (640–642). The role of the surgical pathologist in the evaluation of secondary hyperparathyroidism is basically to identify parathyroid tissue at the time of intraoperative frozen section to allow for the surgeon to remove portions of this tissue for autotransplantation. Secondary hyperparathyroidism is really no different histopathologically from primary hyperparathyroidism. Mitotic activity may occasionally be found in such glands. Usually all four glands are enlarged, although one or two glands may be of very great size (643,644).

Transplanted parathyroid tissue usually takes in the majority of cases, and one can occasionally see part of this tissue removed if hyperfunction again becomes a problem. Such lesions show small nests and islands of vascularized parathyroid tissue growing in muscle or fat, usually having been implanted in the arm (645,646).

Humoral Hypercalcemia of Malignancy or Ectopic Hyperparathyroidism

This syndrome, defined as the presence of hypercalcemia in an individual with a nonparathyroid tumor without bone metastasis, is usually found in association with a malignant tumor (647). Hypercalcemia is relieved by excision of the tumor and returns with its recurrence. This paraneoplastic endocrine syndrome led several investigators to postulate that the neoplasms were producing parathyroid hormone; however, numerous studies have indicated that this is not the case (648). A variety of factors have been suggested including parathyroid hormone itself, osteoclast-activating factor, prostaglandin, vitamin D–related osteolytic sterols, and parathyroid hormone–related protein (PTHrP) (647,649,650). The last of these is more frequently identified. The humoral factors released from a variety of different tumors share the ability to resorb bone and produce hypercalcemia. The parathyroid glands in these patients appear normal or atrophic (531).

Familial Hypocalciuric Hypercalcemia

This disorder, which shows an autosomal dominant pattern of inheritance, is caused by mutations in the calcium ion–sensing receptor (*CaR*) gene located on chromosome 3q. Because of this defect, patients require higher extracellular calcium concentrations to trigger the mutated receptor and to suppress parathyroid hormone secretion (651,652). Clinically, affected individuals have nonprogressive, asymptomatic, and usually mild hypercalcemia. Pathologically, the parathyroid glands may be slightly enlarged, but histologically, they are normal (653).

PARATHYROID GLAND PROLIFERATION: SPECIAL STUDIES

Cytology

Because most parathyroid lesions are not palpable, it is unusual to directly biopsy a parathyroid tumor by FNA (654). However, on occasion, parathyroid lesions present clinically as thyroid nodules or are large enough to be clinically evident. In such cases, an FNA may sample a parathyroid proliferative lesion. The FNA features of parathyroid adenoma include cellular fragments of epithelial cells arranged around vascular cores, organoid or trabecular architecture, and microacini (655). Parathyroid chief cells contain uniform round nuclei; groups of oxyphilic cells are helpful in defining the tissue as parathyroid. If available, immunostains for parathyroid hormone may help; if the possibility of a parathyroid lesion is strongly suspected, portions of the FNA sample can be preserved appropriately for fat stain (656).

Proliferative Markers

Attempts at using immunocytochemical markers of proliferation index (M1B1 for cell cycle–associated Ki-67 antigen) for distinguishing between parathyroid adenomas and hyperplasia have met with varied success (657). Whereas statistically significant differences are found between normal (suppressed "rim") parathyroid tissue and hyperfunctioning glands, similar proliferative indices are noted between adenomas and hyperplasias (658). Loda et al. (659) identified higher numbers of labeled nuclei in adenomas than in hyperplasias by PCNA immunostaining. The labeling index of individual cases of parathyroid tumors shows so much overlap that it cannot be used to distinguish benign from malignant lesions.

Flow Cytometry

Several studies have evaluated ploidy and S phase (proliferative index) by flow cytometry to assess parathyroid proliferations. Normal glands from euparathyroid patients and from patients with adenomas are uniformly diploid. Aneuploidy or tetraploidy is found in some adenomas and some hyperplasias, whereas aneuploidy is often seen in the rare parathyroid carcinomas. Distinguishing adenoma from hyperplasia by flow cytometry is not feasible (660–662).

Molecular Biology

Modern molecular biology techniques primarily using restriction fragment length polymorphisms have shown that most (if not all) parathyroid adenomas are monoclonal proliferations (541,663). In addition, approximately 40% of primary hyperplasias and 60% of secondary hyperplasias (secondary to chronic renal disease) are clonal (664,665). Different laboratories using different probes as markers confirm these findings. The biologic meaning of these results is unclear.

The *PRAD1* oncogene has been implicated in parathyroid tumorigenesis. *PRAD1* (for *p*arathyroid *ade*noma) or *cyclin D1* results from a chromosome inversion that occurs as a dominant clonal event in some parathyroid adenomas. The inversion is created by a break in the vicinity of the parathyroid gene on the short arm of chromosome 11 (band 11p15), another break in the long arm (band 11q 13), rotation of the center piece around the axis of the centromere, and rejoining. *Cyclin D1* overexpression can be detected immunohistochemically in 18% of parathyroid adenomas and in some carcinomas (666–669).

The retinoblastoma (*Rb*) gene is a tumor suppression gene that has growth inhibitory effects in the cell cycle. Inactivation of the *Rb* gene has been associated with loss of an Rb allele by molecular analysis, and immunostaining for Rb protein may assist in the distinction between parathyroid adenomas from carcinomas (670,671). However, caution must be used in interpretation of the results because some parathyroid carcinomas do not show loss of Rb protein and a few adenomas do (669,670,672).

Studies of parathyroid neoplasms (benign and malignant) have not shown *p53* mutations in such lesions. Some studies, however, have shown significant differences between p27 protein expression in parathyroid hyperplasia, adenomas, and carcinomas, suggesting that this cell cycle protein may be useful in distinguishing between these two conditions (673,674). Hunt et al. (675) used molecular genotyping to assess for the loss of heterozygosity across a panel of known tumor suppressor genes in a tissue panel comprised of parathyroid hyperplasia, adenoma, and carcinoma. They found significantly higher loss of alleles for segments of chromosomes 1, 7, 10, and 13 in parathyroid carcinomas than in adenomas and hyperplasia. In addition, a majority of parathyroid carcinomas in this study demonstrated loss of heterozygosity at the loci of the *HRPT2*, *PTEN*, *Rb*, *HRAS*, and *p53* genes (675).

REFERENCES

1. Hoyes AD, Kershaw DR. Anatomy and development of the thyroid gland. *Ear, Nose Throat J* 1985;64:318–333.
2. Ohri AK, Ohri SK, Sing MP. Evidence for thyroid development from the fourth branchial pouch. *J Laryngol Otol* 1994;108:71–73.
3. Sugiyama S. The embryology of the human thyroid gland including ultimobranchial body and others related. *Adv Anat Embryol Cell Biol* 1970;44:6–110.
4. Mansberger AR Jr, Wei JP. Surgical embryology and anatomy of the thyroid and parathyroid glands. *Surg Clin North Am* 1993;73(4):727–746.
5. Chanin LR, Greenberg LM. Pediatric upper airway obstruction due to ectopic thyroid: classification and case reports. *Laryngoscope* 1988;98:422–427.
6. Kaplan M, Kauli R, Lubin E, et al. Ectopic thyroid gland. *J Pediatr* 1978;92:205–209.
7. Kantelip B, Lusson JR, deRiberolles C, et al. Intracardiac ectopic thyroid. *Hum Pathol* 1986;17:1293–1296.
8. Carpenter GR, Emery JL. Inclusions in the human thyroid. *J Anat* 1976;122:77–89.
9. Finkle H, Goldman F. Heterotopic cartilage in the thyroid. *Arch Pathol Lab Med* 1973;95:48–49.
10. Gardner W. Unusual relationships between thyroid gland and skeletal muscle in infants. *Cancer* 1956;6:681–691.
11. Butler J, Tulinius H, Ibanez M, et al. Significance of thyroid tissue in lymph nodes associated with carcinoma of the head, neck or lung. *Cancer* 1967;77:637–643.
12. Roth L. Inclusions of nonneoplastic thyroid tissue within cervical lymph nodes. *Cancer* 1965;18:105–111.
13. Moses D, Thompson N, Nishiyama R, et al. Ectopic thyroid tissue in the neck. *Cancer* 1976;38:361–691.
14. LiVolsi VA. *Surgical Pathology of the Thyroid.* Philadelphia, PA: W.B. Saunders, 1990.
15. Ozaki O, Ito K, Mimura TM, et al. Hemiaplasia of the thyroid associated with Graves' disease: report of three cases and a review of the literature. *Surg Today* 1994;24:164–166.
16. Hegedus L, Perrild H, Poulsen L, et al. The determination of thyroid volume by ultrasound and its relationship to body weight, age, and sex in normal subjects. *J Clin Endocrinol Metab* 1983;56:260–263.
17. Gavilan J, Gavilan C. Recurrent laryngeal nerve: identification during thyroid and parathyroid surgery. *Arch Otolaryngol Head Neck Surg* 1986;112:1286–1288.
18. O'Morchoe P, Han Y, Doyle D, et al. Lymphatic system of the thyroid gland in the rat. *Lymphology* 1987;20:10–19.
19. Brown R, Al-Moussa M, Beck J. Histometry of normal thyroid in man. *J Clin Pathol* 1986;39:475–482.
20. Reid J, Choi C, Oldroyd N. Calcium oxalate crystals in the thyroid: their identification, prevalence, origin and possible significance. *Am J Clin Pathol* 1987;87:443–454.
21. DeLellis R, Nunnemacher G, Wolfe H. C-cell hyperplasia: an ultrastructural analysis. *Lab Invest* 1978;36:237–248.
22. Gould V. Electron microscopy in human medicine. In Johannessen J, ed. *Endocrine Organs.* Volume 10. New York, NY: McGraw-Hill, 1981:29–107.
23. Hazard J. The C-cells (parafollicular cells) of the thyroid gland and medullary thyroid carcinoma. *Am J Pathol* 1977;88:214–249.
24. Hazard J. Thyroiditis: a review. *Am J Clin Pathol* 1955;25:289, 399–442.
25. Volpe R. The pathology of thyroiditis. *Hum Pathol* 1978;9:429–438.
26. LiVolsi V, LoGerfo P. *Thyroiditis.* Boca Raton, FL: CRC Press, 1981.
27. Imai C, Kakihara T, Watanabe A, et al. Acute suppurative thyroiditis as a rare complication of aggressive chemotherapy in children with acute myelogenous leukemia. *Pediatr Hematol Oncol* 2002;19:247–253.
28. Cordray JP, Nys P, Merceron RE, et al. [Frequency of hypothyroidism after De Quervain thyroiditis and contribution of ultrasonographic thyroid volume measurement]. *Ann Med Interne (Paris)* 2001;152:84–88.
29. Eylan E, Zmucky R, Sheba C. Mumps virus and subacute thyroiditis—evidence of a causal association. *Lancet* 1957;1:1062–1063.
30. Woolner L, McConahey W, Beahrs O. Granulomatous thyroiditis (deQuervain's thyroiditis). *J Clin Endocrinol Metab* 1957;17:1202–1221.
31. Lindsay S, Dailey M. Granulomatous or giant cell thyroiditis. *Surg Gynecol Obstet* 1954;98:197–212.
32. Carney J, Moore S, Northcutt R, et al. Palpation thyroiditis (multifocal granulomatous thyroiditis). *Am J Clin Pathol* 1975;64:639–647.
33. Volpe R. Thyroiditis: current views of pathogenesis. *Med Clin North Am* 1975;59:1163–1175.
34. Ban Y, Tozaki T, Tobe T, et al. The regulatory T cell gene FOXP3 and genetic susceptibility to thyroid autoimmunity: an association analysis in Caucasian and Japanese cohorts. *J Autoimmun* 2007;28:201–207.
35. Dittmar M, Kahaly GJ. Polyglandular autoimmune syndromes: immunogenetics and long-term follow-up. *J Clin Endocrinol Metab* 2003;88:2983–2992.
36. Jacobson EM, Tomer Y. The genetic basis of thyroid autoimmunity. *Thyroid* 2007;17:949–961.
37. Jacobson EM, Tomer Y. The CD40, CTLA-4, thyroglobulin, TSH receptor, and PTPN22 gene quintet and its contribution to thyroid autoimmunity: back to the future. *J Autoimmun* 2007;28:85–98.
38. Tomer Y, Menconi F, Davies TF, et al. Dissecting genetic heterogeneity in autoimmune thyroid diseases by subset analysis. *J Autoimmun* 2007;29:69–77.
39. Kurashima C, Hirokawa K. Focal lymphocytic infiltration of thyroids in elderly people. *Survey Synth Pathol Res* 1985;4:457–466.
40. Spjut H, Warren W, Ackerman L. Clinical-pathologic study of 76 cases of recurrent Graves' disease, toxic (nonexophthalmic) goiter, and nontoxic goiter. *Am J Clin Pathol* 1957;27:367–392.
41. Burman K, Baker J. Immune mechanisms in Graves' disease. *Endocr Rev* 1985;6:183–223.
42. Lindsay S, Dailey M, Friedlander J, et al. Chronic thyroiditis: a clinical and pathological study of 354 patients. *J Clin Endocrinol Metab* 1952;12:1578–1600.
43. Hayashi Y, Tamai H, Fukata S, et al. A long term clinical, immunological, and histological follow-up study of patients with goitrous chronic lymphocytic thyroiditis. *J Clin Endocrinol Metab* 1985;61:1172–1178.
44. Berho M, Suster S. Clear nuclear changes in Hashimoto's thyroiditis: a clinicopathologic study of 12 cases. *Ann Clin Lab Sci* 1995;25:513–521.
45. Kotani T, Aratake Y, Hirai K, et al. Apoptosis in thyroid tissue from patients with Hashimoto's thyroiditis. *Autoimmunity* 1995;20:231–236.
46. Iwatani Y, Amino N, Mori H, et al. T lymphocyte subsets in autoimmune thyroid diseases and subacute thyroiditis detected with monoclonal antibodies. *J Clin Endocrinol Metab* 1982;56:251–254.
47. McIntosh RS, Watson PF, Weetman AP. Analysis of the T cell receptor V alpha repertoire in Hashimoto's thyroiditis: evidence for the restricted accumulation of CD8+ T cells in the absence of CD4+ T cell restriction. *J Clin Endocrinol Metab* 1997;82:1140–1146.
48. Thieblemont C, Mayer A, Dumontet C, et al. Primary thyroid lymphoma is a heterogeneous disease. *J Clin Endocrinol Metab* 2002;87:105–111.
49. Ha CS, Shadle KM, Medeiros LJ, et al. Localized non-Hodgkin lymphoma involving the thyroid gland. *Cancer* 2001;91:629–635.
50. Kovacs C, Mant M, Nguyen G, et al. Plasma cell lesions of the thyroid: report of a case of solitary plasmacytoma and a review of the literature. *Thyroid* 1994;4:65–71.
51. Baloch ZW, Solomon AC, LiVolsi VA. Primary mucoepidermoid carcinoma and sclerosing mucoepidermoid carcinoma with eosinophilia of the thyroid gland: a report of nine cases. *Mod Pathol* 2000;13:802–807.
52. Mizukami Y, Michigishi T, Kawato, et al. Chronic thyroiditis: thyroid function and histologic correlations in 601 cases. *Hum Pathol* 1982;23:980–988.
53. Katz S, Vickery A. The fibrous variant of Hashimoto's thyroiditis. *Hum Pathol* 19474;5:161–170.
54. Mizukami Y, Michigishi T, Hashimoto T, et al. Silent thyroiditis: a histologic and immunohistochemical study. *Hum Pathol* 1988;19:423–431.
55. Mittra ES, McDougall IR. Recurrent silent thyroiditis: a report of four patients and review of the literature. *Thyroid* 2007;17:671–675.
56. Weaver D, Batsakis J, Nishiyama R. Relationship of iodine to "lymphocytic goiter." *Arch Surg* 1969;98:183–185.
57. Stenszky V, Kozma L, Balazs C, et al. The genetics of Graves' disease: HLA and disease susceptibility. *J Clin Endocrinol Metab* 1985;61:735–740.
58. Smith B, Hall R. Thyroid stimulating immunoglobulins in Graves' disease and due to autonomous goiter. *J Endocrinol Invest* 1985;8:399–497.
59. Livolsi VA, Merino MJ. Histopathologic differential diagnosis of the thyroid. *Pathol Ann* 1981;16(Pt 2):357–406.
60. Duh YC, Su IJ, Liaw KY, et al. Subpopulations of intrathyroidal lymphocytes in Graves' disease. *J Formos Med Assoc* 1990;89:121–125.
61. Chang D, Wheeler M, Woodcock J, et al. The effect of preoperative Lugol's iodine on thyroid blood flow in patients with Graves' hyperthyroidism. *Surgery* 1987;8:439–447.
62. LiVolsi VA. The pathology of autoimmune thyroid disease: a review. *Thyroid* 1994;4:333–339.

63. Mizukami Y, Michigishi T, Nonomura A, et al. Histologic changes in Graves' thyroid gland after 131I therapy for hyperthyroidism. *Acta Pathol Jpn* 1992;42:419–426.

64. Studer H, Peter H, Gerber H. Toxic nodular goiter. *J Clin Endocrinol Metab* 1985;14: 351–372.

65. Shopsin B, Shenkman L, Blum M, et al. Iodine and lithium-induced hypothyroidism. *Am J Med* 1973;55:695–699.

66. Bocchetta A, Loviselli A. Lithium and thyroid abnormalities. *Clin Pract Epidemol Ment Health* 2006;2:23.

67. Inoue M, Taketani N, Sato T, et al. High incidence of chronic lymphocytic thyroiditis in apparently healthy school children: epidemiological and clinical study. *Endocrinol Jpn* 1975;22:483–489.

68. Alves L, Rose E, Cahill T. Amiodarone and the thyroid. *Ann Intern Med* 1985;102:412.

69. Smyrk T, Goellner J, Brennan M, et al. Pathology of the thyroid in amiodarone associated thyrotoxicosis. *Am J Surg Pathol* 1987;11:197–204.

70. Atkins M, Mier J, Parkinson D, et al. Hypothyroidism after treatment with interleukin-2 and lymphokine-activated killer cells. *N Engl J Med* 1988;318:1557–1563.

71. Carcangui ML, Zampi G, Pupi A, et al. Papillary carcinoma of the thyroid: a clinicopathologic study of 241 cases treated at the University of Florence, Italy. *Cancer* 1985;55:805–828.

72. Bagnasco M, Venuti D, Paolieri F, et al. Phenotypic and functional analysis at the clonal level of infiltrating T lymphocytes in papillary carcinoma of the thyroid: prevalence of cytolytic T cells with natural killer-like or lymphokine-activated killer activity. *J Clin Endocrinol Metab* 1989;69:832–836.

73. Volpe R. The immunoregulatory disturbance in autoimmune thyroid disease. *Autoimmunity* 1988;2:55–72.

74. Woolner L, McConahey W, Beahrs O. Invasive fibrous thyroiditis (Riedel's struma). *J Clin Endocrinol Metab* 1957;17:201–220.

75. Schwaegerle S, Bauer T, Esselstyn C. Riedel's thyroiditis. *Am J Clin Pathol* 1988;90:715–722.

76. Rao C, Ferguson G, Kyle V. Retroperitoneal fibrosis associated with Riedel's struma. *Can Med Assoc J* 1973;108:1019–1021.

77. Hines R, Scheuermann H, Royster H, et al. Invasive fibrous (Riedel's) thyroiditis with bilateral fibrous parotitis. *JAMA* 1970;213:869–871.

78. Papi G, Corrado S, Cesinaro AM, et al. Riedel's thyroiditis: clinical, pathological and imaging features. *Int J Clin Pract* 2002;56:65–67.

79. Comings D, Skubi K, van Eyes J, et al. Familial multifocal fibrosclerosis. *Ann Intern Med* 1967;66:884–892.

80. Harach H, Williams E. Fibrous thyroiditis—an immunopathological study. *Histopathology* 1983;7:739–751.

81. Baloch ZW, Feldman MD, LiVolsi VA. Combined Riedel's Disease and fibrosing Hashimoto's thyroiditis: a report of three cases with two showing coexisting papillary carcinoma. *Endocr Pathol* 2000;11:157–163.

82. Baloch ZW, Saberi M, Livolsi VA. Simultaneous involvement of thyroid by Riedel's [correction of Reidel's] disease and fibrosing Hashimoto's thyroiditis: a case report. *Thyroid* 1998; 8:337–341.

83. Constine L, Donaldson S, McDougall I, et al. Thyroid dysfunction after radiotherapy in children with Hodgkin's disease. *Cancer* 1984;55:878–883.

84. Komorowski R, Hanson G. Morphologic changes in the thyroid following low-dose childhood radiation. *Arch Pathol Lab Med* 1977;101:36–39.

85. Kennedy J, Thomson J, Buchannan W. Amyloid in the thyroid. *QJ Med* 1972;43:127–143.

86. D'Antonio A, Franco R, Sparano L, et al. Amyloid goiter: the first evidence in secondary amyloidosis. Report of five cases and review of literature. *Adv Clin Path* 2000;4:99–106.

87. Goldsmith JD, Lai ML, Daniele GM, et al. Amyloid goiter: report of two cases and review of the literature. *Endocr Pract* 2000;6:318–323.

88. Marasini B, Massarotti M, Cossutta R. Thyroid function, pulmonary arterial hypertension and scleroderma. *Am J Med* 2005;118:322–323.

89. Serup J, Hangdrup H. Thyroid hormones in generalized scleroderma. A controlled study. *Acta Derm Venereol* 1986;66:35–38.

90. Alexander C, Herrara G, Jaffe K, et al. Black thyroid. Clinical manifestations, ultrastructural findings and possible mechanisms. *Hum Pathol* 1985:1672–1678.

91. Doerge DR, Divi RL, Deck J, et al. Mechanism for the anti-thyroid action of minocycline. *Chem Res Toxicol* 1997;10:49–58.

92. Gordon G, Sparano B, Kramer A, et al. Thyroid gland pigmentation and minocycline therapy. *Am J Pathol* 1984;117:98–109.

93. Sherman SI, Angelos P, Ball DW, et al. Thyroid carcinoma. *J Natl Compr Canc Netw* 2007; 5:568–621.

94. Jemal A, Siegel R, Ward E, et al. Cancer statistics, 2007. *CA Cancer J Clin* 2007;57:43–66.

95. Mazzaferi E, Young RL. Papillary thyroid carcinoma: a 10-year follow-up report of the impact of therapy in 576 patients. *Am J Med* 1981;70:511–518.

96. LiVolsi VA. Well differentiated thyroid carcinoma. *Clin Oncol (R Coll Radiol)* 1996;8: 281–288.

97. Mills S, Allen M. Congenital occult papillary carcinoma of the thyroid gland. *Hum Pathol* 1986;17:1179–1181.

98. Mazzaferri EL, Young RL. Papillary thyroid carcinoma: a 10 year follow-up report of the impact of therapy in 576 patients. *Am J Med* 1981;70:511–518.

99. Sherman SI. Thyroid carcinoma. *Lancet* 2003;361:501–511.

100. Williams E, Doniach I, Bjarnson O, et al. Thyroid cancer in an iodide rich area. *Cancer* 1977;39:215–222.

101. Harach H, Escalante D, Onativia A, et al. Thyroid carcinoma and thyroiditis in an endemic goiter region before and after iodine prophylaxis. *Acta Endocrinol (Copenh)* 1985;108:55–60.

102. Block MA, Miller MJ, Horn RC Jr. Carcinoma of the thyroid after external radiation to the neck in adults. *Am J Surg* 1969;118:764–769.

103. Nikiforov Y, Gnepp DR, Fagin JA. Thyroid lesions in children and adolescents after the Chernobyl disaster: implications for the study of radiation tumorigenesis. *J Clin Endocrinol Metab* 1996;81:9–14.

104. Nikiforov YE, Gnepp DR. Pathomorphology of thyroid gland lesions associated with radiation exposure: the Chernobyl experience and review of the literature. *Adv Anat Pathol* 1999;6:78–91.

105. Farbota L, Calandra D, Lawrence A, et al. Thyroid carcinoma in Graves' disease. *Surgery* 1985;98:1148–1152.

106. Vickery A. Thyroid papillary carcinoma. Pathological and philosophical controversies. *Am J Surg Pathol* 1983;7:797–807.

107. Tamimi DM. The association between chronic lymphocytic thyroiditis and thyroid tumors. *Int J Surg Pathol* 2002;10:141–146.

108. Kossev P, Livolsi V. Lymphoid lesions of the thyroid: review in light of the revised European-American lymphoma classification and upcoming World Health Organization classification. *Thyroid* 1999;9:1273–1280.

109. Nikiforova MN, Caudill CM, Biddinger P, et al. Prevalence of RET/PTC 5 arrangements in Hashimoto's thyroiditis and papillary thyroid carcinomas. *Int J Surg Pathol* 2002;10: 15–22.

110. Hunt JL, Baloch Z, Barnes EL, et al. Loss of heterozygosity mutations of tumor suppressor genes in cytologically atypical areas in chronic lymphocytic thyroiditis. *Endocr Pathol* 2002; 13:321–330.

111. Preston-Martin S, Jin F, Duda MJ, et al. A case-control study of thyroid cancer in women under age 55 in Shanghai (People's Republic of China). *Cancer Causes Control* 1993;4: 431–440.

112. Lee ML, Chen GG, Vlantis AC, et al. Induction of thyroid papillary carcinoma cell proliferation by estrogen is associated with an altered expression of Bcl-xL. *Cancer J* 2005;11: 113–121.

113. Cetta F, Toti P, Petracci M, et al. Thyroid carcinoma associated with familial adenomatous polyposis. *Histopathology* 1997;31:231–236.

114. Haibach H, Burman T, Carlson H. Multiple hamartoma syndrome (Cowden's disease) associated with renal cell carcinoma and primary neuroendocrine carcinoma of the skin (Merkel cell carcinoma). *Am J Clin Pathol* 1992;97:705–712.

115. Cetta F, Olschwang S, Petracci M, et al. Genetic alterations in thyroid carcinoma associated with familial adenomatous polyposis: clinical implications and suggestions for early detection. *World J Surg* 1998;22:1231–1236.

116. Cetta F, Dhamo A, Malagnino G, et al. Germ-line and somatic mutations of the APC gene and/or ss catenin gene in the occurrence of FAP associated thyroid carcinoma. *World J Surg* 2007;31:1366–1367.

117. Harach HR, Soubeyran I, Brown A, et al. Thyroid pathologic findings in patients with Cowden disease. *Ann Diagn Pathol* 1999;3:331–340.

118. Dahia PL, Marsh DJ, Zheng Z, et al. Somatic deletions and mutations in the Cowden disease gene, PTEN, in sporadic thyroid tumors. *Cancer Res* 1997;57:4710–4713.

119. Linos D, van Heerden J, Edis A. Primary hyperparathyroidism and nonmedullary thyroid cancer. *Am J Surg* 1982;143:301–303.

120. LiVolsi V, Feind C. Parathyroid adenoma and nonmedullary thyroid carcinoma. *Cancer* 1976;38:1391–1393.

121. Vickery A, Carcangiu M, Johannessen J, et al. Papillary carcinoma. *Semin Diagn Pathol* 1985;2:90–100.

122. Carcangiu M, Zampi G, Pupi A, et al. Papillary carcinoma of the thyroid. A clinicopathologic study of 244 cases treated at the University of Florence, Italy. *Cancer* 1985;55:805–828.

123. Carcangiu M, Zampi G, Rosai J. Papillary thyroid carcinoma. A study of its many morphologic expressions and clinical correlates. *Pathol Annu* 1985;20(Pt 1):1–44.

124. Volante M, Collini P, Nikiforov YE, et al. Poorly differentiated thyroid carcinoma: the Turin proposal for the use of uniform diagnostic criteria and an algorithmic diagnostic approach. *Am J Surg Pathol* 2007;31:1256–1264.

125. Klinck G, Winship T. Psammoma bodies and thyroid cancer. *Cancer* 1959;12:656–662.

126. Johannessen J, Sobrinho-Simoes M. The origin and significance of thyroid psammoma bodies. *Lab Invest* 1980;43:287–296.

127. Hunt JL, Barnes EL. Non-tumor-associated psammoma bodies in the thyroid. *Am J Clin Pathol* 2003;119:90–94.

128. Hapke M, Dehner L. The optically clear nucleus: a reliable sign of papillary carcinoma of the thyroid? *Am J Surg Pathol* 1979;3:31–38.

129. Francis IM, Das DK, Sheikh ZA, et al. Role of nuclear grooves in the diagnosis of papillary thyroid carcinoma. A quantitative assessment on fine needle aspiration smears. *Acta Cytol* 1995;39:409–415.

130. Shurbaji MS, Gupta PK, Frost JK. Nuclear grooves: a useful criterion in the cytopathologic diagnosis of papillary thyroid carcinoma. *Diagn Cytopathol* 1988;4:91–94.

131. LiVolsi VA. Papillary neoplasms of the thyroid. Pathologic and prognostic features. *Am J Clin Pathol* 1992;97:426–434.

132. LiVolsi VA, Merino MJ. Squamous cells in the human thyroid gland. *Am J Surg Pathol* 1978;2:133–140.

133. Vickery AL Jr, Carcangiu ML, Johannessen JV, et al. Papillary carcinoma. *Semin Diagn Pathol* 1985;2:90–100.

134. Mancini A, Rabitti C, Conte G, et al. [Lymphocytic infiltration in thyroid neoplasms. Preliminary prognostic assessments]. *Minerva Chir* 1993;48:1283–1288.

135. de los Santos ET, Keyhani-Rofagha S, Cunningham JJ, et al. Cystic thyroid nodules. The dilemma of malignant lesions. *Arch Intern Med* 1990;150:1422–1427.

136. Sugg SL, Ezzat S, Rosen IB, et al. Distinct multiple RET/PTC gene rearrangements in multifocal papillary thyroid neoplasia. *J Clin Endocrinol Metab* 1998;83:4116–4122.

137. Hunt JL, LiVolsi VA, Baloch ZW, et al. Microscopic papillary thyroid carcinoma compared with clinical carcinomas by loss of heterozygosity mutational profile. *Am J Surg Pathol* 2003; 27:159–166.

138. Crile G, Antunez A, Esselstyn C, et al. The advantages of subtotal thyroidectomy and suppression of TSH in the primary treatment of papillary carinoma of the thyroid. *Cancer* 1985;55:2691–2697.

139. Clark O. Total thyroidectomy: the treatment of choice for patients with differentiated thyroid cancer. *Ann Surg* 1982;196:361–370.

140. Cody H, Shah J. Locally invasive, well differentiated thyroid cancer: 22 years' experience at Memorial Sloan-Kettering Cancer Center. *Am J Surg* 1981;142:480–483.
141. Falvo L, Catania A, D'Andrea V, et al. Prognostic importance of histologic vascular invasion in papillary thyroid carcinoma. *Ann Surg* 2005;241:640–646.
142. Hay I. Nodal metastases from papillary thyroid carcinoma. *Lancet* 1986;2:1283–1284.
143. Mazzaferri E, Young R, Oertel J, et al. Papillary thyroid carcinoma: the impact of therapy in 576 patients. *Medicine (Baltimore)* 1980;56:171–196.
144. Maceri D, Babyak J, Ossakow S. Lateral neck mass: sole presenting sign of metastatic thyroid cancer. *Arch Otolaryngol Head Neck Surg* 1986;112:47–49.
145. Venkatesh YS, Ordonez NG, Schultz PN, et al. Anaplastic carcinoma of the thyroid. A clinicopathologic study of 121 cases. *Cancer* 1990;66:321–330.
146. Ruegemer J, Hay I, Bergstrilh E, et al. Distant metastases in differentiated thyroid carcinoma: a multivariate analysis of prognostic variables. *J Clin Endocrinol Metab* 1988;67: 501–508.
147. Kaneko C, Shamoto M, Niimi H, et al. Studies on intranuclear inclusions and nuclear grooves in papillary thyroid cancer by light, scanning electron and transmission electron microscopy. *Acta Cytol* 1996;40:417–422.
148. Cheung CC, Ezzat S, Freeman JL, et al. Immunohistochemical diagnosis of papillary thyroid carcinoma. *Mod Pathol* 2001;14:338–342.
149. Papotti M, Rodriguez J, Pompa RD, et al. Galectin-3 and HBME-1 expression in well-differentiated thyroid tumors with follicular architecture of uncertain malignant potential. *Mod Pathol* 2004;18:541–546.
150. Barroeta JE, Baloch ZW, Lal P, et al. Diagnostic value of differential expression of CK19, galectin-3, HBME-1, ERK, RET, and p16 in benign and malignant follicular-derived lesions of the thyroid: an immunohistochemical tissue microarray analysis. *Endocr Pathol* 2006;17: 225–234.
151. Mai KT, Ford JC, Yazdi HM, Perkins DG, Commons AS. Immunohistochemical study of papillary thyroid carcinoma and possible papillary thyroid carcinoma-related benign thyroid nodules. *Pathol Res Pract* 2000;196:533–540.
152. Miettinen M, Karkkainen P. Differential reactivity of HBME-1 and CD15 antibodies in benign and malignant thyroid tumours. Preferential reactivity with malignant tumours. *Virchows Arch* 1996;429:213–219.
153. Willgeroth C, Floegel R, Rosler B. [The importance of S-100 protein positive Langerhans cells and Leu-M1 positive tumor cells for prognosis of papillary thyroid cancer]. *Zentralbl Chir* 1992;117:603–606.
154. Joensuu H, Klemi P, Eerola E. DNA aneuploidy in follicular adenomas of the thyroid gland. *Am J Pathol* 1987;124:373–376.
155. Onaran Y, Tezelman S, Gurel N, et al. The value of DNA content in predicting the prognosis of thyroid carcinoma in an endemic iodine deficiency region. *Acta Chirurgica Belgica* 1999;99:30–35.
156. Fusco A, Santoro M, Grieco M, et al. RET/PTC activation in human thyroid carcinomas. *J Endocrinol Invest* 1995;18:127–129.
157. Sheils OM, O'Leary JJ, Sweeney EC. Assessment of ret/PTC-1 rearrangements in neoplastic thyroid tissue using TaqMan RT-PCR. *J Pathol* 2000;192:32–36.
158. Basolo F, Giannini R, Monaco C, et al. Potent mitogenicity of the RET/PTC3 oncogene correlates with its prevalence in tall-cell variant of papillary thyroid carcinoma. *Am J Pathol* 2002;160:247–254.
159. Giordano TJ, Kuick R, Thomas DG, et al. Molecular classification of papillary thyroid carcinoma: distinct BRAF, RAS, and RET/PTC mutation-specific gene expression profiles discovered by DNA microarray analysis. *Oncogene* 2005;24:6646–6656.
160. Ciampi R, Nikiforov YE. RET/PTC rearrangements and BRAF mutations in thyroid tumorigenesis. *Endocrinology* 2007;148:936–941.
161. Jhiang SM, Sagartz JE, Tong Q, et al. Targeted expression of the ret/PTC1 oncogene induces papillary thyroid carcinomas. *Endocrinology* 1996;137:375–378.
162. Fischer AH, Bond JA, Taysavang P, et al. Papillary thyroid carcinoma oncogene (RET/PTC) alters the nuclear envelope and chromatin structure. *Am J Pathol* 1998;153: 1443–1450.
163. Zou M, Shi Y, Farid NR. Low rate of ret proto-oncogene activation (PTC/retTPC) in papillary thyroid carcinomas from Saudi Arabia. *Cancer* 1994;73:176–180.
164. Motomura T, Nikiforov YE, Namba H, et al. RET rearrangements in Japanese pediatric and adult papillary thyroid cancers. *Thyroid* 1998;8:485–489.
165. Nikiforov YE. RET/PTC rearrangement in thyroid tumors. *Endocr Pathol* 2002;13:3–16.
166. Nikiforov YE, Koshoffer A, Nikiforova M, et al. Chromosomal breakpoint positions suggest a direct role for radiation in inducing illegitimate recombination between the ELE1 and RET genes in radiation-induced thyroid carcinomas. *Oncogene* 1999;18:6330–6334.
167. Thomas GA, Bunnell H, Cook HA, et al. High prevalence of RET/PTC rearrangements in Ukrainian and Belarussian post-Chernobyl thyroid papillary carcinomas: a strong correlation between RET/PTC3 and the solid-follicular variant. *J Clin Endocrinol Metab* 1999; 84:4232–42328.
168. Wirtschafter A, Schmidt R, Rosen D, et al. Expression of the RET/PTC fusion gene as a marker for papillary carcinoma in Hashimoto's thyroiditis. *Laryngoscope* 1997;107:95–100.
169. Sheils O, Smyth P, Finn S, et al. RET/PTC rearrangements in Hashimoto's thyroiditis. *Int J Surg Pathol* 2002;10:167–168; discussion 168–169.
170. Elisei R, Romei C, Vorontsova T, et al. RET/PTC rearrangements in thyroid nodules: studies in irradiated and not irradiated, malignant and benign thyroid lesions in children and adults. *J Clin Endocrinol Metab* 2001;86:3211–3216.
171. Di Pasquale M, Rothstein JL, Palazzo JP. Pathologic features of Hashimoto's-associated papillary thyroid carcinomas. *Hum Pathol* 2001;32(1):24–30.
172. Cohen Y, Xing M, Mambo E, et al. BRAF mutation in papillary thyroid carcinoma. *J Natl Cancer Inst* 2003;95:625–627.
173. Fukushima T, Suzuki S, Mashiko M, et al. BRAF mutations in papillary carcinomas of the thyroid. *Oncogene* 2003;22:6455–6457.
174. Xu X, Quiros RM, Gattuso P, et al. High prevalence of BRAF gene mutation in papillary thyroid carcinomas and thyroid tumor cell lines. *Cancer Res* 2003;63:4561–4567.
175. Melillo RM, Castellone MD, Guarino V, et al. The RET/PTC-RAS-BRAF linear signaling cascade mediates the motile and mitogenic phenotype of thyroid cancer cells. *J Clin Invest* 2005;115:1068–1081.
176. Simpson W, McKinney S, Carruthers J, et al. Papillary and follicular thyroid cancer: prognostic factors in 1578 patients. *Am J Med* 1987;83:479–488.
177. Moreno-Egea A, Rodriguez-Gonzales J, Sola-Perez J, et al. Multivariate analysis of histopathological features as prognostic factors in patients with papillary thyroid carcinoma. *Br J Surg* 1995;82:1092.
178. Greene FL. Cancer staging, prognostic factors, and our surgical challenges. *Am Surg* 2005; 71:615–620.
179. Shaha AR. TNM classification of thyroid carcinoma. *World J Surg* 2007;31:879–887.
180. Kjellman P, Learoyd DL, Messina M, et al. Expression of the RET proto-oncogene in papillary thyroid carcinoma and its correlation with clinical outcome. *Br J Surg* 2001;88: 557–563.
181. Basolo F, Molinaro E, Agate L, et al. RET protein expression has no prognostic impact on the long-term outcome of papillary thyroid carcinoma. *Eur J Endocrinol* 2001;145:599–604.
182. Monaco F, Finn SP, Smyth P, et al. Classification of thyroid diseases: suggestions for a revision. *J Clin Endocrinol Metab* 2003;88:1428–1432.
183. Cetta F, Gori M, Raffaelli N, et al. Comment on clinical and prognostic relevance of Ret-PTC activation in patients with papillary thyroid carcinoma. *J Clin Endocrinol Metab* 1999; 84:2257–2258.
184. Xing M, Westra WH, Tufano RP, et al. BRAF mutation predicts a poorer clinical prognosis for papillary thyroid cancer. *J Clin Endocrinol Metab* 2005;90:6373–6379.
185. Saltman B, Singh B, Hedvat CV, et al. Patterns of expression of cell cycle/apoptosis genes along the spectrum of thyroid carcinoma progression. *Surgery* 2006;140:899–905; discussion 905–906.
186. Tallini G, Garcia-Rostan G, Herrero A, et al. Downregulation of p27KIP1 and Ki67/Mib1 labeling index support the classification of thyroid carcinoma into prognostically relevant categories. *Am J Surg Pathol* 1999;23:678–685.
187. Metaye T, Millet C, Kraimps JL, et al. Estrogen receptors and cathepsin D in human thyroid tissue. *Cancer* 1993;72:1991–1996.
188. DeLellis RA, Lloyd RD, Heitz PU, et al., eds. *WHO: Pathology and Genetics. Tumours of Endocrine Organs.* Lyon, France: IARC Press, 2004.
189. Arem R PS, Saliby AH, Sherman SI. Thyroid microcarcinoma: prevalence, prognosis, and management. *Endocr Pract* 1999;5:148–156.
190. Harach HR, Franssila KO. Occult papillary carcinoma of the thyroid appearing as lung metastasis. *Arch Pathol Lab Med* 1984;108:529–530.
191. Falvo L, D'Ercole C, Sorrenti S, et al. Papillary microcarcinoma of the thyroid gland: analysis of prognostic factors including histological subtype. *Eur J Surg Suppl* 2003;588: 28–32.
192. Harach HR, Saravia Day E, Zusman SB. Occult papillary microcarcinoma of the thyroid—a potential pitfall of fine needle aspiration cytology. *J Clin Pathol* 1991;44:205–207.
193. Braga M, Graf H, Ogata A, et al. Aggressive behavior of papillary microcarcinoma in a patient with Graves' disease initially presenting as cystic neck mass. *J Endocrinol Invest* 2002; 25:250–253.
194. Lin KD, Lin JD, Huang HS, et al. Skull metastasis with brain invasion from thyroid papillary microcarcinoma. *J Formos Med Assoc* 1997;96:280–282.
195. Baloch ZW, LiVolsi VA. Microcarcinoma of the thyroid. *Adv Anat Pathol* 2006;13:69–75.
196. Lupoli G, Vitale G, Caraglia M, et al. Familial papillary thyroid microcarcinoma: a new clinical entity. *Lancet* 1999;353:637–639.
197. Rosai J, LiVolsi VA, Sobrinho-Simoes M, et al. Renaming papillary microcarcinoma of the thyroid gland: the Porto proposal. *Int J Surg Pathol* 2003;11:249–251.
198. Chen KTC, Rosai J. Follicular variant of thyroid papillary carcinoma: a clinicopathologic study of six cases. *Am J Surg Pathol* 1977;1:123–130.
199. Tielens ET, Sherman SI, Hruban RH, et al. Follicular variant of papillary thyroid carcinoma. A clinicopathologic study. *Cancer* 1994;73:424–431.
200. Sobrinho-Simoes M, Soares J, Carneiro F, et al. Diffuse follicular variant of papillary carcinoma of the thyroid: report of eight cases of a distinct aggressive type of thyroid tumor. *Surg Pathol* 1990;3:189.
201. Baloch ZW, Livolsi VA. Follicular-patterned lesions of the thyroid: the bane of the pathologist. *Am J Clin Pathol* 2002;117:143–150.
202. Liu J, Singh B, Tallini G, et al. Follicular variant of papillary thyroid carcinoma: a clinicopathologic study of a problematic entity. *Cancer* 2006;107:1255–1264.
203. Williams ED, Abrosimov A, Bogdanova TI, et al. Two proposals regarding the terminology of thyroid tumors. *Int J Surg Pathol* 2000;8:181–183.
204. Baloch ZW, LiVolsi VA. Encapsulated follicular variant of papillary thyroid carcinoma with bone metastases. *Mod Pathol* 2000;13:861–865.
205. Hawk W, Hazard J. The many appearances of papillary carcinoma of the thyroid. *Cleveland Clin Q* 1976;43:207–216.
206. Terry J, St John S, Karkowski F, et al. Tall cell papillary thyroid cancer: incidence and prognosis. *Am J Surg* 1994;168:459–461.
207. Sobrinho-Simoes M, Sambade C, Nesland JM, et al. Tall cell papillary carcinoma. *Am J Surg Pathol* 1989;13:79–80.
208. Rosai J, Carcangui ML, DeLellis RA. In *Tumors of the Thyroid Gland.* Rosai J, Sobin LE, eds. Washington, DC: Armed Forces Institute of Pathology, 1992.
209. Johnson TH, Lloyd RV, Thompson NW, et al. prognostic implications of the tall cell variant of papillary carcinoma. *Am J Surg Pathol* 1988;12:22–27.
210. Flint A, Davenport R, Llyod R. The tall cell variant of papillary carcinoma of the thyroid gland. Comparison with the common form of papillary carcinoma by DNA and morphometric analysis. *Arch Pathol Lab Med* 1991;115:169–171.
211. Ghossein RA, Leboeuf R, Patel KN, et al. Tall cell variant of papillary thyroid carcinoma without extrathyroid extension: biologic behavior and clinical implications. *Thyroid* 2007; 17:655–661.
212. Evans H. Columnar cell carcinoma of the thyroid: a report of two cases of an aggressive variant of thyroid carcinoma. *Am J Clin Pathol* 1986;85:77–80.

213. Evans H. Encapsulated columnar cell neoplasms of the thyroid: a report of four cases suggesting a favorable prognosis. *Am J Surg Pathol* 1996;20:1205–1211.

214. Sobrinho-Simoes M, Nesland JM, Johannessen JV. Columnar-cell carcinoma. Another variant of poorly differentiated carcinoma of the thyroid. *Am J Clin Pathol* 1988;89:264–267.

215. Evans H. Encapsulated papillary neoplasms of the thyroid: a study of 14 cases followed for a minimum of 10 years. *Am J Surg Pathol* 1987;11:592–597.

216. Apel RL, Asa SL, LiVolsi VA. Papillary Hurthle cell carcinoma with lymphocytic stroma. "Warthin-like tumor" of the thyroid. *Am J Surg Pathol* 1995;19:810–814.

217. Baloch ZW, LiVolsi VA. Warthin-like papillary carcinoma of the thyroid. *Arch Pathol Lab Med* 2000;124:1192–1195.

218. Chan JKC, Tsui MS, Tse CH. Diffuse sclerosing variant of papillary thyroid carcinoma. A histological and immunohistochemical study of three cases. *Histopathology* 1987;11: 191–201.

219. Soares J, Limbert E, Sobrinho-Simoes M. Diffuse sclerosing variant of papillary thyroid carcinoma. A clinicopathologic study of 10 cases. *Pathol Res Pract* 1989;185:200–206.

220. Nikiforov YE, Rowland JM, Bove KE, et al. Distinct pattern of ret oncogene rearrangements in morphological variants of radiation-induced and sporadic thyroid papillary carcinomas in children. *Cancer Res* 1997;57:1690–1694.

221. Peters S, Chatten J, LiVolsi V. Pediatric papillary thyroid carcinoma. *Mod Pathol* 1994;7: 55.

222. Furmanchuk A, Averkin J, Egloff B, et al. Pathomorphological findings in thyroid cancers of children from the republic of Belarus: a study of 86 cases occurring between 1986 (post Chernobyl) and 1991. *Histopathology* 1992;21:401–408.

223. Harach HR, Williams ED. Childhood thyroid cancer in England and Wales. *Br J Cancer* 1995;72:777–783.

224. Schroder S, Bocker W, Dralle H, et al. The encapsulated papillary carcinoma of the thyroid: a morphologic subtype of the papillary thyroid carcinoma. *Cancer* 1984;54:90–93.

225. Beckner M, Heffess C, Oertel J. Oxyphilic papillary thyroid carcinomas. *Am J Clin Pathol* 1995;103:280–287.

226. Bisi H, Longatto FA, Asat de Camargo R, et al. Thyroid papillary carcinoma lipomatous type: report of two cases. *Pathologica* 1993;85:761.

227. Chan JKC, Rosai J. Papillary carcinoma of the thyroid with exuberant fasciitis like stroma: report of three cases. *Am J Clin Pathol* 1991;95:309–314.

228. Ostrowski M, Moffat F, Asa S, et al. Myxomatous change in papillary carcinoma of the thyroid. *Surg Pathol* 1989;2:249.

229. Murray D. In *The Thyroid Gland.* Kovacs KA, ed. Malden, MA: Blackwell Science, 1998: 295–380.

230. Khurana KK, Baloch ZW, LiVolsi VA. Aspiration cytology of pediatric solitary papillary hyperplastic thyroid nodule. *Arch Pathol Lab Med* 2001;125:1575–1578.

231. Casey MB, Lohse CM, Lloyd RV. Distinction between papillary thyroid hyperplasia and papillary thyroid carcinoma by immunohistochemical staining for cytokeratin 19, galectin-3, and HBME-1. *Endocr Pathol* 2003;14:55–60.

232. Lever E, Medeiros-Neto G, DeGroot L. Inherited disorders of thyroid metabolism. *Endocr Rev* 1983;4:213–239.

233. Rosenthal D, Carvalho-Guimaraes DP, Knobel M, et al. Dyshormonogenetic goiter: presence of an inhibitor of normal human thyroid peroxidase. *J Endocrinol Invest* 1990;13: 901–904.

234. Medeiros-Neto G, Bunduki V, Tomimori E, et al. Prenatal diagnosis and treatment of dyshormonogenetic fetal goiter due to defective thyroglobulin synthesis. *J Clin Endocrinol Metab* 1997;82:4239–4242.

235. Kennedy J. The pathology of dyshormonogenetic goitre. *J Pathol* 1969;99:251–264.

236. Ghossein RA, Rosai J, Heffess C. Dyshormonogenetic goiter: a clinicopathologic study of 56 cases. *Endocr Pathol* 1997;8:283–292.

237. Kavishwar VS, Phatak AM. Dyshormonogenetic goitre with clear cell change resembling parathyroid adenoma—a case report. *Indian J Pathol Microbiol* 1998;41:469–471.

238. Hamburger J. The autonomously functioning thyroid nodule; Goetsch's disease. *Endocr Rev* 1987;8:439–447.

239. Johnson J. Adenomatous goiters with and without hyperthyroidism. *Arch Surg* 1949;59: 1088–1099.

240. Hamburger J. The autonomously functioning thyroid adenoma. *N Engl J Med* 1983;309: 1312–1313.

241. Hamilton C, Maloof F. Unusual types of hyperthyroidism. *Medicine (Baltimore)* 1973;52: 195–214.

242. Anderson N, Lokich J, McDermott W, et al. Gestational choriocarcinoma and thyrotoxicosis. *Cancer* 1979;44:304–306.

243. Dunzendorfer T, deLas Morenas A, Kalir T, et al. Struma ovarii and hyperthyroidism. *Thyroid* 1999;9:499–502.

244. Zellman H. Iatrogenic and factitious thyroidal disease. *Med Clin North Am* 1979;63: 329–892.

245. Taniyama M, Ishikawa N, Momotani N, et al. Toxic multinodular goitre in a patient with generalized resistance to thyroid hormone who harbours the R429Q mutation in the thyroid hormone receptor beta gene. *Clin Endocrinol (Oxf)* 2001;54:121–124.

246. Al-Moussa M, Berk J. Histometry of thyroids containing few and multiple modules. *J Clin Pathol* 1986;39:483–488.

247. Maloof F, Wang CA, Vickery AL Jr. Nontoxic goiter-diffuse or nodular. *Med Clin North Am* 1975;59:1221–1232.

248. Kraiem Z, Glaser B, Yigla M, et al. Toxic multinodular goiter: a variant of autoimmune hyperthyroidism. *J Clin Endocrinol Metab* 1987;65:659–664.

249. Struder H, Peter H, Gerber H. Morphologic and functional changes in developing goiters. In Hall R, Kobberling J, eds. *Thyroid Disorders Associated with Iodine Deficiency and Excess.* New York, NY: Raven Press, 1987:229–241.

250. Struder H, Ramelli F. Simple goiter and its variants: euthyroid and hyperthyroid. *Endocr Rev* 1982;3:40–61.

251. Hicks D, LiVolsi V, Neidich J, et al. Solitary follicular nodules of the thyroid are clonal proliferations. *Lab Invest* 1989;60:40A.

252. Namba H, Fagin J. Clonal origin of human thyroid tumors; determination by X-chromosome inactivation analysis. *Clin Res* 1989;37:108A.

253. Meissner W, Warren S. *Tumors of the Thyroid Gland.* Washington, DC: Armed Forces Institute of Pathology, 1969.

254. Carney JA, Ryan J, Goellner JR. Hyalinizing trabecular adenoma of the thyroid gland. *Am J Surg Pathol* 1987;11:583–591.

255. de Matos PS, Ferreira AP, de Oliveira Facuri F, et al. Usefulness of HBME-1, cytokeratin 19 and galectin-3 immunostaining in the diagnosis of thyroid malignancy. *Histopathology* 2005;47:391–401.

256. Fonseca E, Nesland J, Sobrinho-Simoes M. Expression of stratified epithelial type cytokeratins in hyalinizing trabecular adenoma supports their relationship with papillary carcinoma of the thyroid. *Histopathology* 1997;31:330–335.

257. Cheung CC, Boerner SL, MacMillan CM, et al. Hyalinizing trabecular tumor of the thyroid: a variant of papillary carcinoma proved by molecular genetics. *Am J Surg Pathol* 2000;24: 1622–1626.

258. Papotti M, Volante M, Giuliano A, et al. RET/PTC activation in hyalinizing trabecular tumors of the thyroid. *Am J Surg Pathol* 2000;24:1615–1621.

259. Nakamura N, Carney JA, Jin L, et al. RASSF1A and NORE1A methylation and BRAFV600E mutations in thyroid tumors. *Lab Invest* 2005;85:1065–1075.

260. Hazard JB, Kenyon R. Atypical adenoma of the thyroid. *Arch Pathol* 1954;58:554–563.

261. Franssila K, Ackerman L, Brown C, et al. Follicular carcinoma. *Semin Diagn Pathol* 1985; 2:101–122.

262. Thompson LD, Wieneke JA, Paal E, et al. A clinicopathologic study of minimally invasive follicular carcinoma of the thyroid gland with a review of the English literature. *Cancer* 2001;91:505–524.

263. LiVolsi V, Asa S. The demise of follicular carcinoma of the thyroid gland. *Thyroid* 1994; 4:233–236.

264. Baloch Z, LiVolsi VA. In *Pathology of the Thyroid Gland.* Livolsi VA, Asa S, eds. Philadelphia, PA: Churchill Livingston, 2002:61–88.

265. Harach HR, Jasani B, Williams ED. Factor VIII as a marker of endothelial cells in follicular carcinoma of the thyroid. *J Clin Pathol* 1977;36:1050–1054.

266. Evans HL. Follicular neoplasms of the thyroid. A study of 44 cases followed for a minimum of 10 years with emphasis on differential diagnosis. *Cancer* 1984;54:535–540.

267. Clark OH, Fredrickson JM, Harvey HK. Thyroid mass. *Head Neck* 1993;15:574–579.

268. Schmidt R, Wang C. Encapsulated follicular carcinoma of the thyroid: diagnosis, treatment and results. *Surgery* 1986;100:1068–1076.

269. Perros P. Recombinant human thyroid-stimulating hormone (rhTSH) in the radioablation of well-differentiated thyroid cancer: preliminary therapeutic experience. *J Endocrinol Invest* 1999;22:30–34.

270. Mazzaferri EL. Treating differentiated thyroid carcinoma: where do we draw the line? *Mayo Clin Proc* 1991;66:105–111.

271. Lang W, Choritz H, Hundeshagen H. Risk factors in follicular thyroid carcinomas. A retrospective follow-up study covering a 14 year period with emphasis on morphological findings. *Am J Surg Pathol* 1986;10:246–255.

272. Cady B, Sedgwick CE, Meissner WA, et al. Changing clinical, pathologic, therapeutic and survival patterns in differentiated thyroid carcinoma. *Ann Surg* 1976;184:541–553.

273. Hruban R, Huvos A, Traganos F, et al. Follicular neoplasms of the thyroid in men older than 50 years of age. A DNA flow cytometric study. *Am J Clin Pathol* 1990;94:527–532.

274. Shaha A, Loree T, Shah JP. Prognostic factors and risk group analysis in follicular carcinoma of the thyroid. *Surgery* 1995;18:1131–1138.

275. Dumitriu L, Stefaneanu L, Tasca C. The anaplastic transformation of differentiated thyroid carcinoma. An ultrastructural study. *Endocrinologie* 1984;22:91–96.

276. Camargo R, Limbert E, Gillam M, et al. Aggressive metastatic follicular thyroid carcinoma with anaplastic transformation arising from a long-standing goiter in a patient with Pendred's syndrome. *Thyroid* 2001;11:981–988.

277. Woolner L. Thyroid carcinoma: pathologic classification with data on prognosis. *Semin Nucl Med* 1971;1:481–502.

278. Baloch ZW, Fleisher S, LiVolsi VA, et al. Diagnosis of "follicular neoplasm": a gray zone in thyroid fine-needle aspiration cytology. *Diagn Cytopathol* 2002;26:41–44.

279. Paphavasit A, Thompson GB, Hay ID, et al. Follicular and Hurthle cell thyroid neoplasms. Is frozen-section evaluation worthwhile? *Arch Surg* 1997;132:674–678; discussion 678–680.

280. Baloch ZW, LiVolsi VA. Intraoperative assessment of thyroid and parathyroid lesions. *Semin Diagn Pathol* 2002;19:219–226.

281. Kahn NF, Perzin KH. Follicular carcinoma of the thyroid: an evaluation of the histologic criteria used for diagnosis. *Pathol Ann* 1983;18(Pt 1):221–253.

282. Lang W, Georgii G. Minimal invasive cancer in the thyroid. *Clin Oncol* 1982;1:527–537.

283. Franssila KO, Ackerman LV, Brown CL, et al. Follicular carcinoma. *Semin Diagn Pathol* 1985;2:101–122.

284. Lida T. The fate and surgical significance of adenoma of the thyroid gland. *Surg Gynecol Obstet* 1974;136:536–540.

285. Evans H. Follicular neoplasms of the thyroid. *Cancer* 1984;54:535–540.

286. Cady B, Sedgwick C, Meissner W, et al. Risk factor analysis in differentiated thyroid cancer. *Cancer* 1979;43:810–820.

287. Oyama T, Vickery AL Jr, Preffer FI, et al. A comparative study of flow cytometry and histopathologic findings in thyroid follicular carcinomas and adenomas. *Hum Pathol* 1994; 25:271–275.

288. Fukunaga M, Shinozaki N, Endo Y, et al. Atypical adenoma of the thyroid. A clinicopathologic and flow cytometric DNA study in comparison with other follicular neoplasms. *Acta Pathol Jpn* 1992;42:632–638.

289. Backdahl M. Nuclear DNA content and prognosis in papillary, follicular, and medullary carcinomas of the thyroid [Doctoral Thesis]. Stockholm, Sweden: Karolinska Medical Institute, 1985.

290. Mase T, Funahashi H, Koshikawa T, et al. HBME-1 immunostaining in thyroid tumors especially in follicular neoplasm. *Endocr J* 2003;50:173–177.

291. Kroll TG, Sarraf P, Pecciarini L, et al. PAX8-PPARgamma1 fusion in oncogene human thyroid carcinoma. *Science* 2000;289:1357–1360.
292. Nikiforov M, Biddinger P, Caudill CM, et al. PAX8-PPAR g rearrangement in thyroid tumors: RT-PCR and immunohistochemical analysis. *Am J Surg Pathol* 2002;26:1016–1023.
293. Villanueva-Siles E, Tanaka K, Wenig BM. Peroxisome proliferator-activated receptor gamma 1 (PPAR-g1) in benign and malignant thyroid lesions: an immunohistochemical study. *Mod Pathol* 2002;15(Abstr):121A.
294. Marques AR, Espadinha C, Catarino AL, et al. Expression of PAX8-PPAR gamma 1 rearrangements in both follicular thyroid carcinomas and adenomas. *J Clin Endocrinol Metab* 2002;87:3947–3952.
295. Gustafson KS, LiVolsi VA, Furth EE, et al. Peroxisome proliferator-activated receptor gamma expression in follicular-patterned thyroid lesions. Caveats for the use of immunohistochemical studies. *Am J Clin Pathol* 2003;120:175–181.
296. Bouras M, Bertholon J, Dutrieux-Berger N, et al. Variability of Ha-ras (codon 12) proto-oncogene mutations in diverse thyroid cancers. *Eur J Endocrinol* 1998;139:209–216.
297. Matsuo K, Tang SH, Fagin JA. Allelotype of human thyroid tumors: loss of chromosome 11q13 sequences in follicular neoplasms. *Mol Endocrinol* 1991;5:1873–1879.
298. Grebe SK, McIver B, Hay ID, et al. Frequent loss of heterozygosity on chromosomes 3p and 17p without VHL or p53 mutations suggests involvement of unidentified tumor suppressor genes in follicular thyroid carcinoma. *J Clin Endocrinol Metab* 1997;82: 3684–3691.
299. Carcangiu ML, Bianchi S, Savino D, et al. Follicular Hurthle cell tumors of the thyroid gland. *Cancer* 1991;68:1944–1953.
300. Sobrinho-Simoes MA, Nesland JM, Holm R, et al. Hurthle cell and mitochondrion-rich papillary carcinomas of the thyroid gland: an ultrastructural and immunocytochemical study. *Ultrastruct Pathol* 1985;8:131–142.
301. Harcourt-Webster J, Stott N. Histochemical study of oxidative and hydrolytic enzymes in the human thyroid. *J Pathol Bacteriol* 1960;80:353–361.
302. Tremblay G, Pearse A. Histochemistry of oxidative enzyme systems in the human thyroid with special reference to Askanazy cells. *J Pathol Bacteriol* 1960;80:353–358.
303. Kendall C, McCluskey E, Naylor J. Oxyphil cells in thyroid disease: a uniform change? *J Clin Pathol* 1986;39:908–912.
304. Baloch ZW, LiVolsi VA. Oncocytic lesions of the neuroendocrine system. *Semin Diagn Pathol* 1999;16:190–199.
305. Thompson N, Dun E, Batsakis J, et al. Hürthle cell lesions of the thyroid gland. *Surg Gynecol Obstet* 1974;139:555–560.
306. Watson R, Brennan M, Goellner J, et al. Invasive Hürthle cell carcinoma of the thyroid: natural history and management. *Mayo Clin Proc* 1984;59:851–855.
307. Gundry S, Burney R, Thompson N, et al. Total thyroidectomy for Hürthle cell neoplasm of the thyroid gland. *Arch Surg* 1983;118:529–553.
308. Bronner MP, LiVolsi VA. Oxyphilic (Askanazy/Hürthle cell) tumors of the thyroid: microscopic features predict biologic behavior. *Surg Pathol* 1988;1:137–149.
309. Baloch ZW, LiVolsi VA. Post fine-needle aspiration histologic alterations of thyroid revisited. *Am J Clin Pathol* 1999;112:311–316.
310. Tollefson H, Shah J, Huvos A. Hürthle cell carcinoma of the thyroid. *Am J Surg* 1975;130: 390–394.
311. Heppe H, Armin A, Calandra D, et al. Hürthle cell tumors of the thyroid gland. *Surgery* 1985;98:1162–1165.
312. Ghossein RA, Hiltzik DH, Carlson DL, et al. Prognostic factors of recurrence in encapsulated Hürthle cell carcinoma of the thyroid gland: a clinicopathologic study of 50 cases. *Cancer* 2006;106:1669–1676.
313. Khafif A, Khafif RA, Attie JN. Hürthle cell carcinoma: a malignancy of low-grade potential. *Head Neck* 1999;21:506–511.
314. McHenry CR, Sandoval BA. Management of follicular and Hürthle cell neoplasms of the thyroid gland. *Surg Oncol Clin North Am* 1998;7:893–910.
315. Abu-Alfa AK, Straus FH 2nd, Montag AG. An immunohistochemical study of thyroid Hürthle cells and their neoplasms: the roles of S-100 and HMB-45 proteins. *Mod Pathol* 1994;7:529–532.
316. Kanthan R, Radhi JM. Immunohistochemical analysis of thyroid adenomas with Hürthle cells. *Pathology* 1998;30:4–6.
317. Nascimento MC, Bisi H, Alves VA, et al. Differential reactivity for galectin-3 in Hürthle cell adenomas and carcinomas. *Endocr Pathol* 2001;12:275–279.
318. Zedenius J, Auer G, Backdahl M, et al. Follicular tumors of the thyroid gland: diagnosis, clinical aspects and nuclear DNA analysis. *World J Surg* 1992;16:589–594.
319. Bronner MP, Clevenger CV, Edmonds PR, et al. Flow cytometric analysis of DNA content in Hürthle cell adenomas and carcinomas of the thyroid. *Am J Clin Pathol* 1988;89:764–769.
320. Stankov K, Landi S, Gioia-Patricola L, et al. GSTT1 and M1 polymorphisms in Hürthle thyroid cancer patients. *Cancer Lett* 2006;240:76–82.
321. Hunt JL. Unusual thyroid tumors: a review of pathologic and molecular diagnosis. *Expert Rev Mol Diagn* 2005;5:725–734.
322. Masood S, Auguste LJ, Westerband A, et al. Differential oncogenic expression in thyroid follicular and Hürthle cell carcinomas. *Am J Surg* 1993;166:366–368.
323. Segev DL, Saji M, Phillips GS, et al. Polymerase chain reaction-based microsatellite polymorphism analysis of follicular and Hürthle cell neoplasms of the thyroid. *J Clin Endocrinol Metab* 1998;83:2036–2042.
324. Maximo V, Soares P, Lima J, et al. Mitochondrial DNA somatic mutations (point mutations and large deletions) and mitochondrial DNA variants in human thyroid pathology: a study with emphasis on Hürthle cell tumors. *Am J Pathol* 2002;160:1857–1865.
325. Fonseca E, Soares P, Cardoso-Oliveira M, et al. Diagnostic criteria in well-differentiated thyroid carcinomas. *Endocr Pathol* 2006;17:109–117.
326. Horn R. Carcinoma of the thyroid. Description of a distinctive morphological variant and report of seven cases. *Cancer* 1951;4:697–707.
327. Hazard J, Hawk W, Crile G. Medullary (solid) carcinoma of the thyroid: a clinicopathologic entity. *J Clin Endocrinol Metab* 1959;19:152–161.
328. Williams E. Histogenesis of medullary carcinoma of the thyroid. *J Clin Pathol* 1966;19: 114–118.
329. Leitz H. C-cells: source of calcitonin. *Curr Top Pathol* 1971;55:109–146.
330. Weston J. The regulation of normal and abnormal neural crest cell development. *Adv Neurol* 1981;29:77–95.
331. Wolfe H, DeLellis R, Voelkel E, et al. Distribution of calcitonin containing cells in the normal neonatal human thyroid gland: a correlation of morphology with peptide content. *J Clin Endocrinol Metab* 1975;41:1076–1081.
332. Wolfe H, Voelkel E, Tashjian A. Distribution of calcitonin containing cells in the normal adult human thyroid gland: a correlation of morphology and peptide content. *J Clin Endocrinol Metab* 1974;38:688–694.
333. O'Toole K, Fenoglio-Preiser C, Pushparaj N. Endocrine changes associated with the human aging process. III. Effect of age on the number of calcitonin immunoreactive cells in the thyroid gland. *Hum Pathol* 1985;16:991–1000.
334. Albores-Saavedra J, LiVolsi VA, Williams ED. Medullary carcinoma. *Semin Diagn Pathol* 1985;2:137–146.
335. Wells SA Jr, Franz C. Medullary carcinoma of the thyroid gland. *World J Surg* 2000;24: 952–956.
336. Eng C, Clayton D, Schuffenecker I, et al. The relationship between specific RET proto-oncogene mutations and disease phenotype in multiple endocrine neoplasia type 2. International RET mutation consortium analysis. *JAMA* 1996;276:1575–1579.
337. Eng C, Mulligan LM. Mutations of the RET proto-oncogene in the multiple endocrine neoplasia type 2 syndromes, related sporadic tumours, and Hirschsprung disease. *Hum Mutat* 1997;9:97–109.
338. Heptulla RA, Schwartz RP, Bale AE, et al. Familial medullary thyroid carcinoma: presymptomatic diagnosis and management in children. *J Pediatr* 1999;135:327–331.
339. Gimm O, Sutter T, Dralle H. Diagnosis and therapy of sporadic and familial medullary thyroid carcinoma. *J Cancer Res Clin Oncol* 2001;127:156–165.
340. Gagel RF, Melvin KE, Tashjian AH Jr, et al. Natural history of the familial medullary thyroid carcinoma-pheochromocytoma syndrome and the identification of preneoplastic stages by screening studies: a five-year report. *Trans Assoc Am Physicians* 1975;88:177–191.
341. Kakudo K, Miyachi A, Ogihara T, et al. Medullary carcinoma of the thyroid with ectopic ACTH syndrome. *Acta Pathol Jpn* 1982;32:793–800.
342. Mertens PR, Goretzki PE, Keck E. cAMP-synthesis in a medullary thyroid carcinoma cell line: response to adrenergic agents and prostaglandins. *Exp Clin Endocrinol Diabetes* 1999; 107:488–495.
343. Sipple J. The association of pheochromocytoma with carcinoma of the thyroid gland. *Am J Med* 1961;31:163–166.
344. Jansson S, Hansson G, Salander H, et al. Prevalence of C-cell hyperplasia and medullary thyroid carcinoma in a consecutive series of pheochromocytoma patients. *World J Surg* 1984;8:493–500.
345. Eng C, Smith DP, Mulligan LM, et al. A novel point mutation in the tyrosine kinase domain of the RET proto-oncogene in sporadic medullary thyroid carcinoma and in a family with FMTC. *Oncogene* 1995;10:509–513.
346. Frich L, Glattre E, Akslen LA. Familial occurrence of nonmedullary thyroid cancer: a population-based study of 5673 first-degree relatives of thyroid cancer patients from Norway. *Cancer Epidemiol Biomarkers Prev* 2001;10:113–117.
347. Feldman GL, Edmonds MW, Ainsworth PJ, et al. Variable expressivity of familial medullary thyroid carcinoma (FMTC) due to a RET V804M (GTG→ATG) mutation. *Surgery* 2000; 128:93–98.
348. Brown R, Colle E, Tashjian A. The syndrome of multiple mucosal neuromas and medullary thyroid carcinoma in childhood. *J Pediatr* 1975;86:77–83.
349. Akama H, Noshiro T, Kimura N, et al. Multiple endocrine neoplasia type 2A with the identical somatic mutation in medullary thyroid carcinoma and pheochromocytoma without germline mutation at the corresponding site in the RET proto-oncogene. *Intern Med* 1999;38:145–149.
350. Carney J, Hales A. Alimentary tract manifestations of multiple endocrine neoplasia, type 2b. *Mayo Clin Proc* 1977;52:543–548.
351. Carney J, Hales A, Pearse A, et al. Abnormal cutaneous innervation in multiple endocrine neoplasia, type 2b. *Ann Intern Med* 1981;94:262–263.
352. Carney J, Roth S, Heath H, et al. The parathyroid glands in multiple endocrine neoplasia, type 2b. *Am J Pathol* 1980;99:387–398.
353. Marsh DJ, Zheng Z, Arnold A, et al. Mutation analysis of glial cell line-derived neurotrophic factor, a ligand for an RET/coreceptor complex, in multiple endocrine neoplasia type 2 and sporadic neuroendocrine tumors. *J Clin Endocrinol Metab* 1997;82:3025–3028.
354. Marsh DJ, Mulligan LM, Eng C. RET proto-oncogene mutations in multiple endocrine neoplasia type 2 and medullary thyroid carcinoma. *Horm Res* 1997;47:168–178.
355. Asa SL. C-cell lesions of the thyroid. *Pathol Case Rev* 1997;2:210–217.
356. Sambade C, Baldaque-Faria A, Cardoso-Oliveira M, et al. Follicular and papillary variants of medullary carcinoma of the thyroid. *Pathol Res Pract* 1988;184:98–107.
357. Harach HR, Williams ED. Glandular (tubular and follicular) variants of medullary carcinoma of the thyroid. *Histopathology* 1983;7:83–97.
358. Schroder S. [Pathological and clinical features of malignant thyroid tumors: classification, immunohistology, prognostic criteria]. *Veroff Pathol* 1988;130:1–159.
359. Huss LJ, Mendelsohn G. Medullary carcinoma of the thyroid gland: an encapsulated variant resembling the hyalinizing trabecular (paraganglioma-like) adenoma of thyroid. *Mod Pathol* 1990;3:581–585.
360. Mendelsohn G, Oertel J. Encapsulated medullary thyroid carcinoma. *Lab Invest* 1981;44: 43a.
361. Kodama T, Okamoto T, Fujimoto Y, et al. C-cell adenoma of the thyroid. A rare but distinct clinical entity. *Surgery* 1988;104:997.
362. Mendelsohn G, Baylin SB, Bigner SH, et al. Anaplastic variants of medullary thyroid carcinoma. A light microscopic and immunohistochemical study. *Am J Surg Pathol* 1980;4: 333–341.

363. Kakudo K, Miyauchi A, Ogihara T, et al. Medullary carcinoma of the thyroid. Giant cell type. *Arch Pathol Lab Med* 1978;102:445–447.
364. Landon G, Ordonez NG. Clear cell variant of medullary carcinoma of the thyroid. *Hum Pathol* 1985;16:844–847.
365. Dominguez-Malagon H, Delgado-Chavez R, Torres-Najera M, et al. Oxyphil and squamous variants of medullary thyroid carcinoma. *Cancer* 1989;63:1183–1188.
366. Zaatari GS, Saigo PE, Huvos AG. Mucin production in medullary carcinoma of the thyroid. *Arch Pathol Lab Med* 1983;107:70–74.
367. Singh ZN, Ray R, Kumar N, et al. Medullary thyroid carcinoma with melanin production—a case report. *Indian J Pathol Microbiol* 1999;42:159–163.
368. Kos M, Separovic V, Sarcevic B. Medullary carcinoma of the thyroid: histomorphological, histochemical and immunohistochemical analysis of twenty cases. *Acta Med Croatica* 1995; 49:195–199.
369. DeLellis RA, Rule AH, Spiler F, et al. Calcitonin and carcinoembryonic antigen as tumor markers in medullary thyroid carcinoma. *Am J Clin Pathol* 1978;70:587–594.
370. Matsubayashi S, Yanaihara C, Ohkubo M, et al. Gastrin-releasing peptide immunoreactivity in medullary thyroid carcinoma. *Cancer* 1984;53:2472–2477.
371. Roth KA, Bensch KG, Hoffman AR. Characterization of opioid peptides in human thyroid medullary carcinoma. *Cancer* 1987;59:1594–1598.
372. Komminoth P, Roth J, Saremasiani P, et al. Polysialic acid of the neural cell adhesion molecule in the human thyroid: a marker for medullary carcinoma and primary C-cell hyperplasia. An immunohistochemical study on 79 thyroid lesions. *Am J Surg Pathol* 1994; 18:399–411.
373. Ravitch MM. Diagnosis and prognosis of medullary carcinoma of the thyroid. *Med Times* 1974;102:131–132.
374. Randolph GW, Maniar D. Medullary carcinoma of the thyroid. *Cancer Control* 2000;7: 253–261.
375. Roman S, Lin R, Sosa JA. Prognosis of medullary thyroid carcinoma: demographic, clinical, and pathologic predictors of survival in 1252 cases. *Cancer* 2006;107:2134–2142.
376. Gilliland FD, Hunt WC, Morris DM, et al. Prognostic factors for thyroid carcinoma. A population-based study of 15,698 cases from the Surveillance, Epidemiology and End Results (SEER) program 1973–1991. *Cancer* 1997;79:564–573.
377. Melvin K, Tashjian A, Miller H. Studies in familial medullary thyroid carcinoma. *Recent Prog Horm Res* 1972;28:399–470.
378. Schroder S, Bocker W, Baisch H, et al. Prognostic factors in medullary thyroid carcinomas. Survival in relation to age, sex, stage, histology, immunocytochemistry, and DNA content. *Cancer* 1988;61:806–816.
379. Matias-Guiu X. Mixed medullary and follicular carcinoma of the thyroid. On the search for its histogenesis. *Am J Pathol* 1999;155:1413–1418.
380. Papotti M, Volante M, Komminoth P, et al. Thyroid carcinomas with mixed follicular and C-cell differentiation patterns. *Semin Diagn Pathol* 2000;17:109–119.
381. Gibson W, Peng T, Croker B. C-cell nodules in adult human thyroid: a common autopsy finding. *Am J Clin Pathol* 1980;73:347–351.
382. DeLellis R, Wolfe H. Pathobiology of the human calcitonin (C) cell: a review. *Pathol Annu* 1981;16(Pt 2):25–52.
383. Carney J, Sizemore G, Hales A. Multiple endocrine neoplasia, type 2b. *Pathobiol Annu* 1978;8:105–153.
384. Perry A, Molberg K, Albores-Saavedra J. Physiologic versus neoplastic C-cell hyperplasia of the thyroid: separation of distinct histologic and biologic entities. *Cancer* 1996;77:750–756.
385. Guyetant S, Wion-Barbot N, Rousselet, et al. C-cell hyperplasia associated with chronic lymphocytic thyroiditis: a retrospective quantitative study of 112 cases. *Hum Pathol* 1994; 25:514–521.
386. Leboulleux S, Baudin E, Travagli JP, et al. Medullary thyroid carcinoma. *Clin Endocrinol (Oxf)* 2004;61:299–310.
387. Albores-Saavedra J, Monforte H, Nadji M, et al. C-cell hyperplasia in thyroid tissue adjacent to follicular cell tumors. *Hum Pathol* 1988;19:795–799.
388. Kaserer K, Scheuba C, Neuhold N, et al. Sporadic versus familial medullary thyroid microcarcinoma: a histopathologic study of 50 consecutive patients. *Am J Surg Pathol* 2001;25: 1245–1251.
389. Kaserer K, Scheuba C, Neuhold N, et al. C-cell hyperplasia and medullary thyroid carcinoma in patients routinely screened for serum calcitonin. *Am J Surg Pathol* 1998;22: 722–728.
390. Krueger JE, Maitra A, Albores-Saavedra J. Inherited medullary microcarcinoma of the thyroid: a study of 11 cases. *Am J Surg Pathol* 2000;24:853–858.
391. Guyetant S, Dupre F, Bigorgne JC, et al. Medullary thyroid microcarcinoma: a clinicopathologic retrospective study of 38 patients with no prior familial disease. *Hum Pathol* 1999; 30:957–963.
392. Akslen LA, LiVolsi VA. Poorly differentiated thyroid carcinoma—it is important. *Am J Surg Pathol* 2000;24:310–313.
393. Hiltzik D, Carlson DL, Tuttle RM, et al. Poorly differentiated thyroid carcinomas defined on the basis of mitosis and necrosis: a clinicopathologic study of 58 patients. *Cancer* 2006; 106:1286–1295.
394. Carcangiu ML, Zampi G, Rosai J. Poorly differentiated ("insular") thyroid carcinoma. A reinterpretation of Langhans' "wuchernde struma." *Am J Surg Pathol* 1984;8:655–668.
395. Justin EP, Seabold JE, Robinson RA, et al. Insular carcinoma: a distinct thyroid carcinoma with associated iodine-131 localization [see comments]. *J Nucl Med* 1991;32:1358–1363.
396. Bal C, Padhy AK, Panda S, et al. "Insular" carcinoma of thyroid. A subset of anaplastic thyroid malignancy with a less aggressive clinical course. *Clin Nucl Med* 1993;18:1056–1058.
397. Nishida T, Katayama S, Tsujimoto M, et al. Clinicopathological significance of poorly differentiated thyroid carcinoma. *Am J Surg Pathol* 1999;23:205–211.
398. Carcangiu ML, Steeper T, Zampi G, et al. Anaplastic thyroid carcinoma. A study of 70 cases. *Am J Clin Pathol* 1985;83:135–158.
399. Getaz E, Shimaoka K, Rao U. Anaplastic carcinoma of the thyroid following external irradiation. *Cancer* 1979;43:2248–2253.
400. Kapp D, LiVolsi V, Sanders M. Anaplastic carcinoma following well differentiated thyroid cancer: etiologic considerations. *Yale J Biol Med* 1982;55:521–528.
401. Venkatesh YS, Ordonez NG, Schultz PN, et al. Anaplastic carcinoma of the thyroid. A clinicopathologic study of 121 cases. *Cancer* 1990;66:321–330.
402. Jaques D, Chambers R, Oertel J. Thyroglossal tract carcinoma. A review of the literature and addition of eighteen cases. *Am J Surg* 1968;120:439–446.
403. Belleannee G, Verdebout J, Feoli F, et al. [Role of cytology and frozen sections in the intraoperative examination of the thyroid: comparison of two experiences]. *Clin Exp Pathol* 1999;47:273–277.
404. Udelsman R, Westra WH, Donovan PI, et al. Randomized prospective evaluation of frozen-section analysis for follicular neoplasms of the thyroid. *Ann Surg* 2001;233:716–722.
405. Kini SR. *Guides to Clinical Aspiration Biopsy Thyroid.* New York, NY: Igaku-Shoin, 1996.
406. Carcangiu ML, Steeper T, Zampi G, et al. Anaplastic thyroid carcinoma. A study of 70 cases. *Am J Clin Pathol* 1985;83:135–158.
407. Kobayashi S, Yamadori I, Ohmori M, et al. Anaplastic carcinoma of the thyroid with osteoclast-like giant cells. An ultrastructural and immunohistochemical study. *Acta Pathol Jpn* 1987;37:807–815.
408. Wan S, Chan J, Tang S. Paucicellular variant of anaplastic thyroid carcinoma. A mimic of Riedel's thyroiditis. *Am J Clin Pathol* 1996;105:388–393.
409. Bronner MP, LiVolsi VA. Spindle cell squamous carcinoma of the thyroid: an unusual anaplastic tumor associated with tall cell papillary cancer. *Mod Pathol* 1991;4:637–643.
410. Nesland JM, Sobrinho-Simoes M, Johannessen JV. Scanning electron microscopy of the human thyroid gland and its disorders. *Scanning Microsc* 1987;1:1797–1810.
411. Miettinen M, Franssila KO. Variable expression of keratins and nearly uniform lack of thyroid transcription factor 1 in thyroid anaplastic carcinoma. *Hum Pathol* 2000;31: 1139–1145.
412. Holting T, Moller P, Tschahargane C, et al. Immunohistochemical reclassification of anaplastic carcinoma reveals small and giant cell lymphoma. *World J Surg* 1990;14:291–294; discussion 295.
413. Matias-Guiu X, LaGuette J, Puras-Gil AM, et al. Metastatic neuroendocrine tumors to the thyroid gland mimicking medullary carcinoma: a pathologic and immunohistochemical study of six cases. *Am J Surg Pathol* 1997;21:754–762.
414. Ozaki O, Sugino K, Mimura T, et al. Primary leiomyosarcoma of the thyroid gland. *Surg Today* 1997;27:177–180.
415. Papi G, Corrado S, LiVolsi VA. Primary spindle cell lesions of the thyroid gland; an overview. *Am J Clin Pathol* 2006;125(Suppl):S95–S123.
416. Tanda F, Massarelli G, Bosincu L, et al. Angiosarcoma of the thyroid: a light, electron microscopic and histoimmunological study. *Hum Pathol* 1988;19:742–745.
417. Lamovec J, Zidar A, Zidanik B. Epithelioid angiosarcoma of the thyroid gland. Report of two cases. *Arch Pathol Lab Med* 1994;118:642–646.
418. Shimizu J, Ishida Y, Takehara A, et al. Salvage surgery for primary non-Hodgkin's lymphoma of the thyroid gland with histopathological complete response to radio-chemotherapy: report of a case. *Surg Today* 2003;33:45–48.
419. Wirtzfeld DA, Winston JS, Hicks WL Jr, et al. Clinical presentation and treatment of non-Hodgkin's lymphoma of the thyroid gland. *Ann Surg Oncol* 2001;8:338–341.
420. Belal AA, Allam A, Kandil A, et al. Primary thyroid lymphoma: a retrospective analysis of prognostic factors and treatment outcome for localized intermediate and high grade lymphoma. *Am J Clin Oncol* 2001;24:299–305.
421. Skacel M, Ross CW, Hsi ED. A reassessment of primary thyroid lymphoma: high-grade MALT-type lymphoma as a distinct subtype of diffuse large B-cell lymphoma. *Histopathology* 2000;37:10–18.
422. Takahashi K, Kashima K, Daa T, et al. Contribution of Epstein-Barr virus to development of malignant lymphoma of the thyroid. *Pathol Int* 1995;45:366–374.
423. Lam KY, Lo CY, Kwong DL, et al. Malignant lymphoma of the thyroid. A 30-year clinicopathologic experience and an evaluation of the presence of Epstein-Barr virus. *Am J Clin Pathol* 1999;112:263–270.
424. Sosna J, Slasky BS, Paltiel O, et al. Multiple myeloma involving the thyroid cartilage: case report. *AJNR Am J Neuroradiol* 2002;23:316–318.
425. Neiman R, Barcos M, Berhard C, et al. Granulocytic sarcoma: a clinicopathologic study of 61 biopsied cases. *Cancer* 1981;48:1426–1437.
426. Allevato PA, Kini SR, Rebuck JW, et al. Signet ring cell lymphoma of the thyroid: a case report. *Hum Pathol* 1985;16:1066–1068.
427. Feigin GA, Buss DH, Paschal B, et al. Hodgkin's disease manifested as a thyroid nodule. *Hum Pathol* 1982;13:774–776.
428. Rappaport H, Thomas L. Myocosis fungoides: the pathology of extracutaneous involvement. *Cancer* 1974;34:1198–1229.
429. Teja K, Sabio H, Langsdon D, et al. Involvement of the thyroid gland in histiocytosis X. *Hum Pathol* 1981;12:1137–1139.
430. Tamouridis N, Deladetsima JK, Kastanias I, et al. Cold thyroid nodule as the sole manifestation of Rosai-Dorfman disease with mild lymphadenopathy, coexisting with chronic autoimmune thyroiditis. *J Endocrinol Invest* 1999;22:866–870.
431. Hanna E. Squamous cell carcinoma in a thyroglossal duct cyst (TGDC): clinical presentation, diagnosis, and management. *Am J Otolaryngol* 1996;17:353–357.
432. Jayaram G, Jayalakshmi P. Follicular adenoma with squamous metaplasia and cystic change: report of a case with fine needle aspiration cytological and histological features. *Malays J Pathol* 1999;21:101–104.
433. Franssila K. Value of histologic classification of thyroid cancer. *Acta Pathol Microbiol Scand Suppl* 1971;225:5–76.
434. Carcangiu ML, Bianchi S. Diffuse sclerosing variant of papillary thyroid carcinoma. Clinicopathologic study of 15 cases. *Am J Surg Pathol* 1989;13:1041–1049.
435. Wenig BM, Adair CF, Heffess CS. Primary mucoepidermoid carcinoma of the thyroid gland: a report of six cases and a review of the literature of a follicular epithelial-derived tumor. *Hum Pathol* 1995;26:1099–1108.

436. Albores-Saavedra J, Gu X, Luna MA. Clear cells and thyroid transcription factor I reactivity in sclerosing mucoepidermoid carcinoma of the thyroid gland. *Ann Diagn Pathol* 2003;7: 348–353.

437. Minagawa A, Iitaka M, Suzuki M, et al. A case of primary mucoepidermoid carcinoma of the thyroid: molecular evidence of its origin. *Clin Endocrinol (Oxf)* 2002;57:551–556.

438. Harach HR. A study on the relationship between solid cell nests and mucoepidermoid carcinoma of the thyroid. *Histopathology* 1985;9:195–207.

439. Chan JK, Albores-Saavedra J, Battifora H, et al. Sclerosing mucoepidermoid thyroid carcinoma with eosinophilia. A distinctive low-grade malignancy arising from the metaplastic follicles of Hashimoto's thyroiditis. *Am J Surg Pathol* 1991;15:438–448.

440. Franssila K, Harach H, Wasenius V. Mucoepidermoid carcinoma of the thyroid. *Histopathology* 1984;8:847–860.

441. Hunt JL, LiVolsi VA, Barnes EL. p63 expression in sclerosing mucoepidermoid carcinomas with eosinophilia arising in the thyroid. *Mod Pathol* 2004;17:526–529.

442. Huang T, Assor D. Primary squamous cell carcinoma of the thyroid gland: a report of four cases. *Am J Clin Pathol* 1971;55:93–98.

443. Simpson W, Carruthers J. Squamous cell carcinoma of the thyroid gland. *Am J Surg* 1988; 156:44–46.

444. Carangiu M, Sibley R, Rosai J. Clear cell change in primary thyroid tumors. *Am J Surg Pathol* 1985;9:705–722.

445. Mortenson J, Woolner L, Bennett W. Secondary malignant tumors of the thyroid gland. *Cancer* 1965;19:306–309.

446. Schroder S, Bocker W. Signet ring cell thyroid tumors: a follicle cell tumor with arrest of folliculogenesis. *Am J Surg Pathol* 1985;9:619–629.

447. Schroder S, Bocker W, Husselman H, et al. Adenolipoma (thyrolipoma) of the thyroid gland: report of two cases and review of the literature. *Virchows Arch (A)* 1984;404:99–103.

448. Fuller R. Hamartomatous adiposity with superimposed amyloidosis of thyroid gland. *J Laryngol Otol* 1963;77:92–93.

449. de la Cruz Vigo F, Ortega G, Gonzalez S, et al. Pathologic intrathyroidal parathyroid glands. *Int Surg* 1997;82:87–90.

450. Harach HR, Vujanic GM. Intrathyroidal parathyroid. *Pediatr Pathol* 1993;13:71–74.

451. Wheeler MH, Williams ED, Wade JS. The hyperfunctioning intrathyroidal parathyroid gland: a potential pitfall in parathyroid surgery. *World J Surg* 1987;11:110–114.

452. Lam KY, Lo CY. Metastatic tumors of the thyroid gland: a study of 79 cases in Chinese patients. *Arch Pathol Lab Med* 1998;122:37–41.

453. Baloch ZW, LiVolsi VA. Tumor-to-tumor metastasis to follicular variant of papillary carcinoma of thyroid. *Arch Pathol Lab Med* 1999;123:703–706.

454. Ivy H. Cancer metastatic to the thyroid gland: a diagnostic problem. *Mayo Clin Proc* 1984; 59:856–859.

455. Czech J, Lichtor T, Carney J, et al. Neoplasms metastatic to the thyroid gland. *Surg Gynecol Obstet* 1982;155:503–505.

456. Miyauchi A, Kuma K, Matsuzuka F, et al. Intrathyroidal epithelial thymoma: an entity distinct from squamous cell carcinoma of the thyroid. *World J Surg* 1985;9:128–135.

457. Chan JK, Rosai J. Tumors of the neck showing thymic or related branchial pouch differentiation: a unifying concept. *Hum Pathol* 1991;22:349–367.

458. Hofman P, Mainguene C, Michiels JF, et al. Thyroid spindle epithelial tumor with thymus-like differentiation (the "SETTLE" tumor). An immunohistochemical and electron microscopic study. *Eur Arch Otorhinolaryngol* 1995;252:316–320.

459. Kirby PA, Ellison WA, Thomas PA. Spindle epithelial tumor with thymus-like differentiation (SETTLE) of the thyroid with prominent mitotic activity and focal necrosis. *Am J Surg Pathol* 1999;23:712–716.

460. Dorfman DM, Shahsafaei A, Miyauchi A. Intrathyroidal epithelial thymoma (ITET)/carcinoma showing thymus-like differentiation (CASTLE) exhibits CD5 immunoreactivity: new evidence for thymic differentiation. *Histopathology* 1998;32:104–109.

461. Dorfman DM, Shahsafaei A, Miyauchi A. Immunohistochemical staining for bcl-2 and mcl-1 in intrathyroidal epithelial thymoma (ITET)/carcinoma showing thymus-like differentiation (CASTLE) and cervical thymic carcinoma. *Mod Pathol* 1998;11:989–994.

462. Newstedt J, Shirkey H. Teratoma of the thyroid region. *Am J Dis Child* 1964;107:88–95.

463. Craver RD, Lipscomb JT, Suskind D, et al. Malignant teratoma of the thyroid with primitive neuroepithelial and mesenchymal sarcomatous components. *Ann Diagn Pathol* 2001;5: 285–292.

464. Hajdu S, Faruque A, Hajdu E, et al. Teratoma of the neck in infants. *Am J Dis Child* 1966; 111:412–416.

465. Hajdu S, Hajdu E. Malignant teratoma of the neck. *Arch Pathol* 1967;83:567–570.

466. Pickelman J, Lee J, Straus F, et al. Thyroid hemangioma. *Am J Surg* 1975;129:331–336.

467. Andrion A, Bellis D, Delsedime L, et al. Leiomyoma and neurilemoma: report of two unusual non-epithelial tumours of the thyroid gland. *Virchows Arch (A)* 1988;413:367–372.

468. Rodriguez I, Ayala E, Caballero C, et al. Solitary fibrous tumor of the thyroid gland: report of seven cases. *Am J Surg Pathol* 2001;25:1424–1428.

469. Mill W, Gowing N, Reeves B, et al. Carcinoma of the lingual thyroid treated with radioactive iodine. *Lancet* 1959;1:76–79.

470. Falvo L, Berni A, Catania A, et al. Sclerosing papillary carcinoma arising in a lingual thyroid: report of a case. *Surg Today* 2005;35:304–308.

471. LiVolsi VA, Perzin KH, Savetsky L. Carcinoma arising in median ectopic thyroid (including thyroglossal duct tissue). *Cancer* 1974;34:1303–1315.

472. Chen F, Sheridan B, Nankervis J. Carcinoma of the thyroglossal duct: case reports and a literature review. *Aust N Z J Surg* 1993;63:614–616.

473. Nussbaum M, Buchwald RP, Ribner A, et al. Anaplastic carcinoma arising from the median ectopic thyroid (thyroglossal duct remnants). *Cancer* 1981;48:2724–2728.

474. Heshmati HM, Fatourechi V, van Heerden JA, et al. Thyroglossal duct carcinoma: report of 12 cases. *Mayo Clin Proc* 1997;72:315–319.

475. Aldasouqi SA. Carcinoma of thyroglossal duct cyst. *Endocr Pract* 2002;8:137.

476. Ferrer C, Ferrandez A, Dualde D, et al. Squamous cell carcinoma of the thyroglossal duct cyst: report of a new case and literature review. *J Otolaryngol* 2000;29:311–314.

477. Maziak D, Borowy ZJ, Deitel M, et al. Management of papillary carcinoma arising in thyroglossal-duct anlage. *Can J Surg* 1992;35:522–525.

478. Fih J, Moore R. Ectopic thyroid tissue and ectopic thyroid carcinoma. *Ann Surg* 1963;157: 212–222.

479. Ersoy E, Taneri F, Tekin E, et al. Preoperative fine-needle aspiration cytology versus frozen section in thyroid surgery. *Endocr Regul* 1999;33:141–144.

480. Chow TL, Venu V, Kwok SP. Use of fine-needle aspiration cytology and frozen section examination in diagnosis of thyroid nodules. *Aust N Z J Surg* 1999;69:131–133.

481. Hamburger JI. Fine needle biopsy diagnosis of thyroid nodules. Perspective. *Thyroidology* 1988;1:21–34.

482. Jayaram G, Razak A, Gan SK, et al. Fine needle aspiration cytology of the thyroid—a review of experience in 1853 cases. *Malays J Pathol* 1999;21:17–27.

483. Leonard N, Melcher DH. To operate or not to operate? The value of fine needle aspiration cytology in the assessment of thyroid swellings. *J Clin Pathol* 1997;50:941–943.

484. Nguyen GK, Lee MW, Ginsberg J, et al. Fine-needle aspiration of the thyroid: an overview. *Cytojournal* 2005;2:12.

485. Silverman JF, West RL, Finley JL, et al. Fine-needle aspiration versus large-needle biopsy or cutting biopsy in evaluation of thyroid nodules. *Diagn Cytopathol* 1986;2:25–30.

486. Renshaw AA. Evidence-based criteria for adequacy in thyroid fine-needle aspiration. *Am J Clin Pathol* 2002;118:518–521.

487. Gharib H. Fine-needle aspiration biopsy of thyroid nodules: advantages, limitations, and effect. *Mayo Clin Proc* 1994;69:44–49.

488. Chow LS, Gharib H, Goellner JR, et al. Nondiagnostic thyroid fine-needle aspiration cytology: management dilemmas. *Thyroid* 2001;11:1147–1151.

489. Tuttle RM, Lemar H, Burch HB. Clinical features associated with an increased risk of thyroid malignancy in patients with follicular neoplasia by fine-needle aspiration. *Thyroid* 1998;8:377–383.

490. Kumar N, Ray C, Jain S. Aspiration cytology of Hashimoto's thyroiditis in an endemic area. *Cytopathology* 2002;13:31–39.

491. Sangalli G, Serio G, Zampatti C, et al. Fine needle aspiration cytology of primary lymphoma of the thyroid: a report of 17 cases. *Cytopathology* 2001;12:257–263.

492. Renshaw A. Interinstitutional review of thyroid fine-needle aspirations. *Diagn Cytopathol* 2002;27:128–129; author reply 130.

493. Hsu C, Boey J. Diagnostic pitfalls in the fine needle aspiration of thyroid nodules. A study of 555 cases in Chinese patients. *Acta Cytol* 1987;31:699–704.

494. Stanley MW. Selected problems in fine needle aspiration of head and neck masses. *Mod Pathol* 2002;15:342–350.

495. Renshaw AA. Follicular lesions of the thyroid. *Am J Clin Pathol* 2001;115:782–785.

496. Schlinkert RT, van Heerden JA, Goellner JR, et al. Factors that predict malignant thyroid lesions when fine-needle aspiration is "suspicious for follicular neoplasm." *Mayo Clin Proc* 1997;72:913–916.

497. Wang HH. Reporting thyroid fine-needle aspiration: literature review and a proposal. *Diagn Cytopathol* 2006;34:67–76.

498. Giorgadze T, Rossi ED, Fadda G, et al. Does the fine-needle aspiration diagnosis of "Hürthle-cell neoplasm/follicular neoplasm with oncocytic features" denote increased risk of malignancy? *Diagn Cytopathol* 2004;31:307–312.

499. Yang YJ, Khurana KK. Diagnostic utility of intracytoplasmic lumen and transgressing vessels in evaluation of Hurthle cell lesions by fine-needle aspiration. *Arch Pathol Lab Med* 2001;125:1031–1035.

500. Elliott DD, Pitman MB, Bloom L, et al. Fine-needle aspiration biopsy of Hürthle cell lesions of the thyroid gland: a cytomorphologic study of 139 cases with statistical analysis. *Cancer* 2006;108:102–109.

501. Fadda G, Mule A, Zannoni GF, et al. Fine needle aspiration of a warthin-like thyroid tumor. Report of a case with differential diagnostic criteria vs. other lymphocyte-rich thyroid lesions. *Acta Cytol* 1998;42:998–1002.

502. Leung CS, Hartwick RW, Bedard YC. Correlation of cytologic and histologic features in variants of papillary carcinoma of the thyroid. *Acta Cytol* 1993;37:645–650.

503. Akerman M, Tennvall J, Biorklund A, et al. Sensitivity and specificity of fine needle aspiration cytology in the diagnosis of tumors of the thyroid gland. *Acta Cytol* 1985;29:850–855.

504. Vojvodich SM, Ballagh RH, Cramer H, et al. Accuracy of fine needle aspiration in the pre-operative diagnosis of thyroid neoplasia. *J Otolaryngol* 1994;23:360–365.

505. Baloch ZW, Puttaswamy K, Brose M, et al. Lack of BRAF mutations in hyalinizing trabecular neoplasm. *Cytojournal* 2006;3:17.

506. Solomon A, Gupta PK, LiVolsi VA, et al. Distinguishing tall cell variant of papillary thyroid carcinoma from usual variant of papillary thyroid carcinoma in cytologic specimens. *Diagn Cytopathol* 2002;27:143–148.

507. Ohori NP, Schoedel KE. Cytopathology of high-grade papillary thyroid carcinomas: tall-cell variant, diffuse sclerosing variant, and poorly differentiated papillary carcinoma. *Diag Cytopathol* 1999;20:19–23.

508. Collins BT, Cramer HM, Tabatowski K, et al. Fine needle aspiration of medullary carcinoma of the thyroid. Cytomorphology, immunocytochemistry and electron microscopy. *Acta Cytol* 1995;39:920–930.

509. Takano T, Miyauchi A, Matsuzuka F, et al. Preoperative diagnosis of medullary thyroid carcinoma by RT-PCR using RNA extracted from leftover cells within a needle used for fine needle aspiration biopsy. *J Clin Endocrinol Metab* 1999;84:951–955.

510. Kudo T, Miyauchi A, Ito Y, et al. Diagnosis of medullary thyroid carcinoma by calcitonin measurement in fine-needle aspiration biopsy specimens. *Thyroid* 2007;17:635–638.

511. Us-Krasovec M, Auersperg M, Bergant D, et al. Medullary carcinoma of the thyroid gland: diagnostic cytopathological characteristics. *Pathologica* 1998;90:5–13.

512. Saunders CA, Nayar R. Anaplastic spindle-cell squamous carcinoma arising in association with tall-cell papillary cancer of the thyroid: a potential pitfall. *Diagn Cytopathol* 1999;21: 413–418.

513. Luze T, Totsch M, Bangerl I, et al. Fine needle aspiration cytodiagnosis of anaplastic carcinoma and malignant haemangioendothelioma of the thyroid in an endemic goitre area. *Cytopathology* 1990;1:305–310.

514. Takashima S, Takayama F, Saito A, et al. Primary thyroid lymphoma: diagnosis of immuno-globulin heavy chain gene rearrangement with polymerase chain reaction in ultrasound-guided fine-needle aspiration. *Thyroid* 2000;10:507–510.

515. Lu JY, Lin CW, Chang TC, et al. Diagnostic pitfalls of fine-needle aspiration cytology and prognostic impact of chemotherapy in thyroid lymphoma. *J Formos Med Assoc* 2001;100:519–525.

516. Michelow PM, Leiman G. Metastases to the thyroid gland: diagnosis by aspiration cytology. *Diagn Cytopathol* 1995;13:209–213.

517. De Micco C, Vasko V, Garcia S, et al. Fine-needle aspiration of thyroid follicular neoplasm: diagnostic use of thyroid peroxidase immunocytochemistry with monoclonal antibody 47. *Surgery* 1994;116:1031–1035.

518. Gasbarri A, Martegani MP, Del Prete F, et al. Galectin-3 and CD44v6 isoforms in the preoperative evaluation of thyroid nodules. *J Clin Oncol* 1999;17:3494–502.

519. van Hoeven KH, Kovatich AJ, Miettinen M. Immunocytochemical evaluation of HBME-1, CA 19-9, and CD-15 (Leu-M1) in fine-needle aspirates of thyroid nodules. *Diagn Cytopathol* 1998;18:93–97.

520. Salvatore G, Giannini R, Faviana P, et al. Analysis of BRAF point mutation and RET/PTC rearrangement refines the fine-needle aspiration diagnosis of papillary thyroid carcinoma. *J Clin Endocrinol Metab* 2004;89:5175–5180.

521. Xing M, Tufano RP, Tufaro AP, et al. Detection of BRAF mutation on fine needle aspiration biopsy specimens: a new diagnostic tool for papillary thyroid cancer. *J Clin Endocrinol Metab* 2004;89:2867–2872.

522. Cohen Y, Rosenbaum E, Clark DP, et al. Mutational analysis of BRAF in fine needle aspiration biopsies of the thyroid: a potential application for the preoperative assessment of thyroid nodules. *Clin Cancer Res* 2004;10:2761–2765.

523. Harlow SP, Duda RB, Bauer KD. Diagnostic utility of DNA content flow cytometry in follicular neoplasms of the thyroid. *J Surg Oncol* 1992;50:1–6.

524. LiVolsi VA, Merino MJ. Worrisome histologic alterations following fine-needle aspiration of the thyroid (WHAFFT). *Pathol Annu* 1994;29:99–120.

525. Kini SR. Post-fine-needle biopsy infarction of thyroid neoplasms: a review of 28 cases. *Diagn Cytopathol* 1996;15:211–220.

526. Pinto RG, Couto F, Mandreker S. Infarction after fine needle aspiration. A report of four cases. *Acta Cytol* 1996;40:739–741.

527. Rastogi A, Jain M, Agarawal T, et al. Parathyroid lipoadenoma: case report and review of the literature. *Indian J Pathol Microbiol* 2006;49:404–406.

528. Gilmour JR. The embryology of the parathyroid glands, the thymus and certain associated remnants. *J Pathol Bacteriol* 1937;45:507–522.

529. Grimelius L, Akerstrom G, Johansson H, et al. Anatomy and histopathology of human parathyroid glands. *Pathol Annu* 1981;16:1–24.

530. Akerstrom G, Malmaeus J, Bergstrom R. Surgical anatomy of human parathyroid glands. *Surgery* 1984;95:14–21.

531. DeLellis RA, ed. *Tumors of the Parathyroid Glands.* Volume Fascicle 6. Washington, DC: Armed Forces Institute of Pathology, 1993.

532. Akerston G, Malmeus J, Bergstrom R. Surgical anatomy of human parathyroid glands. *Surgery* 1984;96:14–21.

533. Cinti S, Balercia G, Zingaretti MC, et al. The normal human parathyroid gland. A histochemical and ultrastructural study with particular reference to follicular structures. *J Submicrosc Cytol* 1983;15:661–679.

534. Dufour DR, Wilkerson SY. The normal parathyroid revisited: percentage of stromal fat. *Hum Pathol* 1982;13:717–721.

535. Dufour DR, Durkowski C. Sudan IV stain. Its limitations in evaluating parathyroid functional status. *Arch Pathol Lab Med* 1982;106:224–227.

536. Dekker A, Dunsford HA, Geyer SJ. The normal parathyroid gland at autopsy: the significance of stromal fat in adult patients. *J Pathol* 1979;128:127–132.

537. Dolgin C, Lo Gerfo P, LiVolsi V, et al. Twenty-five year experience with primary hyperparathyroidism at Columbia Presbyterian Medical Center. *Head Neck Surg* 1979;2:92–98.

538. Farnebo LO. Primary hyperparathyroidism. Update on pathophysiology, clinical presentation and surgical treatment. *Scand J Surg* 2004;93:282–287.

539. Prinz R, Barbato A, Braithwaite S, et al. Prior irradiation and the development of coexistent differentiated thyroid cancer and hyperparathyroidism. *Cancer* 1982;439:874–877.

540. Arnold A, Shattuck TM, Mallya SM, et al. Molecular pathogenesis of primary hyperparathyroidism. *J Bone Miner Res* 2002;17(Suppl 2):N30–N36.

541. Debruyne F, Ostyn F, Delaere P. Distribution of the solitary adenoma over the parathyroid glands. *J Laryngol Otol* 1997;111:459–460.

542. Noguchi S, Motomura K, Inaji H, et al. Clonal analysis of parathyroid adenomas by means of the polymerase chain reaction. *Cancer Lett* 1994;78:93–97.

543. Shundo Y, Nogimura H, Kita Y, et al. Spontaneous parathyroid adenoma hemorrhage. *Jpn J Thorac Cardiovasc Surg* 2002;50:391–394.

544. Sall M, Kissmeyer-Nielsen P, Kiil J. [Cystic parathyroid adenoma. A rare cause of primary hyperparathyroidism]. *Ugeskr Laeger* 2002;164:4291–4292.

545. Govindaraj S, Wasserman J, Rezaee R, et al. Parathyroid adenoma autoinfarction: a report of a case. *Head Neck* 2003;25:695–699.

546. Liechty RD, Teter A, Suba EJ. The tiny parathyroid adenoma. *Surgery* 1986;100:1048–1052.

547. Williams ED. Pathology of the parathyroid glands. *J Clin Endocrinol Metab* 1974;3:285–303.

548. Summers GW. Parathyroid update: a review of 220 cases. *Ear Nose Throat J* 1996;75:434–439.

549. Summers GW. Parathyroid exploration. A review of 125 cases. *Arch Otolaryngol Head Neck Surg* 1991;117:1237–1241.

550. Stojadinovic A, Hoos A, Nissan A, et al. Parathyroid neoplasms: clinical, histopathological, and tissue microarray-based molecular analysis. *Hum Pathol* 2003;34:54–64.

551. Chang YJ, Mittal V, Remine S, et al. Correlation between clinical and histological findings in parathyroid tumors suspicious for carcinoma. *Am Surg* 2006;72:419–426.

552. Szende B, Farid P, Vegso G, et al. Apoptosis and P53, Bcl-2 and Bax gene expression in parathyroid glands of patients with hyperparathyroidism. *Pathol Oncol Res* 2004;10:98–103.

553. DeLellis RA. Parathyroid carcinoma: an overview. *Adv Anat Pathol* 2005;12:53–61.

554. Boehm BO, Rothouse L, Wartofsky L. Metastatic occult follicular thyroid carcinoma. *JAMA* 1976;235:2420–2421.

555. Westra WH, Pritchett DD, Udelsman R. Intraoperative confirmation of parathyroid tissue during parathyroid exploration: a retrospective evaluation of the frozen section. *Am J Surg Pathol* 1998;22:538–544.

556. Giorgadze T, Stratton B, Baloch ZW, et al. Oncocytic parathyroid adenoma: problem in cytological diagnosis. *Diagn Cytopathol* 2004;31:276–280.

557. Erickson LA, Jin L, Papotti M, et al. Oxyphil parathyroid carcinomas: a clinicopathologic and immunohistochemical study of 10 cases. *Am J Surg Pathol* 2002;26:344–349.

558. Ziffer JA, Fajman WA. Ectopic parathyroid gland. Localization with thallium-201 SPECT. *Clin Nucl Med* 1987;12:617–619.

559. Piga M, Serra A, Uccheddu A, et al. Decisive presurgical role of MIBI SPECT/CT in identifying within a calcific thyroid nodule the parathyroid responsible for primary hyperparathyroidism. *Surgery* 2006;140:837–838.

560. Johnson LR, Doherty G, Lairmore T, et al. Evaluation of the performance and clinical impact of a rapid intraoperative parathyroid hormone assay in conjunction with preoperative imaging and concise parathyroidectomy. *Clin Chem* 2001;47:919–925.

561. Roslyn JJ, Mulder DG, Gordon HE. Persistent and recurrent hyperparathyroidism. *Am J Surg* 1981;142:21–25.

562. Gross ND, Wax MK. Unilateral and bilateral surgery for parathyroid disease. *Otolaryngol Clin North Am* 2004;37:799–817, ix–x.

563. Perrier ND, Ituarte PH, Morita E, et al. Parathyroid surgery: separating promise from reality. *J Clin Endocrinol Metab* 2002;87:1024–1029.

564. Harness JK, Ramsburg SR, Nishiyama RH, et al. Multiple adenomas of the parathyroids: do they exist? *Arch Surg* 1979;114:468–474.

565. Tezelman S, Shen W, Shaver JK, et al. Double parathyroid adenomas. Clinical and biochemical characteristics before and after parathyroidectomy. *Ann Surg* 1993;218:300–307; discussion 307–309.

566. Zhou W, Katz MH, Deftos LJ, et al. Metachronous double parathyroid adenomas involving two different cell types: chief cell and oxyphil cell. *Endocr Pract* 2003;9:522–525.

567. Bergson EJ, Heller KS. The clinical significance and anatomic distribution of parathyroid double adenomas. *J Am Coll Surg* 2004;198:185–189.

568. Ogus M, Mayir B, Dinckan A. Mediastinal, cystic and functional parathyroid adenoma in patients with double parathyroid adenomas: a case report. *Acta Chir Belg* 2006;106:736–738.

569. Alveryd A, El-Zawahry MD, Herlitz P, et al. Primary hyperplasia of the parathyroids. *Acta Chir Scand* 1975;141:24–30.

570. Schantz A. The microscopical pathology of primary parathyroid hyperplasia. *Ann Clin Lab Sci* 1979;9:314–318.

571. Awad SS, Miskulin J, Thompson N. Parathyroid adenomas versus four-gland hyperplasia as the cause of primary hyperparathyroidism in patients with prolonged lithium therapy. *World J Surg* 2003;27:486–488.

572. Penner CR, Thompson LD. Primary parathyroid hyperplasia. *Ear Nose Throat J* 2003;82:363.

573. Marsden P, Anderson J, Doyle D, et al. Familial hyperparathyroidism. *Br Med J* 1971;3:87–90.

574. Perrier ND, Villablanca A, Larsson C, et al. Genetic screening for MEN1 mutations in families presenting with familial primary hyperparathyroidism. *World J Surg* 2002;26:907–913.

575. Hunt PS, Poole M, Reeve TS. A reappraisal of the surgical anatomy of the thyroid and parathyroid glands. *Br J Surg* 1968;55:63–66.

576. Thompson NW, Eckhauser FE, Harness JK. The anatomy of primary hyperparathyroidism. *Surgery* 1982;92:814–821.

577. Takahashi F, Denda M, Finch JL, et al. Hyperplasia of the parathyroid gland without secondary hyperparathyroidism. *Kidney Int* 2002;61:1332–1338.

578. Hedback G, Oden A. Parathyroid water clear cell hyperplasia, an O-allele associated condition. *Hum Genet* 1994;94:195–197.

579. Persson S, Hansson G, Hedman I, et al. Primary parathyroid hyperplasia of water-clear cell type. Transformation of water-clear cells into chief cells. *Acta Pathol Microbiol Immunol Scand [A]* 1986;94:391–395.

580. Goshen O, Aviel-Ronen S, Dori S, et al. Brown tumour of hyperparathyroidism in the mandible associated with atypical parathyroid adenoma. *J Laryngol Otol* 2000;114:302–304.

581. Wani S, Hao Z. Atypical cystic adenoma of the parathyroid gland: case report and review of literature. *Endocr Pract* 2005;11:389–393.

582. Fernandez-Ranvier GG, Khanafshar E, Jensen K, et al. Parathyroid carcinoma, atypical parathyroid adenoma, or parathyromatosis? *Cancer* 2007;110:255–264.

583. Yener S, Saklamaz A, Demir T, et al. Primary hyperparathyroidism due to atypical parathyroid adenoma presenting with peroneus brevis tendon rupture. *J Endocrinol Invest* 2007;30:442–444.

584. Fyfe ST, Hoover LA, Zuckerbraun L, et al. Parathyroid carcinoma: clinical presentation and treatment. *Am J Otolaryngol* 1990;11:268–273.

585. Agrawal R, Agarwal A, Kar DK, et al. Parathyroid carcinoma. *J Assoc Physicians India* 2001;49:990–993.

586. Kebebew E. Parathyroid carcinoma. *Curr Treat Options Oncol* 2001;2:347–354.

587. Brown JJ, Mohamed H, Williams-Smith L, et al. Primary hyperparathyroidism secondary to simultaneous bilateral parathyroid carcinoma. *Ear Nose Throat J* 2002;81:395–398, 400–401.

588. Beus KS, Stack BC Jr. Parathyroid carcinoma. *Otolaryngol Clin North Am* 2004;37:845–854, x.

589. Clayman GL, Gonzalez HE, El-Naggar A, et al. Parathyroid carcinoma: evaluation and interdisciplinary management. *Cancer* 2004;100:900–905.

590. Iacobone M, Lumachi F, Favia G. Up-to-date on parathyroid carcinoma: analysis of an experience of 19 cases. *J Surg Oncol* 2004;88:223–228.

591. Wiseman SM, Rigual NR, Hicks WL Jr, et al. Parathyroid carcinoma: a multicenter review of clinicopathologic features and treatment outcomes. *Ear Nose Throat J* 2004;83:491–494.

592. Rodgers SE, Perrier ND. Parathyroid carcinoma. *Curr Opin Oncol* 2006;18:16–22.

593. Thompson SD, Prichard AJ. The management of parathyroid carcinoma. *Curr Opin Otolaryngol Head Neck Surg* 2004;12:93–97.

594. Snover DC, Foucar K. Mitotic activity in benign parathyroid disease. *Am J Clin Pathol* 1981; 75:345–347.

595. Chaitin BA, Goldman RL. Mitotic activity in benign parathyroid disease. *Am J Clin Pathol* 1981;76:363–364.

596. Raizis AM, Becroft DM, Shaw RL, et al. A mitotic recombination in Wilms tumor occurs between the parathyroid hormone locus and 11p13. *Hum Genet* 1985;70:344–346.

597. Kameyama K, DeLellis RA, Lloyd RV, et al. Parathyroid carcinomas: can clinical outcomes for parathyroid carcinomas be determined by histologic evaluation alone? *Endocr Pathol* 2002;13:135–139.

598. Koshiyama M, Fujii H, Konishi M, et al. Recurrent clear cell carcinoma of the ovary changing into producing parathyroid hormone-related protein (PTH-rP) with hypercalcemia. *Eur J Obstet Gynecol Reprod Biol* 1999;82:227–229.

599. Severin MC, Jonas T. Parathyroid carcinoma. *Isr Med Assoc J* 2003;5:604.

600. Busaidy NL, Jimenez C, Habra MA, et al. Parathyroid carcinoma: a 22-year experience. *Head Neck* 2004;26:716–726.

601. Yamaguchi K, Kishikawa H, Shichiri M. [Familial hyperparathyroidism]. *Nippon Rinsho* 1995;53:895–898.

602. Teh BT, Farnebo F, Twigg S, et al. Familial isolated hyperparathyroidism maps to the hyperparathyroidism-jaw tumor locus in 1q21-q32 in a subset of families. *J Clin Endocrinol Metab* 1998;83:2114–2120.

603. Honda M, Tsukada T, Tanaka H, et al. A novel mutation of the MEN1 gene in a Japanese kindred with familial isolated primary hyperparathyroidism. *Eur J Endocrinol* 2000;142: 138–143.

604. Cetani F, Pardi E, Borsari S, et al. Genetic analyses of the HRPT2 gene in primary hyperparathyroidism: germline and somatic mutations in familial and sporadic parathyroid tumors. *J Clin Endocrinol Metab* 2004;89:5583–5591.

605. Tan MH, Morrison C, Wang P, et al. Loss of parafibromin immunoreactivity is a distinguishing feature of parathyroid carcinoma. *Clin Cancer Res* 2004;10:6629–6637.

606. Gill AJ, Clarkson A, Gimm O, et al. Loss of nuclear expression of parafibromin distinguishes parathyroid carcinomas and hyperparathyroidism-jaw tumor (HPT-JT) syndrome-related adenomas from sporadic parathyroid adenomas and hyperplasias. *Am J Surg Pathol* 2006;30:1140–1149.

607. Graber AL, Jacobs K. Familial hyperparathyroidism. Medical and surgical considerations. *JAMA* 1968;204:542–544.

608. Burden RP. Familial hyperparathyroidism. *Proc R Soc Med* 1971;64:1067–1068.

609. Mallette LE, Bilezikian JP, Ketcham AS, et al. Parathyroid carcinoma in familial hyperparathyroidism. *Am J Med* 1974;57:642–648.

610. Rizzoli R, Green J 3rd, Marx SJ. Primary hyperparathyroidism in familial multiple endocrine neoplasia type I. Long-term follow-up of serum calcium levels after parathyroidectomy. *Am J Med* 1985;78:467–474.

611. Todaka M, Yamaguchi K, Miyamura N, et al. Familial primary hyperparathyroidism: study of the pedigree in three generations. *Intern Med* 1992;31:712–715.

612. VanderWalde LH, Haigh PI. Surgical approach to the patient with familial hyperparathyroidism. *Curr Treat Options Oncol* 2006;7:326–333.

613. Calender A, Cougard P. Primary hyperparathyroidism: genetic heterogeneity suggesting different pathogenesis in sporadic and familial forms of parathyroid hyperplasia and tumors. *Eur J Endocrinol* 1996;134:263–266.

614. Ippolito G, Palazzo FF, Sebag F, et al. A single-institution 25-year review of true parathyroid cysts. *Langenbecks Arch Surg* 2006;391:13–18.

615. Fortson JK, Patel VG, Henderson VJ. Parathyroid cysts: a case report and review of the literature. *Laryngoscope* 2001;111:1726–1728.

616. Absher KJ, Truong LD, Khurana KK, et al. Parathyroid cytology: avoiding diagnostic pitfalls. *Head Neck* 2002;24:157–164.

617. Hamy A, Masson S, Heymann MF, et al. [Parathyroid cyst. Report of ten cases]. *Ann Chir* 2002;127:203–207.

618. Makino T, Sugimoto T, Kaji H, et al. Functional giant parathyroid cyst with high concentration of CA19-9 in cystic fluid. *Endocr J* 2003;50:215–219.

619. Perez JA, Poblete MT, Salem C. [Symptomatic parathyroid cysts. Report of one case]. *Rev Med Chil* 2003;131:432–435.

620. Sheikh SS, Massloom HS. Lipoadenoma: is it arising from thyroid or parathyroid? A diagnostic dilemma. *ORL J Otorhinolaryngol Relat Spec* 2002;64:448–450.

621. Fischer I, Wieczorek R, Sidhu GS, et al. Myxoid lipoadenoma of parathyroid gland: a case report and literature review. *Ann Diagn Pathol* 2006;10:294–296.

622. Chow LS, Erickson LA, Abu-Lebdeh HS, et al. Parathyroid lipoadenomas: a rare cause of primary hyperparathyroidism. *Endocr Pract* 2006;12:131–136.

623. Fitko R, Roth SI, Hines JR, et al. Parathyromatosis in hyperparathyroidism. *Hum Pathol* 1990;21:234–237.

624. Baloch ZW, Fraker D, LiVolsi VA. Parathyromatosis as cause of recurrent secondary hyperparathyroidism: a cytologic diagnosis. *Diagn Cytopathol* 2001;25:403–405.

625. Kendrick ML, Charboneau JW, Curlee KJ, et al. Risk of parathyromatosis after fine-needle aspiration. *Am Surg* 2001;67:290–293; discussion 293–294.

626. Lee PC, Mateo RB, Clarke MR, et al. Parathyromatosis: a cause for recurrent hyperparathyroidism. *Endocr Pract* 2001;7:189–192.

627. Reddick RL, Costa JC, Marx SJ. Parathyroid hyperplasia and parathyromatosis. *Lancet* 1977;1:549.

628. Nakazawa H, Rosen P, Lane N, et al. Frozen section experience in 3000 cases. Accuracy, limitations, and value in residency training. *Am J Clin Pathol* 1968;49:41–51.

629. Dehner LP, Rosai J. Frozen section examination in surgical pathology: a retrospective study of one year experience, comprising 778 cases. *Minn Med* 1977;60:83–94.

630. McGarity WC, Mathews WH, Fulenwider JT, et al. The surgical management of primary hyperparathyroidism: a personal series. *Ann Surg* 1981;193:794–804.

631. Dankwa EK, Davies JD. Frozen section diagnosis: an audit. *J Clin Pathol* 1985;38:1235–1240.

632. Baloch ZW, LiVolsi VA. Intraoperative assessment of thyroid and parathyroid lesions. *Semin Diagn Pathol* 2002;19:219–226.

633. Dewan AK, Kapadia SB, Hollenbeak CS, et al. Is routine frozen section necessary for parathyroid surgery? *Otolaryngol Head Neck Surg* 2005;133:857–862.

634. Faquin WC, Roth SI. Frozen section of thyroid and parathyroid specimens. *Arch Pathol Lab Med* 2006;130:1260.

635. King DT, Hirose FM. Chief cell intracytoplasmic fat used to evaluate parathyroid disease by frozen section. *Arch Pathol Lab Med* 1979;103:609–612.

636. Bondeson AG, Bondeson L, Ljungberg O, et al. Fat staining in parathyroid disease—diagnostic value and impact on surgical strategy: clinicopathologic analysis of 191 cases. *Hum Pathol* 1985;16:1255–1263.

637. Westra WH, Pritchett DD, Udelsman R. Intraoperative confirmation of parathyroid tissue during parathyroid exploration: a retrospective evaluation of the frozen section. *Am J Surg Pathol* 1998;22:538–544.

638. Ollila DW, Caudle AS, Cance WG, et al. Successful minimally invasive parathyroidectomy for primary hyperparathyroidism without using intraoperative parathyroid hormone assays. *Am J Surg* 2006;191:52–56.

639. Gil-Cardenas A, Gamino R, Reza A, et al. Is intraoperative parathyroid hormone assay mandatory for the success of targeted parathyroidectomy? *J Am Coll Surg* 2007;204: 286–290.

640. Butterworth PC, Nicholson ML. Surgical anatomy of the parathyroid glands in secondary hyperparathyroidism. *J R Coll Surg Edinb* 1998;43:271–273.

641. Silver J, Kilav R, Naveh-Many T. Mechanisms of secondary hyperparathyroidism. *Am J Physiol Renal Physiol* 2002;283:F367–F376.

642. Lewin E. Parathyroid hormone regulation in normal and uremic rats. Reversibility of secondary hyperparathyroidism after experimental kidney transplantation. *Dan Med Bull* 2004;51:184–206.

643. Malmaeus J, Grimelius L, Johansson H, et al. Parathyroid pathology in hyperparathyroidism secondary to chronic renal failure. *Scand J Urol Nephrol* 1984;18:157–166.

644. Akerstrom G, Malmaeus J, Grimelius L, et al. Histological changes in parathyroid glands in subclinical and clinical renal disease. An autopsy investigation. *Scand J Urol Nephrol* 1984;18:75–84.

645. Salander H, Tisell LE. Latent hypoparathyroidism in patients with autotransplanted parathyroid glands. *Am J Surg* 1980;139:385–388.

646. Walker RP, Paloyan E, Kelley TF, et al. Parathyroid autotransplantation in patients undergoing a total thyroidectomy: a review of 261 patients. *Otolaryngol Head Neck Surg* 1994;111(3 Pt 1):258–264.

647. Cooper Worobey C, Magee CC. Humoral hypercalcemia of malignancy presenting after oncologic surgery. *Kidney Int* 2006;70:225–229.

648. Rodan SB, Insogna KL, Vignery AM, et al. Factors associated with humoral hypercalcemia of malignancy stimulate adenylate cyclase in osteoblastic cells. *J Clin Invest* 1983;72: 1511–1515.

649. Stewart AF. Hyperparathyroidism, humoral hypercalcemia of malignancy, and the anabolic actions of parathyroid hormone and parathyroid hormone-related protein on the skeleton. *J Bone Miner Res* 2002;17:758–762.

650. Fereidooni F, Horvath E, Kovacs K. Humoral hypercalcemia of malignancy due to bipartite squamous cell/small cell carcinoma of the esophagus immunoreactive for parathyroid hormone related protein. *Dis Esophagus* 2003;16:335–338.

651. Schwarz P, Larsen NE, Lonborg Friis IM, et al. Familial hypocalciuric hypercalcemia and neonatal severe hyperparathyroidism associated with mutations in the human Ca2+-sensing receptor gene in three Danish families. *Scand J Clin Lab Invest* 2000;60:221–227.

652. Pidasheva S, D'Souza-Li L, Canaff L, et al. CASRdb: calcium-sensing receptor locus-specific database for mutations causing familial (benign) hypocalciuric hypercalcemia, neonatal severe hyperparathyroidism, and autosomal dominant hypocalcemia. *Hum Mutat* 2004; 24:107–111.

653. Watanabe N, Yamauchi Y, Matsumoto J, et al. [Familial hypocalciuric hypercalcemia with severe neonatal primary hyperparathyroidism]. *Nippon Naika Gakkai Zasshi* 1982;71: 479–484.

654. Abati A, Skarulis MC, Shawker T, et al. Ultrasound-guided fine-needle aspiration of parathyroid lesions: a morphological and immunocytochemical approach. *Hum Pathol* 1995; 26:338–343.

655. Odashiro AN, Nguyen GK. Fine-needle aspiration cytology of an intrathyroid parathyroid adenoma. *Diagn Cytopathol* 2006;34:790–792.

656. Tseng FY, Hsiao YL, Chang TC. Ultrasound-guided fine needle aspiration cytology of parathyroid lesions. A review of 72 cases. *Acta Cytol* 2002;46:1029–1036.

657. Saggiorato E, Bergero N, Volante M, et al. Galectin-3 and Ki-67 expression in multiglandular parathyroid lesions. *Am J Clin Pathol* 2006;126:59–66.

658. Thomopoulou GE, Tseleni-Balafouta S, Lazaris AC, et al. Immunohistochemical detection of cell cycle regulators, Fhit protein and apoptotic cells in parathyroid lesions. *Eur J Endocrinol* 2003;148:81–87.

659. Loda M, Lipman J, Cukor B, et al. Nodular foci in parathyroid adenomas and hyperplasias: an immunohistochemical analysis of proliferative activity. *Hum Pathol* 1994;25:1050–1056.

660. Falkmer UG, Falkmer S. The value of cytometric DNA analysis as a prognostic tool in neuroendocrine neoplastic diseases. *Pathol Res Pract* 1995;191:281–303.

661. Harlow S, Roth SI, Bauer K, et al. Flow cytometric DNA analysis of normal and pathologic parathyroid glands. *Mod Pathol* 1991;4:310–315.

662. Berczi C, Bocsi J, Balazs G, et al. Flow cytometric DNA analysis of benign hyperfunctioning parathyroid glands: significant difference in the S phase fraction and proliferative index between adenomas and hyperplasias. *Pathology* 2002;34:442–445.

663. Sammarelli G, Zannoni M, Bonomini S, et al. A translocation t(4; 13)(q21;q14) as single clonal chromosomal abnormality in a parathyroid adenoma. *Tumori* 2007;93:97–99.

664. Tominaga Y, Kohara S, Namii Y, et al. Clonal analysis of nodular parathyroid hyperplasia in renal hyperparathyroidism. *World J Surg* 1996;20:744–750; discussion 750–752.

665. Shan L, Nakamura Y, Murakami M, et al. Clonal emergence in uremic parathyroid hyperplasia is not related to MEN1 gene abnormality. *Jpn J Cancer Res* 1999;90:965–969.

666. Arnold A, Motokura T, Bloom T, et al. PRAD1 (cyclin D1): a parathyroid neoplasia gene on 11q13. *Henry Ford Hosp Med J* 1992;40:177–180.

667. Motokura T, Arnold A. PRAD1/cyclin D1 proto-oncogene: genomic organization, 5' DNA sequence, and sequence of a tumor-specific rearrangement breakpoint. *Genes Chromosomes Cancer* 1993;7:89–95.

668. Hsi ED, Zukerberg LR, Yang WI, et al. Cyclin D1/PRAD1 expression in parathyroid adenomas: an immunohistochemical study. *J Clin Endocrinol Metab* 1996;81:1736–1739.

669. Tominaga Y, Tsuzuki T, Uchida K, et al. Expression of PRAD1/cyclin D1, retinoblastoma gene products, and Ki67 in parathyroid hyperplasia caused by chronic renal failure versus primary adenoma. *Kidney Int* 1999;55:1375–1383.

670. Cetani F, Pardi E, Viacava P, et al. A reappraisal of the Rb1 gene abnormalities in the diagnosis of parathyroid cancer. *Clin Endocrinol (Oxf)* 2004;60:99–106.

671. Lumachi F, Basso SM, Basso U. Parathyroid cancer: etiology, clinical presentation and treatment. *Anticancer Res* 2006;26:4803–4807.

672. Lloyd RV, Carney JA, Ferreiro JA, et al. Immunohistochemical analysis of the cell cycle-associated antigens Ki-67 and retinoblastoma protein in parathyroid carcinomas and adenomas. *Endocr Pathol* 1995;6:279–287.

673. Ricci F, Mingazzini PL, Sebastiani V, et al. P53 as a marker of differentiation between hyperplastic and adenomatous parathyroids. *Ann Diagn Pathol* 2002;6:229–235.

674. Tokumoto M, Tsuruya K, Fukuda K, et al. Reduced p21, p27 and vitamin D receptor in the nodular hyperplasia in patients with advanced secondary hyperparathyroidism. *Kidney Int* 2002;62:1196–1207.

675. Hunt JL, Carty SE, Yim JH, et al. Allelic loss in parathyroid neoplasia can help characterize malignancy. *Am J Surg Pathol* 2005;29:1049–1055.

Ronald A. DeLellis
Shamlal Mangray

The Adrenal Glands

INTRODUCTION

Diseases of the adrenal glands may be associated with a diverse and highly complex array of clinical syndromes resulting from abnormalities in the production and secretion of steroid hormones or catecholamines. From the vantage point of the surgical pathologist, the complexity of adrenal diseases is magnified by the fact that the same clinical syndromes may develop as a consequence of vastly different pathophysiologic mechanisms. Therefore, gross and microscopic examination of the biopsied or resected adrenal gland must be supplemented by a working knowledge of the pathophysiology of the gland and by familiarity with the clinical and laboratory data in each case. Because morphologic criteria alone may be insufficient to arrive at a correct diagnosis, additional technologies may be necessary to resolve specific problems.

Further complicating the role of the surgical pathologist has been the detection of a variety of mass lesions by computed tomography (CT), magnetic resonance imaging (MRI), or positron emission tomography (PET) in the workup of patients for nonadrenal conditions. The presence of incidental lesions of varying sizes (incidentalomas) has been demonstrated in up to 5% of individuals subjected to abdominal CT studies (1). The vast majority of incidentalomas are of cortical origin, and a proportion of these lesions undergo needle core biopsy or fine-needle aspiration biopsy, posing additional diagnostic challenges.

DEVELOPMENT, ANATOMY, AND PHYSIOLOGY OF THE ADRENAL GLANDS

The adrenal glands are composite endocrine organs located on the superomedial aspects of the kidneys (2). The cortex begins its development at 5 to 6 weeks of gestation (9-mm embryo stage) as a proliferation of cells from the peritoneum at the base of the dorsal mesentery (3). By 8 weeks, the cortical cells separate from the mesothelium and become surrounded by a fibrous capsule. In the fetus, the cortex is divisible into a broad inner zone composed of large eosinophilic cells (provisional zone or fetal cortex) and an outer zone that is destined to become the adult (definitive) cortex. The major secretory product of the fetal cortex is dehydroepiandrosterone sulfate, whereas the cells of the adult cortex produce cortisol, aldosterone, and sex steroids. At birth, the fetal cortex occupies approximately 75% of the cortical volume, but shortly thereafter, it begins to undergo a series of involutional changes that are associated with an approximate 50% reduction in the gland weight (4). The combined weight of the glands at birth is approximately 10 g. Concurrent with the involution of the fetal cortex, the permanent cortex proliferates toward the center of the gland. The fetal cortex progressively decreases in volume and occupies approximately 20% of the cortical volume in the twelfth postgestational week.

In the normal adult, each gland weighs between 4 and 5 g, although greater weights have been recorded in hospitalized patients dying after prolonged illnesses presumably as a result of prolonged stimulation of the glands during stress (2,5). The latter finding correlates with stress-related lipid depletion mediated by increased secretion of adrenocorticotropic hormone (ACTH). Each adrenal gland measures approximately $5 \times 3 \times 1$ cm. The right gland has a roughly pyramidal shape, whereas the left gland has a cresentic shape. The glands have a tripartite structure that consists of head (medial), body (middle), and tail (lateral) portions (6,7). The central vein emerges from the gland at the junction of the head and body of the gland. Within the gland itself, the muscle bundles of the central vein are eccentric and are oriented toward the medulla.

In the fresh state, the outer cortex is bright yellow, whereas the inner cortical zone is brown to tan. The cortex measures approximately 1 mm in thickness in adults and constitutes approximately 90% of the total glandular weight. It consists of the glomerulosa, fasciculata, and reticularis zones (2,8). The glomerulosa comprises up to 15% of the cortical volume and is composed of relatively small lipid-poor cells that synthesize mineralocorticoids. Because this layer is often incomplete, the fasciculata may abut the capsule of the gland directly. The fasciculata is composed of columns of lipid-rich cells, which synthesize both glucocorticoids and sex steroids. This zone occupies 70% to 80% of the cortical volume. Stimulation of the adrenal by ACTH leads to depletion of lipid stores from the fasciculata (2), so that the cells of this layer become compact and eosinophilic (9). In the process of recovery, the lipid content becomes replenished (lipid reversion). The remainder of the cortex is composed of the reticularis, which is capable of synthesis of both glucocorticoids and sex steroids. These cells are characterized by eosinophilic cytoplasm, scanty lipid vacuoles, and prominent deposits of lipochrome pigment, which are responsible for the brown color of the reticularis.

Cortical extrusions are found frequently in the adrenal glands of adults. They are characterized by the presence of nodular groups of cortical cells that extend into the periadrenal fat. Typically, they are attached to the adjacent cortex by a small pedicle and are surrounded by a fibrous capsule; however, they may be completely separated from the gland in some instances.

Focal aggregates of lymphocytes are an incidental finding in the adrenal cortices of normal adults and increase in frequency with the age of the patient (9a). Most of the lymphocytes are of T lineage (10).

The cells of the glomerulosa contain an abundance of smooth endoplasmic reticulum and small amounts of granular endoplasmic reticulum. The mitochondria in this layer tend to be elongated with lamelliform cristae (2,11). In contrast, the mitochondria of the fasciculata and reticularis zones are round to ovoid with a predominance of tubulovesicular cristae. The intermediate filaments of cortical cells include vimentin and variable amounts of low–molecular-weight cytokeratins (12).

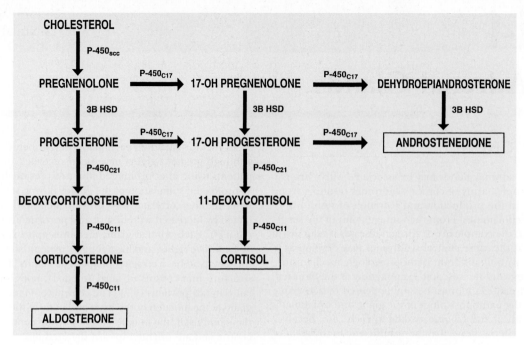

Figure 14.1. Biosynthesis of adrenal steroid hormones.

The precursor of all steroid hormones is cholesterol, which is derived from circulating low-density lipoproteins. After internalization into the cortical cells, the lipoproteins are hydrolyzed with the production of cholesterol esters, which yield cholesterol and free fatty acids (13,14). There are four cytochrome P450 enzymes that are involved in the biosynthesis of adrenal steroids ($P450_{scc}$, $P450_{c17}$, $P450_{c21}$, and $P450_{c11}$). The enzyme 3β-hydroxysteroid dehydrogenase does not belong to the P450 cytochrome family (Fig. 14.1). The synthesis and secretion of glucocorticoids, 18-hydroxysteroids, and androgens are regulated by a complex set of control mechanisms. Hypothalamic corticotropin-releasing hormone (CRH), a 41–amino acid polypeptide, reaches the anterior pituitary gland via the hypophyseal portal system, where it stimulates the release of ACTH (14).

In the adrenal cortex, ACTH stimulates cortical cells by activation of intracytoplasmic cyclases that form cyclic adenosine monophosphate (cAMP) and guanosine monophosphate (GMP) from adenosine triphosphate (ATP) and guanosine triphosphate (GTP), respectively. Both cortisol and ACTH inhibit the release of CRH, and cortisol also inhibits secretion of ACTH. The secretion of ACTH is normally episodic, with the number and duration of episodes increasing to a peak in the early morning and a nadir in the evening. This characteristic pattern is responsible for the circadian rhythm in the secretion of cortisol in healthy individuals (14). The secretion of aldosterone is regulated primarily by the renin-angiotensin system, which operates by volume-regulated changes (14). In addition, aldosterone synthesis and secretion are regulated by potassium ions and, to some extent, by ACTH (15,16).

The intra-adrenal and extra-adrenal paraganglia and the sympathetic nervous system are intimately associated during embryonic development and arise from the neural crest. The cortical anlage is invaded on its medial aspect by primitive sympathetic cells (PSCs) and nerve fibers that originate from the contiguous prevertebral and paravertebral sympathetic tissue in the 14-mm embryo. Some primitive sympathetic cells, however, may penetrate the anlage without associated nerve fibers (17,18). The PSCs are first apparent as nodular aggregates in the cortex, where they may form rosettes or pseudorosettes. Chromaffin cells are identifiable among the primitive sympathetic cells between the 27- and 33-mm stages and gradually increase in number. The nodules of PSCs peak in number and size between 17 and 20 weeks and then decline (Fig. 14.2). Groups of these cells may, however, persist until birth and may also be apparent in early infancy (see section on neuroblastoma). As the medullary chromaffin cells reach their maximum volume, there is a progressive involution of extra-adrenal chromaffin cells.

In the adult, the adrenal medulla occupies 8% to 10% of the gland volume and has an average weight of 0.44 g (5). The major portion of the medulla lies within the head of the gland, whereas the body of the gland contains medullary (chromaffin)

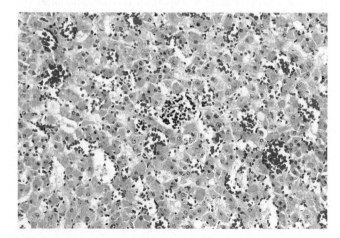

Figure 14.2. Fetal adrenal (16 weeks) with groups of primitive sympathetic cells forming neuroblastic nodules.

cells within its crest and usually within one alar region (6). The average corticomedullary ratio is 5:1 in the head of the gland and 14.7:1 in the body. The tail of the adrenal does not normally contain medullary tissue.

Medullary (chromaffin) cells are typically arranged in small nests and cords that are separated by a rich capillary network. A few medullary cells, particularly those found in the juxtacortical regions, may have enlarged, hyperchromatic nuclei, which increase in number with age (19). In addition, the cytoplasm of medullary cells frequently contains periodic acid-Schiff (PAS)–positive hyaline globules that also tend to be most prominent in juxtacortical regions (20). The most characteristic feature of medullary cells at the ultrastructural level is the presence of membrane-bound secretory granules in which catecholamines and other products are stored. In specimens initially fixed in glutaraldehyde, norepinephrine granules have very dense cores that are separated from their limiting membranes by an irregular lucent space or halo. Epinephrine granules have moderately dense cores that are closely applied to their limiting membranes (21,22). A few medullary cells may also contain intranuclear pseudoinclusions that represent invaginations of the cytoplasm into the nucleus.

In the past, the catecholamine content of chromaffin cells has been demonstrated by a variety of histochemical techniques (23–26), but in current surgical pathology practice, immunohistochemical stains for chromogranins, chromomembrins, synaptophysin, and regulatory peptides are most commonly used (27–30). In addition, antibodies to catecholamine-synthesizing enzymes can be used as markers for medullary cells.

A few ganglion cells are present within the medulla either as single cells or small cell clusters. S-100 protein–positive sustentacular cells are present at the peripheries of the medullary cords and nests and are also evident around the ganglion cells. In addition, a cell type that has been termed the small, intensely

fluorescent cell or small, granule-containing cell is also seen in the medulla of most mammals. These cells may function as interneurons (31). There may also be small collections of lymphocytes and plasma cells within the medulla, but their significance is unknown.

The precursor of the catecholamines is tyrosine, which is converted sequentially to DOPA, dopamine, norepinephrine, and epinephrine by a series of well-characterized enzymatic steps (Fig. 14.3) (32). The major catecholamine product of the medulla is epinephrine, which affects the activities of a wide variety of cells and tissues following its interactions with specific receptors.

In addition to the cortical and medullary cells, hybrid cells showing features of both cell types have been described in the rat. Such hybrid cells, at the ultrastructural level, contain chromaffin granules, mitochondria with tubulovesicular cristae, and relatively abundant smooth endoplasmic reticulum (33,34). However, hybrid cells do not apparently occur in human adrenal glands.

CONGENITAL ANOMALIES, DEVELOPMENTAL DISORDERS, AND METABOLIC ABNORMALITIES

ACCESSORY ADRENALS, ADRENAL FUSION, AND APLASIA

Congenital anomalies of the adrenal gland rarely come to the attention of the surgical pathologist, and the most common is heterotopia (35). Although the term "heterotopia" is commonly used for this condition, a more accurate descriptor is accessory adrenal tissue because, in most cases, orthotopic adrenal gland is also present. Most accessory adrenals consist exclu-

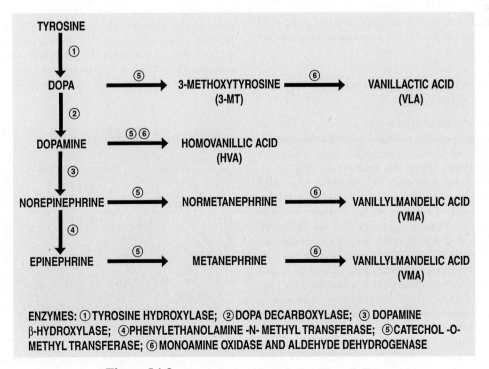

Figure 14.3. Catecholamine biosynthesis and metabolism.

sively of cortical tissue, but a few examples, particularly those in the region of the celiac ganglion, may also contain medulla (36). Accessory adrenal cortex is most frequently found in the retroperitoneal space along the course of the urogenital ridges. In addition, accessory adrenal tissue may also be discovered incidentally just beneath the renal capsule in the upper pole, at the hilar regions of the ovaries and testes, and along the course of the spermatic cord. The studies of MacLennan (37) have shown that adrenal cortical tissue is present in approximately 1% of inguinal hernia sacs from children undergoing inguinal herniorrhaphy. Rare sites of accessory adrenal tissue include pancreas, spleen, liver, mesentery, lung, and brain. Accessory adrenals may undergo hyperplasia in response to increased levels of ACTH and may serve as the site of origin of cortical neoplasms (19,38,39). True heterotopic adrenal glands may be fused with the liver or kidney and are typically surrounded by a common connective tissue capsule (40,41).

Adrenal union (fusion) and adhesion are rare anomalies that are distinguished by the presence (adrenal union) or absence (adhesion) of a connective tissue capsule. Fusion is occasionally associated with midline congenital defects, including spinal dysraphism, indeterminate visceral situs, and the Cornelia de Lange syndrome (42). Fusion of the adrenal glands can occur in patients with bilateral renal agenesis.

Aplasia of the adrenal glands has been reported in association with anencephaly; however, in most instances, the adrenal glands are markedly hypoplastic rather than completely absent (43). In approximately 10% of patients with unilateral renal agenesis, the ipsilateral adrenal gland is also absent. Several types of adrenal hypoplasia have been reported (44). Affected infants typically have signs and symptoms of adrenal insufficiency. In so-called primary hypoplasia, the adult cortex is markedly hypoplastic, but the fetal zone is retained and often demonstrates cytomegalic features. This disorder shows an X-linked pattern of inheritance and has been associated with mutations or deletions of the *DAX-1* gene (Xp21) (36,45,46). The miniature adult type of hypoplasia may appear sporadically or as an inherited abnormality with an autosomal recessive pattern of inheritance. The adrenal glands have a normal architecture despite their small size.

ADRENAL CYTOMEGALY AND BECKWITH-WIEDEMANN SYNDROME

Adrenal *cytomegaly* is characterized by the presence of focal or diffuse collections of markedly enlarged cortical cells containing hyperchromatic and pleomorphic nuclei, occasionally with nuclear pseudoinclusions within the fetal cortex (Fig. 14.4). Cytomegalic cells may measure up to 150 μm in diameter. This is a common finding that has been observed in the normal fetus and in up to 3% of stillborn infants (47,48). Cytomegalic cells may be particularly prominent in infants with the Beckwith-Wiedemann syndrome (BWS) in which the adrenal glands are typically hyperplastic (Fig. 14.5) (36). Characteristic features of BWS, which include macroglossia, prenatal and postnatal overgrowth (gigantism/hemihyperplasia), abdominal wall defects (exomphalos), and pancreatic islet cell hyperplasia leading to hypoglycemia, permit early recognition of the syndrome (Table 14.1). Hemorrhagic adrenal cortical macrocysts may also be found (49,50). Patients with BWS are predisposed to the development of malignant tumors including Wilms tumor, adrenocortical carcinoma, neuroblastoma, hepatoblastoma, and

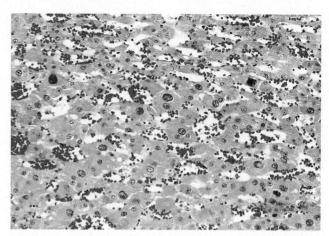

Figure 14.4. Newborn adrenal gland with focal cytomegaly involving cells of the fetal cortex.

pancreaticoblastoma (42,50). Benign adrenal cortical adenomas and ganglioneuromas have also been reported in affected patients (50). An autosomal dominant inheritance is well established in BWS, but approximately 85% of cases are actually sporadic. The molecular basis of this syndrome is complex and involves downregulation of imprinted genes within the chromosome 11p15 regions (*IGF2* and *H19* at domain 1; *CDKN1C*, *KCNQ1*, and *KCNQ1OT1* at domain 2) (50). Other syndromes that predispose to adrenal tumors (Table 14.1) are discussed later under the respective sections.

STORAGE DISEASES

Adrenoleukodystrophy (Addison-Schilder disease) is a rare, X-linked recessive disorder characterized by progressive demyelination of the central and peripheral nervous system and by adrenal cortical insufficiency (51). The disorder is caused by mutations of the gene on chromosome Xq28 encoding an ATP-binding transporter ALDP-adrenoleukodystrophy protein (*ALDP*) that is localized in the peroxisomal membrane. Several mutations have been identified and result in the defective oxidation of very long fatty acids (52). The diagnosis can be estab-

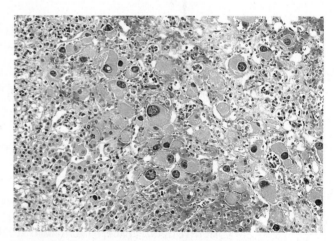

Figure 14.5. Adrenal from newborn with Beckwith-Wiedemann syndrome. There is widespread cytomegaly of the fetal cortex.

TABLE 14.1	Inherited Tumor Syndromes Associated with Adrenal Neoplasia		
Tumor	*Syndrome*	*Gene/s (Chromosome Locus)*	*Extra-Adrenal Features*
Adrenocortical and Neuroblastic Tumors	Beckwith-Wiedemann (OMIM: 130650)	*CDKN1*/NSD1, *KCNQ1*, *KCNQ1OT1*; *IGF2* and *H19* (11p15.5)	Exomphalos, macroglossia, pancreatic islet cell hyperplasia, gigantism/hemihypertrophy, Wilms tumor, hepatoblastoma, pancreaticoblastoma
Adrenocortical Tumors			
Carcinoma	Li-Fraumeni syndrome (OMIM:151623)	*TP53* (17p13.1)	Other neoplasms/cancers
PPNAD	Carney complex (OMIM:160980)	*PRKAR1A* (17q23-q24)	Lentigines and other pigmented skin lesions, myxomas, LCCST of testis, pituitary adenoma, GIST
Adenoma	MEN1 (Wermer syndrome) (OMIM:131100)	*MEN1* (11q13)	Endocrine lesions of parathyroid, pituitary, pancreas, GI tract, skin lesions
Pheochromocytoma	von Hippel-Lindau disease (OMIM:193300)	*VHL* (3p26-p35)	Retinal and cranial hemangioblastoma, RCC, cysts of multiple organs, pancreatic endocrine tumors, ELST of ear
	Familial pheochromocytoma-paraganglioma (OMIM: 115310)	*SDHD, SDHC, SDHB* (1p36.1-p35)	Paraganglioma of abdomen, thorax, head and neck
	MEN2A (Sipple syndrome) (OMIM:171400)	*RET* (10q11.2)	First-degree hyperparathyroidism (hyperplasia), MTC
	MEN2B (OMIM:162300)	*RET* (10q11.2)	Mucosal neuromas, ganglioneuromatosis of intestine, marfanoid habitus, MTC, corneal nerve lesions
	Neurofibromatosis type 1 (OMIM:162200)	*NF1* (17q11.2)	Café-au-lait macules, neurofibromas or plexiform neurofibroma, optic glioma, axillary or inguinal freckling, Lisch nodules, osseous lesions

ELST, endolymphatic sac tumors; GI, gastrointestinal; GIST, gastrointestinal stromal tumor; LCCST, large-cell calcifying Sertoli cell tumor; MEN, multiple endocrine neoplasia; MTC, medullary thyroid carcinoma; OMIM, Online Inheritance in Man (Johns Hopkins University); PPNAD, primary pigmented nodular adrenocortical disease; RCC renal cell carcinoma.

lished by the presence of hexacosanoate and other long-chain fatty acids in cultured skin fibroblasts (53). The adrenal glands in this disorder are grossly atrophic with weights ranging from 1 to 2 g or less, with ballooning and striation of the cells of the inner zona fasciculata and zona reticularis. Groups of ballooned cells form nodules that may undergo degenerative changes with the formation of large cortical vacuoles. At the ultrastructural level, there is proliferation of smooth endoplasmic reticulum and the presence of lamellar inclusions with a trilaminar structure (51). An adult variant with an onset in the second or third decades is known as adrenomyeloneuropathy, a condition that can be associated with unexplained adrenal insufficiency in the absence of neurologic manifestations at first clinical presentation (54). Cortical cells typically appear ballooned and contain linear lamellar inclusions at the ultrastructural level (53,54). A third form of the disease has been reported in women who are carriers of the abnormal gene.

Wolman disease (primary familial xanthomatosis) is a rare lipid storage disorder caused by an autosomal recessive deficiency of lysosomal acid lipase (55). The disease is characterized by the accumulation of triglycerides and cholesterol esters in a variety of tissues including the liver, spleen, and adrenal glands. Most affected individuals die by the age of 6 months. Typically, the adrenal glands are markedly enlarged even though they often retain their normal configurations. The glands often demonstrate multiple foci of calcification in association with necro-

sis and fibrosis (55). Other storage diseases (e.g., Niemann-Pick disease) may result in adrenal enlargement and hypofunction.

CONGENITAL ADRENAL HYPERPLASIA

The syndromes of congenital adrenal hyperplasia (congenital adrenogenital syndromes) result from a series of autosomal recessive enzymatic defects in the biosynthesis of adrenal steroids (56). This group of disorders is caused by deficient activity of one of the following: $P450_{c21}$ (21-hydroxylase), $P450_{c11}$ (11β-hydroxylase), 3β-hydroxysteroid dehydrogenase, $P450_{c17}$ (17-hydroxylase/17,20-lyase), or $P450_{scc}$. On clinical examination, affected patients may have abnormalities of sexual development, salt wasting, hypertension, or acute adrenal insufficiency, depending on the specific defect. In females, common abnormalities associated with these defects include masculinization in utero, postpubertal masculinization, and primary amenorrhea. Males may show signs of precocious puberty or pseudohermaphroditism. The biochemical, genetic, and molecular features of these disorders are discussed in detail elsewhere (56–59).

The most common deficiency affects the enzyme 21-hydroxylase ($P450_{c21}$) and is responsible for approximately 95% of cases of congenital adrenal hyperplasia (56). The worldwide incidence of classic 21-hydroxylase deficiency is 1 in 14,500 births, with a heterozygote frequency of approximately 1 in 60. Affected individuals have evidence of cortisol deficiency, aldosterone deficiency with salt wasting, and excess adrenal androgen production with evidence of virilization. Excess adrenal androgen production is a consequence of the accumulation of 17-hydroxypregnenolone, which is subsequently metabolized to androgenic steroids. Nonclassic 21-hydroxylase deficiency has a frequency of 1 in 100 in certain parts of the United States and is one of the most common autosomal recessive disorders. Affected individuals have mild degrees of cortisol deficiency, normal aldosterone production, and excess production of adrenal androgens. This form of 21-hydroxylase deficiency is most often diagnosed in childhood or early adulthood. A small proportion of individuals with 21-hydroxylase deficiency may have no apparent symptoms.

Deficiency of 11β-hydroxylase (P450$_{c11}$) accounts for approximately 5% of all cases of congenital adrenal hyperplasia and is associated with increased production of androgens and deoxycorticosterone (57–59). As a result, affected individuals typically exhibit signs of hyperandrogenism and hypertension. Deficiency of 17α-hydroxylase is responsible for approximately 1% of cases. External genitalia are female in both sexes. Increased levels of deoxycorticosterone are responsible for the hypertension seen in these patients.

Adrenal hyperplasia in the congenital adrenogenital syndromes results from inadequate production of glucocorticoids, leading to stimulation of the cortex by increased pituitary ACTH production. The adrenal glands become markedly enlarged with a characteristic cerebriform appearance and a tan-brown color (42). On microscopy, cortical cells are lipid depleted. In individuals with deficiency of 20,22-desmolase (P450$_{scc}$), the adrenal glands are pale yellow and are characterized on microscopic examination by vacuolated cells, occasionally with formation of cholesterol clefts and an accompanying giant-cell reaction. These disorders are usually treated by replacement of the deficient steroid hormone and surgical correction of ambiguous genitalia or hypospadias.

Adrenal cortical adenomas and carcinomas may develop, although rarely, in the setting of congenital adrenal hyperplasia (60,61). Testicular tumors can also arise in affected patients. These lesions are not autonomous neoplasms because they are dependent on the presence of elevated levels of ACTH (62). They are commonly bilateral and are most typically located in the hilar regions of the testes. The cell of origin is unknown, but the component cells of these lesions contain abundant eosinophilic cytoplasm, which lacks crystalloids of Reinke. In the series reported by Rutgers et al. (62), the diagnosis of congenital adrenal hyperplasia was made only after the appearance of testicular tumors in 18% of the cases.

HYPOFUNCTIONAL STATES

Hypofunction may occur as the result of a primary disorder of the adrenal cortex or as a secondary change caused by a disorder of the pituitary-hypothalamic axis.

PRIMARY HYPOFUNCTION

Autoimmune Adrenalitis

Inflammation of the adrenals may result from autoimmune mechanisms, infection, or a variety of other causes. Approximately 75% of cases have an autoimmune origin. In idiopathic (autoimmune) Addison disease, the glands are markedly atrophic, and the residual cortical tissue is infiltrated by chronic inflammatory cells, including lymphocytes and plasma cells. As noted in the previous section, focal aggregates of lymphocytes are a normal finding with increasing frequency in the adrenal gland of older patients (10) and should not be misconstrued as evidence of adrenalitis. All layers of the cortex are involved in autoimmune adrenalitis, but the medulla is unaffected. Typically, the capsules of the glands are fibrotic. Both humoral and cell-mediated immune mechanisms have been implicated in the development of autoimmune adrenal hypofunction. Autoantibodies to cortical cells are present in 50% of all patients and in more than 70% of women with newly diagnosed disease. The major targets for autoantibody reactivity are the adrenal cytochrome P450 enzymes (63). Affected patients can also have antibodies to gonadal, gastric parietal, and thyroid follicular cells.

Adrenocortical hypofunction may be associated with hypofunction of other endocrine glands (64). The type I polyglandular autoimmune syndrome is associated with mucocutaneous candidiasis, hypoparathyroidism, adrenal insufficiency, autoimmune thyroiditis, and diabetes mellitus. Alopecia may also be present. This form of the disease has also been termed *autoimmune polyendocrinopathy-candidiasis-ectodermal dystrophy* (*APECED*). Mutations in the *APECED* or autoimmune regulatory gene (21q22.3) have been implicated in the development of this syndrome (65,66). The type II polyglandular autoimmune syndrome is characterized by adrenal insufficiency, autoimmune thyroiditis, and insulin-dependent diabetes mellitus. The type I syndrome is inherited as an autosomal recessive trait, whereas the pattern of inheritance of the type II syndrome is usually dominant.

Tuberculosis and Fungal Diseases

Infectious disorders, including tuberculosis and fungal diseases (e.g., histoplasmosis, North and South American blastomycosis, coccidiomycosis, cryptococcosis), can affect both the cortical and medullary regions of the adrenal glands. Although tuberculosis is now a rare cause of adrenal insufficiency in the United States and Western Europe, it is a common cause in parts of the world where tuberculosis is endemic. In contrast to the shrunken appearance of the adrenal glands in idiopathic Addison disease, the glands in mycobacterial infection are typically enlarged and replaced by caseous material. Infection with *Mycobacterium avium-intracellulare*, on the other hand, is typically associated with the presence of confluent masses of histiocytes containing the acid-fast organisms.

Viruses

Cytomegalovirus (CMV) has been identified in the adrenal glands of a large proportion of patients dying of acquired immunodeficiency syndrome (67). Adrenal cortical necrosis associated with CMV infection can be severe enough to result in acute adrenal insufficiency in some instances. Both herpes simplex and varicella zoster may also involve the adrenal glands and may lead to adrenal cortical insufficiency when they are associated with extensive cortical necrosis.

Amyloidosis

Rarely, amyloid deposition can result in cortical hypofunction (68). Typically, adrenal involvement is associated with extensive systemic amyloid disease of the AA type. The adrenal glands may have a normal shape and size or may be enlarged. In severe cases, the glands are pale tan to yellow. Microscopically, amyloid deposits affect the fasciculata and reticularis zones and are typically present between the cortical cells and capillary endothelium. The cortical cells ultimately become atrophic as a result of the progressive deposition of intercellular amyloid. In patients with AL disease, the amyloid deposits are predominantly vascular in distribution.

Adrenal Hemorrhage

Adrenal hemorrhage may develop in a segmental fashion or may involve the entire adrenal (69). This syndrome may be seen in association with sepsis and shock caused by meningococcal infection or infection with other bacteria, including *Haemophilus influenzae*, *Streptococcus pneumoniae*, and *Pseudomonas aeruginosa* (Waterhouse-Friderichsen syndrome). Typically, the glands are enlarged and hemorrhagic, with necrosis of both cortical and medullary tissue. Adrenal hemorrhage in the Waterhouse-Friderichsen syndrome is regarded as the consequence rather than the cause of shock. Anticoagulant therapy may also be associated with adrenal hemorrhage. Corticomedullary necrosis of milder degrees has been reported in association with hypotension and shock (70). In patients with segmental lesions, examination of the capsular vessels and sinusoids will reveal evidence of thrombus formation. Affected cortical areas show a pattern of ischemic necrosis that ultimately heals by the process of fibrosis.

Miscellaneous Causes of Hypofunction

Rarely, adrenal hypofunction may result from bilateral involvement by tumor, most commonly metastatic carcinoma in which focal lesions of the adrenal glands are demonstrated by imaging studies. A rare case of hypofunction has been reported secondary to involvement by Erdheim-Chester disease, a non-Langerhans histiocytosis that typically involves bone but in which extraskeletal manifestations are present in up to 50% of cases. In this condition, there is diffuse enlargement of the adrenal gland secondary to infiltration by foamy histiocytes (71).

SECONDARY HYPOFUNCTION

Adrenocortical atrophy may be found in association with lesions primarily affecting the adenohypophysis or hypothalamus, leading to diminished secretion of ACTH (2). The administration of exogenous corticosteroids will produce similar changes as a result of suppression of ACTH. The adrenal glands in secondary hypofunctional states are considerably smaller than normal, although the overall configurations of the glands are retained. Typically, the cortex is bright yellow as a result of lipid accumulation in the cortical cells, the capsule is fibrotic, and the medulla is unaffected (Fig. 14.6). The zona glomerulosa is usually of normal thickness in these cases.

HYPERFUNCTIONAL STATES

ADRENOCORTICAL HYPERPLASIA

Hyperplasia of the adrenal cortex, which represents an increased cortical mass resulting from stimulation of the cortex

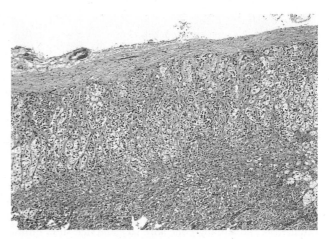

Figure 14.6. Atrophic adrenal gland. The capsule is fibrotic, the cortical layer is atrophic, but the medulla is unaffected.

by ACTH derived from the pituitary gland or from a variety of extrapituitary sources, can be associated with a wide variety of clinical syndromes. Cortical hyperplasia can also selectively involve the zona glomerulosa in patients with so-called idiopathic hyperaldosteronism.

Pituitary/Hypothalamic-Based Hyperplasia (Cushing Disease)

Hyperplasia may be the result of stimulation of the adrenal glands by ACTH-producing pituitary adenomas or of hypothalamic stimulation of the pituitary ACTH cells by CRH (72,73). Basophilic pituitary adenomas were originally observed in association with hypercortisolism by Harvey Cushing in 1932, and this association has been termed Cushing disease or ACTH-dependent Cushing syndrome. Immunohistochemical studies have shown that ACTH-producing pituitary adenomas are considerably more common than had been recognized on light microscopy alone, and many of them have been classified as microadenomas.

Adrenocortical hyperplasia in patients with ACTH-dependent Cushing syndrome can be either diffuse or nodular, and combinations of diffuse and nodular hyperplasia are common. In diffuse hyperplasia, gland weights may be increased only slightly (2). In more advanced cases, the combined average weight varies between 12 and 24 g. The glands have rounded contours, rather than the sharp outlines typical of normal glands. The inner portion of the cortex is widened and often appears pale brown or tan. The outer layers of the cortex are typically yellow. On microscopy, the inner brown zone corresponds to lipid-depleted cells of the fasciculata, whereas the cells of the outer cortex are more characteristically vacuolated (74). The glomerulosa in adults with Cushing disease is often difficult to identify, but in children, the glomerulosa may also appear slightly hyperplastic (75).

In some cases, the cortex may appear nodular with individual nodules measuring less than 0.5 or 1.0 cm in diameter, depending on varying criteria used by different authors (42). This type of change has been referred to as diffuse and micronodular hyperplasia. If the nodules exceed 1 cm in diameter, the hyperplasia is defined as the diffuse and macronodular type.

In diffuse and nodular (micro- or macro-) hyperplasia, multi-

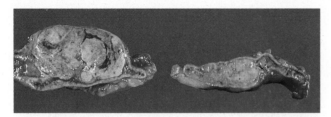

Figure 14.7. Diffuse and nodular adrenocortical hyperplasia associated with adrenocorticotropic hormone–producing pituitary adenoma.

ple cortical nodules are superimposed on a diffusely hyperplastic cortex (Figs. 14.7 and 14.8). Formation of nodules is often asymmetric, and although one adrenal gland may show diffuse and nodular cortical hyperplasia, the contralateral adrenal gland may appear diffusely hyperplastic. The nodules are often composed of admixtures of clear- and compact-type cells. In contrast to the atrophic cortex adjacent to a functioning adenoma, the cortex between or adjacent to the nodules in nodular hyperplasia is diffusely hyperplastic.

Adrenocortical Hyperplasia Associated with Paraneoplastic (Ectopic) Production of Adrenocorticotropic Hormone or Corticotropin-Releasing Hormone

Hyperplasia can be found in association with a variety of neoplasms producing ACTH or CRH (73,76). In most series, bronchial carcinoids and small-cell carcinomas account for the majority of cases. Other tumors associated with the paraneoplastic ACTH syndrome include pancreatic endocrine neoplasms, medullary thyroid carcinoma, thymic carcinoids, and pheochromocytomas. In patients with the paraneoplastic ACTH syndrome associated with bronchogenic small-cell carcinoma or other tumors, the adrenals are usually larger (average combined weight of 20 to 30 g) than those seen in association with diffuse hyperplasia stemming from pituitary ACTH overproduction. The cortex is diffusely hyperplastic and appears tan-brown

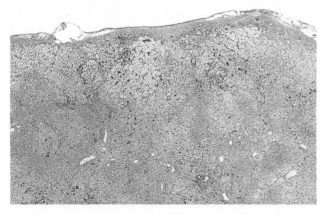

Figure 14.8. Adrenocortical hyperplasia (same case as in Fig. 14.7). The thickened cortex is composed primarily of vacuolated fasciculata cells.

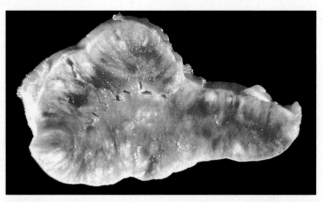

Figure 14.9. Adrenocortical hyperplasia associated with ectopic production of adrenocorticotropic hormone by a bronchogenic carcinoma. The edges of the gland appear rounded, and the darkly colored reticularis zone is irregularly thickened. (From DeLellis RA, Feran Doza M. Diseases of the adrenal glands. In Murphy WM, ed. *Urological Pathology.* Philadelphia, PA: WB Saunders, 1997:539–584, with permission.)

throughout its width (Fig. 14.9) (76a). On microscopy, there is evidence of diffuse hyperplasia of the fasciculata cells, which are characterized by a compact or lipid-depleted appearance (77). Foci of nuclear enlargement and atypia of reticularis cells may be noted, and these features may be particularly striking adjacent to metastatic foci in the glands (19). Both bronchial carcinoids and small-cell bronchogenic carcinomas may also produce CRH. Exceptionally, secretion of both ACTH and CRH from the same tumor has been documented (78).

Adrenocortical Hyperplasia Associated with Hyperaldosteronism

Primary hyperaldosteronism is characterized by the excessive secretion of aldosterone from the adrenal glands and is associated with suppression of plasma renin activity with resultant hypokalemia and hypertension. At least six subtypes of primary hyperaldosteronism have been recognized, including aldosterone-producing adenoma, idiopathic hyperaldosteronism, primary adrenal hyperplasia, aldosterone-producing adrenal cortical carcinoma, aldosterone-producing ovarian tumor, and familial hyperaldosteronism (FH) (79). FH is subdivided into two groups: FH-I (glucocorticoid-remediable hyperaldosteronism) and FH-II (aldosterone-producing adenoma and idiopathic hyperaldosteronism).

Primary hyperaldosteronism is most often associated with adrenocortical adenomas; however, in approximately 40% of cases, the only apparent adrenal abnormality is hyperplasia of the zona glomerulosa with or without the formation of micronodules (7,42,80,81). Generally, biochemical abnormalities in patients with hyperplasia are less severe than in those with adenomas. On histologic examination, hyperplasia of the glomerulosa is characterized by thickening of this cell layer, with tonguelike projections of the glomerulosa extending toward the fasciculata (Fig. 14.10). Micronodules, when present, are usually composed of clear fasciculata-type cells (7,19) and are thought to be a consequence of the associated hypertension. In approximately 10% of cases, it may not be possible to distinguish a micronodule from a true adenoma associated with aldosterone production.

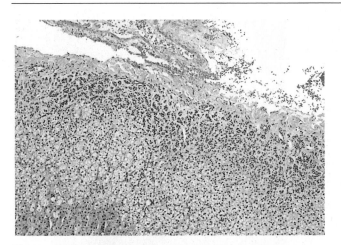

Figure 14.10. Hyperplasia of the zona glomerulosa in a patient with primary hyperaldosteronism.

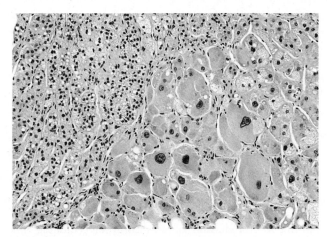

Figure 14.11. Primary pigmented nodular adrenocortical disease. Nodules are composed of large cells with hyperchromatic nuclei.

MACRONODULAR HYPERPLASIA (MASSIVE MACRONODULAR ADRENOCORTICAL DISEASE)

In macronodular hyperplasia with marked adrenal enlargement, the adrenal glands may together weigh up to 180 g, and individual nodules may measure up to 4.0 cm in diameter (36,82,83). Because of the very large size of the glands and confluence of adjacent nodules, the resected adrenal glands may be mistaken for neoplasms. Nodules can be composed of clear cells, compact cells, or admixtures of these cell types. Macronodular hyperplasia is ACTH independent, and this entity can (rarely) involve a single gland (84). The cortex between the nodules is often atrophic, as might be expected in an ACTH-independent process. This entity, which has also been referred to as massive macronodular adrenocortical disease (MMAD), has a bimodal age distribution. A small proportion of patients may present during the first year of life, and this form of the disease may be associated with the McCune-Albright syndrome. Most patients present clinically in the fifth decade, with a male-to-female ratio of 1:1. Rare examples of familial MMAD have also been reported. This disorder has been associated with aberrant (ectopic) expression and regulation of various G-protein–coupled receptors (85).

PRIMARY PIGMENTED NODULAR ADRENOCORTICAL DISEASE— MICROADENOMATOUS HYPERPLASIA OF THE ADRENAL GLAND

Primary pigmented nodular adrenocortical disease (PPNAD) is a rare disorder characterized by the presence of multiple pigmented nodules of cortical cells with intervening atrophic cortical tissue usually seen in association with features of ACTH-independent Cushing syndrome (86–89). The glands may be either smaller than normal or enlarged. Individual nodules, which can vary in color from gray to black, typically measure from 1 to 3 mm in diameter, although larger nodules measuring up to 3 cm in diameter may also be evident (42). The nodules are composed of large, granular eosinophilic cells that often contain enlarged hyperchromatic nuclei with prominent nu-

cleoli (Fig. 14.11). Because of the atypical nuclear features, this entity has also been referred to as micronodular dysplasia. The cells are generally filled with lipochrome pigment, which is responsible for their dark color on gross examination.

The origin of PPNAD is unknown, although some studies have suggested an autoimmune etiology (90). PPNAD arises sporadically or in a familial form that can be associated with Carney complex (CNC), which includes cardiac myxomas, spotty pigmentation, neurofibromatosis, testicular Leydig or Sertoli cell tumors, mammary myxoid fibroadenomas, and cerebral hemangiomas (88,91). CNC may occur sporadically or may be inherited as an autosomal dominant trait. The gene encoding the protein kinase A (PKA) type Iα regulatory subunit, *PRKAR1A*, has been mapped to 17q22-24, and loss of heterozygosity (LOH) studies from patients with CNC have revealed mutations in this gene in approximately 50% of affected individuals. No mutations have been found on 2p16. Studies of sporadic and isolated cases of CNC have also revealed inactivating mutations of *PRKAR1A*. The wild-type alleles could be inactivated by somatic mutations consistent with the hypothesis that the gene belongs to the tumor suppressor class (92,93).

Recently, Horvath et al. (94) reported mutations in the gene encoding phosphodiesterase 11A4 (*PDE11A4*) in cases of PPNAD and other forms of micronodular adrenocortical hyperplasia. LOH and other analyses showed susceptible genes at the 2q31-2q25 locus (94). Phosphodiesterases (PDEs) regulate cyclic nucleotide levels.

The same group subsequently reported that missense mutations of *PDE11A* were present frequently in patients from the general population with adrenal cortical hyperplasia and adenoma, speculating that *PDE11A* genetic defects may be associated with adrenal pathology in a wider clinical spectrum (95).

ADRENAL NEOPLASMS

As in the sections on CNC and BWS, several other syndromes predispose to the development of adrenal tumors (Table 14.1). These include Li-Fraumeni syndrome, multiple endocrine neoplasia (MEN) types 1, 2A, and 2B, familial pheochromocytoma-paraganglioma, neurofibromatosis type 1, and von Hippel-Lindau disease. Unlike BWS, which predisposes to both cortical and medullary tumors, the other syndromes give rise to either cortical or medullary tumors. Although BWS presents early in life, the manifestations of the other syndromes usually occur later in life, but features of MEN2B, which include oral, ocular, and gastrointestinal ganglioneuromatosis associated with a marfanoid habitus, may present at birth or early infancy.

ADRENOCORTICAL NEOPLASMS

ADRENOCORTICAL ADENOMAS

Adrenocortical adenomas are a functionally heterogeneous group of benign neoplasms that can differentiate toward any of the cortical layers (42,96). These tumors can be associated with the overproduction of glucocorticoids (Cushing syndrome), androgenic or estrogenic steroids (adrenogenital syndromes), or mineralocorticoids (Conn syndrome). Mixed syndromes can develop, and cortical adenomas without apparent functional activity are relatively common.

Cushing Syndrome

Tumors associated with Cushing syndrome are typically unilateral and present as sharply circumscribed masses that usually weigh less than 60 g and measure 3 to 4 cm in average diameter. Tumors weighing more than 100 g should be examined with particular care to rule out malignancy (7,19,36). On cross section, adenomas vary from yellow to brown, and occasional examples of heavily pigmented (black) adenomas have been reported (Figs. 14.12 and 14.13). Necrosis is rare in the absence of previous arteriographic or venographic study, but cystic change is relatively common, particularly in larger tumors.

Microscopically, adenomas have pushing borders with a pseudocapsule derived from compression of the adjacent cortex or expansion of the adrenal capsule (9). They are most often composed of small nests, cords, or alveolar arrangements of vacuolated (clear) cells that most closely resemble those of the normal fasciculata. Generally, adenoma cells are somewhat larger than normal cortical cells. Variable numbers of compact-type cells are also evident (Fig. 14.14). Black adenomas are composed exclusively of lipochrome-rich compact cells (Fig. 14.15) (2). Foci of spindle cell growth may be evident in some cases, and *occasional* adenomas may exhibit considerable fibrosis (Fig. 14.16). The nuclear-to-cytoplasmic ratio is generally low, al-

though a few single cells and small cell groups may have enlarged hyperchromatic nuclei. Typically, the nuclei are vesicular with small, distinct nucleoli. Mitotic activity is rare in adenomas. In fine-needle aspiration biopsy specimens, the cells are round to polyhedral with round nuclei and foamy cytoplasm. Numerous naked nuclei in a background of granular to foamy material may be prominent.

On ultrastructural examination, adenoma cells most closely resemble the cells of the normal fasciculata or reticularis (2). The cytoplasm typically contains abundant smooth endoplasmic reticulum and variable numbers of lipid droplets. The mitochondria are round to ovoid with a predominance of tubulovesi-

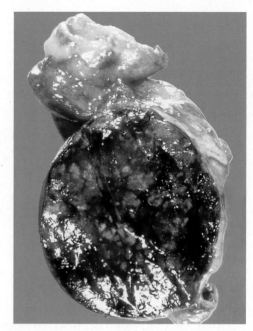

Figure 14.13. Pigmented ("black") adenoma associated with Cushing syndrome. (From DeLellis RA, Feran-Doza M. Diseases of the adrenal glands. In Murphy WM, ed. *Urological Pathology*. Philadelphia, PA: WB Saunders, 1997:539–584, with permission.)

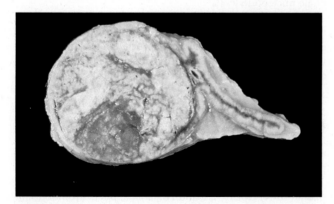

Figure 14.12. Adrenocortical adenoma associated with Cushing disease.

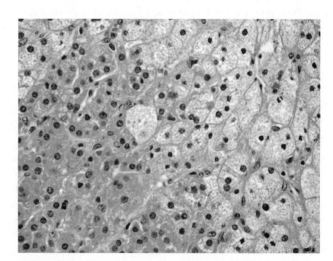

Figure 14.14. Adrenocortical adenoma associated with Cushing syndrome. The tumor is composed of an admixture of clear and compact cells.

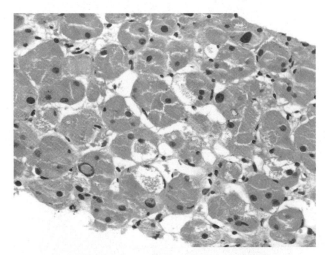

Figure 14.15. Pigmented ("black") adrenocortical adenoma associated with Cushing syndrome. The tumor is composed predominantly of compact cells containing abundant lipochrome pigment.

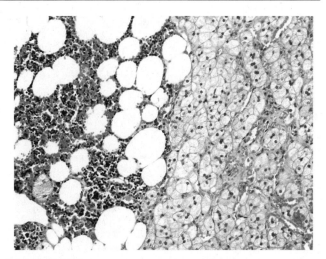

Figure 14.17. Adrenocortical adenoma associated with Cushing syndrome with focal myelolipomatous change.

cular or exclusively vesicular cristae (11). Lamelliform cristae may also be present.

Foci of myelolipomatous change (Fig. 14.17) or calcification may be seen, particularly in larger adenomas (19). The cortex adjacent to functional adenomas and in the contralateral adrenal is typically atrophic, with cortical cells that have a clear or vacuolated cytoplasm. The atrophy, however, does not involve the glomerulosa (81).

X chromosome inactivation analyses have shown that some adenomas are clonal, whereas others are polyclonal. Monoclonal adenomas are larger than polyclonal lesions and have a higher prevalence of nuclear pleomorphism (97). This heterogeneity may reflect different pathogenetic mechanisms or different stages of a common multistep process.

Conn Syndrome

Initial studies suggested that adrenocortical adenomas were responsible for Conn syndrome in up to 90% of cases; however, more recent studies indicate that adenomas are present in a

considerably smaller proportion of cases. Most adenomas associated with hyperaldosteronism measure less than 2.0 cm in diameter and are round to ovoid in configuration (98). Most commonly, they are unilateral, although bilateral tumors have been reported. They are characteristically bright yellow and are generally, but not always, demarcated from the adjacent cortex by a pseudocapsule. The tumor cells are usually arranged in small nests and cords. They can resemble cells of the glomerulosa, fasciculata, or reticularis or combine the features of both glomerulosa and fasciculata cells (hybrid cells) (Fig. 14.18) (19,98). Rarely, black adenomas have been associated with Conn syndrome (99). In patients treated with spironolactone, some cells within the adenoma may contain lamellated eosinophilic inclusions (spironolactone bodies) measuring up to 10 μm in diameter. They are often demarcated from the adjacent cytoplasm by a clear halo (Fig. 14.19). Ultrastructurally, spironolactone bodies most closely resemble myelin figures.

Although most of the tumor cells have relatively small vesicu-

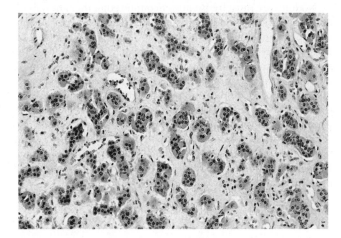

Figure 14.16. Adrenocortical adenoma associated with Cushing syndrome. The stroma shows extensive fibrosis.

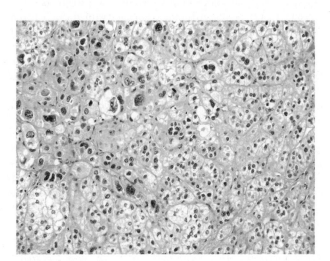

Figure 14.18. Adrenocortical adenoma associated with Conn syndrome. The tumor is composed of an admixture of fasciculata- and glomerulosa-type cells. Cells with enlarged, hyperchromatic nuclei are evident.

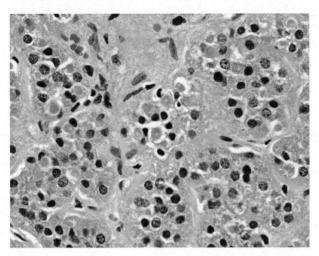

Figure 14.19. Adrenocortical adenoma associated with Conn syndrome. Multiple spironolactone bodies are present with a typical lamellated appearance.

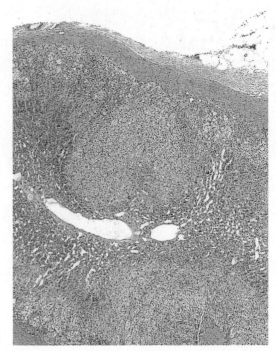

Figure 14.20. Adrenocortical nodule composed of clear cells. Nodules measuring up to 1 cm in diameter were evident in the adrenals of this 75-year-old man. There was no evidence of cortical hyperfunction.

lar nuclei with small but distinct nucleoli, some tumors exhibit considerable variation in nuclear size and shape. At the ultrastructural level, the mitochondria manifest tubular or vesicular cristae, although some may have lamelliform cristae typical of the zona glomerulosa. The fasciculata adjacent to aldosterone-secreting adenomas is of normal thickness. However, hyperplasia of the zona glomerulosa may be present in association with these tumors (98).

Adrenogenital Syndromes

Benign adrenocortical tumors may be associated with syndromes of virilization or feminization, but the presence of a pure adrenogenital syndrome, particularly feminization, should raise the possibility of malignancy. Some authors, in fact, consider all feminizing cortical neoplasms to be potentially malignant. Virilizing adenomas are generally larger than those found in the context of pure Cushing syndrome, and a few adenomas associated with adrenogenital syndromes have weighed up to 500 g (7,19,42). Similar to tumors associated with glucocorticoid overproduction, virilizing adenomas are sharply circumscribed or encapsulated; however, they tend to be red-brown rather than yellow on cross section (19). Smaller tumors have an alveolar pattern of growth, whereas larger tumors tend to have more solid or diffuse growth patterns. Although most tumor cells have a low nuclear-to-cytoplasmic ratio, single cells and small cell groups may exhibit nuclear enlargement and hyperchromasia. The cytoplasm is usually eosinophilic and granular. Rare virilizing tumors contain Reinke crystalloids and have been termed *Leydig cell adenomas* similar to their testicular counterparts (100,101). On ultrastructural examination, the mitochondria are of the tubulolamellar type. Sex steroid–producing adenomas are not associated with atrophy of the adjacent cortex or the contralateral adrenal gland.

Nonfunctional Adrenocortical Adenomas and Cortical Nodules

Adrenocortical nodules are common findings in patients without clinical or biochemical evidence of steroid hormone hyper-

secretion (42). Autopsy studies have revealed cortical nodules in approximately 25% of individuals. The nodules are also commonly detected with abdominal CT and MRI scans and have been grouped among the lesions classified as "incidentalomas." Although cortical nodules are commonly multicentric and bilateral, single nodules measuring up to 2 to 3 cm in diameter may be evident. Smaller nodules are often nonencapsulated (Fig. 14.20), whereas the larger single nodules may be surrounded by a fibrous capsule. The nodules are bright yellow with foci of brownish discoloration and are composed of fasciculata-type cells predominantly. Occasionally, foci of myelolipomatous change or ossification may be evident within the nodules. In contrast to functional adenomas associated with glucocorticoid production, the cortex adjacent to nonfunctional nodules is not atrophic.

Nodules are most frequently encountered in the adrenals of elderly individuals or in patients with essential hypertension or diabetes mellitus. The nodules most likely represent foci of compensatory cortical hyperplasia that have developed in response to focal atrophy of the cortex induced by narrowing of adrenal capsular arterioles (102). Nonfunctional cortical nodules may be particularly prominent in patients with aldosterone-secreting adenomas, presumably as a result of the associated hypertension. Cortical nodularity may also be evident in the zona reticularis. Nodules arising in this zone often appear brown to black because of the presence of lipofuscin pigment. Incidental pigmented nodules may be found in up to one-third of normal adult adrenal glands.

Oncocytic Adenoma (Oncocytoma)

Tumors with oncocytic features (oncocytomas) develop rarely as primary adrenocortical neoplasms. Although some behave

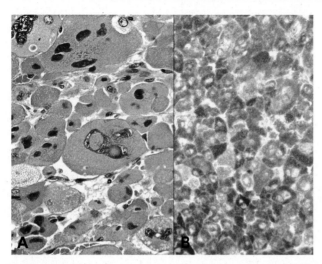

Figure 14.21. Adrenocortical oncocytoma. The cells contain densely granular eosinophilic cytoplasm (**A**) and pleomorphic nuclei with pseudoinclusions. The cytoplasm is positive for melan-A (**B**).

as benign neoplasms, others may be malignant, as discussed in the section on adrenocortical carcinoma. Sasano et al. (103) first described three adrenocortical oncocytomas that were unassociated with clinical syndromes of steroid excess and that lacked steroid hormone synthetic hormones, as determined by immunohistochemical analysis. Subsequent larger series of tumors (104,105) have also shown that the majority of oncocytomas are nonfunctional, but some tumors may be associated with virilization (105,106) or Cushing syndrome (107). A case of a giant oncocytoma arising in retroperitoneal accessory adrenal tissue has been described (108).

Typically, adrenocortical oncocytomas are dark brown, similar to oncocytomas at other sites. They have abundant granular eosinophilic cytoplasm (Fig. 14.21), which corresponds to the presence of numerous mitochondria with both lamellar and tubulovesicular cristae and small, electron-dense inclusions. El-Naggar et al. (109) have reported the presence of both dense matrix inclusions and crystalline inclusions within the mitochondria of a case of oncocytic adrenocortical carcinoma.

ADRENOCORTICAL CARCINOMAS

Adrenocortical carcinomas are rare tumors with an incidence of approximately one to two cases per million population per year. They account for 0.05% to 0.2% of all malignancies. There is a bimodal age distribution, with a small peak in the first two decades and a larger peak in the fifth decade (110). Adrenocortical carcinomas have been reported in approximately 1% of patients with the Li-Fraumeni syndrome, with most affected individuals harboring *p53* mutations at chromosome locus 17p13. These tumors, in fact, may be the only manifestation of this disorder in childhood (111). The frequency of cortical malignancies is also increased in patients with BWS (Table 14.1) and congenital adrenal hyperplasia.

Adrenocortical carcinomas develop somewhat more commonly in women than men in most large clinical series, although some studies have demonstrated a slight male predominance. Some patients may present with abdominal pain, and up to 30% may have a palpable abdominal mass. These tumors may be associated with Cushing syndrome or evidence of sex

steroid overproduction, and mixed syndromes occur more often than with cortical adenomas. Rarely, mineralocorticoid production may be present. A significant proportion of cortical carcinomas (up to 75% in some series) may be unassociated with syndromes of hormone overproduction (112). In some instances, patients may show signs of hypoglycemia as a result of the production of insulin-like growth factors by the tumor or hypercalcemia as a result of the production of parathyroid hormone–related peptide.

As a rule, cortical carcinomas are large tumors weighing more than 100 g in adults; most often, tumor weight is in excess of 750 g (7,113–116). Rarely, however, tumors weighing less than 50 g will metastasize, whereas a small proportion of tumors weighing more than 1000 g may not (42). Benign tumors associated with sex steroid overproduction, however, can weigh considerably more than 100 g. Tumor weight is also a useful predictor of malignancy in children. Tumors weighing more than 500 g in a series of 23 cases reported by Cagle et al. (117) were malignant, whereas only a single tumor weighing less than 500g pursued a malignant course.

On gross examination, most cortical malignancies have a nodular appearance with individual nodules varying from pink to yellow-tan, depending on their lipid content. Carcinomas associated with feminization or virilization tend to be red-brown, whereas those associated with Cushing syndrome are more often yellow-tan. Foci of necrosis, hemorrhage, and calcification are common, particularly in large tumors (Fig. 14.22). The larger tumors often invade contiguous structures, including the kidney and liver.

Adrenocortical carcinomas have alveolar (Fig. 14.23), trabecular, or solid patterns of growth, and admixtures of these patterns are common (19,36,42). Necrosis, particularly in large tumors, may be extensive (Fig. 14.24). Foci of myxoid change, pseudoglandular patterns, and spindle cell growth may be prominent in some tumors (118). Depending on their lipid content, the cytoplasm may vary from vacuolated to eosinophilic. Some tumors may have eosinophilic globular inclusions resembling those seen in pheochromocytomas. Rare cases may exhibit adenosquamous differentiation (119). There may be considerable variation in the appearance of the nuclei. In some instances, they may appear relatively small and uniform (Fig. 14.25), whereas in others, they may exhibit pronounced atypia

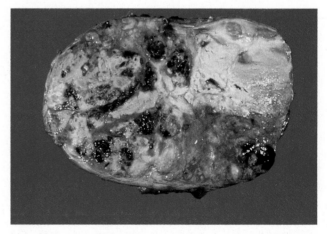

Figure 14.22. Adrenocortical carcinoma. The tumor is extensively necrotic.

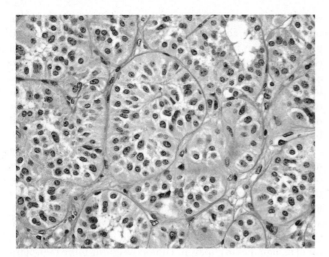

Figure 14.23. Adrenocortical carcinoma. This tumor has an alveolar pattern of growth.

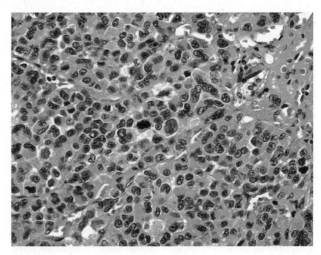

Figure 14.25. Adrenocortical carcinoma. This tumor is composed of small cells.

manifested by pleomorphism (Fig. 14.26), coarse chromatin, and multiple prominent nucleoli. Mitotic activity, including atypical forms (Fig. 14.27), is often prominent. Nuclear pseudo-inclusions, representing invaginations of the cytoplasm into the nucleus (Fig. 14.26), may be particularly striking in some cortical carcinomas.

A subset of adrenocortical carcinomas may be composed of oncocytic cells (105,120–122). Although some of these tumors may be associated with Cushing syndrome or feminizing features (105), others may be nonfunctional. Hoang et al. (121) concluded that large tumor size, extracapsular extension, vascular invasion, necrosis, and metastasis are features of malignancy in these tumors. In the four cases reported by Hoang et al. (121), however, mitotic rate was less than 1 per 10 high-power fields (hpf). Cytologic atypia and mitotic rate, therefore, were not reliable criteria for the prediction of biologic behavior of these neoplasms. Bisceglia et al. (105) have also reviewed the criteria for the distinction of benign and malignant adrenocortical oncocytic tumors. According to these authors, major criteria for malignancy included high mitotic rate, atypical mitoses, and venous invasion, whereas minor criteria included large tumor

size, necrosis, capsular invasion, and sinusoidal invasion. The presence of one major criterion was sufficient for the diagnosis of malignancy, whereas one to four minor criteria were sufficient for a diagnosis of tumors of uncertain malignant potential. The absence of all criteria indicated benignancy.

Very rarely, adrenocortical carcinomas may contain sarcomatous foci (*carcinosarcoma*). In the case reported by Fischler et al. (123), the sarcomatous component had features of rhabdomyosarcoma and stained positively for muscle-specific actin and desmin. Although this tumor was associated with virilization, the case reported by Decorato et al. (124) was nonfunctional.

In fine-needle aspiration biopsy samples, cortical carcinomas generally contain single cells and poorly cohesive cell clusters in a necrotic background. There may be considerable nuclear atypia and mitotic activity, but some cortical carcinomas appear deceptively bland (125). According to Ren et al. (125a), common cytologic features include hypercellularity, necrosis, nuclear pleomorphism, mitotic figures, and prominent nucleoli. Twenty percent of their cases exhibited all five features, whereas necrosis and/or mitoses were found in each case.

There are considerable differences in the reported inci-

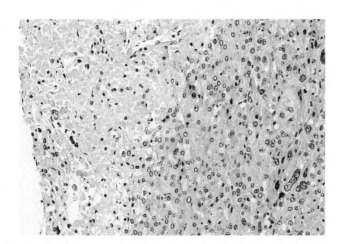

Figure 14.24. Adrenocortical carcinoma. This tumor has a large area of necrosis.

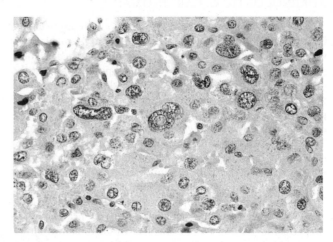

Figure 14.26. Adrenocortical carcinoma associated with virilization. This tumor is composed of eosinophilic cells with marked nuclear pleomorphism. A few intranuclear "pseudoinclusions" are evident.

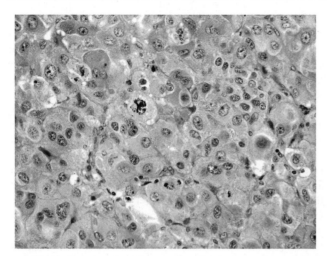

Figure 14.27. Adrenocortical carcinoma. An atypical mitotic figure is present.

dences of keratin positivity in cortical carcinomas, depending on the specificities of the antibodies and the types of tissue preparation (Table 14.2). With microwave retrieval methods, cytokeratin immunoreactivity is present focally in up to 60% of adrenal cortical neoplasms (126,127). Interestingly, all four of the oncocytic carcinomas reported by Hoang et al. (121) were positive for cytokeratins using AE1/AE3 and CAM 5.2 antibodies. Vimentin is evident in most cortical carcinomas following microwave-induced antigen retrieval. Some cortical carcinomas may, therefore, exhibit a vimentin-positive, cytokeratin-negative phenotype, whereas others may coexpress cytokeratins and vimentin (128).

Several other approaches have been used for the identifica-

tion of adrenocortical neoplasms, including antibodies reactive with steroidogenic enzymes and transcription factors that regulate the expression of these genes (129,130). Schröder et al. (131) have developed a monoclonal antibody (D11) that is reactive with normal and neoplastic cortical cells but nonreactive with normal adrenal medullary cells and pheochromocytomas (131). This antibody recognizes several 59-kd proteins that are capable of binding apolipoprotein E. The D11 antibody, however, is not specific for steroid hormone–producing cells because it has also been found in several other tumor types, including hepatocellular carcinoma, renal cell carcinoma, and some cases of bronchogenic carcinoma (132).

The monoclonal antibody A103, which reacts with melan-A, an antigen recognized by cytotoxic T cells and expressed in melanocytes, has also been used for the identification of adrenocortical and other steroid hormone–producing tumors (133). With the exception of melanoma, the only tumors that are consistently reactive with A103 are adrenocortical adenomas and carcinomas, testicular Leydig cell tumors, and ovarian Sertoli-Leydig cell tumors. Antibodies to inhibin A also provide an additional useful approach for the identification of steroid-producing cells. Renshaw and Granter (134) have demonstrated that inhibin A and A103 are both useful for the identification of adrenocortical neoplasms and that A103 is marginally more specific and inhibin A is slightly more sensitive. Calretinin is also expressed in adrenal cortical neoplasms and is a useful adjunct in cases where stains for inhibin A are negative. Jorda et al. (135) demonstrated that 24 of 33 (73%) cortical neoplasms were positive for inhibin A; however, when calretinin was added, the numbers of tumors staining positively for the two markers increased to 94% (31 of 33 cases).

Some adrenocortical carcinomas exhibit evidence of neuroendocrine differentiation, manifested by the presence of immunoreactivity for synaptophysin, neurofilament proteins, and

TABLE 14.2	Differential Diagnosis of Adrenocortical Carcinoma											
Tumor Type	CK[a]	VIM	NF[b]	S-100[c]	EMA[d]	CEA[d]	CHR	SYN[e]	AFP	MEL-A[f]	CAL[g]	INH[h]
Cortical carcinoma	+/−	+	+/−	+/−	−	−	−	+/−	−	+	+	+
Pheochromocytoma	−	+/−	+	+	−	−	+	+	−	−	−	−
Renal cell carcinoma	+	+	−	+/−	+	−	−	−	−	−	−/+	−/+
Hepatocellular carcinoma	+	+/−	−	+/−	+/−	+	−	−	+	−	−	−/+
Metastatic adenocarcinoma	+	+/−	−	+/−	+	+	−	−	−	−	−/+	−
Liposarcoma	−	+	−	+	−	−	−	−	−	−/+	−	−

AFP, alpha-fetoprotein; CAL, calretinin; CEA, carcinoembryonic antigen; CHR, chromogranin; CK, cytokeratin; EMA, epithelial membrane antigen; INH, inhibin; MEL-A, melan-A; NF, neurofilament; SYN, synaptophysin; VIM, vimentin; +, positive; −, negative; +/−, predominantly positive; −/+, predominantly negative.

[a]Although earlier studies had indicated that adrenocortical carcinomas were cytokeratin negative, more recent studies using microwave-induced antigen retrieval reveal positivity in a substantial proportion of cases.

[b]Studies by Miettinen (136) suggest that NF proteins may be present in a subset of adrenocortical carcinomas.

[c]A variety of tumors may exhibit S-100 immunoreactivity within the neoplastic cells, including cortical carcinomas; S-100 positivity in pheochromocytomas is restricted to the sustentacular cells.

[d]The presence of EMA and CEA distinguishes a metastatic adenocarcinoma (positive) from a cortical carcinoma (negative).

[e]Synaptophysin has been demonstrated in up to 90% of cortical carcinomas by Miettinen (136) and Komminoth et al. (137).

[f]The monoclonal antibody A103 reacts with adrenal cortical neoplasms and other steroid hormone–producing tumors, whereas other monoclonal antibodies to melan-A are nonreactive with steroid-producing cells. Although liposarcomas are generally negative for melan-A, Huang and Antonescu (162) have reported positivity in the epithelioid variant of pleomorphic liposarcoma.

[g]Calretinin has been used most extensively for the diagnosis of mesotheliomas; however, up to 20% of adenocarcinomas may also be positive.

[h]Inhibin immunoreactivity is a sensitive marker for adrenal cortical tumors. However, the studies of Renshaw and Granter (134) indicate that positive reactions for this marker may be found rarely in renal cell and hepatocellular carcinomas.

neuron-specific enolase (136,137). The tumors are, however, typically negative for chromogranin/secretogranin proteins. Ultrastructural analysis of some cases showed clusters of membrane-bound secretory granules that measured 150 to 300 nm in diameter and resembled neurosecretory granules. The tumor cells also contained synaptophysin messenger RNA (137). These observations have suggested that adrenocortical carcinomas with evidence of neuroendocrine differentiation could arise from stem cells, which are capable of multidirectional differentiation. In this regard, the studies of Bornstein et al. (33) have shown that hybrid corticomedullary cells exist normally in the rat adrenal cortex.

Recently, Browning et al. (138) reported that D2-40, a marker that is commonly used to highlight lymphatic endothelial cells, was highly specific and sensitive for differentiating adrenocortical tumors from both metastatic renal cell carcinomas and pheochromocytomas. In this series, D2-40 was strongly and diffusely positive in the cells of the neoplastic and nonneoplastic adrenal cortex but was negative in 13 cases of clear-cell renal carcinomas. Normal and neoplastic medullary cells were negative for D2-40.

Ultrastructurally, the mitochondria of cortical carcinomas may be round, ovoid, or elongated. Silva et al. (139) found isolated mitochondria with tubular cristae in virtually every case, but tumors containing a predominance of tubular mitochondria were found in only approximately half of the cases. Although the presence of smooth endoplasmic reticulum has been stressed as an important criterion for the diagnosis of cortical carcinoma, Silva et al. (139) found abundant smooth surface reticulum in only 10% of their cases (Fig. 14.28). The tumor cells also contained stacks of granular endoplasmic reticulum and generally small Golgi regions. A few mitochondria contained dense matrix granules measuring up to 300 nm in diameter. Glycogen deposits have been noted in approximately 20% of cases, and rarely, these deposits may be so abundant that the cells can be mistaken for renal cell carcinoma.

It may be extremely difficult to distinguish between benign and malignant cortical tumors, and different authors have used a variety of parameters to differentiate these groups of neoplasms (113,115,140–146). Hough et al. (115) examined a variety of histologic and clinical features to distinguish metastatic and nonmetastatic cortical tumors. These investigators found that the presence of necrosis (larger than 2 hpf in diameter) and broad fibrous bands were the most useful histologic discriminants. In addition, a diffuse pattern of growth, nuclear hyperchromasia, and vascular invasion were also helpful in making the distinction between benign and malignant cortical neoplasms.

Weiss proposed a system for the distinction of benign and malignant tumors based on the following nine parameters (Table 14.3): high nuclear grade (Fuhrman grade 3 or 4); greater than 5 mitoses per 50 hpf; atypical mitoses; diffuse patterns of growth; necrosis; invasion of venous, sinusoidal, or capsular structures; and clear cells comprising less than 25% of the tumor (113,146). In a series of 43 cases, Weiss (113) found that tumors with fewer than two of these features never metastasized,

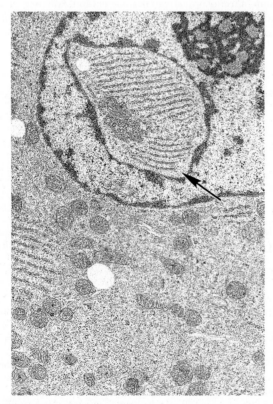

Figure 14.28. Adrenocortical carcinoma associated with virilization. The cells contain abundant smooth endoplasmic reticulum, and the nucleus contains a cytoplasmic "pseudoinclusion" (*arrow*) (10,000×).

TABLE 14.3

Criteria for the Diagnosis of Adrenocortical Carcinoma

Histologic Features	Weiss System (113,147)[a]	Aubert et al. (148)[b] Modification of Weiss System
Venous invasion	1	
High nuclear grade	1	
Necrosis	1	1
Mitoses (>5/50 hpf)	1	2
Diffuse architecture	1	
Capsular invasion	1	1
Atypical mitoses	1	1
Sinusoidal invasion	1	
Clear cells (<25%)	1	2
Threshold for malignancy	>3	≥3

[a]The Weiss system is based on histologic features alone (113,147). High grade refers to grades 3 or 4, according to the criteria used by Fuhrman in the analysis of renal cell carcinoma. The mitotic index is determined by counting the areas with the highest mitotic rates. Capsular invasion is defined as the presence of nests and cords of tumor cells extending into or through the capsule with an accompanying stromal reaction. The architecture is considered diffuse if it involves more than 30% of the area of tumor. With each of these parameters assigned a value of 1, the threshold for malignancy is a total score of >3.

[b]The Aubert system (148) represents a modification of the system proposed by Weiss. In this system, mitotic rate (>5/50 hpf) and cytoplasmic features (clear cells <25%) are each assigned values of 2, whereas the remaining parameters are assigned values of 1. The threshold for malignancy is a score ≥3.

whereas those with more than four almost invariably recurred or metastasized. Subsequently, Weiss et al. (147) lowered the threshold for malignancy from four to three parameters. Aubert et al. (148) confirmed the value of the Weiss system but have proposed a modification based on the most reproducible criteria, including mitotic rate (>5/50 hpf), cytoplasm (<25% clear cells), abnormal mitoses, necrosis, and capsular invasion. The first two features were assigned values of 2, whereas the remainder was assigned values of 1. According to this system, each tumor could be given a score of 0 to 7. The threshold for malignancy remained a score of 3 or more.

The issue of malignancy is even more complicated in the pediatric population in which the criteria of Weiss are less predictive of an aggressive course. As noted earlier, Cagle et al. (117) found tumor weight greater than 500 g to be the most useful determinant in predicting malignant behavior. More recently, Wieneke et al. (149) studied 83 cortical neoplasms in patients less than 20 years of age and found that 23 of 74 cases with a malignant histology based on adaptation of Weiss's criteria had a clinically malignant course. From their analysis, features associated with an increased probability of malignant behavior included tumor weight greater than 400 g, size greater than 10.5 cm, vena cava invasion, capsular and/or vascular invasion, extension into periadrenal soft tissue, confluent necrosis, severe nuclear atypia, greater than 15 mitoses per 20 hpf, and the presence of atypical mitotic figures. Of these, vena cava invasion, necrosis, and mitotic activity independently predicted malignant behavior in multivariate analyses. Because of the added uncertainty in pediatric tumors, Dehner (149a) has suggested labeling tumors fulfilling Weiss's criteria as "atypical adenomas." Recently, Dehner (149b) suggested that adrenocortical neoplasms in children under the age of 2 years were likely to demonstrate "malignant histologic features" but a benign clinical course because they recapitulated or resembled the fetal cortex of the adrenal gland. Additional studies will be required to confirm these findings.

There are no generally accepted criteria for the grading of cortical carcinomas. In an analysis of 42 carcinomas, the only parameter that had a strong statistical association with patient outcome was mitotic rate (147). Patients with tumors containing more than 20 mitoses per 50 hpf had a mean survival of 14 months, whereas patients with tumors with less than 20 mitoses had a mean survival of 58 months. Atypical mitoses, capsular invasion, tumor weight in excess of 250 g, and size in excess of 10 cm each had a marginal association with survival. Other features, including nuclear grade, presence of necrosis, venous or sinusoidal invasion, character of the tumor cell cytoplasm, and architectural pattern, had no impact on survival.

Other methods that have been examined in an effort to predict outcome include DNA content, MIB-1 labeling index, and p53 status (142–144). Initially, carcinomas were shown to be aneuploid and adenomas were shown to be diploid, but subsequent studies demonstrated aneuploidy in some adenomas and diploidy in some carcinomas (145,146). Vargas et al. (150) demonstrated that the mean proliferative fraction, as determined by counting the proportion of MIB-1–positive cells, was 1.49% in adenomas, 20.8% in carcinomas, and 16.6% in recurrent or metastatic tumors. None of 20 benign lesions had an MIB-1 score that exceeded 8%, whereas only 1 of 20 malignancies had a score of less than 8%. Forty-five percent of the carcinomas were positive for p53, whereas none of 20 adenomas was p53 positive. Aubert et al. (148) also observed a statistically signifi-

cant difference in MIB-1 labeling between benign (2.4% ± 1.3%) and malignant (21.2% ± 18.44%) tumors.

In vitro analyses have suggested that any tumor with functional abnormalities, such as the secretion of precursor steroids and blunted or absent response to ACTH, should be considered potentially malignant (151).

Comparative genomic hybridization studies have revealed that genetic alterations are more common in malignant than in benign cortical tumors, whereas they occur rarely in hyperplastic lesions. Losses of 1p21-31, 2q, 3p, 3q, 6q, 9p, and 11q14-qter, and gains of 5q12, 9q32-qter, 12q, and 20q were the most frequent abnormalities present in carcinomas. Gains in 17q, 17p, and 9q32-qter were the most frequent abnormalities in adenomas, whereas gains in two of six cases of cortical hyperplasia involved 17 or 17q (152). Several groups have demonstrated LOH of 11q13 in a significant proportion of adrenal cortical carcinomas; however, none of the tumors demonstrated a mutation in the *MEN1* gene (153,154). LOH of 17p13 and 11p15 has been demonstrated in approximately 80% of cortical carcinomas. Gicquel et al. (155) have further demonstrated that 17p13 LOH and histologic grade were independently associated with tumor recurrence.

Results of gene expression profiling have demonstrated that most significantly upregulated genes in carcinomas include ubiquitin-specific protease 4 (*USP4*) and ubiquitin degradation 1-like (*UFD1L*), which are upregulated at least 40-fold compared with adenomas. Additional genes upregulated in carcinomas include members of the insulin-like growth factor (IGF) family such as *IGF2*, *IGF2R*, *IGFBP3*, and *IGFBP6* (156). Giordano et al. (157) also demonstrated increased expression of *IGF2* in adrenocortical carcinomas. Downregulated genes in carcinomas include chemokine (C-X-C motif) ligand 10 (*CXCL10*), retinoic acid receptor responder 2, aldehyde dehydrogenase family member A1 (*ALD1f1A1*), cytochrome b reductase 1, and glutathione S-transferase A4 (156).

West et al. (158) have demonstrated similar patterns of gene expression in pediatric adrenal cortical tumors. Interestingly, there was a consistent marked decrease in the expression of all major histocompatibility complex (MHC) class II genes in carcinomas compared with adenomas. These results parallel the observations by Marx et al. (159) that pre- and postnatal adrenals do not express MHC class II antigens in contrast to adult adrenals, which do express these antigens.

Adrenocortical carcinomas must be distinguished from a variety of secondary tumors involving the adrenal gland, including renal cell carcinoma, hepatocellular carcinoma, metastatic carcinoma, and liposarcoma. Immunohistochemistry may be of particular value in discriminating cortical carcinomas from these tumor types (12,128,139,160–162), as summarized in Table 14.2.

Didolkar et al. (112) have studied the natural history of a large series of patients with adrenocortical carcinoma. The mean duration of symptoms in patients with or without hormonal manifestations was 6 months. Fifty-two percent of patients had distant metastases at the time of diagnosis, 41% had locally advanced disease, and 7% had tumor confined to the adrenal gland. The overall median survival was 14 months, and the 5-year survival rate was 24%. The median survival of patients with functional tumors was somewhat longer than that of patients with nonfunctional tumors. The most common sites of metastasis were the lungs, followed by retroperitoneal lymph

TABLE 14.4

Staging of Adrenocortical Carcinoma

TNM

T1	Tumor ≤5 cm, no local invasion
T2	Tumor ≥5 cm, no local invasion
T3	Tumor of any size with local invasion but without invasion of adjacent organs
T4	Tumor of any size with invasion of adjacent organs
N0	No regional node
N1	Positive regional nodes
M0	No distant metastases
M1	Distant metastases

Stage Definitions			
Stage I	T1	N0	M0
Stage II	T2	N0	M0
Stage III	T1	N1	N0
	T2	N1	M0
	T3	N0	M0
Stage IV	Any T	Any N	M1
	T3	N1	M0
	T4	N0	M0

TNM, tumor-node-metastasis.

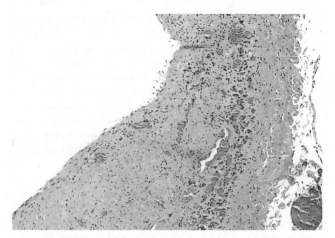

Figure 14.29. Adrenal cyst, endothelial type. The cells lining the cyst were focally positive for the factor VIII–related antigen.

nodes, liver, and bone. The staging of adrenocortical carcinoma is summarized in Table 14.4.

In view of the improvements in sensitivity of imaging modalities, the question arises as to whether there have been improvements in the diagnosis of adrenocortical carcinoma at an earlier stage with resultant improved survival. Paton et al. (163) analyzed data from the Surveillance, Epidemiology and End Results (SEER) database between 1988 and 2002. Of 602 tumors, 3% were less than 5 cm and localized (stage I), 36% were greater than 5 cm and localized (stage II), and 20.3% invaded adjacent structures (stage III). There were distant metastases (stage IV) in 31.4% of cases, and stage was unknown in 8.8%. Although 5-year survival rate was better in localized disease (62%) compared with advanced disease (7%), tumor stage and survival did not improve over the 15-year study period.

OTHER ADRENAL MASS LESIONS

The advent of high-resolution abdominal imaging techniques, including CT and MRI, has markedly increased the rate of discovery of nonfunctional adrenal mass lesions (164–168). As a group, these lesions have been referred to as "incidentalomas," and the differential diagnosis includes primary and metastatic carcinoma, cysts, myelolipomas, a variety of benign tumors, lymphoid hyperplasia, and periadrenal lesions. Nonfunctional cortical adenomas and cortical nodules are also frequently detected by this approach.

CYSTS AND PSEUDOCYSTS

Although adrenal cysts are uncommon, the rate of their detection as a result of CT and MRI scanning has increased dramati-

cally. Most adrenal cysts are unilateral, with a predominance in women. Adrenal cysts may be divided into four major categories, including epithelial cysts, parasitic cysts, endothelial (vascular) cysts, and pseudocysts (Fig. 14.29) (42,169).

The term *pseudocyst* describes a lesion that lacks recognizable endothelial or epithelial cells. Typically, pseudocysts are unilocular. In the series of eight pseudocysts reported by Medeiros et al. (170), seven of the patients were women, with a median age of 41 years. Pseudocysts range in size from 1.8 to 10 cm, but lesions of considerably larger size have been reported. The cyst usually contains hemorrhagic fibrinous material, whereas the wall is composed of dense fibrous tissue with areas of calcification and granulation tissue. Many adrenal pseudocysts probably develop as lymphangioendothelial cysts that undergo episodes of hemorrhage, fibrosis, and hemosiderin deposition with the ultimate disappearance of the endothelial lining (171). This conclusion is based on the occasional presence of residual lining cells that are positive for factor VIII–related antigen. Occasionally, abundant elastic tissue may be present within the cyst wall, further suggesting a vascular origin. True vascular cysts are typically multilocular and are most likely related to pre-existing benign vascular lesions. They are lined by flattened endothelial cells.

True epithelial cysts include retention cysts, some of which are of mesothelial origin, embryonal cysts, and cystic neoplasms. As noted in the other sections, any adrenal neoplasm may contain foci of cystic change. Rarely cystic change may involve a neoplasm almost entirely so that, on imaging studies, it simulates a cyst or pseudocyst, but on pathologic examination, residual mural tumor nodules can be found. Erickson et al. (172) reported 2 adrenocortical carcinomas, 2 adrenocortical adenomas, and 2 pheochromocytomas associated with 6 of 32 pseudocysts from the archives of the Mayo Clinic over a 25-year period. An additional case of pheochromocytoma was associated with an endothelial cyst. Parasitic cysts are the least common adrenal cysts and are most often a result of echinococcal infection.

MYELOLIPOMA

The myelolipoma is an uncommon, benign, tumorlike lesion of the adrenal gland composed of mature adipose tissue ad-

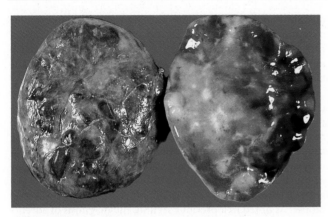

Figure 14.30. Adrenal myelolipoma. The cut surface has a mottled yellow-brown appearance.

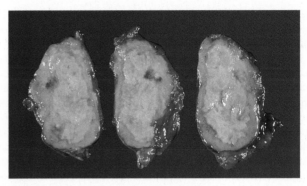

Figure 14.32. Adrenal gland with metastatic adenocarcinoma. This adrenal gland is replaced completely by metastatic tumor.

SECONDARY TUMORS

Secondary involvement of the adrenal glands has been reported in almost 30% of patients with *metastatic tumors* of diverse sites of origin (19), with bilateral involvement in almost 50%. The high frequency of adrenal metastases is most likely related to the rich sinusoidal blood supply of the glands. In most series from the United States and Western Europe, primary tumors of the lung (Figs. 14.32 and 14.33) and breast account for 60% of the cases, followed by primary tumors of the gastrointestinal tract, kidney, skin (melanoma), and thyroid gland. Sites of origin of metastatic tumors differ geographically. For example, in a series of 464 patients from Hong Kong, Lam and Lo (176) noted that the most common primary site was lung (35%) followed by stomach (14%), esophagus (12%), liver/bile ducts (10%), pancreas (6.9%), colon (5.4%), kidney (4.3%), and breast (2.9%). Adrenocortical carcinomas may also occasionally metastasize to the contralateral adrenal gland. Patients with metastatic carcinoma involving one or both adrenal glands may initially be seen for diagnosis of an intra-adrenal mass, and in such cases, the primary tumor may not be evident until the time of autopsy. Overt adrenal insufficiency is uncommon in patients with adrenal metastasis; however, mild degrees of adrenal insufficiency may be present (177). Clinically significant adrenal

mixed with hematopoietic cells. Most myelolipomas appear as unilateral adrenal masses; however, similar lesions may develop in extra-adrenal sites in the retroperitoneum. The mean age at diagnosis is approximately 50 years, and most patients are asymptomatic. Sometimes, however, patients have evidence of flank pain with or without a palpable mass or hematuria. The typical myelolipoma is a nonencapsulated but circumscribed lesion that is bright yellow with foci of tan-brown discoloration (42). These tumors vary considerably in size, from those that are of microscopic dimensions to those that fill the abdomen. At the microscopic level, the lesions are composed of mature adipose tissue with scattered islands of hematopoietic cells (Figs. 14.30 and 14.31) (173). Areas of necrosis, hemorrhage, cyst formation, and calcification or ossification may also be evident, particularly in larger tumors. Foci of myelolipomatous change may be found in cortical adenomas and cortical hyperplasia and within otherwise normal adrenal glands (19,174). As a result, it has been debatable whether myelolipomas are true neoplasms or a reactive process. Bishop et al. (175) recently demonstrated nonrandom X chromosome inactivation in the hematopoietic elements and fat in 8 of 11 myelolipomas from female patients in support of a clonal origin of these tumors.

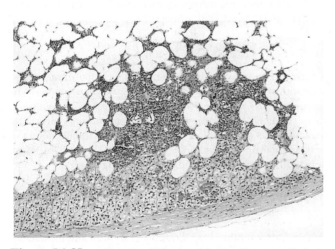

Figure 14.31. Adrenal myelolipoma. Islands of hematopoietic tissue are scattered among the fat cells.

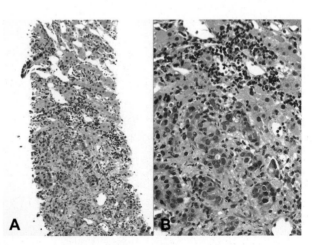

Figure 14.33. Needle biopsy of a pulmonary metastatic adenocarcinoma involving the adrenal gland. Intermingling of metastatic tumor cells with adrenocortical tumor cells can be appreciated at low power (**A**). At high power, gland formation is present (**B**).

hemorrhage secondary to adrenal metastases may occur but is rare (176). Metastases to cortical adenomas (178) and pheochromocytomas (179) have been reported.

On gross examination, metastases may appear as multiple or single firm masses that replace all or part of the glands. Larger metastases frequently exhibit foci of necrosis and hemorrhage and may therefore simulate primary adrenocortical carcinomas. Their microscopic appearances differ according to their sites of origin. Although most such lesions are recognizable as metastases, their distinction from cortical carcinomas may be difficult. Generally, however, metastatic carcinomas can be distinguished from other tumor types on the basis of immunohistochemistry, as described subsequently.

Secondary involvement of the adrenal glands may occur in up to 25% of patients with disseminated *malignant lymphoma* studied at autopsy (42). Both Hodgkin disease and non-Hodgkin lymphomas have been reported, with a somewhat higher frequency for non-Hodgkin lymphomas. Rarely, however, is the lymphomatous involvement associated with adrenal insufficiency. This complication occurs primarily in patients with high-grade tumors (180).

Adrenal involvement can be unilateral or bilateral, and tumors can range in size from those of microscopic dimensions to those that replace the adrenal and adjacent structures. The gross appearance can be identical to that of primary cortical carcinomas. The histologic characteristics vary according to the type of lymphoma. The differential diagnosis includes metastatic carcinoma, primary adrenal cortical carcinoma, metastatic amelanotic melanoma, and pheochromocytoma. Malignant lymphomas can be distinguished from other tumor types on the basis of positive staining for leukocyte common antigen and other markers of lymphoid differentiation. Very rare examples of primary lymphomas of the adrenal glands have also been reported (181–184). Virtually all of the primary adrenal lymphomas have been of the non-Hodgkin large-cell type, including the large-cell angiotrophic type (184). Leukemic involvement of the kidney is typically identified as an incidental finding at autopsy.

Fine-needle aspiration biopsy is an important approach for the differential diagnosis of primary and metastatic adrenal lesions (Fig. 14.34) (185). In a series of 23 cases reported by Katz

and Shirkhoda (168), 10 lesions were identified with fine-needle aspiration cytology as cortical adenomas, and the remainder proved to be metastatic carcinomas. The adenomas had a mean size of 2.5 cm, whereas the metastases averaged 7.8 cm in diameter.

Adrenal biopsy is typically performed when adrenal lesions cannot be accurately characterized with CT, MRI, or PET scanning. However, the pathologic workup of adrenal masses on core needle or fine-needle aspiration biopsies is a challenging process. Foremost, is the determination of whether the biopsy is lesional. In the case of benign adrenocortical nodules or tumors, the lesion may recapitulate the histology of the normal adrenal cortex, precluding a definite diagnosis of neoplasia on biopsy. As noted in a previous section, the diagnosis of adrenocortical carcinoma can be difficult on resection specimens. Because of variability in a neoplasm, the area sampled may only permit a diagnosis of "consistent with adrenocortical neoplasm" to be rendered. Clearly, in functional tumors, differentiation from metastatic tumors or extension from adjacent structures is aided by biochemical studies when available. However, because the majority of cases that are encountered on needle biopsies are nonfunctional tumors, an immunohistochemical approach is used.

Metastatic carcinomas are positive for cytokeratins, whereas cortical tumors may be positive or negative (Fig. 14.35). Most melanomas and sarcomas are negative for cytokeratins; however, some sarcomas (e.g., synovial sarcoma, epithelioid variants of leiomyosarcoma, and liposarcoma) and melanomas may be cytokeratin positive. Accordingly, melan-A, inhibin, and calretinin will be most useful in establishing an adrenocortical origin provided that melanoma can be ruled out. Thyroid transcription factor 1 (TTF-1) is commonly positive in metastatic lung and thyroid carcinomas but negative in non–small-cell primaries of breast, gastrointestinal tract, liver, and kidney. Thyroglobulin (THY) is used to differentiate lung carcinoma (THY negative) from thyroid carcinoma (THY positive). Other commonly used antibodies include gross cystic disease fluid 15 (GCDFP-15) for breast; CDX2 for gastrointestinal primaries; polyclonal carcinoembryonic antigen (pCEA) and HepPar-1 for hepatocellular carcinoma; and CD10 and renal cell carcinoma antigen (RCC), both of which may be expressed in renal cell carcinoma. CD45 is positive in and is used to screen for lymphoreticular and hematopoietic neoplasms. Additional lineage-specific markers are used for further classification into T-cell or B-cell subtypes (CD3 and CD20, respectively).

CONNECTIVE TISSUE TUMORS

A variety of benign and malignant mesenchymal tumors may arise within the adrenal gland, including *hemangiomas, lipomas, leiomyomas, osteomas, neurofibromas, angiomyolipomas,* and *neurilemomas* (19,42,68,186). Among the benign tumors, cavernous hemangiomas are the most common and are usually detected as incidental findings at surgery or autopsy (Fig. 14.36). Most hemangiomas are solitary lesions involving a single adrenal gland. These lesions should be distinguished from adrenal cortical adenomas with degenerative changes and secondary vascular proliferation. The gross and histologic features of adrenal neurofibromas and neurilemomas are the same as those of similar tumors found at other sites. *Leiomyomas* are rare and most likely originate from smooth muscle cells of the central vein. Prevot et al. (187) reported a single case of a solitary fibrous tumor of

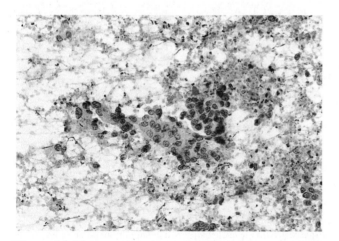

Figure 14.34. Adrenal gland with metastatic bronchogenic adenocarcinoma. In this fine-needle aspiration biopsy sample, clusters of malignant cells are surrounded by necrotic debris.

DIFFERENTIAL DIAGNOSIS OF ADRENAL MASSES

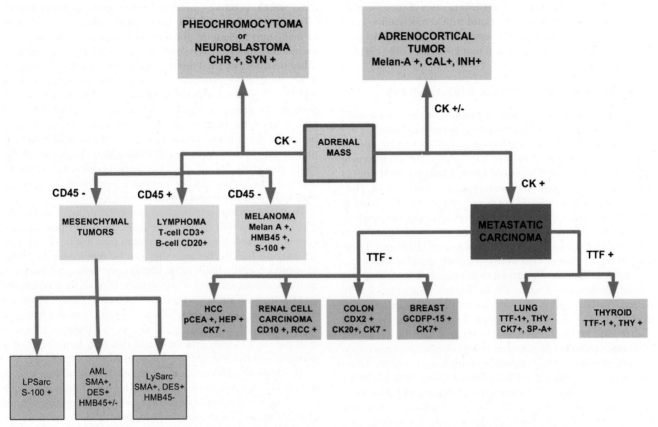

Figure 14.35. Algorithm for immunohistochemical workup of adrenal tumor on needle biopsy. AML, angiomyolipoma; CAL, calretinin; CHR, chromogranin; CK, cytokeratin; DES, desmin; GCDFP, gross cystic disease fluid protein; HEP, hepatocyte; INH, inhibin; LPSarc, liposarcoma; LySarc, leiomyosarcoma; pCEA, polyclonal carcinoembryonic; RCC, renal cell carcinoma; SMA, smooth muscle actin; SP-A, surfactant protein A; SYN, synaptophysin; THY, thyroglobulin; TTF, thyroid transcription factor.

the adrenal gland. The lesion was well circumscribed but not encapsulated and infiltrated the adrenal and surrounding adipose tissue. On microscopic examination, it was seen to be composed of spindle cells that were arranged in small, interlacing fascicles separated by bundles of collagen with focal collections of lymphocytes.

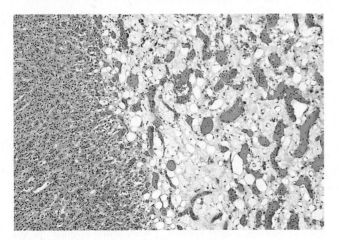

Figure 14.36. Adrenocortical hemangioma.

Rare cases of *calcifying fibrous tumor/pseudotumor* have been reported in the adrenal gland (188,189). This benign mesenchymal tumor occurs predominantly in peripheral soft tissue but has also been described in the serosal surfaces of the pleura and peritoneum. The two reported cases measured 15 and 12 cm. These unencapsulated lesions are composed predominantly of sparsely cellular, hyalinized, fibrotic stroma with haphazardly arranged collagen fibers and foci of dystrophic or psammomatous calcification. Bland, factor XIIIa–positive spindle cells (189) are scattered throughout, as is an inflammatory component. From a radiologic standpoint, calcifying fibrous tumors may simulate neuroblastic tumors.

Although *primary adrenal sarcomas* have been reported, it must be remembered that a primary retroperitoneal sarcoma growing around the adrenal gland may simulate an adrenal primary on imaging studies. Angiosarcomas arising within the adrenal gland are extremely rare. In a series of 10 angiosarcomas reported by Wenig and Heffess (190), the tumors ranged in size from 6 to 10 cm and were composed of spindle-shaped and/or epithelioid cells. A vascular origin was confirmed by the finding of factor VIII–related antigen and CD34 immunoreactivity. Epithelioid angiosarcomas may show focal keratin immunoreactivity, as reported for epithelioid angiosarcomas at other sites. Rarely, extensive hemorrhagic infarction of an adrenal adenoma with the formation of pseudovascular spaces lined by large, atypical fibroblasts may mimic a primary adrenal angiosarcoma (191). Leiomyosarcomas, including cases of pleomorphic leiomyosarcoma of the adrenal gland with osteoclast-like giant cells, and malignant peripheral nerve sheath tumors may rarely develop as primary adrenal gland malignancies (192–194).

RARE TUMORS AND TUMOR-LIKE LESIONS

Adenomatoid tumors occur most commonly in the genital tract, but similar lesions may also arise within the adrenal gland. They are generally small with infiltrative margins and may appear solid or cystic. Rarely, they may have a papillary architecture (195). The histologic features of adrenal adenomatoid tumors are similar to those that have been reported at other sites. They are composed of nests and cords of epithelioid cells forming glands and tubules (Fig. 14.37). In some instances, the epithelioid cells may have a flattened appearance resembling endothelial cells. In the cases described by Simpson (196) and Travis et al. (197), the tumor cells were cytokeratin positive, and ultrastructural analysis demonstrated well-formed desmosomes and extensively developed microvilli, indicating a mesothelial derivation. Further studies have demonstrated that the cells are typically positive for calretinin (198). None of the cases reported to date has been associated with functional activity.

Ovarian thecal metaplasia refers to a focal subcapsular proliferation of spindle cells that resembles ovarian stroma (199). Ovarian thecal metaplasia is an uncommon lesion that has been reported in less than 5% of women undergoing adrenalectomy for metastatic carcinoma of the breast. A similar lesion may occur in men but is exceptionally uncommon. The spindle cells may be surrounded by a collagenous matrix, and groups of cortical cells may be admixed with the spindle cells. Very rarely, gross enlargement of the adrenals may result from similar proliferations of spindle cells (200). Granulosa cell and Leydig cell tumors have also been reported within the adrenal glands (201,202).

Primary adrenal melanomas are rare and controversial tumors with less than 20 cases reported in the literature. Considerably more common is the presence of an occult primary melanoma originating in the skin, mucous membranes, or eyes with metastasis to the adrenal gland (203,204). Dao et al. (204) have proposed that adrenal melanomas can arise from pheochromocytomas, which produce melanin rather than catecholamines. Moreover, they suggest that these tumors should be classified as malignant melanotic pheochromocytomas. It should be remembered, however, that some pheochromocytomas, similar to other neuroectodermal tumors, may contain melanin pigment. Typically, pheochromocytomas are positive for synaptophysin and chromogranin, whereas melanomas are positive for S-100 protein, tyrosinase, melan-A, and HMB-45. Of particular interest has been the observation that approximately one-third of nonmelanotic pheochromocytomas exhibit positivity for the melanoma-specific antibody HMB-45 (205). In three of the cases, less than 5% of the cells were positive for HMB-45, whereas the fourth case demonstrated positivity in approximately 50% of the tumor cells.

As noted earlier, *angiomyolipoma* may be primary within the adrenal gland (186) or may arise from the upper pole of adjacent kidney such that its exact location may not be discernible on imaging studies. Because they can be dominated by HMB-45–positive epithelioid cells, distinction from melanoma is made by absent staining with melan-A. It must be emphasized that the algorithmic approach, summarized in Figure 14.35, is a simplification, because sensitivity and specificity of the different immunohistochemical markers vary, so that despite adequate material on a biopsy, one neoplasm can only be favored over another, without a definitive diagnosis in some cases.

Dysembryonic neoplasms and *adrenocortical blastomas* are exceptionally uncommon. Santonja et al. (206) have reported a single case of a primary adrenal tumor in a 4-year-old boy with features of Wilms tumor. The tumor was composed of blastemal nodules, primitive tubules, glomeruloid structures, and areas resembling sclerotic nephrogenic rests. Molberg et al. (207) have reported a malignant virilizing adrenocortical tumor in a 21-month-old child with elevated alpha-fetoprotein levels. The neoplasm was composed of immature epithelial and mesenchymal elements including slitlike spaces lined by primitive epithelial cells. They felt that the histologic features were reminiscent of the embryonic adrenal cortex so they used the term *adrenocortical blastoma* (207).

Mixed corticomedullary tumors composed of admixtures of cortical and medullary cells are exceptionally rare with less than 10 reported cases (208). Although some of these cases most likely represent collision tumors, others have been characterized by intimate admixtures of cortical and medullary cells.

ADRENAL MEDULLA

NEUROBLASTIC TUMORS

Neuroblastic tumors (NTs) are embryonic neoplasms of the sympathetic nervous system and are the most common solid neoplasms of childhood other than central nervous system tumors. They account for approximately 15% of all neoplasms in children 4 years and younger (mean age, 21 months) (209). NTs have been divided traditionally into three categories: neuroblastoma (NB), ganglioneuroblastoma (GNB), and ganglioneuroma (GN). These categories have been regarded conceptually as a continuum from the most immature to the most mature forms of NT. The epidemiologic and clinical characteristics of NTs are largely related to NBs, which account for the majority of these neoplasms.

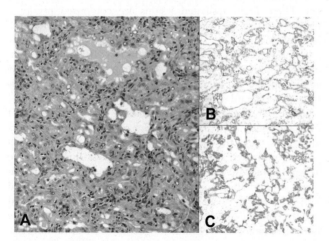

Figure 14.37. Adenomatoid tumor. The tumor is composed of glandular and tubular formations (**A**). Neoplastic cells are positive for cytokeratin (**B**) and calretinin (**C**).

Most NTs occur sporadically, although isolated cases of familial NBs have been recorded (210). They may be found in association with BWS, von Recklinghausen disease, Hirschsprung disease, opsoclonus/myoclonus, heterochromia iridis, watery diarrhea, or Cushing syndrome (42). Rare examples of NTs/NBs have been reported in adults (211–213).

NBs/NTs most commonly develop in relationship to the sympathetic nervous system and most often appear as abdominal masses. The ratio of adrenal to extra-adrenal primary sites is approximately 1.5 to 2:1. The remaining tumors may develop within the head and neck region, mediastinum, or pelvic area. In approximately 10% of cases, it may not be possible to establish the primary site of origin with certainty.

Increased levels of catecholamines and their metabolites are found in most patients with NBs; however, hypertension is present only rarely in affected patients. Rare cases of NB have been associated with cardiogenic shock (214). In advanced stage tumors, increased catecholamine levels and positive bone marrow biopsy results will suffice in making the diagnosis. Mass screening with analysis of urinary catecholamines in infants has been successful in detecting occult cases of NB both in Japan and other countries (215). However, recent studies have suggested that little or no survival advantage has been gained by detecting occult cases in infants (216–218). The patterns of catecholamine secretion as they relate to prognosis are discussed in a subsequent section (219–221).

The concept of in situ NBs was initially proposed by Beckwith and Perrin in 1963 (222) for neuroblastomatous foci confined to the adrenals of newborns. At the microscopic level, these lesions are composed of clusters of immature neuroblasts ranging in size from 0.7 to 9.5 mm, with frequent foci of cystic change. The incidence varies from 0.4% to 2.5% in different autopsy series. This high rate, compared with clinically apparent NBs, has suggested that a substantial number may undergo spontaneous regression, degeneration, or maturation. The distinction between in situ NBs and nodules of normally developing neuroblasts is difficult. Bolande (223) has suggested that neuroblastic nodules measuring more than 2 mm in diameter represent latent NBs. Lesions of smaller diameter, on the other hand, are thought to be an integral part of adrenal morphogenesis (224).

Classification of Neuroblastic Tumors

Several classification and grading schemes have been proposed to correlate morphologic features with prognosis (225–228). A consensus classification that is thought to be prognostically significant, biologically relevant, and reproducible using criteria from previous classification schemes applied to NTs from the Children's Cancer Group (CCG) registry was proposed by member pathologists of the International Neuroblastoma Pathology Committee (INPC). The resulting classification system is largely based on the Shimada classification but also draws from traditional and other recent schemes (229,230).

In the INPC classification (229), NTs are divided into four major categories (Table 14.5): NB (Schwannian stroma-poor NT); GNB, nodular (composite Schwannian stroma-rich/stroma-dominant and stroma-poor NT); GNB, intermixed (Schwannian stroma-rich NT); and GN (Schwannian stroma-dominant NT).

NEUROBLASTOMA (SCHWANNIAN STROMA-POOR NEUROBLASTIC TUMOR)

NBs vary in size from those measuring less than 1 cm in diameter to those that may fill the abdomen or thorax. They are generally soft and white to gray-pink (Fig. 14.38) (19,42,231). However, more differentiated tumors may have a yellow-tan appearance and firmer consistency similar to GN (Fig. 14.39). With increasing size, the tumors typically undergo hemorrhage, necrosis,

TABLE 14.5	Classification of Neuroblastic Tumors	
Joshi (1992)	*Shimada (1984)*	*INPC (1999)*
Neuroblastoma	Stroma-poor NT	Neuroblastoma (Schwannian stroma-poor NT)
Undifferentiated	*Undifferentiated*	*Undifferentiated[a]*
Poorly differentiated		*Poorly differentiated[b]*
Differentiating	*Differentiating*	*Differentiating[c]*
Ganglioneuroblastoma (nodular)	Stroma-rich NT, nodular	Ganglioneuroblastoma, nodular (composite Schwannian stroma-rich/stroma-dominant and stroma-poor NT)[d]
Ganglioneuroblastoma (intermixed)	Stroma-rich NT, intermixed	Ganglioneuroblastoma intermixed (Schwannian stroma-rich NT)[e]
Ganglioneuroblastoma (borderline)	Stroma-rich NT, well differentiated	Ganglioneuroma (Schwannian stroma-dominant NT)
		Maturing[f]
Ganglioneuroma	Ganglioneuroma	*Mature[g]*

INPC, International Neuroblastoma Pathology Committee; NT, neuroblastic tumors.
[a]Undifferentiated neuroblastoma: no ganglionic differentiation (ganglionic differentiation refers to synchronous enlargement of the nucleus and cell body such that the diameter of the cell is twice that of the nucleus) and absence of neuropil.
[b]Poorly differentiated neuroblastoma: <5% ganglionic differentiation, neuropil present, and no or minimal ganglioneuromatous stroma.
[c]Differentiating neuroblastoma: >5% ganglionic differentiation, neuropil present, and <50% ganglioneuromatous stroma.
[d]Ganglioneuroblastoma, nodular: one or more well-defined nodules of neuroblastoma in a background of ganglioneuroma or ganglioneuroblastoma intermixed.
[e]Ganglioneuroblastoma, intermixed: nests of neuroblasts and neuropil intermixed with ganglioneuromatous stroma, as in differentiating neuroblastoma, but >50% ganglioneuromatous stroma.
[f]Maturing ganglioneuroma: individual neuroblasts merge into differentiating ganglion cells without the presence of discrete nests of neuroblasts.
[g]Mature ganglioneuroma: mature ganglion cells and Schwannian stroma.

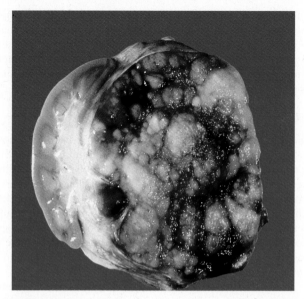

Figure 14.38. Neuroblastoma. The tumor has a nodular appearance with areas of hemorrhage and calcification. The kidney is present just to the left of the tumor.

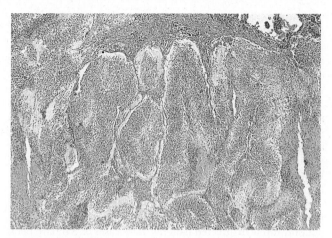

Figure 14.40. Neuroblastoma. This tumor has a lobular appearance on low-power examination.

cyst formation, and calcification; however, cyst formation and hemorrhage may also be evident in small tumors. Adrenal primaries tend to grow toward the midline and can extend to the contralateral adrenal gland. Large, right-sided tumors can invade the liver directly, whereas large, left-sided tumors can invade the pancreatic parenchyma.

NBs are composed of sheets of small cells with hyperchromatic nuclei and scanty cytoplasm. They frequently have a lobular appearance as a result of the presence of thin fibrovascular septa between groups of tumor cells (Fig. 14.40). Depending on the degree of differentiation, there may be a finely fibrillary matrix (neuropil) between the tumor cells. At the ultrastructural level, the neuropil corresponds to masses of unmyelinated axons (232). Homer Wright pseudorosettes are found in approximately 30% of cases (19). The pseudorosettes are composed of one to two layers of neuroblasts arranged around a central space that is filled with tangles of neuritic processes (Fig.

14.41). In tumors in which there is hemorrhage, pseudorosettes or nests of cells may assume a papillary pattern reminiscent of Schiller-Duvall bodies of yolk sac tumors.

In the INPC classification (229), undifferentiated NB lacks neuropil and is characterized by the presence of small to medium-sized cells with thin rims of cytoplasm and indistinct cytoplasmic borders. The nuclei are round to ovoid with coarsely granular (salt and pepper) chromatin and indistinct nucleoli (Fig. 14.42). Caution is needed in not mistaking areas of coagulative necrosis for neuropil. The presence of occasional cells with vesicular nuclei and prominent nucleoli apparently differentiating toward immature ganglion cells is a useful clue in differentiating these tumors from other small blue-cell tumors, including Ewing sarcoma/primitive neuroectodermal tumor (EWS/PNET), rhabdomyosarcoma, desmoplastic small round-cell tumor, blastemal Wilms tumor, and lymphoma. Immunohistochemical and molecular genetic studies are critical in arriving at the correct diagnosis (Table 14.6).

Poorly differentiated NB contains a neuropil background (Fig. 14.41). Most neoplastic cells are undifferentiated, but

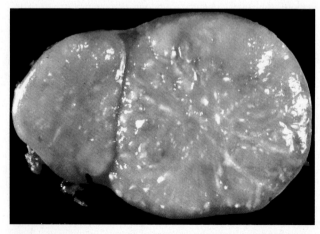

Figure 14.39. Neuroblastoma, differentiating. The tumor has a firm consistency and cut surface reminiscent of ganglioneuroma.

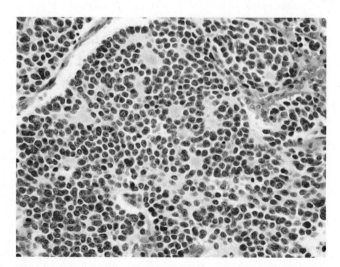

Figure 14.41. Neuroblastoma, poorly differentiated. This tumor contains prominent Homer Wright pseudorosettes and undifferentiated neuroblasts.

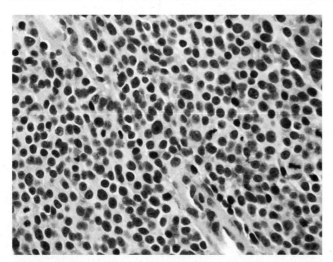

Figure 14.42. Neuroblastoma, undifferentiated. The tumor is composed of undifferentiated neuroblasts with occasional cells with prominent nucleoli that suggest an attempt at differentiation toward immature ganglion cells. Neuropil is absent.

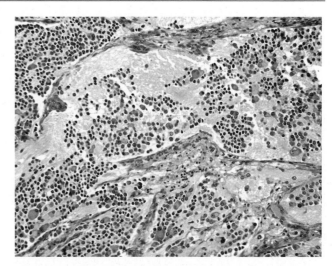

Figure 14.43. Neuroblastoma, differentiating. The tumor has abundant neuropil, Schwannian stroma, and ganglion cells (immature and mature) that constitute less than 50% of tumor cells.

some cells with evidence of ganglionic differentiation (differentiating neuroblasts) are usually present. By definition, differentiating neuroblasts account for less than 5% of the neoplastic cells (229). Maturation is manifested by synchronous differentiation of the nucleus (enlarged eccentric nucleus, vesicular chromatin, and single prominent nucleolus) and cytoplasm that may appear eosinophilic or amphophilic. The cell diameter must be at least twice the nuclear diameter. In some instances, pleomorphic cells containing large nuclei and prominent nucleoli may be present. These pleomorphic cells may occasionally have rhabdoid features and may be mistaken for cells showing ganglionic differentiation. Both undifferentiated and poorly differentiated NBs contain no or minimal ganglioneuromatous stroma.

Differentiating NBs are characterized by the presence of more than 5% of cells showing evidence of ganglionic differentiation. Usually, differentiating NBs contain more abundant neuropil than poorly differentiated NBs, although the most critical feature of the differentiating tumors is the proportion of maturing neuroblasts (Fig. 14.43). Both ganglionic differentiation and Schwannian stromal formation, which are frequently present at the periphery of the tumor, may be prominent in differentiating NBs. By definition, however, these features should comprise less than 50% of the tumor, in contrast to GNB, intermixed in which they represent more than 50% of the tumor (229). Also, distinguishing differentiating NBs from nodular GNB may at times be difficult. Generally, the transitional zone between the NB and ganglioneuroblastomatous component is poorly defined in the differentiating NBs. Of

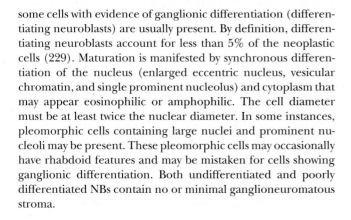

TABLE 14.6	Immunohistochemical Profile of Neuroblastoma and Other Small, Round Blue-Cell Tumors					
Immunoperoxidase Stain	*NB*	*EWS/PNET*	*RMS*	*Wilms (Blastemal)*	*DSRCT*	*Lymphoma*
NB84	++++	+	±	±	++	−
Neurofilament	+++	+	+	±	−	−
NSE	+++	++	+	−	+++	±
Synaptophysin	++	+	−	−	+	−
Chromogranin	+++	−	−	−	±	−
CD57	±	+	+	−	++	±
Vimentin	++	+++	++++	+	+++	++
CD99	−	++++	+	+	+	±
FLI-1	−	+++	−	−	+	+
Desmin	−	−	++++	++	++++	−
Myogenin	−	−	+++	±	−	−
Cytokeratin	−	±	+	±	++++	±
EMA	±	±	±	−	++++	±
CD45	−	−	−	−	−	++++
WT1	±	−	++	+++	++++	−

− to + + + + denotes the relative quantity of cases, *not* the intensity of staining; ± = variably positive.
DSRCT, desmoplastic small round-cell tumor; EWS/PNET, Ewing sarcoma/primitive neuroectodermal tumor; NB, neuroblastoma; RMS, rhabdomyosarcoma.

note, a large-cell variant of NB has been reported in which there is an aggressive clinical behavior (233).

Immunohistochemistry and Ultrastructure

NBs most commonly express the 68-kd neurofilament protein; however, some cases may react positively with antibodies to the 150- and 200-kd neurofilament proteins. GNBs and GNs, however, contain cells that are reactive to antibodies to all three major neurofilament proteins (234–238). The presence of neurofilament proteins may, therefore, provide an important clue in making the distinction between NB and other small, round blue-cell tumors of infancy and childhood (Table 14.6). However, it should be remembered that neurofilament proteins may be present in other small, round blue-cell tumors, including rhabdomyosarcoma (Table 14.6) (239).

Catecholamine-synthesizing enzymes can also be demonstrated in immunohistochemical formats. Neuron-specific enolase (NSE) is present in virtually all NBs; however, this marker may also be present in nonneuroblastic tumors (30). Additional markers that have been used for diagnosis of NBs include chromogranins and secretogranins (240), synaptophysin (Fig. 14.44) (27,241), CD57 (leu-7) (242), ganglioside D2 (243), protein gene product 9.5 (PGP-9.5) (240), microtubule (MAP-1 and MAP-2), tau proteins (238,244), and certain epitopes detectable with NB-directed monoclonal antibodies, including UJ13A (245,246) and HSAN 1.2 (247,248). The UJ13A epitope corresponds to neural adhesion molecule (NCAM/CD56), a family of cell surface glycoproteins involved in direct cell-to-cell adhesion. Antibodies to NCAM/CD56 frequently react with NB (249–251). NB84, a monoclonal antibody raised against NB cells, recognizes a large proportion of NBs as well as EWS/PNETs and desmoplastic small round-cell tumors (252). Although rhabdomyosarcomas and lymphoblastic lymphomas were reported initially to be negative for NB84, Folpe et al. (253) demonstrated positivity for this marker in occasional rhabdomyosarcomas and small-cell osteosarcomas. Immunohistochemical staining with S-100 protein highlights cells in the Schwannian stroma, but the neuroblasts are negative (Fig. 14.45). The anaplastic lymphoma kinase (*ALK*) gene is expressed/activated using reverse transcriptase polymerase chain reaction (RT-PCR) and Western blotting in NB cell lines and frozen tissue from NBs (254). However, immunohistochemical staining of a few of the NBs was weak and cytoplasmic and therefore was of limited clinical utility. Membranous staining with CD99 (detectable by monoclonal antibodies HBA-71, 12E7, and O13), which is typically seen in the EWS/PNET tumor group of PNET tumors, is negative in NBs (255).

NB cells contain scattered ribosomes, small amounts of granular endoplasmic reticulum, few mitochondria, and small Golgi regions (Fig. 14.46). The most poorly differentiated tumors can contain isolated organelles and only a few adherens-type junctions (232,256,257). Cell processes contain intermediate filaments and bundles of microtubules as well as neurosecretory granules and synaptic vesicles. Lysosomal granules may be prominent in some cells. Glycogen deposits are present in approximately 10% of cases (258). Distinction of undifferentiated NB from EWS/PNET is difficult or impossible at the ultrastructural level; accordingly, molecular genetic and biochemical studies are invaluable ancillary studies for this distinction.

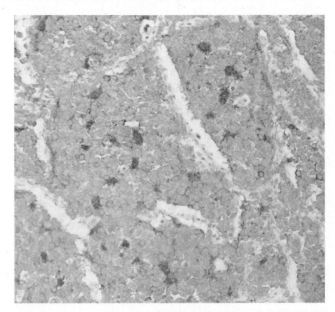

Figure 14.44. Neuroblastoma, poorly differentiated. A synaptophysin immunohistochemical stain shows positive granular cytoplasmic staining of neuroblasts and highlights the Homer Wright pseudorosettes.

Molecular Genetic Features

Several genetic and molecular features are seen in NBs, including *MYCN* gene amplification, chromosome 1p loss, and 17q gain. These parameters and other genetic features are discussed in detail in the section on prognosis (Table 14.7).

Spread and Metastases

NBs can metastasize widely through both lymphatic and vascular routes (19). The most common sites of spread include bone

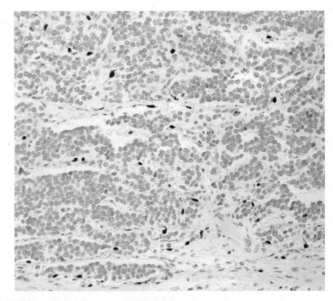

Figure 14.45. Neuroblastoma, poorly differentiated. An immunohistochemical stain for S-100 protein shows positive staining of Schwann cells within the delicate septae, but neuroblasts are negative.

TABLE 14.7	**Molecular Genetic Markers of Small Blue-Cell Tumors in the Differential Diagnosis of Neuroblastoma**	
Neoplasm	*Genetics*	*Comments*
Neuroblastoma	*MYCN* amplification 1p deletion 17q gain	Not specific for neuroblastoma, but are prognostic markers
EWS/PNET	t(11;22)(q24;q12) *EWS/FLI-1* t(21;22)(q22;q12) *EWS/ERG* t(7;22)(p22;q12) *EWS/ETV1* t(17;22)(q12;q12) *EWS/E1AF*	
Rhabdomyosarcoma	*Alveolar* t(2;13)(q35-37;q14) *PAX3/FKHR* t(1;13)(p36;q14) *PAX7/FKHR* *Embryonal* Allelic loss of 11p15; extra 2, 8, 13 Rearrangement of 2, 8, 13, 1p11-1q11, 12q13	*MYCN* amplification may be associated with a worse prognosis *PAX3/FKHR* translocation appears to be associated with decreased survival compared to no translocation or *PAX7/FKHR* translocation
Wilms (blastemal)	No consistent cytogenetic/genetic abnormality in sporadic cases	
Desmoplastic small round-cell tumor	t(11;22)(p13;q12) *EWS/WT1*	
Lymphoma	T-cell β, γ, immunoglobulin heavy or light chain gene rearrangement	

EWS/PNET, Ewing sarcoma/primitive neuroectodermal tumor.

marrow (78%), bone (69%), lymph nodes (42%), and liver (20%), whereas pulmonary and brain metastases are uncommon. Pulmonary metastases have been reported in 3% of cases in one study and are usually associated with widespread disease and unfavorable histology with poor outcome (259). Even in these cases, the metastatic nodules tend to be small. From a clinical standpoint, in the presence of lung nodules, NB is viewed as a less likely primary than other small round-cell tumors such as EWS/PNET. Skin (2%) and testes (2%) may also be involved. Spontaneous regression is well documented. Although the mechanisms responsible for these phenomena are incompletely understood, increasing evidence suggests that genetic prerequisites that are involved include an intact chromosome 1 short arm, lack of *MYCN* amplification, and near triploidy (229).

Differential Diagnosis

The distinction of undifferentiated and poorly differentiated NBs from other small, round blue-cell tumors (Table 14.6) is challenging on routine hematoxylin and eosin–stained sections, particularly in small biopsy samples. EWS/PNET is the most difficult to distinguish from NB because they share morphologic and immunohistochemical features. Both tumors can have a lobular growth pattern and may contain Homer Wright pseudorosettes, but EWS/PNET lacks the neuropil background of poorly differentiated NB. Although both tumors react with antibodies to NSE and synaptophysin, EWS/PNET is almost never positive for chromogranin. CD99 is positive in EWS/PNET, whereas it is negative in NB. Molecular genetic studies are useful adjuncts in making the distinction (Table 14.7); however, these studies may provide conflicting results. For example,

Burchill et al. (260) reported that 2 of 12 cases of typical NB had the EWS/FLI-1 fusion transcript by RT-PCR. In the cases described, serum and urinary markers and histologic features were consistent with NB. Immunohistochemical staining of both tumors revealed positivity for NB84, PGP-9.5, and NSE, whereas CD99 was negative. These observations underscore the need for detailed clinical-pathologic correlation in arriving at a diagnosis, particularly when faced with limited material in biopsy samples. In view of the propensity that NB shows for presenting with metastatic disease, it is a useful approach to consider NB the first diagnosis in cases of small round-cell tumors until proven otherwise, particularly in patients younger than 5 years of age. EWS/PNET typically occurs in an older age group, being uncommon in patients younger than 5 years of age (261).

Rhabdomyosarcoma occurs in the same age group as NB, but the presence of rhabdomyoblasts and strap cells helps in making the distinction. However, as discussed previously, undifferentiated or poorly differentiated NB may have pleomorphic cells with rhabdoid features, but immunohistochemistry will permit their specific identification. Similarly, Wilms tumor occurs in the same age group. Triphasic or epithelial tumors pose less of a diagnostic problem, but blastemal Wilms is more likely to be mistaken for NB on routine sections. This is complicated by small biopsy specimens from large tumors that may show extension between the adrenal gland and kidney. Serum and urinary catecholamines and immunohistochemistry (Table 14.6) are invaluable in making the distinction.

Lymphoblastic lymphoma is another important differential diagnosis when there is bulky disease of the retroperitoneum. The distinction is particularly difficult on small biopsies in which neuropil is not apparent. CD45 can be negative in a subset of these tumors (261a); accordingly, stains for terminal deoxynucleotidyl transferase (TdT) and T and B lymphocytes may be necessary for conclusive exclusion.

GANGLIONEUROBLASTOMA, NODULAR (COMPOSITE SCHWANNIAN STROMA-RICH/ STROMA-DOMINANT AND STROMA-POOR NEUROBLASTIC TUMOR)

Ganglioneuroblastoma, nodular (GNB, nodular) is characterized by a gross appearance in which frequently hemorrhagic NB nodules (Fig. 14.47) are present in a background that may resemble the gross appearance of GNB, intermixed or the glistening tan-pink whorled cut surface of GN. Microscopically, there is usually an abrupt demarcation of the neuroblastic (stroma-poor) component from the stroma-rich (GNB, intermixed) or stroma-dominant (GN) component. Neuroblastic nodules, therefore, have pushing borders and may even have a fibrous pseudocapsule. The neuroblastic nodules most probably develop as a consequence of evolution of one or more aggressive clones within the tumor. This may be the result of newly acquired genetic alterations or the persistence of two or more genetically and biologically different clones (229).

The proportion of both components may vary. The stroma-rich/stroma-dominant component is often located at the periphery, but it can appear as thin or broad septa between contiguous nodules. In rare cases, the neuroblastic component may dominate the tumor, with the stroma-rich/stroma-dominant component being in the periphery. Therefore, examination of the periphery of these tumors is essential for accurate classification because the category of GNB, nodular is grouped in the unfavorable histology group of NTs. The proportion of stroma-rich/stroma-dominant tissue is not critical for the diagnosis. Cases in which GNB, intermixed or GN is found in the sections

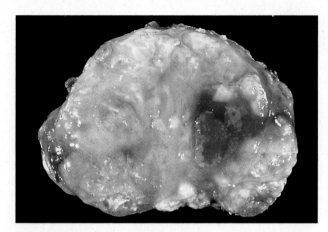

Figure 14.47. Ganglioneuroblastoma, nodular (composite Schwannian stroma-rich/stroma-dominant and stroma-poor neuroblastic tumor).

from the primary site, but NB is found in sections from a metastatic site, are classified as GNB, nodular.

GANGLIONEUROBLASTOMA, INTERMIXED (SCHWANNIAN STROMA-RICH NEUROBLASTIC TUMOR)

Ganglioneuroblastoma, intermixed (GNB, intermixed) can have the same gross appearance as NB or GN depending on the extent of differentiation. It is characterized by the random intermingling of neuroblastic nests within the stroma-rich (ganglioneuromatous) component (Fig. 14.48). Usually a mixture of neuroblastic cells in various stages of differentiation is seen, with differentiating neuroblasts and ganglion cells dominating in a background of abundant neuropil. Therefore, GNB, intermixed differs from GNB, nodular by lacking a macroscopically distinct hemorrhagic nodule, and microscopically, the interface between the stroma-poor and stroma-rich components is infiltrative rather than pushing. GNB, intermixed is distinguished from differentiating NB on the basis of the extent of the ganglio-

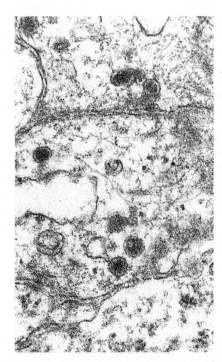

Figure 14.46. Neuroblastoma. The electron micrograph shows cell processes with a few membrane-bound secretory granules (58,000×).

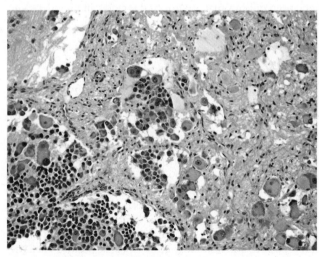

Figure 14.48. Ganglioneuroblastoma, intermixed. The stroma-poor component on the lower left merges in an infiltrative fashion with the stroma-rich component in the upper right.

neuromatous component, which should exceed 50% of the total volume in microscopic field(s) from representative section(s) of the tumor (229). GNB, intermixed, unlike GNB, nodular, is classified as a favorable-histology NT.

GANGLIONEUROMA (SCHWANNIAN STROMA-DOMINANT NEUROBLASTIC TUMOR)

In the INPC classification, GN is subdivided into GN, maturing and GN, mature subtypes (229,230). The GN, maturing subtype was previously classified as "stroma-rich, well-differentiated NT" in the original Shimada classification (227). It is composed predominantly of ganglioneuromatous stroma with a minor component of scattered, evenly or unevenly distributed collections of differentiating neuroblasts and/or maturing ganglion cells in addition to fully mature ganglion cells. Separation from GNB, intermixed is based on the fact that neuroblastomatous foci do not form distinct microscopic nests, but instead, individual neuroblastic cells merge into the ganglioneuromatous stroma.

GN, mature subtype is the prototypic GN of traditional classification schemes. Less than 30% of these tumors occur in the adrenal glands, where they are most commonly asymptomatic (262,263). The remainder develops in the posterior compartment of the mediastinum, retroperitoneum, and other sites. Rarely, they are associated with hypertension, watery diarrhea, and hypokalemia or masculinization (264). Adrenal GNs (GN, mature subtype) are generally smaller than those in the mediastinum or retroperitoneum. They are sharply circumscribed but do not have a true capsule (Fig. 14.49). On cross section, they are gray to tan, and their consistency varies from soft and gelatinous to firm and whorled with an appearance reminiscent of that of a leiomyoma. Microscopically, GN, mature subtype contains varying numbers of mature ganglion cells and Schwann cells together with variable amounts of collagen (Fig. 14.50) (265). A few multinucleated ganglion cells may also be evident. The Schwann cells and collagen are often arranged in interlacing bundles. Ganglion cells may be distributed diffusely throughout the tumor or arranged in small clusters. Fully mature ganglion cells are usually surrounded by satellite cells. Complete maturation requires the absence of a neuroblastomatous component. Because lymphocytes are commonly pres-

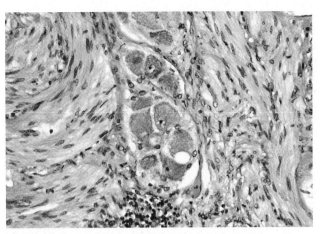

Figure 14.50. Ganglioneuroma. The tumor contains a group of mature ganglion cells surrounded by a Schwann cell–rich stroma.

ent within these tumors, immunohistochemical staining with CD45 may be necessary in some instances to exclude the presence of a neuroblastic component. Surgical excision of GN, mature subtype is usually curative. Very rarely, GN, mature subtype may transform into malignant peripheral nerve sheath tumor either spontaneously or after irradiation for NB or GNB (42).

PROBLEMATIC CASES OF HISTOLOGIC CLASSIFICATION AND GRADING

The preceding discussion summarizes a clear-cut definition of NTs. In practice, categorization may be hampered by small biopsies in which clear distinction of NB, GNB nodular, GNB intermixed, and GN is not possible. In these instances, a diagnosis of "NT unclassifiable" is appropriate, and a multidisciplinary discussion is useful in determining the adequacy of the biopsy. A diagnosis of NB not otherwise specified (NOS) is appropriate when there is poor quality of sections, extensive hemorrhage, cystic degeneration, necrosis, crush artifact, and/or diffuse calcification. These factors may also impede evaluation of neuroblastic differentiation, mitosis-karyorrhexis index (MKI), and mitotic rate. Similarly, a diagnosis of GNB NOS is appropriate when extensive calcification may obscure a stroma-poor nodule (229).

POSTTHERAPEUTIC SPECIMENS

Posttherapeutic resection specimens are difficult to assess. There is usually extensive fibrosis and calcification of specimens from the abdomen or retroperitoneum, complicating the assessment of margins and the presence of residual tumor. Microscopically, necrotic foci, fibrosis, chronic inflammation, and calcification are commonly seen. In residual foci of tumor, the features of both differentiation and nuclear enlargement may be seen. Grading of these tumors with stratification into favorable or unfavorable categories is not performed (229).

PROGNOSIS

The prognosis of NTs is determined by multiple variables, including age, histopathologic features, and stage, as well as a

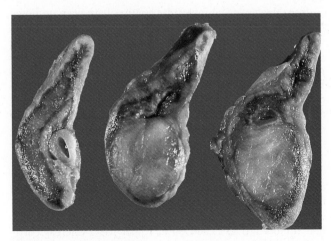

Figure 14.49. Ganglioneuroma. The tumor is sharply circumscribed but not encapsulated.

series of molecular, genetic, and biologic parameters. Age at diagnosis is an important independent prognostic factor, with outcome being inversely related to age at diagnosis (265). The cutoff age of 1 year is used for risk stratification for treatment purposes. This differs from that used in the age-linked histologic grading.

Although the number of mitoses per 10 hpf and calcification have been used to stratify NBs into different prognostic groups (266,267), the INPC adopted the MKI. The number of cells undergoing mitosis and karyorrhexis is expressed as a percentage of 5000 cells and is assessed on high power (400×). MKI is designated as low, intermediate, or high based on counts of less than 100 (<2%), 100 to 200 (2% to 4%), and more than 200 (>4%) mitotic and karyorrhectic cells, respectively (227). There may be variability in the MKI in different fields of a section or variability between sections, but the overall MKI is the average determined by assessing all sections. Of note, MKI should not be assessed adjacent to areas of necrosis. MKI can be assessed in metastatic tumor. The MKI, along with age and grade of NB, is used to assign NBs to favorable and unfavorable histology categories.

Application of the INPC classification to a large group of cases of NTs by Shimada et al. (268) produced stratification into favorable and unfavorable histology prognostic groups similar to the original Shimada classification (Table 14.8) (226). GNB, intermixed and GN were classified as favorable histology NTs (100% 5-year overall survival). GNB, nodular was classified as unfavorable histology (59.1% 5-year overall survival) (268). However, Umehara et al. (269) reported prognostic subsets of GNB, nodular based on the grade of the nodular NB component using the same parameters as those used for favorable and unfavorable histology in NBs. Favorable and unfavorable subsets, with 5-year overall survival rates of 95.0% and 40.7%, respectively, were defined.

Ambros et al. (270) attempted to correlate morphologic features of NB, independent of age, that might be able to identify clinically favorable and unfavorable groups. Prominent nucleoli in undifferentiated and poorly differentiated neuroblasts, cellularity, and nuclear size appeared to have clinical significance.

For the most part, the morphology and biology of NBs are rather homogeneous. However, Sano et al. (271) recently reported a case in a 12-month-old child in which two distinct histologic and biologic clones could be distinguished. Both were poorly differentiated, but one clone had a high MKI and thus an unfavorable histology and the other had a low MKI and thus a favorable histology. *MYCN* was amplified in the unfavorable histology clone and nonamplified in the favorable histology clone. Metastasis to lymph nodes contained the former clone. Because of these findings, they considered this to be a composite NB.

Tumor stage is clearly an important independent prognostic indicator. The currently used staging system is the International Neuroblastoma Staging System (INSS) (Table 14.9) (272,273). Of note, stage 4S is considered essentially localized disease (stages 1 and 2) with limited distant spread. In the revised INSS, stage 4S is restricted to patients younger than 1 year of age. Ikeda et al. (274) found no significant differences in 4-year overall survival rates for patients younger than 1 year of age with stage 1, 2A, 2B, 3, or 4S disease (98.5% survival) versus patients with stage 4 disease (73.1% survival). Similarly, patients older than 1 year of age with stage 1, 2A, 2B, or 3 disease had similar 4-year overall survival rates versus patients with stage 4 disease, in which survival was 48.5%.

Although stage 4 cases are usually associated with progressive disease and a poor outcome, Kushner et al. (275) reported their experience with chronic NB in children diagnosed with stage 4 NB in the first decade of life who had metastatic disease for 5 years or more from diagnosis. As they point out, this represented indolent or smoldering NB, a concept usually limited to adolescents and adults. This phenomenon may be attributed to the expanding repertoire of chemotherapeutic modalities, including biologic therapies, currently in use.

Serum ferritin and lactate dehydrogenase (LDH) have been reported to be useful prognostic markers for NB at diagnosis but lack sensitivity and specificity to monitor disease activity (273). Increased serum ferritin levels (>150 ng/mL) have been associated with advanced stage tumors and poor overall survival (265), but they may also reflect rapid tumor growth and/or large tumor burden. Serum levels of NSE also reflect the extent of disease in patients with these tumors (276). NSE, chromogranin (CGA), and GD2 (tumor-associated ganglioside) are more specific but not as sensitive as serum ferritin levels. Catecholamine levels have also been associated with prognosis (277).

Several genetic and molecular features have been proposed as prognostic indicators in NTs, including *MYCN* amplification, chromosome 1p deletion, ploidy, and gains in chromosome 17q (Table 14.10). *MCYN* amplification (>10 copies of *MYCN*) and ploidy are used routinely for stratification into treatment groups by the Children's Oncology Group. *MYCN* amplification is present in 25% to 30% of NB patients with advanced stage disease and is associated with rapid tumor progression and poor clinical outcome (278–280). *MYCN* amplification is used as a determinant in applying more aggressive treatment protocols for stage 1, 2, and 4S tumors (similar to more advanced stage tumors). *MYCN* amplification is present almost exclusively in NBs, with a smaller proportion in the GNB, nodular category and none in GNB, intermixed and GN categories (281). Five-year overall survival rates for favorable histology nonamplified and amplified tumors are 99% and 50%, respectively, whereas corresponding survival rates for unfavorable histology nonamplified and amplified tumors are 47.1% and 23.0%, respectively. Kobay-

TABLE 14.8

Age-Linked Prognostic Effects Using the INPC Classification

Grade	MKI	Age (years)		
		<1.5	1.5–5	≥5
Undifferentiated	Low	–	–	–
	Intermediate	–	–	–
	High	–	–	–
Poorly differentiated	Low	+	–	–
	Intermediate	+	–	–
	High	–	–	–
Differentiating	Low	+	+	–
	Intermediate	+	–	–
	High	–	–	–

INPC, International Neuroblastoma Pathology Committee; MKI, mitosis-karyorrhexis index.
+, good (favorable histology); –, poor (unfavorable histology).

TABLE 14.9	International Neuroblastoma Staging System	

Stage	Definition	Comments
1	Localized tumor with gross excision, with or without microscopic residual disease; representative ipsilateral lymph nodes negative for tumor microscopically	Nodes attached to and removed with primary tumor may be positive; includes grossly resectable tumor arising in the midline from pelvic ganglia or organ of Zuckerkandl
2A	Localized tumor with incomplete gross excision; representative ipsilateral nonadherent lymph nodes negative for tumor microscopically	Includes a midline tumor that extends beyond one side of the vertebral column and is unresectable
2B	Localized tumor with or without gross excision, with ipsilateral nonadherent lymph nodes positive for tumor; enlarged contralateral lymph nodes must be negative microscopically	Includes a midline tumor that extends beyond one side of the vertebral column and is unresectable with positive ipsilateral lymph node involvement (on side of extension); a thoracic tumor with malignant unilateral pleural effusion
3	Unresectable unilateral tumor infiltrating across the midline with or without regional lymph node involvement; or localized unilateral tumor with contralateral regional lymph node involvement	Includes midline tumor with bilateral extension by infiltration (unresectable) or by lymph node involvement; a tumor of any size with malignant ascites or peritoneal implants
4	Any primary tumor with dissemination to distant lymph nodes, bone, bone marrow, liver, skin, and/or other organs (except as defined for 4S)	
4S	Localized primary tumor (stage 1, 2A, or 2B) with dissemination limited to skin, liver, and/or bone marrow (limited to infants <1 year of age)	Marrow involvement should be minimal (<10% of total nucleated cells identified as malignant on biopsy or aspirate); more extensive involvement should be considered stage 4

Midline is defined as the vertebral column with the vertebral body margin as the limit. Multifocal primary tumors should be staged according to the greatest extent of disease and followed by the subscript letter M.

ashi et al. (282) have suggested that enlarged and prominent nucleoli may indicate presence of *MYCN* amplification in NB. Detection of *MYCN* amplification can be determined with Southern blot, fluorescent in situ hybridization (FISH), and polymerase chain reaction. Recently, Thorner at al. (283) used chromogenic in situ hybridization (CISH) for determining *MYCN* gene copy number in routine tissue sections. Although typically done on frozen tissue, *MYCN* amplification can be assessed from paraffin-embedded tissue by FISH and CISH.

Deletion of chromosome 1p is the most characteristic cytogenetic abnormality described in NBs and has been identified in 30% to 50% of cases (284). Although there has been some debate about whether 1p loss has independent prognostic value,

multivariate analysis has suggested that it is associated with decreased event-free survival (285).

FISH studies have demonstrated unbalanced translocations involving 17q, resulting in gains of 17q. Such unbalanced partial 17q gain is significantly associated with well-established indicators of clinical risk in NB including advanced stage and older age (286). Interestingly, *MYCN* amplification almost never occurs in the absence of 1p allele loss, 17q gain, or both.

Tumors with a near diploid karyotype have a poorer prognosis than those with a hyperdiploid or triploid karyotype (279), and *MYCN* amplification is significantly more frequent in diploid than hyperdiploid tumors (284). Furthermore, chromosome 1p abnormalities, double minutes (DMs), and homo-

TABLE 14.10	Prognostic Subsets of Neuroblastoma Based on Clinical and Biologic Parameters		

Prognostic Feature	Low-Risk Tumors	Intermediate-Risk Tumors	High-Risk Tumors
Age	<1 year	>1 year	1–5 years
Stage (INSS)	1, 2, 4S	3, 4	3, 4
MYCN[a]	1 copy	1 copy	Amplified
DNA ploidy	Hyperdiploid or near triploid	Near diploid or near tetraploid	Near diploid or near tetraploid
Chromosome 1p36	Usually intact	Usually intact	Deletion
Chromosome 17q gain	Absent	Present	Present
TRK-A/C expression	High	Low or absent	Low or absent
TRK-B expression	Truncated	Low or absent	High
Clinical course and survival	Very good response; 5-year survival 95%	Initial response but tendency for relapse; 5-year survival 40%–50%	Rapidly progressive disease; frequently fatal; 5-year survival 25%

INSS, International Neuroblastoma Staging System.
[a]MYCN status correlates with homogeneously staining regions (HSRs) and double minutes (DMs) on chromosome karyotyping.
Modified from Brodeur GM. Neuroblastoma: biological insights into a clinical enigma. *Nat Rev* 2003;3:203–216.

geneous staining regions (HSRs) appear to be more prevalent in diploid and tetraploid tumors (Table 14.10).

Expression of the tyrosine kinase receptor for nerve growth factor, TRK-A, is present in 91% of NBs, and high levels of expression of TRK-A are associated with a good prognosis (280,287,288). Conversely, lack of TRK-A is associated with aggressive behavior. TRK-A expression has been suggested to play a role in differentiation and programmed cell death, which may explain the correlation with behavior. Related neurotrophin receptors, TRK-B and TRK-C, have also been studied. Expression of full-length TRK-B is associated with *MYCN*-amplified tumors, whereas expression of TRK-C, similar to TRK-A, is not expressed in *MYCN*-amplified tumors (Table 14.10).

Other factors that appear to be associated with a better outcome include CD44 expression, high HRAS expression (284,288), LOH of chromosome 11q23 (in stage 4 NBs) (289), and deletions in the region of chromosome 9p22-p24 (290). However, advanced stage and poor prognosis appear to be associated with LOH of chromosome 14q (288), expression of the multidrug resistance genes (*MDR1*) or multidrug resistance–related protein (MRP), high levels of telomerase activity (284,288), bcl-2 overexpression (291–293), and allelic imbalances of chromosomes 8q, 10p11, 12q24, and 19q13 (292,293). In addition, Krams et al. (294) suggested that proliferation index assessed by immunohistochemical staining has greater predictive power than *MYCN* amplification as a single factor.

Studies using *gene expression profiling* have also been used to predict behavior of NBs. Wei et al. (295) identified 19 predictor genes by performing gene expression profiling using cDNA microarrays containing 42,578 clones along with an artificial neural network and were able to predict outcome for 98% of patients in the study group (56 pretreatment samples from 49 NB patients). From the 19 identified genes, 12 are known genes, eight of which are expressed in neural tissue (295). Along with *MYCN*, four other genes were upregulated in the poor outcome group (*DLK1*, *PRSS3*, *ARC*, and *SLIT3*), and three were downregulated (*CNR1*, *ROBO2*, and *BTBD3*). The highest ranked was *DLK1*, a transmembrane protein that activates the Notch signaling pathway and has also been shown to inhibit neuronal differentiation. The authors noted that there was upregulation of the neuron axon repellant gene *SLIT3*, with downregulation of one of its receptors (*ROBO2*) in the poor outcome group, and speculated that NB cells may secrete a substrate to repel connecting axons and potentially prevent differentiation. Of additional interest, one of the genes that is downregulated in the poor prognostic group (*ARH1*) maps to chromosome 1p31. It is a maternally imprinted tumor suppressor gene implicated in ovarian and breast cancer and lies in close proximity to the 1p36 region, the deletion of which has already been noted to be associated with high-risk NBs.

More recently, Asgharzadeh et al. (296) used Affymetrix microarrays to determine the gene expression profiles of 102 patients with untreated primary NBs without *MYCN* amplification but with metastatic disease. They used a supervised method of diagonal linear discriminant analysis to build a multigene model for predicting risk of disease progression. From a 55-gene expression model, they were able to define two subgroups of patients older than 12 months who were classified as having clinically high-risk disease: a low-risk group with a progression-free survival (PFS) of 79% and a high-risk group with a PFS of 16%. The *TrkB* gene was found to be the most statistically significant gene associated with risk of progression.

In summary, a variety of biologic parameters have been reported to influence prognosis of NBs. However, in routine clinical practice, *MYCN* amplification and DNA ploidy are the ones used in conjunction with patient age, tumor histology, and stage to stratify patients into low-, intermediate-, and high-risk treatment groups.

SPECIMEN HANDLING AND REPORTING

The surgical pathologist must be involved in evaluating NTs immediately after surgery so that fresh tissue can be appropriately submitted for genetic and biologic markers. Specimen dimensions and weight are obtained. Although accurate staging of NBs can be quite problematic by gross examination, careful examination of all specimens for the presence or absence of a capsule and the adequacy of margins is mandatory. Specimens should be sectioned at 1.0- to 1.5-cm intervals such that the relationships to identifiable structures are maintained. Fresh tissue should be submitted in culture medium for conventional cytogenetics. Snap-frozen fresh tissue and touch/squash preparations (fixed in acetone or ethanol for 10 to 15 minutes) should be prepared for molecular genetic studies. Tissue fixed in glutaraldehyde is used for ultrastructural examination as needed. Representative sections from all heterogeneous-appearing areas must be submitted, making sure to demonstrate the interface between these areas (to facilitate making the diagnosis of nodular GNB), as well as those areas between tumor and recognizable normal/anatomic structures. In resection specimens, sections to delineate margins are necessary. A black and white photograph, photocopy, or diagram clearly demonstrating a map of the sections should be made (229,297).

The final report should include the following information: site and weight, a specific and descriptive diagnosis based on the INPC classification, and the stage. The results of DNA content studies and the presence or absence of *MYCN* amplification when available, together with cytogenetic results, should be included in the final report.

PHEOCHROMOCYTOMA

Pheochromocytomas (intra-adrenal paragangliomas) are uncommon tumors that have been reported in 0.005% to 0.1% of unselected autopsies (298,299). Their average annual incidence is eight per million person-years in the United States, and they are responsible for less than 0.1% of cases of hypertension. Although they were among the first adrenal tumors to be recognized and described, their clinical significance and treatment were not fully understood until many years later. Manasse (300) described the chromaffin reaction in several of these tumors in 1896, but the term *pheochromocytoma* was introduced by Pick (301) in 1912 to express the fact that the tumors darkened after exposure to potassium dichromate. Approximately 70% of pheochromocytomas arise in the adrenal glands, but tumors of identical morphology and function may also appear in a wide variety of extra-adrenal sites. Although the extra-adrenal tumors have also been designated as pheochromocytomas by some authors, the preferred terminology for such neoplasms is *extra-adrenal paraganglioma*.

In most large series, the majority of pheochromocytomas are sporadic (nonfamilial). Although previous studies indicated that approximately 10% were familial, more recent analyses indicate that a considerably higher proportion have a heritable basis. This distinction is of particular importance because most familial tumors are bilateral and multicentric, whereas most sporadic tumors are unilateral. Familial pheochromocytomas are found in 30% to 50% of patients with types 2A and 2B MEN syndromes, 10% to 20% of patients with von Hippel-Lindau (VHL) disease, and 1% to 5% of patients with von Recklinghausen disease (302).

The clinical manifestations of pheochromocytoma are protean but are generally dominated by signs and symptoms of catecholamine hypersecretion or by the complications of hypertension. Common symptoms include headache, diaphoresis, palpitations, anxiety, chest pain, and weight loss. In most series, hypertension, which may be sustained or paroxysmal, is the most common sign at presentation. A few patients with pheochromocytomas are normotensive, and a few may even be hypotensive. Tachycardia, postural hypotension, and evidence of a hypermetabolic state are also very common. Most pheochromocytomas produce a combination of norepinephrine and epinephrine, with a predominance of norepinephrine. Tumors producing epinephrine exclusively may be associated with hypotension. The diagnosis depends on the presence of increased urinary and plasma levels of catecholamines and their metabolites. Preoperative localization of pheochromocytomas is accomplished most effectively with CT or MRI.

In patients with nonfamilial forms of pheochromocytoma, the right adrenal gland is somewhat more commonly involved than the left. Most nonfamilial tumors are unilateral, sharply circumscribed, solid masses with fibrous pseudocapsules. Most tumors from surgical series measure 3 to 5 cm in diameter, with tumor weights ranging from 70 to 150 g (19). Size and weight variations may be considerable, and even very small tumors can be associated with serious symptoms. The tumors vary in color from gray-white to pink-tan, with foci of congestion (Fig. 14.51). Larger tumors can contain central areas of fibrosis. Occasionally, very large pheochromocytomas undergo cystic degeneration, and they may be difficult to distinguish from nonneoplastic adrenal cysts. Exposure of the cut surfaces of pheochromocytomas to air or bright light often results in darkening of the tumor as a result of the formation of yellow-brown adrenochrome or nonadrenochrome pigments (23). These pigments are similar to those produced after immersion of the tumors in potassium dichromate solutions.

Familial pheochromocytomas are typically bilateral and mul-

ticentric, and the adjacent medulla may appear hyperplastic grossly (303–305). Large tumor masses in patients with familial pheochromocytomas most likely develop as a result of the confluence of multiple small tumor nodules.

Pheochromocytomas are rare in childhood, but they are more likely to be bilateral and multicentric than those in adults (306). Approximately 90% of affected children have sustained hypertension; polydipsia, polyuria, and convulsions are considerably more common in children than in adults. In addition, the rate of metachronous or synchronous extra-adrenal paragangliomas is considerably higher in children than in adults (298). The high rates of bilaterality and multicentricity suggest that many of these cases may represent unrecognized examples of familial pheochromocytomas.

On histologic examination, the tumors are composed of intermediate to large polygonal cells that may be arranged in alveolar, trabecular, or solid patterns. Most pheochromocytomas exhibit admixtures of these growth patterns. In tumors with alveolar arrangements, the groups of tumor cells are surrounded by a capillary-rich framework that results in a characteristic zellballen appearance (Fig. 14.52). In some instances, the capillary channels are prominent enough to result in an angiomatous appearance. Some tumor cells may be arranged in a glandular or acinar pattern. In patients with familial pheochromocytomas, the adjacent medulla is often hyperplastic.

Depending on the fixation, the cytoplasm may be acidophilic, amphophilic, or basophilic and typically has a finely granular texture. A few pheochromocytomas contain abundant cytoplasmic vacuoles resulting from lipid degeneration, and tumors with these features may be particularly difficult to distinguish from adrenal cortical tumors. In some instances, however, extensive cytoplasmic vacuolation is the result of fixation artifacts. Rarely, pheochromocytomas may show oncocytic features (307). Eosinophilic globules, which are typically PAS positive, are evident in a high proportion of cases (Fig. 14.53). Identical structures are usually present in normal adrenal medullary cells, particularly in juxtacortical regions. The globules are most likely derived from the membrane components of secretory granules. Similar globular cytoplasmic inclusions may also appear in the cytoplasm of adrenal cortical carcinoma cells.

Although most pheochromocytomas are composed of intermediate- to large-sized polygonal cells, some tumors may be

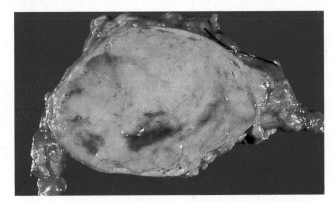

Figure 14.51. Pheochromocytoma. This tumor measures 4.5 cm in diameter and has a fleshy appearance. (From DeLellis RA, Feran-Doza M. Diseases of the adrenal glands. In Murphy WM, ed. *Urological Pathology*. Philadelphia, PA: WB Saunders, 1997:539–584, with permission.)

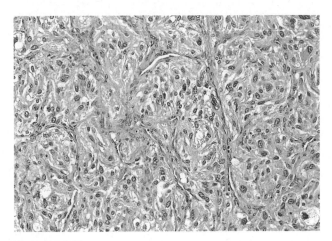

Figure 14.52. Pheochromocytoma. This tumor has a lobular pattern of growth.

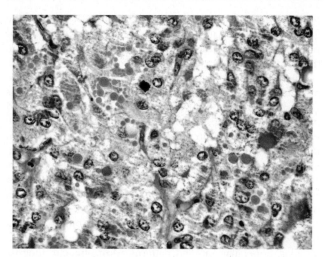

Figure 14.53. Pheochromocytoma. Numerous cytoplasmic hyaline globules are evident in this field.

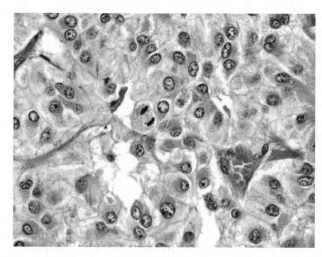

Figure 14.55. Pheochromocytoma. A mitotic figure is present.

composed of spindle cells (Fig. 14.54) or relatively small cells resembling pheochromoblasts. Moreover, very large cells resembling ganglion cells may also be evident in some cases. In addition to chromaffin cells, pheochromocytomas also contain a population of sustentacular cells, which are difficult to recognize in hematoxylin and eosin–stained preparations; however, they can be demonstrated selectively with antibodies to S-100 protein. Typically, the sustentacular cells are present at the peripheries of the cell nests.

The nuclei of pheochromocytoma cells are round to ovoid, with coarsely clumped chromatin and a single prominent nucleolus. Nuclear pseudoinclusions, which represent invaginations of the cytoplasm into the nucleus, may be particularly prominent in some tumors. Similar pseudoinclusions can also be a feature of adrenocortical tumors. Nuclear pleomorphism and hyperchromasia may be particularly prominent in some pheochromocytomas, but this finding does not correlate with malignant behavior. Benign pheochromocytomas can contain mitotic figures (Fig. 14.55). Thirty-five percent of benign tumors compared with 65% of malignant tumors have mitotic

activity (308). Mitotic counts in the malignant tumors (3/30 hpf) were slightly higher than in the benign tumors (1/30 hpf); however, this difference was not statistically significant.

Large tumors frequently display areas of hemorrhage and may show necrosis. The stroma may have areas of myxoid change with foci of lymphocytic infiltration, but the significance of the lymphoid infiltrates is unknown. Amyloid deposits have been identified in up to 70% of pheochromocytomas in some series, whereas other series have reported the presence of amyloid in a significantly smaller proportion of cases (309). Foci of capsular and venous invasion may also be evident, but these features do not correlate with malignant behavior. Brown fat has been reported in the retroperitoneum surrounding pheochromocytomas; this change, however, is not specific (310).

The diagnosis of an adrenal tumor as a pheochromocytoma depends in part on the ability to determine its catecholamine content by biochemical or histochemical methods. The chromaffin reaction is an insensitive procedure for the demonstration of catecholamines—some tumors that contain catecholamines, as determined by biochemical analysis, have shown negative results with the standard chromaffin reaction. Catecholamine-synthesizing enzymes, including tyrosine hydroxylase, dopamine beta-hydroxylase, and phenylethanolamine *N*-methyltransferase, may also be demonstrated in pheochromocytomas using immunohistochemical procedures (26).

Pheochromocytomas are usually positive for vimentin and neurofilament proteins and negative for cytokeratins. However, focal cytokeratin immunoreactivity (AE1/AE3 and CK1) can occur (311). Pheochromocytomas exhibit positivity for chromogranin proteins (Fig. 14.56) and synaptophysin, but synaptophysin is also present in a large proportion of adrenal cortical carcinomas. S-100 protein is restricted to the sustentacular cells and is particularly evident in those areas with a zellballen pattern (Fig. 14.57). Pheochromocytomas may also contain a large array of regulatory peptide products, including leu- and met-enkephalin, endorphins, ACTH, somatostatin, and calcitonin (28,312). The overproduction of these substances may give rise, in rare cases, to syndromes of hormone excess, including Cushing syndrome (313).

Ultrastructurally, pheochromocytomas contain variable numbers of membrane-bound, dense-core, secretory-type gran-

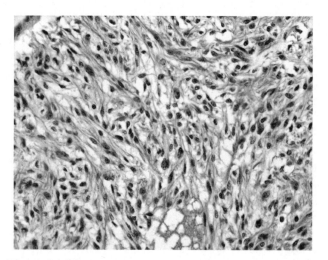

Figure 14.54. Pheochromocytoma. The tumor is composed of spindle cells.

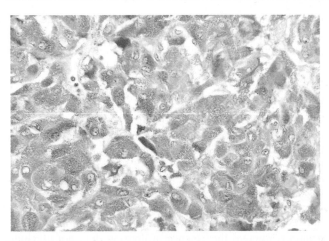

Figure 14.56. Pheochromocytoma. This tumor is stained with antibodies to chromogranin A (immunoperoxidase with diaminobenzidine).

ules (Fig. 14.58) (314–316). In general, tumors that contain a preponderance of norepinephrine secretory granules have highly electron-dense cores separated from their limiting membranes by an electron-lucent halo. Tumors with a preponderance of epinephrine granules demonstrate less dense matrices that are closely applied to their limiting membranes. It is not always possible, however, to determine the catecholamine content on the basis of granule morphology.

Germline mutations in the *ret* proto-oncogene, a member of the transmembrane protein kinase family, are responsible for MEN2A and MEN2B. The mutations, which typically affect exons 10, 11, and 16, convert this proto-oncogene into a dominant activating oncogene. Interestingly, based on a description of an 18-year-old woman with bilateral adrenal tumors ("sarcoma and angiosarcoma") in 1886 and the presence of a germline mutation of the *ret* gene in living relatives, Neumann et al. (317) have made a case for MEN2 in the patient and family of the original description of pheochromocytoma. Approximately 10% of sporadic pheochromocytomas harbor somatic mutations involving the *ret* proto-oncogene (318). LOH surrounding

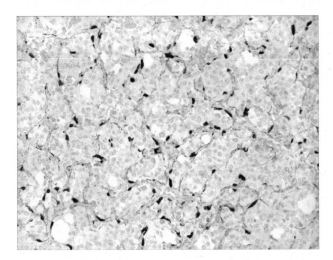

Figure 14.57. Pheochromocytoma. This tumor is stained with antibodies to S-100 protein. Sustentacular cells are present at the peripheries of the tumor cell clusters.

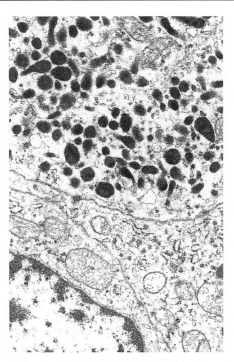

Figure 14.58. Pheochromocytoma. This tumor contains a predominance of epinephrine-type granules (28,000×).

the neurofibromatosis I (NFI) locus and loss of neurofibromin expression are evident in pheochromocytomas from patients with neurofibromatosis (319). These findings support the view that mutations of the neurofibromin gene contribute to the development of pheochromocytomas in patients with von Recklinghausen disease. The *VHL* gene, located on chromosome 3p25, encodes a protein that operates by a mechanism involving transcription elongation that is mediated by interactions with elongation factors B and C. This raises the possibility that the disease may involve oncogenes that are regulated at the level of elongation, such as *c-myc*, *n-myc*, *l-myc*, and *c-fos* (320). In VHL-associated pheochromocytomas, the VHL protein often contains a missense mutation at codon 238. In VHL families without pheochromocytomas, the mutation is more often a nonsense codon, frame shift, or deletion (321). Familial paragangliomas and pheochromocytomas have been reported to arise as a result of mutations in the genes for succinate dehydrogenase subunits D (*SDHD*), B (*SDHB*), or C (*SDHC*) (322).

Neumann et al. (323) demonstrated that 66 of 271 patients (24%) with apparent sporadic pheochromocytomas had germline mutations of one of these genes including *VHL* (45%), *RET* (19.6%), *SDHD* (16.6%), and *SDHB* (18.2%) (323). Interestingly, only 32% of patients who were positive for mutations had multifocal tumors; in addition, 35% of patients presented after the age of 30 years and 17% presented after the age of 40 years. Most true sporadic pheochromocytomas become clinically evident in the fourth to fifth decades.

Comparative genomic hybridization studies have revealed that gene copy alterations in pheochromocytomas and paragangliomas are common. Loss of 1p has been observed in more than 80% of these tumors (324). The minimal region of loss was 1cen-p31. Additional losses have involved 3q22-25, 11p, 3p13-14, 4q, 2q, and 11q22-23, whereas gains were found on 19p, 19q, 17q24-qter, 11cen-q13, and 16p. Dannenberg et al.

(325) reported similar findings and have further demonstrated that losses of 6q and 17p may play an important role in the progression to malignancy. The studies of Petri et al. (326) have demonstrated that although there is frequent loss of the *p53* locus on 17p, the *p53* gene does not appear to play a major role in pheochromocytoma tumorigenesis. Interestingly, deletions of 1p have also been demonstrated in NBs and adrenocortical carcinomas, as discussed in previous sections.

Gene expression profiling studies of pheochromocytomas have revealed consistent downregulation of genes involved in catecholamine metabolism (fumaryl acetate hydrolase and monoamine oxidase), peptide processing (glutaminyl-peptide cyclotransferase and peptidylglycine alpha-amidating monooxygenase), and hormone secretion (synaptophysin-like 3 and secretogranin II) in malignant pheochromocytomas; expression of astrotactin and plexin C1, which are involved in cell adhesion, are also downregulated in these tumors (327,328).

Composite Pheochromocytoma

The terms *composite pheochromocytoma* and *compound tumor of the adrenal medulla* have been used to describe tumors containing pheochromocytoma together with foci of NB, GNB, GN, or malignant peripheral nerve sheath tumor (Fig. 14.59) (42). Composite pheochromocytomas are rare tumors that make up less than 3% of sympathoadrenal pheochromocytomas. Rarely, they may be associated with neurofibromatosis type 1 (329) or MEN2A or MEN2B. The predominant component of the tumor is usually the pheochromocytoma. The possibility of differentiation along more than one cell line has been supported by studies that have shown that normal and neoplastic chromaffin cells are capable of differentiation into ganglion cells under the influence of nerve growth factor (330). It has been suggested that the sustentacular cells of pheochromocytomas could serve as the progenitors of the malignant peripheral nerve sheath component of some composite pheochromocytomas. Many of the reported composite tumors have been associated with signs and symptoms typical of pheochromocytomas, and some have been found in the context of the Verner-Morrison syndrome of watery diarrhea and hypokalemia. A unique case of composite pheochromocytoma consisting of typical pheochromocytoma and neuroendocrine carcinoma has been reported (331).

Malignant Pheochromocytoma

The diagnosis of malignancy in pheochromocytomas is particularly difficult. Differences in criteria have resulted in considerable variation in the reported rates of malignant pheochromocytomas, which have ranged from 2.4% to 14%. With the exception of the presence of lymph node or distant metastases (Fig. 14.60), there are no absolute criteria that distinguish benign from malignant pheochromocytomas reliably. Focal invasion, even when it is extensive, is a poor predictor of metastatic behavior, whereas the absence of invasion does not preclude the development of metastases. In a study of adrenal and extra-adrenal sympathoadrenal paragangliomas, Linnoila et al. (308) noted the following features more frequently in malignant tumors: male predominance, extra-adrenal location, greater tumor weight (mean of 383 g for malignant tumors vs. 73 g for benign tumors), confluent tumor necrosis, and the presence of vascular invasion and/or extensive local invasion. Hyaline globules that were PAS positive were found in 59% of benign tumors and 32% of malignant tumors. Logistic regression analysis of 16 nonhistologic and histologic parameters revealed that four were most predictive of malignancy—extra-adrenal location, coarse nodularity of the primary tumor, confluent tumor necrosis, and absence of cytoplasmic hyaline globules. Although most malignant tumors had two or three of these features, most benign tumors had only one or none.

In a series from the Armed Forces Institute of Pathology, Thompson (311) was unable to demonstrate a statistically significant difference in weight between benign and malignant pheochromocytomas. He developed a system for the assessment of malignancy of pheochromocytomas (Pheochromocytomas of the Adrenal gland Scaled Score [PASS]). In this system, each of the following features was assigned a value of 1: vascular invasion, capsular invasion, profound nuclear pleomorphism, and hyperchromasia. Features assigned a value of 2 included periadrenal adipose tissue invasion, large tumor nests or diffuse growth pattern, focal or confluent necrosis, high cellularity,

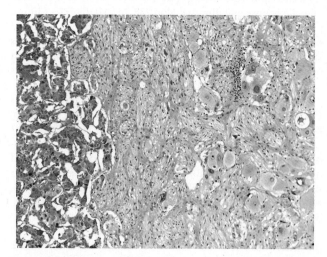

Figure 14.59. Composite tumor (pheochromocytoma/ganglioneuroma) of the adrenal medulla. The pheochromocytoma component on the left shows the typical zellballen arrangement, whereas the ganglioneuroma component on the right shows mature ganglion cells in a Schwannian-dominant stroma.

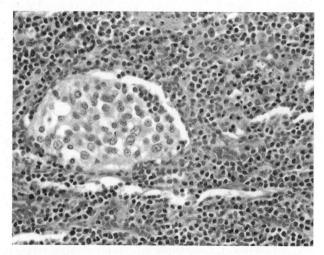

Figure 14.60. Pheochromocytoma metastatic to lymph node.

tumor cell spindling, cellular monotony, mitotic figures in excess of 3 per 10 hpf, and atypical mitoses. Among 50 tumors that were classified as histologically malignant and assigned a PASS ≥ 4, metastases developed in 33 patients, whereas 17 patients were free of metastases. Patients with tumors with a PASS ≤ 3 remained free of metastases, with a mean follow-up time of 14.1 years.

A variety of other parameters have been used for the assessment of malignancy of pheochromocytomas. Clarke et al. (332) reported that a cutoff value of MIB-1 of greater than 3% yielded a specificity of 100% and a sensitivity of 50% in predicting malignancy. The value of S-100 protein for the distinction of benign and malignant pheochromocytomas has been controversial. In general, those tumors with a well-developed zellballen pattern show well-developed staining in the sustentacular cells present at the peripheries of cell nests. Tumors with a large nesting or diffuse growth pattern, however, may be devoid of S-100–positive sustentacular cells. Most malignant pheochromocytomas have a decreased number of sustentacular cells, which undoubtedly reflects the diffuse growth pattern so commonly seen in these tumors. Interestingly, abundant S-100 positivity may be present in sustentacular cells in metastatic tumors, particularly those with a well-developed zellballen pattern.

Cytomorphometry has been used in the differential diagnosis of malignant and benign pheochromocytomas. In a study reported by Lewis (333), benign pheochromocytomas had a mode corresponding to a diploid (2n) DNA content and a wide range of values with nuclei measuring up to 40n. Malignant pheochromocytomas, however, had a hyperdiploid or triploid mode with a smaller range of values.

Recent interest has been focused on the vascular patterns of pheochromocytomas (334). Malignant tumors have an abnormal vascular architecture with an irregular pattern of large vascular volumes flattened between tumor nodules. Benign pheochromocytomas exhibit a regular pattern of short, straight capillaries (335). Correlative molecular studies have shown an increase of EPAS1 (a hypoxia-inducible transcription factor), vascular endothelial growth factor (VEGF), and endothelin receptor, type B (ETB) of 4.5-, 3.5-, and 10-fold, respectively, in malignant versus benign pheochromocytomas. Expression of stromal tenascin has also been suggested as a marker to distinguish benign (predominantly negative) from malignant (strongly positive) pheochromocytomas (336).

Malignant pheochromocytomas are generally slowly growing neoplasms with 5-year survival rates in the range of 40% to 50%. The most common sites of metastatic spread include lymph nodes, bone, and liver. In assessing lymph node metastases, all efforts should be directed to distinguishing concurrent extra-adrenal paragangliomas that compress adjacent lymph nodes from true nodal metastases.

ADRENAL MEDULLARY HYPERPLASIA

Diffuse and nodular hyperplasia of the medulla has been recognized only relatively recently as a distinct clinical and pathologic entity (Figs. 14.61 to 14.64) (305,335,337). This change has been reported in association with MEN2A and MEN2B and VHL disease and has also been noted in a few patients without an apparent familial syndrome. Of the four patients with nonfamilial hyperplasia reported by Rudy et al. (338), three underwent unilateral adrenalectomy, and one underwent bilateral adrenalectomy. In this series, the hyperplasia was diffuse in three cases

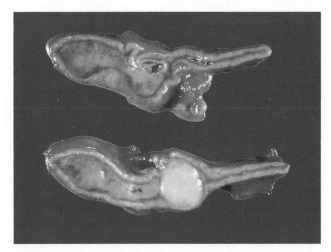

Figure 14.61. Diffuse and nodular hyperplasia. This adrenal was resected from a patient with a type 2A multiple endocrine neoplasm. In addition to the diffuse hyperplasia of the medulla, there is focal nodule formation.

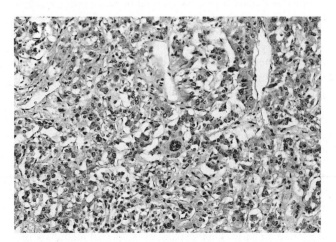

Figure 14.62. Diffuse and nodular hyperplasia (same case as in Fig. 14.61). The focus of nodule formation is on the left, and the diffusely hyperplastic medulla is on the right.

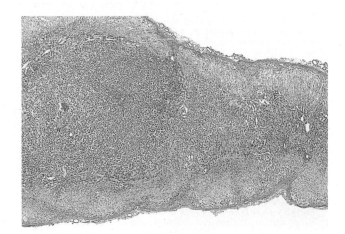

Figure 14.63. Area of diffuse hyperplasia (same case as in Fig. 14.61). There is considerable variation in the size and shape of medullary cells in areas of diffuse hyperplasia.

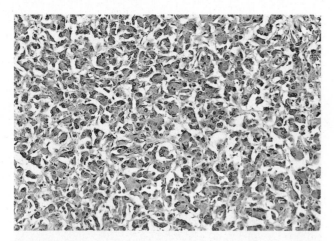

Figure 14.64. Area of nodular hyperplasia (same case as in Fig. 14.61). The foci of nodular hyperplasia show more uniformity in cell size and shape than the adjacent hyperplastic medullary cells.

and diffuse and nodular in the fourth case. The diagnosis of adrenal medullary hyperplasia should be made with considerable care. In the context of cortical atrophy, for example, the medulla may appear more prominent than usual. The diagnosis of medullary hyperplasia should be made only on the basis of increased medullary volume, as determined morphometrically. Other findings suggestive of medullary hyperplasia include the presence of medullary tissue in both alar regions of the gland and extension of the medulla into the tail region. The studies of Naeye (339) have suggested that adrenal medullary hyperplasia may also be found in victims of the sudden infant death syndrome.

Molecular studies of microdissected nodules in patients with MEN2A-associated nodular adrenal medullary hyperplasia have shown that this disorder is a multifocal monoclonal proliferation. Interestingly, the same X chromosome is inactivated in individual nodules from the same patient. This observation has suggested an early clonal expansion of adrenal medullary precursors in these patients (340).

REFERENCES

1. Young WF. The incidentally discovered adrenal mass. *N Engl J Med* 2007;356:601–610.
2. Symington T. The adrenal cortex. In Bloodworth JMB Jr, ed. *Endocrine Pathology General and Surgical*. Baltimore, MD: Williams & Wilkins, 1982:419–472.
3. Seron-Ferre M, Jaffee RB. The fetal adrenal gland. *Annu Rev Physiol* 1981;43:141–162.
4. Beck K, Tygstrup I, Nerup J. The involution of the fetal adrenal cortex: a light microscopic study. *Acta Pathol Microbiol Scand* 1969;76:391–400.
5. Quinan C, Berger AA. Observations on human adrenals with special reference to the relative weight of the normal medulla. *Ann Intern Med* 1933;6:1180–1192.
6. Dobbie JW, Symington T. The human adrenal gland with special reference to the vasculature. *J Endocrinol* 1966;34:479–489.
7. Neville AM, O'Hare MJ. Aspects of structure, function and pathology. In James VHT, ed. *The Adrenal Gland*. New York, NY: Raven Press, 1979:165.
8. Motto P, Muto M, Fujita T. Three dimensional organization of mammalian adrenal cortex. *Cell Tissue Res* 1979;196:23–38.
9. Wieneke JA, Lack EE. The adrenal gland. In Silverberg SG, DeLellis RA, Frable WJ, et al., eds. *Silverberg's Principles and Practice of Surgical Pathology and Cytopathology*. Philadelphia, PA: Churchill Livingstone (Elsevier), 2006:2169.
9a. Lloyd RV, Douglas BR, Young WF. *Atlas of Nontumor Pathology. Endocrine Disease*. Washington, DC: American Registry of Pathology & Armed Forces Institute of Pathology, 2002.
10. Hayashi Y, Hiyoshi T, Takemura T, et al. Focal lymphocytic infiltration in the adrenal cortex of the elderly: immunohistological analysis of infiltrating lymphocytes. *Clin Exp Immunol* 1998;77:101–105.
11. Tannenbaum M. Ultrastructural pathology of the adrenal cortex. In Sommers SC, ed. *Endocrine Pathology Decennial (1966–1975)*. New York, NY: Appleton-Century-Crofts, 1975: 423–472.
12. Miettinen M, Lehto VP, Virtanen I. Immunofluorescence microscopic evaluation of the intermediate filament expression of the adrenal cortex and medulla and their tumors. *Am J Pathol* 1985;118:360–366.
13. Boggaram V, Funkenstein B, Waterman MR, et al. Lipoproteins and the regulation of adrenal steroidogenesis. *Endocr Res* 1985;10:387–409.
14. Bondy P. Disorders of the adrenal cortex. In Wilson JD, Foster DW, eds. *Williams' Textbook of Endocrinology*. Philadelphia, PA: WB Saunders, 1985:816–891.
15. Carey RM, Sen S, Dolan LM, et al. Idiopathic hyperaldosteronism: a possible role for aldosterone stimulation factor. *N Engl J Med* 1984;311:94–100.
16. Sen S, Bumpus FM, Oberfield S, et al. Development and preliminary application of a new assay for aldosterone stimulation factor. *Hypertension* 1983;5(Suppl 1):127–131.
17. Coupland RE. The development and fate of catecholamine secreting endocrine cells. In Parvez H, Parez S. *Biogenic Amines in Development*. Amsterdam, The Netherlands: Elsevier/North Holland, 1980:3–28.
18. Tischler AS. Paraganglia. In Sternberg SS, ed. *Histology for Pathologists*. 2nd edition. Philadelphia, PA: Lippincott-Raven Publishers, 1997.
19. Page DL, DeLellis RA, Hough AJ. Tumors of the adrenal. In *Atlas of Tumor Pathology*. 2nd series, fascicle 23. Washington, DC: Armed Forces Institute of Pathology, 1985.
20. Dekker A, Oehrle JS. Hyaline globules of the adrenal medulla of man. *Arch Pathol* 1971; 91:353–364.
21. Grynszpan-Winograd O. Ultrastructure of the chromaffin cell. In Greep RO, Astwood EB, eds. *Handbook of Physiology*. Washington, DC: American Physiological Society, 1975: 295–308.
22. Fawcett DW, Long JA, Jones AL. The ultrastructure of endocrine glands. *Recent Prog Horm Res* 1969;25:315–380.
23. Sherwin RP. The adrenal medulla paraganglia and related tissues. In Bloodworth JMB, ed. *Endocrine Pathology*. Baltimore, MD: Williams & Wilkins, 1968:256–315.
24. DeLaTorre JC, Surgeon JW. A methodological approach to rapid and sensitive monoamine histofluorescence using a modified glyoxylic acid technique. *Histochemistry* 1976; 45:81–93.
25. Falck B, Owman C. A detailed methodological description of the fluorescence method for the cellular demonstration of biogenic monoamines. *Acta Univ Lund (Sect II)* 1965; 2(7):523.
26. Lloyd RV, Sisson JC, Shapiro B, et al. Immunohistochemical localization of epinephrine, norepinephrine, catecholamine synthesizing enzymes and chromogranin in neuroendocrine cells and tumors. *Am J Pathol* 1986;125:45–54.
27. Gould VE, Lee I, Wiedemann B, et al. Synaptophysin: a novel marker for neurons, certain neuroendocrine cells and their neoplasms. *Hum Pathol* 1986;17:979–983.
28. Hassoun J, Monges G, Giraud P, et al. Immunohistochemical study of pheochromocytomas: an investigation of methionine enkephalin, vasoactive intestinal peptide, somatostatin corticotropin, β-endorphin and calcitonin in 16 tumors. *Am J Pathol* 1984;114:56–63.
29. Lloyd RV, Blaivas M, Wilson BS. Distribution of chromogranin and S-100-protein in normal and abnormal adrenal medullary tissues. *Arch Pathol Lab Med* 1985;109:633–635.
30. Schmechel D. Gamma subunit of the glycolytic enzyme enolase: nonspecific or neuron specific? *Lab Invest* 1985;52:239–242.
31. Kobayashi S, Coupland RE. Two populations of microvesicles in the SGC (small granule chromaffin) cells of the mouse adrenal medulla. *Arch Histol Jpn* 1977;40:251–259.
32. Winkler H, Smith AD. The chromaffin granule and the storage of catecholamines. In Greep RO, Astwood EB, eds. *Endocrinology*. Washington, DC: American Physiological Society, 1975:321–339.
33. Bornstein SR, Ehrhart-Bornstein M, Scherbaum WA. Ultrastructural evidence for corticochromaffin cells in rat adrenals. *Endocr Rev* 1991;129:1113–1115.
34. Kovacs K, Horvath E. Ultrastructural features of corticomedullary cells in a human adrenal cortical adenoma and in rat adrenal cortex. *Anat Anz* 1973;134:387–393.
35. Gutowski T, Gray GF. Ectopic adrenal in inguinal hernia sacs. *J Urol* 1979;121:353–354.
36. Lack EE. *Pathology of the Adrenal Glands*. New York, NY: Churchill Livingstone, 1990.
37. MacLennan A. On the presence of adrenal rests in hernial sac walls. *Surg Gynecol Obstet* 1919;29:387.
38. Burke EF, Gilbert E, Uehling DT. Adrenal rest tumors of the testes. *J Urol* 1973;109: 649–652.
39. Johnson RE, Scheithauer B. Massive hyperplasia of testicular adrenal rests in a patient with Nelson's syndrome. *Am J Clin Pathol* 1982;77:501–507.
40. Dolan MF, Janouski NA. Adrenohepatic union. *Arch Pathol* 1968;86:22.
41. O'Crowley CR, Martland HS. Adrenal heterotopia, rests and the so-called Grawitz tumor. *J Urol* 1943;50:576.
42. Lack EE. *Tumors of the Adrenal Gland and Extra-Adrenal Paraganglia*. Washington, DC: Armed Forces Institute of Pathology, 1997.
43. Benirschke K. Adrenals in anencephaly and hydrocephaly. *Obstet Gynecol* 1956;8:442.
44. Pakravan P, Kenny FM, Depp R, et al. Familial congenital absence of adrenal glands: evaluation of glucocorticoid, mineralocorticoid and estrogen metabolism in the neonatal period. *J Pediatr* 1974;84:74–78.
45. Wise JE, Matalon R, Morgan AM, et al. Phenotypic features of patients with congenital adrenal hypoplasia and glycerol kinase deficiency. *Am J Dis Child* 1987;141:744–747.
46. Burris TP, Guo W, McCabe ER. The gene responsible for congenital adrenal hypoplasia DAX-1, encodes a nuclear hormone receptor that defines a new class within the superfamily. *Recent Prog Horm Res* 1996;54:241.
47. Borit A, Kosek J. Cytomegaly of the adrenal cortex: electron microscopy in Beckwith's syndrome. *Arch Pathol* 1969;88:58–64.
48. Oppenheimer EH. Adrenal cytomegaly: studies by light and electron microscopy in Beckwith's syndrome. *Arch Pathol* 1970;90:57–64.
49. McCawley RG, Beckwith JB, Elias ER, et al. Benign hemorrhagic macrocysts in Beckwith-Wiedemann syndrome. *AJR Am J Roentgenol* 1991;157:549–552.
50. Cohen MM Jr. Beckwith-Wiedemann syndrome: historical clinicopathological and etiopathogenetic perspectives. *Pediatr Dev Pathol* 2005;8:287–304.

51. Ghatak NR, Nochlin D, Peris M. Morphology and distribution of cytoplasmic inclusions in adrenoleukodystrophy. *J Neurol Sci* 1981;50:391–398.

52. Cartier N, Lopez J, Moullier P, et al. Retroviral-mediated gene transfer connects very long chain fatty acid metabolism in adrenoleukodystrophy fibroblasts. *Proc Natl Acad Sci U S A* 1995;92:1674.

53. Powers JM, Schaumberg HH, Johnson AB, et al. A correlative study of the adrenal cortex in adrenoleukodystrophy: evidence for a fatal intoxication with very long chain saturated fatty acids. *Invest Cell Pathol* 1980;3:3–53.

54. Schaumberg HH, Powers JM, Raine CS. Adrenomyeloneuropathy: a probable variant of adrenoleukodystrophy. II. General pathologic, neuropathologic and biochemical aspects. *Neurol Rep* 1977;27:11–14.

55. Wolman M, Sterk VV, Gratt S, et al. Primary familial xanthomatosis with involvement and calcification of adrenal. Report of two more cases in siblings of a previously described infant. *Pediatrics* 1961;28:742–757.

56. White PC, New MI, Dupont D. Congenital adrenal hyperplasia. *N Engl J Med* 1987;316:1519–1524, 1580–1586.

57. Hughes I. Congenital adrenal hyperplasia: phenotype and genotypes. *J Pediatr Endocrinol Metab* 2002;15(Suppl 15):1529–1540.

58. Peter M. Congenital adrenal hyperplasia: 11 beta-hydroxylase deficiency. *Semin Reprod Med* 2002;20:249–254.

59. Auchus RJ. The genetics, pathophysiology and management of deficiencies of $P450_{c17}$. *Endocrinol Metab Clin North Am* 2001;30:101–119.

60. Daeschner GL. Adrenal cortical adenoma arising in a girl with congenital adrenogenital syndrome. *Pediatr Pathol* 1965;36:140–142.

61. Jaursch-Hancke C, Allollio B, Meltzer U, et al. Adrenal cortical carcinoma in patients with untreated congenital adrenal hyperplasia. *Acta Endocrinol* 1988;117:146–147.

62. Rutgers JL, Young RH, Scully RE. The testicular tumor of the adrenogenital syndrome: a report of 6 cases and review of the literature on testicular masses in patients with adrenocortical disorders. *Am J Surg Pathol* 1988;12:503–513.

63. Weetman AP. Autoimmunity to steroid producing cells and familial polyendocrinopathy. *Ballieres Clin Endocrinol Metab* 1995;9:157–174.

64. Neufeld M, MacLaren NK, Blizzard RM. Two types of autoimmune Addison's disease associated with different polyglandular autoimmune syndromes. *Medicine* 1981;60:355–362.

65. Wang CY, Davoodi-Semiromi A, Huang W, et al. Characterization of mutations in patients with autoimmune polyglandular syndrome type I (APSI). *Hum Genet* 1998;103:681–685.

66. Ahomen P. Autoimmune polyendocrinopathy—candidiasis ectodermal dystrophy (APECED): autosomal recessive inheritance. *Clin Genet* 1985;27:535–542.

67. Grinspoon SK, Bilezikian JP. HIV disease and the endocrine system. *N Engl J Med* 1992;327:1360–1365.

68. Wenig BM, Heffess CS, Adair CF. *Atlas of Endocrine Pathology.* Philadelphia, PA: WB Saunders, 1997.

69. Friderichsen C. Waterhouse-Friderichsen syndrome. *Acta Endocrinol* 1955;18:482–492.

70. Kuhajda FP, Hutchins GM. Adrenal corticomedullary junction necrosis: a morphological marker for hypotension. *Am Heart J* 1979;98:294–297.

71. Haroche J, Amoura Z, Toouraine P, et al. Bilateral adrenal infiltration in Erdheim-Chester disease. Report of seven cases and literature review. *J Clin Endocrinol Metab* 2007;92:2007–2012.

72. Burch C. Cushing's disease: a review. *Arch Intern Med* 1985;145:1106–1111.

73. Upton GV, Amatruda TT. Evidence for the presence of tumor peptide with corticotropin-releasing factor like activity in the ectopic ACTH syndrome. *N Engl J Med* 1971;285:419–424.

74. Reibord H, Fisher ER. Electron microscopic study of adrenal cortical hyperplasia in Cushing's syndrome. *Arch Pathol* 1968;86:419–426.

75. Neville AM, Symington T. Bilateral adrenal cortical hyperplasia in children with Cushing's syndrome. *J Pathol* 1972;107:95–106.

76. Carey RM, Varma SK, Drake CR, et al. Ectopic secretion of corticotropin releasing factor as a cause of Cushing's syndrome: a clinical, morphological and biochemical study. *N Engl J Med* 1984;311:13–20.

76a. DeLellis RA, Feran-Doza M. Diseases of the adrenal glands. In Murphy WM, ed. *Urological Pathology.* Philadelphia, PA: WB Saunders, 1997:539–584.

77. Neville AM, Symington T. The pathology of the adrenal in Cushing's syndrome. *J Pathol Bacteriol* 1967;93:19–35.

78. Zarate A, Kovacs K, Flores M, et al. ACTH and CRF-producing bronchial carcinoid associated with Cushing's syndrome. *Clin Endocrinol (Oxf)* 1986;24:523.

79. Young WF. Pheochromocytoma and primary aldosteronism: diagnostic approaches. *Endocrinol Metab Clin North Am* 1997;26:801–827.

80. Bravo EL, Tarazi RC, Dustan HP, et al. The changing clinical spectrum of primary aldosteronism. *Am J Med* 1983;74:641–651.

81. Conn JW, Knopf RF, Nesbit RM. Clinical characteristics of primary aldosteronism from an analysis of 145 cases. *Am J Surg* 1964;107:159.

82. Hidai H, Fuji H, Otsuka K, et al. Cushing's syndrome due to huge adrenocortical multinodular hyperplasia. *Endocrinol Jpn* 1975;22:555–560.

83. Neville AM. The nodular adrenal. *Invest Cell Pathol* 1978;1:99–111.

84. Josse RG, Bear R, Kovacs K, et al. Cushing's syndrome due to unilateral nodular adrenal hyperplasia: a new pathophysiologic entity? *Acta Endocrinol* 1980;93:495–504.

85. Bourdeau I, Stratakis CA. Cyclic AMP dependent signaling aberrations in macronodular adrenal disease. *Ann NY Acad Sci* 2002;968:240–255.

86. Meador CK, Bowdoin B, Owen WC, et al. Primary adrenocortical nodular dysplasia: a rare cause of Cushing's syndrome. *J Clin Endocrinol Metab* 1967;27:1255–1263.

87. Hasleton PS, Ali HH, Anfield C, et al. Micronodular adrenal disease: a light and electron microscopic study. *J Clin Pathol* 1982;35:1078–1085.

88. Schweizer-Cagianut M, Froesch ER, Hedinger C. Familial Cushing's syndrome with primary adrenocortical microadenomatosis (primary adrenocortical nodular dysplasia). *Acta Endocrinol* 1980;94:529–535.

89. Shenoy BV, Carpenter PC, Carney JA. Bilateral primary pigmented nodular adrenocortical disease: rare cause of the Cushing syndrome. *Am J Surg Pathol* 1984;8:335–344.

90. Wulffraat NM, Drexhage HA, Wiersinga WM, et al. Immunoglobulins of patients with Cushing's syndrome due to pigmented adrenocortical micronodular dysplasia simulate in vitro steroidogenesis. *J Clin Endocrinol Metab* 1988;66:601.

91. Carney JA, Young WF. Primary pigmented nodular adrenal cortical disease and its associated conditions. *Endocrinologist* 1992;2:6–21.

92. Groussin L, Jullian E, Perlemoine K, et al. Mutations of the PRKAR1A gene in Cushing's syndrome due to sporadic primary pigmented nodular adrenal cortical disease. *J Clin Endocrinol Metab* 2002;87:4324–4329.

93. Stratakis CA. Mutations of the gene encoding the protein kinase A type Iα regulatory subunit (PRKAR1A) in patients with the "complex of spotty skin pigmentation, myxomas, endocrine overactivity and schwannomas" (Carney complex). *Ann N Y Acad Sci* 2002;968:3–21.

94. Horvarth A, Boikos S, Giatzakis C, et al. A genome wide scan identifies mutations in the gene encoding phosphodiesterase 11A4 (PDE11A) in individuals with adrenocortical hyperplasia. *Nat Genet* 2006;38:794–800.

95. Horvath A, Giatzakas C, Robinson-White A, et al. Adrenal hyperplasia and adenomas are associated with inhibition of phosphodiesterase 11A in carriers of PDE11A sequence variants that are frequent in the population. *Cancer Res* 2006;66:1157S.

96. Bertagna C, Orth DN. Clinical and laboratory findings and results of therapy in 58 patients with adrenocortical tumors admitted to a single medical center (1951–1978). *Am J Med* 1981;71:855–875.

97. Gicquel C, Leblond-Francillard M, Bertagna X, et al. Clonal analysis of human adrenal cortical carcinomas and secreting adenomas. *Clin Endocrinol (Oxf)* 1994;40:465–477.

98. Neville AM, Symington T. Pathology of primary aldosteronism. *Cancer* 1966;19:1854–1868.

99. Caplan RH, Virata RL. Functional black adenoma of the adrenal cortex: a rare cause of primary aldosteronism. *Am J Clin Pathol* 1974;62:97–103.

100. Pollock WJ, McConnell CF, Hilton C, et al. Virilizing Leydig cell adenoma of the adrenal gland. *Am J Surg Pathol* 1986;10:816–822.

101. Ryan JJ, Rezkalla MA, Rizk SN, et al. Testosterone-secreting adrenal adenoma that contained crystalloids of Reinke in an adult female patient. *Mayo Clinic Proc* 1995;70:380–383.

102. Dobbie JM. Adrenal cortical nodular hyperplasia: the aging adrenal. *J Pathol* 1969;99:1–18.

103. Sasano H, Szuki T, Sano T, et al. Adrenocortical oncocytoma: a true nonfunctioning adrenal cortical tumor. *Am J Surg Pathol* 1991;15:949–956.

104. Lin BT, Bonsib SM, Mierau GW, et al. Oncocytic adrenocortical neoplasms: a report of seven cases and review of the literature. *Am J Surg Pathol* 1998;22:603–614.

105. Bisceglia M, Ludovico O, Di Mattia A, et al. Adrenocortical oncocytic tumors: report of 10 cases and review of the literature. *Int J Surg Pathol* 2004;12:231–243.

106. Erlandson RA, Reuter VE. Oncocytic adrenal cortical adenoma. *Ultrastruct Pathol* 1991;15:539–547.

107. Xiao GQ, Pertsemlidis DS, Unger PD. Functioning adrenocortical oncocytoma: a case report and review of the literature. *Ann Diagn Pathol* 2005;9:295–297.

108. Corsi A, Riminucci M, Petrozza V, et al. Incidentally detected giant oncocytoma arising in retroperitoneal heterotopic adrenal tissue. *Arch Pathol Lab Med* 2002;126:1118–1122.

109. El-Naggar AK, Evans DB, Mackay B. Oncocytic adrenal cortical carcinoma. *Ultrastruct Pathol* 1991;15:549–556.

110. Correa P, Chen VW. Endocrine gland cancer. *Cancer* 1995;75:338–352.

111. Sameshima Y, Tsunematsu Y, Watanabe S, et al. Detection of novel germline p53 mutations in diverse cancer prone families identified by selecting patients with childhood adrenocortical carcinoma. *J Natl Cancer Inst* 1992;84:703–710.

112. Didolkar MD, Bescher RA, Elias EG, et al. Natural history of adrenal cortical carcinoma: a clinicopathologic study of 42 patients. *Cancer* 1981;47:2153–2161.

113. Weiss LM. Comparative histological study of 43 metastasizing and nonmetastasizing adrenocortical tumors. *Am J Surg Pathol* 1984;8:163–169.

114. Hutter AM, Kayhoe DE. Adrenal cortical carcinoma: clinical features of 138 patients. *Am J Med* 1966;41:572–592.

115. Hough AJ, Hollifield JW, Page DL, et al. Prognostic factors in adrenal cortical tumors: a mathematical analysis of clinical and morphologic data. *Am J Clin Pathol* 1979;72:390–399.

116. Hajjar RA, Hickey RC, Samaan NA. Adrenal cortical carcinoma: a study of 32 patients. *Cancer* 1975;35:549–554.

117. Cagle PT, Hough A, Pyeher J, et al. Comparison of adrenal cortical tumors in children and adults. *Cancer* 1986;57:2235–2237.

118. Brown FM, Gaffey TA, Wold LE, et al. Myxoid neoplasms of the adrenal cortex: a rare histologic variant. *Am J Surg Pathol* 2000;24:396–401.

119. Drachenberg CB, Lee HK, Gann DS, et al. Adrenal cortical carcinoma with adenosquamous differentiation. Report of a case with immunohistochemical and ultrastructural studies. *Arch Pathol Lab Med* 1995;119:260–265.

120. Alexander A, Paulose KP. Oncocytic variant of adrenal carcinoma presenting as Cushing's syndrome. *J Assoc Physicians India* 1998;46:235–237.

121. Hoang MP, Ayala AG, Albores-Saavedra J. Oncocytic adrenal cortical carcinoma: a morphologic immunohistochemical and ultrastructural study of four cases. *Mod Pathol* 2002;15:973–978.

122. Song SY, Park S, Kim SR, et al. Oncocytic adrenocortical carcinomas: a pathological and immunohistochemical study of four cases in comparison with conventional adrenocortical carcinomas. *Pathol Int* 2004;54:603–610.

123. Fischler DF, Nunez C, Levin HS, et al. Adrenal carcinosarcoma presenting in a woman with clinical signs of virilization: a case report with immunohistochemical and ultrastructural findings. *Am J Surg Pathol* 1992;16:626–631.

124. Decorato JW, Gruber H, Petti M, et al. Adrenal carcinosarcoma. *J Surg Oncol* 1990;45:134–136.

125. DeMay R. *The Art and Science of Cytopathology.* Chicago, IL: ASCP Press, 1996:703–778.

125a. Ren R, Guo M, Sneige N, et al. Fine-needle aspiration of adrenal cortical carcinoma: cytologic spectrum and diagnostic challenges. *Am J Clin Pathol* 2006;126:389–398.

126. Delellis RA, Shin SJ. Diagnostic immunohistochemistry of endocrine tumors. In Dabbs DJ, ed. *Diagnostic Immunohistochemistry*. New York, NY: Churchill Livingstone, 2002:209–240.
127. Shin SJ, Hoda RS, Ying L, et al. Diagnostic utility of the monoclonal antibody A103 in fine needle aspiration biopsies of the adrenal. *Am J Clin Pathol* 2002;10:295–302.
128. Gaffey MJ, Traweek ST, Mills S, et al. Cytokeratin expression in adrenal cortical neoplasia: an immunohistochemical and biochemical study with implications for the differential diagnosis of adrenocortical, hepatocellular and renal cell carcinoma. *Hum Pathol* 1992; 23:144–153.
129. Sasano H, Suzuki T, Nagura H, et al. Steroidogenesis in human adrenocortical carcinoma: biochemical activities, immunohistochemistry and in situ hybridization of steroidogenic enzymes and histopathologic study in 9 cases. *Hum Pathol* 1993;24:397–404.
130. Sasano H, Shizawa S, Suzuki T, et al. Transcription factor adrenal 4 binding protein is a marker of adrenocortical malignancy. *Hum Pathol* 1995;26:1154–1156.
131. Schröder S, Padberg BC, Achilles E, et al. Immunohistochemistry in adrenocortical tumors: a clinicomorphological study of 72 neoplasms. *Virchows Arch A Pathol Anat Histopathol* 1992;420:65–70.
132. Tartour E, Caillou B, Tennenbaum F, et al. Immunohistochemical staining of adrenocortical carcinoma: prediction value of the D11 antibody. *Cancer* 1993;72:3296–3303.
133. Busam KJ, Iversen K, Coplan KA, et al. Immunoreactivity for A103, an antibody to melan-A (Mart-1), in adrenocortical and other steroid tumors. *Am J Surg Pathol* 1998;22:57–63.
134. Renshaw AA, Granter SR. A comparison of A103 and inhibin reactivity in adrenal cortical tumors: distinction from hepatocellular carcinoma and renal tumors. *Mod Pathol* 1998; 11:1160–1164.
135. Jorda M, De MB, Nadji M. Calretinin and inhibin A are useful in separating adrenal cortical neoplasms from pheochromocytomas. *Appl Immunohistochem Mol Morph* 2002;10: 67–70.
136. Miettinen M. Neuroendocrine differentiation in adrenal cortical carcinoma: new immunohistochemical findings supported by electron microscopy. *Lab Invest* 1992;66:169–174.
137. Komminoth P, Roth J, Schröder S, et al. Overlapping expression of immunohistochemical markers and synaptophysin mRNA in pheochromocytomas and adrenocortical carcinomas: implications for the differential diagnosis of adrenal gland tumors. *Lab Invest* 1995; 72:424–431.
138. Browning L, Bailey D, Parlcer A. D2-40 is a sensitive and specific marker in differentiating primary adrenal cortical tumors from both metastatic clear cell renal cell carcinoma and pheochromocytoma. *J Clin Pathol* 2008;61:293–296.
139. Silva EG, Mackay B, Samaan NA, et al. Adrenal cortical carcinomas: an ultrastructural study of 22 cases. *Ultrastruct Pathol* 1982;3:1–7.
140. King DR, Lack EE. Adrenal cortical carcinoma. *Cancer* 1979;44:239–244.
141. Van Slooten H, Schaberg A, Smeenk D, et al. Morphological characteristics of benign and malignant adrenal cortical tumors. *Cancer* 1985;55:766–773.
142. Amberson JB, Vaughn ED, Gray G, et al. Flow cytometric analysis of nuclear DNA from adrenal cortical neoplasms. *Cancer* 1987;59:2091–2095.
143. Bowlby LS, DeBault LE, Abraham SR. Flow cytometric analysis of adrenal cortical tumor DNA: relationship between cellular DNA and histopathologic classification. *Cancer* 1986; 58:1499–1505.
144. Taylor SR, Roederer M, Murphy RF. Flow cytometric DNA analysis of adrenal cortical tumors in children. *Cancer* 1987;59:2059–2063.
145. Cibas ES, Medeiros LJ, Weinberg ES, et al. Cellular DNA profiles of benign and malignant adrenal cortical tumors. *Am J Surg Pathol* 1990;14:948–955.
146. Medeiros LJ, Weiss LM. New developments in the pathological diagnosis of adrenal cortical neoplasms. *Am J Clin Pathol* 1992;97:73–83.
147. Weiss LM, Medeiros LJ, Vickery AL Jr. Pathologic features of prognostic significance in adrenocortical carcinoma. *Am J Surg Pathol* 1989;13:202–206.
148. Aubert S, Wacrenier A, Leroy X, et al. Weiss system revisited. A clinicopathologic and immunohistochemical study of 49 adrenocortical tumors. *Am J Surg Pathol* 2002;26: 1612–1619.
149. Wieneke JA, Thompson LDR, Heffess CS. Adrenal cortical neoplasms in the pediatric population. A clinicopathologic and immunophenotypic analysis of 83 patients. *Am J Surg Pathol* 2003;27:867–881.
149a. Dehner LP. Pediatric adrenocortical neoplasms. On the road to some clarity. *Am J Surg Pathol* 2003;27:1005–1007.
149b. Dehner LP. Adrenal cortical neoplasia in children. Society for Pediatric Pathology Symposium: Endocrine Pathology Annual Meeting, Denver, CO, March, 2008.
150. Vargas MP, Vargas HI, Kleiner DE, et al. Adrenocortical neoplasms: role of prognostic markers MIB-1, p53, and RB. *Am J Surg Pathol* 1997;21:556–562.
151. O'Hare MJ, Monaghan P, Neville AM. The pathology of adrenal cortical neoplasia: a correlated structural and functional approach to the diagnosis of malignant disease. *Hum Pathol* 1979;10:137–154.
152. Zhao J, Speel EMJ, Muletta-Feurer S, et al. Analysis of genomic alterations in sporadic adrenal cortical lesions. Gain of chromosome 17 is an early event in adrenocortical tumorigenesis. *Am J Pathol* 1999;155:1039–1045.
153. Heppner C, Reincke M, Agarwal SK, et al. MEN1 gene analysis in sporadic adrenocortical neoplasms. *J Clin Endocrinol Metab* 1999;84:216–219.
154. Gortz B, Roth J, Speel EJ, et al. MEN1 gene mutation analysis of sporadic adrenocortical lesions. *Int J Cancer* 1999;80:373–379.
155. Gicquel C, Bertagna X, Gaston V, et al. Molecular markers and long term recurrence in a large cohort of patients with sporadic adrenocortical tumors. *Cancer Res* 2001;61: 6762–6767.
156. Velazquez-Fernandez D, Laurell C, Geli J, et al. Expression profiling of adrenocortical neoplasms suggests a molecular signature of malignancy. *Surgery* 2005;138:1087–1094.
157. Giordano TJ, Thomas DG, Kuiche R, et al. Distinct transcriptional profiles of adrenocortical tumors uncovered by microarray analysis. *Am J Pathol* 2003;162:521–531.
158. West AN, Neale GA, Pounds S, et al. Gene expression profiling of childhood adrenocortical tumors. *Cancer Res* 2007;67:600–608.
159. Marx C, Bornstein SR, Wolkersdorfer GW, et al. Relevance of major histocompatibility complex class II expression as a hallmark for the cellular differentiation in the human adrenal cortex. *J Clin Endocrinol Metab* 1997;82:2136–2140.
160. Wick MR, Cherwitz DL, McGlennen RC, et al. Adrenal cortical carcinoma: an immunohistochemical comparison with renal cell carcinoma. *Am J Pathol* 1986;122:343–352.
161. Cote RJ, Cardon-Cardo C, Reuter VE, et al. Immunopathology of adrenal and renal cortical tumors: coordinated changes in antigen expression is associated with neoplastic conversion in the adrenal cortex. *Am J Pathol* 1990;136:1077–1084.
162. Huang HY, Antonescu CR. Epithelioid variant of pleomorphic liposarcoma: a comparative immunohistochemical and ultrastructural analysis of six cases with emphasis on overlapping features with epithelial malignancies. *Ultrastruct Pathol* 2002;26:299–308.
163. Paton BL, Novitsky YW, Zerey M, et al. Outcomes of adrenal cortical carcinoma in the United States. *Surgery* 2006;140:914–920.
164. Belldegrun A, Hussain S, Seltzer SE, et al. Incidentally discovered mass of the adrenal gland. *Surg Gynecol Obstet* 1986;163:203–208.
165. Copeland PM. The incidentally discovered adrenal mass. *Ann Intern Med* 1983;98:940–945.
166. Geelhoed GW, Druy EM. Management of the adrenal "incidentaloma." *Surgery* 1982;92: 866–874.
167. Glazer HS, Weyman PJ, Sagel SS, et al. Nonfunctioning adrenal masses: incidental discovery on computed tomography. *AJR Am J Roentgenol* 1982;39:81–85.
168. Katz RL, Shirkhoda A. Diagnostic approach to incidental adrenal nodules in the cancer patient. *Cancer* 1985;55:1995–2000.
169. Foster DG. Adrenal cysts: review of literature and report of a case. *Arch Surg* 1966;92: 131–143.
170. Medeiros LJ, Levandrowski KB, Vickey AL. Adrenal pseudocyst: a clinical and pathological study of eight cases. *Hum Pathol* 1989;20:660–665.
171. Incze JS, Lui PS, Merriam JC, et al. Morphology and pathogenesis of adrenal cysts. *Am J Pathol* 1979;95:423–432.
172. Erickson LA, Lloyd RV, Hartman R, et al. Cystic adrenal neoplasms. *Cancer* 2004;101: 1537–1544.
173. Selye H, Stone H. Hormonally induced transformation of adrenal into myeloid tissue. *Am J Pathol* 1950;26:211–233.
174. Bennett B, McKenna TJ, Hough AJ, et al. Adrenal myelolipoma associated with Cushing's disease. *Am J Clin Pathol* 1980;73:443–447.
175. Bishop E, Eble JN, Cheng L et al. Adrenal myelolipomas show nonrandom X-chromosome inactivation in hematopoietic elements and fat: support for a clonal origin of myelolipomas. *Am J Surg Pathol* 2006;30:838–843.
176. Lam K-Y, Lo C-Y. Metastatic tumors of the adrenal glands: a 30 year experience in a teaching hospital. *Clin Endocrinol* 2002;56:95–101.
177. Redman BG, Pazdur R, Zingas AP, et al. Prospective evaluation of adrenal insufficiency in patients with adrenal metastasis. *Cancer* 1987;60:103–107.
178. McMahon RF. Tumor-to-tumor metastasis: bladder carcinoma metastasizing to an adrenocortical adenoma. *Br J Urol* 1991;67:216.
179. Lack EE. Pathology of the adrenal and extra-adrenal paraganglia. In *Major Problems in Pathology*. Philadelphia, PA: WB Saunders, 1994:29.
180. Gamelin E, Beldent V, Rousselet M-C, et al. Non-Hodgkin's lymphoma presenting with primary adrenal insufficiency: a disease with an underestimated frequency? *Cancer* 1992; 69:2333–2336.
181. Choi GH, Durishin M, Garbudawala ST, et al. Non-Hodgkin's lymphoma of the adrenal gland. *Arch Pathol Lab Med* 1990;114:883–885.
182. Schnitzer B, Smid D, Lloyd RV. Primary T-cell lymphoma of the adrenal glands with adrenal insufficiency. *Hum Pathol* 1986;17:634–636.
183. Donner LR, Mott FE, Tafur I. Cytokeratin positive, CD45 negative primary centroblastic lymphoma of the adrenal gland: a potential for a diagnostic pitfall. *Arch Pathol Lab Med* 2002;125:1104–1106.
184. Chu P, Costa J, Lackman MF. Angiotropic large cell lymphoma presenting as primary adrenal insufficiency. *Hum Pathol* 1996;27:209–211.
185. Nosher JL, Amorosa JK, Seiman S, et al. Fine needle aspiration of the kidney and adrenal gland. *J Urol* 1982;128:895–899.
186. Lam KY, Lo CY. Adrenal lipomatous tumors: a 30 year clinicopathological experience at a single institution. *J Clin Pathol* 2001;54:707–712.
187. Prevot S, Penna CT, Imbert J-C, et al. Solitary fibrous tumor of the adrenal gland. *Mod Pathol* 1996;9:1170–1174.
188. Eftekhari F, Ater JL, Ayala AG, et al. Calcifying fibrous pseudotumor of the adrenal gland. *Br J Radiol* 2001;74:452–454.
189. Lau SK, Weiss LM. Calcifying fibrous tumor of the adrenal gland. *Hum Pathol* 2007;38: 656–659.
190. Wenig B, Heffess C. Adrenal angiosarcoma; a clinicopathologic and immunocytochemical study. *Lab Invest* 1992;66:39A.
191. Granger JK, Hoan H-Y, Collins C. Massive hemorrhagic functional adrenal adenoma histologically mimicking angiosarcoma: report of a case with immunohistochemical study. *Am J Surg Pathol* 1991;15:699–704.
192. Lack EE, Graham CW, Azumi N, et al. Primary leiomyosarcoma of adrenal gland: case report with immunohistochemical and ultrastructural study. *Am J Surg Pathol* 1991;15:899
193. Candanedo-Gonzalez FA, Chavez TV, Cerubulo-Vasquez A. Pleomorphic leiomyosarcoma of the adrenal gland with osteoclast-like giant cells. *Endocr Pathol* 2005;16:75–82.
194. Zetler PJ, Filipanko JD, Bilbey JH, et al. Primary adrenal leiomyosarcoma in a man with acquired immunodeficiency syndrome (AIDS): further evidence for an increase in smooth muscle tumors related to Epstein Barr virus infection in AIDS. *Arch Pathol Lab Med* 1995; 119:1164–1167.
195. Glantz K, Wegmann W. Papillary adenomatoid tumor of the adrenal gland. *Histopathology* 2000;37:376–377.
196. Simpson PR. Adenomatoid tumor of the adrenal glands. *Arch Pathol Lab Med* 1990;114: 725–727.
197. Travis WD, Lack EE, Azumi N, et al. Adenomatoid tumors of the adrenal gland with ultrastructural and immunohistochemical demonstrations of a mesothelial origin. *Arch Pathol Lab Med* 1990;114:722–727.

198. Isotalo PA, Keeney GL, Sebo TJ, et al. Adenomatoid tumor of the adrenal gland: clinicopathologic study of five cases and review of the literature. *Am J Surg Pathol* 2003;27:969–977.

199. Fidler WJ. Ovarian thecal metaplasia in adrenal glands. *Am J Clin Pathol* 1976;67:318–323.

200. Carney JA. Unusual tumefactive spindle cell lesions in the adrenal glands. *Hum Pathol* 1987;18:980–985.

201. Orselli RC, Bassler TJ. Theca granulosa cell tumor arising in adrenal. *Cancer* 1973;31:474.

202. Pollock WJ, McConnell CF, Hilton C, et al. Virilizing Leydig cell adenoma of adrenal gland. *Am J Surg Pathol* 1986;10:816–822.

203. Carstens PHB, Kuhns JG, Ghazi C. Primary malignant melanomas of the lung and adrenal. *Hum Pathol* 1984;15:910–914.

204. Dao AH, Page DL, Reynold VH, et al. Primary malignant melanoma of the adrenal glands: a report of two cases and review of the literature. *Am Surg* 1990;56:199–203.

205. Unger PD, Hoffman K, Thung SN, et al. HMB-45 reactivity in adrenal pheochromocytomas. *Arch Pathol Lab Med* 1992;116:151–153.

206. Santonja C, Diaz MA, Dehner LP. A unique dysembryonic neoplasm of the adrenal gland composed of nephrogenic rests in a child. *Am J Surg Pathol* 1996;20:118–124.

207. Molberg K, Vuitch F, Stewart D, et al. Adrenocortical blastoma. *Hum Pathol* 1992;23:1187–1190.

208. Wieneke JA, Thompson LA, Heffess CS. Corticomedullary mixed tumor of the adrenal gland. *Ann Diagn Pathol* 2001;5:304–308.

209. Ross JA, Severson RK, Pollock BH, et al. Childhood cancer in the United States: a geographical analysis of cases from the Pediatric Cooperative Clinical Trials Group. *Cancer* 1996;77:201–207.

210. Hardy PC, Nesbit ME Jr. Familial neuroblastoma: report of a kindred with a high incidence of familial tumors. *J Pediatr* 1973;80:74–77.

211. MacKay B, Luna MA, Butler JJ. Adult neuroblastoma. *Cancer* 1976;37:1334–1351.

212. Allan SG, Cornbleet MA, Carmichael J, et al. Adult neuroblastoma: report of three cases and review of the literature. *Cancer* 1986;57:2419–2421.

213. Kaye JA, Warhol NJ, Kretschmar C, et al. Neuroblastoma in adults: three case reports and review of the literature. *Cancer* 1986;58:1149–1157.

214. Chauty A, Raimondo G, Vergeron H, et al. Discovery of a neuroblastoma producing cardiogenic shock in a two-month-old child. *Arch Pediatr* 2002;9:602–605.

215. Sawada T. Past and future of neuroblastoma screening in Japan. *Am J Pediatr Hematol Oncol* 1992;14:320–326.

216. Woods WG, Gao RN, Shuster JJ, et al. Screening of infants and mortality due to neuroblastoma. *N Engl J Med* 2002;346:1041–1046.

217. Schilling FH, Spix C, Berthold F, et al. Neuroblastoma screening at one year of age. *N Engl J Med* 2002;346:1047–1053.

218. Yamato K, Ohta S, Ito E, et al. Marginal decrease in mortality and marked increase in incidence as a result of neuroblastoma screening at 6 months of age: cohort study in seven prefectures in Japan. *J Clin Oncol* 2002;20:1209–1214.

219. Gitlow SE, Bertani LM, Rausen A, et al. Diagnosis of neuroblastoma by qualitative and quantitative determination of catecholamine metabolites in urine. *Cancer* 1970;25:1377–1383.

220. Lang WE, Siegel SE, Shaw KNF, et al. Initial urinary catecholamine metabolite concentrations and prognosis in neuroblastoma. *Pediatr Pathol* 1978;62:77–83.

221. Nakagawara A, Ideda K, Itigashi K, et al. Inverse correlation between N-myc amplification and catecholamine metabolism in children with advanced neuroblastoma. *Surgery* 1990;107:43–49.

222. Beckwith JB, Perrin EV. In situ neuroblastomas: a contribution to the natural history of neural crest tumors. *Am J Pathol* 1963;43:1089–1104.

223. Bolande RP. Developmental pathology. *Am J Pathol* 1979;94:623–683.

224. Turkel SB, Itabashi HH. The natural history of neuroblastic cells in the fetal adrenal gland. *Am J Pathol* 1974;76:225–244.

225. Beckwith JB, Martin RF. Observations on the histopathology of neuroblastomas. *J Pediatr Surg* 1968;3:106–110.

226. Hughes M, Marsden HB, Palmer MK. Histological patterns of neuroblastomas related to prognosis and clinical staging. *Cancer* 1974;34:1706–1711.

227. Shimada H, Chatten J, Newton WA, et al. Histopathologic prognostic factors in neuroblastic tumors: definition of subtypes of ganglioneuroblastoma and an age linked classification of neuroblastomas. *J Natl Cancer Inst* 1984;73:405–413.

228. Joshi VV, Cantor AB, Altshuler G, et al. Age linked prognostic categorization based on a new histologic grading system of neuroblastomas. *Cancer* 1992;69:2197–2211.

229. Shimada H, Ambros IM, Dehner LP, et al. Terminology and morphologic criteria of neuroblastic tumors. Recommendations by the International Neuroblastoma Pathology Committee. *Cancer* 1999;86:349–363.

230. Shimada H, Ambros IM, Dehner LP, et al. The International Neuroblastoma Pathology Classification (the Shimada System). *Cancer* 1999;86:364–372.

231. Russell DS, Rubinstein LJ. *Pathology of Tumors of the Nervous System.* Baltimore, MD: Williams & Wilkins, 1971.

232. Taxy JB. Electron microscopy in the diagnosis of neuroblastoma. *Arch Pathol Lab Med* 1980;104:355–360.

233. Tornoczky T, Kalman E, Kajar PG, et al. Large cell neuroblastoma. A distinct phenotype of neuroadenoma with aggressive clinical behavior. *Cancer* 2004;100:390–397.

234. Moll R, Lee I, Gould V, et al. Immunocytochemical analysis of Ewing's tumors: patterns of expression of intermediate filaments and desmosomal proteins indicate cell type heterogeneity and pluripotential differentiation. *Am J Pathol* 1987;127:288–304.

235. Osborn M, Dirk T, Kaser H, et al. Immunohistochemical localization of neurofilaments and neuron specific enolase in 19 cases of neuroblastoma. *Am J Pathol* 1986;122:433–442.

236. Hachitanda Y, Tsuneyoshi M, Enjoji M. An ultrastructural and immunohistochemical evaluation of cytodifferentiation in neuroblastic tumors. *Mod Pathol* 1989;2:13–19.

237. Mukai M, Torikata C, Iri H, et al. Expression of neurofilament triplet proteins in human neural tumors: an immunohistochemical study of paraganglioma, ganglioneuroma, ganglioneuroblastoma and neuroblastoma. *Am J Pathol* 1985;122:28–35.

238. Molenaar WM, Baker DL, Pleasure D, et al. The neuroendocrine and neural profiles of neuroblastomas, ganglioneuroblastomas and ganglioneuromas. *Am J Pathol* 1990;136:375–382.

239. Hasegawa T, Matsumo Y, Hiroshashi S, et al. Second primary rhabdomyosarcoma in patients with bilateral retinoblastoma: a clinical and immunohistochemical study. *Am J Surg Pathol* 1998;22:1351–1360.

240. Brook FB, Raafat F, Eldeeb BB, et al. Histological and immunohistochemical investigation of neuroblastomas and correlation with prognosis. *Hum Pathol* 1988;19:879–888.

241. Wiedemann B, Franke W. Identification and localization of synaptophysin, an integral membrane glycoprotein of Mr 38,000 characteristic of presynaptic vesicles. *Cell* 1985;41:1017–1028.

242. Wirnsberger GH, Becker H, Ziervogel K, et al. Diagnostic immunohistochemistry of neuroblastic tumors. *Am J Surg Pathol* 1992;16:49–57.

243. Sariola H, Terava H, Rapola J, et al. Cell surface ganglioside D2 in the immunohistochemical detection and differential diagnosis of neuroblastoma. *Am J Clin Pathol* 1991;96:248–252.

244. Artlieb V, Krepler R, Wiche G. Expression of microtubule associated proteins, Map-1 and Map-2, in human neuroblastomas and differential diagnosis of immature neuroblasts. *Lab Invest* 1985;53:684–691.

245. Oppedal BR, Strom-Mathiesen I, Kemshead JT, et al. Bone marrow examination in neuroblastoma patients: a morphological, immunocytochemical and immunohistochemical study. *Hum Pathol* 1989;20:800–805.

246. Reid MM, Wallis JP, McGuckin AG, et al. Routine histological compared to immunohistological examination of bone marrow trephine biopsy specimens in disseminated neuroblastoma. *J Clin Pathol* 1991;44:483–486.

247. Smith RG, Reynolds CP. Monoclonal antibody recognizing a human neuroblastoma-associated antigen. *Diagn Clin Immunol* 1987;5:209–220.

248. Moss TJ, Reynolds CP, Sather HN, et al. Prognostic value of immunocytologic detection of bone marrow metastases in neuroblastoma. *N Engl J Med* 1991;324:219–226.

249. Shipley WR, Hammer RD, Lennington WJ, et al. Paraffin immunohistochemical detection of CD56, a useful marker for neural adhesion molecule (NCAM) in normal and neoplastic fixed tissues. *Appl Immuno* 1997;5:87–93.

250. Wick MR. Immunohistology of neuroendocrine and neuroectodermal tumors. *Semin Diagn Pathol* 2000;17:194–203.

251. Phimister E, Kiely F, Kemshead JT, et al. Expression of neural adhesion molecule (NCAM) isoforms in neuroblastoma. *J Clin Pathol* 1991;44:580–585.

252. Miettinen M, Chatten J, Paetau A, et al. Monoclonal antibody NB84 in the differential diagnosis of neuroblastoma and other small round cell tumors. *Am J Surg Pathol* 1998;22:327–332.

253. Folpe AL, Patterson K, Gown AM. Antineuroblastoma antibody NB84 also identifies a significant subset of other small round blue cell tumors. *Appl Immuno* 1997;5:239–245.

254. Lamant L, Pulford K, Bischof D, et al. Expression of the ALK tyrosine kinase gene in neuroblastomas. *Am J Pathol* 2000;156:1711–1721.

255. Stevenson AJ, Chatten J, Bertoni F, et al. CD99 (p30/32 mic2) neuroectodermal/Ewing's sarcoma antigen, an immunohistochemical marker: review of more than 600 tumors and the literature experience. *Appl Immunohistochem* 1994;2:231–240.

256. Triche T, Askin FB. Neuroblastoma and the differential diagnosis of small-, round-, blue-cell tumors. *Hum Pathol* 1983;14:568–595.

257. Gonzalez-Angulo A, Reyes H, Reyna AN. The ultrastructure of ganglioneuroblastoma. *Neurol Rep* 1965;15:242–252.

258. Triche T, Ross WE. Glycogen-containing neuroblastoma with clinical histopathologic features of Ewing's sarcoma. *Cancer* 1978;41:1425–1432.

259. Kammen BF, Matthay KK, Pacham P, et al. Pulmonary metastases at diagnosis of neuroblastoma in pediatric patients: CT findings and prognosis. *AJR Am J Roentgenol* 2001;176:755–759.

260. Burchill SA, Wheeldon J, Cullinane C, et al. EWS-FLI1 fusion transcripts identified in patients with typical neuroblastoma. *Eur J Cancer* 1997;33:239–243.

261. Kempson RL, Fletcher CDM, Evans HL, et al. Tumors of soft tissues. In *Atlas of Tumor Pathology.* 3rd series, fascicle 30. Washington, DC: Armed Forces Institute of Pathology, 2001.

261a. Ozdermirli M, Farnburg-Smith JC, Hartman DP. Differentiating lymphoblastic lymphoma and Ewing's sarcoma: lymphocyte markers and gene rearrangement. *Mod Pathol* 2001;14:1175–1182.

262. Stout JP. Ganglioneuroma of the sympathetic nervous system. *Surg Gynecol Obstet* 1947;84:101–110.

263. Stowens D. Neuroblastomas and related tumors. *Arch Pathol* 1957;63:451–459.

264. Mack E, Sarto GE, Crummy AB, et al. Virilizing adrenal ganglioneuroma. *JAMA* 1978;239:2273–2274.

265. Evans AE, D'Angio GJ, Propert K, et al. Prognostic factors in neuroblastoma. *Cancer* 1987;59:1853–1859.

266. Joshi VV, Silverman JF. Pathology of neuroblastic tumors. *Semin Diagn Pathol* 1994;11:107–117.

267. Chatten J, Shimada H, Sather HN, et al. Prognostic value of histopathology in advanced neuroblastoma: a report from the Children's Cancer Group. *Hum Pathol* 1988;19:1187–1198.

268. Shimada H, Umehara S, Monobe Y, et al. International neuroblastoma pathology classification for prognostic evaluation of patients with peripheral neuroblastic tumors. A report from the Children's Cancer Group. *Cancer* 2001;92:2451–2461.

269. Umehara S, Nakagawa A, Matthay KK, et al. Histopathology defines prognostic subsets of ganglioneuroblastoma, nodular. A report from the Children's Cancer Group. *Cancer* 2000;89:1150–1161.

270. Ambros IM, Hata J, Joshi VV, et al. Morphologic features of neuroblastoma (schwannian stroma-poor tumors) in clinically favorable and unfavorable groups. *Cancer* 2002;94:1574–1583.

271. Sano H, Gonzalez-Gomez I, Wu SQ, et al. A case of composite neuroblastoma composed of histologically and biologically distinct clones. *Pediatr Dev Pathol* 2007;10:229–232.

272. Brodeur GM, Seeger RC, Barrett A, et al. International criteria for diagnosis, staging, and response to treatment in patients with neuroblastoma. *J Clin Oncol* 1988;6:1874–1881.

273. Brodeur GM, Pritchard J, Berthold F, et al. Revisions of the international criteria for neuroblastoma diagnosis, staging and response to treatment. *J Clin Oncol* 1993;11:1466–1477.

274. Ikeda H, Iehara T, Tsuchida Y, et al. Experience with the international neuroblastoma staging system and pathology classification. *Br J Cancer* 2002;86:1110–1116.

275. Kushner BH, Kramer K, Cheung NKV. Chronic neuroblastoma. Indolent stage 4 disease in children. *Cancer* 2002;95:1366–1375.

276. Zeltzer PM, Marangos PA, Evans AE, et al. Serum neuron specific enolase in children with neuroblastoma: relationship to stage and disease course. *Cancer* 1986;57:1230–1234.

277. Berthold F, Hunnemann DH, Harms D, et al. Serum vanillylmandelic acid/homovanillic acid contributes to prognosis estimation in patients with localized but not with metastatic neuroblastoma. *Eur J Cancer* 1992;28A:1950.

278. Brodeur GM, Seeger RC, Schwab M, et al. Amplification of N-myc in untreated human neuroblastomas correlates with advanced stage disease. *Science* 1984;224:1121–1124.

279. Brodeur GM. Molecular pathology of human neuroblastomas. *Semin Diagn Pathol* 1994;11:118–125.

280. Brodeur GM. Neuroblastoma: biological insights into a clinical enigma. *Nat Rev* 2003;3:203–216.

281. Goto S, Umehara S, Gerbing RB, et al. Histopathology (International Neuroblastoma Pathology Classification) and MYCN status in patents with peripheral neuroblastic tumors. A report from the Children's Cancer Group. *Cancer* 2001;92:2699–2708.

282. Kobayashi C, Monforte-Munoz HL, Gerbing RB, et al. Enlarged and prominent nucleoli may be indicative of MYCN amplification. A study of neuroblastoma (Schwannian Stroma-poor), undifferentiated/poorly differentiated subtype with high mitosis-karyorrhexis index. *Cancer* 2005;103:174–180.

283. Thorner PS, Ho M, Chilton-MacNeill S, et al. Use of chromogenic in situ hybridization to identify MYCN copy number in neuroblastoma using routine tissue sections. *Am J Surg Pathol* 2006;30:635–642.

284. Bown N. Neuroblastoma tumor genetics: clinical and biological aspects. *J Clin Pathol* 2001;54:897–910.

285. Caron H, van Sluis P, de Kraker J, et al. Allelic loss of chromosome 1p as a predictor of unfavorable outcome in patients with neuroblastoma. *N Engl J Med* 1996;334:225–230.

286. Bown N, Cotterill S, Lastowska M, et al. Gain of chromosome arm 17q and adverse outcome in patients with neuroblastoma. *N Engl J Med* 1999;340:1954–1961.

287. Nakagawara A, Arima M, Azar CG, et al. Inverse relationship between trk expression and N-myc amplification in human neuroblastomas. *Cancer Res* 1992;52:1364–1368.

288. Brodeur GM, Maris JM, Yamashiro DJ, et al. Biology and genetics of human neuroblastomas. *J Pediatr Hematol Oncol* 1997;19:93–101.

289. Mora J, Gerald WL, Qin J, et al. Evolving significance of prognostic markers associated with treatment improvement in patients with stage 4 neuroblastoma. *Cancer* 2002;94:2756–2765.

290. Giordani L, Iolascon A, Servedio V, et al. Two regions of deletion in 9p22-p24 in neuroblastoma are frequently observed in favorable tumors. *Cancer Genet Cytogenet* 2002;135:42–47.

291. Ramani R. Expression of bcl-2 gene product in neuroblastoma. *J Pathol* 1994;172:273–278.

292. Chan HSL, Haddad G, Thorner PS, et al. P-glycoprotein expression as a predictor of outcome in therapy for neuroblastoma. *N Engl J Med* 1991;325:1608–1614.

293. Mora J, Cheung NK, Oplanich S, et al. New regions of allelic imbalance identified by genome-wide analysis of neuroblastoma. *Cancer Res* 2002;62:1761–1767.

294. Krams M, Hero B, Berthold F, et al. Proliferation marker KI-S5 discriminates between favorable and adverse prognosis in advanced stages of neuroblastoma with and without MYCN amplification. *Cancer* 2002;94:854–861.

295. Wei JS, Greer BT, Westerman F, et al. Prediction of clinical outcome using gene expression profiling and artificial neural networks for patients with neuroblastoma. *Cancer Res* 2004;64:6883–6891.

296. Asgharzadeh A, Pique-Regi R, Sposto R, et al. Prognostic significance of gene expression profiles of metastatic neuroblastomas lacking gene amplification. *J Natl Cancer Inst* 2006;98:1193–1203.

297. Askin FB, Perlman EJ. Neuroblastoma and peripheral neuroectodermal tumors. *Am J Clin Pathol* 1998;109(Suppl 1):S23–S30.

298. Manger WM, Gifford RW Jr. *Pheochromocytoma.* New York, NY: Springer-Verlag, 1977.

299. Remine WH, Chong GC, Van Heerden JA, et al. Current management of pheochromocytoma. *Ann Surg* 1974;179:741–748.

300. Manasse P. Zur histologie und histogenese der primaren nierengeschwulske. *Arch Pathol Anat Klin Med* 1893;133:391–404.

301. Pick L. Das ganglioma embryonale sympathicum. *Klin Wochenschrv* 1912;49:16–22.

302. Koch CA, Vortmeyer A, Zhuang Z, et al. New insights into the genetics of familial chromaffin cell tumors. *Ann N Y Acad Sci* 2002;970:11–28.

303. Atuk NO, McDonald T, Wood T, et al. Familial pheochromocytoma, hypercalcemia and von Hippel-Lindau disease. *Medicine* 1979;58:209–218.

304. DeLellis RA, Dayal Y, Tischler AS, et al. Multiple endocrine neoplasia (MEN) syndromes: cellular origins and inter-relationships. *Int Rev Exp Pathol* 1986;28:163–215.

305. Carney JA, Sizemore GW, Sheps SG. Adrenal medullary disease in multiple endocrine neoplasia, type 2. *Am J Clin Pathol* 1976;66:279–290.

306. Stackpole RH, Melicow MM, Uson AC. Pheochromocytoma in children. *J Pediatr* 1953;63:315–330.

307. Li M, Wenig BM. Adrenal oncocytic pheochromocytoma. *Am J Surg Pathol* 2000;24:1552–1557.

308. Linnoila RI, Keiser HR, Steinberg SM, et al. Histopathology of benign versus malignant sympathoadrenal paragangliomas: clinicopathologic study of 120 cases including unusual histological features. *Hum Pathol* 1990;21:1168–1180.

309. Steinhoff MN, Wells SA, DeSchryver-Kelskemeti K. Stromal amyloid in pheochromocytomas. *Hum Pathol* 1992;23:33–36.

310. Medeiros LJ, Katsas GG, Balogh K. Brown fat and adrenal pheochromocytoma: association or coincidence? *Hum Pathol* 1985;16:580–589.

311. Thompson LDR. Pheochromocytoma of the adrenal gland scaled score (PASS) to separate benign form malignant neoplasms. A clinicopathologic and immunophenotypic study of 100 cases. *Am J Surg Pathol* 2002;26:551–556.

312. DeLellis RA, Tischler AS, Lee AK, et al. Leu-enkephalin-like immunoreactivity in proliferative lesions of the human adrenal medulla and extra-adrenal paraganglia. *Am J Surg Pathol* 1983;7:29–37.

313. Berenyi MR, Singh G, Gloster ES, et al. ACTH-producing pheochromocytoma. *Arch Pathol Lab Med* 1977;101:31–35.

314. Tannenbaum M. *Ultrastructural Pathology of Adrenal Medullary Tumors.* In Sommers SC, ed. New York, NY: Appleton-Century-Crofts, 1970:145–171.

315. Wantanabe H, Burnstock G, Jarrott B, et al. Mitochondrial abnormalities in human phaeochromocytoma. *Cell Tissue Res* 1976;171:281–288.

316. Yokoyama M, Takayasu H. An electron microscopic study of the human adrenal medulla and pheochromocytoma. *Urol Int* 1969;24:79–95.

317. Neumann HP, Vortmeyer A, Schmidt D, et al. Evidence of MEN-2 in the original description of classic pheochromocytoma. *N Engl J Med* 2007;357:1311–1315.

318. Lindor NM, Honchel R, Khsla S, et al. Mutations in the ret proto-oncogene in sporadic pheochromocytomas. *J Clin Endocrinol Metab* 1995;80:627–629.

319. Gutmann DH, Cole JH, Stone WJ, et al. Loss of neurofibromin in adrenal gland tumors from patients with neurofibromatosis type I. *Genes Chromosomes Cancer* 1993;10:55–58.

320. Krumm A, Meulia T, Groudine M. Common mechanisms for the control of eukaryotic transcriptional elongation. *Bioassays* 1993;15:659–665.

321. Crossey PA, Richards FM, Foster K, et al. Identification of intragenic mutations in the von Hippel-Lindau tumor suppressor gene and correlation with disease phenotype. *Hum Mol Genet* 1994;3:1303–1308.

322. Maher ER, Eng C. The pressure rises: update on the genetics of phaeochromocytoma. *Hum Mol Genet* 2002;11:2347–2354.

323. Neumann HPH, Bausch B, McWhinney S et al. Germ-line mutations in nonsyndromic pheochromocytoma. *N Engl J Med* 2001;346:1459–1466.

324. Edstrom E, Mahlamaki E, Nord B, et al. Comparative genomic hybridization reveals frequent losses of chromosomes 1p and 3q in pheochromocytomas and abdominal paragangliomas, suggesting a common genetic etiology. *Am J Pathol* 2000;156:651–659.

325. Dannenberg H, Speel EJM, Zhao J, et al. Losses of chromosomes 1p and 3q are early genetic events in the development of sporadic pheochromocytomas. *Am J Pathol* 2002;157:353–359.

326. Petri BJ, Speel EJ, Korpershoek E, et al. Frequent loss of 17p, but no p53 mutations or protein overexpression in benign and malignant pheochromocytomas. *Mod Pathol* 2008;21:407–413.

327. Thouennon E, Elkahlom AG, Guillemot J, et al. Identification of potential gene markers and insights into the pathophysiology of pheochromocytoma malignancy. *J Endocrinol Metab* 2007;92:4865–4872.

328. Brouwers FM, Elkahloun AG, Munson PJ. Gene expression profiling of benign and malignant pheochromocytoma. *Ann N Y Acad Sci* 2006;1073:541–556.

329. Kimura N, Watanabe T, Fukase M, et al. Neurofibromin and NF1 gene analysis in composite pheochromocytoma and tumors associated with von Recklinghausen's disease. *Mod Pathol* 2002;15:183–188.

330. Tischler AS, DeLellis RA, Biales B, et al. Nerve growth factor induced neurite outgrowth from normal human chromaffin cell. *Lab Invest* 1980;43:399–409.

331. Juarez D, Brown RW, Ostrowski M, et al. Pheochromocytoma associated with neuroendocrine carcinoma. A new type of composite pheochromocytoma. *Arch Pathol Lab Med* 1999;123:1274–1279.

332. Clarke MR, Weyant RJ, Watson CG, et al. Prognostic markers in pheochromocytoma. *Hum Pathol* 1998;29:522–526.

333. Lewis PD. A cytophotometric study of benign and malignant pheochromocytomas. *Virchows Arch B [Zellpathol]* 1971;9:371–376.

334. Favier J, Plouin PF, Corvol P, et al. Angiogenesis and vascular architecture in pheochromocytomas. Distinctive traits in malignant tumors. *Am J Pathol* 2002;161:1235–1246.

335. DeLellis RA, Wolfe HJ, Gagel RF, et al. Adrenal medullary hyperplasia: a morphometric analysis in patients with familial medullary thyroid carcinoma. *Am J Pathol* 1976;83:177–196.

336. Salmenkivi K, Haglund C, Arola J, et al. Increased expression of tenascin in pheochromocytomas correlates with malignancy. *Am J Surg Pathol* 2001;25:1419–1423.

337. Visser JW, Axt R. Bilateral adrenal medullary hyperplasia: a clinicopathological entity. *J Clin Pathol* 1975;28:298–304.

338. Rudy FR, Bates RD, Cimorelli AJ, et al. Adrenal medullary hyperplasia: a clinicopathologic study of four cases. *Hum Pathol* 1980;11:650–657.

339. Naeye RL. Brainstem and adrenal abnormalities in the sudden infant death syndrome. *Am J Clin Pathol* 1976;66:526–530.

340. Diaz-Cano SJ, de Miguel M, Blanes A, et al. Clonal patterns in pheochromocytomas and MEN2 adrenal medullary hyperplasia: histologic and kinetic correlates. *J Pathol* 2000;192:221–228.

Ernest E. Lack
Jacqueline A. Wieneke

Paragangliomas

Extra-adrenal paraganglia make up part of the dispersed neuroendocrine system (DNS) having a centripetal and roughly symmetrical distribution with extension from the base of the skull down to the pelvic floor. There is brief reference to the presence of a structure reminiscent of paraganglia within soft tissues surrounding large femoral vessels, but it is not well documented (1). These paraganglia can be divided into two groups—paraganglia in the head and neck region (including aorticopulmonary paraganglia), which have a close alignment with the parasympathetic nervous system, and the paraganglia of the sympathoadrenal neuroendocrine system.

The amine precursor uptake and decarboxylation (APUD) cell concept was proposed by Pearse (2,3) in an attempt to unify a broad array of endocrine cells that were presumed to have a common embryologic derivation from neural crest. Although no longer widely accepted, this concept accelerated scientific investigation, particularly in the areas of immunology and molecular pathology (4,5). The term *neuroendocrine* has now come into vogue because it emphasizes the close relationship between the nervous system (e.g., neurons) and endocrine cells (6–8). A wide variety of hormones and regulatory neuropeptides have been identified in normal paraganglia and the tumors arising from them. Some of these substances have an endocrine function through interaction with receptors at distant sites, whereas others mediate a regulatory effect on neighboring cells (paracrine function) or perhaps even an autoregulatory effect on the same cell (autocrine function).

The terminology of paragangliomas is based on the anatomic site of origin rather than the chromaffin or nonchromaffin status of the tumor. The term *pheochromocytoma* has been arbitrarily restricted to an adrenal medullary paraganglioma, although there are extra-adrenal tumors that are functionally and morphologically identical. Because extra-adrenal paragangliomas can arise at such a variety of anatomic sites, one must be aware of other tumors that enter into the differential diagnosis. Accurate recognition of these tumors can be particularly difficult when one is dealing with limited biopsy material or tumor that is partially crushed. Stromal alterations can also cause diagnostic difficulties.

PARAGANGLIA OF THE HEAD AND NECK REGION

EMBRYOLOGY AND PHYSIOLOGY

Paraganglia in the head and neck region are closely aligned with the parasympathetic nervous system and often have a close spatial relationship with neural or vascular structures (Fig. 15.1). Using a cytochemical marker system, glomus type I or chief cells have been shown in the avian carotid body to have embryologic origin from neural crest (9), and presumably, chief cells in humans at various other locations in the head and neck

region have this same embryogenesis. Carotid body and aorticopulmonary paraganglia have been shown in experimental physiologic studies in animals to have a chemoreceptor role, with modulation of respiratory and cardiovascular function in response to changes in arterial partial pressure of oxygen (PO_2), partial pressure of carbon dioxide (PCO_2), pH, and other chemical alterations (10,11). de Castro (12) was the first to propose a chemosensory role for carotid bodies, based on morphologic observations in animals. The physiologic function of other paraganglia in the head and neck region is not known, but their histologic appearance is very similar, thus suggesting a similar role in chemosensation.

Changes in oxygen (O_2) tension are detected by O_2-sensitive K^+ and Ca^{2+} channels, and a suprathreshold increase of cytosolic Ca^{2+} triggers neurotransmitter (i.e., dopamine) release,

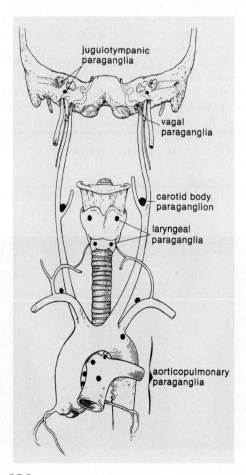

Figure 15.1. Anatomic distribution of paraganglia in the head and neck region, including the base of the heart. Carotid bodies are the largest compact collection of paraganglia; these, along with aorticopulmonary paraganglia, have been shown experimentally to have a physiologic role in chemosensation.

which activates afferent nerve terminals (13). Despite the immense amount of experimental research in animals, the primary chemosensor or transducer is still not known with certainty. Numerous proposals have been put forth. Favored candidates include mitochondria, AMP-activated kinase, hemoxygenase-2, and succinate dehydrogenase (SDH). No single mechanism has been shown to explain the multitude of accumulated data, and it may be that a cascade involving several mechanisms is required to accomplish the necessary homeostatic response to arterial hypoxemia (14–18).

MORPHOLOGY AND ANATOMIC DISTRIBUTION

Carotid bodies are the largest compact collection of paraganglia in the head and neck region; they appear as a small ovoid structure on the medial aspect of the carotid bifurcation on each side of the neck (Fig. 15.2). The average combined weight of carotid bodies in adults without chronic hypoxia or systemic hypertension is approximately 12 mg (19,20). Paraganglia located elsewhere in the head and neck region have a nearly identical histomorphologic picture, but they are smaller and usually lack the compact lobular architecture of the carotid bodies (Fig. 15.3A). The basic anatomic unit of the carotid body is the lobule, which contains clusters ("zellballen") or cords of chief cells (Fig. 15.3B). Within the lobule, a variety of different cells are present, including chief cells and sustentacular or glomus type II cells, as well as pericytes, endothelial cells, and Schwann cells. Chief cells can be vividly depicted by staining for cytoplasmic argyrophilia (Fig. 15.3C) or chromogranin A (Fig. 15.3D), and this organoid arrangement of chief cells is vaguely recapitulated in the neoplasms derived from them. Sustentacular cells are located at the periphery of clusters of chief cells and can be demonstrated by immunostain for S-100 protein (Fig. 15.3E); these cells are typically present in paragangliomas at all anatomic sites in the head and neck region and the sympathoadrenal neuroendocrine system.

Carotid body and other paraganglia contain catecholamines, and chief cells have been shown to have enzymes involved in catecholamine synthesis. The immunophenotype of these endocrine cells and tumors derived from them, however, are remarkably diverse. Paraganglia in the head and neck region are located at a variety of sites, including the middle ear, adventitia of the jugular bulb, ganglion nodosum of the vagus nerve, larynx, and base of the heart (Fig. 15.1). This anatomic distribution in some areas parallels the branchial arch derivatives that in aquatic species correspond to gill arches. In some cases, paragangliomas have been reported at sites where normal paraganglionic tissue has not yet been described in humans. We cite the recent report of the rare occurrence of paraganglioma of the ovary as an example (21).

HYPERPLASIA OF CHEMORECEPTOR PARAGANGLIA

Carotid body enlargement was reported by Arias-Stella (22) in natives born and living in the Peruvian Andes 14,350 feet above sea level. This was confirmed in other studies (23) and also by Saldana et al. (24), who reported a 10-fold increase in incidence of "chemodectomas" at high altitude. An increased incidence of carotid body paragangliomas (CBPs) has been reported in other locations at high altitude (25,26). Carotid body hypertrophy and hyperplasia have also been observed in humans under normobaric conditions, for example, in patients with chronic obstructive pulmonary disease (19,27), systemic hypertension (19), and some cases of cystic fibrosis (Fig. 15.4A,B) and cyanotic congenital heart disease (20,28). Chronic hypoxia leads to hypersensitivity of the carotid bodies with subsequent morphologic and neurochemical changes in the carotid body, including carotid body enlargement, hyperplasia of glomus cells, and neovascularization (29,30). Hyperplasia of vagal paraganglia (31) and aorticopulmonary paraganglia (32) suggests a similar role in chemosensation. Chemoreceptor hyperplasia in most cases is presumably a compensatory response to prolonged and severe hypoxemia (22). Although on rare occasion paragangliomas associated with hypoxemia related to conditions other than high altitude have been reported (33–35), the increased risk of developing a paraganglioma appears to be negligible in patients at sea level, with or without hypoxemia.

PARAGANGLIOMAS OF THE HEAD AND NECK REGION

CAROTID BODY PARAGANGLIOMA

Tumors of this type have been referred to as chemodectomas (*chemeia*, meaning "infusion"; *deschesthai*, meaning "to receive"; and *oma*, meaning "tumor") (36), and this term has been used synonymously for paragangliomas at other sites in the head and neck region. There is no evidence, however, that any of these tumors have a functional role in chemosensation. The first CBP was reported by Marchand (37) in 1891 in a patient who had been operated on by Riegner in 1880. CBPs typically appear as a slow-growing, painless mass near the angle of the mandible (Fig. 15.5A) (32,38–41). In some patients, there may be signs or symptoms of cranial nerve palsy, such as dysphagia or dysphonia; the carotid sinus syndrome is an unusual feature, with bradycardia and syncopal episodes. On rare occasion, CBPs and other head and neck paragangliomas may be functional, with signs or symptoms of excess catecholamine secretion (32, 42,43). The average age at diagnosis is usually in the fifth decade

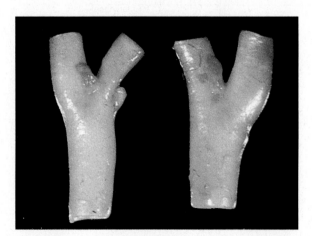

Figure 15.2. Normal carotid body paraganglia are ovoid pink structures on the medial aspect of the carotid bifurcation on both sides. The external carotid artery branches are directed medially, whereas the internal carotid artery and carotid sinus are lateral. The patient was a 12-year-old boy who died of metastatic malignant melanoma. The combined weight of the carotid bodies was 13 mg.

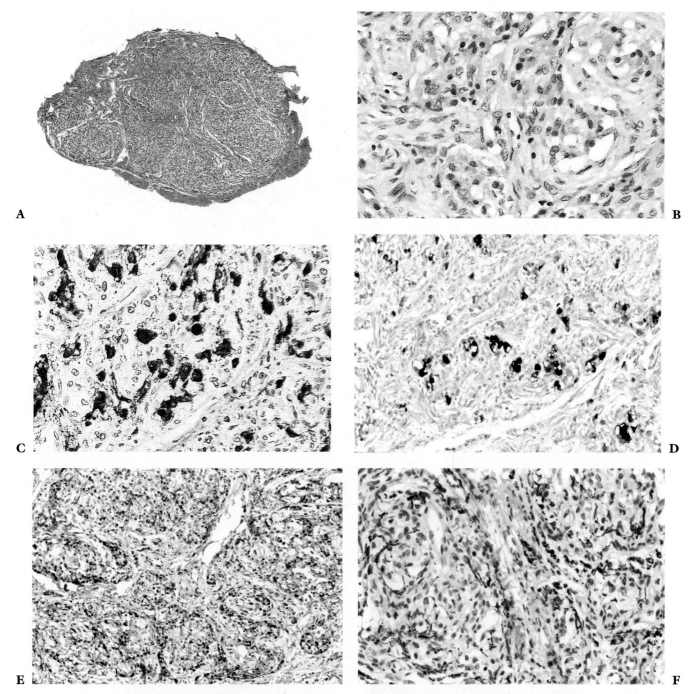

Figure 15.3. **(A)** Carotid body from a 4-month-old child who died of hepatoblastoma. Note the lobular architecture and lack of true encapsulation. **(B)** Closer view of a carotid body lobule showing cords and clusters of chief cells. **(C)** Chief cells in a normal carotid body show an organoid arrangement and marked cytoplasmic argyrophilia (Bodian stain). **(D)** Chief cells are strongly positive for chromogranin immunostaining (avidin-biotin peroxidase method). **(E)** Sustentacular cells are present at the periphery of chief cell clusters and are demonstrated by immunostain for S-100 protein. **(F)** The normal carotid body also stains with antibodies for neurofilament protein.

of life, and the average duration of symptoms is approximately 4 years (41,42). Some series report a roughly equal gender distribution, whereas others show a slightly higher incidence in women (44–46). It has been estimated in the sporadic setting that 4% to 8% of patients with CBPs have bilateral tumors (47,48). CBPs are more often bilateral when arising in a familial setting (45,46). Occasionally there may be multiple paragangliomas at other sites, such as the vagus nerve, orbit, middle ear, and base of the heart (49,50). Preoperative selective angiography may be useful for delineating tumor location (Fig. 15.5B), defining blood supply, and providing a route for selective embolization if this is considered before surgery. Preoperative emboli-

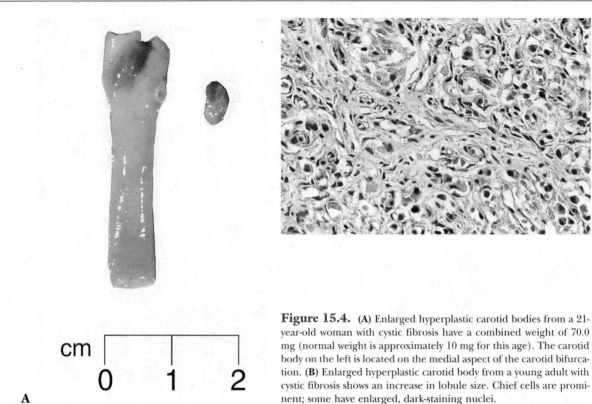

Figure 15.4. **(A)** Enlarged hyperplastic carotid bodies from a 21-year-old woman with cystic fibrosis have a combined weight of 70.0 mg (normal weight is approximately 10 mg for this age). The carotid body on the left is located on the medial aspect of the carotid bifurcation. **(B)** Enlarged hyperplastic carotid body from a young adult with cystic fibrosis shows an increase in lobule size. Chief cells are prominent; some have enlarged, dark-staining nuclei.

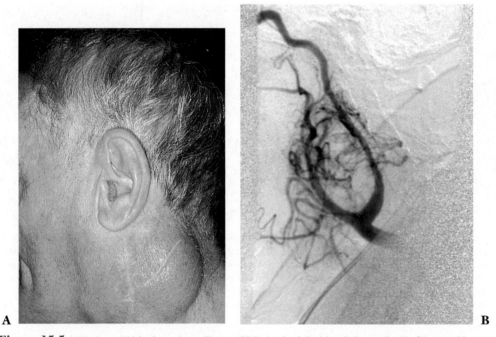

Figure 15.5. **(A)** A carotid body paraganglioma (CBP) in the left side of the neck of a 70-year-old man had been operated on years earlier, but the tumor was not successfully resected. **(B)** Carotid body paraganglioma from a different case is present in early arterial phase of carotid arteriography and causes a widening of carotid bifurcation with "lyre-like" splaying of both branches. Lateral view of carotid angiography.

zation can decrease blood loss in patients with paragangliomas of the head and neck region (46,51) and other sites (52).

JUGULOTYMPANIC PARAGANGLIOMA

Jugulotympanic paraganglioma (JTP) tumors have a predilection for women and arise from microscopic collections of paraganglia, which were described by Guild (53,54) in a study involving serial sectioning of temporal bones; the first case of a patient with JTP was reported by Rosenwasser (55) in 1945. These paraganglia (average of two to three in each temporal bone) may be found along the course of the Jacobsen nerve (tympanic branch of the 9th cranial nerve), the nerve of Arnold (auricular branch of the 10th cranial nerve), the adventitia of the jugular bulb, the osseous canal connecting the jugular fossa to the middle ear cavity, or within the middle ear—usually over the cochlear promontory. The varied locations of these paraganglia and the complex anatomy of this area form the basis for the different clinical presentations of patients with JTP (56). Small tumors arising over the cochlear promontory (tympanic paraganglioma) may arise as an aural polyp, with filling of the middle ear cavity or extension into the external ear canal. JTP can involve the temporal bone, with intracranial extension, or appear as a mass at the base of the skull, with erosion of the jugular foramen. Rarely, these tumors display clinical evidence of malignancy, primarily metastatic disease. The most common site of metastasis includes lymph nodes, skeleton, lungs, and liver (43). The histologic appearance of these tumors is usually not predictive of biologic behavior.

VAGAL PARAGANGLIOMA

These tumors also have a predilection for women in the fourth and fifth decades of life and usually develop as a lateral neck mass with extension up to the base of the skull (41). Vagal paragangliomas (VPs) arise from paraganglia located at the level of or just below the nodose ganglion of the vagus nerve that are usually multiple on either side of the neck (31). They have been referred to as vagal body paraganglia, although they are anatomically dispersed microscopic collections of cells. As with CBPs, these tumors may protrude medially with deviation of oropharyngeal structures, such as the palatine tonsil, or extend even higher up into the nasopharynx. They may also demonstrate intracranial extension (57). Vagus nerve palsy may be apparent and may be accompanied by hoarseness and dysphagia (58).

LARYNGEAL PARAGANGLIOMA

Laryngeal paragangliomas (LPs) arise from microscopic collections of paraganglia distributed on either side of the larynx that form a superior and inferior group (59); these tumors usually evolve from superior laryngeal paraganglia above the anterior part of the vocal cords near the aryepiglottic fold, but they can also develop inferiorly and appear in the subglottic or tracheal area. Hoarseness and dysphagia are the most common complaints (60). In the literature, LPs have been associated with a very high rate of malignancy (61), but most of these "alleged" malignant paragangliomas have undoubtedly been confused

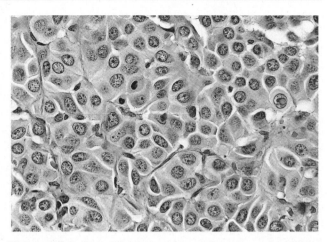

Figure 15.6. A laryngeal atypical carcinoid tumor arose in the submucosa of the aryepiglottic fold. The tumor has a vague nesting pattern that can be confused with a paraganglioma.

with laryngeal atypical carcinoid tumor of the larynx (Fig. 15.6) (62–64). At present, it is believed that true LPs have very limited malignant potential (65,66).

AORTICOPULMONARY PARAGANGLIOMA

Aorticopulmonary paragangliomas (APPs) arise from small collections of paraganglia that are located at various sites, both dorsal and ventral, at the base of the heart in relation to the great vessels (67). Some paraganglia can be found above the aortic arch in relation to the subclavian arteries. APPs can cause symptoms or signs such as hoarseness, dysphagia, chest pain or discomfort, and, rarely, hemoptysis or the superior vena cava syndrome (68). There appears to be a slight predominance among women. The average size of APPs is approximately 7.5 cm (range, 1.2 to 17 cm) (68). Some tumors can involve the pericardium or heart directly (cardiac paragangliomas) (69). A pigmented cardiac paraganglioma has also been reported (70).

OTHER PARAGANGLIOMAS

Paragangliomas have been reported at a variety of other sites in the head and neck region, including the orbit (71–73), nasal cavity (74–76), nasopharynx (77), cheek (78), pineal (79) and sellar regions (80,81), and thyroid gland (82). They have a histologic appearance similar to CBP. Rare examples of primary pulmonary paragangliomas have also been described (83–86). These tumors may arise from intrapulmonary paraganglia, as described by Blessing and Hora (87), although some may be very difficult to distinguish from a bronchial carcinoid tumor. One example has been reported as multicentric metachronous pulmonary and intravagal paragangliomas with an identical immunophenotype; they showed negative results for epithelial markers, as one would expect for paragangliomas (88). A recent case of Cushing syndrome resulting from an adrenocorticotropic hormone (ACTH)–secreting primary pulmonary paraganglioma has been reported (89). A large primary paraganglioma of the lung was reported measuring 13 cm in diameter and is largest of the 17 pulmonary paragangliomas reported thus far in the English-language literature (90).

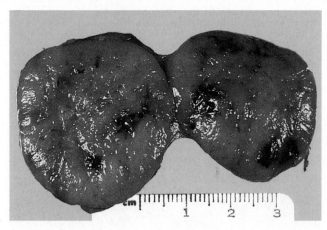

Figure 15.7. The carotid body paraganglioma, on cross section, is tan with a slightly bulging surface and patchy areas of hemorrhage. The tumor measured approximately 3 cm in diameter.

GROSS PATHOLOGY

Paragangliomas are rubbery, firm, and usually well demarcated, with expansile borders (Fig. 15.7). The compressed rim of connective tissue surrounding the tumor is best regarded as a fibrous pseudocapsule. Some tumors, such as JTP, may be small and irregular or fragmented, making gross examination difficult. On cross section, these tumors have a meaty to light tan appearance and, if closely scrutinized, may have punctate to linear vascular markings that are often retracted slightly beneath the cut surface. Sometimes there are intersecting bands of fibrous tissue or intense sclerosis (Fig. 15.8). The average sizes of paragangliomas recorded in one series are as follows: CBPs, 3.8 cm (range, 1.8 to 8.5 cm); VPs, 4.0 cm (range, 2.0 to 6.0 cm); and LP, 2 to 5 cm in diameter (91). The tumor volume was calculated by Nora et al. (92) for CBPs; it ranged from 2.0 to 164 cm^3. Larger tumor volume or size correlates with increasing difficulty of surgical resection and longer duration of tumor.

Some series have shown a correlation of large CBPs with circumferential spread and adherence to carotid vessels, based on the three groups of tumors reported by Shamblin et al. (40). This classification scheme was based on gross vessel-tumor relationship: class I, localized tumors; class II, tumors that were adherent and partially surrounding the carotid vessels; and class III, tumors intimately surrounding the carotid vessels (40,92,93). Mechanical manipulation of tumor during surgery may cause a deep red-brown discoloration as a result of congestion and hemorrhage. Areas of degenerative change with necrosis and cystic alteration are very uncommon; however, foci of ischemic necrosis can be seen in some tumors that have been embolized before surgical removal. On rare occasion, a paraganglioma can invade the lumen of the carotid artery or cause total occlusion of a large vessel (94–96).

MICROSCOPIC PATHOLOGY

In general, the microscopic patterns encountered in head and neck paragangliomas do not allow one to reliably distinguish between tumors arising at different anatomic sites (32,38). The most typical pattern is a discrete or organoid arrangement of neoplastic chief cells often referred to as zellballen (Fig. 15.9) (97). Several different patterns were recognized by LeCompte (98)—the usual (Fig. 15.9), adenoma-like, and angioma-like. The cell cytoplasm is eosinophilic and faintly granular with indistinct borders. Some tumors may have cells with abundant, deeply eosinophilic cytoplasm, thus imparting an oncocytic appearance (32,38). The orientation of neoplastic chief cells within individual cell clusters tends to be haphazard, without polarization along the fibrovascular septa, and there is no formation of true rosettes or acini, as one might see in other endocrine tumors, such as carcinoids. The nesting pattern can vary in size, and it is most vividly accentuated by staining for reticulum (Fig. 15.10). There is a network of supporting cells referred to as sustentacular cells that can be highlighted by immunohistochemical methods with antibodies to S-100 protein. Staining for cytoplasmic argyrophilia can be useful in diagnosis and often shows that the neoplastic chief cells contain myriad pinpoint cytoplasmic granules. This stain is seldom done today.

Nuclear hyperchromasia and pleomorphism can be quite prominent, but these are not reliable criteria for judging malignancy (Fig. 15.11) (32,38). Nuclear pseudoinclusions, repre-

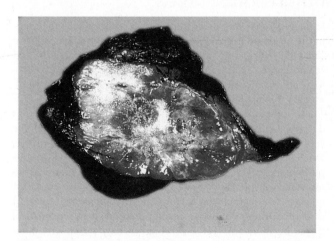

Figure 15.8. Vagal paraganglioma on cross section has areas of pearly white sclerosis. A transected segment of vagus nerve is present on the right side. India ink had been applied to the surface of the tumor.

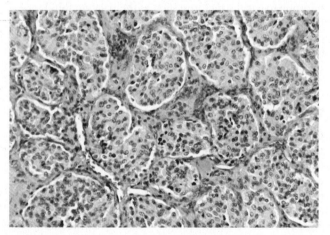

Figure 15.9. The typical histologic pattern for head and neck paragangliomas. Organoid clustering of neoplastic chief cells vaguely recalls the architecture of the normal paraganglion (Fig. 15.3B).

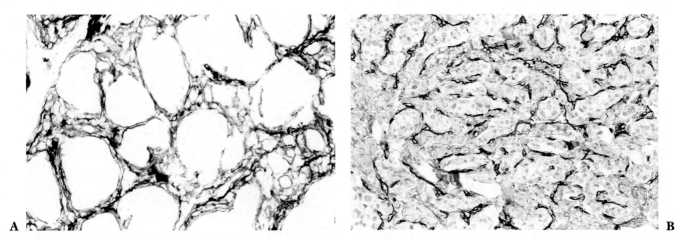

Figure 15.10. **(A)** Staining of the reticulum framework shows a distinct clustering of neoplastic chief cells with variation in the size of nests of cells (reticulin stain). **(B)** CD34 by immunohistochemical technique highlights the vascular supporting network seen in carotid body paraganglioma.

senting invagination of cell cytoplasm, are occasionally seen (Fig. 15.12). A most unusual architectural pattern is a spindle cell or pseudosarcomatous arrangement of cells that, on careful examination, is usually accompanied by a more typical nesting pattern elsewhere in the tumor (Fig. 15.13) (32,91). Large expansile or locally aggressive tumors, such as CBPs or VPs, may incorporate myelinated nerve bundles, but true intraneural growth is seldom seen (Fig. 15.14). Limited biopsy material can hamper accurate diagnosis; an example is the small tympanic paraganglioma, which can appear as an aural polyp (Fig. 15.15A) or a small, hypercellular biopsy specimen of a skull base tumor without an obvious organoid or nesting pattern (Fig. 15.15B). Immunostain for chromogranin A may greatly aid in diagnosis by demonstrating discrete collections of neoplastic chief cells (Fig. 15.15C). It is well known that biopsies of paragangliomas can be hazardous and lead to brisk hemorrhage.

Stromal alterations may be apparent in some paragangliomas and, at times, are so marked as to obscure the true nature of the tumor (32,38). An example is stromal fibrosis with evidence of old hemorrhage (Fig. 15.16A) that may be so extensive

that it causes compression and distortion of nests of neoplastic chief cells (Fig. 15.16B). In some cases, one may find sinusoidal sclerosis, which accentuates the organoid arrangement of tumor cells (Fig. 15.17). Congestion and hemorrhage within the tumor can cause wide spacing of individual zellballen, but more typical diagnostic features can usually be found. Interstitial amyloid deposits were reported in two CBPs by Capella and Solcia (99) on ultrastructural study, but none was illustrated.

Dysmorphic vessels as a result of symmetric or asymmetric myointimal proliferation or thickening may be present, and in some tumors, vascular ectasia or an arborizing pattern can focally simulate a hemangiopericytoma. Chronic inflammatory infiltrates are uncommon. They may be evident as sparse perivascular lymphocytic infiltration, usually at the periphery of the tumor, but rarely, the inflammatory component can be more extensive, with separation of nests of chief cells. It can also simulate a lymph node metastasis, such as Hürthle cell carcinoma of the thyroid (Fig. 15.18A). Necrosis is an unusual morphologic finding, but it may be extensive and confluent if the tumor has been effectively embolized before surgery (Fig. 15.18B).

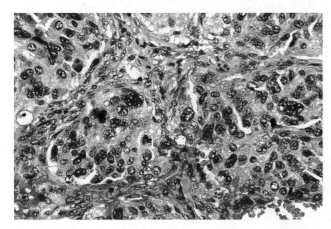

Figure 15.11. Marked nuclear pleomorphism is present in this carotid body paraganglioma from a 21-year-old patient who had bilateral tumors. The family history was unavailable. The patient was alive and free of disease 8 years later.

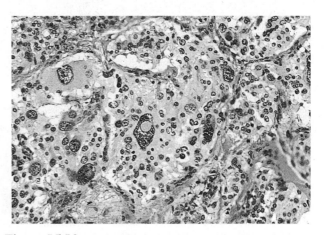

Figure 15.12. Several enlarged nuclei in this clinically benign carotid body paraganglioma show round, pink pseudoinclusions of cell cytoplasm.

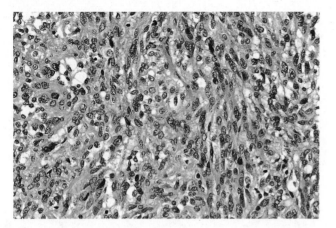

Figure 15.13. A carotid body paraganglioma from a 62-year-old woman has a spindle cell component in this field, with only vague clustering of tumor cells. A more typical pattern was present in other areas. The patient was alive and well 16 years later.

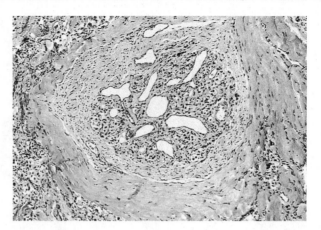

Figure 15.14. A portion of vagal paraganglioma growing within a myelinated nerve bundle.

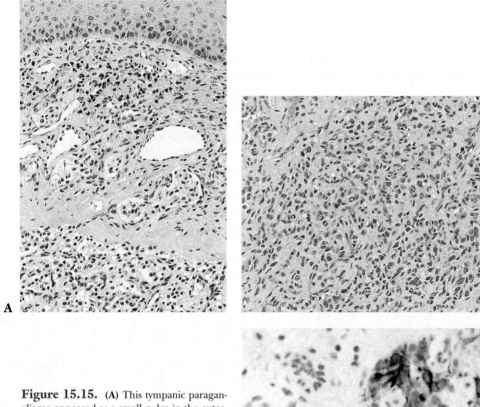

A

B

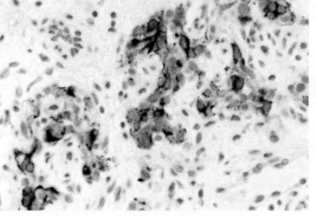

C

Figure 15.15. **(A)** This tympanic paraganglioma appeared as a small polyp in the external auditory canal. The biopsy specimen shows intact squamous epithelium, chronic inflammation, and a vague organoid pattern of underlying tumor. **(B)** A jugulotympanic paraganglioma shows a more disorganized tissue pattern and, if tumor is crushed, can significantly add to diagnostic problems. **(C)** Immunostain for chromogranin highlights the nested or short cord arrangement of chief cells (avidin-biotin-peroxidase method).

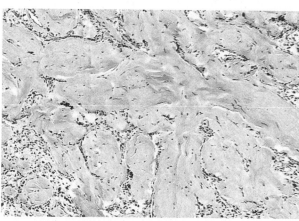

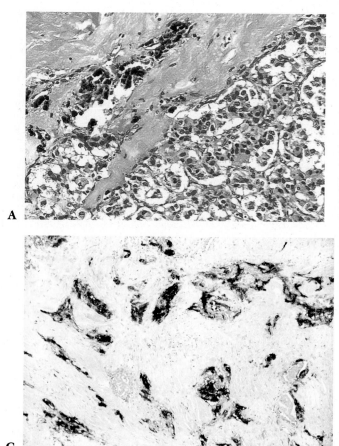

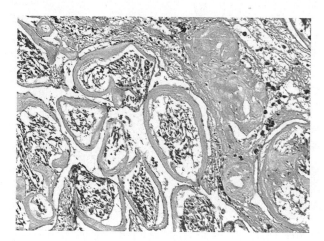

Figure 15.16. **(A)** This carotid body paraganglioma shows stromal fibrosis and evidence of old hemorrhage. Tumor cells are present in distinct clusters typical of a paraganglioma. **(B)** This vagal paraganglioma is intensely sclerotic with compression and distortion of zellballen, which can make diagnosis difficult. **(C)** Chromogranin by immunohistochemical technique highlights the distorted zellballen nested growth of the neoplastic cells within the sclerosis.

SYMPATHOADRENAL NEUROENDOCRINE SYSTEM

The prototype tissues are the adrenal medullae, which synthesize and secrete catecholamines, causing rapid physiologic changes that are dissipated rather quickly. The distribution of extra-adrenal paraganglia (Fig. 15.19) parallels that of the sympathetic nervous system within the abdomen and urinary bladder, thorax, and neck (100), and some paraganglia are located

Figure 15.17. A carotid body paraganglioma shows encirclement of individual zellballen by fibrous tissue representing sinusoidal sclerosis. There is also evidence of old hemorrhage.

within viscera such as the gallbladder and urinary bladder (Fig. 15.20). During fetal life, the chromaffin cells of the adrenal gland are usually inconspicuous, but postnatally, they develop rapidly, becoming structurally similar to medullary cells of the adult gland by the end of the first year of life. Epinephrine is the predominant catecholamine in the normal adrenal medulla, in a ratio of approximately 4:1 relative to norepinephrine (32).

Most of the chromaffin tissue in the fetus is extra-adrenal in location, with the most prominent collections residing on either side of the aorta near the origin of the inferior mesenteric or renal arteries, down to the aortic bifurcation. These paraganglia were described by Zuckerkandl (101,102) in 1901 and referred to as the "aortic bodies"; on macroscopic examination, they may be difficult to distinguish from small lymph nodes or sympathetic ganglia (103). The organs of Zuckerkandl involute after birth; by the age of 6 or 7 years, only microscopic collections of chromaffin cells can be detected (Fig. 15.21) (104). The function of fetal chromaffin tissue in utero is not fully known, but it may have some role in maintenance of vascular tone and blood pressure. Norepinephrine predominates in extra-adrenal chromaffin tissue, such as the organs of Zuckerkandl, and catecholamine content is reported to decline with structural involution (105). The microanatomy of sympathetic paraganglia elsewhere in the abdomen, chest, and other locations is less well defined.

EXTRA-ADRENAL PARAGANGLIOMAS

These tumors arise predominantly in the retroperitoneum anywhere from the upper abdomen to the pelvic floor. One of the

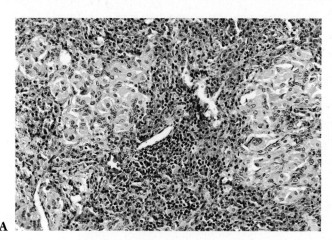

A

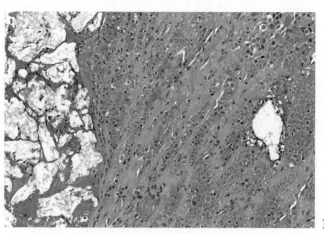

B

Figure 15.18. **(A)** Nests of neoplastic chief cells in this clinically benign carotid body paraganglioma (CBP) are separated by chronic inflammation with lymphocytes and numerous plasma cells. The tumor simulated a metastatic Hurthle cell thyroid carcinoma to a lymph node. **(B)** Clinically benign CBP had been embolized prior to surgery and had extensive areas of ischemic necrosis. Foreign embolic material is present in left half of field.

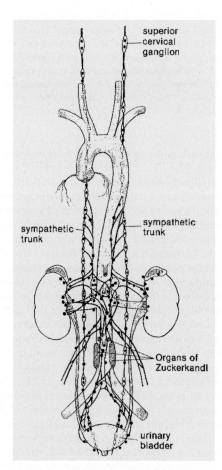

Figure 15.19. Anatomic distribution of the sympathoadrenal neuroendocrine system, with adrenal medullae representing the largest compact collections of paraganglia in adults. Note the multiple separate extra-adrenal paraganglia along the lower part of the aorta, which represent the organs of Zuckerkandl. (Modified from Saeki T, Akiba T, Jon K, et al. An extremely large solitary paraganglioma of the lung: report of a case. *Surg Today* 1999;29:1195–1200.)

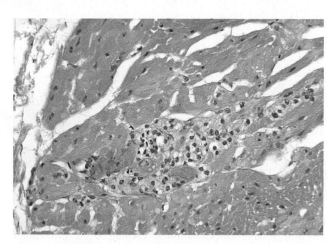

Figure 15.20. A small paraganglion insinuates itself between smooth muscle bundles of musculature of the wall of the urinary bladder.

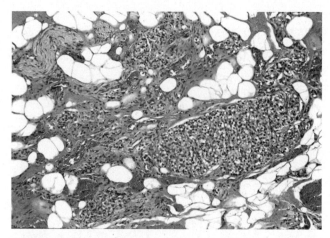

Figure 15.21. A small extra-adrenal paraganglion was discovered incidentally on histologic study of tissue from the retroperitoneum of an adult patient. Chromaffin cells have a delicate lobulated architecture with prominent microvasculature.

more common sites is the anatomic region corresponding to the organs of Zuckerkandl. It has been estimated that 5% to 10% of pheochromocytomas are extra-adrenal in location, mainly in the retroperitoneum but also in the posterior thorax and neck (32,38,106). A higher incidence of extra-adrenal tumors has been reported in childhood (20% to 25%) (107), with the most common locations being the retroperitoneum and head and neck region (108). In the literature review of extra-adrenal paragangliomas (mainly sympathoadrenal neuroendocrine system) by Fries and Chamberlin (109), 71% of tumors were located in the superior or inferior para-aortic area, 9.8% arose in the urinary bladder, 12% were intrathoracic, and 1.2% were cervical.

Other anatomic sites of origin include the gallbladder (110,111), spermatic cord (112,113), prostate gland (114,115), prostatic urethra (116), pancreas (117), and uterus (118). A pigmented or melanotic paraganglioma has also been reported in the uterus (119), but the histopathology is a bit unusual for a typical paraganglioma. These extra-adrenal tumors are often hormonally active, with excess catecholamine secretion. It is worth noting that although functionally active CBPs and other head and neck paragangliomas rarely occur, some paragangliomas reported to be CBPs actually arise from the cervical sympathetic trunk (120,121); because of overlap in histologic features, the distinction may rest with precise anatomic localization. Multifocal paragangliomas can develop at various sites where one might expect to find paraganglionic tissue. An extreme example of paragangliomatosis was reported by Karasov et al. (122) in a patient who had 21 paragangliomas removed between 13 and 17 years of age and had evidence of additional tumors.

GROSS MORPHOLOGY

Most tumors are well circumscribed and, at times, almost encapsulated, ranging in diameter from only a few centimeters to 20.0 cm. The average diameter of extra-adrenal retroperitoneal tumors reported from Memorial Hospital was 9.9 cm, and the functionally active tumors tended to be smaller than the nonfunctional tumors (123). The average size of paragangliomas of the urinary bladder is approximately 2 cm (range, 0.3 to 5.5 cm) (124), and the average size of paravertebral paragangliomas is 5.8 cm (125). Some tumors are red-brown and show areas of hemorrhage on cross section, whereas other foci appear tan to gray-white with a slightly bulging surface. Hemorrhage and cystic degeneration may be marked in some tumors (Fig. 15.22).

MICROSCOPIC PATHOLOGY

The most common architectural pattern in pheochromocytomas and extra-adrenal paragangliomas is an anastomosing cell cord or trabecular arrangement of tumor cells (Fig. 15.23A,B). In a minority of cases, one may see a more discrete, organoid pattern of oval to round clusters of cells similar to head and neck paragangliomas. Occasionally there may be a solid or diffuse growth pattern or even a spindle cell component. Tumor cells have relatively abundant cytoplasm that is lightly acidophilic and finely granular, and some neoplasms may appear "oncocytic." Occasionally, the cytoplasm has an amphophilic or lilac coloration. There may be considerable variation in nuclear size and shape with marked pleomorphism, but again, this is not a reliable feature in terms of diagnosing malignancy (32,38).

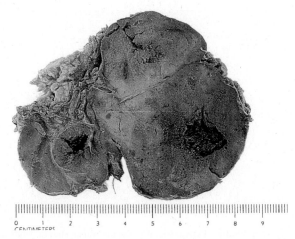

Figure 15.22. A large extra-adrenal paraganglioma from the upper abdomen is dark brown on cross section, with areas of hemorrhage and cystic degeneration.

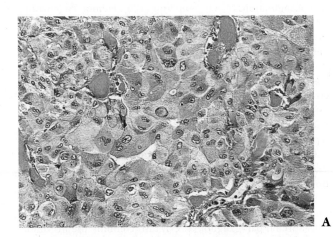

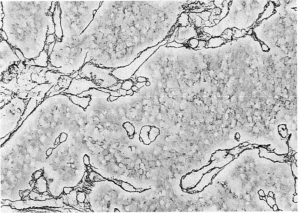

Figure 15.23. **(A)** This extra-adrenal paraganglioma has broad anastomosing cell cords. Tumor cells have copious cytoplasm that is finely granular and amphophilic to lilac in hue. Note the nuclear pseudoinclusion in the center of the field. **(B)** The reticulum framework of the tumor is well defined, with tumor forming anastomosing trabeculae (reticulin stain). Compare with Figure 15.10.

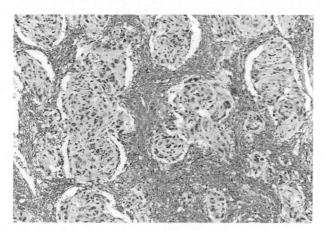

Figure 15.24. Extra-adrenal paraganglioma. Hemorrhage within the tumor separates irregular islands of neoplastic cells.

Nuclear pseudoinclusions are more frequently found in adrenal and extra-adrenal paragangliomas compared with head and neck paragangliomas (Fig. 15.23A); they have been shown to be invaginations of cell cytoplasm (126). Hemorrhage within the tumor can separate clusters of tumor cells (Fig. 15.24) or give a pseudopapillary or pseudoglandular pattern. The chromaffin reaction is positive in most of these tumors, provided the tumor is fixed immediately in the fresh state in appropriate fixatives, such as Orth's, Zenker's, or Helly's fluid. In cases studied at the National Cancer Institute (NCI), the chromaffin reaction was positive for all sympathoadrenal paragangliomas. The reaction depends on the oxidation of epinephrine and norepinephrine to adrenochrome pigments.

Ganglion-like cells may be present in some tumors; when accompanied by a fibrillary stroma resembling neuropil, the tumor may focally resemble a neuroblastoma or ganglioneuroblastoma and is referred to as a composite pheochromocytoma (Fig. 15.25) (32,38). Composite pheochromocytomas and extra-adrenal paragangliomas may also combine the histomorphologic features of a paraganglioma-ganglioneuroma (Fig.

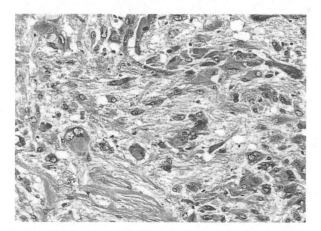

Figure 15.25. Composite pheochromocytoma. This adrenal medullary paraganglioma has large areas with more typical histologic characteristics but also fields where cells resembling ganglion cells are set within a fibrillar stroma similar to neuropil. The tumor here resembles a ganglioneuroblastoma.

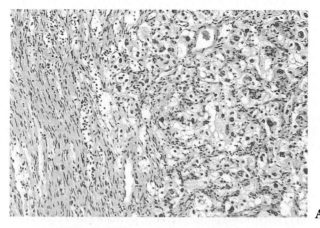

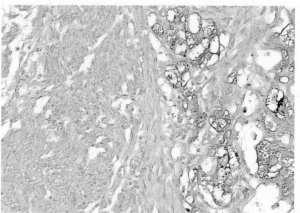

Figure 15.26. **(A)** A composite paraganglioma-ganglioneuroma of the upper abdomen near the celiac axis. The tumor was extra-adrenal in location. A portion of ganglioneuroma is present on the left (ganglion cells are evident in other fields), and paraganglioma is present on the right. **(B)** This paraganglioma shows clusters of argyrophil cells. The ganglioneuroma portion of this composite extra-adrenal tumor is shown on the left (Grimelius stain).

15.26A,B). A composite pheochromocytoma-ganglioneuroma has been reported in association with multiple endocrine neoplasia (MEN) type 2A (127). Composite pheochromocytoma–malignant peripheral nerve sheath tumor has also been reported (128). The occurrence of composite pheochromocytomas reflects the plastic phenotype of cells grown in vitro as well as the close relationship between the endocrine and nervous systems. Common embryogenesis from neural crest may help explain these unusual tumors (32). Rare cases of corticomedullary mixed tumors of the adrenal gland have also been reported (129).

The urinary bladder can also be a primary site for a paraganglioma, and the patient may experience syncope or hypertension with bladder distention and/or micturition (130). These tumors are usually located in the bladder trigone or near the ureteral orifice, followed by the dome and lateral walls. The gross appearance is similar to paragangliomas elsewhere, except that the tumor tends to be smaller in size (Fig. 15.27). These neoplasms may show broad trabeculae growing between and separating bundles of smooth muscle, but this should not by itself be regarded as evidence of malignancy (Fig. 15.28). Occasional cases of malignant paragangliomas of the bladder have been reported (131–133).

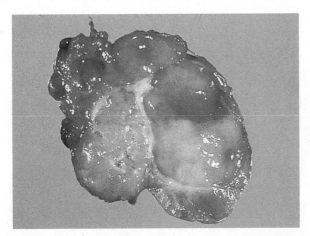

Figure 15.27. This paraganglioma of the urinary bladder is tan and lobulated. Tumors in this location may be only a few centimeters in size.

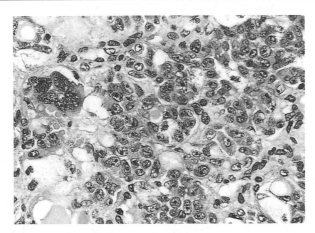

Figure 15.29. Numerous intracytoplasmic hyaline globules in an adrenal cortical carcinoma. Distinguishing it from a paraganglioma can sometimes be very difficult. Identical hyaline globules can be found much more commonly in sympathoadrenal paragangliomas.

Intracytoplasmic hyaline globules are not uncommon; of more than 120 sympathoadrenal paragangliomas studied at the NCI, hyaline globules were identified in 47% of tumors (134). They were also noted in 43% of pheochromocytomas reported elsewhere (135). In some tumors, these hyaline globules are numerous, whereas in other neoplasms, they are very difficult to find on casual inspection. These globules have been related in some fashion to secretory activity by the tumor (136). It should be remembered that virtually identical hyaline globules can be found in some adrenal cortical neoplasms, both benign and malignant—although much less frequently—and this may be a source of misdiagnosis of these tumors, which in some instances, can be difficult to distinguish from pheochromocytomas (Fig. 15.29) (137,138). Hyaline globules are extremely uncommon in head and neck paragangliomas such as CBPs.

Interstitial amyloid has also been reported in a retroperitoneal paraganglioma (139) as well as pheochromocytomas (140). In one study, amyloid was identified in only 9% of pheochromocytomas (141). Pigmented or melanotic pheochromocytomas and extra-adrenal paragangliomas have also been reported (32,142). The gross appearance can be striking, with its jet-black color. Some tumors have not been rigorously investigated to distinguish the precise nature of the pigment, whereas in others, the presence of melanosomes or premelanosomes has been confirmed by ultrastructural examination. In one case, the intracytoplasmic pigment was abundant (Fig. 15.30) and had characteristics of neuromelanin (143).

MULTICENTRIC AND FAMILIAL OCCURRENCE OF TUMORS

Recent molecular and genetic studies have identified germline mutations of six genes that contribute to the development of pheochromocytoma/paraganglioma in patients: *RET, VHL, NF1*, and SDH subunits *SDHB, SDHC*, and *SDHD* (144). Up to one-third of patients with pheochromocytoma/paraganglioma carry one of the germline mutations predisposing them to the disease (145). *RET* gene mutations predispose to MEN. Mutations of the *VHL* gene predispose to von Hippel-Lindau disease, and the *NF1* gene is associated with neurofibromatosis type 1. Mutation of the SDH subunits *SDHB, SDHC*, and *SDHD* predispose to pheochromocytoma/paraganglioma syndromes that otherwise might be regarded as "sporadic" in nature because many of the patients do not display the expected clinical association of multifocal disease, young age, and/or positive family history (144). Since the first report by Chase (146) of the familial occurrence of CBP, numerous patients have been described with familial tumors of the head and neck region. Hereditary deficiency of clotting factors VII and X has also been described in association with familial CBP (147). Several studies indicate an autosomal dominant inheritance pattern, with variable penetrance and expressivity (46,47,148,149). In one study of six generations of a family spanning nearly 200 years, a very high degree of penetrance was found (nearly 100% by 45 years of age), which may be related in part to long-term follow-up and intensive investigations in patients at risk who are clinically asymptomatic (148). The gender incidence of these familial tumors is variable. Sex-linked transmission has been suggested by the findings of some studies showing a marked predominance among women (150).

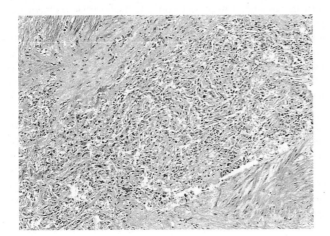

Figure 15.28. Paraganglioma of the urinary bladder. The tumor has grown between bundles of smooth muscle in the wall of the bladder. The pattern seen here is not a reliable criterion of malignancy.

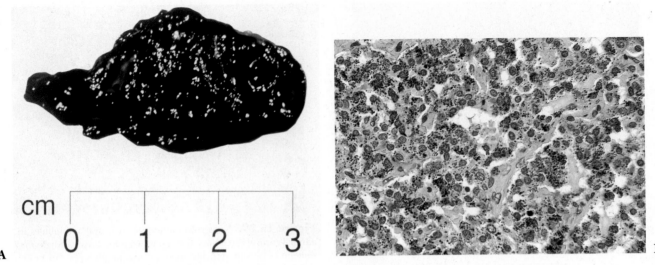

Figure 15.30. (A) Pigmented (black) extra-adrenal paraganglioma. **(B)** Tumor cells contain abundant coarse pigment granules, which had histochemical and ultrastructural features most resembling neuromelanin, a nonenzymatic or oxidative waste product of catecholamine metabolism.

A genomic imprinting hypothesis was proposed to explain pedigrees in which familial paragangliomas were transmitted almost exclusively along the paternal line; based on this theory, the autosomal dominant gene is inactivated during oogenesis in females but becomes activated during spermatogenesis in males (151,152). Approximately one-third of patients with a positive familial history have bilateral CBPs (46,47), and in addition, there may be multicentric paragangliomas, including pheochromocytomas (153). In a review of familial head and neck paragangliomas, 78% of tumors were CBPs, 16% were jugular paragangliomas, 4.5% were VPs, and 1.5% were tympanic paragangliomas (154). Genetic linkage to human chromosomal region 11q23 (*PGL1*) and 11q13 (*PGL2*) has been reported with genomic imprinting and paternal inheritance (155). Sympathoadrenal paragangliomas also occur in families, with the most notable being the MEN syndrome types 2A (MEN2A) and 2B (MEN2B) (32,38,106). MEN2A (Sipple syndrome) has an autosomal dominant mode of inheritance with a high degree of penetrance in the case of medullary carcinoma of the thyroid. MEN2B can be inherited in an autosomal dominant fashion, but a significant number of cases appear to be sporadic in nature. Patients with MEN2B also have a characteristic phenotype and prominent gastrointestinal manifestations with ganglioneuromatosis (32,38,106). Mutations in the *RET* proto-oncogene have been noted in MEN2 kindreds; mutations in the *RET* oncogene have also been associated with some familial forms of Hirschsprung's disease (156,157). A germline mutation in *SDHD* has been reported in familial pheochromocytoma (158) within the same *PGL1* locus on chromosome 11q13 (155). Selective loss of chromosome 11 has also been reported in pheochromocytomas associated with von Hippel-Lindau disease (159). Another genetic alteration has been noted in chromosome 1p, but other chromosomal alterations have been seen involving chromosomes 3, 11, 17, and 19 (160).

Pheochromocytomas in both forms of the MEN2 syndrome are often bilateral and multicentric within the involved gland (161) and are usually preceded by adrenal medullary hyperplasia, which may be nodular or diffuse (162–164). There is also an increased incidence of pheochromocytoma with neuroectodermal syndromes such as von Recklinghausen disease, von Hippel-Lindau disease, and tuberous sclerosis (165). There are relatively few reports of extra-adrenal paragangliomas in these syndromes.

ASSOCIATION WITH OTHER ENDOCRINE DISORDERS

CBPs have been reported in association with the triad described by Carney et al. (166) that consists of extra-adrenal paraganglioma, gastric epithelioid leiomyosarcoma, and pulmonary chondroma. Carney triad (CT) primarily affects young females; in recent literature, the gastric epithelioid leiomyosarcoma component is now included in the gastrointestinal stromal tumor (GIST) category (167,168). Although initially the condition was thought to possibly be familial (169), a familial inheritance pattern has not been definitely confirmed. Recent molecular genetic studies have attempted to elucidate the pathogenetic pathway (170,171). In a review of 24 cases, four patients had a CBP, and three had additional tumors, including an aorticopulmonary paraganglia (APP) that may have been functionally active (172). A review of the association between CBP and paragangliomas outside the head and neck region identified 25 cases—including nine pheochromocytomas, eight intrathoracic paragangliomas, and one APP (173). Head and neck paragangliomas have also been reported in association with papillary carcinoma of the thyroid (174) and hyperparathyroidism caused by either adenoma or hyperplasia (175,176). An unusual complex of tumors, including bilateral CBPs, raises the possibility of a new pattern of MEN syndrome (177,178). Additionally, a new syndrome of familial paraganglioma and GIST, distinct from CT, has been identified. Patients with this syndrome were diagnosed at an average age of 23 years; the tumors were multifocal and inherited in an autosomal dominant pattern with incomplete penetrance (179).

CYTOLOGY AND FINE-NEEDLE ASPIRATION BIOPSY OF PARAGANGLIOMAS

Smears or imprints of resected paragangliomas show irregular clusters of tumor cells with eosinophilic, finely granular cytoplasm and irregularly shaped nuclei that can have finely stippled or densely clumped chromatin (Fig. 15.31A,B). However, the correct diagnosis can be very difficult to make on cytologic evaluation alone, and the nuclear pleomorphism can be so marked that the unwary may be lured into making a diagnosis of malignancy. The cell cytoplasm of adjacent cells may be pulled apart into tapering irregular processes that give a latticelike configuration. Correlation with histologic findings will usually ensure an accurate diagnosis.

Preoperative aspiration of cervical paragangliomas has been done successfully (180–184), but the diagnostic yield may be low, and there is potential for hemorrhage or thrombosis of major vessels. In the series by Engzell et al. (180), one of 13 CBPs was misinterpreted as neurofibroma, two as neurofibrosarcoma, and two as metastatic thyroid carcinoma. These investigators caution that if a CBP is suspected on clinical examination, fine-needle aspiration should not be performed; instead, carotid angiography is recommended. One of the cases reported by Qizilbash and Young (183) was misinterpreted as metastatic squamous cell carcinoma. In the series from Memorial Hospital, needle aspiration was performed uneventfully on 15 patients with CBPs and 4 patients with VPs, leading to the correct diagnosis in 9 patients (41). The finding of much blood alone should raise the possibility of a head and neck paraganglioma. Fine-needle aspiration biopsy may yield material for cell block preparation, which can be used for immunohistochemistry (185).

There are several reports that underscore the potential danger of needle aspiration of catecholamine-producing tumors of the sympathoadrenal neuroendocrine system (186–188). Catecholamine crisis and hemorrhage are the two main complications that lead some to caution against needle aspiration of these tumors. As with head and neck paragangliomas, a mistaken diagnosis of malignancy can also be rendered on the basis of cytologic findings (188).

ELECTRON MICROSCOPIC FEATURES

Paragangliomas of the head and neck region may show an admixture of light and dark cells on ultrastructural study, with intertwining and interdigitation of cytoplasmic processes (Fig. 15.32). There may be rudimentary intercellular attachments, but no true desmosomes are visible. A morphologic hallmark of all paragangliomas is the presence of dense-core neurosecretory granules. The granules tend to be round and regular with a uniform halo (Fig. 15.33), but some may be irregular in shape. Granules range from 120 to 200 nm in diameter (32,38,91,97, 189). The neurosecretory granules in extra-adrenal paragangliomas and pheochromocytomas are usually 150 to 250 nm in diameter. There may be a dimorphic population, with some having a prominent, eccentrically placed lucency adjacent to the dense core and others a narrow halo (Fig. 15.34A,B). The former granule morphologic appearance has been associated with norepinephrine storage, and the latter has been associated with epinephrine (190). Some granules, however, can have an irregular shape—oval, cylindrical, or curved—and the varied immunophenotype indicates that other hormones and neuropeptides may be stored. Granule morphology by itself, therefore, is not indicative of storage of any particular neuropeptide or hormone.

IMMUNOHISTOCHEMISTRY

Paragangliomas in general have a remarkably varied immunophenotype. Catecholamines can be identified in tumor extracts in many cases, and enzymes involved in catecholamine synthesis can be localized immunohistochemically (191). There have been several studies of the immunohistochemical profile of paragangliomas of the head and neck region (192–195). Immunostaining for neuron-specific enolase has been most consistently positive, but it may be nonspecific (Fig. 15.35). Many tumors are positive for serotonin (Fig. 15.36) (193). Immunoreactivity for chromogranin and synaptophysia has been reported in almost all CBPs and pheochromocytomes (Fig 15.37A,B) (194,196). (Fig. 15.36) (193). In one study, adjacent step sections stained for dif-

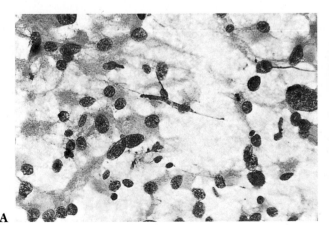
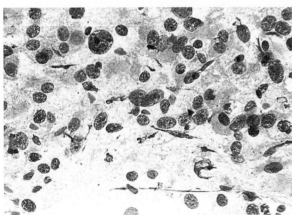

Figure 15.31. (A) Smear/imprint of a carotid body paraganglioma (CBP). Neoplastic chief cells have distinct epithelioid features with irregular strands of eosinophilic cytoplasm. (B) The nuclear chromatin in some CBPs has a grainy or stippled pattern. Note the mild degree of nuclear irregularity (Papanicolaou stain).

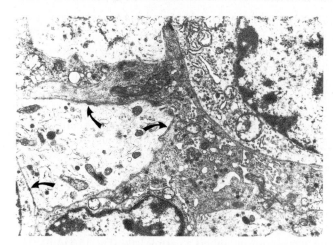

Figure 15.32. Note the complex interdigitation of cytoplasmic processes of light and dark neoplastic chief cells. Neurosecretory granules tend to be more numerous in dark cells. Some tumors apparently do not show this disparity in cellular electron density. Note the rudimentary intercellular attachments (*curved arrows*) (7500×).

ferent hormonal substances strongly suggested reactivity for more than one hormone in a given cell (193).

There have been a variety of other immunoreactive substances identified in CBPs and JTPs; in descending order, these include leu-enkephalin, gastrin, substance P, vasoactive intestinal peptide (VIP), somatostatin, bombesin, α-melanocyte–stimulating hormone, and calcitonin (193). Staining for cytokeratin has been reported occasionally, and investigators caution that this might be a potential source of misdiagnosis unless a panel of markers is used (194,197). The presence of S-100 protein–positive cells (sustentacular cells) encircling nests of tumor cells is a characteristic feature of paragangliomas in general (Fig. 15.37), and in the study by Capella et al. (192), these were estimated to account for 1% to 5% of the entire cell population. Immunostain for neurofilament triplet proteins can also be a useful marker (198–200).

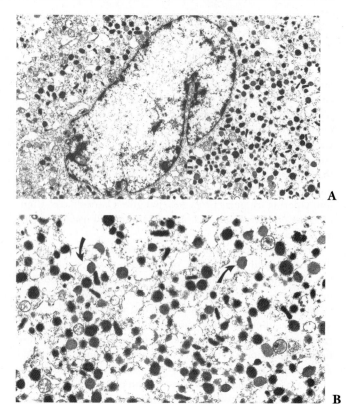

Figure 15.34. **(A)** Paraganglioma with irregular folding of the nucleus and deep invagination of cell cytoplasm. The tumor contained numerous dense-core neurosecretory granules, some of which were elongated and slightly curved (6000×). **(B)** Many neurosecretory granules are round and relatively uniform with a distinct limiting membrane and a thin, clear halo. Other granules have a wide halo with an eccentrically located dense core (*curved arrows*). Note that some granules are elongated or cylindrical in shape (15,000×).

The immunophenotype of sympathoadrenal paragangliomas is also quite varied (201–203). The following immunoprofile of 10 neuropeptides was reported by Linnoila et al. (201): leu-enkephalin (76%), met-enkephalin (75%), somatostatin (67%), bovine pancreatic polypeptide (51%), VIP (43%), sub-

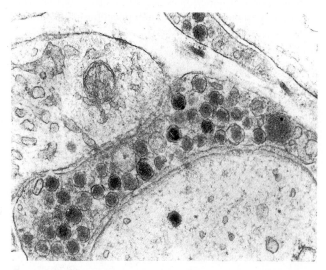

Figure 15.33. A vagal paraganglioma shows interdigitation of cytoplasmic processes of light and dark cells. The dark cell contains numerous dense-core neurosecretory granules that are relatively uniform in size but with some variation in electron density (40,000×).

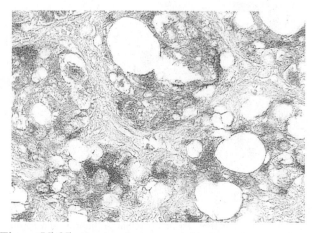

Figure 15.35. Tumor cells are strongly immunoreactive for neuron-specific enolase (streptavidin–alkaline phosphatase method).

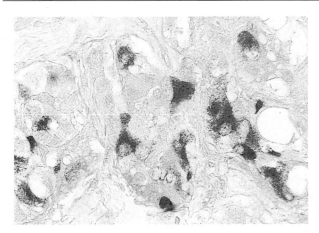

Figure 15.36. Some tumor cells in this CBP were immunoreactive for serotonin (streptavidin–alkaline phosphatase method).

stance P (31%), ACTH (28%), calcitonin (23%), bombesin (15%), and neurotensin (12%). Although there is often no syndrome associated with these tumors—aside from excess catecholamine secretion—a few tumors have elicited ectopic Cushing syndrome as a result of ACTH release (204–207), and watery diarrhea has been reported in several instances, probably as a result of secretion of VIP (208–210). VIP has been localized within composite pheochromocytomas in several studies (208,211), and although synthesis and secretion of VIP have been closely linked with ganglion cell differentiation or maturation within the tumor (212), this does not appear to be an absolute requirement. Survivin has been characterized as a novel neuroendocrine marker for pheochromocytoma but did not reliably distinguish benign from malignant tumors (213). Malignant pheochromocytomas have also been reported to have a higher frequency of p53 and bcl-2 expression, which may be helpful in predicting biologic behavior (214). A recent study suggests that galectin 3 expression in pheochromocytomas may help to distinguish benign from malignant tumors, but further investigation is necessary (215).

Synaptophysin and neuron-specific enolase have been regarded as good immunomarkers for neuroendocrine differentiation, but adrenal cortical adenoma and carcinoma have also been shown to stain positively, which may lead to a misdiagnosis of paraganglioma (Fig. 15.38A,B) (216). Calretinin, inhibin, and melan-A have been shown to be helpful in differentiating adrenal cortical tumors (which should be positive for these markers) from adrenal medullary tumors (which should be negative) (217). In the study by Hamid et al. (218), clinically functional tumors expressed at least two of the following antigens: enkephalin, neuropeptide Y, and tyrosine hydroxylase. None of the nonfunctional tumors possessed more than one of these antigens. A study of 13 CBPs showed immunoreactivity for the oncoprotein c-myc as well as other oncoproteins, such as bcl-2 and c-jun, suggesting that oncogene expression may contribute to genesis of the tumor (219).

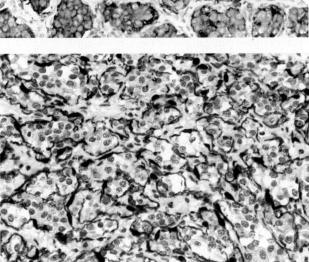

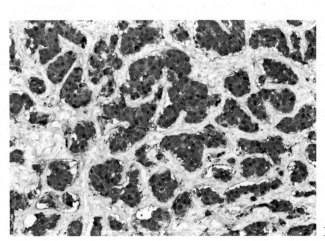

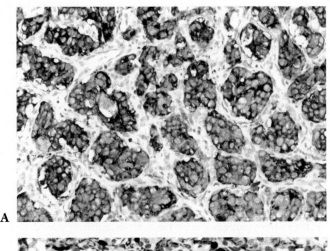

Figure 15.37. Carotid body tumor stains strongly with **(A)** synaptophysin and **(B)** chromogranin by immunohistochemical techniques. **(C)** Jugulotympanic paraganglioma. Sustentacular cells appear as slender stellate cells showing positive nuclear and cytoplasmic staining for S-100 protein. These cells are characteristically located at the periphery of clusters of neoplastic chief cells (avidin-biotin-peroxidase).

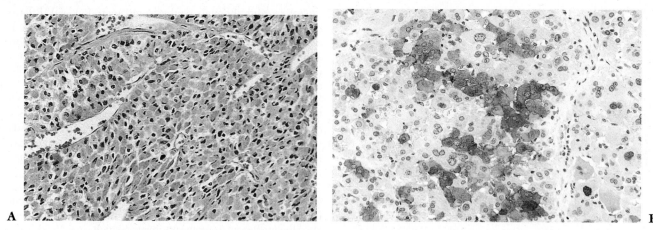

Figure 15.38. **(A)** This adrenal cortical carcinoma was mistakenly diagnosed as an extra-adrenal paraganglioma; tumor arose in the upper quadrant close to the adrenal gland and could have originated from small adrenal cortical rests. Note the trabecular pattern, with tumor cells having abundant, compact (lipid-poor) cytoplasm. **(B)** Immunostaining for synaptophysin was strongly positive in some areas of tumor, but this can be seen in some adrenal cortical neoplasms, both benign and malignant (peroxidase-antiperoxidase stain).

ANALYSIS OF DNA CONTENT

DNA ploidy analysis has been done on paragangliomas of the head and neck region (220–223) and sympathoadrenal paragangliomas (203,224–226), and the results have not been uniformly contributory in predicting biologic behavior. Aneuploid cell populations can be seen in CBPs and VPs and in pheochromocytomas that prove to be clinically benign. With regard to head and neck paragangliomas, several studies indicate that abnormalities of DNA content are sufficiently common in clinically benign tumors that DNA content cannot be used to assess malignant behavior (221,223); moreover, DNA ploidy is not correlated with the familial or sporadic nature of the tumors (223). DNA aneuploidy, however, has been considered an indication that these tumors are true neoplasms. However, a recent study suggests that the sustentacular cell component of the paraganglioma should be regarded as a nonneoplastic cell population rather than a neoplastic cell population like the chief cells/pheochromocytes (227). Image analysis of CBPs and APPs has also shown that it is of little use in differentiating between paragangliomas on the basis of either site of origin or clinical behavior (228).

Hosaka et al. (224) studied 75 pheochromocytomas for DNA content and reported that a normal diploid DNA histogram identified a group of clinically benign tumors, whereas 8 of 26 tumors (31%) with DNA tetraploidy or polyploidy and 7 of 18 tumors (39%) with aneuploid peaks were malignant. Another study, however, showed that aneuploid DNA content was rather common in clinically benign tumors, and this was not considered a specific marker of malignancy (225). The presence of aneuploidy or tetraploidy has also not been shown to be useful as a diagnostic criterion for malignancy in urinary bladder paragangliomas. The likelihood of malignancy of pheochromocytomas has been reported to be greater in tumors with tetraploid and peritetraploid DNA (226); other studies report that flow cytometry is not a reliable predictor of malignant behavior (229).

MALIGNANT PARAGANGLIOMAS

The incidence of malignant paragangliomas varies according to the anatomic site of origin, but one must be cautious in the interpretation of some of the reported data because (a) malignant tumors are more apt to be reported (particularly uncommon tumors), whereas benign tumors are not; (b) in some cases, it may be difficult to distinguish multicentric paragangliomas from metastases; and (c) at some sites (e.g., larynx), a more aggressive neuroendocrine neoplasm may be mistaken for a paraganglioma (32,38).

Based on selected literature reviews, large clinical series, or other reference sources, the following rates of malignancy (as evidenced by regional or distant metastases) have been reported: CBPs, 2% (40,92) and 12% (230); VPs, 10.6% (231); JTPs, 3% (232); LPs, 3% (65,66); pheochromocytomas (adrenal medullary paragangliomas), 2.4% (233), 2.5% (234), 8% (135), and 14% (235); extra-adrenal paragangliomas of the abdomen, 24% to 50% (123,236–238); urinary bladder paragangliomas, less than 7% (124,130); paragangliomas of the posterior mediastinum, 15% (239). As noted by Neville (240), the only absolute criterion for diagnosing malignancy is the presence of tumor at sites where paraganglionic tissue is not normally found. One must also be aware that series of cases including pheochromocytomas and extra-adrenal paragangliomas may show an incidence of malignancy that is greater than the incidence of pheochromocytomas alone.

Reliable prediction of biologic behavior of paragangliomas on the basis of histopathologic features is notoriously difficult. Recent studies of adrenal pheochromocytomas have proposed that variable histologic parameters can indicate a higher likelihood of aggressive clinical behavior (malignancy) with some success (241,242), but this has not been universally accepted (243,244), and additional evaluation will be required to determine sensitivity and specificity of such features. In a study of head and neck paragangliomas at Memorial Hospital, clinically malignant tumors (four CBPs and two VPs) showed a combination of at least two of the following characteristics: necrosis (confluent or central within enlarged zellballen), vascular invasion, and the presence of mitotic figures (91). A recent study that looked at 30 extra-adrenal sympathetic paragangliomas in addition to 116 adrenal pheochromocytomas found some statistical significance when using six factors (histologic pattern, cellularity, coagulation necrosis, vascular/capsular invasion, Ki-67 immunoreactivity, and types of catecholamine produced) (245). Other studies, although considerably smaller, indicate no apparent relationship between clinical behavior and nuclear pleomorphism, mitotic activity, or perineural and vascular invasion (221). In a study of sympathoadrenal paragangliomas at the NCI, logistic regression analysis showed four features to be most predictive of malignancy: extra-adrenal location, coarse nodularity of the primary tumor, confluent tumor necrosis, and absence of hyaline globules. Although malignant tumors were larger in size with a slightly higher mitotic rate and rate of vascular invasion (Fig. 15.39), these attributes were not prognostically significant in the statistical model used (134). Immunohistochemical staining for MIB-1 (Ki-67), a proliferation marker, may be useful in identifying potentially aggressive tumors (229,245,246). A scaled scoring system was applied to pheochromocytomas with evaluation of invasion, large nests or diffuse growth, focal or confluent necrosis, tumor cell spindling, increased mitotic figures (<3/10 hpf scored as 2), atypical mitotic figures, nuclear pleomorphism, and hyperchromasia. Application of this scaled score helped to identify tumors with a more aggressive biologic behavior (241). Another study identified adverse factors such as high 24-hour urinary dopamine levels, extra-adrenal location, and high tumor weight (>80 g) as being associated with malignant behavior (247).

The pattern of metastases reflects both lymphatic and hematogenous dissemination. Some of the more common sites of metastases are regional lymph nodes, liver, lung, and bone (Fig. 15.40A,B). On rare occasions, the initial manifestation is an osteolytic metastasis. Immunohistochemistry has also been used to try to identify malignant paragangliomas. Clinically malignant sympathoadrenal paragangliomas have been shown to express significantly fewer neuropeptides compared with benign tumors; malignant tumors expressed an average of two neuropeptides, in contrast to five for the benign neoplasms (201). A few studies have also suggested a relationship between aggres-

sive or frankly malignant paragangliomas and a diminished number or density of sustentacular cells, as indicated by S-100 protein (248–254) and glial fibrillary acidic protein (251,252) positivity. Exceptions do exist because some examples of metastatic paraganglioma may also contain sustentacular cells, which do not appear significantly diminished in number (220). Other researchers report a lower expression of neuropeptide Y (255) and a diminished number of HLA-DR antigen-positive dendritic cells in aggressive or malignant paragangliomas (256). Increased expression of tenascin (257) and cyclooxygenase-2 (258) has been reported in malignant paragangliomas, but further studies may be needed to better define the utility of these immunomarkers in establishing prognosis. There appears to be an increased risk of malignancy in patients with genetically detected mutation in the *SDHB* and *SDHD* genes (259–261).

Laparoscopic surgery has been used to resect a variety of adrenal tumors, including pheochromocytomas (262). The risk of this procedure can be reduced by accurate preoperative evaluation and pretreatment with alpha-blockers. Recently, a case of putative laparoscopic-induced seeding of pheochromocytoma was reported ("iatrogenic pheochromocytomatosis") (263). The tumor had recurred locally as multiple small tumor nodules in the adrenal bed near the site of the initial laparoscopic resection.

GANGLIOCYTIC PARAGANGLIOMA

Gangliocytic paraganglioma (GP) is a very unusual tumor that has both a ganglioneuroma-like and paraganglioma-like appearance and is typically located within mucosa and muscularis of the second part of the duodenum (264–270). It can also be found in other parts of the duodenum and, rarely, the pylorus and proximal jejunum and appendix (271). A case was even reported in the cauda equina region (272), but this could represent a paraganglioma with neuronal or ganglionic differentiation. Some investigators propose an endodermal or even pancreatic origin for epithelial cells of GPs, with development from ventral primordial rests of pancreas (267). These tumors contain three cell types: spindle cells with the appearance of nerve sheath or Schwann cells, ganglion or ganglion-like cells (Fig. 15.41A), and epithelioid cells arranged in an endocrine growth pattern (Fig. 15.41B). GP is considered to be a benign tumor; a few cases have been associated with regional lymph node involvement, although some doubt exists whether this signifies malignant spread (270,273). An unusual case of pulmonary GP with associated Cushing syndrome has recently been reported (274).

PARAGANGLIOMA OF CAUDA EQUINA REGION

Paragangliomas of the cauda equina are rare tumors with variable attachment to the filum terminale or caudal nerve roots (275–279). These tumors occur in the fourth to seventh decades of life and are slightly more predominant in men; they range in size from 1.5 to 10 cm (average, 3 cm) (278). Most tumors are intradural and extramedullary and often appear grossly encapsulated. Some tumors show neuronal or ganglionic differentiation similar to composite paragangliomas and can resemble a GP (272,275,278). At the microscopic level, these

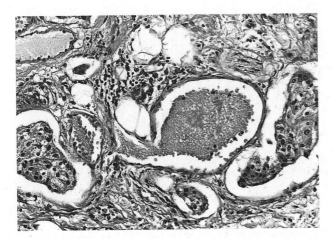

Figure 15.39. Vascular invasion is evident in this clinically malignant extra-adrenal paraganglioma that originated in area of aortic bifurcation.

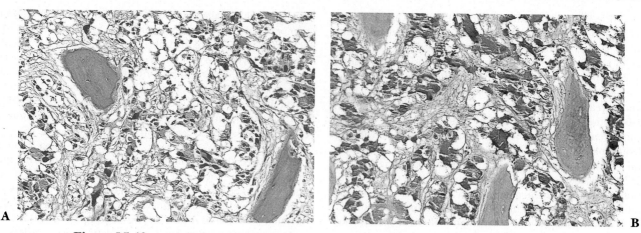

Figure 15.40. **(A)** Malignant carotid body paraganglioma (CBP) metastatic to the ribs. The patient was a 51-year-old man who initially had a 3-cm CBP and cervical lymph node metastases at the time of diagnosis. The patient died 6 years later with metastatic CBP in the liver, ribs, femur, and lymph nodes. **(B)** The tumor cells retain an organoid pattern and show cytoplasmic argyrophilia (Grimelius stain).

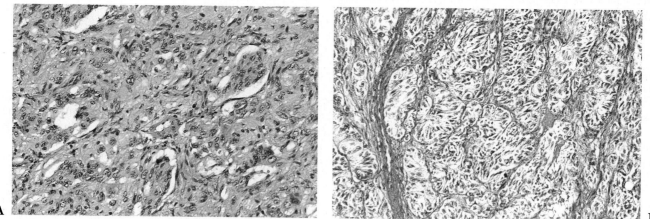

Figure 15.41. **(A)** Ganglioneuroma-like area in a duodenal gangliocytic paraganglioma (GP). A few ganglion-like cells are apparent in this field, with a spindle cell Schwannian component. **(B)** Anastomosing cords of epithelioid cells in a different GP.

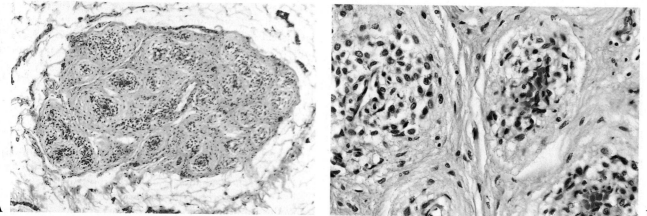

Figure 15.42. **(A)** A normal glomus coccygeum obtained from an adult at autopsy. **(B)** This glomus coccygeum has scattered vascular channels with layering of epithelioid cells. Although there may be a superficial resemblance to a paraganglion or vascular tumor, it is a normal anatomic structure with a blood supply from the median sacral artery.

tumors resemble paragangliomas at other sites, and immunohistochemical study has demonstrated immunoreactivity for neuron-specific enolase, neurofilament protein, and other endocrine substances, such as serotonin and somatostatin; sustentacular cells have also been identified by positive staining for S-100 protein (278). The differential diagnosis includes ependymoma. A report of cytokeratin expression in some of these lesions should be kept in mind to avoid mistaking them for metastatic neuroendocrine carcinoma (280).

GLOMUS COCCYGEUM

The glomus coccygeum is a small, ovoid vascular structure normally located just ventral to the tip of the coccyx and is composed of epithelioid cells arranged in layers around small vascular channels (Fig. 15.42). It was first noted by Luschka (281) and normally consists of a nodule several millimeters in diameter, but there are often smaller satellite nodules. There is no known function for this glomus, and it bears no homology with chemoreceptor tissue, such as the carotid body (also referred to as a glomus) (282). The main importance of the glomus coccygeum to the surgical pathologist is recognition of it as a normal histologic finding in this area; it should not be mistaken for a tumor, such as a glomus tumor or a paraganglioma (283–286).

REFERENCES

1. Smetana HF, Scott WF Jr. Malignant tumors of nonchromaffin paraganglia. *Mil Surgeon* 1951;69:330–349.
2. Pearse AGE. The cytochemistry and ultrastructure of polypeptide hormone–producing cells of the APUD series and the embryologic, physiologic and pathologic implications of the concept. *J Histochem Cytochem* 1969;17:303–313.
3. Pearse AGE. The APUD cell concept and its implications in pathology. *Pathol Annu* 1974;9:27–41.
4. Andrew A. The APUD concept: where has it led us? *Br Med Bull* 1982;38:221–225.
5. Toni R. The neuroendocrine system: organization and homeostatic role. *J Endocrinol Invest* 2004;27(Suppl 6):35–47.
6. Tischler AS, Dichter MA, Biales B, et al. Neural properties of cultured human endocrine tumor cells of proposed neural crest origin. *Science* 1976;192:902–904.
7. Cryer PE. Physiology and pathophysiology of the sympathoadrenal neuroendocrine system. *N Engl J Med* 1980;303:436–444.
8. Wolfe HJ. Endocrine pathology: past, present, and future. In Kovacs K, Asa SL, eds. *Functional Endocrine Pathology.* New York, NY: Blackwell Scientific, 1991:3–14.
9. Pearse AGE, Polak JM, Rost FWD, et al. Demonstration of the neural crest origin of type I (APUD) cells in the avian carotid body, using a cytochemical marker system. *Histochemie* 1973;34:191–203.
10. Heymans C, Bouckhaert JJ, Dautrebande L. Sinus carotidien et reflexes respiratoires. II. Influences respiratoires reflexes de l'acidose, de l'alkalose, de l'anhydride carbonique, de l'ion hydrogene et de l'anoxémie: sinus carotidiens et échanges respiratoires dans les poumons et au dela des poumons. *Arch Int Pharmacodyn Ther* 1930;39:400–450.
11. Comroe JH Jr. The location and function of the chemoreceptors of the aorta. *Am J Physiol* 1939;127:176–191.
12. de Castro F. Sur la structure et l'innervation du sinus carotidien de l'homme et des mammifères: nouveau faits sur l'innervation et la fonction du glomus caroticum. Etudes anatomiques et physiologiques. *Trab Lab Invest Biol Univ Madr* 1928;25:331–380.
13. Montoro RJ, Urena J, Fernández-Chacón R, et al. Oxygen sensing by ion channels and chemotransduction in single glomus cells. *J Gen Physiol* 1996;107:133–143.
14. Acker H. The oxygen sensing signal cascade under the influence of reactive oxygen species. *Philos Trans R Soc Lond B Biol Sci* 2005;360:2201–2210.
15. Kemp PJ. Detecting acute changes in oxygen: will the real sensor please stand up? *Exp Physiol* 2006;92:829–834.
16. Prabhakar NR. O2 sensing at the mammalian carotid body: why multiple O2 sensors and the multiple transmitters? *Exp Physiol* 2006;1:17–23.
17. Baysal BE. A phenotypical perspective on Mammalian oxygen sensor candidates. *Ann NY Acad Sci* 2006;1073:221–233.
18. Ortega-Saenz P, Pascual A, Pirut JI, et al. Mechanisms of acute oxygen sensing by the carotid body: lessons from genetically modified animals. *Respir Physiol Neurobiol* 2007;157:140–147.
19. Smith P, Jago R, Heath D. Anatomical variation and quantitative histology of the normal and enlarged carotid body. *J Pathol* 1982;137:287–304.
20. Lack EE, Perez-Atayde AR, Young JB. Carotid body hyperplasia in cystic fibrosis and cya-
21. notic heart disease: a combined morphometric, ultrastructural and biochemical study. *Am J Pathol* 1985;119:301–314.
21. McCluggage WG, Young RH. Paraganglioma of the ovary: report of three cases of a rare ovarian neoplasm, including two exhibiting inhibin positivity. *Am J Surg Pathol* 2006;30:600–605.
22. Arias-Stella J. Human carotid body at high altitude. *Am J Pathol* 1969;55:82a.
23. Arias-Stella J, Valcarcel J. Chief cell hyperplasia in the human carotid body at high altitudes: physiologic and pathologic significance. *Hum Pathol* 1976;7:361–373.
24. Saldana MJ, Salem LE, Travezan R. High altitude hypoxia and chemodectomas. *Hum Pathol* 1973;4:251–263.
25. Pacheco-Ojeda L, Durango E, Rodriquez C, et al. Carotid body tumors at high altitudes: Quito, Ecuador, 1987. *World J Surg* 1988;12:856–860.
26. Rodriguez-Cuevas S, Lopez-Garza J, Labastida-Almendaro S. Carotid body tumors in inhabitants of altitudes higher than 2000 meters above sea level. *Head Neck* 1998;20:374–378.
27. Heath D, Edwards C, Harris P. Post-mortem size and structure of the human carotid body: its relation to pulmonary disease and cardiac hypertrophy. *Thorax* 1970;25:129–140.
28. Lack EE. Carotid body hypertrophy in patients with cystic fibrosis and cyanotic congenital heart disease. *Hum Pathol* 1977;8:39–51.
29. Wang ZY, Bisgard GE. Chronic hypoxia-induced morphological and neurochemical changes in the carotid body. *Microsc Res Tech* 2002;59:168–177.
30. Prabhakar NR, Jacono FJ. Cellular and molecular mechanisms associated with carotid body adaptations to chronic hypoxia. *High Alt Med Biol* 2005;6:112–120.
31. Lack EE. Hyperplasia of vagal and carotid body paraganglia in patients with chronic hypoxemia. *Am J Pathol* 1978;91:497–516.
32. Lack EE. Tumors of the adrenal glands and extra-adrenal paraganglia. In *Atlas of Tumor Pathology.* 4th series, fascicle 8. Washington, DC: Armed Forces Institute of Pathology, 2007.
33. Chedid A, Jao W. Hereditary tumors of the carotid bodies and chronic obstructive pulmonary disease. *Cancer* 1974;33:1635–1641.
34. Nissenblatt MJ. Cyanotic heart disease: low altitude risk for carotid body tumor? *J Hosp Med J* 1978;142:12–21.
35. Bockelman HW, Arya S, Gilbert EF. Cyanotic congenital heart disease with malignant paraganglioma. *Cancer* 1982;50:2513–2517.
36. Mulligan RM. Chemodectoma in the dog. *Am J Pathol* 1950;26:680–681.
37. Marchand F. Beitrage zur Kenntniss der normalen und pathologischen anatomie der grandula carotica und der nebennieren. *Int Beitr Z Wissensch Med Festschr R Virchow* 1891;1:535–581.
38. Lack EE. *Pathology of Adrenal and Extra-Adrenal Paraganglia. Major Problems in Pathology.* Vol. 29. Philadelphia, PA: WB Saunders, 1994.
39. Oberman HA, Holtz F, Sheffer LA, et al. Chemodectomas (nonchromaffin paragangliomas) of the head and neck. *Cancer* 1968;21:838–851.
40. Shamblin WR, ReMine WH, Sheps SG, et al. Carotid body tumor (chemodectoma): clinicopathologic analysis of ninety cases. *Am J Surg* 1971;122:732–739.
41. Lack EE, Cubilla AL, Woodruff JM, et al. Paragangliomas of the head and neck region. *Cancer* 1977;39:397–409.
42. Pellitteri PK, Rinaldo A, Myssiorek D, et al. Paragangliomas of the head and neck. *Oral Oncol* 2004;40:563–575.
43. Manolidis S, Shohet JA, Jackson CG, et al. Malignant glomus tumors. *Laryngoscope* 1999;109:30–34.
44. Van der May AGL, Jansen FC, Van Baalen JM. Management of carotid body tumors. *Otolaryngol Clin North Am* 2001;34:907–923.
45. Patetsios P, Gable DR, Garrett WV, et al. Management of carotid body paragangliomas and review of a 30-year experience. *Ann Vasc Surg* 2002;16:331–338.
46. Kasper GC, Welling RE, Wladis AR, et al. A multidisciplinary approach to carotid paragangliomas. *Vasc Endovascular Surg* 2006;40:467–474.
47. Grufferman S, Gillman MW, Pasternak LR, et al. Familial carotid body tumors: case report and epidemiologic review. *Cancer* 1980;46:2112–2116.
48. Parry DM, Li FP, Strong LC, et al. Carotid body tumors in humans: genetics and epidemiology. *J Natl Cancer Inst* 1982;68:573–578.
49. Lattes R. Nonchromaffin paraganglioma of ganglion nodosum, carotid body, and aortic arch bodies. *Cancer* 1950;3:667–694.
50. Lattes R, McDonald JJ, Sproul E. Nonchromaffin paraganglioma of carotid body and orbit: report of a case. *Ann Surg* 1954;139:382–384.
51. Kafie FE, Freischlag JA. Carotid body tumors: the role of preoperative embolization. *Ann Vasc Surg* 2001;15:237–242.
52. Rakovich G, Ferraro P, Therasse E, et al. Preoperative embolization in the management of a mediastinal paraganglioma. *Ann Thorac Surg* 2001;72:601–603.
53. Guild SR. A hitherto unrecognized structure, the glomus jugularis, in man. *Anat Rec* 1941;79:28A.
54. Guild SR. The glomus jugulare, a nonchromaffin paraganglion, in man. *Ann Otol Rhinol Laryngol* 1953;62:1045–1071.
55. Rosenwasser H. Carotid body tumor of the middle ear and mastoid. *Arch Otolaryngol* 1945;41:64–67.
56. Jackson CG. Glomus tympanicum and glomus jugulare tumors. *Otolaryngol Clin North Am* 2001;34:941–969.
57. Netterville JL, Jackson CG, Miller FR, et al. Vagal paraganglioma: a review of 46 patients treated during 20-year period. *Arch Otolaryngol Head Neck Surg* 1998;124:1133–1140.
58. Sniezek JC, Netterville JL, Sabri AN, et al. Vagal paragangliomas. *Otolaryngol Clin North Am* 2001;34:925–939.
59. Lawson W, Zak FG. The glomus bodies ("paraganglia") of the human larynx. *Laryngoscope* 1974;803:98–110.
60. Myssiorek D, Halaas Y, Silver C, et al. Laryngeal and sinonasal paragangliomas. *Otolaryngol Clin North Am* 2001;34:971–981.
61. Gallivan MVE, Chun B, Rowden G, et al. Laryngeal paraganglioma: case report with ultrastructural analysis and literature review. *Am J Surg Pathol* 1979;3:85–92.

62. Woodruff JM, Shah JP, Huvos AG, et al. Neuroendocrine carcinomas of the larynx: a study of two types, one of which mimics thyroid medullary carcinoma. *Am J Surg Pathol* 1985;9: 771–790.

63. Woodruff JM, Senie RT. Atypical carcinoid tumor of the larynx: a critical review of the literature. *ORL J Otorhinolaryngol Relat Spec* 1991;53:194–209.

64. Ferlito A, Devaney KO, Rinaldo A. Neuroendocrine neoplasms of the larynx: advances in identification, understanding and management. *Oral Oncol* 2006;42:770–788.

65. Barnes L. Paraganglioma of the larynx: a critical review of the literature. *ORL* 1991;53: 220–234.

66. Myssiorek D, Rinaldo A, Barnes L, et al. Laryngeal paraganglioma: an updated critical review. *Acta Otolaryngol* 2004;124:995–999.

67. Becker AE. The glomera in the region of the heart and great vessels: a microscopic-anatomical and histochemical study [M.D. Thesis]. Amsterdam, The Netherlands: Laboratory of Pathological Anatomy of the University of Amsterdam, 1966.

68. Lack EE, Stillinger RA, Colvin DB, et al. Aortico-pulmonary paraganglioma: report of a case with ultrastructural study and review of the literature. *Cancer* 1979;43:269–278.

69. Johnson TL, Lloyd RV, Shapiro B, et al. Cardiac paragangliomas: a clinicopathologic and immunohistochemical study of four cases. *Am J Surg Pathol* 1985;9:827–834.

70. Mikolaenko I, Galliani CA, Davis GG. Pigmented cardiac paraganglioma. *Arch Pathol Lab Med* 2001;125:680–682.

71. Fisher ER, Hazard JB. Nonchromaffin paraganglioma of the orbit. *Cancer* 1952;5:521–524.

72. Thacker WC, Duckworth JK. Chemodectoma of the orbit. *Cancer* 1969;23:1233–1238.

73. Thorbeck RV, Valentin OIM, Morales MR. Non-chromaffin paraganglioma of the orbit. *Zentralbl Chir* 1986;111:46–49.

74. Veda N, Yoshida A, Fukunishi R, et al. Nonchromaffin paraganglioma in the nose and paranasal sinuses. *Acta Pathol Jpn* 1985;35:489–495.

75. Watson DJ. Nasal paraganglioma. *J Laryngol Otol* 1988;102:526–529.

76. Mevio E, Bignami M, Luinetti O, et al. *Acta Otorhinolaryngol Belg* 2001;55:247–249.

77. Schuller DE, Lucas JG. Nasal paraganglioma: a case report. *Arch Otolaryngol* 1982;108: 667–670.

78. DeLozier HL. Chemodectoma of the cheek: a case report. *Ann Otol Rhinol Laryngol* 1983; 92:109–112.

79. Smith WT, Hughes B, Ermocilla R. Chemodectoma of the pineal region, with observations on the pineal body and chemoreceptor tissue. *J Pathol Bacteriol* 1966;92:69–76.

80. Bilbao JM, Horvath E, Kovacs K, et al. Intrasellar paraganglioma associated with hypopituitarism. *Arch Pathol Lab Med* 1978;102:95–98.

81. Sambaziotis D, Kontogeorgos G, Kovacs K, et al. Intrasellar paraganglioma presenting as nonfunctioning pituitary adenoma. *Arch Pathol Lab Med* 1999;123:429–432.

82. Buss DH, Marshall RB, Baird FG, et al. Paraganglioma of the thyroid gland. *Am J Surg Pathol* 1980;4:589–593.

83. Heppleston AG. A carotid body–like tumour in the lung. *J Pathol Bacteriol* 1958;75: 461–464.

84. Goodman ML, LaForet EG. Solitary primary chemodectomas of the lung. *Chest* 1972;61: 48–50.

85. Singh G, Lee RE, Brooks DH. Primary pulmonary paraganglioma: report of a case and review of the literature. *Cancer* 1977;40:2286–2289.

86. daSilva RA, Gross JL, Haddad FJ, et al. Primary pulmonary paraganglioma: case report and literature review. *Clinics* 2006;61:83–86.

87. Blessing MH, Hora BI. Glomera in der lunge des menschen. *Z Zellforsch Mikrosk Anat* 1968; 87:562–570.

88. Medaline NS, Mendelsohn MG, Esposito M. Multicentric metachronous pulmonary and intravagal paraganglioma: a case report with immunohistochemical findings. *Arch Pathol Lab Med* 1996;120:1137–1140.

89. Dahir KM, Gonzalez A, Revelo MP, et al. Ectopic adrenocorticotropic hormone hypersecretion due to a primary pulmonary paraganglioma. *Endocr Pract* 2004;10:424–428.

90. Saeki T, Akiba T, Jon K, et al. An extremely large solitary paraganglioma of the lung: report of a case. *Surg Today* 1999;29:1195–1200.

91. Lack EE, Cubilla AL, Woodruff JM. Paragangliomas of the head and neck region: a pathologic study of tumors from 71 patients. *Hum Pathol* 1979;10:191–218.

92. Nora JD, Hallett JW Jr, O'Brien PC, et al. Surgical resection of carotid body tumors: long-term survival, recurrence, and metastasis. *Mayo Clin Proc* 1988;63:348–352.

93. Davidge-Pitts KJ, Pantanowitz D. Carotid body tumors. *Surg Annu* 1984;16:203–227.

94. Sacher M, Som PM, Lanzieri CF, et al. Total internal carotid artery occlusion by a benign carotid body tumor: a rare occurrence. *J Comput Tomogr* 1985;9:213–217.

95. Warshawski ST, de Souza FM. The carotid body tumor. *J Otolaryngol* 1989;18:306–310.

96. Roland PS. Malignant paraganglioma with retrograde flow in the internal carotid artery. *Ann Otol Rhinol Laryngol* 1991;100:345–347.

97. Grimley PM, Glenner CG. Histology and ultrastructure of carotid body paragangliomas: comparison with the normal gland. *Cancer* 1967;20:1473–1488.

98. LeCompte PM. Tumors of the carotid body and related structures (chemoreceptor system). In *Atlas of Tumor Pathology*. 1st series, fascicle 16. Washington, DC: Armed Forces Institute of Pathology, 1951.

99. Capella C, Solcia E. Optical and electron microscopical study of cytoplasmic granules in human carotid body, carotid body tumours and glomus jugulare tumours. *Virchows Arch B Cell Pathol* 1971;7:37–53.

100. Coupland RE. *The Natural History of the Chromaffin Cell.* London, United Kingdom: Longmans, Green, 1965.

101. Zuckerkandl E. Ueber nebenorgane des sympathicus im retroperitonaealraum des menschen. *Verh Dtsch Anat Ges* 1901;15:95–107.

102. Zuckerkandl E. The development of the chromaffin organs and of the suprarenal glands. In Keibel F, Mall EP, eds. *Manual of Human Embryology.* Philadelphia, PA: JB Lippincott, 1912:157–159.

103. Lack EE, Kozakewich HPW. Embryology, developmental anatomy, and selected aspects of non-neoplastic pathology. In Lack EE, ed. *Pathology of the Adrenal Glands.* New York, NY: Churchill Livingstone, 1990:1–74.

104. Coupland RE. Post-natal fate of the abdominal para-aortic bodies in man. *J Anat* 1954; 88:455–464.

105. West GB, Shepherd DM, Hunter RB. The function of the organs of Zuckerkandl. *Clin Sci* 1953;12:317–325.

106. Lack EE. Adrenal medullary hyperplasia and pheochromocytoma. In Lack EE, ed. *Pathology of the Adrenal Glands.* New York, NY: Churchill Livingstone, 1990:173–235.

107. Ross JH. Pheochromocytoma. Special considerations in children. *Ped Urol Oncol* 2000;27: 393–402.

108. Tekautz TM, Pratt CB, Jenkins JJ, et al. Pediatric extra adrenal paraganglioma. *J Pediatr Surg* 2003;38:1317–1321.

109. Fries JG, Chamberlin JA. Extra-adrenal pheochromocytoma: literature review and report of a cervical pheochromocytoma. *Surgery* 1968;63:268–279.

110. Miller TA, Weber TR, Appelman HD. Paraganglioma of the gallbladder. *Arch Surg* 1972; 105:637–639.

111. Cho Yu, Kim JY, Choi SK, et al. A case of hemorrhagic gallbladder paraganglioma causing acute cholecystitis. *Yonsei Med J* 2001;42:352–356.

112. Eusebi V, Massarelli G. Pheochromocytoma of the spermatic cord: report of a case. *J Pathol* 1971;105:283–284.

113. Bacchi CE, Schmidt RA, Brandao M, et al. Paraganglioma of the spermatic cord: report of a case with immunohistochemical and ultrastructural studies. *Arch Pathol Lab Med* 1990; 114:899–901.

114. Nielsen VM, Skovgaard N, Kvist N. Phaeochromocytoma of the prostate. *Br J Urol* 1987; 59:478–479.

115. Campodonico F, Bandelloni R, Maffezzini M. Paraganglioma of the prostate in a young adult. *Urology* 2005;66:657.

116. Altavilla G, Cavazzini L, Russo R. Secreting benign paraganglioma of the prostatic urethra. *Tumori* 1983;69:79–82.

117. Parithivel VS, Niazi M, Malhotra AK, et al. Paraganglioma of the pancreas. Literature review and case report. *Dig Dis Sci* 2000;45:438–441.

118. Young TW, Thrasher TV. Nonchromaffin paraganglioma of the uterus. *Arch Pathol Lab Med* 1982;106:608–609.

119. Tavassoli FA. Melanotic paraganglioma of the uterus. *Cancer* 1986;58:942–948.

120. Glenner GG, Crout JR, Roberts WC. A functional carotid-body-like tumor secreting levarterenol. *Arch Pathol* 1962;73:230–240.

121. Crowell WT, Grizzle WE, Siegel AL. Functional carotid paragangliomas: biochemical, ultrastructural, and histochemical correlation with clinical symptoms. *Arch Pathol Lab Med* 1982;106:599–603.

122. Karasov RS, Sheps SG, Carney JA, et al. Paragangliomatosis with numerous catecholamine-producing tumors. *Mayo Clin Proc* 1982;57:590–595.

123. Lack EE, Cubilla AL, Woodruff JM, et al. Extra adrenal paragangliomas of the retroperitoneum: a clinicopathologic study of 12 tumors. *Am J Surg Pathol* 1980;4:109–120.

124. Leestma JE, Price EB Jr. Paragangliomas of the urinary bladder. *Cancer* 1971;28: 1063–1072.

125. Gallivan MVE, Chun B, Rowden G, et al. Intrathoracic paravertebral malignant paraganglioma. *Arch Pathol Lab Med* 1980;104:46–51.

126. DeLellis RA, Suchow E, Wolfe HJ. Ultrastructure of nuclear inclusions in pheochromocytoma and paraganglioma. *Hum Pathol* 1980;11:205–207.

127. Brody S, Leehan RM, Schwaitzberg SD, et al. Composite pheochromocytoma/ganglioneuroma of the adrenal gland associated with multiple endocrine neoplasia 2A: case report with immunohistochemical analysis. *Am J Surg Pathol* 1997;21:102–108.

128. Sakaguchi N, Sano K, Ito M, et al. A case of von Recklinghausen's disease with bilateral pheochromocytoma: malignant peripheral nerve sheath tumor of the adrenal and gastrointestinal autonomic nerve tumors. *Am J Surg Pathol* 1996;20:889–897.

129. Wieneke JA, Thompson LDR, Heffess CS. Corticomedullary mixed tumor of the adrenal gland. *Ann Diagn Pathol* 2001;5:304–308.

130. Cheng L, Leibovich BC, Cheville JC, et al. Paraganglioma of the urinary bladder. Can biologic potential be predicted? *Cancer* 2000;88:844–852.

131. Yoshida S, Nakagomi K, Goto S, et al. Malignant pheochromocytoma of the urinary bladder: effectiveness of radiotherapy in conjunction with chemotherapy. *Int J Urol* 2004;11: 175–177.

132. Kovacs K, Bell D, Gardiner GW, et al. Malignant paraganglioma of the urinary bladder: immunohistochemical study of prognostic indicators. *Endocr Pathol* 2005;16:363–369.

133. Havekes B, Corssmit EP, Hansen JC, et al. Malignant paragangliomas associated with mutations in the succinate dehydrogenase D gene. *J Clin Endocrinol Metab* 2007;92: 1245–1248.

134. Linnoila RI, Keiser HR, Steinberg SM, et al. Histopathology of benign versus malignant sympathoadrenal paragangliomas: clinicopathologic study of 120 cases including unusual histologic features. *Hum Pathol* 1990;21:1168–1180.

135. Medeiros LJ, Wolf BC, Balogh K, et al. Adrenal pheochromocytoma: a clinicopathologic review of 60 cases. *Hum Pathol* 1985;16:580–589.

136. Mendelsohn G, Olson JL. Pheochromocytomas [Letter]. *Hum Pathol* 1978;9:607–608.

137. Lack EE, Travis WD, Oertel JE. Adrenal cortical neoplasms. In Lack EE, ed. *Pathology of the Adrenal Glands.* New York, NY: Churchill Livingstone, 1990:115–171.

138. Lack EE, Mulvihill JJ, Travis WD, et al. Adrenal cortical neoplasms in the pediatric and adolescent age group: clinicopathologic study of 30 cases with emphasis on epidemiological and prognostic factors. *Pathol Annu* 1992;27:1–53.

139. Rey C, Escribano JC, Vidal MT. Retroperitoneal paraganglioma and systemic amyloidosis: a case report. *Cancer* 1979;43:702–706.

140. Steinhoff MM, Wells SA Jr, DeSchryver-Kecskemeti K. Stromal amyloid in pheochromocytomas. *Hum Pathol* 1992;23:33–36.

141. Miranda RN, Wu CD, Nayak RN, et al. Amyloid in adrenal gland pheochromocytomas. *Arch Pathol Lab Med* 1995;119:827–830.

142. Bellezza G, Giansanti M, Cavaliere A, et al. Pigmented "black" pheochromocytoma of the adrenal gland: a case report and review of the literature. *Arch Pathol Lab Med* 2004; 128:125–128.

143. Lack EE, Kim H, Reed K. Pigmented (black) extra-adrenal paraganglioma. *Am J Surg Pathol* 1998;22:265–269.
144. Neumann HP, Cybulla M, Shibata H, et al. New genetic causes of pheochromocytoma: current concepts and the clinical relevance. *Keio J Med* 2005;54:15–21.
145. Elder EE, Elder G, Larsson C. Pheochromocytoma and functional paraganglioma syndrome: no longer the 10% tumor. *J Surg Oncol* 2005;89:193–201.
146. Chase WH. Familial and bilateral tumors of the carotid body. *J Pathol Bacteriol* 1933;36:1–12.
147. Kroll AJ, Alexander B, Cochios F, et al. Hereditary deficiencies of clotting factors VII and X associated with carotid body tumors. *N Engl J Med* 1964;270:6–13.
148. Van Baars F, Cremers C, Van den Broek P, et al. Familial nonchromaffin paragangliomas (glomus tumors). *Acta Otolaryngol* 1981;91:589–593.
149. Sobol SM, Dailey JC. Familial multiple cervical paragangliomas: report of a kindred and review of the literature. *Otolaryngol Head Neck Surg* 1990;102:382–390.
150. Pratt LW. Familial carotid body tumors. *Arch Otolaryngol* 1973;97:334–336.
151. Van der May AGL, Maaswinkel-Mooy PD, Cornelisse CJ, et al. Genomic imprinting in hereditary glomus tumours: evidence for new genetic theory. *Lancet* 1989;2:1291–1294.
152. Baysal BE. Genomic imprinting and environment in hereditary paraganglioma. *Am J Med Genet C Semin Med Genet* 2004;129:85–90.
153. Parkin JL. Familial multiple glomus tumors and pheochromocytomas. *Ann Otol* 1981;90:60–63.
154. van Baars F, van den Broek P, Cremers C, et al. Familial non-chromaffin paragangliomas (glomus tumors): clinical aspects. *Laryngoscope* 1981;91:988–996.
155. Baysal BE. Genetics of familial paragangliomas. *Otolaryngologic Clin North Am* 2001;34:863–879.
156. Blank RD, Sklar CA, Dimich AB, et al. Clinical presentations and RET protooncogene mutations in seven multiple endocrine neoplasia type 2 kindreds. *Cancer* 1996;78:1996–2003.
157. Eng C. The RET proto-oncogene in multiple endocrine neoplasia type 2 and Hirschsprung's disease. *N Engl J Med* 1996;335:943–951.
158. Astuti D, Douglas F, Leonard TWJ, et al. Germline SDHD mutation in familial pheochromocytomas. *Lancet* 2001;357:1181–1182.
159. Lui WO, Chen J, Glasker S, et al. Selective loss of chromosome 11 in pheochromocytomas associated with the VHL syndrome. *Oncogene* 2002;21:1117–1122.
160. Edstrom E, Mahlamaki E, Nord B, et al. Comparative genomic hybridization reveals frequent losses of chromosomes 1p and 3q in pheochromocytomas and abdominal paragangliomas, suggesting a common genetic etiology. *Am J Pathol* 2000;156:651–659.
161. Webb TA, Sheps SG, Carney JA. Differences between sporadic pheochromocytoma and pheochromocytoma in multiple endocrine neoplasia type 2. *Am J Surg Pathol* 1980;4:121–126.
162. Carney JA, Sizemore GW, Tyce GM. Bilateral adrenal medullary hyperplasia in multiple endocrine neoplasia, type 2: the precursor of bilateral pheochromocytoma. *Mayo Clin Proc* 1975;50:3–10.
163. DeLellis RA, Wolfe HJ, Gagel RF, et al. Adrenal medullar hyperplasia: a morphometric analysis in patients with familial medullary thyroid carcinoma. *Am J Pathol* 1976;83:177–190.
164. Carney JA, Sizemore GW, Sheps SG. Adrenal medullary disease in multiple endocrine neoplasia, type 2: pheochromocytoma and its precursors. *Am J Clin Pathol* 1976;66:279–290.
165. Keiser HR, Doppman JL, Robertson CN, et al. Diagnosis, localization, and management of pheochromocytoma. In Lack EE, ed. *Pathology of the Adrenal Glands.* New York, NY: Churchill Livingstone, 1990:237–255.
166. Carney JA, Sheps SG, Go VLW, et al. The triad of gastric leiomyosarcoma, functioning extra-adrenal paraganglioma and pulmonary chondroma. *N Engl J Med* 1977;296:1517–1518.
167. Diment J, Tamborinin E, Casali P, et al. Carney triad: case report and molecular analysis of gastric tumor. *Hum Pathol* 2005;336:112–116.
168. Miettinen M, Lasota J. Gastrointestinal stromal tumors: review on morphology, molecular pathology, prognosis and differential diagnosis. *Arch Pathol Lab Med* 2006;130:1466–1478.
169. Carney JA. Gastric stromal sarcoma, pulmonary chondroma and extra-adrenal paraganglioma (Carney triad): natural history, adrenocortical component and possible familial occurrence. *Mayo Clin Proc* 1999;74:543–552.
170. Matyakhina L, Bei TA, McWhinney SR, et al. Genetics of Carney triad: recurrent losses at chromosome 1 but lack of germline mutations in genes associated with paragangliomas and gastrointestinal stromal tumors. *J Clin Endocrinol Metab* 2007;92:2938–2943.
171. Agaimy A, Pelz AF, Corless CL, et al. Epithelioid gastric stromal tumours of the antrum in young females with the Carney triad: a report of three new cases with mutational analysis and comparative genomic hybridization. *Oncol Rep* 2007;18:9–15.
172. Carney JA. The triad of gastric epithelioid leiomyosarcoma, pulmonary chondroma and functioning extra-adrenal paraganglioma: a five-year review. *Medicine* 1983;62:159–169.
173. Dunn GD, Brown MJ, Sapsford RN, et al. Functioning middle mediastinal paraganglioma (phaeochromocytoma) associated with intercarotid paragangliomas. *Lancet* 1986;1:1061–1064.
174. Albores-Saavedra J, Devián ME. Association of thyroid carcinoma and chemodectoma. *Am J Surg* 1968;116:887–890.
175. Steely WM, Davies RS, Brigham RA. Carotid body tumor and hyperparathyroidism: a case report and review of the literature. *Am Surg* 1987;53:337–338.
176. Palmer FJ, Sawyers TM. Hyperparathyroidism, chemodectoma, thymoma, and myasthenia gravis. *Arch Intern Med* 1978;138:1402–1403.
177. Larraza-Hernandez O, Albores-Saavedra J, Benavides G, et al. Multiple endocrine neoplasia: pituitary adenoma, multicentric papillary thyroid carcinoma, bilateral carotid body paraganglioma, parathyroid hyperplasia, gastric leiomyoma and systemic amyloidosis. *Am J Clin Pathol* 1982;78:527–532.
178. Berg B, Biörklund A, Grimelius L, et al. A new pattern of multiple endocrine adenomatosis: chemodectoma, bronchial carcinoid, GH-producing pituitary adenoma, and hyperplasia of the parathyroid glands and antral and duodenal gastrin cells. *Acta Med Scand* 1976;200:321–326.
179. Carney JA, Stratakis CA. Familial paraganglioma and gastric stromal sarcoma: a new syndrome distinct from the Carney triad. *Am J Med Genet* 2002;108:132–139.
180. Engzell U, Franzen S, Zajicek J. Aspiration biopsy of tumors of the neck. II. Cytologic findings in 13 cases of carotid body tumor. *Acta Cytol* 1971;15:25–30.
181. Jacobs DM, Waisman J. Cervical paraganglioma with intranuclear vacuoles in a fine needle aspirate. *Acta Cytol* 1987;31:29–32.
182. González-Cámpora R, Otal-Salaverri C, Panea-Flores P, et al. Fine needle aspiration cytology of paraganglionic tumors. *Acta Cytol* 1988;32:386–390.
183. Qizilbash AH, Young JEM. *Guides to Clinical Aspiration Biopsy: Head and Neck.* New York, NY: Igaku-Shoin, 1988;279–289.
184. Fleming MV, Oertel YC, Rodriguez ER, et al. Fine-needle aspiration of six carotid body paragangliomas. *Diagn Cytopathol* 1993:9:510–515.
185. Zaharopoulos P. Diagnostic challenges in the fine-needle aspiration diagnosis of carotid body paragangliomas: report of five cases. *Diagn Cytopathol* 2000;23:202–207.
186. Nguyen G-K. Cytopathologic aspects of adrenal pheochromocytoma in a fine needle aspiration biopsy: a case report. *Acta Cytol* 1982;26:354–358.
187. McCorkell SJ, Niles NL. Fine needle aspiration of catecholamine-producing adrenal masses: a possibly fatal mistake. *AJR Am J Roentgenol* 1985;145:113–114.
188. Lambert MA, Hirschowitz L, Russell RCG. Fine needle aspiration biopsy: a cautionary tale. *Br J Surg* 1985;72:364.
189. Grimley PM. Tumors of the extra-adrenal paraganglia system (including chemoreceptors). In *Atlas of Tumor Pathology* 2nd series, fascicle 9. Washington, DC.: Armed Forces Institute of Pathology; 1974.
190. Tannenbaum M. Ultrastructural pathology of adrenal medullary tumors. *Pathol Annu* 1970;5:145–171.
191. Lloyd RV, Sisson JC, Shapiro B, et al. Immunohistochemical localization of epinephrine, norepinephrine, catecholamine-synthesizing enzymes, and chromogranin in neuroendocrine cells and tumors. *Am J Pathol* 1986;125:45–54.
192. Capella C, Riva C, Cornaggia M, et al. Histopathology, cytology and cytochemistry of pheochromocytomas and paragangliomas including chemodectomas. *Pathol Res Pract* 1988;183:176–187.
193. Warren WH, Lee I, Gould VE, et al. Paragangliomas of head and neck: ultrastructural and immunohistochemical analysis. *Ultrastr Pathol* 1985;8:333–343.
194. Johnson TL, Zarbo RJ, Lloyd RV, et al. Paragangliomas of the head and neck: immunohistochemical, neuroendocrine and intermediate filament typing. *Mod Pathol* 1988;1:216–223.
195. McNicol AM. Histopathology and immunohistochemistry of adrenal medullary tumors and paragangliomas. *Endocr Pathol* 2006;17:329–336.
196. Kimura N, Sasano N, Yamada R, et al. Immunohistochemical study of chromogranin in 100 cases of pheochromocytoma, carotid body tumor, medullary thyroid carcinoma and carcinoid tumour. *Virchows Arch A Pathol Anat Histopathol* 1988;413:33–38.
197. Chetty R, Pillay P, Jaichand V. Cytokeratin expression in adrenal phaeochromcytomas and extra-adrenal paragangliomas. *J Clin Pathol* 1998;51:477–478.
198. Lehto V-P, Virtanen I, Miettinen M, et al. Neurofilaments in adrenal and extra-adrenal pheochromocytoma: demonstration using immunofluorescence microscopy. *Arch Pathol Lab Med* 1983;107:492–494.
199. Mukai M, Torikata C, Iri H, et al. Expression of neurofilament triplet proteins in human neural tumors: an immunohistochemical study of paraganglioma, ganglioneuroma, ganglioneuroblastoma, and neuroblastoma. *Am J Pathol* 1986;122:28–35.
200. Miettinen M. Synaptophysin and neurofilament proteins as markers for neuroendocrine tumors. *Arch Pathol Lab Med* 1987;3:813–818.
201. Linnoila RI, Lack EE, Steinberg SM, et al. Decreased expression of neuropeptides in malignant paragangliomas: an immunohistochemical study. *Hum Pathol* 1988;19:41–50.
202. Moyana TN, Kontozoglou T. Urinary bladder paragangliomas: an immunohistochemical study. *Arch Pathol Lab Med* 1988;112:70–72.
203. Grignon DT, Ro JY, Mackay B, et al. Paraganglioma of the urinary bladder: immunohistochemical, ultrastructural and DNA flow cytometric studies. *Hum Pathol* 1991;22:1162–1169.
204. Spark RF, Connolly PB, Gluckin DS, et al. ACTH secretion from a functioning pheochromocytoma. *N Engl J Med* 1979;301:416–418.
205. Dahir KM, Gonzalez A, Revelo MP, et al. Ectopic adrenocorticotropic hormone hypersecretion due to a primary pulmonary paraganglioma. *Endocr Pract* 2004;10:424–428.
206. Otsuka F, Miyoshi T, Murakami K, et al. An extra-adrenal abdominal pheochromocytoma causing ectopic ACTH Syndrome. *Am J Hypertens* 2005;18:1364–1368.
207. Willenberg HS, Feldkamp J, Lehmann R, et al. A case of catecholamine and glucocorticoid excess syndrome due to a corticotropin-secreting paraganglioma. *Ann NY Acad Sci* 2006;1073:52–58.
208. Trump DL, Livingston JN, Baylin SB. Watery diarrhea syndrome in an adult with ganglioneuroma–pheochromocytoma: identification of vasoactive intestinal peptide, calcitonin, and catecholamines and assessment of their biologic activity. *Cancer* 1977;40:1526–1532.
209. Viale G, Dell'Orto P, Moro E, et al. Vasoactive intestinal polypeptide-, somatostatin-, and calcitonin-producing adrenal pheochromocytoma associated with the watery diarrhea (WDHA) syndrome: first case report with immunohistochemical findings. *Cancer* 1985;55:1099–1106.
210. Quarles Van Ufford-Mannesse P, Castro Cabezas M, Vroom TM, et al. A patient with neurofibromatosis type 1 and watery diarrhoea syndrome due to a VIP-producing adrenal phaeochromocytoma. *J Intern Med* 1999;246:231–234.
211. Tischler AS, Dayal Y, Balogh K, et al. The distribution of immunoreactive chromogranins, S-100 protein, and vasoactive intestinal peptide in compound tumors of the adrenal medulla. *Hum Pathol* 1987;18:909–917.
212. Mendelsohn G, Eggleston JC, Olson JL, et al. Vasoactive intestinal peptide and its relationship to ganglion cell differentiation in neuroblastic tumors. *Lab Invest* 1979;41:144–149.

213. Koch CA, Vortmeyer AO, Diallo R, et al. Survivin: a novel neuroendocrine marker for pheochromocytoma. *Eur J Endocrinol* 2002;146:381–388.

214. de Krijger RR, van der Harst E, van der Ham F, et al. Prognostic value of p53, bcl-2 and c-erb-2 protein expression in pheochromocytomas. *J Pathol* 1999;188:51–55.

215. Gimm O, Krause U, Brauckhoff M, et al. Distinct expression of galectin-3 in pheochromocytomas. *Ann NY Acad Sci.* 2006;1073:571–577.

216. Miettinen M. Neuroendocrine differentiation in adrenocortical carcinoma: new immunohistochemical findings supported by electron microscopy. *Lab Invest* 1992;66:169–174.

217. Zhang PJ, Genega EM, Tomaszewski JE, et al. The role of calretinin, inhibin, melan-A, bcl-2 and c-kit in differentiating adrenal cortical and medullary tumors: an immunohistochemical study. *Mod Pathol* 2003;16:591–597.

218. Hamid Q, Verndell IM, Ibrahim NB, et al. Extra-adrenal paragangliomas: an immunohistochemical and ultrastructural report. *Cancer* 1987;60:1776–1781.

219. Wang D-G, Barros D, Sa AAB, et al. Oncogene expression in carotid body tumors. *Cancer* 1996;77:2581–2587.

220. Granger JK, Houn H-Y. Head and neck paragangliomas: a clinicopathologic study with DNA flow cytometric analysis. *South Med J* 1990;83:1407–1412.

221. Barnes L, Taylor SR. Carotid body paragangliomas: a clinicopathologic and DNA analysis of 13 tumors. *Arch Otolaryngol Head Neck Surg* 1990;116:447–453.

222. Sauter ER, Hollier LH, Bolton JS, et al. Prognostic value of DNA flow cytometry in paragangliomas of the carotid body. *J Surg Oncol* 1991;46:151–153.

223. Van der Mey AGL, Cornelisse CJ, Hermans J, et al. DNA flow cytometry of hereditary and sporadic paragangliomas (glomus tumours). *Br J Cancer* 1991;63:298–302.

224. Hosaka Y, Rainwater LM, Grant CS, et al. Pheochromocytoma: nuclear deoxyribonucleic acid patterns studied by flow cytometry. *Surgery* 1986;100:1003–1010.

225. Amberson JB, Vaughan ED Jr, Gray GF, et al. Flow cytometric determination of nuclear DNA content in benign adrenal pheochromocytomas. *Urology* 1987;30:102–104.

226. Garcia-Escudero A, de Miguel-Rodriguez M, Moreno-Fernandez A, et al. Prognostic value of DNA flow cytometry in sympathoadrenal paragangliomas. *Anal Quant Cytol Histol* 2001;23:238–244.

227. Douwes Dekker PB, Corver WE, Hogendoorn PC, et al. Multiparameter DNA flow-sorting demonstrates diploidy and SDHD wild-type gene retention in the sustentacular cell compartment of head and neck paragangliomas: chief cells are the only neoplastic component. *J Pathol* 2004;202:456–462.

228. Mauri MF, Mingazzini P, Sisti S, et al. Histomorphometric and morphologic studies of the carotid body and aortic paragangliomas. *Appl Pathol* 1989;7:310–317.

229. Brown HM, Komorowski RA, Wilson SD, et al. Predicting metastasis of pheochromocytomas using DNA flow cytometry and immunohistochemical markers of cell proliferation. A positive correlation between MIB-1 staining and malignant tumor behavior. *Cancer* 1999;86:1583–1589.

230. Zbaren P, Lehmann W. Carotid body paraganglioma with metastases. *Laryngoscope* 1985;95:450–454.

231. Heinrich MC, Harris AE, Bell WR. Metastatic intravagal paraganglioma: case report and review of the literature. *Am J Med* 1985;78:1017–1024.

232. Zak FG, Lawson W. *The Paraganglionic Chemoreceptor System: Physiology, Pathology, and Clinical Medicine.* New York, NY: Springer-Verlag, 1982.

233. Melicow MM. One hundred cases of pheochromocytoma (107 tumors) at the Columbia-Presbyterian Medical Center 1926–1976: a clinicopathological analysis. *Cancer* 1977;40:1987–2004.

234. Symington T, Goodall AL. Studies in pheochromocytoma. I. Pathological aspects. *Glas Med J* 1953;34:75–96.

235. Van Heerden JA, Sheps SG, Hamberger B, et al. Pheochromocytoma: current status and changing trends. *Surgery* 1982;91:367–373.

236. Olson JR, Abell MR. Nonfunctional nonchromaffin paragangliomas of the retroperitoneum. *Cancer* 1969;23:1358–1367.

237. Glenn F, Gray GF. Functional tumors of the organ of Zuckerkandl. *Ann Surg* 1976;183:578–586.

238. Sclafani LM, Woodruff JM, Brennan MF. Extra adrenal retroperitoneal paragangliomas: natural history and response to treatment. *Surgery* 1990;108:1124–1130.

239. Odze R, Begin LR. Malignant paraganglioma of the posterior mediastinum: a case report and review of the literature. *Cancer* 1990;65:564–569.

240. Neville AM. The adrenal medulla. In Symington T, ed. *Functional Pathology of the Human Adrenal Gland.* Baltimore, MD: Williams & Wilkins, 1969:217–324.

241. Thompson LD. Pheochromocytoma of the adrenal gland scaled score (PASS) to separate benign from malignant neoplasms: a clinicopathologic and immunophenotypic study of 100 cases. *Am J Surg Pathol* 2002;26:551–566.

242. Gao B, Meng F, Bian W, et al. Development and validation of pheochromocytoma of the adrenal gland scaled score for predicting malignant pheochromocytomas. *Urology* 2006;68:282–286.

243. deKrijger RR, van Nederveen FH, Korpershoek E, et al. New developments in the detection of the clinical behavior of pheochromocytomas and paragangliomas. *Endocr Pathol* 2006;17:137–141.

244. Tischler AS, Kimura N, McNicol AM. Pathology of pheochromocytoma and extra-adrenal paraganglioma. *Ann N Y Acad Sci* 2006;1073:557–570.

245. Kimura N, Watanabe T, Noshiro T, et al. Histological grading of adrenal and extra-adrenal pheochromocytomas and relationship to prognosis: a clinicopathological analysis of 116 adrenal pheochromocytomas and 30 extra-adrenal sympathetic paragangliomas including 38 malignant tumors. *Endocr Pathol* 2005;16:23–32.

246. van der Harst E, Bruining HA, Jaap BH, et al. Proliferative index in pheochromocytomas: does it predict the occurrence of metastases? *J Pathol* 2000;191:175–180.

247. John H, Ziegler WH, Hauri D, et al. Pheochromocytomas: can malignant potential be predicted? *Urology* 1999;53:679–685.

248. Lloyd RV, Shapiro B, Sisson JC, et al. Paragangliomas: an immunohistochemical study of pheochromocytomas. *Arch Pathol Lab Med* 1984;108:541–544.

249. Lloyd RV, Blaivas M, Wilson BS. Distribution of chromogranin and S-100 protein in normal and abnormal adrenal medullary tissues. *Arch Pathol Lab Med* 1985;109:633–635.

250. Schroder HD, Johannsen L. Demonstration of S-100 protein in sustentacular cells of pheochromocytomas and paragangliomas. *Histopathology* 1986;10:1023–1033.

251. Kliewer KE, Wen D-R, Cancilla PA, et al. Paragangliomas: assessment of prognosis by histologic, immunohistochemical, and ultrastructural techniques. *Hum Pathol* 1989;20:29–39.

252. Kliewer KE, Cochran AJ. A review of the histology, ultrastructure, immunohistology, and molecular biology of extra-adrenal paragangliomas. *Arch Pathol Lab Med* 1989;113:1209–1218.

253. Bhansali SA, Bojrab DI, Zarbo RJ. Malignant paragangliomas of the head and neck: clinical and immunohistochemical characterization. *Otolaryngol Head Neck Surg* 1991;104:132.

254. Unger P, Hoffman K, Pertsemlidis D, et al. S-100 protein-positive sustentacular cells in malignant and locally aggressive adrenal pheochromocytomas. *Arch Pathol Lab Med* 1991;115:484–487.

255. Helman LJ, Cohen PS, Averbuch SD, et al. Neuropeptide Y expression distinguishes malignant from benign pheochromocytoma. *J Clin Oncol* 1989;7:1720–1725.

256. Furihata M, Ohtsuki Y. Immunohistochemical characterization of HLA-DR-antigen positive dendritic cells in pheochromocytomas and paragangliomas as a prognostic marker. *Virchows Arch A Pathol Anat Histopathol* 1991;418:33–39.

257. Salmenkivi K, Haglund C, Arola J, et al. Increased expression of tenascin in pheochromocytomas correlates with malignancy. *Am J Surg Pathol* 2001;25:1419–1423.

258. Salmenkivi K, Haglund C, Ristimaki A, et al. Increased expression of cyclooxygenase-2 in malignant pheochromocytomas. *J Clin Endocrinal Metab* 2001;86:5615–5619.

259. Fuentes C, Menendez E, Pineda J, et al. The malignant potential of a succinate dehydrogenase subunit B germline mutation. *J Endocrinol Invest* 2006; 29:350–352.

260. Van Nederveen FH, Dinjens WN, Korpershoek E, et al. The occurrence of SDHB gene mutations in pheochromocytoma. *Ann N Y Acad Sci* 2006;1073:177–182.

261. Havekes B, Corssmit EP, Jansen JC, et al. Malignant paragangliomas associated with mutation in the succinate dehydrogenase D gene. *J Clin Endocrinol Metab* 2007;92:1245–1248.

262. Janetschek G, Neumann HP. Laparoscopic surgery for pheochromocytoma. *Urol Clin North Am* 2001;28:97–105.

263. Li ML, Fitzgerald PA, Price DC, et al. Iatrogenic pheochromocytomatosis: a previously unreported result of laparoscopic adrenalectomy. *Surgery* 2001;130:1072–1077.

264. Taylor HB, Helwig EB. Benign nonchromaffin paragangliomas of the duodenum. *Virchows Arch A Pathol Anat Histopathol* 1962;335:356–366.

265. Kepes JJ, Zacharias DL. Gangliocytic paragangliomas of the duodenum: a report of two cases with light and electron microscopic examination. *Cancer* 1971; 27:61–70.

266. Reed RJ, Daroca PL Jr, Harkin JC. Gangliocytic paraganglioma. *Am J Surg Pathol* 1977;1:207–216.

267. Perrone T, Sibley RK, Rosai J. Duodenal gangliocytic paraganglioma: an immunohistochemical and ultrastructural study and a hypothesis concerning its origin. *Am J Surg Pathol* 1985;9:31–41.

268. Hamid QA, Bishop AE, Rode J, et al. Duodenal gangliocytic paragangliomas: a study of 10 cases with immunocytochemical neuroendocrine markers. *Hum Pathol* 1986;17:1151–1157.

269. Scheithauer BW, Nora FE, Lechago J, et al. Duodenal gangliocytic paraganglioma: clinicopathologic and immunocytochemical study of 11 cases. *Am J Clin Pathol* 1986;86:559–565.

270. Burke AP, Helwig EB. Gangliocytic paraganglioma. *Am J Clin Pathol* 1989;92:1–9.

271. van Eeden S, Offerhaus GJA, Peterse HL, et al. Gangliocytic paraganglioma of the appendix. *Histopathology* 2000;36:47–49.

272. Llena J, Wisoff HS, Hirano A. Gangliocytic paraganglioma in cauda equina region with biochemical and neuropathological studies. *J Neurosurg* 1982;56:280–282.

273. Witkiewicz A, Galler A, Yeo CJ, et al. Gangliocytic paraganglioma: case report and review of the literature. *J Gastrointest Surg* 2007;11:1351–1354.

274. Palau MA, Merino MJ, Quezado M. Corticotropin-producing pulmonary gangliocytic paraganglioma associated with Cushing's syndrome. *Hum Pathol* 2006;37:623–626.

275. Böker D-K, Wassman H, Solymosi L. Paragangliomas of the spinal canal. *Surg Neurol* 1983;19:461–468.

276. Lipper S, Decker RE. Paraganglioma of the cauda equina: a histologic, immunohistochemical, and ultrastructural study and review of the literature. *Surg Neurol* 1984;22:415–420.

277. Shuangshoti S, Suwanwela N, Suwanwela C. Combined paraganglioma and glioma of conus medullaris and cauda equina. *J Surg Oncol* 1984;25:162–167.

278. Sonneland PRL, Scheithauer BW, Lechago J, et al. Paraganglioma of the cauda equina region: clinicopathologic study of 31 cases with special reference to immunocytopathology and ultrastructure. *Cancer* 1986;58:1720–1735.

279. Ashkenazi E, Onesti ST, Kader A, et al. Paraganglioma of the filum terminale: case report and literature review. *J Spinal Disord* 1998;11:540–542.

280. Labrousse F, Leboutet MJ, Petit B et al. Cytokeratin expression in paragangliomas of the cauda equine. *Clin Neuropathol* 1999;18:208–213.

281. Luschka H. Ueber die drüsenartige natur des sogenannten ganglion intercaroticum. *Arch F Anat Physiol Wissensch Med Jahrq S* 1862;405–414.

282. Hollinshead WH. A comparative study of the glomus coccygeum and the carotid body. *Anat Rec* 1942;84:1–13.

283. Albrecht S, Zbieranowski I. Incidental glomus coccygeum: when a normal structure looks like a tumor. *Am J Surg Pathol* 1990;14:922–924.

284. Gatalica Z, Wang L, Luci ET, et al. Glomus coccygeum in surgical pathology specimens: small troublemaker. *Arch Pathol Lab Med* 1990;123:905–908.

285. Santos LD, Chow C, Kennerson AR. Glomus coccygeum may mimic glomus tumour. *Pathology* 2002;34:339–343.

286. Rahemtullah A, Szyfelbein K, Zembowicz A. Glomus coccygeum: report of a case and review of the literature. *Am J Dermatopathol* 2005;27:497–499.

CHAPTER

16

Robert W. McKenna
Steven H. Kroft

Disorders of Bone Marrow

THE BONE MARROW BIOPSY PROCEDURE

The bone marrow biopsy is a routine technique in the diagnosis of hematologic disorders, metastatic tumors, and infectious and metabolic diseases. Experience in interpretation of marrow biopsies is a valuable asset to the surgical pathologist. The major indications for a marrow biopsy are listed in Table 16.1 (1–4). A systematic approach to obtaining and processing bone marrow specimens is essential for optimal bone marrow examination and laboratory operations. The process must include good communication with the patient's physician, especially if the physician will perform the biopsy procedure. Advance notice of an impending marrow biopsy and knowledge of clinical findings and differential diagnosis allow for formulation of a diagnostic strategy.

The design of most bone marrow biopsy needles is similar and the principle and technique for using them is basically the same (5). Needles with various-sized lumina are available, including those of small gauge designed specifically for pediatric patients. Users must have a detailed knowledge of the anatomy of the iliac crest and be well trained in the recommended technique for a specific biopsy needle. Inexperienced individuals should perform trephine biopsies under the supervision of a physician thoroughly familiar with the procedure until they have gained adequate experience. The marrow biopsy is a safe procedure in the hands of persons adequately trained who exercise good judgment and proper caution.

Several methods for processing the marrow specimen provide excellent material for microscopic examination. The techniques used are determined by individual preference and suitability for a specific laboratory. The methods described here are those preferred by the authors (4,6).

The biopsy procedure may be performed in a patient's hospital room or in an outpatient clinic using sterile technique. Local anesthesia is used on the skin and periosteum over the intended biopsy site. Prebiopsy sedation is often helpful in pediatric patients and adults who have a high level of anxiety about the procedure. The posterior iliac crest is the preferred anatomic site for the biopsy; the anterior iliac crest may be used as an alternative. The sternum should never be the site for trephine biopsies. Marrow aspirates can be performed on the sternum with a specially designed needle equipped with a guard device to prevent advance of the needle through the sternum. Bilateral iliac crest biopsies are recommended to assess diseases in which diagnostic lesions are likely to be distributed focally, such as lymphomas and metastatic tumors (7–11).

Immediately after obtaining the trephine biopsy specimen, and prior to placing it in fixative, it should be imprinted on several glass slides. In cases where a marrow aspirate is not obtainable, the touch preparations will provide the only material for cytologic study on Romanowsky-stained slides. B5 fixative is recommended for marrow core biopsies. For laboratories that restrict use of mercury-based fixatives, AZF or formalin can be used as a substitute, but significant degradation of section quality may be experienced. Following fixation, the specimen is decalcified and processed by routine histologic techniques. Sections should be no thicker than 4 μm. In cases where lesions are expected to be small and distributed focally, sections should be mounted on the slides at multiple levels of the specimen. Samples from the ribbon can be saved temporarily and used if additional sections are required for histochemical or immunohistochemical (IHC) stains. In most instances, well-prepared paraffin sections are adequate for diagnosis when combined with marrow aspirate smears and appropriate special studies, but some laboratories prefer plastic embedded biopsies, which often provide superior cytologic detail (6,12,13).

The marrow aspirate specimen is preferably obtained a few millimeters from the site of the trephine biopsy through the same skin incision. The major portion of the aspirated specimen can be placed in ethylene diamine tetra-acetic acid (EDTA) anticoagulant and the remainder used to make smears at the patient's bedside. Once smears are made at the bedside, the bone marrow aspirate and trephine biopsy specimens should be transported to the laboratory for processing. In the laboratory, the anticoagulated portion of the bone marrow is separated into fluid and particle portions. Smear preparations can

---

TABLE 16.1

Indications for Bone Marrow Trephine Biopsies

- Assessment of patients with unexplained blood cytopenias
- Suspected diagnoses of lymphoma, leukemia, myeloproliferative or myelodysplastic syndromes, lymphoproliferative disorders, plasma cell dyscrasias, and metastatic tumor
- Monitoring therapy and recurrence of neoplastic disease
- Suspected infectious disease, particularly granulomatous disease, and assessment of fever of unknown origin
- Suspected storage disease, metabolic bone disease, and myelofibrosis
- Evaluation for bone marrow transplant engraftment
- Assessment of patients with AIDS for cytopenias, infections, and malignancy

be made from the nucleated cell layer (buffy coat) of centrifuged marrow fluid and by particle crush techniques. The remaining particles are then aggregated and used to make sections.

SPECIAL PROCEDURES

When the bone marrow is examined with thorough knowledge of the clinical findings, a strategy for optimal use of the available specimens for morphologic assessment and special studies can be devised. In most hematopathology practices, a host of special techniques are available to aid in diagnosis. These include histochemistry, IHC, flow cytometry, cytogenetics/fluorescent in situ hybridization (FISH), and various molecular analyses. Use of a multitechnique approach is not always necessary when morphologic findings are diagnostic but, increasingly, supplemental studies provide needed information not only for diagnosis but also for prognosis assessment and optimal patient management. When flow cytometry or molecular analysis is required, aspirated marrow is collected in EDTA or acid-citrate-dextrose (ACD) tubes and sent for immediate processing. For cytogenetic analysis, heparin anticoagulant is preferred. In cases where a bone marrow aspirate cannot be obtained, cells teased from a fresh trephine biopsy may be used for flow cytometry, cytogenetics, and molecular studies. For infectious disease assessment in patients with a fever of unknown origin or in AIDS cases, microbiologic cultures may be performed on fresh aspirated marrow or trephine biopsies.

HEMATOPOIESIS AND BONE MARROW HISTOLOGY

For most individuals, the bone marrow comprises 3.5% to 6% of total body weight. It is the major organ of hematopoiesis and is both a primary and secondary lymphoid organ that provides an environment for cell development and immunologic interaction (14). The marrow consists of hematopoietic cells and adipose and stromal tissues. The stroma is composed of connective tissue and vascular structures that include arterioles, venules, capillaries, and a system of sinusoids.

Hematopoiesis in the bone marrow begins at mid gestation and is the major site of hematopoiesis by birth. In the first year of life, hematopoiesis occurs in both the axial and radial skeleton. By the mid-teens, the flat bones of the central skeleton usually become the sole sites of hematopoietic marrow. Hematopoiesis consists of two major cell lineages, myeloid and lymphoid. Their common precursor is a bone marrow pluripotent stem cell. Differentiation and maturation of the four types of myeloid cells (granulocytes, monocytes, erythrocytes, and megakaryocytes) and some lymphoid cells occur in the bone marrow; most lymphocytes, however, differentiate and mature primarily outside of the bone marrow.

All types of myeloid cells have a common progenitor. The first precursor of each of the four myeloid lineages is a blast. Neutrophils are in two functional groups in the marrow, the mitotic and storage pools. The earliest precursors (myeloblasts, promyelocytes, and myelocytes) are present in the mitotic pool for 2 to 3 days, where they multiply and mature. The cells of the mitotic pool are mostly found in paratrabecular and perivas-

cular locations. Additional maturation occurs in the storage pool, which is composed of metamyelocytes, bands, and segmented neutrophils. Normally, cells remain in the storage pool for approximately 5 to 7 days. Neutrophils move from the storage pool in a unidirectional fashion, to the blood and finally to the tissues. Monocytes have an origin closely related to that of neutrophils, but maturational stages are less well defined. Histiocytes, the tissue form of monocytes, are commonly observed in bone marrow. As erythroid precursors mature in the bone marrow, they become smaller and richer in hemoglobin. Early precursors are found in randomly distributed cellular islands that are generally perivascular. After extruding their nucleus, erythrocytes spend the final 2 to 3 days in the marrow while their cytoplasm continues to mature. Megakaryocytes are normally present as single cells that are randomly distributed throughout the bone marrow. As they mature, they become progressively larger and increase their nuclear lobes.

The bone marrow provides an environment for lymphocyte development and immunologic interaction. Variable numbers of B-cell precursors (hematogones) are present in bone marrow, most notably in children. However, most lymphocyte development occurs in extramedullary sites, especially in lymph nodes. Immunologic markers can characterize lymphoid maturational stages, but a morphologic developmental sequence is not recognized in lymphocytes to the degree that it is in myeloid cells. Lymphocytes comprise approximately 10% of marrow cells in normal adults. Plasma cells are found primarily in a perivascular distribution and account for approximately 1% to 2% of marrow hematopoietic cells.

Osteoblasts and osteoclasts are found along the endosteal surface of bone trabeculae in trephine biopsies, but are uncommon in normal aspirate smears except in children; they may be found in aspirates in several pathologic conditions. Mast cells are found adjacent to endosteal cells and in perivascular locations and are a minor component in normal bone marrow.

BONE MARROW CELLULARITY

Assessment of marrow cellularity is important for diagnosis and treatment in several clinical conditions. These include evaluation of blood cytopenias, following patients on chemotherapy, and assessing engraftment in marrow transplant recipients. Biopsy sections are preferable to aspirate smears for assessment of cellularity. Aspirate smears are affected by hemodilution and variations in technique. Biopsies from the posterior iliac crest generally reflect the cellularity of the overall hematopoietic marrow (3). However, local marrow insults, particularly radiotherapy, may leave the iliac crest unrepresentative of overall marrow cellularity.

In children in the first decade of life, approximately 80% of ilium bone marrow is hematopoietic and 20% fat, a ratio of 4:1. There is gradual change to a ratio of approximately 1:1 to 1.2:1 by age 30. The cellularity remains relatively stable until the seventh decade, when hematopoietic marrow and bone trabeculae decrease and adipose tissue increases (15–17). There is significant variation in cellularity in different individuals of the same age (3). The proportion of hematopoietic marrow may also vary in different areas of the ilium; in adults the immediate subcortical marrow is often less cellular than deeper areas, a finding that is accentuated with aging (3).

TABLE 16.2

Causes of Pancytopenia

Bone marrow failure
   Aplastic anemia
   Overwhelming infections
   AIDS
Ineffective hematopoiesis
   Megaloblastic anemia
   Myelodysplastic syndrome
   AIDS
Bone marrow replacement/invasion
   Leukemia/lymphoma
   Metastatic tumor
   Myelofibrosis
   Metabolic bone disease
   Storage disease
   Granulomatous/infectious disease
Peripheral destruction
   Hypersplenic syndromes
   Miscellaneous other disorders

PANCYTOPENIA

There are many causes of pancytopenia (Table 16.2), and marrow cellularity and composition differ in relationship to the cause. The marrow is generally hypocellular in cases of pancytopenia caused by a primary production defect. Cytopenias resulting from ineffective hematopoiesis, increased peripheral utilization or destruction of cells, and bone marrow invasive processes are usually associated with a normocellular or hypercellular marrow.

HYPOCELLULAR BONE MARROW

The marrow in severe aplastic anemia is markedly hypocellular with a profound decrease in hematopoietic tissue and a corresponding increase in marrow fat (Fig. 16.1). Macrophages containing hemosiderin are often prominent and increased numbers of lymphocytes, plasma cells, and mast cells are observed. Lymphocytes may be found in loose aggregates or nodules (18).

Scattered erythroid islands are sometimes present and occasional granulocytes and megakaryocytes may be observed. The quantity of residual hematopoietic cells varies with the severity of the aplastic anemia. Careful evaluation of the marrow sections may help in predicting the likelihood of spontaneous recovery; generally, the more severe the aplasia, the less likelihood of recovery (18). When a single blood cell type is diminished due to a primary production defect (e.g., pure red-cell aplasia or amegakaryocytosis), cells of that lineage are decreased or absent but the overall cellularity of the marrow may be only slightly altered.

HYPERCELLULAR BONE MARROW

In a hypercellular bone marrow there is increased hematopoietic tissue and decreased fat. In most cases hypercellularity is a normal physiologic response to increased demand for blood cell production. Physiologic causes include increased granulopoiesis in systemic infections and increased erythropoiesis in hemolytic anemias or following blood loss. Pathologic hypercellularity results from ineffective hematopoiesis, dysplastic hematopoiesis, leukemia, myeloproliferative syndromes, and invasive neoplasms. The cause of the hypercellularity is generally reflected in the composition of the marrow cells.

CELLULARITY IN NEOPLASTIC DISEASE

Determination of marrow cellularity is important at diagnosis and in monitoring patients with leukemia and other hematopoietic neoplasms. The estimated tumor load (percentage of marrow space replaced) is a staging criterion for some malignancies (19–21). Assessment of changes in marrow cellularity in response to chemotherapy is useful in managing treatment. In successful induction chemotherapy for acute leukemia, there is early marrow hypocellularity caused by the cytotoxic effect of the drugs (22,23). In this stage there is predominantly necrotic tissue and proteinaceous debris in the marrow space. Other findings include sinusoidal dilation, degenerative stromal changes, and increased reticulin. In the blood there is marked pancytopenia. If a significant reduction in cellularity is not achieved in the first week of induction chemotherapy, it may

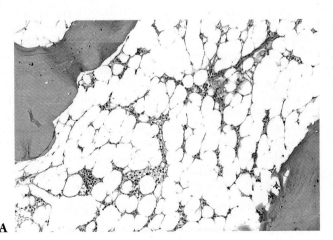

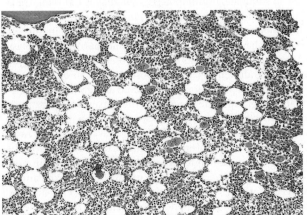

Figure 16.1. **(A)** Bone marrow section from a child with severe aplastic anemia. The marrow is markedly hypocellular with no identifiable hematopoietic cells. **(B)** A nearly normocellular bone marrow following transplantation.

signal resistance to the therapy and portend a worse prognosis (24). With successful induction, regeneration of normal bone marrow begins in the first week or two after the initiation of therapy. If growth factors are not administered, erythroid regeneration is generally first, followed in sequence by granulocyte and megakaryocyte regeneration. In patients treated with G-CSF, granulocyte production occurs most rapidly. Hematopoietic marrow regeneration accelerates in the second and third weeks, with blood counts showing recovery and in some patients approaching normal within 28 days. Slow or asynchronous recovery of blood counts toward normal may indicate resistant disease. However, retarded bone marrow regeneration may also be caused by medications, virus infections (especially cytomegalovirus [CMV], human herpes virus-6 [HHV6], and parvovirus B19), marrow stroma damage, and extraordinary sensitivity to chemotherapy (23,25). With remission and regeneration of normal hematopoietic tissue, the marrow returns to normal or near-normal cellularity; the bone marrow may remain mildly hypocellular in patients on maintenance chemotherapy. If blood cytopenias appear following complete remission of the disease, a bone marrow examination is indicated to determine whether the leukemia has relapsed or the marrow is suppressed by maintenance chemotherapy or other causes (25).

CHANGES IN CELLULARITY FOLLOWING BONE MARROW TRANSPLANT

Assessment of marrow cellularity is important when following hematopoietic stem cell or bone marrow transplant recipients for engraftment and rejection (26). Generally the sequence of change is similar for bone marrow and cord blood or peripheral blood stem cell transplants; the changes are similar to regeneration following chemotherapy, described earlier (22,23). There is usually evidence of significant hematopoiesis in the bone marrow prior to any changes in blood counts, but, for practical reasons, assessment of engraftment is usually done by monitoring blood counts (27). A bone marrow may be performed if blood counts do not recover in the expected time and sequence. In allogeneic transplants, the first good evidence of engraftment of transplanted marrow is found 1 to 2 weeks posttransplant. Growth factor therapy, such as erythropoietin and granulocyte colony-stimulating factor (G-CSF), accelerates the process of regeneration and may alter its sequence. Many patients receive G-CSF to stimulate granulopoiesis immediately following transplantation, and left-shifted granulopoiesis with numerous large promyelocytes and myelocytes are observed early in the engraftment phase; a slight increase in bone marrow myeloblasts and circulating myeloblasts are often observed. There is usually obvious engraftment by 3 weeks posttransplantation, and clusters of erythroid precursors are observed along with abundance of maturing granulocyte precursors; there may be only scattered megakaryocytes. Between 4 and 8 weeks, the marrow cellularity increases and blood counts rise progressively to normal or near-normal levels. The rate of engraftment and return to normocellularity varies from patient to patient. In some cases, engraftment of one or more cell lineages may be unusually retarded. Patients who receive autologous transplants generally recover their blood counts more rapidly than do allogeneic marrow recipients. Declining blood counts after the fourth week posttransplant may be indicative of an infectious complication or graft failure. Recurrence of a neoplastic disease generally occurs somewhat later.

The usual first indication of graft rejection of an allogeneic bone marrow transplant is a decline in erythroid precursors. This may precede, by several days or weeks, the rejection of all of the marrow cell lineages and return to aplasia. Patients with graft-versus-host disease (GVHD) may have increased numbers of lymphocytes, plasma cells, and eosinophils in their marrow; lymphocytic aggregates and granulomas have been noted in some cases (23).

GROWTH FACTORS

Erythropoietin, G-CSF, and granulocyte-monocyte colony-stimulating factor (GM-CSF) are commonly used to enhance hematopoiesis in patients with marrow suppression following chemotherapy or a marrow or stem cell transplant, and in some cases of primary or secondary anemia and neutropenia. Patients treated with G-CSF or GM-CSF exhibit an early predominance of granulopoiesis, which often evolves to granulocytic hyperplasia. There are increased large, toxic-appearing promyelocytes and myelocytes that may occupy much of the marrow space. The blood smear may show a leukemoid reaction with increased and immature neutrophils, eosinophils, and monocytes. Myeloblasts and neutrophils with hyposegmentation or hypersegmentation of nuclei, Döhle bodies, and atypical granulation are frequently observed on blood smears (28). In patients with acute myeloid leukemia (AML), the presence of strikingly left-shifted granulopoiesis, circulating myeloblasts, and dysplastic features in some of the maturing neutrophils may be confused with residual AML in the early post–G-CSF–treated marrow. In a small number of patients, treatment with GM-CSF has been reported to induce increased marrow fibrosis (29). G-CSF and GM-CSF have no effect on red-cell and megakaryocyte recovery. Erythropoietin stimulates erythropoiesis and may induce erythroid hyperplasia in a marrow in early recovery.

SEROUS ATROPHY

Serous atrophy, sometimes referred to as gelatinous transformation of marrow adipose tissue, is usually associated with severe malnutrition (30–33). It may be found in kwashiorkor, anorexia nervosa, cachexia, starvation from other causes, and AIDS. Patients are generally anemic and may have leukopenia or thrombocytopenia. The bone marrow is hypocellular with decreased hematopoietic tissue. Hematopoietic cells are found in clusters within areas of the degenerating fat or in focal uninvolved areas of the marrow. Fat cells are decreased and smaller than normal. The histologic appearance may resemble edema, necrosis, or amyloid (30) (Fig. 16.2). The extracellular gelatinous material is amorphous and faintly eosinophilic. It consists primarily of hyaluronic acid in patients with anorexia and starvation (31). In patients with AIDS, the gelatinous material contains large amounts of sulfated glycosaminoglycan in addition to hyaluronic acid (33). Sulfated glycosaminoglycan has been shown to adversely affect erythropoiesis and may contribute to the anemia in patients with AIDS.

BONE MARROW NECROSIS

Bone marrow necrosis is seen occasionally in patients with infectious diseases, leukemia, lymphoma, metastatic tumor, systemic lupus erythematosus, sickle cell anemia, and miscellaneous other disorders (34–38). The necrosis may involve extensive

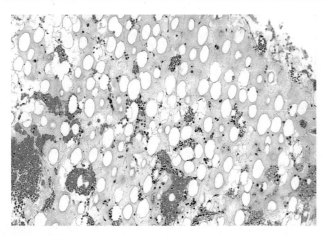

Figure 16.2. Serous atrophy of fat (gelatinous transformation) in a bone marrow biopsy taken from a 36-year-old man with AIDS. Note the reduction in hematopoietic tissue, the small fat cells, and amorphous extracellular material.

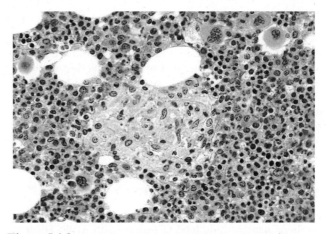

Figure 16.3. A small sarcoid-like granuloma found in a staging bone marrow biopsy for Hodgkin lymphoma. Stains for microorganisms and cultures were negative.

areas of marrow or may affect only focal areas of a malignant tumor or granuloma. In cases of generalized marrow necrosis, the underlying primary disorder is frequently complicated by infection and sepsis.

If necrosis is of recent origin, the individual cells are recognizable in the sections, but show early nuclear and cytoplasmic degenerative changes (e.g., pyknosis, granular cytoplasm). With more advanced necrosis karyolysis occurs; nuclei are not clearly visualized and the cytoplasm is uniformly eosinophilic. With advanced degenerative changes, only amorphous debris remains. Macrophages containing phagocytosed material are often present at this stage. Occasionally patients with lymphoblastic leukemia, chronic myelogenous leukemia, Burkitt lymphoma, and metastatic tumors have extensively necrotic marrow that precludes a diagnosis. An additional marrow biopsy in another anatomic site may reveal viable diagnostic tissue. If not, the biopsy may be repeated after a few days or weeks, when marrow and the neoplastic tissue have regenerated. It is generally important to characterize a bone marrow neoplasm as quickly as possible. Therefore, if at least a few viable cells can be obtained, special studies such as immunophenotyping or molecular analysis should be performed. Some IHC stains are useful on necrotic tissue. Involved tissue in other anatomic sites should always be sought.

INFLAMMATORY DISORDERS OF THE BONE MARROW

GRANULOMAS

Granulomas may be incidental findings in bone marrow trephine biopsies or discovered during the course of evaluation for infectious disease or a fever of unknown origin (FUO). The majority of bone marrow granulomas have no demonstrable infectious etiology. Despite this, appropriate special stains and microbiologic cultures should generally be performed. Most of the granulomas without an infectious etiology consist of epithelioid histiocytes, lymphocytes, occasional giant cells, and eosinophils. They are usually small, focal, and well circumscribed. These nonspecific granulomas have been reported in several

conditions, including sarcoidosis, Hodgkin disease, non-Hodgkin lymphoma, other malignancies, and miscellaneous other conditions (39–45) (Fig. 16.3).

Bone marrow granulomas with an infectious etiology are found in mycobacterial and fungal infections, brucellosis, typhoid fever, Q fever, and viral infections including infectious mononucleosis, cytomegalovirus infections, and herpes zoster (44,46–48). There are no morphologic features that are pathognomonic of a particular infection. Necrosis, commonly present in mycobacterial and histoplasma infections, may also be found in other infections and in granulomas resulting from immune vasculitis. Intracellular yeast can often be identified in hematoxylin and eosin (H&E)-stained sections of granulomas in cryptococcosis and histoplasmosis, but are often few in number and difficult to recognize (47). Appropriate cytochemical stains and cultures for mycobacterium and fungi should always be performed. Cultures of bone marrow aspirates may be positive in several types of infections when the special stains on trephine sections are negative.

Lipid granulomas are a relatively common finding in marrow sections (49). They are usually small and composed of macrophages with lipid vacuoles, lymphocytes, plasma cells, eosinophils, and occasionally giant cells. Large, extracellular lipid deposits may be observed. Lipid granulomas may be adjacent to or incorporated into a loose aggregate of lymphocytes.

Bone marrow aspirate smears are often normal, even when several granulomas are identified on the marrow sections. Occasionally clusters or sheets of histiocytes are observed on the smear. In some mycobacterial and yeast infections, histiocytes may contain intracellular microorganisms.

NONSPECIFIC INFLAMMATORY REACTIONS

Nonspecific inflammatory changes accompany several marrow disorders, including acute and chronic infections, malignant tumors, and collagen-vascular diseases. In acute inflammation, an exudative reaction with increased mature granulocytes, edema, and necrosis is observed. In chronic infections or malignancies, decreased hematopoiesis with increased lymphocytes, plasma cells, and mast cells is more common (50). When the disease process is prolonged, hematopoiesis is diminished and reticulin fibrosis and alterations of vascularity may be present.

REACTIVE MYELOFIBROSIS

Reactive myelofibrosis can occur in infectious and metabolic disorders, neoplastic disease, and secondary to various physical and chemical agents (51–54). The underlying disease process is generally identified in the biopsy sections or is known from the patient's medical history. The fibrosis is confined to the areas involved by the primary disease and may consist of increased reticulin fibers only or variable amounts of collagen. The bone trabeculae may be normal or manifest increased osteoblastic or osteoclastic changes.

ACQUIRED IMMUNODEFICIENCY SYNDROME

Several types of pathologic changes are commonly observed in the bone marrow and blood of patients with AIDS. These include various cytopenias, changes in marrow cellularity, ineffective hematopoiesis, dysplasia, hyperchromatic and bare megakaryocyte nuclei, increased marrow plasma cells, increased histiocytes, serous atrophy, reactive polymorphous lymphohistiocytic lesions, granulomas, and involvement by lymphomas (33,55–64). Most of the changes are found in the more advanced stages of HIV infection. Although none is specific for AIDS, a combination of several is strongly suggestive of the diagnosis. The reactive and other nonneoplastic changes in the marrow can resemble findings in myelodysplastic syndromes, myeloproliferative disorders, or lymphomas. A thorough history and familiarity with the histologic features typical of HIV infection are essential to avoid an erroneous diagnosis of a hematopoietic neoplasm (63).

A bone marrow biopsy may be performed in patients infected with HIV who have blood cytopenias, infectious disease symptomatology, or suspected lymphoma. The marrow cellularity in patients with blood cytopenias may be normal, increased, or decreased depending on the cause; the majority have a normocellular or hypercellular bone marrow (61). A single cell lineage may be hyperplastic in patients with hemolytic anemia or immune thrombocytopenia (65). The cause of blood cytopenias, ineffective hematopoiesis, and myelodysplasia is often multifactorial. A direct effect of HIV infection on bone marrow stem cells may contribute, but altered cytokine regulation of hematopoiesis and autoimmune phenomenon are probably more important (63,66,67). In addition to these factors, many patients

are chronically infected, malnourished, and receiving several drugs, some of which may suppress myelopoiesis and cause dysplasia. For example, azidothymidine (AZT) causes myelosuppression, which may lead to macrocytic anemia and neutropenia. Pancytopenia and a hypocellular bone marrow are uncommonly related to AZT (68). Many agents used to treat secondary infections and neoplasms also cause marrow suppression.

Mycobacterial, histoplasma, and cryptococcal infections are particularly likely to involve the marrow of patients with AIDS; rarely, *Pneumocystis carinii* is found in bone marrow (69) (Figs. 16.4 through 16.6). Granulomas, histiocytic clusters, diffuse histiocytic infiltrates, and marrow necrosis may be observed (56,59,60,62,70). In some cases of *Mycobacterium avium intracellulare* infection, there is no clear evidence of disease in routine sections, but organisms are identified in scattered histiocytes with acid-fast stains. Cultures and special stains for microorganisms may be indicated in patients with AIDS, even when granulomas or necrosis are not observed in the biopsy sections.

Persistent red-cell aplasia in patients with AIDS may be caused by chronic parvovirus B19 infection (71–73). The bone marrow may exhibit red-cell aplasia with scattered giant erythroblasts or normal numbers of variably dysplastic erythroid precursors with intranuclear inclusions that are most apparent on biopsy sections (Fig. 16.7). Documentation of suspected parvovirus B19 infection should be attempted by polymerase chain reaction (PCR) or in situ hybridization techniques on the bone marrow because serologic studies for antibodies to parvovirus are often negative.

Polymorphous reactive lymphohistiocytic lesions are commonly found in marrow sections from patients with AIDS (59,60,62,74). They are composed of a polymorphous population of lymphocytes, plasma cells, epithelioid histiocytes, eosinophils, and endothelial cells. In some cases these lesions replace large areas of the marrow (56,62,74,75). Diffuse histiocytic proliferations such as those seen in the infection (virus)-associated hemophagocytic syndrome (see the section "Histiocytic Proliferations" later in the chapter) may be observed in very ill or terminal patients (76).

Patients with AIDS have an increased incidence of both Hodgkin and non-Hodgkin lymphoma, and the bone marrow is frequently involved. The most common types of non-Hodgkin

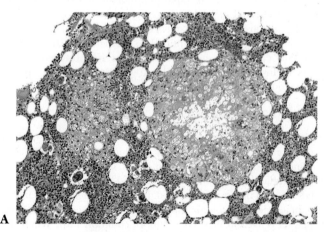

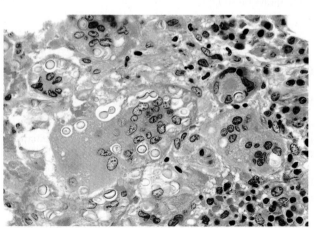

A   B

Figure 16.4. (A) Bone marrow section from a patient with AIDS showing two granulomas. (B) Numerous yeast forms are seen in the cytoplasm of the histiocytes. *Cryptococcus neoformans* was cultured from the marrow.

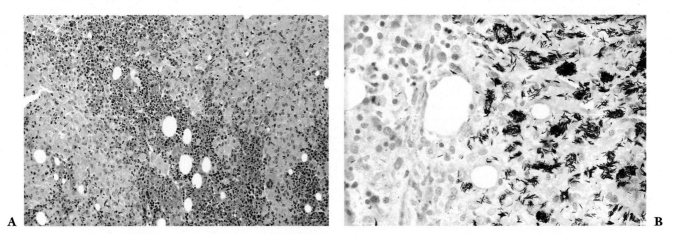

Figure 16.5. **(A)** Bone marrow section from a patient with AIDS. There are sheets of epithelioid histiocytes replacing large areas of the marrow. **(B)** High magnification of an acid-fast stain shows numerous acid-fast organisms that were identified as *Mycobacterium avium intracellulare.*

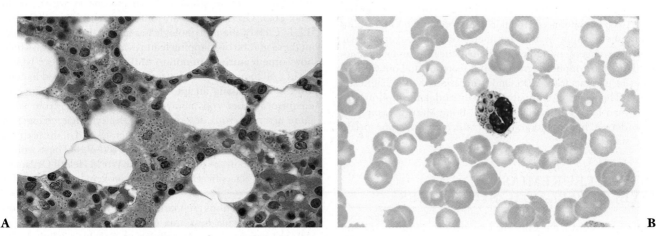

Figure 16.6. **(A)** High magnification of a marrow section from a patient with advanced AIDS showing a cluster of histiocytes containing numerous yeast forms in their cytoplasm. The infection was identified as histoplasmosis. **(B)** A neutrophil on a blood smear from this patient contains several phagocytosed organisms.

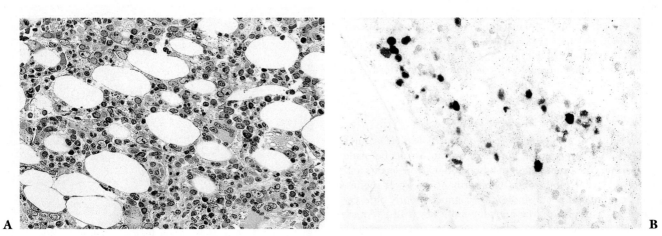

Figure 16.7. **(A)** Bone marrow biopsy from a patient with AIDS and recent onset of severe anemia with reticulocytopenia. The section shows numerous inclusions in the nuclei of erythroid precursors. **(B)** In situ hybridization for parvovirus B19 on the marrow section is positive.

TABLE 16.3	Cytologic Features of Acute Leukemias	
	Acute Myeloid Leukemia	*Acute Lymphoblastic Leukemia*
Blast size	Larger, often uniform	Variable; usually small to medium size
Cytoplasm	Moderately abundant	Usually scant
	Granules often present	Coarse granules sometimes present
Auer rods	Present in 60%–70% of cases	Not present
Chromatin	Usually finely dispersed	Coarse to fine
Nucleoli	1 to 4, often prominent	Absent or 1 or 2, often indistinct
Other cell types	Often dysplastic changes in maturing myeloid cells	Myeloid cells not dysplastic

lymphomas are Burkitt and diffuse large B cell, but other types are less frequently encountered, including peripheral T-cell lymphomas (77–79). Occasionally the marrow is the primary or only diagnostic tissue (77). If the marrow lesions are in any way equivocal in patients with AIDS, caution should be exercised in considering a diagnosis of marrow lymphoma. The florid reactive polymorphous lymphoid infiltrates described previously can be confused with lymphoma, particularly peripheral T-cell lymphoma or Hodgkin lymphoma (62,63,74,75). Immunophenotyping by flow cytometry or IHC and molecular gene rearrangement studies may help in the differential diagnosis. Hodgkin lymphoma involves the marrow in about 50% of cases in patients with AIDS, and is occasionally the diagnostic tissue. The lesions are usually typical of Hodgkin lymphoma, as described later in the chapter (see "Bone Marrow Lymphoid Disorders"), but should always be confirmed with appropriate IHC stains.

ACUTE LEUKEMIAS AND MYELODYSPLASTIC SYNDROMES

The diagnosis of acute leukemia or a myelodysplastic syndrome (MDS) is usually considered because of abnormal blood counts or findings on a blood smear. A bone marrow examination should always be done for confirmation of the diagnosis and to obtain material for supplemental studies.

Optimal morphologic evaluation for leukemias and MDS includes examination of well-prepared blood and bone marrow smears and biopsy sections. Most of the errors in the diagnosis of these disorders result from inadequate specimens or technically poor blood and marrow preparations. In cases of suspected leukemia, the pathologist interpreting the blood and marrow slides should always be equipped with complete clinical information before rendering an opinion.

ACUTE LEUKEMIAS

In cases of AML in which the leukemic blasts exhibit features of myeloid differentiation, the diagnosis can usually be made by morphologic examination of blood and marrow smears and selected cytochemical stains. A minority of cases will require one or more additional studies for diagnosis. Poorly differentiated AML and acute lymphoblastic leukemia (ALL) require immunophenotyping for diagnosis. Bone marrow cytogenetic and molecular studies are performed for the prognostic and treatment information they provide and for their role in the classification of acute leukemias.

Morphology

Morphologic assessment of blood and marrow smears and biopsy sections is important in the distinction of leukemias from other neoplasms and nonneoplastic proliferations; to distinguish AML from ALL; and in the classification of acute leukemia. The usual morphologic features that help distinguish AML and ALL in routine blood and marrow smears are shown in Table 16.3. Overall, there are differences between AML and ALL in each of the morphologic parameters listed in the table, but there may be overlapping features in individual cases, which show some features common to AML and others more typical of ALL. All morphologic features should be considered in composite when making an interpretation. Only the presence of unequivocal Auer rods always distinguishes AML from ALL. There are numerous descriptions of the cytologic changes in blood and marrow smears in acute leukemias and of the features that help define the various categories (80–92). These will be briefly reviewed in the discussion of the World Health Organization (WHO) classification of acute leukemias later in this chapter.

The biopsy sections are markedly hypercellular in the majority of cases of acute leukemia (Fig. 16.8), but occasionally in AML the marrow is normocellular or even hypocellular. The normal distribution and spectrum of maturation of hematopoietic cells is lacking and the marrow is mostly replaced by very immature-appearing cells. Mitotic activity is variable in acute

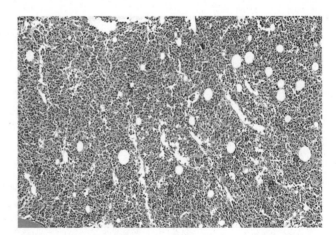

Figure 16.8. A marrow section from an adult male with t(9;22) (Philadelphia chromosome) positive acute lymphoblastic leukemia. The marrow is hypercellular and normal hematopoietic cells are largely replaced by lymphoblasts.

leukemias, but usually mitotic figures are easily found. In ALL the blasts are relatively uniform, whereas in AML the cytologic features vary depending on the percentage of myeloblasts and the lineage differentiation patterns. Myelofibrosis is present in some cases of both AML and ALL, and it may be particularly prominent in acute megakaryoblastic leukemia (84,88). Reticulin fibrosis may preclude obtaining an aspirate specimen. When this occurs, the trephine biopsy sections and touch preparations may be particularly important in the diagnosis.

Cytochemistry

Cytochemical stains on blood and bone marrow smears are helpful in the distinction of AML and ALL, and in the subclassification of AML (88,93). The combination of a myeloperoxidase or Sudan black stain and a nonspecific esterase stain provides the desired information in most instances. The myeloperoxidase or Sudan black reactions are most useful in establishing the identity of AML. The nonspecific esterase stain is used to identify a monocytic component in AML and to distinguish poorly differentiated monoblastic leukemia from AML, minimally differentiated and ALL.

Immunophenotype

Immunophenotyping by flow cytometry is the primary method for distinguishing ALL and AML when the morphology and cytochemistry of the leukemic blasts lack defining features (88,90,94). Immunophenotyping is also vitally important in the classification of ALL (88,94–97). Assessment of blasts for terminal deoxynucleotidyl transferase (TdT) and expression of T-cell–associated antigens (CD2, cytoplasmic CD3, CD5, CD7), and B-cell–associated antigens (e.g., HLADR, CD10, CD19, CD22) will identify and categorize nearly all cases of ALL. Likewise, assessment for myeloid-associated antigens (e.g., CD13, CD14, CD15, CD33, CD36, CD61, CD64) will identify the large majority of cases of AML. Panels must always include several antigens associated with each of the major cell lineages. Loss of antigens or aberrant expression is common in acute leukemias. In many cases, only by analysis of panels of antigen expression can an accurate interpretation be made. Immunophenotyping by IHC stains on bone marrow smears or biopsy sections may be used as an alternative to flow cytometry.

Cytogenetics

Bone marrow cytogenetic studies are essential in the evaluation of patients with acute leukemia and MDS (88,90,93,98–101). Cytogenetic findings are the single most important independent indicator of prognosis, and they define some of the categories of the WHO classification of acute leukemia (80, 102–104). They may also help distinguish between AML and ALL in selected cases, and between an MDS and a nonneoplastic cause of myelodysplasia. Chromosome rearrangements that define specific types of AML and provide important treatment and prognostic information include t(8;21), t(15;17), inv(16), and abnormalities of 11q23. Deletion of chromosome 5q and/or 7q, and monosomy 5 and/or 7 are commonly associated with multilineage dysplasia in de novo AML and therapy-related AML or MDS and a poor prognosis. In patients with precursor B ALL hyperdiploidy with more than 50 chromosomes, t(12; 21), t(1;19), t(9;22), and t(4;11) have important prognostic and therapeutic implications and are categories of the WHO classification (80). Prognostic implications of cytogenetic findings in acute leukemias are shown in Table 16.4.

Molecular Analysis

Molecular studies are valuable in bone marrow diagnosis in several respects. They may establish clonality; detect specific chromosome numerical and structural abnormalities; identify gene mutations or cryptic structural rearrangements that result in fusion genes; and identify viruses associated with neoplasms (105–108). Information provided by detection of molecular translocations and gene mutations contributes directly to the classification of leukemias and may provide valuable treatment and prognostic information. PCR and FISH studies for specific gene segments are also highly sensitive indicators of minimal residual leukemia and early relapse. Probes are available for detection of many of the mutations and fusion genes that identify clinically relevant categories of acute leukemia, myelodysplastic syndromes, and chronic myeloproliferative disorders.

TABLE 16.4	**Prognostic Implications of Cytogenetics in Acute Leukemia: Bone Marrow Chromosome Findings**	
	Chromosome Findings	
Prognostic Group	*Acute Myeloid Leukemia*	*Acute Lymphoblastic Leukemia*
Favorable	inv 16 or t(16;16)	Hyperdiploidy >50
	t(8;21) (adults)	Trisomy 4 and 10
	t(15;17)	Cryptic t(12;21)
	Single miscellaneous defects	
Intermediate	+8	Hyperdiploidy 47–50
	t(9;11) (children)	Normal (diploidy)
	Normal	del (6q)
Unfavorable	−7 or −5, del 7q,	Hypodiploidy—near haploid
	t(11;q23)	Near tetraploid
	inv(3q)	del 17p
	t(6;9)	t(9;22)
	Complex abnormalities	t(11q23) e.g., t(4;11)

TABLE 16.5

Molecular Genetic Abnormalities In Acute Myeloid Leukemia (AML) and Acute Lymphoblastic Leukemia (ALL)

Acute Myeloid Leukemia

Cytogenetic Translocation	Resulting Molecular Genetic Abnormality
t(8;21)(q22;q22)	RUNX1/RUNX1T1
inv(16)(p13;q22)	MYH11X/CBFβ
t(15;17)(q22;q21)	PML/RARα
t(6;9)(p23;q34)	DEK/NUP214
t(9;11)(p22;q23)	MLLT3/MLL

Acute Lymphoblastic Leukemia

Cytogenetic Translocation	Resulting Molecular Genetic Abnormality
t(12;21)(p12;q22)	TEL/AML-1
t(1;19)(q23;p13)	PBX/E2A
t(9;22)(q34;q11)	ABL/BCR (p190)
t(V;11)(V;q23)	V/MLL[a]

[a]In children, the t(4;11)(q21;q23) AF4/MLL is most common.

Examples of some of the most common ones found in acute leukemias are listed in Table 16.5, with corresponding cytogenetic changes, where applicable.

CLASSIFICATION OF ACUTE LEUKEMIAS

The WHO classification of hematopoietic neoplasms is the most widely used for acute leukemia and has largely replaced the French-American-British (FAB) Cooperative Group classification (80). It incorporates morphologic, immunophenotypic, genetic, and clinical features to define categories of acute leukemia that are biologically homogeneous and have clinical relevance. It provides a more precise diagnosis than do former classifications based exclusively on morphology, and introduces important prognostic and treatment correlations. The WHO classification of hematopoietic neoplasms has recently been revised (109). The categories listed in Tables 16.6 and 16.7 and discussed in the text include recent modifications.

ACUTE MYELOID LEUKEMIA

There are four major categories of AML in the WHO classification (80). Those with recurrent genetic abnormalities include AMLs with highly specific biologic and prognostic features. The category of AML with myelodysplasia-related features recognizes a group that has morphologic features or cytogenetic abnormalities of an MDS. These leukemias may arise de novo or as part of the evolution of a preexisting MDS. Therapy-related AML is a category of leukemia occurring in patients who have previously received cytotoxic chemotherapy for another disease. AML not otherwise specified (NOS) includes cases of AML that lack recurrent genetic rearrangements or myelodysplasia-related features and have not received prior cytotoxic drugs. This category is subclassified into traditional morphologic sub-

TABLE 16.6

WHO Classification of Acute Myeloid Leukaemia (AML) and Related Precursor Neoplasms

AML with recurrent genetic abnormalities
  AML with t(8;21)(q22;q22); *RUNX1-RUNX1T1*
  AML with inv(16)(p13.1;q22) or t(16;16)(p13.1;q22); *CBFB/MYH11*
  Acute promyelocytic leukaemia with t(15;17)(q22;q12); *PML/RARA*
  AML with t(9;11)(p22;q23); *MLLT3-MLL*
  AML with t(6;9)(P23;q34); *DEK-NUP214*
  AML with inv(3)(q21;q26.2) or t(3;3)(q21;q26.2); *RPN1-EVI1*
  AML (megakaryoblastic) with t(1;22)(p13;q13); *RBM15-MKL1*
  AML with mutated NPM1
  AML with mutated CEBPA
AML with myelodysplasia-related changes
Therapy-related myeloid neoplasms
Acute myeloid leukaemia, NOS
  AML minimal differentiation
  AML without maturation
  AML with maturation
  Acute myelomonocytic leukaemia
  Acute monoblastic and monocytic leukaemia
  Acute erythroid leukaemias
  Acute megakaryoblastic leukaemia
  Acute basophilic leukaemia
  Acute panmyelosis with myelofibrosis
Myeloid sarcoma
Myeloid proliferations related to Down syndrome
  Transient abnormal myelopoiesis
  Myeloid leukeaemia associated with Down syndrome
Blastic plasmacytoid dendritic cell neoplasm

WHO Classification of Acute Leukaemias of Ambiguous Lineage

  Acute undifferentiated leukaemia
  Mixed phenotype acute leukaemia with t(9;22)(q34;q11.2); *BCR-ABL1*
  Mixed phenotype acute leukaemia with t(v;11q23); *MLL* rearranged
  Mixed phenotype acute leukaemia, B/myeloid, NOS
  Mixed phenotype acute leukaemia, T/myeloid, NOS

---

types. The minimum number of blasts in the blood or bone marrow required for a diagnosis of AML remains at 20% (80) (110–112).

Acute Myeloid Leukemia with Recurrent Genetic Abnormalities

There are seven categories of AML with recurrent genetic abnormalities and two provisional types with specific gene mutations. The genetic findings in this group have prognostic significance. They are described in the following paragraphs.

AML with t(8;21)(q22;q22);(RUNX1-RUNX1T1) exhibits a characteristic morphology, immunophenotype, and clinical findings and constitutes about 5% of AMLs (80,113). The morphologic features are nearly always those of AML with maturation, and include large blasts, frequent and often large Auer rods, and striking dysplasia in the neutrophil lineage. Immunophenotypically, there is usually aberrant expression of the B-lymphocyte–associated antigens CD19, PAX5 and CD79a, and

TABLE 16.7

WHO Classification of Precursor Lymphoid Neoplasms

B lymphoblastic leukaemia/lymphoma
 B lymphoblastic leukaemia/lymphoma, NOS
 B lymphoblastic leukaemia/lymphoma with recurrent genetic
  abnormalities
  B lymphoblastic leukaemia/lymphoma with t(9;22)
   (q34;q11.2); *BCR/ABL1*
  B lymphoblastic leukaemia/lymphoma with t(v;11q23);
   MLL rearranged
  B lymphoblastic leukaemia/lymphoma with t(12;21)(p13;q22);
   TEL-AML1 (ETV6-RUNX1)
  B lymphoblastic leukaemia/lymphoma with hyperdiploidy
  B lymphoblastic leukaemia/lymphoma with hypodiploidy
   (hypodiploid ALL)
  B lymphoblastic leukaemia/lymphoma with t(5;14)(q31;q32);
   IL3-IGH
  B lymphoblastic leukaemia/lymphoma with t(1;19)(q23;
   p13.3); *E2A*-PBX1; *(TCF3-PBX1)*
T lymphoblastic leukaemia/lymphoma

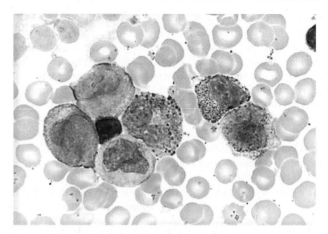

Figure 16.9. A marrow smear from a patient with acute myeloid leukemia and inv(16)(p13;q22) shows the typical myelomonocytic morphology and increased eosinophils with dysplastic granulation.

often expression of CD56 (114–116). AML with a t(8;21) is associated with a relatively favorable prognosis in adult patients.

AML with inv(16)(p13;q22) or t(16;16)(p13;q22);(CBFB-MYH11) generally has the morphologic features of acute myelomonocytic leukemia, with the addition of increased and dysplastic eosinophils in the marrow (117,118) (Fig. 16.9). The dysplastic eosinophils are recognized by an abundance of large, basophilic-staining granules. AML with inv(16) constitutes approximately 8% of cases of adult AML and approximately 25% of cases of acute myelomonocytic leukemia (80,119). The incidence of extramedullary disease is higher (approximately 50%) than for most types of AML; lymphadenopathy and hepatomegaly are particularly common. Myeloid sarcoma concurrent with or preceding bone marrow involvement appears to be more common than in other leukemias. Some investigators have reported a high incidence of central nervous system (CNS) relapse with intracerebral myeloblastomas (120). High complete

remission rates are expected for AML with an inv(16), and the prospect for extended remission is fairly good (121).

Acute promyelocytic leukemia (APL) with t(15;17)(q22;q21); (PML/RARα) comprises about 8% of AMLs and is associated with distinctive biologic and clinical features (80,119). The leukemic cell population is abnormal promyelocytes that usually contain numerous red to purple cytoplasmic granules (80,122) (Fig. 16.10). The granules are often larger and darker-staining than normal and may be so numerous as to obscure the nuclear borders. In some cases a high percentage of the leukemic cells have intensely basophilic cytoplasm. Cells containing multiple Auer rods are found in approximately 90% of cases. The Auer rods may be numerous and intertwined. Large globular inclusions of Auer-like material are found in the cytoplasm of occasional cells. The nuclei of many of the cells are reniform or bilobed. In the microgranular variant of APL, the leukemic cells have sparse or fine granulation and markedly irregular nuclei, which may obscure their identity as abnormal promyelocytes (123). Cells containing multiple Auer rods are usually present but less abundant than in typical hypergranular APL. Both typical hypergranular APL and the microgranular variant have the

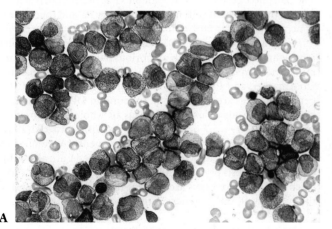
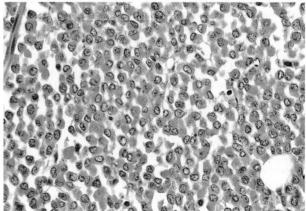

Figure 16.10. **(A)** Intermediate magnification of a marrow aspirate smear from a patient with acute promyelocytic leukemia and t(15;17) showing numerous abnormal hypergranular promyelocytes. **(B)** A marrow section is hypercellular and completely replaced with leukemic promyelocytes.

same characteristic clinical ultrastructural, cytogenetic, and molecular features. They differ only in the size and number of granules in the cytoplasm; the prominence of the abnormal nuclear shape in the predominant leukemic cells; and in the magnitude of the blood leukocyte count. Hypergranular APL is generally associated with leukopenia at presentation, whereas microgranular APL often presents with marked leukocytosis (122).

Ultrastructurally, APL is distinctive by the presence of Auer rods with a specific tubular substructure, markedly dilated endoplasmic reticulum, and stellate complexes of rough endoplasmic reticulum (122,124). The immunophenotype by flow cytometry is also characteristic in most cases and is different from other types of AML, mainly by increased side scatter and lack of expression of human leukocyte antigen DR-1 (HLA-DR) and CD34. The most striking clinical feature in APL is the high frequency of disseminated intravascular coagulation (DIC). In most patients there is severe DIC and hemorrhage prior to or during standard induction chemotherapy. Hemorrhage is the cause of early death in some patients.

The t(15;17) breakpoint regions are at the *PML* gene on band q22 of chromosome 15 and on band q21 in the first intron of the retinoic acid receptor (*RAR*) gene on chromosome 17 (113,125,126). The resulting *PML-RARα* fusion messenger RNA product inhibits maturation of the affected cells, leading to an accumulation of large numbers of abnormal promyelocytes. Treatment with all-*trans* retinoic acid (ATRA) can overcome the maturation blockage in most instances and lead to a temporary complete remission. Treatment with standard induction chemotherapy along with ATRA is required to sustain remission. For adult patients who achieve complete remission, the prognosis is better than for any other category of AML.

Promyelocytic leukemias with t(V;17)(V;q21);(V/RARα) have many of the morphologic and clinical features of APL but have a variant cytogenetic translocation that involves the *RARα* gene on chromosome 17 but not the *PML* gene on 15; t(11;17)(q23; q12) ZBTB16. *RARα* is one of the more common variant translocations (80,124). Morphologically, cases with t(V;17) may have morphologic features intermediate between APL and AML with maturation. As with t(15;17) APL patients with a t(V;17) APL often experience disseminated intravascular coagulation. It is important to distinguish the two because most t(V;17) APLs do not respond to ATRA therapy and often have an aggressive clinical course (126).

AML with t(9;11)(p22;q23) (MLLT3-MLL) is usually monoblastic, monocytic, or myelomonocytic and occurs most frequently in children and young adults (9% to 12% of cases in children and 1% to 2% in adults) (127,128). Translocation 9:11 may also be found in cases of topoisomerase II inhibitor, therapy-related AML, and in biphenotypic leukemias (129). 11q23 (MLL) is involved with several other translocations and partner genes in acute leukemias. De novo AMLs with a t(9;11) are associated with an intermediate prognosis; 11q23 (MLL) leukemias with other translocations/partner genes usually have a poor prognosis (113,130).

AML with t(6;9) (p23;q34) (DEK-CAN) is a rare type of AML that occurs in both children and adults (131,132). There is a wide range of morphologic features and frequently evidence of multilineage dysplasia; basophilia is often present. There are no distinctive immunophenotypic features. Cases with t(6;9) have an overall poor prognosis.

AML with inv(3)(q21;q26) or a t(3;3) presents either de novo or following a myelodysplastic syndrome (133,134). A notable feature is the frequent presentation with normal or elevated platelet counts. Megakaryocytes are increased in the marrow and exhibit dysplastic features. Multilineage dysplasia is a common finding. This is an aggressive type of AML with a poor prognosis.

AML with t(1;22)(p13;q13) (RBM15-MKL1) is a rare form of acute megakaryoblastic leukemia, representing less than 1% of AMLs and most frequently occurring in infants. It is associated with marked organomegaly and prominent myelofibrosis and may have features of a panmyelosis. The pattern of marrow and other organ involvement often resembles that of a metastatic small-cell tumor (135). Recent studies suggest that AML with t(1;22) may respond well to intensive treatment for AML (136).

AML with mutated NPM1 (provisional category) has mutations of the gene that result in aberrant cytoplasmic expression of nucleophosmin, which can be detected by IHC staining (137,138). Mutated MPM1 is one of the most common recurring genetic abnormalities in AML—found in at least 50% of adults with normal conventional banding chromosome analysis—but may also occur in a small number of cases with chromosomal abnormalities (137,139,140,156). There are no specific morphologic or immunophenotypic features, but the leukemia frequently has myelomonocytic or monocytic morphology (137). It occurs most commonly in females (137). AML with mutated NPM1 seems to show a good response to therapy and favorable prognosis unless there is also FLT3-internal tandem duplication mutation, in which case it is associated with a poorer prognosis.

AML with mutated CEBPA (provisional category) is found in approximately 10% of AMLs, and about 70% of these have a normal karyotype (141,142). In most cases the leukemia has features of either AML with maturation or AML without maturation. The importance of the CEBPA mutation is its association with a favorable prognosis, similar to t(8;21) and inv(16) AMLs.

Acute Myeloid Leukemia with Myelodysplasia-Related Changes

AML with myelodysplasia-related features may arise in patients with an MDS or de novo with an MDS-related cytogenetic abnormality or multilineage dysplasia (80, 109). These leukemias increase in incidence with age and are rare in children; they account for approximately one-third of all AMLs (108,143,144). The morphologic features are variable. The blast count is at least 20% of the nucleated cells in the bone marrow, and there is evidence of dysplasia in 50% or more of the maturing cells in two or more lineages and/or an MDS-related cytogenetic abnormality is present. There is frequently an obvious panmyelosis (145). Immunophenotype varies but there is usually expression of panmyeloid markers and aberrant antigen expression is frequent. Cytogenetic findings are similar to those found in MDS and include gains or deletions of major segments or whole chromosomes (e.g., −5 or 5q−, −7 or 7q−, i(17q)/t(17p), −13/del(13q), etc.) and complex cytogenetic rearrangements. A number of translocations involving chromosomes 3, 5, or 11 are also sufficient for diagnosis of AML with myelodysplasia-related features when 20% or more blasts are present (109). The prognosis for this category of AML is generally unfavorable (143).

Therapy-Related Myeloid Neoplasms

Therapy-related AML and MDS occur in patients previously treated with chemotherapy or radiation therapy. Alkylating drugs and the topoisomerase II inhibitors are the agents most commonly implicated (129,146). The median onset of therapy-related AML or MDS is approximately 5 years after initiation of alkylating agents, and 2.5 to 3 years after first use of topoisomerase II inhibitor drugs. In cases associated with alkylating-agent therapy, patients typically present with pancytopenia and features of an MDS. The dysplastic changes in the blood and marrow cells are often severe; however, the marrow myeloblast percentage may be less than 5% (147). In some cases the MDS is followed in a short time by progression to AML. In others, severe bone marrow failure leads to patient demise without evolution to leukemia. Myelofibrosis, hypocellularity, and ringed sideroblasts are encountered more frequently than in de novo AML or MDS. Therapy-related MDS associated with alkylating agents commonly has cytogenetic abnormalities affecting chromosomes 5 or 7 and complex cytogenetic abnormalities. Patients with AML and MDS secondary to alkylating agent drugs generally respond poorly to treatment and have a short survival. The topoisomerase II inhibitor drugs more often lead to acute monocytic or myelomonocytic leukemias and have abnormalities of chromosome 11q23 (MLL); only rarely do they present as an MDS (129,148). Although the initial response to treatment is often favorable in topoisomerase II inhibitor-induced AML, overall prognosis is poor.

Acute Myeloid Leukemia, Not Otherwise Specified

Cases of AML that are not included in one of the three major categories cited previously are classified as AML, not otherwise specified. These are classified morphologically using descriptive terminology from the French-American-British Cooperative Group (FAB) classification (81,85).

AML, minimally differentiated exhibits no definitive evidence of myeloid differentiation by morphology and cytochemistry; the nature of the blasts is determined by immunophenotyping (80). The blasts are agranular, lack Auer rods, and are myeloperoxidase and Sudan-black-B−negative (85). They express one or more panmyeloid antigens, such as CD13, CD33, and CD117, and may express other myeloid lineage-associated antigens. CD34 and TdT are expressed more frequently than for other types of AML (149). CD7, CD2, and CD19 are expressed in a few cases but the blasts generally lack expression of B- and T-lymphocyte−restricted antigens such as CD3 and CD22. Chromosome abnormalities, often complex, are found in most cases, but cytogenetic changes unique to AML, minimally differentiated have not been identified (149,150). The prognosis is usually poor with a shorter survival than for other types of AML.

AML without maturation accounts for about 10% of cases of AML (80,119). The sum of blasts must be 90% or more of the nonerythroid cells in the bone marrow (80,81) (Fig. 16.11). Evidence of maturation to promyelocytes is variable but may be minimal or absent. The cytologic features of the myeloblasts vary considerably from case to case. The blast nucleus may be round or indented, and in some cases exhibits a distinctive invagination (151). Cytoplasmic granulation varies from abundant to virtually absent; Auer rods are found in approximately 50% of cases. In those without Auer rods, at least 3% of the leukemic myeloblasts must be myeloperoxidase or Sudan-black-B−positive.

AML with maturation is the single most common type of AML, comprising about 30% of cases. It may occur at any age but is more common in older individuals (80,81,119). The marrow blast percentage is 20% to 89% of the nonerythroid cells (Fig. 16.12). Granulocytes from promyelocytes to mature neutrophils

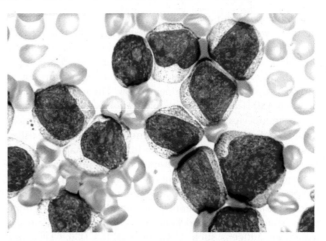

Figure 16.11. A high magnification of a marrow smear from a patient with acute myeloid leukemia without maturation. Nearly all of the leukemic cells have nuclear features of blasts. Cytoplasmic granulation varies from absent to relatively abundant.

comprise more than 10% of cells; monocytes and precursors are less than 20%. The maturing neutrophils often show dysplastic features. In about 70% of cases, Auer rods can be identified (119). Erythroid and megakaryocyte precursors may show evidence of dyspoiesis and a frank panmyelosis is present in some cases. If the dysplastic changes in two or more lineages exceed 50% of the cells, the case should be classified in the WHO category of AML with multilineage dysplasia. Because of the obvious maturation of the leukemic cells, the myeloid nature is not often in question. The blasts and maturing granulocytes are positive for myeloperoxidase and Sudan black B. There are no distinctive immunophenotypic features that characterize AML with maturation. A majority of cases have demonstrable cytogenetic abnormalities typical of AMLs, but there is no common aberration for this category. The prognosis is variable from poor to quite favorable. Those of advanced age and with multilineage dysplasia and unfavorable cytogenetic changes generally respond less well to therapy and have a shorter survival.

Acute myelomonocytic leukemia (AMML) comprises 15% to 25% of AMLs (80,119). Bone marrow myeloblasts and monoblasts/promonocytes number 20% or more, but the sum of myeloblasts

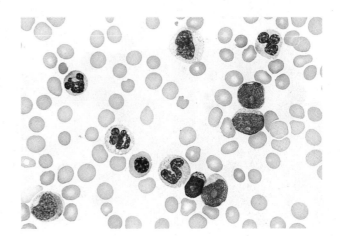

Figure 16.12. An intermediate magnification of a marrow smear illustrates features of acute myeloid leukemia with maturation. The marrow contained about 30% myeloblasts.

and neutrophils and precursors is 80% or less; 20% or more of the marrow cells are in the monocyte lineage (81). If fewer than 20% of the marrow cells are monocytes, the diagnosis may still be AMML if blood monocytes number more than 5×10^9 per L. Both granulocytic and monocytic differentiation is present in varying proportions in the bone marrow. The major difference between AMML and AML with maturation is the proportion of the promonocytes and monocytes, which must be 20% or more in AMML. Early promonocytes cannot always be distinguished from early granulocyte precursors in routine marrow smears. For this reason, an additional requirement of nonspecific esterase reactivity in 20% or more of the cells is included. Auer rods are present in the myeloblast component in approximately 60% of cases. The immunophenotype of AMML generally exhibits a spectrum of myeloid-associated antigens with some monocyte-associated antigens such as CD14, CD11, CD36/CD64, and CD4. There may be two distinctive immunophenotypic populations of granulocytic and monocytic cells. Similar to AML with maturation, cytogenetic abnormalities are common and include rearrangements typical of AML in general. Those with marrow eosinophilia and an inv(16) are classified in the AML with recurrent genetic abnormalities, described previously. AMML occurs in both children and adults. The median age at diagnosis is approximately 50 years. The blood leukocyte count is often markedly elevated. Organomegaly, lymphadenopathy, and other tissue infiltration are commonly present. The prognosis is variable and overall similar to other AMLs.

Acute monoblastic and acute monocytic leukemias comprise about 8% of AMLs when those with a t(9;11) chromosome abnormality are included (152). They are composed of 80% or more leukemic cells in the monocyte lineage (80,81). Acute monoblastic leukemia is seen predominantly in children and young adults. Monoblasts exhibit moderately abundant, variably basophilic cytoplasm, which frequently contains delicate peroxidase-negative azurophilic granules. The nucleus is round with reticular chromatin and one or more prominent nucleoli. Acute monocytic leukemia may be seen in all age groups. The leukemic cells are predominantly promonocytes that show more obvious evidence of monocytic differentiation and maturation (Fig. 16.13). The nuclei are folded or cerebriform with delicate chromatin. The cytoplasm is less basophilic than in monoblasts and contains a variable number of azurophilic granules. Both

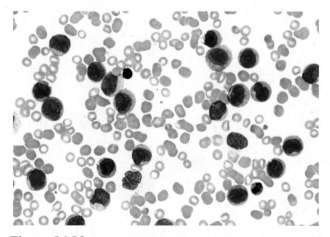

Figure 16.13. An intermediate magnification of a blood smear from a patient with acute monocytic leukemia. There is a marked leukocytosis consisting primarily of promonocytes and scattered monoblasts.

monoblasts and promonocytes are nonspecific esterase-positive. Monoblasts are generally myeloperoxidase-negative but promonocytes may exhibit weak to moderate myeloperoxidase activity. The leukemic monocytes express variable patterns of myeloid antigens, including monocyte-associated antigens such as CD14, CD15, CD11b, CD36, and CD64. Cytogenetic abnormalities are more common in acute monoblastic (approximately 75%) than monocytic (approximately 30%) leukemias.

Acute monoblastic and monocytic leukemias are associated with a high incidence of organomegaly, lymphadenopathy, and other tissue infiltration (e.g., gingival, skin). There is a higher incidence of CNS involvement than for other types of AML. In a few cases the first clinical manifestations of leukemia result from extramedullary tissue infiltrates. Prognosis is poor to intermediate, at least partly resulting from the association of high-risk clinical findings (e.g., high presenting leukocyte counts, extramedullary involvement, 11q23 chromosome abnormalities).

Acute erythroid leukemias are characterized by a predominance of leukemic cells that are erythrocyte precursors. There are two subtypes, *erythroleukemia (erythroid/ myeloid)* and *pure erythroid leukemia* (80,81). In erythroid/myeloid leukemia, 50% or more of all nucleated marrow cells are in the erythroid lineage and 20% or more of the remaining cells (nonerythroid) are myeloblasts; dyserythropoiesis is prominent. The predominant leukemic cells are erythroid precursors including the least mature erythroblasts. The erythroid component is characterized by abnormalities of nuclear development, including megaloblastoid changes, karyorrhexis, and occasional giant erythroblasts with multiple nuclei. The leukemic erythroblasts may contain confluent cytoplasmic vacuoles, which correspond to cytoplasmic glycogen and react positively with the periodic acid-Schiff (PAS) stain. There is often evidence of a panmyelosis with striking megakaryocytic and platelet abnormalities. These cases might preferably be classified as AML with multilineage dysplasia by WHO classification criteria. Auer rods are present in myeloblasts in 50% to 60% of cases (119). The blood smear in erythroid/myeloid leukemia may show striking erythroblastemia. Progression of the disease is frequently marked by an increase in myeloblasts and decrease in erythroblasts.

Pure erythroid leukemia is very rare. The only obvious neoplastic cells are erythroid; a myeloblast component is not apparent (153). The leukemic erythroid cells are predominantly or exclusively proerythroblasts and early basophilic erythroblasts. These cells may constitute 90% or more of the marrow elements. Despite the lack of myeloblasts, these cases should be considered acute leukemia.

The immunophenotype reflects the mixture of myeloid and erythroid precursors in erythroid/myeloid leukemia. The erythroid cells in both subtypes typically express CD36, CD71, hemoglobin A, and glycophorin A; the least mature erythroblasts are often negative for hemoglobin A and glycophorin A. No specific cytogenetic abnormalities are associated with the erythroleukemias, but complex structural rearrangements are common and chromosomes 5 and 7 are frequently involved.

Acute megakaryoblastic leukemia (AMKL) comprises 3% to 5% of AMLs and is found in both adults and children. Fifty percent or more of the leukemic blasts are of megakaryocyte lineage (80). Blasts are usually identified as megakaryocytic by expression of antigens specific for megakaryocytes or by demonstration of platelet peroxidase by electron microscopy. In blood and marrow smears, megakaryoblasts are usually medium-sized to large cells with a high nuclear:cytoplasmic ratio. Nuclear chromatin is dense and homogeneous. There is scanty, variably basophilic cytoplasm, which may be vacuolated. An irregular cytoplasmic border is often noted, and there are occasionally projections resembling budding of atypical platelets. Transition between poorly differentiated blasts and recognizable micromegakaryocytes is often observed. In many cases the majority of the leukemic cells are small blasts with features similar to lymphoblasts. Megakaryoblasts are negative for myeloperoxidase, Sudan black B, and α-naphthyl butyrate esterase; they manifest variable α-naphthyl acetate esterase activity, usually in scattered clumps or granules in cytoplasm. PAS staining also varies from negative to focal or granular positivity to strongly positive staining. In many cases a marrow aspirate is difficult to obtain because of myelofibrosis. The biopsy sections often reveal morphologic evidence of megakaryocytic differentiation that is not appreciated in the smears.

Clues to the lineage of poorly differentiated megakaryoblasts include the presence of circulating micromegakaryocytes; atypical platelets; projections on the surface of the blasts; zoning of the cytoplasm; myelofibrosis; and clusters of small megakaryocytes in sections. More precise identification can be accomplished by immunophenotyping. Megakaryoblasts variably express CD13, CD33, HLADR, and CD71 and mostly express CD36. Some of the blasts express the megakaryocyte-specific antigens CD41 and CD61 in virtually all cases (154). The more differentiated megakaryocytes express factor VIII antigen.

There are no distinctive cytogenetic abnormalities in adults with AMKL. AML t(1;22)(p13;q13) is a category of AML with recurrent genetic abnormalities (described above) that occurs in infants (155).

An extra chromosome 21 has been identified in many cases of AMKL, but is not specific. However, a striking number of children with AMKL have constitutional trisomy 21 (Down syndrome). The incidence of AMKL is 400 times that of the general pediatric population. Neonates and, rarely, older infants with Down syndrome may develop a transient myeloproliferative disorder (TMD). TMD is an abnormal proliferation of myeloid blasts in the blood that resolves without therapeutic intervention in 2 to 14 weeks. TMD and AMKL show similar morphologic features. Most examples of TMD have a major megakaryoblast component, identical to AMKL in Down syndrome. The major clinical difference is age of onset. AMKL rarely occurs in Down syndrome in the first month of life. Blasts in TMD only rarely have cytogenetic abnormalities other than constitutional trisomy 21, whereas those in AMKL often exhibit additional abnormalities. Evidence indicates that TMD is a clonal disorder, and an estimated 15% of TMD patients develop AMKL within 3 years. Mutations in the transcription factor GATA1 have been found in Down syndrome-AMKL and TMD, which suggests that GATA1 mutagenesis represents a very early event in Down syndrome leukemogenesis (156–158). TMD and AMKL are related disorders; AMKL may represent clonal evolution of a spontaneously remitted and dormant TMD (154).

Acute basophilic leukemia is a rare form of AML (80,159). Cases may show obvious basophil differentiation or be cytologically undifferentiated with only ultrastructural evidence suggesting the basophil lineage. The poorly differentiated acute basophilic leukemias would most likely be classified as AML minimally differentiated without confirmation by electron microscopy. Acute basophilic leukemias are myeloperoxidase-negative on light microscopy. The granules stain metachromatically with toluidine blue. Myeloid antigens such as CD13 and CD33 are usually expressed. There are no specific cytogenetic findings but a t(9;22) (Philadelphia chromosome) is frequently found. In some cases of AML with t(6;9), basophils are a predominant component. There are no clinically distinguishing features of acute basophilic leukemia, but it may be more common in children and young adults and carry a poor prognosis (159).

Acute panmyelosis with myelofibrosis is an uncommon form of acute leukemia occurring primarily in adults and rarely in children (80). Patients present with pancytopenia and a multilineage proliferation. There are usually prominent megakaryocytic abnormalities. The degree of fibrosis varies. In most cases there is marked reticulin fibrosis; collagen fibrosis is less common. The disorder shares features with other myeloid disorders with prominent myelofibrosis. At initial presentation it may be difficult to exclude chronic idiopathic myelofibrosis, AMKL, or an MDS with myelofibrosis as diagnostic considerations. The spleen is generally normal or only minimally increased in size. No specific immunophenotypic or cytogenetic features have been described for acute panmyelosis with myelofibrosis. The disease has an aggressive course.

Myeloid sarcomas are tumor masses of neoplastic immature myeloid cells in an extramedullary site. Usually the patient has evidence of myeloid leukemia in the bone marrow and blood but, in some instances, myeloid sarcomas occur without obvious leukemia. The most common sites for myeloid sarcomas are subperiosteal bone, skin, lymph nodes, orbit, spinal canal, and mediastinum (80) (Fig. 16.14). Most types of AML may occasionally present in an extramedullary site, but the monocytic and myelomonocytic leukemias have the highest propensity.

ACUTE LEUKEMIAS OF AMBIGUOUS LINEAGE

In these leukemias the morphologic, cytochemical, and immunophenotypic features of the blasts lack sufficient specificity to classify the leukemias as either myeloid or lymphoblastic. These may be acute, undifferentiated leukemias in which there is lack of expression of lineage differentiation antigens. Other cases may exhibit morphologic and immunophenotypic features of both myeloid and lymphoblastic cells. These may be either bilineal leukemias with separate blast populations—one expressing myeloid characteristics and the other lymphoid—or biphenotypic, in which the blasts express characteristics of both myeloid and lymphoid cells (160) (Fig. 16.15). In addition to mixed immunophenotypes, there may be a mixture of morphologic, cytochemical, and ultrastructural features in these cases. Bilineal leukemias may be synchronous with simultaneous, distinct populations of leukemic cells of more than one lineage or metachronous (lineage switch) in which one lineage is expressed following the other. In the latter case, reappearance of the original clone must be demonstrated to distinguish from the emergence of a secondary (therapy-related) leukemia. There is an increased incidence of chromosome translocations involving 11q23 or a t(9;22) in biphenotypic and bilineal leukemias. The WHO requirements for assigning more than one lineage to a single blast population are shown in Table 16.8 (80, 161).

PRECURSOR LYMPHOID NEOPLASMS

The WHO classification of acute lymphoblastic leukemia (ALL) is based on immunophenotypic and cytogenetic/molecular

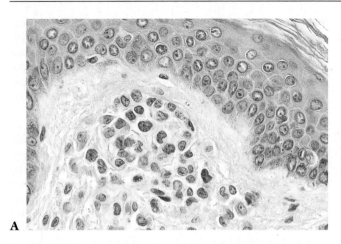

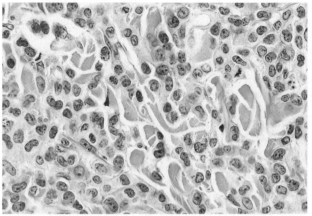

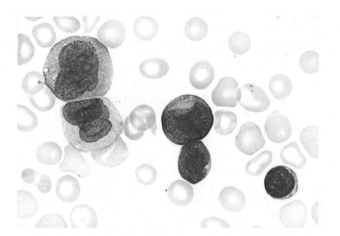

Figure 16.14. Myeloid sarcoma in a biopsy of a skin plaque. **(A)** There is an upper dermal infiltrate. **(B)** The infiltrate extends into the deeper dermis and consists of medium-sized to large hematopoietic cells with fine chromatin and variably prominent nucleoli. **(C)** A lysozyme stain is strongly positive. An IHC stain for CD68 was also positive and stains for B- and T-lymphocyte–associated antigens were all negative. A bone marrow examination revealed a monocytic leukemia.

Figure 16.15. A blood smear from a neonate with bilineal acute leukemia shows two types of leukemic cells, monoblasts/promonocytes and lymphoblasts. Flow cytometry analysis identified two immunophenotypically distinct leukemic blast populations, precursor B lymphoblasts and monoblasts. A t(4;11)(q21;q23) AF4/MLL was found by conventional cytogenetics.

TABLE 16.8

WHO Requirements For Assigning More Than One Lineage To A Single Blast Population

Myeloid lineage
Myeloperoxidase (flow cytometry, immunohistochemistry or cytochemistry)
or
Monocytic differentiation (at least 2 of the following: NSE, CD11c, CD14, CD64, lysozyme)

T lineage
Cytoplasmic CD3 (flow cytometry with antibodies to CD3 epsilon chain; immunohistochemistry using polyclonal anti-CD3 antibody may detect CD3 zeta chain, which is not T-cell specific)
or
Surface CD3 (rare in mixed phenotype acute leukaemias)

B lineage (multiple antigens required)
Strong CD19 with at least 1 of the following strongly expressed; CD79a, cytoplasmic CD22, CD10
or
Weak CD19 with at least 2 of the following strongly expressed: CD79a, cytoplasmic CD22, CD10

findings, and recognizes the major treatment and prognostic groups of childhood ALL (80) (Table 16.7). There are two major immunophenotypic categories, precursor B ALL and precursor T ALL. Within precursor B ALL, there are six subtypes determined by recurrent cytogenetic/molecular abnormalities. Acute lymphoblastic leukemia with a t(9:22)-Philadelphia chromosome-positive ALL is recognized in the classification as a distinctive category of leukemia based on its extremely poor response to treatment.

Precursor B Acute Lymphoblastic Leukemia

Precursor B ALL is the most common of the immunophenotypic categories, accounting for about 85% of cases in children and 75% in adults. The presenting signs and symptoms relate to blood cytopenias resulting from bone marrow failure. Physical findings may include pallor, ecchymoses or petechiae, lymphadenopathy, and organomegaly. In a minority of patients the presenting clinical symptoms are caused by extramedullary leukemic infiltrates. In some of these, the blood and marrow may contain little or no evidence of involvement. In these cases, diagnosis of precursor B lymphoblastic lymphoma is preferred (162,163). Lymph node, CNS, skin, gonadal, renal, bone, and joint involvement are most frequent; the CNS and testicles are major sites of extramedullary relapse, often independent of bone marrow relapse.

The *morphologic* features on blood and marrow smears that distinguish ALL and AML are listed in Table 16.3. The lymphoblasts in precursor B ALL are small to medium-sized, approximately twice the size of normal small lymphocytes, with sparse cytoplasm and a high nuclear:cytoplasmic ratio (Fig. 16.16A). The nucleus is generally round or oval, but a variable number of cells have an indented or convoluted nuclear outline. The chromatin is usually coarsely reticular and quite homogenous. In most cases, nucleoli are small and indistinct or not visualized. The cytoplasm is variably basophilic. Vacuoles are often present, and cytoplasmic granules are found in a small number of cases. In a minority of cases, the predominant lymphoblasts are large. In these, the blast size may be relatively uniform or quite heterogeneous, but most of the lymphoblasts exceed twice the size of a normal small lymphocyte. In the large

blasts, nucleoli are often prominent and vary from one to four; these cells may be difficult to distinguish from myeloblasts.

In biopsy sections the marrow is usually markedly hypercellular (Figs. 16.8, 16.16B) but may be normocellular and, in rare cases, hypocellular. Normal hematopoiesis is markedly reduced and the marrow is replaced by a uniform, diffuse proliferation of lymphoblasts. Occasionally there is only partial marrow involvement in an interstitial pattern. A focal pattern of involvement is rare in ALL at diagnosis but may be observed at relapse (164). Cytoplasm is barely discernible and nuclei are mostly medium-sized with evenly dispersed to moderately dense chromatin and inconspicuous nucleoli. Nuclear contour is often heterogeneous; convoluted cells are usually present and may predominate. Mitotic activity is variable but usually brisk, and mitotic figures are always easy to find.

Immunophenotyping should be performed in all cases of ALL to differentiate it from AML and to distinguish precursor B and precursor T ALL. The profile of antigen expression on the leukemic blasts also serves as an important fingerprint for later assessment for minimal residual disease (165). The lymphoblasts in precursor B ALL express various combinations of the B-lymphocyte–associated antigens CD19, CD22, CD79a, CD24, CD10, and CD9, and several lineage-nonspecific antigens, including CD34, TdT, HLADR, CD38, and CD45 (95,97). μ-immunoglobulin heavy chains (CIg) are present in the cytoplasm of the lymphoblasts in 20% to 25% of precursor B ALLs but, except in rare cases, lymphoblasts lack expression of surface immunoglobulin (SIg). More than 95% of cases of precursor B ALL are TdT-positive and the progenitor cell–associated antigen CD34 is found in about 80%. TdT is useful in differentiating ALL from lymphoproliferative disorders of mature lymphocytes, which are TdT-negative, but more than 90% of precursor T ALLs and 5% to 10% of AMLs also express TdT (166). In virtually all cases of precursor B ALL, the lymphoblasts exhibit incomplete maturation and immunophenotypic asynchrony and aberrancy that deviate from the spectrum of antigen expression typical of normal B-lymphocyte stages of maturation (167). In 30% to 80% of cases, one or more myeloid-associated antigens are detected on the neoplastic lymphoblasts; CD15, CD13, and CD33 appear to be most common (167).

Conventional cytogenetic analysis shows 80% to 90% of cases

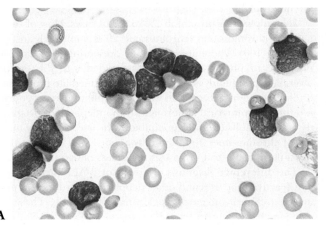
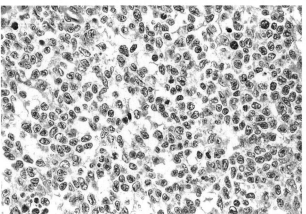

A **B**

Figure 16.16. (**A**) A blood smear from a 3-year-old child with precursor B acute lymphoblastic leukemia. The blasts show typical morphologic features. (**B**) A marrow biopsy section is markedly hypercellular and normal hematopoietic cells are replaced by lymphoblasts.

of precursor B ALL have demonstrable chromosome abnormalities (168,169). The incidence is even higher when FISH techniques are used to supplement conventional studies (170). The major recurrent cytogenetic abnormalities define categories of precursor B ALL in the WHO classification. Chromosome numerical changes are found in about 50% of children and 15% of adults with precursor B ALL. In children, ploidy defines important prognostic groups, but in adults it has little effect on prognosis except in a small group of hypodiploid cases (171,172). The five major chromosome numerical groups of precursor B ALL are hyperdiploid with more than 50; hyperdiploid with 47 to 50; diploid; hypodiploid; and pseudodiploid. Structural changes are always present in pseudodiploid ALL and may be found in the other numerical groups except diploid. Translocations are most important because several recurrent ones are independent indicators of prognosis. The cytogenetic categories of precursor B ALL included in the WHO classification are briefly discussed below.

ALLs with t(9;22)(q34;q11), BCR/ABL (Philadelphia [Ph1] chromosome) arise from a reciprocal translocation involving the cytoplasmic tyrosine-kinase gene ABL on chromosome 9q34 and the BCR (breakpoint cluster region) on chromosome 22q11 (173). The t(9;22) is found in the lymphoblasts of 3% to 5% of children with ALL and approximately 30% of adults, making it the most common structural abnormality in adults with ALL (168,172,174). Translocation (9;22) cases span the spectrum of morphology for ALL. There are no defining cytologic features, but there appears to be a higher proportion of cases with a predominance of large blasts with prominent nucleoli than for other precursor B ALLs, and cytoplasmic granules are more commonly observed (175,176). Translocation (9;22) ALL is characterized by an older age and high presenting leukocyte counts and, in some studies, more frequent organomegaly and CNS involvement (175,177,178). The prognosis is unfavorable in both children and adults.

ALLs with (11q23) abnormalities are found in up to 80% of infants with ALL and approximately 10% of older children and adults (172,179,180). Most of the translocations at 11q23 involve the MLL gene (168,181). There are numerous partner genes in MLL translocations; the AF4 gene at 4q21, which partners in the t(4;11)(q21;q23)-AF4/MLL, is the most frequent, occurring in about 60% of infants, 2% of other children, and 3% to 6% of adults with ALL (102,172). The leukocyte count is typically markedly increased in t(4;11) ALL. In blood and marrow smears, there are no defining cytologic features. In cases of bilineal t(4;11) leukemia, both lymphoblasts and neoplastic myeloid cells (usually monoblasts and promonocytes) are observed (102). The immunophenotype is characteristically that of early precursor B ALL: CD10(−), TdT(+), CD34(+), CD19(+), HLADR(+). The myeloid-associated antigen CD15 is present in the majority of cases and CD13 and CD33 are commonly expressed (102). The presence of an MLL rearrangement is significantly associated with high-risk clinical features: age under 1 year; markedly elevated leukocyte counts; and a relatively high frequency of CNS involvement. The prognosis is among the worst for ALL, with a high rate of relapse and poor overall survival (102,171,179).

t(1;19)(q23;p13), PBX1/E2A is the most frequent translocation identified by conventional cytogenetics in children with precursor B ALL. It is found in 5% to 6% of patients, 25% of CIg-positive cases, and approximately 1% of CIg-negative cases; it is less common in adults (100,168). There are no distinctive

morphologic findings associated with t(1;19) ALL. The immunophenotype of the lymphoblasts is characterized by homogeneous expression of CD19, CD10, CD9, absent CD34, and absent or underexpression of CD20 (182).

High-risk features have been reported in ALL with t(1;19), including high leukocyte counts, more frequent CNS involvement, and black race (172,183). Recent studies, however, have not always corroborated the high frequency of these adverse features (184). The poor prognosis once ascribed to CIg-positive ALL, and attributed specifically to the t(1;19), appears to have been overcome by contemporary therapies (185).

t(12;21)(p13;q22), TEL/AML-1 is a cryptic translocation generally not found by conventional cytogenetic karyotyping because the rearranged segments are too small to be recognized. The translocation is identified by molecular techniques (e.g., PCR or FISH). The TEL/AML-1 fusion is found in 16% to 39% of children and 3% to 4% of adults with precursor B ALL, making it the most common chromosome structural abnormality in childhood ALL (172,186,187). In some patients, t(12;21) is the only cytogenetic aberrancy and the karyotype appears normal. In others, additional abnormalities are present, but high hyperdiploidy (greater than 50 chromosomes) is virtually never observed with t(12;21) (187). There are no distinctive morphologic features associated with t(12;21) ALL and the immunophenotype is generally that of common precursor B ALL. Bright CD10 and HLADR, lack of expression of CD9 and CD20, and frequent expression of the myeloid-associated antigens CD13 and CD33 are characteristic.

Most studies suggest that t(12;21) ALL has an excellent prognosis (186,187). Response to conventional antimetabolite-based therapy is excellent, with remission rates approaching 100% and high event-free and overall survival.

Hyperdiploidy with more than 50 chromosomes is found in 25% to 30% of children and about 5% of adults with precursor B ALL. There are no unique morphologic or immunophenotypic findings in this category. In children, hyperdiploidy greater than 50 is associated with favorable clinical features and an excellent prognosis; long-term, event-free survival is more than 80% (188). There are prognostic variables within hyperdiploidy greater than 50 ALL. Duplication of chromosomes 4 and 10 appears to impart a particularly favorable prognosis (189). Assessment for duplication of these chromosomes can be done by interphase FISH analysis if conventional cytogenetic studies are not available.

Hypodiploidy is present in 2% to 9% of cases. Most of these have 45 chromosomes; chromosome 20 is commonly lost in children (100). There are no specific presenting clinical, morphologic, or phenotypic features associated with this group. Overall, hypodiploidy is considered an intermediate prognostic finding in children, but adults with hypodiploidy do very poorly; it is the one numerical abnormality with independent prognostic value in adults (171). Hypodiploidy with a near-haploid number of chromosomes, found in only about 1% of cases of ALL, has a particularly bad prognosis regardless of age (190).

The differential diagnosis of precursor B ALL includes several reactive processes and other neoplastic disorders that may manifest clinical or morphologic similarity to ALL. These include increased bone marrow hematogones (normal B lymphocyte precursors); reactive lymphocytosis; aplastic anemia; AML; leukemic Burkitt lymphoma (Burkitt cell leukemia) and other non-Hodgkin lymphomas; chronic lymphoproliferative disorders; and metastatic small-cell tumors. The distinctive features of these are discussed in other sections of this chapter.

Precursor T Acute Lymphoblastic Leukemia

Most of the clinical, morphologic, and cytochemical findings in precursor T ALL are quite similar to those of precursor B ALL, described previously. Only features that are distinctive for precursor T ALL will be discussed here.

The median age of children with precursor T ALL is higher than for precursor B ALL and a greater proportion of patients are adults; approximately 80% of patients are male. There is more often significant extramedullary disease; approximately 50% of patients present with a mediastinal mass, and other lymphadenopathy and organomegaly are more frequent as well. Precursor T neoplasms more commonly present as a lymphoma with minimal or no bone marrow involvement (162,163). Relative to precursor B ALL, there is a higher incidence of CNS disease at presentation (12%) and relapse; the median leukocyte count is significantly higher; and there is more often marked leukocytosis (greater than 100×10^9 per L) (191). Morphologic findings in blood and marrow smears in precursor T ALL are generally similar to precursor B ALL.

Marrow biopsy sections also appear similar but, in some cases of precursor T ALL, most of the lymphoblasts are convoluted and the mitotic rate is generally higher, averaging about twice the number of mitotic figures per high-power field found in precursor B ALL (192).

Immunophenotypically, the lymphoblasts in precursor T ALL express variable combinations of T-cell–associated antigens that include CD1a, CD2, CD3, CD4, CD5, CD7, and CD8, as well as several lineage-nonspecific antigens, especially CD45, CD34, and TdT (95,97,193). In children, nearly all cases of precursor T ALL express one or more of the antigens CD7 (approximately 98%), CD5 (approximately 95%), and CD2 (approximately 92%); concurrent expression of these three antigens is found in nearly 85% (191). CD3 is the most specific marker for T-lineage leukemia but is lacking on the cell surface in about two-thirds of cases of precursor T ALL; however, virtually all cases express cytoplasmic CD3 (cCD3). TdT is present in more than 90% of cases, but CD34 is found less commonly than in precursor B ALL in children and in only about one-third of adult cases (194). TdT is valuable in distinguishing precursor T-lymphoblastic leukemia/lymphoma from peripheral T-cell neoplasms, which lack TdT but may express any of the other T-cell–associated antigens except CD1a.

Cytogenetic abnormalities are found in 50% to 60% of cases of precursor T ALL. In about one-third of cases of precursor T ALL, translocations involve the α/δ T-cell receptor loci at 14q11-q13 or the β/γ loci at 7q34; a variety of partner genes may be involved (101). In contrast to precursor B ALL, there is a relative lack of prognostic importance of chromosomal abnormalities in precursor T ALL, and no cytogenetic categories of precursor T ALL have been included in the WHO classification (101,195). The recurring translocations of precursor B ALL are rarely observed in precursor T ALL; hyperdiploidy greater than 50 is also relatively uncommon and is not associated with survival advantage. Conversely, the two most common translocations in precursor T ALL (t[11;14]) and (t[10;14]), are virtually never observed in precursor B ALL (101).

The differential diagnosis includes all of the same entities as listed for precursor B ALL and several peripheral T-cell prolif-

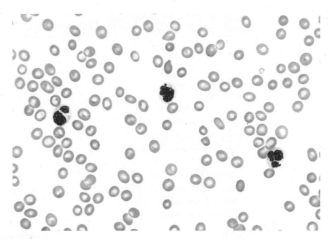

Figure 16.17. A blood smear from a patient with refractory cytopenias with multilineage dysplasia illustrating marked pancytopenia and dysplastic neutrophils.

erations, such as T-prolymphocytic leukemia, adult T-cell leukemia, and Sézary syndrome. These disorders are discussed in the section "T-Cell Lymphomas" below.

The remission rate and survival for patients with precursor T ALL has improved significantly with contemporary therapies. Despite this, the overall prognosis for precursor T ALL is less favorable than for precursor B ALL in children.

MYELODYSPLASTIC SYNDROME

MDS is a bone marrow stem cell disorder resulting in disorderly and ineffective hematopoiesis manifested by irreversible quantitative and qualitative defects in hematopoietic cells (Fig. 16.17). Most patients are over age 50 at diagnosis, but MDS may affect young adults and children. Some patients present with profoundly dysplastic changes and increased myeloblasts, allowing for an immediate diagnosis of MDS. In others, changes are subtle and the diagnosis may be delayed until the patient has been followed for several months and other causes of the cytopenias have been thoroughly evaluated and ruled out. The clinical and morphologic distinction of the more aggressive types of MDS and AML is frequently difficult. The criterion for distinguishing the two is the percentage of myeloblasts in the blood and marrow; a diagnosis of AML is made if there are 20% or more myeloblasts (196). Approximately one-third of patients with MDS develop AML within months.

The features used to define MDS are listed in Table 16.9. There are numerous descriptions of the cytologic features of the MDS in blood and marrow smears (83,85,91,147,197–205).

TABLE 16.9

Features That Define Myelodysplastic Syndrome

Blood cytopenias
Ineffective hematopoiesis
Dyserythropoiesis
Dysgranulopoiesis
Dysmegakaryopoiesis
Increased myeloblasts

TABLE 16.10	Hematologic Findings in Myelodysplastic Syndromes
Blood	*Bone Marrow*
Dyserythropoiesis	
Anemia	Erythroid hyperplasia (occasionally hypoplasia)
Anisopoikilocytosis	Nuclear-cytoplasmic asynchrony
Oval macrocytes	Megaloblastic(oid) chromatin
Hypochromic cells	Karyorrhexis
Dimorphic populations	Multinuclearity
Decreased polychromatophilic cells	Internuclear bridging
Basophilic stippling	Nuclear fragments
Nucleated red blood cells	Ringed sideroblasts
Vacuolated red blood cells	Periodic acid-Schiff–positive erythroblasts
Howell-Jolly bodies	
Dysgranulopoiesis	
Neutropenia	Increased myeloblasts and immature granulocytes
Rarely neutrophilia	Abnormally localized, immature precursors
Immature granulocytes	Maturation defects
Hypogranularity	Hypogranularity
Nuclear hyposegmentation (pseudo–Pelger-	Abnormal granules
Huët change)	Abnormal nuclei
Nuclear "sticks"	Myeloperoxidase-deficient neutrophils
Occasionally hypersegmentation	Increased monocytes
Hypercondensed chromatin	Increased basophils
Circulating myeloblasts (<5%)	
Dysmegakaryopoiesis	
Thrombocytopenia	Increased or decreased megakaryocytes
Large platelets	Clusters of megakaryocytes
Hypogranular platelets	Micromegakaryocytes
Vacuolated platelets	Monolobation or hypolobation
Abnormal platelet granules	Odd-numbered nuclei
Micromegakaryocytes	Multiple, widely separated nuclei
	Hypogranulation

These will be reviewed briefly in the discussion of the WHO categories of MDS. Examples of dysplastic changes for each of the lineages are listed in Table 16.10. The marrow sections in MDS are generally hypercellular (200,206). However, a normocellular or even hypocellular marrow is more common than in acute leukemia (203,207). The proliferative cells are obviously myeloid, with most showing maturation beyond the earliest stages. A panmyelopathy may be apparent or abnormalities of one cell type may predominate. In the refractory anemias, there is usually striking erythroid hyperplasia, and increased storage iron is common. In aggressive forms of MDS, all bone marrow cell lineages may be affected and there is often an increase in the most immature cells. In some cases, myeloblasts and promyelocytes are found in clusters remote from their usual paratrabecular location (Fig. 16.18B). This abnormal localization of immature precursors (ALIP) is a useful diagnostic criterion and has been shown by some investigators to be indicative of an increased likelihood of leukemic transformation (208,209). Increased and dysplastic megakaryocytes are present in many cases. In a minority of patients, the biopsies show increased reticulin; rarely, severe myelofibrosis is observed (210–212). With progression of the MDS, the marrow usually becomes increasingly cellular and more severe dysplastic changes are noted. There is frequently a concurrent increase in myeloblasts and progressively severe bone marrow failure (197–199).

Immunophenotype and Cytogenetics

Immunophenotyping contributes to the diagnosis of MDS in some cases. On flow cytometry analysis there is often aberrant antigen expression on the maturing leukocytes, and side scatter is abnormally diminished because of hypogranularity. IHC on marrow biopsies can aid in determining the blast percentage in some cases where there is a poor aspirate.

As with the acute leukemias, bone marrow cytogenetic studies are important in the diagnosis and as an indicator of prognosis. The finding of bone marrow clonal abnormal (nonconstitutional) cytogenetics is very strong evidence in support of MDS in a patient with cytopenias and dysplasia (213,214). There are no cytogenetic changes that are specific for MDS. The majority of patients show a recurrent loss of chromosome material but reciprocal translocations or inversions may also be found, althoughly less commonly than in AML. Frequent recurring chromosome defects in patients with MDS include complete or partial loss of chromosome 5 or 7, +8, 20q-, and complex chromosome abnormalities (196). 5q- alone or in combination with other chromosome abnormalities appears to be the most

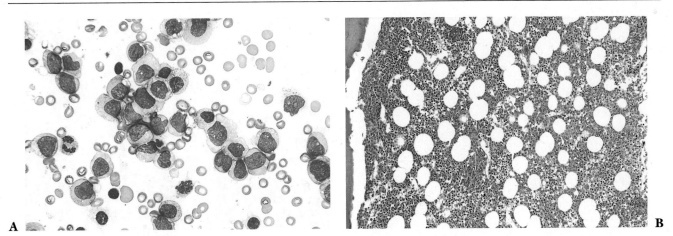

Figure 16.18. **(A)** A bone marrow smear from a 72-year-old man with refractory anemia with excess blasts, type 2. There is a shift toward immaturity, dysplasia in the neutrophil precursors, and increased myeloblasts; the differential count showed 15% blasts. **(B)** The marrow is mildly hypercellular for the patient's age and there is abnormal localization of immature precursors.

common defect. The type of cytogenetic abnormality has prognostic significance (112).

Classification of Myelodysplastic Syndrome

The WHO classification of MDS is shown in Table 16.11 (109,196). The categories are discussed below.

The major manifestation of refractory cytopenias is ineffective hematopoiesis of a single lineage, erythropoiesis, granulopoiesis, or megakaryopoiesis. Refractory anemia is the most common and is characterized by anemia, reticulocytopenia, and erythroid hyperplasia in the bone marrow (83). The anemia may be normocytic or macrocytic with anisopoikilocytosis; oval macrocytes are common. There is no evidence of dysplastic changes in the neutrophils or platelets. Myeloblasts are not identified in the blood smear and monocytes are less than 1.0 $\times 10^9$ per L.

The bone marrow is hypercellular or normocellular with erythroid hyperplasia in most cases; occasionally the marrow is hypoplastic. Dyserythropoiesis may be noted but is usually not severe. Ringed sideroblasts are occasionally observed but they number less than 15% of the erythroblasts. Dysgranulopoiesis and dysmegakaryopoiesis are absent. Myeloblasts are less than

5% in the marrow. A thorough evaluation for other causes of anemia must always be performed before a diagnosis of refractory anemia (RA) is made. In some cases the diagnosis is made only after following the patient for several months and eliminating all other possible causes. Most patients with RA have a chronic course but may require red-cell transfusion support. A small minority evolve to a more aggressive MDS and bone marrow failure or AML.

The clinical and morphologic features of RA with ringed sideroblasts (RARS) are similar to those of RA (83). However, in RARS 15% or more of the bone marrow erythroblasts are ringed sideroblasts. A dimorphic anemia with normal erythrocytes and microcytic or hypochromic poikilocytes is commonly found. Coarse basophilic stippling (including Pappenheimer bodies) is observed in some of the erythrocytes. Neutropenia and thrombocytopenia are not present or are minimal, and there are no dysplastic changes in either lineage. Myeloblasts are not present in the blood and monocytes are less than 1.0 $\times 10^9$ per L.

The bone marrow is hypercellular or normocellular with erythroid hyperplasia and markedly increased iron stores. The numerous ringed sideroblasts are the most prominent feature. Mild to moderate dyserythropoiesis may be observed but dysplastic changes in granulocytes and megakaryocytes are not present. Myeloblasts are rarely increased and never exceed 4%.

Ringed sideroblasts may be observed in any of the other categories of MDS, occasionally exceeding 15% of the erythroblasts. In some cases of refractory cytopenia with multilineage dysplasia (see below), there are 15% or more ringed sideroblasts. This group is distinguished from RARS by the presence of bicytopenia or pancytopenia and dysplastic changes in more than one lineage. It is important to distinguish these cases from RARS because of their more aggressive clinical course.

In refractory cytopenias with multilineage dysplasia (RCMD), there are one or more blood cytopenias and dysplastic changes in 10% or more of the cells in two or more myeloid lineages (196) (Fig. 16.17). Bone marrow and blood myeloblasts are less than 5%. RCMD is distinguished from RA by the significant changes in the granulocyte and platelet/megakaryocytic

TABLE 16.11

WHO Classification of Myelodysplastic Syndromes

Refractory cytopenia with unilineage dysplasia
  Refractory anaemia
  Refractory neutropenia
  Refractory thombocytopenia
Refractory anaemia with ring sideroblasts
Refractory cytopenia with multilineage dysplasia
Refractory anaemia with excess blasts
Myelodysplastic syndrome, associated with isolated del(5q)
Myelodysplastic syndrome, unclassifiable
Childhood myelodysplastic syndrome
  Refractory cytopenia of childhood

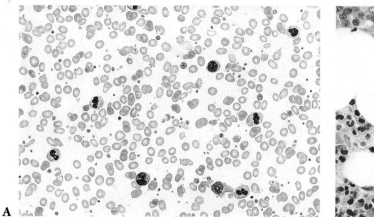
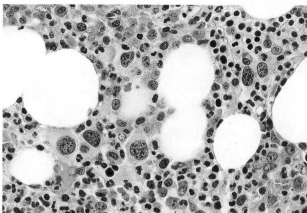

A   B

Figure 16.19. **(A)** A blood smear from a 60-year-old woman with a myelodysplastic syndrome associated with isolated del(5q) chromosome abnormality. There is macrocytic anemia and thrombocytosis. **(B)** The bone marrow section shows several hypolobulated megakaryocyte nuclei.

lineages in addition to the erythrocytes, and differs from RA with excess blasts by having fewer than 5% myeloblasts. In some instances dysgranulopoiesis or dysmegakaryopoiesis are the major abnormalities. RCMD usually has a more aggressive course than RA and a greater propensity for evolution to AML. The clinical course is often similar to that of refractory anemia with excess blasts (RAEB). In many respects this category bridges RA and RAEB.

Pancytopenia or bicytopenia are characteristic of RAEB (83). Dysplastic changes are commonly observed in erythrocytes, granulocytes, and platelets. Nucleated red blood cells and immature granulocytes, including myeloblasts and, occasionally, micromegakaryocytes, may be found in the blood smears. Myeloblasts may constitute up to 19% of the leukocytes in the blood.

The bone marrow is normocellular or hypercellular, and granulocytic or erythroid hyperplasia are present. Myeloblasts are increased to at least 5% but less than 20%. Auer rods may be present. Dyserythropoiesis is more severe than in RA or RARS. Dysgranulopoiesis is often prominent (Fig. 16.18). Megakaryocytic hyperplasia with dysmegakaryopoiesis and megakaryocytic clusters on biopsy sections may be observed. The features that distinguish RAEB from RA and RARS include the severity of the pancytopenia or bicytopenia; dysplastic changes in more than one cell lineage; and the presence of 5% or more myeloblasts in the blood or bone marrow.

RAEB is distinguished from RCMD by the myeloblast percentage. The WHO classification separates RAEB into two types based on blast percentage (196). Type 1 RAEB is characterized by 5% to 9% blasts in the blood or bone marrow. Type 2 RAEB has 10% to 19% blasts in the blood or bone marrow (Fig. 16.18). The basis for this separation into two types stems from the finding that patients with RAEB with 10% or more myeloblasts often have a more aggressive course and a greater propensity for transformation to AML. The presence of Auer rods in a case of MDS, regardless of the blast count, elevates the diagnosis to RAEB type 2.

"MDS Unclassifiable" has features diagnostic of MDS but lacks the typical findings that define RA, RARS, RCMD, and RAEB (196). Most commonly, patients present with isolated neutropenia or thrombocytopenia, and dysplastic changes are confined to neutrophils and precursors or megakaryocytes and platelets.

MDS with isolated del(5q) chromosome abnormality (5q-syndrome) is characterized by macrocytic anemia, often thrombocytosis (approximately 50%), erythroblastopenia, megakaryocyte hyperplasia with nuclear hypolobation, and an isolated interstitial deletion of chromosome 5 (Fig. 16.19). The 5q-syndrome is found predominantly in older women (215). Most patients have a stable clinical course but are often transfusion-dependent.

MYELODYSPLASTIC/MYELOPROLIFERATIVE DISEASES

Some myeloid diseases bridge MDS and chronic myeloproliferative disease (MPD) in their morphologic and clinical features, and do not clearly fit into the categories of either group of disorders. The WHO classification recognizes three myeloid diseases that may have overlapping features of MDS and MPD, which are described below (196) (Table 16.12).

Disorders with diagnostic features of chronic myelomonocytic leukemia (CMML) appear to encompass both myelodysplastic and chronic myeloproliferative diseases. CMML is associated with a broad spectrum of clinical and hematologic presentations (83). Some patients exhibit the typical clinical and morphologic features of MDS, including blood cytopenias, ineffective hematopoiesis, dysplastic changes, and increased blasts. The morphologic features of CMML in these cases may be similar to those of RA, RCMD, or RAEB, with the addition

TABLE 16.12

World Health Organization (WHO) Classification of Myelodysplastic/Myeloproliferative Neoplasms (MDS/MPN)

Chronic myelomonocytic leukaemia
Atypical chronic myeloid leukaemia
   BCR-ABL1 negative
Juvenile myelomonocytic leukaemia
Myelodysplastic/myeloproliferative neoplasm, unclassifiable
Refractory anaemia with ring sideroblasts associated with marked thrombocytosis

of monocytosis of greater than 1.0×10^9 per L. The monocytes may exhibit dysplastic features in blood smears in the form of hyperlobulated nuclei, increased basophilia of the cytoplasm, and abnormal granulation. Blasts and promonocytes comprise fewer than 20% of the nucleated cells in the blood and marrow. Other cases present with marked leukocytosis, with monocytosis, organomegaly, and minimal or no dysplasia or increase in blasts; there is effective hematopoiesis and red-cell and platelet counts may be normal. Regardless of the presenting features in CMML, it is not always predictable whether a case will evolve clinically like MDS or MPD.

Atypical chronic myelogenous leukemia (aCML) is characterized by an increased leukocyte count composed predominantly of cells in the neutrophil lineage. Mature neutrophils predominate but immature granulocytes usually account for more than 10% of the blood leukocytes. Monocytosis may occur but is less than 10% of the leukocytes (216). The bone marrow is hypercellular and there is granulocytic hyperplasia with dysplastic changes. In some cases there is dyserythropoiesis and dysmegakaryopoiesis. Several features of aCML are similar to CML but, unlike CML, basophilia is minimal or lacking; dysplasia is a prominent feature in the neutrophils; and anemia and thrombocytopenia are common (216). The Philadelphia chromosome and rearrangement of the BCR gene are lacking. The prognosis for aCML is similar to an aggressive MDS, with reported median survivals of less than 2 years. Patients may manifest terminal bone marrow failure or AML.

Juvenile myelomonocytic leukemia (JMML) was formerly referred to as juvenile chronic myeloid leukemia (196,217). The designation JMML is more appropriate because its morphologic and clinical features more closely mimic CMML than CML. Approximately 60% of cases are diagnosed in patients less than 2 years of age. However, cases have been diagnosed in children from less than 1 month of age to early adolescence. JMML arises from a stem cell defect that leads to deranged hematopoiesis. The disorder is characterized by leukocytosis in the range of 20 to 30×10^9 per L, composed of granulocytes and monocytes. Immature and dysplastic forms can be identified but dysplasia is usually not prominent. Blasts and promonocytes are fewer than 20% of the blood and bone marrow cells. The bone marrow is hypercellular with granulocytic hyperplasia. The degree of monocyte involvement is variable, from 5% to greater than 30% of the bone marrow cells. In vitro cell culture studies show spontaneous formation of high numbers of abnormal colony-forming units. Hypersensitivity of the neoplastic cells to GM-CSF has also been repeatedly demonstrated.

Other features of JMML are thrombocytopenia, hepatosplenomegaly and lymphadenopathy, skin rash, and an elevated hemoglobin F level. The latter can be a helpful diagnostic clue in the early stages of the disease. Cytogenetic studies are often normal; the most commonly reported abnormality is a monosomy 7. In about 10% of patients there is deletion of the NF1 tumor suppressor gene and an associated neurofibromatosis, type 1 (217).

Unfavorable risk factors in JMML include age greater than 1 year, low platelet counts, elevated hemoglobin F levels, and abnormal cytogenetics. The disease course may wax and wane in some cases, but ultimately most patients succumb to the disease. The only potentially curative treatment modality is allogeneic bone marrow transplant.

CHRONIC MYELOPROLIFERATIVE DISEASES

The chronic myeloproliferative diseases arise from clonal hematopoietic stem cell disorders. They are characterized by effective autonomous proliferation of one or more myeloid lineages resulting in increased numbers of leukocytes, erythrocytes, or platelets in the blood. The elevation in blood counts is often marked. The morphology of the cells is usually normal at least in the early or chronic phase of the disorders. The WHO classification of the chronic myeloproliferative disorders is shown in Table 16.13 (218a,219).

CHRONIC MYELOID LEUKEMIA

The diagnosis of chronic myeloid leukemia (CML) is usually made from examination of a blood smear (216,220,221) (Fig. 16.20A). There is marked leukocytosis, with the entire neutrophil series represented from myeloblasts to segmented neutrophils; neutrophil myelocytes and segmented neutrophils are most numerous. Myeloblasts generally account for less than 5% of the leukocytes. All patients have basophilia and the platelet count is elevated in more than half.

The bone marrow in CML is markedly hypercellular, often with a complete absence of adipose tissue. There is marked granulocytic hyperplasia, primarily of the neutrophil lineage, but an increase in basophils, eosinophils, and sometimes monocytes may be observed (Fig. 16.20B). Megakaryocytes are increased in most cases and may be markedly increased and clustered in biopsy sections; they are typically smaller than normal. This finding can be helpful in distinguishing CML from other chronic myeloproliferative disorders in which megakaryocytes are normal-sized or larger than normal. In some cases the marrow smears and sections are not readily distinguishable from a profound leukemoid reaction (222).

A mild increase in reticulin fibers may be found in marrow biopsy sections in the majority of patients, but prominent myelofibrosis is uncommon at diagnosis (223). Extensive myelofibrosis evolves during the course of the disease in a minority of patients. In these cases, the histopathologic features may be indistinguishable from those of chronic idiopathic myelofibrosis or advanced polycythemia vera. The evolution to myelofibrosis in CML is reported to be a poor prognostic factor.

TABLE 16.13

WHO Classification of Myeloproliferative Neoplasms

Chronic myelogenous leukaemia, *BCR-ABL1* positive
Chronic neutrophilic leukaemia
Polycythemia vera
Primary myelofibrosis
Essential thrombocythemia
Chronic eosinophilic leukaemia, NOS
Mastocytosis
    Cutaneous mastocytosis
    Systemic mastocytosis
    Mast cell leukaemia
    Mast cell sarcoma
    Extracutaneous mastocytoma
Myeloproliferative neoplasm, unclassifiable

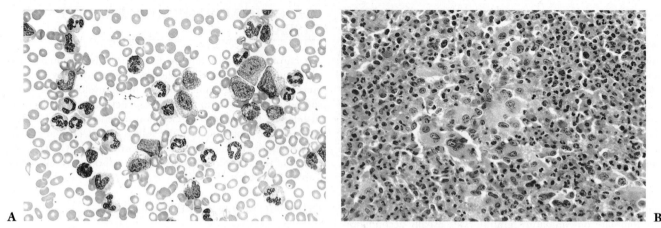

Figure 16.20. **(A)** Blood smear from a patient with chronic myelogenous leukemia (CML). The blood leukocyte count is markedly elevated and consists mostly of neutrophils at various stages of maturation from myeloblasts to segmented neutrophils and basophils. **(B)** Biopsy section from a 48-year-old man with CML. The marrow is markedly hypercellular with predominantly granulocytes at various stages of maturation. Several abnormally small megakaryocytes are present.

Other diagnostic features of CML include a low leukocyte (neutrophil) alkaline phosphatase (LAP) score and the presence of a specific bone marrow chromosome rearrangement, the t(9;22) (q34;q11) (Philadelphia chromosome). The breakpoints of the translocation involve the ABL gene on chromosome 9 and the BCR gene on chromosome 22. These form a chimeric BCR/ABL gene. This fusion gene can be detected by PCR or FISH (224,225). Its presence defines CML and distinguishes it from other chronic myeloproliferative disorders that may share some of the other features of CML (e.g., chronic myelomonocytic leukemia, atypical CML) (216).

The natural course of CML is to evolve to an accelerated or blastic phase in an average of approximately 3 years (226–230). Features of the accelerated phase may include any of the following, singly or in various combinations: blast count of 10% to 19% in the blood or marrow; blood basophils of greater than 20%; persistent thrombocytopenia of less than 100×10^9/L; persistent thrombocytosis of greater than 1000×10^9/L while on therapy; increasing spleen size and leukocyte count while on adequate therapy; marked dysplasia; marked myelofibrosis; and chromosomal evolution (218). When the blastic phase occurs, the blast count is 20% or more and the picture in the marrow and blood changes to those of an acute leukemia of either myeloid or lymphoblastic type (227). In some instances, there is an extramedullary blast proliferation prior to obvious bone marrow blast phase, or the marrow blast phase is focal in biopsy sections (218). The blastic phase is generally poorly responsive to therapy and portends a short survival.

CHRONIC NEUTROPHILIC LEUKEMIA

Chronic neutrophilic leukemia (CNL) is a rare, chronic myeloproliferative disorder characterized by a sustained increase (more than 25×10^9/L) in mature blood neutrophils without an identifiable cause (109,231–233). The marrow is hypercellular with granulocytic hyperplasia; erythroid and megakaryocyte hyperplasia may occur in some cases. There is minimal or no myelodysplasia, and myeloblasts are not increased. Splenomegaly is frequently present resulting from infiltration by mature neutrophils. Cytogenetics are normal in approximately 90% of cases. In cases with cytogenetic abnormalities, changes common

to other myeloid neoplasms are the usual finding, e.g., +8, del(20q), etc. Rare cases of CML with a variant BCR/ABL fusion gene, p230, may exhibit predominantly mature neutrophils in the blood and should not be mistaken for CNL (234).

Several cases of CNL have been reported in association with other neoplasms, most commonly plasma cell myeloma (235,236). None of these cases has had documented clonal cytogenetic changes in the granulocytes, and they may represent secondary proliferations due to abnormal cytokine release by the neoplastic cells (218).

CNL has a chronic course in most instances. Cases undergoing transformation to MDS or AML have been reported (232,233).

CHRONIC EOSINOPHILIC LEUKEMIA AND THE HYPEREOSINOPHILIC SYNDROME

In chronic eosinophilic leukemia (CEL) there is a sustained eosinophilia of greater than 1.5×10^9 per L, increased eosinophils in the marrow, and less than 20% myeloblasts (218a,237b). Causes of reactive eosinophilia must be excluded by clonality, or an increase in myeloblasts should be demonstrated. Other myeloid disorders that may be associated with eosinophilia, such as CML and other MPD, AML, and MDS, must be excluded. In cases where clonality of the eosinophils cannot be demonstrated and there is no increase in myeloblasts, the designation "idiopathic hypereosinophilic syndrome" is preferred.

The degree of eosinophilia is variable from the minimum necessary for a diagnosis to greater than 100×10^9 per L. Most of the eosinophils are mature but scattered, and sometimes numerous immature eosinophils may be present. Dysplastic changes are found in some of the cells but are often similar to findings observed in marked reactive eosinophilia. Neutrophilia is present in some cases. The marrow is hypercellular with a marked increase in eosinophil precursors. Usually neutrophil erythroid and megakaryocyte maturation is normal. Myeloblasts may be increased but, in many cases, are normal in number at first presentation. Dysplastic changes vary from no obvious abnormalities to dysplastic changes in both eosinophils and other lineages.

There are no specific cytogenetic abnormalities in CEL and

idiopathic hypereosinophilic syndrome, but changes common to other myeloid neoplasms such as +8, i(17q) are found in some cases. Chromosome 8p11 rearrangements have been reported in several cases of CEL.

Most patients suffer multiorgan disease due to tissue infiltration by eosinophils and release of cytokines and other factors in the eosinophil granules. The most commonly affected organs are the heart, lungs, CNS, gastrointestinal (GI) tract, and skin. Survival is variable, from relatively short to more than 5 years. Massive splenomegaly, increased blasts, dysplasia, cytogenetic abnormalities, and severe clinical symptoms with organ damage are associated with more aggressive disease (237a,237b).

POLYCYTHEMIA VERA

Polycythemia vera (PV) is a myeloproliferative disorder characterized by panhyperplasia of the bone marrow with erythrocytosis, leukocytosis, and thrombocytosis in the blood (219,238–242). Erythroid and megakaryocytic hyperplasia are the most profound. The hemoglobin, hematocrit, and platelet count are often markedly increased. Clinical criteria for the diagnosis established by the Polycythemia Study Group and expanded in the WHO classification are based on red-cell mass and oxygen saturation, splenomegaly, and other laboratory studies (218,243). Erythropoietin levels are markedly decreased and usually distinguish PV from secondary causes of erythrocytosis. Trephine biopsy sections are usually moderately to markedly hypercellular, with striking erythroid hyperplasia and increased megakaryocytes, many of which are larger than usual and often polymorphic (244–247) (Fig. 16.21). The marrow may show increased vascularity and depleted storage iron. The prominent erythroid hyperplasia distinguishes PV from CML.

Reticulin may be increased in PV, particularly in areas where megakaryocytes are concentrated. There may be a gradual increase in reticulin fibrosis, culminating in advanced myelosclerosis at the terminal stage of disease, at which time the changes in trephine biopsy sections are indistinguishable from chronic idiopathic myelofibrosis. The incidence of transformation of PV to AML is low and appears to be related to the type of therapy used to control the polycythemia (247,248).

The histopathologic changes in PV must be distinguished from those in cases of secondary erythrocytosis. In secondary erythroid hyperplasia, megakaryocytes are not affected, the cellularity may be less than in PV, there is no increase in reticulin, and iron stores are less likely to be depleted. In most instances, PV and secondary erythrocytosis are readily distinguished by the erythropoietin levels and the WHO classification criteria (218).

ESSENTIAL THROMBOCYTHEMIA

Essential thrombocythemia is a chronic myeloproliferative disorder in which the most striking feature is a marked increase in megakaryocytes and florid thrombocytosis (219,242,249–253). The WHO classification criteria for diagnosis include a sustained platelet count of 600×10^9 per L or more; a marrow biopsy showing proliferation mainly of the megakaryocyte lineage with increased numbers of enlarged mature megakaryocytes; and exclusion of other causes of thrombocytosis (218) (Fig. 16.22). The morphology of the platelets on blood smears may be normal, or numerous large, atypical forms may be observed. The bone marrow is normocellular or hypercellular (252). Megakaryocytes show considerable variation in size, similar to those in PV. Increased reticulin is demonstrable in some cases but prominent fibrosis is not a feature.

Thrombocythemia must be distinguished from secondary thrombocytosis and the other chronic myeloproliferative disorders, especially PV. The platelet count is generally not as elevated in secondary thrombocytosis, but the distinction is best made by the clinical findings. Panhyperplasia is present in some cases of essential thrombocythemia, but erythroid precursors are less strikingly increased than in PV and the red-cell mass is normal (252,254). Many cases of essential thrombocythemia cannot be distinguished from PV or other chronic myeloproliferative disorders exclusively on morphologic criteria (255).

CHRONIC IDIOPATHIC MYELOFIBROSIS WITH MYELOID METAPLASIA

Chronic idiopathic myelofibrosis with myeloid metaplasia is a chronic MPD characterized by a panmyelopathy, marrow fibrosis, extramedullary hematopoiesis, and moderate to marked

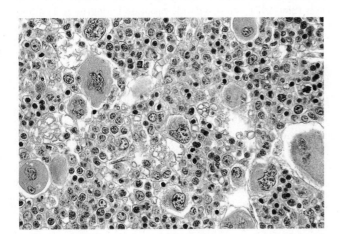

Figure 16.21. Bone marrow trephine biopsy section from a 57-year-old woman with polycythemia vera. The marrow is markedly hypercellularity with a striking increase in erythroid precursors and megakaryocytes.

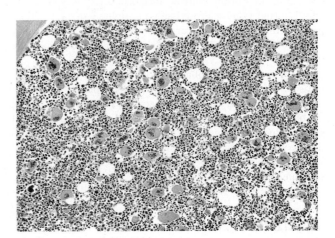

Figure 16.22. Bone marrow section from a patient with essential thrombocythemia. The patient's platelet count was 1.7 million. The marrow is hypercellular and megakaryocytes are markedly increased.

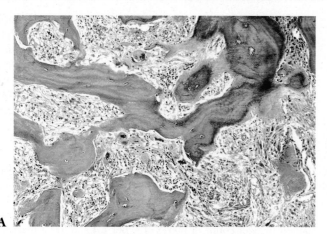
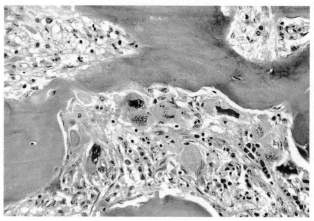

A   **B**

Figure 16.23. **(A)** Chronic idiopathic myelofibrosis in a marrow biopsy from a 70-year-old man. There is myelofibrosis and osteosclerosis. **(B)** A higher magnification shows megakaryocytes and other hematopoietic cells and myelofibrosis.

splenomegaly (218,219,242,256–264) (Fig. 16.23). In the natural course of the disease, the bone marrow becomes increasingly myelosclerotic and in some cases osteosclerotic; normal hematopoietic tissue is gradually reduced. The myelofibrosis appears to be caused by factors produced and released by the abnormal megakaryocytes (265,266). The disease is characterized by a chronic course, often of several years' duration. The designation "malignant myelosclerosis" has been used to describe cases with an unusually rapid clinical course (267).

The histopathology of the marrow reflects the progression of the disease and can be divided into three phases (268). A hypercellular phase is characterized by an increase in hematopoietic elements of the marrow, primarily megakaryocytes and granulocytes. Unusually large and small megakaryocytes may be found in clusters. Increased fibrous connective tissue is not always apparent in the hypercellular phase, but increased reticulin can usually be demonstrated around clusters of megakaryocytes. A patchy phase features alternating areas of hematopoiesis and fibrosis. The phase of obliterative myelosclerosis is characterized by extensive marrow replacement with fibrous connective tissue. The remaining scattered clusters of hematopoietic cells have the appearance of being entrapped and compressed in the fibrotic marrow; megakaryocytes may be markedly distorted. Osteosclerosis is often prominent in this terminal phase of the disease. The marrow histopathologic features may vary among the three phases in biopsies from different anatomic sites (268).

In the hypercellular phase, blood counts are normal or increased; immature granulocytes and atypical platelets are commonly observed. As the marrow becomes increasingly fibrotic, the blood counts drop and more abnormal cells appear in blood smears. Red-cell changes are particularly striking, with abundant teardrop-shaped elliptocytes. Extramedullary hematopoiesis and spleen size increase as the marrow becomes progressively sclerotic.

MASTOCYTOSIS

Mastocytosis encompasses several clinical syndromes that result from an abnormal, clonal proliferation of mast cells in one or

more organs. Mutations of KIT, a proto-oncogene, have been identified in all types of systemic mastocytosis (269,291).

The WHO classification of mastocytosis is shown in Table 16.14 (269,270). Major and minor criteria for diagnosis of systemic mastocytosis are detailed in the WHO classification (270). Diagnosis requires the major criterion plus one minor criterion, or three minor criteria. The major criterion is presence of multifocal, dense infiltrates of 15 or more mast cells in aggregates in marrow biopsies or other extracutaneous organs. These should be confirmed by tryptase or other special stains. The minor criteria include:

- More than 25% of the mast cells in the infiltrate on a biopsy section are spindle-shaped or have atypical morphology, or more than 25% of the mast cells in a marrow aspirate are immature or atypical.
- Detection of a KIT point mutation.
- Mast cells coexpressing CD117 with CD2 and/or CD25.
- Serum tryptase persistently >20 ng/mL (unless there is an associated clonal myeloid disorder).

Bone marrow is the tissue most commonly biopsied to establish the diagnosis of systemic mastocytosis and is involved in most cases (269–277). There is a wide variation in degree and pattern of involvement from case to case. In more than 80% of patients,

TABLE 16.14

Classification of Mastocytosis

Cutaneous mastocytosis
Indolent systemic mastocytosis
Systemic mastocytosis with associated clonal, hematological non-mast-cell lineage disease
Aggressive systemic mastocytosis
Mast cell leukemia
Mast cell sarcoma
Extracutaneous mastocytoma

From: Valent P, Horny HP, Li CY, et al. Mastocytosis. In Jaffe ES, Harris NL, Stein H, et al., eds. *World Health Organization Classification of Tumors. Pathology and Genetics of Tumours of Haematopoietic and Lymphoid Tissues.* Lyon, France: IARC Press, 2001:291–293.

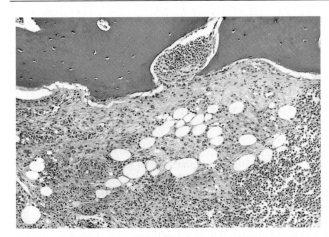

Figure 16.24. Trephine biopsy from a 78-year-old woman with systemic mast cell disease. There is widening and irregularity of the bone trabeculae and a paratrabecular infiltrate.

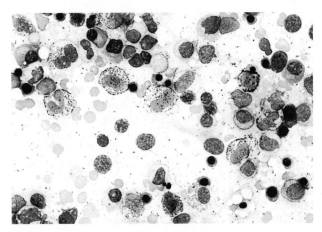

Figure 16.26. A bone marrow smear from a 59-year-old man with mast cell disease and a myelodysplastic syndrome. There are numerous mast cells on the smear.

the pattern of involvement is focal and in less than 20% diffuse (273,275,278). Focal lesions may be paratrabecular, perivascular, or randomly distributed; all three types may be observed in the same biopsy specimen (273,276). The paratrabecular lesions marginate along the trabecular border and are associated with fibrosis and expansion of the trabeculae (Fig. 16.24). The perivascular lesions induce prominent medial and adventitial hypertrophy.

Focal lesions are polycellular or relatively monocellular (273,276,278). Polycellular lesions are usually randomly distributed and characterized by a mixture of mast cells, lymphocytes, eosinophils, neutrophils, histiocytes, endothelial cells, and fibroblasts. The various cell types may be uniformly mixed, but often there is an element of compartmentalization of cell types with a central focus of lymphocytes encircled by mast cells (Fig. 16.25). The mast cells are usually round or oval with abundant eosinophilic cytoplasm.

The monocellular focal lesions are composed primarily of mast cells with occasional lymphocytes and eosinophils. The mast cells are frequently spindle-shaped with pale to lightly eosinophilic cytoplasm. The nuclei are round, oval, elongated, or monocytoid in configuration; these mast cells resemble histiocytes or fibroblasts.

In all types of focal lesions, nucleoli are inconspicuous and mitotic figures absent. The uninvolved portion of the bone marrow may be normocellular or hypercellular with increased granulocytes (273,276).

In diffuse lesions the entire marrow space between trabeculae is replaced. The mast cells vary from round to elongated, and may resemble fibroblasts. They are frequently mixed with neutrophils, eosinophils, and macrophages. Moderate to marked fibrosis is present and normal hematopoietic cells are markedly reduced.

Bone changes are common in both focal and diffuse lesions. Widened, irregular trabeculae are often observed, particularly in areas near paratrabecular lesions. In some cases osteoclasts are increased and are associated with thinning of trabeculae (273,279).

There is a relatively common association of systemic mastocytosis and myeloid neoplasms, including AML, MDS, or MPD (SM-AHNMD). In these cases the bone marrow biopsy shows features of both disorders (276,280,281) (Fig. 16.26). In the rare cases of mast cell leukemia, the marrow is markedly hypercellular with replacement of normal hematopoietic cells by mast cells that are frequently immature-appearing with atypical features (278,282).

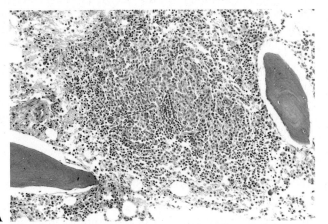

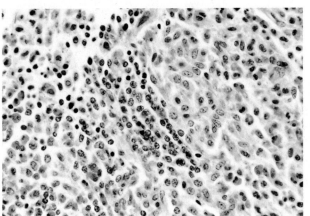

A **B**

Figure 16.25. (A) A polymorphic focal infiltrate in the marrow of a 67-year-old woman with systemic mast cell disease. (B) A higher magnification shows a core of lymphocytes surrounded by mast cells.

Bone marrow aspirate smears usually contain only a few scattered mast cells. The mast cells vary from normal-appearing with round nuclei and densely packed granules, to unusually large cells with abundant cytoplasm and scattered fine granules. When there is a concurrent myeloproliferative process, atypical-appearing mast cells may be found in the marrow smears along with increased myeloblasts and dysplastic hematopoietic cells (278,280,281). In cases of mast cell leukemia, numerous atypical mast cells with decreased granules and irregular-shaped nuclei are found in aspirate smears (273–275,280,282). Mast cells are rarely found in blood smears except in cases of mast cell leukemia (275,281,282).

Recognition of mast cells in a lesion on H&E-stained sections of bone marrow may be problematic because of their morphologic similarity to histiocytes and fibroblasts. When histologic features suggest mastocytosis, the mast cell tryptase and CD117 (c-kit) immunocytochemical stains are the most useful for confirmation of the diagnosis (283). The tryptase stain is highly sensitive and the most specific for mast cells in the bone marrow (Fig. 16.27). CD117 is strongly expressed by mast cells but may also be positive in early myeloid cells. CD33, CD45, CD68, vimentin, lysozyme, α1-antitrypsin, and α1-antichymotrypsin are expressed in normal and most neoplastic mast cells. Mast cells lack myeloperoxidase, CD14, CD15, CD16, CD34, and most B- and T-cell–associated antigens (283–286). Antibodies for several of the chemical mediators produced by mast cells can also be applied by IHC methods (284). Mast cell granules exhibit prominent metachromasia with a Giemsa or toluidine blue stain in both marrow smears and sections (271). The chloroacetate esterase stain may be helpful in identifying mast cells in nondecalcified, formalin-fixed specimens (273,275).

IHC staining or flow cytometry analysis for CD2 and CD25 expression can be particularly useful in distinguishing mast cells in normal or reactive marrow from mastocytosis. Neoplastic mast cells differ from their normal counterparts by the frequent aberrant expression of CD2 and/or CD25 (286–290).

Conditions that merit consideration in the differential diagnosis of systemic mastocytosis in marrow sections include chronic idiopathic myelofibrosis, angioimmunoblastic T-cell lymphoma, hairy cell leukemia, eosinophilic granuloma, and acute promyelocytic leukemia. Familiarity with the histologic features that characterise mast cell lesions and appropriate IHC

stains will provide the distinction from these disorders in nearly all cases.

BONE MARROW LYMPHOID DISORDERS

NON-HODGKIN LYMPHOMA AND CHRONIC LYMPHOPROLIFERATIVE DISORDERS

The pathologic features of the bone marrow biopsy in patients with non-Hodgkin lymphoma (NHL) has been investigated in numerous studies (7,292–313). The incidence of bone marrow involvement at the time of diagnosis is 30% to 53%, and varies widely for the different categories of NHL. The clinical symptomatology in patients with bone marrow involvement also is variable. Many patients with low-grade lymphomas or chronic lymphoproliferative disorders (CLPDs) are completely asymptomatic, whereas patients with aggressive lymphomas more commonly have constitutional symptoms and may have blood cytopenias.

Trephine biopsies are more often positive for NHL than are bone marrow aspirates, but, in the majority of cases, disease is found in both the biopsy and aspirate smears; in a minority of cases the aspirate smears are diagnostic when the sections are negative or equivocal (7–9,11,295,297,314). The aspirated marrow is the best material for several supplementary studies, including immunophenotyping, cytogenetics, and molecular analysis.

The incidence and morphologic features of marrow involvement in relationship to the Rappaport and Lukes-Collins classifications of NHL and the International Working Formulation have been the subjects of numerous reports (75,292–295, 315–320). The International Lymphoma Study Group (ILSG) presented a revised classification of lymphoid neoplasms that incorporated new entities and new diagnostic techniques not considered in the Working Formulation (321). This classification scheme was updated in the 2001 WHO Classification of Hematolymphoid Neoplasms (109). WHO terminology is used in this discussion (Table 16.15). In the following discussion, NHLs and CLPDs that have a high incidence of marrow involvement or that may present major diagnostic problems are emphasized.

The primary diagnosis of NHL is usually established outside of the bone marrow; marrow examination is often performed for staging purposes only. For the CLPDs, the blood and bone marrow examinations often establish the diagnosis. The histologic and cytologic features of each of the categories of NHLs are detailed in Chapter 17, Lymph Nodes; they are discussed here only as they specifically apply to the bone marrow.

The NHLs that most frequently involve the bone marrow are the B-cell categories composed primarily of small cells (with the exception of extranodal marginal zone lymphoma), lymphoblastic lymphoma/leukemia, Burkitt lymphoma, and the various peripheral T-cell lymphomas (295,321–323).

PATTERN AND EXTENT OF MARROW INVOLVEMENT IN BIOPSY SECTIONS

The five major patterns of bone marrow infiltration by NHLs are focal paratrabecular, focal random (nonparatrabecular), interstitial, diffuse, and intrasinusoidal/intravascular (Fig. 16.28A–F). Focal lesions occur more frequently than do intersti-

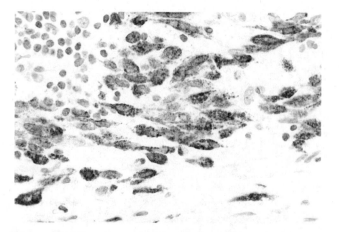

Figure 16.27. A mast cell tryptase stain on a marrow section from a patient with plasma cell myeloma and mastocytosis. The mast cells are elongated and strongly tryptase-positive.

TABLE 16.15

World Health Organization (WHO) Classification of Lymphoid Neoplasms

B-CELL NEOPLASMS

Precursor B-cell neoplasm
  Precursor B lymphoblastic leukemia/lymphoma
Mature B-cell neoplasms
  Chronic lymphocytic leukemia/small lymphocytic lymphoma
  B-cell prolymphocytic leukemia
  Lymphoplasmacytic lymphoma
  Splenic marginal zone lymphoma
  Hairy cell leukemia
  Plasma cell myeloma
  Monoclonal gammopathy of undetermined significance
  Solitary plasmacytoma of bone
  Extraosseous plasmacytoma
  Primary amyloidosis
  Heavy chain diseases
  Extranodal marginal zone B-cell lymphoma of mucosa-associated lymphoid tissue
  Nodal marginal zone B-cell lymphoma
  Follicular lymphoma
  Mantle cell lymphoma
  Diffuse large B-cell lymphoma
  Mediastinal (thymic) large B-cell lymphoma
  Intravascular large B-cell lymphoma
  Primary effusion lymphoma
  Burkitt lymphoma/leukemia
B-cell proliferations of uncertain malignant potential
  Lymphomatoid granulomatosis
  Post-transplant lymphoproliferative disorder, polymorphic

T-CELL AND NATURAL KILLER (NK) CELL NEOPLASMS

Precursor T-cell neoplasms
  Precursor T-lymphoblastic leukemia/lymphoma
  Blastic NK cell lymphoma
Mature T-cell and NK-cell neoplasms
  T-cell prolymphocytic leukemia
  T-cell large granular lymphocytic leukemia
  Aggressive NK-cell leukemia
  Adult T-cell leukemia/lymphoma
  Extranodal NK/T-cell lymphoma, nasal type
  Enteropathy-type T-cell lymphoma
  Hepatosplenic T-cell lymphoma
  Subcutaneous panniculitis-like T-cell lymphoma
  Mycosis fungoides
  Sézary syndrome
  Primary cutaneous anaplastic large cell lymphoma
  Peripheral T-cell lymphoma, unspecified
  Angioimmunoblastic T-cell lymphoma
  Anaplastic large-cell lymphoma
T-cell proliferation of uncertain malignant potential
  Lymphomatoid papulosis

HODGKIN LYMPHOMA

  Nodular lymphocyte predominant Hodgkin lymphoma
  Classical Hodgkin lymphoma
  Nodular sclerosis classic Hodgkin lymphoma
  Lymphocyte-rich classic Hodgkin lymphoma
  Mixed cellularity classic Hodgkin lymphoma
  Lymphocyte-depleted classic Hodgkin lymphoma

tial or diffuse infiltration (295,312). Paratrabecular focal lesions and randomly distributed focal lesions occur with similar frequency. In some cases, both patterns of focal involvement are present in the same biopsy specimen. The number of lesions varies from a single focus to several on each section.

Some categories of NHL have a distinct predilection for a particular pattern of marrow infiltration. For example, the bone marrow lesions of grade 1 and 2 follicular lymphomas are mostly focal and paratrabecular, whereas those of chronic lymphocytic leukemia/small lymphocytic lymphoma are most commonly diffuse or interstitial, uncommonly random focal, and virtually never paratrabecular; Burkitt and lymphoblastic lymphomas generally have an interstitial or diffuse pattern of infiltration (20,294,297,312,315,324,325). Splenic marginal zone lymphoma, hepatosplenic T-cell lymphoma, T-cell large-granular lymphocyte leukemia, and intravascular large-B-cell lymphomas manifest the intravascular or sinusoidal pattern in the bone marrow (326–330).

When the marrow infiltrate is focal in distribution, there is often considerable marrow sparing; in the majority trephines involved by NHL, less than a third of the marrow space is occupied by malignant lymphoma (312). With advanced disease, focal lesions enlarge and may coalesce. With interstitial infiltration, much of the hematopoietic tissue and marrow fat is spared. Diffuse involvement is associated with extensive replacement of normal marrow cells.

MORPHOLOGIC DISCORDANCE OF LYMPH NODE AND BONE MARROW HISTOLOGY

Histologic discordance between the lymph node and bone marrow is noted in 15% to 40% of cases (7,295,296,298,313, 331–334). The more aggressive subtype is usually found in the lymph node. Divergent histologic features are most common with follicular lymphomas and diffuse large-B-cell lymphoma. In a typical discordant pattern, the lymph node exhibits a diffuse large-B-cell lymphoma, whereas the lesions in the bone marrow are paratrabecular infiltrates of small cells. Interestingly, small-cell lymphomatous infiltrates in marrow do not appear to alter the prognosis of diffuse large-B-cell lymphoma (298,313,331,333). In this setting, the morphologically discordant lesions have been shown to be clonally related in two-thirds of cases and apparently unrelated in the remaining third (335,336).

B-CELL NEOPLASMS

PRECURSOR B-LYMPHOBLASTIC LEUKEMIA/LYMPHOMA

Precursor B-lymphoblastic leukemia/lymphoma generally presents as acute leukemia and is discussed in the section "Acute Leukemias and Myelodysplastic Syndromes" earlier in the chapter. Occasional cases manifest primarily as extramedullary lymphoblastic lymphomas and may have minimal or no bone marrow involvement at presentation (163). These share many morphologic features with precursor T-cell lymphoblastic lymphoma/leukemia, which is discussed below.

CHRONIC LYMPHOCYTIC LEUKEMIA/SMALL LYMPHOCYTIC LYMPHOMA

Chronic lymphocytic leukemia/small lymphocytic lymphoma (CLL/SLL) is a clonal proliferation of peripheral, well-differen-

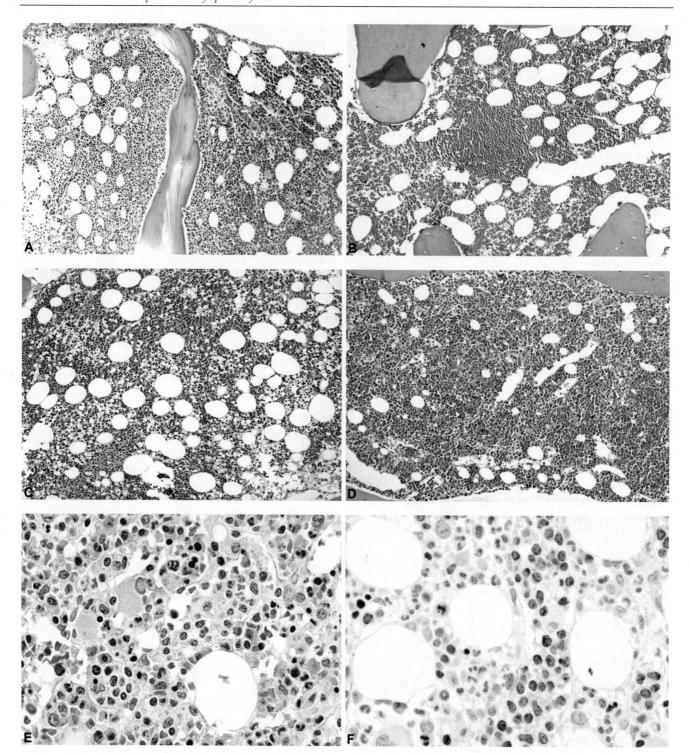

Figure 16.28. Patterns of bone marrow involvement by non-Hodgkin lymphoma (NHL). **(A)** Focal paratrabecular involvement by follicular lymphoma. **(B)** Focal random marrow involvement by mantle cell lymphoma. **(C)** Interstitial marrow involvement by small B-lymphocytic lymphoma/chronic lymphocytic leukemia. **(D)** Diffuse marrow replacement by Burkitt lymphoma. **(E)** Intrasinusoidal pattern of marrow involvement in a patient with hepatosplenic T-cell lymphoma. The clusters of lymphoma cells are within marrow sinuses and encircled by endothelial cells. **(F)** A CD20 immunostain shows the lymphoma cells to have a distinctly intrasinusoidal distribution.

tiated B lymphocytes (109). The diagnosis of CLL/SLL is generally made presumptively from the blood smear of an adult with persistent lymphocytosis. Immunophenotyping should be performed to confirm the diagnosis, however, because other disorders may cytologically mimic CLL (337,338).

In blood and bone marrow smears, the cytology of the lymphocytes is relatively uniform in most cases. The lymphocytes are small to medium-sized with narrow rims of cytoplasm and coarsely clumped chromatin. In a minority of patients there is an admixture of larger lymphocytes with the small lymphocytes, producing a heteromorphous appearance. Such cases are collectively designated "mixed cell type CLL" (339). When more than 10% are present, the designation of "CLL with increased prolymphocytes" (CLL/PL) is sometimes used (339,340); many of these cases are likely CLL in prolymphocytoid transformation. A small number of patients have increased numbers of cleaved nuclei or cells with plasmacytoid features (341,342). Such cases, along with the mixed cell types, are often referred to as "atypical CLL," although the criteria for this designation vary widely.

Four patterns of infiltration may be observed in bone marrow trephine biopsy sections in CLL/SLL: diffuse, interstitial, nodular, and mixed (20,343,344) (Fig. 16.29). With interstitial involvement, the marrow architecture is preserved and the marrow is normocellular or mildly hypercellular; the leukemic lymphocytes are mixed with normal hematopoietic cells. With diffuse involvement, there is extensive, uniform infiltration of the marrow by leukemic lymphocytes; the marrow is markedly hypercellular with a decrease or absence of fat and reduction of normal hematopoietic tissue. The relatively uncommon nodular pattern is characterized by foci of various-sized concentrated lymphocytes randomly dispersed throughout the section between areas of normal marrow; this pattern has been associated with atypical blood cytologic features in one study (345).

The natural history of CLL/SLL can be divided into clinical stages (346,347). The pattern of lymphocytic infiltrate in the marrow parallels the clinical stage of disease and correlates well with prognosis (20,343). The interstitial and nodular patterns of involvement are generally associated with the least advanced stage and the best prognosis, and the diffuse pattern with the most advanced stage and the poorest prognosis (20).

In marrow sections, the lymphocytes are generally small with little cytoplasm. The nuclei are round, have coarse chromatin, and either lack or have small indistinct nucleoli. Mitotic figures are usually not detected. In many cases, individual scattered lymphocytes or small foci of lymphocytes are larger than the predominant cells with less condensed chromatin and prominent nucleoli. These foci of transformed lymphocytes, or proliferation centers, are similar to those in lymph node biopsies from patients with CLL. These areas are most prominent in cases of the mixed-cell types of CLL.

The lymphocytes in CLL have a characteristic immunophenotype that is particularly helpful in distinguishing it from other B-cell lymphoproliferative disorders (339,348–352) (Table 16.16) (Fig. 16.30). The cells express CD5 and CD23 and typically exhibit weak expression of CD20, CD22, and surface immunoglobulin (SIg). They do not express CD10 and usually lack FMC-7 and CD79b.

In a minority of cases of CLL/SLL there is clinical and morphologic transformation to a proliferation of large lymphocytes and an aggressive clinical course. The two most common types

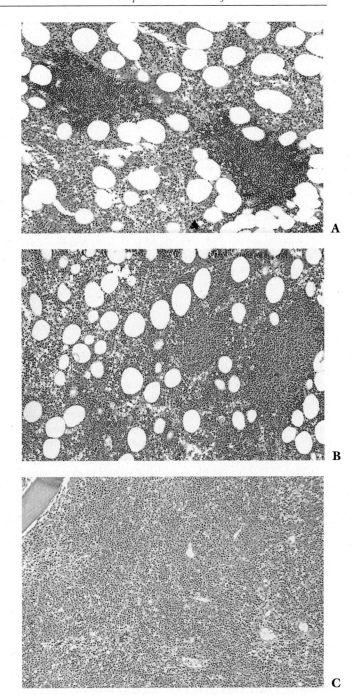

Figure 16.29. Bone marrow biopsy sections from patients with chronic lymphocytic leukemia. An interstitial pattern of involvement is illustrated in Figure 16.28C. **(A)** Nodular pattern of involvement. **(B)** Mixed (interstitial and nodular) involvement. **(C)** Diffuse involvement.

of transformation are prolymphocytoid change and large-cell transformation (Richter syndrome) (339,353–361).

Prolymphocytoid transformation is characterized by a progressive increase in prolymphocytes in the blood. There is generally an increase in the total leukocyte count, accompanied by enlarging lymph nodes and spleen. The prolymphocytes may express the same immunophenotype as the original CLL, or there may be immunophenotypic evolution. The most commonly reported changes in immunophenotype are any combi-

TABLE 16.16		Immunophenotype of B-Cell Chronic Lymphoproliferative Disorders/Low-Grade Non-Hodgkin Lymphomas								
	CD20	*Ig*	*CD5*	*CD10*	*CD23*	*FMC7*	*CD38*	*CD25*	*CD11c*	*CD103*
Chronic lymphocytic leukemia/ small lymphocytic lymphoma	dim+	dim+	+	−	+	−	−/dim+	+/−	−/+	−
Prolymphocytic leukemia	+	+	−/+	−	−/dim+	+	+/−	−	−	−
Lymphoplasmacytoid lymphoma/ leukemia	+	+	−/+	−	−/+	+/−	+/−	−/+	−/+	−
Mantle cell lymphoma	+	+	+	−	−	+	+	−	−	−
Follicular center lymphoma	+	+	−	+	−/+	+	bright+	−	−	−
Marginal zone lymphoma	+	+	−	−	−/+	+	−/dim+	−	+/−	−
Hairy cell leukemia	bright+	bright+	−	−	−/+	+	−	+	bright+	+

Ig, surface immunoglobulin expression.
Modified from: Harris NL, Jaffe ES, Stein H, et al. A revised European-American classification of lymphoid neoplasms: a proposal from the International Lymphoma Study Group. *Blood* 1994;84:1361–1392, and Rozman C, Montserrat E. Chronic lymphocytic leukemia. *N Engl J Med* 1995;333:1052–1057.

nation of stronger expression of SIg, loss of CD5, and expression of FMC-7 (339,356,357).

The bone marrow trephine biopsy sections are markedly hypercellular, with a combination of small lymphocytes and prolymphocytes. The prolymphocytes are slightly larger than the CLL/SLL lymphocytes, with more dispersed chromatin and distinct, often single, central eosinophilic nucleoli. The two populations may be evenly distributed in the marrow, or foci of transformation may be separated by areas of concentrated small lymphocytes.

Classical Richter syndrome is characterized by development of an aggressive large-cell lymphoma with a rapidly enlarging mass and abrupt deterioration of clinical statues. The large-cell lymphoma may be localized to a particular anatomic site; there is evidence of residual CLL/SLL in separate areas (Fig. 16.31). In the majority of cases, the large-cell proliferation is demonstrably clonally related to the original CLL/SLL clone (357, 360–364). In some cases, however, there is an apparent development of a new neoplastic clone. Occasionally, Hodgkin lymphoma develops in a patient with CLL/SLL; this has been termed the *Hodgkin disease variant of Richter syndrome* (359). Rarely, a blastic leukemia or multiple myeloma supervenes in CLL/SLL (365).

B-CELL PROLYMPHOCYTIC LEUKEMIA

B-cell prolymphocytic leukemia (B-PLL) classically occurs primarily in older men and is characterized by marked lymphocytosis, prominent splenomegaly without significant lymphadenopathy, and generally a short survival (339,366–369). In blood and bone marrow smears there is an abundance of prolymphocytes. These are medium to large cells with moderately abundant cytoplasm, a round or oval nucleus with somewhat reticular chromatin, and a large, centrally located vesicular nucleolus (Fig. 16.32). The bone marrow sections show a mixed focal and interstitial or diffuse infiltration of prolymphocytes. The prolymphocytes are medium- to large-sized and have a round to oval nucleus with a prominent single nucleolus and a distinct rim of cytoplasm. A moderate number of mitotic figures may be observed.

The reported genetic and immunophenotypic features of

B-PLL are heterogeneous and it now appears that many, if not most, cases of B-PLL are classifiable as other disorders—most notably, prolymphocytoid transformation of CLL/SLL and leukemic mantle cell lymphoma (370–372). Consequently, the defining attributes and clinicopathologic features of B-PLL are in doubt, and renewed investigation of this entity is warranted.

LYMPHOPLASMACYTIC LYMPHOMA

Lymphoplasmacytic lymphoma (LPL) involves the bone marrow in most patients at the time of diagnosis (373,374). The pattern of involvement is similar to that in CLL/SLL, although up to one-third of cases will demonstrate some degree of paratrabecular infiltration (312,373–375). The dominant cells in most LPL infiltrates of LPL are small lymphocytes with regular nuclei, clumped chromatin, and scanty cytoplasm, closely resembling the neoplastic cells of CLL/SLL. Varying proportions of the lymphocytes have a plasmacytoid appearance, and variable numbers of mature plasma cells and histiocytes are present (Fig. 16.33). The plasma cells may be morphologically atypical. Dutcher bodies (intranuclear, eosinophilic pseudoinclusions consisting of immunoglobulin) are seen in approximately 40% of cases (373). The majority of cases of lymphoplasmacytic lymphoma lack CD5 and CD10; small numbers of cases have been reported to express one of these antigens (374). A monoclonal gammopathy, usually of immunoglobulin M (IgM) type, is associated with some cases of lymphoplasmacytoid lymphoma. The clinical manifestations of Waldenström macroglobulinemia are present in many of these (320, 321,376, 377) (see "Plasma-Cell Neoplasms [Immunosecretory Disorders]" later in the chapter).

SPLENIC MARGINAL ZONE LYMPHOMA

Splenic marginal zone lymphoma (SMZL) is a relatively recently described entity characterized by splenomegaly, leukemic manifestations, and almost invariable involvement of bone marrow (378–381). This entity includes cases previously designated as splenic lymphoma with circulating villous lymphocytes (SLVL). In blood and marrow smears, the neoplastic cells demonstrate variable cytology. Most typically the cells have clumped chroma-

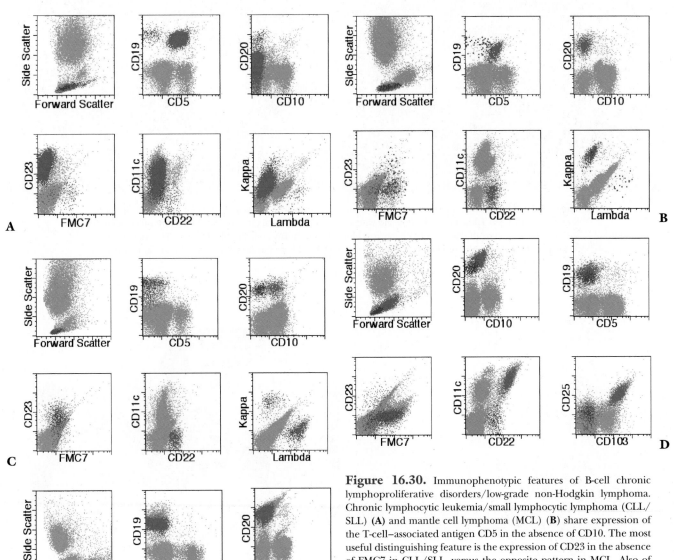

Figure 16.30. Immunophenotypic features of B-cell chronic lymphoproliferative disorders/low-grade non-Hodgkin lymphoma. Chronic lymphocytic leukemia/small lymphocytic lymphoma (CLL/SLL) **(A)** and mantle cell lymphoma (MCL) **(B)** share expression of the T-cell–associated antigen CD5 in the absence of CD10. The most useful distinguishing feature is the expression of CD23 in the absence of FMC7 in CLL/SLL, versus the opposite pattern in MCL. Also of use is the typically dim expression of CD20, CD22, and surface immunoglobulin in CLL/SLL versus normal or bright levels of these antigens in MCL. This example of CLL/SLL also illustrates variable expression of CD11c, a common finding. **(C)** Follicular lymphoma is largely distinguished from other disorders by virtue of CD10 expression in the absence of CD5. Follicular lymphomas are typically FMC7-positive and show varying degrees of CD23 expression. **(D)** Hairy cell leukemia (HCL) cells characteristically have higher forward- and side-light scatter characteristics than do small lymphocytes, similar to the pattern of monocytes. HCL is most commonly CD5- and CD10-negative, although CD10 may be expressed in a minority of cases. Extremely characteristic of HCL is bright coexpression of CD11c, and CD22. HCL cells also express CD103 as well as CD25 in most cases. Finally, HCL typically expresses FMC7 in the absence of CD23. **(E)** Splenic marginal zone lymphoma (SMZL) also lacks CD5 and CD10. As opposed to HCL, SMZL lacks bright coexpression of CD22 and CD11c, although some coexpression of these markers may be seen, as in the present case. Also notice the light scatter characteristics similar to normal mature lymphocytes. SMZL usually (although not always) lacks CD103 expression; CD23 may be expressed in some cases. *Red, neoplastic B-lineage cells; blue, mature polytypic B cells; green, mature T cells.*

tin, small nucleoli, and scant to abundant cytoplasm that is often more basophilic than normal lymphocytes, although it may be gray-blue as well. Large, transformed cells with more dispersed chromatin may be seen. Despite the relationship of SMZL to SLVL, only a minority of cases manifest prominent villous projections. In trephine biopsies, various patterns are seen (326,379–382). In the large majority of cases, one sees focal random infiltrates, but this is often accompanied by interstitial or paratrabecular infiltrates. In addition, in more than 80% of cases there is an intrasinusoidal infiltrate present. Although this pattern can also be seen in other small-B-cell disorders, it is most prominent in SMZL (379). Notably, intrasinusoidal infiltrates are often difficult to appreciate on routine sections, but will be highlighted by IHC for B-cell markers. A very distinctive

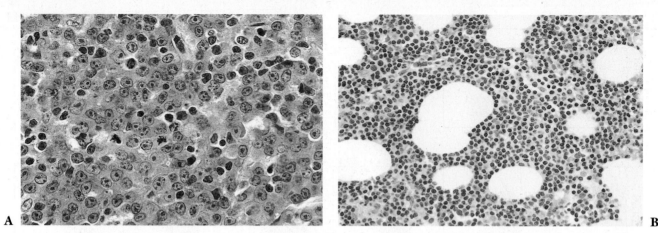

Figure 16.31. Richter transformation in a 68-year-old man with a 6-year history of chronic lymphocytic leukemia (CLL). **(A)** Tibial biopsy section showing a large-cell lymphoma that revealed a t(8;22) on cytogenetic studies. **(B)** Section of an iliac crest bone marrow biopsy taken shortly after the tibial biopsy. The marrow shows a small lymphocyte proliferation identical to the original CLL. There was no t(8;22) in the marrow biopsy from the iliac crest.

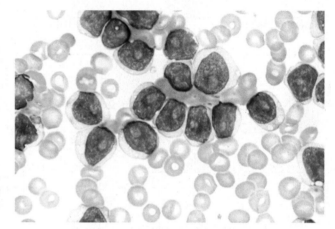

Figure 16.32. Blood smear from a patient with prolymphocytic leukemia. The prolymphocytes are large lymphocytes with moderately abundant cytoplasm, a round or oval nucleus, coarse chromatin, and a large, centrally located vesicular nucleolus.

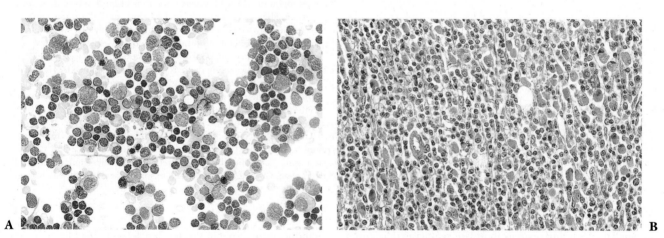

Figure 16.33. **(A)** Marrow aspirate smear from a patient with lymphoplasmacytic lymphoma and Waldenström macroglobulinemia. There are numerous lymphocytes, plasmacytoid lymphocytes, and plasma cells. **(B)** A marrow biopsy section from a different patient with lymphoplasmacytic lymphoma shows a dense infiltrate consisting of plasmacytoid lymphocytes, plasma cells (some with cytoplasmic inclusions), and histiocytes with cytoplasmic inclusions.

644

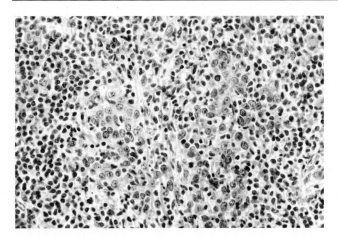

Figure 16.34. Marrow involvement with marginal zone lymphoma illustrating a colonized germinal center.

feature of SMZL infiltrates, although present in only a minority of cases, is the presence of reactive germinal centers within the neoplastic infiltrate (Fig. 16.34). In sections, the neoplastic cells of SMZL are mildly irregular or monocytoid with clumped chromatin, generally indistinct nucleoli, and moderate amounts of pale cytoplasm. SMZL cells are CD5-, CD10-, and CD43-negative (326,341,383). Although they may express CD11c and CD22, they do not show the bright coexpression of these markers that is characteristic of hairy cell leukemia (Table 16.16) (Fig. 16.30). SMZL cells are also generally tartrate-resistant acid phosphatase (TRAP)-negative.

HAIRY CELL LEUKEMIA

Hairy cell leukemia (HCL) is a B-cell chronic lymphoproliferative disorder with distinctive cytologic and histopathologic characteristics (19,384–387). Most patients have splenomegaly and blood cytopenias, usually pancytopenia. The diagnosis is made from blood smears or bone marrow smears and sections, typically supplemented by flow cytometry.

Hairy cells vary from rare to more than 80% of the leukocytes in blood smears. They are slightly larger than lymphocytes and have reticular, rather than clumped, chromatin. The nuclei are usually round but may be indented or folded. Nuclei are generally inconspicuous. Most often, the cytoplasmic border is serrated or shaggy-appearing, with irregular, delicate cytoplasmic strands or broad-blunt cytoplasmic projections.

The number of hairy cells in bone marrow aspirate smears is highly variable and often inconsistent with the degree of involvement observed in trephine biopsy sections. The hairy cells exhibit the same general morphologic features in marrow smears as in blood smears. In many cases, it is difficult to obtain a satisfactory aspirate because of reticulin fibrosis. In these cases, trephine biopsy imprints may provide the only material for cytologic and cytochemical studies. Cytoplasmic projections are not as obvious in trephine imprints as in blood smears.

Trephine biopsy sections virtually always show evidence of HCL if adequate specimens are obtained (19,384). The distribution of the hairy cell infiltrate is either diffuse or patchy, with complete or partial replacement of normal tissue. With extensive diffuse involvement, there may be only an occasional residual hematopoietic island (Fig. 16.35). With patchy infiltrates and partial replacement, there is considerable marrow sparing. The uninvolved marrow is often hypocellular. The patchy lesions are randomly distributed without any predilection for a paratrabecular location. The margins of the infiltrates are often poorly demarcated. Hairy cells may intermingle with normal hematopoietic cells, making them difficult to recognize (384). Occasionally, the marrow trephine in HCL is hypocellular, mimicking aplastic anemia (Fig. 16.36).

In both diffuse and patchy lesions, the hairy cell infiltrate is loosely structured with widely separated nuclei (Fig. 16.35). Large, clear areas surround the individual hairy cells. This distinct histology is a constant finding in the bone marrow lesions and is an important diagnostic feature (384). The nuclei of the hairy cells are mostly round or oval, but some may be indented or cleaved. Occasionally the cells have a distinctly spindled appearance. Nucleoli are usually not discernible and mitotic figures are rarely seen.

Reticulin fibrosis always accompanies HCL (19,384,386). The reticulin stains show deposition of a branching network of fibers. This network forms a tight lattice that may surround nearly every cell.

Hairy cells are TRAP- and fluoride-resistant α-naphthyl butyrate esterase-reactive. These stains and a distinctive immunophenotype (Table 16.16) (Fig. 16.30) distinguish HCL from most

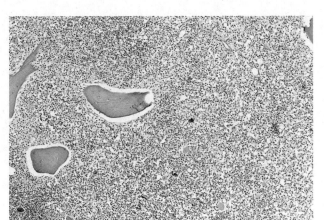 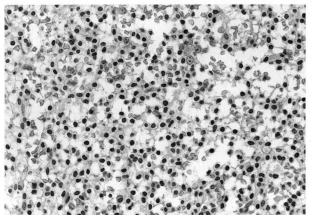

A   B

Figure 16.35. (A) Bone marrow section from a patient with hairy cell leukemia showing extensive marrow involvement. (B) A higher magnification illustrates the characteristic widely separated nuclei.

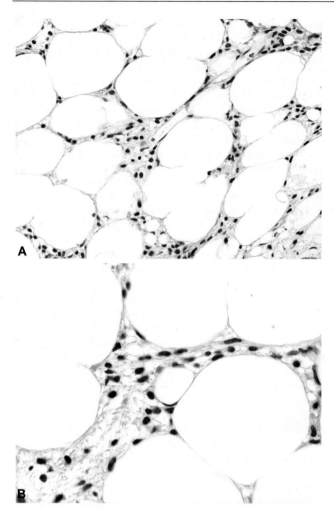

Figure 16.36. (A) The bone marrow trephine from this presenting bone marrow in a patient with hairy cell leukemia is markedly hypocellular, mimicking aplastic anemia. (B) On higher power, there is a population of bland mononuclear cells in the interstitium; CD20 stain (not shown) highlighted virtually all of these.

other hematologic malignancies that may be considered in the differential diagnosis (387). In cases where the bone marrow aspirate yields a dry tap, flow cytometry should be performed on peripheral blood. Even when hairy cells are difficult or impossible to appreciate morphologically in the blood smear, they will be detectable by flow cytometry.

EXTRANODAL MARGINAL ZONE LYMPHOMA OF MUCOSA-ASSOCIATED LYMPHOID TISSUE

The bone marrow is involved in extranodal marginal zone lymphoma (EMZL) in 15% to 20% of cases (323,388–390). Focal random and interstitial infiltrates are seen in more than 80% of involved marrow; paratrabecular lesions are appreciated in nearly half (379). Although intrasinusoidal infiltrates may be seen in more than half of involved marrows, in any given case they are usually rare. The cytologic features of EMZL in marrow are similar to those seen in primary sites.

NODAL MARGINAL ZONE LYMPHOMA

Nodal marginal zone lymphoma (NMZL) is a rare, poorly defined entity that encompasses cases previously designated monocytoid B-cell lymphoma. The marrow appears to be involved in about 30% of cases (388,390–394). Based on few cases, the dominant patterns of bone marrow involvement are focal random and/or paratrabecular. The cytologic features are similar to those of EMZL.

FOLLICULAR LYMPHOMA

Follicular lymphomas of low grade (grades 1 and 2) involve the marrow at diagnosis in 50% to 70% of cases (314,395–397). Grade 3 follicular lymphoma involves the marrow in roughly 10% to 25% of cases (398–401). In trephine biopsy sections, the dominant pattern of marrow infiltration is distinct paratrabecular localization. This is often the only pattern present, although it may be accompanied by random focal infiltrates as well (295,312) (Fig. 16.37). Occasionally one encounters intertrabecular lesions containing neoplastic follicles; rarely, this is the predominant pattern of involvement (402). In most cases the lymphoma cells are predominantly small, cleaved cells or centrocytes, regardless of the lymph node histology (295,315). Transformation of bone marrow lesions from small cleaved to

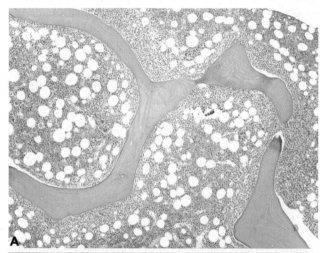

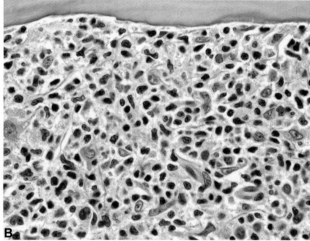

Figure 16.37. (A) Low-power view of this staging bone marrow biopsy from a patient with low-grade follicular lymphoma demonstrates a striking pattern of paratrabecular infiltration. (B) High power demonstrates a predominance of small lymphocytes with centroblastic cytologic features. The lesion also contains endothelial cells and histiocytes.

large cleaved or noncleaved cells may occur after several months or years.

In marrow aspirate smears, the cytologic features of the lymphoma cells encompass a wide morphologic spectrum that includes small cleaved cells, large transformed lymphocytes, and well-differentiated–appearing lymphocytes. The predominant cell is usually of the small-cleaved type, characterized by little or no recognizable cytoplasm and a smooth, uniformly staining nucleus that is frequently deeply indented or cleaved (315,403). The characteristic immunophenotype for follicular center lymphoma is shown in Table 16.16 and Figure 16.30.

Tumor cell representation may be minimal in tissue obtained from bone marrow for immunophenotyping or molecular genotyping because of minimal involvement and the difficulty in removing the neoplastic cells from the marrow. An additional problem with follicular lymphomas is that they may be difficult to evaluate by PCR analysis for B-cell clonality (404). IHC staining of a core biopsy section, combined with the histopathology, is often sufficient to demonstrate marrow involvement.

MANTLE CELL LYMPHOMA

Although classic mantle cell lymphoma (MCL) is cytologically intermediate between CLL/SLL and follicular lymphomas, the wide cytologic spectrum of this tumor has been recently emphasized (338,405–408). MCL may consist of round cells closely resembling CLL/SLL; mildly or highly irregular cells of varying size; large nucleolated cells, sometimes mimicking prolymphocytes; or blastoid cells. The marrow is involved at diagnosis in approximately 60% to 80% of cases (388,407,409–413). Most cases demonstrate a random focal infiltration pattern (Fig. 16.28B), but accompanying interstitial, paratrabecular, or diffuse infiltrates are common as well. Immunophenotyping is a valuable aid to the diagnosis. MCLs are CD5-positive B-cell neoplasms like CLL/SLL. The two differ in that MCLs are characteristically CD23-negative and FMC-7-positive (Table 16.16) (Fig. 16.30). Demonstration of cyclin D1 overexpression by IHC or the t(11;14)(q13;q32) by conventional cytogenetics, FISH, or PCR confirms the diagnosis.

DIFFUSE LARGE-B-CELL LYMPHOMA

Diffuse large-B-cell lymphomas have an incidence of bone marrow involvement of 10% to 20% (388,414–416). The pattern and extent of bone marrow infiltration is highly variable, ranging from minimal small foci to virtual total marrow replacement. The lesions in trephine sections are usually readily recognizable by an obvious destructive pattern and the abnormal cytologic characteristics of the lymphocytes. Rarely, however, subtle interstitial infiltration may be seen (Fig. 16.38). IHC staining of the section with a B-cell marker (e.g., CD20) may assist in tumor cell identification in small or interstitial lesions.

MEDIASTINAL (THYMIC) LARGE-B-CELL LYMPHOMA

This type of large-B-cell lymphoma only rarely involves the marrow at presentation (2% to 4%) (388). The pathologic features of marrow involvement by this tumor have not been described.

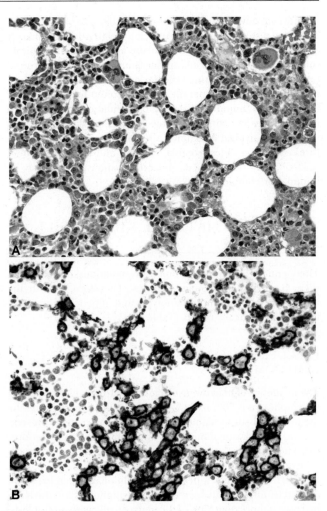

Figure 16.38. **(A)** This staging trephine biopsy from a patient with diffuse large-cell lymphoma manifests no obvious neoplastic infiltrates. However, there are scattered large, nucleolated cells in the interstitium of uncertain lineage. **(B)** A CD20 stain highlights an unusual interstitial pattern of infiltration by large-cell lymphoma.

INTRAVASCULAR LARGE-B-CELL LYMPHOMA

This unique form of aggressive lymphoma produces almost exclusively intravascular infiltrates in a variety of organs. Morphologically evident bone marrow involvement is uncommon but, when present, the neoplastic cells infiltrate in an exclusively sinusoidal distribution (330). A variant form of this lymphoma that is seen predominantly in Asia has a high rate of morphologic bone marrow involvement (417).

BURKITT LYMPHOMA

Burkitt lymphoma involves marrow in roughly 35% of adults and 23% of children at diagnosis (418–420). Many patients without initial involvement will manifest marrow invasion later in their course. The pattern is nearly always diffuse or interstitial, and the degree of involvement is usually extensive (320,312) (Fig. 16.28D). Even with extensive involvement, the "starry sky" pattern commonly observed in lymph nodes is usually absent (421). There may be small foci or expansive areas of necrosis; in some cases the entire section consists of necrotic tissue. The lymphoma cells have round or oval nuclei with two to four nucleoli. There is a distinct rim of cytoplasm, and cell borders are sharply defined. Mitotic figures are usually numerous. In aspirate smears, the lymphoma cells are medium to large, with a round or oval nucleus containing reticular or slightly condensed chromatin. Nucleoli are generally small but often multiple. There is a moderate amount of deeply basophilic cytoplasm, which in most cases contains a variable number of sharply defined vacuoles. In atypical Burkitt lymphomas, aberrant cytologic features, such as a more irregular nucleus and more prominent nucleoli, may be observed, and cytoplasmic vacuoles may be minimal or completely lacking (320).

T-CELL AND NATURAL KILLER CELL NEOPLASMS

These entities have varying clinical presentations, but several of them have similar cytologic features. Therefore, as with the B-cell disorders, immunophenotypic and genetic characterization is diagnostically useful (Table 16.17).

PRECURSOR T-LYMPHOBLASTIC LEUKEMIA/ LYMPHOMA

The incidence of marrow involvement by T-lineage lymphoblastic lymphomas is 50% to 60% (295–297). Bone marrow may be the primary tissue available for examination in patients presenting with a mediastinal mass and no peripheral lymphadenopathy. The histologic, cytologic, and immunophenotypic features of lymphoblastic lymphoma are identical to those of ALL (192,422,423). The distinction has traditionally been based on clinical features and the percentage of lymphoblasts in the bone marrow. If more than 25% of the marrow cells are lymphoblasts, the case is generally considered ALL.

The pattern of marrow infiltration is nearly always interstitial (295,297). The degree of involvement varies from occasional lymphoma cells recognizable only in smear preparations, to 25% of the bone marrow cells. Nuclear convolution and a high mitotic rate are prominent features (192). In bone marrow smears, the lymphoblasts are identical to those of ALL (82) (see "Acute Leukemias and Myelodysplastic Syndromes" in this chapter).

BLASTIC NATURAL KILLER CELL LYMPHOMA

This rare tumor, which has also been referred to as CD4+/ CD56+ hematodermic neoplasm, is an aggressive blastic tumor that usually presents in skin, with variable blood and bone marrow involvement (424,425). The infiltration pattern and cytologic features in blood and marrow are similar to ALL. The neoplastic cells express CD56, CD4, CD45, and CD43, and may express TdT, but usually lack other lymphoid and myeloid antigens. Recent data indicate that this tumor arises from a population of plasmacytoid dendritic cells, and thus the current terminology for this neoplasm is a misnomer (426,427).

T-CELL PROLYMPHOCYTIC LEUKEMIA

T-cell prolymphocytic leukemia (T-PLL) is a rare disorder. Patients typically present with splenomegaly, hepatomegaly, and lymphadenopathy. Cutaneous lesions and serous effusions are relatively common (337,339,368,428). The disease has an aggressive course (368). The leukocyte count is usually markedly elevated and consists of cells resembling prolymphocytes. In most cases the neoplastic lymphocytes are medium-sized with coarse chromatin and a single prominent nucleolus. In about half the cases the nucleus is round or oval; in the remainder there is nuclear irregularity with folds and convolutions. A small-cell variant of T-PLL has been described (337,368). The immunophenotype for T-CLL/T-PLL is shown in Table 16.17. There are no specific immunophenotypic features. Most cases express CD4 and lack CD8, although cases expressing both CD4 and CD8, and, rarely, only CD8, are encountered. The expression of CD7 by the neoplastic cells in nearly all cases helps distinguish this neoplasm from Sézary syndrome and adult T-cell leukemia/ lymphoma. A cytogenetic abnormality involving an inv(14) (q11; q32) is found in approximately 75% of cases of T-PLL; in 50% there is a trisomy 8q (368).

T-CELL LARGE-GRANULAR LYMPHOCYTE LEUKEMIA

The major hematologic findings in cases of T-cell large-granular lymphocyte leukemia (T-LGLL) are lymphocytosis and neutropenia; anemia and thrombocytopenia are present in some patients (429–433). The lymphocytes have abundant cytoplasm that contains varying numbers of coarse azurophilic granules.

TABLE 16.17	**Immunophenotype of T-Cell Lymphoproliferative Disorders/Non-Hodgkin Lymphomas**									
	CD2	*CD3*	*CD4*	*CD5*	*CD7*	*CD8*	*CD16*	*CD25*	*CD56*	*CD57*
T-cell prolymphocytic leukemia	+	+	+/−[a]	+	+	−/+[a]	−	−	−	−
Mycosis fungoides/Sézary syndrome	+	+	+	+	−	− (rare +)[b]	−	− (rare +)	−	−
Adult T-cell lymphoma/leukemia	+	+	+	+	−	−	−	+	−	−
T-cell large-granular lymphocytic leukemia	+	+	−	−	+	+	+	−	−	+
Natural killer cell large-granular lymphocytic leukemia	+	−	−	−	+	+	+	+	+/−	+/−

[a]Minority of cases express both subset markers.
[b]Rare CD8(−) cases are CD4(−) and not coexpressant.
Modified from: Harris NL, Jaffe ES, Stein H, et al. A revised European-American classification of lymphoid neoplasms: a proposal from the International Lymphoma Study Group. *Blood* 1994;84:1361–1392.

The nucleus is round or oval with coarse chromatin and generally lacks a nucleolus.

The bone marrow smears show a moderate increase in lymphocytes with the same features as those in the blood. Neutrophil precursors may be normal or moderately decreased. The maturation sequence is generally normal (429). In trephine biopsy sections, the marrow is normocellular or hypercellular. The neoplastic infiltrates are subtle interstitial and intrasinusoidal lesions (Fig. 16.39); the latter finding, highlighted by IHC for CD3, CD8, TIA-1, or granzyme B, is not seen in normal marrows (329). Interestingly, the focal lymphoid aggregates that are often seen in the marrow in T-LGLL are likely reactive because they are largely composed of CD4+ cells. The lymphocytes show mature cytologic features.

T-LGLL cells demonstrate a CD3+/CD8+ immunophenotype (433–435) (Table 16.17). The cells also typically express the NK-associated markers CD57 and CD16, but uncommonly express CD56. It has recently been demonstrated that all T-LGLL cases show aberrant antigen expression relative to normal CD8+ T cells (434,435). The majority of cases manifest clonal T-cell antigen receptor gene rearrangements. Despite evidence of clonality, most cases do not progress, and occasionally patients experience a spontaneous regression of their dis-

ease (429). A minority of cases behave as aggressive lymphoproliferative disorders. Although indolent CD3− NK-cell proliferations exist (436,437), they are not well defined and currently are not included in the WHO classification.

AGGRESSIVE NATURAL KILLER CELL LEUKEMIA

This is rare, aggressive systemic leukemia/lymphoma derived from natural killer (NK) cells (438). Like extranodal NK/T-cell lymphomas of nasal type, these tumors demonstrate immunophenotypic features of NK cells: they lack surface CD3, but express CD2 and CD56. Also, like their localized counterparts, most cases contain Epstein-Barr virus sequences and lack T-cell receptor gene rearrangements. Patients typically present with systemic symptoms, hepatosplenomegaly, and a leukemic picture. The neoplastic cells may resemble normal large-granular lymphocytes in that they contain azurophilic cytoplasmic granules, but they will demonstrate overt atypical features such as hyperchromatism, nuclear irregularity, or distinct nucleoli.

ADULT T-CELL LEUKEMIA/LYMPHOMA

Adult T-cell lymphoma/leukemia (ATL/L) is an aggressive T-cell lymphoma variant with a unique geographic distribution. It is endemic in Japan and the Caribbean basin and is seen sporadically in the United States and Europe (439–441). It is uniformly associated with the human T-cell lymphoma-leukemia virus type 1 (HTLV-1). The disease has its onset in adulthood. There is frequently skin involvement, lymphadenopathy, and hepatosplenomegaly. Hypercalcemia is found in about one-third of patients. There is a high incidence of bone marrow and blood involvement. The leukocyte count in ATL/L spans a broad range, and the abnormal cells vary from 10% to 90% in blood smears. The leukemic cells are heteromorphous from small to large, with a characteristic lobated nucleus, coarse chromatin, and scant cytoplasm (Fig. 16.40). Nucleoli are small and inconspicuous. The trephine biopsy sections show minimal to heavy infiltration. The infiltrate is interstitial or diffuse, occasionally with poorly demarcated focal accentuation. The lymphocytes are pleomorphic and predominantly medium-sized to small with irregular nuclear borders. ATL/L may be difficult

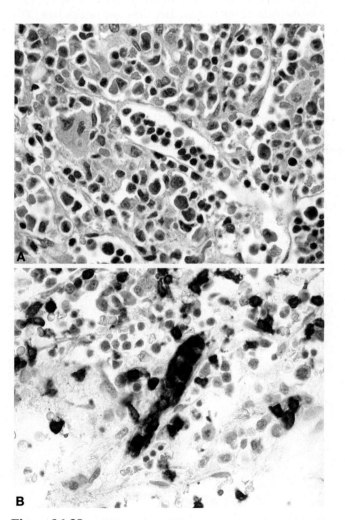

Figure 16.39. (A) This marrow biopsy contains intrasinusoidal infiltrates of small lymphocytes. (B) The intrasinusoidal infiltrates are highlighted by a CD3 stain.

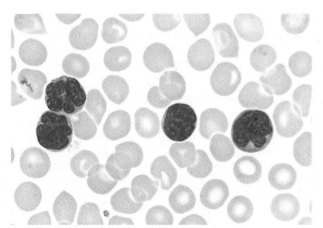

Figure 16.40. Blood smear from a patient with adult T-cell leukemia/lymphoma. Some of the lymphoma cells are markedly convoluted, typical of this disorder.

to distinguish from T-PLL and Sézary syndrome. HTLV-I serology and immunophenotyping are useful aids in the differential diagnosis (321) (Table 16.17).

ENTEROPATHY-TYPE T-CELL LYMPHOMA

Little data regarding the incidence and features of marrow involvement are available for this neoplasm. In one study, 2 of 24 cases (8%) involved the bone marrow at presentation (442). Literature descriptions of the pathologic features of this tumor in bone marrow are not available, but we have encountered several cases with a subtle, interstitial pattern of infiltration.

EXTRANODAL NATURAL KILLER/T-CELL LYMPHOMA, NASAL TYPE

The bone marrow is involved in fewer than 10% of cases at presentation is uncommon in nasal NK/T cell lymphomas, although it may be higher (10% to 25%) in those presenting at nonnasal sites (443–447). The marrow involvement may be extremely subtle, requiring special studies such as IHC for CD56 or EBER in situ hybridization for detection.

HEPATOSPLENIC T-CELL LYMPHOMA

Hepatosplenic T-cell lymphoma (HSTCL) involves the marrow in nearly all cases (448–450). This distinctive and aggressive form of peripheral T-cell lymphoma is typified by presentation in young adult males as hepatosplenomegaly (328,448–452). The infiltrates in spleen, liver, and bone marrow show a distinctly intrasinusoidal distribution (Fig. 16.28E,F) (449–451). Cytologically, the neoplastic cells are usually medium in size, with regular nuclei, inconspicuous nucleoli, and small to moderate amounts of cytoplasm, although variable degrees of nuclear irregularity may also be seen. Most cases express the γ/δ T-cell receptor and CD56, but lack CD4 and CD8. A minority of cases with identical clinicopathologic features express the α/β T-cell receptor. An isochromosome 7q is seen in virtually all γ/δ-expressing tumors, as well some α/β-expressing cases (452,453).

SUBCUTANEOUS PANNICULITIS-LIKE T-CELL LYMPHOMA

This rare form of peripheral T-cell lymphoma does not involve the bone marrow directly. It is notable, however, for its propensity to be associated with a systemic hemophagocytic syndrome, which may be evident on bone marrow examination (454,455).

MYCOSIS FUNGOIDES/SÉZARY SYNDROME

Mycosis fungoides and Sézary syndrome are cutaneous T-cell lymphomas. They may involve the bone marrow and blood as advanced-stage manifestations. Sézary syndrome is characterized by erythroderma, lymphadenopathy, and circulating atypical cells. With disease progression, visceral organs become infiltrated. There is bone marrow infiltration in 12% to 40% of cases of mycosis fungoides/Sézary syndrome, usually of minimal degree and most often in patients with Sézary syndrome (456–459). The number of atypical lymphoid cells in the blood is variable. Large and small Sézary cell variants have been described; both are characterized by striking nuclear convolutions

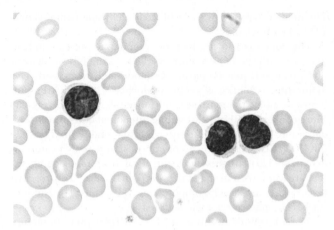

Figure 16.41. Blood smear from a patient with Sézary syndrome. The Sézary cells show typical cerebriform convolution.

that give the nucleus a cerebriform appearance; only the large variant is specific for mycosis fungoides/Sézary syndrome (456) (Fig. 16.41). The immunophenotype may be helpful in differentiating Sézary syndrome from other leukemic chronic lymphoproliferative disorders (Table 16.17). Sézary cells express CD4 and other pan–T-cell antigen, lack CD8, and usually lack CD7.

PERIPHERAL T-CELL LYMPHOMA, UNSPECIFIED

This group of lymphomas is heterogeneous and likely includes multiple distinct entities. Overall, they invole the bone marrow in 30% to 40% of cases (460–463). The pattern of marrow involvement for the peripheral T-cell lymphomas is about equally split between diffuse and randomly focal; occasionally, focal paratrabecular lesions are encountered (75,322,464). Typically, the lesions may consist of a heteromorphous lymphocyte population and a polycellular infiltrate of eosinophils, plasma cells, neutrophils, endothelial cells, and epithelioid histiocytes (Fig. 16.42). There may be prominent vascularity and reticulin fibrosis. The reactive cell component is mixed with the lymphoma cells. In some T-cell lymphomas, diffuse bone marrow infiltrates

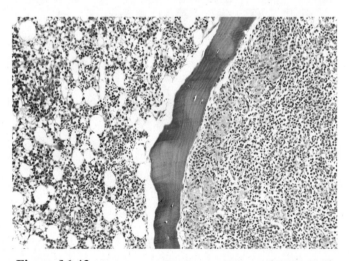

Figure 16.42. Bone marrow involvement with a peripheral T-cell lymphoma with epithelioid histiocytes. The marrow to the *right* of the trabecula is replaced by tumor; the area to the *left* is spared.

may blend uniformly with the normal hematopoietic cells and may be difficult to discern even when there is extensive marrow disease (75,322,465). In these cases, the overall picture may suggest a myeloproliferative disorder. The epithelioid histiocytes are often found in clusters and may impart a granulomatous appearance. In some large T-cell lymphomas, large lymphocytes and immunoblasts predominate and the reactive cell infiltrate is not a prominent feature.

Pleomorphic focal lesions of peripheral T-cell lymphoma are randomly distributed and usually poorly circumscribed. They can be difficult to distinguish from lymphohistiocytic reactive lesions, particularly those commonly found in the bone marrow of patients with AIDS or an autoimmune disease (59,60,74, 75,322). In some cases the marrow histology may be indistinguishable from a reactive polymorphous lymphohistiocytic lesion, T-cell–rich large-B-cell lymphoma, or Hodgkin lymphoma (75). IHC on bone marrow sections, immunophenotyping of aspirated marrow, and molecular analysis for T-cell receptor and immunoglobulin gene rearrangements may be helpful in the differential diagnosis (322,464).

Lymphoma cells are found in aspirate smears in at least half of the cases with bone marrow disease (75). Interpretation of the smears may be difficult because of the heterogeneity of the lymphocytes, many of which exhibit cytologic features of mature or reactive lymphocytes.

ANGIOIMMUNOBLASTIC T-CELL LYMPHOMA

Angioimmunoblastic T-cell lymphoma (AILT) involves bone marrow in 60% to 80% of cases (466–468). The lesions vary from focal to diffuse; focal lesions may be random or paratrabecular. They are similar in composition to the lymph node infiltrates and are typically composed of a mixture of immunoblasts, plasmacytoid cells, lymphocytes of varying size and cytologic features, eosinophils, histiocytes, and blood vessels. The marrow infiltrates of AILT are not morphologically distinct from those of peripheral T-cell lymphoma, unspecified. Flow cytometry studies identifies an aberrant CD4+ T-cell population in most cases (469). The neoplastic cells in most cases express CD10, a feature unique to this neoplasm among peripheral T-cell lymphomas (469,470).

ANAPLASTIC LARGE-CELL LYMPHOMA

Systemic anaplastic large-cell lymphoma (ALCL) involves the marrow in approximately 15% of cases (471–473). Involvement may be diffuse, focal, random, or even in the form of single cells in the interstitium (Fig. 16.40). The last pattern may be extremely subtle, and IHC for CD30, epithelial membrane antigen, or anaplastic lymphoma kinase (ALK) may be necessary to reliably detect bone marrow involvement in some cases (471). As in primary sites, ALCL cells may vary considerably in size and cytology. Usually at least some of the cells will possess a horseshoe-shaped, wreathlike, or embryoid nucleus with a distinct eosinophilic paranuclear zone ("hallmark cells"). The infiltrate may be cohesive-appearing, mimicking an epithelial neoplasm, or may occasionally be embedded in fibrosis, mimicking Hodgkin lymphoma. In smears, ALCL cells are large and pleomorphic, often with multiple or lobated nuclei, prominent nucleoli, and deeply basophilic, vacuolated cytoplasm, occasionally with a few azurophilic granules (Fig. 16.43).

POSTTHERAPY BONE MARROW IN NON-HODGKIN LYMPHOMA AND MINIMAL RESIDUAL DISEASE

Morphologic changes following chemotherapy vary for the different types of NHL. Bone marrow lesions in low-grade lymphomas diminish in size with response to chemotherapy, but may not resolve completely; morphologic detection of residual disease is relatively common. Transformation to a more aggressive histopathologic type may occur in some low-grade lymphomas. Complete resolution of marrow lesions is observed with effective response to chemotherapy for high-grade lymphomas. Repopulation of the marrow with normal hematopoietic tissue follows. Bone marrow relapse is morphologically similar to the original lymphoma.

For T-cell and B-cell NHLs, demonstration of clonality by immunophenotypic or molecular genotypic analysis may be useful in identification of morphologically undetectable or equivocal early relapse or minimal residual disease in the bone marrow (474–483). However, these techniques may give false-negative results in certain diagnostic settings. For example, follicular lymphomas are characteristically paratrabecular. When foci are

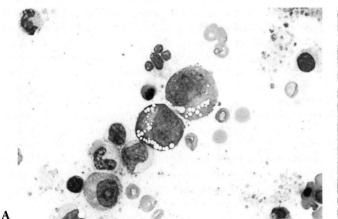

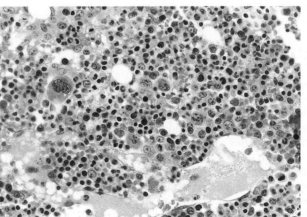

A **B**

Figure 16.43. Marrow involvement by anaplastic large-cell lymphoma (ALCL). **(A)** A marrow aspirate smear shows two large lymphoma cells with typical cytologic features of ALCL. **(B)** Scattered individual ALCL cells and small clusters are observed in the biopsy section.

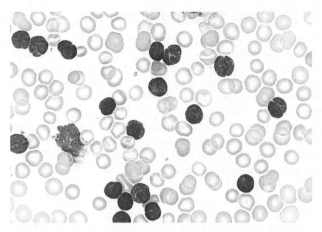

Figure 16.44. Blood smear showing involvement with follicular small cleaved cell lymphoma.

minimal in a trephine section, tumor cell representation may be minimal in cytologic material obtained for immunophenotyping or molecular genotyping. Follicular lymphomas also may be difficult to evaluate by PCR analysis for B-cell clonality as a result of high levels of somatic hypermutation (404). Poor representation of large-cell lymphomas in cell suspensions due to their fragile nature also may be a problem in flow cytometric immunophenotyping (484). IHC staining of a trephine biopsy section with appropriate markers is sufficient to demonstrate low-level marrow involvement in some cases.

BLOOD INVOLVEMENT BY NON-HODGKIN LYMPHOMA

Circulating lymphoma cells are found in blood smears in 10% to 25% of cases overall, and in 40% to 50% of cases with bone marrow involvement (295,297,485–487). Blood involvement is rare in cases without marrow disease (295,297). The degree of blood involvement is generally related to the extent of marrow disease (297). The incidence of circulating lymphoma cells is highest for the chronic lymphoproliferative disorders, lymphoblastic lymphomas/leukemias, and some of the T-cell disorders and follicular center lymphomas, but virtually every category of NHL manifests blood involvement in some cases (485,488) (Fig. 16.44).

HODGKIN LYMPHOMA

Bone marrow involvement is present at the time of diagnosis in 5% to 15% of cases of Hodgkin lymphoma (HL) (489–494). Constitutional symptoms, bulky disease, splenic involvement, high erythrocyte sedimentation rate, increased lactate dehydrogenase, increased alkaline phosphatase, and decreased blood counts are all predictive of bone marrow involvement (489,492–495). Most commonly, marrow involvement is a manifestation of disseminated disease and is detected in random iliac crest trephine biopsies. Direct extension to the marrow from adjacent lymph nodes in otherwise localized HL is rare.

Marrow biopsies are far more likely to be positive for HL than aspirate smears, and bilateral iliac crest biopsies provide a higher yield than a single biopsy (7). Evidence of HL is uncom-

monly found in aspiration smears because the fibrosis in the lesions prevents neoplastic cells from being aspirated. Reed-Sternberg (RS) cells are virtually never seen in aspirate smears in the absence of disease in the core biopsy (492,494). When marrow disease is extensive, attempts at aspiration may yield a "dry tap."

The bone marrow biopsy is a component of staging protocols for HL. The following are the histopathologic criteria for diagnosis of marrow involvement in patients with proven HL on a lymph node biopsy (496):

1. HL may be diagnosed when typical RS cells or their mononuclear variant are found in one of the characteristic cellular environments of HL.
2. The presence of atypical histiocytes that lack the nuclear features of RS cells in a typical background for HL, or in focal or diffuse areas of fibrosis, is strongly suggestive of marrow involvement.
3. Fibrosis or necrosis alone should be considered suspicious for HL.

In some marrow lesions, RS cells are the predominant cell type, whereas in others examination of multiple sections may be necessary to find a single example. RS cells are always found in a stromal reaction characteristic of HL and not in areas of otherwise normal marrow. In suspicious lesions, IHC staining with the RS cell-reactive markers, CD15 (Leu-M1) and CD30 (Ki-1), LCA (which is negative in RS cells), and T-cell and B-cell markers can aid in identification and characterization of suspicious cells. When lesions are identified that are suspicious for HL but typical RS cells or variants are not found after serial sectioning and appropriate immunostaining, the trephine biopsy should be repeated unless there is other definitive evidence of advanced disease.

The extent of bone marrow involvement in biopsy specimens varies from small lesions occupying less than one-third of the marrow space, to complete marrow replacement. In 70% to 80% of cases there is diffuse involvement, with Hodgkin tissue occupying entire areas between bone trabeculae and usually replacing large contiguous portions of marrow (Fig. 16.45) (491). The cellular infiltrate in diffuse lesions may be uniformly distributed or localized between broad sheets of sparsely cellular, loose, or dense connective tissue. Focal, small, isolated lesions that are completely encircled by normal marrow tissue or paratrabecular in location are found in 20% to 30% of cases (Fig. 16.46). These are usually polycellular with a uniform cell mixture throughout the lesion. Both diffuse and focal lesions may be found in the same biopsy. All of the various histologic patterns of infiltrate found in lymph nodes may also be observed in the bone marrow. Reticulin or collagen is always present and is most prominent in cases with extensive diffuse involvement (491).

The areas of marrow adjacent to Hodgkin tissue often show nonspecific changes, such as hypoplasia or granulocytic hyperplasia (491,497). Increased plasma cells, erythroid hyperplasia, eosinophilic and granulocytic hyperplasia, and increased megakaryocytes may be observed in patients without marrow involvement (498). These nonspecific changes are not related to pathologic stages of disease or other prognostic factors.

The highest incidence of bone marrow involvement is found with mixed cellularity HL and the rare lymphocyte-depletion type (491,497). Less than 10% of patients with nodular sclerosis HL have marrow disease at diagnosis, and only rare cases of

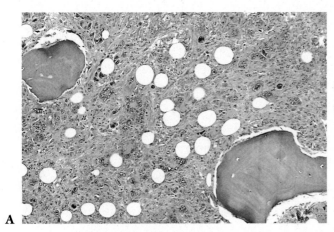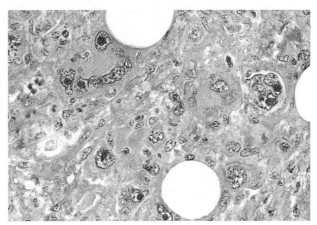

Figure 16.45. (A) Bone marrow involvement by Hodgkin disease. The pattern of involvement is diffuse. There is complete replacement of the hematopoietic marrow and fat. (B) A higher magnification shows typical and variant Reed-Sternberg cells in a polycellular infiltrate.

lymphocyte-predominant HL and lymphocyte-rich classic HL involve the bone marrow (499,500). Classic HL cannot be reliably classified in bone marrow biopsies. The small size of the specimen precludes evaluation of the complete histologic pattern. Furthermore, the histopathology of HL may differ significantly in lymph nodes and bone marrow from the same patient (489,501).

POSTTREATMENT BIOPSIES IN HODGKIN LYMPHOMA

Posttherapy bone marrow examination may be useful in assessing a patient's response to chemotherapy and monitoring for recurrent disease. The histopathology of posttreatment residual HL and relapse is generally similar to that of pretreatment lesions, but changes may occur. In some cases, there is progression to more aggressive-appearing histologic features with relapse; increased numbers of RS cells, fibrosis, and depletion of lymphocytes may be observed. Necrosis of Hodgkin tissue is more often present following chemotherapy than in pretreatment biopsies (491). Usually only part of the lesion is necrotic

with patches of amorphous eosinophilic material containing karyorrhectic and karyolytic cells. Occasionally, granulomas secondary to opportunistic infections, such as cryptococcosis, are found mixed with or separate from Hodgkin tissue (491). The myelofibrotic component of Hodgkin tissue is reversible with successful chemotherapy and often shows complete resolution (490).

DIFFERENTIAL DIAGNOSIS OF HODGKIN LYMPHOMA

In some patients the initial diagnosis of HL is made from a bone marrow biopsy taken for evaluation of blood cytopenias, fever of unknown origin, or organomegaly. In these cases, particular caution must be exercised. Bone marrow lesions in peripheral T-cell lymphomas and T-cell–rich large-B-cell lymphomas often simulate HL, and occasionally the marrow lesions in follicular lymphomas show fibrosis, a histiocyte proliferation, and a pleomorphic cell population that may be confused with HL (75,502). RS-like cells have been observed in the marrow in both peripheral T-cell and follicular lymphomas. The cytol-

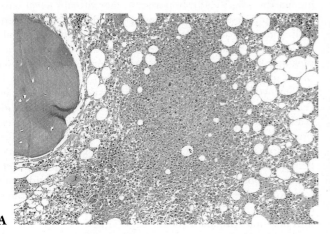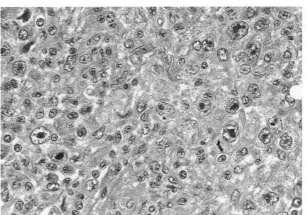

Figure 16.46. (A) Bone marrow biopsy showing focal involvement with Hodgkin disease. The lesion is encircled by normal marrow. (B) A high magnification of the lesion shows numerous mononuclear Reed-Sternberg cell variants.

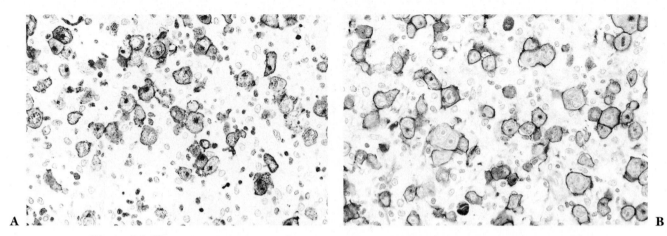

Figure 16.47. IHC stains on a bone marrow involved with classic Hodgkin lymphoma. **(A)** A positive CD15 reaction in the Reed-Sternberg cells. **(B)** A positive CD30 reaction in similar cells.

ogy of the neoplastic cells on marrow smears or biopsy imprints may help distinguish these disorders from HL (75,315,403). IHC studies using a panel of antibodies to T- and B-cell–associated antigens and to antigens expressed by RS cells (e.g., CD15 [Leu-M1] and CD30) may clarify the diagnosis in problematic cases (13,320,464,503) (Fig. 16.47) (Table 16.18). Bone marrow lesions of nodular lymphocyte predominant HL are probably not distinguishable from T-cell/histiocyte-rich large-B-cell lymphoma (500); clarifying this differential diagnosis requires a lymph node biopsy.

Other bone marrow lesions such as granulomas, polymorphous reactive lymphoid infiltrates, myelofibrosis, mast cell disease, eosinophilic granuloma, and other histiocytic proliferative disorders may mimic HL histologically (292,320). RS-like cells have been described in some of these disorders (504,505). The diagnostic features of each of these are described elsewhere in this chapter.

LYMPHOMA-LIKE LESIONS

REACTIVE LYMPHOID LESIONS

Reactive lymphoid lesions have been identified in 18% to 47% of bone marrow biopsy specimens (506–510). They are particu-

larly common in older age groups, increasing in frequency with age after about age 50. They are found in patients with a variety of unrelated disorders, as well as in healthy persons (507,511,512). In many geriatric individuals, reactive lymphocytic bone marrow lesions are of unknown significance. In younger individuals, they are often associated with an inflammatory process or immune disorder (507,512).

In marrow biopsy sections, reactive lymphoid lesions range from 50 to 1000 μm in diameter and vary in number from a solitary focus in one section to several on each section of a trephine biopsy. They are randomly distributed in the marrow. They may be categorized into four morphologic types:

- Focal benign lymphoid aggregates
- Reactive polymorphous lymphohistiocytic lesions
- Lymphoid follicles with germinal centers
- Systemic polyclonal immunoblastic proliferations

The most common are focal benign lymphoid aggregates. They consist of loosely arranged, well-differentiated lymphocytes of varying size; histiocytes, plasma cells, mast cells, and eosinophils may be found as minor components. Small blood vessels or endothelial cells are often present (292,506,507,510,513). Focal benign lymphoid aggregates are usually small, round to oval, well circumscribed, and clearly demarcated from the surrounding marrow (Fig. 16.48). Importantly, they virtually never have a truly paratrabecular localization, although they may tangentially abut bony trabeculae. These are the lesions commonly encountered in marrow biopsies from older individuals, but they may be found in all age groups. There is no association with a specific disease process.

Reactive polymorphous lymphohistiocytic lesions are polycellular, consisting of a heteromorphous population of lymphocytes, including small lymphocytes, transformed lymphocytes, lymphocytes with irregular nuclei, plasma cells, epithelioid histiocytes, eosinophils, mast cells, and endothelial cells. They may be multiple with poorly defined margins and occupy relatively large portions of marrow (Fig. 16.49). These florid lesions are commonly observed in the marrow of patients with immune disorders such as AIDS, rheumatoid arthritis, and in association with immune cytopenias (56–59,62,507,512).

Germinal centers are randomly distributed and often single on a marrow section (Fig. 16.50). They consist of a mantle of small lymphocytes encircling a germinal center composed of

---

TABLE 16.18

Usual IHC Profile of Neoplastic Cells in Hodgkin Lymphoma and Non-Hodgkin Lymphoma That May Simulate Hodgkin Lymphoma in Bone Marrow

	CD15	CD30	LCA	CD3	CD20	EMA
Classic HL	+	+	−	−	−/+	−
LP HL	−	−	+	−	+	+
ALCL	−	+	+	−/+	−	+
T-cell–rich LBCL	−	−	+	−	+	−
PTCL-NOS	−	−	+	+	−	−

ALCL, anaplastic large-cell lymphoma; EMA, epithelial membrane antigen; HL, Hodgkin lymphoma; LBCL, large-B-cell lymphoma; LCA, leukocyte commonantigen; LP, lymphocyte-predominant; NHL, non-Hodgkin lymphoma, PTCL-NOS, peripheral T-cell lymphoma/not otherwise specified.

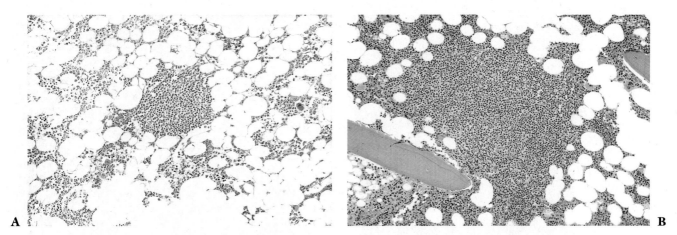

Figure 16.48. **(A)** A reactive lymphocytic aggregate in the bone marrow of an older adult woman. The aggregate is small, round, well circumscribed, and loosely structured. **(B)** A lesion from the marrow of a woman with a splenic marginal zone lymphoma. The lesion is larger than the reactive aggregate, irregularly shaped, with infiltrating margins, and consists of a monomorphous population of tightly concentrated lymphocytes.

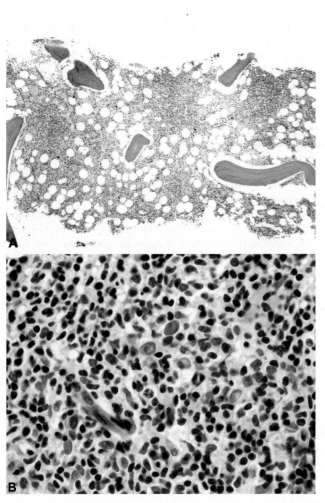

Figure 16.49. **(A)** Low-power view of a core biopsy of a patient with common variable immune deficiency showing several reactive polymorphous lymphohistiocytic lesions. **(B)** High-power view revealing a polymorphous cellular composition.

large transformed lymphocytes, scattered histiocytes, and frequent mitotic figures (292,514). These are most common in young patients who have an immune or inflammatory disorder, in particular AIDS and systemic lupus erythematosous.

In systemic polyclonal immunoblastic proliferations the bone marrow, lymph nodes, and other tissues are involved. The reaction may be florid with lesions consisting of polyclonal lymphocytes, plasma cells, and immunoblasts observed throughout the aspirate smears and core biopsies (Fig. 16.51) (515). The peripheral blood smears typically show leukocytosis dominated by reactive lymphocytes and plasma cells. Most patients present with an acute systemic illness, including fever, lymphadenopathy, and hepatosplenomegaly. The pathogenesis of the disorder is unknown. Some patients experience a dramatic response to corticosteroid therapy.

Bone marrow aspirate smears from patients with reactive lymphoid lesions may be normal or show increased lymphocytes and other reactive cells. A spectrum of morphologic features from relatively uniform small and medium-sized lymphocytes to a heteromorphous population of transformed lymphocytes may be observed. Increased numbers of histiocytes, mast cells, and plasma cells are present in some cases.

The reactive lymphoid lesions in bone marrow are important because of their morphologic similarity to some of the neoplastic lymphoproliferative disorders. They are most problematic in lymphoma staging biopsies and in following patients with a lymphoma. Occasionally, florid reactive lymphoid lesions are encountered in marrow biopsies from patients undergoing evaluation for blood cytopenias, constitutional symptoms, or poorly accessible mass lesions. In these cases their distinction from lymphoma is essential. Histologic criteria for distinguishing reactive lymphoid lesions from lymphoma are listed in Table 16.19. Biopsies that contain several, or have unusually large, lymphocytic aggregates may resemble involvement with small lymphocytic, mantle cell, marginal zone, or follicular lymphomas (Fig. 16.48). The florid, polymorphous, lymphohistiocytic reactive lesions often occupy large portions of the marrow section and have poorly defined borders; they may resemble a peripheral T-cell lymphoma, T-cell–rich large-B-cell lymphoma, or HL. The lymphohistiocytic lesions found in marrow sections

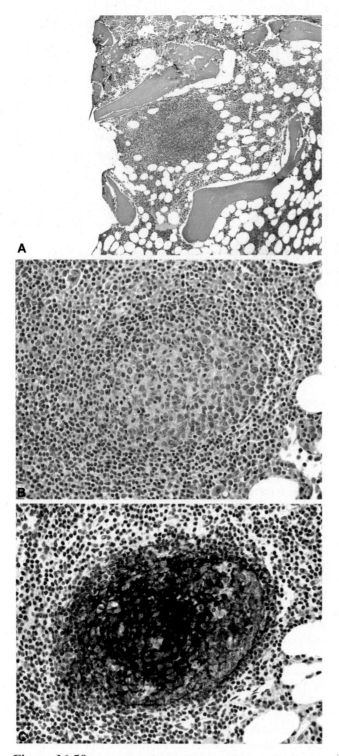

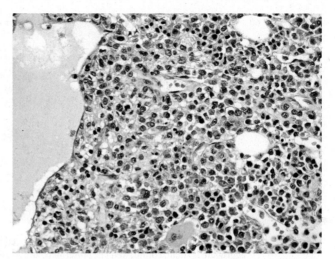

Figure 16.51. This trephine biopsy image from a patient with systemic polyclonal immunoblastic proliferation demonstrates a prominent parasinusoidal infiltrate of plasma cells and immunoblasts.

Figure 16.50. Low (**A**) and high (**B**) magnification of a reactive germinal center in the staging trephine biopsy of a 27-year-old man with diffuse large-B-cell lymphoma. (**C**) A CD21 stain highlights a sharply defined follicular dendritic cell meshwork.

from patients with AIDS may be indistinguishable from peripheral T-cell lymphoma (56,62,75,322) (Fig. 16.49). However, T-cell lymphomas are rarely encountered in patients with AIDS, and the diagnosis should be made cautiously and with the aid of other confirmatory evidence. The systemic polyclonal immu-

noblastic proliferations can potentially be confused with large-cell lymphoma with immunoblastic features or plasma cell myeloma.

In some instances, the distinction between benign and malignant lymphoid lesions in the bone marrow cannot be made solely on morphologic grounds. Immunophenotyping, cytogenetic studies, or molecular genotypic analysis may be necessary to distinguish florid reactive lymphocytic proliferations from lymphoma (322,516–523)

INCREASED LYMPHOCYTE PROGENITOR CELLS (HEMATOGONES)

Bone marrow specimens from young children or, less commonly, adult patients may contain increased numbers of small, lymphoid-appearing, hematopoietic progenitor cells. These cells have been referred to as hematogones in the literature (167,524–529). They often have morphologic features in common with the lymphoblasts of acute lymphoblastic leukemia/lymphoma. In bone marrow smears, they range in size from 10 to 20 μm and have a smudged, homogeneous chromatin pattern. The nucleus may be indented but usually lacks a distinct nucleolus. Cytoplasm is sparse, deeply basophilic, and devoid of granules or vacuoles (Fig. 16.52). In trephine biopsy sections, these cells are diffusely dispersed and resemble small or medium-sized lymphocytes but with slightly less dense and more homogeneous nuclear chromatin.

Hematogones may be found in bone marrow smears in large numbers in normal infants and children with a number of disorders, including congenital and immune cytopenias, neoplastic disorders, immune thrombocytopenic purpura, and in regenerative marrows following chemotherapy or bone marrow transplantation (524–529). In rare cases, as many as 70% of the bone marrow cells are hematogones. Hematogones express a reproducible spectrum of B-cell precursor-associated antigens, including CD34, TdT, CD19, CD22, CD10, and CD20 (167, 524–526,528,529). They are heterogeneous in their expression of these antigens and show the characteristic pattern of B-lymphocyte maturation (Fig. 16.53). This is in contrast to a more homogeneous and aberrant pattern of antigen expression of

TABLE 16.19	Distinction Between Reactive Lymphoid Lesions and Malignant Lymphoproliferative Disorders in Marrow Sections

Benign	*Malignant*
Randomly distributed	Frequently paratrabecular
Usually well circumscribed	Often irregular shape with infiltration into adjacent marrow
Polymorphous with small lymphocytes, plasma cells, immunoblasts, histiocytes, and endothelial cells; cellular atypia less common	Most commonly homogeneous in NHL, heterogeneous in HL; cellular atypia (cleaved or convoluted nuclei, nucleoli, etc.)
Vascularity is frequently prominent	Vascularity is not usually prominent (except in HL and a few NHLs)
Germinal centers are occasionally present	Germinal centers are not present
No lymphoma cells are present in marrow smears and imprints	Lymphoma cells may be present in smear and imprints

the neoplastic lymphoblasts in lymphoblastic lymphoma and ALL (167). Immunophenotyping by multicolor flow cytometry is often critical when a differential diagnosis includes hematogones versus neoplastic lymphoblasts. IHC may also be useful; clusters of more than five TdT and/or CD34+ cells are usually not seen in florid hematogone proliferations, and usually CD20+ cells outnumber CD34- or TdT-positive cells (530). It is important that the pathologist be knowledgeable about the conditions in which these normal lymphoid progenitor cells are increased.

GRANULOMAS

Granulomas are discussed in detail in the "Inflammatory Disorders of the Bone Marrow" section earlier in the chapter. They are considered here only as a lesion that may simulate lymphoma in the bone marrow. Nonspecific granulomas have been observed in the marrow in approximately 7% of patients whose marrow biopsies were negative for HL at the time of staging (491) (Fig. 16.3). They appear to be slightly less common in patients with NHL (40,43). When bone marrow granulomas are unusually large or confluent, lack giant cells, and have an

eosinophil component, they may resemble HL or a peripheral T-cell lymphoma. They are distinguished from Hodgkin tissue by the predominance of epithelioid histiocytes and Langhans-type giant cells and the absence of typical RS cells or variants. The cytologic features of the lymphocytes and comparison with lymphoma tissue from lymph nodes are important in distinguishing atypical granulomas from a peripheral T-cell lymphoma.

PLASMA CELL NEOPLASMS

The plasma cell neoplasms are proliferations of clonal immunoglobulin-producing cells. The cells are generally recognizable as plasma cells or plasmacytoid lymphocytes and produce a single class of immunoglobulin or polypeptide subunit of immunoglobulin that is detectable in the serum or urine as a monoclonal protein (M-protein). The diagnosis of these disorders is made by a combination of the morphologic, immunologic, radiographic, and clinical features. The WHO classification of the plasma cell neoplasms is shown in Table 16.20 (109). Waldenström macroglobulinemia and the heavy-chain diseases are immunosecretory disorders generally associated with lymphoplasmacytic proliferations; they are not listed with the plasma cell neoplasms but are separate categories of the WHO classification. They are discussed briefly in this section because of their many features in common with the plasma cell neoplasms.

PLASMA CELL MYELOMA (MULTIPLE MYELOMA)

Plasma cell myeloma is the most common of the plasma cell neoplasms. It is characterized by disseminated marrow infiltration by neoplastic plasma cells and a serum or urine M-protein (531–537). The following studies should be performed on patients suspected of having myeloma (532):

- Serum and urine protein electrophoresis
- Serum and urine protein immunofixation electrophoresis
- Serum and urine protein quantification
- Radiographic skeletal survey
- Bone marrow examination

Several systems have been devised that define criteria for a diag-

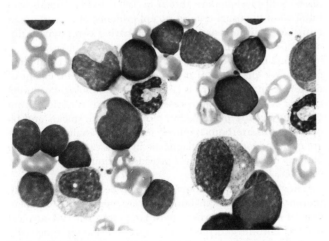

Figure 16.52. Bone marrow smear from a 2-year-old healthy bone marrow transplant donor with increased hematogones (B-lymphocyte precursors).

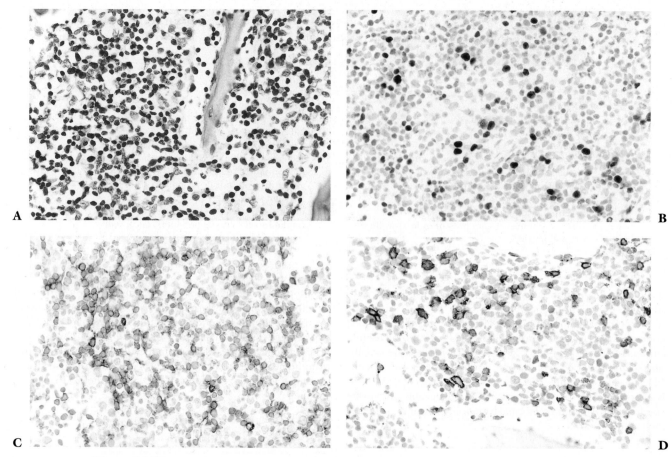

Figure 16.53. Marrow biopsy section from a 2-month-old child with thrombocytopenia and a cytomegalovirus infection. **(A)** The marrow contains more than 60% lymphoid cells. **(B)** A TdT immunostain is positive in scattered cells. **(C)** CD10 stains the majority of the lymphoid cells. **(D)** CD20 is positive in scattered cells. This pattern of staining is typical of hematogones, which show a maturation spectrum with scattering of the most immature (TdT +) cells, and differentiates hematogones from neoplastic lymphoblasts.

TABLE 16.20

World Health Organization (WHO) Classification of Plasma Cell Neoplasms

Plasma cell myeloma (multiple myeloma)
Plasma cell myeloma variants
   Nonsecretory myeloma
   Asymptomatic (smoldering) myeloma
   Plasma cell leukemia
Plasmacytomas
   Solitary plasmacytoma of bone
   Extraosseous (extramedullary) plasmacytoma
Immunoglobulin deposition diseases
   Primary amyloidosis
   Systemic light and heavy chain deposition diseases
Osteosclerotic myeloma (POEMS syndrome)
Heavy chain diseases (HCD)
   γ-HCD
   μ-HCD
   α-HCD

POEMS, polyneuropathy, organomegaly, endocrinopathy, monoclonal protein, skin changes.

---

nosis of myeloma (79,109,532,534,535,538–540). These use a combination of clinical, radiographic, and pathological findings. The most significant criterion in determining whether a patient is treated for myeloma is end-organ damage. The newly revised WHO classification criteria for diagnosis of symptomatic plasma cell myeloma are shown in Table 16.21. Patients who fulfill all of the usual criteria except evidence of related organ or tissue impairment are diagnosed as having asymptomatic myeloma (see "Variants of Plasma Cell Myeloma" below).

A bone marrow examination should always be performed to confirm the diagnosis of myeloma and evaluate the extent of disease, even when there is convincing immunologic or radiographic evidence. In many cases the diagnosis is obvious from the bone marrow examination alone. Aspirate smears and biopsy sections are both required for optimal evaluation. They are each independently diagnostic in most cases, but in some patients only one of the two provides definitive morphologic evidence.

The diagnosis of myeloma can usually be made based on the morphologic features in bone marrow preparations independent of other criteria when there are more than 10% atypical plasma cells with morphologic features outside the range of a reactive process, infiltrative sheets of plasma cells, or a very high percent of plasma cells on a hypercellular section or aspirate (542).

TABLE 16.21

Diagnostic Criteria for Symptomatic Plasma Cell Myeloma

M-protein in serum or urine[a]
Bone marrow clonal plasma cells or plasmacytoma[b]
Related organ or tissue impairment[c]

[a]No level of serum or urine M-protein is included. M-protein in most cases is >30 g/L of IgG or >25 g/L of IgA or >1 g/24 hr of urine light chain, but some patients with symptomatic myeloma have levels lower than these.
[b]Monoclonal plasma cells usually exceed 10% of nucleated cells in the marrow, but no minimal level is designated because about 5% of patients with symptomatic myeloma have fewer than 10% marrow plasma cells.
[c]The most important criteria for symptomatic myeloma is evidence of end-organ damage manifested by anemia, hypercalcemia, lytic bone lesions, renal insufficiency, hyperviscosity, amyloidosis or recurrent infections.
Modified from: Criteria for the classification of monoclonal gammopathies, multiple myeloma and related disorders: a report of the International Myeloma Working Group. *Br J Haematol* 2003;121: 749–757.

In biopsy sections, the pattern of the plasma cell infiltrate may be interstitial, focal, or diffuse (21,531) (Fig. 16.54). The extent of marrow involvement varies from a small increase in plasma cells in a normocellular marrow, to hypercellularity with complete marrow replacement. The pattern of involvement is directly related to the extent of disease. With the interstitial and focal patterns, there is often considerable marrow sparing and preservation of normal hematopoiesis. With diffuse involvement, expansive areas of the marrow are replaced and hematopoiesis is markedly suppressed. Typically there is progression from interstitial and focal disease in early myeloma, to diffuse involvement in advanced stages of the disease (21,531,535).

Myelomas with markedly atypical plasma cell morphology may be difficult to recognize in core biopsies. Cases of plasmablastic myeloma, myelomas with lymphoid-appearing plasma cells, and those with lobulated nuclei or markedly pleomorphic plasma cells may be particularly problematic (531,534,543,544). Cytologic examination of the cells in aspirate smears is essential for diagnosis in these cases. Occasionally, cytoplasmic inclusions in the myeloma cells are the most striking feature on the bone marrow section. The inclusions are often found in large plasma cells that appear distorted by crystalline or globular material (531). In a minority of cases of myeloma, the bone marrow lesions are fibrotic (531,545). Coarse fibrosis has been reported to correlated with extensive diffuse marrow involvement and aggressive disease (21).

In marrow smears, the plasma cells vary from normal-appearing to primitive plasmablasts barely recognizable as plasma cells (534). In most cases of myeloma, the neoplastic cells are easily recognized as plasma cells (Fig. 16.55). They are often larger than normal but may be normal-sized or even small. Moderate to abundant basophilic cytoplasm is usual. A spectrum of cytoplasmic changes may be observed, including vacuoles, granules, hyaline inclusions, small or large crystalline inclusions, and fraying and shedding at the cytoplasmic boarder. The nucleus is larger than normal in most cases and the nuclear chromatin is less condensed. Nucleoli are variable, but in immature myelomas they are particularly prominent.

Several studies have addressed the significance of plasma cell morphology in myeloma. Most have been aimed at relating cytology to prognosis by separating cases into morphologic categories (21,543,546). One classification defines mature, intermediate, immature, and plasmablastic types of myeloma (543). Myelomas consisting mostly of plasmablastic cells are the least cytologically mature and most aggressive (21,109,543,547). The other morphologic categories do not appear to correlate well with prognosis.

The minimum percentage of plasma cells in a marrow smear necessary for diagnosis of myeloma is generally placed at 10%. However, because the distribution of plasma cells in the marrow is often focal, there may be discrepancies between the plasma cell number in aspirate smears and trephine biopsy sections. In one study, 6% of cases of myeloma had less than 5% plasma cells in the marrow aspirates, but the biopsy sections showed focal infiltration with clusters or sheets of plasma cells (531). In another report, nearly 40% of patients had less than 10% marrow plasma cells at presentation (535). Furthermore, a reactive plasmacytosis in excess of 10% in a normocellular bone marrow may occur in several conditions, including viral infections and immune reactions to drugs (531,535). These conditions are usually distinguished from plasma cell myeloma by the lack of an M-protein in the serum or urine.

IHC studies for κ- and λ-light chains and plasma cell–associated antigens such as CD138 are useful in assessing the quantity of plasma cells and in distinguishing between reactive and neoplastic proliferations (548,549) (Fig. 16.56). In some instances, CD138 or κ and λ stains help distinguish myeloma from other neoplasms. Demonstration of a light chain excess of either κ or λ in the marrow plasma cells of 16:1 or greater is significantly associated with myeloma. Ratios of less than 16:1 are generally found in monoclonal gammopathy of undetermined significance (MGUS). Reactive plasmacytosis usually has a normal κ:λ ratio but may overlap with some cases of MGUS (548).

PRECURSOR LESION: MONOCLONAL GAMMOPATHY OF UNDETERMINED SIGNIFICANCE

M-proteins are found in approximately 3% of individuals over the age of 50 and in more than 5% of individuals past 70 without evidence of myeloma, macroglobulinemia, amyloidosis, or a lymphoproliferative disease (550–554). These are usually designated MGUS. The criteria for diagnosis of an MGUS are shown on Table 16.22.

There are two distinctive types of MGUS: non-IgM MGUS, which has plasma cell features and may progress to a malignant plasma cell neoplasm; and IgM MGUS, which generally has lymphoplasmacytic features and can progress to lymphoma. In non-IgM MGUS, the proportion of plasma cells in marrow smears varies from 1% to 10%, with a median of approximately 3% (531). The plasma cell morphology is usually normal, but changes (including cytoplasmic inclusions and visible nucleoli) may be observed. In trephine biopsy sections, the marrow is normocellular and there is minimal plasma cell infiltration. The plasma cells are interstitial and evenly distributed or found in small clusters, often concentrated around blood vessels. The plasma cells express the same monotypic cytoplasmic Ig as the M-protein but the clone is often small and in a background of

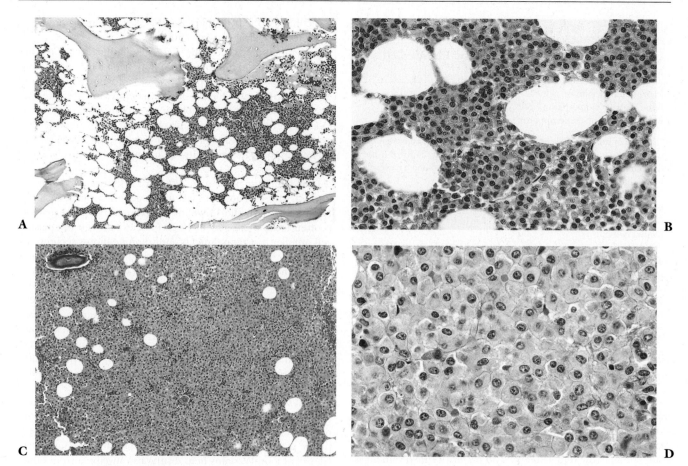

Figure 16.54. Bone marrow biopsy sections showing patterns of involvement by plasma-cell myeloma. **(A)** Interstitial pattern of involvement by plasma cell myeloma. **(B)** A high magnification of the section illustrated in **(A)** shows atypical plasma cells. **(C)** Marrow biopsy section showing diffuse involvement and extensive replacement of the marrow by myeloma. **(D)** A high magnification of the biopsy illustrated in **(C)** shows myeloma cells with somewhat immature nuclei and abundant cytoplasm.

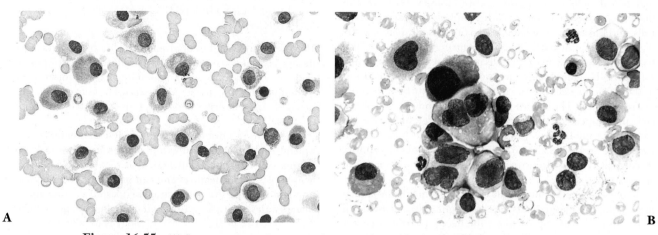

Figure 16.55. **(A)** Bone marrow aspirate smear from a patient with plasma cell myeloma. The smears contained mostly plasma cells with atypical features. **(B)** Bone marrow smear from a patient with a serum immunoglobulin A monoclonal spike. The smear contains numerous atypical pleomorphic plasma cells.

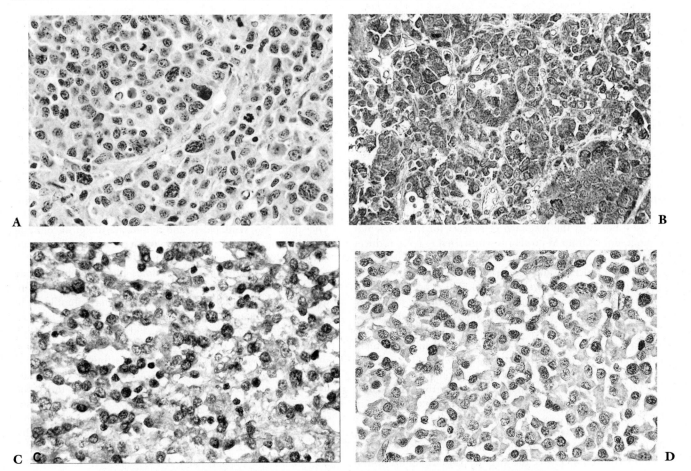

Figure 16.56. **(A)** Marrow section from a patient with a pleomorphic tumor and a monoclonal spike. The differential diagnosis included a lymphoma or metastatic tumor in addition to plasma cell myeloma. **(B)** An IHC stain for CD138 is strongly positive, supporting the diagnosis of plasma cell myeloma. **(C)** and **(D)** Immunoperoxidase stains on marrow sections from a patient with marrow plasmacytosis and a serum monoclonal immunoglobulin spike. The immunoperoxidase studies support the diagnosis of plasma cell myeloma. **(C)** Anti-κ reacts with nearly all of the plasma cells. **(D)** Anti-λ antibody shows no reactivity in the plasma cells.

normal plasma cells, so that monotypic Ig is not always detectable by routine IHC (548,549). Flow cytometry analysis generally identifies two populations of plasma cells, one with an aberrant immunophenotype (either CD19−/CD56+ or CD19−/CD56−) and one with a normal immunophenotype (CD19+, CD56−, CD38 bright). (555,556)

TABLE 16.22

Diagnostic Criteria for Monoclonal Gammopathy of Undetermined Significance

M-protein in serum <30 g/L
Bone marrow clonal plasma cells <10% and low level of plasma cell infiltration in a trephine biopsy
No lytic bone lesions
No myeloma-related organ or tissue impairment
No evidence of other B-cell proliferative disorder

Modified from: Criteria for the classification of monoclonal gammopathies, multiple myeloma and related disorders: a report of the International Myeloma Working Group. *Br J Haematol* 2003;121: 749–757.

MGUS must be distinguished from a malignant plasma cell dyscrasia. In most cases this is not difficult because the percentage of plasma cells in the marrow and the quantity of the M-protein are less than required for a diagnosis of myeloma and there is no evidence of end-organ damage. In cases of MGUS with an unusually high M-protein or moderately increased plasma cells, the distinction from an asymptomatic myeloma may be more problematic.

For most persons with MGUS, the course is stable and there is no increase in M-protein or evidence of progression to a malignant disorder. In approximately 25% of individuals, however, there is eventual progression to a plasma cell myeloma, amyloidosis, Waldenström macroglobulinemia, or other lymphoproliferative disorder (541,554,557,558). The interval from the recognition of the MGUS to diagnosis of a malignancy averages about 10 years. Risk of progression is about 1% per year, is indefinite, and persists even after 30 years (559–561). MGUS should be considered a preneoplastic condition. Patients must be followed indefinitely for evidence of disease progression (562,563). Size and type of M-protein and serum-free light-chain ratio are the most significant clinical risk factors for progression (541,559,562). Patients with an IgM or an IgA MGUS are at greater risk of progression to a malignant disorder than are those with IgG MGUS (554,560,561,564). IgM MGUS progresses to lymphoma or Waldenström macroglobulinemia rather than to plasma cell myeloma (554,564).

VARIANTS OF PLASMA CELL MYELOMA

Nonsecretory myeloma accounts for 1% to 3% of myelomas. No M-protein is detected in the serum or urine on immunofixation electrophoresis (109,541,565–568). In most cases of nonsecretory myeloma, an M-protein can be identified in the cytoplasm of the myeloma cells by IHC stains for κ- and λ-light chains and, in up to two-thirds of patients, increased serum-free light chains and/or an abnormal free–light chain ratio is detectable, suggesting that they are minimally secretory (569). In about 15% of cases, however, the myeloma cells react for neither κ nor λ, suggesting that no M-protein is synthesized ("non-producer myeloma"). There is reportedly a lower incidence of renal failure and hypercalcemia and less depression of normal polyclonal Ig compared to other myelomas (541,570). The diagnosis is generally made by morphologic criteria and demonstration of light chain restriction by κ- and λ-IHC stains on a marrow biopsy.

Asymptomatic ("smoldering") myelomas manifest the diagnostic criteria for myeloma but no related organ or tissue impairment (end-organ damage) is present (Table 16.22) (109,541,551, 571–574). They resemble MGUS clinically but are much more likely to progress to symptomatic myeloma (109,551,561,571, 575–577). The criteria for asymptomatic myeloma are listed in Table 16.23.

About 8% of patients with plasma cell myeloma are initially asymptomatic (576). The majority has between 10% and 20% bone marrow plasma cells; the atypical plasma cells are found in clusters or aggregates in the marrow sections. Patients may have stable disease for long periods but the incidence of eventual progression to symptomatic myeloma or amyloidosis is 51% at 5 years, 66% at 10 years, and 73% at 15 years; median time to progression is 4.8 years (576). Patients with asymptomatic myelomas are not usually treated until they become symptomatic.

In *plasma cell leukemia* (PCL) the number of neoplastic plasma cells in the blood is greater than 20% of the total leukocytes, or the absolute count exceeds 2.0×10^9 per L (109, 578–581). Primary PCL is found in 2% to 5% of cases of myeloma (581–586). The cytologic features of the circulating plasma cells are similar to the spectrum found in other myelomas, but large and pleomorphic plasma cells are unusual; frequently, many of the plasma cells are small with relatively little cytoplasm (587). The bone marrow is hypercellular and diffusely infiltrated. PCL is more frequently encountered in patients with IgD, IgE, or light chain–only myeloma. but any immunoglobulin type may present with or evolve to a PCL (582,588). Patients with PCL more often have lymphadenopathy, organomegaly, and renal failure than those with other myelomas; osteolytic lesions and bone pain are less frequent. PCL is an aggressive neoplasm. Patients have a poor response to therapy and usually a short survival (578,579,582–586).

PLASMACYTOMAS

Solitary plasmacytoma of bone is a localized plasma cell tumor of cytologically mature or immature plasma cells (589–591). The spine, ribs, skull, pelvis, and femurs are the most common sites of involvement. Patients most often present with bone pain at the site of the lesion or with a pathologic fracture.

The criteria for diagnosis of solitary plasmacytoma include the presence of a single bone lesion with histology consistent with a plasma cell tumor, absence of a plasma cell infiltrate in random bone marrow biopsies, no evidence of other bone lesions by radiographic examination, and absence of other clinical manifestations that could be attributable to myeloma (541,592). A low quantity of M-protein is found in serum or urine in 24% to 72% of patients (541,575,592,593). Plasmacytomas are usually easily recognizable in tissue sections unless the plasma cells are very poorly differentiated (e.g., plasmablastic or anaplastic), in which case confirmation of a clonal plasma cell lesion can be accomplished by IHC staining or in situ hybridization studies for kappa and lambda light chains.

The usual course is progression to multiple myeloma within 2 to 10 years, but approximately one-third of patients remain disease free for more than 10 years (541,589–591). New bone lesions, generalized marrow plasmacytosis, and an increasing M-protein evolve in those with progression to myeloma.

Solitary extramedullary (extraosseous) plasmacytomas are most common in the mucous membranes of the upper air passages but may arise in a variety of other sites. These tumors require the same diagnostic criteria as those in the bone. Extramedullary plasmacytomas are more easily confused with other neoplasms, particularly lymphomas. Careful microscopic and IHC studies are important for correct diagnosis. Patients with extramedullary plasmacytomas may have local recurrence. They infrequently evolve to multiple myeloma (~15%); approximately 70% of patients are disease-free at 10 years (589, 590,594–596).

MONOCLONAL IMMUNOGLOBULIN DEPOSITION DISEASES

Monoclonal immunoglobulin deposition diseases are plasma cell dyscrasias that are characterized by deposition of immunoglobulins in visceral and soft tissues, resulting in compromised organ function (597,598). These plasma cell neoplasms are part of the spectrum of plasma cell myeloma but they produce an immunoglobulin that accumulates in tissues prior to developing a large tumor burden. Patients typically do not fulfill the criteria for plasma cell myeloma at the time of the diagnosis.

Primary Amyloidosis

Primary amyloidosis is a plasma cell neoplasm in which the fibril amyloid protein is produced by monoclonal plasma cells and

---

TABLE 16.23

Diagnostic Criteria for Asymptomatic (Smoldering) Myeloma

M-protein in serum at myeloma levels (>30 g/L)
  and/or
10% or more clonal plasma cells in bone marrow
No related organ or tissue impairment (end-organ damage or bone lesions) or myeloma-related symptoms

Modified from: Criteria for the classification of monoclonal gammopathies, multiple myeloma and related disorders: a report of the International Myeloma Working Group. *Br J Haematol* 2003;121: 749–757.

consists of whole or fragments of immunoglobulin light chains (AL amyloid), which are deposited in tissues and form a β-pleated sheet structure that binds Congo red dye with characteristic birefringence (599–602). Primary amyloidosis is associated with plasma cell myeloma in approximately 20% of cases. In the remaining cases the diagnostic criteria for myeloma are lacking, but a moderate increase in clonal plasma cells is usually present in the bone marrow. An M-protein is found in the serum and/or urine in more than 80% of patients (599).

Marrow biopsy sections vary from having no identifiable pathologic changes to overt myeloma or extensive replacement of the hematopoietic marrow with amyloid. Less than half of the nonmyeloma cases are diagnosed by marrow examination (603,604). Subcutaneous fat aspiration and rectal biopsies are each diagnostic in about 80% of cases (605). The most common finding is a mild increase in plasma cells. If adequate-sized vessels are included in the biopsy section, amyloid may be recognized in a thickened vessel. The amyloid deposits outside of a vessel wall may be perivascular or have no association with vessels. Occasionally most of the bone marrow biopsy is replaced with amyloid (Fig. 16.57). Amyloid may be detected in a Congo red–stained marrow section; under polarized light it produces a characteristic apple-green birefringence (531,599). IHC techniques using antiamyloid fibril antibodies may be used to characterize amyloid and to distinguish primary and secondary amyloidosis (597,599,606,607). Extensive extra-vessel deposits of amyloid in the bone marrow may resemble serous atrophy of fat (Fig. 16.2). The clinical history, laboratory findings, and Congo red stain should readily distinguish the two processes.

In the marrow aspirate smears there are less than 10% plasma cells in the majority of cases (599). The plasma cells may be morphologically normal or any of a spectrum of changes described for cases of plasma cell myeloma may be observed. Vacuolated plasma cells resembling those often found in μ-heavy chain disease are present in some cases (531,534). When there is extensive amyloid deposition in bone marrow, lightly eosinophilic to basophilic proteinaceous material may be scattered on the smears in various-sized clumps.

Monoclonal Light and Heavy Chain Deposition Diseases

These disorders are plasma cell tumors that secrete an abnormal light or, less often, heavy chain or both, which deposits in tissues causing organ dysfunction. These disorders include light chain deposition disease (LCDD) (608–611), heavy chain deposition disease (HCDD) (612–614), and light and heavy chain deposition disease (LHCDD) (611). The deposits differ from amyloid by absence of amyloid β-pleated sheets, lack of binding of Congo red, and no amyloid P-component. There is a monoclonal gammopathy in 75% of cases, with or without myeloma; in 80% of cases the light chain is κ. Bone marrow plasmacytosis is present in most cases. Renal glomeruli are most prominently affected (598).

OSTEOSCLEROTIC MYELOMA

Osteosclerotic myeloma (POEMS syndrome) is characterized by one or more sclerotic bone lesions with features of a plasmacytoma. The lesions consist of focally thickened trabecular bone and paratrabecular fibrosis with entrapped plasma cells, which may be elongated due to distortion by bands of fibrous tissue. Away from the lesions, the marrow usually contains fewer than 5% plasma cells. These lesions are often a component of a rare syndrome comprising a constellation of clinical findings that includes polyneuropathy, organomegaly, endocrinopathy, monoclonal protein, and skin changes (POEMS syndrome). Not all patients with osteosclerotic myeloma have all of these features, but the diagnosis of POEMS syndrome should be considered in any patient with osteosclerotic myeloma and polyneuropathy (615–617). Some patients have lymphadenopathy with the features of the plasma cell variant of Castleman disease (618).

HEAVY CHAIN DISEASE

Heavy chain diseases are a group of syndromes characterized by the production of an M-protein composed of incomplete heavy chains of IgG, IgA, or IgM type that are devoid of light chains (321,619,620). The protein abnormality is usually associated with a lymphoproliferative or lymphoplasmacytic disorder.

Gamma Chain Disease

The bone marrow is involved in 30% to 60% of patients with gamma chain disease (620). About 40% of patients have an underlying hematologic malignancy similar to Waldenström macroglobulinemia (lymphoplasmacytic lymphoma) with a pleomorphic lymphoplasmacellular proliferation in the bone marrow, lymph nodes, and spleen (621,622). In about 15% of cases there is a predominance of plasma cells. Occasionally, gamma chain disease is found with chronic lymphocytic leukemia (CLL) or a large-cell lymphoma. In some cases, there is no evidence of a lymphoproliferative disorder (621,622). The clinical course varies from indolent to aggressive (321,620).

μ-Chain Disease

The majority of patients with μ-chain disease have a long history of CLL (619,623,624). In trephine biopsy sections, the microscopic features are similar to those of other cases of CLL. Two-thirds of patients with μ-chain disease have a distinct population of vacuolated plasma cells in the bone marrow smears (619, 623). Occasionally, patients present with a lymphoma, immunoblastic transformation of CLL, myeloma, or amyloidosis. In more than half of the patients with μ-chain disease, the prolifer-

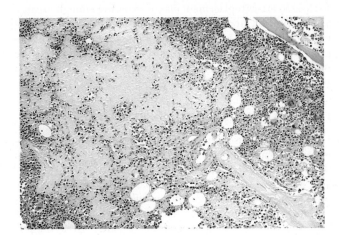

Figure 16.57. A bone marrow section from a patient with primary amyloidosis showing extensive replacement of marrow with deposits of amyloid.

ative cells produce monoclonal light chains that do not assemble with the heavy chain. The light chains are excreted in the urine as Bence Jones protein. μ-chain disease is slowly progressive (321).

α-Chain Disease

The lymphoproliferative disorder associated with α-chain disease involves the GI tract, mainly the small intestine and mesenteric lymph nodes. It is a variant of marginal zone B-cell lymphoma of mucosa-associated lymphoid tissue (MALT) type (321). The bone marrow is usually normal, but α-chain–secreting plasma cells may be identified (619,625).

WALDENSTRÖM MACROGLOBULINEMIA

Waldenström macroglobulinemia is an IgM monoclonal gammopathy generally associated with a lymphoproliferative disorder of lymphoplasmacytic, or small lymphocytic, type; rare cases have been described in association with follicular lymphoma (321,531,534,626–630). The clinical manifestations result from tumor infiltration of bone marrow, lymph nodes, and spleen, or from the affects of the secreted IgM. The monoclonal IgM may lead to hyperviscosity, cryoglobulinemia, and cold agglutinin anemia from circulating IgM, and neuropathy, glomerular disease, and amyloidosis from its deposition in tissues (629).

A lymphoproliferative process involving the bone marrow is found in approximately 90% of cases of Waldenström macroglobulinemia (376,531,626,629–631). The pattern of involvement and cytology of the neoplastic cells are usually typical for the type of lymphoma, usually lymphoplasmacytic lymphoma (Fig. 16.33; see description in the section "B-Cell Neoplasms" in this chapter). The extent of disease varies from a few focal lesions to extensive marrow replacement.

Intranuclear inclusions (Dutcher bodies) in the lymphocytes are commonly observed in the sections and may be numerous (531). Their presence is suggestive but not pathognomonic of lymphoplasmacytic lymphoma/Waldenström macroglobulinemia. In some cases, the plasma cells and histiocytes contain abundant cytoplasmic inclusions that stain intensely with the PAS reaction (531).

The percentage of lymphocytes in bone marrow smears varies from normal to more than 90%. They usually have the cytologic features of well-differentiated small lymphocytes and plasmacytoid lymphocytes. Plasma cells, mast cells, and histiocytes are increased in most cases (534). Neoplastic lymphocytes are found on blood smears in patients with CLL and often in cases of lymphoplasmacytic lymphoma.

HISTIOCYTIC PROLIFERATIONS

The histiocytic proliferations that involve bone marrow consist of several reactive and neoplastic conditions, including storage histiocyte diseases, Langerhans cell histiocytosis, the hemophagocytic syndromes, and malignant histiocyte disorders.

STORAGE HISTIOCYTE DISORDERS

Storage histiocyte disorders result from inborn errors of metabolism leading to hyperplasia of the monocyte-macrophage system and accumulation of large quantities of storage material in the cytoplasm of histiocytes. Storage histiocytes in tumor-like masses or as individual scattered cells may be present in bone marrow.

GAUCHER DISEASE

Gaucher disease is the most prevalent lysosomal storage disorder and the one most likely to be diagnosed on a bone marrow biopsy (632–634). Marrow sections show dispersed small focal collections of Gaucher cells, numerous focal collections, or total replacement of the marrow (Fig. 16.58). The Gaucher cells are large histiocytes with abundant cytoplasm and a small nucleus. Their characteristic cytologic feature is the striated or fibrillary cytoplasm that often resembles wrinkled tissue paper (633–635). Hemosiderin pigment is commonly observed in the cytoplasm. Gaucher cells react strongly with tartrate-resistant acid phosphatase, nonspecific esterase, and PAS stains (633–636).

Cells morphologically similar to Gaucher cells are observed in small numbers in bone marrow smears from patients with chronic myelogenous leukemia, acute leukemias, and congenital dyserythropoietic anemia (637,638). In addition, macrophages containing atypical mycobacteria in the setting of HIV may also cytologically resemble Gaucher cells. In the appropriate clinical setting, however, the distinctive cytologic features of the histiocytes are virtually diagnostic of Gaucher disease.

NIEMANN-PICK DISEASE

Patients with Niemann-Pick disease (sphingomyelin cholesterol lipidosis) have hepatosplenomegaly and foamy histiocytes in the bone marrow (639). Bone marrow sections are usually diffusely involved. The extent of marrow replacement varies from a few scattered foamy histiocytes to vast accumulations. The histiocytes are large with a single nucleus and abundant vacuolated cytoplasm. They are often found in abundance near the thin edge of bone marrow smears. In blood smears, lymphocytes with numerous sharply defined lipid vacuoles may be observed (633). Cells morphologically similar to Niemann-Pick histiocytes are found in other conditions in which lipids accumulate in the cytoplasm of histiocytes (e.g., hyperlipidemia).

In other metabolic diseases such as oxalosis and cystinosis, crystals may be deposited in the bone marrow. The crystals are found in histiocytes, giant cells, and extracellularly (640). In oxalosis, marrow replacement may be extensive enough to cause a myelophthisic anemia (640). Several other rare storage diseases are associated with morphologic changes in marrow histiocytes and other hematopoietic cells (633). These changes are usually identified in blood and marrow smears but may not be recognized in sections.

LANGERHANS CELL HISTIOCYTOSIS

Langerhans cell histiocytosis (LCH), previously known as histiocytosis X, is a localized or systemic proliferation of histiocytic dendritic cells with the features of Langerhans cells (642,643). The WHO recognizes three main variants: unifocal, multifocal/unisystem, and multifocal/multisystem (641). Although differing in clinical severity, these have common histopathological features. Older designations of clinical variants such as Letterer-Siwe disease and Hand-Schuller-Christian disease are presently obsolete. The primary diagnosis of LCH is rarely made on bone marrow biopsies, but the marrow is commonly examined to

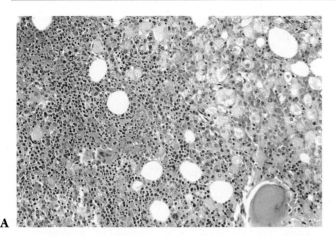

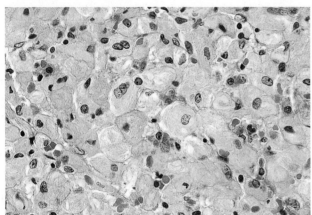

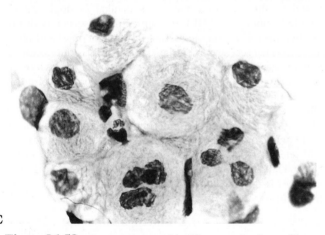

Figure 16.58. Bone marrow trephine biopsy section from a 29-year-old woman with mild splenomegaly and pancytopenia. (**A**) The marrow is involved by a patchy infiltrate of Gaucher cells. (**B**) High magnification showing several Gaucher histiocytes with typical striated cytoplasm. (**C**) A bone marrow aspirate contains clusters of typical Gaucher cells on the thin edge of the buffy coat smear.

assess the extent of disease; marrow trephine specimens often contain LCH lesions in cases with multifocal or generalized marrow involvement (644–647).

In marrow sections, lesions of LCH vary from small focal clusters of Langerhans histiocytes to large lesions that occupy all of the marrow space (648). The lesions may be composed almost exclusively of histiocytes, but in most cases there is a mixture of multinucleate giant cells, plasma cells, eosinophils,

lymphocytes, and neutrophils (Fig. 16.59). Some of the lesions resemble granulomas. Langerhans histiocytes have a characteristic indented or grooved nucleus with delicate chromatin and inconspicuous nucleoli (646). Occasionally in aggressive cases, the Langerhans cells demonstrate prominent nucleoli. The cytoplasm is eosinophilic and may contain hemosiderin granules. The marrow smears are generally nondiagnostic but may contain increased histiocytes scattered as single cells or concentrated at the edge of the smear.

Single bone lesions are the most frequent finding in localized LCH (eosinophilic granuloma) (649). The lesions are uncommon in the ilium and it is unusual to diagnose an eosinophilic granuloma in a random posterior iliac crest needle biopsy. Localized LCH is usually identified by radiographic studies, and bone biopsies are obtained by directed needle or open biopsy techniques. The histologic characteristics are essentially the same as those found in generalized LCH.

In rare cases, other histiocytoses or other polycellular lesions in bone marrow such as granulomas, Hodgkin disease, and mast cell disease may be considered in the differential diagnosis of LCH. The characteristic nuclear indentation of the histiocytes, lack of prominent nucleoli, and the lipid and pigment in the cytoplasm should identify cases of LCH. When the histopathology is equivocal, Langerhans cells can be differentiated from other histiocytes by their histochemical, IHC, and ultrastructural profile. Most importantly, they coexpress S-100 and CD1a (646,651–653); this combination is essentially diagnostic of LCH in the appropriate setting. In contrast to normal Langerhans cells, they frequently express CD68 (650). In addition, they are generally negative for lysozyme (650). In rare cases, identification of Birbeck granules by electron microscopy may be required to confirm the diagnosis of LCH (651,652).

INFECTION (VIRUS)-ASSOCIATED HEMOPHAGOCYTIC SYNDROME

Patients with infection-associated hemophagocytic syndrome (IAHS) have fever, severe constitutional symptoms, and blood cytopenias, usually pancytopenia (654–656). A viral etiology has been demonstrated in many cases, but other infections may occasionally cause similar changes. The clinical and pathologic manifestations appear to result from a defective immune response to the infection (657–660). Systemic reactive hemophagocytic syndromes may also be seen in association with malignant disease, particularly some variants of T-cell lymphoma (455,661,662). The most striking feature in the bone marrow is histiocytic hyperplasia with phagocytosis of red cells, platelets, and nucleated hematopoietic cells (Fig. 16.60A). The histiocytes are cytologically mature with a low nuclear:cytoplasmic ratio, abundant cytoplasm, condensed chromatin, and inconspicuous or absent nucleoli. The cytoplasm of the histiocytes may be filled with intact or degenerating phagocytosed cells, or may contain vacuoles of varying size.

The histiocytic hyperplasia is usually most evident in buffy coat smears of marrow; the histiocytes are concentrated at the thin edge of the smear. In the marrow sections, histiocytes are both diffusely scattered and in distinct clusters. The marrow is usually hypocellular with decreased granulopoiesis and erythropoiesis; megakaryocytes are generally normal or increased. Evidence of extensive destruction of the marrow with focal areas of necrosis is often seen (Fig. 16.60B). Reactive lymphocytic

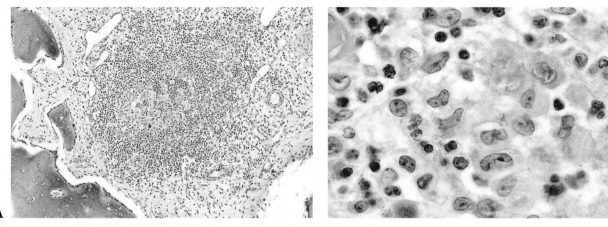

Figure 16.59. Bone marrow trephine biopsy section from a patient with Langerhans cell histiocytosis. **(A)** Low magnification of a large focal lesion consisting of Langerhans histiocytes admixed with various reactive cells. **(B)** A higher magnification illustrates some of the typical features of Langerhans cells. Note the folded or grooved nucleus in most of the cells.

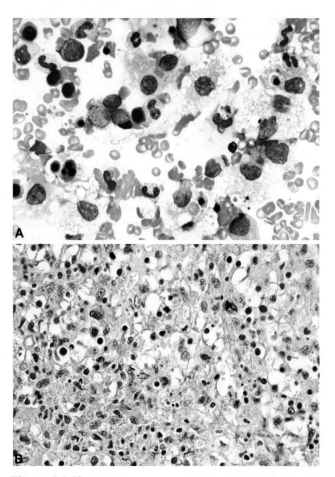

Figure 16.60. **(A)** Bone marrow smear from a 5-year-old boy with an infection (virus)-associated hemophagocytic syndrome. There is marked histiocytic hyperplasia. The histiocytes are mature-appearing and many show hemophagocytosis. **(B)** A bone marrow section from this patient shows evidence of marrow destruction and histiocytic hyperplasia with hemophagocytosis. Normal hematopoietic cells are markedly reduced.

aggregates and granulomatous lesions are present in some cases. Histiocytic hyperplasia and hemophagocytosis are also observed in lymph nodes, spleen, and liver (654,655).

IAHS may be mistaken for a malignant histiocytic process. However, careful attention to the cytologic features of the proliferating histiocytes reveals benign features: low nuclear:cytoplasmic ratio, abundant cytoplasm, evenly dispersed chromatin, and inconspicuous nucleoli (Fig. 16.60A). A constellation of clinical and morphologic features similar to those in IAHS is found in the syndrome known as familial hemophagocytic lymphohistiocytosis (FHL) (658,663); this disorder is distinguished from IAHS on the basis of early age of onset and often an autosomal-recessive inheritance pattern. It is due to inherited impairment of NK- and T-cell cytotoxic function as a result of inherited mutations in several different genes involved in cell killing (664–666). The defective cytotoxic activity results in failure to downregulate cellular immune activation. IAHS and FHL have in common immune deficiency and defective immune regulation with depressed T-cell and NK-cell cytotoxicity and elevation of interferon-γ and tumor necrosis factor (659,660,667,668). Abnormal cytokine production by T lymphocytes is the likely cause of the histiocytic hyperplasia and hemophagocytosis.

MALIGNANT HISTIOCYTE DISORDERS

The entities of malignant histiocytosis and true histiocytic lymphoma, defined as tumors of mature phagocytic histiocytes, have all but disappeared in recent years because of improved diagnostic techniques, particularly IHC and molecular pathology. Most cases previously diagnosed as true histiocytic malignancies have, on reexamination, been reclassified as a variety of lesions, particularly reactive hemophagocytic syndromes, anaplastic large-cell lymphoma, and other NHLs (669–672). Thus, previous data regarding clinical and pathologic features of true histiocytic malignancies can no longer be considered accurate.

Among the remaining lesions that are likely to be classified as true histiocytic malignancies, most appear to represent extramedullary deposits of acute monocytic leukemias (myeloid sarcomas). These leukemias have a well-known tendency to involve

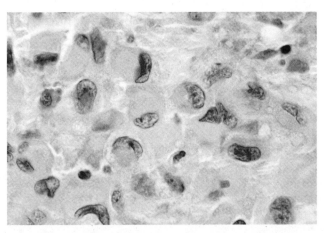

Figure 16.61. Cohesive bone marrow infiltrate of malignant histiocytic-appearing cells with abundant cytoplasm with inclusion like perinuclear zones and eccentric, highly irregular nuclei. In smears the perinuclear zones corresponded to localized cytoplasmic vacuolization with evidence of phagocytic activity. Small numbers of these cells were found circulating in peripheral blood. This patient progressed over the next several months to an acute monocytic leukemia. Although most of the leukemic cells were more typical monoblasts and promonocytes, a population of histiocytic-appearing cells remained, and transitional forms were evident.

extramedullary sites, and may initially present in such locations in the absence of overt blood and bone marrow involvement (673). Although immature monocytic proliferations (AML M5a) are unlikely to be confused with true histiocytic neoplasms, those consisting of promonocytes (M5b) can have a deceptively mature appearance in tissue. These lesions should be considered myeloid sarcomas (674). In marrow, immature monocytic proliferations obviously should be considered acute leukemia.

Very rarely, acute monocytic leukemia initially presents with bone marrow lesions composed of cells having features of mature histiocytes, including cohesive growth, abundant cytoplasm with indented nuclei, and phagocytic activity (Fig. 16.61). Over time, these lesions will declare themselves as acute leukemias and are best considered as such (675,676). Useful differential diagnostic points include fine, blast-like chromatin, myelodysplasia, and an admixture of more typical myelomonocytic blasts.

Malignancies of mature histiocytes (excluding LCH and dendritic cell sarcomas) are exceedingly rare, and should be diagnosed as such with extreme caution, and only after the application of stringent diagnostic criteria (677).

METASTATIC TUMORS

Assessment of the bone marrow for metastatic tumor may be important in staging, monitoring response to therapy, and identifying recurrent disease (678,679). In some instances the initial diagnosis of a malignant solid-tissue tumor is made from a marrow biopsy taken for evaluation of abnormal blood counts, a chest or abdominal mass, or other symptomatology. The marrow core biopsy is more often positive for metastatic disease than the marrow aspirate, but both should always be performed; metastatic tumor cells may occasionally be found in aspirate smears only (680,681). Histologic identification of the type of

metastatic neoplasm is much more likely with biopsy sections than with smear preparations. The cytologic features of a metastatic tumor in marrow aspirate smears are generally insufficiently distinctive to allow more than generic characterization.

HISTOPATHOLOGY OF BONE MARROW METASTASIS

The distribution of metastases in trephine biopsy sections may be focal, diffuse, or a mixture of both. The extent of involvement varies from minute foci present in one or two sections to total replacement of normal hematopoietic elements. Small foci of metastatic tumor are usually sharply separated from normal hematopoietic cells and are readily recognized as clusters of cells foreign to the marrow. Bone marrow adjacent to metastatic tumor may be entirely normal or may manifest nonspecific changes such as generalized hyperplasia, increased eosinophils, lymphocytes, granulocytes, or plasma cells (682). With diffuse and extensive involvement, confluent metastatic tumor may comprise virtually all of the cellular elements of the bone marrow biopsy. The histologic features of the metastasis may be identical to those of the primary lesion or more or less differentiated.

Changes in the bone trabeculae are common and may be present even in the absence of identifiable tumor cells (683,684). Most commonly, there is destruction of bone with osteopenia and increased osteoclastic activity. Less frequently, metastases induce osteoblastic, osteosclerotic reactions with markedly thickened and irregularly shaped bone trabeculae (Fig. 16.62). Adenocarcinoma of the breast and prostate are most notorious for producing osteoblastic lesions (685) (Fig. 16.59).

Myelofibrosis is a feature common to most metastatic lesions in bone marrow (686). The degree of fibrosis is highly variable, ranging from a mild increase in reticulin fibers encircling clusters of neoplastic cells to extensive collagenous fibrosis (Figs. 16.63 and 16.64). Carcinomas from the breast and prostate may be particularly fibrotic. Extensive myelofibrosis may mask the underlying neoplasm and be confused with other processes such as primary myelofibrosis. In these cases a careful search for metastatic tumor in several sections or repeat biopsies may be necessary if there is not a known primary neoplasm. The myelofibrosis may be completely reversed with successful therapy for the underlying malignancy (687).

Metastatic disease is the most common cause of necrosis in bone marrow (35,678,688). Necrotic tissue may be patchy and scattered throughout a lesion, or the entire biopsy specimen may be necrotic (34). Diagnosis and characterization of a metastatic tumor may not be possible when necrosis is extensive. Unexplained bone marrow necrosis is an indication for additional biopsies at adjacent sites.

Special techniques applicable to bone marrow specimens, including histochemistry, IHC, and, rarely, electron microscopy, may be used to characterize a poorly differentiated metastatic tumor in a patient without a known primary (689,690). IHC is a particularly valuable tool for this purpose and may also be used to highlight minute foci of metastatic tumor that are not apparent in hematoxylin and eosin–stained marrow sections (690,691). The IHC stains used for characterization of specific tumor types are detailed in other chapters.

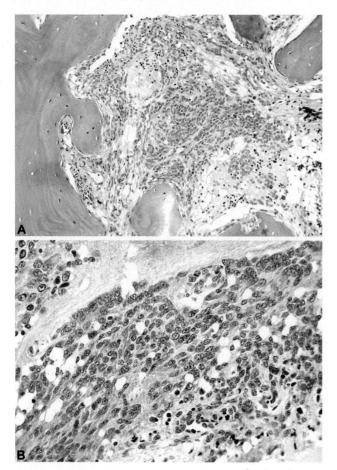

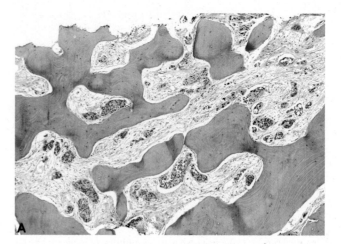

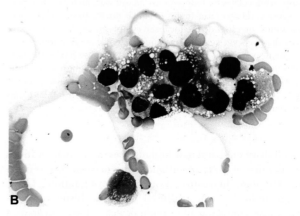

Figure 16.62. Metastatic neuroblastoma. **(A)** Osteoblastic bone changes with replacement of normal marrow with tumor cells. **(B)** The neoplastic cells exhibit a positive neuron-specific enolase immunostain.

Figure 16.63. **(A)** Low magnification of a bone marrow biopsy section showing an osteoblastic lesion of metastatic carcinoma of the breast. There is a marked desmoplastic reaction with scattered tumor clumps. **(B)** A marrow aspirate smear from the same case shows a clump of tumor cells.

CYTOLOGY IN ASPIRATE SMEARS

The marrow aspirate specimens from patients with bone marrow metastases are often of poor quality because of fibrosis, osteosclerosis, and necrosis. In some cases, small clusters of metastatic tumor are found in only one or two of several marrow aspirate smears, whereas in others they are abundant in all of the smears and may be the predominant cell population. Metastatic tumor cells are generally concentrated in various-sized clusters toward the thin edge and lateral aspects of the smear (Figs. 16.63 and 16.65). These areas should be carefully examined when marrow metastasis is a consideration. Clusters of osteoblasts and individual osteoclasts are occasionally found in smears and should not be mistaken for neoplastic cells.

BONE MARROW METASTASIS IN ADULTS

Carcinomas of the breast, prostate, lung, and GI tract have the highest frequency of bone marrow metastasis in adults (678–680,685,692,693). In female patients, infiltrating ductal carcinoma of the breast is the most common; the incidence of marrow metastasis in patients with nonlocalized breast carcinoma varies between 6% and 57% (679,692–695). Approximately two-thirds of the patients have osteoblastic lesions, one-

fifth have osteolytic lesions, and in the remainder there are no apparent radiographic bone changes (693).

In male patients, carcinomas of the lung and prostate are most commonly associated with bone marrow metastasis (680,692). The incidence of marrow involvement at diagnosis in patients with carcinoma of the lung is 5% to 21% and varies with the histologic-type, small-cell carcinoma having the highest incidence (692,696,697). Prostatic carcinoma has been found in bone marrow biopsies in 13% to 20% of patients prior to treatment (692,698). Poorly differentiated prostatic carcinomas are more likely to involve the bone marrow than moderately differentiated or well-differentiated subtypes (698).

GI malignancies are the fourth most common to metastasize to the bone marrow; 3% to 4% of patients with GI cancers have marrow involvement at diagnosis (692). Carcinomas of the stomach and colon are the most likely to involve the marrow.

Several other tumors occasionally metastasize to the bone marrow early in the clinical course, including melanoma, renal cell carcinoma, thyroid adenocarcinoma, pancreatic adenocarcinoma, ovarian and testicular cancers, transitional cell carcinomas, lymphoepitheliomas, rhabdomyosarcoma, and Ewing sarcoma. A long list of other malignant neoplasms occasionally or rarely metastasize to the bone marrow, generally late in the course of the disease.

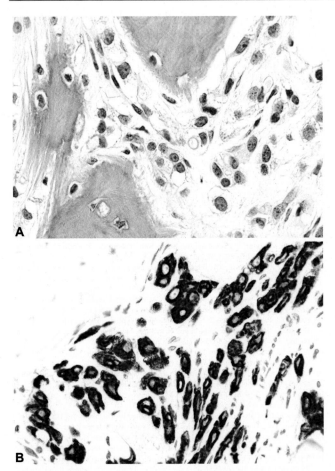

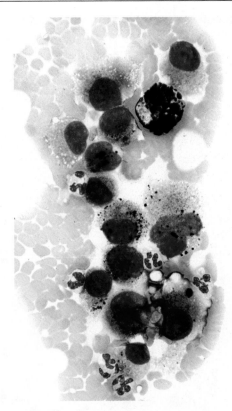

Figure 16.65. Bone marrow aspirate smear showing a metastatic cluster of malignant melanoma cells. Dark, granular pigment is present in the cytoplasm of the tumor cells. The pigment is an identifying characteristic in this case. The cytologic characteristics of metastatic tumor cells in smears are usually not distinctive enough to identify the primary tumor in bone marrow smears.

Figure 16.64. **(A)** Bone marrow involvement by metastatic carcinoma of the breast. There are blastic bone changes and a desmoplastic reaction around tumor cells. **(B)** An AE1/AE3 immunostain shows a strongly positive reaction in the neoplastic cells.

BONE MARROW METASTASIS IN CHILDREN

Neuroblastoma is the most common solid-tissue tumor in children, and in 50% to 60% of cases manifests bone marrow infiltration at diagnosis (692,699,700) (Fig. 16.62). The incidence of marrow involvement is less in patients under 1 year of age than in older children. Several other childhood malignancies have a relatively high incidence of marrow metastasis, including ganglioneuroblastoma, rhabdomyosarcoma (15% to 20%), Ewing sarcoma (13% to 36%), and retinoblastoma (23% to 50%) (692,699,700) (Fig. 16.66). Osteosarcoma, fibrosarcoma, and various carcinomas in children may involve the bone marrow late in the course. Nephroblastomas, hepatoblastomas, and CNS tumors—except for medulloblastomas—rarely, if ever metastasize to the marrow (692,699,701).

DIFFERENTIAL DIAGNOSIS

In most cases, a metastatic lesion in a marrow biopsy is easily recognized as such, even when a primary neoplasm is not apparent, but occasionally a metastatic tumor simulates a hematopoietic malignancy.

In adults, tumors that elicit marrow fibrosis may be mistaken for primary myelofibrosis. Compounding this problem are the frequent presence of a leukoerythroblastic reaction in blood smears in the setting of bone marrow metastasis, and the occasional resemblance of metastatic tumor deposits to clusters of highly atypical megakaryocytes so characteristic of primary myelofibrosis. However, the peripheral blood in patients with metastatic tumor generally lacks the teardrop poikilocytosis, atypical platelets, and circulating megakaryocytes seen in primary myelofibrosis. In addition, the spleen is usually not enlarged and the marrow lacks such features as intrasinusoidal hematopoiesis and prominent megakaryocytic hyperplasia. In equivocal cases, IHC is usually definitive.

In both adults and children, occasional metastatic tumors, particularly those of the "small blue cell" variety, are quite dyscohesive in smears, mimicking either malignant lymphoma or acute leukemia. The latter problem is exacerbated by the cytologic resemblance of many of these tumors to hematolymphoid blasts in smear preparations. However, the peripheral blood is not involved, and careful examination of aspirate smears usually reveals some evidence of cellular cohesion. Furthermore, the infiltrate in the core biopsy usually demonstrates more obvious cohesion than in the smears. An unusual pitfall is the admixture of small lymphocytes with metastatic tumor cells, producing a morphologic resemblance to a benign or atypical lymphoid aggregate; IHC is invaluable in such cases.

METABOLIC BONE DISEASES

Bone changes are found in a wide variety of inherited and acquired metabolic diseases. The pathology of these disorders is

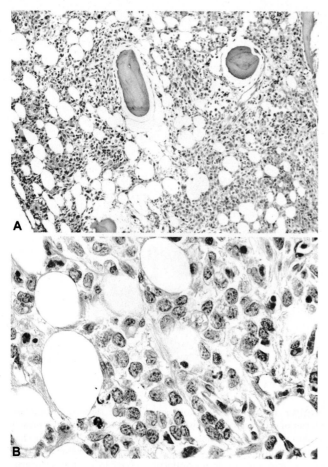

Figure 16.66. Low **(A)** and high **(B)** magnifications of metastatic rhabdomyosarcoma in the marrow of an 11-year-old boy. The tumor exhibits an interstitial pattern of involvement with focal clustering.

discussed in other chapters of this book. Bone marrow biopsies are uncommonly performed for diagnosis of primary bone diseases, although in some instances they can be diagnostic.

Bone pathology is usually encountered fortuitously in a biopsy during the course of evaluation for a hematologic disorder. In rare instances, blood cytopenias result from encroachment on the marrow space by bone trabeculae altered by metabolic bone disease. Bone diseases that may be diagnosed from a trephine biopsy include osteoporosis, osteomalacia, Paget disease of bone, hyperparathyroid and renal osteodystrophy, and osteopetrosis (702) (Fig. 16.67).

REFERENCES

1. Ellman L. Bone marrow biopsy in the evaluation of lymphoma, carcinoma and granulomatous disorders. *Am J Med* 1976;60:1–7.
2. Burkhardt R, Frisch B, Bartl R. Bone biopsy in haematological disorders. *J Clin Pathol* 1982;35:257–284.
3. Frisch B, Lewis SM, Burkhardt R, et al. *Biopsy Pathology of Bone and Bone Marrow.* New York: Raven Press, 1985:1–17.
4. Brynes RK, McKenna RW, Sundberg RD. Bone marrow aspiration and trephine biopsy. An approach to a thorough study. *Am J Clin Pathol* 1978;70:753–759.
5. Jamshidi K, Swaim WR. Bone marrow biopsy with unaltered architecture: a new biopsy device. *J Lab Clin Med* 1971;77:335–342.
6. Brunning RD, McKenna RW. Bone marrow specimen processing. In Brunning RD, McKenna RW, eds. *Tumors of the Bone Marrow. Atlas of Tumor Pathology.* Washington, DC: Armed Forces Institute of Pathology, 1994:475–489.
7. Brunning RD, Bloomfield CD, McKenna RW, et al. Bilateral trephine bone marrow biopsies in lymphoma and other neoplastic diseases. *Ann Intern Med* 1975;82:365–366.
8. Haddy TB, Parker RI, Magrath IT. Bone marrow involvement in young patients with non-Hodgkin's lymphoma: the importance of multiple bone marrow samples for accurate staging. *Med Pediatr Oncol* 1989;17:418–423.
9. Juneja SK, Wolf MM, Cooper IA. Value of bilateral bone marrow biopsy specimens in non-Hodgkin's lymphoma. *J Clin Pathol* 1990;43:630–632.
10. Ebie N, Loew JM, Gregory SA. Bilateral trephine bone marrow biopsy for staging non-Hodgkin's lymphoma—a second look. *Hematol Pathol* 1989;3:29–33.
11. Barekman CL, Fair KP, Cotelingam JD. Comparative utility of diagnostic bone-marrow components: a 10-year study. *Am J Hematol* 1997;56:37–41.
12. Beckstead JH, Halverson PS, Ries CA, et al. Enzyme histochemistry and IHC on biopsy specimens of pathologic human bone marrow. *Blood* 1981;57:1088–1098.
13. Kubic VL, Brunning RD. IHC evaluation of neoplasms in bone marrow biopsies using monoclonal antibodies reactive in paraffin-embedded tissue. *Mod Pathol* 1989;2:618–629.
14. Brunning RD, McKenna RW. Normal bone marrow. In Brunning RD, McKenna RW, eds. *Tumors of the Bone Marrow. Atlas of Tumor Pathology.* Third Series, Fascicle 9. Washington, DC: Armed Forces Institute of Pathology, 1994:2–18.
15. Hartsock RJ, Smith EB, Petty CS. Normal variations with aging of the amount of hematopoietic tissue in bone marrow from the anterior iliac crest. *Am J Clin Pathol* 1965;43:326–331.
16. Mauch P, Botnick LE, Hannon EC, et al. Decline in bone marrow proliferative capacity as a function of age. *Blood* 1982;60:245–252.
17. Williams L, Udupa KB, Lipschutz DA. Age and erythropoiesis. *Clin Res* 1981;29:864a.
18. Frisch B, Lewis SM, Burkhardt R, et al. *Biopsy Pathology of Bone and Bone Marrow.* New York: Raven Press, 1985:47–57.
19. Bartl R, Frisch B, Hill W, et al. Bone marrow histology in hairy cell leukemia. Identification of subtypes and their prognostic significance. *Am J Clin Pathol* 1983;79:531–545.
20. Rozman C, Montserrat E, Rodriguez-Fernandez JM, et al. Bone marrow histologic pattern—the best single prognostic parameter in chronic lymphocytic leukemia: a multivariate survival analysis of 329 cases. *Blood* 1984;64:642–648.
21. Bartl R, Frisch B, Fateh-Moghadam A, et al. Histologic classification and staging of multiple

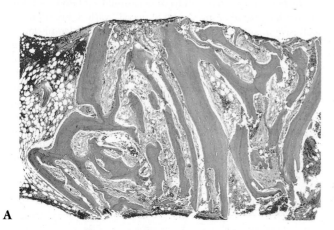

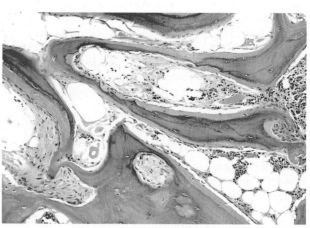

Figure 16.67. Low **(A)** and high **(B)** magnifications of bone changes secondary to hyperparathyroidism due to a parathyroid adenoma. The bone marrow biopsy was performed for evaluation of blood cytopenias.

myeloma. A retrospective and prospective study of 674 cases. *Am J Clin Pathol* 1987;87: 342–355.
22. Dick FR, Burns CP, Weiner GJ, et al. Bone marrow morphology during induction phase of therapy for acute myeloid leukemia (AML). *Hematol Pathol* 1995;9:95–106.
23. Foucar K, Dick F. Interpretation of post chemotherapy and post transplantation bone marrow specimens. In Knowles D, ed. *Neoplastic Hematopathology*. Baltimore: Williams & Wilkins, 1992:1439–1457.
24. Steinherz PG, Gaynon PS, Breneman JC, et al. Cytoreduction and prognosis in acute lymphoblastic leukemia—the importance of early marrow response: report from the Children's Cancer Group. *J Clin Oncol* 1996;14:389–398.
25. Damon LE, Rugo HS, Ries CA, et al. Post-remission cytopenias following intense induction chemotherapy for acute myeloid leukemia. *Leukemia* 1994;8:535–541.
26. van den berg H, Kluin PM, Zwaan FE, et al. Histopathology of bone marrow reconstitution after allogeneic bone marrow transplantation. *Histopathology* 1989;15:363–373.
27. Naeim F, Smith GS, Gale RP. Morphologic aspects of bone marrow transplantation in patients with aplastic anemia. *Hum Pathol* 1978;9:295–308.
28. Schmitz LL, McClure JS, Litz CE, et al. Morphologic and quantitative changes in blood and marrow cells following growth factor therapy. *Am J Clin Pathol* 1994;101:67–75.
29. Antin JH, Weinberg DS, Rosenthal DS. Variable effect of recombinant human granulocyte-macrophage colony-stimulating factor on bone marrow fibrosis in patients with myelodysplasia. *Exp Hematol* 1990;18:266–270.
30. Tavassoli M, Eastlund DT, Yam LT, et al. Gelatinous transformation of bone marrow in prolonged self-induced starvation. *Scand J Haematol* 1976;16:311–319.
31. Seaman JP, Kjeldsberg CR, Linker A. Gelatinous transformation of the bone marrow. *Hum Pathol* 1978;9:685–692.
32. Clarke BE, Brown DJ, Xipell JM. Gelatinous transformation of the bone marrow. *Pathology* 1983;15:85–88.
33. Mehta K, Gascon P, Robboy S. The gelatinous bone marrow (serous atrophy) in patients with acquired immunodeficiency syndrome. Evidence of excess sulfated glycosaminoglycan. *Arch Pathol Lab Med* 1992;116:504–508.
34. Brown CH 3rd. Bone marrow necrosis. A study of seventy cases. *Johns Hopkins Med J* 1972; 131:189–203.
35. Kiraly JF 3rd, Wheby MS. Bone marrow necrosis. *Am J Med* 1976;60:361–368.
36. Conrad ME, Carpenter JT. Bone marrow necrosis. *Am J Hematol* 1979;7:181–189.
37. Cowan JD, Rubin RN, Kies MS, et al. Bone marrow necrosis. *Cancer* 1980;46:2168–2171.
38. Eide J. Bone infarcts in bacterial endocarditis. *Hum Pathol* 1982;13:631–634.
39. Kadin ME, Donaldson SS, Dorfman RF. Isolated granulomas in Hodgkin's disease. *N Engl J Med* 1970;283:859–861.
40. Kim H, Dorfman RF. Morphological studies of 84 untreated patients subjected to laparotomy for the staging of non-Hodgkin's lymphomas. *Cancer* 1974;33:657–674.
41. Rigberg LA, Robinson MJ, Espiritu CR. Chlorpropamide-induced granulomas. A probable hypersensitivity reaction in liver and bone marrow. *JAMA* 1976;235:409–410.
42. Browne PM, Sharma OP, Salkin D. Bone marrow sarcoidosis. *JAMA* 1978;240:2654–2655.
43. Yu NC, Rywlin AM. Granulomatous lesions of the bone marrow in non-Hodgkin's lymphoma. *Hum Pathol* 1982;13:905–910.
44. Bodem CR, Hamory BH, Taylor HM, et al. Granulomatous bone marrow disease. A review of the literature and clinicopathologic analysis of 58 cases. *Medicine (Baltimore)* 1983;62: 372–383.
45. Bhargava V, Farhi DC. Bone marrow granulomas: clinicopathologic findings in 72 cases and review of the literature. *Hematol Pathol* 1988;2:43–50.
46. Okun DB, Sun NC, Tanaka KR. Bone marrow granulomas in Q fever. *Am J Clin Pathol* 1979;71:117–121.
47. Davies SF, McKenna RW, Sarosi GA. Trephine biopsy of the bone marrow in disseminated histoplasmosis. *Am J Med* 1979;67:617–622.
48. Farhi DC, Mason UG 3rd, Horsburgh CR, Jr. The bone marrow in disseminated mycobacterium avium-intracellulare infection. *Am J Clin Pathol* 1985;83:463–468.
49. Rywlin AM, Ortega R. Lipid granulomas of the bone marrow. *Am J Clin Pathol* 1972;57: 457–462.
50. Frisch B, Lewis SM, Burkhardt R, et al. *Biopsy Pathology of Bone and Bone Marrow*. New York: Raven Press, 1985:58–71.
51. Burston J, Pinniger JL. The reticulin content of bone marrow in hematological disorders. *Br J Haematol* 1963;9:172–184.
52. Bauermeister DE. Quantitation of bone marrow reticulin—a normal range. *Am J Clin Pathol* 1971;56:24–31.
53. Hernandez Nieto L, Muncunill J, Rozman C, et al. [Secondary myelofibrosis and/or osteosclerosis. An assessment of 400 biopsies]. *Sangre (Barc)* 1978;23:402–410.
54. Duhamel G, Stachowiak J. [Bone marrow fibrosis in malignant hemopathies and cancers. Histological study of 2786 biopsies]. *Sem Hop* 1981;57:111–116.
55. Schneider DR, Picker LJ. Myelodysplasia in the acquired immune deficiency syndrome. *Am J Clin Pathol* 1985;84:144–152.
56. Castella A, Croxson TS, Mildvan D, et al. The bone marrow in AIDS. A histologic, hematologic, and microbiologic study. *Am J Clin Pathol* 1985;84:425–432.
57. Sandhaus LM, Scudder R. Hematologic and bone marrow abnormalities in pediatric patients with human immunodeficiency virus (HIV) infection. *Pediatr Pathol* 1989;9:277–288.
58. Danova M, Riccardi A, Brugnatelli S, et al. Bone marrow morphology and proliferative activity in acquired immunodeficiency syndrome. *Haematologica* 1989;74:365–369.
59. Karcher DS, Frost AR. The bone marrow in human immunodeficiency virus (HIV)-related disease. Morphology and clinical correlation. *Am J Clin Pathol* 1991;95:63–71.
60. Diebold J, Tabbara W, Marche C, et al. [Bone marrow changes at several stages of HIV infection, studied on bone marrow biopsies in 85 patients]. *Arch Anat Cytol Pathol* 1991; 39:137–146.
61. Aboulafia DM, Mitsuyasu RT. Hematologic abnormalities in AIDS. *Hematol Oncol Clin North Am* 1991;5:195–214.
62. Osborne BM, Guarda LA, Butler JJ. Bone marrow biopsies in patients with the acquired immunodeficiency syndrome. *Hum Pathol* 1984;15:1048–1053.
63. Bain BJ. The haematological features of HIV infection. *Br J Haematol* 1997;99:1–8.
64. Moses A, Nelson J, Bagby GC, Jr. The influence of human immunodeficiency virus-1 on hematopoiesis. *Blood* 1998;91:1479–1495.
65. Abrams DI, Kiprov DD, Goedert JJ, et al. Antibodies to human T-lymphotropic virus type III and development of the acquired immunodeficiency syndrome in homosexual men presenting with immune thrombocytopenia. *Ann Intern Med* 1986;104:47–50.
66. Zauli G, Davis BR, Re MC, et al. tat protein stimulates production of transforming growth factor-beta 1 by marrow macrophages: a potential mechanism for human immunodeficiency virus-1-induced hematopoietic suppression. *Blood* 1992;80:3036–3043.
67. Moses AV, Williams S, Heneveld ML, et al. Human immunodeficiency virus infection of bone marrow endothelium reduces induction of stromal hematopoietic growth factors. *Blood* 1996;87:919–925.
68. Pluda JM, Mitsuya H, Yarchoan R. Hematologic effects of AIDS therapies. *Hematol Oncol Clin North Am* 1991;5:229–248.
69. Nichols L, Florentine B, Lewis W, et al. Bone marrow examination for the diagnosis of mycobacterial and fungal infections in the acquired immunodeficiency syndrome. *Arch Pathol Lab Med* 1991;115:1125–1132.
70. Cohen RJ, Samoszuk MK, Busch D, et al. Occult infections with *M. intracellulare* in bone-marrow biopsy specimens from patients with AIDS. *N Engl J Med* 1983;308:1475–1476.
71. Frickhofen N, Abkowitz JL, Safford M, et al. Persistent B19 parvovirus infection in patients infected with human immunodeficiency virus type 1 (HIV-1): a treatable cause of anemia in AIDS. *Ann Intern Med* 1990;113:926–933.
72. van Elsacker-Neile AM, Kroon FP, van der Ende ME, et al. Prevalence of parvovirus B19 infection in patients infected with human immunodeficiency virus. *Clin Infect Dis* 1996; 23:1255–1260.
73. Crook TW, Rogers BB, McFarland RD, et al. Unusual bone marrow manifestations of parvovirus B19 infection in immunocompromised patients. *Hum Pathol* 2000;31:161–168.
74. Mead JH, Mason TE. Lymphoma versus AIDS. *Am J Clin Pathol* 1983;80:546–547.
75. Hanson CA, Brunning RD, Gajl-Peczalska KJ, et al. Bone marrow manifestations of peripheral T-cell lymphoma. A study of 30 cases. *Am J Clin Pathol* 1986;86:449–460.
76. Rule S, Reed C, Costello C. Fatal haemophagocytic syndromes in HIV-antibody positive patient. *Br J Haematol* 1991;79:127.
77. Ziegler JL, Beckstead JA, Volberding PA, et al. Non-Hodgkin's lymphoma in 90 homosexual men. Relation to generalized lymphadenopathy and the acquired immunodeficiency syndrome. *N Engl J Med* 1984;311:565–570.
78. Levine AM. Acquired immunodeficiency syndrome-related lymphoma. *Blood* 1992;80: 8–20.
79. Knowles D, Chadburn A. Lymphadenopathy and the lymphoid neoplasms associated with the acquired immune deficiency syndrome (AIDS). In Knowles D, ed. *Neoplastic Hematopathology*. Baltimore: Williams & Wilkins, 1992:773–835.
80. Jaffe ES, Harris NL, Stein H, et al. World Health Organization Classification of Tumors. In Jaffe ES, Harris NL, Stein H, et al., eds. *Pathology and Genetics of Tumours of Haematopoietic and Lymphoid Tissues*. Lyon, France: IARC Press, 2001:75–117.
81. Bennett JM, Catovsky D, Daniel MT, et al. Proposals for the classification of the acute leukaemias. French-American-British (FAB) Co-operative Group. *Br J Haematol* 1976;33: 451–458.
82. Bennett JM, Catovsky D, Daniel MT, et al. The morphological classification of acute lymphoblastic leukaemia: concordance among observers and clinical correlations. *Br J Haematol* 1981;47:553–561.
83. Bennett JM, Catovsky D, Daniel MT, et al. Proposals for the classification of the myelodysplastic syndromes. *Br J Haematol* 1982;51:189–199.
84. Bennett JM, Catovsky D, Daniel MT, et al. Criteria for the diagnosis of acute leukemia of megakaryocyte lineage (M7). A report of the French-American-British Cooperative Group. *Ann Intern Med* 1985;103:460–462.
85. Bennett JM, Catovsky D, Daniel MT, et al. Proposed revised criteria for the classification of acute myeloid leukemia. A report of the French-American-British Cooperative Group. *Ann Intern Med* 1985;103:620–625.
86. Bennett JM, Catovsky D, Daniel MT, et al. Proposal for the recognition of minimally differentiated acute myeloid leukaemia (AML-MO). *Br J Haematol* 1991;78:325–329.
87. Behm FG. Morphologic and cytochemical characteristics of childhood lymphoblastic leukemia. *Hematol Oncol Clin North Am* 1990;4:715–741.
88. Brunning RD, McKenna RW. Acute lymphoblastic leukemias. In Brunning RD, McKenna RW, eds. *Tumors of the Bone Marrow. Atlas of Tumor Pathology*. Washington, DC: Armed Forces Institute of Pathology, 1994:100–142.
89. Gassmann W, Loffler H, Thiel E, et al. Morphological and cytochemical findings in 150 cases of T-lineage acute lymphoblastic leukaemia in adults. German Multicentre ALL Study Group (GMALL). *Br J Haematol* 1997;97:372–382.
90. Barnard DR, Kalousek DK, Wiersma SR, et al. Morphologic, immunologic, and cytogenetic classification of acute myeloid leukemia and myelodysplastic syndrome in childhood: a report from the Children's Cancer Group. *Leukemia* 1996;10:5–12.
91. Foucar K. Acute myeloid leukemia. In Foucar K, ed. *Bone Marrow Pathology*. Chicago: ASCP Press, 1995:189–224.
92. McKenna RW. Acute myeloid leukemia. In Kjeldsberg CK, ed. *Practical Diagnosis of Hematological Disorders*. Chicago: ASCP Press, 1995:381.
93. Foucar K. Acute myelogenous leukemia. In Foucar K, ed. *Bone Marrow Pathology*, 2nd edition Chicago: ASCP Press, 2001:262–312.
94. Traweek ST. Immunophenotypic analysis of acute leukemia. *Am J Clin Pathol* 1993;99: 504–512.
95. Borowitz MJ. Immunologic markers in childhood acute lymphoblastic leukemia. *Hematol Oncol Clin North Am* 1990;4:743–765.
96. Pui CH, Behm FG, Crist WM. Clinical and biologic relevance of immunologic marker studies in childhood acute lymphoblastic leukemia. *Blood* 1993;82:343–362.
97. Borowitz MJ, DiGiuseppe JA. *Acute Lymphoblastic Leukemia*. Philadelphia: Lippincott Williams & Wilkins, 2001.
98. Morphologic, immunologic and cytogenetic (MIC) working classification of the acute

myeloid leukaemias. Second MIC Cooperative Study Group. *Br J Haematol* 1988;68: 487–494.

99. Abshire TC, Buchanan GR, Jackson JF, et al. Morphologic, immunologic and cytogenetic studies in children with acute lymphoblastic leukemia at diagnosis and relapse: a Pediatric Oncology Group study. *Leukemia* 1992;6:357–362.
100. Pui CH, Crist WM, Look AT. Biology and clinical significance of cytogenetic abnormalities in childhood acute lymphoblastic leukemia. *Blood* 1990;76:1449–1463.
101. Schneider NR, Carroll AJ, Shuster JJ, et al. New recurring cytogenetic abnormalities and association of blast cell karyotypes with prognosis in childhood T-cell acute lymphoblastic leukemia: a pediatric oncology group report of 343 cases. *Blood* 2000;96:2543–2549.
102. Pui CH, Frankel LS, Carroll AJ, et al. Clinical characteristics and treatment outcome of childhood acute lymphoblastic leukemia with the t(4;11)(q21;q23): a collaborative study of 40 cases. *Blood* 1991;77:440–447.
103. Rubin CM, Le Beau MM, Mick R, et al. Impact of chromosomal translocations on prognosis in childhood acute lymphoblastic leukemia. *J Clin Oncol* 1991;9:2183–2192.
104. Rubnitz JE, Shuster JJ, Land VJ, et al. Case-control study suggests a favorable impact of TEL rearrangement in patients with B-lineage acute lymphoblastic leukemia treated with antimetabolite-based therapy: a Pediatric Oncology Group study. *Blood* 1997;89: 1143–1146.
105. Cline MJ. The molecular basis of leukemia. *N Engl J Med* 1994;330:328–336.
106. Russell NH. Biology of acute leukaemia. *Lancet* 1997;349:118–122.
107. Sawyers CL. Molecular genetics of acute leukaemia. *Lancet* 1997;349:196–200.
108. Head DR. Revised classification of acute myeloid leukemia. *Leukemia* 1996;10:1826–1831.
109. Swerdlow SH, Campo E, Harris NL, et al. *WHO Classification of Tumours of Haematopoietic and Lymphoid Tissues.* Lyon, France: IARC Press, 2008.
110. Estey E, Pierce S, Kantarjian H, et al. Treatment of myelodysplastic syndromes with AML-type chemotherapy. *Leuk Lymphoma* 1993;11[Suppl 2]:59–63.
111. Estey E, Thall P, Beran M, et al. Effect of diagnosis (refractory anemia with excess blasts, refractory anemia with excess blasts in transformation, or acute myeloid leukemia [AML]) on outcome of AML-type chemotherapy. *Blood* 1997;90:2969–2977.
112. Greenberg P, Cox C, LeBeau MM, et al. International scoring system for evaluating prognosis in myelodysplastic syndromes. *Blood* 1997;89:2079–2088.
113. Caligiuri MA, Strout MP, Gilliland DG. Molecular biology of acute myeloid leukemia. *Semin Oncol* 1997;24:32–44.
114. Hurwitz CA, Gore SD, Stone KD, et al. Flow cytometric detection of rare normal human marrow cells with immunophenotypes characteristic of acute lymphoblastic leukemia cells. *Leukemia* 1992;6:233–239.
115. Kita K, Nakase K, Miwa H, et al. Phenotypical characteristics of acute myelocytic leukemia associated with the t(8;21)(q22;q22) chromosomal abnormality: frequent expression of immature B-cell antigen CD19 together with stem cell antigen CD34. *Blood* 1992;80: 470–477.
116. Tiacci E, Pileri S, Orleth A, et al. PAX5 expression in acute leukemias: higher B-lineage specificity than CD79a and selective association with t(8;21)-acute myelogenous leukemia. *Cancer Res* 2004; 64:7399–7404.
117. Marlton P, Keating M, Kantarjian H, et al. Cytogenetic and clinical correlates in AML patients with abnormalities of chromosome 16. *Leukemia* 1995;9:965–971.
118. Le Beau MM, Larson RA, Bitter MA, et al. Association of an inversion of chromosome 16 with abnormal marrow eosinophils in acute myelomonocytic leukemia. A unique cytogenetic-clinicopathological association. *N Engl J Med* 1983;309:630–636.
119. Stanley M, McKenna RW, Ellinger G, et al. Classification of 358 cases of acute myeloid leukemia by FAB criteria: analysis of clinical and morphologic features. In Bloomfield CD, ed. *Chronic and Acute Leukemias in Adults.* Boston: Martinus Nijhoff, 1985:147–174.
120. Holmes R, Keating MJ, Cork A, et al. A unique pattern of central nervous system leukemia in acute myelomonocytic leukemia associated with inv(16)(p13q22). *Blood* 1985;65: 1071–1078.
121. Marcucci G, Mrozek K, Ruppert AS, et al. Prognostic factors and outcome of core binding factor acute myeloid leukemia patients with t(8;21) differ from those of patients with inv(16): a Cancer and Leukemia Group B study. *J Clin Oncol* 2005;23:5705–5717.
122. McKenna RW, Parkin J, Bloomfield CD, et al. Acute promyelocytic leukaemia: a study of 39 cases with identification of a hyperbasophilic microgranular variant. *Br J Haematol* 1982; 50:201–214.
123. Golomb HM, Rowley JD, Vardiman JW, et al. "Microgranular" acute promyelocytic leukemia: a distinct clinical, ultrastructural, and cytogenetic entity. *Blood* 1980;55:253–259.
124. Parkin JL, Brunning RD. Unusual configurations of endoplasmic reticulum in cells of acute promyelocytic leukemia. *J Natl Cancer Inst* 1978;61:341–348.
125. de Thé H, Chomienne C, Lanotte M, et al. The t(15;17) translocation of acute promyelocytic leukaemia fuses the retinoic acid receptor alpha gene to a novel transcribed locus. *Nature* 1990;347:558–561.
126. Melnick A, Licht JD. Deconstructing a disease: RAR-alpha, its fusion partners, and their roles in the pathogenesis of acute promyelocytic leukemia. *Blood* 1999;93:3167–3215.
127. Forestier E, Heim S, Blennow E, et al. Cytogenetic abnormalities in childhood acute myeloid leukaemia: a Nordic series comprising all children enrolled in the NOPHO-93-AML trial between 1993 and 2001. *Br J Haematol* 2003;121:566–577
128. Byrd JC, Mrozek K, Dodge RK, et al. Pretreatment cytogenetic abnormalities are predictive of induction success, cumulative incidence of relapse, and overall survival in adult patients with de novo acute myeloid leukemia: results from Cancer and Leukemia Group B (CALGB 8461). *Blood* 2002;100:4325–4336
129. Pui CH, Relling MV, Rivera GK, et al. Epipodophyllotoxin-related acute myeloid leukemia: a study of 35 cases. *Leukemia* 1995;9:1990–1996.
130. Rubnitz JE, Raimondi SC, Tong X, et al. Favorable impact of the t(9;11) in childhood acute myeloid leukemia. *J Clin Oncol* 2002;20:2302–2309.
131. Pearson MG, Vardiman JW, Le Beau MM, et al. Increased numbers of basophils may be associated with a t(6:9) in ANLL. *Am J Hematol* 1985;18:393–403.
132. Slovak ML, Gundacker H, Bloomfield CD, et al. A retrospective study of 69 patients with t(6;9)(p23;q34) AML emphasizes the need for a prospective, multicenter initiative for rare poor prognosis myeloid malignancies. *Leukemia* 2006;20:1295–1297.
133. Bitter MA, Neilly ME, Le Beau MM, et al. Rearrangements of chromosome 3 involving bands 3q21 and 3q26 are associated with normal or elevated platelet counts in acute non lymphocytic leukemia. *Blood* 1985;66:1362–1370.
134. Secker-Walker LM, Metha A, Bain B. Abnormalities of 3q21 and 3q26 in myeloid malignancy: a United Kingdom Cancer Cytogenetic Group Study. *Br. J Haematol* 1995;91: 490–501.
135. Bernstein J, Dastugue N, Haas OA, et al. Nineteen cases of the t(1;22)(q13;q13) acute megakaryoblastic leukaemia of infants/children and a review of 39 cases: report from a t(1;22) study group. *Leukaemia* 2000;14:216–218.
136. Duchayne E, Fenneteau O, Pages MP, et al. Acute megakaryoblastic leukaemia: a national clinical and biological study of 53 adult and childhood cases by the Groupe Francais d'Hematologie Cellulaire (GFHC). *Leuk Lymphoma* 2003;44:49–58.
137. Falini B, Mecucci C, Tiacci E, et al. Cytoplasmic nucleophosmin in acute myelogenous leukemia with a normal karyotype. *N Engl J Med* 2005;352:254–266.
138. Falini B, Nicoletti I, Martelli MF, et al. Acute myeloid leukemia carrying cytoplasmic/ mutated nucleophosmin (NPMc+ AML): biologic and clinical features. *Blood* 2007;109: 874–885.
139. Chou WC, Tang JL, Lin LI, et al. Nucleophosmin mutations in de novo acute myeloid leukemia: the age-dependent incidences and the stability during disease evolution. *Cancer Res* 2006;66:3310–3316.
140. Cazzaniga G, Dell'Oro MG, Mecucci C, et al. Nucleophosmin mutations in childhood acute myelogenous leukemia with normal karyotype. *Blood* 2005;106:1419–1422.
141. Bienz M, Ludwig M, Leibundgut EO, et al. Risk assessment in patients with acute myeloid leukemia and a normal karyotype. *Clin Cancer Res* 2005;11:1416–1424.
142. Frohling S, Schlenk RF, Stolze I, Bihlmayr J, et al. CEBPA mutations in younger adults with acute myeloid leukemia and normal cytogenetics: prognostic relevance and analysis of cooperating mutations. *J Clin Oncol* 2004;22:624–633.
143. Arber DA, Stein AS, Carter NH, et al. Prognostic impact of acute myeloid leukemia classification. Importance of detection of recurring cytogenetic abnormalities and multilineage dysplasia on survival. *Am J Clin Pathol* 2003;119:672–680.
144. Leith CP, Kopecky KJ, Godwin J, et al. Acute myeloid leukemia in the elderly: assessment of multidrug resistance (MDR1) and cytogenetics distinguishes biologic subgroups with remarkably distinct responses to standard chemotherapy. A Southwest Oncology Group study. *Blood* 1997;89:3323–3329.
145. Gahn B, Haase D, Unterhalt M, et al. De novo AML with dysplastic hematopoiesis: cytogenetic and prognostic significance. *Leukemia* 1996;10:946–951.
146. Ellis M, Ravid M, Lishner M. A comparative analysis of alkylating agent and epipodophyllotoxin-related leukemias. *Leuk Lymphoma* 1993;11:9–13.
147. Michels SD, McKenna RW, Arthur DC, et al. Therapy-related acute myeloid leukemia and myelodysplastic syndrome: a clinical and morphologic study of 65 cases. *Blood* 1985;65: 1364–1372.
148. Pedersen-Bjergaard J, Philip P, Larsen SO, et al. Therapy-related myelodysplasia and acute myeloid leukemia. Cytogenetic characteristics of 115 consecutive cases and risk in seven cohorts of patients treated intensively for malignant diseases in the Copenhagen series. *Leukemia* 1993;7:1975–1986.
149. Venditti A, Del Poeta G, Buccisano F, et al. Minimally differentiated acute myeloid leukemia (AML-M0): comparison of 25 cases with other French-American-British subtypes. *Blood* 1997;89:621–629.
150. Cuneo A, Ferrant A, Michaux JL, et al. Cytogenetic profile of minimally differentiated (FAB M0) acute myeloid leukemia: correlation with clinicobiologic findings. *Blood* 1995; 85:3688–3694.
151. Anastasi J, Kolitz J, Baer MR, et al. Two distinct subtypes of AML without differentiation (FAB-M1): analysis of 74 cases from CALGB studies 9621 & 9720. *Mod Pathol* 2000;13: 142a.
152. Haferlach T, Schoch C, Schnittger S, et al. Distinct genetic patterns can be identified in acute monoblastic and acute monocytic leukaemia (FAB AML M5a and M5b): a study of 124 patients. *Br J Haematol* 2002;118:426–431.
153. Garand R, Duchayne E, Blanchard D, et al. Minimally differentiated erythroleukaemia (AML M6 'variant'): a rare subset of AML distinct from AML M6. Groupe Francais d'Hematologie Cellulaire. *Br J Haematol* 1995;90:868–875.
154. Karandikar NJ, Aquino DB, McKenna RW, et al. Transient myeloproliferative disorder and acute myeloid leukemia in Down syndrome. An immunophenotypic analysis. *Am J Clin Pathol* 2001;116:204–210.
155. Bernstein J, Dastugue N, Haas OA, et al. Nineteen cases of the t(1;22)(p13;q13) acute megakaryoblastic leukaemia of infants/children and a review of 39 cases: report from a t(1;22) study group. *Leukemia* 2000;14:216–218.
156. Mundschau G, Gurbuxani S, Gamis AS, et al. Mutagenesis of GATA1 is an initiating event in Down syndrome leukemogenesis. *Blood* 2003;101:4298–4300.
157. Xu G, Nagano M, Kanezaki R, et al. Frequent mutations in the GATA-1 gene in the transient myeloproliferative disorder of Down's syndrome. *Blood* 2003;June 19 (Epub ahead of print).
158. Rainis L, Bercovich D, Strehl S, et al. Mutations in exon 2 of GATA1 are early events in megakaryocytic malignancies associated with trisomy 21. *Blood* 2003;102:981–986.
159. Peterson LC, Parkin JL, Arthur DC, et al. Acute basophilic leukemia. A clinical, morphologic, and cytogenetic study of eight cases. *Am J Clin Pathol* 1991;96:160–170.
160. Hurwitz CA, Mirro J, Jr. Mixed-lineage leukemia and asynchronous antigen expression. *Hematol Oncol Clin North Am* 1990;4:767–794.
161. Killick S, Matutes E, Powles RL, et al. Outcome of biphenotypic acute leukemia. *Haematologica* 1999;84:699–706.
162. Lin P, Jones D, Dorfman DM, et al. Precursor B-cell lymphoblastic lymphoma: a predominantly extranodal tumor with low propensity for leukemic involvement. *Am J Surg Pathol* 2000;24:1480–1490.
163. Maitra A, McKenna RW, Weinberg AG, et al. Precursor B-cell lymphoblastic lymphoma.

A study of nine cases lacking blood and bone marrow involvement and review of the literature. *Am J Clin Pathol* 2001;115:868–875.

164. Golembe B, Ramsay NK, McKenna R, et al. Localized bone marrow relapse in acute lymphoblastic leukemia. *Med Pediatr Oncol* 1979;6:229–234.
165. Neale GA, Coustan-Smith E, Pan Q, et al. Tandem application of flow cytometry and polymerase chain reaction for comprehensive detection of minimal residual disease in childhood acute lymphoblastic leukemia. *Leukemia* 1999;13:1221–1226.
166. Hutton JJ, Coleman MS, Moffitt S, et al. Prognostic significance of terminal transferase activity in childhood acute lymphoblastic leukemia: a prospective analysis of 164 patients. *Blood* 1982;60:1267–1276.
167. McKenna RW, Washington LT, Aquino DB, et al. Immunophenotypic analysis of hematogones (B-lymphocyte precursors) in 662 consecutive bone marrow specimens by 4-color flow cytometry. *Blood* 2001;98:2498–2507.
168. Ferrando AA, Look AT. Clinical implications of recurring chromosomal and associated molecular abnormalities in acute lymphoblastic leukemia. *Semin Hematol* 2000;37:381–395.
169. Williams DL, Raimondi S, Rivera G, et al. Presence of clonal chromosome abnormalities in virtually all cases of acute lymphoblastic leukemia. *N Engl J Med* 1985;313:640–641.
170. Gozzetti A, Le Beau MM. Fluorescence in situ hybridization: uses and limitations. *Semin Hematol* 2000;37:320–333.
171. Secker-Walker LM, Prentice HG, Durrant J, et al. Cytogenetics adds independent prognostic information in adults with acute lymphoblastic leukaemia on MRC trial UKALL XA. MRC Adult Leukaemia Working Party. *Br J Haematol* 1997;96:601–610.
172. Faderl S, Kantarjian HM, Talpaz M, et al. Clinical significance of cytogenetic abnormalities in adult acute lymphoblastic leukemia. *Blood* 1998;91:3995–4019.
173. Gordon MY. Biological consequences of the BCR/ABL fusion gene in humans and mice. *J Clin Pathol* 1999;52:719–722.
174. Secker-Walker LM, Craig JM, Hawkins JM, et al. Philadelphia positive acute lymphoblastic leukemia in adults: age distribution, BCR breakpoint and prognostic significance. *Leukemia* 1991;5:196–199.
175. Faderl S, Kantarjian HM, Thomas DA, et al. Outcome of Philadelphia chromosome-positive adult acute lymphoblastic leukemia. *Leuk Lymphoma* 2000;36:263–273.
176. Brunning RD, Parkin JL, McKenna RW. *Acute Lymphoblastic Leukemia.* Boston: Martinus Nijhoff, 1984.
177. Preti HA, O'Brien S, Giralt S, et al. Philadelphia-chromosome-positive adult acute lymphocytic leukemia: characteristics, treatment results, and prognosis in 41 patients. *Am J Med* 1994;97:60–65.
178. Crist W, Carroll A, Shuster J, et al. Philadelphia chromosome positive childhood acute lymphoblastic leukemia: clinical and cytogenetic characteristics and treatment outcome. A Pediatric Oncology Group study. *Blood* 1990;76:489–494.
179. Behm FG, Raimondi SC, Frestedt JL, et al. Rearrangement of the MLL gene confers a poor prognosis in childhood acute lymphoblastic leukemia, regardless of presenting age. *Blood* 1996;87:2870–2877.
180. Chen CS, Sorensen PH, Domer PH, et al. Molecular rearrangements on chromosome 11q23 predominate in infant acute lymphoblastic leukemia and are associated with specific biologic variables and poor outcome. *Blood* 1993;81:2386–2393.
181. Dimartino JF, Cleary ML. Mll rearrangements in haematological malignancies: lessons from clinical and biological studies. *Br J Haematol* 1999;106:614–626.
182. Borowitz MJ, Hunger SP, Carroll AJ, et al. Predictability of the t(1;19)(q23;p13) from surface antigen phenotype: implications for screening cases of childhood acute lymphoblastic leukemia for molecular analysis: a Pediatric Oncology Group study. *Blood* 1993;82: 1086–1091.
183. Crist WM, Carroll AJ, Shuster JJ, et al. Poor prognosis of children with pre-B acute lymphoblastic leukemia is associated with the t(1;19)(q23;p13): a Pediatric Oncology Group study. *Blood* 1990;76:117–122.
184. Maitra A, Schneider NR, Kroft SK, et al. t(1;19) Acute lymphoblastic leukemia (ALL) revisited. *Mod Pathol* 2001;14:171A.
185. Chessels JM, Swansbury GJ, Reeves BR. Cytogenetics and prognosis in childhood lymphoblastic leukaemia: results of MRC UKALL X. *Br J Haematol* 1997;99:93–100.
186. Rubnitz JE, Downing JR, Pui CH, et al. TEL gene rearrangement in acute lymphoblastic leukemia: a new genetic marker with prognostic significance. *J Clin Oncol* 1997;15: 1150–1157.
187. Shurtleff SA, Buijs A, Behm FG, et al. TEL/AML1 fusion resulting from a cryptic t(12; 21) is the most common genetic lesion in pediatric ALL and defines a subgroup of patients with an excellent prognosis. *Leukemia* 1995;9:1985–1989.
188. Trueworthy R, Shuster J, Look T, et al. Ploidy of lymphoblasts is the strongest predictor of treatment outcome in B-progenitor cell acute lymphoblastic leukemia of childhood: a Pediatric Oncology Group study. *J Clin Oncol* 1992;10:606–613.
189. Harris MB, Shuster JJ, Carroll A, et al. Trisomy of leukemic cell chromosomes 4 and 10 identifies children with B-progenitor cell acute lymphoblastic leukemia with a very low risk of treatment failure: a Pediatric Oncology Group study. *Blood* 1992;79:3316–3324.
190. Heerema NA, Nachman JB, Sather HN, et al. Hypodiploidy with less than 45 chromosomes confers adverse risk in childhood acute lymphoblastic leukemia: a report from the Children's Cancer Group. *Blood* 1999;94:4036–4045.
191. Pui CH, Behm FG, Singh B, et al. Heterogeneity of presenting features and their relation to treatment outcome in 120 children with T-cell acute lymphoblastic leukemia. *Blood* 1990;75:174–179.
192. McKenna RW, Parkin J, Brunning RD. Morphologic and ultrastructural characteristics of T-cell acute lymphoblastic leukemia. *Cancer* 1979;44:1290–1297.
193. Borowitz MJ, Dowell BL, Boyett JM, et al. Monoclonal antibody definition of T cell acute leukemia: a Pediatric Oncology Group study. *Blood* 1985;65:785–788.
194. Czuczman MS, Dodge RK, Stewart CC, et al. Value of immunophenotype in intensively treated adult acute lymphoblastic leukemia: cancer and leukemia Group B study 8364. *Blood* 1999;93:3931–3939.
195. Heerema NA, Sather HN, Sensel MG, et al. Frequency and clinical significance of cytogenetic abnormalities in pediatric T-lineage acute lymphoblastic leukemia: a report from the Children's Cancer Group. *J Clin Oncol* 1998;16:1270–1278.
196. Jaffe ES, Harris NL, Stein H, et al. World Health Organization Classification of Tumors. In Jaffe ES, Harris NL, Stein H, et al., eds. *Pathology and Genetics of Tumours of Haematopoietic and Lymphoid Tissues.* Lyon, France: IARC Press, 2001:47–73.
197. Vallespi T, Torrabadella M, Julia A, et al. Myelodysplastic syndromes: a study of 101 cases according to the FAB classification. *Br J Haematol* 1985;61:83–92.
198. Foucar K, Langdon RM 2nd, Armitage JO, et al. Myelodysplastic syndromes. A clinical and pathologic analysis of 109 cases. *Cancer* 1985;56:553–561.
199. Recommendations for a morphologic, immunologic, and cytogenetic (MIC) working classification of the primary and therapy-related myelodysplastic disorders. Report of the workshop held in Scottsdale, Arizona, USA, on February 23–25, 1987. Third MIC Cooperative Study Group. *Cancer Genet Cytogenet* 1988;32:1–10.
200. Brunning RD, McKenna RW. Myelodysplastic syndromes. In Brunning RD, McKenna RW, eds. *Tumors of the Bone Marrow. Atlas of Tumor Pathology.* Washington, DC: Armed Forces Institute of Pathology, 1994:143–194.
201. Kouides PA, Bennett JM. Morphology and classification of the myelodysplastic syndromes and their pathologic variants. *Semin Hematol* 1996;33:95–110.
202. Michels SD, Saumur J, Arthur DC, et al. Refractory anemia with excess of blasts in transformation hematologic and clinical study of 52 patients. *Cancer* 1989;64:2340–2346.
203. Nand S, Godwin JE. Hypoplastic myelodysplastic syndrome. *Cancer* 1988;62:958–964.
204. Rosati S, Anastasi J, Vardiman J. Recurring diagnostic problems in the pathology of the myelodysplastic syndromes. *Semin Hematol* 1996;33:111–126.
205. Farhi DC. Myelodysplastic syndromes and acute myeloid leukemia. Diagnostic criteria and pitfalls. *Pathol Annu* 1995;30(Pt 1):29–57.
206. Frisch B, Schlag R, Bartl R, et al. Histologic characteristics of myelodysplasia. *Verh Dtsch Ges Pathol* 1983;67:132–135.
207. Yoshida Y, Oguma S, Uchino H, et al. Refractory myelodysplastic anaemias with hypocellular bone marrow. *J Clin Pathol* 1988;41:763–767.
208. Tricot G, De Wolf-Peeters C, Vlietinck R, et al. Bone marrow histology in myelodysplastic syndromes. II. Prognostic value of abnormal localization of immature precursors in MDS. *Br J Haematol* 1984;58:217–225.
209. Delacretaz F, Schmidt PM, Piguet D, et al. Histopathology of myelodysplastic syndromes. The FAB classification (proposals) applied to bone marrow biopsy. *Am J Clin Pathol* 1987; 87:180–186.
210. Sultan C, Sigaux F, Imbert M, et al. Acute myelodysplasia with myelofibrosis: a report of eight cases. *Br J Haematol* 1981;49:11–16.
211. Lambertenghi-Deliliers G, Orazi A, Luksch R, et al. Myelodysplastic syndrome with increased marrow fibrosis: a distinct clinico-pathological entity. *Br J Haematol* 1991;78: 161–166.
212. Maschek H, Georgii A, Kaloutsi V, et al. Myelofibrosis in primary myelodysplastic syndromes: a retrospective study of 352 patients. *Eur J Haematol* 1992;48:208–214.
213. Fenaux P, Morel P, Lai JL. Cytogenetics of myelodysplastic syndromes. *Semin Hematol* 1996; 33:127–138.
214. Suciu S, Kuse R, Weh HJ, et al. Results of chromosome studies and their relation to morphology, course, and prognosis in 120 patients with de novo myelodysplastic syndrome. *Cancer Genet Cytogenet* 1990;44:15–26.
215. Mathew P, Tefferi A, Dewald GW, et al. The 5q- syndrome: a single-institution study of 43 consecutive patients. *Blood* 1993;81:1040–1045.
216. Bennett JM, Catovsky D, Daniel MT, et al. The chronic myeloid leukaemias: guidelines for distinguishing chronic granulocytic, atypical chronic myeloid, and chronic myelomonocytic leukaemia. Proposals by the French-American-British Cooperative Leukaemia Group. *Br J Haematol* 1994;87:746–754.
217. Arico M, Biondi A, Pui CH. Juvenile myelomonocytic leukemia. *Blood* 1997;90:479–488.
218a. Jaffe ES, Harris NL, Stein H, et al. World Health Organization Classification of Tumors. In Jaffe ES, Harris NL, Stein H, et al., eds. *Pathology and Genetics of Tumours of Haematopoietic and Lymphoid Tissues.* Lyon, France: IARC Press, 2001:17–45.
218b. Schooley RT, Flaum MA, Gralnick HR, et al. A clinicopathologic correlation of the idiopathic hypereosinophilic syndrome. II. Clinical manifestations. *Blood* 1981;58:1021–1026.
219. Tefferi A, Thiele J, Orazi A, et al. Proposals and rationale for revision of the World Health Organization diagnostic criteria for polycythemia vera, essential thrombocythemia, and primary myelofibrosis: recommendations from an ad hoc international expert panel. *Blood* 2007;110:1092–1097.
220. Cortes JE, Talpaz M, Kantarjian H. Chronic myelogenous leukemia: a review. *Am J Med* 1996;100:555–570.
221. Tefferi A, Litzow MR, Noel P, et al. Chronic granulocytic leukemia: recent information on pathogenesis, diagnosis, and disease monitoring. *Mayo Clin Proc* 1997;72:445–452.
222. Georgii A, Vykoupil KF, Buhr T, et al. Chronic myeloproliferative disorders in bone marrow biopsies. *Pathol Res Pract* 1990;186:3–27.
223. Dekmezian R, Kantarjian HM, Keating MJ, et al. The relevance of reticulin stain-measured fibrosis at diagnosis in chronic myelogenous leukemia. *Cancer* 1987;59:1739–1743.
224. Gordon MY, Goldman JM. Cellular and molecular mechanisms in chronic myeloid leukaemia: biology and treatment. *Br J Haematol* 1996;95:10–20.
225. Melo JV. The molecular biology of chronic myeloid leukaemia. *Leukemia* 1996;10:751–756.
226. Lee SJ. Chronic myelogenous leukaemia. *Br J Haematol* 2000;111:993–1009.
227. Muehleck SD, McKenna RW, Arthur DC, et al. Transformation of chronic myelogenous leukemia: clinical, morphologic, and cytogenetic features. *Am J Clin Pathol* 1984;82:1–14.
228. Kantarjian HM, Dixon D, Keating MJ, et al. Characteristics of accelerated disease in chronic myelogenous leukemia. *Cancer* 1988;61:1441–1446.
229. Derderian PM, Kantarjian HM, Talpaz M, et al. Chronic myelogenous leukemia in the lymphoid blastic phase: characteristics, treatment response, and prognosis. *Am J Med* 1993; 94:69–74.
230. Schmetzer HM, Gerhartz HH. Immunological classification of chronic myeloid leukemia

distinguishes chronic phase, imminent blastic transformation, and acute lymphoblastic leukemia. *Exp Hematol* 1997;25:502–508.

231. You W, Weisbrot IM. Chronic neutrophilic leukemia. Report of two cases and review of the literature. *Am J Clin Pathol* 1979;72:233–242.
232. Zittoun R, Rea D, Ngoc LH, et al. Chronic neutrophilic leukemia. A study of four cases. *Ann Hematol* 1994;68:55–60.
233. Hasle H, Olesen G, Kerndrup G, et al. Chronic neutrophilic leukaemia in adolescence and young adulthood. *Br J Haematol* 1996;94:628–630.
234. Pane F, Frigeri F, Sindona M, et al. Neutrophilic-chronic myeloid leukemia: a distinct disease with a specific molecular marker (BCR/ABL with C3/A2 junction). *Blood* 1996; 88:2410–2414.
235. Cehreli C, Undar B, Akkoc N, et al. Coexistence of chronic neutrophilic leukemia with light chain myeloma. *Acta Haematol* 1994;91:32–34.
236. Standen GR, Jasani B, Wagstaff M, et al. Chronic neutrophilic leukemia and multiple myeloma. An association with lambda light chain expression. *Cancer* 1990;66:162–166.
237a. Bain BJ. Eosinophilic leukaemias and the idiopathic hypereosinophilic syndrome. *Br J Haematol* 1996;95:2–9.218a.
237b. Weller PF, Bubley GJ. The idiopathic hypereosinophilic syndrome. *Blood* 1994;83: 2759–2779.
238. Spivak JL. Polycythemia vera: myths, mechanisms, and management. *Blood* 2002;100: 4272–4290.
239. Anger B, Haug U, Seidler R, et al. Polycythemia vera. A clinical study of 141 patients. *Blut* 1989;59:493–500.
240. Green AR. Pathogenesis of polycythaemia vera. *Lancet* 1996;347:844–845.
241. Murphy S. Polycythemia vera. *Dis Mon* 1992;38:153–212.
242. Thiele J, Kvasnicka HM, Orazi A. Bone marrow histopathology in myeloproliferative disorders—current diagnostic approach. *Semin Hematol* 2005;42:184–195.
243. Wasserman LR. The treatment of polycythemia vera. *Semin Hematol* 1976;13:57–78.
244. Vykoupil KF, Thiele J, Stangel W, et al. Polycythemia vera. I. Histopathology, ultrastructure and cytogenetics of the bone marrow in comparison with secondary polycythemia. *Virchows Arch [A] Pathol Anat Histol* 1980;389:307–324.
245. Lucie NP, Young GA. Marrow cellularity in the diagnosis of polycythaemia. *J Clin Pathol* 1983;36:180–183.
246. Thiele J, Holgado S, Choritz H, et al. Density distribution and size of megakaryocytes in inflammatory reactions of the bone marrow (myelitis) and chronic myeloproliferative diseases. *Scand J Haematol* 1983;31:329–341.
247. Ellis JT, Peterson P, Geller SA, et al. Studies of the bone marrow in polycythemia vera and the evolution of myelofibrosis and second hematologic malignancies. *Semin Hematol* 1986;23:144–155.
248. Landaw SA. Acute leukemia in polycythemia vera. *Semin Hematol* 1986;23:156–165.
249. Nimer SD. Essential thrombocythemia: another "heterogeneous disease" better understood? *Blood* 1999;93:415–416.
250. Hehlmann R, Jahn M, Baumann B, et al. Essential thrombocythemia. Clinical characteristics and course of 61 cases. *Cancer* 1988;61:2487–2496.
251. Mitus AJ, Schafer AI. Thrombocytosis and thrombocythemia. *Hematol Oncol Clin North Am* 1990;4:157–178.
252. Murphy S, Peterson P, Iland H, et al. Experience of the Polycythemia Vera Study Group with essential thrombocythemia: a final report on diagnostic criteria, survival, and leukemic transition by treatment. *Semin Hematol* 1997;34:29–39.
253. Thiele J, Moedder B, Kremer B, et al. Chronic myeloproliferative diseases with an elevated platelet count (in excess of 1,000,000/microliter): a clinicopathological study on 46 patients with special emphasis on primary (essential) thrombocythemia. *Hematol Pathol* 1987; 1:227–237.
254. Fialkow PJ, Faguet GB, Jacobson RJ, et al. Evidence that essential thrombocythemia is a clonal disorder with origin in a multipotent stem cell. *Blood* 1981;58:916–919.
255. Adams JA, Barrett AJ, Beard J, et al. Primary polycythaemia, essential thrombocythaemia and myelofibrosis—three facets of a single disease process? *Acta Haematol* 1988;79:33–37.
256. Reilly JT. Pathogenesis of idiopathic myelofibrosis: present status and future directions. *Br J Haematol* 1994;88:1–8.
257. Varki A, Lottenberg R, Griffith R, et al. The syndrome of idiopathic myelofibrosis. A clinicopathologic review with emphasis on the prognostic variables predicting survival. *Medicine (Baltimore)* 1983;62:353–371.
258. Visani G, Finelli C, Castelli U, et al. Myelofibrosis with myeloid metaplasia: clinical and haematological parameters predicting survival in a series of 133 patients. *Br J Haematol* 1990;75:4–9.
259. Weinstein IM. Idiopathic myelofibrosis: historical review, diagnosis and management. *Blood Rev* 1991;5:98–104.
260. Ward HP, Block MH. The natural history of agnogenic myeloid metaplasia (AMM) and a critical evaluation of its relationship with the myeloproliferative syndrome. *Medicine (Baltimore)* 1971;50:357–420.
261. Cervantes F, Pereira A, Esteve J, et al. Identification of 'short-lived' and 'long-lived' patients at presentation of idiopathic myelofibrosis. *Br J Haematol* 1997;97:635–640.
262. Ozen S, Ferhanoglu B, Senocak M, et al. Idiopathic myelofibrosis (agnogenic myeloid metaplasia): clinicopathological analysis of 32 patients. *Leuk Res* 1997;21:125–131.
263. Pereira A, Cervantes F, Brugues R, et al. Bone marrow histopathology in primary myelofibrosis: clinical and haematologic correlations and prognostic evaluation. *Eur J Haematol* 1990;44:95–99.
264. Sekhar M, Prentice HG, Popat U, et al. Idiopathic myelofibrosis in children. *Br J Haematol* 1996;93:394–397.
265. Moore MAS. Pathogenesis in myelofibrosis. In Hoffman AV, ed. *Recent Advances in Haematology*. Edinburgh, UK: Churchill Livingstone, 1982:136–139.
266. Castro-Malaspina H, Moore MA. Pathophysiological mechanisms operating in the development of myelofibrosis: role of megakaryocytes. *Nouv Rev Fr Hematol* 1982;24:221–226.
267. Lubin J, Rozen S, Rywlin M. Malignant myelosclerosis. *Arch Intern Med* 1976;136:141–145.
268. Frisch B, Lewis SM, Burkhardt R, et al. *Biopsy Pathology of Bone and Bone Marrow*. New York: Raven Press, 1985:108–145.
269. Valent P, Horny HP, Escribano L, et al. Diagnostic criteria and classification of mastocytosis: a consensus proposal. *Leuk Res* 2001;25:603–625.
270. Valent P, Horny HP, Li CY, et al. Mastocytosis. In Jaffe ES, Harris NL, Stein H, et al., eds. *World Health Organization Classification of Tumors. Pathology and Genetics of Tumours of Haematopoietic and Lymphoid Tissues*. Lyon, France: IARC Press, 2001:291–302.
271. Lennert K, Parwaresch MR. Mast cells and mast cell neoplasia: a review. *Histopathology* 1979;3:349–365.
272. Hutchinson RM. Mastocytosis and co-existent non-Hodgkin's lymphoma and myeloproliferative disorders. *Leuk Lymphoma* 1992;7:29–36.
273. Brunning RD, McKenna RW, Rosai J, et al. Systemic mastocytosis. Extracutaneous manifestations. *Am J Surg Pathol* 1983;7:425–438.
274. Webb TA, Li CY, Yam LT. Systemic mast cell disease: a clinical and hematopathologic study of 26 cases. *Cancer* 1982;49:927–938.
275. Travis WD, Li CY, Bergstralh EJ, et al. Systemic mast cell disease. Analysis of 58 cases and literature review. *Medicine (Baltimore)* 1988;67:345–368.
276. Brunning RD, McKenna RW. Mast cell disease. In Brunning RD, McKenna RW, eds. *Tumors of the Bone Marrow. Atlas of Tumor Pathology*. Washington, DC: Armed Forces Institute of Pathology, 1994:419–437.
277. Parker RI. Hematologic aspects of mastocytosis. I: Bone marrow pathology in adult and pediatric systemic mast cell disease. *J Invest Dermatol* 1991;96:47S–51S.
278. Horny HP, Parwaresch MR, Lennert K. Bone marrow findings in systemic mastocytosis. *Hum Pathol* 1985;16:808–814.
279. Udoji WC, Razavi SA. Mast cells and myelofibrosis. *Am J Clin Pathol* 1975;63:203–209.
280. Horny HP, Ruck M, Wehrmann M, et al. Blood findings in generalized mastocytosis: evidence of frequent simultaneous occurrence of myeloproliferative disorders. *Br J Haematol* 1990;76:186–193.
281. Travis WD, Li CY, Yam LT, et al. Significance of systemic mast cell disease with associated hematologic disorders. *Cancer* 1988;62:965–972.
282. Travis WD, Li CY, Hoagland HC, et al. Mast cell leukemia: report of a case and review of the literature. *Mayo Clin Proc* 1986;61:957–966.
283. Li WV, Kapadia SB, Sonmez-Alpan E, et al. IHC characterization of mast cell disease in paraffin sections using tryptase, CD68, myeloperoxidase, lysozyme, and CD20 antibodies. *Mod Pathol* 1996;9:982–988.
284. Horny HP, Reimann O, Kaiserling E. Immunoreactivity of normal and neoplastic human tissue mast cells. *Am J Clin Pathol* 1988;89:335–340.
285. Valent P. 1995 Mack-Forster Award Lecture [Review]. Mast cell differentiation antigens: expression in normal and malignant cells and use for diagnostic purposes. *Eur J Clin Invest* 1995;25:715–720.
286. Jordan JH, Walchshofer S, Jurecka W, et al. IHC properties of bone marrow mast cells in systemic mastocytosis: evidence for expression of CD2, CD117/Kit, and bcl-x(L). *Hum Pathol* 2001;32:545–552.
287. Orfao A, Escribano L, Villarrubia J, et al. Flow cytometric analysis of mast cells from normal and pathological human bone marrow samples: identification and enumeration. *Am J Pathol* 1996;149:1493–1499.
288. Escribano L, Orfao A, Villarrubia J, et al. Immunophenotypic characterization of human bone marrow mast cells. A flow cytometric study of normal and pathological bone marrow samples. *Anal Cell Pathol* 1998;16:151–9
289. Escribano L, Orfao A, Diaz-Agustin B, et al. Indolent systemic mast cell disease in adults: immunophenotypic characterization of bone marrow mast cells and its diagnostic implications. *Blood* 1998;91:2731–2736.
290. Horny HP, Valent P. Histopathological and IHC aspects of mastocytosis. *Int Arch Allergy Immunol* 2002;127:115–117
291. Nagata H, Worobec AS, Oh CK, et al. Identification of a point mutation in the catalytic domain of the protooncogene c-kit in peripheral blood mononuclear cells of patients who have mastocytosis with an associated hematologic disorder. *Proc Natl Acad Sci USA* 1995;92:10560–10564.
292. Brunning RD, McKenna RW. Bone marrow manifestations of malignant lymphoma and lymphoma-like conditions. *Pathol Annu* 1979;14 Pt 1:1–59.
293. Dick F, Bloomfield CD, Brunning RD. Incidence cytology, and histopathology of non-Hodgkin's lymphomas in the bone marrow. *Cancer* 1974;33:1382–1398.
294. Stein RS, Ultmann JE, Byrne GE, Jr., et al. Bone marrow involvement in non-Hodgkin's lymphoma: implications for staging and therapy. *Cancer* 1976;37:629–636.
295. Foucar K, McKenna RW, Frizzera G, et al. Bone marrow and blood involvement by lymphoma in relationship to the Lukes—Collins classification. *Cancer* 1982;49:888–897.
296. Bartl R, Hansmann ML, Frisch B, et al. Comparative histology of malignant lymphomas in lymph node and bone marrow. *Br J Haematol* 1988;69:229–237.
297. Lai HS, Tien HF, Hsieh HC, et al. Bone marrow involvement in non-Hodgkin's lymphoma. *Taiwan Yi Xue Hui Za Zhi* 1989;88:114–121.
298. Conlan MG, Bast M, Armitage JO, et al. Bone marrow involvement by non-Hodgkin's lymphoma: the clinical significance of morphologic discordance between the lymph node and bone marrow. Nebraska Lymphoma Study Group. *J Clin Oncol* 1990;8:1163–1172.
299. Cousar JB, Glick AD, York JC, et al. Peripheral blood and bone marrow involvement by non-Hodgkin's lymphoma: morphological, immunological and cytochemical features. *Prog Clin Pathol* 1984;9:173–196.
300. Navone R, Pich A, Fiammotto M, et al. Bone marrow histopathology and prognosis in malignant lymphomas. *Tumori* 1992;78:176–180.
301. Wong KF, Chan JK, Ng CS, et al. Large cell lymphoma with initial presentation in the bone marrow. *Hematol Oncol* 1992;10:261–271.
302. Lambertenghi-Deliliers G, Annaloro C, Soligo D, et al. Incidence and histological features of bone marrow involvement in malignant lymphomas. *Ann Hematol* 1992;65:61–65.
303. Lee WI, Lee JH, Kim IS, et al. Bone marrow involvement by non-Hodgkin's lymphoma. *J Korean Med Sci* 1994;9:402–408.

304. Ponzoni M, Li CY. Isolated bone marrow non-Hodgkin's lymphoma: a clinicopathologic study. *Mayo Clin Proc* 1994;69:37–43.

305. Heinz R, Hopfinger G, Tuchler H. Outcome of patients with low-grade B cell non-Hodgkin lymphoma and initial bone marrow involvement: data of a single institution. *Leukemia* 1997;11[Suppl 2]:S52–S54.

306. Naughton MJ, Hess JL, Zutter MM, et al. Bone marrow staging in patients with non-Hodgkin's lymphoma: is flow cytometry a useful test? *Cancer* 1998;82:1154–1159.

307. Yan Y, Chan WC, Weisenburger DD, et al. Clinical and prognostic significance of bone marrow involvement in patients with diffuse aggressive B-cell lymphoma. *J Clin Oncol* 1995; 13:1336–1342.

308. Heinz R, Hopfinger G, Tuchler H. Outcome of patients with low-grade B cell non-Hodgkin lymphoma and initial bone marrow involvement: data of a single institution. *Leukemia* 1997;11:S52–S54.

309. Pittaluga S, Tierens A, Dodoo YL, et al. How reliable is histologic examination of bone marrow trephine biopsy specimens for the staging of non-Hodgkin lymphoma? A study of hairy cell leukemia and mantle cell lymphoma involvement of the bone marrow trephine specimen by histologic, IHC, and polymerase chain reaction techniques. *Am J Clin Pathol* 1999;111:179–184.

310. Pezzella F, Munson PJ, Miller KD, Goldstone AH, Gatter KC. The diagnosis of low-grade peripheral B-cell neoplasms in bone marrow trephines. *Br J Haematol* 2000;108:369–376.

311. Buhr T, Langer F, Schlue J, et al. Reliability of lymphoma classification in bone marrow trephines. *Br J Haematol* 2002;118:470–476.

312. Arber DA, George TI. Bone marrow biopsy involvement by non-Hodgkin's lymphoma: frequency of lymphoma types, patterns, blood involvement, and discordance with other sites in 450 specimens. *Am J Surg Pathol* 2005;29:1549–1557.

313. Chung R, Lai R, Wei P, et al. Concordant but not discordant bone marrow involvement in diffuse large B-cell lymphoma predicts a poor clinical outcome independent of the International Prognostic Index. *Blood* 2007;110:1278–1282.

314. Luoni M, Declich P, De Paoli AP, et al. Bone marrow biopsy for the staging of non-Hodgkin's lymphoma: bilateral or unilateral trephine biopsy? *Tumori* 1995;81:410–413.

315. McKenna RW, Bloomfield CD, Brunning RD. Nodular lymphoma: bone marrow and blood manifestations. *Cancer* 1975;36:428–440.

316. Rappaport H. Tumors of the hematopoietic system. In Brunning RD, McKenna RW, eds. *Atlas of Tumor Pathology.* Section III. Fascicle 8. Washington, DC: Armed Forces Institute of Pathology, 1966.

317. Lukes RJ, Collins RD. A functional classification of malignant lymphomas. In Rebuck JW, Berard CW, Abel MR, eds. *The Reticuloendothelial System.* Baltimore: Williams & Wilkins, 1975:213–242.

318. National Cancer Institute sponsored study of classifications of non-Hodgkin's lymphomas: summary and description of a working formulation for clinical usage. The Non-Hodgkin's Lymphoma Pathologic Classification Project. *Cancer* 1982;49:2112–2135.

319. McKenna RW, Hernandez JA. Bone marrow in malignant lymphoma. *Hematol Oncol Clin North Am* 1988;2:617–635.

320. Brunning RD, McKenna RW. Bone marrow lymphoma. In Brunning RD, McKenna RW, eds. *Tumors of the Bone Marrow. Atlas of Tumor Pathology.* Washington, DC: Armed Forces Institute of Pathology, 1994:369–408.

321. Harris NL, Jaffe ES, Stein H, et al. A revised European-American classification of lymphoid neoplasms: a proposal from the International Lymphoma Study Group. *Blood* 1994;84: 1361–1392.

322. Gaulard P, Kanavaros P, Farcet JP, et al. Bone marrow histologic and IHC findings in peripheral. T-cell lymphoma: a study of 38 cases. *Hum Pathol* 1991;22:331–338.

323. Thieblemont C, Berger F, Dumontet C, et al. Mucosa-associated lymphoid tissue lymphoma is a disseminated disease in one third of 158 patients analyzed. *Blood* 2000;95: 802–806.

324. Desablens B, Claisse JF, Piprot-Choffat C, et al. Prognostic value of bone marrow biopsy in chronic lymphoid leukemia. A study of 98 initial bone marrow biopsies. *Nouv Rev Fr Hematol* 1989;31:179–182.

325. Henrique R, Achten R, Maes B, et al. Guidelines for subtyping small B-cell lymphomas in bone marrow biopsies. *Virchows Arch* 1999;435:549–558.

326. Franco V, Florena AM, Campesi G. Intrasinusoidal bone marrow infiltration: a possible hallmark of splenic lymphoma. *Histopathology* 1996;29:571–575.

327. Costes V, Duchayne E, Taib J, et al. Intrasinusoidal bone marrow infiltration: a common growth pattern for different lymphoma subtypes. *Br J Haematol* 2002;119:916–922.

328. Vega F, Medeiros LJ, Bueso-Ramos C, et al. Hepatosplenic gamma/delta T-cell lymphoma in bone marrow. A sinusoidal neoplasm with blastic cytologic features. *Am J Clin Pathol* 2001;116:410–419.

329. Morice WG, Kurtin PJ, Tefferi A, et al. Distinct bone marrow findings in T-cell granular lymphocytic leukemia revealed by paraffin section immunoperoxidase stains for CD8, TIA-1, and granzyme B. *Blood* 2002;99:268–274.

330. Estalilla OC, Koo CH, Brynes RK, et al. Intravascular large B-cell lymphoma. A report of five cases initially diagnosed by bone marrow biopsy. *Am J Clin Pathol* 1999;112:248–255.

331. Fisher DE, Jacobson JO, Ault KA, et al. Diffuse large cell lymphoma with discordant bone marrow histology. Clinical features and biological implications. *Cancer* 1989;64: 1879–1887.

332. Kluin PM, van Krieken JH, Kleiverda K, et al. Discordant morphologic characteristics of B-cell lymphomas in bone marrow and lymph node biopsies. *Am J Clin Pathol* 1990;94: 59–66.

333. Hodges GF, Lenhardt TM, Cotelingam JD. Bone marrow involvement in large-cell lymphoma. Prognostic implications of discordant disease. *Am J Clin Pathol* 1994;101:305–311.

334. Crisan D, Mattson JC. Discordant morphologic features in bone marrow involvement by malignant lymphomas: use of gene rearrangement patterns for diagnosis. *Am J Hematol* 1995;49:299–309.

335. Kremer M, Spitzer M, Mandl-Weber S, et al. Discordant bone marrow involvement in diffuse large B-cell lymphoma: comparative molecular analysis reveals a heterogeneous group of disorders. *Lab Invest* 2003;83:107–114.

336. Wright B, Asplund S, McKenna R, et al. Large B-cell lymphoma with discordant marrow involvement: an immunophenotypic analysis of 11 cases [Abstract]. *Mod Pathol* 2002;15: 270A.

337. Hoyer JD, Ross CW, Li CY, et al. True T-cell chronic lymphocytic leukemia: a morphologic and immunophenotypic study of 25 cases. *Blood* 1995;86:1163–1169.

338. Nelson BP, Variakojis D, Peterson LC. Leukemic phase of B-cell lymphomas mimicking chronic lymphocytic leukemia and variants at presentation. *Mod Pathol* 2002;15: 1111–1120.

339. Bennett JM, Catovsky D, Daniel MT, et al. Proposals for the classification of chronic (mature) B and T lymphoid leukaemias. French-American-British (FAB) Cooperative Group. *J Clin Pathol* 1989;42:567–584.

340. Dighiero G, Travade P, Chevret S, et al. B-cell chronic lymphocytic leukemia: present status and future directions. French Cooperative Group on CLL. *Blood* 1991;78:1901–1914.

341. Matutes E, Morilla R, Owusu-Ankomah K, et al. The immunophenotype of splenic lymphoma with villous lymphocytes and its relevance to the differential diagnosis with other B-cell disorders. *Blood* 1994;83:1558–1562.

342. Frater JL, McCarron KF, Hammel JP, et al. Typical and atypical chronic lymphocytic leukemia differ clinically and immunophenotypically. *Am J Clin Pathol* 2001;116:655–664.

343. Pangalis GA, Roussou PA, Kittas C, et al. Patterns of bone marrow involvement in chronic lymphocytic leukemia and small lymphocytic (well differentiated) non-Hodgkin's lymphoma. Its clinical significance in relation to their differential diagnosis and prognosis. *Cancer* 1984;54:702–708.

344. Brunning RD, McKenna RW. Small lymphocytic leukemias and related disorders. In Brunning RD, McKenna RW, eds. *Tumors of the Bone Marrow. Atlas of Tumor Pathology.* Washington, DC: Armed Forces Institute of Pathology, 1994:255–322.

345. Bonato M, Pittaluga S, Tierens A, et al. Lymph node histology in typical and atypical chronic lymphocytic leukemia. *Am J Surg Pathol* 1998;22:49–56.

346. Rai KR, Sawitsky A, Cronkite EP, et al. Clinical staging of chronic lymphocytic leukemia. *Blood* 1975;46:219–234.

347. Chronic lymphocytic leukaemia: proposals for a revised prognostic staging system. Report from the International Workshop on CLL. *Br J Haematol* 1981;48:365–367.

348. Freedman AS. Immunobiology of chronic lymphocytic leukemia. *Hematol Oncol Clin North Am* 1990;4:405–429.

349. Geisler CH, Larsen JK, Hansen NE, et al. Prognostic importance of flow cytometric immunophenotyping of 540 consecutive patients with B-cell chronic lymphocytic leukemia. *Blood* 1991;78:1795–1802.

350. Kroft SH, Finn WG, Peterson LC. The pathology of the chronic lymphoid leukaemias. *Blood Rev* 1995;9:234–250.

351. Finn WG, Thangavelu M, Yelavarthi KK, et al. Karyotype correlates with peripheral blood morphology and immunophenotype in chronic lymphocytic leukemia. *Am J Clin Pathol* 1996;105:458–467.

352. Moreau EJ, Matutes E, A'Hern RP, et al. Improvement of the chronic lymphocytic leukemia scoring system with the monoclonal antibody SN8 (CD79b). *Am J Clin Pathol* 1997; 108:378–382.

353. Richter MN. Generalized reticular cell sarcoma of lymph nodes associated with lymphatic leukemia. *Am J Pathol* 1928;4:285–292.

354. Enno A, Catovsky D, O'Brien M, et al. 'Prolymphocytoid' transformation of chronic lymphocytic leukaemia. *Br J Haematol* 1979;41:9–18.

355. Foucar K, Rydell RE. Richter's syndrome in chronic lymphocytic leukemia. *Cancer* 1980; 46:118–134.

356. Kjeldsberg CR, Marty J. Prolymphocytic transformation of chronic lymphocytic leukemia. *Cancer* 1981;48:2447–2457.

357. Melo JV, Catovsky D, Galton DA. The relationship between chronic lymphocytic leukaemia and prolymphocytic leukaemia. II. Patterns of evolution of 'prolymphocytoid' transformation. *Br J Haematol* 1986;64:77–86.

358. Trump DL, Mann RB, Phelps R, et al. Richter's syndrome: diffuse histiocytic lymphoma in patients with chronic lymphocytic leukemia. A report of five cases and review of the literature. *Am J Med* 1980;68:539–548.

359. Brecher M, Banks PM. Hodgkin's disease variant of Richter's syndrome. Report of eight cases. *Am J Clin Pathol* 1990;93:333–339.

360. Matolcsy A, Inghirami G, Knowles DM. Molecular genetic demonstration of the diverse evolution of Richter's syndrome (chronic lymphocytic leukemia and subsequent large cell lymphoma). *Blood* 1994;83:1363–1372.

361. Robertson LE, Pugh W, O'Brien S, et al. Richter's syndrome: a report on 39 patients. *J Clin Oncol* 1993;11:1985–1989.

362. McDonnell JM, Beschorner WE, Staal SP, et al. Richter's syndrome with two different B-cell clones. *Cancer* 1986;58:2031–2037.

363. Lane PK, Townsend RM, Beckstead JH, et al. Central nervous system involvement in a patient with chronic lymphocytic leukemia and non-Hodgkin's lymphoma (Richter's syndrome), with concordant cell surface immunoglobulin isotypic and immunophenotypic markers. *Am J Clin Pathol* 1988;89:254–259.

364. Kroft SH, Dawson DB, McKenna RW. Large cell lymphoma transformation of chronic lymphocytic leukemia/small lymphocytic lymphoma. A flow cytometric analysis of seven cases. *Am J Clin Pathol* 2001;115:385–395.

365. Foon KA, Gale RP. Clinical transformation of chronic lymphocytic leukemia. *Nouv Rev Fr Hematol* 1988;30:385–388.

366. Galton DA, Goldman JM, Wiltshaw E, et al. Prolymphocytic leukaemia. *Br J Haematol* 1974; 27:7–23.

367. Stone RM. Prolymphocytic leukemia. *Hematol Oncol Clin North Am* 1990;4:457–471.

368. Matutes E, Brito-Babapulle V, Swansbury J, et al. Clinical and laboratory features of 78 cases of T-prolymphocytic leukemia. *Blood* 1991;78:3269–3274.

369. Melo JV, Catovsky D, Gregory WM, et al. The relationship between chronic lymphocytic leukaemia and prolymphocytic leukaemia. IV. Analysis of survival and prognostic features. *Br J Haematol* 1987;65:23–29.

370. Catovsky D, Montserrat E, Muller-hermelink HK, Harris NL. B-cell prolymphocytic leukae-

mia. In Jaffe ES, Harris NL, Stein H, et al., eds. *World Health Organization Classification of Tumours Pathology and Genetics of Tumours of Haematopoietic and Lymphoid Tissues.* Lyon, France: IARC Press, 2001:131–132.

371. Schlette E, Bueso-Ramos C, Giles F, Glassman A, Hayes K, Medeiros LJ. Mature B-cell leukemias with more than 55% prolymphocytes. A heterogeneous group that includes an unusual variant of mantle cell lymphoma. *Am J Clin Pathol.* 2001;115:571–581.

372. Ruchlemer R, Parry-Jones N, Brito-Babapulle V, et al. B-prolymphocytic leukaemia with t(11;14) revisited: a splenomegalic form of mantle cell lymphoma evolving with leukaemia. *Br J Haematol* 2004;125:330–336.

373. Andriko JA, Aguilera NS, Chu WS, et al. Waldenstrom's macroglobulinemia: a clinicopathologic study of 22 cases. *Cancer* 1997;80:1926–1935.

374. Owen RG, Barrans SL, Richards SJ, et al. Waldenstrom macroglobulinemia. Development of diagnostic criteria and identification of prognostic factors. *Am J Clin Pathol* 2001;116:420–428.

375. Mansoor A, Medeiros LJ, Weber DM, et al. Cytogenetic findings in lymphoplasmacytic lymphoma/Waldenstrom macroglobulinemia. Chromosomal abnormalities are associated with the polymorphous subtype and an aggressive clinical course. *Am J Clin Pathol* 2001;116:543–549.

376. Pangalis GA, Nathwani BN, Rappaport H. Malignant lymphoma, well differentiated lymphocytic: its relationship with chronic lymphocytic leukemia and macroglobulinemia of Waldenstrom. *Cancer* 1977;39:999–1010.

377. Owen RG, Barrans SL, Richards SJ, et al. Waldenstrom macroglobulinemia. Development of diagnostic criteria and identification of prognostic factors. *Am J Clin Pathol* 2001;116:420–428.

378. Hammer RD, Glick AD, Greer JP, et al. Splenic marginal zone lymphoma. A distinct B-cell neoplasm. *Am J Surg Pathol* 1996;20:613–626.

379. Kent SA, Variakojis D, Peterson LC. Comparative study of marginal zone lymphoma involving bone marrow. *Am J Clin Pathol* 2002;117:698–708.

380. Audouin J, Le Tourneau A, Molina T, et al. Patterns of bone marrow involvement in 58 patients presenting primary splenic marginal zone lymphoma with or without circulating villous lymphocytes. *Br J Haematol* 2003;122:404–412.

381. Chacon JI, Mollejo M, Munoz E, et al. Splenic marginal zone lymphoma: clinical characteristics and prognostic factors in a series of 60 patients. *Blood* 2002;100:1648–1654.

382. Franco V, Florena AM, Stella M, et al. Splenectomy influences bone marrow infiltration in patients with splenic marginal zone cell lymphoma with or without villous lymphocytes. *Cancer* 2001;91:294–301.

383. Isaacson PG, Matutes E, Burke M, et al. The histopathology of splenic lymphoma with villous lymphocytes. *Blood* 1994;84:3828–3834.

384. Burke JS. The value of the bone-marrow biopsy in the diagnosis of hairy cell leukemia. *Am J Clin Pathol* 1978;70:876–884.

385. Paoletti M, Bitter MA, Vardiman JW. Hairy-cell leukemia. Morphologic, cytochemical, and immunologic features. *Clin Lab Med* 1988;8:179–195.

386. Naeim F, Smith GS. Leukemic reticuloendotheliosis. *Cancer* 1974;34:1813–1821.

387. Katayama I, Aiba M. Tartrate-resistant acid phosphatase reaction. *Am J Clin Pathol* 1980;73:143.

388. The Non-Hodgkin's Lymphoma Classification Project. A clinical evaluation of the International Lymphoma Study Group classification of non-Hodgkin's lymphoma. *Blood* 1997;89:3909–3918.

389. Zucca E, Conconi A, Pedrinis E, et al. Nongastric marginal zone B-cell lymphoma of mucosa-associated lymphoid tissue. *Blood* 2003;101:2489–2495.

390. Nathwani BN, Anderson JR, Armitage JO, et al. Marginal zone B-cell lymphoma: a clinical comparison of nodal and mucosa-associated lymphoid tissue types. Non-Hodgkin's Lymphoma Classification Project. *J Clin Oncol* 1999;17:2486–2492.

391. Camacho FI, Algara P, Mollejo M, et al. Nodal marginal zone lymphoma: a heterogeneous tumor: a comprehensive analysis of a series of 27 cases. *Am J Surg Pathol* 2003;27:762–771.

392. Arcaini L, Paulli M, Boveri E, et al. Splenic and nodal marginal zone lymphomas are indolent disorders at high hepatitis C virus seroprevalence with distinct presenting features but similar morphologic and phenotypic profiles. *Cancer* 2004;100:107–115.

393. Oh SY, Ryoo BY, Kim WS, et al. Nodal marginal zone B-cell lymphoma: analysis of 36 cases. Clinical presentation and treatment outcomes of nodal marginal zone B-cell lymphoma. *Ann Hematol* 2006;85:781–786.

394. Traverse-Glehen A, Felman P, Callet-Bauchu E, et al. A clinicopathological study of nodal marginal zone B-cell lymphoma. A report on 21 cases. *Histopathology* 2006;48:162–173.

395. Federico M, Vitolo U, Zinzani PL, et al. Prognosis of follicular lymphoma: a predictive model based on a retrospective analysis of 987 cases. Intergruppo Italiano Linfomi. *Blood* 2000;95:783–789.

396. Canioni D, Brice P, Lepage E, et al. Bone marrow histological patterns can predict survival of patients with grade 1 or 2 follicular lymphoma: a study from the Groupe d'Etude des Lymphomes Folliculaires. *Br J Haematol* 2004;126:364–371.

397. Solal-Celigny P, Roy P, Colombat P, et al. Follicular lymphoma international prognostic index. *Blood* 2004;104:1258–1265.

398. Bartlett NL, Rizeq M, Dorfman RF, Halpern J, Horning SJ. Follicular large-cell lymphoma: intermediate or low grade? *J Clin Oncol* 1994;12:1349–1357.

399. Wendum D, Sebban C, Gaulard P, et al. Follicular large-cell lymphoma treated with intensive chemotherapy: an analysis of 89 cases included in the LNH87 trial and comparison with the outcome of diffuse large B-cell lymphoma. Groupe d'Etude des Lymphomes de l'Adulte. *J Clin Oncol* 1997;15:1654–1663.

400. Rodriguez J, McLaughlin P, Hagemeister FB, et al. Follicular large cell lymphoma: an aggressive lymphoma that often presents with favorable prognostic features. *Blood* 1999;93:2202–2207.

401. Ott G, Katzenberger T, Lohr A, et al. Cytomorphologic, IHC, and cytogenetic profiles of follicular lymphoma: 2 types of follicular lymphoma grade 3. *Blood* 2002;99:3806–3812.

402. Torlakovic E, Torlakovic G, Brunning RD. Follicular pattern of bone marrow involvement by follicular lymphoma. *Am J Clin Pathol* 2002;118:780–786.

403. Spiro S, Galton DA, Wiltshaw E, et al. Follicular lymphoma: a survey of 75 cases with special reference to the syndrome resembling chronic lymphocytic leukaemia. *Br J Cancer* 1975;31[Suppl 2]:60–72.

404. Segal GH, Jorgensen T, Scott M, et al. Optimal primer selection for clonality assessment by polymerase chain reaction analysis: II. Follicular lymphomas. *Hum Pathol* 1994;25:1276–1282.

405. Wasman J, Rosenthal NS, Farhi DC. Mantle cell lymphoma. Morphologic findings in bone marrow involvement. *Am J Clin Pathol* 1996;106:196–200.

406. Swerdlow SH, Zukerberg LR, Yang WI, et al. The morphologic spectrum of non-Hodgkin's lymphomas with BCL1/cyclin D1 gene rearrangements. *Am J Surg Pathol* 1996;20:627–640.

407. Cohen PL, Kurtin PJ, Donovan KA, et al. Bone marrow and peripheral blood involvement in mantle cell lymphoma. *Br J Haematol* 1998;101:302–310.

408. Wong KF, So CC, Chan JK. Nucleolated variant of mantle cell lymphoma with leukemic manifestations mimicking prolymphocytic leukemia. *Am J Clin Pathol* 2002;117:246–251.

409. Pittaluga S, Verhoef G, Criel A, et al. Prognostic significance of bone marrow trephine and peripheral blood smears in 55 patients with mantle cell lymphoma. *Leuk Lymphoma* 1996;21:115–125.

410. Samaha H, Dumontet C, Ketterer N, et al. Mantle cell lymphoma: a retrospective study of 121 cases. *Leukemia* 1998;12:1281–1287.

411. Oinonen R, Franssila K, Teerenhovi L, et al. Mantle cell lymphoma: clinical features, treatment and prognosis of 94 patients. *Eur J Cancer* 1998;34:329–336.

412. Argatoff LH, Connors JM, Klasa RJ, et al. Mantle cell lymphoma: a clinicopathologic study of 80 cases. *Blood* 1997;89:2067–2078.

413. Weisenburger DD, Vose JM, Greiner TC, et al. Mantle cell lymphoma. A clinicopathologic study of 68 cases from the Nebraska Lymphoma Study Group. *Am J Hematol* 2000;64:190–196.

414. Colomo L, Lopez-Guillermo A, Perales M, et al. Clinical impact of the differentiation profile assessed by immunophenotyping in patients with diffuse large B-cell lymphoma. *Blood* 2003;101:78–84.

415. Moller MB, Pedersen NT, Christensen BE. Diffuse large B-cell lymphoma: clinical implications of extranodal versus nodal presentation—a population-based study of 1575 cases. *Br J Haematol* 2004;124:151–159.

416. Winter JN, Weller EA, Horning SJ, et al. Prognostic significance of Bcl-6 protein expression in DLBCL treated with CHOP or R-CHOP: a prospective correlative study. *Blood* 2006;107:4207–4213.

417. Murase T, Nakamura S, Kawauchi K, et al. An Asian variant of intravascular large B-cell lymphoma: clinical, pathological and cytogenetic approaches to diffuse large B-cell lymphoma associated with haemophagocytic syndrome. *Br J Haematol* 2000;111:826–834.

418. McMaster ML, Greer JP, Greco FA, Johnson DH, Wolff SN, Hainsworth JD. Effective treatment of small-noncleaved-cell lymphoma with high-intensity, brief-duration chemotherapy. *J Clin Oncol* 1991;9:941–946.

419. Soussain C, Patte C, Ostronoff M, et al. Small noncleaved cell lymphoma and leukemia in adults. A retrospective study of 65 adults treated with the LMB pediatric protocols. *Blood* 1995;85:664–674.

420. Cairo MS, Sposto R, Perkins SL, et al. Burkitt's and Burkitt-like lymphoma in children and adolescents: a review of the Children's Cancer Group experience. *Br J Haematol* 2003;120:660–670.

421. Brunning RD, McKenna RW, Bloomfield CD, et al. Bone marrow involvement in Burkitt's lymphoma. *Cancer* 1977;40:1771–1779.

422. Barcos MP, Lukes RJ. Malignant lymphoma of convoluted lymphocytes: a new entity of possible T-cell type. In Sink LF, Godden JO, eds. *Conflicts in Childhood Cancer.* New York: Alan R. Liss, 1975:147–178.

423. Nathwani BN, Kim H, Rappaport H. Malignant lymphoma, lymphoblastic. *Cancer* 1976;38:964–983.

424. Petrella T, Dalac S, Maynadie M, et al. CD4+ CD56+ cutaneous neoplasms: a distinct hematological entity? Groupe Francais d'Etude des Lymphomes Cutanes (GFELC). *Am J Surg Pathol* 1999;23:137–146.

425. DiGiuseppe JA, Louie DC, Williams JE, et al. Blastic natural killer cell leukemia/lymphoma: a clinicopathologic study. *Am J Surg Pathol* 1997;21:1223–1230.

426. Petrella T, Comeau MR, Maynadie M, et al. 'Agranular CD4+ CD56+ hematodermic neoplasm' (blastic NK-cell lymphoma) originates from a population of CD56+ precursor cells related to plasmacytoid monocytes. *Am J Surg Pathol* 2002;26:852–862.

427. Feuillard J, Jacob MC, Valensi F, et al. Clinical and biologic features of CD4(+)CD56(+) malignancies. *Blood* 2002;99:1556–1563.

428. Valbuena JR, Herling M, Admirand JH, et al. T-cell prolymphocytic leukemia involving extramedullary sites. *Am J Clin Pathol* 2005;123:456–464.

429. McKenna RW, Arthur DC, Gajl-Peczalska KJ, et al. Granulated T cell lymphocytosis with neutropenia: malignant or benign chronic lymphoproliferative disorder? *Blood* 1985;66:259–266.

430. Loughran TP, Jr. Starkebaum G. Large granular lymphocyte leukemia. Report of 38 cases and review of the literature. *Medicine (Baltimore)* 1987;66:397–405.

431. Oshimi K. Granular lymphocyte proliferative disorders: report of 12 cases and review of the literature. *Leukemia* 1988;2:617–627.

432. Agnarsson BA, Loughran TP, Jr., Starkebaum G, et al. The pathology of large granular lymphocyte leukemia. *Hum Pathol* 1989;20:643–651.

433. Loughran TP, Jr. Clonal diseases of large granular lymphocytes. *Blood* 1993;82:1–14.

434. Morice WG, Kurtin PJ, Leibson PJ, et al. Demonstration of aberrant T-cell and natural killer-cell antigen expression in all cases of granular lymphocytic leukaemia. *Br J Haematol* 2003;120:1026–1036.

435. Lundell R, Hartung L, Hill S, et al. T-cell large granular lymphocyte leukemias have multiple phenotypic abnormalities involving pan-T-cell antigens and receptors for MHC molecules. *Am J Clin Pathol* 2005;124:937–946.

436. Chan WC, Link S, Mawle A, et al. Heterogeneity of large granular lymphocyte proliferations: delineation of two major subtypes. *Blood* 1986;68:1142–1153.

437. Chan WC, Gu LB, Masih A, et al. Large granular lymphocyte proliferation with the natural killer-cell phenotype. *Am J Clin Pathol* 1992;97:353–358.

438. Cheung MM, Chan JK, Wong KF. Natural killer cell neoplasms: a distinctive group of highly aggressive lymphomas/leukemias. *Semin Hematol* 2003;40:221–232.
439. Uchiyama T, Yodoi J, Sagawa K, et al. Adult T-cell leukemia: clinical and hematologic features of 16 cases. *Blood* 1977;50:481–492.
440. Jaffe ES, Blattner WA, Blayney DW, et al. The pathologic spectrum of adult T-cell leukemia/lymphoma in the United States. Human T-cell leukemia/lymphoma virus-associated lymphoid malignancies. *Am J Surg Pathol* 1984;8:263–275.
441. Tajima K. The 4th nation-wide study of adult T-cell leukemia/lymphoma (ATL) in Japan: estimates of risk of ATL and its geographical and clinical features. The T- and B-cell Malignancy Study Group. *Int J Cancer* 1990;45:237–243.
442. Gale J, Simmonds PD, Mead GM, et al. Enteropathy-type intestinal T-cell lymphoma: clinical features and treatment of 31 patients in a single center. *J Clin Oncol* 2000;18: 795–803.
443. Wong KF, Chan JK, Cheung MM, et al. Bone marrow involvement by nasal NK cell lymphoma at diagnosis is uncommon. *Am J Clin Pathol* 2001;115:266–270.
444. Kwong YL, Chan AC, Liang R, et al. CD56+ NK lymphomas: clinicopathological features and prognosis. *Br J Haematol* 1997;97:821–829.
445. Chan JK, Sin VC, Wong KF, et al. Nonnasal lymphoma expressing the natural killer cell marker CD56: a clinicopathologic study of 49 cases of an uncommon aggressive neoplasm. *Blood* 1997;89:4501–4513.
446. Cheung MM, Chan JK, Wong KF. Natural killer cell neoplasms: a distinctive group of highly aggressive lymphomas/leukemias. *Semin Hematol* 2003;40:221–232.
447. Chim CS, Ma SY, Au WY, et al. Primary nasal natural killer cell lymphoma: long-term treatment outcome and relationship with the International Prognostic Index. *Blood* 2004; 103:216–221.
448. Wong KF, Chan JK, Matutes E, et al. Hepatosplenic gamma delta T-cell lymphoma. A distinctive aggressive lymphoma type. *Am J Surg Pathol* 1995;19:718–726.
449. Cooke CB, Krenacs L, Stetler-Stevenson M, et al. Hepatosplenic T-cell lymphoma: a distinct clinicopathologic entity of cytotoxic gamma delta T-cell origin. *Blood* 1996;88: 4265–4274.
450. Belhadj K, Reyes F, Farcet JP, et al. Hepatosplenic gammadelta T-cell lymphoma is a rare clinicopathologic entity with poor outcome: report on a series of 21 patients. *Blood* 2003; 102:4261–4269.
451. Vega F, Medeiros LJ, Bueso-Ramos C, et al. Hepatosplenic gamma/delta T-cell lymphoma in bone marrow. A sinusoidal neoplasm with blastic cytologic features. *Am J Clin Pathol* 2001;116:410–419.
452. Macon WR, Levy NB, Kurtin PJ, et al. Hepatosplenic alphabeta T-cell lymphomas: a report of 14 cases and comparison with hepatosplenic gammadelta T-cell lymphomas. *Am J Surg Pathol* 2001;25:285–296.
453. Alonsozana EL, Stamberg J, Kumar D, et al. Isochromosome 7q: the primary cytogenetic abnormality in hepatosplenic gammadelta T cell lymphoma. *Leukemia* 1997;11:1367–1372.
454. Willemze R, Jansen PM, Cerroni L, et al. Subcutaneous panniculitis-like T-cell lymphoma: definition, classification, and prognostic factors: an EORTC Cutaneous Lymphoma Group Study of 83 cases. *Blood* 2008;111:838–845.
455. Gonzalez CL, Medeiros LJ, Braziel RM, et al. T-cell lymphoma involving subcutaneous tissue. A clinicopathologic entity commonly associated with hemophagocytic syndrome. *Am J Surg Pathol* 1991;15:17–27.
456. Salhany KE, Greer JP, Cousar JB, et al. Marrow involvement in cutaneous T-cell lymphoma. A clinicopathologic study of 60 cases. *Am J Clin Pathol* 1989;92:747–754.
457. Graham SJ, Sharpe RW, Steinberg SM, et al. Prognostic implications of a bone marrow histopathologic classification system in mycosis fungoides and the Sezary syndrome. *Cancer* 1993;72:726–734.
458. Marti RM, Estrach T, Reverter JC, et al. Utility of bone marrow and liver biopsies for staging cutaneous T-cell lymphoma. *Int J Dermatol* 1996;35:450–454.
459. Sibaud V, Beylot-Barry M, Thiebaut R, et al. Bone marrow histopathologic and molecular staging in epidermotropic T-cell lymphomas. *Am J Clin Pathol* 2003;119:414–423.
460. Magrini U, Castello A, Boveri E, et al. Histopathology of bone marrow involvement in T-cell lymphomas. *Leukemia* 1991;5:24–25.
461. Lopez-Guillermo A, Cid J, Salar A, et al. Peripheral T-cell lymphomas: initial features, natural history, and prognostic factors in a series of 174 patients diagnosed according to the R.E.A.L. Classification. *Ann Oncol* 1998;9:849–855
462. Kim K, Kim WS, Jung CW, et al. Clinical features of peripheral T-cell lymphomas in 78 patients diagnosed according to the Revised European-American lymphoma (REAL) classification. *Eur J Cancer* 2002;38:75–81.
463. Gallamini A, Stelitano C, Calvi R, et al. Peripheral T-cell lymphoma unspecified (PTCL-U): a new prognostic model from a retrospective multicentric clinical study. *Blood* 2004; 103:2474–2479.
464. White DM, Smith AG, Whitehouse JM, et al. Peripheral T cell lymphoma: value of bone marrow trephine immunophenotyping. *J Clin Pathol* 1989;42:403–408.
465. Auger MJ, Nash JR, Mackie MJ. Marrow involvement with T cell lymphoma initially presenting as abnormal myelopoiesis. *J Clin Pathol* 1986;39:134–137.
466. Schnaidt U, Vykoupil KF, Thiele J, et al. Angioimmunoblastic lymphadenopathy. Histopathology of bone marrow involvement. *Virchows Arch A Pathol Anat Histol* 1980;389:369–380.
467. Ghani AM, Krause JR. Bone marrow biopsy findings in angioimmunoblastic lymphadenopathy. *Br J Haematol* 1985;61:203–213.
468. Pautier P, Devidas A, Delmer A, et al. Angioimmunoblastic-like T-cell non Hodgkin's lymphoma: outcome after chemotherapy in 33 patients and review of the literature. *Leuk Lymphoma* 1999;32:545–552
469. Chen W, Kesler MV, Karandikar NJ, McKenna RW, Kroft SH. Flow cytometric features of angioimmunoblastic T-cell lymphoma. *Cytometry B Clin Cytom* 2006;70B:142–148.
470. Attygalle A, Al-Jehani R, Diss TC, et al. Neoplastic T cells in angioimmunoblastic T-cell lymphoma express CD10. *Blood* 2002;99:627–633.
471. Fraga M, Brousset P, Schlaifer D, et al. Bone marrow involvement in anaplastic large cell lymphoma. IHC detection of minimal disease and its prognostic significance. *Am J Clin Pathol* 1995;103:82–89.
472. Tilly H, Gaulard P, Lepage E, et al. Primary anaplastic large-cell lymphoma in adults: clinical presentation, immunophenotype, and outcome. *Blood* 1997;90:3727–3734.
473. Weisenburger DD, Anderson JR, Diebold J, et al. Systemic anaplastic large-cell lymphoma: results from the non-Hodgkin's lymphoma classification project. *Am J Hematol* 2001;67: 172–178.
474. Coad JE, Olson DJ, Christensen DR, et al. Correlation of PCR-detected clonal gene rearrangements with bone marrow morphology in patients with B-lineage lymphomas. *Am J Surg Pathol* 1997;21:1047–1056.
475. Duggan PR, Easton D, Luider J, Auer IA. Bone marrow staging of patients with non-Hodgkin lymphoma by flow cytometry: correlation with morphology. *Cancer* 2000;88: 894–899.
476. Gebhard S, Benhattar J, Bricod C, et al. Polymerase chain reaction in the diagnosis of T-cell lymphoma in paraffin-embedded bone marrow biopsies: a comparative study. *Histopathology* 2001;38:37–44.
477. Palacio C, Acebedo G, Navarrete M, et al. Flow cytometry in the bone marrow evaluation of follicular and diffuse large B-cell lymphomas. *Haematologica* 2001;86:934–940.
478. Braunschweig R, Baur AS, Delacretaz F, et al. Contribution of IgH-PCR to the evaluation of B-cell lymphoma involvement in paraffin-embedded bone marrow biopsy specimens. *Am J Clin Pathol* 2003;119:634–642.
479. Gomyo H, Shimoyama M, Minagawa K, et al. Morphologic, flow cytometric and cytogenetic evaluation of bone marrow involvement in B-cell lymphoma. *Haematologica* 2003;88: 1358–1365.
480. Stacchini A, Demurtas A, Godio L, et al. Flow cytometry in the bone marrow staging of mature B-cell neoplasms. *Cytometry B Clin Cytom* 2003;54:10–18.
481. Perea G, Altes A, Bellido M, et al. Clinical utility of bone marrow flow cytometry in B-cell non-Hodgkin lymphomas (B-NHL). *Histopathology* 2004;45:268–274.
482. Lassmann S, Gerlach UV, Technau-Ihling K, et al. Application of BIOMED-2 primers in fixed and decalcified bone marrow biopsies: analysis of immunoglobulin H receptor rearrangements in B-cell non-Hodgkin's lymphomas. *J Mol Diagn* 2005;7:582–591.
483. Schmidt B, Kremer M, Gotze K, et al. Bone marrow involvement in follicular lymphoma: comparison of histology and flow cytometry as staging procedures. *Leuk Lymphoma* 2006; 47:1857–1862.
484. Bertram HC, Check IJ, Milano MA. Immunophenotyping large B-cell lymphomas. Flow cytometric pitfalls and pathologic correlation. *Am J Clin Pathol* 2001;116:191–203.
485. Bain B, Matutes E, Robinson D, et al. Leukaemia as a manifestation of large cell lymphoma. *Br J Haematol* 1991;77:301–310.
486. Nakano M, Kawanishi Y, Kuge S, et al. Clinical and prognostic significance of monoclonal small-cells in the peripheral blood and bone marrow of various B-cell lymphomas. *Blood* 1992;79:3253–3260.
487. Bain BJ, Catovsky D. The leukaemic phase of non-Hodgkin's lymphoma. *J Clin Pathol* 1995;48:189–193.
488. Anderson MM, Ross CW, Singleton TP, et al. Ki-1 anaplastic large cell lymphoma with a prominent leukemic phase. *Hum Pathol* 1996;27:1093–1095.
489. Bartl R, Frisch B, Burkhardt R, et al. Assessment of bone marrow histology in Hodgkin's disease: correlation with clinical factors. *Br J Haematol* 1982;51:345–360.
490. Myers CE, Chabner BA, De Vita VT, et al. Bone marrow involvement in Hodgkin's disease: pathology and response to MOPP chemotherapy. *Blood* 1974;44:197–204.
491. O'Carroll DI, McKenna RW, Brunning RD. Bone marrow manifestations of Hodgkin's disease. *Cancer* 1976;38:1717–1728.
492. Munker R, Hasenclever D, Brosteanu O, et al. Bone marrow involvement in Hodgkin's disease: an analysis of 135 consecutive cases. German Hodgkin's Lymphoma Study Group. *J Clin Oncol* 1995;13:403–409.
493. Macintyre EA, Vaughan Hudson B, Linch DC, et al. The value of staging bone marrow trephine biopsy in Hodgkin's disease. *Eur J Haematol* 1987;39:66–70.
494. Howell SJ, Grey M, Chang J, et al. The value of bone marrow examination in the staging of Hodgkin's lymphoma: a review of 955 cases seen in a regional cancer centre. *Br J Haematol* 2002;119:408–411.
495. Spector N, Nucci M, Oliveira De Morais JC, et al. Clinical factors predictive of bone marrow involvement in Hodgkin's disease. *Leuk Lymphoma* 1997;26:171–176.
496. Rappaport H, Berard CW, Butler JJ, et al. Report of the Committee on Histopathological Criteria Contributing to Staging of Hodgkin's Disease. *Cancer Res* 1971;31:1864–1865.
497. Neiman RS, Rosen PJ, Lukes RJ. Lymphocyte-depletion Hodgkin's disease. A clinicopathological entity. *N Engl J Med* 1973;288:751–755.
498. Te Velde J, Den Ottolander GJ, Spaander PJ, et al. The bone marrow in Hodgkin's disease: the non-involved marrow. *Histopathology* 1978;2:31–46.
499. Diehl V, Sextro M, Franklin J, et al. Clinical presentation, course, and prognostic factors in lymphocyte-predominant Hodgkin's disease and lymphocyte-rich classical Hodgkin's disease: report from the European Task Force on Lymphoma Project on Lymphocyte-Predominant Hodgkin's Disease. *J Clin Oncol* 1999;17:776–783.
500. Khoury JD, Jones D, Yared MA, et al. Bone marrow involvement in patients with nodular lymphocyte predominant Hodgkin lymphoma. *Am J Surg Pathol* 2004;28:489–495.
501. Macavei I, Galatar N. Bone marrow biopsy (BMB). III. Bone marrow biopsy in Hodgkin's disease (HD). *Morphol Embryol (Bucur)* 1990;36:25–32.
502. Colon-Otero G, McClure SP, Phyliky RL, et al. Peripheral T-cell lymphoma simulating Hodgkin's disease with initial bone marrow involvement. *Mayo Clin Proc* 1986;61:68–71.
503. Warnke R, Weiss L, Chan J, et al. Classic Hodgkin's disease. In Warnke R, Weiss L, Chan J, et al., eds. *Tumors of Lymph Node and Spleen.* Third series. Fascicle 14. Washington, DC: Armed Forces Institute of Pathology, 1995:277–304.
504. Strum SB, Park JK, Rappaport H. Observation of cells resembling Sternberg-Reed cells in conditions other than Hodgkin's disease. *Cancer* 1970;26:176–190.
505. McKenna RW, Brunning RD. Reed-Sternberg-like cells in nodular lymphoma involving the bone marrow. *Am J Clin Pathol* 1975;63:779–785.
506. Maeda K, Hyun BH, Rebuck JW. Lymphoid follicles in bone marrow aspirates. *Am J Clin Pathol* 1977;67:41–48.

507. Rywlin AM, Ortega RS, Dominguez CJ. Lymphoid nodules of bone marrow: normal and abnormal. *Blood* 1974;43:389–400.

508. Liu PI, Takanari H, Yatani R, et al. Comparative studies of bone marrow from the United States and Japan. *Ann Clin Lab Sci* 1989;19:345–351.

509. Kemona A, Dzieciol J, Sulik M, et al. [Lymphocytic aggregations in the bone marrow: their occurrence and morphologic analysis]. *Patol Pol* 1989;40:219–225.

510. Brunning RD, McKenna RW. Lesions simulating lymphoma. In Brunning RD, McKenna RW, eds. *Tumors of the Bone Marrow. Atlas of Tumor Pathology*. Third series. Fascicle 9. Washington, DC: Armed Forces Institute of Pathology, 1994:409–438.

511. Cervantes F, Pereira A, Marti JM, et al. Bone marrow lymphoid nodules in myeloproliferative disorders: association with the nonmyelosclerotic phases of idiopathic myelofibrosis and immunological significance. *Br J Haematol* 1988;70:279–282.

512. Rosenthal NS, Farhi DC. Bone marrow findings in connective tissue disease. *Am J Clin Pathol* 1989;92:650–654.

513. Crocker J, Jones EL, Curran RC. Study of nuclear sizes in the centres of malignant and benign lymphoid follicles. *J Clin Pathol* 1983;36:1332–1334.

514. Farhi DC. Germinal centers in the bone marrow. *Hematol Pathol* 1989;3:133–136.

515. Peterson LC, Kueck B, Arthur DC, et al. Systemic polyclonal immunoblastic proliferations. *Cancer* 1988;61:1350–1358.

516. Chilosi M, Pizzolo G, Fiore-Donati L, et al. Routine immunofluorescent and histochemical analysis of bone marrow involvement of lymphoma/leukaemia: the use of cryostat sections. *Br J Cancer* 1983;48:763–775.

517. Ellison DJ, Hu E, Zovich D, et al. Immunogenetic analysis of bone marrow aspirates in patients with non-Hodgkin lymphomas. *Am J Hematol* 1990;33:160–166.

518. Liang R, Chan VV, Chan TK, et al. Immunoglobulin gene rearrangement in the peripheral blood and bone marrow of patients with lymphomas of the mucosa-associated lymphoid tissues. *Acta Haematol* 1990;84:19–23.

519. Sandhaus LM, Voelkerding KV, Dougherty J, et al. Combined utility of gene rearrangement analysis and flow cytometry in the diagnosis of lymphoproliferative disease in the bone marrow. *Hematol Pathol* 1990;4:135–148.

520. Sangster G, Crocker J, Nar P, et al. Benign and malignant (B cell) focal lymphoid aggregates in bone marrow trephines shown by means of an immunogold-silver technique. *J Clin Pathol* 1986;39:453–457.

521. Horny HP, Wehrmann M, Griesser H, et al. Investigation of bone marrow lymphocyte subsets in normal, reactive, and neoplastic states using paraffin-embedded biopsy specimens. *Am J Clin Pathol* 1993;99:142–149.

522. Bluth RF, Casey TT, McCurley TL. Differentiation of reactive from neoplastic small-cell lymphoid aggregates in paraffin-embedded marrow particle preparations using L-26 (CD20) and UCHL-1 (CD45RO) monoclonal antibodies. *Am J Clin Pathol* 1993;99:150–156.

523. Ben-Ezra JM, King BE, Harris AC, et al. Staining for Bcl-2 protein helps to distinguish benign from malignant lymphoid aggregates in bone marrow biopsies. *Mod Pathol* 1994;7:560–564.

524. Muehleck SD, McKenna RW, Gale PF, et al. Terminal deoxynucleotidyl transferase (TdT)-positive cells in bone marrow in the absence of hematologic malignancy. *Am J Clin Pathol* 1983;79:277–284.

525. Longacre TA, Foucar K, Crago S, et al. Hematogones: a multiparameter analysis of bone marrow precursor cells. *Blood* 1989;73:543–552.

526. van den Doel LJ, Pieters R, Huismans DR, et al. Immunological phenotype of lymphoid cells in regenerating bone marrow of children after treatment for acute lymphoblastic leukemia. *Eur J Haematol* 1988;41:170–175.

527. Kobayashi SD, Seki K, Suwa N, et al. The transient appearance of small blastoid cells in the marrow after bone marrow transplantation. *Am J Clin Pathol* 1991;96:191–195.

528. Davis RE, Longacre TA, Cornbleet PJ. Hematogones in the bone marrow of adults. Immunophenotypic features, clinical settings, and differential diagnosis. *Am J Clin Pathol* 1994;102:202–211.

529. Leitenberg D, Rappeport JM, Smith BR. B-cell precursor bone marrow reconstitution after bone marrow transplantation. *Am J Clin Pathol* 1994;102:231–236.

530. Rimsza LM, Larson RS, Winter SS, et al. Benign hematogone-rich lymphoid proliferations can be distinguished from B-lineage acute lymphoblastic leukemia by integration of morphology, immunophenotype, adhesion molecule expression, and architectural features. *Am J Clin Pathol* 2000;114:66–75.

531. Reed M, McKenna RW, Bridges R, et al. Morphologic manifestations of monoclonal gammopathies. *Am J Clin Pathol* 1981;76:8–23.

532. Kyle RA. Diagnostic criteria of multiple myeloma. *Hematol Oncol Clin North Am* 1992;6:347–358.

533. Bataille R. New insights in the clinical biology of multiple myeloma. *Semin Hematol* 1997;34:23–28.

534. Brunning RD, McKenna RW. Plasma cell dyscrasias and related disorders. In Brunning RD, McKenna RW, eds. *Tumors of the Bone Marrow. Atlas of Tumor Pathology*. Third series. Fascicle 9. Washington, DC: Armed Forces Institute of Pathology, 1994:323–367.

535. Sukpanichnant S, Cousar JB, Leelasiri A, et al. Diagnostic criteria and histologic grading in multiple myeloma: histologic and immunohistologic analysis of 176 cases with clinical correlation. *Hum Pathol* 1994;25:308–318.

536. Hallek M, Bergsagel PL, Anderson KC. Multiple myeloma: increasing evidence for a multistep transformation process. *Blood* 1998;91:3–21.

537. Kyle RA, Greipp PA. Plasma cell dyscrasias: current status. *Crit Rev Oncol Hematol* 1988;8:93–152.

538. Lukes RJ, Tindle BH. Immunoblastic lymphadenopathy. A hyperimmune entity resembling Hodgkin's disease. *N Engl J Med* 1975;292:1–8.

539. Durie BG, Salmon SE. A clinical staging system for multiple myeloma. Correlation of measured myeloma cell mass with presenting clinical features, response to treatment, and survival. *Cancer* 1975;36:842–854.

540. Durie BG. Staging and kinetics of multiple myeloma. *Semin Oncol* 1986;13:300–309.

541. Criteria for the classification of monoclonal gammopathies, multiple myeloma and related disorders: a report of the International Myeloma Working Group, *Br J Haematol* 2003;121:749–757.

542. Dick FR. Plasma cell myeloma and related disorders with monoclonal gammopathy. In Koepke JA, ed. *Laboratory Hematology*. New York: Churchill Livingstone, 1984:445–481.

543. Greipp PR, Raymond NM, Kyle RA, et al. Multiple myeloma: significance of plasmablastic subtype in morphological classification. *Blood* 1985;65:305–310.

544. Zukerberg LR, Ferry JA, Conlon M, et al. Plasma cell myeloma with cleaved, multilobated, and monocytoid nuclei. *Am J Clin Pathol* 1990;93:657–661.

545. Krzyzaniak RL, Buss DH, Cooper MR, et al. Marrow fibrosis and multiple myeloma. *Am J Clin Pathol* 1988;89:63–68.

546. Greipp PR, Leong T, Bennett JM, et al. Plasmablastic morphology—an independent prognostic factor with clinical and laboratory correlates: Eastern Cooperative Oncology Group (ECOG) myeloma trial E9486 report by the ECOG Myeloma Laboratory Group. *Blood* 1998;91:2501–2507.

547. Carter A, Hocherman I, Linn S, et al. Prognostic significance of plasma cell morphology in multiple myeloma. *Cancer* 1987;60:1060–1065.

548. Peterson LC, Brown BA, Crosson JT, et al. Application of the immunoperoxidase technic to bone marrow trephine biopsies in the classification of patients with monoclonal gammopathies. *Am J Clin Pathol* 1986;85:688–693.

549. Wolf BC, Brady K, O'Murchadha MT, et al. An evaluation of immunohistologic stains for immunoglobulin light chains in bone marrow biopsies in benign and malignant plasma cell proliferations. *Am J Clin Pathol* 1990;94:742–746.

550. Singh J, Dudley AW Jr., Kulig KA. Increased incidence of monoclonal gammopathy of undetermined significance in blacks and its age-related differences with whites on the basis of a study of 397 men and one woman in a hospital setting. *J Lab Clin Med* 1990;116:785–789.

551. Kyle RA. Monoclonal gammopathy of undetermined significance and smoldering multiple myeloma. *Eur J Haematol Suppl* 1989;51:70–75.

552. Kyle RA. Monoclonal gammopathy of undetermined significance (MGUS). *Baillieres Clin Haematol* 1995;8:761–781.

553. Kyle RA, Therneau TM, Rajkumar SV, et al. Prevalence of monoclonal gammopathy of undetermined significance, *N Engl J Med* 2006, 354:1362–1369

554. Kyle RA, Rajkumar SV. Monoclonal gammopathy of undetermined significance, *Br J Haematol* 2006, 134:573–589

555. Cheanu H, Wang H-Y, Chen W, et al. Immunophenotypic studies of monoclonal gammopathy of undetermined significance. *Clin Pathol* 2008;8:13.

556. Ocqueteau M, Orfao A, Almeida J, et al. Immunophenotypic characterization of plasma cells from monoclonal gammopathy of undetermined significance patients. Implications for the differential diagnosis between MGUS and multiple myeloma, *Am J Pathol* 1998, 152:1655–1665.

557. Kyle RA. Monoclonal gammopathy of undetermined significance and solitary plasmacytoma. Implications for progression to overt multiple myeloma. *Hematol Oncol Clin North Am* 1997;11:71–87.

558. Vuckovic J, Ilic A, Knezevic N, et al. Prognosis in monoclonal gammopathy of undetermined significance. *Br J Haematol* 1997;97:649–651.

559. Kyle RA, Therneau TM, Rajkumar SV, et al. Long-term follow-up of 241 patients with monoclonal gammopathy of undetermined significance: the original Mayo Clinic series 25 years later. *Mayo Clin Proc* 2004;79:859–866.

560. Kyle RA, Rajkumar SV. Monoclonal gammopathies of undetermined significance: a review. *Immunol Rev* 2003;194:112–139.

561. Kyle RA, Therneau TM, Rajkumar SV, et al. A long-term study of prognosis in monoclonal gammopathy of undetermined significance. *N Engl J Med* 2002;346:564–569 .

562. Pasqualetti P, Festuccia V, Collacciani A, et al. The natural history of monoclonal gammopathy of undetermined significance. A 5- to 20-year follow-up of 263 cases. *Acta Haematol* 1997;97:174–179.

563. Blade J. On the "significance" of monoclonal gammopathy of undetermined significance. *Mayo Clin Proc* 2004;79:855–856.

564. Kyle RA, Therneau TM, Rajkumar SV, et al. Long-term follow-up of IgM monoclonal gammopathy of undetermined significance. *Blood* 2003;102: 3759–3764.

565. Cavo M, Galieni P, Gobbi M, et al. Nonsecretory multiple myeloma. Presenting findings, clinical course and prognosis. *Acta Haematol* 1985;74:27–30.

566. Dreicer R, Alexanian R. Nonsecretory multiple myeloma. *Am J Hematol* 1982;13:313–318.

567. Bosman C, Fusilli S, Bisceglia M, et al. Oncocytic nonsecretory multiple myeloma. A clinicopathologic study of a case and review of the literature. *Acta Haematol* 1996;96(1):50–56.

568. Bourantas K. Nonsecretory multiple myeloma. *Eur J Haematol* 1996;56(1–2):109–111.

569. Drayson M, Tang LX, Drew R, et al. Serum free light-chain measurements for identifying and monitoring patients with nonsecretory multiple myeloma. *Blood* 2001;97:2900–2902.

570. Smith DB, Harris M, Gowland E, et al. Non-secretory multiple myeloma: a report of 13 cases with a review of the literature. *Hematol Oncol* 1986;4:307–313.

571. Kyle RA, Greipp PR. Smoldering multiple myeloma. *N Engl J Med* 1980;302:1347–1349.

572. Greipp PR, Kyle RA. Clinical, morphological, and cell kinetic differences among multiple myeloma, monoclonal gammopathy of undetermined significance, and smoldering multiple myeloma. *Blood* 1983;62:166–171.

573. Witzig TE, Kyle RA, O'Fallon WM, et al. Detection of peripheral blood plasma cells as a predictor of disease course in patients with smouldering multiple myeloma. *Br J Haematol* 1994;87:266–272.

574. International Myeloma Working Group. Criteria for the classification of monoclonal gammopathies, multiple myeloma and related disorders: a report of the International Myeloma Working Group. *Br J Haematol* 2003;121(5):749–757.

575. Dimopoulos MA, Moulopoulos LA, Maniatis A, et al. Solitary plasmacytoma of bone and asymptomatic multiple myeloma. *Blood* 2000;96:2037–2044.

576. Kyle RA, Remstein ED, Therneau TM, et al. Clinical course and prognosis of smoldering (asymptomatic) multiple myeloma. *N Engl J Med* 2007, 356:2582–2590.

577. Kyle RA, Therneau TM, Rajkumar SV, et al. A long-term study of prognosis in monoclonal gammopathy of undetermined significance. *N Engl J Med* 2002;346(8):564–569.

578. Kosmo MA, Gale RP. Plasma cell leukemia. *Semin Hematol* 1987;24:202–208.

579. Noel P, Kyle RA. Plasma cell leukemia: an evaluation of response to therapy. *Am J Med* 1987;83:1062–1068.

580. Dimopoulos MA, Palumbo A, Delasalle KB, et al. Primary plasma cell leukaemia. *Br J Haematol* 1994;88:754–759.

581. Kyle RA, Maldonado JE, Bayrd ED. Plasma cell leukemia. Report on 17 cases. *Arch Intern Med* 1974;133:813–818.

582. Garcia-Sanz R, Orfao A, Gonzalez M, et al. Primary plasma cell leukemia: clinical, immunophenotypic, DNA ploidy, and cytogenetic characteristics. *Blood* 1999;93(3):1032–1037.

583. Dimopoulos MA, Palumbo A, Delasalle KB, et al. Primary plasma cell leukaemia. *Br J Haematol* 1994;88(4):754–759.

584. Avet-Loiseau H, Daviet A, Brigaudeau C, et al. Cytogenetic, interphase and multicolor fluorescence in situ hybridization analyses in primary plasma cell leukemia. A study of 40 cases at diagnosis, on behalf of the Intergroupe Francophone du Myelome and the Groupe Francais de Cytogenetique Hematologique. *Blood* 2001;97:822–825.

585. Dimopoulos MA, Palumbo A, Delasalle KB, et al. Primary plasma cell leukaemia. *Br J Haematol* 1994, 88:754–759.

586. McKenna RW, Kyle RA, Kuehl WM, et al. Plasma cell neoplasms. In Swerdlow SH, Campo E, Harris NL, et al. WHO classification of Tumours of Haematopoietic and lymphoid tissues. Lyon, France: IARC Press, 2008:200–213.

587. Brunning RD, McKenna RW. Plasma cell dyscrasias and related disorders. In Brunning RD, McKenna RW, eds. *Atlas of Tumor Pathology. Tumors of the Bone Marrow.* Washington, DC: Armed Forces Institute of Pathology, 1994;323–367.

588. Hegewisch S, Mainzer K, Braumann D. IgE myelomatosis. Presentation of a new case and summary of literature. *Blut* 1987;55:55–60.

589. Wiltshaw E. The natural history of extramedullary plasmacytoma and its relation to solitary myeloma of bone and myelomatosis. *Medicine (Baltimore)* 1976;55:217–238.

590. Bataille R. Localized plasmacytomas. *Clin Haematol* 1982;11:113–122.

591. Dimopoulos MA, Moulopoulos A, Delasalle K, et al. Solitary plasmacytoma of bone and asymptomatic multiple myeloma. *Hematol Oncol Clin North Am* 1992;6:359–369.

592. Soutar R, Lucraft H, Jackson G, et al. Guidelines on the diagnosis and management of solitary plasmacytoma of bone and solitary extramedullary plasmacytoma. *Br J Haematol* 2004;124:717–726.

593. Wilder RB, Ha CS, Cox JD, et al. Persistence of myeloma protein for more than one year after radiotherapy is an adverse prognostic factor in solitary plasmacytoma of bone. *Cancer* 2002;94:1532–1537.

594. Galieni P, Cavo M, Avvisati G, et al. Solitary plasmacytoma of bone and extramedullary plasmacytoma: two different entities? *Ann Oncol* 1995;6:687–691.

595. Lin BT, Weiss LM. Primary plasmacytoma of lymph nodes. *Hum Pathol* 1997;28:1083–1090.

596. Dimopoulos MA, Hamilos G. Solitary bone plasmacytoma and extramedullary plasmacytoma. *Curr Treat Options Oncol* 2002;3:255–259.

597. Feiner HD. Pathology of dysproteinemia: light chain amyloidosis, non-amyloid immunoglobulin deposition disease, cryoglobulinemia syndromes, and macroglobulinemia of Waldenstrom. *Hum Pathol* 1988;19:1255–1272.

598. Buxbaum J. Mechanisms of disease: monoclonal immunoglobulin deposition. Amyloidosis, light chain deposition disease, and light and heavy chain deposition disease. *Hematol Oncol Clin North Am* 1992;6:323–346.

599. Kyle RA, Greipp PR. Amyloidosis (AL). Clinical and laboratory features in 229 cases. *Mayo Clin Proc* 1983;58:665–683.

600. Kyle RA, Greipp PR, O'Fallon WM. Primary systemic amyloidosis: multivariate analysis for prognostic factors in 168 cases. *Blood* 1986;68:220–224.

601. Kyle RA, Linos A, Beard CM, et al. Incidence and natural history of primary systemic amyloidosis in Olmsted County, Minnesota, 1950 through 1989. *Blood* 1992;79:1817–1822.

602. Gillmore JD, Hawkins PN, Pepys MB. Amyloidosis: a review of recent diagnostic and therapeutic developments. *Br J Haematol* 1997;99:245–256.

603. Wolf BC, Kumar A, Vera JC, et al. Bone marrow morphology and immunology in systemic amyloidosis. *Am J Clin Pathol* 1986;86:84–88.

604. Wu SS, Brady K, Anderson JJ, et al. The predictive value of bone marrow morphologic characteristics and immunostaining in primary (AL) amyloidosis. *Am J Clin Pathol* 1991;96:95–99.

605. Kyle RA, Gertz MA. Primary systemic amyloidosis: clinical and laboratory features in 474 cases. *Semin Hematol* 1995;32:45–59.

606. Linke RP, Nathrath WBJ, Eulitz M. *Classification of Amyloid Syndromes from Tissue Sections Using Antibodies against Various Amyloid Fibril Proteins: Report of 142 Cases.* New York: Plenum, 1986.

607. Feiner HD. Pathology of dysproteinemia: light chain amyloidosis, non-amyloid immunoglobulin deposition disease, cryoglobulinemia syndromes, and macroglobulinemia of Waldenstrom. *Hum Pathol* 1988;19:1255–1272.

608. Randall, RE, Williamson WC, Mullinax F, et al. Manifestations of systemic light chain deposition. *Am J Med* 1976;60(2):293–299.

609. Preud'Homme, JL, Aucouturier P, Touchard G, et al. Monoclonal immunoglobulin deposition disease (Randall type). Relationship with structural abnormalities of immunoglobulin chains. *Kidney Int* 1994;46(4):965–972.

610. Gallo G, Goni F, Boctor F, et al. Light chain cardiomyopathy. Structural analysis of the light chain tissue deposits. *Am J Pathol* 1996;148(5):1397–1406.

611. Buxbaum J. Mechanisms of disease: monoclonal immunoglobulin deposition. Amyloidosis, light chain deposition disease, and light and heavy chain deposition disease. *Hematol Oncol Clin North Am* 1992;6(2):323–346.

612. Aucouturier P, Khamlichi AA, Touchard G, et al. Brief report: heavy-chain deposition disease. *N Engl J Med* 1993;329(19):1389–1393.

613. Kambham N, Markowitz GS, Appel GB, et al. Heavy chain deposition disease: the disease spectrum. *Am J Kidney Dis* 1999;33(5):954–962.

614. Herzenberg AM, Lien J, Magil AB. Monoclonal heavy chain (immunoglobulin G3) deposition disease: report of a case. *Am J Kidney Dis* 1996;28(1):128–131.

615. Miralles GD, O'Fallon JR, Talley NJ. Plasma-cell dyscrasia with polyneuropathy. The spectrum of POEMS syndrome. *N Engl J Med* 1992;327:1919–1923.

616. Soubrier MJ, Dubost JJ, Sauvezie BJ. POEMS syndrome: a study of 25 cases and a review of the literature. French Study Group on POEMS Syndrome. *Am J Med* 1994;97:543–553.

617. Schey S. Osteosclerotic myeloma and 'POEMS' syndrome. *Blood Rev* 1996;10:75–80.

618. Dispenzieri A, Kyle RA, Lacy MQ, et al. POEMS syndrome: definitions and long-term outcome. *Blood* 2003;101:2496–2506.

619. Seligmann M, Mihaesco E, Preud'homme JL, et al. Heavy chain diseases: current findings and concepts. *Immunol Rev* 1979;48:145–167.

620. Wahner-Roedler DL, Witzig TE, Loehrer LL, Kyle RA. Gamma-heavy chain disease: review of 23 cases. *Medicine (Baltimore)* 2003;82:236–250.

621. Kyle RA, Greipp PR, Banks PM. The diverse picture of gamma heavy-chain disease. Report of seven cases and review of literature. *Mayo Clin Proc* 1981;56:439–451.

622. Fermand JP, Brouet JC, Danon F, et al. Gamma heavy chain "disease": heterogeneity of the clinicopathologic features. Report of 16 cases and review of the literature. *Medicine (Baltimore)* 1989;68:321–335.

623. Franklin EC. Mu-chain disease. *Arch Intern Med* 1975;135:71–72.

624. Wahner-Roedler DL, Kyle RA. Mu-heavy chain disease: presentation as a benign monoclonal gammapathy. *Am J Hematol* 1992;40:56–60.

625. Price SK. Immunoproliferative small intestinal disease: a study of 13 cases with alpha heavy-chain disease. *Histopathology* 1990;17:7–17.

626. Bartl R, Frisch B, Mahl G, et al. Bone marrow histology in Waldenstrom's macroglobulinaemia. Clinical relevance of subtype recognition. *Scand J Haematol* 1983;31:359–375.

627. Harris NL, Bhan AK. B-cell neoplasms of the lymphocytic, lymphoplasmacytoid, and plasma cell types: immunohistologic analysis and clinical correlation. *Hum Pathol* 1985;16:829–837.

628. Kyle RA, Garton JP. The spectrum of IgM monoclonal gammapathy in 430 cases. *Mayo Clin Proc* 1987;62:719–731.

629. Dimopoulos MA, Alexanian R. Waldenstrom's macroglobulinemia. *Blood* 1994;83:1452–1459.

630. Fonseca R, Hayman S. Wadenstrom macroglobulinaemia. *Br J Haematol* 2007 138:700–720.

631. Feiner HD, Rizk CC, Finfer MD, et al. IgM monoclonal gammapathy/Waldenstrom's macroglobulinemia: a morphological and immunophenotypic study of the bone marrow. *Mod Pathol* 1990;3:348–356.

632. Barranger JA, Ginns EI. *Glucosylceramide Lipidoses: Gaucher's Disease.* New York: McGraw-Hill, 1989.

633. Brunning RD. Morphologic alterations in nucleated blood and marrow cells in genetic disorders. *Hum Pathol* 1970;1:99–124.

634. Peters SP, Lee RE, Glew RH. Gaucher's disease, a review. *Medicine (Baltimore)* 1977;56:425–442.

635. Lee RE. *The Pathology of Gaucher Disease.* New York: Alan R. Liss, 1982.

636. Parkin J, Brunning RD. *Pathology of the Gaucher Cell.* New York: Alan R. Liss, 1982.

637. Dosik H, Rosner F, Sawitsky A. Acquired lipidosis: Gaucher-like cells and "blue cells" in chronic granulocytic leukemia. *Semin Hematol* 1972;9:309–316.

638. Van Dorpe A, Broeckaert-van O, Desmet V, et al. Gaucher-like cells and congenital dyserythropoietic anaemia, type II (HEMPAS). *Br J Haematol* 1973;25:165–170.

639. Spence MW, Callahan JW. Sphingomyelin-cholesterol lipidoses: the Niemann-Pick group of disease. In Scriver CR, Beaudet AL, Sly WS, et al., eds. *The Metabolic Basis of Inherited Disease.* New York: McGraw-Hill, 1989:1655–1676.

640. McKenna RW, Dehner LP. Oxalosis. An unusual cause of myelophthisis in childhood. *Am J Clin Pathol* 1976;66:991–997.

641. Weiss LM, Grogan TM, Muller-Hermelink HK, et al. Langerhans cell histiocytosis. In Jaffe ES, Harris NL, Stein H, et al., eds. *World Health Organization Classification of Tumours Pathology and Genetics of Tumours of Haematopoietic and Lymphoid Tissues.* Lyon, France: IARC Press, 2001.

642. Willman CL, Busque L, Griffith BB, et al. Langerhans'-cell histiocytosis (histiocytosis X)—a clonal proliferative disease. *N Engl J Med* 1994;331:154–160.

643. Yu RC, Chu C, Buluwela L, et al. Clonal proliferation of Langerhans cells in Langerhans cell histiocytosis. *Lancet* 1994;343:767–768.

644. Favara BE, McCarthy RC, Mierau GW. Histiocytosis X. *Hum Pathol* 1983;14:663–676.

645. Favara BE. Langerhans' cell histiocytosis pathobiology and pathogenesis. *Semin Oncol* 1991;18:3–7.

646. Dehner LP. Morphologic findings in the histiocytic syndromes. *Semin Oncol* 1991;18:8–17.

647. Risdall RJ, Dehner LP, Duray P, et al. Histiocytosis X (Langerhans' cell histiocytosis). Prognostic role of histopathology. *Arch Pathol Lab Med* 1983;107:59–63.

648. McClain K, Ramsay NK, Robison L, et al. Bone marrow involvement in histiocytosis X. *Med Pediatr Oncol* 1983;11:167–171.

649. Nauert C, Zornoza J, Ayala A, et al. Eosinophilic granuloma of bone: diagnosis and management. *Skeletal Radiol* 1983;10:227–235.

650. Hage C, Willman CL, Favara BE, et al. Langerhans' cell histiocytosis (histiocytosis X): immunophenotype and growth fraction. *Hum Pathol* 1993;24:840–845.

651. Ide F, Iwase T, Saito I, et al. IHC and ultrastructural analysis of the proliferating cells in histiocytosis X. *Cancer* 1984;53:917–921.

652. Mierau GW, Favara BE. S-100 protein IHC and electron microscopy in the diagnosis of Langerhans cell proliferative disorders: a comparative assessment. *Ultrastruct Pathol* 1986;10:303–309.

653. Emile JF, Wechsler J, Brousse N, et al. Langerhans' cell histiocytosis. Definitive diagnosis with the use of monoclonal antibody O10 on routinely paraffin-embedded samples. *Am J Surg Pathol* 1995;19:636–641.

654. Risdall RJ, McKenna RW, Nesbit ME, et al. Virus-associated hemophagocytic syndrome: a benign histiocytic proliferation distinct from malignant histiocytosis. *Cancer* 1979;44:993–1002.

655. McKenna RW, Risdall RJ, Brunning RD. Virus associated hemophagocytic syndrome. *Hum Pathol* 1981;12:395–398.

656. Histiocytic medullary reticulosis. *Lancet* 1983;1:455–456.

657. McClain K, Gehrz R, Grierson H, et al. Virus-associated histiocytic proliferations in children. Frequent association with Epstein-Barr virus and congenital or acquired immunodeficiencies. *Am J Pediatr Hematol Oncol* 1988;10:196–205.

658. Henter JI, Elinder G, Ost A. Diagnostic guidelines for hemophagocytic lymphohistiocytosis. The FHL Study Group of the Histiocyte Society. *Semin Oncol* 1991;18:29–33.

659. Egeler RM, Shapiro R, Loechelt B, et al. Characteristic immune abnormalities in hemophagocytic lymphohistiocytosis. *J Pediatr Hematol Oncol* 1996;18:340–345.

660. Ohga S, Matsuzaki A, Nishizaki M, et al. Inflammatory cytokines in virus-associated hemophagocytic syndrome. Interferon-gamma as a sensitive indicator of disease activity. *Am J Pediatr Hematol Oncol* 1993;15:291–298.

661. Wong KF, Chan JK. Reactive hemophagocytic syndrome—a clinicopathologic study of 40 patients in an Oriental population. *Am J Med* 1992;93:177–180.

662. Falini B, Pileri S, De Solas I, et al. Peripheral T-cell lymphoma associated with hemophagocytic syndrome. *Blood* 1990;75:434–444.

663. Loy TS, Diaz-Arias AA, Perry MC. Familial erythrophagocytic lymphohistiocytosis. *Semin Oncol* 1991;18:34–38.

664. Janka GE. Familial and acquired hemophagocytic lymphohistiocytosis. *Eur J Pediatr* 2007; 166:95–109.

665. Filipovich AH. Hemophagocytic lymphohistiocytosis and related disorders. *Curr Opin Allergy Clin Immunol* 2006;6:410–415.

666. Stepp SE, Dufourcq-Lagelouse R, Le Deist F, et al. Perforin gene defects in familial hemophagocytic lymphohistiocytosis. *Science* 1999;286:1957–1959.

667. Arico M, Janka G, Fischer A, et al. Hemophagocytic lymphohistiocytosis. Report of 122 children from the International Registry. FHL Study Group of the Histiocyte Society. *Leukemia* 1996;10:197–203.

668. Henter JI, Elinder G, Soder O, et al. Hypercytokinemia in familial hemophagocytic lymphohistiocytosis. *Blood* 1991;78:2918–2922.

669. Egeler RM, Schmitz L, Sonneveld P, et al. Malignant histiocytosis: a reassessment of cases formerly classified as histiocytic neoplasms and review of the literature. *Med Pediatr Oncol* 1995;25:1–7.

670. Arai E, Su WP, Roche PC, et al. Cutaneous histiocytic malignancy. IHC re-examination of cases previously diagnosed as cutaneous "histiocytic lymphoma" and "malignant histiocytosis." *J Cutan Pathol* 1993;20:115–120.

671. van der Valk P, van Oostveen JW, Stel HV, et al. Phenotypic and genotypic analysis of large-cell lymphomas, formerly classified as true histiocytic lymphoma: identification of an unusual group of tumors. *Leuk Res* 1990;14:337–346.

672. Wilson MS, Weiss LM, Gatter KC, et al. Malignant histiocytosis. A reassessment of cases previously reported in 1975 based on paraffin section immunophenotyping studies. *Cancer* 1990;66:530–536.

673. Hutchison RE, Kurec AS, Davey FR. Granulocytic sarcoma. *Clin Lab Med* 1990;10:889–901.

674. Brunning RD, Matutes E, Flandrin G, et al. Acute myeloid leukaemia, not otherwise categorised. In Jaffe ES, Harris NL, Stein H, et al., eds. *World Health Organization Classification of Tumours. Pathology and Genetics of Tumours of Haematopoietic and Lymphoid Tissues.* Lyon, France: IARC Press, 2001:91–105.

675. Laurencet FM, Chapuis B, Roux-Lombard P, et al. Malignant histiocytosis in the leukaemic stage: a new entity (M5c-AML) in the FAB classification? *Leukemia* 1994;8:502–506.

676. Esteve J, Rozman M, Campo E, et al. Leukemia after true histiocytic lymphoma: another type of acute monocytic leukemia with histiocytic differentiation (AML-M5c)? *Leukemia* 1995;9:1389–1391.

677. Hornick JL, Jaffe ES, Fletcher CD. Extranodal histiocytic sarcoma: clinicopathologic analysis of 14 cases of a rare epithelioid malignancy. *Am J Surg Pathol* 2004;28:1133–1144.

678. Frisch B, Bartl R, Mahl G, et al. Scope and value of bone marrow biopsies in metastatic cancer. *Inv Metastasis* 1984;4[Suppl 1]:12–30.

679. Gale PF, Mckenna RW. Monitoring metastasis in bone marrow. In Stoll BA, ed. *Screening and Monitoring of Cancer.* Chichester, England: John Wiley, 1985:265–283.

680. Singh G, Krause JR, Breitfeld V. Bone marrow examination: for metastatic tumor: aspirate and biopsy. *Cancer* 1977;40:2317–2321.

681. Savage RA, Hoffman GC, Shaker K. Diagnostic problems involved in detection of metastatic neoplasms by bone-marrow aspirate compared with needle biopsy. *Am J Clin Pathol* 1978;70:623–627.

682. Jakoubkova J, Hermanska Z, Bek V. Reaction of the bone marrow in malignant tumours of the kidney and testis. *Neoplasma* 1970;17:427–431.

683. Cramer SF, Fried L, Carter KJ. The cellular basis of metastatic bone disease in patients with lung cancer. *Cancer* 1981;48:2649–2660.

684. Galasko CS. Mechanisms of lytic and blastic metastatic disease of bone. *Clin Orthop* 1982; 20–27.

685. Keen JC, Davidson NE. The biology of breast carcinoma. *Cancer* 2003;97:825–833.

686. Rubins JM. The role of myelofibrosis in malignant leukoerythroblastosis. *Cancer* 1983;51: 308–311.

687. Kiang DT, McKenna RW, Kennedy BJ. Reversal of myelofibrosis in advanced breast cancer. *Am J Med* 1978;64:173–176.

688. Colvin BT, Revell PA, Ibbotson RM, et al. Necrosis of bone marrow and bone in malignant disease. *Clin Oncol* 1980;6:265–272.

689. Osborne MP, Asina S, Wong GY, et al. Immunofluorescent monoclonal antibody detection of breast cancer in bone marrow: sensitivity in a model system. *Cancer Res* 1989;49: 2510–2513.

690. Moss TJ, Reynolds CP, Sather HN, et al. Prognostic value of immunocytologic detection of bone marrow metastases in neuroblastoma. *N Engl J Med* 1991;324:219–226.

691. Bitter MA, Fiorito D, Corkill ME, et al. Bone marrow involvement by lobular carcinoma of the breast cannot be identified reliably by routine histological examination alone. *Hum Pathol* 1994;25:781–788.

692. Anner RM, Drewinko B. Frequency and significance of bone marrow involvement by metastatic solid tumors. *Cancer* 1977;39:1337–1344.

693. Ridell B, Landys K. Incidence and histopathology of metastases of mammary carcinoma in biopsies from the posterior iliac crest. *Cancer* 1979;44:1782–1788.

694. Ingle JN, Tormey DC, Tan HK. The bone marrow examination in breast cancer: diagnostic considerations and clinical usefulness. *Cancer* 1978;41:670–674.

695. Landys K. Prognostic value of bone marrow biopsy in breast cancer. *Cancer* 1982;49: 513–518.

696. Hansen HH, Muggia FM, Selawry OS. Bone-marrow examination in 100 consecutive patients with bronchogenic carcinoma. *Lancet* 1971;2:443–445.

697. Hirsch F, Hansen HH, Dombernowsky P, et al. Bone-marrow examination in the staging of small-cell anaplastic carcinoma of the lung with special reference to subtyping. An evaluation of 203 consecutive patients. *Cancer* 1977;39:2563–2567.

698. Duchek M, Lingardh G, Saterborg NE, et al. Bone marrow examination as a diagnostic tool in carcinoma of the prostate. *Int Urol Nephrol* 1975;7:59–64.

699. Delta BG, Pinkel D. Bone marrow aspiration in children with malignant tumors. *J Pediatr* 1964;64:542–546.

700. Finklestein JZ, Ekert H, Isaacs H, Jr., et al. Bone marrow metastases in children with solid tumors. *Am J Dis Child* 1970;119:49–52.

701. Marsden HB, Lennox EL, Lawler W, et al. Bone metastases in childhood renal tumours. *Br J Cancer* 1980;41:875–879.

702. Frisch B, Lewis SM, Burkhardt R, et al. *Biopsy Pathology of Bone and Bone Marrow.* New York: Raven Press, 1985:88–107.

John B. Cousar
William R. Macon
Thomas L. McCurley
Steven H. Swerdlow

CHAPTER 17

Lymph Nodes

Lymph nodes are organized into anatomic and functional sub-compartments and serve as the critical meeting place for antigens derived from pathogens, antigen-presenting cells, and naïve B- and T-cells. They are the site of clonal expansion and differentiation of lymphocytes necessary for an effective adaptive immune response. Lymphocyte proliferation and differentiation (somatic mutation, class switching, etc.) also may lead to the translocations and point mutations underlying most lymphomas (1–3).

Nodes may be the only site of disease; however, many nodal diseases are related to abnormalities in the organ associated with the abnormal node. Nodal diseases are complex because of the large number of diseases reaching nodes via lymph and because of the inherent complexity of the immune system and its own diseases. Nevertheless, there is an order and predictability to node diseases; in general, they follow the same rules in terms of tissue analysis and diagnosis that apply to other tissues. The basic questions pathologists first attempt to answer when studying node biopsies are addressed in the introductory section: Is the process reactive or neoplastic, and what is the general characterization of the neoplastic process? Discussions of these questions follow sections on guidelines and basic techniques in node examination and a brief description of classification of node diseases.

NODE EXAMINATION: GUIDELINES AND BASIC TECHNIQUES

Most mistakes in node examination are made because of (a) pathologists' unfamiliarity with certain nodal diseases, (b) inadequate sampling, or (c) improper processing of nodal specimens. Improper processing is the culprit in most cases—despite attestations by hematopathologists that recognition of many nodal diseases depends on ideal tissue processing.

Ideal processing requires fresh, intact tissue and a laboratory protocol that is followed in all biopsies. Success of biopsy (in terms of reaching the correct diagnosis) is greatly facilitated by consulting surgeons who are experienced in evaluating lymphadenopathy and cognizant of the importance of node biopsy. Node biopsy is deceptive in its apparent simplicity. All nodes are not affected equally in a given patient. Disease often increases nodal fragility, and removal of intact nodes in these cases requires skill and patience. A protocol modified from that developed by Collins (4) for handling fresh tissue has the following essential components:

1. Frozen sections are not usually performed on nodes suspected of being involved by a lymphoproliferative process. Diagnostic material may be irretrievably damaged by freezing. Touch imprints are strongly recommended as an alternative for ensuring that diagnostic material has been obtained and for guiding immunologic, molecular genetic, and cytogenetic studies, if needed.

2. Nodes are cut across the long axis; node poles are used for cultures and cell-suspension flow cytometry studies.

3. Representative samples are routinely frozen and stored for immunologic and molecular genetic studies. Fresh material should also be obtained for cytogenetic studies, particularly in cases such as Burkitt lymphoma, anaplastic large-cell lymphoma, and others.

4. In the past, fixatives containing mercuric chloride (i.e., B5 fixative) were used to accentuate sharp nuclear detail, but these are less commonly employed today due to problems in disposing of mercury. Neutral buffered formalin and zinc formalin solutions are acceptable, as long as fixation time is adequate and sections are thin. Sections stained with hematoxylin and eosin (H&E) are routinely prepared.

5. All immunologic, molecular, and cytogenetic data are integrated with histopathologic findings to produce a final diagnosis in the final report. Separate interpretations of immunologic/genetic and histopathologic data often lead to mistaken diagnoses at worst and clinical confusion at best.

6. Phenotypic analyses are not performed routinely on all node biopsies. Immunohistochemistry (IHC) of paraffin-embedded tissue sections is an essential component of many nodal examinations, especially in diagnosing large-cell lymphomas, including diffuse large-B-cell lymphoma and anaplastic large-cell lymphoma, many cases of Hodgkin lymphoma (HL), lymphomas with plasmacytic differentiation, and subclassification of neoplastic proliferations of small lymphocytes. (Fig. 17.1) In addition, IHC is an important adjunct

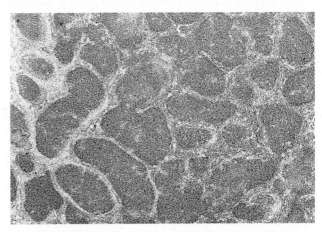

Figure 17.1. Lymph node, follicular lymphoma. The potential of immunoperoxidase for identifying lymphoid populations in situ is illustrated. Anti-CD20, a B-cell marker, delineates the follicular architecture. This marker is very helpful in evaluating B-cell processes. Paraffin immunoperoxidase with diaminobenzidine substrate.

for evaluating suspected T-cell lymphomas and to rule out B-cell lymphomas with a high percentage of reactive T-cells. Phenotyping is not necessary for diagnosis of most follicular lymphomas, but it may be useful in assessing recurrences. Some of the most useful antibodies for evaluating lymphomas by IHC are given in Table 17.1, and several recent reviews (5,6) on the application of IHC in the diagnosis of lymphomas are available.

Flow cytometric evaluation is valuable and available to most community hospitals. This technique is particularly helpful for analyzing small lymphocytic infiltrates and leukemic processes. Sampling errors and excessive cell fragility may minimize its sensitivity in phenotyping large-cell lymphomas; the various HLs are more specifically recognized by IHC techniques.

7. Polymerase chain reaction (PCR) has rapidly moved from a research technique to a very valuable method in clinical hematology, with applications ranging from detection to molecular characterization and management of various disorders (7). Because large quantities of relatively pure DNA sequences may be produced, this technique sets new standards for sensitivity and perhaps for specificity. The starting material for amplification can be crude DNA rather than purified; it is noteworthy that PCR has been successfully performed on an extremely small number of cells (approximately 100) as well as on paraffin-embedded biopsy specimens.

DNA is stable in tissues for long periods, and its presence can be verified in archival material, whereas RNA detection requires optimal tissue preparation and fixation.

PCR has been used to detect mutant genes, oncogenes, and minimal residual malignancy. It is perhaps in the latter area that the sensitivity of PCR is most apparent; PCR has detected tumor DNA equivalent to the presence of 0.001% tumor cells. The technique has been particularly useful in recognizing the presence of residual disease in follicular lymphoma and chronic myeloid leukemia.

The extreme sensitivity of PCR does have a negative aspect. The slightest contamination of starting materials, reagents, or equipment can lead to amplification of unwanted DNA and false results. However, PCR is now widely used in clinical practice as well as research institutes for diagnosis and management of hematologic disorders. The most frequently used PCR-based tests for evaluation of primary lymph node disorders are T-cell receptor gamma and immunoglobulin heavy chain gene rearrangement assays to determine T- or B-cell clonality, respectively.

8. Conventional karyotyping is valuable in detecting translocations that, in part, define certain lymphomas, such as t(11;14)(q13;q32) in mantle cell lymphoma, t(14;18)(q32;q21) in follicular lymphomas, and translocations involving the MYC gene at chromosome 8q24 in Burkitt lymphoma. In addition, karyotyping will detect other translocations, deletions, etc. that are indicative of more complex molecular changes.

Fluorescence in situ hybridization (FISH) is being employed more frequently because it can be performed on metaphases of intact cell nuclei and is applicable to paraffin-embedded tissues. FISH is especially helpful in detection of the translocations associated with mantle cell lymphoma and Burkitt lymphoma.

9. Fine-needle aspiration (FNA) of nodes, despite inherent sampling problems, has the potential to provide rapid diagnosis in those patients with carcinomas, some infections, and some lymphomas. FNA is particularly useful in patients who are not suitable candidates for excisional biopsies (8). Material from FNA can be used for essentially all of the special studies obtainable on larger biopsies, and virtually all node groups can be sampled. The diagnostic accuracy of FNA has been summarized as ranging from 83% to 96% in lymphadenopathy of all types, 80% to 90% in lymphomas, and 90% to 96% in carcinomas (8). Subclassification of lymphomas and grading, however, seem particularly challenging on FNA-obtained samples, given the legendary difficulties in these areas using traditional samples. FNA has been especially useful in evaluating recurrence in deep-seated nodes in patients previously diagnosed as having lymphoma.

The Association of Directors of Anatomic and Surgical Pathology recently developed recommendations for the reporting of lymphoid neoplasms which include background clinical information, gross description, diagnostic information, and immunophenotypic, molecular, viral, and cytogenetic ancillary data (9).

CLASSIFICATION OF NODE DISEASES

Reactive states are most logically categorized by the various etiologic factors responsible for adenopathy. The recognition of specific reactive disorders is greatly facilitated by analyzing histopathologic abnormalities in relation to architectural features (see "Reactive Adenopathy").

Various classifications of malignant lymphomas have been used during the past 25 years. In 1994, the International Lymphoma Study Group proposed a classification of lymphoid neoplasms that appear to be distinct entities, based on morphologic, immunologic, and genetic features (10). Many of these entities have characteristic clinical symptoms. This system was named the Revised European-American Classification of Lymphoid Neoplasms, or REAL.

The World Health Organization (WHO) developed a new classification of lymphomas and leukemias in 2001, which was based in part on the earlier REAL classification (11). This classification has gained wide acceptance. The WHO classification was updated in 2008 and Table 17.2 is a partial listing of the classification, which only B-cell, T/NK-cell, Hodgkin, and histiocytic/dendritic cell neoplasms and immunodeficiency-associated proliferation includes (11a). Only nodal lymphomas are discussed in detail in this chapter; the reader is referred to other appropriate chapters for discussion of extranodal lymphomas and leukemias. The approach of the WHO classification is comparable to those of the systems used to classify all other neoplasms and has the following advantages:

1. Lymphomas are neoplasms of the immune system; an understanding of their appearance, behavior, and pathogenesis will ultimately come from coordinated analyses of the biology of normal cells and their neoplastic counterparts.

2. The WHO classification is based on integrating histopathologic, immunologic, molecular genetic, and cytogenetic data to reach diagnoses. Although many lymphomas have characteristic and, in many cases, specific histopathologic features, ancillary data in other cases provide useful additional information or are required for diagnosis. Using this approach, many types of lymphoma have distinct clinical expressions.

TABLE 17.1		Commonly Used Antibodies in Immunohistochemical Procedures in Paraffin-Embedded Tissue Sections and Corresponding Reactivity Patterns[a]	
Category	*CD Antigen or Antibody*	*Reactivity in Normal Cells*	*Reactivity in Hematopoietic-Lymphoid Neoplasms*
Pan-leukocyte	CD45	B cells, most T cells, macrophages, and granulocytes	Most non-Hodgkin lymphomas and leukemias
B-cell–related	CD10	Precursor B cells, follicular-center B cells, and some follicular-center T cells	Many precursor B lymphoblastic leukemias/lymphomas; some precursor T lymphoblastic leukemias/lymphomas; many follicular lymphomas; Burkitt lymphoma; some DLBCL; angioimmunoblastic T-cell lymphoma
	CD20	B cells	Most B NHL, L&H RS cell in LPHL; RS cells in some cases of classic HL
	CD21	Mantle and marginal zone B cells, FDC	Some mantle and marginal lymphomas; follicular dendritic cell tumors
	CD23	Mantle zone B cells; some FDC	Chronic lymphocytic leukemia/small lymphocytic lymphoma
	CD45RA	B cells and subset of T cells	B-cell NHL; L&H cells in LPHL; some T-cell lymphoid and myeloid leukemias
	CD79a	B cells	Most B-cell NHL and many B-cell leukemias
	CD138	Plasma cells; some epithelial cells and fibroblasts	Plasma cell neoplasms; some variants of DLBCL
	Bcl-6	Mainly germinal center B cells; some T cells	Follicular lymphoma; Burkitt lymphoma, some DLBCL; some T-cell lymphomas, L&H cells of LPHL
	MUM1	Plasma cells; rare germinal-center B cells; some T cells	Plasma cell neoplasms; many DLBCL; Hodgkin lymphoma; ALCL; primary effusion lymphoma
	PAX5	Many B cells	Most B-NHL; L&H cells in LPHL; RS cells in classic Hodgkin lymphoma; some acute myeloid leukemias
	Anti-immunoglobulin heavy and light chains	B cells, plasma cells	B-cell NHL and plasma cell neoplasms
T-cell–related	CD1a	Cortical thymocytes and Langerhans cells	Precursor T-cell lymphoblastic leukemia/lymphoma; Langerhans cell histiocytosis
	CD2	T and NK cells	Many T-cell lymphomas and leukemias
	CD3	T cells	Most T-cell neoplasms
	CD5	T cells and subset of small B cells	Many T-cell lymphomas and leukemias and subset of diffuse small-B-cell neoplasms, such as small lymphocytic lymphoma/chronic lymphocytic leukemia and mantle cell lymphoma
	CD7	Most T cells and NK cells	Many T-cell lymphomas and leukemias
	CD43	T cells, some macrophages, granulocytes, and plasma cells	Most T-cell lymphomas; some B-cell lymphomas; acute myeloid leukemias, and plasma cell neoplasms
	CD45RO	Most T cells, some macrophages, some myeloid cells	Most T-cell lymphomas; some B-cell lymphomas
	CD57	Some NK cells, subset of T cells	Some NK- and T-cell lymphomas/leukemias and some lymphoblastic lymphomas
	βF1 (β chain of T-cell receptor)	T cells	Many T-cell lymphomas
Hodgkin-related	CD15	Granulocytes and some macrophages	RS cells in most cases of NS, MC, and LDHL; some T and B large-cell lymphomas; some carcinomas
	CD30	Activated B and T cells, plasma cells	RS cells in most cases of NS, MC, and LDHL; most cases of ALCL; other T- and B-cell NHL
Miscellaneous	CD34	Progenitor cells	Some acute myeloid leukemias and some precursor lymphoblastic leukemias/lymphomas
	CD56	NK cells, few T cells	Many NK-cell neoplasms
	CD68	Macrophages and granulocytes	True malignant histocytosis; many myeloid leukemias
	S-100	Langerhans cells, IDRC, sometimes FDC	Langerhans cell histiocytes, sinus histiocytosis with massive lymphadenopathy; rare T-cell lymphomas, myeloid leukemias
	Tdt	Precursor marrow cells, cortical thymocytes	Most precursor B- or T-lymphoblastic leukemias/lymphomas; some acute myeloid leukemias
	Ki-67	Proliferating cells (not in GO phase of cell cycle)	Proliferating cells

(continued)

TABLE 17.1	Commonly Used Antibodies in Immunohistochemical Procedures in Paraffin-Embedded Tissue Sections and Corresponding Reactivity Patterns[a] *(continued)*		
Category	CD Antigen or Antibody	Reactivity in Normal Cells	Reactivity in Hematopoietic-Lymphoid Neoplasms
	Myeloperoxidase	Myeloid cells	Myeloid leukemias
	bcl-2	Nonfollicular-center B cells, T cells	Most follicular lymphomas; many other diffuse NHL and leukemias
	Epithelial membrane antigen	Various epithelia, plasma cells	L&H RS cells in LPHL; plasma cell neoplasms; anaplastic large-cell lymphoma; some other B and T large-cell NHL and many epithelial tumors
	Cyclin D1	Minimal to no expression in normal lymphoid cells	Mantle cell lymphoma, hairy cell leukemia, and some cases of myeloma
	ALK1	No expression in normal tissue	Most cases of T or null ALCL; rare cases of DLBCL
	CXCL13	Some T cells, dendritic cells and histiocytes in germinal centers; some T cells, histiocytes in paracortex	
	Langerin (CD207)	Langerhans cells	Langerhans cell neoplasms

ALCL, anaplastic large-cell lymphoma; DLBCL, diffuse large-B-cell lymphoma; FDC, follicular dendritic cell; LDHL, lymphocyte-depletion Hodgkin lymphoma; L&H, lymphocytic and histiocytic; LPHL, lymphocyte-predominance Hodgkin lymphoma; MC, mixed cellularity; NHL, non-Hodgkin lymphoma; NK, natural killer; NS, nodular sclerosis; RS, Reed-Sternberg.
[a]Modified from: Arber DA, Cousar JB. Hematopoietic tumors: principles of pathologic diagnosis. In *Wintrobe's Clinical Hematology.* 12th ed. (2009).

Furthermore, virtually all current research on lymphomas is of a multiparameter nature and particularly deals with immunologic, molecular genetic, or karyotypic features.

3. All classifications of lymphomas are incomplete; the number of significant clinical-pathologic entities yet to be recognized is unknown, and classifications must have a conceptual framework that facilitates incorporation of newly recognized entities in relationship to their presumed cell of origin.

DIFFERENTIATION BETWEEN REACTIVE AND NEOPLASTIC STATES

Neoplasms arising in nodes resemble other malignant neoplasms in that lymphomas are clonal; usually produce invasive tumorous masses that destroy architecture; and are often composed of monomorphic growths. Neoplastic cells may show cytologic atypia. In contrast, reactive states are usually not clonal; they distort rather than efface architecture (Fig. 17.2); they contain polymorphic mixtures of cells; and they show minimal, if any, cytologic atypia.

One of the most reliable criteria of malignancy is the presence of mass lesions detected by low-magnification examination (Fig. 17.3). Lymphoproliferative processes that fail to produce mass lesions and architectural effacement should be considered benign unless there is clear cytologic or immunologic evidence of malignancy. Note that some lymphomas partially involve nodes; portions of nodes may be normal when lymphoma is present elsewhere.

High-magnification features suggesting a benign process include mixtures of cell types; in contrast, monomorphic processes are likely to be neoplastic. Dysplasia may be recognized in well-prepared material and is an indicator of malignancy (Fig. 17.4).

There are many exceptions to these general rules. In practice, we diagnose malignancy only when there is convincing histopathologic evidence; the recognition of such diagnostic

lesions is greatly facilitated by thorough familiarity with the various reactive and neoplastic disorders covered in this chapter.

Immunologic and molecular genetic studies are particularly useful in evaluating small lymphocytic infiltrates. Clonal processes (as inferred by light-chain restriction or abnormal phenotypes or demonstrated by gene rearrangements) are generally thought to be neoplastic, but the increasing sensitivity of these immunophenotypic and genotypic tests may make them less specific as indicators of malignancy. Caution is always advised in the overinterpretation of clonality because nagging exceptions exist with many of these guidelines. Aneuploidy or abnormal karyotypes indicate malignancy but often are not routinely assessed.

GUIDELINES FOR DIFFERENTIATION BETWEEN HODGKIN LYMPHOMA AND OTHER LYMPHOMAS

HL is the term applied to several clinical-pathologic entities. There are histopathologic and clinical differences between these groups, and the immunologic features of the neoplastic cells in the subtypes vary as well. The features held in common by these neoplasms are distinctive reaction patterns (referring not only to the low-magnification appearance but also to the reactive cellular components) and the presence of various dysplastic tumor cells; for example, Reed-Sternberg (RS) cells or their variants. Of these two, the reaction pattern is more distinctive because dysplastic cells similar in appearance (and perhaps with identical immunologic features) may be found in a variety of reactive states and non-Hodgkin lymphoma (NHL). There is no specific structural or functional marker of RS cells, and it seems unlikely that such a marker will be found in the future. We emphasize, therefore, the importance of recognizing reaction patterns in diagnosing and classifying HL.

For instance, in nodular lymphocyte-predominant HL

TABLE 17.2	**2008 World Health Organization Classification of B-Cell, T–Cell, NK-cell, and Histiocytic/Dendritic Neoplasms**

Precursor Lymphoid Neoplasms

B-lymphoblastic leukaemia/lymphoma
B-lymphoblastic leukaemia/lymphoma, not otherwise specified
B-lymphoblastic leukaemia/lymphoma with recurrent genetic abnormalities
   B-lymphoblastic leukaemia/lymphoma with t(9;22)(q34;q11.2); BCR-ABL1
   B-lymphoblastic leukaemia/lymphoma with t(V;11q23); MLL rearranged
   B-lymphoblastic leukaemia/lymphoma with t(12;21)(p13;q22); TEL-AML-1 (ETV6-RUNX1)
   B-lymphoblastic leukaemia/lymphoma with hyperdiploidy
   B-lymphoblastic leukaemia/lymphoma with hypodiploidy (hypodiploid ALL)
   B-lymphoblastic leukaemia/lymphoma with t(5;14)(q31;q32); (IL3-IGH)
   B-lymphoblastic leukaemia/lymphoma with t(1;19)(q23;p13.3); (E2A-PBX1; TCF3/PBX1)
T-lymphoblastic leukaemia/lymphoma

Mature B-Cell Neoplasms

Chronic lymphocytic leukemia /small-cell lymphocytic lymphoma
B-cell prolymphocytic leukemia
Splenic B-cell marginal zone lymphoma
Hairy cell leukemia
Splenic lymphoma/leukemia, unclassifiable
   Splenic diffuse red pulp small-B-cell lymphoma[a]
   Hairy cell leukemia—variant[a]
Lymphoplasmacytic lymphoma
   Waldenström macroglobulinemia
Heavy chain diseases
  Alpha heavy chain disease
  Gamma heavy chain disease
  Mu heavy chain disease
Plasma cell myeloma
Solitary plasmacytoma of bone
Extraosseous plasmacytoma
Extranodal marginal zone lymphoma of mucosa-associated lymphoid tissue (MALT lymphoma)
Nodal marginal zone lymphoma
   Pediatric nodal MZL
Follicular lymphoma
   Pediatric follicular lymphoma
Primary cutaneous follicle center lymphoma
Mantle cell lymphoma
Diffuse large B-cell lymphoma (DLBCL), not otherwise specified
   T-cell/histiocyte-rich large-B-cell lymphoma
   Primary DLBCL of the CNS
   EBV+ DLBCL of the elderly
   DLBCL associated with chronic inflammation
Lymphomatoid granulomatosis
Primary mediastinal (thymic) large-B-cell lymphoma
Intravascular large-B-cell lymphoma
   Primary cutaneous DLBCL, leg type
ALK positive large B-cell lymphoma
Plasmablastic lymphoma
Large-B-cell lymphoma arising in HHV8-associated multicentric Castleman disease
Primary effusion lymphoma
Burkitt lymphoma
B-cell lymphoma, unclassifiable, with features intermediate between diffuse large B-cell lymphoma and Burkitt lymphoma
B-cell lymphoma, unclassifiable, with features intermediate between diffuse large B-cell lymphoma and classical Hodgkin lymphoma

Mature T-Cell and NK-Cell Neoplasms

T-cell prolymphocytic leukemia
T-cell large granular lymphocytic leukemia
Chronic lymphoproliferative disorder of NK-cells[9]
Aggressive NK-cell leukemia
Systemic EBV+ T-cell lymphoproliferative disease of childhood

(continued)

TABLE 17.2	2008 World Health Organization Classification of B-Cell, T-Cell, NK-Cells, and Histiocytic/Dendritic Neoplasms

Hydroa vacciforme-like lymphoma
Adult T-cell leukemia/lymphoma
Extranodal NK/T-cell lymphoma, nasal type
Enteropathy-associated T-cell lymphoma
Hepatosplenic T-cell lymphoma
Subcutaneous panniculitis-like T-cell lymphoma
Mycosis fungoides
Sézary syndrome
Primary cutaneous CD30 positive T-cell lymphoproliferative disorders lymphomatoid & papulosis
    Primary cutaneous anaplastic large-cell lymphoma
Primary cutaneous gamma-delta T-cell lymphoma
Primary cutaneous CD8-positive aggressive epidermotropic cytotoxic T-cell lymphoma[a]
Primary cutaneous CD4 positive small/medium T-cell lymphoma[a]
Peripheral T-cell lymphoma, not otherwise specified
Angioimmunoblastic T-cell lymphoma
Anaplastic large-cell lymphoma, ALK positive
Anaplastic large-cell lymphoma, ALK negative[a]

Hodgkin Lymphoma

Nodular lymphocyte-predominant Hodgkin lymphoma
Classic Hodgkin lymphoma
    Nodular-sclerosis classic Hodgkin lymphoma
    Lymphocyte-rich classic Hodgkin lymphoma
    Mixed-cellularity classic Hodgkin lymphoma
    Lymphocyte-depleted classic Hodgkin lymphoma

Histiocytic and Dendritic Cell Neoplasms

Histiocytic sarcoma
Langerhans cell histiocytosis
Langerhans cell sarcoma
Interdigitating dendritic cell sarcoma
Follicular dendritic cell sarcoma
Fibroblastic reticular cell tumor
Indeterminate dendritic cell tumor
Disseminated juvenile xanthogranuloma

PostTransplant Lymphoproliferative Disorders (PTLD)

Early lesions
    Plasmacytic hyperplasia PTLD
    Infectious mononucleosis-like
Polymorphic PTLD
Monomorphic PTLD (B- and T/NK-cell types)[b]
Classical Hodgkin lymphoma type PTLD[b]

[a]These are provisional entities[b] for which the WHO Working Group felt there was insufficient, evidence to fully recognize as distinct diseases at this time.
[b]These lesions are classified according to the leukaemic or lymphome to which they correspond.

(NLPHL), the low-magnification appearance is distinctive. The combination of large nodules and a compressed adjacent uninvolved node is almost, in itself, diagnostic of NLPHL. Cellular components in this disease include small lymphocytes, scattered histiocytes, a few giant cells, and lymphocytic and histiocytic (L&H) RS cell variants.

Most cases of nodular-sclerosing classic HL (NSHL) show characteristic cellular nodules demarcated by broad bands of refractile connective tissue when viewed with polarized light. The composition of the cellular nodules is quite variable; there are considerable differences in the number of RS cells as well as the

type and number of reacting cells. Sheets of mononuclear RS cell variants are particularly troublesome because they may lead to mistaken diagnoses of metastatic carcinoma or some of the NHLs.

IHC may be very helpful in diagnosing HL, although the findings are not specific. In NLPHL, the reacting component contains numerous B cells, and the L&H variants are typically positive for CD45 (leukocyte common antigen [LCA]) and negative for CD15. In NSHL, RS cell variants are usually CD45−, CD15+, and CD30+ (membrane and Golgi staining pattern). Reactive lymphocytes are usually T cells.

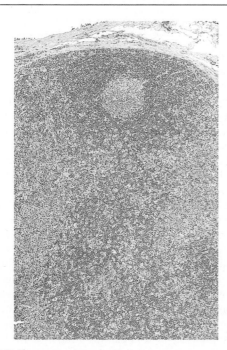

Figure 17.2. Lymph node, infectious mononucleosis. This low-magnification view shows expansion of an interfollicular area surrounding a preserved follicular center.

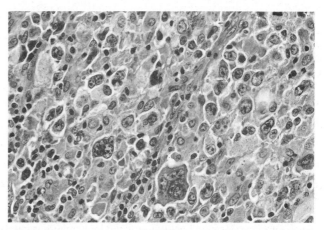

Figure 17.4. Lymph node, malignant lymphoma. This high-magnification photomicrograph shows dysplasia of transformed lymphocytes with abnormal nuclear profiles. Cells with these atypical nuclear configurations usually are not seen in reactive processes.

HL is usually easily distinguished from NHL using the criteria described herein; the most reliable feature is the growth pattern of the lymphoma. NLPHL and NSHL have characteristic low-magnification appearances, as do follicular lymphomas producing neoplastic follicles (Fig. 17.5). Pathologists must also be aware of the typical sclerosing growth pattern in follicular lymphomas. It must be emphasized that the low-magnification appearance of these three lymphomas is virtually diagnostic, but in some cases IHC is necessary to differentiate HL from other lymphomas. Diffuse processes are more troublesome and are described in more detail in the sections dealing with the various NHLs.

Certain cytologic criteria are helpful in distinguishing HL from other lymphomas. In most B-cell NHLs, a uniform appearance of the predominant cell and the inapparent reactive component indicate an NHL. Many lymphomas, as well as reactive processes, contain large transformed lymphocytes that may resemble RS cells. There are no specific cytologic features that identify binucleate or dysplastic cells as RS cells, although prominent nucleoli are often impressive in RS cells. The appropriate reaction pattern is a more reliable indicator of HL than the cytologic features of RS cells.

Immunologic studies are often helpful in recognizing lymphomas other than HL because most of them have B-cell features and are thereby recognizable by monotypic surface or

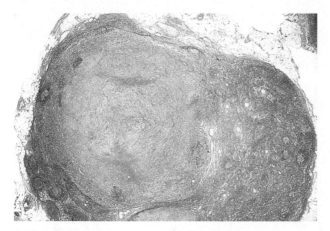

Figure 17.3. Lymph node, nodular-sclerosing Hodgkin lymphoma. This low-magnification view shows a clearly defined nodule of tumor with consolidation and compression of adjacent nodal tissue. Lesions of this type are highly suggestive of malignant lymphomas.

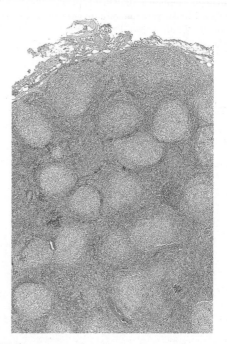

Figure 17.5. Lymph node, follicular lymphoma. Neoplastic follicular nodules, as shown in this low-magnification photomicrograph, are diagnostic of follicular-center cell lymphomas; their recognition allows specific histopathologic and immunologic characterization of an important type of malignant lymphoma.

cytoplasmic immunoglobulin. NHLs usually confused with HL on the basis of immunologic studies are peripheral T-cell lymphomas and certain B-cell lymphomas containing high percentages of T lymphocytes (T-cell–rich B-cell lymphomas). The former is confused with HL because of the high percentage of reacting T cells in HL, whereas the latter is confused with HL because the monotypic B-cell population is not detectable or is obscured by the high percentage of T cells.

GUIDELINES FOR DIFFERENTIATION AMONG LYMPHOMAS, CARCINOMAS, HISTIOCYTOSES, AND LEUKEMIAS

Diagnosis of carcinomas, histiocytoses, and leukemias has been enormously facilitated by IHC procedures. Most carcinomas are identified (Fig. 17.6) and even classified with these techniques. The great majority of histiocytoses, dendritic neoplasms, and myeloid sarcomas require immunoperoxidase stains, such as CD1a, S-100, Langerins (CD207), CD68, CD21, and myeloperoxidase, to confirm the histopathologic impression.

By light microscopy, the correct diagnosis may be suggested by the cohesion of carcinoma cells and the involvement of lymphatics; by the tendency of leukemic infiltrates to surround lymphoid aggregates; and by sinus involvement in histiocytoses. The last feature is not specific because both carcinomas and certain lymphomas show preferential sinus involvement. Phagocytosis of erythrocytes is not a specific marker of malignant histiocytes.

REACTIVE ADENOPATHY

Reactive adenopathy is significant because of its incidence; because some patients have clinical or histopathologic features that mimic malignant lymphoma; and, finally, because reactive adenopathy may precede lymphoma (12). Histopathologic examination in reactive adenopathy has been supplemented by immunopathologic and molecular genetic techniques for identification of cell phenotypes, etiologic agents, and clonality. Such studies have increased the precision of diagnosis in many cases, but have also raised questions as to whether clonal processes are always neoplastic and polyclonal ones are always benign (13,14). The answer to both questions is "No." Rare patients with follicular hyperplasias have lymphoid cells that mark monotypically and yet have a benign clinical course with resolution of adenopathy (15,16). Small, circulating, clonal T-cell populations and benign monoclonal gammopathies are very common in the elderly (17,18). On the other hand, B-cell lymphomas in renal transplant patients may be immunophenotypically polyclonal and are notoriously aggressive (19). Molecular genetic studies have demonstrated clonal proliferations of B or T lymphocytes in histopathologically reactive lesions in Sjögren syndrome (20) and HIV infection (21). These studies might identify the patients at greatest risk for lymphoma, but clonal proliferations do not always progress to malignancy (14,22).

Reactive processes are best analyzed by their architectural features rather than etiologic factors (Table 17.3). Processes causing follicular hyperplasia are considered together, as are

Figure 17.6. Lymph node, metastatic carcinoma. **(A)** The diffuse growth of metastatic carcinoma in this node biopsy can be confused with malignant lymphoma. **(B)** The neoplastic cells show negative results for CD45 (leukocyte common antigen) (*left*) and strongly positive results for cytokeratin (*right*). Paraffin immunoperoxidase stain with diaminobenzidine substrate.

A

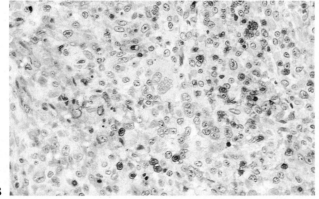

B

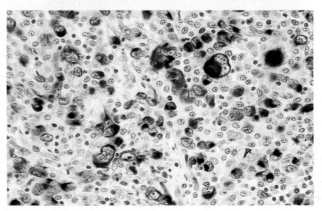

TABLE 17.3	Reactive Processes in Relation to Etiologic Factor and Architectural Distortion

Etiologic Factor	*Architectural Distortion*
Infections	Reactive states with follicular hyperplasia
Viral-associated adenitis (infectious mononucleosis, postvaccinal, herpes zoster, cytomegalovirus, measles, HIV)	Nonspecific follicular hyperplasia and progressive transformation of germinal center
Secondary syphilis	Rheumatoid arthritis
Toxoplasmosis	Sjögren syndrome
Cat-scratch disease	Adult-onset Still disease
Various granulomatous processes	Systemic lupus erythematosus
Whipple disease	Kimura disease
Rheumatologic/immunologic	Histiocytic necrotizing lymphadenitis (Kikuchi-Fujimoto disease)
Rheumatoid arthritis	Cat-scratch disease
Lupus erythematosus	Toxoplasmosis
Sjögren syndrome	Syphilis
Immunodeficiency states	HIV infection
Infarction, some cases	Angiofollicular hyperplasia (Castleman disease)
Adult-onset Still disease	Reactive states with interfollicular hyperplasia
Drug-induced	Whipple disease
Dilantin	Viral adenitis
Unknown cause	Posttransplant lymphoproliferative disorder
Sarcoidosis	Virus-associated hemophagocytic syndrome
Angiofollicular hyperplasia	Hemophagocytic lymphohistiocytosis
Inflammatory pseudotumor	Dermatopathic lymphadenopathy
Dermatopathic lymphadenopathy	Sinus histiocytosis with massive adenopathy
Sinus histiocytosis with massive adenopathy	Reactive states causing diffuse architectural effacement
Necrotizing adenitis	Drug reactions
Kimura disease	Sarcoidosis
	Infarction
	Vasoproliferative lesions

HIV, human immunodeficiency virus.

those with prominent interfollicular expansion and those producing diffuse architectural changes.

REACTIVE STATES WITH FOLLICULAR HYPERPLASIA

Nonspecific Follicular Hyperplasia and Progressive Transformation of Germinal Centers

Follicular hyperplasia reflects a normal response of lymph nodes to antigenic stimulation. Hyperplastic follicles are usually spherical to oval in shape and are confined to the cortex, but, with prolonged stimulation, involve the medulla and may assume more serpentine forms. The low-power appreciation of intact architecture, specifically the absence of follicular crowding and preserved mantle zones coupled with zonation (dark and light zones in follicles with retained tingible body macrophages), are features helpful in distinguishing exuberant reactions from follicular lymphoma.

Patients with progressive transformation of germinal centers are often asymptomatic adolescents or young adults and have isolated enlarged nodes up to 5 cm or more in size. These nodes exhibit exuberant follicular hyperplasia with scattered large follicles (four to five times normal size) in which the germinal center is broken up and infiltrated by small B lymphocytes. On CD21 staining, the follicular dendritic meshwork is dispersed and fragmented. The borders of these giant follicles are often indistinct and may be surrounded by wreaths of histiocytes. The absence of variant RS cells, the overall preservation of architecture, and the background of unremarkable hyperplastic follicles are all features helpful in distinguishing this variant of follicular hyperplasia from NLPHL (23–26).

Rheumatoid Arthritis

Generalized adenopathy occurs in many patients with rheumatoid arthritis and may be accompanied by weight loss, anemia, and fever. Lymph nodes show architectural preservation with large hyperplastic follicles in both the cortex and medulla, surrounded by impressive aggregates of interfollicular plasma cells. Russell bodies may be prominent. Intrasinus polymorphonuclear leukocytes may be present (27,28). Occasionally, lymph nodes may be partially effaced by extracellular hyaline material that is periodic acid-Schiff (PAS)-positive and Congo red-negative (29). Longitudinal studies have suggested that patients with rheumatoid arthritis have a modestly increased risk of malignant lymphoma (30). This risk may be related, in part, to the increased use of methotrexate in these patients (31). Several reports have described malignant lymphomas with diverse histologic features, including HL and large-B-cell lymphomas, arising in patients with rheumatoid arthritis who are receiving methotrexate. These lymphomas are often associated with Epstein-Barr virus (EBV) infection and sometimes resolve with discontinuation of methotrexate (32,33).

More recently, the use of tumor necrosis factor (TNF) inhibitors has been associated with lymphoma. TNF inhibitors also disrupt formation of follicular centers, leading to a loss of normal architecture. This may lead to a misdiagnosis of lymphoma (34,35).

Adult-Onset Still Disease

Several histologic patterns have been described in adult-onset Still disease, including follicular hyperplasia resembling rheumatoid arthritis (36) as well as changes resembling histiocytic necrotizing lymphadenitis (37). One report described partial effacement of nodal architecture by a paracortical proliferation that included large immunoblasts and mimicked malignant lymphoma in seven of eight patients (38).

Sjögren Syndrome

Patients with Sjögren syndrome may have adenopathy similar to that in rheumatoid arthritis, with follicular hyperplasia and interfollicular plasmacytosis. Immunoperoxidase studies in these patients (and in patients with rheumatoid arthritis) show polytypic marking of plasma cells for immunoglobulin heavy and light chains. In other patients, lymphoid proliferations that fail to meet criteria for malignancy develop at nodal and extranodal sites and have been labeled "pseudolymphomas." Lymph nodes from such patients may show partial obliteration of nodal architecture by heterogeneous interfollicular infiltrates of macrophages, plasma cells, small lymphocytes, and immunoblasts. The sinuses may be distorted by lymphocytes with small central nuclei and clear cytoplasm, similar in cytologic features to the marginal zone or monocytoid B-cells described in nodal marginal zone lymphoma. Evolution to lymphoma is indicated by architectural effacement and expanding masses of these monocytoid B cells or by the presence of monotypic collections of plasma cells and plasmacytoid lymphocytes demonstrated by IHC. Monotypism of B cells in these cases may be missed in immunologic studies on cell suspensions (39).

Patients with Sjögren syndrome have an increased risk of lymphoma (40). Lymphomas complicating Sjögren syndrome are almost always B-cell neoplasms, usually low grade and often extranodal, with features of mucosa-associated lymphoid tissue (MALT)/marginal zone lymphomas. These indolent lymphomas frequently transform to more aggressive large-cell lymphomas (41,42).

Systemic Lupus Erythematosus

Many patients with systemic lupus erythematosus (SLE) have cervical adenopathy, whereas generalized adenopathy is less common. Nodes show architectural preservation with variably sized follicles and interfollicular expansion with plasma cells and immunoblasts. Frequently, there are sharply circumscribed areas of paracortical necrosis with few neutrophilic leukocytes and no granulomatous response (Fig. 17.7). Necrosis may be present within follicular centers, occasionally associated with hematoxylin bodies (43). Immunohistochemical studies of the paracortical zones surrounding areas of necrosis demonstrate CD11b+ and CD15+ histiocytes and CD8+ T cells (44). The absence of neutrophilic or granulomatous inflammation distinguishes this process from cat-scratch disease and lymphogranu-

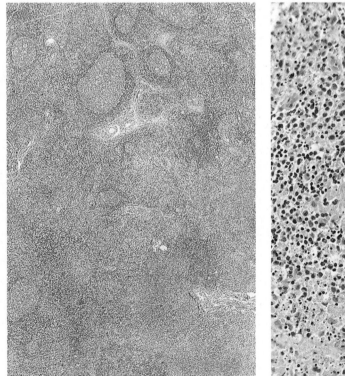
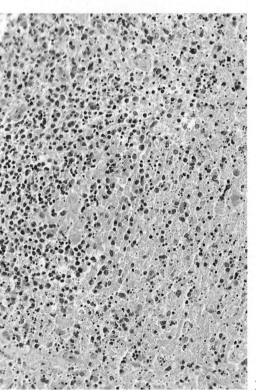

A   **B**

Figure 17.7. Lymph node, systemic lupus erythematosus. **(A)** Nodes usually show follicular hyperplasia and areas of parenchymal necrosis (*lower right*). **(B)** Areas of necrosis show dustlike nuclear fragments, often with hematoxylin bodies (not apparent at this magnification).

loma venereum. The histopathologic characteristics of SLE adenopathy are similar to those of histiocytic necrotizing lymphadenitis; however, follicular hyperplasia and interfollicular plasma cells are more prominent in SLE, and immunoblastic proliferations mimicking lymphomas may be more impressive in histiocytic necrotizing lymphadenitis. Hematoxylin bodies are seen only in SLE. Of note is that this pattern of nongranulomatous cortical necrosis with karyorrhexes has also been described in tuberculosis (45).

Histiocytic Necrotizing Lymphadenitis (Kikuchi-Fujimoto Disease)

Initially described as a disease of young Oriental women, histiocytic necrotizing lymphadenitis is now recognized with increasing frequency in men and in all parts of the world. Patients usually show initial signs of fever and painless cervical adenopathy, often accompanied by leukopenia (46). Nodes usually show partially effaced architecture with large, discrete areas of eosinophilic necrosis with abundant nuclear debris surrounded by transformed lymphocytes, histiocytes, and plasmacytoid monocytes (47). Plasmacytoid dendritic cells (previously called plasmacytoid T cells or plasmacytoid monocytes) are CD4+ mononuclear cells two to three times the size of small lymphocytes, with round nuclei, open chromatin, small nucleoli, and variable cytoplasm (48). The transformed lymphocytes are predominantly CD8+ T cells with a cytotoxic phenotype and are associated with apoptosis of neighboring cells (49). Granulocytes are notably absent and follicular centers are usually not hyperplastic. In a few cases, foamy histiocytes may dominate. These histiocytes may resemble signet ring cells of adenocarcinoma (50).

The absence of granulocytes in areas of necrosis and the lack of follicular hyperplasia differentiate these cases from lymphadenitis caused by cat-scratch disease and other bacterial infections. Early-stage lesions without overt necrosis may be distinguished from malignant lymphoma by (a) the focal nature of the lymph node involvement with incomplete architectural effacement; (b) the presence of plasmacytoid dendritic cells at the periphery of the lesion; and (c) bland cytologic features of the mixed-cell population in areas of involvement (51). The origin of Kikuchi-Fujimoto disease is unknown. Although viruses such as human herpesvirus 6, EBV, and hepatitis B have been linked to Kikuchi-Fujimoto disease, these associations have not been confirmed (52,53).

Kimura Disease

Kimura disease commonly appears in young Asian men as a deep, subcutaneous cervical mass with regional lymph node involvement (54–56). In soft tissue, there is proliferation of thin-walled vessels with tissue eosinophilia. Lymph nodes show follicular hyperplasia with variable interfollicular eosinophilia, polykaryocytes, and proliferation of thin-walled vessels. Nodal and extranodal soft tissue lymphoid follicles show folliculolysis with infiltration by eosinophils. Late lesions may become sclerotic with collections of Charcot-Leyden crystals. The major consideration in the differential diagnosis is angiolymphoid hyperplasia with eosinophilia—a disease that characteristically involves the skin (not nodes) of older Caucasian men in the form of multiple small papules. Blood vessels in angiolymphoid hyperplasia are thick-walled and lined by plump endothelial cells.

Cat-Scratch Disease

Regional lymphadenopathy (axillary, cervical, inguinal) in cat-scratch disease appears about 3 weeks after primary exposure. Early lesions show interfollicular microabscesses associated with proliferation of monocytoid B cells, and plasmacytoid dendritic cells as well as reactive hyperplasia of secondary follicular centers (57,58). Small clusters of epithelioid histiocytes surrounding necrotic foci contain central polymorphonuclear leukocytes (Fig. 17.8). Giant cells are occasionally noted. Capsulitis is often prominent. Suppurative foci may drain through the node cap-

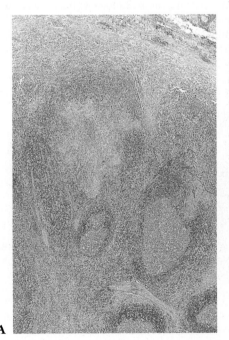

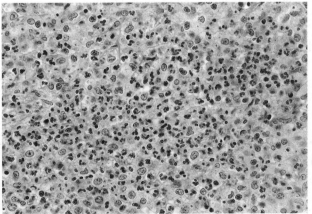

Figure 17.8. Lymph node, cat-scratch disease. **(A)** There is partial architectural distortion in most cases of cat-scratch disease. Capsulitis with subcapsular granulomas is almost invariably present, as in this case. Focal areas of necrosis lie just below the capsule (*center*). **(B)** At high magnification, the necrotic area is rich in polymorphonuclear leukocytes.

sule into perinodal soft tissue (59). Affected nodes sometimes contain pleomorphic small rods on Warthin-Starry silver stain, which are particularly abundant around small blood vessels and lymphatics before suppuration (60).

Cases of clinically overt cat-scratch disease have serologic and molecular genetic evidence of infection with *Bartonella henselae* (61). The histopathologic features of cat-scratch disease are similar to those described in lymphogranuloma venereum, tularemia, and *Yersinia* infections. In addition, similar findings are seen in immunocompetent young children (age younger than 4 years) with *Mycobacterium avian-intracellulare* infection (62). Patients with cat-scratch disease may show signs of extranodal disease, with necrotizing granulomatous lesions in liver, spleen, or bone; these extranodal lesions are seen in patients who appear to be immunologically intact and in patients with immunodeficiency (63,64). *Bartonella henselae* infection in HIV-positive patients can produce a pattern of reaction dominated by a tumor-like proliferation of small vessels (see "Bacillary Angiomatosis").

Toxoplasmosis

Cervical lymph nodes, particularly posterior cervical nodes, are most commonly enlarged in toxoplasmosis. Lymph nodes show a classic triad of (a) follicular hyperplasia; (b) irregular clusters of epithelioid histiocytes, which may invade follicular centers; and (c) collections of parafollicular/monocytoid B cells that distort the subcapsular peritrabecular architecture (Fig. 17.9). The clusters of epithelioid histiocytes rarely form tight, sarcoid-type granulomas or become necrotic. The causative protozoan parasite stains with H&E, but it is rarely evident except in immunocompromised patients with overwhelming infection (65–67). Isolated patients have focal areas of vascular proliferation that mimic Kaposi sarcoma (KS) in areas of resolving toxoplasmosis (68). Recent molecular genetic and serologic studies have confirmed the sensitivity and specificity of histologic findings in the diagnosis of toxoplasmosis (69).

Syphilis

Nodes draining primary syphilitic lesions (usually inguinal, less commonly cervical) characteristically are enlarged but painless.

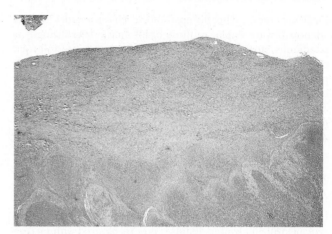

Figure 17.10. Lymph node, syphilis. A low-magnification photomicrograph shows marked capsular thickening with moderately dense fibrosis and a plasmacytic infiltrate.

Nodes evidence follicular hyperplasia with large secondary follicles, inter- and intrafollicular plasmacytosis, and a prominent capsulitis with proliferation of small blood vessels, fibroblasts, and plasma cells (Fig. 17.10). Granulomas or small collections of histiocytes, with or without giant cells, may be seen in the interfollicular areas. Patients with secondary syphilis may have generalized adenopathy with the features just described, although capsulitis may be absent. Warthin-Starry stains in primary and secondary types demonstrate spirochetes, which are most numerous in and around small blood vessels (70,71). Patients with HIV infection may have negative results on serologic studies despite identification of spirochetes in tissue sections (72).

HIV Infection

Patients with HIV infection may have persistent generalized lymphadenopathy associated with a stable clinical course before progressing to symptoms of the acquired immunodeficiency syndrome (AIDS). The pathologic features of lymph node enlargement in early HIV infection are predominantly hyperplasia of follicular centers; these centers may have a dumbbell, serpentine, or serrated configuration (Fig. 17.11). The follicles contain

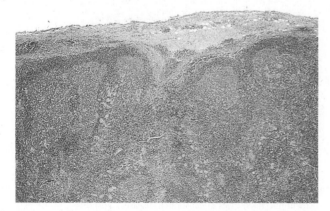

Figure 17.9. Lymph node, toxoplasmosis. At low magnification, there is mild capsular inflammation and scarring, proliferation of parafollicular/monocytoid lymphocytes, and scattered aggregates of histiocytes within hyperplastic follicles.

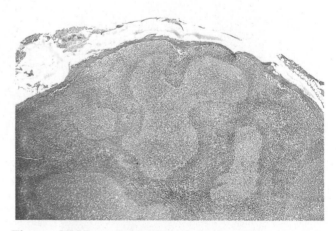

Figure 17.11. Lymph node, acquired immunodeficiency syndrome-related complex. Serpentine hyperplastic follicles are shown.

numerous tingible-body macrophages and plasma cells. Mantle zones are frequently scant or even absent, creating "naked" germinal centers. Other germinal centers may be disrupted by central or peripheral infiltrates of small lymphocytes (folliculolysis).

The interfollicular areas show vascular proliferation and contain more numerous plasma cells, granulocytes, and macrophages, either singly or in clusters. Hyperplasia of monocytoid B lymphocytes (similar to that seen in toxoplasmosis) is a common finding. Parenchymal hemorrhage and Warthin-Finkeldey–like giant cells have also been described (73). Immunopathologic analysis of lymph node tissue usually shows a depressed ratio of CD4 to CD8 lymphocytes, with a characteristic infiltration of CD8 lymphocytes into follicular centers (74). These CD8 T cells have an activated cytotoxic phenotype and may play a role in the loss of follicular dendritic cells that is seen in advanced disease (75).

Lymph nodes, with progression of HIV infection, show involution and loss of follicular centers, with intrafollicular hyalinized vessels resembling those seen in the hyaline-vascular type of angiofollicular hyperplasia (Castleman disease). Other areas of the same node may show residual hyperplasia, with both interfollicular and intrafollicular plasma cells mimicking the plasma cell variant of angiofollicular hyperplasia. These histologic changes may be accompanied by constitutional symptoms similar to those seen in multicentric Castleman disease. Many of these patients have evidence of co-infection with human herpesvirus-8 (HHV8) (76,77) (see "Castleman Disease"). The disappearance of follicles, lymphocyte depletion, and vascular proliferation in the terminal states of HIV infection may mimic immunoblastic lymphoma (78) (Fig. 17.12).

Nodes from patients with HIV infection may contain fungi or atypical mycobacteria without the usual histopathologic indicators of these infections (Figs. 17.13 and 17.14). When PCR is used, HIV viral DNA is readily evident in formalin-fixed, paraffin-embedded lymph node tissue in all pathologic stages of lymph node involvement (79).

Angiofollicular Hyperplasia (Castleman Disease)

A disease of unsettled complexity and morbidity, angiofollicular hyperplasia (castleman disease) as originally described presented as large, single masses in mediastinal biopsy specimens from asymptomatic patients. Three histologic variants of Castleman disease (CD) are currently recognized. The hyaline-vascular form of angiofollicular hyperplasia is characterized by numerous small, involuted follicular centers evenly distributed throughout the node parenchyma, resembling a "bag of marbles." The follicles are often surrounded by concentric layers of small lymphocytes, referred to as "onion skinning." These atretic follicles also display penetration by prominent central vessels with hyalinized walls and plump endothelial cells (Fig. 17.15). The interfollicular areas show proliferation of small vessels surrounded by a cuff of collagen and an absence of sinuses, with variable numbers of plasma cells and immunoblasts. Residual lymph node is usually found at the periphery of the mass. The plasma cell variant of angiofollicular hyperplasia is distinguished by follicular hyperplasia with sheets of interfollicular plasma cells; this variant is more likely to be associated with constitutional symptoms and generalized adenopathy (80). Recently a third plasmablastic variant of CD has been described.

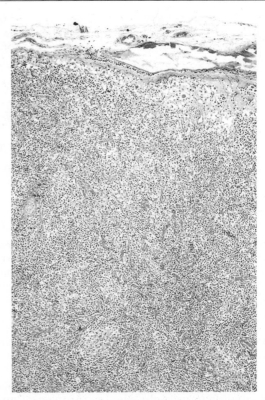

Figure 17.12. Lymph node, acquired immunodeficiency syndrome–related complex. In advanced stages, lymph nodes may become more depleted, as in this case. There is loss of follicular centers and partial alteration of nodal architecture. Hypervascularity is present in this node, but there is no morphologic evidence of Kaposi sarcoma.

It usually occurs in patients with morphologic and clinical features of the plasma cell variant. This form is distinguished by mantle zone infiltration by large numbers of plasmablasts (cells with large vesicular nuclei containing one to two prominent nucleoli and a moderate amount of amphophilic cytoplasm) (81).

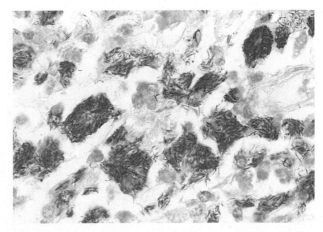

Figure 17.13. Lymph node, acquired immunodeficiency syndrome–related complex, secondary infection by tuberculosis. On Fite stain, innumerable acid-fast bacilli are visible in a node showing architectural distortion, lymphocyte depletion, and proliferation of macrophages.

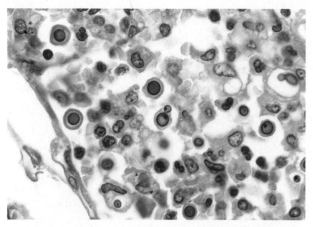

Figure 17.14. Lymph node, acquired immunodeficiency syndrome–related complex, secondary infection by cryptococcosis. At high magnification, typical cryptococci are present in a node showing lymphocytic depletion and no granulomatous reaction despite the presence of innumerable cryptococci.

Two clinical presentations of CD may occur. Unicentric (localized) CD, most often of the hyaline-vascular variant, usually occurs in HIV-negative patients who are asymptomatic aside from a single enlarged lymph node or mass lesion. These patients are usually treated with surgical excision alone. The multicentric (systemic) form of CD, more often of the plasma cell variant (or plasmablastic variant), is often associated with HIV and HHV8 infection. These patients may have generalized adenopathy, fever, hypergammaglobulinemia, and multiple organ dysfunction. Anemia, thrombocytopenia, hepatomegaly, abnormal liver function, pleural effusions, and peripheral neuropathy have also been described. On histologic examination, nodes usually show features of the plasma cell variant of angiofollicular hyperplasia, although a minority exhibit changes of the hyaline-vascular form. Unlike patients with localized disease, who have a good prognosis (cure following resection), patients with systemic angiofollicular hyperplasia often have a progressive course, complicated by infection, Kaposi sarcoma, or lymphoma (82,83).

Plasma cells in angiofollicular hyperplasia are usually polytypic. Monotypic marking of interfollicular plasma cells (usually lambda-predominant) in a few patients does not typically portend evolution to lymphoma (84,85). In contrast, plasmablasts in the plasmablastic variant are IgM λ-restricted and may coalesce to form microlymphomas (81,86).

IHC studies show a follicular dendritic cell network similar to that of normal or reactive follicular centers in the plasma cell variant, whereas the hyaline vascular variant frequently demonstrates either an expanded or disrupted network of multiple tight collections of follicular dendritic cells (87). The follicular dendritic cells identified on IHC may exhibit dysplastic features (nuclear enlargement and prominent nucleoli) in both the hyaline vascular and plasma cell variants (88). Gene rearrangement studies as a rule do not show clonal rearrangements of either the T- or B-cell receptor genes (89).

The pathogenesis of CD is complex. The role of interleukin-6 (IL-6) is suggested by the finding of increased IL-6 production by germinal centers in angiofollicular hyperplasia (90). Serum IL-6 appears to correlate with systemic manifestations of disease (91). One study demonstrated elevated levels of both IL-6 and IL-1β in five patients with clinical features of POEMS syndrome (polyneuropathy, organomegaly, endocrinopathy, M-protein, and skin changes); four had multicentric CD (92). HHV8 sequences have been identified in almost all HIV-positive patients with pathologic features of multicentric Castleman disease and in a few HIV negative patients. IHC studies using antibodies to HHV8 LNA (latent nuclear antigens) show nuclear staining of lambda-restricted plasmablasts, and mantle zone plasmablasts in multicentric CD (86,93). These patients may develop clonal disease and frank plasmablastic lymphoma.

REACTIVE STATES WITH INTERFOLLICULAR HYPERPLASIA

Whipple Disease

Whipple disease is a multisystem process usually dominated by signs of intestinal malabsorption. Either intra-abdominal or peripheral lymph nodes may be submitted for examination, often with the clinical suspicion of cancer. Whipple disease is rare and may be difficult to recognize in those laboratories that do not use PAS stains routinely. Nodal architecture is obscured by an ill-defined granulomatous process associated with large clear

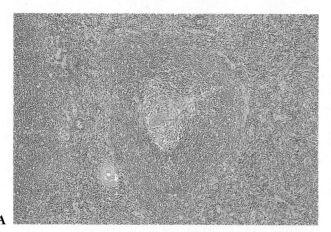

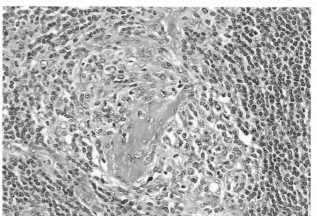

A   B

Figure 17.15. Lymph node, angiofollicular hyperplasia. **(A)** At low power, an atretic follicle exhibiting a penetrating, prominent central hyalinized vessel is surrounded by concentric layers of small lymphocytes. **(B)** High power demonstrates the sclerotic vessel.

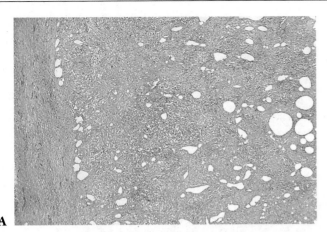
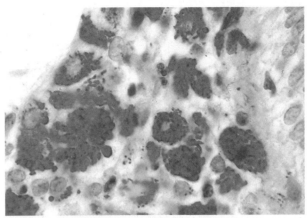

A **B**

Figure 17.16. Lymph node, Whipple disease. **(A)** Nodal architecture is usually obscured by an ill-defined granulomatous reaction with numerous distended intervening clear spaces containing lipid. **(B)** Numerous intensely staining macrophages that show positive results with periodic acid-Schiff are present throughout the lymph node.

spaces (lipid). In all lymph nodes, interfollicular macrophages on H&E-stained sections have abundant bubbly or frothy cytoplasm. PAS stains show intensely positive, diastase-resistant particles that have sickle shapes, average 2 to 3 μm in their greatest dimension, and have a brilliant magenta hue (Fig. 17.16). Whipple disease should not be diagnosed unless there is massive involvement of the node accompanied by intense PAS staining because small aggregates of PAS-positive macrophages are nonspecific. Electron microscopic features of intracytoplasmic bacilliform bodies are characteristic (94). The DNA of the causative agent *Tropheryma whippelii* can be easily demonstrated with PCR using paraffin-embedded tissue in patients with atypical histologic and/or clinical features (95–97).

Viral Adenitis with Emphasis on Infectious Mononucleosis

Infectious mononucleosis is classically a disease of adolescents and young adults characterized by fever, tonsillitis, cervical adenopathy, and mild hepatitis. Epstein-Barr virus (EBV) infects B lymphocytes and causes them to proliferate and differentiate to plasma cells. The immune response to the virus is dominated by CD8 + cytotoxic T cells that account for the majority of "atypical" lymphocytes in peripheral blood. On histopathologic evaluation, there is distortion of lymph node architecture resulting from varying degrees of follicular hyperplasia, with the follicles having a mottled or ragged perimeter; the interfollicular areas are expanded by numerous immunoblasts, small lymphocytes, and a few plasma cells. Large lymphocytes fill the subcapsular and peritrabecular sinuses (Figs. 17.2 and 17.17). Histiocytes may be present, although they do not form large aggregates encroaching on follicular centers, as seen in toxoplasmosis. A minority of patients have focal interfollicular necrosis.

Immunoblasts may be binucleate, mimicking RS cells of HL, or become so numerous as to suggest a large-cell or immunoblastic lymphoma (98–101). Recognition of this process as reactive is dependent upon low-magnification evidence of partial architectural preservation with hyperplasia of all nodal compartments. The process lacks the nodular distortion of architecture characteristic of HL on low magnification. On high power, the cellular mix, including fibroblasts, eosinophils, and neutrophils

of classic HL is not seen. Phenotypically, immunoblasts are mixed B and T cells, with the former dominating. B immunoblasts are CD20 +, MUM1 +, CD10 − and Bcl-6 −. CD8 T cell dominates CD4 cells. Epstein-Barr virus-encoded RNA (EBER) is positive primarily in interfollicular immunoblasts (102). The RS-like immunoblasts are usually CD20-positive and CD15- and CD30-positive. Without clinical history and immunophenotypic/molecular genetic studies for clonality, lesions dominated by immunoblasts may be very difficult to differentiate from aggressive NHL. Lymphadenopathy with similar histopathologic changes may complicate drug reactions, vaccination with live virus, and other viral infections, including cytomegalovirus, herpes simplex, and herpes zoster (103,104). Lesions of herpes simplex frequently show small areas of necrosis with viral inclusions (105).

Post-Transplant Lymphoproliferative Disorder

Post-transplant lymphoproliferative disorder (PTLD) is a life-threatening complication of both solid organ and bone marrow transplantation. The incidence ranges from 1% to 10% and is influenced by the type of transplant and the particular immunosuppressive protocol. Most cases of PTLD have been linked to EBV infection by serologic tests and molecular studies of involved tissues. PTLD often occurs at extranodal sites (central nervous system, lung, small bowel) and may involve the allograft in a histologic pattern mimicking rejection (106–109). The majority of cases are B-cell proliferations; however a minority of cases of PTLD is T-cell lymphomas (110,111). Approximately 15% to 20% of PTLD is not associated with EBV infection (112,113).

The pathologic spectrum of PTLD is broad (114). Plasmacytic hyperplasia (PH) or infectious mononucleosis-like PTLD characteristically occurs early in the posttransplant period, is more common in children and young adults, and frequently involves lymph nodes and tonsillar tissue. Plasma cell hyperplasia may be admixed with a few immunoblasts that do not show cytologic atypia. Both plasma cell hyperplasia and the infectious mononucleosis-like lesions demonstrate architectural preservation. These lesions are genetically and immunophenotypically polyclonal, with EBV-latent membrane protein demon-

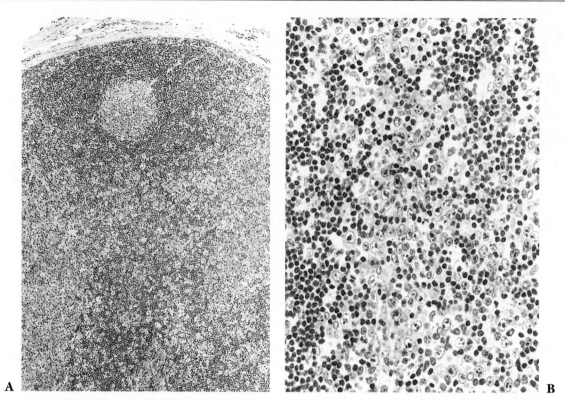

Figure 17.17. Lymph node, infectious mononucleosis. **(A)** Germinal centers show somewhat ragged margins with striking interfollicular expansion by a mixed infiltrate, including numerous transformed lymphocytes with abundant cytoplasm and prominent nucleoli. **(B)** Sheets of transformed lymphocytes may mimic a malignant lymphoma, but partial preservation of nodal architecture can be demonstrated focally in all.

strable by IHC. Resolution with reduction in immunosuppression is the most common outcome.

Polymorphic PTLD is more clinically aggressive and is characterized by architectural effacement by a mixed population of immunoblasts, plasma cells, and lymphocytes, pleomorphic in size and cytology. There may be necrosis and significant cytologic atypia. These cases are usually clonal by immunoglobulin heavy chain gene rearrangement studies, although immunophenotypic studies may be either clonal or polyclonal. EBV-associated antigens are usually detected by IHC. Detection of EBER with in situ hybridization may be helpful distinguishing PTLD (numerous cells positive) from rejection (0 to few cells positive) in transplanted organs.

Monomorphic PTLD meets morphologic criteria for malignant lymphoma, most commonly diffuse large-B-cell lymphoma, with Burkitt lymphoma, plasmacytic neoplasms, and T-cell lymphomas constituting most of the remaining cases. These lymphomas are usually EBV-associated with clonality easily demonstrated by immunophenotyping and genetic studies (114–117).

Prognosis is related to stage, performance status site, histologic features, EBV status (worse in primary infection), and clonality as defined by flow cytometry or molecular genetic studies of EBV termini and immunoglobulin gene rearrangements. Lesions at the more benign end of the spectrum may respond to reduction in immunosuppressive therapy alone (116,118–120).

Hemophagocytic Lymphohistiocytosis

Hemophagocytic lymphohistiocytosis (HLH) is characterized by fever, cytopenia, hepatosplenomegaly, abnormal liver func-

tion tests, hypertriglyceridemia, and hypofibrinogenemia. Erythrophagocytosis must be present in bone marrow, lymph nodes, or spleen (121). Patients with HLH have high levels of circulating cytokines, including interferon gamma, interleukin-2, and TNF-α, that may contribute to macrophage activation (122).

HLH includes cases that have a genetic basis and characteristically present in infants and young children with a virulent clinical course (123). Acquired forms of HLH were originally described by Risdall et al. as a complication of viral infection (usually EBV) in immunocompromised patients (124).

Defects in the perforin gene have been described in many of the patients with the autosomal recessive form of HLH (125). HLH may also follow EBV infection in male patients with germline mutations in SH2DIA in X-linked lymphoproliferative disease (126).

The acquired secondary forms of HLH have not only been described complicating viral infections following immunosuppression, but also in patients with autoimmune disease (e.g., Still disease), other nonviral infections, and with the use of certain drugs as well as in NHL (e.g., panniculitic T-cell lymphoma) (127). HLH has also been well described as complicating both acute and chronic EBV infection in patients who are not apparently immunocompromised or are without any identifiable genetic predisposition (120,121,128,129).

Lymph node biopsy in patients with HLH reveals intact architecture, with infiltration of cortex, sinuses, and paracortex by histiocytes that are cytologically benign and filled with erythrocytes and, occasionally, small numbers of lymphocytes and neutrophils. The interfollicular areas may show vascular proliferation, more numerous plasma cells, and immunoblasts. Follicular centers may be atrophic or depleted.

It is important to recognize that hemophagocytosis in tissue sections without the clinical features of HLH is a common finding in a variety of circumstances, including posttransfusion (130). HPS is usually distinguishable from malignant histiocytosis by its clinical context, benign histiocyte cytologic features, and architectural preservation. Patients with peripheral T-cell lymphomas may have a similar explosive clinical picture, with prominent erythrophagocytosis by macrophages. These patients, however, have infiltrates in marrow, spleen, liver, and lymph nodes of cytologically atypical T cells accompanied by benign-appearing histiocytes (131–133).

Dermatopathic Lymphadenopathy

Patients with various skin diseases may show signs of regional adenopathy. Lymph node architecture is distorted by focal nodular expansions of the subcapsular paracortical areas by aggregates of histiocytes, interdigitating reticulum cells, and Langerhans cells with elongated grooved nuclei (Fig. 17.18). Melanin is usually present in the cytoplasm of cells and as extracellular deposits. Admixed with the histiocytes are small lymphocytes, many of which have folded or cerebriform nuclei. Distinguishing dermatopathic lymphadenopathy from focal involvement of lymph nodes by mycosis fungoides may be particularly difficult (see "Mycosis Fungoides/Sézary Syndrome" below).

Sinus Histiocytosis with Massive Adenopathy (Rosai-Dorfman Disease)

Sinus histiocytosis with massive adenopathy (SHMA) usually occurs in young patients and produces prominent bilateral painless cervical adenopathy, often accompanied by fever, leukocytosis, anemia, and polyclonal hypergammaglobulinemia. Extranodal involvement is not uncommon. On histopathologic examination, lymph nodes show capsular fibrosis and packing of sinuses by histiocytes that are sometimes multinucleate. Histiocytes may exhibit mild to moderate cytologic atypia with nuclear pleomorphism and prominent nucleoli. A distinctive histopathologic feature is emperipolesis—the presence of lymphocytes, red blood cells, and a few plasma cells within vacuoles in the cytoplasm of many histiocytes (134,135) (Fig. 17.19). Marked plasmacytosis is usually noted in connective tissue between the sinuses. Residual germinal centers may be hyperplastic or sparse to absent. Macrophages in SHMA are positive for S-100, CD68, and CD14, but differ phenotypically from Langerhans cells in that most are CD1a− (136). Patients with localized nodal disease usually have a chronic indolent course. Extranodal involvement of liver, kidney, and the lower respiratory tract as well as signs of overt immune dysfunction are associated with a poor prognosis. Patients may die as a direct result of infiltrative disease, but no cases of transformation to malignancy have been reported (137). Studies of human androgen receptor polymorphisms in women with SHMA have found evidence of polyclonal patterns of X-chromosome inactivation (138).

REACTIVE STATES CAUSING DIFFUSE ARCHITECTURAL EFFACEMENT

Drug Reactions with Emphasis on Phenytoin Reactions

In 1959, Saltzstein and Ackerman (139) described the cases of 82 patients who suffered lymphadenopathy while receiving anticonvulsant therapy. Most patients had started either mephenytoin (Mesantoin) or phenytoin (Dilantin) 1 to 6 weeks before experiencing tender bilateral cervical lymphadenopathy accompanied by fever, eosinophilia, and a variety of skin changes, ranging from morbilliform rashes to exfoliative dermatitis. Lymph node biopsy findings of early lesions were characterized by architectural preservation and residual follicular centers with interfollicular expansion by a mixed infiltrate of immunoblasts, plasma cells, and eosinophils with varying degrees of vascular proliferation. In more advanced lesions, the lymph nodes dem-

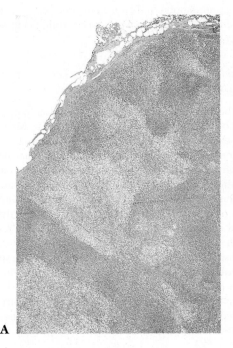

A

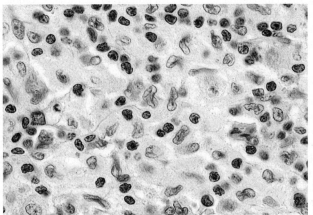

B

Figure 17.18. Lymph node, dermatopathic lymphadenopathy. **(A)** Pale-staining nodules are prominent in the cortex of the node. **(B)** The pale-staining cortical nodules are composed, in part, of histiocytes with conspicuous linear nuclear grooves, a cytologic feature of Langerhans cells.

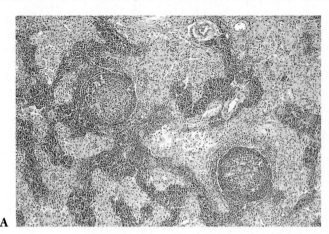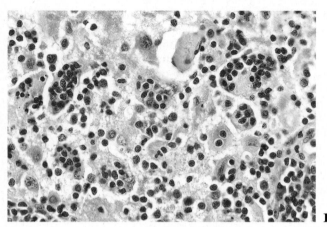

A **B**

Figure 17.19. Lymph node, sinus histiocytosis with massive lymphadenopathy. **(A)** This low-magnification photomicrograph shows distention of sinuses with pale-staining histiocytes and interspersed medullary cords in which numerous plasma cells are present. **(B)** A high-magnification photomicrograph shows numerous lymphocytes in some of the macrophages.

onstrated complete obliteration of architecture with changes similar to those in immunoblastic lymphadenopathy. Some lymph nodes showed focal necrosis. In patients with early or advanced lesions, adenopathy and other symptoms resolved within 1 to 2 weeks after discontinuing drugs. Fatal cases developed pancytopenia or polyarteritis nodosa.

A later series from the Armed Forces Institute of Pathology described 15 cases with reactive changes that fell into two major histologic patterns (140). Nine cases that arose during the first 18 months of therapy showed prominent immunoblastic hyperplasia in the paracortical area, associated with follicular hyperplasia in five. Some patients exhibited disrupted follicular centers, obliterative vasculitis, and focal architectural effacement. Eosinophilia was present in all cases. The second histologic pattern, seen in 4 patients, consisted of paracortical hyperplasia accompanied by atrophic follicular centers. This pattern occurred late after initiation of phenytoin therapy. NHL developed in 2 of the 15 patients. Such an evolution to HL and NHL has been described in patients on long-term phenytoin therapy (141,142). Similar reactive changes in lymph nodes have been described with other drugs, including sulfa derivatives, penicillin, and quinidine (143,144).

Sarcoidosis

Sarcoidosis is a multisystem granulomatous disease of unknown cause characterized by bilateral hilar adenopathy, pulmonary infiltrates, and ocular and skin lesions. Young black women are often affected. Peripheral lymphadenopathy is present in most patients. Histopathologic features are distinctive and consist of total effacement of nodal architecture by epithelioid granulomas that are compact and sharply demarcated from intervening small lymphocytes (Fig. 17.20).

Granulomas may show rare small foci of necrosis and contain Langhans giant cells. Schaumann and asteroid bodies may be present. Granulomas may be surrounded or replaced by dense hyalinized connective tissue. Follicular centers are absent or rare in involved lymph nodes. Special stains and cultures must be performed to exclude infection by fungi and tubercle bacilli. Sarcoid-type granulomas may coexist in both involved and uninvolved lymph nodes of patients with HL and NHL (145) and

in patients with nonhematologic malignancies (146). Immunopathologic studies demonstrate increased numbers of activated helper (CD4+) lymphocytes at sites of injury in the lung or lymph node, with a paradoxical depression of these cells in peripheral blood (147).

Lymph Node Infarction

Lymph node infarction is uncommon and may result from infection, vasculitis, or trauma (e.g., postmediastinoscopy) (148); in a substantial minority of cases, infarction may be the initial symptom of malignant lymphoma. Lymphomas associated with lymph node infarction are typically diffuse large-B-cell lymphomas, but they also include follicular lymphoma, T-cell lymphomas, and HL. The diagnosis of lymphoma in patients with infarction is universally made within 2 years (149,150). Because the capsule is often spared, serial sectioning may reveal viable lymphomatous tissue in subcapsular or extracapsular locations. Clonal immunoglobulin heavy chain gene rearrangement may be evident on DNA extracted from necrotic tissue in patients with B-cell lymphomas (151).

Vasoproliferative and Spindle Cell Lesions of Lymph Node, including Kaposi Sarcoma

Several benign lesions in lymph nodes are dominated by proliferation of spindle cells and vascular channels. Many of these lesions are seen in immunosuppressed patients. The following discussion emphasizes histologic features that may help in distinguishing these reactive lesions from Kaposi sarcoma (KS). In HIV-infected patients, KS is typically lymphadenopathic or extracutaneous. It frequently involves capsular and subcapsular regions of lymph node, forming nodular masses that extend into and efface the underlying parenchyma. Usually, small vessels with plump and atypical endothelial cells alternate with areas of spindle cell proliferation containing slitlike spaces with extravasated erythrocytes and hemosiderin. The tumor often contains plasma cells. Mitotic figures are common (Fig. 17.21). The remaining lymph node may show typical features of HIV-associated adenopathy (152,153). PCR confirms the presence of HHV8 DNA in more than 95% of cases (154).

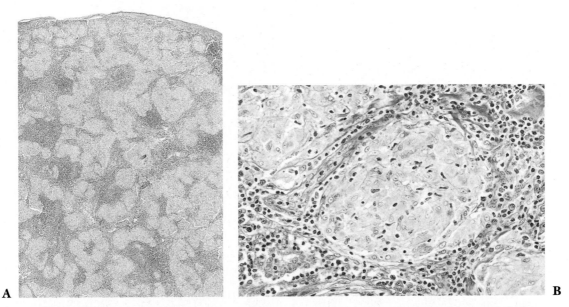

Figure 17.20. Lymph node, sarcoidosis. **(A)** This low-magnification photomicrograph shows a typical advanced stage of sarcoidosis. Granulomas are homogeneous in size, show no necrotizing changes, and produce architectural distortion with back-to-back granulomas across the node. Follicular centers are usually not present or are solitary. **(B)** The granulomas are usually sharply demarcated and lack necrosis.

Inflammatory Pseudotumor of Lymph Nodes

Patients are commonly young adults with localized adenopathy accompanied by fever and other signs of systemic inflammatory disease. Lesions involve the connective tissue framework of the node (capsule, sinuses, hilum) and are composed of small blood vessels, fibroblasts, and inflammatory cells, including plasma cells, neutrophils, eosinophils, and macrophages. Intranodal areas of fibroblastic proliferation are prominent; extension into perinodal soft tissues with accompanying obliterative vasculitis is common (Fig. 17.22) (155,156). Many of the spindle cells show a phenotype suggestive of a macrophage (CD45+, CD68+, HDA-DR+) (157). Inflammatory pseudotumor is distinguished from KS by the absence of dense spindle cell proliferation in the parenchymal portions of the node; extravasated erythrocytes and slitlike vascular spaces are also usually not pres-

ent. Lymphomas with prominent vascularity are excluded by the absence of cytologic atypia and monomorphism.

Mycobacterial Spindle Cell Pseudotumor

Mycobacterial spindle cell pseudotumor is almost always seen in patients with HIV infection and may involve many sites, including skin, spleen, and lymph nodes. In lymph nodes, there is partial or complete alteration of nodal architecture by a proliferation of cytologically bland spindle cells, often producing a storiform pattern. Although some spindle cells are vacuolated, multinucleated giant cells and foamy histiocytes are not present. The spindle cells mark as macrophages with CD45, CD68, and HDA-DR. Vessels are lined by plump endothelial cells. Numerous acid-fast bacilli are evident on Ziehl-Neelsen stain. The star-

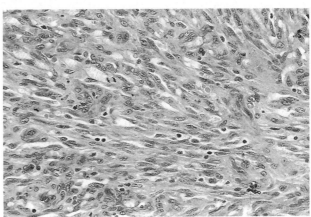

Figure 17.21. Lymph node with Kaposi sarcoma. **(A)** Low magnification showing subcapsular vascular tumor. **(B)** At high magnification there are dense spindle cell fascicles with slitlike vascular spaces, extravasated erythrocytes, extracellular hemosiderin, and prominent mitotic figures.

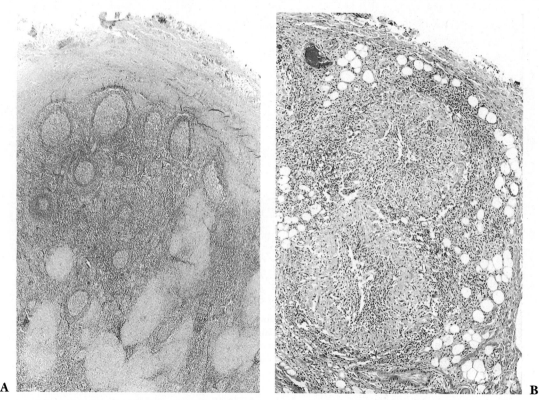

Figure 17.22. Lymph node, inflammatory pseudotumor. **(A)** On low magnification there is capsular thickening and foci of intranodal fibrosis. **(B)** There is often an associated obliterative vasculitis in perinodal vessels.

tling ability of this proliferative lesion to mimic neoplastic spindle cell tumors suggests that acid-fast stains should be a part of the evaluation of any spindle cell lesion lacking nuclear atypia in immunodeficient patients (158,159).

Vascular Transformation of Lymph Node Sinuses

Vascular transformation of lymph node sinuses is usually found incidentally after resection of a nearby tumor. The lesion is confined to the subcapsular and medullary sinuses and consists of proliferating anastomosing vessels of varying caliber, with foci of sclerosis (160). Extravasated erythrocytes may be present. Similar lesions are described in the literature as nodal angiomatosis (161). The lesion is distinguished from KS by the absence of parenchymal involvement, lack of well-formed spindle cell fascicles, and maturation to distinct vascular channels at the capsular aspect of the lymph node (162).

Bacillary Angiomatosis

Bacillary angiomatosis is caused by *Bartonella henselae* infection and occurs in immunosuppressed patients. It may appear in the form of red to violaceous skin lesions mimicking KS. In lymph nodes, the architecture is focally effaced by large, pale nodules composed of an exuberant proliferation of small vessels lined by plump endothelial cells. The cytoplasm of endothelial cells is pale and finely vacuolated. Between the blood vessels is a deeply eosinophilic granular material that on Warthin-Starry stains clusters of small bacilli (162). Interstitial neutrophils vary in number. Molecular genetic techniques have shown that *B. henselae* is the causative agent (163,164).

Palisaded Myofibroblastoma (Intranodal Hemorrhagic Spindle Cell Tumor with Amianthoid Fibers)

Palisaded myofibroblastoma arises almost exclusively in lymph nodes in the groin and is composed of interlacing fascicles of spindle cells that surround large mats of eosinophilic material (amianthoid fibers). These tumors may be highly vascularized, with associated hemorrhagic foci, and compress adjacent node parenchyma. Spindle cells show focal nuclear palisading mimicking neurilemoma. These neoplasms differ from KS in their lack of cytologic atypia, insignificant mitotic activity, and absence of slitlike vascular spaces (165,166). Reported cases of intranodal leiomyoma have been found to be composed of cytologically similar cells, but they lack nuclear palisading and amianthoid fibers (167).

HODGKIN LYMPHOMA

HL is a malignant neoplasm of the lymphoid system, meeting the usual criteria for malignancies, including the potential to spread to many sites and the production of large tumorous masses containing dysplastic cells (RS cells) (Fig. 17.23). HL has been the subject of controversy, principally surrounding the precise nature of the RS cell (168). This controversy is probably due, in part, to (a) the heterogeneity of HL; (b) difficulties in separating RS cells from the associated abundant reactive component; (c) mistaking RS cells for activated histiocytes; and (d) the loss of antigenic determinants on the larger RS cells. Although clonality often is difficult to demonstrate in HL, many recent studies have proven the clonal nature and B-cell lineage of this neoplasm (169–171).

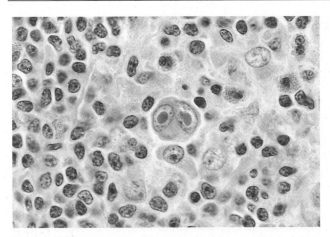

Figure 17.23. Lymph node, Hodgkin lymphoma. A diagnostic binucleate Reed-Sternberg cell with eosinophilic inclusionlike nucleoli.

HL is distinctive among the lymphomas for the extent and variety of the reactive components. Whether this reaction is a reflection of variation in the host or an oncogenic event is uncertain; nevertheless, it seems likely that in HL we are witnessing immunologic reactions to neoplastic induction.

CLASSIFICATION OF HODGKIN LYMPHOMA

The Lukes-Butler classification of HL (172), modified at the Rye Conference (173) in 1966, described the criteria for the four familiar subtypes of HL: lymphocyte-predominant, nodular sclerosing, mixed cellularity, and lymphocyte-depleted. The REAL classification separated the nodular lymphocyte-predominant (NLP) subtype from so-called classic HL based on the immunophenotypic and genotypic differences discussed later herein (10). Classic HL includes nodular-sclerosis, mixed-cellularity, and lymphocyte-depleted subtypes as well as "lymphocyte-rich classic HL," which is similar to lymphocyte-predominant HL but has the phenotype more characteristic of classic HL. The REAL classification of HL was carried forward to the 2001 WHO classification of HL (11) and the 2008 WHO classification (11a), summarized in Table 17.2.

THE IMMUNOPHENOTYPE AND GENOTYPE OF THE REED-STERNBERG CELL

Most current studies indicate the RS cells of HL are lymphocytic in nature and, in the great majority of cases, are of B-cell origin.

RS cells in NLPHL possess B-cell phenotypic features (174,175) and are reported to show clonal immunoglobulin gene rearrangements using sensitive PCR techniques (176). Recent studies demonstrate that immunoglobulin gene rearrangements in L&H variant cells of NLPHL possess some features in common with germinal center cells. In fact, L&H cells can be considered neoplastic germinal center cells, as evidenced by the high load of somatic hypermutation in the variable region of the heavy chain gene (177–179) and the frequent occurrence of *bcl-6* rearrangements (180).

The nature of the RS cell in classic HL is a bit more enigmatic (181). The B-cell origin of classic HL is suggested by studies demonstrating coexpression of CD15 and CD20 by RS cells in some cases (182), and molecular analyses showing clonal B-cell

populations (183). Classic RS cells are derived from germinal center or activated postgerminal center B cells as shown by their rearranged and hypermutated immunoglobulin genes (184) and appear to have lost the B-cell specific gene expression program (185). This latter feature helps explain why classic RS cells demonstrate absent or weak expression of most B-cell–associated immunophenotypic markers.

PRACTICAL CONSIDERATIONS IN THE DIAGNOSIS OF HODGKIN LYMPHOMA

Although past difficulties in the identification of RS cells may be due in part to heterogeneity in the study population, difficulties may also stem from abnormal/absent antigen expression in the malignant lymphoid cells. The practical significance of this point becomes more evident with the expanded use of IHC to distinguish between HL and NHL. Individual RS cells in some unequivocal cases of HL may show B-cell staining with specific antibodies to CD20 (182). Therefore, B-cell marking of RS cells in HL can occur and should not be used as the sole reason to exclude a diagnosis of HL in any particular case. Immunophenotypic characterization has been further complicated by observed phenotypic changes of RS cells over time in sequential biopsies. Such changes in phenotype mostly appear to be due to technical variations in tissue fixation and staining, and can be minimized with antigen retrieval procedures and sensitive immunoperoxidase techniques (186).

Because specific immunohistochemical markers are not available for identification of RS cells, IHC reactivities are considered secondary to morphologic features in establishing a diagnosis of HL. Until such markers become available, the following steps are useful in establishing the diagnosis of HL:

1. Detection of the growth pattern and reactive component specific for each type of HL (see subsequent discussion on "Pathologic Features of Hodgkin Lymphoma").
2. Detection of dysplastic cells (RS cells) in areas of consolidation in node or spleen.
3. In borderline cases, proof by IHC tests that RS cells are CD45−, CD15+, and CD30+ in classic HL (Fig. 17.24) and do not contain monotypic immunoglobulin by routine immunophenotypic studies.

CLINICAL FEATURES OF HODGKIN LYMPHOMA

HL usually presents with painless peripheral adenopathy involving cervical and supraclavicular nodes; less frequently, there is involvement of axillary and inguinal nodes. HL typically causes enlargement of single or contiguous nodes as opposed to the diffuse adenopathy seen in NHL. Constitutional symptoms, including fever, night sweats, and weight loss, may be present. Adjacent nodal groups are usually affected as the disease progresses. Involvement of extranodal sites, such as the spleen, liver, or bone marrow, is less common in HL than in NHL. The incidence of HL in HIV-positive patients is higher, although not to the same extent as NHL. HL most often is diagnosed at stage III or IV in HIV-positive patients and progresses in a more aggressive fashion. These differences in clinical presentation and prognosis may be the result of the altered cellular immunity in acquired immunodeficiency (187). Patients with a history of EBV infection or positive EBV serology are apparently at higher risk of HL, and the EBV genome has been found in diseased

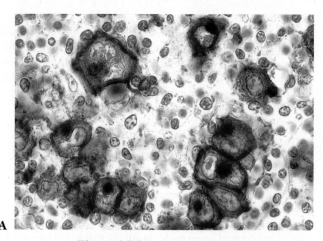
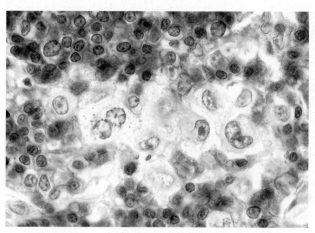

Figure 17.24. Lymph node, nodular-sclerosing Hodgkin lymphoma. **(A)** Clusters of Reed-Sternberg cells and variants react with anti-CD15 (Leu-M1). **(B)** Reed-Sternberg cells in the same case show negative results for CD45 (leukocyte common antigen), in contrast to positive surrounding small lymphocytes. Immunoperoxidase stain with diaminobenzidine substrate.

tissues in approximately one-half of HL cases (188). There appears to be an even stronger correlation between EBV and HL in pediatric patients (189). The following are clinical features specific for each subtype of HL.

Nodular Lymphocyte-Predominant Hodgkin Lymphoma

Nodular lymphocyte-predominant Hodgkin lymphoma (NLPHL) comprises approximately 5% of HL cases (190,191). Although NLPHL occurs in all age groups, the peak incidence is in young adult men (192). Most patients are asymptomatic and have localized disease; approximately 80% of patients are diagnosed in stage I or II; stage IV is rare (190,192). Cervical and axillary nodes are more commonly involved than inguinal or femoral nodes (190,192,193). The prognosis of NLPHL is very favorable. Due to the generally favorable prognosis and low-grade nature of the disease, timing of therapy is the subject of controversy, particularly in patients presenting in low clinical stage (194,195).

Lymphocyte-Rich Classic Hodgkin Lymphoma

Lymphocyte-rich classic Hodgkin lymphoma (LRCHL) often presents similarly to NLPHL, frequently with low stage (196,197). Prognosis is also similar to NLPHL. LRCHL occurs with approximately half the frequency of LPHL. Differences in presentation include a slightly older affected patient population for LRCHL. Mediastinal involvement also occurs with twice the frequency in LRCHL when compared to LPHL (195).

Nodular-Sclerosis Hodgkin Lymphoma

Nodular-sclerosis Hodgkin lymphoma (NSHL) comprises 60% or more of HL cases seen at referral centers (190,191). NSHL is most prevalent in young adults, often appearing as cervical or supraclavicular adenopathy with a mediastinal mass. NSHL develops in women at a rate equal to or greater than that seen in men. Sixty percent of patients have stage I or II disease at diagnosis, and approximately 35% of patients have stage III disease (191).

Mixed-Cellularity Hodgkin Lymphoma

Mixed-cellularity HL (MCHL) makes up approximately 30% of HL cases (191,198). MCHL is more frequent in patients with HIV disease (11). Slightly more than 50% of patients are first seen with stage III or IV disease, and subdiaphragmatic disease is common.

Lymphocyte-Depleted Hodgkin Lymphoma

Approximately 1% to 5% of HL cases are classified as lymphocyte-depleted HL (LDHL) (190,191,198). Most patients with LDHL experience symptoms of fever, weight loss, or night sweats (199,200). LDHL affects an older population more than do the other subtypes of HL, with a median age of onset in the late fifties (200). Almost one-half of these patients have peripheral adenopathy, but approximately 90% have evidence of subdiaphragmatic disease or organomegaly. Because a high proportion of patients have marrow involvement, the diagnosis of LDHL can be made on marrow biopsy alone in some patients (201). Liver involvement is also seen. Other abnormalities in these patients include anemia, thrombocytopenia, peripheral lymphopenia, and abnormal liver function tests (199,200). Like MCHL, this subtype is often associated with HIV disease (202).

PATHOLOGIC FEATURES OF HODGKIN LYMPHOMA

Nodular Lymphocyte-Predominant Hodgkin Lymphoma

HISTOPATHOLOGIC FEATURES. LPHL is divided into two histopathologic subtypes: lymphocytic and histiocytic (L&H) nodular and L&H diffuse (198,203). Currently the WHO classification recognizes only the nodular type and requires at least a partially nodular growth pattern for diagnosis (11). Whether the diffuse type is a distinct entity is controversial.

Small lymphocytes predominate in the reactive component in both types and are intermixed with varying numbers of histiocytes. Eosinophils, neutrophils, and "diagnostic" or "classic" RS cells are rare. In fact, the diagnosis of LPHL is doubtful if diagnostic RS cells are found easily; the number of such cells

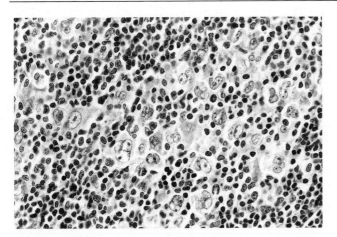

Figure 17.25. Lymph node, nodular lymphocyte-predominant Hodgkin lymphoma. Lymphocytic and histiocytic variants of a Reed-Sternberg cell with clear cytoplasm and hyperlobated, popcorn nuclei are intermixed with small lymphocytes and histiocytes.

should be fewer than one per histologic section (204). In LPHL, L&H variants of RS cells are conspicuous. These mononuclear cells resemble large transformed lymphocytes, with hyperlobated nuclei and finely granular chromatin ("popcorn nuclei"). There is a small amount of pale cytoplasm, and nucleoli are characteristically small (11,198,203) (Fig. 17.25).

In the nodular subtype of LPHL, there is almost total obliteration of the nodal architecture by a vaguely nodular process (198,203). Often, an attenuated rim of residual node is compressed against the nodal capsule (Fig. 17.26). Some cases have a few delicate bands of connective tissue, suggesting the sclerosing patterns in NSHL, but LPHL nodules are composed principally of small, round lymphocytes with varying numbers of epithelioid histiocytes. The histiocytes often form small aggregates and may resemble sarcoid granulomas. L&H variants of RS cells may be numerous and are principally seen in the nodules. "Diagnostic" or "classic" RS cells are rare or nonexistent and are not required for the diagnosis of NLPHL in cases meeting the histopathologic criteria described here. The nodular growth

pattern and predominance of small lymphocytes may suggest follicular lymphoma (203), a diagnosis readily excluded by the absence of the monomorphism and nuclear irregularity characteristic of centrocytes typically seen in follicular lymphomas. Immunophenotypic studies are also useful in this differential.

Variant growth patterns of NLPHL have been described in addition to the typical B-cell–rich nodular pattern (205). Variants include cases with prominent extranodular L&H cells and other cases with nodules rich in T cells. In some cases of NLPHL, a partially diffuse growth pattern rich in reactive T cells with scattered L&H cells is seen, resembling T-cell–rich diffuse large-B-cell lymphoma. The detection of at least one typical nodule of NLPHD is sufficient to exclude T-cell–rich diffuse large-B-cell lymphoma in such cases.

There is a very modest (approximately 5%) increased incidence of NHL, usually diffuse large-B-cell lymphoma, in patients with NLPHL, which can occur either concurrently with or subsequently to the diagnosis of HL. In many cases, a clonal relationship between the L&H cells of NLPHL and the diffuse large-B-cell lymphoma can be demonstrated (206).

Diffuse LPHL is rare, and its existence as a distinct subtype of HL is the subject of controversy. It differs from nodular LPHL by having an essentially diffuse growth pattern without a thin rim of compressed nodal tissue (199,203). Some cases diagnosed as diffuse LPHL may contain a few very ill-defined nodules that are difficult to identify without using IHC markers, such as CD21, to highlight follicular dendritic cell networks. The reactive component is similar in morphologic features to that in NLPHL, although the histiocytic component may be less apparent. L&H variants of RS cells are present.

Nodes from patients with NLPHL may show a distinctive follicular center abnormality termed *progressive transformation of germinal centers* (PTGC) (23,26). PTGC may occur in patients with antecedent or concurrent NLPHL as well as in patients in whom NLPHL later develops. There is also a subset of patients with PTGC who never develop NLPHL. Germinal centers in PTGC are unusually large. There is breakdown of the interface between the mantle zones and germinal centers, producing a scalloped, serpentine, or blurred border. As the lesion progresses, there is extensive infiltration of germinal centers by small lymphocytes, until single or small groups of large, transformed cells are completely surrounded by small lymphocytes. The resulting enlarged and distorted germinal center is reminiscent of nodular NLPHL but lacks RS cell variants.

IMMUNOHISTOCHEMICAL FEATURES. The association of NLPHL with PTGC was the first predictor that NLPHL is a germinal center proliferation (26). L&H cells are commonly CD45+ and express many B-cell–associated antigens, including CD20, CD79a, Bcl-6, J-chain, and PAX-5 (207–209). Epithelial membrane antigen expression is seen on L&H cells in about 50% of cases of NLPHL, but EBER transcripts are virtually always absent. L&H cells are CD15− and CD30−, in contrast to the RS cells of classic HL. Caution is advised in evaluating CD30 staining because activated mononuclear CD30+ cells, usually a bit smaller than L&H cells, are frequently seen in reactive lymphoid tissue and are easily mistaken for L&H cells (208).

The small lymphocytes in NLPHL are predominantly polytypic B cells with a mantle zone phenotype (IgM+, IgD+), but T lymphocytes may be prominent in some cases (175). Cells immediately surrounding L&H variants are T lymphocytes,

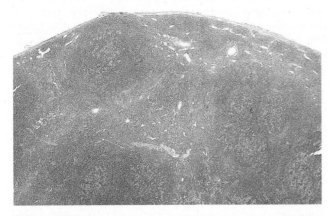

Figure 17.26. Lymph node, nodular, lymphocyte-predominant Hodgkin lymphoma (NLPHL). An attenuated rim of residual normal node (*top*) is often present in nodular NLPHL. The vaguely nodular growth pattern and compressed adjacent normal node seen at low magnification are features highly suggestive of Nodular NLPHL.

which in many cases, T cells are CD4+ and CD57+. NLPHL shows prominent networks of dendritic reticulum cells within the nodules, a feature which is highlighted by immunohistochemical stains for CD21 or CD35.

CLASSIC HODGKIN LYMPHOMA

HISTOPATHOLOGIC FEATURES

Lymphocytic-Rich Classic Hodgkin Lymphoma

Some cases of HL may be difficult to classify due to a background rich in small lymphocytes similar to LPHL, but contain RS cells which demonstrate a phenotype like that seen in classic HL (208,210). The WHO classification has incorporated a category LRCHL for such cases, which in the past were classified either as LPHL, cellular phase of NSHL, or MCHL.

LCRHL shows more commonly a nodular growth pattern or, rarely, a diffuse growth (208). The nodules often contain small, atretic germinal centers that are eccentrically located in an expanded mantle zone. The RS cells usually are embedded within the mantle zone or at the periphery of the follicle. "Classic" RS cells are found in many cases, and cells resembling L&H cells can also be seen.

Nodular-Sclerosis Hodgkin Lymphoma

The classic histopathologic criteria for NSHL are (a) prominent nodularity, (b) presence of lacunar RS cell variants, and (c) birefringent broad collagen bands (198,203). Nodal architecture is obliterated by relatively large nodules of tumor partly or totally encircled by dense connective tissue bands that are birefringent when viewed under polarized light (Figs. 17.3 and 17.27). In early lesions, fibrosis may involve only the capsule of

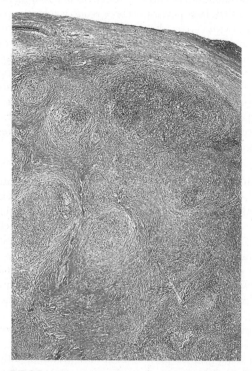

Figure 17.27. Lymph node, nodular-sclerosis Hodgkin lymphoma. Characteristic nodules of tumor surrounded by dense connective tissue are apparent on this low-magnification view.

the node, but broad bands of sclerosis develop and intersect the fibrotic capsule as the lesion progresses (198,203).

The RS cells typically seen in NSHL are termed *lacunar variants* (211). These variants possess large, multilobated, or irregular nuclei with finely dispersed chromatin; nucleoli are usually small. The cytoplasm of lacunar cells is pale, eosinophilic, or "water clear." In formalin-fixed material, the cytoplasm displays a retraction artifact from surrounding cells, and the cell nucleus is surrounded by an empty space. Cytoplasmic retraction does not occur in tissues fixed in Zenker fixative or B5, and "lacunar cells" must be identified on the basis of their nuclear features and pale cytoplasm (Fig. 17.28).

There is considerable variation in the histologic features of NSHL, especially in the reactive component as well as in the number and distribution of RS cells (198,203). NSHL usually contains a reactive component of small lymphocytes, plasma cells, and numerous eosinophils and histiocytes; rarely, large numbers of polymorphonuclear leukocytes predominate. Large geographic zones of necrosis are often seen. RS cells and the lacunar variants are readily identified and have a tendency to form clusters. Mononuclear RS cell variants may predominate in some cases. RS cells showing necrosis with intense cytoplasmic eosinophilia are called "mummified" or "zombie" cells (212).

Previously, the presence of nodules and lacunar cells without fibrous bands was often referred to as the cellular phase of NSHL (198,203). However, this term is imprecisely defined and probably should be avoided. Some cases of NSHL may also show large sheets of RS cells and mononuclear variants, with little or no reactive component, which frequently surround areas of necrosis. This appearance is termed the *syncytial variant* (213) or *monomorphic growth pattern* of NSHL (Fig. 17.29) (214). This lesion may be confused with the reticular form of LDHL, large-cell NHL, and even metastatic melanocytic or germ cell tumors. In the syncytial or monomorphic variant, lacunar cells are often present, and there is usually a history of NSHL or another area of the biopsy that shows more classic NS histologic features (213,214). A rare fibroblastic variant of HL, seen most often as a component of NSHL, is characterized by a fibrohistiocytic proliferation that may obscure RS cells and be misdiagnosed as a spindle cell neoplasm (215). Several systems have been proposed for the grading of NSHL; most notable is that of the British National Lymphoma Investigation (216). In this system, NSHL is graded based on the numbers of RS cells relative to the reactive component. Grade I NSHL is defined as having 75% or more nodules composed of a mixed reactive infiltrate, with only scattered RS cells present. Grade II NSHL possesses greater than 25% of nodules with increased RS cells, which is further defined as a sheet of RS cells or variants occupying a diameter of at least one high-power (40×) field. Syncytial NSHL is thus a grade II NSHL. Grading of NSHL is not typically used for clinical purposes at this time, but is used as a parameter in investigative studies (11).

Mixed-Cellularity Hodgkin Lymphoma

The original Rye classification MCHL category included cases that were in transition between LPHL and LDHL as well as cases that did not fulfill all the diagnostic criteria of the other subtypes (198,203). The WHO classification regards MCHL as a true subtype and not a "wastebasket" category (11). Most cases of MCHL show a diffuse obliteration of nodal architecture without

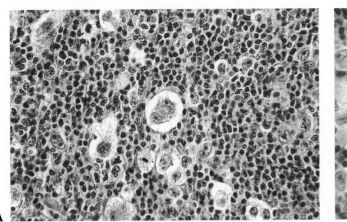
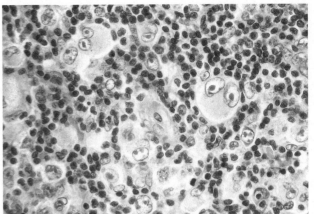

A
B

Figure 17.28. Lymph node, nodular-sclerosis Hodgkin lymphoma. **(A)** Lacunar Reed-Sternberg cells in formalin-fixed paraffin sections show extensive cytoplasmic retraction artifact. **(B)** In mercuric chloride–fixed material, lacunar Reed-Sternberg cells do not show retraction artifact but, rather, abundant amounts of water-clear cytoplasm.

capsular thickening or broad bands of parenchymal fibrosis. "Classic" RS cells are easily found, often in a background of small lymphocytes, eosinophils, histiocytes, plasma cells, or neutrophils (Fig. 17.30).

Some cases of MCHL display an interfollicular growth pattern (Fig. 17.31). Such cases may be difficult to distinguish from peripheral T-cell lymphomas. Classic RS cells are usually not present in peripheral T-cell lymphomas, but some binucleate cells may be seen. The small lymphocytes in MCHL should not display dysplastic features, but such cytologic nuances are of marginal value in individual cases. IHC is helpful in that the large cells in peripheral T-cell lymphomas should mark as T cells; in MCHL, the RS cells usually do not mark as T cells and are often PAX-5+. CD15 reactivity in dysplastic cells is often helpful in the recognition of HL; rare cases of peripheral T-cell lymphomas, however, may be CD15+ (217).

Interfollicular MCHL may resemble infectious mononucleosis (13) and other types of viral adenitis. Distinguishing between interfollicular HL and viral adenitis can be very difficult, especially if few RS cells are present. Mononucleosis often causes

interfollicular expansion (see previous section on "Reactive Adenopathy"), and binucleate cells resembling RS cells may be seen (101). Interfollicular consolidation with a discrete mass effect is the most reliable morphologic criterion for interfollicular HL; in viral adenitis, there is a more even expansion of the interfollicular regions of the node. Although these histologic features are reasonably specific, all young adults with isolated cervical adenopathy should undergo routine serologic studies for mononucleosis.

MCHL may also be associated with a prominent granulomatous reaction (218). These cases are frequently difficult to recognize because focus is often on the granulomas. Focal consolidation of the node, resulting from interfollicular infiltration of eosinophils, plasma cells, macrophages, and lymphocytes, suggests the diagnosis. Mononuclear and RS cells may be difficult to find, but appropriate IHC studies facilitate confirmation of the diagnosis. MCHL may also show foci of cellular depletion and diffuse fibrosis.

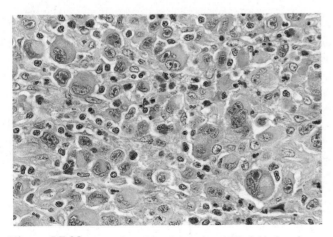

Figure 17.29. Lymph node, nodular-sclerosis Hodgkin lymphoma. A monomorphic or syncytial growth pattern is present, with sheets of lacunar Reed-Sternberg cells and variants. There is little or no reactive component.

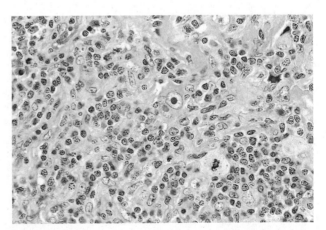

Figure 17.30. Lymph node, mixed-cellularity Hodgkin lymphoma disease. Diagnostic Reed-Sternberg cells are usually found without difficulty in mixed-cellularity Hodgkin lymphoma. The reactive component consists of small, round lymphocytes, histiocytes, plasma cells, and eosinophils.

Figure 17.31. Lymph node, mixed-cellularity Hodgkin lymphoma (MCHL). Some cases of MCHL show a striking interfollicular growth pattern. These lesions may be difficult to diagnose if few Reed-Sternberg cells are present.

Lymphocyte-Depleted Hodgkin Lymphoma

The biologic hallmark of LDHL is a collapse of cell-mediated immunity, a process reflected in histologic sections as a depletion of the reactive component of the neoplasm (219). In the past, two subtypes of LDHL—diffuse fibrosis and reticular LDHL (198,203)—were recognized and, at times, coexisted in the same patient. The WHO classification (Table 17.2) does not subdivide the LDHL. Although the morphologic appearance of LDHL is varied, a unifying feature is the relative predominance of RS cells compared with the depletion of background lymphocytes (11).

In some cases there is a diffuse fibrosis background. Sections show a hypocellular background and abundant disorderly connective tissue admixed with a PAS-positive fibrinoid material that is not birefringent (Fig. 17.32). Nodal architecture is completely obliterated. RS cells may be rare and difficult to identify. Initial biopsy specimens obtained in patients with LDHL may be from the liver or marrow. At these sites, the foci of involve-

ment may show small areas of fibrosis, fibrinoid change, and cellular depletion; multiple sections may be required to find RS cells (201).

Other cases of LDHL have little in the way of a reactive component but are distinguished by the presence of numerous large RS cells (198,203) with bizarre cytologic features. The sheetlike growth of bizarre RS cells is responsible for the older term *Hodgkin sarcoma*. These cases of LDHL have histologic and cytologic similarities to various other large-cell neoplasms, including anaplastic large-cell lymphoma (ALCL; see "Anaplastic Large-Cell Lymphoma" below), malignant histiocytoses, large-cell carcinomas, malignant melanoma, and the monomorphic variant of NSHL (219). In most situations, LDHL is readily differentiated from the previously mentioned neoplasms by a comprehensive IHC battery (Table 17.1).

Immunophenotypic Features of Classic Hodgkin Lymphoma

The RS cells of classic HL usually express CD15, CD30, and are negative for CD45 by paraffin IHC, in contrast to the L&H cells of NLPH (220–222) (Fig. 17.24). CD30 positivity of RS cells is seen in virtually all cases of classic HL, whereas CD15 expression is present in about 60% to 90% (5). CD15 expression is not unique to RS cells of classic HL and can be seen in granulocytes, cytomegalovirus cells (223), rare cases of peripheral T-cell lymphomas, and some carcinomas. CD30 expression is even less specific for classic HL RS cells and can be demonstrated in a variety of other reactive lymphoid and nonlymphoid cells, as well as other types of large-cell lymphomas, both B- and T-cell types.

The detection of EBV-encoded latent membrane protein 1 (LMP1) or RNA (EBER-1) by IHC or in situ hybridization, respectively, is seen in RS cells in approximately 50% of cases of classic HL, most often in MCHL and in HL associated with HIV disease.

The B-cell origin of classic HL is demonstrated by the expression of B-cell antigens such as CD20 (182) and CD79a in RS cells in up to 40% of cases. However, CD20 staining is often weaker and more variable than typically seen in cases of large-

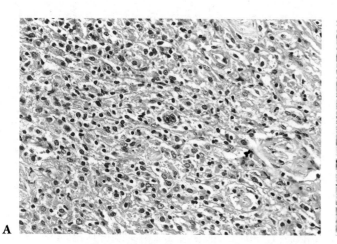

A

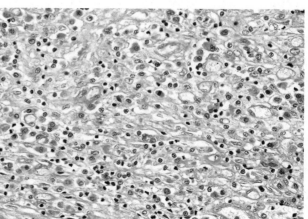

B

Figure 17.32. Lymph node, lymphocyte-depleted Hodgkin lymphoma. **(A)** Diagnostic Reed-Sternberg cells may be difficult to find in the diffuse fibrosis variant of lymphocyte-depleted Hodgkin lymphoma, although variants may be abundant. **(B)** Deposition of a fibrinoid material that is positive on periodic acid-Schiff is usually seen.

B-cell lymphomas or NLPHL, likely due to the loss of the B-cell–specific gene expression program in classic HL (185). Likewise, classic HL cells usually express PAX-5 (B-cell–specific activator protein) in a nuclear pattern, but at an intensity that is less than background reactive B cells, a feature that facilitates the recognition of RS cells (5).

The differentiation of classic HL from large B-cell NHL usually can be made on the basis of CD45, CD20, CD15, and CD30 expression. Differentiation from T/null anaplastic large-cell lymphoma is accomplished with T-cell, PAX-5, and ALK-1 immunostaining.

B-CELL NEOPLASMS

More than 80% of non-Hodgkin lymphomas are of B-cell origin in the United States and Europe (224). As described several decades ago in the functional lymphoma classifications of Lukes/Collins (225) and Kiel (226), and expanded upon more recently in the REAL (10) and WHO (11a) lymphoma classifications (Table 17.2), most, although not all, can be related to normal B-cell compartments based on their anatomic location, architectural and cytologic characteristics, and immunophenotype. Genotypic and karyotypic features are also useful in better understanding these neoplasms, in their recognition and precise classification, and in prognostication in selected circumstances. Many of the B-cell lymphomas composed of small, nontransformed cells can be recognized from histopathology alone, although immunophenotypic confirmation is useful and will help avoid unnecessary errors. It is important to remember that the WHO classification is not purely a "cell of origin" classification and that each entity recognized is identified, in part, because it is considered to be a distinct clinicopathologic entity. With some entities, clinical information is also critical in making a precise diagnosis.

B-cell development begins with the commitment of primitive blasts to the B-lineage and rearrangement of the immunoglobulin genes, accumulation of cytoplasmic μ-heavy chain (pre-B cells), and then development into small surface immunoglobulin-positive prefollicular/naïve B cells. The latter make up the mantle zone cells in organized lymphoid tissue and a subpopulation of the recirculating small lymphocytes. These naïve B cells have unmutated immunoglobulin genes. Some normally express the T-cell–associated CD5 antigen, but others do not. B cells then enter follicular centers where they undergo somatic mutation of the immunoglobulin genes, antigenic selection, and heavy chain class switching that lead to antibodies of varied affinities and greater antibody diversity. The numerous follicular center cells that are not selected undergo apoptosis/programmed cell death. Morphologically, the cells entering the follicular centers transform into rapidly dividing, intermediate-sized, transformed (noncleaved) follicular center cells or centroblasts. Transformed lymphoid cells, like those exposed to a mitogen, are intermediate to large with dispersed chromatin and nucleoli. These cells divide and then either die or, if selected, develop into the more dormant cleaved follicular center cells or centrocytes and potentially other transformed follicular center cells or centroblasts and immunoblasts. Most follicular center B cells are CD5−, CD10+, and Bcl-6+. Late follicular center cells lose their Bcl-6 positivity and become positive for MUM-1/IRF4 (227). Follicular centers also include many CD4+, often CD57+, follicular helper T cells in their "pale

zones" and antigen-presenting CD21+, partially CD23+ follicular dendritic cells. B cells, now with their immunoglobulin genes mutated, then leave the follicles to become either memory-type B cells or plasma cells. Although B immunoblasts also may exit the follicular centers and be found in interfollicular areas, in the absence of neoplasia, both cleaved and transformed follicular center cells should be restricted to the follicles. The memory-type B cells include both many recirculating small lymphocytes as well as many of the cells of the marginal zone, a B-cell compartment most prominent in the spleen and mesenteric lymph nodes. Although memory B cells generally have mutated Ig genes without ongoing mutational activity, some may once again undergo additional mutations (possibly by re-entering follicles) and some appear to be unmutated.

The B-cell lymphomas can be thought of as clonal proliferations with partial or total blocks in this maturational sequence and accumulations of one or more B-cell type. Some are made up predominantly of nontransformed, slowly dividing cells ("small B-cell lymphoid neoplasms"); others largely of transformed more rapidly dividing cells (Burkitt and large-B-cell lymphomas); some have greater admixtures of the former two cell types; and a minority are composed of true lymphoblasts (the B-lymphoblastic leukemia/lymphomas). In general, because of similar morphologic appearances and overlapping phenotypic features, it is often impossible with routine diagnostic studies (and sometimes even with very sophisticated studies) to separate the different types of transformed cells, whereas most small B-cell lymphomas can be more easily recognized. It is largely for this reason, at the current time, that most diffuse B-cell lymphomas of large transformed cells are lumped into a single, very heterogeneous category. This category is utilized even when a precise cell type can be identified, such as the diffuse large-B-cell lymphomas that are clonally related to classic follicular lymphomas. The 2008 WHO classification separates some of these large-B-cell types into meaningful subsets (Table 17.2). Finally, there are B-cell neoplasms composed exclusively or largely of the B-cell effectors, the plasma cells.

Many principles of lymphoma biology that are important to recognize were illustrated several decades ago by the studies of the lymphomas of follicular center cell origin and highlighted in the Lukes/Collins classification (225,228):

1. Histopathologic features, in some circumstances, can be used to identify a precise type of lymphoma and cell of origin (Figs. 17.5, 17.33).
2. Lymphomas with different appearances and behaviors can arise from a single functional subpopulation. Follicular centers, for example, give rise to indolent tumors (grade 1 follicular lymphoma) and aggressive neoplasms (a subset of diffuse large-B-cell lymphoma [DLBCL] and Burkitt lymphoma [BL]).
3. B-cell lymphomas can contain neoplastic cells at various stages of the cell cycle. All lymphomas contain a dividing component (e.g., transformed follicular center cells or centroblasts), but these cells may be in the minority, such as in follicular lymphomas with predominantly cleaved cells or centrocytes.
4. Some B-cell lymphomas, such as follicular lymphoma and BL, are strongly associated with specific genotypic/karyotypic abnormalities. They also often have characteristic, although not necessarily specific, immunophenotypic profiles.

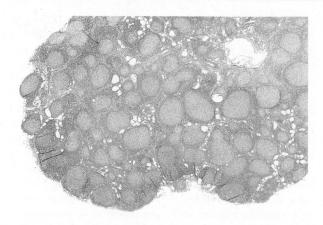

Figure 17.33.   Lymph node, follicular lymphoma. The nodal architecture is effaced by a predominantly follicular lymphoid proliferation. Note the crowding of the follicles and lack of cortical/medullary distinction.

5. Progression of indolent to aggressive lymphomas, usually with a marked increase in the size of the dividing component, occurs and is often associated with secondary genotypic abnormalities, such as IP53 mutation.
6. Lymphomas of follicular center cell origin often contain numerous admixed T cells, most of which are often CD4+ T-helper cells. This reacting component, which can represent the majority of cells present in a B-cell lymphoma, may have important regulatory functions in terms of neoplastic B-cell growth and differentiation, since under normal conditions T cells control B-cell functions.

This section covers the nodal B-cell lymphomas as categorized in the WHO classification (Tables 17.2 and 17.4). Those considered to be of extranodal type are discussed largely or exclusively in other chapters. The major B-cell lymphoma types not included in this chapter are extranodal marginal zone B-cell lymphoma of mucosa-associated lymphoid tissue (MALT lymphoma), splenic marginal zone lymphoma, and the extranodal plasmacytic neoplasms. Although not classic "extranodal lymphomas," many of the lymphomas discussed in this chapter can present at extranodal sites, including some with a propensity for certain extranodal sites, such as mantle cell lymphomas that can present in the gastrointestinal tract as multiple lymphomatous polyposis.

CHRONIC LYMPHOCYTIC LEUKEMIA/SMALL LYMPHOCYTIC LYMPHOMA

Definition

Chronic lymphocytic leukemia (CLL)/small lymphocytic lymphoma (SLL) is a lymphoid neoplasm in which small, usually round, B lymphocytes with a characteristic immunophenotypic profile predominate (226,229,230). They presumably arise in either marrow or lymph nodes, and many cases have significant peripheral blood involvement. At least in lymph nodes, there are typically admixed collections of prolymphocytes/paraimmunoblasts. Lacking nodal involvement, there must be a monoclonal lymphocytosis with a CLL phenotype of $\geq 5 \times 10/L$ in

the peripheral blood. Variants of CLL, called "CLL of mixed-cell type" by the French-American-British (FAB) cooperative group, are recognized with one type having "pleomorphic lymphocytes" but less than 10% prolymphocytes in the peripheral blood ("atypical" CLL), and the other CLL with increased (10% to 55%) prolymphocytes in the peripheral blood (CLL/PL) (231). Prolymphocytes are larger than typical small lymphocytes, and have more abundant basophilic cytoplasm and prominent nucleoli.

Histopathologic Features

Rare follicular centers or sinuses may remain, but nodal architecture is usually completely and diffusely effaced (Figs. 17.34, 17.35). The predominant cells are monomorphic small lymphocytes with relatively round nuclei, clumped chromatin, and scant cytoplasm. Approximately 90% of cases contain ill-defined, pale-staining proliferation centers or pseudofollicles in which there are slightly larger cells with dispersed chromatin and more cytoplasm. Some of the larger cells have distinct nucleoli ("paraimmunoblasts"); classic immunoblasts are uncommon. Mitotic figures are found almost exclusively in proliferation centers. Proliferation centers are a very useful histologic finding because they are found only in CLL/SLL. Occasional CLL/SLLs may appear somewhat nodular, raising the differential diagnosis of a follicular lymphoma. Overt plasmacytic differentiation in CLL/SLL is uncommon; however, plasmacytoid features may be present. Histopathologic characteristics are not predictive of the likelihood of a leukemic phase in CLL/SLL. Cases of the "mixed-cell type" of CLL/SLL have been associated with lymph nodes with large numbers of paraimmunoblasts and prolymphocytes and very large proliferation centers and/or nuclear irregularities in the neoplastic cells (232).

Interfollicular SLL (I-SLL) is a variant of CLL/SLL, not specifically identified in the WHO classification, in which there are residual follicular centers and, often, at least some patent sinuses (233,234). Sometimes the proliferation centers encircle the reactive follicles, raising the possibility of a nodal marginal zone lymphoma. In other cases, the extensive architectural retention makes distinguishing I-SLL from a reactive lymph node challenging until immunophenotypic studies are performed. Recognizing the proliferation centers, however, is a very useful histologic feature in these circumstances to help distinguish I-SLL from a reactive hyperplasia.

Immunologic/Genotypic/Karyotypic Features

CLL/SLL is a monoclonal B-cell neoplasm with a characteristic CD5+, CD10−, CD23+, FMC7− phenotype (229,230,235–237). Except for CD19, most pan-B-cell antigens are only weakly expressed or are undetectable (e.g., CD20, CD22, CD79b) (229,237,238). Surface immunoglobulin of the IgM/IgD type is usually present, although it is scanty and difficult to detect. CD11c expression may be present. Most CLL/SLLs can be identified immunophenotypically using paraffin section immunostains, even though immunoglobulin staining will give completely negative results in most laboratories (239). Useful panels include antibodies to CD5, CD10, CD23, CD43, Bcl-2, and cyclin D1(240). Most lymph nodes affected by B-CLL/SLL contain less than 15% T cells, predominantly CD4 (230). Peripheral

TABLE 17.4	Differential Diagnosis of Major B-Cell Lymphomas[a]		
Type of Lymphoma	Histopathologic Features	Immunophenotype[b]	Genotype/Karyotype[bd]
CLL/SLL	Diffuse architectural effacement by small lymphocytes and paler proliferation centers that include paraimmunoblasts	SIg weak +, CIg[c], CD5+, CD10−, CD23+, FMC7−, CD43 usually +, cyclin D1−, bcl-2+	Chromosome 13q14 and 11q deletions; trisomy 12, especially in "atypical" CLL
LPL	Partial or complete architectural effacement by small lymphocytes, plasmacytoid, and plasma cells; may have mantle zone growth pattern and intact sinuses; must exclude other B-cell lymphomas with plasmacytic differentiation; Dutcher bodies common	SIg+, CIg+, CD5−, CD10−	Uncertain
MCL	Diffuse, vaguely nodular or mantle zone proliferation of relatively small lymphocytes with slightly irregular to cleft nuclei; some cases more blastic or with larger cells; transformed cells absent	SIg+, CD5+, CD10−, CD23−, FMC7 usually +, CD43 usually +, cyclin D1+, bcl-2+	CCND1 (cyclin D1/bcl-1) rearrangement (t[11; 14])([q13;q32]) in virtually all cases. ATM gene abnormalities
FL	Architectural effacement by a proliferation that, at least in part, forms closely packed follicular nodules; predominantly small cleaved cells/centrocytes in most cases but others have more numerous transformed cells/centroblasts (see text for discussion of grading); diffuse areas with numerous transformed cells should be separately designated	SIg usually +, CD5−, usually CD10+, bcl-6+, CD43 usually −, follicles bcl-2+	bcl-2 (t[14; 18][q32;q21]) rearrangement in ~85% of cases.
NMZL	Partial or complete architectural effacement by pale-appearing nontransformed marginal zone-like/parafollicular/monocytoid B cells that may grow around reactive follicles. Plasmacytic differentiation and follicular colonization can be seen; must exclude nodal involvement by MALT lymphoma	SIg+, CIg variable, CD5−, CD10−, bcl-2+, cyclin D1−.	Trisomy 3, trisomy 18, 1q21, or 1q34 structural abnormalities
DLBCL	Diffuse architectural effacement by transformed lymphoid cells (centroblastic, immunoblastic, plasmablastic, anaplastic)	SIg and CIg variable, CD5−, CD10 variable, bcl-2 variable	Minority have bcl-2 or bcl-6 rearrangements. Rare c-myc rearrangements
BL	Diffuse architectural effacement by relatively small amphophilic/basophilic/pyroninophilic transformed lymphoid cells with a high mitotic rate and starry-sky appearance; rarely follicular in part	SIg+, CD5−, CD10+, bcl-6+, bcl-2−	c-myc rearrangements (most often (t[8;14][q24;q32])

[a]Beware of exceptions to the generalizations expressed in this table.
[b]In all cases, pan-B-cell antigens (especially CD19 and CD20) are positive and there are clonal immunoglobulin gene rearrangements demonstrable by Southern blot or PCR analysis.
[c]See text for full discussion of genotypic/karyotypic findings. Table includes only the major abnormalities most specifically associated with each neoplasm.
[d]CIg may be documented using sensitive methods or in cases with some plasmacytoid differentiation.
CLL/SLL, chronic lymphocytic leukemia/small lymphocytic lymphoma; LPL, lymphoplasmacytic lymphoma; MCL, mantle cell lymphoma; FL, follicular lymphoma; NMZL, nodal marginal zone B-cell lymphoma; DLBCL, diffuse large-B-cell lymphoma; BL, Burkitt lymphoma; SIg, surface immunoglobulin; CIg, cytoplasmic immunoglobulin.

blood studies, however, often show an inversion of the CD4:CD8 ratio.

Expression of CD38, an activation antigen, is variably expressed in CLL (241–245). Although not useful diagnostically, when present in more than 20% to 30% of peripheral blood CLL cells, it is associated with an adverse prognosis (241–245). More recently, expression of ZAP-70 and absence of MUM-1 proteins have also been associated with an adverse prognosis (246–248).

CLL/SLL may be distinguished from hairy cell leukemia and from most follicular and marginal zone B-cell lymphomas by its CD5 positivity and CD10 negativity. Immunophenotypic distinction from mantle cell lymphoma (MCL) is based on the usually very weak surface immunoglobulin staining, CD23 positivity,

FMC7 negativity, and lack of cyclin D1 staining. The presence of the T-cell–associated CD43 antigen on the neoplastic B cells is useful in helping diagnose a B-cell neoplasm and, in many cases, along with CD10 and Bcl-6 negativity, is helpful in distinguishing CLL/SLLs from most follicular lymphomas (249). It is worth noting that peripheral blood studies will show clonal B cells with a CLL phenotype in 3.5% of adults with normal white blood cell counts (250).

Trisomy 12 is present in about 10% to 30% of CLL/SLL (232,251,252). It may be detected by routine karyotypic studies, but it is more readily shown using interphase cytogenetic studies. Trisomy 12 is associated with cases of "atypical" CLL (mixed type and/or atypical phenotype) and is much less common in typical CLL/SLL (232,251,252). A more common cytogenetic

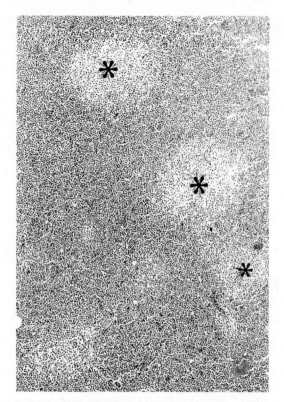

Figure 17.34. Lymph node, B-cell chronic lymphocytic leukemia/small lymphocytic lymphoma. The nodal architecture is diffusely effaced by a proliferation of small lymphocytes. Note the paler-staining proliferation centers that have ill-defined borders (*asterisk*).

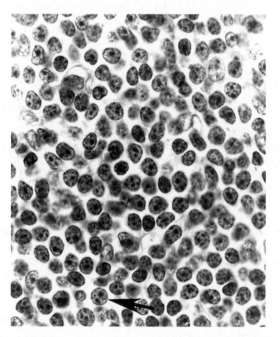

Figure 17.35. Lymph node, B-cell chronic lymphocytic leukemia/small lymphocytic lymphoma. Many of the lymphocytes are small and have round nuclei with clumped chromatin and little cytoplasm. Note the slightly larger lymphocytes with more dispersed chromatin and medium-sized nucleoli (*arrow*). The latter cells, which are most frequently found in proliferation centers, also have slightly more cytoplasm than the predominant small lymphocytes.

abnormality, seen in up to about half of B-CLL/SLL, is chromosome 13q14 deletions or, sometimes, translocations (251–253). Deletion 11q22-23 has been reported in up to 27% of patients and, in contrast to chromosome 13 abnormalities, is associated with an adverse prognosis (245,251,252,254). Cases of CLL/SLL may have other karyotypic abnormalities, including del6q21 and 17p13, either with or without the more common abnormalities (232,251,252). 17p deletions are another adverse prognostic indicator (245,251,254). A minority also have ATM (ataxia telangiectasia mutated) gene mutations (255).

Originally considered a neoplasm of naïve B cells, it is now recognized that many cases of CLL/SLL have mutated immunoglobulin (Ig) genes (230,232–234,246–249). These latter cases have a better prognosis than CLL/SLL with unmutated Ig genes. A specific subset of mutated cases that use the *VH3-21* gene, however, have a survival more like the unmutated cases (250). Gene profiling studies have suggested that both the mutated and unmutated subtypes are most closely related to memory-type B cells (246,247,250). Zap-70 expression and, in some but not all studies, CD38 expression correlate with the unmutated cases (241–244,246,248,256,257). Currently, assessment of mutational status is not a widely used practical laboratory test.

Clinical Features

CLL/SLL is a typically indolent but incurable neoplasm with many patients surviving for 15 years or longer. There is a subset of patients with a more aggressive clinical course who succumb to their disease just a few years after diagnosis, despite aggressive therapy (229). The NHL classification project reports a 5-year overall survival rate of 51%, but other series demonstrate longer median survivals (224,243,244). Clinical staging systems, such as the Rai (258) and Binet (259) and other prognostic indicators have been used to identify those patients with a higher risk of more aggressive disease (229).

Approximately 3% to 10% of CLL patients experience the development of a second, more aggressive-appearing lymphoma, and this event is termed *Richter syndrome* or *Richter transformation*, in tribute to Dr. Maurice Richter who first recognized the entity (260).

Richter syndrome is often heralded by a sudden clinical deterioration, fever, weight loss, and enlargement of lymph node masses (261). This transformation often portends a poor prognosis. It is likely that Richter transformation represents at least two separate phenomena (262): the progression of CLL/SLL to a clonally related aggressive lymphoma; or the development of a clonally unrelated second lymphoma in patients with CLL/SLL.

The aggressive lymphoma in Richter syndrome usually is a DLBCL that often, but not always, can be demonstrated to have a clonal relationship to the CLL/SLL. A smaller number of cases of CLL/SLL show signs of transformation that are morphologically and immunophenotypically more like Hodgkin lymphoma (263–267). A similar phenomenon seen in rare cases of CLL/SLL is the emergence of scattered RS-like cells in the background of CLL/SLL. The HL-like cases have a better prognosis than the classic DLBCL Richter syndrome (268). Transformation in CLL/SLL may also be reflected by increasing numbers (15% to 90%) of prolymphocytes in the peripheral blood (269,270). Lymph nodes do not necessarily reflect this type of transformation.

Incidental lymphomas are discovered in a small percentage

of patients who undergo radical lymph node dissection for staging of various carcinomas. The most common type of lymphoma found in these patients is CLL/SLL (271).

LYMPHOPLASMACYTIC LYMPHOMA

Definition

Lymphoplasmacytic lymphoma (LPL) is a B-cell neoplasm composed of small, relatively round lymphocytes, plasmacytoid lymphocytes, and plasma cells (272,273). Cases of other well-defined lymphomas with plasmacytic differentiation and CLL/SLL with plasmacytoid features must be excluded. LPL can be leukemic and may be associated with Waldenström macroglobulinemia; similar-appearing neoplasms may produce IgG or IgA.

Histopathologic Features

Nodal architecture is either partially or completely effaced by a proliferation of small, round lymphocytes with little cytoplasm, variable numbers of plasmacytoid lymphocytes, and well-developed plasma cells. Plasmacytoid lymphocytes often have slightly eccentric nuclei, some pyroninophilic cytoplasm, and what appear to be PAS-positive "nuclear inclusions" known as Dutcher bodies (Fig. 17.36). These are actually cytoplasmic Ig surrounded by a narrow rim of the nucleus. Similar inclusions may also be found in the cytoplasm (Russell bodies) with the nucleus barely, if at all, visible. Transformed cells are relatively sparse in many cases but can be moderately numerous in some, raising the differential diagnosis of a diffuse large-B-cell lymphoma (273). Intact and sometimes dilated sinuses, as well as increased mast cells and hemosiderin, are often present. Some cases closely resemble reactive lymph nodes. LPL can surround reactive-appearing follicular centers, producing a mantle zone growth pattern or have a vaguely nodular growth pattern. Some cases have numerous epithelioid histiocytes and may be confused with HL (274). Amyloid may be present. LPL must be distinguished from follicular lymphomas and marginal zone lymphomas (of nodal and MALT type), which may also show marked plasmacytic differentiation (275–277). LPL also may be confused with T-cell lymphomas containing numerous reactive plasma cells.

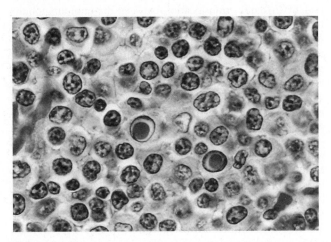

Figure 17.36. Lymph node, lymphoplasmacytic lymphoma. Note the two Dutcher bodies (nuclear invaginations that are periodic acid-Schiff positive) and plasmacytoid lymphocytes.

Immunologic/Genotypic/Karyotypic Features

Monoclonal surface and cytoplasmic immunoglobulin, usually of the IgM/IgD type, is detectable in LPL. Paraffin-section immunoperoxidase studies are very useful, both in documenting the plasmacytic nature of the lymphoid cells and in demonstrating their monotypic cytoplasmic immunoglobulin. LPL typically has a CD5−, CD10−, pan-B-cell antigen-positive phenotype. Because some cells may be CD20−, CD79a stains may be useful here to mark more of the plasmacytoid cells. Most cases do not demonstrate Bcl-2 expression. There may be numerous admixed T cells. Older studies demonstrated a t(9;14) translocation in one-half of cases (278,279); however, more recent investigations have failed to find any cases with this translocation, perhaps relating to different diagnostic criteria (280,281). Therefore, the t(9;14) should not be considered a cytogenetic characteristic of this disease (282). Other chromosomal abnormalities can be found, including 6q deletions (280,281). Other authors (283) have suggested that deletion of 6q is not a characteristic marker of nodal LPL and that nodal and marrow-based cases may be different in their cytogenetic findings. Some cases of LPL are associated with hepatitis C virus infection (284).

Clinical Features

LPL is a usually indolent lymphoma reported by some to be more aggressive than CLL/SLL (95,226). The NHL classification project, however, reports a 59% 5-year overall survival rate (224). Most cases of LPL demonstrate a serum IgM paraprotein level of >3 g/dL. Cases with more numerous admixed transformed cells have more chromosomal abnormalities and may be more aggressive (273,281). Some cases show transformation to a overt DLBCL. Some transformed LPLs are purely immunoblastic proliferations, whereas others are pleomorphic and contain RS-like cells (226,269).

MANTLE CELL LYMPHOMA

Definition

MCL is a B-cell lymphoma, believed to be derived from inner mantle zone cells, that is composed of small cleaved and slightly irregular lymphocytes (which resemble centrocytes) *without* transformed cells, paraimmunoblasts, or proliferation centers (226,285–291). Growth around hyperplastic follicular centers (mantle zone pattern) is present in only a minority of cases. Clinically important aggressive variants are composed of cells that resemble lymphoblasts (blastoid) or sometimes cells of DLBCL (pleomorphic). MCLs are characterized by their t(11;14)(q13;q32) translocation involving the CCND1 (cyclin D1) and immunoglobulin heavy chain (IgH) genes and their expression of cyclin D1.

Histopathologic Features

Lymph nodes show complete or partial architectural effacement by a very monotonous-appearing infiltrate of small lymphocytes (Figs. 17.37 through 17.39). Four growth patterns are observed. The most common is a diffuse growth, followed by either vaguely nodular, mantle zone, or (rarely) follicular-appearing growth patterns. The classic cytology of the infiltrate is small to medium-sized cells with condensed chromatin and indented nuclei (291–294). Other much less common cytologic

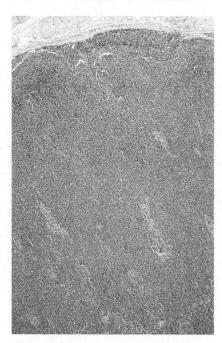

Figure 17.37. Lymph node, mantle cell lymphoma. At low power, note the dense, homogeneous diffuse growth pattern.

variants include small-cell (CLL-like), pleomorphic (often resembling DLBCL), and blastoid, with dispersed nuclear chromatin and a high mitotic rate (resembling lymphoblastic lymphomas). The latter two types often are lumped together as "blastoid" variants. Prominent hyalinized blood vessels are frequently present. An extremely important feature is the virtual absence of paraimmunoblasts and centroblasts. Likewise, proliferation or growth centers, as seen in SLL, are not present. Occasional cases are composed of cells that resemble those of marginal zone B-cell lymphomas, and some cases with a follicular-appearing growth pattern can suggest the diagnosis of follicular lymphoma. Lymph nodes in which there is a mantle zone growth pattern and intact sinuses may be easily dismissed as simply showing reactive hyperplasia. Close inspection will reveal more typical areas in all of these circumstances.

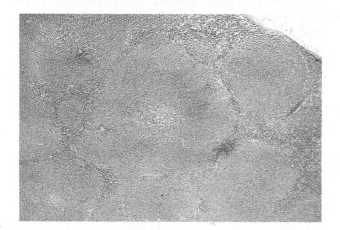

Figure 17.38. Lymph node, mantle cell lymphoma. This case demonstrates a prominent mantle zone growth pattern around residual follicular centers. Note that in some areas the growth is just vaguely nodular.

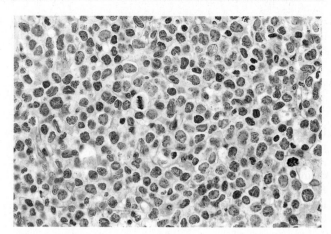

Figure 17.39. Lymph node, mantle cell lymphoma. At high magnification, several mitoses are evident. Also note the absence of transformed cells, an unusual finding in other small cleaved cell lymphomas.

Immunologic/Genotypic/Karyotypic Features

MCLs are monoclonal B-cell proliferations traditionally considered to be of prefollicular B cells with unmutated immunoglobulin genes (295). More recently, a subset with mutated immunoglobulin genes has been described (296,297). The neoplastic B cells are usually CD5+, CD10−, CD23−, often FMC7+, CD43+, Bcl-6−, and express at least moderate amounts of IgM/IgD surface immunoglobulin (236,237,239,286–288,291, 298,299). Bcl-2 immunostains can be used to highlight the negative hyperplastic germinal centers, present in cases with a mantle zone growth pattern, that are surrounded by the Bcl-2 protein-positive lymphoma. Even cases without a mantle zone growth pattern demonstrate loose meshworks of follicular dendritic cells using antibodies against CD21 or CD35. An extremely important feature of MCL is the expression of cyclin D1 in almost all cases, as detected using paraffin-section immunostains (300–302). Aside from aiding in the classification of a B-cell lymphoma, this critical stain can be extremely helpful in demonstrating relatively subtle nodal involvement in cases with significant architectural preservation. Hairy cell leukemia and a minority of myelomas also express cyclin D1 protein. The cyclin D1 overexpression in MCL (and myeloma) results from a t(11;14)(q13;q32) translocation between the immunoglobulin heavy chain and CCND1 (cyclin D1, *BCL-1*) genes (286,288, 303–305). This translocation can be documented in approximately 70% of cases using Southern blot analysis with multiple probes and restriction enzymes, and in almost all cases using FISH analysis (286,288,303–307). Many cases also have ATM gene point mutations and/or deletions (308,309). MCL may also show a variety of secondary genotypic abnormalities involving cell cycle regulatory genes (TP53, p15/p16, and other cyclin-dependent kinase inhibitors) that are often associated with more aggressive or blastoid disease (286,288,310–313). Many other cytogenetic abnormalities also are present in varying proportions of cases, including some well known to be associated with CLL, such as trisomy 12 or 13q14 deletions (312,314). Some, such as trisomy 12 and karyotypic complexity, are associated with an adverse prognosis (312). A recent study (315) using gene expression profiling has demonstrated a characteristic MCL proliferation gene expression signature and a novel small subset of cases that lacked cyclin D1 expression.

These cases have the typical morphologic features of MCL but lack t(11;14) and fail to express cyclin D1. Instead, cases expressed either cyclin D2 or cyclin D3 (316).

Clinical Features

MCL is associated with median survivals of 3 to 5 years and is considered by many to be incurable, like the more indolent lymphomas (291,317,318). The NHL classification project found MCL to be among the most aggressive of the NHLs, with a 27% 5-year overall survival rate (224). More indolent cases have been noted—they are most likely to have a low mitotic rate; more small, round lymphocytes; and, possibly, a mantle zone or vaguely nodular growth pattern (285,289,317,318). MCL is usually disseminated at diagnosis, and peripheral blood involvement is not uncommon (279,281,308). Unlike follicular lymphomas, MCLs do not undergo transformation to traditional DLBCL (226,285). They may, however, lose their mantle zone growth pattern and, with an increase in cell size and chromatin dispersal, show transformation to the blastoid/pleomorphic variant (285,317). Analysis of the expression of proliferation signature genes in MCL has shown a strong association with survival (315).

FOLLICULAR LYMPHOMAS

Definition

Follicular lymphoma (FL), one of the most common lymphomas in the Western world, is a neoplasm composed of varying proportions of follicular center B cells (centrocytes and centroblasts) that has, at least in part, a follicular growth pattern (228,319). The number of centroblasts/large transformed cells is used to subclassify the FL into three grades. It is important to distinguish FL from follicular colonization that occurs with many other small-B-cell neoplasms. Follicular colonization refers to the infiltration of neoplastic non–follicular center B cells into intact follicles. It is also important to recognize that in cases of follicular lymphoma with diffuse areas composed of many centroblasts/large transformed cells, a diagnosis of DLBCL is also made even if present in association with an FL (see subsequent detailed discussion).

Histopathologic Features

FLs are most easily recognized at low magnification based on partial or complete nodal architectural effacement by numer-ous, closely packed follicular nodules that frequently appear homogeneous with numerous centrocytes (228,319) (Figs. 17.5 and 17.33). Neoplastic follicular nodulation is often ill-defined and frequently, but not always, lacks a mantle zone. Polarization into dark and light zones—characteristic of reactive germinal centers—is not seen. Centrocytes have clefted to angulated nuclei with clumped chromatin and without nucleoli. Some neoplastic centrocytes may have exaggerated clefts as a manifestation of dysplasia and appear cerebriform or multilobated. Centrocytes are variably sized, including some with nuclei larger than a histiocyte nucleus. Varying proportions of centroblasts are also always present, and their numbers are used to determine the grade of the FL (see subsequent discussion of grading). Centroblasts have round to sometimes irregularly shaped nuclei with vesicular chromatin and usually several nucleoli that often lie adjacent to the nuclear membrane. Occasional cases have only transformed centroblasts.

Recognition of interfollicular involvement is another very useful common histopathologic finding, although the interfollicular cells are often smaller, have less cytoplasm, and are sometimes less cleaved-appearing than those in the follicles. Similarly, capsular infiltration by centrocytes, often with a single-file growth pattern, is a diagnostically useful feature in helping to exclude follicular hyperplasia. Occasional cases have only intrafollicular involvement (''in-situ'' follicular lymphoma) and even partially involved follicles are sometimes observed (320). Normal mantles may remain, and, in rare cases, there are irregular invaginations of mantle zone cells into the neoplastic follicles, creating a floral-like pattern and mimicking progressively transformed germinal centers (321). Variably sized and shaped follicles are not reliable indicators of a benign process. The features most useful in the distinction of FL from follicular hyperplasia are listed in Table 17.5.

FL may demonstrate morphologic and phenotypic differentiation to pale marginal zone–type B cells, a feature that may be associated with an adverse prognosis (322). Some cases reported in the past may represent marginal zone lymphomas with follicular colonization. Plasmacytic differentiation also occurs in a small proportion (<5%) of cases, and some patients may even have monoclonal paraproteins (275,276). Immunophenotypic studies are required to confirm that the plasma cells are part of the neoplastic process because reactive plasma cells can also be present in follicular lymphomas. The presence of moderate numbers of plasma cells in up to almost 10% of FL means that they cannot be used to strongly favor a reactive process.

TABLE 17.5	Histopathologic Distinction of Follicular Hyperplasia from Follicular Lymphomas
Follicular Hyperplasia	*Follicular Lymphoma*
Well-separated follicles predominantly in nodal cortex, with preservation of normal architecture	Abnormal crowding of follicles and extension through entire nodal pulp, with marked destruction of normal architecture
Heterogeneity of follicular center cells and frequent presence of tingible-body macrophages and mitotic figures	Homogeneity of follicular center cells—usually homogeneous centrocytes, often without many tingible-body macrophages or mitotic figures
Normal-appearing follicular center cells	Dysplastic follicular center cells
Centrocytes cells restricted to follicles	Infiltration of centrocytes into interfollicular area or capsule

Other types of immunoglobulin accumulation that can occur in cells of an FL include several small cytoplasmic inclusions or massive single globules that distort the nucleus and give the cells a signet ring appearance (275). Cases with PAS-positive inclusions have been associated with IgM production, and those with clear, vacuolated cytoplasm are associated with IgG (323). Most cases of "signet ring cell" lymphomas have been FL. FL occasionally contains PAS-positive extracellular material (often in follicular nodules) that may be mistaken for amyloid.

Another histopathologic feature seen in some FLs is prominent sclerosis within or sometimes between the follicles (226,324). Sometimes the sclerosis is most prominent in areas with numerous large centrocytes, and it also may be seen in areas of extranodal extension. The sclerosis is usually denser than the more delicate compartmentalization of peripheral T-cell lymphomas, whereas the bands in NSHL are typically more dense and circumscribed. Some FL lymphomas have total nodal necrosis (Fig. 17.40). Residual lymphoma may be apparent at the periphery of the necrotic area only after multiple recuts.

Grading

Criteria for grading FL have varied greatly over the past few decades, with reproducible grading of FL very difficult even when set criteria are agreed upon. Nevertheless, because of the great cytologic variation in FL, grading often is required. Grading in the past often relied on estimating the proportion of large or large transformed cells or counting "large" cells. The WHO classification recommends counting the number of intrafollicular centroblasts in 10 40× (0.159-mm^2) fields and determining the average number per high-power field (319). This number is used to divide FL into three grades (1, 2, 3a, 3b) (Fig. 17.41). The specific criteria, including issues relating to field of view size, are in Table 17.6. In some cases, visual estimation of counts is straightforward so that actual counting is not necessary. For example, some FLs contain extremely few centroblasts and in others there are virtually no centrocytes. Furthermore, it is important to recognize that the most important decision to make is grade 3 versus grade 1 or 2, because there are no clinically significant differences between grades 1 and 2. However, there is clinical relevance in distinguishing grade

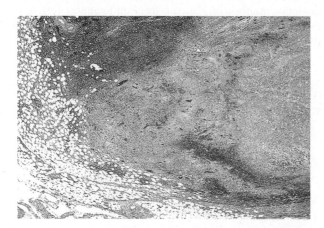

Figure 17.40. Lymph node, follicular lymphoma, grade I. Massive necrosis is demonstrated on the right side, whereas a lymphomatous infiltrate is noted on the left. Such infiltrates may be completely obscured by necrosis in some cases.

3 FLs from grades 1 and 2 (low grades) and the suggestion that there are clinical and biologic differences between grades 3a and 3b. Although the WHO grading strategy relies on an average number of centroblasts per high-power field, if there are clearly distinct areas with different grades, they should be separately reported.

The WHO also recommends reporting the degree of a follicular growth pattern. Cases are called "follicular" if more than 75% of their area contains neoplastic follicular structures; "follicular and diffuse" if 25% to 75% is follicular; or "focally follicular" if less than 25% is follicular. The approximate proportion for the latter two categories is also supposed to be specified. As noted above, cases with diffuse areas that are not grade 1 or 2 are diagnosed as DLBCL in addition to whatever type of FL is present. In these cases the proportional area occupied by the DLBCL should be stated. Entirely diffuse (nonfollicular) proliferations of centrocytes and less frequent centroblasts occasionally are seen on small biopsy sections. This phenomenon usually represents a diffuse area of FL in which the follicular component has not been biopsied.

Immunologic/Genotypic/Karyotypic Features

FLs are B-cell neoplasms with clonally rearranged immunoglobulin genes that often show significant and ongoing somatic mutation, as is typical of germinal center B cells (234,295). FLs express pan-B-cell antigens, including strong CD20, and either have monotypic surface immunoglobulin or, much less often, are surface immunoglobulin-negative. They usually express IgM, IgD, or IgG; only a few cases are IgA-positive. Lack of a demonstrable population of light chain class-restricted B cells in cell suspension studies is often the result of numerous polyclonal interfollicular B cells or to the scarcity of detectable surface or cytoplasmic immunoglobulin (325). FLs, like normal germinal center B cells, are usually positive for CD10 and Bcl-6 (a transcriptional repressor found in follicular center cells and a subset of T cells) and negative for CD5 and CD43 (236,239,249,299,325–328). Although caution is advised, finding numerous CD10+ mature B cells outside of follicles in paraffin-section immunostains supports the diagnosis of a follicular lymphoma rather than a follicular hyperplasia. Conversely, CD10 expression may be downregulated in the interfollicular neoplastic cells. Follicular large-cell lymphomas are usually CD10+ and CD5− but express immunoglobulin in only 65% of cases (328).

In contrast to normal follicles, most FLs, especially of grade 1 type, also show expression of the antiapoptotic protein Bcl-2 (238,329–331). Demonstrating Bcl-2 reactivity in cells marking as germinal center B cells is an important way in which paraffin-section immunostains are used to further support the diagnosis of an FL. Caution is advised because many normal nongerminal center B cells as well as many other types of lymphoma are also Bcl-2 protein-positive. FLs often have numerous admixed T cells, which can predominate. The T cells frequently have a normal CD4:CD8 ratio. Even if the T cells are numerous, these FLs are not considered to represent T-cell–rich B-cell lymphomas. Although T cells are usually most numerous in the interfollicular areas, some cases have many intrafollicular T cells.

Up to 85% of all FLs and 100% of so-called small cleaved cell (grade 1) type have a characteristic t(14;18)(q32;q21) translocation (332–335). This can be documented using conven-

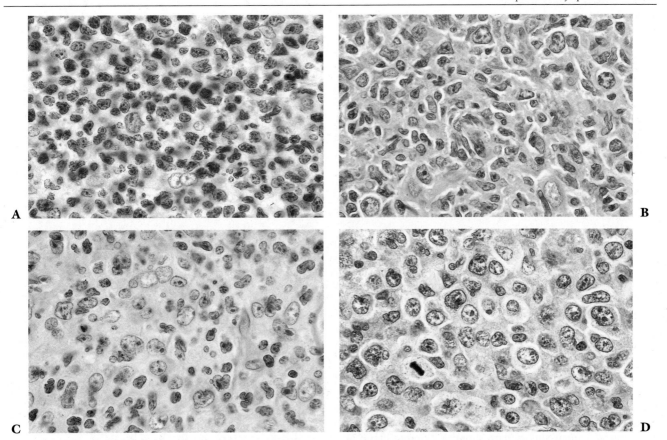

Figure 17.41. Lymph nodes, follicular lymphomas. Grading. **(A)** Follicular lymphoma, grade 1. There are numerous centrocytes and infrequent centroblasts. Note also the binucleate follicular dendritic cell at *bottom*. **(B)** Follicular lymphoma, grade 2. There are many variably sized centrocytes with a moderate number of admixed centroblasts. **(C)** Follicular lymphoma, grade 3a. There are many centroblasts with admixed centrocytes. A pale binucleate follicular dendritic cell is also seen at the *top*. **(D)** Follicular lymphoma, grade 3b. There is a relatively pure population of centroblasts with nucleoli that are often adjacent to the nuclear membrane.

TABLE 17.6

WHO Classification Recommendation for Grading of Follicular Lymphomas

Grade	Criteria[a]
1–2	0–15 centroblasts/hpf
3a	>15 centroblasts/hpf with admixed centrocytes
3b	>15 centroblasts/hpf[b]

hpf, high-power field. Ten random but representative intrafollicular fields should be counted.

[a]The numbers listed in this table are for a 40× hpf of 0.159 mm². A correction must be made for smaller or large fields as calculated based on the ocular field of view. Either a different number of fields can be counted, a different divisor used after 10 fields are counted, or different ranges used. With a 22-mm ocular field of view, the ranges are 0 to 7, 8 to 22, and >22 centroblasts/hpf.

tional cytogenetics, FISH analysis using fresh or paraffin-embedded material, and Southern blot or PCR genotypic studies (332–336). The FISH methodology appears to be the most sensitive technique. The t(14;18) translocation involves the immunoglobulin heavy chain and *bcl-2* genes, with breakpoints in the *bcl-2* gene occurring at the major, minor, or sometimes other breakpoint sites. Many other recurrent chromosomal defects have been described in follicular lymphomas, some associated with an increased number of cells or centroblasts, a leukemic blood picture, and/or a poor prognosis (337–339). FLs do not have CCND1 (cyclin D1) gene rearrangements, and most do not have *myc* rearrangements.

Clinical Features

FLs are among the most indolent of lymphomas; the NHL classification project has reported a 5-year overall survival rate of 72% (224). Most patients have advanced disease and are conventionally considered incurable. Reported cures may be seen in the infrequent patients with limited-stage disease and also possibly in patients with grade 3 FL. FLs have a propensity to transform over time. Centrocyte-rich FLs develop increasing numbers of centroblasts and tend to become diffuse (224,269,340–342). The true incidence of such transformation is difficult to determine. Of those patients with FL grade 1 who undergo repeat biopsy, approximately 20% to 40% have a dif-

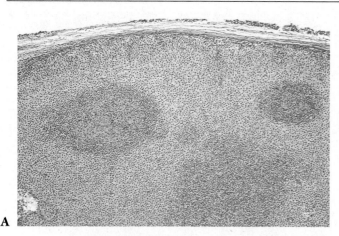
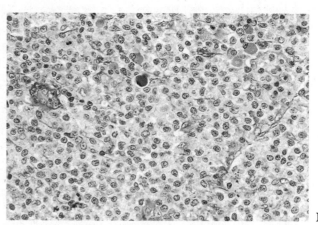

Figure 17.42.   Lymph node, nodal marginal zone B-cell lymphoma. **(A)** This low-magnification view shows a typical growth pattern for nodal marginal zone B-cell lymphomas. Residual follicles are noted, with a distinct subcapsular and perifollicular growth of cells with small nuclei and abundant cytoplasm. **(B)** On PAS stains, numerous plasmacytoid cells are seen, a feature found in a minority of cases. In addition, small lymphocytes with abundant cytoplasm are present.

fuse growth pattern, and approximately 10% to 40% show cytologic progression. One autopsy series reported that 63% of cases became diffuse and 43% showed cytologic transformation (342). Transformation to DLBCL is most common, but conversion to Burkitt lymphomas is also possible. Transformation is usually associated with a poor prognosis. It apparently involves the original neoplastic clone in most cases, but immunoglobulin gene rearrangement studies have shown a different clone in others. Interpretation of these studies is difficult because clonal evolution can be misinterpreted as the presence of a new and unrelated clone.

FLs occur rarely in children and often are morphologically similar to those seen in adults, but important differences are reported (343–345). Pediatric patients are more frequently male, present with early-stage disease, commonly have a grade 3 morphology, and often lack Bcl-2 protein expression and t(14; 18). The primary site of disease is usually cervical nodes or tonsil. However, testicular disease is well documented.

NODAL MARGINAL ZONE LYMPHOMA

Definition

Nodal marginal zone B-cell lymphoma (NMZL) is an uncommon, lymph node–based small-B-cell lymphoma composed of cells considered to be of marginal zone type (346–350). In many cases, the neoplastic B cells show a close morphologic resemblance to monocytoid/parafollicular B cells seen frequently in toxoplasmic lymphadenitis, although derivation of NMZL from this population is controversial (351–353). NMZL is not distinguishable from nodal involvement by extranodal marginal zone lymphoma of mucosa-associated lymphoid tissue (MALT) type (an extranodal lymphoma not discussed in this chapter) (354). Although it is sometimes difficult, NMZL must also be distinguished from splenic marginal zone lymphoma, which is discussed in Chapter 18, The Spleen (355–358). A subtype of NMZL that more closely resembles SMZL has been described (288).

Histopathologic Features

Lymph nodes in NMZL often show a sinus, parafollicular, and usually interfollicular distribution of neoplastic cells that resem-

ble parafollicular/monocytoid B cells (Fig. 17.42). Parafollicular or monocytoid B cells are small lymphocytes with abundant pale cytoplasm found in a parafollicular distribution in certain reactive states, such as toxoplasmosis or AIDS/AIDS-related complex. They are two to three times the size of small lymphocytes and have round to irregularly shaped nuclei with clumped chromatin and moderately abundant pale cytoplasm. A small-cell variant of NMZL has also been reported, with cells more like nonmonocytoid nodal marginal zone cells (350).

Benign hyperplastic follicular centers are a distinctive part of NMZL and may lead to an erroneous diagnosis of reactive adenopathy. Neoplastic plasmacytoid or frank plasma cells are present in up to 61% of cases (359), occasionally in sufficient numbers to suggest a diagnosis of lymphoplasmacytic lymphoma or plasmacytoma. In cases with marked plasmacytic differentiation, unless the presence of marginal zone-type B cells is minimal, the diagnosis of a NMZL would be made. FL may have a marginal zone B cell component but those cases are still diagnosed as an FL (322,349). Nodal involvement by an extranodal marginal zone B-cell lymphoma of mucosa-associated lymphoid tissue (MALT) type also must be excluded, largely based on clinical findings because it would be histologically indistinguishable. In some cases, genotypic/karyotypic findings might also be useful.

Immunologic/Genotypic/Karyotypic Features

NMZLs contain monoclonal B cells; bear IgM or, less often, IgG; and lack expression of CD5, CD10, CD25, and usually CD11c (346–349). Most NMZL cells are Bcl-2 protein–positive, like normal marginal zone cells but unlike normal parafollicular/monocytoid B cells that are negative or only variably Bcl-2-positive (329). Three neoplasms that resemble NMZL histologically may be differentiated by special stains: HCL marks with CD103, CD11c, and usually CD25; MCL is usually positive for CD5 and cyclin D1; and mastocytosis is recognizable histochemically or with a tryptase IHC. Genotypic studies demonstrate clonal immunoglobulin gene rearrangement but no specific oncogene abnormalities. Some cytogenetic abnormalities are reportedly similar to those in marginal zone lymphomas of the MALT type and include variable proportions of cases with trisomy 3, trisomy 18, and structural 1q21 or 1q34 abnormalities (360); however, the t(11;18) seen in approximately one-third of MALT lymphomas is absent (361).

Clinical Features

NMZLs are indolent lymphomas of adults that infrequently transform to aggressive, higher-grade DLBCLs (346,348–350). The NHL classification project has reported a 5-year survival rate of 57% (224). Although quite rare, NMZL occurs in children and young adults(362). A word of caution: Attygalle et al. (363) have described cases of atypical marginal zone hyperplasia of tonsils and appendices of children that morphologically and immunophenotypically mimic lymphoma, but molecular studies and clinical follow-up suggest a reactive condition.

DIFFUSE LARGE-B-CELL LYMPHOMA

Diffuse large-B-cell lymphoma (DLBCL) is a heterogeneous category that includes most diffuse lymphomas composed of large, transformed B cells. A neoplastic large B cell is generally defined based on a nuclear size, which is greater than twice the size of a normal lymphocyte or equal to or greater than the nucleus of a macrophage (11). Six morphologic variants were recognized in the 2001 WHO classification: centroblastic, immunoblastic, T-cell/histiocyte-rich, anaplastic, plasmablastic, and DLBCL with expression of full-length ALK (anaplastic lymphoma-kinase). Use of the broader category DLBCL was promoted because, in many cases, it is impossible to be more precise and because of problems with reproducibly distinguishing the different DLBCL variants. In the 2008 WHO classification (Table 17.2), more emphasis is directed at recognizing the subcategories of T-cell/histiocyte-rich large-B-cell lymphoma, plasmablastic, and ALK-positive DLBCL, with the latter two being separately designated. New subcategories of DLBCL include DLBCL associated with chronic inflammation and EBV+ DLBCL of the elderly. Primary mediastinal (thymic) large-B-cell lymphoma, intravascular large-B-cell lymphoma, primary effusion lymphoma, and lymphomatoid granulomatosis continue to be separately designated and are not included among the other DLBCLs. Four new large-B-cell neoplasms are designated in the 2008 classification; they include primary cutaneous DLBCL, leg type; large-B-cell lymphoma arising in HHV8-associated multicentric Castleman disease; B-cell lymphoma, unclassifiable, with features intermediate between DLBCL and Burkitt lymphoma; and B-cell lymphoma, unclassifiable, with features intermediate between DLBCL and classic Hodgkin lymphoma. The remainder of this section will concentrate on the more general features of nodal DLBCL. More specific variants and newer entities will be discussed separately.

Histopathologic Features

DLBCLs usually have a predominance of large, transformed lymphoid cells with vesicular chromatin. Those of centroblastic type are predominantly composed of neoplastic cells that resemble large, transformed follicular center cells or centroblasts, and have nuclei usually larger than histiocyte nuclei with round to oval but sometimes more irregular nuclear contours. Nuclear chromatin is dispersed and vesicular with one to several moder-

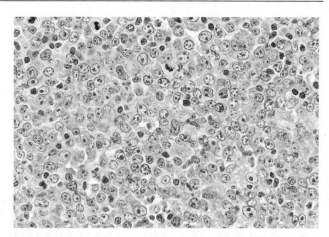

Figure 17.43. Lymph node, diffuse large-B-cell lymphoma. Note the numerous large cells with their dispersed chromatin and moderately prominent nucleoli. Some of the cells have nucleoli that lie close to the nuclear membrane, as is typical of centroblasts.

ately prominent nucleoli, often lying adjacent to the nuclear membrane (228,364,365) (Fig. 17.43). Some cases may have many (>30%) cells with multilobated nuclei.

Many DLBCLs contain at least some immunoblasts, which are defined as large, transformed cells with more prominent central nucleoli and amphophilic/pyroninophilic/basophilic cytoplasm (227,364–366). DLBCL of immunoblastic type shows a marked predominance of immunoblasts (greater than 90%), sometimes with plasmacytic differentiation (Fig. 17.44). The plasmacytic differentiation is recognized by the presence of eccentric nuclei and abundant pyroninophilic cytoplasm, sometimes with a perinuclear hof. Variable numbers of mature plasma cells may be present. Differentiation from the plasmablastic variant or myeloma may require immunophenotypic studies and clinical correlation.

The anaplastic variant has large pleomorphic cells that raise the differential diagnosis of an anaplastic large-cell lymphoma (364). There may even be an intrasinus growth pattern that, in addition, suggests the differential diagnosis of metastatic carci-

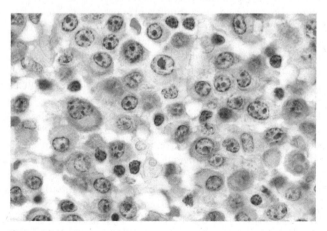

Figure 17.44. Lymph node, diffuse large-B-cell lymphoma, immunoblastic type. In this high-magnification photomicrograph, there are numerous large immunoblasts with amphophilic cytoplasm, often eccentric nuclei, and distinct plasmacytic differentiation.

noma and certain histiocytic proliferations. Other nonanaplastic DLBCLs may also grow within sinuses (such as "microvillous B-cell lymphoma"). Microvillous lymphoma of B-cell origin is a large, transformed cell lymphoma with a sinus growth pattern that is not specifically recognized in the WHO classification (367). Ultrastructural studies demonstrate surface villi on the neoplastic cells. Diffuse involvement of lymph nodes is also seen.

Immunologic/Genotypic/Karyotypic Features

Most DLBCLs express variable numbers of pan-B-cell antigens (CD19, CD20, CD22, CD79a, PAX-5), with the exception of those of plasmablastic type (see below) or those with ALK expression (see below) (364). Some also lack HLA-DR. CD20 expression, seen in many but not all cases, is important to document because of the widespread use of a therapeutic anti-CD20 antibody (Rituximab). However, in contrast to FL, DLBCLs are more likely to be surface immunoglobulin-negative. Some, but not all, DLBCLs contain cytoplasmic immunoglobulin. The detailed phenotype of DLBCL is quite variable. Some cases mark like typical FL (CD5−, CD10+, Bcl-6+, Bcl-2+), whereas others lack various combinations of CD10, Bcl-2, and Bcl-6. MUM-1 (multiple myeloma oncogene 1 transcription factor) expression, a marker of late germinal center or postgerminal center B-cells, is seen in many DLBCLs while the acquisition of the plasma cell-associated CD138 antigen is present in a small number of cases (5,326,364,368–370). Plasmablastic lymphomas (see "Plasmablastic Lymphomas" below) generally lack CD45 and CD20 expression but express plasma cell–associated markers such as CD138 (364,371). CD5 expression is seen infrequently and is reported to be an adverse prognostic indicator (372). It is important in CD5+ cases that one rules out the possibility of a blastoid mantle cell lymphoma or Richter transformation of CLL/SLL.

Like FLs, DLBCLs have clonally rearranged immunoglobulin genes that are mutated, often with ongoing mutations (373–376). Genotypic studies may fail to find a clonal population of B cells in the T-cell–rich cases, presumably because of their small numbers. bcl-2 gene rearrangements are present in approximately 20% to 40% of cases, with a higher proportion in DLBCL that represent transformed FL. bcl-6 gene rearrangements are reported in a similar proportion of cases (326, 370,377–389). Mutations in one or more other proto-oncogenes including *PIM1*, *MYC*, and *PAX5* are seen in approximately three-fourths of DLBCL, and are also believed to play a role in the pathogenesis of these lymphomas (390). c-myc gene rearrangements are described in a small number of DLBCL, including transformed FL. Cases with both bcl-2 and c-myc translocations are associated with a very adverse prognosis (385,391).

Gene expression profiling that looks at the mRNA expression of thousands of genes has rekindled great interest in subdividing the clinically heterogeneous DLBCL. Although still a research tool, it is expected that these studies will become of greater practical importance. Use of the customized cDNA "lymphochip" has led to the recognition of first two (392) and now three types of DLBCLs (393). One has a gene expression profile most like germinal center B cells; one is most like activated B cells (ABC); and the third is more heterogeneous and simply called "type 3." The germinal center subtype is where one finds the cases with a t(14;18); those most likely to have a

germinal center–like phenotype; and those with a "monomorphic centroblastic" morphologic appearance (as opposed to cases with more immunoblastic cells) (393,394). The germinal center B-cell subtype is associated with a longer survival. Gene expression profiling has also been used to find more limited numbers of genes that can be used to predict prognosis in DLBCL (393,395). A "gene expression-based outcome predictor score" was developed based on analysis of 17 genes used to assess germinal center B-cell signature, MHC class II signature, lymph node signature (genes associated with extracellular matrix, connective-tissue growth factor, macrophages, and NK cells), proliferation signature score, and *BMP6* (393). Other investigators found a 13-gene predictor model using oligonucleotide gene profiling for separating two clinically distinct groups of DLBCLs (395). IHC surrogates for the genotypic germinal center B-cell and activated B-cell groups have been proposed. The most widely cited is that of Hans et al. (396), which utilized antibodies to CD10, Bcl-6, and MUM-1 to distinguish two clinically significant groups.

Clinical Features

DLBCLs are aggressive lymphomas that develop in both children and adults (224). About one-half are stage III or IV at diagnosis. The NHL classification project reports an overall 5-year survival rate of 46% (224). Although controversial, DLBCL of centroblastic type may have a better prognosis, and those of immunoblastic type a worse one (364,397,398). A history of an immune disorder has been reported in 31% of patients diagnosed with immunoblastic lymphomas, and a previous lymphoproliferative malignancy has been reported in 13% (399). Some patients have monoclonal serum paraproteins (399). Other variants that may be associated with a more aggressive course include T-cell/histiocyte–rich and ALK-positive cases (364,400). Clinical factors are also very important in prognostication of DLBCL, with the international prognostic index (IPI) score often used. The IPI score is based on an assessment of age (≤60 vs. >60), performance status, lactate dehydrogenase (LDH) (≤normal vs. >normal), extranodal sites (0–1 vs. >1), and stage (I/II vs. III/IV) (401).

Numerous phenotypic and genotypic markers, variably expressed in DLBCL, have been studied with the hope of identifying those predictive of clinical outcome. For example, Bcl-2 expression has been associated with an adverse prognosis in DLBCL, whereas strong Bcl-6 expression was predictive of a better prognosis in some studies (364,369,370,397,402–405). Gene expression profiling of DLBCL (see above) has identified a germinal center B-cell signature subgroup that predicts a more favorable outcome. Most of these studies were based on cohorts of patients with DLBCL treated with CHOP (cyclophosphamide, doxorubicin, vincristine, and prednisone). However, with the recent addition of Rituximab to the CHOP regimen for treatment of DLBCL, the prognostic impact of many of the markers has been minimized (406–409). Nonetheless, determination of germinal center versus nongerminal center origin is still prognostically important in the postrituximab era.

Comments on Important Variants of Diffuse Large-B-Cell Lymphoma

T-cell/histiocyte–rich, large-B-cell lymphoma (TCHRBCL). Criteria defining TCHRBLL vary; however, the WHO classification defines these cases as having a limited number of scattered large

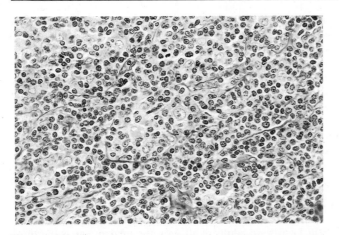

Figure 17.45. Lymph node, diffuse large-B-cell lymphoma with T-cell/histiocyte–rich large-B-cell features. At high magnification, many small lymphocytes are evident, and only isolated large transformed cells are present. There is one in the center of the field. Paraffin-section immunostains must be used to identify the small cells as T cells and the large cells as B cells.

atypical B cells, few small B cells, and a predominance of T cells often with or without admixed histocytes (364,410–412) (Figs. 17.45 and 17.46). The large B cells may resemble centroblasts, L&H cells of NLPHL, or RS cells of classic HL. The small background T cells may have irregular nuclear contours.

The large B cells of most cases of TCHRBCL are CD45+ and CD20+. Bcl-6 positivity is frequently seen in the nuclei of the neoplastic cells. Epithelial membrane antigen and CD30 are variably expressed and expression of CD15, CD10, Bcl-2, and latent infection by EBV is less commonly seen (410,413,414). The background small T cells are commonly CD3+, CD8+ and TIA1+ (413,415). There is an absence of follicular dendritic cell networks when studied with anti-CD21 or CD35.

Differentiation of TCHRBCL from some cases of HL, particularly NLPHL, may be difficult and is an area of controversy (410,413,416). The presence of nodularity (including CD21/CD35-positive dendritic networks), admixed small B cells and numerous CD57+ T cells with rosettes around cells resembling L&H RS-cell variants all favor a diagnosis of NLPHL. Some cases of TCHRBCL also may be associated with FL.

Clinically, TCHRBCL predominantly affects men, usually presents in advanced stages with B symptoms, and pursues a more aggressive course than that of some other types of DLBCLs (413,417).

Epstein-Barr virus–positive diffuse large-B-cell lymphoma of the elderly. EBV is associated with a variety of lymphoproliferative disorders, including endemic BL, lymphomatoid granulomatosis, plasmablastic lymphoma, NK/T-cell lymphoma of nasal type, lymphomas arising in patients with congenital or acquired immunodeficiencies, some cases of classic HL, and peripheral T-cell lymphomas.

A Japanese study recently reported cases of EBV-associated B-cell lymphoproliferative disorders arising in patients older than 50 years and without evidence of predisposing immunodeficiencies (418,419). Extranodal disease was common. Biopsied material often shows diffuse and polymorphic proliferations of varying numbers of centroblasts, immunoblasts, and RS-like cells, often with a background of small lymphocytes, plasma cells, and histocytes. Necrosis and angioinvasion can be seen. Two morphologic groups are recognized: a large-cell lymphoma and a polymorphic lymphoproliferative subtype. Typically, the tumor cells express CD20. In situ hybridization for EBER and IHC staining for LMP-1 is present in the large atypical cells. CD30 positivity is frequently seen in the larger cells.

The clinicopathologic features of these cases is similar to immunodeficiency-related lymphoproliferative disorders; however, the patients lack evidence of apparent immunodeficiency. The disease course is often aggressive, despite chemotherapy.

Diffuse large-B-cell lymphoma associated with chronic inflammation. It is now recognized that chronic inflammatory stimulation may play a role in the development of large-cell lymphomas in some patients (420). This is best illustrated by the pleural lymphomas reported to arise in patients with long-standing pleural chronic inflammation resulting from artificial pneumothorax for the treatment of tuberculosis. The lymphomas are termed *pyothorax-associated pleural lymphomas* (421–423). These neoplasms are CD20+ DLBCLs, often with immunoblastic morphology and frequent plasmacytoid differentiation. The presence of EBV genomes in the nuclei of tumor cells can be detected by in situ hybridization for EBER and IHC for LMP-1 (424). Although artificial pneumothorax is no longer utilized for the treatment of tuberculosis, similar lymphomas have been described in association with a variety of other chronic inflammatory conditions, including long-standing osteomyelitis, chronic venous ulcers of the skin, and metallic knee prothesis implants (424,425).

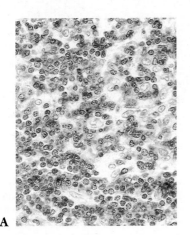
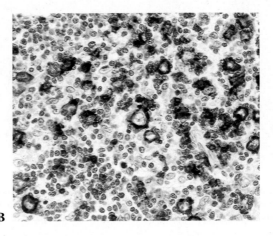

A   **B**

Figure 17.46. Lymph node, diffuse large-B-cell lymphoma with T-cell/histiocyte–rich large-B-cell features. **(A)** Numerous T cells are shown with the pan-T marker anti-CD45RO (UCHL-1). A large cell in the center does not mark. **(B)** Pan-B antibody anti-CD20 shows scattered large cells marking strongly. Numerous negative small lymphocytes are also visible (paraffin immunoperoxidase with diaminobenzidine substrate).

PRIMARY MEDIASTINAL (THYMIC) LARGE-B-CELL LYMPHOMA

Definition

Mediastinal (thymic) large-B-cell lymphoma (PMBCL) is a locally invasive, frequently sclerotic DLBCL that usually involves the thymus at diagnosis and that may be derived from thymic B cells (426–432). The major differential diagnoses include HL, other NHLs, thymoma, and seminoma/dysgerminoma.

Histopathologic Features

PMBCLs are often large or bulky and infiltrate adjacent mediastinal structures and organs. They demonstrate a diffuse proliferation of cytologically variable, medium to large-sized lymphoid cells that have oval, angulated, cleaved, or even multilobated nuclei with generally dispersed chromatin and often a moderate amount of pale cytoplasm (426–428,430,431) (Fig. 17.47). The latter accounts for the old term of *clear-cell lymphoma*. It is important to recognize that in a moderate number of cases the neoplastic cells do not have classic, large, transformed-appearing nuclei. RS-like cells can be present. Some cases may have numerous histiocytes or a predominance of relatively small lymphocytes, raising the differential of a marginal zone lymphoma. Frequently there is diffuse compartmentalizing, fine interstitial, or bandlike sclerosis. Residual thymic tissue sometimes with epithelial proliferation can be seen (432).

Immunologic/Genotypic/Karyotypic Features

PMBCLs are typically composed of surface immunoglobulin negative CD5-negative, often CD10-negative, B cells that express pan–B-cell antigens, and, like thymic medullary B cells, do not express CD21 (426,427,429,431). Many cases are at least weakly CD30-positive. CD23 may be expressed. In contrast to most other B-cell lymphomas, many, but not all, cases express the MAL protein (429,433). In contrast to classic HL, the large cells are CD45-positive and CD15-negative, and they express immunoglobulin transcription factors BOB.1 and Oct-2 (429). Genotypic studies reveal clonal immunoglobulin gene rearrangements. Many cases show characteristic karyotypic/genotypic abnormalities, including 9p gains and amplification of the *REL* gene (426,433–436). The frequency of class I/II HLA antigen expression and *bcl-6* mutations and expression are controversial, with the proportion that have features suggesting a follicular or postfollicular phenotype/genotype extremely variable (429, 436,437). Recent studies have shown that the molecular signature of PMBCL is more like that of classic HL than other DLBCLs (438,439). These studies suggest that PMBCL may be related to nodular sclerosis HL and could explain the occurence of cases with features intermediate between the two, termed by some as *mediastinal gray zone lymphoma* (440).

Clinical Features

MBCLs arise in adults of all ages; the median age is the third or fourth decade, and, in most series, there is a female predominance (224,426,430,431,441,442). Patients have initial signs of a mediastinal mass, superior vena cava syndrome, and symptomatic tracheobronchial compression. Most cases do not have extrathoracic involvement at diagnosis. The lymph nodes are affected in a minority of patients. More than one-half of patients are diagnosed at stage I or II, and marrow involvement is uncommon. The NHL classification project reports a 5-year overall survival rate of 50% (224). Relapses are frequently extranodal and are found at unusual sites, including the kidney, breast, adrenal cortex, ovaries, liver, pancreas, gastrointestinal tract, and central nervous system.

INTRAVASCULAR LARGE-B-CELL LYMPHOMA

Intravascular large-B-cell lymphoma (IVL), which is known by many different names, including *angiotrophic large-cell lymphoma* and *malignant angioendotheliomatosis*, is a large transformed cell lymphoma with a striking intravascular growth pattern (443–445) (Fig. 17.48). Phenotypic studies demonstrate B-cell antigen and sometimes CD5 expression. Rare, histologically similar cases are of T-cell origin and must be separately classified (446). This clinically aggressive lymphoma frequently involves the skin and nervous system. Hemophagocytosis is frequently

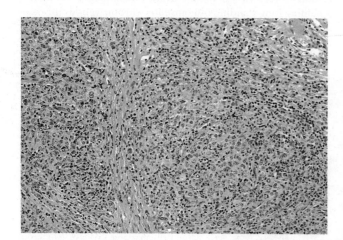

Figure 17.47. Mediastinal mass, mediastinal (thymic) large-B-cell lymphoma. Note the presence of sclerosis and mostly large lymphoid cells with a moderate amount of cytoplasm.

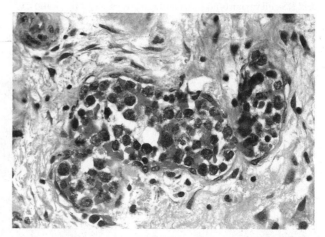

Figure 17.48. Lymph node with intravascular large-B-cell lymphoma. High magnification shows a vascular space in the soft tissue adjacent to a lymph node. The intravascular distribution of large cells is typical of this particular neoplasm.

associated with IVL in Japanese and other Asian groups, but is absent in Western patients (447). Lymph nodes may show focal or diffuse architectural effacement without a prominent intravascular component.

ANAPLASTIC LYMPHOMA KINASE-POSITIVE DIFFUSE LARGE-B-CELL LYMPHOMA

DLBCL with expression of anaplastic lymphoma kinase (ALK) is a rare variant of DLBCL, initially described in 1997 by Delsol et al. (400). ALK+ DLBCL usually demonstrates an immunoblastic or plasmablastic morphology with a diffuse or intrasinusoidal growth pattern (448). Necrosis is frequent and RS-like cells are occasionally seen. The neoplastic cells have a characteristic phenotype, usually lacking pan-B-cell markers (CD20 and CD79a) but expressing plasma cell–associated markers CD38 and CD138. Monotypic cytoplasmic IgA and epithelial membrane antigen (EMA) positivity is seen in most cases. CD45 is variably expressed, as are CD4 and CD57. Most ALK+ DLBCLs lack CD30 positivity. Of paramount importance is the expression of ALK, usually showing granular *cytoplasmic* staining as a result of a t(2;17) (p23;q23) translocation involving the *ALK* and clathrin genes (449,450). Less frequently, the classic t(2;5) (p23;q35) translocation involving the nucleophosmin gene at 5q35 is seen with a corresponding nuclear and cytoplasmic ALK positivity.

PLASMABLASTIC LYMPHOMA

Plasmablastic lymphoma (PBL) probably is a heterogeneous group of aggressive large-B-cell lymphomas that express a plasmacytic phenotype, absent or weak for CD45 and CD20, and positive for terminal markers of B-cell differentiation (MUM1/CD138/EMA-positive) (451,452). PBL was originally described as a variant of DLBCL, often presenting in the oral cavity of HIV+ patients and referred to as PBL of oral mucosa type (453). The tumor is composed of immunoblastic, large, transformed lymphoid cells with absent or weak expression of CD45 and CD20 and strong reactivity with plasma cell markers CD38 and CD138. Most cases are EBV+ but HHV8-negative. Similar cases occur outside of the oral cavity and in HIV-negative patients with other underlying immunodificiencies or in elderly individuals (451,454). The clinical behavior is highly aggressive, with many patients dying in less than 12 months after diagnosis.

Other large-B-cell lymphomas may show a plasmablastic morphology and phenotype, including cases arising in HIV-negative nonimmunocompromised patients. Considerable overlap exists with extramedullary "plasmablastic" myelomas and plasmacytomas, ALK+ DLBCL, HHV8+ plasmablastic lymphomas associated with multicentric Castleman disease, and HHV8+ extracavitary variant of primary effusion lymphoma (451).

PRIMARY EFFUSION LYMPHOMA

Primary effusion (body cavity-based) lymphoma (PEL) is a very aggressive large-B-cell lymphoma that grows principally in body cavities rather than forming solid tumor masses (455,456). It is most commonly seen in HIV-positive patients but also develops in nonimmunosuppressed, often elderly, patients (455–457). The large transformed cells often appear immunoblastic or ana-

plastic and lack B- or T-cell–associated surface antigens; genotypic studies demonstrate their B-cell lineage. PELS are HHV8 (KS herpesvirus)- and variably EBV-positive.

LARGE-B-CELL LYMPHOMA ARISING IN HUMAN HERPESVIRUS-8–ASSOCIATED MULTICENTRIC CASTLEMAN DISEASE

Human herpesvirus-8 (HHV8), also known as Kaposi sarcoma-associated virus, is associated with the pathogenesis of several lymphoproliferations, including primary effusion lymphoma and multicentric Castleman disease (MCD). Several plasmablastic proliferations have been identified in MCD (81,86, 458,459). In some cases of MCD, HHV8+ plasmablasts or immunoblasts that express monotypic IgM lambda have been identified in the expanded mantle zones, leading to the term *plasmablastic Castleman disease*. Additional cases have shown small clusters of immunoblasts in the follicles (called *microlymphomas*), whereas others demonstrate frank plasmablastic lymphomas.

BURKITT LYMPHOMA

Definition

Burkitt lymphoma (BL) is a rapidly dividing lymphoma composed of very uniform, relatively small transformed B cells with a distinct phenotype and with a *myc* translocation (460). The 2008 WHO recognized three clinical variants: enderdic, sporadic, and immunodeficiency associated. Classic BL includes the EBV-related endemic cases found in Africa and Papua, New Guinea, and the less frequent EBV-related, nonendemic or sporadic cases are found worldwide (461). A variant of BL with plasmacytoid differentiation is also recognized, which occurs most frequently in HIV-infected patients (226,365,460). B-cell acute lymphoblastic leukemia (also known as ALL, FAB type L3) is now grouped with BL and known as the Burkitt leukemia variant (460).

Histopathologic Features

BL shows diffuse architectural effacement in most cases, but with focal follicle formation in a minority of cases (228,365,462). There is a uniform and homogeneous proliferation of transformed lymphoid cells with round nuclei smaller than those of normal histiocytes, dispersed chromatin, several small nucleoli, and a small amount of very amphophilic, pyroninophilic cytoplasm (Fig. 17.49). A high mitotic rate and a "starry sky" appearance resulting from the presence of numerous tingible-body macrophages are typically noted. The neoplastic cells of BL with plasmacytic differentiation often have a single central nucleolus and monotypic cytoplasmic immunoglobulin. The term *Burkitt-like* or *atypical Burkitt* should not be used anymore (452,460). Currently, it is believed that classic BL and atypical (Burkitt-like) BL (Fig. 17.50). represent the same entity but with more cytologic variation seen in the latter and illustrating the relatively wide morphologic spectrum of BL (460).

Immunologic/Genotypic/Karyotypic Features

BL is a B-cell neoplasm considered to be of follicular or postfollicular center cell origin (463,464). Most BLs are surface Ig+,

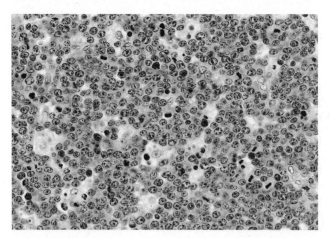

Figure 17.49. Lymph node, Burkitt lymphoma. There is a very homogeneous infiltrate of small noncleaved follicular center cells that have several nucleoli and amphophilic cytoplasm. Numerous mitotic figures are present. The macrophages create a "starry sky" appearance at low power.

CD10+, Bcl-6+, CD43+ but CD5−, CD23−, Bcl-2−, CD138− and Tdt− (460,465). Another important feature of BL is that nearly 100% of nuclei of the neoplastic cells are Ki-67-positive. Cytoplasmic immunoglobulin may be present. The t(8;14) (q24; q32) that represents a translocation between *myc* and the immunoglobulin heavy chain gene is characteristic of BL, although it is also reported in some DLBCLs (460,466–469). Approximately 20% of BLs show variant *myc* translocations that involve the immunoglobulin kappa or lambda light chain genes on chromosomes 2p11 and 22q11, respectively. Most endemic BLs have breakpoints far upstream from the actual *myc* gene, whereas most nonendemic cases have breakpoints within or close to the gene (468,469). BLs also demonstrate *myc* mutations in many or all cases (463,467,470). It is important to realize that a *myc* translocation is not specific to BL, and other B-cell lymphoma-associated translocations, such as t(14;18) and those involving *Bcl*-6, are absent in BL. Almost all African/endemic

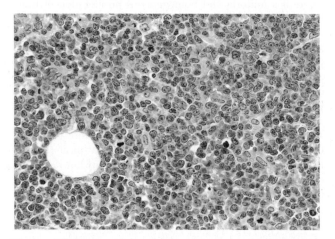

Figure 17.50. Lymph node, Burkitt lymphoma. The tumor cells here are more pleomorphic and in the past this case would have been called atypical Burkitt lymphoma.

BLs, BL in HIV+ patients, and a smaller number of sporadic BLs (approximately 10% to almost 40%) are associated with EBV (468,471–473).

Clinical Features

BL is a very aggressive but potentially curable lymphoma frequently seen in children (460,471,472). It often presents at extranodal sites such as the jaw in African children or in the gastrointestinal tract in the United States. Nodal presentations occur especially in adults. It can also have a leukemic presentation. It is important to distinguish BL from DLBCL because most patients will be treated differently. The NHL classification project reports a 5-year overall survival rate of 44% for BL (224).

BURKITT LYMPHOMA VERSUS DIFFUSE LARGE-B-CELL LYMPHOMA OR B-CELL LYMPHOMA, UNCLASSIFIABLE WITH FEATURES INTERMEDIATE BETWEEN BL AND DLBCL

Although the features of BL and DLBCL are distinctive in many ways, at times they overlap in morphologic, immunophenotypic, and cytogenetic characteristics. For example, BL may have a minor component of large lymphoid cells, and DLBCL may have frequent small to medium-sized cells, a starry sky pattern, a high proliferation index, evidence of a *myc*-rearrangement, and a CD20+, CD10+, Bcl-6+, Bcl-2+ phenotype (465,474). This overlap is confounded by the necessity to accurately diagnose each of these entities to avoid overtreating DLBCL or undertreating BL.

This differentiation is usually more problematic in adults than in children. Lymphomas with Burkitt morphology are more frequent in children and appear to be more homogeneous with respect to the clinical picture, immunophenotype, cytogenetics, and favorable response to short-duration, high-intensity chemotherapy. Those cases intermediate between BL and DLBCL, which occur in children, probably do not differ clinically (475). In adults, on the other hand, very few if any cases of classic BL are found and more often one sees cases with (a) Burkitt-like morphology but atypical phenotypic or genotypic/cytogenetic features; (b) cytologic features that are more variable than comfortably acceptable for atypical BL; or (c) both (452,476–478). An example of atypical features includes (a) the presence of larger cells with more prominent nucleoli; (b) Bcl-2 positivity in neoplastic cells and a proliferation index (Ki-67 positivity) between 80% and 95%; and (c) the presence of other translocations in addition to *myc*, such as *BCL*-2 translocations. Recent gene profiling studies have revealed a molecular signature that defines a homogeneous group of BL (479,480). However, within this group, the morphologic, immunophenotypic, and cytogenetic features are somewhat heterogeneous, suggesting the criteria we use to diagnose BL are not infallible (452). Some of these studies suggest that there are indeed cases that are intermediate between BL and DLBCL.

Several authors (452,465) suggest that when confronted with a high-grade B-cell lymphoma, one should diagnose BL when the morphology is "acceptable (but not necessarily typical)"; the phenotype is monotypic sIg+, CD20+, CD10+, Bcl-6+, Bcl-2−, Tdt−; Ki-67 positivity is essentially 100%; and a *myc* (but not a *bcl-2* or *bcl-6*) translocation is present. If there is a departure from these criteria, then the diagnosis is a high-grade B-cell lymphoma, not otherwise specified (NOS). A major unresolved question is how these high-grade B-cell lymphomas with some (but not all) features of BL should be treated. Clearly, these neoplasms act aggressively but whether treatment should be more like that for BL or for DLBCL awaits further study.

DIFFUSE LARGE-B-CELL LYMPHOMA VERSUS CLASSIC HODGKIN LYMPHOMA OR B-CELL LYMPHOMA, UNCLASSIFIED, WITH FEATURES INTERMEDIATE BETWEEN DLBCL AND CHL

It is not surprising that rare cases of B-cell lymphoma with features intermediate between DLBCL and classic Hodgkin lymphoma (CHL) exist. In fact, gene profiling studies have shown that the molecular signature of one type of B-cell NHL—primary mediastinal large-B-cell lymphoma—differs from that of other types of DLBCLs but shares features with CHL (438). Likewise, there are reports of mediastinal lymphomas with morphological features of DLBCLs and immunophenotypic characteristics of CHL, and vice versa. Additionally, some cases show immunophenotypic features (CD30+, CD15+, and strong CD20+) intermediate between CHL and DLBCL (439,440, 481). These observations have led to the concept of "mediastinal gray zone lymphomas," which have features transitional between nodular sclerosing classic HL and primary mediastinal large-B-cell lymphoma (440). Rare cases of T-cell/histiocyte–rich large-B-cell lymphoma overlapping with CHL also have been described (410).

In difficult cases such as these, attempts should be made to distinguish CHL from DLBC, using IHC and cytogenetic and molecular techniques. In some cases this may be impossible and the category B-cell lymphoma unclassified with features intermediate between DLBCL and HL can be used (452).

GENERAL APPROACH TO THE DIAGNOSIS OF T-CELL AND NATURAL KILLER-CELL LYMPHOMAS

As with other malignancies, the surgical pathologist must first establish that a lymphoproliferative process is neoplastic by careful histopathologic examination. Once the lesion is recognized as a malignant lymphoma, characteristic features may suggest a T-cell lineage. The most common growth pattern for T-cell lymphomas in lymph nodes is a diffuse lymphoid infiltrate that completely effaces the architecture (482). Rarely, follicular, perifollicular, and paracortical nodular growth patterns can be seen (482a,483,484). Some nodal peripheral T-cell lymphomas (PTCLs), such as anaplastic large-cell lymphoma (ALCL), show interfollicular or sinus infiltrates (482).

The morphologic pattern of complete effacement of nodal architecture by a diffuse lymphocytic infiltrate in which numerous evenly dispersed, ill-defined, small clusters of epithelioid histiocytes are the predominant feature represents malignant lymphoma in 99% of cases (Fig. 17.51) (485). Most cases with this low-magnification appearance are PTCLs (unspecified type, lymphoepithelioid cell variant, and angioimmunoblastic types), followed by HL (mixed-cellularity and lymphocyte-predominant types) and B-cell lymphomas with plasmacytic differentiation (lymphoplasmacytic lymphoma). Rare reactive cases have

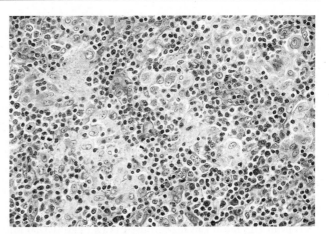

Figure 17.51. Lymph node, peripheral T-cell lymphoma, unspecified (lymphoepithelioid cell [Lennert] lymphoma cytologic category). Numerous reactive epithelioid histiocytes are scattered throughout the neoplastic lymphoid infiltrate.

included Whipple disease and chronic miliary tuberculosis. Lymphadenitis with focal epithelioid cell reactions caused by toxoplasmosis, infectious mononucleosis, and syphilis can be excluded because of the preservation of nodal architecture and other criteria.

Certain cytologic features of the neoplastic cells may suggest the presence of T-cell lymphoma. Precursor T-cell lymphoblastic leukemia/lymphoblastic lymphoma cells often have convoluted nuclei. Mycosis fungoides generally is composed of tumor cells with cerebriform nuclei. Adult T-cell leukemia/lymphoma (ATLL) may have circulating cells with cloverleaf nuclei. Other PTCLs often have a spectrum of neoplastic cell sizes in the same tissue. Nuclear pleomorphism is not unusual, and clear cytoplasm is often found. Occasionally, tumor cells may resemble RS cells; however, HL generally has a dichotomy of cell sizes and a more polymorphic reactive cell background.

There are no precise histopathologic or cytologic markers for T-cell malignancies, in contrast to the features of follicular nodulation and plasmacytic differentiation seen in some B-cell neoplasms. Furthermore, some B-cell lymphomas may exhibit many of the morphologic features associated with PTCLs, particularly T-cell–rich B-cell lymphomas (TCRBLs) (411). Therefore, T-cell neoplasms are diagnosed most easily when morphologic characteristics can be correlated with immunophenotypic data.

Flow cytometry is useful in diagnosing T-cell malignancies but generally cannot prove T-cell clonality, unless quantification of TCR β-chain variable region (Vβ) family usage is compared to established normal values (486). An aberrant T-cell phenotype (e.g., loss or diminished or heightened expression of T-cell antigens normally expressed, or expression of antigens not usually present) implies T-cell clonality (487,488). An abnormal phenotype by flow cytometry is seen in up to 90% of PTCLs (488). CD3 is the most common abnormally expressed antigen, followed by CD7 and CD5; CD2 expression is the most stable (487,488). NK-cell–associated antigen (CD11b, CD11c, CD16, CD56, and CD57) expression is important in the diagnosis of NK-cell lymphomas and NK-like PTCLs and is easily recognized by flow cytometry (111,489).

Because many biopsy specimens are fixed before any fresh tissue is apportioned for flow cytometry, paraffin IHC is generally very useful for phenotyping T/NK-cell lymphomas (490).

Many T-cell and NK-cell–associated antigens can now be detected in paraffin-embedded tissues, including CD2, CD3, CD4, CD5, CD7, CD8, CD43, CD45RO, CD56, CD57, and TCR beta chains (Table 17.1). A panel of antibodies that includes two T-cell lineage-related markers and at least one highly sensitive and highly specific B-cell marker will mark at least 95% of T-cell lymphomas (Fig. 17.52) (491–493). Polyclonal CD3 will also mark NK-cell lymphomas because this antibody detects cytoplasmic CD3ε (489). CD20 rarely marks T-cell lymphomas (494), but may mark nonneoplastic large-B-cells scattered throughout some PTCLs (495); these latter cases should not be confused with TCRBLs (496,497).

Important nonlineage markers are CD15, CD30, LCA (CD45), and EMA. CD15 is an effective antibody for labeling RS cells in HL, but it can mark some PTCLs (498). CD30 will mark RS cells as well as neoplastic cells of ALCL (499). CD45 and EMA are useful in distinguishing epithelial neoplasms from lymphomas, but it should be remembered that some ALCLs lack CD45 expression, and most ALCLs, NLPHLs, and multiple myeloma cases are positive for EMA (500–502). Cytokeratin should be an antibody used with EMA if the differential diagnosis is ALCL versus metastatic carcinoma, but even then some ALCLs may have cytoplasmic cytokeratin positivity (502).

Molecular genetic analysis is not needed for the diagnosis of most T-cell lymphomas, but gene rearrangement studies may be useful in the context of unusual cases. Southern blotting to detect TCR gene rearrangements can demonstrate T-cell clonality in unfixed tissues, but not all T-cell lymphomas exhibit these rearrangements by this method (503). PCR to detect TCR gene rearrangements is a more sensitive means of identifying T-cell clonality than Southern blotting and can be used for paraffin-embedded tissue (504). However, the limits of specificity must be appreciated. Clonal TCR gene rearrangements are not lineage-specific and can be detected in some B-cell lymphomas and myeloid leukemias. Reactive processes can also be associated with clonal TCR gene rearrangements, particularly in peripheral blood, bone marrow, and skin specimens.

Gene expression profiling studies have shown that different T-cell lymphoma types, such as PTCL, unspecified, precursor T-cell lymphoblastic lymphoma, angioimmunoblastic T-cell lymphoma and ALCL, can be distinguished by expression signatures (505–507).

T-CELL LYMPHOBLASTIC LYMPHOMA

Definition

Precursor T-cell lymphoblastic lymphomas are highly aggressive malignancies of immature (precursor) T-cells that frequently appear in the form of an anterior mediastinal tumor. If untreated, the neoplasm quickly disseminates to involve viscera, the central nervous system, and bone marrow, with the development of a leukemic phase that resembles T-cell acute lymphoblastic leukemia (T-ALL).

Histopathologic Features

Involved nodes are often effaced by a diffuse lymphomatous infiltrate (Fig. 17.53), but there may be residual islands of normal tissue. Capsular and perinodal soft-tissue infiltrates may be extensive. Tingible-body macrophages may impart a starry sky appearance similar to that seen in BL. Neoplastic lymphocytes are small to intermediate-sized, contain scanty cytoplasm, and have irregular and often convoluted nuclei best seen by fine focusing (Fig. 17.54). The chromatin is dispersed and blastlike; nucleoli are usually indistinct, unlike BL. Mitotic figures are numerous. These morphologic features are indistinguishable from those of disseminated T-ALL (508) and the uncommon B-cell lymphoblastic lymphomas (509,510). The latter are more likely to have cutaneous and osteolytic bone involvement and

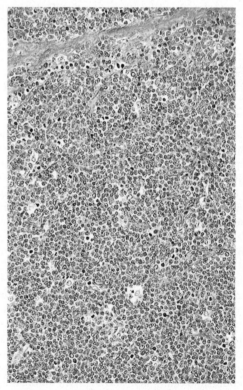

Figure 17.53. Lymph node, T-cell lymphoblastic lymphoma. The normal architecture is diffusely effaced. The capsule of the node (*above*) is also infiltrated.

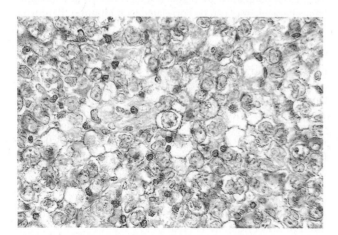

Figure 17.52. Lymph node, peripheral T-cell lymphoma, unspecified. Paraffin immunoperoxidase using anti-CD3 and diaminobenzidine substrate. Note the membrane positivity of most of the large cells.

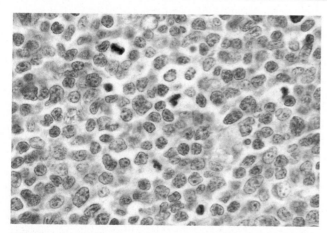

Figure 17.54. Lymph node, T-cell lymphoblastic lymphoma. Neoplastic cells have scanty cytoplasm, irregular nuclear configurations, finely dispersed chromatin, and indistinct nucleoli; mitotic figures are present.

rarely affect the mediastinum. In rare cases of T-cell lymphoblastic lymphoma, eosinophilia has heralded the subsequent development of myeloid malignancy (511).

Immunologic and Molecular Genetic Features

T-cell lymphoblastic lymphomas are generally CD7+ and CD3+, and some correspond to early (CD1−, cytoplasmic CD3+, CD4−, CD8−), common (CD1+, cytoplasmic CD3+, CD4+, CD8+), or late (CD1−, surface CD3+, CD4+, or CD8+) thymocytes (512). Cytoplasmic CD3 is the most specific early marker of a T-cell phenotype and is also seen in T-ALL (513,514). Tdt is present in virtually all T-cell lymphoblastic lymphomas, but only 25% of these lymphomas express common ALL antigen (CD10). HLA-DR expression is absent in almost all cases, unlike B-ALL and most nonlymphoid leukemias. Occasionally, lymphoblastic lymphomas express NK-cell–associated antigens and may be of true NK-cell lineage (515).

Varying patterns of TCR gene rearrangements can be seen in T-cell lymphoblastic lymphomas, and the incidence of Notch1 mutations is approximately 50%, which is similar to that in T-ALL (516). Expression of HOXA9 or TLXI transcripts in adults may define a subset of T-cell lymphoblastic lymphomas with a superior clinical outcome (516). The FIP1L1-PDGFRA fusion gene can be detected in some cases of eosinophilia-associated T-cell lymphoblastic lymphoma, which may have therapeutic significance (517).

Clinical Features

T-cell lymphoblastic lymphoma generally occurs in children and young adults, most often males, in the form of anterior mediastinal masses, often accompanied by supradiaphragmatic lymphadenopathy. Pleural or pericardial effusions and bone marrow and peripheral blood involvement are common. A smaller peak in incidence occurs in older adults, who less frequently have mediastinal and marrow involvement (518). The NHL classification project reports a 26% 5-year overall survival rate for T-cell lymphoblastic lymphoma (224).

The overlap of clinicopathologic features of T-cell lympho-

blastic lymphoma and T-ALL is so considerable that it may be impossible to distinguish between the two for individual T-cell neoplasms. Extensive mediastinal and peripheral lymph node involvement with limited bone marrow and peripheral blood disease favors a diagnosis of T-cell lymphoblastic lymphoma, whereas the presence of more than 25% lymphoblasts in the marrow is considered T-ALL. Overlap cases may be diagnosed as T-cell lymphoblastic leukemia/lymphoblastic lymphoma.

PERIPHERAL T-CELL LYMPHOMAS, NOT OTHERWISE SPECIFIED

Definition

PTCLs, not otherwise specified (NOS) are post-thymic (mature) T-cell malignancies that are yet to be well defined in terms of their classification into distinct entities (519). These PTCLs are among the most common nodal T-cell lymphomas (520).

Histopathologic Features

The growth pattern is generally diffuse. A variety of other morphologic features may also be seen, including neoplastic lymphocytes of varying size that often have clear cytoplasm; large tumor cells that may have hyperlobated nuclei, be multinucleated, or resemble RS cells; many reactive epithelioid histiocytes; delicate connective tissue bands that segregate cells into clusters; and hypervascularity (Figs. 17.55, 17.56) (520a).

T-zone lymphoma and lymphoepithelioid cell (Lennert) lymphoma are considered variants among PTCL, unspecified in the WHO classification (519). T-zone lymphoma has an interfollicular growth pattern with sparing of secondary lymphoid

Figure 17.55. Lymph node, peripheral T-cell lymphoma, unspecified. The characteristic uniform, diffuse growth pattern is best appreciated at low magnification. This homogeneous effacement, similar from area to area, is characteristic of unspecified peripheral T-cell lymphomas.

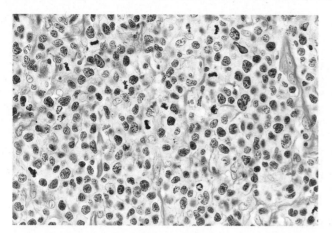

Figure 17.56. Lymph node, peripheral T-cell lymphoma, NOS. Neoplastic cells, are often pleomorphic and have clear cytoplasm. Small groups of tumor cells are compartmentalized by delicate connective tissue that is PAS positive.

follicles. Lennert lymphoma is characterized by numerous clusters of epithelioid histiocytes that are relatively evenly dispersed throughout tissues obliterated by a lymphomatous infiltrate composed primarily of small T-cells (Fig. 17.51) (485). It is imperative that pathologists focus attention on the destructive lymphoid infiltrate rather than on the histiocytes, which may cause misinterpretation as a reactive process. As mentioned previously, other PTCLs and some cases of HL and B-cell lymphomas can resemble Lennert lymphoma.

Immunologic and Molecular Genetic Features

T-cell phenotypes are often aberrant (521), and most express TCR gene rearrangements. Most nodal PTCLs, NOS have a TCRαβ phenotype, although rare nodal γδ T-cell lymphomas have been reported (522). Occasionally, nodal PTCLs, NOS, usually with pleomorphic cytologic features, express a cytotoxic (TIA-1+, granzyme B+, and/or perforin-positive)/NK-like (CD11b+, CD16+, CD56+, and/or CD57+) T-cell phenotype (490,523–525). Many posttransplant PTCLs fall within this spectrum of cytotoxic/NK-like T-cell lymphomas (111,526). Cytotoxic /NK-like PTCLs often have a very aggressive clinical course (111), and they are usually CD4−, CD8+ or CD4−, CD8−; the latter phenotypic features may serve as clues for testing for cytotoxic granules or NK-cell–associated antigen expression.

Pathogenetic chromosomal abnormalities in PTCLs, NOS are largely unknown (527). However, a small number of PTCLs, NOS that are preferentially localized in lymphoid follicles and have a CD3+, CD4+, CD5+, CD10+, and Bcl-6+ phenotype have a t(5;9)(q33;q22) that fuses ITK and SYK (528). This translocation results in a fusion protein with constitutive activation of the SYK tyrosine kinase. Despite the lack of a t(5;9), most T-cell lymphomas express SYK protein as detected by IHC or flow cytometry (529). On the other hand, nonneoplastic T cells appear to lack SYK expression, an attribute that may help distinguish reactive processes from T-cell lymphomas (529).

Clinical Features

PTCLs, NOS usually develop in adults, although cases have been reported in children. Patients typically have generalized lym-

phadenopathy, advanced-stage disease, and B symptoms (fever, weight loss, and night sweats). Most PTCLs, NOS are considered moderately aggressive and are treated with multiagent chemotherapy. The NHL classification project reports a 25% 5-year survival rate for all types of PTCLs except anaplastic large-cell lymphoma (ALCL) (224).

ANGIOIMMUNOBLASTIC T-CELL LYMPHOMA

Definition

Angioimmunoblastic T-cell lymphoma (AITL) is a common primary nodal subtype of PTCL (520) that is moderately aggressive.

Histopathologic Features

The nodal architecture in AITL is usually effaced by a diffuse lymphoproliferation that often extends through the capsule into the perinodal soft tissue (Fig. 17.57) (530). A striking feature is the arborizing proliferation of high endothelial venules with hyalinized PAS-staining walls (Fig. 17.58) accompanied by

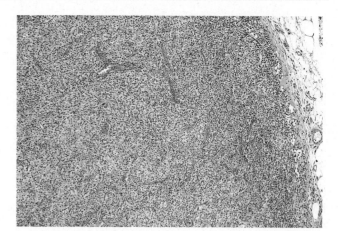

Figure 17.57. Lymph node, angioimmunoblastic T-cell lymphoma. The architecture is effaced by a diffuse lymphomatous infiltrate.

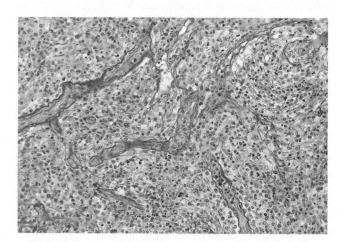

Figure 17.58. Lymph node, angioimmunoblastic T-cell lymphoma. A characteristic feature is the presence of arborizing high endothelial venules with hyalinized walls that are periodic acid-Schiff–positive. Clear cell clusters are usually seen around the vessels.

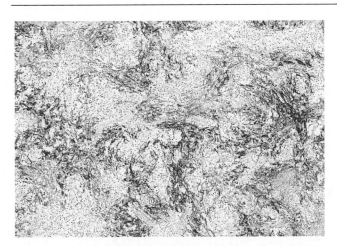

Figure 17.59. Lymph node, angioimmunoblastic T-cell lymphoma. A dense meshwork of follicular dendritic cells and their processes are stained with anti-CD21 in this paraffin immunoperoxidase section with diaminobenzidine substrate.

an irregular meshwork of proliferating follicular dendritic cells that surrounds the vessels (530). There is a mixed population of small lymphocytes and immunoblasts, the latter often having clear cytoplasm and clustering around vessels (Fig. 17.58) (530). Epithelioid histiocytes, plasma cells, and eosinophils are present in the background in variable proportions. Some AITLs do not completely efface the lymph node but contain depleted lymphoid follicles or, uncommonly, hyperplastic follicles (530).

Immunologic, Cytogenetic, and Molecular Genetic Features

The tumor cells in AITL have a CD4+ and CD10+ phenotype, and show attributes of follicular T-helper cells (531–538). Aberrant T-cell antigen expression is common. The follicular dendritic cell meshworks are highlighted by stains for CD21 (Fig. 17.59) (531). Approximately 75% of AILs have TCR gene rearrangements. After microdissection, the clonally rearranged TCR genes are confined to the CD10+ population (531). Trisomy 3, trisomy 8, and an additional X chromosome are the most frequently found karyotypic abnormalities (539). EBV-infected B-cell immunoblasts, some resembling RS cells, are increased in number as compared to normal lymph nodes and other PTCLs (530).

Clinical Features

AITL typically appears in adults who have B symptoms, generalized lymphadenopathy, skin rash, polyclonal hypergammaglobulinemia, and various autoimmune symptoms. Although they have been the subject of controversy, angioimmunoblastic lymphadenopathy with dysproteinemia (AILD) and immunoblastic lymphadenopathy (IBL) are now accepted by many as forms of AITL because the clinicopathologic features are similar for each and because most cases of AILD and IBL show T-cell clonality and nonrandom chromosomal abnormalities (530).

ANAPLASTIC LARGE-CELL LYMPHOMA

Definition

ALCL, a common nodal PTCL (520), is typically characterized by an infiltrate of highly pleomorphic large lymphocytes that express strong reactivity with antibodies directed against CD30, a T-cell activation-associated antigen (540). ALCL is undergoing reappraisal, however, because it has a broad spectrum of morphologic characteristics and because expression of CD30 no longer defines the disease. Primary ALCL arises de novo and can be subdivided into systemic (nodal) and cutaneous forms (Table 17.7) (541). Secondary ALCL represents a morphologic (and immunologic) transformation of another lymphoma, such as mycosis fungoides (542). Primary nodal ALCL is often associated with the t(2;5) (p23;q35) chromosomal abnormality (see later discussion).

Histopathologic Features

Nodal ALCL preferentially infiltrates sinuses and extends into the paracortical region, often sparing lymphoid follicles (Fig. 17.60). The neoplastic large cells seem cohesive and usually have great variability in nuclear appearance, including some that are horseshoe- or doughnut-shaped or are multinucleated with a resemblance to the RS cells of HL. There are dispersed chromatin, prominent nucleoli, and often a perinuclear eosinophilic region. The cytoplasm is abundant and the mitotic rate is frequently brisk. These so-called hallmark cells are numerous in the common variant of ALCL and are also seen in fewer numbers in the small-cell and lymphohistiocytic variants (543–545). The common variant of ALCL may be misdiagnosed as metastatic carcinoma or malignant histiocytosis because of the bizarre cytologic features of the tumor cells. Small-cell and lymphohistiocytic variants, which tend to have a poorer prog-

TABLE 17.7	Classification of CD30+ Anaplastic Large-Cell Lymphomas (ALCLs) and Associated Clinicopathologic Features		
ALCL Type	*t(2;5)/p80 or ALK1*	*Predominant Age Group*	*Prognosis*
Primary systemic (nodal)	Positive	Children and young adults	Good[a]
Primary systemic (nodal)	Negative	Older adults	Poor
Primary cutaneous	Negative	Adults	Good
Secondary	Negative	Adults	Poor

[a]The small-cell and lymphohistiocytic variants of ALCL tend to have a poorer prognosis than the pleomorphic (common) subtype.

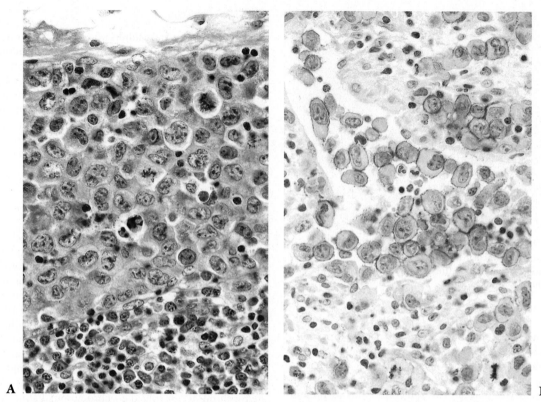

Figure 17.60. Lymph node, anaplastic large-cell lymphoma. **(A)** Note the growth of anaplastic large cells in the subcapsular sinus and the adjacent plasma cell reaction. **(B)** Paraffin immunoperoxidase with anti-CD30 (Ber H2) demonstrates the characteristic cytoplasmic membrane positivity.

nosis than the common variant, may be misdiagnosed as inflammatory processes unless the perivascular hallmark cells are evident.

Immunologic, Cytogenetic, Molecular Genetic Features

The tumor cells of ALCL are always CD30+, generally with both cytoplasmic and Golgi region staining on IHC (Fig. 17.60). It should be remembered, however, that CD30 may be seen in the neoplastic cells of other T-cell or B-cell lymphomas and in RS cells of HL (499,546). Embryonal carcinoma, seminoma, and pancreatic carcinoma may also have some CD30 positivity (547–549). Furthermore, CD30 is expressed in some florid immunoblastic reactions, such as in infectious mononucleosis (550,551). Most ALCLs have a T-cell phenotype or genotype, but 10% to 20% lack T-cell and B-cell antigens (null cell type). The latter lymphomas are grouped with T-cell ALCL, whereas large-cell NHLs that are CD30+ and express only B-cell antigens are included as part of the DLBCL category in the WHO classification. Most ALCLs contain cytotoxic granule-associated protein expression suggestive of a cytotoxic lymphocyte origin (552). EMA is often expressed by tumor cells of ALCL, particularly the primary nodal cases (541,553).

The t(2;5) (p23;q35) chromosomal abnormality, which fuses part of the nucleophosmin (*NPM*) gene on chromosome 5q35 to a portion of the anaplastic lymphoma kinase (*ALK*) gene on chromosome 2p23, producing a novel NPM-ALK protein, is present in approximately 60% of primary nodal ALCL (554–556). This translocation may also be recognized by molec-

ular techniques or by IHC detection of the unique fusion protein by antibodies p80[NPM/ALK] and ALK1 (556–560). Approximately 70% to 80% of ALK1+ ALCLs have cytoplasmic and nuclear staining that identifies the NPM/ALK fusion protein (559). The vast majority of the remaining ALK1+ ALCLs have cytoplasmic staining only, which indicates variant translocations involving *ALK* and partner genes other than *NPM*, such as tropomyosin 3 (*TPM3*) on chromosome 1 (t[1;2] [q25;p23]); *TRK*-fused gene (*TFG*) on chromosome 3 (t[2;3] [p23;q21]); *ATIC* (encoding for 5-aminoimidazole-4-carboxamideribonucleotide) on chromosome 2 (inv[2] [p23 q35]); the clathrin heavy chain (*CLTC*) gene on chromosome 17 (t[2;17] [p23;q11-qter]); tropomyosin 4 and MYH9 on chromosome 22 (t[2;22] [p23;q11.2]) (561–568). A rare variant translocation involving the moesin (*MSN*) gene on the X chromosome (t[2;X] [p23; q11–12]) produces a distinctive cytoplasmic membrane ALK1 staining pattern (569).

Gene expression profiling can distinguish ALK1+ and ALK1− systemic ALCLs, suggesting they are two different entities (570–572).

Clinical Features

Primary nodal ALCL is a moderately aggressive tumor that generally occurs in young patients who have peripheral lymphadenopathy and extranodal disease that may include dissemination to skin (541,573). Patients with primary systemic ALCL who have genetic or phenotypic evidence of t(2;5) generally have a good prognosis (Table 17.7). Distinguishing this group of patients from those with systemic CD30+, ALK− T-cell lymphomas is necessary because the latter patients, who tend to be older, apparently have a poor prognosis similar to those with PTCL, unspecified (558,574–576). The NHL classification projects a 5-year overall survival rate of 77% for all types of ALCLs, regardless of whether there is evidence of t(2;5) (224).

Additional Comment

Primary cutaneous ALCL typically develops in adults and remains localized (541). This form of ALCL is often indolent and may be an extension of lymphomatoid papulosis type A. Primary cutaneous ALCLs usually lack EMA, ALK1, and t(2;5), suggesting that it has a different pathogenetic mechanism from primary nodal ALCL (541,556,577). Clusterin expression does not distinguish secondary cutaneous involvement by systemic ALCL from primary cutaneous ALCL (578).

ADULT T-CELL LEUKEMIA/LYMPHOMA

Adult T-cell leukemia/lymphoma (ATLL) is a peripheral T-cell neoplasm caused by human T-cell lymphotropic virus type I (HTLV-I). Most cases occur where the virus is endemic: southwestern Japan, the Caribbean islands, New Guinea, and parts of central Africa and South America. Some cases have been reported in the United States, particularly in the southeast, and in Europe, where most patients are immigrants from endemic areas. HTLV-I is transmitted by blood transfusions, needle sharing, sexual intercourse, and from mother to child through the placenta or breast milk. There is usually a latency period of several decades before clinical features of ATLL appear, with a lifetime risk of 1% to 5% for HTLV-I antibody-seropositive individuals (579).

There are four clinical subtypes of ATLL: acute, chronic, lymphomatous, and smoldering (580). The acute form is most common (55% to 65% of patients with ATLL) and is characterized by lymphadenopathy, organomegaly, skin lesions, elevated white blood cell count, hypercalcemia, elevated lactate dehydrogenase level, isolated lytic bone lesions, and a rapidly fatal course. Lymph nodes are generally effaced by a diffuse infiltrate of pleomorphic lymphocytes varying in size, which makes it difficult to distinguish from other pleomorphic PTCLs by morphologic features alone. Cutaneous infiltrates are usually dermal, but epidermotropism with formation of Pautrier microabscesses may develop, which may be difficult to differentiate from mycosis fungoides (581). Bone marrow infiltrates are diffuse and may be less impressive than the degree of peripheral blood involvement. Circulating tumor cells have hyperlobated nuclei, sometimes with a cloverleaf shape (Fig. 17.61). The tumor cells are generally CD4+ and CD25+ and express FoxP3, a phenotype consistent with a derivation from regulatory T-cells (Treg) responsible for suppressing T-cell expressor function (582). The neoplastic cells often lack CD7 but express other T-cell antigens. ATLL exhibits TCR gene rearrangements and clonal integration of HTLV-I genomes (583).

The lymphomatous subtype is the second most common form of ATLL (20% to 25% of cases) and is manifest by prominent lymphadenopathy without significant peripheral blood involvement. Nodal infiltrates are similar to those described for the acute form. The chronic subtype of ATLL is associated with an increased white blood cell count and occasionally with slight lymphadenopathy and organomegaly. Patients with the smoldering subtype have few ATLL cells in the peripheral blood

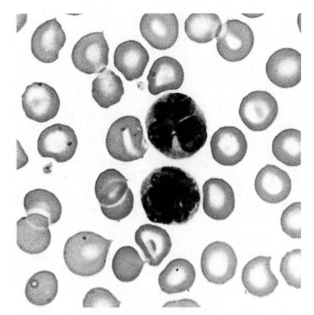

Figure 17.61. Peripheral blood, adult T-cell leukemia/lymphoma. Neoplastic cells have distinct multilobated nuclei (Wright stain).

and may have skin lesions, slight lymphadenopathy, organomegaly, and marrow infiltrates. Chronic and smoldering ATLL may evolve into the acute form after years of indolent disease.

NATURAL KILLER-CELL LYMPHOMAS

NK-cell lymphomas rarely occur outside East Asia, and most have extranodal location (sinonasal, skin, gastrointestinal tract, and testes). They are usually associated with EBV and often display angiocentric characteristics (489,584). A few NK-cell neoplasms arise as lymphoblastic lymphomas, as mentioned previously. Occasionally, NK-cell neoplasms appear in the form of aggressive, nonlymphoblastic leukemia/lymphoma that now and then involves nodes (585,586). The tumor cells are frequently pleomorphic large lymphocytes that contain azurophilic cytoplasmic granules on Romanovsky-type–stained touch imprints or smears. The neoplastic cells lack surface CD3 (but may express cytoplasmic CD3 when antibodies to the epsilon component of CD3 are used) and αβ and γδ chains of the TCR, and do not rearrange their TCR genes. Rarely, extranodal NK/T-cell lymphoma, nasal type has a primary nodal presentation, and these cases have many of the pathologic features characteristic of the nasal tumors (587,588).

NODAL INVOLVEMENT BY PRIMARY EXTRANODAL PERIPHERAL T-CELL AND NK-CELL LYMPHOMAS

Primary extranodal PTCLs and NK-cell lymphomas may infiltrate lymph nodes localized around the principal site of disease, or may show widely disseminated nodal involvement. Patterns of lymph node involvement by specific types of extranodal PTCLs are described here.

Mycosis Fungoides/Sézary Syndrome

Lymph nodes are the most common site of extracutaneous involvement by mycosis fungoides/Sézary syndrome (MF/SS).

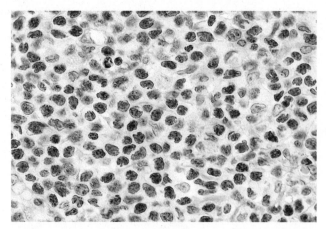

Figure 17.62. Lymph node involved by cutaneous mycosis fungoides/Sézary syndrome. Homogeneous aggregates of cerebriform lymphocytes, recognized by their extreme nuclear folding, are present.

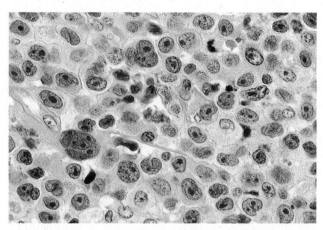

Figure 17.63. Lymph node involved by transformed-cell variant of mycosis fungoides/Sézary syndrome. The neoplastic cells have features of immunoblasts: large cells with abundant cytoplasm, dispersed chromatin, and prominent central nucleoli.

Lymphadenopathy, particularly in the axillary and inguinal areas, is present in approximately 70% of patients with MF/SS, and nodal involvement has been documented in more than 60% of autopsied cases (589,590). Nodal changes in patients with MF/SS have three basic patterns: nonspecific reactive type, dermatopathic lymphadenopathy, and frank lymphomatous involvement (591). Nonspecific patterns are generally follicular or paracortical lymphoid hyperplasia. Dermatopathic lymphadenopathy has been described earlier in this chapter (see "Dermatopathic Lymphadenopathy"). Nodes affected by MF/SS show either partial or complete architectural effacement by atypical lymphocytes, which often have cerebriform nuclei but may have immunoblastic features (Figs. 17.62 and 17.63) (592).

Two principal classification schemes for lymph nodes from patients with MF/SS have been developed following the National Cancer Institute (NCI) and Dutch criteria (Table 17.8) (593,594). The NCI classification grades lymph nodes on a scale of 0 to 4, where LN-0 equates with nodes with nonspecific reactive changes. Grades LN-1 through LN-3 correspond to dermatopathic lymphadenopathy: LN-1 has only scattered atypical lymphocytes in the paracortex; LN-2 has atypical lymphocytes singly or in clusters of three to six cells admixed with histiocytes; and LN-3 has numerous small and large atypical lymphocytes singly or in aggregates of 15 or more cells that separate paracortical histiocytes. LN-4 corresponds to frank lymphoma with either partial or complete effacement of the node.

In the Dutch scheme, categories I and II correspond to dermatopathic lymphadenopathy. Category I encompasses nodes with cerebriform lymphocytes having a maximum nuclear diameter less than 7.5 μm; they are considered to be uninvolved by

MF/SS. Category II nodes have cerebriform lymphocytes with nuclear diameters exceeding 7.5 μm, thought to be representative of early involvement by MF/SS. Categories III and IV correspond to frank lymphoma, with the former representing partial effacement.

Clinical studies of the NCI and Dutch classifications have shown each to be associated with poorer survival rates with increasing levels of morphologic changes in nodes. Molecular genetic studies on nodes classified by these two systems have produced similar results (Table 17.8) (595,596), with Dutch categories I/NCI LN-1 and LN-2 showing no molecular evidence of involvement by MF/SS and categories III and IV/LN-4 demonstrating consistent T-cell clonality. The morphologic gray zone for predicting nodal involvement/T-cell clonality is category II/LN-3, where TCR gene rearrangements were present in 46% of cases studied; survival was better for patients without clonality in this group, which suggests that molecular analysis is a useful adjunct for evaluating nodes in patients with MF/SS who have dermatopathic lymphadenopathy without any effacement of architecture but with evidence of enlarged cerebriform lymphocytes.

Other Primary Extranodal Peripheral T-Cell Lymphomas and NK-Cell Lymphomas in Nodes

Enteropathy-type T-cell lymphomas commonly involve intra-abdominal lymph nodes, particularly within the mesentery. The neoplastic infiltrates consist of small intrasinus aggregates or sheets of tumor cells that may expand the paracortex (597,598).

TABLE 17.8	Morphologic Patterns of Lymph Node Changes in Patients with Mycosis Fungoides with Associated Classification and T-Cell Clonality		
Morphologic Pattern	*NCI Classification*	*Dutch Classification*	*T-Cell Clonality*
Nonspecific reactive	LN-0	—	—
Dermatopathic lymphadenopathy	LN-1 and LN-2	Category I	
	LN-3	Category II	46%
Frank lymphoma, partial or complete effacement	LN-4	Category III or IV	94%

Hepatosplenic T-cell lymphomas may affect splenic hilar nodes and other intra-abdominal nodes. It is usually exemplified by partial interfollicular and sinus infiltrates of tumor cells (77,599).

Subcutaneous panniculitis-like T-cell lymphomas rarely involve lymph nodes (600,601), and no good descriptions of nodal infiltrates exist. Extranodal NK/T-cell lymphomas, nasal type are T-cell or true NK-cell lymphomas that usually arise in the sinonasal area or skin and may rarely involve nodes. The nodes are often effaced by lymphocytes of variable size and nuclear atypia. Perivascular and intravascular infiltrates that are angiodestructive are usually present and associated with areas of parenchymal necrosis (602).

HISTIOCYTIC NEOPLASMS

Histiocytes include cells from both the monocyte/macrophage series and the Langerhans cell/dendritic cell series (603). Monocytes and macrophages are the principal phagocytic cells of the mononuclear phagocyte and immunoregulatory effector (M-PIRE) system, whereas Langerhans cells, follicular dendritic cells (FDCs), and interdigitating dendritic cells (IDCs) are the major antigen-presenting cells of the M-PIRE system. Histiocytic proliferations may be classified by the cell types of either the phagocytic or antigen-presenting series and further subdivided according to their reactive or neoplastic nature (Table 17.9). The main histiocytic neoplasm that can involve lymph nodes is histiocytic sarcoma (HS) (604). The Langerhans cell/dendritic cell neoplasms that can be seen in lymph nodes include Langerhans cell histiocytosis, Langerhans cell sarcoma, FDC sarcoma/tumor, and IDC sarcoma/tumor (604).

HISTIOCYTIC SARCOMA

HS is rare and has apparently been overly diagnosed. Most cases previously diagnosed as malignant histiocytosis and histiocytic medullary reticulosis (605,606) have been subsequently shown to be PTCLs, particularly of the ALCL type (607–609). HS is an extremely aggressive disease that generally appears in adults and leads to B symptoms, lymphadenopathy, hepatosplenomegaly, and peripheral blood cytopenias. The diagnosis should be made only when there is unequivocal histopathologic evidence of neoplasia (some widespread, fatal histiocytic proliferations may not be malignant) and the neoplastic cells are proved to be of monocyte/macrophage origin by cytochemical, immunophenotypic, genotypic, and ultrastructural studies.

Lymph nodes may be obliterated or show expansion of sinuses by neoplastic histiocytes (Fig. 17.64) that spare follicles or islands of lymphoid tissue. Tumor cells display varying degrees of pleomorphism and often have reniform nuclei and abundant eosinophilic cytoplasm. Tumor giant cells may be seen. Necrosis is common and erythrophagocytosis may be present. Tumor cells on touch imprints show diffuse positivity with nonspecific esterase, which is partially or totally inhibited by fluoride, and with acid phosphatase, which is not resistant to tartrate. These cells contain lysosomes associated with such enzymes as lysozyme, alpha$_1$-antitrypsin, and alpha$_1$-antichymotrypsin. They variably express cell surface antigens such as CD4, CD11b, CD14, CD15, CD18, CD25, CD35, CD45, CD68, CD163, and MAC-387. CD1a, S-100, and Langerin generally show negative results. Immunoglobulin and TCR gene rearrangements should be absent. Ultrastructural features of malignant histiocytes include abundant surface activity, microfilaments, short segments of rough endoplasmic reticulum, and scattered haloed granules. Birbeck granules are absent. The differential diagnosis of HS includes metastatic carcinoma, large-cell lymphomas with a sinus growth pattern (ALCL and microvillous B-cell lymphomas), and some reactive histiocytic proliferations. Occasional HSs develop as a transdifferentiation of a pre-existing B-cell neoplasm (610,611).

LANGERHANS CELL HISTIOCYTOSIS AND SARCOMA

Langerhans cell histiocytosis (LCH) has previously been diagnosed as histiocytosis X. It is a syndrome of variable biologic behavior that predominantly affects children and encompasses Letterer-Siwe disease, Hand-Schüller-Christian disease, and eosinophilic granuloma (612–614). All forms of this syndrome are associated with a clonal proliferation of Langerhans histiocytes (615). Lymphadenopathy may be the initial and only manifestation of LCH, but skin or bone involvement often accompanies lymphadenopathy. On rare occasions, Langerhans cell histiocytes are associated with a variety of malignant neoplasms (616).

Lymph node architecture is partially preserved, with retention of normal or hypoplastic germinal centers. Sinuses are distended by benign-appearing histiocytes with abundant pale eosinophilic cytoplasm and vesicular nuclei with an indented "coffee bean" appearance. Nucleoli are absent or small. Nuclear atypia is not seen. Multinucleated giant cells are usually present. Admixed eosinophils may form aggregates with central necrosis. On ultrastructural examination, histiocytes are seen to contain the characteristic Birbeck or Langerhans granules. On immunologic studies, these Langerhans cells express many of the antigens common to monocytes/macrophages but are distinguished from them by strong marking with antibodies to CD1a, S-100, and Langerin (617).

Langerhans cell sarcoma is also a neoplasm of Langerhans cells and is distinguished from LCH by its overtly malignant

---

TABLE 17.9

Histiocytic Proliferations Involving Lymph Nodes

Disease by Cell Type

Monocyte/Macrophage
  Reactive
    Viral-associated hemophagocytic syndrome
    Sinus histiocytosis with massive lymphadenopathy (Rosai Dorfman disease)
  Neoplastic
    Acute monocytic leukemia
    Histiocytic sarcoma
Langerhans Cell/Dendritic Cell
  Reactive
    Dermatopathic lymphadenopathy
  Neoplastic
    Langerhans cell histiocytosis
    Langerhans cell sarcoma
    Follicular dendritic cell sarcoma/tumor
    Interdigitating cell sarcoma/tumor

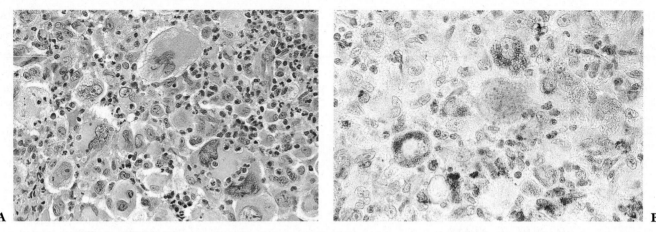

Figure 17.64. Lymph node, histiocytic sarcoma. **(A)** Pleomorphic tumor cells, including some multinucleated giant T cells, are associated with a mixed inflammatory background. **(B)** Paraffin immunoperoxidase with anti-CD68 (KP-1) demonstrates cytoplasmic positivity characteristic of histiocytes.

cytologic features and higher-grade clinical behavior (618). It may arise de novo or from pre-existing LCH (619).

DENDRITIC CELL SARCOMAS

Follicular Dendritic Cell Sarcoma/Tumor

FDC sarcomas/tumors are rare, and the terminology is meant to reflect the variable cytologic features and clinical behavior among these neoplasms. Most arise in the superficial lymph nodes of adults, but intra-abdominal, oral, and soft-tissue types are described (620,621). These tumors may arise as a complication of the hyaline vascular variant of Castleman disease (621,622). Growth patterns are typically storiform/whorled (Fig. 17.65), fascicular, or solid. Occasional cases may show nodular (follicle-like) or trabecular patterns. The neoplastic FDCs often appear syncytial because of their interwoven cell processes. Individual cells are usually spindly but can be oval, polygonal, or multinucleated. The nuclei exhibit dispersed chromatin and small, but distinct, nucleoli (Fig. 17.65). Small

lymphocytes (T cells) tend to be sprinkled about FDC sarcomas, and perivascular lymphocyte cuffing is common. IHC studies are essential for diagnosis, and there should be staining with at least two FDC markers, such as CD21, CD35, R4/23, KiM4, KiM4p, Ki-FDC1p, and CNA42. Clusterin is a highly sensitive and specific marker of FDC sarcomas/tumors as compared to other dendritic cells and neoplasms (623,624). These tumors are frequently positive for EMA, HLA-DR, and vimentin; occasionally positive for CD45, CD68, S-100, and muscle-specific actin; rarely positive for CD20; and negative for cytokeratin and vascular markers. Ultrastructural studies are desirable but not essential; such studies show that FDC sarcomas/tumors have long, villous cytoplasmic processes, and desmosomes (Fig. 17.66). Birbeck granules are absent.

Interdigitating Dendritic Cell Sarcoma/Tumor

IDC sarcomas/tumors are even more rare than FDC sarcomas/ tumors (623,625). The terminology, again, reflects the variable cytologic features and clinical behavior among these neoplasms.

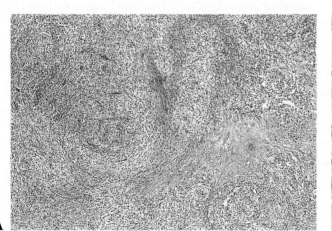
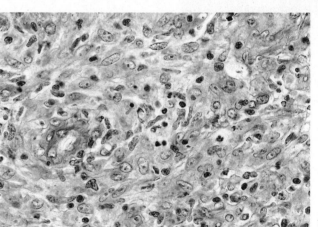

Figure 17.65. Lymph node, follicular dendritic cell sarcoma/tumor. **(A)** The nodal architecture is effaced by a neoplasm that produces a nodular and whorled growth pattern. **(B)** The neoplasm is composed of oval and spindle-shaped cells with dispersed chromatin and small nucleoli. The tumor cells were CD21 and CD35 positive by IHC (not shown).

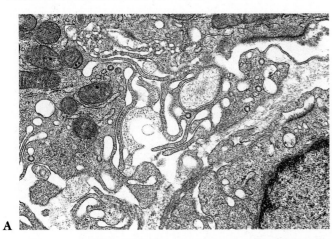
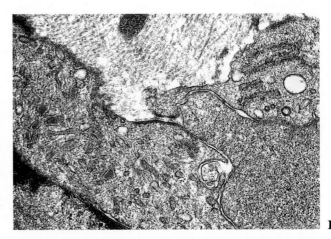

A   B

Figure 17.66. Lymph node, follicular dendritic cell sarcoma/tumor. Electron micrographs of cytoplasmic processes (**A**) and desmosomes (**B**) characteristic of follicular dendritic cells (13,050×).

They typically arise as widespread lymphadenopathy in adults. Tumor infiltrates are most frequently paracortical, with sparing of lymphoid follicles, or sinusoidal. The neoplastic IDCs are generally pleomorphic large cells that often have a bizarre, grooved nucleus and abundant pale/eosinophilic cytoplasm. Tumor giant cells may be present. The neoplastic cells express S-100, are negative for CD1a and Langerin, and lack FDC markers. On ultrastructural study, the IDCs have interdigitating cytoplasmic processes but no junctional complexes or Birbeck granules.

OTHER NEOPLASMS

METASTATIC TUMORS IN LYMPH NODES

Metastatic carcinomas, melanomas, and sarcomas are usually easily recognized from histopathologic evidence or strongly suspected on clinical grounds, but poorly differentiated neoplasms of this type may resemble malignant lymphomas (including HL) or malignant histiocytosis (MH). Cohesion of tumor cells, sinus involvement, and clearly defined interfaces with normal lymphoid tissue are all strongly suggestive of carcinomas. In many cases, however, IHC or ultrastructural examination is required for diagnosis. Electron microscopy often provides very specific information about the type of neoplastic cell, although most laboratories now rely on IHC procedures.

IHC techniques are appealing because of their availability to community hospitals and their alleged specificity. In practice, their reliability must be established by the usual quality controls and the experience of studying known neoplasms. Very few antibodies are as specific as claimed. An exception seems to be CD45 (LCA), which rarely gives false-positive staining. A battery of antibodies should be used for characterization of neoplasms; use of a single antibody is hazardous.

There are several specific neoplasms in which nodal metastases may closely mimic malignant lymphomas. Nasopharyngeal carcinoma may occur in children and young adults; patients often show initial signs of cervical adenopathy without a readily apparent mass in the nasopharynx. Nodal involvement by nasopharyngeal carcinoma may be misinterpreted as nodular-sclerosing classic HL (NSHL) because of its fibrotic tissue reac-

tion, eosinophilia, and small clusters of tumor cells (Figs. 17.67, 17.68) or NHL (626–628). Metastatic melanoma may be mistaken for immunoblastic B-cell lymphomas or lymphocyte-depleted HL and has also been shown to have a granulomatous reaction (629). Breast carcinoma, particularly lobular carcinoma, often infiltrates nodes without evidence of gland formation and may be confused with malignant lymphomas or histiocytic proliferations. Inguinal and abdominal nodes are frequently sites for metastasis by seminoma. Seminoma cells resemble transformed lymphocytes to some degree, but the cytoplasm of seminoma cells, unlike most lymphomas, is PAS-positive, and the nodal stroma may show a granulomatous response to metastatic seminoma (Fig. 17.69) (630).

LEUKEMIC INVOLVEMENT OF LYMPH NODES

Nodes may be involved in both lymphoid and myeloid leukemias, including megakaryoblastic leukemia (631), during acute as well as chronic phases of these diseases. Nodal involvement may be the presenting manifestation, but it is more commonly part of a widespread infiltrative process. Although histopatho-

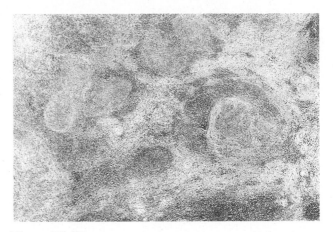

Figure 17.67. Lymph node, metastatic nasopharyngeal carcinoma. The low-magnification appearance is often nodular, mimicking that of nodular-sclerosing Hodgkin lymphoma. The reaction to nasopharyngeal carcinoma may be rich in macrophages and eosinophils as well.

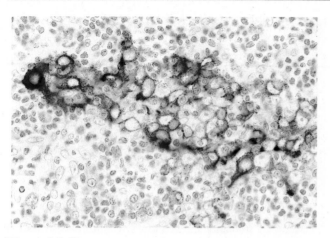

Figure 17.68. Lymph node, metastatic nasopharyngeal carcinoma. Small focus of carcinoma is identified by staining for cytokeratin.

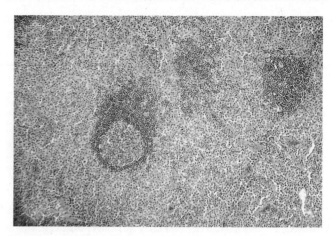

Figure 17.70. Lymph node, myeloid sarcoma. A characteristic growth pattern of leukemia is shown, with marked distortion of the cortex and paracortical areas and partial preservation of follicles.

logic features offer useful clues to the correct diagnosis, precise identification of the neoplastic cell in many cases requires multiparameter analysis, including immunophenotypic studies.

Histopathologic Features

MYELOID LEUKEMIAS. Lymphadenopathy may be the initial manifestation of acute myeloid leukemias; marrow involvement in some cases may not be detected for months or years. Nodal architecture may be partially or completely effaced.

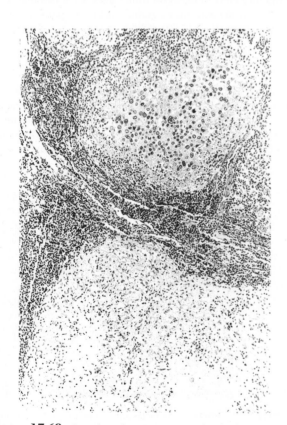

Figure 17.69. Lymph node, metastatic seminoma. Note the focus of metastatic tumor (*top*) and adjacent characteristic granulomatous inflammation.

Prominent infiltrates in the medullary and paracortical areas of nodes are the rule, and small islands of cortical lymphocytes or follicular centers are almost always present (Fig. 17.70). Blasts have distinct cytoplasmic borders, dispersed chromatin, and small nucleoli. In some cases, eosinophilic myelocytes are indicators of the leukemic nature of the infiltrate (632) but are not present in the more primitive myeloid and monocytic neoplasms. Antibodies to myeloperoxidase and CD33 are quite helpful, especially when the only material available is paraffin-embedded (633,634). Lymphadenopathy is a common manifestation of the blast crisis of chronic myeloid leukemias (635–637). Some of these cases show prominent megakaryocytic differentiation and may be confused with Hodgkin disease.

LYMPHOID LEUKEMIAS. Patients with acute lymphocytic leukemias may have widespread adenopathy and hepatosplenomegaly at diagnosis; node biopsies are occasionally the initial diagnostic procedure. Nodal architecture is usually effaced by infiltrates of primitive cells resembling those described for T-cell lymphoblastic lymphoma. Marrow involvement is virtually always present (in contrast to apparently negative marrow examination in some myeloid leukemias). Recognition of the neoplastic phenotype is dependent on multiparameter evaluation. The nodal changes in CLL have been discussed previously. Abdominal lymphadenopathy is occasionally noted in hairy cell leukemia, as described earlier (638).

REFERENCES

1. Murphy K, Travers P, Walport M. Immunobiology. In Janeway C, ed. *Janeway's Immunobiology.* 7th ed. New York: Garland Science, 2007:8–23.
2. Kuppers R, Dalla-Favera R. Mechanisms of chromosomal translocations in B cell lymphomas. *Oncogene* 2001;20:5580–5594.
3. Liso A, Capello D, Marafioti T, et al. Aberrant somatic hypermutation in tumor cells of nodular-lymphocyte-predominant and classic Hodgkin lymphoma. *Blood* 2006;108: 1013–1020.
4. Collins RD. Lymph node examination. What is an adequate workup? *Arch Pathol Lab Med* 1985;109:797–799.
5. Higgins RA, Blankenship JE, Kinney MC. Application of immunohistochemistry in the diagnosis of non-Hodgkin and Hodgkin lymphoma. *Arch Pathol Lab Med* 2008;132: 441–461.
6. Falini B, Mason DY. Proteins encoded by genes involved in chromosomal alterations in lymphoma and leukemia: clinical value of their detection by immunocytochemistry. *Blood* 2002;99:409–426.
7. Cossman J, Fend F, Staudt L, et al. Application of molecular genetics to the diagnosis and

classification of malignant lymphoma. In Knowles DM, ed. *Neoplastic Hematopathology.* 2nd ed. Philadelphia: Lippincott Williams & Wilkins, 2001: 365–390.

8. Das DK. Lymph nodes. In Bibbo M, ed. *Comprehensive Cytopathology.* Philadelphia: WB Saunders, 1991: 671–702.

9. Recommendations for the reporting of lymphoid neoplasms: a report from The Association of Directors of Anatomic and Surgical Pathology. *Virchows Arch A Pathol Anat Histol* 2002;441:314–319.

10. Harris NL, Jaffe ES, Stein H, et al. A revised European-American classification of lymphoid neoplasms: a proposal from the International Lymphoma Study Group. *Blood* 1994;84: 1361–1392.

11. Jaffe E, Harris N, Steen H, et al. Pathology and genetics of tumours of haematopoietic and lymphoid tissue. In Jaffe E, Harris N, Steen H, et al, eds. *Pathology and Genetics of Tumours of Haematopoietic and Lymphoid Tissues. World Health Organization Classification of Tumours.* Lyon, France: IARC Press, 2001.

11a. Swerdlow SH, Campo E, Harris NL, et al. (Eds.) *WHO Classification of Tumors of Haematopoietic and Lymphoid Tissues.* Lyon, France: IARC Press, 2008.

12. Dorfman RF, Warnke R. Lymphadenopathy simulating the malignant lymphomas. *Hum Pathol* 1974;5:519–550.

13. Davey MP, Waldmann TA. Clonality and lymphoproliferative lesions. *N Engl J Med* 1986; 315:509–511.

14. Collins RD. Is clonality equivalent to malignancy: specifically, is immunoglobulin gene rearrangement diagnostic of malignant lymphoma? *Hum Pathol* 1997;28:757–759.

15. Levy N, Nelson J, Meyer P, et al. Reactive lymphoid hyperplasia with single class (monoclonal) surface immunoglobulin. *Am J Clin Pathol* 1983;80:300–308.

16. Palutke M, Schnitzer B, Mirchandani I, et al. Increased numbers of lymphocytes with single class surface immunoglobulins in reactive hyperplasia of lymphoid tissue. *Am J Clin Pathol* 1982;78:316–323.

17. Chamberlain WD, Falta MT, Kotzin BL. Functional subsets within clonally expanded CD8(+) memory T cells in elderly humans. *Clin Immunol* 2000;94:160–172.

18. Lust JA, Donovan KA. Biology of the transition of monoclonal gammopathy of undetermined significance (MGUS) to multiple myeloma. *Cancer Control* 1998;5:209–217.

19. Hanto DW, Frizzera G, Purtilo DT, et al. Clinical spectrum of lymphoproliferative disorders in renal transplant recipients and evidence for the role of Epstein-Barr virus. *Cancer Res* 1981;41:4253–4261.

20. Fishleder A, Tubbs R, Hesse B, et al. Uniform detection of immunoglobulin-gene rearrangement in benign lymphoepithelial lesions. *N Engl J Med* 1987;316:1118–1121.

21. Alonso ML, Richardson ME, Metroka CE, et al. Chromosome abnormalities in AIDS-associated lymphadenopathy. *Blood* 1987;69:855–858.

22. Lipford EH, Smith HR, Pittaluga S, et al. Clonality of angioimmunoblastic lymphadenopathy and implications for its evolution to malignant lymphoma. *J Clin Invest* 1987;79: 637–642.

23. Burns BF, Colby TV, Dorfman RF. Differential diagnostic features of nodular L&H Hodgkin's disease, including progressive transformation of germinal centers. *Am J Surg Pathol* 1984;8:253–261.

24. Nguyen PL, Ferry JA, Harris NL. Progressive transformation of germinal centers and nodular lymphocyte predominance Hodgkin's disease: a comparative immunohistochemical study. *Am J Surg Pathol* 1999;23:27–33.

25. Osborne BM, Butler JJ. Clinical implications of progressive transformation of germinal centers. *Am J Surg Pathol* 1984;8:725–733.

26. Poppema S, Kaiserling E, Lennert K. Hodgkin's disease with lymphocytic predominance, nodular type (nodular paragranuloma) and progressively transformed germinal centres—a cytohistological study. *Histopathology* 1979;3:295–308.

27. Nosanchuk JS, Schnitzer B. Follicular hyperplasia in lymph nodes from patients with rheumatoid arthritis. A clinicopathologic study. *Cancer* 1969;24:243–254.

28. Kondratowicz GM, Symmons DP, Bacon PA, et al. Rheumatoid lymphadenopathy: a morphological and immunohistochemical study. *J Clin Pathol* 1990;43:106–113.

29. McCluggage WG, Bharucha H. Lymph node hyalinisation in rheumatoid arthritis and systemic sclerosis. *J Clin Pathol* 1994;47:138–142.

30. Santana V, Rose NR. Neoplastic lymphoproliferation in autoimmune disease: an updated review. *Clin Immunol Immunopathol* 1992;63:205–213.

31. Gridley G, McLaughlin JK, Ekbom A, et al. Incidence of cancer among patients with rheumatoid arthritis. *J Natl Cancer Inst* 1993;85:307–311.

32. Kamel OW, Gelb AB, Shibuya RB, et al. Leu 7 (CD57) reactivity distinguishes nodular lymphocyte predominance Hodgkin's disease from nodular sclerosing Hodgkin's disease, T-cell-rich B-cell lymphoma and follicular lymphoma. *Am J Pathol* 1993;142:541–546.

33. Kamel OW, van de Rijn M, LeBrun DP, et al. Lymphoid neoplasms in patients with rheumatoid arthritis and dermatomyositis: frequency of Epstein-Barr virus and other features associated with immunosuppression. *Hum Pathol* 1994;25:638–643.

34. Askling J, Klareskog L, Hjalgrim H, et al. Do steroids increase lymphoma risk? A case-control study of lymphoma risk in polymyalgia rheumatica/giant cell arteritis. *Ann Rheum Dis* 2005;64:1765–1768.

35. Wolfe F, Michaud K. Lymphoma in rheumatoid arthritis: the effect of methotrexate and anti-tumor necrosis factor therapy in 18,572 patients. *Arthritis Rheum* 2004;50:1740–1751.

36. Bujak JS, Aptekar RG, Decker JL, et al. Juvenile rheumatoid arthritis presenting in the adult as fever of unknown origin. *Medicine (Baltimore)* 1973;52:431–444.

37. Ohta A, Matsumoto Y, Ohta T, et al. Still's disease associated with necrotizing lymphadenitis (Kikuchi's disease): report of 3 cases. *J Rheumatol* 1988;15:981–983.

38. Valente RM, Banks PM, Conn DL. Characterization of lymph node histology in adult onset Still's disease. *J Rheumatol* 1989;16:349–354.

39. McCurley TL, Collins RD, Ball E. Nodal and extranodal lymphoproliferative disorders in Sjogren's syndrome: a clinical and immunopathologic study. *Hum Pathol* 1990;21:482–492.

40. Kassan SS, Thomas TL, Moutsopoulos HM, et al. Increased risk of lymphoma in sicca syndrome. *Ann Intern Med* 1978;89:888–892.

41. Shin SS, Sheibani K, Fishleder A, et al. Monocytoid B-cell lymphoma in patients with Sjogren's syndrome: a clinicopathologic study of 13 patients. *Hum Pathol* 1991;22:422–430.

42. Royer B, Cazals-Hatem D, Sibilia J, et al. Lymphomas in patients with Sjogren's syndrome are marginal zone B-cell neoplasms, arise in diverse extranodal and nodal sites, and are not associated with viruses. *Blood* 1997;90:766–775.

43. Fox RA. The lymph nodes in disseminated lupus erythematosus. *Am J Pathol* 1943;19: 73–79.

44. Medeiros LJ, Kaynor B, Harris NL. Lupus lymphadenitis: report of a case with immunohistologic studies on frozen sections. *Hum Pathol* 1989;20:295–299.

45. Sanpavat A, Wannakrairot P, Assanasen T. Necrotizing non-granulomatous lymphadenitis: a clinicopathologic study of 40 Thai patients. *Southeast Asian J Trop Med Public Health* 2006; 37:563–570.

46. Norris AH, Krasinskas AM, Salhany KE, et al. Kikuchi-Fujimoto disease: a benign cause of fever and lymphadenopathy. *Am J Med* 1996;101:401–405.

47. Pileri S, Kikuchi M, Helbron D, et al. Histiocytic necrotizing lymphadenitis without granulocytic infiltration. *Virchows Arch A Pathol Anat Histol* 1982;395:257–271.

48. Kikuchi M. Histiocytic necrotizing lymphadenitis (Kikuchi-Fujimoto disease) in Japan. *Am J Surg Pathol* 1991;15:197–198.

49. Felgar RE, Furth EE, Wasik MA, et al. Histiocytic necrotizing lymphadenitis (Kikuchi's disease): in situ end-labeling, immunohistochemical, and serologic evidence supporting cytotoxic lymphocyte-mediated apoptotic cell death. *Mod Pathol* 1997;10:231–241.

50. Kuo TT. Kikuchi's disease (histiocytic necrotizing lymphadenitis). A clinicopathologic study of 79 cases with an analysis of histologic subtypes, immunohistology, and DNA ploidy. *Am J Surg Pathol* 1995;19:798–809.

51. Chamulak GA, Brynes RK, Nathwani BN. Kikuchi-Fujimoto disease mimicking malignant lymphoma. *Am J Surg Pathol* 1990;14:514–523.

52. Cho KJ, Lee SS, Khang SK. Histiocytic necrotizing lymphadenitis. A clinico-pathologic study of 45 cases with in situ hybridization for Epstein-Barr virus and hepatitis B virus. *J Korean Med Sci* 1996;11:409–414.

53. Hollingsworth HC, Peiper SC, Weiss LM, et al. An investigation of the viral pathogenesis of Kikuchi-Fujimoto disease. Lack of evidence for Epstein-Barr virus or human herpesvirus type 6 as the causative agents. *Arch Pathol Lab Med* 1994;118:134–140.

54. Kuo TT, Shih LY, Chan HL. Kimura's disease. Involvement of regional lymph nodes and distinction from angiolymphoid hyperplasia with eosinophilia. *Am J Surg Pathol* 1988;12: 843–854.

55. Hui PK, Chan JK, Ng CS, et al. Lymphadenopathy of Kimura's disease. *Am J Surg Pathol* 1989;13:177–186.

56. Li TJ, Chen XM, Wang SZ, et al. Kimura's disease: a clinicopathologic study of 54 Chinese patients. *Oral Surg Oral Med Oral Pathol Oral Radiol Endod* 1996;82:549–555.

57. Vermi W, Facchetti F, Riboldi E, et al. Role of dendritic cell-derived CXCL13 in the pathogenesis of Bartonella henselae B-rich granuloma. *Blood* 2006;107:454–462.

58. Kojima M, Morita Y, Shimizu K, et al. Plasmacytoid monocytes in cat scratch disease with special reference to the histological diversity of suppurative lesions. *Pathol Res Pract* 2006; 202:17.22.

59. Campbell JA. Cat-scratch disease. *Pathol Annu* 1977;12 Pt 1:277–292.

60. Wear DJ, Margileth AM, Hadfield TL, et al. Cat scratch disease: a bacterial infection. *Science* 1983;221:1403–1405.

61. Scott MA, McCurley TL, Vnencak-Jones CL, et al. Cat scratch disease: detection of Bartonella henselae DNA in archival biopsies from patients with clinically, serologically, and histologically defined disease. *Am J Pathol* 1996;149:2161–2167.

62. Kommareddi S, Abramowsky CR, Swinehart GL, et al. Nontuberculous mycobacterial infections: comparison of the fluorescent auramine-O and Ziehl-Neelsen techniques in tissue diagnosis. *Hum Pathol* 1984;15:1085–1089.

63. Delahoussaye PM, Osborne BM. Cat-scratch disease presenting as abdominal visceral granulomas. *J Infect Dis* 1990;161:71–78.

64. Lamps LW, Gray GF, Scott MA. The histologic spectrum of hepatic cat scratch disease. A series of six cases with confirmed Bartonella henselae infection. *Am J Surg Pathol* 1996;20: 1253–1259.

65. Dorfman RF, Remington JS. Value of lymph-node biopsy in the diagnosis of acute acquired toxoplasmosis. *N Engl J Med* 1973;289:878–881.

66. Sheibani K, Fritz RM, Winberg CD, et al. "Monocytoid" cells in reactive follicular hyperplasia with and without multifocal histiocytic reactions: an immunohistochemical study of 21 cases including suspected cases of toxoplasmic lymphadenitis. *Am J Clin Pathol* 1984; 81:453–458.

67. Gray GF, Jr., Kimball AC, Kean BH. The posterior cervical lymph node in toxoplasmosis. *Am J Pathol* 1972;69:349–358.

68. Rousselet MC, Saint-Andre JP, Beaufils JM, et al. Benign vascular proliferation in a lymph node following acute toxoplasmosis. A differential diagnosis from Kaposi's sarcoma. *Arch Pathol Lab Med* 1988;112:1264–1266.

69. Lin MH, Kuo TT. Specificity of the histopathological triad for the diagnosis of toxoplasmic lymphadenitis: polymerase chain reaction study. *Pathol Int* 2001;51:619–623.

70. Turner DR, Wright DJM. Lymphadenopathy in early syphilis. *J Pathol* 1973;110:305–308.

71. Hartsock RJ, Halling LW, King FM. Luetic lymphadenitis: a clinical and histologic study of 20 cases. *Am J Clin Pathol* 1970;53:304–314.

72. Gregory N, Sanchez M, Buchness MR. The spectrum of syphilis in patients with human immunodeficiency virus infection. *J Am Acad Dermatol* 1990;22:1061–1067.

73. Chadburn A, Metroka C, Mouradian J. Progressive lymph node histology and its prognostic value in patients with acquired immunodeficiency syndrome and AIDS-related complex. *Hum Pathol* 1989;20:579–587.

74. Garcia CF, Lifson JD, Engleman EG, et al. The immunohistology of the persistent generalized lymphadenopathy syndrome (PGL). *Am J Clin Pathol* 1986;86:706–715.

75. Sunila I, Vaccarezza M, Pantaleo G, et al. Activated cytotoxic lymphocytes in lymph nodes from human immunodeficiency virus (HIV) 1-infected patients: a light and electronmicroscopic study. *Histopathology* 1997;30:31–40.

76. Soulier J, Grollet L, Oksenhendler E, et al. Kaposi's sarcoma-associated herpesvirus-like DNA sequences in multicentric Castleman's disease. *Blood* 1995;86:1276–1280.

77. Salhany KE, Feldman M, Kahn MJ, et al. Hepatosplenic gammadelta T-cell lymphoma:

ultrastructural, immunophenotypic, and functional evidence for cytotoxic T lymphocyte differentiation. *Hum Pathol* 1997;28:674–685.

78. Ewing EP, Jr., Chandler FW, Spira TJ, et al. Primary lymph node pathology in AIDS and AIDS-related lymphadenopathy. *Arch Pathol Lab Med* 1985;109:977–981.

79. Shibata D, Brynes RK, Nathwani B, et al. Human immunodeficiency viral DNA is readily found in lymph node biopsies from seropositive individuals. Analysis of fixed tissue using the polymerase chain reaction. *Am J Pathol* 1989;135:697–702.

80. Keller AR, Hochholzer L, Castleman B. Hyaline-vascular and plasma-cell types of giant lymph node hyperplasia of the mediastinum and other locations. *Cancer* 1972;29:670–683.

81. Dupin N, Diss TL, Kellam P, et al. HHV-8 is associated with a plasmablastic variant of Castleman disease that is linked to HHV-8-positive plasmablastic lymphoma. *Blood* 2000; 95:1406–1412.

82. Frizzera G. Systemic Castleman's disease. *Am J Surg Pathol* 1991;15:192.

83. Weisenburger DD, Nathwani BN, Winberg CD, et al. Multicentric angiofollicular lymph node hyperplasia: a clinicopathologic study of 16 cases. *Hum Pathol* 1985;16:162–172.

84. Moller P, Moldenhauer G, Momburg F, et al. Mediastinal lymphoma of clear cell type is a tumor corresponding to terminal steps of B cell differentiation. *Blood* 1987;69:1087–1095.

85. Ohyashiki JH, Ohyashiki K, Kawakubo K, et al. Molecular genetic, cytogenetic, and immunophenotypic analyses in Castleman's disease of the plasma cell type. *Am J Clin Pathol* 1994;101:290–295.

86. Du MQ, Liu H, Diss TC, et al. Kaposi sarcoma-associated herpesvirus infects monotypic (IgM lambda) but polyclonal naive B cells in Castleman disease and associated lymphoproliferative disorders. *Blood* 2001;97:2130–2136.

87. Nguyen DT, Diamond LW, Hansmann ML, et al. Castleman's disease. Differences in follicular dendritic network in the hyaline vascular and plasma cell variants. *Histopathology* 1994;24:437–443.

88. Menke DM, Tiemann M, Camoriano JK, et al. Diagnosis of Castleman's disease by identification of an immunophenotypically aberrant population of mantle zone B lymphocytes in paraffin-embedded lymph node biopsies. *Am J Clin Pathol* 1996;105:268–276.

89. Soulier J, Grollet L, Oksenhendler E, et al. Molecular analysis of clonality in Castleman's disease. *Blood* 1995;86:1131–1138.

90. Yoshizaki K, Matsuda T, Nishimoto N, et al. Pathogenic significance of interleukin-6 (IL-6/BSF-2) in Castleman's disease. *Blood* 1989;74:1360–1367.

91. Leger-Ravet MB, Peuchmaur M, Devergne O, et al. Interleukin-6 gene expression in Castleman's disease. *Blood* 1991;78:2923–2930.

92. Gherardi RK, Belec L, Fromont G, et al. Elevated levels of interleukin-1 beta (IL-1 beta) and IL-6 in serum and increased production of IL-1 beta mRNA in lymph nodes of patients with polyneuropathy, organomegaly, endocrinopathy, M protein, and skin changes (POEMS) syndrome. *Blood* 1994;83:2587–2593.

93. Dupin N, Fisher C, Kellam P, et al. Distribution of human herpesvirus-8 latently infected cells in Kaposi's sarcoma, multicentric Castleman's disease, and primary effusion lymphoma. *Proc Natl Acad Sci U S A* 1999;96:4546–4551.

94. Haubrich WS, J.H.L. W, Sieracki JC. Unique morphologic features of Whipple's disease. *Gastroenterology* 1960;39:454–468.

95. Wilson KH, Blitchington R, Wilson JA. Phylogeny of the Whipple's-disease-associated bacterium. *Lancet* 1991;338:474–475.

96. Muller C, Petermann D, Stain C, et al. Whipple's disease: comparison of histology with diagnosis based on polymerase chain reaction in four consecutive cases. *Gut* 1997;40:425–427.

97. Ramzan NN, Loftus E, Jr., Burgart LJ, et al. Diagnosis and monitoring of Whipple disease by polymerase chain reaction. *Ann Intern Med* 1997;126:520–527.

98. Salvador AH, Harrison EG, Jr., Kyle RA. Lymphadenopathy due to infectious mononucleosis: its confusion with malignant lymphoma. *Cancer* 1971;27:1029–1040.

99. Gowing NF. Infectious mononucleosis: histopathologic aspects. *Pathol Annu* 1975;10:1–20.

100. Childs CC, Parham DM, Berard CW. Infectious mononucleosis. The spectrum of morphologic changes simulating lymphoma in lymph nodes and tonsils. *Am J Surg Pathol* 1987; 11:122–132.

101. Tindle BH, Parker JW, Lukes RJ. "Reed-Sternberg cells" in infectious mononucleosis? *Am J Clin Pathol* 1972;58:607–617.

102. Segal GN, Kjeldsberg CR, Smith GP, et al. CP30 antigen expression in Florid immunoblastic proliferations. A clinicopathologic study of 14 cases. *Am J Clin Pathol* 1994;102:292–298.

103. Hartsock RJ. Postvaccinial lymphadenitis. Hyperplasia of lymphoid tissue that simulates malignant lymphomas. *Cancer* 1968;21:632–649.

104. Patterson SD, Larson EB, Corey L. Atypical generalized zoster with lymphadenitis mimicking lymphoma. *N Engl J Med* 1980;302:848–851.

105. Miliauskas JR, Leong AS. Localized herpes simplex lymphadenitis: report of three cases and review of the literature. *Histopathology* 1991;19:355–360.

106. Swerdlow SH. Post-transplant lymphoproliferative disorders: a morphologic, phenotypic and genotypic spectrum of disease. *Histopathology* 1992;20:373–385.

107. Craig FE, Gulley ML, Banks PM. Posttransplantation lymphoproliferative disorders. *Am J Clin Pathol* 1993;99:265–276.

108. Opelz G, Henderson R. Incidence of non-Hodgkin lymphoma in kidney and heart transplant recipients. *Lancet* 1993;342:1514–1516.

109. Cohen JI. Epstein-Barr virus lymphoproliferative disease associated with acquired immunodeficiency. *Medicine (Baltimore)* 1991;70:137–160.

110. van Gorp J, Doornewaard H, Verdonck LF, et al. Posttransplant T-cell lymphoma. Report of three cases and a review of the literature. *Cancer* 1994;73:3064–3072.

111. Macon WR, Williams ME, Greer JP, et al. Natural killer-like T-cell lymphomas: aggressive lymphomas of T-large granular lymphocytes. *Blood* 1996;87:1474–1483.

112. Swerdlow SH. Classification of the posttransplant lymphoproliferative disorders: from the past to the present. *Semin Diagn Pathol* 1997;14:2–7.

113. Cockfield SM, Preiksaitis J, Harvey E, et al. Is sequential use of ALG and OKT3 in renal transplants associated with an increased incidence of fulminant posttransplant lymphoproliferative disorder? *Transplant Proc* 1991;23:1106–1107.

114. Harris N, Swerdlow S, Frizzera G, et al. Post Transplant Lymphoproliferative disorders. In Jaffe E, Harris N, Steen H, et al., eds. *Pathology and Genetics of Tumours of Haematopoietic and Lymphoid Tissues. World Health Organization Classification of Tumours.* Lyon, France: IARC Press, 2001:264–269.

115. Frizzera G, Hanto DW, Gajl-Peczalska KJ, et al. Polymorphic diffuse B-cell hyperplasias and lymphomas in renal transplant recipients. *Cancer Res* 1981;41:4262–4279.

116. Nalesnik MA, Jaffe R, Starzl TE, et al. The pathology of posttransplant lymphoproliferative disorders occurring in the setting of cyclosporine A-prednisone immunosuppression. *Am J Pathol* 1988;133:173–192.

117. Knowles DM, Cesarman E, Chadburn A, et al. Correlative morphologic and molecular genetic analysis demonstrates three distinct categories of posttransplantation lymphoproliferative disorders. *Blood* 1995;85:552–565.

118. Locker J, Nalesnik M. Molecular genetic analysis of lymphoid tumors arising after organ transplantation. *Am J Pathol* 1989;135:977–987.

119. Chen JM, Barr ML, Chadburn A, et al. Management of lymphoproliferative disorders after cardiac transplantation. *Ann Thorac Surg* 1993;56:527–538.

120. Leblond V, Dhedin N, Mamzer Bruneel MF, et al. Identification of prognostic factors in 61 patients with posttransplantation lymphoproliferative disorders. *J Clin Oncol* 2001;19:772–778.

121. Henter JI, Elinder G, Ost A. Diagnostic guidelines for hemophagocytic lymphohistiocytosis. The FHL Study Group of the Histiocyte Society. *Semin Oncol* 1991;18:29–33.

122. Osugi Y, Hara J, Tagawa S, et al. Cytokine production regulating Th1 and Th2 cytokines in hemophagocytic lymphohistiocytosis. *Blood* 1997;89:4100–4103.

123. Filipovich AH. Hemophagocytic lymphohistiocytosis: a lethal disorder of immune regulation. *J Pediatr* 1997;130:337–338.

124. Risdall RJ, McKenna RW, Nesbit ME, et al. Virus-associated hemophagocytic syndrome: a benign histiocytic proliferation distinct from malignant histiocytosis. *Cancer* 1979;44:993–1002.

125. Stepp SE, Dufourcq-Lagelouse R, Le Deist F, et al. Perforin gene defects in familial hemophagocytic lymphohistiocytosis. *Science* 1999;286:1957–1959.

126. Sayos J, Wu C, Morra M, et al. The X-linked lymphoproliferative-disease gene product SAP regulates signals induced through the co-receptor SLAM. *Nature* 1998;395:462–469.

127. Reiner AP, Spivak JL. Hematophagic histiocytosis. A report of 23 new patients and a review of the literature. *Medicine (Baltimore)* 1988;67:369–388.

128. Kasahara Y, Yachie A, Takei K, et al. Differential cellular targets of Epstein-Barr virus (EBV) infection between acute EBV-associated hemophagocytic lymphohistiocytosis and chronic active EBV infection. *Blood* 2001;98:1882–1888.

129. Quintanilla-Martinez L, Kumar S, Fend F, et al. Fulminant EBV(+) T-cell lymphoproliferative disorder following acute/chronic EBV infection: a distinct clinicopathologic syndrome. *Blood* 2000;96:443–451.

130. Suster S, Hilsenbeck S, Rywlin AM. Reactive histiocytic hyperplasia with hemophagocytosis in hematopoietic organs: a reevaluation of the benign hemophagocytic proliferations. *Hum Pathol* 1988;19:705–712.

131. Jaffe ES. Post-thymic T-cell lymphomas. In Jaffe ES, ed. *Surgical pathology of the lymph nodes and related organs.* 2nd edition. Philadelphia: WB Saunders; 1995 pp. 344–389.

132. Jaffe ES, Costa J, Fauci AS, et al. Malignant lymphoma and erythrophagocytosis simulating malignant histiocytosis. *Am J Med* 1983;75:741–749.

133. Falini B, Pileri S, De Solas I, et al. Peripheral T-cell lymphoma associated with hemophagocytic syndrome. *Blood* 1990;75:434–444.

134. Rosai J, Dorfman RF. Sinus histiocytosis with massive lymphadenopathy: a pseudolymphomatous benign disorder. Analysis of 34 cases. *Cancer* 1972;30:1174–1188.

135. Foucar E, Rosai J, Dorfman R. Sinus histiocytosis with massive lymphadenopathy (Rosai-Dorfman disease): review of the entity. *Semin Diagn Pathol* 1990;7:19–73.

136. Paulli M, Rosso R, Kindl S, et al. Immunophenotypic characterization of the cell infiltrate in five cases of sinus histiocytosis with massive lymphadenopathy (Rosai-Dorfman disease). *Hum Pathol* 1992;23:647–654.

137. Foucar E, Rosai J, Dorfman RF. Sinus histiocytosis with massive lymphadenopathy. Current status and future directions. *Arch Dermatol* 1988;124:1211–1214.

138. Paulli M, Bergamaschi G, Tonon L, et al. Evidence for a polyclonal nature of the cell infiltrate in sinus histiocytosis with massive lymphadenopathy (Rosai-Dorfman disease). *Br J Haematol* 1995;91:415–418.

139. Saltzstein SL, Ackerman LV. Lymphadenopathy induced by anticonvulsant drugs and mimicking clinically and pathologically malignant lymphomas. *Cancer* 1959;12:164–182.

140. Abbondanzo SL, Irey NS, Frizzera G. Dilantin-associated lymphadenopathy. *Am J Surg Pathol* 1995;19:675–686.

141. Li FP, Willard DR, Goodman R, et al. Malignant lymphoma after diphenylhydantoin (dilantin) therapy. *Cancer* 1975;36:1359–1362.

142. Garcia-Suarez J, Dominguez-Franjo P, Del Campo F, et al. EBV-positive non-Hodgkin's lymphoma developing after phenytoin therapy. *Br J Haematol* 1996;95:376–379.

143. Delage C, Lagace R. Maladie serique avec hyperplasie ganglionnaire pseudolymphomateuse secondaire a la prise de salicylazosulfapyridine. *Union Med Can* 1975;104:579–584.

144. Gay RG, Fielder KL, Grogan TM. Quinidine-induced reactive lymphadenopathy. *Am J Med* 1987;82:143–145.

145. Mitchell DN, Scadding JG, Heard BE, et al. Sarcoidosis: histopathological definition and clinical diagnosis. *J Clin Pathol* 1977;30:395–398.

146. Hunsaker AR, Munden RF, Pugatch RD, et al. Sarcoidlike reaction in patients with malignancy. *Radiology* 1996;200:255–261.

147. Viale G, Codecasa L, Bulgheroni P, et al. T-cell subsets in sarcoidosis: an immunocytochemical investigation of blood, bronchoalveolar lavage fluid, and prescalenic lymph nodes from eight patients. *Hum Pathol* 1986;17:476–481.

148. Miller RR, Nelems B. Mediastinal lymph node necrosis: a newly recognized complication of mediastinoscopy. *Ann Thorac Surg* 1989;48:247–250.

149. Maurer R, Schmid U, Davies JD, et al. Lymph-node infarction and malignant lymphoma: a multicentre survey of European, English and American cases. *Histopathology* 1986;10:571–588.

150. Cleary KR, Osborne BM, Butler JJ. Lymph node infarction foreshadowing malignant lymphoma. *Am J Surg Pathol* 1982;6:435–442.

151. Laszewski MJ, Belding PJ, Feddersen RM, et al. Clonal immunoglobulin gene rearrangement in the infarcted lymph node syndrome. *Am J Clin Pathol* 1991;96:116–120.
152. Dorfman RF. Kaposi's sarcoma. With special reference to its manifestations in infants and children and to the concepts of Arthur Purdy Stout. *Am J Surg Pathol* 1986;10 Suppl 1: 68–77.
153. Finkbeiner WE, Egbert BM, Groundwater JR, et al. Kaposi's sarcoma in young homosexual men: a histopathologic study with particular reference to lymph node involvement. *Arch Pathol Lab Med* 1982;106:261–264.
154. Moore PS, Chang Y. Detection of herpesvirus-like DNA sequences in Kaposi's sarcoma in patients with and without HIV infection. *N Engl J Med* 1995;332:1181–1185.
155. Davis RE, Warnke RA, Dorfman RF. Inflammatory pseudotumor of lymph nodes. Additional observations and evidence for an inflammatory etiology. *Am J Surg Pathol* 1991;15: 744–756.
156. Perrone T, De Wolf-Peeters C, Frizzera G. Inflammatory pseudotumor of lymph nodes. A distinctive pattern of nodal reaction. *Am J Surg Pathol* 1988;12:351–361.
157. Menke DM, Griesser H, Araujo I, et al. Inflammatory pseudotumors of lymph node origin show macrophage- derived spindle cells and lymphocyte-derived cytokine transcripts without evidence of T-cell receptor gene rearrangements. Implications for pathogenesis and classification as an idiopathic retroperitoneal fibrosis-like sclerosing immune reaction. *Am J Clin Pathol* 1996;105:430–439.
158. Umlas J, Federman M, Crawford C, et al. Spindle cell pseudotumor due to Mycobacterium avium-intracellulare in patients with acquired immunodeficiency syndrome (AIDS). Positive staining of mycobacteria for cytoskeleton filaments. *Am J Surg Pathol* 1991;15: 1181–1187.
159. Chen KT. Mycobacterial spindle cell pseudotumor of lymph nodes. *Am J Surg Pathol* 1992; 16:276–281.
160. Chan JK, Warnke RA, Dorfman R. Vascular transformation of sinuses in lymph nodes. A study of its morphological spectrum and distinction from Kaposi's sarcoma. *Am J Surg Pathol* 1991;15:732–743.
161. Fayemi AO, Toker C. Nodal angiomatosis. *Arch Pathol* 1975;99:170–172.
162. Chan JK, Lewin KJ, Lombard CM, et al. Histopathology of bacillary angiomatosis of lymph node. *Am J Surg Pathol* 1991;15:430–437.
163. Relman DA, Loutit JS, Schmidt TM, et al. The agent of bacillary angiomatosis. An approach to the identification of uncultured pathogens. *N Engl J Med* 1990;323:1573–1580.
164. LeBoit PE. Bacillary angiomatosis. *Mod Pathol* 1995;8:218–222.
165. Weiss SW, Gnepp DR, Bratthauer GL. Palisaded myofibroblastoma. A benign mesenchymal tumor of lymph node. *Am J Surg Pathol* 1989;13:341–346.
166. Suster S, Rosai J. Intranodal hemorrhagic spindle-cell tumor with "amianthoid" fibers. Report of six cases of a distinctive mesenchymal neoplasm of the inguinal region that simulates Kaposi's sarcoma. *Am J Surg Pathol* 1989;13:347–357.
167. Starasoler L, Vuitch F, Albores-Saavedra J. Intranodal leiomyoma. Another distinctive primary spindle cell neoplasm of lymph node. *Am J Clin Pathol* 1991;95:858–862.
168. Taylor CR, Riley CR. Molecular morphology of Hodgkin lymphoma. *Appl Immunohistochem Mol Morphol* 2001;9:187–202.
169. Weiss LM, Strickler JG, Hu E, et al. Immunoglobulin gene rearrangements in Hodgkin's disease. *Hum Pathol* 1986;17:1009–1014.
170. Braeuninger A, Kuppers R, Strickler JG, et al. Hodgkin and Reed-Sternberg cells in lymphocyte predominant Hodgkin disease represent clonal populations of germinal center-derived tumor B cells. *Proc Natl Acad Sci U S A* 1997;94:9337–9342.
171. Marafioti T, Hummel M, Foss HD, et al. Hodgkin and reed-sternberg cells represent an expansion of a single clone originating from a germinal center B-cell with functional immunoglobulin gene rearrangements but defective immunoglobulin transcription. *Blood* 2000;95:1443–1450.
172. Lukes RJ, Butler JJ. The pathology and nomenclature of Hodgkin's disease. *Cancer Res* 1966;26:1063–1083.
173. Lukes RJ, Craver LF, Hall TC, et al. Report of the nomenclature committee. *Cancer Res* 1966;26:1311.
174. Poppema S. The diversity of the immunohistological staining pattern of Sternberg-Reed cells. *J Histochem Cytochem* 1980;28:788–791.
175. Timens W, Visser L, Poppema S. Nodular lymphocyte predominance type of Hodgkin's disease is a germinal center lymphoma. *Lab Invest* 1986;54:457–461.
176. Ohno T, Stribley JA, Wu G, et al. Clonality in nodular lymphocyte-predominant Hodgkin's disease. *N Engl J Med* 1997;337:459–465.
177. Marafioti T, Hummel M, Anagnostopoulos I, et al. Origin of nodular lymphocyte-predominant Hodgkin's disease from a clonal expansion of highly mutated germinal-center B cells. *N Engl J Med* 1997;337:453–458.
178. Kuppers R, Rajewsky K, Braeuninger A, et al. L&H cells in lymphocyte-predominant Hodgkin's disease. *N Engl J Med* 1998;338:763–764; author reply 764–765.
179. Chan WC. Cellular origin of nodular lymphocyte-predominant Hodgkin's lymphoma: immunophenotypic and molecular studies. *Semin Hematol* 1999;36:242–252.
180. Wlodarska I, Nooyen P, Maes B, et al. Frequent occurrence of BCL6 rearrangements in nodular lymphocyte predominance Hodgkin lymphoma but not in classic Hodgkin lymphoma. *Blood* 2003;101:706–710.
181. Poppema S. Immunobiology and pathophysiology of hodgkin lymphomas. *Hematology Am Soc Hematol Educ Program* 2005:231–238.
182. Zuckerberg L, Collins A, Ferry J, et al. Coexpression of CD15 and CD20 by Reed-Sternberg cells in Hodgkin's disease. *Am J Pathol* 1991;139:475–483.
183. Kamel OW, Chang PP, Hsu FJ, et al. Clonal VDJ recombination of the immunoglobulin heavy chain gene by PCR in classical Hodgkin's disease. *Am J Clin Pathol* 1995;104:419–423.
184. Kanzler H, Kuppers R, Hansmann ML, et al. Hodgkin and Reed-Sternberg cells in Hodgkin's disease represent the outgrowth of a dominant tumor clone derived from (crippled) germinal center B cells. *J Exp Med* 1996;184:1495–1505.
185. Schwering I, Brauninger A, Klein U, et al. Loss of the B-lineage-specific gene expression program in Hodgkin and Reed-Sternberg cells of Hodgkin lymphoma. *Blood* 2003;101: 1505–1512.
186. Vasef MA, Alsabeh R, Medeiros LJ, et al. Immunophenotype of Reed-Sternberg and Hodgkin's cells in sequential biopsy specimens of Hodgkin's disease: a paraffin-section immunohistochemical study using the heat-induced epitope retrieval method. *Am J Clin Pathol* 1997;108:54–59.
187. Knowles DM, Chamulak GA, Subar M, et al. Lymphoid neoplasia associated with the acquired immunodeficiency syndrome (AIDS). The New York University Medical Center experience with 105 patients (1981–1986). *Ann Intern Med* 1988;108:744–753.
188. Shibata D, Hansmann ML, Weiss LM, et al. Epstein-Barr virus infections and Hodgkin's disease: a study of fixed tissues using the polymerase chain reaction. *Hum Pathol* 1991;22: 1262–1267.
189. Andriko JA, Aguilera NS, Nandedkar MA, et al. Childhood Hodgkin's disease in the United States: an analysis of histologic subtypes and association with Epstein-Barr virus. *Mod Pathol* 1997;10:366–371.
190. Keller AR, Kaplan HS, Lukes RJ, et al. Correlation of histopathology with other prognostic indicators in Hodgkin's disease. *Cancer* 1968;22:487–499.
191. Desforges JF, Rutherford CJ, Piro A. Hodgkin's disease. *N Engl J Med* 1979;301:1212–1222.
192. Trudel MA, Krikorian JG, Neiman RS. Lymphocyte predominance Hodgkin's disease. A clinicopathologic reassessment. *Cancer* 1987;59:99–106.
193. Mauch P, Greenberg H, Lewin A, et al. Prognostic factors in patients with subdiaphragmatic Hodgkin's disease. *Hematol Oncol* 1983;1:205–214.
194. Aster JC. Lymphocyte-predominant Hodgkin's disease: how little therapy is enough? *J Clin Oncol* 1999;17:744–746.
195. Diel V, Sextro M, Franklin J, et al. Clinical presentation, course, and prognostic factors in lymphocyte predominant Hodgkin's disease and lymphocyte rich classical Hodgkin's disease: report from the European task force on lymphoma project on lymphocyte predominant hodgkin's disease. *J Clin Oncol* 1999;17:776–783.
196. Shimabukuro-Vornhagen A, Haverkamp H, Engert A, et al. Lymphocyte-rich classical Hodgkin's lymphoma: clinical presentation and treatment outcome in 100 patients treated within German Hodgkin's Study Group trials. *J Clin Oncol* 2005;23:5739–5745.
197. de Jong D, Bosq J, MacLennan KA, et al. Lymphocyte-rich classical Hodgkin lymphoma (LRCHL): clinico-pathological characteristics and outcome of a rare entity. *Ann Oncol* 2006;17:141–145.
198. Lukes RJ, Butler JJ, Hicks EB. Natural history of Hodgkin's disease as related to its pathologic picture. *Cancer* 1966;19:317.344.
199. Neiman RS, Rosen PJ, Lukes RJ. Lymphocyte-depletion Hodgkin's disease. A clinicopathological entity. *N Engl J Med* 1973;288:751–755.
200. Greer JP, Kinney MC, Cousar JB, et al. Lymphocyte-depleted Hodgkin's disease. Clinicopathologic review of 25 patients. *Am J Med* 1986;81:208–214.
201. Kinney MC, Greer JP, Stein RS, et al. Lymphocyte-depletion Hodgkin's disease. Histopathologic diagnosis of marrow involvement. *Am J Surg Pathol* 1986;10:219–226.
202. Tirelli U, Errante D, Dolcetti R, et al. Hodgkin's disease and human immunodeficiency virus infection: clinicopathologic and virologic features of 114 patients from the Italian Cooperative Group on AIDS and Tumors. *J Clin Oncol* 1995;13:1758–1767.
203. Lukes RJ. Criteria for involvement of lymph node, bone marrow, spleen, and liver in Hodgkin's disease. *Cancer Res* 1971;31:1755–1767.
204. Butler JJ. The Lukes-Butler classification of Hodgkin's disease revisited. In Bennett JM, ed. *Controversies in the Management of Lymphomas.* Boston: Martinus Nijhoff; 1983 pp. 1–18.
205. Fan Z, Natkunam Y, Bair E, et al. Characterization of variant patterns of nodular lymphocyte predominant hodgkin lymphoma with immunohistologic and clinical correlation. *Am J Surg Pathol* 2003;27:1346–1356.
206. Wickert RS, Weisenburger DD, Tierens A, et al. Clonal relationship between lymphocytic predominance Hodgkin's disease and concurrent or subsequent large-cell lymphoma of B lineage. *Blood* 1995;86:2312–2320.
207. von Wasielewski R, Georgii A, Werner M, et al. Lymphocyte-predominant Hodgkin's disease: an immunohistochemical analysis of 208 reviewed Hodgkin's disease cases from the German Hodgkin Study Group. *Am J Pathol* 1997;150:793–803.
208. Anagnostopoulos I, Hansmann ML, Franssila K, et al. European Task Force on Lymphoma project on lymphocyte predominance Hodgkin disease: histologic and immunohistologic analysis of submitted cases reveals 2 types of Hodgkin disease with a nodular growth pattern and abundant lymphocytes. *Blood* 2000;96:1889–1899.
209. Krenacs L, Wellmann A, Sorbara L, et al. Cytotoxic cell antigen expression in anaplastic large cell lymphomas of T- and null-cell type and Hodgkin's disease: evidence for distinct cellular origin. *Blood* 1997;89:980–989.
210. Ashton-Key M, Thorpe PA, Allen JP, et al. Follicular Hodgkin's disease. *Am J Surg Pathol* 1995;19:1294–1299.
211. Anagnostou D, Parker JW, Taylor CR, et al. Lacunar cells of nodular sclerosing Hodgkin's disease: an ultrastructural and immunohistologic study. *Cancer* 1977;39:1032–1043.
212. Jackson H, Parker F. Hodkin's disease. XI. Pathology. *N Engl J Med* 1944;231:35.
213. Strickler JG, Michie SA, Warnke RA, et al. The "syncytial variant" of nodular sclerosing Hodgkin's disease. *Am J Surg Pathol* 1986;10:470–477.
214. Casey TT, Cousar JB, Mangum M, et al. Monomorphic lymphomas arising in patients with Hodgkin's disease. Correlation of morphologic, immunophenotypic, and molecular genetic findings in 12 cases. *Am J Pathol* 1990;136:81–94.
215. Warnke RA, Weiss LM, Chan JKC, et al. *Tumors of the Lymph Nodes and Spleen.* 3rd series, Fascicle 14. Washington, DC: Armd Forces Institute of Pathology, 1995.
216. MacLennan KA, Bennett MH, Tu A, et al. Relationship of histopathologic features to survival and relapse in nodular sclerosing Hodgkin's disease. A study of 1659 patients. *Cancer* 1989;64:1686–1693.
217. Weiczorek R, Burke JS, Knowles DM 2nd. Leu M1 antigen expression in T-cell neoplasia. *Am J Pathol* 1985;121:374–380.
218. Sacks EL, Donaldson SS, Gordon J, et al. Epithelioid granulomas associated with Hodgkin's disease: clinical correlations in 55 previously untreated patients. *Cancer* 1978;41: 562–567.

219. Kinney MC, Greer JP, Collins RD. Assessment of lymphocyte depleted Hodgkin's disease, reticular variant, by monoclonal antibodies. *Mod Pathol* 1991;4:75A.

220. Casey TT, Cousar JB, Salhany KE, et al. Evaluation of paraffin section immunoperoxidase in the differentiation of Hodgkin's disease from non-Hodgkin's lymphomas, and T cell from B cell neoplasms. *Lab Invest* 1987;56:11A.

221. Pinkus GS, Thomas P, Said JW. Leu-M1—a marker for Reed-Sternberg cells in Hodgkin's disease. An immunoperoxidase study of paraffin-embedded tissues. *Am J Pathol* 1985;119: 244–252.

222. Swerdlow SH, Wright SA. The spectrum of Leu-M1 staining in lymphoid and hematopoietic proliferations. *Am J Clin Pathol* 1986;85:283–288.

223. Rushin JM, Riordan GP, Heaton RB, et al. Cytomegalovirus-infected cells express Leu-M1 antigen. A potential source of diagnostic error. *Am J Pathol* 1990;136:989–995.

224. A clinical evaluation of the International Lymphoma Study Group classification of non-Hodgkin's lymphoma. The Non-Hodgkin's Lymphoma Classification Project. *Blood* 1997; 89:3909–3918.

225. Lukes RJ, Collins RD. Tumors of the hematopoietic system. In Hartman WH, Sorbin LH, eds. *Atlas of Tumor Pathology*. Washington DC: Armed Forces Institute of Pathology, 1988.

226. Lennert K, Feller AC. Histopathology of non-Hodkin's lymphomas (based on the Kiel classification). Berlin: Springer-Verlag; 1992.

227. Falini B, Fizzotti M, Pucciarini A, et al. A monoclonal antibody (MUM1p) detects expression of the MUM1/IRF4 protein in a subset of germinal center B cells, plasma cells, and activated T cells. *Blood* 2000;95:2084–2092.

228. Lukes RJ, Collins RD. Immunologic characterization of human malignant lymphomas. *Cancer* 1974;34:suppl:1488–1503.

229. Muller-Hermelink H, Catovsky D, Montserrat E, et al. Chronic lymphocytic leukaemia/small lymphocytic lymphoma. In Jaffe E, Harris N, Steen H, et al., eds. *Pathology and Genetics of Tumours of Haematopoietic and Lymphoid Tissues. World Health Organization Classification of Tumours*. Lyon, France: IARC Press, 2001:127–130.

230. Swerdlow SH, Murray LJ, Habeshaw JA, et al. Lymphocytic lymphoma/B-chronic lymphocytic leukaemia—an immunohistopathological study of peripheral B lymphocyte neoplasia. *Br J Cancer* 1984;50:587–599.

231. Bennett JM, Catovsky D, Daniel MT, et al. Proposals for the classification of chronic (mature) B and T lymphoid leukaemias. French-American-British (FAB) Cooperative Group. *J Clin Pathol* 1989;42:567–584.

232. Bonato M, Pittaluga S, Tierens A, et al. Lymph node histology in typical and atypical chronic lymphocytic leukemia. *Am J Surg Pathol* 1998;22:49–56.

233. Ellison DJ, Nathwani BN, Cho SY, et al. Interfollicular small lymphocytic lymphoma: the diagnostic significance of pseudofollicles. *Hum Pathol* 1989;20:1108–1118.

234. Bahler DW, Levy R. Clonal evolution of a follicular lymphoma: evidence for antigen selection. *Proc Natl Acad Sci U S A* 1992;89:6770–6774.

235. Matutes E, Owusu-Ankomah K, Morilla R, et al. The immunological profile of B-cell disorders and proposal of a scoring system for the diagnosis of CLL. *Leukemia* 1994;8: 1640–1645.

236. Zukerberg LR, Medeiros LJ, Ferry JA, et al. Diffuse low-grade B-cell lymphomas. Four clinically distinct subtypes defined by a combination of morphologic and immunophenotypic features. *Am J Clin Pathol* 1993;100:373–385.

237. DiGiuseppe JA, Borowitz MJ. Clinical utility of flow cytometry in the chronic lymphoid leukemias. *Semin Oncol* 1998;25:6–10.

238. Moreau EJ, Matutes E, A'Hern RP, et al. Improvement of the chronic lymphocytic leukemia scoring system with the monoclonal antibody SN8 (CD79b). *Am J Clin Pathol* 1997; 108:378–382.

239. Chen CC, Raikow RB, Sonmez-Alpan E, et al. Classification of small B-cell lymphoid neoplasms using a paraffin section immunohistochemical panel. *Appl Immunohistochem Mol Morphol* 2000;8:1–11.

240. Coelho Siqueira SA, Ferreira Alves VA, Beitler B, et al. Contribution of immunohistochemistry to small B-cell lymphoma classification. *Appl Immunohistochem Mol Morphol* 2006;14: 1–6.

241. Hamblin TJ, Davis Z, Gardiner A, et al. Unmutated Ig V(H) genes are associated with a more aggressive form of chronic lymphocytic leukemia. *Blood* 1999;94:1848–1854.

242. Hamblin TJ, Orchard JA, Gardiner A, et al. Immunoglobulin V genes and CD38 expression in CLL. *Blood* 2000;95:2455–2457.

243. Hamblin TJ, Orchard JA, Ibbotson RE, et al. CD38 expression and immunoglobulin variable region mutations are independent prognostic variables in chronic lymphocytic leukemia, but CD38 expression may vary during the course of the disease. *Blood* 2002;99: 1023–1029.

244. Damle RN, Wasil T, Fais F, et al. Ig V gene mutation status and CD38 expression as novel prognostic indicators in chronic lymphocytic leukemia. *Blood* 1999;94:1840–1847.

245. Krober A, Seiler T, Benner A, et al. V(H) mutation status, CD38 expression level, genomic aberrations, and survival in chronic lymphocytic leukemia. *Blood* 2002;100:1410–1416.

246. Wiestner A, Cho HJ, Asch AS, et al. Rituximab in the treatment of acquired factor VIII inhibitors. *Blood* 2002;100:3426–3428.

247. Chang CC, Lorek J, Sabath DE, et al. Expression of MUM1/IRF4 correlates with clinical outcome in patients with B-cell chronic lymphocytic leukemia. *Blood* 2002;100:4671–4675.

248. Bosch F, Villamor N, Crespo M, et al. ZAP-70 expression is a reliable surrogate for immunoglobulin variable region mutations in chronic lymphocytic leukemia (abstract). *Blood* 2002; 100:169a.

249. Arber DA, Weiss LM. CD43: a review. *Appl Immunohistochem* 1993;1:88–96.

250. Rawstron AC, Green MJ, Kuzmicki A, et al. Monoclonal B lymphocytes with the characteristics of "indolent" chronic lymphocytic leukemia are present in 3.5% of adults with normal blood counts. *Blood* 2002;100:635–639.

251. Dohner H, Stilgenbauer S, James MR, et al. 11q deletions identify a new subset of B-cell chronic lymphocytic leukemia characterized by extensive nodal involvement and inferior prognosis. *Blood* 1997;89:2516–2522.

252. Fegan CD, Davies FE. Karyotypic and molecular abnormalities in chronic lymphocytic leukaemia. *J Clin Pathol Mol Pathol* 1996;49:185–191.

253. Matutes E, Oscier D, Garcia-Marco J, et al. Trisomy 12 defines a group of CLL with atypical morphology: correlation between cytogenetic, clinical and laboratory features in 544 patients. *Br J Haematol* 1996;92:382–388.

254. Stilgenbauer S, Lichter P, Dohner H. Genetic features of B-cell chronic lymphocytic leukemia. *Rev Clin Exp Hematol* 2000;4:48–72.

255. Stankovic T, Stewart GS, Fegan C, et al. Ataxia telangiectasia mutated-deficient B-cell chronic lymphocytic leukemia occurs in pregerminal center cells and results in defective damage response and unrepaired chromosome damage. *Blood* 2002;99:300–309.

256. Ghia P, Guida G, Stella S, et al. The pattern of CD38 expression defines a distinct subset of chronic lymphocytic leukemia (CLL) patients at risk of disease progression. *Blood* 2003; 101:1262–1269.

257. Chen L, Widhopf G, Huynh L, et al. Expression of ZAP-70 is associated with increased B-cell receptor signaling in chronic lymphocytic leukemia. *Blood* 2002;100:4609–4614.

258. Rai KR, Sawitsky A, Cronkite EP, et al. Clinical staging of chronic lymphocytic leukemia. *Blood* 1975;46:219–234.

259. Binet JL, Auquier A, Dighiero G, et al. A new prognostic classification of chronic lymphocytic leukemia derived from a multivariate survival analysis. *Cancer* 1981;48:198–206.

260. Richter M. *Am J Clin Pathol* 1928;4:285–291.

261. Robertson LE, Pugh W, O'Brien S, et al. Richter's syndrome: a report on 39 patients. *J Clin Oncol* 1993;11:1985–1989.

262. Hamblin TJ. Richter's syndrome—the downside of fludarabine? *Leuk Res* 2005;29: 1103–1104.

263. Ohno T, Smir BN, Weisenburger DD, et al. Origin of the Hodgkin/Reed-Sternberg cells in chronic lymphocytic leukemia with ''Hodgkin's transformation''. *Blood* 1998;91: 1757–1761.

264. Choi H, Keller RH. Coexistence of chronic lymphocytic leukemia and Hodgkin's disease. *Cancer* 1981;48:48–57.

265. Hansmann ML, Fellbaum C, Hui PK, et al. Morphological and immunohistochemical investigation of non-Hodgkin's lymphoma combined with Hodgkin's disease. *Histopathology* 1989;15:35–48.

266. Momose H, Jaffe ES, Shin SS, et al. Chronic lymphocytic leukemia/small lymphocytic lymphoma with Reed-Sternberg-like cells and possible transformation to Hodgkin's disease. Mediation by Epstein-Barr virus. *Am J Surg Pathol* 1992;16:859–867.

267. Mao Z, Quintanilla-Martinez L, Raffeld M, et al. IgVH mutational status and clonality analysis of Richter's transformation: diffuse large-B-cell lymphoma and Hodgkin lymphoma in association with B-cell chronic lymphocytic leukemia (B-CLL) represent 2 different pathways of disease evolution. *Am J Surg Pathol* 2007;31:1605–1614.

268. Brecher M, Banks PM. Hodgkin's disease variant of Richter's syndrome. Report of eight cases. *Am J Clin Pathol* 1990;93:333–339.

269. York JC, Glick AD, Cousar JB, et al. Changes in the appearance of hematopoietic and lymphoid neoplasms: clinical, pathologic, and biologic implications. *Hum Pathol* 1984;15: 11–38.

270. Enno A, Catovsky D, O'Brien M, et al. 'Prolymphocytoid' transformation of chronic lymphocytic leukaemia. *Br J Haematol* 1979;41:9–18.

271. He H, Cheng L, Weiss LM, et al. Clinical outcome of incidental pelvic node malignant B-cell lymphomas discovered at the time of radical prostatectomy. *Leuk Lymphoma* 2007; 48:1976–1980.

272. Berger F, Isaacson P, Piris M, et al. Lymphoplasmacytic lymphoma/Waldenstrom macroglobulinemia. In Jaffe E, Harris N, Steen H, et al., eds. *Pathology and Genetics of Tumours of Haematopoietic and Lymphoid Tissues. World Health Organization Classification of Tumours*. Lyon, France: IARC Press, 2001:132–134.

273. Andriko JA, Swerdlow SH, Aguilera NI, et al. Is lymphoplasmacytic lymphoma/immunocytoma a distinct entity? A clinicopathologic study of 20 cases. *Am J Surg Pathol* 2001;25: 742–751.

274. Patsouris E, Noel H, Lennert K. Lymphoplasmacytic/lymphoplasmacytoid immunocytoma with a high content of epithelioid cells. Histologic and immunohistochemical findings. *Am J Surg Pathol* 1990;14:660–670.

275. Keith TA, Cousar JB, Glick AD, et al. Plasmacytic differentiation in follicular center cell (FCC) lymphomas. *Am J Clin Pathol* 1985;84:283–290.

276. Pileri S, Rivano MT, Gobbi M, et al. Neoplastic and reactive follicles within B-cell malignant lymphomas. A morphological and immunological study of 30 cases. *Hematol Oncol* 1985; 3:243–260.

277. Davis GG, York JC, Glick AD, et al. Plasmacytic differentiation in parafollicular (monocytoid) B-cell lymphoma. A study of 12 cases. *Am J Surg Pathol* 1992;16:1066–1074.

278. Iida S, Rao PH, Nallasivam P, et al. The t(9;14)(p13;q32) chromosomal translocation associated with lymphoplasmacytoid lymphoma involves the PAX-5 gene. *Blood* 1996;88: 4110–4117.

279. Iida S, Rao PH, Ueda R, et al. Chromosomal rearrangement of the PAX-5 locus in lymphoplasmacytic lymphoma with t(9;14)(p13;q32). *Leuk Lymphoma* 1999;34:25–33.

280. Schop RF, Kuehl WM, Van Wier SA, et al. Waldenstrom macroglobulinemia neoplastic cells lack immunoglobulin heavy chain locus translocations but have frequent 6q deletions. *Blood* 2002;100:2996–3001.

281. Mansoor A, Medeiros LJ, Weber DM, et al. Cytogenetic findings in lymphoplasmacytic lymphoma/Waldenstrom macroglobulinemia. Chromosomal abnormalities are associated with the polymorphous subtype and an aggressive clinical course. *Am J Clin Pathol* 2001;116:543–549.

282. Lin P, Medeiros LJ. Lymphoplasmacytic lymphoma/waldenstrom macroglobulinemia: an evolving concept. *Adv Anat Pathol* 2005;12:246–255.

283. Cook JR, Aguilera NI, Reshmi S, et al. Deletion 6q is not a characteristic marker of nodal lymphoplasmacytic lymphoma. *Cancer Genet Cytogenet* 2005;162:85–88.

284. Viswanatha DS, Dogan A. Hepatitis C virus and lymphoma. *J Clin Pathol* 2007;60: 1378–1383.

285. Swerdlow SH, Habeshaw JA, Murray LJ, et al. Centrocytic lymphoma: a distinct clinicopathologic and immunologic entity. A multiparameter study of 18 cases at diagnosis and relapse. *Am J Pathol* 1983;113:181–197.

286. Swerdlow SH, Williams ME. From centrocytic to mantle cell lymphoma: a clinicopathologic and molecular review of 3 decades. *Hum Pathol* 2002;33:7–20.
287. Swerdlow S, Berger F, Isaacson P, et al. Mantle cell lymphoma. In Jaffe E, Harris N, Steen H, et al., eds. *Pathology and Genetics of Tumours of Haematopoietic and Lymphoid Tissues. World Health Organization Classification of Tumours.* Lyon, France: IARC Press, 2001:168–170.
288. Campo E, Raffeld M, Jaffe ES. Mantle-cell lymphoma. *Semin Hematol* 1999;36:115–127.
289. Argatoff LH, Connors JM, Klasa RJ, et al. Mantle cell lymphoma: a clinicopathologic study of 80 cases. *Blood* 1997;89:2067–2078.
290. Lardelli P, Bookman MA, Sundeen J, et al. Lymphocytic lymphoma of intermediate differentiation. Morphologic and immunophenotypic spectrum and clinical correlations. *Am J Surg Pathol* 1990;14:752–763.
291. Zucca E, Stein H, Coiffier B. European Lymphoma Task Force (ELTF): report of the workshop on mantle cell lymphoma (MCL). *Ann Oncol* 1994;5:507–511.
292. Swerdlow SH, Zukerberg LR, Yang WI, et al. The morphologic spectrum of non-Hodgkin's lymphomas with BCL1/cyclin D1 gene rearrangements. *Am J Surg Pathol* 1996;20:627–640.
293. Tiemann M, Schrader C, Klapper W, et al. Histopathology, cell proliferation indices and clinical outcome in 304 patients with mantle cell lymphoma (MCL): a clinicopathological study from the European MCL Network. *Br J Haematol* 2005;131:29–38.
294. Yatabe Y, Suzuki R, Matsuno Y, et al. Morphological spectrum of cyclin D1-positive mantle cell lymphoma: study of 168 cases. *Pathol Int* 2001;51:747–761.
295. Hummel M, Tamaru J, Kalvelage B, et al. Mantle cell (previously centrocytic) lymphomas express VH genes with no or very little somatic mutations like the physiologic cells of the follicle mantle. *Blood* 1994;84:403–407.
296. Du MQ, Diss TC, Xu CF, et al. Ongoing immunoglobulin gene mutations in mantle cell lymphomas. *Br J Haematol* 1997;96:124–131.
297. Walsh S, Thorselius M, Johnson A, et al. Mantle cell lymphoma—new insights based on immunoglobulin variable heavy chain gene analysis (abstract). *Blood* 2002;100:168a.
298. Zucca E, Bertoni F, Bosshard G, et al. Clinical significance of bcl-2 (MBR)/JH rearrangement in the peripheral blood of patients with diffuse large-B-cell lymphomas. *Ann Oncol* 1996;7:1023–1027.
299. Harris NL, Nadler LM, Bhan AK. Immunohistologic characterization of two malignant lymphomas of germinal center type (centroblastic/centrocytic and centrocytic) with monoclonal antibodies. Follicular and diffuse lymphomas of small-cleaved-cell type are related but distinct entities. *Am J Pathol* 1984;117:262–272.
300. Swerdlow SH, Yang WI, Zukerberg LR, et al. Expression of cyclin D1 protein in centrocytic/mantle cell lymphomas with and without rearrangement of the BCL1/cyclin D1 gene. *Hum Pathol* 1995;26:999–1004.
301. Zukerberg LR, Yang WI, Arnold A, et al. Cyclin D1 expression in non-Hodgkin's lymphomas. Detection by immunohistochemistry. *Am J Clin Pathol* 1995;103:756–760.
302. Yang WI, Zukerberg LR, Motokura T, et al. Cyclin D1 (Bcl-1, PRAD1) protein expression in low-grade B-cell lymphomas and reactive hyperplasia. *Am J Pathol* 1994;145:86–96.
303. Medeiros LJ, Van Krieken JH, Jaffe ES, et al. Association of bcl-1 rearrangements with lymphocytic lymphoma of intermediate differentiation. *Blood* 1990;76:2086–2090.
304. Vaandrager JW, Schuuring E, Zwikstra E, et al. Direct visualization of dispersed 11q13 chromosomal translocations in mantle cell lymphoma by multicolor DNA fiber fluorescence in situ hybridization. *Blood* 1996;88:1177–1182.
305. Williams ME, Westermann CD, Swerdlow SH. Genotypic characterization of centrocytic lymphoma: frequent rearrangement of the chromosome 11 bcl-1 locus. *Blood* 1990;76:1387–1391.
306. Remstein ED, Kurtin PJ, Buno I, et al. Diagnostic utility of fluorescence in situ hybridization in mantle-cell lymphoma. *Br J Haematol* 2000;110:856–862.
307. Li JY, Gaillard F, Moreau A, et al. Detection of translocation t(11;14)(q13;q32) in mantle cell lymphoma by fluorescence in situ hybridization. *Am J Pathol* 1999;154:1449–1452.
308. Camacho E, Hernandez L, Hernandez S, et al. ATM gene inactivation in mantle cell lymphoma mainly occurs by truncating mutations and missense mutations involving the phosphatidylinositol-3 kinase domain and is associated with increasing numbers of chromosomal imbalances. *Blood* 2002;99:238–244.
309. Schaffner C, Idler I, Stilgenbauer S, et al. Mantle cell lymphoma is characterized by inactivation of the ATM gene. *Proc Natl Acad Sci U S A* 2000;97:2773–2778.
310. Hernandez L, Fest T, Cazorla M, et al. p53 gene mutations and protein overexpression are associated with aggressive variants of mantle cell lymphomas. *Blood* 1996;87:3351–3359.
311. Pinyol M, Hernandez L, Cazorla M, et al. Deletions and loss of expression of p16INK4a and p21Waf1 genes are associated with aggressive variants of mantle cell lymphomas. *Blood* 1997;89:272–280.
312. Cuneo A, Bigoni R, Rigolin GM, et al. Cytogenetic profile of lymphoma of follicle mantle lineage: correlation with clinicobiologic features. *Blood* 1999;93:1372–1380.
313. Williams M, Woytowitz D, Finkelstein S, et al. MTS1/MTS2 (p15/p16) deletions and p53 mutations in mantle cell (centrocytic) lymphoma. *Blood* 1995;86:747a.
314. Korz C, Pscherer A, Benner A, et al. Evidence for distinct pathomechanisms in B-cell chronic lymphocytic leukemia and mantle cell lymphoma by quantitative expression analysis of cell cycle and apoptosis-associated genes. *Blood* 2002;99:4554–4561.
315. Rosenwald A, Wright G, Wiestner A, et al. The proliferation gene expression signature is a quantitative integrator of oncogenic events that predicts survival in mantle cell lymphoma. *Cancer Cell* 2003;3:185–197.
316. Fu K, Weisenburger DD, Greiner TC, et al. Cyclin D1-negative mantle cell lymphoma: a clinicopathologic study based on gene expression profiling. *Blood* 2005;106:4315–4321.
317. Norton AJ, Matthews J, Pappa V, et al. Mantle cell lymphoma: natural history defined in a serially biopsied population over a 20-year period. *Ann Oncol* 1995;6:249–256.
318. Bookman MA, Lardelli P, Jaffe ES, et al. Lymphocytic lymphoma of intermediate differentiation: morphologic, immunophenotypic, and prognostic factors. *J Natl Cancer Inst* 1990; 82:742–748.
319. Nathwani B, Harris N, Weisenburger D, et al. Follicular lymphoma. In Jaffe E, Harris N, Steen H, et al., eds. *Pathology and Genetics of Tumours of Haematopoietic and Lymphoid Tissues. World Health Organization Classification of Tumours.* Lyon, France: IARC Press, 2001: 162–167.
320. Cong P, Raffeld M, Teruya-Feldstein J, et al. In situ localization of follicular lymphoma: description and analysis by laser capture microdissection. *Blood* 2002;99:3376–3382.
321. Osborne BM, Butler JJ. Follicular lymphoma mimicking progressive transformation of germinal centers. *Am J Clin Pathol* 1987;88:264–269.
322. Nathwani BN, Anderson JR, Armitage JO, et al. Clinical significance of follicular lymphoma with monocytoid B cells. Non-Hodgkin's Lymphoma Classification Project. *Hum Pathol* 1999;30:263–268.
323. Kim H, Dorfman RF, Rappaport H. Signet ring cell lymphoma. A rare morphologic and functional expression of nodular (follicular) lymphoma. *Am J Surg Pathol* 1978;2:119–132.
324. Waldron JA, Jr., Newcomer LN, Katz ME, et al. Sclerosing variants of follicular center cell lymphomas presenting in the retroperitoneum. *Cancer* 1983;52:712–720.
325. Swerdlow SH, Murray LJ, Habeshaw JA, et al. B- and T-cell subsets in follicular centroblastic/centrocytic (cleaved follicular center cell) lymphoma: an immunohistologic analysis of 26 lymph nodes and three spleens. *Hum Pathol* 1985;16:339–352.
326. King BE, Chen C, Locker J, et al. Immunophenotypic and genotypic markers of follicular center cell neoplasia in diffuse large-B-cell lymphomas. *Mod Pathol* 2000;13:1219–1231.
327. Arber D. CD10: a review. *Appl Immunohistochem* 1997;5:125–140.
328. Garcia CF, Warnke RA, Weiss LM. Follicular large cell lymphoma. An immunophenotype study. *Am J Pathol* 1986;123:425–431.
329. Hernandez AM, Nathwani BN, Nguyen D, et al. Nodal benign and malignant monocytoid B cells with and without follicular lymphomas: a comparative study of follicular colonization, light chain restriction, bcl-2, and t(14;18) in 39 cases. *Hum Pathol* 1995;26:625–632.
330. Utz GL, Swerdlow SH. Distinction of follicular hyperplasia from follicular lymphoma in B5-fixed tissues: comparison of MT2 and bcl-2 antibodies. *Hum Pathol* 1993;24:1155–1158.
331. Wang T, Lasota J, Hanau CA, et al. Bcl-2 oncoprotein is widespread in lymphoid tissue and lymphomas but its differential expression in benign versus malignant follicles and monocytoid B-cell proliferations is of diagnostic value. *Apmis* 1995;103:655–662.
332. Yunis JJ, Frizzera G, Oken MM, et al. Multiple recurrent genomic defects in follicular lymphoma. A possible model for cancer. *N Engl J Med* 1987;316:79–84.
333. Horsman DE, Gascoyne RD, Coupland RW, et al. Comparison of cytogenetic analysis, southern analysis, and polymerase chain reaction for the detection of t(14; 18) in follicular lymphoma. *Am J Clin Pathol* 1995;103:472–478.
334. Albinger-Hegyi A, Hochreutener B, Abdou MT, et al. High frequency of t(14;18)-translocation breakpoints outside of major breakpoint and minor cluster regions in follicular lymphomas: improved polymerase chain reaction protocols for their detection. *Am J Pathol* 2002;160:823–832.
335. Akasaka T, Akasaka H, Yonetani N, et al. Refinement of the BCL2/immunoglobulin heavy chain fusion gene in t(14;18)(q32;q21) by polymerase chain reaction amplification for long targets. *Genes Chromosomes Cancer* 1998;21:17.29.
336. Paternoster SF, Brockman SR, McClure RF, et al. A new method to extract nuclei from paraffin-embedded tissue to study lymphomas using interphase fluorescence in situ hybridization. *Am J Pathol* 2002;160:1967–1972.
337. Viardot A, Moller P, Hogel J, et al. Clinicopathologic correlations of genomic gains and losses in follicular lymphoma. *J Clin Oncol* 2002;20:4523–4530.
338. Horsman DE, Connors JM, Pantzar T, et al. Analysis of secondary chromosomal alterations in 165 cases of follicular lymphoma with t(14;18). *Genes Chromosomes Cancer* 2001;30: 375–382.
339. Ott G, Katzenberger T, Lohr A, et al. Cytomorphologic, immunohistochemical, and cytogenetic profiles of follicular lymphoma: 2 types of follicular lymphoma grade 3. *Blood* 2002;99:3806–3812.
340. Oviatt DL, Cousar JB, Collins RD, et al. Malignant lymphomas of follicular center cell origin in humans. V. Incidence, clinical features, and prognostic implications of transformation of small cleaved cell nodular lymphoma. *Cancer* 1984;53:1109–1114.
341. Cullen MH, Lister TA, Brearley RI, et al. Histological transformation of non-Hodgkin's lymphoma: a prospective study. *Cancer* 1979;44:645–651.
342. Risdall R, Hoppe RT, Warnke R. Non-Hodgkin's lymphoma: a study of the evolution of the disease based upon 92 autopsied cases. *Cancer* 1979;44:529–542.
343. Finn LS, Viswanatha DS, Belasco JB, et al. Primary follicular lymphoma of the testis in childhood. *Cancer* 1999;85:1626–1635.
344. Lorsbach RB, Shay-Seymore D, Moore J, et al. Clinicopathologic analysis of follicular lymphoma occurring in children. *Blood* 2002;99:1959–1964.
345. Pileri SA, Sabattini E, Rosito P, et al. Primary follicular lymphoma of the testis in childhood: an entity with peculiar clinical and molecular characteristics. *J Clin Pathol* 2002;55: 684–688.
346. Isaacson P, Nathwani B, Piris M, et al. Nodal marginal zone B-cell lymphoma. In Jaffe E, Harris N, Steen H, et al., eds. *Pathology and Genetics of Tumours of Haematopoietic and Lymphoid Tissues. World Health Organization Classification of Tumours.* Lyon, France: IARC Press, 2001:161.
347. Cousar JB, McGinn DL, Glick AD, et al. Report of an unusual lymphoma arising from parafollicular B-lymphocytes (PBLs) or so-called "monocytoid" lymphocytes. *Am J Clin Pathol* 1987;87:121–128.
348. Sheibani K, Burke JS, Swartz WG, et al. Monocytoid B-cell lymphoma. Clinicopathologic study of 21 cases of a unique type of low-grade lymphoma. *Cancer* 1988;62:1531–1538.
349. Ngan BY, Warnke RA, Wilson M, et al. Monocytoid B-cell lymphoma: a study of 36 cases. *Hum Pathol* 1991;22:409–421.
350. Nizze H, Cogliatti SB, von Schilling C, et al. Monocytoid B-cell lymphoma: morphological variants and relationship to low-grade B-cell lymphoma of the mucosa-associated lymphoid tissue. *Histopathology* 1991;18:403–414.
351. Camacho FI, Garcia JF, Sanchez-Verde L, et al. Unique phenotypic profile of monocytoid B cells: differences in comparison with the phenotypic profile observed in marginal zone B cells and so-called monocytoid B cell lymphoma. *Am J Pathol* 2001;158:1363–1369.
352. Conconi A, Bertoni F, Pedrinis E, et al. Nodal marginal zone B-cell lymphomas may arise from different subsets of marginal zone B lymphocytes. *Blood* 2001;98:781–786.
353. Camacho FI, Algara P, Mollejo M, et al. Nodal marginal zone lymphoma: a heterogeneous tumor: a comprehensive analysis of a series of 27 cases. *Am J Surg Pathol* 2003;27:762–771.

354. Isaacson P, Muller-Hermelink H, Piris M, et al. Extranodal marginal zone B-cell lymphoma of mucosa-associated lymphoid tissue (MALT lymphoma). In Jaffe E, Harris N, Steen H, et al., eds. *Pathology and Genetics of Tumours of Haematopoietic and Lymphoid Tissues. World Health Organization Classification of Tumours.* Lyon, France: IARC Press, 2001:157–160.
355. Bahler DW, Pindzola JA, Swerdlow SH. Splenic marginal zone lymphomas appear to originate from different B cell types. *Am J Pathol* 2002;161:81–88.
356. Chacon JI, Mollejo M, Munoz E, et al. Splenic marginal zone lymphoma: clinical characteristics and prognostic factors in a series of 60 patients. *Blood* 2002;100:1648–1654.
357. Hammer RD, Glick AD, Greer JP, et al. Splenic marginal zone lymphoma. A distinct B-cell neoplasm. *Am J Surg Pathol* 1996;20:613–626.
358. Isaacson P, Piris M, Catovsky D, et al. Splenic marginal zone lymphoma. In Jaffe E, Harris N, Steen H, et al., eds. *Pathology and Genetics of Tumours of Haematopoietic and Lymphoid Tissues. World Health Organization Classification of Tumours.* Lyon, France: IARC Press, 2001: 135–137.
359. Traverse-Glehen A, Felman P, Callet-Bauchu E, et al. A clinicopathological study of nodal marginal zone B-cell lymphoma. A report on 21 cases. *Histopathology* 2006;48:162–173.
360. Dierlamm J, Pittaluga S, Wlodarska I, et al. Marginal zone B-cell lymphomas of different sites share similar cytogenetic and morphologic features. *Blood* 1996;87:299–307.
361. Remstein ED, James CD, Kurtin PJ. Incidence and subtype specificity of API2-MALT1 fusion translocations in extranodal, nodal, and splenic marginal zone lymphomas. *Am J Pathol* 2000;156:1183–1188.
362. Taddesse-Heath L, Pittaluga S, Sorbara L, et al. Marginal zone B-cell lymphoma in children and young adults. *Am J Surg Pathol* 2003;27:522–531.
363. Attygalle AD, Liu H, Shirali S, et al. Atypical marginal zone hyperplasia of mucosa-associated lymphoid tissue: a reactive condition of childhood showing immunoglobulin lambda light-chain restriction. *Blood* 2004;104:3343–3348.
364. Gatter K, Warnke R. Diffuse large-B-cell lymphoma. In Jaffe E, Harris N, Steen H, et al., eds. *Pathology and Genetics of Tumours of Haematopoietic and Lymphoid Tissues. World Health Organization Classification of Tumours.* Lyon, France: IARC Press, 2001:171–174.
365. Hui PK, Feller AC, Lennert K. High-grade non-Hodgkin's lymphoma of B-cell type. I. Histopathology. *Histopathology* 1988;12:127–143.
366. Schneider DR, Taylor CR, Parker JW, et al. Immunoblastic sarcoma of T- and B-cell types: morphologic description and comparison. *Hum Pathol* 1985;16:885–900.
367. Kinney MC, Glick AD, Stein H, et al. Comparison of anaplastic large cell Ki-1 lymphomas and microvillous lymphomas in their immunologic and ultrastructural features. *Am J Surg Pathol* 1990;14:1047–1060.
368. Dogan A, Bagdi E, Munson P, et al. CD10 and BCL-6 expression in paraffin sections of normal lymphoid tissue and B-cell lymphomas. *Am J Surg Pathol* 2000;24:846–852.
369. Natkunam Y, Warnke RA, Montgomery K, et al. Analysis of MUM1/IRF4 protein expression using tissue microarrays and immunohistochemistry. *Mod Pathol* 2001;14:686–694.
370. Skinnider BF, Horsman DE, Dupuis B, et al. Bcl-6 and Bcl-2 protein expression in diffuse large-B-cell lymphoma and follicular lymphoma: correlation with 3q27 and 18q21 chromosomal abnormalities. *Hum Pathol* 1999;30:803–808.
371. Gaidano G, Cerri M, Capello D, et al. Molecular histogenesis of plasmablastic lymphoma of the oral cavity. *Br J Haematol* 2002;119:622–628.
372. Yamaguchi M, Seto M, Okamoto M, et al. De novo CD5+ diffuse large-B-cell lymphoma: a clinicopathologic study of 109 patients. *Blood* 2002;99:815–821.
373. Stevenson F, Sahota S, Zhu D, et al. Insight into the origin and clonal history of B-cell tumors as revealed by analysis of immunoglobulin variable region genes. *Immunol Rev* 1998;162:247–259.
374. Ottensmeier CH, Thompsett AR, Zhu D, et al. Analysis of VH genes in follicular and diffuse lymphoma shows ongoing somatic mutation and multiple isotype transcripts in early disease with changes during disease progression. *Blood* 1998;91:4292–4299.
375. Lossos IS, Okada CY, Tibshirani R, et al. Molecular analysis of immunoglobulin genes in diffuse large-B-cell lymphomas. *Blood* 2000;95:1797–1803.
376. Kuppers R, Rajewsky K, Hansmann ML. Diffuse large cell lymphomas are derived from mature B cells carrying V region genes with a high load of somatic mutation and evidence of selection for antibody expression. *Eur J Immunol* 1997;27:1398–1405.
377. Weiss LM, Warnke RA, Sklar J, et al. Molecular analysis of the t(14;18) chromosomal translocation in malignant lymphomas. *N Engl J Med* 1987;317:1185–1189.
378. Pescarmona E, De Sanctis V, Pistilli A, et al. Pathogenetic and clinical implications of Bcl-6 and Bcl-2 gene configuration in nodal diffuse large-B-cell lymphomas. *J Pathol* 1997; 183:281–286.
379. Raghoebier S, Kramer MH, van Krieken JH, et al. Essential differences in oncogene involvement between primary nodal and extranodal large cell lymphoma. *Blood* 1991;78: 2680–2685.
380. Jacobson JO, Aisenberg AC, Lamarre L, et al. Mediastinal large cell lymphoma. An uncommon subset of adult lymphoma curable with combined modality therapy. *Cancer* 1988;62: 1893–1898.
381. Kramer MH, Hermans J, Wijburg E, et al. Clinical relevance of BCL2, BCL6, and MYC rearrangements in diffuse large-B-cell lymphoma. *Blood* 1998;92:3152–3162.
382. Rao PH, Houldsworth J, Dyomina K, et al. Chromosomal and gene amplification in diffuse large-B-cell lymphoma. *Blood* 1998;92:234–240.
383. Offit K, Lo Coco F, Louie DC, et al. Rearrangement of the bcl-6 gene as a prognostic marker in diffuse large-cell lymphoma. *N Engl J Med* 1994;331:74–80.
384. Bastard C, Deweindt C, Kerckaert JP, et al. LAZ3 rearrangements in non-Hodgkin's lymphoma: correlation with histology, immunophenotype, karyotype, and clinical outcome in 217 patients. *Blood* 1994;83:2423–2427.
385. Vitolo U, Gaidano G, Botto B, et al. Rearrangements of bcl-6, bcl-2, c-myc and 6q deletion in B-diffuse large-cell lymphoma: clinical relevance in 71 patients. *Ann Oncol* 1998;9:55–61.
386. Muramatsu M, Akasaka T, Kadowaki N, et al. Rearrangement of the BCL6 gene in B-cell lymphoid neoplasms: comparison with lymphomas associated with BCL2 rearrangement. *Br J Haematol* 1996;93:911–920.
387. Liang R, Chan WP, Kwong YL, et al. High incidence of BCL-6 gene rearrangement in diffuse large-B-cell lymphoma of primary gastric origin. *Cancer Genet Cytogenet* 1997;97: 114–118.
388. Michaud GY, Gascoyne RD, McNeil BK, et al. Bcl-6 and lymphoproliferative disorders. *Leuk Lymphoma* 1997;26:515–525.
389. Lo Coco F, Bihui YH, Florigio L, et al. Rearrangements of the BCL6 gene in diffuse large cell non-Hodgkin's lymphoma. *Blood* 1994;83:1757–1759.
390. Pasqualucci L, Neumeister P, Goossens T, et al. Hypermutation of multiple proto-oncogenes in B-cell diffuse large-cell lymphomas. *Nature* 2001;412:341–346.
391. Macpherson N, Lesack D, Klasa R, et al. Small noncleaved, non-Burkitt's (Burkit-Like) lymphoma: cytogenetics predict outcome and reflect clinical presentation. *J Clin Oncol* 1999;17:1558–1567.
392. Alizadeh AA, Eisen MB, Davis RE, et al. Distinct types of diffuse large-B-cell lymphoma identified by gene expression profiling. *Nature* 2000;403:503–511.
393. Rosenwald A, Wright G, Chan WC, et al. The use of molecular profiling to predict survival after chemotherapy for diffuse large-B-cell lymphoma. *N Engl J Med* 2002;346:1937–1947.
394. Huang JZ, Sanger WG, Greiner TC, et al. The t(14;18) defines a unique subset of diffuse large-B-cell lymphoma with a germinal center B-cell gene expression profile. *Blood* 2002; 99:2285–2290.
395. Shipp MA, Ross KN, Tamayo P, et al. Diffuse large-B-cell lymphoma outcome prediction by gene-expression profiling and supervised machine learning. *Nat Med* 2002;8:68–74.
396. Hans CP, Weisenburger DD, Greiner TC, et al. Confirmation of the molecular classification of diffuse large-B-cell lymphoma by immunohistochemistry using a tissue microarray. *Blood* 2004;103:275–282.
397. Loeffler M, Shipp M, Stein H. 2 Report on the workshop: "Clinical consequences of pathology and prognostic factors in aggressive NHL." *Ann Hematol* 2001;80(Suppl 3): B8–12.
398. Engelhard M, Brittinger G, Huhn D, et al. Subclassification of diffuse large-B-cell lymphomas according to the Kiel classification: distinction of centroblastic and immunoblastic lymphomas is a significant prognostic risk factor. *Blood* 1997;89:2291–2297.
399. Levine AM, Taylor CR, Schneider DR, et al. Immunoblastic sarcoma of T-cell versus B-cell origin: I. Clinical features. *Blood* 1981;58:52–61.
400. Delsol G, Lamant L, Mariame B, et al. A new subtype of large-B-cell lymphoma expressing the ALK kinase and lacking the 2; 5 translocation. *Blood* 1997;89:1483–1490.
401. A predictive model for aggressive non-Hodgkin's lymphoma. The International Non-Hodgkin's Lymphoma Prognostic Factors Project. *N Engl J Med* 1993;329:987–994.
402. Barrans SL, Carter I, Owen RG, et al. Germinal center phenotype and bcl-2 expression combined with the International Prognostic Index improves patient risk stratification in diffuse large-B-cell lymphoma. *Blood* 2002;99:1136–1143.
403. Hermine O, Haioun C, Lepage E, et al. Prognostic significance of bcl-2 protein expression in aggressive non-Hodgkin's lymphoma. Groupe d'Etude des Lymphomes de l'Adulte (GELA). *Blood* 1996;87:265–272.
404. Hill ME, MacLennan KA, Cunningham DC, et al. Prognostic significance of BCL-2 expression and bcl-2 major breakpoint region rearrangement in diffuse large cell non-Hodgkin's lymphoma: a British National Lymphoma Investigation Study. *Blood* 1996;88:1046–1051.
405. Gascoyne RD, Adomat SA, Krajewski S, et al. Prognostic significance of Bcl-2 protein expression and Bcl-2 gene rearrangement in diffuse aggressive non-Hodgkin's lymphoma. *Blood* 1997;90:244–251.
406. Sehn LH. Optimal use of prognostic factors in non-Hodgkin lymphoma. *Hematology Am Soc Hematol Educ Program* 2006:295–302.
407. Wilson KS, Sehn LH, Berry B, et al. CHOP-R therapy overcomes the adverse prognostic influence of BCL-2 expression in diffuse large-B-cell lymphoma. *Leuk Lymphoma* 2007;48: 1102–1109.
408. Winter JN, Weller EA, Horning SJ, et al. Prognostic significance of Bcl-6 protein expression in DLBCL treated with CHOP or R-CHOP: a prospective correlative study. *Blood* 2006; 107:4207–4213.
409. Nyman H, Adde M, Karjalainen-Lindsberg ML, et al. Prognostic impact of immunohistochemically defined germinal center phenotype in diffuse large-B-cell lymphoma patients treated with immunochemotherapy. *Blood* 2007;109:4930–4935.
410. Lim MS, Beaty M, Sorbara L, et al. T-cell/histiocyte-rich large-B-cell lymphoma: a heterogeneous entity with derivation from germinal center B cells. *Am J Surg Pathol* 2002;26: 1458–1466.
411. Macon WR, Williams ME, Greer JP, et al. T-cell-rich B-cell lymphomas. A clinicopathologic study of 19 cases. *Am J Surg Pathol* 1992;16:351–363.
412. Ramsey AD, Smith WJ. T-cell-rich B-cell lymphoma. *Am J Surg Pathol* 1988;12:433–443.
413. Fraga M, Sanchez-Verde L, Forteza J, et al. T-cell/histiocyte-rich large-B-cell lymphoma is a disseminated aggressive neoplasm: differential diagnosis from Hodgkin's lymphoma. *Histopathology* 2002;41:216–229.
414. Achten R, Verhoef G, Vanuytsel L, et al. Histiocyte-rich, T-cell-rich B-cell lymphoma: a distinct diffuse large-B-cell lymphoma subtype showing characteristic morphologic and immunophenotypic features. *Histopathology* 2002;40:31–45.
415. Felgar RE, Steward KR, Cousar JB, et al. T-cell-rich large-B-cell lymphomas contain non-activated CD8+ cytolytic T cells, show increased tumor cell apoptosis, and have lower Bcl-2 expression than diffuse large-B-cell lymphomas. *Am J Pathol* 1998;153:1707–1715.
416. Rudiger T, Gascoyne RD, Jaffe ES, et al. Workshop on the relationship between nodular lymphocyte predominant Hodgkin's lymphoma and T cell/histiocyte-rich B cell lymphoma. *Ann Oncol* 2002;13 Suppl 1:44–51.
417. Abramson JS. T-cell/histiocyte-rich B-cell lymphoma: biology, diagnosis, and management. *Oncologist* 2006;11:384–392.
418. Oyama T, Ichimura K, Suzuki R, et al. Senile EBV+ B-cell lymphoproliferative disorders: a clinicopathologic study of 22 patients. *Am J Surg Pathol* 2003;27:16–26.
419. Oyama T, Yamamoto K, Asano N, et al. Age-related EBV-associated B-cell lymphoproliferative disorders constitute a distinct clinicopathologic group: a study of 96 patients. *Clin Cancer Res* 2007;13:5124–5132.
420. Smedby KE, Baecklund E, Askling J. Malignant lymphomas in autoimmunity and inflam-

mation: a review of risks, risk factors, and lymphoma characteristics. *Cancer Epidemiol Biomarkers Prev* 2006;15:2069–2077.

421. Iuchi K, Ichimiya A, Akashi A, et al. Non-Hodgkin's lymphoma of the pleural cavity developing from long-standing pyothorax. *Cancer* 1987;60:1771–1775.
422. Nakatsuka S, Yao M, Hoshida Y, et al. Pyothorax-associated lymphoma: a review of 106 cases. *J Clin Oncol* 2002;20:4255–4260.
423. Aozasa K. Pyothorax-associated lymphoma. *J Clin Exp Hematop* 2006;46:5–10.
424. Copie-Bergman C, Niedobitek G, Mangham DC, et al. Epstein-Barr virus in B-cell lymphomas associated with chronic suppurative inflammation. *J Pathol* 1997;183:287–292.
425. Cheuk W, Chan AC, Chan JK, et al. Metallic implant-associated lymphoma: a distinct subgroup of large-B-cell lymphoma related to pyothorax-associated lymphoma? *Am J Surg Pathol* 2005;29:832–836.
426. Banks P, Warnke R. Mediastinal (thymic) large-B-cell lymphoma. In Jaffe E, Harris N, Steen H, et al., eds. *Pathology and Genetics of Tumours of Haematopoietic and Lymphoid Tissues. World Health Organization Classification of Tumours.* Lyon, France: IARC Press, 2001: 175–176.
427. de Leval L, Ferry JA, Falini B, et al. Expression of bcl-6 and CD10 in primary mediastinal large-B-cell lymphoma: evidence for derivation from germinal center B cells? *Am J Surg Pathol* 2001;25:1277–1282.
428. Paulli M, Strater J, Gianelli U, et al. Mediastinal B-cell lymphoma: a study of its histomorphologic spectrum based on 109 cases. *Hum Pathol* 1999;30:178–187.
429. Pileri SA, Gaidano G, Zinzani PL, et al. Primary mediastinal B-cell lymphoma: high frequency of BCL-6 mutations and consistent expression of the transcription factors OCT-2, BOB.1, and PU.1 in the absence of immunoglobulins. *Am J Pathol* 2003;162:243–253.
430. Perrone T, Frizzera G, Rosai J. Mediastinal diffuse large-cell lymphoma with sclerosis. A clinicopathologic study of 60 cases. *Am J Surg Pathol* 1986;10:176–191.
431. Addis BJ, Isaacson PG. Large cell lymphoma of the mediastinum: a B-cell tumour of probable thymic origin. *Histopathology* 1986;10:379–390.
432. Chan JK. Mediastinal large-B-cell lymphoma: new evidence in support of its distinctive identity. *Adv Anat Pathol* 2000;7:201–209.
433. Copie-Bergman C, Plonquet A, Alonso MA, et al. MAL expression in lymphoid cells: further evidence for MAL as a distinct molecular marker of primary mediastinal large-B-cell lymphomas. *Mod Pathol* 2002;15:1172–1180.
434. Joos S, Otano-Joos MI, Ziegler S, et al. Primary mediastinal (thymic) B-cell lymphoma is characterized by gains of chromosomal material including 9p and amplification of the REL gene. *Blood* 1996;87:1571–1578.
435. Bentz M, Barth TF, Bruderlein S, et al. Gain of chromosome arm 9p is characteristic of primary mediastinal B-cell lymphoma (MBL): comprehensive molecular cytogenetic analysis and presentation of a novel MBL cell line. *Genes Chromosomes Cancer* 2001;30: 393–401.
436. Tsang P, Cesarman E, Chadburn A, et al. Molecular characterization of primary mediastinal B cell lymphoma. *Am J Pathol* 1996;148:2017.2025.
437. Capello D, Vitolo U, Pasqualucci L, et al. Distribution and pattern of BCL-6 mutations throughout the spectrum of B-cell neoplasia. *Blood* 2000;95:651–659.
438. Savage KJ, Monti S, Kutok JL, et al. The molecular signature of mediastinal large-B-cell lymphoma differs from that of other diffuse large-B-cell lymphomas and shares features with classical Hodgkin lymphoma. *Blood* 2003;102:3871–3879.
439. Calvo KR, Traverse-Glehen A, Pittaluga S, et al. Molecular profiling provides evidence of primary mediastinal large-B-cell lymphoma as a distinct entity related to classic Hodgkin lymphoma: implications for mediastinal gray zone lymphomas as an intermediate form of B-cell lymphoma. *Adv Anat Pathol* 2004;11:227–238.
440. Traverse-Glehen A, Pittaluga S, Gaulard P, et al. Mediastinal gray zone lymphoma: the missing link between classic Hodgkin's lymphoma and mediastinal large-B-cell lymphoma. *Am J Surg Pathol* 2005;29:1411–1421.
441. Lazzarino M, Orlandi E, Paulli M, et al. Treatment outcome and prognostic factors for primary mediastinal (thymic) B-cell lymphoma: a multicenter study of 106 patients. *J Clin Oncol* 1997;15:1646–1653.
442. Cazals-Hatem D, Lepage E, Brice P, et al. Primary mediastinal large-B-cell lymphoma. A clinicopathologic study of 141 cases compared with 916 nonmediastinal large-B-cell lymphomas, a GELA ("Groupe d'Etude des Lymphomes de l'Adulte") study. *Am J Surg Pathol* 1996;20:877–888.
443. Gatter K, Warnke R. Intravascular large-B-cell lymphoma. In Jaffe E, Harris N, Steen H, et al., eds. *Pathology and Genetics of Tumours of Haematopoietic and Lymphoid Tissues. World Health Organization Classification of Tumours.* Lyon, France: IARC Press, 2001:177–178.
444. Wick MR, Mills SE. Intravascular lymphomatosis: clinicopathologic features and differential diagnosis. *Semin Diagn Pathol* 1991;8:91–101.
445. Demirer T, Dail DH, Aboulafia DM. Four varied cases of intravascular lymphomatosis and a literature review. *Cancer* 1994;73:1738–1745.
446. Sepp N, Schuler G, Romani N, et al. "Intravascular lymphomatosis" (angioendotheliomatosis): evidence for a T-cell origin in two cases. *Hum Pathol* 1990;21:1051–1058.
447. Ferreri AJ, Dognini GP, Campo E, et al. Variations in clinical presentation, frequency of hemophagocytosis and clinical behavior of intravascular lymphoma diagnosed in different geographical regions. *Haematologica* 2007;92:486–492.
448. Reichard KK, McKenna RW, Kroft SH. ALK-positive diffuse large-B-cell lymphoma: report of four cases and review of the literature. *Mod Pathol* 2007;20:310–319.
449. Chikatsu N, Kojima H, Suzukawa K, et al. ALK+, CD30-, CD20- large-B-cell lymphoma containing anaplastic lymphoma kinase (ALK) fused to clathrin heavy chain gene (CLTC). *Mod Pathol* 2003;16:828–832.
450. De Paepe P, Baens M, van Krieken H, et al. ALK activation by the CLTC-ALK fusion is a recurrent event in large-B-cell lymphoma. *Blood* 2003;102:2638–2641.
451. Colomo L, Loong F, Rives S, et al. Diffuse large-B-cell lymphomas with plasmablastic differentiation represent a heterogeneous group of disease entities. *Am J Surg Pathol* 2004; 28:736–747.
452. Prakash S, Swerdlow SH. Nodal aggressive B-cell lymphomas: a diagnostic approach. *J Clin Pathol* 2007;60:1076–1085.
453. Delecluse HJ, Anagnostopoulos I, Dallenbach F, et al. Plasmablastic lymphomas of the oral cavity: a new entity associated with the human immunodeficiency virus infection. *Blood* 1997;89:1413–1420.
454. Borenstein J, Pezzella F, Gatter KC. Plasmablastic lymphomas may occur as post-transplant lymphoproliferative disorders. *Histopathology* 2007;51:774–777.
455. Banks P, Warnke R. Primary effusion lymphoma. In Jaffe E, Harris N, Steen H, et al., eds. *Pathology and Genetics of Tumours of Haematopoietic and Lymphoid Tissues. World Health Organization Classification of Tumours.* Lyon, France: IARC Press, 2001:179–180.
456. Nador RG, Cesarman E, Chadburn A, et al. Primary effusion lymphoma: a distinct clinicopathologic entity associated with the Kaposi's sarcoma-associated herpes virus. *Blood* 1996; 88:645–656.
457. Said JW, Tasaka T, Takeuchi S, et al. Primary effusion lymphoma in women: report of two cases of Kaposi's sarcoma herpes virus-associated effusion-based lymphoma in human immunodeficiency virus-negative women. *Blood* 1996;88:3124–3128.
458. Oksenhendler E, Boulanger E, Galicier L, et al. High incidence of Kaposi sarcoma-associated herpesvirus-related non-Hodgkin lymphoma in patients with HIV infection and multicentric Castleman disease. *Blood* 2002;99:2331–2336.
459. Seliem RM, Griffith RC, Harris NL, et al. HHV-8+, EBV+ multicentric plasmablastic microlymphoma in an HIV+ man: the spectrum of HHV-8+ lymphoproliferative disorders expands. *Am J Surg Pathol* 2007;31:1439–1445.
460. Leoncini L, Raphael M, Stein H, et al. Burkitt lymphoma. In Swerdlow SH, Campo E, Hams ML, et al. (Eds.) *WHO Classification of Tumors of Haemopoietic and Lymphoid Tissues.* Lyon, France: IARC Press, 2008.
461. Yano T, van Krieken JH, Magrath IT, et al. Histogenetic correlations between subcategories of small noncleaved cell lymphomas. *Blood* 1992;79:1282–1290.
462. Singh N, Wright DH. The value of immunohistochemistry on paraffin wax embedded tissue sections in the differentiation of small lymphocytic and mantle cell lymphomas. *J Clin Pathol* 1997;50:16–21.
463. Chapman CJ, Mockridge CI, Rowe M, et al. Analysis of VH genes used by neoplastic B cells in endemic Burkitt's lymphoma shows somatic hypermutation and intraclonal heterogeneity. *Blood* 1995;85:2176–2181.
464. Tamaru J, Hummel M, Marafioti T, et al. Burkitt's lymphomas express VH genes with a moderate number of antigen-selected somatic mutations. *Am J Pathol* 1995;147:1398–1407.
465. Ferry JA. Burkitt's lymphoma: clinicopathologic features and differential diagnosis. *Oncologist* 2006;11:375–383.
466. Dalla-Favera R, Bregni M, Erikson J, et al. Human c-myc onc gene is located on the region of chromosome 8 that is translocated in Burkitt lymphoma cells. *Proc Natl Acad Sci U S A* 1982;79:7824–7827.
467. Magrath IT, K. B. Pathogenesis of small noncleaved cell Lymphomas (Burkitt's Lymphoma). In Magrath IT, ed. *The Non-Hodgkin's Lymphomas.* Vol 1 London: Arnold; 1997 pp. 385–409.
468. Shiramizu B, Barriga F, Neequaye J, et al. Patterns of chromosomal breakpoint locations in Burkitt's lymphoma: relevance to geography and Epstein-Barr virus association. *Blood* 1991;77:1516–1526.
469. Pelicci PG, Knowles DM, 2nd, Magrath I, et al. Chromosomal breakpoints and structural alterations of the c-myc locus differ in endemic and sporadic forms of Burkitt lymphoma. *Proc Natl Acad Sci U S A* 1986;83:2984–2988.
470. Bhatia K, Spangler G, Hamdy N, et al. Mutations in the coding region of c-myc occur independently of mutations in the regulatory regions and are predominantly associated with myc/Ig translocation. *Curr Top Microbiol Immunol* 1995;194:389–398.
471. Wright D, McKeever P, Carter R. Childhood non-Hodgkin lymphomas in the United Kingdom: findings from the UK Children's Cancer Study Group. *J Clin Pathol* 1997;50: 128–134.
472. Sandlund JT, Downing JR, Crist WM. Non-Hodgkin's lymphoma in childhood. *N Engl J Med* 1996;334:1238–1248.
473. de The G. The etiology of Burkitt's lymphoma and the history of the shaken dogmas. *Blood Cells* 1993;19:667–673; discussion 674–665.
474. Harris NL, Horning SJ. Burkitt's lymphoma—the message from microarrays. *N Engl J Med* 2006;354:2495–2498.
475. Kelly DR, Nathwani BN, Griffith RC, et al. A morphologic study of childhood lymphoma of the undifferentiated type. The Pediatric Oncology Group experience. *Cancer* 1987;59: 1132–1137.
476. Haralambieva E, Boerma EJ, van Imhoff GW, et al. Clinical, immunophenotypic, and genetic analysis of adult lymphomas with morphologic features of Burkitt lymphoma. *Am J Surg Pathol* 2005;29:1086–1094.
477. Cogliatti SB, Novak U, Henz S, et al. Diagnosis of Burkitt lymphoma in due time: a practical approach. *Br J Haematol* 2006;134:294–301.
478. McClure RF, Remstein ED, Macon WR, et al. Adult B-cell lymphomas with Burkitt-like morphology are phenotypically and genotypically heterogeneous with aggressive clinical behavior. *Am J Surg Pathol* 2005;29:1652–1660.
479. Hummel M, Bentink S, Berger H, et al. A biologic definition of Burkitt's lymphoma from transcriptional and genomic profiling. *N Engl J Med* 2006;354:2419–2430.
480. Dave SS, Fu K, Wright GW, et al. Molecular diagnosis of Burkitt's lymphoma. *N Engl J Med* 2006;354:2431–2442.
481. Garcia JF, Mollejo M, Fraga M, et al. Large-B-cell lymphoma with Hodgkin's features. *Histopathology* 2005;47:101–110.
482. Pinkus G, Said J. Peripheral T-cell lymphomas. In Knowles D, ed. *Neoplastic Hematopathology.* Philadelphia: Lippincott Williams & Wilkins, 2001:1091–1125.

482a. de Leval L, Sanio E, Longtine J, et al. Peripheral T-cell lymphoma with follicular involvement and a CD4+/bcl-6+ phenotype. *Am J Surg Pathol* 2001;25:359–400.

483. Rudiger T, Ichinohasama R, Ott MM, et al. Peripheral T-cell lymphoma with distinct perifollicular growth pattern: a distinct subtype of T-cell lymphoma? *Am J Surg Pathol* 2000; 24:117–122.
484. Macon WR, Williams ME, Greer JP, et al. Paracortical nodular T-cell lymphoma. Identification of an unusual variant of peripheral T-cell lymphoma. *Am J Surg Pathol* 1995;19: 297–303.

485. Patsouris E, Noel H, Lennert K. Histological and immunohistological findings in lympho-epithelioid cell lymphoma (Lennert's lymphoma). *Am J Surg Pathol* 1988;12:341–350.

486. Morice WG, Kimlinger T, Katzmann JA, et al. Flow cytometric assessment of TCR-Vbeta expression in the evaluation of peripheral blood involvement by T-cell lymphoprolifera-tive disorders: a comparison with conventional T-cell immunophenotyping and molecular genetic techniques. *Am J Clin Pathol* 2004;121:373–383.

487. Picker LJ, Weiss LM, Medeiros LJ, et al. Immunophenotypic criteria for the diagnosis of non-Hodgkin's lymphoma. *Am J Pathol* 1987;128:181–201.

488. Jamal S, Picker LJ, Aquino DB, et al. Immunophenotypic analysis of peripheral T-cell neoplasms. A multiparameter flow cytometric approach. *Am J Clin Pathol* 2001;116:512–526.

489. Emile JF, Boulland ML, Haioun C, et al. CD5-CD56 + T-cell receptor silent peripheral T-cell lymphomas are natural killer cell lymphomas. *Blood* 1996;87:1466–1473.

490. Macon WR, Salhany KE. T-cell subset analysis of peripheral T-cell lymphomas by paraffin section immunohistology and correlation of CD4/CD8 results with flow cytometry. *Am J Clin Pathol* 1998;109:610–617.

491. Macon WR, Casey TT, Kinney MC, et al. Leu-22 (L60). A more sensitive marker than UCHL1 for peripheral T-cell lymphomas, particularly large-cell types. *Am J Clin Pathol* 1991;95:696–701.

492. Kurtin PJ, Roche PC. Immunoperoxidase staining of non-Hodgkin's lymphoma for T-cell lineage associated antigens in paraffin sections. *Am J Surg Pathol* 1993;17:898–904.

493. Chadburn A, Knowles DM. Paraffin-resistant antigens detectable by antibodies L26 and polyclonal CD3 predict the B- or T-cell lineage of 95% of diffuse aggressive non-Hodgkin's lymphomas. *Am J Clin Pathol* 1994;102:284–291.

494. Quintanilla-Martinez L, Preffer F, Rubin D, et al. CD20 + T-cell lymphoma. Neoplastic transformation of a normal T-cell subset. *Am J Clin Pathol* 1994;102:483–489.

495. Higgins JP, van de Rijn M, Jones CD, et al. Peripheral T-cell lymphoma complicated by a proliferation of large B cells. *Am J Clin Pathol* 2000;114:236–247.

496. Macon WR, Cousar JB, Collins RD. Clarifying statements on T-cell-rich B-cell lymphomas. *Am J Surg Pathol* 1995;19:850–851.

497. Chan WC. T-cell-rich B-cell lymphoma: what is new? What is cool? *Am J Clin Pathol* 1997;108:489–491.

498. Arber DA, Weiss LM. CD15: a review. *Appl Immunohistochem* 1993;1:17.30.

499. Chang KL, Arber DA, Weiss LM. CD30: a review. *Appl Immunohistochem* 1993;1:244–255.

500. Weiss LM, Arber DA, Chang KL. CD45: a review. *Appl Immunohistochem* 1993;1:166–181.

501. Perkins SL, Kjeldsberg CR. Immunophenotyping of lymphomas and leukemias in paraffin-embedded tissues. *Am J Clin Pathol* 1993;99:362–373.

502. Gustmann C, Altmannsberger M, Osborn M, et al. Cytokeratin expression and vimentin content in large cell anaplastic lymphomas and other non-Hodgkin's lymphomas. *Am J Pathol* 1991;138:1413–1422.

503. Weiss LM, Picker LJ, Grogan TM, et al. Absence of clonal beta and gamma T-cell receptor gene rearrangements in a subset of peripheral T-cell lymphomas. *Am J Pathol* 1988;130:436–442.

504. van Krieken JH, Langerak AW, Macintyre EA, et al. Improved reliability of lymphoma diagnostics via PCR-based clonality testing: report of the BIOMED-2 Concerted Action BHM4-CT98–3936. *Leukemia* 2007;21:201–206.

505. Piccaluga PP, Agostinelli C, Califano A, et al. Gene expression analysis of peripheral T cell lymphoma, unspecified, reveals distinct profiles and new potential therapeutic tar-gets. *J Clin Invest* 2007;117:823–834.

506. Martinez-Delgado B, Melendez B, Cuadros M, et al. Expression profiling of T-cell lym-phomas differentiates peripheral and lymphoblastic lymphomas and defines survival re-lated genes. *Clin Cancer Res* 2004;10:4971–4982.

507. Ballester B, Ramuz O, Gisselbrecht C, et al. Gene expression profiling identifies molecular subgroups among nodal peripheral T-cell lymphomas. *Oncogene* 2006;25:1560–1570.

508. Nathwani BN, Kim H, Rappaport H. Malignant lymphoma, lymphoblastic. *Cancer* 1976;38:964–983.

509. Nathwani BN, Diamond LW, Winberg CD, et al. Lymphoblastic lymphoma: a clinicopatho-logic study of 95 patients. *Cancer* 1981;48:2347–2357.

510. Sander CA, Jaffe ES, Gebhardt FC, et al. Mediastinal lymphoblastic lymphoma with an immature B-cell immunophenotype. *Am J Surg Pathol* 1992;16:300–305.

511. Abruzzo LV, Jaffe ES, Cotelingam JD, et al. T-cell lymphoblastic lymphoma with eosino-philia associated with subsequent myeloid malignancy. *Am J Surg Pathol* 1992;16:236–245.

512. Bernard A, Boumsell L, Reinherz EL, et al. Cell surface characterization of malignant T cells from lymphoblastic lymphoma using monoclonal antibodies: evidence for pheno-typic differences between malignant T cells from patients with acute lymphoblastic leuke-mia and lymphoblastic lymphoma. *Blood* 1981;57:1105–1110.

513. Mori N, Oka K, Yoda Y, et al. Leu-4 (CD3) antigen expression in the neoplastic cells from T-ALL and T-lymphoblastic lymphoma. *Am J Clin Pathol* 1988;90:244–249.

514. Gouttefangeas C, Bensussan A, Boumsell L. Study of the CD3-associated T-cell receptors reveals further differences between T-cell acute lymphoblastic lymphoma and leukemia. *Blood* 1990;75:931–934.

515. Swerdlow SH, Habeshaw JA, Richards MA, et al. T lymphoblastic lymphoma with LEU-7 positive phenotype and unusual clinical course: a multiparameter study. *Leuk Res* 1985;9:167–173.

516. Baleydier F, Decouvelaere AV, Bergeron J, et al. T cell receptor genotyping and HOXA/TLX1 expression define three T lymphoblastic lymphoma subsets which might affect clinical outcome. *Clin Cancer Res* 2008;14:692–700.

517. Metzgeroth G, Walz C, Score J, et al. Recurrent finding of the FIP1L1-PDGFRA fusion gene in eosinophilia-associated acute myeloid leukemia and lymphoblastic T-cell lymphoma. *Leukemia* 2007;21:1183–1188.

518. Quintanilla-Martinez L, Zukerberg LR, Harris NL. Prethymic adult lymphoblastic lym-phoma. A clinicopathologic and immunohistochemical analysis. *Am J Surg Pathol* 1992;16:1075–1084.

519. Ralfkiaer E, Muller-Hermelink H, Jaffe E. Peripheral T-cell lymphoma, unspecified. In Jaffe E, Harris N, Steen H, et al., eds. *Pathology and Genetics of Tumours of Haematopoietic*

and Lymphoid Tissues. World Health Organization Classification of Tumours. Lyon, France: IARC Press, 2001:227–229.

520. Harris NL, Jaffe ES, Stein H, et al. Lymphoma classification proposal: clarification. *Blood* 1995;85:857–860.

520a. Waldron JA, Leech JM, Glicic AD, et al. Malignant lymphoma of peripheral T lymphocyte origin: immunologic, pathologic, and clinical features in six patients. *Cancer* 1977;40:1604–1607.

521. Went P, Agostinelli C, Gallamini A, et al. Marker expression in peripheral T-cell lym-phoma: a proposed clinical-pathologic prognostic score. *J Clin Oncol* 2006;24:2472–2479.

522. Saito T, Matsuno Y, Tanosaki R, et al. Gamma delta T-cell neoplasms: a clinicopathological study of 11 cases. *Ann Oncol* 2002;13:1792–1798.

523. Boulland ML, Kanavaros P, Wechsler J, et al. Cytotoxic protein expression in natural killer cell lymphomas and in alpha beta and gamma delta peripheral T-cell lymphomas. *J Pathol* 1997;183:432–439.

524. Yamashita Y, Yatabe Y, Tsuzuki T, et al. Perforin and granzyme expression in cytotoxic T-cell lymphomas. *Mod Pathol* 1998;11:313–323.

525. Kagami Y, Suzuki R, Taji H, et al. Nodal cytotoxic lymphoma spectrum: a clinicopathologic study of 66 patients. *Am J Surg Pathol* 1999;23:1184–1200.

526. Hanson MN, Morrison VA, Peterson BA, et al. Posttransplant T-cell lymphoproliferative disorders—an aggressive, late complication of solid-organ transplantation. *Blood* 1996;88:3626–3633.

527. Nelson M, Horsman DE, Weisenberger DD, et al. Cytogenetic abnormalities and clinical correlations in peripheral T-cell lymphoma. *Br J Haematol* 2008;141:461–469.

528. Streubel B, Vinatzer U, Willheim M, et al. Novel t(5;9)(q33;q22) fuses ITK to SYK in unspecified peripheral T-cell lymphoma. *Leukemia* 2006;20:313–318.

529. Feldman A, Sun D, Law M, et al. Overexpression of Syk tyrosine kinase in peripheral T-cell lymphomas. *Leukemia* 2008;22:1139–1143.

530. Dogan A, Attygalle AD, Kyriakou C. Angioimmunoblastic T-cell lymphoma. *Br J Haematol* 2003;121:681–691.

531. Attygalle A, Al-Jehani R, Diss TC, et al. Neoplastic T cells in angioimmunoblastic T-cell lymphoma express CD10. *Blood* 2002;99:627–633.

532. Ree HJ, Kadin ME, Kikuchi M, et al. Bcl-6 expression in reactive follicular hyperplasia, follicular lymphoma, and angioimmunoblastic T-cell lymphoma with hyperplastic ger-minal centers: heterogeneity of intrafollicular T-cells and their altered distribution in the pathogenesis of angioimmunoblastic T-cell lymphoma. *Hum Pathol* 1999;30:403–411.

533. Grogg KL, Attygalle AD, Macon WR, et al. Angioimmunoblastic T-cell lymphoma: a neo-plasm of germinal-center T-helper cells? *Blood* 2005;106:1501–1502.

534. Grogg KL, Attygalle AD, Macon WR, et al. Expression of CXCL13, a chemokine highly upregulated in germinal center T-helper cells, distinguishes angioimmunoblastic T-cell lymphoma from peripheral T-cell lymphoma, unspecified. *Mod Pathol* 2006;19:1101–1107.

535. Dupuis J, Boye K, Martin N, et al. Expression of CXCL13 by neoplastic cells in angioimmu-noblastic T-cell lymphoma (AITL): a new diagnostic marker providing evidence that AITL derives from follicular helper T cells. *Am J Surg Pathol* 2006;30:490–494.

536. Dorfman DM, Brown JA, Shahsafaei A, et al. Programmed death-1 (PD-1) is a marker of germinal center-associated T cells and angioimmunoblastic T-cell lymphoma. *Am J Surg Pathol* 2006;30:802–810.

537. de Leval L, Rickman DS, Thielen C, et al. The gene expression profile of nodal peripheral T-cell lymphoma demonstrates a molecular link between angioimmunoblastic T-cell lym-phoma (AITL) and follicular helper T (TFH) cells. *Blood* 2007;109:4952–4963.

538. Piccaluga PP, Agostinelli C, Califano A, et al. Gene expression analysis of angioimmuno-blastic lymphoma indicates derivation from T follicular helper cells and vascular endothe-lial growth factor deregulation. *Cancer Res* 2007;67:10703–10710.

539. Schlegelberger B, Zhang Y, Weber-Matthiesen K, et al. Detection of aberrant clones in nearly all cases of angioimmunoblastic lymphadenopathy with dysproteinemia-type T-cell lymphoma by combined interphase and metaphase cytogenetics. *Blood* 1994;84:2640–2648.

540. Stein H, Mason DY, Gerdes J, et al. The expression of the Hodgkin's disease associated antigen Ki-1 in reactive and neoplastic lymphoid tissue: evidence that Reed-Sternberg cells and histiocytic malignancies are derived from activated lymphoid cells. *Blood* 1985;66:848–858.

541. de Bruin PC, Beljaards RC, van Heerde P, et al. Differences in clinical behaviour and immunophenotype between primary cutaneous and primary nodal anaplastic large cell lymphoma of T-cell or null cell phenotype. *Histopathology* 1993;23:127–135.

542. Kaudewitz P, Stein H, Dallenbach F, et al. Primary and secondary cutaneous Ki-1 + (CD30 +) anaplastic large cell lymphomas. Morphologic, immunohistologic, and clinical-characteristics. *Am J Pathol* 1989;135:359–367.

543. Chott A, Kaserer K, Augustin I, et al. Ki-1-positive large cell lymphoma. A clinicopathologic study of 41 cases. *Am J Surg Pathol* 1990;14:439–448.

544. Kinney MC, Collins RD, Greer JP, et al. A small-cell-predominant variant of primary Ki-1 (CD30) + T-cell lymphoma. *Am J Surg Pathol* 1993;17:859–868.

545. Pileri S, Falini B, Delsol G, et al. Lymphohistiocytic T-cell lymphoma (anaplastic large cell lymphoma CD30 + /Ki-1 + with a high content of reactive histiocytes). *Histopathology* 1990;16:383–391.

546. Pallesen G. The diagnostic significance of the CD30 (Ki-1) antigen. *Histopathology* 1990;16:409–413.

547. Pallesen G, Hamilton-Dutoit SJ. Ki-1 (CD30) antigen is regularly expressed by tumor cells of embryonal carcinoma. *Am J Pathol* 1988;133:446–450.

548. Hittmair A, Rogatsch H, Hobisch A, et al. CD30 expression in seminoma. *Hum Pathol* 1996;27:1166–1171.

549. Schwarting R, Gerdes J, Durkop H, et al. BER-H2: a new anti-Ki-1 (CD30) monoclonal antibody directed at a formol-resistant epitope. *Blood* 1989;74:1678–1689.

550. Segal GH, Kjeldsberg CR, Smith GP, et al. CD30 antigen expression in florid immunoblas-tic proliferations. A clinicopathologic study of 14 cases. *Am J Clin Pathol* 1994;102:292–298.

551. Abbondanzo SL, Sato N, Straus SE, et al. Acute infectious mononucleosis. CD30 (Ki-1) antigen expression and histologic correlations. *Am J Clin Pathol* 1990;93:698–702.

552. Felgar RE, Salhany KE, Macon WR, et al. The expression of TIA-1 + cytolytic-type granules and other cytolytic lymphocyte-associated markers in CD30 + anaplastic large cell lym-

phomas (ALCL): correlation with morphology, immunophenotype, ultrastructure, and clinical features. *Hum Pathol* 1999;30:228–236.

553. Delsol G, Al Saati T, Gatter KC, et al. Coexpression of epithelial membrane antigen (EMA), Ki-1, and interleukin-2 receptor by anaplastic large cell lymphomas. Diagnostic value in so-called malignant histiocytosis. *Am J Pathol* 1988;130:59–70.

554. Kaneko Y, Frizzera G, Edamura S, et al. A novel translocation, t(2;5) (p23;q35), in childhood phagocytic large T-cell lymphoma mimicking malignant histiocytosis. *Blood* 1989; 73:806–813.

555. Le Beau MM, Bitter MA, Larson RA, et al. The t(2;5) (p23;q35): a recurring chromosomal abnormality in Ki-1-positive anaplastic large cell lymphoma. *Leukemia* 1989;3:866–870.

556. Morris SW, Kirstein MN, Valentine MB, et al. Fusion of a kinase gene, ALK, to a nucleolar protein gene, NPM, in non-Hodgkin's lymphoma. *Science* 1994;263:1281–1284.

557. Wellmann A, Otsuki T, Vogelbruch M, et al. Analysis of the t(2;5)(p23;q35) translocation by reverse transcription-polymerase chain reaction in CD30+ anaplastic large-cell lymphomas, in other non-Hodgkin's lymphomas of T-cell phenotype, and in Hodgkin's disease. *Blood* 1995;86:2321–2328.

558. Nakamura S, Shiota M, Nakagawa A, et al. Anaplastic large cell lymphoma: a distinct molecular pathologic entity: a reappraisal with special reference to p80(NPM/ALK) expression. *Am J Surg Pathol* 1997;21:1420–1432.

559. Pulford K, Lamant L, Morris SW, et al. Detection of anaplastic lymphoma kinase (ALK) and nucleolar protein nucleophosmin (NPM)-ALK. proteins in normal and neoplastic cells with the monoclonal antibody ALK1. *Blood* 1997;89:1394–1404.

560. Benharroch D, Meguerian-Bedoyan Z, Lamant L, et al. ALK-positive lymphoma: a single disease with a broad spectrum of morphology. *Blood* 1998;91:2076–2084.

561. Falini B, Pulford K, Pucciarini A, et al. Lymphomas expressing ALK fusion protein(s) other than NPM-ALK. *Blood* 1999;94:3509–3515.

562. Lamant L, Dastugue N, Pulford K, et al. A new fusion gene TPM3-ALK in anaplastic large cell lymphoma created by a (1;2)(q25;p23) translocation. *Blood* 1999;93:3088–3095.

563. Hernandez L, Pinyol M, Hernandez S, et al. TRK-fused gene (TFG) is a new partner of ALK in anaplastic large cell lymphoma producing two structurally different TFG-ALK translocations. *Blood* 1999;94:3265–3268.

564. Wlodarska I, De Wolf-Peeters C, Falini B, et al. The cryptic inv(2) (p23q35) defines a new molecular genetic subtype of ALK-positive anaplastic large-cell lymphoma. *Blood* 1998;92:2688–2695.

565. Touriol C, Greenland C, Lamant L, et al. Further demonstration of the diversity of chromosomal changes involving 2p23 in ALK-positive lymphoma: 2 cases expressing ALK kinase fused to CLTCL (clathrin chain polypeptide-like). *Blood* 2000;95:3204–3207.

566. Meech SJ, McGavran L, Odom LF, et al. Unusual childhood extramedullary hematologic malignancy with natural killer cell properties that contains tropomyosin 4—anaplastic lymphoma kinase gene fusion. *Blood* 2001;98:1209–1216.

567. Cools J, Wlodarska I, Somers R, et al. Identification of novel fusion partners of ALK, the anaplastic lymphoma kinase, in anaplastic large-cell lymphoma and inflammatory myofibroblastic tumor. *Genes Chromosomes Cancer* 2002;34:354–362.

568. Lamant L, Gascoyne RD, Duplantier MM, et al. Non-muscle myosin heavy chain (MYH9): a new partner fused to ALK in anaplastic large cell lymphoma. *Genes Chromosomes Cancer* 2003;37:427–432.

569. Tort F, Pinyol M, Pulford K, et al. Molecular characterization of a new ALK translocation involving moesin (MSN-ALK) in anaplastic large cell lymphoma. *Lab Invest* 2001;81:419–426.

570. Thompson MA, Stumph J, Henrickson SE, et al. Differential gene expression in anaplastic lymphoma kinase-positive and anaplastic lymphoma kinase-negative anaplastic large cell lymphomas. *Hum Pathol* 2005;36:494–504.

571. Lamant L, de Reynies A, Duplantier MM, et al. Gene-expression profiling of systemic anaplastic large-cell lymphoma reveals differences based on ALK status and two distinct morphologic ALK+ subtypes. *Blood* 2007;109:2156–2164.

572. Salaverria I, Bea S, Lopez-Guillermo A, et al. Genomic profiling reveals different genetic aberrations in systemic ALK-positive and ALK-negative anaplastic large cell lymphomas. *Br J Haematol* 2008;140:516–526.

573. Kadin ME, Sako D, Berliner N, et al. Childhood Ki-1 lymphoma presenting with skin lesions and peripheral lymphadenopathy. *Blood* 1986;68:1042–1049.

574. Falini B, Pileri S, Zinzani PL, et al. ALK+ lymphoma: clinico-pathological findings and outcome. *Blood* 1999;93:2697–2706.

575. Gascoyne RD, Aoun P, Wu D, et al. Prognostic significance of anaplastic lymphoma kinase (ALK) protein expression in adults with anaplastic large cell lymphoma. *Blood* 1999;93:3913–3921.

576. ten Berge RL, de Bruin PC, Oudejans JJ, et al. ALK-negative anaplastic large-cell lymphoma demonstrates similar poor prognosis to peripheral T-cell lymphoma, unspecified. *Histopathology* 2003;43:462–469.

577. DeCoteau JF, Butmarc JR, Kinney MC, et al. The t(2;5) chromosomal translocation is not a common feature of primary cutaneous CD30+ lymphoproliferative disorders: comparison with anaplastic large-cell lymphoma of nodal origin. *Blood* 1996;87:3437–3441.

578. Lae ME, Ahmed I, Macon WR. Clusterin is widely expressed in systemic anaplastic large cell lymphoma but fails to differentiate primary from secondary cutaneous anaplastic large cell lymphoma. *Am J Clin Pathol* 2002;118:773–779.

579. Sarma PS, Gruber J. Human T-cell lymphotropic viruses in human diseases. *J Natl Cancer Inst* 1990;82:1100–1106.

580. Shimoyama M. Diagnostic criteria and classification of clinical subtypes of adult T-cell leukaemia-lymphoma. A report from the Lymphoma Study Group (1984–87). *Br J Haematol* 1991;79:428–437.

581. Jaffe ES, Blattner WA, Blayney DW, et al. The pathologic spectrum of adult T-cell leukemia/lymphoma in the United States. Human T-cell leukemia/lymphoma virus-associated lymphoid malignancies. *Am J Surg Pathol* 1984;8:263–275.

582. Karube K, Ohshima K, Tsuchiya T, et al. Expression of FoxP3, a key molecule in CD4CD25 regulatory T cells, in adult T-cell leukaemia/lymphoma cells. *Br J Haematol* 2004;126:81–84.

583. Yoshida M, Seiki M, Yamaguchi K, et al. Monoclonal integration of human T-cell leukemia provirus in all primary tumors of adult T-cell leukemia suggests causative role of human T-cell leukemia virus in the disease. *Proc Natl Acad Sci U S A* 1984;81:2534–2537.

584. Jaffe ES. Classification of natural killer (NK) cell and NK-like T-cell malignancies. *Blood* 1996;87:1207–1210.

585. Imamura N, Kusunoki Y, Kawa-Ha K, et al. Aggressive natural killer cell leukaemia/lymphoma: report of four cases and review of the literature. Possible existence of a new clinical entity originating from the third lineage of lymphoid cells. *Br J Haematol* 1990;75:49–59.

586. Sun T, Brody J, Susin M, et al. Aggressive natural killer cell lymphoma/leukemia. A recently recognized clinicopathologic entity. *Am J Surg Pathol* 1993;17:1289–1299.

587. Chim CS, Ma ES, Loong F, et al. Diagnostic cues for natural killer cell lymphoma: primary nodal presentation and the role of in situ hybridisation for Epstein-Barr virus encoded early small RNA in detecting occult bone marrow involvement. *J Clin Pathol* 2005;58:443–445.

588. Takahashi E, Asano N, Li C, et al. Nodal T/NK-cell lymphoma of nasal type: a clinicopathological study of six cases. *Histopathology* 2008;52:585–596.

589. Bunn PA, Jr., Huberman MS, Whang-Peng J, et al. Prospective staging evaluation of patients with cutaneous T-cell lymphomas. Demonstration of a high frequency of extracutaneous dissemination. *Ann Intern Med* 1980;93:223–230.

590. Winkler CF, Bunn PA, Jr. Cutaneous T-cell lymphoma: a review. *Crit Rev Oncol Hematol* 1983;1:49–92.

591. Wood GS, Matthews MJ. Diagnosis of T-cell malignant lymphoproliferative disorders in the skin. In Jaffe ES, ed. *Surgical Pathology of the Lymph Nodes and Related Organs.* 2nd edition Philadelphia: WB Saunders, 1995:413–447.

592. Salhany KE, Cousar JB, Greer JP, et al. Transformation of cutaneous T cell lymphoma to large cell lymphoma. A clinicopathologic and immunologic study. *Am J Pathol* 1988;132:265–277.

593. Sausville EA, Eddy JL, Makuch RW, et al. Histopathologic staging at initial diagnosis of mycosis fungoides and the Sezary syndrome. Definition of three distinctive prognostic groups. *Ann Intern Med* 1988;109:372–382.

594. Sheffer E, Meijer CJLM, van Vloten WA, et al. Dermatopathic lymphadenopathy and lymph node involvement in mycosis fungoides. *Cancer* 1980;45:137–148.

595. Lynch JW, Jr., Linoilla I, Sausville EA, et al. Prognostic implications of evaluation for lymph node involvement by T-cell antigen receptor gene rearrangement in mycosis fungoides. *Blood* 1992;79:3293–3299.

596. Bakels V, Van Oostveen JW, Geerts ML, et al. Diagnostic and prognostic significance of clonal T-cell receptor beta gene rearrangements in lymph nodes of patients with mycosis fungoides. *J Pathol* 1993;170:249–255.

597. Isaacson P, Wright DH. Malignant histiocytosis of the intestine. Its relationship to malabsorption and ulcerative jejunitis. *Hum Pathol* 1978;9:661–677.

598. Loughran TP, Jr., Kadin ME, Deeg HJ. T-cell intestinal lymphoma associated with celiac sprue. *Ann Intern Med* 1986;104:44–47.

599. Macon WR, Levy NB, Kurtin PJ, et al. Hepatosplenic alphabeta T-cell lymphomas: a report of 14 cases and comparison with hepatosplenic gammadelta T-cell lymphomas. *Am J Surg Pathol* 2001;25:285–296.

600. Mehregan DA, Su WP, Kurtin PJ. Subcutaneous T-cell lymphoma: a clinical, histopathologic, and immunohistochemical study of six cases. *J Cutan Pathol* 1994;21:110–117.

601. Salhany KE, Macon WR, Choi JK, et al. Subcutaneous panniculitis-like T-cell lymphoma: clinicopathologic, immunophenotypic, and genotypic analysis of alpha/beta and gamma/delta subtypes. *Am J Surg Pathol* 1998;22:881–893.

602. Takeshita M, Akamatsu M, Ohshima K, et al. Angiocentric immunoproliferative lesions of the lymph node. *Am J Clin Pathol* 1996;106:69–77.

603. Cline MJ. Histiocytes and histiocytosis. *Blood* 1994;84:2840–2853.

604. Pileri SA, Grogan TM, Harris NL, et al. Tumours of histiocytes and accessory dendritic cells: an immunohistochemical approach to classification from the International Lymphoma Study Group based on 61 cases. *Histopathology* 2002;41:1–29.

605. Byrne GE, Rappaport H. Malignant histiocytosis. *Gann Monogr Cancer Res* 1973;15:145–162.

606. Scott RB, Robb-Smith AHT. Histiocytic medullary reticulosis. *Lancet* 1939;2:194–198.

607. Weiss LM, Trela MJ, Cleary ML, et al. Frequent immunoglobulin and T-cell receptor gene rearrangements in "histiocytic" neoplasms. *Am J Pathol* 1985;121:369–373.

608. Wilson MS, Weiss LM, Gatter KC, et al. Malignant histiocytosis. A reassessment of cases previously reported in 1975 based on paraffin section immunophenotyping studies. *Cancer* 1990;66:530–536.

609. Cattoretti G, Villa A, Vezzoni P, et al. Malignant histiocytosis. A phenotypic and genotypic investigation. *Am J Pathol* 1990;136:1009–1019.

610. Feldman AL, Minniti C, Santi M, et al. Histiocytic sarcoma after acute lymphoblastic leukaemia: a common clonal origin. *Lancet Oncol* 2004;5:248–250.

611. Feldman AL, Arber DA, Pittaluga S, et al. Clonally related follicular lymphomas and histiocytic/dendritic cell sarcomas: evidence for transdifferentiation of the follicular lymphoma clone. *Blood* 2008;111:5433–5439.

612. Favara BE, McCarthy RC, Mierau GW. Histiocytosis X. *Hum Pathol* 1983;14:663–676.

613. Reid H, Fox H, Whittaker JS. Eosinophilic granuloma of lymph nodes. *Histopathology* 1977;1:31–37.

614. Malone M. The histiocytoses of childhood. *Histopathology* 1991;19:105–119.

615. Willman CL, Busque L, Griffith BB, et al. Langerhans'-cell histiocytosis (histiocytosis X)—a clonal proliferative disease. *N Engl J Med* 1994;331:154–160.

616. Egeler RM, Neglia JP, Puccetti DM, et al. Association of Langerhans cell histiocytosis with malignant neoplasms. *Cancer* 1993;71:865–873.

617. Lau S, Chu P, Weiss L. Immunohistochemical expression of Langerin in Langerhans cell histiocytosis and non-Langerhans cell histiocytic disorders. *Am J Surg Pathol* 2008;32:615–619.

618. Ferringer T, Banks PM, Metcalf JS. Langerhans cell sarcoma. *Am J Dermatopathol* 2006;28:36–39.

619. Lee JS, Ko GH, Kim HC, et al. Langerhans cell sarcoma arising from Langerhans cell histiocytosis: a case report. *J Korean Med Sci* 2006;21:577–580.

620. Perez-Ordonez B, Erlandson RA, Rosai J. Follicular dendritic cell tumor: report of 13 additional cases of a distinctive entity. *Am J Surg Pathol* 1996;20:944–955.

621. Chan JK, Fletcher CD, Nayler SJ, et al. Follicular dendritic cell sarcoma. Clinicopathologic analysis of 17 cases suggesting a malignant potential higher than currently recognized. *Cancer* 1997;79:294–313.

622. Chan JK, Tsang WY, Ng CS. Follicular dendritic cell tumor and vascular neoplasm complicating hyaline-vascular Castleman's disease. *Am J Surg Pathol* 1994;18:517–525.

623. Grogg KL, Lae ME, Kurtin PJ, et al. Clusterin expression distinguishes follicular dendritic cell tumors from other dendritic cell neoplasms: report of a novel follicular dendritic cell marker and clinicopathologic data on 12 additional follicular dendritic cell tumors and 6 additional interdigitating dendritic cell tumors. *Am J Surg Pathol* 2004;28:988–998.

624. Grogg KL, Macon WR, Kurtin PJ, et al. A survey of clusterin and fascin expression in sarcomas and spindle cell neoplasms: strong clusterin immunostaining is highly specific for follicular dendritic cell tumor. *Mod Pathol* 2005;18:260–266.

625. Rousselet MC, Francois S, Croue A, et al. A lymph node interdigitating reticulum cell sarcoma. *Arch Pathol Lab Med* 1994;118:183–188.

626. Giffler RF, Gillespie JJ, Ayala AG, et al. Lymphoepithelioma in cervical lymph nodes of children and young adults. *Am J Surg Pathol* 1977;1:293–302.

627. Zarate-Osorno A, Jaffe ES, Medeiros LJ. Metastatic nasopharyngeal carcinoma initially presenting as cervical lymphadenopathy. A report of two cases that resembled Hodgkin's disease. *Arch Pathol Lab Med* 1992;116:862–865.

628. Carbone A, Micheau C. Pitfalls in microscopic diagnosis of undifferentiated carcinoma of nasopharyngeal type (lymphoepithelioma). *Cancer* 1982;50:1344–1351.

629. Coyne JD, Banerjee SS, Menasce LP, et al. Granulomatous lymphadenitis associated with metastatic malignant melanoma. *Histopathology* 1996;28:470–472.

630. Richter HJ, Leder LD. Lymph node metastases with PAS-positive tumor cells and massive epithelioid granulomatous reaction as diagnostic clue to occult seminoma. *Cancer* 1979; 44:245–249.

631. Hirose Y, Masaki Y, Shimoyama K, et al. Granulocytic sarcoma of megakaryoblastic differentiation in the lymph nodes terminating as acute megakaryoblastic leukemia in a case of chronic idiopathic myelofibrosis persisting for 16 years. *Eur J Haematol* 2001;67:194–198.

632. Neiman RS, Barcos M, Berard C, et al. Granulocytic sarcoma: a clinicopathologic study of 61 biopsied cases. *Cancer* 1981;48:1426–1437.

633. Hoyer JD, Grogg KL, Hanson CA, et al. CD33 detection by immunohistochemistry in paraffin-embedded tissues: a new antibody shows excellent specificity and sensitivity for cells of myelomonocytic lineage. *Am J Clin Pathol* 2008;129:316–323.

634. Pinkus GS, Pinkus JL. Myeloperoxidase: a specific marker for myeloid cells in paraffin sections. *Mod Pathol* 1991;4:733–741.

635. Boggs DR. The pathogenesis and clinical patterns of blastic crisis of chronic myeloid leukemia. *Semin Oncol* 1976;3:289–296.

636. Peterson LC, Bloomfield CD, Brunning RD. Blast crisis as an initial or terminal manifestation of chronic myeloid leukemia. A study of 28 patients. *Am J Med* 1976;60:209–220.

637. Theologides A. Unfavorable signs in patients with chronic myelocytic leukemia. *Ann Intern Med* 1972;76:95–99.

638. Vardiman JW, Variakojis D, Golomb HM. Hairy cell leukemia: an autopsy study. *Cancer* 1979;43:1339–1349.

The Spleen

Many surgical pathologists approach the spleen with trepidation, thus indirectly reinforcing the old axiom that the spleen is an organ of mystery. The reason may be related to the fact that many pathologists initially learn splenic pathology at postmortem examination; at autopsy, spleens frequently are autolyzed and the normal histologic landmarks are obscured. In contrast, in surgically resected spleens that are properly fixed, the splenic white and red pulp are readily distinguished, thereby allowing a systematic means of morphologic analysis.

In previous reviews, the white and red pulp of the spleen formed the basis for pathologic diagnosis (1,2). The conditions most commonly seen in Western surgical pathology laboratories were divided into those disorders that most frequently affected these two compartments. This system of microscopic examination, however, does not include some systemic conditions (e.g., amyloidosis), or many infectious disorders (e.g., malaria) that are uncommon in North America and Europe. Moreover, some pathologic conditions do not obey this arbitrary division, and these may involve both the white and red pulp. These conditions encompass the various pathologic alterations attending splenic trauma, including the development of splenosis (3,4). In some cases, an exception to the general disease category is present such that one compartment is involved when the general disease category usually affects the opposite compartment (5). Despite these exceptions, this approach remains valid, particularly for the problem of idiopathic hypersplenism, and it thus forms the basis of organization in this chapter. This chapter is not concerned with a reiteration of the normal anatomy, electron microscopic features, physiology, and immunohistology of the spleen, for which ample studies and reviews are available (6–11).

PROCESSING THE SPLEEN

A major factor that allows for proper pathologic evaluation of the surgically resected spleen is that the pathologist receives the specimen immediately following splenectomy when it is still fresh. Spleens that are simply deposited in fixative prior to examination do not adequately fix because the capsule impedes penetration of the fixative. Upon receipt of the fresh splenic specimen and following removal of the hilar fat and nodes, as well as weighing and measuring, the spleen is sectioned with a sharp knife. Depending on the clinical condition and whether gross photographs are required, the spleen may be cut either in the long or short axis. Regardless, the cuts should be at intervals of 3 to 5 mm, with examination of both sides of the splenic slices for macroscopic lesions, such as nodules, infarcts, and hemorrhage (12). At this time, the tissue may be allocated for any special studies that are required, such as immunophenotypic, molecular genetic and cytogenetic analyses, and electron microscopy.

My policy is to prepare the tissue blocks immediately rather than to wait for fixation. Surgically removed spleens usually are sufficiently firm to obtain satisfactorily thin blocks. That the tissue blocks not be large is imperative so that the histotechnologist can prepare technically adequate slides. Sections approximately $2.0 \times 1.5 \times 0.2$ cm typically are an ideal "postage stamp" size. Depending on the clinical situation, tissue from the first block may be employed for imprints. This tissue should be blotted with a towel to remove excess blood before imprints are obtained.

The number of tissue blocks varies depending on the size of the spleen, macroscopic findings, and the clinical setting. Generally, I submit from 2 to 10 blocks for histologic studies. The choice of fixative is optional; the only requirement is sufficiently thin tissue blocks and time for adequate fixation. In practice, half the cassettes are placed in formalin and the remainder in B5 solution. After approximately 30 minutes to 1 hour, the blocks should be trimmed if adequately thin sections were not initially obtained. At this time, the slowness of the penetration of the fixative into the splenic parenchyma (probably because of blood within the tissues) becomes obvious. Overnight fixation is recommended; however, depending on when the specimen was received and the urgency of the case, pilot sections may be sent for processing the same night.

If the spleen harbors a lymphoid neoplasm, the guidelines proposed by the Association of Directors of Anatomic and Surgical Pathology for the splenic pathology report are recommended, including the employment of the World Health Organization (WHO) classification (12,13).

DISORDERS PREDOMINATING IN THE SPLENIC WHITE PULP

In the histologic examination of a spleen, the surgical pathologist should determine on low magnification whether the pathologic process primarily involves the white or red pulp, and whether the architecture appears intact. For those disorders disposed to affect mainly the white pulp, expansion of the white pulp is observed. The expanded white pulp will appear as a nodule or series of nodules against the diffuse red pulp background. The term *nodular* is employed simply as a description in this context and does not imply a follicular lymphoma (FL). The scope and pattern of nodular expansion are diverse, depending on the etiology and the extent of the disease. The major disorders leading to an enlarged white pulp are analogous to the disorders leading to lymphadenopathy. Essentially, white pulp expansion is either the result of lymphoid hyperplasia or a malignant lymphoproliferative disorder (Table 18.1).

REACTIVE FOLLICULAR HYPERPLASIA

Secondary germinal centers within the splenic white pulp are normally found in children, but they are unusual in adults, in

TABLE 18.1

Disorders Predominating in Splenic White Pulp

Reactive Hyperplasia

Follicular
    Rheumatoid arthritis (Felty syndrome)
    Immune thrombocytopenic purpura
    Thrombotic thrombocytopenic purpura
    Acquired hemolytic anemias
    Systemic Castleman disease
    AIDS
    Localized form
    Idiopathic antigenic stimulation
Nonfollicular
    Acute infections
    Graft rejection
    Idiopathic antigenic stimulation

Malignant Lymphomas and Related Lymphoproliferative Disorders

Chronic lymphocytic leukemia or small lymphocytic lymphoma
Lymphoplasmacytic lymphoma
    Waldenström macroglobulinemia
    Plasma cell myeloma and/or plasmacytoma
Mantle cell lymphoma
Marginal zone lymphoma; +/− villous lymphocytes
Follicular lymphoma
Large-B-cell lymphoma
    T-cell– or histiocyte-rich
T-cell lymphoma
    Peripheral
    Angioimmunoblastic
    Anaplastic large cell
    Mycosis fungoides
Hodgkin lymphoma
Prolymphocytic leukemia

AIDS, acquired immunodeficiency syndrome.

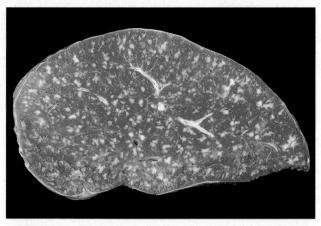

Figure 18.1. Enlarged spleen due to idiopathic reactive follicular hyperplasia of the white pulp. The nodular appearance of the white pulp on the cut surface is indistinguishable from the macroscopic appearance of many lymphomas.

Reactive follicular hyperplasia, however, is rarely an isolated pathologic finding. Unlike the situation in lymphomas, the antigenically stimulated white pulp usually is accompanied by a proliferation of mature lymphocytes and plasma cells in the red pulp as a probable manifestation of antibody production against a specific hematopoietic element (1,14). Light microscopic evidence of granulocytic phagocytosis is not apparent in spleens removed from patients with Felty syndrome; however, the red pulp sinuses and cords are expanded with increased numbers of macrophages (15).

In immune thrombocytopenic purpura (ITP), foamy macrophages or ceroid-laden histiocytes may be observed within the red pulp cords, attributable to the increased phagocytosis of platelets (Fig. 18.2) (16,17). The more numerous ceroid histiocytes within the red pulp are most likely related to a relative sphingomyelinase deficiency (18). Scanning electron microscopy of spleens removed from patients with ITP reveals changes in the microcirculatory pathways that consist of increased vascularization of the white pulp and marginal zones and absence of the marginal sinuses (19). These microcirculatory changes

whom reactive follicles imply antigenic stimulation. Reactive follicular hyperplasia of the white pulp is the predominant morphologic abnormality in spleens that is associated with blood cytopenias and hypersplenism. The cytopenia is a reduction in all major hematopoietic lines or a decrease in one specific hematopoietic element, such as the diminished neutrophils found in Felty syndrome. Reactive follicular hyperplasia also may be the major pathologic abnormality in spleens from patients with hypersplenism in whom the hypersplenic state does not precisely correspond to a well-defined clinical condition and in whom the cause of the antigenic stimulus is unknown. Such spleens may be dramatically enlarged, and the splenic cut surface may contain multiple pale-tan nodules indistinguishable macroscopically from lymphoma (Fig. 18.1). Spleens with idiopathic reactive follicular hyperplasia and Felty syndrome may weigh more than 1000 g (5,14).

The reactive follicles in the splenic white pulp are similar to reactive follicles in lymph nodes in that they often vary in both size and shape. This observation, coupled with a mixed follicular center-cell population and tingible-body macrophages, serves to distinguish reactive follicular hyperplasia of the spleen from FL. At times, reactive follicles may be impossible to distinguish from the follicles of early-stage grade 2 FL; immunologic studies may be necessary for an accurate diagnosis.

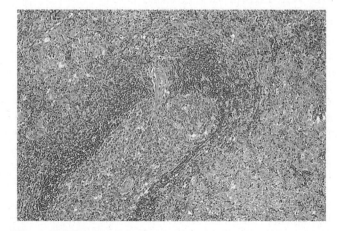

Figure 18.2. Reactive follicular hyperplasia of the white pulp. This is common in immune thrombocytopenic purpura. The pale cells in the red pulp are ceroid-filled histiocytes, which are the result of increased platelet phagocytosis.

likely increase the exposure of platelets to splenic macrophages and add to increased platelet destruction in ITP. Splenectomy is effective in most patients with ITP because this procedure impedes the clearance of autoantibody-coated platelets by receptors on splenic macrophages, as well as impeding the interactions between T and B cells that are involved in the synthesis of antiplatelet antibodies (20).

Although reactive follicular hyperplasia of the splenic white pulp and plasmacytosis of the red pulp, together with some degree of ceroid histiocytosis and even extramedullary hematopoiesis, are the recognized features of ITP, not all of these findings are apparent in many cases. Reactive follicular hyperplasia may be minimal to nonexistent despite a well-established clinical diagnosis. The morphologic absence of lymphocytic stimulation in ITP has been suggested to be a consequence of prior steroid therapy (21). Platelet phagocytosis, however, will persist and may be evident in touch imprints (21). In ITP, patients whose spleens exhibit neither prominent secondary reactive follicular hyperplasia nor ceroid histiocytosis have a significantly poorer response to splenectomy, leading to the conclusion that the thrombocytopenia in such patients may result from a different mechanism of action (22). When the constellation of morphologic findings is not present in a setting of clinically established ITP, a descriptive diagnosis is advised. A description is especially relevant in ITP spleens that are morcellated in the course of a laparoscopic splenectomy (23).

Secondary germinal centers and B-cell hyperplasia of the white pulp also are commonly prominent in thrombotic thrombocytopenic purpura (TTP) (24). The reactive follicles often are accompanied by periarteriolar concentric fibrosis, which suggests an immunologic role in this condition. In TTP, arterial thrombi and hyaline subendothelial deposits of platelet and platelet-related material are the most characteristic pathologic alterations. In this context, hemophagocytosis, iron deposition in histiocytes, and extramedullary hematopoiesis are other common findings in TTP spleens.

Other causes of splenic reactive follicular hyperplasia include the rare cases of systemic Castleman disease, the acquired immunodeficiency syndrome (AIDS), and an unusual localized tumorous form (25–27). In systemic Castleman disease, the spleen exhibits changes of the hyaline-vascular and plasma cell type similar to the changes found in Castleman disease involving lymph nodes (25). In some cases of nonspecific florid reactive follicular hyperplasia of the spleen, isolated white pulp segments also may have hyaline vascular changes indistinguishable from those seen in systemic Castleman disease.

Most descriptions of the spleen from patients with AIDS are derived from postmortem studies in which the spleen itself is characterized frequently by lymphoid depletion, with atrophy of the marginal zone, signs of opportunistic infections, and often deposition of perivascular para-amyloid material (26,28,29). Nonetheless, splenic AIDS cases may exhibit florid lymphoid hyperplasia in which plasmacytosis and immunoblastic proliferation affecting the white and red pulp are also seen (30). Some cases of ITP may be related to the prodromal phase of AIDS; the spleens from these cases exhibit reactive follicular hyperplasia (31). Moreover, the degree of reactive follicular hyperplasia is more prominent and splenic weights are greater in comparison to patients with ITP who do not have AIDS (32).

The localized form of reactive lymphoid hyperplasia is characterized by isolated tumor-type nodules on the splenic cut surface (27). Although the macroscopic appearance suggests a lymphoma (particularly because the majority of cases originally

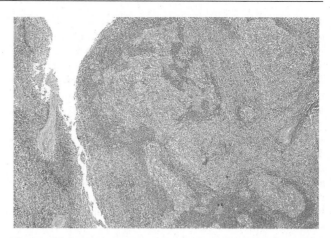

Figure 18.3. Localized lymphoid hyperplasia of the spleen formed by coalescing germinal centers.

were derived from spleens obtained at staging laparotomy for lymphoma), microscopic studies indicate that the nodules are a result of focal coalescence of white pulp germinal centers (Fig. 18.3); a localized diffuse proliferation of lymphocytes, plasma cells, and immunoblasts that is often associated with sclerosis; or a combination of both patterns (27).

REACTIVE NONFOLLICULAR HYPERPLASIA

Reactive lymphoid hyperplasia of the splenic white pulp in which secondary germinal centers are absent is analogous to diffuse lymphoid hyperplasia found in lymph nodes. The hyperplastic white pulp may be composed mainly of small lymphocytes, but, most frequently, a range of lymphoid transformation that includes plasma cells and immunoblasts is discovered. This form of hyperplasia may be observed in acute infections, such as viral infections like AIDS, and graft rejection, but, frequently, the etiology is unknown (1).

The most blatant examples of reactive nonfollicular lymphoid hyperplasia that I have observed occurred in two cases of acute ITP (Fig. 18.4) (5). Both cases were associated with

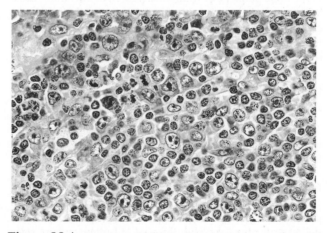

Figure 18.4. Reactive nonfollicular hyperplasia in a patient with acute immune thrombocytopenic purpura. The reactive nonfollicular hyperplasia is characterized by a diffuse proliferation of small lymphocytes, plasmacytoid lymphocytes, and numerous immunoblasts in the white pulp.

florid immunoblastic proliferation involving both the white and red pulp in the presence of immunoblastic infiltration of the subintima of trabecular veins and the splenic capsule. The immunoblastic proliferation resembled an acute viral infection, such as infectious mononucleosis (33), but the presence of a viral infection (including infectious mononucleosis) could not be demonstrated.

Because reactive nonfollicular hyperplasia is relatively unusual, it may be misdiagnosed as lymphoma. The confusion is not surprising because nests and clusters of immunoblasts often dominate nonfollicular hyperplasia. The observation of an overall heterogeneous lymphocytic population with an orderly range of lymphocytic transformation aids in the distinction from lymphoma. In florid examples of nonfollicular hyperplasia, however, the histologic diagnosis requires supplementation by immunophenotypic markers and frequently by gene rearrangement studies.

MALIGNANT LYMPHOMAS AND RELATED LYMPHOPROLIFERATIVE DISORDERS

The main question posed by clinicians whenever a spleen is removed for "idiopathic hypersplenism" is whether an underlying lymphoma is present. In fact, lymphomas restricted to the spleen are uncommon. Most patients who have lymphoma that is first discovered in the spleen have the simultaneous involvement of splenic hilar or abdominal lymph nodes (34). In one series, only 17 of 500 splenectomy specimens (3.4%) with malignant lymphoma were identified as primary lymphoma of the spleen (35). Similarly, only 65 of 1280 (5%) sequential splenectomy specimens were found to contain primary lymphoma (36). Large-B-cell lymphoma was the most common type of primary splenic lymphoma that was encountered, with marginal zone lymphoma (MZL) being second in frequency (36). Other series also have documented MZL as the most frequent form of primary splenic low-grade lymphoma (37,38).

Among patients with known lymphomas, including Hodgkin lymphoma (HL), data from the staging laparotomy studies indicate that the spleen is affected in approximately 40% of patients; for patients with FL, the prevalence of splenic involvement increases to 56% (39,40). Although lymphomas develop mainly in the white pulp, the distributional pattern of the various histologic types is diverse yet frequently pathognomonic (41). In the case of many lymphomas, the red pulp is infiltrated secondarily; for some large-cell lymphomas, the red pulp is the dominant site of involvement (Table 18.2).

Chronic Lymphocytic Leukemia or Small Lymphocytic Lymphoma

The histologic and immunophenotypic features of chronic lymphocytic leukemia (CLL) are identical to those described for small lymphocytic lymphoma (SLL), so both disorders are categorized as a single entity in the WHO classification (13,13a). Prior to the recognition of splenic marginal zone lymphoma (SMZL), historically, SLL was the most common type found in patients with primary lymphoma in the spleen (34). Because the majority of patients with this type of lymphoma have stage IV disease, splenic involvement is common (13,42). In cases of CLL, splenectomy usually is performed because of hypersplenism or autoimmune phenomena and progressive or refractory disease in patients with splenomegaly (43).

TABLE 18.2

Distributional Patterns of Malignant Lymphomas in the Spleen

Uniform multicentric involvement of white pulp
   Follicular
Irregular expansion of white pulp with secondary involvement of
   red pulp
   Chronic lymphocytic leukemia or small lymphocytic lymphoma
   Lymphoplasmacytic
   Mantle cell
   Marginal zone
   Large-B-cell
      T-cell– or histiocyte-rich
   T-cell
      Peripheral
      Angioimmunoblastic
      Anaplastic
      Mycosis fungoides
   Hodgkin
Early localization to periarteriolar lymphoid sheath or marginal
   zone
   Marginal zone
   Peripheral T-cell
      + / − epithelioid histiocytes (Lennert type)
   Large-B-cell
   Mycosis fungoides
   Hodgkin
Diffuse infiltration of red pulp
   Chronic lymphocytic leukemia or small lymphocytic lymphoma
   Splenic diffuse red pulp small B-cell
   Peripheral T-cell
   Hepatosplenic T-cell
   S-100 protein-positive T-cell
   Mycosis fungoides
   Large-B-cell

The diagnosis generally is not difficult to determine. In CLL or SLL, the splenic white pulp areas, including the marginal zones and T-cell regions, are randomly expanded and effaced by a proliferation of small, round lymphocytes (41,44). On the cut surface, the white pulp is prominent and the nodules are asymmetric. Frequently, adjacent expanded white pulp nodules coalesce, and simultaneous diffuse invasion of the red pulp cords and sinuses is generally observed (Fig. 18.5); infiltration of the trabeculae and the subendothelium also occurs (45). In some cases, the involvement of the red pulp may be so widespread that the white pulp component is obscured. These unusual cases can be difficult to distinguish from hairy cell leukemia (HCL), but immunophenotypic studies, specifically the finding of CD5 and CD23 expression in paraffin sections in CLL or SLL, coupled with a lack of DBA.44 and cyclin D1 reactivity aid in the diagnosis (46,47).

Other circumstances in which the diagnosis of CLL or SLL of the spleen may be challenging are encountered. One such situation may be the consequence of epithelioid granulomas developing in both splenic white and red pulp. If the granulomas are sufficiently extensive, they may mask the underlying lymphoma (48). Epithelioid granulomas may also manifest in other splenic small-B-cell lymphomas, including SMZL, lymphoplasmacytic lymphoma (LPL), and lymphomas that are not

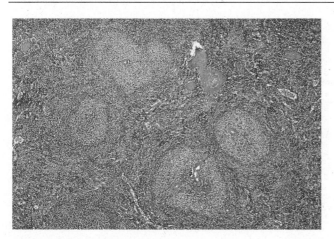

Figure 18.5. Expanded and merging white pulp in chronic lymphocytic leukemia or small lymphocytic lymphoma with concomitant infiltration of the red pulp.

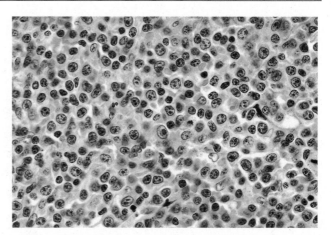

Figure 18.6. Admixed large cells (prolymphocytes and paraimmunoblasts) forming a proliferation center in the white pulp. Proliferation centers are common in chronic lymphocytic leukemia or small lymphocytic lymphoma, and should not be confused with a follicular grade 2 or a large–cell lymphoma.

otherwise classifiable (44,49). A second source of diagnostic difficulty is encountered in patients whose spleens weigh less than 300 to 400 g and in those whose spleens are removed at exploratory laparotomy. Under these conditions, white pulp enlargement may be extremely subtle, and associated germinal centers may be present (37). Because the small lymphocytes are indistinguishable from normal-appearing reactive lymphocytes, cytological evaluation is not helpful in this situation. A diagnosis of malignancy may be suspected because of secondary spread to the splenic red pulp, but immunologic markers are usually required to determine monoclonality. The finding of CD5 and CD23 coexpression also is helpful (46). Use of a silver nitrate immunoperoxidase double-staining technique is another method to facilitate the diagnosis of CLL or SLL and to separate such cases from reactive lymphoid hyperplasia (45).

A third problem in establishing a diagnosis of CLL or SLL is seen in cases in which the formation of proliferation centers in the white pulp occurs (44,50). The admixture of larger lymphocytes, specifically prolymphocytes and paraimmunoblasts in the proliferation centers, frequently leads to the misdiagnosis of follicular grade 2 lymphoma or even large-cell lymphoma (Fig. 18.6); unlike what is found in these other lymphomas, the admixed small lymphocytes in CLL or SLL are round and they are devoid of atypia. The large lymphocytes found in CLL or SLL of the spleen are identical to those reported in their nodal counterparts. If the number of large cells is relatively small, they likely have no bearing on prognosis; however, the evidence in lymph nodes suggests that focal aggregates of large cells may be a poor prognostic factor (51). On occasion, we have seen spleens in which the number of large cells was so great that it indicated transformation of CLL or SLL to large-cell lymphoma analogous to Richter syndrome. In splenic Richter syndrome, often a strict compartmentalization of the residual CLL or SLL and the large-cell lymphoma is present; the small lymphocytes of CLL or SLL are confined to the red pulp, whereas large–cell lymphoma replaces the white pulp (Fig. 18.7) (37).

Lymphoplasmacytic Lymphoma

Lymphoplasmacytic lymphoma (LPL) and its clinical counterpart, Waldenström macroglobulinemia, is composed of a variable mixture of small lymphocytes, plasmacytoid lymphocytes, and plasma cells, including cells with Dutcher bodies, without CD5 and CD23 expression (13,13a,52). In the spleen, the distributional features are histologically indistinguishable from CLL or SLL. The white pulp is irregularly enlarged as a result of lymphoma. The T-cell areas are often infiltrated, epithelioid histiocytes may be prominent, and nodules may form in the red pulp (Fig. 18.8) (37,41). In some cases, the red pulp is diffusely infiltrated with loss of the white pulp and the characteristic nodular pattern of most splenic lymphomas (37,53). The absence of proliferation centers and the lack of CD5 and CD23 expression serves to distinguish LPL from cases of CLL or SLL with plasmacytoid cells (54). LPL is more difficult to distinguish from SMZL, specifically from those cases of SMZL that exhibit plasmacytoid features, because of overlapping immunophenotypic, as well as morphologic, features (55). Both entities are composed of small lymphocytes, lymphoplasmacytoid cells, and plasma cells with similar distributional features in the spleen. Whereas the presence of a pale corona surrounding residual reactive or colonized germinal centers and the identification of marginal zone lymphocytes is stated to distinguish SMZL from LPL, the differential diagnosis is onerous and whether LPL and SMZL actually are distinct lymphomas remains controversial (52,54–56).

Primary plasmactyomas of the spleen are rare and splenic involvement by systemic plasma cell myeloma is also uncommon, although splenomegaly is found in the context of plasma cell leukemia (50,57). Primary splenic plasmacytomas cause massive splenomegaly, and spontaneous rupture may develop (50). Tumor nodules form owing to expanded white pulp segments and nodular aggregates of plasma cells in the red pulp, but, as with LPL, the red pulp may be diffusely infiltrated. The plasma cells range from mature forms to plasmablasts and both binucleated and multinucleated plasma cells are encountered (57). Cytoplasmic monotypic immunoglobulin expression is readily detectable. Distinguishing plasmacytoma from large-cell immunoblastic lymphoma of the plasmacytoid type may be problematic, but plasmacytomas usually are reactive for CD79a and CD138, whereas they generally do not express CD20.

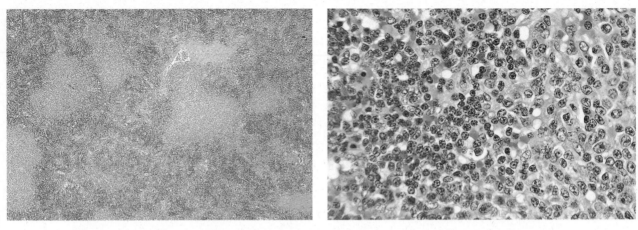

Figure 18.7. Richter syndrome with initial manifestation in the spleen. **(A)** Large-B-cell lymphoma is confined to the white pulp, whereas the residual chronic lymphocytic leukemia (CLL) or small lymphocytic lymphoma (SLL) is limited to the intervening red pulp. **(B)** Interface of large-cell lymphoma in the white pulp and the small, round lymphocytes of CLL or SLL in the red pulp.

Mantle Cell Lymphoma

Mantle cell lymphoma (MCL) is a clinically aggressive lymphoma of small lymphocytes that is thought to arise from naïve pregerminal center cells localized in primary follicles or the lymphocyte corona or mantle zone surrounding secondary follicles (58–60). Although they bear some histologic and immunophenotypic similarities to CLL or SLL, including coexpression of CD5 and CD43, MCL does not have proliferation centers and it generally fails to react for CD23 (58,59). Moreover, almost all cases of MCL contain the t(11;14) chromosomal translocation with virtual universal overexpression of cyclin D1 protein that is independent of demonstrable bcl-1/PRAD-1 rearrangements (58–60).

Many patients with MCL have splenomegaly and advanced-stage disease on initial examination (59). In one series, 42% of patients with primary small-B-cell lymphoma in the spleen were diagnosed as having the mantle cell type (38). Patients with MCL who present with splenomegaly and without lymphade-

nopathy generally manifest a leukemic phase, whereas those with the blastoid variant may develop spontaneous splenic rupture (61,62). In some patients with the splenomegalic form of MCL, the peripheral blood and spleen contain nucleolated cells to mimic prolymphocytic leukemia (PLL) (63); unlike PLL, the MCL cases harbor the t(11;14) translocation and express cyclin D1. In the spleen of patients with MCL, the white pulp is irregularly expanded by a proliferation of small lymphocytes with dense chromatin, indistinct nucleoli, and variable nuclear membrane irregularities (Fig. 18.9) (44). The expanded white pulp may result in confluent tumor nodules or enlarged lymphocytic coronas that surround the residual secondary germinal centers and frequently obliterate the marginal zones. The red pulp cords and sinuses are also often infiltrated and the lymphoma frequently forms small nodules in the red pulp (37,38,44). In the splenic cases of MCL that simulate PLL, the lymphomatous cell population is more heterogeneous and includes intermediate-sized cells with coarse, clumped chromatin and single cen-

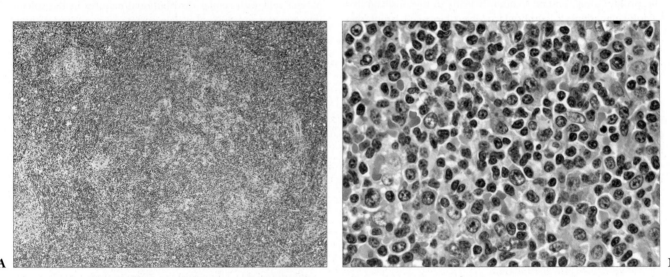

Figure 18.8. Lymphoplasmacytic lymphoma. **(A)** The white pulp is expanded by the lymphoma and clusters of epithelioid histiocytes. **(B)** Heterogeneous population of small lymphocytes, plasmacytoid lymphocytes, plasma cells, and some immunoblasts is typical of lymphoplasmacytic lymphoma. Monoclonal lambda light chain restriction was detected by IHC and by flow cytometry.

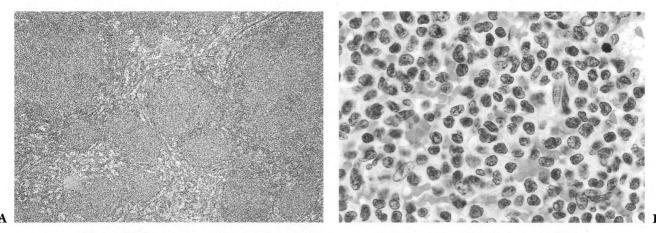

Figure 18.9. Markedly enlarged white pulp in mantle cell lymphoma. **(A)** The coalescing white pulp segments form asymmetrical tumor nodules. **(B)** Irregular nuclear contours and dense chromatin are found in neoplastic mantle cells.

tral, small, prominent eosinophilic nucleoli, in addition to the more typical lymphocytes of MCL (63). In some case of splenic MCL, marginal zonelike differentiation—in which cells with more abundant pale-staining cytoplasm are evident—may occur, suggesting SMZL (64); this diagnostic issue is particularly relevant in cases with associated residual germinal centers. The relative monomorphous cytologic appearance, together with cyclin D1 reactivity, should establish the diagnosis of MCL.

The presence of residual germinal centers in the spleen also may lead to an erroneous diagnosis of reactive follicular hyperplasia. In MCL, however, adjacent white pulp segments coalesce; this observation, when coupled with frequent secondary involvement of the red pulp and nuclear atypia in the proliferating lymphocytes surrounding the germinal centers, serves to distinguish MCL in the spleen from reactive follicular hyperplasia on histologic examination. Immunologic studies demonstrating monoclonality and cyclin D1 expression confirm the diagnosis.

Marginal Zone Lymphoma

Splenic marginal zone lymphoma (SMZL) is a recently described low-grade lymphoma that probably encompasses many primary splenic lymphomas that previously were regarded as CLL or SLL and LPL, making SMZL currently the most common primary low-grade lymphoma of the spleen (36,38,65). SMZL exhibits histologic heterogeneity, but this lymphoma usually exhibits a marginal zone or a biphasic pattern, and, less commonly, a possible diffuse red pulp pattern (66). The marginal zone pattern is characterized by the expansion of the marginal zone of the splenic white pulp due to a proliferation a marginal zone lymphocytes, together with varying numbers of larger, blastlike cells and plasma cells (38,65–69). Marginal zone lymphocytes are small to medium-sized cells with ovoid to reniform-shaped nuclei and a characteristically abundant pale-staining cytoplasm that differentiates them from adjacent mantle zone lymphocytes. Splenic marginal zone lymphocytes resemble monocytoid B cells, and cases of disseminated nodal MZL and extranodal MZL of mucosa-associated lymphoid tissue (MALT) have in fact been reported in the spleen, where they involve the splenic marginal zone and are indistinguishable from primary SMZL (70,71).

In SMZL, the marginal zones are expanded and the neoplastic marginal zone lymphocytes surround, encroach upon, and frequently invade attenuated rims of mantle zone lymphocytes and secondary germinal centers, if these are present (Fig. 18.10). This

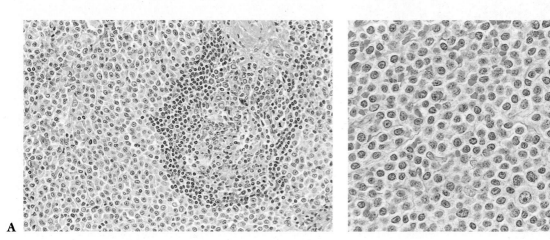

Figure 18.10. Splenic marginal zone lymphoma. **(A)** The marginal zone cells encircle the residual germinal centers. Note the attenuated cuff of dark-staining mantle zone lymphocytes. **(B)** Marginal zone lymphocytes have abundant pale-staining cytoplasm, and they are virtually identical to monocytoid B cells in their histologic features. An occasional large cell is admixed with the marginal zone lymphocytes.

marginal zone pattern may be observed in both massively enlarged spleens and spleens of normal weight in the presumed early phase of the lymphoma (72). In the latter case, replacement of the T cells in the periarteiolar lymphoid sheaths by the neoplastic B cells of SMZL often occurs. The early or supposedly indolent forms of SMZL must be distinguished from cases of marginal zone hyperplasia, such as found in ruptured spleens (3); making this distinction on histologic examination may be formidable, and ancillary studies, such as immunohistochemistry (IHC) and immunoglobulin gene rearrangement studies, are often required (73).

In contrast to SMZL in low-weight spleens, in markedly enlarged spleens residual mantle zone lymphocytes and germinal centers are completely obliterated and are replaced by neoplastic marginal zone lymphocytes forming relatively monomorphous tumor nodules in the white pulp. Red pulp infiltration is usually present and, in a few cases, predominant red pulp involvement has been described with massive, diffuse infiltration of the red pulp leading to destruction of white pulp and the splenic architecture (Fig. 18.11) (66,69,74). The morphologic features of SMZL displaying a diffuse red pulp pattern of infiltration are similar to those of HCL and its variant form. Unlike HCL, the SMZL cases usually do not express CD25, CD103, CD123, cyclin D1, or annexin A1 (47,75–77).

In the 2008 WHO lymphoma classification, cases that formerly were regarded as the diffuse red pulp variant of SMZL are placed in the provisional category of splenic diffuse red pulp small B-cell lymphoma (13a).

In other cases, SMZL has a distinct lymphoplasmacytic component; such cases often are associated with a monoclonal gammopathy and autoimmune hemolytic anemia (55); as discussed above, the lymphoplasmacytic form of SMZL is exceedingly difficult to differentiate from splenic LPL (55,56). In still other cases of SMZL, increased numbers of blasts or large cells are found, and frank transformation to large-B-cell lymphoma may develop (55,67,78,79).

The biphasic pattern of SMZL comprises cases in which the white pulp manifests a prominent central core of small lymphocytes, similar to the cells of MCL, that is surrounded by a peripheral zone of marginal zone–type cells; both zones are considered part of the same neoplastic clone (80,81). The inclusion of biphasic cases in an expanded definition of SMZL arose out of a review of the splenic histologic findings of 37 cases documented as splenic lymphoma with villous lymphocytes (SLVL) (80). In that study, all of the cases of SLVL, including those with a biphasic appearance, were interpreted as being identical to SMZL; these cases currently are categorized as a leukemic form of SMZL (13,80,81).

SLVL is a chronic lymphoproliferative disorder that predominantly develops in older adult men. Consistent massive splenomegaly and circulating atypical lymphocytes with cytoplasmic villous projections that often are localized to one pole of the cell are observed (82). A monoclonal spike is found in the serum or urine in about one-third of patients. About 15% of patients have translocation of t(11;14)(q13;q32) and rearrangement of the *bcl-1* locus with increased expression of cyclin D1; the latter patients usually have a more aggressive clinical course and actually are leukemic MCL cases simulating SMZL or SLVL, including the biphasic pattern (Fig. 18.12) (38,64,83,84).

SMZL is a B-cell neoplasm expressing various B-cell antigens, IgM and IgD monoclonal immunoglobulin, and bcl-2 protein; CD5, CD10, CD23, CD43, and cyclin D1 generally are not reactive (38,65,69,81–84). The absence of CD5 and CD43 expression, as well as cyclin D1, eliminates CLL or SLL and MCL from the diagnosis, and lack of CD10 excludes FL (38,55,64,84). Despite similar cytologic features, immunophenotypic profiles, and a shared designation as "marginal zone," it is of interest that SMZL differs genetically from its extranodal namesake. Similar to node-based MZL, but unlike extranodal MZL of MALT, the splenic cases do not have detectable t(11;18) translocations or *API2-MALT1* fusion transcripts (85). Patients with SMZL, however, display a variety of karyotype abnormalities, and one, specifically a 7q31 deletion, appears to be characteristic and is associated with an absence of somatic mutations and

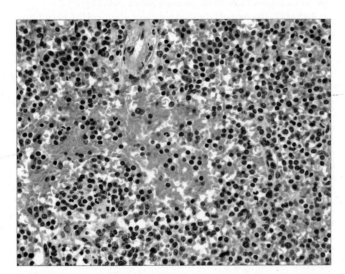

Figure 18.11. Diffuse pattern of red pulp infiltration is described in some cases of splenic marginal zone lymphoma. The histologic features are virtually indistinguishable from hairy cell leukemia and hairy cell leukemia variant. In the 2008 WHO lymphoma classification, such cases are placed in the provisional category of splenic diffuse red pulp small B-cell lymphoma or as splenic lymphoma/leukemia, unclassifiable.

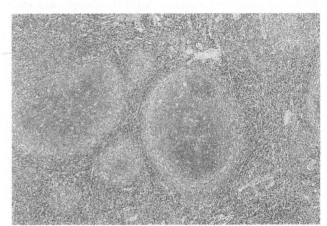

Figure 18.12. Lymphoproliferative disorder with a biphasic appearance of the white pulp due to an enlarged core of dark-staining lymphocytes surrounded by a nonexpanded rim of paler-staining marginal zone cells. The biphasic appearance mainly is equated with splenic marginal zone lymphoma. This case, however, proved to be mantle cell lymphoma in which the neoplastic B cells were CD5+, CD23– and cyclin D1 was expressed.

a shorter survival, as opposed to patients with mutations of the rearranged immunoglobulin heavy chain variable (*IgV$_H$*) genes (81,86). The employment of cDNA microarray analysis demonstrates that SMZL has a largely homogeneous signature and verifies that shorter survival is affiliated with unmutated *IgV$_H$* genes, as well as expression of CD38 and a set of NF-κB pathway genes (87); p53 overexpression is another adverse prognostic factor (88). In general, SMZL is an indolent lymphoma (89). In a report of 309 patients, the 5-year cause-specific survival rate was 76% (90). Hepatitis C virus may play a role in the lymphomagenesis of SMZL or SLVL, and some patients benefit from antiviral therapy (91).

Splenic Diffuse Red Pulp Small B-Cell Lymphoma

Although clearly not a disorder of the white pulp, splenic diffuse red pulp small B-cell lymphoma is a provisional category of indolent lymphoma in the 2008 WHO lymphoma classification scheme (13a). This form of lymphoma encompasses the cases that were formerly designated as the diffuse red pulp variant of SMZL and more recently reported as splenic red pulp lymphoma with numerous basophilic villous lymphocytes (66,69, 74,91a). Such lymphomas are associated with peripheral blood involvement, often with villous type-lymphocytes, as well as bone marrow involvement. In the spleen, the red pulp cords and sinuses are diffusely infiltrated by small to medium-sized, generally round lymphocytes admixed with occasional large cells (Fig. 18.11). Similar to HCL and hairy cell leukemia variant (HCL-V), pseudosinuses and red cell lakes may be present and the white pulp usually is atrophic or obliterated. The neoplastic lymphocytes express CD20 and DBA.44, but unlike HCL, they are CD11c, CD25, CD103, CD123 and annexin A1 negative (13a,75–77). Similar to SMZL, splenic diffuse red pulp small B-cell lymphoma does not express CD5, CD10 or CD23. The cells are IgG positive and may also express IgD. TRAP staining is not found (13a). Cases often exhibit IgH mutations (91a). Complex cytogenetic alterations have been described, but this lymphoma does not exhibit del 7q or t(11; 14) (13a). Although splenic diffuse red pulp small B-cell lymphoma is a provisional category in the new WHO system, and while usually CD103 negative, it displays considerable overlap with HCL-V so that additional cases and further investigations are required to further delineate these uncommon lymphomas and/or leukemias. Cases that do not satisfy the proposed criteria for either splenic diffuse red pulp small B-cell lymphoma or HCL-V are probably best interpreted as splenic B-cell lymphoma/leukemia, unclassifiable (13a).

Follicular Lymphoma

Involvement of the spleen by lymphomas with a follicular architecture in lymph nodes is morphologically distinctive. Because these lymphomas usually involve multiple lymphoid sites initially, FL in the spleen, specifically the grade 1 and grade 2 types, similarly embrace virtually every splenic lymphoid site in a multicentric pattern (1,92). With extensive disease, the splenic cut surface is peppered by uniformly expanded white pulp nodules that allow ready diagnosis on microscopic examination. The uniform multicentric pattern, when it is coupled with grade 1 or grade 2 cytology, generally implies, but does not absolutely equate with, a follicular architecture in nodes. In the spleen,

the neoplastic follicles frequently contain extracellular hyaline deposits (44).

The era of splenectomy for pathologic staging of non-Hodgkin lymphoma has passed, but examination of those spleens demonstrated that almost one-third were involved by lymphoma, although the spleens were not palpable on clinical evaluation (40). The spleens usually were of normal weight and, even though obviously expanded white pulp was absent on either gross or low-power microscopic examination, a detailed pathologic analysis demonstrated that practically every white pulp segment contained a central core of neoplastic cells, usually centrocytes (Fig. 18.13) (92).

In this context, grade 2 cases are more difficult to diagnose with confidence because they resemble reactive follicular hyperplasia (1). Such lymphoma cases, however, usually lack tingible-body macrophages; the mantle zone is often diminished or obliterated; no associated plasmacytosis in the red pulp exists; and, paradoxically, the distribution in the white pulp is usually more homogeneous than that observed in hyperplasia. Again, immunologic markers, such as bcl-2 protein reactivity, are an important adjunct for reaching the diagnosis.

In some spleens involved by FL, the marginal zones, regardless of weight, are often conspicuous and may resemble SMZL (1,37,44,64). The splenic cases containing FL with marginal zone differentiation are similar to cases in lymph nodes (93,94). Those cases with concurrent FL and marginal zone differentiation usually exhibit coalescence of adjacent marginal zones. In addition, the central follicular component of the expanded white pulp strongly expresses bcl-2 protein in comparison to the weak reactivity of the peripheral marginal zone component; the t(14;18) translocation may be detected (93,94). Molecular genetic studies, however, demonstrate that both components have the same clonal sequences, and together with the *bcl*-2 rearrangements, indicate that such cases are of follicular center cell origin (95).

Large-B-Cell Lymphoma

Large-B-cell lymphoma is the most common primary lymphoma in the spleen (36). Similar to SMZL, hepatitis C virus may have a role in the lymphomagenesis of splenic large-B-cell lymphoma (91,96). Classically, it appears as a large tumor mass or a series of large, confluent nodules extensively replacing the splenic parenchyma and secondarily invading the red pulp (Fig. 18.14) (1,35,97,98). The lymphoma frequently breaches the capsule to invade contiguous organs (99). The distribution appears completely random, and the neoplastic cells are often adjacent to uninvolved segments of white pulp (37,41).

Primary splenic large-B-cell cases include not only those with large coalescent tumor masses but also those with multiple, discrete monomorphous nodules in the centers of the white pulp (Fig. 18.15), an association with CLL or SLL, FL of grade 1 or 2 type, or SMZL, and a centroblastic or immunoblastic plasmacytoid cytology (97,98). Some large-B-cell lymphomas may manifest initially in the marginal zone, resulting in the formation of crescent-shaped infiltrates around intact follicles (50,100).

Although these histologic features provide guidelines, immunologic analysis is mandatory for an absolute discrimination between B-cell and T-cell large-cell lymphomas in the spleen. For example, T-cell and/or histiocyte-rich large-B-cell lym-

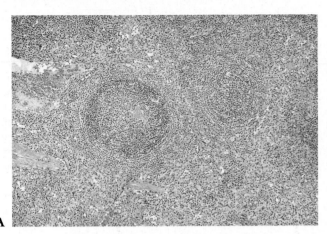

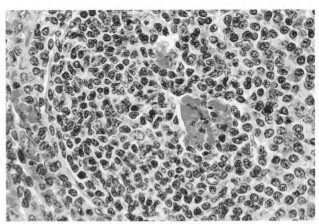

A   B

Figure 18.13. Follicular lymphoma. **(A)** Multicentric involvement of the white pulp is a characteristic feature of follicular lymphomas. Note the intact and relatively discrete peripheral maginal zone. **(B)** The center of every malpighian body in this normal-weight spleen is composed of centrocytes.

phomas may involve the spleen (5,98,101,102). T-cell and/or histiocyte-rich large-B-cell lymphoma cases in which the spleen is the initial site of disease mimic reactive inflammatory lesions, as well as peripheral T-cell lymphoma (PTCL) and HL (Fig. 18.16) (5,101,102). Lymphomas of T-cell and/or histiocyte-rich large-B-cell type form a series of micronodules engaging the white pulp. The nodules are composed of scattered large B cells set among abundant T cells and histiocytes. Paraffin-section immunophenotypic studies are invaluable in these cases and they demonstrate that the micronodules comprise numerous CD3-reactive T cells, CD68-positive histiocytes, and randomly dispersed large cells expressing CD20 with immunoglobulin light chain restriction (101). The prognosis in these cases is poor.

Rare cases of large-B-cell lymphoma may also primarily reposit in the splenic red pulp with diffuse infiltration of the cords and, occasionally, the sinuses (97,98,103). In addition to B-cell antigens, the diffuse red pulp splenic large-cell lymphoma cases may coexpress CD5 (103,104). If the large B cells are predominately distributed in the red pulp sinuses, such cases may represent a version of intravascular large-B-cell lymphoma, and, principally in Asia, may be affiliated with a hemophagocytic syndrome and aggressive clinical behavior (105,106). Currently,

the diagnosis of splenic involvement by intravascular large-B-cell lymphoma requires confirmation by the detection of extrasplenic intravascular lymphoma (107).

T-Cell Lymphoma

Splenic lymphomas of peripheral T-cell origin, including those with a mixed cellular composition and those with epithelioid histiocytes (Lennert lymphoma), are uncommon in contrast to those of B-cell lineage, and they may be confined to the periarteriolar lymphoid sheaths (Fig. 18.17) and/or marginal zones (41,50,97,108,109). At the latter site, epithelioid histiocytes form a ringlike array around the white pulp. Cases without epithelioid histiocytes may form seemingly indiscriminate tumor nodules. Among immunologically verified PTCLs in the spleen, histologic features favoring a T-cell phenotype include not only epithelioid histiocytes and confinement of the lymphoma to the splenic T zones (periarteriolar lymphoid sheaths) or periphery of the marginal zones, but also clear-cell or polymorphous cytology (97). More commonly, however, neoplastic T cells diffusely invade the red pulp without the involvement

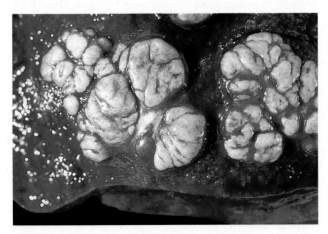

Figure 18.14. Large-cell lymphoma. Tumor masses are typical of large-cell lymphoma in the spleen.

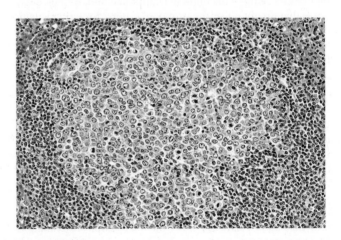

Figure 18.15. Large-cell lymphoma replacing the center of a malpighian body. This is an indication of a follicular grade 3 lymphoma of B-cell lineage.

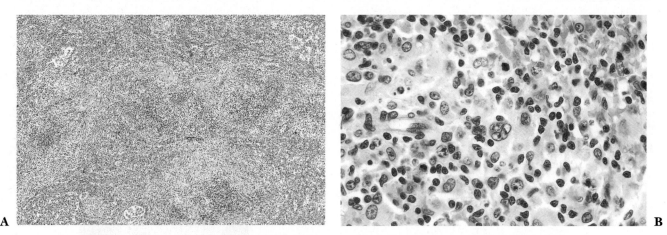

Figure 18.16. T-cell and/or histiocyte-rich, large-B-cell lymphoma presenting in a 2000-g spleen. **(A)** The white pulp is variably enlarged with coalescence of adjoining white pulp segments to form micronodules. **(B)** Detail of the enlarged white pulp reveals a polymorphous cell population dominated by small lymphocytes together with atypical large cells, including Reed-Sternberg–like cells. The small lymphocytes reacted with T-cell antibodies, whereas the large cells, including the Reed-Sternberg–like cells, expressed B-cell antigens. No expression of the Hodgkin lymphoma–associated antigens, CD15 and CD30, was seen.

of white pulp or obvious formation of tumor masses (Fig. 18.18) (109–111); many such cases are of the hepatosplenic T-cell type (112).

Hepatosplenic T-cell lymphomas are rare, clinically aggressive lymphomas sometimes arising in immunocompromised patients, in which neoplastic medium-sized to large lymphocytes infiltrate the splenic sinuses and, occasionally, the cords, as well as the sinuses of the liver and bone marrow (109,111–116). The hepatosplenic T-cell cases may show extensive tumor necrosis and hemophagocytosis. Phagocytosis may be performed by the neoplastic-appearing cells or by true, albeit reactive, histiocytes (109–111,114–116). The immunophenotype is characteristic in that, in addition to T-lineage markers, the neoplastic lymphocytes commonly express natural killer (NK)-cell antigen CD56, and the cytotoxic granule-associated protein TIA1, but do not express CD4, CD8 and no Epstein-Barr virus (EBV) sequences (109,113–116). Most cases are of γδ T-cell type and display an isochrome 7q (114–116); however, identical-appearing hepa-

tosplenic T-cell lymphomas of αβ type develop and those cases may also have isochrome 7q (117).

Other T-cell lymphomas found in the spleen are angioimmunoblastic T-cell lymphoma (AILT), anaplastic large cell lymphoma (ALCL), S-100 protein-positive PTCL, and mycosis fungoides. Although splenomegaly is reported in about half the patients with AILT, descriptions of splenic AILT are uncommon, and, as in lymph nodes, AILT may be easily confused with nonfollicular atypical hyperplasia (118,119). In AILT, white pulp expansion usually is accompanied by increased vascularity and a concomitant polymorphous infiltrate into the red pulp (119). Unless cases of presumptive AILT are associated with cytologic atypia or cellular monomorphism, distinguishing them from an atypical form of reactive lymphoid hyperplasia is problematic, and gene rearrangement studies may be required (120). Monoclonal or oligoclonal T cells are found in most cases. The neoplastic T cells in AILT also have been discovered to express CD10, which may be used to distinguish AILT from

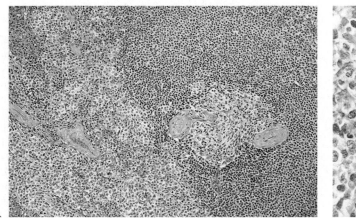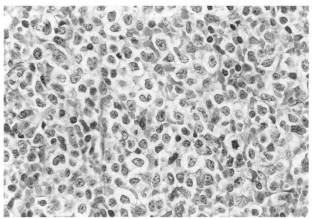

Figure 18.17. Peripheral T-cell lymphoma. **(A)** This peripheral T-cell lymphoma of the large, clear-cell type concentrates around the periarteriolar lymphoid sheath. At the right of the photograph, the splenic B zone with a germinal center is relatively intact. **(B)** Detail of the neoplastic large cells with clear cytoplasm.

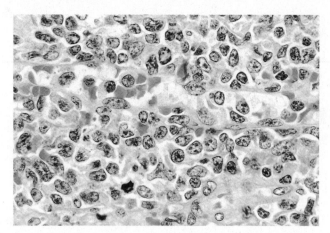

Figure 18.18. Hepatosplenic T-cell lymphoma. Lymphomas, particularly the hepatosplenic T-cell type, may diffusely invade the splenic red pulp without the formation of white pulp nodules. This case has a T-cell phenotype and also involved the sinuses of the liver and bone marrow. The same diffuse red pulp pattern also can occur in large-cell lymphoma of B-cell type.

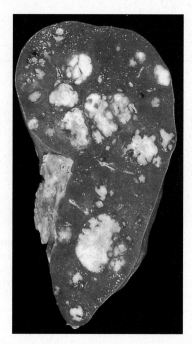

Figure 18.19. Hodgkin lymphoma. Irregularly sized and distributed nodules are characteristic of Hodgkin lymphoma in the spleen. The number of macroscopic nodules has a bearing on prognosis. See text for details.

other PTCLs (121). AILT is thought to arise from germinal center T cells (122). Primary splenic presentation of ALCL is rare, but if the spleen is involved, ALCL usually forms fleshy tumor nodules (109). ALCL cases have been described in association with spontaneous splenic rupture (123) and with symptoms of a splenic abscess (124). S-100 protein-positive PTCL is an uncommon form of PTCL (109); in the spleen, this lymphoma exhibits diffuse red pulp infiltration by medium-sized or large lymphocytes. In addition to expressing T lineage markers and S-100 protein, the neoplastic lymphocytes are frequently CD56-positive (109).

Mycosis fungoides (MF) is another form of T-cell lymphoma that occasionally manifests in the spleen. In a pilot study during the era of staging laparotomy, most cases of MF were discovered to concentrate in the splenic T-dependent zones, but, like aggressive PTCL, heterogeneity is seen among these cases (125). For example, some cases of MF form irregular nodules throughout the white and red pulp, whereas other cases diffusely infiltrate the red pulp cords and sinuses (125).

Hodgkin Lymphoma

HL with an initial diagnosis in the spleen is rare, but this is the one lymphoma in which splenectomy occasionally remains part of current staging procedures—not only for clinical investigational purposes, but also specifically for those patients with low clinical stage disease in whom pathologic staging affects therapy (126,127). Characteristically, spleens involved by HL contain scattered haphazard nodules with a miliary distribution (Fig. 18.19), but, at staging, only a solitary focus as small as 1 mm in diameter may be present (128). These foci may not be noticed unless the spleen is meticulously sectioned according to the earlier descriptions. Because the number of splenic nodules containing HL is related to the prognosis, counting the macroscopic nodules and indicating in the report whether fewer than five nodules are found are important (129).

The diagnosis of HL in the spleen is dependent on the identical histologic criteria that are employed in assessing the lymph nodes; however, even in advanced cases, Reed-Sternberg cells

may be difficult to identify in the spleen. Similar to the lymph nodes, focal or early lesions are localized in the periarteriolar lymphoid sheaths and marginal zones (130). That epithelioid sarcoid-type granulomas may be seen in up to 9% of HL cases and that they may even form macroscopic nodules has been documented (131). The discovery of granulomas does not indicate involvement of the spleen by HL, because these granulomas may be found in cases with no association with HL.

Subclassification of HL in the spleen is optional. Moreover, because some cases of mixed cellularity HL have considerable fibrosis (whereas cases of known nodular sclerosing HL may lack apparent lacunar cells in the spleen), subclassification may be inaccurate (1). Because subclassification of HL is not a factor in therapy, I tend not to subclassify (39).

Prolymphocytic Leukemia

Splenomegaly is the major physical finding in *prolymphocytic leukemia* (PLL), a malignancy that shares features with CLL. The general histologic distribution in the spleen is similar to that of CLL, but many more intermediate-sized to large prolymphocytes, in which the heterochromatin is more dispersed, are observed and small nucleoli are present (Fig. 18.20) (132,133). Paraimmunoblast-type cells also are evident. Making the distinction between PLL and prolymphocytoid transformation of CLL is tenuous on histologic grounds without a clinical history (50). Most cases of PLL have a B-cell phenotype, and, unlike CLL, strong expression of surface immunoglobulin and usually no reactivity for CD5 are found. As discussed earlier, prolymphocyte-like cells may be observed in the splenomegalic variant of MCL and, in contrast to B-PLL, the MCL cases express cyclin D1 as well as seat the t(11;14) translocation (63). B-PLL is biologically heterogeneous with respect to IgV_H mutations, ZAP-

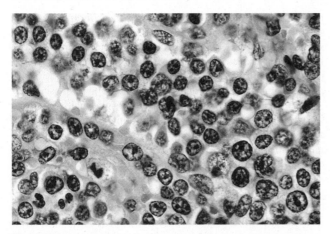

Figure 18.20. B-cell prolymphocytic leukemia. The heterogeneous lymphocytic population in this leukemia is dominated by medium to large prolymphocytes. The cytologic characteristics are morphologically similar to the prolymphocytoid transformation of chronic lymphocytic leukemia.

70, and CD38 expression, exhibiting a pattern that is reported to be distinct from that of other lymphoproliferative disorders (134).

T-PLL accounts for 20% of cases of PLL (135). Immunologically verified T-PLL is similar in its morphologic features to B-PLL in the spleen, although the T-cell cases have been suggested to involve the splenic red pulp preferentially and to embrace more nuclear membrane irregularities (50,135,136). In the spleen, cases of T-PLL also invade the splenic capsule, the fibrous trabeculae, and any residual white pulp; these cases express T-cell antigens, including CD5 and CD45RO, but do not react for cytotoxic granule proteins or NK-cell markers (136).

DISORDERS PREDOMINATING IN THE SPLENIC RED PULP

The major disorders that predominantly affect the red pulp of the spleen are multiple, ranging from those leading to congestion and hypersplenism to leukemias and primary nonhematopoietic neoplasms (Table 18.3). If an expanded white pulp is regarded as imparting a nodular configuration to the spleen, an expanded red pulp results in diminution of white pulp and a diffuse morphologic appearance (Fig. 18.21).

CONGESTION

A congested spleen is a major pathologic finding in patients with hypersplenism. The concepts of Rappaport (137) regarding two major pathophysiologic mechanisms as the basis of congestion are particularly worthwhile. For the various hemolytic anemias, whether congenital or acquired, the red cells are the major site of pathologic changes, whereas the red pulp cords are essentially normal (138). For example, splenectomy in the spectrin/ankyrin type of hereditary spherocytosis prolongs the survival of the red cells because they lose their deformability more slowly than do red cells from patients who do not undergo splenectomy (139). In hereditary spherocytosis or elliptocytosis, the spleen characteristically shows marked congestion of the cords, whereas the sinuses appear empty (Fig. 18.22) (137). Hemosiderosis is minimal, but prominent sinusoidal endothelial cells

are often encountered. In the acquired hemolytic anemias, the morphologic findings are essentially similar, although increased hemosiderin deposition, extramedullary hematopoiesis, and erythrophagocytosis with a pronounced neutrophilic reaction are frequently observed (140). As a reflection of the immunologic basis of some acquired hemolytic anemias, the white pulp may appear enlarged and it may be associated with increased numbers of reactive small lymphocytes, plasma cells, and a few immunoblasts in the red pulp cords.

Fibrocongestive splenomegaly secondary to portal hypertension, regardless of the source, is the prototype of the other proposed mechanism of congestion. In this condition, the splenic cords are abnormal, whereas the hematopoietic elements are normal (137). As a result of the amplified portal pressure, blood pools in the cords, leading to a reactive (or

TABLE 18.3

Disorders Predominating in Splenic Red Pulp

Congestion
  Congenital and acquired hemolytic anemias
  Fibrocongestive splenomegaly
Infections
  Infectious mononucleosis
  Acute septic splenitis
  Bacillary angiomatosis
Histiocytic proliferations
  Lipid histiocytoses
    Ceroid histiocytosis
    Gaucher disease
  Hemophagocytic syndromes
  Histiocytic and dendritic cell neoplasms
    Histiocytic sarcoma
    Langerhans cell histiocytosis
    Interdigitating dendritic cell sarcoma or tumor
    Follicular dendritic cell sarcoma or tumor
Leukemias, myeloproliferative diseases, and myelodysplastic syndromes
  Chronic myelogenous leukemia
  Myeloid metaplasia
    Primary myelofibrosis
    Secondary
  Myelodysplasia
  Hairy cell leukemia
  Splenic B-cell lymphoma/leukemia, unclassifiable
    Splenic diffuse red pulp small B-cell lymphoma
    Hairy cell leukemia variant
  T-cell large-granular lymphocyte leukemia
  Systemic mastocytosis
Nonhematopoietic tumors
  Developmental
    Cysts
    Hamartomas
  Vascular neoplasms
    Hemangiomas
    Lymphangiomas
    Littoral cell angiomas
    Angiosarcomas
  Nonvascular sarcomas
    Malignant fibrous histiocytoma
  Metastases
  Inflammatory pseudotumor
    Mycobacterial spindle cell pseudotumor
  Sclerosing angiomatoid nodular transformation

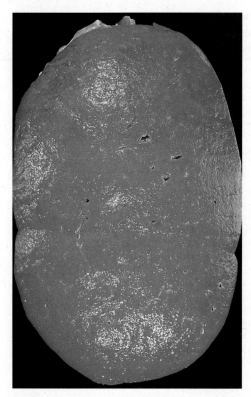

Figure 18.21. A diffusely enlarged red pulp without evident white pulp. This is characteristic of most leukemias and other disorders predominating in the red pulp (chronic myelogenous leukemia).

secondary) proliferation of cordal macrophages. With time, the cords widen and, later, deposition of reticulin and fibrous connective tissue develops. Focal hemorrhages may occur, causing enhanced hemosiderin deposition and formation of siderotic nodules (Gamna-Gandy bodies).

INFECTIONS

Infectious Mononucleosis

Infectious mononucleosis is the best known model of an infectious condition producing expansion of the splenic red pulp,

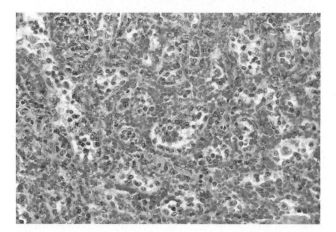

Figure 18.22. Hereditary elliptocytosis. In this condition, like hereditary spherocytosis, the red pulp cords are congested, whereas the sinuses appear deceptively empty.

probably as a result of the tendency of this condition to cause splenic rupture (Fig. 18.23). Rupture of the spleen in infectious mononucleosis has been postulated to result from increased intrasplenic pressure stemming from congestion, and weakening of the capsule as a consequence of infiltration by immunoblasts (141). As with reactive nonfollicular hyperplasia of the white pulp, immunoblastic proliferation is the major histologic feature of infectious mononucleosis. In infectious mononucleosis, however, the proliferating immunoblasts have a predominant distribution in the red pulp. The immunoblasts in the expanded red pulp often result in a disturbing morphologic appearance (142). The red pulp expansion, which results from infiltration of the cords and sinuses by immunoblasts, simulates leukemia, including the tendency for mononucleosis to infiltrate the subintima of intratrabecular veins (33). In addition to an appropriate clinical history, immunoblastic reactivity with both B-cell and T-cell antibodies and lack of positivity for various leukemia markers aid in the diagnosis (143).

Reactivity with both B-cell and T-cell antibodies also serves to distinguish infectious mononucleosis from large-cell lymphoma predominating in the red pulp, including ALCL; similarly to the situation with ALCL, the immunoblasts of acute infectious mononucleosis frequently express the CD30 antigen (143). Moreover, unusual cases are seen with florid immunoblastic proliferation predominating in the splenic red pulp in patients who do not have typical serologic evidence of infectious mononucleosis; these cases generally also exhibit hemophagocytosis (144). In order to solidify a reactive diagnosis, in situ hybridization studies to detect EBV DNA and gene rearrangement studies to demonstrate an absence of B-cell and T-cell clonality may be necessary (145,146).

Acute Septic Splenitis

Acute septic splenitis is a nonspecific term to describe other conditions that cause alterations in the spleen similar to those of infectious mononucleosis. The major differences in acute splenitis are (a) an absence of capsular invasion by immunoblasts, and (b) the generally increased numbers of neutrophils in the red pulp (2). In both conditions, the white pulp is inconspicuous.

Bacillary Angiomatosis

Bacillary angiomatosis is a distinct vascular proliferative disease predominantly involving the skin and lymph nodes of immunocompromised patients, mainly those with AIDS (147,148). This disorder, which is caused by the organism *Bartonella henselae*, may also affect the spleen (149,150). The spleen may show signs of a proliferation of histiocytoid endothelial cells forming vascular channels associated with the presence of granular material; this material can be proven to be bacillary organisms with a Warthin-Starry stain and IHC (150). In some cases, the spleen may manifest peliosis or even rupture (151,152).

HISTIOCYTIC PROLIFERATIONS

Because the red pulp, particularly the cords, is rich in macrophages and is also a major site of phagocytosis of senescent hematopoietic elements, it is not surprising that it is the primary site of histiocytic proliferation in various pathologic conditions.

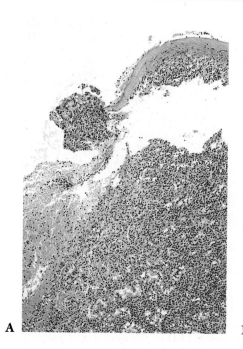

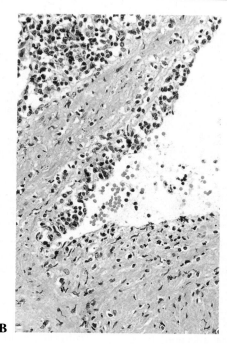

Figure 18.23. Infectious mononucleosis. **(A)** Capsular rupture is a common cause for splenectomy in infectious mononucleosis. Note the expanded cellular red pulp even at this magnification, which is due to proliferating immunoblasts. **(B)** Invasion of the subintima of trabecular veins in infectious mononucleosis is indistinguishable from the pattern observed in most leukemias in the spleen.

Lipid Histiocytoses

Ceroid or sea-blue histiocytosis and Gaucher disease are the major lipid histiocytoses that involve the splenic red pulp. *Ceroid* is a general term employed to describe numerous conditions in which a proliferation of benign histiocytes with abundant, foamy, vacuolated cytoplasm exists (153). These histiocytes are found diffusely in the splenic cords, and, at times they may be so numerous as to widely separate the white pulp. However, unlike neoplastic diseases in the red pulp, the white pulp is not diminished in size. The foamy cytoplasm is a result of the accumulation of a variety of phospholipids, particularly sphingomyelin (154). Ceroid histiocytes react with fat stains and acid-fast stains, as well as with periodic acid-Schiff (PAS) combined with diastase; they also autofluoresce (155).

Ceroid histiocytosis develops in a number of clinical settings, including inherited lipidoses, hyperlipoproteinemia, light chain deposition disease, and chronic myelogenous leukemia (CML), but it is best known in the context of ITP because of the excess phagocytosis of platelets and accumulation of their lipid-rich membranes (16,17,153,156). In ITP, the number of ceroid histiocytes is generally small, but the phagocytosis of platelets is easily seen on touch-imprint preparations and particularly by electron microscopy, where an abundance of myelinic figures is often seen within histiocytic lysosomes (Fig. 18.24) (17,21,155).

Ceroid histiocytosis may also be associated with a primary disorder, the sea-blue histiocyte syndrome (154). This syndrome is thought to be an inherited autosomal recessive disorder and is probably related to adult Niemann-Pick disease (157). The ceroid histiocytes in the primary syndrome are identical in morphologic characteristics to those found in other conditions.

Gaucher disease has a distributional pattern similar to that of ceroid histiocytosis, but the number of histiocytes is generally greater (Fig. 18.25). Spleens from patients with Gaucher disease often are massively enlarged, weighing up to 10,000 g and with a mean volume of 19.8 times normal (158,159). Consequently, the red pulp cords are markedly expanded by the pale-staining

histiocytes. In Gaucher disease, the cytoplasm has a fine, fibrillar appearance (160). This pattern represents the accumulation of glucocerebroside because of a defect in lysosomal glucocerebrosidase (158). Unlike ceroid histiocytosis, the histiocytes in Gaucher disease fail to stain with phospholipid stains, acid-fast stains, or basic dyes, and they have less intense reactivity with PAS; conversely, in contrast to ceroid-containing histiocytes, Gaucher cells stain for iron (155). Gaucher-like cells may occasionally be observed in the red pulp of spleens in patients with chronic hematologic disorders, including CML. Electron microscopy, however, reveals differences from Gaucher cells (160). The pathogenesis probably is the excess catabolism of phagocytosed granulocytes and the secondary depletion of glu-

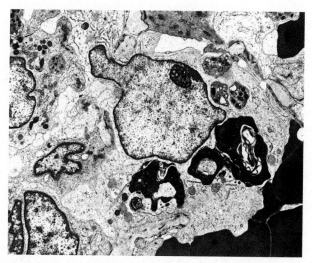

Figure 18.24. Immune thrombocytopenic purpura. Phagocytosed platelets are found within the cordal macrophages in immune thrombocytopenic purpura. The dark-staining myelinic figures in the cytoplasm are probably degraded platelets; this accounts for the ceroid or foamy histiocytes seen by light microscopy (6000×).

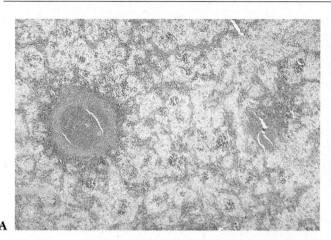
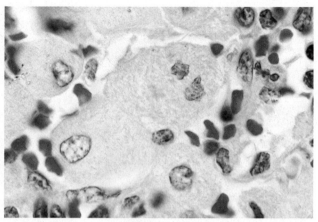

A   B

Figure 18.25.   Gaucher disease. **(A)** The red pulp cords are expanded by lipid-filled histiocytes. Unlike malignant disorders affecting the red pulp, the white pulp remains intact. The identical pattern may be observed in florid ceroid histiocytosis. **(B)** Detail of the fine, fibrillar cytoplasm of Gaucher cells.

cocerebrosidase. Pseudo-Gaucher cells also are reported in patients with AIDS and with mycobacterial infection (161).

Histiocytic and Dendritic Cell Neoplasms

Histiocytic sarcoma is a rare, clinically aggressive neoplasm that most commonly arises in extranodal sites, such as gastrointestinal tract, soft tissue, and skin (162–165). It may develop in patients with follicular lymphoma and, despite the morphologic and immunophenotypic disparities, both tumors can be clonally related (166). The initial involvement of the spleen is extremely uncommon and, as with histiocytic sarcoma in general, this should be diagnosed only after the exclusion of a large-B-cell or T-cell lymphoma, including ALCL (162–168). Histiocytic sarcoma cases react for CD45, CD68, CD163, generally lysozyme and CD4, and, to a lesser extent, S-100 protein. In the spleen, the neoplastic histiocytes form tumor masses in the red pulp (167,168). Historically, histiocytic neoplasms in the spleen had usually been regarded as examples of malignant histiocytosis; however, the term *malignant histiocytosis* currently is limited to cases of disseminated histiocytic sarcoma (13,163).

Paradoxically, hemophagocytosis, a hallmark of histiocytes, is the exception in histiocytic sarcoma (162,163,165,168). In the context of a lymphoma, usually one of T-cell lineage, hemophagocytosis in the spleen generally represents phagocytosis by benign reactive histiocytes, and it often is an indication of a hemophagocytic syndrome (110,111,169). The hemophagocytic syndromes may be precipitated by a viral infection, such as EBV (169). Unlike histiocytic sarcoma or malignant histiocytosis, the histiocytes in the viral-associated hemophagocytic syndrome and those associated with familial hemophagocytic lymphohistiocytosis do not exhibit cytologic atypia (169–171).

Langerhans cell histiocytosis (LCH) in the spleen is not a problem to surgical pathologists because involvement of the spleen is rare and it generally is not described in the unifocal and multifocal cases (172). In the spleen, LCH usually is found only at autopsy and in the acute disseminated syndrome associated with fatal thrombocytopenia due to hypersplenism (173). As an exception, we reviewed one case of adult LCH presenting

with spontaneous splenic rupture (Fig. 18.26). In this case, the distributional features of LCH in the spleen were identical to those of classic malignant histiocytosis, but the cytologic and immunologic characteristics differed, including the reactivity of the Langerhans cells, which reacted with antibodies directed against S-100, vimentin, CD1a, and CD68. Langerhans cell sarcoma can involve the spleen, but the histologic features of this rare, cytologically malignant variant of LCH have not been described in the spleen (163).

Interdigitating dendritic cell (IDC) sarcoma or tumor, an exceedingly uncommon neoplasm, has been suspected and reported in the spleen (174,175). The sarcoma or tumor forms cohesive cell aggregates and confluent masses in the red pulp with impingement of the white pulp (Fig. 18.27). The neoplastic cells are large, with copious amounts of cytoplasm and variable nuclear pleomorphism. They are arranged in sheets and fascicles, and associated erythrophagocytosis can occur. By electron microscopy, the tumor cells possess complex, interdigitating cell processes (174,175). In concert with IDC sarcoma or tumor in the lymph nodes, the malignant cells express S-100 and CD68, but not CD1a (163).

Follicular dendritic cell (FDC) sarcoma or tumor is characterized by the consistent expression of FDC markers, such as CD21 and CD35, but it has variable expression of epithelial membrane antigen, S-100, and CD68 and no reactivity for CD1a (163). FDC sarcoma or tumor also expresses clusterin and podoplanin (D2-40) (176,177). This rare neoplasm usually is discovered in the lymph nodes and extranodal sites, where it is composed of oval and spindle-shaped cells distributed in fascicles and sheets with frequent focal storiform and whorled patterns (178). Occasional cases engage the spleen (163). To date, the largest series of FDC sarcoma or tumor in the spleen consisted of three cases in which the neoplasm mimicked an inflammatory pseudotumor because of an admixture of lymphocytes and plasma cells, in addition to spindle cells (179). In contrast to inflammatory pseudotumor, the FDC neoplasms exhibit nuclear atypia, and they are immunoreactive for CD21 and CD35; unlike conventional FDC sarcoma or tumor, the inflammatory pseudotumor-like cases are EBV-associated (179). Chromosomal aberrations embracing loss of Xp have been described in FDC sarcoma or tumor, including a case that presented in the spleen (180).

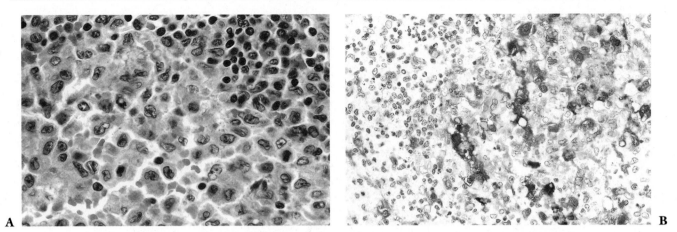

Figure 18.26. Langerhans cell histiocytosis presenting as a ruptured spleen in an adult. **(A)** The paler-staining Langerhans cells in the red pulp impinge upon residual lymphocytes in the white pulp. **(B)** Strong reactivity for S-100 is present in the cytoplasm of the Langerhans cells.

LEUKEMIAS, MYELOPROLIFERATIVE DISEASES, AND MYELODYSPLASTIC SYNDROMES

Chronic Myelogenous Leukemia

Chronic myelogenous leukemia (CML) is the prototype for the malignant disorders that mainly affect the splenic red pulp. This disease diffusely infiltrates the red pulp cords and sinuses, and it generally obliterates the splenic white pulp (2). The diffuse red pulp infiltration imparts a homogeneous solid appearance to the splenic parenchyma, with a lack of visible nodules on cut section that is in contrast to what is seen in most lymphomas (Fig. 18.21). In CML, the infiltrate is polymorphous and includes myeloid cells in all stages of differentiation with an occasional increase in eosinophils and eosinophilic myelocytes (Fig. 18.28). Reactivity with a battery of monoclonal antibodies, such as myeloperoxidase, CD33, CD34, CD68, and CD117 confirms the diagnosis. These reactions are particularly valuable in cases in which the spleen is the initial site of blast crisis prior to any clinical or bone marrow manifestations (2). The blast crisis of CML in the spleen is diagnosed by the morphologic recognition

of immature cells with verification of the diagnosis by IHC means (181). Cytochemical stains also may be done on touch imprints of the spleen. In spleens from CML patients, loss of heterozygosity studies demonstrate frequent allelic losses (182). Caution is required in patients who receive granulocyte colony-stimulating factor because such patients may develop striking myeloid hyperplasia in the spleen to simulate myelogenous leukemia (183).

Myeloid Metaplasia

In the splenic red pulp, the distributional features of myeloid metaplasias, specifically primary myelofibrosis, are similar to those described for CML. In primary myelofibrosis, megakaryocytes, granulocyte precursors, and nucleated red cells may be observed predominantly in the red pulp sinuses in varying proportions (Fig. 18.29) (2). The megakaryocytes occasionally form clusters and may exhibit bizarre morphologic features (181). Reactivity with CD42b or CD63 accentuates the abnormal megakaryocytes. Identical to CML, allelic losses are discovered in the

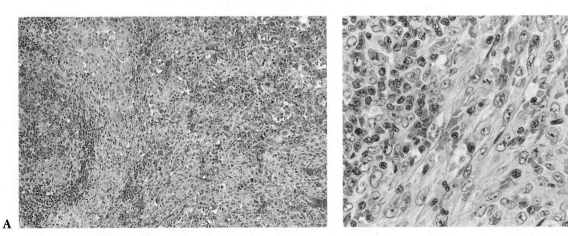

Figure 18.27. Interdigitating dendritic cell sarcoma/tumor. **(A)** The white pulp (*left*) is invaded and diminished in size as a result of diffuse infiltration by malignant cells from the red pulp in a case of interdigitating dendritic cell sarcoma/tumor. **(B)** The malignant cells are large and pleomorphic, and they have a focal fusiform configuration.

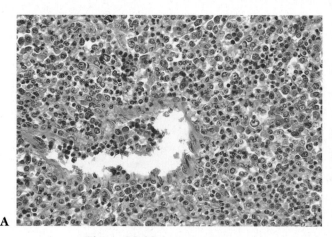

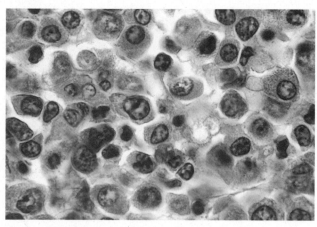

A   **B**

Figure 18.28. Chronic myelogenous leukemia. **(A)** The red pulp cords and sinuses typically are infiltrated, and the white pulp is obliterated in chronic myelogenous leukemia. **(B)** Myeloid cells in all stages of differentiation, including eosinophilic myelocytes, are evident in the red pulp.

spleens with primary myelofibrosis (182); however, in contrast to CML, spleens from primary myelofibrosis exhibit the V617F mutation in the *Janus kinase 2* gene (184). As well as diffuse infiltration of the red pulp sinuses, the pattern of extramedullary hematopoiesis in chronic idiopathic myelofibrosis may also be nodular, and, in a minority of cases, immature myeloid precursors predominate. The observation of myeloid immaturity correlates with decreased survival (185).

Although extramedullary hematopoiesis is observed in cases of CML, all of the three main hematopoietic cell lines generally do not proliferate in relatively equal proportions. In secondary or reactive myeloid metaplasia, such as seen in the spleens from ITP patients, a single cell type of extramedullary hematopoiesis usually predominates, but this finding often is subtle and inconsistent (181,186). For example, extramedullary hematopoiesis may be pronounced in the TTP/hemolytic uremic syndrome and in post-bone marrow transplant spleens. Under these conditions, the extramedullary hematopoiesis may be accompanied by immature histologic features to mimic a myeloproliferative disorder (24,181). However, as opposed to a neoplastic myeloid process, in the benign-associated reactive cases the foci of extramedullary hematopoiesis do not express CD34 or CD117 (181).

Myelodysplastic Syndromes

Patients with myelodysplastic syndromes (MDSs) generally do not have splenomegaly, and information concerning splenic pathologic alterations is limited. In one report of 13 patients with MDS, four histologic patterns in the spleen were described (187). The patterns included a predominance of erythrophagocytosis, another with plasmacytosis of the red pulp, a third characterized by extramedullary hematopoiesis, and one containing a monocytic infiltrate associated with an expanded red pulp found in patients with chronic myelomonocytic leukemia. Clusters of immature large cells were discovered in the red pulp of several cases, and some of those patients evolved into acute myeloid leukemia (187). The spleens from two other patients with MDS also were reported to contain increased immature CD34-positive cells, as well as atypical megakaryocytes including small hypolobated forms (181).

Personal experience with a splenectomy specimen from a patient with long-standing MDS who was diagnosed with refractory anemia and a 5q- abnormality revealed a markedly enlarged red pulp due to diffuse infiltration by atypical mononuclear cells (Fig.18.30). Characterization of the atypical cells by both

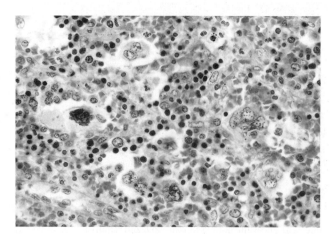

Figure 18.29. Primary myelofibrosis. In this condition, extramedullary hematopoiesis of all three main hematopoietic cell lines is found in the red pulp sinuses.

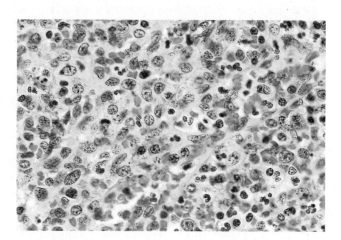

Figure 18.30. Acute myelomonocytic leukemia. This was discovered in the splenic red pulp from a patient with a documented myelodysplastic syndrome, specifically refractory anemia and the 5q- abnormality.

flow cytometry and immunoperoxidase stains indicated that they correlated with acute myelomonocytic leukemia.

Hairy Cell Leukemia

Splenomegaly is frequently the initial symptom in patients with hairy cell leukemia (HCL). The patients often suffer from hypersplenism, and their spleens have a median weight of 1000 g. Although splenectomy is no longer the standard therapy for patients with HCL, the pathologic features in the spleen are distinctive. As in CML, the red pulp cords and sinuses are infiltrated diffusely (Fig. 18.31). The white pulp may be completely obliterated, or it may appear atrophic and encroached upon by the infiltrating hairy cells. The subendothelium of the trabecular veins is consistently infiltrated (188). The hairy cells in the spleen are cytologically bland and homogeneous. Mitotic figures are uncommon. The nuclei usually are oval or reniform, and the cytoplasm is characteristically abundant and lucent, often with well-delineated cell borders (188). The presence of variably dilated sinuses filled with red cells ("lakes") and lined by hairy cells ("pseudosinuses") is another characteristic morphologic feature of spleens involved by HCL (189). In rare cases, the blood lakes may be so prominent as to resemble a cavernous hemangioma. The red cell lakes, however, are not pathognomonic of HCL, and, on occasion, may be found in other leukemias involving the spleen, such as CLL (188). Extramedullary megakaryopoiesis also may be found occasionally in the splenic red pulp in HCL. Because patients with HCL are prone to develop infections, including those caused by atypical acid-fast bacilli, cases of HCL in the spleen may be masked by the presence of large, necrotizing granulomas (188).

Although these morphologic criteria usually serve to distinguish HCL from other leukemias in the spleen, they may not be valid for patients with HCL and only minimally enlarged or normal-weight spleens. Under these circumstances, the infiltration of the red pulp is subtle, and the hairy cells are frequently identified only adjacent to fibrous trabeculae, where they form small aggregates (188). In some cases, immunohistologic studies are required for a definitive diagnosis (190). In sections, the hairy cells express B-cell antigens, including CD20 and CD79a, but not CD5, CD10, or CD23. They also react with monoclonal

antibody DBA.44, express cyclin D1, and are tartrate-resistant acid phosphatase (TRAP)-positive (47,191). CD123, annexin A1, and the T-cell associated transcription factor T-bet are newer markers that expedite the diagnosis of HCL in paraffin sections (76,77,192). Employing flow cytometry, the hairy cells strongly express CD11c, CD25, and CD103 (193).

Splenic B-cell Lymphoma/Leukemia, Unclassifiable

Splenic B-cell lymphoma/leukemia, unclassifiable obviously accommodates splenic small B-neoplasms that do not fulfill the canons of a well-defined clinicopathologic entity, as well as the newly proposed provisional category of splenic diffuse red pulp small B-cell lymphoma and also hairy cell leukemia variant (HCL-V) (13a). As discussed earlier, splenic diffuse red pulp small B-cell lymphoma embraces the cases that were formerly proposed as the diffuse red pulp variant of SMZL and those cases that were more recently interpreted as splenic red pulp lymphoma with numerous basophilic villous lymphocytes (66,69,74,91a). Splenic diffuse red pulp small B-cell lymphoma is morphologically indistinguishable from HCL and HCL-V (66,74,194,195). The diffuse distributional features (Fig 18.11), including the presence of red cell lakes, as well as the absence of tumor nodules in the white pulp, are identical in these conditions; however, splenic diffuse red pulp small B-cell lymphoma frequently exhibits more cytologic polymorphism containing occasional larger, blast-type lymphocytes with conspicuous nucleoli (13a). Splenic diffuse red pulp small B-cell lymphoma and HCL share immunophenotypic markers including the expression of CD103 in a minority of the splenic diffuse red pulp small B-cell lymphoma cases (91a,195). Cyclin D1, CD123, and annexin A1 facilitate the diagnosis since these three markers are usually negative in splenic diffuse red pulp small B-cell lymphoma, whereas they are positive in HCL (13a,47,76,77).

HCL-V can contain red cell lakes and also simulates HCL by its diffuse red pulp pattern of leukemic infiltration in the spleen and occasional TRAP positivity (194,195). The immunophenotype of HCL-V equally mimics HCL with the expression of DBA.44, CD11c and CD103, but, unlike typical HCL, the variant cells are CD25 negative and do not express CD123 or annexin A1 (76,77,194). In point of fact, the most challenging differential diagnosis in the spleen rests not between HCL and HCL-V or HCL and splenic diffuse red pulp small B-cell lymphoma, but between HCL-V and splenic diffuse red pulp small B-cell lymphoma; moreover, it remains contentious whether HCL-V and splenic diffuse red pulp small B-cell lymphoma are actually discrete malignancies. In both neoplasms, the histologic features in the spleen and immunophenotype are interchangeable as is a frequently similar pattern of sinusoidal bone marrow involvement, although the coexpression of preswitched with postswitched immunoglobulin heavy chain isotypes found in HCL-V appears different (194,196).

T-Cell Large-Granular Lymphocyte Leukemia

T-cell large-granular lymphocyte leukemia (T-LGL) is a heterogenous disorder resulting from the clonal proliferation of large-granular lymphocytes; these most commonly are CD3+, TCRαβ+, CD4−, CD8+, and NK-related antigen CD57+. CD5 and CD7 expression is often aberrant, with frequent dim or absent expression of these antigens (197). In tissue sections,

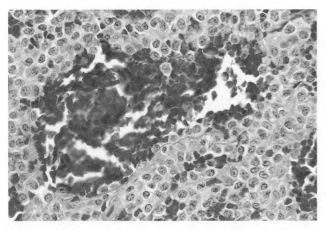

Figure 18.31. Hairy cell leukemia. Massive diffuse invasion of the red pulp cords and sinuses is typical in hairy cell leukemia. The hairy cells are homogeneous on cytologic examination, they have abundant pale cytoplasm, and they line dilated sinuses or red cell lakes.

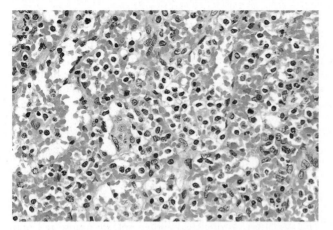

Figure 18.32. T-cell large-granular lymphocyte leukemia. Similar to hairy cell leukemia (HCL), the red pulp is diffusely infiltrated in T-cell large-granular lymphocyte leukemia. In contrast to HCL, no red cell lakes are present and the white pulp contains reactive follicles.

no reactivity is found for CD5 and CD45RO, but the cytotoxic-granule–associated protein TIA1 is consistently expressed (136). However, deviations from this immunophenotype do occur and multiparameter studies are often required for diagnosis (198,199). Patients with T-LGL generally have an indolent clinical course with chronic, often severe neutropenia and auto-immune features (199,200). Splenomegaly is a common clinical finding. T-LGL in the spleen is reported to reposit mainly in the red pulp (136,201,202). The red pulp cords and sinuses are infiltrated by the proliferating, usually medium-sized, round lymphocytes (Fig. 18.32). The white pulp is not involved, but it often displays prominent germinal centers; associated plasmacytosis is seen in the red pulp (201). In the spleen, T-LGL differs from reactive follicular hyperplasia, such as that found in Felty syndrome, by the monomorphous CD3+, CD8+ lymphocytic infiltrate in the red pulp cords and sinuses. The T-cell infiltrate in the red pulp and lack of red cell lakes are unlike that found in the spleens involved by HCL, as are the preserved, hyperplastic germinal centers in the white pulp; in HCL, the splenic white pulp is almost always atrophic and over-

run by the hairy cell infiltrate (188,195). Atrophy and loss of the white pulp are similarly present in hepatosplenic T-cell lymphoma, in contrast to T-LGL. Both T-LGL and hepatosplenic T-cell lymphoma share immunophenotypic features, but the hepatosplenic T-cell lymphoma cases tend to be CD8− and have isochrome 7q (109,116).

A CD3+, CD56+ aggressive form of T-LGL has been described in which massive splenomegaly occurs due to extensive diffuse infiltration of the red pulp by the lymphoid cells, similar to that seen in the more indolent form of T-LGL (203). The CD3+, CD56+ variant may overlap with hepatosplenic T-cell lymphoma and the rare cases of S-100 protein-positive PTCL (109,204). T-LGL also may transform to a large-cell form of PTCL that coexpresses CD30 (205).

Systemic Mastocytosis

Systemic mastocytosis is a rare disorder that is characterized by a systemic neoplastic proliferation of mast cells and by the frequent detection of the D816V mutation of *c-kit* in the malignant mast cells (206). In this disease, up to 72% of patients have clinically enlarged spleens (207–209). Rarely, the spleen will be the sole anatomic site that is diagnostic of mastocytosis (210). Mast cell infiltration of the spleen is frequently accompanied by fibrosis, which can be observed on the splenic cut surface on macroscopic examination. The fibrous connective tissue can have a diffuse distribution, or it can appear around the mast cell infiltrates (Fig. 18.33). The infiltrating mast cells tend to concentrate in the red pulp, particularly around trabeculae and the capsule (207,208). They also can affect the parafollicular and follicular regions of the white pulp, and, in some cases, they diffusely invade the red pulp. Although neoplastic mast cells may cytologically resemble hairy cells in tissue sections, their tendency to aggregate and to form nodules, even within the red pulp, aids in distinguishing them from cases of HCL. Metachromatic stains and a combination of reactivity for mast cell tryptase, as well as for CD2, CD25, CD43, CD68, CD117, and histidine decarboxylase confirm the diagnosis (206,211–213).

NONHEMATOPOIETIC TUMORS

Nonhematopoietic tumors are a group of disparate lesions that generally are distributed throughout the splenic red pulp, al-

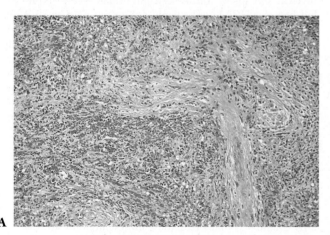

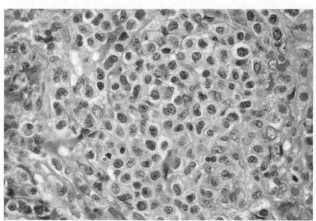

Figure 18.33. Systemic mastocytosis. **(A)** An irregular proliferation of fibrous connective tissue is seen adjacent to the mast cell aggregates. **(B)** The neoplastic mast cells resemble hairy cells, but the fibrous connective tissue reaction and the nodular aggregates help to distinguish between mast cells and hairy cells in the spleen.

though they may form tumor nodules or masses. Most of these lesions are relatively uncommon, and they usually are an incidental finding. They may, however, result in diagnostic confusion because, on occasion, patients with these lesions do present with hypersplenism.

Developmental Lesions

Benign cysts of the spleen are unusual and they typically do not create diagnostic problems. They are lined by either squamous epithelium or mesothelial-type cells. Cysts with an epithelial lining are regarded as true cysts, whereas those in which a cellular lining is absent are considered false cysts (214). The squamous-lined epithelial cysts are the most common splenic cyst; they are thought to result from metaplasia in mesothelial cysts, which, in turn, are postulated to stem from trauma (215). Cases reported as solitary splenic lymphangiomas are also mesothelial cysts. In contrast to lymphangiomas, the lining cells in such cysts do not express vascular markers, such as factor VIII–related antigen, CD31, or CD34; rather, they react for cytokeratin and the mesothelial-associated antibody HBME-1 (216).

Splenic hamartomas usually are discovered as incidental, well-circumscribed nodules in the splenic red pulp (217). Approximately 15% of patients present with symptoms and these mostly develop in association with larger hamartomatous nodules (218); hamartomas are reported to vary from 0.3 cm to 20 cm in size. In contrast to lymphoma, splenic hamartomas are red, unencapsulated, and frequently hemorrhagic. White pulp and fibrous trabeculae usually are not found within hamartomas, but extramedullary hematopoiesis may be discerned. The hamartomas are composed of a disorganized series of anastomotic channels lined and supported by endothelial-type cells (130,214,217). A haphazard stroma is interspersed between the endothelial cells. The stroma is often loose and embraces macrophages, lymphocytes, erythrocytes, spindle cells, and an inconstant degree of fibrosis (218). The stromal cells in splenic hamartomas may occasionally appear bizarre with large oval to irregular nuclei, but they are without mitotic activity (219). The bizarre cells generally have a negative IHC profile; however, one case report described reactivity for both desmin and cytokeratin in the bizarre cells to suggest that they are a type of fibroblastic reticulum cell (220). In the context of a hamartoma, the bizarre stromal cells should not be construed as malignant. Nonetheless, a malignant neoplasm that was composed of fibroblastic reticulum cells has been reported in the spleen (221). Splenic hamartomas may appear remarkably similar to hemangiomas, but they can be differentiated by the use of immunologic markers, such as the expression of vascular antigens, including factor VIII and CD31, as well as CD8 by the hamartomatous endothelium; hemangiomas express factor VIII and CD31, but lack CD8 (222).

Vascular Neoplasms

Vascular neoplasms are the most common primary nonhematopoietic tumors of the spleen, and they are mainly analogous to their counterparts in other sites. The neoplasms include hemangiomas, lymphangiomas, littoral cell angiomas, and angiosarcomas (223). Many hemangiomas are localized and generally measure 4 cm or less in diameter; however, splenic involvement may form part of a pattern of generalized angiomatosis and

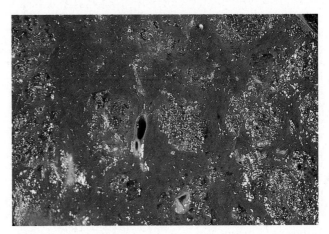

Figure 18.34. Multiple spongelike nodular hemangiomas on the cut surface of this 790-g spleen.

diffuse involvement of the splenic red pulp with a predominantly cavernous, or a less common capillary hemangiomatous pattern may be observed (Fig. 18.34) (223,224). The diffuse splenic hemangiomas may be CD68-positive (222,223). In most cases, the lesions are found only incidentally; occasionally, however, patients may develop hemorrhage and even hypersplenism (137). Lymphangiomas of the spleen usually are part of the spectrum of disseminated lymphangiomatosis. The lumens of lymphangiomas contain proteinaceous material rather than red cells, and the endothelium may form small papillary projections (223). As was already noted, the so-called solitary subcapsular splenic lymphangiomas are actually mesothelial cysts (216).

Littoral cell angiomas are unique splenic vascular neoplasms composed of anastomosing vascular channels that resemble splenic sinuses and that often have papillary projections and cystlike spaces (225). The endothelial cells frequently detach into the vascular spaces (Fig. 18.35) and evidence hemophagocytosis. In addition to factor VIII–related antigen expression, which is seen in normal splenic sinus endothelium, the lining

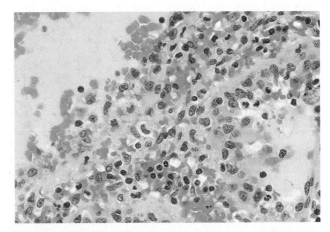

Figure 18.35. Littoral cell angioma. Such cases are characterized by enlarged vascular channels that are lined by papillary-type endothelial cells, which frequently desquamate into the lumens. The lining cells express histiocytic antigens as well as vascular markers, including factor VIII–related antigen and CD31.

cells of littoral cell angioma also express histiocytic markers, such as CD68, CD163, and lysozyme (225,226). Unlike other splenic vascular tumors, littoral cell angiomas express CD31, but not CD34 (222,223). The clinical behavior of patients with littoral cell angioma appears benign, although cases of seemingly malignant littoral cell tumors have been reported, with some examples being designated as *littoral cell hemangioendothelioma* to reflect transitional attributes between angioma and angiosarcoma (227–229).

Angiosarcomas of the spleen are rare aggressive neoplasms with a high metastatic rate; fewer than 150 primary cases have been reported (214,223,230,231). The most dramatic presentation is splenic rupture, which is seen in approximately 13% to 33% of cases. Angiosarcomas can form large hemorrhagic tumor nodules or masses in the splenic red pulp, or a series of diffuse, spongelike anastomosing channels that are lined by characteristic atypical, budded endothelial cells (Fig. 18.36). They also can simulate a cavernous hemangioma; normal splenic sinuses; or another sarcoma, such as Kaposi sarcoma (230–232). Splenic angiosarcomas mark for various vascular antigens and occasionally CD34 and CD8 (222). They also can express histiocytic antigens to suggest that some angiosarcomas may originate from splenic lining cells (231).

Other primary splenic vascular malignant neoplasms, including those of uncertain malignant potential—specifically, Kaposi sarcoma, hemangiopericytoma, and angioendothelioma—are even less common than splenic angiosarcomas (233–236). Nonvascular primary sarcomas of the spleen are extremely rare, with malignant fibrous histiocytoma being the most common type reported (237).

Metastases

Metastases to the spleen from various neoplasms, including lung, gastrointestinal tract, breast, ovary, and malignant melanoma, are usually discovered at autopsy. In one study of 1280 consecutive splenectomy specimens, 1.3% of the spleens contained a metastasis, and, in the same study, metastases were discovered in 9.8% of 122 of the diagnostic splenectomy specimens (36). With modern medical imaging techniques, the prevalence of splenic metastases appears to be escalating (238). Rarely, metastases cause clinical symptoms, including those re-

lated to splenomegaly. One series described seven such cases in which splenic enlargement or rupture resulted from metastatic carcinoma from the placenta, colon, lung, pancreas, and ovary (239). Another report described metastatic carcinoma of the breast in the spleen that presented as ITP (240). Metastases to the spleen may appear as diffuse infiltrates in the red pulp; more typically, they form tumor nodules.

Inflammatory Pseudotumor

Inflammatory pseudotumors of the spleen are unusual lesions that involve the splenic red pulp and form prominent, well delineated, nodular masses, thus replacing the parenchyma to simulate malignant lymphomas (241). The nodules have a median size of 6.2 cm and, in some cases, more than one nodular mass is present (218). The mass lesions are composed of a heterogeneous proliferation of various reactive cells with a typical zonal distribution; they are delineated by variably dense, benign-appearing, spindle-shaped fibrous tissue. Central necrosis and hemorrhage with cholesterol formation may be observed. These areas are surrounded by lymphocytes, sheets of plasma cells, fibroblasts, and even epithelioid granulomas. The lymphocytes are mainly of T-cell lineage (241). The spindle cells are mostly vimentin+ fibroblasts, but some spindle cells are myofibroblasts that express smooth muscle actin, whereas others are CD68+ spindled histiocytes (218,242). The spindle cells also may be EBV+ ; in one case, the EBV genome was proven to be clonal (242,243). The pathologic features are similar to those of inflammatory myofibroblastic tumors in soft tissue, except that the lesions in the spleen do not react for anaplastic lymphoma kinase (218,244). As was already discussed, inflammatory pseudotumors must be distinguished from a malignant process, such as FDC sarcoma or a tumor with a prominent chronic inflammatory cell reaction (179).

Another benign, spindle-shaped lesion has been described in the spleen in patients with AIDS; it is designated mycobacterial spindle cell pseudotumor (245). In this pseudotumor, clusters of spindle cells form nodules in the red pulp. The spindle cells are of histiocytic lineage and abundant acid-fast bacilli are demonstrable in the cytoplasm.

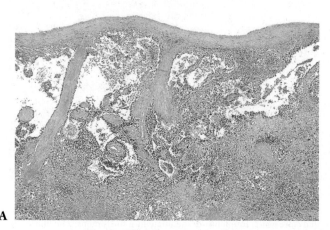
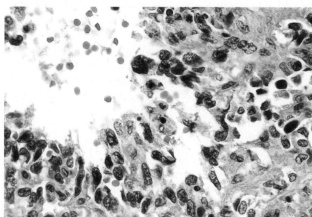

A   **B**

Figure 18.36. Angiosarcoma of the spleen. **(A)** Dilated anastomosing vascular channels in angiosarcoma of the spleen. **(B)** The neoplastic endothelial cells are clearly budded and atypical.

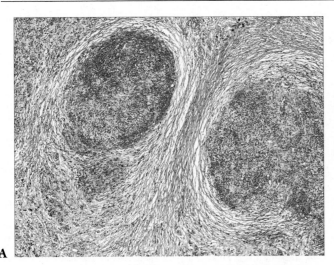
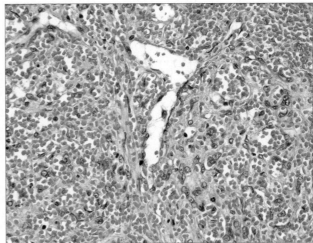

A   B

Figure 18.37. Sclerosing angiomatoid nodular transformation (SANT). **(A)** SANT is composed of a series of angiomatoid nodules set in a dense, collagenized stroma. **(B)** Detail of the vascular spaces in an angiomatoid nodule that contains many erythrocytes.

Sclerosing Angiomatoid Nodular Transformation

Sclerosing angiomatoid nodular transformation (SANT) is a recently described nonneoplastic vascular lesion of the spleen that has been proposed to represent an unusual transformation of the red pulp in response to an exaggerated stromal proliferation (246). Occasionally, such cases were reported in the past as a variant of a splenic hamartoma, for example, cord capillary hemangioma (218). Most frequently, SANT is discovered as an incidental finding. The lesions appear as a solitary, well-circumscribed, unencapsulated, round to bosselated mass ranging from 3 to 17 cm (246). SANT comprises a series of angiomatoid nodules embedded in a dense fibrosclerotic stroma (Fig. 18.37). The angiomatoid nodules are composed of slitlike, variably irregular vascular spaces that are lined by ovoid, benign-appearing endothelial cells; the vascular lumens are either empty or contain erythrocytes. Lymphocytes and plasma cells are frequently found in the angiomatoid nodules (246). The internodular stroma is dense fibrous or fibromyxoid tissue that is often hyalinized and may contain dystrophic calcifications as well as chronic inflammatory cells. IHC studies reveal that the angiomatoid nodules recapitulate the splenic red pulp embracing sinuses (CD31+, CD8+, CD34−), capillaries (CD31+, CD8−, CD34+), and small veins (CD31+, CD8−, CD34−) (246). The histologic and immunophenotypic features of SANT differ from other angiomatous splenic lesions, such as hemangiomas (including littoral cell angiomas), and from inflammatory pseudotumors. They also differ from a splenic hamartoma, although the likelihood that SANT is a sclerotic variety of hamartoma, or even a sclerotic version of an inflammatory pseudotumor or an organized hematoma, cannot be entirely excluded (246). In rendering a diagnosis of SANT, metastatic carcinoma must be considered in the differential diagnosis because a splenic metastasis can form a series of sclerotic vascular nodules to mimic SANT.

REFERENCES

1. Burke JS. Surgical pathology of the spleen: an approach to the differential diagnosis of splenic lymphomas and leukemias. Part I. Diseases of the white pulp. *Am J Surg Pathol* 1981;5:551–563.

2. Burke JS. Surgical pathology of the spleen: an approach to the differential diagnosis of splenic lymphoma and leukemias. Part II. Diseases of the red pulp. *Am J Surg Pathol* 1981; 5:681–694.

3. Fahri DC, Ashfaq R. Splenic pathology after traumatic injury. *Am J Clin Pathol* 1996;105: 474–478.

4. Carr NJ, Turk EP. The histological features of splenosis. *Histopathology* 1992;21:549–553.

5. Burke JS. Splenic lymphoid hyperplasia versus lymphomas/leukemias: a diagnostic guide. *Am J Clin Pathol* 1993;99:486–493.

6. van Krieken JHJM, te Velde J. Normal histology of the human spleen. *Am J Surg Pathol* 1988;12:777–785.

7. Burke JS, Simon GT. Electron microscopy of the spleen. I. Anatomy and microcirculation. *Am J Pathol* 1970;58:127–155.

8. Chadburn A. The spleen: anatomy and anatomical function. *Semin Hematol* 2000;37(Suppl 1):13–21.

9. Mebius RE, Kraal G. Structure and function of the spleen. *Nat Rev Immunol* 2005;5: 606–616.

10. Nolte MA, Arens R, Kraus M, et al. B cells are crucial for both development and maintenance of the splenic marginal zone. *J Immunol* 2004;172:3620–3627.

11. Kraus MD. Splenic histology and histopathology: an update. *Semin Diagn Pathol* 2003;20: 84–93.

12. Jaffe ES, Banks PM, Nathwani B, et al. Recommendations for the reporting of lymphoid neoplasms: a report from the Association of Directors of Anatomic and Surgical Pathology. The Ad Hoc Committee on Reporting of Lymphoid Neoplasms. *Hum Pathol* 2002;33: 1064–1068.

13. Jaffe ES, Harris NL, Stein H, et al. *Pathology and Genetics of Tumours of Haematopoietic and Lymphoid Tissues.* Lyon, France: IARC Press, 2001.

13a. Swerdlow SH, Campo E, Harris NL, et al. *WHO Classification of Tumours of Haematopoietic and Lymphoid Tissues*, 4th ed. Lyon, France: IARC Press, 2008.

14. Laszlo J, Jones R, Silberman HR, et al. Splenectomy for Felty's syndrome: clinicopathological study of 27 patients. *Arch Intern Med* 1978;183:597–602.

15. van Krieken JHJM, Breedveld FS, te Velde J. The spleen in Felty's syndrome: a histological, morphometrical, and immunohistochemical study. *Eur J Haematol* 1988;40:58–64.

16. Tavassoli M, McMillan R. Structure of the spleen in idiopathic thrombocytopenic purpura. *Am J Clin Pathol* 1975;64:180–191.

17. Lasser A. Diffuse histiocytosis of the spleen and idiopathic thrombocytopenic purpura (ITP): histochemical and ultrastructural studies. *Am J Clin Pathol* 1983;80:529–533.

18. Hom BL, Belles Q, Oishi N. Splenic histiocytosis in idiopathic thrombocytopenic purpura: a relative sphingomyelinase deficiency? *Hum Pathol* 1985;16:1175–1177.

19. Schmidt EE, MacDonald IC, Groom AC. Changes in splenic microcirculatory pathways in chronic idiopathic thrombocytopenic purpura. *Blood* 1991;78:1485–1489.

20. Cooper N, Bussel J. The pathogenesis of immune thrombocytopaenic purpura. *Br J Haematol* 2006;133:364–374.

21. Hassan NMR, Neiman RS. The pathology of the spleen in steroid-treated immune thrombocytopenic purpura. *Am J Clin Pathol* 1985;84:433–438.

22. Chang C-S, Li C-L, Cha SS. Chronic idiopathic thrombocytopenic purpura: splenic pathologic features and their clinical correlation. *Arch Pathol Lab Med* 1993;117:981–985.

23. Marcaccio MJ. Laparoscopic splenectomy in chronic idiopathic thrombocytopenic purpura. *Semin Hematol* 2000;37:267–274.

24. Saracco SM, Fahri DC. Splenic pathology in thrombotic throbocytopenic purpura. *Am J Surg Pathol* 1990;14:223–229.

25. Weisenburger DD, Nathwani BN, Winberg CD, et al. Multicentric angiofollicular lymph node hyperplasia: pathology of the spleen. *Am J Surg Pathol* 1988;12:176–181.

26. Diaz LK, Murphy RL, Phair JP, et al. The AIDS autopsy spleen: a comparison of the pre–anti-retroviral and highly active anti-retroviral therapy eras. *Mod Pathol* 2002;15: 406–412.

27. Burke JS, Osborne BM. Localized reactive lymphoid hyperplasia of the spleen simulating malignant lymphoma: a report of seven cases. *Am J Surg Pathol* 1983;7:373–380.
28. Wilkins BS, Davis Z, Lucas SB. et al. Splenic marginal zone atrophy and progressive CD8+ T-cell lymphocytosis in HIV infection: a study of adult post-mortem spleens from Côte d'Ivoire. *Histopathology* 2003;42:173–185.
29. Markowitz GS, Factor SM, Borczuk AC. Splenic para-amyloid material: a possible vasculopathy of the acquired immunodeficiency syndrome. *Hum Pathol* 1998;29:371–376.
30. Falk S, Müller H, Stutte H-J. The spleen in acquired immunodeficiency syndrome (AIDS). *Pathol Res Pract* 1988;183:425–433.
31. Rousselet MC, Audouin J, Le Tourneau A, et al. Idiopathic thrombocytopenic purpura in patients at risk for acquired immunodeficiency syndrome: histopathologic study, immunohistochemistry, and ultrastructural study on six spleens. *Arch Pathol Lab Med* 1988;112: 1242–1250.
32. Marti M, Feliu E, Campo E, et al. Comparative study of spleen pathology in drug abusers with thrombocytopenia related to human immunodeficiency virus infection and in patients with idiopathic thrombocytopenic purpura: a morphometric, immunohistochemical, and ultrastructural study. *Am J Clin Pathol* 1993;100:633–642.
33. Gowing NFC. Infectious mononucleosis: histopathologic aspects. *Pathol Annu* 1975;10: 1–20.
34. Kraemer BB, Osborne BM, Butler JJ. Primary splenic presentation of malignant lymphoma and related disorders: a study of 49 cases. *Cancer* 1984;54:1606–1619.
35. Falk S, Stutte HJ. Primary malignant lymphomas of the spleen: a morphologic and immunohistochemical analysis of 17 cases. *Cancer* 1990;66:2612–2619.
36. Kraus MD, Fleming MD, Vonderheide RH. The spleen as a diagnostic specimen: a review of 10 years' experience at two tertiary care institutions. *Cancer* 2001;91:2001–2009.
37. Arber DA, Rappaport H, Weiss LM. Non-Hodgkin's lymphoproliferative disorders involving the spleen. *Mod Pathol* 1997;10:18.32.
38. Pittaluga S, Verhoef G, Criel A, et al. "Small" B-cell non-Hodgkin's lymphomas with splenomegaly at presentation are either mantle cell lymphoma or marginal zone lymphoma: a study based on histology, cytology, immunohistochemistry, and cytogenetic analysis. *Am J Surg Pathol* 1996;20:211–223.
39. Kaplan HS. *Hodgkin's Disease*, 2nd edition. Cambridge, MA: Harvard University Press, 1980.
40. Goffinet DR, Warnke R, Dunnick NR, et al. Clinical and surgical (laparotomy) evaluation of patients with non-Hodgkin's lymphomas. *Cancer Treat Rep* 1977;61:981–992.
41. van Krieken JHJM, Feller AC, te Velde J. The distribution of non-Hodgkin's lymphoma in the lymphoid compartments of the human spleen. *Am J Surg Pathol* 1989;13:757–765.
42. The Non-Hodgkin's Lymphoma Pathologic Classification Project. A clinical evaluation of the International Lymphoma Study Group classification of non-Hodgkin's lymphoma. *Blood* 1997; 89:3909–3918.
43. Ruchlemer R, Wotherspoon AC, Thompson JN, et al. Splenectomy in mantle cell lymphoma with leukaemia: a comparison with chronic lymphocytic leukaemia. *Br J Haematol* 2002;118:952–958.
44. Kansal R, Ross CW, Singleton TP, et al. Histopathologic features of splenic small B-cell lymphomas. A study of 42 cases with a definitive diagnosis by the World Health Organization classification. *Am J Clin Pathol* 2003;120:335–347.
45. Edelman M, Evans L, Zee S, et al. Splenic micro-anatomical localization of small lymphocytic lymphoma/chronic lymphocytic leukemia using a novel combined silver nitrate and immunoperoxidase technique. *Am J Surg Pathol* 1997;21:445–452.
46. de Leon ED, Alkan S, Huang JC, et al. Usefulness of an immunohistochemical panel in paraffin-embedded tissues for the differentiation of B-cell non-Hodgkin's lymphomas of small lymphocytes. *Mod Pathol* 1998;11:1046–1051.
47. Miranda RN, Briggs RC, Kinney MC, et al. Immunohistochemical detection of cyclin D1 using optimized conditions is highly specific for mantle cell lymphoma and hairy cell leukemia. *Mod Pathol* 2000;13:1308–1314.
48. Braylan RC, Long JC, Jaffe ES, et al. Malignant lymphoma obscured by concomitant extensive epithelioid granulomas. *Cancer* 1977;39:1146–1155.
49. Soma LA, Gollin SM, Remstein ED, et al. Splenic small B-cell lymphoma with *IHG/BCL3* translocation. *Hum Pathol* 2006;37:218.230.
50. Falk S, Stutte, HJ. Morphologic manifestations of malignant lymphomas in the spleen: a histologic and immunohistochemical study of 500 biopsy cases. *Prog Surg Pathol* 1992;12: 49–95.
51. Ben-Ezra J, Burke JS, Swartz WG, et al. Small lymphocytic lymphoma: a clinicopathologic analysis of 268 cases. *Blood* 1989;73:579–587.
52. Andriko J-AW, Swerdlow SH, Aguilera NI, et al. Is lymphoplasmacytic lymphoma/immunocytoma a distinct entity? A clinicopathologic study of 20 cases. *Am J Surg Pathol* 2001; 25:742–751.
53. Audouin J, Diebold J, Schvartz H, et al. Malignant lymphoplasmacytic lymphoma with prominent splenomegaly (primary lymphoma of the spleen). *J Pathol* 1988;155:17–33.
54. Krause MD. Lymphoplasmacytic lymphoma/Waldenström macroglobulinemia: one disease or three? *Am J Clin Pathol* 2001;116:799–801.
55. Van Huyen J-PD, Molina T, Delmer A, et al. Splenic marginal zone lymphoma with or without plasmacytic differentiation. *Am J Surg Pathol* 2000;24:1581–1592.
56. Berger F, Traverse-Glehen A, Felman P, et al. Clinicopathologic features of Waldenström's macroglobulinemia and marginal zone lymphoma: are they distinct or the same entity? *Clin Lymphoma* 2005;5:220–224.
57. Horny H-P, Saal J, Kaiserling E. Primary splenic presentation of plasma cell dyscrasia: report of two cases. *Hematol Pathol* 1992;6:155–160.
58. Pittaluga S, Wlodarska I, Stul MS, et al. Mantle cell lymphoma: a clinicopathologic study of 55 cases. *Histopathology* 1995;26:17–24.
59. Campo E, Raffeld M, Jaffe ES. Mantle-cell lymphoma. *Semin Hematol* 1999;36:115–127.
60. Swerdlow SH, Williams ME. From centrocytic to mantle cell lymphoma: a clinicopathologic and molecular review of 3 decades. *Hum Pathol* 2002;33:7–20.
61. Angelopoulou MK, Siakantariz MP, Vassilakopoulos TP, et al. The splenic form of mantle cell lymphoma. *Eur J Haematol* 2002;68:12–21.
62. Oinonen R, Franssila K, Elonen E. Spontaneous splenic rupture in two patients with a blastoid variant of mantle cell lymphoma. *Ann Hematol* 1997;74:33–35.
63. Ruchlemer R, Parry-Jones N, Brito-Babapulle V, et al. B-prolymphocytic leukaemia with t(11;14) revisited: a splenomegalic form of mantle cell lymphoma evolving with leukaemia. *Br J Haematol* 2004;125:330–336.
64. Piris MA, Mollejo M, Campo E, et al. A marginal zone pattern may be found in different varieties of non-Hodgkin's lymphoma: the morphology and immunohistology of splenic involvement by B-cell lymphomas simulating splenic marginal zone lymphoma. *Histopathology* 1998;33:230–239.
65. Schmid C, Kirkham N, Diss T, et al. Splenic marginal zone cell lymphoma. *Am J Surg Pathol* 1992;16:455–466.
66. Papadaki T, Stamatopoulos K, Belessi C, et al. Splenic marginal-zone lymphoma: one or more entities? A histologic, immunohistochemical, and molecular study of 42 cases. *Am J Surg Pathol* 2007;31:438–446.
67. Mollejo M, Menarguez J, Lloret E, et al. Splenic marginal zone lymphoma: a distinctive type of low-grade B-cell lymphoma. A clinicopathologic study of 13 cases. *Am J Surg Pathol* 1995;19:1146–1157.
68. Pawade J, Wilkins BS, Wright DH. Low-grade B-cell lymphomas of the splenic marginal zone: a clinicopathological and immunohistochemical study of 14 cases. *Histopathology* 1995;27:129–137.
69. Hammer RD, Glick AD, Greer JP, et al. Splenic marginal zone lymphoma: a distinct B-cell neoplasm. *Am J Surg Pathol* 1996; 20:613–626.
70. Fend F, Kraus-Huonder B, Müller-Hermelink H-K, et al. Monocytoid B-cell lymphoma: its relationship to and possible cellular origin from marginal zone cells. *Hum Pathol* 1993; 24:336–339.
71. Du M-Q, Peng H-Z, Dogan A, et al. Preferential dissemination of B-cell gastric mucosa-associated lymphoid tissue (MALT) lymphoma to the splenic marginal zone. *Blood* 1997; 90:4071–4077.
72. Rosso R, Neiman RS, Paulli M, et al. Splenic marginal zone cell lymphoma: report of an indolent variant without massive splenomegaly presumably representing an early phase of the disease. *Hum Pathol* 1995;26:39–46.
73. Kroft SH, Singleton TP, Dahiya M, et al. Ruptured spleens with expanded marginal zones do not reveal occult B-cell clones. *Mod Pathol* 1997;10:1214–12220.
74. Mollejo M, Algara P, Mateo MS, et al. Splenic small B-cell lymphoma with predominant red pulp involvement: a diffuse variant of splenic marginal zone lymphoma? *Histopathology* 2002;40:22–30.
75. Melo JV, Hegde U, Parreira A, et al. Splenic B cell lymphoma with circulating villous lymphocytes: differential diagnosis of B cell leukaemias with large spleens. *J Clin Pathol* 1987;40:642–651.
76. Del Giudice I, Matutes E, Morilla R, et al. The diagnostic value of CD123 in B-cell disorders with hairy or villous lymphocytes *Haematologica*. 2004;89:303–308.
77. Falini B, Tiacci E, Liso A, et al. Simple diagnostic assay for hairy cell leukaemia by immunocytochemical detection of annexin A1 (ANXA1). *Lancet* 2004;363:1869–1870.
78. Lloret E, Mollejo M, Mateo MS, et al. Splenic marginal zone lymphoma with increased number of blasts: an aggressive variant? *Hum Pathol* 1999;30:1153–1160.
79. Camacho FI, Mollejo M, Mateo M-S, et al. Progression to large B-cell lymphoma in splenic marginal zone lymphoma: a description of a series of 12 cases. *Am J Surg Pathol* 2001;25: 1268–1276.
80. Isaacson PG, Matutes E, Burke M, et al. The histopathology of splenic lymphoma with villous lymphocytes. *Blood* 1994;84:3828–3834.
81. Dogan A, Isaacson PG. Splenic marginal zone lymphoma. *Semin Diagn Pathol* 2003;20: 121–127.
82. Matutes E, Morilla R, Owusu-Ankomah K, et al. The immunophenotype of splenic lymphoma with villous lymphocytes and its relevance to the differential diagnosis with other B-cell disorders. *Blood* 1994;83:1558–1562.
83. Jadayel D, Matutes E, Dyer MJS, et al. Splenic lymphoma with villous lymphocytes: analysis of BCL-1 rearrangements and expression of the cyclin D1 gene. *Blood* 1994;83:3664–3671.
84. Savilo E, Campo E, Mollejo M, et al. Absence of cyclin D1 protein expression in splenic marginal zone lymphoma. *Mod Pathol* 1998;11:601–606.
85. Remstein ED, James CD, Kurtin PJ. Incidence and subtype specificity of *API2-MALT1* fusion transcripts in extranodal, nodal, and splenic marginal zone lymphomas. *Am J Pathol* 2000;156:1183–1188.
86. Algara P, Mateo MS, Sanchez-Beato M, et al. Analysis of the IgV_H somatic mutations in splenic marginal zone lymphoma defines a group of unmutated cases with frequent 7q deletion and adverse clinical course. *Blood* 2002;99:1299–1304.
87. Ruiz-Ballesteros E, Mollejo M, Rodriguez A, et al. Splenic marginal zone lymphoma: proposal of new diagnostic and prognostic markers identified after tissue and cDNA microarray analysis. *Blood* 2005;106:1831–1838.
88. Chacón JI, Mollejo M, Muñoz E, et al. Splenic marginal zone lymphoma: clinical characteristics and prognostic factors in a series of 60 patients. *Blood* 2002;100:1648–1654.
89. Franco V, Florena AM, Iannitto E. Splenic marginal zone lymphoma. *Blood* 2003;101: 2464–2472.
90. Arainci L, Lazzarino M, Colombo N, et al. Splenic marginal zone lymphoma: a prognostic model for clinical use. *Blood* 2006;107:4643–4649.
91. Saadoun D, Suarez F, Lefere F, et al. Splenic lymphoma with villous lymphocytes, associated with type II cryoglobulinemia and HCV infection: a new entity? *Blood* 2005;105:74–76.

91a. Traverse-Glehen A, Baseggio L, Callet-Bauchu E, et al. Splenic red pulp lymphoma with numerous basophilic villous lymphocytes: a distinct clinicopathologic and molecular entity? *Blood* 2008,1:2253-2260.

92. Kim H, Dorman RF. Morphological studies of 84 untreated patients subjected to laparotomy for the staging of non-Hodgkin's lymphomas. *Cancer* 1974;33:657–674.

93. Hernandez AM, Nathwani BN, Nguyen D, et al. Nodal benign and malignant monocytoid B cells with and without follicular lymphomas: a comparative study of follicular colonization, light chain restriction, bcl-2, and t(14;18) in 39 cases. *Hum Pathol* 1995;26:625–632.
94. Schmid U, Cogliatti SB, Diss TC, et al. Monocytoid/marginal zone B-cell differentiation in follicle centre cell lymphoma. *Histopathology* 1996;29:201–208.
95. Abou-Elella A, Shafer MT, Wan XY, et al. Lymphomas with follicular and monocytoid B-cell components: evidence for a common clonal origin from follicle center cells. *Am J Clin Pathol* 2000;114:516–522.
96. Takeshita M, Sakai H, Okamura S, et al. Splenic large B-cell lymphoma in patients with hepatitis C virus infection. *Hum Pathol* 2005;36:878–885.
97. Stroup R, Burke JS, Sheibani K, et al. Splenic involvement by aggressive malignant lymphomas of B-cell and T-cell types: a morphologic and immunophenotypic study. *Cancer* 1992;69:413–420.
98. Mollejo M, Algara P, Mateo M, et al. Large B cell lymphoma presenting in the spleen: identification of different clinicopathologic conditions. *Am J Surg Pathol* 2003;27:895–902.
99. Harris NL, Aisenberg AC, Meyer JE, et al. Diffuse large cell (histiocytic) lymphoma of the spleen; clinical and pathologic characteristics of ten cases. *Cancer* 1984;54:2460–2467.
100. Alkan S, Ross CW, Hanson CA, et al. Follicular lymphoma with involvement of the splenic marginal zone: a pitfall in the differential diagnosis of splenic marginal zone lymphoma. *Hum Pathol* 1996;27:503–506.
101. Dogan A, Burke JS, Goteri G, et al. Micronodular T-cell/histiocyte-rich large B-cell lymphoma of the spleen: histology, immunophenotype and differential diagnosis. *Am J Surg Pathol* 2003;27:903–911.
102. Li S, Mann KP, Holden JT. T-cell-rich B-cell lymphoma presenting in the spleen: a clinicopathologic analysis of 3 cases. *Int J Surg Pathol* 2004;12:31–37.
103. Morice WG, Rodriguez FJ, Hoyer JD, et al. Diffuse large B-cell lymphoma with distinctive patterns of splenic and bone marrow involvement: clinicopathologic features of two cases. *Mod Pathol* 2005;18:495–502.
104. Kroft SH, Howard MS, Picker LJ, et al. De novo CD5+ diffuse large B-cell lymphomas: a heterogenous group containing an unusual form of splenic lymphoma. *Am J Clin Pathol* 2000;114:523–533.
105. Kobrich U, Falk S, Karhoff M, et al. Primary large cell lymphoma of the splenic sinuses: a variant of angiotropic B-cell lymphoma (neoplastic angioendotheliomatosis). *Hum Pathol* 1992;23:1184–1187.
106. Murase T, Nakamura S, Kawauchi K, et al. An Asian variant of intravascular large B-cell lymphoma: clinical, pathological and cytogenetic approaches to diffuse large B-cell lymphoma associated with haemophagocytic syndrome. *Br J Haematol* 2000;111:826–834.
107. Ponzoni M, Ferreri AJM, Campo E, et al. Definition, diagnosis, and management of intravascular large B-cell lymphoma: proposals and perspectives from an international consensus meeting. *J Clin Oncol* 2007;25:3168–3173.
108. Burke JS, Butler JJ. Malignant lymphoma with a high content of epithelioid histiocytes (Lennert's lymphoma). *Am J Clin Pathol* 1976;66:1–9.
109. Chan JKC. Splenic involvement by peripheral T-cell and NK-cell neoplasms. *Semin Diagn Pathol* 2003;20:105–120.
110. Jaffe ES, Costa J, Fauci AS, et al. Malignant lymphoma and erythrophagocytosis simulating malignant histiocytosis. *Am J Med* 1983;75:741–749.
111. Falini B, Pileri S, De Solas I, et al. Peripheral T-cell lymphoma associated with hemophagocytic syndrome. *Blood* 1990; 75:434–444.
112. Farcet JP, Gaulard P, Marolleau JP, et al. Hepatosplenic T-cell lymphoma: Sinusal/sinusoidal localization of malignant cells expressing the T-cell receptor γδ. *Blood* 1990;75: 2213–2219.
113. Cooke CB, Krenacs L, Stetler-Stevenson M, et al. Hepatosplenic T-cell lymphoma: a distinct clinicopathologic entity of cytotoxic γδ T-cell origin. *Blood* 1996;88:4265–4274.
114. Salhany KE, Feldman M, Kahn MJ, et al. Hepatosplenic γδ T-cell lymphoma: ultrastructural, immunophenotypic, and functional evidence for cytotoxic T lymphocyte differentiation. *Hum Pathol* 1997;28:674–685.
115. Belhadj K, Reyes F, Farcet JP, et al. Hepatosplenic γδ T-cell lymphoma is a rare clinicopathologic entity with poor outcome: report on a series of 21 patients. *Blood* 2003;102: 4261–4269.
116. Vega F, Medeiros LJ, Gaulard P. Hepatosplenic and other γδ T-cell lymphomas. *Am J Clin Pathol* 2007;127:869–880.
117. Macon WR, Levy NB, Kurtin PJ, et al. Hepatosplenic αβ T-cell lymphomas: a report of 14 cases and comparison with hepatosplenic γδ T-cell lymphomas. *Am J Surg Pathol* 2001; 25:285–296.
118. Lachenal F, Berger F, Ghesquières H et al. Angioimmunoblastic T-cell lymphoma: clinical and laboratory features at diagnosis in 77 patients. *Medicine* 2007;86:282–292
119. Nathwani BN, Rappaport H, Moran EM, et al. Malignant lymphoma arising in angioimmunoblastic lymphadenopathy. *Cancer* 1978;41:578–606.
120. Smith JL, Hodges E, Quin CT, et al. Frequent T and B cell oligoclones in histologically and immunophenotypically characterized angioimmunoblastic lymphadenopathy. *Am J Pathol* 2000;156:661–669.
121. Attygalle AD, Chaung SS, Diss TC, et al. Distinguishing angioimummnoblastic T-cell lymphoma from peripheral T-cell lymphoma, unspecified, using morphology, immunophenotype and molecular genetics. *Histopathology* 2007;50:498–508.
122. Roncador G, Garcia Verdes-Montenegro JF, Tedoldi S, et al. Expression of two markers of germinal center T cells (SAP and PD-1) in angioimmunoblastic T-cell lymphoma. *Haematologica* 2007:92:1059–1066.
123. Hebeda KM, MacKenzie MA, van Krieken JH. A case of anaplastic lymphoma kinase-positive anaplastic large cell lymphoma presenting with spontaneous rupture: an extremely unusual presentation. *Virchows Arch* 2000;437:459–464.
124. Sakadamis A, Ballas K, Denga K, et al. Primary anaplastic large cell lymphoma of the spleen presenting as a splenic abscess. *Leuk Lymphoma* 2001;42:1419–1421.
125. Variakojis D, Rosas-Uribe A, Rappaport H. Mycosis fungoides: pathologic findings in staging laparotomies. *Cancer* 1974; 33:1589–1600.
126. Rueffer U, Sieber M, Stemberg M, et al. Spleen involvement in Hodgkin's lymphoma: assessment and risk profile. *Ann Hematol* 2003;82:390–396.
127. Leibenhaut MK, Hoppe RT, Efron B, et al. Prognostic indicators of laparotomy findings in clinical stage I-II supradiaphragmatic Hodgkin's disease. *J Clin Oncol* 1989;7:81–91.
128. Kadin ME, Glatstein E, Dorfman RS. Clinicopathologic studies of 117 untreated patients subjected to laparotomy for the staging of Hodgkin's disease. *Cancer* 1971;27:1277–1294.
129. Hoppe RT, Rosenberg SA, Kaplan HS, et al. Prognostic factors in pathological stage IIIA Hodgkin's disease. *Cancer* 1980;46:1240–1246.
130. Butler JJ. Pathology of the spleen in benign and malignant conditions. *Histopathology* 1983; 7:453–474.
131. Sacks EL, Donaldson SS, Gordon J, et al. Epithelioid granulomas associated with Hodgkin's disease. *Cancer* 1978;41:562–567.
132. Bearman RM, Pangalis GA, Rappaport H. Prolymphocytic leukemia: clinical, histopathological, and cytochemical observations. *Cancer* 1978;42:2360–2372.
133. Lampert I, Catovsky D, March GW, et al. The histopathology of prolymphocytic leukemia with particular reference to the spleen: a comparison with chronic lymphocytic leukemia. *Histopathology* 1980;4:3–19.
134. Del Giudice I, Davis Z, Matutes E, et al. IgVH genes mutation and usage, ZAP-70 and CD38 expression provide new insights on B-cell prolymphocytic leukemia (B-PLL). *Leukemia* 2006;20:1231–1237.
135. Matutes E, Brito-Babapulle V, Swansbury J, et al. Clinical and laboratory features of 78 cases of T-prolymphocytic leukemia. *Blood* 1991;78:3269–3274.
136. Osuji N, Matutes E, Catovsky D, at al. Histopathology of the spleen in T-cell large granular lymphocyte leukemia and T-cell prolymphocytic leukemia: a comparative review. *Am J Surg Pathol* 2005;29:935–941.
137. Rappaport H. The pathologic anatomy of the splenic red pulp. In Lennert K, Harms D, eds. *The Spleen.* Berlin: Springer-Verlag, 1970:24–41.
138. Da Costa L, Mohandas N, Sorette M, et al. Temporal differences in membrane loss lead to distinct reticulocyte features in hereditary spherocytosis and in autoimmune hemolytic anemia. *Blood* 2001;98:2894–2899.
139. Reliene R, Mariani M, Zanella A, et al. Splenectomy prolongs in vivo survival of erythrocytes differently in spectrin/ankyrin- and band 3–deficient hereditary spherocytosis. *Blood* 2002;100:2208–2215.
140. Chang C-S, Li C-Y, Liang Y-H, et al. Clinical features and splenic pathologic changes in patients with autoimmune hemolytic anemia and congenital hemolytic anemia. *Mayo Clin Proc* 1993;68:757–762.
141. Carter RK, Penman HG. *Infectious Mononucleosis.* Oxford: Blackwell Scientific, 1969.
142. Childs CC, Parham DM, Berard CW. Infectious mononucleosis: the spectrum of morphologic changes simulating lymphoma in lymph nodes and tonsils. *Am J Surg Pathol* 1987; 11:122–132.
143. Reynolds DJ, Banks PM, Gulley ML. New characterization of infectious mononucleosis and a phenotypic comparison with Hodgkin's disease. *Am J Pathol* 1995;146:379–388.
144. Ross CW, Schnitzer B, Weston BW, et al. Chronic active Epstein-Barr virus infection and virus-associated hemophagocytic syndrome. *Arch Pathol Lab Med* 1991;115:470–474.
145. Shin SS, Berry GJ, Weiss LM. Infectious mononucleosis: diagnosis by in situ hybridization in two cases with atypical features. *Am J Surg Pathol* 1991;15:625–631.
146. Plumbley JA, Fan H, Eagan PA, et al. Lymphoid tissues from patients with infectious mononucleosis lack monoclonal B and T cells. *J Mol Diagn* 2002;4:37–43.
147. LeBoit PE, Berger TG, Egbert BM, et al. Bacillary angiomatosis: the histopathology and differential diagnosis of a pseudoneoplastic infection in patients with human immunodeficiency virus disease. *Am J Surg Pathol* 1989;13:909–920.
148. Chan JKC, Lewin KJ, Lombard CM, et al. Histopathology of bacillary angiomatosis of lymph node. *Am J Surg Pathol* 1991;15:430–437.
149. Agan BK, Dolan MJ. Laboratory diagnosis of Bartonella infections. *Clin Lab Med* 2002;22: 937–962.
150. Reed JA, Brigati DJ, Flynn SD, et al. Immunocytochemical identification of *Rochalimaea henselae* in bacillary (epithelioid) angiomatosis, parenchymal bacillary peliosis, and persistent fever with bacteremia. *Am J Surg Pathol* 1992;16:650–657.
151. Perkocha LA, Geaghan SM, Yen TSB, et al. Clinical and pathological features of bacillary peliosis hepatis in association with human immunodeficiency virus infection. *N Engl J Med* 1990;323:1581–1586.
152. Daybell D, Paddock CD, Zaki SR, et al. Disseminated infection with Bartonella henselae as a cause of spontaneous splenic rupture. *Clin Infect Dis* 2004;39:e21–24.
153. Rywlin AM, Hernandez JA, Chastain DE, et al. Ceroid histiocytosis of spleen and bone marrow in idiopathic thrombocytopenic purpura (ITP): a contribution to the understanding of the sea-blue histiocyte. *Blood* 1971;37:587–593.
154. Sawitsky A, Rosner F, Choksky S. The sea-blue histiocyte syndrome, a review: genetic and biochemical studies. *Semin Hematol* 1972;9:285–297.
155. Reidbord HR, Horvat BL, Fisher ER. Splenic lipidosis: histochemical and ultrastructural differentiation with special reference to the syndrome of the sea-blue histiocyte. *Arch Pathol* 1972;93:518.524.
156. de Lajarte-Thirouard AS, Molina T, Audouin J, et al. Spleen localization of light chain deposition disease associated with sea blue histiocytosis, revealed by spontaneous rupture. *Virchows Arch* 1999;434:463–465.
157. Long RG, Lake BD, Pettit JE, et al. Adult Niemann-Pick disease: its relationship to the syndrome of the sea-blue histiocyte. *Am J Med* 1977;62:627–635.
158. Fleshner PR, Aufses AH, Grabowski GA, et al. A 27-year experience with splenectomy for Gaucher's disease. *Am J Surg* 1991;161:69–75.
159. Charrow J, Andersson HC, Kaplan P, et al. The Gaucher registry: demographics and disease characteristics of 1698 patients with Gaucher disease. *Arch Intern Med* 2000;160: 2835–2843.
160. Lee RE, Peters SD, Glew RH. Gaucher's disease: clinical, morphologic, and pathogenetic considerations. *Pathol Annu* 1977; 72:309–339.

161. Dunn P, Kuo MC, Sun CF. Psudo-Gaucher cells in mycobactrial infection: a report of two cases. *J Clin Pathol* 2005;58:1113–1114.
162. Copie-Bergman C, Wotherspoon AC, Norton AJ, et al. True histiocytic lymphoma: a morphologic, immunohistochemical, and molecular genetic study of 13 cases. *Am J Surg Pathol* 1998:22:1386–1392.
163. Pileri SA, Grogan TM, Harris NL, et al. Tumours of histiocytes and accessory dendritic cells: an immunohistochemical approach to classification from the International Lymphoma Study Group based on 61 cases. *Histopathology* 2002;41:1–29.
164. Hornick JL, Jaffe ES, Fletcher CD. Extranodal histiocytic sarcoma: clinicopathologic analysis of 14 cases of a rare epithelioid malignancy. *Am J Surg Pathol* 2004:28:1133–1144.
165. Vos JA, Abbondanzo SL, Barekman CL, et al. Histiocytic sarcoma: a study of five cases including the histiocyte marker CD163. *Mod Pathol* 2005;18:693–704.
166. Feldman AL, Arber DA, Pittalliga S, et al. Clonally related follicular lymphomas and histiocytic/dendritic cell sarcomas: evidence for transdifferentiation of the follicular lymphoma clone *Blood* 2008;111:5433-5439.
167. Franchino C, Reich C, Distenfeld A, et al. A clinicopathologically distinctive primary splenic histiocytic neoplasm: demonstration of its histiocytic derivation by immunophenotypic and molecular genetic analysis. *Am J Surg Pathol* 1988;12:398–404.
168. Audouin J, Vercelli-Retta J, Le Tourneau A, et al. Primary histiocytic sarcoma of the spleen associated with erythrophagocytic histiocytosis. *Pathol Res Pract* 2003;199:107–112.
169. Quintanilla-Martinez L, Kumar S, Fend F, et al. Fulminant EBV+ T-cell lymphoproliferative disorder following acute/chronic EBV infection: a distinct clinicopathologic syndrome. *Blood* 2000;96:443–451.
170. Favara BE. Hemophagocytic lymphohistiocytosis: a hemophagocytic syndrome. *Semin Diagn Pathol* 1992;9:63–74.
171. Öst Å, Nilsson-Ardnor S, Henter J-I. Autopsy findings in 27 children with hemophagocytic lymphohistiocytosis. *Histopathology* 1998;31:310–316.
172. Lieberman PH, Jones CR, Steinman RM, et al. Langerhans cell (eosinophilic) granulomatosis: a clinicopathologic study encompassing 50 years. *Am J Surg Pathol* 1996;20:519–552.
173. Nezelof C, Frileux-Herbert F, Cronier et al. Disseminated histiocytosis X: analysis of prognostic factors based on a retrospective study of 50 cases. *Cancer* 1979;44:1824–1838.
174. Turner RR, Wood GS, Beckstead JH, et al. Histiocytic malignancies: morphologic, immunologic, and enzymatic heterogeneity. *Am J Surg Pathol* 1984:8:485–500.
175. Kawachi K, Nakatani Y, Inayama Y, et al. Interdigitating dendritic cell sarcoma of the spleen: report of a case with a review of the literature. *Am J Surg Pathol* 2002;26:530–537.
176. Grogg KL, Macon WR, Kurtin PJ, et al. A survey of clusterin and fascin expression in sarcomas and spindle cell neoplasms: strong clusterin immunostaining is highly specific for follicular dendritic cell tumor. *Mod Pathol* 2005;18:260–266.
177. Yu H, Gibson JA, Pinkus GS, et al. Podoplanin (D2–40) is a novel marker for follicular dendritic cell tumors. *Am J Clin Pathol* 2007;128:776–782.
178. Chan JKC, Fletcher CDM, Nayler SJ, et al. Follicular dendritic cell sarcoma: clinicopathologic analysis of 17 cases suggesting a malignant potential higher than currently recognized. *Cancer* 1997;79:294–313.
179. Cheuk W, Chan JKC, Shek TWH, et al. Inflammatory pseudotumor-like follicular dendritic cell tumor: a distinctive low-grade malignant intra-abdominal neoplasm with consistent Epstein-Barr virus association. *Am J Surg Pathol* 2001;25:721–731.
180. Sander B, Middel P, Gunawan B, et al. Follicular dendritic cell sarcoma of the spleen. *Hum Pathol* 2007;38:668–672.
181. O'Malley DP, Kim YS, Perkins SL, et al. Morphologic and immunohistochemical evaluation of splenic hematopoietic proliferations in neoplastic and benign disorders. *Mod Pathol* 2005;18:1550–1561.
182. O'Malley DP, Orazi A, Wang M, et al. Analysis of loss of heterozygosity and X chromosome inactivation in spleens with myeloproliferative disorders and acute myeloid leukemia. *Mod Pathol* 2005;18:1562–1568.
183. Vasef MA, Neiman RS, Meletiou SD, et al. Marked granulocytic proliferation induced by granulocyte colony–stimulating factor in the spleen simulating a myeloid leukemic infiltrate. *Mod Pathol* 1998;11:1138–1141.
184. Hsieh P-P, Olsen RJ, O'Malley DP, et al. The role of Janus Kinase 2 V617F mutation in extramedullary hematopoiesis of the spleen in neoplastic myeloid disorders. *Mod Pathol* 2007;20:929–935.
185. Mesa RA, Li C-Y, Schroeder G, et al. Clinical correlates of splenic histopathology and splenic karyotype in myelofibrosis with myeloid metaplasia. *Blood* 2001;97:3665–3667.
186. O'Malley DP. Benign extramedullary myeloid proliferations. *Mod Pathol* 2007;20:405–415.
187. Kraus MD, Bartlett NL, Fleming MD, et al. Splenic pathology in myelodysplasia: a report of 13 cases with clinical correlation. *Am J Surg Pathol* 1998;22:1255–1266.
188. Burke JS, Rappaport H. The diagnosis and differential diagnosis of hairy cell leukemia in bone marrow and spleen. *Semin Oncol* 1985;11:334–346.
189. Nanba K, Soban E, Bowling MC, et al. Splenic pseudosinuses and hepatic angiomatous lesions: distinctive features of hairy cell leukemia. *Am J Clin Pathol* 1977;67:415–426.
190. Burke JS, Sheibani K, Winberg CD, et al. Recognition of hairy cell leukemia in a spleen of normal weight: the contribution of immunohistologic studies. *Am J Clin Pathol* 1987; 87: 276–281.
191. Hoyer JD, Li CY, Yam YT, et al. Immunohistochemical demonstration of acid phosphatase isoenzyme 5 (tartrate-resistant) in paraffin sections of hairy cell leukemia and other hematologic disorders. *Am J Clin Pathol* 1997;108:308–315.
192. Jõhrens K, Stein H, Anagnostopoulos I. T-bet transcription factor detection facilitates the diagnosis of minimal hairy cell leukemia infiltrates in bone marrow trephines. *Am J Surg Pathol* 2007;31:1181–1185.
193. Matutes E, Morilla R, Owusu-Ankomah K, et al. The immunophenotype of hairy cell leukemia (HCL). Proposal for a scoring system to distinguish HCL from B-cell disorders with hairy or villous lymphocytes. *Leuk Lymphoma* 1994;14(Suppl 1):57–61.
194. Matutes E, Wotherspoon A, Catovsky D. The variant form of hairy cell leukaemia. *Best Pract Res Clin Haematol* 2003;16:41–56.
195. Sharpe RW, Bethel KJ. Hairy cell leukemia: diagnostic pathology. *Hematol Oncol Clin N Am* 2006;20:1023–1049.
196. Cessna MH, Hartung L, Tripp S, et al. Hairy cell leukemia variant: fact or fiction. *Am J Clin Pathol* 2005;123:132–138.
197. Lundell R, Hartung L, Hill, S, et al. T-cell large granular lymphocyte leukemias have multiple phenotypic abnormalities involving pan–T-cell antigens and receptors for MHC molecules. *Am J Clin Pathol* 2005;124:937–946.
198. Semenzato G, Zambello R, Starkebaum G, et al. The lymphoproliferative disease of granular lymphocytes: updated criteria for diagnosis. *Blood* 1997;89:256–260.
199. Lamy T, Loughran TP. Current concepts: large granular lymphocyte leukemia. *Blood Rev* 1999;13:230–240.
200. Lamy T, Loughran TP. Clinical features of large granular lymphocyte leukemia. *Semin Hematol* 2003;40:185–195.
201. Agnarsson BA, Loughran TP, Starkebaum G, et al. The pathology of large granular lymphocyte leukemia. *Hum Pathol* 1989;20:643–651.
202. O'Malley DP. T-cell large granular leukemia and related proliferations. *Am J Clin Pathol* 2007;127:850–859.
203. Gentile TC, Uner AH, Hutchison RE, et al. CD3+, CD56+ aggressive variant of large granular lymphocyte leukemia. *Blood* 1994;84:2315–2321.
204. Kingma DW, Raffeld M, Jaffe ES. Differential diagnosis of CD3+, CD56+ T-cell leukemia [Letter]. *Blood* 1995;85:1675–1676.
205. Matutes E, Wotherspoon AC, Parker NE, et al. Transformation of T-cell large granular lymphocyte leukaemia into a high-grade T-cell lymphoma. *Br J Haematol* 2001;115: 801–806.
206. Horny HP, Sotlar K, Valent P. Mastocytosis: state of the art. *Pathobiology* 2007;74:121–132.
207. Brunning RD, McKenna RW, Rosai J, et al. Systemic mastocytosis: extracutaneous manifestations. *Am J Surg Pathol* 1983;7:425–438.
208. Travis WD, Li CY. Pathology of the lymph node and spleen in systemic mast cell disease. *Mod Pathol* 1988;1:4–14.
209. Horny HP, Ruck MT, Kaiserling E. Spleen findings in generalized mastocytosis: a clinicopathologic study. *Cancer* 1992;70:459–468.
210. Wimazal F, Schwarzmeier J, Sotlar K, et al. Splenic mastocytosis: report of two cases and detection of the transforming somatic C-KIT mutation D816V. *Leuk Lymphoma* 2004;45: 723–729.
211. Yang F, Tran T-A, Carlson JA, et al. Paraffin section immunophenotype of cutaneous and extracutaneous mast cell disease: comparison to other hematopoietic neoplasms. *Am J Surg Pathol* 2000;24:703–709.
212. Valent P, Horny H, Escribano L, et al. Diagnostic criteria and classification of mastocytosis: a consensus proposal. *Leuk Res* 2001:25:603–625.
213. Krauth MT, Agis H, Aichberger KJ, et al. Immunohistochemical detection of histidine decarboxylase in neoplastic mast cells in patients with systemic mastocytosis. *Hum Pathol* 2006;37:439–447.
214. Garvin DF, King FM. Cysts and nonlymphomatous tumors of the spleen. *Pathol Annu* 1981; 16:61–80.
215. Bürrig K-F. Epithelial (true) splenic cysts: pathogenesis of the mesothelial and so-called epidermoid cyst of the spleen. *Am J Surg Pathol* 1988;12:275–281.
216. Arber DA, Strickler JG, Weiss LM. Splenic mesothelial cysts mimicking lymphangiomas. *Am J Surg Pathol* 1997;21:334–338.
217 Falk S, Stutte HJ. Hamartomas of the spleen: a study of 20 biopsy cases. *Histopathology* 1989;14:603–612.
218. Krishnan J, Frizzera G. Two splenic lesions in need of clarification: hamartoma and inflammatory pseudotumor. *Semin Diagn Pathol* 2003;20:94–104.
219. Cheuk W, Lee AKC, Arora N, et al. Splenic hamartoma with bizarre stromal cells. *Am J Surg Pathol* 2005;29:109–114.
220. Laskin WB, Alasadi R, Variakojis D. Splenic hamartoma [Letter]. *Am J Surg Pathol* 2005; 29:1114–1115.
221. Martel M, Sarli D, Colecchia M, et al. Fibroblastic reticular cell tumor of the spleen: report of a case and review of the entity. *Hum Pathol* 2003;34:954–957.
222. Arber DA, Stickler JG, Chen Y-Y, et al. Splenic vascular tumors: a histologic, immunophenotypic, and virologic study. *Am J Surg Pathol* 1997;21:827–835.
223. Kutok JL, Fletcher CDM. Splenic vascular tumors. *Semin Diagn Pathol* 2003;20:128–139.
224. Steininger H, Pfofe D, Marquardt L, et al. Isolated diffuse hemangiomatosis of the spleen: case report and review of literature. *Pathol Res Pract* 2004;200:479–485.
225. Falk S, Stutte HJ, Frizzera G. Littoral cell angioma: a novel splenic vascular lesion demonstrating histiocytic differentiation. *Am J Surg Pathol* 1991;15:1023–1033.
226. Nguyen TT, Scwartz EJ, West RB, et al. Expression of CD163 (hemoglobin scavenger receptor) in normal tissues, lymphomas, carcinomas, and sarcomas is largely restricted to the monocyte/macrophage lineage. *Am J Surg Pathol* 2005;29:617–624.
227. Rosso R, Paulli M, Gianelli U, et al. Littoral cell angiosarcoma of the spleen: case report with immunohistochemical and ultrastructural analysis. *Am J Surg Pathol* 1995;19: 1203–1208.
228. Ben-Izhak O, Bejar J, Ben-Eliezer S, et al. Splenic littoral cell haemangioendothelioma: a new low-grade variant of malignant littoral cell tumour. *Histopathology* 2001;39:469–475.
229. Fernandez S, Cook GW, Arber DA. Metastasizing splenic littoral cell hemangioendothelioma. *Am J Surg Pathol* 2006;30:1036–1040.
230. Falk S, Krishnan J, Meis JM. Primary angiosarcoma of the spleen: a clinicopathologic study of 40 cases. *Am J Surg Pathol* 1993;17:959–970..
231. Neuhauser TS, Derringer GA, Thompson LDR, et al. Splenic angiosarcoma: a clinicopathologic and immunophenotypic study of 28 cases. *Mod Pathol* 2000;13:978–987.
232. Mikami T, Saegusa M, Akino F, et al. A Kaposi-like variant of splenic angiosarcoma lacking association with human herpesvirus 8. *Arch Pathol Lab Med* 2002;126:191–194.
233. Sarode VR, Datta BN, Savitri K, et al. Kaposi's sarcoma of spleen with unusual clinical and histologic features. *Arch Pathol Lab Med* 1991;115:1042–1044.
234. Neill JSA, Park HK. Hemangiopericytoma of the spleen. *Am J Clin Pathol* 1991;95:680–683.
235. Suster S. Epithelioid and spindle cell hemangioendothelioma of the spleen: report of a distinctive splenic vascular neoplasm of childhood. *Am J Surg Pathol* 1992;16:785–792.

236. Kraus MD, Dehner LP. Benign vascular neoplasms of the spleen with myoid and angioen-dotheliomatous features. *Histopathology* 1999;35:328–336.

237. Wick MR, Scheithauer BW, Smith SL, et al. Primary nonlymphoreticular malignant neo-plasms of the spleen. *Am J Surg Pathol* 1982;6:229–242.

238. Compérat E, Bardier-Dupas A, Camparo P, et al. Splenic metastases: clinicopathologic presentation, differential diagnosis, and pathogenesis. *Arch Pathol Lab Med* 2007;131:965–969.

239. Lam KY, Tang V. Metastatic tumors to the spleen: a 25-year clinicopathologic study. *Arch Pathol Lab Med* 2000;124:526–530.

240. Cummings OW, Mazur MT. Breast carcinoma diffusely metastatic to the spleen: a report of two cases presenting as idiopathic thrombocytopenic purpura. *Am J Clin Pathol* 1992;97:484–489.

241. Thomas RM, Jaffe ES, Zarate-Osorno A, et al. Inflammatory pseudotumor of the spleen: a clinicopathologic and immunophenotypic study of eight cases. *Arch Pathol Lab Med* 1993;117:921–926.

242. Neuhauser TS, Derringer GA, Thompson LDR, et al. Splenic inflammatory myofibroblas-tic tumor (inflammatory pseudotumor): a clinicopathologic and immunophenotypic study of 12 cases. *Arch Pathol Lab Med* 2001;125:379–385.

243. Lewis JT, Gaffney RL, Casey MB, et al. Inflammatory pseudotumor of the spleen associated with a clonal Epstein-Barr virus genome. Case report and review of the literature. *Am J Clin Pathol* 2003;120:56–61.

244. Kutok JL, Pinkus GS, Dorfman DM, et al. Inflammatory pseudotumor of lymph node and spleen: an entity biologically distinct from inflammatory myofibroblastic tumor. *Hum Pathol* 2001;32:1382–1387.

245. Suster S, Moran CA, Blanco M. Mycobacterial spindle-cell pseudotumor of the spleen. *Am J Clin Pathol* 1994;101:539–542.

246. Martel M, Cheuk W, Lombardi L, et al. Sclerosing angiomatoid nodular transformation (SANT): report of 25 cases of a distinctive benign splenic lesion. *Am J Surg Pathol* 2004;28:1268–1279.

CHAPTER

19

Richard J. Zarbo

The Jaws and Oral Cavity

Pathologic diagnosis of diseases of the jaws and oral cavity is greatly facilitated by understanding the gross and microscopic anatomy of the region. Communication with clinicians, especially dentists and oral surgeons, is enhanced by understanding and use of oral- and dental-related terminology rather than lay terms. For instance, it is preferable to use the term *gingiva* (subdivided into marginal or free gingiva, attached or hard gingiva, and loose or movable gingiva/mucosa) rather than *gums*. The space between the marginal gingiva and the tooth is called the gingival sulcus, and insufficient dental hygiene supports the growth of numerous microorganisms in this microenvironment, leading to gingival and periodontal diseases described later in this chapter. Another example of appropriate terminology is use of the term *buccal mucosa* instead of *cheek*.

Although all intraoral epithelium is of a stratified squamous type, there are regional histologic variations, such as nonkeratinized, parakeratinized, and orthokeratinized, as well as morphologic variations, such as filiform, fungiform, vallate, and nodular. These histologic nuances are well described in histology texts. Knowledge of the normal histology of the jaws, teeth and periodontium, and remnants of tooth formation are important to the understanding of inflammatory, developmental, and neoplastic odontogenic cysts and tumors.

During fetal development, epithelial invaginations from alveolar mucosa, known as dental laminae, give rise to enamel organs and, subsequently, to teeth. The dental lamina gives rise to 20 deciduous or primary teeth during the second month in utero and, subsequently, to 32 permanent teeth through distal extensions from the deciduous tooth buds (Fig. 19.1). Once tooth formation is complete, remnants of the epithelium involved in tooth formation persist indefinitely in the tooth-bearing areas of the jaws and gingiva. Epithelial remnants in the periodontium around the roots of teeth are known as rests of Malassez, those in overlying gingiva are called rests of Serres, and those over the crowns of unerupted teeth are called reduced enamel epithelia. They are the sources of odontogenic cysts and most odontogenic tumors (1).

These residual odontogenic rests may be encountered in histologic evaluation of extracted teeth or in sections of tooth-bearing jaws. Odontogenic rests are typically round or strandlike in form (Fig. 19.2). Acanthotic or hyperplastic variations may be confused with a neoplastic squamous proliferation (Fig. 19.3). Rests are distinguished by their bland cytology and lack of ameloblastic differentiation of peripheral columnar cells with nuclear polarization and central stellate reticulum–like zones.

ORAL MUCOSAL LESIONS

GINGIVITIS

Gingivitis is a painless inflammatory reaction limited to the soft tissues around the teeth. It is seen as redness of the gingiva and is caused by dental plaque, a biofilm composed mainly of streptococcal bacteria (*Streptococcus sanguinis* and *Streptococcus mutans*) and anaerobes, salivary polymers, and bacterial extracellular matrix products at the marginal gingiva and in the gingival sulcus (2). Plaque-associated gingivitis generally progresses through three histologic stages: initial neutrophilic infiltrate, early T-cell–dominated lymphoid infiltrate, and late-stage infiltration by abundant B cells and plasma cells (2). Gingivitis may also be modified by nutritional deficiency (vitamins B and C),

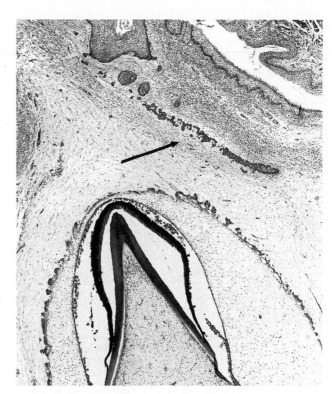

Figure 19.1. The dental lamina (*arrow*), responsible for the formation of the deciduous tooth present below, trails off from the overlying oral epithelium from which it was derived. The resulting scattered epithelial rests located in gingiva and bone, as they fragment, are potential sources of odontogenic cysts and tumors.

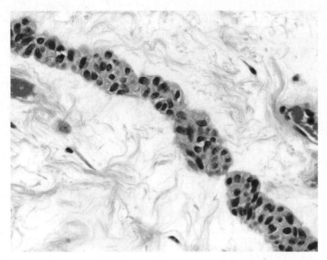

Figure 19.2. Strandlike odontogenic rest derived from the dental lamina was located adjacent to an odontogenic cyst.

endocrine imbalances of adolescence or pregnancy, generalized infection, or drugs (e.g., phenytoin).

ACUTE NECROTIZING GINGIVITIS

An acute, necrotizing form of plaque-associated gingivitis is known by several names including acute necrotizing gingivitis (ANG), acute necrotizing ulcerative gingivitis (ANUG), ulcerative stomatitis, Vincent disease, and Vincent stomatitis. This infection is caused by fusospirochetal microbes (fusospirochetal gingivitis) usually in association with predisposing factors, such as poor oral hygiene, smoking, and stress (3,4). It occurs almost exclusively in younger age groups of late teens to midtwenties. The clinical appearance is that of highly inflamed, sore, bleeding gingiva with interdental gingival necrosis covered by a gray pseudomembrane that is easily removed, leaving exposed, raw bleeding tissue. This results in a characteristic fetid odor (trench mouth) and an accumulation of detritus. Histologically,

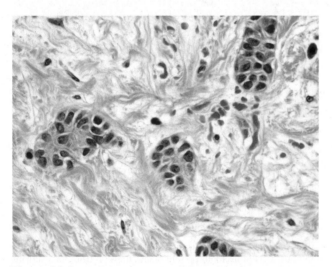

Figure 19.3. Acanthomatous odontogenic rests show squamous differentiation that, although bland, may suggest squamous neoplasia, primary or metastatic to the jaws.

there is necrosis of the interdental gingival papillae overlying acute purulent inflammation. ANG lesions heal with scarring and blunting of the interdental papillae. Chronic recurrent forms of ANG do occur.

PERIODONTITIS

Periodontitis is bacterial-related inflammation of the tissues of the periodontium that support the teeth, thereby resulting in loss of supporting bone, loose teeth, and eventual tooth loss (5). Periodontal disease is induced by the activity of a mixed bacterial biofilm growing under anaerobic conditions. Viruses may also play a synergistic role with bacteria in the initiation and progression of periodontitis (6). The most commonly recognized bacterial pathogens are Gram-negative anaerobes—*Actinobacillus actinomycetemcomitans*, *Bacteroides forsythus*, *Campylobacter* species, *Capnocytophaga* species, *Eikenella corrodens*, *Fusobacterium nucleatum*, *Porphyromonas gingivalis*, *Prevotella intermedia*, and oral spirochetes like *Treponema denticola*. Although gingivitis is inflammation limited to the gingiva and results in no bone loss, it may progress to the periodontal ligament and the surrounding alveolar bone forming the tooth socket. When the attachment of the gingival sulcus epithelium to the tooth is lost, the subjacent periodontal ligament becomes involved in the inflammatory process. Eventually, periodontal fibers that attach the tooth to bone are lost, and the formation of a so-called periodontal pocket begins along the tooth root. This creates an occult microenvironment for subgingival bacteria and their products to drive the periodontal destructive process. Bacterial plaque within pockets serves as a nidus for mineralization and calcifies to form dental calculus that is adherent to the tooth roots. Histologically, the inflammatory process is mostly chronic with superimposed acute inflammation. Occasionally, a periodontal abscess may form in a pocket. Risk factors for periodontal disease include poor oral hygiene, genetic predisposition, smoking, and diabetes mellitus (7–9).

Treatment of periodontal disease includes enhanced personal daily dental hygiene to mechanically remove plaque, regular professional scaling and planing of the root surfaces to remove subgingival plaque and calculus, antiseptic mouthwashes to alter bacterial flora, and periodontal surgery to reduce pocket depth and make them more hygienic.

PYOGENIC GRANULOMA

Pyogenic granuloma, a common red tumorlike mass of the gingiva is a well-vascularized lesion (granulation tissue) (10). Pyogenic granuloma is a misnomer because it is neither pus producing nor granulomatous. Histologically, two types of proliferations have been called pyogenic granuloma: either a uniform granulation tissue mass or a lobular capillary proliferation with intervening fibrous connective tissue. Ulceration may or may not be present (11).

Pyogenic granulomas are reactive lesions whose growth may be modified by hormonal changes associated with pregnancy and puberty. Pyogenic granulomas may be included in some generalized gingival hyperplasias, which are associated with bacterial plaque and subgingival calculus. Generalized lesions may also be modified (enhanced) by hormonal imbalances, drugs (oral contraceptives, phenytoin, cyclosporine, nifedipine, other calcium channel blockers, and epidermal growth factor recep-

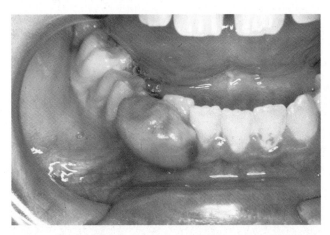

Figure 19.4. Peripheral giant-cell granuloma. The reactive lesion forms an expansile gingival mass.

PERIPHERAL FIBROMA (FOCAL FIBROUS HYPERPLASIA)

This is the result of focal chronic gingival inflammation and represents a localized hyperplastic fibrous mass in the free or attached gingiva. Synonyms used include focal fibrous hyperplasia, peripheral ossifying fibroma, fibroid epulis (old), and fibroepithelial polyp (12). Peripheral fibromas can contain insignificant islands of ossification and are designated peripheral ossifying fibroma. Occasionally peripheral fibromas contain stellate and multinucleated fibroblasts and have been designated giant-cell fibromas. Yet another variant is the peripheral *odontogenic* fibroma containing strands of odontogenic epithelium and small calcifications. Unlike the other peripheral fibromas, it has a slight propensity for recurrence and is described in more detail under the section on benign mesenchymal odontogenic tumors. The reactive nature of peripheral fibromas and their variants is in contradistinction to the central ossifying fibromas of the jaws, which are fibro-osseous neoplasms.

PERIPHERAL GIANT-CELL GRANULOMA

Microscopically, peripheral giant-cell granuloma (PGCG) is the gingival soft tissue counterpart of central giant-cell lesion (reparative granuloma) located within the jaws (13). The peripheral lesion is reactive in nature, whereas the central lesion is of disputed behavior. Clinically, PGCG is a localized erythematous mass of the gingiva similar in clinical appearance to pyogenic granuloma (Fig. 19.4). PGCG may erode subjacent alveolar bone and periodontal membrane. Histologically, PGCG is a lobular mass of fibroblasts with numerous, often clustered osteoclast-like giant cells associated with hemorrhage and hemosiderin (Fig. 19.5A,B). Occasional bone formation is found. In edentulous or partly edentulous patients, the lesions may show

tor inhibitor therapies), leukemia, and genetic factors. Lesions usually occur in children and young adults or pregnant women at the second or third trimester as a "pregnancy tumor" of the gingiva. They commonly involve the oral mucosa (especially maxillary labial gingiva) or skin of the head, neck, extremities, and upper trunk. In the oral cavity, it involves, in decreasing order, the gingiva, lips, tongue, buccal mucosa, and alveolus.

Pyogenic granulomas characteristically evolve relatively rapidly over a few weeks and commonly ulcerate and bleed. They are usually associated with gingivitis in the area (Fig. 19.4). Occasionally untreated lesions may become fibrotic. The lesions are treated by simple excision with removal of any initiating factors (e.g., calculus, foreign body). Occasional recurrences are seen, but there is no malignant potential.

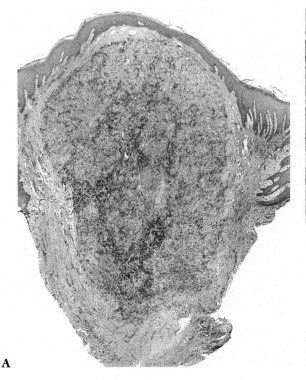

A

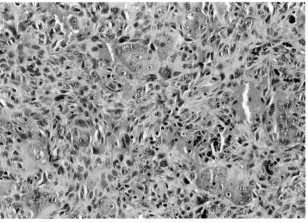

B

Figure 19.5. Peripheral giant-cell granuloma. **(A)** A cellular, hemorrhagic mass expands the gingiva. **(B)** Scattered multinucleate giant cells with old and new hemorrhage are noted in a fibroblastic stroma.

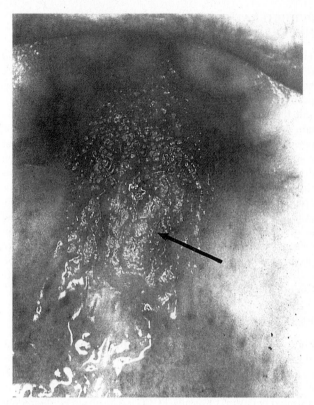

Figure 19.6. Inflammatory papillary hyperplasia. "Papillary" mucosa seen in the arch of the palate (*arrow*) resulted from an ill-fitting denture.

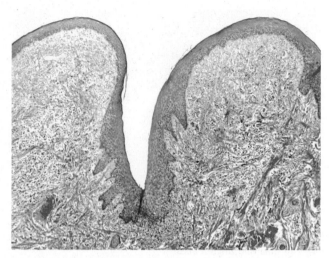

Figure 19.7. Inflammatory papillary hyperplasia. Formerly known as palatal papillomatosis, this is a coarsely exophytic mucosal hyperplasia of combined epithelial and mesenchymal components.

a characteristic erosion of alveolar bone. The treatment of PGCG is surgical excision. This includes a thorough curettage of the base of the lesion extending into the adjacent periodontal membrane or periosteum because PGCG may recur if not completely excised.

INFLAMMATORY PAPILLARY (DENTURE) HYPERPLASIA

This is a benign papillary hyperplastic lesion of the oral mucosa commonly affecting the palate, where it is also known as palatal papillomatosis (Fig. 19.6). The lesions are associated with ill-fitting dentures or partial dentures in adults and occur 10 times more often in those who wear prostheses at night and/or have poor oral hygiene (14,15).

This is not a true papilloma but rather a combined epithelial and mesenchymal reactive hyperplasia. Mucosal epithelial hyperplasia, which may be in a pseudoepitheliomatous pattern, overlies hyperplastic submucosal fibrous tissue (Fig. 19.7). Occasionally, denture trauma can result in trapped islands of hyperplastic squamous mucosa embedded in the fibrous connective tissue of the submucosa. Other secondary chronic inflammatory changes may be seen in the accessory salivary glands in the palate, with sialofibrosis, acinar atrophy, and ductal sialometaplasia. There is no epithelial dysplasia and no premalignant risk associated with the lesion. Inflammatory papillary hyperplasia is treated by complete excision and avoided by construction of a well-fitting denture or partial denture.

ORAL PAPILLOMA

The most common benign intraoral squamous epithelial neoplasm is the solitary papilloma. The usual sites are posterior aspect of the hard and soft palates and uvula (34%), dorsum and lateral tongue borders (24%), gingiva (12%), lower lips (12%), and buccal mucosa (6%) (16).

These lesions are white to pink cauliflowerlike surface epithelial proliferations. Three-fourths of such lesions are less than 1 cm in size. No gender preference is observed, and the average age of occurrence is approximately 38 years (16). The presence of human papillomavirus (HPV) antigens has been verified by the immunoperoxidase method in approximately 50% of oral papillomas. However, the koilocytotic epithelial changes associated with HPV infection are not always evident. HPV-6 and -11 DNA sequences have been identified in most, but not all, intraoral papillomas by in situ hybridization (17). Interestingly, a minority of cases of inflammatory papillary hyperplasia, described earlier, have also tested positive for HPV-6 by in situ hybridization (17). Despite sensitive polymerase chain reaction (PCR) for multiple HPV types, HPV DNA is not detectable in many esophageal squamous papillomas, which suggests that some oral papillomas may yet represent forms of reactive epithelial hyperplasia secondary to mucosal injury and repair but not associated with HPV as a promoter (18).

Histologically, the solitary squamous papilloma is a localized exophytic growth consisting of multiple papillary epithelial projections supported by delicate fibrovascular cores. Hyperkeratosis characterizes 82% of papillomas; 72% are surfaced by parakeratin, and the remainder is surfaced by orthokeratin or combinations of the two (16). Atypical epithelial changes may be encountered; these include hyperplasia of the basilar and parabasilar layers, hyperplasia of the prickle and granular cell layers, individual cell keratinization, and abnormal mitoses. A diagnosis of frank squamous dysplasia or papillary squamous carcinoma should be entertained in the context of a solitary squamous epithelial proliferation with papillary architecture and a significant degree of cytologic atypia and maturation abnormalities. In human immunodeficiency virus (HIV)/acquired immunodeficiency syndrome (AIDS) patients, a small percentage of oral warts (papillomas) may show histologic features of dysplasia. Progression of these lesions to squamous cell carcinoma has not been documented.

Differential diagnosis of solitary intraoral papilloma-like proliferations includes condyloma acuminatum, which is characterized by a more cauliflowerlike acanthosis, and verruca vulgaris, which is noted for its cup-shaped margins and hyperkeratinized spires with a prominent keratohyalin granular layer. Both of these lesions are also associated with HPV.

With the exception of HIV/AIDS patients, multiple papillary proliferations rarely develop in the oral cavity. Multiple lesions may be seen in HPV-associated juvenile papillomatosis of the upper aerophagic pathway and HPV-associated focal epithelial hyperplasia (Heck disease). The latter was described in 1965 by Archard et al. (19) as discrete, recurrent papillary lesions on the oral mucosa in Indian children and is now recognized in other parts of the world. Histologically, the lesions are composed of localized areas of mucosal epithelial hyperplasia characterized by marked acanthosis and parakeratosis. HPV types 1, 13, and 32 have been found in these proliferations (17).

Multiple oral papillomas that affect the lips and, less commonly, the intraoral mucosal sites are seen in focal dermal hypoplasia. Other manifestations of this X-linked dominant disorder include hypoplasia of hair, nails, or teeth; linear areas of hypoplasia of the skin; ulcers caused by congenital absence of skin; fatty herniation; bilateral syndactyly with a characteristic "lobster claw" deformity; colobomas of the iris and choroid; and strabismus (20).

Papillary lymphoid hyperplasia of the tonsils results in the clinical appearance of tonsils studded by papillary surface excrescences. This morphologic picture can be confused with epithelial papillomas on clinical examination, but microscopically, this is an unusual form of lymphoid hyperplasia surfaced by unremarkable epithelium (21). Nodular lymphoid hyperplasia may also be seen in the lateral tongue and floor of the mouth.

Oral papillomas are treated by simple excision. A low rate (4%) of recurrence and/or multiple lesions is observed (16), although the rate is higher in HIV/AIDS patients.

INTRAORAL AND OROPHARYNGEAL SQUAMOUS CELL CARCINOMA

Worldwide, oral cancer is the sixth most prevalent cancer, ranking eighth in developed countries and third in the developing world. The frequency of oral cavity malignancies has held constant over the years in the United States, accounting for an estimated 3% of all malignant tumors in men and a lesser percentage in women (22). However, the incidence of tonsillar and base of tongue cancers in the United States has increased annually since 1973 (23,24). This is likely the result of behavioral risk factors that include viruses in addition to the accepted chemical carcinogens of smoking and alcohol. Squamous cell carcinoma (SCC) of varying grades of differentiation and some unusual microscopic variants account for more than 90% of the intraoral malignancies. The overall 5-year survival rate for oral cancer when all stages are considered has shown little improvement over the past several decades, hovering at approximately 50%. It is important to note that the oral cancer 5-year survival rate in American blacks is significantly lower than that in whites. This difference has been attributed, in part, to lifestyle habits, clinical stage at diagnosis, and access to healthcare (22,25,26).

GENERAL CONSIDERATIONS

The typical demographic profile of an individual with oral SCC is that of a man in the fifth to eighth decade of life who is a smoker and a drinker. Most patients are older than 50 years. Rarely, SCC occurs in younger people. In a report of SCC of the head and neck in persons younger than 40 years of age, Mendez et al. (27) found that 41% of the neoplasms were in the oral cavity and that the incidence in women was 35% higher than that of the general population.

ETIOLOGY

Most cases of oral cavity and oropharyngeal SCC are associated with lifestyle habits of smoking and drinking. An estimated 50% of cases of oral cancer in American men are attributable to excessive consumption of tobacco and alcohol (28). The most significant etiologic agent associated with the development of oral SCC is tobacco. The risk of oral cancer increases with larger amounts and longer durations of tobacco use (29). In Western countries, tobacco use usually takes the form of cigarette, cigar, or pipe smoking. Other forms of tobacco use, such as snuff dipping and tobacco chewing, are arguably associated with a slight increased incidence of oral SCC. However, when smokeless tobacco is combined with betel nut leaf and slaked lime as is commonly done in India and Southeast Asia, oral cancer rates are markedly increased. Carcinogens in tobacco are believed to act as initiators, as well as promoters, in the transformation process because the relative risk declines after cessation of smoking (29). Carcinogen exposure in chronic marijuana smoking has been suggested in the young patient without other risk factors, and more recently, a history of regular marijuana use has been associated with oropharyngeal cancer (30,31).

Another important etiologic factor is alcohol consumption. Alcohol appears to act synergistically with tobacco as either a cocarcinogen (increasing the risk) or a promoter (decreasing the lag time) of neoplastic transformation. According to Rothman (32), heavy smoking alone carries a twofold to threefold increased risk of oral cancer, whereas the risk is two to six times greater in the heavy drinker compared with the nondrinker; the rate increases with the amount of tobacco smoked. The risk of development of SCC in the heavy drinker and smoker is 15 times greater than the risk in those who neither smoke nor drink. A study in young adults less than age 46 years indicates an oral and pharyngeal cancer risk of 20-fold for heavy smokers, 5-fold for heavy drinkers, and almost 50-fold for those with heavy combined smoking and drinking habits (33). Oral carcinomas arising in nonusers of tobacco and alcohol (13% in one series of 109 cancers) tend to affect older women, to spare the floor of the mouth, to be found at earlier stages, and to lack an association with second primary malignancies (34).

The dominant and synergistic role of chemical toxins in tobacco and alcohol in the causation of most head and neck squamous cancers is undisputed, but other factors appear to play a role. Chief among these is the probable pathogenetic role of oncogenic HPV virus infection in the development of some head and neck cancers. Oncogenic HPV infections are causative of most cervical squamous neoplasia (35). Genomic DNA of oncogenic HPV has been detected in roughly one-quarter of all SCCs worldwide but in almost three-quarters of oropharyngeal tonsillar and tongue-based cancers (30,36). High-risk HPV types 16 and 18 and, far less commonly, low-risk HPV types 6 and 11 have been found in oral carcinomas. HPV-16 is the most prevalent type detected, with tonsillar carcinomas having the highest prevalence (37). Interestingly, although the histologic observation of koilocytosis has been noted in more than 65% of oral cavity carcinomas, it does not appear to correlate with presence of HPV DNA by PCR testing (38).

Epidemiologic evidence points to a role for exposure to and infection with HPV-16 in the development of a subgroup of oropharyngeal SCCs. After controlling for other accepted risk factors like smoking and alcohol, high-risk sexual behaviors appear to place individuals at higher risk for these HPV-associated oropharyngeal cancers (30). These are mainly younger, non-smoking white females. In multivariate analysis, 55% of oropharyngeal cancer cases have been attributed to HPV-16 exposure alone (30). This proportion may be even higher if other high-risk HPV types (types 18, 31, 33, and 35) are evaluated. Heavy tobacco and alcohol use remain important risk factors for oropharyngeal cancers, but lack of synergy with exposure to HPV suggests that these chemical agents do not act as cofactors in HPV-mediated carcinogenesis.

Oral cancers, like other malignancies, arise from the accumulation of genetic events that disturb cell cycle control, proliferation, motility, survival, and tumor-related angiogenesis. Molecular genetic evidence indicates that there are distinctive molecular alterations in the tumors of smokers compared with those of nonsmokers, suggesting different mechanisms of tumorigenesis for morphologically similar head and neck SCCs (39). HPV appears to act early as an initiator of proliferation or in the early stage of carcinogenesis in a subset of oral cancers (40). HPV carcinogenesis affects cell control of transcription and the cell cycle via the E6 and E7 viral oncoproteins that bind to and inactivate the tumor suppressor proteins p53 and pRb (retinoblastoma gene product) and activate telomerase.

A separate viral-mediated pathway of carcinogenesis for some oral/oropharyngeal cancers presents a public health opportunity. Some have suggested that HPV vaccination of both girls and boys might be effective in reducing the incidence of some head and neck cancers because exposure to HPV can precede the appearance of cancer by 10 years or more (30). At this time, there appears to be no indication for HPV laboratory testing of oral precursor lesions or carcinomas.

HPV-16–positive oral cavity and oropharyngeal tumors appear to represent a distinct disease process with a more favorable survival (41). In the series by Gillison et al. (42), those with HPV-positive SCCs had a more favorable prognosis, with a 59% reduced risk of death from cancer compared with patients with HPV-negative tumors.

There may be more to your parents' admonition to "brush your teeth" than the avoidance of restorative dentistry bills. Independent risk associations for oral and oropharyngeal cancers have been noted for poor long-term oral hygiene and dental status as reflected in tooth loss, infrequent tooth brushing, and infrequent dental visits (30,43). Recent studies suggest that periodontal pockets may act as a reservoir for HPV and that chronic periodontitis, a chronic bacterial infection, may be associated with tongue cancer independent of smoking history (44,45).

Independent increased risk associations are also noted for those with a history of head and neck SCC in a first-degree relative or sibling, suggesting a specific genetic basis for some cases. A kindred with a germline mutation of the tumor suppressor *p16* gene, which is normally responsible for a protein inhibitor of cell proliferation, may represent the genetic basis of a familial predisposition to the development of head and neck SCC (46).

Other more controversial risk factors include the chronic use of alcohol-based mouthwashes; oral mechanical irritation, such as chronic trauma from ill-fitting dentures and jagged teeth; and the potentially precancerous conditions of syphilitic glossitis, severe iron deficiency (sideropenic dysphagia or Plummer-Vinson syndrome), oral submucous fibrosis, lichen planus, and discoid lupus erythematosus (47).

CLINICAL APPEARANCE AND HISTOLOGIC CORRELATES OF PRECURSORS TO ORAL SQUAMOUS CELL CARCINOMA

Oral squamous mucosa responds to chronic injury or carcinogenic stimuli by either hyperplasia or atrophy. Lesions related to chronic irritation are focal hyperkeratosis and represent the most common oral white lesions. Other white lesions in which the causes are unknown are called idiopathic leukoplakias. These lesions cannot be scraped off, reversed by the removal of irritants, or ascribed to another disease entity. Most oral idiopathic leukoplakias are found on the buccal mucosa, mandibular and maxillary alveolar ridges, and sulci, palate, and lip (48). Various clinical types of idiopathic leukoplakia are recognized; among these are the homogeneous, speckled, and verruciform types (Fig. 19.8). This white thickening of the normally thin pink mucosa is caused by the expansion of the keratin layer (hyperkeratosis) and/or the prickle cell layer (acanthosis) (Fig. 19.9).

Idiopathic leukoplakia is a clinical term and should not be used microscopically because it encompasses many microscopic

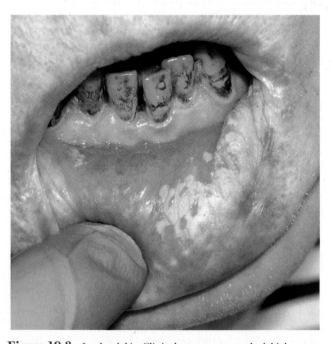

Figure 19.8. Leukoplakia. Clinical appearance on the labial mucosa of the lower lip presenting as patchy, homogeneous, well-demarcated, raised white plaques was found to be hyperkeratosis without epithelial atypia on biopsy. (Courtesy of Dr. Eric Carlson, Department of Oral and Maxillofacial Surgery, University of Tennessee Graduate School of Medicine, Knoxville, TN.)

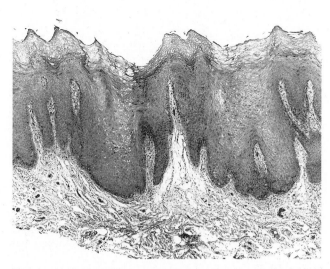

Figure 19.9. Leukoplakia—histologic appearance. Most exhibit varying degrees of epithelial thickening with acanthosis and hyperkeratosis but without dysplasia.

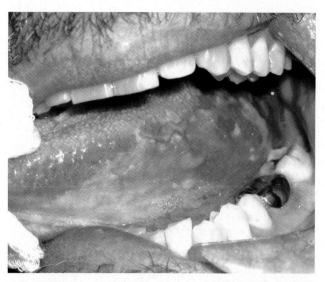

Figure 19.10. Erythroplakia—clinical appearance (lateral border of tongue). (Courtesy of Dr. Eric Carlson, Department of Oral and Maxillofacial Surgery, University of Tennessee Graduate School of Medicine, Knoxville, TN.)

lesions. Approximately 80% of idiopathic leukoplakias are diagnosed as hyperkeratosis. Dysplasias make up approximately 12% of idiopathic leukoplakias, carcinoma in situ (CIS) makes up approximately 3%, and invasive carcinomas make up approximately 5%. Transformation rates of all idiopathic leukoplakias are between 5% and 15% (48–52). Significantly higher rates of malignant transformation are observed in speckled (mixed red and white) leukoplakias and verrucous-papillary hyperkeratotic lesions known as proliferative verrucous leukoplakia (52–54). More than 75% of intraoral SCCs arise in a horseshoe-shaped area of the mouth that is defined by the floor of the mouth, the lateral-ventral tongue, and the soft palate–retromolar trigone-anterior tonsillar pillar region. These high-risk regions are constantly bathed in the salivary pool, with the potential for concentrated intraoral exposure to carcinogens. White lesions arising in these areas should be viewed with great suspicion. Nonetheless, all oral idiopathic leukoplakias should be biopsied because microscopy cannot be predicted from clinical appearance.

Erythroplakia, or "red patch," is a particularly ominous oral mucosal lesion (Fig. 19.10), representing carcinoma in 51% of cases, severe dysplasia or CIS in 40% of cases, and mild to moderate dysplasia in 9% of cases (55). These bright red, velvety patches correspond to thinned, atrophic epithelium with prominent subepithelial vascular telangiectasia and inflammation (Fig. 19.11). The lesion tends to be located predominantly in the cancer-prone areas of the floor of the mouth (28%), the retromolar trigone (19%), the mandibular gingiva and sulcus (12.5%), the ventral and/or lateral tongue (12.5%), and the palate (12.5%) (55).

SQUAMOUS DYSPLASIA AND CARCINOMA IN SITU

Dysplasia refers to abnormal epithelial growth that is characterized by features of cytologic, maturational, and architectural changes. These disturbances may comprise some or all of the features defined by the World Health Organization (WHO) Collaborating Center for Oral Precancerous Lesions in 1978, and refined more recently by the WHO in 2005 (47,56), and shown in Table 19.1. The former criterion of the presence of more

than one layer of cells having a basaloid appearance (basal/parabasal cell hyperplasia) has been eliminated. Histologic recognition of hyperplasia versus an early precursor lesion (dysplasia) is not always a reproducible observation, as acknowledged in the 2005 WHO publication (56): "There is a challenge in the recognition of the earliest manifestations of dysplasia and no single combination of the above features allows for consistent distinction between hyperplasia and the earliest stages of dysplasia. Dysplasia is a spectrum and no criteria exist to precisely divide this spectrum into mild, moderate and severe categories." In fact, given the 16 histologic variables of dysplasia described by the WHO, any of which can be observed in reactive squamous epithelium, there would be 560 combinations of any three histologic criteria to observe. Clearly, the requirement to reproducibly diagnose and grade squamous dysplasia is a challenge to the practicing pathologist.

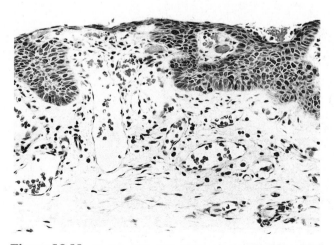

Figure 19.11. Erythroplakia—histologic appearance. Most exhibit high-grade dysplasia or carcinoma in situ. The red appearance correlates with a thin epithelium and telangiectatic superficial vessels.

TABLE 19.1

Histologic Features of Squamous Dysplasia

ARCHITECTURE
   Irregular epithelial stratification
   Loss of polarity of basal cells
   Drop-shaped rete ridges
   Abnormally superficial mitoses
   Premature keratinization in single cells (dyskeratosis)
   Keratin pearls within rete pegs
CYTOLOGY
   Abnormal variation in nuclear size (anisonucleosis)
   Abnormal variation in nuclear shape (nuclear pleomorphism)
   Abnormal variation in cell size (anisocytosis)
   Abnormal variation in cell shape (cellular pleomorphism)
   Increased nuclear-to-cytoplasmic ratio
   Increased nuclear size
   Atypical mitotic figures
   Increased number and size of nucleoli
   Hyperchromasia

From: Barnes L, Eveson JW, Reichart P, et al. *World Health Organization Classification of Tumours. Pathology and Genetics of Head and Neck Tumours.* Lyon, France: IARC Press, 2005.

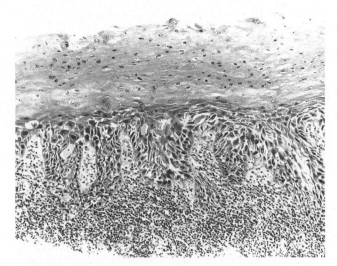

Figure 19.13. Lichenoid dysplasia. The hyperkeratotic epithelium has irregular rete ridges and a dense, hugging subepithelial band of lymphocytes, like that seen in lichen planus. Note the significant dysplasia in the lower zone that is marked by the disordered proliferation of keratinocytes with pleomorphic, hyperchromatic nuclei.

Nevertheless, the intent of histologic grading of dysplasia is to convey to the clinician a sense of the risk of development of subsequent carcinoma. In the oral cavity, biopsy samples showing only CIS have the same age and sex distribution as the invasive oral carcinomas, with a similar grouping at the high-risk sites of the floor of the mouth, the tongue, and the lips (57). Most biopsy samples containing CIS are taken from locations adjacent to an invasive cancer, and therefore, the presumption is that moderate and severe degrees of dysplasia, if they are sequential, carry increasing risk. However, the relationship of increasing degrees of oral squamous dysplasia to the subsequent progression to invasive carcinoma is not well defined. In fact, some invasive cancers do not develop from an in situ continuum but rather arise as "drop-off" or "drop-down" cancers from apparently normal or minimally atypical surface epithelium (Fig. 19.12).

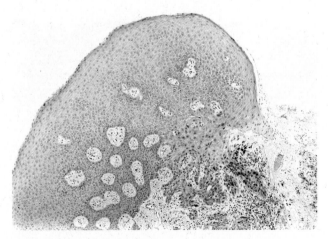

Figure 19.12. "Drop-off" or "drop-down" cancers. These invade from morphologically hyperplastic or nondysplastic overlying epithelium.

Histologic grading of epithelial abnormalities arising in the upper aerodigestive tract mucosa is notoriously subjective for several reasons. These include the absence of an accepted single standardized scheme or quantitative criteria for classification; the recognition that the lesser grades recognized as dysplasia may not be neoplastic at all but may rather represent reversible, reactive mucosal change; the realization that mild to moderate degrees of squamous dysplasia arising in the mucosa with lichenoid inflammatory features may be masked and difficult to discern as truly dysplastic (Fig. 19.13); and the understanding that many lesions are keratinized and that they therefore never meet the CIS criteria for full-thickness abnormal proliferation. To acknowledge the histologic uncertainty in identifying true neoplasia from a reversible reactive process in cases of low-grade abnormalities or mild "dysplasia" (58), some pathologists prefer to use the term *squamous atypia* rather than *dysplasia*. However, the following caveat from WHO 1997 (59), which was lost in the 2005 WHO publication, acknowledges that histologic appearances are imperfect predictors and should be remembered when attempting to convey to the clinician the importance of a squamous abnormality in certain oral mucosal sites: "slight degrees of epithelial dysplasia do not indicate any great danger for the patient (although special reference should be made to certain high risk sites, such as *floor of mouth and ventral surface of tongue where importance should be attached to even slight dysplasia*)."

Despite these shortcomings discussed earlier and the fact that histologic grading cannot be reliably shown to offer significant prognostic value, the custom is to classify oral epithelial abnormalities into three grades of dysplasia based on a combination of the level of proliferation of cytologically atypical keratinocytes within the mucosa, the degree of cytologic atypia, the maturation, and the architectural abnormalities (60). Figures 19.14, 19.15, and 19.16 illustrate mild, moderate, and severe dysplasia, respectively. A full-thickness proliferation of undifferentiated basaloid cells (classic CIS), as is commonly seen in the cervical intraepithelial neoplasia, is rarely seen in the head and neck mucosa (Fig. 19.17).

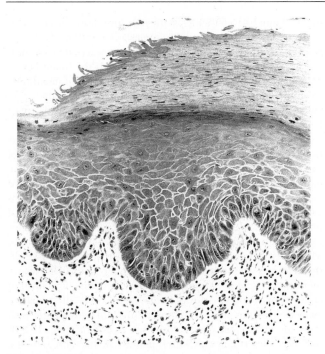

Figure 19.14. Mild squamous dysplasia. Hyperkeratotic squamous epithelium with normal maturation and enlarged, hyperchromatic, cytologically atypical keratinocytes and increased numbers of mitotic figures is limited to the basal lower one-third zone of the mucosa.

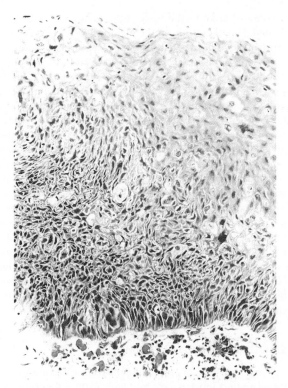

Figure 19.16. Severe keratinizing squamous dysplasia. Although surface keratinization is present, cells with significant nuclear pleomorphism are found throughout the mucosa and are more densely concentrated in the lower epithelium. Loss of the normal orderly mosaic pattern of maturation, increased numbers of mitotic figures at higher levels, and dyskeratotic cells in the middle and deep mucosa occur.

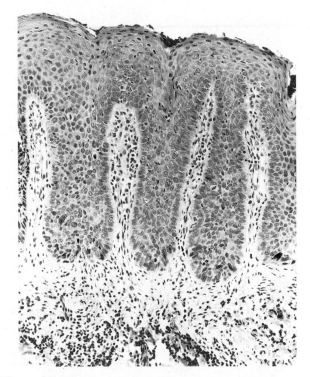

Figure 19.15. Moderate squamous dysplasia. Elongated rete processes contain a disordered proliferation of crowded basaloid cells with nuclear pleomorphism, hyperchromatism, and enhanced mitotic activity extending into the mid zones of the mucosa.

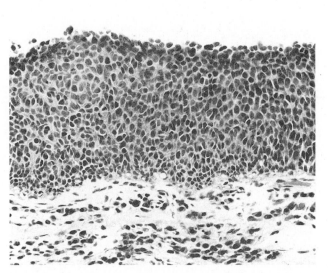

Figure 19.17. Squamous carcinoma in situ (CIS). This tonsil biopsy shows the histologic features of classic CIS, which is rarely encountered in the head and neck mucosa. Full-thickness proliferation of basaloid cells lacking surface keratinization, basal organization, and the normal equidistant mosaic pattern of nuclear orientation is observed.

Severe dysplasias in the upper tract mucosa are commonly thickened, hyperkeratotic epithelium in which marked nuclear abnormalities, abnormal mitoses, disordered maturation with loss of orientation, and dyskeratosis confined to the lower portion of the epithelium can be seen; these are seldom full thickness in their extent (Fig. 19.16). Shafer and Waldron (57) have suggested that the presence of single-cell keratinization and/or keratin pearl formation in oral CIS is often a hallmark of transition to invasive carcinoma. This biopsy finding of deep keratinization warrants careful examination for invasion. Some evidence from studies of laryngeal glottic mucosa indicates that severe keratinizing dysplasias may exhibit as high a rate of progression to invasive carcinoma as does classic CIS at that site. For this reason, the suggestion has been that both of these high-grade forms be categorized under the rubric of squamous intraepithelial neoplasia grade III to standardize the terminology and histologic criteria connoting the high risk of malignant transformation (61). In the oral cavity mucosa, whether these two high-grade histologic abnormalities of severe keratinizing dysplasia versus classic CIS carry different rates or periods of progression is not known.

MICROINVASIVE CARCINOMA

The primary purpose of identifying microinvasive carcinoma is to convey to the clinician a morphologic feature that should be predictive of biologic behavior and direct therapeutic intervention. However, no consensus exists on the definition of the depth or histologic form of invasion that constitutes microinvasive, early, or superficially invasive squamous carcinoma in the head and neck region. The assessment of tumor thickness or depth of invasion using Breslow-type measurements, excluding the layers of surface keratin and parakeratin, has consistently shown statistical significance and independent power in predicting the rate of cervical lymph node metastasis, recurrence, and survival (Fig. 19.18) (62–68). In a study of SCC from mixed oral cavity and oropharyngeal sites, tumors with depths of invasion of less than 4 mm had a metastatic rate of 8.3%, those with invasion

of 4 to 8 mm had a 35% metastatic rate, and those with invasion greater than 8 mm had an 83% metastatic rate (66). However, the least depth of invasion predictive of cervical node metastasis was a 2-mm invasive cancer. Therefore, with the limited available data, a 1- to 2-mm distance from the basement membrane to define microinvasive carcinoma appears reasonable, provided that no extension into muscle or cartilage or evidence of lymphovascular space invasion is present.

The assessment of microinvasion requires well-oriented sections that are perpendicular to the mucosa to define either of two histologic patterns of extension. The first frankly invasive pattern is that of discontinuous, often irregularly contoured nests of dysplastic epithelium in the underlying stroma that is usually associated with a host desmoplastic edematous stromal fibrosis (Fig. 19.19). The second pattern of invasion is analogous to the discrimination of actinic keratosis from SCC of skin, in which a criterion of depth of contiguous extension is used. In the head and neck mucosa, this is a much more subjective assessment that is dependent on well-oriented sections. This form of attached or "incipient" invasion may be very well differentiated, as is seen in verrucous carcinoma, or frankly dysplastic with cytologic atypia and dyskeratosis that is evident (Fig. 19.20). Although describing this latter pattern of invasion into the stroma is appropriate for directing therapy, the biologic behavior compared with the frankly invasive pattern is undefined.

Several notable pitfalls are seen in the interpretation of invasion. The first is use of tangential sections of markedly thickened, high-grade dysplastic mucosa as a sign of invasion. Dysplastic squamous mucosa in the head and neck region may often be markedly thickened, but it still may not be invasive. Tangen-

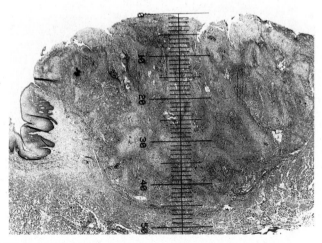

Figure 19.18. Measurement of tumor thickness or depth of invasion. Demonstrated in this 4.7-mm invasive squamous cell carcinoma of the lateral tongue, this is a statistically significant and independent factor in predicting the rate of cervical lymph node metastasis, recurrence, and survival.

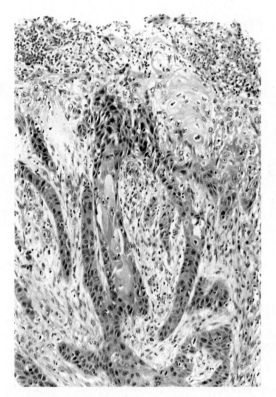

Figure 19.19. Microinvasion characterized by discontinuous, often irregularly contoured nests of dysplastic epithelium in the underlying stroma associated with a host desmoplastic, edematous stromal fibrosis.

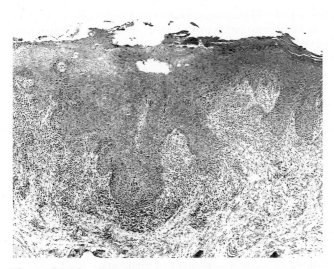

Figure 19.20. Microinvasion. In well-oriented sections of attached epithelial patterns, microinvasion can be inferred by deep contiguous extension into underlying stroma.

tial sectioning may exaggerate this thickness, lending the appearance of a mass. In addition, tangential sectioning with exaggeration and elongation of the rete often populated by an apparently increased proportion of darker basal cells may mimic invasion. Furthermore, the well-contoured, detached epithelial foci without desmoplasia in the underlying stroma are often not invasive. Deeper levels through the block may "stand" the section up and show that foci that were previously "detached" and appeared invasive are nonetheless attached to the overlying epithelium. Another pitfall is overcalling invasion by misinterpreting the extension of CIS into the underlying minor salivary gland ducts and mucous glands. This spread of CIS is recognized by the rounded, filled ductal contours and preserved but expanded lobular salivary gland architecture. These features can be confirmed with immunohistochemical stains for residual native basal and myoepithelial cells. It is advisable to section oral biopsies with atypical epithelium at several levels because many head and neck lesions are histopathologically heterogeneous.

MULTIPLE PRIMARIES

Patients with head and neck cancer are prone to the development of multiple synchronous and metachronous malignancies involving both upper and lower aerodigestive tracts. Of those patients with initial signs of oral cavity SCC, 27% have ultimately had second primary cancers (69). The occurrence of a second primary cancer is an unfavorable prognostic factor, resulting in an overall 5-year survival rate of 17% compared with a 35% survival rate in patients with only a single head and neck cancer (70). Until now, the prevailing explanation for the increased frequency of second head and neck mucosal malignancies in this population has been that of field cancerization. This proposal by Slaughter et al. (71) in 1953 postulated a multiclonal origin such that multiple, separate cancers develop in these patients from independent neoplastic events in a mucosa that has been widely activated by common exposure to carcinogens such as tobacco and alcohol. More recently, based on molecular evidence, some multiple, geographically and temporally sepa-

rate squamous cancers have been proposed to arise from an initial single cancer clone that spreads laterally within the mucosa and appear as separate "primaries" but, in essence, are the extensions of one tumor (72–75). These studies somewhat negate the reliance on previously accepted histologic criteria for the diagnosis of a second primary SCC. These criteria had required biopsy proof that two synchronous tumors were anatomically separated by an intervening nonneoplastic mucosa or that a metachronous tumor had an in situ mucosal origin. Typically, however, the reappearance of tumor at or near the site of a previously treated carcinoma is not usually taken as evidence of surface origin. When the tumor is located in the deeper portions of the submucosa, its reappearance is presumed to represent persistence of the original tumor (76).

TUMOR-NODE-METASTASIS STAGING

Tumor staging parameters of primary tumor size and the extent of invasion; the size, number, and laterality of positive cervical lymph nodes; and the presence of distant metastases remain the most important factors influencing therapeutic decisions and predicting outcome in patients with oral SCC. Staging is accomplished with the tumor-node-metastasis (TNM) staging classification (77). The requirements of the pathologic classification system, which is designated pTNM and which verifies the clinical classification (cTNM), specify that resection of the primary tumor or biopsy must be adequate to evaluate the highest pathologic tumor (pT) category and that removal of regional nodes must be an effective means of validating the absence of regional lymph node metastasis and of evaluating the highest pathologic node (pN) category. For pathologic metastasis (pM), microscopic examination of a distant metastasis is required. Notable changes from the last edition include describing T4 lesions as T4a (resectable) and T4b (unresectable), so that advanced-stage disease is classified as stage IVA, advanced resectable disease; stage IVB, advanced unresectable disease; and stage IVC, advanced distant metastatic disease. Moreover, a descriptor has been added to designate nodal metastasis in the upper neck as (U) and lower neck as (L), but this has no influence on nodal staging.

The unified TNM staging classification of lip, oral cavity, and oropharynx sites defines primary tumor (T) extent using not only size of tumor in greatest dimension (T1 to T3) but also local extension of disease in T4 categories:

TX, primary tumor cannot be assessed.
T0, no evidence of primary tumor.
Tis, carcinoma in situ.
T1, tumor of 2 cm or less in greatest dimension.
T2, tumor more than 2 cm but not more than 4 cm in greatest dimension.
T3, tumor more than 4 cm in greatest dimension.
T4a (lip), tumor invading through the cortical bone, inferior alveolar nerve, floor of mouth, or skin (chin or nose).
T4a (oral cavity), tumor invading through cortical bone into the deep (extrinsic) muscle of the tongue (genioglossus, hyoglossus, palatoglossus, and styloglossus), maxillary sinus, or skin of face.
T4b (lip and oral cavity), tumor invades the masticator space, pterygoid plate, or skull base or encases the internal carotid artery.

Note that superficial erosion alone of the bone and/or tooth socket by primary gingival tumor is not sufficient to classify a tumor as T4.

REGIONAL LYMPH NODE METASTASIS

Several types of neck dissections may be encountered, classified as (a) radical neck dissection; (b) modified radical neck dissection, with internal jugular vein and/or sternocleidomastoid muscle spared; (c) selective neck dissection as specified by the surgeon as (i) supraomohyoid neck dissection, (ii) posterolateral neck dissection, (iii) lateral neck dissection, or (iv) central compartment neck dissection or other; and (d) extended radical neck dissection as specified by the surgeon.

The presence and number of regional lymph node metastases are the strongest predictors of survival in oral cavity SCC. The importance of these parameters as prognostic indicators lies in the recognition that cancer deaths in many patients stem from uncontrolled regional disease in the cervical lymph nodes that is often associated with local recurrence at the primary site.

The size and level of involved lymph nodes correlate with prognosis (78). Therefore, the surgical pathology report should document lymph node involvement by anatomic subdivisions of the submental, submandibular, or anterior triangle; the subdigastric–upper jugular, midjugular, low jugular, posterior cervical, or posterior triangle; and the supraclavicular regions.

The surgical pathologic documentation of extracapsular lymph node spread of SCC in neck dissections is another significant prognostic indicator of survival (Fig. 19.21). The survival rate of patients with oral cavity SCC with metastases and intact lymph node capsules is 33% at 5 years compared with an 11% survival rate in patients with extracapsular infiltration into adjacent soft tissues (79). The communication of this finding in the surgical pathology report is important because it often modifies the treatment plan to include regional radiotherapy, radioactive seed implantation, or chemotherapy.

It is accepted that both clinical and routine pathologic staging underestimate the presence of lymph node metastases. Given that elective neck dissection for early oral cancers is an unsettled clinical issue, some have resorted to sentinel lymph node biopsy for direction. Roughly 20% of clinically negative

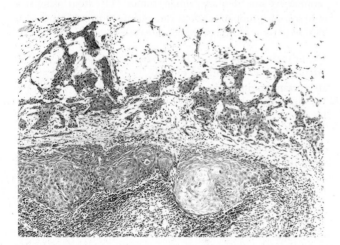

Figure 19.21. Extracapsular spread of squamous cell carcinoma from a cervical lymph node metastasis. This significant histologic finding is associated with lower survival rates.

necks (N0) will have metastases detected histologically, and routine pathologic techniques provide a negative predictive value of 96% in the assessment of neck nodes (80,81). In two single-institution studies, sentinel lymph node biopsy was used to up-stage 32% to 35% of clinical N0 necks to positive necks, leading to therapeutic neck dissection for this subset of patients (82,83). This would include histopathologic findings of isolated tumor cells, micrometastases less than 2 mm, and macrometastases greater than 2 mm. The sensitivity of sentinel node examination in predicting lymph node metastasis in oral and oropharyngeal carcinomas in another study was 89%, leaving an 11% false-negative rate, which is similar to the experience in breast cancer (84,85). Currently, the use of sentinel lymph node biopsy for head and neck cancer is not standard therapy, and the prognostic significance of immunohistochemically demonstrated occult nodal micrometastases is not known. The role of sentinel node biopsy for head and neck cancers in lieu of elective neck dissection awaits multi-institutional trial validation.

The TNM classification of regional lymph node (N) involvement for oral cavity and oropharyngeal tumors is based on single versus multiple node involvement, greatest size dimension of involved node, and ipsilateral versus bilateral node involvement, specified as follows:

NX, regional lymph nodes cannot be assessed.

N0, no regional lymph node metastasis.

N1, metastasis in a single ipsilateral lymph node that is 3 cm or less at its greatest dimension.

N2, metastasis in a single ipsilateral lymph node that is more than 3 cm but not more than 6 cm in greatest dimension; or in multiple ipsilateral lymph nodes, none of which is more than 6 cm in greatest dimension; or in bilateral or contralateral lymph nodes, none of which is more than 6 cm in greatest dimension.

N2a, metastasis in a single ipsilateral lymph node of more than 3 cm but not more than 6 cm.

N2b, metastasis in multiple ipsilateral lymph nodes with none being more than 6 cm.

N2c, metastasis in bilateral or contralateral lymph nodes with none being more than 6 cm.

N3, metastasis in a lymph node that is more than 6 cm in greatest dimension.

Note: midline nodes are considered ipsilateral nodes.

DISTANT METASTASIS

In contrast to the 1923 autopsy study by Crile (86), which showed a 1% rate of distant metastasis, a significant rate of systemic metastases from oral cavity SCC is now recognized (87). This rate of distant metastasis ranges from 31% in patients who die of oral carcinoma after initially having negative results on neck dissections to 59% in patients with pathologically staged positive regional lymph node metastases (79). The most probable explanation is that improvements in local and regional tumor control have led to longer survival and thereby opportunities, especially in those with recurrent disease, for the metastatic cascade to be successfully completed and clinically recognized.

In the TNM classification, distant metastasis (M) is designated as follows:

Mx, the presence of distant metastasis cannot be assessed.

M0, no distant metastasis.

M1, distant metastasis.

The combinations of increasing T, N, and M stages result in the following stage groupings for lip, oral cavity, oropharynx, and hypopharynx sites:

Stage 0: Tis, N0, M0.

Stage I: T1, N0, M0.

Stage II: T2, N0, M0.

Stage III: T1 or T2, N1, M0; T3, N0 or N1, M0.

Stage IVA: T1 or T2 or T3, N2, M0; T4a, N0 or N1 or N2, M0.

Stage IVB: any T, N3, M0; T4b, any N, M0.

Stage IVC: any T, any N, M1.

HISTOPATHOLOGIC PARAMETERS OF PROGNOSTIC SIGNIFICANCE

Numerous studies of histopathologic features of tumor and host response parameters in oral SCC have shown variable prognostic significance. Although some studies have found tumor grade to be predictive of regional lymph node metastasis, the assessments of tumor grade encompassing traditional histologic and cytologic features of differentiation are not highly reproducible. Therefore, the tumor grade is of limited clinical value in comparison with the clinical staging parameters. Also because most SCCs are moderately differentiated, no apparent correlation of grade with tumor size has been found.

Two of the more important histopathologic observations in oral SCC are the pattern or mode of tumor invasion within the stroma and the depth or thickness of tumor invasion. The patterns of noncohesive, irregular, jagged small cords and infiltrative, widespread single cells (Fig. 19.22) are associated with a higher rate of regional lymph node metastasis than are patterns composed of well-defined, blunt pushing borders or thick, rounded invasive cords of tumor (Fig. 19.23) (62,66,88–91). When the pattern of invasion is subjected to multivariate analysis, it is a significant histologic feature that surpasses that of the conventional tumor grade as a prognostic indicator (62). Depth

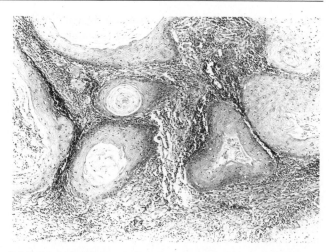

Figure 19.23. A more favorable invasive histologic pattern. Composed of well-defined, blunt, pushing borders or thick, rounded, invasive cords of tumor, this pattern is a more favorable prognostic indicator.

of invasion is an independent predictor of lymph node metastasis for cancers of numerous oral sites.

Additional microscopic findings associated with increased rates of cervical lymph node metastasis and poor prognosis that are recommended for inclusion in the surgical pathology report by the Association of Directors of Anatomic and Surgical Pathology (92) are the presence of angiolymphatic invasion (Fig. 19.24) (62,66,93) and perineural invasion (94). Other assessments of lymph node reaction patterns and host inflammatory and desmoplastic response have added no consistent or independent discriminating information (66). In the upcoming sections, the significance of these histopathologic parameters as they pertain to the specific oral cavity and oropharyngeal sites of SCC is elaborated.

EVALUATION OF RESECTION MARGINS

The pathologic evaluation and documentation of the completeness of primary excision margins provide significant informa-

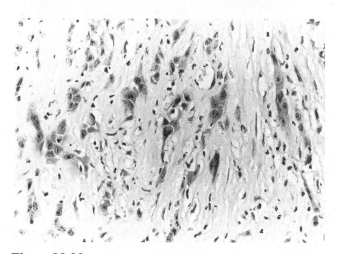

Figure 19.22. An unfavorable histologic pattern of invasion. Characterized by noncohesive, irregular, jagged small cords and infiltrative, widespread single cells, this pattern is associated with a higher rate of regional lymph node metastasis.

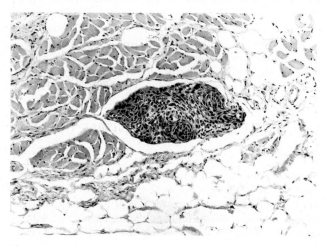

Figure 19.24. A focus of angiolymphatic invasion in tongue muscle. Found away from the small primary carcinoma that was associated with cervical lymph node metastases, this microscopic finding predicts a poor prognosis.

tion for the intraoperative and postsurgical treatment options and prognosis. The definition of a positive margin is usually restricted to the finding of invasive carcinoma at the microscopic margin (95,96). The observations of CIS and a close margin of less than 5 mm from the resection line are noteworthy because patients with high-grade dysplasia and close margins also appear to be at risk for locally recurrent carcinoma (97).

When defining a positive margin as either in situ or invasive SCC, Byers et al. (95) have noted an 80% local recurrence rate for oral cavity and oropharynx tumors with positive margins, compared with rates of 12% for oral cavity SCC and 18% for oropharyngeal cancers with initially free margins (95). In some studies, the frequency of positive margins in head and neck cancer appears to correlate with increased tumor size or the stage of disease and, therefore, with the potential to resect the tumor surgically without sacrificing vital structures or the tissue required for closure (96). Postoperative radiotherapy for positive margins appears to be ineffectual, and the 2-year survival rate is dismal in this group of patients (95,96).

The intraoperative consultation assessment of margin adequacy is a time-consuming endeavor but has been shown to be reliable and accurate and represents a prime opportunity for assuring surgical eradication of the disease. In practice, techniques of sectioning margins include full-thickness, serial, and bread-loaf types, with inked surgical margins, as well as parallel, shave margins from the edges. The latter are often used in the examination of separately submitted marginal tissue and additional tissue taken from previously positive or close margins.

SITE-SPECIFIC CONSIDERATIONS

No distinct histopathologic differences in SCC have been identified for the various intraoral sites. In general, larger oral cavity and oropharyngeal tumors exhibit a higher rate of metastasis such that the risk from tumors less than 3 cm is low, the risk from tumors that are 3 to 4 cm is intermediate, and the risk from tumors more than 4 cm is the highest (98). An analysis of 898 SCCs of the oral cavity and oropharynx has shown that same-size tumors of the lip, floor of the mouth, buccal mucosa, hard palate, and gingiva have approximately the same risk for metastasis to the regional lymph nodes (98). Some site-specific differences in biologic behavior are recognized that may relate to innate biologic differences, the associated clinical symptoms leading to timely diagnosis at earlier stages, and variations in local anatomy that are associated with lymphatic drainage. These differences and other pertinent histopathologic observations for SCC involving specific intraoral sites are enumerated in the following sections.

SQUAMOUS CELL CARCINOMA OF THE LIP

The most common oral cancer, which accounts for 42% of all cases, is SCC of the lip (99). Roughly 90% of these SCCs arise in the lower lip, usually along the mucocutaneous junction or vermilion border. Unlike other oral SCCs, chronic sunlight exposure is a prime etiologic agent, in addition to tobacco exposure in the form of pipe and cigarette smoking and poor oral hygiene. The pattern of metastasis from lower lip SCC is to the ipsilateral submandibular and submental lymph nodes, with potential for bilateral metastases in midline lesions. The lym-

phatic drainage from SCCs of the upper lip is to the preauricular and infraparotid lymph nodes. The rate of metastasis from SCCs of the lip is directly related to size, with a 5% rate of metastasis in SCCs less than 2 cm, 50% in tumors of 2 to 4 cm, and 73% in SCCs larger than 4 cm. Other pathologic observations that are predictive of subsequent regional metastasis include a high tumor grade, tumor thickness of more than 6 mm, an aggressive pattern of invasion, and the presence of perineural invasion (63). These histologic parameters are best assessed in the deeper portions of the neoplasm. The survival rates for patients with lip SCC decline with advancing tumor size, the presence of lymph node metastases, and high tumor grade.

SQUAMOUS CELL CARCINOMA OF THE TONGUE

SCC of the tongue accounts for 22% of intraoral SCCs, which is practically equal to the total incidence of SCC at all other sites of intraoral carcinoma if the lips are excluded (99). The neoplasm most often develops as an area of leukoplakia, chronic ulcer, or erythroplakia on the lateral aspect of the middle one-third of the tongue (Fig. 19.25). SCC involving the anterior two-thirds, or the mobile tongue, has a higher tendency to metastasize than do other intraoral carcinomas, with the exception of carcinomas of the tongue base (posterior one-third) and oropharynx, which exhibit the most aggressive behavior (98). Overall, 70% of patients with carcinoma of the tongue have unilateral or bilateral metastases at their first examination. Tongue SCC characteristically metastasizes to the ipsilateral subdigastric, submandibular, and midjugular lymph nodes. Bilateral nodal involvement is more common in tumors of the midline and base

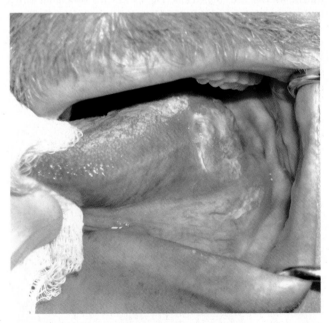

Figure 19.25. Squamous cell carcinoma of the ventral-lateral tongue. This tumor appears as a raised, hyperkeratotic mass extending from the posterior lateral tongue surface to the ventral tongue border at the floor of the mouth. Note: separate patch of leukoplakia in the floor of the mouth. (Courtesy of Dr. Eric Carlson, Department of Oral and Maxillofacial Surgery, University of Tennessee Graduate School of Medicine, Knoxville, TN.)

of the tongue, as opposed to lateral tongue tumors. Whereas most intraoral primary SCCs metastasize initially to the nearest draining nodes (level I or II) with progressive overflow to neighboring nodes, tongue cancers may show a more aggressive pattern with skip lesions and peppering of lymph nodes (100). Tongue base cancers may show isolated level IV metastasis and, overall, have a high rate of level IV nodal involvement that translates to a worse 5-year survival (101). Because of their posterior location and, at times, endophytic growth pattern, the patients usually are not aware of early-stage tongue base carcinomas; 90% are first evaluated in the advanced stages III and IV, compared with 37% of patients with mobile tongue cancers (102).

Histologically, posterior tongue SCCs tend to be less differentiated than those arising in the mobile tongue, but the microscopic pattern or mode of invasion is the feature that predicts for nodal metastasis. Also, pathologic determination of depth of invasion is a significant predictor of regional lymph node metastasis for tongue cancers. Assessment of tumor thickness is a very good indicator of the presence of occult cervical node metastasis and of poor outcomes in early-stage I/II oral tongue cancer (103). Tongue cancers that exceed 5 mm in tumor depth have a metastatic rate of approximately 51% to 65% compared with approximately 6% to 8% for those less than or equal to 5 mm (104,105).

SQUAMOUS CELL CARCINOMA OF THE FLOOR OF MOUTH

The third most common site of intraoral SCC is the floor of the mouth, which comprises 17% of intraoral carcinomas (99). This is the most common site of intraoral carcinoma in African Americans (106). The area of the floor of the mouth that is most often affected is the anterior region of the caruncles of the submaxillary gland and the lingual frenum, where it can appear as either an elevated leukoplakia or a velvety erythroplakic lesion. On the initial examination, SCC of the floor of the mouth has invaded one or more contiguous structures in 75% of cases (107). The submandibular triangle and subdigastric lymph nodes are most commonly involved, but submental nodes are rarely affected, even in anterior tumors. In tumors of the floor of the mouth, palpable nodes designated as positive on clinical examination have shown a false-positive rate of up to 56%; in tumors with negative results on clinical evaluation, the false-negative rate is 24% after histologic examination (108). This high rate of erroneous clinical assessment is attributed to confusion with the obstructive enlargement of the sublingual and submandibular glands, as well as to reactive lymph node hyperplasia caused by inflammation.

In general, the frequency of lymph node metastasis is related to the tumor size, with most notable differences being seen between T1 and T3 and T4 tumors. Histopathologic assessment of the pattern of invasion and the depth of tumor invasion in T2 lesions of the floor of the mouth appears to have discriminatory power in predicting lymph node metastasis, with no metastases being noted from superficially invasive tumors and a 44% rate of metastases with confluent, nodular, or deeply invasive cancers (108). Histologic measurements of the tumor thickness, independent of tumor size, may be a stronger predictor for the subsequent development of nodal metastases from the floor of the mouth, with a 2% metastatic rate from SCCs measuring less than 1.5 mm compared with a 33% rate for tumor thicknesses

of 1.6 to 3.5 mm and a 60% rate for lesions thicker than 3.6 mm (64). The importance of tumor thickness has been corroborated by another study applying multivariate analysis to cancers of the floor of the mouth and tongue that showed that tumor thickness less than 2 mm was the most significant favorable predictor of recurrence and survival (67).

SQUAMOUS CELL CARCINOMA OF THE GINGIVA

Carcinoma of the gingiva accounts for 6% of intraoral carcinomas and usually occurs in the mandibular bicuspid and molar areas (99). In nonedentulous patients, the lesions develop at the free gingival margin, whereas, in edentulous patients, the lesions are located on the alveolar ridge (Fig. 19.26). Carcinoma of the gingiva is often clinically misdiagnosed as one of the many inflammatory lesions of the periodontium (e.g., pyogenic granuloma, PGCG, localized gingivitis/periodontitis), papilloma, or even fibroid epulis (inflammatory hyperplasia).

SCC of the gingiva is usually a well-differentiated carcinoma that tends to invade bone. These patients often have loose teeth because of tumor invasion of adjacent periodontal ligament and alveolar bone. Metastasis is often to the submandibular lymph nodes, where it may demonstrate a less differentiated histopathologic appearance. Although rarely seen, the gingiva (and hard palate) is the intraoral site of predilection for melanoma.

SQUAMOUS CELL CARCINOMA OF THE BUCCAL MUCOSA

SCC of the buccal mucosa accounts for 2% of intraoral carcinomas (99). Buccal mucosal carcinoma, like SCC arising at other oral cavity sites, predominates among men. Some American series from southern states, however, are heavily weighted toward women because of the more commonplace habit of tobacco chewing or oral snuff dipping (109). Many of these people have

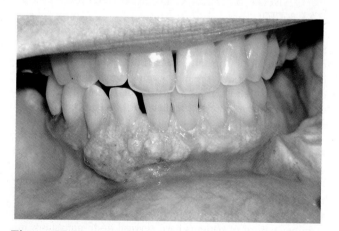

Figure 19.26. Squamous cell carcinoma of gingiva. In this nonedentulous patient, the hyperkeratotic cancer involves the anterior mandibular gingiva from left canine to central incisor and extends to the junction at the buccal sulcus. (Courtesy of Dr. Eric Carlson, Department of Oral and Maxillofacial Surgery, University of Tennessee Graduate School of Medicine, Knoxville, TN.)

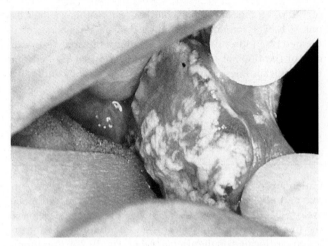

Figure 19.27. Classic verrucous carcinoma of the buccal mucosa. It appears as a raised, granular, red and white hyperkeratotic plaque-like mass.

verrucous carcinoma in the buccal mucosa (Fig. 19.27) or gingiva. SCC of the buccal mucosa may extend to involve the contiguous soft tissue and bony structures that is directly related to tumor size. Regional metastasis, which is usually limited to the submandibular lymph nodes, is typically a late-stage phenomenon.

In addition to tumor stage, observations of anterior-posterior tumor location and histopathologic factors have prognostic value. Five-year cure rates decline with more posterior buccal mucosal sites: 40% for tumors located in the anterior buccal, 17% for the middle third, and 10% for the posterior third (110). The rates of recurrence and survival are significantly related to a depth of invasion less than 3 mm and tumor thickness of less than 6 mm (111). The latter observation is an independent variable in predicting survival regardless of stage.

SQUAMOUS CELL CARCINOMA OF THE PALATE

SCC arising from the oral surfaces of the palate is more commonly localized to the soft palate (112). It accounts for 5.5% of intraoral SCC but is the most common malignant neoplasm of the palate (99,112). A male predominance of 2.5 to 1 is observed, with no gender predilection between the hard and soft palates. More than half of palatal SCCs extend beyond the anatomic confines of the palate at the initial examination (113). The resection specimens of hard palate should be decalcified to evaluate the extent of invasion into underlying bone. The lymphatic drainage pathway of the hard and soft palates is through the retromolar triangle to the lymph nodes of the internal jugular chain, the submandibular, and the retropharyngeal regions. A third of patients have cervical node metastases initially, with a similar incidence for both hard and soft palate lesions. Bilateral cervical metastases and distant metastases are uncommon. The tumor size and histologic grade correlate with survival, but the stage of the disease at presentation is the most important prognostic indicator (112,113).

SQUAMOUS CELL CARCINOMA OF THE OROPHARYNX

Anatomically, the oropharynx has been subdivided into the palatine arch and the oropharynx proper. The palatine arch is the superior wall of the oropharynx; it is composed of the soft palate, uvula, anterior tonsillar pillars (glossopalatine folds), and retromolar trigone. The oropharynx proper has an anterior wall, consisting of the posterior third (or base) of the tongue, the intervening vallecula, and the lingual surface of the epiglottis, which is sometimes included with laryngeal tumors; a lateral wall, comprising the palatine tonsils or tonsillar fossa, the posterior tonsillar pillars (pharyngopalatine folds), and the glossotonsillar sulcus; and a posterior wall, made up of the posterior and lateral oropharyngeal walls from the soft palate to the level of the hyoid bone, including the pharyngoepiglottic fold (114). Oropharyngeal carcinomas are more aggressive than palatine arch carcinomas, and they exhibit a distant metastatic rate twice that of the palatine tumors (115).

In general, SCC arising in the oropharynx has a tendency to be less differentiated than the more proximally located intraoral carcinomas. The oropharynx lymphatic drainage includes the jugulodigastric, retropharyngeal, and parapharyngeal lymph node groups. In addition, an increased incidence of bilateral and contralateral cervical metastases is seen from these posterior sites because of the richer lymphatic drainage. This, in turn, is reflected in the poorer overall survival rates for patients with oropharyngeal primaries (116).

SQUAMOUS CELL CARCINOMA OF THE TONSIL

In the United States, the tonsil is the most common primary site of SCC in the oropharynx, followed by the base of the tongue, the soft palate and/or uvula, and the pharyngeal wall (117). Tonsillar SCC has a demographic profile and associated etiologic factors similar to those of intraoral carcinomas. Although this cancer is rare, when it develops in adults younger than 40 years of age, it carries a much poorer prognosis (118). More recent studies have shown that HPV-16–positive tonsillar carcinomas tend to arise in younger individuals without smoking or drinking risk factors and exhibit a better overall and disease-specific survival compared with HPV-negative tonsillar carcinomas (37). A poor prognosis is also associated with an advanced stage, which is related to large tumor size, presence of regional lymph node metastasis, and involvement of the base of the tongue (119). The tumor's pattern of invasion and mitotic index as assessed by histopathologic observations are correlated with survival, although these microscopic features are of lesser prognostic value (62).

Tonsillar carcinomas have a high overall rate of lymph node metastasis. They usually metastasize to the ipsilateral subdigastric lymph nodes, but they also involve the middle and lower jugular nodes, as well as the posterior cervical triangle nodes (119). Occasionally, node metastases may exhibit a cystic and, at times, deceptively bland histologic appearance that simulates a branchial cyst or a branchiogenic carcinoma (120). The latter entity is exceedingly rare, and blind tonsillar or nasopharyngeal biopsies have led to the correct diagnosis of metastatic carcinoma in many purported cases. The tonsil is also notable for being the primary site of undifferentiated carcinomas of the nasopharyngeal type, which have biologic behavior and increased radiosensitivity that are similar to nasopharyngeal lymphoepitheliomas.

UNUSUAL VARIANTS OF SQUAMOUS CELL CARCINOMA

VERRUCOUS CARCINOMA

Verrucous carcinoma (VC) of the oral cavity was first described by Friedell and Rosenthal (121) in 1941 and was further elaborated as a locally invasive, nonmetastasizing variant of SCC by Ackerman (121a) in 1948. It accounts for approximately 5% of oral cancers. The name of this clinicopathologic entity derives from its exophytic, warty clinical appearance (Fig. 19.27).

Clinical Features

In the oral cavity, the most common sites of occurrence of VC in decreasing order are the buccal mucosa, gingiva, tongue, palate, and tonsillar pillar. The average demographic profile is the same as most patients with oral cancer, with a predominance being seen among men late in the seventh decade of life (122). The oral tumors range from 1 to 10 cm in size (123). The tumor may extend by blunt invasion into the surrounding soft tissue and periosteum, and it may invade bone. Common symptoms include difficult mastication (because of a mass), ulcer, pain, and tenderness.

At one time, the association between long-term smokeless tobacco use and VC was thought to be quite strong (122), but this has not been substantiated with controlled clinical studies. Nonetheless, smokeless tobacco use is generally regarded as a risk factor for oral cancer, although the level of risk has likely been exaggerated. However, it has been well substantiated that intense smokers are at significant risk for developing verrucous and other types of oral SCCs (122,123). Alcohol abuse has not been implicated as a major etiologic agent in oral VC. Nearly 40% of 159 VCs tested have been HPV positive, with 47% involving HPV-6/-11, 35.3% involving HPV-16/-18, and 17.7% involving HPV-2 (124).

Morphologic Features

On clinical examination, VC appears as a relatively well-circumscribed, elevated, nodular mass with a surface that may be pebbled, papillary, verrucous, or smooth. Depending on the degree of surface keratinization, the VC varies in color from white to red to admixtures of both. The histologic picture of the tumor is well-differentiated squamous epithelium that exhibits orderly maturation in both upward and downward hyperplastic growth. The exophytic surface is covered by abundant orthokeratin and/or parakeratin that also fill the crevices of deep surface invaginations (Fig. 19.28). Because the lesions are well differentiated, superficial biopsies often do not yield a diagnosis. Clinical correlation can be of great value because lesions tend to be more impressive visually than microscopically. Typically, the epithelial downgrowth is made up of broad, blunt rete pegs that appear to be "pushing" into submucosa (Fig. 19.29). The advancing edge of the squamous epithelium is very well differentiated and may contain many mitotic figures that are rarely atypical. Unless the lesion is acutely inflamed, cytologic atypia

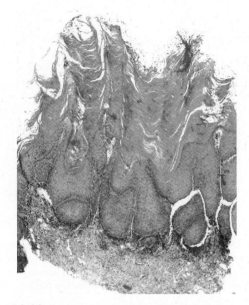

Figure 19.28. Verrucous carcinoma—histologic appearance. This is a well-differentiated squamous epithelium with hyperkeratotic exophytic surface and downward-pushing rete pegs. Minimal cytologic atypia is present, and the lamina propria contains a persistent lymphoplasmacytic inflammatory cell infiltrate.

is minimal. The lamina propria commonly contains a mild to moderate chronic inflammatory cell infiltrate.

In 104 oral VCs, Medina et al. (125) identified 21 (20%) hybrid oral tumors that were characterized by VC patterns with foci of less differentiated infiltrating SCCs. This finding within an otherwise typical VC should lead to a diagnosis of "VC with a coexisting focus of SCC" to alert the clinician to the risk of metastasis (Fig. 19.30). Observing strict histologic criteria, VC is locally invasive but is unlikely to metastasize unless there is evidence of transformation to a conventional invasive SCC. Trauma and infection of bulky VCs may result in the reactive enlargement of regional lymph nodes, thus mimicking meta-

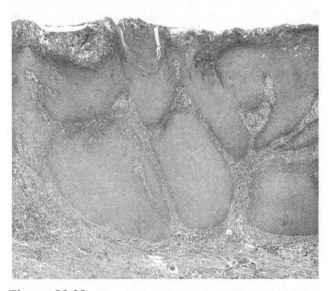

Figure 19.29. Verrucous carcinoma. Well-differentiated, large, blunt rete pegs "push" into the stroma at the same level.

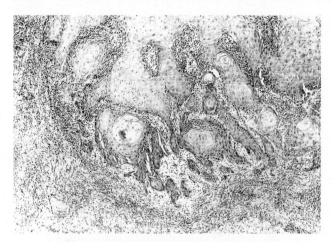

Figure 19.30. Focus of less-differentiated conventional squamous cell carcinoma with an infiltrating margin arising at the base of a verrucous carcinoma. The presence of coexisting foci of squamous cell carcinoma signals the potential for metastasis from this verrucous carcinoma.

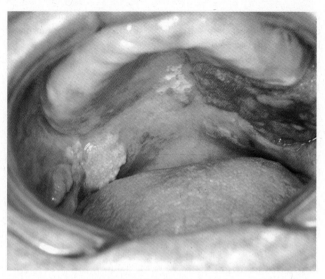

Figure 19.31. Proliferative verrucous leukoplakia. Widespread raised, granular, white and red hyperkeratotic plaques extending across the bilateral posterior edentulous alveolar ridges and palate appear similar to verrucous carcinoma. (Courtesy of Dr. Eric Carlson, Department of Oral and Maxillofacial Surgery, University of Tennessee Graduate School of Medicine, Knoxville, TN.)

static disease. Some recurrences of VC have been noted to take the form of less differentiated, nonverrucal carcinomas (125).

Differential Diagnosis

The clinical and histologic differential diagnosis of VC includes benign and malignant squamous proliferations. The benign lesions that should be considered are condyloma acuminatum, robust broad-based squamous papilloma, intraoral keratoacanthoma, pseudoepitheliomatous hyperplasia, and hyperkeratoses (leukoplakias) with warty, exophytic surfaces (proliferative verrucous leukoplakia and verrucous hyperplasia). Malignant lesions simulating VC include hyperkeratotic, bulky squamous dysplasias and well-differentiated SCCs exhibiting a papillary or verrucoid surface growth.

Broad-based squamous papillomas may be hyperkeratotic and have somewhat thick, club-shaped rete ridges, but they do not demonstrate acanthotic, downward "pushing" into underlying submucosa. Rarely seen oral keratoacanthomas exhibit the same architecture as their actinic cutaneous counterparts, most notable a symmetric cup-shaped morphology with a central keratin plug. The base may exhibit a blunt edge as is seen in VC, but it often has irregular tongues of epithelium that mimic invasion patterns of well-differentiated SCC. Intraoral pseudoepitheliomatous hyperplasia is typically seen in association with granular cell tumors, papillary hyperplasia of the palate, mycotic infections, and hyperplastic gingivitis. Although this form of hyperplasia may occasionally be hyperkeratotic, its irregular and pseudoinfiltrative character differs from the broad, pushing margins of VC.

Although hyperkeratotic white lesions (leukoplakias) may have a shaggy, verrucoid surface simulating VC superficially, they do not show any expansion into submucosa. The intraoral hyperkeratoses known as proliferative verrucous leukoplakia and verrucous hyperplasia represent slow-growing, persistent, irreversible, and often multifocal proliferations that simulate VC on clinical (Fig. 19.31) and histologic grounds (Fig. 19.32) (126). These lesions are entirely exophytic and superficial to the adjacent normal epithelium, lacking the downward proliferation of the rete pegs beyond the level of the adjacent squamous

mucosa. This is best evaluated in complete excisional biopsy specimens taken from the margins of the lesion. Proliferative verrucous leukoplakia is, however, a premalignant lesion that can transform into VC or SCC. It exhibits a significant association with coexisting VC (29%); conventional SCC, either coexisting or separate (10% to 37%); and epithelial dysplasia (26% to 66%) (127,128). With long-term follow-up, Silverman and Gorsky (54) have demonstrated the high-risk precancerous nature of proliferative verrucous leukoplakia, with SCC developing in 70% of patients in a mean time of 7.7 years. Interestingly,

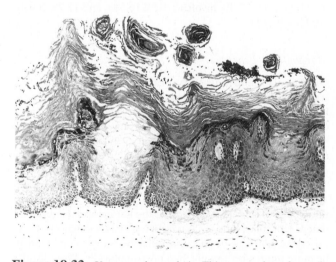

Figure 19.32. Verrucous hyperplasia. This mature, hyperkeratotic proliferation from a proliferative verrucous leukoplakia lesion is entirely exophytic, and it lacks downward proliferation of the rete pegs beyond the level of the adjacent squamous mucosa. Verrucous hyperplasia appears to be a premalignant precursor to many forms of squamous neoplasia.

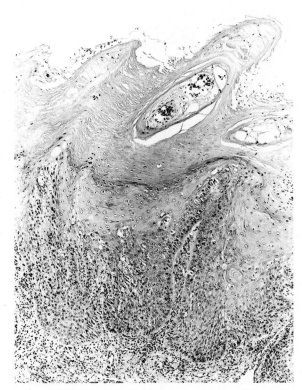

Figure 19.33. Verrucoid dysplasia. A hyperkeratotic, verrucoid surface growth pattern may be common to both squamous dysplasias and invasive carcinomas. Moderate to marked cytologic atypia seen at the base of the proliferation distinguishes this from verrucous carcinoma.

oral examples of proliferative verrucous leukoplakia have tested negative for HPV by PCR (129,130).

Some well-differentiated squamous dysplasias (Fig. 19.33) and SCCs demonstrate a hyperkeratotic, verrucoid surface architecture. They are distinguished from VC by moderate to marked cytologic atypia that usually is seen at the base of the proliferation. The carcinomas have an irregular infiltrative pattern of stromal invasion rather than the blunt, pushing border of VC. The discrimination from papillary SCC is described in the section "Papillary Squamous Cell Carcinoma."

Treatment and Prognosis

Surgical excision continues to be the most effective form of therapy, providing tumor control in 82% of patients after the initial surgical procedure and in 94% of patients after the surgical salvage of recurrences (125). Radiation therapy alone or combined with surgery has been used to treat selected oral cavity tumors, usually in unsuitable surgical candidates or as palliation in the case of advanced bulky disease. This treatment has resulted in favorable overall responses, but the effectiveness is diminished in larger tumors. The customary proscription against using irradiation is attributed to the cases of anaplastic transformation (dedifferentiation) of VC that have occurred after radiation therapy, but this outcome has been well documented in only four cases (131). This rare adverse outcome has been challenged as a concern in choosing radiation therapy as a therapeutic option, especially in light of the recognition of spontaneous transformation to SCC of a significant number of untreated or surgically excised tumors. The well-differentiated histologic appearance and slow growth of VC appears to render chemotherapy ineffectual.

PAPILLARY SQUAMOUS CELL CARCINOMA

As Batsakis and Suarez (132) noted, "there is no uniformly accepted clinicopathologic definition of papillary squamous cell carcinoma of the upper aerodigestive tract." The term *papillary SCC (PSCC)* has been applied with different criteria by numerous authors attempting to describe the histologic features of malignant, exophytic squamous proliferations that are not VC or exophytic conventional SCC. The term has been used for purely in situ proliferations that are suggested to be invasive based on the formation of a significant mass lesion (133) and those that only have documented invasion within the papillary cores or at the base of the lesion (134). The former criterion is reasonable, given the difficulty in demonstrating invasion in maloriented sections. However, many of the lesions designated as PSCC are noninvasive, and they represent a form of squamous CIS that, in combination with the exophytic nature of the growth, likely explains the more favorable stage-corrected outcome. I believe that the clinician and patient are best served by restricting a definitive diagnosis of PSCC to malignant-appearing papillary proliferations that contain invasive carcinoma within the papillary cores or the base of the lesion and applying a diagnosis of papillary CIS or papillary dysplasia to noninvasive forms.

Clinical Features

PSCC is a rare form of invasive cancer found anywhere in the upper aerodigestive tract, with most arising in the larynx, sinonasal tract, hypopharynx, and oral cavity (134–136). The demographics of patients are similar to those of patients with conventional SCC. The clinical, demographic, and etiologic associations, as well as the main sites, of intraoral PSCC are not well defined. Although laryngeal lesions are described in a large series as de novo malignancies (136), as yet, neither the possible precursor relationship of a pre-existing or coexisting papilloma component nor the rate of concomitant or subsequent invasive squamous carcinoma has been adequately defined. Approximately one-third of PSCC cases tested have been HPV positive for either low-risk types 6 and 11 or high-risk types 16 and 18 (134–136). Although no definitive statement can be made about the prognosis of oral PSCC, generalizations about this histologic form of SCC from other head and neck sites indicate that laryngeal tumors, especially those with a filiform rather than broad exophytic architecture, have a more favorable prognosis than do conventional SCCs of a similar stage (132,136).

Morphologic Features

PSCC may present in two morphologic forms. The first is an exophytic broad-based, cauliflowerlike growth, and the second is a filiform pattern composed of multiple, slender, fingerlike papillary projections. The latter simulates the fibrovascular, frondlike growth pattern of a papilloma. PSCC is usually a nonkeratinizing, cytologically atypical epithelial proliferation, and it is only minimally hyperkeratotic.

Two histologic types of epithelial proliferations are recognized based on the maturation of the proliferating epithelial

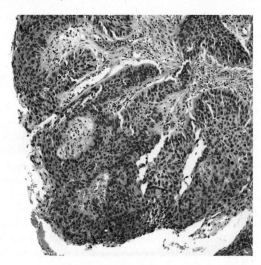

Figure 19.34. Papillary squamous cell carcinoma. Nonkeratinizing type composed of proliferating transitional cell–like dysplastic basal- and parabasal-type cells.

cells. The first type is undifferentiated and transitional cell–like, and it is composed of nonkeratinizing dysplastic basal- and parabasal-type cells (Fig. 19.34). This most closely mimics classic small-cell CIS in its full-thickness proliferation of uncommitted cells and is seen more often in the tonsillar-oropharyngeal region. The second histologic form of PSCC displays various degrees of keratinization in dysplastic epithelium (Fig. 19.35). Careful histologic examination of the fibrovascular cores and the base of all dysplastic papillary squamous lesions should be performed to assess for stromal and lymphovascular space invasion (Fig. 19.36). Both the typical keratinizing cordlike and the nonkeratinizing ribbonlike patterns of invasive squamous carcinoma arising in PSCC can be seen.

Differential Diagnosis

The papillary growth pattern of PSCC invokes a clinical and histologic differential diagnosis of dysplasia arising within solitary papilloma or papillomatosis, VC, and conventional SCC.

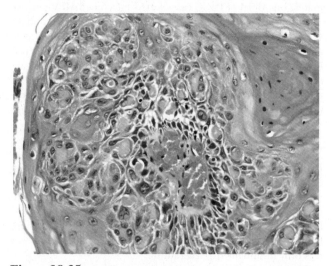

Figure 19.35. Papillary squamous cell carcinoma. Keratinizing type may show varying degrees of keratinization.

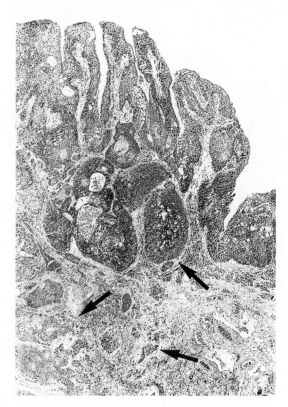

Figure 19.36. Papillary squamous cell carcinoma. The exophytic, dysplastic squamous proliferation has the fibrovascular frondlike growth pattern of a papilloma, and it contains an invasive component with pushing and infiltrative carcinoma at the base of the lesion (*arrows*).

Either solitary papilloma or papillomatosis (usually recurrent adult or juvenile disease) may demonstrate degrees of squamous dysplasia mimicking the dysplastic papillary component of PSCC. The clinical history of papillomatosis extending into adulthood can be extremely helpful in correlating these persistent dysplasias that do not appear to progress to invasive cancer with long-term follow-up (135). Without that clinical history, PSCC and dysplastic papilloma and/or papillomatosis are histologically indistinguishable; therefore, the criterion of invasion to diagnose PSCC is important. This simplifies the diagnostic process and obviates an overdiagnosis of carcinoma in a dysplastic lesion.

The cytologically well-differentiated VC is discriminated from PSCC by the latter's fibrovascular-based growth pattern, as well as the presence of significant cytologic atypia and the lack of hyperkeratosis. Although VC may exhibit a papillary, verrucous architecture, the surface commonly has spires of keratin, and the base has a more sessile attachment and confluent, downward "pushing" growth. Some carcinomas may display hybrid PSCC-VC features, and these are probably best diagnosed as well-differentiated squamous carcinomas. These are usually broad-based cancers that have a verrucoid surface growth and demonstrate varying degrees of cytologic atypia.

Treatment and Prognosis

Papillary dysplasia or noninvasive PSCC is treated by complete surgical excision. The treatment of invasive PSCC is based on the stage of the invasive component.

SPINDLE CELL CARCINOMA

Spindle cell carcinoma (SpCC) designates a microscopic variant of SCC in which spindled epithelial tumor cells resemble a sarcoma on histologic examination. Past controversies over the cell of origin and the cellular composition have resulted in numerous other appellations, including SCC with sarcoma-like stroma, sarcomatoid or pseudosarcomatous SCC, and pseudosarcoma. Interestingly, the term *carcinosarcoma* has not been favored for tumors of the upper aerodigestive tract, but it is applied to these tumors in the esophagus. These unusual tumors are now accepted to have a monoclonal origin and to be the result of a histologic spectrum of mesenchymal metaplasias of carcinoma. This is supported by the immunohistochemical and molecular DNA typing of identical p53 status in both epithelial and spindle cell components (137). More recently, microsatellite marker analysis has been used to demonstrate early genetic abnormalities common to conventional SCC in 70% of matched microdissected epithelial and sarcoma-like components, and additional distinctive genetic changes in 20% of cases support the evolution of the sarcomatoid component from the SCC (138).

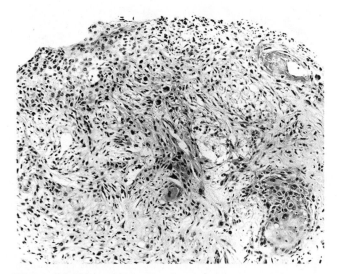

Figure 19.37. Spindle cell carcinoma—pseudosarcoma pattern. In situ and superficially invasive squamous cell carcinoma overlies a mass composed of an atypical spindle cell proliferation.

Clinical Features

Most cases in the head and neck arise in the oral cavity and larynx. Oral cases predominantly involve the vermilion portion of the lower lip, tongue, alveolar ridge, and gingiva. The most common signs/symptoms associated with these tumors in the oral cavity are pain, swelling, and nonhealing ulcers (139). The mean age of appearance for SpCC is the sixth decade of life. It has a male predominance, similar to that found in common SCC arising in the upper aerodigestive tract (139–141). The predisposing factors are the same as well, including tobacco use, alcohol abuse, poor oral hygiene, and previous irradiation to the site in which the tumor arose (140).

Patients diagnosed with SpCC have a significant incidence (17%) of multiple synchronous and metachronous primary carcinomas in the upper aerodigestive tract (141). This rate is, again, within the same range of the 10% to 27% reported for common SCCs of the head and neck region.

Morphologic Features

The macroscopic growth pattern in two-thirds of the cases is that of a polypoid mass protruding from the mucosal surface. Less commonly, the tumors appear as sessile, ulcerated growths. The tumors vary in size from less than 1 to 8 cm. The exophytic tumors may be attached by a broad base or by a narrow pedicle, giving the impression that they may be easily "snared." The polypoid tumors often ulcerate so that the majority of the tumor exposed for biopsy is devoid of malignant epithelium. In this case, the squamous component is often minimal, and it is noted more frequently at the base or pedicle of the tumor.

The microscopic diagnosis of SpCC requires identification of a biphasic histologic picture that consists of squamous carcinoma and a malignant spindle cell stroma. Two basic histologic variants are observed. The first is a superficially invasive or an in situ SCC that is overlying and seemingly separate from the atypical spindle cell proliferation (Fig. 19.37). This has been designated the histologic pattern of "pseudosarcoma." The second histologic variant is an infiltrative SCC admixed within the sarcomatoid component (Fig. 19.38). This has been labeled the

"carcinosarcoma" pattern. Separate classification into these two histologic growth patterns is artificial, and it is not indicative of either histogenesis or biologic potential; rather, it is a reflection of the spectrum of the mesenchymal metaplasia of the carcinoma.

All of the histologic grades of infiltrative squamous carcinoma can be encountered in these tumors. The overlying epithelium may have areas of squamous CIS, atypical squamous hyperplasia, or VC. Light microscopic transitions from the squamous component, whether infiltrative or surface epithelium, to the undifferentiated spindle cells are occasionally observed and are viewed as morphologic evidence of mesenchymal metaplasia or as a variant growth pattern of the carcinoma (Fig. 19.39).

The sarcomatoid element can also exhibit highly variable histologic features. A granulation tissue–like component can compose most of the tumor, or it may be limited to the surface in the superficially necrotic polypoid variants. More commonly,

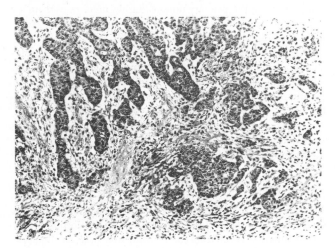

Figure 19.38. Spindle-cell carcinoma—carcinosarcoma pattern. Infiltrative squamous cell carcinoma is diffusely admixed within the sarcomatoid component.

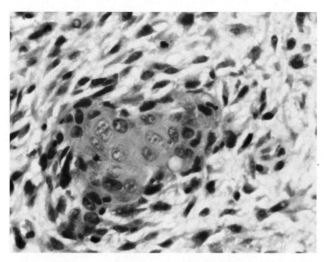

Figure 19.39. Spindle cell carcinoma. Light microscopic transition between malignant epithelial nest and malignant spindled cells is shown.

various sarcoma-like patterns—an edematous myxoid stroma with atypical bipolar spindle cells or plump epithelioid cells admixed with inflammatory cells and blood vessels—or a densely cellular proliferation resembling fibrosarcoma, hemangiopericytoma, or malignant fibrous histiocytoma are found. Admixtures of these sarcomatous patterns may appear within the same tumor. Some patterns defy classification. A few cells may contain deeply eosinophilic cytoplasm, superficially resembling rhabdomyoblasts. However, mixed rhabdomyosarcoma and SCC is rare. Histologic features of the malignant giant-cell tumor of soft parts with numerous osteoclast-like giant cells have been reported. Pleomorphic malignant giant cells and foreign body–type giant cells are encountered more frequently. The sarcomatous stroma may also exhibit foci of neoplastic chondroid, cartilage, osteoid, and osseous bony metaplasia.

The histologic characteristics of metastases may be markedly variable. Many are purely SCC; however, purely spindle cell metastases and mixed epithelial-sarcomatous patterns may also be encountered. Some metastases contain malignant cartilage or bone, verifying the neoplastic nature of these heterologous components in the primary tumors. Rarely, metastases from an SpCC may contain anatomically separate deposits of pure carcinoma and sarcoma (140,141).

By ultrastructure, the spindled cells bear occasional epithelial features of tonofilament bundles and primitive desmosome attachments (141). The immunoprofile of cytokeratin and vimentin positivity in the spindled cells is diagnostically helpful, but up to half of these tumors may be cytokeratin negative. Another potentially misleading feature is the presence of the myogenic markers desmin and muscle-specific actin in the spindled components (142).

Differential Diagnosis

The chief differential diagnoses of SpCC are true superficial sarcomas and benign but atypical reactive angiofibroblastic or myofibroblastic proliferations involving the mucosa. Because sarcomas and reactive pseudosarcomatous proliferations arising from the submucosa in the upper aerodigestive tract are exceedingly rare, the assumption that a polypoid mucosal malignant

spindle cell proliferation is an SpCC is reasonable unless convincing evidence to the contrary is present. Although some SpCC biopsy specimens reveal only the monophasic sarcomatoid component, the histologic identification of the carcinomatous elements is the sine qua non (despite the advent of diagnostic immunocytochemistry) of an SpCC diagnosis for two reasons. First, only 50% of biphasic SpCCs demonstrate cytokeratin-positive spindle cells, which often are focal in distribution (141). Second, SpCCs show bona fide histologic patterns of mesenchymal metaplasia, as well as immunocytochemical smooth muscle actin and desmin intermediate-filament staining that agrees with the findings of electron microscopic studies of myofibroblastic differentiation. These findings may lead to an erroneous diagnosis of sarcoma in nonrepresentative small biopsies (142).

Nearly half of the head and neck sarcomas are rhabdomyosarcomas, and although rhabdomyoblastic differentiation has been described, in SpCC, it is exceedingly rare. "Pseudomalignant" or bizarre granulation tissue and ulcerated irradiation reactions can be worrisome mimics of the sarcomatoid component of SpCC. The histologic features of marked cytologic atypia in stromal and endothelial cells with a granulation tissue–like reaction can be common to both, especially in SpCC arising after irradiation. The presence of atypical mitotic figures and DNA aneuploidy in pseudomalignant granulation tissue makes the distinction difficult as well (143). Inflammatory myofibroblastic tumors in the head and neck are also uncommon, and these are described as polypoid mucosal masses that occur mostly in the larynx (144). These loosely organized spindled and stellate cells set in a myxoid or fibrous stroma are only mildly pleomorphic, and they demonstrate the vimentin and smooth muscle actin cytoskeleton consistent with myofibroblasts. Because of the immunohistochemical overlap with cytokeratin-negative SpCC, the histologic documentation of a malignant squamous component in SpCC is often necessary to discriminate these neoplastic and pseudoneoplastic spindle cell entities in the differential diagnoses.

Treatment and Prognosis

SpCCs of the oral cavity are highly aggressive neoplasms, with a 61% mortality rate and a mean survival that ranges from 10 months to less than 2 years (139,141). The tumor size, gross appearance (polypoid or ulceroinfiltrative), grade of carcinoma, histologic features of sarcoma, depth of invasion, and prior irradiation bear no relationship to survival (139). Local recurrence and presence of cervical lymph node metastases are significant in predicting a fatal outcome for oral cavity tumors (139). The most effective treatment is surgical resection using the current approach to the more common forms of SCC. Primary radiation therapy alone has resulted in 80% failure rates for these tumors in the oral cavity (139).

ADENOSQUAMOUS CARCINOMA

Adenosquamous carcinoma of the upper aerodigestive tract was first described by Gerughty et al. (145) in 1968. Although this entity is rare, it is worth identifying because of its clinically aggressive nature, which results in determinate survival rates of 32% at 3 years, 13% at 5 years, and 4.5% at 10 years (146). This malignancy has a tendency for early neck node metastasis, frequent local recurrence, and occasional distant metastasis, most often to lung. Most patients die from their disease within 2 to 3 years (146).

The biphasic histologic features are diagnostic, but they leave uncertainty regarding whether the adenosquamous carcinoma is derived from surface mucosa (SCC variant) or from the minor salivary glands and ducts as initially proposed (minor salivary gland malignancy). Derivation from surface epithelium is currently favored. Adenosquamous carcinoma has been reported in the tongue, floor of the mouth, palate, tonsil, nasal cavity, and larynx (145–147). The involvement of major salivary glands has not been described.

Clinical Features

Possible predisposing risk factors have not been well defined, but alcohol and tobacco abuse have been noted in one series (146). Based on a review of 58 cases by Keelawat et al. (146), the male predominance is 4.3 to 1, with an average age at diagnosis of 60.8 years (range, 34 to 81 years). In the oral cavity, the clinical appearance of adenosquamous carcinoma is usually that of a small, 0.2- to 1-cm, erythroplakic ulcer or indurated submucosal nodule (145). In the larynx, however, it may manifest as a larger exophytic and ulcerated tumor with the involvement of contiguous anatomic sites (146,147).

Morphologic Features

The histologic features of adenosquamous carcinoma consist of the following three distinct and separate components of varying degrees of differentiation: (a) adenocarcinoma, (b) SCC, and (c) a mixed histologic pattern of glandular mucous cell and squamous differentiation mimicking mucoepidermoid carcinoma (Fig. 19.40). Most cases are dominated by the squamous component with adenocarcinoma evident in the deeper regions (148). Abundantly keratinized "glassy" cells may be a feature of the squamous component. A careful examination of the overlying surface epithelium may show foci of dysplasia, CIS, or invasive SCC. This may result in an appearance of either downward extension of multifocal CIS involving the salivary gland

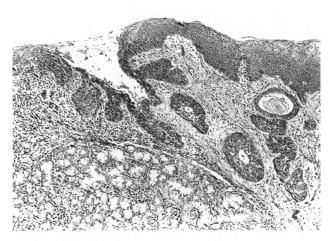

Figure 19.41. A component of adenosquamous carcinoma. Multifocal carcinoma in situ involves the salivary gland ducts and the overlying mucosal epithelium.

ducts (Fig. 19.41) or upward extension of the intraductal carcinoma to involve the overlying mucosal epithelium in the form of squamous CIS. By either mechanism, extensive permeation of the existing ductal-glandular framework occurs in all directions, with widespread invasion of the adjacent submucosal soft tissue. The glandular component can be brought out by immunostaining for CEA, CK7, and CAM5.2 (148). Perineural invasion is common. Metastases from adenosquamous carcinoma usually display all three components of adenocarcinoma, squamous carcinoma, and mixed carcinoma.

The intracellular mucin content can be demonstrated with mucicarmine, periodic acid-Schiff with diastase, and Alcian blue (pH 2.5 and 1.0) stains. The mucosubstances produced by adenosquamous carcinoma appear to be neutral glycoproteins, acidic sialomucins, and sulfomucins. This is similar to the spectrum of mucins that are synthesized by the minor salivary glands and that are present in mucoepidermoid carcinomas.

The differential diagnosis of adenosquamous carcinoma presents several problems because the various histologic components are distinct and they may be present in separate foci. For these reasons, small incisional biopsy specimens can be misleading because they can show only SCC or what appears to be mucoepidermoid carcinoma. A significant mucosal in situ squamous carcinoma component may also lead to the perception of squamous carcinoma with an origin from the surface epithelium and the involvement of underlying minor gland ducts. At times, the correct diagnosis may be apparent only in resection specimens.

Differential Diagnosis

Mucoepidermoid carcinoma is commonly confused on histologic examination with adenosquamous carcinoma. Mucoepidermoid carcinoma, thought to be of salivary excretory duct origin, exhibits a histologic spectrum of proliferating cell types that is similar to that of adenosquamous carcinoma. In contrast to adenosquamous carcinoma, mucoepidermoid carcinomas, even those that are high grade, do not demonstrate anaplastic nuclear features or in situ squamous carcinoma involving the overlying mucosa and rarely form true keratin pearls. High-grade intraoral mucoepidermoid carcinoma is also noted to be

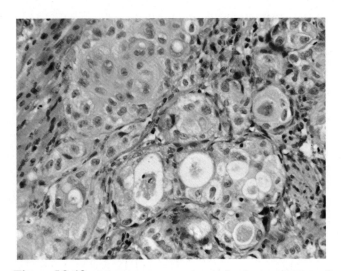

Figure 19.40. Adenosquamous carcinoma that features patterns of admixed squamous (*above*) and glandular differentiation (*below*).

biologically aggressive, with recurrence rates of 30% to 80% and a 20% 5-year survival rate (149,150). In contrast to the often small (<1 cm) and lethal adenosquamous carcinomas, mucoepidermoid carcinomas less than 2.5 cm in size, regardless of the grade, are rarely fatal (151).

Acantholytic or adenoid variants of SCC, although rare in the oral cavity, also feature in the differential diagnosis of adenosquamous carcinoma. These pseudoglandular carcinomas are characterized by foci of squamous carcinoma with a loss of tumor cell cohesion that leaves a peripheral single layer of cuboidal cells and single or clumped acantholytic tumor cells lying free in the resulting clefts. Although eosinophilic fluid may be present in these alveolar spaces, mucin cannot be demonstrated, and the ultrastructural examination fails to disclose glandular features. An adenoid pattern appears to be a feature that is inherent to the neoplasm because it persists even in lymph node metastases (152). The biologic behavior, although worse than that of skin carcinomas with identical histologic manifestations, seems similar to the common forms of squamous carcinoma of the upper aerodigestive tract.

Basaloid SCC also enters the differential diagnosis because it displays surface carcinoma, glandlike spaces, and foci of squamous differentiation. Its more distinguishing features are discussed in detail in the section "Basaloid Squamous Cell Carcinoma."

Necrotizing sialometaplasia of the minor salivary glands (see Chapter 20) can also be confused with both adenosquamous carcinoma and mucoepidermoid carcinoma because of the intraductal proliferation of metaplastic squamous epithelium containing trapped mucous cells and the pseudoepitheliomatous hyperplasia of the ulcerated surface mucosa.

Treatment and Prognosis

The treatment of adenosquamous carcinoma is surgical resection. Nearly 78% of cases present with stage III and IV disease (146). The high incidence (71%) of regional lymph node metastases from even small primaries indicates that neck dissection and/or cervical radiotherapy should be considered. The pathologic features of submucosal invasiveness in concert with mucosal squamous carcinoma may alter the surgical approach in favor of complete excision. Despite small tumor size, regional and distant metastatic disease develops in 80% of patients with tumors less than 1 cm in size (145). Approximately half of patients are dead of disease at a mean time interval of 23 months (148).

BASALOID SQUAMOUS CELL CARCINOMA

Basaloid SCC (BSCC) was first recognized as a distinct pathologic entity in 1986 by Wain et al. (153). In the oral cavity, this tumor has a predilection for the base of the tongue and the tonsil, but it also arises in the larynx and hypopharynx. HPV has not been demonstrated in BSCC (154).

Clinical Features

In the series of 40 BSCCs reported by Banks et al. (155), the median age of patients was 62 years (range, 27 to 88 years), and there was a marked male predominance (88%); nearly all of these individuals were smokers (92%) and drinkers (88%). BSCC appears to be a highly aggressive cancer; 68% of patients

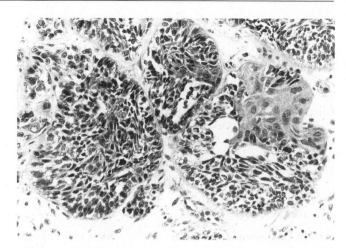

Figure 19.42. Basaloid squamous cell carcinoma. Nests composed of small basaloid cells with moderately pleomorphic, densely hyperchromatic nuclei, scanty cytoplasm, and peripheral nuclear palisading show abrupt foci of squamous differentiation.

have regional metastases on the initial examination, and 77% are categorized as having clinical stage III and IV disease. The favored site of distant metastasis is the lung.

Morphologic Features

BSCC is distinguished on histologic inspection by lobules, nests, and cribriform patterns of basaloid cells that commonly have abrupt foci of squamous differentiation within the nests (Fig. 19.42). At the periphery, the basaloid component may exhibit nuclear palisading (Fig. 19.43). Necrosis is typical, taking the form of single-cell necrosis and central comedo necrosis in larger nests. Conventional SCC is usually present in combination with or separate from the basaloid patterns and as squamous CIS of the overlying mucosa. Direct continuity with surface CIS in some cases argues for BSCC originating from the surface epithelium. The small basaloid cells have moderately pleomorphic, densely hyperchromatic nuclei with scanty cytoplasm, and they usually contain mitotic figures. Larger cells with

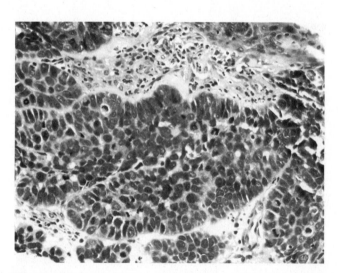

Figure 19.43. Basaloid squamous cell carcinoma. Nuclei palisade at the periphery of basaloid nests. Numerous atypical mitoses are evident.

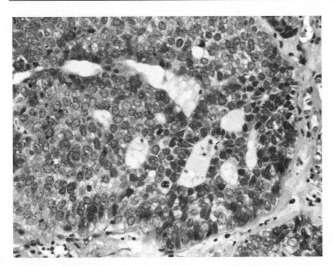

Figure 19.44. Basaloid squamous cell carcinoma. Pseudoglandular spaces contain a pale mucinous material mimicking adenoid cystic carcinoma.

more cytoplasm, vesicular nuclei, and small nucleoli can be seen as well. Some nests show small pseudoglandular spaces that contain material that stains with periodic acid-Schiff and Alcian blue, thereby mimicking adenoid cystic carcinoma (Fig. 19.44). An associated hyalinized eosinophilic or myxoid-appearing stroma in a cylindromatous pattern may also be seen (Fig. 19.45) (153,155).

Differential Diagnosis

The histologic differential diagnosis is typically between adenoid cystic carcinoma and small-cell carcinoma, but it can also include adenosquamous carcinoma, salivary basal cell neoplasms, and a composite or collision carcinoma of SCC with adenoid cystic carcinoma or small-cell carcinoma. Adenoid cystic carcinomas, even the high-grade solid variant, lack the degree of nuclear pleomorphism, the foci of squamous differentia-

tion, the high-grade dysplasia, the in situ squamous carcinoma of the surface epithelium, and the extensive necrosis seen in BSCC. Cribriform and pseudoglandular patterns with a hyalinized stroma are common to both neoplasms, but most adenoid cystic carcinomas exhibit myoepithelial differentiation and stain for muscle-specific actin, which is absent in BSCC (155). Immunostaining for p63 appears to reveal distinct diagnostic patterns distinguishing the myoepithelial phenotype of adenoid cystic carcinoma from the diffusely staining cells of BSCC (156).

Adenosquamous carcinoma most closely shares the histologic features of in situ SCC and admixtures of basaloid nests of tumor-forming glandular spaces, as well as SCC. However, the neoplastic involvement of excretory ducts and mucinous goblet cells within the tumor nests that are reminiscent of mucoepidermoid carcinoma are not observed in BSCC. Although foci of keratinization may be seen in basal cell adenomas, basal cell adenocarcinomas, and high-grade mucoepidermoid carcinomas, these salivary gland tumors lack the high-grade nuclear abnormalities of BSCC, as well as the frank squamous carcinoma and the intramucosal neoplasia.

Intraoral small-cell (undifferentiated) carcinoma, which is believed to derive from the minor salivary glands, may rarely exhibit focal squamous or ductal differentiation and rosette formation that simulate BSCC. Unlike BSCC, small-cell carcinoma can secondarily involve the surface epithelium in a focal manner, but it does not arise from surface epithelium and does not demonstrate an in situ surface component or cribriform patterns. Primary salivary gland small-cell carcinomas are now recognized to have immunohistochemical evidence of neuroendocrine differentiation despite a lack of evidence of dense-core granules in some tumors on electron microscopy (157). Although the majority of BSCCs stain for neuron-specific enolase and S-100 protein, the small-cell proliferation of BSCC lacks ultrastructural neuroendocrine features, and BSCC lacks the neuroendocrine antigens chromogranin and synaptophysin on immunoperoxidase staining (153,155). The foci of squamous differentiation and the intimate association of invasive SCC within nests of BSCC argue against a coincidence of separately arising squamous, small-cell, or adenoid cystic carcinomas.

Treatment and Prognosis

Most patients with BSCC are treated by radical surgery combined with radiation or chemotherapy. Of those patients dying of BSCC, the median survival time from diagnosis is 18 months. The 5-year disease-free survival rate of 40% for patients with BSCC of the oral cavity is similar to the rate of those with conventional SCC when matched for high stage at diagnosis regardless of degree of differentiation (155,158).

CYSTS OF THE JAWS

Cysts of the jaws are divided into two major categories, namely odontogenic and nonodontogenic (or developmental) (Fig. 19.46). Only a few cysts of the region have distinctive histologic features allowing diagnosis without clinicoradiologic correlation. The majority has a generic nonkeratinized squamous epithelial lining requiring reference to clinical/radiographic information to arrive at a specific name (e.g., dentigerous cyst or periapical [radicular] cyst). The epithelial lining of odontogenic cysts is derived from either reduced enamel epithelium

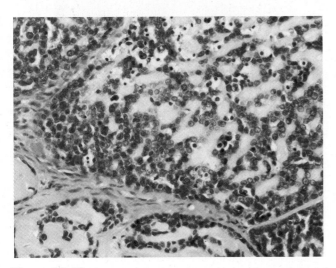

Figure 19.45. Basaloid squamous cell carcinoma. Accumulation of hyalinized matrix and cylindromatous pattern simulate poorly differentiated adenoid cystic carcinoma.

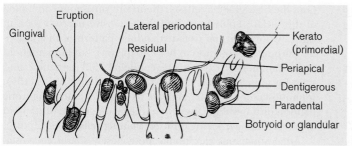

Figure 19.46. Odontogenic cysts of the jaws and their typical location. These are illustrated in the maxilla.

overlying the crown of an unerupted tooth (remnants of the enamel organ), rests of Malassez (epithelial remnants from tooth root formation), or rests of Serres (remnants of the dental lamina).

There has been some reconsideration of odontogenic cyst taxonomy based on more experience with biologic behavior related to surgical therapy and newer genetic evaluations. More recently, odontogenic keratocyst has been reclassified by the WHO as a cystic neoplasm (keratocystic odontogenic tumor), and calcifying odontogenic cyst (COC or Gorlin cyst) has been reclassified as calcifying cystic odontogenic tumor (CCOT) (56). This terminology is not universally applied at this time.

ODONTOGENIC CYSTS

Periapical Cyst (Radicular Cyst)

Periapical or radicular cyst is the most common odontogenic cyst. It results from severe pulpal inflammation that leads to pulp necrosis and periapical inflammation (a sequela of dental caries or tooth trauma). The cyst epithelial lining is derived from inflammatory stimulation of epithelial rests (rests of Malassez) in the apical periodontal membrane that remain after the development of roots of teeth. The teeth most often affected are the maxillary incisors and the mandibular molars. Periapical cysts are seldom found in association with deciduous teeth. These cysts do not usually cause pain or swelling but are often found during routine dental radiographic examination. They are seldom greater than 1 cm in diameter. The radiographic appearance is a periapical round (spheroidal) or pear-shaped radiolucency with a radiopaque margin (focal sclerosing osteitis or condensing osteitis) (Fig. 19.47).

These cysts are typically lined by hyperplastic, nonkeratinized stratified squamous epithelium. Infrequently, focal keratinization, goblet cells, and Rushton bodies (acellular hyalinized oval structures) may be seen microscopically in the epithelium (Fig. 19.48). Rushton bodies are hyaline eosinophilic structures of variable shape and size that may also appear basophilic with calcium salt deposition (159). The precise nature of these hyaline bodies has not been determined (i.e., whether produced by the epithelium itself or representing a byproduct of blood breakdown). The cyst wall is fibrotic and contains a mixed chronic inflammatory cell infiltrate.

It should be noted that the periapical cyst is preceded by a nonspecific chronic inflammatory lesion known as a periapical granuloma. This nonspecific "dental" granuloma is in contradistinction to a "medical" granuloma that is characterized by a focal macrophage infiltrate. The pathogenesis of a periapical cyst is presumably related to inflammatory stimulation (associated with the periapical granuloma) of the rests of Malassez that

proliferate to provide a protective epithelial barrier between the root apex and surrounding bone.

Treatment of periapical cysts (20%) and granulomas (80%) is the mainstay of an endodontic practice. Periapical granulomas resolve following root canal therapy (replacing necrotic dental pulp with inert material), and cysts only resolve following enucleation of the epithelial lining. The problem for the clinician, however, is that differentiation between these two lesions can only be determined by microscopic examination. Nonetheless, endodontists typically treat all periapical lesions with root canal fillings. Those that resolve are presumed to have been granulomas, and those that persist (probable cysts) are enucleated.

Residual Cyst

"Residual cyst" is the name given to a periapical cyst that persists in the jaws after the involved tooth is extracted. This requires knowledge that the jaw cyst occurs in the region of a previously removed nonvital tooth.

Dentigerous Cyst

The dentigerous (tooth-bearing) cyst is an odontogenic cyst associated with the crown of an unerupted tooth. The cyst devel-

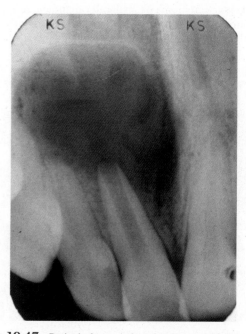

Figure 19.47. Periapical cyst. A dental radiograph demonstrates a large periapical lucency resulting from trauma and pulpal necrosis of the central incisor.

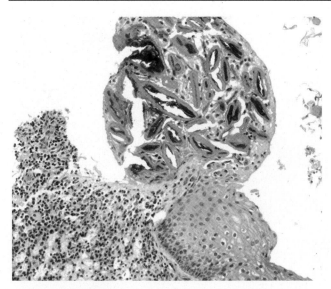

Figure 19.48. Periapical cyst. Chronically inflamed stratified squamous cyst lining containing hyaline Rushton bodies that are focally calcified.

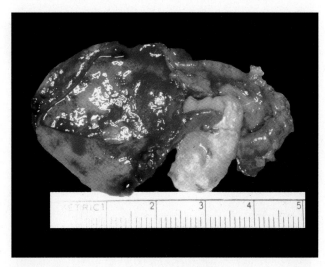

Figure 19.50. Dentigerous cyst. Unerupted tooth is usually removed with the cyst. Here the crown of the impacted molar in Figure 19.49 lies within cyst membrane.

ops from fluid accumulation between the reduced ameloblastic epithelium and tooth crown (160). The stimulation for the proliferation of this epithelium is unknown. Because there is no specific histology, the diagnosis is predicated on knowledge of clinical history, radiograph, or the pathologic specimen of a tooth with an attached pericoronal cystic membrane. These cysts are typically discovered on routine radiographic examination, but larger cysts may be symptomatic. Most dentigerous cysts are unilocular, although multilocular lesions are not uncommon. Complications include displacement of adjacent teeth, jaw expansion and possibly fracture in large lesions, and, rarely, neoplastic transformation to ameloblastoma (Fig. 19.49).

Grossly, the cyst wall is usually thin, and if submitted intact with the impacted tooth, it will envelop the crown and be at-

tached to the tooth at the enamel-cementum junction. Dentigerous cysts are typically lined by nonspecific stratified epithelium and are minimally inflamed. Frequently, a moderate to intense secondary chronic inflammatory cell infiltrate is seen in the presence of capsular fibrosis (Fig. 19.50). Occasionally, only the two normal residual layers of reduced enamel epithelium, seen microscopically as eosinophilic columnar cells with dark nuclei, are found lining a hyperplastic fibrous wall of a pericoronal lesion (Fig. 19.51). Strictly speaking, this is not a dentigerous cyst because the epithelium is not stratified squamous in type. This should be designated as a hyperplastic dental follicle. Treatment of dentigerous cyst is extraction of the impacted tooth and enucleation of the cyst wall. Microscopy is required to confirm the clinical diagnosis and to rule out ameloblastomatous transformation.

Paradental Cyst

Paradental cyst is a form of dentigerous cyst that is found in the bifurcation of an erupting mandibular molar (Fig. 19.52A,B)

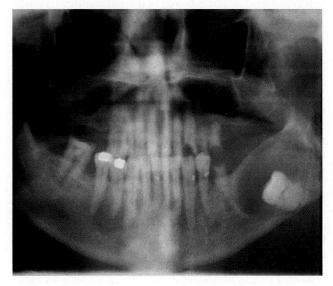

Figure 19.49. Dentigerous cyst. Panographic x-ray shows a large expansile cyst pushing the unerupted permanent molar to the angle of the mandible with erosion of the inferior cortex.

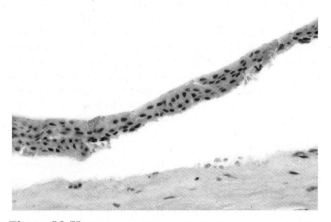

Figure 19.51. Reduced enamel epithelium is a normal structure associated with an unerupted tooth and recognized as two layers of compressed eosinophilic, columnar cells derived from the ameloblast layers.

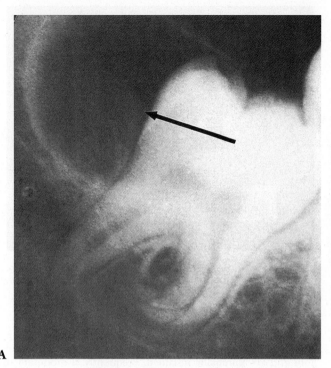

A

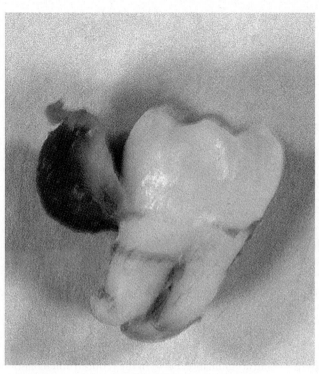

B

Figure 19.52. Paradental cyst. **(A)** A dental radiograph shows a typical distal coronal position of a mandibular paradental cyst *(arrow)*. **(B)** The corresponding gross specimen shows the cyst attached at the coronal top third of the tooth root on the distal surface.

(161). The cysts are usually 1 to 2 cm in diameter and attached to the cemento-enamel junction and the coronal one-third of the roots. Although it is associated with the crown of a tooth, unlike the dentigerous cyst, the paradental cyst does not have the potential to expand greatly or cause displacement of teeth. Histologically, it exhibits features of a dentigerous cyst. A secondary chronic inflammatory infiltrate may be present. The treatment is enucleation.

Eruption Cyst

This is another form of dentigerous cyst, seen mainly in children in association with erupting primary or deciduous teeth. Seward (162) reported that these cysts occurred in 11% of children during the eruption of deciduous incisors and in 30% of infants during the eruption of deciduous cuspids and molars. The cyst is apparent clinically as a bluish, compressible, dome-shaped expansion of the alveolar ridge over the erupting tooth. The tooth erupts through the lesion without treatment. Rarely, it is necessary to speed the eruption process along by excising a superficial portion of the cyst overlying the tooth.

Gingival Cyst of the Newborn

Gingival cysts, also known as Bohn nodules, are congenital odontogenic cysts, usually multiple, occurring in newborns. They arise from dental lamina remnants in the gingiva overlying the edentulous ridge and appear as whitish, firm nodules as a result of keratin accumulation. Similar-appearing cysts occurring in the midline palate along the line of fusion of the palatal and nasal processes are termed Epstein pearls or palatine cysts of the newborn. A thin layer of squamous or cuboidal epithe-lium usually lines gingival cysts. These cysts are not usually treated because they involute or rupture and fuse into the oral cavity epithelium in the first few months of life.

Gingival Cyst of the Adult

Gingival cyst of the adult also arises from dental lamina rests forming a soft tissue swelling. It is usually found in the mandibular premolar and maxillary incisor-canine regions where it can be seen in the dental papilla between teeth or along the edentulous gingival ridge. The histology of this soft tissue cyst is similar to the intrabony lateral periodontal cyst (12). Simple excision is curative.

Lateral Periodontal Cyst

Lateral periodontal cyst is an uncommon developmental odontogenic cyst arising from dental lamina rests in alveolar bone between the roots of vital mandibular canines and premolars (Fig. 19.53) (163). It is usually found as an incidental radiographic finding in males more than 21 years of age. It presents radiographically as an oval- or triangular-shaped, unilocular radiolucency. Lateral periodontal cysts neither resorb roots nor form a soft tissue swelling. They are lined by thin epithelium (two to three cells thick) with focal thickenings. Cells making up the focal thickenings usually have clear cytoplasm and form scattered mounds of epithelium protruding into the lumen or sitting in the wall (Fig. 19.54). Treatment by enucleation is curative.

Botryoid Odontogenic Cyst

A polycystic variant of the lateral periodontal cyst, bearing the same histology, is the extremely uncommon botryoid odonto-

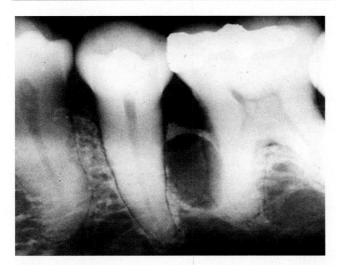

Figure 19.53. Lateral periodontal cyst. Radiograph shows a unilocular radiolucency between the lateral roots of the mandibular second premolar and first molar teeth. (Courtesy of Dr. Joseph Regezi.)

genic cyst that is thought to have an increased potential for recurrence. This is most likely related to the incomplete removal of the polycystic lesion.

Odontogenic Keratocyst (Keratocystic Odontogenic Tumor)

The odontogenic keratocyst (OKC) is a potentially recurring and destructive cyst that occurs over a broad age range and that has a unique and defining histology and genetic syndromic associations. Approximately 5% of those afflicted have the stigmata of the nevoid basal cell carcinoma syndrome (NBCCS) (164). Gorlin and Goltz (165) described NBCCS in 1960, with multiple OKCs and multiple basal cell carcinomas of skin as major components. The syndrome is caused by an autosomal dominant gene with variable expressivity and high penetrance. The other more common components of the syndrome include

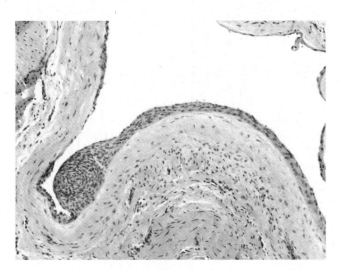

Figure 19.54. Lateral periodontal cyst. Distinctive features are a thin lining with occasional mounds of epithelium protruding into the lumen.

jaw, skull, and skeletal anomalies and skin (commonly dyskeratotic pitting of the hands and feet), internal organ, and central nervous system defects and tumors (Fig. 19.55).

More recently, the neoplastic nature of OKC has been defined by molecular genetic studies in sporadic and NBCCS-associated OKC lesions showing allelic loss in the *PTCH* gene on chromosome 9q22.3-q31. This mutation in the *PTCH* gene leads to overexpression of bcl-1 and TP53 in NBCCS. In OKC, loss of heterozygosity in additional tumor suppressor genes *p16*, *p53*, and *MCC* also supports a neoplastic origin (166). Therefore, the term *keratocystic odontogenic tumor (KCOT)* has been proposed by the WHO in 2005 to replace OKC (56).

OKC usually appears as a single or multiple, unilocular or multilocular radiolucency in the posterior mandible or maxilla; it has also been reported in the anterior maxilla (167). Histologically, the cyst demonstrates a thin, flat (without rete) stratified squamous epithelial lining of five to eight cells in thickness bearing a corrugated, parakeratinized surface. A distinguishing feature (but also common to calcifying odontogenic cyst and cystic ameloblastoma) is the presence of cuboidal to columnar basal cells with darkly stained nuclei that are well defined in a palisade and often with nuclei polarized away from the basement membrane (Fig. 19.56). The lining may become hyperplastic when secondarily inflamed, and mitoses may be seen. Dysplasia in OKC has been noted, but transformation to SCC is rare (168,169). Within a usually noninflammatory fibrous connective wall are undulating, tortuous projections of the cyst lining and daughter (satellite) cysts that may be derived from odontogenic rests within the wall (Fig. 19.57). Epithelial budding from the cyst lining may also be evident. The lumen may accumulate keratin, but this is quite variable. When the cyst is heavily inflamed, as is often the case when a large cyst is initially treated by decompression (marsupialization) before cystectomy, the distinctive histologic features are lost, and squamous hyperplasia and metaplasia occur (170). Lining epithelium tucked in crevices away from the inflammation may yet be revealing of the distinctive histology of OKC (Fig. 19.58).

It has been demonstrated that OKC from patients with the NBBCS compared with matched controls have a greater number of satellite cysts, solid islands of epithelial proliferation, odontogenic rests within the capsule, and mitotic figures in the epithelium of the main cavity, suggesting a greater growth potential in syndrome cysts (164). Jaw cysts lined by orthokeratinizing squamous epithelium and lacking basal epithelial features of OKC should not be classified as OKC because they are not seen in NBBCS and have a lower recurrence rate. These keratinizing cysts are not a distinct entity but are thought to represent other specific types of odontogenic cysts that may keratinize (e.g., dentigerous cyst, periapical cyst) (Fig. 19.59).

The most important feature concerning OKC is its potential for recurrence and destructive growth. Recurrences result from persistent disease related to incomplete removal of the cyst lining or the development of a new cyst in the same region from odontogenic rests at a more remote time. Given variation in removal methods and their success and the propensity for multiple cysts in those with syndromic association, reported recurrence rates have been quite variable. Recurrence rates range from 26% to 43% (168,171). Multiple OKCs and those arising in the NBCCS have a higher propensity for recurrence, as do multilocular cysts, cysts enucleated in several pieces, and those with clinically observable infection with fistula or perforated boney wall (171).

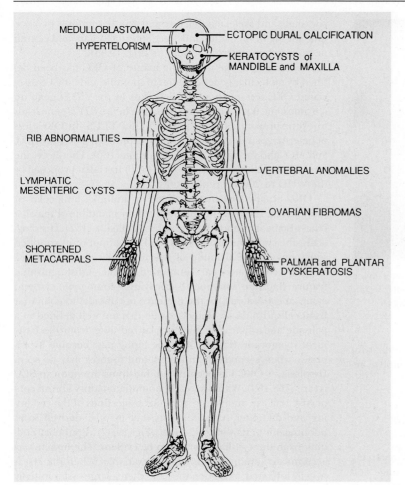

Figure 19.55. An illustration of the major components of the nevoid basal cell carcinoma syndrome (NBCCS).

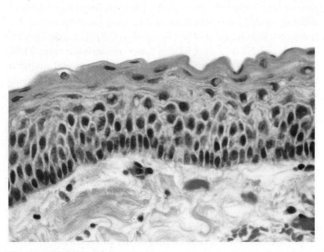

Figure 19.56. Odontogenic keratocyst. A thin, flat cyst is lined with a corrugated, parakeratinized surface with palisaded and often polarized cuboidal to columnar basal cells.

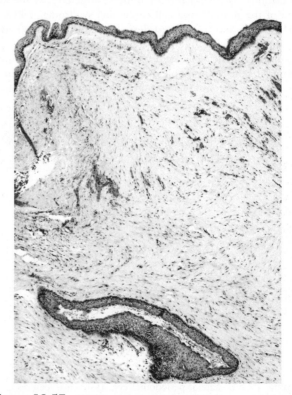

Figure 19.57. Odontogenic keratocyst. Daughter cyst is located within the wall of the main cyst.

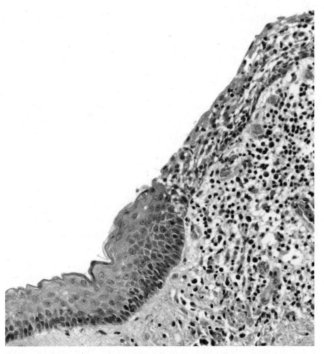

Figure 19.58. Odontogenic keratocyst. After marsupialization, this inflamed cyst is lined mostly by nondiagnostic squamous epithelium, but histologic features of keratocyst are still evident at one edge (*left*).

Calcifying Odontogenic Cyst (Calcifying Cystic Odontogenic Tumor)

Like OKC, the calcifying odontogenic cyst (COC) has been reclassified as a benign cystic neoplasm, the calcifying cystic odontogenic tumor (CCOT), by the WHO (56). This cystic tumor may have distinct clinical and radiographic appearances. It exhibits a spectrum of cystic and solid histology bearing a common and distinctive ameloblastoma-like odontogenic epithelium that produces keratin in the form of "ghost cells." These cells may calcify, and this is quite variable. When first described by Gorlin et al. (172) (Gorlin cyst), it was proposed as a possible analogy to the cutaneous "shadow cell" producing calcifying epithelioma of Malherbe. The lesion most often develops as a painless enlargement of the mandible or maxilla, usually in the

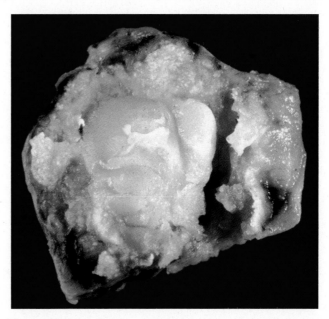

Figure 19.60. Calcifying odontogenic cyst. This enucleated cyst appears grossly solid and is filled with an odontoma associated with dentin matrix and ghost cell keratin.

incisor-cuspid region. It may also arise as a purely extraosseous tumor. COC occurs over a broad age range without gender predilection. When occurring as a cystic lesion, the average age of presentation is 33 years. One-fourth of COCs are associated with an odontoma, usually occurring in younger patients (average age, 16 years), and are more solid in gross appearance (Fig. 19.60). Radiographically, COCs are usually unilocular, well-circumscribed radiolucencies and may have variable radiopacities depending on the degree of calcification (Fig. 19.61).

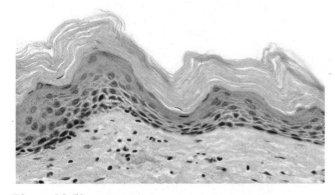

Figure 19.59. Nonspecific keratinizing odontogenic cyst. This cyst lacks the basal epithelial features and corrugated, parakeratinized surface of keratocyst. It does not share the same biologic potential for recurrence as the odontogenic keratocyst.

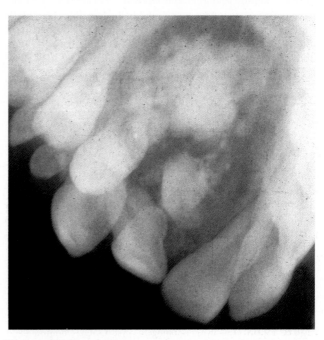

Figure 19.61. Calcifying odontogenic cyst. Radiograph reveals a large maxillary cyst containing numerous opacities and an odontoma shown in Figure 19.60.

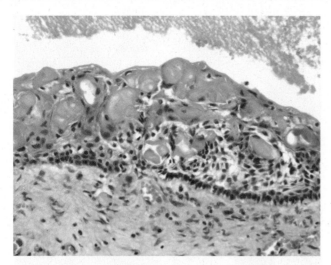

Figure 19.62. Calcifying odontogenic cyst. Epithelial lining with ameloblastic basal epithelial features contains numerous ghost cells.

One-third of COCs are associated with an unerupted tooth. Besides odontoma or an unerupted tooth, COC may be associated with an ameloblastoma or ameloblastic fibroma.

Histologically, the epithelium has features similar to cystic ameloblastoma, with a distinct layer of palisaded and polarized basal cells bearing hyperchromatic nuclei, and an overlying loose layer resembling stellate reticulum. The diagnostic elements are pale, eosinophilic ghost cells, scattered or forming masses within the epithelium or the wall or filling the lumen (Fig. 19.62). Some ghost cells may keratinize, calcify, or elicit a stromal foreign body giant-cell reaction. A homogeneous eosinophilic deposit within the wall adjacent to the epithelium is quite variably seen and has been referred to as dentinoid or dysplastic dentin. Cysts filled with a mixture of eosinophilic ghost cell keratin and an odontoma with associated dental hard tissue matrix may appear more solid histologically (Fig. 19.63). The main differential diagnoses of cystic COC are OKC and unicystic ameloblastoma because of similar ameloblastic epithelium. The presence of ghost cells differentiates the COC. The

more solid and less cystic variant of COC is synonymous with the term *dentinogenic ghost cell tumor*, currently applied in the WHO classification to convey its neoplastic nature. The very rare odontogenic malignancy with ghost cell differentiation is termed *odontogenic ghost cell carcinoma*. The treatment of COC is enucleation and curettage. Recurrence is rare. Solid and infiltrative central lesions may have a higher recurrence rate, and therefore, a resection margin similar to that considered for ameloblastoma may be appropriate.

Glandular Odontogenic Cyst

Glandular odontogenic cyst is rare. Since being declared an entity in 1988, the glandular odontogenic cyst has been problematic for pathologists to diagnose and begs the question of its true existence as an entity (173). Other synonyms used have been sialo-odontogenic cyst, mucin-producing cyst, mucoepidermoid odontogenic cyst, and polymorphous odontogenic cyst. The chief issues are (a) whether some degree of mucinous metaplasia within the lining of an otherwise classifiable odontogenic cyst is acceptable; (b) whether mucinous differentiation is an indicator of more aggressive behavior (recurrence); (c) at what threshold the term *glandular odontogenic cyst* is invoked to signify such, suggesting a more aggressive approach or closer follow-up; and (d) whether these proliferations represent early histologic forms of central cystic low-grade mucoepidermoid carcinoma. The fact that some "recurrences" have been later diagnosed as low-grade mucoepidermoid carcinoma would lend credence to the latter interpretation (174).

The majority of glandular odontogenic cysts have occurred as multilocular radiolucencies in the anterior mandible. The epithelial lining is usually a flat squamous lining bearing variable surface cuboidal or columnar cells, some with cilia, and mucous cells within the lining. Intraepithelial arcades may be formed of these various cell types (Fig. 19.64). The lining may also be thin, resembling lateral periodontal or multilocular botryoid odontogenic cysts with the mural thickenings of clear cells. The histologic similarity to low-grade mucoepidermoid carcinoma is one of threshold, and appropriate levels should be made to assure complete histologic sampling and evaluation. Because of the increased frequency of local recurrence, treatment by enucleation and curettage is favored (175). A diagnosis

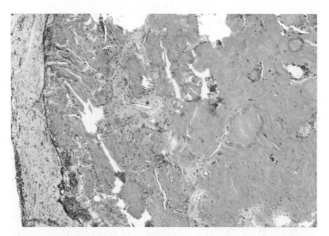

Figure 19.63. Calcifying odontogenic cyst (COC). Odontoma and associated dentin matrix admixed with accumulated ghost cell keratin contribute to the solid appearance of this COC. Distinctive epithelial lining is present at the periphery.

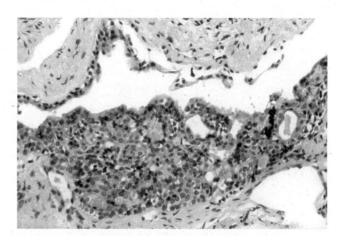

Figure 19.64. Glandular odontogenic cyst. Cyst lining is thin (*above*) but hyperplastic with intraepithelial arcades and scattered mucous cells (*below*).

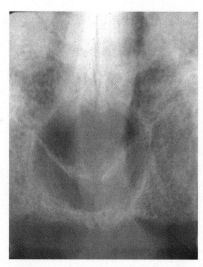

Figure 19.65. Nasopalatine canal cyst. Radiograph shows characteristic intrabony heart-shaped lucency superior to the maxillary central incisors.

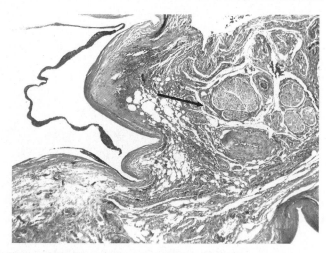

Figure 19.67. Nasopalatine canal cyst. This cyst is lined by a thin, stratified, squamous epithelial lining adjacent to a prominent neurovascular bundle (*arrow*).

of mucoepidermoid carcinoma may warrant jaw resection to achieve a tumor margin.

NONODONTOGENIC CYSTS

Nasopalatine Canal Cyst

The most frequently encountered nonodontogenic cyst is the nasopalatine canal cyst. It can develop entirely within bone, within the incisive papilla of the anterior palatal gingiva, or partially within bone and soft tissue of the region. The epithelium is derived from the remnants of the paired embryonal nasopalatine ducts. These are vestigial oronasal ducts that in other animal species function as accessory olfactory organs in the incisive canal of the anterior maxilla (176). Nasopalatine canal cysts occur most often in the fourth to sixth decades and usually present with swelling and/or drainage. On radiograph, the intrabony cyst characteristically appears as a heart-shaped radiolucency that is superior and posterior to the maxillary central incisors (Fig. 19.65). It is accessed via the palate for removal (Fig. 19.66). Histologically, it is lined by stratified squamous

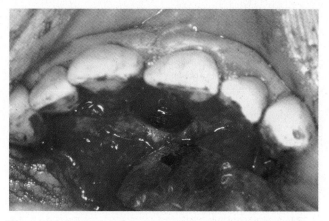

Figure 19.66. Nasopalatine canal cyst. Palatal defect is seen behind maxillary central incisors at surgical removal by enucleation and curettage.

epithelium and/or pseudostratified columnar respiratory epithelium. Clues to diagnosis can be found in the connective tissue wall of the cyst where a prominent neurovascular bundle and, occasionally, islands of cartilage are found (Fig. 19.67).

Median Palatine Cyst

The median palatine cyst is located within the palate and is believed to be a posteriorly situated nasopalatine cyst. On palatal radiograph, there is a well-circumscribed midline radiolucency that is usually in the molar region. Histologically, the cyst is lined by stratified squamous and/or respiratory epithelium. The treatment is enucleation.

Nasolabial Cyst

The pathogenesis of this cyst is unknown, although it has been suggested that it has its origin from remnants of the nasolacrimal ducts. It is found in the soft tissues of the upper lip and/or lateral aspect of the nose (177). It can develop bilaterally on occasion. It predominates among blacks and women. Histologically, the cyst is usually lined by stratified squamous or pseudostratified epithelium. Enucleation is the treatment of choice.

Globulomaxillary Lesion

The globulomaxillary lesion is a nonspecific designation for any lesion occurring between the maxillary lateral incisor and the cuspid. The historic concept of a fissural cyst derived from entrapped epithelium within mesenchyme during embryogenesis and formation of the anterior maxilla is no longer accepted (178). Globulomaxillary radiolucencies may represent an inflammatory lesion (periapical granuloma), odontogenic cyst (periapical cyst, lateral periodontal cyst, OKC, or COC), odontogenic tumor (odontogenic myxoma), or nonodontogenic lesion (central giant-cell lesion). The most common is a laterally displaced periapical cyst. Biopsy is required to establish a diagnosis and define treatment (179).

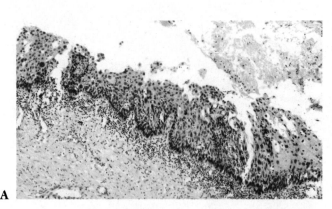

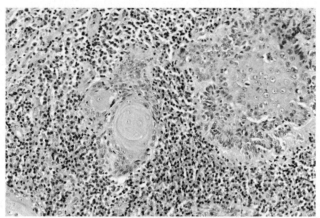

A   B

Figure 19.68. Carcinoma arising in odontogenic cyst. **(A)** Marked squamous dysplasia in the lining of a recurrent maxillary dentigerous cyst. **(B)** Nests of squamous cell carcinoma infiltrate the inflamed cyst wall.

CARCINOMA ARISING IN ODONTOGENIC CYSTS

Carcinoma rarely arises in odontogenic cysts. Because the origin of the epithelium is odontogenic, these carcinomas are designated under the broad heading of odontogenic carcinoma. The WHO classification includes the designations of primary intraosseous SCC derived from keratocystic odontogenic tumor (OKC) and the more general designation of primary intraosseous SCC derived from odontogenic cysts (Fig. 19.68A,B) (56). Primary intraosseous SCC–solid type is also thought to be derived from odontogenic epithelial remnants and would be the term of choice if there is no clear-cut evidence of origin from the lining of an odontogenic cyst or in association with another odontogenic tumor. Most are moderately to well-differentiated SCCs that are indistinguishable from metastatic SCC to the jaws unless origin from a cyst lining can be documented (180). Fewer are identified as intraosseous mucoepidermoid carcinoma of cyst origin (181). Most are incidental radiographic findings with no specific appearance, mimicking a variety of odontogenic cysts.

ODONTOGENIC TUMORS

In the United States, odontogenic tumors account for approximately 9% of all tumors of the oral cavity. Although the 2005 WHO classification of benign (Table 19.2) and malignant (Table 19.3) odontogenic tumors seems complex, it is helpful in histologically categorizing numerous entities as proliferations that are of odontogenic epithelial, mesenchymal, or mixed epithelial and mesenchymal differentiation with or without the formation of dental hard tissues (56). Some odontogenic tumors mimic epithelial stages of tooth development histologically, like ameloblastoma, whereas others, like odontogenic myxomas, by virtue of location in the tooth-forming regions of the jaws, are assumed to be of odontogenic origin.

BENIGN ODONTOGENIC EPITHELIAL TUMORS

Odontoma

Odontomas are the most common tumorlike lesions of the jaws, representing hamartomatous malformations. Odontomas are usually detected as incidental jaw findings in the tooth-bearing

regions of children and adolescents, but some may attain a larger size, resulting in painless jaw swelling. Two types are recognized, although the differences are insignificant. The complex type simulates an osteoma on radiograph as an opaque mass (Fig. 19.69) surrounded by a radiolucent zone and is composed of an irregular arrangement of enamel, dentin, and cementum (Fig. 19.70). The compound type is composed of rudimentary small teeth (Fig. 19.71). Typically, those that appear like small teeth (compound odontomas) can be diagnosed without microscopic examination. In addition to the dental hard tissues, loose stroma containing reduced enamel epithelium,

TABLE 19.2

World Health Organization Histologic Classification of Benign Odontogenic Tumors

Odontogenic epithelium with mature, fibrous stroma without odontogenic ectomesenchyme
　Ameloblastoma, solid/multicystic type
　Ameloblastoma, extraosseous/peripheral type
　Ameloblastoma, desmoplastic type
　Ameloblastoma, unicystic type
　Squamous odontogenic tumor
　Calcifying epithelial odontogenic tumor
　Adenomatoid odontogenic tumor
　Keratocystic odontogenic tumor (odontogenic keratocyst)
Odontogenic epithelium with odontogenic ectomesenchyme, with or without hard tissue formation
　Ameloblastic fibroma
　Ameloblastic fibrodentinoma
　Ameloblastic fibro-odontoma
　Odontoma
　　Odontoma, complex type
　　Odontoma, compound type
　Odontoameloblastoma
　Calcifying cystic odontogenic tumor (calcifying odontogenic cyst)
　Dentinogenic ghost cell tumor
Mesenchyme and/or odontogenic ectomesenchyme with or without odontogenic epithelium
　Odontogenic fibroma
　Odontogenic myxoma/myxofibroma
　Cementoblastoma

TABLE 19.3

World Health Organization Histologic Classification of Malignant Odontogenic Tumors

ODONTOGENIC CARCINOMAS
Metastasizing (malignant) ameloblastoma
Ameloblastic carcinoma–primary type
Ameloblastic carcinoma–secondary type (dedifferentiated), intraosseous
Ameloblastic carcinoma–secondary type (dedifferentiated), peripheral
Primary intraosseous squamous cell carcinoma–solid type
Primary intraosseous squamous cell carcinoma derived from keratocystic odontogenic tumor
Primary intraosseous squamous cell carcinoma derived from odontogenic cysts
Clear-cell odontogenic carcinoma
Ghost cell odontogenic carcinoma
ODONTOGENIC SARCOMAS
Ameloblastic fibrosarcoma
Ameloblastic fibrodentinosarcoma and fibro-odontosarcoma

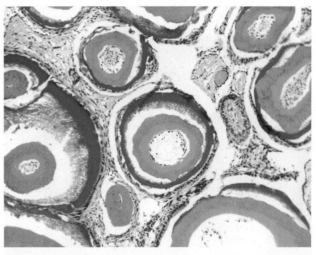

Figure 19.70. Complex odontoma. Numerous disorganized profiles of dentin, enamel, and pulpal tissues compose the mass lesion microscopically.

cords of odontogenic epithelium with calcifications, and ghost cells may be seen. The last microscopic feature can also be seen in other odontogenic tumors and cysts (182). Odontomas are treated by enucleation and curettage.

Ameloblastoma

Ameloblastoma is a benign yet locally aggressive intraosseous odontogenic tumor occurring most often in the posterior mandible (80%), followed by posterior maxilla (20%). Ameloblastoma may rarely arise as a peripheral extraosseous tumor of the overlying gingival soft tissue mostly of the posterior jaw and ascending ramus or rarely the buccal mucosa.

Within the jaws, intraosseous ameloblastomas affect both sexes in all age groups, with the highest incidence in those age 30 to 50 years (average age, 39 years). The neoplasm is often associated with an impacted tooth or is derived from the wall of

a dentigerous cyst. On radiograph, ameloblastomas are usually multiloculated radiolucencies corresponding to the most common solid/multicystic type, seen at gross examination in Figure 19.72. Most ameloblastomas are solid/multicystic growths. Occasionally they may present as a cystic lesion, designated unicystic type (183–187). This is to be differentiated from a dominant cystic component occurring in an otherwise conventional solid ameloblastoma.

The tumor is believed to be derived from one of several sources of odontogenic epithelium, including enamel organ, odontogenic rests, and linings of odontogenic cysts. There are numerous histologic variants of solid ameloblastoma, but all are of similar biologic behavior. Unicystic ameloblastomas and peripheral (gingival) ameloblastomas exhibit less aggressive behavior than solid tumors. Histologically, the common theme of the epithelium of all variants is resemblance to the enamel organ with peripheral ameloblastic columnar cells surrounding

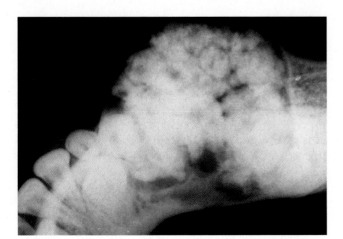

Figure 19.69. Complex odontoma. Radiograph shows a large, expansile, mottled radiopaque lesion of the jaw without resemblance to teeth.

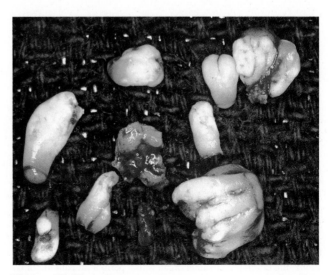

Figure 19.71. Compound odontoma. Single or multiple, small, often misshapen teeth comprising the compound-type odontoma are readily recognized on gross examination.

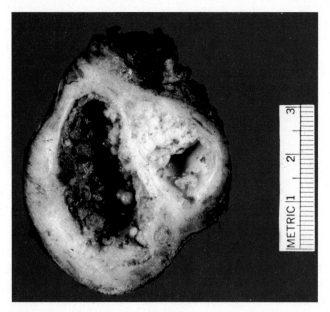

Figure 19.72. Ameloblastoma. Gross inspection of this resection specimen shows the cystic and solid growth nature of conventional ameloblastoma.

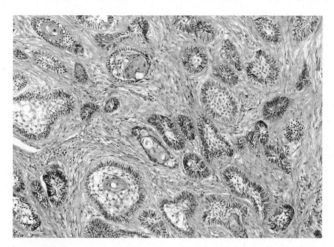

Figure 19.74. Ameloblastoma—follicular histologic type.

areas of edematous stellate reticulum–like cells (Fig. 19.73), illustrated best in the more common follicular variant (Fig. 19.74) (188). Other histologic types or patterns include plexiform (Fig. 19.75), spindle cell (Fig. 19.76), basal cell (Fig. 19.77), and desmoplastic (Fig. 19.78) types. Other histologic changes of keratinization and granular cell change within stellate reticulum give rise to designations of acanthomatous (Fig. 19.73) and granular cell type (Fig. 19.79), respectively (189). The desmoplastic type has been distinguished separately in the WHO classification because of specific clinical, radiographic, and histologic features. Ameloblastic features in some purely cystic ameloblastomas may be so subtle that they simulate a bland odontogenic cyst. Histologic criteria for the diagnosis of ameloblastoma include well-differentiated epithelium with min-

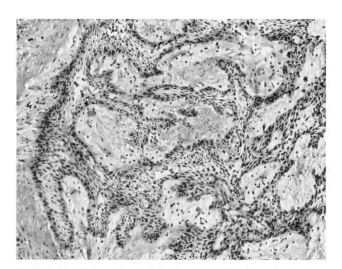

Figure 19.75. Ameloblastoma—plexiform histologic type.

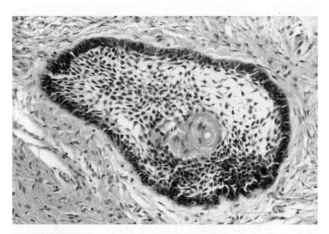

Figure 19.73. Ameloblastoma. Characteristic histologic features resemble the developing enamel organ with a peripheral palisade of columnar cells surrounding edematous epithelium resembling stellate reticulum. A focus of keratinization is present (acanthomatous ameloblastoma).

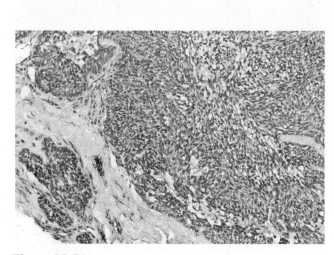

Figure 19.76. Ameloblastoma—spindle cell histologic type.

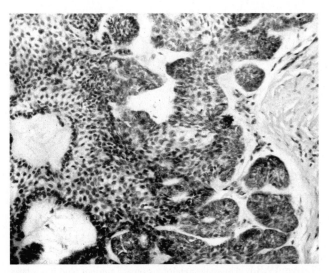

Figure 19.77. Ameloblastoma—basal cell histologic type.

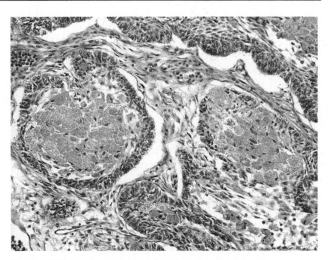

Figure 19.79. Ameloblastoma—granular cell histologic type.

imal or no atypia, with few if any mitoses, composed of nests, strands, plexiform networks, and cyst linings, with peripheral palisaded columnar cells having dark stained basal nuclei polarized away from the basement membrane, vacuolated basilar cell cytoplasm, an edematous spindled stellate reticulum–like region, and budding of epithelium from nests (Fig. 19.80) (190). Another histologic feature of ameloblastoma is that the stroma is fibrous without any inductive mesenchymal effect that may be diagnostic of other odontogenic tumors such as ameloblastic fibroma. No dental hard tissues are found in ameloblastomas.

Treatment by resection with 1- to 1.5-cm boney margins is curative, but more conservative enucleation and curettage, which may be appropriate palliative therapy for some, results in a very high recurrence rate (191). Although intraosseous ameloblastoma is histologically benign and locally aggressive, it only rarely metastasizes.

Peripheral Ameloblastoma

Peripheral ameloblastoma develops in the gingival soft tissue overlying the maxilla or mandible, but, on occasion, it can occur in the buccal mucosa. It is a tumor of adulthood, presenting at a higher mean age (early 50s) compared with conventional intraosseous ameloblastoma (187,192). The peripheral ameloblastoma is strictly a soft tissue proliferation and does not invade bone, although there may be superficial erosion. The same histologic types may be encountered as in conventional ameloblastoma. It must be distinguished from a conventional intraosseous ameloblastoma that perforates the cortex of the jaw to secondarily present in the gingiva. Peripheral ameloblastoma may be mimicked by peripheral odontogenic fibroma with an extensive epithelial proliferation or squamous odontogenic tumor. It is thought to be the same as entities described as gingival basal cell carcinoma (192) and odontogenic gingival epithelial hamartoma (193). Unlike the intraosseous ameloblastoma, peripheral ameloblastoma is cured by conservative excision.

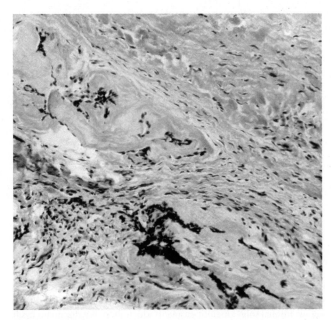

Figure 19.78. Ameloblastoma—desmoplastic histologic type.

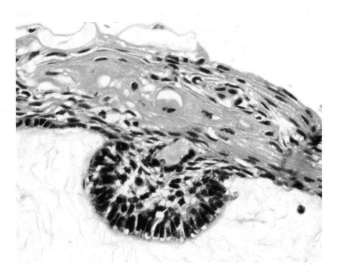

Figure 19.80. Unicystic ameloblastoma. Budding from epithelial nests, here from the cyst lining, is a feature of ameloblastoma mimicking the dental lamina during odontogenesis.

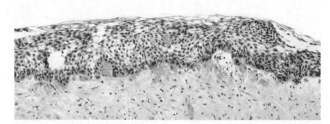

Figure 19.81. Unicystic ameloblastoma. This is a simple cystic type in which the cyst lining demonstrates an edematous stellate reticulum zone overlying the subtle palisading of the low columnar basal cells.

Unicystic Ameloblastoma

The uncommon unicystic ameloblastoma is important to note because the specimen is usually obtained by enucleation of a presumed dentigerous cyst but pathologic evaluation may reveal infiltration that will determine whether further therapy or close follow-up is indicated. Most unicystic ameloblastomas arise in the setting of an unerupted tooth and occur at a mean of 16 years of age, whereas those unassociated with a tooth occur later, at a mean of 35 years (194). The most common location is in the posterior mandibular molar region associated with a third molar. On radiograph, the lesion is a sharply circumscribed, unilocular radiolucency. If not in the pericoronal location of a dentigerous cyst, it may resemble a variety of odontogenic cysts. The designation and precise definition of this entity is still somewhat controversial. Some prefer the term cystic or cystogenic ameloblastoma and accept multicystic examples (195). Most would agree that is a diagnosis made in retrospect with specimen in hand.

There are three histologic variations of unicystic ameloblastoma. First, it may appear as a simple cyst with the ameloblastic epithelial features of peripheral palisading of columnar cells with polarized dark nuclei. An overlying edematous stellate reticulum–like zone is helpful when present (Fig. 19.81). Keratinization may occur but not have the type diagnostic of OKC or COC (Fig. 19.82). The diagnostic features may be focal. The second type is the luminal type containing an intraluminal polypoid plexiform growth but no tumor growing within the wall

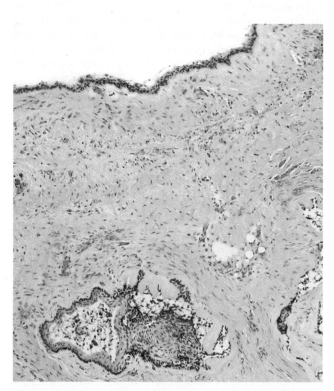

Figure 19.83. Unicystic ameloblastoma. Luminal type has a large polypoid nodule of ameloblastoma arranged in a plexiform pattern protruding into the lumen of the cyst.

(Fig. 19.83). The third pattern, and the most important to document depending on depth of invasion because it may require further therapy, is the mural type containing infiltrating ameloblastomatous epithelium within the wall (Fig. 19.84). This must be differentiated from a conventional solid ameloblastoma in which there is a dominant cystic or multicystic component. Unicystic ameloblastoma, despite conservative removal, has a more favorable prognosis compared to conventional solid/multicystic ameloblastoma (196).

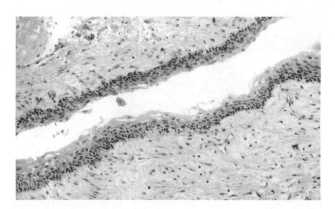

Figure 19.82. Unicystic ameloblastoma. More prominent palisaded basal cells and parakeratinization of the cyst lining are featured.

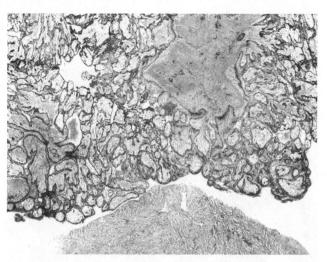

Figure 19.84. Unicystic ameloblastoma. Mural type has nests of ameloblastoma infiltrating the wall. This must be differentiated from a conventional solid ameloblastoma in which there is a dominant cystic component.

Ameloblastic Fibroma, Ameloblastic Fibrodentinoma, and Ameloblastic Fibro-Odontoma

These three rare, benign tumors are mixed odontogenic neoplasms composed of bland strands and islands of odontogenic epithelium embedded in a pulplike, myxoid, cellular connective tissue stroma resembling odontogenic mesenchyme. In normal odontogenesis, the analogous odontogenic mesenchyme of the dental papilla results from an inductive stimulus by the oral epithelium-derived dental lamina, causing the mesenchyme to condense and proliferate. The mesenchymal-derived odontoblasts in turn form the dentin matrix, and the residual dental papilla becomes the dental pulp housed within the tooth.

These odontogenic tumors occur in the early teenage years as a well-circumscribed radiolucency usually associated with a malpositioned or an unerupted tooth arising mostly in the posterior mandible (197). Grossly and microscopically, the tumors are lobulated with a fibrous capsule (Fig. 19.85). These neoplasms are distinguished in the following manner. Histologically, the connective tissue component of each is identical and is composed of an immature, myxoid spindle cell stroma. The amount of epithelium is variable and is composed of thin ribbons and anastomosing cords with ameloblastic features of peripheral palisaded columnar cells (Fig. 19.86). The amount of enclosed stellate reticulum–like areas is also variable but usually minimal. When no hard tissue is present, the tumor is classified as ameloblastic fibroma (AF). If dentin is formed, the designation of ameloblastic fibrodentinoma (AFD) applies. When dentin and enamel hard tissues are formed, the tumor is called ameloblastic fibro-odontoma (AFO). Unlike ameloblastoma, conservative enucleation and curettage is effective therapy for AF, with a low but acceptable recurrence rate. Recurrence of AFO is rare.

The myxoid stroma of a hyperplastic dental follicle containing proliferating odontogenic rests may mimic AF, and diagnosis should be made after correlation with a radiographic image (cyst around the crown of an unerupted tooth) (Fig. 19.87). Differential diagnosis should also include odontoameloblastoma, a rare variant of true ameloblastoma containing odontoma-like dental hard tissues that behaves like conventional ameloblastoma.

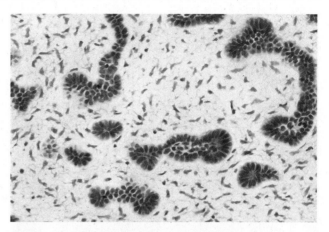

Figure 19.86. Ameloblastic fibroma (AF). Epithelial and stromal proliferation is common to the mixed odontogenic neoplasms of AF, ameloblastic fibro-odontoma, and fibrodentinoma.

Calcifying Epithelial Odontogenic Tumor (Pindborg Tumor)

The calcifying epithelial odontogenic tumor (CEOT) was previously called Pindborg tumor after the oral pathologist who originally reported it (198). It is rare, presents in adults with an average age of 40 years, and has a preference for the mandibular premolar-molar region (199). An even more uncommon peripheral variant has been described (200). CEOT is a locally expansive tumor behaving much like ameloblastoma, although it is considered to be somewhat less aggressive. Radiographically the tumor can resemble a unilocular dentigerous cyst when associated with an impacted tooth. Other appearances include a multilocular radiolucency, mixed radiolucent-radiopaque image with small radiopacities, and a densely radiopaque lesion (Fig. 19.88). Histologically, the tumor is composed of strands, islands, and sheets of polyhedral, eosinophilic epithelial cells (Fig. 19.89). Intercellular bridges may be noted between the well-defined cell borders (Fig. 19.90). The cytologic features

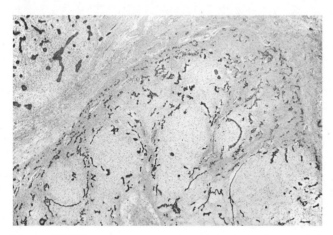

Figure 19.85. Ameloblastic fibroma. Well-circumscribed, lobular masses of myxoid stroma, separated by fibrous connective tissue, contain interspersed strands of branching odontogenic epithelium.

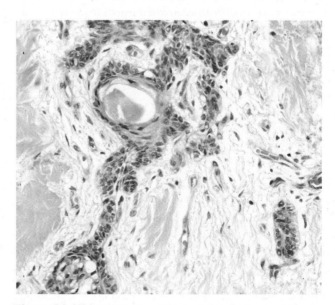

Figure 19.87. Proliferating odontogenic rests in the myxoid stroma of a hyperplastic dental follicle may mimic ameloblastic fibroma.

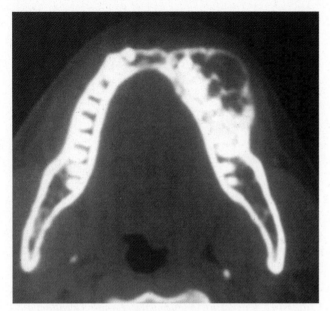

Figure 19.88. Pindborg tumor. Radiographic image of a mixed radiopaque-radiolucent, expansile, multilocular tumor of the mandible is shown.

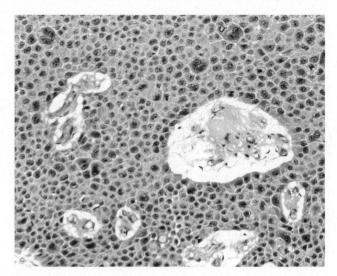

Figure 19.90. Pindborg tumor. Intercellular bridges and nuclear atypia are noted in this example.

are usually bland, but cells with binucleate, trinucleate, and markedly pleomorphic, hyperchromatic nuclei can be seen (Fig. 19.90). A histologic variant is dominated by glycogen-containing clear cells (199). Eosinophilic hyaline deposits can be found within epithelial nests and among the epithelial masses that stain like amyloid with Congo red and thioflavin-T stains (Fig. 19.89). This epithelium-derived "amyloid" may undergo dystrophic calcification, occasionally in a psammoma-like Liesegang ring pattern (Fig. 19.91). The CEOT is effectively treated like an ameloblastoma.

Adenomatoid Odontogenic Tumor

Adenomatoid odontogenic tumor (AOT) occurs preferentially in the anterior tooth-bearing area of the maxilla (incisor-cuspid area). AOT arises over a broad age range, but most patients

(70%) present in the second decade of life (201). Most AOTs are associated with an unerupted permanent tooth, usually the maxillary canine tooth, and therefore, in the younger age group, they simulate a dentigerous cyst or keratocyst on radiographic examination. The presence of stromal calcifications in AOT may raise other radiographic differential diagnoses. A rare peripheral variant has been described in the anterior maxillary gingiva (202).

Histologically, the tumor is well encapsulated, presenting as a cyst often containing a tooth within the cystic space. The wall is usually thickened with a proliferation of epithelium-forming solid masses (Fig. 19.92) composed of whorled nodules of spindled cells and columnar cells with polarized nuclei forming rosettes and ductlike tubular structures (Fig. 19.93). Trabecular and cribriform patterns can be seen as well. Eosinophilic amorphous material (often calcified) can be found within and between tumor cells, as well as in ductlike structures (Fig. 19.94).

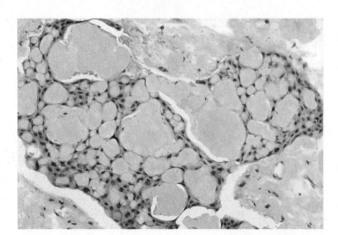

Figure 19.89. Pindborg tumor. Strands and sheets of polyhedral, eosinophilic epithelial cells and associated eosinophilic hyaline matrix with staining characteristics of amyloid are shown.

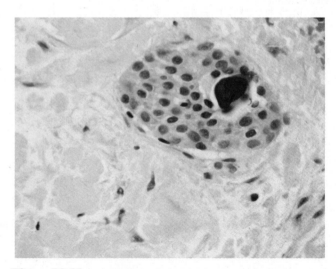

Figure 19.91. Pindborg tumor. Tumor nest containing small calcification resembling a psammoma body is surrounded by extensive amyloid matrix.

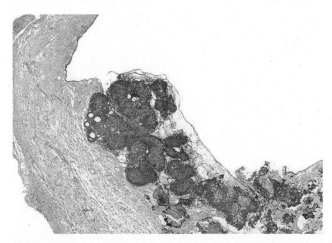

Figure 19.92. Adenomatoid odontogenic tumor. Within the fibrotic wall of the cyst are nodular masses of epithelium and matrix that calcifies.

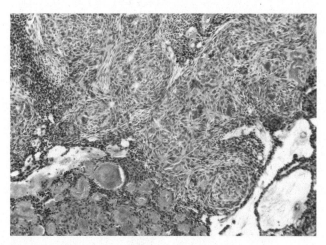

Figure 19.94. Adenomatoid odontogenic tumor. Eosinophilic amorphous material is seen between tumor cells and in ductlike structures.

Occasionally, the calcification is seen in concentric rings similar to Liesegang rings.

AOT is probably best classified as a hamartoma rather than a true neoplasm; it is not related to ameloblastoma. Despite its ability to expand to a very large size with local destruction, the proper therapy for AOT, unlike that for the ameloblastoma, is conservative, consisting of enucleation and curettage. Recurrences are very rare (203).

Squamous Odontogenic Tumor

Squamous odontogenic tumor (SOT) is a rare neoplasm that occurs in the alveolar process of the jaws (204). It may even less frequently occur in soft tissue as a peripheral variant. SOTs occur over a broad age range, and 20% are multiple (205,206). The typical radiograph shows a well-circumscribed radiolucency approximating the roots of the teeth. SOT is composed of is-

lands of well-differentiated squamous epithelium with no pleomorphism or mitotic activity in a fibrous connective tissue stroma (Fig. 19.95). The mature epithelial islands are round to oval, are of varying size and shape, and often bear a peripheral flattened layer of low cuboidal cells. Epithelial nests may exhibit microcystic change and laminar calcifications. The chief histologic differential diagnosis is ameloblastoma (acanthomatous type) and SCC (primary intraosseous or metastatic). SOT-like islands of epithelium may also arise in the wall of odontogenic cysts (Fig. 19.96). Recurrences of SOT are rare after conservative surgery.

Benign Odontogenic Mesenchymal Tumors

ODONTOGENIC FIBROMA. The rare odontogenic fibroma may present in peripheral or central locations. Two histologic forms are recognized: epithelium-poor lesions and epithelium-rich lesions (207–209). The peripheral odontogenic fibroma is a well-circumscribed gingiva mass usually found in the mandibular gingival. The central or intrabony counterpart of the odontogenic fibroma appears as a painless, expansile, unilocular, or

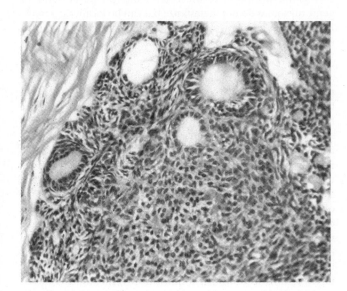

Figure 19.93. Adenomatoid odontogenic tumor. Rosettes and ductlike tubular structures are present in the whorled nodules of spindled and columnar cells.

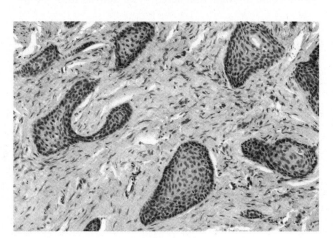

Figure 19.95. Squamous odontogenic tumor. Islands of well-differentiated squamous epithelium with no pleomorphism or mitotic activity in a fibrous connective tissue stroma are shown.

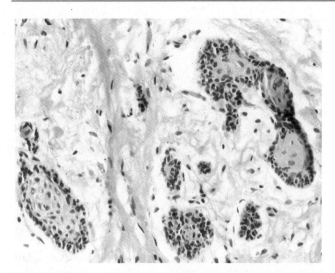

Figure 19.96. Odontogenic rests can be found in the wall of odontogenic cysts, where they may proliferate and undergo squamous metaplasia, thereby mimicking squamous odontogenic tumor.

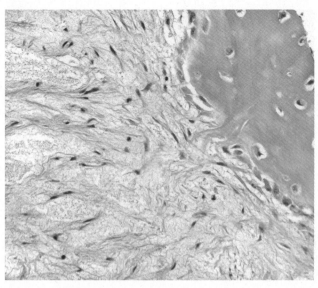

Figure 19.98. Odontogenic myxoma. Innocuous appearance of sparse, bland stellate and spindled cells in a myxomatous stroma showing resorption of bone (*right*) as the locally aggressive tumor infiltrates marrow spaces.

multilocular radiolucency and may be associated with the crown of an unerupted tooth. Odontogenic fibromas occur over a broad age range and favor the mandibular premolar region. The epithelium-rich type has a background of cellular fibroblastic stroma containing strands of bland odontogenic epithelium of variable amount and focal calcifications (Fig. 19.97). Variants may also contain multinucleated giant cells similar to central giant-cell granuloma and even granular or clear cells. The epithelium-poor type is dominated by less cellular connective tissue resembling a dental follicle with occasional epithelial islands and calcifications. Both central and peripheral odontogenic fibromas are treated conservatively by local enucleation and curettage. Recurrence rates are undefined but are likely low.

ODONTOGENIC MYXOMA. Odontogenic myxoma is the third most common odontogenic tumor and presents over a broad age range (210). This gelatinous neoplasm occurs only in the jaws, and therefore, the term "odontogenic" is applied. Rare peripheral examples in gingiva have been described (211). Odontogenic myxoma is believed to be derived from odonto-

genic mesenchyme. Odontogenic epithelial nests are rarely found on microscopic examination, and they are not required for diagnosis. Most arise in the mandibular molar region as painless expansions that may perforate the cortex when large. Radiographically they may appear as a unilocular or multilocular, "soap bubble" or "honeycomb" lucency. Histologically, odontogenic myxoma is an unencapsulated, infiltrative neoplasm of sparse, bland stellate or spindled cells in a myxomatous stroma (Fig. 19.98). The term *myxofibroma* is used when the lesion is more collagenized than myxoid. The ground substance-rich character of this neoplasm may mimic a hyperplastic dental follicle (Fig. 19.99), the dental papilla (pulp) of a developing tooth, or even a nasal polyp, but clinical and radiographic correlation will point to the correct interpretation. Odontogenic myxomas do not metastasize but can be locally aggressive. Permeation of marrow spaces and inadequate removal contribute to recurrence rates of approximately 25%.

CEMENTOBLASTOMA. Cementoblastoma is a true neoplasm attached to the root of a tooth that produces cementum-like tissue. Cementoblastomas have been reported to occur from 8 to 44 years of age (average age, 20 years). The favored site of involvement is the mandibular first molar (212). They usually cause a painful swelling in association with a vital tooth. Radiographically, cementoblastoma presents as a well-defined radiopaque density in continuity with the root of a tooth and surrounded by a thin radiolucency. The normal thin lucency of the periodontal ligament space normally defining the root outline is obliterated, and there may be root resorption. Cementoblastoma is composed of dense, acellular and cellular cemental tissue, attached to the tooth root. The cellular osteoid-like cementum exhibits a range of calcification in a fibrous, highly vascularized stroma. Multinucleate cementoclasts and reversal lines may be abundant (Fig. 19.100). Histologically, the mass appears identical to osteoblastoma, with the only distinction being its attachment to a tooth root (Fig. 19.101). If the

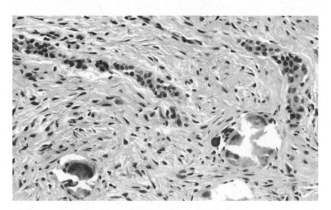

Figure 19.97. Peripheral odontogenic fibroma. This gingival tumor is characterized by a cellular fibroblastic stroma containing strands of bland odontogenic epithelium and focal calcifications.

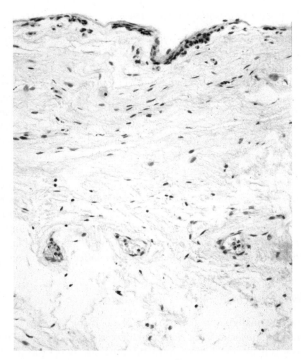

Figure 19.99. Dental follicle. Myxoid stroma of the soft tissue surrounding the developing tooth may mimic odontogenic myxoma out of context. Note the thin reduced enamel epithelium lining the surface of the dental follicle.

mass is biopsied or removed without the attached tooth, it is important to correlate the histology with the dental radiograph to confirm attachment to a tooth root to exclude osteosarcoma from the differential diagnosis. Cementoblastomas have a tendency to recur unless completely removed with the tooth.

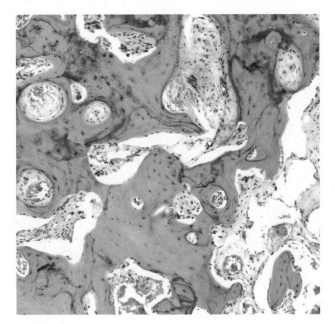

Figure 19.100. Cementoblastoma. Trabecular arrangement of cementum, indistinguishable from bone, exhibits numerous reversal lines. Note the loose, highly vascular stroma.

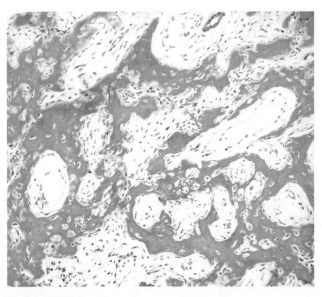

Figure 19.101. Cementoblastoma. Cellular cementum in a highly vascular stroma mimics osteoblastoma with the exception of a cemental mass component attached to a tooth root.

MALIGNANT EPITHELIAL ODONTOGENIC TUMORS

Odontogenic Carcinoma

Odontogenic carcinoma is a generic term for several rare epithelial malignancies derived from the dental lamina (Table 19.3) (213,214). Despite treatment by surgical resection with free margins, the prognosis is often poor.

Metastasizing (Malignant) Ameloblastoma

Metastases, usually to lungs, derived from a histologically benign ameloblastoma are termed *metastasizing (malignant) ameloblastoma* (Fig. 19.102). The diagnosis can only be made from

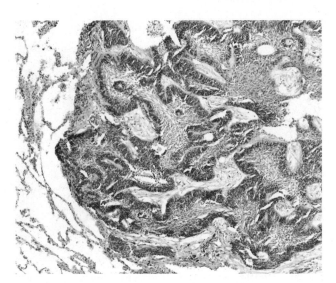

Figure 19.102. Metastasizing (malignant) ameloblastoma. A pulmonary nodule of metastatic ameloblastoma derived from a histologically benign primary ameloblastoma is shown.

the histologic documentation of the benign-appearing metastasis, not the well-differentiated, benign-appearing primary ameloblastoma. They occur at a mean age of 30 years, but arise over a broad age range (4 to 75 years), more often in mandible than maxilla. Metastases of this nature have occurred over a wide time interval, from 1 to 30 years after therapy of the initial ameloblastoma, with 30% occurring 10 years after treatment. They may also occur after numerous recurrences of a primary jaw ameloblastoma (215).

Ameloblastic Carcinoma

In contrast, a cytologically atypical, primary ameloblastoma is designated ameloblastic carcinoma. The diagnosis is not related to whether the neoplasm is productive of metastases or not. Some may result in metastases resembling ameloblastoma. Ameloblastic carcinoma has a similar age demographic, occurring at a mean age of 30 years (range, 15 to 84 years). These malignancies usually show rapid and destructive growth with perforation of cortical plates and extension into adjacent soft tissues (213,214).

Two forms are recognized: a primary de novo type and a secondary (dedifferentiated) type arising in a pre-existing benign ameloblastoma, either intraosseous or peripheral in location (56). Histologically, these odontogenic carcinomas retain the cytomorphologic features of ameloblastoma, with a peripheral palisade of columnar cells and a resemblance to the stellate reticulum in the large islands of tumor, but evince degrees of nuclear hyperchromatism, pleomorphism, mitoses, necrosis, or perineural invasion (Fig. 19.103). Clear-cell, spindle cell, and basal cell features may predominate. These carcinomas are usually the result of (a) tumor of long duration, (b) multiple local jaw recurrences or surgical procedures, or (c) radiation therapy.

Both metastasizing (malignant) ameloblastoma and ameloblastic carcinoma are locally aggressive neoplasms that metastasize late in their course to the lungs, cervical lymph nodes, vertebra, other bones, and viscera. The prognosis for both types of malignancies is poor, with approximately half of patients dying of disease (213,214).

Clear-Cell Odontogenic Carcinoma

Formerly called clear-cell odontogenic tumor, this lesion has been reclassified a malignancy because of increased documentation of biologic behavior (56,216,217). It is rare and arises over a wide age range, with a mean age of 60 years (218). Histologically, it presents a nested pattern with islands of clear cells with well-demarcated cell borders and zones of dark staining basaloid cells with scant eosinophilic cytoplasm (Fig. 19.104). Narrow bands of fibrous stroma course through the tumor. Cells abutting the fibrous bands may show ameloblastomatous features of palisading and nuclear polarization. The clear cells have a cytokeratin- and EMA-positive and vimentin- and S-100 protein–negative immunophenotype. Some cells contain glycogen, but all cells are mucin negative. The main differential diagnoses to entertain are clear-cell variant of calcifying epithelial odontogenic tumor (198), a central clear-cell salivary gland neoplasm, and metastatic clear-cell melanoma or renal cell carcinoma.

Ghost Cell Odontogenic Carcinoma

This rare malignancy has features of calcifying cystic odontogenic tumor (calcifying odontogenic cyst) and dentinogenic ghost cell tumor. Unlike most odontogenic neoplasms, it is more common in the maxilla. The tumor can be cystic and solid and composed of mitotically active, cytologically atypical epithelium producing the pathognomonic ghost cells either singly or in clusters. The neoplasm has the potential to be highly aggressive with local destruction, recurrence, and metastasis (219).

Primary Intraosseous Squamous Cell Carcinoma

This central jaw carcinoma is thought to be derived from odontogenic epithelial remnants. Three types are recognized: (a) de novo SCC, and SCC arising from (b) an odontogenic cyst (Fig. 19.68) or (c) a benign odontogenic tumor (56). Because there are no distinguishing features, unless there is clear derivation

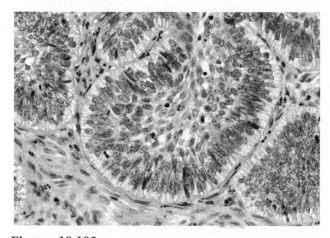

Figure 19.103. Ameloblastic carcinoma. Features of ameloblastoma are retained with a peripheral palisade of columnar cells and a resemblance to the stellate reticulum in the islands of tumor that display nuclear atypia, mitoses, and single-cell necrosis.

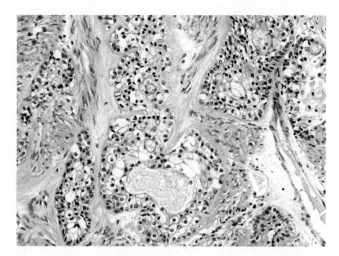

Figure 19.104. Clear-cell odontogenic carcinoma. Nests are composed of atypical clear cells with well-demarcated cell borders and zones of dark staining basaloid cells with scant eosinophilic cytoplasm. Peripheral cells show ameloblastomatous features of palisading and nuclear polarization.

from a pre-existing odontogenic cyst or tumor, the possibility of metastatic SCC to the jaws must be excluded.

MALIGNANT MESENCHYMAL ODONTOGENIC TUMORS

Odontogenic Sarcomas

Malignant transformation of the stroma of an ameloblastic fibroma to produce an ameloblastic fibrosarcoma is rare (220). It is preceded by multiple surgical procedures for recurrence after initial curettage or local excision. Approximately one-third of odontogenic sarcomas arise in a pre-existing ameloblastic fibroma. Histologically, this odontogenic sarcoma resembles ameloblastic fibroma with benign cords and rests of odontogenic epithelium in a hypercellular, fibrous connective tissue. However, the stromal cells are hyperchromatic and pleomorphic with the numerous mitotic figures typical of a fibrosarcoma. Other extremely rare histologic variants may produce dental hard tissues as well (ameloblastic fibrodentinosarcoma and fibro-odontosarcoma). All are low-grade sarcomas that are locally aggressive with low metastatic potential.

Fibro-Osseous Lesions

These intraosseous lesions are discussed as a group for the purpose of microscopic differential diagnosis because they may have common histologic features but they represent distinct clinical entities that require clinical and radiographic correlation to distinguish. The WHO classification of fibro-osseous lesions of the jaws is presented in Table 19.4. This group of lesions has experienced an evolution in concept and terminology over the past 40 years (221–224).

Ossifying Fibroma

Ossifying fibroma is the name given to jaw tumors that may have a variety of histologic appearances but are composed of islands/trabeculae/reticulae of bone in a benign fibroblastic proliferation. They arise in various clinical settings and locations. In the usual type of ossifying fibroma, the tumor is well demarcated but may expand the bony cortex of the jaw. It appears radiolucent and/or radiodense depending on the stage of development, amount of hard tissue produced, and degree

of calcification. Ossifying fibromas occur at a mean age of 35 years, with a female predilection, and anywhere in the tooth-bearing regions of the jaws but mostly in the posterior mandible (221). However, they may also arise in non–tooth-bearing mandibular ramus. The so-called juvenile variant of ossifying fibroma is most commonly encountered in the maxilla and the walls of the paranasal sinuses (vide supra). Ossifying fibromas, usually multiple, are a common component of the rare hereditary hyperparathyroidism-jaw tumor syndrome in which there is a mutation of the endocrine tumor gene *HRPT2* on chromosome 1q encoding parafibromin (225–227).

The radiographic appearance begins as a small, round well-demarcated radiolucency that, with maturation and mineralization of the osteoid zones, becomes a mixed radiolucent/opaque image (Fig. 19.105). Some eventually become dominantly radiopaque lesions. Although the surgeon may appreciate the tumor to be clinically encapsulated because of its circumscription, on removal, there is no true capsule. Histologically, ossifying fibroma is characterized by a benign, variably fibrocellular stroma with variably shaped profiles of woven and lamellar bone that may coalesce into anastomosing patterns (Fig. 19.106). A variation on the usual histology, of no biologic significance, in which rounded or cementum-like droplets of acellular osteoid are seen, has been called cementifying fibroma or cemento-ossifying fibroma (Fig. 19.107). Cementum cannot be distinguished from bone, and the cementum-like pattern of osteoid/bone may also be found in extragnathic bone tumors, so that descriptive designation is now considered part of the histologic spectrum of ossifying fibroma.

Some regions of an ossifying fibroma may display histologic

TABLE 19.4
Bone-Related Tumors and Lesions of the Jaws
Ossifying fibroma
Fibrous dysplasia
Osseous dysplasias
Periapical osseous dysplasia (formerly periapical cemental dysplasia)
Focal osseous dysplasia (formerly focal cemento-osseous dysplasia)
Florid osseous dysplasia
Familial gigantiform cementoma
Central giant-cell lesion
Cherubism
Aneurysmal bone cyst
Simple bone cyst

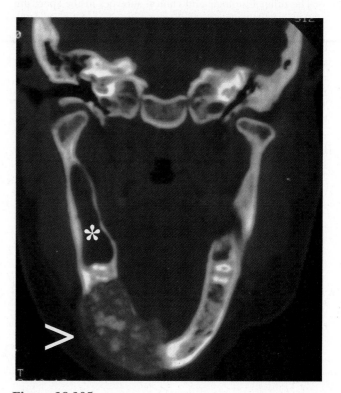

Figure 19.105. Ossifying fibroma. Computed tomography image demonstrates a well-demarcated, expansile lucent ossifying fibroma containing mottled densities in the mid/anterior mandible (*arrowhead*). The lytic lesion just posterior (*asterisk*) is a separate dentigerous cyst.

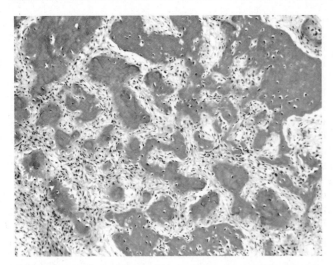

Figure 19.106. Ossifying fibroma. The classic histology of a benign fibrocellular stroma containing variably shaped profiles of woven and lamellar bone that coalesce into anastomosing patterns is shown.

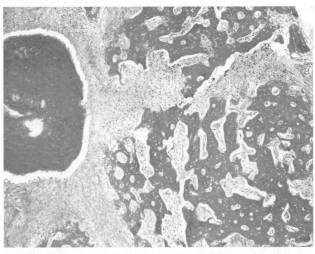

Figure 19.108. Ossifying fibroma. The anastomosing trabecular pattern in a fibrocellular stroma (*right*) is present next to a pattern of large, round masses in a denser, less cellular stroma (*left*).

maturation (Fig. 19.108). Older lesions may be dominated by large coalescent calcified masses with little fibrocellular stroma or set in a densely fibrotic stroma (Fig. 19.109). At one time, it was thought that osteoblastic rimming around the osseous profiles was a diagnostic discriminant from the similar-appearing proliferations of fibrous dysplasia, but this is not the case (Fig. 19.110) (228). The latter lesion may look identical histologically but is distinguished by a different clinical presentation and radiographic image showing indistinct margins.

The other histologic and clinical subtypes in the spectrum of ossifying fibroma include the rarer variants occurring in the younger age groups in the maxilla, juvenile active ossifying fibroma, and in the walls of the paranasal sinuses, juvenile aggressive or active or psammomatoid ossifying fibroma. The use of the term *juvenile* reflects the average age of 20 years for the former subtype and an even younger mean age range of 8.5 to 12 years for the latter subtype (229,230). Both have a fibrocellular stroma, as in the usual ossifying fibroma. However, the juvenile trabecular variant is a mimic of osteosarcoma because of bands of cellular osteoid and trabeculae of immature bone that

may form a lattice, as well as the presence of mitotic figures (Fig. 19.111).

The juvenile psammomatoid variant contains innumerable, small, so-called *ossicles* that resemble psammoma bodies (Fig. 19.112). However, unlike true psammoma bodies, these mineralized deposits range from acellular to sparsely cellular and may fuse to form trabeculae with reversal lines. Given the favored location in the paranasal sinuses, an extracranial meningioma may therefore be raised in differential diagnosis because of the resemblance of the psammomatoid bodies. Multinucleate giant cells, cystic change, and hemorrhage resembling aneurysmal bone cyst may be present in both "juvenile" variants.

Ossifying fibromas are benign, slow-growing neoplasms with a low recurrence rate. Treatment either by enucleation and curettage or by resection is tailored to tumor size, location, the desire to preserve vital structures, and the ability to remove the tumor without incurring a high risk of recurrence. The

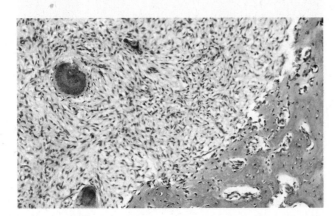

Figure 19.107. Ossifying fibroma. The pattern of rounded or cementum-like acellular osteoid deposits, here coexisting with the trabecular pattern, has been called cementifying fibroma or cemento-ossifying fibroma in the past.

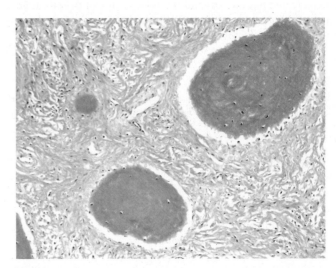

Figure 19.109. Ossifying fibroma. Large calcified masses in a densely fibrotic stroma typify older lesions that appear more radiopaque.

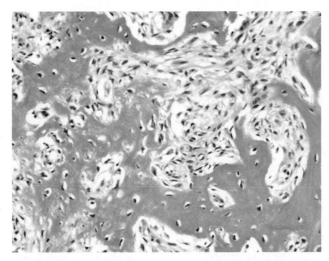

Figure 19.110. Ossifying fibroma. Immature cellular osteoid in this ossifying fibroma appears to arise from the cellular stroma without prominent osteoblastic rimming.

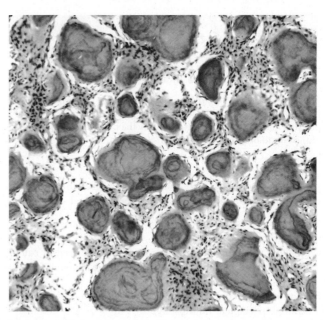

Figure 19.112. Ossifying fibroma, juvenile psammomatoid variant. Innumerable small so-called *ossicles* that resemble psammoma bodies dominate the pattern. However, unlike true psammoma bodies, these mineralized deposits range from acellular to sparsely cellular and may fuse to form trabeculae with reversal lines.

"aggressive" biologic behavior of the "juvenile" variants appears to be a consequence of increased likelihood to encounter recurrences in sinonasal-based tumors initially treated conservatively. In the hereditary hyperparathyroidism-jaw tumor syndrome, "recurrent" tumors may represent development of a new ossifying fibroma rather than persistent/recurrent disease.

FIBROUS DYSPLASIA

Fibrous dysplasia in the jaws more often affects the maxilla than mandible and presents in children and young adults (223). Clinically, there is usually painless facial swelling and asymmetry that may result in displaced teeth. The radiographic appearance is unlike ossifying fibroma and is characterized by radiodense opacities with a "ground glass" appearance that blend into the

adjacent normal bone. Histologically, there is a fibrocellular stroma with scattered trabeculae of woven bone, without osteoblastic rimming. However, older lesions showing maturation to lamellar bone may exhibit osteoblastic rimming. The etiology of fibrous dysplasia has been shown to be the result of a mutation in the *GNAS1* gene affecting proliferation and differentiation of preosteoblasts (231). Lesions of fibrous dysplasia may cease to grow with skeletal maturation.

OSSEOUS DYSPLASIAS

Osseous dysplasias are a difficult spectrum of lesions for the general pathologist to diagnose without clinical and radiographic correlation to the periapical region of a vital tooth or the tooth-bearing region of the jaws. They favor the mandible of middle-aged black females (221). Most are radiolucent initially, with progression to mixed and more radiodense lesions in older stages. The lesions are separated from the tooth root and surrounding bone by a radiolucent zone.

Simply, these are fibro-osseous lesions histologically resembling the spectrum of usual-type ossifying fibromas with cementum-like osseous deposits, woven and trabecular bone in a fibrocellular stroma, but without encapsulation. They are given different names in various clinical settings, including *periapical osseous dysplasia*, formerly periapical cemental dysplasia (anterior mandible involving a limited number of adjacent vital teeth) (Fig. 19.113); *focal osseous dysplasia* or focal cemento-osseous dysplasia (limited involvement in the posterior jaw); *florid osseous dysplasia* (bilateral extensive lesions in the mandible or all four jaw quadrants usually in middle-aged black females) (Fig. 19.114); and *familial gigantiform cementoma* (autosomal dominant lesion involving younger ages and causing jaw expansion). On radiographic and histologic evaluation, the following

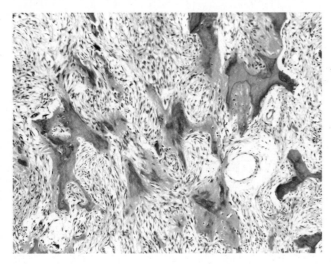

Figure 19.111. Ossifying fibroma, juvenile trabecular variant. Bands of cellular osteoid and trabeculae of immature bone in a fibrocellular stroma may form a lattice, and the presence of mitotic figures may mimic osteosarcoma.

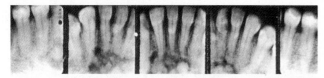

Figure 19.113. Periapical osseous dysplasia. Calcifying osteoid/cemental deposits and fibrocellular stroma at the root apexes of multiple, vital mandibular anterior teeth typify the radiographic appearance of mixed radiolucent/opaque lesions.

three phases of the most frequently encountered form, periapical osseous (cemental) dysplasia, can be observed:

1. Osteolytic stage, characterized by periapical fibrosis (periapical radiolucency)
2. Osteoblastic (cementoblastic) stage, characterized by calcification of the periapical fibrosis (periapical mixed radiolucency-opacity) (Fig. 19.115)
3. Mature stage, characterized by an excessive amount of calcification (periapical radiopacity)

The osseous dysplasias are usually not biopsied and do not require treatment. The larger forms, florid osseous dysplasia and familial gigantiform cementoma, may resemble ossifying fibroma radiographically and contain sclerotic bone masses that may become secondarily infected and require therapy (221,232).

GIANT-CELL LESIONS

CENTRAL GIANT-CELL LESION

Central giant-cell lesion (CGCL) is a localized, destructive lesion of the jaws that has been known historically as central giant-cell granuloma or reparative giant-cell granuloma. Although CGCL is considered benign, recurrences are seen, and lesions may be clinically aggressive. It occurs over a broad age range, with most arising in those under the age of 30 years. The mandibular premolar-molar region is the most common site of involvement, but CGCL may also arise in the ascending ramus, condyle, maxilla, and maxillary sinus (233,234). Radiographically, CGCL may appear as a well-defined, expansile unilocular or multilocular

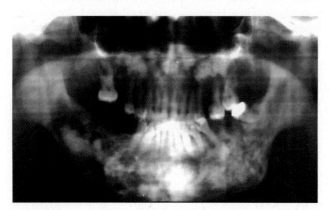

Figure 19.114. Florid osseous dysplasia. Panographic radiograph shows extensive, mostly radiopaque lesions involving all four jaw quadrants in this middle-aged black female.

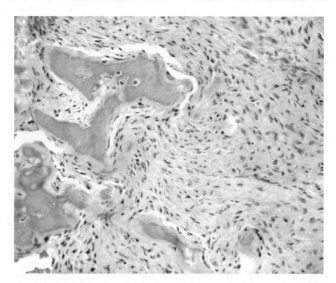

Figure 19.115. Periapical osseous dysplasia. Rarely biopsied, this lesion was at the osteolytic stage presenting as periapical lucency and histologically dominated by periapical fibrosis with little immature bone formation.

radiolucency, especially when large, that may resorb tooth roots. Histologically, CGCL is a proliferation of fibroblastic spindled cells with patchy areas of fresh and remote hemorrhage, in which there are clustered osteoclast-like giant cells (Fig. 19.116). The spindle cells may show mitotic activity and areas of metaplastic bone formation.

The main differential diagnosis is the histologically identical brown tumor of hyperparathyroidism that can be distinguished by abnormal levels of serum calcium and parathyroid hormone. Biopsies of the autosomal dominant condition cherubism may also be histologically identical to CGCL, but the clinical and radiographic appearances are diagnostic. Aneurysmal bone cyst often enters the differential diagnosis of giant-cell lesion of the jaws because of the osteoclast-like giant cells lining the fibrous septa of the blood-filled spaces. Although it may be a primary lesion, aneurysmal bone cyst can be a secondary finding in

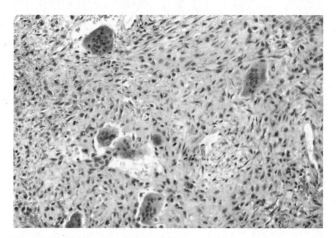

Figure 19.116. Central giant-cell lesion. The histologic appearance of fibroblastic spindled cells with patchy areas of fresh hemorrhage, hemosiderin, and clustered osteoclast-like giant cells is identical to that of the brown tumor of hyperparathyroidism.

CGCL. Scattered giant cells may also be found in the non–epithelial-lined, thin, myxomatous wall of the simple bone cyst of the mandible. Giant-cell tumor, as found in long bone, is probably not seen in the jaws. Nonetheless, the possible neoplastic nature of CGCL of the jaws awaits genetic evaluation.

REFERENCES

1. Robinson BG. Development and growth of the teeth. In Sicher H, ed. *Orban's Oral Histology and Embryology*. St. Louis, MO: Mosby, 1962:41.
2. Page RC. Gingivitis. *J Clin Periodontol* 1986;13:345–355.
3. Johnson BD, Engel D. Acute necrotizing ulcerative gingivitis. *J Periodontol* 1986;57:141–150.
4. Sabiston CB Jr. A review and proposal for the etiology of acute necrotizing gingivitis. *J Clin Periodontol* 1986;13:727–734.
5. Page RC. Current understanding of the aetiology and progression of the periodontal disease. *Int Dent J* 1986;36:153–161.
6. Cappuyns I, Gugerli P, Mombelli A. Viruses in periodontal disease: a review. *Oral Dis* 2005;11:219–229.
7. Grossi SG, Genco RJ, Machtei EE, et al. Assessment of risk for periodontal disease II. Risk indicators for alveolar bone loss. *J Periodontol* 1995;66:23–29.
8. Hart TC. Genetic risk factors for early-onset periodontal diseases. *J Periodontol* 1996;67:355–366.
9. Seppala B, Ainamo J. A site-by-site follow-up study on the effect of controlled versus poorly controlled insulin-dependent diabetes mellitus. *J Clin Periodontol* 1994;21:161–165.
10. Kerr DA. Granuloma pyogenicum. *Oral Surg Oral Med Oral Pathol* 1951;4:158–176.
11. Mills SE, Cooper PH, Fechner RE. Lobular capillary hemangioma: the underlying lesion of pyogenic granuloma. *Am J Surg Pathol* 1980;4:471–479.
12. Buchner A, Hansen LS. The histomorphologic spectrum of the gingival cyst in the adult. *Oral Surg Oral Med Oral Pathol* 1979;48:532–539.
13. Mirabile R, Brown AS, Gisser S. Giant cell granuloma of the palate. *Plast Reconstr Surg* 1986;77:479–481.
14. Lowe WD, Forka FA, Mixson RJ. Etiology of mucosal inflammation with dentures. *J Prosthet Dent* 1967;18:515–527.
15. Yrastova JA. Inflammatory papillary hyperplasia of the palate. *J Oral Surg* 1963;21:330–336.
16. Abbey LM, Page DG, Sawyer D. The clinical and histomorphologic features of a series of 464 oral squamous cell papillomas. *Oral Surg Oral Med Oral Pathol* 1980;49:419–428.
17. Syrjanen SM, Syrjanen KJ, Lamberg MA. Detection of human papillomavirus DNA in oral mucosal lesions using in situ DNA-hybridization applied on paraffin sections. *Oral Surg Oral Med Oral Pathol* 1986;62:660–667.
18. Carr NJ, Bratthauer GL, Lichy JD, et al. Squamous cell papillomas of the esophagus. A study of 23 lesions for human papillomavirus by in situ hybridization and the polymerase chain reaction. *Hum Pathol* 1994;25:536–540.
19. Archard HO, Heck JW, Stanley HR. Focal epithelial hyperplasia: an unusual oral mucosal lesion found in Indian children. *Oral Surg Oral Med Oral Pathol* 1965;20:201–212.
20. Goltz RW, Peterson WCJ, Gorlin R, et al. Focal dermal hypoplasia. *Arch Dermatol* 1962;86:708–717.
21. Carrillo-Farga J, Abbud-Neme F, Deutsch E. Lymphoid papillary hyperplasia of the palatine tonsils. *Am J Surg Pathol* 1983;7:579–582.
22. American Cancer Society. Cancer statistics 2006. Accessed at http://www.cancer.org/docroot/PRO/content/PRO_1_1_Cancer_Statistics_2006_presentation.asp.
23. Frisch M, Hjalgrim H, Jaeger AB, et al. Changing patterns of tonsillar squamous cell carcinoma in the United States. *Cancer Causes Control* 2000;11:489–495.
24. Shiboski CH, Schmidt BL, Jordan RC. Tongue and tonsil carcinoma: increasing trends in the U.S. population ages 20–44 years. *Cancer* 2005;103:1843–1849.
25. Boring CC, Squires TS, Heath CW. Cancer statistics for African Americans. *CA Cancer J Clin* 1992;42:7–18.
26. Jemal A, Thomas A, Murray T, et al. Cancer statistics, 2002. *CA Cancer J Clin* 2002;52:23–47.
27. Mendez PJ, Maves MD, Panje WR. Squamous cell carcinoma of the head and neck in patients under 40 years of age. *Arch Otolaryngol* 1985;111:762–764.
28. Rothman KJ, Keller AZ. The effect of joint exposure to alcohol and tobacco on risk of cancer of the mouth and pharynx. *J Chron Dis* 1972;25:711–716.
29. Cann CI, Fried MP, Rothman KJ. Epidemiology of squamous cell cancer of the head and neck. *Otolaryngol Clin North Am* 1985;18:367–388.
30. D'Souza G, Kreimer AR, Viscidi R, et al. Case-control study of human papillomavirus and oropharyngeal cancer. *N Engl J Med* 2007;356:1944–1956.
31. Zhang ZE, Morgenstern H, Spitz MR, et al. Marijuana use and increased risk of squamous cell carcinoma of the head and neck. *Cancer Epidemiol Biomarkers Prev* 1999;8:1071–1078.
32. Rothman KJ. The proportion of cancer attributable to alcohol consumption. *Prev Med* 1980;9:174–179.
33. Rodriquez T, Altieri A, Chatenoud L, et al. Risk factors for oral and pharyngeal cancer in young adults. *Oral Oncol* 2004;40:207–213.
34. Wey PD, Lotz MJ, Triedman LJ. Oral cancer in women nonusers of tobacco and alcohol. *Cancer* 1987;60:1644–1650.
35. Bosch FX, Manos MM, Munoz N, et al. Prevalence of human papillomavirus in cervical cancer: a worldwide perspective. International Biological Study of Cervical Cancer (IBSCC) Study Group. *J Natl Cancer Inst* 1995;87:796–802.
36. Kreimer AR, Clifford GM, Boyle P, et al. Human papillomavirus types in head and neck squamous cell carcinomas worldwide: a systematic review. *Cancer Epidemiol Biomarkers Prev* 2005;14:467–475.
37. Syrjanen SM. HPV infections and tonsillar carcinoma. *J Clin Pathol* 2004;57:449–455.
38. Al-Qahtani K, Brousseau V, Paczeny D, et al. Koilocytosis in oral squamous cell carcinoma: what does it mean? *J Otolaryngol* 2007;36:26–31.
39. Koch WM, Lango M, Sewell D, et al. Head and neck cancer in nonsmokers: a distinct clinical and molecular entity. *Laryngoscope* 1999;109:1544–1551.
40. Sugiyama M, Bhawal UK, Dohmen T, et al. Detection of human papillomavirus-16 and HPV-18 DNA in normal, dysplastic and malignant oral epithelium. *Oral Surg Oral Med Oral Pathol Radiol Endod* 2003;95:594–600.
41. Ringstrom E, Peters E, Hasegawa M, et al. Human papillomavirus type 16 and squamous cell carcinoma of the head and neck. *Clin Cancer Res* 2002;8:3187–3192.
42. Gillison M, Koch WM, Capone RB, et al. Evidence for a causal association between human papillomavirus and a subset of head and neck cancers. *J Natl Cancer Inst* 2000;92:709–720.
43. Rosenquist K, Wennerberg J, Schildt EB, et al. Oral status, oral infections and some lifestyle factors as risk factors for oral and oropharyngeal squamous cell carcinoma. A population-based case-control study in southern Sweden. *Acta Otolaryngol* 2005;125:1327–1336.
44. Hornia M, Willberg J, Ruokonen H, et al. Marginal periodontium as a potential reservoir of human papillomavirus in oral mucosa. *J Peridontol* 2005;76:358–363.
45. Tezel M, Sullivan MA, Reid ME, et al. Chronic periodontitis and the risk of tongue cancer. *Arch Otolaryngol Head Neck Surg* 2007;133:450–454.
46. Yu KK, Zanation AM, Moss JR, et al. Familial head and neck cancer: molecular analysis of a new clinical entity. *Laryngoscope* 2002;112:1587–1593.
47. Kramer IR, Lucas RB, Pindborg JJ, et al. Definition of leukoplakia and related lesions: an aid to studies on oral precancer. *Oral Surg Oral Med Oral Pathol* 1978;46:518–539.
48. Waldron CA, Shafer WG. Leukoplakia revisited: a clinicopathologic study of 3,256 oral leukoplakias. *Cancer* 1975;36:1386–1392.
49. Einhorn J, Wersall J. Incidence of oral carcinoma in patients with leukoplakia of the oral mucosa. *Cancer* 1967;20:2189–2193.
50. Mashberg A. Erythroplasia vs leukoplasia in the diagnosis of early asymptomatic oral squamous carcinoma. *N Engl J Med* 1977;297:109–110.
51. Pindborg JJ, Jolst O, Renstrup G, et al. Studies in oral leukoplakia: a preliminary report on the period prevalence of malignant transformation in leukoplakia based on a follow-up study of 248 patients. *J Am Dent Assoc* 1968;76:767–771.
52. Silverman S, Gorsky M, Lozada F. Oral leukoplakia and malignant transformation: a follow-up study of 257 patients. *Cancer* 1984;53:563–568.
53. Mashberg A. Erythroplasia: the earliest sign of asymptomatic oral cancer. *J Am Dent Assoc* 1978;96:615–620.
54. Silverman SJ, Gorsky M. Proliferation verrucous leukoplakia: a follow-up study of 54 cases. *Oral Surg Oral Med Oral Pathol Oral Radiol Endod* 1997;84:154–157.
55. Shafer WG. Oral carcinoma in situ. *Oral Surg Oral Med Oral Pathol* 1975;39:227–238.
56. Barnes L, Eveson JW, Reichart P, et al. *World Health Organization Classification of Tumours. Pathology and Genetics of Head and Neck Tumours*. Lyon, France: IARC Press, 2005.
57. Shafer WG, Waldron CA. Erythroplakia of the oral cavity. *Cancer* 1975;36:1021–1028.
58. Krutchkoff DJ, Eisenberg E, Anderson C. Dysplasia of oral mucosa: a unified approach of proper evaluation. *Mod Pathol* 1991;4:113–119.
59. Pindborg JJ, Reichart PA, Smith CJ, et al. *World Health Organization (WHO) International Histological Classification of Tumours*. Berlin, Germany: Springer-Verlag, 1997:24–26.
60. Sudbo J, Bryne M, Johannessen AC, et al. Comparison of histological grading and large-scale genomic status (DNA ploidy) as prognostic tools in oral dysplasia. *J Pathol* 2001;194:303–310.
61. Crissman JD, Zarbo RJ. Dysplasia, in situ carcinoma, and progression to invasive squamous cell carcinoma of the upper aerodigestive tract. *Am J Surg Pathol* 1989;13:5–16.
62. Crissman JD, Liu WY, Gluckman JL, et al. Prognostic value of histopathologic parameters in squamous cell carcinoma of the oropharynx. *Cancer* 1984;54:2995–3001.
63. Frierson HF, Cooper PH. Prognostic factors in squamous cell carcinoma of the lower lip. *Hum Pathol* 1986;17:346–354.
64. Mohit-Tabatabai MA, Sobel HJ, Ruch BF, et al. Relation of thickness of floor of mouth stage I and II cancers to regional metastasis. *Am J Surg* 1986;152:351–353.
65. Moore C, Kuhns JG, Greenberg RA. Thickness as prognostic aid in upper aerodigestive tract cancer. *Arch Surg* 1986;121:1410–1414.
66. Shingaki S, Suzuki I, Nakajima T, et al. Evaluation of histopathologic parameters in predicting cervical lymph node metastasis of oral and oropharyngeal carcinoma. *Oral Surg Oral Med Oral Pathol* 1988;66:683–688.
67. Spiro RH, Huvos AG, Wong GY, et al. Predictive value of tumor thickness in squamous carcinoma confined to the tongue and floor of the mouth. *Am J Surg* 1986;152:345–350.
68. Thompson SH. Cervical lymph node metastases of oral carcinoma related to the depth of invasion of the primary lesion. *J Surg Oncol* 1986;31:120–122.
69. Tepperman BS, Fitzpatrick PJ. Second respiratory and upper digestive tract cancers after oral cancer. *Lancet* 1981;2:547–549.
70. Gluckman JL, Crissman JD. Survival rates in 548 patients with multiple neoplasms of the upper aerodigestive tract. *Laryngoscope* 1983;91:71–74.
71. Slaughter DP, Southwick HW, Smejkal W. Field cancerization in oral stratified squamous epithelium: clinical implication of multicentric origin. *Cancer* 1953;6:963–968.
72. Bedi GC, Westra WH, Gabrielson E, et al. Multiple head and neck tumors: evidence for a common clonal origin. *Cancer Res* 1996;56:2484–2487.
73. Califano J, van der Riet P, Westra W, et al. Genetic progression model for head and neck cancer: implications for field cancerization. *Cancer Res* 1996;56:2488–2492.
74. Carey TE. Field cancerization: are multiple primary cancers monoclonal or polyclonal? *Ann Med* 1996;28:183–188.
75. Worsham MJ, Wolman SR, Carey TE, et al. Common clonal origin of synchronous primary head and neck squamous cell carcinomas: analysis by tumor karyotypes and fluorescence in situ hybridization. *Hum Pathol* 1995;26:251–261.
76. Zarbo RJ, Crissman JD. The surgical pathology of the head and neck cancer. *Semin Oncol* 1988;15:10–19.
77. Greene FL, Page DL, Fleming ID, et al. *AJCC Cancer Staging Manual*. Philadelphia, PA: Lippincott Williams & Wilkins, 2002.

78. Platz H, Fries R, Hudec M, et al. The prognostic relevance of various factors at the time of the first admission of the patient: retrospective DOSAK study on carcinoma of the oral cavity. *J Maxillofac Surg* 1983;11:3–12.
79. Kalnins IK, Leonard AG, Sako K, et al. Correlation between prognosis and degree of lymph node involvement in carcinoma of the oral cavity. *Am J Surg* 1977;134:450–454.
80. Civantos F, Zitsch R, Bared A. Sentinel node biopsy in oral squamous cell carcinoma. *J Surg Oncol* 2007;96:330–336.
81. Woolgar JA. Pathology of the N0 neck. *Br J Oral Maxillofac Surg* 1999;37:205–209.
82. Ross G, Shoaib R, Soutar DS, et al. The use of sentinel node biopsy to upstage the clinically N0 neck in head and neck cancer. *Arch Otolaryngol Head Neck Surg* 2002;128:1287–1291.
83. Stoeckli SJ, Pfaltz M, Steinert H, et al. Histopathological features of occult metastasis detected by sentinel lymph node biopsy in oral and oropharyngeal squamous cell carcinoma. *Laryngoscope* 2002;112:111–115.
84. Nieuwenhuis EJ, van der Waal I, Leemand CR, et al. Histopathological validation of the sentinel node concept in oral and oropharyngeal squamous cell carcinomas. *Head Neck* 2005;27:150–158.
85. Pargaonkar AS, Beissner RS, Snyder S, et al. Evaluation of immunohistochemistry and multiple-level sectioning in sentinel lymph nodes from patients with breast cancer. *Arch Pathol Lab Med* 2003;127:701–705.
86. Crile GW. Carcinoma of the jaws, tongue, cheek and lips: general principles involved in operations and results obtained at Cleveland Clinic. *Surg Gynecol Obstet* 1923;36:159–162.
87. Carlson ER, Ord RA. Vertebral metastases from oral squamous cell carcinoma. *J Oral Maxillofac Surg* 2002;60:858–862.
88. Ross GL, Soutar DS, MacDonald DG, et al. Improved staging of cervical metastases in clinically node-negative patients with head and neck squamous cell carcinoma. *Ann Surg Oncol* 2004;11:213–218.
89. Sawair FA, Irwin CR, Gordon DJ, et al. Invasive front grading: reliability and usefulness in the management of oral squamous cell carcinoma. *J Oral Pathol Med* 2003;32:1–9.
90. Sparano A, Weinstein G, Chalian A, et al. Multivariate predictors of occult neck metastasis in early oral tongue cancer. *Otolaryngol Head Neck Surg* 2004;131:472–476.
91. Yamamoto E, Miyakawa A, Kohama GI. Mode of invasion and lymph node metastasis in squamous cell carcinoma of the oral cavity. *Head Neck Surg* 1984;6:938–946.
92. Zarbo RJ, Barnes L, Crissman JD, et al. Recommendations for the reporting of specimens containing oral cavity and oropharynx neoplasms. *Mod Pathol* 2000;13:1028–1041.
93. Poleksic S, Kalwaic HJ. Prognostic value of vascular invasion in squamous cell carcinoma of the head and neck. *Plast Recronstr Surg* 1978;61:234–240.
94. Carter RL, Tanner NS, Clifford P, et al. Perineural spread in squamous cell carcinomas of the head and neck: a clinicopathologic study. *Clin Otolaryngol* 1979;4:271–281.
95. Byers RM, Bland KI, Borlase B, et al. The prognostic and therapeutic value of frozen section determinations in the surgical treatment of squamous carcinoma of the head and neck. *Am J Surg* 1978;136:525–528.
96. Zieske LA, Johnson JT, Myers EN, et al. Squamous cell carcinoma with positive margins: surgery and postoperative irradiation. *Arch Otolaryngol Head Neck Surg* 1986;112:863–866.
97. Looser KG, Shah JP, Strong EW. The significance of positive margins in surgically resected epidermoid carcinomas. *Head Neck Surg* 1978;1:107–111.
98. Shear M, Hawkins DM, Far HW. The prediction of lymph node metastases from oral squamous carcinoma. *Cancer* 1976;37:1901–1907.
99. Krolls SO, Hoffman S. Squamous cell carcinoma of the oral soft tissues: a statistical analysis of 14,253 cases by age, sex and race of patients. *J Am Dent Assoc* 1976;92:571–574.
100. Woolgar JA. Histological distribution of cervical lymph node metastases from intraoral/oropharyngeal squamous cell carcinoma. *Br J Oral Maxillofac Surg* 1999;37:175–180.
101. Lim YC, Koo BS, Lee JY, et al. Distribution of cervical lymph node metastases in oropharyngeal carcinoma: therapeutic implications for the N0 neck. *Laryngoscope* 2006;116:1148–1152.
102. Spiro RH, Strong EW. Surgical treatment of the tongue. *Surg Clin North Am* 1974;54:759–765.
103. O-Charoenrat P, Pillai G, Patel S, et al. Tumour thickness predicts cervical nodal metastases and survival in early oral tongue cancer. *Oral Oncol* 2003;39:386–390.
104. Fukano H, Matsuura H, Hasegawa Y, et al. Depth of invasion as a predictive factor for cervical lymph node metastases in tongue carcinoma. *Head Neck* 1997;19:205–210.
105. Veness MJ, Morgan GJ, Sathiyaseelan Y, et al. Anterior tongue cancer and the incidence of cervical lymph node metastases with increasing tumour thickness: should elective treatment to the neck be standard practice in all patients? *ANZ J Surg* 2005;75:101–105.
106. Lefall AD, White JE. Cancer of the oral cavity in Negroes. *Surg Gynecol Obstet* 1965;120:70–72.
107. Harrold CC. Management of cancer of the floor of the mouth. *Am J Surg* 1971;122:487–493.
108. Crissman JD, Gluckman JL, Whiteley J, et al. Squamous-cell carcinoma of the floor of the mouth. *Head Neck Surg* 1980;3:2–7.
109. Brown RL, Suh JM, Scarborough JE, et al. Snuff dippers intra-oral cancer: clinical characteristics and response to the therapy. *Cancer* 1965;18:2–13.
110. Cernea P, Billet J. Epitheliomas of the buccal mucosa: study of 60 cases. *Rev Stomatol (Paris)* 1962;63:222–232.
111. Urist M, O'Brien CJ, Soong SJ, et al. Squamous cell carcinoma of the buccal mucosa: analysis of prognostic factors. *Am J Surg* 1987;154:411–414.
112. Eneroth CM, Hjertman L, Moberger G. Squamous cell carcinomas of the palate. *Acta Otolaryngol* 1972;73:418–427.
113. Evans JF, Shah JP. Epidermoid carcinoma of the palate. *Am J Surg* 1981;142:451–455.
114. Stell PM. Tumours of the oropharynx. *Clin Otolaryngol* 1976;1:71–90.
115. Merino OR, Lindberg RD, Fletcher GH. An analysis of distant metastases from squamous cell carcinoma of the upper respiratory and digestive tracts. *Cancer* 1977;40:145–151.
116. Rubin P. Cancer of the head and neck. *JAMA* 1971;217:940–942.
117. Weller SA, Goffinet DR, Goode RL, et al. Carcinoma of the oropharynx: results of megavoltage radiation therapy in 305 patients. *Am J Roentgenol Rad Ther Nucl Med* 1976;126:236–247.
118. Johnston WD, Byers RM. Squamous cell carcinoma of the tonsil in young adults. *Cancer* 1977;39:632–636.
119. Martin H, Sugarbaker E. Cancer of the tonsil. *Am J Surg* 1941;52:158–197.
120. Micheau C, Cachin Y, Caillou B. Cystic metastases in the neck revealing occult carcinoma of the tonsil: a report of 6 cases. *Cancer* 1974;33:228–233.
121. Friedell HL, Rosenthal LM. The etiologic role of chewing tobacco in cancer of the mouth: report of eight cases treated with radiation. *JAMA* 1941;116:2130–2135.
121a. Ackerman LV. Verrucous carcinoma of the oral cavity. *Surgery* 1948;23:670–678.
122. Shafer WG. Verrucous carcinoma. *Int Dent J* 1972;22:451–459.
123. Kraus FT, Perez-Mesa C. Verrucous carcinoma: clinical and pathologic study of 105 cases involving oral cavity, larynx and genitalia. *Cancer* 1966;19:26–38.
124. Syrjanen SM. Human papillomavirus (HPV) in head and neck cancer. Review. *J Clin Virol* 2005;32S:S59–S66.
125. Medina JE, Dichtel W, Luna MA. Verrucous squamous carcinomas of the oral cavity. *Arch Otolaryngol* 1984;110:437–440.
126. Hansen LS, Olsen JA, Silverman S Jr. Proliferative verrucous leukoplakia. *Oral Surg Oral Med Oral Pathol* 1985;60:285–298.
127. Shear M, Pindborg JJ. Verrucous hyperplasia of the oral mucosa. *Cancer* 1980;46:1855–1862.
128. Slootweg PJ, Muller H. Verrucous hyperplasia or verrucous carcinoma. *J Maxillofac Surg* 1983;11:13–19.
129. Bagan JV, Jimenez Y, Murillo J, et al. Lack of association between proliferative verrucous leukoplakia and human papillomavirus infection. *J Oral Maxillo Surg* 2007;65:46–49.
130. Fettig A, Pogrel MA, Silverman SJ, et al. Proliferative verrucous leukoplakia of the gingiva. *Oral Surg Oral Med Oral Pathol Oral Radiol Endod* 2000;90:723–730.
131. McDonald JS, Crissman JD, Gluckman JL. Verrucous carcinoma of the oral cavity. *Head Neck Surg* 1982;5:22–28.
132. Batsakis JG, Suarez P. Papillary squamous carcinoma: will the real one please stand up? *Adv Anat Pathol* 2000;7:2–8.
133. Wenig BM. Squamous cell carcinoma of the upper aerodigestive tract. Precursors and problematic variants. *Mod Pathol* 2002;15:229–254.
134. Crissman JD, Kessis T, Shah KV, et al. Squamous papillary neoplasia of the adult upper aerodigestive tract. *Hum Pathol* 1988;19:1387–1396.
135. Suarez PA, Adler-Storthz K, Luna MA, et al. Papillary squamous cell carcinomas of the upper aerodigestive tract: a clinicopathologic and molecular study. *Head Neck* 2000;22:360–368.
136. Thompson LD, Wenig BM, Heffner DK, et al. Exophytic and papillary squamous cell carcinoma of the larynx: a clinicopathologic series of 104 cases. *Otolaryngol Head Neck Surg* 1999;120:718–724.
137. Ansari-Lari MA, Hoque M, Califano J, et al. Immunohistochemical p53 expression patterns in sarcomatoid carcinomas of the upper respiratory tract. *Am J Surg Pathol* 2002;26:1024–1031.
138. Choi HR, Sturgis E, Rosenthal D, et al. Sarcomatoid carcinoma of the head and neck: molecular evidence for evolution and progression from conventional squamous cell carcinomas. *Am J Surg Pathol* 2003;27:1216–1220.
139. Ellis GL, Corio RL. Spindle cell carcinoma of the oral cavity: a clinicopathologic assessment of fifty-nine cases. *Oral Surg Oral Med Oral Pathol* 1980;50:523–534.
140. Leventon GS, Evans HL. Sarcomatoid squamous cell carcinoma of the mucous membranes of the head and neck: a clinicopathologic study of 20 cases. *Cancer* 1981;48:994–1003.
141. Zarbo RJ, Crissman JD, Venkat H, et al. Spindle-cell carcinomas of the upper aerodigestive tract mucosa. *Am J Surg Pathol* 1986;10:741–753.
142. Nakhleh RE, Zarbo RJ, Ewing S, et al. Myogenic differentiation in spindle cell (sarcomatoid) carcinomas of the upper aerodigestive tract. *Appl Immunohistochem* 1993;1:58–68.
143. Weidner N, Askin FB, Berthrong M, et al. Bizarre (pseudomalignant) granulation-tissue reactions following ionizing-radiation exposure: a microscopic, immunohistochemical and flow-cytometric study. *Cancer* 1987;59:1509–1514.
144. Wenig BM, Devaney K, Bisceglia M. Inflammatory myofibroblastic tumor of the larynx. A clinicopathologic study of eight cases simulating a malignant spindle cell neoplasm. *Cancer* 1995;76:2217–2229.
145. Gerughty RM, Hennigar GR, Brown RM. Adenosquamous carcinoma of the nasal, oral and laryngeal cavities: a clinicopathologic survey of ten cases. *Cancer* 1968;22:1140–1155.
146. Keelawat S, Liu CZ, Roehm PC, et al. Adenosquamous carcinoma of the upper aerodigestive tract: a clinicopathologic study of 12 cases and review of the literature. *Am J Otolaryngol* 2002;23:160–168.
147. Ferlito A. A pathologic and clinical study of adenosquamous carcinoma of the larynx: report of four cases and review of the literature. *Acta Otorhinolaryngol Belg* 1976;30:380–389.
148. Alos L, Castillo M, Nadal A, et al. Adenosquamous carcinoma of the head and neck: criteria for diagnosis in a study of 12 cases. *Histopathology* 2004;44:570–579.
149. Eversole LP. Mucoepidermoid carcinoma of minor salivary glands: report of 17 cases with follow-up. *J Oral Surg* 1972;30:107–112.
150. Melrose RJ. Mucoepidermoid tumors of the intraoral minor salivary glands: a clinicopathologic study of 54 cases. *J Oral Pathol* 1973;2:314–325.
151. Evans HL. Mucoepidermoid carcinoma of salivary glands: a study of 69 cases with special attention to histologic grading. *Am J Clin Pathol* 1984;81:696–701.
152. Takagi M, Sakota Y, Takayama S, et al. Adenoid squamous cell carcinoma of the oral mucosa: report of two autopsy cases. *Cancer* 1977;40:2250–2255.
153. Wain SL, Kier R, Vollmer RT, et al. Basaloid-squamous carcinoma of the tongue, hypopharynx, and larynx: report of 10 cases. *Hum Pathol* 1986;17:1158–1166.
154. Cabanillas R, Rodrigo JP, Ferlito A, et al. Is there an epidemiological link between human papillomavirus DNA and basaloid squamous cell carcinoma of the pharynx? *Oral Oncol* 2007;43:327–332.
155. Banks ER, Frierson HF, Mills SE, et al. Basaloid squamous cell carcinoma of the head and neck: a clinicopathologic and immunohistochemical study of 40 cases. *Am J Surg Pathol* 1992;16:939–946.
156. Emanuel P, Wang B, Wu M, et al. p63 immunohistochemistry in the distinction of adenoid cystic carcinoma from basaloid squamous cell carcinoma. *Mod Pathol* 2005;18:645–650.

157. Gnepp DR, Wick MR. Small cell carcinoma of the major salivary glands: an immunohisto-chemical study. *Cancer* 1990;66:185–192.

158. de Sampaio Goes FC, Oliveira DT, Dorta RG, et al. Prognoses of oral basaloid squamous cell carcinoma and squamous cell carcinoma: a comparison. *Arch Otolaryngol Head Neck Surg* 2004;130:83–86.

159. Yamaguchi A. Hyaline bodies of odontogenic cysts: histological, histochemical and electron microscopic studies. *J Oral Pathol* 1980;9:221–234.

160. Lucas RB. Pathology of tumors of the oral tissues. In *Cysts of the Oral Tissues*. New York, NY: Churchill Livingstone, 1984:357–391.

161. Ackerman G, Cohen MA, Altini M. The paradental cyst: a clinicopathologic study of 50 cases. *Oral Surg Oral Med Oral Pathol* 1987;64:308–312.

162. Seward MH. Eruption cyst: an analysis of its clinical features. *J Oral Surg* 1973;31:31–35.

163. Standish SM, Shafer WG. The lateral periodontal cyst. *J Periodontol* 1958;29:27–33.

164. Woolgar JA, Rippin JS, Browne RM. The odontogenic keratocyst and its occurrence in the nevoid basal cell carcinoma syndrome. *Oral Surg Oral Med Oral Pathol* 1987;64:727–730.

165. Gorlin RJ, Goltz RW. Multiple nevoid basal cell epithelioma, jaw cysts and syndrome. *N Eng J Med* 1960;262:908–914.

166. Agaram NP, Collins BM, Barnes L, et al. Molecular analysis to demonstrate the odontogenic keratocysts are neoplastic. *Arch Pathol Lab Med* 2004;128:313–317.

167. Woo SB, Eisenbud L, Kleiman M, et al. Odontogenic keratocysts in the anterior maxilla: report of two cases, one simulating a nasopalatine cyst. *Oral Surg Oral Med Oral Pathol* 1987;64:463–465.

168. Ahlfors E, Larsson A, Sjogren S. The odontogenic keratocyst: a benign cystic tumor? *J Oral Maxillo Surg* 1984;42:10–19.

169. MacLeod RI, Soames JV. Squamous cell carcinoma arising in an odontogenic keratocyst. *Br J Oral Maxillofac Surg* 1988;26:52–57.

170. Marker P, Brondum N, Clausen PP, et al. Treatment of large odontogenic keratocysts by decompression and later cystectomy. A long-term follow-up study of 23 cases. *Oral Surg Oral Med Oral Pathol Oral Radiol Endod* 1996;82:122–131.

171. Forsell K, Forsell H, Kahnberg KE. Recurrence of keratocysts. A long term follow-up study. *Int J Maxillofac Surg* 1988;17:25–28.

172. Gorlin RJ, Pindborg JJ, Redman RS, et al. The calcifying odontogenic cyst: a new entity and possible analogue of the cutaneous calcifying epithelioma of Malherbe. *Cancer* 1964;17:723–729.

173. Gardner DG, Kessler HP, Morency R, et al. The glandular odontogenic cyst: an apparent entity. *Oral Surg Oral Med Oral Pathol* 1988;17:359–366.

174. Marx RE, Stern D. *Oral and Maxillofacial Pathology: A Rationale for Diagnosis and Treatment.* Chicago, IL: Quintessence Publishing Co., 2003:609.

175. Patron M, Colmenero C, Larrauri J. Glandular odontogenic cyst: a clinicopathological analysis of three cases. *Oral Surg Oral Med Oral Pathol* 1991;72:71–74.

176. Abrams AM, Howell FV, Bullock WK. Nasopalatine cysts. *Oral Surg Oral Med Oral Pathol* 1963;16:306–332.

177. Walsh-Waring GP. Nasoalveolar cysts: aetiology, presentation, and treatment. *J Laryngol Otolaryngol* 1967;81:263–271.

178. Christ TF. The globulomaxillary cyst: an embryologic misconception. *Oral Surg Oral Med Oral Pathol* 1970;30:515–526.

179. Wysocki GP. The differential diagnosis of globulomaxillary radiolucencies. *Oral Surg Oral Med Oral Pathol* 1981;51:281–286.

180. Waldron CA, Mustoc TA. Primary intraosseous carcinoma of the mandible with probable origin in an odontogenic cyst. *Oral Surg Oral Med Oral Pathol* 1989;67:716–724.

181. Eversole LP, Sabes WR, Rovin S. Aggressive growth and neoplastic potential of odontogenic cysts with special reference to central epidermoid and mucoepidermoid carcinomas. *Cancer* 1975;35:270–282.

182. Sedano HO, Pindborg JJ. Ghost cell epithelium in odontomas. *J Oral Pathol* 2003;4:27–30.

183. Baden E. Odontogenic tumors. *Pathol Annu* 1971;6:475–568.

184. Larsson A, Almeren H. Ameloblastoma of the jaws: an analysis of a consecutive series of all cases reported to the Swedish Cancer Registry during 1958–1971. *Acta Pathol Microbiol Scand* 1978;86A:337–349.

185. McClatchey KD. Tumors of the dental lamina: a selective review. *Semin Diagn Pathol* 1987;4:200–204.

186. Mehlisch DR, Dahlin DC, Masson JK. Ameloblastoma: a clinicopathologic report. *J Oral Surg* 1972;30:9–22.

187. Reichart PA, Philipsen HP, Sonner S. Biological profile of 3677 cases. *Eur J Cancer B Oral Oncol* 1995;31B:86–99.

188. Regezi JA, Kerr DA, Courtney RM. Odontogenic tumors: an analysis of 706 cases. *Oral Surg Oral Med Oral Pathol* 1978;36:771–778.

189. Waldron CA, El-Mofty SK. A histopathologic study of 116 ameloblastomas with special reference to the desmoplastic variant. *Oral Surg Oral Med Oral Pathol* 1987;63:441–451.

190. Vickers RA, Gorlin RJ. Ameloblastoma: delineation of early histopathologic features of neoplasia. *Cancer* 1970;26:699–710.

191. Carlson ER, Marx RE. The ameloblastoma-primary curative surgical management. *J Oral Maxillofac Surg* 2006;64:484–494.

192. Gardner DG. Peripheral ameloblastoma: a study of 21 cases, including 5 reported as basal cell of the gingiva. *Cancer* 1977;39:1625–1633.

193. Baden E, Moskow BS, Moskow R. Odontogenic gingival epithelial hamartoma. *J Oral Surg* 1968;26:702–714.

194. Philipsen HP, Reichart PA. Unicystic ameloblastoma: a review of 193 cases from the literature. *Oral Oncol* 1998;34:317–325.

195. Rosenstein T, Pogrel MA, Smith RA, et al. Cystic ameloblastoma—behavior and treatment of 21 cases. *J Oral Maxillofac Surg* 2001;59:1311–1316.

196. Carlson ER. Chapter 30: odontogenic cysts and tumors. In Miloro M, ed. *Peterson's Principles of Oral and Maxillofacial Surgery.* Hamilton, British Columbia, Canada: Decker, 2004:575–596.

197. Philipsen HP, Reichart PA, Praetorius F. Mixed odontogenic tumors and odontomas: considerations on interrelationship. Review of the literature and presentation of 134 new cases of odontomas. *Oral Oncol* 1997;33:86–99.

198. Pindborg JJ. Calcifying epithelial odontogenic tumor. *Cancer* 1958;11:838–843.

199. Philipsen HP, Reichart PA. Calcifying epithelial odontogenic tumour: biological profile bases on 181 cases from the literature. *Oral Oncol* 2000;3:17–26.

200. Houston GD, Fowler CB. Extraosseous calcifying epithelial odontogenic tumor: report of two cases and review of the literature. *Oral Surg Oral Med Oral Pathol Oral Radiol Endod* 1997;83:577–583.

201. Courtney RM, Kerr DA. The odontogenic adenomatoid tumor. *Oral Surg Oral Med Oral Pathol* 1975;39:424–435.

202. Toida M, Hyodo I, Okuda T, et al. Adenomatoid odontogenic tumor: report of two cases and survey of 126 cases in Japan. *J Oral Maxillo Surg* 1990;48:404–408.

203. Philipsen HP, Reichart PA, Nikai H. The adenomatoid odontogenic tumour (AOT): an update. *Oral Med Pathol* 1998;2:55–60.

204. Pullon PA, Shafer WG, Elzay RP, et al. Squamous odontogenic tumor. Report of six cases of a previously undescribed lesion. *Oral Surg Oral Med Oral Pathol* 1975;40:616–630.

205. Baden E, Doyle J, Meso M, et al. Squamous odontogenic tumor. *Oral Surg Oral Med Oral Pathol* 1993;75:733–738.

206. Goldblatt LI, Brannon RB, Ellis GL. Squamous odontogenic tumor. *Oral Surg Oral Med Oral Pathol* 1982;54:187–195.

207. Dunlap CL. Odontogenic fibroma. *Semin Diagn Pathol* 1999;16:293–296.

208. Farman AG. The peripheral odontogenic fibroma. *Oral Surg Oral Med Oral Pathol* 1975;40:82–92.

209. Gardner DG. The central odontogenic fibroma: an attempt at clarification. *Oral Surg Oral Med Oral Pathol* 1980;50:425–532.

210. Kaffe I, Naor H, Buchner A. Clinical and radiological features of odontogenic myxoma of the jaws. *Dentomaxillofac Radiol* 1997;26:299–303.

211. Shimoyama T, Horie N, Kato T, et al. Soft tissue myxoma of the gingiva: report of a case and review of the literature of soft tissue myxoma in the oral region. *J Oral Sci* 2000;42:107–109.

212. Brannon RB, Fowler CB, Carpenter WM, et al. Cementoblastoma: an innocuous neoplasm? A clinicopathologic study of 44 cases and review of the literature with special emphasis on recurrence. *Oral Surg Oral Med Oral Pathol Oral Radiol Endod* 2002;93:311–320.

213. Corio RL, Goldblatt LI, Edwards PA, et al. Ameloblastic carcinoma: a clinicopathologic study and assessment of eight cases. *Oral Surg Oral Med Oral Pathol* 1987;64:570–576.

214. Slootweg PJ, Muller H. Malignant ameloblastoma or ameloblastic carcinoma. *Oral Surg Oral Med Oral Pathol* 1984;57:168–176.

215. Zarbo RJ, Marunick MT, Johns R. Malignant ameloblastoma, spindle cell variant. *Arch Pathol Lab Med* 2003;127:352–355.

216. Hansen LS, Eversole LP, Green TL, et al. Clear cell odontogenic tumor: a new histologic variant with aggressive potential. *Head Neck Surg* 1985;8:115–123.

217. Waldron CA, Small IA, Silverman H. Clear cell ameloblastoma: an odontogenic carcinoma. *J Oral Maxillofac Surg* 1985;43:707–717.

218. Mosqueda-Taylor A, Meneses-Garcia A, Ruiz-Godoy Rivera LM, et al. Clear cell odontogenic carcinoma of the mandible. *J Oral Pathol Med* 2002;31:439–441.

219. Lu Y, Xuan M, Takata T, et al. Odontogenic ghost cell carcinoma: report of four new cases and review of the literature. *J Oral Pathol Med* 1999;28:323–329.

220. Wood RW, Markle TL, Barker BF, et al. Ameloblastic fibrosarcoma. *Oral Surg Oral Med Oral Pathol* 1988;66:74–77.

221. Brannon RB, Fowler CB. Benign fibro-osseous lesions: a review of current concepts. *Adv Anat Pathol* 2001;8:126–142.

222. Hamner JE, Scofield HH, Coryn J. Benign fibro-osseous jaw lesions of periodontal membrane origin: an analysis of 249 cases. *Cancer* 1968;22:861–878.

223. Waldron CA. Fibro-osseous lesions of the jaws. *J Oral Maxillofac Surg* 1993;51:828–835.

224. Waldron CA, Giansante JD. Benign fibro-osseous lesions of the jaws: a clinical-radiologic-histologic review of sixty-five cases. II. Benign fibro-osseous lesions of periodontal membrane origin. *Oral Surg Oral Med Oral Pathol* 1973;35:340–350.

225. Carpten JD, Robbins CM, Villablanca A, et al. HRPT2, encoding parafibromin, is mutated in hyperparathyroidism-jaw tumor syndrome. *Nat Genet* 2002;32:676–680.

226. Hobbs MR, Pole AR, Pidwirny G, et al. Hyperparathyroidism-jaw tumor syndrome: the HRPT2 focus is within a 0.7 cM region on chromosome 1q. *Am J Hum Genet* 1999;64:518–525.

227. Szabo J, Heath B, Hill VM, et al. Hereditary hyperparathyroidism-jaw tumor syndrome: the endocrine tumor gene HRPT2 maps to chromosome 1q21-q31. *Am J Hum Genet* 1995;56:944–950.

228. Fechner RE. Problematic lesions of the craniofacial bones. *Am J Surg Pathol* 1989;13:17–30.

229. El Mofty S. Psammomatoid and trabecular juvenile ossifying fibroma of the craniofacial skeleton: two distinct clinicopathologic entities. *Oral Surg Oral Med Oral Pathol Oral Radiol Endod* 2002;93:296–304.

230. Johnson LC, Yousefi M, Vinh TN, et al. Juvenile active ossifying fibroma. Its nature, dynamics and origin. *Acta Otolaryngol* 1991;488:1–40.

231. Cohen MJ, Howell RE. Etiology of fibrous dysplasia and McCune-Albright syndrome. *Int J Oral Maxillofac Surg* 1999;28:366–371.

232. Young SK, Markowitz NR, Sullivan S, et al. Familial gigantiform cementoma: classification and presentation of a large pedigree. *Oral Surg Oral Med Oral Pathol Oral Radiol Endod* 1989;68:740–747.

233. Kaffe I, Ardekian L, Taicher S, et al. Radiologic features of central giant cell granuloma of the jaws. *Oral Surg Oral Med Oral Pathol Oral Radiol Endod* 1996;81:720–726.

234. Whitaker SB, Waldron CA. Central giant cell lesions of the jaws. A clinical, radiologic and histopathologic study. *Oral Surg Oral Med Oral Pathol Oral Radiol Endod* 1993;75:199–208.

CHAPTER 20

Stacey E. Mills

Salivary Glands

EMBRYOLOGY

Salivary glands are of ectodermal derivation and arise from the solid epithelial buds of the oral mucosa. Beginning in the fifth week, the parotid anlage appears, followed by the submandibular primordia in the sixth week and the sublingual primordia in the eighth. The salivary anlage has duct buds lined by ciliated cells and myoepithelial cells. The salivary units undergo elongation, branching, and differentiation into acinar cells and intercalated ducts. The production of saliva begins during the postnatal period under the stimulation of feeding. As the salivary glands mature, their connective tissue stroma progressively diminishes when compared to the glandular elements, and the myoepithelial cells decrease in number. Condensation of the surrounding mesenchyme, which leads to encapsulation, occurs earlier and is more complete in the submandibular and sublingual glands, as compared to the parotid gland. This allows for mixing of parotid buds and lymphoid tissue during embryonic development, giving rise to the frequent presence of intraparotid lymph nodes and, conversely, salivary gland inclusions within lymph nodes adjacent to the parotid gland (Fig. 20.1). As will be discussed later, this intimate association of lymphoid and salivary tissue accounts for the development of Warthin tumors, sebaceous lymphadenomas, and lymphoepithelial cysts virtually exclusively in the parotid and periparotid tissues.

HISTOLOGY

Both the major and minor salivary glands possess acinar and ductal systems. These glands may be of the serous, mucous, or mixed seromucous type. The parotid and the Ebner glands of the tongue are exclusively of the serous makeup (Fig. 20.2). The palatal salivary glands and those situated at the base and the lateral border of the tongue are predominantly of the mucinous type (Fig. 20.3). The submandibular and sublingual salivary glands have both serous and mucinous components (Fig. 20.4), with mucous cells being more prominent in the latter. Mixed salivary glands are also found among the minor salivary glands present in the lip, cheek, and the apex of the tongue, although most minor salivary glands are exclusively mucinous in type.

Saliva is formed by the acinar cells; it is high in amylase content when secreted by the serous glands, and it contains acidic and neutral sialomucin if it is formed by the mucinous acini. The serous acinar cells display intracytoplasmic periodic acid-Schiff (PAS)–positive secretory granules. Large basally located intercellular capillaries characterize these acinar cells. The mucinous acinar cells are arranged around an empty lumen, and they have a well-rounded, basally located nucleus. Myoepithelial cells surround the individual acini and contract during secretion.

The intricate duct system is composed of intercalated, striated, and interlobular ducts. The intercalated duct is quite

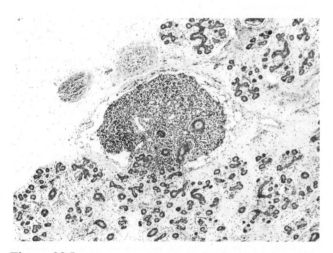

Figure 20.1. This fetal parotid gland shows lack of encapsulation and the close association of developing lymphoid tissue with salivary acini.

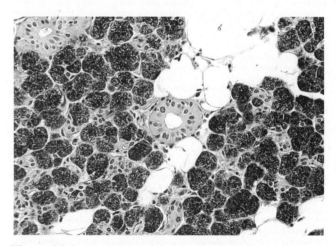

Figure 20.2. Normal parotid composed exclusively of serous acini.

This is a revision of the salivary gland chapter authored by Dr. Andrew Huvos and colleagues since the inception of *Diagnostic Surgical Pathology*. The editor assumed responsibility for this chapter following Dr. Huvos' death. It is an honor to update his work.

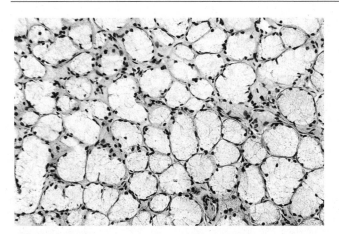

Figure 20.3. Mucous glands making up minor salivary gland tissue.

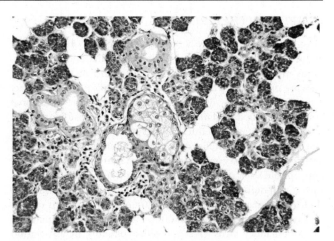

Figure 20.5. A nest of cells with sebaceous metaplasia appears to bud from a salivary gland duct.

short, and it is lined by a single layer of cuboidal epithelial cells that are backed by myoepithelial cells on the outside. The striated ducts are lined by a columnar epithelium featuring a luminal brush border. The most important function of these ducts is active saliva secretion. The interlobular ducts form the terminal portion of the duct system. Depending on the circumference of these ducts, multiple stratified layers of epithelial cells are present. Elastic and collagen fibers surround the periphery, facilitating the active transport of the saliva through the system.

Scattered sebaceous cells arising from intercalated and striated ducts are a normal occurrence in the parotid gland (Fig. 20.5). Oncocytic metaplasia in salivary glands is a common finding with advancing age.

Heterotopic salivary gland tissue has been identified in a wide variety of anatomic sites, including the following: the external and middle ear, the mastoid region, the thyroglossal duct, the thyroid capsule, and even the parathyroid glands. By far, cervical (periparotid) lymph nodes are the most common sites for the benign salivary gland inclusions. The embryologic basis for this is discussed earlier. Intramandibular salivary gland tissue may appear on the lingual surface of the bone within surface

indentations, most often situated in the angle of the mandible. These heterotopic salivary rests explain the rare occurrence of salivary tumors arising within the mandibular bone.

NONNEOPLASTIC PROCESSES

MUCOCELE

Mucoceles (mucous retention and extravasation cysts) arising from the minor salivary glands are common. Favored sites in the submucosa of the oral cavity are the lower lip, the cheeks, the dorsal surface of the tip of the tongue, and the floor of the mouth. In superficial locations, the cyst is well circumscribed, blue-white, and feels like a tiny nodule. Large nodules are distinctly unusual. Viscous fluid erupts if the cyst spontaneously ruptures. Without proper evacuation, repeated rupture and reformation are often the case.

Microscopically, the cyst wall is made up of compressed connective tissue with a denuded epithelial lining and granulation tissue. Chronic inflammatory cells usually infiltrate the surrounding connective tissue. The minor salivary glands in close proximity to the cystic space are also affected by this inflammatory reaction, and the salivary ductules in this location are often ectatic. An incomplete, stratified squamous epithelial lining is rarely observed within the cyst.

RANULA

A ranula is a collection of extravasated mucin from the sublingual glands that presents as a cyst of the floor of the mouth (1). The term is derived from the Latin word for little frog (*rana*) and is based on its likeness to the throat pouch of frogs. A ranula may be extraoral (also called a cervical or plunging ranula), and it may even extend to the supraclavicular area, upper mediastinum, or skull base (2).

The exact etiology of these mucous cysts is not clearly established. Inflammation, trauma, and mechanical obstruction have all been invoked in the pathogenesis of mucous cysts.

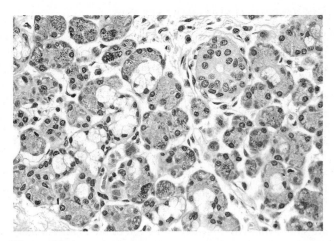

Figure 20.4. Normal submandibular gland composed of serous and mucous components.

LYMPHOEPITHELIAL CYST

Most lymphoepithelial cysts occur in the region of the parotid gland where they appear to arise from cystic dilatation and squamous metaplasia of intranodal salivary gland inclusions. The cysts are usually lined by flattened to stratified squamous epithelium, surrounded by lymphoid stroma (Fig. 20.6). Occasional cysts may be lined by glandular epithelium. The resultant microscopic image may be identical to that of a second branchial cleft cyst, and lymphoepithelial cysts are often misdiagnosed as such. True cysts of the second branchial cleft must be located in the appropriate area of the lateral neck and are often associated with a well-defined sinus tract. In our experience, lymphoepithelial cysts are far more common than branchial cleft cysts.

Lymphoepithelial cysts are often encountered in human immunodeficiency virus (HIV)–positive patients in association with the striking lymphoid hyperplasia seen early in the course of that disease. The term *cystic lymphoid hyperplasia* has been applied to this condition. Typically, these patients have a single cyst or multiple cysts lined by a flattened epithelium and surrounded by a prominent lymphoid infiltrate with germinal centers. The pathogenesis of cystic lymphoid hyperplasia remains unresolved (3). Cyst formation may be caused by obstruction of the ducts by the lymphoid infiltrate (4).

SCLEROSING POLYCYSTIC ADENOSIS

Sclerosing polycystic adenosis is a recently described, mass-forming lesion with a striking predilection for the parotid gland (5,6). Grossly, there is a mass several centimeters in diameter with a sclerotic, variably cystic appearance. Microscopically, there is a mixture of cystic, sclerotic stroma with entrapped glands and inflammatory changes. Apocrine metaplasia is a common finding, as are areas of complex ductal hyperplasia reminiscent of mammary ductal hyperplasia. Intraductal necrosis may be present, and areas of epithelial atypia are commonly seen. The exact nature of this process remains unclear, but one recent study showed clonality in six cases, suggesting that this may represent a neoplastic process (7).

MISCELLANEOUS CYSTS

The rarely observed submandibular salivary gland cyst is often lined by flattened epithelium. Parotid duct cysts occur mostly

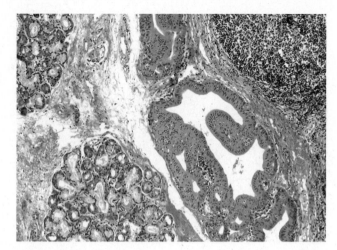

Figure 20.7. This small oncocytic cyst was an incidental finding in a submandibular gland resected as part of a radical neck dissection.

in elderly men. They vary from 1 to 3 cm in size, and they are unilocular. Histologically, they closely resemble the mucous cysts of minor salivary glands (8). The lining of salivary duct cysts can exhibit epithelial proliferation and various types of metaplasia (goblet cell, clear cell, squamous cell, and oncocytic) (Fig. 20.7), or rarely, they can even give rise to a malignancy. The lumen may contain calcospherites or crystalline deposits in addition to retained mucus.

ONCOCYTOSIS/DIFFUSE ONCOCYTIC HYPERPLASIA

Rarely, diffuse oncocytosis may affect the parotid gland with complete oncocytic transformation of the ductal and acinar epithelium. It is always unilateral and occurs almost exclusively in the elderly. Nodular adenomatous (oncocytic) hyperplasia diffusely involves the salivary ducts. The multifocal nodular oncocytic foci may measure up to 1 cm in diameter, and they have a solid trabecular growth pattern. These nodular hyperplastic areas may, on occasion, progress into an oncocytoma.

NECROTIZING SIALOMETAPLASIA

Necrotizing sialometaplasia is an infarctive, inflammatory, metaplastic process that can occur wherever there are seromucinous glands. Typically, there is vascular compromise leading to necrosis of ducts and glandular acini with secondary inflammatory changes and eventual repopulation of the acini by metaplastic squamous epithelium. Often there is a history of prior surgery or trauma. As a spontaneous process, necrotizing sialometaplasia most commonly involves the palatal minor salivary glands. The blood vessels supplying this region are not large and are subject to trauma as a result of compression against the hard palate during mastication. In this location, it is generally encountered in white men with a mean age of 46 years (9).

Regardless of location or causation, the microscopic features are stereotypical and related to the age of the lesion. Initially, there is infarction of seromucinous glands with extravasation of luminal contents and a surrounding acute and chronic in-

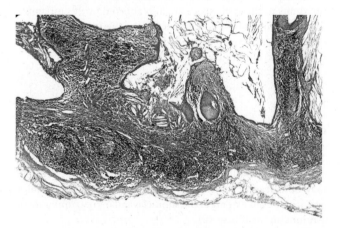

Figure 20.6. A lymphoepithelial cyst composed of keratinizing squamous epithelium with a prominent lymphoid stroma. Centrally, a small cyst rupture has produced cholesterol clefts.

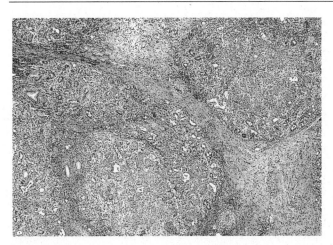

Figure 20.8. Necrotizing sialometaplasia showing preservation of lobular architecture.

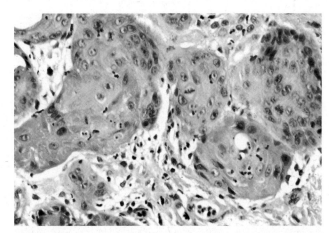

Figure 20.10. At higher magnification, the nests of squamous cells in necrotizing sialometaplasia can exhibit worrisome pleomorphism and mitotic activity.

flammatory reaction (Fig. 20.8). Within a few days, the necrotic acini become filled with metaplastic squamous cells (Fig. 20.9) that may show prominent mitotic activity and mild cytologic atypia (Fig. 20.10). The squamous cells often coexist with residual noninfarcted mucous cells, creating a pattern that may be confused with mucoepidermoid carcinoma. Because necrotizing sialometaplasia is a process superimposed on pre-existent normal salivary acini, it retains a lobular pattern at low magnification. Mucoepidermoid carcinoma, in contrast, does not have a lobular pattern, tends to be infiltrative, is usually not inflamed, and is composed of varying combinations of basal, intermediate, clear, squamous, mucous, and oncocytic cells.

RADIATION-RELATED CHANGE

Salivary glands, particularly their serous acini, are relatively sensitive to radiation therapy, accounting for the dry mouth frequently encountered after radiation to the head and neck. Submandibular glands included in radical neck dissections will often show marked atrophy with variable degrees of chronic inflammation if there has been a protracted interval (several months) between radiation therapy and resection. More

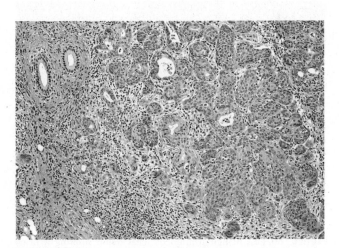

Figure 20.9. Necrotizing sialometaplasia exhibiting squamous metaplasia with prominent inflammatory infiltrate.

acutely, radiation-related changes are ischemic in nature and identical to the changes of necrotizing sialometaplasia described earlier, with the additional imposition of radiation-related atypia. The latter consists of cells with enlarged, often densely hyperchromatic, "smudged" nuclei and similarly increased amounts of cytoplasm such that the nuclear-to-cytoplasmic ratio remains nearly normal. As with other causes of necrotizing sialometaplasia, confusion with mucoepidermoid carcinoma or even squamous cell carcinoma is possible, particularly on frozen sections, and the superimposed radiation atypia may add to this confusion. Attention to the low magnification pattern with maintenance of the lobular architecture, inflammation, and lack of other cell types (e.g., basal, intermediate, oncocytic) will allow distinction.

ACUTE SIALADENITIS

Salivary gland tissue is relatively resistant to bacterial infection, although acute suppurative sialadenitis may occasionally be encountered, often secondary to a variety of predisposing conditions including trauma, immunosuppression, and duct obstruction caused by sialolithiasis. Responsible agents are usually staphylococcal or streptococcal species, although Gram-negative organisms may also be involved.

Historically, viral sialadenitis has most commonly been caused by mumps virus, although coxsackie species, enteric cytopathic human orphan (ECHO) viruses, Epstein-Barr virus (EBV), and cytomegalovirus, among others, have also been encountered. With the advent of vaccination, mumps parotiditis has become rare in much of the world. Although seldom biopsied, even when more common, the microscopic changes of mumps parotiditis have been described as interstitial edema with dense lymphoplasmacytic infiltrate, swelling and vacuolization of acinar cells, and dilation of ductal lumina as a result of accumulation of secretions and desquamated lining cells (10).

CHRONIC SIALADENITIS

Lymphocytic infiltration of a salivary gland as an isolated finding unassociated with Sjögren syndrome or other autoimmune disease is most likely a result of chronic duct obstruction secondary

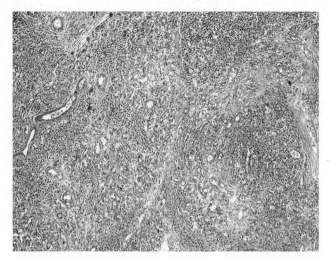

Figure 20.11. Low-power view of chronic sclerosing sialadenitis (Kuttner tumor) shows inflammatory cells and periductal fibrosis.

to sialolithiasis. Over time, there is progressive glandular atrophy with varying degrees of fibrosis and chronic inflammation. The latter is much less intense than in autoimmune-related conditions.

A specific variant of chronic sialadenitis, termed *chronic sclerosing sialadenitis* or Kuttner tumor, deserves mention (11). This process almost exclusively involves the submandibular gland and usually produces a palpable mass clinically mimicking a neoplasm. Microscopically, the lobular architecture is usually preserved, but a lymphoplasmacytic infiltrate surrounds the ducts with accompanying periductal fibrosis (Figs. 20.11 and 20.12) (12). As the process progresses, the salivary acini proximal to the duct obstruction become atrophic. Reactive lymphoid follicles may be present. The overall appearance is similar to that of sclerosing autoimmune pancreatitis, and this process now appears to be a member of the growing family of immunoglobulin (Ig) G4–related sclerosing diseases (12). Immunohistochemistry documents a predominance of T cells (except in germinal centers) with prominent IgG4-positive

plasma cells. A mucosa-associated lymphoma tissue (MALT)–type lymphoma has been reported in the setting of chronic sclerosing sialadenitis (13).

GRANULOMATOUS SIALADENITIS

Virtually any granuloma-producing process can affect the salivary glands. In addition, involvement of intraparotid lymph nodes by a granulomatous process will be clinically indistinguishable from disease of the parotid parenchyma. Sarcoidosis is commonly encountered in these locations, and infections with fungi or mycobacteria are occasionally seen. Cat scratch disease frequently involves the neck region and may produce necrotizing granulomatous inflammation in intraparotid lymph nodes. Approximately 2% to 3% of patients with cat scratch disease will present with parotid gland swelling and pain (14).

SJÖGREN SYNDROME

The San Diego diagnostic criteria for primary Sjögren syndrome are as follows: keratoconjunctivitis sicca, xerostomia, extensive lymphocytic infiltrate on minor salivary gland biopsy, and laboratory evidence of a systemic autoimmune disorder (15). Specific exclusions are pre-existing lymphoma, graft-versus-host disease, acquired immunodeficiency syndrome (AIDS), and sarcoidosis. The patients may develop primary biliary cirrhosis, sclerosing cholangitis, pancreatitis, interstitial nephritis, interstitial lymphocytic pneumonitis, and peripheral vasculitis.

Microscopic examination of the enlarged salivary glands, both major and minor, may reveal a lymphoepithelial sialadenitis, also known as *benign lymphoepithelial lesion* (BLL). This is characterized by heavy infiltration of the ductal epithelium by lymphocytes of marginal zone or monocytoid B-cell type. The result is the formation of cellular aggregates commonly known as epimyoepithelial islands (Fig. 20.13), although the myoepithelial component of these predominantly epithelial structures may be sparse or absent by immunohistochemistry. BLL must be distinguished from lymphoepithelioma-like undifferentiated carcinoma of the salivary gland, also referred to somewhat am-

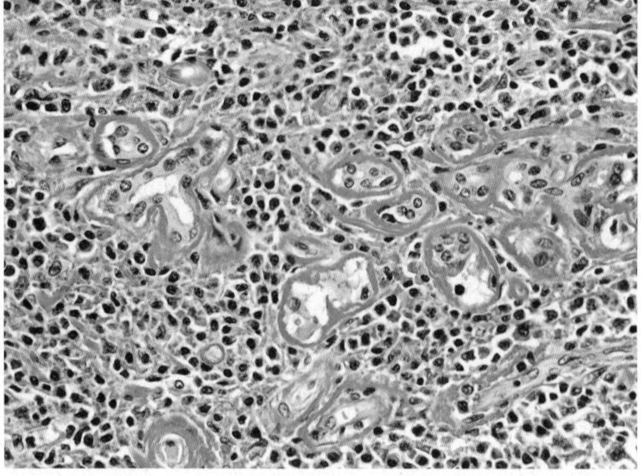

Figure 20.12. At higher magnification, the periductal fibrosis in chronic sclerosing sialadenitis is prominent, and the inflammatory infiltrate can be seen to be predominantly plasmacytic.

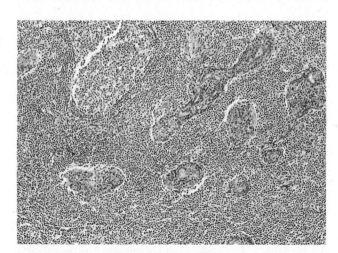

Figure 20.13. Benign lymphoepithelial lesion showing a heavy lymphocytic infiltration with a germinal center and epimyoepithelial islands.

biguously as a *malignant lymphoepithelial lesion*. This entity and its distinction from BLL are discussed in more detail later under the section on malignant salivary gland neoplasms.

B-cell clones are detected in more than 50% of BLL, but they do not correlate with morphologic or clinical evidence of lymphoma (16). Patients with BLL have a 44-fold increased risk of developing salivary gland or extrasalivary lymphoma, of which 80% are the marginal zone and/or MALT type (3). Salivary gland lymphomas are discussed later.

For a minor salivary gland biopsy specimen to be diagnostic of Sjögren syndrome, it should contain at least four lobules with at least two foci of lymphocytes per 4 mm^2; a focus is defined as a cluster of 50 or more lymphocytes (17). The labial salivary gland biopsy has a sensitivity of 70% to 83%, and it is most useful in patients with partial San Diego criteria, not in patients in whom the index of suspicion is low (18).

The terms *Mikulicz disease* and *Mikulicz syndrome* have been used in the past for salivary or lacrimal gland swellings resulting from Sjögren syndrome and various other conditions. These terms and designations are so obscure and ambiguous that they should not be used (19).

GENERAL COMMENTS ON SALIVARY NEOPLASIA

Salivary gland neoplasms occur frequently enough that even pathologists in small practices can expect to encounter them from time to time. Yet, they are infrequent enough that pathologists in large, high-volume medical centers often feel uncomfortable diagnosing them. This discomfort is compounded by the fact that a broad spectrum of tumors arises in this location, there is considerable morphologic overlap between some subtypes, and a substantial minority of tumors do not fit easily into existing diagnostic categories.

Fine-needle aspiration is a useful adjunct for presumptively or, in many instances, definitively diagnosing salivary gland neoplasms. Definitively diagnosing a salivary gland tumor on frozen section may vary from extremely easy to impossible. Experienced ear, nose, and throat (ENT) surgeons are aware of this difficulty, and most use frozen sections only to assess margin status and not to provide a definitive diagnosis. Even when a definitive diagnosis cannot be made on frozen section, some assessment can be provided about the nature of the lesion based on standard histologic features such as the cellularity, pleomorphism, and nature of the margin (encapsulated, pushing, or diffusely invasive). Thus, it should be perfectly acceptable, if frozen section interpretation is requested, to render diagnoses such as "low-grade neoplasm, adenoma versus low-grade carcinoma" or "high-grade carcinoma, await permanents for definitive classification."

BENIGN EPITHELIAL NEOPLASMS

MIXED TUMOR ("PLEOMORPHIC ADENOMA")

Although the terms *benign mixed tumor* or simply *mixed tumor* are the preferred designations for this entity, the unfortunate designation of *pleomorphic adenoma* is entrenched in the pathology literature as a classic example of nosologic imprecision. "Pleomorphic" is used by pathologists to indicate nuclear vari-

ability, a feature not commonly encountered in this neoplasm. The more appropriate designation would have been *polymorphic adenoma* to correctly identify the variable cell types seen in these lesions.

Mixed tumors typically present as a painless, persistent swelling, and they can occur at any age. They are most common in adults during the third through fifth decades of life, but they may be found during childhood. Rare bilateral synchronous or metachronous and even familial mixed tumors have been reported (20). Approximately 75% of mixed tumors arise in the parotid gland. The rest occur in the submandibular gland (approximately 5% to 10%) and the minor salivary glands (approximately 10%). The most common minor salivary gland sites are the palate (approximately 60% to 65%), cheek (15%), tongue, and floor of mouth (approximately 10%). Occasionally, mixed tumors arise in intraparotid or periparotid lymph nodes or in the heterotopic salivary gland tissues (21). Approximately 70% of all tumors in the parotid gland are mixed tumors. This compares with 50% of the submandibular salivary gland tumors and 45% of the minor salivary gland tumors. The vast majority (>90%) of mixed tumors arise in the superficial portion of the parotid gland, whereas the rest present in the deep lobe occupying the parapharyngeal space. These tumors of the deep lobe result in oropharyngeal swelling that is often misdiagnosed as unrelated to the parotid gland, and the patients are subjected to intraoral biopsy. It should be noted that tumors histologically similar or identical to salivary gland mixed tumors may occasionally arise from closely related glands of the breast, skin (chondroid syringoma), or ceruminal glands of the external ear.

On gross examination, the lesional tissue is made up of nodules connected by a delicate network of fibrous connective tissue (Figs. 20.14 and 20.15). Multicentric tumor at the time of initial surgery is virtually nonexistent, but conversely, improperly resected tumor will often recur as multicentric nodules, a pattern referred to as *satellitosis*. This multifocal recurrence is a result of improper initial resection of the tumor by a "shelling out" procedure that leaves tiny pseudopod-like transcapsular processes of the tumor in the adjacent salivary gland. Such recurrences may be quite difficult to eradicate and can be avoided by performing a superficial parotidectomy or, if necessary for large or deep lesions, a more complete resection. After proper resection, the recurrence rate is low (≤2%) (22,23).

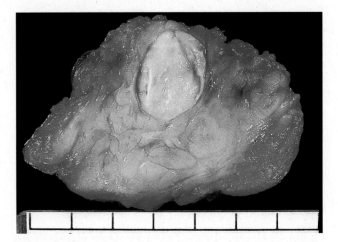

Figure 20.14. Mixed tumor of the parotid gland. The tumor is encapsulated with a smooth, shiny cut surface.

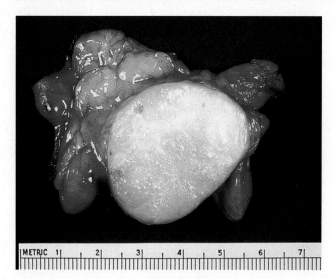

Figure 20.15. A well-circumscribed mixed tumor from the submandibular gland. The cut surface is traversed by delicate fibrous septa.

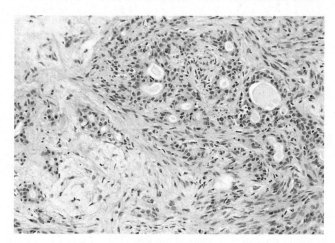

Figure 20.17. Cord-like tubular structures in a mixed tumor with only minimal stroma present.

Grossly, mixed tumors appear sharply demarcated or encapsulated. The appearance of their cut surface varies tremendously depending on the epithelial and stromal elements present. Areas of chondroid differentiation are often easily visible and allow virtual diagnosis on gross examination. Small cysts may be present grossly, and some may appear hemorrhagic.

Microscopic examination confirms the capsule seen grossly, but as noted earlier, fingerlike projections of tumor can often be found extending through the capsule for a short distance into the surrounding stroma. The presence and extent of these pseudopods of extracapsular growth do not correlate with recurrence rate, provided that proper resection technique is used.

The complex and highly variable histologic patterns seen in mixed tumors are a result of the interplay of the epithelial and stromal elements (Fig. 20.16) (24). The epithelial components may form trabeculae, tubules, ductules, nonkeratinizing squamous cell aggregates, keratinizing squamous cysts, mucous cysts, aggregates of plasmacytoid or spindled myoepithelial cells, scat-

tered sebaceous cells, or sheets of nondescript epithelium. Some ductal structures may display hyperplastic epithelial linings with cribriforming. The ductules typically include both epithelial and myoepithelial components (Fig. 20.17) (25,26).

The stromal elements are nearly as variable as the epithelial and may include mucoid, myxoid, fibroblastic, cartilaginous, osseous, and lipogenic elements. The osseous component may be replete with hematopoietic bone marrow. It has been postulated that mixed tumor is a fundamentally epithelial (or myoepithelial) neoplasm with a propensity for multifocal stromal metaplasia. Often, the epithelial and stromal components are so delicately intertwined that their separation from each other is not feasible. Ultrastructural studies of this blurred epithelial-stromal junction have shown "transitional cells" with both epithelial and mesenchymal properties in this region, with modulation to more definite epithelial or stromal elements at respective edges of the junction. The amount of epithelium versus stroma varies tremendously from lesion to lesion. Some mixed tumors are predominantly stromal and often highly cartilaginous. Others are so lacking in stromal elements as to border on the appearance of a monomorphic adenoma. Often, when epithelial elements are predominant, particularly when they assume a nearly sheetlike pattern, the lesion may display high cellularity that leads to concern for malignancy (cellular mixed tumor) (Fig. 20.18). Areas of squamous metaplasia combined with mucinous differentiation may cause the unwary to classify the lesion as a mucoepidermoid carcinoma.

Cytogenetic and molecular studies in mixed tumors have repeatedly shown chromosomal abnormalities involving the long arm of chromosomes of 8 and 12 (27). Translocations in these regions probably promote tumor development or progression through the activation of proto-oncogenes. Loss of heterozygosity has been implicated as an early event in the development of mixed tumor (28).

WARTHIN TUMOR

Warthin tumor, or papillary cystadenoma lymphomatosum, represents 15% of epithelial salivary gland tumors. It is almost exclusively a tumor of the parotid gland and periparotid lymph nodes. Rare reports in the submandibular gland may represent

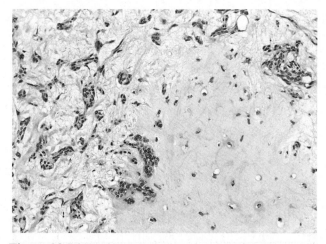

Figure 20.16. Mixed tumor. An intimate mixture of epithelial and stromal elements is seen in this mixed tumor. The stroma exhibits cartilaginous differentiation.

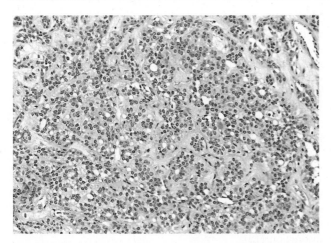

Figure 20.18. Cellular mixed tumor. Because of its extreme cellularity, this tumor may be mistaken for a malignant tumor.

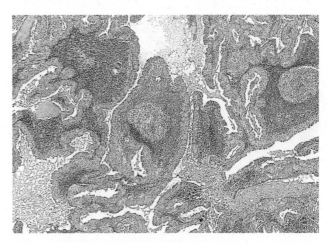

Figure 20.19. Warthin tumor with a partly cystic appearance. It is lined by oncocytic cells and a lymphoid stroma.

origin in the closely adjacent tail of the parotid gland. Cases reported in unusual locations such as the larynx invariably represent oncocytic cysts with a smattering of chronic inflammation. The reason for the sharp localization to the parotid and periparotid lymph nodes relates to the unique admixture of salivary and lymphoid elements in this region during embryologic development (see earlier "Embryology" section).

Studies suggest a strong association of Warthin tumor with smoking (29,30). This tumor more commonly affects men in their sixth and seventh decades of life, but the incidence in females is increasing, probably because of the increase in smoking in women (31). Bilateral or multifocal tumor involvement is observed in approximately 10% of patients (32). However, because bilateral involvement is so uncommon in salivary neoplasia, Warthin tumor is by far the most common bilateral tumor in this location.

The typical Warthin tumor is well delineated and, on average, is 2 cm in greatest dimension. The cut surface is frequently cystic, with cyst contents that may be mucinous, proteinaceous, or even resemble used (dark) motor oil. Because of the cystic aspects and the occasional presence of friable amorphous material in the central or cystic regions, a branchial cleft cyst or even caseating tuberculous lymphadenitis may be part of the differential diagnosis. Some of the lesions are tiny and are incidental histologic findings at parotid resections for unrelated reasons.

The histologic appearance of Warthin tumor is one of the most distinctive images in all of surgical pathology. An oncocytic epithelial component and a prominent lymphoid stroma with well-developed follicles (Fig. 20.19) blend together in this tumor. The oncocytic epithelial elements have (by definition) strikingly eosinophilic granular cytoplasm as a result of large numbers of mitochondria. This component consists of two or occasionally multiple layers of cells, which often form papillary projections into the cystic lumina (Fig. 20.20). The cystic spaces may contain cast-off epithelial cells, inflammatory cells, crystalline structures, or corpora amylacea. Apocrine or squamous metaplasia of the luminal epithelium may also be present focally. The latter is often associated with areas of infarction and, if prominent, may lead to confusion with squamous or mucoepidermoid carcinoma.

The lymphoid stroma closely resembles a normal lymph

node, and it is composed of T and B cells with occasional germinal centers. Immunohistochemical characterization of Ig reveals that approximately 50% of the B lymphocytes contain IgG, with roughly 33% containing IgA. The lymphoid stroma can serve as a metastatic site for carcinoma or melanoma, or it may give rise to malignant lymphomas. Carcinomas can, on rare occasion, develop in the epithelium of a Warthin tumor. Among these, adenocarcinomas, squamous carcinomas, and undifferentiated carcinomas have been reported (33).

Cytogenetic studies on a small series of cases revealed 6p rearrangements and t(11;19) as being specific for Warthin tumor (34).

BASAL CELL ADENOMA

Approximately 70% of basal cell adenomas occur in the parotid gland, with the remainder arising in the submandibular gland and a variety of sites in the oral cavity, including the upper lip. Although the age range is broad, most patients are in their sixth decade of life or older. Grossly, these are sharply circumscribed, encapsulated masses that resemble hyperplastic lymph nodes. The exception is the uncommon membranous variant, which

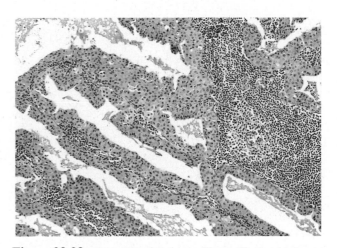

Figure 20.20. Typical Warthin tumor. The papillary projection exhibits oncocytic lining cells and an underlying lymphoid stroma.

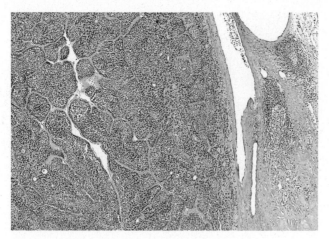

Figure 20.21. Basal cell adenoma showing encapsulation and closely packed tumor nests.

closely resembles and may be associated with a nearby dermal eccrine cylindroma. These membranous tumors are often multinodular in the parotid and lack well-formed capsules.

Microscopically, uniform basal cells form, in order of decreasing frequency, solid, trabecular, tubular, or membranous structures (Fig. 20.21). With the exception of approximately half of the membranous subtype lesions, a distinct capsule should be present and is important for distinguishing this entity from basal cell adenocarcinoma and adenoid cystic carcinoma (see "Basal Cell Adenocarcinoma" and "Adenoid Cystic Carcinoma" sections later in this chapter). The tumor cells are clearly separated from the nonmucoid stroma by a well-defined basement membrane (Fig. 20.22). Peripheral cell palisading is characteristic and is best seen in the larger nests of the solid pattern. The cells within the more central portions of the solid nests often have more cytoplasm and show varying degrees of squamoid differentiation ranging from only slightly more prominent eosinophilic cytoplasm to overt keratin pearl formation. The trabecular pattern is often mixed with the solid pattern. It can be thought of as elongated solid nests that vary in size down to thin structures only two cells in thickness. The tubular pattern consists of the trabecular pattern with superimposed ductlike lumina. In many instances,

the cells are haphazardly arranged around the openings such that they appear to represent extracellular spaces rather than true glandular lumina. In other foci, however, a distinctly glandlike cell orientation is present. The membranous pattern consists of nests similar to those of the solid pattern but with interposed hyaline stroma within, around, and between the nests of basaloid cells. The multinodular pattern seen grossly in approximately half of these cases will be reflected microscopically as multiple, nonencapsulated nodules (35–37).

Immunohistochemically, the tumor cells are reactive for carcinoembryonic antigen (CEA), epithelial membrane antigen (EMA), cytokeratin, and, focally, S-100 protein (38). Two recent markers noted to be positive in adenoid cystic carcinomas, KIT and CD43, may also be seen in basal cell adenomas (and basal cell adenocarcinomas), rendering them of little value in this distinction (12).

CANALICULAR ADENOMA

Canalicular adenoma is closely related to basal cell adenoma, and cases with hybrid microscopic features are occasionally encountered. Indeed, the distinction has often been confused in the literature. Although lumping the two together under such terms as *basal cell adenoma* or even *monomorphic adenoma* will cause no harm to the patient, there are sufficient clinicopathologic differences to warrant pathologic distinction. Canalicular adenoma is a tumor of adults that approximately three-fourths of the time occurs in the seromucinous glands of the upper lip (35). Grossly, there may be a single encapsulated nodule, a well-demarcated but unencapsulated nodule, or a distinctly multinodular growth pattern. Microscopically, the tumor displays elongated tubules or ducts lined by small cuboidal to columnar cells with scant to moderate amounts of eosinophilic cytoplasm, a morphologic spectrum that clearly encompasses basaloid cells. Scattered mucous or oncocytic cells may be present (35). Papillary structures and psammoma bodies have also been described. The cords of cells form intermittent expansions with "canal-like" lumina that create a beaded pattern (Fig. 20.23). The stroma typically has a loose myxoid quality with prominent vascularity. Canalicular adenomas are positive for cytokeratin and S-100 protein and, focally, for glial fibrillary acidic protein (GFAP) (39).

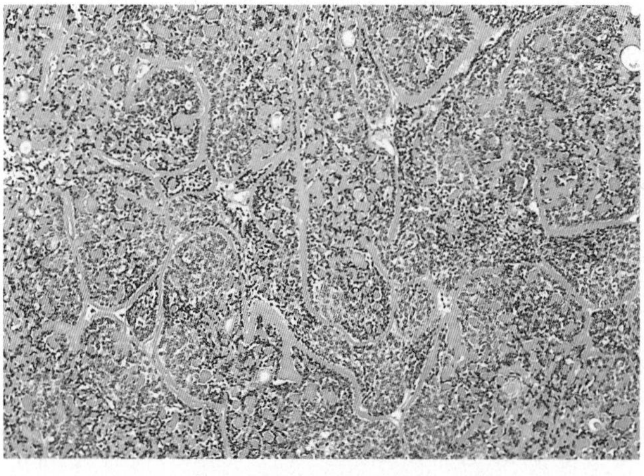

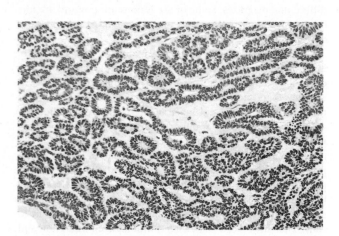

Figure 20.23. Canalicular adenoma arising in the upper lip, the most common location of occurrence. The budding ductular elements appear in a canalicular configuration.

Figure 20.22. Basal cell adenoma with basement membrane material separating tumor nests.

ONCOCYTOMA

Oncocytic cells are recognized components of a wide variety of salivary gland neoplasms including Warthin tumor, mucoepidermoid carcinoma, acinic cell carcinoma, mixed tumor, and multiple other benign and malignant processes. It is doubtful that any salivary gland neoplasm is completely free of their presence as a scattered component. They are also frequent in nonneoplastic conditions including incidental foci of oncocytic metaplasia and oncocytic cysts of the seromucinous glands, particularly in the false vocal cords.

Benign tumors composed entirely of oncocytes (oncocytomas) account for approximately 1% of all salivary gland neoplasms (40). Most involve the parotid, followed by the submandibular gland and minor salivary glands from the lower lip, palate, pharynx, and oral mucosa. In addition, approximately 5% arise in salivary rests in periparotid lymph nodes (40). Oncocytomas occur in middle-aged and older adults, with a mean age of 58 years. Approximately 20% of all patients have a history of radiation therapy to the face or upper torso or long-term occupational radiation exposure that occurred 5 or more years before tumor discovery (40). Patients with previous radiation exposure are, on average, 20 years younger at tumor discovery than are those without a documented history. The exact nature of oncocytomas with regard to the neoplastic role of nuclear versus mitochondrial DNA is a fascinating but unresolved topic.

On gross examination, oncocytomas are usually 3 to 4 cm in size, possess a well-defined capsule, and have a light brown to mahogany color. Larger lesions may show a lobular or mutinodular pattern (Fig. 20.24). Microscopically, the oncocytic cells are arranged in a solid (Fig. 20.25) or trabecular pattern. Microcyst formation is rarely observed. By definition, oncocytes have ample, distinctly granular acidophilic cytoplasm that ultrastructurally corresponds to large numbers of cytoplasmic mitochondria to the virtual exclusion of other organelles. The nuclei are small and pyknotic. Rarely, oncocytomas present with large polyhedral clear cells in an organoid distribution, separated by a thin fibrovascular stroma. Occasional clear cells may be encountered in oncocytomas, and tumors with a predominantly clear-cell component are referred to by the apparent oxymoron of *clear-cell oncocytoma*. The optically clear-cell appearance is a

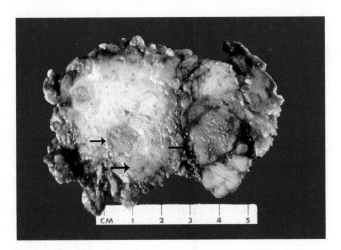

Figure 20.24. Oncocytoma of the parotid gland has a distinctly multinodular growth pattern. Each nodule has a brown to mahogany color.

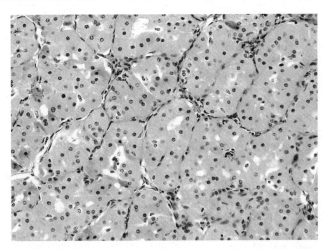

Figure 20.25. Oncocytoma of the parotid with a solid growth pattern.

result of fixation artifact or intracytoplasmic glycogen, in addition to the numerous mitochondria (41,42).

Histochemical studies demonstrate phosphotungstic acid hematoxylin (PTAH)–positive cytoplasmic staining. PAS staining before and after diastase digestion demonstrates granular cytoplasmic positivity that represents the numerous, tightly packed mitochondria. Antimitochondrial antibodies will show strong positivity in oncocytomas, but this stain is seldom needed for diagnosis. By electron microscopy, the mitochondria have elongated cristae and a partial lamellar internal structure (43). The nuclei of the oncocytes are irregular, and they contain inclusions and glycogen granules.

The clear-cut separation of oncocytic adenomatous (nodular) hyperplasia of the parotid gland from a multinodular oncocytoma (a true neoplasm) is not always possible because the two entities overlap histologically (44–46). The multinodular feature may impart an undeserved sinister, malignant appearance to the lesion. In our experience, these nodules are separated by normal salivary gland, whereas the rare oncocytic carcinoma has multinodularity with intervening fibrotic or desmoplastic stroma (see "Oncocytic Carcinoma" section later in this chapter).

Oncocytomas only rarely recur, and when they do, recurrences are often multiple and bilateral, suggesting that they, in reality, represent new lesions arising in multifocal nodular oncocytic hyperplasia. The differential diagnosis of oncocytoma includes the extremely rare oncocytic carcinoma discussed later and a wide variety of salivary gland lesions that can have at least a minor oncocytic component. In our experience, acinic cell carcinomas and mucoepidermoid carcinomas with prominent oncocytes, also discussed later, present the greatest diagnostic challenges. In both cases, careful search for other diagnostic cell types will allow distinction. With the exception of focal clear-cell change, oncocytomas should have a monomorphous appearance.

MYOEPITHELIOMA

Cells with myoepithelial differentiation figure prominently in a wide variety of salivary gland neoplasms, and immunohistochemical markers for this differentiation (e.g., p63, smooth muscle actin, calponin, CD10, etc.) can be valuable in differentiating tumors with myoepithelial cells from those without. Although recognition of myoepithelial *differentiation* has significant diagnostic practicality, this feature tells us nothing about the *origin* of the neoplastic cells, and complex lineage charts for salivary neoplasms based on the flawed assumption that differentiation equates with origin are of no practical value.

Benign salivary gland tumors composed entirely of myoepithelial cells (i.e., myoepitheliomas) are rare encapsulated or sharply demarcated neoplasms. Approximately 50% of such lesions involve the parotid gland, 40% arise in minor salivary glands, and a few affect the submandibular salivary gland (47–50). The vast majority of the intraoral minor salivary gland lesions are of palatal origin. The incidence in males and females is equal. The lesions present as asymptomatic, slowly growing masses in patients who have an average age of 40 years (age range, 6 to 81 years).

Several distinct cell types are encountered in these tumors, including spindle cells, plasmacytoid (hyaline) cells, and, possibly, clear cells. Each is associated with a different group of differential diagnoses. Mixtures of cell types in a single tumor are common. The spindle cell tumors usually exhibit cellular growth with little or no ground substance (Fig. 20.26). The neoplastic cells form storiform, swirling, herringbone, or fascicular patterns. The differential diagnosis accordingly includes benign fibrous histiocytoma, leiomyoma, benign fibroblastic lesions, and benign peripheral nerve sheath tumor.

In the plasmacytoid or hyaline cell variant, the tumor cells are distributed in nests and groups that are separated by an abundant myxoid stroma containing hyaluronic acid and lacking mucin (Fig. 20.27). The individual cells are polygonal to round and typically have prominent glassy (nongranular) eosinophilic cytoplasm, often with eccentrically placed nuclei. The resultant appearance may mimic a plasma cell proliferation or any of a variety of neoplasms noted to have a "rhabdoid" phenotype, including malignant melanoma. The glassy cytoplasm corresponds ultrastructurally to aggregates of intermediate filaments. In our experience, these are predominantly vimentin rather than actin, and immunohistochemical evidence of myoepithelial differentiation may be difficult or impossible in some cases (51).

Myoepithelial cells can have completely clear cytoplasm and are most commonly encountered in epithelial-myoepithelial

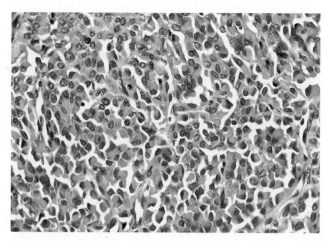

Figure 20.27. The plasmacytoid or hyaline cell variant of myoepithelioma consists of sheets of epithelioid cells with glassy eosinophilic cytoplasm and eccentric nuclei. The resemblance to plasma cells is obvious.

carcinoma. However, the existence of a pure clear-cell myoepithelioma is questionable, and we have not encountered, or at least recognized, an example. Diagnosis would require an encapsulated or sharply demarcated, benign-appearing (and acting) neoplasm with immunohistochemical or ultrastructural demonstration of myoepithelial differentiation. Entities to be excluded in the differential diagnosis would include the extremely rare clear-cell adenoma, a lesion of glycogen-filled epithelial cells lacking myoepithelial differentiation; the hyalinizing clear-cell carcinoma, also lacking myoepithelial differentiation; and an epithelial-myoepithelial carcinoma with prominent clear cells.

Myoepitheliomas are closely related to salivary gland mixed tumors. The latter tumors may contain all of the cell types seen in myoepitheliomas, and we have encountered multiple cases in which the distinction of myoepithelioma from mixed tumor rested solely on the presence of a small focus of stromal (often cartilaginous) differentiation. This distinction has little or no clinical importance.

SEBACEOUS ADENOMA AND LYMPHADENOMA

These tumors are rare, and they occur almost exclusively in the parotid gland and periparotid lymph nodes (52–54). The localization of sebaceous adenoma to this location may relate to the predilection of the parotid to show sebaceous metaplasia, a rare finding in other salivary tissues (55). In addition to this factor, the sharp localization of lymphadenoma to this region, as with Warthin tumor and lymphoepithelial cyst, is a result of the unique intermingling of salivary and lymphoid tissue in the parotid and periparotid lymph nodes. The average age of patients with sebaceous neoplasms is approximately 60 years, but they can occur from the second through the ninth decades of life. The tumors vary in size from 1 to 3 cm in diameter, and they are well encapsulated or at least sharply circumscribed. The clinical behavior is entirely benign, and local recurrence is virtually unheard of. There have been isolated reports of carcinomas arising in sebaceous lymphadenomas, and these have been referred to as *sebaceous lymphadenocarcinomas*. Examples that we have encountered resembled basal cell adenocarcinoma, described later.

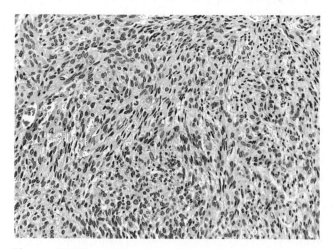

Figure 20.26. Myoepithelioma of parotid gland. The tumor cells have a spindled and plasmacytoid appearance.

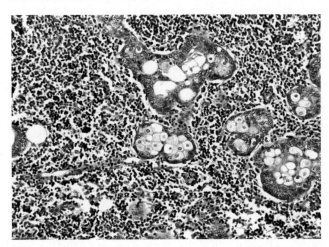

Figure 20.28. Sebaceous lymphadenoma consists of nests of sebaceous and basaloid cells in a prominent lymphoid stroma.

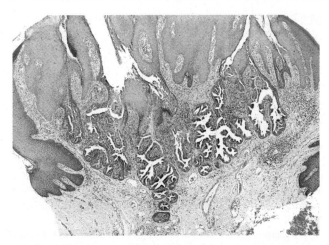

Figure 20.29. Sialadenoma papilliferum consists of complex proliferating ducts opening onto a reactive surface epithelium. Moderate inflammation surrounds the deeper portions of the lesion.

Sebaceous adenomas and lymphadenomas are usually solid, but on occasion, they may have a cystic quality. The well-differentiated sebaceous cells show minimal, if any, cellular pleomorphism, unlike sebaceous carcinomas discussed later. They have practically no tendency for local invasion. In sebaceous lymphadenoma, in addition to the sebaceous cell nests, a background of lymphoid follicles and lymphocytes is seen (Fig. 20.28). In our experience, the large majority of cells in sebaceous adenomas have distinctly sebaceous differentiation with prominent foamy cytoplasm. In contrast, sebaceous lymphadenomas are typically composed primarily of more nonspecific ductal or basaloid epithelial cells with only scattered small nests of sebaceous cells. In some cases, the sebaceous nests may be quite rare.

Although some sebaceous lymphadenomas are clearly within the parotid gland and probably arise from intraparotid lymph nodes, others are distinct from the parotid, although immediately adjacent to it, and appear to arise from salivary inclusions within periparotid nodes. The latter scenario leads to the potential to misdiagnose the lesion as a metastatic carcinoma. We have encountered several sebaceous lymphadenomas in periparotid lymph nodes submitted for consultation with a diagnosis of metastatic mucoepidermoid carcinoma, with the sebaceous cells being misinterpreted as mucinous.

Lesions similar to sebaceous lymphadenoma except completely lacking sebaceous nests have been referred to as simply *lymphadenomas.* These may represent basal cell adenomas involving lymphoid tissue. Fortunately, these lesions are rare because they can be difficult to distinguish from BLL when present within the parotid gland and from a metastatic carcinoma when present in a periparotid lymph node. In the former situation, the sharp circumscription or encapsulation of the lesion with surrounding normal salivary gland should allow distinction from the more diffuse involvement of BLL. In the latter situation, the small size of the cell nests, the paucity of mitotic figures, and the lack of pleomorphism should suggest the diagnosis.

DUCTAL PAPILLOMAS

The term *ductal papilloma* currently encompasses three benign and probably related tumors predominantly arising in the minor salivary glands: sialadenoma papilliferum, inverted ductal papilloma, and intraductal papilloma (56). These occur in the sixth to eighth decades of life and are slightly more common

in men. *Sialadenoma papilliferum* has an exophytic surface and is usually mistaken clinically for a squamous papilloma. It shows a strong predilection for the minor salivary glands of the palate. Microscopically, it has a cauliflowerlike surface that merges at its base with underlying often cystically dilated minor salivary gland ducts (Fig. 20.29). The lining of the complex papillary structures varies from columnar glandular epithelium to keratinizing squamous cells. A mild to intense mixed inflammatory infiltrate is located in the fibrovascular cores of the papilla. The appearance greatly resembles syringocystadenoma papilliferum of the skin adnexae. *Inverted ductal papilloma* has an endophytic growth that is contiguous with the surface epithelium but does not extend above it (Fig. 20.30). It consists of a mixture of squamous and basaloid cells, often in a ribbonlike growth pattern, that project into a cystic space, representing a dilated salivary gland duct. *Intraductal papilloma* is characterized by complex branching papillary fronds within a cystic expansion of a salivary gland duct. The epithelium is predominantly columnar or cuboidal with scattered mucous cells (57).

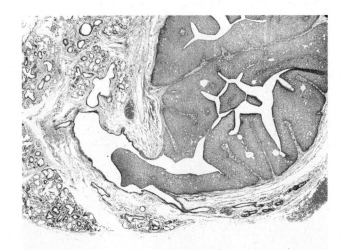

Figure 20.30. Inverted ductal papilloma. A minor salivary gland duct is grossly expanded by a proliferation of nonkeratinizing squamous cells. The lesion is contiguous with the squamous surface mucosa just beyond the top of the image.

MALIGNANT SALIVARY GLAND NEOPLASMS

ADENOID CYSTIC CARCINOMA

Adenoid cystic carcinoma accounts for approximately 10% of all salivary gland tumors. It is the most common malignant tumor of the submandibular and minor salivary glands (58). The ages of patients range from 20 to 84 years, with a median age of 52 years (59). Among the 264 adenoid cystic carcinomas studied at Memorial Sloan-Kettering Cancer Center, 45 (17%) arose in the parotid, and 41 (15.5%) involved the submandibular gland (59). The rest were in minor salivary gland sites. Intramandibular adenoid cystic carcinomas are rare occurrences (60,61).

The tumor grossly appears solid and circumscribed, but microscopically, it extends well beyond the grossly visible and palpable limits of the lesion (Fig. 20.31). This infiltrative capacity is a hallmark of this salivary gland carcinoma. Spreading along nerve sheaths with associated severe pain is often noted (Fig. 20.32). Facial nerve paralysis may be the first presenting symptom, appearing before the lesion becomes otherwise obvious. The usual clinical course is lengthy, often spanning decades, with multiple late local recurrences after operative intervention (59). Occasional patients have a rapid demise. Although adenoid cystic carcinomas may involve lymph nodes by direct extension, particularly when they arise in the submandibular gland, embolic lymph node metastases are rare. A review of a large registry of these tumors at our institution revealed only two examples of small, solitary metastases to regional nodes. Clearly, radical neck dissection should not be a component of normal treatment. In contrast, hematogenous tumor spread, often to the lungs, is quite characteristic. Lung metastases, although clearly identifiable on routine chest radiographs, may remain stable for years.

Three histologic patterns are typically encountered in these tumors: cribriform, tubular, and solid (62–64). Multiple patterns are often present in a single tumor. The cribriform, or classic, pattern consists of basaloid epithelial cells forming sharply demarcated nests containing multiple extracellular

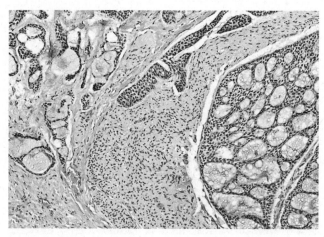

Figure 20.32. Adenoid cystic carcinoma. The perineural invasion of this carcinoma is the hallmark of this lesion.

spaces (Fig. 20.33). The spaces contain PAS-positive connective tissue mucin or eosinophilic hyaline-like material. The cells surrounding the spaces are haphazardly oriented or stretched out around them, indicating that these are extracellular spaces and not true glandular lumina with radially oriented, polarized surrounding cells (Fig. 20.34). This can be confirmed ultrastructurally. This pattern is encountered, at least focally, in the majority of adenoid cystic carcinomas.

The tubular pattern is characterized by smaller ductlike arrays of basaloid epithelial cells surrounding a single central lumenlike space (Fig. 20.35). The surrounding stroma is typically fibrous or hyalinized. The lumenlike space may contain PAS-positive mucin or hyaline material or appear nearly empty. Close examination shows that the cells surrounding the spaces are haphazardly oriented, as in the cribriform pattern, and these again represent extracellular spaces rather than true glandular lumina. Approximately 20% to 30% of adenoid cystic carcinomas contain this pattern.

The solid pattern is the least frequently encountered (Fig. 20.36) and is most often mixed with one of the other variants. It consists of solid nests of basaloid cells, often in a hyalinized stroma. The cells should be cytologically similar or identical to

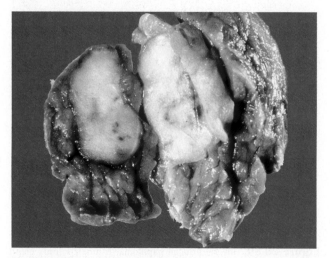

Figure 20.31. Adenoid cystic carcinoma of the parotid gland has deceptively well-delineated outlines. Microscopically, the tumor extends well beyond the grossly apparent edges of the tumor.

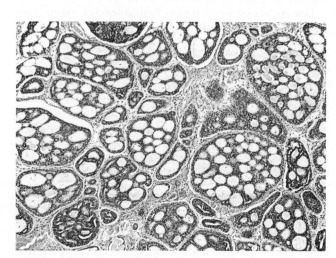

Figure 20.33. The classic cribriform pattern of adenoid cystic carcinoma.

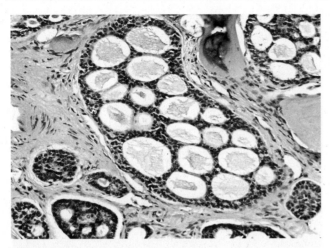

Figure 20.34. Adenoid cystic carcinoma. At higher magnification, the cells are haphazardly arranged around the extracellular spaces.

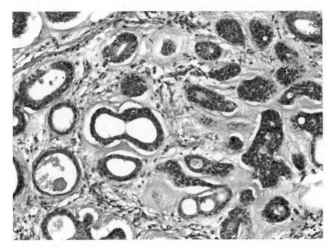

Figure 20.35. The tubular pattern of adenoid cystic carcinoma may be confused with a variety of other neoplasms, including polymorphous low-grade adenocarcinoma.

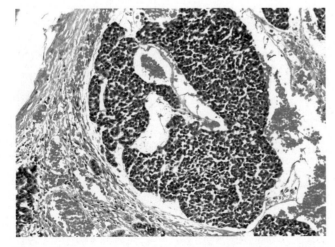

Figure 20.36. The solid variant of adenoid cystic carcinoma should consist of cells highly similar or identical to those of the more typical variants. Marked pleomorphism and necrosis are not features of this pattern.

those seen in the cribriform and tubular patterns. Nuclei should be relatively uniform with dark, coarse nuclear chromatin. Mitotic rate may be slightly increased in this variant, but marked nuclear pleomorphism, enlarged nuclei with prominent nucleoli, or substantial areas of necrosis should lead to alternate diagnostic considerations.

Some studies have emphasized that histologic pattern correlates with prognosis (tubular = best, cribriform = intermediate, and solid = worst) (63,64). However, two large studies and our own experience with a substantial number of these lesions failed to duplicate these prognostic assertions (58,59). This discrepancy may relate to diagnostic misadventures at each end of the morphologic spectrum. Polymorphous low-grade adenocarcinoma (PLGA) is an indolent neoplasm that often has a distinctly tubular growth pattern. Misinterpretation as a tubular adenoid cystic carcinoma would improve the apparent prognosis of that variant. Conversely, the solid pattern of adenoid cystic carcinoma is relatively nonspecific, and similar or identical patterns can be seen in basaloid squamous cell carcinomas, sinonasal undifferentiated carcinomas, and high-grade neuroendocrine carcinomas. These lesions are highly aggressive, and their misinterpretation as the solid variant would greatly decrease the apparent prognosis of the latter subtype.

In reality, predicting the prognosis of these tumors is difficult or impossible on an individual basis. Statistically important prognostic factors include the size and site of the primary tumor and the presence of metastases. Of these, the clinical stage is not surprisingly the most reliable guide (65). Proliferative activity measured by MIB-1 (Ki-67 antigen) has been found to be higher in those cases in which treatment failed, and it may provide additional information on the short-term prognosis (66). The p53 oncoprotein may also be an adverse prognostic marker in adenoid cystic carcinoma (67). In a limited study, it was detected more frequently in recurrent tumors than in primary ones, which may be a reflection of its involvement in the later stages of tumor progression (68). KIT expression has been demonstrated in the majority of adenoid cystic carcinomas (69), but the mutation associated with sensitivity to imatinib mesylate does not appear to be present in these tumors.

The prototypical cribriform pattern is easy to diagnose. As mentioned earlier, the tubular pattern may be confused with PLGA. Attention to cytologic detail usually will allow distinction. PLGA is a tumor of larger cells with more prominent eosinophilic cytoplasm than the distinctly basaloid cells of adenoid cystic carcinoma. Many of the tubules in PLGA have cells oriented radially around them, indicating true ductal or luminal differentiation. As its name implies, PLGA is noted for its histologic variability (and cytologic uniformity). Many of the patterns present are well beyond the spectrum of adenoid cystic carcinoma. Immunohistochemically, adenoid cystic carcinomas typically express KIT and stain weakly for S-100 protein. PLGA shows a reverse pattern, with weak staining for KIT and strong positivity for S-100 protein. Recently, CD43 has been touted as a marker for adenoid cystic carcinoma, but this antigen requires more complete study in salivary neoplasia (12).

Fortunately, the solid variant of adenoid cystic carcinoma is uncommon and rarely occurs in pure form. If the cells in the solid nests vary more than minimally from the cells of the more typical cribriform pattern, if there is obvious necrosis, if the mitotic rate is extremely high, or if abrupt squamous differentiation is noted, strong consideration should be given to other basaloid neoplasms. In our experience, squamous differentiation in particular is extremely rare in salivary adenoid cystic carcinomas and, conversely, is a classic feature of basaloid squamous cell carcinoma. This distinction is important because the latter tumor frequently metastasizes to regional lymph nodes, and a formal lymph node dissection is often warranted. High-grade "solid" carcinoma may arise through "dedifferentiation" in recurrent adenoid cystic carcinoma, and these high-grade solid nests should be clearly distinguished from the solid variant of conventional adenoid cystic carcinoma.

Other lesions may be confused with adenoid cystic carcinoma. Mixed tumors occasionally have a membranous pattern that can be difficult to distinguish from adenoid cystic carcinoma, and the cells in this pattern may be more basaloid, adding to the confusion. Searching for more typical microscopic patterns will usually allow diagnosis, and markers such as KIT and CD43 may be of value for their tendency to be positive in adenoid cystic carcinoma. Distinction from epithelial-myoepithelial carcinoma relies on the (usually) distinct biphasic pattern of the latter, although we have seen composite examples of these two tumors on several occasions. Distinction from basal cell adenoma is rarely a problem and rests on the encapsulation of the latter benign tumor.

MUCOEPIDERMOID CARCINOMA

These tumors represent approximately 5% of all salivary gland tumors, with approximately 67% arising in the parotid gland and 33% arising in the minor salivary glands (70–73). Mucoepidermoid carcinoma is the third most frequently encountered minor salivary gland tumor (10%), preceded only by mixed tumor and adenoid cystic carcinoma. Occasional examples may arise within the mandibular or maxillary bones (60). Women are affected slightly more often than men. The incidence tends to peak at approximately the fifth decade, but it should be noted that this tumor is the most common salivary gland malignancy in childhood. On occasion, mucoepidermoid carcinomas may arise in intraparotid or periparotid lymph nodes, or they may be associated with a Warthin tumor.

The low-grade tumors are well-circumscribed, often cystic masses. Slow painless growth is quite characteristic. High-grade variants are poorly delineated, solid masses that may be fixed to the surrounding soft tissues. They are often painful as a result of facial nerve involvement. Lymph node metastases are a sure clinical sign that one is dealing with a high-grade tumor.

On gross examination, the lesions vary from smooth to irregular contours and measure 3 to 5 cm in average size. Both solid and cystic areas are discernible on cut section (Fig. 20.37). The cystic spaces contain mucus or hemorrhagic material. Histologic examination, by definition, shows multiple cell types. The most common are squamous cells, mucous cells, cuboidal intermediate cells, and basaloid cells. The squamous cells form solid nests, often with individual cell keratinization and intercellular bridging. This component often predominates in higher grade tumors. The mucous cells may be diffusely dispersed, or they may form small clusters partly lining the cystic spaces. Mucous cells often predominate in low-grade tumors, and occasional examples will consist of a single large cyst lined by bland mucus-producing cells with only a small mural nodule of other cell types to allow for correct diagnosis. If the mucinous secretions escape into adjacent salivary gland tissues, a foreign body giant-cell reaction is elicited that may make a proper diagnosis more

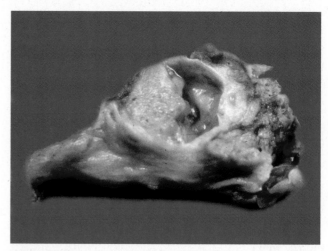

Figure 20.37. Low-grade mucoepidermoid carcinomas may have a distinctly cystic gross appearance.

difficult. Occasionally, mucoepidermoid carcinomas are composed of prominent clear cells (74) or prominent oncocytic cells (75–77).

Histologic criteria used in grading mucoepidermoid carcinomas include nuclear atypia, intracystic components, mitotic activity, perineural invasion, and necrosis (78,79). One study proposed the addition of the characterization of the invasive front, the lymphatic and/or vascular invasion, and the bony invasion as criteria for grading (80). In low-grade mucoepidermoid carcinomas, well-formed glandular or microcystic structures are present; they are lined by a single layer of mucus-secreting columnar cells (Fig. 20.38) (72). In some areas, these cystic spaces are bordered by papillary infoldings that are formed by intermediate, basaloid, or squamous cells. In these low-grade malignant lesions, microcysts that coalesce into macrocysts may be quite prominent.

Intermediate-grade malignant lesions are usually characterized by solidly growing areas of squamous, intermediate, basaloid cells or clear cells or by papillary cystic infoldings (Fig.

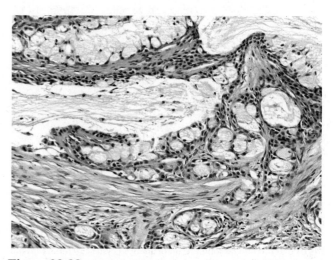

Figure 20.38. Low-grade mucoepidermoid carcinoma. This example consists of cystic spaces lined by mucous cells, nonkeratinizing squamous (intermediate) cells, and scattered basaloid cells.

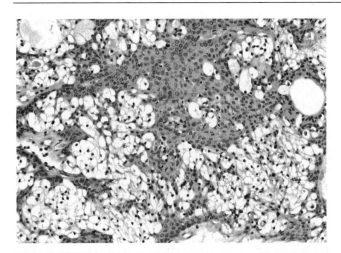

Figure 20.39. This intermediate-grade mucoepidermoid carcinoma consists of solid nests of clear and nonkeratinizing squamous cells. Only scattered mucous cells are present.

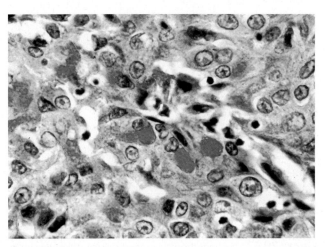

Figure 20.41. Mucous cells may not be obvious in high-grade mucoepidermoid carcinomas, and a mucin stain may be helpful to distinguish the lesion from a squamous cell carcinoma (periodic acid-Schiff stain with diastase).

20.39) (81). Variations in the size and shape of the carcinoma cells, prominent nucleoli, and abundant mitotic figures are easily recognizable. Obvious invasion, including perineural extension, focal necrosis, increased mitotic figures, and greater pleomorphism are also more evident in high-grade tumors (Fig. 20.40) (79). Metastases in patients with high-grade tumors show varying proportions of squamous or mucin-producing cells that do not necessarily reflect the ratios observed in the primary salivary gland lesion.

In a study of more than 350 patients with mucoepidermoid carcinoma, of those with low-grade tumors, 92%, 90%, and 82% were alive and well at 5, 10, and 15 years after treatment, respectively. When the tumor was high-grade malignant, only 49%, 42%, and 33% of the patients were alive and well at 5, 10, and 15 years after treatment, respectively (72). Both stage and grade must be considered to arrive at a proper treatment decision (72). For instance, 90% of stage I, intermediate-grade, or high-grade mucoepidermoid carcinomas can be successfully treated by less than radical excision. However, a lethal clinical outcome, including distant metastases, may be observed with some low-grade mucoepidermoid carcinomas that were extensive (stage

III) when they were first noticed (72). H-ras mutations may contribute to the development of mucoepidermoid carcinoma, and they seem to be correlated with tumor grade (82).

In the differential diagnosis of mucoepidermoid carcinomas, various sebaceous neoplasms, clear-cell tumors, and squamous cell carcinoma must be ruled out. The rare sclerosing form of mucoepidermoid carcinoma may be mistaken for chronic sialadenitis (83). Similarly, necrotizing sialometaplasia of a minor salivary gland origin may present diagnostic difficulties. Before the diagnosis of a rare primary squamous cell carcinoma of the salivary glands can be confirmed, mucoepidermoid carcinoma and metastatic squamous cell carcinoma must be excluded (Fig. 20.41) (84).

ACINIC CELL CARCINOMA

Acinic cell carcinomas represent approximately 2% of salivary gland tumors, with approximately 90% arising in the parotid gland (85–93). The rest involve the submandibular and the minor salivary glands (85,86). This tumor is more common in women, and the peak incidence is in the fifth and sixth decades of life. Rarely, it may arise in ectopic salivary gland tissue involving periparotid lymph nodes, or it may be multiple or bilateral. On gross examination, the lesional tissue is often well delineated, solid, and yellow, gray, or brown in color. Occasionally, cysts may be grossly visible (Fig. 20.42). Distinction from other salivary gland neoplasms, benign or malignant, is not possible grossly.

Microscopically, the classic acinar tumor cells resemble the serous cellular elements of the normal parotid gland with finely granular, basophilic cytoplasm (Figs. 20.43 and 20.44). In addition to the classic serous cells, the lesional tissue may be composed of clear cells, oncocytic cells, basaloid cells, and nonspecific-appearing ductal cells (Fig. 20.45). These varied cell types may be arranged in equally varied growth patterns, including solid, acinar, microcystic, papillary cystic, and follicular (87). The end result is a tumor with a very wide spectrum of appearances, such that considerable caution must be applied to avoid overdiagnosis because these patterns and cell types can be seen in a wide variety of other salivary neoplasms. Although it is im-

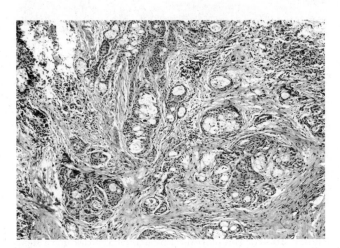

Figure 20.40. This high-grade mucoepidermoid carcinoma exhibits obvious invasion with stromal desmoplasia.

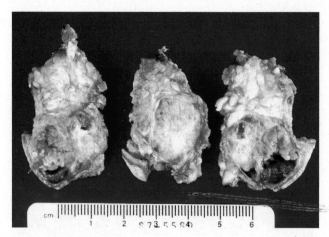

Figure 20.42. Sections through a superficial parotidectomy for an acinic cell carcinoma reveal a sharply demarcated tumor with a partially cystic appearance.

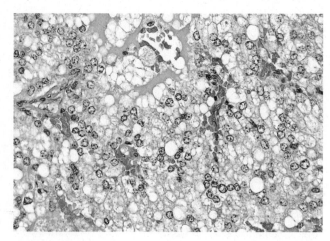

Figure 20.45. Acinic cell carcinoma in which the majority of the tumor cells have clear cytoplasm.

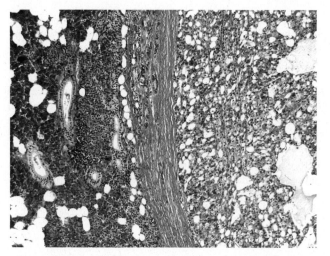

Figure 20.43. Microscopically, this acinic cell carcinoma is separated from the adjacent normal parotid gland (*left*) by a well-formed fibrous capsule.

portant to recognize this morphologic spectrum, subclassification based on cell type and architecture appears to have no prognostic value and is usually not fruitful because several patterns are often present in the same tumor.

Acinic cell carcinoma is a well-differentiated tumor that typically lacks overt cytologic features of malignancy. The presence of prominent nuclear pleomorphism, high mitotic rate, or necrosis should prompt consideration of other entities, and if these findings are focal in an otherwise typical acinic cell carcinoma, they may represent areas of "dedifferentiation" (Fig. 20.46). Dedifferentiated acinic cell carcinoma is a highly aggressive tumor that requires adjuvant treatment (88,89). Some acinic cell carcinomas contain a prominent lymphoid stroma, and extreme examples may be confused with lymph node metastases.

That the ultrastructural appearance is a close replica of the cellular morphology observed by optical means is not surprising (90). The cellular characteristics of the serous types of cells include well-formed endoplasmic reticulum, developed Golgi apparatus, and secretory granules of various sizes and densities (91). Although ductular cell differentiation may be seen in

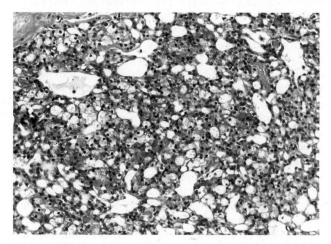

Figure 20.44. At higher magnification, the cells of acinic cell carcinoma have predominantly basophilic cytoplasm and resemble normal serous salivary cells. Small microcystic spaces are also noted.

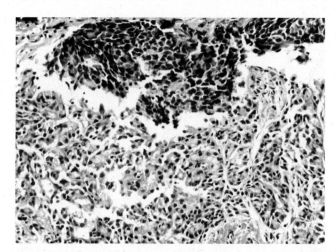

Figure 20.46. This otherwise typical acinic cell carcinoma shows an area (*upper*) of higher grade carcinoma with small-cell features. This phenomenon has been referred to as "dedifferentiation."

some otherwise typical acinic cell carcinomas, a myoepithelial component is not present. Immunohistochemical stains using antibodies against amylase or antichymotrypsin will highlight acinar differentiation, but these cells are the easiest to recognize on routine hematoxylin and eosin (H&E)–stained sections. In their absence, a simple PAS stain will often suffice and show strong granular cytoplasmic positivity in the acinar cell type. Myoepithelial markers are typically absent.

Forecasting the clinical behavior of an acinic cell neoplasm based solely on histologic appearance is difficult or impossible. If the tumor is well encapsulated and shows no intratumoral vascular permeation, it is less likely to recur than if these features are present (86). Overall, local recurrence develops in 20% of cases. Regional lymph node metastases and distant metastases are present in 10% and 6% of patients, respectively (86), but formal lymph node dissection is not indicated unless there is obvious clinical involvement. Some studies have emphasized a histologic spectrum ranging from well-differentiated to poorly differentiated tumors with an apparently good prognostic correlation (92). In our experience, poorly differentiated acinic cell carcinomas are rare, and many (if not most) of these tumors would be better classified as adenocarcinoma not otherwise specified (NOS) or dedifferentiated acinic cell carcinoma. Overall, the 5-year survival rate for patients with acinic cell carcinoma is 83% (93). This figure may represent an overreporting of problematic cases. In our experience, death from disease is extremely rare in tumors lacking dedifferentiation.

POLYMORPHOUS LOW-GRADE ADENOCARCINOMA

PLGA, also known as lobular carcinoma, terminal duct carcinoma, or trabecular carcinoma, almost exclusively involves the minor salivary glands, particularly those of the palate (94–101). This tumor is twice as common in women compared with men, and the average age at diagnosis is 57 years (100). Frequently, the tumors present as slowly enlarging, painless palatal masses or swellings (49%). PLGA is now considered the most common glandular malignancy of the palate, replacing adenoid cystic carcinoma. Before the recognition of PLGA, this tumor was undoubtedly misdiagnosed as adenoid cystic carcinoma, accounting for the historically excellent prognosis of "adenoid cystic carcinoma" when it involved the palate. The buccal mucosa, lip, retromolar triangle, cheek, and tongue may also be involved, as well as seromucinous gland from other locations (94,102). Involvement of major salivary glands is extremely rare and virtually always occurs in the parotid gland in the setting of a carcinoma arising in a pre-existent mixed tumor.

The tumors range in size from 1 to 5 cm and usually have intact overlying mucosa. True to its designation, this adenocarcinoma has diverse architectural patterns but uniform, bland cytologic features (Figs. 20.47 to 20.50). The grossly well-delineated lesional borders lack capsule formation, and peripheral infiltration into the adjacent soft tissues or bone usually occurs in a single file pattern. Perineural involvement by carcinoma cells is often seen (Fig. 20.50), although not to the degree encountered in adenoid cystic or salivary duct carcinomas. A pronounced papillary growth pattern may be present. We have referred to pure or nearly pure papillary tumors of this type as *low-grade papillary adenocarcinomas of salivary origin* (LPASO) (103). Long-term follow-up suggests that cases with more than a focal

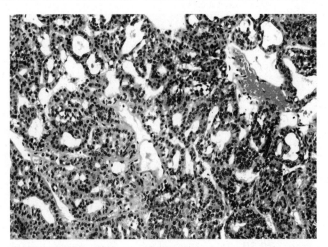

Figure 20.47. This polymorphous low-grade adenocarcinoma arising in the palate has a complex cribriform pattern with little intervening stroma. The cells are larger and more eosinophilic than those of adenoid cystic carcinoma.

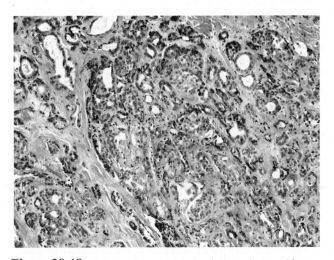

Figure 20.48. Polymorphous low-grade adenocarcinoma with more prominent sclerotic stroma.

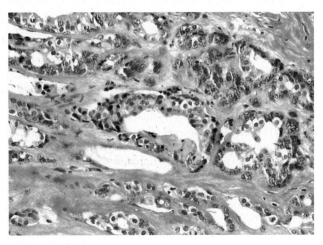

Figure 20.49. At higher magnification, the cells of polymorphous low-grade adenocarcinoma have relatively uniform nuclei and a quite low mitotic rate.

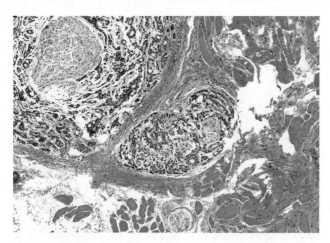

Figure 20.50. This polymorphous low-grade adenocarcinoma shows prominent perineural invasion, a common finding in this tumor.

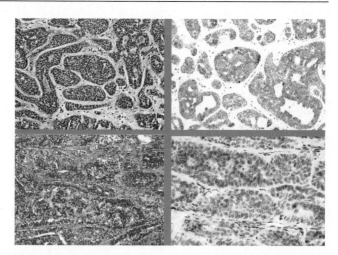

Figure 20.51. Adenoid cystic carcinoma (*upper*) compared with polymorphous low-grade adenocarcinoma (PLGA) (*lower*). The hematoxylin and eosin images on the left show the distinctly more basaloid nature of the adenoid cystic carcinoma cells. CD117 reactivity on the right is much stronger in adenoid cystic carcinoma (*upper*) than in PLGA (*lower*).

area of papillary growth have a higher incidence of cervical node metastases (103,104).

The monomorphous cells of PLGA are cuboidal or low columnar with oval or elongated uniform basophilic nuclei. The cytoplasm is modest in amount and usually eosinophilic. Intralesional necrosis unrelated to prior biopsy is rare, and mitotic figures are infrequent. We encountered an example of PLGA that underwent histologic transformation to a high-grade carcinoma after a prolonged course with several recurrences (105). This was characterized by nuclear pleomorphism, enlarged nucleoli, increased mitotic activity, and the presence of necrosis.

Because of its variegated microscopic appearance, PLGA is often mistaken for a mixed tumor or an adenoid cystic carcinoma. Mixed tumors do not feature vascular, perineural, or bony invasion, whereas such behavior is common in PLGA. The tubular pattern of adenoid cystic carcinoma is most likely to cause confusion. Tubule formation is one of many patterns encountered in PLGA, and in this tumor, the cells are often polarized around the central tubular lumen, resembling a true gland. This is unlike the haphazard orientation seen in adenoid cystic carcinoma. The distinction between adenoid cystic carcinoma and PLGA is ultimately based on both cytologic and histologic characteristics (106). Eosinophilic cytoplasm with rounded nuclear outlines characterizes PLGA; in contrast, the cells of adenoid cystic carcinoma have basophilic cytoplasm and angulated darkly staining nuclei.

Immunohistochemical studies show consistent reactivity to EMA and more variable staining for CEA in PLGA. In adenoid cystic carcinoma, these two cell markers are equally intensely positive in the luminal cells. In our experience, the best markers for distinguishing PLGA from adenoid cystic carcinoma have been CD117 and S-100 protein. Staining for CD117 is typically stronger and more diffuse in adenoid cystic carcinoma than in PLGA (Fig. 20.51), with S-100 protein showing the reverse. Smooth muscle actin has also been noted to be stronger in adenoid cystic carcinoma (107–109). The role of CD43 in this distinction awaits further study (12).

The practical significance in separating these two tumor entities lies in the relative malignant potential of both. Adenoid cystic carcinoma has a much more aggressive clinical behavior because it tends to feature multiple recurrences, more aggressive local invasion, and a much higher frequency of vascular

metastases (lungs and bone). Interestingly, cytogenetic similarities do exist between PLGA and adenoid cystic carcinoma. Both share various abnormalities involving chromosome 12, including the same t(6;12)(p21;q13) (110).

SALIVARY DUCT CARCINOMA

Salivary duct carcinoma is an aggressive neoplasm occurring primarily in the parotid gland of middle-aged and elderly males (Fig. 20.52). Most salivary duct carcinomas (80%) occur in the parotid gland, and only 5% arise in intraoral minor salivary glands. Patients present with a mass, and many have facial nerve involvement. The outcome is unfavorable, and approximately half of these patients develop local recurrences. Lymph node metastases are common, and nearly two-thirds of patients develop distant metastases to the brain, liver, adrenals, and lungs. Even with aggressive therapy, the mortality rate is 77% at a mean interval of 3 years after diagnosis (111,112). The prognosis is

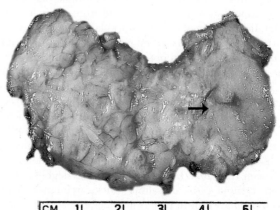

Figure 20.52. Salivary duct carcinoma of the parotid gland (*arrow*). This tumor is a soft, fleshy mass with slightly ill-defined borders.

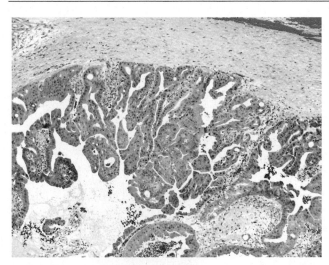

Figure 20.53. Salivary duct carcinoma showing a distinctly papillary intraductal-like pattern. The cells have eosinophilic, apocrine cytoplasm.

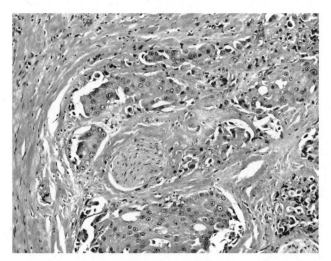

Figure 20.55. The more overtly invasive component of salivary duct carcinoma has irregular nests of apocrine cells in dense fibrous stroma. Perineural invasion is present in the center of the field.

related to tumor size and the presence of metastases, and it is not influenced by the results of ancillary studies, such as DNA ploidy and proliferative fractions (113). The treatment consists of radical excision and lymphadenectomy with radiation therapy or chemotherapy.

The comedocarcinoma-like component of this tumor imparts a striking resemblance to intraductal carcinoma of the breast and clearly separates this malignancy from other salivary gland tumors. Although this pattern may appear to represent intraductal growth (carcinoma in situ), in many instances, it represents a pattern of invasive growth because it can be seen in perineural spaces or distant metastases. Myoepithelial markers may be used to document examples of true intraductal growth (see below). The intraductal-like component can have a papillary, comedo-like, or cribriform pattern (Figs. 20.53 and 20.54). The more obviously infiltrating component may have a papillary appearance but more commonly resembles nonspe-

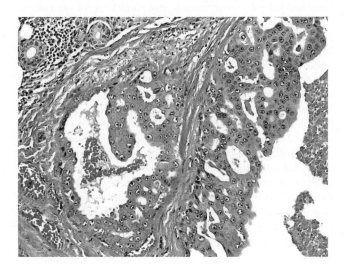

Figure 20.54. Salivary duct carcinoma with intraductal comedonecrosis (*right*). The apocrine cells have prominent nucleoli and closely resemble apocrine breast cells.

cific adenocarcinoma in a densely sclerotic stroma (Fig. 20.55). Cytologically, the cells often have an apocrine appearance with large nuclei and prominent nucleoli. The cytoplasm is moderately abundant and eosinophilic. Mitotic figures are common. Perineural spread along branches of the facial nerve is often extensive, making complete resection difficult or impossible. Mucinous (114), micropapillary (115), and sarcomatoid (116) variants have been described. The micropapillary variant has been noted to have an extremely poor prognosis, and the sarcomatoid variant may be difficult to differentiate from a carcinosarcoma.

Since the initial description by Chen in 1983 (117), there have been multiple reports of a variant of salivary duct carcinoma exhibiting pure intraductal growth, confirmed by immunohistochemistry, and having, as would be expected, an excellent prognosis (12,118–120). In fact, if properly defined, no patient has developed a metastasis or died of this disease, regardless of the nuclear grade (12). Terms applied to this lesion have included *low-grade salivary duct carcinoma, intraductal carcinoma*, and *low-grade cribriform cystadenocarcinoma*. The last is the World Health Organization's 2005 designation for this lesion, but we agree with Cheuk and Chan (12), Weinreb et al. (118), and others that this term is confusing and should be avoided. Likewise, labeling these lesions as low-grade salivary duct carcinoma is likely to cause clinician confusion with the much more aggressive conventional salivary duct carcinoma. We prefer the term *intraductal carcinoma*. This should be diagnosed only after thorough sampling and immunohistochemical studies for myoepithelial markers to confirm its purely in situ nature. Nuclear grade is not a feature of this diagnosis. Small foci of microinvasion should be noted and thus far do not appear to affect prognosis. We have encountered three cases of pure intraductal carcinoma of the parotid gland in our practice and all appear to have been cured by wide excision.

Despite its resemblance to breast carcinoma, including its reactivity for gross cystic disease fluid protein, salivary duct carcinoma is different because it is positive for androgen receptor, it may be positive for prostate-specific antigen and prostatic acid phosphatase (PAP), and it only rarely is reactive for estrogen and progesterone receptors (121–123). The inactivation of the tumor suppressor gene *p16* may play a role in the development of salivary duct carcinoma (124).

MALIGNANCY ASSOCIATED WITH MIXED TUMOR

The term *malignant mixed tumor* is ambiguous and should not be used without appropriate modifiers, if at all. There are three clinicopathologically distinct scenarios under which mixed tumors have been associated with more aggressive or overtly malignant behavior. These are so-called *benign metastasizing mixed tumor, carcinoma arising in a mixed tumor,* and *salivary carcinosarcoma* or *true malignant mixed tumor.* Each of these entities will be briefly discussed.

Benign Metastasizing Mixed Tumor

Rarely, mixed tumors of entirely normal histologic appearance have metastasized (125,126), and the term *benign metastasizing mixed tumor* has been applied to these lesions. Most of the metastasizing tumors arose in the parotid, followed by the submandibular gland and the minor salivary glands (127), a distribution virtually identical to that of mixed tumors in general. With rare exception, all of the primary mixed tumors recurred locally at least once before distant metastases were noted. The sites of metastases are most commonly bone and lungs, but metastases to regional lymph nodes, skin, kidney, retroperitoneum, oral cavity, pharynx, brain, and, in one case, an old abdominal scar have been reported. The metastases may become clinically apparent synchronously with the local recurrence, or they may develop many decades after resection(s) of the primary tumor. Retrospective analysis of the histologic appearance of these tumors has thus far failed to identify features predictive of this incongruous clinical behavior.

As with other benign metastasizing entities such as leiomyoma of the uterus and giant-cell tumor of bone, almost all patients with benign metastasizing mixed tumors have an entirely benign clinical course. They remain alive and well without disease or disease progression for many years after the metastases are first noted. There have been rare but well-documented reports of aggressive behavior, including a rapid death resulting from a normal-appearing metastasizing mixed tumor in an immunosuppressed patient (128). Examples of aggressive behavior in immunocompetent patients are extremely rare. They should be viewed with skepticism, and strong consideration should be given to possible misdiagnosis.

Carcinoma Arising in Mixed Tumor

These neoplasms are mixtures of benign mixed tumor and a distinct second component of carcinoma (129–132). The clinical presentation follows one of three pathways. Most commonly, an asymptomatic salivary gland swelling, presumably the benign component, is present for many years and then suddenly enlarges and becomes painful, signaling the development of the malignant component with neural invasion. Alternatively, following one or more local recurrences of a benign mixed tumor, the subsequent recurrence consists of a carcinoma. Residual benign mixed tumor may or may not be identifiable. Finally, salivary gland symptomatology may be noted for less than a year, and the resection documents a benign mixed tumor with associated carcinoma, with both components apparently originating almost simultaneously.

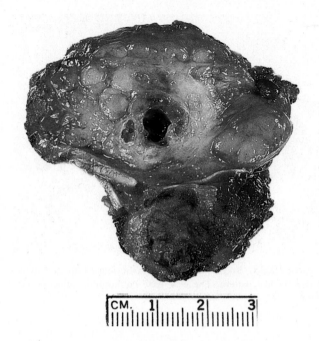

Figure 20.56. Malignant mixed tumor of the parotid gland with a multinodular appearance, central hemorrhage, and necrosis.

Malignant transformation occurs in approximately 2% to 7% of mixed tumors (133,134). These most commonly involve the parotid gland (73%). The submandibular gland (16%) and the minor salivary glands (11%) are sites that are less frequently noted. The patients range in age from 7 to 86 years (median age, 54 years). More women (54%) than men are affected by this tumor.

On gross examination, the tumors usually appear to be well encapsulated, but in some areas, the capsule may be either infiltrated or is clearly disrupted by the lesion (Fig. 20.56). Some of the tumors are entirely solid and gritty on cut section, whereas others may show areas of necrosis and hemorrhage. Occasionally a distinctly biphasic appearance can be seen grossly with translucent or chondroid elements marking the benign component and yellow or hemorrhagic tissue marking the area of malignancy. The tumor size varies considerably, but 80% of the lesions measure more than 3 cm in diameter. Infrequently, the lesions are freely movable (38%); the rest show skin ulceration and fixation to the underlying soft tissues or bone.

Increased cellularity, local recurrence, multiple tumor nodules, an apparent lack of encapsulation, and small foci of capsular penetration are not indicative of malignancy (135). More reliable features of transformation into a malignant tumor are overtly invasive growth, necrosis, vascular permeation, perineural extension, and prominent cytologic atypia associated with abnormal mitotic figures. Large areas of hyalinized scarlike fibrosis within a mixed tumor should lead to careful examination for a malignant component. The earliest microscopic evidence of a malignant transformation is often characterized by aggregates of large, hyperchromatic, cytologically atypical cells embedded in this hyalinized stroma (Figs. 20.57 and 20.58) (136).

Although the malignant component has often been reported to resemble a de novo salivary gland carcinoma such as salivary duct carcinoma, adenoid cystic carcinoma, PLGA, or myoepi-

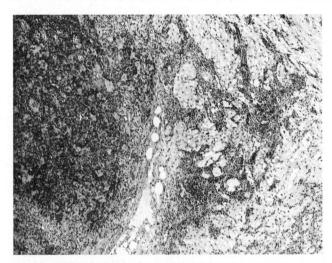

Figure 20.57. Carcinoma arising in mixed tumor. The typical mixed tumor component (*right*) consists of strands of small cells in a myxoid stroma and contrasts sharply with the far more cellular malignant component on the left side of the image.

thelial carcinoma (137), in our experience, the malignant component is typically poorly differentiated, high grade, and rarely resembles a de novo salivary carcinoma (Fig. 20.58). It is often best described as simply *high-grade (adeno)carcinoma NOS.* The growth pattern of the malignant component may be solid, glandular, squamous, or spindle cell or rarely may contain giant cells.

Once a diagnosis of carcinoma has been made, it is of prognostic importance to assess the degree of invasion, if any, beyond the confines of the pre-existent mixed tumor. Unfortunately, this is not always as straightforward as it sounds because the edge of the benign component is not always clear cut. Tortoledo et al. (137) noted that invasion of more than 8 mm past the benign component was associated with a very bad prognosis (137). Conversely, it has been noted that when the malignant component is confined to the pre-existent mixed tumor (the term *carcinoma in situ* has been applied somewhat imprecisely

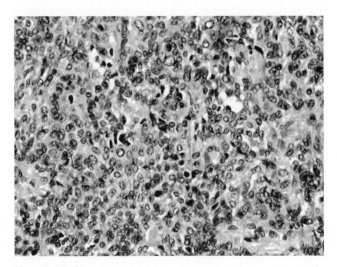

Figure 20.58. The malignant component of carcinoma arising in a mixed tumor rarely resembles a de novo salivary carcinoma and more often consists of poorly differentiated cellular neoplasms.

to these lesions), the patients do not develop metastatic disease (131,138). We have encountered several dozen such cases in consultation over the years and have yet to encounter one that subsequently behaved in a malignant fashion. This raises the issue of proper terminology. In our own practice, we have used the diagnosis of *carcinoma arising in and confined to a pre-existent mixed tumor* for these lesions, accompanied by a note indicating that the literature and our own experience strongly suggests benign behavior for these cases.

At the other extreme from the above are tumors in which the specimen consists almost entirely of high-grade carcinoma. A history of a stable tumor of long duration followed by sudden enlargement may strongly suggest a prior benign component with malignant transformation, but documenting it microscopically may be difficult or impossible when the malignancy overgrows and destroys the benign elements. It seems likely that many high-grade salivary tumors not fitting well into other diagnostic categories represent this phenomenon. Others may represent salivary duct carcinomas with destruction of the characteristic in situ component of these tumors (see above).

Not surprisingly, metastases from carcinomas arising in mixed tumors consist of the carcinomatous component, and features of a mixed tumor are rare. Cervical lymph node involvement early in the clinical course is present in only approximately 12% of patients. If one considers the entire course of the disease, at least 25% of patients eventually develop metastases (130,131).

Carcinosarcoma

Carcinosarcoma is by far the rarest of the three forms of malignant or aggressive behavior associated with mixed tumors (139–143). Fewer than 50 cases have been described, most as case reports. The term *true mixed tumor* has also been applied to these neoplasms. In many other organ systems, the concept of carcinosarcoma has been replaced by the concept of a fundamentally carcinomatous tumor with mesenchymal differentiation (sarcomatoid carcinoma). We strongly suspect that approach is appropriate in the salivary gland as well, but for our purposes here, we will continue to use the term *carcinosarcoma*. These are high-grade malignancies showing both malignant epithelial and stromal elements. The former typically consist of high-grade adenocarcinomas without features of conventional de novo salivary gland carcinoma. Squamous cell carcinoma may also be present. The sarcomatous component consists of overtly malignant stromal elements that may resemble fibrosarcoma, malignant fibrous histiocytoma (i.e., sarcoma NOS), chondrosarcoma, osteosarcoma, liposarcoma, or even rhabdomyosarcoma (Fig. 20.59). Metastases typically include both epithelial and stromal elements and most commonly involve the lung, followed by regional lymph nodes. The majority of patients die of disease with an average survival of approximately 2 years (142). Salivary carcinosarcomas have been described arising in benign mixed tumors.

EPITHELIAL-MYOEPITHELIAL CARCINOMA

Although this form of carcinoma is said to represent less than 0.5% of all salivary gland neoplasms (144–147), our own experience suggests that it is considerably more common and often underdiagnosed. The patients are, on average, in their mid-60s. It is twice as common in women as in men. More than 80%

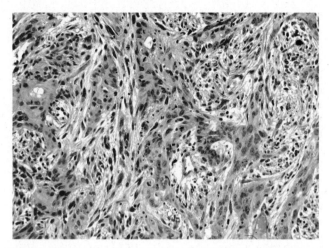

Figure 20.59. This carcinosarcoma (sarcomatoid carcinoma) consists of cohesive epithelial nests mixed with a malignant spindle cell stroma.

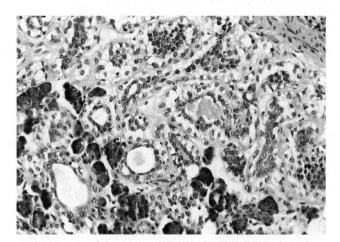

Figure 20.61. Epithelial-myoepithelial carcinoma. In the classic appearance of this tumor, shown here, a rim of clear myoepithelial cells surrounds an inner layer of smaller ductal lining cells.

occur in the parotid gland, with the rest occurring in the submandibular and minor salivary glands. Slowly progressive swelling with or without facial nerve palsy are the cardinal symptoms at presentation. Epithelial-myoepithelial carcinoma behaves as a low-grade malignancy with a high likelihood for local recurrence (148,149). Regional lymph node metastases and distant blood-borne metastatic spread to lungs and kidneys have been reported.

On histologic examination, a well-defined fibrous capsule surrounds a multinodular growth pattern (Fig. 20.60). Not infrequently, the capsule is focally absent or is breached by nests of tumor cells. In the classic form of this tumor (the one usually illustrated), two tumor cell types are present in a characteristic orientation producing a distinct and easy to recognize biphasic appearance (Fig. 20.61). Small cuboidal cells with amphophilic cytoplasm and eccentric small nuclei form ductlike structures with central lumen formation. These ductal epithelial cells contain PAS-positive material that is not removable by diastase. Mucin production is not demonstrable. Surrounding these cells is a layer of larger oval or polyhedral myoepithelial cells with clear cytoplasm on H&E-stained sections. Glycogen is demon-

strable in the cytoplasm by PAS staining. PAS-positive basement membrane may be seen ensheathing tumor cell nests in an organoid growth pattern. Intratumoral hyalinization and cystification may be prominent features. The mitotic rate is usually low, with most mitotic figures noted in the clear-cell component.

In tumors having the above stereotypical appearance, the diagnosis is straightforward, once considered. However, in many epithelial-myoepithelial carcinomas, the ductal component is difficult to spot in H&E-stained sections and is often hidden in an overgrowth of the clear-cell, myoepithelial component (Fig. 20.62). Immunohistochemistry may be of considerable value in such cases. The ductal epithelial cells react for cytokeratin, EMA, and occasionally S-100 protein. The clear myoepithelial cells will demonstrate variable cytokeratin reactivity with strong reactivity for S-100 protein, smooth muscle actin, p63, CD10, calponin, and other myoepithelial markers (146,150).

A recent large review has documented several unusual variants of epithelial-myoepithelial carcinoma including ancient change, Verocay-like bodies, sebaceous differentiation, oncocytic differentiation, dedifferentiation, myoepithelial "anaplasia," and tumors with a clear-cell ductal and myoepithelial ("double clear") appearance (150). The differential diagnosis of epithelial-myoepithelial carcinoma includes the large list of salivary neoplasms that may contain focal or more diffuse clear cells. In most instances, attention to more characteristic microscopic areas will allow distinction. The hyalinizing clear-cell carcinoma discussed later is most often confused with this tumor in our experience, but it lacks any evidence of myoepithelial differentiation. Whenever attempting to diagnose clear-cell tumors arising in salivary glands, the possibility of a metastasis from a clear-cell carcinoma of the kidney should also be given serious diagnostic consideration.

BASAL CELL ADENOCARCINOMA

Basal cell adenocarcinoma is the malignant counterpart of basal cell adenoma. Isolated cases had been reported under a variety of names, but the first well-documented series defining this entity was published less than 20 years ago (151). This tumor ac-

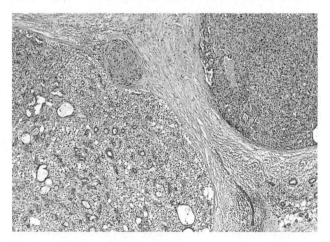

Figure 20.60. Epithelial-myoepithelial carcinoma of the parotid gland with a multinodular growth pattern.

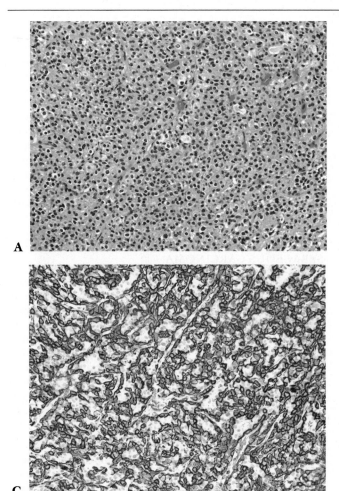

A

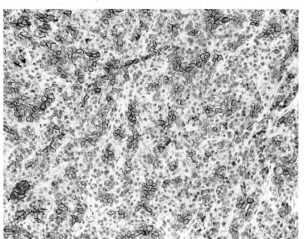

B

C

Figure 20.62. In this epithelial-myoepithelial carcinoma, the two elements are not easily distinguished in a hematoxylin and eosin–stained section (**A**). Immunohistochemical staining for cytokeratin (**B**) and smooth muscle actin (**C**) outlines the two cell populations.

counts for approximately 2% of salivary malignancies and occurs chiefly in the parotid gland of elderly individuals (median age, 60 years) (152). In a series of 25 cases from the Armed Forces Institute of Pathology (AFIP), seven patients developed local recurrences, three patients developed regional lymph node metastases, and one patient developed pulmonary metastases (152). One patient died of local spread, but the patient with pulmonary disease was alive and well 7 years after initial resection. Vascular invasion has, so far, not been associated with a worsened prognosis. Basal cell adenocarcinoma appears to be a low-grade, favorable malignancy that must be distinguished from more aggressive salivary neoplasms such as adenoid cystic carcinoma on the one hand and basal cell adenoma on the other hand.

The central portions of a basal cell adenocarcinoma are usually indistinguishable from a basal cell adenoma, and the critical diagnostic feature for the former is the presence of an infiltrative growth pattern (Fig. 20.63). The lesion may be partially encapsulated, but at least focal invasion into the adjacent salivary gland, often with "cancerization" of adjacent acini (Fig. 20.64), perineural invasion, and intravascular growth (Fig. 20.65) signify that the tumor is malignant. Thus, distinction of this lesion from basal cell adenoma is not possible on fine-needle aspiration. Although any of the growth patterns seen in basal cell adenoma may be encountered in the corresponding adenocarcinoma, in our experience with perhaps a dozen of these cases, almost all were of the "solid" type, often with cen-

tral areas of abrupt keratinization. It should be remembered that the membranous pattern of basal cell adenoma may be multifocal without a well-formed capsule, but this pattern lacks true destructive invasion, acinar cancerization, and vascular or perineural invasion. Occasional basal cell adenocarcinomas will show more nuclear pleomorphism and mitotic figures than a

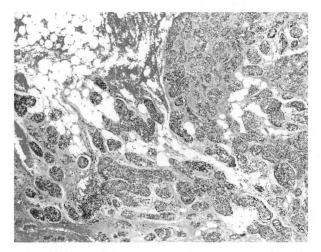

Figure 20.63. Basal cell adenocarcinoma differs from basal cell adenoma by lacking encapsulation and demonstrating invasion into adjacent tissues.

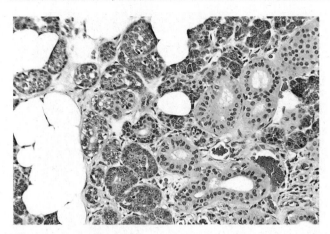

Figure 20.64. Basal cell adenocarcinoma exhibiting "cancerization" of salivary acini at the infiltrating edges of the lesion.

basal cell adenoma, but these features cannot be counted on to be present. Immunohistochemistry and electron microscopy do not aid in distinguishing basal cell adenoma from basal cell adenocarcinoma (153). These tumors express many of the same markers (e.g., KIT, etc.) seen in adenoid cystic carcinoma. Ductal and myoepithelial cells are prominent in both.

Distinction of this variant of adenocarcinoma from adenoid cystic carcinoma is based on morphologic features. Adenoid cystic carcinoma lacks the biphasic appearance with more basaloid peripheral palisaded cells and larger central cells, often with keratinization. Basal cell adenocarcinoma lacks well-formed cribriform spaces with extracellular mucin in pseudocystic spaces. Both tumors may have sclerotic stroma and perineural invasion, although the degree of the latter is typically much more prominent in adenoid cystic carcinoma.

ONCOCYTIC CARCINOMA

Oncocytic carcinoma is a rare, often aggressive, infiltrative neoplasm (Fig. 20.66). As in oncocytoma, the tumor cells have abundant granular eosinophilic cytoplasm as a result of numerous mitochondria. The nuclei may be enlarged, hyperchromatic, and pleomorphic, but we have also encountered examples in which the cells exhibited no significant cytologic atypia, yet the

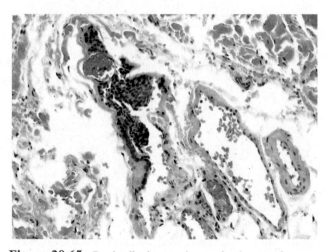

Figure 20.65. Basal cell adenocarcinoma showing vascular space invasion.

tumor had produced regional metastases (154–158). In our experience, these tumors are often multinodular, with the nodules separated by dense fibrous stroma. Destructive invasion of adjacent acini may be seen, along with perineural and vascular permeation. Several potential pitfalls merit brief discussion. First, this is a diagnosis of exclusion because acinic cell carcinomas, mucoepidermoid carcinomas, and, less commonly, other salivary gland carcinomas may have prominent oncocytic components. The tumors should be thoroughly sampled to exclude these elements. Second, care should be taken not to overinterpret salivary gland inclusions with oncocytic metaplasia in periparotid lymph nodes as metastatic disease. Finally, as discussed earlier, oncocytomas may occur in the setting of multifocal oncocytic metaplasia. These should not be misinterpreted as infiltrative growth.

SEBACEOUS CARCINOMA

Sebaceous carcinoma is a rare neoplasm. These carcinomas are easy to distinguish from much more common sebaceous adenomas because of their invariably pleomorphic tumor cells with clear invasion into adjacent structures (Fig. 20.67). Most are located in the parotid, presenting clinically as a painful mass with facial nerve paralysis (159). The tumors vary in size from less than 1 cm to approximately 6 cm. The treatment often requires total parotidectomy and involves sacrificing the facial nerve coupled with adjuvant radiation therapy. The mean survival time is approximately 5 years (160,161).

MYOEPITHELIAL CARCINOMA

Myoepithelial carcinoma, the malignant counterpart of myoepithelioma, is a rare neoplasm that occurs primarily in the parotid gland. The mean age of patients is 55 years. It is characterized grossly by multinodularity, necrosis, and lack of encapsulation. The histologic hallmarks of malignancy are cytologic atypia and infiltration into adjacent structures. Myoepithelial carcinoma is composed of varying proportions of spindled, epithelioid, plasmacytoid, and clear cells set against a mucoid or myxoid background (Fig. 20.68). The majority of the tumor should express myoepithelial differentiation by either immunohistochemistry or electron microscopy. Myoepithelial carcinomas have varied clinical outcomes, and they are fully capable of resulting in local recurrence, distant metastases (Fig. 20.69), and tumor-related death. Wide excision is the mode of treatment.

In our experience, these tumors have a predominantly spindle cell pattern, although plasmacytoid variants may also be encountered (Fig. 20.68). Immunohistochemical confirmation is almost invariably required to confirm myoepithelial differentiation and exclude other mesenchymal neoplasms. The antibody panel used also should include epithelial markers (e.g., cytokeratin, EMA, etc.). Any ductal differentiation, either by light microscopy or immunohistochemistry, should lead to strong consideration of an epithelial-myoepithelial carcinoma. Lesions with prominent clear cells initially considered to represent myoepithelial carcinomas are often epithelial-myoepithelial carcinomas with areas of myoepithelial overgrowth.

LYMPHOEPITHELIOMA-LIKE UNDIFFERENTIATED CARCINOMA

The parotid or, less commonly, the submandibular gland may give rise to an undifferentiated carcinoma that is morphologically indistinguishable from a nasopharyngeal "lymphoepithelioma" (Fig. 20.70) (162–164). Origin in minor salivary gland

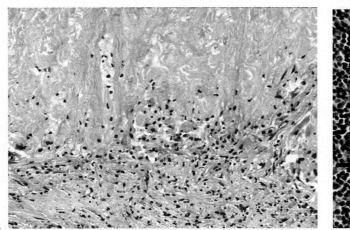
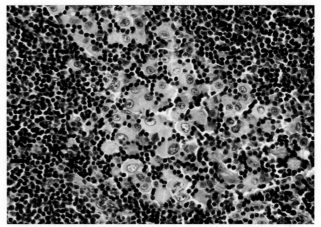

Figure 20.66. This oncocytic carcinoma exhibited extensive necrosis with only a few viable cells present at the edges of the primary tumor **(A)**. The associated lymph node metastasis showed more obvious viable tumor **(B)**.

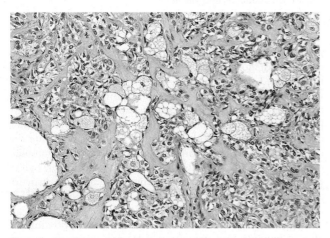

Figure 20.67. Sebaceous carcinoma. The tumor is composed of irregular nests of moderately pleomorphic sebaceous cells with conspicuously clear, finely vacuolated cytoplasm.

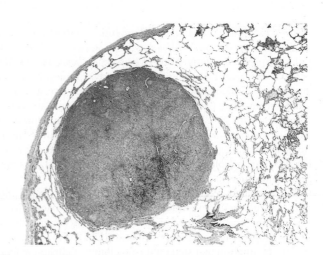

Figure 20.69. Metastatic myoepithelial carcinoma involving the lung.

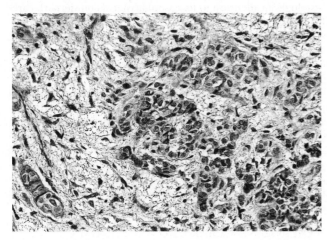

Figure 20.68. Myoepithelial carcinoma. The plasmacytoid cells appear in a myxoid background.

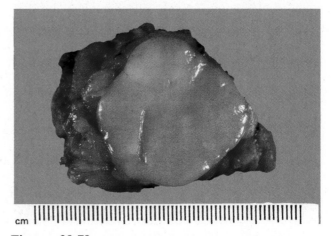

Figure 20.70. Undifferentiated, lymphoepithelioma-like carcinoma of the parotid gland. The tumor has sharply demarcated margins and grossly resembles a lymphoma.

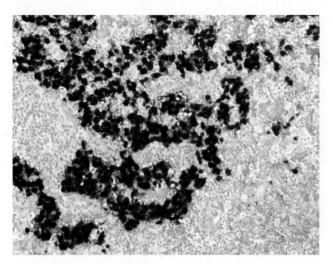

Figure 20.71. Undifferentiated, lymphoepithelioma-like carcinoma shows extensive Epstein-Barr virus RNA by in situ hybridization in the large neoplastic epithelial cells (blue staining).

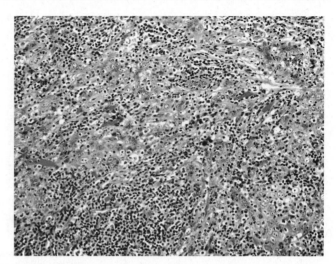

Figure 20.73. The neoplastic cells of undifferentiated, lymphoepithelioma-like carcinoma have large, vesicular, but relatively uniform nuclei. Mitotic figures are typically easily identified. Cell borders are indistinct. The epithelial cells are mixed in a complex fashion with the reactive lymphoplasmacytic elements.

tissue is extremely rare (165). Although the confusing term of *malignant lymphoepithelial lesion* has been applied to these tumors, we prefer the designation of *lymphoepithelioma-like undifferentiated carcinoma.* This tumor is particularly common in Asians and native Alaskan Eskimos (163) but can involve any geoethnic group. The patients range in age from teenagers to the elderly. As with its nasopharyngeal counterpart, this tumor is strongly associated with EBV, as can often be demonstrated by in situ hybridization (Fig. 20.71). There is no clear-cut relationship between this neoplasm and chronic sialadenitis (BLL) or Sjögren syndrome.

On histologic examination, the normal salivary acini and ducts are replaced by a diffuse reactive lymphoplasmacytic infiltrate admixed with neoplastic epithelial cells occurring singly or in multiple epithelial islands and nests (Fig. 20.72). Although initial examination may suggest the possibility of chronic sialadenitis (BLL), on closer inspection, the nests are larger, more irregular, and often coalescent, unlike the much smaller epimy-

oepithelial islands of chronic sialadenitis. At higher magnification, the neoplastic cells are clearly malignant with considerably enlarged but morphologically and chromatically uniform, ovoid to elongated vesicular nuclei and variably prominent nucleoli (Fig. 20.73). When present in nests, the cells have indistinct borders such that the vesicular nuclei appear to float in a cytoplasmic syncytium. Variable numbers of lymphocytes, plasma cells, and occasionally other inflammatory cells permeate the cell nests. Mitotic figures, including atypical forms, are numerous. Perineural invasion can be found in approximately half of cases (162). Tonofilaments may be demonstrated ultrastructurally, but squamous or glandular differentiation is completely absent at the light microscopic level.

Regional lymph node metastases develop in approximately 40% of patients, and systemic metastases develop in approximately 20% (162). Reported overall mortality rates have ranged from 17% to 86%, but prognosis appears to be better than initially thought. Some patients in initial series may have had nasopharyngeal carcinomas with salivary gland metastases, the prognosis for which is quite poor. Indeed, because this tumor is histologically identical to its nasopharyngeal counterpart, careful clinical evaluation is mandatory to rule out the presence of a primary nasopharyngeal carcinoma (166). It has also been suggested that this tumor may follow a more aggressive clinical course in Eskimos compared with Asians and other geo-ethnic groups (162).

In addition to the distinction from BLL and metastatic nasopharyngeal carcinoma, consideration should be given to the possibility of a large-cell lymphoma. We have encountered large B-cell lymphomas involving the parotid gland as coalescent aggregates of cells that were virtually indistinguishable from the cell nests of undifferentiated carcinoma (see Fig. 20.83). Appropriate lymphoid markers (e.g., CD20, CD3, LCA, etc.), along with broad-spectrum epithelial markers (e.g., cytokeratins, EMA), will allow for this clinically important distinction (Fig. 20.74).

HYALINIZING CLEAR-CELL CARCINOMA

This low-grade malignancy has a predilection to arise in the oral cavity, especially in the base of the tongue, of adult women

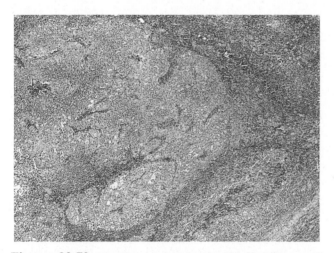

Figure 20.72. Undifferentiated, lymphoepithelioma-like carcinoma. A large component of tumor (*left*) is surrounded by a brisk lymphoplasmacytic reaction (*right*).

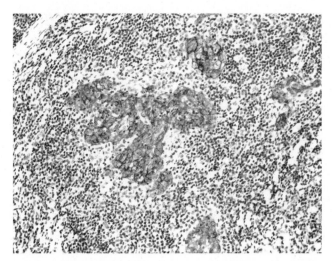

Figure 20.74. Cytokeratin confirms the epithelial nature of the neoplastic cells in undifferentiated, lymphoepithelioma-like carcinoma.

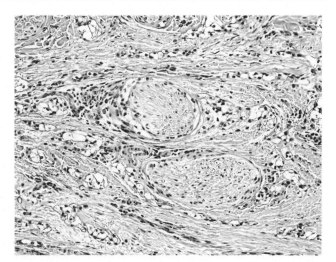

Figure 20.76. Hyalinizing clear-cell carcinoma exhibiting prominent perineural invasion.

(167). Histologically, it is composed of broad hyaline bands in the stroma and infiltrating nests or cords of monomorphous clear cells containing cytoplasmic glycogen (Fig. 20.75). Perineural invasion is readily identified (Fig. 20.76), but vascular invasion is not seen. Myoepithelial differentiation is lacking immunohistochemically. Local recurrences may follow incomplete excision, and occasional patients have developed regional lymph node metastases. The classic lesion has not, thus far, been associated with mortality. However, O'Regan et al. (168) described an otherwise typical case with minor foci of high-grade carcinoma, and that patient followed an aggressive course with widespread metastases and death within 1 year of diagnosis.

SMALL-CELL UNDIFFERENTIATED (NEUROENDOCRINE) CARCINOMA

Small-cell undifferentiated carcinoma (SCUC) represents approximately 1% to 2% of all salivary gland tumors. Patients are typically in the fourth to sixth decades of life, and slightly more men than women are affected. SCUC involving the larynx, sinonasal region, oral cavity, or pharynx is often thought to arise from minor salivary glands, but mucosal origin is difficult to exclude. Origin within major salivary glands, usually the parotid gland, is much easier to document (Figs. 20.77 and 20.78).

On histologic examination, the tumors resemble oat cell carcinoma of the lung. Sheets, strands, and nests of oval tumor cells with hyperchromatic, coarsely granular nuclei and scant cytoplasm are seen (Fig. 20.78). The mitotic rate is high, vascular and perineural invasion are common, and large areas of infarct-like intralesional necrosis are often present. The typical crush artifact that is characteristic of pulmonary oat cell carcinomas is less often observed in the salivary gland lesions. In our experience, these tumors are often associated with a better differentiated neoplastic component.

Although not strictly required for the diagnosis, neuroendocrine differentiation can typically be demonstrated in salivary SCUC based on immunoreactivity for chromogranin, synapto-

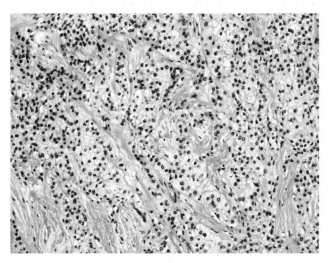

Figure 20.75. Hyalinizing clear-cell carcinoma with variably sized nests and cords of polygonal to round tumors cells. The cytoplasm is clear with a periodic acid-Schiff–positive staining reaction but without mucin production.

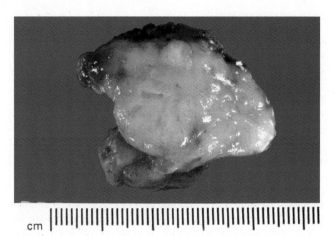

Figure 20.77. Small-cell undifferentiated (neuroendocrine) carcinoma has a soft fleshy gross appearance, similar to that of lymphoma. In larger tumors, areas of necrosis and hemorrhage are common.

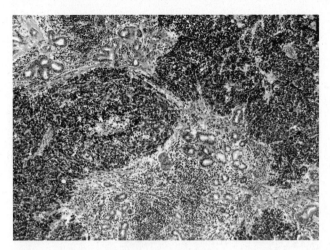

Figure 20.78. Small-cell undifferentiated (neuroendocrine) carcinoma is composed of closely packed cells with granular chromatin and scant cytoplasm. The tumor infiltrates residual parotid gland ducts and acini.

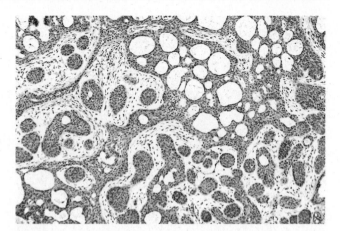

Figure 20.79. Sialoblastoma or embryoma. The tumor forms sheets of basaloid cells with focal ductal differentiation. The tumor cells are uniform without mitotic figures or pleomorphism.

physin, neuron-specific enolase, or CD57 (169–174). Ultrastructural examination will demonstrate sparse neurosecretory granules.

Patients with salivary SCUC have a better chance of survival than do patients with analogous pulmonary neoplasms. Regional lymph node metastases are less common in salivary SCUC than in their pulmonary counterpart. The estimated 2- and 5-year survival rates for salivary SCUC are 70% and 46%, respectively. This relatively good survival, coupled with an approximately 75% positivity rate for CK20, has led to the suggestion that most salivary SCUCs are Merkel-like carcinomas with a similar prognosis (175,176). CK20-negative tumors may have worse prognosis (175).

Isolated examples of large-cell neuroendocrine carcinoma of the salivary glands have been reported. Nagao et al. (174) described two patients, both of whom ultimately died of disease. The histologic features were identical to those of pulmonary large-cell neuroendocrine carcinoma.

SIALOBLASTOMA

Sialoblastoma (salivary embryoma) is a rare congenital or perinatal salivary gland tumor with fewer than three dozen reported cases (177), although some additional cases may have been described under such terms as *congenital basal cell adenoma*. Sialoblastoma is composed of primitive basaloid or epithelioid cells in a ductular, organoid, or cribriform pattern within a fibrous or partly myxoid stroma (Fig. 20.79). Mitotic figures and occasional necrosis can impart a worrisome histologic picture. Conservative surgical management is advocated for this tumor (178). In one series of seven patients seen in consultation and probably biased toward problematic examples, three patients experienced recurrence, and one developed pulmonary metastases (177). Features associated with more benign behavior included semi-encapsulation and cytologically benign basaloid cells with intervening stroma (177). Unfavorable features included anaplastic basaloid cells, minimal stroma, and pushing or infiltrative invasion at the periphery of the tumor (177).

CRIBRIFORM ADENOCARCINOMA

This recently described entity occurs in the tongue. Microscopically, it resembles the solid and follicular variants of papillary thyroid carcinoma. The tumor cells have overlapping nuclei with a ground-glass quality, but they are negative for thyroglobulin (179).

HIGH-GRADE PAPILLARY CYSTADENOCARCINOMA

This rare tumor arises in the major salivary gland, but it has also been reported in the lip, palate, buccal mucosa, and tongue (180). It seems likely that this entity is now better interpreted as an *intraductal carcinoma* (see "Salivary Duct Carcinoma" section earlier in this chapter).

ADENOCARCINOMA NOT OTHERWISE SPECIFIED

The various otherwise unclassified adenocarcinomas represent approximately 4% to 9% of all major salivary gland neoplasms (181). This proportion has decreased with the recognition of subtypes that used to fall into this category (e.g., salivary duct carcinoma, polymorphous low-grade carcinoma, epithelial-myoepithelial carcinoma, etc.) (182). These unclassified adenocarcinomas are a heterogeneous group exhibiting clinical behaviors ranging from relatively low grade to virulently aggressive.

High-grade variants may be composed of small, irregular glands lined by clearly malignant cells with variable eosinophilic cytoplasm (Fig. 20.80). The stroma in such cases is typically abundant, rich in collagen, and often hyalinized. Tumors with this appearance resemble so-called scirrhous carcinoma of the breast, and we suspect that these are salivary duct carcinomas in which the more typical ductlike pattern was not sampled or was overgrown by the more infiltrative tumor. Mucin-producing adenocarcinomas may contain large pools of extracellular mucin or may exhibit prominent signet ring cells. Some of these may represent examples of the mucin-rich variant of salivary duct carcinoma lacking more diagnostic areas. In other tumors, a papillary growth pattern with or without mucin production is featured (Fig. 20.81). Trabecular or solid adenocarcinomas lacking clear-cut gland formation may also been seen.

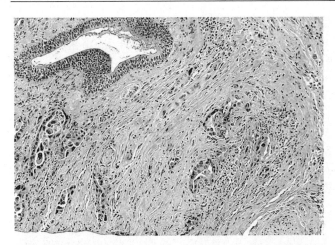

Figure 20.80. High-grade adenocarcinoma with irregular infiltrating glandular structures and cords of tumor cells.

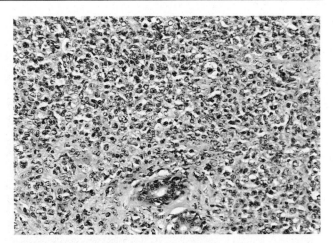

Figure 20.82. Diffuse large-cell lymphoma with poorly cohesive cells around the salivary ducts.

Although this category is shrinking with the recognition of new tumors and their variants, this remains a viable diagnosis and probably always will. It is certainly preferable to inappropriately "pigeonholing" unusual-appearing tumors into a more definitive category. In particular, care should be taken to avoid labeling a nonspecific-appearing carcinoma as an acinic cell carcinoma if it lacks the characteristic features of that tumor.

MALIGNANT LYMPHOMA

In most instances, lymphomas associated with salivary glands arise from intraglandular or periglandular lymph nodes. The subtypes and biologic behaviors of these tumors are those of nodal lymphomas in general, and they are discussed in the chapter on lymph nodes. A lymphoma of salivary parenchymal origin is less common (183–186). These lymphomas may arise in salivary glands without any pre-existent diseases, or they may accompany other disease conditions, such as chronic lymphadenitis, Sjögren disease, chronic sclerosing sialadenitis (Kuttner tumor), or Warthin tumor. Overall, lymphomas represent approximately 1% to 4% of all salivary gland neoplasms (187,188).

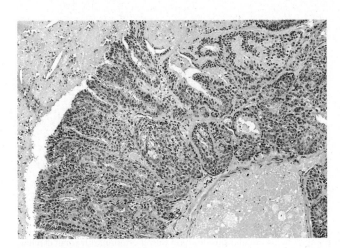

Figure 20.81. High-grade papillary adenocarcinoma with cystic spaces and slender projections.

The parotid gland is the most commonly involved site, and the submandibular gland is affected in approximately 15% of cases. The peak age of occurrence is in the sixth to seventh decades of life.

Lymphomas arising within the salivary parenchyma fall into two broad categories: lymph node–type lymphomas and MALT (marginal zone) lymphomas. Nodal-type B-cell lymphomas are primarily either follicular lymphomas (35%) or diffuse large B-cell lymphomas (30%) (Fig. 20.82). Approaches to the diagnosis of these tumors are reviewed in the lymph node chapter. Although the diagnosis of large B-cell lymphoma is typically straightforward in the salivary glands, we have encountered occasional examples in which the lymphoid cells formed cohesive aggregates that were indistinguishable from the cell nests of lymphoepithelioma-like undifferentiated carcinoma (Fig. 20.83).

Salivary MALT lymphomas often arise in a setting of pre-existent Sjögren disease. Broad strands of marginal zone or monocytoid B cells around lymphoepithelial lesions and monotypic Ig detection by immunohistochemistry are considered diagnostic of MALT lymphoma (Fig. 20.84) (3). These tumors have an excellent long-term prognosis, although they may recur after a protracted interval and can also involve the contralateral gland and other anatomic sites. Primary plasmacytoma or Hodgkin disease of the salivary glands is extremely rare. Occasional T-cell lymphomas may arise in this location. Recently we have seen several examples of senile EBV-associated B-cell lymphoproliferative disorder in the region of the parotid gland (189). These were characterized by extensive necrosis, a polymorphous infiltrate not readily identifiable as neoplastic, and only scattered atypical immunoblast-like cells. Rare granulomas were present, raising the issue of a mycobacterial or fungal infection. In situ hybridization for EBV RNA was strongly positive.

The prognosis of lymphoma arising in the salivary gland is generally agreed to be more favorable than that arising in nodal sites (186,190). This is probably related to the frequently encountered nodular growth pattern or the low-grade histology and the initially low stage of the lymphoma at the time of diagnosis. To establish a suspected diagnosis of a salivary gland lymphoma, the clinician should preferably examine not only a biopsy of the salivary gland but also the adjacent lymph nodes. Ideally, fresh tissue should also be sent for flow cytometry.

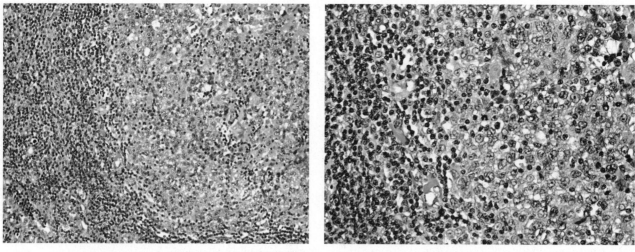

Figure 20.83. This large B-cell lymphoma of the parotid gland formed cohesive nests of neoplastic cells distinct from a surrounding population of small lymphocytes (**A**). Cytologically, the neoplastic cells were very similar to those of lymphoepithelioma-like carcinoma (**B**). Distinction required immunohistochemistry.

BENIGN STROMAL NEOPLASMS

VASCULAR LESIONS

Most vascular tumors arising in salivary glands are hemangiomas. They usually affect the parotid glands of newborns and infants, but they may involve any salivary gland and can occasionally occur in adults (191,192). Half of the parotid tumors in infancy are hemangiomas; girls are affected more often than boys (193–195). The tumors usually arise in the superficial lobe of the parotid, imparting a blue tinge to the overlying skin. In infants, these are often capillary proliferations with prominent increased cellularity and a high mitotic rate (Fig. 20.85). These features, coupled with invasion-like extension into adjacent structures, may lead to confusion with angiosarcoma. The term *benign infantile hemangioendothelioma* (196) has been applied to these tumors. Most congenital and infantile tumors regress spontaneously after approximately 1 year. In older patients, the tumors may be of cavernous type. Phleboliths and thrombosis may be associated with the enlarged vascular spaces.

Salivary gland lymphangiomas are much rarer than hemangiomas (197,198). The soft, jellylike tumors predominantly infiltrate the periglandular soft tissues, especially those inferior to the parotid glands or the submandibular salivary glands, but they also involve the gland itself. Cystic lymphangiomas may also occur (199).

LIPOMA

Most salivary gland lipomas arise in the parotid, and only very rarely can one be found involving the submandibular salivary gland (Fig. 20.86). Salivary gland lipoma appears most frequently during the fifth and sixth decades of life (200,201). In contrast to lipomatous infiltration or lipomatosis, a lipoma is an encapsulated tumor. On gross examination, lipomas are soft

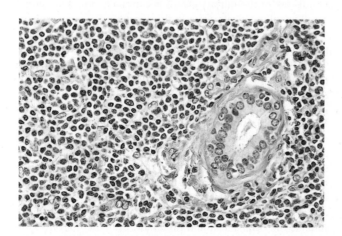

Figure 20.84. Mucosa-associated lymphoid tissue lymphoma composed of monocytoid B cells.

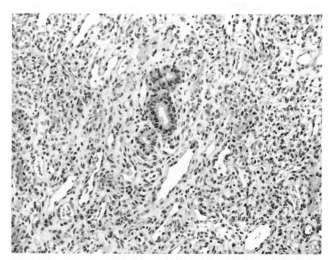

Figure 20.85. Benign infantile hemangioma the parotid gland as a highly cellular vascular proliferation with predominantly small capillary lumina. Mitotic figures are often readily apparent at higher magnification.

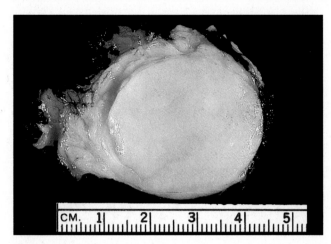

Figure 20.86. Lipoma of the parotid gland forms as a well-circumscribed, bright yellow mass.

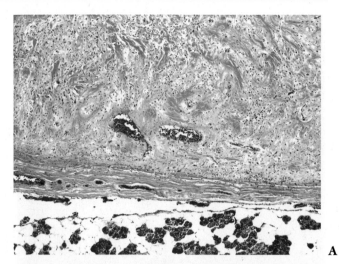

and yellow, and clinically, they may be confused with a Warthin tumor. They grow by lesional tissue expansion, displacing the glandular parenchyma; therefore, surgical removal is easy and complete. Lipomatosis is associated with diabetes, cirrhosis, chronic alcoholism, malnutrition, and hormonal disturbance (202).

BENIGN PERIPHERAL NERVE SHEATH TUMOR

Schwannomas (neurilemomas) (Fig. 20.87) and neurofibromas rarely involve the salivary glands (203,204). The clinical complaint is usually a slowly enlarging parotid mass without functional abnormality. Although the lesion may be closely associated with a branch of the facial nerve, if it is encapsulated (schwannoma) and does not invade the nerve, it may be resected with nerve sparing.

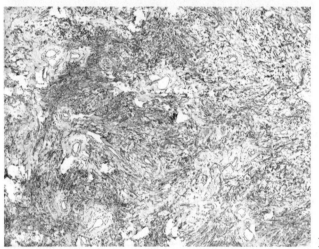

Figure 20.88. Solitary fibrous tumor forms an encapsulated densely fibrotic mass within the parotid gland **(A)**. The tumor cells are strongly positive for CD34 **(B)**.

SOLITARY FIBROUS TUMOR

Solitary fibrous tumors continue to be described throughout the body, including the salivary glands (Fig. 20.88) (205). These tumors often have a distinctly hemangiopericytoma-like appearance, and undoubtedly, some tumors reported as salivary hemangiopericytomas, before recognition of solitary fibrous tumor, represent examples of the latter entity (206–208). Immunohistochemical studies with CD34 and smooth muscle markers should aid in the differential diagnosis.

SARCOMAS OF SALIVARY GLANDS

Sarcomas involving salivary glands and immediately adjacent soft tissues are extremely rare, but multiple variants have been reported (Fig. 20.89) (209–211). Malignant peripheral nerve sheath tumors, fibrosarcomas (210), Ewing sarcomas, synovial sarcomas, angiosarcomas (212), and others have been reported. Immunohistochemistry is mandatory to rule out the possibility that some of these spindle cell or pleomorphic malignant neo-

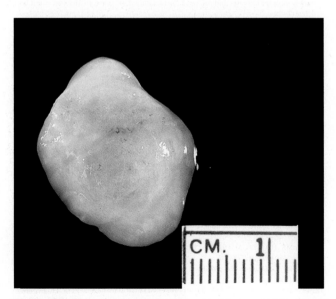

Figure 20.87. Benign peripheral nerve sheath tumor of the parotid gland. The tumor has well-defined margins and a glistening, lobulated, light yellow cut surface.

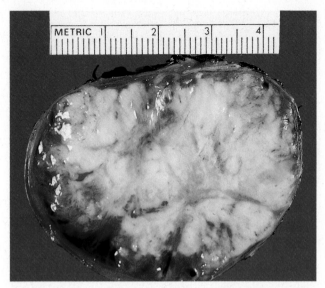

Figure 20.89. Undifferentiated sarcoma ("malignant fibrous histiocytoma") of the submandibular gland. The tumor has virtually replaced the entire gland, and extensive necrosis and hemorrhage are present.

plasms are not spindle cell (sarcomatoid) carcinomas, myoepithelial carcinomas, or malignant melanomas.

METASTATIC LESIONS

The parotid parenchyma, the intraparotid lymph nodes, or, less frequently, the submandibular gland can harbor a metastatic tumor (213). Primary tumors from the head and neck region account for two-thirds of these cases, of which 60% are squamous carcinomas and 15% are melanomas (Fig. 20.90) (214). Distant primary sites include the lung, kidney, breast, and colon. Metastatic renal carcinoma is part of the differential diagnosis when the pathologist is faced with a clear-cell malignancy (Fig.

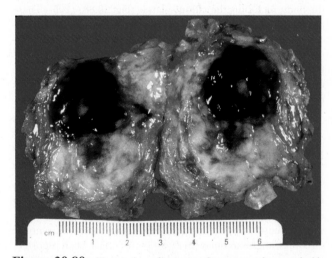

Figure 20.90. Metastatic malignant melanoma produces a darkly pigmented mass within the parotid gland.

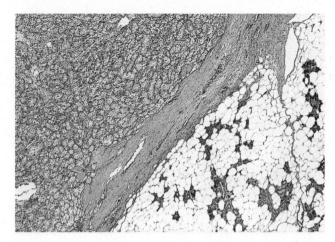

Figure 20.91. Metastatic renal cell carcinoma in the parotid gland.

20.91) (215). In select cases, the appropriate use of immunohistochemical stains can greatly aid in the diagnosis of metastatic lesions.

REFERENCES

1. Morton RP, Bartley JR. Simple sublingual ranulas: pathogenesis and management. *J Otolaryngol* 1995;24:253–254.
2. Batsakis JG, McClatchey KD. Cervical ranulas. *Ann Otol Rhinol Laryngol* 1988;97:561–562.
3. Harris NL. Lymphoid proliferations of the salivary glands. *Am J Clin Pathol* 1999;111:S94–S103.
4. Maiorano E, Favia G, Viale G. Lymphoepithelial cysts of salivary glands: an immunohistochemical study of HIV-related and HIV-unrelated lesions. *Hum Pathol* 1998;29:260–265.
5. Smith BC, Ellis GL, Slater LJ, et al. Sclerosing polycystic adenosis of major salivary glands. A clinicopathologic analysis of nine cases. *Am J Surg Pathol* 1996;20:161–170.
6. Gnepp DR, Wang LJ, Brandwein-Gensler M, et al. Sclerosing polycystic adenosis of the salivary gland: a report of 16 case. *Am J Surg Pathol* 2006;30:154–164.
7. Skalova A, Gnepp DR, Simpson RH, et al. Clonal nature of sclerosing polycystic adenosis of salivary glands demonstrated by using the polymorphism of the human androgen receptor (HUMARA) locus as a marker. *Am J Surg Pathol* 2006;30:939–944.
8. Pieterse AS, Seymour AE. Parotid cysts. An analysis of 16 cases and suggested classification. *Pathology* 1981;13:225–234.
9. Brannon RB, Fowler CB, Hartman KS. Necrotizing sialometaplasia. A clinicopathologic study of sixty-nine cases and review of the literature. *Oral Surg Oral Med Oral Pathol* 1991;72:317–325.
10. Werning JT. Infectious and systemic diseases. In Ellis GL, Auclair PL, Gnepp DR, eds. *Surgical Pathology of the Salivary Glands.* Philadelphia, PA: Saunders, 1991:50.
11. Chann JK. Kuttner tumor (chronic sclerosing sialadenitis) of the submandibular gland: an underrecognized entity. *Adv Anat Pathol* 1998;5:239–251.
12. Cheuk W, Chan JK. Advances in salivary gland pathology. *Histopathology* 2007;51:1–20.
13. Ochoa ER, Harris NL, Pilch BZ. Marginal zone B-cell lymphoma of the salivary gland arising in chronic sclerosing sialadenitis (Kuttner tumor). *Am J Surg Pathol* 2001;25:1546–1550.
14. Watkinson JC, Hornung EA, Fagg NLK. Cat-scratch disease: an unusual cause of parotid pain (a case report and literature review). *J Laryngol Otol* 1988;102:562–564.
15. Fox RI, Robinson CA, Curd JG, et al. Sjögren's syndrome. Proposed criteria for classification. *Arthritis Rheum* 1986;29:577–585.
16. Carbone A, Gloghini A, Ferlito A. Pathological features of lymphoid proliferations of the salivary glands: lymphoepithelial sialadenitis versus low-grade B-cell lymphoma of the MALT type. *Ann Otol Rhinol Laryngol* 2000;109:1170–1175.
17. Greenspan J, Daniels T, Talal N, et al. The histopathology of Sjögren's syndrome in labial biopsies. *Oral Surg Oral Med Oral Pathol* 1974;37:217–230.
18. Lee M, Rutka JA, Slomovic AR, et al. Establishing guidelines for the role of minor salivary gland biopsy in clinical practice for Sjögren's syndrome. *J Rheumatol* 1998;25:247–253.
19. Daniels TE. Salivary histopathology in diagnosis of Sjögren's syndrome. *Scand J Rheumatol* 1986;61:36–43.
20. Ahn MS, Hayashi GM, Hilsinger RL, et al. Familial mixed tumors of the parotid gland. *Head Neck* 1999;21:772–775.
21. Batsakis JG. Heterotopic and accessory salivary tissues. *Ann Otol Rhinol Laryngol* 1986;95:434–435.
22. Leverstein H, van der Wal JE, Tiwari RM, et al. Surgical management of 246 previously untreated pleomorphic adenomas of the parotid gland. *Br J Surg* 1997;84:399–403.
23. McGurk M, Renehan A, Gleave EN, et al. Clinical significance of the tumour capsule in the treatment of parotid pleomorphic adenomas. *Br J Surg* 1996;83:1747–1749.
24. Erlandson RA, Cordon-Cardo C, Higgins PJ. Histogenesis of benign pleomorphic ade-

noma (mixed tumor) of the major salivary glands: an ultrastructural and immunohisto-chemical study. *Am J Surg Pathol* 1984;8:803–820.

25. Kahn HJ, Baumal R, Marks A, et al. Myoepithelial cells in salivary gland tumors: an immu-nohistochemical study. *Arch Pathol Lab Med* 1985;109:190–195.

26. Buchner A, David R, Hansen LS. "Hyaline cells" in pleomorphic adenoma of salivary gland origin. *Oral Surg Oral Med Oral Pathol* 1981;52:506–512.

27. Roijer E, Kas K, Van de Ven W, et al. Mapping of the 8q12 translocation breakpoint to a 40-kb region in a pleomorphic adenoma with an ins (8;3) (q12;p21.3p14.1). *Cytogenet Cell Genet* 1997;76:23–26.

28. Gillenwater A, Hurr K, Wolf P, et al. Microsatellite alterations at chromosome 8q loci in pleomorphic adenoma. *Otolaryngol Head Neck Surg* 1997;117:448–452.

29. Pinkston JA, Cole P. Cigarette smoking and Warthin's tumor. *Am J Epidemiol* 1996;144: 183–187.

30. Yoo GH, Eisele DW, Askin FB, et al. Warthin's tumor: a 40-year experience at the Johns Hopkins hospital. *Laryngoscope* 1994;104:799–803.

31. Lamelas J, Terry JH, Alfonso AE. Warthin's tumor: multicentricity and increasing inci-dence in women. *Am J Surg* 1987;154:347–351.

32. Eveson JW, Cawson RA. Warthin's tumor (cystadenolymphoma) of salivary glands. A clini-copathologic investigation of 278 cases. *Oral Surg Oral Med Oral Pathol* 1986;61:256–262.

33. Damjanov I, Sneff EM, Delerme AN. Squamous cell carcinoma arising in Warthin's tumor of the parotid gland. A light, electron microscopic, and immunohistochemical study. *Oral Surg Oral Med Oral Pathol* 1983;55:286–289.

34. Martins C, Fonseca I, Roque L, et al. Cytogenetic characterisation of Warthin's tumour. *Oral Oncol* 1997;33:344–347.

35. Kratochvil FJ. Canalicular adenoma and basal cell adenoma. In Ellis GL, Auclair PL, Gnepp DR, eds. *Surgical Pathology of the Salivary Glands*. Philadelphia, PA: Saunders, 1991: 202–224.

36. Headington JT, Batsakis JG, Beals TF, et al. Membranous basal cell adenoma of the par-otid, dermal cylindromas, and trichoepitheliomas. Comparative histochemistry and ultra-structure. *Cancer* 1977;39:2460–2469.

37. Batsakis JG, Brannon RB. Dermal analogue tumours of major salivary glands. *J Laryngol Otol* 1981;95:155–164.

38. Ferreiro JA. Immunohistochemistry of basal cell adenoma of the major salivary glands. *Histopathology* 1994;24:539–542.

39. Ferreiro JA. Immunohistochemical analysis of salivary gland canalicular adenoma. *Oral Surg Oral Med Oral Pathol* 1994;78:761–765.

40. Brandwein MS, Huvos AG. Oncocytic tumors of major salivary glands. A study of 68 cases with follow-up of 44 patients. *Am J Surg Pathol* 1991;15:514–528.

41. Davy CL, Dardick I, Hammond E, et al. Relationship of clear cell oncocytoma to mitochon-drial-rich (typical) oncocytomas of parotid salivary gland. An ultrastructural study. *Oral Surg Oral Med Oral Pathol* 1994;77:469–479.

42. Seifert G. Classification and differential diagnosis of clear and basal cell tumors of the salivary glands. *Semin Diagn Pathol* 1996;13:95–103.

43. Johns ME, Regezi JA, Batsakis JG. Oncocytic neoplasms of salivary glands: an ultrastruc-tural study. *Laryngoscope* 1977;87:862–871.

44. Blank C, Eneroth CM, Jakobsson PA. Oncocytoma of the parotid gland: neoplasm or nodular hyperplasia? *Cancer* 1970;25:919–925.

45. Ghandur-Mnaymneh L. Multinodular oncocytoma of the parotid gland: a benign lesion simulating malignancy. *Hum Pathol* 1984;15:485–486.

46. Srensen M, Baunsgaard P, Fredriksen P, et al. Multifocal adenomatous oncocytic hyperpla-sia of the parotid gland (unusual clear cell variant in two female siblings). *Pathol Res Pract* 1986;181:254–259.

47. Luna MA, Mackay B, Gamez-Araujo J. Myoepithelioma of the palate. Report of a case with histochemical and electron microscopic observations. *Cancer* 1973;32:1429–1435.

48. Chaudhry AP, Satchidanand S, Peer R, et al. Myoepithelial cell adenoma of the parotid gland: a light and ultrastructural study. *Cancer* 1982;49:288–293.

49. Sciubba JJ, Brannon RB. Myoepithelioma of salivary glands: report of 23 cases. *Cancer* 1982;49:562–572.

50. Chaudhry AP, Cutler IS, Satchidanand S, et al. Glycogen-rich tumor of the oral minor salivary glands. A histochemical and ultrastructural study. *Cancer* 1983;52:105–111.

51. Franquemont DW, Mills SE. Plasmacytoid monomorphic adenoma of salivary glands. Ab-sence of myogenous differentiation and comparison to spindle cell myoepithelioma. *Am J Surg Pathol* 1993;17:146–153.

52. Pageaut G, Opperman A, Carbillet JP. "Sebaceous" metaplasia of the normal, inflamma-tory and tumorous parotid gland. *Anat Pathol* 1969;17:101–105.

53. Wasan SM. Sebaceous lymphadenoma of the parotid gland. *Cancer* 1971;28:1019–1022.

54. Baratz M, Loewenthal M, Rozin M. Sebaceous lymphadenoma of the gland. *Arch Pathol Lab Med* 1976;100:269–270.

55. Batsakis JG, el-Naggar AK. Sebaceous lesions of salivary glands and oral cavity. *Ann Otol Rhinol Laryngol* 1990;99:416–418.

56. Brannon RB, Sciubba JJ, Giulani M. Ductal papillomas of salivary gland origin: a report of 19 cases and a review of the literature. *Oral Surg Oral Med Oral Pathol Oral Radiol Endod* 2001;92:68–77.

57. Ellis GL, Auclair PL. Ductal papillomas. In Ellis GL, Auclair PL, Gnepp DR, eds. *Surgical Pathology of the Salivary Glands*. Philadelphia, PA: Saunders, 1991:238–251.

58. Spiro RH, Huvos AG, Strong EW. Adenoid cystic carcinoma of salivary origin: a clinico-pathological study of 242 cases. *Am J Surg* 1974;128:512–520.

59. Spiro RH, Huvos AG, Strong EW. Adenoid cystic carcinoma: factors influencing survival. *Am J Surg* 1979;138:579–583.

60. Brookstone MS, Huvos AG. Central salivary gland tumors of the maxilla and mandible: a clinicopathologic study of 11 cases with an analysis of the literature. *J Oral Maxillofac Surg* 1992;50:229–236.

61. Brookstone M, Huvos AG, Spiro RH. Central adenoid cystic carcinoma of the mandible. *J Oral Maxillofac Surg* 1990;48:1329–1333.

62. Nochomovitz LE, Kahn LB. Adenoid cystic carcinoma of the salivary gland and its histo-logic variants. A clinicopathologic study of 30 cases. *Oral Surg* 1977;44:394–404.

63. Perzin KH, Gullane P, Clairmont AC. Adenoid cystic carcinoma arising in salivary glands. A correlation of histologic features and clinical course. *Cancer* 1978;42:265–282.

64. Santucci M, Bondi R. Histologic prognostic correlations in adenoid cystic carcinoma of major and minor salivary glands of the oral cavity. *Tumori* 1986;72:293–300.

65. Spiro RH, Huvos AG. Stage means more than grade in adenoid cystic carcinoma. *Am J Surg* 1992;164:623–628.

66. Nordgard S, Franzen G, Boysen M, et al. Ki-67 as a prognostic marker in adenoid cystic carcinoma assessed with the monoclonal antibody MIB1 in paraffin sections. *Laryngoscope* 1997;107:531–536.

67. Zhu QR, White FH, Tipoe GL. p53 oncoprotein accumulation in adenoid cystic carcinoma of parotid and palatine salivary glands. *Pathology* 1997;29:154–158.

68. Papadaki H, Finkelstein SD, Kounelis S, et al. The role of p53 mutation and protein expression in primary and recurrent adenoid cystic carcinoma. *Hum Pathol* 1996;27: 567–572.

69. Holst VA, Marshall CE, Moskaluk CA, et al. KIT protein expression and analysis of c-kit gene mutation in adenoid cystic carcinoma. *Mod Pathol* 1999;12:956–960.

70. Stewart FW, Foote FW, Becker WF. Muco-epidermoid tumors of salivary glands. *Ann Surg* 1945;122:820–844.

71. Eversole LR. Mucoepidermoid carcinomas: review of 815 reported cases. *J Oral Surg* 1970; 28:490–494.

72. Spiro RH, Huvos AG, Berk R, et al. Mucoepidermoid carcinoma of salivary gland origin. *Am J Surg* 1978;136:461–468.

73. Nascimento AG, Amaral LP, Prado LA, et al. Mucoepidermoid carcinoma of salivary glands: a clinicopathologic study of 46 cases. *Head Neck Surg* 1986;8:409–417.

74. Miura K, Ishimaru Y, Yoshimura T. Light and electron microscopic study of mucoepider-moid tumor of clear cell type. *Acta Pathol Jpn* 1986;36:1419–1427.

75. Ferreiro JA, Stylopoulos N. Oncocytic differentiation in salivary gland tumours. *J Laryngol Otol* 1995;109:569–571.

76. Hamed G, Shmookler BM, Ellis GL, et al. Oncocytic mucoepidermoid carcinoma of the parotid gland. *Arch Pathol Lab Med* 1994;118:313–314.

77. Parwar-Jahan B, Huberman RM, Donovan DT, et al. Oncocytic mucoepidermoid carci-noma of the salivary glands. *Am J Surg Pathol* 1999;23:523–529.

78. Goode RK, Auclair PL, Ellis GL. Mucoepidermoid carcinoma of the major salivary glands. Clinical and histopathologic analysis of 234 cases with evaluation of grading criteria. *Cancer* 1998;82:1217–1224.

79. Auclair PL, Goode RK, Ellis GL. Mucoepidermoid carcinoma of intraoral salivary glands. Evaluation and application of grading criteria in 143 cases. *Cancer* 1992;69:2021–2030.

80. Brandwein MS, Ivanov K, Wallace DI, et al. Mucoepidermoid carcinoma. A clinicopatho-logic study of 80 patients with special reference to histological grading. *Am J Surg Pathol* 2001;25:835–845.

81. Dardick I, Daya D, Hardie J, et al. Mucoepidermoid carcinoma: ultrastructural and histoge-netic aspects. *J Oral Pathol* 1984;13:342–358.

82. Yoo J, Robinson RA. H-ras gene mutations in salivary gland mucoepidermoid carcinomas. *Cancer* 2000;88:518–523.

83. Muller S, Barnes L, Goodurn WJ Jr. Sclerosing mucoepidermoid carcinoma of the parotid. *Oral Surg Oral Med Oral Pathol Oral Radiol Endod* 1997;83:685–690.

84. Shemen LJ, Huvos AG, Spiro RH. Squamous carcinoma of salivary origin. *Head Neck Surg* 1987;9:235–240.

85. Abrams AM, Cornyn J, Scofield HH, et al. Acinic cell adenocarcinoma of the major salivary glands: a clinicopathologic study of 77 cases. *Cancer* 1965;18:1145–1162.

86. Spiro RH, Huvos AG, Strong EW. Acinic cell carcinoma of salivary origin: a clinicopatho-logic study of 67 cases. *Cancer* 1978;41:924–935.

87. Ellis GL, Corio RL. Acinic cell adenocarcinoma. A clinicopathologic analysis of 294 cases. *Cancer* 1983;52:542–549.

88. Stanley RJ, Weiland LH, Olsen KD, et al. Dedifferentiated acinic cell (acinous) carcinoma of the parotid gland. *Otolaryngol Head Neck Surg* 1988;98:155–161.

89. Henley JD, Geary WA, Jackson CL, et al. Dedifferentiated acinic cell carcinoma of the parotid gland: a distinct rarely described entity. *Hum Pathol* 1997;28:869–873.

90. Gustafsson H, Carlsoo B, Henriksson R. Ultrastructural morphometry and secretory behav-ior of acinic cell carcinoma. *Cancer* 1985;55:1706–1710.

91. Erlandson RA, Tandler B. Ultrastructure of acinic cell carcinoma of the parotid gland. *Arch Pathol* 1972;93:130–140.

92. Batsakis JG, Chinn EK, Weimert TA, et al. Acinic cell carcinoma: a clinicopathologic study of thirty-five cases. *J Laryngol Otol* 1979;93:325–340.

93. Hoffman HT, Karnell LH, Robinson RA, et al. National Cancer Data Base report on cancer of the head and neck: acinic cell carcinoma. *Head Neck* 1999;21:297–309.

94. Batsakis JG, Pinkston GR, Luna MA, et al. Adenocarcinomas of the oral cavity: a clinico-pathologic study of terminal duct carcinomas. *J Laryngol Otol* 1983;97:825–835.

95. Matsuba HM, Mauney M, Simpson JR, et al. Adenocarcinomas of major and minor salivary gland origin: a histopathologic review of treatment failure patterns. *Laryngoscope* 1988;98: 784–788.

96. Slootweg PJ, Muller H. Low-grade adenocarcinoma of the oral cavity: a comparison be-tween the terminal duct and the papillary type. *J Craniomaxillofac Surg* 1987;15:359–364.

97. Anderson C, Krutchkoff D, Pedersen C, et al. Polymorphous low grade adenocarcinoma of minor salivary gland: a clinicopathologic and comparative immunohistochemical study. *Mod Pathol* 1990;3:76–82.

98. Gnepp DR, Chen JC, Warren C. Polymorphous low-grade adenocarcinoma of minor sali-vary gland: an immunohistochemical and clinicopathologic study. *Am J Surg Pathol* 1988; 12:461–468.

99. Evans HL, Batsakis JG. Polymorphous low-grade adenocarcinoma of minor salivary glands: a study of 14 cases of a distinctive neoplasm. *Cancer* 1984;53:935–942.

100. Castle JT, Thompson LD, Fommelt RA, et al. Polymorphous low grade adenocarcinoma. A clinicopathologic study of 164 cases. *Cancer* 1999;86:207–219.

101. Perez-Ordonez B, Linkov I, Huvos AG. Polymorphous low-grade adenocarcinoma of minor salivary glands: a study of 17 cases with emphasis on cell differentiation. *Histopathology* 1998;32:521–529.

102. Merchant WJ, Cook MG, Eveson JW. Polymorphous low-grade adenocarcinoma of parotid gland. *Br J Oral Maxillofac Surg* 1996;34:328–330.

103. Mills SE, Garland TA, Allen MS Jr. Low grade papillary adenocarcinoma of palatal salivary gland origin. *Am J Surg Pathol* 1984;8:367–374.

104. Evans HL, Luna MA. Polymorphous low-grade adenocarcinoma. A study of 40 cases with long-term follow up and an evaluation of the importance of papillary areas. *Am J Surg Pathol* 2000;24:1319–1328.

105. Pelkey TJ, Mills SE. Histologic transformation of polymorphous low-grade adenocarcinoma of salivary gland. *Am J Clin Pathol* 1999;111:785–791.

106. Simpson RH, Clarke TJ, Sarsfield PT, et al. Polymorphous low-grade adenocarcinoma of the salivary glands: a clinicopathological comparison with adenoid cystic carcinoma. *Histopathology* 1991;19:121–129.

107. Penner CR, Folpe AL, Budnic SD. C-kit expression distinguishes salivary gland adenoid cystic carcinoma from polymorphous low-grade adenocarcinoma. *Mod Pathol* 2002;15:687–691.

108. Beltran D, Faquin WC, Gallagher G, et al. Selective immunohistochemical comparison of polymorphous low-grade adenocarcinoma and adenoid cystic carcinoma. *J Oral Maxillofac Surg* 2006;64:414–423.

109. Mino M, Pilch BZ, Faquin WC. Expression of KIT (CD117) in neoplasms of the head and neck; an ancillary marker of adenoid cystic carcinoma. *Mod Pathol* 2003;16:1224–1231.

110. Martins C, Fonseca I, Roque L, et al. Cytogenetic similarities between two types of salivary gland carcinomas: adenoid cystic carcinoma and polymorphous low-grade adenocarcinoma. *Cancer Genet Cytogenet* 2001;128:130–136.

111. Lewis JE, McKinney BC, Weiland LH, et al. Salivary duct carcinoma: clinicopathologic and immunohistochemical review of 26 cases. *Cancer* 1996;77:223–230.

112. Guzzo M, DiPalma S, Grandi C, et al. Salivary duct carcinoma: clinical characteristics and treatment strategies. *Head Neck* 1997;19:126–133.

113. Felix A, El-Naggar AK, Press MF, et al. Prognostic significance of biomarkers (c-erB-2, p53, proliferating cell nuclear antigen, and DNA content) in salivary duct carcinoma. *Hum Pathol* 1996;27:561–566.

114. Simpson RHW, Prasad AR, Lewis JE, et al. Mucin-rich variant of salivary duct carcinoma. A clinicopathologic and immunohistochemical study of four cases. *Am J Surg Pathol* 2003;27:1070–1079.

115. Nagao T, Gaffey TA, Visscher DW, et al. Invasive micropapillary salivary duct carcinoma. A distinct histologic variant with biologic significance. *Am J Surg Pathol* 2004;28:319–326.

116. Henley JD, Seo IS, Dayan D, et al. Sarcomatoid salivary duct carcinoma of the parotid gland. *Hum Pathol* 2000;31:208–213.

117. Chen KT. Intraductal carcinoma of the minor salivary gland. *J Laryngol Otol* 1983;97:189–191.

118. Weinreb H, Tabanda-Lichauco R, Van der Kwast T, et al. Low-grade intraductal carcinoma of salivary gland. Report of 3 cases with marked apocrine differentiation. *Am J Surg Pathol* 2006;30:1014–1021.

119. Brandwein-Gensler M, Hille J, Wang BY, et al. Low-grade salivary duct carcinoma. Description of 16 cases. *Am J Surg Pathol* 2004;28:1040–1044.

120. Cheuk W, Miliauskas JR, Chan JK. Intraductal carcinoma of the oral cavity: a case report and reappraisal of the concept of pure ductal carcinoma in situ in salivary duct carcinoma. *Am J Surg Pathol* 2004;28:266–270.

121. Barnes L, Rao U, Contis L, et al. Salivary duct carcinoma. II. Immunohistochemical evaluation of 13 cases for estrogen and progesterone receptors, cathepsin D, and c-erB-2 protein. *Oral Surg Oral Med Oral Pathol* 1994;78:74–80.

122. Kapadia SB, Barnes L. Expression of androgen receptor, gross cystic disease fluid protein, and CD44 in salivary duct carcinoma. *Mod Pathol* 1998;11:1033–1038.

123. Fan CY, Wang J, Barnes EL. Expression of androgen receptor and prostatic specific markers in salivary duct carcinoma: an immunohistochemical analysis of 13 cases and review of the literature. *Am J Surg Pathol* 2000;24:579–586.

124. Cerilli LA, Swartzbaugh JR, Saadut R, et al. Analysis of chromosome 9p21 deletion and p16 gene mutation in salivary gland carcinomas. *Hum Pathol* 1999;30:1242–1246.

125. Roussel JG, Van Dongen JA, Delemarre JF. The metastasizing pleomorphic adenoma of the salivary glands. In Hellman K, Eccles SA, eds. *Treatment of Metastasis: Problems and Prospects*. Philadelphia, PA: Taylor and Francis, 1985:53–56.

126. Sim DW, Maran AG, Harris D. Metastatic salivary pleomorphic adenoma. *J Laryngol Otol* 1990;104:45–47.

127. Qureshi AA, Gitelis S, Templeton AA, et al. "Benign" metastasizing pleomorphic adenoma. A case report and review of literature. *Clin Orthop* 1994;308:192–198.

128. Sampson BA, Jarcho JA, Winter GL. Metastasizing mixed tumor of the parotid gland: a rare tumor with unusually rapid progression in a cardiac transplant patient. *Mod Pathol* 1998;11;1142–1145.

129. Lewis JE, Olsen KD, Sebo T. Carcinoma ex pleomorphic adenoma: pathologic analysis of 73 cases. *Hum Pathol* 2001;32:596–604.

130. Spiro RH, Huvos AG, Strong EW. Malignant mixed tumor of salivary origin: a clinicopathologic study of 146 cases. *Cancer* 1977;39:388–396.

131. LiVolsi VA, Perzin KH. Malignant mixed tumors arising in salivary glands. I. Carcinomas arising in benign mixed tumors: a clinicopathologic study. *Cancer* 1977;39:2209–2230.

132. Nagao K, Matsuzaki O, Saiga H, et al. Histopathologic studies on carcinoma in pleomorphic adenoma of the parotid gland. *Cancer* 1981;48:113–121.

133. Phillips PP, Olsen KD. Recurrent pleomorphic adenoma of the parotid gland: report of 126 cases and a review of the literature. *Ann Otol Rhinol Laryngol* 1995;104:100–104.

134. Righi PD, Li YQ, Deutsch M, et al. The role of the p53 gene in the malignant transformation of pleomorphic adenomas of the parotid gland. *Anticancer Res* 1994;14:2253–2257.

135. Zachariades N. Carcinoma in pleomorphic adenoma. Review of the literature and report of a case. *J Oral Med* 1986;41:121–123.

136. Auclair PL, Ellis GL. Atypical features in salivary gland mixed tumors: their relationship to malignant transformation. *Mod Pathol* 1996;9:652–657.

137. Tortoledo ME, Luna MA, Batsakis JG. Carcinomas, ex pleomorphic adenoma, and malignant mixed tumors. Histomorphologic indexes. *Arch Otolaryngol* 1984;110:172–176.

138. Brandwein M, Huvos AG, Dardick I, et al. Noninvasive and minimally invasive carcinoma ex mixed tumor: a clinicopathologic and ploidy study of 12 patients with major salivary tumors of low (or no?) malignant potential. *Oral Surg Oral Med Oral Pathol Oral Radiol Endod* 1996;81:655–664.

139. Stephen J, Batsakis JG, Luna A, et al. True malignant mixed tumors (carcinosarcoma) of salivary glands. *Oral Surg Oral Med Oral Pathol* 1986;61:597–602.

140. Bleiweiss I, Huvos AG, Lara J, et al. Carcinosarcoma of the submandibular salivary gland: immunohistochemical findings. *Cancer* 1992;69:2031–2035.

141. Toynton SC, Wilkins MJ, Cook HT, et al. True malignant mixed tumour of a minor salivary gland. *J Laryngol Otol* 1994;108:76–79.

142. Gnepp DR, Wenig BM. Malignant mixed tumors. In Ellis GL, Auclair PL, Gnepp DR, eds. *Surgical Pathology of the Salivary Glands*. Philadelphia, PA: Saunders, 1991:350–368.

143. Kwon MY, Gu M. True malignant mixed tumor (carcinosarcoma) of parotid gland with unusual mesenchymal component: a case report and review of the literature. *Arch Pathol Lab Med* 2001;125:812–815.

144. Corio RL, Sciubba JJ, Brannon RB, et al. Epithelial-myoepithelial carcinoma of intercalated duct origin: a clinicopathologic and ultrastructural assessment of sixteen cases. *Oral Surg Oral Med Oral Pathol* 1982;53:280–287.

145. Lampe H, Ruby RR, Greenway RE, et al. Epithelial-myoepithelial carcinoma of the salivary gland. *J Otolaryngol* 1984;13:247–251.

146. Luna MA, Ordonez NG, Mackay B, et al. Salivary epithelial-myoepithelial carcinomas of intercalated ducts: a clinical, electron microscopic, and immunocytochemical study. *Oral Surg Oral Med Oral Pathol* 1985;59:482–490.

147. Palmer RM. Epithelial-myoepithelial carcinoma: an immunocytochemical study. *Oral Surg Oral Med Oral Pathol* 1985;59:511–515.

148. Cho KJ, El-Naggar AK, Ordonez NG, et al. Epithelial-myoepithelial carcinoma of salivary glands. A clinicopathologic, DNA flow cytometric, and immunohistochemical study of Ki-67 and HER-2/neu oncogene. *Am J Clin Pathol* 1995;103:432–437.

149. Fonseca I, Soares J. Epithelial-myoepithelial carcinoma of the salivary glands. A study of 22 cases. *Virchows Arch A Pathol Anat Histol* 1993;422:389–396.

150. Seethala RR, Barnes EL, Hunt JL. Epithelial-myoepithelial carcinoma: a review of the clinicopathologic spectrum and immunophenotypic characteristics in 61 tumors of the salivary glands and upper aerodigestive tract. *Am J Surg Pathol* 2007;31:44–57.

151. Ellis GL, Wiscovitch JG. Basal cell adenocarcinomas of the major salivary glands. *Oral Surg Oral Med Oral Pathol* 1990;69:461–469.

152. Ellis GL, Auclair PL. Basal cell adenocarcinoma. In Ellis GL, Auclair PL, Gnepp DR, eds. *Surgical Pathology of the Salivary Glands*. Philadelphia, PA: Saunders, 1991:441–454.

153. Quddus MR, Henley JD, Afify AM, et al. Basal cell adenocarcinoma of the salivary gland. An ultrastructural and immunohistochemical study. *Oral Surg Oral Med Oral Pathol Oral Radiol Endod* 1999;87:485–492.

154. Mair IW, Johannessen TA. Benign and malignant oncocytoma of the parotid gland. *Laryngoscope* 1972;82:638–642.

155. Lee SC, Roth LM. Malignant oncocytoma of the parotid gland. A light and electron microscopic study. *Cancer* 1976;37:1606–1614.

156. Ross CF. Malignant oncocytoma ("oxyphilic granular-cell tumour") of the parotid gland. *Clin Oncol* 1976;2:253–260.

157. Laurian N, Zohar Y, Kende L. Malignant oncocytoma. *J Laryngol Otol* 1977;91:805–858.

158. Chu W, Strawitz JG. Oncocytoma of the parotid gland with malignant change. *Arch Surg* 1978;113:318–319.

159. Granstrom G, Aldenborg F, Jeppsson PH. Sebaceous carcinoma of the parotid gland: report of a case and review of the literature. *J Oral Maxillofac Surg* 1987;45:731–733.

160. Gnepp DR. Sebaceous neoplasms of salivary gland origin: a review. *Pathol Annu* 1983;18:71–102.

161. Gnepp DR, Brannon R. Sebaceous neoplasms of salivary gland origin. Report of 21 cases. *Cancer* 1984;53:2155–2170.

162. Saw D, Iau WH, Ho J, et al. Malignant lymphoepithelial lesions of the salivary glands. *Hum Pathol* 1986;17:914–923.

163. Redondo C, Garcia A, Vasquez F. Malignant lymphoepithelial lesion of the parotid gland. *Cancer* 1981;48:289–292.

164. Amaral AL, Nascimento AG. Malignant lymphoepithelial lesion of the submandibular gland. *Oral Surg Oral Med Oral Pathol* 1984;58:184–190.

165. Worley NK, Daroca PJ, Jr. Lymphoepithelial carcinoma of the minor salivary gland. *Arch Otolaryngol Head Neck Surg* 1997;123:638–640.

166. Wanamaker JR, Kraus DH, Biscotti CV, et al. Undifferentiated nasopharyngeal carcinoma presenting as a parotid mass. *Head Neck* 1994;16:589–593.

167. Milchgrub S, Gnepp DR, Vuitch F, et al. Hyalinizing clear cell carcinoma of salivary gland. *Am J Surg Pathol* 1994;18:74–82.

168. O'Regan E, Shandilya M, Gnepp DR, et al. Hyalinizing clear cell carcinoma of salivary gland: an aggressive variant. *Oral Oncol* 2004;40:348–352.

169. Wirman JA, Battifora HA. Small cell undifferentiated carcinoma of salivary gland origin: an ultrastructural study. *Cancer* 1976;37:1840–1848.

170. Gnepp DR, Ferlito A, Hyams V. Primary anaplastic small cell (oat cell) carcinoma of the larynx: review of the literature and report of 18 cases. *Cancer* 1983;51:1731–1745.

171. Gnepp DR, Wick MR. Small cell carcinoma of the major salivary glands. An immunohistochemical study. *Cancer* 1990;66:185–192.

172. Perez-Ordonez B, Caruana SM, Huvos AG, et al. Small cell neuroendocrine carcinoma of the nasal cavity and paranasal sinuses. *Hum Pathol* 1998;29:826–832.

173. Woodruff JM, Huvos AG, Erlandson RA, et al. Neuroendocrine carcinomas of the larynx. A study of two types, one of which mimics thyroid medullary carcinoma. *Am J Surg Pathol* 1985;9:771–790.

174. Nagao T, Sugano I, Ishida Y, et al. Primary large-cell neuroendocrine carcinoma of the

174. parotid gland: immunohistochemical and molecular analysis of two cases. *Mod Pathol* 2000;13:554–561.
175. Nagao T, Gaffey TA, Olsen KD, et al. Small cell carcinoma of the major salivary glands: clinicopathologic study with emphasis on cytokeratin 20 immunoreactivity and clinical outcome. *Am J Surg Pathol* 2004;28:762–770.
176. Chan JC, Suster S, Wenig BM, et al. Cytokeratin 20 immunoreactivity distinguishes Merkel cell (primary cutaneous neuroendocrine) carcinomas and salivary gland small cell carcinomas from small cell carcinomas of various sites. *Am J Surg Pathol* 1997;21:226–234.
177. Williams SB, Ellis GL, Warnock GR. Sialoblastoma: a clinicopathologic and immunohistochemical study of 7 cases. *Ann Diagn Pathol* 2006;10:320–326.
178. Brandwein M, Al-Naief NS, Manwani D, et al. Sialoblastoma: clinicopathological/immunohistochemical study. *Am J Surg Pathol* 1999;23:342–348.
179. Michal M, Skalova A, Simpson RH, et al. Cribriform adenocarcinoma of the tongue: a hitherto unrecognized type of adenocarcinoma characteristically occurring in the tongue. *Histopathology* 1999;35:495–501.
180. Pollett A, Perez-Ordonez B, Jordan RC, et al. High-grade papillary cystadenocarcinoma of the tongue. *Histopathology* 1997;31:185–188.
181. Spiro RH, Strong EW, Huvos AG. Adenocarcinoma of salivary origin. *Am J Surg* 1982;144:423–431.
182. Batsakis JG, El-Naggar AK, Luna MA. "Adenocarcinoma, not otherwise specified": a diminishing group of salivary carcinomas. *Ann Otol Rhinol Laryngol* 1992;101:102–104.
183. Nichols RD, Rebuck JW, Sullivan JC. Lymphoma and the parotid gland. *Laryngoscope* 1982;92:365–369.
184. Schmid U, Helbron D, Lennert K. Primary malignant lymphomas localized in salivary glands. *Histopathology* 1982;6:673–687.
185. Watkin GT, MacLennan KA, Hobsley M. Lymphomas presenting as lumps in the parotid region. *Br J Surg* 1984;71:701–702.
186. Gleeson MJ, Bennett MH, Cawson RA. Lymphomas of salivary glands. *Cancer* 1986;58:699–704.
187. Mehle ME, Kraus DH, Wood BG, et al. Lymphoma of the parotid gland. *Laryngoscope* 1993;103:17–21.
188. Balm AJ, Delaere P, Hilgers FJ, et al. Primary lymphoma of mucosa associated lymphoid tissue (MALT) in the parotid gland. *Clin Otolaryngol* 1993;18:528–532.
189. Oyama T, Ichimura K, Suzuki R, et al. Senile EBV+ B-cell lymphoproliferative disorders: a clinicopathologic study of 22 patients. *Am J Surg Pathol* 2003;27:16–26.
190. Hjorth L, Donunberby H, Kruse S, et al. Primary malignant lymphoma of the salivary glands. *Tumori* 1986;72:491–497.
191. Batsakis JG. Vascular tumors of the salivary glands. *Ann Otol Rhinol Laryngol* 1986;95:649–650.
192. Hughes RG, Oates J. Capillary haemangioma of the parotid in an adult: an unusual case and a review of the literature. *J Laryngol Otol* 1997;111:588–589.
193. Goldman RL, Perzik SL. Infantile hemangioma of the parotid gland: a clinicopathological study of 15 cases. *Arch Otolaryngol* 1969;90:605–608.
194. Martinez-Mora J, Boix-Ochoa J, Tresserra L. Vascular tumors of the parotid region in children. *Surg Gynecol Obstet* 1971;133:937–973.
195. Faber RG, Ibrahim SZ, Drew DS, et al. Vascular malformations of the parotid region. *Br J Surg* 1978;65:171–175.
196. Nagao K, Matsuzaki O, Shigematsu H, et al. Histopathologic studies of benign infantile hemangioendothelioma of the parotid gland. *Cancer* 1980;46:2250–2256.
197. Kornblutt AD, Ilse H, Haurbrich J. Parotid lymphangioma: a congenital tumor. *J Otorhinolaryngol Relat Spec* 1973;35:303–314.
198. Takato T, Nakatsuka T, Ohhara Y. Lymphangioma of the parotid gland. *Ann Plast Surg* 1984;13:353–356.
199. Stenson KM, Mishelle J, Toriumi DM. Cystic hygroma of the parotid gland. *Ann Otol Rhinol Laryngol* 1991;100:518–520.
200. Walts AE, Perzik SL. Lipomatous lesions of the parotid area. *Otolaryngology* 1976;102:230–232.
201. Baker SE, Jensen JL, Correll RW. Lipomas of the parotid gland. *Oral Surg Oral Med Oral Pathol* 1981;52:167–171.
202. Saleh HA, Ram B, Harmse JL, et al. Lipomatosis of the minor salivary glands. *J Laryngol Otol* 1998;112:895–897.
203. Avery AP, Sprinkle PM. Benign intraparotid schwannomas. *Laryngoscope* 1972;82:199–203.
204. Tsutsumi T, Oku T, Komatsuzaki A. Solitary plexiform neurofibroma of the submandibular salivary gland. *J Laryngol Otol* 1996;110:1173–1175.
205. Ferreiro JA, Nascimento AG. Solitary fibrous tumor of the major salivary glands. *Histopathology* 1996;28:261–264.
206. Yamaguchi KT, Krugman ME, Barr RJ, et al. Hemangiopericytoma of the parotid gland with a review of the literature. *J Otolaryngol* 1977;6:431–435.
207. Massarelli G, Tanda F, Fois V, et al. Hemangiopericytoma of the parotid gland. Report of a case and review of the literature. *Virchows Arch A Pathol Anat Histol* 1980;386:81–89.
208. Farr HW, Carandang CM, Huvos AG. Malignant vascular tumors of the head and neck. *Am J Surg* 1970;120:501–504.
209. Benjamin E, Wells S, Fox H, et al. Malignant fibrous histiocytomas of the salivary glands. *J Clin Pathol* 1982;35:946–953.
210. Auclair P, Langloss JM, Weiss SW, et al. Sarcomas and sarcomatoid neoplasms of the major salivary gland regions. A clinicopathologic and immunohistochemical study of 67 cases and review of the literature. *Cancer* 1986;58:1305–1315.
211. Luna MA, Tortoledo ME, Ordonez NG, et al. Primary sarcomas of the major salivary glands. *Arch Otolaryngol Head Neck Surg* 1991;117:302–306.
212. Fanburg-Smith J, Furlong M, Childers E. Oral and salivary gland angiosarcoma: a clinicopathologic study of 209 cases. *Mod Pathol* 2003;16:666–675.
213. Seifert G, Hennings K, Caselitz J. Metastatic tumors to the parotid and submandibular glands. Analysis and differential diagnosis of 108 cases. *Pathol Res Pract* 1986;181:684–692.
214. Renaut AJ. Melanoma arising within the parotid salivary gland. A case report and review of management. *Eur J Surg Oncol* 1996;22:201–202.
215. Melnick SJ, Amazon K, Denison V. Metastatic renal cell carcinoma presenting as a parotid tumor: a case report with immunohistochemical findings and a review of the literature. *Hum Pathol* 1989;20:195–197.

The Nose, Paranasal Sinuses, and Nasopharynx

The nasal cavity, paranasal sinuses, and nasopharynx are sites for a wide variety of tumors and nonneoplastic conditions. The large number of diseases affecting these structures is, in major part, a result of the many specialized tissues, each with its own associated aberrations, that exist in this region. Basic knowledge of the anatomy and histologic features of this area is of value because many conditions show a strong predilection for a specific anatomic location. For example, angiofibromas and lymphoepitheliomas develop almost exclusively in the nasopharynx, lobular capillary hemangiomas and schneiderian papillomas involve the nasal cavity, intestinal-type adenocarcinomas typically occur in the paranasal sinuses, and olfactory neuroblastomas arise from the superior portion of the nasal cavity.

REVIEW OF ANATOMY

NASAL CAVITY

The nasal cavity is divided into the nares by the nasal septum and, at the anterior extreme, the columella. Each cavity is wedge-shaped, being narrow superiorly and wider inferiorly (1,2). The anterior portion of each nasal cavity is the vestibule (Fig. 21.1). The choana forms the posterior border of each cavity, separating it from the nasopharynx. The nasal turbinates are the lateral walls of each nasal cavity, and the cribriform plate forms the superior boundary. The lower portion of the vestibule is lined by skin containing adnexal structures, including hair. Posterior to the vestibule, the nasal cavity, except for its uppermost portion, is lined by thick, highly vascularized, ciliated columnar epithelium. This mucosa, in conjunction with that of the paranasal sinuses, is often referred to as the schneiderian membrane. Goblet cells may be present in the surface mucosa, and secretions from the seromucinous glands beneath the sur-

face drain into the nasal cavity through small ducts. Areas of squamous metaplasia may occasionally be found, particularly on the anterior surface of the middle and lower turbinates and the anterior nasal septum (1).

The superior one-third of the nasal septum, the superior turbinate, and the cribriform plate are covered with thinner olfactory mucosa. The latter develops at the embryonic stage from the respiratory mucosa. The specialized receptor cells of the olfactory mucosa have neuroendocrine features and grow through the cribriform plate to establish contact with the central nervous system. In infants, the olfactory mucosa is uniform and sharply demarcated; in adults, however, progressive atrophy leads to an irregular, patchy distribution with intervening islands of respiratory epithelium (3).

PARANASAL SINUSES

The paranasal sinuses are diverticula of the nasal cavity that extend into neighboring bones (Fig. 21.2). The ethmoid sinuses begin development in fetal life and are well developed at birth. The frontal, maxillary, and sphenoid sinuses, in contrast, are small or rudimentary at birth. The maxillary and sphenoid sinuses develop rapidly during childhood and reach essentially adult configuration after permanent dentition is acquired. The frontal sinuses begin development in childhood and continue to enlarge through puberty. The mucosa of the paranasal sinuses is in continuity with the nasal cavity and consists of identical, pseudostratified, ciliated columnar epithelium. Typically, it is only approximately half as thick as the nasal mucosa, with fewer associated goblet cells and seromucinous glands.

NASOPHARYNX

The nasopharynx is the part of the respiratory passage that lies above and behind the soft palate (Fig. 21.1). It has anterior, posterior, and lateral walls (4). The anterior wall is perforated by the posterior nares (choanae). The posterior wall is an arch

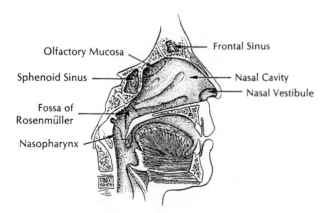

Figure 21.1. This midline sagittal section demonstrates the contours of the nasal cavity, limits of the nasopharynx (*straight dashed lines*), and region of olfactory mucosa (*curved dashed line*).

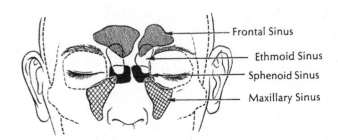

Figure 21.2. The paranasal sinuses are projected onto the face. The frontal sinuses are most anterior, the maxillary sinuses lie under the cheek, the ethmoid sinuses are between the orbits, and the sphenoid sinuses are most posterior, at the base of the brain.

that includes the roof of the nasopharynx; it also comprises the posterior portion against the base of the skull. The posterior wall extends inferiorly to the level of the free border of the soft palate, at which point the oropharynx begins. The ostium of the eustachian tube, located in the lateral wall, is surrounded by a mucosa-covered cartilaginous prominence. Posterior to this ostium is the pharyngeal recess or fossa of Rosenmüller.

The nasopharyngeal mucosa in the adult has a surface area of approximately 50 cm². Approximately 60% is lined by stratified squamous epithelium, and most of the remainder is covered by ciliated columnar epithelium (4). Squamous epithelium lines the inferior half of the anterior and posterior walls; it also lines the anterior half of the lateral walls. Ciliated epithelium is present around the nasal choanae and over the roof of the posterior wall. The remainder of the nasopharynx, including the posterior lateral walls and the middle third of the posterior wall, has alternating islands of squamous and ciliated epithelium. There also may be focal areas of "transitional," or intermediate, epithelium. The latter term is preferred because, although the epithelium resembles urothelium on light microscopy, it lacks the specialized ultrastructural features of urinary tract mucosa. Intermediate epithelial cells are less polyhedral than squamous cells, yet they are rounder than columnar ciliated cells and their nonciliated precursors. Intermediate epithelium tends to be concentrated as a wavy ring at the junction of the nasopharynx and oropharynx. Oncocytic metaplasia of the seromucinous glands of the nasopharynx is occasionally an incidental finding in nasopharyngeal biopsies. A few cases have resulted in clinically visible masses, and they may produce symptoms by obstructing the eustachian tube (5).

INFLAMMATORY LESIONS

INFECTIONS

Tissue from patients with common viral and bacterial infections of the upper airway is not seen by the surgical pathologist. However, biopsies of tissue changes caused by infectious diseases that are destructive, involve large areas of mucosa, or result in a mass may be performed.

FUNGI

A variety of fungi affect the nose and sinuses, which may constitute the sole site of infection. Mucormycosis (phycomycosis) is a life-threatening opportunistic infection by organisms of the order Mucorales. Broad nonseptate hyphae, readily seen on hematoxylin and eosin–stained sections, spread along nerves, across tissue planes, and into blood vessels. Inflammation ranges from negligible to large numbers of neutrophils and histiocytes within granulation tissue.

Aspergillus organisms are septate hyphae that branch at 45 degrees. Fungus balls can occur in the antrum of immunocompetent people and can elicit a minimal inflammatory reaction of granulation tissue with microabscesses or multinucleated giant cells. Invasive aspergillosis occurs in immunosuppressed and immunocompetent persons (6). Extension into the retroorbital region, cranial vault, or parapharyngeal space can be fatal (7). Putative allergic reactions to *Aspergillus* species (not culture proven) have been characterized by pathologic evidence of "allergic mucin" (8,9). The mucin is often so tena-

cious that it requires curettage for adequate removal, and recurrent disease is common (10). Bone erosion may be present on radiography, but it is caused by pressure remodeling rather than destruction by fungal invasion (10). The mucin contains eosinophils, Charcot-Leyden crystals, and hyphae. The mucin and infiltrate are often laminated. Culture-proven infection by *Curvularia lunata* and the dematiaceous fungi *Drechslera, Bipolaris,* and *Exserohilum* has also resulted in an inflammatory response with the appearance of allergic mucin (11,12). The dematiaceous fungi may be identified by their positive staining with a Fontana-Masson melanin stain (12).

Cryptococcosis (13) and actinomycosis (14) are extremely unusual infections of the nose. Other invasive fungal infections may be caused by *Zygomycetes* (15), *Pseudallescheria boydii* (16), *Paecilomyces* species (17), *Alternaria* species (18), *Cladosporium trichoides* (19), and *Fusarium* (20). Fungi causing noninvasive sinusitis include *Pseudallescheria boydii, Sporothrix schenckii, Penicillium meliniiu, Stemphylium mucosporideum, Candida* species (21), and *Chrysosporium pruinosum* (22). Organisms are usually visible on hematoxylin and eosin–stained sections, but they may be focal and sparse, requiring methenamine silver to facilitate diagnosis. Inflammatory reactions are purulent, granulomatous, or mixed. The inflammation serves only to alert one to the possibility of an infectious process. It has no diagnostic specificity.

TUBERCULOSIS

Tuberculosis of the sinonasal mucosa is an uncommon manifestation of hematogenous spread; even more rarely, it develops in the nose (23). The septum and inferior turbinate are preferentially involved by either an ulcerated or polypoid lesion. Septal perforation can occur. On microscopic examination, the granulomas are usually poorly formed and almost never necrotic. Sometimes, epithelioid histiocytes intermixed with lymphocytes and plasma cells are the only inflammatory response. It is uncommon to identify organisms in tissue sections, and the diagnosis usually must be established by culture.

LEPROSY

Leprosy affects the nasal mucosa in 95% of patients and sometimes is the initial manifestation of disease (24). As with some other granulomatous inflammations, the inferior turbinate and the septum are the favored sites. In the early stage, there may be only a small number of histiocytes and lymphocytes, with a predominance of plasma cells (Figs. 21.3 and 21.4). Later, the histiocytes form broad sheets containing many foam cells (25). The tuberculoid form of leprosy, with well-formed granulomas, is uncommon in the nose.

RHINOSPORIDIOSIS

The organisms of rhinosporidiosis are huge, thick-walled sporangia that contain up to several thousand spores (Fig. 21.5) (26). They elicit an inflammatory response of neutrophils, lymphocytes, and plasma cells (27).

RHINOSCLEROMA

Rhinoscleroma may be confused with leprosy because rhinoscleroma is also characterized by foamy histiocytes (Mikulicz

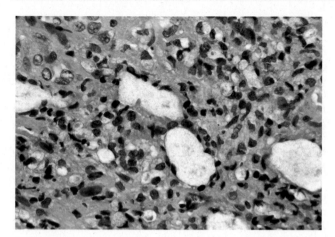

Figure 21.3. Nasal leprosy consists of large, foamy histiocytes, without visible nuclei in this microscopic field, in association with a mixed inflammatory infiltrate.

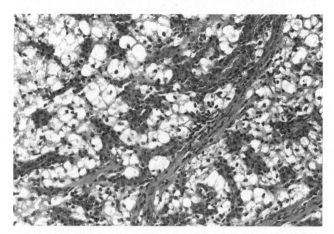

Figure 21.6. Nasal rhinoscleroma contains a large number of foamy histiocytes in a plasma-cell–rich inflammatory background. The appearance may be indistinguishable on light microscopy from leprosy. (Courtesy of J. C. Watts, MD.)

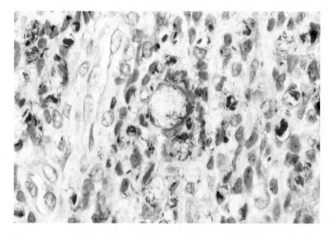

Figure 21.4. Acid-fast stain from the case seen in Figure 21.3 shows numerous acid-fast organisms, some forming aggregates.

cells) intermixed with plasma cells (Fig. 21.6) (28). The organisms of leprosy are acid-fast (Fig. 21.4), whereas rhinoscleroma is caused by Gram-negative rods (*Klebsiella rhinoscleroma*) (Fig. 21.7).

MIDFACIAL NECROTIZING LESION ("LETHAL MIDLINE GRANULOMA")

Midfacial necrotizing lesion ("lethal midline granuloma") is a clinical designation for one or more infiltrative, often destructive, mucosal lesions of the upper aerodigestive tract (29). This is not a pathologic diagnosis because many diseases, including infections and neoplasms, have clinically similar initial symptoms (30). The three pathologic entities that cause the most diagnostic difficulty are Wegener granulomatosis, natural killer (NK)/T-cell lymphoma, and so-called idiopathic midline destructive disease. These conditions must be sharply separated because of markedly different prognoses and therapies. All are difficult to diagnose on punch biopsies because the only tissue obtained is often secondarily inflamed, ulcerated mucosa. Deep incisional biopsies are usually necessary to obtain sufficient tis-

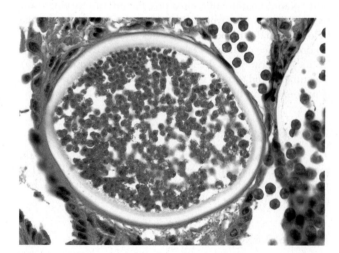

Figure 21.5. A large, thick-walled sporangium of rhinosporidiosis contains hundreds of spores.

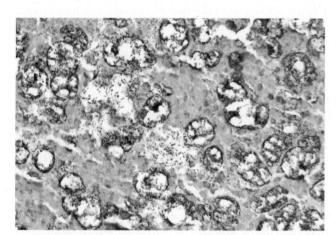

Figure 21.7. Large numbers of rod-shaped bacillary organisms are seen in this Steiner stain from the lesion depicted in Figure 21.6.

sue, given the spotty nature of diagnostic areas in Wegener granulomatosis and NK/T-cell lymphoma. Similarly, the diagnosis of idiopathic midline destructive disease requires generous sampling because it is a diagnosis of exclusion.

Clinical Features

The clinical signs of Wegener granulomatosis, NK/T-cell lymphoma, and idiopathic midline destructive disease share similarities. Patients most often complain of rhinorrhea and sinus pain. The mucosa of the nose, paranasal sinus, oral cavity, and nasopharynx is thickened in variable combinations. Lesions of the nasopharynx often result in otitis media or mastoiditis as a result of eustachian tube involvement. Regardless of the site, the affected mucosa is focally ulcerated. Of the three, Wegener granulomatosis is the least destructive of underlying cartilage or bone in the early stages of disease. On the other hand, patients with NK/T-cell lymphoma and idiopathic midline destructive disease often have a perforated nasal septum, perforated palate, erosion of the bone of the antrum, or ulceration of the skin overlying the nose or antrum (31).

Morphologic Characteristics

Wegener granulomatosis is characterized by necrotizing vasculitis involving arterioles, small arteries, and veins. The affected vessels are often situated in a broad sheet of extravascular inflammatory cells that makes their detection difficult. An elastic stain is sometimes useful, especially when the vessel lumen has been obliterated by inflammatory cells and thrombus. All stages of vasculitis are present, ranging from acute to healed. The acute vasculitis is characterized by a predominantly neutrophilic infiltrate of the vessel wall, accompanied by patchy fibrinoid necrosis. The inflammation and necrosis can involve small sectors or the entire circumference. Vessels with healed vasculitis have narrowed or obliterated lumina with concentric rims of perivascular collagen (Fig. 21.8). Variable numbers of lymphocytes, plasma cells, or histiocytes are in the wall and surrounding stroma.

Giant cells unassociated with granulomas are usually evident in Wegener granulomatosis, but they may be sparse. Granulomas are rarely well formed, and they most often consist of ill-defined aggregates of mononuclear or multinucleated histiocytes associated with nuclear debris. The giant cells or granulomas may be far from vessels, adjacent to a vessel with vasculitis, or within the vessel wall. Rarely, a granuloma may be centered around fragmented elastic tissue representing the remnants of a totally destroyed vessel.

Patchy foci of necrotic connective tissue and inflammatory cells are invariably present, given adequate tissue sampling. The necrosis is of the coagulative type and may contain degenerating neutrophils (Fig. 21.9). The necrotic areas can have a rim of giant cells with epithelioid or palisaded, spindle-shaped mononuclear histiocytes. The necrotic foci may have a geographic, "punched out" appearance or may be serpiginous. Some researchers consider this type of necrosis and histiocytic response sufficient for the diagnosis, even in the absence of vasculitis (32). In addition to the neutrophils and histiocytes, the extravascular tissue has lymphocytes, plasma cells, and eosinophils. Eosinophils are numerous in a minority of cases and are almost totally absent in others.

Biopsies from the head and neck region, usually the nasal cavity, have been considered to be fully diagnostic in 20% to 41% of patients with Wegener granulomatosis (33,34). Colby et al. (35) noted that biopsies were diagnostic or suggestive of Wegener granulomatosis in approximately 70% of cases. Devaney et al. (33) have proposed the following criteria for the diagnosis of Wegener granulomatosis in head and neck biopsies: (a) The finding of all three microscopic features (granulomatous inflammation, necrosis, and vasculitis) is considered diagnostic if the patient has additional clinical features of involvement of the lung, kidney, or both. (b) If two of the three microscopic features are present, the biopsy is considered diagnostic only if both the lungs and kidneys show clinical signs of disease; if only one additional site is involved, the biopsy is termed "probable." (c) When only one of the three microscopic features is present, the biopsy is considered suggestive if there is pulmonary and renal involvement or suspicious if only one of these sites is affected. (d) If none of the three microscopic features is present, the biopsy is considered nonspecific, even when there is clinical evidence of pulmonary and renal disease (33).

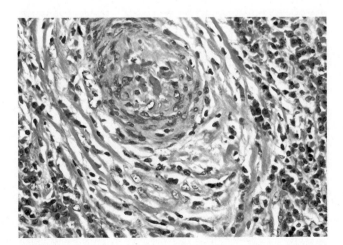

Figure 21.8. Clinically active Wegener granulomatosis can exhibit arteritis at all stages, including a healing phase seen here. The lumen has been obliterated by proliferating fibrous tissue, and there is concentric fibrous tissue surrounding the vessel.

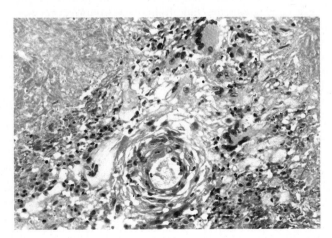

Figure 21.9. Wegener granulomatosis has geographic areas of necrosis that may be rimmed in part by multinucleated giant cells. An inflamed vessel is present.

If necrotizing vasculitis is the only change, one must be careful to distinguish it from secondary inflammation of the vessel wall resulting from some other cause. Similarly, transmigration of neutrophils can mimic vasculitis. In neither instance, however, is fibrinoid necrosis seen. When there is necrosis of the extravascular tissues, with or without giant cells or granulomas, infection must be considered. Stains for acid-fast organisms and fungi are warranted, accompanied by cultures.

Approximately two-thirds of patients with Churg-Strauss syndrome have nasal polyps or mucosal crusting. At the microscopic level, the tissue has discrete necrotizing granulomas with numerous eosinophils that may form microabscesses. In one series, angiitis was absent in the sinonasal lesions (36). Because Wegener granulomatosis sometimes has large numbers of eosinophils and minimal angiitis, the distinction from Churg-Strauss syndrome may rest mainly on clinical grounds.

Another entity that can be confused with Wegener granulomatosis is NK/T-cell lymphoma because the latter often has a considerable inflammatory component. In addition, the atypical lymphocytes tend to be angiocentric, infiltrate the vessel wall, and superficially mimic vasculitis (37). The majority of the cells in the vessel wall, however, are atypical lymphocytes, and the vessel is not necrotic. NK/T-cell lymphoma of the upper respiratory tract has been referred to by a variety of terms, including midline malignant reticulosis and polymorphic reticulosis. These lesions are described in detail in the later section on NK/T-cell lymphoma. The pulmonary lesion of so-called lymphomatoid granulomatosis (38,39) can secondarily involve the upper respiratory tract, producing lesions that are similar to primary NK/T-cell lymphomas in many morphologic features, including a distinctly angiocentric growth pattern. Although previously thought to be synonymous with these lesions, lymphomatoid granulomatosis is now believed to represent a distinctly different process, a T-cell–rich B-cell lymphoma.

Idiopathic midline destructive disease (IMDD) is characterized by normal-appearing acute and chronic inflammatory cells with variable amounts of necrosis. Atypical lymphocytes are absent, thus eliminating the possibility of NK/T-cell lymphoma. The inflammatory cells occasionally infiltrate the walls of small vessels, but fibrinoid necrosis is absent, which distinguishes it from Wegener granulomatosis. Eosinophils are inconspicuous. Multinucleated giant cells and granulomas have been described in a few cases of IMDD. In instances where the pathologic findings are ambiguous, the clinical differences from Wegener granulomatosis, emphasized by Tsoskos et al. (40), may be influential in reaching the correct clinicopathologic diagnosis. Cocaine users can have a midfacial destructive syndrome that closely mimics IMDD (Fig. 21.10). Although some have suggested a less fulminant course in cocaine abusers (41), it seems likely that many examples of IMDD represent unrecognized cases of cocaine abuse. Indeed, whether IMDD represents a distinct entity or heterogeneous group of cases remains unclear.

SARCOIDOSIS

Approximately 5% of patients with sarcoidosis have upper airway disease, and the nose is rarely the first site of involvement (42,43). As with tuberculosis, the nasal septum and inferior turbinate are the preferred sites. The nonnecrotic granulomas of sarcoid and tuberculosis can be identical at the light microscopic level (Fig. 21.11).

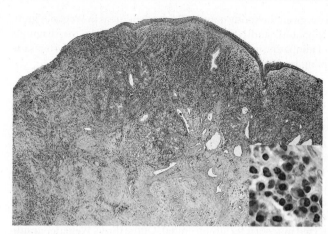

Figure 21.10. Cocaine abuse. This nasal biopsy from a long-term cocaine user shows dense submucosal inflammation, predominantly plasma cells (*inset*) with focal mucosal ulceration at the upper left. Vasculitis is not present.

NONINFECTIOUS GRANULOMATOUS REACTIONS

Steroid injections of the nasal mucosa can produce granulomas with palisades of histiocytes surrounding an amorphous area. The amorphous zone probably is the residual injected substance (44). Nonnecrotic granulomas are occasionally found in otherwise unremarkable inflammatory nasal polyps and sometimes in relation to small nasal ulcers. The granulomas, which are of unknown origin, are usually just beneath the epithelium, may resolve spontaneously, and do not recur after excision (45). Nasal granulomas have been reported in a patient with Crohn disease (46). Cholesterol granulomas of the sinuses consist of (a) a foreign-body giant-cell reaction around empty, needle-shaped spaces and (b) a chronic inflammatory reaction with hemosiderin. As with cholesterol granulomas of the middle ear, hemorrhage is the presumed pathogenesis, although a specific cause is rarely identified (47). Cholesteatoma, a foreign-body giant-cell response to keratin, has been described in the maxillary antrum (45).

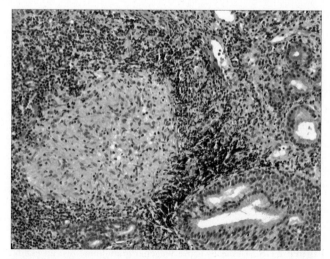

Figure 21.11. Nasal sarcoidosis. A well-formed noncaseating granuloma is present along with dense chronic inflammation, adjacent to seromucinous glands of the nasal mucosa.

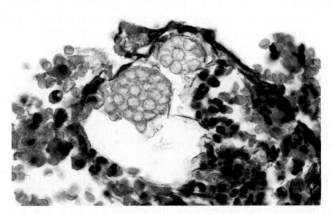

Figure 21.12. Myospherulosis consists of aggregates of altered erythrocytes surrounded by a membrane.

MYOSPHERULOSIS

Myospherulosis is an inflammatory and fibrous reaction that surrounds encysted, degenerating erythrocytes (Fig. 21.12) (48,49). This iatrogenic condition follows surgical procedures when an oil-based hemostatic packing has been used. Symptomatic reaction to the oil may necessitate reoperation (50). The encysted erythrocytes mimic *Prototheca* but do not stain with methenamine silver.

MUCOCELE

Mucoceles of the paranasal sinuses are generally considered to arise from obstruction of the ostium as a result of inflammation, trauma, osteoma, or, occasionally, a neoplasm (51). Two-thirds of mucoceles are in the frontal sinus, and most of the rest are in the anterior ethmoid sinus. The resected mucosa is either normal or compressed ciliated epithelium that sometimes has squamous metaplasia. Mucus may be extravasated in the lamina propria, where it can be phagocytosed by histiocytes (mucophages).

NONSECRETORY CYST

Rarely, cysts of the antrum will be lined by fibroblasts. They have been termed nonsecretory cysts and are thought to originate from edema beneath the mucous membrane stemming from infection or allergy. The accumulation of fluid forms multiple spaces that eventually coalesce into a single cyst lined by flattened fibroblasts rather than epithelium (52).

NECROTIZING SIALOMETAPLASIA

Necrosis of seromucinous glands with secondary squamous metaplasia after surgery on the nose or sinuses produces the microscopic image of necrotizing sialometaplasia (53). The benign, although focally atypical, cytologic appearance of the cells and, more importantly, maintenance of the acinar architecture distinguish necrotizing sialometaplasia from either squamous carcinoma or mucoepidermoid carcinoma. This entity is illustrated and discussed in detail in Chapter 20.

NASAL POLYPS

Polyps of the nasal cavity and paranasal sinuses are nonneoplastic stromal and epithelial proliferations of uncertain pathogene-

sis. Although all nasal and paranasal polyps share morphologic similarities, there are three clinically—and, to a lesser extent, microscopically—distinctive subtypes.

INFLAMMATORY POLYPS

Clinical Features

Inflammatory polyps are by far the most common. They are almost invariably multiple and typically bilateral, and they involve both the nasal cavity and the paranasal sinuses. To find them in patients less than 20 years of age is distinctly uncommon; most patients are more than 30 years old. An association with asthma or chronic rhinitis, often with negative skin allergen tests, is well established. Approximately 14% of patients with nasal polyps manifest aspirin intolerance, usually in the form of a bronchospastic, asthmatic reaction (54). The presumed mechanism of bronchospasm is a defect in prostaglandin metabolism.

Morphologic Characteristics

On gross inspection, these polyps have a translucent, moist, or edematous cut surface. Most have broad bases of attachment. Areas of opacity should be sectioned to exclude other processes, such as inverted papilloma. At the microscopic level, nasal polyps are localized outgrowths of lamina propria resulting from the accumulation of edema-like fluid with varying degrees of fibroblastic proliferation and inflammation (Fig. 21.13). Mucous glands are embedded in the stroma, particularly in the distal portion of the polyp. The glands vary greatly in number but are typically less numerous than those in normal mucosa. They have a distinctly tubular configuration, connect to the surface of the polyp, and probably arise secondarily after the polyp has begun to form (55). Polyps with prominent glandular elements should not be mistaken for low-grade adenocarcinoma (56) or polypoid mixed tumors of the salivary type (57). The basement membrane underlying the surface mucosa is markedly thickened in most, but not all, inflammatory polyps. The amount and composition of the inflammatory component

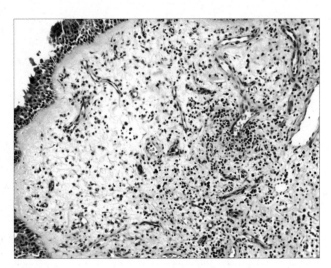

Figure 21.13. Inflammatory nasal polyp. The edematous stroma contains capillaries and a mixed inflammatory infiltrate with prominent eosinophils.

are highly variable. There may be a predominance of neutrophilic, eosinophilic, or lymphoplasmacytic elements. Attempts to differentiate "allergic" nasal polyps from inflammatory polyps on the basis of tissue eosinophilia have given inconsistent results.

NASAL POLYPS IN CYSTIC FIBROSIS

Clinical Features

Inflammatory nasal polyps are rare in childhood, except in children with cystic fibrosis. In the latter population, they are seen in up to 20% of children (58). The majority of polyps occur in patients with documented disease, but there are examples of nasal polyps occurring up to 12 years before the diagnosis of cystic fibrosis (59). For this reason, it is important to suspect this condition in any child with an inflammatory-type nasal polyp. Rarely, nasal polyps may be the initial manifestation in adults with cystic fibrosis.

Morphologic Characteristics

Nasal polyps in cystic fibrosis closely resemble inflammatory polyps, but there are minor differences that, when taken in aggregate, usually allow the pathologist to make the distinction (60). Polyps in cystic fibrosis lack basement membrane thickening and submucosal hyalinization, and they usually contain few stromal eosinophils. More important, the mucous glands, cysts, and blanket contain predominantly acid mucin, manifested as a blue or purple-blue coloration with combined Alcian blue/periodic acid-Schiff stain (60). In contrast, the neutral mucin in inflammatory polyps stains red or purple-red (Fig. 21.14). Goblet cells in both conditions contain acid mucin.

ANTROCHOANAL POLYPS

Clinical Features

Antrochoanal polyps originate from a wall of the maxillary antrum. They extend via a long stalk through a large primary or accessory maxillary ostium into the nasal cavity. With continued growth, they often pass through the choana and into the nasopharynx (61–65). Large antrochoanal polyps may even be visible in the back of the oropharynx. In contrast to typical nasal polyps, antrochoanal polyps are less common (4% to 6% of all nasal polyps) and frequently occur in childhood (61–63). Approximately 90% are solitary (63).

Morphologic Characteristics

Resected antrochoanal polyps have a long, narrow stalk, and the body of the polyp is usually firm and fibrous (Fig. 21.15). On microscopic examination, the surface mucosa is thin and usually lacks the thickened basement membrane of inflammatory polyps. The stroma is variable, but frequently, it is less edematous and more fibrotic, and it contains fewer glands than that of typical nasal polyps. Large vascular spaces may be present. Stromal inflammation is patchy, and only approximately 20% of antrochoanal polyps contain prominent eosinophils (61).

STROMAL ATYPIA IN POLYPS

Most, if not all, polyps of the nasal cavity and paranasal sinuses have scattered, mildly atypical stromal cells (66,67). Occasionally, such polyps contain sufficient numbers of pleomorphic or overtly bizarre stromal cells to lead to its confusion with a sarcoma (66–68). Atypical cells are most numerous in polyps from younger individuals (66) or in polyps with a prominent fibrous stroma (67). Antrochoanal polyps may develop marked degrees of this change, perhaps because of their frequent occurrence in childhood and typically fibrous stroma (69). Similar, overtly bizarre pseudomalignant changes have been described in granulation tissue removed from the paranasal sinuses after radiation therapy (70).

The atypical stromal cells tend to be concentrated in the submucosal region or near small vascular channels. They are characteristically spindled and have variably enlarged, angu-

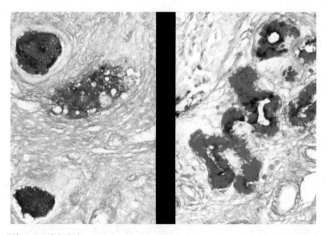

Figure 21.14. The predominantly acid mucin in a nasal polyp of cystic fibrosis stains blue to purple-blue with the Alcian blue/periodic acid–Schiff stain (*left*). The neutral mucin in an inflammatory nasal polyp stains red to purple-red with the Alcian blue/periodic acid–Schiff stain (*right*).

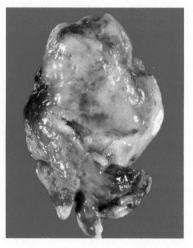

Figure 21.15. The cut surface of an antrochoanal polyp has a fibrous appearance, unlike the more edematous inflammatory polyp.

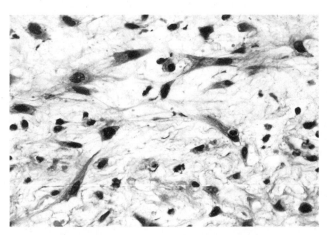

Figure 21.16. Scattered, atypical stromal cells with hyperchromatic, enlarged nuclei and prominent cytoplasm may be seen in nasal polyps of all types. The atypical cells resemble "radiation fibroblasts" and must not be confused with a sarcoma.

lated, dark nuclei (Fig. 21.16). Nuclear chromatin may have a bubbly appearance or may be densely hyperchromatic. A few cells may have small, distinct nucleoli. Eosinophilic cytoplasm is usually abundant and parallels nuclear size, such that the nucleus-to-cytoplasm ratio tends to remain constant. Despite their individually alarming appearance, the cells are haphazardly arranged in otherwise typical, fibrous to edematous stroma. There is no increased cellularity or neovascularity, and mitotic figures are extremely rare or absent. Confusion with sarcoma, particularly rhabdomyosarcoma, is avoided if these features are noted and if the low-power pattern of a polyp with stromal glands is observed. Immunocytochemical studies of the atypical cells have documented fibrohistiocytic features (68).

SQUAMOUS AND SCHNEIDERIAN PAPILLOMAS

Papillomas of the nose and paranasal sinuses include lesions lined with mature squamous epithelium and the histologically diverse schneiderian papillomas. Papillomas lined with mature squamous epithelium usually develop in the vestibule of the nose, where they originate from skin. Rarely, the nasopharynx is involved in patients with extensive juvenile papillomatosis (71).

The schneiderian papillomas have many names, reflecting their different microscopic features. The major types are fungiform papilloma, inverted papilloma, and oncocytic schneiderian papilloma. The latter has often been referred to as cylindrical-cell papilloma, whereas fungiform papilloma and inverted papilloma have often been called transitional cell papilloma or, simply, papillomatosis. The role of human papillomavirus (HPV) in the development of schneiderian papillomas has been the subject of numerous studies. In situ hybridization and polymerase chain reaction (PCR) studies have shown papillomavirus DNA in almost all fungiform papillomas and in a minority of inverted papillomas (72–75). Cylindrical-cell papillomas have been negative for HPV DNA (72,73,76). Epstein-Barr virus (EBV) has not been detected in schneiderian papillomas (73).

CLINICAL FEATURES

The schneiderian papillomas develop in patients who are mainly between 30 and 50 years of age, with men being affected twice as often as women. Unilateral nasal obstruction is the most common complaint, but epistaxis, facial pain, purulent discharge, and proptosis may also occur. The latter symptom has been reported only with inverted papilloma and reflects its ability to erode bone by pressure. Although the papillomas are often multifocal, bilaterality is rare. All three types have a recurrence rate of 50% to 70% (usually within 1 to 2 years) if treated only by local excision. The recurrences are usually microscopically identical to the original lesion unless carcinoma has supervened. However, some authors report greater atypia and a higher rate of mitoses in recurrences (77). The recurrence rate can be reduced to approximately 5% for papillomas involving the lateral nose and antrum by performing a medial maxillectomy (78). The rate of recurrence has not been consistently related to the histologic features.

MORPHOLOGIC CHARACTERISTICS

On gross inspection, all three types of schneiderian papillomas are soft to moderately firm, with a granular or finely clefted surface (Fig. 21.17). The cell types in fungiform and inverted papilloma are the same, but the two differ architecturally, in their site of origin and in their association with carcinoma. Fungiform papilloma arises almost exclusively on the nasal septum, whereas the inverted form predominantly affects the lateral wall of the nose and/or the paranasal sinuses. Fungiform papilloma is not associated with carcinoma, whereas inverted papilloma is (vide infra) (79–81).

There is some architectural overlap between fungiform and inverted papilloma. Generally, fungiform papilloma has connective tissue stalks that form an exophytic architecture (Fig. 21.18). By contrast, inverted papilloma has invaginations of the surface epithelium into the underlying stroma (Fig. 21.19). Nonetheless, some inverted papillomas will have an exophytic surface in addition to the invaginations, and fungiform papilloma can have sporadic invaginations. The epithelium of fungi-

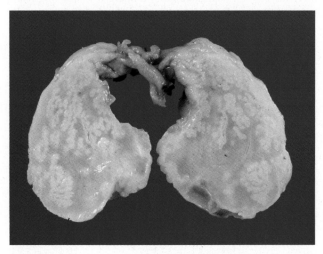

Figure 21.17. Inverted papilloma. The stroma is edematous much like an inflammatory polyp, but the epithelial invaginations are clearly evident.

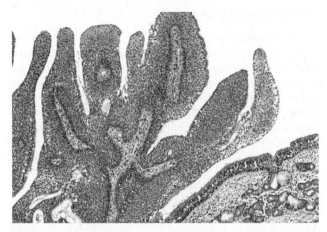

Figure 21.18. The epithelium of a fungiform papilloma has a serpiginous configuration without the deep invaginations of inverted papilloma. On cytologic examination, the epithelium is identical to that of an inverted papilloma. Normal respiratory epithelium is seen at the right.

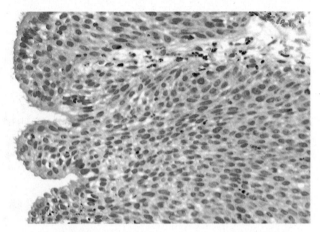

Figure 21.20. Inverted papilloma and fungiform papilloma are often lined by intermediate or ciliated epithelium. Mucous cells may be interspersed.

form and inverted papilloma includes squamous, ciliated columnar, intermediate, and mucus-secreting cells.

Nonkeratinizing squamous epithelium is most common, followed by intermediate epithelium (Fig. 21.20). These epithelial types range from 5 to 30 cells in thickness. Ciliated epithelium has the appearance of normal respiratory mucosa, although ciliated cells occasionally form a single layer on top of intermediate or squamous cells. The mucous cells have distended cytoplasm with an eccentric nucleus. They usually are seen individually but occasionally form small clusters. All epithelial types may be present in a single papilloma. Mitotic figures are usually few in number and are located in the basal or parabasal region, but they may be more numerous and can be found in the upper half of the epithelium as well. Atypical forms are absent.

Nuclear pleomorphism is prominent in approximately 10% of inverted papillomas, mainly as a few isolated cells at any depth within the epithelium. Sometimes, atypical nuclei form larger aggregates in the inner third of the mucosa. Neutrophils can be scattered throughout the epithelial layer as single cells or microabscesses. This inflammation imparts a disquieting histologic appearance to the lesion, especially when it is accompa-

nied by nuclear abnormalities. The stroma is variably fibrous, edematous, or vascular. Inflammatory cells can be absent or abundant. Plasma cells, lymphocytes, and neutrophils predominate, but eosinophils are sometimes numerous. Unlike inflammatory polyps, seromucinous glands are not present, except at the base of the lesion, where it arises from the mucosa.

The differential diagnosis of inverted and fungiform papilloma includes nonkeratinizing squamous carcinoma when it has either a papillary architecture or narrow, serpiginous ribbons of invading epithelium. On cytologic examination, however, papillary carcinoma has widespread, severe nuclear abnormalities (Figs. 21.21 and 21.22), and often the cells have a partially clear cytoplasm. Papillary squamous carcinoma frequently has scattered small, round nests of mature squamous epithelium.

Oncocytic schneiderian papilloma has areas of intermediate-cell proliferation identical to inverted papilloma, and the low-power architectures of these two papillomas are indistinguishable. In contrast to inverted papilloma, however, the majority of the cells in oncocytic papilloma have a finely granular eosinophilic cytoplasm and less sharply defined cell borders (Figs. 21.23 and 21.24). The outermost layer is often ciliated, and the cells rarely form a layer more than six to eight cells thick.

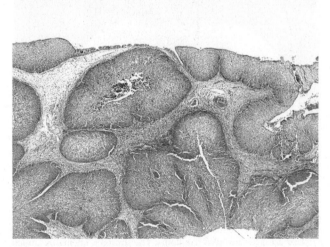

Figure 21.19. This inverted papilloma consists of deeply invaginated nests of benign, predominantly squamous epithelium.

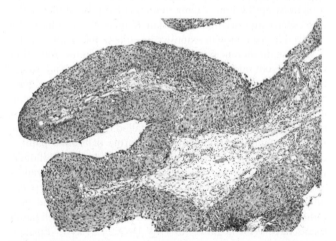

Figure 21.21. This nasal papillary carcinoma has well-developed fibrovascular cores and superficially resembles a fungiform papilloma.

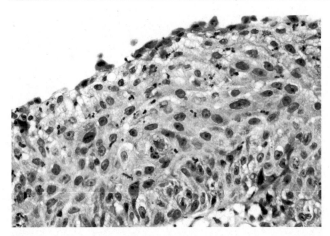

Figure 21.22. A higher-power view of the epithelium seen in Figure 21.17 shows mildly pleomorphic, hyperchromatic, and somewhat disorganized squamous cells. A suprabasal mitotic figure is present.

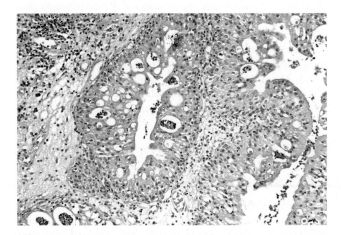

Figure 21.23. Oncocytic schneiderian papilloma has irregularly distributed strips of eosinophilic cells with interspersed mucous cells and acute inflammation.

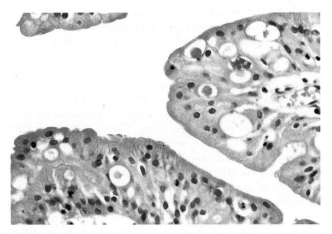

Figure 21.24. Inspissated mucin lies within the clear spaces of the mucous cells.

Oncocytic papilloma frequently contains numerous cells with sharply delimited, inspissated mucin droplets (81).

The differential diagnosis of oncocytic papilloma includes inflammatory polyp. When there are many neutrophils in the epithelium and stroma of oncocytic papilloma, the resemblance to an inflammatory polyp is enhanced. Inflammatory polyps, however, do not have the oncocytic epithelial cells or mucous inclusions. The numerous vacuoles containing inspissated mucus superficially resemble rhinosporidiosis. The organisms of rhinosporidiosis, however, involve both the epithelium and underlying stroma. Moreover, they are not accompanied by oncocytic epithelium. When the mucosa of oncocytic papilloma is cut tangentially, the numerous small lumina may mimic adenocarcinoma. However, adenocarcinomas of the nose or paranasal sinuses rarely have eosinophilic cytoplasm. The lack of nuclear atypia in oncocytic papilloma further distinguishes it from carcinoma.

For practical purposes, inverted and oncocytic papillomas are not metastasizing lesions in the absence of carcinoma. Two patients with inverted papilloma have had lesions in the neck (82,83). It is debatable whether these represent true metastases, implants in lymph nodes, or papillary transformation of a branchial-cleft epithelial remnant. Rarely, inverted papilloma extends up the eustachian tube and involves the middle ear and mastoid (84).

The association of carcinoma with inverted and oncocytic papillomas is indisputable. Invasive squamous cell carcinoma occurs in approximately 6% to 14% of patients with these papillomas (85–87). In our experience, as well as that of others, the oncocytic variants seem most prone to undergo malignant transformation (85,87). Patients with carcinoma have a mean age 9 to 13 years older than the mean age of all patients with inverted papilloma (88). The carcinoma may be within the papilloma at the time the patient is first seen or may arise after an interval that may or may not have included recurrent papillomas. Metachronous carcinoma may or may not be associated with a papilloma. There are no criteria to predict which papillomas will be followed by carcinoma. The rate at which papillomas recur and the length of time between recurrences do not correlate with the risk of subsequent carcinoma. The carcinomas are mostly of the squamous cell type (89), but spindle cell (90), clear-cell (91), high-grade mucoepidermoid (81,91), and sinonasal undifferentiated carcinomas (92) have also been described. All tissue removed from a patient with inverted or oncocytic papilloma should be submitted for microscopic examination so as not to overlook small foci of carcinoma.

RESPIRATORY EPITHELIAL ADENOMATOID HAMARTOMA

The term *respiratory epithelial adenomatoid hamartoma* (*REAH*) was coined by Wenig and Heffner (93) to refer to a proliferation of glandular spaces lined by ciliated epithelium and, less often, goblet cells. The glands are situated in a stromal background resembling inflammatory polyp, replete with edema and chronic inflammatory cells (Figs. 21.25 and 21.26). The lesion arises most often on the posterior nasal septum, but it may occur in the lateral nasal mucosa, the nasopharynx, or the paranasal sinuses. The patients of Wenig and Heffner were 27 to 82 years of age, with a median age of 58 years. Many had a history of chronic rhinosinusitis. One patient had an inverted papilloma in continuity with the REAH, and one had a solitary fibrous

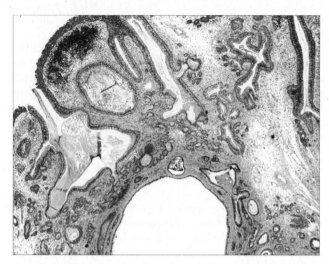

Figure 21.25. Respiratory epithelial adenomatoid hamartoma has the low-power appearance of an inflammatory polyp but contains large numbers of irregular glands.

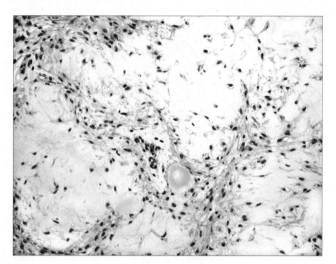

Figure 21.27. Chondromesenchymal hamartoma. Loose chondromyxoid tissue forms a distinctly lobular pattern.

tumor in the contralateral nasal fossa. REAH did not recur during the follow-up time of 4 months to 5 years. The tumors measured as large as 4.9 cm, but the destructive growth of schneiderian papillomas was absent. There have been scattered additional descriptions of this lesion as case reports, but the author's experience suggests that this entity is relatively common and often interpreted as an inflammatory polyp with prominent epithelium or as a schneiderian papilloma. Although initially considered to be nonneoplastic, one recent study has suggested otherwise (94).

CHONDROMESENCHYMAL HAMARTOMA

Chondromesenchymal hamartomas almost always arise in children less than 3 months of age (95). Most involve the nasal

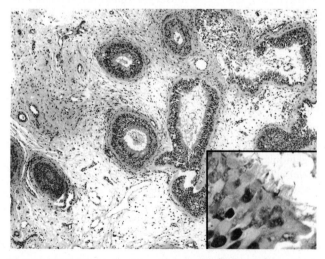

Figure 21.26. Respiratory epithelial adenomatoid hamartoma. At higher magnification, the glands resemble respiratory bronchial mucosa, complete with cilia (*inset*).

cavity, but the sinuses may also be affected. Patients usually present with a mass or difficulty breathing. The lesions are well circumscribed and do not recur if completely excised. Histologically, there is a proliferation of various mesenchymal elements, predominantly hyaline cartilage, often in a lobular pattern (Fig. 21.27). The intervening stroma is composed of bland spindled cells and can appear either hypercellular or myxoid. Osteoclast-like giant cells can be present, as can vascular proliferation.

SQUAMOUS CELL CARCINOMA

NOSE AND PARANASAL SINUSES

Carcinoma of the nose and paranasal sinuses accounts for only approximately 3% of head and neck neoplasms. Approximately 58% develop in the maxillary antrum, 30% develop in the nasal cavity, 10% develop in the ethmoid, and 1% develop in the sphenoid and frontal sinuses (96). Squamous cell carcinoma of the nasal cavity is related to cigarette smoking (97,98) and industrial exposure to nickel ore (99). Job-related exposures to chromium, isopropyl alcohol, and radium also have been associated with sinonasal squamous cell carcinoma (100). Thorotrast has been linked with squamous cell carcinoma of the maxillary antrum (101). Although chronic recurrent sinusitis with secondary squamous metaplasia has been suggested as a factor in the development of sinonasal carcinoma, it is quite possible that, in many such cases, an occult carcinoma is responsible for the recurrent infections, rather than the reverse.

The role (if any) of HPV and EBV in the development of the conventional type of squamous cell carcinomas of the nose and paranasal sinuses remains to be clarified. DNA from HPV types 16 and 18 has been detected, using the highly sensitive PCR, in one study in 14% of squamous cell carcinomas of the sinonasal region (102). Using this technique, however, apparently normal mucosa in the ear, nose, and throat region also has been noted to contain HPV DNA, raising questions about the significance of this finding. Similarly, although EBV RNA has been confirmed by in situ hybridization in undifferentiated nasopharyngeal carcinomas (and related neoplasms), the finding of EBV by PCR in conventional squamous cell carcinomas is of questionable significance, given the high prevalence of latent EBV in normal lymphocytes. The possible relationship between schneiderian papillomas and the subsequent development of sinonasal carcinoma has been discussed.

Clinical Features

Squamous cell carcinoma of both the nasal cavity and paranasal sinuses shows a male predominance of approximately 2:1 (103). Most patients are in their sixth or seventh decade of life, and cases in patients under 40 years of age are extremely rare. Nasal lesions cause obstruction, rhinorrhea, epistaxis, or pain. An origin in the paranasal sinuses produces symptoms identical to those of chronic sinusitis (96). Regardless of the mode of therapy (surgery, radiation, and/or chemotherapy), recurrences are common; death is usually a result of local spread. The prognosis varies with stage (103).

Nasal cavity carcinoma is associated with a high rate (6% to 28%) of second primary neoplasms (97,103). Other neoplasms may antedate, postdate, or occur concurrently with nasal carcinoma. Approximately 40% of the second primaries involve the head and neck, with the remainder developing at sites such as lung, breast, and gastrointestinal tract (103). In contrast, carcinoma of the maxillary antrum carries a 5% incidence of a second primary carcinoma in the contralateral antrum but no increased rate of occurrence of carcinoma at other sites (104).

Morphologic Characteristics

The majority of sinonasal squamous cell carcinomas are focally keratinizing, easily diagnosable lesions (Fig. 21.28). Nonkeratinizing carcinomas occasionally occur in this region; rarely, undifferentiated carcinomas (lymphoepithelioma) analogous to those of the nasopharynx may develop. Nonkeratinizing carcinomas have been referred to by a variety of terms, including transitional cell carcinoma, intermediate-cell carcinoma, and schneiderian carcinoma. In our experience, these neoplasms are difficult to recognize as a morphologically distinctive group, and we prefer to view them as within the spectrum of squamous cell carcinoma. Nonkeratinizing carcinomas do tend to grow as large cell nests and anastomosing cords of cells, often with only mild cellular pleomorphism. Such carcinomas may be confused, on cursory examination, with fungiform or inverted nasal papillomas because of their architectural similarities. Closer inspection will reveal a degree of mitotic activity and pleomorphism beyond that seen in papillomas. Some larger nests of carcinoma may also have central, comedo-like necrosis.

Unusual variants of squamous cell carcinoma, such as spindle cell carcinoma or sarcomatoid carcinoma, have been described in the sinonasal region (105). These are described and illustrated in the subsequent chapter on laryngeal pathology. If islands of conventional carcinoma are present, the diagnosis is straightforward. Biopsies containing only spindle cells may

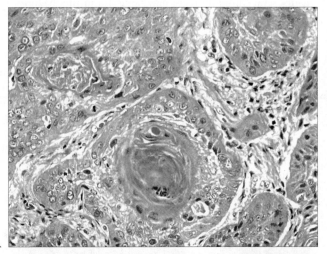

A

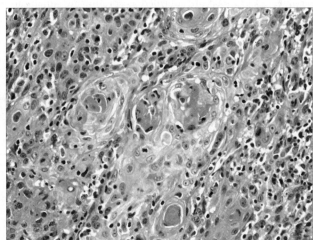

B

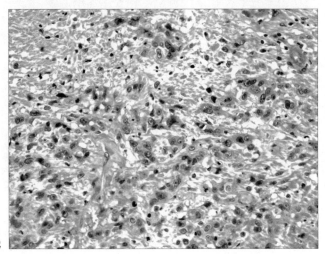

C

Figure 21.28. Sinonasal squamous cell carcinoma. **(A)** Well-differentiated squamous cell carcinoma forms large, regular nests with minimal pleomorphism and central keratin pearl formation. **(B)** In moderately differentiated squamous cell carcinoma, the nests are more irregular with greater pleomorphism. **(C)** Poorly differentiated squamous cell carcinoma consists of individual malignant cells, some with keratinization, infiltrating the stroma.

be difficult or impossible to distinguish from sarcoma or amelanotic melanoma on hematoxylin and eosin–stained sections. Immunocytochemistry may demonstrate focal epithelial differentiation in the spindle cell component (105). Although it may be tempting to label high-grade spindle cell lesions in this region lacking evidence of epithelial or specific mesenchymal differentiation as sarcomas, experience indicates that their behavior is that of a high-grade carcinoma. These tumors are discussed in more detail in relation to the larynx and oral cavity.

Verrucous carcinoma of the nasal cavity and paranasal sinuses has been reported (106) but is much less common than its morphologically identical oral and laryngeal counterparts. Manivel et al. (107) reported two unusual sinonasal and nasopharyngeal carcinomas containing areas of endodermal sinus (yolk sac) tumor, replete with α_1-antitrypsin and α-fetoprotein expression.

NASOPHARYNX

In the United States, 78% to 90% of malignant neoplasms arising in the nasopharynx are nonglandular carcinomas (108). In some areas of Asia, where nasopharyngeal carcinomas are much more common, they account for up to 98% of all nasopharyngeal malignancies (108,109). Acquiring an understanding of these tumors was hampered by a lack of uniform nomenclature before 1978, when the World Health Organization published its classification scheme. Under this system, nonglandular nasopharyngeal carcinomas are subtyped as keratinizing squamous cell carcinoma (type 1), nonkeratinizing carcinoma (type 2), and undifferentiated carcinoma (lymphoepithelioma). The morphologic criteria for these groups are discussed later in this chapter.

Clinical Features

Many nasopharyngeal carcinomas arise near the eustachian tube opening in the fossa of Rosenmüller. Initial complaints are often caused by middle-ear obstruction (e.g., otitis, hearing loss) or local invasion (e.g., headache, cranial nerve deficits, epistaxis) (110–112). Approximately 50% to 80% of patients with undifferentiated carcinoma are initially seen with cervical lymph node metastases from an occult primary (110,111); 25% have bilateral nodal involvement (110,111). Involved lymph nodes are typically posterior to the sternocleidomastoid at the level of the angle of the jaw (111). Examination of the nasopharynx may show entirely normal features, may reveal fullness or surface granularity, or may demonstrate an obvious carcinoma. In patients with a normal-appearing nasopharynx, random biopsies yield diagnostic tissue in 70% of cases; the remainder may require rebiopsy (111).

Squamous cell carcinoma and nonkeratinizing carcinoma are rare in childhood (108,112). In contrast, undifferentiated carcinoma often occurs in children and shows a distinctly bimodal age distribution, with peaks in the second and sixth decades (108,111–115). All forms of nasopharyngeal carcinoma have a male predominance of approximately 2.5 to 3:1 (108,111,112). Nasopharyngeal carcinoma is treated exclusively with radiation; survival correlates with the stage of disease and its histologic type. Keratinizing squamous cell carcinomas are the least radiation sensitive and have the poorest prognosis; there were no 5-year survivors reported in one series (110). Nonkeratinizing carcinomas have been reported variously as having a survival rate intermediate between keratinizing and undifferentiated carcinoma (110) or as behaving like undifferentiated carcinoma (108). In several large historical series, patients treated with radiation therapy for undifferentiated carcinoma had the following 5-year survival rates, according to stage: stage I (confined to the nasopharynx), 50% to 60%; stage II (cervical node involvement), 20% to 30%; and stage III (invasion of surrounding structures), 5% to 20% (108,110,111). More recent studies using combined platinum-based chemotherapy and radiation therapy have reported overall 5-year survival rates of 70% to 90% for these patients (116).

In Hong Kong, nasopharyngeal carcinoma accounts for 18% of all malignant neoplasms (117), as opposed to approximately 2% in the United States. Racial susceptibility tends to remain constant in those emigrating to other countries. Chinese patients in Singapore have significantly higher rates of the histocompatibility antigens HLA-A2 and HLA-BW46 (118). In addition, the incidence of nasopharyngeal carcinomas may be lower in patients with blood group A (119). The association between EBV infection and nasopharyngeal carcinoma of the undifferentiated and nonkeratinizing type is well established (108,120–125). EBV genomic RNA has been repeatedly demonstrated in the neoplastic epithelial cells of undifferentiated (and some nonkeratinizing) nasopharyngeal carcinomas using an in situ hybridization technique (Fig. 21.29) (108,114,124). The detection of serum antibodies against viral proteins, particularly immunoglobulin A (IgA) and immunoglobulin G (IgG) directed against viral capsid antigen, may be useful in the diagnosis of metastases from occult primary tumors (120–122).

Morphologic Characteristics

Squamous cell carcinoma (keratinizing) of the nasopharynx is defined as a tumor having squamous differentiation in the form of intercellular bridges or keratinization over most of its extent (108). These tumors seldom pose diagnostic difficulties except for rare "adenoid" or acantholytic forms that may be confused with adenocarcinoma (123) or even angiosarcoma. Nonkeratinizing nasopharyngeal carcinoma has cells at differing levels of maturation but lacking light microscopic evidence of squamous differentiation. Nuclei vary in size, shape, and chromatin distri-

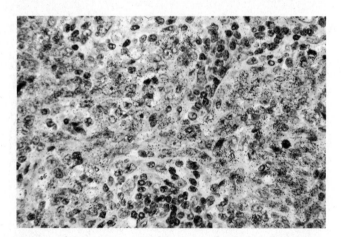

Figure 21.29. In situ hybridization for Epstein-Barr virus RNA in this undifferentiated carcinoma shows positivity (black silver grains) overlying the neoplastic epithelial cells but not the smaller lymphoid component. (Courtesy of L. M. Weiss, MD.)

bution. Tumor cells have well-defined cell margins that interdigitate in a "pavement stone" pattern. There is no evidence of mucin production or glandular differentiation (108). Variable numbers of lymphocytes, eosinophils (126), and plasma cells may be present in the stroma.

Undifferentiated nasopharyngeal carcinoma (lymphoepithelioma) consists of cytologically uniform cells with ovoid vesicular nuclei, prominent nucleoli, and indistinct cell borders resulting in a syncytial pattern. Spindle cells may sometimes be present, and there may be scattered effete cells with shrunken, hyperchromatic nuclei. An inflammatory infiltrate rich in lymphocytes and occasionally containing prominent eosinophils (126) is usually a component of lymphoepithelioma, but the diagnosis is based solely on the nature of the neoplastic epithelial component. The inflammatory and neoplastic elements in lymphoepithelioma may interact to produce two microscopic patterns named for their initial describers (127,128).

In the Regaud pattern, the neoplastic cells form well-defined, cohesive cell nests and cords separated by inflammation (Fig. 21.30). The cohesive nature of the cell nests allows for its ready recognition as a carcinoma, and diagnosis is straightforward (113). In the Schmincke pattern, however, the inflammatory component permeates the cell nests to a much greater degree, separating and isolating the carcinoma cells in a "sea" of polymorphic inflammation that is predominantly lymphoid (Fig. 21.31). Such lesions may be difficult or impossible to distinguish from lymphoma on hematoxylin and eosin–stained sections (113,129), particularly when the lesion appears as a lymph node metastasis from an occult primary. The two patterns have no prognostic differences, and mixtures of both patterns are common.

The use of immunocytochemical markers to distinguish undifferentiated carcinoma from lymphoma is discussed in the section on lymphoplasmacytic proliferations (Figs. 21.32 and 21.33). Standard light microscopic features are also useful in this regard. Even in Schmincke pattern tumors, isolated, delicate cytoplasmic strands can be seen connecting separated cells, and a careful search should be made for more cohesive cell nests. Lymph node metastases with the Schmincke pattern can mimic Hodgkin disease in terms of both clinical characteristics (because of their typical bilaterality and presence in young patients) and microscopic features (because the neoplastic cells

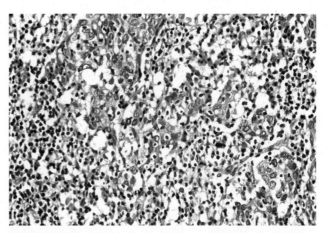

Figure 21.31. In the Schmincke pattern of undifferentiated carcinoma (lymphoepithelioma), the neoplastic cells are dispersed in the surrounding inflammation. Distinguishing it from lymphoma may be impossible without special techniques.

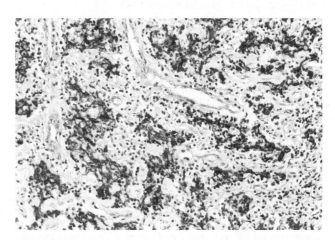

Figure 21.32. Undifferentiated carcinoma. In contrast to Figure 21.33, the larger neoplastic cells stain for cytokeratin, and the inflammatory infiltrate is nonreactive (anticytokeratin immunoperoxidase).

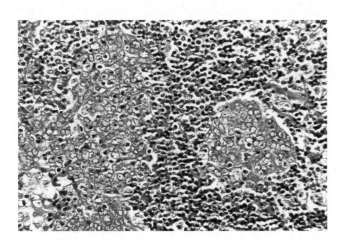

Figure 21.30. In the Regaud pattern of undifferentiated carcinoma (lymphoepithelioma), the neoplastic cells form cohesive nests. Confusion with lymphoma is unlikely.

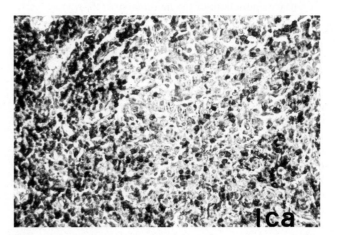

Figure 21.33. This undifferentiated carcinoma (lymphoepithelioma) demonstrates prominent staining for leukocyte common antigen (LCA, CD45) confined to the inflammatory component. Larger neoplastic cells in the center of the field are unstained (anti-LCA immunoperoxidase).

somewhat resemble mononuclear Reed-Sternberg cells in a polymorphic inflammatory background) (113,129). In contrast to Reed-Sternberg cells, undifferentiated carcinoma cells (a) are always mononuclear, (b) have thin chromatin rims and smaller nucleoli, and (c) lack pericellular clearing (lacunae) (113). Verrucous carcinoma may rarely arise in the nasopharynx (130,131). Its clinicopathologic features are identical to those of the more common verrucous carcinomas of the larynx and oral cavity.

VARIANTS OF ADENOCARCINOMA

Adenocarcinomas account for approximately 10% to 20% of all sinonasal malignancies (96,132,133). These tumors can be divided into two main groups: salivary-type neoplasms and a heterogeneous group of distinctive, nonsalivary adenocarcinomas.

SALIVARY-TYPE ADENOCARCINOMAS

Of the salivary-type tumors, adenoid cystic carcinoma is most common in the sinonasal and nasopharyngeal region (56). The maxillary antrum is the most typical site (134), but involvement of the nasal cavity, nasopharynx, and ethmoid and sphenoid sinuses is also typical (134,135). Frontal sinus tumors are unusual. Mucoepidermoid carcinoma is the second most common salivary-type adenocarcinoma of the upper aerodigestive tract (56). The morphologic appearance and clinical behavior of these tumors are discussed in more detail in the chapter on salivary gland neoplasms (Chapter 20).

NONSALIVARY ADENOCARCINOMAS

Adenocarcinomas of the sinonasal region that do not resemble salivary-type neoplasms may be subdivided into low-grade adenocarcinomas (56) and intestinal-type adenocarcinomas (56, 136). The clinicopathologic features of each group differ markedly, warranting careful distinction. Additionally, low-grade papillary adenocarcinomas have been described that arose from the surface epithelium of the nasopharynx (137).

LOW-GRADE ADENOCARCINOMA

Clinical Features

Low-grade sinonasal adenocarcinomas affect males and females with equal frequency and occur in a broad age range (age range, 9 to 75 years; median age, 54 years) (56). The distribution of lesions in one study was as follows: nasal cavity, 22%; nasal septum, 18%; ethmoid or nasoethmoid, 30%; maxillary or nasomaxillary, 13%; and multiple locations, 18% (56). There is no known association with carcinogens. Patients with low-grade carcinoma have a good prognosis. Recurrences develop in 30% of cases but do not indicate intractable disease (56). In one study, after a median follow-up interval of more than 6 years, 78% of patients were disease free (56). Death from disease is a result of uncontrollable local invasion rather than metastases. None of the nine patients with low-grade nasopharyngeal adenocarcinoma reported by Wenig et al. (137) experienced metastases, although one tumor recurred locally after radiation therapy.

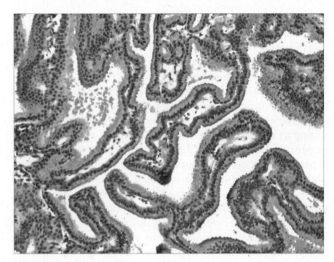

Figure 21.34. Low-grade sinonasal adenocarcinoma forms papillary structures lined by uniform, bland cells.

Morphologic Characteristics

Low-grade sinonasal adenocarcinomas are a morphologically heterogeneous group. In some, the architectural and cytologic uniformity frequently leads to misdiagnosis as an adenoma or a papilloma (137). In the majority of cases, small glands are lined by a single layer of cuboidal or columnar cells, often in a back-to-back arrangement without intervening stroma (Figs. 21.34 and 21.35) (56). Some glands are cystically dilated, and others contain papillary infoldings. Nuclei vary in size from case to case but tend to be uniform within a given lesion. Mitotic figures are generally rare but may occasionally be abundant (56). Most tumors contain both intracellular and extracellular mucin, and they can be seen to originate from surface mucosa. Some neoplasms included under the rubric of low-grade adenocarcinoma consist of cells with basophilic cytoplasm in small, acinar-like nests. Such lesions are indistinguishable from acinic cell carcinoma of the salivary gland type (56) and should probably be segregated from the other, nonsalivary tumors in this group.

Low-grade sinonasal adenocarcinoma must be distinguished from intestinal-type adenocarcinoma, which is described in the

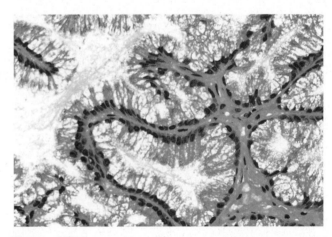

Figure 21.35. Low-grade sinonasal adenocarcinoma consists of glands lined by columnar cells with uniform nuclei. There is no nuclear stratification.

next section, because of the more aggressive clinical course of the latter lesion. Making the distinction is usually straightforward, given the nuclear stratification and colonic appearance of the intestinal neoplasms. In addition, intestinal-type tumors are more pleomorphic than low-grade adenocarcinomas on cytologic examination—with the exception of rare nasal neoplasms resembling normal intestinal mucosa. Oncocytic schneiderian papillomas may also be confused with low-grade adenocarcinoma. Heffner et al. (56) list the following differentiating features: (a) stratified epithelium in papillomas as opposed to single-layered cells in adenocarcinoma; (b) true glandular lumina in adenocarcinoma; and (c) more abundant, myxomatous stroma in papillomas. The complex papillary pattern, vesicular nuclei, and focal psammoma bodies seen in some low-grade nasopharyngeal adenocarcinomas can mimic a metastatic papillary carcinoma of the thyroid gland (137). However, the primary nasopharyngeal neoplasms lack positivity for thyroglobulin (137).

INTESTINAL-TYPE ADENOCARCINOMA

Clinical Features

After adenoid cystic carcinoma, the second most common glandular neoplasm of the sinonasal region is composed of cells mimicking normal, adenomatous, or carcinomatous intestinal mucosa (56,136–143). Although the histologic spectrum is broad, as described later, the clinical features are stereotypical and are only slightly affected by the microscopic form of intestinal differentiation. Nasal intestinal-type adenocarcinoma has a strong association with long-term exposure to fine hardwood dusts in the woodworking industry (142,144–147); in such populations, the incidence approaches 1000 times that of the general public (144). Approximately 20% of cases occur in patients with industrial wood-dust exposure. Exposure to leather dust has also been incriminated (148). With the advent of widespread dust control measures in the workplace, the incidence of occupationally related tumors appears to be declining.

There are minor clinical differences between intestinal-type adenocarcinomas occurring sporadically and those arising in woodworkers (136). Tumors related to industrial dust exposure are found predominantly in men (85% to 95%), show a striking predilection for the ethmoid sinus (146,147), and have a slightly better prognosis (50% at 5 years) (147). Tumors arising sporadically frequently develop in women, often arise in the maxillary antrum (20% to 50%), and have a poorer prognosis (20% to 40% at 5 years) (136). In both groups, the clinical course may be quite protracted; 5-year survival does not indicate cure. Local recurrences are common (53%) (136), and death usually results from uncontrollable local disease with intracranial extension or exsanguination. Metastasis to regional lymph nodes takes place in approximately 8% of cases, and distant metastases are seen in approximately 13% of cases (136).

Although all forms of intestinal-type neoplasia in the sinonasal region are at least locally aggressive, studies have suggested that grading these lesions provides additional prognostic information (149–151). Kleinsasser and Schroeder (149) divided intestinal-type sinonasal adenocarcinomas into the papillary-tubular type, grades I to III; the goblet cell type; the signet ring cell type; and the mixed or transitional type. Their study, and the subsequent studies by Franquemont et al. (150) and Franchi

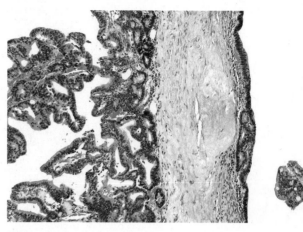

Figure 21.36. Intestinal-type sinonasal adenocarcinoma has a papillary configuration resembling adenomatous polyp of the colon.

et al. (151), showed a somewhat better prognosis for the well-differentiated papillary-tubular neoplasms.

Morphologic Characteristics

These neoplasms recapitulate the entire range of appearances assumed by normal and neoplastic large and small intestinal mucosa. At the exquisitely well-differentiated end of the spectrum are tumors that resemble normal intestinal mucosa replete with goblet, resorptive, Paneth, and argentaffin cells, along with well-formed villi and muscularis mucosae (138,143). Although it is tempting to label such proliferations as benign heterotopias, they are highly aggressive, invasive lesions (143). The papillary tumors consist of elongated fronds lined by stratified columnar and goblet cells reminiscent of intestinal villous or tubular adenoma (Fig. 21.36). Papillary tumors may be invasive or intramucosal (136,140).

The most common form of sinonasal intestinal-type adenocarcinoma resembles conventional colonic adenocarcinoma (Fig. 21.37). In this variant, glands lined by more pleomorphic columnar cells are often back to back, vary in size, and invade the underlying stroma. Intracellular mucin is present focally,

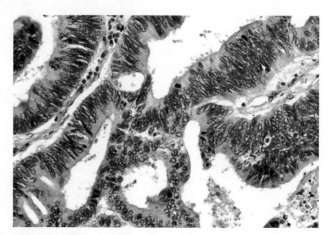

Figure 21.37. Intestinal-type sinonasal adenocarcinoma is indistinguishable from adenocarcinoma of the colon. Atypical, stratified epithelium lines well-formed glands.

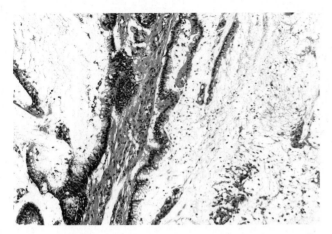

Figure 21.38. Some intestinal-type sinonasal adenocarcinomas have broad areas of extracellular mucin and resemble colloid carcinoma.

but goblet cells are not prominent (136,140). In less differentiated tumors, solid sheets of tumor cells may be present, with only scattered glandular lumina (136). Completing the analogy to intestinal neoplasms are the less typical mucinous tumors (136,140). The predominant pattern in this variant consists of large glands distended with mucin or pools of extracellular mucin containing small clusters of neoplastic cells (Fig. 21.38). Signet ring cells form a minor component or, rarely, predominate (140). The resemblance of intestinal-type adenocarcinoma to normal and neoplastic intestinal epithelium is not limited to the light microscopic manifestations. Ultrastructural studies have confirmed the presence of resorptive, goblet, Paneth, and argentaffin cells identical to their intestinal counterparts (143,152,153), and intestinal-type hormones have been documented on immunocytochemical evidence (152). Newer markers of intestinal differentiation, CDX-2 and MUC-2 (Fig. 21.39), are positive in these tumors (154). Although these markers are

of value in the distinction from low-grade adenocarcinoma, they do not establish primary sinonasal origin.

The rare intestinal-type adenocarcinoma resembling normal intestinal mucosa, as well as the papillary form resembling villous adenoma, can easily be recognized as a primary nasal lesion. Intestinal epithelium with this histologic picture is not capable of metastasis. In contrast, there are no morphologic features to clearly distinguish nasal tumors resembling conventional or mucinous adenocarcinoma from a metastasis. Immunohistochemical studies may be of some limited value in this regard. In one study, primary sinonasal intestinal-type tumors were less often strongly positive for carcinoembryonic antigen than histologically analogous colonic neoplasms (2 of 12 cases vs. 12 of 12 cases), and the sinonasal tumors had a stronger tendency to display neuroendocrine differentiation (9 of 12 cases vs. rare cells in 3 of 12 cases), as manifest by chromogranin reactivity (155). In a review of 82 tumors metastatic to the nose and paranasal sinuses, 5 tumors were primary in the gastrointestinal tract; in some patients, the sinonasal lesion was the initial clinical manifestation (156). Therefore, it is reasonable to perform barium radiographic studies on patients suspected of having primary sinonasal adenocarcinoma resembling colonic carcinoma.

NEURAL, NEUROECTODERMAL, AND NEUROENDOCRINE TUMORS

OLFACTORY NEUROBLASTOMA

Clinical Features

Olfactory neuroblastoma is an uncommon neoplasm that arises from the olfactory mucosa in the superior portion of the nasal cavity (157–164). A variety of other terms have been applied to these neoplasms, including esthesioneuroblastoma, esthesioneurocytoma, esthesioneuroma, and esthesioneuroepithelioma. Evidence for its origin from the olfactory epithelium is

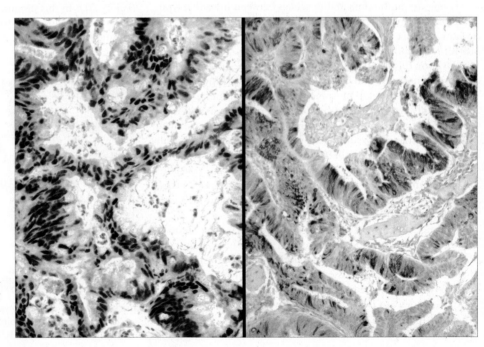

Figure 21.39. Intestinal-type adenocarcinoma. The tumor shows strong nuclear staining for CDX-2 (*left*) and strong cytoplasmic staining for MUC-2 (*right*).

based on the absolute localization of these tumors to this region. The mitotically active reserve cell is the putative cell of origin. During embryologic development, this cell gives rise to both neuronal and epithelial (sustentacular) cells. In adults the reserve cells supply new sustentacular cells, but it is unknown whether olfactory neuronal cells can regenerate in humans (2). Examples of olfactory neuroblastoma have been documented to contain low levels of catecholamines without systemic symptoms (165) and to produce vasopressin with secondary hypertension and hyponatremia (166).

Olfactory neuroblastomas affect patients across a broad age range, with bimodal peaks at approximately 15 and 55 years of age (157). There is no gender bias (157). Presenting symptoms are usually obstruction or hemorrhage (158). Physical examination demonstrates a large, often polypoid mass high in the nasal cavity or ethmoid sinus. The Kadish staging system is applied to these tumors (162):

1. Stage A: disease confined to the nasal cavity
2. Stage B: disease confined to the nasal cavity and paranasal sinuses
3. Stage C: local or distant spread beyond the nasal cavity or sinuses

Stage B disease is most common and occurs in 40% to 50% of cases (157,158). The prognosis has correlated with stage in some reports (157,162), with 5-year survival rates of 75%, 68%, and 41% for stages A, B, and C disease, respectively, in one large study (157). In another study, complete tumor resection was of more prognostic value than Kadish stage (158).

The division of olfactory neuroblastomas into subtypes, based on morphologic features (particularly the degree of epithelial vs. neuronal differentiation), has been of prognostic value in some studies (167,168), but most reports have been unable to correlate morphologic characteristics and prognosis (159–161,163,164). In our own experience, necrosis was the only morphologic feature tending to show prognostic correlation (poorer survival if present) (158). Complete surgical excision, often supplemented by radiation therapy or chemotherapy, appears to offer the highest apparent cure rate of approximately 75% (158). Long disease-free intervals do not indicate cure because recurrences or metastases can develop after more than a decade. Among patients with recurrence, 68% have local disease, 22% have nodal involvement, and 16% have distant spread (157).

Morphologic Characteristics

The proper diagnosis of olfactory neuroblastoma requires a carefully obtained, preferably incisional biopsy because the tumor cells are easily distorted by crush artifact. Initial diagnosis on frozen section is seldom possible and should be avoided because of the artifact in subsequent permanent sections from the frozen tissue. The clinical features, especially the tumor's location, usually lead experienced otolaryngologists to be highly suspicious.

At low power, the tumor exhibits two major growth patterns (Fig. 21.40). Most commonly, it forms irregular, circumscribed nests of cells separated by stroma. Less often, the tumor grows as a diffuse sheet of cells with a prominent background of capillaries but little intervening stroma (158). The neoplastic cells have small, round nuclei with coarse punctate to fine chromatin and very little cytoplasm. Most often there is only mild to moderate nuclear pleomorphism (Fig. 21.41). Mitotic figures are extremely variable; they can be virtually absent, or there can be more than 10 per high-power field. Occasionally, olfactory neuroblastomas contain areas of divergent differentiation, such as adenocarcinoma (169) or even rhabdomyoblasts.

In our experience, as well as that of others (170), the key microscopic feature for a definitive diagnosis is the presence of a fibrillary intercytoplasmic background (Fig. 21.42). Such fibrils can be seen on hematoxylin and eosin–stained sections in approximately 86% of cases (158) and correspond to neuronal cell processes. Another, less common diagnostic feature is the presence of Flexner-type or Homer Wright–type rosettes. The

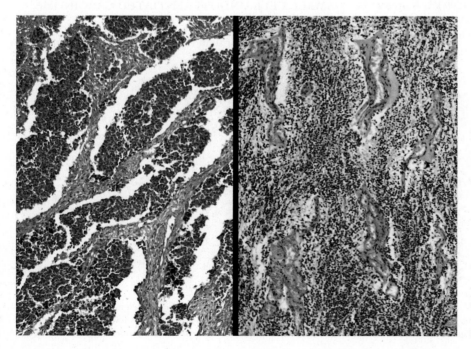

Figure 21.40. Olfactory neuroblastoma typically exhibits a nested growth pattern (*left*) or a diffuse pattern of growth with prominent vascularity (*right*).

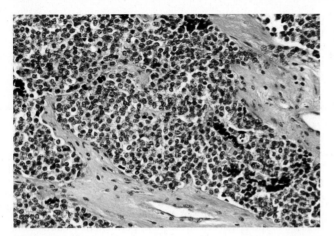

Figure 21.41. A nest of olfactory neuroblastoma showing uniform nuclei with punctuate, coarse chromatin.

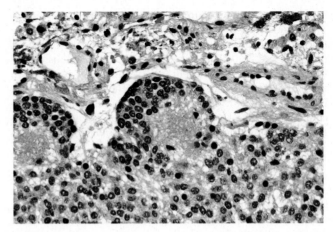

Figure 21.43. Neurofibrillary aggregates in olfactory neuroblastoma are rimmed by irregular clusters of neuroblasts.

former are glandlike structures that are too infrequent to be of much diagnostic value. Homer Wright rosettes, also termed *pseudorosettes*, are annular arrays of cells surrounding central zones of fibrils (Fig. 21.43). They are most common in cases that contain a prominent fibrillary background (158). Ganglion cells are rarely seen in olfactory neuroblastoma, but when present, they also have diagnostic value (158). Ganglion cells may be more prominent following radiation or chemotherapy.

Ancillary techniques can be used to diagnose olfactory neuroblastoma lacking fibrils, rosettes, or ganglion cells on hematoxylin and eosin–stained sections. Diagnostic ultrastructural features include dense-core granules and cell processes containing neurofilaments and/or neurotubules (171–176). Formaldehyde fume–induced fluorescence has been documented in olfactory neuroblastoma, but it requires fresh tissue and experience with the technique (165,168,176). Immunohistochemical staining is a valuable diagnostic adjunct. Between 84% and 100% of olfactory neuroblastomas react for neuron-specific enolase (159,177). Synaptophysin is found in 64% to 100% of cases (177,178). Neurofilament protein (200 kd) is present in approximately 73% of cases (159,177,179), but antibodies to this protein typically do not function well in paraffin-embedded tissue. A similar percentage of tumors contain S-100 protein

(159,177). The latter is present in Schwann-like cells that are preferentially located at the periphery of neoplastic cell nests (Fig. 21.44) (159,177) and usually are absent in areas of more diffuse growth. In our experience, the presence of S-100 protein–positive cells around cell nests is extremely helpful diagnostically. The scattered nature of the S-100–positive cells and their location should avoid confusion with the more diffuse S-100 staining in malignant melanoma. To add to the potential for confusion, isolated olfactory neuroblastomas may contain melanin pigment and stain focally with HMB-45 (178). A clear-cell variant has also been described (Fig. 21.45). Most olfactory neuroblastomas also contain microtubule-associated protein-2 (Fig. 21.46) and the class III beta-tubulin isotype (177). Approximately one-third of olfactory neuroblastomas contain cytokeratin (CK) (159,177), a potential source of confusion with nasopharyngeal-type carcinomas. Epithelial membrane antigen (EMA) is typically absent (177). Olfactory neuroblastoma is not related to primitive neuroectodermal tumors (PNET) and is negative for CD99 (180).

SMALL-CELL UNDIFFERENTIATED CARCINOMA

Carcinomas indistinguishable from pulmonary oat cell carcinoma occasionally arise in the nasal cavity but are more com-

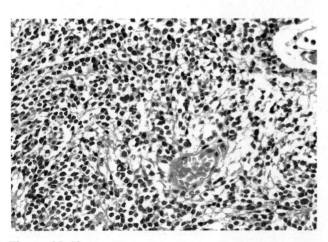

Figure 21.42. An olfactory neuroblastoma growing in the diffuse pattern with a fibrillary intercytoplasmic background.

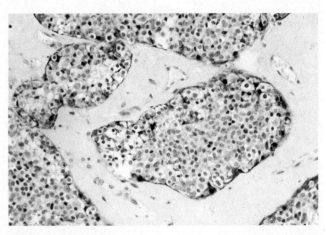

Figure 21.44. Cells at the periphery of cell nests in olfactory neuroblastoma frequently stain for S-100 protein. A few cells within the nests are also staining (anti–S-100 protein immunoperoxidase).

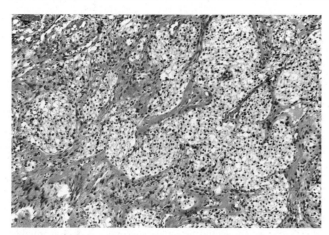

Figure 21.45. Olfactory neuroblastoma, clear-cell variant. Rare olfactory neuroblastomas are composed of cells with clear cytoplasm. Note the prominent vascularity common in all forms of this tumor, which in this variant may add to confusion with metastatic renal cell carcinoma.

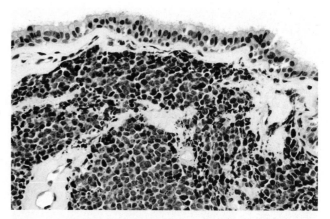

Figure 21.47. Small-cell undifferentiated (neuroendocrine) carcinoma infiltrates beneath intact sinonasal mucosa.

SINONASAL UNDIFFERENTIATED CARCINOMA

A clinicopathologically distinctive neoplasm, undifferentiated on light microscopy, with varying degrees of neuroendocrine differentiation has been designated sinonasal undifferentiated carcinoma (186–188). Other examples have been reported as anaplastic carcinoma (189).

Clinical Features

Both young adults and the elderly are affected. The median age in one study was 58 years (range, 20 to 81 years), and there was a male-to-female predominance of 3:1 (187). Seven of eight patients in one study were smokers (186). Symptoms are multiple and are related to a sinonasal mass. Physical examination usually finds a large tumor obstructing a nasal cavity and invading surrounding structures, including the nasopharynx. Involvement of the nasal cavity, maxillary antrum, and ethmoids is most common; extension into the sphenoid sinus, frontal sinus, orbit, and cranial cavity is also typical. Surgical resection is difficult or impossible, and radiation and chemotherapy have been of

mon in the paranasal sinuses (181–184). The biologic behavior of these tumors differs from their pulmonary counterparts in that aggressive local disease, rather than dissemination, dominates the clinical picture. Of eight reported cases, five patients died of disease (median survival, 11 months), two were alive at 1 year, and one was alive at 8 years. In some instances, an origin from minor salivary glands seems likely (181).

On light microscopy, these are anaplastic small-cell carcinomas with the typical features of pulmonary oat cell carcinoma (Fig. 21.47). Cells have (a) little visible cytoplasm; (b) densely hyperchromatic, pleomorphic nuclei; and (c) a high rate of mitosis. Large areas of necrosis are common. Dense-core granules and cell processes are seen on ultrastructural inspection (184). Neuroendocrine markers such as CD56 or synaptophysin will show variable positivity, and CK will often display the typical dotlike perinuclear staining seen with similar tumors in the lung (Fig. 21.48). An unusual small-cell undifferentiated neoplasm with some features of small-cell undifferentiated carcinoma, but also showing divergent mesenchymal differentiation, has been described in the sinonasal region following radiation therapy for bilateral retinoblastoma (185).

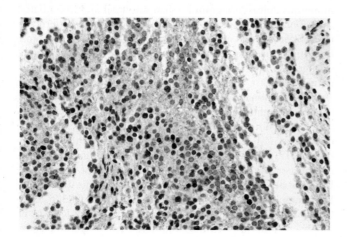

Figure 21.46. The fibrillary background in olfactory neuroblastoma demonstrates prominent staining for microtubule-associated protein (MAP)-2 (anti–MAP-2 immunoperoxidase).

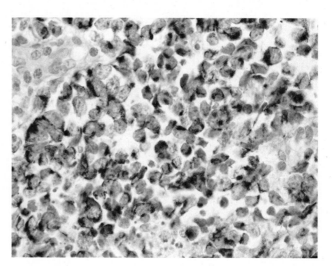

Figure 21.48. Small-cell undifferentiated (neuroendocrine) carcinoma displays punctate dotlike perinuclear positivity for cytokeratin, a surrogate marker of neuroendocrine differentiation.

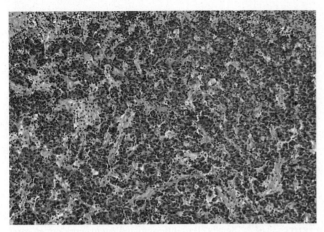

Figure 21.49. Sinonasal undifferentiated carcinoma. The tumor forms ribbons and cords of medium-sized cells with no evidence of glandular or squamous differentiation.

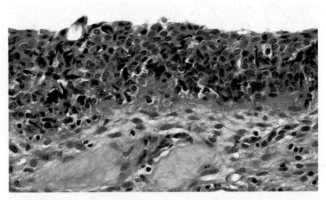

Figure 21.51. Sinonasal undifferentiated carcinoma. Highly atypical cells are present within the surface mucosa. It is unclear whether this is secondary involvement or a distinct form of carcinoma in situ.

little additional value. The median survival time in one study of 16 patients was 18 months, with only 1 long-term (10-year) disease-free survivor (187).

Morphologic Characteristics

These tumors consist of nests, trabeculae, ribbons, and sheets of medium-sized polygonal cells, often with an "organoid" appearance (Fig. 21.49). Nuclei are round to oval, slightly to moderately pleomorphic, and hyperchromatic. Chromatin varies from diffuse to coarsely granular. Nucleoli are typically large, but in some cases, they may be inconspicuous. Most cells have small to moderate amounts of eosinophilic cytoplasm (Fig. 21.50). Mitotic figures are numerous, and vascular permeation is usually extensive. Individual cell necrosis and central necrosis of cell nests are common. Homer Wright rosettes, intercellular fibrils, and argyrophil granules are absent, as is squamous or glandular differentiation. Some sinonasal undifferentiated carcinomas involve the overlying surface mucosa (Fig. 21.51). Whether this represents carcinoma in situ or secondary spread is not clear.

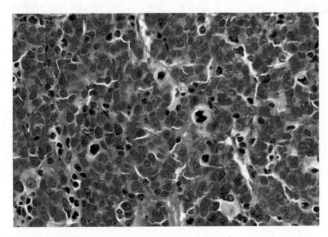

Figure 21.50. Sinonasal undifferentiated carcinoma. The neoplastic cells have moderate amounts of eosinophilic cytoplasm with often prominent nucleoli and a very high mitotic rate.

Immunocytochemical stains for CK and EMA are positive for one or both markers in virtually all cases (187). From 18% to 50% of cases are positive for neuron-specific enolase (186,187), and electron microscopic studies document rare dense-core granules occurring singly in individual cells (186). Immunohistochemistry and in situ hybridization are negative for EBV protein or RNA (187).

Differential diagnostic considerations include olfactory neuroblastoma, lymphoepithelioma, small-cell undifferentiated carcinoma, lymphoma, malignant melanoma, and rhabdomyosarcoma. The microscopic features of sinonasal undifferentiated carcinoma usually allow for its ready distinction from lymphoma, melanoma, and rhabdomyosarcoma. In difficult cases, immunocytochemical stains for leukocyte common antigen (LCA, CD45), S-100 protein, and a myogenous marker such as myoglobin, muscle-specific actin, or desmin may be of value in making these distinctions.

Olfactory neuroblastoma should be distinguished from sinonasal undifferentiated carcinoma because of the much better prognosis of the former tumor. Olfactory neuroblastoma consists of uniform to mildly pleomorphic cells, frequently with an intercellular fibrillary background. Rosettes and ganglion cells are also diagnostic of this disease. On ultrastructural examination, olfactory neuroblastoma contains cell processes and more numerous dense-core granules than sinonasal undifferentiated carcinoma. S-100–positive Schwann-like cells are scattered in neuroblastoma and are lacking in undifferentiated carcinoma. Both tumors can stain for CK, but the staining is more common, stronger, and more diffuse in sinonasal undifferentiated carcinoma (159,186).

Unlike sinonasal undifferentiated carcinoma, the cells of lymphoepithelioma have uniform nuclei with a dispersed, vesicular chromatin pattern. Lymphoepithelioma grows as single cells or syncytial-like sheets in a prominent inflammatory stroma. Trabecular or "organoid" growth patterns, common in sinonasal undifferentiated carcinoma, are not seen (187). Differential CK expression may be of value in this distinction. Lymphoepithelioma has been shown to express CK5/6, CK8, CK13, and CK19 and will often be positive for EBV RNA by in situ hybridization. Sinonasal undifferentiated carcinomas express CK7, CK8, and CK19 and lack EBV RNA (188). Small-cell undifferentiated (oat cell) carcinoma may be related to sinonasal undifferentiated carcinoma but is distinguished by its smaller cell size, densely hyperchromatic nuclei, and dotlike perinuclear staining for CK.

MALIGNANT MELANOMA

Clinical Features

Approximately 1% of all malignant melanomas arise in the nasal cavity and paranasal sinuses. Origin from the nasal cavity is several times more common than from the sinuses, although both sites are often involved. Within the nasal cavity, inception in the anterior septum, inferior turbinate, and middle turbinate is most common. Melanoma of the paranasal sinuses usually involves the antrum (80%) followed by the ethmoid. Frontal and sphenoid sinuses are rarely, if ever, primary sites, although they may frequently be affected by direct extension. Primary melanoma of the nasopharynx is extremely rare.

Males and females are equally affected (190,191). The ages range from adolescence through the elderly, but most patients are more than 50 years old. Symptoms are nonspecific. Physical examination typically demonstrates a sessile or polypoid mass that is often pigmented. Complete excision is the treatment of choice; radiation and chemotherapy have had little or no value as adjuvant treatment. The prognosis is poor, as is typical of mucosal melanomas at other sites; the 5-year survival rate is approximately 35%, and median survival time is 36 months (190,191).

Morphologic Characteristics

Approximately 70% of upper respiratory tract malignant melanomas contain intracytoplasmic melanin pigment (192); diagnosis in such cases is straightforward. The remaining 30% are nonpigmented lesions that cause considerable diagnostic consternation. Common microscopic patterns encountered in sinonasal malignant melanoma include (in order of decreasing frequency) small blue cell (Fig. 21.52), spindle cell (Fig. 21.53), epithelioid (Fig. 21.54), and pleomorphic (193). Junctional change, a helpful diagnostic feature, is present in only approximately one-third of cases because of frequent surface ulceration (193). A nesting or theque-like growth pattern is suggestive of the diagnosis, but it is also seen in only approximately one-third

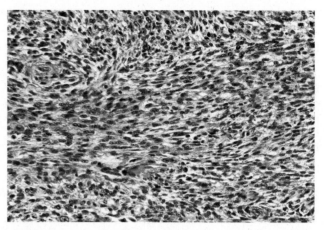

Figure 21.53. Sinonasal malignant melanoma, spindle cell variant. In the absence of pigment or other growth patterns, this variant is indistinguishable from a spindle cell sarcoma.

of cases (193). Sinonasal malignant melanomas with a small-cell pattern may be confused with olfactory neuroblastoma and other small-cell neoplasms. Strong immunohistochemical staining for S-100 protein, vimentin, HMB-45, melan-A, and tyrosinase is of diagnostic value (192,193). Isolated sinonasal malignant melanomas may contain scattered cells that stain positive for CK and EMA, but diffuse staining, as seen in carcinomas, is absent (193). As discussed earlier, both olfactory neuroblastomas (159,177) and sometimes carcinomas (194) can contain S-100–positive cells.

PARAGANGLIOMA

The paraganglia associated with the vagus nerve occasionally give rise to a paraganglioma, which appears as a mass in the region of the fossa of Rosenmüller (195). These are typically slow-growing lesions that remain symptomatic for several years (196). Biopsy may be associated with copious hemorrhage. Paragangliomas also occur in the nasal cavity, although infrequently (196). The clinicopathologic features of paragangliomas are

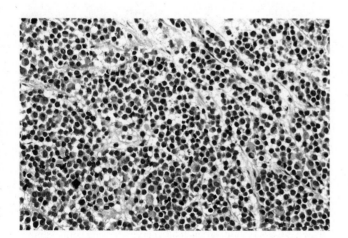

Figure 21.52. Sinonasal malignant melanoma, small-cell variant. The tumor consists of small, uniform cells lacking pigment and resembling malignant lymphoma.

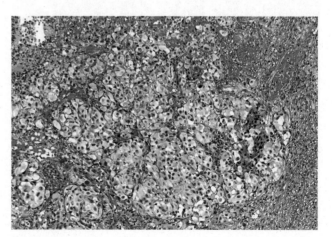

Figure 21.54. Sinonasal malignant melanoma, epithelioid variant. This form more closely resembles cutaneous melanoma and often has prominent nucleoli. Confusion with carcinoma is still a common problem, however.

discussed in detail elsewhere in this text. Making the microscopic distinction from other nasal and nasopharyngeal neoplasms is not difficult once the possibility is considered and the characteristic nesting (Zellballen) growth pattern is recognized. The nests of paraganglioma, like those of olfactory neuroblastoma, are often surrounded by S-100–positive, Schwann-like cells. Confusion is easily avoided, however, given that the cells of paraganglioma have more prominent cytoplasm; smaller, more closely packed cell nests; and absent or extremely rare mitotic figures.

DISPLACED NEURAL AND RELATED LESIONS

Neoplasms and ectopias derived from central nervous system elements may arise as a mass in the nasopharynx, nasal cavity, or sinuses. Considerable diagnostic difficulty may result, primarily at the time of frozen section, because of failure to consider this group of lesions.

PITUITARY ADENOMA

Approximately 10% of pituitary adenomas invade beyond the sella, and approximately 2% develop as a mass in the upper aerodigestive tract (197). Much less commonly, ectopic pituitary adenomas, not in continuity with the intrasellar pituitary, may be found in the nasal cavity or sphenoid sinus (198–202). Such lesions presumably arise from Rathke pouch remnants. In fact, tiny asymptomatic nests of pituitary tissue are present in the roof of the nasopharynx in 95% to 100% of patients (203,204) and have been termed the *pharyngeal pituitary* (203).

The microscopic features of ectopic pituitary adenomas are identical to their intrasellar counterparts, described elsewhere. Small, distorted biopsy samples may be difficult to distinguish from nasopharyngeal paraganglioma, olfactory neuroblastoma, or other small-cell neoplasms (Fig. 21.55). Pituitary adenomas may have the nesting, or zellballen, architecture typical of para-

ganglioma. The cells of pituitary adenoma tend to be smaller than those of paraganglioma, with less cytoplasm and more uniform nuclei. Olfactory neuroblastomas have a fibrillary intercytoplasmic background and larger, more pleomorphic nuclei than pituitary adenoma. In difficult cases, immunocytochemical staining for pituitary endocrine products may be of value.

CRANIOPHARYNGIOMA

Craniopharyngioma rarely arises as a nasopharyngeal or sphenoid sinus lesion (205–207). The morphologic features are identical to those of its intrasellar counterpart described elsewhere. More commonly, tumors resembling (or identical to) adamantinomatous craniopharyngiomas arise in the nasal cavity or paranasal sinuses without apparent connection to the sella. These lesions are also microscopically identical to ameloblastomas of the jaw and are generally labeled as sinonasal ameloblastomas (Fig. 21.56) (208). They are typically cured following complete resection.

GLIAL HETEROTOPIA

Clinical Features

The unfortunate term *nasal glioma* is often given to heterotopic central nervous system tissue. Glial heterotopias are variants of encephalocele and are not true neoplasms (209–213). Most are present at birth or are clinically manifest within the first few years of life. Approximately 60% are in the subcutaneous tissue of the nose, 30% are in the nasal cavity, and the rest are mixed cutaneous and nasal cavity lesions (210). Occasionally, glial heterotopias are found in the paranasal sinus (209) or the nasopharynx (214). In approximately 80% of cases, there is no connection to the central nervous system; 20% maintain a small fibrous or glial attachment (210,211).

Morphologic Characteristics

At the microscopic level, mature astrocytes usually predominate, and the gliosis is associated with varying degrees of stromal

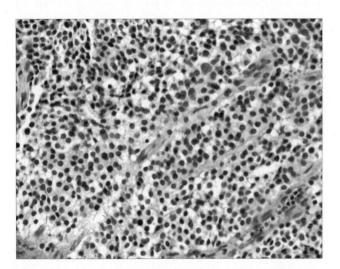

Figure 21.55. Pituitary adenoma may involve the nasopharynx by direct invasion from the sella or as an apparent ectopic primary. Confusion with olfactory neuroblastoma and other small-cell tumors is a frequent problem.

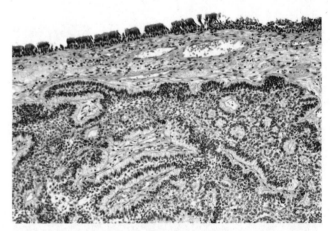

Figure 21.56. Sinonasal ameloblastoma underlying normal sinonasal mucosa. Distinction of this lesion from an adamantinomatous craniopharyngioma requires clinicoradiographic correlation. These tumors are also histologically identical to ameloblastomas of the jaw.

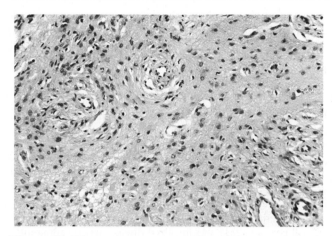

Figure 21.57. Glial heterotopia. This consists of extracranial glial tissue that occasionally connects to the central nervous system.

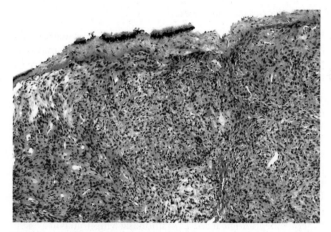

Figure 21.58. Sinonasal meningioma. Nests of meningotheliomatous meningioma grow beneath intact (but partially denuded) sinonasal mucosa. There was no identifiable central nervous system attachment.

fibrosis (Fig. 21.57). Gemistocytic or mildly atypical astrocytes may be present. Neuronal cells are generally sparse or absent (209), but in rare instances, they may be prominent (215). The distinction from typical encephalocele is based on the absence of a well-formed central nervous system connection; however, in some instances, poorly formed connections make this differentiation challenging. Unlike teratomas with neural elements, glial heterotopias are mature, predominantly or exclusively neuroglial lesions. A single case of an oligodendroglioma arising in glial heterotopia has been described (216).

MENINGIOMA

Clinical Features

Approximately 20% of intracranial meningiomas extend beyond the cranial cavity, and approximately 3% secondarily involve the upper respiratory tract (217). Nonetheless, most meningiomas of the sinonasal region appear to be true extracranial neoplasms (218–220). In some instances, it may be impossible to make the distinction between extracranial and intracranial origin. Both primary and secondary meningiomas of the upper respiratory tract prefer the paranasal sinuses, followed by the nasal cavity (219). The age range is broad, there may be a slight female predominance, and there is a bias for primary lesions to affect the left side of the body (218–220). Symptoms are nonspecific and varied, but mass, nasal obstruction, and epistaxis are common (219,220). Primary extracranial lesions have a good prognosis, but intracranial lesions invading into the upper respiratory tract may be difficult to eradicate (219).

Morphologic Characteristics

At the microscopic level, most meningiomas in this region have had a meningothelial pattern (Fig. 21.58) (219,220). Transitional cell meningiomas may be confused with cemento-ossifying fibromas (COF). The latter entity tends to be more cellular and has clearly fibroblastic stromal cells; the spherical calcifications often contain cells, distinguishing them from laminated psammoma bodies of meningioma (219). Sinonasal meningiomas may be confused with neurilemomas. Meningiomas almost invariably express vimentin and EMA; a small minority also label for CK and S-100 protein (220,221). Because this staining pattern overlaps with that of neurilemoma, immunohistochemistry is of limited value in making this distinction (221). Other lesions in the differential diagnosis of meningioma include fibrous histiocytoma, neurofibroma, and salivary myoepithelioma (219).

LYMPHOPLASMACYTIC PROLIFERATIONS

LYMPHOID HYPERPLASIA

Tumefactive lymphoid hyperplasia (pseudolymphoma) in the head and neck region most commonly affects the major salivary glands, thyroid gland, and orbit. There are rare descriptions of pseudolymphomas in the nasopharynx (222) and nasal cavity (223). Features of lymphoid hyperplasia include germinal center formation with tingible bodies, a mixed inflammatory cell infiltrate, cytologic evidence of normal lymphoid cells, benign neighboring lymph nodes on microscopic evaluation, and polyclonality for light chains (224). The diagnosis of lymphoid hyperplasia or pseudolymphoma as a specific entity should be approached with caution because identical reactions can be seen surrounding carcinomas and lymphomas or can stem from an infection. Reactive inflammatory proliferations contain a variable plasma cell component. When the latter cells predominate, the terms *plasma cell granuloma* (225) and *inflammatory pseudotumor* are applied.

LYMPHOMA

Clinical Features

Non-Hodgkin lymphomas are the most common nonepithelial malignancies arising in the sinonasal region (226). Clinical features are nonspecific and relate to obstruction, mass effect, or hemorrhage (226–232). The age range is broad, although most patients are elderly (227). Sinonasal lymphomas are typically bulky lesions involving multiple sinuses and the nasal cavity. Extension into the nasopharynx is common. A distinctly polypoid appearance is often noted on physical examination, and radiographic destruction of sinonasal walls is almost invariably present (227). Overall 5-year survival rate for limited disease (stages I and II) is approximately 55% (227,230).

Morphologic Characteristics

Lymphomas arising in the paranasal sinuses are usually of the diffuse, large-cell type (227–229,231,232). Up to 50% may have immunoblastic features (227,231,233). Nodular subtypes are extremely rare (228). In our experience, the majority of paranasal sinus lymphomas in the United States have been of the B-cell phenotype, including the typical immunoblastic forms (227,233). Primary nasal cavity lesions may more often be of NK/T subtype (see section on NK/T-cell lymphoma later in this chapter). In Asia, where T-cell lymphomas in general are far more common, sinonasal lymphomas are predominantly of the T-cell type (230,234). Moreover, some studies from the United States have also shown a high percentage of T-cell subtypes (229,231).

The morphologic features of sinonasal lymphomas are essentially identical to analogous subtypes arising in lymph nodes and described in detail elsewhere. Distinguishing lymphoma from lymphoepithelioma or other small-cell neoplasms in the sinonasal region can be impossible in some instances, even when strict morphologic criteria are applied by experienced observers. In such cases, immunohistochemical staining for EMA (238,239), CK (Fig. 21.32) (240–243), and LCA (CD45) (Fig. 21.33) (235–238) is helpful. If staining for these markers is negative, antibodies directed against specific differentiation markers can be applied to evaluate other diagnostic possibilities, including embryonal rhabdomyosarcoma, melanoma, or olfactory neuroblastoma. One recognized source of error is the staining of some anaplastic large-cell lymphomas and, occasionally, T-cell lymphomas with EMA (239). There also have been rare reports of lymphomas staining focally for CK, but strong, diffuse staining coupled with EMA positivity is compelling evidence of epithelial differentiation.

Some sinonasal lymphomas, particularly those of T-cell lineage, may stimulate the overlying mucosa to undergo florid squamous cell hyperplasia that proliferates downward to engulf the neoplastic lymphoid cells (231,244). The resultant biphasic appearance may lead to an erroneous diagnosis of lymphoepithelioma or a mixed carcinoma and lymphoma (Fig. 21.59). Immunohistochemical stains are of no value in such cases. Correct diagnosis requires knowledge of this phenomenon coupled with recognition that the epithelial component, although florid, lacks cytologic features of malignancy.

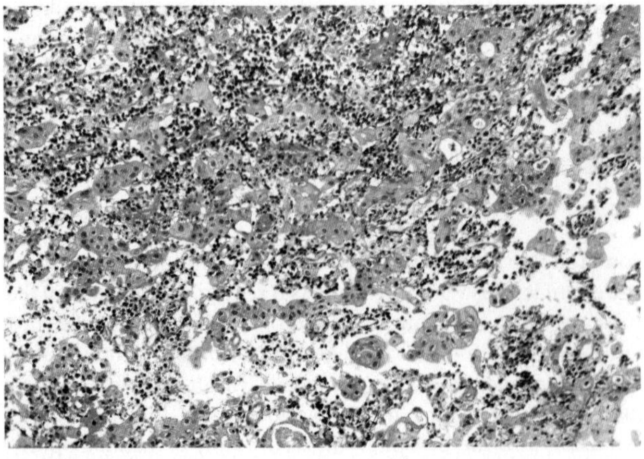

PLASMACYTOMA

Clinical Features

Extramedullary plasma cell neoplasms are uncommon, but approximately 90% occur in the head and neck, and at least 75% involve the sinonasal region (245–252). In this location, they account for 4% of nonepithelial tumors (251). Symptoms are nonspecific. The age range is broad, but it peaks in the seventh decade; 95% of patients are more than 40 years old (252). There is a male predominance of up to 4:1.

Extramedullary plasmacytomas may pursue one of several clinical courses (251): (a) localized disease may be apparently cured by surgery and/or radiation; (b) local disease can recur but may eventually be eradicated; (c) local disease may persist and cause death by uncontrolled growth; or (d) disseminated disease (multiple myeloma) may develop. The presence of disseminated disease at the time of diagnosis should be excluded by careful evaluation. Most patients with primary extramedullary disease will not have a monoclonal spike on serum or urine electrophoresis (252). Regional lymph node involvement is present in approximately 25% of cases (246,248) but does not adversely affect prognosis (245,246,248). Local control is usually achieved with surgery or radiation for patients with isolated or regional disease. Reported 5-year survival rates range from 31% to 82% (245,246,249–251,253). Disseminated disease (multiple myeloma) develops in 11% to 50% of patients from months to decades after initial diagnosis (245,246,253).

Morphologic Characteristics

Well-differentiated lesions are composed of minimally deviant plasma cells (Fig. 21.60). The distinction between plasmacytoma and plasma cell granuloma is based on (a) the exclusion of other inflammatory cell types, (b) the presence of mildly atypical nuclei lacking the range of maturation from immunoblasts to mature plasma cells seen in reactive lesions, and

Figure 21.59. Sinonasal malignant lymphoma, particularly of the T-cell type, may stimulate intense squamous hyperplasia. In this example, irregular islands of benign squamous epithelium are interspersed within malignant lymphoma.

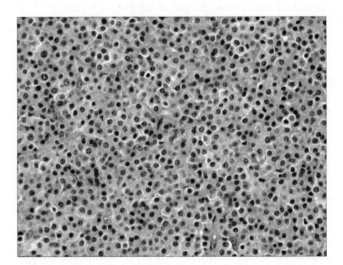

Figure 21.60. Sinonasal plasmacytoma. Well-differentiated plasma cells may be mistaken for olfactory neuroblastoma, myoepithelioma, malignant melanoma, and other entities.

(c) most importantly, immunocytochemical monoclonality for immunoglobulin light chains or heavy chains (253).

Distinguishing poorly differentiated plasmacytomas from large B-cell lymphomas with immunoblastic features may occasionally be difficult. The presence of more mature, albeit neoplastic, plasma cells supports the designation of plasmacytoma (253). Other hematopoietic neoplasms to be considered in the differential diagnosis include Waldenström macroglobulinemia and granulocytic sarcoma (253). Waldenström macroglobulinemia is an invariably disseminated lymphoproliferative disorder with an associated monoclonal immunoglobulin M (IgM) gammopathy. It is polymorphic, with plasma cells, lymphocytes, and plasmacytoid cells in varying proportions. Granulocytic sarcomas can be recognized by their eosinophilic myelocytes or a positive chloroacetate esterase stain (253). Plasmacytomas can also be confused with malignant melanoma (253), olfactory neuroblastoma (254), and pituitary adenoma, which are discussed in detail elsewhere in this chapter. It should be remembered that reactive and neoplastic plasma cells stain immunocytochemically for EMA (239) and often fail to stain for LCA (CD45) (235,236).

NK/T-CELL LYMPHOMA

Clinical Features

The upper respiratory tract is a common site for the development of an unusual, polymorphous angiocentric lymphoma that has been referred to by a wide variety of terms, including midline malignant reticulosis, polymorphic reticulosis, nasal T-cell lymphoma, lymphomatoid granulomatosis, and angiocentric immunoproliferative lesion (30,37,226,255–258).

In the past, the proliferative cells of this lesion have been variously interpreted as polyclonal B cells (259–261), T cells (234,258,262–264), and true histiocytes (265). Patients have been shown to have impairment of T-lymphocyte function (260,266), and a strong association with EBV has been noted (258,261,264,267,268). More recently, it has become clear that lesions of this type arising in the head and neck are NK/T-cell lymphomas (269–277). The currently preferred term applied to these lesions is e*xtranodal NK/T-cell lymphoma, nasal type,* but for brevity, here we will refer to them simply as NK/T-cell lymphoma. Polymorphous lymphoid lesions arising in the lung and secondarily involving the head and neck appear to be distinct, T-cell–predominant, B-cell lymphomas (275). The latter lesions are the ones most associated with the old term *lymphomatoid granulomatosis.* Much of the previous difficulty regarding typing of these lesions or even convincingly identifying them as neoplasms relates to the fact that neoplastic NK/T cells show no rearrangements of heavy or light immunoglobulin chains and express germline T-cell receptors.

On immunohistochemical examination, the neoplastic NK/T cells are noted for their CD56 positivity (71%) and CD57 negativity (276). The neoplastic cells also typically express CD45RO and CD43, as well as some T antigens including CD2 and CD3 (cytoplasmic, not surface). Almost all NK/T-cell lymphomas contain large amounts of EBV RNA by in situ hybridization (Fig. 21.61). Some publications have lumped NK/T-cell lymphomas with conventional T-cell lymphomas. Purported angiocentric lymphomas lacking CD56 immunoreactivity and displaying T-cell receptor gene rearrangements are most likely more conventional lymphomas rather than true NK/T-cell neoplasms.

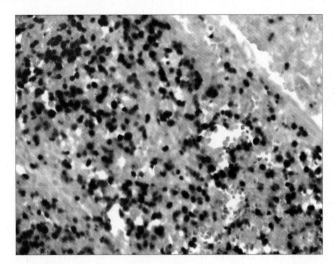

Figure 21.61. Nasal natural killer/T-cell lymphoma. The lesion demonstrates strong reactivity for Epstein-Barr virus RNA by in situ hybridization.

NK/T-cell lymphomas of the head and neck affect patients in a broad age range, with a peak in the fifth decade of life (228). Localized disease may be effectively treated with high-dose radiation therapy; there is a 77% complete remission rate. Approximately 35% of patients with complete remissions experience localized or disseminated recurrent disease. Regional lymph nodes, skin, lung, and brain have been reported as sites of disseminated disease. Disease-free survival at 5 years has ranged from 46% to 63%. A hemophagocytic syndrome, also associated with EBV, has been noted in some patients with sinonasal NK/T-cell lymphomas. This complication is typically fatal.

Morphologic Characteristics

At the microscopic level, NK/T-cell lymphomas are composed of a polymorphic infiltrate of inflammatory cells. Normal-appearing lymphocytes, plasma cells, a few neutrophils, and scattered atypical lymphoid cells are present (Figs. 21.62 and 21.63). The last cells are the diagnostic subpopulation (30,37,

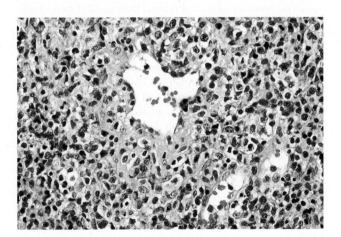

Figure 21.62. The wall of a blood vessel has been expanded by the polymorphic infiltrate of nasal-type natural killer/T-cell lymphoma. At this low magnification, cells with perinuclear clearing are apparent.

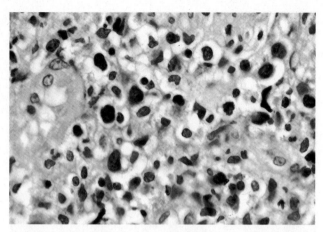

Figure 21.63. A higher magnification demonstrates the polymorphic nature of the infiltrate in nasal-type natural killer/T-cell lymphoma. Scattered, atypical lymphoid cells with enlarged nuclei are apparent. One of the latter cells in the center of the field exhibits perinuclear clearing.

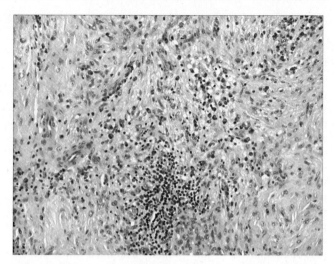

Figure 21.64. Follicular dendritic cell tumor. The tumor consists of sweeping fascicles of relatively uniform spindle cells with associated inflammation.

38,255). The atypical cells usually have enlarged, hyperchromatic, convoluted nuclei with scant basophilic cytoplasm. Frequently, they are surrounded by a zone of clearing, an artifact of formalin fixation that is helpful in spotting these cells at low magnification (Fig. 21.63). The angiocentric quality of the lesion may be masked in biopsy specimens containing large numbers of inflammatory cells, foci of necrosis, and proliferating capillaries. Deep biopsies are usually necessary for diagnosis. Superficial biopsy specimens contain predominantly granulation tissue and acute inflammation.

The characteristics distinguishing angiocentric lymphoma from Wegener granulomatosis and IMDD are included in the section dealing with midfacial necrotizing lesions. NK/T-cell lymphoma differs from conventional lymphoma in that it is more polymorphic, usually has a paucity of atypical cells, and often exhibits prominent angiocentricity.

DENDRITIC CELL TUMORS

Follicular dendritic cell tumor often occurs at extranodal sites and frequently involves the upper aerodigestive tract (278–281). These tumors of antigen-presenting cells occur slightly more frequently in women and over a broad age range. Nearly half recur or metastasize, and the most frequent site of metastasis is the lung. Approximately 5% of patients have died of their disease.

Histologically, these are hypercellular proliferations composed of plump spindled and epithelioid cells, often in a syncytial growth pattern with indistinct cell borders (Fig. 21.64). The nuclei are round to oval and have wrinkled nuclear membranes, typically with vesicular-appearing chromatin and without prominent nucleoli. Mitotic activity can vary greatly but is usually low. Tumor cells are intermixed with numerous small lymphocytes, and coagulative necrosis has been seen in 30% of cases.

The differential diagnosis for follicular dendritic cell tumors includes other spindle cell neoplasms such as sarcomatoid carcinoma and malignant melanoma, among others. By immunohistochemistry, the neoplastic cells of follicular dendritic cell tumors are reactive for CD21, CD35, clusterin, and fascin in most cases (278,281). Although most examples will react with antibodies to EMA, CK immunoreactivity is rare.

Interdigitating dendritic cell tumors should be distinguished from the follicular variant because the former have a more variable prognosis and sometimes present with disseminated disease (280). Histologically, the two tumors may closely resemble each other; however the neoplastic cells of the interdigitating variant often appear more epithelioid (Fig. 21.65). Neoplastic cells in the interdigitating variant are reactive for S-100 protein and not for CD21 (278,280). The former reactivity often leads to a misdiagnosis of spindle cell malignant melanoma, but other, more specific melanocytic markers will be nonreactive.

VASCULAR LESIONS

ANGIOFIBROMA

Clinical Features

Angiofibromas are uncommon tumors that have sharply defined clinical features (282–287). Nasal obstruction and epi-

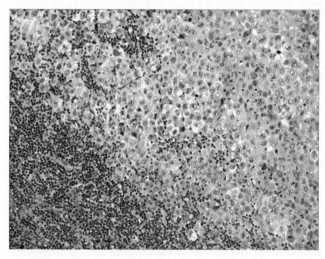

Figure 21.65. Interdigitating dendritic cell tumor. The cells appear more epithelioid and pleomorphic than in Figure 21.64.

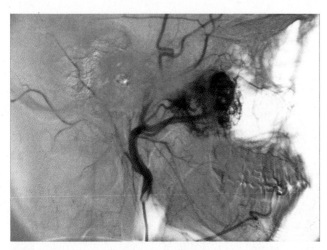

Figure 21.66. Nasopharyngeal angiofibroma. This carotid artery angiogram highlights the highly vascular nature of a nasopharyngeal angiofibroma.

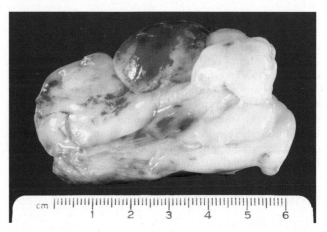

Figure 21.67. Nasopharyngeal angiofibroma. On gross inspection, nasopharyngeal angiofibromas are fibrous masses with a circumscribed, deceptively avascular appearance.

staxis are nearly always present. These tumors originate from the lateral nasopharynx or, rarely, the extreme posterior portion of the nasal cavity (Fig. 21.66). There is a marked predilection for adolescent boys, with a peak at approximately 15 years of age (286). Tumors occasionally arise in very young boys or middle-aged men. The occurrence of angiofibroma in females is the subject of controversy. In four large studies, there were no female patients in a total of 216 cases (283–286). Review of purported female cases often indicates erroneous diagnoses (282).

Angiofibromas have been shown to possess testosterone receptors (288) and to lack estrogen or progesterone receptors (288,289). In anecdotal cases, testosterone administration has produced clinical enlargement (290,291). Estrogen administration often decreases tumor size and blood loss at the time of surgery (289). The presumed mechanism is feedback inhibition by estrogen of gonadotropin-releasing hormone (289). In more recent studies, antibodies directed against testosterone receptor protein have been shown to label the stromal and endothelial cells in routinely processed, paraffin-embedded tissue specimens from angiofibromas (292).

The overall prognosis of angiofibroma is good, although large tumors may extend into the nasal cavity, pterygomaxillary fossa, cheek, maxillary antrum, or orbit; rarely, they extend intracranially. Such extensions make complete surgical excision—the treatment of choice—difficult or impossible. Residual disease after incomplete resection may progress, remain stable, or occasionally regress. Radiation therapy is of value in unresectable cases; however, postirradiation sarcoma is a well-recognized, albeit rare, complication (291,293,294). Chemotherapy for unresectable lesions has also been successful (295). The overall reported mortality, as a result of exsanguination or intracranial extension, has ranged from 0% to 9% (285,286). The higher rate comes from a large referral center (286) and reflects a bias toward difficult cases. Reports of metastasizing "angiofibroma" or sarcomatous change without radiation therapy represent misdiagnosed sarcomas (296,297).

Morphologic Characteristics

On gross inspection, resected angiofibromas are well-circumscribed but unencapsulated, firm fibrous masses. The cut sur-

face is tan-gray and distinctly fibrous (Fig. 21.67). Larger blood vessels may be visible near the base of resection, but much of the lesion appears deceptively avascular. The histologic hallmark of angiofibroma is a partially collagenized fibrous stroma containing numerous irregular vascular spaces that vary in size from small slits to dilated lumens (Fig. 21.68). Usually these vascular spaces are seen only as defects in the stroma lined by a single layer of endothelial cells. Vessels with thicker walls, devoid of elastic tissue, may also be present. In our experience and that of Sternberg (282), the relationship of vessels to stroma varies within the mass. In the central portions of an angiofibroma, the stromal elements are more prominent, and the vascular element is less obvious. At the periphery, vessels are more closely packed, smaller, and uniform in size, with little stromal fibrosis. Diagnosis based on biopsies from such regions may not be possible. This is particularly true when there is ulceration because the associated inflammation results in a pattern indistinguishable from granulation tissue.

Collagen deposition is haphazard, with randomly intersecting collagen strands. The stromal cells frequently have a stellate

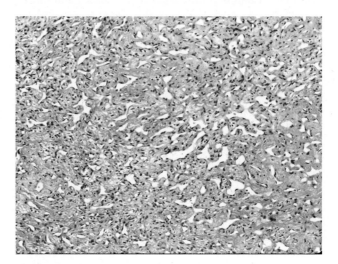

Figure 21.68. Nasopharyngeal angiofibroma. The tumor has haphazardly arranged, small vascular spaces; prominent, irregular collagen fibers; and stellate stromal cells.

configuration, unlike the bipolar appearance of fibroblasts in aggressive fibromatosis. The nuclei vary from small pyknotic structures to large vesicular forms with prominent nucleoli. Multinucleated stromal cells may be common, and cells with prominent eosinophilic cytoplasm resembling the "ganglion-like" cells of proliferative myositis may also be found. Stromal mitotic figures are extremely rare. Ultrastructural studies have demonstrated that the stromal cells are myofibroblasts (285,298,299). In addition, these cells contain highly characteristic intranuclear dense granules that apparently represent tightly bound RNA protein complexes (300).

LOBULAR CAPILLARY HEMANGIOMA

Clinical Features

This distinctive vascular proliferation most commonly involves the skin and is the underlying vascular anomaly of so-called pyogenic granuloma. It may also develop intravenously (301) or within the subcutis (302). In the respiratory tract, lobular capillary hemangioma arises exclusively in the nasal cavity and predominantly on the septum (303). Patients less than 18 years of age are typically male (82%), and patients in the reproductive age range are frequently female (86%) and often pregnant (303). Regression after delivery in pregnant patients has been noted. Despite these clinical features, estrogen and progesterone receptors have not been detected in lobular capillary hemangiomas (304). Bleeding is the most common complaint, and there is seldom a history of antecedent trauma. Simple excision is usually curative, with only an occasional recurrence.

Morphologic Characteristics

The essential histologic feature is a lobular arrangement of capillaries, often surrounding a larger central vessel (Fig. 21.69). The capillaries vary from tightly packed clusters of endothelial cells with barely visible lumina to larger, obviously vascular spaces (Fig. 21.70). Mitotic rates in the closely packed endothelial cells may be very high, but atypical forms are not seen. Surrounding the endothelial cells is a second population of spindled, pericytic cells exhibiting positivity for muscle-specific actin (304). Confusion with angiosarcoma or angiofibroma is

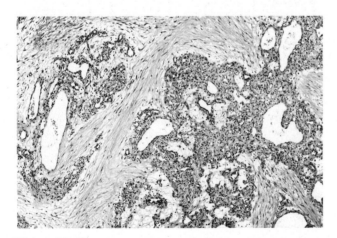

Figure 21.69. Lobular capillary hemangioma. The lobules consist of compact clusters of endothelial and pericytic cells with capillary lumina of varying sizes.

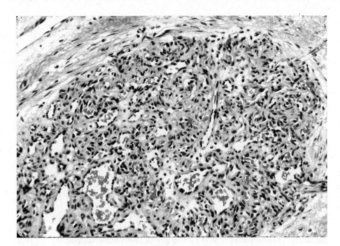

Figure 21.70. Lobular capillary hemangioma. A characteristic lobule contains irregular anastomosing vascular channels with prominent endothelial cells. Confusion with angiosarcoma is avoided by noting the low-power lobular architecture.

unlikely if the location of the lesion and its low-power architecture are considered. Secondary changes in lobular capillary hemangioma include mucosal ulceration with surface granulation tissue, prominent stromal inflammation, and papillary endothelial hyperplasia in large vascular spaces (303).

GLOMANGIOPERICYTOMA

According to pathology legend, when asked near the end of his career if he had any regrets, Dr. Arthur Purdy Stout, one of the pioneers of surgical pathology, reportedly replied, "Yes, I wish that I had never described hemangiopericytoma." Whether the attribution is true or not, the sentiment expressed is valid. Lauren Ackerman, another pioneer in the field, once described hemangiopericytoma as, "the diagnosis of the diagnostically destitute." The term *hemangiopericytoma* has been applied far too freely to many spindle cell proliferations having little or no evidence of pericytic differentiation and exhibiting only a nonspecific pattern of gaping, branching, "staghorn" vascular spaces. In the upper aerodigestive tract, many lesions previously given this designation are now recognized to be solitary fibrous tumors (see later section on solitary fibrous tumor). Other lesions, particularly those described as *hemangiopericytoma-like tumor* or *sinonasal-type hemangiopericytoma*, probably do represent neoplasms with true pericytic differentiation and appear related to glomus tumors (305–309). The term *glomangiopericytoma* has been suggested for these lesions (310).

Clinical Features

Glomangiopericytomas most frequently arise in the nasal cavities or, less often, the paranasal sinuses (308–311). They can arise at any age and are slightly more common in women. Patients present with nonspecific symptoms such as obstruction and epistaxis. The tumors behave very well, and more than 95% of patients have no recurrence after initial surgical resection. Rare cases do behave more aggressively, however, and can eventually lead to the death of the patient.

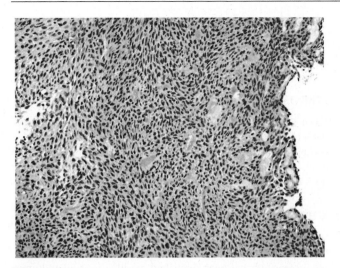

Figure 21.71. Sinonasal glomangiopericytoma is a spindle cell neoplasm containing small, irregular vascular spaces and little stromal collagen.

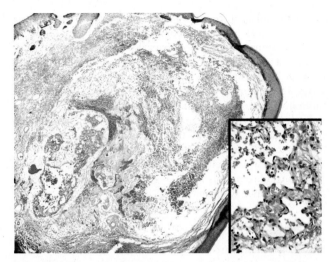

Figure 21.73. Vascular nasal polyp. This vascular nasal polyp has undergone thrombosis and recanalization with papillary endothelial hyperplasia (*inset*). Overdiagnosis of this benign reaction accounts for many examples of "polypoid angiosarcoma" of the sinonasal region.

Morphologic Characteristics

Grossly, the lesions are typically described as polypoid and free of surface ulceration (305,306,308,311). Histologically, these are cellular neoplasms composed of spindle-shaped, ovoid, or polygonal cells that grow in fascicular, storiform, whorled, palisaded, and reticular patterns (Fig. 21.71). The neoplastic cells have indistinct cell borders with a small amount of eosinophilic cytoplasm. Nuclei have blunt ends and rarely display more than mild atypia. Mitotic figures are infrequent. Numerous small, thin-walled vessels course through the tumors and typically have a "staghorn" appearance (Fig. 21.72). Occasionally these vessels may be surrounded by a small cuff of acellular fibrosis. Mast cells, eosinophils, and extravasated red cells are usually present.

Immunohistochemically, the neoplastic cells react with antibodies to smooth muscle actin, muscle-specific actin, and factor XIIIa (308). Of note, the neoplastic cells do not react with antibodies to CKs, desmin, CD34, S-100 protein, bcl-2, factor VIII,

and CD31. The immunophenotype of these tumors is extremely helpful and allows for their ready distinction from histologically similar tumors such as solitary fibrous tumors and the vast variety of vascular, smooth muscle, neural, and other mesenchymal tumors that may be considered in the differential diagnosis.

OTHER VASCULAR TUMORS

Hemangiomas (nonlobular) occasionally arise within the nasal cavity but are extremely rare in the paranasal sinuses or nasopharynx (287). The soft tissue and bones of the facial region may be involved as a component of diffuse angiomatosis (287). Vascular glomus tumors develop in the nasal cavity and prefer the nasal septum (287,312); they are cured by simple excision. Angiosarcomas of this region are uncommon and appear as bleeding polypoid masses (287); they have been said to differ from angiosarcomas at more conventional sites in that they develop at a younger age and have a lower incidence of recurrence or metastasis and a lower mortality rate (313). We have encountered antrochoanal and nasal polyps with stromal atypia and a prominent vascular component with exuberant papillary endothelial hyperplasia (Fig. 21.73). Such lesions may be confused with angiosarcoma unless the low-power architecture is considered. Overdiagnosis of papillary endothelial hyperplasia in nasal lesions could account for the reportedly indolent prognosis of nasal "angiosarcoma."

FIBROUS AND FIBROHISTIOCYTIC LESIONS

FIBROMATOSIS

Clinical Features

The fibromatoses are clinicopathologically related, well-differentiated fibroblastic and myofibroblastic proliferations that locally invade, recur after incomplete excision, and never metastasize (314). Aggressive or desmoid-type fibromatosis involves

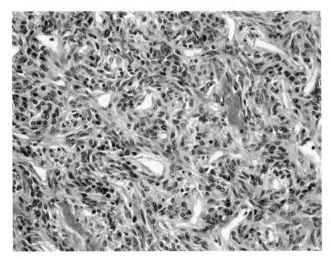

Figure 21.72. Sinonasal glomangiopericytoma. In this example, the vascular spaces are more prominent, and their cuffing by the neoplastic cells is clearly visible.

the head and neck region in approximately 12% of all cases (315). The neck is the most common site, but the nasal cavity, paranasal sinuses, and nasopharynx also are affected (316,317). All ages are susceptible, and there is no gender bias for this location. Symptoms relate to a mass, nasal obstruction, or epistaxis. The anatomic constraints of this region, along with the infiltrative nature of the tumor, often make complete excision difficult or impossible. Incompletely excised lesions can remain stable but typically recur; the rate of regrowth varies from months to more than a decade. Spontaneous regression is rare and tends to occur in children with multiple fibromatoses (316). Aggressive fibromatosis in this region is also seen as a component of Gardner syndrome (315).

Morphologic Characteristics

Excised specimens are firm, fibrous masses with grossly infiltrative margins. On microscopic examination, they are composed of well-differentiated, collagenized fibrous tissue. The spindle-shaped fibroblasts are arranged in bundles and broad fascicles. Herringbone patterns are not seen, but storiform arrays can sometimes form. The fibroblastic nuclei are uniform and, when cut longitudinally, have sharply pointed ends. Chromatin is dense or occasionally vacuolated. Nucleoli are absent or small, and mitotic figures are rare. At the periphery of the lesion, infiltration of surrounding structures is apparent (Fig. 21.74).

Fibromatoses should be distinguished from other fibrous lesions, including nasal fibromas and fibrosarcomas (see later sections). Incorrect diagnosis as a scar is common, particularly on small biopsies submitted without clinical history. The collagenized, fibrous bundles of fibromatosis tend to be broad and dense, and they intersect at angles. Scar tissue is composed of finer, parallel arrays of collagen. Neurofibromas may produce polypoid tumors in the nasal cavity or sinuses (318). On histologic examination, the examples we have encountered have been of the nonplexiform type, S-100 positive by immunoperoxidase, and composed of delicate, spindle-shaped cells interlacing in a loose, focally myxoid stroma. Fibrous proliferations containing intralesional osteoid and having radiographic evidence of bone involvement are probably fibro-osseous tumors

or the infiltrating margin of an intraosseous fibromatosis (desmoplastic fibroma). Distinguishing between fibromatosis and angiofibroma is based on the stellate stromal cells and characteristic vascularity of the latter.

FIBROMA

Nasal fibroma is a small, localized, slightly raised nodule less than 1 cm in size and typically located on the nasal septum or vestibule (316). It is invariably asymptomatic. At the microscopic level, it is composed of mature, hypocellular fibrous tissue that does not invade the surrounding tissue. Excision is curative.

SOLITARY FIBROUS TUMOR

Solitary fibrous tumor is a benign fibroblastic lesion that frequently involves the pleura ("benign fibrous mesothelioma") but increasingly has been described in wide variety of anatomic sites (319,320). In the head and neck region, it often arises in the nasal cavity or paranasal sinuses. The usual appearance is as a polypoid intranasal mass in a middle-aged patient. There is no gender preference. There may be erosion of adjacent structures, but the tumors do not metastasize. Local excision is almost invariably curative.

Microscopic examination shows a patternless proliferation of spindled fibroblasts in a variably collagenized background (Fig. 21.75). Blood vessels are prominent, may have dense perivascular sclerosis (Fig. 21.76), and may form areas resembling hemangiopericytoma. The spindle cells express vimentin but are negative or only weakly positive for muscle-specific actin, desmin, S-100 protein, factor VIII–related antigen, and neurofilament (319–321). The tumors have been shown to be strongly positive for CD34 (Fig. 21.75) (322,323). This finding may be of some diagnostic usefulness because neurofibromas, schwannomas, fibrosarcomas, and hemangiopericytomas have shown absent or weak staining for CD34 (322). CD99 and bcl-2 are also frequently positive in these tumors.

FIBROSARCOMA

Fibrosarcomas in the upper aerodigestive tract are rare tumors that have clinical features similar to those of aggressive fibro-

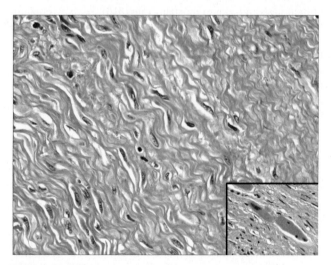

Figure 21.74. Aggressive fibromatosis. The lesion consists of hypocellular spindled cells in a densely collagenized stroma. Infiltration at its periphery is demonstrated by engulfment of skeletal muscle (*inset*).

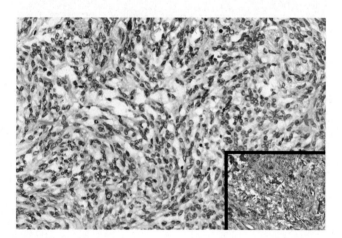

Figure 21.75. Solitary fibrous tumor. The tumor consists of haphazardly arranged spindle cells. In other regions, stromal collagen was more prominent. These tumors are typically strongly positive for CD34 (*inset*).

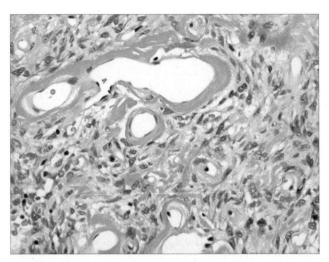

Figure 21.76. Solitary fibrous tumor. This example shows more prominent stromal collagen with a perivascular accentuation.

matosis. Unlike fibromatosis, fibrosarcoma is a hypercellular proliferation of fibroblasts, often oriented in a herringbone pattern (Fig. 21.77). Mitotic figures are easily found. Fibrosarcomas in this region tend to grow slowly, with only a 10% metastatic rate (316,324). Rarely, this tumor arises as a late complication of radiation therapy (325,326). Distinguishing fibrosarcoma from sarcomatoid carcinoma or amelanotic melanoma may sometimes be difficult, but these tumors lack the herringbone growth pattern often seen in fibrosarcoma. Immunohistochemical markers for epithelial (e.g., EMA, CK) or melanocytic differentiation (e.g., S-100, HMB-45, melan-A, etc.) may aid in this distinction, although many sarcomatoid carcinomas will lack epithelial marker positivity. Fibrosarcomas should label only for vimentin.

FIBROUS HISTIOCYTOMA

The concept of fibrous histiocytoma, particularly the malignant form, continues to undergo revision, and most (some would

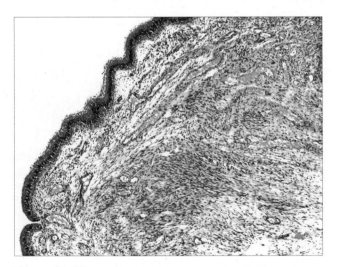

Figure 21.77. Sinonasal fibrosarcoma. This cellular spindle cell proliferation forms a polypoid mass beneath intact mucosa. Sweeping fascicles of cells are present, but a "herringbone" pattern is not obvious.

say all) lesions formerly placed in this diagnostic category have now been shown to exhibit more definitive directions of differentiation. The few remaining cases have simply been labeled as *undifferentiated sarcoma*. Perzin and Fu (327) reported 9 fibrous histiocytomas of the nasal cavity and paranasal sinuses and reviewed 12 additional cases, including nasopharyngeal lesions. The clinical features and prognosis were similar to those of fibrosarcoma, except that regional lymph node metastases developed in approximately 25% of cases (327). This raises the strong possibility that this group included some sarcomatoid carcinomas. In our experience, malignant fibrous histiocytoma in the head and neck has become a virtual nonentity. After exclusion of sarcomatoid malignant melanoma and other pleomorphic sarcomas, the remaining tumors appear to represent sarcomatoid carcinomas. Approximately half will demonstrate epithelial differentiation immunohistochemically, but even those that do not behave clinically as high-grade carcinomas.

OTHER FIBROUS LESIONS

Nodular fasciitis may affect the head and neck region, primarily as a subcutaneous lesion (328,329). Orbital involvement is common (330,331), and we have encountered an example in the nasopharynx. The histologic features are identical to those of nodular fasciitis in more typical locations (328,329). Rarely, a fibroinflammatory proliferation identical in morphologic features to sclerosing mediastinitis arises in the nasal cavity or sinuses (332). These lesions are characterized by a mixture of proliferating, variably collagenized fibrous tissue with acute and chronic inflammation. Invasion of adjacent structures is visible microscopically, although grossly the lesions appear to be circumscribed (332). The distinction between this lesion and aggressive fibromatosis is based on the lack of an intrinsic inflammatory element in aggressive fibromatosis.

OTHER BENIGN SOFT TISSUE NEOPLASMS

Benign soft tissue neoplasms arising in the mucosa of the upper airway include leiomyomas (333), schwannomas (318,334), neurofibromas (318,334), chondromas (335), lipomas (336), and rhabdomyomas (337). The diagnostic criteria are identical to those of neoplasms in other soft tissues and will not be reiterated here, with one exception. Rhabdomyomas are benign neoplasms of striated muscle that have a preference for the head and neck. They are divided into fetal and adult types based on histologic features rather than patient age, as the name might imply. Fetal rhabdomyomas have been reported in the nasopharynx and nose (337). They consist of immature, slender muscle fibers and more primitive spindle-shaped mesenchymal cells. The lack of pleomorphism and mitotic figures and the greater maturation of muscle at the periphery of the tumors distinguish the lesion from rhabdomyosarcoma.

Adult rhabdomyomas are usually located in the floor of the mouth and soft palate but have been reported in the nasopharynx (337). The cytoplasm is often clear as a result of large quantities of glycogen. This imparts a vacuolated appearance, sometimes resulting in so-called spider cells. Striations are sparse; however, the eosinophilic, finely granular cytoplasm resembles striated muscle, and Z-bands may be found on ultrastructural examination. Immunohistochemical markers for skeletal muscle will confirm the diagnosis but are seldom necessary.

MISCELLANEOUS SOFT TISSUE SARCOMAS

Virtually every soft tissue sarcoma can arise in the nose, sinuses, or nasopharynx. Their diagnostic criteria are the same as those detailed in the chapter on soft tissue tumors (see Chapter 5). Angiosarcoma, malignant hemangiopericytoma, malignant fibrous histiocytoma, and fibrosarcoma are briefly discussed elsewhere in this chapter. Other sarcomas occasionally encountered in the upper airway include synovial sarcoma (338), leiomyosarcoma (333,339), malignant peripheral nerve sheath tumor (318), and rhabdomyosarcoma. The last is by far the most common.

RHABDOMYOSARCOMA

Rhabdomyosarcoma in the head and neck arises, in descending order, in the orbit, nasopharynx, middle ear/mastoid, and nose/paranasal sinuses (340). Symptoms depend on the location and include epistaxis, rhinorrhea, ear pain, or proptosis. Mucosal tumors consist of small red nodules or a polypoid mass (sarcoma botryoides). Approximately 75% of the patients are 12 years of age or younger, but examples are seen in adolescents, young adults (341), or even the elderly. Approximately 85% of rhabdomyosarcomas in the head and neck are embryonal in type, including sarcoma botryoides variants producing grossly polypoid mucosal masses. Most of the rest are of the alveolar subtype, with rare examples of the spindle cell or pleomorphic variants. The embryonal variant is more common in younger children, whereas older children and adolescents have a higher frequency of the alveolar subtype.

As discussed in more detail in the chapter on soft tissue, it has now been clearly documented that the light microscopic variants of rhabdomyosarcoma have distinctive cytogenetic abnormalities. The t(2;13) and, less commonly, t(1;13) translocations are well documented for the alveolar subtype and are distinct from a spectrum of cytogenetic abnormalities seen in embryonal variants.

Microscopically, embryonal rhabdomyosarcoma frequently has alternating hypercellular and hypocellular fields. The stroma is sparsely collagenized or myxoid. Most tumor cells have small, round or oval nuclei and scanty cytoplasm. Occasional larger, elongated cells may have abundant, deeply eosinophilic cytoplasm with cross-striations. Anaplasia, defined as the presence of markedly hyperchromatic nuclei at least three times larger than adjacent cells and clearly abnormal mitotic figures, may be focally present (342).

Alveolar rhabdomyosarcoma has fibrous septa lined by a single row of round tumor cells, with additional tumor cells lying free between the septa. Multinucleated tumor cells with peripheral nuclei may occasionally be present. Alveolar rhabdomyosarcoma may have solid areas consisting of closely packed round cells identical in cytologic characteristics to those lining the septa (Fig. 21.78) (343). The solid areas tend to be at the periphery of otherwise more typical alveolar rhabdomyosarcomas and are a clue that an alveolar pattern may be present somewhere in the tumor. The therapeutic failure rate is higher for alveolar rhabdomyosarcoma than for embryonal tumors (344,345).

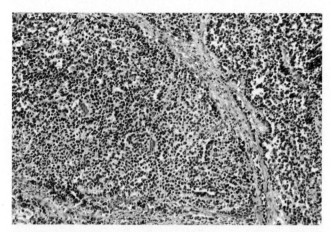

Figure 21.78. Alveolar rhabdomyosarcoma, solid variant. There are nests of tumor cells demarcated by fibrous septa. Histologic recognition of this pattern as an alveolar variant has been supported by cytogenetic studies showing the characteristic t(2;13) translocation.

The diagnosis can often be substantiated by immunohistochemical staining or on ultrastructural study (Figs. 21.79 and 21.80) (346–348). In one study, desmin was present in 100% of cases, fast myosin was present in 65%, slow myosin was present in 40%, and myoglobin was present in 65% (349). More recently, two new markers, myogenin and myoD1, have been shown to be sensitive and highly specific for skeletal muscle differentiation (350,351). Care must be taken to ensure that cells staining for myogenous markers are actually cells of rhabdomyosarcoma. Necrotic skeletal muscle and its associated antigens can be phagocytosed by nonmyogenous tumor cells and histiocytes at the edge of an invading soft tissue tumor, leading to false-positive reactions (352).

After chemotherapy or radiation therapy, rhabdomyosarcoma can have a population of cells with large quantities of eosinophilic cytoplasm that appear to have matured (Fig. 21.81). Even this cytologic "differentiation" is a sign of active, persistent tumor and has been found in metastases at autopsy (353). Possible hypotheses for this phenomenon have been discussed by Molenaar et al. (354). It is prognostically important

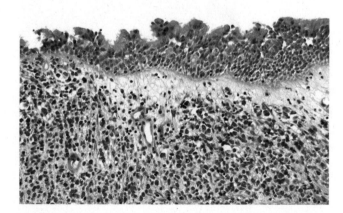

Figure 21.79. Embryonal rhabdomyosarcoma lies beneath respiratory epithelium. The tumor is focally separated from the surface by uninvolved stroma. The small-cell pattern is nonspecific.

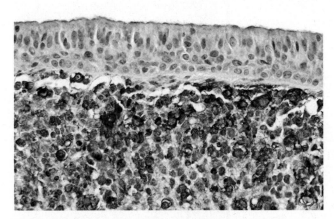

Figure 21.80. Embryonal rhabdomyosarcoma demonstrates strong staining for muscle-specific antigen (MSA).

to separate rhabdomyosarcoma into three anatomic groups: the orbit, the parameningeal area (which includes nose, sinuses, and nasopharynx), and other head/neck sites. The survival rates for these groups are 90%, 45%, and 75%, respectively (342).

The differential diagnosis of rhabdomyosarcoma includes fetal rhabdomyoma, peripheral PNET (Ewing sarcoma), malignant lymphoma, olfactory neuroblastoma, and sinonasal undifferentiated carcinoma. These can often be distinguished by light microscopy. Nevertheless, immunohistochemistry may be crucial, and sometimes electron microscopy is helpful. The cells of PNET are more uniform than those of rhabdomyosarcoma, have a negligible amount of cytoplasm (355), and strongly express CD99 as a result of their characteristic t(11;22) translocation. Malignant lymphoma consists of noncohesive cells that stain for LCA (CD45). Olfactory neuroblastoma usually expresses synaptophysin and often has S-100 protein–positive cells around cell nests. On ultrastructure examination, olfactory neuroblastoma usually exhibits long, interdigitating cell processes and dense-core secretory granules. Distinguishing it from sinonasal undifferentiated carcinoma has been discussed in an earlier section.

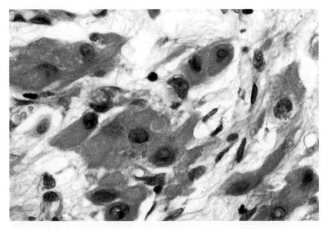

Figure 21.81. Embryonal rhabdomyosarcoma. Nearly all of the cells of this postchemotherapy embryonal rhabdomyosarcoma have a large quantity of eosinophilic cytoplasm. Only a few cells in the original tumor had conspicuous quantities of cytoplasm.

The myxomatous stroma of rhabdomyosarcoma may lead to an erroneous diagnosis of myxoma. Myxomas virtually never occur in children. The finding of a tumor (especially in a child) with a predominantly myxomatous background should stimulate a prolonged search for cells showing muscle differentiation and the use of appropriate immunohistochemical studies for muscle differentiation.

TERATOCARCINOSARCOMA

Teratocarcinosarcomas are rare tumors arising in the nose, paranasal sinuses, or nasopharynx and composed of a wide variety of cellular components of highly variable maturity and pleomorphism. These lesions may contain neuroepithelial tissue, glands, squamous nests, myxoid stroma, cartilaginous islands, osteoid, skeletal muscle, or smooth muscle (Fig. 21.82) (356). Any element may range from overtly immature or malignant to virtually normal in appearance. One reported lesion of the nasopharynx diagnosed as blastoma may be more akin to teratocarcinosarcoma (357). We also believe that some lesions reported as olfactory neuroblastomas with widely divergent differentiation may actually represent teratocarcinosarcomas. Approximately 67% of patients die of this disease within 3 years, usually because of uncontrollable local growth. These tumors have been shown to express a variety of immunohistochemical markers including vimentin, CD99, neuron-specific enolase, CK, EMA, glial fibrillary acidic protein (GFAP), chromogranin, and synaptophysin (358).

OSSEOUS TUMORS

Expansile osseous neoplasms or nonneoplastic conditions of the craniofacial bones, especially the maxilla, may encroach on the upper airway passages. Most lesions are diagnostically straightforward, using the same microscopic criteria applied to lesions elsewhere in the skeleton. Nevertheless, some conditions pose problems in interpretation. For example, giant-cell granuloma, aneurysmal bone cyst, giant-cell tumor, benign fibrous histiocytoma, and fibro-osseous lesions have considerable histologic overlap. In one report, a patient had a lesion of the ethmoid bones that was variously diagnosed by experienced bone pathologists as giant-cell granuloma, giant-cell tumor, aneurysmal bone cyst with areas of giant-cell granuloma, and fibro-osseous lesion (359). Only a few publications have acknowledged this problem (360,361).

GIANT-CELL TUMOR

Giant-cell tumors of craniofacial bones are extremely rare (362). A few well-documented cases have been reported, which had the diagnostic mononuclear cell background identical to that of giant-cell tumor of long bones (363). Several cases of giant-cell tumor in patients with Paget disease have been reported, but these more closely resemble giant-cell granuloma (364) (see next section).

GIANT-CELL GRANULOMA AND ANEURYSMAL BONE CYST

Giant-cell granuloma (giant-cell reparative granuloma) and aneurysmal bone cyst are discussed together because of the consid-

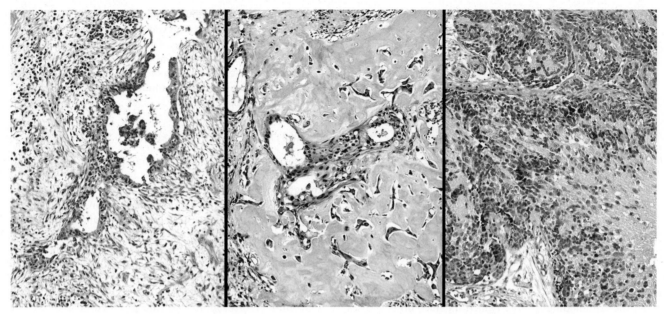

Figure 21.82. Teratocarcinosarcoma. These rare lesions are noted for the wide spectrum of their microscopic appearances. This example contains neoplastic glands in a spindle cell matrix (*left*), neoplastic glands in a chondro-osseous matrix (*center*), and areas of immature neural differentiation with neuroblasts, ganglion-like cells, and neuropil (*right*).

erable overlap in their histologic features. Furthermore, there are no demographic differences between giant-cell granuloma and aneurysmal bone cyst. The age range and slight predilection for women is similar for both lesions. Giant-cell granuloma consists of spindle, ovoid, or round histiocyte-like cells set in well-vascularized fibrous tissue (Fig. 21.83). The cells are mononuclear, binuclear, and trinuclear and may form giant cells with approximately 10 to 20 nuclei. The giant cells may aggregate in groups of 6 to 12 cells, areas for which the word granuloma is appropriate. The giant cells have a propensity to invade vascular channels and often line them. Osteoid is formed within the center as well as the periphery of the lesion. It consists of metaplastic woven bone and lamellar trabeculae.

Mature trabeculae are lined by osteoblasts and sometimes osteoclasts. Mitotic figures are often numerous to the point of

being alarming (365). Extravasation of blood is focally prominent and is considered by some to be the cause of this lesion. This seems unlikely in view of the large number of traumatized facial bones, coupled with the localized hemorrhage resulting from a dental extraction—situations rarely followed by giant-cell granuloma. Moreover, extravasated blood is commonly seen in benign lesions, such as fibrous dysplasia (FD), as well as in benign and malignant neoplasms.

This histologic description also applies to the broad septa and solid areas that are present in aneurysmal bone cyst, including the propensity for giant cells to line vascular spaces. It is arbitrary whether one concentrates on the more solid areas and labels a lesion as a giant-cell granuloma or concentrates on the vascular component and considers it to be an aneurysmal bone cyst (Fig. 21.84). In this context, the radiographic features can

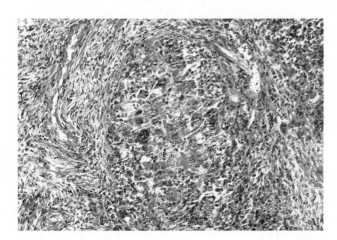

Figure 21.83. Giant-cell granuloma has a predominantly fibrous background. Mononuclear and multinucleated giant cells form an ill-defined aggregate centrally. Many capillaries are evident.

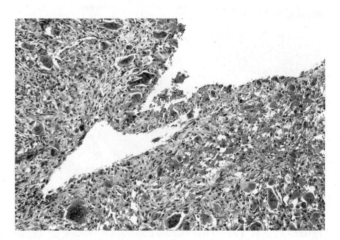

Figure 21.84. Giant-cell granulomas may have large, thin-walled vessels. These may form gaping vascular spaces (*upper right*) characteristic of aneurysmal bone cyst.

influence the pathologic interpretation. For example, involvement of contiguous bones is more typical of aneurysmal bone cyst. Moreover, a solid variant of aneurysmal bone cyst has been reported in the facial bones, and it can affect several adjacent bones synchronously (366). In retrospect, some lesions called giant-cell granuloma are better classified as solid aneurysmal bone cyst (367).

The practical importance of separating giant-cell granuloma from either cystic or solid aneurysmal bone cyst is minimal. Both giant-cell granuloma and aneurysmal bone cyst have a propensity for recurrence that is variably reported to be in the range of 15% to 26%. As with aneurysmal bone cyst of long bones, there may be an underlying lesion, such as FD, associated with aneurysmal bone cyst of the facial bones (368,369).

FIBRO-OSSEOUS LESIONS

Lesions with fibrous and osseous components include FD, ossifying fibroma (OF), and COF. COFs in the extragnathic facial bones are frequently called psammomatoid OF (370). Johnson et al. (371) used the term *juvenile active OF* for psammomatoid OF whether it arose in the gnathic or extragnathic bones. Slootweg et al. (372,373) have used the phrase *juvenile OF* for what they believe is a unique lesion with an osteoblast-rich stroma and delicate strands of osteoid.

FD and OF lie on a broad and continuous microscopic spectrum (360,374), as do FDs (Fig. 21.85) and COFs (Fig. 21.86) (375). FD is at one end of the spectrum for both pairs of lesions. It is characterized by trabeculae of woven bone that are irregularly shaped, branching, and often curvilinear. Rimming of osteoblasts at the edges of the trabeculae is rarely seen. These features constitute the usual histologic definition of FD. At the other end of one of the pairs of spectra are the conventional features of OF, with trabeculae of lamellar bone prominently lined by osteoblasts. The fully developed COF has sharply defined, rounded, calcified spherules and nonlinear trabeculae of bone. On the one hand, many lesions have mixtures of woven bone and lamellar bone intermediate between FD and OF (374), and on the other hand, composites of OF and COF can be distinguished on histologic grounds alone (373,376,377).

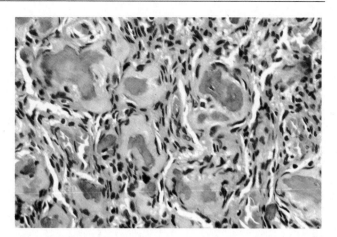

Figure 21.86. Cemento-ossifying fibromas have sharply defined, irregularly shaped, calcified spherules set in a densely fibrotic stroma.

Not surprisingly, many pathologists, including the author, find this a challenging area. In fact, Voytek et al. (375) believed that there were neither histologic nor radiographic features that consistently differentiated FD and COF.

Regarding FD and OF, Boysen et al. (378) stated that the "differential diagnosis of fibrous dysplasia versus ossifying fibroma rests on a radiographic criterion after the histopathologist has verified the fibro-osseous nature of the lesion" (Fig. 21.85). OF has well-circumscribed margins and often a "punched-out" appearance on the radiograph. Conversely, FD has radiographically ill-defined borders and a ground glass or orange peel quality. When fibro-osseous lesions are divided using these radiographic features, clinical differences emerge, including different locations in the facial bones, ages of the patients, and, most important, rates of recurrence (379,380). FD recurs in approximately 20% of patients, whereas recurrence of OF is rare (381,382). Parenthetically, FD of the craniofacial bones shows greater microscopic variation than FD in other locations (383). Furthermore, there is a tendency for maturation in recurrent FD of the facial bones, in contrast to FD of the long bones (384).

MYXOMA

Myxomas of the skeleton are almost completely limited to the maxilla and mandible, strongly suggesting an association with odontogenic structures (385–387). The maxillary lesions often encroach on the nose or antrum, resulting in airway obstruction, drainage, or, rarely, epistaxis. The soft tissues and bone are usually involved simultaneously, and it may be arbitrary regarding which is the true primary site. Generally the tumor cells are uniform spindle cells lying in a myxoid background with a modest number of blood vessels (Fig. 21.87). Some foci are more cellular, with collagen replacing the mucoid areas. Large, bizarre nuclei are sometimes seen, but these apparently are not associated with a higher risk of recurrence or more aggressive behavior (388). Treatment of choice is complete surgical excision. Recurrence rate is approximately 25% (386). The differential diagnosis includes fibromatosis and low-grade fibrosarcoma. Fibromatosis has collagen throughout the lesion. Low-grade fibrosarcoma is far more cellular, and the nuclei are more uniformly atypical.

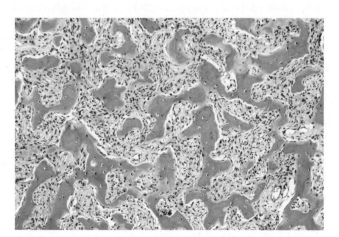

Figure 21.85. A fibro-osseous lesion from the zygomatic arch of a 15-year-old boy has interconnecting trabeculae of bone with focal osteoblastic rimming. On histologic grounds, this resembles an ossifying fibroma, but the radiograph and age of the patient are typical of fibrous dysplasia.

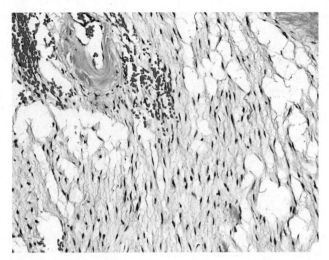

Figure 21.87. Maxillary myxoma. Bland, hypocellular spindled cells are dispersed in a myxoid matrix containing scattered blood vessels, some with fibrotic walls (*upper left*).

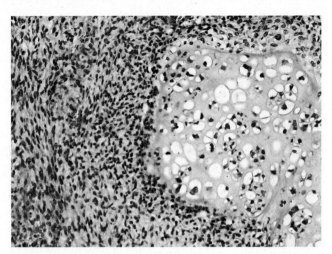

Figure 21.88. Mesenchymal chondrosarcoma. Dense spindle cell stroma, much like that of monophasic synovial sarcoma, contains a well-demarcated island of atypical cartilage.

OSTEOMA

Osteomas are most common in the frontal sinuses, followed in decreasing frequency by the ethmoid, antrum, and sphenoid sinuses. Osteomas may also develop in the mandible, either within the medulla or protruding from the cortex. Most osteomas are of the compact or "ivory" type, consisting of dense lamellar bone with a small amount of intervening fibrous tissue that only rarely has hematopoietic elements. Small, normal osteoblasts are sparse. From time to time, there are small areas resembling fibro-osseous lesions (389). Multiple osteomas of the mandible or calvarium raise the possibility of Gardner syndrome. The pathogenesis of osteomas is controversial; some hypotheses view them as benign neoplasms, developmental anomalies, the end stage of FD, or sclerosing reactions to an inflammatory process. Removal is necessary only when there is symptomatic obstruction of the sinus ostium.

OSTEOSARCOMA

Gnathic osteosarcomas differ somewhat from osteosarcomas of long bones in that they are heavily weighted by chondroblastic lesions and do not usually metastasize (390). These favorable features do not hold true, however, for osteosarcoma in Paget disease (391), osteosarcoma subsequent to therapeutic radiation (392), or osteosarcoma involving the extragnathic craniofacial bones (393).

MESENCHYMAL CHONDROSARCOMA

Approximately 15% of mesenchymal chondrosarcomas occur in craniofacial bones (394). When the maxilla or base of the skull is involved, there is encroachment on the upper airway. The tumor has a population of small cells that may be confused with rhabdomyosarcoma and PNET (Ewing sarcoma). The presence of an hemangiopericytoma-like pattern helps differentiate it from these tumors, as do the cartilaginous and occasionally

osteoid foci in mesenchymal chondrosarcoma (Fig. 21.88). Moreover, the radiographic location of the tumor, centered in the bone, favors mesenchymal chondrosarcoma rather than rhabdomyosarcoma, although the latter sometimes erodes into bone.

OTHER INTRAOSSEOUS LESIONS

Other lesions that sometimes involve the maxilla include desmoplastic fibroma (395), chondroblastoma (396), hemangioma (397), PNET (Ewing sarcoma) (398), chondrosarcoma (335), and parosteal osteosarcoma (399). Tumors also arise in the small bones of the face. Osteoblastomas of the ethmoid bone (362) and hemangioma of the nasal bone are examples (400). Odontogenic tumors may also encroach on the maxillary antrum (401).

CHORDOMA

Chordomas sometimes appear as a mass in the nasopharynx or nasal cavity (402). The cells have a vacuolated cytoplasm and are situated in a myxoid stroma. Chordoma may be mistaken for adenocarcinoma, especially if there are tumor cells with a single vacuole. Because chordomas express epithelial cell markers, such as CK and EMA, immunohistochemical stains are not of value (403,404). Nonetheless, close study will usually permit the diagnosis. Chordomas do not form glands, and the multivacuolated (physaliphorous) cells seen in most chordomas are not typical of adenocarcinoma (Fig. 21.89).

Some chordomas contain areas indistinguishable on light microscopy from cartilage; the term *chondroid chordoma* has been applied to these neoplasms. In addition, purely cartilaginous neoplasms may arise in the spheno-occipital region. There has been considerable debate in the literature regarding the method and clinical importance of distinguishing these three related tumors—the classic chordoma, the so-called chondroid chordoma, and low-grade chondrosarcoma (404–406). Part of the debate has focused on whether chondroid chordomas are true chordomas with chondroid or chondroid-like differentiation or chondrosarcomas with foci resem-

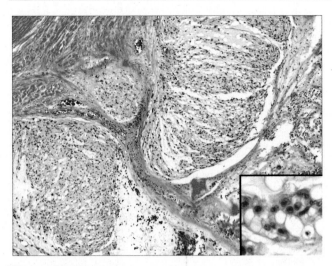

Figure 21.89. Nasal chordoma. Nests of relatively bland eosinophilic cells are embedded in a loose myxoid matrix. At higher magnification (*inset*), the cells have prominent cytoplasmic vacuoles.

bling chordoma (403,406). It is now clear that so-called chondroid chordomas, like conventional chordomas, contain CK-positive cells and should be considered to represent chordoma variants (407–410).

A second debate has centered on the clinical significance of this distinction. Initial studies suggested that patients with chondroid chordomas had a conspicuously prolonged survival compared with individuals with conventional chordomas (405). Another, newer study from the same institution now indicates no significant differences in survival for patients with CK-positive "classic" chordomas, chondroid chordomas with CK positivity, and CK-negative, low-grade chondrosarcomas (407). In the same study, the patient's age did show a strong correlation with survival. Patients younger than 40 years of age did significantly better than older individuals (407).

High-grade sarcomas occasionally arise at the site of previously excised chordomas. The sarcoma usually has a nonspecific appearance with a prominent spindle cell component. These neoplasms have been referred to as dedifferentiated chordomas, and they are associated with a poor prognosis (411,412).

REFERENCES

1. Walike JW. Anatomy of the nasal cavities. *Otolaryngol Clin North Am* 1973;6:609–621.
2. Mills SE, Gaffey MJ, Frierson HF, Jr. Tumors of the upper aerodigestive tract and ear. In *Atlas of Tumor Pathology*, 3rd series. Washington, DC: Armed Forces Institute of Pathology, 1997:1–14.
3. Nakashima T, Kimmelman CP, Snow JB, Jr. Structure of human fetal and adult olfactory neuroepithelium. *Arch Otolaryngol* 1984;110:641–646.
4. Ali MY. Histology of the human nasopharyngeal mucosa. *J Anat* 1965;99:657–672.
5. Morin GV, Shank EC, Burgess LPA, et al. Oncocytic metaplasia of the pharynx. *Otolaryngol Head Neck Surg* 1991;105:86–91.
6. Garrish MT, Podnos SD, Meyerhoff WL. Chronic progressive aspergillosis in an immunocompetent host. *Otolaryngol Head Neck Surg* 1987;96:565–568.
7. McGill TJ, Simpson G, Healy GB. Fulminant aspergillosis of the nose and paranasal sinuses: a new clinical entity. *Laryngoscope* 1980;90:748–754.
8. Katzenstein A-LA, Sale SR, Greenberger PA. Pathologic findings in allergic aspergillus sinusitis: a newly recognized form of sinusitis. *Am J Surg Pathol* 1983;7:439–443.
9. Waxman JE, Spector JG, Sale SR, Katzenstein A-LA. Allergic aspergillus sinusitis: concepts in diagnosis and treatment of a new clinical entity. *Laryngoscope* 1987;97:261–266.
10. Kupferberg SB, Bent JP III, Kuhn FA. Prognosis of allergic fungal sinusitis. *Otolaryngol Head Neck Surg* 1997;117:25–41.
11. MacMillan RH III, Cooper PH, Body BA, et al. Allergic fungal sinusitis due to *Curvularia lunata*. *Hum Pathol* 1987;18:960–964.
12. Freidman GC, Hartwick RWJ, Ro JY, et al. Allergic fungal sinusitis: report of three cases associated with dematiaceous fungi. *Am J Clin Pathol* 1991;96:368–372.
13. Briggs DR, Barney PL, Bahu RM. Nasal cryptococcosis. *Arch Otolaryngol* 1974;100:390–392.
14. Thomas GG, Toohill RJ, Lehman RH. Nasal actinomycosis following heterograft: a case report. *Arch Otolaryngol* 1974;100:377–378.
15. Dworzack DL, Pollock AS, Hodges GR, et al. Zygomycosis of the maxillary sinus and palate caused by *Basidiobolus haptosporus*. *Arch Intern Med* 1978;138:1274–1276.
16. Gluckman SJ, Reis K, Abrutyn E. *Allescheria (Petriellidium) boydii* sinusitis in a compromised host. *J Clin Microbiol* 1977;5:481–484.
17. Rowley SD, Strom CG. *Paecilimyces fungus* infection of the maxillary sinus. *Laryngoscope* 1982;92:332–334.
18. Shugar MA, Montgomery WW, Hyslop NE. Alternaria sinusitis. *Ann Otol Rhinol Laryngol* 1981;90:251–254.
19. Brown JW III, Nadell J, Sanders CV, et al. Brain abscess caused by *Cladosporium trichoides* (*Bantianum*): a case with paranasal sinus involvement. *South Med J* 1976;69:1519–1521.
20. Valenstein P, Schell WA. Primary intranasal *Fusarium* infection: potential for confusion with rhinocerebral zygomocosis. *Arch Pathol Lab Med* 1986;110:751–754.
21. Morgan MA, Wilson WR, Neel HB III, et al. Fungal sinusitis in healthy and immunocompromised individuals. *Am J Clin Pathol* 1984;82:597–601.
22. Phillips P, Rippon JW, Stein L, et al. Fungal sinusitis caused by *Chrysosporium pruinosum*. *Otolaryngol Head Neck Surg* 1987;96:577–579.
23. Waldman SR, Levine HL, Sebek BA. Nasal tuberculosis: a forgotten entity. *Laryngoscope* 1981;91:11–16.
24. Pollack JD, Pincus RL, Lucente FE. Leprosy of the head and neck. *Otolaryngol Head Neck Surg* 1987;97:93–96.
25. McDougall AC, Rees RJW, Weddel AGM, et al. The histopathology of lepromatous leprosy of the nose. *J Pathol* 1975;115:215–226.
26. Kannan-Kutty M, Teh E-C. *Rhinosporidium seeberi*: an ultrastructural study of its endosporulation phase and trophocyte phase. *Arch Pathol* 1975;99:51–54.
27. Jiminez JF, Young DE, Hough AJ Jr. Rhinosporidiosis: a report of two cases from Arkansas. *Am J Clin Pathol* 1984;82:611–615.
28. Berger SA, Pollock AA, Richmond AS. Isolation *of Klebsiella ozaenae* and *Klebsiella rhinoscleromatis* in a general hospital. *Am J Clin Pathol* 1977;67:499–502.
29. Batsakis JG, Luna MA. Midfacial necrotizing lesions. *Semin Diagn Pathol* 1987;4:90–116.
30. Crissman JD, Weiss MA, Gluckman J. Midline granuloma syndrome: a clinicopathologic study of 13 patients. *Am J Surg Pathol* 1982;6:335–346.
31. Tsoskos M, Fauci AS, Costa J. Idiopathic midline destructive disease (IMDD): a subgroup of patients with the "midline granuloma" syndrome. *Am J Clin Pathol* 1982;77:162–168.
32. Fienberg R. The protracted superficial phenomenon in pathergic (Wegener's) granulomatosis. *Hum Pathol* 1981;12:458–467.
33. Devaney KO, Travis WD, Hoffman G, et al. Interpretation of head and neck biopsies in Wegener's granulomatosis: a pathologic study of 136 biopsies from 70 patients. *Am J Surg Pathol* 1990;14:555–564.
34. Del Buono EA, Flint A. Diagnostic usefulness of nasal biopsy in Wegener's granulomatosis. *Hum Pathol* 1991;22:107–110.
35. Colby TV, Tazelaar HD, Specks U, et al. Nasal biopsy in Wegener's granulomatosis. *Hum Pathol* 1991;22:101–104.
36. Olsen KD, Neel HB III, DeRemee RA. Nasal manifestations of allergic granulomatosis and angiitis (Churg-Strauss syndrome). *Otolaryngol Head Neck Surg* 1980;88:85–89.
37. Fechner RE, Lamppin DW. Midline malignant reticulosis: a clinicopathologic entity. *Arch Otolaryngol* 1972;95:467–476.
38. DeRemee RA, Weiland LH, McDonald TJ. Polymorphic reticulosis, lymphomatoid granulomatosis: two diseases or one? *Mayo Clin Proc* 1978;53:634–640.
39. Crissman JD. Midline malignant reticulosis and lymphomatoid granulomatosis: a case report. *Arch Pathol Lab Med* 1979;103:561–564.
40. Tsoskos M, Fauci AS, Costa J. Letter. *Am J Clin Pathol* 1982;78:137–138.
41. Sercarz JA, Strasnick B, Newman A, et al. Midline nasal destruction in cocaine abusers. *Otolaryngol Head Neck Surg* 1991;105:694–701.
42. Postma D, Fry TL, Malenbaum BT. The nose, minor salivary glands, and sarcoidosis. *Arch Otolaryngol* 1984;110:28–30.
43. Gordon WN, Cohn AM, Greenberg SD, et al. Nasal sarcoidosis. *Arch Otolaryngol* 1976;102:11–14.
44. Wolff M. Granulomas in nasal mucous membranes following local steroid injections. *Am J Clin Pathol* 1974;62:775–782.
45. Coup AJ, Hopper IP. Granulomatous lesions in nasal biopsies. *Histopathology* 1980;4:293–308.
46. Kinnear WJM. Crohn's disease affecting the nasal mucosa. *J Otolaryngol* 1985;14:399–400.
47. Graham J, Michaels L. Cholesterol granuloma of the maxillary antrum. *Clin Otolaryngol* 1978;3:155–160.
48. Rosai J. The nature of myospherulosis of the upper respiratory tract. *Am J Clin Pathol* 1978;69:475–481.
49. Travis WD, Li C-Y, Weiland LH. Immunostaining for hemoglobin in two cases of myospherulosis. *Arch Pathol Lab Med* 1986;110:763–765.
50. Wheeler TM, Sessions RB, McGavran MH. Myospherulosis: a preventable nasal and paranasal entity. *Arch Otolaryngol* 1980;106:272–274.
51. Natvig K, Larsen TE. Mucocele of paranasal sinuses: a retrospective clinical and histological study. *J Laryngol Otol* 1978;92:1075–1082.
52. Allard RHB, van der Kwast WAM, van der Waal I. Mucosal antral cyst: review of literature and report of a radiographic survey. *Oral Surg* 1981;51:2–9.
53. Johnston WH. Necrotizing sialometaplasia involving the mucous glands of the nasal cavity. *Hum Pathol* 1977;8:589–592.
54. Settipane GA, Chafee FH. Nasal polyps in asthma and rhinitis: a review of 6,037 cases. *J Allergy Clin Immunol* 1977;59:17–21.
55. Tos M, Morgensen C. Mucous glands in nasal polyps. *Arch Otolaryngol* 1977;103:407–413.

56. Heffner DK, Hyams VJ, Hauck KW, et al. Low-grade adenocarcinoma of the nasal cavity and paranasal sinuses. *Cancer* 1982;50:312–322.

57. Compagno J, Wong RT. Intranasal mixed tumors (pleomorphic adenomas): a clinicopathologic study of 40 cases. *Am J Clin Pathol* 1977;68:213–238.

58. Taylor B, Evans JNG, Hope GA. Upper respiratory tract in cystic fibrosis: ear-nose-throat survey of 50 children. *Arch Dis Child* 1974;49:133–136.

59. Kulczycki LL, Mueller H, Shwachman H. Respiratory allergy in patients with cystic fibrosis. *JAMA* 1961;175:358–364.

60. Oppenheimer EH, Rosenstein BJ. Differential diagnosis of nasal polyps in cystic fibrosis and atopy. *Lab Invest* 1979;40:445–449.

61. Heck WE, Hallberg OE, Williams HL. Antrochoanal polyp. *Arch Otolaryngol* 1950;52:538–548.

62. Hardy G. The choanal polyp. *Ann Otol Rhinol Laryngol* 1957;66:306–326.

63. Sirola R. Choanal polyps. *Acta Otolaryngol* 1966;61:42–48.

64. Crowe JE, Sumner TE, Ramquist NA, et al. Antrochoanal polyps. *South Med J* 1982;75:674–676.

65. Berg O, Carenfelt C, Silfversward C, et al. Origin of the choanal polyp. *Arch Otolaryngol Head Neck Surg* 1988;114:1270–1271.

66. Compagno J, Hyams VJ, Lepore ML. Nasal polyposis with stromal atypia: review and follow-up study of 14 cases. *Arch Pathol Lab Med* 1976;100:224–226.

67. Klenoff BH, Goodman ML. Mesenchymal cell atypicality in inflammatory polyps. *J Laryngol* 1977;91:751–756.

68. Kindblom L-G, Angervall L. Nasal polyps with atypical stroma cells: a pseudosarcomatous lesion. *Acta Pathol Microbiol Immunol Scand [A]* 1984;92:65–72.

69. Smith CJ, Echevarria R, McLelland CA. Pseudosarcomatous changes in antrochoanal polyps. *Arch Otolaryngol* 1974;99:228–230.

70. Weidner N, Askin FB, Berthrong M, et al. Bizarre (pseudomalignant) granulation-tissue reactions following ionizing-radiation exposure: a microscopic, immunohistochemical, and flow-cytometric study. *Cancer* 1987;59:1509–1514.

71. Brodsky L, Siddiqui SY, Stanievich JF. Massive oropharyngeal papillomatosis causing obstructive sleep apnea in a child. *Arch Otolaryngol Head Neck Surg* 1987;113:882–884.

72. Werner JS, Sherris D, Kasperbauer J, et al. Relationship of human papillomavirus to Schneiderian papillomas. *Laryngoscope* 1999;109:21–26.

73. Gaffey MJ, Frierson HF, Weiss LM, et al. Human papillomavirus and Epstein-Barr virus in sinonasal Schneiderian papillomas. An in situ hybridization and polymerase chain reaction study. *Am J Clin Pathol* 1996;106:475–482.

74. Weber RS, Shillitoe EJ, Robbins KT, et al. Prevalence of human papillomavirus in inverted nasal papillomas. *Arch Otolaryngol Head Neck Surg* 1988;114:23–26.

75. Syrjänen S, Happonen R, Virolainen E, et al. Detection of human papillomavirus (HPV) structural antigens and DNA types in inverted papillomas and squamous cell carcinomas of the nasal cavities and paranasal sinuses. *Acta Otolaryngol (Stockh)* 1987;104:334–341.

76. Kintanar EB, Sarkar FH, Plieth DA, et al. Cylindrical cell sinonasal papillomas: HPV typing by polymerase chain reaction. *Mod Pathol* 1991;4(Abstr):65A.

77. Christensen WN, Smith RRL. Schneiderian papillomas: a clinicopathologic study of 67 cases. *Hum Pathol* 1986;17:393–400.

78. Calceterra TC, Thompson JW, Paglia DE. Inverting papillomas of the nose and paranasal sinuses. *Laryngoscope* 1980;90:53–58.

79. Hyams VJ. Papillomas of the nasal cavity and paranasal sinuses: a clinicopathologic study of 315 cases. *Ann Otol Rhinol Laryngol* 1971;80:192–207.

80. Weissler MC, Montgomery WW, Turner PA, et al. Inverted papilloma. *Ann Otol Rhinol Laryngol* 1986;95:215–221.

81. Barnes L, Bedetti C. Oncocytic schneiderian papilloma: a reappraisal of cylindrical cell papilloma of the sinonasal tract. *Hum Pathol* 1984;15:344–351.

82. Schoub L, Timme AH, Uyss CJ. A well-differentiated inverted papilloma of the nasal space associated with lymph node metastases. *S Afr Med J* 1973;47:1663–1665.

83. Fechner RE, Sessions RB. Inverted papilloma of the lacrimal sac, the paranasal sinuses and the cervical region. *Cancer* 1977;40:2303–2308.

84. Stone DM, Berktold RE, Ranganathan C, et al. Inverted papilloma of the middle ear and mastoid. *Otolaryngol Head Neck Surg* 1987;97:416–418.

85. Kaufman MR, Brandwein MS, Lawson W. Sinonasal papillomas: clinicopathologic review of 40 patients with inverted and oncocytic schneiderian papillomas. *Laryngoscope* 2002;112:1372–1377.

86. Smith O, Gullane PJ. Inverting papilloma of the nose: analysis of 48 cases. *J Otolaryngol* 1987;16:154–156.

87. Ward BE, Fechner RE, Mills SE. Carcinoma arising in oncocytic schneiderian papilloma. *Am J Surg Pathol* 1990;14:364–369.

88. Benninger MS, Roberts JK, Sebek BA, et al. Inverted papillomas and associated squamous cell carcinoma. *Otolaryngol Head Neck Surg* 1990;103:457–461.

89. Fechner RE. Pathologic quiz case 2: cylindrical cell papilloma with invasive, nonkeratinizing squamous carcinoma. *Arch Otolaryngol* 1981;107:454–457.

90. Ridolfi FL, Lieberman PH, Erlandson RA, et al. Schneiderian papillomas: a clinicopathologic study of 30 cases. *Am J Surg Pathol* 1977;1:43–53.

91. Snyder RN, Perzin KH. Papillomatosis of the nasal cavity and paranasal sinuses (inverted papilloma, squamous papilloma): a clinicopathologic study. *Cancer* 1972;30:668–690.

92. Kapadia SB, Barnes L, Pelzman K, et al. Carcinoma ex oncocytic schneiderian (cylindrical cell) papilloma. *Am J Otolaryngol* 1993;14:332–338.

93. Wenig BM, Heffner DK. Respiratory epithelial adenomatoid hamartomas of the sinonasal tract and nasopharynx: a clinicopathologic study of 31 cases. *Ann Otol Rhinol Laryngol* 1995;104:639–645.

94. Ozolek JA, Hunt JL. Tumor suppressor gene alterations in respiratory epithelial adenomatoid hamartoma (REAH): comparison to sinonasal adenocarcinoma and inflamed sinonasal mucosa. *Am J Surg Pathol* 2006;30:1576–1580.

95. McDermott MB, Ponder TB, Dehner LP. Nasal chondromesenchymal hamartoma: an upper respiratory tract analogue of the chest wall mesenchymal hamartoma. *Am J Surg Pathol* 1998;22:425–433.

96. Lewis JS, Castro EB. Cancer of the nasal cavity and paranasal sinuses. *J Laryngol Otol* 1972;86:255–262.

97. Beatty CW, Pearson BW, Kern EB. Carcinoma of the nasal septum: experience with 85 cases. *Otolaryngol Head Neck Surg* 1982;90:90–94.

98. Bosch A, Vallecillo L, Frias Z. Cancer of the nasal cavity. *Cancer* 1976;37:1458–1463.

99. Virtue JA. The relationship between the refining of nickel and cancer of the nasal cavity. *Can J Otolaryngol* 1972;1:37–42.

100. Rousch GC. Epidemiology of cancer of the nose and paranasal sinuses: current concepts. *Head Neck Surg* 1979;2:3–11.

101. Goren AD, Harley N, Eisenbud L, et al. Clinical and radiobiologic features of Thorotrast-induced carcinoma of the maxillary sinus: a case report. *Oral Surg Oral Med Oral Pathol* 1980;49:237–242.

102. Furuta Y, Takasu T, Asai T, et al. Detection of human papillomavirus DNA in carcinomas of the nasal cavities and paranasal sinuses by the polymerase chain reaction. *Cancer* 1992;69:353–357.

103. Barnes L, Verbin RS, Gnepp DR. Diseases of the nose, paranasal sinuses, and nasopharynx. In Barnes L, ed. *Surgical Pathology of the Head and Neck.* New York, NY: Marcel Dekker, 1985:403–451.

104. Shibuya H, Amagasa T, Hanai A, et al. Second primary carcinomas in patients with squamous cell carcinoma of the maxillary sinus. *Cancer* 1986;58:1122–1125.

105. Piscioli F, Aldovini D, Bondi A, et al. Squamous cell carcinoma with sarcoma-like stroma of the nose and paranasal sinuses: report of two cases. *Histopathology* 1984;8:633–639.

106. Hanna GS, Ali MH. Verrucous carcinoma of the nasal septum. *J Laryngol Otol* 1987;101:184–187.

107. Manivel C, Wick MR, Dehner LP. Transitional (cylindric) cell carcinoma with endodermal sinus tumor-like features of the nasopharynx and paranasal sinuses: clinicopathologic and immunohistochemical study of two cases. *Arch Pathol Lab Med* 1986;110:198–202.

108. Shanmugaratnam K, Chan SH, de-The G, et al. Histopathology of nasopharyngeal carcinoma: correlations with epidemiology, survival rates and other biological characteristics. *Cancer* 1979;44:1029–1044.

109. Yeh S. A histological classification of carcinomas of the nasopharynx with critical review as to the existence of lymphoepitheliomas. *Cancer* 1962;15:895–920.

110. Bloom SM. Cancer of the nasopharynx: a study of ninety cases. *J Mt Sinai Hosp* 1969;36:277–298.

111. Creely JJ Jr., Lyons GD Jr., Trail ML. Cancer of the nasopharynx: a review of 114 cases. *South Med J* 1973;66:405–409.

112. Easton JM, Levine PH, Hyams VJ. Nasopharyngeal carcinoma in the United States: a pathologic study of 177 US and 30 foreign cases. *Arch Otolaryngol* 1980;106:88–91.

113. Giffler RF, Gillespie JJ, Ayala AG, et al. Lymphoepithelioma in cervical lymph nodes of children and young adults. *Am J Surg Pathol* 1977;1:293–302.

114. Hawkins EP, Krischer JP, Smith BE, et al. Nasopharyngeal carcinoma in children: a retrospective review and demonstration of Epstein-Barr viral genomes in tumor cell cytoplasm: a report of the Pediatric Oncology Group. *Hum Pathol* 1990;21:805–810.

115. Sham JST, Poon YF, Wei WI, et al. Nasopharyngeal carcinoma in young patients. *Cancer* 1990;65:2606–2610.

116. Ayan I, Kaytan E, Ayan N. Childhood nasopharyngeal carcinoma: from biology to treatment. *Lancet Oncol* 2003;4:13–21.

117. Digby KH, Fook WL, Che YT. Nasopharyngeal malignancy. *Br J Surg* 1941;28:517–537.

118. Simons MJ, Wee GB, Goh EH, et al. Immunogenetic aspects of nasopharyngeal carcinoma. IV. Increased risk in Chinese of nasopharyngeal carcinoma associated with a Chinese-related HLA profile (A2, Singapore 2). *J Natl Cancer Inst* 1976;57:977–980.

119. Clifford P. Blood groups and nasopharyngeal carcinoma. *Lancet* 1970;2:48–49.

120. Pearson GR, Weiland LH, Neel HB III, et al. Application of Epstein-Barr virus (EBV) serology to the diagnosis of North American nasopharyngeal carcinoma. *Cancer* 1983;51:260–268.

121. Ringborg U, Henle W, Henle G, et al. Epstein-Barr virus–specific serodiagnostic tests in carcinomas of the head and neck. *Cancer* 1983;52:1237–1243.

122. Tamada A, Makimoto K, Yamabe H, et al. Titers of Epstein-Barr virus–related antibodies in nasopharyngeal carcinoma in Japan. *Cancer* 1984;53:430–440.

123. Zaatari GS, Santoianni RA. Adenoid squamous cell carcinoma of the nasopharynx and neck region. *Arch Pathol Lab Med* 1986;110:542–546.

124. Weiss LM, Movahed LA, Butler AE, et al. Analysis of lymphoepithelioma and lymphoepithelioma-like carcinomas for Epstein-Barr viral genomes by in situ hybridization. *Am J Surg Pathol* 1989;13:625–631.

125. Gaffey MJ, Weiss LM. Association of Epstein-Barr virus with human neoplasia. *Pathol Annu* 1992;27:55–74.

126. Looi L-M. Tumor-associated tissue eosinophilia in nasopharyngeal carcinoma: a pathologic study of 422 primary and 138 metastatic tumors. *Cancer* 1987;59:466–470.

127. Regaud C, Reverchon L. Sur un cas d'epithelioma epidermoide developpé dans le massif maxillaire superieur. *Rev Laryngol Otol Rhinol (Bord)* 1921;42:369–378.

128. Schmincke A. Über lympho-epitheliale Geschwülste. *Beitr Pathol Anat Allg Pathol* 1921;68:161–170.

129. Carbone A, Micheau C. Pitfalls in microscopic diagnosis of undifferentiated carcinoma of nasopharyngeal type (lymphoepithelioma). *Cancer* 1982;50:1344–1351.

130. Wolff AP, Ossoff RH, Clemis JD. Four unusual neoplasms of the nasopharynx. *Otolaryngol Head Neck Surg* 1980;88:753–759.

131. Jahn AF, Walter JB, Farkashidy J. Verrucous carcinoma of the nasopharynx: a clinicopathologic case report. *J Otolaryngol* 1980;9:84–89.

132. Robin PE, Powell DJ, Stansbie JM. Carcinoma of the nasal cavity and paranasal sinuses: incidence and presentation of different histological types. *Clin Otolaryngol* 1979;4:431–456.

133. Weber AL, Stanton AC. Malignant tumors of the paranasal sinuses: radiologic, clinical, and histopathologic evaluation of 200 cases. *Head Neck Surg* 1984;6:761–776.

134. Rafla S. Mucous gland tumors of paranasal sinuses. *Cancer* 1969;24:683–691.

135. Marsh WL Jr., Allen MS Jr. Adenoid cystic carcinoma: biologic behavior in 38 patients. *Cancer* 1979;43:1463–1473.

136. Barnes L. Intestinal-type adenocarcinoma of the nasal cavity and paranasal sinuses. *Am J Surg Pathol* 1986;10:192–202.
137. Wenig BM, Hyams VJ, Heffner DK. Nasopharyngeal papillary adenocarcinoma: a clinicopathologic study of a low-grade carcinoma. *Am J Surg Pathol* 1988;12:946–953.
138. Jarvi O. Heterotopic tumors with an intestinal mucous membrane structure in the nasal cavity. *Acta Otolaryngol* 1945;33:471–485.
139. Simard LC, Jean A. Adenocarcinoma with argentaffin cells of the nasal cavity, giving widespread metastases. *Cancer* 1953;6:699–703.
140. Batsakis JG, Sueper RH. Adenocarcinoma of the nasal and paranasal cavities. *Arch Otolaryngol* 1963;77:625–633.
141. Sanchez-Casis G, Devine KD, Weiland LH. Nasal adenocarcinomas that closely simulate colonic carcinomas. *Cancer* 1971;28:714–720.
142. Ironside P, Matthews J. Adenocarcinoma of the nose and paranasal sinuses in woodworkers in the state of Victoria, Australia. *Cancer* 1975;36:1115–1121.
143. Mills SE, Fechner RE, Cantrell RW. Aggressive sinonasal lesion resembling normal intestinal mucosa. *Am J Surg Pathol* 1982;6:803–809.
144. Acheson ED, Cowdell RH, Hadfield E, et al. Nasal cancer in woodworkers in the furniture industry. *Br Med J* 1968;2:587–596.
145. Brinton LA, Blot WJ, Stone BJ, et al. A death certificate analysis of nasal cancer among furniture workers in North Carolina. *Cancer Res* 1977;37:3473–3474.
146. Hadfield EH. A study of adenocarcinoma of the paranasal sinuses in woodworkers in the furniture industry. *Ann R Coll Surg Engl* 1970;46:301–319.
147. Klintenberg C, Olofsson J, Hellquist H, et al. Adenocarcinoma of the ethmoid sinuses: a review of 28 cases with special reference to wood dust exposure. *Cancer* 1984;54:482–488.
148. Acheson ED, Cowdell RH, Jolles B. Nasal cancer in the Northhamptonshire boot and shoe industry. *Br Med J* 1970;1:385–393.
149. Kleinsasser O, Schroeder H-G. Adenocarcinomas of the inner nose after exposure to wood dust: morphological findings and relationships between histopathology and clinical behavior in 79 cases. *Arch Otorhinolaryngol* 1988;245:1–15.
150. Franquemont DW, Fechner RE, Mills SE. Histologic classification of sinonasal intestinal-type adenocarcinoma. *Am J Surg Pathol* 1991;15:368–375.
151. Franchi A, Gallo O, Santucci M. Clinical relevance of the histological classification of sinonasal intestinal-type adenocarcinomas. *Hum Pathol* 1999;30:1140–1145.
152. Batsakis JG, Mackay B, Ordonez G. Enteric-type adenocarcinoma of the nasal cavity: an electron microscopic and immunocytochemical study. *Cancer* 1984;54:855–860.
153. Schmid KO, Auback L, Albegger K. Endocrine-amphicrine enteric carcinoma of the nasal mucosa. *Virchows Arch A Pathol Anat Histopathol* 1979;383:329–343.
154. Cathro HP, Mills SE. Immunophenotypic differences between intestinal-type and low-grade papillary sinonasal adenocarcinomas: an immunohistochemical study of 22 cases utilizing CDX2 and MUC2. *Am J Surg Pathol* 2004;28:1026–1032.
155. McKinney CD, Mills SE, Franquemont DW. Sinonasal intestinal-type adenocarcinoma: immunohistochemical profile and comparison with colonic adenocarcinoma. *Mod Pathol* 1995;8:421–426.
156. Bernstein JM, Montgomery WW, Balogh K, Jr. Metastatic tumors to the maxilla, nose, and paranasal sinuses. *Laryngoscope* 1966;76:621–650.
157. Elkon D, Hightower SI, Lim ML, et al. Esthesioneuroblastoma. *Cancer* 1979;44:1087–1094.
158. Mills SE, Frierson HF Jr. Olfactory neuroblastoma: a clinicopathologic study of 21 cases. *Am J Surg Pathol* 1985;9:317–327.
159. Taxy JB, Bharani NK, Mills SE, et al. The spectrum of olfactory neural tumors: a light-microscopic, immunohistochemical and ultrastructural analysis. *Am J Surg Pathol* 1986;10:687–695.
160. Djalilian M, Zujko RD, Weiland LH, et al. Olfactory neuroblastoma. *Surg Clin North Am* 1977;57:751–762.
161. Oberman HA, Rice DH. Olfactory neuroblastomas: a clinicopathologic study. *Cancer* 1976;38:2494–2502.
162. Kadish S, Goodman M, Wang CC. Olfactory neuroblastoma: a clinical analysis of 17 cases. *Cancer* 1976;37:1571–1576.
163. Lewis JS, Hutter RVP, Tollefsen HR, et al. Nasal tumors of olfactory origin. *Arch Otolaryngol* 1965;81:169–174.
164. Bailey BJ, Barton S. Olfactory neuroblastoma: management and prognosis. *Arch Otolaryngol* 1975;101:1–5.
165. Micheau C, Guerinot F, Bohuon C, et al. Dopamine-B-hydroxylase and catecholamines in an olfactory esthesioneuroma. *Cancer* 1975;35:1309–1312.
166. Singh W, Ramage C, Best P, et al. Nasal neuroblastoma secreting vasopressin: a case report. *Cancer* 1980;45:961–966.
167. Gerard-Marchant R, Micheau C. Microscopical diagnosis of olfactory esthesioneuromas: general review and report of five cases. *J Natl Cancer Inst* 1965;35:75–82.
168. Silva EG, Butler JJ, Mackay B, et al. Neuroblastomas and neuroendocrine carcinomas of the nasal cavity: a proposed new classification. *Cancer* 1982;50:2388–2405.
169. Miller DC, Goodman ML, Pilch BZ, et al. Mixed olfactory neuroblastoma and carcinoma: a report of two cases. *Cancer* 1984;54:2019–2028.
170. Obert GJ, Devine KD, McDonald JR. Olfactory neuroblastomas. *Cancer* 1960;13:205–215.
171. Chaudhry AP, Haar JG, Koul A, et al. Olfactory neuroblastoma (esthesioneuroblastoma): a light and ultrastructural study of two cases. *Cancer* 1979;44:564–579.
172. Kahn LB. Esthesioneuroblastoma: a light and electron microscopic study. *Hum Pathol* 1974;5:364–371.
173. Mackay B, Luna MA, Butler JJ. Adult neuroblastoma: electron microscopic observations in nine cases. *Cancer* 1976;37:1334–1351.
174. Osamura RY, Fine G. Ultrastructure of the esthesioneuroblastoma. *Cancer* 1976;38:173–179.
175. Taxy JB, Hidvegi DF. Olfactory neuroblastoma: an ultrastructural study. *Cancer* 1977;39:131–138.
176. Judge DM, McGavran MH, Trapukdi S. Fume-induced fluorescence in diagnosis of nasal neuroblastoma. *Arch Otolaryngol* 1976;102:97–98.
177. Frierson HF Jr., Ross GW, Mills SE, et al. Olfactory neuroblastoma: additional immunohistochemical characterization. *Am J Clin Pathol* 1990;94:547–553.
178. Wick MR, Stanley SJ, Swanson PE. Immunohistochemical diagnosis of sinonasal melanoma, carcinoma, and neuroblastoma with monoclonal antibodies HMB-45 and anti-synaptophysin. *Arch Pathol Lab Med* 1988;112:616–620.
179. Trojanowski JQ, Lee V, Pillsbury N, et al. Neuronal origin of human esthesioneuroblastoma demonstrated with anti-neurofilament monoclonal antibodies. *N Engl J Med* 1982;307:159–161.
180. Devany K, Wenig BM, Abbondanzo SL. Olfactory neuroblastoma and other round cell lesions of the sinonasal region. *Mod Pathol* 1996;9:658–663.
181. Koss LG, Spiro RH, Hajdu S. Small cell (oat cell) carcinoma of minor salivary gland origin. *Cancer* 1972;30:737–741.
182. Raychowdhuri RN. Oat-cell carcinoma and paranasal sinuses. *J Laryngol Otolaryngol* 1965;79:253–255.
183. Rejowski JE, Campanella RS, Block LJ. Small cell carcinoma of the nose and paranasal sinuses. *Otolaryngol Head Neck Surg* 1982;90:516–517.
184. Weiss MD, deFries HO, Taxy JB, et al. Primary small cell carcinoma of the paranasal sinuses. *Arch Otolaryngol* 1983;109:341–343.
185. Frierson HF, Jr., Ross GW, Stewart FM, et al. Unusual sinonasal small-cell neoplasms following radiotherapy for bilateral retinoblastomas. *Am J Surg Pathol* 1989;13:947–954.
186. Frierson HF Jr., Mills SE, Fechner RE, et al. Sinonasal undifferentiated carcinoma: an aggressive neoplasm derived from schneiderian epithelium and distinct from olfactory neuroblastoma. *Am J Surg Pathol* 1986;10:771–779.
187. Cerilli LA, Holst VA, Brandwein MS, et al. Sinonasal undifferentiated carcinoma. Immunohistochemical profile and lack of EBV association. *Am J Surg Pathol* 2001;25:156–163.
188. Franchi A, Moroni M, Massi D, et al. Sinonasal undifferentiated carcinoma, nasopharyngeal-type undifferentiated carcinoma, and keratinizing and nonkeratinizing squamous cell carcinoma express different cytokeratin patterns. *Am J Surg Pathol* 2002;26:1597–1604.
189. Helliwell TR, Yeoh LH, Stell PM. Anaplastic carcinoma of the nose and paranasal sinuses: light microscopy, immunohistochemistry and clinical correlation. *Cancer* 1986;58:2038–2045.
190. Patel SG, Prasad ML, Escrig M, et al. Primary mucosal malignant melanoma of the head and neck. *Head Neck* 2002;24:247–257.
191. Brandwein MS, Rothstein A, Lawson W, et al. Sinonasal melanoma. A clinicopathologic study of 25 cases and literature meta-analysis. *Arch Otolaryngol Head Neck Surg* 1997;123:290–296.
192. Prasad ML, Jungbluth AA, Iversen K, et al. Expression of melanocytic differentiation markers in malignant melanomas of the oral and sinonasal mucosa. *Am J Surg Pathol* 2001;25:782–787.
193. Franquemont DW, Mills SE. Sinonasal malignant melanoma: a clinicopathologic and immunohistochemical study of 14 cases. *Am J Clin Pathol* 1991;96:689–697.
194. Drier JK, Swanson PE, Cherwitz DL, et al. S100 protein immunoreactivity in poorly differentiated carcinomas: immunohistochemical comparison with malignant melanoma. *Arch Lab Med* 1987;111:447–452.
195. House JM, Goodman ML, Gacek RR, et al. Chemodectomas of the nasopharynx. *Arch Otolaryngol* 1972;96:138–141.
196. Lack EE, Cubilla AL, Woodruff JM, et al. Paragangliomas of the head and neck region: a clinical study of 69 patients. *Cancer* 1977;39:397–409.
197. Kay S, Lees JK, Stout AP. Pituitary chromophobe tumors of the nasal cavity. *Cancer* 1950;3:695–704.
198. Rasmussen P, Lindholm J. Ectopic pituitary adenoma. *Clin Endocrinol* 1979;11:69–74.
199. Kammer H, George R. Cushing's disease in a patient with ectopic pituitary adenoma. *JAMA* 1981;246:2722–2741.
200. Davis JM, Weber A. Pituitary adenoma presenting as a sphenoid sinus lesion. *Ann Otol Rhinol Laryngol* 1980;89:483–484.
201. Gillespie CA, Walker JS, Burch WM, et al. Cushing's syndrome secondary to ectopic pituitary adenoma in the sphenoid sinus. *Otolaryngol Head Neck Surg* 1987;96:569–572.
202. Chessin H, Urdaneta N, Smith H, et al. Chromophobe adenoma manifesting as a nasopharyngeal mass. *Arch Otolaryngol* 1976;102:631–633.
203. Melchionna RH, Moore RA. The pharyngeal pituitary gland. *Am J Pathol* 1938;14:763–772.
204. McGrath P. Extrasellar adenohypophyseal tissue in the female. *Australas Radiol* 1970;14:241–247.
205. Podoshin L, Rolan L, Altman MM, et al. Pharyngeal craniopharyngioma. *J Laryngol Otol* 1970;84:93–99.
206. Prasad U, Kwi NK. Nasopharyngeal craniopharyngioma. *J Laryngol Otol* 1975;89:445–452.
207. Illum P, Elbrond O, Nehen AM. Surgical treatment of nasopharyngeal craniopharyngioma: radical removal by the transpalatal approach. *J Laryngol Otol* 1977;91:227–233.
208. Schafer DR, Thompson LD, Smith BC, et al. Primary ameloblastoma of the sinonasal tract: a clinicopathologic study of 24 cases. *Cancer* 1998;82:667–674.
209. Genut AA, Miranda FG, Garcia JH. Organized cerebral heterotopia in the ethmoid sinus: a case report. *J Neurol Sci* 1976;28:339–344.
210. Karma P, Rasanen O, Karja J. Nasal gliomas: a review and report of two cases. *Laryngoscope* 1977;87:1169–1179.
211. Kubo K, Garrett WS Jr., Musgrave RH. Nasal gliomas. *Plast Reconstr Surg* 1973;52:47–51.
212. Lampertico P, Ibanez ML. Nasal glioma (encephalochoristoma nasofrontalis). *Arch Otolaryngol* 1964;79:628–631.
213. Walker EA, Jr., Resler DR. Nasal glioma. *Laryngoscope* 1963;73:93–107.
214. Barnes L, Peel RL, Verbin RS. Tumors of the nervous system. In Barnes L, ed. *Surgical Pathology of the Head and Neck.* New York, NY: Marcel Dekker, 1985:659–724.
215. Mirra SS, Pearl GS, Hoffman JC, et al. Nasal "glioma" with prominent neuronal component: report of a case. *Arch Pathol Lab Med* 1981;105:540–541.
216. Bossen EH, Hudson WR. Oligodendroglioma arising in heterotopic brain tissue of the soft palate and nasopharynx. *Am J Surg Pathol* 1987;11:571–574.
217. Farr HW, Gray GF, Vrana M, et al. Extracranial meningioma. *J Surg Oncol* 1973;5:411–420.

218. Ho K-L. Primary meningioma of the nasal cavity and paranasal sinuses. *Cancer* 1980;46:1442–1447.
219. Perzin KH, Pushparaj N. Nonepithelial tumors of the nasal cavity, paranasal sinuses, and nasopharynx: a clinicopathologic study. XIII: Meningiomas. *Cancer* 1984;54:1860–1869.
220. Thompson LD, Gyure KA. Extracranial sinonasal tract meningiomas: a clinicopathologic study of 30 cases with review of the literature. *Am J Surg Pathol* 2000;24:640–650.
221. Winek RR, Scheithauer BW, Wick MR. Meningioma, meningeal hemangiopericytoma (angioblastic meningioma), peripheral hemangiopericytoma, and acoustic schwannoma: a comparative immunohistochemical study. *Am J Surg Pathol* 1989;13:251–261.
222. Mabry RL. Lymphoid pseudotumor of the nasopharynx and larynx. *J Laryngol Otol* 1967; 81:441–443.
223. Rimarenko S, Schwartz IS. Polypoid nasal pseudolymphoma. *Am J Clin Pathol* 1985;83: 507–509.
224. Saltzstein SL. Extranodal malignant lymphomas and pseudolymphomas. *Pathol Annu* 1969; 9:159–184.
225. Seide MJ, Cleary KR, van Tassel P, et al. Plasma cell granuloma of the nasal cavity treated by radiation therapy. *Cancer* 1991;67:929–932.
226. Fu Y-S, Perzin KH. Nonepithelial tumors of the nasal cavity, paranasal sinuses and nasopharynx: a clinicopathologic study. X. Malignant lymphomas. *Cancer* 1979;43:611–621.
227. Frierson HF, Jr., Mills SE, Innes DJ, Jr. Non-Hodgkin's lymphomas of the sinonasal region: histologic subtypes and their clinicopathologic features. *Am J Clin Pathol* 1984;81:721–727.
228. Cuadra-Garcia I, Proulx GM, Wu CL, et al. Sinonasal lymphoma: a clinicopathologic analysis of 58 cases from the Massachusetts General Hospital. *Am J Surg Pathol* 1999;23: 1356–1369.
229. Quraishi MS, Bessell EM, Clark D, et al. Non-Hodgkin's lymphoma of the sinonasal tract. *Laryngoscope* 2000;110:1489–1492.
230. Hanna E, Wanamaker J, Adelstein D, et al. Extranodal lymphomas of the head and neck. A 20-year experience. *Arch Otolaryngol Head Neck Surg* 1997;123:1318–1323.
231. Ferry JA, Sklar J, Zukerberg LR, et al. Nasal lymphoma: a clinicopathologic study with immunophenotypic and genotypic analysis. *Am J Surg Pathol* 1991;15:268–279.
232. Campo E, Cardesa A, Alos L, et al. Non-Hodgkin's lymphomas of the nasal cavity and paranasal sinuses: an immunohistochemical study. *Am J Clin Pathol* 1991;96:184–190.
233. Frierson HF, Jr., Innes DJ, Jr., Mills SE, et al. Immunophenotypic analysis of sinonasal non-Hodgkin's lymphomas. *Hum Pathol* 1989;20:636–642.
234. Chan JKC, Ng CS, Lau WH, et al. Most nasal/nasopharyngeal lymphomas are peripheral T-cell neoplasms. *Am J Surg Pathol* 1987;11:418–429.
235. Warnke RA, Gatter KC, Fallini B, et al. Diagnosis of human lymphoma with monoclonal antileukocyte antibodies. *N Engl J Med* 1983;309:1275–1281.
236. Kurtin PJ, Pinkus GS. Leukocyte common antigen: a diagnostic discriminant between hematopoietic and nonhematopoietic neoplasms in paraffin sections using monoclonal antibodies. Correlation with immunologic studies and ultrastructural localization. *Hum Pathol* 1985;16:353–365.
237. Lauder I, Holland D, Mason DY, et al. Identification of large cell undifferentiated tumors in lymph nodes using leukocyte common and keratin antibodies. *Histopathology* 1984;8: 259–272.
238. Sloane JP, Ormerod MG. Distribution of epithelial membrane antigen in normal and neoplastic tissues and its value in diagnostic tumor pathology. *Cancer* 1981;47:1786–1795.
239. Pinkus GS, Kurtin PJ. Epithelial membrane antigen: a diagnostic discriminant in surgical pathology. Immunohistochemical profile in epithelial, mesenchymal, and hematopoietic neoplasms using paraffin sections and monoclonal antibodies. *Hum Pathol* 1985;16: 929–940.
240. Taxy JB, Hidvegi DF, Battifora H. Nasopharyngeal carcinoma: antikeratin immunohistochemistry and electron microscopy. *Am J Clin Pathol* 1985;83:320–325.
241. Madri JA, Barwick KW. An immunohistochemical study of nasopharyngeal neoplasms using keratin antibodies: epithelial versus nonepithelial neoplasms. *Am J Surg Pathol* 1982; 6:143–149.
242. Zeigels-Weissman J, Nadji M, Penneys NS, et al. Prekeratin immunohistochemistry in the diagnosis of undifferentiated carcinoma of the nasopharyngeal type. *Arch Pathol Lab Med* 1984;108:588–589.
243. Shi S-R, Goodman ML, Bhan AK, et al. Immunohistochemical study of nasopharyngeal carcinoma using monoclonal keratin antibodies. *Am J Pathol* 1984;117:53–63.
244. Krasne DL, Warnke RA, Weiss LM. Malignant lymphoma presenting as pseudoepitheliomatous hyperplasia: a report of two cases. *Am J Surg Pathol* 1988;12:835–842.
245. Miller FR, Lavertu P, Wanamaker JR, et al. Plasmacytomas of the head and neck. *Otolaryngol Head Neck Surg* 1998;119:614–618.
246. Webb NE, Harrison EG, Masson JK, et al. Solitary extramedullary myeloma (plasmacytoma) of the upper part of the respiratory tract and oropharynx. *Cancer* 1962;15: 1142–1155.
247. Batsakis JG, Fries GT, Goldman RT, et al. Upper respiratory tract plasmacytoma. *Arch Otolaryngol* 1964;79:613–618.
248. Poole AG, Marchetta FC. Extramedullary plasmacytoma of the head and neck. *Cancer* 1968;22:14–21.
249. Kotner LM, Wang CC. Plasmacytoma of the upper air and food passages. *Cancer* 1972;30: 414–418.
250. Castro EB, Lewis JS, Strong EW. Plasmacytoma of paranasal sinuses and nasal cavity. *Arch Otolaryngol* 1973;97:326–329.
251. Fu Y-S, Perzin KH. Nonepithelial tumors of the nasal cavity, paranasal sinuses and nasopharynx: a clinicopathologic study. IX. Plasmacytomas. *Cancer* 1978;42:2399–2406.
252. Medini E, Rao Y, Levitt SH. Solitary extramedullary plasmacytoma of the upper respiratory and digestive tracts. *Cancer* 1980;45:2893–2896.
253. Kapadia SB, Desai U, Cheng VS. Extramedullary plasmacytoma of the head and neck: a clinicopathologic study of 20 cases. *Medicine* 1982;61:317–329.
254. Abrams RA, Wilson JF, Komorowski RA, et al. Esthesioneuroblastoma masquerading as extramedullary plasmacytoma. *Cancer* 1987;60:88–89.
255. Kassel SH, Echevarria RA, Guzzo FP. Midline malignant reticulosis (so-called lethal midline granuloma). *Cancer* 1969;23:920–935.
256. Katzenstein A-LA, Carrington CB, Liebow AA. Lymphomatoid granulomatosis: a clinicopathologic study of 152 cases. *Cancer* 1979;43:360–373.
257. Stamenkovic I, Toccanier M-F, Kapanci Y. Polymorphic reticulosis (lethal midline granuloma) and lymphomatoid granulomatosis: identical or distinct entities? *Virchows Arch A Pathol Anat Histopathol* 1981;390:81–91.
258. Medeiros LJ, Peiper SC, Elwood L, et al. Angiocentric immunoproliferative lesions: a molecular analysis of eight cases. *Hum Pathol* 1991;22:1150–1157.
259. Bender BL, Jaffe R. Immunoglobulin production in lymphomatoid granulomatosis and relation to other "benign" lymphoproliferative disorders. *Am J Clin Pathol* 1980;73:41–47.
260. Petras RE, Tubbs RR, Gephart GN, et al. T lymphocyte proliferation in lymphomatoid granulomatosis. *Cleve Clin Q* 1985;52:137–146.
261. Mittal K, Neri A, Feiner H, et al. Lymphomatoid granulomatosis in the acquired immunodeficiency syndrome: evidence of Epstein-Barr virus infection and B-cell clonal selection without *myc* rearrangement. *Cancer* 1990;65:1345–1349.
262. Ishii Y, Yamanaka N, Ogawa K, et al. Nasal T-cell lymphoma as a type of so-called "lethal midline granuloma." *Cancer* 1982;50:2336–2340.
263. Nichols PW, Koss M, Levine AM, et al. Lymphomatoid granulomatosis: a T-cell disorder? *Am J Med* 1982;72:467–471.
264. Bleiweiss IJ, Strauchen JA. Lymphomatoid granulomatosis of the lung: report of a case and gene rearrangement studies. *Hum Pathol* 1988;19:1109–1112.
265. Yamamura T, Asada K, Mike N, et al. Immunohistochemical and ultrastructural studies on disseminated skin lesions of midline malignant reticulosis. *Cancer* 1986;58:1281–1285.
266. Sordillo PP, Epremian B, Koziner B, et al. Lymphomatoid granulomatosis: an analysis of clinical and immunologic characteristics. *Cancer* 1982;49:2070–2076.
267. Veltri RW, Raich PC, McClung JE, et al. Lymphomatoid granulomatosis and Epstein-Barr virus. *Cancer* 1982;50:1513–1517.
268. Katzenstein A-LA, Peiper SC. Detection of Epstein-Barr virus genomes in lymphomatoid granulomatosis: analysis of 29 cases by polymerase chain reaction technique. *Mod Pathol* 1990;3:435–441.
269. Strickler JG, Meneses MF, Habermann TM, et al. Polymorphic reticulosis: a reappraisal. *Hum Pathol* 1994;25:659–665.
270. Tanaka Y, Sasaki Y, Kurozumi H, et al. Angiocentric immunoproliferative lesion associated with chronic active Epstein-Barr virus infection in an 11-year-old boy: clonotopic proliferation of Epstein-Barr virus-bearing CD4? T lymphocytes. *Am J Surg Pathol* 1994;18:623–631.
271. Medeiros LJ, Jaffe ES, Chen YY, et al. Localization of Epstein-Barr viral genomes in angiocentric immunoproliferative lesions. *Am J Surg Pathol* 1992;16:439–447.
272. Jaffe ES, Chan JKC, Su I-J, et al. Report of the workshop on nasal and related extranodal angiocentric T/natural killer cell lymphomas: definitions, differential diagnosis, and epidemiology. *Am J Surg Pathol* 1996;20:103–111.
273. Jaffe ES. Nasal and nasal-type NK/T cell lymphoma: a unique form of lymphoma associated with Epstein-Barr virus. *Histopathology* 1995;27:581–583.
274. Jaffe ES. Classification of natural killer (NK) cell and NK-like T-cell malignancies. *Blood* 1996;87:1207–1210.
275. Myers JL, Kurtin PJ, Katzenstein A-LA, et al. Lymphomatoid granulomatosis: evidence of immunophenotypic diversity and relationship to Epstein-Barr virus infection. *Am J Surg Pathol* 1995;19:1300–1312.
276. Nakamura S, Suchi T, Koshikawa T, et al. Clinicopathologic study of CD56 (NCAM)-positive angiocentric lymphoma occurring in sites other than the upper and lower respiratory tract. *Am J Surg Pathol* 1995;19:284–286.
277. Petrella T, Delfau-Larue M-H, Caillot D, et al. Nasopharyngeal lymphomas: further evidence for a natural killer cell origin. *Hum Pathol* 1996;27:827–833.
278. Pileri SA, Grogan TM, Harris NL, et al. Tumours of histiocytes and accessory dendritic cells: an immunohistochemical approach to classification from the International Lymphoma Study Group based on 61 cases. *Histopathology* 2002;41:1–29.
279. Chan JK, Tsang WY, Ng CS, et al. Follicular dendritic cell tumors of the oral cavity. *Am J Surg Pathol* 1994;18:148–157.
280. Gaertner EM, Tsokos M, Derringer GA, et al. Interdigitating dendritic cell sarcoma. A report of four cases and review of the literature. *Am J Clin Pathol* 2001;115:589–597.
281. Shia J, Chen W, Tang LH, et al. Extranodal follicular dendritic cell sarcoma: clinical, pathologic, and histogenetic characteristics of an underrecognized disease entity. *Virchows Arch* 2006;449:148–158.
282. Sternberg SS. Pathology of juvenile nasopharyngeal angiofibroma: a lesion of adolescent males. *Cancer* 1954;7:15–28.
283. Hubbard EM. Nasopharyngeal angiofibromas. *Arch Pathol* 1958;65:192–204.
284. Apostol JV, Frazell EL. Juvenile nasopharyngeal angiofibroma: a clinical study. *Cancer* 1965;18:869–878.
285. McGavran MH, Sessions DG, Dorfman RF, et al. Nasopharyngeal angiofibroma. *Arch Otolaryngol* 1969;90:68–78.
286. Neel HB, Whicker JH, Devine KD, et al. Juvenile angiofibroma: review of 120 cases. *Am J Surg* 1973;126:547–556.
287. Fu Y-S, Perzin KH. Non-epithelial tumors of the nasal cavity, paranasal sinuses, and nasopharynx: a clinicopathologic study. I. General features and vascular tumors. *Cancer* 1974; 33:1275–1288.
288. Lee DA, Rao BR, Meyer JS, et al. Hormonal receptor determination in juvenile nasopharyngeal angiofibromas. *Cancer* 1980;46:547–551.
289. Johns ME, MacLeod RM, Cantrell RW. Estrogen receptors in nasopharyngeal angiofibromas. *Laryngoscope* 1980;90:628–634.
290. Johnson S, Kloster JH, Schiff M. The action of hormones on juvenile nasopharyngeal angiofibroma. *Acta Otolaryngol* 1966;61:153–160.
291. Batsakis JG, Klopp CT, Newman W. Fibrosarcoma arising in a "juvenile" nasopharyngeal angiofibroma following extensive radiation therapy. *Am Surgeon* 1955;21:786–793.
292. Gown AM, Morihara J, Davie P, et al. Androgen receptor expression in angiofibromas of the nasopharynx. *Mod Pathol* 1993;6(Abstr):81A.

293. Spagnolo DV, Papadimitriou JM, Archer M. Postirradiation malignant fibrous histiocytoma arising in juvenile nasopharyngeal angiofibroma and producing alpha-1-antitrypsin. *Histopathology* 1984;8:339–352.
294. Chen KTK, Bauer FW. Sarcomatous transformation of nasopharyngeal angiofibroma. *Cancer* 1982;49:369–371.
295. Goepfert H, Cangir A, Lee Y-Y. Chemotherapy for aggressive juvenile nasopharyngeal angiofibroma. *Arch Otolaryngol* 1985;111:285–289.
296. Hormia M, Koskinen O. Metastasizing nasopharyngeal angiofibroma: a case report. *Arch Otolaryngol* 1969;89:523–526.
297. Gisselsson L, Lindgren M, Stenram U. Sarcomatous transformation of a juvenile, nasopharyngeal angiofibroma. *Acta Pathol Microbiol Scand* 1958;42:305–312.
298. Svoboda DJ, Kirchner F. Ultrastructure of nasopharyngeal angiofibromas. *Cancer* 1966; 19:1949–1962.
299. Taxy JB. Juvenile nasopharyngeal angiofibroma: an ultrastructural study. *Cancer* 1977;39: 1044–1054.
300. Topilko A, Zakrzewski A, Pichard E, et al. Ultrastructural cytochemistry of intranuclear dense granules in nasopharyngeal angiofibroma. *Ultrastruct Pathol* 1984;6:221–228.
301. Cooper PH, McAllister HA, Helwig EB. Intravenous pyogenic granuloma: a study of 18 cases. *Am J Surg Pathol* 1979;3:221–228.
302. Cooper PH, Mills SE. Subcutaneous granuloma pyogenicum: lobular capillary hemangioma. *Arch Dermatol* 1982;118:30–33.
303. Mills SE, Cooper PH, Fechner RE. Lobular capillary hemangioma: the underlying lesion of pyogenic granuloma. A study of 73 cases from the oral and nasal mucous membranes. *Am J Surg Pathol* 1980;4:471–479.
304. Nichols GE, Gaffey MJ, Mills SE, et al. Lobular capillary hemangioma: an immunohistochemical study including steroid hormone receptor status. *Am J Clin Pathol* 1992;97: 770–775.
305. Compagno J, Hyams VJ. Hemangiopericytoma-like intranasal tumors: a clinicopathologic study of 23 cases. *Am J Clin Pathol* 1976;66:672–683.
306. Eichhorn JH, Dickersin GR, Bhan AK, et al. Sinonasal hemangiopericytoma: a reassessment with electron microscopy, immunohistochemistry, and long-term follow-up. *Am J Surg Pathol* 1990;14:856–866.
307. Compagno J. Hemangiopericytoma-like tumors of the nasal cavity: a comparison with hemangiopericytoma of soft tissues. *Laryngoscope* 1978;88:460–469.
308. Thompson LD, Miettinen M, Wenig BM. Sinonasal-type hemangiopericytoma: a clinicopathologic and immunophenotypic analysis of 104 cases showing perivascular myoid differentiation. *Am J Surg Pathol* 2003;27:737–749.
309. Tse LL, Chan JK. Sinonasal haemangiopericytoma-like tumour: a sinonasal glomus tumour or a haemangiopericytoma? *Histopathology* 2002;40:510–517.
310. Thompson LDR, Fanburg-Smith JC, Wenig BM. Borderline and low malignant potential tunours of soft tissues. In Barnes L, Eveson JW, Reichart P, et al., eds. *Pathology and Genetics of Head and Neck Tumours.* Lyon, France: IARC Press; 2005:43–45.
311. el-Naggar AK, Batsakis JG, Garcia GM, et al. Sinonasal hemangiopericytomas. A clinicopathologic and DNA content study. *Arch Otolaryngol Head Neck Surg* 1992;118:134–137.
312. Potter AJ, Khatib G, Peppard SB. Intranasal glomus tumor. *Arch Otolaryngol* 1984;110: 755–756.
313. Bankaci M, Myers EN, Barnes L, et al. Angiosarcoma of the maxillary sinus: literature review and case report. *Head Neck Surg* 1979;1:274–280.
314. Allen PW. The fibromatoses: a clinicopathologic classification based on 140 cases. *Am J Surg Pathol* 1977;1:255–270, 305–321.
315. Masson JK, Soule EH. Desmoid tumors of the head and neck. *Am J Surg* 1966;112:615–622.
316. Fu Y-S, Perzin KH. Nonepithelial tumors of the nasal cavity, paranasal sinuses, and nasopharynx: a clinicopathologic study. VI. Fibrous tissue tumors (fibroma, fibromatosis, fibrosarcoma). *Cancer* 1976;37:2912–2928.
317. Conley J, Healey WV, Stout AP. Fibromatosis of the head and neck. *Am J Surg* 1966;112: 609–614.
318. Perzin KH, Panyu H, Wechter S. Nonepithelial tumors of the nasal cavity, paranasal sinuses and nasopharynx: a clinicopathologic study. XII. Schwann cell tumors (neurilemoma, neurofibroma, malignant schwannoma). *Cancer* 1982;50:2193–2202.
319. Zukerberg LR, Rosenberg AE, Randolph G, et al. Solitary fibrous tumor of the nasal cavity and paranasal sinuses. *Am J Surg Pathol* 1991;15:126–130.
320. Witkin GB, Rosai J. Solitary fibrous tumor of the upper respiratory tract: a report of six cases. *Am J Surg Pathol* 1991;15:842–848.
321. Gunhan O, Yildiz FR, Celasun B, et al. Solitary fibrous tumour arising from sublingual gland: report of a case. *J Laryngol Otol* 1994;108:998–1000.
322. Hanau CA, Miettinen M. Solitary fibrous tumor: histological and immunohistochemical spectrum of benign and malignant variants presenting at different sites. *Hum Pathol* 1995; 26:440–449.
323. Westra WH, Gerald WL, Rosai J. Solitary fibrous tumor: consistent CD34 immunoreactivity and occurrence in the orbit. *Am J Surg Pathol* 1994;18:992–998.
324. Rockley TJ, Liu KC. Fibrosarcoma of the nose and paranasal sinuses. *J Laryngol Otol* 1986; 100:1417–1420.
325. Nageris B, Elidan J, Sherman Y. Fibrosarcoma of the vocal fold: a late complication of radiotherapy. *J Laryngol Otol* 1994;108:993–994.
326. Lalwani AK, Jackler RK, Gutin PH. Lethal fibrosarcoma complicating radiation therapy for benign glomus jugulare tumor. *Am J Otol* 1993;14:398–402.
327. Perzin KH, Fu Y-S. Non-epithelial tumors of the nasal cavity, paranasal sinuses and nasopharynx: a clinicopathologic study. XI. Fibrous histiocytomas. *Cancer* 1980;45:2616–2626.
328. Bernstein KE, Lattes R. Nodular (pseudosarcomatous) fasciitis, a nonrecurrent lesion: clinicopathologic study of 134 cases. *Cancer* 1982;49:1668–1678.
329. Shimizu S, Hashimoto H, Enjoji M. Nodular fasciitis: an analysis of 250 cases. *Pathology* 1984;16:161–166.
330. Font RL, Zimmerman LE. Nodular fasciitis of the eye and adnexa: a report of ten cases. *Arch Ophthalmol* 1966;75:475–481.
331. Levitt JM, deVeer JA, Oguzhan MC. Orbital nodular fasciitis. *Arch Ophthalmol* 1969;81: 235–237.
332. Wold LE, Weiland LH. Tumefactive fibro-inflammatory lesions of the head and neck. *Am J Surg Pathol* 1983;7:477–482.
333. Fu Y-S, Perzin KH. Nonepithelial tumors of the nasal cavity, paranasal sinuses, and nasopharynx: a clinicopathologic study. IV. Smooth muscle tumors (leiomyoma, leiomyosarcoma). *Cancer* 1975;35:1300–1308.
334. Robitaille Y, Seemayer TA, El Deiry A. Peripheral nerve tumors involving paranasal sinuses: a case report and review of the literature. *Cancer* 1975;35:1254–1258.
335. Fu Y-S, Perzin KH. Non-epithelial tumors of the nasal cavity, paranasal sinuses, and nasopharynx: a clinicopathologic study. III. Cartilaginous tumors (chondroma, chondrosarcoma). *Cancer* 1974;34:453–463.
336. Fu Y-S, Perzin KH. Non-epithelial tumors of the nasal cavity, paranasal sinuses, and nasopharynx: a clinicopathologic study. VIII. Adipose tissue tumors (lipoma and liposarcoma). *Cancer* 1977;40:1314–1317.
337. Fu Y-S, Perzin KH. Nonepithelial tumors of the nasal cavity, paranasal sinuses, and nasopharynx: a clinicopathologic study. V. Skeletal muscle tumors (rhabdomyoma and rhabdomyosarcoma). *Cancer* 1976;37:364–376.
338. Moore DM, Berke GS. Synovial sarcoma of the head and neck. *Arch Otolaryngol Head Neck Surg* 1987;113:311–313.
339. Kuruvilla A, Wenig BM, Humphrey DM, et al. Leiomyosarcoma of the sinonasal tract: a clinicopathologic study of nine cases. *Arch Otolaryngol Head Neck Surg* 1990;116:1278–1286.
340. Sutow WW, Lindberg RD, Gehan EA, et al. Three-year relapse-free survival rates in childhood rhabdomyosarcoma of the head and neck: report from the Intergroup Rhabdomyosarcoma Study. *Cancer* 1982;49:2217–2221.
341. Nakhleh RE, Swanson PE, Dehner LP. Juvenile (embryonal and alveolar) rhabdomyosarcoma of the head and neck in adults: a clinical, pathologic, and immunohistochemical study of 12 cases. *Cancer* 1991;67:1019–1024.
342. Hawkins HK, Camacho-Velasquez JV. Rhabdomyosarcoma in children: correlation of form and prognosis in one institution's experience. *Am J Surg Pathol* 1987;11:531–542.
343. Tsokos M, Triche TJ. Immunocytochemical and ultrastructural study of primitive, "solid variant" rhabdomyosarcoma. *Lab Invest* 1986;54:65a.
344. Shimada H, Newton WA, Jr., Soule EH, et al. Pathology of fatal rhabdomyosarcoma: report from intergroup rhabdomyosarcoma study (IRS-I and IRS-II). *Cancer* 1987;59:459–465.
345. Harms D, Schmidt D, Treuner J. Soft-tissue sarcomas of childhood: a study of 262 cases including 169 cases of rhabdomyosarcoma. *Z Kinderchir* 1985;40:140–145.
346. Scupham R, Gilbert EF, Wilde J, et al. Immunohistochemical studies of rhabdomyosarcoma. *Arch Pathol Lab Med* 1986;110:818–821.
347. Tsokos M. The role of immunocytochemistry in the diagnosis of rhabdomyosarcoma. *Arch Pathol Lab Med* 1986;110:776–778.
348. Osborn M, Hill C, Altmannsberger M, et al. Monoclonal antibodies to titin in conjunction with antibodies to desmin separate rhabdomyosarcomas from other tumor types. *Lab Invest* 1986;55:101–108.
349. Eusebi V, Ceccarelli C, Gorza L, et al. Immunocytochemistry of rhabdomyosarcoma: the use of four different markers. *Am J Surg Pathol* 1986;10:293–299.
350. Cessna MH, Zhou H, Perkins SL, et al. Are myogenin and myoD1 expression specific for rhabdomysarcoma? A study of 150 cases, with emphasis on spindle cell mimics. *Am J Surg Pathol* 2001;25:1150–1157.
351. Folpe AL. MyoD1 and mygenin expression in human neoplasia: a review and update. *Adv Anat Pathol* 2002;9:198–203.
352. Eusebi V, Bondi A, Rosai J. Immunohistochemical localization of myoglobin in nonmuscular cells. *Am J Surg Pathol* 1984;8:51–55.
353. Gaiger AM, Soule EH, Newton WA. Pathology of rhabdomyosarcoma: experience of the intergroup rhabdomyosarcoma study, 1972–1978. In *Sarcomas of Soft Tissue and Bone in Childhood.* 1981;56:19–28 (National Cancer Institute Monograph).
354. Molenaar WM, Oosterhuis JW, Kamps WA. Cytologic "differentiation" in childhood rhabdomyosarcomas following polychemotherapy. *Hum Pathol* 1984;15:973–979.
355. Dickman PS, Triche TJ. Extraosseous Ewing's sarcoma versus primitive rhabdomyosarcoma: diagnostic criteria and clinical correlation. *Hum Pathol* 1986;17:881–893.
356. Heffner DK, Hyams VJ. Teratocarcinosarcoma (malignant teratoma?) of the nasal cavity and paranasal sinuses: a clinicopathologic study of 20 cases. *Cancer* 1984;53:2140–2154.
357. Meinecke R, Bauer F, Skouras J, et al. Blastomatous tumors of the respiratory tract. *Cancer* 1976;38:818–823.
358. Pai SA, Naresh KN, Masih K, et al. Teratocarcinosarcoma of the paranasal sinuses: a clinicopathologic and immunohistochemical study. *Hum Pathol* 1998;29:718–722.
359. DeMello DE, Archer CR, Blair JD. Ethmoidal fibro-osseous lesion in a child: diagnostic and therapeutic problems. *Am J Surg Pathol* 1980;4:595–601.
360. Fechner RE. Problematic lesions of the craniofacial bones. *Am J Surg Pathol* 1989;13(Suppl 1):17–30.
361. Barnes L, Kapadia SB. The biology and pathology of selected skull base tumors. *J Neurooncol* 1994;20:213–240.
362. Fu Y-S, Perzin KH. Non-epithelial tumors of the nasal cavity, paranasal sinuses and nasopharynx: a clinicopathologic study. II. Osseous and fibroosseous lesions including osteoma, fibrous dysplasia, ossifying fibroma, osteoblastoma, giant cell tumor, and osteosarcoma. *Cancer* 1974;33:1289–1305.
363. Wolfe JT III, Scheithauer BW, Dahlin DC. Giant-cell tumor of the sphenoid bone: review of ten cases. *J Neurosurg* 1983;59:322–327.
364. Upchurch KS, Simmon LS, Schiller AL. Giant cell reparative granuloma of Paget's disease of bone: a unique clinical entity. *Ann Intern Med* 1983;98:35–40.
365. Waldron CA, Shafer WG. The central giant cell reparative granuloma of the jaws: an analysis of 38 cases. *Am J Clin Pathol* 1966;45:437–447.
366. Sanerkin NG, Mott MG, Roylance J. An unusual intraosseous lesion with fibroblastic, osteoclastic, osteoblastic, aneurysmal and fibromyxoid elements: "solid" variant of aneurysmal bone cyst. *Cancer* 1983;51:2278–2286.

367. Fechner RE, Fitz-Hugh GS, Pope TL Jr. Extraordinary growth of giant cell reparative granuloma during pregnancy. *Arch Otolaryngol* 1984;110:116–119.

368. Struthers PJ, Shear M. Aneurysmal bone cyst of the jaws. I. Clinicopathologic features. *Int J Oral Surg* 1984;13:85–91.

369. Struthers PJ, Shear M. Aneurysmal bone cyst of the jaws. II. Pathogenesis. *Int J Oral Surg* 1984;13:92–100.

370. Margo CE, Ragsdale BD, Perman KI, et al. Psammomatoid (juvenile) ossifying fibroma of the orbit. *Ophthalmology* 1985;92:150–159.

371. Johnson LC, Yousefi M, Vinh TN, et al. Juvenile active ossifying fibroma: its nature, dynamics and origin. *Acta Otolaryngol (Stockh)* 1991;488(Suppl):1–40.

372. Slootweg PJ, Muller H. Juvenile ossifying fibroma: report of four cases. *J Craniomaxillofac Surg* 1990;18:125–129.

373. Slootweg PJ, Panders AK, Koopmans R, et al. Juvenile ossifying fibroma: an analysis of 33 cases with emphasis on histopathological aspects. *J Oral Pathol* 1994;23:385–388.

374. Waldron CA. Fibro-osseous lesions of the jaws. *J Oral Maxillofac Surg* 1993;51:828–835.

375. Voytek TM, Ro JY, Edeiken J, et al. Fibrous dysplasia and cemento-ossifying fibroma: a histologic spectrum. *Am J Surg Pathol* 1995;19:775–781.

376. Slootweg PJ, Muller H. Differential diagnosis of fibro-osseous jaw lesions: a histological investigation on 30 cases. *J Craniomaxillofac Surg* 1990;18:210–214.

377. Slootweg PJ, Panders AK, Nikkels PGJ. Psammomatoid ossifying fibroma of the paranasal sinuses: an extragnathic variant of cemento-ossifying fibroma. Report of three cases. *J Craniomaxillofac Surg* 1993;21:294–297.

378. Boysen ME, Olving JH, Vaten K, et al. Fibro-osseous lesions of the cranio-facial bones. *J Laryngol Otol* 1979;93:793–807.

379. Langdon JD, Rapidis AD, Patel MF. Ossifying fibroma: one disease or six? An analysis of 39 fibro-osseous lesions of the jaws. *Br J Oral Surg* 1976;14:1–11.

380. Shafer WG, Hine MK, Levy BM. *A Textbook of Oral Pathology.* 4th edition. Philadelphia, PA: WB Saunders, 1983:143.

381. Waldron CA, Giansanti JS. Benign fibro-osseous lesions of the jaws: a clinical-radiologic-histologic review of sixty-five cases. I. Fibrous dysplasia of the jaws. *Oral Surg* 1973;35:190–201.

382. Waldron CA, Giansanti JS. Benign fibro-osseous lesions of the jaws: a clinical-radiologic-histologic review of sixty-five cases. II. Benign fibro-osseous lesions of periodontal ligament origin. *Oral Surg* 1973;35:340–350.

383. Harris WH, Dudley HR, Barry RJ. The natural history of fibrous dysplasia: an orthopaedic, pathological, and roentgenographic study. *J Bone Joint Surg* 1962;44A:207–233.

384. Slootweg PJ. Maxillofacial fibro-osseous lesions: classification and differential diagnosis. *Semin Diagn Pathol* 1996;13:104–112.

385. Fu Y-S, Perzin KH. Non-epithelial tumors of the nasal cavity, paranasal sinuses and nasopharynx: a clinico-pathologic study. VII. Myxoma. *Cancer* 1977;39:195–203.

386. Barker BF. Odontogenic myxoma. *Semin Diagn Pathol* 1999;16:297–301.

387. Slootweg PJ, Wittkampf ARM. Myxoma of the jaws: an analysis of 15 cases. *J Maxillofac Surg* 1986;14:46–52.

388. Dahlin DC, Unni KK. *Bone Tumors: General Aspects and Data on 8,542 Cases.* 4th edition. Springfield, IL: Charles C. Thomas, 1986:502.

389. Dahlin DC, Unni KK. *Bone Tumors: General Aspects and Data on 8,542 Cases.* 4th edition. Springfield, IL: Charles C. Thomas, 1986:84.

390. Clark JL, Unni KK, Dahlin DC, et al. Osteosarcoma of the jaw. *Cancer* 1983;51:2311–2316.

391. Huvos AG, Butler A, Bretsky SS. Osteogenic sarcoma associated with Paget's disease of bone: a clinicopathologic study of 65 patients. *Cancer* 1983;52:1489–1495.

392. Huvos AG, Woodard HQ, Cahan WG, et al. Postradiation osteogenic sarcoma of bone and soft tissues: a clinicopathologic study of 66 patients. *Cancer* 1985;55:1244–1255.

393. Nora FE, Unni KK, Pritchard DJ, et al. Osteosarcoma of the extragnathic craniofacial bones. *Mayo Clin Proc* 1983;58:268–272.

394. Huvos AG, Rosen G, Dabska M, et al. Mesenchymal chondrosarcoma: a clinicopathologic analysis of 35 patients with emphasis on treatment. *Cancer* 1983;51:1230–1237.

395. Graudal N. Desmoplastic fibroma of bone: case report and literature review. *Acta Orthop Scand* 1984;55:215–219.

396. Al-Dewachi AS, Al-Naib N, Sangal BC. Benign chondroblastoma of the maxilla: a case report and review of chondroblastomas in cranial bones. *Br J Oral Surg* 1980;18:150–156.

397. Har-El G, Levy R, Avidor I, et al. Haemangioma of the zygoma presenting as a tumour in the maxillary sinus. *J Maxillofac Surg* 1987;14:161–164.

398. Ferlito A. Primary Ewing's sarcoma of the maxilla: a clinicopathological study of four cases. *J Laryngol Otol* 1978;92:1007–1024.

399. Marks MP, Marks SC, Segall HD, et al. Case report 420: parosteal osteosarcoma. *Skeletal Radiol* 1987;16:246–251.

400. Pope TL Jr., Fechner RE, Keats TE. Case report 367: hemangioma of nasal bone. *Skeletal Radiol* 1986;15:327–329.

401. Waldron CA. Odontogenic tumors and selected jaw cysts. In Gnepp DR, ed. *Pathology of the Head and Neck.* New York, NY: Churchill Livingstone, 1988:431–433.

402. Perzin KH, Pushparaj N. Nonepithelial tumors of the nasal cavity, paranasal sinuses, and nasopharynx: a clinicopathologic study. XIV. Chordomas. *Cancer* 1986;57:784–796.

403. Salisbury JR, Isaacson PG. Demonstration of cytokeratin and an epithelial membrane antigen in chordomas and human fetal notochord. *Am J Surg Pathol* 1985;9:791–797.

404. Meis JM, Giraldo AA. Chordoma: an immunohistochemical study of 20 cases. *Arch Pathol Lab Med* 1988;112:553–556.

405. Heffelfinger MJ, Dahlin DC, MacCarty CS, et al. Chordomas and cartilaginous tumors of the skull base. *Cancer* 1973;32:410–420.

406. Brooks JJ, LiVolsi VA, Trojanowski JQ. Does chordoid chordoma exist? *Acta Neuropathol (Berl)* 1987;72:229–235.

407. Mitchell A, Scheithauer BW, Unni KK, et al. Chordoma and chondroid neoplasms of the spheno-occiput: an immunohistochemical study of 41 cases with prognostic and nosologic implications. *Cancer* 1993;72:2943–2949.

408. Jeffrey PB, Biava CG, Davis RL. Chondroid chordoma: a hyalinized chordoma without cartilaginous differentiation. *Am J Clin Pathol* 1995;103:271–279.

409. Wojno KJ, Hruban RH, Garin-Chesa P, et al. Chondroid chordomas and low-grade chondrosarcomas of the craniospinal axis: an immunohistochemical analysis of 17 cases. *Am J Surg Pathol* 1992;16:1144–1152.

410. Miettinen M, Karaharju E, Jarvinen H. Chordoma with a massive spindle-cell sarcomatous transformation: a light- and electron-microscopic and immunohistological study. *Am J Surg Pathol* 1987;11:563–570.

411. Meis JM, Raymond AK, Evans HL, et al. "Dedifferentiated" chordoma: a clinicopathologic and immunohistochemical study of three cases. *Am J Surg Pathol* 1987;11:516–525.

412. Hruban RH, Traganos F, Reuter VE, et al. Chordomas with malignant spindle cell components: a DNA flow cytometric and immunohistochemical study with histogenetic implications. *Am J Pathol* 1990;137:435–447.

CHAPTER

22

Edward B. Stelow

The Larynx

ANATOMY AND HISTOLOGY

The larynx lies between the hypopharynx and the trachea. For the purposes of discussion, it is generally subdivided based on relative location to the glottis into the supraglottic, glottic, and subglottic larynx (1–4). The true vocal cords and anterior commissure comprise the glottis. The supraglottic larynx is then defined as larynx above the true cords and includes the epiglottis, the false cords (ventricular bands), the aryepiglottic folds, and the arytenoid cartilages. The subglottic larynx is defined as the larynx below the true cords, ending at the trachea (usually defined as the inferior edge of the cricoid cartilage).

The epithelium lining the larynx varies throughout life and from patient to patient. The newborn larynx is lined almost completely by a columnar ciliated epithelium with occasional mucinous cells except over the true cords, where it is lined by a nonkeratinized squamous epithelium (5). Patchy nonkeratinized squamous epithelium is often present in adults throughout their larynges, frequently covering the posterior portion of the epiglottis and even portions of the subglottis (Fig. 22.1) (1). The larynges of smokers may be entirely covered by squamous epithelium. A stratified, transitional-type epithelium is sometimes seen between areas of squamous metaplasia and columnar epithelium that may be sometimes confused with dysplasia. Numerous seromucinous glands are present immediately beneath the epithelium, except in the true cord where they are either greatly diminished in number or not seen at all (Fig. 22.2) (6). These glands are sometimes seen deep within laryngeal skeletal muscle and extend through the elastic cartilage of the epiglottis through its numerous fenestrations.

The lamina propria of the larynx is composed of a loose stromal tissue with numerous small vessels, lymphatic channels, and nerves. The vocal cord is an exception, and although some small capillaries are seen here, few, if any, lymphatic channels can be found (1). A few scattered inflammatory cells, including mast cells, are sometimes seen. Adipose tissue is intermingled with the lamina propria stroma and the skeletal muscle of the larynx. Two pairs of paraganglia are normally present within the larynx (7). The superior paraganglia are supraglottic and located within the false cords, whereas the inferior paraganglia are usually found near the cricoid cartilage.

The laryngeal framework is then comprised of the laryngeal cartilages, ligaments, and intrinsic and extrinsic muscles (1). The cartilages include the thyroid cartilage, a shield-shaped structure that forms most of the anterior surface of the larynx; the cricoid cartilage, the only complete ring of cartilage in the tracheobronchial tract that forms most of the posterior support of the larynx; the paired arytenoid cartilages, the mobile cartilages that articulate with the cricoid cartilage allowing for phon-

ation; and the epiglottis. The epiglottis is elastic cartilage, whereas the others are hyaline cartilages that ossify as individuals grow older.

The most prominent ligament is the vocal cord ligament, which runs just over the intrinsic muscle of the true cord (the thyroarytenoid muscle) and connects the thyroid and arytenoid cartilages. It appears as a white band by laryngoscopy and can frequently be seen in biopsies of the vocal cords lying immediately beneath the sparsely vascular submucosal stromal tissue (Reinke space). Other dense ligaments anchor the thyroid and cricoid cartilages together and tether the arytenoids to the cri-

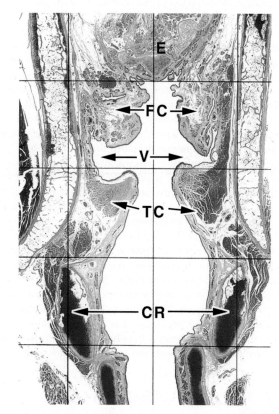

Figure 22.1. A mid larynx coronal section of a normal larynx in an adult male (grid: 1 cm). The upper edge of the cricoid cartilage lies 1 cm below the true vocal cords at the mid larynx. The epiglottic epithelium is stratified and squamous. The epithelium in the false cords is ciliated columnar, while the epithelium in the true cords is stratified squamous. The epithelium of the upper half is ciliated columnar, and the epithelium of the lower half is stratified squamous. Abbreviations: *E*, epiglottis; *FC*, false cords; *TC*, true cords; *V*, ventricle.

This chapter was originally authored by Drs. Kirchner and Carter. It has been an honor to update it.

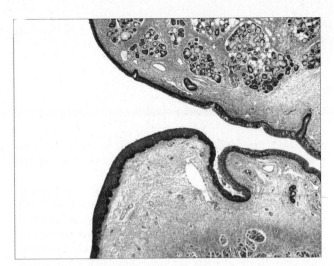

Figure 22.2. The false (upper) and true (lower) vocal cords. The true vocal cords are covered by a metaplastic squamous epithelium and lack subepithelial seromucinous glands.

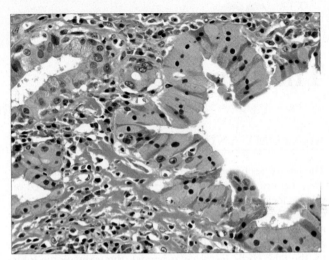

Figure 22.3. Oncocytic metaplasia can involve the laryngeal seromucinous glands and ducts. This does not imply neoplasia.

coid cartilage. Between the various cartilages, joint spaces lined by synovium are present.

The muscles of the larynx may be either extrinsic, those connecting the larynx to other structures, or intrinsic. Extrinsic muscles include the omohyoid and sternohyoid muscles (the hyoid bone, although not actually a portion of the larynx, is connected to it by ligaments) and the sternothyroid and thyrohyoid muscles. Intrinsic muscles include the cricothyroid, posterior and lateral cricoarytenoids, and the thyroarytenoids. The extrinsic muscles of the larynx help to move it primarily during swallowing, whereas the intrinsic muscles function primarily for vocalization.

The superior and inferior laryngeal arteries supply the larynx (1). The superior laryngeal artery and cricothyroid arteries are branches of the superior thyroid artery, which arises from the external carotid. The inferior laryngeal artery is a branch of the inferior thyroid artery, which arises from the thyrocervical trunk of the subclavian artery. The arteries are accompanied by veins, the superior and inferior laryngeal veins, which drain into the superior and inferior thyroid veins, respectively. The lymphatic system then drains along the vascular system of the larynx, with the supraglottic larynx draining superiorly and the subglottic larynx draining inferiorly. The superior laryngeal lymphatic system then empties into jugulodigastric and midjugular nodes, whereas the inferior laryngeal lymphatic system empties into the pretracheal, paratracheal, and inferior jugular nodes.

NONNEOPLASTIC LESIONS OF THE LARYNX

The larynx is most often biopsied because of suspicion of malignancy. Many biopsies will be diagnosed as conventional squamous cell carcinomas; however, many nonneoplastic pathologies also involve the larynx.

METAPLASIA AND HYPERPLASIA

Several metaplastic lesions occur within the larynx that clinically mimic malignancy. Necrotizing sialometaplasia is a metaplastic condition of the seromucinous glands that may develop sponta-

neously or secondary to injury, often iatrogenic (8–10). Characteristically, the seromucinous glands show a mixture of necrosis and squamous metaplasia. Cytologic atypia is sometimes present, especially in lesions developing after radiation therapy. Unlike squamous cell carcinoma, necrotizing sialometaplasia usually retains a lobular architecture, and admixed normal seromucinous glands are usually present. Chondroid metaplasia of the vocal cord is common, usually affecting the mid or posterior portions of the cord (11,12). The lesions are typically surrounded by dense elastic tissue that blends into the surrounding stroma and do not have the lobular growth pattern typical of chondroid neoplasms. Oncocytic metaplasia of the seromucinous glands is also common and does not imply salivary gland–type neoplasia (Fig. 22.3) (13,14). It is often seen with nonneoplastic laryngeal cysts (discussed later).

Pseudoepitheliomatous hyperplasia is a reactive hyperplasia of the squamous epithelium that can occur throughout the body (15). It may be associated with wide variety of neoplastic or inflammatory conditions but is especially noted with granular cell tumors (16,17). Histologically, it is characterized by downgrowths of the squamous epithelium into the underlying stroma, generally with quite elongated and jagged rete. Although some mild architectural and cytologic disturbance may be present with focal abrupt keratinization and mild cytologic atypia, individual cell dyskeratosis and marked cytologic atypia should not be seen.

CONTACT ULCER

Contact ulcer or laryngeal granuloma is a relatively common lesion that typically involves the posterior portion of one or both sides of the glottis (18–23). Most lesions are traumatic and develop secondary to many causes including, but not limited to, endotracheal intubation, acid reflux (peptic contact ulcer), and vocal cord abuse related to shouting, coughing, and so on. Patients tend to be older than 30 years of age, and most are men. They present with hoarseness, low-pitched voices, frequent coughing, and even severe pain. The posterior vocal cords are usually ulcerated; however, some lesions can have a marked nodular or polypoid appearance simulating neoplasia. Although the epithelium is frequently ulcerated and covered

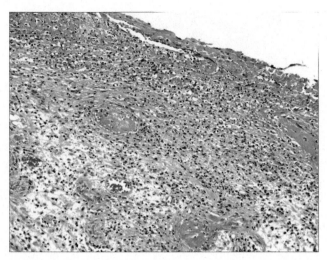

Figure 22.4. This typical contact ulcer is composed of granulation tissue covered by a fibrinous exudate. True lobular capillary hemangiomas of the larynx are rare or nonexistent.

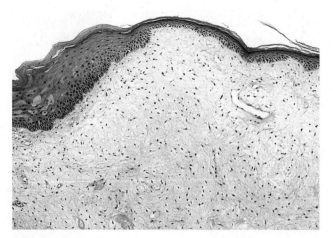

Figure 22.5. Vocal cord polyp. This true cord lesion has a polypoid appearance similar to that seen in Figure 22.6, but the thin-walled dilated vessels are less prominent. The submucosa is edematous and myxoid.

with a fibrinous exudate, lesions can be covered by a proliferative epithelium that may resemble pseudoepitheliomatous hyperplasia. Abundant granulation tissue is seen either at the ulcer site or immediately beneath the squamous epithelium and comprises the bulk of these lesions (Fig. 22.4). Occasional atypical stromal cells are sometimes seen; however, stromal mitotic figures are rare.

VOCAL CORD POLYPS AND NODULES

Vocal cord polyps or singer's nodules occur with equal frequency in men and women and can be found at any age (some have noted the lesions to be more common in men) (24–26). The patients present with hoarseness frequently after abusing their voices (overly enthusiastic bowlers appear to have been especially at risk). The lesions are usually unilateral, located on the anterior third of the vocal cord, and less than 5 mm in size. Histologically, the overlying squamous epithelium is most often intact and is sometimes hyperplastic or atrophic. The underlying stroma is paucicellular because of edema or, less commonly, fibrin deposition. Rarely the stroma may appear hyaline or myxoid (Fig. 22.5). Dilated vessels are frequently seen with a mild amount of chronic inflammation and hemosiderin-laden macrophages (Fig. 22.6). Occasional cases have been noted to have atypical stromal cells.

Vocal cord nodules are similar histologically to vocal cord polyps; however, they tend to be bilateral and occur slightly more posteriorly at the border of the anterior and middle third of the vocal cord (24). Reinke edema may be either unilateral or bilateral and usually is described as a sessile swelling. Both lesions share the histologic features typical of vocal cord polyps.

NONNEOPLASTIC CYSTS

Nonneoplastic cysts of the larynx include laryngoceles, saccular cysts, and ductal cysts (27–30). Although laryngoceles and saccular cysts have a similar histology, they occur in slightly different clinical situations. Laryngoceles are cystic dilatations of the saccule of Morgani, communicate with the larynx, and are air-filled. Those that are "internal" are limited to the larynx. These

extend from the saccule posterosuperiorly into the area of the false cord and aryepiglottic fold. "External" laryngoceles extend through the opening in the thyrohyoid membrane into the soft tissues of the neck. Laryngoceles are less common than saccular cysts and develop in either sex at any age. Patients present with hoarseness or cough and, when the lesion extends into the neck, a mass. Histologically, laryngoceles are lined by a columnar, ciliated epithelium and may be surrounded by chronic inflammation. Focally, the epithelium can appear more oncocytic (Fig. 22.7).

Saccular cysts also occur at the laryngeal saccule; however, they do not communicate with the larynx and are filled with mucin (28,29). Saccular cysts are either lateral and extend posterosuperiorly into the false cord and aeroepiglottic fold or even through the thyrohyoid membrane or are anterior and extend medially and posteriorly and thus protrude into the laryngeal lumen. Like laryngoceles, saccular cysts can occur at any age and may even be congenital. The cysts are generally lined by a ciliated, columnar epithelium that may have squamous or oncocytic metaplasia.

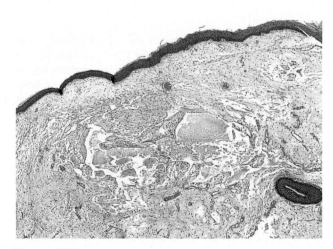

Figure 22.6. Vocal cord polyp. The keratinizing squamous epithelium of the true cord overlies a highly vascular submucosal mass.

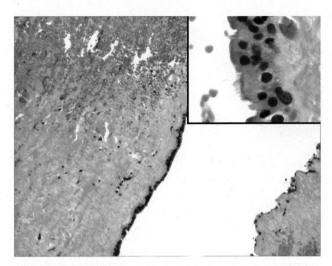

Figure 22.7. This laryngocele lined by a single layer of metaplastic oncocytic epithelium (*inset*) with underlying chronically inflamed, fibrous tissue.

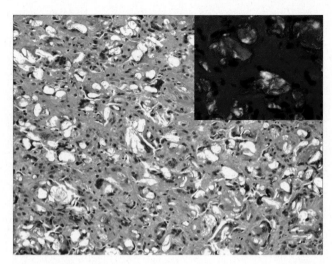

Figure 22.8. "Teflonoma." This laryngeal mass was composed of numerous foreign body–type giant cells, many of which contained foreign, polarizable material (*inset*).

Ductal cysts occur throughout the larynx and are thought to result from the retention of mucus within the ducts of the submucosal seromucinous glands (28,30). These cysts are much more common than saccular cysts and are lined by a columnar or cuboidal mucinous epithelium that can have squamous or oncocytic metaplasia. Because these frequently involve the supraglottic larynx, they are occasionally associated with tonsillar tissue.

FOREIGN BODY REACTION

Foreign body reactions within the larynx are most often iatrogenic (22,31–34). The most extensively studied reaction is that secondary to Teflon injection used to restore glottic competence. A resultant foreign body reaction may form a mass that bulges into the larynx. Histologically, clusters and sheets of multinucleated foreign body–type giant cells containing birefringent clear material are present with intermixed chronic inflammation and fibrosis (Fig. 22.8). Other material, including silicone, Gore-Tex, and titanium, may be used for vocal cord medialization and can result in similar changes.

SARCOIDOSIS

Between 1% and 5% of patients with sarcoidosis will have symptomatic involvement of their larynges (35–37). Clinically, the supraglottic larynx is most frequently affected, and the lesions may appear edematous, granular, or even nodular. The histologic features are classic for sarcoid with numerous noncaseating granulomata with occasional Schaumann or asteroid bodies (Fig. 22.9).

AUTOIMMUNE DISEASE

Systemic autoimmune disease such as rheumatoid arthritis and systemic lupus erythematosus can involve larynx, as can autoimmune disease that primarily affects mucosa and skin. Although involvement of the larynx usually only occurs in well-developed disease, it can sometimes represent the initial presentation of the disease. Because such cases are rare, other disease is usually suspected clinically.

Up to one-quarter of patients with rheumatoid arthritis have involvement of the larynx, and a characteristic synovitis can be demonstrated in biopsy specimens of the cricothyroid and cricoarytenoid joints (38). Rheumatoid nodules may involve the larynx, and it is these lesions that are most likely to be sampled by biopsy (39). These have the typical appearance of necrobiotic collagen nodules with central fibrinoid necrosis surrounded by palisading histiocytes with some lymphocytes and occasional multinucleated giant cells.

Wegener granulomatosis involves the upper or lower respiratory tract, and laryngeal disease occurs in up to 25% of patients affected (22,37,40,41). Here, it may progress to subglottic stenosis. The histologic features are similar to those seen elsewhere. Although necrosis, vasculitis, and granulomata are considered diagnostic of the disease, the three are seldom seen together in biopsy specimens. In fact, many cases will show only nonspecific acute and chronic inflammation.

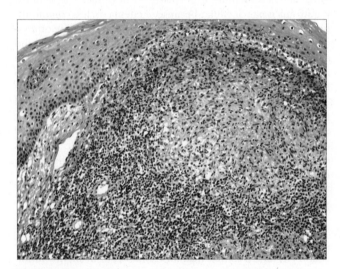

Figure 22.9. Sarcoidosis can sometimes present in the larynx. Here, biopsies will show noncaseating granulomatous inflammation as they do elsewhere.

Relapsing polychondritis is a rheumatic disease characterized by episodic and progressive inflammation of cartilage (42,43). It may involve multiple structures throughout the body but most frequently affects the external ear, joints, eye, respiratory tract, nose, and inner ear. Involvement of laryngeal cartilages and the epiglottis can lead to severe airway compromise as the cartilaginous support of the airway fails. The diagnosis of relapsing polychondritis is generally based on clinical criteria; however, histologic findings are also often a requirement. Histologically, the cartilage usually shows a loss of basophilia or metachromasia with perichondrial acute and chronic inflammation. Cartilage destruction and its replacement by fibrous tissue are also seen.

Several other autoimmune diseases affect the larynx. Systemic lupus erythematosus can be associated with laryngeal rheumatoid nodules (44). Diffuse acute and chronic inflammation may also be seen with hematoxylin bodies and lupus erythematosus (LE) cells, and although less common, a vasculitis with fibrinoid necrosis may also be seen. Sjögren syndrome may also involve the larynx and, as with lupus, can be associated with rheumatoid nodules (45,46). The disease may also be associated with more conventional-appearing vocal cord polyps possibly secondary to a lack of secretions. An intense infiltrate composed of lymphocytes and plasma cells can also be seen with the disease. Bullous pemphigoid and pemphigus vulgaris may both involve the larynx (47,48). The histologic features are similar to those seen elsewhere. Finally, Crohn disease rarely involves the upper aerodigestive tract and larynx (49). It is histologically characterized by nonspecific chronic inflammation; rarely, noncaseating granulomata may be seen.

DEPOSITION AND OTHER

Patients with long-term hyperuricemia eventually develop soft tissue deposits of crystallized uric acid (Gout). Rarely, these have been reported in the larynx (50–52). Patients have typically complained of hoarseness and dysphagia and are noted clinically to have mass lesions, often involving the cords, that limit their mobility. Histologically, pseudoepitheliomatous hyperplasia may be present overlying deposits of an amorphous negatively birefringent crystalline material that is surrounded by a foreign body–type reaction.

Amyloid deposition within the larynx may be localized or secondary to systemic disease (53–58). In the upper aerodigestive tract, amyloid deposits are sometimes seen with extramedullary plasmacytomas (59). Patients vary widely in age, with the mean age at presentation in the fourth or fifth decades of life. They typically present with progressive hoarseness. The lesions are usually described as supraglottic or transglottic and range from firm, elevated, smooth lesions to polypoid mass-like lesions that have a tan-yellow to red-grey cut surface. Histologically, these lesions characteristically have abundant amorphous, eosinophilic material deposited extracellularly within the lamina propria; prominent periglandular or perivascular deposition is sometimes seen. Scattered lymphocytes and plasma cells are frequently noted with occasional macrophages and rare giant cells. Congo red or methyl violet histochemical staining can be used to confirm the diagnosis of typically light chain amyloid. Light chain restriction can sometimes be demonstrated in the plasma cell population and predicts recurrent disease. The diagnosis should obviously instigate further workup for systemic causes of amyloid deposition.

Eosinophilic angiocentric fibrosis can involve the larynx, and rare cases have been reported to cause breathing difficulties (60). Like the cases in the nasal cavities or paranasal sinuses, these lesions have abundant fibrosis that appears to wrap around small blood vessels. Numerous eosinophils are seen with occasional lymphocytes.

The larynx may be involved by tracheopathia osteoplastica, a bizarre condition that most commonly affects men over the age of 50 years (61,62). Patients may present with hemoptysis, cough, hoarseness, or wheezing. The mucosa will appear cobblestone as hard, irregular nodules project into the laryngeal and tracheal lumina. Histologically, islands of hyaline cartilage and lamellar bone are present immediately beneath a metaplastic squamous epithelium.

Subglottic laryngeal stenosis is most often acquired; however, occasional cases may be congenital (63–65). Causes include trauma, prolonged intubation, burns, surgery, radiotherapy, infection, autoimmune disease, neoplasia, sarcoid, amyloidosis, and, possibly, gastroesophageal reflux. Patients usually have difficulty breathing, and children may be noted to have feeding abnormalities or abnormal crying. The larynx will appear markedly narrowed, sometimes by an apparent mass lesion. Histologically, sections usually show a nonspecific fibrosis with dense eosinophilic collagen, fibroblasts, and variable chronic inflammatory infiltrate. Clinical history may be helpful for determining the etiology of the disease.

Hamartomas of the larynx are extremely rare (66). They appear somewhat reminiscent of respiratory epithelial adenomatous hamartomas of the nasal cavity with a disorganized proliferation of respiratory epithelium, seromucinous glands, smooth muscle, and cartilage.

INFECTIOUS DISEASE

The larynx may be infected by a great host of organisms that more commonly involve the lungs or sinonasal area. Many of these entities present as mass lesions, and an infectious etiology is often unsuspected. Pathologists, however, should be well aware of these lesions because the correct diagnosis can spare a patient unnecessary treatment.

Mycobacterial Infections

Since the advent of effective antituberculosis treatments, laryngeal involvement has only seldom been reported, and when reported, it has been described as a clinical and gross mimic of laryngeal carcinoma (37,67–70). Laryngeal disease shares the histologic features of tuberculosis found elsewhere, with caseating granulomatous inflammation and Langhans giant cells. Histochemical staining for acid-fast bacilli can sometimes be helpful.

The larynx is the second most common site in the head and neck after the sinonasal area to be involved by leprosy (37). Laryngeal leprosy presents with painless ulcerated and nodular lesions located supraglottically that later progress to involve the glottis. Histologically, the process is similar to that noted in the nasal area and is usually composed of a mixture of chronic inflammatory cells and large, foamy macrophages. *Mycobacterium leprae* (Hansen bacillus) may be identified by histochemical staining for acid-fast bacilli.

Fungal Infections

Fungal infections of the larynx are uncommon, are frequently associated with widespread disease, and are most often found in immunocompromised patients. Laryngeal *histoplasmosis* may present as either multiple nodular or ulcerated lesions of the vocal cords (37,71). A mixture of acute and chronic inflammation is usually present with numerous large macrophages with abundant granular cytoplasm with or without well-formed granulomata. The overlying epithelium is often ulcerated; however, marked pseudoepitheliomatous hyperplasia may be present and should not be confused with squamous cell carcinoma. Although the organisms can frequently be seen on routine, hematoxylin and eosin (H&E)–stained material, silver or periodic acid-Schiff (PAS) staining also can be used to highlight their presence.

Patients with laryngeal blastomycosis typically present with hoarseness, with or without coexistent pulmonary or cutaneous lesions (37,72,73). It is typically described as erythematous, irregular, and granular lesions that may also appear verrucoid. Histologically, these lesions are characterized by pseudoepitheliomatous hyperplasia with mixed acute and chronic inflammation, Langhans giant cells, intraepithelial microabscesses, and granulomata, some of which may be suppurative. The causative organism, *Blastomyces dermatitidis*, can usually be identified with H&E-stained material or with silver or PAS stain.

Other fungal organisms may also involve the larynx, and infections secondary to *Coccidioides immitis*, *Cryptococcus neoformans*, *Candida albicans*, *Aspergillus* species, *Rhinosporidium seeberi*, and *Paracoccidioides* have been reported (74–80). Each of these may be seen in immunocompromised patients with or without more widespread disease. Occasionally, they may present in apparently immunocompetent patients without evidence of disease elsewhere. Patients typically present with hoarseness and have granular and sometimes exophytic lesions involving the larynx. As with other fungal infections, pseudoepitheliomatous hyperplasia is often present. A mixed inflammatory infiltrate is typically seen that can involve the epithelium. Fungal organisms may be identified on routine and special stains (Fig. 22.10). A mucicarmine stain can be used to highlight the capsule of *Cryptococcus neoformans*.

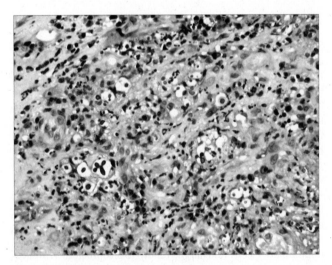

Figure 22.10. A periodic acid-Schiff stain demonstrates numerous yeasts in this case of laryngeal *Cryptococcus*.

Bacterial Infections

Bacterial infection of the supraglottic larynx and hypopharynx is now rare thanks to vaccinations for *Haemophilus influenzae* and *Corynebacterium diphtheriae* (81,82). Histologically, *Haemophilus influenzae* infection will show abundant acute inflammation. Patients with diphtheria have ulceration of the oral cavity, pharynx, and larynx with pseudomembrane formation. Histologically, the pseudomembranes contain fibrin, neutrophils, cell debris, and bacteria, whereas the underlying stromal tissues are edematous with acute inflammation.

Secondary and tertiary syphilis rarely involves the larynx (37,75). Histologically, secondary syphilis is characterized by a thinned epithelium or epithelial hyperplasia (condyloma latum) with a dense lymphoplasmacytic infiltrate, sometimes with granulomas. Tertiary syphilis is characterized by gummas, which are destructive and painless necrotic lesions. Histologically, these are characterized by necrotizing, granulomatous inflammation. A lymphoplasmacytic vasculitis may be noted in both secondary and tertiary forms of disease. Spirochetes may be identified in earlier lesions with silver stains (Warthin-Starry, Dieterle, etc.).

The larynx is rarely involved by rhinoscleroma secondary to infection by *Klebsiella rhinoscleromatis* (83). Patients usually also have sinonasal disease; however, isolated laryngeal infection has been reported. The histologic features are similar to those of the sinonasal area. Rare cases of laryngeal infection secondary to *Actinomyces* have been reported (84). Histologically, these lesions characteristically have sulfur granules (basophilic clusters of bacteria with a peripheral, more eosinophilic zone of radiating filaments) surrounded by acute inflammation and granulation tissue.

SQUAMOUS PAPILLOMA

Squamous papillomas of the larynx are warty growths that are categorized according to their number (solitary or multiple) and the age of the patient affected (juvenile or adult) (85–95). Most laryngeal papillomatosis occurs in younger patients. These lesions usually are located in the region of the true vocal cords; however, they may be found throughout the larynx and throughout the oropharynx, trachea, and even lung. They often recur after resection and may cause obstruction. Rarely, patients with long-term disease develop well-differentiated squamous cell carcinomas, often without other risk factors for laryngeal or pulmonary squamous cell carcinoma (96,97). Some have developed in patients who received radiation therapy for their disease. Most juvenile lesions and many of the adult lesions are etiologically related to infection of the mucosa with human papillomavirus (HPV) types 6 and 11, although some have been associated with HPV types 16 or 18 (86,98). Indeed, rather limited evidence has been used to claim that patients with lesions associated with HPV-16 or -18 are at higher risk for developing subsequent malignancy (99). In cases of juvenile papillomatosis, it is thought that infection occurs at birth, whereas with adults, it is believed that the infection may occur at a later age.

Grossly, the lesions are variably sized but are usually smaller than 1 cm in greatest dimension. Histologically, they are characterized by a branched fibrovascular core covered with maturing

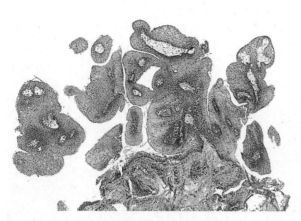

Figure 22.11. Numerous fragments of papilloma from a 4-year-old child; they are characteristically composed of a squamous epithelium covering fibrovascular cores.

stratified squamous epithelium (Fig. 22.11). Keratosis is generally not seen. Koilocytic change is sometimes present; however, intraepithelial dysplasia is infrequent, and severe or full-thickness dysplasia is very uncommon and should suggest a diagnosis of papillary carcinoma (Fig. 22.12).

The differential diagnosis should include other squamoproliferative lesions, especially squamous cell carcinoma, and some cases of laryngeal papillomas in older individuals may be very difficult to separate from papillary squamous cell carcinomas or verrucous carcinomas. Indeed, reported solitary papillomas in adults associated with malignancy likely represent sampling errors rather than progression of disease from a true papilloma. Thus, clinical follow-up and complete excision are recommended for any adult with a solitary papillary lesion that shows any degree of atypia (88,90,93). In general, malignancies are destructive or will show invasion; however, history is often unavailable, and invasion may be difficult to assess with small biopsies. Papillary squamous cell carcinoma should show full-thickness cytologic atypia. Verrucous carcinomas will not, by definition, show severe cytologic atypia but often show keratinization.

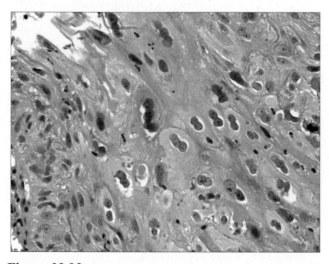

Figure 22.12. This laryngeal papilloma showed marked human papillomavirus (HPV) cytopathic effect with prominent koilocytes.

PRECURSOR LESIONS OF SQUAMOUS CELL CARCINOMA

As with squamous cell carcinoma of the cervix, squamous cell carcinoma of the larynx develops through progressive, worsening intraepithelial lesions prior to becoming invasive (100–110). Clinically, precursor lesions may appear white or red (or speckled) by endoscopy and are termed *leukoplakia* and *erythroplakia*. Although these clinical lesions do not correspond with definitive histologic features, speckled and red lesions (i.e., erythroplakia) are more likely to show squamous dysplasia and be associated with concurrent squamous cell carcinoma or the eventual development of squamous cell carcinoma. The data regarding the risk of these lesions progressing to malignancy are varied, and it is estimated that somewhere between 5% and 20% of clinically apparent intraepithelial lesions will develop into invasive malignancies. Studies that have quantified the amount of intraepithelial dysplasia have found that worsening dysplasia is associated with increased risk.

The World Health Organization (WHO) currently uses a five-tier system for the grading of intraepithelial neoplasia of the larynx and classifies these lesions as hyperplasia, mild dysplasia, moderate dysplasia, severe dysplasia, and carcinoma in situ (105). Although the descriptions of these lesions sound somewhat similar to the progressive abnormalities seen with cervical specimens, these lesions are not histologically identical, and only rarely does laryngeal intraepithelial dysplasia show a progressively basaloid appearance akin to cervical intraepithelial neoplasia. Indeed, many laryngeal squamous cell carcinomas are associated with intraepithelial lesions that do not appear to meet the criteria for carcinoma in situ or even severe dysplasia.

The WHO classification scheme uses two histologic parameters for the diagnosis of squamous precursor lesions of the upper aerodigestive tract—architectural and cytologic atypia. Architectural disturbance is the result of disturbed cellular maturation. This is manifest histologically through lack of typical nuclear polarization, non–basally located mitotic figures, dyskeratosis, and abrupt, early keratinization. Unlike with cervical intraepithelial neoplasia, dyskeratotic cells are very helpful for the diagnosis of squamous intraepithelial neoplasia of the larynx and may be one of the few histologic clues of dysplasia. The identification of drop-shaped rete ridges can also be helpful, especially for the diagnosis of higher grade, dysplastic lesions. Atypical cytologic features include anisonucleosis and nuclear pleomorphism, anisocytosis and cytologic pleomorphism, increased nuclear size and increased nuclear-to-cytoplasmic ratios, nuclear hyperchromasia, prominent nucleoli, and atypical mitotic figures. The greater the degree of architectural disturbance and cytologic atypia are, the higher the grade of dysplasia.

Squamous hyperplasia is characterized by an increase in epithelial thickness (i.e., increased numbers of cells) and, often, keratosis (Fig. 22.13). The cells may be located throughout the epithelium or appear somewhat localized. These lesions should be devoid of architectural or cytologic atypia. Although considered to be a precursor lesion, the risk for the eventual development of squamous cell carcinoma in patients with these lesions is low. Mild dysplasia shows minimal architectural and cytologic atypia. Most of the lesions described as mild dysplasia appear to show some basal cell hyperplasia with cytologic atypia confined to the lower one-third of the epithelium (Fig. 22.14). Moderate dysplasia is characterized by a greater degree of architec-

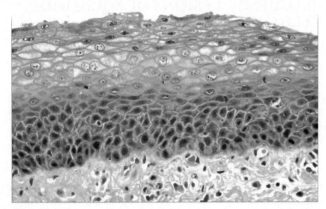

Figure 22.13. Squamous hyperplasia of the larynx. The squamous epithelium is thickened primarily as a result of increased numbers of basaloid cells. Cytologic atypia is not seen

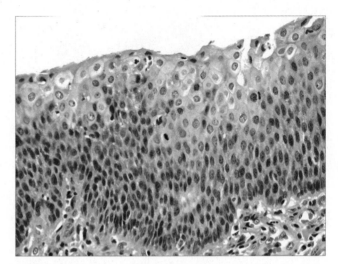

Figure 22.15. This example of moderate dysplasia shows lack of maturation of the epithelial cells into the middle third of the squamous epithelium with occasional mitotic figures.

tural disturbance than mild dysplasia, with architectural changes extending into the middle one-third of the epithelium (Fig. 22.15). However, the atypia may also be more pronounced; if it is severe, such lesions may be categorized as severe dysplasia. Lesions with severe dysplasia have architectural disturbances that extend to more than two-thirds of the thickness of the squamous epithelium with marked cytologic atypia (Fig. 22.16). Finally, carcinoma in situ is defined as malignant transformation without actual invasion. Histologically, full-thickness architectural disturbance should be accompanied by severe cytologic atypia (Fig. 22.17).

Progressive molecular abnormalities have been shown to correlate with progressive histologic atypia and the risk of subsequent invasive squamous cell carcinoma (111,112). Worsening atypia correlates with aneuploidy, which has been shown to correlate with progression (102,113). Loss of heterozygosity (LOH) studies have shown that the losses at 3p and 9p are likely early events in the development of squamous cell carcinoma of the upper aerodigestive tract and that such losses correlate with the risk for malignant transformation (114–116). Furthermore, it

has been shown that additional molecular abnormalities increase the risk even more. Much attention has also been paid to *p53* mutations, which are common in precursor lesions and are associated with increased risk for the development of invasive disease; however other tumor suppressor genes, including but not limited to *p16, p14, p12, p21, p27, MGMT,* and retinoblastoma (*RB*) have been shown to be mutated or lost by other means to some degree in precursor and malignant lesions of the larynx (114,116–119). Cyclin D1 overexpression has also been noted, as has overexpression of epidermal growth factor receptor (EGFR) (120).

Ancillary studies are usually not very helpful for diagnosing precursor lesions, likely because of the heterogeneous molecular events that can lead to squamous cell carcinoma of the larynx. Most reports have used immunohistochemistry with antibodies directed toward proteins that are lost or gained secondary to genetic alterations such as those just mentioned.

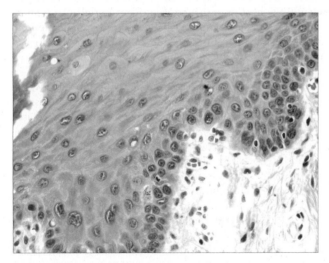

Figure 22.14. Mild dysplasia of the laryngeal squamous epithelium is characterized by subtle cytologic atypia restricted to the more basal cells.

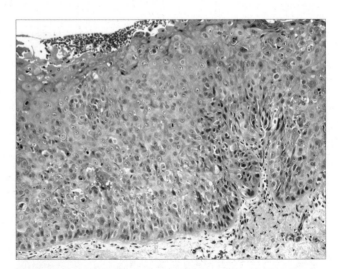

Figure 22.16. Severe squamous dysplasia. The squamous epithelium is thickened, and squamous atypia is present throughout nearly the entire thickness.

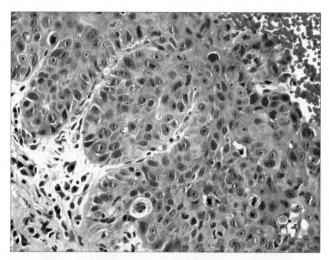

Figure 22.17. Squamous cell carcinoma in situ. Malignant squamous cells have replaced the entirety of the laryngeal epithelium. Invasion is not seen.

Immunostaining for p53 protein has often been touted as useful, as mutations of the gene are frequent and generally lead to an accumulation of defective protein (121). Proliferation markers such as ki67 may also be helpful, and substantial nuclear labeling above the basal layer of the epithelium may be associated with intraepithelial neoplasia (122). Immunostaining for the p21 protein, a target gene that can be activated by p53, may also be helpful, although results have been mixed. Although some authors have attempted to use the expression of various keratins to assist in the diagnosis, the results have proven to be too mixed or inconsistent to be of much use (121).

Verrucous hyperplasia is a term used to describe a verrucous and keratotic form of squamous hyperplasia that can show varying degrees of cytologic atypia (123,124). These lesions are more aggressive than conventional forms of intraepithelial neoplasia and are more likely to progress to malignancy. Histologically, they are characterized by folded, keratotic, hyperplastic squamous epithelium. Unlike verrucous carcinomas, these lesions are not yet invasive, and the bases of the lesions should not appear deeper than the surrounding normal squamous epithelium. Furthermore, although often without cytologic atypia, these lesions may show cytologic atypia, which should not be seen with verrucous carcinoma.

SQUAMOUS CELL CARCINOMA

Squamous cell carcinoma accounts for the vast majority of laryngeal malignancies. It was predicted that a little more than 12,000 people would be diagnosed with laryngeal cancer in the United States in 2008 and that nearly 3700 people would die from the disease (125). This equates to an age-adjusted incidence rate of 3.6 per 100,000 people per year and an age-adjusted mortality rate of 1.3 per 100,000 people per year. Less than 5% of patients diagnosed are less than 45 years of age, and cancer of the larynx is approximately five times more common in men.

Laryngeal squamous cell carcinoma is a smoking-related disease, and it is estimated that, with smoking, there is a 10-fold increased relative risk for laryngeal carcinoma (126–130). Alco-

hol consumption, as with other head and neck carcinomas, also plays a role because patients who drink heavily and smoke are at a much increased risk for the development of laryngeal squamous cell carcinoma. The risk of other possible factors in the development of this disease, including oncogenic viruses, asbestos exposure, familial susceptibilities, and gastroesophageal reflux, remains unclear, but it is likely trivial (131–133). With the decline of per capita cigarette consumption in the United States since the 1960s, the incidence of laryngeal cancer has also declined, although the decline in disease incidence trails by approximately 15 years (134–136). Mortality rates have also followed suit, roughly mirroring the changes in incidence. Indeed, the incidence and mortality rates for laryngeal cancer in the United States are now roughly 70% of what they were in 1975. These changes suggest that current multimodality therapies have done little to change the mortality rate of laryngeal squamous cell carcinoma. Furthermore, the 5-year survival rates for the disease have changed little and even slightly worsened over the past 20 years.

Staging parameters have, in general, been developed to predict outcome. As with cancer at many sites, the localization of a laryngeal cancer plays a key role in its staging and outcome. According to the National Cancer Institute (NCI), approximately 47% of laryngeal squamous cell carcinomas are localized at the time of diagnosis, 42% have metastasized to lymph nodes or directly spread from their primary site, and 7% have metastasized distally (125); the corresponding 5-year relative survival rates are 81%, 50%, and 24%, respectively.

The current American Joint Committee on Cancer (AJCC) staging system for laryngeal squamous cell carcinoma subdivides the tumors based on their relationship to the glottis (137). The node (N) and metastasis (M) statuses throughout the larynx are determined using the same criteria. N1 metastases are those confined to a single ipsilateral lymph node and 3 cm or less in size. N2a metastases are those confined to a single ipsilateral lymph node and between 3 and 6 cm in size. N2b disease is defined by the presence of multiple ipsilateral lymph node metastases, all less than 6 cm in size. N2c disease is defined as metastases to bilateral or contralateral nodes, all less than 6 cm in size. N3 metastases are those lymph node metastases that are greater than 6 cm in greatest dimension. All distant metastases are simply classified as M1.

The tumor (T) portion of the staging parameters for laryngeal carcinoma varies depending on the site of the primary tumor (137). This reflects the anatomy of the larynx, which in turn likely influences the behavior of laryngeal tumors. Examples of this include the frequent involvement of the pre-epiglottic space by supraglottic carcinomas likely secondary to the fenestrations that pass through the epiglottis. Another example includes the infrequent metastasis of small glottic tumors, perhaps secondary to the relative lack of lymphatics at the site.

Because the glottis is a relatively small structure, tumors can sometimes involve the glottis and either or both the supraglottic and subglottic larynx. This is especially reflected in the cases that now come to laryngectomy, as smaller glottic tumors are frequently treated with radiation alone. Tumors should be categorized based on the location of the bulk of the tumor with the caveats that many transglottic tumors should be considered glottic and those tumors extending more than 1 cm below the glottis should be categorized as subglottic. Fortunately, the definitions of the higher T categories are rather similar, regardless of the subclassification of the tumor. The AJCC cancer staging atlas well illustrates the various T levels and can be very helpful when one is staging a laryngeal squamous cell carcinoma (138). Because the T component includes a clinical aspect, it can be relatively confusing for pathologists, and some cases can even be staged pathologically differently from the way they had been staged clinically. With difficult cases, it is incumbent upon the pathologist to ascertain necessary clinical information, usually the status of vocal cord mobility.

Patients present with clinical symptoms related to the site of laryngeal involvement by tumor. Those glottic tumors or subglottic/supraglottic tumors involving the glottis often present with hoarseness. Patients with supraglottic tumors can present with difficulty swallowing, sore throats, referred pain to their ears, and lymph node metastases. Those with subglottic tumors sometimes present with difficulty breathing or metastases.

The treatment of laryngeal squamous cell carcinoma varies depending on the site involved and the stage. Although current treatments seem not to have improved survival rates, they are associated with much less morbidity than previous treatments. Localized, smaller tumors, especially T1 or T2 malignancies, can frequently be treated with radiation alone or, sometimes, laser excision, with more extensive surgery reserved for patients who fail the initial therapy (139,140). Higher stage malignancies require partial or total laryngectomy with subsequent radiation therapy (141,142). Conversely, some patients may receive radiation therapy and even chemotherapy, with surgery used as a salvage therapy (143,144). Patients with laryngeal cancer are frequently also treated with isotretinoin to reduce the up to 25% risk for the development of a second primary malignancy (145).

Grossly, squamous cell carcinomas of the larynx are almost always described as fungating, white-tan masses, often with ulceration (Figs. 22.18 to 22.21). Rarely, the lesions appear flat. Other than with small, poorly oriented superficial biopsies, the diagnosis of laryngeal conventional squamous cell carcinoma rarely poses any difficulty for pathologists. The tumors are composed of infiltrative, irregular nests of squamous cells that show varying degrees of intracellular and extracellular keratin formation. With better differentiated tumors, increased differentia-

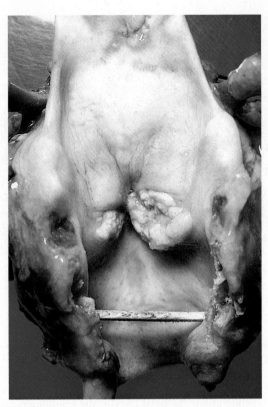

Figure 22.19. Glottic T3 invasive squamous cell carcinoma of the right true cord. The left vocal cord shows premalignant changes. Despite its size, the carcinoma does not cross the ventricle and does not involve the ventricular band.

tion is usually present toward the center of the nests, with the most peripheral cells having a basaloid phenotype and the more central cells having more abundant eosinophilic cytoplasm. Extracellular keratin, commonly intermixed with necrotic debris, is often identified at the centers of the nests (Fig. 22.22). The squamous nests can vary considerably in size, with some appearing large and cystic. Single-cell infiltration may be present, espe-

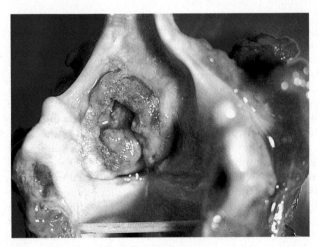

Figure 22.18. Supraglottic cancer originating in the angle between the epiglottis and false cord. This is a common type of supraglottic lesion, which is usually resected by total laryngectomy. This specimen shows a deep vertical cleft in the substance of the tumor.

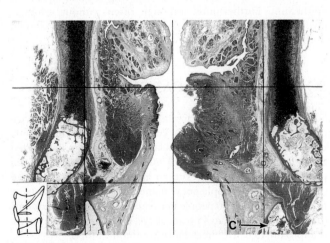

Figure 22.20. Coronal section of specimen in Figure 22.19. Cancer has infiltrated the thyroarytenoid muscle, but it has not crossed the ventricle, leaving the false cord free of tumor.

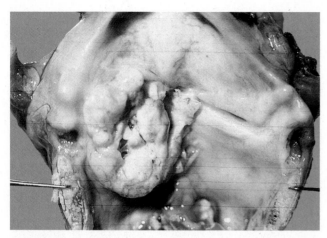

Figure 22.21. Typical transglottic carcinoma extending across the ventricle and involving both the ventricular band and the true cord.

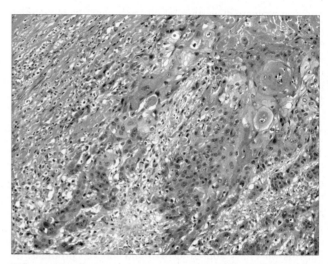

Figure 22.23. This laryngeal moderately differentiated squamous cell carcinoma shows less organized differentiation with more cytologic atypia. Occasional small groups of squamous cells and singe cells infiltrate away from the tumor in the lower portion of this photomicrograph.

cially with higher grade tumors (Fig. 22.23). The surrounding stroma usually has some degree of chronic inflammation, often with stromal desmoplasia. The nuclei of the neoplastic cells show moderate to marked differences in shape and size with irregular contours and vesicular to granular, malignant-appearing chromatin. Prominent nucleoli are usually seen, and mitotic figures, including atypical mitotic figures, can usually be found. Necrosis of both individual tumor cells and of large portions of tumor is frequently seen with laryngeal squamous cell carcinomas.

Several histologic parameters are generally reported with cases of laryngeal squamous cell carcinomas that have been shown to have variable prognostic significance. These generally include grade (sometimes recorded from the advancing tumor front), the presence or absence of perineural and angiolymphatic invasion, and margin status (146–150). (Regardless of the fact that most pathologists do not use "standardized" and "objective" criteria for grading, grading frequently conforms to such stated criteria.) Some have suggested that tumor border

configuration and degree and character of the inflammatory infiltrate may also be important, as well as the presence of extracapsular extension seen with lymph node metastases (148,151,152). Although not a histologic parameter per se, a measurement of tumor depth of invasion may also provide prognostic information (153).

There are no specific immunohistochemical markers of laryngeal squamous cell carcinomas, and these tumors react with antibodies akin to squamous cell carcinomas from other sites. Conventional squamous cell carcinomas are invariably reactive with antibodies to cytokeratins, with better differentiated tumors expressing higher weight keratins and poorly differentiated tumors expressing lower molecular weight keratins. Immunostaining with antibodies to p63 can also be helpful for the diagnosis of these lesions and can assist the pathologist in distinguishing some tumors with other lesions. However, salivary gland–type tumors frequently also express the antigen.

Cytogenetic and molecular abnormalities associated with laryngeal squamous cell carcinomas have been shown by some to have prognostic value and have been used by some to assist in the diagnosis of difficult biopsies. The findings are similar, although somewhat more advanced, than those seen in preinvasive disease (see previous discussions). Cytogenetically, laryngeal squamous cell carcinomas frequently show gains of 3q, 5p, 8q, 11q13, and 17q with losses of 3p (154,155). *p53* and *p16* genes are inactivated in some cases of laryngeal squamous cell carcinomas, as is *RB*, although in a smaller percentage of cases (114). *EGFR* is amplified in up to 25% of cases (120). The prognostic information that can be gained from studying cytogenetic or molecular markers and even ploidy remains controversial (156,157). Such abnormalities are not frequently investigated or reported in general practice.

VARIANTS OF SQUAMOUS CELL CARCINOMA

All common variants of squamous cell carcinoma have been reported to involve the larynx. These include verrucous carci-

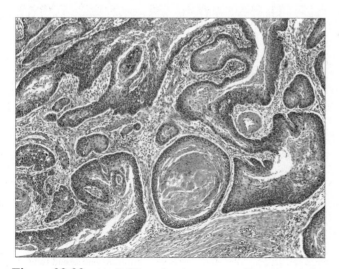

Figure 22.22. A well-differentiated squamous cell carcinoma of the larynx with large squamous nests showing central maturation and abundant extracellular keratin formation.

noma, sarcomatoid or spindle cell carcinoma, basaloid squamous cell carcinoma, adenosquamous carcinoma, papillary squamous cell carcinoma, adenoid squamous cell carcinoma, and undifferentiated carcinomas. Distinguishing these malignancies from conventional squamous cell carcinomas and other malignancies is important for several reasons that will be discussed with each particular variant.

VERRUCOUS CARCINOMA

The larynx is the second most common site within the upper aerodigestive tract after the mouth to be involved by verrucous carcinoma (158–163). Here, these lesions typically involve the vocal cords and are much more common in men, usually coming to attention in the sixth and seventh decades of life. Most patients present with hoarseness. As with conventional squamous cell carcinomas, these tumors arise most frequently in patients who have abused alcohol and tobacco products. Although numerous studies have been published regarding the etiologic role of HPV with these lesions, its role, if any, is still debated (117,164–166). p53 protein accumulation has been demonstrated by immunohistochemistry with increased proliferative activity (117,167). LOH studies have shown fewer abnormalities with these tumors compared with other more poorly differentiated squamous cell carcinomas, and deletions of 9p have been noted (168).

Grossly, the tumors are white and papillary or fungating (Fig. 22.24) (158–160,163,169). The size of the lesions can vary, and tumors can become very large with extensive invasion and destruction of the laryngeal tissues. Histologically, the tumors are composed of a thickened and folded squamous epithelium frequently with abundant keratosis and parakeratosis extending from the filiform peaks of the surface (Fig. 22.25). The tumor bases are circumscribed and composed of broad tongues of squamous epithelium that extend deeper than the surrounding nonneoplastic epithelium into the subepithelial tissues (Fig. 22.26). Invasive, irregular nests of squamous cells should not be seen. Chronic inflammation and, rarely, foreign body–type giant cells are present in the surrounding stroma. Cytologically, little, if any, atypia should be present, with normal maturation and mitotic activity limited to the basal levels of the neoplasm. Occasional dyskeratotic cells are sometimes seen within the epithelium.

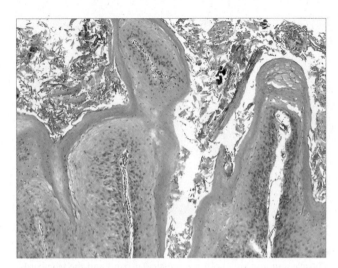

Figure 22.25. Verrucous carcinoma. The tumor's surface is verrucoid with abundant parakeratosis. The base infiltrated the stroma with a circumscribed and pushing border.

Verrucous hyperplasia should be distinguished from both benign and other malignant lesions (15,123,124). Unlike benign lesions, such as verrucous hyperplasia, verrucous carcinoma is destructive and, as mentioned, extends deeper than the surrounding epithelium. Furthermore, somewhat counterintuitively, verrucous carcinoma frequently shows less cytologic atypia than verrucous hyperplasia, which often shows some degree of dysplasia. Unlike with conventional squamous cell carcinomas, no infiltrating nests of tumor should be present. Indeed, if a tumor has any infiltrating nests, it should not be diagnosed as verrucous carcinoma because it may metastasize.

When strict criteria are applied for the diagnosis of verrucous carcinoma, the lesions have an excellent prognosis, and less than 10% of patients die from their tumors; none develops metastases. Indeed, neck dissection is not warranted for true verrucous carcinoma. Some have suggested that radiation ther-

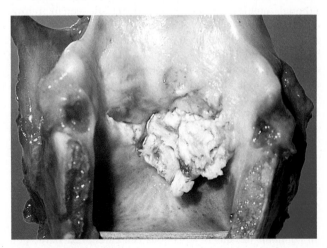

Figure 22.24. Verrucous carcinoma of the right vocal cord.

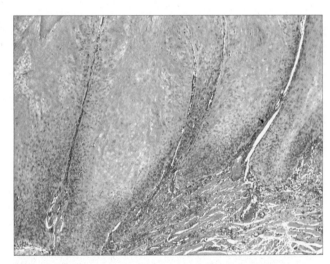

Figure 22.26. Verrucous carcinomas infiltrate with broad tongues of squamous epithelium. Irregular infiltrating nests of squamous cells should not be seen. The neoplastic cells show little cytologic atypia, although occasional dyskeratotic cells are sometimes seen.

apy may be as effective as resection; however, others have noted frequent failure with radiation therapy; some even believe that radiation therapy predisposes the tumor to anaplastic transformation (158).

SPINDLE CELL CARCINOMA

The larynx is the most frequent site within the upper aerodigestive tract to be involved by spindle cell or sarcomatoid carcinoma (170–176). These tumors arise in a cohort of patients similar to conventional squamous cell carcinomas of the larynx and affect mostly men with a mean age of presentation in the seventh decade of life. Although once debated, most now accept that the mesenchymal components of these tumors are neoplastic and share the molecular abnormalities of the epithelial components of the malignancies, when present (172,177,178). The tumors are poorly differentiated and show LOH frequencies similar to other poorly differentiated squamous cell carcinomas of the upper aerodigestive tract (168). A specific marker on the short arm of chromosome 4 was shown to be more commonly lost in these tumors compared to other squamous cell carcinoma variants.

Most patients have smoking histories, and heavy alcohol use is common (173,174,176). Radiation exposure has also been linked to a spindle cell phenotype, especially after treatment of a previous conventional squamous cell carcinoma. Approximately 70% of these tumors are glottic, and nearly 60% present at low stage (AJCC T1). Because so many tumors are glottic and low stage, it is not surprising that the majority of patients present with hoarseness. Approximately 20% of patients die with disease.

Nearly all laryngeal spindle cell carcinomas are exophytic and present as polypoid masses (173,174,176). Most cases have ulcerated surfaces, typically covered with necrotic fibrinoid material; when surface epithelium is present, epithelial dysplasia is often seen. Consistent with the tumor's appellation, the majority of tumor cells show a mesenchymal phenotype and are spindled and fusiform (Fig. 22.27). The degree of cellularity and cellular atypia can vary, although most cases have been noted to have mild to moderate cellularity and mild to moderate

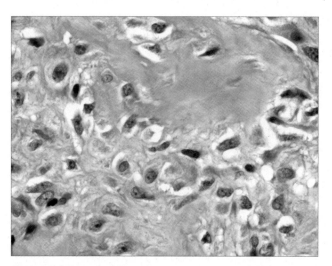

Figure 22.28. Spindle cell carcinoma of the larynx. Focal osteoid formation was seen with this tumor. Specific mesenchymal differentiation should not lead one from a diagnosis of spindle cell carcinoma.

cellular pleomorphism. Necrosis is only occasionally present, although mitotic figures are frequent. A variety of growth patterns can also be seen, including nodular fasciitis–like, fibromatosis-like, storiform, herringbone, and fascicular growth patterns. Furthermore, osteocartilaginous regions and giant cells, including osteoclast-like giant cells, can also be seen (Fig. 22.28). Frequently, a minor squamous component can be found that appears to "blend" into the spindle cell component.

In short, spindle cell carcinomas of the larynx can mimic any number of mesenchymal lesions. Indeed, with any lesion of the larynx believed to be mesenchymal, one should carefully consider a spindle cell carcinoma. A diligent search should be made for a squamous component, either invasive or intraepithelial. Immunohistochemistry can also be helpful because between 50% and 75% of laryngeal spindle cell carcinomas will show immunoreactivity for at least one epithelial antigen (171,174,175). A pankeratin cocktail may be the most helpful immunostain to perform. Recently, some have suggested that p63 immunostaining may also be of assistance because these tumors are frequently immunoreactive (179). Unfortunately, some spindle cell carcinomas may lack histologic and immunohistochemical evidence of epithelial differentiation (especially when only biopsy is available for review). Indeed, immunoreactivity with antibodies to mesenchymal antigens, especially smooth muscle antigen (SMA), may even be noted.

PAPILLARY SQUAMOUS CELL CARCINOMA

Papillary squamous cell carcinoma is a rare variant of squamous cell carcinoma that most frequently involves the larynx when it involves the upper aerodigestive tract (180–183). Like all laryngeal squamous cell carcinomas, these occur most frequently in older men. Because these lesions resemble laryngeal papillomas and cervical dysplasia, some have suggested that HPV may play some role in their development. Grossly, papillary squamous cell carcinomas appear exophytic and somewhat warty. Histologically, they are composed of numerous papillary and filiform stromal projections covered by a stratified squamous epithelium that shows full-thickness dysplasia akin to that seen in cervical

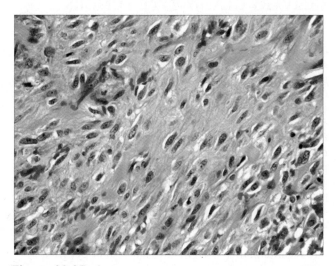

Figure 22.27. Spindle cell carcinomas typically have a moderate degree of cytologic atypia.

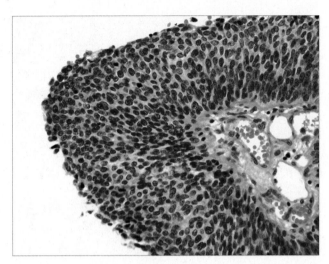

Figure 22.29. Papillary squamous cell carcinoma of the larynx. These malignancies are very exophytic and composed of numerous filiform fronds. The fronds are covered by squamous cell carcinoma in situ, distinctly resembling high-grade squamous intraepithelial lesion of the cervix.

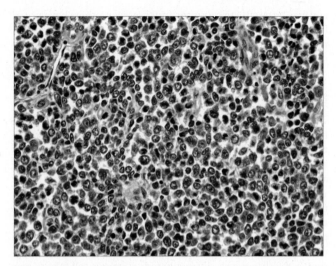

Figure 22.31. Undifferentiated carcinoma. Undifferentiated carcinomas sometimes arise in the larynx. These tumors may be associated with Epstein-Barr virus infection and with a lymphoid infiltrate. This tumor was found to harbor a t(15;19).

squamous cell carcinoma in situ replete with a complete lack of maturation, cytologic atypia, and numerous mitotic figures present throughout the entire thickness of the epithelium (Fig. 22.29). Because of the complex, exophytic nature of these tumors, true tissue invasion may be hard to identify, especially with biopsy material. When present, invasion should appear similar to conventional squamous cell carcinoma. Invasive lesions behave similar, stage for stage, to matched conventional squamous cell carcinomas.

OTHER VARIANTS

Other variants of squamous cell carcinoma have also been found in the larynx including basaloid squamous cell carcinomas, adenosquamous carcinomas, adenoid squamous cell carcinomas, and undifferentiated carcinomas (Figs. 22.30 and 22.31)

(184–192). Although basaloid squamous cell carcinomas of the oropharynx have been linked etiologically to human papillomavirus, those of the larynx may not be (193). Laryngeal squamous cell carcinomas can focally show glandular differentiation and should be diagnosed as adenosquamous carcinomas and not confused with mucoepidermoid carcinomas. Laryngeal squamous cell carcinomas rarely show an adenoid phenotype. Such cases need to be distinguished from glandular and vascular neoplasia. Finally, some laryngeal squamous cell carcinomas can appear undifferentiated. Lesions akin to those of the nasopharynx with a prominent chronic inflammatory component and sometimes associated with Epstein-Barr virus (EBV) infection have been noted in the larynx. Other undifferentiated carcinomas, including those associated with chromosomal rearrangements of the gene encoding nuclear protein of the testis (*NUT*) have been described here (194).

SALIVARY GLAND–TYPE TUMORS

Seromucinous glands are present throughout the larynx except in the region of the true cord, and thus, it is not surprising that salivary gland–type neoplasms occur within the larynx. Nonetheless, they are rare, and less than 3% of laryngeal neoplasms resemble those typically identified in the major salivary glands (195). Most are malignant. In a large series of laryngeal salivary gland–type neoplasms seen at the Armed Forces Institute of Pathology, adenoid cystic carcinomas, mucoepidermoid carcinomas, pleomorphic adenomas, and oncocytic lesions comprised the majority of cases (195). Smaller series and case reports suggest that virtually any type of salivary gland–type neoplasm can arise in the larynx (196–209). Unfortunately, because adenoid cystic carcinomas and mucoepidermoid carcinomas are frequently misclassified as basaloid squamous cell carcinomas and adenosquamous carcinomas (and vice versa), the literature regarding these lesions leaves much to be desired.

Pleomorphic adenomas or benign mixed tumors are the most common benign salivary gland–type neoplasms of the lar-

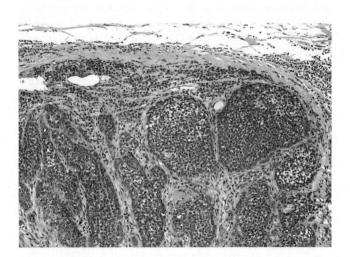

Figure 22.30. Basaloid squamous cell carcinomas are less common in the larynx than they are in the oropharynx. They are composed of nests of basaloid squamous cells that sometimes have central "comedoform" necrosis.

ynx (195,206,207,209,210). As with other portions of the upper aerodigestive tract, pleomorphic adenomas here typically contain less stromal tissue than those seen in the major salivary glands, are circumscribed but not encapsulated, and often have a significant squamous component. Most of these tumors are benign; however, rare cases of malignant mixed tumors or carcinomas and ex-pleomorphic adenomas have been reported.

Adenoid cystic carcinomas likely represent the most common malignant salivary gland–type neoplasm of the larynx (195–197,199,201,203,205,207,208,211). These may occur anywhere within the larynx; however, the subglottic area is most frequently involved. Patients present at any age and of either sex with shortness of breath, hoarseness, and pain, depending on the location of the tumor. Histologically, they are identical to those seen elsewhere and show tubular, solid, and cribriform growth patterns, frequently with perineural invasion (Fig. 22.32). Up to 50% recur, and tumors can metastasize to the lung; they rarely, if ever, metastasize to lymph nodes. Adenoid cystic carcinomas must be distinguished from basaloid squamous cell carcinomas, which more frequently involve the supraglottic larynx and frequently metastasize to lymph nodes. Basaloid squamous cell carcinomas are associated with intra-epithelial neoplasia, focal clear-cut squamous differentiation, and more cytologic atypia.

Mucoepidermoid carcinomas are the second most commonly reported salivary gland–type neoplasms of the larynx (187,195,199,203,211,212). They occur in either sex at any age, and patients present with hoarseness or other mass-related symptoms. Careful attention should be applied to distinguish these tumors from adenosquamous carcinomas of the larynx. Unlike adenosquamous carcinomas, mucoepidermoid carcinomas should show glandular and epidermoid or squamous differentiation throughout. Adenosquamous carcinomas, instead, are predominantly squamous and generally of higher grade and are associated with squamous intraepithelial neoplasia.

Other reported benign salivary gland–type tumors of the larynx include myoepitheliomas and oncocytic lesions (13,14, 195). Of note here, most of the reported oncocytic tumors likely represent oncocytic metaplasia of nonneoplastic cysts, and only rarely have lesions resembling oncocytomas been reported. Other reported laryngeal salivary gland–type malignancies include acinic cell carcinomas, myoepithelial carcinomas, malignant mixed tumors, salivary duct carcinomas, and clear-cell carcinomas (198,200–202,213,214).

NEUROENDOCRINE CARCINOMAS

Neuroendocrine carcinomas of the larynx are uncommon, although they may be the second most frequent epithelial malignancy of the larynx, occurring as often or slightly more often than salivary gland–type neoplasms (215–217). They occur more frequently in older individuals and in men and are most often supraglottic and submucosal. The WHO currently subclassifies these tumors as well-differentiated (carcinoid), moderately differentiated (atypical carcinoid), and small-cell carcinomas with or without other epithelial components (218).

Well-differentiated neuroendocrine carcinomas or "carcinoid tumors" are much less common than moderately differentiated neoplasms and show a striking predilection for men (215,216). These tumors resemble pulmonary carcinoid tumors and should be devoid of necrosis with minimal cytologic atypia or mitotic activity (Fig. 22.33). The surface epithelium is usually intact and uninvolved by the lesion. The neoplastic cells grow in organoid nests and trabeculae, frequently with gland formation, and have round to oval nuclei with finely granular chromatin. It is important to distinguish these tumors from the more common moderately differentiated neuroendocrine carcinomas because they rarely metastasize and are associated with a much better 5-year survival (>90%).

Moderately differentiated neuroendocrine carcinomas or "atypical carcinoid tumors" of the larynx comprise the bulk of

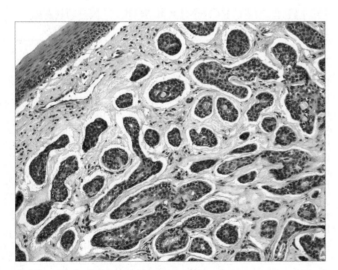

Figure 22.32. Adenoid cystic carcinoma of the larynx. Although the overlying epithelium is metaplastic, atypia is not present. Laryngeal adenoid cystic carcinomas show the same growth patterns as elsewhere, frequently exhibiting a tubular and cribriform growth pattern.

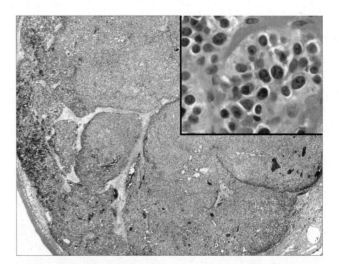

Figure 22.33. Well-differentiated neuroendocrine carcinomas of the larynx are uncommon and appear similar to pulmonary carcinoid tumors. They exhibit organoid, trabecular, nested, and, sometimes, glandular growth patterns and are composed of epithelioid cells with round to oval nuclei (*inset*). They lack necrosis and significant mitotic activity.

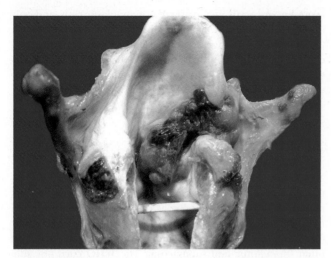

Figure 22.34. Moderately differentiated neuroendocrine carcinoma. Neuroendocrine carcinomas of the larynx are typically supraglottic. This tumor was also polypoid and hemorrhagic.

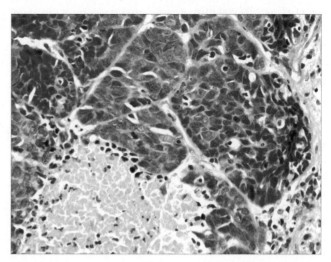

Figure 22.36. Small-cell carcinoma of the larynx. These tumors resemble pulmonary small-cell carcinomas histologically and behave poorly. They are composed of small- to medium-sized epithelioid cells with little cytoplasm. Abundant necrosis, both confluent and single cell, is present with numerous mitotic figures.

laryngeal neuroendocrine neoplasia (Fig. 22.34) (215,216, 219–221). The tumors show typical neuroendocrine growth patterns (e.g., trabecular, nested, organoid, etc.); however, unlike well-differentiated neuroendocrine carcinomas, they are sometimes associated with necrosis and have increased mitotic activity and cytologic atypia (Fig. 22.35). The prognosis for these lesions is guarded with a 5-year survival rate of approximately 50%. They are frequently associated with lymph node metastases or metastases at other sites.

Small-cell carcinomas of the larynx are also rare and can be associated with squamous cell carcinomas or adenocarcinomas (215,216,219,222,223). Histologically, they share the features of small-cell carcinomas seen elsewhere, with high nuclear-to-cytoplasmic ratios, abundant mitotic figures and apoptotic bodies, necrosis, nuclear molding, the Azzopardi effect, and fre-

quent crush artifact (Fig. 22.36). Patients typically have metastases and are not surgical candidates. As with small-cell carcinomas elsewhere, these tumors have a dismal prognosis with reported 5-year survival rates of less than 5%.

Laryngeal neuroendocrine carcinomas should almost always react with antibodies to keratins and neuroendocrine antigens such as CD56, neuron-specific enolase (NSE), chromogranin, and synaptophysin (216,224). Some have noted frequent reactivity with antibodies to calcitonin, especially with moderately differentiated tumors (219). As in the lung, immunostaining these cases with antibodies to p63 may be helpful for distinguishing them from squamous cell carcinomas, which should be immunoreactive.

OTHER NEUROENDOCRINE, NEURAL, AND NEUROECTODERMAL TUMORS

PARAGANGLIOMAS

Paragangliomas of the larynx are almost always sporadic and benign, although both familial and malignant cases have been reported (215,216,221,225–228). They occur more often in women. These lesions are also more frequently supraglottic, and this has suggested to some that the superior paired paraganglia of the larynx more frequently develop tumors than the inferior paraganglia. In the report by Lack et al. (227) of 69 head and neck paragangliomas, only one arose in the larynx. These lesions are identical to paragangliomas found elsewhere with nested ("zellballen"), large epithelioid cells surrounded by spindled sustentacular cells (Fig. 22.37). The tumors typically are immunoreactive with antibodies to synaptophysin and chromogranin but not with antibodies to cytokeratins (216,221, 225,229). Sustentacular cells can be highlighted with antibody to S-100 protein. Keratin and S-100 protein immunostaining may be used to distinguish paragangliomas from neuroendocrine carcinomas because neuroendocrine carcinomas should

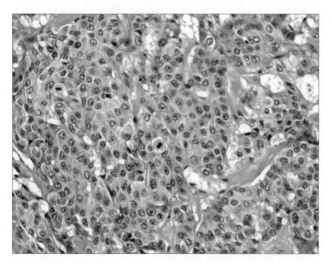

Figure 22.35. This moderately differentiated neuroendocrine carcinoma of the larynx showed more atypia than a typical well-differentiated neuroendocrine carcinoma. Areas of necrosis (not pictured) were found, as were frequent mitotic figures.

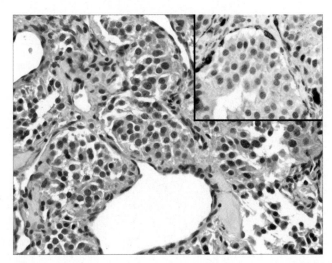

Figure 22.37. Supraglottic laryngeal paraganglioma. These tumors are composed of nested epithelioid cells. An S-100 protein immunostain can be used to highlight the sustentacular cells that surround the nests of neuroendocrine cells (*inset*).

be immunoreactive with antibodies to keratins and should not have sustentacular cells (230).

NEURAL AND NERVE SHEATH TUMORS

Although uncommon, neural or nerve sheath tumors have been described in the larynx (17,231–236). These lesions typically present as submucosal masses and should be diagnosed with the same criteria applied with specimens from other parts of the body. Traumatic neuromas, although not thought to be neoplastic, have been described here, as have the submucosal neuromas of multiple endocrine neoplasia type 2. Lack et al. (236) described two laryngeal granular cell tumors of the larynx in his series of 110 cases. These lesions are similar to granular cell tumors elsewhere and are composed of large histiocytoid cells with granular cytoplasm and small nuclei (Fig. 22.38). As at other sites, the lesions are frequently associated with

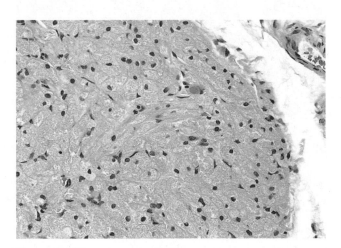

Figure 22.38. Granular cell tumor of true cord. It is composed of large, polygonal cells with granular eosinophilic cytoplasm that resemble histiocytes. The nuclear morphology is bland.

pseudoepitheliomatous hyperplasia. The neoplastic cells show Schwann cell differentiation and react with antibodies to S-100 but not with antibodies to cytokeratins (237–239). Schwannomas or neurilemomas have also been reported in the larynx, as have solitary neurofibromas and neurofibromas associated with neurofibromatosis type 1. Rare cases of malignant peripheral nerve sheath tumors of the larynx have been reported, as have laryngeal primitive neuroectodermal tumors.

MELANOCYTIC LESIONS

Primary melanocytic neoplasia of the larynx is very uncommon. Only melanoma occurs with any frequency (240–243). The majority of patients (>80%) diagnosed with laryngeal melanoma are men, and the average age of diagnosis is in the seventh decade of life. Most are supraglottic, and patients typically present with hoarseness or symptoms secondary to a mass lesion. The tumors are polypoid and infiltrate the submucosal tissues. Most laryngeal melanomas exhibit a solid pattern of growth; however, other growth patterns associated with melanomas can be seen. An in situ component is not usually seen with laryngeal melanomas. The neoplastic cells are pleomorphic, epithelioid, or spindle shaped and have atypical, hyperchromatic nuclei with pseudoinclusions and prominent nucleoli. Abundant mitotic activity and necrosis are also seen. Patients most often die of disease. Obviously other forms of neoplasia, especially poorly differentiated squamous cell carcinomas, need to be excluded. Laryngeal melanomas should be immunoreactive with antibodies to S-100 and to more specific melanocytic antigens such as HMB-45. Cytokeratin immunoreactivity should not be seen. Other melanocytic lesions, including nevi, have only extremely rarely been reported to involve the larynx.

MESENCHYMAL NEOPLASIA

Most laryngeal neoplasia is epithelial. That said, a vast array of mesenchymal neoplasia has been reported to occur in the larynx. Pathologists should be especially careful to distinguish these tumors from epithelial malignancies that have a mesenchymal phenotype (e.g., spindle cell carcinoma).

FATTY TUMORS

Fatty tumors of the larynx are rare and often involve the larynx through direct extension (244–248). Lipomas and liposarcomas usually involve the supraglottic larynx, often with involvement of the hypopharynx. Patients present with obstructive symptoms such as snoring. Lipomas, with lobules of mature, nonatypical lipocytes, are less common than liposarcomas. These tumors are benign, and only rare recurrence has been reported. Rare variants of lipoma (e.g., spindle cell lipoma) have also been reported to involve the larynx, as has hibernoma. Liposarcomas are more common and occur much more often in men. These present as polypoid or exophytic masses and are unencapsulated and infiltrative. They are almost always well differentiated (atypical lipomatous tumors) and are composed of lobules of variably sized lipocytes separated by broad fibrous

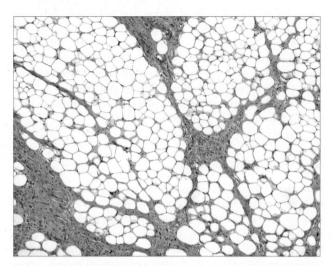

Figure 22.39. Liposarcomas of the larynx are typically well differentiated (atypical lipomatous tumors). These are composed of lobules of mature-appearing adipocytes separated by fibrous bands. Atypical stromal cell are typically seen within the fibrous bands, and lipoblasts can usually be found.

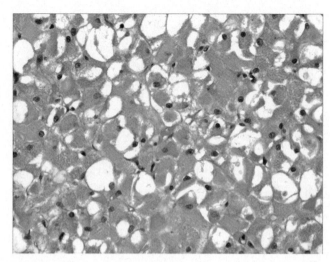

Figure 22.40. Adult rhabdomyoma. This tumor is composed of large, polygonal eosinophilic and clear cells. The differential diagnosis for these tumors usually includes granular cell tumor. Rhabdomyomas should be immunoreactive with antibodies to muscle antigens.

bands (Fig. 22.39). Both the lipocytes and stromal cells of the fibrous bands show cellular atypia, and rare lipoblasts are seen. These tumors frequently recur but do not metastasize. Rarely, recurrences have been noted to have dedifferentiation. Other liposarcoma variants, including myxoid liposarcomas and pleomorphic liposarcomas, have rarely been reported to involve the larynx.

MYOGENOUS TUMORS

Rare laryngeal tumors show myogenous differentiation, both skeletal and smooth (249–255). Extracardiac rhabdomyomas frequently involve the upper aerodigestive tract, often the larynx (250–252,255). Adult rhabdomyomas occur in older adults with a mean age of presentation in the seventh decade. The tumors occur more often in men and usually present as unifocal polypoid masses, although multifocal and sessile lesions have been reported. Grossly, the lesions are tan to red-brown, circumscribed, and fleshy on cut section. Histologically, adult rhabdomyomas are composed of unencapsulated lobules of large polygonal cells (Fig. 22.40). The neoplastic cells have abundant eosinophilic, granular, or vacuolated cytoplasm with small, round nuclei with prominent nucleoli. Cross-striations and crystalline structures are often present. Mitotic figures and necrosis are only rarely seen. Immunohistochemically, neoplastic cells react with antibodies to muscle-specific actin (MSA), desmin, and myoglobin. S-100 protein immunoreactivity is also frequently noted and can lead one to erroneously diagnose this lesion as a granular cell tumor. The tumors are benign and do not metastasize, although nearly half have been reported to recur. Fetal rhabdomyomas present at any age but tend to occur in younger patients than adult rhabdomyomas, with most cases presenting in the first 5 years of life. The lesions are more common in boys and present as polypoid obstructive masses that grossly appear circumscribed with gray-white to tan-pink, mucoid cut surfaces. Histologically, the tumors are well demarcated but unencapsulated and composed of haphazardly arranged,

immature skeletal muscle cells with cross-striations (Fig. 22.41). More mature cells can also be present akin to those seen in adult rhabdomyomas (Kapadia et al. [250] referred to these as cases with intermediate differentiation). These tumors can show a wide range of differentiation and also may contain immature-appearing spindled cells. Mitotic figures are frequently noted; however, marked nuclear atypia and necrosis should not be seen. As with adult rhabdomyomas, neoplastic cells react with antibodies to MSA, desmin, and myoglobin and frequently with antibodies to S-100 protein and SMA. These lesions do not metastasize and only rarely recur.

Other neoplasms of the larynx showing myogenous differentiation include rhabdomyosarcomas and smooth muscle tumors (249,252–254). Both embryonal and alveolar rhabdomyosarcomas have been reported in the larynx. Leiomyomas have been reported within the larynx and can have prominent vascularity

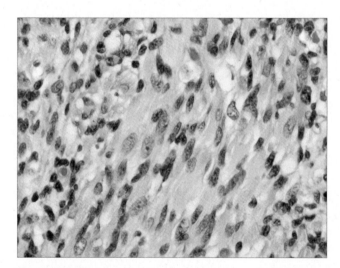

Figure 22.41. Fetal rhabdomyomas are composed of less mature-appearing, spindle cell skeletal muscle cells; cross-striations are typically seen.

(vascular leiomyoma) or epithelioid or pleomorphic cells (epithelioid leiomyoma). Rare leiomyosarcomas have also been reported in the larynx replete with cytologic atypia, necrosis, and increased mitotic activity. The criteria used to distinguish these lesions from leiomyomas have obviously not been agreed upon, although cases showing more indeterminate features have not been reported.

FIBROBLASTIC AND MYOFIBROBLASTIC TUMORS

Many neoplasms showing fibroblastic or myofibroblastic differentiation have been reported to involve the larynx (256–261). These include rare cases of extra-abdominal fibromatosis that have been reported in the head and neck, occasionally primarily affecting the larynx. Solitary fibrous tumors have rarely been noted. Wenig et al. (260) reported a series of eight cases of inflammatory myofibroblastic tumor. These lesions were polypoid, frequently arose from the true vocal cord, did not show invasive growth, and were composed of spindled cells in a loose, myxoid background containing mixed inflammatory cells (Fig. 22.42). None of the cases experienced recurrence, although the follow-up time ranged from only 1 to 3 years. Adult-type fibrosarcomas and undifferentiated high-grade pleomorphic sarcomas with and without giant cells have been reported within the larynx. Here, one should be reminded that before a diagnosis of a mesenchymal tumor of the larynx is made, especially that of a fibroblastic or myofibroblastic malignancy, spindle cell carcinoma should be excluded.

VASCULAR TUMORS

Laryngeal hemangiomas occur in children and adults (262–264). In children, they are usually subglottic, and patients present with obstructive symptoms. These tumors have features typical of juvenile capillary hemangiomas. Younger lesions are lobular and very cellular with closely packed capillaries lined by plump endothelial cells. Many of the capillaries do not have discernible lumina. With older lesions, the capillaries dilate and become ectatic, separated by a less cellular fibrous stroma. In

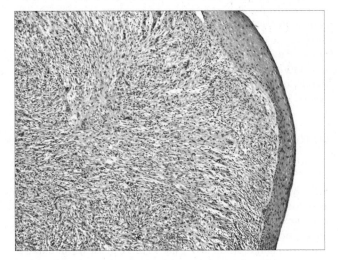

Figure 22.42. A subepithelial recurrence of a laryngeal inflammatory myofibroblastic tumor. This example has a loose, storiform growth pattern akin to nodular fasciitis.

adults, most hemangiomas occur in men in the glottic or supraglottic larynx and have features of cavernous hemangiomas. These are poorly circumscribed and are typically composed of dilated thin-walled vessels lined by flattened endothelium. Lobular capillary hemangiomas akin to those in the mouth or nose do not usually occur in the larynx, and some have noted that such lesions described in the literature more likely represent abundant granulation tissue (265). Cervical lymphangiomas or cystic hygromas can sometimes involve the larynx (263,266). These are poorly circumscribed, spongy tumors composed of dilated lymphatic channels sometimes surrounded by chronic inflammatory cells. Rare cases of intravascular or extravascular papillary endothelial hyperplasia have been reported in the larynx (267).

Most malignant vascular tumors of the larynx are angiosarcomas (268,269). These are rare and occur mostly in the supraglottic or glottic larynx usually in older adults. They typically have high-grade cytology and are either epithelioid or vasiform. Some have arisen in patients with previous radiation therapy, and the tumors typically kill the patients. Kaposi sarcomas and hemangioendotheliomas have also been reported in the larynx (270,271). Immunohistochemistry is sometimes needed for the diagnosis of these lesions, and most tumors will react with antibodies to factor VIII–related antigen, CD31, or CD34 (272,273). Kaposi sarcoma is frequently associated with human herpesvirus-8 (HHV8) infection, which can be identified with immunohistochemistry (274).

CARTILAGINOUS TUMORS

Cartilaginous tumors are the most common mesenchymal neoplasms of the larynx, and they represent approximately 1% of all laryngeal tumors (275–282). Chondrosarcomas are much more common than chondromas; indeed, one should be very hesitant regarding the diagnosis of chondroma in the larynx (see later discussion). Laryngeal chondrosarcomas are more common in older men, and the mean age of presentation reported in the huge series and review of the literature by Thompson and Gannon (276) was in the early seventh decade of life. More than 70% arise from the cricoid cartilage, and 10% to 20% arise from the thyroid cartilage. Patients typically present with hoarseness or difficulty breathing.

As mentioned, the vast majority of cartilaginous neoplasms of the larynx are chondrosarcomas. Whether true chondromas occur in the larynx and whether they can be diagnosed as such is debated. Thompson and Gannon (276) noted that in 62% of their more than 100 chondrosarcomas, a benign chondroma was associated with the lesion. This alone may be enough reason not to unequivocally diagnose chondroma at biopsy. Indeed, the diagnosis of well-differentiated chondrosarcoma rather than chondroma simply connotes a propensity for recurrence and, although unlikely, a small chance of dedifferentiation and poor behavior. Grossly, chondrosarcomas can vary greatly in size, and lesions smaller than 1 cm and larger than 10 cm have been reported (Fig. 22.43). They appear lobular, gray-blue, and myxoid and typically infiltrate soft tissues. Most chondrosarcomas of the larynx are chondrocytic and low grade, but occasional myxoid chondrosarcomas or, less commonly, dedifferentiated chondrosarcomas have been noted (Fig. 22.44). Recurrence is not infrequent, with rates ranging between 18% and 45% in the literature. Tumor grade and completeness of

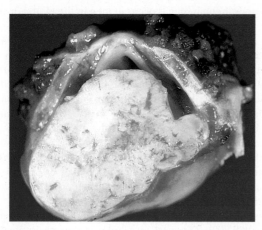

Figure 22.43. Chondrosarcoma of the larynx. A cross section of the larynx demonstrates a massive cartilaginous tumor arising in the posterior cricoid and virtually filling the airway.

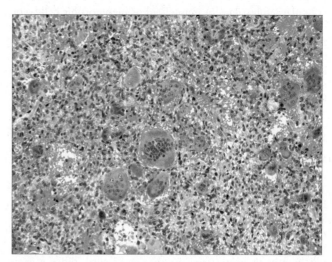

Figure 22.45. Giant-cell tumors of the larynx frequently involve the cricoid cartilage and are histologically identical to giant-cell tumors seen in other bones. The are composed of evenly distributed multinucleated giant cells that contain 20 or more nuclei each with bland, oval, or spindled mononuclear cells.

resection contribute. Metastases are uncommon, as is death from tumor, with more than 90% of patients achieving survival.

OSSEOUS AND OTHER BONE TUMORS

Osseous or other bone tumors of the larynx are very rare. Osteosarcomas are the most common of these tumors (283–285). Unlike conventional osteosarcomas of long bones, these lesions occur in older individuals with a median age of approximately 63 years. Patients typically present with hoarseness, dyspnea, and obstruction. Although approximately one-third of cases have been noted to arise from the cricoid or thyroid cartilages, more than half have arisen from soft tissue, mostly from the glottis. These osteosarcomas are typically high grade with cytologic atypia and numerous mitotic figures. Osteoid production is essential for the diagnosis. Occasional osteoclast-type giant cells and cartilage formation are also sometimes seen. These

tumors behave poorly, and more than half of the patients die secondary to the disease. As with other mesenchymal tumors, it is essential to distinguish these lesions from sarcomatoid carcinomas (see previous discussion). That these osteosarcomas present in older individuals, often in the glottis, raises some question about the legitimacy of at least some of the reported cases.

Giant-cell tumor of the larynx is a rare benign tumor that recapitulates giant-cell tumor of bone (286,287). Within the larynx, these tumors present in adults over a wide age range (23 to 62 years) and are much more common in men. Most have arisen from the thyroid or cricoid cartilages, and patients typically present with hoarseness or obstruction. Tumors have averaged approximately 4 cm in greatest dimension and are grossly infiltrative, sometimes with associated hemorrhage or cystic degeneration. Microscopically, the lesions are identical to those of the bone and are composed of innumerable giant cells admixed with histiocytes and fibroblasts (Fig. 22.45). The giant cells have numerous (often >20) bland nuclei, similar to those of the surrounding spindled cells. Mitotic figures are often noted. Patients with giant-cell tumors of the larynx do well, and the tumors do not recur after resection or other treatment. Rarely, other bone tumors have been reported to involve the larynx, including aneurysmal bone cyst (288).

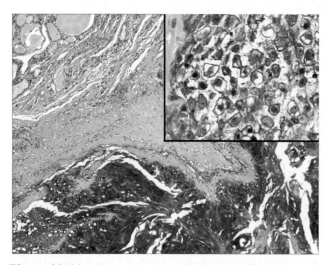

Figure 22.44. This laryngeal chondrosarcoma is low grade and has a typical lobular growth pattern as it extends toward the thyroid gland. A higher power image (*inset*) shows it to be more cellular than typical nonneoplastic cartilage. Many laryngeal low-grade chondrosarcomas do not appear this cellular.

OTHER MESENCHYMAL TUMORS

Synovial sarcoma has rarely been reported to involve the larynx (289). In a large series from the Armed Forces Institute of Pathology, approximately 4% of synovial sarcomas were found to arise within the larynx or pharynx (although other authors report significantly lower percentages) (290). Within the larynx, most synovial sarcomas arise at or near the aryepiglottic folds. These typically occur in young adults often in the third or fourth decades of life, although they can occur at any age. The histologic appearance of these tumors is akin to that seen elsewhere, and both monophasic and biphasic variants have been reported.

The diagnosis can frequently be confirmed by ancillary methods demonstrating the classic t(X;18)(p11;p11) (291). Synovial sarcomas of the larynx behave as they do elsewhere, and approximately 50% of patients will eventually develop metastases. Other sarcomas uncommonly noted in the larynx or neck include alveolar soft part sarcoma and epithelioid sarcoma (292,293).

HEMATOLYMPHOID NEOPLASIA

Most hematolymphoid neoplasia has been reported within the larynx, including predominantly cutaneous or mucosal lymphomas such as mycoses fungoides (294–296). The most common malignant hematolymphoid lesions to involve the larynx are diffuse large B-cell lymphomas and extramedullary plasmacytomas.

Extraosseous plasmacytomas are monoclonal proliferations of plasma cells that occur at extraosseus sites in older patients without concomitant bone marrow involvement (297–300). Up to 20% of these patients, however, have a monoclonal gammopathy. Furthermore, up to 25% of cases recur after surgery, and 15% of patients eventually are found to have myeloma. Although these are relatively uncommon tumors, they have a predilection for the head and neck and frequently involve the mucosa of the upper aerodigestive tract. At these sites, approximately 11% of plasmacytomas involve the larynx. Histologically, extraosseous plasmacytomas characteristically are composed of sheets of plasma cells with abundant amphophilic cytoplasm and eccentrically placed round to oval nuclei with granular (clock-faced) chromatin (Fig. 22.46). Occasional cases will have cells that show more cytologic atypia or have a more "plasmablastic" phenotype with larger nuclei, finer chromatin, and more prominent nucleoli. Mott cells and Russell bodies are frequently encountered. Neoplastic cells often fail to express some of the typical B-cell antigens such as CD19 and CD20. They typically express CD79a, CD38, and CD138 and will show light chain restriction by immunohistochemistry or in situ hybridization. The tumors may be hard to distinguish from extranodal marginal zone lymphomas with plasmacytic differentiation.

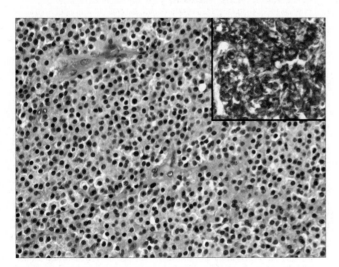

Figure 22.46. Extramedullary plasmacytoma. These tumors are composed of sheets of plasma cells. Ancillary methods (*inset*: kappa-immunostain) will demonstrate light chain restriction.

METASTASES

The larynx is infrequently involved by metastatic malignancies (301–303). Rarely do such cases represent the initial presentation of the disease. In a large review of secondary tumors of the larynx, the most common sites of the primary malignancies were skin (melanoma), kidney, breast, lung, and prostate, in that order (303). Any malignancies from surrounding sites can directly invade the larynx. This is especially true with thyroid malignancies such as anaplastic carcinomas (304).

REFERENCES

1. Mills SE. Larynx and pharynx. In Mills SE, ed. *Hisology for Pathologists.* 3rd edition. Philadelphia, PA: Lippincott Williams & Wilkins, 2007:431–444.
2. Stell PM, Gregory I, Watt J. Morphology of the human larynx. II. The subglottis. *Clin Otolaryngol Allied Sci* 1980;5:389–395.
3. Stell PM, Gregory I, Watt J. Morphometry of the epithelial lining of the human larynx. I. The glottis. *Clin Otolaryngol Allied Sci* 1978;3(1):13–20.
4. Stell PM, Gudrun R, Watt J. Morphology of the human larynx. III. The supraglottis. *Clin Otolaryngol Allied Sci* 1981;6(6):389–393.
5. Hopp ES. The development of the epithelium of the larynx. *Laryngoscope* 1955;65(7):475–499.
6. Nassar VH, Bridger GP. Topography of the laryngeal mucous glands. *Arch Otolaryngol* 1971;94(6):490–498.
7. Lawson W, Zak FG. The glomus bodies ("paraganglia") of the human larynx. *Laryngoscope* 1974;84(1):98–111.
8. Abrams AM, Melrose RJ, Howell FV. Necrotizing sialometaplasia. A disease simulating malignancy. *Cancer* 1973;32(1):130–135.
9. Fechner RE. Necrotizing sialometaplasia: a source of confusion with carcinoma of the palate. *Am J Clin Pathol* 1977;67(4):315–317.
10. Wenig BM. Necrotizing sialometaplasia of the larynx. A report of two cases and a review of the literature. *Am J Clin Pathol* 1995;103(5):609–613.
11. Hill MJ, Taylor CL, Scott GB. Chondromatous metaplasia in the human larynx. *Histopathology* 1980;4(2):205–214.
12. Iyer PV, Rajagopalan PV. Cartilaginous metaplasia of soft tissues in the larynx. Case report and literature review. *Arch Otolaryngol* 1981;107(9):573–575.
13. Gallagher JC, Puzon BQ. Oncocytic lesions of the larynx. *Ann Otol Rhinol Laryngol* 1969;78(2):307–318.
14. Lundgren J, Olofsson J, Hellquist H. Oncocytic lesions of the larynx. *Acta Otolaryngol* 1982;94(3–4):335–344.
15. Schrader M, Laberke HG. Differential diagnosis of verrucous carcinoma in the oral cavity and larynx. *J Laryngol Otol* 1988;102(8):700–703.
16. Agarwal RK, Blitzer A, Perzin KH. Granular cell tumors of the larynx. *Otolaryngol Head Neck Surg* 1979;87(6):807–814.
17. Compagno J, Hyams VJ, Ste-Marie P. Benign granular cell tumors of the larynx: a review of 36 cases with clinicopathologic data. *Ann Otol Rhinol Laryngol* 1975;84(3 Pt 1):308–314.
18. Barton RT. Observation on the pathogenesis of laryngeal granuloma due to endotracheal anesthesia. *N Engl J Med* 1953;248(26):1097–1099.
19. Holinger PH, Johnston KC. Contact ulcer of the larynx. *JAMA* 1960;172:511–515.
20. Miko TL. Peptic (contact ulcer) granuloma of the larynx. *J Clin Pathol* 1989;42(8):800–804.
21. Ward PH, Zwitman D, Hanson D, et al. Contact ulcers and granulomas of the larynx: new insights into their etiology as a basis for more rational treatment. *Otolaryngol Head Neck Surg* 1980;88(3):262–269.
22. Wenig BM, Devaney K, Wenig BL. Pseudoneoplastic lesions of the oropharynx and larynx simulating cancer. *Pathol Annu* 1995;30 (Pt 1):143–187.
23. Wenig BM, Heffner DK. Contact ulcers of the larynx. A reacquaintance with the pathology of an often underdiagnosed entity. *Arch Pathol Lab Med* 1990;114(8):825–828.
24. Dikkers FG, Nikkels PG. Benign lesions of the vocal folds: histopathology and phonotrauma. *Ann Otol Rhinol Laryngol* 1995;104(9 Pt 1):698–703.
25. Kambic V, Radsel Z, Zargi M, et al. Vocal cord polyps: incidence, histology and pathogenesis. *J Laryngol Otol* 1981;95(6):609–618.
26. Kleinsasser O. Pathogenesis of vocal cord polyps. *Ann Otol Rhinol Laryngol* 1982;91(4 Pt 1):378–381.
27. Canalis RF, Maxwell DS, Hemenway WG. Laryngocele—an updated review. *J Otolaryngol* 1977;6(3):191–199.
28. DeSanto LW, Devine KD, Weiland LH. Cysts of the larynx—classification. *Laryngoscope* 1970;80(1):145–176.
29. Holinger LD, Barnes DR, Smid LJ, et al. Laryngocele and saccular cysts. *Ann Otol Rhinol Laryngol* 1978;87(5 Pt 1):675–685.
30. Newman BH, Taxy JB, Laker HI. Laryngeal cysts in adults: a clinicopathologic study of 20 cases. *Am J Clin Pathol* 1984;81(6):715–720.
31. Schmidt PJ, Wagenfeld D, Bridger MW, et al. Teflon injection of the vocal cord: a clinical and histopathologic study. *J Otolaryngol* 1980;9(4):297–302.
32. Stein J, Eliachar I, Myles J, et al. Histopathologic study of alternative substances for vocal fold medialization. *Ann Otol Rhinol Laryngol* 2000;109(2):221–226.
33. Ustundag E, Boyaci Z, Keskin G, et al. Soft tissue response of the larynx to silicone, Gore-Tex, and irradiated cartilage implants. *Laryngoscope* 2005;115(6):1009–1014.

34. Varvares MA, Montgomery WW, Hillman RE. Teflon granuloma of the larynx: etiology, pathophysiology, and management. *Ann Otol Rhinol Laryngol* 1995;104(7):511–515.

35. Devine KD. Sarcoidosis and sarcoidosis of the larynx. *Laryngoscope* 1965;75:533–569.

36. Neel HB 3rd, McDonald TJ. Laryngeal sarcoidosis: report of 13 patients. *Ann Otol Rhinol Laryngol* 1982;91(4 Pt 1):359–362.

37. Pillsbury HC 3rd, Sasaki CT. Granulomatous diseases of the larynx. *Otolaryngol Clin North Am* 1982;15(3):539–551.

38. Bridger MW, Jahn AF, van Nostrand AW. Laryngeal rheumatoid arthritis. *Laryngoscope* 1980;90(2):296–303.

39. Sorensen WT, Moller-Andersen K, Behrendt N. Rheumatoid nodules of the larynx. *J Laryngol Otol* 1998;112(6):573–574.

40. Devaney KO, Travis WD, Hoffman G, et al. Interpretation of head and neck biopsies in Wegener's granulomatosis. A pathologic study of 126 biopsies in 70 patients. *Am J Surg Pathol* 1990;14(6):555–564.

41. Hoare TJ, Jayne D, Rhys Evans P, et al. Wegener's granulomatosis, subglottic stenosis and antineutrophil cytoplasm antibodies. *J Laryngol Otol* 1989;103(12):1187–1191.

42. Batsakis JG, Manning JT. Relapsing polychondritis. *Ann Otol Rhinol Laryngol* 1989;98(1 Pt 1):83–84.

43. Damiani JM, Levine HL. Relapsing polychondritis—report of ten cases. *Laryngoscope* 1979;89(6 Pt 1):929–946.

44. Smith GA, Ward PH, Berci G. Laryngeal lupus erythematosus. *J Laryngol Otol* 1978;92(1):67–73.

45. Barrs DM, McDonald TJ, Duffy J. Sjogren's syndrome involving the larynx: report of a case. *J Laryngol Otol* 1979;93(9):933–936.

46. Prytz S. Vocal nodules in Sjogren's syndrome. *J Laryngol Otol* 1980;94(2):197–203.

47. Block LJ, Caldarelli DD, Holinger PH, et al. Pemphigus of the air and food passages. *Ann Otol Rhinol Laryngol* 1977;86(5 Pt 1):584–587.

48. Frangogiannis NG, Gangopadhyay S, Cate T. Pemphigus of the larynx and esophagus. *Ann Intern Med* 1995;122(10):803–804.

49. Gianoli GJ, Miller RH. Crohn's disease of the larynx. *J Laryngol Otol* 1994;108(7):596–598.

50. Goodman M, Montgomery W, Minette L. Pathologic findings in gouty cricoarytenoid arthritis. *Arch Otolaryngol* 1976;102(1):27–29.

51. Guttenplan MD, Hendrix RA, Townsend MJ, et al. Laryngeal manifestations of gout. *Ann Otol Rhinol Laryngol* 1991;100(11):899–902.

52. Marion RB, Alperin JE, Maloney WH. Gouty tophus of the true vocal cord. *Arch Otolaryngol* 1972;96(2):161–162.

53. Bartels H, Dikkers FG, van der Wal JE, et al. Laryngeal amyloidosis: localized versus systemic disease and update on diagnosis and therapy. *Ann Otol Rhinol Laryngol* 2004;113(9):741–748.

54. Berg AM, Troxler RF, Grillone G, et al. Localized amyloidosis of the larynx: evidence for light chain composition. *Ann Otol Rhinol Laryngol* 1993;102(11):884–889.

55. Godbersen GS, Leh JF, Hansmann ML, et al. Organ-limited laryngeal amyloid deposits: clinical, morphological, and immunohistochemical results of five cases. *Ann Otol Rhinol Laryngol* 1992;101(9):770–775.

56. Lewis JE, Olsen KD, Kurtin PJ, et al. Laryngeal amyloidosis: a clinicopathologic and immunohistochemical review. *Otolaryngol Head Neck Surg* 1992;106(4):372–377.

57. Pribitkin E, Friedman O, O'Hara B, et al. Amyloidosis of the upper aerodigestive tract. *Laryngoscope* 2003;113(12):2095–2101.

58. Thompson LD, Derringer GA, Wenig BM. Amyloidosis of the larynx: a clinicopathologic study of 11 cases. *Mod Pathol* 2000;13(5):528–535.

59. Michaels L, Hyams VJ. Amyloid in localised deposits and plasmacytomas of the respiratory tract. *J Pathol* 1979;128(1):29–38.

60. Fageeh NA, Mai KT, Odell PF. Eosinophilic angiocentric fibrosis of the subglottic region of the larynx and upper trachea. *J Otolaryngol* 1996;25(4):276–278.

61. Smid L, Lavrencak B, Zargi M. Laryngo-tracheo-bronchopathia chondro-osteoplastica. *J Laryngol Otol* 1992;106(9):845–848.

62. Young RH, Sandstrom RE, Mark GJ. Tracheopathia osteoplastica: clinical, radiologic, and pathological correlations. *J Thorac Cardiovasc Surg* 1980;79(4):537–541.

63. Benjamin B, Jacobson I, Eckstein R. Idiopathic subglottic stenosis: diagnosis and endoscopic laser treatment. *Ann Otol Rhinol Laryngol* 1997;106(9):770–774.

64. Grillo HC, Mark EJ, Mathisen DJ, et al. Idiopathic laryngotracheal stenosis and its management. *Ann Thorac Surg* 1993;56(1):80–87.

65. Jindal JR, Milbrath MM, Shaker R, et al. Gastroesophageal reflux disease as a likely cause of "idiopathic" subglottic stenosis. *Ann Otol Rhinol Laryngol* 1994;103(3):186–191.

66. Zapf B, Lehmann WB, Snyder GG 3rd. Hamartoma of the larynx: an unusual cause for stridor in an infant. *Otolaryngol Head Neck Surg* 1981;89(5):797–799.

67. Bailey CM, Windle-Taylor PC. Tuberculous laryngitis: a series of 37 patients. *Laryngoscope* 1981;91(1):93–100.

68. Bull TR. Tuberculosis of the larynx. *Br Med J* 1966;2(5520):991–992.

69. Hunter AM, Millar JW, Wightman AJ, et al. The changing pattern of laryngeal tuberculosis. *J Laryngol Otol* 1981;95(4):393–398.

70. Thaller SR, Gross JR, Pilch BZ, et al. Laryngeal tuberculosis as manifested in the decades 1963–1983. *Laryngoscope* 1987;97(7 Pt 1):848–850.

71. Bennett DE. Histoplasmosis of the oral cavity and larynx. A clinicopathologic study. *Arch Intern Med* 1967;120(4):417–427.

72. Blair PA, Gnepp DR, Riley RS, et al. Blastomycosis of the larynx. *South Med J* 1981;74(7):880–882.

73. Dumich PS, Neel HB 3rd. Blastomycosis of the larynx. *Laryngoscope* 1983;93(10):1266–1270.

74. Benson-Mitchell R, Tolley N, Croft CB, et al. Aspergillosis of the larynx. *J Laryngol Otol* 1994;108(10):883–885.

75. Brandwein MS, Kapadia SB, Gnepp DR. Nonsquamous pathology of the larynx, hypopharynx, and trachea. In Gnepp DR, ed. *Diagnostic Surgical Pathology of the Head and Neck*. Philadelphia, PA: WB Saunders, 2001:239–323.

76. Ganesan S, Harar RP, Dawkins RS, et al. Invasive laryngeal candidiasis: a cause of stridor in the previously irradiated patient. *J Laryngol Otol* 1998;112(6):575–578.

77. Kheir SM, Flint A, Moss JA. Primary aspergillosis of the larynx simulating carcinoma. *Hum Pathol* 1983;14(2):184–186.

78. Platt MA. Laryngeal coccidioidomycosis. *JAMA* 1977;237(12):1234–1235.

79. Smallman LA, Stores OP, Watson MG, et al. Cryptococcosis of the larynx. *J Laryngol Otol* 1989;103(2):214–215.

80. Ward PH, Berci G, Morledge D, et al. Coccidioidomycosis of the larynx in infants and adults. *Ann Otol Rhinol Laryngol* 1977;86(5 Pt 1):655–660.

81. Goutas N, Simopoulou S, Papazoglou K, et al. A fatal case of diphtheria. *Pediatr Pathol* 1994;14(3):391–395.

82. Senior BA, Radkowski D, MacArthur C, et al. Changing patterns in pediatric supraglottitis: a multi-institutional review, 1980 to 1992. *Laryngoscope* 1994;104(11 Pt 1):1314–1322.

83. Jay J, Green RP, Lucente FE. Isolated laryngeal rhinoscleroma. *Otolaryngol Head Neck Surg* 1985;93(5):669–673.

84. Brandenburg JH, Finch WW, Kirkham WR. Actinomycosis of the larynx and pharynx. *Otolaryngology* 1978;86(5):ORL-739–ORL-742.

85. Abramson AL, Steinberg BM, Winkler B. Laryngeal papillomatosis: clinical, histopathologic and molecular studies. *Laryngoscope* 1987;97(6):678–685.

86. Bauman NM, Smith RJ. Recurrent respiratory papillomatosis. *Pediatr Clin North Am* 1996;43(6):1385–1401.

87. Doyle DJ, Gianoli GJ, Espinola T, et al. Recurrent respiratory papillomatosis: juvenile versus adult forms. *Laryngoscope* 1994;104(5 Pt 1):523–527.

88. Friedberg SA, Stagman R, Hass GM. Papillary lesions of the larynx in adults. A pathologic study. *Ann Otol Rhinol Laryngol* 1971;80(5):683–692.

89. Kashima HK, Mounts P, Shah K. Recurrent respiratory papillomatosis. *Obstet Gynecol Clin North Am* 1996;23(3):699–706.

90. Kashima HK, Shah F, Lyles A, et al. A comparison of risk factors in juvenile-onset and adult-onset recurrent respiratory papillomatosis. *Laryngoscope* 1992;102(1):9–13.

91. Lampertico P, Russell WO, Maccomb WS. Squamous papilloma of upper respiratory epithelium. *Arch Pathol* 1963;75:293–302.

92. Lindeberg H, Elbrond O. Laryngeal papillomas: clinical aspects in a series of 231 patients. *Clin Otolaryngol Allied Sci* 1989;14(4):333–342.

93. Lindeberg H, Oster S, Oxlund I, et al. Laryngeal papillomas: classification and course. *Clin Otolaryngol Allied Sci* 1986;11(6):423–429.

94. Quick CA, Foucar E, Dehner LP. Frequency and significance of epithelial atypia in laryngeal papillomatosis. *Laryngoscope* 1979;89(4):550–560.

95. Wiatrak BJ. Overview of recurrent respiratory papillomatosis. *Curr Opin Otolaryngol Head Neck Surg* 2003;11(6):433–441.

96. Helmuth RA, Strate RW. Squamous carcinoma of the lung in a nonirradiated, nonsmoking patient with juvenile laryngotracheal papillomatosis. *Am J Surg Pathol* 1987;11(8):643–650.

97. Guillou L, Sahli R, Chaubert P, et al. Squamous cell carcinoma of the lung in a nonsmoking, nonirradiated patient with juvenile laryngotracheal papillomatosis. Evidence of human papillomavirus-11 DNA in both carcinoma and papillomas. *Am J Surg Pathol* 1991;15(9):891–898.

98. Levi JE, Delcelo R, Alberti VN, et al. Human papillomavirus DNA in respiratory papillomatosis detected by in situ hybridization and the polymerase chain reaction. *Am J Pathol* 1989;135(6):1179–1184.

99. Moore CE, Wiatrak BJ, McClatchey KD, et al. High-risk human papillomavirus types and squamous cell carcinoma in patients with respiratory papillomas. *Otolaryngol Head Neck Surg* 1999;120(5):698–705.

100. Blackwell KE, Fu YS, Calcaterra TC. Laryngeal dysplasia. A clinicopathologic study. *Cancer* 1995;75(2):457–463.

101. Crissman JD. Laryngeal keratosis and subsequent carcinoma. *Head Neck Surg* 1979;1(5):386–391.

102. Crissman JD, Fu YS. Intraepithelial neoplasia of the larynx. A clinicopathologic study of six cases with DNA analysis. *Arch Otolaryngol Head Neck Surg* 1986;112(5):522–528.

103. Crissman JD, Zarbo RJ. Dysplasia, in situ carcinoma, and progression to invasive squamous cell carcinoma of the upper aerodigestive tract. *Am J Surg Pathol* 1989;13(Suppl 1):5–16.

104. Gale N, Kambic V, Michaels L, et al. The Ljubljana classification: a practical strategy for the diagnosis of laryngeal precancerous lesions. *Adv Anat Pathol* 2000;7(4):240–251.

105. Gale N, Pilch BZ, Sidransky D, et al. Epithelial precursor lesions. In Barnes L, Eveson JE, Reichart P, eds. *Pathology and Genetics of Head and Neck Tumors*. Lyon, France: IARC Press, 2005:140–143.

106. Hellquist H, Cardesa A, Gale N, et al. Criteria for grading in the Ljubljana classification of epithelial hyperplastic laryngeal lesions. A study by members of the Working Group on Epithelial Hyperplastic Laryngeal Lesions of the European Society of Pathology. *Histopathology* 1999;34(3):226–233.

107. Myssiorek D, Vambutas A, Abramson AL. Carcinoma in situ of the glottic larynx. *Laryngoscope* 1994;104(4):463–467.

108. Spayne JA, Warde P, O'Sullivan B, et al. Carcinoma-in-situ of the glottic larynx: results of treatment with radiation therapy. *Int J Radiat Oncol Biol Phys* 2001;49(5):1235–1238.

109. Henry RC. The transformation of laryngeal leucoplakia to cancer. *J Laryngol Otol* 1979;93(5):447–459.

110. Norris CM, Peale AR. Keratosis of the larynx. *J Laryngol Otol* 1963;77:635–647.

111. Califano J, van der Riet P, Westra W, et al. Genetic progression model for head and neck cancer: implications for field cancerization. *Cancer Res* 1996;56(11):2488–2492.

112. Califano J, Westra WH, Meininger G, et al. Genetic progression and clonal relationship of recurrent premalignant head and neck lesions. *Clin Cancer Res* 2000;6(2):347–352.

113. Hellquist H, Olofsson J, Grontoft O. Carcinoma in situ and severe dysplasia of the vocal cords. A clinicopathological and photometric investigation. *Acta Otolaryngol* 1981;92:543–555.

114. Scholnick SB, Sun PC, Shaw ME, et al. Frequent loss of heterozygosity for Rb, TP53, and chromosome arm 3p, but not NME1 in squamous cell carcinomas of the supraglottic larynx. *Cancer* 1994;73(10):2472–2480.

115. Sun PC, el-Mofty SK, Haughey BH, et al. Allelic loss in squamous cell carcinomas of the larynx: discordance between primary and metastatic tumors. *Genes Chromosomes Cancer* 1995;14(2):145–148.
116. Jares P, Fernandez PL, Nadal A, et al. p16MTS1/CDK4I mutations and concomitant loss of heterozygosity at 9p21–23 are frequent events in squamous cell carcinoma of the larynx. *Oncogene* 1997;15(12):1445–1453.
117. Lopez-Amado M, Garcia-Caballero T, Lozano-Ramirez A, et al. Human papillomavirus and p53 oncoprotein in verrucous carcinoma of the larynx. *J Laryngol Otol* 1996;110(8): 742–747.
118. Hirai T, Hayashi K, Takumida M, et al. Reduced expression of p27 is correlated with progression in precancerous lesions of the larynx. *Auris Nasus Larynx* 2003;30(2):163–168.
119. Jeannon JP, Soames JV, Aston V, et al. Molecular markers in dysplasia of the larynx: expression of cyclin-dependent kinase inhibitors p21, p27 and p53 tumour suppressor gene in predicting cancer risk. *Clin Otolaryngol Allied Sci* 2004;29(6):698–704.
120. Almadori G, Bussu F, Cadoni G, et al. Molecular markers in laryngeal squamous cell carcinoma: towards an integrated clinicobiological approach. *Eur J Cancer* 2005;41(5): 683–693.
121. Coltrera MD, Zarbo RJ, Sakr WA, et al. Markers for dysplasia of the upper aerodigestive tract. Suprabasal expression of PCNA, p53, and CK19 in alcohol-fixed, embedded tissue. *Am J Pathol* 1992;141(4):817–825.
122. Pignataro L, Capaccio P, Pruneri G, et al. The predictive value of p53, MDM-2, cyclin D1 and Ki67 in the progression from low-grade dysplasia towards carcinoma of the larynx. *J Laryngol Otol* 1998;112(5):455–459.
123. Batsakis JG, Suarez P, el-Naggar AK. Proliferative verrucous leukoplakia and its related lesions. *Oral Oncol* 1999;35(4):354–359.
124. Murrah VA, Batsakis JG. Proliferative verrucous leukoplakia and verrucous hyperplasia. *Ann Otol Rhinol Laryngol* 1994;103(8 Pt 1):660–663.
125. National Cancer Institute. Cancer Stat Fact Sheets: Cancer of the Larynx. Available at: http://seer.cancer.gov/statfacts/html/laryn.html.
126. Brugere J, Guenel P, Leclerc A, et al. Differential effects of tobacco and alcohol in cancer of the larynx, pharynx, and mouth. *Cancer* 1986;57(2):391–395.
127. Flanders WD, Rothman KJ. Interaction of alcohol and tobacco in laryngeal cancer. *Am J Epidemiol* 1982;115(3):371–379.
128. Lewin F, Norell SE, Johansson H, et al. Smoking tobacco, oral snuff, and alcohol in the etiology of squamous cell carcinoma of the head and neck: a population-based case-referent study in Sweden. *Cancer* 1998;82(7):1367–1375.
129. Luce D, Guenel P, Leclerc A, et al. Alcohol and tobacco consumption in cancer of the mouth, pharynx, and larynx: a study of 316 female patients. *Laryngoscope* 1988;98(3): 313–316.
130. Tuyns AJ, Esteve J, Raymond L, et al. Cancer of the larynx/hypopharynx, tobacco and alcohol: IARC international case-control study in Turin and Varese (Italy), Zaragoza and Navarra (Spain), Geneva (Switzerland) and Calvados (France). *Int J Cancer* 1988;41(4): 483–491.
131. Mork J, Moller B, Glattre E. Familial risk in head and neck squamous cell carcinoma diagnosed before the age of 45: a population-based study. *Oral Oncol* 1999;35(4):360–367.
132. Trizna Z, Schantz SP. Hereditary and environmental factors associated with risk and progression of head and neck cancer. *Otolaryngol Clin North Am* 1992;25(5):1089–1103.
133. Yu KK, Zanation AM, Moss JR, et al. Familial head and neck cancer: molecular analysis of a new clinical entity. *Laryngoscope* 2002;112(9):1587–1593.
134. Sturgis EM, Cinciripini PM. Trends in head and neck cancer incidence in relation to smoking prevalence: an emerging epidemic of human papillomavirus-associated cancers? *Cancer* 2007;110(7):1429–1435.
135. Carvalho AL, Nishimoto IN, Califano JA, et al. Trends in incidence and prognosis for head and neck cancer in the United States: a site-specific analysis of the SEER database. *Int J Cancer* 2005;114(5):806–816.
136. Hoffman HT, Porter K, Karnell LH, et al. Laryngeal cancer in the United States: changes in demographics, patterns of care, and survival. *Laryngoscope* 2006;116(9 Pt 2 Suppl 111): 1–13.
137. Greene FL, Page DL, Fleming ID, et al., eds. Head and neck sites. In *AJCC Cancer Staging Manual*. 6th edition. New York, NY: Springer, 2002:17–88.
138. Greene FL, Compton CC, Fritz AG, et al., eds. Head and neck sites. In *AJCC Cancer Staging Atlas*. New York, NY: Springer, 2006:11–74.
139. Mendenhall WM, Amdur RJ, Morris CG, et al. T1-T2N0 squamous cell carcinoma of the glottic larynx treated with radiation therapy. *J Clin Oncol* 2001;19(20):4029–4036.
140. Steiner W. Results of curative laser microsurgery of laryngeal carcinomas. *Am J Otolaryngol* 1993;14(2):116–121.
141. Arriagada R, Eschwege F, Cachin Y, et al. The value of combining radiotherapy with surgery in the treatment of hypopharyngeal and laryngeal cancers. *Cancer* 1983;51(10): 1819–1825.
142. Tupchong L, Scott CB, Blitzer PH, et al. Randomized study of preoperative versus postoperative radiation therapy in advanced head and neck carcinoma: long-term follow-up of RTOG study 73-03. *Int J Radiat Oncol Biol Phys* 1991;20(1):21–28.
143. MacKenzie RG, Franssen E, Balogh JM, et al. Comparing treatment outcomes of radiotherapy and surgery in locally advanced carcinoma of the larynx: a comparison limited to patients eligible for surgery. *Int J Radiat Oncol Biol Phys* 2000;47(1):65–71.
144. Forastiere AA, Goepfert H, Maor M, et al. Concurrent chemotherapy and radiotherapy for organ preservation in advanced laryngeal cancer. *N Engl J Med* 2003;349(22):2091–2098.
145. Hong WK, Lippman SM, Itri LM, et al. Prevention of second primary tumors with isotretinoin in squamous-cell carcinoma of the head and neck. *N Engl J Med* 1990;323(12): 795–801.
146. Bradford CR, Wolf GT, Fisher SG, et al. Prognostic importance of surgical margins in advanced laryngeal squamous carcinoma. *Head Neck* 1996;18(1):11–16.
147. Gallo A, Manciocco V, Tropiano ML, et al. Prognostic value of resection margins in supracricoid laryngectomy. *Laryngoscope* 2004;114(4):616–621.
148. Ozdek A, Sarac S, Akyol MU, et al. Histopathological predictors of occult lymph node metastases in supraglottic squamous cell carcinomas. *Eur Arch Otorhinolaryngol* 2000; 257(7):389–392.
149. Fagan JJ, Collins B, Barnes L, et al. Perineural invasion in squamous cell carcinoma of the head and neck. *Arch Otolaryngol Head Neck Surg* 1998;124(6):637–640.
150. Bryne M, Jenssen N, Boysen M. Histological grading in the deep invasive front of T1 and T2 glottic squamous cell carcinomas has high prognostic value. *Virchows Arch* 1995;427(3): 277–281.
151. Oosterkamp S, de Jong JM, Van den Ende PL, et al. Predictive value of lymph node metastases and extracapsular extension for the risk of distant metastases in laryngeal carcinoma. *Laryngoscope* 2006;116(11):2067–2070.
152. Thompson AC, Bradley PJ, Griffin NR. Tumor-associated tissue eosinophilia and long-term prognosis for carcinoma of the larynx. *Am J Surg* 1994;168(5):469–471.
153. Yilmaz T, Hosal S, Gedikoglu G, et al. Prognostic significance of depth of invasion in cancer of the larynx. *Laryngoscope* 1998;108(5):764–768.
154. Huang Q, Yu GP, McCormick SA, et al. Genetic differences detected by comparative genomic hybridization in head and neck squamous cell carcinomas from different tumor sites: construction of oncogenetic trees for tumor progression. *Genes Chromosomes Cancer* 2002;34(2):224–233.
155. Hermsen M, Guervos MA, Meijer G, et al. New chromosomal regions with high-level amplifications in squamous cell carcinomas of the larynx and pharynx, identified by comparative genomic hybridization. *J Pathol* 2001;194(2):177–182.
156. Hermsen M, Alonso Guervos M, Meijer G, et al. Chromosomal changes in relation to clinical outcome in larynx and pharynx squamous cell carcinoma. *Cell Oncol* 2005;27(3): 191–198.
157. Narayana A, Vaughan AT, Gunaratne S, et al. Is p53 an independent prognostic factor in patients with laryngeal carcinoma? *Cancer* 1998;82(2):286–291.
158. Ferlito A. Diagnosis and treatment of verrucous squamous cell carcinoma of the larynx: a critical review. *Ann Otol Rhinol Laryngol* 1985;94(6 Pt 1):575–579.
159. Ferlito A, Recher G. Ackerman's tumor (verrucous carcinoma) of the larynx: a clinicopathologic study of 77 cases. *Cancer* 1980;46(7):1617–1630.
160. Maurizi M, Cadoni G, Ottaviani F, et al. Verrucous squamous cell carcinoma of the larynx: diagnostic and therapeutic considerations. *Eur Arch Otorhinolaryngol* 1996;253(3):130–135.
161. McCaffrey TV, Witte M, Ferguson MT. Verrucous carcinoma of the larynx. *Ann Otol Rhinol Laryngol* 1998;107(5 Pt 1):391–395.
162. Orvidas LJ, Olsen KD, Lewis JE, et al. Verrucous carcinoma of the larynx: a review of 53 patients. *Head Neck* 1998;20(3):197–203.
163. Ryan RE, Jr., DeSanto LW, Devine KD, et al. Verrucous carcinoma of the larynx. *Laryngoscope* 1977;87(12):1989–1994.
164. Abramson AL, Brandsma J, Steinberg B, et al. Verrucous carcinoma of the larynx. Possible human papillomavirus etiology. *Arch Otolaryngol* 1985;111(11):709–715.
165. Brandsma JL, Steinberg BM, Abramson AL, et al. Presence of human papillomavirus type 16 related sequences in verrucous carcinoma of the larynx. *Cancer Res* 1986;46(4 Pt 2): 2185–2188.
166. Fliss DM, Noble-Topham SE, McLachlin M, et al. Laryngeal verrucous carcinoma: a clinicopathologic study and detection of human papillomavirus using polymerase chain reaction. *Laryngoscope* 1994;104(2):146–152.
167. Gimenez-Conti IB, Collet AM, Lanfranchi H, et al. p53, Rb, and cyclin D1 expression in human oral verrucous carcinomas. *Cancer* 1996;78(1):17–23.
168. Choi HR, Roberts DB, Johnigan RH, et al. Molecular and clinicopathologic comparisons of head and neck squamous carcinoma variants: common and distinctive features of biological significance. *Am J Surg Pathol* 2004;28(10):1299–1310.
169. Kraus FT, Perezmesa C. Verrucous carcinoma. Clinical and pathologic study of 105 cases involving oral cavity, larynx and genitalia. *Cancer* 1966;19(1):26–38.
170. Batsakis JG, Rice DH, Howard DR. The pathology of head and neck tumors: spindle cell lesions (sarcomatoid carcinomas, nodular fasciitis, and fibrosarcoma) of the aerodigestive tracts, Part 14. *Head Neck Surg* 1982;4(6):499–513.
171. Ellis GL, Langloss JM, Heffner DK, et al. Spindle-cell carcinoma of the aerodigestive tract. An immunohistochemical analysis of 21 cases. *Am J Surg Pathol* 1987;11(5):335–342.
172. Lewis JE, Olsen KD, Sebo TJ. Spindle cell carcinoma of the larynx: review of 26 cases including DNA content and immunohistochemistry. *Hum Pathol* 1997;28(6):664–673.
173. Olsen KD, Lewis JE, Suman VJ. Spindle cell carcinoma of the larynx and hypopharynx. *Otolaryngol Head Neck Surg* 1997;116(1):47–52.
174. Thompson LD, Wieneke JA, Miettinen M, et al. Spindle cell (sarcomatoid) carcinomas of the larynx: a clinicopathologic study of 187 cases. *Am J Surg Pathol* 2002;26(2):153–170.
175. Zarbo RJ, Crissman JD, Venkat H, et al. Spindle-cell carcinoma of the upper aerodigestive tract mucosa. An immunohistologic and ultrastructural study of 18 biphasic tumors and comparison with seven monophasic spindle-cell tumors. *Am J Surg Pathol* 1986;10(11): 741–753.
176. Leventon GS, Evans HL. Sarcomatoid squamous cell carcinoma of the mucous membranes of the head and neck: a clinicopathologic study of 20 cases. *Cancer* 1981;48(4):994–1003.
177. Ansari-Lari MA, Hoque MO, Califano J, et al. Immunohistochemical p53 expression patterns in sarcomatoid carcinomas of the upper respiratory tract. *Am J Surg Pathol* 2002; 26(8):1024–1031.
178. Rizzardi C, Frezzini C, Maglione M, et al. A look at the biology of spindle cell squamous carcinoma of the oral cavity: report of a case. *J Oral Maxillofac Surg* 2003;61(2):264–268.
179. Lewis JS, Ritter JH, El-Mofty S. Alternative epithelial markers in sarcomatoid carcinomas of the head and neck, lung, and bladder-p63, MOC-31, and TTF-1. *Mod Pathol* 2005; 18(11):1471–1481.
180. Suarez PA, Adler-Storthz K, Luna MA, et al. Papillary squamous cell carcinomas of the upper aerodigestive tract: a clinicopathologic and molecular study. *Head Neck* 2000;22(4): 360–368.
181. Thompson LD, Wenig BM, Heffner DK, et al. Exophytic and papillary squamous cell carcinomas of the larynx: a clinicopathologic series of 104 cases. *Otolaryngol Head Neck Surg* 1999;120(5):718–724.

182. Ereno C, Lopez JI, Sanchez JM, et al. Papillary squamous cell carcinoma of the larynx. *J Laryngol Otol* 2001;115(2):164–166.

183. Ferlito A, Devaney KO, Rinaldo A, et al. Papillary squamous cell carcinoma versus verrucous squamous cell carcinoma of the head and neck. *Ann Otol Rhinol Laryngol* 1999;108(3):318–322.

184. Ferlito A, Altavilla G, Rinaldo A, et al. Basaloid squamous cell carcinoma of the larynx and hypopharynx. *Ann Otol Rhinol Laryngol* 1997;106(12):1024–1035.

185. Banks ER, Frierson HF, Jr., Mills SE, et al. Basaloid squamous cell carcinoma of the head and neck. A clinicopathologic and immunohistochemical study of 40 cases. *Am J Surg Pathol* 1992;16(10):939–946.

186. Alos L, Castillo M, Nadal A, et al. Adenosquamous carcinoma of the head and neck: criteria for diagnosis in a study of 12 cases. *Histopathology* 2004;44(6):570–579.

187. Damiani JM, Damiani KK, Hauck K, et al. Mucoepidermoid-adenosquamous carcinoma of the larynx and hypopharynx: a report of 21 cases and a review of the literature. *Otolaryngol Head Neck Surg* 1981;89(2):235–243.

188. Fujino K, Ito J, Kanaji M, et al. Adenosquamous carcinoma of the larynx. *Am J Otolaryngol* 1995;16(2):115–118.

189. Gerughty RM, Hennigar GR, Brown FM. Adenosquamous carcinoma of the nasal, oral and laryngeal cavities. A clinicopathologic survey of ten cases. *Cancer* 1968;22(6):1140–1155.

190. Ferlito A, Devaney KO, Rinaldo A, et al. Mucosal adenoid squamous cell carcinoma of the head and neck. *Ann Otol Rhinol Laryngol* 1996;105(5):409–413.

191. Sone M, Nakashima T, Nagasaka T, et al. Lymphoepithelioma-like carcinoma of the larynx associated with an Epstein-Barr viral infection. *Otolaryngol Head Neck Surg* 1998;119(1):134–137.

192. Tardio JC, Cristobal E, Burgos F, et al. Absence of EBV genome in lymphoepithelioma-like carcinomas of the larynx. *Histopathology* 1997;30(2):126–128.

193. D'Souza G, Kreimer AR, Viscidi R, et al. Case-control study of human papillomavirus and oropharyngeal cancer. *N Engl J Med* 2007;356(19):1944–1956.

194. Stelow EB, Bellizzi AM, Taneja T, et al. NUT rearrangement in undifferentiated carcinomas of the upper aerodigestive tract. *Am J Surg Pathol* 2008;32(6):828–834.

195. Heffner DK. Sinonasal and laryngeal salivary gland lesions. In Ellis GL, Auclair PL, Gnepp DR, eds. *Surgical Pathology of the Salivary Glands. Volume 25, Major Problems in Pathology.* Philadelphia, PA: WB Saunders Company, 1991:544–559.

196. Batsakis JG, Luna MA, el-Naggar AK. Nonsquamous carcinomas of the larynx. *Ann Otol Rhinol Laryngol* 1992;101(12):1024–1026.

197. Cohen J, Guillamondegui OM, Batsakis JG, et al. Cancer of the minor salivary glands of the larynx. *Am J Surg* 1985;150(4):513–518.

198. Crissman JD, Rosenblatt A. Acinous cell carcinoma of the larynx. *Arch Pathol Lab Med* 1978;102(5):233–236.

199. Fechner RE. Adenocarcinoma of the larynx. *Can J Otolaryngol* 1975;4(2):284–289.

200. Ferlito A. Acinic cell carcinoma of minor salivary glands. *Histopathology* 1980;4(3):331–343.

201. Ganly I, Patel SG, Coleman M, et al. Malignant minor salivary gland tumors of the larynx. *Arch Otolaryngol Head Neck Surg* 2006;132(7):767–770.

202. Goel MM, Agrawal SP, Srivastava AN. Salivary duct carcinoma of the larynx: report of a rare case. *Ear Nose Throat J* 2003;82(5):371–373.

203. Mahlstedt K, Ussmuller J, Donath K. Malignant sialogenic tumours of the larynx. *J Laryngol Otol* 2002;116(2):119–122.

204. Nascimento AG, Amaral AL, Prado LA, et al. Adenoid cystic carcinoma of salivary glands. A study of 61 cases with clinicopathologic correlation. *Cancer* 1986;57(2):312–319.

205. Olofsson J, van Nostrand AW. Adenoid cystic carcinoma of the larynx: a report of four cases and a review of the literature. *Cancer* 1977;40(3):1307–1313.

206. Som PM, Nagel BD, Feuerstein SS, et al. Benign pleomorphic adenoma of the larynx. A case report. *Ann Otol Rhinol Laryngol* 1979;88(1 Pt 1):112–114.

207. Spiro RH, Koss LG, Hajdu SI, et al. Tumors of minor salivary origin. A clinicopathologic study of 492 cases. *Cancer* 1973;31(1):117–129.

208. Stillwagon GB, Smith RR, Highstein C, et al. Adenoid cystic carcinoma of the supraglottic larynx: report of a case and review of the literature. *Am J Otolaryngol* 1985;6(4):309–314.

209. MacMillan RH 3rd, Fechner RE. Pleomorphic adenoma of the larynx. *Arch Pathol Lab Med* 1986;110(3):245–247.

210. Zakzouk MS. Pleomorphic adenoma of the larynx. *J Laryngol Otol* 1985;99(6):611–616.

211. Ferlito A. Malignant laryngeal epithelial tumors and lymph node involvement: therapeutic and prognostic considerations. *Ann Otol Rhinol Laryngol* 1987;96(5):542–548.

212. Ferlito A, Recher G, Bottin R. Mucoepidermoid carcinoma of the larynx. A clinicopathological study of 11 cases with review of the literature. *ORL J Otorhinolaryngol Relat Spec* 1981;43(5):280–299.

213. Nistal M, Yebenes-Gregorio L, Esteban-Rodriguez I, et al. Malignant mixed tumor of the larynx. *Head Neck* 2005;27(2):166–170.

214. Seo IS, Tomich CE, Warfel KA, et al. Clear cell carcinoma of the larynx. A variant of mucoepidermoid carcinoma. *Ann Otol Rhinol Laryngol* 1980;89(2 Pt 1):168–172.

215. Batsakis JG, el-Naggar AK, Luna MA. Neuroendocrine tumors of larynx. *Ann Otol Rhinol Laryngol* 1992;101(8):710–714.

216. Ferlito A, Barnes L, Rinaldo A, et al. A review of neuroendocrine neoplasms of the larynx: update on diagnosis and treatment. *J Laryngol Otol* 1998;112(9):827–834.

217. Mills SE. Neuroectodermal neoplasms of the head and neck with emphasis on neuroendocrine carcinomas. *Mod Pathol* 2002;15(3):264–278.

218. Barnes L. Neuroendocrine tumors. In Barnes L, Eveson JE, Reichart P, et al, eds. *Pathology and Genetics of Head and Neck Tumours.* Lyon, France: IARC Press, 2005:135–139.

219. Woodruff JM, Huvos AG, Erlandson RA, et al. Neuroendocrine carcinomas of the larynx. A study of two types, one of which mimics thyroid medullary carcinoma. *Am J Surg Pathol* 1985;9(11):771–790.

220. Mills SE, Johns ME. Atypical carcinoid tumor of the larynx. A light microscopic and ultrastructural study. *Arch Otolaryngol* 1984;110(1):58–62.

221. Milroy CM, Rode J, Moss E. Laryngeal paragangliomas and neuroendocrine carcinomas. *Histopathology* 1991;18(3):201–209.

222. Gnepp DR, Ferlito A, Hyams V. Primary anaplastic small cell (oat cell) carcinoma of the larynx. Review of the literature and report of 18 cases. *Cancer* 1983;51(9):1731–1745.

223. Mills SE, Cooper PH, Garland TA, et al. Small cell undifferentiated carcinoma of the larynx. Report of two patients and review of 13 additional cases. *Cancer* 1983;51(1):116–120.

224. Salim SA, Milroy C, Rode J, et al. Immunocytochemical characterization of neuroendocrine tumours of the larynx. *Histopathology* 1993;23(1):69–73.

225. Barnes L. Paraganglioma of the larynx. A critical review of the literature. *ORL J Otorhinolaryngol Relat Spec* 1991;53(4):220–234.

226. Lack EE, Cubilla AL, Woodruff JM. Paragangliomas of the head and neck region. A pathologic study of tumors from 71 patients. *Hum Pathol* 1979;10(2):191–218.

227. Lack EE, Cubilla AL, Woodruff JM, et al. Paragangliomas of the head and neck region: a clinical study of 69 patients. *Cancer* 1977;39(2):397–409.

228. Myssiorek D, Rinaldo A, Barnes L, et al. Laryngeal paraganglioma: an updated critical review. *Acta Otolaryngol* 2004;124(9):995–999.

229. Johnson TL, Zarbo RJ, Lloyd RV, et al. Paragangliomas of the head and neck: immunohistochemical neuroendocrine and intermediate filament typing. *Mod Pathol* 1988;1(3):216–223.

230. Achilles E, Padberg BC, Holl K, et al. Immunocytochemistry of paragangliomas—value of staining for S-100 protein and glial fibrillary acid protein in diagnosis and prognosis. *Histopathology* 1991;18(5):453–458.

231. Cummings CW, Montgomery WW, Balogh K, Jr. Neurogenic tumors of the larynx. *Ann Otol Rhinol Laryngol* 1969;78(1):76–95.

232. Rahbar R, Litrovnik BG, Vargas SO, et al. The biology and management of laryngeal neurofibroma. *Arch Otolaryngol Head Neck Surg* 2004;130(12):1400–1406.

233. Stanley RJ, Scheithauer BW, Weiland LH, et al. Neural and neuroendocrine tumors of the larynx. *Ann Otol Rhinol Laryngol* 1987;96(6):630–638.

234. Willcox TO, Jr., Rosenberg SI, Handler SD. Laryngeal involvement in neurofibromatosis. *Ear Nose Throat J* 1993;72(12):811–812, 815.

235. Rosen FS, Pou AM, Quinn FB, Jr. Obstructive supraglottic schwannoma: a case report and review of the literature. *Laryngoscope* 2002;112(6):997–1002.

236. Lack EE, Worsham GF, Callihan MD, et al. Granular cell tumor: a clinicopathologic study of 110 patients. *J Surg Oncol* 1980;13(4):301–316.

237. Filie AC, Lage JM, Azumi N. Immunoreactivity of S100 protein, alpha-1-antitrypsin, and CD68 in adult and congenital granular cell tumors. *Mod Pathol* 1996;9(9):888–892.

238. Mazur MT, Shultz JJ, Myers JL. Granular cell tumor. Immunohistochemical analysis of 21 benign tumors and one malignant tumor. *Arch Pathol Lab Med* 1990;114(7):692–696.

239. Nathrath WB, Remberger K. Immunohistochemical study of granular cell tumours. Demonstration of neurone specific enolase, S 100 protein, laminin and alpha-1-antichymotrypsin. *Virchows Arch A Pathol Anat Histopathol* 1986;408(4):421–434.

240. Nandapalan V, Roland NJ, Helliwell TR, et al. Mucosal melanoma of the head and neck. *Clin Otolaryngol Allied Sci* 1998;23(2):107–116.

241. Wenig BM. Laryngeal mucosal malignant melanoma. A clinicopathologic, immunohistochemical, and ultrastructural study of four patients and a review of the literature. *Cancer* 1995;75(7):1568–1577.

242. Curtiss C, Kosinski AA. Primary melanoma of the larynx; report of a case and review of the literature. *Cancer* 1955;8(5):961–963.

243. Reuter VE, Woodruff JM. Melanoma of the larynx. *Laryngoscope* 1986;96(4):389–393.

244. El-Monem MH, Gaafar AH, Magdy EA. Lipomas of the head and neck: presentation variability and diagnostic work-up. *J Laryngol Otol* 2006;120(1):47–55.

245. Golledge J, Fisher C, Rhys-Evans PH. Head and neck liposarcoma. *Cancer* 1995;76(6):1051–1058.

246. Wenig BM. Lipomas of the larynx and hypopharynx: a review of the literature with the addition of three new cases. *J Laryngol Otol* 1995;109(4):353–357.

247. Wenig BM, Heffner DK. Liposarcomas of the larynx and hypopharynx: a clinicopathologic study of eight new cases and a review of the literature. *Laryngoscope* 1995;105(7 Pt 1):747–756.

248. Wenig BM, Weiss SW, Gnepp DR. Laryngeal and hypopharyngeal liposarcoma. A clinicopathologic study of 10 cases with a comparison to soft-tissue counterparts. *Am J Surg Pathol* 1990;14(2):134–141.

249. Hicks J, Flaitz C. Rhabdomyosarcoma of the head and neck in children. *Oral Oncol* 2002;38(5):450–459.

250. Kapadia SB, Meis JM, Frisman DM, et al. Fetal rhabdomyoma of the head and neck: a clinicopathologic and immunophenotypic study of 24 cases. *Hum Pathol* 1993;24(7):754–765.

251. Kapadia SB, Meis JM, Frisman DM, et al. Adult rhabdomyoma of the head and neck: a clinicopathologic and immunophenotypic study. *Hum Pathol* 1993;24(6):608–617.

252. Kleinsasser O, Glanz H. Myogenic tumours of the larynx. *Arch Otorhinolaryngol* 1979;225(2):107–119.

253. Matsumoto T, Nishiya M, Ichikawa G, et al. Leiomyoma with atypical cells (atypical leiomyoma) in the larynx. *Histopathology* 1999;34(6):532–536.

254. McKiernan DC, Watters GW. Smooth muscle tumours of the larynx. *J Laryngol Otol* 1995;109(1):77–79.

255. Willis J, Abdul-Karim FW, di Sant'Agnese PA. Extracardiac rhabdomyomas. *Semin Diagn Pathol* 1994;11(1):15–25.

256. Allen PW. The fibromatoses: a clinicopathologic classification based on 140 cases. *Am J Surg Pathol* 1977;1(3):255–270.

257. Coffin CM, Watterson J, Priest JR, et al. Extrapulmonary inflammatory myofibroblastic tumor (inflammatory pseudotumor). A clinicopathologic and immunohistochemical study of 84 cases. *Am J Surg Pathol* 1995;19(8):859–872.

258. Dotto JE, Ahrens W, Lesnik DJ, et al. Solitary fibrous tumor of the larynx: a case report and review of the literature. *Arch Pathol Lab Med* 2006;130(2):213–216.

259. Frankenthaler R, Ayala AG, Hartwick RW, et al. Fibrosarcoma of the head and neck. *Laryngoscope* 1990;100(8):799–802.

260. Wenig BM, Devaney K, Bisceglia M. Inflammatory myofibroblastic tumor of the larynx.

A clinicopathologic study of eight cases simulating a malignant spindle cell neoplasm. *Cancer* 1995;76(11):2217–2229.

261. Mirra M, Calo S, Salviato T, et al. Aggressive fibromatosis of the larynx: report of a new case in an adult patient and review of the literature. *Pathol Res Pract* 2001;197(1):51–55; discussion 56–58.

262. Bridger GP, Nassar VH, Skinner HG. Hemangioma in the adult larynx. *Arch Otolaryngol* 1970;92(5):493–498.

263. Coffin CM, Dehner LP. Vascular tumors in children and adolescents: a clinicopathologic study of 228 tumors in 222 patients. *Pathol Annu* 1993;28(Pt 1):97–120.

264. Seikaly H, Cuyler JP. Infantile subglottic hemangioma. *J Otolaryngol* 1994;23(2):135–137.

265. Fechner RE, Cooper PH, Mills SE. Pyogenic granuloma of the larynx and trachea. A causal and pathologic misnomer for granulation tissue. *Arch Otolaryngol* 1981;107(1):30–32.

266. Emery PJ, Bailey CM, Evans JN. Cystic hygroma of the head and neck. A review of 37 cases. *J Laryngol Otol* 1984;98(6):613–619.

267. Sezgin S, Kotiloglu E, Kaya H, et al. Extravascular papillary endothelial hyperplasia of the larynx: a case report and review of the literature. *Ear Nose Throat J* 2005;84(1):52–53.

268. Mark RJ, Tran LM, Sercarz J, et al. Angiosarcoma of the head and neck. The UCLA experience 1955 through 1990. *Arch Otolaryngol Head Neck Surg* 1993;119(9):973–978.

269. Sciot R, Delaere P, Van Damme B, et al. Angiosarcoma of the larynx. *Histopathology* 1995; 26(2):177–180.

270. Abramson AL, Simons RL. Kaposi's sarcoma of the head and neck. *Arch Otolaryngol* 1970; 92(5):505–508.

271. Boscaino A, Errico ME, Orabona P, et al. Epithelioid hemangioendothelioma of the larynx. *Tumori* 1999;85(6):515–518.

272. Loos BM, Wieneke JA, Thompson LD. Laryngeal angiosarcoma: a clinicopathologic study of five cases with a review of the literature. *Laryngoscope* 2001;111(7):1197–1202.

273. Traweek ST, Kandalaft PL, Mehta P, et al. The human hematopoietic progenitor cell antigen (CD34) in vascular neoplasia. *Am J Clin Pathol* 1991;96(1):25–31.

274. Robin YM, Guillou L, Michels JJ, et al. Human herpesvirus 8 immunostaining: a sensitive and specific method for diagnosing Kaposi sarcoma in paraffin-embedded sections. *Am J Clin Pathol* 2004;121(3):330–334.

275. Casiraghi O, Martinez-Madrigal F, Pineda-Daboin K, et al. Chondroid tumors of the larynx: a clinicopathologic study of 19 cases, including two dedifferentiated chondrosarcomas. *Ann Diagn Pathol* 2004;8(4):189–197.

276. Thompson LD, Gannon FH. Chondrosarcoma of the larynx: a clinicopathologic study of 111 cases with a review of the literature. *Am J Surg Pathol* 2002;26(7):836–851.

277. Devaney KO, Ferlito A, Silver CE. Cartilaginous tumors of the larynx. *Ann Otol Rhinol Laryngol* 1995;104(3):251–255.

278. Lewis JE, Olsen KD, Inwards CY. Cartilaginous tumors of the larynx: clinicopathologic review of 47 cases. *Ann Otol Rhinol Laryngol* 1997;106(2):94–100.

279. Thome R, Thome DC, de la Cortina RA. Long-term follow-up of cartilaginous tumors of the larynx. *Otolaryngol Head Neck Surg* 2001;124(6):634–640.

280. Brandwein M, Moore S, Som P, et al. Laryngeal chondrosarcomas: a clinicopathologic study of 11 cases, including two "dedifferentiated" chondrosarcomas. *Laryngoscope* 1992; 102(8):858–867.

281. Finn DG, Goepfert H, Batsakis JG. Chondrosarcoma of the head and neck. *Laryngoscope* 1984;94(12 Pt 1):1539–1544.

282. Huizenga C, Balogh K. Cartilaginous tumors of the larynx. A clinicopathologic study of 10 new cases and a review of the literature. *Cancer* 1970;26(1):201–210.

283. Athre RS, Vories A, Mudrovich S, et al. Osteosarcomas of the larynx. *Laryngoscope* 2005; 115(1):74–77.

284. Madrigal FM, Godoy LM, Daboin KP, et al. Laryngeal osteosarcoma: a clinicopathologic analysis of four cases and comparison with a carcinosarcoma. *Ann Diagn Pathol* 2002;6(1): 1–9.

285. Topaloglu I, Isiksacan V, Ulusoy S, et al. Osteosarcoma of the larynx. *Otolaryngol Head Neck Surg* 2004;131(5):789–790.

286. Devaney KO, Ferlito A, Rinaldo A. Giant cell tumor of the larynx. *Ann Otol Rhinol Laryngol* 1998;107(8):729–732.

287. Wieneke JA, Gannon FH, Heffner DK, et al. Giant cell tumor of the larynx: a clinicopathologic series of eight cases and a review of the literature. *Mod Pathol* 2001;14(12):1209–1215.

288. Della Libera D, Redlich G, Bittesini L, et al. Aneurysmal bone cyst of the larynx presenting with hypoglottic obstruction. *Arch Pathol Lab Med* 2001;125(5):673–676.

289. Roth JA, Enzinger FM, Tannenbaum M. Synovial sarcoma of the neck: a follow-up study of 24 cases. *Cancer* 1975;35(4):1243–1253.

290. Weiss SW, Goldblum JR. *Malignant Soft Tissue Tumors of Uncertain Type. Soft Tissue Tumors.* St. Louis, MO: Mosby, 2001:1483–1571.

291. Sandberg AA, Bridge JA. Updates on the cytogenetics and molecular genetics of bone and soft tissue tumors. Synovial sarcoma. *Cancer Genet Cytogenet* 2002;133(1):1–23.

292. Kuhel WI, Monhian N, Shanahan EM, et al. Epithelioid sarcoma of the neck: a rare tumor mimicking metastatic carcinoma from an unknown primary. *Otolaryngol Head Neck Surg* 1997;117(6):S210–S213.

293. Altug T, Inci E, Guvenc MG, et al. Alveolar soft part sarcoma of the larynx. *Eur Arch Otorhinolaryngol* 2007;264(4):445–449.

294. Morgan K, MacLennan KA, Narula A, et al. Non-Hodgkin's lymphoma of the larynx (stage IE). *Cancer* 1989;64(5):1123–1127.

295. Swerdlow JB, Merl SA, Davey FR, et al. Non-Hodgkin's lymphoma limited to the larynx. *Cancer* 1984;53(11):2546–2549.

296. Kuhn JJ, Wenig BM, Clark DA. Mycosis fungoides of the larynx. Report of two cases and review of the literature. *Arch Otolaryngol Head Neck Surg* 1992;118(8):853–858.

297. Alexiou C, Kau RJ, Dietzfelbinger H, et al. Extramedullary plasmacytoma: tumor occurrence and therapeutic concepts. *Cancer* 1999;85(11):2305–2314.

298. Batsakis JG, Fries GT, Goldman RT, et al. Upper respiratory tract plasmacytoma. *Arch Otolaryngol* 1964;79:613–618.

299. Batsakis JG, Medeiros JL, Luna MA, et al. Plasma cell dyscrasias and the head and neck. *Ann Diagn Pathol* 2002;6(2):129–140.

300. Vega F, Lin P, Medeiros LJ. Extranodal lymphomas of the head and neck. *Ann Diagn Pathol* 2005;9(6):340–350.

301. Abemayor E, Cochran AJ, Calcaterra TC. Metastatic cancer to the larynx. Diagnosis and management. *Cancer* 1983;52(10):1944–1948.

302. Batsakis JG, Luna MA, Byers RM. Metastases to the larynx. *Head Neck Surg* 1985;7(6): 458–460.

303. Ferlito A, Caruso G, Recher G. Secondary laryngeal tumors. Report of seven cases with review of the literature. *Arch Otolaryngol Head Neck Surg* 1988;114(6):635–639.

304. Djalilian M, Beahrs OH, Devine KD, et al. Intraluminal involvement of the larynx and trachea by thyroid cancer. *Am J Surg* 1974;128(4):500–504.

The Ear and Temporal Bone

NORMAL DEVELOPMENT AND STRUCTURE

The ear is the sense organ for hearing and for balance. The ear can be considered as three distinct regions or compartments: the external ear, the middle ear and temporal bone, and the inner ear. The embryology, anatomy, and histology of the ear are complex, so they are briefly discussed here. For a more in-depth discussion of the embryology, anatomy, and histology of the ear, the reader is referred to additional texts (1–6).

EXTERNAL EAR

The external ear develops from the first branchial groove. The external auricle (pinna) forms from the fusion of the auricular hillocks or tubercles—a group of mesenchymal tissue swellings from the first and second branchial arches—that lie around the external portion of the first branchial groove (1). The external auditory canal is considered a normal remnant of the first branchial groove. The tympanic membrane forms from the first and second branchial pouches and the first branchial groove (1). The ectoderm of the first branchial groove gives rise to the epithelium on the external side; the endoderm from the first branchial pouch gives rise to the epithelium on the internal side; and the mesoderm of the first and second branchial pouches gives rise to the connective tissue lying between the external and internal epithelia (1).

The outer portion of the external ear includes the auricle or pinna leading into the external auditory canal, with its medial limit being the external aspect of the tympanic membrane. Histologically, the auricle is essentially a cutaneous structure composed of keratinizing, stratified squamous epithelium with associated dermal adnexal structures, including hair follicles, sebaceous glands, and eccrine sweat glands. The subcutaneous tissue is composed of fibroconnective tissue, fat, and elastic-type fibrocartilage that gives the auricle its structural support. In addition to the dermal adnexal structures, the outer third of the external canal is noteworthy for the presence of modified apocrine glands called *ceruminal glands* that replace the eccrine glands seen in the auricular dermis. Ceruminal glands produce cerumen, and they are arranged in clusters composed of cuboidal cells with eosinophilic cytoplasm often containing a granular, golden-yellow pigment. These cells have secretory droplets along their luminal border. In the inner portion of the external auditory canal, ceruminal glands, as well as the other adnexal structures, are absent. Similar to the auricle, the external auditory canal is lined by keratinizing squamous epithelium that extends to include the entire canal and that covers the external aspect of the tympanic membrane. The inner two-thirds of the external auditory canal contains bone rather than cartilage.

MIDDLE EAR

The middle ear space develops from invagination of the first branchial pouch (pharyngotympanic tube) from the primitive pharynx. The eustachian tube and tympanic cavity develop from the endoderm of the first branchial pouch; the malleus and incus develop from the mesoderm of the first branchial arch (Meckel cartilage), and the stapes develops from the mesoderm of the second branchial arch (Reichert cartilage) (1).

The middle ear or tympanic cavity contents include the ossicles (malleus, incus, and stapes), eustachian tube, tympanic cavity proper, epitympanic recess, mastoid cavity, and the chorda tympani of the facial nerve (7th cranial nerve). The middle ear, as well as the external ear, functions as a conduit for sound conduction for the auditory part of the internal ear. The anatomic limits of the middle ear include the following: (a) a lateral or internal aspect made up by the tympanic membrane and the squamous portion of the temporal bone; (b) a medial aspect bordered by the petrous portion of the temporal bone; (c) a superior (roof) delimited by the tegmen tympani, a thin plate of bone separating the middle ear space from the cranial cavity; (d) an inferior (floor) aspect bordered by a thin plate of bone separating the tympanic cavity from the superior bulb of the internal jugular vein; (e) an anterior aspect delimited by a thin plate of bone separating the tympanic cavity from the carotid canal housing the internal carotid artery; and (f) a posterior aspect delimited by the petrous portion of the temporal bone, which contains the mastoid antrum and mastoid air cells. Histologically, the lining of the middle ear is a respiratory epithelium varying from ciliated epithelium in the eustachian tube to a flat, single, cuboidal epithelium in the tympanic cavity and mastoid. The epithelium lining the eustachian tube becomes pseudostratified as it approaches the pharyngeal end. Under normal conditions, no glandular elements are found within the middle ear. The eustachian tubes contain a lymphoid component, particularly in children, that is referred to as Gerlach tubal tonsil. The ossicular articulations are typical synovial joints.

INNER EAR

The first division of the ear that develops is the inner ear, which appears toward the end of the first month of gestation (1,2). The membranous labyrinth, including the utricle, saccule, semicircular ducts, and cochlear duct, arises from the otic vesicle (otocyst). The otic vesicle forms from the invagination of the surface ectoderm located on either side of the neural plate into the mesenchyme. This invagination eventually loses its connection with the surface ectoderm. The bony labyrinth, including the vestibule, semicircular canals, and cochlea arises from the mesenchyme around the otic vesicle (1,2).

The internal ear is embedded within the petrous portion of the temporal bone, and it consists of the structures of the membranous and osseous labyrinth and the internal auditory canal in which the vestibulocochlear (8th) nerve runs. The internal ear is the sense organ for hearing and balance. The anatomy and histology of this region are complex and beyond the scope of this chapter. The reader is referred to specific texts detailing the anatomy and histology of the inner ear (4,5). Similarly, the interested reader is referred to other texts that describe the role of the auditory and vestibular systems in the physiologic aspects of hearing and balance (7–9).

RESECTION SPECIMENS

Most surgical specimens taken from the ear are small, so they are handled in a similar manner to small biopsies of other regions of the body. Less often, the surgical pathologist may be confronted with larger resection specimens of the external ear or auditory canal for a cutaneous-type neoplasm (e.g., squamous cell carcinoma, malignant melanoma). This type of resection may include the pinna, deep external auditory canal, tympanic membrane, and portions of the middle ear. Orientation of the specimen with the identification of the surgical margins of resection is essential for the proper sectioning of the specimen. Occasionally, the surgical pathologist may be confronted with a more complex (radical) resection specimen of the ear that includes not only the external ear and portions of the middle ear but also the entire middle ear space, as well as portions of the inner ear. Such procedures include petrosectomy and tympanomastoidectomy, which provide anatomically complex specimens that require close interaction with the neuro-otologic surgeon for specimen orientation; determination of the site of lesion; and, perhaps most importantly, the identification of the surgical margins of resection. These larger procedures invariably include portions of rather thick bone, which necessitate extensive decalcification. In some surgical procedures of the ear, smaller and less thick bone is excised (e.g., stapedectomy), for which only brief decalcification is required. Resection specimens of stapes superstructure or of the whole stapes should be oriented for embedding after decalcification so that the outline of the whole ossicle is revealed in the section.

NONNEOPLASTIC LESIONS OF THE EAR AND TEMPORAL BONE

The classification of nonneoplastic lesions of the ear and temporal bone is detailed in Table 23.1.

CONGENITAL ABNORMALITIES OF THE EAR

The ear, including the external, middle, and internal ear, is often the target for congenital anomalies. These congenital abnormalities occur as an isolated defect or in combination with other aural and extra-aural abnormalities, and they vary from cosmetic defects to complete hearing loss. A complete discussion of the developmental defects of the ear is beyond the scope of this chapter; the interested reader is referred to other texts that discuss this subject (10–12). This section includes the more common developmental abnormalities the surgical pathologist is likely to encounter in daily practice.

ACCESSORY TRAGI

Accessory tragi, which are also referred to as accessory or supernumerary ears, accessory auricle, and polyotia, appear at birth;

TABLE 23.1
Classification of Nonneoplastic Lesions of the Ear and Temporal Bone

External Ear

Developmental (accessory tragi; first branchial cleft anomalies, others)
Infectious and inflammatory
   Keloid
   Epidermal and sebaceous cysts
   Idiopathic cystic chondromalacia
   Chondrodermatitis nodularis helicis chronicus
   Angiolymphoid hyperplasia with eosinophilia/Kimura disease
Autoimmune systemic diseases
   Relapsing polychondritis
   Gout
   Wegener's granulomatosis
Others
   Exostosis
   Synovial chondromatosis

Middle and Inner Ear, Including Temporal Bone

Developmental and congenital anomalies
Infectious (otitis media) and inflammatory
Otic or aural polyp
Cholesteatoma
Langerhans cell histiocytosis (eosinophilic granuloma)
Heterotopias (central nervous system tissue; salivary gland)
Otosclerosis
Paget disease
Ménière disease
Others

they may be solitary or multiple, unilateral or bilateral, sessile or pedunculated, soft or cartilaginous, skin-covered nodules or papules. They are located on the skin surface, often anterior to the auricle; clinically, they may be mistaken for a papilloma. Histologically, accessory tragi recapitulate the normal external auricle and include the skin, cutaneous adnexal structures, and a central core of cartilage (Fig. 23.1). Squamous papillomas

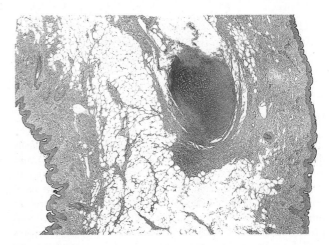

Figure 23.1. Accessory tragus. Histologically, accessory tragi have the appearance of the normal external auricle, as the presence of skin (including keratinizing squamous epithelium), cutaneous adnexal structures, and a central core of cartilage demonstrate.

lack cutaneous adnexal structures and cartilage (13). Accessory tragi are thought to be related to the second branchial arch anomalies. Accessory tragi may occur independent of other congenital anomalies, but they may be observed in association with cleft palate or lip, mandibular hypoplasia, or other anomalies such as Goldenhar syndrome (oculoauriculovertebral dysplasia) (10).

BRANCHIAL CLEFT ANOMALIES

First Branchial Cleft Anomalies

CLINICAL FEATURES. First branchial cleft anomalies typically occur in the area of the external ear and include cysts, sinuses, and fistulas (14). In comparison to second branchial cleft anomalies, first branchial cleft anomalies are uncommon, representing only 1% to 8% of all branchial apparatus defects. First branchial cleft anomalies may be identified in a variety of locations, including preauricular, postauricular, or infraauricular sites; at the angle of the jaw; associated with the ear lobe; and in the external auditory canal or involving the parotid gland. Involvement of the external auditory canal may result in otalgia or otorrhea. Parotid involvement may result in an intraparotid or periparotid mass. The majority of first branchial cleft anomalies are cysts representing more than two-thirds (68%) of these anomalies (14,15). Sinuses and fistulas equally make up the remainder of these lesions. The fistula tract in first branchial cleft anomalies may extend from the skin over or through the parotid and open in the external auditory canal.

PATHOLOGIC FEATURES. Some authors believe that first branchial cleft lesions can be divided into two types (16,17). Type I lesions contain only ectodermal elements, including keratinizing squamous epithelium without adnexal structures or cartilage, duplicating the membranous external auditory canal. Type II lesions show both ectodermal and mesodermal elements, including keratinized squamous epithelium, cutaneous adnexa, and cartilage, thereby duplicating the external auditory canal and pinna. Olsen et al. (14) believed that the histology between types I and II overlapped and, therefore, recommended that these anomalies should be classified into cyst, sinus, or fistula.

INFECTIOUS AND INFLAMMATORY LESIONS OF THE EXTERNAL AND MIDDLE EAR REGION

Necrotizing Malignant External Otitis

CLINICAL FEATURES. Necrotizing malignant external otitis (NEO) is a virulent, potentially fatal form of external otitis related to *Pseudomonas aeruginosa* infection.

NEO primarily affects older patients. The typical clinical setting is that of a diabetic patient or a patient who is chronically debilitated or immunologically deficient, although NEO may occur in nondebilitated patients (18–20). NEO originates in the external auditory canal with the initial symptoms of an acute otitis externa. With the progression of disease, pain, purulent otorrhea, and swelling occur. If it is left untreated, the infectious process may extend into the surrounding soft tissue structures (cellulitis), the cartilage (chondritis), bone (osteomyelitis), the base of the skull, and the middle ear space, leading to cranial nerve palsies, meningitis, intracranial venous thrombosis, or brain abscess.

The pathogenesis of NEO is related to tissue ischemia secondary to an underlying predisposing pathologic state (diabetic angiopathy) and a migratory defect of polymorphonuclear leukocytes related to systemic disease. These host factors that impede the inflammatory response to infection, when combined with the destructive properties of *P. aeruginosa*, are thought to be responsible for the lethal potential of NEO (18). By virtue of its endotoxins and exotoxins, neurotoxins, collagenases, and elastases, the organism is capable of causing rapid extensive tissue necrosis and necrotizing vasculitis that compounds the destruction (18).

Antibiotics, surgical debridement, and control of diabetes mellitus in patients suffering from that disease are the treatments of choice. Mortality rates may exceed 75% if the diagnosis and treatment are delayed (21). Death may result from extensive spread of the infection to adjacent structures, including intracranial involvement. Cures can be achieved with early recognition and aggressive treatment.

PATHOLOGIC FEATURES. The changes of NEO are most pronounced in the osseous portion of the external canal where the destructive infection usually begins. In this area, the skin becomes ulcerated, leaving a layer of thick granulation tissue covering the exposed and irregularly eroded bone, usually along the anterior and inferior surfaces of the external auditory canal (22). Necrotic tissue is abundant in fully developed NEO, and it may, along with purulent exudate, obstruct the canal. The histologic appearance of NEO is dominated by the presence of necrotic material and exuberant granulation tissue. If the epithelium remains, it is ulcerated, with pseudoepitheliomatous hyperplasia adjacent to denuded areas. Diffuse, heavy, acute, and chronic inflammation is seen in the subcutis, and a necrotizing vasculitis is commonly present. The bone and cartilage are necrotic, with acute and chronic inflammatory cells massively infiltrating the adjacent viable bone. Sequestra of nonviable bone or cartilage may be seen. The dermis is eventually replaced by acellular collagen. Gram-negative bacilli are easily demonstrated by tissue Gram stain.

The infectious nature of NEO is usually evident from the clinical course and the histologic findings. The presence of squamous pseudoepitheliomatous hyperplasia may suggest a squamous cell carcinoma. Conversely, squamous cell carcinoma, if it is associated with extensive necrosis, may elude diagnosis by biopsy, yielding only necroinflammatory material such as one finds in NEO. Occasionally, the clinical presentation of squamous cell carcinoma of the external auditory canal may closely mimic NEO (23,24), or the two diseases may occur concurrently (25).

Otitis Media

CLINICAL FEATURES. Otitis media is either an acute or chronic infectious disease of the middle ear space. Otitis media is predominantly, but not exclusively, a childhood disease. The most common organisms implicated in causing disease are *Streptococcus pneumoniae* and *Haemophilus influenzae*. Otoscopic examination reveals a hyperemic, opaque, bulging tympanic membrane with limited mobility; purulent otorrhea may be present. Bilateral involvement is not uncommon. The middle ear infection is believed to result from infection via the eustachian tube either at the time of or following pharyngitis (bacterial or viral).

In general, otitis media is managed medically. However, tissue is removed for histopathologic examination at times.

In the antibiotic era, complications associated with otitis media are not generally seen. However, if it is left unchecked, the complications of otitis media include acute mastoiditis, suppurative labyrinthitis (inflammation of the inner ear), meningitis, and brain abscess (26).

PATHOLOGIC FEATURES. No specific macroscopic features are present. The tissue specimens usually are received as multiple small fragments of soft to rubbery granulation tissue. If tympanosclerosis is present, the tissues may be firm to hard, consisting of calcific debris. In general, all of the tissue fragments should be processed for histologic examination. The histology of otitis media varies depending on the disease state (27). Acute otitis media is virtually never a surgical disease. The middle ear mucosa, which is also referred to as the *mucoperiosteum*, responds to infection with inflammation, hyperemia, polypoid thickening, and edema. The inflammatory infiltrate in acute otitis media is predominantly composed of polymorphonuclear leukocytes with a variable admixture of chronic inflammatory cells. Secretory otitis media refers to otitis media in which associated effusion is present behind an intact tympanic membrane. The exudate may be serous, hemorrhagic, fibrinous, mucoid, purulent, or an admixture of types (28). The inflammatory infiltrate in acute otitis media is composed of polymorphonuclear leukocytes. Acute otitis media usually heals by resorption by the mucoperiosteum. However, localized destruction of the middle ear ossicles may occur. Further, granulation tissue may develop, resulting in scar formation. Fibrosing osteitis is seen in areas of bone destruction that may result in reactive sclerotic bone.

Acute inflammatory cells may be superimposed in a case of chronic otitis media (COM). The histologic changes in COM include a variable amount of chronic inflammatory cells consisting of lymphocytes, histiocytes, plasma cells, and eosinophils. Multinucleated giant cells and foamy histiocytes may be present. The middle ear low cuboidal epithelium may or may not be seen. However, glandular metaplasia (Fig. 23.2), a response of

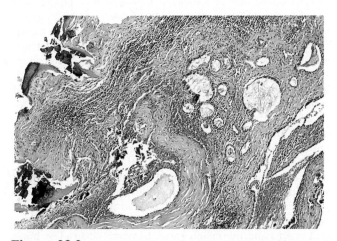

Figure 23.2. Chronic otitis media. The histologic features of chronic otitis media include a background of chronic inflammation composed of lymphocytes with fibrosis and hemorrhage; scattered, unevenly distributed metaplastic glands of variable size and shape that contain thin (serous) fluid and that are separated by abundant stromal tissue are seen. Foci of calcification (tympanosclerosis) are present. In the lower right of the illustration, the normal middle ear low cuboidal epithelium is seen.

the middle ear epithelium to the infectious process, may be present. The glands tend to be more common in nonsuppurative otitis media than in suppurative otitis media. The metaplastic glands are unevenly distributed in the tissue specimens, they are variably shaped, and they are separated by abundant stromal tissue. The glands are lined by columnar to cuboidal epithelium, with or without cilia or goblet cell metaplasia. Glandular secretions may or may not be present, so the glands may appear empty or they may contain varying secretions, including thin (serous) or thick (mucoid) fluid content. The identification of cilia is confirmatory of middle ear glandular metaplasia because this feature is not found in association with middle ear adenomas (29). Furthermore, the haphazard arrangement of the glands in the background of changes of COM should allow the observer to differentiate metaplastic from neoplastic glands.

In addition to the inflammatory cell infiltrate and glandular metaplasia, other histopathologic findings that usually are seen in association with COM or that represent its sequelae include fibrosis, granulation tissue, tympanosclerosis, cholesterol granulomas, and reactive bone formation. Due to the presence of scar tissue, the middle ear ossicles may be destroyed (partially or totally), or they may become immobilized. Perforation of the tympanic membrane pars tensa may occur, with the resulting ingrowth of squamous epithelium potentially leading to the development of cholesteatoma.

Tympanosclerosis represents dystrophic mineralization (calcification or ossification) of the tympanic membrane or middle ear that is associated with recurrent episodes of otitis media (29). The incidence of tympanosclerosis in otitis media varies from 3% to 33% (30). Tympanosclerosis of the tympanic membrane can be seen in children following myringotomy and tube insertion. In this setting, the tympanosclerotic foci may or may not be permanent. Tympanosclerosis of the middle ear typically affects older patients; it represents the irreversible accumulation of mineralized material, and is associated with conductive hearing loss (31,32).

On gross examination, tympanosclerotic foci may be localized or diffuse, and they appear as white nodules or plaques. Histologically, dense clumps of mineralized, calcified, or ossified material or debris can be seen within the stromal tissues or in the middle (connective tissue) aspect of the tympanic membrane (Fig. 23.2). Tympanosclerosis may cause scarring and ossicular fixation.

Cholesterol granulomas represent a foreign body granulomatous response to cholesterol crystals that are derived from the rupture of red blood cells and the resulting breakdown of the lipid layer of the erythrocyte cell membrane. Cholesterol granulomas arise in the middle ear and mastoid in any condition in which hemorrhage occurs in combination with interference in drainage and ventilation of the middle ear space (33). Cholesterol granuloma of the middle ear may present as idiopathic hemotympanum; patients may also complain of hearing loss and tinnitus. The involvement of the petrous apex is more likely to be associated with sensorineural hearing loss, headaches, and cranial nerve deficits; rarely, bone erosion with the involvement of the posterior or middle cranial fossa has been reported (34,35).

The histology of cholesterol granulomas includes the presence of irregular, clear-appearing spaces surrounded by histiocytes or multinucleated giant cells (foreign body granuloma)

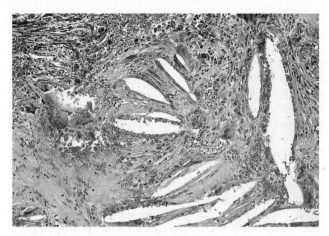

Figure 23.3. Cholesterol granuloma. It appears as empty, irregularly shaped clefts or spaces surrounded by histiocytes and multinucleated giant cells. Fresh hemorrhage and hemosiderin pigment are readily apparent.

(Fig. 23.3). Cholesterol granulomas are not related to cholesteatomas, but they may occur in association with them.

DIFFERENTIAL DIAGNOSIS. The pathologic alterations are generally straightforward, but secondary changes, such as glandular metaplasia of the surface epithelium, which is the result of chronic infection, may occur and might be confused with a true gland-forming neoplasm. The differential diagnosis of the glandular metaplasia seen in otitis media includes middle ear adenoma. The haphazard arrangement of the glands occurring in the background of changes of COM and the presence of cilia should allow one to differentiate metaplastic from neoplastic glands.

Miscellaneous Infections

SPECIFIC CAUSES. Uncommonly, otitis media may be caused by tuberculosis (36); syphilis (37); fungi, including *Candida, Mucor, Cryptococcus,* and *Aspergillus* (38); and actinomycosis (39). The setting for some of these infections, particularly mycoses, is often in patients who are diabetic or debilitated. In patients infected with human immunodeficiency virus (HIV) or who suffer from acquired immunodeficiency syndrome (AIDS), *Pneumocystis carinii* may be seeded by pulmonary lesions to the middle ear and temporal bone (40). In this setting, the initial clinical presentation may occur as an aural polyp that, on histologic examination, shows characteristic foamy exudate containing the causative organisms. Viruses, including herpes, cytomegalovirus, rubella, rubeola, and mumps, can infect this region, and they may result in labyrinthitis and sensorineural hearing loss (41,42).

DIFFERENTIAL DIAGNOSIS. Myospherulosis is an iatrogenic-induced pseudomycotic lesion resulting from the interaction of red blood cells and petrolatum-based ointments (43). Common sites of occurrence in the head and neck region include the nasal cavity and paranasal sinuses, and occasionally the middle ear (44). Typically, before the development of a mass, patients give a history of recent surgery, followed by packing of the area with a petrolatum-based ointment. Histologi-

cally, myospherulosis is characterized by the presence of cysts devoid of an epithelial lining (pseudocysts) that are embedded within fibrotic tissue, with an associated chronic inflammatory infiltrate composed of lymphocytes, histiocytes, giant cells, and plasma cells. The pseudocysts contain round, saclike structures called *parent bodies*; these parent bodies, in turn, contain numerous spherules or endobodies. Special stains for fungi are invariably negative, and they assist in differentiating myospherulosis from fungal infections (e.g., rhinosporidiosis, coccidioidomycosis). Treatment is symptomatic.

Labyrinthitis

Labyrinthitis is inflammation of the inner ear, and it includes pathologic changes of the labyrinth that arise in response to a variety of injuries, including infectious, inflammatory, and traumatic insults. Labyrinthitis can occur due to complications of otitis media and meningitis, or from seeding of microorganisms via the vascular system.

Based on the pathologic changes seen, labyrinthitis can be classified into serous, suppurative, chronic, viral, or ossifying (45). The clinical manifestations of labyrinthitis depend on the severity and extent of the pathologic changes, which vary from the transient, mild vertigo that might accompany an upper aerodigestive tract infection, to the severe vertigo with nystagmus and profound sensorineural hearing loss that is caused by suppurative labyrinthitis (45,46). *Serous labyrinthitis,* the mildest form of labyrinthitis, represents reactive changes in response to an irritant to the region as might occur secondary to either acute or chronic otitis media but without direct bacterial invasion of the inner ear. In contrast, *suppurative labyrinthitis* is the result of bacterial invasion of the inner ear that originates in the middle ear and/or temporal bone region (tympanogenic labyrinthitis) or from the meninges (meningogenic labyrinthitis). *Chronic labyrinthitis* may be focal or diffuse, and it results from a local osteitis of the otic capsule as a consequence of a previous acute suppurative labyrinthitis or from of a chronic inflammatory process of the membranous labyrinth. This type of labyrinthitis may be associated with sudden or gradual loss of hearing and balance. *Ossifying labyrinthitis* is the end stage of suppurative labyrinthitis; it is characterized by new bone formation in the labyrinth, which likely represents an osseous metaplasia. *Viral labyrinthitis* is the result of generalized viral infection, such as mumps, measles, and cytomegalovirus infection, with involvement of the scala media and vestibular end organs and resulting sensorineural hearing loss.

In serous labyrinthitis, granular eosinophilic material accumulates within the labyrinth and/or perilymphatic spaces. Mild endolymphatic hydrops may be seen. In suppurative labyrinthitis, an acute inflammatory infiltrate that includes polymorphonuclear leukocytes is present in the perilymphatic spaces and surrounding tissues, and it contains identifiable bacterial colonies. Gram stain may be of assistance in the identification of bacteria. With time, necrosis and the destruction of the sensory end organs and the membranous labyrinth occur. The histologic changes in ossifying labyrinthitis include ossification of the labyrinthian structures in the absence of an inflammatory infiltrate. The designation of labyrinthitis for this process is liberally applied. Viral labyrinthitis produces viral cytopathic changes in the scala media (stria vascularis, tectorial membrane, and organ of Corti) with associated cellular swelling, degeneration, cyst formation, and destruction.

Complications of labyrinthitis include extension and involvement of the intracranial structures, including meningitis, venous thrombophlebitis, intracranial abscess, facial nerve paralysis, and otic hydrocephalus.

Inflammatory Otic or Aural Polyp

CLINICAL FEATURES. Otic (aural) polyp is an inflammatory polypoid proliferation that originates from the middle ear mucosa secondary to COM. Despite its origin from the middle ear, otic polyps may cause perforation of the tympanic membrane with extension into the external auditory canal. In this situation, the polyp may appear to be originating from the external auditory canal (47). In large polyps completely obstructing the external ear, radiographic studies are an invaluable aid in identifying the origin of the polyp. Otic polyps may occur at any age, but they are most common in children. Symptoms include otorrhea, conductive hearing loss, and/or a mass protruding from the external auditory canal. In this situation, the polyp may appear to be originating from the external auditory canal. In longstanding cases, destruction (partial or complete) of the ossicles may occur. In the absence of an infectious etiology, local surgical excision is curative.

PATHOLOGIC FEATURES. The gross appearance of otic polyps is that of a polypoid, soft to rubbery, tan-white to pink-red–appearing lesion. The polypoid mass is composed of a cellular infiltrate that primarily consists of a chronic inflammatory cell infiltrate, including mature lymphocytes, plasma cells, histiocytes, and eosinophils (Fig. 23.4) (47–49). Russell bodies or Mott cells containing large eosinophilic immunoglobules can be seen, and they are indicative of a benign plasma cell proliferation. Polymorphonuclear leukocytes may be present. The stroma includes granulation tissue varying in appearance from edematous and richly vascularized to fibrous with a decreased vascular component. Multinucleated giant cells, cholesterol granulomas, and calcific debris (tympanosclerosis) may be present. An overlying epithelium may not be seen; however, when it is present, it appears as pseudostratified columnar or cuboidal cells with or without cilia. Foci of squamous metaplasia and a glandular metaplastic proliferation may also be seen. Special stains for microorganisms are indicated to rule out an infectious etiology.

DIFFERENTIAL DIAGNOSIS. In general, the presence of a mixed cell population of chronic inflammatory cells indicates that the polyp is benign, so a diagnosis of a malignant lymphoproliferative process is not an issue. Rarely, lymphomatous or leukemic involvement of the middle ear and temporal bone occurs secondary to systemic disease. The dense plasma cell component may lead to consideration of a plasmacytoma. Although plasma cell dyscrasia may occur in this site in rare instances (50), the presence of mature plasma cells, Russell bodies, and polyclonality by immunohistochemistry (IHC) should preclude a diagnosis of plasmacytoma. The cellular component in otic polyps may be very dense, and it may obscure an underlying neoplastic process (e.g., rhabdomyosarcoma, Langerhans cell granulomatosis, carcinoma).

Malakoplakia

Malakoplakia, an inflammatory disease that usually involves the genitourinary tract, may rarely occur in the middle ear (51,52). Malakoplakia, which is derived from Greek, means "soft plaque." The light microscopic features include the presence of solid sheets of histiocytes with slightly granular to vacuolated cytoplasm (so-called Hansemann cells) admixed with inflammatory cells, including lymphocytes, plasma cells, and neutrophils. Intracytoplasmic, diastase-resistant, periodic acid-Schiff (PAS)-positive, targetoid inclusion bodies termed *Michaelis-Gutmann bodies* can be seen within occasional cells (Fig. 23.5). These inclusions or calcospherites can also be seen extracellularly, and they contain calcium and frequently iron salts, thereby showing reactivity to a von Kossa stain for calcium and a Prussian blue stain for iron. Malakoplakia is believed to represent an unusual host response to infection with a variety of organisms, and, ultrastructurally, phagolysosomes that have ingested breakdown products of bacteria, such as *Escherichia coli*, have been found.

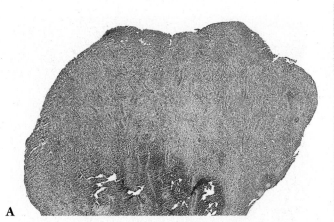

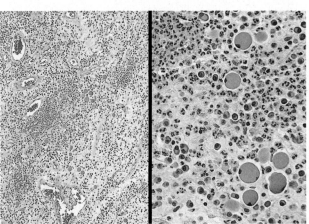

A   B

Figure 23.4. Otic (aural) polyp. **(A)** This polyp, which was protruding from the external auditory canal, appears as an exophytic or polypoid mass with surface ulceration, a dense, inflammatory cell infiltrate, and granulation tissue. **(B)** This otic (aural) polyp is composed of a cellular infiltrate primarily consisting of an admixture of mature lymphocytes, plasma cells, and polymorphonuclear leukocytes (*left panel*); Russell bodies, which are also referred to as Mott cells, containing large eosinophilic immunoglobules can be seen (*right panel*).

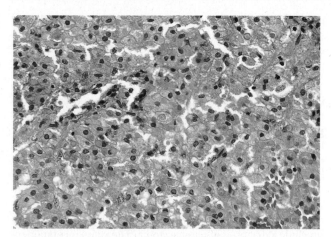

Figure 23.5. Malakoplakia of the middle ear. This is characterized by the presence of solid sheets of histiocytes with a slightly granular to vacuolated cytoplasm (so-called Hansemann cells); a Michaelis-Gutmann body appears as an intracytoplasmic targetoid basophilic inclusion.

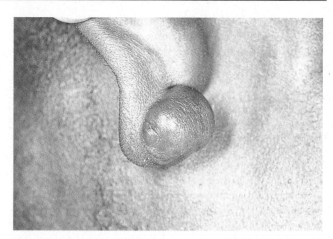

Figure 23.6. Keloid appearing as a polypoid mass covered by thin, glistening, hairless skin.

Acquired Nonneoplastic Lesions of the External and Middle Ear (Keloid)

CLINICAL FEATURES. The term *keloid* is derived from the Greek word *chele*, which means "crab claw." It describes the tendency for these lesions to extend beyond the site of injury. Keloids are not true neoplasms; rather, they are an exaggerated reaction to trauma that represents one extreme of the spectrum of reparative reactions of the skin. Keloids are common among young black women who have had their ears pierced (53). Surgical excision is the treatment of choice, although Cheng et al. (53) reported a recurrence rate of 40% following simple surgical resection. Intralesional steroid injections alone provide response rates of 50% to 100%, with recurrence rates of 5% to 50% at 5 years (54,55). When surgery is followed by steroid injection or radiation therapy, the recurrence rates are consistently below 50% (56–59). Intralesional injection of interferon has been shown to reduce the size by 50%, and this response appears to be limited to the area treated (60,61).

PATHOLOGIC FEATURES. Grossly, keloids are often polypoid in appearance, and they are covered by thin, glistening, hairless skin (Fig. 23.6). The size is variable, usually measuring less than 2 cm; however, they may attain a diameter of several centimeters (53,62). The histology includes haphazardly arranged fascicles of hyalinized collagenous fibers with scattered fibroblasts and myofibroblasts (Fig. 23.7). The proliferation is not encapsulated; instead, it blends subtly with the surrounding dermal fibrous tissue. The collagen bundles are often separated by dermal mucosubstances, which creates an "edematous" appearance. Keloids are poorly vascularized, containing widely scattered, dilated blood vessels. The overlying epidermis is thin and atrophic, without dermal adnexal structures. A foreign body giant-cell reaction is uncommon, except in those patients treated with corticosteroid injection. Pools of amorphous, mucin-like material may also be seen following steroid injection.

DIFFERENTIAL DIAGNOSIS. The differential diagnosis includes hypertrophic scar, dermatofibroma, and dermatofibrosarcoma protuberans. In contrast to keloids, hypertrophic scars lack the dense, hyalinized collagenous fibers; they have more delicate fibrillar collagen; and their arrangement of the collagen and fibroblastic cells is more orderly, often with an orientation parallel to the skin surface. Mature hypertrophic scars generally do not have an abundance of mucosubstances, and, thus, they have a more compact microscopic appearance (63). Further, keloids may recur after excision whereas hypertrophic scars do not. The extremely low cellularity of keloids distinguishes them from dermatofibromas and dermatofibrosarcoma protuberans. The latter also have hyperplasia of the overlying epidermis. Kuo et al. (64) described an unusual variant of dermatofibroma that was characterized by keloid-type changes and termed it *keloidal dermatofibroma*.

Chondrodermatitis Nodularis Helicis Chronicus (Winkler Disease)

CLINICAL FEATURES. Chondrodermatitis nodularis helicis chronicus (CNHC) is an idiopathic, nonneoplastic ulcerative lesion of the auricle. CNHC usually affects men in the late middle-aged and older age groups, and is considered uncommon in

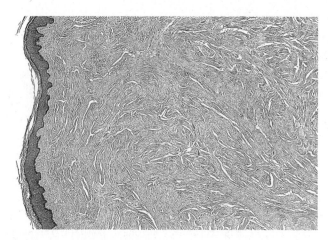

Figure 23.7. Keloid. Histologically, keloids are characterized by the presence of haphazard fascicles of hyalinized collagen that blend with the surrounding dermal fibers. The overlying cutaneous epithelium is thin and devoid of hair follicles.

women (65,66). Patients present with spontaneously occurring, unilateral painful nodules. Even gentle manipulation may precipitate excruciating pain, eventually prompting patients to seek treatment. CNHC most frequently occurs along the superior portion of the helix; lateral helical, antihelical, and antitragal involvement are also seen. They typically appear as round, reddish, tender areas usually measuring less than 1 cm in diameter. Clinically, many cases are considered carcinomas (66).

The etiology of CNHC is not known, but several theories have been suggested, including cold exposure, actinic damage, local trauma, and degenerative change with pressure necrosis. Because the skin of the auricle is quite thin, with little subcutaneous fat, the area may be unusually sensitive to injury. In addition, the vascular supply to the area is somewhat deficient, with the avascular cartilage depending on the dermal circulation for its sustenance. These anatomic features may predispose the auricle to the development of CNHC. Winkler (67) considered the underlying pathologic event to be a cartilaginous-based process. However, the etiology appears to be linked to a primary cutaneous alteration as the cutaneous changes are more significant and they are a more constant feature. The development of CNHC is likely multifactorial, and it includes actinic damage.

Complete surgical excision—wedge excision (68) or cartilage excision alone (69)—is the treatment of choice, and it is curative. In a minority of patients, trials with injection of glucocorticoids directly into the lesion have been effective in eradicating the lesion. Although the lesion has no malignant potential, differentiating these from basal cell carcinoma and squamous cell carcinoma frequently requires biopsy.

PATHOLOGIC FEATURES. CNHC usually appears as a dome-shaped, discrete nodule with a scale crust covering a central area of ulceration that ranges in diameter from 3 to 18 mm, with an average of 7 mm. Rarely, CNHC may achieve diameters of 2 to 3 cm. Histologically, the central portion of the involved epidermis is ulcerated, while the adjacent epithelium shows acanthosis, hyperkeratosis, parakeratosis, and pseudoepitheliomatous hyperplasia (Fig. 23.8). The base of the ulcer shows granulation tissue with a pronounced capillary proliferation, edema, fibrinoid necrosis, and an acute and/or chronic inflammatory cell infiltrate (65). The granulation tissue and inflammatory process usually involves the perichondrium and cartilage. Pain is thought to result from this perichondrial involvement. The dermis lacks cutaneous adnexal structures in the area of the lesion, and the vasculature appears telangiectatic. Foci of fibrinoid eosinophilic material or, in some cases, frank necrobiosis of the collagen may be present. Occasionally, palisading histiocytes are seen in association with necrobiotic collagen. The changes in the auricular cartilage deep to the ulcer range from mild perichondritis through variable degrees of degenerative changes that are characterized by edema and loss of chondrocytes, with smudging (i.e., loss of basophilia) and hyalinization of the chondroid matrix. The necrotic material from the dermis (and even, occasionally, fragments of degenerated cartilage) may protrude into the ulcer crater. Calcification and ossification of the underlying cartilage may be present (70).

DIFFERENTIAL DIAGNOSIS. CNHC is frequently misdiagnosed as a cutaneous malignancy, particularly as basal cell carcinoma or squamous cell carcinoma. Metzger and Goodman (65) noted a clinical diagnosis of either a malignant or premalignant lesion in 80% of the cases they reviewed. Unfortunately,

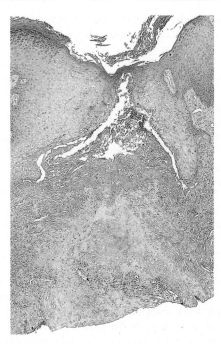

Figure 23.8. Chondrodermatitis nodularis helicis chronicus. The central portion of the involved epidermis is ulcerated, with acanthosis and hyperkeratosis of the adjacent epithelium and granulation tissue along the base of the lesion. This extends to and involves the subjacent perichondrium and cartilage. Perichondrial involvement is associated with pain.

the same mistake may be perpetuated by microscopic examination, particularly if the epidermal hyperplastic changes are misinterpreted as representing either squamous cell carcinoma or a hypertrophic actinic keratosis. Careful attention to the extensive dermal changes and usually some degree of cartilaginous alterations, along with the well-demarcated nature of the epidermal proliferation and the lack of cytologic atypia in the adjacent epidermis, should help in excluding a squamous neoplasm in cases of CNHC.

Idiopathic Cystic Chondromalacia of the Auricular Cartilage or Auricular or Endochondral Pseudocyst

CLINICAL FEATURES. Idiopathic cystic chondromalacia (ICC) is a benign cystic degeneration of the auricular cartilage that is of unknown etiology. ICC typically occurs in young and middle-aged adult males, but, in uncommon instances, it does occur in women (71,72). These lesions arise as unilateral, painless swellings of the cartilage without overlying ulceration or erythema over weeks to years. They are occasionally bilateral (73). Although they may arise anywhere on the auricle, the scaphoid fossa is the most common site (80%) (74).

Although trauma has been implicated in causing these lesions, no definitive connection to a prior traumatic event has been made, and the origin(s) for this condition remain unknown. Engel (75), the first to describe them in the English literature, believed that these lesions were secondary to repeated minor trauma. He attributed them to the habit of sleeping on hard pillows, although he could not substantiate his claim. Others have also believed that these lesions were traumatic in origin, citing the wearing of motorcycle helmets, stereo headphones, the Italian birthday custom of having one's auricle pulled, and the habit of sleeping on hard pillows (71,76–79). Auricular pseudocysts may arise within the potential plane left during embryonic fusion of the auricular hillocks. Ischemic necrosis of the cartilage or the abnormal release of lysosomal enzymes by chondrocytes may also be cofactors (73,78).

Complete surgical excision without distortion of the underlying cartilaginous framework is the treatment of choice. Due to the potential for surgical-related deformity, full-thickness resection is not advocated. In addition to the obvious cosmetic concerns, long-standing lesions may result in deformity of the ear. Steroid injection alone has been unsuccessful, and it may result in cartilage deformity. Incision and drainage or curettage has shown variable success. Needle aspiration alone results in the rapid reaccumulation of fluid; however, when this is combined with bolster suture compression, long-term follow-up has shown an absence of recurrences (80).

PATHOLOGIC FEATURES. The gross appearance of ICC is that of a fluid-filled, distended mass. The excised tissue may include only a fragment of the cyst wall, or, less often, it is a full-thickness excision of the ear. An intact cyst usually contains fluid that has been described as "olive oil–like" (75). The cyst wall consists of a 1- to 2-mm rim of cartilage. The cyst lining may be a smooth and glistening cartilaginous surface or may include roughened, rust-colored patches. The cyst is usually an elongated cleft, but multifocal cystic degeneration may be seen.

Histologically, the changes are restricted to the cartilage, within which irregular-shaped cystic areas are seen (Fig. 23.9). The cysts lack a cell lining and they generally are devoid of content. An epithelial lining is absent, hence the term *pseudocyst*. The cyst is the result of the loss of cartilage. The cystic cleft is often centrally placed in the cartilaginous plate. A rim of fibrous tissue along the inner rim of the cyst, or a granulation tissue reaction composed of fibrovascular tissue, may be observed, and scattered chronic inflammatory cells can be seen in association with the cysts. In long-standing cases, fibrous tissue may essentially obliterate the cystic space. Some examples of cystic chondromalacia are characterized by a distinctly proliferative cartila-

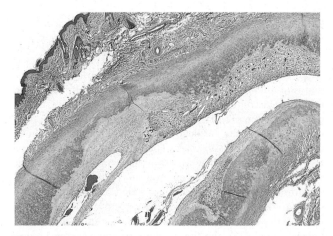

Figure 23.9. Idiopathic cystic chondromalacia. Histologically, idiopathic cystic chondromalacia is characterized by the cystic degeneration of the auricular cartilage. The cysts result in the loss of cartilage. The cysts, which lack a true epithelial lining (pseudocysts), are composed of fibrous tissue along the inner rim of the cyst and granulation tissue within the wall adjacent to the cartilage.

ginous response in which a thickened cartilaginous wall develops.

DIFFERENTIAL DIAGNOSIS. Slight cytologic atypia may be seen; however, the orderly nature of the proliferation and the associated central cystic degeneration facilitate the exclusion of malignancy neoplasia (72). The differential diagnosis may also include relapsing polychondritis, subperichondral hematoma, and CNHC.

Angiolymphoid Hyperplasia with Eosinophilia

Angiolymphoid hyperplasia with eosinophilia (ALHE) has been a controversial lesion with regard to its classification (reactive proliferation or neoplastic process) and its relationship to Kimura disease. Categorizing ALHE with a group of neoplastic lesions, including epithelioid hemangioma, hemangioendothelioma of bone, and epithelioid hemangioendothelioma, has been suggested (81). However, the behavior of ALHE and the evidence for a reactive etiology militate against this approach. ALHE shares features with Kimura disease, but the clinical and histologic differences allow these entities to be separated. Recent studies have also supported the separation of the two as distinct clinicopathologic entities (81–86) (Table 23.2).

CLINICAL FEATURES. ALHE represents a benign angiomatous subcutaneous proliferation with a predilection for the external ear (auricle and external canal), as well as other head and neck sites, including the scalp and forehead (87,88). ALHE most frequently occurs in the third to fifth decades of life; no gender predilection is evident. The symptoms include pruritus and bleeding following scratching. Regional lymphadenopathy and peripheral eosinophilia are uncommon, but they may be present. A history of trauma is elicited in a number of cases, and the demonstration of immunoglobulin deposits in the vessels, as well as the microscopic impression of vascular damage, has led several observers to favor a reactive or reparative etiology (87–89). Hormonal influences may play a role in some cases, as the association with pregnancy in some patients and the age and gender distribution of the disease may suggest. Human herpesvirus-8 (HHV8) has not been identified in association with ALHE (90). Local surgical excision or desiccation are the treatments of choice for ALHE, and these are curative. Recurrences are occasionally seen. Medical regimens, including intralesional or systemic steroids, have been used with some success in treating the symptoms, but they have not been curative. An investigational protocol of intralesional vincristine, bleomycin, and fluorouracil has not been proven to be of value (91).

PATHOLOGIC FEATURES. ALHE is characterized by single or multiple, pink to red-brown indurated cutaneous papules or subcutaneous nodules. These lesions measure from a few millimeters to 1 cm in diameter. Clusters of papules may coalesce to form large, plaquelike lesions (87,88). Histologically, ALHE is characterized by a nodular vascular proliferation that is accompanied by a variably dense lymphoid infiltrate that is rich in eosinophils (Fig. 23.10). The process is circumscribed but not encapsulated, and it may involve the subcutis, dermis, or both. The vascular component varies in size from capillary to medium-sized arteries and veins, and the vascular spaces are lined by plump-appearing (epithelioid) endothelial cells with pleomorphism, hyperchromatic nuclei, copious eosinophilic

TABLE 23.2	Angiolymphoid Hyperplasia with Eosinophilia versus Kimura Disease	
	ALHE	*Kimura Disease*
Gender	M = F or F > M	M > F
Peak incidence	Third to fifth decades	Second to third decade
Head and neck site	Periauricular, forehead	Postauricular, scalp
Lymphadenopathy	Absent to rare	Common
Peripheral eosinophilia	<25%	>50%
Location	More superficial; situated in subcutaneous dermis	More deeply situated; extending to the subcutaneous fat, fascia, and skeletal muscle
Histology	Nodular vascular proliferation lined by plump-appearing (epithelioid) endothelial cells with pleomorphic changes and hyperchromatic nuclei; accompanied by a prominent inflammatory cell infiltrate with variable admixture of lymphocytes, histiocytes, plasma cells, and eosinophils	Vascular component is sparse with minimal epithelioid endothelial changes; lymphoid proliferation predominates, but prominent eosinophilic cell infiltrate (including eosinophilic microabscesses) can be seen; associated fibrosis is present

ALHE, angiolymphoid hyperplasia with eosinophilia.

cytoplasm, and inconspicuous nucleoli (81,84,87). Frequently, the endothelial cells protrude into the vessel lumen in a "hobnail" fashion, creating a cobblestonelike appearance (83). A lobular arrangement of the proliferating vessels, as is seen in hemangiomas, may be evident; however, the distribution of vessels is more haphazard in some lesions. The vessels vary from irregular, poorly canalized, thin-walled spaces to rounded, well-formed vessels with thickened walls. In some cases, evidence of disruption or damage to some of the involved vessels is present. An admixture of lymphocytes, histiocytes, and eosinophils characterizes the inflammatory component. On occasion, eosinophils may be few or absent.

Kimura Disease

CLINICAL FEATURES. In contrast to ALHE, Kimura disease primarily occurs in Asians; it tends to affect males; it is often associated with regional lymphadenopathy and peripheral eo-sinophilia; and it is characterized by larger lesions that are predominantly subcutaneous nodules with a tendency to occur in locations other than the head and neck (92).

PATHOLOGIC FEATURES. Kimura disease shares many histologic features with ALHE. However, subtle histologic differences are seen. In Kimura disease, the lymphoid proliferation predominates and the vascular component is sparse, exhibiting minimal epithelioid endothelial changes (Fig. 23.11). Kimura disease is usually located much deeper than ALHE, often extending to the fascia and to skeletal muscle, and the subcutaneous fat is usually quite fibrotic. Eosinophils are always numerous in Kimura disease, but they may be sparse or even absent in ALHE.

DIFFERENTIAL DIAGNOSIS. The differential diagnosis for ALHE and Kimura disease includes lobular capillary hemangioma and angiosarcoma. ALHE is distinguished from hemangi-

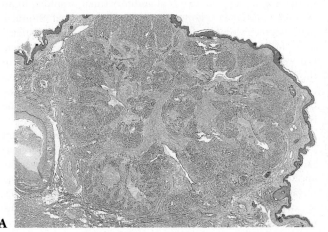
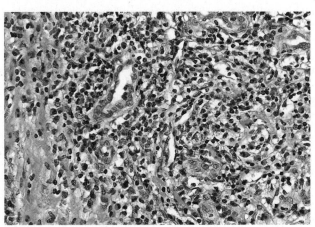

A   **B**

Figure 23.10. Angiolymphoid hyperplasia with eosinophilia. **(A)** This lesion is characterized by a dermal-situated, nodular-appearing proliferation composed of granulation-like tissue with a patchy inflammatory cell infiltrate that is accompanied by haphazardly arranged, small-caliber–sized, irregularly shaped blood vessels. **(B)** The vascular spaces are lined by plump-appearing pleomorphic (epithelioid) endothelial cells with hyperchromatic nuclei. The inflammatory component is characterized by an admixture of mature lymphocytes, numerous eosinophils, and scattered histiocytes.

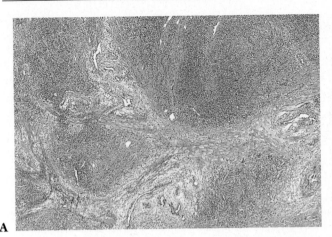
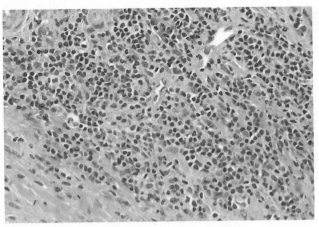

A   B

Figure 23.11. Kimura disease. **(A)** This lesion was deeply situated in the subcutis, and shows a nodular proliferation of inflammatory cells separated by fibrous tissue. **(B)** A mature lymphoid cell proliferation predominates with scattered eosinophils; the vascular component is sparse and lacks the epithelioid endothelial changes seen in angiolymphoid hyperplasia with eosinophilia.

oma by the prominence of the epithelioid endothelial features and by the associated lymphoplasmacytic and eosinophilic infiltrate. Angiosarcoma is a diffusely infiltrative lesion composed of anastomosing vascular channels that are lined by pleomorphic cells with increased mitotic activity. The presence of the characteristic inflammatory infiltrate of ALHE is not found in angiosarcoma.

Exostosis

CLINICAL FEATURES. Exostoses are localized overgrowths of bone that classically are described as reactive lesions consisting of a compact proliferation of layers of bone of varied size and appearance, including nodular, moundlike, pedunculated, or flat protuberances on the surface of a bone. Broad-based lesions are referred to as *exostosis*, whereas pedunculated lesions have been termed *osteoma.*

Exostoses are broad-based outgrowths of bone arising from the wall of the external auditory canal. Exostoses usually are multiple and bilateral (93). External auditory canal exostoses tend to remain asymptomatic until they reach a size sufficient to interfere with the normal egress of cerumen and exfoliated skin. Most canal exostoses are asymptomatic but external auditory canal obstruction may occur, causing recurrent episodes of external otitis, conductive hearing loss, and tinnitus (94). Exostoses of the external auditory canal affect cold-water swimmers and surfers (93), with the highest incidence being found in Australia and New Zealand (95). Medical treatment resolves the symptomatic external otitis and related hearing loss. For patients who do not respond to medical treatment, transmeatal surgical excision is the treatment of choice (94).

PATHOLOGIC FEATURES. The gross appearance of exostoses is usually better appreciated by the surgeon because only fragments are available to the pathologist in most cases. The intact exostosis is a broad-based, moundlike, bony proliferation that is similar in color and texture to the normal cortical bone. A layer of periosteum with overlying thin skin covers the bone. The periosteal layers resemble the skin of an onion, and they usually lack trabecular architecture or marrow spaces.

DIFFERENTIAL DIAGNOSIS. The chief differential diagnosis is osteoma, which is much less common in this location. The distinction between exostosis and osteoma usually is readily made on the basis of the clinical presentation. Some controversy exists regarding the ability to distinguish between the two lesions histologically. Some observers consider the lesions to differ histologically (93,96,97), whereas others do not find the microscopic features sufficiently distinctive to allow separation (98).

Synovial Chondromatosis

CLINICAL FEATURES. Synovial chondromatosis is a reactive process of unknown pathogenesis that is characterized by the formation of multiple cartilaginous nodules in the synovium. Many become detached and float within the joint space. Other terms for synovial chondromatosis include *synovial osteochondromatosis* and *synovial chondrometaplasia* (98,99).

Synovial chondromatosis of the temporomandibular joint (TMJ) may involve the external auditory canal, resulting in an asymptomatic mass lesion (100–103). TMJ synovial chondromatosis affects women, and it generally occurs in adults. Patients with TMJ synovial chondromatosis may present with preauricular swelling and limited motion of the joint with deviation of the mandible. The radiographic features of synovial chondromatosis include the presence of numerous radiopaque loose bodies within the region of the joint, but destruction of bone is absent (104,105).

Intraoperatively, the lesion is usually confined to the joint space and is easily enucleated. On occasion, the tumor may extend beyond the joint capsule into the parotid gland, the auditory canal, the temporal bone, or the cranium (106). Conservative surgical management is the treatment of choice (107). Reported cases of synovial chondrosarcoma have suggested the possibility of malignant transformation of synovial chondromatosis (108,109). Cell proliferation studies of synovial chondromatosis have shown proliferative activity that is intermediate between enchondromas and chondrosarcomas (110).

Synovial chondromatosis is a condition in which foci of the cartilage develop in the synovial membrane of a joint, apparently through metaplasia of the sublining connective tissue of the synovial membrane. Recent studies have shown clonal chromosomal alterations in synovial chondromatosis, suggesting that this is a neoplastic lesion rather than a metaplastic and/or reactive process (111).

PATHOLOGIC FEATURES. The synovium may be diffusely studded with innumerable nodules. The nodules are polypoid or pedunculated with a delicate stalk, and they vary in size from as small as 1 mm to as large as 3 cm. The external surface varies from smooth to convoluted and granular.

Histologically, synovial chondromatosis consists of nodules of mature cartilage of varying cellularity that are found within the synovium and that lie loosely in the joint space. The cartilage may appear atypical, with hypercellularity, hyperchromasia, binucleated chondrocytes, and an increased mitotic rate (Fig. 23.12). Calcification and ossification may be present.

DIFFERENTIAL DIAGNOSIS. The presence of increased cellularity with atypical features, including binucleated chondrocytes, may suggest a diagnosis of chondrosarcoma. In such examples, correlation with the radiographic appearance is essential to differentiate these lesions. The radiographic features of synovial chondromatosis include the presence of numerous radiopaque loose bodies within the region of the joint (104,105).

Cholesteatoma (Keratoma)

Cholesteatoma is a pseudoneoplastic lesion of the middle ear characterized by invasive growth and the presence of stratified squamous epithelium that forms a saclike accumulation of keratin within the middle ear space. Despite their invasive growth, cholesteatomas are not considered to be true neoplasms. The term *cholesteatoma* is a misnomer in that it is not a neoplasm and it does not contain cholesterol (112). As such, the designation of *keratoma* would be more accurate but the term *cholesteatoma* is entrenched in the literature. Other designations include *epidermal cyst* or *epidermal inclusion cyst of the middle ear* (113,114).

CLINICAL FEATURES. Cholesteatomas occur more frequently in men than in women, and they are most common in the third to fourth decades of life. The middle ear space is the most usual site of occurrence. Initially, cholesteatomas may remain clinically silent until extensive invasion of the middle ear space and mastoid has occurred. Symptoms include hearing loss, malodorous discharge, and pain, and they may be associated with a polyp arising in the attic of the middle ear or with the perforation of the tympanic membrane. Otoscopic examination may reveal the presence of white debris within the middle ear, which is considered diagnostic.

Complete surgical excision of all histologic components of the cholesteatoma is the treatment of choice. If the cholesteatoma is not completely excised, it can have progressive and destructive growth, including widespread bone destruction, which may lead to hearing loss, facial nerve paralysis, labyrinthitis, meningitis, or brain abscess.

PATHOGENESIS. The majority of cholesteatomas are acquired; they arise either de novo without a history of middle ear disease or following a middle ear infection; a small percentage of cases are congenital. The latter have also been referred to as epidermoid cysts (114,115). The pathogenesis is thought to occur via the migration of squamous epithelium from the external auditory canal or the external surface of the tympanic membrane into the middle ear. The mechanism by which the epithelium may enter the middle ear probably is by a combination of events, including perforation of the tympanic membrane (particularly in its superior aspect, which is referred to as the pars flaccida or Shrapnell membrane) following an infection, coupled with the invagination or retraction of the tympanic membrane into the middle ear as a result of long-standing negative pressure on the membrane secondary to blockage or obstruction of the eustachian tube. Other theories by which cholesteatomas are thought to occur include traumatic implantation, squamous metaplasia of the middle ear epithelium, and congenital derivation.

Cholesteatoma of the petrous apex is an epidermoid cyst of this location, and it bears no relation to cholesteatoma of the middle ear. It likely is of congenital origin, but no cell rests have been discovered that may explain the origin of these lesions. The symptoms usually relate to the involvement of the 7th and 8th cranial nerves in the cerebellopontine angle (115).

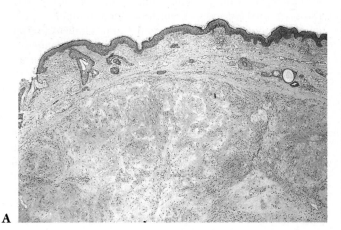
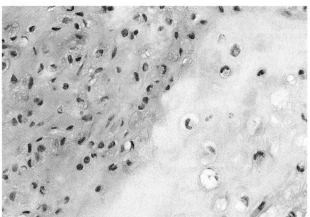

Figure 23.12. Synovial chondromatosis of the temporomandibular joint. **(A)** It involves the external auditory canal and appears histologically as subcutaneous nodules of cartilage. **(B)** At higher magnification, the cartilage may appear atypical with hypercellularity, nuclear hyperchromasia, pleomorphism, and binucleated chondrocytes.

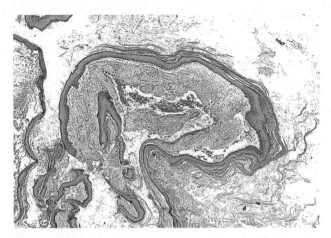

Figure 23.13. Cholesteatoma. The histologic diagnosis of cholesteatoma is based on the finding of keratinizing squamous epithelium within the middle ear space.

PATHOLOGIC FEATURES. Cholesteatomas appear as cystic, white to pearly appearing masses of varying size that contain creamy or waxy granular material (116). The histologic diagnosis is made based on the presence of stratified keratinizing squamous epithelium, subepithelial fibroconnective or granulation tissue, and keratin debris (Fig. 23.13) (116). The essential diagnostic feature is the keratinizing squamous epithelium. *The presence of keratin debris alone is not diagnostic of a cholesteatoma.* The keratinizing squamous epithelium is cytologically bland, and it shows cellular maturation without evidence of dysplasia. In spite of its benign histology, cholesteatomas are invasive and they have widespread destructive capabilities. The destructive properties of cholesteatomas result from a combination of interrelated reasons, including mass effect with pressure erosion of the surrounding structures from the cholesteatoma and the production of collagenase, which has osteodestructive capabilities (117). Collagenase is produced by both the squamous epithelial and the fibrous tissue components of the cholesteatoma.

Keratosis obturans (KO) results when the normal self-cleaning mechanism of keratin maturation and lateral extrusion from the external auditory canal is defective, causing the accumulation of keratin debris deep within the bony aspect of the external auditory canal. The etiology of KO remains unclear. KO most commonly occurs in the first two decades of life, and the symptoms generally relate to conductive hearing loss due to the keratin plug. Pain is a common finding. The keratin debris may exert pressure effects on the bony canal wall, resulting in widening of the external auditory canal, bone remodeling, and inflamed epithelium. The histologic appearance is that of tightly packed keratin squames in a lamellar pattern. The treatment for KO is debridement of the keratin plug. In contrast to KO, external ear canal cholesteatomas generally occur in individuals who are older; it presents with otorrhea and unilateral chronic pain; it does not produce a conductive hearing loss; and it is composed of loosely packed, irregularly arranged keratin squames histologically (117).

DIFFERENTIAL DIAGNOSIS. The histologic diagnosis of cholesteatomas is relatively straightforward in the presence of keratinizing squamous epithelium. In contrast to cholesteatomas, squamous cell carcinoma shows dysplastic or overtly malig-

nant cytologic features with a prominent desmoplastic stromal response to its infiltrative growth. Cholesteatomas do not transform into squamous cell carcinomas.

In an attempt to determine whether cholesteatomas were low-grade squamous carcinomas, Desloge et al. (118) performed DNA analysis on human cholesteatomas to determine whether ploidy abnormalities were present. In ten cases with interpretable data, nine were euploid and one was aneuploid. These authors concluded that, due to a lack of overt genetic instability, cholesteatomas could not be considered to be malignant neoplasms. Molecular genetic evaluation has found genes induced or upregulated in cholesteatoma, including genes involved in cell proliferation and differentiation (e.g., calgranulin A, calgranulin B, psoriasin, thymosin beta-10) and genes involved in cell invasion (e.g., cathepsin C, cathepsin D, cathepsin H) (119). Keratinocyte growth factor (KGF), a mesenchymal cell–derived paracrine growth factor that specifically stimulates epithelial cell proliferation, is present in cholesteatomas with KGFR protein and mRNA localized in the epithelium in 72% of cases and with significant correlation between KGF+/KGFR+ expression and recurrence (120). KGF and KGFR may play a role in enhanced epithelial cell proliferative activity and recurrence of cholesteatomas (120). Angiogenesis and angiogenic growth factors have been reported to be present in cholesteatoma (121). Sudhoff et al. (121) reported a close relationship between the density of capillaries, degree of inflammation, and expression of the angiogenic factors and the increased number of microvessels in cholesteatomas. Further, these authors suggest that angiogenesis enables and supports the sustained migration of keratinocytes into the middle ear cavity, representing a pivotal factor in the destructive behavior of middle ear cholesteatoma (121). Cholesterol granuloma is not synonymous with cholesteatoma. These entities are distinctly different pathologic entities that should not be confused with one another (113).

Langerhans Cell Histiocytosis, Langerhans Cell (Eosinophilic) Granulomatosis, and Eosinophilic Granuloma

Langerhans cell histiocytosis (LCH) is a clonal proliferation of Langerhans cells occurring as an isolated lesion or as part of a systemic (multifocal) proliferation (122,123). The designation of LCH replaced the previous nomenclature of the group of diseases termed *histiocytosis X*, which included eosinophilic granuloma, Letterer-Siwe syndrome, and Hand-Schüller-Christian disease. Lieberman et al. (124) suggested the designation of *Langerhans cell (eosinophilic) granulomatosis* to indicate that the Langerhans cell represents a cellular component of the dendritic cell system rather than a tissue macrophage (histiocyte).

CLINICAL FEATURES. LCH most commonly occurs in the second to third decades of life, and it tends to arise in males. The lesions are most often osseous. The most frequent osseous sites involved are those in the skull, including the middle ear and the temporal bone (125). In patients with middle ear and temporal bone involvement, the symptoms include aural discharge, swelling of the temporal bone area, otitis media, bone pain, otalgia, loss of hearing, and vertigo. A single or multiple sharply circumscribed osteolytic lesion(s) can be seen by radiographic studies.

Surgical excision (curettage) and low-dose radiation therapy (500 to 1500 rads) are the treatments of choice. The prognosis

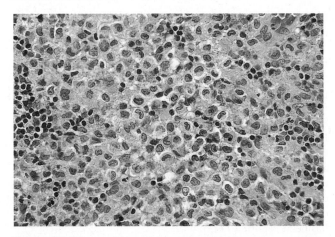

Figure 23.14. Langerhans cell histiocytosis. This condition is characterized by a sheetlike proliferation of Langerhans cells, which are the cells with lobulations and/or indentations of the nuclear membrane (reniform nuclei); admixed eosinophils are present.

is considered very good. Recurrence, which may be part of a systemic or multifocal process, generally occurs within 6 months of the diagnosis. Failure of a new bone lesion to occur within 1 year of diagnosis is considered a cure. Chemotherapy is used for multifocal and systemic disease. In general, the younger the patient is at the onset of disease and the more extensive the involvement (i.e., multiple sites including bone and viscera), the worse the prognosis.

PATHOLOGIC FEATURES. Histologically, LCH is characterized by a proliferation of Langerhans cells (LCs), which are arranged in sheets, nests, or clusters and are composed of cells with reniform nuclei characterized by nuclear membrane lobations or indentations (Fig. 23.14). The nuclei have vesicular chromatin with inconspicuous to small, centrally located basophilic nucleoli and a moderate amount of eosinophilic cytoplasm. The LCs may show mild pleomorphism, and mitotic figures are uncommon. An inflammatory cell infiltrate that primarily consists of eosinophils accompanies the LCs. Other inflammatory cells are present, including polymorphonuclear leukocytes, plasma cells, and lymphocytes. In addition, foamy

histiocytes and multinucleated giant cells may also be observed. These histiocytes may show phagocytosis of mononuclear cells.

The diagnosis of Langerhans cell (eosinophilic) granulomatosis (LCG) is facilitated by an IHC evaluation. LCs are diffusely immunoreactive with S-100 protein (126,127) and CD1a (Fig. 23.15) (128). On electron microscopy, elongated granules referred to as Langerhans or Birbeck granules can be seen within the cytoplasm of the LCs (129). The foamy histiocytes and multinucleated giant cells are S-100 protein– and CD1a-negative, but they do react for CD68 (KP1).

DIFFERENTIAL DIAGNOSIS. The histologic differential diagnosis of LCG includes extranodal sinus histiocytosis with massive lymphadenopathy (Rosai-Dorfman disease) and non-Hodgkin malignant lymphoma. Rosai-Dorfman disease may occasionally involve the ear and temporal bone region (130). Like LCs, the cells of Rosai-Dorfman disease are S-100 protein–reactive; they differ from LCs in that they are nonreactive for CD1a. Differentiating LCH from a malignant lymphoproliferative disease is usually not problematic by light microscopy. If necessary, IHC stains help in differentiating LCH from a malignant lymphoma.

Heterotopias, or Choristomas, of the Middle Ear and Mastoid

Heterotopias, which are also referred to as *choristomas* and *ectopias*, are characterized by the presence of normal-appearing tissue(s) in an anatomic location in which they normally are not found. Heterotopias that occur in the middle ear include salivary gland tissue and neuroglial tissue. Salivary gland choristomas may present with unilateral conductive hearing loss; they tend to occur more often in women; and they are seen over a wide age range (131–133). Salivary gland choristomas often arise in conjunction with facial nerve and ossicular chain anomalies (134). The combination of facial nerve and ossicular chain anomalies may be explained as a second branchial arch developmental abnormality. True neuronal heterotopias in which isolated neuroglial tissue is located in the middle ear and temporal bone without continuity with the central nervous system are rare, but they have been reported (135,136).

Neuroglial tissues in the middle ear and mastoid generally represent an acquired encephalocele with herniation of the brain into the middle ear and mastoid via compromise of the

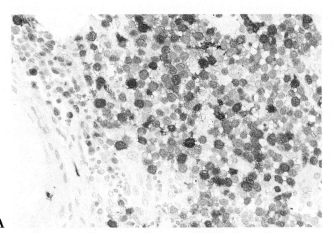

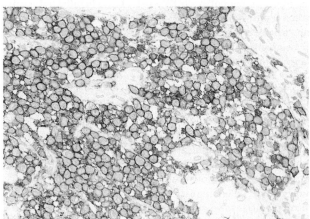

Figure 23.15. Langerhans cells. These are immunoreactive with for S-100 protein (**A**) and CD1a (**B**).

tegmen, a thin bony shell that separates the middle ear and mastoid cavity from the temporal lobe. The tegmen may be compromised or destroyed secondary to trauma or prior surgery, by a complication of otitis media, or due to a congenital defect (137). Potential complications include brain abscess. Conservative surgical removal is the treatment of choice. However, choristomas often adhere to dehiscent facial nerve. If complete surgical resection will compromise the integrity of the facial nerve, then incomplete resection is justified. Biopsy for diagnostic purposes followed by observation is an alternative to surgical excision. Rarely, salivary gland ectopia may produce a neoplastic proliferation (mixed tumor) (138,139).

PATHOLOGIC FEATURES. Choristomas appear as lobulated, nonpulsatile, soft tissue masses lying in the middle ear space with an intact tympanic membrane. Microscopically, the salivary tissues are composed of an admixture of seromucous glands and adipose tissue. A neuroglial heterotopia includes a heterogeneous population of cells, with glial cells, histiocytes, and mature lymphocytes. Reactive alterations of the neuroglial tissue (gliosis) may be present. In addition, granulation tissue and keratinizing squamous epithelium (cholesteatoma) may be found. IHC confirmation of neuroglial tissues includes reactivity for glial fibrillary acidic protein (GFAP).

DIFFERENTIAL DIAGNOSIS. In COM, a fibrillary stroma is often present that may simulate the appearance of the neurofibrillary matrix. Reactivity for GFAP assists in confirming or excluding neuroglial tissues. The differential diagnosis also includes a glial neoplasm.

AUTOIMMUNE, SYSTEMIC, AND DEGENERATIVE DISEASES

Relapsing Polychondritis

Relapsing polychondritis (RP) is an uncommon systemic episodic or relapsing disease that is characterized by the progressive degeneration of cartilaginous structures throughout the body. RP is also referred to as *polychondropathia* (140).

CLINICAL FEATURES. RP primarily occurs in whites, and it affects men and women equally. RP may occur at any age, but the symptoms are most frequent in the fifth to seventh decades of life. The auricular cartilage is involved, usually bilaterally, in nearly 90% of patients with RP (141,142). The affected ear is erythematous, swollen, and very tender. In advanced cases, the pinna may be distorted as a result of destruction of the cartilage. The overlying skin is not ulcerated. The disease manifestations relapse with marked variability in both the severity and frequency of occurrence. The progression of disease may result in "cauliflower" ears and "saddle" nose deformities. The involvement of the audiovestibular system may result in hearing loss (conductive, sensorineural, or mixed) (143). Other cartilaginous sites, as well as noncartilaginous locations of the body, may be involved, including arthropathy (large and small joints), laryngotracheal and bronchial chondritis, nasal chondritis, cardiovascular complications (valvular insufficiency, aneurysm), ocular manifestations (episcleritis, conjunctivitis, retinopathy), and cutaneous involvement (oral and genital ulcers) (144,145).

The current clinical diagnostic criteria for RP are defined by three or more of the following: (a) recurrent chondritis of both auricles; (b) nonerosive inflammatory arthritis; (c) chondritis of nasal cartilages; (d) ocular inflammation, including conjunctivitis, keratitis, scleritis and/or episcleritis, and/or uveitis; (e) chondritis of the upper respiratory tract that involves the larynx and/or tracheal cartilages; and (f) cochlear and/or vestibular damage manifested by sensorineural hearing loss, tinnitus, and/or vertigo. The diagnosis can be confirmed when one or more of the above criteria occur in association with histologic confirmation or by the presence of chondritis in two or more separate anatomic locations that responds to steroids and/or dapsone. The laboratory findings are nonspecific, including an elevated erythrocyte sedimentation rate; mild leukocytosis; and normochromic, normocytic anemia. The presence of elevated antineutrophil cytoplasmic antibody (ANCA) titers has been reported (145).

The etiology of RP has not been clearly elucidated; however, evidence has implicated an autoimmune process. In association with RP, some patients suffer from other autoimmune disorders, including systemic lupus erythematosus, rheumatoid arthritis, scleroderma, Sjögren syndrome, Reiter syndrome, glomerulonephritis, autoimmune thyroid disease, ulcerative colitis, pernicious anemia, and Raynaud syndrome (142,145,146). Patients with RP have been known to have factors in their serum that react with cartilage (147). Circulating antibodies to type II collagen (148) with titers reflecting severity of disease and the documentation of immunofluorescent localization of immune complex components at the perichondral-cartilaginous interface have been reported in patients with RP (149,150). Patients with RP have immune complexes of immunoglobulins and complement detected in the biopsy specimens taken from the inflamed cartilage of the involved ear(s) (151). No evidence exists to support either a hereditary or familial predisposition.

The treatment of RP depends on the stage. In the acute stages of disease, corticosteroids are used. In more advanced stages, immunosuppressive agents may be used. The prognosis is variable and unpredictable, with some patients having a prolonged course and others suffering from a more aggressive and fulminant disease. Death may occur, most often as the result of respiratory tract or cardiovascular system involvement.

PATHOLOGIC FEATURES. The histologic findings in RP include perichondrial inflammation with a mixed infiltrate of lymphocytes, plasma cells, polymorphonuclear leukocytes, and occasional eosinophils that blurs the interface between the perichondrium and the auricular cartilage (Fig. 23.16). Loss of the usual basophilia occurs in the cartilage, which assumes an eosinophilic appearance with hematoxylin and eosin (H&E) staining. At the advancing edge of the inflammation, loss of chondrocytes and destruction of the lacunar architecture are observed. As cartilage is destroyed, it is eventually replaced by fibrous tissue. The immunomicroscopic findings include the diffuse granular deposition of immunoglobulin G (IgG) and complement protein 3 (C3) in the perichondrial fibrous tissue (152).

Tophaceous Gout

Gout is a disorder of purine metabolism or of the renal excretion of uric acid. Monosodium urate precipitates as deposits (tophi) throughout the body.

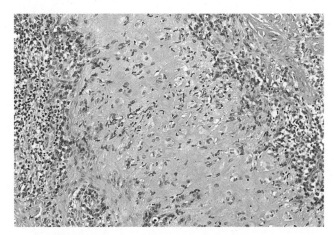

Figure 23.16. Relapsing polychondritis. The histologic features associated with relapsing polychondritis include a mixed inflammatory cell infiltrate extending into the cartilage, with blurring or obliteration of the interface between the cartilaginous plate and the adjacent fibroconnective tissues. The involved cartilage shows a loss of its normal basophilic appearance.

CLINICAL FEATURES. Gout may occur as an inherited or acquired disease (153,154). Primary gout, which represents 90% of cases, is an inherited error of metabolism that results from either an enzymatic defect in purine synthesis or a defect in the renal excretion of uric acid. Secondary or acquired gout, which comprises the remaining 10%, occurs secondary to disorders that increase the production of uric acid (e.g., leukemias) or that decrease the excretion of uric acid (e.g., chronic renal failure).

The laboratory findings include the presence of elevated urinary uric acid. Additionally, leukocytosis and an increased erythrocyte sedimentation rate are often observed. The measurement of 24-hour urinary uric acid excretion helps the clinician determine whether uric acid overproduction is a cause of the hyperuricemia (153,154). In normal body tissues, sodium urate is deposited (tophi) but, in urine with a lower pH, uric acid is precipitated (153,154). The treatment is directed toward the systemic disorder. One of the more common sites of gouty tophi is the helix of the ear. In this location, tophi may present as variably painful, skin-covered, firm nodules.

PATHOLOGIC FEATURES. Histologically, gouty tophi are composed of needle-shaped aggregates of urate crystals with a surrounding foreign body giant-cell reaction. If a diagnosis of gout is suspected, the resected tissue should be fixed in absolute alcohol or any nonaqueous fixative because the urate crystals are water-soluble.

DIFFERENTIAL DIAGNOSIS. Tophaceous gout may share similar features with tophaceous pseudogout. The designation of *pseudogout* was initially coined by McCarty et al. (155) to describe the presence of calcium pyrophosphate dihydrate crystal deposition in the synovial fluid of patients with gout-like symptoms but without sodium urate crystals. Other designations include *tumoral calcium pyrophosphate dihydrate deposition (CPPD) disease* (156), *chondrocalcinosis*, and *pyrophosphate arthropathy*. More recently, this disease has been designated as *CPPD crystal deposition disease* (157). Histologically, tophaceous pseudogout is characterized by the presence of a variably cellular, chondroid-

appearing tissue in which crystalline material is found. The crystalline material appears rhomboid or needle-shaped, and, under polarized light microscopy, the crystals show weak positive birefringence. In decalcified material, the crystals may be lost. A foreign body granulomatous reaction can be seen in association with the crystal deposition. Chondroid metaplasia is often present in and around the areas of CPPD deposition. Some evidence indicates that metaplastic chondrocytes may play a role in the initial precipitation of CPPD crystals. Synovial chondrometaplasia may be seen in patients with pyrophosphate arthropathy. The metaplastic chondrocytes may show cytologic atypia that could lead to a diagnosis of chondrosarcoma. This is particularly true in decalcified sections from which CPPD crystals are lost. In contrast to pseudogout, radiographic calcification in gouty tophi is relatively uncommon. In addition, the identification of the specific positive birefringence of the calcium pyrophosphate crystals that is seen in tophaceous pseudogout is not a feature of gouty tophi.

Wegener Granulomatosis

Wegener granulomatosis is a systemic necrotizing vasculitis that typically involves the kidneys, lung, and upper aerodigestive tract.

CLINICAL FEATURES. Otologic involvement by Wegener granulomatosis (WG) occurs in 20% to 60% of patients who have disease at these more usual sites (158–160). The most common otologic manifestations include unilateral or bilateral otitis media (serous or suppurative); perforation of the tympanic membrane; and sensorineural hearing loss (161). Cutaneous involvement of the external ear can include perforation of the ear lobes and external otitis (158,160,162). Facial palsy may occur as the initial manifestation of disease (159). The involvement of the middle ear may occur secondary to nasopharyngeal and sinonasal disease via the eustachian tube, or it may be due to direct involvement by disease.

Antineutrophil cytoplasmic autoantibodies (ANCAs) should be elevated in the active phase of WG. Two distinct staining patterns of ANCA positivity are found, including cytoplasmic (C-ANCA) and perinuclear (P-ANCA). WG is associated with C-ANCA and, infrequently, with P-ANCA (163–165); P-ANCA is more often associated with rheumatic diseases. Patients with generalized WG have a 60% to 100% C-ANCA positivity, whereas patients with limited WG have a 50% to 67% C-ANCA positivity (163,164). C-ANCA results can be utilized in establishing a diagnosis of WG in clinically suspect lesions in which the biopsies are not entirely diagnostic; false-positive results are uncommon. C-ANCA titers correlate with disease activity and recurrent disease. Proteinase-3 (PR-3) is a neutral serine proteinase present in azurophil granules of human polymorphonuclear leukocytes and monocyte lysosomal granules. PR-3 serves as the major target antigen of antineutrophil cytoplasmic antibodies with a cytoplasmic staining pattern (c-ANCA) in WG (166,167). ANCAs with specificity for PR3 are characteristic for patients with WG. Patients with WG demonstrate a significantly higher percentage of mPR3+ neutrophils than do healthy controls and patients with other inflammatory diseases. The detection of ANCAs directed against proteinase 3 (PR3-ANCA) is highly specific for WG (166,167). ANCA positivity is found only in about 50% of the patients with localized WG, whereas PR3-ANCA positivity is seen in 95% of the patients with generalized WG (167). The pathogenesis of vascular injury in WG is ascribed to antineutrophil cytoplasmic antibodies directed mainly against PR-3, and the interaction of ANCAs with neutrophilic ANCA antigens is necessary for the development of ANCA-associated diseases. In patients with WG, high expression of PR3 on the surface of nonprimed neutrophils is associated with an increased incidence and rate of relapse.

Combined corticosteroid and immunosuppressive therapy may result in long-term remissions, and treatment is capable of reversing the hearing loss and facial palsy if the diagnosis can be established and management can be initiated early in the disease course.

PATHOLOGIC FEATURES. The histologic features are similar to those described in the lungs, kidney, or upper aerodigestive tract. Elevated serum levels of ANCAs are of great assistance in those cases in which the diagnosis is suspected but the histology may not be definitively diagnostic of WG (163,165).

DIFFERENTIAL DIAGNOSIS. Other autoimmune or systemic diseases that may involve the middle or inner ear include polyarteritis nodosa and rheumatoid arthritis. Polyarteritis nodosa is a necrotizing vasculitis of small and medium-sized muscular arteries. The aural-related symptoms include otitis media with effusion (168,169). Sensorineural hearing loss may be the initial presentation, or it may develop after the diagnosis has already been established (169). The histologic diagnosis is dependent on the presence of necrotizing vasculitis. The treatment includes corticosteroids and immunosuppressant agents. The manifestations of rheumatoid arthritis of the audiovestibular system include conductive hearing loss resulting from the involvement of the incudomalleal and incudostapedial articulations (170). High-dose salicylates used in combination with steroids and nonsteroidal anti-inflammatory agents (NSAIDs) are the treatment of choice.

Otosclerosis

Otosclerosis is a disorder of the bony labyrinth and stapedial footplate that exclusively occurs in humans; it is of unknown etiology.

CLINICAL FEATURES. Otosclerosis affects women more often than men, and a family history is present in more than 50% of cases. The prevalence of otosclerosis varies with race; it is more common in whites than in blacks, Asians, or Native Americans (171). Otosclerosis primarily causes conductive hearing loss that usually begins in the second and third decades of life and slowly progresses. The extent of the hearing loss directly correlates with the degree of stapedial footplate fixation. For patients with otosclerosis also to have vestibular disturbances is not uncommon (172,173). Otosclerosis usually involves both ears; however, unilateral disease can occur in up to 15% of cases (174). Although many theories appear in the literature, the etiology of otosclerosis is unclear. Hereditary factors are often cited. Surgical management of the conductive hearing loss caused by stapes fixation (stapedectomy) is the treatment of choice.

PATHOLOGIC FEATURES. Histologically, the initial alterations include the resorption of bone around blood vessels. Cellular fibrovascular tissue replaces the resorbed bone, resulting

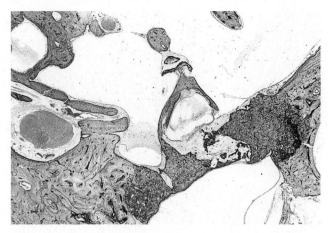

Figure 23.17. Otosclerosis of the stapedial footplate. This entity is characterized by densely sclerotic bone resulting in fixation of the stapes.

in the softening of the bone (otospongiosis). Immature bone is laid down with continuous active resorption and remodeling. The new bone is rich in ground substance and is deficient in collagen, but, over time, more mature bone with increased collagen and less ground substance is produced, resulting in densely sclerotic bone. This process most often begins anterior to the oval window, eventually involving the footplate of the stapes (Fig. 23.17). Stapedial involvement causes fixation of the stapes and the inability to transmit sound waves, resulting in conductive hearing loss. Similar pathologic involvement of the inner ear may produce sensorineural hearing loss.

Paget Disease of Bone (Osteitis Deformans)

Paget disease is a chronic, progressive disorder of unknown etiology.

CLINICAL FEATURES. The skull and temporal bone are involved in approximately 70% of cases (175). Other sites of involvement include the external auditory canal, the tympanic membrane, the eustachian tube, the ossicles, the oval window, the round window, the internal auditory canal, the cochlea, and the endolymphatic sac (175). It is slightly more common in men than in women. Paget disease affects approximately 3% of the population older than 40 years of age, and as high as 11% of the population older than 80 years of age (176). The symptoms include hearing loss, tinnitus, and vertigo. The facial nerve is spared. The hearing loss is sensorineural; mixed sensorineural and conductive; or, less often, only conductive. The hearing losses are progressive and result from involvement of the osseous portion of the external auditory canal, of the ossicles, and/or of the cochlea and labyrinth. Sarcomatous transformation occurs in roughly 1% of cases, usually as an osteosarcoma. Osteosarcomas arising in Paget disease are highly malignant, with 5-year survival rates of less than 10% (177,178).

PATHOLOGIC FEATURES. Paget disease is characterized by three histologic phases. In the first or osteolytic phase, excessive osteoclastic activity results in bone resorption. In the second mixed or combined phase, new bone formation (osteoblastic activity) predominates over bone resorption (osteoclastic activity), with deposition of new bone next to areas of bone resorption. In the third or osteoblastic phase, increased new bone that is characterized by dense, irregular masses showing a mosaic pattern of cement lines is observed.

DIFFERENTIAL DIAGNOSIS. The differential diagnosis includes otosclerosis. Features in Paget disease that assist in separating this from otosclerosis include a later age of onset, greater sensorineural hearing loss, enlarging calvaria, and enlargement and tortuosity of the superficial temporal artery and its anterior branches (176).

Ménière Disease or Endolymphatic Hydrops, Idiopathic Endolymphatic Hydrops, or Lermoyez Syndrome

Ménière disease is an idiopathic disorder of the inner ear associated with a symptom complex of spontaneous, episodic attacks of vertigo; sensorineural hearing loss; tinnitus; and a sensation of aural fullness.

CLINICAL FEATURES. The incidence of Ménière disease varies in the literature from 157 per 100,000 people in England to 46 per 100,000 in Sweden to 7.5 per 100,000 in France (170). Ménière disease occurs slightly more frequently in women than in men (1.6:1). The peak incidence is in the fifth to seventh decades of life, but it may occur in children as well as in older individuals (ninth and tenth decades). The onset of the vertigo is frequently sudden, reaching maximum intensity within a few minutes and lasting for an hour or more. It then either subsides completely or continues as a sensation of unsteadiness for hours to days.

The etiology is uncertain, although the incidence of Ménière disease is noted to be increased in patients with certain genetically acquired major histocompatibility complexes (MHCs), including human leukocyte antigen (HLA) B8/DR3 and Cw7, which suggests a possible autoimmune etiology (180–182). Familial occurrences of Ménière disease have been reported (183,184), although the role that genetic inheritance plays in the mode of transmission is variable.

Ménière disease appears to be due to changes in the anatomy of the membranous labyrinth as a consequence of the overaccumulation of endolymph (endolymphatic hydrops) at the expense of the perilymphatic space (184,185). Endolymph, which is produced by the stria vascularis in the cochlea and by cells in the vestibular labyrinth, circulates in a radial and longitudinal fashion. In patients with Ménière disease, the absorption of endolymph by the endolymphatic sac is believed to be inadequate (174–184).

Medical management is the mainstay of therapy. The therapy is aimed at the reduction of symptoms, and is therefore empiric and supportive. Optimally, management should resolve the vertigo, tinnitus, and hearing loss. The current management is directed at relieving vertigo, the most debilitating of symptoms. Therapy includes prophylaxis via the reduction of endolymph accumulation by dietary modification, intermittent dehydration, and diuretics; the enhancement of the microcirculation of the ear using vasodilators (e.g., betahistidine, adenosine triphosphate, isosorbide); and reduction in immunoreactivity using steroids, immunoglobulin, and allergy therapy (186). Symptomatic therapies include antivertiginous medications, antiemetics, sedatives, antidepressants, and psychiatric management. Improvements in 60% to 80% of patients have been re-

ported (181,187). Surgical treatment is reserved for those patients who have failed medical management (approximately 10% of patients), and includes shunting or decompression of the endolymphatic sac, labyrinthectomy, or sectioning of the vestibular nerve (186). Combined corticosteroid and immunosuppressive therapy may result in long-term remissions, and this combination is capable of reversing the hearing loss and facial palsy if the diagnosis can be established and the treatment is initiated early in the disease course.

PATHOLOGIC FEATURES. In the early stages of the disease, endolymphatic hydrops primarily involves the cochlear duct and saccule, but, in the later stages, the entire endolymphatic system is involved. Alterations of the membranous labyrinth include dilatation, outpouching, rupture, and collapse. Fistulae (unhealed ruptures) may occur. Severe cytoarchitectural and atrophic changes may occur, including the loss of neurons in the cochlea.

Neoplasms of the Ear and Temporal Bone

The classification of neoplastic lesions of the ear and temporal bone is detailed in Table 23.3. The most common lesions of the external ear have a cutaneous origin; these include basal cell carcinoma, squamous cell carcinoma, verrucous carcinoma, malignant melanoma, Merkel cell carcinoma, keratoacanthoma, squamous papilloma, and others. The reader is referred to the chapter on neoplasms of the skin found elsewhere in this text for a more complete discussion of these entities. This chapter focuses instead on neoplasms that are unique or that are primarily localized to the ear and temporal bone.

BENIGN EPITHELIAL NEOPLASMS OF THE EXTERNAL EAR

Ceruminal Gland Adenoma

Ceruminal gland tumors are benign tumors of cerumen-secreting modified apocrine glands (ceruminal glands) located in the external auditory canal. These glands are located in the dermis of the cartilaginous (inner) portion of the external auditory canal. In general, ceruminal gland neoplasms are uncommon, but they represent one of the more common tumors of the external auditory canal. The generic designation of *ceruminoma* should be avoided. Ceruminal gland neoplasms should be specifically diagnosed according to tumor type. The classification of ceruminal gland neoplasms includes benign and malignant tumors. The benign ceruminal gland tumors include ceruminal gland adenoma (ceruminoma), pleomorphic adenoma, and syringocystadenoma papilliferum (188). The malignant ceruminal gland tumors include ceruminal gland adenocarcinoma, adenoid cystic carcinoma, and mucoepidermoid carcinoma (188).

CLINICAL FEATURES. Ceruminal gland adenomas tend to affect men more than women, and they occur over a wide age range; they are seen most frequently in the fourth to sixth decades of life. The symptoms include a slow-growing external auditory canal mass or blockage; hearing difficulty; and, infrequently, otic discharge (188–192). For all benign ceruminal gland neoplasms, complete surgical excision, which is curative,

TABLE 23.3	Classification of Neoplasms of the Ear and Temporal Bone

External Ear

Benign	Malignant
Epithelial/neuroectodermal/ mesenchymal	Epithelial/neuroectodermal/mesenchymal
Keratoacanthoma	Basal cell carcinoma
Ceruminal gland neoplasms	Squamous cell carcinoma and variants (verrucous
Seborrheic keratoses	carcinoma, spindle cell squamous carcinoma,
Squamous papilloma	adenoid squamous cell carcinoma)
Melanocytic nevi	Ceruminal gland adenocarcinomas
Dermal adnexal neoplasms	Malignant melanoma
Pilomatrixoma (calcifying epithelioma	Merkel cell carcinoma
of Malherbe)	Atypical fibroxanthoma (superficial malignant fibrous
Neurilemoma/neurofibroma	histiocytoma)
Osteoma; chondroma	
Hemangioma	
Others	

Middle and Inner Ear

Benign	Malignant
Epithelial	Epithelial
Middle ear adenoma	Middle ear adenocarcinoma
Middle ear papilloma	Primary squamous cell carcinoma
Others	Mesenchymal
Neuroectodermal/mesenchymal	Rhabdomyosarcoma
Jugulotympanic paraganglioma	Vascular (angiosarcoma; Kaposi sarcoma)
Meningioma	Lymphoproliferative (malignant lymphoma; plasmacy-
Acoustic neuroma	toma)
Others	Secondary tumors
Indeterminant	Squamous cell carcinoma from other head and neck
Endolymphatic sac papillary tumor	sites; breast carcinoma; pulmonary adenocarci-
	noma malignant melanoma; renal cell carcinoma,
	prostatic adenocarcinoma, others

is the treatment of choice. Recurrences can develop, and they are related to inadequate surgical excision.

PATHOLOGIC FEATURES. The gross appearance of ceruminal gland neoplasms includes skin-covered, circumscribed, polypoid, or rounded masses from 1 to 4 cm in diameter. Ulceration is uncommon, and it may suggest a malignant neoplasm. Histologically, ceruminal gland adenomas are unencapsulated but well-demarcated glandular proliferations. The glands vary in size and they may have various combinations of growth patterns, including solid, cystic, and papillary. A cribriform or back-to-back glandular pattern is commonly seen. The glands are composed of two cell layers. The inner or luminal epithelial cell is cuboidal or columnar with eosinophilic cytoplasm and the decapitation-type secretion (apical "snouts") characteristic for apocrine cells, whereas the outer cell layer, which is of myoepithelial differentiation, is spindled with hyperchromatic nuclei (Fig. 23.18). A golden yellow-brown, granular-appearing pigment can be seen in the cells of the inner lining; this represents cerumen. Cellular pleomorphism and mitotic figures can be seen but they are not prominent.

Diastase-resistant, PAS-positive, or mucicarmine-positive intracytoplasmic or intraluminal material may be seen. IHC stains show the luminal cells to be strongly and diffusely immunoreactive with CK7, as well as with CD117 positivity (192). The basal cells are CK5/6-, S-100 protein-, and p63-positive (192). Ultra-

structure evaluation includes the presence of epithelial (apocrine cell) and myoepithelial cell differentiation. Epithelial cells show features of apocrine cells, including apocrine caps, microvilli, cell junctions, secretory granules, vacuoles, lipid droplets, and siderosomes (193).

Ceruminal gland pleomorphic adenomas are uncommon tumors. The histologic composition is similar to that of pleomorphic adenomas of salivary gland origin, including a variable admixture of epithelial and myoepithelial components set in a myxoid to chondromyxoid stroma. Syringocystadenoma papilliferum is a benign tumor of apocrine gland origin that usually occurs on the scalp and face area, but that may originate from ceruminal glands in the external auditory canal. The histologic makeup is similar to that of tumors of the more common cutaneous sites.

BENIGN MESENCHYMAL TUMORS OF THE EXTERNAL EAR

Mesenchymal tumors of the external auditory canal are rare; they include osteoma (194), chondroma (195), leiomyoma (196), schwannoma (197), and myxomas (198). In contrast to exostosis, osteomas are true neoplasms of bone that are capable of unlimited growth. Osteomas occur in the external auditory canal and present as an asymptomatic solitary mass. Histologi-

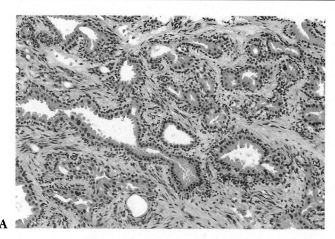

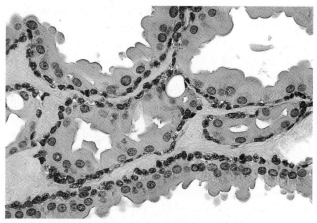

A   B

Figure 23.18. Ceruminal gland adenoma. **(A)** This adenoma is characterized by unencapsulated glandular proliferations in which the glands vary in size and shape; it may include a back-to-back glandular pattern of growth. **(B)** The glands are composed of two cell layers, including inner (luminal) epithelial cells that vary in appearance from cuboidal to columnar with an eosinophilic cytoplasm and decapitation-type secretion (apical "snouts") characteristic of apocrine-derived cells, and an outer layer of spindle-shaped cells with hyperchromatic nuclei representing myoepithelial cells. Intracytoplasmic granular, golden yellow to brown-appearing pigment (cerumen) is seen within the inner (luminal) epithelial cells.

cally, osteomas are composed of mature bone with associated intraosseous fibrovascular tissue.

Myxomas of the external ear and external auditory canal have been described in an autosomal dominant syndrome complex that includes myxomas in other locations, most notably cardiac sites; spotty pigmentation; endocrine tumors; and schwannomas (198). Myxomas are characterized by the presence of sparse cellularity and a paucity of blood vessels. The lesion consists chiefly of mucoid material in which a loose framework of reticulin fibers is suspended. The cellular component consists of a population of spindled to stellate cells with tiny pyknotic nuclei and delicate cytoplasmic process. Cellular pleomorphism is not seen. A pseudocapsule of condensed reticulin fibers and compressed host tissue, particularly skeletal muscle, surrounds the periphery of the tumor. The myxoid matrix in myxoma stains with Alcian blue and is hyaluronidase-sensitive. Mucicarmine and colloidal iron also stain the material. The cellular component of myxomas is vimentin-positive but does not express skeletal muscle antigens or S-100 protein. Although soft tissue myxomas lack a discrete capsule, they rarely recur after excision.

Myxoid change occurs in a variety of benign neoplasms, including neurofibroma, neurilemoma, and lipoma, and it may mimic myxoma, especially in limited biopsy material. Of greater concern is the histologic pattern in myxomas, which may mimic myxoid soft tissue malignancies. These particularly embryonal rhabdomyosarcoma, as well as myxoid malignant fibrous histiocytoma, myxoid liposarcoma, and myxoid chondrosarcoma, are much more common in this location. In contrast to myxoma, sarcomas display much greater cellularity and a richer vascular pattern. Furthermore, the cytologic features differ. Cellular pleomorphism and increased numbers of mitotic figures are seen in sarcomas. Differentiated cell types, such as multinucleated giant cells in myxoid malignant fibrous histiocytoma, lipoblasts in liposarcoma, rhabdomyoblasts in rhabdomyosarcoma, and atypical chondroblasts in chondrosarcoma, are distinctive features.

MALIGNANT NEOPLASMS OF THE EXTERNAL EAR

Squamous Cell Carcinoma of the External Auditory Canal

CLINICAL FEATURES. Squamous cell carcinoma (SCC) accounts for approximately 15% of all primary cutaneous carcinomas of the external ear and auditory canal (199). SCC of the external ear is more common in men than in women, whereas SCC of the external auditory canal is more common in women than in men (200,201). SCC in both of these sites is most frequent in the seventh to eighth decades of life. SCC of the external ear presents as a nonhealing sore, whereas SCC of the external auditory canal may present with symptoms mimicking those of a COM, including pain, hearing deficits, and otorrhea (bloody or purulent).

The treatment for SCC of these sites is complete surgical excision. In general, early detection and complete removal result in a good prognosis. SCC of the external auditory canal often requires a radical procedure (mastoidectomy or temporal bone resection). Radiation therapy may be indicated, depending on the extent of disease. The prognosis is dependent on the extent of disease and the presence or absence of metastases. SCC of the ear has unusually high recurrence and metastatic rates (18.7% and 11%, respectively) that are more than twice the rates observed in squamous cell carcinomas of other cutaneous sites (202).

The histologic differentiation does not correlate with the prognosis. Regional lymph node metastases are infrequently seen, and death is generally attributed to the invasion of regional structures, particularly intracranial extension. The presence of a malignancy should be considered in patients with chronic ear infections who suddenly have a change in symptoms, including pain, bleeding, or facial paralysis. A large study of SCCs of the skin by Rowe et al. linked several pathologic factors to a propensity for local recurrence and metastases (202). These included a diameter greater than 2 cm, a depth greater than 4 mm, poor differentiation, perineural invasion, development within a scar, previously treated squamous carcinoma in the site, and host immunosuppression.

PATHOLOGIC FEATURES. SCCs of the external ear often are polypoid, rubbery to firm nodules that frequently have ulceration. In general, SCCs in this region tend to be well differentiated, and they are composed of infiltrating nests of cells with keratinization in the form of keratin pearls or individual cell keratinization and intercellular bridges. Nuclear atypia is present, but it is quite variable. Increased mitotic activity is present, and it may include atypical forms. Frequently, invasive growth is seen, varying from superficial invasion with irregular budding of the basal epithelium from the skin surface, to the more obvious invasion characterized by irregular tongues of tumor projecting downward from the surface epithelium and irregular strands of atypical epithelial cells extending between the dermal collagen fibers. Moderately differentiated squamous cell carcinoma lacks keratin pearls, but does have scattered individual keratinized cells. In poorly differentiated SCC, keratinization is extremely difficult to identify, and the classification as SCC is based on features such as associated squamous epithelial dysplasia, a pavementlike squamoid cellular pattern, or foci in which intercellular bridges or some evidence of keratinization is seen.

Spindle cell squamous carcinoma (SCSC) or sarcomatoid carcinoma is a morphologic variant that may occur on the external ear. SCSCs are characterized by an infiltrative tumor with interlacing bundles or a fascicular growth pattern composed of spindle-shaped and epithelioid cells with pleomorphic and hyperchromatic nuclei, increased nuclear:cytoplasmic ratios, variable amphophilic to eosinophilic cytoplasm, and increased mitotic activity with atypical forms. Surface ulceration is often present. In the presence of an intact surface epithelium, the tumor's direct continuity with the overlying epithelium may be seen. Helpful histologic features in determining the epithelial differentiation of these tumors include the presence of surface epithelial dysplasia, infiltrating nests of differentiated SCC, or the presence of cytokeratin immunoreactivity in the spindle cells. However, these findings are not infrequently absent. Some SCSCs may exhibit evidence of divergent differentiation with the production of chondroid or osteoid matrix (191–203).

Adenoid squamous cell carcinoma is an unusual variant of SCC, with a propensity to occur on the face and scalp and especially on the periauricular area (204). The "adenoid" designation refers to a pseudoglandular appearance that results from tumor cell acantholysis (Fig. 23.19) (205). The islands of tumor cells show central acantholysis, in which cohesiveness is lost and the tumor cells crumble apart, leaving a relatively intact peripheral rim of more cohesive tumor cells and simulating the presence of a glandular lumen. The acantholytic cells in the false "lumen" often show the deeply eosinophilic cytoplasm that is common in exfoliated dyskeratotic cells. The tumor can usually be seen emanating from dysplastic surface epithelium, further supporting its squamous origins. The glandlike spaces often contain some amorphous basophilic material; however, histochemically, no evidence of epithelial mucin is found.

IHC is not usually required in the diagnosis of SCCs of the pinna and external auditory canal, except in the SCSCs. SCSC is reactive for cytokeratin or epithelial membrane antigen (EMA) (cell membrane staining pattern), as well as p63 (nuclear staining), though the staining may be focal. Vimentin, although it is not specific, is almost always reactive as well. The tumor cells

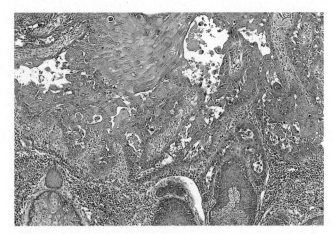

Figure 23.19. Preauricular adenoid squamous cell carcinoma. The associated acantholysis creates a pseudoglandular appearance.

do not mark for S-100 protein or with melanocytic markers (e.g., HMB-45, tyrosinase, MelanA).

DIFFERENTIAL DIAGNOSIS. The differential diagnosis of SCC of the external ear and auditory canal includes seborrheic keratosis, especially those that are inflamed. SCSC must be differentiated from cutaneous malignant melanoma and malignant fibrous histiocytoma.

Ceruminal Gland Adenocarcinoma

Ceruminal gland adenocarcinoma is a malignant neoplasm of cerumen-secreting modified apocrine glands (ceruminal glands) located in the external auditory canal.

CLINICAL FEATURES. The demographics of ceruminal gland adenocarcinomas are similar to those of ceruminal gland adenomas. In contrast to ceruminal gland adenoma, patients with ceruminal gland adenocarcinomas have associated pain more often (188,190,206,207).

For ceruminal gland adenocarcinoma, en bloc surgical resection is the treatment of choice. Middle ear or temporal bone involvement necessitates more radical surgery (206). Supplemental radiation therapy is recommended. Metastases are rare, and they include regional lymph nodes and the lung (190,206). For ceruminal gland adenoid cystic carcinoma and mucoepidermoid carcinoma, wide surgical resection with or without supplemental radiation therapy is the recommended treatment (207). The prognosis for ceruminal gland adenoid cystic carcinoma generally is similar to its salivary gland counterpart, including relatively good short-term (i.e., 5-year) survival but poor long-term (i.e., 10-year to 20-year) survival (206,207).

PATHOLOGIC FEATURES. Histologically, features that may assist in differentiating the ceruminal gland adenocarcinomas from the adenomas include a loss of the glandular double cell layer, with identification of only the inner or luminal epithelial cell; the presence of cell pleomorphism with nuclear anaplasia; increased mitotic activity; and invasive growth (Fig. 23.20). However, well-differentiated ceruminal gland adenocarcinomas may appear similar to their benign counterparts, and these are differentiated only on the basis of invasive growth. At the other

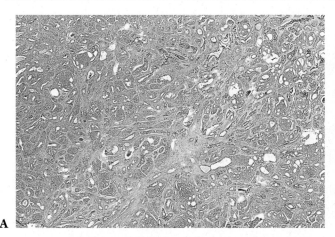
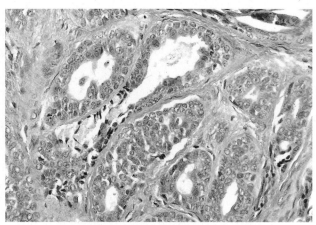

A   **B**

Figure 23.20. Ceruminal gland adenocarcinoma. **(A)** This external auditory canal glandular lesion is infiltrative with a complex growth, including cribriform and solid patterns. **(B)** At higher magnification, the glands are characterized by the presence of cellular pleomorphism with nuclear anaplasia and by the loss of the dual cell layers seen in ceruminal gland adenomas.

end of the spectrum, poorly differentiated ceruminal adenocarcinomas do occur; these are recognized on the basis of their localization in the external auditory canal. In addition to the more conventional type of ceruminal gland adenocarcinomas, other types of ceruminal gland malignant tumors include adenoid cystic carcinoma and mucoepidermoid carcinoma. These tumors are morphologically identical to their salivary gland counterparts.

DIFFERENTIAL DIAGNOSIS. Given the proximity of the parotid gland to the external auditory canal, the differential diagnosis for ceruminal gland adenoid cystic carcinoma and mucoepidermoid carcinoma includes the direct extension of similar tumors of primary parotid origin. Therefore, parotid gland adenoid cystic carcinoma and mucoepidermoid carcinoma should be excluded before such tumors are diagnosed as being of primary ceruminal gland origin. The same applies for ceruminal gland pleomorphic adenoma. Wolf et al. (191) have also cautioned about misdiagnosing a benign dermal eccrine cylindroma of the external auditory canal as an adenoid cystic carcinoma.

Atypical Fibroxanthoma or Superficial Malignant Fibrous Histiocytoma

Atypical fibroxanthoma (AFX) is a pleomorphic, predominantly dermal mesenchymal tumor found on actinic-damaged cutaneous sites of older patients, or are found in younger patients and involve the superficial soft tissues of the extremities and trunk (208). Synonyms include superficial (low-grade) malignant fibrous histiocytoma, pseudosarcoma of skin, and pseudosarcomatous dermatofibroma.

CLINICAL FEATURES. AFX occurs in two clinical forms, neither having a specific gender predilection. The most common form, accounting for approximately 75% of cases, affects elderly patients and commonly involves the head and neck (ears, cheeks, nose). A less common form, accounting for approximately 25% of cases, affects younger patients and commonly involves superficial sites on the limbs and trunk. Both forms

most often present as an asymptomatic solitary growth on the affected body site; bleeding, pruritus, and pain may occur.

The etiology is related to actinic damage. The presence of *p53* mutations supports the role of ultraviolet radiation damage in the development of AFX (209).

Conservative but complete surgical excision is the treatment of choice. The prognosis is excellent. Local recurrence, which is uncommon, is related to incomplete excision. Recurrent tumors may present as a large mass in the deep soft tissue; these neoplasms should be considered and treated as bona fide malignant fibrous histiocytomas (208). AFX has been reported to metastasize, but these cases may, in fact, represent malignant fibrous histiocytoma (MFH) (208).

PATHOLOGIC FEATURES. AFX of the ear presents as an asymptomatic, firm nodule measuring from 1 to 2 cm in diameter, and it frequently has associated ulceration. Histologically, AFX is an unencapsulated but generally circumscribed spindle cell neoplasm arising in the dermis. The cellular component is varied, including a spectrum of elongated, spindle-shaped to pleomorphic cells with hyperchromatic nuclei and bizarre, multinucleated cells (Fig. 23.21). The larger cells may have foamy cytoplasm that is reminiscent of lipid-rich histiocytic cells. In some cases, a pleomorphic component may be absent. AFX may also appear as a predominantly spindle-cell, nonpleomorphic tumor (210). Increased mitotic figures, including atypical forms, are readily identified. Areas may exhibit a storiform pattern, but this is not usually prominent. Junctional activity is absent. Superficial areas adjacent to the tumor show solar elastosis and vascular proliferation; prominent stromal sclerosis may be present (211). A chronic inflammatory infiltrate may accompany the tumor. Vascular invasion may be seen, but necrosis is uncommon.

Unusual variants include clear-cell and granular-cell (212,213). The clear-cell variant of AFX is characterized by sheets of large cells with foamy cytoplasms and hyperchromatic, polypoid nuclei with frequent mitoses, including atypical mitoses (212). The clear cells express CD68 but not CD3, CD20, CD34, S-100 protein, muscle-specific actin, factor XIIIa, Melan-A, carcinoembryonic antigen, or cytokeratin (212). Differentia-

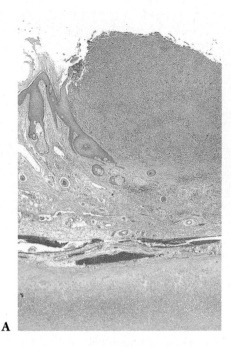

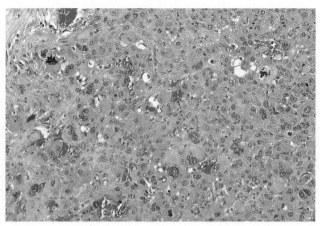

Figure 23.21. Atypical fibroxanthoma (AFX) of the ear. **(A)** An ulcerated, circumscribed cellular lesion is seen in the superficial aspect of the auricular skin. **(B)** The cellular component of AFX includes markedly pleomorphic cells with hyperchromatic nuclei; bizarre, multinucleated cells; and increased mitotic figures, including atypical mitoses. Cells with foamy-appearing cytoplasm that are reminiscent of lipid-rich histiocytic cells are present.

tion from balloon-cell melanoma, sebaceous carcinoma, pleomorphic liposarcoma, chordoma, parachordoma, tricholemmal carcinoma, and clear-cell squamous cell carcinoma is predicated on differentiating IHC staining. Multinucleated, osteoclastic-like giant cells, as well as osteoid, may rarely be present (214).

Uncommonly, pigmentation may occur. These lesions have been termed *pigmented atypical fibroxanthoma* (215). Pigmented AFX can be easily mistaken for malignant melanoma clinically and histopathologically. The pigmentation is believed to represent hemorrhage, with neoplastic cells ingesting and degrading erythrocytes following intratumoral hemorrhage and to accumulate hemosiderin in their cytoplasm; pigment stains for iron.

IHC is extremely valuable in the differential diagnosis of AFX. In AFX, there is variable staining for CD68 (KP1), muscle-specific actin, and smooth muscle actin (216,217). CD99 reactivity is present (218). No immunoreactivity is seen for cytokeratins, S-100 protein (except for scattered, nonneoplastic dendritic cells), desmin, and melanoma markers (e.g., HMB-45, Melan-A) (210,216,217). Aberrant HMB45 and MART-1 (melanoma antigen recognized by T cells-1) staining have been reported limited to the large, multinucleated cells with vacuolated cytoplasm (219).

Ultrastructural studies have shown evidence of fibrohistiocytic and myofibroblastic features and, to a lesser extent, features of Langerhans cells (220). Features indicative of epithelial differentiation (e.g., prominent intercellular bridges, tonofibrils) or melanocytic differentiation (e.g., premelanosome, melanosomes) are absent.

Deletions on chromosomes 9p and 13q have been identified, representing similar genetic alterations as seen in undifferentiated high-grade pleomorphic sarcoma; this suggests a common pathogenetic pathway (221). However, statistically significant differences of genetic alterations between AFX and undifferentiated high-grade pleomorphic sarcoma concerning deletions on 1q, 3p, 5q, 11p, and 11q; gains on 7q, 12q; and high-level gains on 5p and 11q have been found (221). These

genetic differences may contribute to the different biological behavior of these two tumors.

DIFFERENTIAL DIAGNOSIS. The differential diagnosis of AFX includes SCSC and spindle cell malignant melanoma. This distinction has been previously discussed in those sections. AFX must be differentiated from leiomyosarcoma. IHC stains should allow the pathologist to separate AFX from leiomyosarcoma, with the latter tumor showing reactivity for desmin (210). The relationship of AFX to *superficial* MFH may be academic because both are associated with a good prognosis following complete surgical resection (208). If a tumor has the histologic features of AFX but is large (greater than 2 cm in diameter) and extensively infiltrative, and has necrosis or vascular invasion, then it should be considered a malignant fibrous histiocytoma (MFH) (208). This distinction is important because therapy for MFH includes surgery with supplemental irradiation.

NEOPLASMS OF THE MIDDLE EAR AND TEMPORAL BONE

BENIGN TUMORS OF THE MIDDLE EAR AND TEMPORAL BONE

Middle Ear Adenoma

CLINICAL FEATURES. Middle ear adenoma (MEA) is a benign glandular neoplasm originating from the middle ear mucosa (222,223). MEA occurs equally in both genders and over a wide age range, but it is most common in the third to fifth decades of life. Any portion of the middle ear may be affected, including the eustachian tube, mastoid air spaces, ossicles, and chorda tympani nerve. The most common symptom is unilateral conductive hearing loss, but fullness, tinnitus, and dizziness may also occur. Pain, otic discharge, and facial nerve paralysis rarely occur; if they are present, they may be indicative of a malignant process. In the majority of cases, otoscopic examination identifies an intact tympanic membrane with a tumor that is confined to the middle ear space with possible extension to the mastoid. Occasionally, the adenoma perforates through the tympanic membrane with extension into and presentation as an external auditory canal mass. No etiologic factors related to the development of MEA are known. MEAs are not associated with a history of COM. Concurrent cholesteatomas may be seen with MEA, but no known association exists between these two lesions.

The treatment for all MEAs is complete surgical excision. Surgery may be conservative if the lesion is small and confined to the middle ear, or more radical (mastoidectomy) for larger lesions associated with more extensive structural involvement. A recurrent tumor is a function of inadequate excision. Some MEAs may be locally aggressive, and they may rarely invade vital structures, causing death; however, metastatic disease does not occur. In general, the clinical, radiologic, and pathologic findings are indicative of a benign tumor. Nevertheless, the histologic appearance is not always predictive of the clinical behavior.

PATHOLOGIC FEATURES. MEAs are gray-white to red-brown, rubbery to firm masses free of significant bleeding on manipulation. Histologically, MEAs are unencapsulated lesions with gland or tubule formation, as well as solid, sheetlike, trabecular, cystic, and cribriform growth patterns (Fig. 23.22). The neoplastic glands occur individually or have back-to-back growth. The glands are composed of a single layer of cuboidal to columnar cells with a varying amount of eosinophilic cytoplasm and a round to oval hyperchromatic nucleus. Nucleoli may be seen and, generally, are eccentrically located. The cells may have a prominent plasmacytoid appearance that is particularly evident in the more solid areas of growth, but also in the cells forming the glandular structures (Fig. 23.23). A paranuclear clear zone is not present. Cellular pleomorphism may be prominent but mitotic figures are uncommon. The stromal component is sparse and it may appear fibrous or myxoid.

Histochemical stains show the presence of intraluminal, but not intracytoplasmic, mucin-positive material. PAS-positive material is not present. On IHC evaluation (Table 23.4), the neoplastic cells are cytokeratin-positive, including diffusely positive for AE1/AE3, CAM 5.2, and CK7, and exhibit focal and weak CK20 reactivity (224). Neuroendocrine differentiation may be

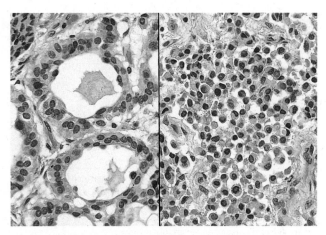

Figure 23.23. Middle ear adenoma. The neoplastic cells in the glandular (*left*) and solid (*right*) components show plasmacytoid features.

seen (see next section), as seen by chromogranin, synaptophysin, and neuron-specific enolase immunoreactivity. Serotonin and human pancreatic polypeptide also may be present. S-100 protein and vimentin staining may be present. Desmin and actin are negative.

Middle Ear Adenomas with Neuroendocrine Differentiation

In some MEAs, the cells may have dispersed or stippled nuclear chromatin with the "salt and pepper" pattern seen in neuroendocrine tumors (Fig. 23.24) and/or demonstrate architectural characteristics seen in association with neuroendocrine neoplasms (e.g., ribbons, cords, organoid growth).

Immunoreactivity for one or more neuroendocrine markers, including chromogranin and synaptophysin, is present (Fig. 23.24; Table 23.4). In addition, neuron-specific enolase, serotonin, and human pancreatic polypeptide also may be present. Despite the presence of vasoactive compounds in these tumors, carcinoid syndrome is extraordinarily rare in association with these middle ear neoplasms. These MEAs with neuroendocrine differentiation have been termed *carcinoid tumors of the middle ear* (224–228), as well as *neuroendocrine adenoma* (224). However, these so-called carcinoid tumors are better viewed as part of the histologic spectrum of MEA (229,230), albeit one with neuroendocrine differentiation, rather than as representing a distinct middle ear neoplasm separate from MEA. El-Naggar et al. (230) showed the presence of chromogranin-positive cells within hyperplastic but not in nonneoplastic middle ear epithelium overlying an MEA, which supports the inclusion of middle ear glandular tumors with neuroendocrine differentiation within the spectrum of MEA. Nevertheless, the issue whether to classify these tumors as MEA with neuroendocrine differentiation or carcinoid tumors (also referred to as *well-differentiated neuroendocrine carcinomas*) remains controversial. The controversy relates to the biologic behavior of these tumors. On the basis of long-term follow-up, the overwhelming majority of these tumors have a benign biologic course, supporting the classification of these tumors as part of the histologic spectrum of MEA, albeit with neuroendocrine differentiation, rather than representing a distinct middle ear neoplasm separate from MEA. However, Ramsey et al. (231) report locally recurrent tumor (which may be

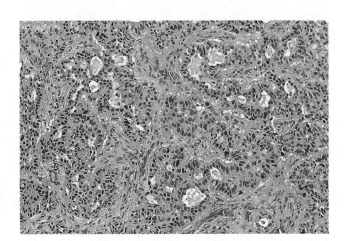

Figure 23.22. Middle ear adenoma composed of a diffuse gland-forming proliferation. The glands may appear individually or they may have back-to-back growth.

TABLE 23.4		Immunohistochemical Reactivity of Middle Ear Neoplasms								
Neoplasm	*CK*	*EMA*	*CG*	*SYN*	*S-100*	*NSE*	*GFAP*	*VIM*	*DES*	*Myf4*
MEA	+	+	−	−	−	−	−	−	−	−
MEA-NE	+	+	+	+	v	+	−	−	−	−
JTP	−	−	+	+	+[a]	+	−	−	−	−
MEN	−	+	−	−	−	−	−	+	−	−
AN	−	−	−	−	+	+	−	−	−	−
ESPT	v	v	−	−	v	v	v	v	−	+
RMS	−	−	−	−	−	−	−	+	+	+

[a]Positive in the peripherally situated sustentacular cells.
MEA, middle ear adenoma; NE, neuroendocrine features; JTP, jugulotympanic paraganglioma; MEN, meningioma; AN, acoustic neuroma; ESPT, endolymphatic sac papillary tumor; RMS, rhabdomyosarcoma; CK, cytokeratin; EMA, epithelial membrane antigen; CG, chromogranin; SYN, synaptophysin; NSE, neuron-specific enolase; GFAP, glial fibrillary acidic protein; VIM, vimentin; DES, desmin.
+, positive; −, negative; v, variably positive.
Adapted from Wenig BM. Immunohistochemistry of middle ear neoplasms. In Wenig BM, ed. *Atlas of Head and Neck Pathology.* 2nd ed. St. Louis: Elsevier, 2008:812.

a function of inadequate initial excision) or regional metastasis, asserting that at least some of these middle ear neoplasms are carcinoid tumors/well-differentiated neuroendocrine carcinomas.

DIFFERENTIAL DIAGNOSIS. The differential diagnosis of MEA primarily includes jugulotympanic paraganglioma, meningioma, and acoustic neuroma. The pathologic features of these other tumor types are discussed in their respective sections. Glandular metaplasia may occur in the setting of COM. In contrast to MEA, the glandular proliferation in COM is focal or haphazardly arrayed, and it occurs in the presence of histologic features of COM, including chronic inflammation with fibrosis and calcifications (tympanosclerosis). MEA may perforate the tympanic membrane, and it may appear to represent a neoplasm of the external auditory canal, such as a ceruminal gland adenoma. The histologic features of these two tumor types are distinctly different, so they should allow easy distinction. In contrast to the rare middle ear adenocarcinoma, MEA lacks marked cellular pleomorphism, increased mitotic activity, necrosis, or invasion of the bone and other soft tissue structures.

Some confusion exists in the literature regarding MEA and its relationship to the endolymphatic sac papillary tumor (ESPT). As is discussed in "Endolymphatic Sac Papillary Tumor" below, the pathologic features and clinical course of ESPT differ decidedly from those of MEA.

Jugulotympanic Paraganglioma

Jugulotympanic paraganglioma (JTP) is a benign neoplasm that arises from the extra-adrenal neural crest-derived paraganglia specifically located in the middle ear or temporal bone region. Synonyms include glomus jugulare tumor or glomus tympanicum tumor.

CLINICAL FEATURES. JTPs are considered the most common tumor of the middle ear (222,223). They affect women more often than men, and they are most common in the fifth

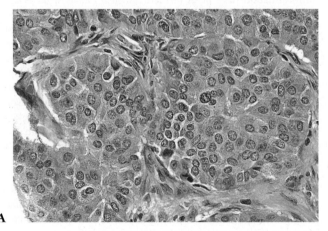
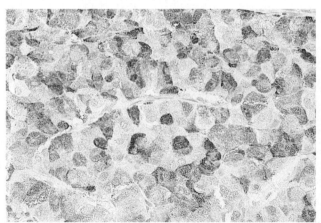

A   **B**

Figure 23.24. Middle ear adenoma with neuroendocrine differentiation. **(A)** This middle ear adenoma shows foci of solid cell nests with an organoid growth pattern and nuclei with dispersed nuclear chromatin that is suggestive of neuroendocrine differentiation. **(B)** In addition to cytokeratin immunoreactivity (not shown), these foci were immunoreactive for chromogranin (seen in this illustration) and synaptophysin (not shown).

to seventh decades of life. The majority (85%) of JTPs arise in the jugular bulb, resulting in a mass lesion in the middle ear or external auditory canal (222). Approximately 12% originate from the Jacobson nerve (tympanic branch of the glossopharyngeal nerve) and present as a middle ear tumor (222). Roughly 3% begin from the Arnold nerve (posterior auricular branch of the vagus nerve) and arise in the external auditory canal (222). The most common symptom is conductive hearing loss. Other symptoms include tinnitus, fullness, otic discharge, pain, hemorrhage, facial nerve abnormalities, and vertigo. JTPs are often locally invasive neoplasms that destroy the adjacent structures, including the temporal bone and mastoid (222,232). Neurologic abnormalities, including cranial nerve palsies, cerebellar dysfunction, dysphagia, and hoarseness, may be seen, and these correlate to the invasive capabilities of this neoplasm. Computed tomography scan shows a soft tissue mass often with evidence of extensive destruction of adjacent structures. Because JTPs are vascularized lesions, carotid angiography will show the lesion fed by branches of nearby large arteries. By MR imaging, tumors larger than 2 cm have a unique salt-and-pepper pattern of hyperintensity and hypointensity on T1-weighted and T2-weighted imaging.

JTPs may be familial (233). Familial JTPs may be multifocal, including the jugulotympanic and carotid bodies. An autosomal dominant pattern of inheritance is favored. Genetic analysis has shown linkage with two different loci, including 11q13.1 and 11q22.3-q23 (234,235).

Jugular and tympanic paragangliomas have been reported as a single entity (i.e., temporal bone paragangliomas) but their distinction has important clinical and therapeutic implications; as such, classification schemes based on site of origin (Table 23.5) or based on site and origin and extent of tumor involvement have been developed (Table 23.6) (236).

Complete surgical excision is the treatment of choice; however, the location and invasive nature of these lesions often

TABLE 23.5

Classification of Temporal Bone Paragangliomas

Class A	Tumors arising along the tympanic plexus on the middle ear promontory
Class B	Tumors arising from the inferior tympanic canal of the hypotympanum; may invade the middle ear and mastoid; cortical bone over jugular bulb is intact; carotid canal is intact
Class C	Tumors arising in dome of jugular bulb and involving the overlying cortical bone
C1	Tumors eroding the carotid canal but not involving the carotid artery
C2	Tumors involving the vertical carotid canal
C3	Tumors involving the horizontal carotid canal; foramen lacerum is free of tumor
C4	Tumors involving the foramen lacerum and the cavernous sinus
Class D	Tumors with intracranial extension of posterior fossa
De1	Extradural tumor of less than 2 cm medial dural displacement
De2	Extradural tumor of more than 2 cm medial dural displacement
Di1	Intradural tumor of less than 2 cm
Di2	Intradural tumor of more than 2 cm
Di3	Neurosurgically unresectable tumor

TABLE 23.6

Glassock-Jackson Classification of Glomus Tumors

Glomus Tympanicum

Type I	Small mass limited to promontory
Type II	Tumor completely filling the middle ear space
Type III	Tumor filling the middle ear and extending into the mastoid
Type IV	Tumor filling the middle ear, extending into the mastoid or through the tympanic membrane to fill the external auditory canal; may also extend anterior to the internal carotid artery

Glomus Jugulare

Type I	Small tumor involving the jugular bulb, middle ear, and mastoid
Type II	Tumor extending under the internal auditory canal; may have intracranial extension
Type III	Tumor extending into petrous apex; may have intracranial extension
Type IV	Tumor extending beyond the petrous apex into the clivus or infratemporal fossa; may have intracranial extension

preclude complete resection. Unresectable paragangliomas include those with extensive skull base involvement or intracranial extension, and patients who might be poor surgical candidates include medically infirm and elderly. In such cases, radiation therapy is a useful adjunct to surgery. Radiotherapy results in a decrease or ablation of vascularity and promotes fibrosis. Radiotherapy has been primarily used to treat jugular paragangliomas of the temporal bone. Because there is rarely total resolution of the tumor following radiotherapy, successful treatment of paragangliomas with radiotherapy is defined as local control in the form of stability or regression of tumor size, and nonprogression or improvement of neurologic symptoms (236,237). Preoperative embolization is useful in decreasing the vascularity of the tumor and facilitating surgical resection. Postembolization angiography should document absence of tumor "blush" with continued patency of the external carotid systems; not all paragangliomas should be embolized. The decision is dependent on the location and extent of tumor, and the experience of the surgeon and interventional radiologist. Local recurrences can be seen in up to 50% of cases. The histologic appearance of paragangliomas does not correlate to the biologic behavior of the tumor. Intracranial extension may occur in up to 15% of cases (238). Functioning JTPs, which are evidenced by endocrinopathic manifestations, do occur but they are extremely uncommon. Malignant JTPs also occur; they are associated with histologic criteria of malignancy, including increased mitotic activity; necrosis that is usually seen within the center of the cell nests; and vascular invasion. They may metastasize to cervical lymph nodes, lungs, and liver (239,240). In general, DNA ploidy studies by image analysis are not predictive of the behavior of paragangliomas (241).

PATHOLOGIC FEATURES. Grossly, JTPs are polypoid, red, friable masses that are identified behind an intact tympanic

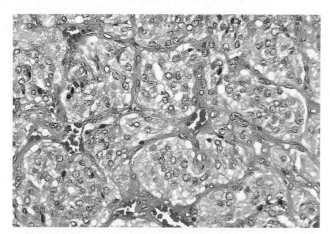

Figure 23.25. Jugulotympanic paraganglioma. This lesion shows the classic organoid or cell nest growth pattern, including round or oval cells with uniform nuclei, a dispersed chromatin pattern, and abundant eosinophilic granular or vacuolated cytoplasm. The sustentacular cells are located at the periphery of the cell nests, but these are difficult to identify by light microscopy.

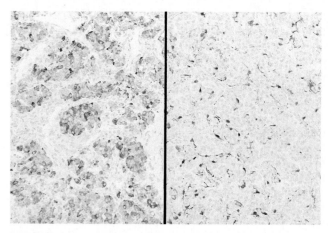

Figure 23.26. Paraganglioma. The immunohistochemical antigenic profile of paragangliomas includes chromogranin positivity in the chief cells (*left*) and S-100 protein staining localized to the peripheral sustentacular cells (*right*).

membrane or within the external auditory canal. They vary in size from a few millimeters to a large mass that completely fills the middle ear space. The histologic appearance of all extra-adrenal paragangliomas is the same. The hallmark feature is the presence of cell nests or a so-called zellballen pattern (Fig. 23.25). The stroma surrounding and separating the nests is composed of prominent fibrovascular tissue. Although this pattern is characteristic of paragangliomas, it can be seen in other tumors, including other neuroendocrine tumors, melanomas, and carcinomas. Paragangliomas are predominantly composed of chief cells, which are round or oval cells with uniform nuclei; a dispersed chromatin pattern; and abundant eosinophilic, granular, or vacuolated cytoplasm. The sustentacular cells, which represent modified Schwann cells, are located at the periphery of the cell nests, appearing as spindle-shaped, basophilic cells, but these are difficult to identify by light microscopy. Cellular and nuclear pleomorphism can be seen, but these features are not indicative of malignancy. Mitotic figures and necrosis are infrequently identified. Paragangliomas lack glandular or alveolar differentiation.

The diagnosis of JTP is facilitated by IHC stains. The IHC profile includes chromogranin and synaptophysin positivity in the chief cells and S-100 protein staining localized to the peripheral sustentacular cells (Fig. 23.26). Vimentin is variably reactive in both the chief cells and sustentacular cells. Epithelial markers, including cytokeratin, as well as HMB-45 and mesenchymal markers (desmin and other markers of myogenic differentiation), are negative. Rare examples of apparently cytokeratin-reactive paragangliomas have been reported (242). The ultrastructural evaluation shows the presence of neurosecretory granules (243).

Paragangliomas are often readily identified by light microscopic evaluation. However, in certain instances, they may be difficult to differentiate from other tumors. Not infrequently, middle ear and temporal paragangliomas do not show the characteristic cell nest appearance. This "loss" of the organoid growth may be artifactually induced by surgical manipulation ("squeezing") of the tissue during removal. The absence of the typical growth pattern may result in diagnostic confusion with

other middle ear tumors (Fig. 23.27). Reticulin staining may better delineate the cell nest growth pattern, with staining of the fibrovascular cores surrounding the neoplastic nests (Fig. 23.27). In addition, the tumor cells are argyrophilic (Churukian-Schenk). Argentaffin (Fontana), mucicarmine, and PAS stains are negative. In addition to the loss of an organoid pattern of growth, JTPs may be associated with a dense, fibrous stroma and an appearance of infiltrative growth (Fig. 23.28). These findings may result in an erroneous interpretation as a malignant neoplasm. Typical immunoreactive staining patterns for chromogranin and S-100 protein (Fig. 23.28) should allow for a correct diagnosis.

DIFFERENTIAL DIAGNOSIS. The differential diagnosis of JTP primarily includes middle ear adenoma, meningioma, and acoustic neuroma. If the histology is not distinctive in separating JTP from these other tumors, the IHC reactivity differentiates these tumors (Table 23.4).

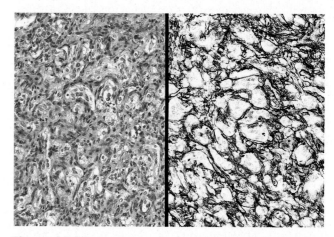

Figure 23.27. Jugulotympanic paragangliomas. The typical organoid growth pattern may be obscured or lost (*left*); reticulin stains may be helpful in delineating the cell nest growth pattern by staining of the fibrovascular stroma surrounding the neoplastic nests (*right*).

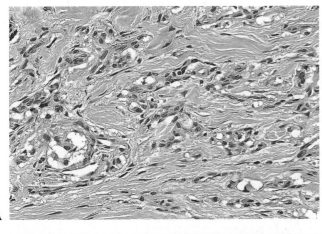

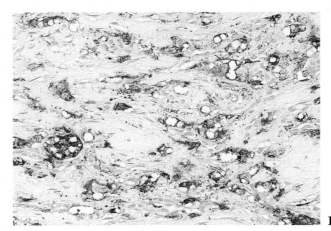

A   B

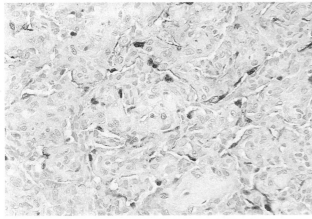

Figure 23.28. Jugulotympanic paragangliomas. Not infrequently, the tumors are associated with a densely fibrotic stroma (**A**). This finding in conjunction with the absence of the typical organoid growth pattern may suggest other tumor types and possible consideration of a malignant neoplasm. Typical immunoreactive staining patterns for chromogranin (**B**) and S-100 protein (**C**) should allow one to make the correct diagnosis.

C

Acoustic Neuroma

Acoustic neuroma (AN) is a benign neoplasm that originates from Schwann cells, specifically from the 8th cranial nerve. Synonyms include *neurilemoma, acoustic schwannoma,* and *benign peripheral nerve sheath tumor.*

CLINICAL FEATURES. AN accounts for up to 10% of all intracranial neoplasms and represents up to 90% of all cerebellopontine angle tumors (222,223). ANs are more common in women than in men, and they may affect any age; they are, however, most common in the fourth to seventh decades of life. The majority of ANs involve the superior or vestibular portion rather than the cochlear portion of the 8th cranial nerve. Symptoms include progressive (sensorineural) hearing loss, tinnitus, and loss of equilibrium. With progression, the tumor enlarges, and it may compress adjacent cranial nerves (5th, 7th, 9th, 10th, 11th), the cerebellum, and the brainstem, leading to facial paresthesia and numbness, headaches, nausea, vomiting, diplopia, and ataxia. Up to 8% may be bilateral (244–248), a potential indicator of neurofibromatosis type 2 (NF-2) (247,248). NF-2 is an autosomal dominant condition. The gene for NF-2 has been mapped to the long arm of chromsome 22 (22q12). The hallmark of NF-2 is bilateral acoustic neuromas (249). Patients with NF-2 have an increased incidence of developing a meningioma. Patients with NF-2 also experience increased incidence of multiple, separate-occurring meningiomas in intra- and extracranial meningiomas. Symptoms of neurofibromatosis may be seen in up to 16% of patients, and those with neurofibromatosis

who develop acoustic neuromas generally are symptomatic at an earlier age (second decade) and have a higher incidence of bilateral acoustic neuromas. Patients with acoustic neuroma (or meningioma) who are under 30 years of age should raise concern for a diagnosis of NF-2. The radiologic features of AN include flaring, asymmetric widening, or erosion of the internal auditory canal. Tumors as small as 1 cm or less are capable of being detected with computed tomography (CT) or magnetic resonance imaging (MRI).

Complete surgical excision is the treatment of choice, and is usually curative. AN may result in death secondary to the herniation of the brainstem in patients with untreated or large neoplasms. Malignant ANs are exceedingly rare; if they are present, neurofibromatosis should be suspected.

PATHOLOGIC FEATURES. The gross appearance of AN includes a circumscribed, tan-white, rubbery to firm mass that may appear yellow and can show cystic change. The tumor ranges in size from a few millimeters up to 4 to 5 cm at its greatest diameter. Histologically, the tumors are unencapsulated and are similar in appearance to benign schwannomas of all other locations. The cellular component includes elongated and twisted nuclei with indistinct cytoplasmic borders. The cells are arranged in short, interlacing fascicles, and whorling or palisading of nuclei called Verocay bodies may be seen (Fig. 23.29). The cellularity varies, and some benign schwannomas can be highly cellular (so-called cellular schwannoma). Mitotic figures are usually sparse in number. Cellular pleomorphism with hyperchromasia can be identified, but it is not a feature of the malignancy.

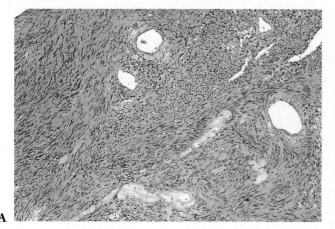

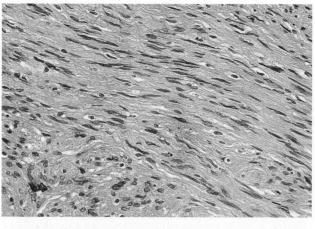

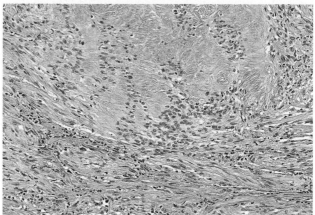

Figure 23.29. Acoustic neuroma. **(A)** The tumor is unencapsulated and shows a fascicular growth of spindle-shaped cells; vascular hyalinization is present. **(B)** The cellular component includes elongated and twisted-appearing nuclei with indistinct cytoplasmic borders. **(C)** Nuclear palisading (Verocay bodies) may be seen.

Retrogressive changes, including cystic degeneration, necrosis, hyalinization, calcification, and hemorrhage, may also be seen. Schwannomas have prominent vascularity composed of large vessels with thickened (hyalinized) walls.

IHC evaluation shows the presence of diffuse, intense S-100 protein reactivity (Table 23.4). No immunoreactivity for cytokeratin or the neuroendocrine markers chromogranin and synaptophysin is present.

Meningioma

Meningiomas are benign neoplasms arising from arachnoid cells forming the arachnoid villi that are seen in relation to the dural sinuses.

CLINICAL FEATURES. Meningiomas represent from 13% to 18% of all intracranial tumors, and they are the second most common tumor of the cerebellopontine angle (222,223). Meningiomas are more common in women than in men, and they are most often seen in the fifth decade of life (250). They infrequently occur in children. The occurrence of a meningioma outside the central nervous system (CNS) is considered ectopic, and it can be divided into those tumors with no identifiable CNS connection (primary) and those with a CNS connection (secondary). The development of primary meningiomas in the middle ear and temporal bone results either from direct extension or from the presence of ectopic arachnoid cells. The middle ear and temporal bone are the most common sites of ectopically located meningiomas in the head and neck region. Sites

of involvement include the internal auditory canal, jugular foramen, geniculate ganglion, the roof of the eustachian tube, and the sulcus of the greater petrosal nerve (222). The clinical presentation of middle ear meningiomas includes progressive hearing loss, loss of equilibrium, headaches, cerebellar dysfunction, and cranial nerve abnormalities. Meningiomas may be associated with neurofibromatosis type 2. Patients with NF-2 have an increased incidence of developing a meningioma. Patients with NF-2 also experience increased incidence of multiple, separate-occurring meningiomas in intra- and extracranial meningiomas. Patients with a meningioma (or acoustic neuroma) who are under 30 years of age should raise concern for a diagnosis of NF-2. The radiologic findings include a soft tissue mass with variable vascularity. A pathognomonic feature for meningioma in this location is the presence of speckled calcification in a soft tissue mass.

Complete surgical excision is the treatment of choice, and is curative. Malignant change rarely, if ever, occurs. A diagnosis of middle ear meningioma should be made only after clinical evaluation has excluded secondary extension from an intracranial neoplasm (251).

PATHOLOGIC FEATURES. The histologic features of middle ear and temporal bone meningioma are similar to their intracranial counterparts (Fig. 23.30). The IHC antigenic profile of meningiomas includes reactivity for EMA and vimentin. In contrast to middle ear adenomas, meningiomas are generally nonreactive for cytokeratin, and, in contrast to JTPs, meningiomas

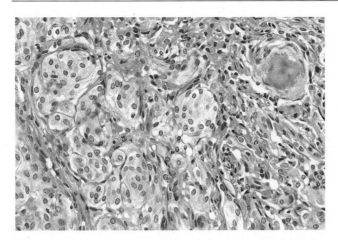

Figure 23.30. Meningioma of the internal auditory canal showing a cell nest or lobular growth separated by fibrovascular tissue. The cells are composed of round to oval or spindle-shaped nuclei with pale-staining cytoplasm and indistinct cell borders; the nuclei show a characteristic punched-out or empty appearance resulting from intranuclear cytoplasmic inclusions. At the upper right is a psammoma body, a helpful diagnostic feature that is seen in this tumor.

are nonreactive for neuroendocrine markers (i.e., chromogranin and synaptophysin) (Table 23.4).

Endolymphatic Sac Papillary Tumor

The endolymphatic sac papillary tumor (ESPT) is an uncommon but distinct neoplasm that possibly is a manifestation of von Hippel-Lindau (VHL) syndrome (252,253). ESPT has had a variety of names, including *adenoma of endolymphatic sac; adenoma and/or adenocarcinoma of temporal bone or mastoid; low-grade adenocarcinoma of probable endolymphatic sac origin; papillary adenoma of temporal bone; aggressive papillary tumor of temporal bone; aggressive papillary middle ear tumor*; and, more recently, the *Heffner tumor* (254,255).

CLINICAL FEATURES. There is no gender predilection. ESPT occurs over a wide age range from the second through eighth decades of life. The most common symptom is unilateral hearing loss ranging from 6 months to 18 years in duration; the hearing loss is most frequently sensorineural rather than conductive, but mixed types of hearing loss also occur. Other symptoms include tinnitus, vertigo, ataxia, and cranial nerve deficits. CT scan and MRI may show a lytic temporal bone lesion measuring from 4 to 6 cm. The center of the lesion most often is seen at or near the posterior-medial face of the petrous bone. Extension of tumor to the posterior cranial cavity has led to suggestions that the tumor took origin from the cerebellopontine angle; extension results in cerebellar involvement and evidence of compression and/or shifting of the 4th ventricle, brain stem, or pineal gland. Angiographic studies show a vascular or hypervascular lesion. The diagnosis of this tumor is based on clinical, radiographic, and pathologic correlation. A diagnosis of ESPT should prompt the clinician to consider the possibility that the patient has VHL syndrome (252,253). VHL is an autosomal dominant disorder with variable expression. Tumor suppressor gene for VHL has been identified at chromosome 3p25-p26 (256). Patients with VHL have a predisposition to the

TABLE 23.7

Neoplasms Associated with von Hippel-Lindau Syndrome

Retinal angiomas
Cerebellar and spinal hemangioblastomas
Endolymphatic sac papillary tumor
Renal cysts and cystadenomas
Pancreas: microcystic adenoma; endocrine tumors
Pheochromocytoma
Epididymal cyst and cystadenoma

development of numerous CNS and abdominal organ tumors (Table 23.7).

An endolymphatic sac origin for these tumors is supported by the following: (a) early clinical manifestations of vestibular disease, including sensorineural hearing loss, tinnitus and episodic vertigo; (b) radiographic features showing a tumor in the posterior-medial petrous ridge, a site where the endolymphatic sac is located; (c) identification of an in situ tumor (i.e., originating from within the endolymphatic sac); and (d) the morphologic, IHC, and ultrastructural similarities of the tumor with the normal endolymphatic sac epithelium (254).

Radical surgery, including mastoidectomy and temporal bone resection that may necessitate sacrifice of cranial nerves, is the treatment of choice, and is potentially curative. Local recurrence results following inadequate surgical removal, and operative morbidity may be high. Despite its relatively slow growth, these neoplasms are capable of widespread infiltration and destruction, and they may be lethal (257). The prognosis is dependent on the extent of disease and the adequacy of the resection. Earlier detection, when the tumors are relatively small and confined, may decrease the operative-associated morbidity, and it may be curative.

PATHOLOGIC FEATURES. The histopathologic appearance of ESPT is quite variable. The papillary structures are generally not complex in their growth. The neoplastic cells vary in look, from flattened or attenuated-appearing cells to columnar-appearing cells (Fig. 23.31). Most often, only a single row of cells is present. Occasionally, the surface epithelial cells may have an appearance that suggests a double layer of cells (epithelial and myoepithelial); however, the "outer" row of cells in all probability represents a stromal element because these cells have not been shown to be immunoreactive with epithelial markers (257). The epithelial cells have uniform nuclei that are usually situated either in the center of the cells or toward the luminal aspect, and they have a pale eosinophilic to clear-appearing cytoplasm. The latter may predominate in any given tumor. Cell borders may be seen but, not infrequently, the neoplastic cells lack a distinct cell membrane (Fig. 23.31). In some cases, hypercellular areas with crowded, variably sized cystic glandular spaces that contain eosinophilic (colloid-like) material are noted (Fig. 23.32). The latter appear remarkably similar to thyroid tissue. In all cases, pleomorphism is minimal and mitotic activity and necrosis are rarely present.

A granulation tissue reaction is seen in association with the neoplastic cells, and it includes the small vascular spaces lying in close proximity to the surface epithelium and/or within the stroma of the papillary fronds. Due to the absence of a distinct

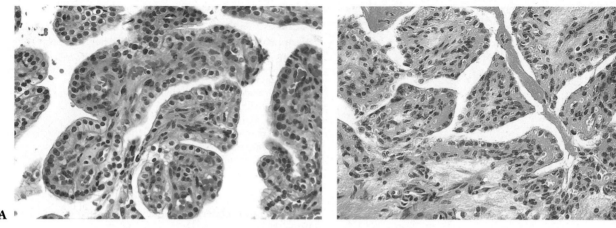

A **B**

Figure 23.31. Endolymphatic sac papillary tumor characterized by a papillary growth pattern. **(A)** In this example, the epithelial component is distinctly composed of a single layer of cuboidal to columnar-appearing cells with delineated cell borders. **(B)** At times, the epithelial component may not be as readily apparent due to indistinct cell borders, and the overall process may be mistaken for granulation tissue.

cell membrane around the neoplastic cells, a sharp demarcation separating the neoplastic cells from the subjacent granulation tissue is not observed. This appearance may create diagnostic confusion such that the neoplastic proliferation is not appreciated and the entire process is viewed as reactive. This interpretation is further enhanced by the stromal presence of a mixed inflammatory cell infiltrate, fibrosis, vascular proliferation, fresh hemorrhage and/or hemosiderin (within the neoplastic cells or within macrophages), cholesterol granulomas, and dystrophic calcification. Dystrophic calcification does not include laminated calcific concretions (psammomatous bodies).

Intracytoplasmic diastase-sensitive, PAS-positive material may be present. The colloid-like luminal material stains strongly with PAS either with or without diastase digestion. Intracytoplasmic and intraluminal mucin staining is rarely positive. Iron stains are positive. ESPTs are diffusely cytokeratin-positive, and they also show variable reactivity for EMA, S-100 protein, vimen-

tin, neuron-specific enolase (NSE), GFAP, Ber-EP4, synaptophysin, and Leu-7 (Table 23.4). Thyroglobulin immunoreactivity is not seen. Ultrastructurally, ESPTs show the presence of intercellular junctional complexes, microvilli, basement membrane material, rough endoplasmic reticulum, intracytoplasmic glycogen, and secretory granules (257).

DIFFERENTIAL DIAGNOSIS. The differential diagnosis includes MEA. However, the clinical, radiographic, and pathologic features that are unique to ESPT should allow for distinction. The same would apply for the other common neoplasms of the middle ear and temporal bone. The differential diagnosis also includes choroid plexus papilloma and metastatic carcinoma of thyroid gland or renal origin. Choroid plexus papillomas are intracranial (i.e., intraventricular) tumors with histologic features that are different from those of ESPT (254). The absence of thyroglobulin reactivity differentiates ESPT from

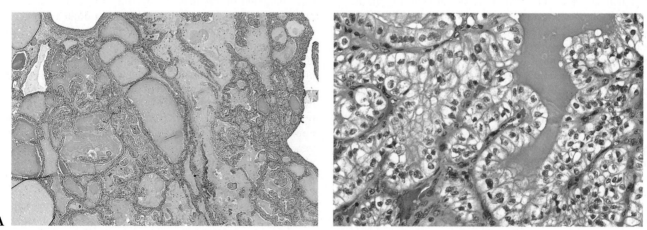

A **B**

Figure 23.32. Endolymphatic sac papillary tumor. **(A)** This inner ear tumor localized to the petrous apex shows the appearance of a thyroid lesion, including variably sized cystic spaces that contain eosinophilic (colloid-like) material. **(B)** At higher magnification, the presence of a papillary architecture, colloid-like material, and variability in the nuclear size and shape with dispersed to clear-appearing nuclear chromatin and an occasional intranuclear inclusion mimics the histology of a thyroid papillary carcinoma. Thyroglobulin and thyroid transcription factor-1 staining were negative.

metastatic thyroid papillary carcinoma. Metastatic renal cell carcinoma does not have the IHC antigenic features seen in ESPT.

OTHER BENIGN TUMORS OF THE MIDDLE EAR AND TEMPORAL BONE

Although other primary benign tumors are uncommon, a number can be found in the middle ear or temporal bone. Middle ear papillary epithelial neoplasms that are histologically identical to sinonasal or Schneiderian papillomas have been reported (258). Other uncommon primary benign tumors of the middle ear and temporal bone are primarily mesenchymal, including hemangiomas (259–260), lipoma (262,263), osteoma (264–266), osteoblastoma (267), chondroblastoma (268), and teratomas (269).

MALIGNANT NEOPLASMS OF THE MIDDLE EAR

Middle Ear Squamous Cell Carcinoma

Middle ear squamous cell carcinoma (ME-SCC) is a rarely occuring primary malignant neoplasm with squamous differentiation that originates from the middle ear mucosal epithelium (270,271).

CLINICAL FEATURES. ME-SCC is most common in the sixth to seventh decades of life. There is no gender predilection. The majority of patients have a long history of COM, which is usually longer than 20 years in duration. Early symptoms include pain with radiation to the scalp and face, and hearing impairment; late symptoms include facial palsies and vertigo. ME-SCC should be suspected in patients with long-standing COM who suddenly present with pain out of proportion to the clinical extent of disease and/or with an onset or increase of otorrhea that is often hemorrhagic, and/or in those patients in whom clinical resolution following therapeutic doses of antibiotics is lacking.

The development of ME-SCC is also linked to radiation treatment for intracranial neoplasms and radiation therapy for middle ear inflammatory conditions, although the latter is no longer used. High-risk human papillomavirus types 16 and 18 identified in middle ear squamous cell carcinomas raises HPV as a possible etiologic factor in the development of ME-SCC, although a direct cause and effect have not been established (272). Although concomitant cholesteatomas can be seen in up to 25% of cases, there is no correlation between cholesteatomas and the development of an ME-SCC.

Radical surgery with radiation therapy is the treatment of choice. In advanced disease, chemotherapy may be of benefit. The prognosis is poor, with 5-year and 10-year survival rates of 39% and 21%, respectively (270). Metastases may occur but these are considered uncommon.

PATHOLOGIC FEATURES. The histology of ME-SCC is similar to that of squamous carcinomas of other sites. The tumors vary from well to poorly differentiated, and they include infiltrative malignant cells with associated keratinization and/or intercellular bridges.

DIFFERENTIAL DIAGNOSIS. The differential diagnosis includes cholesteatoma and metastatic SCC. Cholesteatomas do not have the dysplastic cytologic changes seen in squamous carcinoma. The secondary involvement of this area may occur by SCC originating from a distant site and metastasizing to the middle ear and temporal bone. Alternatively, a cutaneous SCC from an adjacent site (e.g., external ear, nasopharynx, parotid gland, skin) can directly invade the middle ear or temporal bone.

Middle Ear Adenocarcinoma

Middle ear adenocarcinomas are extremely rare malignant glandular neoplasms arising from the middle ear mucosa (273).

CLINICAL FEATURES. Middle ear adenocarcinoma has no gender predilection and occurs over a wide age range between the second and sixth decades of life. Symptoms are typically present for many years, and include progressive hearing loss and a unilateral draining ear; pain and vestibular manifestations are uncommon.

In the majority of cases, otoscopic examination will identify an intact tympanic membrane with tumor confined to the middle ear space with possible extension to the mastoid; occasionally, and similar to the middle ear adenoma, the adenocarcinoma will perforate through the tympanic membrane with extension into and presentation as an external auditory canal mass. Middle ear adenocarcinomas may attain a large size, filling the middle ear space and encasing the ossicles. There is no association between chronic otitis media and the development of these adenocarcinomas. Before rendering a diagnosis of primary middle ear adenocarcinoma, a metastasis to this region from a separate primary adenocarcinoma should be excluded.

Complete surgical excision is the treatment of choice. In general, these are slow-growing neoplasms that are locally aggressive but do not metastasize. Death may occur as a result of direct intracranial extension.

PATHOLOGIC FEATURES. Histologically, middle ear adenocarcinomas are similar in many respects to adenomas, but they have increased cellular pleomorphism, greater mitotic activity, and extensive infiltration of the surrounding structures.

Rhabdomyosarcoma

Rhabdomyosarcoma (RMS) is a malignant neoplasm showing skeletal muscle differentiation.

CLINICAL FEATURES. In the head and neck, RMS is primarily (but not exclusively) a disease of children, in whom it represents the most common aural-related malignant neoplasm. No gender predilection is observed. RMS of the middle ear and mastoid presents as painless, unilateral otitis media that is unresponsive to antibiotic therapy. At diagnosis, approximately one-third of patients have associated neurologic findings, the most common of which are facial nerve deficits; neuropathies of the 3rd and 5th through 12th cranial nerves may also occur.

An international classification of RMS proposed four groups based on the prognosis. They are as follows (274):

I: Superior prognosis (botryoid RMS and spindle cell RMS)
II: Intermediate prognosis (embryonal RMS)
III: Poor prognosis (alveolar RMS and undifferentiated RMS)
IV: Subtypes whose prognosis is not presently evaluable (RMS with rhabdoid features).

RMS is treated by a combination of surgery, radiation therapy, and chemotherapy. This combined therapeutic approach has greatly enhanced survival for pediatric patients with head and neck RMS (275). Prognosis is determined by clinical stage, histologic classification, age, and site of origin (276). Adverse outcomes accounting for prognostic differences related to anatomic sites have been linked to late detection of tumor, large tumor size, difficulties during surgical excision, meningeal involvement with or without spinal fluid spread, and metastatic disease. A problem specifically related to middle ear and mastoid RMS is the delay in diagnosis due to misinterpretation of the biopsy specimen as inflammatory polyps or as granulation tissue (275); this delay in diagnosis may result in more advanced-stage disease, placing patients at greater risk for treatment failure due to uncontrollable local disease.

Poor prognostic findings include meningeal involvement (277). Regional lymph node metastasis and distant hematogenous metastasis to the lungs and bones may also occur.

PATHOLOGIC FEATURES. RMS of the middle ear and mastoid most often appears as an aural (external or middle ear) polypoid lesion that is similar in appearance to an aural polyp. The majority of RMS of the middle ear and mastoid are of the embryonal type, which includes botryoid RMS. The next most common histologic type is alveolar RMS. Other histologic types, including pleomorphic RMS, rarely occur. IHC staining is important in the diagnosis of RMS (Table 23.4). The reader is referred to several other chapters in this text for a more detailed discussion of the pathologic findings of rhabdomyosarcoma.

OTHER MALIGNANT TUMORS OF THE MIDDLE EAR AND TEMPORAL BONE

Although other malignant tumors are rare, a number can originate in the middle ear or temporal bone. They are uncommon, with approximately 1% to 2% of all osteosarcomas occurring in this location (278,279). Osteosarcomas of the skull often arise in the setting of Paget disease of bone, or fibrous dysplasia, or secondary to radiation therapy (278,279). Osteosarcomas of the skull are aggressive tumors with a tendency to metastasize to the lungs and brain and with 5-year survivals of less than 15% (278–280). Chondrosarcomas of the temporal bone are rare. The petrous apex and the posteromedial aspect of the temporal bone are perhaps the most common sites of occurrence (281). Chondrosarcomas in this location are not necessarily lethal tumors, as one study reported disease-free survival with a follow-up to 8 years in 76% of patients (281).

Other malignancies of the middle ear and temporal bones include malignant lymphomas (non-Hodgkin and Hodgkin), leukemias, and plasma cell dyscrasias (282). Involvement by a malignant hematolymphoid neoplasm is often secondary to primary disease elsewhere.

Secondary Tumors

Metastatic tumors secondarily involving the middle ear and temporal bone originate from virtually every site. The more common malignant tumors metastasizing to this region originate from the breast, lungs, and kidneys (283,284), followed by malignant melanoma and prostatic adenocarcinoma. Metastatic disease to the temporal bone occurs via hematogenous spread, but it may also occur by direct extension from a nearby primary tumor (e.g., SCC), meningeal carcinomatosis, or leptomeningeal extension from an intracranial primary neoplasm.

REFERENCES

1. Moore KL, Persaud TVN. The eye and ear. In Moore ML, Persaud TVN, eds. *The Developing Human: Clinically Oriented Embryology.* 7th edition. Philadelphia: WB Saunders, 2003: 465–483.
2. Dayal VS, Farkashidy J, Kokshanian A. Embryology of the ear. *Can J Otolaryngol* 1973;2: 136–142.
3. Hollinshead WH. The ear. In Hollinshead WH, ed. *Anatomy for Surgeons.* 3rd edition. Philadelphia: Harper and Row, 1982:159–221.
4. Schuknecht HF. Anatomy. In Schuknecht HF, ed. *Pathology of the Ear.* 2nd edition. Philadelphia: Lea & Febiger, 1993:31–74.
5. Nager GT. Anatomy. In Nager GT, ed. *Pathology of the Ear and Temporal Bone.* Baltimore: Williams & Wilkins, 1993:3–187.
6. Wenig BM, Michaels LM. The ear and temporal bone. In Mills SE, ed. *Histology for Pathologists.* 3rd edition. Philadelphia; Lippincott Williams & Wilkins; 2007:371–401.
7. Baloh RW, Honrubia V. Vestibular physiology. In Cummings CW, Frederickson JM, Harker LA, et al., eds. *Otolaryngology—Head and Neck Surgery.* 3rd edition. St. Louis: Mosby, 1998: 2584–2622.
8. Lysakowski A, McCrea RA, Tomlinson RD. Anatomy of vestibular end organs and neural pathways. In Cummings CW, Frederickson JM, Harker LA, et al., eds. *Otolaryngology—Head and Neck Surgery.* 3rd edition. St. Louis: Mosby, 1998:2561–2583.
9. Schuknecht HF. Pathophysiology. In Schuknecht HF, ed. *Pathology of the Ear.* 2nd edition. Philadelphia: Lea & Febiger, 1993:77–113.
10. Schuknecht HF. Developmental defects. In Schuknecht HF, ed. *Pathology of the Ear.* 2nd edition. Philadelphia: Lea & Febiger, 1993:115–189.
11. Nager GT. Dysplasia of the external and middle ear. In Nager GT, ed. *Pathology of the Ear and Temporal Bone.* Baltimore: Williams & Wilkins, 1993:83–118.
12. Nager GT. Dysplasia of the osseous and membranous cochlea and vestibular labyrinth. In Nager GT, ed. *Pathology of the Ear and Temporal Bone.* Baltimore: Williams & Wilkins, 1993:119–146.
13. Brownstein MH, Wanger N, Helwig EB. Accessory tragi. *Arch Dermatol* 1971;104:625–631.
14. Olsen KD, Maragos NE, Weiland LH. First branchial cleft anomalies. *Laryngoscope* 1980; 90:423–436.
15. Greenway RE, Hurst L, Fenton NA. An unusual first branchial cleft cyst. *J Laryngol* 1981; 10:219–225.
16. Work WP. Newer concepts of first branchial cleft defects. *Laryngoscope* 1972;81:1581–1593.
17. Aronsohn RS, Bataskis JG, Rice DH, Work WP. Anomalies of the first branchial cleft. *Arch Otolaryngol* 1976;102:737–740.
18. Nager GT. Necrotizing ("malignant") granulomatous external otitis and osteomyelitis. In Nager GT, ed. *Pathology of the Ear and Temporal Bone.* Baltimore: Williams & Wilkins, 1993:192–206.
19. Weinroth SE, Schessel D, Tuazon CU. Malignant otitis externa in AIDS patients: case report and review of the literature. *Ear Nose Throat J* 1994;73:772–774.
20. Shpitzer T, Stern Y, Cohen O, et al. Malignant external otitis in nondiabetic patients. *Ann Otol Rhinol Laryngol* 1993;102:870–872.
21. Damiani JM, Damiani KK, Kinney SE. Malignant external otitis with multiple cranial nerve involvement. *Am J Otol* 1979;1:115–120.
22. Bernheim J, Sade J. Histopathology of the soft parts in 50 patients with malignant external otitis. *J Laryngol Otol* 1989;103:366–368.
23. Al-Shihabi BA. Carcinoma of the temporal bone presenting as malignant otitis externa. *J Laryngol Otol* 1992;106:908–910.
24. Grandis JR, Hirsch BE, Yu VL. Simultaneous presentation of malignant external otitis and temporal bone cancer. *Arch Otolaryngol Head Neck Surg* 1993;119:687–689.
25. Chandler JR. Pathogenesis and treatment of facial paralysis due to malignant otitis externa. *Ann Otol Rhinol Laryngol* 1972;81:1–11.
26. Friedmann I. The pathology of acute and chronic infections of the middle ear cleft. *Ann Otol Rhinol Laryngol* 1971;80:390–396.
27. Nager GT. Acute and chronic otitis media (tympanomastoiditis) and their regional and endocranial complications. In Nager GT, ed. *Pathology of the Ear and Temporal Bone.* Baltimore: Williams & Wilkins, 1993:220–297.
28. Goycoolea MV, Hueb MM, Ruah C. Definitions and terminology. *Otolaryngol Clin North Am* 1991;24:757–761.
29. Wenig BM. Otitis media. In Wenig BM, ed. *Atlas of Head and Neck Pathology.* 2nd edition. St. Louis: Saunders Elsevier, 2008:740–745.
30. Barnes EL, Peel RL. Tympanosclerosis. In Barnes L, ed. *Diseases of the External Auditory Canal, Middle Ear, and Temporal Bone.* 2nd edition. New York: Marcel Dekker, 2001:557–599.
31. Bhaya MH, Schachern PA, Morizono T, et al. Pathogenesis of tympanosclerosis. *Otolaryngol Head Neck Surg* 1993;109:413–420.
32. Gibb AG, Pang YT. Current considerations in the etiology and diagnosis of tympanosclerosis. *Eur Arch Otorhinolaryngol* 1994;251:439–451.
33. Nager GT, Vanderveen TS. Cholesterol granuloma involving the temporal bone. *Ann Otol Rhinol Laryngol* 1976;85:204–209.
34. Nager GT. Cholesterol granulomas. In Nager GT, ed. *Pathology of the Ear and Temporal Bone.* Baltimore: Williams & Wilkins, 1994:914–939.
35. Thedinger BA, Nadol JB Jr, Montgomery WW, et al. Radiographic diagnosis, surgical treatment, and long-term follow-up of cholesterol granulomas of the petrous apex. *Laryngoscope* 1989;99:896–907.
36. Windle-Taylor PC, Bailey CM. Tuberculous otitis media: a series of 22 patients. *Laryngoscope* 1980;90:1039–1044.

37. McNulty JS, Fassett RL. Syphilis: an otolaryngolic perspective. *Laryngoscope* 1981;91: 889–905.
38. McGill TJI. Mycotic infections of the temporal bone. *Arch Otolaryngol* 1978;104:140–144.
39. Leek JH. Actinomycosis of the tympanomastoid. *Laryngoscope* 1974;84:290–301.
40. Sandler ED, Sandler JM, Leboit P, et al. Pneumocystis carinii otitis media in AIDS: a case report and review of the literature regarding extrapulmonary pneumocystosis. *Otolaryngol Head Neck Surg* 1990;103:817–821.
41. Schuknecht HF. Infections. In Schuknecht HF, ed. *Pathology of the Ear.* 2nd edition. Philadelphia: Lea & Febiger, 1993:191–253.
42. Wilson WR. The relationship of herpesvirus family to sudden hearing loss: a prospective clinical study and literature review. *Laryngoscope* 1986;96:870–877.
43. Rosai J. The nature of myospherulosis of the upper respiratory tract. *Am J Clin Pathol* 1978;69:475–481.
44. Kyriakos M. Myospherulosis of the paranasal sinuses, nose and middle ear: a possible iatrogenic disease. *Am J Clin Pathol* 1977;67:118–130.
45. Hawke M, Jahn AF. Labyrinthitis. In Hawke M, ed. *Diseases of the Ear: Clinical and Pathologic Aspects.* Philadelphia: Lea & Febiger, 1987:5.27–5.32.
46. Bassiouni M, Paparella MM. Labyrinthitis. In Paparella MM, Shumrick DA, Gluckman JL, et al., eds. *Otolaryngology.* 3rd edition. Philadelphia: WB Saunders, 1991:1601–1618.
47. Hyams VJ, Batsakis JG, Michaels L. Inflammatory polyps of the middle ear. In Hartmann WH, Sobin LH, eds. *Tumors of the Upper Respiratory Tract and Ear. Atlas of Tumor Pathology.* Fascicle 25, second series. Washington, DC: Armed Forces Institute of Pathology, 1988: 301.
48. Gaafar H, Maher A, Al-Ghazzawi E. Aural polypi: a histopathological and histochemical study. *ORL J Otorhinolaryngol Relat Spec* 1982;44:108–115.
49. Wenig BM. Otitis media. In Wenig BM, ed. *Atlas of Head and Neck Pathology.* 2nd edition. St. Louis: Saunders Elsevier, 2008:745–746.
50. Marks PV, Brookes GB. Myelomatosis presenting as an isolated lesion in the mastoid. *Laryngoscope* 1985;99:903–906.
51. Azadeh B, Ardehali S. Malakoplakia of middle ear: a case report. *Histopathology* 1983;7: 129–134.
52. Azadeh B, Dabiri S, Moshfegh I. Malakoplakia of the middle ear. *Histopathology* 1991;19: 276–278.
53. Cheng LH. Keloid of ear lobe. *Laryngoscope* 1972;82:673–681.
54. Griffith BH, Monroe CW, McKinney P. A follow-up study on the treatment of keloids with triamcinolonec acetonide. *Plast Reconstr Surg* 1970;46:145–150.
55. Kiil J. Keloids treated with topical injections of triamcinolone acetonide (Kenalog). Immediate and long-term results. *Scand J Plast Reconstr Surg* 1977;11:169–172.
56. Escarmant P, Zihmermann S, Amar A, et al. The treatment of 783 keloid scars by iridium 192 interstitial radiation after surgical excision. *Int J Radiat Oncol Biol Phys* 1993;26: 245–257.
57. Sallstrom KO, Larson O, Heden P, et al. Treatment of keloids with surgical excision and postoperative x-ray radiation. *Scand J Plast Reconstr Surg Hand Surg* 1989;23:211–215.
58. Stucker FJ, Shaw GY. An approach to management of keloids. *Arch Otolaryngol Head Neck Surg* 1992;188:63–67.
59. Tang YW. Intra and postoperative steroid injections for keloids and hypertrophic scars. *Br J Plast Surg* 1992;45:371–373.
60. Granstein RD, Rook A, Flotte TJ. Controlled trial of intralesional recombinant interferon γ in the treatment of keloidal scarring. *Arch Dermatol* 1990;126:1295–1302.
61. Larrabee WF, Jr., East CA, Jaffe HS, et al. Intralesional interferon γ treatment for keloids and hypertrophic scars. *Arch Otolaryngol Head Neck Surg* 1990;116:1159–1162.
62. Murray JC, Pollack SV, Pinnel SR. Keloids: a review. *J Am Acad Dermatol* 1981;4:461–470.
63. Blackburn WR, Cosman B. Histologic basis of keloid and hypertrophic scar differentiation. *Arch Pathol* 1966;82:65–71.
64. Kuo TT, Hu S, Chan HL. Keloidal dermatofibroma: report of 10 cases of a new variant. *Am J Surg Pathol* 1998;22:564–568.
65. Metzger SA, Goodman ML. Chondrodermatitis helicis: a clinical re-evaluation and pathological review. *Laryngoscope* 1976;86:1402–1412.
66. Shuman R, Helwig EB. Chondrodermatitis helicis. *Am J Clin Pathol* 1954;24:126–144.
67. Winkler M. Knotchenformige erkrankung am helix (Chondrodermatitis nodularis chronica helicis). *Arch Dermatol Syphilol* 1915;212:278–285.
68. Kitchens GG. Auricular wedge resection and reconstruction. *Ear Nose Throat* 1989;68: 673–683.
69. Lawrence CM. The treatment of chondrodermatitis nodularis with cartilage removal alone. *Arch Dermatol* 1991;127:530–535.
70. Goette DK. Chondrodermatitis nodularis chronica helicis: a perforating necrobiotic granuloma. *J Am Acad Dermatol* 1980;2:148–154.
71. Hansen JE. Pseudocysts of the auricle in Caucasians. *Arch Otolaryngol Head Neck Surg* 1967; 85:13–14.
72. Heffner DK, Hyams VJ. Cystic chondromalacia (endochondral pseudocyst) of the auricle. *Arch Pathol Lab Med* 1986;110:740–743.
73. Lazar RH, Heffner DK, Huges GB, Hyams VK. Pseudocyst of the auricle: a review of 21 cases. *Otolaryngol Head Neck Surg* 1986;94:360–361.
74. Kontis TC, Goldstone A, Brown M, Paull G. Pathological quiz: auricular pseudocyst. *Arch Otolaryngol Head Neck Surg* 1992;118:1128–1130.
75. Engel D. Pseudocysts of the auricle in Chinese. *Arch Otolaryngol* 1966;83:197–202.
76. Borroni G, Brazzeli V, Merlino M. Pseudocyst of the auricle. A birthday ear pull. *Br J Dermatol* 1991;125:292–294.
77. Glamb R, Kim R. Pseudocyst of the auricle. *J Am Acad Dermatol* 1984;11:58–63.
78. Grabski WJ, Salasche SJ, McCollough ML, et al. Pseudocyst of the auricle associated with trauma. *Arch Dermatol* 1989;125:528–530.
79. Choi S, Lam KH, Chan KW, et al. Endochondral pseudocyst of the auricle in Chinese. *Arch Otolaryngol* 1984;110:792–796.
80. Ophir D, Marshak G. Needle aspiration and pressure sutures for auricular pseudocyst. *Plast Reconstr Surg* 1991;87:783–784.
81. Rosai J, Gold J, Landy R. The histiocytoid hemangioma: a unifying concept embracing several previously described entities of skin, soft tissues, large vessels, bone and heart. *Hum Pathol* 1979;10:707–730.
82. Allen PW, Ramakrishna B, MacCormac LB. The histiocytoid hemangiomas and other controversies. *Pathol Ann* 1992;27:51–87.
83. Chun SI, Goo H. Kimura's disease and angiolymphoid hyperplasia with eosinophilia: clinical and histopathologic differences. *J Am Acad Dermatol* 1992;27:954–958.
84. Googe PB, Harris NL, Mihm MC. Kimura's disease and angiolymphoid hyperplasia with eosinophilia: two distinct histopathological entities. *J Cutan Pathol* 1987;14:263–271.
85. Kuo TT, Shih LY, Chan HL. Kimura's disease: involvement of regional lymph nodes and distinction from angiolymphoid hyperplasia with eosinophilia. *Am J Surg Pathol* 1988;12: 843–854.
86. Urabe A, Tsuneyoshi M, Enjoji M. Epithelioid hemangioma verses Kimura's disease: a comparative clinicopathologic study. *Am J Surg Pathol* 1987;11:758–766.
87. Barnes L, Koss W, Nieland ML. Angiolymphoid hyperplasia with eosinophilia: a disease that may be confused with malignancy. *Head Neck Surg* 1980;2:425–434.
88. Olsen TG, Helwig EB. Angiolymphoid hyperplasia with eosinophilia. A clinicopathologic study of 116 patients. *J Am Acad Dermatol* 1985;12:781–796.
89. Fetsch JF, Weiss SW. Observations concerning the pathogenesis of epithelioid hemangioma (angiolymphoid hyperplasia). *Mod Pathol* 1991;4:449–455.
90. Bhattacharjee P, Hui P, McNiff J. Human herpesvirus-8 is not associated with angiolymphoid hyperplasia with eosinophilia. *Cutan Pathol* 2004;31:612–615.
91. Baum DW, Sams WM, Monheit GD. Angiolymphoid hyperplasia with eosinophilia. The disease and a comparison of treatment modalities. *J Dermatol Surg Oncol* 1982;8:966–970.
92. Kung IT, Gibson JB, Bonnatyne PM. Kimura's disease: a clinicopathological study of 21 cases and its distinction from angiolymphoid hyperplasia with eosinophilia. *Pathology* 1984; 16:39–44.
93. Shuknecht H. Exostoses of the external auditory canal. In Shuknecht H, ed. *Pathology of the Ear.* 2nd edition. Philadelphia: Lea & Febiger, 1993:398–399.
94. Whitaker SR, Cordier A, Kosjakov S, Charbonneau R. Treatment of external auditory canal exostoses. *Laryngoscope* 1998;108:195–199.
95. Fisher EW, McManus TC. Surgery for external auditory canal exostoses and osteomata. *J Laryngol Otol* 1994;108:106–110.
96. Graham MD. Osteomas and exostoses of the external auditory canal. A clinical, histopathological, and scanning electron microscopic study. *Ann Otol* 1979;88:566–572.
97. Nager GT. Osteomas and exostoses. In Nager GT, ed. *Pathology of the Ear and Temporal Bone.* Baltimore: Williams & Wilkins, 1993:483–493.
98. Fenton JE, Turner J, Fagan PA. A histopathologic review of temporal bone exostoses and osteomata. *Laryngoscope* 1996;106:624–628.
99. Villacin AB, Brigham LN, Bullough PG. Primary and secondary synovial chondrometaplasia: histopathologic and clinicoradiologic differences. *Hum Pathol* 1979;10:439–451.
100. Allias-Montmayeur F, Durroux R, Dodart L, et al. Tumours and pseudotumorous lesions of the temporomandibular joint: a diagnostic challenge. *J Laryngol Otol* 1997;111:776–781.
101. Nussenbaum B, Roland PS, Gilcrease MZ, Odell DS. Extra-articular synovial chondromatosis of the temporomandibular joint: pitfalls in diagnosis. *Arch Otolaryngol Head Neck Surg* 1999;125:1394–1397.
102. Psimopoulou M, Karakasis D, Magoudi D, et al. Synovial chondromatosis of the temporomandibular joint. *Br J Oral Maxillofac Surg* 1998;36:317–318.
103. Wu CW, Chen YK, Lin LM, et al. Primary synovial chondromatosis of the temporomandibular joint. *J Otolaryngol* 2004;33:114–119.
104. Deahl ST, Ruprecht A. Asymptomatic radiographically detected chondrometaplasia in the temporomandibular joint. *Oral Surg Oral Med Oral Pathol* 1991;72:371–374.
105. Yu Q, Yang J, Wang P, Shi H, et al. CT features of synovial chondromatosis in the temporomandibular joint. *Oral Surg Oral Med Oral Pathol Oral Radiol Endod* 2004;97:524–528.
106. Karlis V, Glickman RS, Zaslow M. Synovial chondromatosis of the temporomandibular joint with intracranial extension. *Oral Surg Oral Med Oral Pathol Oral Radiol Endod* 1998; 86:664–666.
107. Bell G, Sharp CW, Fourie LR, et al. Conservative surgical management of synovial chondromatosis. *Oral Surg Oral Med Oral Pathol Oral Radiol Endod* 1997;84:592–593.
108. Davis RI, Hamilton A, Biggart JD. Primary synovial chondromatosis: a clinicopathologic review and assessment of malignant potential. *Hum Pathol* 1998;29:683–688.
109. Ichikawa T, Miyauchi M, Nikai H, et al. Synovial chondrosarcoma arising in the temporomandibular joint. *J Oral Maxillofac Surg* 1998;56:890–894.
110. Davis RI, Foster H, Arthur K, et al. Cell proliferation studies in primary synovial chondromatosis. *J Pathol* 1998;184:18–23.
111. Sciot R, Dal Cin P, Bellemans J, et al. Synovial chondromatosis: clonal chromosome changes provide further evidence for a neoplastic disorder. *Virchows Arch* 1998;433: 189–191.
112. Ferlito A, Devaney KO, Rinaldo A, et al. Ear cholesteatoma versus cholesterol granuloma. *Ann Otol Rhinol Laryngol* 1997;106:79–85.
113. Michaels L. Pathology of cholesteatomas: a review. *J R Soc Med* 1979;72:366–369.
114. Schuknecht HF. Cholesteatoma. In Schuknecht HF, ed. *Pathology of the Ear.* 2nd ed. Philadelphia: Lea & Febiger, 1993:204–206.
115. Michaels L. An epidermoid formation in the developing middle ear: possible source of cholesteatoma. *J Laryngol Otol* 1986;15:169–174.
116. Abramson M, Moriyama H, Huang CC. Histology, pathogenesis, and treatment of cholesteatoma. *Otol Rhinol Laryngol* 1984;112:125–128.
117. Piepergerdes MC, Kramer BM, Behnke EE. Keratosis obturans and external auditory canal cholesteatoma. *Laryngoscope* 1980;90:383–391.
118. Desloge RB, Carew JF, Finstad CL, et al. DNA analysis of human cholesteatomas. *Am J Otol* 1997;18:155–159.
119. Tokuriki M, Noda I, Saito T, et al. Gene expression analysis of human middle ear cholesteatoma using complementary DNA arrays. *Laryngoscope* 2003;113:808–814.

120. Yamamoto-Fukuda T, Aoki D, Hishikawa Y, et al. Possible involvement of keratinocyte growth factor and its receptor in enhanced epithelial-cell proliferation and acquired recurrence of middle-ear cholesteatoma. *Lab Invest* 2003;83:123.136.
121. Sudhoff H, Dazert S, Gonzales AM, et al. Angiogenesis and angiogenic growth factors in middle ear cholesteatoma. *Am J Otol* 2000;21:793–798.
122. Willman CL. Detection of clonal histiocytes in Langerhans cell histiocytosis: biology and clinical significance. *Br J Cancer Suppl* 1994;23:S29–S33.
123. Willman CL, Busque L, Griffith BB, et al. Langerhans'-cell histiocytosis (histiocytosis X)—a clonal proliferative disease. *N Engl J Med* 1994;331:154–160.
124. Lieberman PH, Jones CR, Steinman RM, et al. Langerhans cell (eosinophilic) granulomatosis: a clinicopathologic study encompassing 50 years. *Am J Surg Pathol* 1997;20:519–552.
125. Appling D, Jenkins HA, Parton GA. Eosinophilic granuloma in the temporal bone and skull. *Otolaryngol Head Neck Surg* 1983;91:358–365.
126. Azumi N, Sheibani K, Swartz WG, et al. Antigenic phenotype of Langerhans cell histiocytosis: an immunohistochemical study demonstrating the value of LN-2, LN-3 and vimentin. *Hum Pathol* 1988;19:1376–1382.
127. Beckstead JH, Wood GS, Turner RR. Histiocytosis X cells and Langerhans cells: enzyme histochemical and immunologic similarities. *Hum Pathol* 1984;15:826–833.
128. Emile JF, Wechsler J, Brousse N, et al. Langerhans' cell histiocytosis. Definitive diagnosis with the use of monoclonal antibody O10 on routinely paraffin-embedded samples. *Am J Surg Pathol* 1995;19:636–641.
129. Ide F, Iwase T, Saito I, et al. Immunohistochemical and ultrastructural analysis of the proliferating cells in histiocytosis X. *Cancer* 1984;53:917–921.
130. Wenig BM, Abbondanzo SL, Childers E, et al. Extranodal sinus histiocytosis with massive lymphadenopathy (Rosai-Dorfman disease) of the head and neck. *Hum Pathol* 1993;24: 483–492.
131. Bottrill ID, Chawla OP, Ramsay AD. Salivary gland choristoma of the middle ear. *J Laryngol Otol* 1992;106:630–632.
132. Cannon CR. Salivary gland choristoma of the middle ear. *Am J Otol* 1980;1:250–251.
133. Kenneth KL, Gruskin P, Carberry JN. Salivary gland choristoma of the middle ear. *Arch Pathol Lab Med* 1982;106:39–40.
134. Kartush JM, Graham MD. Salivary gland choristoma of the middle ear: a case report and review of the literature. *Laryngoscope* 1984;94:228–230.
135. Gulya AJ, Gassock ME III, Pensak ML. Neural choristoma of the middle ear. *Otolaryngol Head Neck Surg* 1987;97:52–56.
136. Wazen J, Silverstein H, McDaniel A, et al. Brain tissue heterotopia in the eighth cranial nerve. *Otolaryngol Head Neck Surg* 1987;96:373–378.
137. Glassock ME III, Dickins JRE, Jackson CR, et al. Surgical management of brain tissue herniation into the middle ear and mastoid. *Laryngoscope* 1979;89:1743–1754.
138. Moore PJ, Benjamin BNP, Kan AE. Salivary gland choristoma of the middle ear. *Int J Pediatr Otorhinolaryngol* 1984;8:91–95.
139. Saeed YM, Bassis ML. Mixed tumor of the middle ear. A case report. *Arch Otolaryngol* 1971; 93:433–434.
140. Jaksch-Wartenhorst R. Polychondropathia. *Wien Arch Intern Med* 1923;6:93–100.
141. Damiani JM, Levine HL. Relapsing polychondritis—report of ten cases. *Laryngoscope* 1979; 89:929–946.
142. McAdam LP, O'Hanlan MA, Bluestone R, et al. Relapsing polychondritis: prospective study of 23 patients and a review of the literature. *Medicine* 1976;55:193–215.
143. Cody DT, Sones DA. Relapsing polychondritis: audiovestibular manifestations. *Laryngoscope* 1971;81:1208–1222.
144. McCaffrey TV, McDonald TJ, McCaffrey LA. Head and neck manifestations of relapsing polychondritis: review of 29 cases. *Otolaryngol* 1978;86:473–478.
145. Schumacher HR, Jr. Relapsing polychondritis. In Goldman L, Bennett JC, eds. *Cecil Textbook of Medicine.* 21st edition. Philadelphia: WB Saunders, 2000:1550.
146. Harisdangkul V, Johnson WW. Association between relapsing polychondritis and systemic lupus erythematosus. *South Med J* 1994;87:753–757.
147. Dolan DL, Lemmon GB, Jr., Teitelbaum SL. Relapsing polychondritis: analytical literature review and studies on pathogenesis. *Am J Med* 1966;41:285–299.
148. Ebringer B, Rook G, Swana T, et al. Autoantibodies to cartilage and type II collagen in relapsing polychondritis and other rheumatic diseases. *Ann Rheum Dis* 1981;40:473–479.
149. Valenzuela R, Cooperrider PA, Gogate P, et al. Relapsing polychondritis: immunomicroscopic findings in cartilage of ear biopsy specimens. *Hum Pathol* 1980;11:19–22.
150. Helm TN, Valenzuela R, Glanz S, et al. Relapsing polychondritis: a case diagnosed by direct immunofluorescence and coexisting with pseudocyst of the auricle. *J Am Acad Dermatol* 1992;26:315–318.
151. Irani BS, Martin-Hirsch DP, Clark D, et al. Relapsing polychondritis—a study of four cases. *J Laryngol Otol* 1992;106:911–914.
152. Lang B, Rothenfusser A, Lanchbury JS, et al. Susceptibility to relapsing polychondritis is associated with HLA-DR4. *Arthritis Rheum* 1993;36:660–664.
153. Grahame R, Scott JT. Clinical survey of 354 patients with gout. *Ann Rheum Dis* 1970;29: 461–468.
154. Resnick D, Nikiyama G. Gouty arthritis. In Resnick D, Niwayama G, eds. *Diagnosis of Bone and Joint Disorders.* 2nd edition. Philadelphia: WB Saunders, 1988:1618–1671.
155. McCarty DJ, Hollander JL. Identification of urate crystals in gouty synovial fluid. *Ann Intern Med* 1961;54:452–460.
156. Ishida T, Dorfman HD, Bullough PG. Tophaceous pseudogout (tumoral calcium pyrophosphate dihydrate crystal deposition disease). *Hum Pathol* 1995;26:587–593.
157. Vargas A, Teruel J, Trull J, et al. Calcium pyrophosphate dihydrate crystal deposition disease presenting as a pseudotumor of the temporomandibular joint. *Eur Radiol* 1997; 7:1452–1453.
158. Illum P, Thorling K. Otologic manifestations of Wegener's granulomatosis. *Laryngoscope* 1982;92:801–804.
159. Kornblut AD, Wolff SM, Fauci AS. Ear disease in patients with Wegener's granulomatosis. *Laryngoscope* 1982;92:713–717.
160. McCaffrey TV, McDonald TJ, Facer GW, et al. Otologic manifestations of Wegener's granulomatosis. *Otolaryngol Head Neck Surg* 1980;88:586–593.
161. Okamura H, Ohtani I, Anzai T. The hearing loss in Wegener's granulomatosis: relationship between hearing loss and serum ANCA. *Auris Nasus Larynx* 1992;19:1–6.
162. Fauci AS, Haynes BF, Katz P, et al. Wegener's granulomatosis: prospective clinical and therapeutic experience with 85 patients for 21 years. *Ann Intern Med* 1983;98:76–85.
163. Nolle B, Specks U, Ludemann J, et al. Anticytoplasmic autoantibodies: their immunodiagnostic value in Wegener's granulomatosis. *Ann Int Med* 1989;111:28–40.
164. DeRemee RA. Antineutrophil cytoplasmic autoantibody-associated diseases: a pulmonologist's perspective. *Am J Kidney Dis* 1991;18:180–183.
165. Specks U, Wheatley CL, McDonald TJ, et al. Anticytoplasmic autoantibodies in the diagnosis and follow-up of Wegener's granulomatosis. *Mayo Clin Proc* 1989;64:28–36.
166. Braun MG, Csernok E, Gross WL, et al. Proteinase 3, the target antigen of anticytoplasmic antibodies circulating in Wegener's granulomatosis. Immunolocalization in normal and pathologic tissues. *Am J Pathol* 1991;139:831–838.
167. Csernok E, Holle J, Hellmich B, et al. Evaluation of capture ELISA for detection of antineutrophil cytoplasmic antibodies directed against proteinase 3 in Wegener's granulomatosis: first results from a multicentre study. *Rheumatology (Oxford)* 2004;43:174–180.
168. McDonald TJ, Remee RA. Wegener's granulomatosis. *Laryngoscope* 1983;93:220–231.
169. Wolf M, Kronenberg J, Engelberg S, et al. Rapidly progressive hearing loss as a symptom of polyarteritis nodosa. *Am J Otolaryngol* 1987;8:105–108.
170. Gussen R. Atypical ossicle joint lesions in rheumatoid arthritis with sicca syndrome (Sjögren's syndrome). *Arch Otolaryngol* 1977;103:284–286.
171. House JW. Otosclerosis. In Cummings CW, Frederickson JM, Harker LA, et al., eds. *Otolaryngology—Head and Neck Surgery.* 3rd ed. St. Louis: Mosby, 1998:3126–3135.
172. Cody DT, Baker HL Jr. Otosclerosis: vestibular symptoms and sensorineural hearing loss. *Ann Otol Rhinol Laryngol* 1978;87:778–796.
173. Morales-Garcia C. Cochleo-vestibular involvement in otosclerosis. *Acta Otolaryngol (Stockh)* 1972;73:484–492.
174. Schuknecht HF. Otosclerosis. In Schuknecht HF, ed. *Pathology of the Ear.* 2nd edition. Philadelphia: Lea & Febiger, 1993:365–379.
175. Schuknecht HF. Paget's disease. In Schuknecht HF, ed. *Pathology of the Ear.* 2nd edition. Philadelphia: Lea & Febiger, 1993:379–390.
176. Davies DG. Paget's disease of the temporal bone: a clinical and histopathological survey. *Acta Otolaryngol Suppl (Stockh)* 1968;242:7–47.
177. Haibach H, Farrell C, Dittrich FJ. Neoplasms arising in Paget's disease of bone: a study of 82 cases. *Am J Clin Pathol* 1985;83:594–600.
178. Wick MR, McLeod RA, Siegel GP, et al. Sarcomas of bone arising complicating osteitis deformans (Paget's disease). Fifty years' experience. *Am J Surg Pathol* 1981;5:47–59.
179. Nager GT. Ménière's disease. In Nager GT, ed. *Pathology of the Ear and Temporal Bone.* Baltimore: Williams & Wilkins, 1994:1213–1228.
180. Morrison AW, Mowbray JF, Williamson R, et al. On genetic and environmental factors in Ménière's disease. *Am J Otol* 1994;15:35–39.
181. Ruckenstein MJ, Rutka JA, Hawke M. The treatment of Ménière's disease: Torok revisited. *Laryngoscope* 1991;101:211–218.
182. Xenellis J, Morrison AW, McClowskey D, Festenstein H. HLA antigen in the pathogenesis of Ménière's disease. *J Laryngol Otol* 1986;100:21–24.
183. Birgerson L, Gustavson K, Stahle J. Familial Ménière's disease: a genetic investigation. *Am J Otol* 1987;8:323–826.
184. Paparella MM. The cause (multifactorial inheritance) and pathogenesis (endolymphatic malabsorption) of Ménière's disease and its symptoms (mechanical and chemical). *Acta Otolaryngol (Stockh)* 1985;99:445–451.
185. Klis SFL, Buijs J, Smoorenburg GF. Quantification of the relationship between electrophysiologic and morphologic changes in experimental endolymphatic hydrops. *Ann Otol Rhinol Laryngol* 1990;99:566–570.
186. Schessel DA, Minor LB, Nedzelski J. Ménière's disease and other peripheral vestibular disorders. In Cummings CW, Frederickson JM, Harker LA, et al., eds. *Otolaryngology—Head and Neck Surgery.* 3rd ed. St. Louis: Mosby, 1998:2672–2705.
187. Torok N. Old and new in Ménière's disease. *Laryngoscope* 1977;87:1870–1877.
188. Hyams VJ, Batsakis JG, Michaels L. Adenomatous neoplasms of ceruminal gland origin. In Hartmann W, Sobin, LS, eds. *Tumors of the Upper Respiratory Tract and Ear. Atlas of Tumor Pathology.* Fascicle 25, second series. Washington, DC: Armed Forces Institute of Pathology, 1988:285–291.
189. Wetli CV, Prado V, Millard M, et al. Tumors of ceruminous glands. *Cancer* 1972;29: 1169–1178.
190. Pulec JL. Glandular tumors of the external auditory canal. *Laryngoscope* 1977;87: 1601–1612.
191. Wolf BA, Gluckman JL, Wirman JA. Benign dermal cylindroma of the external auditory canal: a clinicopathologic report. *Am J Otolaryngol* 1985;6:35–38.
192. Thompson LD, Nelson BL, Barnes EL. Ceruminous adenomas: a clinicopathologic study of 41 cases with a review of the literature. *Am J Surg Pathol* 2004;28:308–318.
193. Schenk P, Handisurya A, Steurer M. Ultrastructural morphology of a middle ear ceruminoma. *ORL J Otorhinolaryngol Relat Spec* 2002;64:358–363.
194. Tran LP, Grunfast KM, Selesnick SH. Benign lesions of the external auditory canal. *Otolaryngol Clin North Am* 1996;29:807–825.
195. Johnson IJ, Tadpatrikar MH, Sharp JF. Chondroma of the external auditory canal. *J Laryngol Otol* 1998;112: 278–279.
196. Petschenik AJ, Linstrom CJ, McCormick SA. Leiomyoma of the external auditory canal. *Am J Otol* 1996;17:133–136.
197. Lewis WB, Mattucci KF, Smilari T. Schwannoma of the external auditory canal: an unusual finding. *Int Surg* 1995;80:287–290.
198. Ferreiro JA, Carney JA. Myxomas of the external ear and their significance. *Am J Surg Pathol* 1994;18:274–280.
199. Byers R, Kesler K, Redmon B, et al. Squamous carcinoma of the external ear. *Am J Surg* 1983;146:447–450.

200. Conley J, Schuller DE. Malignacies of the ear. *Laryngoscope* 1976;86:1147–1163.

201. Johns ME, Headington JT. Squamous cell carcinoma of the external auditory canal. A clinicopathologic study of 20 cases. *Arch Otolaryngol Head Neck Surg* 1974;100:45–49.

202. Rowe DE, Carroll RJ, Day CL. Prognostic factors for local recurrence, metastasis, and survival rates in squamous cell carcinoma of the skin, ear, and lip. *J Am Acad Dermatol* 1992;26:976–990.

203. Wick MR, Fitzgibbon J, Swanson PE. Cutaneous sarcomas and sarcomatoid neoplasms of the skin. *Sem Diagn Pathol* 1993;10:148–158.

204. Johnson WC, Helwig EB. Adenoid squamous cell carcinoma: adenoacanthoma. *Cancer* 1996;19:1639–1650.

205. Nappi O, Wick MR, Pettinato G, et al. Pseudovascular adenoid squamous cell carcinoma of the skin. *Am J Surg Pathol* 1992;16:429–438.

206. Hicks GW. Tumors arising from the glandular structures of the external auditory canal. *Laryngoscope* 1983;93:326–340.

207. Perzin KH, Gullane P, Conley J. Adenoid cystic carcinoma involving the external auditory canal. A clinicopathological study of 16 cases. *Cancer* 1982;50:2873–2883.

208. Weiss SW, Goldblum JR. Malignant fibrohistiocytic tumors. In Weiss SW, Goldblum JR, eds. *Enzinger and Weiss's Soft Tissue Tumors.* 4th edition. St. Louis: Mosby, 2001:535–569.

209. Dei Tos AP, Maestro R, Doglioni C, et al. Ultraviolet induced p53 mutations in atypical fibroxanthoma. *Am J Pathol* 1994;145:11–17.

210. Calonje E, Wadden C, Wilson-Jones E, Fletcher CD. Spindle-cell non-pleomorphic atypical fibroxanthoma: analysis of a series and delineation of a distinctive variant. *Histopathol* 1993;22:247–254.

211. Bruecks AK, Medlicott SA, Trotter MJ. Atypical fibroxanthoma with prominent sclerosis. *J Cutan Pathol* 2003;30:336–339.

212. Crowson AN, Carlson-Sweet K, Macinnis C, et al. Clear cell atypical fibroxanthoma: a clinicopathologic study. *J Cutan Pathol* 2002;29:374–381.

213. Orosz Z, Kelemen J, Szentirmay Z. Granular cell variant of atypical fibroxanthoma. *Pathol Oncol Res* 1996;2:244–247.

214. Orlandi A, Bianchi L, Ferlosio A, et al. The origin of osteoclast-like giant cells in atypical fibroxanthoma. *Histopathology* 2003;42:407–410.

215. Diaz-Cascajo C, Weyers W, Borghi S. Pigmented atypical fibroxanthoma: a tumor that may be easily mistaken for malignant melanoma. *Am J Dermatol* 2003;25:1–5.

216. Ma CK, Zarbo RJ, Gown AM. Immunohistochemical characterization of atypical fibroxanthoma and dermatofibrosarcoma protuberans. *Am J Clin Pathol* 1992;97:478–483.

217. Longacre TA, Smoller BR, Rouse RV. Atypical fibroxanthoma. Multiple immunohistologic profiles. *Am J Surg Pathol* 1993;17:1199–1209.

218. Monteagudo C, Calduch L, Navarro S, et al. CD99 immunoreactivity in atypical fibroxanthoma: a common feature of diagnostic value. *Am J Clin Pathol* 2002;117:126–131.

219. Smith-Zagone MJ, Prieto VG, Hayes RA, et al. HMB-45 (gp103) and MART-1 expression within giant cells in an atypical fibroxanthoma: a case report. *J Cutan Pathol* 2004;31: 284–286.

220. Barr RJ, Wueker RB, Graham JH. Ultrastructure of atypical fibroxanthoma. *Cancer* 1977; 40:736–743.

221. Mihic-Probst D, Zhao J, Saremaslani P, et al. CGH analysis shows genetic similarities a and differences in atypical fibroxanthoma and undifferentiated high grade pleomorphic sarcoma. *Anticancer Res* 2004;24:19–26.

222. Hyams VJ, Batsakis JG, Michaels L. Neoplasms of the middle ear. In Hartmann W, Sobin LS, eds. *Tumors of the Upper Respiratory Tract and Ear. Atlas of Tumor Pathology.* Fascicle 25, second series. Washington, DC: Armed Forces Institute of Pathology, 1986:306–330.

223. Mills SE, Frierson H Jr, Gaffney M. Neoplasms of the middle ear. In Rosai J, Sobin LS, eds. *Tumors of the Upper Respiratory Tract and Ear. Atlas of Tumor Pathology.* Fascicle 25, second series. Washington, DC: Armed Forces Institute of Pathology, 2001:383–450.

224. Torske KR, Thompson LD. Adenoma versus carcinoid tumor of the middle ear: a study of 48 cases and review of the literature. *Mod Pathol* 2002;15:543–555.

225. Stanley MW, Horwitz CA, Levinson RM, Sibley RK. Carcinoid tumors of the middle ear. *Am J Clin Pathol* 1987;87:592–600.

226. Latif MA, Madders DJ, Shaw PA. Carcinoid tumour of the middle ear associated with systemic symptoms. *J Laryngol Otol* 1987;101:480–486.

227. Manni J, Faverly DR, van Haelst UJ. Primary carcinoid tumor of the middle ear: report of four cases and a review of the literature. *Arch Otolaryngol Head Neck Surg* 1992;118: 1341–1347.

228. Faverly DR, Manni J, Smedts F, et al. Adenocarcinoid or amphicrine tumors of the middle ear. *Pathol Res Pract* 1992;188:162–171.

229. Batsakis JG. Adenomatous tumors of the middle ear. *Ann Otol Rhinol Laryngol* 1989;98: 749–752.

230. El-Naggar AK, Pflatz M, Ordóñez NG, et al. Tumors of the middle ear and endolymphatic sac. *Pathol Annual* 1994;29:199–231.

231. Ramsey MJ, Nadol Jr JB, Pilch BZ, et al. Carcinoid tumor of the middle ear: clinical features, recurrences, and metastases. *Laryngoscope* 2005;115:1660–1666.

232. Larson TC, Reese DF, Baker HL, et al. Glomus tympanicum chemodectomas: radiographic and clinical characteristics. *Radiology* 1987;163:801–806.

233. Lemaire M, Persu A, Hainaut P, et al. Hereditary paraganglioma. *J Intern Med* 1999;246: 113–116.

234. Bikhazi PH, Messina L, Mhatre AN, et al. Molecular pathogenesis in sporadic head and neck paraganglioma. *Laryngoscope* 2000;110:1346–1348.

235. Petropoulos AE, Luetje CM, Camarata PJ, et al. Genetic analysis in the diagnosis of familial paragangliomas. *Laryngoscope* 2000;110:1225–1229.

236. Persky MS, Hu KS, Berenstein A. Paragangliomas of the head and neck. In Harrison LB, Sessions RB, Hong WK, eds. *Head and Neck Cancer. A Multidisciplinary Approach.* 2nd ed. Philadelphia: Lippincott Williams & Wilkins, 2004:678–713.

237. Hu K, Persky MS. Multidisciplinary management of paragangliomas of the head and neck, Part 1. *Oncology* 2003;17:983–993.

238. Spector GJ, Ciralsky RH, Ogura JH. Glomus tumors in the head and neck. III. Analysis of clinical manifestations. *Ann Rhinol Otol Laryngol* 1975;84:73–79.

239. Taylor DM, Alford BR, Greenberg SD. Metastases of glomus jugulare tumors. *Arch Otolaryngol* 1965;82:5–13.

240. Johnstone PA, Foss RD, Desilets DJ. Malignant jugulotympanic paraganglioma. *Arch Pathol Lab Med* 1990;114: 976–979.

241. Barnes L, Taylor SR. Carotid body paragangliomas. A clinicopathologic and DNA analysis of 13 cases. *Arch Otolaryngol Head Neck Surg* 1990;116:447–453.

242. Johnson TL, Zarbo RJ, Lloyd RV, et al. Paragangliomas of the head and neck: immunohistochemical neuroendocrine and intermediate filament typing. *Modern Pathol* 1998;1: 216–223.

243. Kliewer KE, Wen DR, Cancilla PA, et al. Paragangliomas: assessment of prognosis by histologic, immunohistochemical, and ultrastructural techniques. *Hum Pathol* 1989;20: 29–39.

244. Erickson LS, Sorenson GD, McGavran MH. A review of 140 acoustic neuromas (neurilemmoma). *Laryngoscope* 1965;75:601–627.

245. Kasantikul V, Netsky MG, Glassock ME III, et al. Acoustic neurilemmoma. Clinicoanatomical study of 103 patients. *J Neurosurg* 1980;52:28–35.

246. Martuza RL, Ojemann RG. Bilateral acoustic neuromas: clinical aspects, pathogenesis and treatment. *Neurosurgery* 1982;10:1–12.

247. Anand T, Byrnes DP, Walby AP, et al. Bilateral acoustic neuromas. *Clin Otolaryngol* 1993; 18:365–371.

248. Moffat DA, Irving RM. The molecular genetics of vestibular schwannomas. *J Laryngol Otol* 1995;109:381–384.

249. Kishore A, O'Reilly BF. A clinical study of vestibular schwannomas in type 2 neurofibromatosis. *Clin Otolaryngol* 2000;25:561–565.

250. Thompson LD, Bouffard JP, Sandberg GD, et al. Primary ear and temporal bone meningiomas: a clinicopathologic study of 36 cases with a review of the literature. *Mod Pathol* 2003; 16:236–245.

251. Rietz DR, Ford CN, Kurtycz DF, et al. Significance of apparent intratympanic meningiomas. *Laryngoscope* 1983;93:1397–1404.

252. Megerian CA, McKenna MJ, Nuss RC, et al. Endolymphatic sac tumors: histopathologic confirmation, clinical characterization, and implication in von Hippel-Lindau disease. *Laryngoscope* 1995;105:801–808.

253. Manski TJ, Heffner DK, Glenn GM, et al. Endolymphatic sac tumors: the basis of morbid hearing loss in von Hippel-Lindau disease. *JAMA* 1997;277:1461–1466.

254. Wenig BM, Heffner DK. Endolymphatic sac tumors: fact or fiction? *Adv Anat Pathol* 1996; 3:378–387.

255. Batsakis JG, El-Naggar AK. Papillary neoplasms (Heffner's tumors) of the endolymphatic sac. *Ann Otol Rhinol Laryngol* 1993;102:648–651.

256. Sgambati MT, Stolle C, Choyke PL, et al. Mosaicism in von Hippel-Lindau disease: lessons from kindreds with germline mutations identified in offspring with mosaic parents. *Am J Hum Genet* 2000;66:84–91.

257. Heffner DK. Low-grade adenocarcinoma of probable endolymphatic sac origin. A clinicopathologic study of 20 cases. *Cancer* 1989;64:2292–2302.

258. Wenig BM. Schneiderian papillomas of the middle ear. *Ann Otol Rhinol Laryngol* 1996; 105:226–233.

259. Andrade JM, Gehris CW, Jr., Breitnecker R. Cavernous haemangioma of the tympanic membrane. A case report. *Am J Otol* 1993;4:198–199.

260. Jackson CG, Levine SC, McKennan KX. Hemangioma of the middle ear. *Am J Otol* 1987; 8:131–132.

261. Eby TL, Fisch U, Malek MS. Facial nerve management in temporal bone hemangiomas. *Am J Otol* 1992;13:223–232.

262. Olson JE, Glassock ME, III, Britton BH. Lipomas of the internal auditory canal. *Arch Otolaryngol* 1978;104:431–436.

263. Huang TS. Primary intravestibular lipoma. *Ann Otol Rhinol Laryngol* 1989;98:393–395.

264. Ishikawa T, Saito H, Takahashi K. Osteoma of the mastoid. *Arch Otorhinolaryngol* 1997; 217:93–97.

265. Denia A, Perez F, Canalis RR, et al. Extracanalicular osteomas of the temporal bone. *Arch Otolaryngol* 1979;105:706–709.

266. Marlowe FI, Dave U, Wolfson RJ. Giant osteoma of the mastoid. *Am J Otolaryngol* 1980;1: 191–193.

267. Potter C, Conner GH, Sharkey FE. Benign osteoblastoma of the temporal bone. *Am J Otol* 1983;4:318–322.

268. Bertoni F, Unni KK, Beabout JW, et al. Chondroblastoma of the skull and facial bones. *Am J Clin Pathol* 1987;88:1–9.

269. Silverstein H, Griffin WL Jr, Balough K Jr. Teratoma of the middle ear and mastoid process. A case with aberrant innervation of the facial musculature. *Arch Otolaryngol* 1967; 85:243–248.

270. Hyams VJ, Batsakis JG, Michaels L. Squamous cell carcinoma of the middle ear. In Hartmann WH, Sobin LH, eds. *Tumors of the Upper Respiratory Tract and Ear. Atlas of Tumor Pathology.* Fascicle 25, second series. Washington, DC: Armed Forces Institute of Pathology, 1986:326–327.

271. Kenyon GS, Marks PV, Scholtz CL, et al. Squamous cell carcinoma of the middle ear. A 25-year retrospective study. *Ann Otol Rhinol Laryngol* 1985;94:273–277.

272. Tsai ST, Li C, Jun YT, et al. High prevalence of human papillomavirus types 16 and 18 in middle ear carcinomas. *Int J Cancer* 1997;71:208–212.

273. Hyams VJ, Batsakis JG, Michaels L. Adenocarcinoma of the middle ear. In Hartmann, WH, Sobin LH, eds. *Tumors of the Upper Respiratory Tract and Ear. Atlas of Tumor Pathology.* Fascicle 25, second series. Washington, DC: Armed Forces Institute of Pathology, 1986: 320–323.

274. Newton WA, Gehan EA, Webber BL, et al. Classification of rhabdomyosarcomas and related sarcomas. Pathologic aspects and proposal for a new classification—an Intergroup Rhabdomyosarcoma Study. *Cancer* 1995;76:1073–1085.

275. Kraus DH, Saenz NC, Gollamudi S, et al. Pediatric rhabdomyosarcoma of the head and neck. *Am J Surg* 1997;174:556–560.

276. Parham DM, Barr FG. Embryonal rhabdomyosarcoma. In Fletcher CDM, Unni KK, Mertens F, eds. *World Health Organization Classification of Tumours, Pathology, and Genetics. Tumours of Soft Tissue and Bone.* Lyon, France: IARC Press, 2002:146–149.

277. Raney RB Jr, Tefft M, Newton WA, et al. Improved prognosis with cranial soft tissue sarcomas arising in nonorbital parameningeal sites. A report from the Intergroup Rhabdomyosarcoma Study. *Cancer* 1987;59:147–155.

278. Nora FE, Unni KK, Pritchard DJ. Osteosarcoma of extragnathic craniofacial bones. *Mayo Clin Proc* 1983;58:268–272.

279. Huvos AG, Sandaresan N, Bretsky SS. Osteogenic sarcoma of the skull. A clinicopathologic study of 19 patients. *Cancer* 1985;56:1214–1221.

280. Caron AS, Hajdu S I, Strong EW. Osteogenic sarcoma of the facial and cranial bones. A review of forty-three cases. *Am J Surg* 1971;122:719–725.

281. Coltera MC, Googe PB, Harrist TJ, et al. Chondrosarcoma of the temporal bone. Diagnosis and treatment in 13 cases and review of the literature. *Cancer* 1986;58:2689–2696.

282. Schuknecht HF. Neoplastic growths. In Schuknecht HF, ed. *Pathology of the Ear.* Philadelphia: Lea & Febiger, 1993:447–498.

283. Hill BA, Kohut RI. Metastatic adenocarcinoma of the temporal bone. *Arch Otolaryngol* 1976;102:568–571.

284. Berlinger NT, Koutroupas S, Adams G, et al. Patterns of involvement of the temporal bone in metastatic and systemic malignancy. *Laryngoscope* 1980;90:619–627.

Gordon K. Klintworth
Thomas J. Cummings

The Eye and Ocular Adnexa

Numerous diseases affect the eye and ocular adnexa, and, in many cases, prompt and careful communication with the ophthalmologist who submitted the specimens is essential if a meaningful diagnosis is to be provided. Awareness of the proper techniques for processing eyes is also essential for the successful evaluation of ocular specimens by the surgical pathologist. Knowledge of normal ocular anatomy is necessary to interpret many of the diverse pathologic changes that involve these structures. For a review of normal ophthalmic anatomy and histology, the reader should consult one of the available texts (1–3). This chapter reviews some of the more common lesions excised by ophthalmologists that can be successfully diagnosed by the general surgical pathologist. A complete discussion of all surgical ophthalmic pathology specimens is beyond the scope of this survey. The reader is referred elsewhere for detailed descriptions of ophthalmic diseases (www.The EyePathologist.com) (4–6).

A major manifestation of cranial ("giant cell" or "temporal") arteritis is retinal ischemia, and, in the absence of prompt treatment, this can rapidly lead to irreversible blindness resulting from retinal infarction. For diagnostic purposes, ophthalmologists frequently perform biopsies of the temporal artery (7–9). See Index for additional information on cranial arteritis.

THE GLOBE

The globe is excised surgically (enucleated) for many reasons, including significant ocular trauma or infection; blindness in the eye; an eye that is severely scarred and painful (phthisis bulbi); chronic glaucoma that is unresponsive to therapy; and suspicion of primary intraocular neoplasms. Although biopsy techniques have been developed for evaluating intraocular tumors (10) and certain chorioretinal inflammatory conditions (11), the diagnosis of many of these disorders is made clinically without histopathologic confirmation.

A wide variety of tumors can arise from different ocular structures (12). Some are benign (Table 24.1). Malignant intraocular tumors include retinoblastoma, melanoma, and metastatic neoplasms, which are discussed elsewhere in this chapter under the specific structures in which they occur.

TRAUMA

The eye is excised after severe ocular trauma if no potential for visual recovery exists. Blunt trauma to the eye may rupture the eyeball, especially at the junction of the cornea and sclera or immediately posterior to the insertion of the rectus muscles where the sclera is thinnest. Potential complications of ocular trauma include blood within the anterior chamber (hyphema) with associated corneal discoloration that is caused by hemoglobin deposition (corneal blood staining), and separation of the

ciliary body from the iris (iridodialysis) or sclera (cyclodialysis), as well as cataracts, retinal detachments, and choroidal rupture.

FOREIGN BODIES

Foreign bodies commonly enter the eye as projectiles or as fragments accompanying branches or other sharp objects that per-

TABLE 24.1
Benign Intraocular Tumors
Choroid
Ganglioneuroma
Hemangioma (cavernous)
Inflammatory pseudotumor
Leiomyoma
Neurofibroma
Nevi
Osteoma
Schwannoma
Ciliary body
Adenoma of pigmented or nonpigmented epithelium
Hemangioma
Leiomyoma
Mesectodermal leiomyoma
Neurofibroma
Nevi
Iris
Adenoma of pigment epithelium
Cysts
Pigment epithelial
Stromal
Traumatic epithelial
Granular cell tumor
Hemangioma
Juvenile xanthogranuloma
Leiomyoma
Neurofibroma
Nevi
Xanthoma
Optic nerve
Pilocytic astrocytoma
Glioneuroma
Drusen
Medulloepithelioma
Melanocytoma
Meningioma
Retina
Adenoma of pigment epithelium
Astrocytic hamartoma
Glioneuroma
Hemangioma (capillary, cavernous, and racemose)
"Massive retinal gliosis"
Retinocytoma

forate the globe. Vegetable matter, hair, and skin may enter the intraocular tissues after an explosive or perforating injury. These agents incite an inflammatory reaction that occasionally may be granulomatous in nature.

Some sterile foreign objects do not incite intraocular inflammation or cause specific adverse effects, whereas others cause a significant tissue response. Intraocular foreign bodies containing iron are particularly toxic to the retina, and they may cause a diffuse deposition of iron throughout the eye (13). Copper-rich foreign bodies incite a significant intraocular acute inflammatory reaction (14). Other metals such as lead, zinc, nickel, aluminum, and mercury may also evoke intraocular inflammation. Energy-dispersive x-ray microanalysis is often helpful in identifying the composition of intraocular foreign bodies (15).

INFLAMMATION

Inflammation of the eye may involve the intraocular contents but spare the sclera and cornea (endophthalmitis), or it may affect the cornea and sclera in addition to the ocular contents (panophthalmitis). Both endophthalmitis and panophthalmitis may follow ocular trauma, surgery, or the hematogenous spread of a systemic infection. The distinction between endophthalmitis and panophthalmitis is clinically important because infections causing panophthalmitis potentially expose the patient's orbit to microorganisms, whereas, in infectious endophthalmitis, the cornea and sclera encase the intraocular infection, similar to an encapsulated abscess.

In both endophthalmitis and panophthalmitis, a profuse polymorphonuclear leukocytic infiltration is present, and intraocular hemorrhage may also be seen. The involved intraocular tissues are usually necrotic and disorganized, and the causal bacteria or fungi may be identified with special stains. A mild endophthalmitis due to *Propionibacterium acnes* sometimes follows cataract extraction (16,17). It has a minimal inflammatory reaction. A wide variety of organisms can cause intraocular inflammation (Table 24.2) (16–22).

Aside from sympathetic uveitis, granulomatous inflammation of the eye occurs in some conditions (Table 24.3). An important granulomatous endophthalmitis occurs around the lens as part of an immunologic reaction to lens proteins (phacoanaphylactic endophthalmitis) (23,24).

PHTHISIS BULBI

Numerous pathologic processes eventually culminate in an atrophic disorganized eye. Because such eyes with phthisis bulbi

---

TABLE 24.2

Infectious Organisms Isolated in Endophthalmitis

Bacillus	*Propionibacterium acnes*
Clostridium perfringens	*Proteus*
Escherichia coli	*Pseudomonas*
Haemophilus influenzae	*Salmonella typhimurium*
Klebsiella	*Serratia marcescens*
Listeria monocytogenes	*Staphylococcus aureus*
Mycobacterium	*Staphylococcus epidermidis*
Neisseria meningitidis	*Streptococcus*
Nocardia asteroides	

TABLE 24.3

Causes of Intraocular Granulomatous Inflammation

Bacteria	Idiopathic
Mycobacterium tuberculosis	Sarcoidosis
Treponema pallidum	Vogt-Koyanagi-Harada syndrome
Fungi	Immunologic disorders
Aspergillus	Juvenile rheumatoid arthritis
Blastomyces dermatitidis	Sympathetic uveitis
Candida	Parasites
Coccidioides immitis	*Taenia solium (Cysticercus cellulosae)*
Histoplasma capsulatum	*Toxocara canis*
Sporothrix schenckii	

---

almost always contain significant amounts of lamellar bone, decalcification is usually required before the globe can be cut and submitted for tissue processing. The intraocular ossification can be detected on radiographic examination of the enucleated eye (25). The bone usually contains marrow with adipose tissue and blood vessels and occasionally megakaryocytes, as well as erythrocytic and myelocytic lineage precursors (26). Phthisical eyes usually manifest extensive scleral thickening, chronic retinal detachment, and the intraocular contents are markedly disorganized. A fibrous diaphragm often extends circumferentially from the ciliary body behind the lens (cyclitic membrane). As a rule, a histologic examination of phthisical eyes fails to disclose evidence of the initial condition that led to this condition. Rarely, phthisical eyes have contained an unsuspected intraocular melanoma, lymphoma, or adenocarcinoma (27).

GLAUCOMA

The term *glaucoma* refers to a group of disorders that develop an optic neuropathy that is accompanied by a distinct excavation of the optic nerve head and an incremental loss of visual-field sensitivity. In most cases, the intraocular pressure is increased, and, most notably, this damages the retina and optic nerve. Several types of glaucoma are recognized and are classified as follows: primary glaucoma, which is not associated with significant antecedent ocular disease; and secondary glaucoma, which is due to some ocular pathologic process. Primary glaucoma can result from a blockage of the drainage of the aqueous humor distal to the anterior chamber angle (primary open-angle glaucoma) and from a narrow anterior chamber angle (primary narrow-angle glaucoma) (28). Increased intraocular pressure, abnormal visual fields, and optic nerve damage are secondary effects of glaucoma.

Some surgical procedures used in the treatment of glaucoma result in excised tissue specimens that are submitted for pathologic evaluation at some institutions. For example, a small fragment of the trabecular meshwork is often excised (trabeculectomy) to enhance the drainage of aqueous humor from the eye to decrease intraocular pressure. This procedure produces a minute fragment of tissue that is often less than 1 mm in diameter. The processing of such specimens is not clinically important, but communication between the surgical pathologist and the histotechnician responsible for embedding such specimens is essential for proper tissue orientation; the use of a dissecting microscope is required. Light or transmission electron microscopic examination of trabeculectomy specimens is often unre-

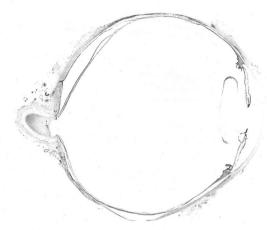

Figure 24.1. Marked cupping of the optic disc. This eye was surgically excised (enucleated) because of glaucoma.

warding, but the trabecular meshwork, melanin pigment, Schlemm canal, ciliary muscle, or the peripheral cornea may be disclosed (29).

In end-stage glaucoma, the painful blind eyes may require enucleation. Morphologic evidence of increased intraocular pressure includes atrophy of the nerve fiber and ganglion cell layer and excavation of the optic nerve disc (glaucomatous cupping of the optic disc) (Fig. 24.1). A peculiar degeneration of an atrophic optic nerve is characterized by an accumulation of hyaluronic acid that stains positively with the Hale colloidal iron technique or the Alcian blue stain (Schnabel cavernous atrophy). An examination of a glaucomatous eye may also disclose the cause of congenital or secondary glaucoma. For example, fibrocollagenous adhesions may be present between the posterior surface of the peripheral cornea and the iris (peripheral anterior synechiae), and this may have obstructed the aqueous humor outflow.

CORNEA

EVALUATION OF CORNEAL TISSUE

Most surgically excised corneal specimens represent tissue obtained at the time of a full-thickness corneal transplant (penetrating keratoplasty). Less often, lamellar keratoplasty (a partial-thickness corneal graft) and corneal biopsy specimens (30) are submitted for histopathologic evaluation. During corneal grafts, tissue is surgically removed from the cornea with the aid of a trephine so that a button approximately 8 mm in diameter is obtained. The manner by which corneal tissue is processed depends on the suspected pathologic process. Most specimens are fixed in formalin and processed for light microscopy according to standard procedures. Certain specimens, however, need special handling to ensure that the correct diagnosis is made. For example, some corneal disorders, such as Schnyder corneal dystrophy and other lipid keratopathies, need special fixatives or frozen sections to preserve the abnormal accumulations. Meesmann, Thiel-Behnke, and Reis-Bücklers corneal dystrophy require transmission electron microscopy for a morphologic diagnosis, but these dystrophies can now be diagnosed with molecular genetic techniques by using DNA from blood, tissue, or buccal swabs (31,32).

For histopathologic evaluation, a representative cross section through the center of each corneal button that includes any opacification or other abnormalities should usually be processed. Because the normal monolayer of corneal endothelium at the back of the cornea is easily disrupted, corneal specimens should be handled with care and should be cut with a sharp razor so that the lesion of interest is present within the portion of cornea submitted for microscopic examination.

CORNEAL GRAFTS

Indications for Corneal Grafts

Frequent indications for penetrating keratoplasty include corneal endothelial decompensation (bullous keratopathy); keratoconus; certain corneal dystrophies; failed corneal grafts; chronic keratitis, which is most often caused by herpes simplex; and corneal scarring resulting from acute nonspecific keratitis (33,34).

Graft Failure

Most currently performed corneal transplants are successful, and they provide long-term improvements in visual acuity for individuals with certain corneal diseases. In contrast to grafts of most tissues or organs, those involving the cornea are usually successful without compatibility matching of donor and recipient tissues (35). Some fail for various reasons, including endothelial decompensation (discussed under "Bullous Keratopathy"), recurrent disease (36–39), immunologic graft rejection (40–43), or improper surgical technique. The donor–host margin of the previous corneal graft can often be identified in tissue sections by finding defects through all or part of the peripheral corneal tissue, especially in the Bowman layer and Descemet membrane. Epithelial irregularities, stromal vascularization, endothelial cell loss, and retrocorneal fibrous membranes often characterize failed corneal grafts, but a pronounced stromal inflammatory infiltrate is rarely evident. Unlike Fuchs endothelial corneal dystrophy, the basic abnormality of the macular, lattice, granular, and the other corneal dystrophies may recur in the corneal grafts (36–39,44).

NONSPECIFIC RESPONSES

Different pathologic processes cause nonspecific histopathologic responses, and these may be evident in the corneal tissue. For example, intraepithelial vesicles and bullae between the epithelium and Bowman layer may follow corneal edema, especially of the epithelium (Fig. 24.2). An aberrant basal lamina develops within the corneal epithelium during the healing of some injuries (Fig. 24.2). Fibrous tissue, sometimes with blood vessels and mononuclear inflammatory cells, may accumulate between the epithelium and Bowman layer (pannus) (Fig. 24.3).

Blood vessels are present in the superficial or deep stroma of the normally avascular cornea in numerous pathologic states associated with inflammation. With aging, corneal endothelial cells diminish in number, and Descemet membrane thickens. A diffuse, irregular thickening of Descemet membrane accompanies some long-standing degenerative changes of the endothelial layer. Fibrous retrocorneal membranes between the Des-

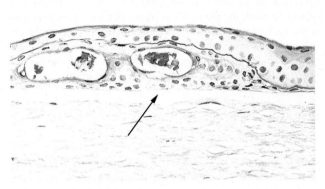

Figure 24.2. Basement membrane material within the epithelial layer of the cornea. Also present are two intraepithelial cysts. Note that Bowman layer (*arrow*) does not react positively with the periodic acid-Schiff stain.

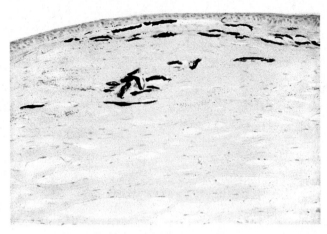

Figure 24.4. Calcific band keratopathy. Linear deposits of calcium phosphate are present within the superficial corneal stroma (von Kossa stain).

cemet membrane and the corneal endothelium may follow grafts or various inflammatory processes of the cornea (45).

CALCIFIC BAND KERATOPATHY

Under a variety of circumstances, calcium is deposited in the cornea (46–49), particularly in the Bowman layer and the superficial corneal stroma (calcific band keratopathy) (Fig. 24.4). In its early stages, a faint basophilic stippling of Bowman layer typifies calcific band keratopathy, and, in advanced cases, the entire thickness of the Bowman layer is involved.

CHRONIC ACTINIC KERATOPATHY (CLIMATIC DROPLET KERATOPATHY)

Amorphous globules of protein accumulate in the superficial stroma of the interpalpebral portion of the cornea in an entity known by numerous terms, including *chronic actinic keratopathy* (50), *climatic droplet keratopathy* (51), and *spheroidal degeneration* (52). The condition, which initially involves the periphery of the cornea, varies in severity and increases in incidence and

intensity with age. It is particularly pronounced in individuals exposed over long periods to excessive ultraviolet light. Similar globules can accumulate nonspecifically in corneas with various underlying disorders ("spheroidal degeneration").

BULLOUS KERATOPATHY

The corneal endothelium helps to maintain proper hydration of the cornea. Meaningful injury to this monolayer of cells, which does not regenerate significantly in humans, may result in corneal epithelial and stromal edema, subepithelial bullae, and decreased visual acuity. The many causes of this so-called bullous keratopathy include immunologic rejection of the corneal endothelium, and Fuchs corneal dystrophy. Bullous keratopathy also may be precipitated by cataract extraction (aphakic bullous keratopathy), sometimes after the combined implantation of a prosthetic intraocular lens (pseudophakic bullous keratopathy) (53). Descemet-stripping endothelial keratoplasty (DSEK) is a technique currently being performed in eyes with corneal endothelial decompensation and failed penetrating keratoplasty (54,55).

Corneal buttons removed from patients with bullous keratopathy manifest intraepithelial vesicles, bullae between the epithelium and the Bowman layer, and markedly fewer endothelial cells than normal. An intraepithelial basement membrane and a mild subepithelial pannus may also be present. Mild degrees of stromal edema are difficult to discern histologically, but increased corneal thickness in association with an absence of the normal artifactual clefts between the collagen lamellae in routinely processed tissue sections is suggestive of corneal edema.

KERATOCONUS

Noninflammatory thinning of the central corneal stroma takes place in keratoconus, causing a cone-shaped cornea (56). Scarring and astigmatism associated with this disorder often prevent adequate refractive correction and decrease visual acuity. A brown, stainable intraepithelial iron arc or ring frequently surrounds the conical portion of the cornea (Fleischer ring). Numerous breaks in the Bowman layer that are associated with the thinning of the central corneal stroma characterize advanced

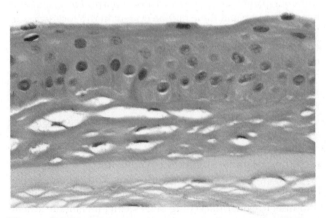

Figure 24.3. Collagenous tissue between the corneal epithelium and Bowman layer (pannus).

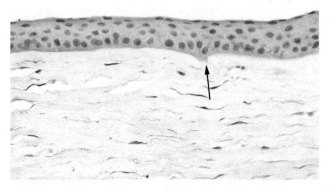

Figure 24.5. Keratoconus. Focal disruptions of Bowman layer (*arrow*) are common.

cases (56) (Fig. 24.5). The endothelium in corneas with keratoconus is usually unremarkable, but endothelial cell loss may accompany ruptures of Descemet membrane ("corneal hydrops"). Rarely, keratoconus recurs in the graft (57).

CORNEAL DYSTROPHIES

The corneal dystrophies are a heterogeneous group of inherited bilateral corneal disorders (Table 24.4). The prevalence of the different corneal dystrophies varies in different countries and even within the different parts of some countries. Fuchs endothelial dystrophy accounts for most corneal dystrophy specimens submitted for pathologic examination in the United States. Other corneal specimens that reach the pathology laboratory have macular, lattice, or granular corneal dystrophy. Many of these diseases have been mapped to specific chromosomes, and the genes have been identified in many of them. Space restrictions prevent a description of all corneal dystrophies. For details, the reader is referred elsewhere (31,32).

Fuchs Corneal Dystrophy

Fuchs corneal dystrophy is characterized by the presence of multiple wartlike excrescences on the Descemet membrane (cornea guttae) (Fig. 24.6) and the histologic features of bullous keratopathy. The centrally located cornea guttae are morphologically identical with the structures that form in the peripheral cornea with normal aging (Hassall-Henle bodies). However, Hassall-Henle bodies are too peripheral in location to be observed in specimens obtained during a routine penetrating keratoplasty. Cornea guttae are not specific for Fuchs corneal dystrophy; they are also found in macular corneal dystrophy (described under "Macular Corneal Dystrophy") and in some cases of interstitial keratitis and keratoconus. The presence of inconspicuous ghost vessels in the most posterior corneal stroma distinguishes interstitial keratitis from Fuchs corneal dystrophy.

Macular Corneal Dystrophy

Corneas from patients with macular corneal dystrophy are characterized by an accumulation of a keratan sulfate-related glycosaminoglycan within both the fibroblasts and the endothelium of the cornea, as well as among the collagen lamellae and in the Descemet membrane. The Hale colloidal iron technique and the Alcian blue stain are particularly useful in coloring the abnormal accumulations (58) that result from a mutation in the *CHST6* gene on human chromosome 16 (16q22.1) (31) (Fig. 24.7).

Corneal Dystrophies with Amyloid Deposition

The inherited corneal dystrophies with amyloid deposition are characterized by irregular linear opacities resulting from stromal amyloid deposition (Fig. 24.8) in corneas with an unremarkable Descemet membrane and endothelium. Amyloid is apparently localized to the cornea in most cases of lattice corneal dystrophy, but, in one type (lattice corneal dystrophy type 2) it is a manifestation of a systemic disease (familial amyloid polyneuropathy type 3, Finnish or Meretoja type). Like deposits of amyloid elsewhere, the corneal deposits in the lattice corneal dystrophies react positively with the Congo red stain and with other methods for amyloid. Lattice corneal dystrophy type 1 is caused by specific mutations in the *TGFBI* gene, and affected individuals often have recurrent epithelial erosions and subepithelial amyloid or collagenous plaques. The amyloid in this dystrophy reacts with antibodies to the transforming growth factor-β–induced protein (59).

Amyloid also accumulates in the corneal stroma in numerous nonspecific, long-standing ocular disorders, including trauma, keratoconus, trachoma, uveitis, the retinopathy of prematurity, phlyctenular keratoconjunctivitis, sympathetic ophthalmia, and glaucoma (62). In most of the corneal amyloidoses, the nature of the amyloid remains unknown, but, in lattice corneal dystrophy type 1, mutant transforming growth factor-β–induced protein is a major component (59). In lattice corneal dystrophy type 2, the amyloid is derived from a part of mutant gelsolin (60,61). A significant amount of lactoferrin accumulates within the cornea in gelatinous droplike dystrophy of the cornea (familial subepithelial corneal amyloidosis) (62), an inherited corneal disorder due to a mutation in the *TACSTD2* (formerly known as *MISI*) gene on human chromosome 1 (1p32) (31).

Granular Corneal Dystrophy

In granular corneal dystrophy, abnormal subepithelial and anterior stromal deposits appear bright red with the Masson trichrome stain (Fig. 24.9). The posterior stroma, Descemet membrane, and corneal endothelium are usually unaffected. This dystrophy results from a mutation in the *TGFBI* (*BIGH3*) gene (31,58), and the corneal deposits react with antibodies to transforming growth factor-β–induced protein (63). The *TGFBI* mutation responsible for granular corneal dystrophy type 1 is usually R55W and it differs from those causing granular corneal dystropy type 2 and type 3 (Reis-Bücklers corneal dystrophy) (32,33).

KERATITIS CAUSED BY ORGANISMS

Bacteria, fungi, viruses, or protozoa (64–68) (Table 24.5) frequently infect the cornea, and, especially if corneal perforation is imminent, corneal transplantation may be performed on such tissue. Corneal biopsies are occasionally used to identify the offending organism in acute keratitis (30). Those who wear contact lenses are particularly susceptible to keratitis from *Pseudomonas* species (69) and *Acanthamoeba* (70,71). Keratitis caused

TABLE 24.4	Significant Features and Predominant Corneal Layer Affected in Some Corneal Dystrophies

Epithelium
  Meesmann dystrophy
    Autosomal dominant inheritance
    Mutation in *KRT3* or *KRT12* gene on chromosome 12 (12q) or 17 (17q)
    Intraepithelial microcysts
    Peculiar substance evident by transmission electron microscopy
    Diagnosis possible with molecular genetic analysis on DNA
    Microcystic, map dot, and fingerprint dystrophy
    Usually nonspecific reaction, but may be familial
    Intraepithelial basement membrane and microcysts
Bowman layer and superficial stroma
  Granular corneal dystrophy type 3 (Reis-Bücklers dystrophy)
    Autosomal dominant inheritance
    Most cases due to R124L mutation in *TGFBI* gene on chromosome 5 (5q31)
  Thiel-Behnke dystrophy
    Subepithelial "curly" fibers by transmission electron microscopy
    Most cases due to R555Q mutation in *TGFBI* gene on chromosome 5 (5q31)
    Also maps to chromosome 10 (10q23–q24)
    Focal loss of epithelial basement membrane and Bowman layer
  Gelatinous droplike cornea dystrophy (familial subepithelial amyloidosis)
    Autosomal recessive inheritance
    Most cases due to mutation in *TACSTD2* gene on chromosome 1 (1p32)
    Subepithelial amyloid deposits that contain lactoferrin
Stroma
  Granular corneal dystrophy type 1
    Autosomal dominant inheritance
    Most cases due to R555W mutation in *TGFBI* gene on chromosome 5 (5q31)
    Discrete deposits of mutated transforming growth factor-β–induced protein
    Deposits appear red with Masson trichrome stain
  Granular corneal dystrophy type 2 (Avellino corneal dystrophy)
    Autosomal dominant inheritance
    Corneal deposits similar to granular corneal dystrophy plus amyloid
    Due to R124H mutation in *TGFBI* gene on chromosome 5 (5q31)
  Macular corneal dystrophy
    Autosomal recessive inheritance
    Due to mutation in *CHST6* gene on chromosome 16 (16q22.1)
    Basic defect—a deficiency of a specific carbohydrate sulfotransferase
    Low sulfated keratan-sulfate–related glycosaminoglycan deposits throughout stroma, Descemet membrane, and endothelium; corneal guttae usually present
    Accumulations react with colloidal iron and Alcian blue
    Type I
      Deposits do not react with antibody to keratan sulfate
      Serum keratan sulfate very low or absent
    Type IA
      Keratocytes react with antibody to keratan sulfate
      Serum keratan sulfate very low or absent
    Type II
      Deposits react with antibody to keratan sulfate
      Serum keratan sulfate normal

Lattice dystrophy
  Type I
    Autosomal dominant inheritance
    Most cases due to R124C mutation in *TGFBI* on chromosome 5 (5q31)
    Lesions limited to cornea
  Type II
    Autosomal dominant inheritance
    Mutation in *GSN* gene on chromosome 9 (9q34)
    Associated with familial amyloid polyneuropathy (Meretoja or Finnish type)
    Amyloid derived from fragment of mutated gelsolin
Schnyder corneal dystrophy (central stromal crystalline dystrophy)
  Due to mutation in the *UBIAD1* gene on chromosome 1 (1p34p32)
  Crystals of cholesterol ester in anterior stroma
Fleck dystrophy (speckled, cloudy dystrophy)
  Autosomal dominant inheritance
  Due to mutation in the *PIP5K3* gene on chromosome 2 (2q35)
  Individual keratocytes react with colloidal iron and Alcian blue stains
Endothelium
  Fuchs endothelial corneal dystrophy
    Females affected more often than males (4:1)
    Sometimes autosomal dominant inheritance
    Some cases with early onset caused by mutation in *COL8A2* gene on chromosome 1 (1p34.3–p32.3); other cases have been mapped to chromosomes 13 (13pTel–3q12.13) and 18 (18q21.2–q21.32)
    Epithelial cysts and edema
    Stromal edema
    Thickened Descemet membrane
    Corneal guttae
    Diminished number of endothelial cells
  Posterior polymorphous dystrophy
    Autosomal dominant or recessive inheritance
    Some cases due to mutation in *COL8A2* gene on chromosome 1 (1p34.3–p32.3); others due to *TCF8* mutation on chromosome 10 (10p11.2)
    Disease also maps to chromosome 20 (20q12–q13) where *VSX1* mutations implicated, but disputed
    Abnormal Descemet membrane
    Multilayered epithelial cells line posterior cornea
  Congenital hereditary endothelial dystrophy type 1 (CHED type 1)
    Autosomal dominant inheritance
    Maps to chromosome 20 (20q12–q13.1)
    Edematous epithelium
    Loss of Bowman layer
    Thickening of stroma and Descemet membrane
    Diminished number of endothelial cells
  Congenital hereditary endothelial dystrophy type 2 (CHED type 2)
    Autosomal recessive inheritance
    Due to mutation in *SLC4A11* gene on chromosome 20 (20p13–p12)
    Edematous epithelium
    Loss of Bowman layer
    Corneal stroma much thicker than in CHED type 1
    Thickening of Descemet membrane
    Diminished number of endothelial cells

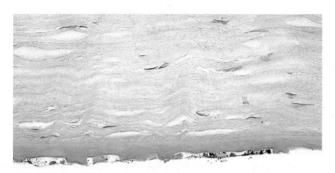

Figure 24.6. Fuchs corneal dystrophy. Excrescences form over the peripheral and central part of Descemet membrane. The corneal endothelial cells are diminished in number, and Descemet membrane is also often abnormally thickened.

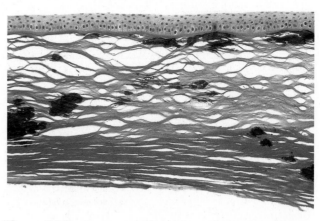

Figure 24.9. Granular corneal dystrophy. Abnormal collections of mutated transforming growth factor-β–induced protein accumulate within the corneal stroma. This material appears bright red with the Masson trichrome stain.

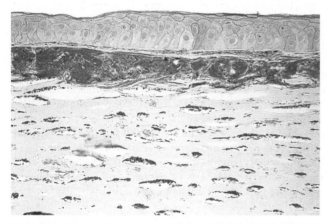

Figure 24.7. Macular corneal dystrophy. Extracellular stromal deposits of glycosaminoglycans are found. Similar material is also present within the corneal fibroblasts (keratocytes) (Hale colloidal iron).

by the microfilaria of the nematode *Onchocerca volvulus* is a leading cause of blindness worldwide, but affected individuals are rarely treated in the United States (72). Caterpillar hairs can also cause keratitis (73).

Although the pathogenic agent influences the nature of the tissue reaction in acute ulcerative keratitis, the histopathologic features are strikingly similar in most instances; these include destruction of the corneal epithelium, Bowman layer, and stroma, as well as necrosis and a prominent polymorphonuclear leukocytic infiltrate. With corneal perforation, discontinuities of Descemet membrane develop, and inflammatory debris adheres to the posterior surface of the cornea. The causative microorganism is often difficult to detect in tissue sections without the aid of special stains. Colonies of some bacteria, such as *Streptococcus viridans*, may produce crystalline-like stromal opacities in the absence of an inflammatory cell infiltrate ("infectious pseudocrystalline keratopathy") (74).

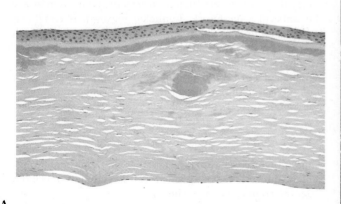

A

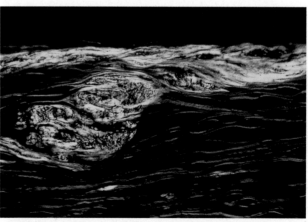

B

Figure 24.8. Lattice corneal dystrophy. **(A)** Amyloid accumulation is shown within the corneal stroma in a variant of lattice corneal dystrophy type 1. In this photomicrograph, amyloid is evident immediately beneath the Bowman layer and within the anterior corneal stroma. **(B)** The amyloid is birefringent and exhibits apple-green dichroism after being stained with Congo red.

TABLE 24.5

Some Infectious Organisms in Keratitis

Viruses
   Human herpesvirus-1 (herpes simplex virus type 1)
   Human herpesvirus-3 (varicella-zoster virus)
   Human herpesvirus-5 (cytomegalovirus)
Bacteria
   Escherichia coli   *Pseudomonas aeruginosa*
   Haemophilus influenzae   *Staphylococcus aureus*
   Klebsiella   *Staphylococcus epidermidis*
   Mycobacterium   *Streptococcus pneumoniae*
   Neisseria gonorrhoeae   Other streptococci
   Proteus   *Treponema pallidum*
Fungi
   Aspergillus
   Candida   *Myrathecium*
   Cladosporium   *Paecilomyces*
   Curvularia   *Petriellidium boydii*
   Fusarium   *Phialophora*
Protozoa
   Acanthamoeba
   Nosema

Acanthamoeba

Keratitis caused by *Acanthamoeba* (*A. castellani*, *A. culbertsoni*, *A. polyphaga*, or *A. rhysodes*) is a well recognized complication in those who wear contact lenses. This protozoan can be recognized in hematoxylin and eosin (H&E)-stained sections, but special stains (calcofluor white, periodic acid-Schiff, methenamine silver, Giemsa), immunofluorescent techniques, and transmission electron microscopy have been advocated for the diagnosis of amebic keratitis (Fig. 24.10). Amebic cysts and trophozoites are most often found near areas of stromal necrosis (75,76). In the absence of specific immunohistochemical (IHC) methods, the differentiation of trophozoites from reactive corneal fibroblasts may be difficult.

Herpes Simplex

Human herpesvirus-1 (herpes simplex type 1) is the most common viral cause of clinically significant corneal disease (77).

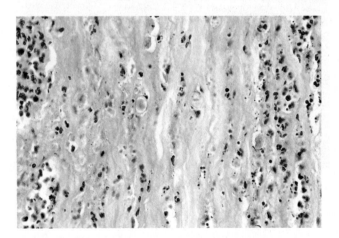

Figure 24.10. Acanthamoebic keratitis. Amebic keratitis is characterized by numerous stromal polymorphonuclear leukocytes and necrotic tissue. The amebae are evident within the affected tissue.

The histopathologic features of long-standing keratitis resulting from this virus are nonspecific. The epithelium may be irregular in thickness. Bowman layer is frequently disrupted, and pannus formation is often present. Neovascularization and an infiltrate of mononuclear inflammatory cells that is composed primarily of lymphocytes may be present in the corneal stroma. Rarely, a granulomatous infiltrate is present in the deep stroma or surrounding Descemet membrane. Granulomatous keratitis is not specific for herpes simplex, and it may also occur in juvenile xanthogranuloma, sarcoidosis, leprosy, and other conditions.

Herpes simplex may incite a hypersensitivity reaction, which accounts for most of the tissue damage (78). In chronic or recurrent herpes simplex keratitis, viral cultures of corneal tissue are usually negative, and viral inclusions are rarely identified in tissue sections. Transmission electron microscopy, immunocytochemical methods, in situ hybridization, and the polymerase chain reaction (PCR) may be helpful in establishing the diagnosis in some cases (79).

RHEUMATOID ARTHRITIS

Individuals with rheumatoid arthritis are susceptible to a spontaneous thinning of the peripheral or central corneal stroma (80–82). Thinning of the peripheral cornea is more common, but the central corneal melts cause perforation more frequently. In some instances, a full-thickness perforation develops, whereas, in others, the stromal tissue loss occurs in the presence of an intact Descemet membrane (descemetocele). The pathogenesis of this disorder remains elusive, and corneal specimens from patients with rheumatoid arthritis keratopathy are characterized by a loss of stromal tissue, often without a conspicuous associated inflammatory infiltrate.

EPITHELIAL INGROWTH

Sometimes after a penetrating corneal wound resulting from an accident, a cataract extraction, or another ocular surgical procedure, the epibulbar epithelium grows through the wound and into the anterior chamber (83,84). This may replace the corneal endothelium (Fig. 24.11), causing bullous keratopathy. It may also cause intractable glaucoma if the epithelium invades the trabecular meshwork. Epithelial ingrowth is easily diagnosed in pathologic specimens in which the normally single-layered corneal endothelium is replaced by several layers of squamous epithelium. In subtle cases, immunocytochemical staining for cytokeratin facilitates the diagnosis, because the endothelial cells lining the cornea and trabecular meshwork do not contain histochemically detectable keratin.

NEOPLASMS

Tumors of the cornea are rare, and they almost invariably represent the direct spread of squamous cell carcinoma or melanoma from the conjunctiva or eyelid.

SCLERA

From the standpoint of surgical pathology, most scleral specimens are related to inflammatory reactions (85). A necrotizing scleritis is often part of a systemic collagen autoimmune disease (86,87). Primary and metastatic tumors of the sclera are exceed-

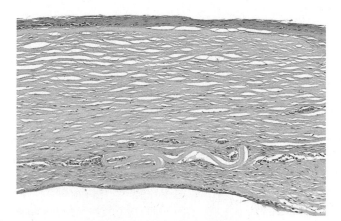

Figure 24.11. Transformation of corneal endothelium to stratified squamous epithelium. Epithelium derived from the conjunctiva has entered the eye through a traumatic wound. This ingrowth of aberrant squamous epithelium may extend along the posterior surface of the cornea and into the anterior chamber angle. Collagenous tissue is often present between remnants of Descemet membrane and the ectopic squamous epithelium. Neovascularization of the posterior corneal stroma is also evident in this photomicrograph. Histochemical markers for cytokeratins are useful in selected cases of epithelial ingrowth.

ingly rare, but uveal melanomas frequently spread by growing through the emissary channels in the sclera. A leiomyoma has been reported to extend across the sclera (88).

CONJUNCTIVA

Conjunctival tissue is usually biopsied for congenital abnormalities (89,90); inflammatory lesions, such as suspected sarcoidosis (91,92); tumors; or possible systemic metabolic diseases (93). Specimens from the conjunctiva are often extremely small, and communication between the surgeon and pathologist is therefore critical to ensure proper orientation when the precise orientation is important. The specimen should be spread out on a flat surface in the operating room, and the relevant landmarks should be labeled. When the surgical margins of resection must be evaluated, the specimen should be allowed to adhere to a level surface during fixation to prevent the specimen from curling.

DEVELOPMENTAL ABNORMALITIES

Nonneoplastic masses composed of tissues not normally found in conjunctiva sometimes form, especially at the junction of the conjunctiva and the cornea (corneoscleral limbus). Such choristomas include epibulbar dermoids, dermolipomas, and complex choristomas.

Epibulbar Dermoids

Epibulbar dermoids are characterized by dense, fibrocollagenous tissue containing sebaceous glands, hair follicles, and sweat glands, and they are covered by epidermis. They are frequently located in the inferotemporal conjunctiva. These choristomas are usually isolated lesions, but they are sometimes associated with other ocular abnormalities (colobomas of the iris and cili-

ary body), Goldenhar syndrome (pretragal auricular appendages, blind-ended preauricular fistulae, vertebral anomalies) (90), or the organoid nevus syndrome (linear nevus sebaceus of Jadassohn, Solomon syndrome) (94,95).

Dermolipomas and Complex Choristomas

Adipose connective tissue may constitute a major component of an epibulbar choristoma (dermolipoma). Less commonly, varying amounts of cartilage, lacrimal tissue, smooth muscle, adipose tissue, and even neural tissue are also present within the mass (complex choristomas).

CYSTS

Dermoid Cysts

Like dermoid cysts elsewhere, those of the conjunctiva are lined by a stratified squamous epithelium, and they contain cutaneous adnexal structures (96).

Inclusion Cysts

Inclusion cysts of the conjunctiva usually have a one-cell or two-cell lining of nonkeratinizing epithelium that contains goblet cells (97).

INFLAMMATION

Conjunctivitis is usually not a source of ophthalmic surgical pathology specimens. Certain changes in the conjunctival tissue in chronic conjunctivitis are nonspecific. The mucin-secreting goblet cells of the normal conjunctival epithelium often become numerous, and a hyperplastic epithelium may acquire papillary folds. Small islands of epithelium may become isolated and may form retention cysts that eventually calcify. In long-standing conjunctivitis, epithelial atrophy and keratinization with stromal scarring may occur.

Ligneous Conjunctivitis

The woody induration of the eyelid and conjunctiva that accompanies some cases of bilateral pseudomembranous conjunctivitis is occasionally excised, but it recurs relentlessly. The lesions in this rare ligneous conjunctivitis contain a considerable amount of fibrin but also immunoglobulins (98). The condition is caused by homozygous mutations in the *PLG* gene on human chromosome 6 (6q26) that encodes for plasminogen (99).

Ocular Cicatricial Pemphigoid

Ocular cicatricial pemphigoid, a mucocutaneous autoimmune disorder, frequently affects individuals older than 50 years of age. The condition affects women more often than men. The conjunctiva is involved in more than half of the cases, but this usually occurs 10 years after the onset of cutaneous or another mucosal disease (100,101). Epithelial erosions and bullae form in the conjunctiva early in the course of the disorder, but, later, the eye becomes scarred and dry.

Conjunctival tissue from patients with suspected ocular cicatricial pemphigoid should be submitted in a fixative suitable for immunofluorescent studies. A pathognomonic linear depo-

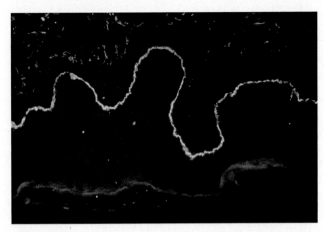

Figure 24.12. Ocular cicatricial pemphigoid. Linear deposits of immunoglobulin G (IgG) (pictured), as well as immunoglobulin A (IgA), accumulate along the basement membrane of the conjunctival epithelium.

sition of immunoglobulin A (IgA) and IgG along the conjunctival basal lamina occurs in ocular cicatricial pemphigoid (Fig. 24.12). Light microscopy of conjunctival biopsies late in the course of the disease discloses nonspecific epithelial and stromal scarring, perivascular infiltrates of lymphocytes, plasma cells, and occasional eosinophils. A cicatricial conjunctivitis can be a paraneoplastic manifestation of a nonocular carcinoma (102).

Sarcoidosis

The ocular tissues are involved in up to 38% of patients with sarcoidosis (92). Because of its common involvement in sarcoidosis, a biopsy frequently is performed on the conjunctiva to establish a tissue diagnosis of sarcoidosis (91). When sarcoidosis is present, light microscopy reveals the typical nonnecrotizing granulomatous inflammation in the absence of stainable microorganisms. Because the granulomatous inflammation of sarcoidosis may be focal, step sections through the entire specimen are often indicated in cases of clinically suspected sarcoidosis.

Other Granulomatous Conjunctivitis

Other causes of granulomatous inflammation, such as tuberculosis, cat-scratch fever (103,104), tularemia, syphilis, or other infections, and foreign bodies (105) may involve the conjunctiva, and these must be considered in the differential diagnosis. In contrast to sarcoidosis, the granulomatous inflammation in tuberculosis, cat-scratch fever, and tularemia is characterized by extensive necrosis.

NEOPLASMS

Benign: Squamous Papilloma

Squamous papillomas of the conjunctiva occur in diverse clinical settings, and they probably lack malignant potential (Fig.

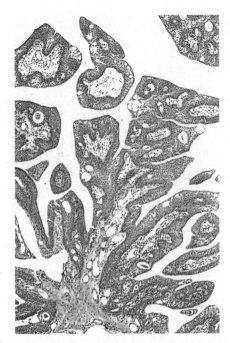

Figure 24.13. Conjunctival papillomas. Lobules of squamous epithelium surrounding a fibrovascular core characterize these papillomas histologically.

24.13). In children, conjunctival papillomas are often bilateral, and they recur after excision ("recurrent conjunctival papillomatosis"). Characteristically, these pedunculated lesions are composed of papillomatous fronds of squamous epithelium that cover a fibrovascular core. Human papillomavirus has been implicated in the development of these lesions in younger individuals (106–108).

In adults, papillomas are usually solitary and unilateral, and they may be confused clinically with squamous cell carcinoma. Inverted papillomas of the conjunctiva are rare (109).

Premalignant: Intraepithelial Neoplasms or Dysplasia and Intraepithelial Carcinoma

Dysplasia of the conjunctival epithelium is characterized by acanthosis, loss of cellular polarity, and cellular pleomorphism, and it resembles dysplasia of the uterine cervix microscopically. Depending on the extent of the epithelial abnormalities, conjunctival dysplasia can be designated as mild, moderate, or severe. In intraepithelial carcinoma, atypical cells extend throughout the entire epithelial thickness, but the lesion does not extend beneath the basal lamina of the conjunctival epithelium. The adjacent corneal epithelium may become involved. Because dysplasia and intraepithelial carcinoma represent a spectrum of change, the nature of which depends on tissue sampling, these lesions are often designated intraepithelial neoplasia (110,111).

Malignant: Squamous Cell Carcinoma

Squamous cell carcinoma of the conjunctiva usually grows in a papillary or exophytic manner (Fig. 24.14). It is characterized histopathologically by cellular atypia throughout the entire thickness of the epithelium, and by individual neoplastic cells

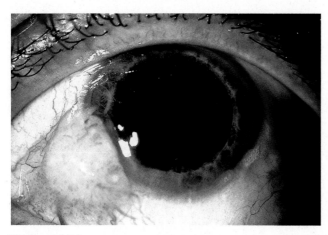

Figure 24.14. Squamous cell carcinoma of the conjunctiva. These most often arise at the corneoscleral limbus.

or nests of tumor cells that extend into the underlying stroma. The epithelium is sometimes keratinized. When the carcinoma is large, it may invade the globe or the orbit (112); however, conjunctival carcinoma is rarely responsible for death.

Pigmented Squamous Cell Carcinoma

Occasionally, squamous cell carcinoma of the conjunctiva is jet black and, clinically, it mimics a melanoma. However, in contrast to malignant melanocytic neoplasms, the pigmented squamous cell carcinoma occurs in heavily pigmented individuals. Insufficient tumors of this type have been documented to evaluate their biologic behavior, but it seems to be the same as that of conjunctival nonpigmented squamous cell carcinomas (113).

Mucoepidermoid Carcinoma

Mucoepidermoid carcinoma of the conjunctiva resembles squamous cell carcinoma in appearance but contains mucus-secreting cells and intraepithelial mucin. The mucin may not be readily apparent without the use of special stains, such as Alcian blue, Hale colloidal iron technique, or mucicarmine. This tumor must be differentiated from the more common squamous cell carcinoma of the conjunctiva, as it is more likely to invade the eye and orbit (114,115).

Spindle Cell Carcinoma

Spindle cell carcinoma rarely arises in the conjunctiva, but it pursues a more aggressive clinical course than the usual conjunctival squamous carcinoma (116). The tumor must be differentiated from spindle-shaped sarcomas, and both immunohistocytochemistry and transmission electron microscopy may be helpful in this regard. IHC staining of tissue sections discloses the presence of intracytoplasmic cytokeratin within the tumor, and ultrastructural studies reveal that tumor cells possess epithelial features, such as desmosomes and tonofibrils.

Melanocytic Lesions

Increased conjunctival melanotic pigmentation may be congenital or acquired, and, because various forms of conjunctival pigmentation are premalignant or malignant, they often create a diagnostic challenge for the pathologist (117,118). Acquired conjunctival melanosis may develop in previously normal eyes (primary acquired conjunctival melanosis), or it may be the result of inflammation or a neoplasm of the conjunctiva, as well as of a metabolic (e.g., Addison disease) or a toxic state (secondary acquired conjunctival melanosis).

Nevocellular Nevi

Nevocellular nevi are common in the conjunctiva. They are frequently pigmented, but are not necessarily so, and they may involve the subepithelial tissues (subepithelial nevi), the subepithelium and epithelium (compound nevi), or the base of the epithelium (junctional nevi). In contrast to their counterparts in the skin, compound and subepithelial nevi are frequently associated with a substantial mononuclear inflammatory infiltrate in the conjunctival stroma and epithelial inclusion cysts. Occasionally, enlargement of these epithelial cysts may lead to the clinical suspicion of a conjunctival malignancy. The epithelial hyperplasia should not be confused with invasive squamous cell carcinoma. Junctional nevi are most commonly present in children.

Ephelis or Freckle

Congenital pigmentation of the conjunctival epithelium (ephelis or freckle) does not evolve into a melanoma.

Congenital Ocular Melanocytosis and Oculodermal Melanocytosis (Nevus of Ota)

Congenital discoloration of the subepithelial tissues of the conjunctiva may be associated with congenital pigmentation of the uvea and other parts of the eye (ocular melanocytosis), and a benign clinical course usually ensues. If the skin of the eyelids or the periorbital area is also affected, the condition is known as oculodermal melanocytosis (nevus of Ota), which may carry a very slight risk of uveal melanoma (119).

PREMALIGNANT: PRIMARY ACQUIRED MELANOSIS

Primary acquired melanosis (PAM) is a unilateral premalignant acquired variety of conjunctival pigmentation that slowly affects the conjunctiva in middle-aged people of European ancestry. PAM is characterized by an evolving spectrum of varying degrees of intraepithelial melanocytic hyperplasia (benign acquired melanosis) or dysplasia (melanocytic dysplasia) and a variable subepithelial mononuclear cell infiltrate and vascular engorgement. Biopsies are occasionally performed on the lesions to establish a tissue diagnosis or because of the clinical suspicion of a melanoma. Tissue sampling is important in evaluating the conjunctiva because different parts of the same conjunctiva may manifest different degrees of the disorder, and parts may portray melanoma (120).

When the individual melanocytes are confined to the basal epithelium, the patient's risk of developing melanoma is about 20% (120). However, if nests or pagetoid spread of atypical cells is present, approximately 90% of such lesions eventually develop into a melanoma (120).

MALIGNANT

Conjunctival melanomas are uncommon, and they are typically pigmented. They may arise from PAM, nevocellular nevi, or apparently normal conjunctiva, but the nature of the initial lesion does not seem to be of prognostic importance. Conjunctival melanomas are often apparently multicentric, especially when they are preceded by PAM. In a series of 131 patients with conjunctival melanomas followed up for a median period of at least 8 years, about 25% of patients died from metastases (121).

LYMPHOID TUMORS

Reactive Lymphoid Hyperplasia

Reactive lymphoid hyperplasia may be difficult to distinguish from lymphoma. Features suggestive of reactive lymphoid lesions include a population of well-differentiated lymphocytes with occasional plasma cells, macrophages, eosinophils, and germinal follicles, which are often irregular in shape and distribution, within a stroma that contains scant fibrous tissue. These reactive germinal follicles often contain tingible bodies in macrophages and significant mitotic activity.

Although some lymphocytes are present in the conjunctiva of apparently healthy persons, a large number of lymphocytes (especially when they are arranged in lymphoid follicles with germinal centers) suggests reactive lymphoid hyperplasia. Other features of reactive conjunctival lymphoid hyperplasia include a prominent vascularity with hyperplastic, plump vascular endothelial cells and a polymorphic, immunophenotypically polyclonal population of mononuclear cells (122).

Lymphoma

Lymphocytic proliferations in the conjunctiva typically produce salmon-colored masses; from the standpoint of therapy and prognosis, these lesions remain an enigma to the clinician and pathologist.

The lymphoid tissue of the conjunctiva and, arguably, also of the orbit forms part of the mucosa-associated lymphoid tissue (MALT). The conjunctiva-associated lymphoid system consists of immunocompetent cells together with specialized conjunctival epithelial and dendritic antigen-presenting cells. Most lymphomas arising from the conjunctiva and orbit resemble other MALT-derived lymphomas. They remain localized for a long time, and they are often preceded by an apparent reactive inflammatory stage. Conjunctival and orbital lymphomas are usually composed of well-differentiated small lymphocytes, and they occur as isolated lesions or in association with a systemic lymphoma. They are usually composed of a monoclonal population of B lymphocytes (Fig. 24.15) (123), and fewer than 15% are of the follicular or nodular type. The cell population of orbital lymphomas is rarely derived from T cells (124). Orbital lymphomas usually express a restriction of κ-light or λ-light chains; although monoclonal lymphomatous masses are generally regarded as neoplastic, not all of those in the orbit or conjunctiva progress to systemic disease. Furthermore, some polyclonal masses that are considered to represent benign reactive lymphoid hyperplasia by an immunocytochemical evaluation express B-lymphocyte clonality on molecular genetic analysis (125). Orbital involvement in Burkitt lymphoma (126) is com-

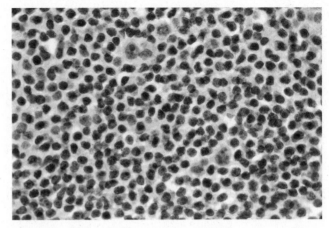

Figure 24.15. Lymphoid tumor of the conjunctiva and orbit. These are often composed of monoclonal populations of small lymphocytes that express B-cell antigens.

mon in Africa, but the orbit is rarely involved in Hodgkin disease (127).

These conjunctival lymphoid tumors are difficult to compartmentalize as benign or malignant. Their malignant potential is often difficult, if not impossible, to predict by using routine light microscopy, IHC (128), and even molecular biologic studies for immunoglobulin and T cell–receptor gene rearrangements (129). Most lymphomas of the conjunctiva are composed of well-differentiated small–B lymphocytes and they usually are first seen as isolated lesions, and remain so; sometimes, however, an associated systemic lymphoma exists at the time of the conjunctival presentation or on subsequent follow-up. Some conjunctival and other ocular adnexal MALT lymphomas have a chromosomal translocation involving the *IGH* and *MALT1* genes (t14,18)(q32;q21)(128).

When a lymphoma of the orbit or conjunctiva is suspected because of the clinical appearance or as a result of a histopathologic evaluation with frozen sections at the time of surgery, fresh tissue from conjunctival and orbital lymphoid tumors should be appropriately prepared for the immunohistopathologic evaluation of the lymphocyte populations, flow cytometry, and molecular biologic analysis of immunoglobulin and possibly T cell–receptor gene rearrangement. However, the practical value of these potentially useful but costly techniques remains questionable.

OTHER TUMORS

Benign

Other benign tumors of the conjunctiva include hereditary benign intraepithelial dyskeratosis (130).

Malignant

Other malignant neoplasms that occasionally arise in the conjunctiva include rhabdomyosarcoma (131); leiomyosarcoma (132); and Kaposi sarcoma, which most frequently develops in patients with AIDS (133). Malignant neoplasms of the orbit and eyelid may also extend to the conjunctiva.

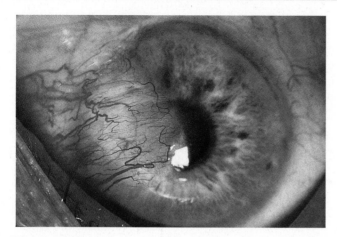

Figure 24.16. Pterygium. This is an abnormal growth of fibrovascular tissue over the surface of the cornea.

Nonneoplastic Growths

PINGUECULA. Extensive conjunctival elastosis can produce an elevated whitish-yellow lesion near the corneal border. Because of its clinical resemblance to fat, this mass is called a pinguecula. It is rarely removed surgically; when it is, it is mainly for cosmesis. A prominent foreign-body giant-cell reaction sometimes surrounds and incorporates the elastotic material (134). Such an actinic granuloma may lead the pathologist to suspect microorganisms.

PTERYGIUM. Vascularized conjunctival tissue may grow horizontally over the cornea in a triangular fashion. In most parts of the world, this pterygium is almost always associated with an underlying actinic elastosis of the conjunctiva (135), and it is thought to be the result of long-term solar (actinic) irradiation (Fig. 24.16).

Pterygia are often excised when they compromise the visual axis or induce corneal astigmatism, and occasionally when they are unsightly. Pterygia frequently recur after excision but they do not undergo malignant transformation. Histologically, pterygia are composed of vascularized connective tissue, usually with solar elastosis and a peculiar corkscrew configuration of individual collagen fibers. In the cornea, the Bowman layer may be focally destroyed. The contiguous corneal epithelium may be atrophic or thickened and dysplastic. The conjunctival epithelium frequently contains more mucus-secreting goblet cells than is normal, and, in keeping with its history of being sun-induced, it is occasionally dysplastic or it may have intraepithelial carcinoma.

CARUNCLE

The caruncle is the fleshy nodular prominence in the nasal portion of the interpalpebral fissure. It is lined by conjunctival epithelium, and it contains cutaneous adnexal structures. Sebaceous gland hyperplasia (136), sebaceous carcinoma (137), oncocytoma (138), and other tumors arise from the caruncle in rare instances. Conjunctival tumors may extend into the caruncle.

EYELIDS

Several pathologic processes involving the eyelids are treated by the ophthalmologist, and a high percentage of surgically excised ophthalmic specimens submitted for histopathologic evaluation are obtained from this site. Tissue excised during cosmetic blepharoplasty, blepharoptosis repair, or other reparative eyelid surgery may also be submitted for pathologic evaluation, but this does not usually disclose any noteworthy abnormalities. Surgically excised tissue from the eyelid in the floppy-eyelid syndrome (139) does not have any specific light-microscopic features. Other cutaneous disorders affecting the eyelid are identical to those found elsewhere in the skin; these are discussed in Chapters 1, 2, and 3. As in other parts of the body, certain tumors of the eyelid, such as keratoacanthoma and sebaceous tumors, may be associated with visceral carcinomas, especially of the colon (Muir-Torre syndrome) (140,141).

INFLAMMATORY REACTIONS

Chalazion

A chalazion is a localized, acute, lipogranulomatous, inflammatory process within the eyelid that is sometimes encapsulated. After an obstruction of any cause, the ducts draining the sebaceous glands (meibomian glands) within the eyelid may rupture, releasing material that presumably incites the reaction. Several factors, including inspissated secretions, infections, or neoplasms, may lead to the ductal obstruction. Specimens submitted for pathologic examination are usually curettings and sometimes biopsies of discrete masses. Most ophthalmologists do not submit suspected chalazia for pathologic evaluation after initial excision or curettage; however, because chalazia and sebaceous carcinoma are sometimes indistinguishable clinically, a histopathologic evaluation is imperative for recurrent chalazia. The characteristic histopathologic feature is a mixed inflammatory cell infiltrate composed of polymorphonuclear leukocytes, lymphocytes, plasma cells, macrophages, epithelioid cells, and, often, multinucleated giant cells (Fig. 24.17). Although this microscopic appearance may resemble that of other granulomatous processes, such as sarcoidosis, tuberculosis, or fungal infec-

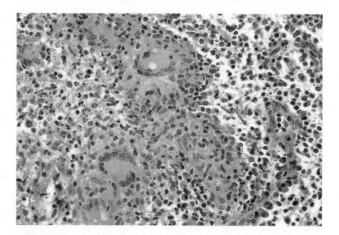

Figure 24.17. Chalazion. The granulomatous inflammation is characteristic. Microorganisms are not associated with this process, which presumably follows the release of lipids from obstructed sebaceous glands within the eyelid.

tions, special stains for microorganisms are usually not justified in the typical case in view of the low yield of specific causal agents for the cost.

Pyogenic Granuloma

Exuberant granulation tissue (pyogenic granuloma) may form on the eyelid after trauma or surgical incisions.

Hordeolum or Stye

An acute suppurative inflammation of the sebaceous glands or follicles of the eyelid (hordeolum, or stye) is usually due to *Staphylococcus.* An internal hordeolum affects the meibomian glands, whereas an external hordeolum involves the Moll or Zeiss glands and the adjacent hair follicles and cilia. Because hordeola are generally responsive to medical therapy, they are rarely subjected to biopsy or excision.

Sarcoidosis

The characteristic nonnecrotizing granulomatous inflammation of sarcoidosis may involve the eyelid, and such lesions need to be differentiated from the much more common chalazia.

Other Inflammatory Lesions

Uncommon inflammatory lesions of the eyelid include necrotizing fasciitis, juvenile xanthogranuloma, pseudorheumatoid nodules, and necrobiotic xanthogranuloma with paraproteinemia (142–145).

INFECTIONS AND INFESTATIONS

Viruses

MOLLUSCUM CONTAGIOSUM. Molluscum contagiosum is caused by a poxvirus, and it commonly produces small nodules on the eyelid. When the eyelid margins are affected, they are occasionally excised because they may release virions onto the ocular surface, and these elicit a noninfectious conjunctivitis (146). Microscopically, lobules of acanthotic epithelium surround the characteristic intracytoplasmic inclusion bodies (molluscum bodies) (Figs. 24.18 and 24.19).

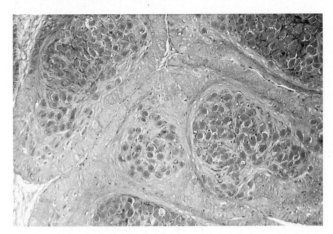

Figure 24.19. Numerous molluscum bodies representing accumulations of pox virus.

VERRUCA VULGARIS. Verruca vulgaris, which is caused by the DNA papovavirus known as human papillomavirus, may involve the eyelid skin; the lesions are often excised, especially for cosmetic reasons. Histologically, these papillomatous lesions manifest hyperkeratosis, acanthosis, and parakeratosis. Infected cells in the granular epithelial layer are often vacuolated, with a paucity of keratohyaline granules and clear perinuclear halos.

Mites: Demodicosis

The eyelids commonly contain mites within the hair follicles (*Demodex folliculorum*) or sebaceous glands (*Demodex brevis*) (Fig. 24.20). Although these organisms may incite inflammation, they are frequently evident in eyelid tissue excised for unrelated reasons from individuals without blepharitis. They are found with increasing incidence with age. In one study, *Demodex* was identi-

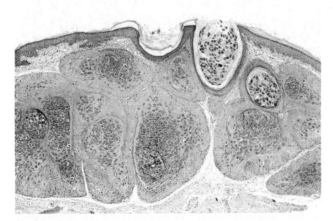

Figure 24.18. Lobules of acanthotic eyelid epithelium in molluscum contagiosum.

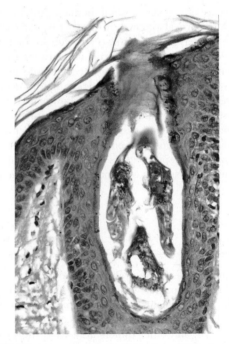

Figure 24.20. *Demodex folliculorum* is common in the hair follicles of the eyelids. These mites do not usually incite an inflammatory reaction.

fied in all eyelid specimens from patients older than 70 years (147).

Nematodes

Nematodes, such as the guinea worm (*Dracunculus medinensis*), *Gnathostoma spinigerum,* and other round worms, sometimes produce lesions in the eyelid or orbit in tropical countries (148).

NONNEOPLASTIC MASSES

Amyloid

Deposits of amyloid in the dermis and subcutis of the eyelid, which are frequently perivascular in location, are characteristic of systemic amyloidosis (149).

Cysts

EPIDERMAL INCLUSION CYSTS. In the eyelid, epidermal inclusion cysts lined by squamous epithelium and containing accumulations of keratin may be congenital, or they may follow trauma or surgery. A marked granulomatous reaction may occur if the cyst ruptures.

HIDROCYSTOMAS (SUDORIFEROUS CYSTS). Hidrocystomas (sudoriferous cysts) arise from the sweat glands of the eyelids. Apocrine hidrocystomas develop in the eyelid from obstructed ducts of modified sweat glands (glands of Moll), and multiple cysts often occur at the eyelid margin (150). A double layer of columnar cells with eosinophilic cytoplasm that often manifest prominent papillary projections lines the cysts. Some regard the apocrine hidrocystoma as a variant of the papillary cystadenoma, as opposed to a true retention cyst.

The eccrine hidrocystoma is a true retention cyst. The cyst is lined by two layers of epithelium, but it does not have papillary infoldings.

DERMOID CYSTS. Dermoid cysts may occur in the eyelids, but they are much more common in the orbit. Indeed, even when they are present in the eyelid, many of these developmentally derived cysts, which contain masses of keratin surrounded by a layer of squamous epithelium, represent an extension of an orbital lesion. Adnexal structures, such as sweat and sebaceous glands and hair follicles, are usually evident in the cyst wall. Should the cyst rupture, a marked granulomatous response may ensue.

NEOPLASMS

Benign

Common benign epithelial tumors of the eyelid include seborrheic keratosis, squamous cell papillomas, inverted follicular keratoses, keratoacanthomas, skin tags, nevocellular nevi, and xanthelasmas (151). Although the keratoacanthoma has the potential to involute spontaneously, it may exhibit aggressive behavior with deep perineural invasion (152). Less commonly encountered eyelid lesions are hyperplasia or adenomas of the sebaceous glands, trichilemmoma, papillary oncocytoma, and choristomas, as well as other tumors of sweat glands, hair folli-

TABLE 24.6
Tumors of the Eyelids

Benign	
Epithelial	Pleomorphic adenoma
Squamous cell papilloma	Syringoma
Keratoacanthoma	Trichoepithelioma
Seborrheic keratosis	Trichofolliculoma
Inverted follicular keratosis	Trichilemmoma
Melanocytic: nevocellular nevi	Developmental: phakomatous
Vascular	choristoma
Hemangioma	Cysts
Capillary	Dermoid cysts
Cavernous	Epidermal inclusion cysts
Lymphangioma	Sudoriferous cysts
Glomus tumor	(apocrine and eccrine
Adnexal	hidrocystomas)
Apocrine gland adenoma	Mesenchymal
Eccrine acrospiroma	Fibrous histiocytoma
Oncocytoma	Xanthelasma
Pilomatrixoma	Miscellaneous:
	granular cell tumor
Malignant	
Epithelial carcinoma	Eccrine sweat gland
Basal cell	Mucinous sweat gland
Sebaceous cell	Miscellaneous
Squamous cell	Mycosis fungoides
Melanocytic: melanoma	Merkel cell tumor
Vascular: angiosarcoma	Metastatic
Adnexal carcinoma	Carcinoma
Apocrine gland	Melanoma

cles, blood vessels, nerves, and mesenchymal tissue (Table 24.6) (153–157). A myxoma rarely occurs on the eyelid but, when it does, the surgical pathologist has an opportunity to recognize a treatable life-threatening disorder. Myomas of the eyelid and conjunctiva may be part of Carney syndrome (spotty pigmentation of the skin, overactivity of endocrine glands, and myxoma of the heart) (158).

Premalignant

Actinic keratoses and intraepithelial squamous cell carcinoma of the eyelid occasionally evolve into invasive squamous cell carcinoma. Xeroderma pigmentosum and prior radiation therapy to the eyelid, as occurs in the treatment of paranasal sinus malignant neoplasms, also predispose the individual to basal cell and squamous cell carcinomas (159,160). Malignant melanoma of the eyelid may also develop in patients with xeroderma pigmentosum (161).

Malignant

BASAL CELL CARCINOMA. Basal cell carcinomas account for approximately 90% of all eyelid malignancies in the United States, and they more commonly develop on the lower eyelid (151,162). These tumors may be ulcerated, pigmented, superficial, or sclerosing. Several studies indicate that when basal cell carcinomas of the eyelid are excised under frozen-section control of the surgical margins of resection, the incidence of tumor recurrence is significantly reduced (162). This is thus one of the indications for frozen sections in surgical ophthalmic pathology.

SQUAMOUS CELL CARCINOMA. In the Western hemisphere, squamous cell carcinomas account for 9% of all malignancies in the eyelid (163); the lower eyelid is more commonly affected. They rarely invade the eye or orbit or metastasize from this location.

SEBACEOUS CELL CARCINOMA. Although sebaceous cell carcinoma rarely arises from the skin in other parts of the body, it is an important neoplasm of the eyelids, where it accounts for approximately 1% to 3% of the malignant epithelial lesions of the eyelid in the United States (164) (Fig. 24.21). Sebaceous carcinoma may originate in the meibomian glands of the connective tissue plate of the eyelids (tarsus), the glands of the eyelashes (glands of Zeiss), the skin of the eyelid, or in the caruncle. The tumor most often originates in the upper eyelid, but the lower eyelid is involved in about one-third of cases. In approximately 10% of cases, the tumor apparently begins multicentrically.

Several morphologic patterns of sebaceous carcinoma are recognized (165,166). The bulk of the tumor may consist of distinct nests of neoplastic cells (lobular variant). The tumor lobules may manifest central necrosis that is reminiscent of the comedocarcinoma of the breast (comedocarcinoma pattern). A papillary pattern also may be evident, and combinations of any of these morphologic subtypes may occur (mixed pattern).

Sebaceous cell carcinomas manifest varying degrees of differentiation. Mitotic figures may be sparse in well-differentiated tumors, which contain cells with abundant foamy, finely vacuolated cytoplasm and well-defined cellular borders (Fig. 24.22). Such cells with sebaceous differentiation tend to be most conspicuous in the center of tumor lobules (167). As the degree of cellular differentiation decreases, the tumor cells manifest marked pleomorphism, prominent nucleoli, and numerous mitotic figures. In anaplastic sebaceous carcinomas, the scant cytoplasm of some tumor cells makes identifying the vacuoles of sebaceous differentiation difficult. Stains for lipids, such as Oil Red O, on frozen material may help to establish sebaceous differentiation, but, because many poorly differentiated neoplasms accumulate stainable lipid, the presence of lipid is not pathognomonic for sebaceous carcinoma. In some cases, poorly differentiated sebaceous carcinoma may be difficult to distinguish from squamous cell carcinoma or basal cell carcinoma.

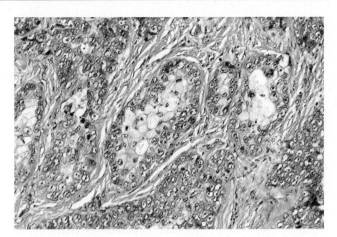

Figure 24.22. Sebaceous carcinoma. The intracytoplasmic vacuolation within the neoplastic cells is highly suggestive of this neoplasm.

Use of an IHC panel of antibodies against epithelial membrane antigen, cytokeratins (CAM5.2), and BCD-225 glycoprotein (BRST-1) may be helpful (168).

Sebaceous carcinoma commonly invades adjacent structures by intraepithelial spread (169), and the neoplastic intraepithelial cells resemble the pagetoid spread of breast carcinoma in the skin of the nipple. Individual or small clusters of intraepithelial neoplastic cells contain a vacuolated, foamy cytoplasm that reacts positively with lipid stains.

Sebaceous carcinoma should always be considered in the differential diagnosis of eyelid tumors because this potentially lethal neoplasm is commonly misdiagnosed by both clinicians and pathologists (170). A delayed diagnosis can lead to a disastrous effect on the ultimate outcome for the patient, and failure to diagnose the tumor often culminates in litigation. In about one-third of patients, the tumor recurs locally after excision, and about 20% of patients eventually die of metastases (167).

MELANOMA. Primary melanomas of the eyelid are rare, accounting for less than 1% of all eyelid malignancies (171). Most have a nodular pattern.

OTHER PRIMARY MALIGNANT TUMORS. Rarely, a variety of other primary malignant neoplasms arise from the eyelid. These tumors, which are identical to comparable tumors elsewhere, include mucous sweat gland adenocarcinoma and other neoplasms of sweat glands (172–174), angiosarcomas (175), lymphomas (176), and Merkel cell tumors (177).

Metastatic Carcinoma

Carcinomas rarely metastatize to the eyelid but, when they do, the primary tumor usually arises in the breast, lung, or kidney (178). Metastatic breast carcinoma in the eyelid is occasionally composed of individual cells with a histiocytoid appearance suggestive of macrophages, and the neoplasm occasionally becomes evident before the patient is known to have a malignant neoplasm elsewhere (179). Especially with renal cell carcinoma, the metastasis is sometimes the first detectable evidence of the tumor (180).

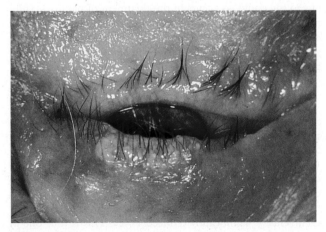

Figure 24.21. Sebaceous cell carcinoma of the eyelid. This potentially lethal neoplasm may cause induration of the eyelid margins.

LENS

Numerous abnormalities are recognized in the lens (181), but surgically removed tissue relates mainly to cataracts and prosthetic intraocular lenses.

CATARACT

A cataract is an opacity of the crystalline lens that decreases visual acuity. Some cataracts appear in infancy or in childhood, but most develop in older individuals. Cataractous changes may affect the nucleus, cortex, or subcapsular regions of the lens. By the time vision becomes impaired, all of these zones of the lens may be affected. Senile cataractous lenses may be yellowish, and some may appear brown. Cataractous changes in the lens nucleus are characterized histologically by the presence of homogeneous eosinophilic lens fibers (Fig. 24.23). Cortical lens abnormalities include vacuolization of the superficial cortical fibers, and both extracellular clefts and eosinophilic globules of variable size (Morgagnian globules) are frequently evident between lens fibers. Unlike those in the normal lens, the epithelial cells migrate posteriorly beyond the lens equator in certain cataracts (posterior subcapsular cataracts). Posterior epithelial migration may be difficult to detect if only fragmented lens material is submitted for evaluation. However, the greater thickness of the anterior lens capsule relative to the posterior capsule may aid in this determination.

After the removal of the cataractous lens by contemporary methods, the posterior lens capsule is usually left within the eye (extracapsular cataract extraction). In the past, and much less often today, the entire lens is extracted with its capsule (intracapsular cataract extraction). Present-day techniques of cataract removal use high-frequency sound waves to disintegrate the lens (phacoemulsification) before the lens constituents are aspirated. In many institutions, especially after phacoemulsification, lens material is not submitted for histopathologic examination. Light microscopy rarely discloses useful information of benefit to patient care, in view of the lens damage occurring during both surgical removal and tissue processing. However, the examination of lens material in the pathology laboratory may be warranted in specific cases, such as inherited cataracts, develop-

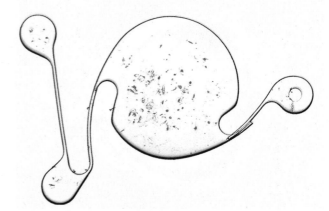

Figure 24.24. Prosthetic intraocular lenses are composed of a central optic with peripheral extensions ("haptics") and are occasionally removed surgically. Multinucleated giant cells are commonly present on both the optic and haptics of prosthetic intraocular lenses.

mental lens anomalies, and traumatic cataracts with medicolegal implications.

PROSTHETIC INTRAOCULAR LENSES

After most cataract extractions in adults, a prosthetic intraocular lens made of polymethylmethacrylate is placed in the eye, often in the space enclosed by the lens capsule. Numerous types of prosthetic intraocular lenses are available, but most are composed of a central optical zone (the "optic") and peripheral extensions that secure the lens within the eye ("haptics") (182). These prostheses usually remain in place for the remainder of the patient's life, but, under certain conditions, they are removed (e.g., if they are not securely in place and injure the cornea [pseudophakic bullous keratopathy] or iris mechanically, or if they provoke intraocular inflammation) (183). Prosthetic lenses are flat, and they can be mounted in their entirety on glass slides so that their surface can be examined by light microscopy (Fig. 24.24). Multinucleated giant cells; mononuclear and other inflammatory cells; fragments of lens capsule; and melanin granules, which may be found within macrophages, are often adherent to the optic or haptics or to both of the extracted prosthetic intraocular lenses.

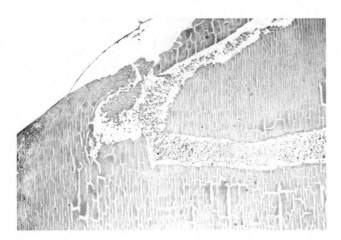

Figure 24.23. Common age-related cataract. Cortical extracellular clefts and globules are present in many cataractous lenses, as illustrated here.

RETINA

RETINOBLASTOMA

Most retinoblastomas occur sporadically, but about 30% to 40% are inherited (184). The inherited examples of this most frequent intraocular malignancy of children are often bilateral, and they may be associated with a similar tumor in the pineal gland or above the pituitary gland (trilateral retinoblastoma) (185,186). The average age at which retinoblastomas are diagnosed in the United States is 24 months, but some patients may be older than 5 years (187). Patients with retinoblastoma often have a white pupil (leukocoria), strabismus, decreased visual acuity, glaucoma, or a red and painful eye. Currently, the diagnosis can usually be made clinically with considerable accuracy based on ophthalmologic, ultrasonographic, and radiographic

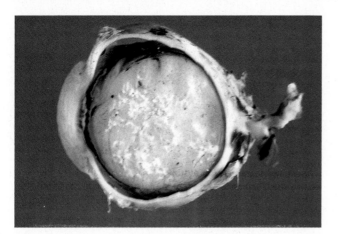

Figure 24.25. Retinoblastoma. It may grow to a large size and fill most of the eye.

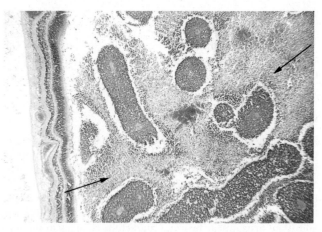

Figure 24.27. Retinoblastoma. Necrosis is often present in retinoblastomas (*arrow*). Viable neoplastic cells frequently surround the blood vessels. Nonneoplastic retina is present at the left side of this photomicrograph.

observations. The management of affected patients depends on tumor size and its intraocular location relative to the equator of the eye. Radiotherapy, chemotherapy, cryotherapy, photocoagulation, and enucleation are used to treat retinoblastomas.

Retinoblastomas are usually creamy white with chalky areas of calcification and yellowish necrotic regions (Fig. 24.25). Retinoblastomas may grow inward toward the vitreous cavity (endophytic retinoblastoma), outward toward the choroid (exophytic retinoblastoma), or in a mixed endophytic and exophytic pattern. Rarely, retinoblastomas thicken the retina diffusely without forming a discrete mass (diffusely infiltrative retinoblastoma) (188). The tumor frequently spreads intraocularly, producing multiple retinal and vitreous seedings that are often apparent on macroscopic examination.

The microscopic appearance of retinoblastomas varies with the degree of differentiation. Small, undifferentiated cells with scant cytoplasm and hyperchromatic nuclei make up the bulk of many retinoblastomas. Tumor cells may surround a central glycosaminoglycan-containing lumen that is delineated by a distinct eosinophilic circle, which has been shown by transmission electron microscopy to be composed of terminal bars analogous to those constituting the outer limiting membrane of the normal retina (Flexner-Wintersteiner rosettes) (Fig. 24.26) (189).

The nuclei of the neoplastic cells are displaced away from the lumen of the Flexner-Wintersteiner rosettes. Less frequently, the cells in retinoblastomas, in common with some neuroblastomas and medulloblastomas, form rosettes that lack a well-defined lumen (Homer Wright rosettes). Some well-differentiated tumor cells exhibiting photoreceptor differentiation are aligned in patterns reminiscent of the fleur-de-lis (fleurette) (190).

Necrosis is common in retinoblastomas, and it usually surrounds cores of viable perivascular tumor cells (Fig. 24.27). Prominent foci of calcification are common in these necrotic regions. The DNA released from the necrotic cells may precipitate and adhere to intraocular blood vessels, the lens capsule, and the trabecular meshwork (191,192).

Retinoblastomas may invade the optic nerve (193) and may extend along it toward the brain (Fig. 24.28), or individual neoplastic cells may reach the cerebrospinal fluid by penetrating into the subarachnoid space surrounding the optic nerve. Thus, the surgical pathologist should pay careful attention to the sur-

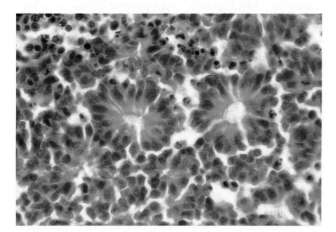

Figure 24.26. Retinoblastoma is composed of small hyperchromatic tumor cells with scant cytoplasm, and the tumor cells often surround a central lumen that is lined by basement membrane material (Flexner-Wintersteiner rosettes).

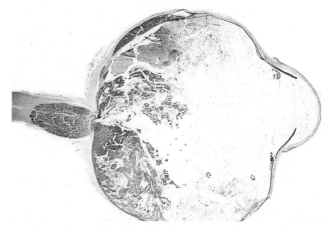

Figure 24.28. Retinoblastoma. Histologic evaluation of the surgical margin of resection at the optic nerve is crucial in every suspected case of retinoblastoma. This is a common way by which retinoblastoma spreads extraocularly.

gical margin of resection of the optic nerve in eyes enucleated for suspected retinoblastomas. The extent of optic nerve invasion relative to the lamina cribrosa correlates directly with the prognosis (194). Retinoblastomas infrequently spread extraocularly through scleral channels that contain blood vessels and nerves (emissarial canals), but the spread mainly occurs through the optic nerve and choroid (195).

Other Tumors

Astrocytomas, medulloepitheliomas, adenomas, and adenocarcinomas of the retinal pigment epithelium, and metastatic tumors uncommonly occur within the retina (196).

IRIS, CILIARY BODY, AND CHOROID

SYMPATHETIC UVEITIS

Sympathetic uveitis, a rare cause of uveitis after trauma or surgery, affects both eyes and is thought to represent an autoimmune response to retinal antigens (197,198). Granulomatous inflammation of the iris, ciliary body, and choroid is characteristic, and the retina is usually spared. After injury to one eye, the other eye usually becomes involved within 2 to 12 weeks. However, cases developing from 5 days to 12 years after injury have been reported (198). Sympathetic uveitis may eventually culminate in blindness. Enucleation of an injured eye within the first 2 weeks of injury usually prevents the development of sympathetic uveitis.

MELANOMA

Intraocular malignant melanomas arise from melanocytes of the uveal tract (iris, ciliary body, and choroid). This tumor is the most common primary intraocular malignant neoplasm in the United States, Western Europe, and some other countries, but intraocular melanomas, like those of the skin, are rare in Africa and Asia. These tumors are diagnosed clinically with ophthalmoscopic, fluorescein angiographic, and ultrasonographic methods, and biopsies are rarely performed. Contemporary methods of treating uveal-tract melanomas include surgical excision of the eye, thermoradiotherapy, iridocyclectomy, tumor resection, radiotherapy, or photocoagulation. Most enucleations for this melanocytic tumor are for choroidal melanomas and, less commonly, for tumors confined to the ciliary body.

In the laboratory, eyes with suspected melanoma should be transilluminated in a darkened area with a focal light source to document the location of the intraocular tumor. Furthermore, the adjacent sclera and the contiguous muscle and connective tissue should be carefully examined for evidence of extraocular tumor extension (Fig. 24.29). In contrast to retinoblastomas, intraocular melanomas commonly spread through scleral emissarial canals, but they rarely extend into the optic nerve. Optic nerve invasion by melanomas occurs virtually only in blind glaucomatous eyes.

Uveal tract melanomas are usually solitary, discrete unilateral tumors containing variable amounts of dark brown to black pigmentation, but some are amelanotic (Fig. 24.30). Occasionally, the melanoma diffusely infiltrates the uvea without forming an obvious mass (12).

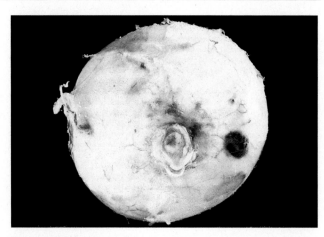

Figure 24.29. Melanoma. The extraocular spread of melanoma occurs through channels in the sclera that contain blood vessels and nerves. When tumor extends through such emissarial canals, pigmented neoplastic cells may be evident on the scleral aspect of the enucleated specimen.

A major classification of uveal melanomas (revised Callender classification) recognizes four distinct cell types within these tumors (199,200). Some cells are spindle-shaped with indistinct cell borders and slender nuclei (occasionally with a prominent longitudinal fold in the nuclear membrane) that lack nucleoli (spindle A cells). Other spindle-shaped cells have plumper nuclei with small distinct nucleoli (spindle B cells) (Fig. 24.31). The third cell type (epithelioid cell) is polygonal and larger than the spindle variants; it has one or more prominent nucleoli; and it frequently contains mitotic figures (Fig. 24.32). A fourth cell type (intermediate cells) is similar to epithelioid cells, but it may be smaller and it has indefinite margins. Spindle A and B cells grow in a cohesive manner, and evidence of mitotic activity is rarely, if ever, identified within them. Most primary intraocular melanomas contain variable numbers of spindle A and B cells and epithelioid cells. Tumors composed entirely of epithelioid cells account for only about 3% of all intraocular melanomas.

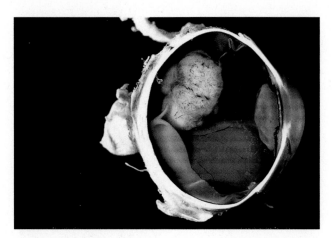

Figure 24.30. Choroidal melanoma. Intraocular melanomas are often mushroom-shaped and not conspicuously pigmented, such as that pictured. The retina adjacent to a choroidal melanoma is frequently detached from the retinal pigment epithelium by a protein-rich exudate.

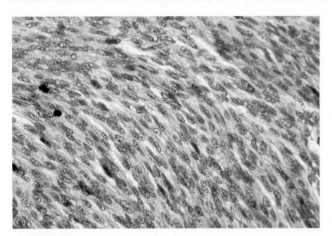

Figure 24.31. Uveal melanoma. The spindle-B-cell melanoma is composed predominantly of spindle-shaped tumor cells with prominent nucleoli.

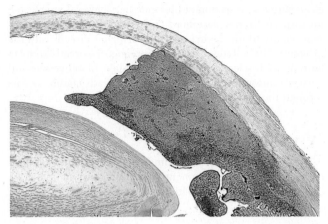

Figure 24.33. Melanoma of the anterior uvea. A melanoma in this location may invade the anterior chamber of the eye and the aqueous humor drainage pathway angle, causing intractable glaucoma.

The retina overlying a choroidal melanoma often atrophies, and a protein-rich eosinophilic exudate frequently separates the adjacent sensory retina from the retinal pigment epithelium. Necrosis and tumor cells containing abundant cytoplasmic lipid ("balloon degeneration") may be identified in some melanomas.

The prognosis of uveal melanomas is related to several factors, including tumor size, extrascleral extension, cell type, mitotic activity, lymphocytic infiltration (201), and perhaps fibrovascular loops (200,202–204). The 10-year death rate of patients with small (less than 11 mm) intraocular tumors is lower than that seen with larger (greater than 15 mm) tumors (19% and 65%, respectively) (205). As one might expect, the extraocular extension of an ocular melanoma has a higher incidence of orbital recurrence than do those tumors restricted to within the eye.

The mortality of patients with intraocular melanomas varies with the prominent cell type. In a study of 90 patients with spindle A-cell melanomas followed for at least 5 years, 11 deaths were attributed to the tumor (206). The 15-year mortality rate of uveal melanomas is as follows: spindle B-cell melanomas, 20%; mixed-cell melanomas (combination of spindle and epithelioid cells), 60%; and the rare pure epithelioid melanomas, about 75%. The outcome of individuals with surgically excised eyes for mixed-cell melanomas appears to be unaffected by the absolute percentage of epithelioid cells within the tumor (199). Even a few epithelioid cells in a melanoma composed predominantly of spindle B cells indicate a more unfavorable course than that seen in a melanoma consisting entirely of spindle cells. The most convenient morphometric benchmark of long-term survival is the mean size of the 10 largest nucleoli (202). The presence of vascular loops has not been found to be a strong indicator of poor outcome (202).

Iris melanomas have a more benign course than do melanomas arising elsewhere in the eye, and they rarely result in death. They are usually managed by observation for growth over time or local resection; enucleation for iris melanomas is typically restricted to cases with intractable glaucoma (Fig. 24.33) (207); and, in many of these cases, the melanomas arise in the ciliary body.

OTHER UVEAL TUMORS

Metastatic carcinoma is more common than primary intraocular neoplasms, and it occasionally is the first indication of the neoplasm. Eyes with metastatic carcinoma are sometimes enucleated for a suspected intraocular melanoma. Patients with the Sturge-Weber syndrome are especially prone to choroidal hemangiomas (208,209). Uncommon tumors of the ciliary epithelium include the medulloepithelioma (210), adenoma, and adenocarcinoma (211).

Other rare uveal tumors include leiomyosarcoma, rhabdomyosarcoma, lymphoma, mesenchymoma (212), and leiomyoma (213). Many reported intraocular leiomyomas may actually be melanomas (214). Some tumors are not neoplasms but, rather, are hamartomas of choristomas. For example, ectopic lacrimal tissue may be present in the eye (215).

ORBIT

In certain clinical settings, the orbit is surgically explored, and a biopsy is performed or abnormal tissue is excised. Congenital

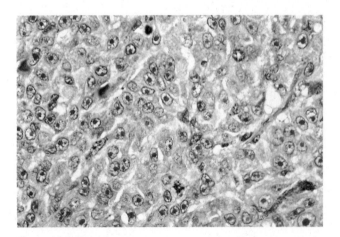

Figure 24.32. Intraocular melanoma. The epithelioid melanoma is composed of epithelioid cells with abundant eosinophilic cytoplasm and prominent nucleoli. The presence of such cells indicates a more unfavorable prognosis than do melanomas that are composed primarily of spindle-shaped tumor cells.

abnormalities, primary and metastatic tumors, inflammatory masses, and thyroid ophthalmopathy (Graves disease) form expanding masses within the orbit and produce proptosis (Tables 24.7 and 24.8) (216,217). Clinical examination, computed tomography, magnetic resonance imaging, and cytopathologic examination of fine needle aspirates are frequently used to diagnose orbital lesions (218).

DEVELOPMENTAL ANOMALIES

Dermoid Cysts

Dermoid cysts commonly develop within the bones or soft tissue of the orbit. Although they are presumably present before birth, they may not become clinically evident until after the age of 20 years. Like dermoid cysts elsewhere, they are lined by stratified squamous epithelium with dermal appendages, and they contain desquamated epithelial cells, keratin, and other products of the epithelium (Fig. 24.34). A marked granulomatous inflammatory reaction with multinucleated giant cells occurs if the cyst ruptures, and this reaction may be the only tissue component biopsied.

Other Developmental Anomalies

Teratomas, meningoceles, meningoencephaloceles, ectopic brain tissue, and choristomatous cysts may also occur in the orbit (219–223). A carcinoma may arise from an orbital choristomatous cyst (224).

MUCOCELES

Mucoceles of the frontal and ethmoid sinuses occasionally extend into the orbit and require surgical repair (225). They are noteworthy for the presence of the ciliated columnar epithelium characteristic of paranasal sinus mucosa, and an abundant mononuclear inflammatory cell infiltrate in the adjacent connective tissue.

INFLAMMATION

Inflammatory Pseudotumors

OVERVIEW. The imprecise term *pseudotumor* is well entrenched in the ophthalmic literature despite its shortcomings. The designation *pseudotumor* refers to an idiopathic inflammatory process of the orbit that often involves the extraocular muscles, the adjacent adipose tissue, and sometimes the lacrimal gland (226). Patients with orbital inflammatory pseudotumors often develop ocular pain, proptosis, and decreased ocular motility.

Many inflammatory pseudotumors are composed predominantly of lymphocytes; others consist of a cytologically benign mononuclear inflammatory infiltrate composed of lymphocytes, plasma cells, macrophages, and rare eosinophils. The stroma is composed of dense fibrous tissue, and lymphoid follicles are occasionally evident.

Wegener granulomatosis often involves the orbit (227,228) and must be considered in the differential diagnosis of inflammatory pseudotumors, especially because the customary triad of vasculitis, tissue necrosis, and granulomatous inflammation is frequently absent in well-defined cases of Wegener granulo-

TABLE 24.7

Relative Incidence of Expanding Lesions of the Orbit Examined at the Institute of Ophthalmology, London

	Number of Cases	Percentage (%)
Inflammatory	183	12.3
Nonspecific	169	
Sarcoidosis	11	
Fasciitis	3	
Fibrous tissue tumors	20	1.32
Fibrous histiocytoma (benign)	8	
Fibrous histiocytoma (malignant)	6	
Fibrosarcoma	6	
Histiocytic tumors	9	0.6
Xanthogranuloma	5	
Histiocytosis X	4	
Adipose tissue tumors	10	0.7
Lipoma	3	
Liposarcoma	7	
Muscle tumors	78	5.3
Rhabdomyosarcoma	78	
Vascular tumors	231	15.6
Capillary hemangioma	26	
Cavernous hemangioma	101	
Malformations	93	
Hemangiopericytoma	7	
Angiosarcoma	4	
Bone and cartilage tumors	10	0.6
Chondroma	1	
Chondrosarcoma	2	
Benign osteoblastoma	3	
Aneurysmal bone cyst	2	
Osteoma	2	
Peripheral nerve tumors	93	6.3
Neurofibroma	36	
Schwannoma	45	
Granular cell	7	
Malignant	5	
Optic nerve tumors	109	7.3
Astrocytoma (juvenile)	33	
Malignant astrocytoma	2	
Meningioma	74	
Germ cell tumors	100	6.7
Dermoid cyst	99	
Teratoma	1	
Lymphoid tumors	353	23.8
Lymphoid hyperplasia	151	
Lymphoma (non-Hodgkin)	142	
Indeterminate	60	
Lacrimal gland tumors	132	8.9
Pleomorphic adenoma	76	
Adenocarcinoma	16	
Adenoid cystic carcinoma	39	
Mucoepidermoid	1	
Secondary tumors	113	7.6
Local spread	56	
Metastases	57	
Miscellaneous	49	3.3
Mucocele	7	
Cholesterol granuloma	9	
Others	33	2.2

From: Garner A, Klintworth GK. Tumors of the orbit, optic nerve, and lacrimal sac. In Garner A, Klintworth GK, eds. *Pathobiology of Ocular Disease.* 2nd ed. New York: Marcel Dekker, 1994:1523–1606, with permission. Generally, similar percentages were also encountered in a series of 1264 patients with orbital tumors and simulating lesions (217).

TABLE 24.8

Frequency of Orbital Tumors in Children Based on Several Series

	Number of Cases	Percentage (%)
Dermoid cyst	134	37.4
Hemangioma	42	11.7
Rhabdomyosarcoma	31	8.7
Glioma of optic nerve	20	5.6
Neurofibroma	14	3.9
Neuroblastoma	12	3.4
Lymphangioma	10	2.8
Inflammatory pseudotumor	9	2.5
Leukemia and lymphoma	9	2.5
Lipoma	7	2.0
Meningioma (orbit and or sphenoid ridge)	8	2.2
Schwannoma	6	1.7
Microphthalmos with cyst	5	1.4
Teratoma	4	1.1
Prominent palpebral lobe of lacrimal gland	4	1.1
Retinoblastoma	–	–
Orbital recurrence	4	1.1
Orbital presentation	2	0.6
Undifferentiated sarcoma	3	0.8
Epithelial or "sebaceous" cysts	3	0.8
Noninflammatory pseudotumor	3	0.8
Arteriovenous malformation	3	0.8
Ectopic lacrimal gland	2	0.6
Epibulbar, eyelid, and orbital osseous choristoma	2	0.6
Dermolipoma	2	0.6
Lacrimal gland duct cyst	2	0.6
Alveolar soft-part sarcoma	2	0.6
Fibrous dysplasia	1	–
Neurosarcoma	1	–
Metastatic embryonal sarcoma	1	–
Pleomorphic adenoma of lacrimal gland	1	–
Benign adenomatous epithelial hyperplasia of sweat or lacrimal gland	1	–
Osteoma	1	–
Meningoencephalocele	1	–
Amyloidosis	1	–
Eosinophilic granuloma	1	–
Malignant teratoid epithelioma of optic nerve	1	–
"Metastatic" astrocytoma	1	–
Posttraumatic hemorrhagic cyst	1	–
Myxosarcoma	1	–
Prolapsed orbital fat	1	–
Total	**358**	**100**

Modified from: Garner A, Klintworth GK. Tumors of the orbit, optic nerve, and lacrimal sac. In Garner A, Klintworth GK, eds. *Pathobiology of Ocular Disease*. 2nd ed. New York: Marcel Dekker, 1994:1523–1606, with permission.

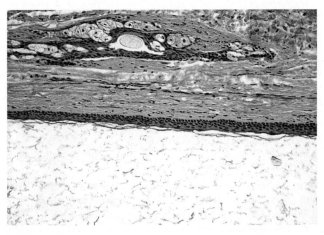

Figure 24.34. Orbital dermoid cyst. The dermoid cyst is lined by stratified squamous epithelium and its wall contains cutaneous appendages, such as sweat glands and hair follicles. If a dermoid cyst ruptures, the release of the cyst contents may incite a granulomatous response.

matosis. This is particularly true if a biopsy is performed on only a small portion of the orbital lesion (228). Other inflammatory disorders that may involve the orbit are Rosai-Dorfman disease (229) and Erdheim-Chester disease (230). An important infection of the eye that commonly leads to orbital exenteration is rhino-orbital-cerebral mucormycosis (231).

VARIANTS OF INFLAMMATORY PSEUDOTUMOR. Less commonly, orbital inflammatory pseudotumors manifest other histologic characteristics. For example, a lipogranulomatous lesion that probably represents fat necrosis may develop. Another variant of the inflammatory pseudotumor is characterized by proliferating fibroblasts in a collagenous or myxomatous stroma that is reminiscent of nodular fasciitis. Vascularity is prominent, but the inflammatory cell infiltrate is scant and mitotic activity is inconspicuous. Foci of dense connective tissue without a significant inflammatory cell infiltrate characterize yet another type of orbital pseudotumor (232). Such fibrosclerosis may be associated with mediastinal or retroperitoneal fibrosis, Reidel thyroiditis, or sclerosing cholangitis (233–235). An idiopathic granulomatous orbital inflammation that has been designated *sarcoidosis limited to the orbit* is related to other inflammatory orbital pseudotumors rather than to sarcoidosis (236). Other orbital lesions that contain numerous lymphoid cells include reactive lymphoid hyperplasia, lymphomas, and Waldenström macroglobulinemia.

Tumors

ANGIOMAS. *Capillary Hemangioma.* Capillary hemangiomas, which are characterized by thin-walled vessels lined by endothelial cells, are most common in the pediatric population (237). The tumor is usually not encapsulated, and mitotic activity may be conspicuous, leading to undue concern about its malignant potential.

Cavernous Hemangioma. Cavernous hemangiomas usually occur in adults, and they contain large blood-filled, endothelium-lined channels (Fig. 24.35) (238). Thrombi frequently form within the lumens of cavernous hemangiomas, and these occasionally calcify.

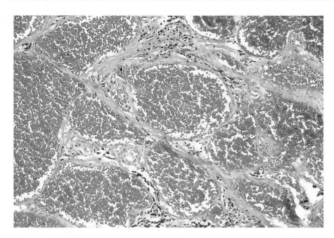

Figure 24.35. Cavernous hemangioma of the orbit. This vascular tumor usually occurs in adults.

Lymphangioma. The normal orbit is traditionally stated to lack lymphatics, but evidence for such vessels in the orbit does exist (239). Nevertheless, orbital lymphangiomas have been reported in children, and they contain thin-walled vessels that lack pericytes or smooth muscle (Fig. 24.36) (240). Lymphocytic foci, occasionally with germinal centers, are present in the connective tissue stroma of lymphangiomas.

Hemangiopericytoma. As in other tissues, orbital hemangiopericytomas may be benign or malignant, but most are slow-growing. They may recur and metastasize if they are incompletely excised (241).

MESENCHYMAL TUMORS. *Fibrous Histiocytoma.* The fibrous histiocytoma, which occurs in adults, is the most common mesenchymal tumor of the orbit (242). It lacks a true capsule, and is composed of spindle-shaped cells that are arranged in a storiform pattern. Scattered giant cells may be identified. Although it most often is benign, locally aggressive and malignant variants of the fibrous histiocytoma are also recognized (242).

Rhabdomyosarcoma. Orbital rhabdomyosarcomas most often

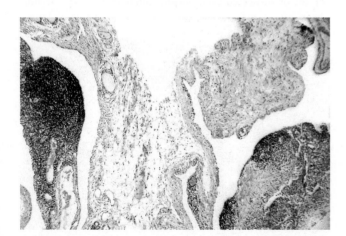

Figure 24.36. Orbital lymphangioma. The orbital lymphangioma is characterized by endothelium-lined spaces that do not contain significant cellular elements of blood, and that are surrounded by a fibrovascular connective tissue stroma, which may contain prominent lymphoid tissue.

develop in childhood (243) and rarely in adults (244). This neoplasm is thought to arise from a pluripotential mesenchymal cell, and they therefore are usually not associated with a particular extraocular muscle. Embryonal, alveolar, and pleomorphic histologic patterns occur (245).

LYMPHOID TUMORS. Lymphoid hyperplasia and lymphomas are common in the orbit. Because they resemble similar conjunctival lesions, with which they are sometimes associated, they are discussed elsewhere (see "Conjunctiva" earlier in this chapter).

OTHER TUMORS. A diverse group of solid tumors may arise in the orbital soft tissues, including benign and malignant vascular, osseous, and neural neoplasms. These tumors include alveolar soft part sarcoma, angiosarcoma, Ewing sarcoma, fibrosarcoma, germ cell tumors, Langerhans cell granulomatosis, leiomyosarcoma, malignant nerve sheath tumor, mesenchymal chondrosarcoma, osteosarcoma, primitive neuroectodermal tumor, solitary fibrous tumor, and osteosarcoma (246–250).

The relative frequency of these masses differs in the pediatric and adult populations (Tables 24.7 and 24.8). Tumors may extend into the orbit from the intraocular tissues, conjunctiva, eyelid, paranasal sinuses, nose, and oropharynx, whereas others may metastasize to the orbit from distant sites.

OPTIC NERVE

OVERVIEW

A biopsy is seldom intentionally performed on the optic nerve for diagnostic purposes because optic nerve neoplasms can rarely be removed or sampled without sacrificing visual function. The surgical pathologist most often encounters lesions of the optic nerve during an examination of enucleation or exenteration specimens. Laminated calcific structures (psammoma bodies) are often found in close association with aggregates of meningothelial cells. Calcified acellular globular concretions of nerve fibers (drusen) may develop at the optic nerve head or deeper within the nerve anterior to the lamina cribrosa.

NEOPLASMS

Primary tumors of the optic nerve are uncommon. They include pilocytic astrocytomas, meningiomas, metastatic neoplasms, medulloepitheliomas, and secondary tumors. The optic nerve choristoma is probably malformative rather than neoplastic (251).

Gliomas

Most optic nerve gliomas are juvenile pilocytic astrocytomas (252,253). These most often occur in individuals between the ages of 2 and 6 years, and they are frequently associated with neurofibromatosis type 1. An arachnoidal hyperplasia adjacent to an optic nerve astrocytoma must be distinguished from a meningioma, especially in a small biopsy. A glioblastoma multiforme (malignant astrocytoma) rarely arises in the optic nerve in adults (254).

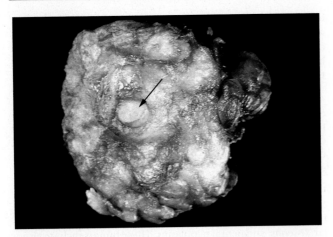

Figure 24.37. Discrete lobular orbital meningioma surrounding a portion of normal optic nerve (*arrow*).

Meningioma

Meningiomas may arise from the optic nerve meninges, but orbital meningiomas more often represent an extension from the cranial meninges (Figs. 24.37 and 24.38). Within the orbit, particularly in younger individuals, a meningioma must be differentiated from a juvenile ossifying fibroma (255).

Medulloepithelioma

The medulloepithelioma is a benign or malignant neoplasm believed to arise from the neuroepithelium of the embryonic optic cup. It is a curiosity in the optic nerve (256).

Metastatic Neoplasms

Tumors from distant tissues rarely metastasize to the optic nerve; when they do, they usually are not seen as surgical pathology specimens.

Secondary Tumors

Secondary tumors that have spread into the optic nerve from the globe, such as retinoblastomas, are more common than primary optic nerve neoplasms.

LACRIMAL GLAND

Located in the superotemporal aspect of the orbit, the nonencapsulated lacrimal gland contributes secretions to the tear film. Occasional lymphocytes and plasma cells are interspersed among the acini of the normal lacrimal gland, and they are not necessarily pathologic. Most lacrimal gland lesions prompting biopsy or excision are tumors or inflammatory masses (257–259). Excisional biopsies of lacrimal gland lesions are preferable to incisional biopsies because of the significant risk for recurrence when tumors such as pleomorphic adenomas are incised.

INFLAMMATION

Dacryoadenitis

Surgically excised specimens from clinically enlarged lacrimal glands sometimes reveal dacryoadenitis. Obstruction of the lacrimal ducts by dacryoliths may also enlarge the lacrimal gland, producing a dacryops (260).

Sarcoidosis

The lacrimal gland is commonly involved in sarcoidosis, and lacrimal gland biopsies have been advocated for diagnostic purposes in some cases of suspected sarcoidosis (Fig. 24.39) (261).

NEOPLASMS

Benign

PLEOMORPHIC ADENOMA. The most common epithelial neoplasm of the lacrimal gland is the pleomorphic adenoma (mixed tumor). It is composed of both glandular epithelial and mesenchymal elements and is usually encapsulated (Fig. 24.40). Foci of squamous metaplasia are occasionally associated with the neoplastic epithelium. The mesenchymal component, which is presumed to develop from metaplastic myoepithelial cells, is often myxomatous in appearance, but bone, cartilage, and fat may also be present. Excisional, rather than incisional, biopsies of suspected pleomorphic adenomas of the lacrimal

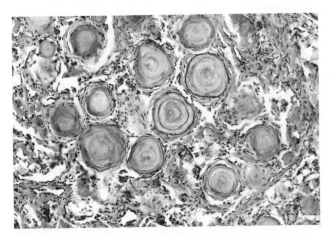

Figure 24.38. Optic nerve sheath meningiomas. Calcified psammoma bodies may occur within these meningiomas.

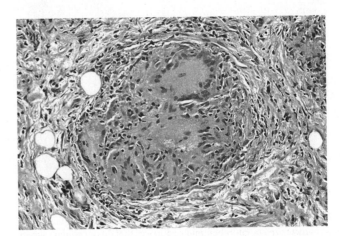

Figure 24.39. Sarcoidosis of the lacrimal gland. This inflammatory mass may totally obliterate the normal structure of the gland. Multinucleated giant cells are a characteristic feature of sarcoidosis.

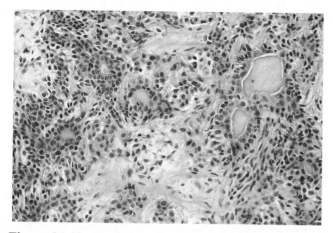

Figure 24.40. Pleomorphic adenoma of the lacrimal gland. This tumor is composed of cytologically benign epithelial and mesenchymal elements. The mesenchymal component of this tumor is frequently myxomatous in appearance.

gland should be performed because the tumor frequently recurs after incomplete excision with the implantation of tumor within the orbit. The surgical margins of excision should be carefully examined because mixed tumors frequently recur if they are incompletely excised (262).

LYMPHOID HYPERPLASIA AND LYMPHOMAS. Lymphoid lesions of the lacrimal gland are discussed with those in the conjunctiva and other parts of the orbit (see ''Conjunctiva'' earlier in this chapter).

Malignant

ADENOID CYSTIC CARCINOMA. Adenoid cystic carcinoma is the most common malignant tumor of the lacrimal gland (263). Several distinct histopathologic patterns are recognized, including the cribriform, sclerosing, basaloid, comedocarcinoma, and tubular subtypes (Fig. 24.41) (264,265). Extension of the basaloid variant of the adenoid cystic carcinoma into the

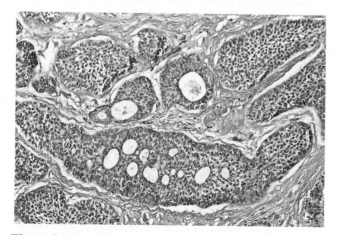

Figure 24.41. Adenoid cystic carcinoma of the lacrimal gland. This malignant tumor may have a basaloid appearance similar to basal cell carcinomas. Areas of cribriform change with focal tumor necrosis are often found.

eyelid may be mistaken for a primary basal cell carcinoma in this location. Despite its highly aggressive behavior, the individual neoplastic cells often possess a surprisingly bland cytologic appearance. Perineural invasion is common in adenoid cystic tumors of the lacrimal gland, and it signifies the route of spread toward the brain.

MALIGNANT MIXED TUMORS. Malignant transformation of a mixed tumor most often results in an adenocarcinoma. Less often, foci of adenoid cystic carcinoma, squamous cell carcinoma, undifferentiated carcinoma, sebaceous carcinoma, or sarcoma are identified (264,266).

OTHER MALIGNANT TUMORS. Mucoepidermoid carcinoma (267) and acinic carcinoma (268) rarely arises in the lacrimal gland.

LACRIMAL DRAINAGE APPARATUS

The lacrimal drainage apparatus transports tears to the nose and comprises the puncta, canaliculi, lacrimal sac, and nasolacrimal duct. Most pathologic processes occurring in these structures are inflammatory, and they are usually not treated surgically. Any obstruction to the distal part of the lacrimal drainage apparatus can dilate the lacrimal sac. Sometimes, a lacrimal sac cyst (dacryocele) is present at birth as a congenital anomaly (269).

NEOPLASMS

Neoplasms of the lacrimal drainage apparatus are uncommon; they include primary as well as secondary tumors arising in the adjacent eyelid, nose, paranasal sinuses, and orbit (270,271) (Table 24.9). Most primary benign and malignant tumors of the lacrimal sac are epithelial in origin (270,272,273).

TABLE 24.9
Tumors of the Lacrimal Sac
Benign
Inflammatory tumors
Granuloma
Pseudotumor
Papillomas
Squamous cell
Transitional cell
Mixed squamous and transitional cell
Oncocytic adenoma
Fibrous histiocytoma
Schwannoma
Malignant
Carcinomas
Squamous cell
Transitional cell
Adenocarcinomas
Mucoepidermoid
Angiosarcoma
Lymphoma
Melanoma
Malignant tumors from adjacent structures

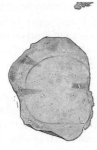

Figure 24.42. Dacryolith. The dacryolith is a concretion found in the lacrimal sac. It often has a laminated appearance, and it may contain degenerating epithelial cells and leukocytes.

Lacrimal Sac Papillomas

Lacrimal sac papillomas are aggregates of cytologically benign transitional epithelial cells, often with numerous interspersed polymorphonuclear leukocytes (271).

Lacrimal Sac Carcinoma

Lacrimal sac carcinomas are composed of either atypical transitional epithelial or squamous cells (271).

Other Tumors of the Lacrimal Sac

Rare tumors of the lacrimal sac include schwannomas (274), benign and malignant oncocytic tumors (275,276), hemangiopericytoma (277), fibrous histiocytoma (278), mucoepidermoid carcinoma (279), melanoma (280), and angiosarcoma (281).

DACRYOLITHS

Dacryoliths are calculi that form in the lacrimal sac; they are caused by microorganisms, especially *Arachnia* (*Actinomyces*) *propionica*. They appear as laminated, somewhat basophilic structures in routinely processed tissue sections (Fig. 24.42) (282).

REFERENCES

1. Bron AJ, Tripathi RC, Tripathi BJ. *Wolff's Anatomy of the Eye and Orbit*. 8th edition London: Chapman & Hall, 1997.
2. Jakobiec FA. *Ocular Anatomy, Embryology, and Teratology*. New York: Harper & Row, 1982.
3. Klintworth GK, Cummings TJ. Normal eye and ocular adnexa. In Mills SE, ed. *Histology for Pathologists*. Philadelphia: Lippincott Williams & Wilkins, 2007:347–370.
4. Eagle RC. *Eye Pathology: An Atlas and Basic Text*. Philadelphia: WB Saunders Company, 1999.
5. Klintworth GK, Garner A. *Garner and Klintworth's Pathobiology of Ocular Disease*. 3rd edition New York: Informa Healthcare, 2008.
6. Spencer WH. *Ophthalmic Pathology: An Atlas and Textbook*. 4th edition Philadelphia: WB Saunders, 1996.
7. McDonnell PJ, Moore GW, Miller NR, et al. Temporal arteritis. A clinicopathologic study. *Ophthalmology* 1986;93:518–530.
8. Mitchell BM, Font RL. Detection of varicella zoster virus DNA in some patients with giant cell arteritis. *Invest Ophthalmol Vis Sci* 2001;42:2572–2577.
9. Dasgupta B, Hassan N. Giant cell arteritis: recent advances and guidelines for management. *Clin Exp Rheumatol* 2007;25:S62–S65.
10. Shields JA, Shields CL, Donoso LA. Management of posterior uveal melanoma. *Surv Ophthalmol* 1991;36:161–195.
11. Chan CC, Palestine AG, Davis JL, et al. Role of chorioretinal biopsy in inflammatory eye disease. *Ophthalmology* 1991;98:1281–1286.
12. Font RL, Croxatto JO, Rao NA. *AFIP Atlas of Tumor Pathology. Tumors of the Eye and Ocular Adnexa*. Fourth series, fascicle 5. Washington, DC: American Registry of Pathology, 2006.
13. Burger PC, Klintworth GK. Experimental retinal degeneration in the rabbit produced by intraocular iron. *Lab Invest* 1974;30:9–19.
14. Rosenthal AR, Appleton B, Hopkins JL. Intraocular copper foreign bodies. *Am J Ophthalmol* 1974;78:671–678.
15. Chu CT, Klintworth GK. Applications of energy dispersive microprobe analysis in ophthalmic pathology. In Ingram P, Shelburne JD, Roggli VL, LeFurgey A, eds. *Biomedical Applications of Microprobe Analysis*. New York: Academic Press, 1999:401–444.
16. Chien AM, Raber IM, Fischer DH, et al. Propionibacterium acnes endophthalmitis after intracapsular cataract extraction. *Ophthalmology* 1992;99:487–490.
17. Meisler DM, Zakov ZN, Bruner WE, et al. Endophthalmitis associated with sequestered intraocular *Propionibacterium acnes*. *Am J Ophthalmol* 1987;104:428–429.
18. Margo CE, Mames RN, Guy JR. Endogenous *Klebsiella* endophthalmitis. Report of two cases and review of the literature. *Ophthalmology* 1994;101:1298–1301.
19. McManaway JW, III, Weinberg RS, Coudron PE. Coryneform group A-4 endophthalmitis. An experimental animal model. *Invest Ophthalmol Vis Sci* 1991;32:2696–2699.
20. Rehany U, Dorenboim Y, Lefler E, et al. *Clostridium bifermentans* panophthalmitis after penetrating eye injury. *Ophthalmology* 1994;101:839–842.
21. Weber DJ, Hoffman KL, Thoft RA, et al. Endophthalmitis following intraocular lens implantation: report of 30 cases and review of the literature. *Rev Infect Dis* 1986;8:12–20.
22. Lemley CA, Han DP. Endophthalmitis: a review of current evaluation and management. *Retina* 2007;27:662–680.
23. Marak GE, Jr. Phacoanaphylactic endophthalmitis. *Surv Ophthalmol* 1992;36:325–339.
24. Rathinam SR, Rao NA. Sympathetic ophthalmia following postoperative bacterial endophthalmitis: a clinicopathologic study. *Am J Ophthalmol* 2006;141:498–507.
25. Klintworth GK. Radiographic abnormalities in eyes with retinoblastoma and other disorders. *Br J Ophthalmol* 1978;62:365–372.
26. Finkelstein EM, Boniuk M. Intraocular ossification and hematopoiesis. *Am J Ophthalmol* 1969;68:683–690.
27. Saeed MU, Chang BY, Khandwala M, et al. Twenty-year review of histopathological findings in enucleated/eviscerated eyes. *J Clin Pathol* 2006;59:153–155.
28. Grierson I. Anterior segment changes in glaucoma. In Garner A, Klintworth GK, eds. *Pathobiology of Ocular Disease*. New York: Marcel Dekker, 2007:397–426.
29. Taylor HR. A histologic survey of trabeculectomy. *Am J Ophthalmol* 1976;82:733–735.
30. Lee P, Green WR. Corneal biopsy. Indications, techniques, and a report of a series of 87 cases. *Ophthalmology* 1990;97:718–721.
31. Klintworth GK. The molecular genetics of the corneal dystrophies—current status. *Front Biosci* 2003;8:d687–d713.
32. Weiss JS, Møller MU, Lish W, et al. The IC3D classification of the corneal dystrophies. *Cornea* 27 (Suppl) 2008;S1–S42.
33. Kang PC, Klintworth GK, Kim T, et al. Trends in the indications for penetrating keratoplasty, 1980–2001. *Cornea* 2005;24:801–803.
34. Lindquist TD, McNeill JI, Wilhelmus KR. Indications for keratoplasty. *Cornea* 1994;13:105–107.
35. The collaborative corneal transplantation studies (CCTS). Effectiveness of histocompatibility matching in high-risk corneal transplantation. The Collaborative Corneal Transplantation Studies Research Group. *Arch Ophthalmol* 1992;110:1392–1403.
36. Klintworth GK, Ferry AP, Sugar A, et al. Recurrence of lattice corneal dystrophy type 1 in the corneal grafts of two siblings. *Am J Ophthalmol* 1982;94:540–546.
37. Klintworth GK, Reed J, Stainer GA, et al. Recurrence of macular corneal dystrophy within grafts. *Am J Ophthalmol* 1983;95:60–72.
38. Meisler DM, Fine M. Recurrence of the clinical signs of lattice corneal dystrophy (type I) in corneal transplants. *Am J Ophthalmol* 1984;97:210–214.
39. Stuart JC, Mund ML, Iwamoto T, et al. Recurrent granular corneal dystrophy. *Am J Ophthalmol* 1975;79:18–24.
40. Chandler JW, Gebhardt BM, Kaufman HE. Immunologic protection of rabbit corneal allografts: preparation and in vitro testing of heterologous "blocking" antibody. *Invest Ophthalmol* 1973;12:646–653.
41. Khodadoust AA, Silverstein AM. Transplantation and rejection of individual cell layers of the cornea. *Invest Ophthalmol* 1969;8:180–195.
42. Khodadoust AA, Silverstein AM. The survival and rejection of epithelium in experimental corneal transplants. *Invest Ophthalmol* 1969;8:169–179.
43. Panda A, Vanathi M, Kumar A, et al. Corneal graft rejection. *Surv Ophthalmol* 2007;52:375–396.
44. Klintworth GK. Genetic disorders of the cornea. In Klintworth GK, Garner A, eds. *Garner and Klintworth's Pathobiology of Ocular Disease*. New York: Informa Healthcare, 2008.
45. Snip RC, Kenyon KR, Green WR. Retrocorneal fibrous membrane in the vitreous touch syndrome. *Am J Ophthalmol* 1975;79:233–244.
46. Fine BS, Berkow JW, Fine S. Corneal calcification. *Science* 1968;162:129–130.
47. Freddo TF, Leibowitz HM. Bilateral acute corneal calcification. *Ophthalmology* 1985;92:537–542.
48. O'Connor GR. Calcific band keratopathy. *Trans Am Ophthalmol Soc* 1972;70:58–81.
49. Porter R, Crombie AL. Corneal and conjunctival calcification in chronic renal failure. *Br J Ophthalmol* 1973;57:339–343.
50. Klintworth GK. Chronic actinic keratopathy—a condition associated with conjunctival elastosis (pingueculae) and typified by characteristic extracellular concretions. *Am J Pathol* 1972;67:327–348.
51. Gray RH, Johnson GJ, Freedman A. Climatic droplet keratopathy. *Surv Ophthalmol* 1992;36:241–253.
52. Garner A, Fraunfelder FT, Barras TC, et al. Spheroidal degeneration of cornea and conjunctiva. *Br J Ophthalmol* 1976;60:473–478.
53. Taylor DM, Atlas BF, Romanchuk KG, et al. Pseudophakic bullous keratopathy. *Ophthalmology* 1983;90:19–24.
54. Covert DJ, Koenig SB. Descemet stripping and automated endothelial keratoplasty (DSAEK) in eyes with failed penetrating keratoplasty. *Cornea* 2007;26:692–696.
55. Price MO, Price FW. Descemet's stripping endothelial keratoplasty. *Curr Opin Ophthalmol* 2007;18:290–294.

56. Scroggs MW, Proia AD. Histopathological variation in keratoconus. *Cornea* 1992;11:553–559.
57. Bechrakis N, Blom ML, Stark WJ, et al. Recurrent keratoconus. *Cornea* 1994;13:73–77.
58. Klintworth GK, Oshima E, al Rajhi A, et al. Macular corneal dystrophy in Saudi Arabia: a study of 56 cases and recognition of a new immunophenotype. *Am J Ophthalmol* 1997;124:9–18.
59. Streeten BW, Qi Y, Klintworth GK, et al. Immunolocalization of beta ig-h3 protein in 5q31-linked corneal dystrophies and normal corneas. *Arch Ophthalmol* 1999;117:67–75.
60. de la CA, Tolvanen R, Boysen G, et al. Gelsolin-derived familial amyloidosis caused by asparagine or tyrosine substitution for aspartic acid at residue 187. *Nat Genet* 1992;2:157–160.
61. Kivela T, Tarkkanen A, Frangione B, et al. Ocular amyloid deposition in familial amyloidosis, Finnish: an analysis of native and variant gelsolin in Meretoja's syndrome. *Invest Ophthalmol Vis Sci* 1994;35:3759–3769.
62. Klintworth GK, Valnickova Z, Kielar RA, et al. Familial subepithelial corneal amyloidosis—a lactoferrin-related amyloidosis. *Invest Ophthalmol Vis Sci* 1997;38:2756–2763.
63. Klintworth GK, Valnickova Z, Enghild JJ. Accumulation of beta Ig-h3 gene product in corneas with granular dystrophy. *Am J Pathol* 1998;152:743–748.
64. Paschal JF, Holland GN, Sison RF, et al. *Mycobacterium fortuitum* keratitis. Clinicopathologic correlates and corticosteroid effects in an animal model. *Cornea* 1992;11:493–499.
65. Telahun A, Waring GO, Grossniklaus HE. *Mycobacterium gordonae* keratitis. *Cornea* 1992;11:77–82.
66. Davis RM, Font RL, Keisler MS, et al. Corneal microsporidiosis. A case report including ultrastructural observations. *Ophthalmology* 1990;97:953–957.
67. Schwartz DA, Visvesvara GS, Diesenhouse MC, et al. Pathologic features and immunofluorescent antibody demonstration of ocular microsporidiosis (*Encephalitozoon hellem*) in seven patients with acquired immunodeficiency syndrome. *Am J Ophthalmol* 1993;115:285–292.
68. Thomas PA, Geraldine P. Infectious keratitis. *Curr Opin Infect Dis* 2007;20:129–141.
69. Hassman G, Sugar J. Pseudomonas corneal ulcer with extended-wear soft contact lenses for myopia. *Arch Ophthalmol* 1983;101:1549–1550.
70. Moore MB, McCulley JP, Luckenbach M, et al. *Acanthamoeba* keratitis associated with soft contact lenses. *Am J Ophthalmol* 1985;100:396–403.
71. Thebpatiphat N, Hammersmith KM, Rocha FN, et al. *Acanthamoeba* keratitis: a parasite on the rise. *Cornea* 2007;26:701–706.
72. Anderson J, Fuglsang H. Ocular onchocerciasis. *Trop Dis Bull* 1977;74:257–272.
73. Teske SA, Hirst LW, Gibson BH, et al. Caterpillar-induced keratitis. *Cornea* 1991;10:317–321.
74. Sridhar MS, Sharma S, Garg P, et al. Epithelial infectious crystalline keratopathy. *Am J Ophthalmol* 2001;131:255–257.
75. Moshari A, McLean IW, Dodds MT, et al. Chorioretinitis after keratitis caused by *Acanthamoeba*: case report and review of the literature. *Ophthalmology* 2001;108:2232–2236.
76. Kumar R, Lloyd D. Recent advances in the treatment of *Acanthamoeba* keratitis. *Clin Infect Dis* 2002;35:434–441.
77. Kaye SB, Baker K, Bonshek R, et al. Human herpesviruses in the cornea. *Br J Ophthalmol* 2000;84:563–571.
78. Metcalf JF, Kaufman HE. Herpetic stromal keratitis-evidence for cell-mediated immunopathogenesis. *Am J Ophthalmol* 1976;82:827–834.
79. Cook SD, Hill JH. Herpes simplex virus: molecular biology and the possibility of corneal latency. *Surv Ophthalmol* 1991;36:140–148.
80. Akpek EK, Demetriades A, Gottsch JD. Peripheral ulcerative keratitis after clear corneal cataract extraction(1). *J Cataract Refract Surg* 2000;26:1424–1427.
81. Kervick GN, Pflugfelder SC, Haimovici R, et al. Paracentral rheumatoid corneal ulceration. Clinical features and cyclosporine therapy. *Ophthalmology* 1992;99:80–88.
82. Jones RR, Maguire LJ. Corneal complications after cataract surgery in patients with rheumatoid arthritis. *Cornea* 1992;11:148–150.
83. Feder RS, Krachmer JH. The diagnosis of epithelial downgrowth after keratoplasty. *Am J Ophthalmol* 1985;99:697–703.
84. Daneshvar H, Brownstein S, Mintsioulis G, et al. Epithelial ingrowth following penetrating keratoplasty: a clinical, ultrasound biomicroscopic and histopathological correlation. *Can J Ophthalmol* 2000;35:222–224.
85. Riono WP, Hidayat AA, Rao NA. Scleritis: a clinicopathologic study of 55 cases. *Ophthalmology* 1999;106:1328–1333.
86. Rao NA, Marak GE, Hidayat AA. Necrotizing scleritis. A clinico-pathologic study of 41 cases. *Ophthalmology* 1985;92:1542–1549.
87. Watson PG, Hayreh SS. Scleritis and episcleritis. *Br J Ophthalmol* 1976;60:163–191.
88. Shields CL, Shields JA, Varenhorst MP. Transscleral leiomyoma. *Ophthalmology* 1991;98:84–87.
89. Sugar HS. The oculoauriculovertebral dysplasia syndrome of Goldenhar. *Am J Ophthalmol* 1966;62:678–682.
90. Mansour AM, Wang F, Henkind P, et al. Ocular findings in the facioauriculovertebral sequence (Goldenhar-Gorlin syndrome). *Am J Ophthalmol* 1985;100:555–559.
91. Nichols CW, Eagle RC, Jr., Yanoff M, et al. Conjunctival biopsy as an aid in the evaluation of the patient with suspected sarcoidosis. *Ophthalmology* 1980;87:287–291.
92. Obenauf CD, Shaw HE, Sydnor CF, et al. Sarcoidosis and its ophthalmic manifestations. *Am J Ophthalmol* 1978;86:648–655.
93. Libert J. Conjunctival biopsy. *Bull Soc Belge Ophtalmol* 1983;208 Pt 1:297–302.
94. Shields JA, Shields CL, Eagle RC, Jr., et al. Ocular manifestations of the organoid nevus syndrome. *Ophthalmology* 1997;104:549–557.
95. Shields JA, Shields CL, Eagle RC, Jr., et al. Ophthalmic features of the organoid nevus syndrome. *Trans Am Ophthalmol Soc* 1996;94:65–86.
96. Jakobiec FA, Bonanno PA, Sigelman J. Conjunctival adnexal cysts and dermoids. *Arch Ophthalmol* 1978;96:1404–1409.
97. Williams BJ, Durcan FJ, Mamalis N, et al. Conjunctival epithelial inclusion cyst. *Arch Ophthalmol* 1997;115:816–817.
98. Holland EJ, Chan CC, Kuwabara T, et al. Immunohistologic findings and results of treatment with cyclosporine in ligneous conjunctivitis. *Am J Ophthalmol* 1989;107:160–166.
99. Schuster V, Seidenspinner S, Zeitler P, et al. Compound-heterozygous mutations in the plasminogen gene predispose to the development of ligneous conjunctivitis. *Blood* 1999;93:3457–3466.
100. Mondino BJ, Ross AN, Rabin BS, et al. Autoimmune phenomena in ocular cicatricial pemphigoid. *Am J Ophthalmol* 1977;83:443–450.
101. Sacks EH, Jakobiec FA, Wieczorek R, et al. Immunophenotypic analysis of the inflammatory infiltrate in ocular cicatricial pemphigoid. Further evidence for a T cell-mediated disease. *Ophthalmology* 1989;96:236–243.
102. Lam S, Stone MS, Goeken JA, et al. Paraneoplastic pemphigus, cicatricial conjunctivitis, and acanthosis nigricans with pachydermatoglyphy in a patient with bronchogenic squamous cell carcinoma. *Ophthalmology* 1992;99:108–113.
103. Ulrich GG, Waecker NJ, Jr., Meister SJ, et al. Cat scratch disease associated with neuroretinitis in a 6-year-old girl. *Ophthalmology* 1992;99:246–249.
104. Wear DJ, Malaty RH, Zimmerman LE, et al. Cat scratch disease bacilli in the conjunctiva of patients with Parinaud's oculoglandular syndrome. *Ophthalmology* 1985;92:1282–1287.
105. Weinberg JC, Eagle RC, Jr., Font RL, et al. Conjunctival synthetic fiber granuloma. A lesion that resembles conjunctivitis nodosa. *Ophthalmology* 1984;91:867–872.
106. Lass JH, Jenson AB, Papale JJ, et al. Papillomavirus in human conjunctival papillomas. *Am J Ophthalmol* 1983;95:364–368.
107. McDonnell JM, McDonnell PJ, Mounts P, et al. Demonstration of papillomavirus capsid antigen in human conjunctival neoplasia. *Arch Ophthalmol* 1986;104:1801–1805.
108. Odrich MG, Jakobiec FA, Lancaster WD, et al. A spectrum of bilateral squamous conjunctival tumors associated with human papillomavirus type 16. *Ophthalmology* 1991;98:628–635.
109. Streeten BW, Carrillo R, Jamison R, et al. Inverted papilloma of the conjunctiva. *Am J Ophthalmol* 1979;88:1062–1066.
110. Erie JC, Campbell RJ, Liesegang TJ. Conjunctival and corneal intraepithelial and invasive neoplasia. *Ophthalmology* 1986;93:176–183.
111. Pe'er J. Ocular surface squamous neoplasia. *Ophthalmol Clin North Am* 2005;18:1–13.
112. Iliff WJ, Marback R, Green WR. Invasive squamous cell carcinoma of the conjunctiva. *Arch Ophthalmol* 1975;93:119–122.
113. Salisbury JA, Szpak CA, Klintworth GK. Pigmented squamous cell carcinoma of the conjunctiva. A clinicopathologic ultrastructural study. *Ophthalmology* 1983;90:1477–1481.
114. Rao NA, Font RL. Mucoepidermoid carcinoma of the conjunctiva: a clinicopathologic study of five cases. *Cancer* 1976;38:1699–1709.
115. Gamel JW, Eiferman RA, Guibor P. Mucoepidermoid carcinoma of the conjunctiva. *Arch Ophthalmol* 1984;102:730–731.
116. Schubert HD, Farris RL, Green WR. Spindle cell carcinoma of the conjunctiva. *Graefes Arch Clin Exp Ophthalmol* 1995;233:52–53.
117. Folberg R, Jakobiec FA, Bernardino VB, et al. Benign conjunctival melanocytic lesions. Clinicopathologic features. *Ophthalmology* 1989;96:436–461.
118. Jakobiec FA, Folberg R, Iwamoto T. Clinicopathologic characteristics of premalignant and malignant melanocytic lesions of the conjunctiva. *Ophthalmology* 1989;96:147–166.
119. Nik NA, Glew WB, Zimmerman LE. Malignant melanoma of the choroid in the nevus of Ota of a black patient. *Arch Ophthalmol* 1982;100:1641–1643.
120. Folberg R, McLean IW, Zimmerman LE. Primary acquired melanosis of the conjunctiva. *Hum Pathol* 1985;16:129–135.
121. Folberg R, McLean IW, Zimmerman LE. Malignant melanoma of the conjunctiva. *Hum Pathol* 1985;16:136–143.
122. Sigelman J, Jakobiec FA. Lymphoid lesions of the conjunctiva: relation of histopathology to clinical outcome. *Ophthalmology* 1978;85:818–843.
123. Knowles DM, Jakobiec FA, McNally L, et al. Lymphoid hyperplasia and malignant lymphoma occurring in the ocular adnexa (orbit, conjunctiva, and eyelids): a prospective multiparametric analysis of 108 cases during 1977 to 1987. *Hum Pathol* 1990;21:959–973.
124. Lauer SA, Fischer J, Jones J, et al. Orbital T-cell lymphoma in human T-cell leukemia virus-I infection. *Ophthalmology* 1988;95:110–115.
125. Jakobiec FA, Neri A, Knowles DM. Genotypic monoclonality in immunophenotypically polyclonal orbital lymphoid tumors. A model of tumor progression in the lymphoid system. The 1986 Wendell Hughes lecture. *Ophthalmology* 1987;94:980–994.
126. Weisenthal RW, Streeten BW, Dubansky AS, et al. Burkitt lymphoma presenting as a conjunctival mass. *Ophthalmology* 1995;102:129–134.
127. Fratkin JD, Shammas HF, Miller SD. Disseminated Hodgkin's disease with bilateral orbital involvement. *Arch Ophthalmol* 1978;96:102–104.
128. Lagoo, AS. Tumors of lymphoid tissue. In Klintworth GK, Garner A. (Eds).*Garner and Klintworth's Pathobiology of Ocular Disease*. 3rd edition New York: Informa Healthcare, 2008.
129. McNally L, Jakobiec FA, Knowles DM. Clinical, morphologic, immunophenotypic, and molecular genetic analysis of bilateral ocular adnexal lymphoid neoplasms in 17 patients. *Am J Ophthalmol* 1987;103:555–568.
130. Allingham RR, Seo B, Rampersaud E, et al. A duplication in chromosome 4q35 is associated with hereditary benign intraepithelial dyskeratosis. *Am J Hum Genet* 2001;68:491–494.
131. Shields CL, Shields JA, Honavar SG, et al. Primary ophthalmic rhabdomyosarcoma in 33 patients. *Trans Am Ophthalmol Soc* 2001;99:133–142.
132. White VA, Damji KF, Richards JS, et al. Leiomyosarcoma of the conjunctiva. *Ophthalmology* 1991;98:1560–1564.
133. Kurumety UR, Lustbader JM. Kaposi's sarcoma of the bulbar conjunctiva as an initial clinical manifestation of acquired immunodeficiency syndrome. *Arch Ophthalmol* 1995;113:978.
134. Proia AD, Browning DJ, Klintworth GK. Actinic granuloma of the conjunctiva. *Am J Ophthalmol* 1983;96:116–118.
135. Austin P, Jakobiec FA, Iwamoto T. Elastodysplasia and elastodystrophy as the pathologic bases of ocular pterygia and pinguecula. *Ophthalmology* 1983;90:96–109.
136. Shields CL, Shields JA. Tumors of the conjunctiva and cornea. *Surv Ophthalmol* 2004;49:3–24.
137. Snow SN, Larson PO, Lucarelli MJ, et al. Sebaceous carcinoma of the eyelids treated by

mohs micrographic surgery: report of nine cases with review of the literature. *Dermatol Surg* 2002;28:623–631.

138. Biggs SL, Font RL. Oncocytic lesions of the caruncle and other ocular adnexa. *Arch Ophthalmol* 1977;95:474–478.
139. Netland PA, Sugrue SP, Albert DM, et al. Histopathologic features of the floppy eyelid syndrome. Involvement of tarsal elastin. *Ophthalmology* 1994;101:174–181.
140. Jakobiec FA, Zimmerman LE, La Piana F, et al. Unusual eyelid tumors with sebaceous differentiation in the Muir-Torre syndrome. Rapid clinical regrowth and frank squamous transformation after biopsy. *Ophthalmology* 1988;95:1543–1548.
141. Demirci H, Nelson CC, Shields CL, et al. Eyelid sebaceous carcinoma associated with Muir-Torre syndrome in two cases. *Ophthal Plast Reconstr Surg* 2007;23:77–79.
142. Codere F, Lee RD, Anderson RL. Necrobiotic xanthogranuloma of the eyelid. *Arch Ophthalmol* 1983;101:60–63.
143. Kronish JW, McLeish WM. Eyelid necrosis and periorbital necrotizing fasciitis. Report of a case and review of the literature. *Ophthalmology* 1991;98:92–98.
144. Ross MJ, Cohen KL, Peiffer RL, Jr., et al. Episcleral and orbital pseudorheumatoid nodules. *Arch Ophthalmol* 1983;101:418–421.
145. Schwartz TL, Carter KD, Judisch GF, et al. Congenital macronodular juvenile xanthogranuloma of the eyelid. *Ophthalmology* 1991;98:1230–1233.
146. Thygeson P. Observations on conjunctival neoplasms masquerading as chronic conjunctivitis or keratitis. *Trans Am Acad Ophthalmol Otolaryngol* 1969;73:969–978.
147. Roth AM. Demodex folliculorum in hair follicles of eyelid skin. *Ann Ophthalmol* 1979;11:37–40.
148. Croxatto JO, Garner A. Ocular disease due to helminths. In Klintworth GK, Garner A, eds. *Garner and Klintworth's Pathobiology of Ocular Disease.* 3rd edition New York: Informa Healthcare, 2008.
149. Olsen KE, Sandgren O, Sletten K, et al. Primary localized amyloidosis of the eyelid: two cases of immunoglobulin light chain-derived proteins, subtype lambda V respectively lambda VI. *Clin Exp Immunol* 1996;106:362–366.
150. Singh AD, McCloskey L, Parsons MA, et al. Eccrine hidrocystoma of the eyelid. *Eye* 2005;19:77–79.
151. Font RL. Eyelids and lacrimal drainage system. In Spencer WH, ed. *Ophthalmic Pathology: An Atlas and Textbook.* Philadelphia: WB Saunders, 1996:2219–2437.
152. Grossniklaus HE, Wojno TH, Yanoff M, et al. Invasive keratoacanthoma of the eyelid and ocular adnexa. *Ophthalmology* 1996;103:937–941.
153. Ellis FJ, Eagle RC, Jr., Shields JA, et al. Phakomatous choristoma (Zimmerman's tumor). Immunohistochemical confirmation of lens-specific proteins. *Ophthalmology* 1993;100:955–960.
154. Gordon AJ, Patrinely JR, Knupp JA, et al. Complex choristoma of the eyelid containing ectopic cilia and lacrimal gland. *Ophthalmology* 1991;98:1547–1550.
155. Grossniklaus HE, Knight SH. Eccrine acrospiroma (clear cell hidradenoma) of the eyelid. Immunohistochemical and ultrastructural features. *Ophthalmology* 1991;98:347–352.
156. Hidayat AA, Font RL. Trichilemmoma of eyelid and eyebrow. A clinicopathologic study of 31 cases. *Arch Ophthalmol* 1980;98:844–847.
157. Rodgers IR, Jakobiec FA, Krebs W, et al. Papillary oncocytoma of the eyelid. A previously undescribed tumor of apocrine gland origin. *Ophthalmology* 1988;95:1071–1076.
158. Kennedy RH, Flanagan JC, Eagle RC, Jr., et al. The Carney complex with ocular signs suggestive of cardiac myxoma. *Am J Ophthalmol* 1991;111:699–702.
159. Martin H, Strong E, Spiro RH. Radiation-induced skin cancer of the head and neck. *Cancer* 1970;25:61–71.
160. Gaasterland DE, Rodrigues MM, Moshell AN. Ocular involvement in xeroderma pigmentosum. *Ophthalmology* 1982;89:980–986.
161. Lynch HT, Anderson DE, Smith JL, Jr., et al. Xeroderma pigmentosum, malignant melanoma, and congenital ichthyosis. A family study. *Arch Dermatol* 1967;96:625–635.
162. Doxanas MT, Green WR, Iliff CE. Factors in the successful surgical management of basal cell carcinoma of the eyelids. *Am J Ophthalmol* 1981;91:726–736.
163. Reifler DM, Hornblass A. Squamous cell carcinoma of the eyelid. *Surv Ophthalmol* 1986;30:349–365.
164. Kass LG, Hornblass A. Sebaceous carcinoma of the ocular adnexa. *Surv Ophthalmol* 1989;33:477–490.
165. Shields JA, Demirci H, Marr BP, et al. Sebaceous carcinoma of the ocular region: a review. *Surv Ophthalmol* 2005;50:103–122.
166. Pereira PR, Odashiro AN, Rodrigues-Reyes AA, et al. Histopathological review of sebaceous carcinoma of the eyelid. *J Cutan Pathol* 2005;32:496–501.
167. Rao NA, Hidayat AA, McLean IW, et al. Sebaceous carcinomas of the ocular adnexa: a clinicopathologic study of 104 cases, with five-year follow-up data. *Hum Pathol* 1982;13:113–122.
168. Sinard JH. Immunohistochemical distinction of ocular sebaceous carcinoma from basal cell and squamous cell carcinoma. *Arch Ophthalmol* 1999;117:776–783.
169. Margo CE, Lessner A, Stern GA. Intraepithelial sebaceous carcinoma of the conjunctiva and skin of the eyelid. *Ophthalmology* 1992;99:227–231.
170. Wolfe JT, III, Yeatts RP, Wick MR, et al. Sebaceous carcinoma of the eyelid. Errors in clinical and pathologic diagnosis. *Am J Surg Pathol* 1984;8:597–606.
171. Grossniklaus HE, McLean IW. Cutaneous melanoma of the eyelid. Clinicopathologic features. *Ophthalmology* 1991;98:1867–1873.
172. Cooper PH. Carcinomas of sweat glands. *Pathol Annu* 1987;22 Pt 1:83–124.
173. Snow SN, Reizner GT. Mucinous eccrine carcinoma of the eyelid. *Cancer* 1992;70:2099–2104.
174. Wright JD, Font RL. Mucinous sweat gland adenocarcinoma of eyelid: a clinicopathologic study of 21 cases with histochemical and electron microscopic observations. *Cancer* 1979;44:1757–1768.
175. Girard C, Johnson WC, Graham JH. Cutaneous angiosarcoma. *Cancer* 1970;26:868–883.
176. Dresner MS, Kincaid MC. Lymphoma of the eyelid. *JAMA* 1991;266:29.
177. Kivela T, Tarkkanen A. The Merkel cell and associated neoplasms in the eyelids and periocular region. *Surv Ophthalmol* 1990;35:171–187.
178. Arnold AC, Bullock JD, Foos RY. Metastatic eyelid carcinoma. *Ophthalmology* 1985;92:114–119.
179. Hood CI, Font RL, Zimmerman LE. Metastatic mammary carcinoma in the eyelid with histiocytoid appearance. *Cancer* 1973;31:793–800.
180. Kindermann WR, Shields JA, Eiferman RA, et al. Metastatic renal cell carcinoma to the eye and adnexae: a report of three cases and review of the literature. *Ophthalmology* 1981;88:1347–1350.
181. Eagle RC, Spencer WH. Lens. In Spencer WH, ed. *Ophthalmic Pathology: An Atlas and Textbook.* Philadelphia: WB Saunders, 1996:372–437.
182. Apple DJ, Mamalis N, Loftfield K, et al. Complications of intraocular lenses. A historical and histopathological review. *Surv Ophthalmol* 1984;29:1–54.
183. Hall JR, Muenzler WS. Intraocular lens replacement in pseudophakic bullous keratopathy. *Trans Ophthalmol Soc U K* 1985;104(Pt 5):541–545.
184. Gamm DM, Kulkarni AD, Albert DM. Retinoblastoma. In Klintworth GK, Garner A, eds. *Garner and Klintworth's Pathobiology of Ocular Disease.* 3rd edition New York: Informa Healthcare, 2008.
185. Provenzale JM, Gururangan S, Klintworth GK. Trilateral retinoblastoma: clinical and radiological progression. *Am J Roentgenol* 2004;183:505–511.
186. Holladay DA, Holladay A, Montebello JF, et al. Clinical presentation, treatment, and outcome of trilateral retinoblastoma. *Cancer* 1991;67:710–715.
187. Shields CL, Shields JA, Shah P. Retinoblastoma in older children. *Ophthalmology* 1991;98:395–399.
188. Materin MA, Shields CL, Shields JA, et al. Diffuse infiltrating retinoblastoma simulating uveitis in a 7-year-old boy. *Arch Ophthalmol* 118:442–443, 2000.
189. Ts'o MO, Fine BS, Zimmerman LE. The Flexner-Wintersteiner rosettes in retinoblastoma. *Arch Pathol* 1969;88:664–671.
190. Ts'o MO, Zimmerman LE, Fine BS. The nature of retinoblastoma. I. Photoreceptor differentiation: a clinical and histopathologic study. *Am J Ophthalmol* 1970;69:339–349.
191. Mullaney J. Retinoblastomas with DNA precipitation. *Arch Ophthalmol* 1969;82:454–456.
192. Datta BN. DNA coating of blood vessels in retinoblastomas. *Am J Clin Pathol* 1974;62:94–96.
193. Shields CL, Shields JA, Baez K, et al. Optic nerve invasion of retinoblastoma. Metastatic potential and clinical risk factors. *Cancer* 1994;73:692–698.
194. Rootman J, Hofbauer J, Ellsworth RM, et al. Invasion of the optic nerve by retinoblastoma: a clinicopathological study. *Can J Ophthalmol* 1976;11:106–114.
195. MacKay CJ, Abramson DH, Ellsworth RM. Metastatic patterns of retinoblastoma. *Arch Ophthalmol* 1984;102:391–396.
196. Cummings TJ, Klintworth GK. Tumors of the retina. In McLendon RE, Rosenblum MK, Bigner DD, eds. *Russell and Rubinstein's Pathology of Tumors of the Nervous System.* London: Hodder Arnold, 2006:623–650.
197. Jakobiec FA, Marboe CC, Knowles DM, et al. Human sympathetic ophthalmia. An analysis of the inflammatory infiltrate by hybridoma-monoclonal antibodies, immunochemistry, and correlative electron microscopy. *Ophthalmology* 1983;90:76–95.
198. Lubin JR, Albert DM, Weinstein M. Sixty-five years of sympathetic ophthalmia. A clinicopathologic review of 105 cases (1913–1978). *Ophthalmology* 1980;87:109–121.
199. Schwent BJ, Grossniklaus, HE. Tumors of melanocytes. In Klintworth GK, Garner A, eds. *Garner and Klintworth's Pathobiology of Ocular Disease.* 3rd edition New York: Informa Healthcare, 2008.
200. McLean IW, Saraiva VS, Burnier MN, Jr. Pathological and prognostic features of uveal melanomas. *Can J Ophthalmol* 2004;39:343–350.
201. Whelchel JC, Farah SE, McLean IW, et al. Immunohistochemistry of infiltrating lymphocytes in uveal malignant melanoma. *Invest Ophthalmol Vis Sci* 1993;34:2603–2606.
202. McLean IW, Keefe KS, Burnier MN. Uveal melanoma. Comparison of the prognostic value of fibrovascular loops, mean of the ten largest nucleoli, cell type, and tumor size. *Ophthalmology* 1997;104:777–780.
203. McLean MJ, Foster WD, Zimmerman LE. Prognostic factors in small malignant melanomas of choroid and ciliary body. *Arch Ophthalmol* 1977;95:48–58.
204. Folberg R, Rummelt V, Parys-van Ginderdeuren R, et al. The prognostic value of tumor blood vessel morphology in primary uveal melanoma. *Ophthalmology* 1993;100:1389–1398.
205. Zimmerman LE, McLean IW. Metastatic disease from untreated uveal melanomas. *Am J Ophthalmol* 1979;88:524–534.
206. McLean IW, Zimmerman LE, Evans RM. Reappraisal of Callender's spindle a type of malignant melanoma of choroid and ciliary body. *Am J Ophthalmol* 1978;86:557–564.
207. Char DH, Crawford JB, Kroll S. Iris melanomas. Diagnostic problems. *Ophthalmology* 1996;103:251–255.
208. Shields JA, Stephens RF, Eagle RC, Jr., et al. Progressive enlargement of a circumscribed choroidal hemangioma. A clinicopathologic correlation. *Arch Ophthalmol* 1992;110:1276–1278.
209. Witschel H, Font RL. Hemangioma of the choroid. A clinicopathologic study of 71 cases and a review of the literature. *Surv Ophthalmol* 1976;20:415–431.
210. Shields JA, Eagle RC, Jr., Shields CL, et al. Congenital neoplasms of the nonpigmented ciliary epithelium (medulloepithelioma). *Ophthalmology* 1996;103:1998–2006.
211. Shields JA, Eagle RC, Jr., Shields CL, et al. Acquired neoplasms of the nonpigmented ciliary epithelium (adenoma and adenocarcinoma). *Ophthalmology* 1996;103:2007–2016.
212. Pe'er J, Neudorfer M, Ron N, et al. Panuveal malignant mesenchymoma. *Arch Pathol Lab Med* 1995;119:844–848.
213. Shields JA, Shields CL, Eagle RC, Jr., et al. Observations on seven cases of intraocular leiomyoma. The 1993 Byron Demorest Lecture. *Arch Ophthalmol* 1994;112:521–528.
214. Foss AJ, Pecorella I, Alexander RA, et al. Are most intraocular "leiomyomas" really melanocytic lesions? *Ophthalmology* 1994;101:919–924.
215. Shields JA, Eagle RC, Jr., Shields CL, et al. Natural course and histopathologic findings of lacrimal gland choristoma of the iris and ciliary body. *Am J Ophthalmol* 1995;119:219–224.
216. Hufnagel TJ, Hickey WF, Cobbs WH, et al. Immunohistochemical and ultrastructural studies on the exenterated orbital tissues of a patient with Graves' disease. *Ophthalmology* 1984;91:1411–1419.

217. Shields JA, Shields CL, Scartozzi R. Survey of 1264 patients with orbital tumors and simulating lesions: the 2002 Montgomery Lecture, part 1. *Ophthalmology* 2004;111:997–1008.
218. Midena E, Segato T, Piermarocchi S, et al. Fine needle aspiration biopsy in ophthalmology. *Surv Ophthalmol* 1985;29:410–422.
219. Consul BN, Kulshrestha OP. Orbital meningocele. *Br J Ophthalmol* 1965;49:374–376.
220. Suwanwela C, Suwanwela N. A morphological classification of sincipital encephalomeningoceles. *J Neurosurg* 1972;36:201–211.
221. Terry A, Patrinely JR, Anderson RL, et al. Orbital meningoencephalocele manifesting as a conjunctival mass. *Am J Ophthalmol* 1993;115:46–49.
222. Ide CH, Davis WE, Black SP. Orbital teratoma. *Arch Ophthalmol* 1978;96:2093–2096.
223. Berlin AJ, Rich LS, Hahn JF. Congenital orbital teratoma. *Childs Brain* 1983;10:208–216.
224. Holds JB, Anderson RL, Mamalis N, et al. Invasive squamous cell carcinoma arising from asymptomatic choristomatous cysts of the orbit. Two cases and a review of the literature. *Ophthalmology* 1993;100:1244–1252.
225. Iliff CE. Mucoceles in the orbit. *Arch Ophthalmol* 1973;89:392–395.
226. Kennerdell JS, Dresner SC. The nonspecific orbital inflammatory syndromes. *Surv Ophthalmol* 1984;29:93–103.
227. Bullen CL, Liesegang TJ, McDonald TJ, et al. Ocular complications of Wegener's granulomatosis. *Ophthalmology* 1983;90:279–290.
228. Kalina PH, Lie JT, Campbell RJ, et al. Diagnostic value and limitations of orbital biopsy in Wegener's granulomatosis. *Ophthalmology* 1992;99:120–124.
229. Zimmerman LE, Hidayat AA, Grantham RL, et al. Atypical cases of sinus histiocytosis (Rosai-Dorfman disease) with ophthalmological manifestations. *Trans Am Ophthalmol Soc* 1988;86:113–135.
230. Spraul CW, Grossniklaus HE, Lang GK. Bilateral adult periocular xanthogranuloma. *Klin Monatsbl Augenheilkd* 1997;211:342–344.
231. Yohai RA, Bullock JD, Aziz AA, et al. Survival factors in rhino-orbital-cerebral mucormycosis. *Surv Ophthalmol* 1994;39:3–22.
232. Rootman J, McCarthy M, White V, et al. Idiopathic sclerosing inflammation of the orbit. A distinct clinicopathologic entity. *Ophthalmology* 1994;101:570–584.
233. Comings DE, Skubi KB, Van Eyes J, et al. Familial multifocal fibrosclerosis. Findings suggesting that retroperitoneal fibrosis, mediastinal fibrosis, sclerosing cholangitis, Riedel's thyroiditis, and pseudotumor of the orbit may be different manifestations of a single disease. *Ann Intern Med* 1967;66:884–892.
234. DuPont HL, Varco RL, Winchell CP. Chronic fibrous mediastinitis simulating pulmonic stenosis, associated with inflammatory pseudotumor of the orbit. *Am J Med* 1968;44:447–452.
235. Richards AB, Shalka HW, Roberts FJ, et al. Pseudotumor of the orbit and retroperitoneal fibrosis. A form of multifocal fibrosclerosis. *Arch Ophthalmol* 1980;98:1617–1620.
236. Mombaerts I, Schlingemann RO, Goldschmeding R, et al. Idiopathic granulomatous orbital inflammation. *Ophthalmology* 1996;103:2135–2141.
237. Haik BG, Karcioglu ZA, Gordon RA, et al. Capillary hemangioma (infantile periocular hemangioma). *Surv Ophthalmol* 1994;38:399–426.
238. Orcutt JC, Wulc AE, Mills RP, et al. Asymptomatic orbital cavernous hemangiomas. *Ophthalmology* 1991;98:1257–1260.
239. Dickinson AJ, Gausas RE. Orbital lymphatics: do they exist? *Eye* 2006;20:1145–1148.
240. Iliff WJ, Green WR. Orbital lymphangiomas. *Ophthalmology* 1979;86:914–929.
241. Croxatto JO, Font RL. Hemangiopericytoma of the orbit: a clinicopathologic study of 30 cases. *Hum Pathol* 1982;13:210–218.
242. Font RL, Hidayat AA. Fibrous histiocytoma of the orbit. A clinicopathologic study of 150 cases. *Hum Pathol* 1982;13:199–209.
243. Kassel SH, Copenhaver R, Arean VM. Orbital rhabdomyosarcoma. *Am J Ophthalmol* 1965;60:811–818.
244. Newton WA, Jr., Soule EH, Hamoudi AB, et al. Histopathology of childhood sarcomas, Intergroup Rhabdomyosarcoma Studies I and II: clinicopathologic correlation. *J Clin Oncol* 1988;6:67–75.
245. Karcioglu ZA, Hadjistilianou D, Rozans M, et al. Orbital rhabdomyosarcoma. *Cancer Control* 2004;11:328–333.
246. Dutton JJ, Tawfik HA, DeBacker CM, et al. Multiple recurrences in malignant peripheral nerve sheath tumor of the orbit: a case report and a review of the literature. *Ophthal Plast Reconstr Surg* 2001;17:293–299.
247. Dorfman DM, To K, Dickersin GR, et al. Solitary fibrous tumor of the orbit. *Am J Surg Pathol* 1994;18:281–287.
248. Jacobs JL, Merriam JC, Chadburn A, et al. Mesenchymal chondrosarcoma of the orbit. Report of three new cases and review of the literature. *Cancer* 1994;73:399–405.
249. Kivela T, Tarkkanen A. Orbital germ cell tumors revisited: a clinicopathological approach to classification. *Surv Ophthalmol* 1994;38:541–554.
250. Brannan PA, Schneider S, Grossniklaus HE, et al. Malignant mesenchymoma of the orbit: case report and review of the literature. *Ophthalmology* 2003;110:314–317.
251. Giannini C, Reynolds C, Leavitt JA, et al. Choristoma of the optic nerve: case report. *Neurosurgery* 2002;50:1125–1128.
252. Cummings TJ, Provenzale JM, Hunter SB, et al. Gliomas of the optic nerve: histological, immunohistochemical (MIB-1 and p53), and MRI analysis. *Acta Neuropathol (Berl)* 2000;99:563–570.
253. Dutton JJ. Gliomas of the anterior visual pathway. *Surv Ophthalmol* 1994;38:427–452.
254. Manor RS, Israeli J, Sandbank U. Malignant optic glioma in a 70-year-old patient. *Arch Ophthalmol* 1976;94:1142–1144.
255. Margo CE, Ragsdale BD, Perman KI, et al. Psammomatoid (juvenile) ossifying fibroma of the orbit. *Ophthalmology* 1985;92:150–159.
256. Green WR, Iliff WJ, Trotter RR. Malignant teratoid medulloepithelioma of the optic nerve. *Arch Ophthalmol* 1974;91:451–454.
257. Massry GG, Harrison W, Hornblass A. Clinical and computed tomographic characteristics of amyloid tumor of the lacrimal gland. *Ophthalmology* 1996;103:1233–1236.
258. Vangveeravong S, Katz SE, Rootman J, et al. Tumors arising in the palpebral lobe of the lacrimal gland. *Ophthalmology* 1996;103:1606–1612.
259. Croxatto JO. Tumors of the lacrimal gland and lacrimal drainage apparatus. In Klintworth GK, Garner A, eds. *Garner and Klintworth's Pathobiology of Ocular Disease.* 3rd edition New York: Informa Healthcare, 2008.
260. Brownstein S, Belin MW, Krohel GB, et al. Orbital dacryops. *Ophthalmology* 1984;91:1424–1428.
261. Weinreb RN, Yavitz EQ, O'Connor GR, et al. Lacrimal gland uptake of gallium citrate Ga 67. *Am J Ophthalmol* 1981;92:16–20.
262. Paulino AF, Huvos AG. Epithelial tumors of the lacrimal glands: a clinicopathologic study. *Ann Diagn Pathol* 1999;3:199–204.
263. Lee DA, Campbell RJ, Waller RR, et al. A clinicopathologic study of primary adenoid cystic carcinoma of the lacrimal gland. *Ophthalmology* 1985;92:128–134.
264. Font RL, Smith SL, Bryan RG. Malignant epithelial tumors of the lacrimal gland: a clinicopathologic study of 21 cases. *Arch Ophthalmol* 1998;116:613–616.
265. Gamel JW, Font RL. Adenoid cystic carcinoma of the lacrimal gland: the clinical significance of a basaloid histologic pattern. *Hum Pathol* 1982;13:219–225.
266. Witschel H, Zimmerman LE. Malignant mixed tumor of the lacrimal gland. A clinicopathologic report of two unusual cases. *Albrecht Von Graefes Arch Klin Exp Ophthalmol* 1981;216:327–337.
267. Levin LA, Popham J, To K, et al. Mucoepidermoid carcinoma of the lacrimal gland. Report of a case with oncocytic features arising in a patient with chronic dacryops. *Ophthalmology* 1991;98:1551–1555.
268. Rosenbaum PS, Mahadevia PS, Goodman LA, et al. Acinic cell carcinoma of the lacrimal gland. *Arch Ophthalmol* 1995;113:781–785.
269. Mansour AM, Cheng KP, Mumma JV, et al. Congenital dacryocele. A collaborative review. *Ophthalmology* 1991;98:1744–1751.
270. Pe'er J, Hidayat AA, Ilsar M, et al. Glandular tumors of the lacrimal sac. Their histopathologic patterns and possible origins. *Ophthalmology* 1996;103:1601–1605.
271. Ryan SJ, Font RL. Primary epithelial neoplasms of the lacrimal sac. *Am J Ophthalmol* 1973;76:73–88.
272. Stefanyszyn MA, Hidayat AA, Pe'er JJ, et al. Lacrimal sac tumors. *Ophthal Plast Reconstr Surg* 1994;10:169–184.
273. Pe'er JJ, Stefanyszyn M, Hidayat AA. Nonepithelial tumors of the lacrimal sac. *Am J Ophthalmol* 1994;118:650–658.
274. Sen DK, Mohan H, Chatterjee PK. Neurilemmoma of the lacrimal sac. *Eye Ear Nose Throat Mon* 1971;50:179–180.
275. Aurora AL. Oncocytic metaplasia in a lacrimal sac papilloma. *Am J Ophthalmol* 1973;75:466–468.
276. Peretz WL, Ettinghausen SE, Gray GF. Oncocytic adenocarcinoma of the lacrimal sac. *Arch Ophthalmol* 1978;96:303–304.
277. Roth SI, August CZ, Lissner GS, et al. Hemangiopericytoma of the lacrimal sac. *Ophthalmology* 1991;98:925–927.
278. Marback RL, Kincaid MC, Green WR, et al. Fibrous histiocytoma of the lacrimal sac. *Am J Ophthalmol* 1982;93:511–517.
279. Bambirra EA, Miranda D, Rayes A. Mucoepidermoid tumor of the lacrimal sac. *Arch Ophthalmol* 1981;99:2149–2150.
280. Farkas TG, Lamberson RE. Malignant melanoma of the lacrimal sac. *Am J Ophthalmol* 1968;66:45–48.
281. Harry J, Ashton N. The pathology of tumours of the lacrimal sac. *Trans Ophthalmol Soc UK* 1969;88:19–35.
282. Seal DV, McGill J, Flanagan D, et al. Lacrimal canaliculitis due to Arachnia (*Actinomyces*) propionica. *Br J Ophthalmol* 1981;65:10–13.

CHAPTER

25

Arthur S. Patchefsky

Nonneoplastic Pulmonary Disease

The lung reacts in a relatively limited way to diverse injurious agents, some of which are known but many are still unknown. These patterns of injury may reflect damage to any part of the lung anatomy, such as the alveolocapillary membrane, the airways, the blood vessels, or combinations of these structures. Histologically, many etiologically specific diseases have similar tissue reactions. This recognition aids the formation of a differential diagnosis (Table 25.1). Diffuse interstitial pulmonary fibrosis, for example, may be seen in such different conditions as rheumatoid arthritis, sarcoidosis, or environmental pneumoconioses (e.g., asbestosis). This is only one of several nonspecific reaction patterns seen in lung biopsy material. The evaluation of lung biopsies, therefore, requires the fullest cooperation between clinician, radiologist, and pathologist if meaningful information about the cause, pathogenesis, and clinical course is to be predicted from microscopic examination. This chapter discusses the surgical pathology (i.e., biopsy pathology) of nonneoplastic pulmonary diseases that are likely to be seen by the surgical pathologist in day-to-day practice.

When infections are excluded, lung biopsy specimens for diffuse infiltrative pulmonary disease are most likely to be from patients with idiopathic interstitial pulmonary fibrosis or sarcoidosis (1). Most other conditions, such as primary pulmonary hypertension, amyloidosis, pulmonary angiitis, and eosinophilic granuloma (EG), although they are of extreme interest, are relatively rare and thus are only occasionally encountered in ordinary clinical experience. However, having a working familiarity with them is important.

The development of a systematic method of microscopic examination of lung biopsy material is useful so that all facets of the pulmonary microanatomy are evaluated. Attention should be focused on the contents of the alveolar space, the condition of the alveolar septal membrane, the conducting airways, and the pulmonary arteries, veins, and lymphatics. In this way, the architectural distribution of pathologic findings (i.e., predominantly intra-alveolar, interstitial, airway, or vascular) is easier to assess, particularly for persons with limited experience. Various combinations of the pulmonary microanatomy may be affected by certain disease states simultaneously. Some conditions that primarily affect the pulmonary interstitium also cause damage to the small airways, and vice versa. For example, usual interstitial pneumonia (UIP) and diffuse alveolar damage may also show areas of involvement of bronchioles. Conversely, idiopathic bronchiolitis obliterans may also cause interstitial inflammation and fibrosis in the alveolar septa adjacent to the inflamed bronchioles. At times, the terminal airways and interstitium may be almost equally involved by diseases such as

hypersensitivity pneumonitis (HP) (2). Such overlapping patterns should always be kept in mind, particularly when reviewing small biopsy material. The degree and balance of these morphologic changes form the basis for the histologic diagnosis, but, unfortunately, they often impart little about specific etiology.

Several lung biopsy techniques are in use; each has advantages and drawbacks. Transbronchial lung biopsy is extremely useful and accurate in the diagnosis of pulmonary infections and certain diffuse lung diseases such as sarcoidosis (3,4). This biopsy method is less accurate, however, for many other diffuse pulmonary conditions because the small biopsy sample may not accurately represent the lung tissue (5). On the other hand, open lung biopsy may be as equally unrewarding if the sample is not representative of the disease process or if it is taken from only subpleural lung tissue. Biopsy specimens of the tip of the lingula or other peripheral sites often show advanced fibrosis, which may not necessarily be representative of the deeper pulmonary parenchyma (1). The use of video-assisted transthoracic surgery (VATS) has made obtaining larger tissue samples from multiple areas of the lung easier (6). In general, the idea that more tissue is better remains true when one considers the optimal amount of lung biopsy material for diagnosis. However, even with open biopsies, certain histologic artifacts, age-related changes, and nonspecific incidental findings must be recognized (7). Among the most common are mechanical compression or fresh hemorrhage due to the biopsy procedure, and rounded clear spaces in the alveoli that can be mistaken for interstitial fibrosis, alveolar hemorrhage, or lipid pneumonia (Fig. 25.1).

Preoperative discussion between pulmonary specialist, pathologist, and surgeon is important to facilitate the appropriate handling of the tissue by the laboratory. A lung biopsy from an acutely ill, immunocompromised patient is treated in a different manner than one from an immunologically normal patient with a slowly progressive diffuse interstitial process.

When an open biopsy is performed, doing a frozen section as an intraoperative consultation is useful so that a judgment can be made about the representation of the disease process in the biopsy. This also ensures that the material arrives in the pathology laboratory fresh and that appropriate bacterial, fungal, or viral cultures and touch preparations can be obtained if necessary. Conditions such as *Pneumocystis carinii* pneumonia, which may require immediate therapy, can thus be rapidly diagnosed. Specialized techniques for mineral analysis, electron microscopy, flow cytometry, or immunofluorescence may also be ordered under the appropriate circumstances (e.g., Goodpasture syndrome, lymphoid lesions, or suspected pneumoconiosis) (8).

TABLE 25.1	Patterns of Injury
Predominant Reaction Pattern	*Examples of Diseases*
Interstitial inflammation and fibrosis	DIP, UIP, NSIP, DAD, eosinophilic granuloma, asbestosis, amyloidosis, sarcoidosis, hypersensitivity pneumonitis
Intra-alveolar reaction	DIP, pulmonary alveolar proteinosis, infections, hypersensitivity pneumonitis, chronic eosinophilic pneumonia[a]
Small-airway disease	Constrictive bronchiolitis, respiratory bronchiolitis, follicular bronchiolitis, cellular bronchiolitis, diffuse pan-bronchiolitis, peribronchiolar metaplasia (Lambertosis), mycoplasma and viral infection, hypersensitivity pneumonitis, eosinophilic pneumonia[a]
Large-airway disease	Allergic bronchopulmonary aspergillosis, bronchocentric granulomatosis, tuberculosis,[a] fungi,[a] Wegener granulomatosis[a]
Vasculitis with granulomatosis	Wegener granulomatosis,[a] necrotizing sarcoidal granulomatosis,[a] Churg-Strauss syndrome,[a] bronchocentric granulomatosis,[a] tuberculosis[a]
Small-vessel disease	Primary pulmonary hypertension, thromboembolic disease, polyarteritis nodosa, veno-occlusive disease,[a] Churg-Strauss syndrome, microscopic polyangiitis[a]
Hemorrhage	Goodpasture[a] syndrome, SLE, immune complex glomerulonephritis, idiopathic pulmonary hemosiderosis, Wegener granulomatosis, microscopic polyangiitis[a]
Lymphoreticular infiltrates	Lymphocytic interstitial pneumonia,[a] pseudolymphoma, malignant lymphoma,[a] hypersensitivity pneumonitis
Pulmonary eosinophilia	Chronic eosinophilic pneumonia,[a] Churg-Strauss syndrome,[a] bronchocentric granulomatosis[a]

[a]May have sarcoid-like granulomas.
DAD, diffuse alveolar damage; DIP, desquamative interstitial pneumonia; SLE, systemic lupus erythematosus; UIP, usual interstitial pneumonia; NSIP, nonspecific interstitial pneumonia; RB-ILD, respiratory bronchiolitis-interstitial lung disease.

In most instances, however, the pathologist's most important diagnostic tool is well-prepared paraffin sections stained with good-quality hematoxylin and eosin (H&E), trichrome, and elastic tissue stains, correlated with thorough knowledge of the clinical and laboratory findings, the radiographic studies, and CT scans. The following discussion generally follows the histologic classification proposed by the American Thoracic and European Respiratory Societies for the interstitial pneumonia (9)

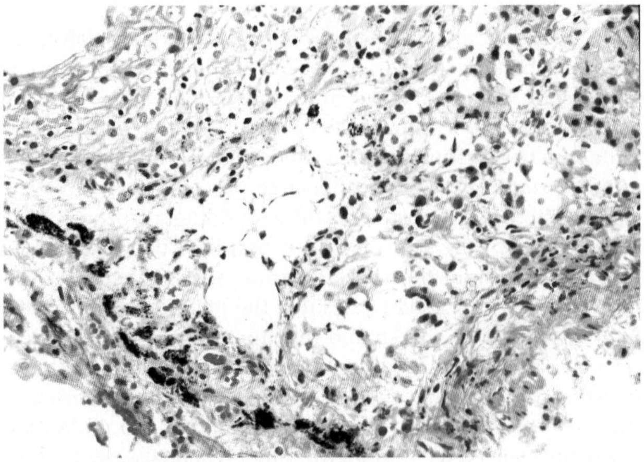

Figure 25.1. Transbronchial lung biopsy showing commonly seen "bubble artifact" resulting from the effects of tissue manipulation. Absence of histiocytes and alveolar cell hyperplasia rules out lipid pneumonia.

(Table 25.2). This classification emphasizes the close liaison necessary between the pathologist and clinical specialists to arrive at an accurate clinical diagnosis.

DIFFUSE INTERSTITIAL PULMONARY FIBROSIS

Diffuse interstitial inflammation and fibrosis is a common reaction to many injurious agents; therefore, each case presents its own diagnostic riddle. Microscopic clues about possible etiology are generally lacking. Complete details about potential etiologic factors such as drug administration, work or environmental exposure, family history, or other associated diseases must always be obtained because they might define each individual case with a specific cause. Broad disease categories, as well as diseases associated with interstitial fibrosis, are listed in Table 25.3. UIP is perhaps the most common condition encountered in biopsies for diffuse interstitial pulmonary fibrosis (10,11). Most often, the etiology is unknown; however, in approximately 40% of cases the onset is heralded by a viral-like illness, although a viral etiology has been elusive. In many cases, low titers of serum antinuclear antibodies (ANAs) or rheumatoid factors are encountered, which are suggestive of an underlying subclinical collagen disease diathesis (9). Cigarette smoking has been shown to be a risk factor (12,13), as has exposure to wood and metal dust (14).

Clinically, UIP most commonly affects patients in middle to old age. The gradual onset of exertional dyspnea, which usually occurs insidiously over months or years, is the cardinal feature

---

TABLE 25.2	Histologic and Clinical Classification of Idiopathic Interstitial Pneumonias[a]
Histologic Patterns	*Clinical-Radiologic-Pathologic Diagnosis*
Usual interstitial pneumonia	Idiopathic pulmonary fibrosis/cryptogenic fibrosing alveolitis
Nonspecific interstitial pneumonia	Nonspecific interstitial pneumonia (provisional)[b]
Organizing pneumonia	Cryptogenic organizing pneumonia[c]
Diffuse alveolar damage	Acute interstitial pneumonia
Respiratory bronchiolitis	Respiratory bronchiolitis interstitial lung disease
Desquamative interstitial pneumonia	Desquamative interstitial pneumonia
Lymphoid interstitial pneumonia	Lymphoid interstitial pneumonia

[a]Unclassifiable interstitial pneumonia: some cases are unclassifiable for a variety of reasons.
[b]This group represents a heterogeneous group with poorly characterized clinical and radiologic features that need further study.
[c]COP is the preferred term, but it is synonymous with idiopathic BOOP.

of the disease. This slowly progressive clinical course is an important feature that immediately separates UIP from more acute causes of diffuse interstitial lung disease. Physiologically, the earliest change is a reduction in diffusing capacity that occurs at first only with exercise, but later at rest also. However, impaired oxygen diffusion across the fibrotic alveolar septa accounts for only a small component of the arterial oxygen unsaturation. The major cause is alteration in the ventilation perfusion relationship that stems from the ventilation of underperfused lung tissue as a result of capillary destruction, and perfusion of underventilated alveoli that is brought about by the profound structural alteration of the lung architecture. Early in the disease, airway function is normal; however, as interstitial fibrosis progresses, obstructive abnormality of the small airways may be present because of peribronchiolar fibrosis. Lung volumes are normal early in the course but with progressive fibrosis the lung volume becomes diminished (15).

Radiologically, a diffuse bilateral pattern of interstitial abnormality that is most prominent in the lower lung fields is characteristic but not specific (16). Mid- and upper-zone involvement alone or in varying combinations also occurs. As the condition worsens, progressive fibrosis is associated with (a) shrinkage of the lungs with elevation of the diaphragm, and (b) progressive radiographic evidence of "honeycomb lung." High-resolution computed tomography (CT) scans show ground-glass opacities, traction bronchiectasis, and subpleural honeycomb changes (17).

The histologic hallmark of UIP is the finding of irregularly distributed areas of interstitial fibrosis with active fibroblastic proliferation that alternate with near-normal lung and advanced cystic honeycombing (Fig. 25.2). The mildest histologic changes are characterized by a modest interstitial infiltrate of lymphocytes and plasma cells, which is accompanied by accumulations of mononuclear histiocytes and lymphocytes within the alveolar space. The alveolar lining cells undergo hyperplasia and they may become prominent. As the condition progresses, interstitial fibrosis becomes increasingly more severe, whereas chronic inflammatory cells diminish. Characteristically, inflammation is only a minor component of the process. A pronounced alteration of the pulmonary architecture with dilation of the alveolar ducts and alveoli, diminished pulmonary capillaries, and marked interstitial fibrosis occurs over time (18–21). Hyperplastic smooth muscle proliferates around terminal bronchioles, becoming insinuated within the peribronchial interstitium and alveolar wall that is formed from indigenous myofibroblasts (Fig. 25.3) (22). This is a compensatory mechanism for overcoming increased lung stiffness (decreased compliance). Extreme examples have been termed *muscular cirrhosis* (23).

As fibrosis progresses and the capillary bed is gradually destroyed, pulmonary arteries and arterioles undergo medial hypertrophy; physiologically, this is reflected by pulmonary hypertension (Fig. 25.4) (21). On low-power microscopy, the process seems to progress at different rates in different areas. Zones of end-stage fibrosis alternate with areas of interstitial inflamma-

TABLE 25.3	Lung Disease Associated with Diffuse Interstitial Fibrosis
Category of Disease	*Examples*
Idiopathic pulmonary fibrosis	Usual interstitial pneumonia; nonspecific interstitial pneumonia
Smoking-related damage	Desquamative interstitial pneumonia; respiratory bronchiolitis-interstitial pneumonia
Diffuse alveolar damage	Radiation pneumonitis; chemotherapy; shock; viral pneumonia
Collagen vascular disease	Rheumatoid arthritis; lupus; scleroderma
Pneumoconiosis	Asbestosis
Granulomatous disease	Sarcoidosis; berylliosis
Hypersensitivity pneumonitis	Farmer's lung; bird fancier's lung; humidifier lung
Histiocytosis	Eosinophilic granuloma
Miscellaneous	Veno-occlusive disease; lymphoid interstitial pneumonia; neurofibromatosis; drugs

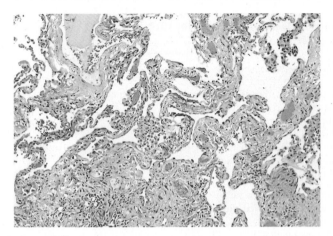

Figure 25.2. Usual interstitial pneumonia (UIP). Irregular distribution of interstitial fibrosis is seen on low-power magnification.

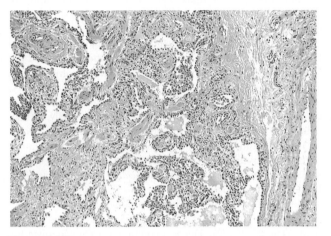

Figure 25.3. Usual interstitial pneumonia (UIP). Interstitial fibrosis is accompanied by dilatation of the alveolar ducts. Chronic inflammatory cells are present in the interstitium along with increased smooth muscle.

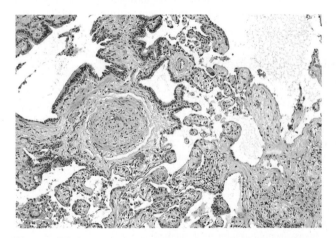

Figure 25.4. Usual interstitial pneumonia (UIP). Hyperplasia of pulmonary artery occurs in established chronic interstitial fibrosis.

tion. Focal areas of new cellular collagen formation are often seen apposed to fibrotic alveolar septae, which indicate areas of disease activity and reflect the progressive nature of the process (Fig. 25.5). These fibrogenic foci are the hallmark of active UIP; they result from damage to alveolar epithelium and basement membrane, resulting in organization of submicroscopic amounts of fibrin and the proliferation of fibroblasts and myofibroblasts (21,24). Qualitatively similar findings can be seen in other types of fibrosing lung diseases, such as hypersensitivity pneumonia (HP), eosinophilic granuloma (EG), and nonspecific interstitial pneumonia (NSIP), but usually not to the extent seen in UIP. Recently, focal areas that resemble eosinophilic pneumonia have been described (25).

The pathogenesis of UIP is largely unknown, but recent observations have led to the conclusion that inflammation per se may not be as important a factor as was previously thought. In fact, most cases show relatively little inflammation. Emphasis has now switched to the roles of alveolar lining cell damage and fibroblast-myofibroblastic proliferation that is modulated by a growing array of cytokines and growth factors in the production of interstitial fibrosis (25–33).

Alveolar lining cells have been shown to express numerous fibrogenic cytokines and growth factors, such as transforming growth factor-β, platelet-derived growth factor, tumor necrosis factor-α, endothelin-1, and connective tissue growth factor, among others. Injury and activation of these cells is believed to be pivotal in the pathogenesis of lung injury and interstitial fibrosis.

Another covalent mechanism is the induction of a procoagulant environment by the synthesis of plasminogen activator inhibitor-1 and tissue factor by alveolar epithelium, resulting in increased alveolar fibrin and inhibition of matrix metaloproteinase necessary for the breakdown of extracellular matrix. Increased activation of fibroblasts also occurs. In addition, the fibroblasts and myofibroblasts themselves provide an array of tissue metaloproteinase inhibitors that results in diminished breakdown of extracellular matrix proteins and thus contributes to the increased interstitial collagen seen in UIP (25–33). For now, this process is not completely understood and there is abundant ongoing investigation regarding pathogenesis.

Ultrastructurally, the normal population of alveolar type I cells is replaced by hyperplastic alveolar type II cells that line the alveolar surface. Polymorphonuclear leukocytes, lymphocytes, plasma cells, and macrophages occupy the interstitium, and the alveolar space is filled with degenerating macrophages, type II pneumocytes, and cellular debris (particularly free lamellar bodies, lipid, and small amounts of fibrin). Eventually, collagen and elastic fibers increase and the intra-alveolar and interstitial exudate decreases. These ultrastructural features are reflected in the progressive changes noted by light microscopy (34).

The prognosis of UIP is poor. The disease is slowly progressive and the average survival is about 4 to 5 years, although variation is seen among patients. Diminished survival is associated with older age, cigarette smoking, severe shortness of breath, decreased pulmonary function, severity of imaging studies, and greater numbers of fibroblastic foci (35–37). Some patients experience acute deterioration that correlates pathologically with the superimposition of acute lung injury qualitatively similar to diffuse alveolar damage (DAD), the so-called accelerated phase of UIP (38,39). Overall, only approximately 20% of patients have shown objective improvement with steroid treatment, but the lack of controlled pathologic studies makes analy-

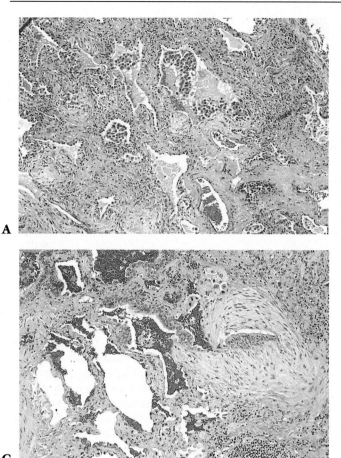

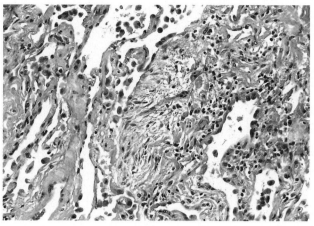

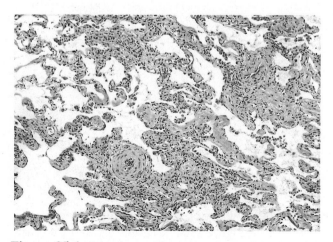

Figure 25.5. Usual interstitial pneumonia (UIP). **(A)** The area of active fibrogenesis (fibroblast foci) shows nodules of young collagen causing interstitial widening, and is associated with interstitial fibrosis. **(B)** A higher magnification of fibroblast focus shows the parallel alignment of fibroblasts to the axis of the alveolar septum. This is the hallmark of UIP. **(C)** Fibroblast foci involve the terminal bronchioles.

sis of retrospective series difficult. (21,35,36,38). Cyclophosphamide and other chemotherapeutic drugs have been used, as has colchicine in cases unresponsive to steroids (39). Interferons and newer drugs targeted against growth factors and fibroblasts and that encourage epithelial regeneration as well as several other novel genetic approaches are currently being investigated (31,40).

Pathologically, two collagen diseases may sometimes be associated with morphologic clues to etiology. In some patients with UIP associated with rheumatoid arthritis, prominent lymphoid nodules that are usually located around bronchioles may be seen (41). This finding, when combined with fibrinous pleuritis or bronchiolitis obliterans, may implicate rheumatoid disease.

Another condition is scleroderma, which, besides showing UIP, may also show lymphoid nodules or may be associated with mucinous changes or laminated fibrosis of the media in pulmonary arteries that appear out of proportion to the degree of interstitial fibrosis (Fig. 25.6) (42). These lung manifestations may sometimes precede the overt signs of collagen disease by several years.

The possibility of pneumoconiosis should always be considered in any otherwise cryptic case of UIP, and attempts to isolate asbestos and identify other minerals may be necessary (Fig. 25.7) (8). The pathologist should remember, however, that patients exposed to asbestos might also have pulmonary fibrosis that is caused by idiopathic UIP (43).

Adverse drug reaction should also be considered and a thorough drug history should be obtained in UIP patients as well

as in those having most other varieties of active or chronic lung injury (44).

Transbronchial lung biopsy is often nondiagnostic in cases of UIP. The problem of sample size and representation, as well as the inherently nonspecific nature of interstitial inflammation and fibrosis, always exists. Open or VATS biopsy has long been the gold standard for the diagnosis of most diffuse interstitial lung diseases (45). A recent study, however, suggests that the

Figure 25.6. Scleroderma. The pulmonary arteriole shows pronounced medial thickening. The lung parenchyma shows UIP.

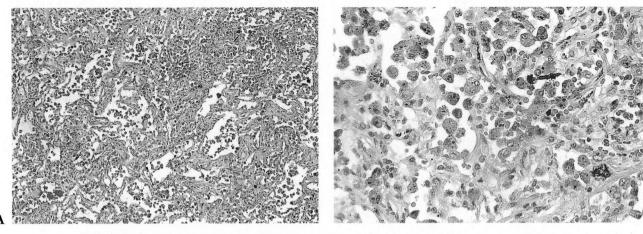

Figure 25.7. Asbestosis. **(A)** Severe diffuse fibrosis of interstitium is accompanied by collections of pigment-laden macrophages in the alveoli. The patient was suspected of having UIP. **(B)** A careful search of the sections revealed several asbestos bodies.

diagnosis of UIP can be confirmed by transbronchial biopsy in one-third of patients if adequate material is obtained (46).

NONSPECIFIC INTERSTITIAL PNEUMONIA

Katzenstein and Fiorelli and others have reported an important group of cases of diffuse interstitial lung disease with certain similarities to UIP but which nonetheless differ histologically and have a better prognosis (47–49). They termed these cases *nonspecific interstitial pneumonia,* or NSIP—an appellation that has been retained.

The central feature distinguishing NSIP from UIP is the uniformity of the pathologic process throughout the biopsy, compared with the variability of findings that characterizes UIP. In NSIP, the biopsy slide looks almost the same from end to end, whereas in UIP, areas of cystic honeycombing alternate with active fibroblastic foci and relatively normal lung.

NSIP has been described as having both a cellular and fibrotic phase. Cellular NSIP demonstrates mild to moderate diffuse interstitial inflammation that is composed predominantly of lymphocytes and plasma cells with little fibrosis (Fig. 25.8).

Fibrotic NSIP shows diffuse uniform interstitial fibrosis with much less inflammation. Both types reveal temporal uniformity under the microscope. Secondary changes such as epithelioid cell granulomas, lymphoid aggregates, isolated foci of organizing pneumonia, and rare fibroblastic foci identical to those of UIP have been observed. This latter feature, which helps define UIP, should only rarely be seen as isolated foci in NSIP.

Such varied findings have led to the speculation that NSIP most likely comprises a heterogeneous group of cases including HP, bronchiolitis obliterans with organizing pneumonia (BOOP), collagen diseases, drug reactions, or nonrepresentative sampling of UIP—each of which can show foci indistinguishable from NSIP (20). More recent series have alternatively suggested that NSIP is a specific entity with earlier age of onset, less advanced imaging studies, and without significant honeycomb change (50,51).

The prognosis of NSIP is much better than that of UIP. Fatalities are rare in cellular NSIP, whereas the mortality of patients with fibrotic NSIP is worse, up to 60%, which still has a much better prognosis than UIP (21,36,52).

Finally, acquired immune deficiency syndrome (AIDS) patients may demonstrate NSIP as a noninfectious cause of diffuse

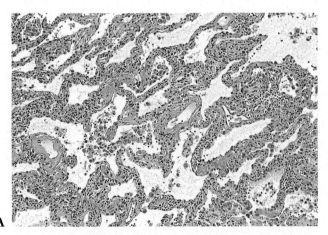

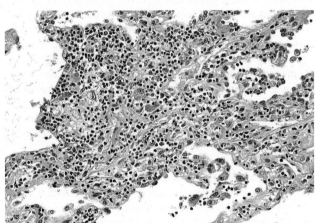

Figure 25.8. Nonspecific interstitial pneumonia, cellular phase. **(A)** Diffuse, uniform lymphocytic infiltration is present in the interstitium. **(B)** Lymphocytic infiltrates are accompanied by hyperplasia of alveolar type II cells and alveolar macrophages.

infiltrative lung disease. Therefore, a thorough investigation into the etiology of each case should be undertaken (52).

DESQUAMATIVE INTERSTITIAL PNEUMONIA

For many years, controversy existed regarding whether desquamative interstitial pneumonia (DIP) was an early phase of UIP or an entirely separate entity, with strong advocacy on both sides (53–55). Currently, most authorities believe that DIP evolves through a different mechanism than UIP and that it represents one phase in a spectrum of smoking-related diffuse lung disease characterized by the accumulation of pulmonary macrophages in the alveolar space (56,57).

Clinically, DIP occurs, on average, a decade earlier than UIP. A strong link to tobacco use exists; almost invariably, the patients are cigarette smokers. The precise mechanism of the disease is, however, unknown. The symptoms are characterized by the gradual onset of shortness of breath on exertion, and cough. Chest radiography and CT reveal bilateral ground-glass opacities that are concentrated in the lower lung fields. Peripheral areas of interstitial fibrosis occur in one-half of cases (58). In some cases, the chest radiograph appears normal.

The prognosis of DIP is much better than that for UIP. Most patients recover after smoking cessation, and steroids are effective for treatment. Only a few patients experience progression to significant interstitial fibrosis. In recent studies, the survival of patients without honeycombing was 100% (21,36).

Pathologically, the alveolar space is filled with mononuclear histiocytes that have eosinophilic cytoplasm along with smaller numbers of alveolar type II cells (Fig. 25.9). The cytoplasm of these cells may stain positively with periodic acid-Schiff (PAS) after diastase, and may contain finely dispersed brown pigment that stains with Prussian blue (55). Hyperplasia of alveolar type II cells along the alveolar membrane is present, and this may be a prominent feature. Scattered lymphocytes and plasma cells infiltrate the alveolar wall and accumulate among the intra-alveolar cells, together with rare polymorphonuclear leukocytes and eosinophils. Reactive lymphoid aggregates around the terminal bronchioles may be seen in some cases. The pathologic

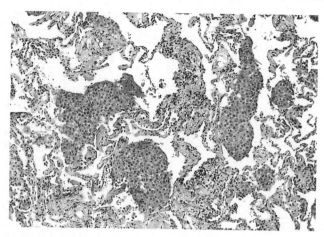

Figure 25.10. Desquamative interstitial pneumonia reaction adjacent to an area of hypersensitivity pneumonia.

changes are generally diffuse and uniform throughout the biopsy sample, but focal areas of interstitial fibrosis that are accompanied by a reciprocal decrease of the interstitial and intra-alveolar cells may be found. Unlike UIP, fibroblastic foci are not observed.

Ultrastructurally, most intra-alveolar cells seen in DIP are macrophages that are derived mostly from the bone marrow and, to a lesser extent, those of the pulmonary interstitium (56). The alveolar membrane in typical cases shows a slight increase of collagen, as well as increased numbers of lymphocytes and macrophages. Hyperplastic type II pneumocytes lining the alveoli are easily recognized by their prominent lamellar bodies, which contain surfactant. The alveolar space contains cellular debris and free lamellar bodies, and these may be phagocytosed by intra-alveolar macrophages.

It is important to recognize that DIP can also be a nonspecific reaction pattern of the lung in several other pulmonary conditions, and that a DIP-like pattern can be seen adjacent to areas that are otherwise diagnostic of such conditions as EG or HP (Fig. 25.10) (Table 25.4) (59). Foci that are histologically indistinguishable from DIP may also be seen in patients with asbesto-

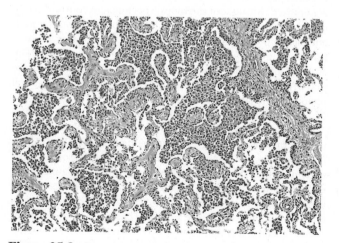

Figure 25.9. Desquamative interstitial pneumonia (DIP). The alveolar spaces are filled with macrophages, and mild chronic alveolitis is seen.

TABLE 25.4
Desquamative Interstitial Pneumonia and Similar Reactions
Specific lung diseases that can mimic idiopathic DIP
Collagen disease (i.e., rheumatoid arthritis, systemic lupus erythematosus)
Pneumoconiosis (caused by asbestos, tungsten carbide)
Drug reactions
Conditions having a DIP-like reaction associated with an independent primary disease
Eosinophilic granuloma
Hypersensitivity pneumonia
Chronic eosinophilic pneumonia
Lung tumors
Pulmonary alveolar proteinosis
Cigarette smoking (respiratory bronchiolitis)
DIP, desquamative interstitial pneumonia.

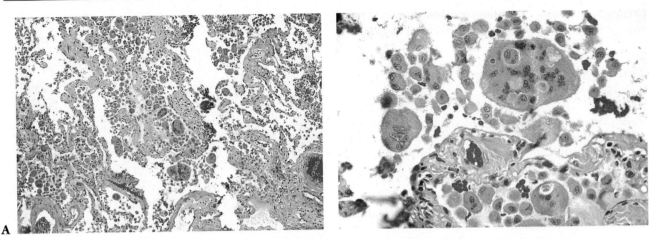

Figure 25.11. Giant-cell interstitial pneumonia. **(A)** Numerous multinucleated histiocytes in alveolar space are surrounded by diffuse interstitial fibrosis. **(B)** Some giant cells are phagocytosing mononuclear histiocytes, a characteristic feature.

sis, in aluminum workers, in those with drug reactions, or in patients with cobalt pneumoconiosis (60–62). In patients with industrial exposure to hard metals, diffuse interstitial lung disease that is characterized by large numbers of intra-alveolar macrophages, similar to those seen in DIP, may develop, but it is accompanied by multinucleated giant cells that phagocytose other histiocytes. This *giant-cell interstitial pneumonia* is extremely rare, and some consider it a specific response to hard metal exposure (Fig. 25.11) (63).

DIFFUSE ALVEOLAR DAMAGE

Diffuse alveolar damage (DAD) is an acute exudative interstitial pulmonary reaction resulting from many different etiologies (Table 25.5) (64–66). In some patients, the cause may be multifactorial, with several factors acting either simultaneously or consecutively—particularly mechanical ventilation with high O_2 concentration (67). DAD is the pathologic counterpart of the adult respiratory distress syndrome.

Clinically, the onset of symptoms is abrupt, generally occurring over 1 or 2 days and consisting of severe dyspnea that is accompanied by fever and cough, in contrast to the slow, insidi-

ous evolution of UIP. This is an important clinical feature that helps to separate DAD from more chronic fibrosing lung diseases. Radiographically, the condition is almost always bilateral and diffuse, and often has the appearance of pulmonary edema (68).

The histologic pattern is characterized by an early exudative phase and a later organizing phase. As DAD progresses to organization, more nodular or confluent radiographic densities are found, reflecting this stage of evolution. The early reaction shows protein-rich edema in the alveolar space, with fibrin-rich eosinophilic hyaline membranes along the surface of the alveolar septa (Fig. 25.12). This exudative reaction is not seen in UIP except as a superimposed, usually terminal event that coincides with rapid clinical deterioration often referred to as the accelerated phase of UIP (38,39). Accompanying the exudate and swelling there is hyperplasia of alveolar type II cells, which often show increased nuclear size and hyperchromasia and which thus may appear atypical. The degree of epithelial hyperplasia is much greater than that of UIP. The alveolar septa show varying amounts of interstitial edema that is usually accompanied by scant numbers of lymphocytes, plasma cells, and a few polymorphonuclear leukocytes. The tissue reaction of DAD is mostly generalized throughout the biopsy specimen, in contrast to UIP in which it is patchier. Intra-alveolar hemorrhage may be present focally but is generally not severe. Thrombi may be seen within pulmonary capillaries, arterioles, and arteries (Fig. 25.13). Large numbers of acute inflammatory cells may indicate that DAD is superimposed on another process, such as bacterial pneumonia or alveolar capillaritis (69).

In lesions of 1 to several weeks' duration, a phase of organization may ensue that can result in complete resolution of the process or that may progress to interstitial fibrosis (Fig. 25.14). Histologically, the picture is usually uniform, but some biopsy specimens may show a mixed pattern of acute exudation along with areas of organization indicative of repeated bouts of lung injury. Squamous metaplasia due to terminal bronchiolar injury often accompanies the more advanced changes. This sometimes may be mistaken for malignancy. Fibrosis results from the incorporation of proteinaceous exudates by the apposition of newly formed collagen onto the preexisting alveolar framework. Collagen synthesis within the alveolar septal membrane also occurs

TABLE 25.5

Causes of Diffuse Alveolar Damage

Etiology	Examples of Disease
Infections	Virus, *Pneumocystis carinii*
Trauma	Smoke inhalation; blast injury
Drugs, toxins	Chemotherapy; paraquat, amiodarone
Oxygen toxicity	Respirator lung
Shock	Septic; hemorrhagic; other causes
Radiation therapy	Radiation pneumonitis
Collagen disease	Acute lupus pneumonitis
Unknown	Acute interstitial pneumonia; idiopathic diffuse alveolar damage
Miscellaneous	Cardiopulmonary bypass; near-drowning; uremia; others

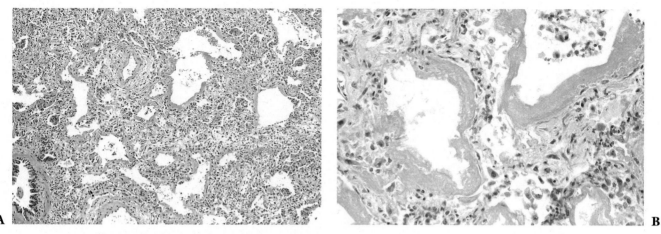

Figure 25.12. Diffuse alveolar damage (DAD). **(A)** The acute exudative phase showing protein-rich hyaline membranes, interstitial edema, and inflammation. The process is uniform throughout the biopsy. **(B)** Higher magnification demonstrates the hyalin membranes in acute DAD.

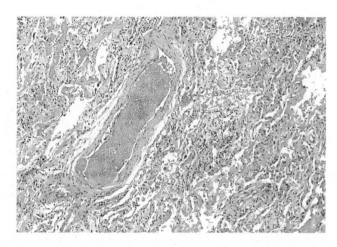

Figure 25.13. Diffuse alveolar damage (DAD). Intra-arterial thrombosis is a common feature.

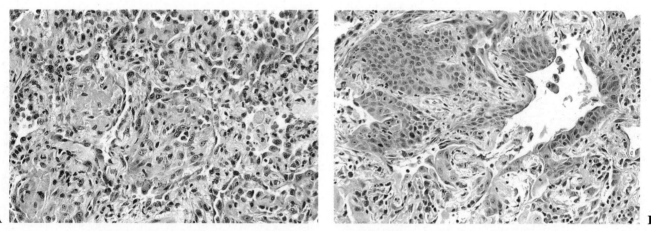

Figure 25.14. Diffuse alveolar damage (DAD). **(A)** The organizing phase showing protein-rich intra-alveolar edema and fibrous organization of the intra-alveolar exudates. The residual alveoli are compressed to slitlike spaces lined by hyperplastic alveolar lining cells that overlie the organizing foci. **(B)** Squamous metaplasia is common in organizing phase of DAD.

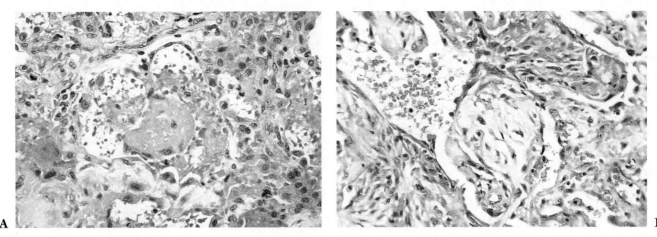

A   B

Figure 25.15. Diffuse alveolar damage (DAD). **(A)** Proteinaceous exudates showing apposition to the markedly edematous interstitium. The exudates are infiltrated by inflammatory cells and are covered by a layer of epithelial cells. **(B)** In the later phase of organization, macrophages and fibroblasts are seen within the newly formed collagen of intra-alveolar exudates. The epithelial covering is more prominent. This may resolve with restitution of normal lung architecture, or it may be incorporated into the alveolar septum, resulting in interstitial fibrosis.

(Fig. 25.15). In addition, fibrosis may also result from so-called collapse induration that is caused by nonexpansion of the alveolar space that is secondary to the loss of pulmonary surfactant and the direct apposition of damaged alveolar septa without the restitution of normal architecture (70,71). Interstitial fibrosis may occur rapidly over a period of several days, or it may progress slowly over several months. Rapidly evolving DAD, which is usually seen in young, previously healthy adults and which has no known etiology, has been termed *acute interstitial pneumonia* (AIP); it is directly analogous to the Hamman-Rich syndrome first reported in the 1940s (Fig. 25.16) (72–74). This disease is fulminant and progressive, and the mortality rate is high. AIP may progress to diffuse fibrosis, and survivors can have persistent abnormalities of pulmonary function (75).

Alveolar ducts are commonly involved in all stages of the evolution of DAD, which is characterized morphologically by rounded organizing plugs of exudate in the terminal bronchioles that can be confused with bronchiolitis obliterans. When fibrosis is established, the alveolar septa are densely fibrotic,

and the late changes are difficult to differentiate from other causes of diffuse interstitial pulmonary fibrosis. However, residual hyperplasia and atypia of alveolar lining cells and remnants of hyaline membranes may be a clue to preexisting DAD (Fig. 25.17).

Unlike UIP, which is chronic and progressive over several years, DAD may fully resolve either in the acute, protein-rich phase or even after biopsy shows organization and fibrosis (76). Death occurs in roughly 40% to 50% of cases, usually after several weeks or months (76). Those patients who recover may show little, if any, residual pulmonary functional disability (75,76). Some patients, however, may show persistent radiographic abnormalities with residual functional impairment (76). In summary, most patients with DAD either die or improve over a relatively short period of time, whereas patients with UIP generally run a much more protracted clinical course with little or no improvement in pulmonary function.

The specific etiology of DAD may be obvious (e.g., near-

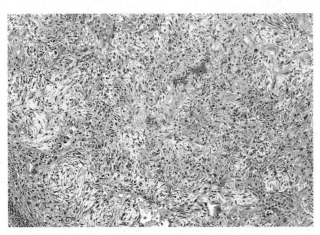

Figure 25.16. Acute interstitial pneumonia. The organizing phase of DAD is most often observed.

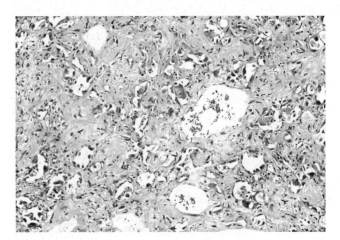

Figure 25.17. Diffuse alveolar damage (DAD). The fibrotic phase shows marked hyperplasia and atypia of alveolar lining cells. This has been busulfan-induced.

drowning; subsequent to cardiopulmonary bypass; following radiation therapy; or after drug therapy, such as with chemotherapeutic agents or amiodarone (77). In many cases, the cause is unknown, as in AIP. Regardless of the inciting cause, a sequence of events that is the result of a complex interplay among the damaging effects of leukocyte enzymes, the inactivation of pulmonary repair mechanisms (α_1-antitrypsin), the depletion of surfactant, the activation of blood coagulation factors, and fibrinolysis result in damage to the endothelial cell basement membrane and alveolar type I cells (76). Basement membrane and endothelial injuries are responsible for the protein-rich hyaline membranes and edema that typify the pattern of DAD. The roles of tumor necrosis factor, interleukins, and other cytokines have been postulated in the pathogenesis of this condition (23,76). The process is reversible but may result in death from (a) impairment of gas exchange through fluid exudates in the early stages or (b) organization and fibrosis.

Many cases require assisted ventilation with high concentrations of oxygen to maintain respiratory function, which may itself induce similar histologic changes. The degree of clinical hypoxemia is related to the prognosis (75).

Secondary bacterial infections resulting from colonization of the protein-rich exudates may alter the clinical course and pathologic findings in some cases. On the other hand, in immunocompromised patients, organisms such as cytomegalovirus (CMV) and *P. carinii* may directly produce a DAD pattern of injury (78). At the ultrastructural level, similarities exist between UIP and DAD that may indicate quantitative differences in the intensity of injury rather than separate pathogenic mechanisms (23,55).

Severe acute respiratory syndrome (SARS) is a particularly virulent form of viral lung infection caused by coronavirus (79). The microscopic pattern is DAD. The disease was first reported in China in 2002 (79), but soon spread throughout Asia and elsewhere. The virus is highly contagious and mortality rates are high. It attacks many epithelial organs, primarily the lung and GI tract, but also renal tubules, heart, liver, nerves, and cells of the immune system (80–82). It can be identified in tissue by polymerase chain reaction (PCR) or in situ hybridization (80–82).

Patients characteristically have severe myalgia, chills, and fever with acute respiratory distress syndrome with or without watery diarrhea. Autopsy has shown the dominant pulmonary changes are acute or organizing DAD (80–82). Recently described outbreaks seem to have abated, fortunately.

HYPERSENSITIVITY PNEUMONIA (EXTRINSIC ALLERGIC ALVEOLITIS)

Hypersensitivity pneumonitis (HP) is the pulmonary manifestation of hypersensitivity to several categories of inhaled antigens from various plant sources, such as moldy hay, grain, sugar cane, bark, cheese, or even cork dust. Animal proteins from the feces of pigeons or parakeets or from the feathers of turkeys or ducks have also been implicated, and certain drugs may also produce this reaction (Table 25.6) (83). In some cases, the offending antigen is not uncovered and the disease is recognized by the characteristic histologic changes. The varying types of exposure are reflected in the numerous names given to patients with HP, including bird-fancier's lung, farmer's lung, maple bark-stripper's lung, humidifier lung, and others.

TABLE 25.6

Causes of Hypersensitivity Pneumonia

Etiology	Example of Disease
Thermophilic actinomycetes	Farmer's lung; grain-handler's lung; humidifier lung; air-conditioner lung; mushroom-worker's lung; bagassosis
Saprophytic fungal spores	Maple-bark-stripper's lung; malt-worker's lung; sequoiosis; cheese-worker's lung; suberosis
Animal and bird proteins	Bird-fancier's lung; chicken-handler's lung; turkey-handler's lung; rodent-handler's lung; duck fever; pituitary snuff-taker's lung
Drugs	Methotrexate
Unknown antigens	

The disease is immunologically mediated by the combined effects of circulating immune complexes and the cell-mediated immunity to the inhaled antigens. Most of the lymphocytes in the tissue reaction are CD3-positive, CD8-positive T-suppressor cells derived from both the lung and the peripheral blood (83,84). The pathogenesis is not fully understood but appears to be related to repeated antigenic exposure, which stimulates chemotaxis and sensitizes T lymphocytes and macrophages, resulting in granuloma formation. Immune complexes result in the fixation of complement to the tissues and the subsequent inflammation. The end result is the elaboration of growth factors that stimulate fibroblasts to produce collagen (83–85). This mechanism of fibrosis is thought to differ from that of UIP (24–30).

In sensitized individuals exposed to a large challenge, an acute febrile illness is marked by the abrupt onset of dyspnea and cough; chest pain develops within 4 to 6 hours. This acute hypersensitivity reaction usually resolves spontaneously without sequelae after the offending agent is withdrawn. Few lung biopsy samples have been examined from this acute reaction (86).

However, chronic insidious exposure to low levels of sensitizing antigen may lead to diffuse interstitial lung disease, which, in some cases, may progress to interstitial fibrosis and honeycomb lung. The histologic pattern and variability of HP is important to recognize because clinical suspicion may be low in some patients. The correct interpretation of lung biopsy material can lead to the identification of the inciting antigenic agent and the prevention of progressive lung disease.

The inflammatory process is concentrated around small airways, and it affects the interstitium, the alveolar space, and the bronchioles in an uneven distribution in the lung biopsy sample (2,87,88). Thus, focal areas may show patchy interstitial pneumonia along with areas of more confluent, solid inflammatory infiltration that alternates with relatively spared areas (Fig. 25.18). Poorly circumscribed epithelioid granulomas containing multinucleated histiocytes are often, but not invariably, present in biopsy material (Fig. 25.19). These are usually distributed preferentially around distal airways, in the interstitium, and within alveolar spaces. The interstitial infiltrate is composed predominantly of lymphocytes and plasma cells, along with fewer numbers of polymorphonuclear leukocytes and rare eosinophils. Histiocytes with pink or foamy clear cytoplasm may

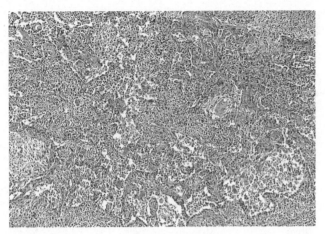

Figure 25.18. Hypersensitivity pneumonia. The solid zone of inflammation showing chronic inflammatory infiltrates that impart the appearance of an organizing lymphocytic-rich pneumonia. Note the presence of isolated multinucleated giant cells.

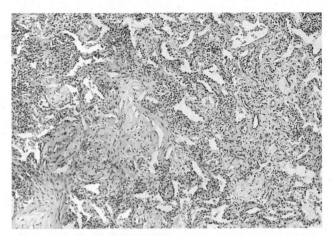

Figure 25.20. Bronchiolitis obliterans in hypersensitivity pneumonia. This patient was a pigeon breeder.

be seen in small clusters within the interstitium, the presence of which is sometimes an important diagnostic clue. Nodules of organizing fibroblasts, histiocytes, and inflammatory cells are often seen within the lumen of distal airways, resulting in bronchiolitis obliterans. This may dominate the histologic pattern in some cases and may obscure the other features (Fig. 25.20). Interstitial fibrosis is usually minimal. Trapped cellular debris is

often transformed into collections of foam cells and cholesterol clefts in the distal airways and alveoli secondary to bronchiolar obstruction. Thus, the combination of chronic interstitial inflammation, poorly formed epithelioid granulomas (often related to bronchioles), and bronchiolitis obliterans make up the characteristic diagnostic features.

Intra-alveolar edema and proteinaceous exudates are generally inconspicuous. This gives the overall histologic pattern a dry, cellular appearance rather than an exudative one. Varying

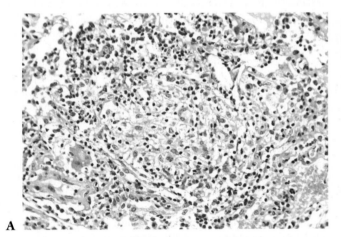

A

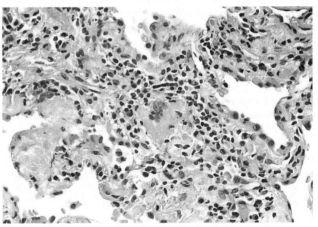

B

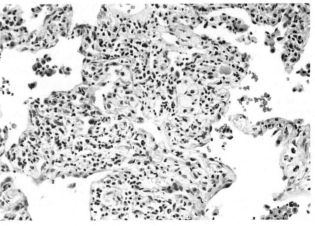

C

Figure 25.19. Hypersensitivity pneumonia. **(A)** These poorly formed interstitial granulomas can be seen in approximately 30% of cases. **(B)** This multinucleated giant cell is found in widened interstitium. Note chronic inflammatory cells and hyperplasia of alveolar lining cells. **(C)** Interstitial foam cells are also present.

degrees of interstitial and peribronchiolar fibrosis resulting from organization of bronchiolitis obliterans and interstitial inflammation may occur, depending on the age of the process. A review of the ultrastructural features of this disease has been published (89).

The symptoms usually consist of fever, cough, malaise, and shortness of breath. The chest x-ray findings usually show diffuse, bilateral, interstitial infiltrates. A diffuse, patchy, reticular pattern may be present on the CT scan (90). The pulmonary function tests characteristically reflect diffusing impairment, restrictive lung disease, and small-airway obstruction, which results from the interstitial inflammation, fibrosis, and bronchiolitis obliterans.

Precipitating serum immunoglobulin G (IgG) antibodies to the offending agent are usually present; together with the history of exposure and pathologic findings; these are extremely useful in diagnosis (76,79). However, precipitating antibodies by themselves are not diagnostic of HP because many people are sensitized to a variety of agents yet they never develop lung disease (91). Thus, the presence of the antibodies cannot be used as an absolute criterion for diagnosis without other accompanying features. On the other hand, the absence of precipitating antibodies may suggest a different disease process. Patients with HP may have inherent differences in their immunologic response to inhaled antigens, compared to that of sensitized individuals without disease (92).

The diagnosis of HP is greatly aided by thorough clinical–pathologic correlation. Even transbronchial biopsy, which usually shows an incomplete histologic picture, can be of value in the appropriate clinical and radiographic setting. The prognosis generally is good and the disease may respond well to steroid treatment (83,86,87). Nevertheless, the best treatment is the identification of the offending antigen and the removal of the agent from the patient's environment. Some patients, particularly bird fanciers, have repeated bouts of antigenic exposure that result in chronic pulmonary impairment and honeycomb lung (2).

Another condition caused by the toxic effects of large doses of inhaled organic dusts, which is usually seen after the unloading of grain silos, is *pulmonary mycotoxicosis* (or *organic dust syndrome*) (93,94). Unlike HP, this condition is not mediated by hypersensitivity but presumably by a direct effect on the lungs, causing acute bronchopneumonia with polymorphonuclear cells, DIP, or DAD, which may progress to organization (93,94). Numerous fungal organisms can be seen histologically, and cultures have shown a mixed variety of fungi, including *Fusarium* and *Penicillium*. Complete recovery is the rule. The disease is separate from *silo-filler's disease*, which is seen in patients after they have filled grain silos; it is caused by the toxic effect of oxides of nitrogen, producing acute bronchiolitis obliterans (95,96).

HONEYCOMB LUNG

Honeycomb lung is the final common pathway of the many different diseases that progress to chronic interstitial fibrosis. The patients usually have a long history of progressively worsening dyspnea and chest radiograph findings. Radiographs and CT scans show severe interstitial fibrosis, diffuse cystic changes with bleb formation, and shrunken lungs with elevation of the diaphragm (97). Pulmonary function shows severe restrictive lung disease, diffusion impairment, small lung volumes, and small-airway disease secondary to peribronchial fibrosis.

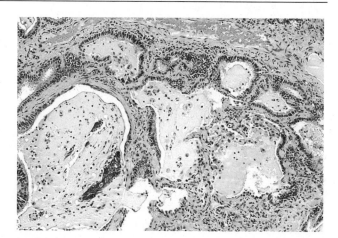

Figure 25.21. Honeycomb lung. Marked interstitial fibrosis and cystic transformation of the pulmonary parenchyma are seen with bronchial-type metaplasia and retained mucus in the nonfunctioning distal airspaces.

Pathologically, the lungs are spongy, stiff, and fibrotic, with readily discernible cystic changes that are apparent to the naked eye on gross inspection of open lung biopsy material (98). Microscopically, dense interstitial and peribronchial scarring is seen along with diminished or absent alveolar capillaries, marked medial hyperplasia of pulmonary arteries and arterioles, and increased peribronchial and interstitial smooth muscle. Loss of surface area for gas exchange is reflected in cystic dilation of alveolar ducts and alveoli with subsequent loss of alveolar membrane surface (Fig. 25.21). This profound restructuring results in diffuse cystic transformation and metaplasia of the alveolar lining to mucinous or columnar epithelium, which often shows cytologic atypia. Such patients are at increased risk of development of adenocarcinoma of the lung (65). The terminal bronchi and dilated alveoli may contain abundant mucus and acute inflammatory cells. Precise characterization of the underlying lung disease may be impossible, unless (a) previous biopsy material is available or (b) less advanced histologic changes are present in other areas of the biopsy.

PULMONARY EOSINOPHILIC REACTIONS

The pulmonary eosinophilias are presumed hypersensitivity reactions that are characterized by tissue and blood eosinophilia. The inciting agents are most commonly fungi, parasites, or drugs, or they may be unknown (99). Several related clinical syndromes are observed. These are Löffler syndrome, tropical eosinophilia, acute eosinophilic pneumonia, chronic eosinophilic pneumonia (CEP), allergic bronchopulmonary aspergillosis (ABPA), and bronchocentric granulomatosis (BCG) (100,101).

Löffler syndrome is a transient febrile illness marked by (a) evanescent diffuse pulmonary infiltrates, and (b) blood eosinophilia that runs a short, self-limiting course. Lung biopsy usually is not necessary for diagnosis, and relatively few examples have been seen (Fig. 25.22).

Tropical eosinophilia is a result of the circulating microfilaria of *Wuchereria bancrofti*, which circulate through the pulmonary capillaries and cause an immediate type of eosinophil-rich

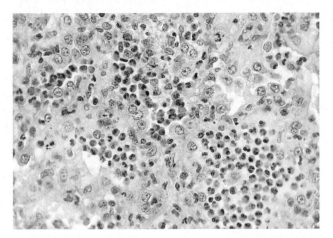

Figure 25.22. Löffler syndrome. This patient had diffuse bilateral interstitial infiltrates on chest radiograph, blood eosinophilia, and fever. The alveoli are heavily infiltrated by eosinophils and macrophages.

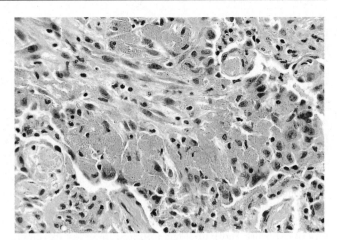

Figure 25.24. Chronic eosinophilic pneumonia. Note the organizing proteinaceous intra-alveolar exudate.

hypersensitivity reaction. The disease is rarely seen outside of tropical regions. Lung biopsy may show rare microfilaria within the pulmonary capillaries that is associated with acute and chronic eosinophilic pneumonia, but, often, no organisms are seen (102).

Acute eosinophilic pneumonia is rare. The rapid onset of fever, chills, and diffuse lung infiltrates is observed. Interestingly, blood eosinophilia is unusual. The histologic picture combines features of DAD and tissue eosinophilia. The condition responds well to steroids (103,104).

CHRONIC EOSINOPHILIC PNEUMONIA

Chronic eosinophilic pneumonia (CEP) is generally a reaction to drugs or fungi, most often *Aspergillus,* and it is characterized by a prolonged febrile illness accompanied by cough, weight loss, and generalized disability (105,106). Many patients have a history of chronic asthma. Peripheral blood eosinophilia is common but is not seen in all cases. Chest radiography and CT reveal a pattern of bilateral patchy infiltrates that is more pronounced in the peripheral portions of the lung, with relative sparing of the central hilar zones (the so-called photographic

negative of pulmonary edema) (105,106). This characteristic pattern, however, is not always observed, and sometimes a peripherally located patchy process with a tendency to wax and wane in sequential chest radiographs is observed.

Histologically, the tissue reaction is patchy and exudative, and has the appearance of pneumonic consolidation with a pronounced intra-alveolar and terminal bronchiolar pattern of involvement (Fig. 25.23) (107). Distal bronchi and bronchioles may be distended by a thick mucus that may contain cellular debris or intact polymorphonuclear cells, eosinophils, and sometimes Charcot-Leyden crystals.

The intra-alveolar exudate is composed of prominent numbers of eosinophils, lymphocytes, plasma cells, and macrophages, as well as proteinaceous exudates and edema fluid in many cases (Fig. 25.24). Focal necrosis of the cellular exudate may be seen, along with collections of granular eosinophilic debris in instances where the eosinophils predominate. The interstitium is widened by eosinophils, plasma cells, and lymphocytes. Paradoxically, eosinophils may be relatively sparse in some cases, which possibly is a reflection of chronicity, fluctuations in the intensity of the immunologic reaction, or the effects of steroids.

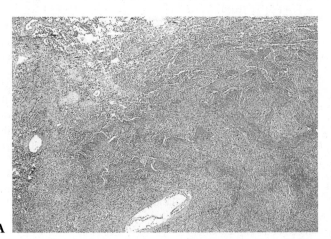

A   B

Figure 25.23. Chronic eosinophilic pneumonia. **(A)** Protein-rich intra-alveolar edema gives the lesion an exudative appearance. **(B)** The intra-alveolar and interstitial pattern of involvement is composed of isolated giant cells, chronic inflammatory cells, and eosinophils.

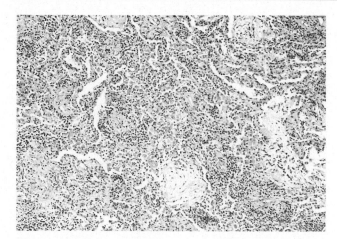

Figure 25.25. Bronchiolitis obliterans in chronic eosinophilic pneumonia. Moderate numbers of eosinophils are present within the organizing bronchiolar exudate.

Bronchiolitis obliterans is commonly present in CEP (Fig. 25.25). In occasional cases, poorly formed epithelioid granulomas may also be found within alveolar exudates, around blood vessels, or within the interstitium. The blood vessels may be infiltrated by inflammatory cells, including eosinophils, giving the impression of vasculitis; however, vascular necrosis is not observed (Fig. 25.26).

In some cases, intra-alveolar macrophages may be numerous around patchy foci of CEP; in such cases, differentiation from DIP may be challenging, particularly with small biopsy material. Attention to the history of atopy, laboratory findings of blood eosinophilia, and the chest radiograph minimize the risk of error. EG may sometimes cause diagnostic difficulty but, unlike CEP, the infiltrate is mainly interstitial and is composed of characteristic Langerhans cells. Diagnostic areas of EG may be few or scattered, however, so they may be missed by transbronchial biopsy. In some cases of CEP where the numbers of eosinophils may not be prominent, diagnostic confusion with chronic infectious pneumonias, HP, BOOP, or small-airway disease may also be a problem. Histologically, HP usually shows more of an interstitial pattern of involvement and less intra-alveolar edema than does CEP. Quite often, HP appears predominantly lymphoplas-

macytic, whereas CEP looks more exudative and edematous. An asthmatic history, as well as tissue and blood eosinophilia, is unusual in HP. All patients with CEP should be investigated for parasites and fungal allergy. A complete drug history should be obtained. The condition usually responds dramatically to steroid therapy, most often with complete resolution of the disease; however, 20% to 30% of patients may relapse (100).

ALLERGIC BRONCHOPULMONARY ASPERGILLOSIS

Allergic bronchopulmonary aspergillosis (ABPA) is caused by hypersensitivity to noninvasive *Aspergillus* organisms (or other fungi) that occupy the lumen of bronchi, usually in mucus or within mucous plugs (102). Clinically, asthma, blood eosinophilia, wheezing, cough, and sometimes hemoptysis are common findings (108). ABPA is a common condition in which the radiographic and pathologic features of CEP may be seen. Microscopically, in addition to the findings of CEP that have already been described, the major bronchi may show thick, tenacious plugs of mucus, sloughing of bronchial epithelial cells, and degenerating cellular debris within the bronchial lumen (so-called allergin mucin). Rarely, fungal hyphae can be histologically detected within the mucous material with the aid of special stains. With chronicity, bronchiectasis may develop. The histologic changes of chronic asthmatic bronchitis with eosinophilic infiltration, thickened epithelial basement membrane, and mucous gland hyperplasia may also be seen. CEP often dominates the pathologic picture. Rarely, however, the biopsy may show changes that are almost entirely limited to the small bronchi and to peribronchial tissue (Fig. 25.27). In such cases, a careful search for viral inclusions in the bronchial epithelial cells is necessary to exclude viral bronchitis.

BRONCHOCENTRIC GRANULOMATOSIS

Bronchocentric granulomatosis (BCG) was originally thought to be part of the spectrum of pulmonary angiitis and granulomatosis, but it has come to be regarded as an immunologic reaction pathogenetically related to CEP and ABPA (109). Indeed, there is significant clinical, radiographic, and pathologic overlap with these other eosinophilic conditions. A history of asthma is fre-

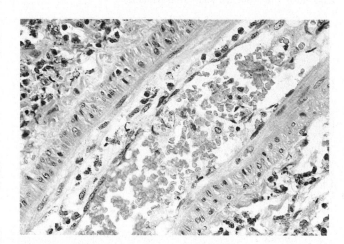

Figure 25.26. Chronic eosinophilic pneumonia. The subendothelial vascular infiltrate is composed of eosinophils.

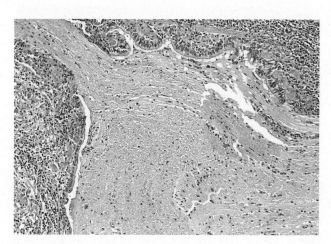

Figure 25.27. Allergic bronchopulmonary aspergillosis. The small bronchus shows hyperplasia and increased thick mucus. The bronchus is infiltrated by eosinophils and chronic inflammatory cells.

quently present, and most cases are due to hypersensitivity to *Aspergillus* or other fungi. In some instances, the cause is unknown. These patients commonly have cough, fever, and patchy consolidations on chest x-ray examination. Single or multiple tumor-like infiltrates in the upper lobes, as well as diffuse infiltrates or atelectasis, may also be seen. The symptoms are usually not severe, and some patients may be entirely asymptomatic. Since the initial reports, only an additional few cases have been recorded.

Pathologically, the lumens of large and medium-sized bronchi are heavily infiltrated by inflammatory cells, and the central necrosis of the exudate forms a granulomatous reaction that often obliterates the bronchial structure. This can best be observed at low-power magnification, in which the absence of bronchi next to the elastic pulmonary arteries is readily discernible (Fig. 25.28). Elastic stains are sometimes helpful in detecting the fragmented bronchial elastic tissue within the mass of inflammatory tissue adjacent to these blood vessels. Inflammation of the pulmonary arteries is usually of a minor degree and is suggestive of passive infiltration of the blood vessel rather than a true vasculitis. Fibrinoid necrosis of blood vessels is not seen, which is a helpful feature in distinguishing BCG from Wegener granulomatosis (WG).

The inflammatory infiltrate is composed predominantly of polymorphonuclear leukocytes, plasma cells, and lymphocytes; however, eosinophils may be abundant, especially in patients with a history of asthma who have fungal hypersensitivity. The center of the granulomatous inflammation is composed of granular necrotic debris, sometimes containing the remnants of eosinophils and other inflammatory cells. Rarely, isolated or degenerating fungal hyphae are present. The periphery of the granuloma shows palisaded histiocytes, sometimes with multinucleated giant cells, imparting the appearance of granulomatous infection (Fig. 25.29). In patients with tissue eosinophilia, the lung parenchyma often shows CEP adjacent to the granulomatous bronchocentric lesion (Fig. 25.30). In cases without eosinophilia, the inflammatory infiltrate has the appearance of nonspecific chronic pneumonitis (109). Varying degrees of bronchiolitis obliterans may also be present, as well as occasional noncaseating sarcoid-like granulomas.

Recognition that the histology of BCG is a reaction pattern that can be seen in several diseases is important (Table 25.7).

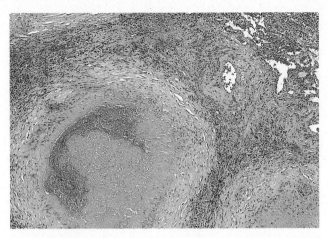

Figure 25.29. Bronchocentric granulomatosis. The granulomatous inflammation completely effaces the bronchus but spares the adjacent artery. Central necrosis, palisaded histiocytes, and a giant cell are seen. The similarity to tuberculosis is striking.

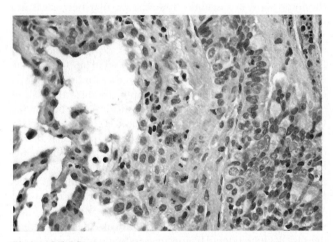

Figure 25.30. Bronchocentric granulomatosis. The eosinophils are adjacent to the bronchial wall in this patient.

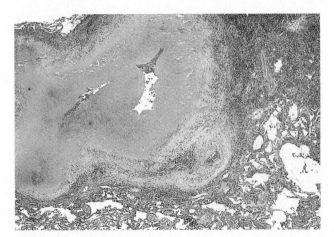

Figure 25.28. Bronchocentric granulomatosis. The bronchus is obliterated by a necrotic inflammatory reaction that is composed predominantly of cellular debris. The artery at the upper right is not involved.

TABLE 25.7
Lung Lesions That May Have a "Bronchocentric" Granuloma Pattern
Bronchocentric granulomatosis
Tuberculosis
Fungal infection
Wegener granulomatosis
Cystic fibrosis
Rheumatoid arthritis

Thus, in patients with a history of asthma, blood and tissue eosinophilia, and positive serum precipitins to *Aspergillus,* the etiology may be clear. However, a similar histologic pattern without eosinophilia may be seen in some cases associated with rheumatoid arthritis, pulmonary tuberculosis, histoplasmosis, or other fungi or in cystic fibrosis (110,111). In addition, some patients with WG may also have a predominantly bronchocentric pattern of disease (112). Such possibilities should always be kept in mind in patients without asthma or in those in whom the pathogenesis is uncertain. Stains for acid-fast and fungus organisms to help exclude a potential infectious etiology in non-asthmatic patients, and careful attention to the nature and extent of blood vessel inflammation helps to differentiate the condition from WG. Negative culture results, special stains, and the absence of vasculitis are essential to the diagnosis. However, problematic cases are encountered; in these, the clinical course of the patient defines the diagnosis. BCG usually responds well to steroids. A localized granulomatous form of semi-invasive aspergillosis has been described that is not associated with allergic pneumonitis that requires antifungal therapy (113).

BRONCHIOLITIS OBLITERANS WITH ORGANIZING PNEUMONIA (CRYPTOGENIC ORGANIZING PNEUMONIA)

Bronchiolitis obliterans with organizing pneumonia (BOOP) is an inflammatory reaction in the terminal bronchioles, alveolar ducts, and alveoli, and is a common pattern of injury seen in many different pulmonary conditions (Table 25.8) (114,115).

TABLE 25.8

Conditions Showing Bronchiolitis Obliterans

Condition	Examples
Bronchiolitis obliterans as the dominant histologic pattern	
Infectious pneumonia	Mycoplasma; viral pneumonia
Postobstructive pneumonia	Tumors
Toxic inhalants	N_2O; others
Graft-versus-host reaction	Obliterative bronchiolitis in bone marrow and heart-lung transplant recipients
Drug reactions	Chemotherapy; penicillamine
Hypersensitivity pneumonia	
Unknown	30% to 50% of cases
Bronchiolitis obliterans associated with other conditions	
Diffuse interstitial pneumonias	DAD; UIP
Collagen disease	Rheumatoid arthritis; Wegener granulomatosis
Hypersensitivity pneumonia	
Chronic eosinophilic pneumonia	
LIP, WDL, LYG	
Organizing pneumonia	Bacteria, mycoplasma
Others	Cystic fibrosis; bronchocentric granulomatosis

DAD, diffuse alveolar damage; LIP, lymphocytic interstitial pneumonia; LYG, lymphomatoid granulomatosis; UIP, usual interstitial pneumonia; WDL, well-differentiated lymphocytic lymphoma.

Some of these may be readily apparent clinically and histologically, examples of which are HP, CEP, and organizing bacterial pneumonia. Sometimes, however, the histologic pattern of bronchiolitis obliterans may far exceed any recognizable diagnostic features of pulmonary hypersensitivity or infection. BOOP may be seen as the primary pathologic reaction to infectious agents, such as mycoplasma and bacterial and viral pneumonia; to the inhalation of toxic fumes, such as oxides of nitrogen (silo filler's disease); or in collagen disease (9,114–116). In about half the cases, however, the etiology cannot be determined (116). The term *cryptogenic organizing pneumonia* (COP) is favored for this process in Europe and more recently here in the United States (9,115). Each case of BOOP requires a thorough investigation of the history of exposure, infection, or associated clinical disease to aid in defining its cause, which generally is not apparent from examination of the biopsy specimen.

The histologic pattern is distinctive if not etiologically specific. Chronic inflammatory cells and plugs of loose, matrix-rich connective tissue are distributed throughout terminal bronchi, bronchioles, alveolar ducts, and alveolar spaces (Fig. 25.31). These areas may vary in their stage of organization from case to case, but they are usually uniform in any one biopsy (Fig. 25.32). Alveoli adjacent to involved airways hold foamy macrophages, inflammatory cells, and cellular debris sometimes containing cholesterol clefts. This reaction, which is seen focally within the alveolar space, is a clue indicating that obstruction of small-terminal airways has occurred. The alveolar septa show varying amounts of chronic interstitial inflammation and alveolar collapse around involved distal airways. The disease is patchy in distribution, with substantial areas of uninvolved lung. Cases secondary to hypersensitivity may show moderate to large numbers of eosinophils.

Clinically, some patients may have an acute febrile illness with dyspnea and wheezing, whereas others have a less abrupt, more insidious syndrome of progressive shortness of breath. Radiographically, the pattern is variable, ranging from diffuse and bilateral reticulonodular disease to an intra-alveolar pattern to cases showing patchy pneumonic consolidation (117). CT scan may show bilateral consolidation (118). The prognosis is

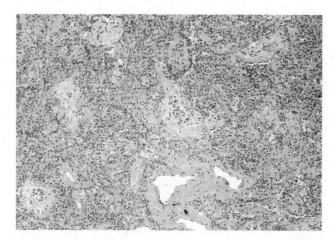

Figure 25.31. Bronchiolitis obliterans with organizing pneumonia (BOOP). Replacement of the terminal bronchioles by loose connective tissue is seen. Mild chronic inflammation of the alveolar septa and the collapse of alveolar spaces are seen, which imparts a solid appearance to the process.

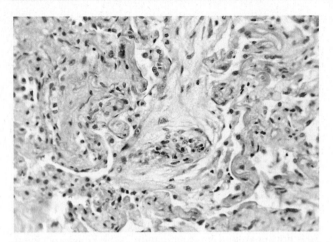

Figure 25.32. Bronchiolitis obliterans with organizing pneumonia (BOOP). A plug of young fibrous tissue occupies the lumen of a terminal bronchiole and alveolar duct.

usually excellent and, in most patients, steroids are effective in ameliorating the condition (114,116). Approximately three-fourths of patients survive for 5 years (115). Some cases may be steroid-resistant, however, leading to relapse and death.

A helpful diagnostic clue to BOOP is seen on low-power microscopy, which shows the patchy distribution of organizing pneumonia and intraluminal connective tissue plugs that obliterate the terminal airways. The paucity of normal-appearing bronchioles in the histologic picture indicates the terminal bronchiolar distribution of the inflammatory process.

SMALL-AIRWAY DISEASE

The concept of small-airway disease has undergone revision and increased emphasis, with multiple categories now identified (Table 25.9).

RESPIRATORY BRONCHIOLITIS AND RESPIRATORY BRONCHIOLITIS-INTERSTITIAL LUNG DISEASE

Respiratory bronchiolitis (RB) and respiratory bronchiolitis-interstitial lung disease (RB-ILD) are thought to be closely related

TABLE 25.9

Small-Airway Disease

Category of Disease	Cause
Respiratory bronchiolitis	Smoking
Bronchiocentric interstitial lung	End-stage bronchiolar injury disease (peribronchiolar metaplasia)
Constrictive-obliterative bronchiolitis	Lung and bone marrow transplant rejection; drugs (gold, penicillin); postinfections; toxic inhalants (popcorn lung)
Panbronchiolitis	Virus HTLV-1
Cellular bronchiolitis	Infectious; idiopathic
Follicular bronchiolitis	Lymphoproliferative; autoimmune
Unclassified bronchiolitis	

to DIP because, like DIP, it is essentially only seen in cigarette smokers and it shares the microscopic finding of macrophage accumulation in distal airway structures.

RB and RB-ILD are often seen incidentally in lung tissue removed for a wide variety of reasons, but may be the reason for lung biopsy in patients who present with shortness of breath clinically. Radiographic abnormalities are mild and nonspecific, consisting of bilateral ground-glass opacities similar to DIP. Many patients have normal chest radiographs. The symptoms usually regress after cessation of smoking (57,58).

Histologically, RB-ILD is characterized by localized chronic inflammation of the terminal bronchioles and alveolar ducts, with focal interstitial inflammation and fibrosis that are adjacent to the involved airways (Fig. 25.33). The alveolar ducts and alveolar spaces are filled with histiocytes similar to those seen in DIP, but the distribution is predominantly peribronchiolar (RB). These cells often contain intracytoplasmic, brown-black, geometrically shaped particles (smoker's granules) that have been formed from the products of cigarette smoke. RB-ILD shows more advanced interstitial fibrosis. RB-ILD commonly accompanies other smoking-related diseases, such as EG and lung cancer. Cigarette smoking may therefore be the cause of established interstitial fibrosis seen in lung biopsy material, either

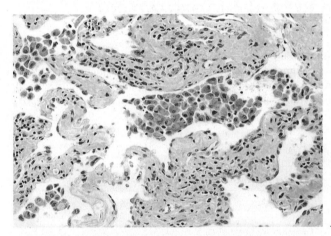

A

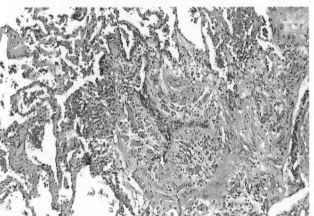

B

Figure 25.33. Respiratory bronchiolitis-interstitial lung disease (RB-ILD). **(A)** The terminal bronchiole shows interstitial fibrosis and intraluminal smoker's macrophages. **(B)** In respiratory bronchiolitis, the thickened terminal bronchus demonstrate chronic inflammation and interstitial fibrosis is seen adjacent to the bronchus. The focal accumulation of macrophages is present.

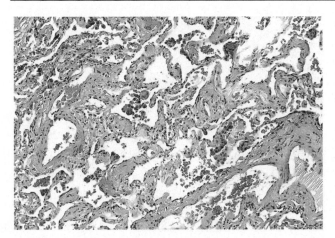

Figure 25.34. Respiratory bronchiolitis-interstitial lung disease (RB-ILD). Significant interstitial fibrosis is seen in association with isolated collections of intra-alveolar macrophages.

as a cofactor with other causes or independently (Fig. 25.34) (119).

BRONCHIOLOCENTRIC INTERSTITIAL LUNG DISEASE (PERIBRONCHIOLAR METAPLASIA)

Bronchiolocentric interstitial lung disease is a recently proposed entity; its histologic hallmark is the presence of fibrosis of terminal bronchioles that extend to include the interstitium of adjacent alveolar walls (Fig. 25.35). This results in zonal areas of discrete airway-based interstitial fibrosis that largely spares the rest of the interstitium. The epithelium overlying the fibrous areas is often ciliated columnar and conforms to bronchiolar metaplasia or "Lambertosis," referring to the canals of Lambert through which the ciliated cells are considered to migrate into alveolar spaces. Some have called this process *peribronchiolar metaplasia*. When it occurs alone, it presents a distinctive histologic appearance. Both obstructive and diffusion impairment are observed. However, it is often associated with a wide variety of chronic fibrosing interstitial lung diseases, including smok-

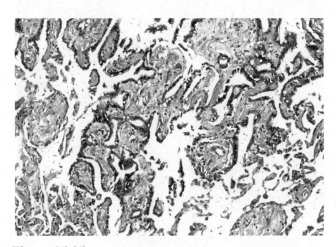

Figure 25.35. Peribronchiolar metaplasia. Fibrosis and distortion of terminal bronchiole extends into adjacent alveolar septae and is accompanied by ciliated bronchial metaplasia of benign epithelium. The process ends sharply, resulting in a bronchiolocentric pattern.

ing, environmental exposure, organic dusts, and collagen disease. As such, it is considered by many as a nonspecific end-stage pattern of terminal airway injury. The prognosis is variable. Some series report 50% mortality, whereas others record no deaths (120–122).

OBLITERATIVE/CONSTRICTIVE BRONCHIOLITIS

In patients who have undergone allogeneic bone marrow and lung transplantation, a particular type of obliterating bronchiolitis may develop; most cases are thought to be secondary to a graft-versus-host reaction (123,124). However, similar findings have been described in patients who have had autologous marrow transplantation—a finding that casts some doubt about the role of graft-versus-host reaction (125). Cytomegalovirus (CMV), human leukocyte antigen (HLA) mismatch, and autoimmunity are thought to play a role in some cases (126).

The same disease process may be seen as a complication of rheumatoid arthritis or the administration of penicillamine or gold; inflammatory bowel disease; and as idiopathic disease (114–116,127). Inflammatory bowel disease can also be associated with a variety of ulcerative and inflammatory lesions of the larger bronchi and trachea (128–130). The histologic picture exclusively involves terminal bronchi and bronchioles, which show lymphocytic infiltration, sloughing of the epithelium, and gradual replacement of the bronchial wall by fibrous tissue that eventually results in total fibrous obliteration. The alveoli become hyperdistended (Fig. 25.36). The term *obliterative* or *constrictive bronchiolitis* has been proposed to aid in separating this from BOOP, which is the more common condition (131). This distinction is important because the prognosis of BOOP is generally favorable, whereas that of obliterative bronchiolitis is poor.

Some transplant recipients may indeed have BOOP as the result of infection, aspiration, or airway obstruction. Lung biopsies in such cases show the characteristic findings of BOOP rather than those of obliterative bronchiolitis (131). An expanding list of etiologic agents for obliterative bronchiolitis includes popcorn (popcorn worker's lung) or potato chip workers exposed to diacetyl as a flavoring agent (132,133).

Diffuse panbronchiolitis is a rare condition that usually affects Japanese and other Asians, but it has occasionally been reported in non-Asian patients in the United States as well (134,135) (Fig. 25.37). A direct association with HLA BW54 exists (136). The cause is unknown but HTLV-1 infection has been suggested. Middle-aged males predominate. The patients complain of dyspnea and cough and often have chronic sinusitis.

Pathologically, the hallmark of this condition is the presence of collections of foamy histiocytes in the pulmonary interstitium and the accompanying chronic and sometimes acute inflammation involving terminal bronchioles. *Pseudomonas* infection is often associated with diffuse panbronchiolitis, and antibiotics are effective in slowing the course of the disease, which is usually chronic and progressive.

Cellular bronchiolitis is characterized by acute inflammation in the bronchiolar lumen surrounded by chronic inflammation of the wall (Fig. 25.38). Unlike follicular bronchiolitis, germinal centers are usually not seen. The etiology is unknown but is suspected to be infectious, although no constant organism has been identified. Steroids are effective.

Follicular bronchiolitis is included as a category of small-

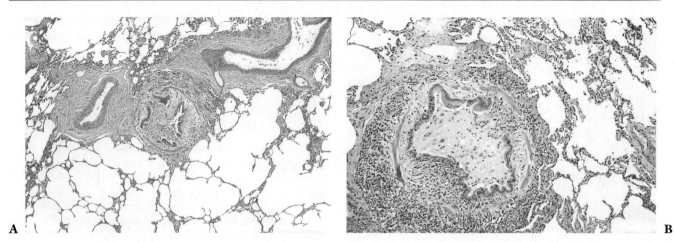

Figure 25.36.   Bone marrow transplant recipient. **(A)** This patient shows fibrous thickening and inflammation of the bronchiole. The alveoli are distended. **(B)** Fibrosis and inflammation of the bronchiole with focal disruption of the epithelial lining are present.

airway disease and is discussed elsewhere in this chapter with the lymphocytic infiltrations.

Finally, there is a group of cases that defy morphologic classification and should best be diagnosed descriptively, with attempts to correlate clinical findings and exposure history.

EOSINOPHILIC GRANULOMA

Alternative terms are *Langerhans cell granulomatosis* and *histiocytosis X* (137). EG is a disease of unknown etiology; it is characterized histologically by tissue infiltration with localized collections or sheets of eosinophilic histiocytes (Langerhans cells)

and eosinophils. Ultrastructurally, the histiocytes contain specific pentilaminar intracytoplasmic structures (Birbeck granules) that impart specificity to the Langerhans cells (Fig. 25.39) (138). The disease may be localized to a single site, or it may involve several different organs simultaneously or progressively. Pulmonary involvement is seen in approximately 20% of cases with multicentric disease, which may also involve bone, skin, lymph nodes, spleen, pituitary gland, and other areas. The lung is the only organ of involvement in more than 50% of cases (139,140).

Clinically, a significant number of patients are asymptomatic, despite an abnormal chest radiograph (139). In others, the clinical findings may vary in their severity from relatively mild dys-

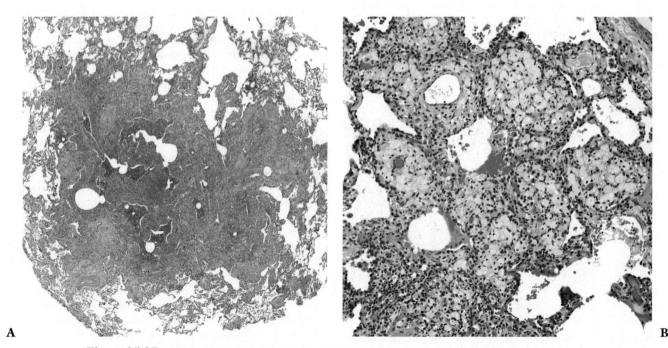

Figure 25.37.   Diffuse panbronchiolitis. **(A)** Bronchiolocentric pattern of inflammation. **(B)** Extensive interstitial foam cell infiltrates around diseased terminal airway are the histologic hallmarks of this disease. Figure courtesy of Dr. Douglas Flieder.

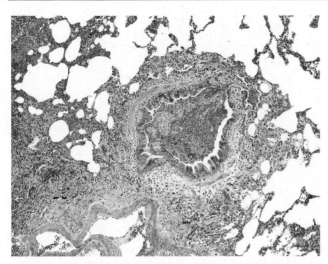

Figure 25.38. Cellular bronchiolitis. Altered bronchiole with intraluminal acute inflammatory exudate and chronic mural inflammation. Surrounding lung shows distended airspaces.

pnea to severe shortness of breath, hemoptysis, and pleuritic chest pain associated with spontaneous pneumothorax. Blood eosinophilia is not seen.

Radiologically, the disease usually shows diffuse and bilateral interstitial or reticulonodular infiltrates that are more pronounced in the periphery of the lung fields than they are in the central zones. It is more common in the upper and middle lung fields than in the bases, but the distribution is variable. Rare cases may show single or multiple nodules that are suggestive of malignancy (140,141). In chronic cases, cysts that are predominantly located in the subpleural regions and are accompanied by interstitial fibrosis are seen. High-resolution CT scans show characteristic and highly specific findings of interstitial infiltrates and thin-walled cysts (141). The etiology is unknown, but the association of EG with cigarette smoking is significant; almost all patients are current or past smokers. In fact, a diagnosis of EG should be suspect in a nonsmoker.

Recent molecular studies have shown the clonal nature of the Langerhans cells of EG in extrapulmonary sites (142–144). Approximately half of pulmonary EG may be clonal by HUMARA assay, although doubt has been expressed as to whether this reflects a neoplastic process (145). Pathologically, the lung infiltrates are patchy and are located around the bronchioles, in the interstitium as intraseptal, perivascular, or peribronchial collections of Langerhans cells that have somewhat glassy pink cytoplasm with indistinct cell borders, lending a syncytial quality to the infiltrate. The nuclei are distinctive, and show longitudinal coffee-bean grooves and an undulating or indented nuclear membrane. These Langerhans cells or histiocytosis X cells are necessary for the diagnosis of EG (Fig. 25.40). Immunohistochemically, the nucleus and cytoplasm stain positively with antibodies to S-100 protein, which is sometimes a useful tool in differentiating Langerhans cells from pulmonary macrophages. HLA-DR and CD1-A are also positive but are they less sensitive (146). Because a variety of inflammatory conditions may contain reactive Langerhans cells, however, caution should be exercised in diagnosing EG, particularly in transbronchial biopsies, unless Langerhans cells are seen as groups or sheets within the interstitium (147).

The pattern of interstitial infiltration may occasionally be diffuse throughout the biopsy, but it more often shows a patchy, stellate, or crablike distribution with a more central bronchiolar component that spreads into the adjacent interstitium. On low-power magnification, this architecture is characteristic of EG (Fig. 25.41). Eosinophilic leukocytes are almost always present but their numbers may vary from case to case; in older lesions, they are fewer in number or even absent. The surrounding lung tissue commonly shows smoking-related changes that are characteristic of RB-ILD or, in exceptional cases, DIP. The alveoli contain varying numbers of pulmonary macrophages containing pigmented smoker's granules and eosinophils that are sometimes accompanied by hemosiderin. Compared with Langerhans cells, these cells have darker cytoplasm and sharper

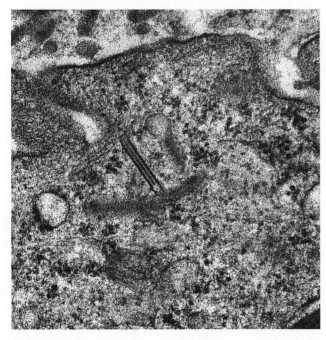

Figure 25.39. Pulmonary eosinophilic granuloma. An electron micrograph shows a Birbeck granule in the cytoplasm of a Langerhans cell from a patient with this condition (90,000×).

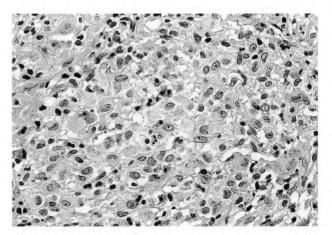

Figure 25.40. Eosinophilic granuloma showing a syncytial growth pattern. Cytoplasmic borders are indistinct. The nuclei are elongated and grooved, with undulating nuclear membranes. Numerous eosinophils are seen.

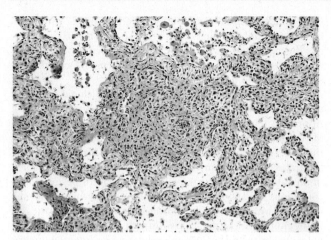

Figure 25.41. Nodule of eosinophilic granuloma. The central area shows collections of Langerhans cells, whereas the more peripheral portion shows interstitial infiltration and eosinophils.

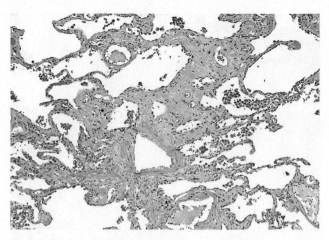

Figure 25.43. Healed phase of pulmonary eosinophilic granuloma. The stellate scar of interstitial fibrosis is characteristic.

cell borders; they lack the characteristic grooved nuclei; and they are negative with immunoperoxidase staining for S-100. They do, however, react with macrophage markers such as CD68. Confusion with DIP may be a problem, particularly in transbronchial or poorly representative open lung biopsies. Considering the possibility of EG is wise under such circumstances when one is confronted with DIP-like changes. This problem may be compounded because both DIP and EG patients may clinically be asymptomatic, and the chest radiographs in the two conditions may at times be similar.

As the disease progresses, Langerhans cells and eosinophils diminish, and chronic inflammation and fibrosis replace the cellular phase (Fig. 25.42). Active cellular foci of intra-alveolar fibrosis, which are similar to those seen in other fibrosing lung diseases, may also be present in EG (148). Older lesions may show acellular stellate scars that are often located in the subpleural region of the lung biopsy. These may show the remnants of burned-out EG containing foamy histiocytes, smoker's pigment, or hemosiderin-laden macrophages. In the appropriate clinical and radiographic setting, these stellate areas of fibrosis are char-

acteristic of the healed phase of the disease (Fig. 25.43). A careful search may disclose the diagnostic cellular features of EG.

The prognosis of EG is generally favorable, with few fatalities resulting from the pulmonary form (142). A significant number of patients undergo spontaneous regression even without treatment. Chest x-ray abnormalities may persist, however, and from 10% to 20% of patients may steadily progress to respiratory failure (139,141). Steroids or chemotherapy may be effective in some cases, but their role is difficult to assess because of the generally excellent prognosis of the disease.

Eosinophilic pleuritis is a nonspecific pleural reaction of sometimes abundant eosinophils mixed with mesothelial cells that is seen in specimens that have usually been resected for the treatment of pneumothorax of any cause (Fig. 25.44). It has been confused with EG, and care should be taken in such clinical situations (149). Eosinophilic vasculitis has been described in subpleural blood vessels in this condition (150).

Malakoplakia is another rare example of histiocytic infiltration of the lung. This disease usually fills and destroys the alveoli rather than involving the interstitium, as occurs in EG (151,152). In the more usual locations, such as the urinary blad-

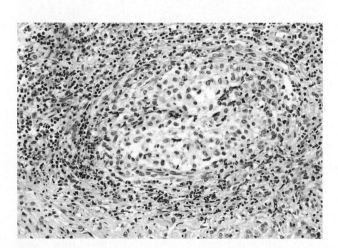

Figure 25.42. Eosinophilic granuloma. The isolated focus is almost obscured by the surrounding inflammatory reaction.

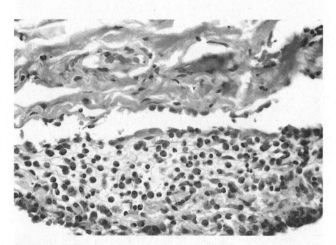

Figure 25.44. Eosinophilic pleuritis. This specimen is from spontaneous pneumothorax secondary to emphysema. Pleural lining is hyperplastic and reactive, and the pleura is infiltrated by eosinophils and chronic inflammatory cells.

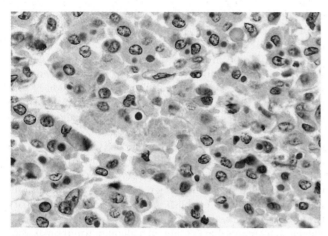

Figure 25.45. Pulmonary malakoplakia showing collections of histiocytes in alveoli. The Michaelis-Guttmann body is seen as the dark-staining intracytoplasmic body just to the left of center.

der or kidney, the common causative organism is *Escherichia coli*, whereas in the lung *Rhodococcus equis* has been isolated in more than 70% of cases. The organism is an animal pathogen that causes an opportunistic infection in patients suffering from severe immunosuppression, most commonly AIDS. The lung disease usually takes the form of nodular masses or infiltrates that may cavitate.

Microscopically, malakoplakia is composed of intra-alveolar collections of pink or foamy histiocytes that often contain intracellular PAS-positive bacteria, mixed with lymphocytes, plasma cells, and polymorphonuclear cells (Fig. 25.45). The pathognomonic Michaelis-Gutmann bodies are deeply staining round or oval structure that measure between 5 and 20 μm in diameter and have a laminated or targetoid appearance. They contain iron and calcium, and stain positively with von Kossa and Prussian blue stains (Fig. 25.46). Treatment with the appropriate antibiotics is usually successful. Malakoplakia must be differentiated from atypical mycobacterial infection in immunosuppressed patients. In the latter, foamy histiocytes that contain organisms may have a bluish cast, in contrast to malakoplakia. Positive acid-fast stains clearly distinguish these conditions (153).

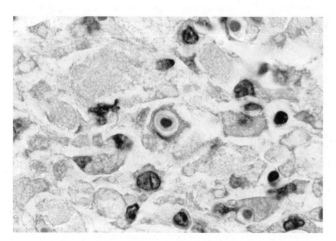

Figure 25.46. Michaelis-Guttmann body. It shows laminated or targetoid appearance.

Whipple disease, Erdheim-Chester disease, and Gaucher disease have also been reported as rare causes of interstitial pulmonary histiocytic infiltration, and are manifestations of more systemic involvement (154–156).

LYMPHOCYTIC INFILTRATIONS

Pulmonary lymphoid lesions are rare. Currently, the great majority are thought to represent indolent malignant lymphomas of the bronchial-associated lymphoid tissue (BALT) system (157–159). Although this chapter is primarily concerned with benign nonneoplastic lung diseases, the benign lymphocytic lung infiltrates cannot be presented meaningfully without a discussion of their differential diagnosis from malignant lymphoma (Table 25.10).

BENIGN LYMPHOID INFILTRATES

The benign lymphoid infiltrates are divided into diffuse and nodular hyperplasia of BALT, lymphocytic interstitial pneumonia (LIP), and nodular lymphoid hyperplasia (NLH) (160,161). More recently, follicular bronchitis—bronchiolitis (FB) has been recognized as the earliest stage of BALT hyperplasia (162).

Clinically, FB is seen in patients having a background of congenital or acquired immunodeficiency, especially AIDS; collagen diseases, particularly rheumatoid arthritis and Sjögren syndrome; and idiopathic cases (163). The symptoms are mild, consisting mainly of shortness of breath; radiographically, diffuse bilateral interstitial and finely reticular infiltrates are seen. Pathologically, the characteristic picture consists of cellular lymphoid nodules that are aggregated in and around distal bronchi and bronchioles; these are composed of small lymphocytes with germinal centers and plasma cells that may compress the lumen (Fig. 25.47). No significant infiltration of the adjacent alveolar septa occurs unless there is coexisting LIP. Steroids and chemotherapy are usually effective treatment, but the disease may be persistent.

Patients with LIP fall into similar clinical groups, as do those with FB. Most cases can be correlated to immunosuppression, particularly AIDS; collagen diseases, with or without Sjögren syndrome; pulmonary drug reactions; or cases of an idiopathic nature (164). Children, most commonly those with AIDS, may

TABLE 25.10
Classification of Pulmonary Lymphoid Infiltrates
Benign
Lymphoid interstitial pneumonia (interstitial lymphoid hyperplasia), follicular bronchiolitis
Pseudolymphoma (nodular lymphoid hyperplasia)
Malignant
Low grade BALT lymphoma
Other low-grade lymphoma
High grade lymphoma
Lymphomatoid granulomatosis
Hodgkin disease
Transitional
Epstein-Barr virus-associated lymphoproliferative lesions in transplant recipients and AIDS

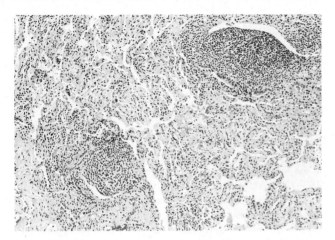

Figure 25.47. Follicular bronchitis-bronchiolitis in a patient with Sjögren syndrome. Lymphoid nodules compress and obliterate bronchioles.

be affected (165). Epstein-Barr virus (EBV) has been detected in both children and adults with AIDS-related LIP by in situ hybridization or PCR, but it is not usually seen in non-AIDS patients (165,166). The clinical, radiographic, and pathologic findings of LIP are difficult to analyze from the older literature because criteria for its separation from low-grade pulmonary lymphoma were based on obsolete morphologic concepts. However, more objective evidence does exist that LIP is indeed a polyclonal lymphoid proliferation and that it is a form of benign lymphoid hyperplasia (163). Clinically, these patients most often manifest shortness of breath and cough. The chest radiograph shows bilateral diffuse reticular or reticular nodular infiltrates that are most prominent at the bases. Polyclonal gammopathy is a common laboratory finding. The clinical course of LIP is difficult to evaluate from the older literature, but recent studies that define LIP by molecular and immunologic methods show that clinical progression to diffuse interstitial fibrosis is much more common than is a response to steroids or chemotherapy (163,167).

Pathologically, LIP shows features of FB, but infiltration of the alveolar septa by lymphocytes and plasma cells occurs as

well. These appear entirely benign and they seemingly percolate through the interstitium without causing the densely cellular and monotonous pattern of low-grade lymphoma, nor is lymphangitic distribution prominent (Fig. 25.48). Germinal centers are common, and epithelioid granulomas may be seen. The visceral pleura may show mild infiltration, but invasion of lymphocytes into the parietal pleura is not part of the histologic picture, whereas it may be a feature of some malignant lymphomas. Rarely, diffuse interstitial fibrosis may rarely be observed in chronic cases. Histologically, biopsies that show the combined features of FB and LIP are common (164).

The place of nodular lymphoid hyperplasia (NLH) of BALT within the spectrum of the benign pulmonary lymphoid infiltrates is difficult to establish. The concept of pulmonary lymphoid infiltrates, as it was reported by Saltstein, evolved from the misconceptions that extranodal malignant lymphomas were multinodular diseases that involved the regional lymph nodes and that they did not contain reactive germinal centers (162). Now that these have been dispelled, many think that most cases that were previously reported in the literature as hyperplastic pulmonary lymphoid infiltrates were most likely lymphomas.

The older reports of NLH from the literature suggest that approximately half of the patients are asymptomatic and that most manifest a solitary discrete mass on chest radiograph (164,168). Multiple nodules have been reported in a minority of patients. The survival of the reported patients has been excellent following surgical resection, with no patients dying of disease. However, recurrences in the lung have been described, as has malignant transformation (164).

Despite some skepticism, a recent review of 14 cases of benign NLH that were studied by immunohistochemistry and molecular techniques revealed a uniform group of patients. Their condition was characterized by usually solitary, well-circumscribed, solid nodules composed of benign-appearing lymphoid cells with prominent reactive germinal centers, preserved mantle and marginal zones, and numerous mature plasma cells with Russell bodies in the interfollicular areas. Fibrosis was commonly seen within the nodule and surrounding germinal centers, and epithelioid granulomas were occasionally observed (Fig. 25.49). The infiltrate is a mixture of polyclonal B cells and T cells. Histologically, the maturation of cells from the germinal centers outward to interfollicular plasma cells re-

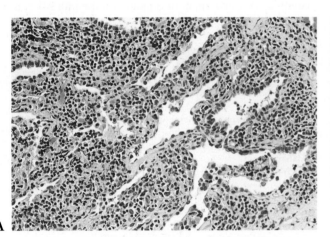

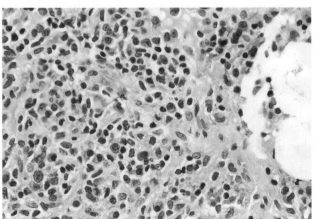

A   B

Figure 25.48. Lymphocytic interstitial pneumonia. **(A)** A lymphoid infiltrate is present in the interstitium in this pneumonia. **(B)** Delicate infiltration of alveolar septa by benign lymphocytes, plasma cells, and histiocytes occurs. The infiltrate lacks the expansile monotony of lymphoma. This patient has rheumatoid arthritis.

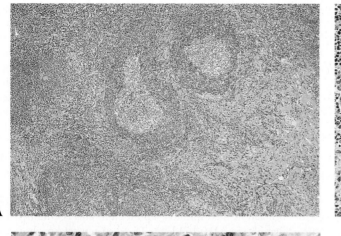

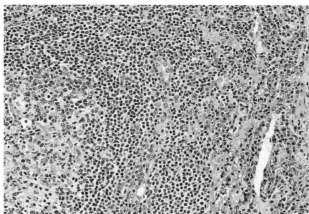

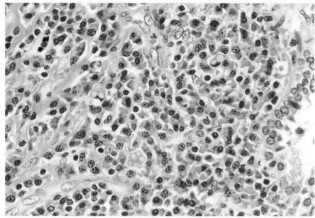

Figure 25.49. Nodular lymphoid hyperplasia. **(A)** The hyperplastic germinal center is surrounded by fibrosis. **(B)** An orderly maturation of cells is seen from the germinal center to preserved mantle lymphocytes to mature plasma cells. **(C)** This detail view shows mature lymphocytes and plasma cells with Russell bodies.

capitulates that of a hyperplastic lymph node. In contrast to LIP, these patients did not have immunosuppression or collagen disease. No recurrences were observed in this group after surgical removal (160).

PULMONARY LYMPHOMA

The benign lymphoid infiltrates (FB, LIP, NLH) must be differentiated from low-grade pulmonary lymphoma, in which 70% to 80% are thought to be derived from pre-existing BALT (157,159). This disease most often affects men and women of middle age or older. As in NLH, 50% of patients are asymptomatic, and the disease is discovered after a routine chest radiograph examination. Others have shortness of breath, cough, and chest pain. Sjögren syndrome has been reported in some cases (169). Radiographically, 70% of cases show solitary nodules or infiltrates (157,159,170). The rest are more diffuse. Bilateral lung involvement is seen in 20% of patients. The tumors range in size from a few centimeters to those that opacify the lung (159,170).

Pleural effusion has been reported in almost 30% of patients, whereas cavitation and mediastinal lymphadenopathy are rare. A monoclonal gammopathy can be seen in roughly one-fifth of cases (159). Histologically, low-grade BALT lymphoma most often shows solid masses or sheets of cells that infiltrate around veins, arteries, and the interlobular connective tissue septa and pleura. This results in a micronodular pattern that is best observed at low power and that often coalesces into more solid,

larger lymphoid nodules (Fig. 25.50). Sometimes the histologic pattern shows predominantly perivascular lymphoid infiltrates that have been termed *lymphatic tracking*; these are seen in approximately 75% of cases of low-grade pulmonary lymphoma (171). Although this can also be seen to some extent in benign hyperplasia of BALT, it is useful for identifying low-grade pulmonary lymphoma when it is a major part of the histologic picture (Fig. 25.51) (163). The recognition that significant

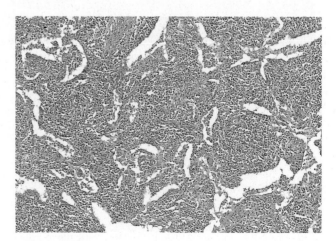

Figure 25.50. Low-grade bronchus-associated lymphoid tissue lymphoma showing interstitial multinodular pattern of infiltration. Note the monotony of the cells and effacement of lung architecture.

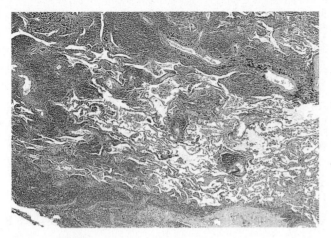

Figure 25.51. Low-grade bronchus-associated lymphoid tissue (BALT) lymphoma. Lymphatic tracking is prominent in this case of low-grade BALT lymphoma.

numbers of reactive plasma cells can be present is important; germinal centers are seen in up to 70% of cases, epithelioid granulomas in 20%, and granulomatous vasculitis in rare instances (Fig. 25.52) (172).

Particular attention should be paid to the morphologic characteristics of the lymphoid infiltrate itself in separating benign lymphoid infiltrates from low-grade malignant lymphoma. In lymphomas, the lymphocytes grow in monotonous sheets that obliterate portions of the pulmonary architecture. Cytologically, the nuclei may deviate only minimally from those of normal lymphocytes, but in some cases the tumors are composed of centrocyte-like cells having hyperchromatic cleaved or lobulated nuclear outlines (173). These cells are smaller than the classic centrocyte (cleaved cell) of follicular-center-cell lymphoma, and they are closer in size to the normal lymphocyte. Other tumors show sheets of pale, monotonous monocytoid lymphocytes, whereas still others have a plasmacytoid appearance with or without Dutcher bodies. Rare examples may show combinations of several of these phenotypes (Fig. 25.53) (169,173). Vascular invasion that obliterates the small arteries and veins is also a feature of lymphoma (Fig. 25.54).

The lymphoepithelial lesion (LEL) consists of the lymphocytic infiltration of respiratory epithelium, and is common in BALT lymphoma (159,169,173). These structures are thought to reflect the arrangement between antigen-processing epithelium and antibody-producing lymphoid cells of the immunologically active, mucosal-associated lymphoid tissue (MALT) system, in a manner analogous to Peyer patches (Fig. 25.55). LELs may also be seen in cases of BALT hyperplasia but, when numerous and containing CD43-positive B cells, they are characteristic of BALT lymphoma (159,163,174). Another common histologic finding is the colonization of germinal centers by small lymphocytic tumor cells. This can lead to the obliteration of the germinal centers, leaving a vaguely nodular architecture that can be easily mistaken for follicular-center-cell lymphoma. This phenomenon, as well as LELs, can be observed with the aid of

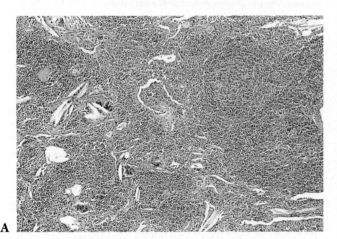

A

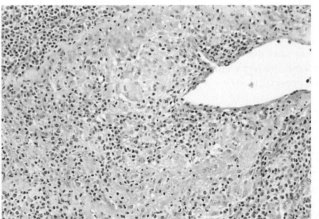

B

C

Figure 25.52. Low-grade lymphoma. **(A)** Several germinal centers are present in this view. **(B)** Granulomatous vasculitis is seen in low-grade BALT lymphoma. **(C)** A small granuloma is present next to the germinal center.

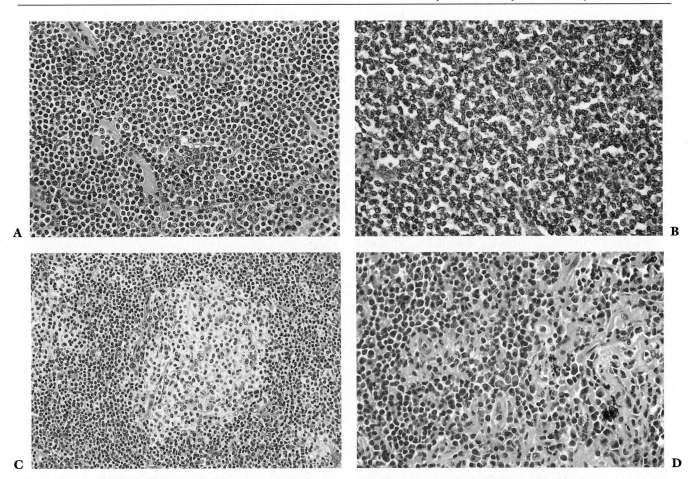

Figure 25.53. Low-grade bronchus-associated lymphoid tissue (BALT) lymphoma. **(A)** This lymphoma is composed predominantly of small, round lymphocytes. Occasional large, transformed cells are characteristic of this tumor. **(B)** This tumor is composed of centrocyte-like cells. **(C)** This focus consists of monocytoid cells in low-grade BALT lymphoma. **(D)** This mixture of lymphocytes and plasma cells is another example of BALT lymphoma.

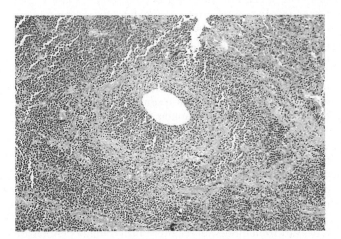

Figure 25.54. Low-grade bronchus-associated lymphoid tissue (BALT) lymphoma. This is an example of vascular invasion.

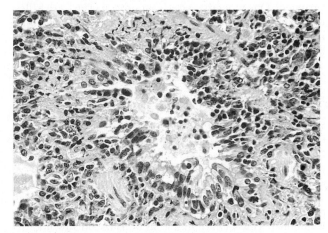

Figure 25.55. Lymphoepithelial lesion in low-grade bronchus-associated lymphoid tissue (BALT) lymphoma. The lymphocytes show an intimate association to the epithelium and infiltrate the bronchiole.

immunohistochemical (IHC) stains for cytokeratin and for CD21, which decorates the dendritic reticulum cell framework of the germinal center. Immunologically, the cells of low-grade BALT lymphoma are CD20-positive B cells that characteristically lack CD5 and CD10. This tends to separate them from follicular-center-cell lymphomas, which are CD10-positive and CD5-negative (157,159,169,172,175). Staining of paraffin sections with κ and λ light chains has shown light chain restriction more often in some studies than others (159,169,172).

Most cases of low-grade BALT lymphoma contain significant numbers of benign polyclonal plasma cells and reactive T cells. One paper has suggested that LIP and low-grade lymphoma may be differentiated from each other by the observation that the lymphocytes that infiltrate the alveolar septa in LIP are T cells, whereas those in low-grade lymphoma are B cells (163). A useful adjunct to IHC is flow cytometry, which can be extremely accurate in immunophenotyping the tumor (168). In addition, flow cytometry of peripheral blood is an often overlooked technique that can detect a small circulating monoclonal cell population; it may help to establish the diagnosis of low-grade lymphoma in problematic cases (168). Recently, giant lamellar bodies have been described in BALT lymphoma but not in reactive lymphoid hyperplasia (176).

The histologic differential diagnosis between low-grade BALT lymphoma and benign lymphoid hyperplasia can be difficult, particularly in small biopsies. Significantly, cases of reactive FB and LIP are far more common in the clinical setting of immunosuppression and collagen disease than are cases of malignant lymphoma. The diagnosis of reactive BALT hyperplasia in the absence of such clinical associations should therefore be suspect. Another aspect of the differential diagnosis is the observation that not all cases of low-grade lymphoma show evidence of light chain restriction by IHC, or of immunoglobulin gene rearrangement by PCR, particularly in paraffin sections (157,169). Hence, in some cases, the observation of clinical progression of disease may run counter to benign IHC or PCR results.

The prognosis of low-grade pulmonary BALT lymphoma is excellent. The clinical course appears to be more a feature of the slow natural history of the disease than a response to specific treatment. One series showed a 5-year survival of 96% regardless of whether patients received chemotherapy, radiation therapy, combinations, or no treatment at all (157,159). Other studies have reported 10-year survival rates of between 72% and 85% (157,159,168,177). This prolonged natural history has raised some questions about whether all cases of clonally defined low-grade BALT lymphoma are obligatory malignancies. Some have speculated that at least some of these cases might actually represent the equivalent of an in situ tumor of the lymphoid system or a nonobligatory premalignant precursor lesion (178). This has some practical aspects in that (a) low-grade BALT lymphomas that are not progressive may be observed without treatment; and (b) surgery may apparently cure small, localized lesions. Chemotherapy and radiation therapy may then be used as treatment for those patients who demonstrate progressive lymphoma. This seems reminiscent of Saltzstein's pseudolymphoma concept, which may have been close to the mark in its clinical approach to these low-grade lesions (161).

Diffuse large-cell lymphoma has been shown to evolve from low-grade BALT lymphoma as a manifestation of the disease progression. However, large-cell lymphomas may be seen without any evidence of a preexisting lesion (157). They usually are

solitary lung masses, and the patients have localizing or systemic symptoms (157,172). Approximately 50% of patients survive 5 years. Hodgkin disease is extremely rare as a primary tumor of the pulmonary parenchyma. It almost always is a manifestation of either direct invasion of the lung from the mediastinum or secondary pulmonary recurrence after treatment failure. Nodular sclerosis is the most common subtype.

LYMPHOMATOID GRANULOMATOSIS

Lymphomatoid granulomatosis (LYG) was originally thought to represent part of the spectrum of pulmonary angiitis and granulomatosis, but it has come to be recognized as a form of pulmonary lymphoma or perhaps, in some cases, an immunoproliferative process akin to those observed in organ transplant recipients (179–184). The term *lymphomatoid granulomatosis* persists, however, by convention. Clinically, the involvement of the central and peripheral nervous system and skin is common. This may precede lung disease; may follow it by months or years; or may occur simultaneously with it. Hilar and mediastinal lymph node involvement is unusual. However, when this does occur, the separation of classic lymphoma from LYG becomes semantic (181,184). These patients are usually ill with fever, cough, hemoptysis, weight loss, and generalized disability. Radiographically, the disease rarely appears as a single nodule; instead, it manifests as multiple nodules that are suggestive of pulmonary metastases. Sometimes, more generalized pneumonic consolidations or interstitial infiltrates are observed.

Histologically, LYG is an angiocentric, angioinvasive, and angiodestructive lesion (Fig. 25.56). Most commonly, nodular, often necrotic, infiltrates of large, pleomorphic, mitotically active lymphoid cells are present (Fig. 25.57). However, the cell population may vary greatly from case to case, as well as within the lung biopsy material of individual cases. Some patients show differences in tumor morphology in different organs that are biopsied simultaneously; alternatively, progressive anaplasia has been demonstrated in biopsy specimens obtained at varying time intervals, whether of the lung or elsewhere (182). Common to all cases, however, is the admixture of benign inflammatory cells, which are composed of lymphocytes, plasma cells, histiocytes, and, more rarely, eosinophils and polymorphonuclear cells, with the neoplastic elements. This imparts the appearance of an inflammatory process, which may obscure the malignant nature of the condition.

Attention to the blood vessels shows that cytologically atypical lymphoid cells invade and efface the vessel wall, causing obliteration of the lumen that is similar to the growth pattern seen in other malignant lymphomas (Fig. 25.58). This characteristic angioinvasion may account, in part, for the necrosis of the solid infiltrates that is often seen. Within such areas, coagulative infarct-like necrosis of tumor cells can be appreciated by observing the ghost outlines of the individual lymphoid elements. Fibrinoid or caseous necrosis of lung tissue is usually not observed, and fibrinoid necrosis of blood vessels is absent. The infiltrate of LYG may show a wide morphologic spectrum. Cases vary from those with relatively small lymphocytes that are mixed with reactive elements, to those with more homogeneous populations of large, pleomorphic, mitotically active cells. Quite often, mixtures of both large and small cells are observed, and individual cases have been demonstrated to change over time from lesions containing relatively small, atypical lymphoid cells

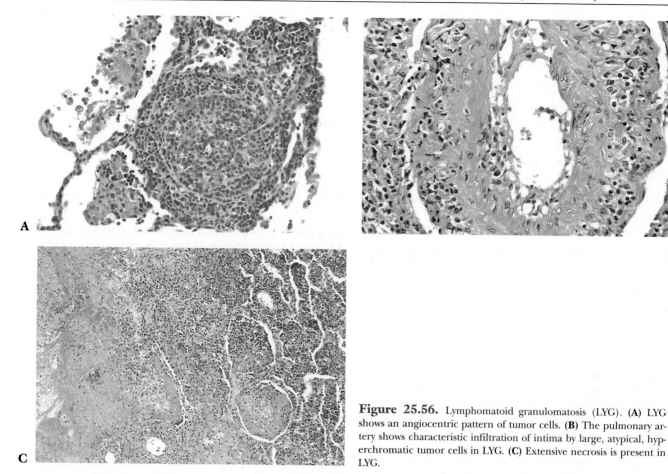

Figure 25.56. Lymphomatoid granulomatosis (LYG). **(A)** LYG shows an angiocentric pattern of tumor cells. **(B)** The pulmonary artery shows characteristic infiltration of intima by large, atypical, hyperchromatic tumor cells in LYG. **(C)** Extensive necrosis is present in LYG.

with abundant inflammation to lesions with many malignant large cells. Jaffe has suggested the term *angioimmunoproliferative lesion* (AIL) for this process, which she grades I, II, and III in ascending order of malignancy (180,185). Others have attempted similar classification schemes (186,187).

Such observations suggest that LYG may evolve through a phase of EBV-mediated immunologic induction, at first characterized by an immunoproliferative lesion that, through clonal selection, becomes a malignant lymphoma containing large

numbers of EBV-positive cells (180,184). This early phase has been termed *benign lymphocytic angiitis and granulomatosis* by Saldana et al. and AIL grade I by Jaffe (Fig. 25.59) (180,182,185). Although LYG was until recently suspected of being a T-cell lymphoma (188), the observation has been made that the majority of cases show a monoclonal population of actively proliferating large B cells containing portions of EBV genome, similar to the picture seen in examples of post-transplantation immunoproliferative disorder or EBV-driven, T-cell–rich, B-cell lym-

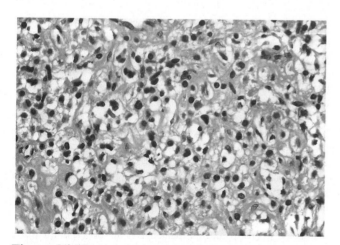

Figure 25.57. Lymphomatoid granulomatosis (LYG) showing a mixture of small and large atypical lymphoid cells.

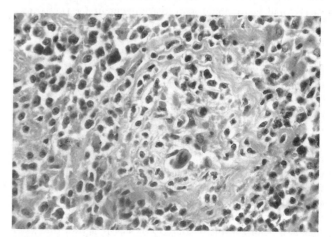

Figure 25.58. Lymphomatoid granulomatosis (LYG). The blood vessel is totally effaced by atypical pleomorphic lymphoid infiltrate.

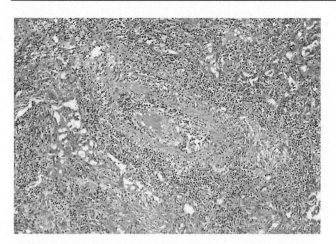

Figure 25.59. Low-grade lymphomatoid granulomatosis. This is variously called *benign lymphocytic angiitis* or *angioimmunoproliferative lesion grade I*. Note the angioinvasive nature of this process, which is composed predominantly of small lymphoid cells.

phoma (184,186,187,189–192). The numerous T cells that often overshadow the large-B-cell population have been shown to be polyclonal (190). A minority of LYG cases, however, do show evidence of T-cell gene rearrangements and do not contain EBV (187,190,193). Therefore, the entity known as LYG appears to be a heterogeneous group of T-cell and B-cell lymphomas or, in cases with more benign histology, immunoproliferations, some of which may be in the process of malignant transformation. Microscopically, the diagnosis is often confounded by the presence of a secondary inflammatory response with focal bronchiolitis obliterans, acute inflammation, and a reactive lymphocyte-plasma-cell response. Multinucleated giant cells or granulomas may rarely be observed in some cases.

The appearance of skin nodules and the microscopic examination of skin biopsy material may precede the development of pulmonary disease (183). These infiltrates may have an inflammatory appearance with (a) lymphocytic infiltration of the vessel wall, (b) eosinophils, and (c) fat necrosis in the deep dermis that is suggestive of a vasculitis or panniculitis. Cytologically, aberrant lymphocytes can usually be detected; however, this should raise suspicion about the true nature of the lesion. These may be positive for EBV by in situ hybridization, and they have clonal heavy chain gene rearrangement (194). In cases with simultaneous skin and lung involvement, skin biopsy alone may be diagnostic.

Systemically, profound immunologic alterations commonly occur in LYG; these are characterized by reversal of the helper-to-suppressor T-cell ratio of the blood and cutaneous anergy (182,193). This latter phenomenon can easily be tested clinically and is a helpful diagnostic aid. LYG has also been described in AIDS patients (195). The prognosis of LYG is poor. Most cases are resistant to chemotherapy and patients die within 1 to 2 years (182,184,196). Some patients, however, may show prolonged survival after intensive combination chemotherapy, and some remissions have even occurred spontaneously or after minimal treatment with steroids (182,184), or, more recently, with rituximab (197). Bone marrow or stem cell transplantation may aid in long-term survival (198). The prognosis has been observed to be the best in cases containing a predominance of small cells; conversely, it is worse in those cases made up

predominantly of large cells (184,196). *Posttransplant lymphoproliferative lesions* in the lung are histologically identical to LYG, and they may share common pathogenetic mechanisms. Both have been shown to contain evidence of EBV proteins and genetic material in proliferating B lymphocytes. Posttransplant lymphoproliferative disease (PTLD) is seen most commonly after heart and lung transplantation, but it has been seen in kidney and liver transplantation cases (186,199,200).

PULMONARY HYALINIZING GRANULOMA

Pulmonary hyalinizing granuloma (PHG) is a rare, tumor-like lung nodule with a characteristic histologic pattern of thick, hyalinized collagen bands arranged in whorls, parallel arrays, or vague storiform patterns (Fig. 25.60). The changes are morphologically identical to those of sclerosing mediastinitis, and patients having both conditions, as well as retroperitoneal fibrosis and Riedel struma, have been described (201–205). Plasma cells and lymphocytes frequently are found between the collagen bands, and germinal centers may be seen at the periphery of the lesion. The nature of this condition is unknown, but autoimmune phenomena have been described in enough cases to imply a pathogenetic role. The possibility that PHG might be a form of immunoproliferation is suggested by its coexistence with malignant lymphoma, multiple myeloma, and amyloidosis in a patient (206). It has also been described with Castleman disease (207).

Clinically, the condition may be asymptomatic, but most patients complain of cough, shortness of breath, and chest pain. Radiographically, multiple, often bilateral nodules that mimic metastatic carcinoma are most often observed. Solitary lesions and infiltrates are less common (201). The course may be one of progressive enlargement of the nodules, particularly in patients with bilateral disease, and new nodules may appear during the period of observation. Single nodules are usually cured by local resection. The prognosis is reasonably favorable; no deaths have thus far been described as a result of this condition, but the disease may be progressive. A unique case of PHG accompanied by mediastinal, retroperitoneal, pericardial-pleural, and widespread soft-tissue fibrosing lesions has been described (207).

INFLAMMATORY PSEUDOTUMOR (INFLAMMATORY MYOBLASTIC TUMOR, PLASMA CELL GRANULOMA)

Inflammatory pseudotumor (IPT) has evoked controversy ever since it was reported by Bahadori and Liebow in 1973 (208). They described 40 patients, two-thirds of whom were younger than 30 years of age, with mostly single tumor-like masses in the lung. A mixture of plasma cells, lymphocytes, histiocytes, and spindle mesenchymal cells characterized these masses microscopically. Since then, several other large series of lung cases have been reported (209–214). This entity has also been recognized in a wide range of extrapulmonary sites (212). Although it can occur at any age, a high incidence is observed in the pediatric age group, and the peak age of all cases is in the third decade. Most patients are asymptomatic, but approximately 25% may have symptoms of cough, dyspnea, fever, hemoptysis,

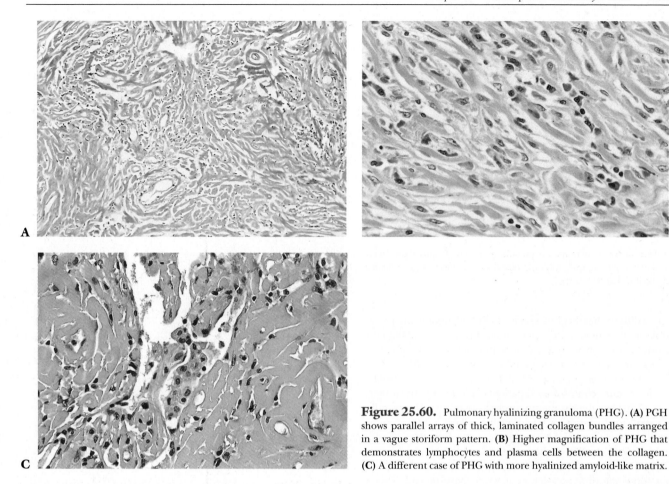

Figure 25.60. Pulmonary hyalinizing granuloma (PHG). **(A)** PGH shows parallel arrays of thick, laminated collagen bundles arranged in a vague storiform pattern. **(B)** Higher magnification of PHG that demonstrates lymphocytes and plasma cells between the collagen. **(C)** A different case of PHG with more hyalinized amyloid-like matrix.

or chest pain. Clubbing of the fingers has been reported. Some patients may have hypergammaglobulinemia, leukocytosis, or anemia that is reversible when the lesion is removed (209).

Radiologically, the most common finding is a single, well-circumscribed mass; only 3% of cases are bilateral. Examples of predominantly endobronchial growth have been reported. Rare cases may involve the lung and mediastinum simultaneously (208). Histologically, wide variation is seen among cases, which has led to conflicting opinions regarding the inflammatory or neoplastic nature of this lesion. Some cases are composed predominantly of bland fibroblast and myofibroblast spindle cells arranged either in interlacing fascicles or in a storiform pattern with only a minor component of inflammatory cells (Fig. 25.61). Other cases show a predominance of mature plasma cells and lymphocytes that are mixed with histiocytes and only a minor mesenchymal component (Fig. 25.62). Dense fibrosis or myxomatous stroma is seen in some cases (Fig. 25.63). All varieties appear as solid, space-occupying, tumor-like masses that may invade the blood vessels and bronchi and may show direct extension to adjacent structures (213). The spindle cells stain positive with antibodies to vimentin and actin; rarely, occasional cells stain with desmin, which is consistent with fibroblasts and myofibroblasts. Plasma cells are polyclonal (212,214).

Debate exists about the inflammatory or neoplastic nature of IPT, with a shift currently in favor of the term *inflammatory myofibroblastic tumor* (215,216). The spindle cells of some examples of pulmonary and extrapulmonary IPT have been shown to possess a persistent abnormality involving chromosome 2p23 at the *ALK* gene locus, which is consistent with a neoplasm

(217). This gene product, the ALK-1 protein, can be stained by IHC, a feature that is also seen with anaplastic large-cell lymphoma (218). Tumors in lung can be ALK-1–positive or –negative (215). Surgical resection is most often curative but, in rare cases, patients have died as the result of local recurrence or direct extension or metastasis to the heart, mediastinum, pleura, bone, brain, and other organs (209,212,215). The best predictor for recurrence is the circumscription or invasiveness of the lesion and the completeness of resection.

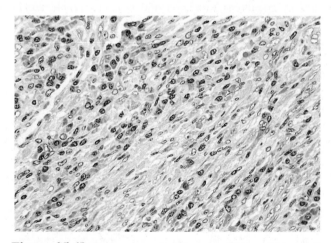

Figure 25.61. Inflammatory pseudotumor. This pseudotumor is composed of fascicles of bland, spindled mesenchymal cells (fibroblasts and myofibroblasts), accompanied by small numbers of plasma cells.

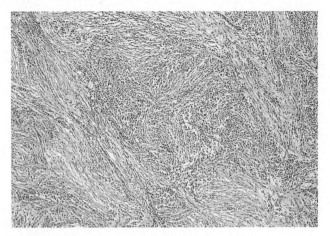

Figure 25.62. Inflammatory pseudotumor. It is composed predominantly of plasma cells with only rare spindle cells, but it shows a fascicular and storiform architecture.

The differential diagnosis includes BOOP, organizing pneumonia, endogenous lipid pneumonia, benign and malignant fibrous histiocytoma, other primary and metastatic spindle cell tumors, and mycobacterial pseudotumor (Fig. 25.64) (219). This last condition can look a great deal like IPT, but it is usually seen in immunocompromised patients and it contains numerous acid-fast bacilli or sometimes other organisms. The spindle cells stain for histiocyte markers such as CD68, rather than as myofibroblasts. Benign fibrous histiocytoma has been considered analogous to IPT by some researchers, whereas malignant fibrous histiocytoma shows the microscopic features of homologous soft-tissue tumors. Wick et al. (220) have recently called attention to inflammatory sarcomatoid carcinomas that share many features with IPT but show a greater degree of atypia and mitoses, and stain with epithelial markers.

PULMONARY ANGIITIS AND GRANULOMATOSIS

Pulmonary angiitis and granulomatosis is a group of conditions originally described by Liebow, who thought these entities were reasonably homogeneous because of shared morphologic features of granuloma formation and vasculitis (Table 25.11)

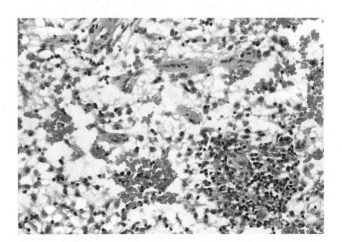

Figure 25.63. Myxoid variant of the inflammatory pseudotumor.

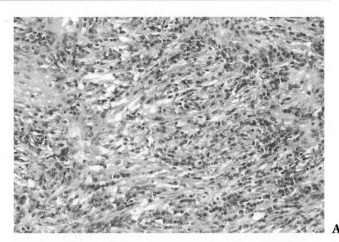

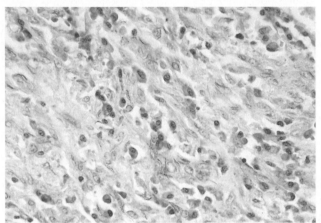

Figure 25.64. Mycobacterial pseudotumor of lung. **(A)** In this pseudotumor, the resemblance to Figure 25.58 should be noted. **(B)** Acid-fast organisms are found in the lesion.

TABLE 25.11

Pulmonary Lesions Showing the Histologic Pattern of Angiitis and Granulomatosis

Morphologic Classification	Pathogenesis
Wegener granulomatosis, Churg-Strauss granulomatosis	Immunologically mediated vasculitis and granuloma
Bronchocentric granulomatosis	Part of bronchopulmonary aspergillosis; eosinophilic pneumonia spectrum of hypersensitivity
Necrotizing sarcoidal granulomatosis	Possibly a form of nodular sarcoidosis or hypersensitivity pneumonitis
Lymphomatoid granulomatosis	Malignant lymphoma of lung
Rheumatoid nodule	Rheumatoid arthritis
Dirofilaria immitis granuloma	Parasite
Infectious granuloma	Tuberculosis, fungi
Unknown etiology	—

—, not available.

(183,221). These conditions included LYG, BCG, WG, and necrotizing sarcoidal granulomatosis (NSG). This group has since been shown to be etiologically heterogeneous in that LYG has come to be recognized as a malignant lymphoma, and BCG has been identified as part of the group of hypersensitivity pulmonary reactions to *Aspergillus* and other fungi (92,159,160). Finally, most experts consider that NSG represents a variant form of nodular sarcoidosis (221–223). Thus, of the entities Liebow originally described, only Wegener granulomatosis remains.

WEGENER GRANULOMATOSIS

WG remains the paradigm of the angiitis and granulomatosis group (224). It is characterized clinically by the inflammatory involvement of the upper respiratory tract and lung, as well as glomerulonephritis. Systemic vasculitis and granulomatosis may often involve peripheral nerves and the central nervous system, the orbit, skin, ear, breast, and other sites as well. The disease most commonly occurs in middle age, but all ages may be affected (182,183,224).

A limited or attenuated form that is confined to the lung is often observed, but unity with the more generalized WG has been demonstrated by cases in which glomerulonephritis has developed after many years of apparently localized respiratory tract involvement (225–227). Similarly, lung involvement has developed after many years in some patients who initially had only localized upper respiratory tract involvement (228). The factors that influence the rate and sites of progression are not understood. However, the observation that has repeatedly been made is that patients with primarily lower respiratory tract granulomatous disease without renal involvement have a better prognosis than do those with glomerulonephritis early in their course (225). Clinically, patients with the predominantly pulmonary form (limited WG) may have fever, cough, chest pain, and hemoptysis. Some patients, however, have relatively few symptoms or are asymptomatic cases, which were discovered by chest x-ray examination alone (182). Radiologically, nodular masses, often with cavitation, are seen commonly in the lower lobes, but less well-defined infiltrates may also be observed (182,225,229). Usually, they are bilateral and multiple, but they may be confined to one lung. Solitary lesions are rare but have been observed (182,225,228,230). One useful radiographic clue is the observation of waxing and waning pulmonary infiltrates and nodules that appear or progress in one area of the lung while resolving in another (227). This radiographic picture tends to rule out infection, but it is not specific and it can also be seen in LYG as well as in pulmonary hypersensitivity reactions (105,227). The CT scans largely correlate with the chest radiograph, but they can also show feeder vessels associated with the infiltrates (231).

Pathologically, necrotic granulomatous inflammation showing central liquefaction necrosis is characteristic of the lesion. The necrosis contains amorphous pink material, nuclear debris, and inflammatory cells, and is surrounded by a rim of palisaded histiocytes and giant cells. Lymphocytes, plasma cells, polymorphonuclear leukocytes, and small to moderate numbers of eosinophils are also present. The overall shape of the necrotic granuloma tends to have a geographic appearance because of the residual islands of viable tissue within the necrosis and the outer angulated contour of the granuloma (Fig. 25.65). The necrotic center gives the impression of being liquefied rather

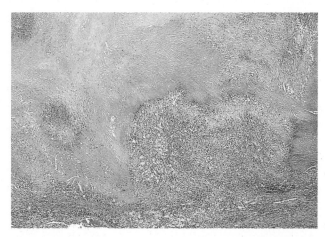

Figure 25.65. Wegener granulomatosis (WG). Necrotizing granuloma with a necrobiotic center, geographic shape, and outer zone of solid-appearing chronic inflammation are seen.

than having a more solid, infarct-like appearance as seen in LYG. Often, fibrinoid necrosis or microabscess-like collections of inflammatory cells are seen in the necrotic granuloma (Fig. 25.66).

Inflammatory vasculitis outside of the necrotic granuloma is important in the diagnosis, and Liebow thought this is the primary mode of lung injury (Fig. 25.67) (225). In some cases, however, vasculitis is not seen. An alternative explanation for the absence of vasculitis is that the formation of the necrotizing granuloma may be the primary tissue reaction, or that the vasculitis is simultaneous or a secondary phenomenon (228). Sampling error may explain some cases. The vasculitis in WG shows edema of the vessel wall and transmural infiltration by polymorphonuclear cells, eosinophils, and plasma cells. It often is eccentric, involving only a portion of the circumference of the vessel (Fig. 25.68). Granulomatous vasculitis may be seen but it is unusual (232). Fibrinoid necrosis of the vessel, when present, is a diagnostic clue to WG; it may, however, not always be seen (Fig. 25.69) (182,225,232). Quite often, the blood vessel involvement is more indolent and is composed of chronic inflammatory cells and fibrosis. The significance of pulmonary vasculitis should be interpreted with some caution, however, because vasculitis without fibrinoid necrosis can be seen in 60% of cases of proven pulmonary tuberculosis and, to a lesser extent, in fungal infection (233). Vasculitis should therefore not be automatically equated with WG. In some cases, the diagnosis of WG rests on clinical and radiographic correlation and on the exclusion of mycobacterial and fungal infection by the appropriate cultures, and the careful examination of special stains. However, some cases in which the diagnosis of WG is only presumptive do remain; in these, the pathologist has to settle for a diagnosis of "consistent with or suggestive of WG" while he or she awaits the results of mycobacterial and fungal cultures or serologic tests, such as those for serum antineutrophilic cytoplasmic antibodies (ANCAs) (234). Close clinical observation may be necessary in some such patients who are acutely ill and who may require immediate cytotoxic therapy for the presumptive diagnosis of WG.

WG may rarely present as a solitary, sometimes cavitating nodule. Such lesions are usually resected to exclude a malignant tumor. Because tuberculosis or fungal diseases are much more

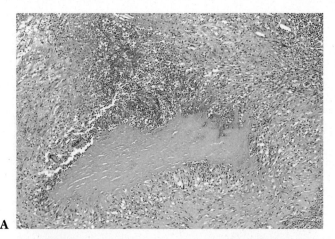

A

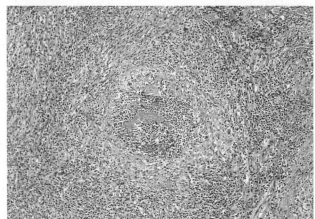

B

Figure 25.66. Wegener granulomatosis (WG). **(A)** The central portion of necrobiotic granuloma demonstrates fibrinoid necrosis, pallisaded histiocytes, and polymorphonuclear cells. **(B)** WG shows a microabscess-like collection of polymorphonuclear cells in the necrotic, inflamed tissue.

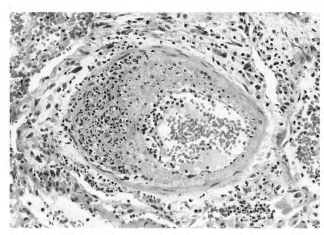

Figure 25.68. Wegener granulomatosis (WG). The active vasculitis shows acute inflammatory cells involving a portion of the pulmonary artery.

likely than WG to manifest as a single nodule, these cases are diagnostic problems. In such instances, unless the classic clinical, histologic, and laboratory findings of WG are present, the diagnosis of WG should be regarded with caution and chemotherapy should be withheld until a visible recurrent lesion is found or the disease progresses to other sites (233). As in some localized infectious granulomas, solitary WG may not recur after surgical removal (227). On the other hand, more generalized involvement by WG of the upper respiratory tract and elsewhere has been observed many years after the excision of a solitary granulomatous lesion that was originally thought to be infectious or of unknown etiology. Whenever the pathologist is confronted with a granulomatous process in the lung, the appropriate cultures and special stains must always be included as part of the workup. *This cannot be overemphasized.* The topic of granulomatous lung disease has recently been addressed in an excellent comprehensive review (235).

Some variations from the classic histology of WG described previously do exist. A less common form of WG in the lung is manifested by acute inflammation of the alveolar septal capillar-

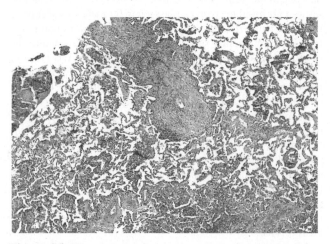

Figure 25.67. Wegener granulomatosis (WG). Vasculitis is present outside of the edge of the granuloma, which is seen at the lower portion of the figure.

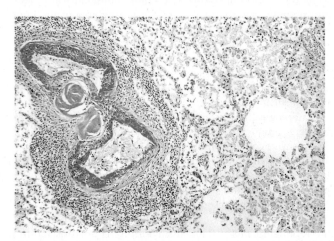

Figure 25.69. Fulminating Wegener granulomatosis. Fibrinoid necrosis of pulmonary arteries is present in this case.

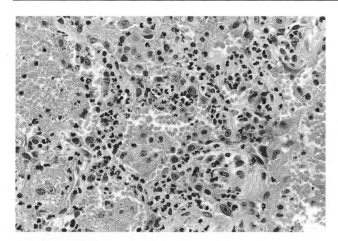

Figure 25.70. Wegener granulomatosis (WG). Acute capillaritis with intra-alveolar hemorrhage is present.

ies, with or without large arteries and veins (Fig. 25.70) (234). Polymorphonuclear leukocytes showing nuclear breakdown may fill the capillary lumen, infiltrate the alveolar septa, and focally spill over into the alveolar space. This capillaritis may be focal or may be more generalized in the biopsy sample; it is associated with the appearance of fresh intra-alveolar hemorrhage. Evidence of older hemorrhage may be present as well, as demonstrated by the intra-alveolar organization and hemosiderin-laden macrophages. Chronic interstitial inflammation may sometimes confuse the histologic picture and overshadow the vessel involvement. Such cases often manifest as hemoptysis, sometimes severe, and tend to be acutely ill. The chest radiograph tends to show more diffuse interstitial or alveolar patterns rather than nodules. Capillaritis may be observed as the primary lung involvement or in patients who have recurrent WG after having initially had more typical nodular or cavitating pulmonary lesions. Other conditions such as microscopic polyangiitis, lupus, or the various hemorrhagic syndromes may also show pulmonary capillaritis; therefore, this finding is not specific for WG without other supporting clinical or pathologic evidence (233,234,236,237). Some cases of WG show a BOOP-like pattern that is accompanied by the usual type of vasculitis, whereas other cases may show large numbers of eosinophils (Fig. 25.71)

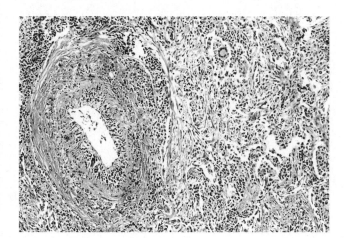

Figure 25.71. Wegener granulomatosis (WG). The bronchiolitis obliterans with organizing pneumonia (BOOP) pattern is seen adjacent to the vasculitis.

(238,239). Rarely, a bronchocentric pattern of involvement is observed (239).

The cause of WG is unknown. Speculation about an infectious agent has long existed but this remains unproven (233). Immunologic mechanisms are thought to play an important role. The serum ANCA test has revolutionized the diagnosis of WG (240). The following two manifestations indicate a positive test result: the C-ANCA, which shows diffuse cytoplasmic staining of neutrophil or monocyte cytoplasm, and the P-ANCA, which stains the cell cytoplasm in a perinuclear distribution. C-ANCA is directed against neutrophil serene proteinase 3 and it gives a positive result in almost 90% of active generalized WG and roughly 60% of active limited WG (234,240). It is not entirely specific, however, because in rare instances, diverse conditions such as inflammatory bowel disease, pulmonary embolism, and collagen vascular disease, among others, may show a positive result (234,240,241). P-ANCA detects myeloperoxidase and it is less common in WG; it more often is present in cases of Churg-Strauss syndrome, microscopic polyarteritis, inflammatory bowel disease, and crescentic glomerulonephritis (234, 242). C-ANCA may play a role in the pathogenesis of WG. Serum titers can be used to follow remissions and exacerbations and to monitor the course of the disease.

In all cases of suspected pulmonary WG, complete study of the patient with attention to the upper airway and kidney is important. In occasional instances, occult disease elsewhere strengthens a presumptive diagnosis of WG that is based on lung biopsy. In some cases, the detection and treatment of silent glomerulonephritis prevent serious progressive renal damage.

Biopsies of the upper airways or skin may show granulomatous inflammation or vasculitis, but they often demonstrate only nonspecific inflammatory changes (Fig. 25.72). In the appropriate clinical setting, these findings can be extremely useful in documenting extrapulmonary disease. Cyclophosphamide and prednisone are effective in controlling both the localized and systemic forms of this disease, resulting in a complete remission rate of approximately 75% (224,226). Bactrim also has been effective in some cases of limited WG (224).

NECROTIZING SARCOIDAL GRANULOMATOSIS

As stated earlier, most regard this entity as a form of sarcoidosis. NSG usually has mild symptoms of low-grade fever, cough, and rarely hemoptysis. The chest radiograph may show a single nodule or multiple bilateral nodules, sometimes with cavitation. Hilar lymph node enlargement is variable (183,221,222). Multiple noncaseating, sarcoid-like granulomas are present; histologically, these may coalesce and form a large nodular collection of granulomatous inflammation.

Sometimes necrosis with cavitation occurs within these foci, similar to that seen in infectious granulomas (222). Other cases show more solid areas of inflammation without necrosis and fewer granulomas (Fig. 25.73). The pulmonary arteries characteristically show giant-cell vasculitis (Fig. 25.74). This can take the form of discrete, sarcoid-like granulomas within the vessel wall, or it may be similar to the vasculitis seen in giant-cell arteritis with radially arranged giant cells without discrete granuloma formation. Both types of vascular lesions may be associated with chronic lymphocytic infiltration, mural fibrosis, and obliteration of the lumen. The similarity to sarcoidosis is illustrated by some cases that show typical sarcoid-like granulomas in the adjacent interstitial tissue, within the alveoli, or next to the inter-

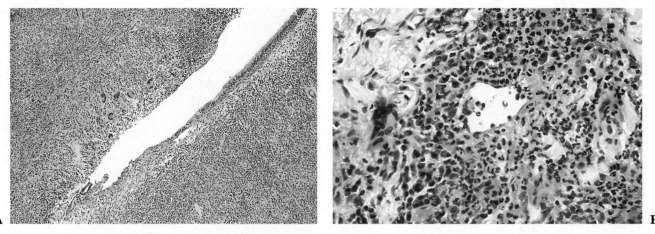

Figure 25.72. Wegener granulomatosis (WG). **(A)** This paranasal sinus biopsy from a patient with WG demonstrates multinucleated giant cells and chronic inflammation. **(B)** This skin biopsy from a patient with WG shows a focus of granulomatosis inflammation and vasculitis in the dermis.

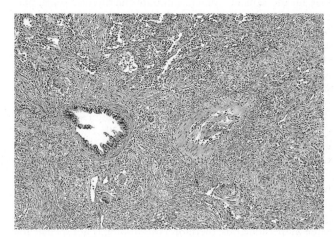

Figure 25.73. Necrotizing sarcoidal granulomatosis. Confluent chronic inflammation shows focal vascular involvement and isolated giant cells.

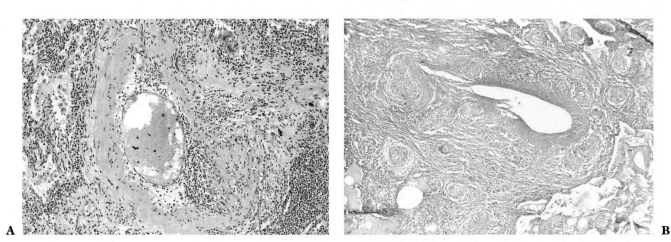

Figure 25.74. Necrotizing sarcoidal granulomatosis (NSG). **(A)** Granulomatous vasculitis is seen in this case of NSG. **(B)** Granulomatous vasculitis involves the entire circumference of the wall of this pulmonary artery.

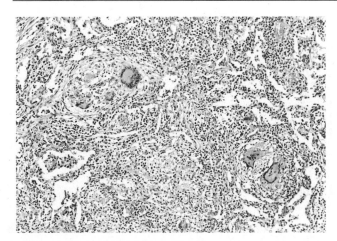

Figure 25.75. Necrotizing sarcoidal granulomatosis (NSG). The isolated intraparenchymal granulomas suggest a relationship to sarcoidosis.

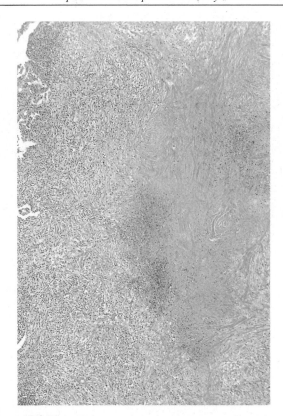

Figure 25.76. Solitary necrotizing granuloma in patient with active rheumatoid arthritis.

lobular connective tissue septa and blood vessels of the lung (Fig. 25.75) (221). Other cases that have been described as NSG have a more necrotizing granulomatous appearance, similar to WG or infection. The involvement of the hilar lymph nodes by sarcoid-like granulomas is unusual but it has been observed, as have rare examples of uveitis or other forms of extrapulmonary involvement (243–246). NSG, like sarcoidosis, is a diagnosis of exclusion. The pathologist must take care to exclude tuberculosis or fungal infection in each case (221,235). The prognosis is generally excellent and the condition responds well to steroid therapy, or it may be cured by surgery.

RHEUMATOID ARTHRITIS

Patients with rheumatoid arthritis may have several different forms of lung disease, including UIP, NSIP, follicular bronchitis, LIP, pulmonary vasculitis, amyloidosis, or pleural effusion (41,247–249). Single or multiple nodular granulomas may also develop in the lung, and these may be confused with infections or WG (225,247). The classic rheumatoid granuloma tends to be round in shape and to have a zone of palisaded histiocytes that are arranged perpendicularly to a necrobiotic center, a pattern similar to that seen in the subcutaneous nodule. The vasculitis is usually not as pronounced as in WG, and it generally is located within or adjacent to the rheumatoid nodule rather than in areas of the lung away from the granuloma, as is seen in some cases of WG. The rheumatoid nodule is often located in the periphery of the lung and it may encroach on the visceral pleura. Clinically, joint disease is usually active and the serum titer of rheumatoid factor is high. However, as it occurs in WG, the pulmonary nodule of rheumatoid arthritis may develop at various times during the course of the disease (247). Some rheumatoid nodules may be indistinguishable from WG histologically, and the precise classification of these cases is difficult (Fig. 25.76) (225). In some instances, the adjacent lung tissue may show UIP or NSIP, with or without lymphoid nodules, which is more suggestive of rheumatoid arthritis. In other cases, however, the clinical course helps to define the lesion. As in WG and NSG, cases of suspected rheumatoid nodule should be thoroughly studied for the possibility of an infectious origin because steroid therapy for arthritis may accelerate lung disease that is

caused by mycobacteria or fungi. Caplan syndrome is seen in patients with rheumatoid nodules who also have coal worker's pneumoconiosis (250). The lesion appears histologically as a rheumatoid nodule with abundant carbon and silica material within the necrotic center. In modern times, it is rarely seen.

DIROFILARIA

Parasites may also cause a pulmonary reaction that can easily be mistaken for infectious or noninfectious granulomatous disease. *Dirofilaria immitis,* the dog heartworm, may infest the human as a secondary end-stage host. It is most common in the southern coastal states, but may also be seen elsewhere. In humans, immature worms die in the right ventricle and embolize into the pulmonary arterial circulation, where they evoke a necrotizing granulomatous response with vasculitis in the lung tissue (Fig. 25.77) (251,252). This vasculitis may contain giant cells that mimic NSG or WG. Often, only by pure luck are the pale eosinophilic shadows of the poorly staining dead worms seen within the necrotic granuloma. Usually these are few in number and are easily overlooked or may not even be in the histologic sections. In humans, the disease is self-limiting. Most cases are asymptomatic, coming to attention only because of the investigation of a solitary peripheral pulmonary nodule that is seen on x-ray study. The identification of the organism within the granuloma immediately clarifies the cause of the granulomatous process.

ALLERGIC ANGIITIS AND GRANULOMATOSIS OF CHURG-STRAUSS

Allergic angiitis and granulomatosis of Churg-Strauss (CS) is a rare condition usually seen in people with chronic asthma

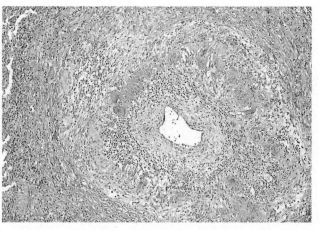

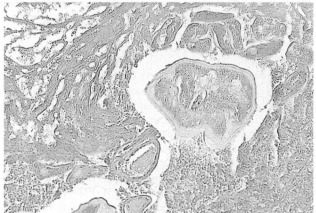

Figure 25.77. Dirofilariasis. **(A)** A single necrotic granuloma is found in the lung. **(B)** Granulomatous vasculitis is seen in lung tissue outside of the granuloma. **(C)** This is a cross section of a parasite seen in one section of this case.

(253–256). It is a multisystemic disease that clinically is characterized by fever, generalized systemic involvement, and blood eosinophilia, which usually comprises more than 10% of the white blood count. Rare cases without asthma have been reported (257). Pathologically, tissue eosinophilia, vasculitis, and granuloma formation in many organ systems, particularly in the lung, skin, heart, nervous system, and gastrointestinal tract, are seen (254–256). The patients may either have an acutely fulminating or a chronic febrile illness that predominantly affects the lung. An occasional case without pulmonary disease is seen as a fever of unknown origin. An indolent cutaneous form of the disease may also occur.

The pulmonary lesion characteristically shows eosinophilic pneumonia with eosinophilic vasculitis (Fig. 25.78). Small granulomas with multinucleated giant cells and fibrinoid necrosis and giant cells in blood vessels are usually present (Fig. 25.79). The finding of small microscopic granulomas surrounded by eosinophils and composed of a bright red central body of collagen necrosis that sometimes contains fragmented eosinophils and eosinophilic granular debris is tantamount to a diagnosis of CS granulomatosis. These characteristically show radially arranged histiocytes and giant cells that are palisaded around fibrinoid material and that are often located within or adjacent to small arteries or arterioles. This eosinophilic microgranuloma enables histologic recognition of the syndrome in biopsy specimens of the skin, lymph nodes, liver, or any other site (Fig. 25.80).

Other associated histologic features in lung biopsy material are fibrin-rich edema, lymphocytic infiltration, scattered iso-

lated giant cells, sarcoid-like granulomas, and focal fibrosis. Eosinophilic microabscesses sometimes containing Charcot-Leyden crystals may also be present. Larger bronchi may show the changes of chronic asthma with eosinophils, mucous cell hyperplasia, and a thickened eosinophilic basement membrane. In lung tissue, the disease sometimes has the overall appearance of a fibrin-rich pneumonia with eosinophilia and vasculitis that is similar to CEP. Less commonly, nodular necrotic lesions similar to those seen in WG or rheumatoid nodules are observed.

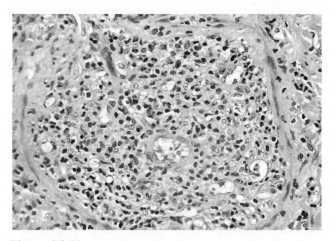

Figure 25.78. Churg-Strauss syndrome. The blood vessel is heavily infiltrated by eosinophils and chronic inflammatory cells.

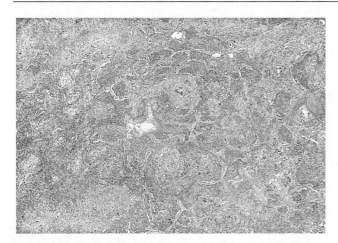

Figure 25.79. Churg-Strauss syndrome. The loosely formed giant-cell granuloma is associated with fibrin-rich exudative inflammation in the lung.

In WG or rheumatoid nodules, however, the tissue eosinophilia is not usually pronounced; blood eosinophilia is not usually seen; and the patient generally does not have an asthmatic background. Also unlike WG, the triad of upper-airway destruction, lung involvement, and glomerulonephritis is uncommon. Some have suggested that CS may have a prevasculitic phase, which is recognizable clinically by the characteristic signs but with only tissue eosinophilia microscopically (254).

Upper-airway disease in CS, when it occurs, is usually characterized by allergic rhinitis with rhinorrhea rather than by an ulcerating, destructive lesion. Furthermore, renal disease, when it occurs, is usually mild without glomerular crescents or fibrinoid necrosis (254,256).

The disease usually responds dramatically to steroids or chemotherapy with full recovery in the majority of patients, but relapses and fatalities may occur. Recently, new cases of CS have emerged following the prescription of steroid-sparing leukotrien receptor antagonists for the treatment of chronic asthma. The suspicion is that previously suppressed CS may become

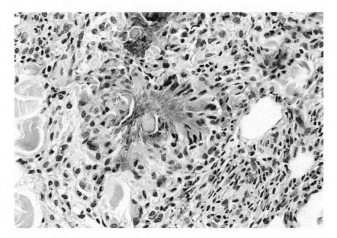

Figure 25.80. Churg-Strauss syndrome. This skin biopsy shows microscopic granuloma composed of collagen necrosis in the center, granular eosinophilic debris, palisaded histiocytes, and numerous eosinophils.

manifest after steroids are tapered and the newer medication is used (258).

P-ANCA is found in slightly less than half of patients with CS, in contrast to WG, where 90% of active cases will demonstrate elevated titers of C-ANCA. Recent studies have suggested that CS patients with P-ANCA have significantly higher incidence of severe renal disease, peripheral neuropathy, lung hemorrhage, and both pulmonary and extrapulmonary vasculitis, whereas P-ANCA–negative cases show eosinophilic cardiomyopathy, nasal polyps, and eosinophilic GI infiltrates. The supposition is that P-ANCA–associated CS has a different pathogenesis than do negative cases with a discernible difference in clinical manifestations. Interestingly, about 10% of cases will demonstrate C-ANCA, similar to WG, which suggests some overlap syndromes (259,260).

An important point in differential diagnosis is that when granulomas and tissue eosinophilia are encountered, consider that coccidioidomycosis can sometimes be associated with significant numbers of eosinophils (261).

POLYARTERITIS NODOSA

Polyarteritis nodosa is rarely the cause of clinical lung disease. Associated asthma and peripheral blood eosinophilia may also be present, but the evidence of serious multisystemic disease usually far overshadows the pulmonary findings. In lung tissue, eosinophils may be prominent; in addition, vasculitis involving predominantly the bronchial arteries is present, with fibrinoid necrosis (262). However, large necrotic granulomas are not seen, and neither are the characteristic microgranulomas of CS syndrome.

MICROSCOPIC POLYANGIITIS

Microscopic polyangiitis (MP) is a more recently defined entity that, with WG and CS, forms a group of pulmonary and systemic vasculitides characterized by a paucity of immune deposits in the walls of blood vessels detected by immunomicroscopy. These entities have therefore been termed *pauci-immune vasculitis* (263).

MP most often affects the lung as diffuse intra-alveolar hemorrhage, and the kidneys as necrotizing glomerulonephritis. It has been recognized as the most common cause of the pulmonary-renal syndrome, far more so than Goodpasture syndrome. The disease is commonly associated with systemic findings in the form of fever, muscle, joint, upper respiratory, and skin involvement. Unlike WG, necrotizing granulomatosis inflammation is usually not observed and P-ANCA rather than C-ANCA titers are elevated in the serum in up to 80% of cases.

Pathologically, the lung shows evidence of intra-alveolar hemorrhage and acute capillaritis that is similar to the capillaritis form of WG. Vasculitis involving larger vessels is less common. The intra-alveolar hemorrhage may be fresh but hemosiderin is usually present. Organizing foci of hemorrhage similar to BOOP are seen in cases of some standing. Other cases show the pattern of DAD in addition to vessel inflammation. Attention to the presence of capillaritis and, clinically, to the systemic nature of MP should aid the morphologic interpretation of such cases. Confusion with the capillaritis form of WG can be expected and clear separation is not always possible, but for differences in serum ANCA. The prognosis is guarded; approximately

68% of cases survive 5 years (264). Treatment consists of cytoxan and prednisone.

PULMONARY HEMORRHAGE

Pulmonary hemorrhage may be a manifestation of severe systemic disease complicated by a bleeding diathesis; it may be secondary to mechanical or functional pulmonary venous obstruction; it may be associated with various intrinsic pulmonary diseases; it has been seen with extramedullary hematopoiesis in the lungs; or it may be the result of a primary pulmonary hemorrhagic syndrome (265) (Table 25.12). Four conditions are generally considered to be primary forms of diffuse intra-alveolar hemorrhage. Three of these—Goodpasture syndrome, microscopic polyangiitis, and hemorrhage associated with immune complex glomerulonephritis—affect the kidney and lung, whereas the fourth, idiopathic pulmonary hemosiderosis, does not.

Goodpasture syndrome combines sometimes massive pulmonary hemorrhage with glomerulonephritis, which usually is of the rapidly progressive crescentic type (237,263). It is mediated by a circulating cytotoxic antibody that reacts to the basement membrane of both the pulmonary capillary and the glomerulus. This antibody is usually of the IgG class, and it fixes complement in a linear pattern along the basement membrane of both the alveolus and the glomerulus, as immunofluorescent microscopy demonstrates. The initial event stimulating this reaction is unknown, but autoimmunity to type IV collagen basement membrane material is thought to play an important role. A few patients have been reported who have minimal or absent renal disease (266).

Clinically, the disease predominates in young men; however, the age range is wide and the condition may be seen in children. Hemoptysis is a common symptom. Most patients have mild anemia and progressive azotemia.

Histologically, the alveoli are filled with fresh blood and hemosiderin-laden macrophages. This latter finding is helpful in distinguishing intrapulmonary hemorrhage from biopsy-related bleeding. The alveolar septa show mild hyperplasia as

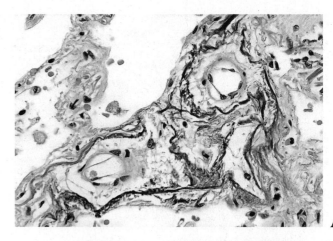

A

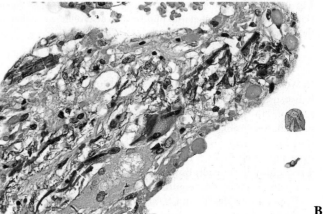

B

Figure 25.81. Pulmonary hemorrhage. **(A)** The pulmonary vein shows iron deposited in the elastica. **(B)** Foreign-body–type giant-cell reaction to fragmented iron-laden elastic fibers.

well as slight thickening of the alveolar lining cells, and sometimes a sparse lymphocytic infiltrate or focal acute capillaritis. Evidence of organization of the intra-alveolar blood is a common finding. Precipitation of iron in vessels as well as a giant-cell reaction (endogenous pneumoconiosis) can be observed. These histologic changes are not specific and can also be seen with other causes of alveolar hemorrhage (Fig. 25.81).

Immunofluorescent microscopy is required to differentiate Goodpasture syndrome from hemorrhage associated with immune complex glomerulonephritis and idiopathic pulmonary hemosiderosis. In immune complex disease, the circulating antibody complexes are fixed in a granular pattern along the basement membrane, in contrast to the linear pattern of Goodpasture syndrome (237). In idiopathic pulmonary hemosiderosis and microscopic polyangiitis, no antibody is detected. The prognosis of Goodpasture syndrome is not favorable, and these patients require plasmapheresis and chemotherapy.

Idiopathic pulmonary hemosiderosis is a diagnosis of exclusion after all other causes of pulmonary hemorrhage have been ruled out. This disease is the most common cause of lung hemorrhage in children. By definition, no circulating antibody to basement membrane material or immune complexes is present, and renal disease is absent. Immunofluorescent microscopy is negative. Otherwise, this condition can be histologically very similar to Goodpasture syndrome in the lung biopsy material (237). The alveoli characteristically are filled with hemosiderin-

TABLE 25.12	
Pulmonary Hemorrhage	
Cause	*Examples of Disease*
Bleeding diathesis	Leukemia; cancer chemotherapy
Venous hypertension	Mitral stenosis; pulmonary veno-occlusive disease
Infection	Aspergillosis; mucormycosis
Tumor	Lung cancer; vascular tumors
Collagen diseases	Systemic lupus exthematosus; Wegener granulomatosis; rheumatoid arthritis; microscopic polyangiitis
Diffuse alveolar damage	Respirator lung; *Pneumocystis carinii*; others.
Pulmonary hemorrhagic syndrome	Goodpasture syndrome; idiopathic pulmonary hemosiderosis; immune complex glomerulonephritis; microscopic polyangiitis

laden macrophages and fresh blood but, unlike in Goodpasture, capillaritis is not observed. Most cases are eventually fatal after several years, but in some patients many years pass between bouts of pulmonary hemorrhage. The etiology of this condition is not understood.

The alveolar capillaritis type of WG, MP, systemic lupus erythematosus (SLE), rheumatoid arthritis, Behçet syndrome, Henoch-Schönlein purpura (HSP), and others may also be associated with significant pulmonary hemorrhage (234,237, 267). Clinical and laboratory findings are often necessary to define the disease category accurately in these cases (237). Organizing alveolar hemorrhage can sometimes be mistaken for BOOP. Attention to the presence of hemosiderin and the clinical finding of hemoptysis are useful in differentiating these conditions.

PULMONARY HYPERTENSION

Many conditions are associated with pulmonary hypertension, and they are etiologically heterogeneous. They include congenital heart defects, acquired cardiac valvular disease, collagen vascular disease, liver cirrhosis, emphysema, and chronic alveolar hypoxia caused by obesity, to name a few. Recently, the World Health Organization (WHO) attempted to classify the condition by primary and secondary causes (268,269) (Table 25.13). Most lung biopsies, however, are performed to diagnose or to evaluate pulmonary hypertension of unknown cause. Patients with cryptogenic pulmonary hypertension usually fall into one of three categories: primary plexogenic hypertension, thrombotic pulmonary hypertension, or pulmonary veno-occlusive disease (PVOD). All of these are rare. Several good comprehensive reviews on the subject have been published (238,268, 270–272).

PRIMARY PLEXOGENIC HYPERTENSION

Primary plexogenic hypertension (PPHT) is of unknown etiology; it occurs predominantly in young women. Rare familial causes are observed (238). Clinically, it is characterized by progressive shortness of breath, angina pectoris, syncope, and the

potential for sudden death. Right ventricular hypertrophy and cardiac failure are common accompaniments of progressive PPHT. The symptoms usually evolve insidiously, and most patients die within several years after diagnosis. Organ transplantation is the only treatment for intractable cases, but a subset of patients with a more protracted clinical course and a more favorable outcome does appear to exist. PPHT has been reported with various collagen diseases, and some patients may have high titers of serum ANAs (235,273). Association with AIDS as well as sickle cell anemia have been recognized (274–276). A genetic lesion has been described in both familial and sporadic cases (268,277). The pathogenesis of PPHT is unknown. Evidence for the role of sex hormones is suggested by the demonstration of progesterone receptors in the lesions, whereas human herpesvirus-8 (HHV8) has been associated with some cases (278,279). Some have suggested it is a monoclonal proliferation of endothelial cells (280,281).

The chest radiograph reflects pulmonary hypertension, with prominence of the pulmonary arterial trunk and right ventricle. Focal alveolar infiltrates may be present as the result of intra-alveolar hemorrhage.

Heath and Edwards have described a sequence of pathologic changes in the small muscular pulmonary arteries and arterioles in patients with congenital heart disease; these have been used to gauge the severity of PPHT (282). Not all cases of PPHT show each of the pathologic findings described in the classic sequence, however, and Wagenvoort has cautioned against too much reliance on strict application of the grading scheme in patients without heart disease (275). The earliest finding is muscularization of pulmonary arterioles and medial hypertrophy of muscular pulmonary arteries (Fig. 25.82). Muscular arterioles within alveolar septae are a useful sign of this. Wagenvoort and Wagenvoort have suggested that, when a calibrated eyepiece is used, if the medial thickness of the vessel wall exceeds 7% of the outside diameter, chronic pulmonary hypertension may be suspected (283). Care should be taken, however, not to confuse normal, age-related medial intimal thickening with pathologic changes (284). As hypertension progresses, intimal hyperplasia of arteries occurs and the vessels show medial muscle hypertrophy as well as cellular intimal hyperplasia that gradually causes attenuation of the vascular lumen. Progressive changes show a more marked narrowing of the vascular lumen in addition to subintimal fibrosis that has a concentric, onion-ring appearance and that is associated with marked reduplication of the internal elastic membrane. At this stage, the arteries and arterioles have the appearance of rigid, noncompliant tubes (Fig. 25.83).

Dilatation and plexiform lesions produced by aneurysmal dilatation of small arteries, and the formation of eccentrically located glomeruloid nodules containing capillary-like channels indicate the presence of severe hypertension (Fig. 25.84). Histologically, these lesions define PPHT and they may form, along with organizing thrombosis, as an attempt to shunt blood past the high-pressure arterial circulation into the venous side. Fresh fibrin thrombi may be seen within the plexiform lesions; in addition, evidence of old or recent intra-alveolar hemorrhage is commonly observed. Recent evidence suggests that abnormal endothelial proliferation is a major feature of this disease (281,285). Least commonly seen in PPHT is evidence of acute arteritis, with or without fibrinoid necrosis that is similar to that seen in polyarteritis nodosa (Fig. 25.85). This is usually associated clinically with extreme degrees of pulmonary hyper-

TABLE 25.13

Causes of Pulmonary Hypertension

Disease Category	*Examples of Disease*
Cardiac disease	Congenital left-to-right shunts; acquired valvular disease; left atrial myxoma; acquired cardiac shunts
Mediastinal disease	Fibrosing mediastinitis; tumors
Intrinsic lung disease	Emphysema; interstitial fibrosis; honeycomb lung; drug abuser's lung
Primary pulmonary hypertension	Pulmonary veno-occlusive disease Plexogenic hypertension Thrombotic hypertension
Miscellaneous	Obesity; high-altitude dwellers; chronic liver disease; adverse drug reactions and toxins; drug-abuser's lung; pulmonary emboli.

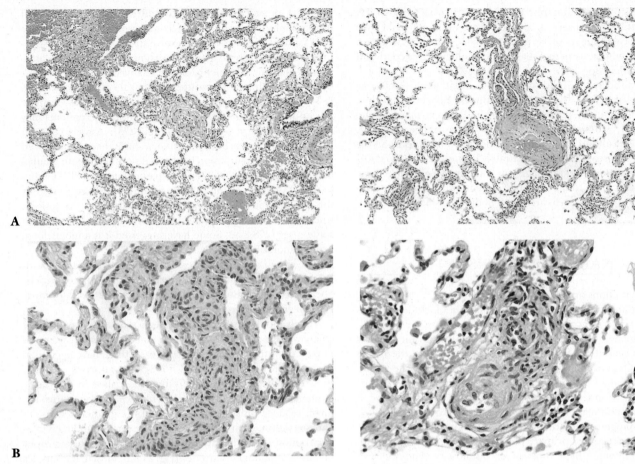

Figure 25.82. Primary pulmonary hypertension. **(A)** Medial thickening and hypertrophy of small pulmonary artery accentuates these structures on low power. **(B)** Marked hypertrophy of the small pulmonary artery is seen.

Figure 25.84. Early plexiform lesion. **(A)** This lesion is adjacent to hyperplastic artery. **(B)** Higher magnification of another lesion showing sievelike vascular channels that appear to be outside the vessel wall.

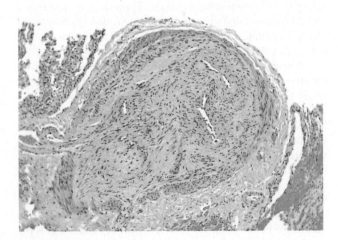

Figure 25.83. Primary pulmonary hypertension. Pronounced fibrous and muscular proliferation of the pulmonary artery is seen in this advanced lesion.

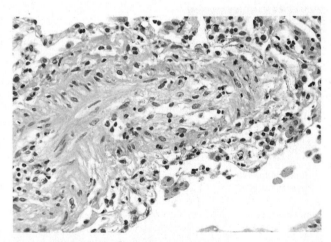

Figure 25.85. Inflammatory infiltration in a hyperplastic pulmonary artery. Fibrinoid necrosis is not seen.

tension. Plexiform changes and arteritis reflect the likelihood of a poor response to therapy and a short survival.

The vascular changes of PPHT and those of secondary pulmonary hypertension resulting from left-to-right cardiac shunts are identical, so knowledge of the cardiac status is necessary before such changes can be attributed to PPHT.

Therapy has been relatively unsuccessful in PPHT. It consists of potent vasodilator drugs, anticoagulation, and supportive measures. Less than half of patients survive 5 years (286). Recently, heart-lung transplantation has been successful (287). Both an adverse reaction to drugs such as aminorex, L-tryptophan, and fenfluramine and toxic oil syndrome may produce pulmonary hypertension that histologically mimics PPHT (288,289).

THROMBOTIC PULMONARY HYPERTENSION

Whether thrombotic pulmonary hypertension and PPHT are the same disease is the subject of some debate (241). As in PPHT, thrombotic pulmonary hypertension is more common in young women, and, clinically, clearly separating the two diseases is often impossible (290). The histologic changes are primarily related to the presence of recent and organized intravascular thrombi. Fresh fibrin thrombi are, however, surprisingly rare (290). Eccentric intimal fibrous plaques and bands, fibrous septa, and multichanneled organized thrombi within the small arteries and arterioles are evidence of thrombosis with organization, and these are the histologic hallmarks of the disease. Sometimes, however, the differentiation of a complex recanalized thrombus from the plexiform lesion of PPHT is difficult (Fig. 25.86). Complicating matters further is the realization that some patients with PPHT may have pulmonary thrombi or emboli (275,282,283). Mild to moderate medial hypertrophy of pulmonary arteries and arterioles is seen in patients with thrombotic disease, suggesting the role of vasospasm in the pathogenesis of the pulmonary hypertension. Likely, in situ thrombosis rather than actual emboli is responsible for this condition, which is also postulated to be an important factor in PPHT (291). Marked intimal fibroplasia, plexiform lesions, and arteritis do not occur as the result of thrombotic disease; when they are present, they tend to implicate PPHT. However, problems in differentiating these two conditions frequently occur.

A small group of patients does appear to suffer from repeated bouts of pulmonary emboli in large vessels that result in pulmonary hypertension. Their age tends to be older, and no sex prevalence similar to that seen in PPHT or thrombotic hypertension is present (292,293).

PULMONARY VENO-OCCLUSIVE DISEASE

PVOD is a rare cause of pulmonary hypertension that results from progressive fibrous obliteration of the pulmonary veins (294–296). The disease is most often seen in children and young adults without any sex predominance, in contrast to PPHT. It has been recorded after chemotherapy for cancer, bone marrow or renal transplantation, scleroderma, or a viral-like illness (297). The disease is usually fatal. Clinically, gradually increasing dyspnea, often with progressive cyanosis; clubbing of the fingers; hemoptysis; and syncope are seen. Radiographically, evidence of increased interstitial markings, pleural effusion, and Kerley lines (which indicate interstitial edema and congestion) are noted, as are findings of right-heart hypertrophy and failure.

Pathologically, the alveolar septa appear prominent and thickened as a result of capillary congestion (298). Evidence of old hemorrhage is seen in the form of collections of hemosiderin-laden macrophages in the alveolar spaces and hemosiderosis of the interstitium. Focal interstitial lymphocytic infiltrates and interstitial fibrosis may be seen as well; together, these combine to give the low-power microscopic appearance of a chronic fibrosing interstitial process. The examination of small and medium-sized pulmonary veins, however, reveals fibrous intimal thickening by dense collagen or by a peculiarly edematous, concentrically laminated, loose connective tissue within the intima and media (Fig. 25.87). The vein lumen is greatly narrowed or it may show total fibrous occlusion. This is best seen with the aid of elastic stains, which outline the changes within parenchymal veins and those within the connective tissue of the subpleural area and perilobular septa (Fig. 25.88).

Evidence of venous thrombosis may be present in the form of fibrin clots or fibrous septa, but this is unusual. Other associated features are mild arterial hypertrophy, recent and recanalized arterial thrombi, venous infarcts, dilation of the lymphatics, and fibrosis of interlobar septae (Fig. 25.89) (299). Reduplication

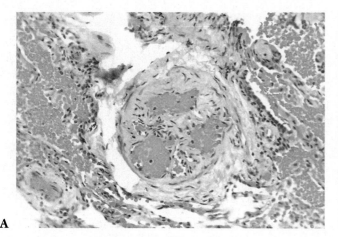
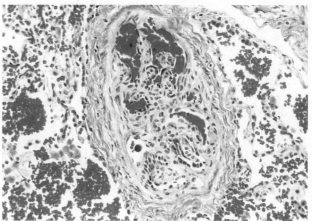

A   **B**

Figure 25.86. Thrombotic pulmonary hypertension. **(A)** Fibrous septa are seen in the small pulmonary artery. **(B)** The recanalized thrombus shows similarity to the plexiform lesion (Trichrome).

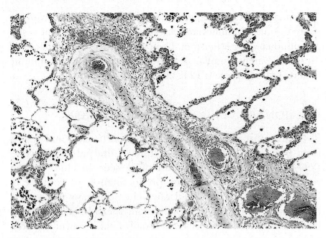

Figure 25.87. Pulmonary veno-occlusive disease. Fibrosis and thickening of pulmonary vein accentuates this structure.

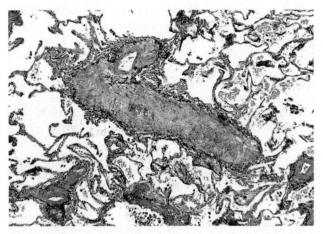

Figure 25.88. Pulmonary veno-occlusive disease. The elastic stain outlines the single external elastic membrane of the fibrosed pulmonary veins.

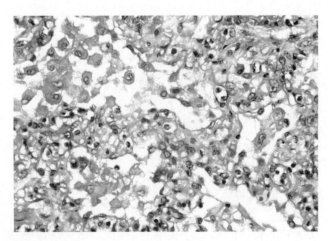

Figure 25.89. Pulmonary veno-occlusive disease. Prominence and dilatation of the alveolar capillaries is seen.

of the elastica within medium-sized pulmonary veins (arterialization) results from the venous obstruction and the transmission of elevated pressures. The use of elastic tissue stains is essential in diagnosing PVOD. These stains outline the internal and external elastic membranes of the arteries and the single external elastic membranes of veins. The totally obliterated veins can sometimes be appreciated only with these special stains. Otherwise, PVOD can be mistaken for UIP or other hemorrhagic and fibrosing processes. Rarely, elastic fibers may be seen within foreign-body giant-cell granulomas as the result of fragmentation and disorganization of the lung framework (so-called endogenous pneumoconiosis) (Fig. 25.81) (300). However, this can be due to many causes of lung hemorrhage and is therefore not specific.

Although medial hypertrophy of arteries is common in both PPHT and PVOD, the severe intimal fibrosis of arteries, the plexiform lesions, and the arteritis seen in PPHT help to differentiate these two conditions. Conversely, severe congestion of the alveolar capillaries and the characteristic occlusive venous fibrosis are pathognomonic of PVOD, and these are not seen in PPHT (Fig. 25.90). In contrast to PPHT, interstitial fibrosis of the lung has been observed following PVOD. A helpful clinical clue that is not always present is the finding of an elevated pulmonary capillary wedge pressure in PVOD, which is not seen in PPHT.

OTHER CAUSES

Pulmonary capillary hemangiomatosis is a rare cause of pulmonary hypertension. Histologically, it is characterized by the proliferation of benign-appearing capillaries in the alveolar septa, interlobar connective tissue, and pleura that appear to compress pulmonary veins, along with evidence of recent hemorrhage and hemosiderosis. Occlusion of small pulmonary veins also occurs. The disease is poorly understood. Some believe it to be a variant of PVOD, with which it may be confused clinically and pathologically (301). The prognosis is poor, similar to PVOD (302).

Lung lesions in intravenous drug abusers result from the injection of insoluble fillers of oral medications, which, when injected intravenously, lodge within the small pulmonary arteries and lead to thrombosis (303). They are usually incidental

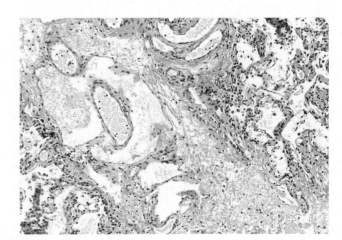

Figure 25.90. Pulmonary veno-occlusive disease. Dilated lymphatics surround the intraseptal veins.

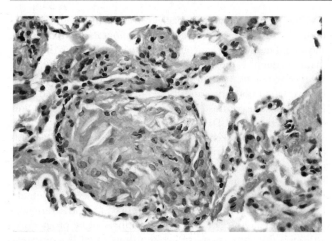

Figure 25.91. Foreign-body granuloma obliterating a small pulmonary artery in an intravenous drug abuser.

findings at autopsy or in surgical biopsy material taken for other reasons. Rarely, however, this condition may clinically be the cause of significant pulmonary hypertension. Microscopically, the characteristic lesion consists of fresh or organizing arterial thrombi containing this foreign material. Perivascular foreign-body granulomas are also commonly seen (Fig. 25.91). Both the vessels and perivascular granulomas contain birefringent foreign material that has the configuration of starch, talc, or other materials. These findings may be associated with acute vasculitis or with interstitial inflammation and fibrosis that, at times, may mimic a primary interstitial pneumonia (Fig. 25.92).

PULMONARY LYMPHANGIOMYOMATOSIS

Lymphangiomyomatosis (LAM) is a rare condition characterized by a peculiar and histologically unique pattern of interstitial smooth-muscle proliferation in the lung that, qualitatively, bears close similarity to that seen in angiomyolipoma of the kidney. It may be associated with the full expression of tuberous sclerosis or with similar smooth-muscle proliferations of the abdominal or thoracic lymphatic ducts and lymph nodes in combi-

nation with renal angiomyolipomas, or it may occur only in the lung (295,304–306). Molecular genetic studies have shown similar allelic loss, most often in the *TSC1* and *TSC2* genes in both patients with tuberous sclerosis complex (TSC)-associated renal angiomyolipoma and isolated pulmonary LAM—confirming the relationship between these conditions (307,308,309). Only 1% to 3% of patients with TSC have full-blown pulmonary LAM, but recent studies using high-resolution CT scans have shown that more than 20% of TSC patients have some evidence of subclinical lung disease (310,311). Unlike tuberous sclerosis, pulmonary LAM occurs almost exclusively in women who are usually in their childbearing years. Only one male patient with coexistent TSC has been described (312). Shortness of breath, cough, and repeated pneumothorax are the most common presentations as well as the predominant cause of disability. Hemoptysis and chylous pleural effusions also occur.

Radiographically, the chest film may be normal. More commonly, a pattern of interstitial fibrosis or reticulonodular densities is seen, sometimes with cysts and blebs. Unlike the more common interstitial processes, however, the lungs may appear expanded or normal in size rather than shrunken. This results from the smooth-muscle proliferation around the bronchioles, which leads to air trapping. High-resolution CT scans show numerous thin-walled cysts throughout the lungs. These can be seen even in patients with normal chest radiographs (313). Physiologically, the finding of severe diffusion impairment with evidence of air trapping and expanded lung volumes in a young woman is the characteristic diagnostic picture.

Pathologically, a lacy pattern of round and spindled smooth-muscle proliferation within the interstitium and around the bronchi, bronchioles, veins, and lymphatics is seen. These appear to spin off the muscle coat of these structures and to extend into the walls of adjacent alveolar ducts and alveoli in a whorled pattern that gives this process its unique histologic appearance (Fig. 25.93). The muscle cells themselves often contain optically clear cytoplasm and abundant intracytoplasmic glycogen (Fig. 25.94). Air trapping and overdistention occurs as the result of bronchiolar obstruction, which may lead to cystic blebs and pneumothorax (Fig. 25.95). Venous and lymphatic obstruction may also occur from (a) muscle proliferation, which causes lo-

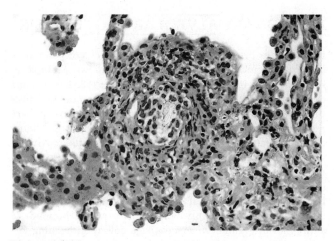

Figure 25.92. Drug abuser. Partially polarized foreign material in the artery lumen is associated with acute vasculitis.

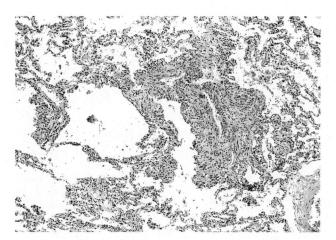

Figure 25.93. Lymphangioleiomyomatosis. Smooth-muscle proliferation is associated with focal cystic change. The muscle is intimately related to the blood vessels and distal airways, and it seems to spin off these structures.

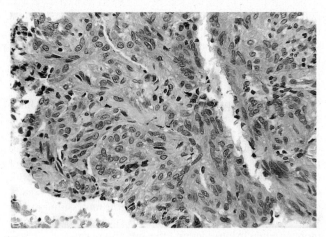

Figure 25.94. Lymphangioleiomyomatosis. Detail of whorled smooth muscle in the wall of the blood vessel gives the pattern of a hamartoma.

calized pulmonary hemorrhage and hemoptysis; or (b) lymphatic cysts, which may rupture into the pleural space, causing chylous pleural effusion. The process is patchy and haphazard in its distribution within the biopsy, and the lung tissue between the foci of involvement may be normal or may show collections of hemosiderin-filled macrophages with some chronic inflammation. The smooth muscle stains positively with melanoma antigen HMB45, a feature shared with both angiomyolipoma and clear-cell tumor of the lung (314,315). All three of these lesions may be found in patients with TSC (314).

The disease is progressive and the prognosis is poor. Death may occur rapidly (i.e., within 1 year) or the disease may be more protracted, with the patient surviving more than 10 years. The 10-year survival has ranged from 30% to 70% in some series (316,317). LAM may contain estrogen and progesterone receptors, and some patients have responded to antiestrogen therapy; however, no drug is entirely effective (318). A grading system that is based on 101 cases has been proposed; it correlates the percentage of cystic and solid architecture with prognosis (317). The 10-year survival ranged from 52% to 100% in this series, depending on the grade of the lesion. Heart-lung transplanta-

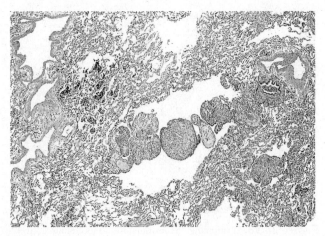

Figure 25.95. Lymphangioleiomyomatosis. Cystic blebs contain smooth muscle. The intervening lung is relatively normal-appearing except for foci of hemosiderin-filled macrophages in the alveoli.

tion has been a recent approach to treatment (319). Interestingly, the disease has recurred in lung allografts, with evidence showing that the muscle proliferation originated from the transplant recipient rather than from the donor lung (320). Rare cases of *metastatic endometrial stromal sarcoma* may become cystic, causing pneumothorax, and these must be differentiated from LAM (321). In contrast to LAM, this is HMB45-negative and often positive with CD10.

Another lesion seen in the lungs of patients with TSC with or without LAM is a bland multifocal proliferation of alveolar type II pneumocystis; this lesion, which measures only a few millimeters, is termed *micronodular pneumocyte hyperplasia* (MPH) (Fig. 25.96) (322–325). It is most commonly seen in women. Unlike LAM, stains for hormone receptors and HMB45 are negative. Most examples of MPH do not appear to be progressive, although the clinical course is often dominated by coexisting LAM. Rare cases of MPH may lead to respiratory failure (326).

LAM must be distinguished from *benign metastasizing leiomyomas of lung.* This condition is also seen predominantly in female patients and is also hormonally dependent; however, this disease has a much better prognosis. Histologically, the smooth-muscle proliferation is composed of single or multiple nodules that are localized rather than diffuse. Cysts and blebs usually are not a feature in this disorder. Most authors regard the entity as well-differentiated leiomyosarcoma that has metastasized to the lung, usually from a "benign" tumor of the uterus resected long ago (327,328). Recent studies have suggested that these cases are a genetically unique subset of uterine myomas (329). Similar to LAM, estrogen receptors have been demonstrated (330). A hamartomatous interstitial smooth-muscle hyperplasia of the lungs that is associated with severe pulmonary hypertension, is seen in men, and is not associated with LAM or TSC has been described (331).

Finally, LAM must be differentiated from *diffuse pulmonary lymphangiomatosis* (332). This condition can be seen in men, women, and children. The symptoms most commonly are wheezing and shortness of breath. Pathologically, the lesion is characterized by prominent lymphatic vessels in the pleura and connective tissue septa that are accompanied by variable degrees of smooth muscle proliferation, the appearance of which may be kaposiform. Chylothorax may occur but cysts, pneumothorax, and HMB45 positivity are not seen. The disease may be progressive and may lead to death.

PULMONARY ALVEOLAR PROTEINOSIS

Ever since its first description, the pathogenesis of pulmonary alveolar proteinosis (PAP) has remained unknown. Multiple associated factors have been described, however (333–335). Some cases have been observed following exposure to inorganic dusts such as silica, aluminum, and fiberglass, among others, and are regarded as a secondary phenomenon (336–338). Areas identical to idiopathic PAP have been seen around tuberculous lesions or in patients with immunosuppression or leukemia (339–341). The pathologic changes are thought to reflect an imbalance between the production of surfactant by alveolar type II cells and the inability of defective lung macrophages to remove this material (342), which results from the presence of antibodies to granulocyte-macrophage colony stimulating factor (GM-SCF). GM-SCF is found in both serum and lavage fluid of DAD patients, which inhibits macrophage function (343).

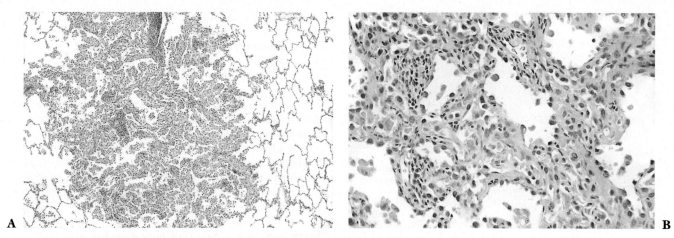

Figure 25.96. Micronodular pneumocyte hyperplasia. **(A)** Multiple small nodules of cuboidal type II pneumocyte proliferation. **(B)** No mitoses or nuclear atypia are observed. Note how some alveolar lining cells appear in slightly widened interstitium; these are characteristic features.

PAP is seen in adults of all ages, but infants and children may also be affected (344). The majority of patients are cigarette smokers (345). Clinically, shortness of breath, cough, sputum production, and fever are observed. Radiographically, a predominantly bilateral perihilar and bibasilar infiltration that often resembles pulmonary edema is seen on the chest radiograph. Unilateral disease has, however, also been seen. Occasional patients may have a normal chest radiograph. High-resolution CT findings reveal bilateral ground-glass, abnormal thickening of interlobar septae (335).

Pathologically, the alveoli are filled with homogeneous pink-red, PAS-positive, granular material with cholesterol clefts as well as with the ghost outlines of degenerated macrophages and alveolar type II cells (Fig. 25.97). The alveolar septa are normal except for occasional areas of mild lymphocytic infiltration. Alveolar type II cells may be prominent in areas and sometimes show foamy transformation of the cytoplasm (Fig. 25.98). Ultrastructurally, the intra-alveolar exudate is seen to contain lamellar bodies in various stages of dissolution, along with cellular debris and lipid particles. The intra-alveolar exudate has been demonstrated to be rich in surfactant (346).

This condition represents still another type of pulmonary

reaction pattern that is not actually a specific disease. In most clinical cases the etiology is unknown. The proteinaceous material is an excellent culture medium for microorganisms, and infection with such organisms as *Nocardia*, mycobacteria, *Aspergillus*, or others may complicate the clinical course. The frothy intra-alveolar exudates of *P. carinii* may closely resemble PAP, and special stains should be conducted if there is any doubt about the diagnosis. PAP can be identified by lung biopsy or by bronchopulmonary lavage with ultrastructural analysis of the lavage fluid, which shows large numbers of lamellar bodies. Since the introduction of bronchoalveolar lavage as treatment, few cases are progressive (347). Lavage is effective and it may be repeated if relapse occurs. Steroids should not be administered (333,347).

SARCOIDOSIS

Sarcoidosis is a common multisystemic granulomatous disease of unknown etiology that, in more than 90% of cases, affects the lungs. It is one of the most common conditions for which

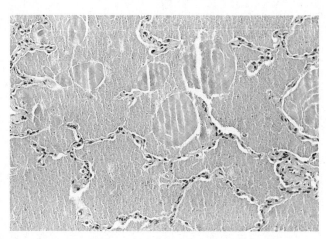

Figure 25.97. Pulmonary alveolar proteinosis (PAP). Characteristic granular proteinaceous material fills the alveoli.

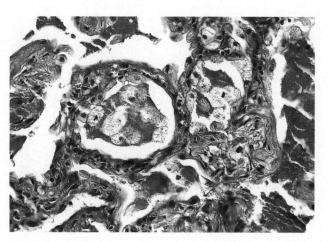

Figure 25.98. Pulmonary alveolar proteinosis (PAP). Foamy degeneration and dissolution of the intra-alveolar macrophages are seen with periodic acid-Schiff stain (PAS).

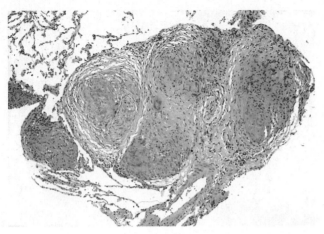

Figure 25.99. Sarcoidosis. Characteristic hard granulomas are seen in this transbronchial biopsy. The concentric, laminated fibrosis of the granuloma is a common feature.

a lung biopsy is performed (348). An infectious cause has long been sought, and familial and environmental case clusters have been reported (349). Using molecular probes for mycobacteria and HHV8, recent studies have shown a positive association in some cases (350–353). A recently proposed provocative theory suggests that foreign environmental particles, too small to see with ordinary microscopy, are causal in genetically prone individuals (354).

Pathologically, sarcoidosis is characterized by noncaseating epithelioid cell granulomas, which, in the lungs, involve primarily the pleura, the connective tissue septa, and the interstitium around pulmonary vessels and bronchi (Fig. 25.99). The distribution of the granulomas appears to follow the pathways of the pulmonary lymphatic circulation, and it thus is preferentially located around the blood vessels and within the connective tissue framework of the lung (Fig. 25.100) (355). Granulomatous angiitis is common (356).

Because of the nonspecific nature of the granulomatous reaction, the diagnosis of sarcoidosis rests with careful assessment of the clinical, radiographic, and pathologic aspects of each case. Clinically, most patients are young, ranging from 20 to 40

years of age, but the disease can occur at any age. It is more common in African Americans. Approximately half the patients are asymptomatic, and the diagnosis is made after a biopsy for an abnormal chest radiograph. Other patients may have an active febrile illness that is marked by severe dyspnea, or they may have uveitis or erythema nodosum. Dyspnea and cough are the most common symptoms of lung disease. Approximately 2% of cases may slowly progress to a fibrotic process that may lead to interstitial fibrosis, honeycomb lung, and death (357).

Radiographically, the pattern is variable. The most common abnormality is hilar adenopathy, which is seen in 50% of cases; 30% show both hilar adenopathy and parenchymal infiltrates, and 12% parenchymal infiltrates only. A normal chest radiograph is found in 8% of cases (357). High-resolution CT reveals small nodules in almost all cases (358). Cases with established fibrosis may have evidence of honeycombing with cysts and bullae.

Laboratory tests are sometimes helpful in diagnosis. Approximately 80% of patients with active sarcoidosis have elevated angiotensin-converting enzyme in the serum, but this is not specific because it can be seen in a small percentage of other conditions as well (359). The bronchial lavage fluid contains increased numbers of CD4-positive T-helper lymphocytes, and reflects increased number of these cells in affected tissue (360). Cutaneous anergy is commonly seen, and the B-cell hyperactivity is reflected by the associated polyclonal hypergammaglobulinemia that is commonly seen in the serum.

Pathologically, the granulomas are small and are composed of epithelioid histiocytes and multinucleated giant cells that sometimes contain nonspecific birefringent crystalline, asteroid, or Schaumann bodies. The histiocytes are tightly packed and the granulomas discretely marginated, often with a few lymphocytes mixed in. The outer borders often show concentric laminated collagen, giving them an onion-skin appearance. Focal necrosis may occur within the center. The granulomas may occur singly or may form nodular collections (Fig. 25.101). Sometimes necrosis and, more rarely, cavitation may occur within the larger confluent areas, making differentiation from infection difficult. These nodular cases are considered to be NSG by most observers (348). A mild lymphocytic interstitial alveolitis in the alveolar septa may accompany the granulomas in about two-thirds of patients; this is thought to precede the

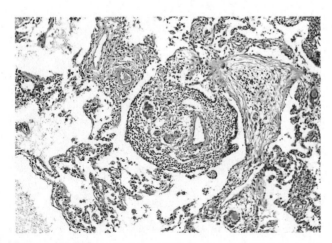

Figure 25.100. Active sarcoidosis. Perivascular granuloma associated with chronic interstitial inflammation and bronchiolitis obliterans are present.

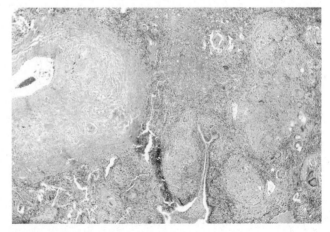

Figure 25.101. Sarcoidosis. Confluent epithelioid granulomas and granulomatous vasculitis are seen.

formation of the epithelioid granulomas, and it decreases over time (361). The granulomas themselves may resolve completely or they may form nodular hyaline scars. Severe interstitial fibrosis with cystic blebs may be a result of progressive sarcoidosis, and, in advanced cases, clinical and radiographic correlation is necessary to arrive at a correct diagnosis. The finding of hyalinized granulomas in such cases is extremely helpful. Unlike its sensitivity for other chronic diffuse interstitial lung disease, transbronchial lung biopsy is highly accurate in making the diagnosis of pulmonary sarcoidosis (2,362). The finding of the characteristic granuloma in the appropriate clinical setting in a transbronchial biopsy is diagnostic, whereas a nonspecific fibrotic or inflammatory biopsy should not dissuade the clinician from the diagnosis if the clinical suspicion for sarcoidosis is high. In such cases, a repeat biopsy is then indicated.

Noncaseating sarcoid-like granulomas may also be seen in such diverse conditions as lymphoid pulmonary infiltrates, lung tissue adjacent to carcinoma, mycobacterial or fungal infections, and HP, as well as in most other types of pulmonary hypersensitivity or angiitis and granulomatosis. In HP, the granulomas are often composed of more loosely arranged epithelioid cells, and they have a tendency to be associated more with airways than with blood vessels, fibrous septa, or pleura, in contrast to sarcoidosis. *Berylliosis* is histologically indistinguishable from sarcoidosis, and a history of exposure and mineral analysis of biopsied tissue are required for diagnosis. Difficulties in diagnosis may also occur from transbronchial lung biopsies taken from areas adjacent to tumors because the biopsy may misleadingly sample a granulomatous reaction and not the neoplasm.

The prognosis of sarcoidosis is excellent. Less than 3% of these patients die; almost all deaths result from cardiac or pulmonary involvement (349,363,364). Steroids are effective in improving symptoms and controlling the inflammatory reaction. However, they are usually only used in patients with severe symptoms or with advanced-stage disease; in those with critical findings, such as involvement of the eye or severe hypercalcemia; or in patients with life-threatening cardiac disease. Their efficacy in preventing pulmonary fibrosis is unproven (349). Antimalarial agents, chemotherapeutic drugs, and nonsteroidal anti-inflammatory drugs (NSAIDs) have also been tried (365).

The diagnosis of sarcoidosis is one of exclusion. Special stains for infectious agents should be performed in all cases and the lung biopsy should be cultured whenever possible. The diagnosis can usually be made by obtaining representative transbronchial biopsy material that shows multiple noncaseating granulomas with little associated inflammatory reaction in the lung. Lymph node, skin, or liver biopsy may also offer diagnostic material in the appropriate clinical and radiographic setting.

A recently described low-grade pulmonary infection by atypical mycobacteria that occurs in immunocompetent patients who are exposed to the organism through the use of contaminated hot tubs has been amusingly dubbed *hot tub lung*. Clinically, patients have cough, fever, and dyspnea. Microscopically, small, noncaseating granulomas that are associated with bronchioles with adjacent interstitial inflammation are observed (Fig. 25.102). Special stains for organisms are usually negative, but the cultures have been positive in almost all cases. The disease responds well to antimycobacterial chemotherapy. Distinction of this infection from sarcoidosis and HP is obviously important (366,367).

AMYLOIDOSIS

Pulmonary amyloidosis can take the form of localized primary tracheobronchial involvement, nodular parenchymal masses, or diffuse interstitial septal amyloidosis that accompanies primary amyloidosis or paraproteinemia secondary to plasma-cell myeloma or Waldenström macroglobulinemia (light chain–derived [AL] amyloid). It is also seen as part of secondary amyloidosis (protein A–derived [AA] amyloid) (368–371).

The most common form is nodular intraparenchymal amyloidosis. Such patients are usually elderly and asymptomatic, and they have no evidence of paraproteinemia or systemic disease. They come to medical attention because of an abnormal chest radiograph that shows single or multiple tumor-like masses (372). Microscopically, glassy pink collections of amyloid form nodular masses of one to several centimeters. Foreign-body giant cells may appear to phagocytose the amyloid material (Fig. 25.103). Ossification and calcification of the amyloid may occasionally be seen. The amyloid exhibits the tinctorial quality of apple-green, Congo-red birefringence with polarized microscopy, and has the ultrastructural qualities of amyloid fibrils. In

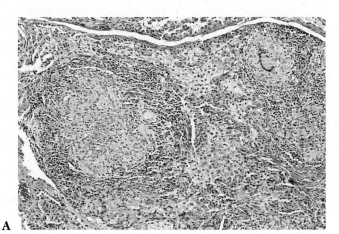
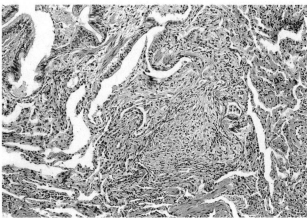

A   B

Figure 25.102. "Hot tub lung." **(A)** Small granuloma are associated with chronic interstitial inflammation. **(B)** Bronchiolitis obliterans with granulomatous inflammation is seen.

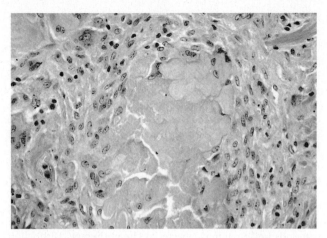

Figure 25.103. Nodular amyloidosis showing a giant-cell reaction to the amyloid material.

some cases, plasma cells may show clonal restriction of light chains, suggesting low-grade immunoproliferation (372).

Tracheobronchial amyloidosis affects the submucosa of the airways as diffuse narrowing or nodular single or multiple tumor-like collections (371). The patients may present with hemoptysis, obstructive pneumonitis, atelectasis, or asthma-like symptoms that are related to bronchial obstruction. The diagnosis is usually made from bronchus biopsy material (Fig. 25.104). Death may result from massive bleeding (373,374).

Diffuse septal amyloidosis predominantly involves the alveolar septa as diffuse interstitial deposits that may lead to physiologic abnormalities identical to those seen in advanced UIP or other forms of diffuse lung fibrosis. The pulmonary arteries are also infiltrated, and, rarely, pulmonary hypertension may result. This condition is most commonly associated with generalized systemic amyloidosis. Cardiac involvement with congestive heart failure and pulmonary edema may confuse the clinical picture, which may mimic primary heart disease. The survival rate is poor and no effective treatment exists. Histologic differentiation of diffuse septal amyloidosis from interstitial fibrosis usually is not a problem. Rare cases of light chain deposition disease have shown Congo-red–negative granular deposits of light chains

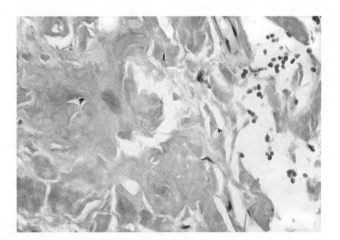

Figure 25.104. Tracheobronchial amyloidosis. Fragments of glassy pink amyloid are seen in this bronchial biopsy material.

that have the light microscope appearance of amyloid. Such cases may sometimes be associated with true amyloid (375).

LUNG BIOPSY IN THE IMMUNOCOMPROMISED HOST

In the adult immunocompromised patient, infiltrative lung disease is most commonly a byproduct of (a) AIDS, (b) leukemia or lymphoma, (c) anticancer chemotherapy, or (d) the administration of drugs in organ transplant recipients. Such patients are often severely ill with diffuse pulmonary infiltrates, fever, and severe shortness of breath with hypoxia, and they often represent medical emergencies.

Several excellent reviews on the infectious agents seen in immunocompromised patients have been published (376–378). The numerous and varied organisms that can cause pulmonary infection in such individuals can be roughly predicted by the categories of host immunodeficiency (376,377). Thus, AIDS patients with severe T-cell deficiency and relatively intact B-cell function are likely to have *P. carinii* pneumonia or *Mycobacterium avium intracellulare*, fungi, toxoplasmosis, or CMV infection. Bacterial infections are most likely to occur in patients with leukemia, and their occurrence is proportionate to the degree of leukopenia. They are also seen in patients who receive high doses of corticosteroids for connective tissue disease or glomerulonephritis. *Aspergillus* infection often complicates the recovery of renal transplant recipients. In all patients, particularly those with AIDS, simultaneous infections with several organisms are common, and the search for causative agents should not cease after one pathogen is found (378).

Several noninvasive techniques available for the identification of organisms, such as bronchoscopy with culture and bronchoalveolar lavage (376,379), which are good for identifying bacteria by cultural methods. Transbronchial biopsy combined with smear and culture is an extremely accurate diagnostic method for uncovering more unusual and opportunistic infections. Adequate material showing alveoli should be present. Nevertheless, even if the biopsy seems inadequate, special stains for *P. carinii* and mycobacteria should be performed because these organisms may rarely be present in fluid or blood adherent to tissue fragments, or deeper cuts may finally show a small amount of lung tissue. Depending on the severity of the clinical situation, an open lung biopsy can be conducted.

In about half of the cases of lung biopsy in immunocompromised hosts, nonspecific findings of hemorrhage or interstitial inflammation with or without hyaline membranes are uncovered, and special stains for organisms are negative (377, 380,381). Such findings usually indicate chemotherapy toxicity, radiation pneumonitis, possible viral infection, pulmonary hemorrhage, nonspecific interstitial pneumonia, or DAD as the cause of pulmonary infiltration. In approximately one-third of cases, pulmonary infiltrates may be due to a new unrelated cause, such as cardiac edema, pulmonary emboli, or aspiration (377). Recurrent leukemia or lymphoma may be identified in the immunocompromised patient.

Conflicting data are available regarding the significance of nonspecific findings in biopsies from immunocompromised patients. Studies have shown that despite a nondiagnostic biopsy, empiric treatment with antibiotics gives the same overall survival as that seen in patients in whom a specific diagnosis of an infectious agent can be made (382). Other studies, however, have shown the opposite, namely, the finding of a specific organism and the application of a specific treatment afford a better outlook (126). Despite the conflicting information, most physicians would rather treat a known organism with specific therapy. *P. carinii* infection is the most common pneumonia in AIDS patients. Bronchoalveolar lavage gives a high yield of diagnosis, with bronchial brushings and induced sputum specimens showing decreasing sensitivity (383,384). Several staining procedures may be used to detect organisms. The most useful are the methenamine silver, Giemsa, and Gram-Weigert techniques. The latter two do not require incubation with silver compounds; they are rapid; and they can be performed by personnel with little technical training, making them ideal for cases that require immediate interpretation during off-peak hours (385).

The lung reaction to *P. carinii* in AIDS patients, as well as in other immunocompromised individuals, may take several forms. The classic pink intra-alveolar exudate may be seen but, commonly, the nonspecific pattern of DAD with hyaline membranes is observed, often without the characteristic frothy intra-alveolar exudates. Foci of organization of the fibrin-rich exudate may be present, evidencing chronicity. Another pattern is a nonspecific interstitial pneumonia without protein-rich edema or hyaline membranes. Granulomatous and cavitary lesions, as well as microcalcifications, have also been described (Fig. 25.105) (386–388). A monoclonal immunofluorescent antibody technique may increase diagnostic accuracy (389,390). *P. carinii* may disseminate widely to other organs besides the lungs (391,392).

Mycobacterium avium-intracellulare (MAI) is also a common pathogen, particularly in AIDS cases. Granulomas may not be observed in these cases; instead, either an intense intra-alveolar and parenchymal infiltration by foamy histiocytes or a proteinaceous exudative reaction is observed. Special stains show high numbers of intracytoplasmic acid-fast bacilli within the intraalveolar exudate (393–395). Tuberculosis is also a common infection in the AIDS population. Unlike in the immunocompetent patient, tuberculosis in these individuals may not show granulomas (396). Intracellular fungi, such as histoplasmosis, may cause a similar nongranulomatous reaction. Because little pathologic change may be observed in severely immunocompromised hosts, all biopsy samples from AIDS patients, regardless of the tissue reaction, should have special stains performed for *P. carinii*, fungi, and mycobacteria.

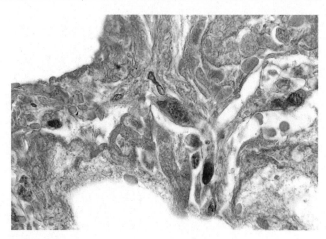

Figure 25.106. Pulmonary toxoplasmosis in a patient receiving anticancer chemotherapy. The cytoplasm of epithelial cells is filled with organisms.

Toxoplasmosis is sometimes observed in AIDS patients as well as in those receiving anticancer drugs (397,398). This intracellular parasite may cause focal parenchymal necrosis similar to that seen in certain viral infections of the herpes group. Furthermore, it may cause a diffuse interstitial pneumonia. The free organisms may be observed in the necrotic tissue, the alveolar lining cells, or the endothelial cells or within the cytoplasm of histiocytes. Cystic forms are not as commonly observed. Methenamine silver, Gram-Weigert, or Giemsa stains may highlight the organisms. Toxoplasmosis, however, can often be recognized in well-prepared H&E-stained sections (Fig. 25.106). Microsporidiosis and cryptosporidiosis may also be seen as pulmonary involvement in AIDS patients (399,400).

CMV and, more rarely, other herpesviruses commonly infect the immunocompromised patient. The characteristic intranuclear and basophilic intracytoplasmic inclusions of CMV are diagnostic; these may be found in alveolar lining cells, cells lying free in the alveoli, bronchial cells, and endothelial cells (Fig. 25.107). They are often easily located, but some cases have only rare inclusions and others none at all in the biopsy sample (401). Serologic and IHC methods are helpful in such cases.

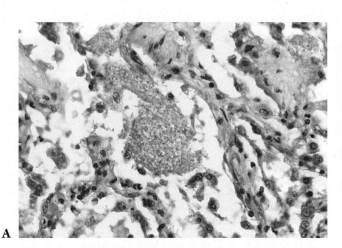

A

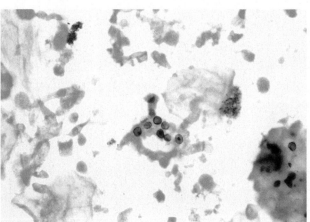

B

Figure 25.105. *Pneumocystis carinii* pneumonia. **(A)** The characteristic pink, frothy intra-alveolar exudate is seen in this patient with AIDS. **(B)** The methenamine silver stain shows the cup-and-saucer–shaped organisms.

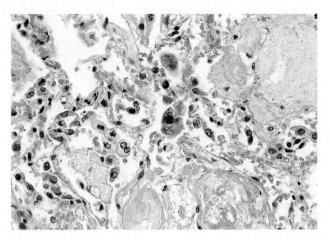

Figure 25.107. Cytomegalovirus pneumonia. The enlarged intra-alveolar cell shows the diagnostic large intranuclear inclusion. The lung tissue shows diffuse alveolar damage.

DAD or focal necrotizing pneumonitis may accompany infection with CMV, and this virus frequently accompanies other infections, particularly those with *P. carinii,* in the immunocompromised patient (402).

Legionnaire disease is commonly seen as the result of corticosteroid administration in renal transplant recipients (403). The organism *Legionella pneumophila* is a small, Gram-negative bacillus that is best seen with silver impregnation techniques such as the Dieterle stain (404). Accurate diagnosis can be made by immunofluorescent microscopy (405). Radiographically, patchy pneumonia with or without consolidation is observed, and pleural effusion is common. Histologically, acute bronchopneumonia is present with acute intra-alveolar exudation of polymorphonuclear leukocytes and histiocytes within fibrin-rich edema fluid. The exudate in the alveoli frequently has a dirty appearance because of fragmentation and degeneration of polymorphonuclear cells within the protein-rich background (Fig. 25.108). Antibiotic therapy is effective but the mortality rate is high in immunocompromised patients. Nematodes such as *Strongyloides* are rare causes of lung disease in AIDS patients (406). Infection by *Strongyloides stercoralis* may be disseminated, and it can be fatal in immunocompromised hosts. The examina-

tion of sputum may disclose the organism in patients with pneumonia (407).

Infection with common bacterial pathogens, as well as more esoteric forms such as *Nocardia, Actinomycetes, Serratia,* and *Rhodococcus* may also be found in the immunocompromised host (408). *R. equis* may be the cause of pulmonary malakoplakia, especially in AIDS patients (see Figs. 25.45 and 25.46). *Bacillary angiomatosis* is a pseudoneoplastic vascular proliferation that is also seen in AIDS patients; it affects many body sites, including the lungs and bronchi. It is caused by *Bartonella* species, which is closely related or identical to the organism that causes cat-scratch fever. Antibiotics are effective (409,410). Most often, the combination of transbronchial lung biopsy, along with bronchial brushing and lavage rather than open lung biopsy, are used to identify specific infections. At least two slides with multiple cuts should be examined. Methenamine silver (pneumocystis) and acid-fast stains have the greatest yield of organisms in AIDS cases. Touch preparations are useful in identifying organisms such as *P. carinii* or toxoplasmosis, and may be rapidly stained by using the Gram-Weigert technique. Although electron microscopy is of little value in identifying infectious organisms, evidence of viral infection may sometimes be found in cases that are otherwise negative by other techniques.

TRANSBRONCHIAL BIOPSY FOR DIFFUSE LUNG DISEASE

The diagnostic accuracy of transbronchial biopsy (TBB) for diffuse lung diseases is less accurate than for infections and is dependent, first of all, on the disease process itself, and second, on the sample obtained (Table 25.14). In one study, this is

TABLE 25.14

Transbronchial Lung Biopsy in Diffuse Noninfectious Lung Disease

Probability of Positive Diagnosis	*Disease*
Excellent due to histologic specificity	Sarcoidosis
	LAM
	EG
	PAP
	EP
	DAD
Inaccurate due to the nonspecific nature of the changes or high sampling error	DIP
	UIP
	NSIP
	BOOP
	Small-airway disease
	RB-ILD
	HP
	Hemorrhagic syndrome
	Vasculitis

BOOP, bronchiolitis obliterans with organizing pneumonia; DAD, diffuse alveolar damage; DIP, desquamative interstitial pneumonia; EG, eosinophilic granuloma; EP, eosinophilic pneumonia; HP, hypersensitivity pneumonitis; LAM, lymphangiomyomatosis; NSIP, nonspecific interstitial pneumonia; PAP, pulmonary alveolar proteinosis; RB-ILD, respiratory bronchiolitis-interstitial lung disease; UIP; usual interstitial pneumonia.

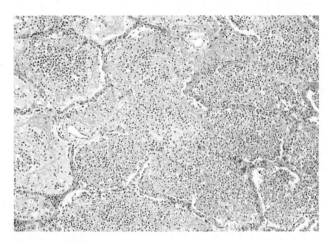

Figure 25.108. Legionnaire disease showing extensive acute pneumonia, alveoli filled with polymorphonuclear cells, and debris.

exemplified by a positive diagnosis in only about 30% of more than 900 cases (411). Most findings in TBB reflect any number of nonspecific reaction patterns. Nevertheless, these still can lead to a specific or highly probable diagnosis provided the histologic findings are coordinated with clinical, radiographic, and laboratory data. Some pathologic entities can be readily diagnosed microscopically because their appearance is disease-specific. These include LAM, EG, PAP, and sarcoidosis (although the sarcoid-like granuloma is nonspecific, an accurate diagnosis can be made in up to 90% of cases with appropriate clinical input). DAD and pulmonary eosinophilia can be added to this category, although the positive diagnosis rate is nowhere near that of sarcoidosis (411).

Some diseases, such as HP (which combines lymphocyte-plasma cell interstitial infiltrates, BOOP, and granuloma), UIP, or one of the alveolar hemorrhagic syndromes, are unlikely to be sampled adequately. Even so, sometimes the combination of nonspecific histologic findings and highly characteristic clinical features may allow a presumptive diagnosis. In doubtful cases, VATS is usually the next step.

REFERENCES

1. Gaensler EA, Carrington CB. Open biopsy for chronic diffuse infiltrative lung disease: clinical, roentgenographic, and physiological correlations in 502 patients. *Ann Thorac Surg* 1980;30:411–426.
2. Perez-Padilla R, Gaxiola M, Salas J, et al. Bronchiolitis in chronic pigeon breeder's disease. Morphologic evidence of a spectrum of small airway lesions in hypersensitivity pneumonitis induced by avian antigens. *Chest* 1996;110:371–377.
3. Gilman MJ, Wang KP. Transbronchial lung biopsy in sarcoidosis. An approach to determine the optimal number of biopsies. *Am Rev Respir Dis* 1980;122:721–724.
4. Katzenstein AL, Askin FB. Interpretation and significance of pathologic findings in transbronchial lung biopsy. *Am J Surg Pathol* 1980;4:223–234.
5. Wall CP, Gaensler EA, Carrington CB, et al. Comparison of transbronchial and open biopsies in chronic infiltrative lung diseases. *Am Rev Respir Dis* 1981;123:280–285.
6. McCarthy JF, Hurley JP, Wood AE. The diverse potential of thoracoscopic assisted surgery. *Int Surg* 1997;82:29–31.
7. Colby TV, Yousem SA. Pulmonary histology for the surgical pathologist. *Am J Surg Pathol* 1988;12:223–239.
8. Ruttner JR, Spycher MA, Sticher H. The detection of etiologic agents in interstitial pulmonary fibrosis. *Hum Pathol* 1973;4:497–512.
9. American Thoracic Society. Idiopathic pulmonary fibrosis: diagnosis and treatment. International consensus statement. American Thoracic Society (ATS), and the European Respiratory Society (ERS). *Am J Respir Crit Care Med* 2000;161:646–664.
10. Coultas DB, Zumwalt RE, Black WC, et al. The epidemiology of interstitial lung diseases. *Am J Respir Crit Care Med* 1994;150:967–972.
11. Demedts M, Costabel U. ATS/ERS international multidisciplinary consensus classification of the idiopathic interstitial pneumonias. *Eur Respir J* 2002;19:794–796.
12. Baumgartner KB, Samet JM, Stidley CA, et al. Cigarette smoking: a risk factor for idiopathic pulmonary fibrosis. *Am J Respir Crit Care Med* 1997;155:242–248.
13. Baumgartner KB, Samet JM, Coultas DB, et al. Occupational and environmental risk factors for idiopathic pulmonary fibrosis: a multicenter case-control study. Collaborating Centers. *Am J Epidemiol* 2000;152:307–315.
14. Hubbard R, Lewis S, Richards K, et al. Occupational exposure to metal or wood dust and aetiology of cryptogenic fibrosing alveolitis. *Lancet* 1996;347:284–289.
15. Erbes R, Schaberg T, Loddenkemper R. Lung function tests in patients with idiopathic pulmonary fibrosis. Are they helpful for predicting outcome? *Chest* 1997;111:51–57.
16. Grenier P, Chevret S, Beigelman C, et al. Chronic diffuse infiltrative lung disease: determination of the diagnostic value of clinical data, chest radiography, and CT and Bayesian analysis. *Radiology* 1994;191:383–390.
17. Akira M, Sakatani M, Ueda E. Idiopathic pulmonary fibrosis: progression of honeycombing at thin-section CT. *Radiology* 1993;189:687–691.
18. Liebow A. Definition and classification of interstitial pneumonias in human pathology. *Pro Respir Res* 1975;8:1–33.
19. Scadding JG, Hinson KF. Diffuse fibrosing alveolitis (diffuse interstitial fibrosis of the lungs). Correlation of histology at biopsy with prognosis. *Thorax* 1967;22:291–304.
20. Katzenstein AL, Zisman DA, Litzky LA, et al. Usual interstitial pneumonia: histologic study of biopsy and explant specimens. *Am J Surg Pathol* 2002;26:1567–1577.
21. Travis WD, Matsui K, Moss J, et al. Idiopathic nonspecific interstitial pneumonia: prognostic significance of cellular and fibrosing patterns: survival comparison with usual interstitial pneumonia and desquamative interstitial pneumonia. *Am J Surg Pathol* 2000;24:19–33.
22. Coalson JJ. The ultrastructure of human fibrosing alveolitis. *Virchows Arch A Pathol Anat Histol* 1982;395:181–199.
23. Davies D, MacFarlane A, Darke CS, et al. Muscular hyperplasia ("cirrhosis") of the lung and bronchial dilatations as features of chronic diffuse fibrosing alveolitis. *Thorax* 1966;21:272–289.
24. Kuhn C. The pathogenesis of pulmonary fibrosis. *Monogr Pathol* 1993:78–92.
25. Crystal RG, Bitterman PB, Mossman B, et al. Future research directions in idiopathic pulmonary fibrosis: summary of a National Heart, Lung, and Blood Institute working group. *Am J Respir Crit Care Med* 2002;166:236–246.
26. Gauldie J, Kolb M, Sime PJ. A new direction in the pathogenesis of idiopathic pulmonary fibrosis? *Respir Res* 2002;3:1.
27. Leask A, Holmes A, Abraham DJ. Connective tissue growth factor: a new and important player in the pathogenesis of fibrosis. *Curr Rheumatol Rep* 2002;4:136–142.
28. Phan SH. The myofibroblast in pulmonary fibrosis. *Chest* 2002;122:286S–289S.
29. Pardo A, Selman M. Idiopathic pulmonary fibrosis: new insights in its pathogenesis. *Int J Biochem Cell Biol* 2002;34:1534–1538.
30. Selman M, King TE, Pardo A. Idiopathic pulmonary fibrosis: prevailing and evolving hypotheses about its pathogenesis and implications for therapy. *Ann Intern Med* 2001;134:136–151.
31. Selman M, Pardo A. Idiopathic pulmonary fibrosis: an epithelial/fibroblastic cross-talk disorder. *Respir Res* 2002;3:3.
32. Yousem SA. Eosinophilic pneumonia-like areas in idiopathic usual interstitial pneumonia. *Mod Pathol* 2000;13:1280–1284.
33. Krein PM, Winston BW. Roles for insulin-like growth factor I and transforming growth factor-beta in fibrotic lung disease. *Chest* 2002;122:289S–293S.
34. Hammar SP, Winterbauer RH, Bockus D, et al. Idiopathic fibrosing alveolitis: a review with emphasis on ultrastructural and immunohistochemical features. *Ultrastruct Pathol* 1985;9:345–372.
35. King TE, Jr., Schwarz MI, Brown K, et al. Idiopathic pulmonary fibrosis: relationship between histopathologic features and mortality. *Am J Respir Crit Care Med* 2001;164:1025–1032.
36. Nicholson AG, Colby TV, du Bois RM, et al. The prognostic significance of the histologic pattern of interstitial pneumonia in patients presenting with the clinical entity of cryptogenic fibrosing alveolitis. *Am J Respir Crit Care Med* 2000;162:2213–2217.
37. Veeraraghavan S, Nicholson AG, Wells AU. Lung fibrosis: new classifications and therapy. *Curr Opin Rheumatol* 2001;13:500–504.
38. Akira M, Hamada H, Sakatani M, et al. CT findings during phase of accelerated deterioration in patients with idiopathic pulmonary fibrosis. *Am J Roentgenol* 1997;168:79–83.
39. Kondoh Y, Taniguchi H, Kawabata Y, et al. Acute exacerbation in idiopathic pulmonary fibrosis. Analysis of clinical and pathologic findings in three cases. *Chest* 1993;103:1808–1812.
40. Nicod LP. Pirfenidone in idiopathic pulmonary fibrosis. *Lancet* 1999;354:268–269.
41. Yousem SA, Colby TV, Carrington CB. Lung biopsy in rheumatoid arthritis. *Am Rev Respir Dis* 1985;131:770–777.
42. Harrison NK, Myers AR, Corrin B, et al. Structural features of interstitial lung disease in systemic sclerosis. *Am Rev Respir Dis* 1991;144:706–713.
43. Gaensler EA, Jederlinic PJ, Churg A. Idiopathic pulmonary fibrosis in asbestos-exposed workers. *Am Rev Respir Dis* 1991;144:689–696.
44. Myers JL. Diagnosis of drug reactions in the lung. *Monogr Pathol* 1993:32–53.
45. Walker WA, Cole FH, Jr., Khandekar A, et al. Does open lung biopsy affect treatment in patients with diffuse pulmonary infiltrates? *J Thorac Cardiovasc Surg* 1989;97:534–540.
46. Berbescu EA, Katzenstein AL, Snow JL, Zisman DA. Transbronchial biopsy in usual interstitial pneumonia. *Chest* 2006;129:1126–1131.
47. Katzenstein AL, Fiorelli RF. Nonspecific interstitial pneumonia/fibrosis. Histologic features and clinical significance. *Am J Surg Pathol* 1994;18:136–147.
48. Katzenstein AL, Myers JL. Idiopathic pulmonary fibrosis: clinical relevance of pathologic classification. *Am J Respir Crit Care Med* 1998;157:1301–1315.
49. Nagai S, Kitaichi M, Itoh H, et al. Idiopathic nonspecific interstitial pneumonia/fibrosis: comparison with idiopathic pulmonary fibrosis and BOOP. *Eur Respir J* 1998;12:1010–1019.
50. Monaghan H, Wells AU, Colby TV, et al. Prognostic implications of histologic patterns in multiple surgical lung biopsies from patients with idiopathic interstitial pneumonias. *Chest* 2004;125:522–526.
51. Daniil ZD, Gilchrist FC, Nicholson AG, et al. A histologic pattern of nonspecific interstitial pneumonia is associated with a better prognosis than usual interstitial pneumonia in patients with cryptogenic fibrosing alveolitis. *Am J Respir Crit Care Med* 1999;160:899–905.
52. Suffredini AF, Ognibene FP, Lack EE, et al. Nonspecific interstitial pneumonitis: a common cause of pulmonary disease in the acquired immunodeficiency syndrome. *Ann Intern Med* 1987;107:7–13.
53. Carrington CB, Gaensler EA, Coutu RE, et al. Natural history and treated course of usual and desquamative interstitial pneumonia. *N Engl J Med* 1978;298:801–809.
54. Liebow A, Steer A, Billingsley J. Desquamative interstitial pneumonia. *Am J Med* 1965;39:369–404.
55. Patchefsky AS, Israel HL, Hoch WS, et al. Desquamative interstitial pneumonia: relationship to interstitial fibrosis. *Thorax* 1973;28:680–693.
56. Myers JL, Veal CF, Jr., Shin MS, et al. Respiratory bronchiolitis causing interstitial lung disease. A clinicopathologic study of six cases. *Am Rev Respir Dis* 1987;135:880–884.
57. Yousem SA, Colby TV, Gaensler EA. Respiratory bronchiolitis-associated interstitial lung disease and its relationship to desquamative interstitial pneumonia. *Mayo Clin Proc* 1989;64:1373–1380.
58. Hartman TE, Primack SL, Swensen SJ, et al. Desquamative interstitial pneumonia: thin-section CT findings in 22 patients. *Radiology* 1993;187:787–790.
59. Bedrossian CW, Kuhn C, 3rd, Luna MA, et al. Desquamative interstitial pneumonia-like reaction accompanying pulmonary lesions. *Chest* 1977;72:166–169.
60. Bone RC, Wolfe J, Sobonya RE, et al. Desquamative interstitial pneumonia following long-term nitrofurantoin therapy. *Am J Med* 1976;60:697–701.
61. Coates EO, Jr., Watson JH. Diffuse interstitial lung disease in tungsten carbide workers. *Ann Intern Med* 1971;75:709–716.
62. Freed JA, Miller A, Gordon RE, et al. Desquamative interstitial pneumonia associated with chrysotile asbestos fibres. *Br J Ind Med* 1991;48:332–337.

63. Ohori NP, Sciurba FC, Owens GR, et al. Giant-cell interstitial pneumonia and hard-metal pneumoconiosis. A clinicopathologic study of four cases and review of the literature. *Am J Surg Pathol* 1989;13:581–587.
64. Katzenstein AL, Bloor CM, Leibow AA. Diffuse alveolar damage—the role of oxygen, shock, and related factors. A review. *Am J Pathol* 1976;85:209–228.
65. Turner-Warwick M, Lebowitz M, Burrows B, et al. Cryptogenic fibrosing alveolitis and lung cancer. *Thorax* 1980;35:496–499.
66. Tomashefski JF, Jr. Pulmonary pathology of the adult respiratory distress syndrome. *Clin Chest Med* 1990;11:593–619.
67. Nash G, Blennerhassett JB, Pontoppidan H. Pulmonary lesions associated with oxygen therapy and artifical ventilation. *N Engl J Med* 1967;276:368–374.
68. Rubenfeld GD, Caldwell E, Granton J, et al. Interobserver variability in applying a radiographic definition for ARDS. *Chest* 1999;116:1347–1353.
69. Gaudin PB, Askin FB, Falk RJ, et al. The pathologic spectrum of pulmonary lesions in patients with anti-neutrophil cytoplasmic autoantibodies specific for anti-proteinase 3 and anti-myeloperoxidase. *Am J Clin Pathol* 1995;104:7–16.
70. Katzenstein AL, Myers JL, Mazur MT. Acute interstitial pneumonia. A clinicopathologic, ultrastructural, and cell kinetic study. *Am J Surg Pathol* 1986;10:256–267.
71. Burkhardt A. Alveolitis and collapse in the pathogenesis of pulmonary fibrosis. *Am Rev Respir Dis* 1989;140:513–524.
72. Katzenstein AL. Pathogenesis of "fibrosis" in interstitial pneumonia: an electron microscopic study. *Hum Pathol* 1985;16:1015–1024.
73. Olson J, Colby TV, Elliott CG. Hamman-Rich syndrome revisited. *Mayo Clin Proc* 1990;65:1538–1548.
74. Vourlekis JS, Brown KK, Cool CD, et al. Acute interstitial pneumonitis. Case series and review of the literature. *Medicine (Baltimore)* 2000;79:369–378.
75. Lamy M, Fallat RJ, Koeniger E, et al. Pathologic features and mechanisms of hypoxemia in adult respiratory distress syndrome. *Am Rev Respir Dis* 1976;114:267–284.
76. Ware LB, Matthay MA. The acute respiratory distress syndrome. *N Engl J Med* 2000;342:1334–1349.
77. Myers JL, Kennedy JI, Plumb VJ. Amiodarone lung: pathologic findings in clinically toxic patients. *Hum Pathol* 1987;18:349–354.
78. Askin FB, Katzenstein AL. Pneumocystis infection masquerading as diffuse alveolar damage: a potential source of diagnostic error. *Chest* 1981;79:420–422.
79. Peiris JS, Yuen KY, Osterhaus AD, et al. The severe acute respiratory syndrome. *N Engl J Med* 2003;349:2431–2441.
80. Gu J, Korteweg C. Pathology and pathogenesis of severe acute respiratory syndrome. *Am J Pathol* 2007;170:1136–1147.
81. Guo Y, Korteweg C, McNutt MA, et al. Pathogenetic mechanisms of severe acute respiratory syndrome. *Virus Res* 2008;133:4–12.
82. Ye J, Zhang B, Xu J, et al. Molecular pathology in the lungs of severe acute respiratory syndrome patients. *Am J Pathol* 2007;170:538–545.
83. Ando M, Suga M. Hypersensitivity pneumonitis. *Curr Opin Pulm Med* 1997;3:391–395.
84. Semenzato G, Zambello R, Trentin L, et al. Cellular immunity in sarcoidosis and hypersensitivity pneumonitis. Recent advances. *Chest* 1993;103:139S–143S.
85. Pepys J. Hypersensitivity diseases of the lungs due to fungi and organic dusts. *Monogr Allergy* 1969;4:1–147.
86. Ando M, Suga M, Kohrogi H. A new look at hypersensitivity pneumonitis. *Curr Opin Pulm Med* 1999;5:299–304.
87. Coleman A, Colby TV. Histologic diagnosis of extrinsic allergic alveolitis. *Am J Surg Pathol* 1988;12:514–518.
88. Kawanami O, Basset F, Barrios R, et al. Hypersensitivity pneumonitis in man. Light- and electron-microscopic studies of 18 lung biopsies. *Am J Pathol* 1983;110:275–289.
89. Reijula K, Sutinen S. Ultrastructure of extrinsic allergic bronchiolo-alveolitis. *Pathol Res Pract* 1986;181:418–429.
90. Adler BD, Padley SP, Muller NL, et al. Chronic hypersensitivity pneumonitis: high-resolution CT and radiographic features in 16 patients. *Radiology* 1992;185:91–95.
91. Arnow PM, Fink JN, Schlueter DP, et al. Early detection of hypersensitivity pneumonitis in office workers. *Am J Med* 1978;64:236–242.
92. Selman M, Chapela R, Raghn G. Hypersensitivity pneumonitis: clinical manifestations, diagnosis, pathogenesis and therapeutic strategies. *Semin Respir Med* 1993;14:353–364.
93. Lougheed MD, Roos JO, et al. Desquamative interstitial pneumonitis and diffuse alveolar damage in textile workers. Potential role of mycotoxins. *Chest* 1995;108:1196–1200.
94. Perry LP, Iwata M, Tazelaar HD, et al. Pulmonary mycotoxicosis: a clinicopathologic study of three cases. *Mod Pathol* 1998;11:432–436.
95. Douglas WW, Hepper NG, Colby TV. Silo-filler's disease. *Mayo Clin Proc* 1989;64:291–304.
96. Zwemer FL, Jr., Pratt DS, May JJ. Silo filler's disease in New York State. *Am Rev Respir Dis* 1992;146:650–653.
97. Genereux GP. The end-stage lung: pathogenesis, pathology, and radiology. *Radiology* 1975;116:279–289.
98. Scadding JG. Diffuse pulmonary alveolar fibrosis. *Thorax* 1974;29:271–281.
99. Allen JN, Davis WB. Eosinophilic lung diseases. *Am J Respir Crit Care Med* 1994;150:1423–1438.
100. Crofton J, Livingstone J, Oswald N, et al. Pulmonary eosinophilia. *Thorax* 1952;7:1–35.
101. Katzenstein AL, Liebow AA, Friedman PJ. Bronchocentric granulomatosis, mucoid impaction, and hypersensitivity reactions to fungi. *Am Rev Respir Dis* 1975;111:497–537.
102. Marshall BG, Wilkinson RJ, Davidson RN. Pathogenesis of tropical pulmonary eosinophilia: parasitic alveolitis and parallels with asthma. *Respir Med* 1998;92:1–3.
103. Allen JN, Pacht ER, Gadek JE, et al. Acute eosinophilic pneumonia as a reversible cause of noninfectious respiratory failure. *N Engl J Med* 1989;321:569–574.
104. Pope-Harman AL, Davis WB, Allen ED, et al. Acute eosinophilic pneumonia. A summary of 15 cases and review of the literature. *Medicine (Baltimore)* 1996;75:334–342.
105. Carrington CB, Addington WW, Goff AM, et al. Chronic eosinophilic pneumonia. *N Engl J Med* 1969;280:787–798.
106. Jederlinic PJ, Sicilian L, Gaensler EA. Chronic eosinophilic pneumonia. A report of 19 cases and a review of the literature. *Medicine (Baltimore)* 1988;67:154–162.
107. Bosken CH, Myers JL, Greenberger PA, et al. Pathologic features of allergic bronchopulmonary aspergillosis. *Am J Surg Pathol* 1988;12:216–222.
108. Cockrill BA, Hales CA. Allergic bronchopulmonary aspergillosis. *Annu Rev Med* 1999;50:303–316.
109. Koss MN, Robinson RG, Hochholzer L. Bronchocentric granulomatosis. *Hum Pathol* 1981;12:632–638.
110. Hellems SO, Kanner RE, Renzetti AD, Jr. Bronchocentric granulomatosis associated with rheumatoid arthritis. *Chest* 1983;83:831–832.
111. Myers JL, Katzenstein AL. Granulomatous infection mimicking bronchocentric granulomatosis. *Am J Surg Pathol* 1986;10:317–322.
112. Yousem SA. Bronchocentric injury in Wegener's granulomatosis: a report of five cases. *Hum Pathol* 1991;22:535–540.
113. Binder RE, Faling LJ, Pugatch RD, et al. Chronic necrotizing pulmonary aspergillosis: a discrete clinical entity. *Medicine (Baltimore)* 1982;61:109–124.
114. Epler GR, Colby TV, McLoud TC, et al. Bronchiolitis obliterans organizing pneumonia. *N Engl J Med* 1985;312:152–158.
115. Lohr RH, Boland BJ, Douglas WW, et al. Organizing pneumonia. Features and prognosis of cryptogenic, secondary, and focal variants. *Arch Intern Med* 1997;157:1323–1329.
116. Gosink BB, Friedman PJ, Liebow AA. Bronchiolitis obliterans. Roentgenologic-pathologic correlation. *Am J Roentgenol Radium Ther Nucl Med* 1973;117:816–832.
117. Bellomo R, Finlay M, McLaughlin P, et al. Clinical spectrum of cryptogenic organising pneumonitis. *Thorax* 1991;46:554–558.
118. Lee KS, Kullnig P, Hartman TE, et al. Cryptogenic organizing pneumonia: CT findings in 43 patients. *AJR Am J Roentgenol* 1994;162:543–546.
119. Auerbach O, Garfinkel L, Hammond EC. Relation of smoking and age to findings in lung parenchyma: a microscopic study. *Chest* 1974;65:29–35.
120. Cordier JF. Challenges in pulmonary fibrosis. 2: Bronchiolocentric fibrosis. *Thorax* 2007;62:638–649.
121. Yousem SA, Dacic S. Idiopathic bronchiolocentric interstitial pneumonia. *Mod Pathol* 2002;15:1148–1153.
122. Fukuoka J, Franks TJ, Colby TV, et al. Peribronchiolar metaplasia: a common histologic lesion in diffuse lung disease and a rare cause of interstitial lung disease: clinicopathologic features of 15 cases. *Am J Surg Pathol* 2005;29:948–954.
123. Holland HK, Wingard JR, Beschorner WE, et al. Bronchiolitis obliterans in bone marrow transplantation and its relationship to chronic graft-v-host disease and low serum IgG. *Blood* 1988;72:621–627.
124. Urbanski SJ, Kossakowska AE, Curtis J, et al. Idiopathic small airways pathology in patients with graft-versus-host disease following allogeneic bone marrow transplantation. *Am J Surg Pathol* 1987;11:965–971.
125. Paz HL, Crilley P, Patchefsky A, et al. Bronchiolitis obliterans after autologous bone marrow transplantation. *Chest* 1992;101:775–778.
126. Schlesinger C, Meyer CA, Veeraraghavan S, et al. Constrictive (obliterative) bronchiolitis: diagnosis, etiology, and a critical review of the literature. *Ann Diagn Pathol* 1998;2:321–334.
127. Ward H, Fisher KL, Waghray R, et al. Constrictive bronchiolitis and ulcerative colitis. *Can Respir J* 1999;6:197–200.
128. Camus P, Piard F, Ashcroft T, et al. The lung in inflammatory bowel disease. *Medicine (Baltimore)* 1993;72:151–183.
129. Shad JA, Sharieff GQ. Tracheobronchitis as an initial presentation of ulcerative colitis. *J Clin Gastroenterol* 2001;33:161–163.
130. Vasishta S, Wood JB, McGinty F. Ulcerative tracheobronchitis years after colectomy for ulcerative colitis. *Chest* 1994;106:1279–1281.
131. Abernathy EC, Hruban RH, Baumgartner WA, et al. The two forms of bronchiolitis obliterans in heart-lung transplant recipients. *Hum Pathol* 1991;22:1102–1110.
132. Hendrick DJ. "Popcorn worker's lung" in Britain in a man making potato crisp flavouring. *Thorax* 2008;63:267–268.
133. Schachter EN. Popcorn worker's lung. *N Engl J Med* 2002;347:360–361.
134. Homer RJ, Khoo L, Smith GJ. Diffuse panbronchiolitis in a Hispanic man with travel history to Japan. *Chest* 1995;107:1176–1178.
135. Iwata M, Colby TV, Kitaichi M. Diffuse panbronchiolitis: diagnosis and distinction from various pulmonary diseases with centrilobular interstitial foam cell accumulations. *Hum Pathol* 1994;25:357–363.
136. Sugiyama Y, Kudoh S, Maeda H, et al. Analysis of HLA antigens in patients with diffuse panbronchiolitis. *Am Rev Respir Dis* 1990;141:1459–1462.
137. Lieberman PH, Jones CR, Steinman RM, et al. Langerhans cell (eosinophilic) granulomatosis. A clinicopathologic study encompassing 50 years. *Am J Surg Pathol* 1996;20:519–552.
138. Vassallo R, Ryu JH, Colby TV, et al. Pulmonary Langerhans'-cell histiocytosis. *N Engl J Med* 2000;342:1969–1978.
139. Colby TV, Lombard C. Histiocytosis X in the lung. *Hum Pathol* 1983;14:847–856.
140. Friedman PJ, Liebow AA, Sokoloff J. Eosinophilic granuloma of lung. Clinical aspects of primary histiocytosis in the adult. *Medicine (Baltimore)* 1981;60:385–396.
141. Fichtenbaum CJ, Kleinman GM, Haddad RG. Eosinophilic granuloma of the lung presenting as a solitary pulmonary nodule. *Thorax* 1990;45:905–906.
142. Travis WD, Borok Z, Roum JH, et al. Pulmonary Langerhans cell granulomatosis (histiocytosis X). A clinicopathologic study of 48 cases. *Am J Surg Pathol* 1993;17:971–986.
143. Egeler RM. Clonality in Langerhan's cell histiocytosis. *BMJ* 1995;310:804–805.
144. Willman CL, Busque L, Griffith BB, et al. Langerhans'-cell histiocytosis (histiocytosis X)—a clonal proliferative disease. *N Engl J Med* 1994;331:154–160.
145. Yousem SA, Colby TV, Chen YY, et al. Pulmonary Langerhans' cell histiocytosis: molecular analysis of clonality. *Am J Surg Pathol* 2001;25:630–636.
146. Hage C, Willman CL, Favara BE, et al. Langerhans' cell histiocytosis (histiocytosis X): immunophenotype and growth fraction. *Hum Pathol* 1993;24:840–845.
147. Hammar S, Bockus D, Remington F, et al. The widespread distribution of Langerhans

cells in pathologic tissues: an ultrastructural and immunohistochemical study. *Hum Pathol* 1986;17:894–905.
148. Fukuda Y, Basset F, Soler P, et al. Intraluminal fibrosis and elastic fiber degradation lead to lung remodeling in pulmonary Langerhans cell granulomatosis (histiocytosis X). *Am J Pathol* 1990;137:415–424.
149. Askin FB, McCann BG, Kuhn C. Reactive eosinophilic pleuritis: a lesion to be distinguished from pulmonary eosinophilic granuloma. *Arch Pathol Lab Med* 1977;101:187–191.
150. Luna E, Tomashefski JF, Jr., Brown D, et al. Reactive eosinophilic pulmonary vascular infiltration in patients with spontaneous pneumothorax. *Am J Surg Pathol* 1994;18:195–199.
151. Crouch E, White V, Wright J, et al. Malakoplakia mimicking carcinoma metastatic to lung. *Am J Surg Pathol* 1984;8:151–156.
152. Kwon KY, Colby TV. Rhodococcus equi pneumonia and pulmonary malakoplakia in acquired immunodeficiency syndrome. Pathologic features. *Arch Pathol Lab Med* 1994;118: 744–748.
153. Klatt EC, Jensen DF, Meyer PR. Pathology of *Mycobacterium avium*-intracellulare infection in acquired immunodeficiency syndrome. *Hum Pathol* 1987;18:709–714.
154. Winberg CD, Rose ME, Rappaport H. Whipple's disease of the lung. *Am J Med* 1978;65: 873–880.
155. Smith RL, Hutchins GM, Sack GH, Jr., et al. Unusual cardiac, renal and pulmonary involvement in Gaucher's disease. Intersitial glucocerebroside accumulation, pulmonary hypertension and fatal bone marrow embolization. *Am J Med* 1978;65:352–360.
156. Egan AJ, Boardman LA, Tazelaar HD, et al. Erdheim-Chester disease: clinical, radiologic, and histopathologic findings in five patients with interstitial lung disease. *Am J Surg Pathol* 1999;23:17–26.
157. Cadranel J, Wislez M, Antoine M. Primary pulmonary lymphoma. *Eur Respir J* 2002;20: 750–762.
158. Isaacson P, Wright DH. Extranodal malignant lymphoma arising from mucosa-associated lymphoid tissue. *Cancer* 1984;53:2515–2524.
159. Li G, Hansmann ML, Zwingers T, et al. Primary lymphomas of the lung: morphological, immunohistochemical and clinical features. *Histopathology* 1990;16:519–531.
160. Abbondanzo SL, Rush W, Bijwaard KE, et al. Nodular lymphoid hyperplasia of the lung: a clinicopathologic study of 14 cases. *Am J Surg Pathol* 2000;24:587–597.
161. Saltzstein S. Pulmonary malignant lymphomas and pseudolymphomas: classification, therapy and prognosis. *Cancer* 1963;16:928–955.
162. Yousem SA, Colby TV, Carrington CB. Follicular bronchitis/bronchiolitis. *Hum Pathol* 1985;16:700–706.
163. Nicholson AG, Wotherspoon AC, Diss TC, et al. Reactive pulmonary lymphoid disorders. *Histopathology* 1995;26:405–412.
164. Koss MN. Pulmonary lymphoid disorders. *Semin Diagn Pathol* 1995;12:158–171.
165. Saldana M, Mones J. Lymphoid interstitial pneumonia in HIV infected individuals. *Prog Surg Pathol* 1992;12:181–215.
166. Malamon-Mitsi V, Tsai M, Gal A, et al. Lymphoid interstitial pneumonia not associated with HIV infection. Role of Epstein-Barr virus. *Mod Pathol* 1992;5:487–491.
167. Swigris JJ, Berry GJ, Raffin TA, et al. Lymphoid interstitial pneumonia: a narrative review. *Chest* 2002;122:2150–2164.
168. Koss MN, Hochholzer L, Nichols PW, et al. Primary non-Hodgkin's lymphoma and pseudolymphoma of lung: a study of 161 patients. *Hum Pathol* 1983;14:1024–1038.
169. Nicholson AG, Wotherspoon AC, Diss TC, et al. Pulmonary B-cell non-Hodgkin's lymphomas. The value of immunohistochemistry and gene analysis in diagnosis. *Histopathology* 1995;26:395–403.
170. Cordier JF, Chailleux E, Lauque D, et al. Primary pulmonary lymphomas. A clinical study of 70 cases in nonimmunocompromised patients. *Chest* 1993;103:201–208.
171. Colby TV, Carrington CB. Pulmonary lymphomas: current concepts. *Hum Pathol* 1983;14: 884–887.
172. Fiche M, Caprons F, Berger F, et al. Primary pulmonary non-Hodgkin's lymphomas. *Histopathology* 1995;26:529–537.
173. Isaacson PG, Spencer J. Malignant lymphoma of mucosa-associated lymphoid tissue. *Histopathology* 1987;11:445–462.
174. Begueret H, Vergier B, Parrens M, et al. Primary lung small B-cell lymphoma versus lymphoid hyperplasia: evaluation of diagnostic criteria in 26 cases. *Am J Surg Pathol* 2002; 26:76–81.
175. Wotherspoon AC, Soosay GN, Diss TC, et al. Low-grade primary B-cell lymphoma of the lung. An immunohistochemical, molecular, and cytogenetic study of a single case. *Am J Clin Pathol* 1990;94:655–660.
176. Perry L, Florio R, Dewar A, et al. Giant lamellar bodies as a feature of pulmonary low-grade MALT lymphomas. *Histopathology* 2000;36:240–244.
177. Kurtin PJ, Myers JL, Adlakha H. Histopathology. Pathologic and clinical features of primary pulmonary extranodal marginal zone B-cell lymphoma of MALT type. *Am J Surg Pathol* 2001;25:997–1008.
178. Collins RD. Is clonality equivalent to malignancy: specifically, is immunoglobulin gene rearrangement diagnostic of malignant lymphoma? *Hum Pathol* 1997;28:757–759.
179. Polish LB, Cohn DL, Ryder JW, Histopathology. Pulmonary non-Hodgkin's lymphoma in AIDS. *Chest* 1989;96:1321–1326.
180. Lipford EH, Jr., Margolick JB, Longo DL, et al. Angiocentric immunoproliferative lesions: a clinicopathologic spectrum of post-thymic T-cell proliferations. *Blood* 1988;72: 1674–1681.
181. Colby TV, Carrington CB. Pulmonary lymphomas simulating lymphomatoid granulomatosis. *Am J Surg Pathol* 1982;6:19–32.
182. Saldana MJ, Patchefsky AS, Israel HI, et al. Pulmonary angiitis and granulomatosis. The relationship between histological features, organ involvement, and response to treatment. *Hum Pathol* 1977;8:391–409.
183. Liebow AA. The J. Burns Amberson lecture—pulmonary angiitis and granulomatosis. *Am Rev Respir Dis* 1973;108:1–18.
184. Jaffe ES, Wilson WH. Lymphomatoid granulomatosis: pathogenesis, pathology and clinical implications. *Cancer* Surv 1997;30:233–248.
185. Jaffe ES. Pulmonary lymphocytic angiitis: a nosologic quandary. *Mayo Clin Proc* 1988;63: 411–413.
186. Katzenstein AL, Peiper SC. Detection of Epstein-Barr virus genomes in lymphomatoid granulomatosis: analysis of 29 cases by the polymerase chain reaction technique. *Mod Pathol* 1990;3:435–441.
187. Myers JL, Kurtin PJ, Katzenstein AL, et al. Lymphomatoid granulomatosis. Evidence of immunophenotypic diversity and relationship to Epstein-Barr virus infection. *Am J Surg Pathol* 1995;19:1300–1312.
188. Medeiros LJ, Peiper SC, Elwood L, et al. Angiocentric immunoproliferative lesions: a molecular analysis of eight cases. *Hum Pathol* 1991;22:1150–1157.
189. Guinee D, Jr., Jaffe E, Kingma D, et al. Pulmonary lymphomatoid granulomatosis. Evidence for a proliferation of Epstein-Barr virus infected B-lymphocytes with a prominent T-cell component and vasculitis. *Am J Surg Pathol* 1994;18:753–764.
190. Guinee DG, Jr., Perkins SL, Travis WD, et al. Proliferation and cellular phenotype in lymphomatoid granulomatosis: implications of a higher proliferation index in B cells. *Am J Surg Pathol* 1998;22:1093–1100.
191. Nicholson AG, Wotherspoon AC, Diss TC, et al. Lymphomatoid granulomatosis: evidence that some cases represent Epstein-Barr virus-associated B-cell lymphoma. *Histopathology* 1996;29:317–324.
192. Wilson WH, Kingma DW, Raffeld M, et al. Association of lymphomatoid granulomatosis with Epstein-Barr viral infection of B lymphocytes and response to interferon-alpha 2b. *Blood* 1996;87:4531–4537.
193. Morice WG, Kurtin PJ, Myers JL. Expression of cytolytic lymphocyte-associated antigens in pulmonary lymphomatoid granulomatosis. *Am J Clin Pathol* 2002;118:391–398.
194. Beaty MW, Toro J, Sorbara L, et al. Cutaneous lymphomatoid granulomatosis: correlation of clinical and biologic features. *Am J Surg Pathol* 2001;25:1111–1120.
195. Haque AK, Myers JL, Hudnall SD, et al. Pulmonary lymphomatoid granulomatosis in acquired immunodeficiency syndrome: lesions with Epstein-Barr virus infection. *Mod Pathol* 1998;11:347–356.
196. Katzenstein AL, Carrington CB, Liebow AA. Lymphomatoid granulomatosis: a clinicopathologic study of 152 cases. *Cancer* 1979;43:360–373.
197. Jordan K, Grothey A, Grothe W, et al. Successful treatment of mediastinal lymphomatoid granulomatosis with rituximab monotherapy. *Eur J Haematol* 2005;74:263–266.
198. Lemieux J, Bernier V, Martel N, et al. Autologous hematopoietic stem cell transplantation for refractory lymphomatoid granulomatosis. *Hematology* 2002;7:355–358.
199. Medeiros LJ, Jaffe ES, Chen YY, et al. Localization of Epstein-Barr viral genomes in angiocentric immunoproliferative lesions. *Am J Surg Pathol* 1992;16:439–447.
200. Armitage JM, Kormos RL, Stuart RS, et al. Posttransplant lymphoproliferative disease in thoracic organ transplant patients: ten years of cyclosporine-based immunosuppression. *J Heart Lung Transplant* 1991;10:877–886; discussion 886–887.
201. Engleman P, Liebow AA, Gmelich J, et al. Pulmonary hyalinizing granuloma. *Am Rev Respir Dis* 1977;115:997–1008.
202. Dent RG, Godden DJ, Stovin PG, et al. Pulmonary hyalinising granuloma in association with retroperitoneal fibrosis. *Thorax* 1983;38:955–956.
203. Gans SJ, van der Elst AM, Straks W. Pulmonary hyalinizing granuloma. *Eur Respir J* 1988; 1:389–391.
204. Yousem SA, Hochholzer L. Pulmonary hyalinizing granuloma. *Am J Clin Pathol* 1987;87: 1–6.
205. Drasin H, Blume MR, Rosenbaum EH, et al. Pulmonary hyalinizing granulomas in a patient with malignant lymphoma, with development nine years later of multiple myeloma and systemic amyloidosis. *Cancer* 1979;44:215–220.
206. Atagi S, Sakatani M, Akira M, et al. Pulmonary hyalinizing granuloma with Castleman's disease. *Intern Med* 1994;33:689–691.
207. Kuramochi S, Kawai T, Yakumaru K, et al. Multiple pulmonary hyalinizing granulomas associated with systemic idiopathic fibrosis. *Acta Pathol Jpn* 1991;41:375–382.
208. Bahadori M, Liebow AA. Plasma cell granulomas of the lung. *Cancer* 1973;31:191–208.
209. Berardi RS, Lee SS, Chen HP, et al. Inflammatory pseudotumors of the lung. *Surg Gynecol Obstet* 1983;156:89–96.
210. Gal AA, Koss MN, McCarthy WF, et al. Prognostic factors in pulmonary fibrohistiocytic lesions. *Cancer* 1994;73:1817–1824.
211. Matsubara O, Tan-Liu NS, Kenney RM, et al. Inflammatory pseudotumors of the lung: progression from organizing pneumonia to fibrous histiocytoma or to plasma cell granuloma in 32 cases. *Hum Pathol* 1988;19:807–814.
212. Pettinato G, Manivel JC, De Rosa N, et al. Inflammatory myofibroblastic tumor (plasma cell granuloma). Clinicopathologic study of 20 cases with immunohistochemical and ultrastructural observations. *Am J Clin Pathol* 1990;94:538–546.
213. Hong HY, Castelli MJ, Walloch JL. Pulmonary plasma cell granuloma (inflammatory pseudotumor) with invasion of thoracic vertebra. *Mt Sinai J Med* 1990;57:117–121.
214. Barbareschi M, Ferrero S, Aldovini D, et al. Inflammatory pseudotumour of the lung. Immunohistochemical analysis on four new cases. Histol Histopathol 1990;5:205–211.
215. Coffin CM, Hornick JL, Fletcher CD. Inflammatory myofibroblastic tumor: comparison of clinicopathologic, histologic, and immunohistochemical features including ALK expression in atypical and aggressive cases. *Am J Surg Pathol* 2007;31:509–520.
216. Moran CA, Suster S. Unusual non-neoplastic lesions of the lung. *Semin Diagn Pathol* 2007; 24:199–208.
217. Yousem SA, Shaw H, Cieply K. Involvement of 2p23 in pulmonary inflammatory pseudotumors. *Hum Pathol* 2001;32:428–433.
218. Cook JR, Dehner LP, Collins MH, et al. Anaplastic lymphoma kinase (ALK) expression in the inflammatory myofibroblastic tumor: a comparative immunohistochemical study. *Am J Surg Pathol* 2001;25:1364–1371.
219. Sekosan M, Cleto M, Senseng C, et al. Spindle cell pseudotumors in the lungs due to *Mycobacterium tuberculosis* in a transplant patient. *Am J Surg Pathol* 1994;18:1065–1068.
220. Wick MR, Ritter JH, Nappi O. Inflammatory sarcomatoid carcinoma of the lung: report of three cases and clinicopathologic comparison with inflammatory pseudotumors in adult patients. *Hum Pathol* 1995;26:1014–1021.

221. Churg A, Carrington CB, Gupta R. Necrotizing sarcoid granulomatosis. *Chest* 1979;76:406–413.
222. Koss MN, Hochholzer L, Feigin DS, et al. Necrotizing sarcoid-like granulomatosis: clinical, pathologic, and immunopathologic findings. *Hum Pathol* 1980;11:510–519.
223. Popper HH, Klemen H, Colby TV, et al. Necrotizing sarcoid granulomatosis—is it different from nodular sarcoidosis? *Pneumologie* 2003;57:268–271.
224. Yi ES, Colby TV. Wegener's granulomatosis. *Semin Diagn Pathol* 2001;18:34–46.
225. Carrington CB, Liebow A. Limited forms of angiitis and granulomatosis of Wegener's type. *Am J Med* 1966;41:497–527.
226. Cassan SM, Coles DT, Harrison EG, Jr. The concept of limited forms of Wegener's granulomatosis. *Am J Med* 1970;49:366–379.
227. Israel HL, Patchefsky AS, Saldana MJ. Wegener's granulomatosis, lymphomatoid granulomatosis, and benign lymphocytic angiitis and granulomatosis of lung. Recognition and treatment. *Ann Intern Med* 1977;87:691–699.
228. Fienberg R. The protracted superficial phenomenon in pathergic (Wegener's) granulomatosis. *Hum Pathol* 1981;12:458–467.
229. Churg A. Pulmonary angiitis and granulomatosis revisited. *Hum Pathol* 1983;14:868–883.
230. Katzenstein AL, Locke WK. Solitary lung lesions in Wegener's granulomatosis. Pathologic findings and clinical significance in 25 cases. *Am J Surg Pathol* 1995;19:545–552.
231. Kuhlman JE, Hruban RH, Fishman EK. Wegener granulomatosis: CT features of parenchymal lung disease. *J Comput Assist Tomogr* 1991;15:948–952.
232. Hoffman GS, Kerr GS, Leavitt RY, et al. Wegener granulomatosis: an analysis of 158 patients. *Ann Intern Med* 1992;116:488–498.
233. Ulbright TM, Katzenstein AL. Solitary necrotizing granulomas of the lung: differentiating features and etiology. *Am J Surg Pathol* 1980;4:13–28.
234. Schultz DR, Diego JM. Antineutrophil cytoplasmic antibodies (ANCA) and systemic vasculitis: update of assays, immunopathogenesis, controversies, and report of a novel de novo ANCA-associated vasculitis after kidney transplantation. *Semin Arthritis Rheum* 2000;29:267–285.
235. El-Zammar OA, Katzenstein AL. Pathological diagnosis of granulomatous lung disease: a review. *Histopathology* 2007;50:289–310.
236. Griffin MT, Robb JD, Martin JR. Diffuse alveolar haemorrhage associated with progressive systemic sclerosis. *Thorax* 1990;45:903–904.
237. Travis WD, Colby TV, Lombard C, et al. A clinicopathologic study of 34 cases of diffuse pulmonary hemorrhage with lung biopsy confirmation. *Am J Surg Pathol* 1990;14:1112–1125.
238. Uner AH, Rozum-Slota B, Katzenstein AL. Bronchiolitis obliterans-organizing pneumonia (BOOP)-like variant of Wegener's granulomatosis. A clinicopathologic study of 16 cases. *Am J Surg Pathol* 1996;20:794–801.
239. Yousem SA, Lombard CM. The eosinophilic variant of Wegener's granulomatosis. *Hum Pathol* 1988;19:682–688.
240. Nolle B, Specks U, Ludemann J, et al. Anticytoplasmic autoantibodies: their immunodiagnostic value in Wegener granulomatosis. *Ann Intern Med* 1989;111:28–40.
241. Davenport A, Lock RJ, Wallington TB, et al. Clinical significance of anti-neutrophil cytoplasm antibodies detected by a standardized indirect immunofluorescence assay. *Q J Med* 1994;87:291–299.
242. Ballieux BE, Zondervan KT, Kievit P, et al. Binding of proteinase 3 and myeloperoxidase to endothelial cells: ANCA-mediated endothelial damage through ADCC? *Clin Exp Immunol* 1994;97:52–60.
243. Beach RC, Corrin B, Scopes JW, et al. Necrotizing sarcoid granulomatosis with neurologic lesions in a child. *J Pediatr* 1980;97:950–953.
244. Saldana MJ. Necrotizing sarcoid granulomatosis: clinicopathologic observations in 24 patients [Meeting abstract]. *Lab Invest* 1978;38:364.
245. Singh N, Cole S, Krause PJ, et al. Necrotizing sarcoid granulomatosis with extrapulmonary involvement. Clinical, pathologic, ultrastructural, and immunologic features. *Am Rev Respir Dis* 1981;124:189–192.
246. Dykhuizen RS, Smith CC, Kennedy MM, et al. Necrotizing sarcoid granulomatosis with extrapulmonary involvement. *Eur Respir J* 1997;10:245–247.
247. Hunninghake GW, Fauci AS. Pulmonary involvement in the collagen vascular diseases. *Am Rev Respir Dis* 1979;119:471–503.
248. Walker WC, Wright V. Pulmonary lesions and rheumatoid arthritis. *Medicine (Baltimore)* 1968;47:501–520.
249. Tansey D, Wells AU, Colby TV, et al. Variations in histological patterns of interstitial pneumonia between connective tissue disorders and their relationship to prognosis. *Histopathology* 2004;44:585–596.
250. Gough J, Rivers D, Seal RM. Pathological studies of modified pneumoconiosis in coal miners with rheumatoid arthritis (Caplan's syndrome). *Thorax* 1955;10:9–18.
251. Asimacopoulos PJ, Katras A, Christie B. Pulmonary dirofilariasis. The largest single-hospital experience. *Chest* 1992;102:851–855.
252. Nicholson CP, Allen MS, Trastek VF, et al. Dirofilaria immitis: a rare, increasing cause of pulmonary nodules. *Mayo Clin Proc* 1992;67:646–650.
253. Churg J, Strauss L. Allergic granulomatosis, allergic angiitis and periarteritis nodosa. *Am J Pathol* 1951;27:277–301.
254. Churg A. Recent advances in the diagnosis of Churg-Strauss syndrome. *Mod Pathol* 2001;14:1284–1293.
255. Conron M, Beynon HL. Churg-Strauss syndrome. *Thorax* 2000;55:870–877.
256. Katzenstein AL. Diagnostic features and differential diagnosis of Churg-Strauss syndrome in the lung. A review. *Am J Clin Pathol* 2000;114:767–772.
257. Jessurun J, Azevedo M, Saldana M. Allergic angiitis and granulomatosis (Churg-Strauss syndrome): report of a case with massive thymic involvement in a nonasthmatic patient. *Hum Pathol* 1986;17:637–639.
258. Wechsler ME, Finn D, Gunawardena D, et al. Churg-Strauss syndrome in patients receiving montelukast as treatment for asthma. *Chest* 2000;117:708–713.
259. Kallenberg CG. Churg-Strauss syndrome: just one disease entity? *Arthritis Rheum* 2005;52:2589–2593.
260. Sable-Fourtassou R, Cohen P, Mahr A, et al. Antineutrophil cytoplasmic antibodies and the Churg-Strauss syndrome. *Ann Intern Med* 2005;143:632–638.
261. Lombard CM, Tazelaar HD, Krasne DL. Pulmonary eosinophilia in coccidioidal infections. *Chest* 1987;91:734–736.
262. Matsumoto T, Homma S, Okada M, et al. The lung in polyarteritis nodosa: a pathologic study of 10 cases. *Hum Pathol* 1993;24:717–724.
263. Lombard CM, Colby TV, Elliott CG. Surgical pathology of the lung in anti-basement membrane antibody-associated Goodpasture's syndrome. *Hum Pathol* 1989;20:445–451.
264. Lauque D, Cadranel J, Lazor R, et al. Microscopic polyangiitis with alveolar hemorrhage. A study of 29 cases and review of the literature. Groupe d'Etudes et de Recherche sur les Maladies "Orphelines" Pulmonaires (GERM"O"P). *Medicine (Baltimore)* 2000;79:222–233.
265. Ozbudak IH, Shilo K, Hale S, et al. Alveolar airspace and pulmonary artery involvement by extramedullary hematopoiesis: a unique manifestation of myelofibrosis. *Arch Pathol Lab Med* 2008;132:99–103.
266. Kelly PT, Haponik EF. Goodpasture syndrome: molecular and clinical advances. *Medicine (Baltimore)* 1994;73:171–185.
267. Myers JL, Katzenstein AA. Microangiitis in lupus-induced pulmonary hemorrhage. *Am J Clin Pathol* 1986;85:552–556.
268. Farber HW, Loscalzo J. Pulmonary arterial hypertension. *N Engl J Med* 2004;351:1655–1665.
269. Clarke B. The pathology of pulmonary arterial hypertension. *Curr Diagn Pathol* 2002;8:412–420.
270. Pietra GG. Histopathology of primary pulmonary hypertension. *Chest* 1994;105:2S–6S.
271. Wagenvoort C, Mooi W. *Vascular Diseases*. New York: Springer-Verlag; 1994.
272. Bjornsson J, Edwards WD. Primary pulmonary hypertension: a histopathologic study of 80 cases. *Mayo Clin Proc* 1985;60:16–25.
273. Burke AP, Farb A, Virmani R. The pathology of primary pulmonary hypertension. *Mod Pathol* 1991;4:269–282.
274. Mesa RA, Edell ES, Dunn WF, et al. Human immunodeficiency virus infection and pulmonary hypertension: two new cases and a review of 86 reported cases. *Mayo Clin Proc* 1998;73:37–45.
275. Wagenvoort CA. Grading of pulmonary vascular lesions—a reappraisal. *Histopathology* 1981;5:595–598.
276. Barnett CF, Hsue PY, Machado RF. Pulmonary hypertension: an increasingly recognized complication of hereditary hemolytic anemias and HIV infection. *JAMA* 2008;299:324–331.
277. Runo JR, Loyd JE. Primary pulmonary hypertension. *Lancet* 2003;361:1533–1544.
278. Cool CD, Rai PR, Yeager ME, et al. Expression of human herpesvirus 8 in primary pulmonary hypertension. *N Engl J Med* 2003;349:1113–1122.
279. Barberis MC, Veronese S, Bauer D, et al. Immunocytochemical detection of progesterone receptors. A study in a patient with primary pulmonary hypertension. *Chest* 1995;107:869–872.
280. Lee SD, Shroyer KR, Markham NE, et al. Monoclonal endothelial cell proliferation is present in primary but not secondary pulmonary hypertension. *J Clin Invest* 1998;101:927–934.
281. Voelkel NF, Cool C. Pathology of pulmonary hypertension. *Cardiol Clin* 2004;22:343–351, v.
282. Heath D, Edwards J. The pathology of hypertensive pulmonary vascular disease. A description of six grades of structural changes in the pulmonary arteries with special reference to congenital cardiac septal defects. *Circulation* 1958;18:533–547.
283. Wagenvoort C, Wagenvoort N. *Pathology of Pulmonary Hypertension.* New York: John Wiley, 1977.
284. Warnock ML, Kunzmann A. Changes with age in muscular pulmonary arteries. *Arch Pathol Lab Med* 1977;101:175–179.
285. Richter A, Yeager ME, Zaiman A, et al. Impaired transforming growth factor-beta signaling in idiopathic pulmonary arterial hypertension. *Am J Respir Crit Care Med* 2004;170:1340–1348.
286. Humbert M, Sitbon O, Simonneau G. Treatment of pulmonary arterial hypertension. *N Engl J Med* 2004;351:1425–1436.
287. Whyte RI, Robbins RC, Altinger J, et al. Heart-lung transplantation for primary pulmonary hypertension. *Ann Thorac Surg* 1999;67:937–941; discussion 941–942.
288. Simonneau G, Fartoukh M, Sitbon O, et al. Primary pulmonary hypertension associated with the use of fenfluramine derivatives. *Chest* 1998;114:195S–199S.
289. Gomez-Sanchez MA, Mestre de Juan MJ, Gomez-Pajuelo C, et al. Pulmonary hypertension due to toxic oil syndrome. A clinicopathologic study. *Chest* 1989;95:325–331.
290. Wagenvoort C. Lung biopsies in the differential diagnosis of thrombo-emboli versus primary pulmonary hypertension. *Pro Respir Res* 1980;13:16–21.
291. Rich S, Levitsky S, Brundage BH. Pulmonary hypertension from chronic pulmonary thromboembolism. *Ann Intern Med* 1988;108:425–434.
292. Goldhaber SZ. Pulmonary embolism death rates. *Am Heart J* 1988;115:1342–1343.
293. Moser KM, Bloor CM. Pulmonary vascular lesions occurring in patients with chronic major vessel thromboembolic pulmonary hypertension. *Chest* 1993;103:685–692.
294. Heath D, Scott O, Lynch J. Pulmonary veno-occlusive disease. *Thorax* 1971;26:663–674.
295. Holcomb BW, Jr., Loyd JE, Ely EW, et al. Pulmonary veno-occlusive disease: a case series and new observations. *Chest* 2000;118:1671–1679.
296. Veeraraghavan S, Koss MN, Sharma OP. Pulmonary veno-occlusive disease. *Curr Opin Pulm Med* 1999;5:310–313.
297. Seguchi M, Hirabayashi N, Fujii Y, et al. Pulmonary hypertension associated with pulmonary occlusive vasculopathy after allogeneic bone marrow transplantation. *Transplantation* 2000;69:177–179.
298. Carrington CB, Liebow AA. Pulmonary veno-occlusive disease. *Hum Pathol* 1970;1:322–324.
299. Katz DS, Scalzetti EM, Katzenstein AL, et al. Pulmonary veno-occlusive disease presenting with thrombosis of pulmonary arteries. *Thorax* 1995;50:699–700.

300. Pai U, McMahon J, Tomashefski JF, Jr. Mineralizing pulmonary elastosis in chronic cardiac failure. "Endogenous pneumoconiosis" revisited. *Am J Clin Pathol* 1994;101:22–28.
301. Almagro P, Julia J, Sanjaume M, et al. Pulmonary capillary hemangiomatosis associated with primary pulmonary hypertension: report of 2 new cases and review of 35 cases from the literature. *Medicine (Baltimore)* 2002;81:417–424.
302. Eltorky MA, Headley AS, Winer-Muram H, et al. Pulmonary capillary hemangiomatosis: a clinicopathologic review. *Ann Thorac Surg* 1994;57:772–776.
303. Tomashefski JF, Jr., Hirsch CS. The pulmonary vascular lesions of intravenous drug abuse. *Hum Pathol* 1980;11:133–145.
304. Basset F, Soler P, Marsac J, et al. Pulmonary lymphangiomyomatosis: three new cases studied with electron microscopy. *Cancer* 1976;38:2357–2366.
305. Corrin B, Liebow AA, Friedman PJ. Pulmonary lymphangiomyomatosis. A review. *Am J Pathol* 1975;79:348–382.
306. Hancock E, Osborne J. Lymphangioleiomyomatosis: a review of the literature. *Respir Med* 2002;96:1–6.
307. Carsillo T, Astrinidis A, Henske EP. Mutations in the tuberous sclerosis complex gene TSC2 are a cause of sporadic pulmonary lymphangioleiomyomatosis. *Proc Natl Acad Sci U S A* 2000;97:6085–6090.
308. Strizheva GD, Carsillo T, Kruger WD, et al. The spectrum of mutations in TSC1 and TSC2 in women with tuberous sclerosis and lymphangiomyomatosis. *Am J Respir Crit Care Med* 2001;163:253–258.
309. Yu J, Astrinidis A, Henske EP. Chromosome 16 loss of heterozygosity in tuberous sclerosis and sporadic lymphangiomyomatosis. *Am J Respir Crit Care Med* 2001;164:1537–1540.
310. Costello LC, Hartman TE, Ryu JH. High frequency of pulmonary lymphangioleiomyomatosis in women with tuberous sclerosis complex. *Mayo Clin Proc* 2000;75:591–594.
311. Moss J, Avila NA, Barnes PM, et al. Prevalence and clinical characteristics of lymphangioleiomyomatosis (LAM) in patients with tuberous sclerosis complex. *Am J Respir Crit Care Med* 2001;164:669–671.
312. Aubry MC, Myers JL, Ryu JH, et al. Pulmonary lymphangioleiomyomatosis in a man. *Am J Respir Crit Care Med* 2000;162:749–752.
313. Muller NL, Chiles C, Kullnig P. Pulmonary lymphangiomyomatosis: correlation of CT with radiographic and functional findings. *Radiology* 1990;175:335–339.
314. Flieder DB, Travis WD. Clear cell "sugar" tumor of the lung: association with lymphangioleiomyomatosis and multifocal micronodular pneumocyte hyperplasia in a patient with tuberous sclerosis. *Am J Surg Pathol* 1997;21:1242–1247.
315. Kimura N, Watanabe M, Date F, et al. HMB-45 and tuberin in hamartomas associated with tuberous sclerosis. *Mod Pathol* 1997;10:952–959.
316. Matsui K, Beasley MB, Nelson WK, et al. Prognostic significance of pulmonary lymphangioleiomyomatosis histologic score. *Am J Surg Pathol* 2001;25:479–484.
317. Taylor JR, Ryu J, Colby TV, et al. Lymphangioleiomyomatosis. Clinical course in 32 patients. *N Engl J Med* 1990;323:1254–1260.
318. Chu SC, Horiba K, Usuki J, et al. Comprehensive evaluation of 35 patients with lymphangioleiomyomatosis. *Chest* 1999;115:1041–1052.
319. Boehler A, Speich R, Russi EW, et al. Lung transplantation for lymphangioleiomyomatosis. *N Engl J Med* 1996;335:1275–1280.
320. Bittmann I, Rolf B, Amann G, et al. Recurrence of lymphangioleiomyomatosis after single lung transplantation: new insights into pathogenesis. *Hum Pathol* 2003;34:95–98.
321. Aubry MC, Myers JL, Colby TV, et al. Endometrial stromal sarcoma metastatic to the lung: a detailed analysis of 16 patients. *Am J Surg Pathol* 2002;26:440–449.
322. Guinee D, Singh R, Azumi N, et al. Multifocal micronodular pneumocyte hyperplasia: a distinctive pulmonary manifestation of tuberous sclerosis. *Mod Pathol* 1995;8:902–906.
323. Lantuejoul S, Ferretti G, Negoescu A, et al. Multifocal alveolar hyperplasia associated with lymphangioleiomyomatosis in tuberous sclerosis. *Histopathology* 1997;30:570–575.
324. Muir TE, Leslie KO, Popper H, et al. Micronodular pneumocyte hyperplasia. *Am J Surg Pathol* 1998;22:465–472.
325. Popper HH, Juettner-Smolle FM, Pongratz MG. Micronodular hyperplasia of type II pneumocytes—a new lung lesion associated with tuberous sclerosis. *Histopathology* 1991;18:347–354.
326. Cancellieri A, Poletti V, Corrin B. Respiratory failure due to micronodular type II pneumocyte hyperplasia. *Histopathology* 2002;41:263–265.
327. Burkhardt A, Otto HF, Kaukel E. Multiple pulmonary (hamartomatous?) leiomyomas. Light and electron microscopic study. *Virchows Arch A Pathol Anat Histol* 1981;394:133–141.
328. Horstmann JP, Pietra GG, Harman JA, et al. Spontaneous regression of pulmonary leiomyomas during pregnancy. *Cancer* 1977;39:314–321.
329. Nucci MR, Drapkin R, Cin PD, et al. Distinctive cytogenetic profile in benign metastasizing leiomyoma: pathogenetic implications. *Am J Surg Pathol* 2007;31:737–743.
330. Jautzke G, Muller-Ruchholtz E, Thalmann U. Immunohistological detection of estrogen and progesterone receptors in multiple and well differentiated leiomyomatous lung tumors in women with uterine leiomyomas (so-called benign metastasizing leiomyomas). A report on 5 cases. *Pathol Res Pract* 1996;192:215–223.
331. Kay JM, Kahana LM, Rihal C. Diffuse smooth muscle proliferation of the lungs with severe pulmonary hypertension. *Hum Pathol* 1996;27:969–974.
332. Tazelaar HD, Kerr D, Yousem SA, et al. Diffuse pulmonary lymphangiomatosis. *Hum Pathol* 1993;24:1313–1322.
333. Prakash UB, Barham SS, Carpenter HA, et al. Pulmonary alveolar phospholipoproteinosis: experience with 34 cases and a review. *Mayo Clin Proc* 1987;62:499–518.
334. Rosen S, Castleman B, Liebow A. Pulmonary alveolar proteinosis. *N Engl J Med* 1958;258:1123–1142.
335. Wang BM, Stern EJ, Schmidt RA, et al. Diagnosing pulmonary alveolar proteinosis. A review and an update. *Chest* 1997;111:460–466.
336. Buechner HA, Ansari A. Acute silico-proteinosis. A new pathologic variant of acute silicosis in sandblasters, characterized by histologic features resembling alveolar proteinosis. *Dis Chest* 1969;55:274–278.
337. Miller RR, Churg AM, Hutcheon M, et al. Pulmonary alveolar proteinosis and aluminum dust exposure. *Am Rev Respir Dis* 1984;130:312–315.
338. Trapnell BC, Whitsett JA, Nakata K. Pulmonary alveolar proteinosis. *N Engl J Med* 2003;349:2527–2539.
339. Bedrossian CW, Luna MA, Conklin RH, et al. Alveolar proteinosis as a consequence of immunosuppression. A hypothesis based on clinical and pathologic observations. *Hum Pathol* 1980;11:527–535.
340. Lakshminarayan S, Schwarz MI, Stanford RE. Unsuspected pulmonary alveolar proteinosis complicating acute myelogenous leukemia. *Chest* 1976;69:433–435.
341. Witty LA, Tapson VF, Piantadosi CA. Isolation of mycobacteria in patients with pulmonary alveolar proteinosis. *Medicine (Baltimore)* 1994;73:103–109.
342. Kitamura T, Tanaka N, Watanabe J, et al. Idiopathic pulmonary alveolar proteinosis as an autoimmune disease with neutralizing antibody against granulocyte/macrophage colony-stimulating factor. *J Exp Med* 1999;190:875–880.
343. Tazawa R, Hamano E, Arai T, et al. Granulocyte-macrophage colony-stimulating factor and lung immunity in pulmonary alveolar proteinosis. *Am J Respir Crit Care Med* 2005;171:1142–1149.
344. Wallot M, Wagenvoort C, deMello D, et al. Congenital alveolar proteinosis caused by a novel mutation of the surfactant protein B gene and misalignment of lung vessels in consanguineous kindred infants. *Eur J Pediatr* 1999;158:513–518.
345. Goldstein LS, Kavuru MS, Curtis-McCarthy P, et al. Pulmonary alveolar proteinosis: clinical features and outcomes. *Chest* 1998;114:1357–1362.
346. Crouch E, Persson A, Chang D. Accumulation of surfactant protein D in human pulmonary alveolar proteinosis. *Am J Pathol* 1993;142:241–248.
347. Ramirez R. Alveolar proteinosis: importance of pulmonary lavage. *Am Rev Respir Dis* 1971;103:666–678.
348. Ma Y, Gal A, Koss MN. The pathology of pulmonary sarcoidosis: update. *Semin Diagn Pathol* 2007;24:150–161.
349. Statement on sarcoidosis. Joint Statement of the American Thoracic Society (ATS), the European Respiratory Society (ERS) and the World Association of Sarcoidosis and Other Granulomatous Disorders (WASOG) adopted by the ATS Board of Directors and by the ERS Executive Committee, February 1999. *Am J Respir Crit Care Med* 1999;160:736–755.
350. DiAlberti L, Piatelli A, et al. Human herpes virus 8 variants in sarcoid tissues. *Lancet* 1997;350:1655–1661.
351. Kon OM, du Bois RM. Mycobacteria and sarcoidosis. *Thorax* 1997;52(Suppl 3): S47–S51.
352. Osaki M, Adachi H, Gomyo Y, et al. Detection of mycobacterial DNA in formalin-fixed, paraffin-embedded tissue specimens by duplex polymerase chain reaction: application to histopathologic diagnosis. *Mod Pathol* 1997;10:78–83.
353. Popper HH, Klemen H, Hoefler G, et al. Presence of mycobacterial DNA in sarcoidosis. *Hum Pathol* 1997;28:796–800.
354. Heffner DK. The cause of sarcoidosis: the Centurial enigma solved. *Ann Diagn Pathol* 2007;11:142–152.
355. Lacronique JG, Bernaudin J, Soler P, et al. Alveolitis and granulomas: sequential course in pulmonary sarcoidosis. In Chretien J, Marsac, J, Saltiel JC, eds. Sarcoidosis and Other Granulomatous Disoreders. Paris: Pergamon, 1986.
356. Takemura T, Matsui Y, Oritsu M, et al. Pulmonary vascular involvement in sarcoidosis: granulomatous angiitis and microangiopathy in transbronchial lung biopsies. *Virchows Arch A Pathol Anat Histopathol* 1991;418:361–368.
357. James DG, Neville E, Siltzbach LE. A worldwide review of sarcoidosis. *Ann NY Acad Sci* 1976;278:321–334.
358. Grenier P, Valeyre D, Cluzel P, et al. Chronic diffuse interstitial lung disease: diagnostic value of chest radiography and high-resolution CT. *Radiology* 1991;179:123–132.
359. Papadopoulos KI, Melander O, Orho-Melander M, et al. Angiotensin converting enzyme (ACE) gene polymorphism in sarcoidosis in relation to associated autoimmune diseases. *J Intern Med* 2000;247:71–77.
360. Hunninghake GW, Crystal RG. Pulmonary sarcoidosis: a disorder mediated by excess helper T-lymphocyte activity at sites of disease activity. *N Engl J Med* 1981;305:429–434.
361. Rosen Y, Athanassiades TJ, Moon S, et al. Nongranulomatous interstitial pneumonitis in sarcoidosis. Relationship to development of epithelioid granulomas. *Chest* 1978;74:122–125.
362. Hsu RM, Connors AF, Jr., Tomashefski JF, Jr. Histologic, microbiologic, and clinical correlates of the diagnosis of sarcoidosis by transbronchial biopsy. *Arch Pathol Lab Med* 1996;120:364–368.
363. Huang CT, Heurich AE, Sutton AL, et al. Mortality in sarcoidosis. A changing pattern of the causes of death. *Eur J Respir Dis* 1981;62:231–238.
364. Perry A, Vuitch F. Causes of death in patients with sarcoidosis. A morphologic study of 38 autopsies with clinicopathologic correlations. *Arch Pathol Lab Med* 1995;119:167–172.
365. Baughman RP, Costabel U, du Bois RM. Treatment of Sarcoidosis. *Clin Chest Med* 2008;29:533–548.
366. Kahana LM, Kay JM, Yakrus MA, et al. Mycobacterium avium complex infection in an immunocompetent young adult related to hot tub exposure. *Chest* 1997;111:242–245.
367. Khoor A, Leslie KO, Tazelaar HD, et al. Diffuse pulmonary disease caused by nontuberculous mycobacteria in immunocompetent people (hot tub lung). *Am J Clin Pathol* 2001;115:755–762.
368. da Costa P, Corrin B. Amyloidosis localized to the lower respiratory tract: probable immunoamyloid nature of the tracheobronchial and nodular pulmonary forms. *Histopathology* 1985;9:703–710.
369. Page DL, Isersky C, Harada M, et al. Immunoglobulin origin of localized nodular pulmonary amyloidosis. *Res Exp Med (Berl)* 1972;159:75–86.
370. Utz JP, Swensen SJ, Gertz MA. Pulmonary amyloidosis. The Mayo Clinic experience from 1980 to 1993. *Ann Intern Med* 1996;124:407–413.
371. Hui AN, Koss MN, Hochholzer L, et al. Amyloidosis presenting in the lower respiratory tract. Clinicopathologic, radiologic, immunohistochemical, and histochemical studies on 48 cases. *Arch Pathol Lab Med* 1986;110:212–218.
372. Ihling C, Weirich G, Gaa A, et al. Amyloid tumors of the lung—an immunocytoma? *Pathol Res Pract* 1996;192:446–452.
373. Thompson PJ, Citron KM. Amyloid and the lower respiratory tract. *Thorax* 1983;38:84–87.
374. Toyoda M, Ebihara Y, Kato H, et al. Tracheobronchial AL amyloidosis: histologic, immu-

nohistochemical, ultrastructural, and immunoelectron microscopic observations. *Hum Pathol* 1993;24:970–976.

375. Stokes MB, Jagirdar J, Burchstin O, et al. Nodular pulmonary immunoglobulin light chain deposits with coexistent amyloid and nonamyloid features in an HIV-infected patient. *Mod Pathol* 1997;10:1059–1065.

376. Matthay RA, Greene WH. Pulmonary infections in the immunocompromised patient. *Med Clin North Am* 1980;64:529–551.

377. Rosenow EC, 3rd, Wilson WR, Cockerill FR, 3rd. Pulmonary disease in the immunocompromised host. 1. *Mayo Clin Proc* 1985;60:473–487.

378. Wilson WR, Cockerill FR, 3rd, Rosenow EC, 3rd. Pulmonary disease in the immunocompromised host. 2. *Mayo Clin Proc* 1985;60:610–631.

379. Colby TV, Weiss RL. Current concepts in the surgical pathology of pulmonary infections. *Am J Surg Pathol* 1987;11(Suppl 1):25–37.

380. Haverkos HW, Dowling JN, Pasculle AW, et al. Diagnosis of pneumonitis in immunocompromised patients by open lung biopsy. *Cancer* 1983;52:1093–1097.

381. Leight GS, Jr., Michaelis LL. Open lung biopsy for the diagnosis of acute, diffuse pulmonary infiltrates in the immunosuppressed patient. *Chest* 1978;73:477–482.

382. Rossiter SJ, Miller C, Churg AM, et al. Open lung biopsy in the immunosuppressed patient. Is it really beneficial? *J Thorac Cardiovasc Surg* 1979;77:338–345.

383. Pitchenik AE, Ganjei P, Torres A, et al. Sputum examination for the diagnosis of *Pneumocystis carinii* pneumonia in the acquired immunodeficiency syndrome. *Am Rev Respir Dis* 1986;133:226–229.

384. Rorat E, Garcia RL, Skolom J. Diagnosis of *Pneumocystis carinii* pneumonia by cytologic examination of bronchial washings. *JAMA* 1985;254:1950–1951.

385. Nicastri A, Hutter R, Collins H. *Pneumocystis carinii* pneumonia in an adult. Emphasis on antimortem morphologic diagnosis. *NY J Med* 1965;65:2149–2154.

386. Blumenfeld W, Basgoz N, Owen WF, Jr., et al. Granulomatous pulmonary lesions in patients with the acquired immunodeficiency syndrome (AIDS) and *Pneumocystis carinii* infection. *Ann Intern Med* 1988;109:505–507.

387. Lee MM, Schinella RA. Pulmonary calcification caused by *Pneumocystis carinii* pneumonia. A clinicopathological study of 13 cases in acquired immune deficiency syndrome patients. *Am J Surg Pathol* 1991;15:376–380.

388. Liu YC, Tomashefski JF, Jr., Tomford JW, et al. Necrotizing *Pneumocystis carinii* vasculitis associated with lung necrosis and cavitation in a patient with acquired immunodeficiency syndrome. *Arch Pathol Lab Med* 1989;113:494–497.

389. Homer KS, Wiley EL, Smith AL, et al. Monoclonal antibody to *Pneumocystis carinii*. Comparison with silver stain in bronchial lavage specimens. *Am J Clin Pathol* 1992;97:619–624.

390. Stager CE, Fraire AE, Kim HS, et al. Modification of the fungi-fluor and the genetic systems fluorescent antibody methods for detection of *Pneumocystis carinii* in bronchoalveolar lavage specimens. *Arch Pathol Lab Med* 1995;119:142–147.

391. Cote RJ, Rosenblum M, Telzak EE, et al. Disseminated *Pneumocystis carinii* infection causing

extrapulmonary organ failure: clinical, pathologic, and immunohistochemical analysis. *Mod Pathol* 1990;3:25–30.

392. Dembinski AS, Smith DM, Goldsmith JC, et al. Widespread dissemination of *Pneumocystis carinii* infection in a patient with acquired immune deficiency syndrome receiving long-term treatment with aerosolized pentamidine. *Am J Clin Pathol* 1991;95:96–100.

393. Chester AC, Winn WC, Jr. Unusual and newly recognized patterns of nontuberculous mycobacterial infection with emphasis on the immunocompromised host. *Pathol Annu* 1986;21(Pt 1):251–270.

394. Marchevsky A, Damsker B, Gribetz A, et al. The spectrum of pathology of nontuberculous mycobacterial infections in open-lung biopsy specimens. *Am J Clin Pathol* 1982;78:695–700.

395. Reyes JM, Putong PB. Association of pulmonary alveolar lipoproteinosis with mycobacterial infection. *Am J Clin Pathol* 1980;74:478–485.

396. Murray J, Mill J. Pulmonary infectious complications of human immunodeficiency virus infection. *Am Rev Respir Dis* 1990:1356–1372, 1582–1596.

397. Catterall JR, Hofflin JM, Remington JS. Pulmonary toxoplasmosis. *Am Rev Respir Dis* 1986; 133:704–705.

398. Remington JS. Toxoplasmosis in the adult. *Bull NY Acad Med* 1974;50:211–227.

399. Remadi S, Dumais J, Wafa K, et al. Pulmonary microsporidiosis in a patient with the acquired immunodeficiency syndrome. A case report. *Acta Cytol* 1995;39:1112–1116.

400. Travis WD, Schmidt K, MacLowry JD, et al. Respiratory cryptosporidiosis in a patient with malignant lymphoma. Report of a case and review of the literature. *Arch Pathol Lab Med* 1990;114:519–522.

401. Shulman HM, Hackman RC, Sale GE, et al. Rapid cytologic diagnosis of cytomegalovirus interstitial pneumonia on touch imprints from open-lung biopsy. *Am J Clin Pathol* 1982; 77:90–94.

402. Abdallah PS, Mark JB, Merigan TC. Diagnosis of cytomegalovirus pneumonia in compromised hosts. *Am J Med* 1976;61:326–332.

403. Saravolatz LD, Burch KH, Fisher E, et al. The compromised host and Legionnaires' disease. *Ann Intern Med* 1979;90:533–537.

404. Chandler FW, Hicklin MD, Blackmon JA. Demonstration of the agent of Legionnaires' disease in tissue. *N Engl J Med* 1977;297:1218–1220.

405. Joly JR, Ramsay D. Use of monoclonal antibodies in the diagnosis and epidemiologic studies of legionellosis. *Am J Med* 1987;83:561–574.

406. Williams J, Nunley D, Dralle W, et al. Diagnosis of pulmonary strongyloidiasis by bronchoalveolar lavage. *Chest* 1988;94:643–644.

407. Maayan S, Wormser GP, Widerhorn J, et al. Strongyloides stercoralis hyperinfection in a patient with the acquired immune deficiency syndrome. *Am J Med* 1987;83:945–948.

408. Russell GM, Mills AE. Pulmonary malakoplakia related to *Rhodococcus equi* occurring in the acquired immunodeficiency syndrome. *Med J Aust* 1994;160:308–309.

409. Slater LN, Min KW. Polypoid endobronchial lesions. A manifestation of bacillary angiomatosis. *Chest* 1992;102:972–974.

410. Finet JF, Abdalsamad I, Bakdach H, et al. Intrathoracic localization of bacillary angiomatosis. *Histopathology* 1996;28:183–185.

411. Churg A. Transbronchial biopsy: nothing to fear. *Am J Surg Pathol* 2001;25:820–822.

Pulmonary Neoplasms

GENERAL COMMENTS

Surgical pathology, not only of lung tumors but also of tumors in general, has changed since the mid-1970s. An increasing number of cases of early-stage lung cancer and atypical proliferative lesions are observed as a result of clinicians' efforts to detect small lung cancers (1–4). Newer techniques, particularly immunohistochemistry (IHC) and molecular biology, have produced a large amount of information on tumor histogenesis, differentiation, and proliferation that has been widely applied to tumor subtyping (5,6). Newer entities have been added, such as localized bronchioloalveolar carcinoma, which has come to be understood as in situ adenocarcinoma of the lung (7); large-cell neuroendocrine carcinoma (LCNEC), which is considered one type of neuroendocrine tumor of the lung (8); and bronchioloalveolar atypical adenomatous hyperplasia (or adenoma), which is defined as a precancerous or preinvasive form of adenocarcinoma (3,4,9–13).

New therapeutic procedures have been introduced; one such representative technique is sleeve resection of the bronchus to preserve one lobe, and another is the application of video-assisted thoracic surgery to many different thoracic operations (e.g., simple wedge resection to lobectomy and pneumonectomy). Especially since the introduction of computer tomography (CT) screening for detection of lung carcinoma, many small lesions can now be detected, and reduction operations such as wedge resection or segmentectomy are now performed frequently (14). Laser therapy or brachytherapy is a choice of treatment for tumors of the major bronchus. However, this has also created the problem of laser-induced atypism in nonneoplastic epithelial cells—a feature that often causes diagnostic difficulty for pathologists (11). From a review of the progress made in surgical pathology, a more scientific basis is thought to have been given to pathologic diagnosis based on sections stained with hematoxylin and eosin.

SEGMENTAL ANATOMY OF BRONCHI AND LUNG

Because lung cancer originates in bronchi and bronchioloalveoli, understanding the course and branching of these airways and remembering the names of each branch are necessary. The current terminology for the bronchi that is used throughout the world was developed in Japan primarily for bronchography and fiberoptic bronchoscopy (Figs. 26.1 and 26.2). In Japan, the lobar bronchus has been called the *first-order bronchus*, and the segmental bronchus has been termed the *second-order bronchus*, according to Ikeda (15). For a description of lesions, the recommendation is to state at least the number of the subsegmental bronchus and the order of bronchi involved in the tumor because clinically manifest lung cancers of peripheral origin almost always involve more than two bronchi.

MATERIALS FOR DIAGNOSIS

Cytology Materials

The materials for cytologic diagnosis include the following: (a) sputum smears; (b) smears prepared from bronchial washing, scraping, or brushing of the lesion; (c) smears prepared from fine-needle aspiration, either through a fiberoptic bronchoscope or through the chest wall; (d) pleural effusion; and (e) pleural washing after surgical resection of the lung tumor (16). Materials obtained by using a fine needle and by curettage or brushing are often scant, and these must be fixed immediately to avoid drying artifacts, which may result in a false-positive diagnosis.

Biopsy Materials

Materials obtained under fiberoptic bronchoscopic guidance are often extremely small, and they are sometimes crushed, particularly in the case of small-cell carcinoma. In crushed specimens of small-cell carcinoma, the free cells present around the tissue fragments may be of help in establishing a histologic diagnosis because they are often well preserved. In small tissue fragments, differentiated tumor features (e.g., a tubular structure or keratinization) may not be present. Therefore, the diagnosis of large-cell carcinoma based on small tissue fragments may not agree with that based on tissue from a resected lung tumor. Tissues obtained by transbronchial lung biopsy should preferably be placed in saline solution or fixative under negative pressure so that collapsed alveolar spaces may become inflated. A Surecut (modified Menghini; TSK Laboratory, Tokyo, Japan) or Tru-cut needle (Baxter Healthcare, Valencia, California, United States) can be used for percutaneous needle biopsy. The tissue obtained by these needles can be diagnosed with relative ease because of their larger gauge, although the incidence of complications (such as air thrombosis) may increase (17). Forceps used for transbronchial lung biopsy and needles used for biopsy should be washed to obtain cytologic preparations.

Surgical Materials

Specimens obtained either by lobectomy or pneumonectomy should be carefully examined for tumor involvement at the surgical resection lines, including the resected end of a bronchus; the extrapulmonary peribronchial and perivascular soft tissue; and the surfaces covering the tumor, such as the pleura, thoracic wall, or diaphragm. In the case of sleeve lobectomy, both of the resected ends of the bronchus should be carefully identified and examined. Resected lymph nodes should be submitted to the pathology laboratory in groups numbered as shown in Figure 26.3 (18). The material obtained by wedge, segmental, or partial resection, either by video-assisted thoracic surgery or by conventional thoracotomy, should be placed in saline solution under negative pressure after the removal of staples, and

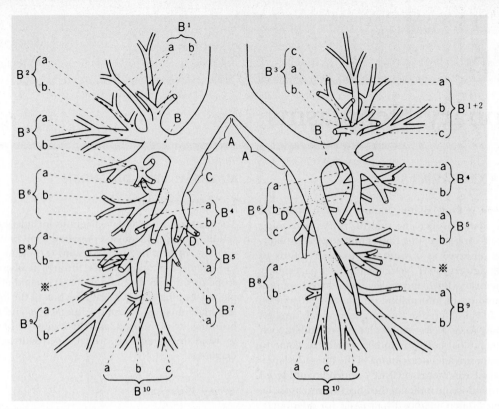

Figure 26.1. Nomenclature of bronchi by the Japanese Committee on the Nomenclature for Bronchial Branching, which is based on that of Jackson-Huber or Boyden. Anterior view. *A*, main bronchus; *B*, truncus superior; *C*, truncus intermedius; *D*, truncus inferior; *B1–10*, segmental bronchi; *a, b*, and *c*, subsegmental bronchi. From: Ikeda S. *Atlas of Flexible Bronchofiberscopy*. Tokyo: Igaku-Shoin, 1974:58–61, with permission.

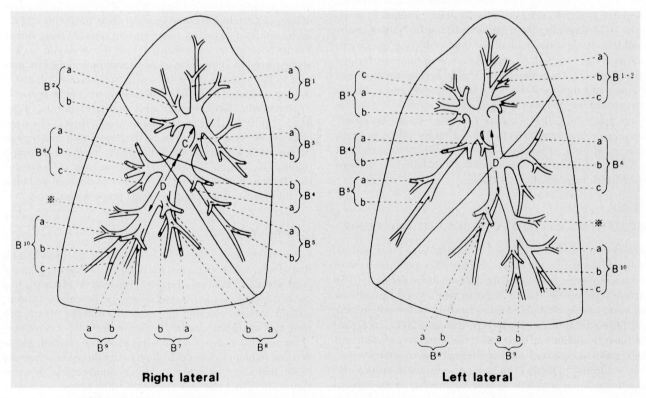

Right lateral   **Left lateral**

Figure 26.2. Nomenclature of bronchi by the Japanese Committee on the Nomenclature for Bronchial Branching, which is based on that of Jackson-Huber or Boyden as in Figure 26.1. Right lateral and left lateral views. From: Ikeda S. *Atlas of Flexible Bronchofiberscopy*. Tokyo: Igaku-Shoin, 1974:58–61, with permission.

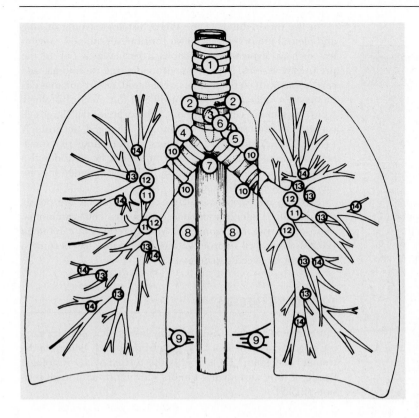

Figure 26.3. Mapping of intrapulmonary, pulmonary hilar, and mediastinal lymph nodes. *1*, superior mediastinal or highest mediastinal; *2*, paratracheal; *3*, pretracheal (*3a*, anterior mediastinal; *3p*, retrotracheal); *4*, tracheobronchial; *5*, subaortic or Botallo; *6*, para-aortic (ascending aorta); *7*, subcarinal; *8*, paraesophageal (below carina); *9*, pulmonary ligament; *10*, hilar; *11*, interlobar; *12*, lobar (upper, middle, and lower lobes); *13*, segmental; and *14*, subsegmental.

then in fixative. Before removal of staples, a touch specimen or a washing specimen of the cut surface should be obtained for cytologic diagnosis of the resected end of the material.

Frozen Section Materials

At the time of frozen section diagnosis during surgery, pathologists must be cautious about distinguishing between dysplasia and carcinoma in situ of the bronchial mucosa, and between bronchioloalveolar atypical adenomatous hyperplasia or bronchioloalveolar carcinoma of the nonmucinous type and small invasive adenocarcinoma. It is also important to discriminate atypical adenomatous hyperplasia from nonmucinous-type bronchioloalveolar carcinoma. Biologically, however, the two lesions have an extremely favorable prognosis and, from a practical viewpoint, there is no need to distinguish between them. It must also be kept in mind that lymph nodes with metastasis may be very small in cases of adenocarcinoma.

The correct diagnosis of a frozen section is based on sufficient knowledge of the pulmonary lesions, great care, and careful sampling. Sampling errors are sometimes encountered in extensively cavitated cancer, in which at least two areas must be selected for sectioning, including one through the wall of an involved bronchus. Insufficient knowledge of lung tumors may lead to erroneous diagnosis of adenocarcinoma when the pathologist observes the presence of atypical papillary proliferation at the periphery of the "sclerosing hemangioma." In such cases, the gross features are most helpful because sclerosing hemangioma is spheric with well-defined borders, and it can be enucleated. The distinction between primary and metastatic

tumors may, at times, be extremely difficult; this is discussed on page 1085.

In any event, an appropriate diagnosis or decision regarding surgical procedures must be obtained by surgeons immediately after rapid frozen sectioning during thoracic surgery so they can avoid having to perform a repeated thoracotomy after the examination of permanent paraffin sections.

REPORT ON SURGICAL MATERIALS

Table 26.1 shows an example of a report on the results of a pathologic examination of a resected lung specimen. Some items are considered important regarding a decision on postoperative chemotherapy in patients with the following pathologic disease status: tumor (T) 1,2; node (N) 0,1; metastasis (M) 0.

At present, in research-oriented hospitals, fresh tumor tissues are often requested for use in (a) the analysis of genetic molecular changes and their products; (b) the determination of nuclear DNA content and ploidy; (c) cell culture; and (d) enzyme and hormone analysis. Pathologists must be prepared to cooperate in projects that have been judged to be important. Needless to say, however, an adequate amount of tissue for pathologic diagnosis, small pieces for electron microscopy, and a piece for IHC with dimensions of $1 \times 1 \times 0.2$ cm must be reserved. The acetone, methylbenzoate, and xylene (AMeX) method has been found to be superior to other fixation procedures for the preservation of DNA, RNA, and antigenicity, which is lost through usual formalin fixation (19,20). Methanol fixation is also recommended when performing DNA and RNA analysis. If the tumor is sufficiently large, we routinely store at least 1 g of the tumor and nontu-

TABLE 26.1

Example of a Report on the Results of a Pathologic Examination of a Resected Lung Specimen

Primary site:
Tumor size: _ × _ × _ cm
Resected end of bronchus: negative or positive for tumor
Other surgical margin: negative or positive for tumor
Involved bronchi:
Involved segments:
Histological diagnosis: Squamous cell carcinoma
                          Small-cell carcinoma
                          Adenocarcinoma   BAC subtype (%)
                                           Papillary subtype (%)
                                           Acinar subtype (%)
                                           Solid subtype (%)
                                           Others (%)
                          Large-cell carcinoma
                          Others
Lymphatic permeation: negative/positive
Vascular invasion: negative/positive
Pleural involvement: p0/p1/p2/p3^a (lateral/medial/
    interlobar/diaphragm)
Intrapulmonary metastases: absent/present
Pleural dissemination: absent/present
Pathologic stage: pT N M
Nuclear atypia: slight/moderate/marked
Mitotic index: low/intermediate/high^b
Therapeutic effect: none/mild/moderate/marked
Lymph nodes (no. positive/no. examined)
#1(/)   #6(/)   #11(/)
#2(/)   #7(/)   #12(/)
#3(/)   #8(/)   #13(/)
#4(/)   #9(/)   #14(/)
#5(/)   #10(/)
Total (/)
n0/n0(+)/n1/n2

^{a}p0, pleura uninvolved; p1, tumor has destroyed the elastic layer but is not exposed on the pleural surface; p2, tumor is exposed on pleural surface; p3, tumor involves parietal pleura or other pulmonary lobe.
^{b}Low, ≤5/10 high-power fields; intermediate, 6–15/10 high-power fields; high, ≥16/10 high-power fields.

morous lung tissues frozen at −20 °C or preferably at −80 °C for future study.

HISTOLOGIC CLASSIFICATION

Lung tumors have been categorized according to the World Health Organization (WHO) classification, which has been revised in 1999 (21), and in 2004 (22). In the 1970s and 1980s, several cytologic subtypes were recognized in adenocarcinoma; in particular, papillary adenocarcinoma was found to be composed of several carcinomas of the following different cell types: a mucus-producing (goblet) cell type, a bronchiolar nonciliated cell (Clara cell) type, a type II alveolar epithelial cell type, and a bronchial surface epithelial cell type producing either no mucin or only scant amounts of it. The last type of cell appears to have a tendency to differentiate as a ciliated columnar cell. In addition, a bronchial gland cell type, which is tubular in most instances, is occasionally observed (23–25).

In the third edition of the WHO histologic typing of lung and pleural tumors and its minor revision, several new categories, such as atypical adenomatous hyperplasia as one of the preinvasive lesions, large-cell neuroendocrine carcinoma, and carcinomas with pleomorphic, sarcomatoid, or sarcomatous elements, were added, and the subtyping of four major histologic types (squamous cell carcinoma, adenocarcinoma, large-cell carcinoma, and small-cell carcinoma) changed accordingly (Table 26.2). A group of investigators recommended that small-cell carcinoma with a large-cell component be considered a subtype of small-cell carcinoma, and it is now included in combined small-cell carcinoma (22).

Electron microscopically, large-cell carcinomas are poorly differentiated adenocarcinoma, squamous cell carcinoma, neuroendocrine carcinoma, or undifferentiated carcinoma (26,27). Large-cell neuroendocrine carcinoma has become a subtype of large-cell carcinoma.

LUNG TUMORS

Lung tumors are composed of many histologic types with varying degrees of malignancy, ranging from entirely benign to extremely malignant. Table 26.2 is the revised WHO histologic typing of lung and pleural tumors with minor additional revision (21,22).

BENIGN EPITHELIAL TUMORS

Tumors in this group present no problems in surgical pathology (Fig. 26.4), except for differential diagnosis between mixed squamous and glandular papilloma and mucoepidermoid carcinoma. Pleomorphic adenoma and mucinous cystadenoma may arise also in distal bronchi, although this is rare (Fig. 26.5). Other bronchial gland adenomas include oncocytoma and mucous gland adenoma (28,29). Papillary adenoma consisting of type II alveolar epithelial cells or Clara cells has been reported to arise in the periphery of the lung (30). Alveolar adenoma is also a peripheral solitary nodule consisting of small cystic spaces lined by type II alveolar epithelial cells and containing fluid (31).

PREINVASIVE LESIONS: DYSPLASIA AND CARCINOMA IN SITU

With the increasing efforts on the part of clinicians to find lung cancer in the early stage, the chances of observing such lesions as dysplasia and carcinoma in situ have correspondingly increased. Usually, dysplasia and carcinoma in situ involve lesions in the bronchi, but those occurring in alveoli are also dealt with here.

Bronchial Dysplasia and Carcinoma in Situ

The criteria for these lesions are similar to those of lesions occurring in the uterine cervix and oral cavity (Figs. 26.6 and 26.7). However, the histologic appearance of these lesions is not identical because the tissue of origin is quite different. The diagnostic points used in differentiating carcinoma in situ from dysplasia in the bronchus have not yet been standardized. Therefore, much more experience is needed to reach agreement in most cases. To treat a lesion such as carcinoma in situ,

TABLE 26.2	World Health Organization (WHO) Histologic Classification of Lung and Pleural Tumors

Epithelial tumors	Well-differentiated fetal adenocarcinoma	*Mesothelial tumors*
Benign	Mucinous ("colloid") adenocarcinoma	Benign
Papillomas	Mucinous cystadenocarcinoma	Adenomatoid tumor
Squamous cell papilloma	Signet-ring adenocarcinoma	Malignant
Exophytic	Clear-cell adenocarcinoma	Epithelioid mesothelioma
Inverted	Large-cell carcinoma	Sarcomatoid mesothelioma
Glandular papilloma	Variant: large-cell neuroendocrine carcinoma	Desmoplastic mesothelioma
Mixed squamous and glandular papilloma	Combined large-cell neuroendocrine carcinoma	Biphasic mesothelioma
Adenoma		*Miscellaneous tumors*
Alveolar adenoma	Basaloid carcinoma	Hamartoma
Papillary adenoma	Lymphoepithelioma-like carcinoma	Sclerosing hemangioma
Adenoma of salivary-gland type	Clear-cell carcinoma	Clear-cell tumor
Mucous gland adenoma	Large-cell carcinoma with rhabdoid phenotype	Germ-cell tumors
Pleomorphic adenoma		Teratoma, mature
Mucinous cystadenoma	Adenosquamous carcinoma	Teratoma, immature
Preinvasive lesions	Carcinomas with pleomorphic, sarcomatoid, or sarcomatous elements	Other germ-cell tumors
Squamous dysplasia		Thymoma
Carcinoma in situ	Carcinomas with spindle and/or giant cells	Malignant melanoma
Atypical adenomatous hyperplasia	Pleomorphic carcinoma	*Lymphoproliferative diseases*
Diffuse idiopathic pulmonary neuroendocrine cell	Spindle cell carcinoma	Lymphoid interstitial pneumonia
	Giant-cell carcinoma	Nodular lymphoid hyperplasia
Hyperplasia	Carcinosarcoma	Low-grade marginal zone B-cell lymphoma of the mucosa-associated lymphoid tissue (MALT)
Malignant	Pulmonary blastoma	
Squamous cell carcinoma	Carcinoid tumor	
Variants	Typical carcinoid	Lymphomatoid granulomatosis
Papillary	Atypical carcinoid	*Secondary tumors*
Clear cell	Carcinomas of salivary-gland type	*Unclassified tumors*
Small cell	Mucoepidermoid carcinoma	*Tumor-like lesions*
Basaloid	Adenoid cystic carcinoma	Tumorlet
Small-cell carcinoma	Unclassified carcinoma	Multiple meningothelioid nodules
Variant: combined small-cell carcinoma	*Soft tissue tumors*	Langerhans cell histiocytosis
Adenocarcinoma	Localized fibrous tumor	Inflammatory pseudotumor (inflammatory myofibroblastic tumor)
Adenocarcinoma with mixed subtypes	Epithelioid hemangioendothelioma	
Acinar	Pleuropulmonary blastoma	Localized organizing pneumonia
Papillary	Chondroma	Amyloid tumor (nodular amyloid)
Bronchioloalveolar carcinoma	Calcifying fibrous pseudotumor of the pleura	Hyalinizing granuloma
Nonmucinous		Lymphangioleiomyomatosis
Mucinous	Congenital peribronchial myofibroblastic tumor	Micronodular pneumocyte hyperplasia
Mixed mucinous and nonmucinous or indeterminate cell type		Endometriosis
	Diffuse pulmonary lymphangiomatosis	Bronchial inflammatory polyp
Solid adenocarcinoma with mucin	Desmoplastic round cell tumor	
Variants		

From: Travis WD, Colby TV, Corrin B, et al. *WHO Histological Typing of Lung and Pleural Tumors.* 3rd ed. Geneva: World Health Organization, 1999, with permission.

a confirmatory diagnosis from at least two competent pathologists is preferred.

Atypical Adenomatous Hyperplasia, and Bronchioloalveolar Carcinoma in the Distal Lung

Diagnostic difficulty is also experienced with lesions that may be called atypical adenomatous hyperplasia and well-differentiated bronchioloalveolar carcinoma of the nonmucinous type (3,4,9–13). In these lesions, cuboidal cells with rather uniform nuclei and scant cytoplasm replace alveolar lining cells (Fig. 26.8). However, the cell density is not sufficiently high, and the cells and nuclei are not sufficiently atypical, for the lesion to be called cancer; almost no mitotic figures are seen. Thus, conflicting views exist concerning the nature of this lesion. Discrimi-

nation between atypical adenomatous hyperplasia (a precancerous lesion) and bronchioloalveolar carcinoma (carcinoma in situ) is sometimes very difficult; morphologic criteria for differentiating between the two lesions were recently reported (32) and are shown in Table 26.3. The 5-year survival rate of patients with both lesions is extremely favorable, and there is no discernible difference in survival. However, current staging criteria seem to indicate differences.

Diffuse Idiopathic Pulmonary Neuroendocrine Cell Hyperplasia

Diffuse idiopathic pulmonary neuroendocrine cell hyperplasia is an extremely rare condition, comprising neuroendocrine cell hyperplasia confined to the bronchiolar epithelium associated

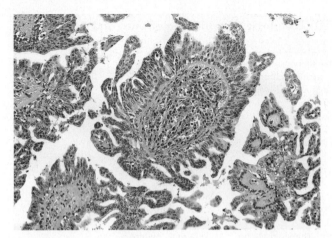

Figure 26.4. Glandular papilloma of bronchus. The papillary lesion is covered by two layers of pseudostratified columnar cells without cilia. This is an extremely rare type of papilloma.

with obliterative bronchiolar fibrosis in the absence of airway inflammation or diffuse interstitial fibrosis. A subset of patients has multiple tumorlets and one or more peripheral carcinoid tumors. Therefore, it is considered to be a preneoplastic lesion (22).

MALIGNANT EPITHELIAL TUMORS

Squamous Cell Carcinoma

Squamous cell carcinoma is the most frequently occurring lung cancer in Western countries, and is the type of cancer most strongly related to cigarette smoking. A marked male predominance in its incidence is seen, with a male-to-female ratio of between 6.6 and 15 to 1. One study in the United States, however, indicated that the rates of squamous cell, small-cell, and large-cell carcinomas among men are declining—a finding reflecting changes in cigarette smoking patterns (33).

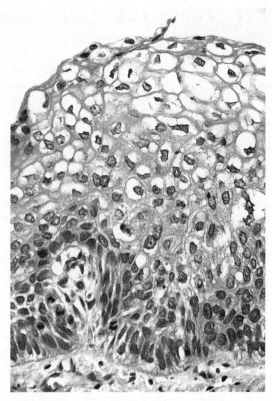

Figure 26.6. Squamous dysplasia. The ciliated respiratory epithelium has been replaced by thick, stratified squamous epithelium with moderate nuclear atypia and koilocytosis in the superficial layers.

GROSS FEATURES. *Overview.* At least 50% of all squamous cell carcinomas arise in a major bronchus (main to segmental bronchus), where the tumor shows both endobronchial and invasive growth into the peribronchial soft tissue, lung parenchyma, and nearby lymph nodes; it often compresses the pulmonary artery and vein (Fig. 26.9). Endobronchial tumor growth

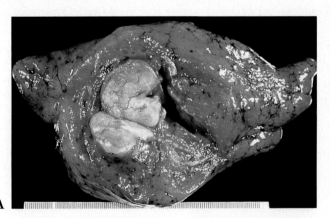
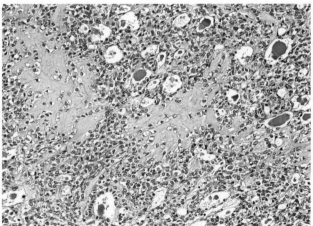

Figure 26.5. Pleomorphic adenoma. **(A)** The bisected tumor in S6 discloses a well-defined border and is not related to any visible bronchi. **(B)** Histologically, the tumor is composed of nests and trabeculae of epithelial cells, with occasional lumina containing secretion and myxomatous or chondromatous areas. Pleomorphic adenoma is most often seen in the trachea and major bronchi; peripheral origin is extremely rare. From: Kameya T. Salivary gland type tumors. In National Cancer Center Hospital. *Cancer of the Lung: Diagnosis and Treatment.* Vol. 1. Tokyo: Kodansha, 1983:179–190 [in Japanese], with permission.

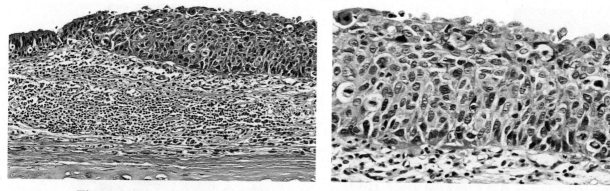

Figure 26.7. Squamous cell carcinoma in situ. Stratified epithelium more than 10 cells thick is composed of polygonal cells with an increased nuclear-to-cytoplasmic (N:C) ratio and nuclear atypia, but it does not show invasive growth; the carcinoma ends abruptly at the normal epithelium. Mitotic figures are scattered. **(A)** Low-power view. **(B)** High-power view.

often results in secondary changes in the distal lung, such as atelectasis, lipid pneumonia, and bronchopneumonia. Squamous cell carcinoma of peripheral origin reveals a nodular growth form with well-defined borders that often show extensive coagulation necrosis and, at times, cavitation. Secondary changes in the distal lung parenchyma may obscure the border of the tumor. Grossly, squamous cell carcinoma of peripheral origin can be roughly divided into the following two types: (a) tumor with central or subpleural fibrosis with anthracosis, with which pleural indentation is often associated (although the indentation is not as sharp or conspicuous as that seen in adenocarcinoma because of a dense fibrotic tissue reaction at the site of indentation [Fig. 26.10]); and (b) tumor without scar, in which the cut surface reveals either no anthracotic pigments or only a scant amount. The former is the result of a growth characteristic involving the filling of alveolar spaces, whereas the latter is formed through compression-type tumor growth.

Early squamous cell carcinoma. If a possibility of cure can be predicted with high accuracy from the gross and microscopic findings, and if the gross and microscopic findings can be defined as those representative of cases with a 5-year survival rate of more than 90%, then the term *early carcinoma* can be used.

Early lung cancer of the hilar type can be defined as follows (34):

1. Tumor arises in a major bronchus (up to the bifurcation of the segmental bronchus into subsegmental bronchi). (One group has suggested inclusion of the subsegmental bronchi among the major or hilar bronchi because they are visible with a fiberoptic bronchoscope.)
2. Tumor is confined to the wall of a bronchus.
3. No lymph node metastasis is present.

Most squamous cell carcinomas confined to the walls of bronchi are free of lymph node metastasis. When metastasis is present, it does not extend beyond the hilar nodes.

Such early carcinomas of the hilar type are found to be squamous in most instances, and they can be divided grossly into the following subtypes (Fig. 26.11) (34):

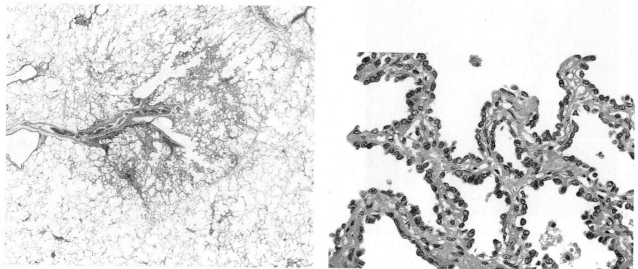

Figure 26.8. Atypical adenomatous hyperplasia. The alveolar lining cells are increased in size with mildly atypical and slightly pleomorphic nuclei. Alveolar septa show slight thickening. No mitotic figures are seen. **(A)** Histologic section. **(B)** High-power view.

TABLE 26.3

Proposed Diagnostic Criteria of Atypical Adenomatous Hyperplasia

Atypical adenomatous hyperplasia (AAH) is a clearly demarcated alveolar-displacing proliferative lesion of the peripheral airway epithelium, and its septa are slightly thicker than normal alveolar walls. The lesions are generally no more than 5 mm in size, but at times large lesions may also be found. They are sometimes associated with collapsed foci within the lesions, lymphocytic infiltration, or follicle formation.

However, in cases in which it would seem impossible to differentiate between AAH and cancer, if the lesion fulfills three or more of the following histologic criteria, it may be deemed as being at least carcinoma in situ.

Marked cell stratification

High cell density and marked overlapping of nuclei

Coarse nuclear chromatin and presence of nucleolus

Tumor cells growing in a wooden-peg-like arrangement or in a true papillary pattern

Tumor cell height greater than the height of the epithelial cells in the surrounding terminal bronchus

From: Minami Y, Matsuno Y, Iijima T, et al. Prognostication of small-sized primary pulmonary adenocarcinomas by histopathological and karyometric analysis. *Lung Cancer* 2005;48:339–348.

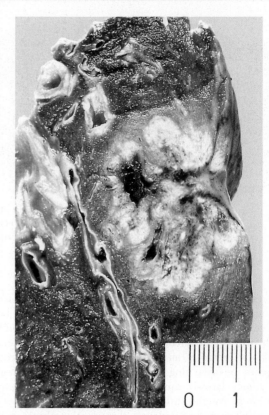

Figure 26.10. Squamous cell carcinoma of peripheral origin. A well-defined tumor shows cavitation in some areas and fibrosis in others, a pattern associated with pleural indentation and fibrosis. Superiorly, the tumor merges into foci of lipid pneumonia. From: National Cancer Center Hospital. *Cancer of the Lung: Diagnosis and Treatment.* Vol. 1. Tokyo: Kodansha, 1983:168–190 [in Japanese], with permission.

1. Polypoid type (frequently arising at the bronchial spur).
2. Nodular type (arising at any site and having a tendency to form a localized tumor and to show vertical invasive growth).
3. Superficially infiltrating type (in situ and microinvasive-type growth often involving a wide area but exhibiting little tendency to produce bronchial stenosis).
4. Combination of these types.

To determine the border of the growth grossly, changes in the pattern of longitudinal mucosal folds are of great help, particularly in deciding the extent of a superficially infiltrating type of tumor, which often shows thickening and fusion of the folds.

Five-year survival of patients with early squamous cell carcinoma of the hilar type is more than 90%, but this neoplasm is frequently found in association with a second squamous cell carcinoma of the bronchus. This finding may result, in part, from the detailed pathologic studies of the lung with early squamous cell carcinoma.

Pathologic T1, N0, M0 squamous cell carcinoma of the peripheral type is not always associated with good prognosis, and the 5-year survival is less than 90%. Because lymph node involvement is quite low in peripheral squamous cell carcinoma of 2 cm or less in diameter (35), early squamous cell carcinoma of the peripheral type should be defined as T1, N0, M0 with a tumor 2 cm or less in diameter. However, small carcinomas such as these are infrequently encountered in practice, probably be-

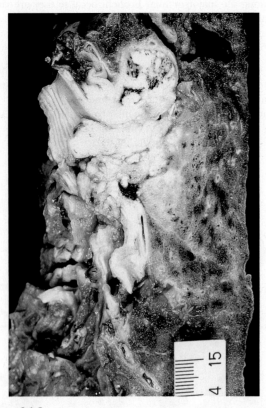

Figure 26.9. Squamous cell carcinoma of a major bronchus. A polypoid tumor arising in the truncus superior of the left lung projects into the main bronchus, invades the peribronchial soft tissue and lung parenchyma, and directly involves a lymph node. The surrounding lung parenchyma displays lipid pneumonia. From: National Cancer Center Hospital. *Cancer of the Lung: Diagnosis and Treatment.* Vol. 1. Tokyo: Kodansha, 1983:168–190 [in Japanese], with permission.

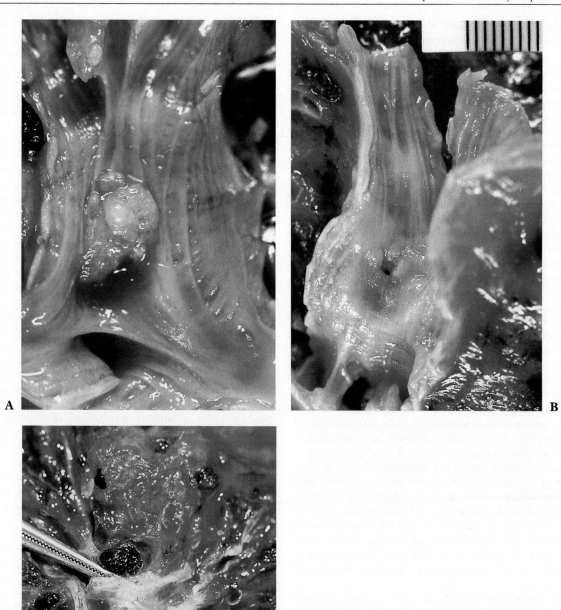

Figure 26.11. Squamous cell carcinoma of major bronchi in the early stage (confined to within the bronchial wall). **(A)** A polypoid growth arises at the spur between B1 + 2 and B3. Note the longitudinal and transverse mucosal folds in the bronchi—good markers of tumor invasion that are distorted or lost on involvement of squamous cell carcinoma. **(B)** A nodular growth, 7 mm in diameter, is seen around the orifice of B*. **(C)** Superficially infiltrating-type tumor involving B3, B3b, and B3c. Longitudinal mucosal folds are thickened and fused in some areas. The tumor extended for 5.2 cm along B1 + 2. **(B)** is from: Kameya T. Salivary gland type tumors. In National Cancer Center Hospital. *Cancer of the Lung: Diagnosis and Treatment.* Vol. 1. Tokyo: Kodansha, 1983:179–190 [in Japanese], with permission.

cause of the rather rapid growth of squamous cell carcinoma compared with that of adenocarcinoma.

HISTOLOGIC CHARACTERISTICS. Compared with such a lesion in the uterine cervix, bronchial carcinoma in situ often displays more frequent and more evident squamous differentiation. However, most invasive squamous cell carcinomas of the lung are moderately to poorly differentiated (Fig. 26.12), and a well-differentiated carcinoma is infrequent in comparison with carcinoma of stratified squamous epithelial origin, such as that of the oral cavity, pharynx, and esophagus.

Another characteristic of squamous cell carcinoma of the lung is its intraepithelial in situ–like extension along the bronchus. As a rule, neither small-cell carcinoma nor adenocarcinoma replaces the bronchial epithelium to any considerable extent; instead, it tends to grow beneath the epithelium. This feature is useful for deciding the histologic type of lung cancer in a small biopsy specimen, particularly when keratinization and intercellular bridges are not evident. At the advancing border of squamous cell carcinoma, tumor cells usually grow by either destroying alveoli or filling alveolar spaces. Infrequently, however, the tumor cells spread beneath a layer of type II alveolar epithelial cells and on the epithelial side of the basement membrane (36), thus preserving narrowed alveolar spaces within the tumor and producing a pattern that mimics the features of adenosquamous carcinoma.

Minor differences in the cytologic characteristics are found between squamous cell carcinoma of the hilar type and that of the peripheral type, which may be reflected in the gross features and prognosis. That mucin-containing cells are frequently seen in squamous cell carcinoma of the lung has been noted (37). Not only mucin-producing cells but also cells reactive with antibody to the secretory component are considered to possess glandular characteristics. In studies with these two markers, glandular cell characteristics were seen in 10% of hilar-type squamous cell carcinomas and in 60% of peripheral-type tumors (38). In other words, more than 50% of peripheral squamous cell carcinomas are actually adenosquamous carcinomas in the strict sense.

The variants in squamous cell carcinoma include papillary, clear-cell, small-cell, and basaloid patterns. The papillary pat-

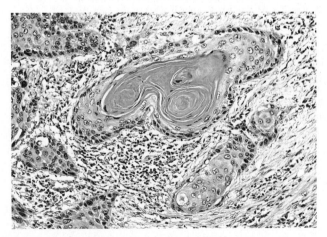

Figure 26.12. Histology of squamous cell carcinoma. Geographic nests are composed of polygonal cells with intercellular bridges and keratinization. The stroma is fibrous.

tern is seen in squamous cell carcinoma with endobronchial, exophytic growth. The small-cell variant can be differentiated from combined small-cell carcinoma with a squamous cell component by the morphologic characteristics of small tumor cells, which show the nuclear features of a non–small-cell carcinoma. The basaloid variant displays peripheral palisading of nuclei at the edge of tumor cell nests of squamous cell carcinoma (39).

BIOLOGIC BEHAVIOR. Squamous cell carcinoma of the hilar type occasionally shows intraepithelial spread that may extend to the resection line. Therefore, examining the mucosa of the resected end by frozen sectioning at the time of surgery is important. Particular attention should be paid in the case of sleeve resection, in which two resected ends are present, and each should be identified correctly. If the resection line is positive for tumor and additional resection is impossible, metal clips should be placed for postoperative irradiation because (a) squamous cell carcinoma of the lung tends to remain within the thoracic cavity; and (b) cure can be expected if the remaining amount of tumor is small.

Peripheral-type squamous cell carcinoma may involve the thoracic wall, mediastinum, and diaphragm. However, pleural carcinomatosis from squamous cell carcinoma occurs only rarely. Therefore, pleural effusion may not be cancerous but may instead be reactive, and cytologic examination should always be conducted to confirm the nature of the effusion.

Hypercalcemia that is not caused by bone metastasis is often associated with squamous cell carcinoma of the lung. This was thought to be caused by hypercalcemic agents, such as osteoclast-activating factor and prostaglandin, produced by tumor cells. However, more recent studies have disclosed that such hypercalcemia results from the parathyroid hormone–related protein produced by the tumor in most such cases (40,41).

Small-Cell Carcinoma

Small-cell carcinoma of the lung has attracted considerable attention from basic scientists, pathologists, and clinicians because of its complex pathobiologic characteristics and high degree of malignancy in spite of its high sensitivity to antitumor agents and radiation. Many excellent and exciting studies concerning small-cell carcinoma of the lung, including reviews, were published in the 1980s (42–47).

Pathologically, this neoplasm was originally classified as mediastinal sarcoma. In 1926, Barnard (48) became the first to classify it as bronchogenic carcinoma, and, after the detailed description by Azzopardi (49), it became an established entity. However, after 1968, electron microscopic analysis of this tumor favored a neuroendocrine nature with regard to histogenesis and function (50–52). Since the 1980s, however, the concept of a bronchial epithelial neoplasm of endodermal stem cell origin with some neuroendocrine characteristics has prevailed, and this seems the most likely possibility (45,53).

MORPHOLOGIC VARIATION. *Gross features.* This tumor arises not only in the major bronchi but also in the peripheral portion of the lung. Tumors arising in a major bronchus may spread subepithelially along its long axis. Replacement of the bronchial epithelium, which is often present in squamous cell carcinoma, is hardly ever seen in small-cell carcinoma. Therefore, the lining of the bronchus is nodular but smooth and glistening, with longitudinal mucosal folds of bronchi climbing

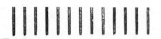

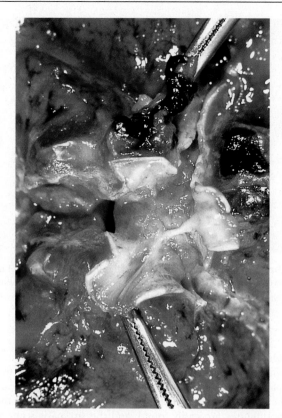

Figure 26.13. Small-cell carcinoma involving major bronchi. The surface of the nodular tumor is smooth, and a few longitudinal mucosal folds climb up and taper off over the nodular tumor—a finding indicating subepithelial tumor growth.

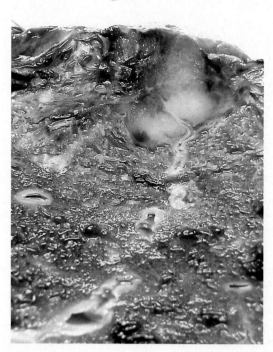

Figure 26.14. Small-cell carcinoma of peripheral lung origin. This well-defined tumor shows no obvious foci of necrosis and a fleshy cut surface.

up and tapering off on the nodular tumor, instead of the fusion and disruption of the folds that are apparent in squamous cell carcinoma (Fig. 26.13) (54). In the more advanced stage, nodular growth involving the lung parenchyma is seen, sometimes distant from the main tumor, producing more than two nodules, although these may be connected with each other by subepithelial growth in the bronchus.

Tumors arising in the periphery of the lung show solid nodular growth with a fairly well-defined border and a fleshy, medullary cut surface (Fig. 26.14). Central fibrosis with anthracosis may occur. Early mediastinal lymph node involvement is a well-known phenomenon that may be extremely extensive and that is, on rare occasions, associated with an undetectable primary focus.

Microscopic features. Small-cell carcinoma is characterized by the diffuse growth of small cells with the following features: (a) hyperchromatic, finely granular nuclei; (b) inconspicuous nucleoli; (c) a thin nuclear membrane; (d) scant, faintly stained, and, at times, very finely granular cytoplasm; and (e) ill-defined cell borders (Fig. 26.15). The stroma is delicate, vascular, and scant, with rare lymphocytic infiltration. Mitotic figures and individual cell necrosis are frequently seen. Occasionally, the tumor cells form rosettes, trabeculae, and nests of various sizes with a peripheral radial arrangement of the cells. Foci of epithelial differentiation, such as squamous cell and glandular differentiation, may be seen, and these are more evident on immunostaining for cytokeratin and secretory components (Fig. 26.16). The typical small cell described earlier was

termed an *oat cell*, and, if the cell size was somewhat increased, it was called the *intermediate cell type*. The latter frequently forms cell nests. Both subtypes are grouped together as small-cell carcinoma in the third WHO edition (21). If squamous, glandular, or "large" cells are readily seen, the neoplasm is designated *combined small cell carcinoma*.

The tumor may show extensive areas of coagulation necrosis, in which DNA deposits may be seen in necrotic blood vessel

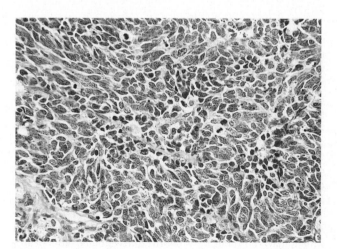

Figure 26.15. Histology of small-cell carcinoma, pure. A diffuse growth of small tumor cells is noted; these cells possess hyperchromatic nuclei, inconspicuous nucleoli, and scant cytoplasm. The cell border is indistinct.

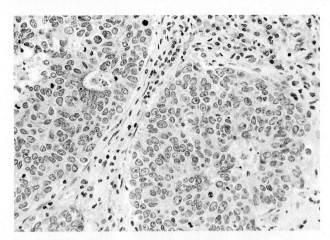

Figure 26.16. Small-cell carcinoma with a rosettelike structure. A rosettelike structure reveals a positive reaction to antikeratin antibody, but most small cells are unstained (antikeratin antibody).

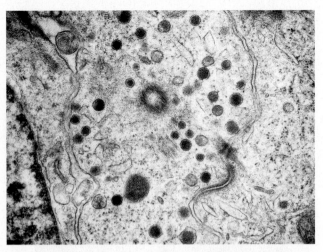

Figure 26.17. Ultrastructure of small-cell carcinoma. Typical neurosecretory-type granules of 100 to 150 nm in diameter are present in a cytoplasmic process and beneath the cell membrane. Desmosomes with tonofibrils and centrioles also are seen.

walls (Azzopardi's sign), but it is not pathognomonic for small-cell carcinoma.

Immunohistochemical findings. IHC findings are described in detail later. In brief, however, the most frequently used neuroendocrine markers for small-cell carcinoma are neural cell adhesion molecule (N-CAM) (CD56), chromogranin A, and synaptophysin (55). If the diagnosis of small-cell carcinoma is very difficult on the basis of morphologic characteristics alone, then IHC staining for these antigens should be performed. If some of the tumor cells are positive for at least one of the antigens, then a diagnosis of small-cell carcinoma is supported, but these markers can also be found in typical and atypical carcinoids, large-cell neuroendocrine carcinoma, and, rarely, in adenocarcinoma. Besides these antigens, the tumor cells often stain positively with either polyclonal or monoclonal antibodies to enzymes, such as aromatic l-amino acid decarboxylase (AADC; l-Dopa decarboxylase), neuron-specific (or γ) enolase (NSE), and creatine kinase BB (CK-BB, brain form); to peptide hormones, such as gastrin-releasing peptide (GRP or bombesin), calcitonin, and various pituitary and brain-gut peptide hormones (5,45,56); and to other antigenic substances such as Leu-7 (57).

Electron microscopic findings. The most characteristic ultrastructural feature of small-cell carcinoma is the presence of membrane-bound secretory granules of 100 to 200 nm in diameter with an electron-dense core. These granules are neurosecretory granules, and they are often present in the cytoplasmic processes and beneath the cell membrane (Fig. 26.17) (50,51). Other organelles are poorly developed, but a few bundles of tonofibrils may be associated with occasional desmosomes. Several cells may form a small glandular space in which microvilli and junctional complexes may be present (Fig. 26.18). Abortive cilia and basal bodies are seen occasionally. These ultrastructural features indicate dual characteristics (neuroendocrine and epithelial) in small-cell lung carcinoma (5,45).

Small-cell carcinoma without a neuroendocrine phenotype may be called *undifferentiated small cell carcinoma* (5), some of which may represent very poorly differentiated adenocarcinoma, squamous cell carcinoma, or large-cell carcinoma.

SMALL-CELL CARCINOMA VERSUS ATYPICAL CARCINOID. Some typical small-cell carcinomas resemble carcinoid tumor

histologically because they are composed of solid nests and trabeculae of small, round to polygonal cells with round, finely stippled nuclei and a small amount of finely granular eosinophilic cytoplasm (Fig. 26.19). Rosettes may frequently be seen, mitotic figures are easily found, and the stroma is scant and vascular. Distinction between the two is often difficult by histologic examination of sections stained with hematoxylin and eosin (H&E). Therefore, if areas more suggestive of small-cell carcinoma are apparent (i.e., they have an increased degree of nuclear atypism, frequent mitotic figures [more than 20 per 10 high-power fields], and extensive areas of necrosis), diagnosing this as small-cell carcinoma is safe. Spindling of the nuclei does not necessarily indicate small-cell carcinoma because spindle cell carcinoid may be found in the periphery of the lung.

Immunohistochemically, an intense and diffuse reaction is more usual in carcinoid tumor than in small-cell carcinoma for enzymes, peptide hormones, chromogranin A, and Grimelius

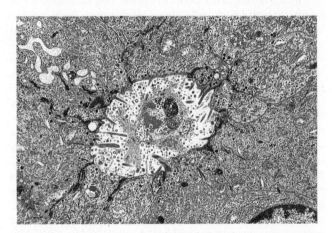

Figure 26.18. Ultrastructure of small-cell carcinoma. Several tumor cells form a minute lumen with long, slender microvilli. Cell attachments mimicking junctional complexes are seen. Dense-core granules of the neurosecretory type are seen beneath the free cell border at the lumen.

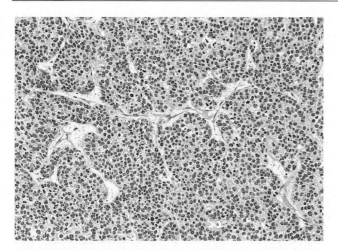

Figure 26.19. Small-cell carcinoma versus atypical carcinoid. Nests of small tumor cells are intimately associated with delicate blood vessels. Both the histologic and cytologic characteristics resemble those of carcinoid tumor. However, mitotic figures are frequent; the patient died after 10 months, with widespread metastasis.

silver staining. The one peptide that is present in some carcinoids and that has not been detected so far in small-cell carcinoma is pancreatic polypeptide (58).

Electron microscopically, neurosecretory-type granules are easily found and are often numerous in carcinoid tumors. They tend to be larger than those found in small-cell carcinoma (44).

INTERPRETATION OF BRONCHIAL BIOPSY SPECIMENS. Bronchial biopsy specimens, particularly those obtained through a flexible fiberoptic bronchoscope, are quite often crushed (Fig. 26.20). In such specimens, the pathologist has to look for intact areas, which may be extremely small. In some cases, single free tumor cells apart from tissue fragments are of help in making a cytologic diagnosis. In these cells, to an experienced eye, the chromatin pattern is different from that of lymphoma cells. To avoid misdiagnosis, endoscopists are advised to prepare cytologic smears at the time of tissue biopsy. Cytology may be superior to histology for making a distinction between small cell and non–small-cell carcinoma. IHC markers for small-cell carcinoma (CD56, chromogranin A, and synaptophysin) and lymphocytes (CD26, CD79a, CD3, etc.) are also useful for distinguishing between small-cell carcinoma and lymphoma, even if the specimen is crushed and cannot be examined morphologically in detail.

Undifferentiated carcinoma of the small-cell type previously described, as well as poorly differentiated adenocarcinoma or squamous cell carcinoma composed of small cells, could also, at times, be identified as such in biopsy specimens on the basis of the nuclear and cytoplasmic features. Another important method for distinguishing between small-cell carcinoma and squamous cell carcinoma made up of small cells is determining the mode of invasion and host reaction to the tumor. The replacement of bronchial epithelium by tumor cells may be seen in cases of squamous cell carcinoma, which shows patterns of in situ carcinoma. This type of growth is not seen in small-cell carcinoma, which often invades tissue beneath the bronchial epithelium. The covering epithelium may show squamous metaplasia or dysplasia. The lymphocytes are sparse in and around the nests of infiltrating small-cell carcinoma.

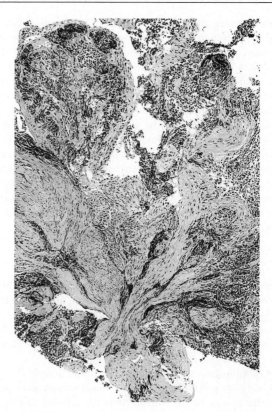

Figure 26.20. Biopsy fragment obtained through a fiberoptic bronchoscope. Cells in the upper half are fairly well preserved, but those in the lower half show crushing artifacts.

CLINICAL ASPECTS. Small-cell carcinoma is said to constitute 25% to 37% of all lung cancers in the United States and Europe, but its frequency at the National Cancer Center Hospital, Tokyo, is 19.2% in autopsy materials and only 3.8% of surgical cases. The male-to-female ratio is 4:1, and it is said to be strongly associated with cigarette smoking. However, we have had cases in female nonsmokers. Small-cell carcinoma is known to metastasize early to the regional lymph nodes and distant organs. Retrograde lymphatic spread involving the peripheral portion of the lung is not infrequently seen. This could be one of the sources of tumor recurrence after a complete response to chemotherapy and radiotherapy.

The postoperative 5-year survival rate used to be extremely low, close to zero. However, along with advances in the chemotherapy of solid tumors, 3-year survivors are gradually increasing in number, particularly in cases of disease that is limited to the thoracic cavity (59).

The outcome of efforts to detect this disease in the early stage has so far been disappointing, particularly in cases of the hilar type. However, more cases of pT1, N0-1, M0 tumors in a peripheral location are being detected and treated surgically, and such patients have shown a considerably better prognosis. Formerly, surgical treatment was not indicated in small-cell carcinoma, but now patients with T1-2, N0-1, M0 disease may be treated surgically as long as the surgery is preceded and followed by intensive chemotherapy.

That small-cell carcinoma produces amine and peptide hormones and that it may be associated with Cushing syndrome or Schwartz-Bartter syndrome are very well known (56,60–62). Therefore, some have been considered it to be an ectopic hormone-producing tumor. However, IHC investigation has disclosed the presence of the following: (a) immunoreactive GRP, calcitonin, and other active peptides in the Kulchitsky cells of the adult bronchus; and (b) immunoreactive adrenocorticotropic hormone (ACTH) in the cells of the diseased lung (63). Therefore, the hormone production should be considered to be eutopic rather than ectopic.

GRP is now believed to be an autocrine growth factor for small-cell carcinoma (64). Study on small-cell carcinoma is still progressing at the molecular level, including oncogenes, antioncogenes, or suppressor genes, such as *RB* gene, *p53* gene, and an as-yet unidentified gene in chromosome 3p, and antigenic substances recognized by monoclonal antibodies. Application of the results of these studies to diagnosis and treatment is expected in the near future.

Adenocarcinoma

Adenocarcinoma of the lung is the most frequent lung cancer occurring in Japan and some Asian countries, and is said to be increasing in the United States and other economically well-developed nations (33,65,66). The male-to-female ratio is about 2:1, and the average age at the time of diagnosis is somewhat lower than that for squamous cell carcinoma.

Grossly, most adenocarcinomas arise in the periphery of the bronchial tree, and differentiated adenocarcinoma often penetrates the pleura to disseminate into the pleural cavity, frequently producing effusion; conversely, poorly differentiated adenocarcinoma directly invades the thoracic wall through fibrous adhesion. Adenocarcinoma also frequently involves the lymphatics, but lymph nodes with metastases may not enlarge. Among the various histologic types of lung cancer, the incidence of intrapulmonary metastasis is highest in adenocarcinoma, occurring not only through the lymphatics and blood vessels but also through the airway. Hematogenous metastasis is also frequently seen in many organs. However, with the recent introduction of CT screening, very early adenocarcinomas that do not show lymph node metastasis, pleural invasion, or vascular invasion are now being detected more often.

Although adenocarcinoma is subdivided histologically into acinar (tubular), papillary, bronchioloalveolar, and solid carcinoma with mucus formation by the WHO classification (21,22), it is very complicated from the standpoint of cytologic differentiation and proliferative activity.

CYTOLOGIC CLASSIFICATION, ULTRASTRUCTURAL CHARACTERISTICS, AND MARKER SUBSTANCES. From a cytologic viewpoint, the papillary and bronchioloalveolar types, particularly by the WHO classification, consist of various tumor cells, such as peg-shaped cells that could well be of Clara cell type; cuboidal cells with a dome-shaped free cell border suggestive of type II alveolar epithelial cells; tall columnar cells producing little or no mucus; and mucus-producing columnar cells. Therefore, classifying the tumor not only from its histologic structure but also from cytologic appearance (i.e., the direction of tumor cell differentiation) is important for reaching a better understanding of the biology and clinical behavior of a given tumor. Experience shows that many adenocarcinomas that are less than 1.5 cm in diameter are composed of tumor cells of a single cell type, whereas larger tumors often consist of two cell types or more, because of metaplastic changes in tumor cells from one cell type to another, such as Clara cell type to mucus-producing

cell (25), which are complicated by anaplastic changes in tumor cells. The direction of differentiation can be assumed by light microscopic observation and is confirmed by ultrastructural and sometimes IHC findings. Adenocarcinoma cells are supposed to differentiate toward any of the various epithelial cells seen in the bronchus and bronchioloalveoli. For the sake of convenience, we subclassify adenocarcinoma of the lung into the following six cytologic types (11,25):

1. Bronchial surface cell type with little or no mucus production
2. Goblet cell type
3. Bronchial gland cell type
4. Clara cell type
5. Type II alveolar epithelial cell type
6. Mixed cell type or indeterminate cell type

Bronchial surface cell type with little or no mucus production. This cell type arises either in cartilage-bearing bronchus showing endobronchial polypoid growth (Fig. 26.21) or in the distal airway (67). It is composed of tall columnar cells arranged in a papillary and tubular fashion; these cells resemble ciliated columnar cells, although no cilia are visible (Fig. 26.22). Ultrastructurally, the cytoplasm is rich in mitochondria and smooth-surfaced vesicles but is devoid of secretory granules. Although cilia are very rarely observed, basal bodies may be seen at the free cell border, a finding indicating that the cells differentiate toward ciliated cells (Fig. 26.23). This type of adenocarcinoma comprises about 8% of our adenocarcinoma cases.

Goblet cell type. The tumor cells resemble goblet cells of the bronchial epithelium, in which the cytoplasm is filled with mucus, frequently displacing the nuclei to the basal portion

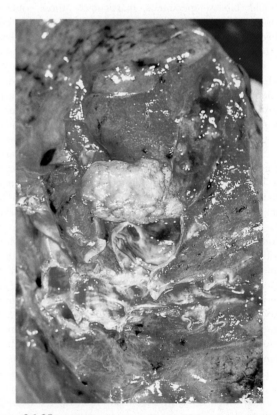

Figure 26.21. Adenocarcinoma of bronchial surface epithelial cell type, showing endobronchial growth in the fourth-order bronchus of B1b.

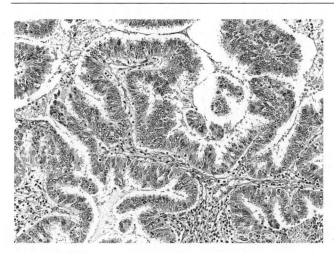

Figure 26.22. Histology of the true papillary adenocarcinoma shown in Figure 26.24. Papillary growth is made up of tall columnar cells with no cilia that somewhat resemble ciliated columnar cells and their own fibrous stroma.

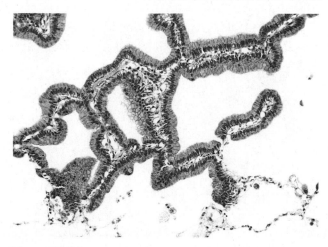

Figure 26.24. Bronchioloalveolar carcinoma of goblet cell type. Alveolar lining cells have been replaced by tall columnar cells with abundant mucus and basal nuclei. This is a mucous type of bronchioloalveolar carcinoma.

(Fig. 26.24). They are most frequently arranged in a bronchioloalveolar pattern with a lobar pneumonia-like gross feature (Fig. 26.25); infrequently, they are arranged in a papillary pattern with nodular tumor growth. Ultrastructurally, the cytoplasm is filled with mucous granules of rather low electron density, and it varies in internal structure. The lateral cell membrane shows interdigitation. Immunohistochemically, this cell type is negative for lactoferrin, a bronchial gland marker, but is often positive for lysozyme.

Bronchial gland cell type. Cuboidal or polygonal cells often containing mucin are arranged in acini, tubules or ductal structures, cribriform patterns, or solid nests (Fig. 26.26A). In solid nests, individual mucin-containing cells may show a signet ring form (Fig. 26.26B). Electron microscopically (23,24), the mu-

cous granules vary in density, and granules suggestive of the serous type also may be encountered. Characteristically present in the cytoplasm of the gland cell–type tumor cells are oval fibrillar structures, which may be found, although infrequently, in nonneoplastic bronchial gland but not in goblet cells or goblet cell-type tumor cells. The cells bordering the nests may resemble myoepithelial cells with myofibril-like fibrillar structures. Immunohistochemically, this type of tumor is often positive for lactoferrin (68,69). It arises in the cartilage-bearing

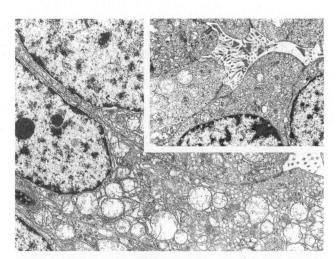

Figure 26.23. Ultrastructure of the adenocarcinoma shown in Figures 26.24 and 26.25. Tall columnar cells are rich in mitochondria and smooth endoplasmic reticulum, but they have no secretory granules. No cilia are present, but microvilli are seen. However, as shown in the inset, basal bodies are seen rather frequently. From: Kameya T. Salivary gland type tumors. In: National Cancer Center Hospital. *Cancer of the Lung: Diagnosis and Treatment.* Vol. 1. Tokyo: Kodansha, 1983:179–190 [in Japanese], with permission.

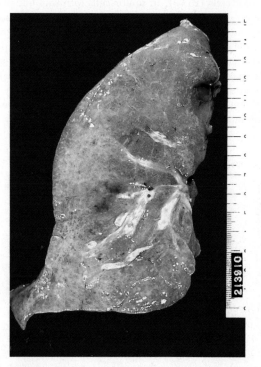

Figure 26.25. Cut surface of the tumor shown in Figure 26.27. The entire lobe is the site of tumor growth, retaining the configuration of a pulmonary lobe, and the bronchi and vessels are intact. The cut surface is extremely mucinous. This is an example of bronchioloalveolar carcinoma of lobar pneumonia type.

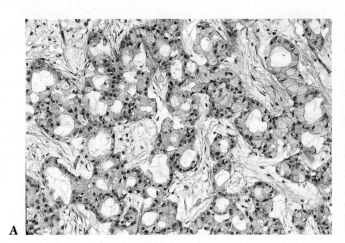

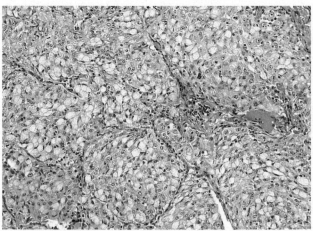

A   B

Figure 26.26. Acinar (tubular) adenocarcinoma of the bronchial gland cell type. **(A)** Neoplastic tubules are composed of cuboidal cells with abundant mucus that resemble the acini of bronchial glands. **(B)** Tumor cells in solid nests are of the signet ring form.

bronchus as an endobronchial polypoid tumor; it also arises in the distal airway and forms a nodular tumor. It accounts for only about 5% of adenocarcinoma cases.

Clara cell type. Peg-shaped cells or low columnar cells with tongue-shaped projections into the spaces are arranged in a papillary pattern (Fig. 26.27). More precisely, they form (a) tubular structures in and around the central or subpleural fibrotic focus; (b) papillary structures in the midzone of the tumor; and (c) a bronchioloalveolar pattern at the periphery or advancing border of the tumor (25). The fibrotic focus is the result of the collapse of the alveoli previously occupied by the tumor cells (25,70). In tumor cells with slight atypia, the nuclei are oval with a thick nuclear membrane, granular chromatin, and inconspicuous nucleoli; in tumors with increased atypia, the nuclei are irregular and pleomorphic with prominent nucleoli. The mitotic figures increase in number as the degree of cell atypia advances. Intranuclear eosinophilic inclusion bodies are frequently seen (71). Differentiation from tumor cells of the type II alveolar epithelial cell type may be difficult or even impossible, at times, by light microscopy. Both

cell types may coexist in a single tumor. Ultrastructurally, the peg-shaped tumor cells possess microvilli on the free cell surface, scattered rough endoplasmic reticulum, and round, electron-dense secretory granules ranging from 200 to 900 nm in diameter with an occasional fingerprint-like inner structure (Fig. 26.28) (25,72,73). Clara cell 10-kd protein (CC10) is the dominant product from Clara cells (74), and it has been thought to have immunomodulatory and anti-inflammatory activity. Reports have indicated that the downregulation of CC10 contributes to carcinogenesis (75). Immunohistochemically, CC10 is detected in many Clara cell–type adenocarcinomas but not in atypical adenomatous hyperplasia.

Grossly, a sharp indentation of the pleura is directed toward the central fibrosis with anthracosis. Peripherally, the tumor is ivory in color, with ill-defined borders in a differentiated tumor,

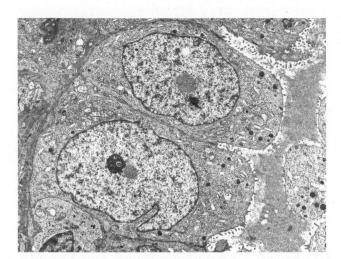

Figure 26.28. Ultrastructure of Clara cell adenocarcinoma. Low columnar epithelial cells project into the lumen from the level of cell junctions. Dense secretory granules of 300 to 400 nm in diameter and rough endoplasmic reticulum are noted in the cytoplasm, and tubular nuclear inclusions and a basal lamina are present. From: Shimosato Y. Pathology of lung cancer. In Hansen HH, Rorth M, eds. *Lung Cancer.* Amsterdam: Excerpta Medica, 1980:27–48, with permission.

Figure 26.27. Papillary adenocarcinoma of Clara cell type. Low columnar, peg-shaped cells are arranged in a papillary fashion. Some pathologists classified this type as bronchioloalveolar carcinoma.

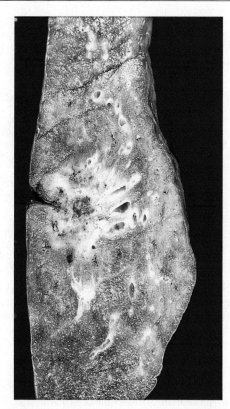

Figure 26.29. Gross features of papillary adenocarcinoma of Clara cell type. A nodular tumor is centrally fibrotic and is associated with sharp pleural indentation. The border is blurred. An increased number of bronchi and vessels at the periphery of the tumor indicates their convergence toward the center of the tumor. This phenomenon, as well as pleural indentation, is the result of shrinkage or cicatricial contracture of the tumor.

but it has well-defined scalloped borders in poorly differentiated portions (Fig. 26.29). Clara cell–type adenocarcinoma is the most common type of adenocarcinoma, accounting for more than 50% of cases (some authors have reported up to 84%) (73).

Type II alveolar epithelial cell type. Individual cells are cuboidal to low columnar with a dome-shaped free cell border; their cytoplasm is often finely vacuolated, with the vacuoles probably corresponding to cytoplasmic lamellar inclusion bodies (Fig. 26.30). These cells are arranged in papillary or bronchioloalveolar patterns, and, grossly, the tumor reveals a solitary nodular form or, rarely, diffuse lobar distribution (Fig. 26.31).

Electron microscopically, the presence of lamellar inclusion bodies in the cytoplasm is characteristic (Fig. 26.32) (25,73,76). Immunohistochemically, surfactant apoprotein is the marker substance (76), although it is also positively stained in tumors that are considered to be of the Clara cell type, the bronchial surface epithelial cell type with little or no mucus, or the bronchial gland cell type (77).

Cytologic subtyping is often impossible in poorly differentiated adenocarcinoma.

HISTOLOGIC CLASSIFICATION OF ADENOCARCINOMA. Adenocarcinomas of the lung frequently reveal mixed histology (i.e., combination of any one of bronchioloalveolar, papillary, acinar, and solid growth patterns) and they are divided into five

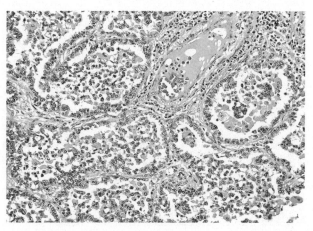

Figure 26.30. Adenocarcinoma of alveolar type II epithelial cell type. Cuboidal cells replace the alveolar lining, and the septa show slight fibrous thickening. Alveolar spaces contain many exfoliated tumor cells.

major subtypes including adenocarcinoma with mixed subtypes (Table 26.2) (21,22).

Acinar and papillary adenocarcinomas may be seen in their pure form but more often they are mixed with other components, including a bronchioloalveolar pattern. Acinar adenocarcinoma roughly corresponds to adenocarcinoma of the bronchial gland cell type (23,24,68,69). However, adenocarcinoma

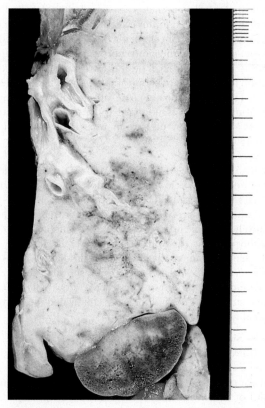

Figure 26.31. Gross features of the alveolar type II epithelial cell-type adenocarcinoma shown in Figure 26.33. It is not mucinous but it does show lobar pneumonia-type growth. However, lobar distribution of predominantly bronchioloalveolar carcinoma of this type is much less frequent than that of the goblet cell type.

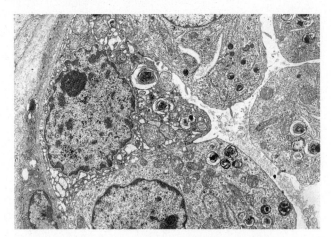

Figure 26.32. Ultrastructure of type II alveolar epithelial cell–type adenocarcinoma. Many osmiophilic lamellar bodies are seen in the cytoplasm. A few electron-dense granules, which could be lysosomes, resemble Clara cell granules. The basal lamina is distinct.

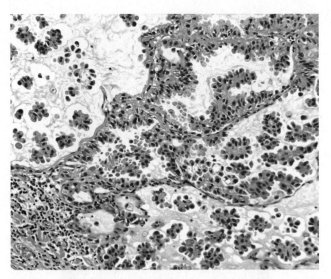

Figure 26.33. Micropapillary adenocarcinoma. A micropapillary cluster (MPC) is a nest without fibrovascular core in it, and it is floating in the brochioloalveolar space. This is also called the pseudopapillary structure. Adenocarcinomas with MPC components have an unfavorable prognosis.

with tubular structures made up of tumor cells of Clara cell and/or type II alveolar epithelial cell type is also called *acinar adenocarcinoma*. Papillary adenocarcinoma is composed predominantly of papillary structures, in which the following two distinct types are seen: one consists of Clara cell and/or type II alveolar epithelial cell–type tumor cells lining alveoli and displaying secondary and tertiary papillary branches (78,79) (adenocarcinoma, predominantly bronchioloalveolar, but with complicated papillary branches associated with thickened alveolar septae are included in this category) (Fig. 26.27); the other consists of tall columnar cells of the bronchial surface epithelial cell type, which have their own fibrous stroma (true papillary adenocarcinoma; Fig. 26.22) (67). Miyoshi et al. have drawn attention to the structure known as the "micropapillary cluster" (MPC). The MPC is a floating nest without a fibrovascular core, and is also known as a pseudopapillary structure. Adenocarcinomas with MPC components have an unfavorable prognosis (Fig. 26.33) (80).

NOGUCHI'S CLASSIFICATION. Among the five histologic subtypes of adenocarcinoma, bronchioloalveolar carcinoma is a special subtype because it mimics atypical adenomatous hyperplasia, which is a preinvasive form of adenocarcinoma and has a relatively favorable prognosis. Many adenocarcinomas contain this subtype in the early phase. Noguchi et al. classified small-sized adenocarcinomas (less than 2 cm in diameter) into two groups (7) (Table 26.4), one group showing replacement growth and the other showing destructive growth of preexisting alveolar structures. Both of them are subdivided into three histological types as follows:

Tumors Showing Replacement Growth

Type A: Localized Bronchioloalveolar Carcinoma

Tumors of this type are solitary and show growth by replacement of alveolar lining cells with minimal or mild thickening of the alveolar septa (Fig. 26.34A). The tumors lack fibrotic foci. Histologically, they are well-differentiated localized bronchioloalveolar carcinomas, and the individual cells resemble Clara cells, type II pneumocytes, or goblet cells. With the recent advances in CT technology, many type A adenocarcinomas are now being detected and sometimes

it is difficult to discriminate type A adenocarcinoma from atypical adenomatous hyperplasia. Minami et al. have proposed criteria for distinguishing them (32).

Type B: Localized Bronchioloalveolar Carcinoma with Foci of Alveolar Structural Collapse

The overall microscopic appearance of these tumors is similar to that of type A, showing a replacement growth pattern (Fig. 26.34B). However, the tumors contain fibrotic foci due to alveolar collapse. This tumor type is sometimes difficult to distinguish from type C tumors. The fibrosis in this tumor is due to alveolar collapse without cellular growth and elastic fiber staining is very useful for diagnosis of this type.

Type C: Localized Bronchioloalveolar Carcinoma with Foci of Active Fibroblastic Proliferation

This type constitutes the largest group of small-sized adenocarcinoma. Tumors also show a replacement growth pattern, but foci of active fibroblastic proliferation are detectable (Fig. 26.34C). In these foci, large nuclei of the proliferating fibroblasts and endothelial cells of small ves-

TABLE 26.4

Histologic Classification of Small-Sized Adenocarcinoma (Noguchi's Classification)

Replacement type (lepidic type) adenocarcinoma
    Type A: Localized bronchioloalveolar carcinoma (LBAC)
    Type B: LBAC with focal collapse of the alveolar structure
    Type C: LBAC with focus of fibroblastic proliferation
Nonreplacement type (nonlepidic type) adenocarcinoma
    Type D: Poorly differentiated adenocarcinoma
    Type E: Tubular or acinar adenocarcinoma
    Type F: True papillary adenocarcinoma

From: Noguchi M, Morikawa A, Kawasaki M, et al. Small adenocarcinoma of the lung. Histologic characteristics and prognosis. *Cancer* 1995;75:2844–2852.

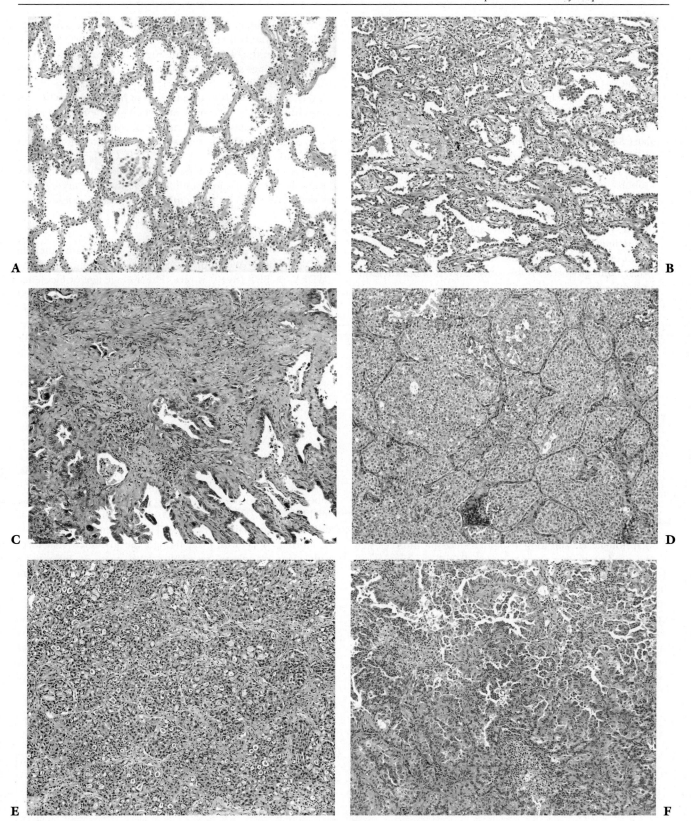

Figure 26.34. Noguchi's classification is applied for small-sized adenocarcinoma less than 2 cm in diameter. (**A**) Type A carcinoma is localized bronchioloalveolar carcinoma. (**B**) Type B carcinoma is localized bronchioloalveolar carcinoma with collapse of alveolar structure. (**C**) Type C carcinoma is localized bronchioloalveolar carcinoma with a focus of fibroblastic proliferation. (**D**) Type D carcinoma is solid adenocarcinoma with mucin production. (**E**) Type E carcinoma is tubular or acinar adenocarcinoma. (**F**) Type F carcinoma is true papillary carcinoma. See Figures 26.35 and Table 26.4.

sels are prominent (83). These actively proliferating fibroblasts are absent in the foci of alveolar collapse that are seen in type B. The nuclei of tumor cells located in the foci of active fibroblastic proliferation are larger and show a more atypical structure than those in the peripheral region where tumors show growth by replacement of alveolar lining cells. Type C is called focally (or minimally) invasive bronchioloalveolar carcinoma (32,84,85,86).

Tumors Showing Nonreplacement Growth

Type D: Poorly Differentiated Adenocarcinoma

These tumors show largely solid growth, and papillary and tubular growth patterns are minor components (Fig. 26.34D). Histologically, their classification is almost the same as that of "solid adenocarcinoma with mucin" in the third WHO classification (21) (Table 26.2). Therefore, it is sometimes difficult to distinguish these tumors from large-cell carcinoma histologically. Macroscopically, they show a clear boundary between the cancer and the noncancerous parenchyma.

Type E: Tubular Adenocarcinoma

This tumor type consists of acinar, tubular, and cribriform structures, and tumor cells with a signet ring appearance may be present (Fig. 26.34E). This type is classified as "acinar adenocarcinoma" in the third WHO classification (Table 26.2). This specific type of adenocarcinoma is thought to originate from or differentiate toward bronchial gland cells. The tumor boundary is always distinct.

Type F: Papillary Adenocarcinoma with a Compressive Growth Pattern

These tumors show papillary growth. However, they do not grow by replacing the alveolar lining cells, but instead show expansive and destructive growth (Fig. 26.34F). This type is classified as "papillary adenocarcinoma" in the third WHO classification (21). Accordingly, they show a clear boundary between the cancer and the noncancerous parenchyma macroscopically.

This histologic classification (Noguchi's classification) is well correlated with patient prognosis and CT findings. Type A and B tumors have an extremely favorable prognosis, and patients have a 5-year survival rate 100% (7). Type C tumors are similar to type A and B and show replacement growth of alveolar lining cells but the 5-year survival rate is 75% (Fig. 26.35). Compared to replacement-type adenocarcinomas, type D, E, and F tumors have a poor prognosis and the 5-year survival rate of patients with type D tumors is 50%. On the other hand, a histologic replacement growth pattern corresponds to the feature *ground*

glass opacity evident by CT (Fig. 26.36). Therefore, type A, B, and C tumors and other nonreplacement-type tumors can be distinguished on the basis of CT findings. These histologic and radiologic findings suggest malignant progression of peripheral-type adenocarcinomas from atypical adenomatous hyperplasia (AAH), types A and B to type C. Loss of heterozygosity for various chromosomes on which important suppressor genes are located accumulates, and activated expression of matrix metalloproteinase (MMP)-2 increases during the course of malignant progression from type A to type C (81,82). On the basis of these findings, type A and B adenocarcinomas with an extremely favorable prognosis are candidates for limited surgery such as wedge resection or segmentectomy, or careful observation alone.

VARIANTS OF ADENOCARCINOMA. The variants include five subtypes. Well-differentiated fetal adenocarcinoma (WDFA) or PET (8–10) is rare. The average age of incidence is in the fifth decade. Grossly, the tumor is nonencapsulated but well defined, and it is not related to visible bronchi. Histologically, the tumor grows expansively, and is composed of irregular tubular structures consisting of columnar epithelial cells with irregularly dispersed oval nuclei and clear cytoplasm, which are continuous with morular structures composed of polygonal cells with scant cytoplasm (Fig. 26.37). The nuclei in morulae are often optically clear or they resemble ground glass, and they are rich in biotin (87), whereas cytoplasm in some morular cells is argyrophilic, often containing chromogranin A, synaptophysin, and N-CAM. The stroma is fibrous with no cellular atypia. The prognosis is much better than that of biphasic blastoma. Mutations in the *p53* gene were not seen in any of nine WDFAs, but they were seen in 5 of 12 biphasic blastomas (88). The subtype that had been referred to as adenocarcinoma of the fetal lung type (Fig. 26.38) (89,90), although it is very rare, is different from WDFA or PET (8). The difference is the absence of morular structures, even though the glandular structures with clear cytoplasm resemble those seen in pulmonary blastoma and WDFA. This subtype is now classified as clear-cell adenocarcinoma in the revised classification.

Mucinous adenocarcinoma, mucinous cystadenocarcinoma, and signet ring adenocarcinoma resemble the tumors of the same name in the gastrointestinal tract. Signet ring carcinoma is a special form of bronchial gland–type adenocarcinoma, as was previously described (Fig. 26.26) (68,69). Adenocarcinomas with spindle cell or giant-cell components (or both) are catego-

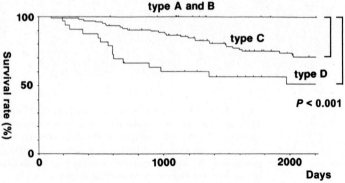

Figure 26.35. Five-year survival rate of each type of small-sized adenocarcinoma (Noguchi's classification). Type A and B adenocarcinoma shows 100% 5-year survival rate but is decreased to 75% for type C. And even if the size is less than 2 cm, 5-year survival rate is only 50%.

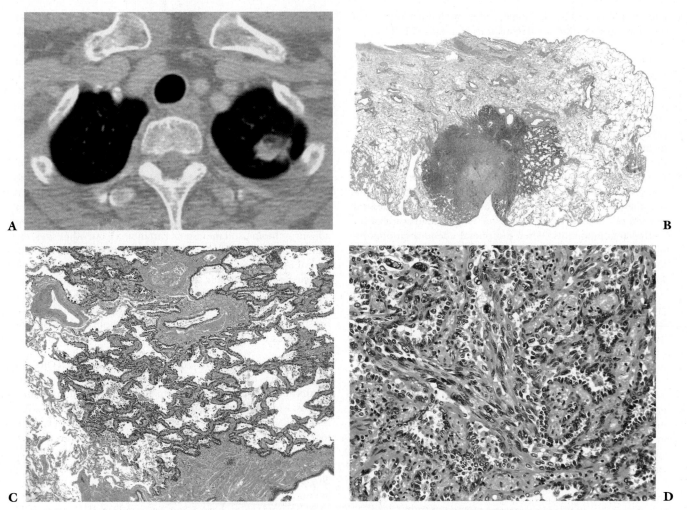

A   B

C   D

Figure 26.36. Correlation between histolopathologic feature and CT appearance. Noguchi's type C adeno-carcinoma. Replacement growth (lepidic growth) of type C adenocarcinoma corresponds to ground-glass opac-ity (GGO) in CT. **(A)** CT. **(B)** Histologic section. **(C)** Bronchioloalveolar carcinoma (BAC). **(D)** Invasive lesion.

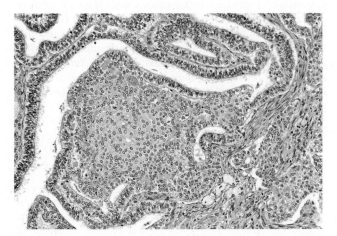

Figure 26.37. Pulmonary endodermal tumor resembling fetal lung (well-differentiated fetal adenocarcinoma, WDFA). Columnar epithe-lial cells forming irregular tubules are continuous with morulae consist-ing of polygonal cells with occasional clear nuclei.

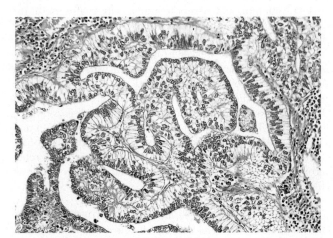

Figure 26.38. Histology of clear-cell adenocarcinoma. Tall colum-nar cells with clear cytoplasm are arranged in a papillary fashion. Nuclei are apically situated. Similar papillotubular structures are also seen in pulmonary blastoma and in well-differentiated fetal adenocarcinoma (WDFA).

rized as pleomorphic carcinoma under carcinomas with pleomorphic, sarcomatoid, or sarcomatous elements (21,22).

BIOPSY INTERPRETATION. Because most adenocarcinomas arise in the periphery of the lung, tissue or cells from those tumors must be obtained by either a transbronchial or a percutaneous route. Therefore, the size of tissue or the number of cells obtained is often extremely small, and this can make interpretation difficult, particularly when cell atypia is mild. This means that sometimes a decision cannot be made on whether the specimen represents atypical adenomatous hyperplasia (3,4,9–13) or quite well-differentiated papillary or bronchioloalveolar carcinoma when the specimen is obtained from the periphery of a tumor. If tissue is obtained from the central portion of a tumor, the fibrous tissue may contain scant or no epithelial components. When peripheral adenocarcinoma invades proximal bronchi, tumor cell nests are frequently seen in the subepithelial layer or in the lymphatics, and these rarely spread intraepithelially.

Adenocarcinomas arising in cartilage-bearing bronchi are of either surface epithelial or bronchial gland cell type. In the latter case, the biopsy specimen may disclose only bronchial mucosa with or without hyperplastic or metaplastic changes because carcinoma tends to grow beneath the bronchial epithelium.

DIFFERENTIATION FROM MESOTHELIOMA OF THE MONOPHASIC EPITHELIAL TYPE. Peripheral-type adenocarcinoma may spread diffusely into, as well as obliterate, the pleural cavity, in which the subpleural primary focus remains small and inconspicuous at times. Such an adenocarcinoma simulates epithelial-type mesothelioma, both grossly and microscopically.

If the tumor cells do not produce mucin, as in the case of the Clara cell or type II alveolar epithelial cell types, differentiation from mesothelioma may become extremely difficult. Even in such instances, conventional approaches (i.e., gross features, histology, and histochemistry of mucosubstances) are of prime importance. However, electron microscopy also may be of great help. The microvilli are often long and slender in mesothelioma, with the ratio of length to diameter often exceeding 10 (91). IHC, using antibodies to carcinoembryonic antigen (CEA), vimentin, and adenocarcinoma cells, is also useful for the differential diagnosis (92). In other words, expression of CEA, surfactant apoprotein, and thyroid transcription factor-1 (TTF-1) is absent or weaker in mesothelioma (93–96); also, some monoclonal antibodies are unreactive with mesothelioma but are reactive with adenocarcinoma (97,98). Mesothelioma-binding antibodies such as thrombomodulin, calretinin, and WT1 are also useful (99–102). For additional discussion, see Chapter 27, The Pleura, and the review article by Ordóñez and Mackay (103), who stated that although no method is consistently reliable, a carefully selected and cautiously interpreted group of immunostains often strongly indicate one tumor or the other.

DIFFERENTIATION FROM METASTATIC ADENOCARCINOMAS IN THE LUNG. The cytologic features and histologic arrangement of tumor cells of the Clara cell and/or type II alveolar epithelial cell types are so characteristic that diagnosis of primary lung cancer can be established with ease in most well-differentiated or moderately differentiated tumors. However, adenocarcinoma metastatic from organs with myoepithelial

cells, such as the breast and salivary gland, may be very similar to some adenocarcinomas of the bronchial gland cell type, and, although rare, some primary lung adenocarcinomas resemble colonic and endometrial adenocarcinomas. If such tumors are solitary in the lung, treating the tumor as a primary adenocarcinoma (unless proved otherwise) is advisable. Adenocarcinoma of the pancreas and endocervix may spread like bronchioloalveolar carcinoma of the goblet cell type, but the presence of coagulation necrosis in the tumor suggests a metastatic, rather than a primary, lesion.

A monoclonal antibody against surfactant apoprotein is useful for the differential diagnosis of primary versus metastatic adenocarcinoma because positive immunostaining almost definitely indicates primary lung origin (77,104). TTF-1 has been found to be valuable in distinguishing between primary lung adenocarcinoma and metastatic carcinoma from other sites, excluding the thyroid gland (95,96). Cytokeratin 7 (CK7), CK20, and villin IHC profiles are useful in the differential diagnosis of primary versus metastatic adenocarcinoma because the primary adenocarcinoma reveals a unique profile of CK7 positivity (98%), CK20 negativity (86%), and villin positivity (without a brush-border pattern; 68%) (see "Immunohistochemistry of Malignant Lung Tumors") (105–107).

BIOLOGIC BEHAVIOR AND PROGNOSTIC FACTORS. In lung cancers, as in other cancers, the three most important factors affecting the prognosis of patients are distant organ metastasis, lymph node metastasis, and pleural involvement—that is, the "TNM factors." Other than the TNM factors, histopathologic findings such as lymphatic and vascular invasion, mitotic index, cell atypia, micropapillary structures, the proportion of bronchioloalveolar carcinoma at the largest cut surface, and Noguchi's classification are associated with poor prognosis of adenocarcinoma (7,108).

Many molecules have been reported as IHC prognostic markers, including CEA, Cox2, EGFR, pEGFR, p27, p53, TTF-1, and γH2AX (109–116). Among these, however, only CEA expression has been shown to be a statistically significant prognostic marker for small-sized adenocarcinomas.

FUNCTION. Besides the production of mucin and surfactant, about 9% of adenocarcinomas are said to contain immunoreactive peptide hormones, such as calcitonin and GRP (117). Some adenocarcinomas are also immunohistochemically positive for NCAM, chromogranin A, and/or synaptophysin, which are markers for small-cell carcinoma. An ectopic function more specific for adenocarcinoma is the production of salivary gland–type amylase (118,119). The incidences of hypertrophic osteoarthropathy and estrogen production are said to be higher in adenocarcinoma cases in comparison with other forms of lung cancer (21).

Large-Cell Carcinoma

The histologic diagnosis of large-cell carcinoma is made after the exclusion of squamous cell carcinoma, small-cell carcinoma, adenocarcinoma, and other lung cancers of specific type. The male-to-female ratio in affected cases is 4 or 5:1, which lies between the ratios of squamous cell carcinoma and adenocarcinoma.

GROSS FEATURES. Large-cell carcinoma arises more frequently in the periphery of the lung, and it may invade the thoracic wall if it is untreated. Typical undifferentiated large-cell carcinoma forms a spherical tumor with well-defined borders, and it has a bulging, fleshy, homogeneous, rather sarcomatous cut surface. Anthracotic pigments are not seen because of compressive growth. However, some large-cell carcinomas resemble poorly differentiated adenocarcinoma or squamous cell carcinoma grossly.

HISTOLOGIC FEATURES. Most large-cell carcinomas are composed of solid nests of polygonal cells with vesicular nuclei, prominent nucleoli, moderately abundant cytoplasm, well-defined cell borders, and rather scant fibrovascular stroma (Fig. 26.39). Carcinomas with frequent mucin-producing cells are classified as adenocarcinoma according to the WHO criteria, but those with occasional or a few mucin-producing cells are placed in the large-cell category. Large-cell carcinomas are either cytocohesive or incohesive. In the latter case, marked infiltration of inflammatory cells, which consist of both lymphoid cells and polymorphonuclear leukocytes, is present.

The WHO has defined five histological variants of large-cell carcinoma: large-cell neuroendocrine carcinoma (LCNEC); basaloid carcinoma; lymphoepithelioma-like carcinoma; clear-cell carcinoma; and large-cell carcinoma with a rhabdoid phenotype (Table 26.2) (21,22). Variants other than LCNEC are rare. Basaloid carcinoma is similar to basaloid squamous cell carcinoma but lacks squamous cell characteristics (39). Lymphoepithelioma-like carcinoma is histologically similar to carcinoma of the same name in the epipharynx and thymus, has shown a geographic distribution similar to epipharyngeal lymphoepithelioma, and has the Epstein-Barr virus genome by in situ hybridization (120). Large-cell carcinoma with the rhabdoid phenotype is made up of large cells containing eosinophilic globular cytoplasmic inclusions, which are vimentin-positive (121). Rhabdoid cells may also be present in poorly differentiated adenocarcinomas.

Giant-cell carcinoma, which was a variant of large-cell carcinoma in the second edition of the WHO classification, is now classified in the category of carcinomas with pleomorphic, sarcomatoid, or sarcomatous elements (21,22).

ULTRASTRUCTURAL AND IMMUNOHISTOCHEMICAL CHARACTERISTICS. Ultrastructurally, many large-cell carcino-

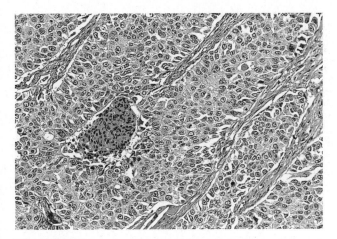

Figure 26.39. Large-cell carcinoma. Large polygonal cells with vesicular nuclei, prominent nucleoli, and rich cytoplasm show diffuse growth accompanied by scant fibrovascular stroma.

mas can be classified as adenocarcinoma (roughly 50%), adenosquamous carcinoma (15%), and squamous cell carcinoma (11%) (27). The incidence of undifferentiated carcinoma (19%) would probably decrease if more samples were examined electron microscopically. Differentiation toward neuroendocrine cells with neurosecretory-type granules has been observed in one case of 27, although it appears to be more frequent in Western countries (26).

Immunohistochemically, some tumors (37%) react positively with DAKO cytokeratin antibody, and other tumors (33%) possess an immunoreactive secretory component (DAKO). A tumor with neuroendocrine-type granules was shown to be positive for calcitonin (27).

INTERPRETATION OF BRONCHIAL BIOPSY SPECIMENS. Because large-cell carcinomas are generally considered poorly differentiated forms of adenocarcinoma, squamous cell carcinoma, or neuroendocrine carcinoma, and all major histologic types of lung cancers may contain foci with features of large-cell carcinoma, a diagnosis of large-cell carcinoma cannot be made from small bronchial biopsy specimens. The same can be said concerning metastatic tumors in lymph nodes. In those instances, the diagnosis must be poorly differentiated carcinoma consisting of large-cell components.

CLINICAL ASPECTS AND BIOLOGIC BEHAVIOR. The 5-year survival rate of patients with large-cell carcinoma is quite close to that for adenocarcinoma. Therefore, a discrepancy in the diagnosis of large-cell carcinoma and poorly differentiated adenocarcinoma does not mean much from a practical viewpoint. The diagnosis of large-cell carcinoma from small biopsy specimens indicates that the tumor is large-cell carcinoma, poorly differentiated squamous cell carcinoma, or adenocarcinoma with large-cell components. The incidence of large-cell carcinoma varies from one institution to another, partly because of variations in the details of histologic examination. Its incidence in autopsy materials is generally higher than that in surgical materials because postmortem changes may obscure the glandular structures. Furthermore, the responses to antitumor agents and radiation may also be similar and fairly good in these tumors.

A sign occasionally noted in cases of large-cell carcinoma and poorly differentiated carcinoma with a predominant large-cell component is leukocytosis in the absence of infection. The white blood cell count may exceed 100,000 cells per mm^3. This results from the production of colony-stimulating factor by the tumor (122). The xenotransplantation of such tumors into athymic nude mice induces leukocytosis, in which the white blood cell count returns to a normal level within a week after removal of the transplanted tumor (123). Patients with large (giant)-cell carcinoma also may develop hepatosplenomegaly without metastasis, which also regresses after the removal of the primary tumor. This phenomenon is probably the result of hypervolemia. In rare instances, this tumor produces human chorionic gonadotropin, and gynecomastia may occur (139).

Large-Cell Neuroendocrine Carcinoma

The revised WHO classification of lung and pleural tumors recommended inclusion of large-cell neuroendocrine carcinoma (LCNEC) in the category of large-cell carcinoma (21,22). LCNEC is defined as a large-cell carcinoma showing histologic

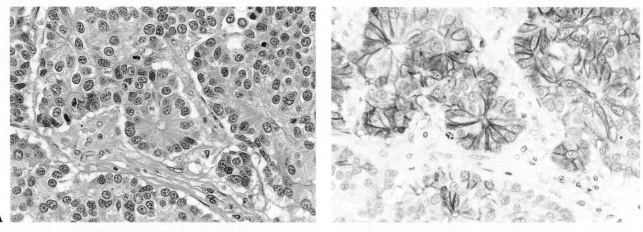

A   **B**

Figure 26.40. Large-cell neuroendocrine carcinoma. **(A)** Histology of a large-cell neuroendocrine carcinoma with a rosettelike structure is shown. **(B)** The cell membrane of large tumor cells is positive for neural cell adhesion molecule (immunostaining).

features such as organoid nesting, trabeculae, and rosette-like and palisading patterns that suggest neuroendocrine differentiation and in which the latter can be confirmed by IHC or electron microscopy. The tumor cells are generally large with moderate to abundant cytoplasm, vesicular to finely granular nuclei, and, often, prominent nucleoli (Fig. 26.40). In distinguishing large-cell neuroendocrine carcinoma from atypical carcinoid, in addition to histology, the mitotic count is useful (21,22), with 2 to 10 mitotic figures per 10 high-power fields in atypical carcinoids and a larger number in LCNEC.

Various terms proposed for non–small-cell lung cancers with neuroendocrine properties are encountered occasionally, including neuroendocrine carcinoma of intermediate cell type, non–small-cell carcinoma with neuroendocrine features, and large-cell neuroendocrine carcinoma (26,125–127). The marker substances used for determination of neuroendocrine properties vary among investigators, and include chromogranin A, N-CAM (CD56), synaptophysin, GRP, neurofilament, NSE, and Leu-7, as well as neurosecretory granules. Expression of TTF-1 and BCL-2 protein is reported to be closely associated with neuroendocrine differentiation in both small-cell carcinoma and large-cell neuroendocrine carcinoma (128,129). NSE and Leu-7 may be positive in nonneuroendocrine cells, and these should be excluded as neuroendocrine markers. The WHO has recommended that CD56, chromogranin A, and synaptophysin be used to confirm the diagnosis of LCNEC immunohistochemically. Interpretation of granules at the ultrastructural level must also be performed cautiously; not only the structure but also the location should be examined carefully. On the basis of these data, together with those of others (130,131), it can be concluded that many large-cell carcinomas are, in fact, poorly differentiated squamous cell carcinomas, adenocarcinomas, or neuroendocrine carcinomas.

Together with LCNEC, neuroendocrine (NE) tumors of the lung include four histological subtypes: LCNEC, typical carcinoid, atypical carcinoid, and small-cell carcinoma. The clinicopathologic differences among these four tumor types are still not fully characterized. However, Asamura et al. examined 366 NE tumors in Japanese patients clinicopathologically, and reported that the 5-year survival rate was 96.2% for those with typical carcinoid, 77.8% for atypical carcinoid, 40.3% for

LCNEC, and 35.7% for small-cell carcinoma (8). LCNEC and small-cell carcinoma are the two most highly malignant NE tumors and show no significant difference in prognosis. However, the question of whether large-cell neuroendocrine carcinoma should be treated similarly to small-cell carcinoma remains to be decided until further cases have been accumulated.

Adenosquamous Carcinoma

Adenosquamous carcinoma, a mixture of adenocarcinoma and squamous cell carcinoma (Fig. 26.41), comprises about 3.5% of surgically resected lung cancers. It arises both in the hilar region (major bronchi) and in the periphery of the lung. Theoretically, the following four types exist: (a) collision of adenocarcinoma and squamous cell carcinoma, in which the gross features and serial chest radiographs, if available, may be of great help; (b) adenocarcinoma showing squamous metaplasia in areas; (c) tumors composed of bipotential cells showing glandular cell differentiation in some areas and squamous cell differentiation in others; and (d) mucoepidermoid tumor with marked cell atypia or of a less differentiated form. Tumors of types (a)

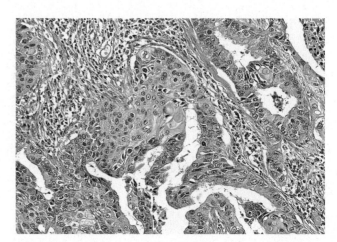

Figure 26.41. Adenosquamous carcinoma. At the upper left, a focus of metaplastic squamous cell change is evident in a neoplastic gland.

TABLE 26.5	Histology of Metastases in Lymph Nodes in Cases of Adenosquamous Carcinoma, According to the Amount of Each Component					
			No. Cases with Lymph Node Metastases by Histology			
Area (%) Occupied by	Total Number of Cases (Male:Female)	Subtotal	Ad	Sq	Adsq	Undiff
Ad > 80, 20 > Sq	5 (3:2)	3	2	1	0	0
80 > Ad > 50, 50 > Sq > 20	9 (6:3)	6	4	1	0	1
Ad > Sq	9 (9:0)	7	4	1	1	1
50 > Ad > 20, 80 > Sq > 50	10 (6:4)	2	2	0	0	0
20 > Ad, Sq > 80	16 (13:3)	11	1	6	3	0
Ad > Undiff > Sq	3 (3:0)	3	1	0	1	1
Total	52	32	14	9	5	3

Ad, adenocarcinoma; Adsq, adenosquamous carcinoma; Sq, squamous cell carcinoma; Undiff, undifferentiated carcinoma.

through (c) supposedly originate in bronchial or bronchioloalveolar cells, but a tumor of type (d) is of bronchial gland origin, and it should therefore not be included in the category of adenosquamous carcinoma.

In any of those instances, both components should be recognized without difficulty and should lead to a diagnosis of adenosquamous carcinoma, with each comprising at least 10% of the whole tumor according to the revised WHO classification (21,22). If either adenocarcinoma or squamous cell carcinoma is the minor component of the tumor, the histologic diagnosis is made on the basis of the histologic characteristics of the major component, and the presence of the minor component is merely described. In our series, about 90% of cases were peripheral in origin. The histology of lymph node metastasis cannot always be predicted from the histology of the primary focus, as Table 26.5 shows. However, the adenocarcinomatous component tends to metastasize more frequently, unless the squamous cell carcinoma component is predominant in the primary

tumor. Analyses of 56 cases of surgically resected adenosquamous carcinomas revealed that the outcome was significantly poorer than that of adenocarcinomas and squamous cell carcinomas, particularly in stages I and II, and that the amount of the adenocarcinoma component did not affect the survival rate (132). The finding that the histologic subtype of adenosquamous carcinoma is one of the independent prognostic determinants may be explained by the general observation that adenosquamous carcinoma of the lung is almost always composed of tumor cells with moderate to severe nuclear atypia.

Carcinoma with Pleomorphic, Sarcomatoid, and Sarcomatous Elements

This new category, in the revised WHO classification, consists of a group of poorly differentiated non–small-cell carcinomas that contain a component of sarcoma or sarcoma-like elements (Fig. 26.42). These tumors include (a) carcinoma with spindle

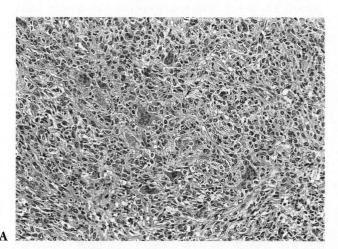
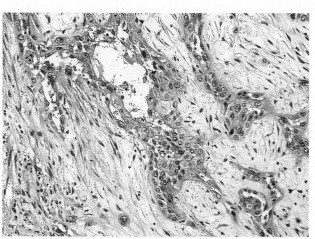

A
B

Figure 26.42. Histology of spindle cell squamous carcinoma (pleomorphic carcinoma). **(A)** The tumor is composed of spindle-shaped to polygonal cells displaying diffuse sarcomatous growth in which osteoclast-like giant cells are scattered. **(B)** In small areas, tumor cells are arranged in solid nests with a slight tendency toward keratinization. The transition between the two was apparent. From: Kameya T. Salivary gland type tumors. In National Cancer Center Hospital. *Cancer of the Lung: Diagnosis and Treatment.* Vol. 1. Tokyo: Kodansha, 1983: 179–190 [in Japanese], with permission.

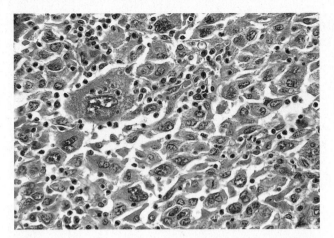

Figure 26.43. Giant-cell carcinoma. Polygonal cells with marked pleomorphism, occasionally possessing multiple nuclei, are growing cytoincohesively, admixed with many lymphoid cells. The giant tumor cells display cannibalism.

and/or giant cells, (b) carcinosarcoma, and (c) pulmonary blastoma. Carcinomas with spindle and/or giant cells consist of three subtypes—in other words, any of the subtypes of non–small-cell carcinoma containing spindle cells and/or giant cells and carcinoma consisting only of spindle cells and giant cells.

GIANT-CELL CARCINOMA. Giant-cell carcinoma contains mononucleated or multinucleated giant cells, is often cytoincohesive (Fig. 26.43), and is occasionally associated with features of adenocarcinoma, which should be diagnosed as pleomorphic adenocarcinoma with giant cells, in some areas. Leukocytosis resulting from the colony-stimulating factor produced by the tumor may also occur in giant-cell carcinoma, as it does in some large-cell carcinomas (122,123).

Giant-cell carcinoma is often more resistant to treatment compared with large-cell carcinoma. This difference may be explained by the difference in the degree of organelle development, which is generally rather poor in large-cell carcinoma but which may be well developed in giant-cell carcinoma.

A metastatic site occasionally seen in cases of giant-cell carcinoma is the small intestine. Patients in whom the discovery of the primary tumor is made only after the appearance of intestinal symptoms and signs are also seen.

CARCINOSARCOMA AND PULMONARY BLASTOMA. *Carcinosarcoma* is defined as a tumor composed of carcinoma and sarcoma. The sarcomatous component in many so-called carcinosarcomas consists of spindle-shaped cells and resembles fibrosarcoma (133). This component is now considered to be the sarcomatous transformation of a carcinomatous component, and such a tumor is diagnosed as pleomorphic carcinoma with areas showing sarcomatous features. Therefore, carcinosarcoma, in a narrow sense, can be defined as a tumor with sarcomatous components that displays differentiation toward tissues such as bone, cartilage, and striated muscle of monoclonal origin (21,22,134,135) (Fig. 26.44). Such tumors arise either in the major bronchi or in the peripheral lung.

Pulmonary blastoma, which received the designation of *embryoma* by Barnard (136), is considered a specific form of carcinosarcoma. This tumor, which is defined by Spencer (137), resembles fetal lung and is composed of tubular structures simulating tubules in the pseudoglandular stage and immature mesenchymal components, which may differentiate toward striated muscle, smooth muscle, cartilage, or a combination of these (Fig. 26.45). The tubules are composed of cuboidal to columnar cells with clear cytoplasm and hyperchromatic nuclei, which may be located near the apical portion of the cells.

Grossly, this is a nodular tumor occurring in the periphery of the lung and sometimes projecting into the bronchial lumen. It is seen more frequently in the main cancer-prone age group, but it has been reported in patients from all age groups. The prognosis appears to be related to the stage at the time of resection. Drawing a line between carcinosarcoma and pulmonary blastoma may sometimes be difficult.

Pleuropulmonary blastoma, which is seen in children younger than 10 years, is a cystic or solid sarcoma. The cysts are lined by metaplastic epithelium, and they produce a pseudobiphasic pattern. The tumor shows features of chondrosarcoma, leiomyosarcoma, rhabdomyosarcoma, liposarcoma, undifferentiated

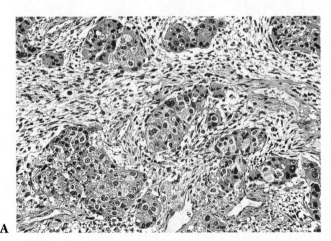

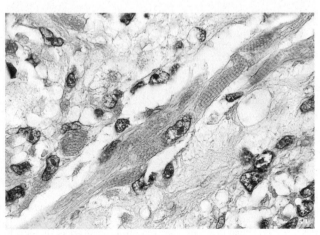

A   **B**

Figure 26.44. Carcinosarcoma. **(A)** Solid epithelial cell nests are supported by spindle cell sarcomatous tissue. **(B)** Within areas of sarcomatous growth, cells with eosinophilic cytoplasm and definite cross-striations, indicating rhabdomyosarcoma, are seen.

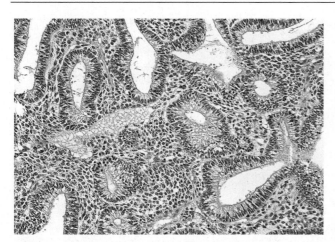

Figure 26.45. Pulmonary blastoma. Tubules lined by tall columnar cells with irregularly dispersed nuclei are supported by immature mesenchymal cells. The cytoplasm of epithelial cells is often clear.

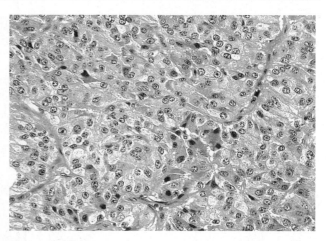

Figure 26.47. Carcinoid tumor. Solid nests of polygonal cells with uniform oval nuclei and finely granular cytoplasm are supported by a vascular stroma.

sarcoma, and mixtures thereof, and it is now classified as a soft tissue tumor (21,22,138,139).

Carcinoid Tumors

Carcinoid tumors are considered tumors of low-grade malignancy. They constitute about 1% to 2% of all lung tumors. Carcinoid tumors often arise in persons who are younger than is usual for lung cancers, and the male-to-female ratio is about 1:1. The tumor is considered to arise from Kulchitsky cells, which belong to the diffuse endocrine system (140,141).

Most of these tumors arise in the main to segmental bronchi, but tumors of peripheral origin are occasionally seen. Grossly, the tumor is polypoid and endobronchial in the major bronchi (Fig. 26.46), bicameral or iceberg-shaped in the intermediate-sized bronchi, and solid and nodular in the periphery of the lung. The tumor is well defined, with a smooth, sometimes lobulated or granular, ivory to pink, glistening cut surface. Necrotic foci are rarely seen.

Histologically, it is made up of nests, trabeculae, and mosaic patterns of medium-sized polygonal cells with oval to spheric, rather uniform, finely granular nuclei, and lightly eosinophilic granular to clear cytoplasm (Fig. 26.47). Rosettes and small acinar structures with or without mucin may be present. Mitotic figures are rare. Peripherally situated tumors may be composed of spindle-shaped cells (142) (Fig. 26.48). The stroma is vascular and scant, and amyloid deposits with bone formation may be seen.

The argentaffin reaction is often negative, but argyrophilia is noted in almost every case. Antigenic substances found in small-cell carcinoma, such as enzymes, amine and peptide hormones, and chromogranin A, are also present in carcinoid tumors, with the IHC reaction being more intense and diffuse in comparison with small-cell carcinoma. Pancreatic polypeptide has so far been demonstrated in some carcinoid tumors but not in small-cell carcinoma (58). The following two other antigenic substances were found in bronchial carcinoid tumor: N-CAM (CD56) (143), which has been detected in all cases examined so far, and S-100 protein, which is present in the sustentacular cells situated at the border of cell nests in approxi-

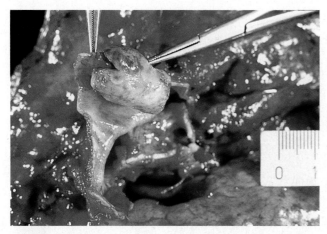

Figure 26.46. Gross features of carcinoid tumor. An endobronchial polypoid growth, the tip of which is hemorrhagic, is shown. From: National Cancer Center Hospital. *Cancer of the Lung: Diagnosis and Treatment.* Vol. 1. Tokyo: Kodansha, 1983:168–190 [in Japanese], with permission.

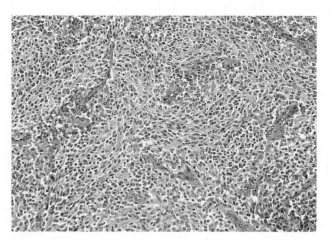

Figure 26.48. Carcinoid tumor of spindle cell type. Short, spindle-shaped cells with uniform, oval nuclei display diffuse growth with a streaming pattern.

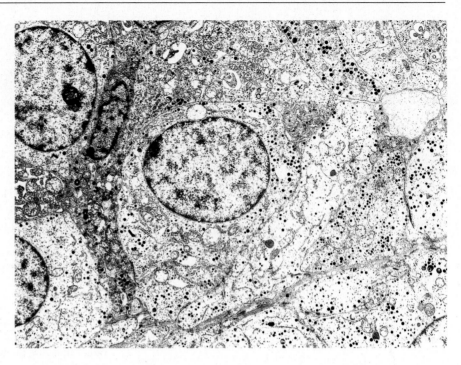

Figure 26.49. Ultrastructure of carcinoid tumor. Tumor cells contain many neurosecretory-type granules. They are rather large for those of small cell carcinoma.

mately 40% of cases (144). BCL-2 protein, which is expressed in most small-cell carcinomas, is expressed infrequently in carcinoid tumor (128,129).

Electron microscopically, membrane-bound, electron-dense granules of 100 to 400 nm in diameter are seen in the cytoplasm beneath the cell membrane, often at the base (Fig. 26.49). Microvilli and junctional complexes are seen in rosettes (44).

Endobronchial polypoid carcinoid tumors are often covered by bronchial epithelium, which may show squamous metaplasia. Therefore, sputum cytology is often negative. Aspiration or scraping cytology reveals uniform tumor cells with no pleomorphism, which may be missed by inexperienced cytologists.

The lung distal to the tumor may show atelectasis, obstructive pneumonia, or bronchiectasis. If the tumor is completely removed, most patients survive for more than 5 years, with a 5-year survival rate of 85% to 95%. Lymph node metastasis has been said to be present in 20% to 50% of cases (145,146), but it was rare in our series. Distant organ metastases were seen in the liver, kidney, bone (osteoplastic), and adrenal gland. Its growth is slow, and, in one case, a tumor took 7 years to grow from 1.2 cm to 2.5 cm in greatest dimension.

Carcinoid syndrome is usually absent when the tumor is confined to the lung, but it may develop several months to several years postoperatively with the appearance of distant organ metastases. Cases associated with Cushing syndrome or acromegaly have been encountered (147,148).

Atypical carcinoid tumor is the name given to the type of tumor showing anaplasia with an increased number of mitotic figures and foci of coagulation necrosis (Fig. 26.50); this tumor has a poorer prognosis than is the case for typical carcinoid tumor

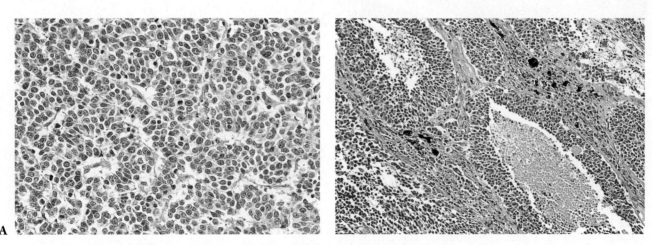

A   B

Figure 26.50. Atypical carcinoid. **(A)** In this field, the tumor appears as typical carcinoid, but a few mitotic figures are seen. **(B)** Elsewhere, foci of coagulation necrosis and foci resembling small-cell carcinoma with increased mitotic activity are seen. The patient died of unknown causes 4 years after surgical treatment.

(149). The number of mitoses was originally described to be 5 to 10 per 10 high-power fields, but the revised WHO classification recommends a wider range of 2 to 10 per 10 high-power fields (21,22). According to this classification, *typical carcinoid* is defined as a tumor with fewer than 2 mitoses per 10 high-power fields and lacking necrosis. It may display cytologic atypia, increased cellularity, and lymphatic invasion, whereas *atypical carcinoid* is defined as a tumor with 2 to 10 mitoses per 10 high-power fields and/or with foci of necrosis, which are usually punctate. Cytologic atypia, nucleoli, increased cellularity, disorganized architecture, and lymphatic invasion may be seen, but the most important criterion is the mitotic count. By these criteria, the 5-year and 10-year survival rates were 87% and 87%, respectively, for typical carcinoid and 56% and 35%, respectively, for atypical carcinoid (150). Histologic differentiation from small-cell carcinoma may be difficult at times, but the mitotic count is also useful.

Bronchial Gland Carcinomas

Adenocarcinoma differentiating toward the *bronchial gland* was described in Fig. 26.26. In this section, special tumors resembling salivary gland tumors are covered, including adenoid cystic carcinoma, mucoepidermoid carcinoma, and malignant mixed tumors. These tumors are rare and, histologically, are identical to tumors of the same name in the salivary gland.

Adenoid cystic carcinoma arises in the trachea and main bronchi (151). The following two types are found on the basis of gross features: one is nodular, projecting into the tracheobronchial lumen in a polypoid fashion; and the other shows diffuse subepithelial growth along the long axis of the bronchus (Fig. 26.51A). This tumor grows infiltratively beyond the grossly recognizable tumor border. Therefore, confirmation of complete removal by frozen section is required. Lymph node and distant

organ metastases are seen in 15% to 35% of cases. If the tumor is removed completely, the chance of cure is high. Because tumor growth is slow, patients with this disease may survive for years. Acinar (or tubular) adenocarcinoma with a cribriform pattern should not be diagnosed as adenoid cystic carcinoma.

Mucoepidermoid carcinoma is another rare tumor; it is seen in young persons, and it shows no sex predilection (151,152). It arises in the main to segmental bronchi and shows endobronchial polypoid growth (Fig. 26.52A). The prognosis is excellent after complete tumor removal of low-grade histology. However, mucoepidermoid carcinoma with a high grade of malignancy has been reported (152,153). In such a case, the pathologist must discriminate between *mucoepidermoid carcinoma* and *adenosquamous carcinoma*. The former term should be used for tumors of possible bronchial gland origin.

Acinic cell tumor of the bronchus, which is also a low-grade malignant bronchial gland tumor, is extremely rare (154). Other rare bronchial gland tumors (carcinomas) include epithelial-myoepithelial tumor (carcinoma) (adenomyoepithelioma) and myoepithelial carcinoma (155–157). Carcinoma in pleomorphic adenoma has not been reported, but a case of malignant mixed tumor showing a mixture of adenosquamous carcinoma, chondrosarcomatous areas, and myxomatous areas was reported (158).

A difficulty may be encountered in establishing the histologic diagnosis of small bronchial biopsy specimens obtained from carcinoid tumor, acinar adenocarcinoma with slight nuclear atypia, adenoid cystic carcinoma, or bronchial gland adenoma when the characteristic features are not present. In such cases, larger pieces of tissue are required. IHC and electron microscopy are helpful for the differential diagnosis. The prognosis is worse in adenoid cystic carcinoma, followed by carcinoid tumor and mucoepidermoid tumor, although it is much better than in adenocarcinoma and squamous cell carcinoma.

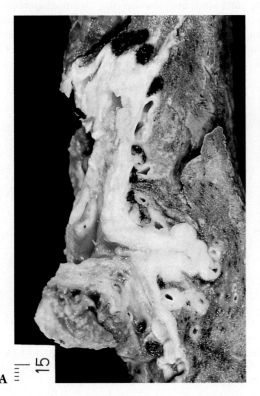
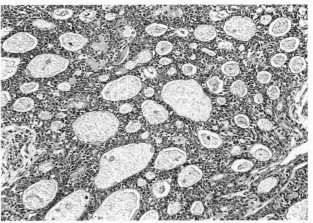

Figure 26.51. Adenoid cystic carcinoma. **(A)** Gross view. The tumor grows subepithelially along the bronchi. The bronchial lining is nodular but smooth, and the wall is markedly thickened. **(B)** Histologic view. A typical cribriform pattern is made up of small tumor cells, and microcystic spaces contain connective tissue mucin, which became hyalinized in areas.

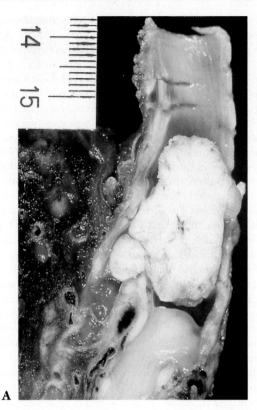

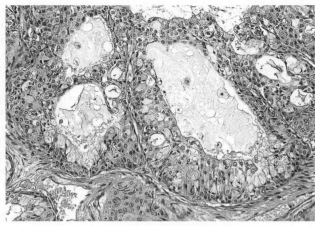

Figure 26.52. Mucoepidermoid carcinoma. **(A)** Gross view. A polypoid tumor sits at the spur between the basal truncus and B6. **(B)** Histologic view. Cystically dilated spaces containing mucus are seen within nests of squamous and intermediate cells. Mucus-containing columnar tumor cells also can be identified.

MISCELLANEOUS TUMORS AND TUMOR-LIKE LESIONS

Mesothelioma, localized fibrous tumor, malignant lymphoma including *MALToma,* and *soft tissue sarcoma* are described in detail in Chapters 27, 25, and 5, respectively. One of the soft tissue sarcomas, *intravascular sclerosing bronchioloalveolar tumor,* which is seen as multiple slow-growing lung tumors with occasional metastasis to the lymph nodes and distant organs (159), must be mentioned here. This tumor is now considered endothelial because of the presence of both immunoreactive factor VIII and Weibel-Palade bodies, and is called *malignant angioendothelioma* or *epithelioid hemangioendothelioma* or *sarcoma* (160) (Fig. 26.53). An identical tumor is known to occur in the liver and other sites.

A very rare tumor was reported. It consisted of *plasmacytoma* of the lung with lymph node and pleural metastases associated with nodular deposits of immunoglobulin (Fig. 26.54) (161).

Primary *malignant melanoma* of the lung is also known to occur (162,163). In one such case, many Fontana-Masson–positive melanocytes were seen in the bronchial epithelium, distant from the main nodule (158). Of course, ruling out the possibility of metastases from other sites is necessary before one can make a diagnosis of primary malignant melanoma of the bronchus.

Multiple *meningothelioid nodule (arachnoid nodule),* which was previously called *chemodectoma* or *paraganglioma* (21,164,165), is frequently microscopic in size and multiple, and it is often detected incidentally at the time of histologic examination of the lung for other diseases. Histologically, it is considered hyperplastic rather than neoplastic because of its relation to veins and nerves; electron microscopically, it resembles meningeal arachnoid granulations.

Benign clear-cell (sugar) tumor of the lung is a peripherally located tumor composed of sheets of clear cells with a fine vascular stroma that possess small, uniform nuclei and have abundant glycogen in the cytoplasm (Fig. 26.55) (166). Recently, this tumor has come to be considered to present a family of tumors showing perivascular epithelioid cell differentiation (PEComas) which includes angiomyolipoma, lymphangiomyomatosis, clear-cell "sugar" tumor of the lung, and a group of rare, morphologically and immunophenotypically similar lesions arising at a variety of visceral and soft tissue sites (167). PEComa is characteristically immunoreactive with both antimelanocytic an-

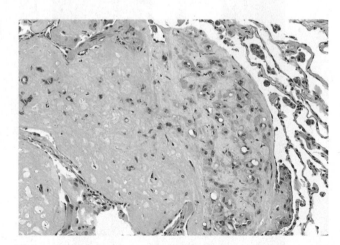

Figure 26.53. Epithelioid hemangioendothelioma. Small clusters of epithelioid cells, some of which possess vacuolated cytoplasm, are embedded in fibromyxoid matrix. The peripheral portion of the tumor is more cellular than the central portion.

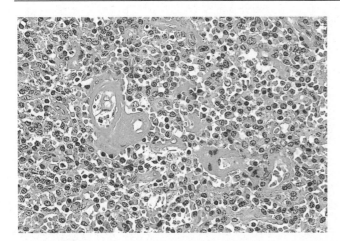

Figure 26.54. Plasmacytoma. The atypical plasma cells proliferate diffusely, and eosinophilic deposits are seen in and around the vessel. This tumor involved the pleura and lymph nodes.

tibodies (HMB-45 and/or melan-A) and anti–smooth muscle antibodies (smooth muscle actin and desmin).

Primary *intrapulmonary meningioma* is rare, and, histologically and immunohistochemically, it is similar to intracranial meningioma, with positive staining for epithelial membrane antigen (EMA) and vimentin (11,168). Other rare benign tumors include lipoma, granular cell tumor, and pulmonary capillary hemangiomatosis.

Sclerosing Hemangioma

Sclerosing hemangioma is a round to oval, well-defined, nonencapsulated lesion arising in the periphery of the lung, the cut surface of which varies from ivory-colored solid to hemorrhagic (Fig. 26.56). It can be shelled out when an attempt at removal is made by wedge resection. Histologically, it is variegated in appearance, with cuboidal cells that are arranged in a papillary fashion in the peripheral portion of the tumor and round to polygonal medium-sized cells with rather clear cytoplasm that are arranged in sheets in some areas. Small vessels with hyalinized walls and small spaces lined by cuboidal cells are scattered

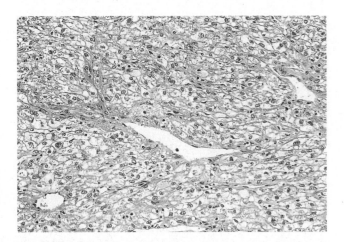

Figure 26.55. PEComa. Plump, short, spindle-shaped cells with abundant clear cytoplasm and small, uniform nuclei grow diffusely. Sinusoid-like vessels are well developed.

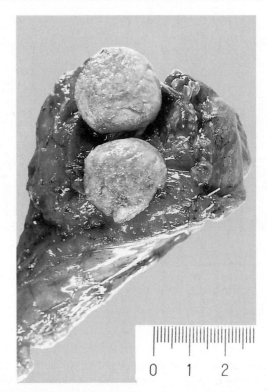

Figure 26.56. Gross features of sclerosing hemangioma. The bisected spheric tumor shows a tan, bulging cut surface, and it appears as though it would be shelled out readily.

in sclerotic areas, and, in angiomatous areas, spaces filled with red blood cells and a few macrophages are lined with flat to cuboidal cells (Fig. 26.57). Foamy macrophages and mast cells are frequently found.

Immunohistochemically and electron microscopically, cells covering or lining the papillary and tubular structures and located in the angiomatous areas are found to have the characteristics of type II alveolar epithelial cells, but the nature of the polygonal cells with the clear cytoplasm has not yet been settled.

Some investigators had considered this lesion to be angiomatous neoplasia (169), but more recently, much support has been lent to the idea that this is a tumor related to type II alveolar epithelial cells (170). Other theories include mesothelioma (171) and hamartoma. A case showing numerous tumors (172), a case with microscopic lymph node metastasis (151,172,173), and a case with pleural involvement were reported, all of which support the theory that this tumor is an alveolar epithelial cell neoplasm. By their monoclonality, the derivation of both the surface lining cuboidal cells and pale polygonal cells was shown to be from the same cell (174), and they possessed immunoreactive TTF-1 (175). From these data, it is reasonable to consider that sclerosing hemangioma is an epithelial neoplasm derived from the primitive respiratory epithelium or an incompletely differentiated type II pneumocyte or Clara cell (175).

Sclerosing hemangioma is found more often as a coin lesion in the lower lung field in middle-aged women. It appears to grow very slowly, and it is symptomless in many instances.

Inflammatory Pseudotumor

Inflammatory pseudotumor is a tumorous lesion that develops after nonspecific inflammation. It occurs in any age group, in-

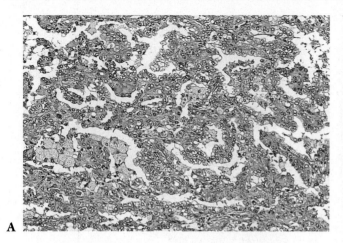

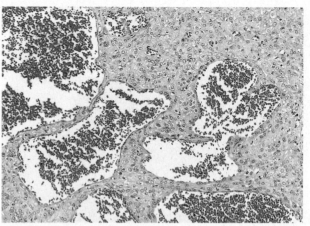

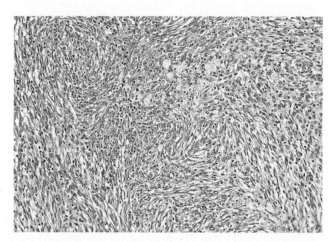

Figure 26.57. Sclerosing hemangioma. **(A)** At the periphery, slightly atypical type II pneumocytes proliferate in papillary fashion. **(B)** In a hemangiomatous area, blood-containing spaces are lined by flat epithelial cells instead of by endothelial cells. Diffuse growth of polygonal cells, a component of sclerosing hemangioma, is also seen. **(C)** Within a sclerotic area, small spaces are lined by cuboidal cells. Both the flat epithelial cells in **(B)** and the cuboidal cells in **(C)** are surfactant apoprotein-positive type II alveolar epithelial cells.

cluding children. It appears as a grossly benign soft tissue tumor with a well-defined nonencapsulated border (Fig. 26.58). It is called *plasma cell granuloma* when the infiltration of plasma cells and lymphocytes is conspicuous and *fibroxanthoma* when it is composed of fibrous tissue with foamy histiocytes (Fig. 26.59) (176,177). It is also called *inflammatory myofibroblastic tumor.* However, fibrous histiocytoma may be diagnosed as pseudotumor.

Tumorlet

Tumorlets are microscopic lesions consisting of solid nests of small cells somewhat resembling oat cells; these lesions are often

multiple, and they are frequently associated with bronchiolar epithelium (178,179). Individual cells are argyrophilic, and they contain dense-core granules of neurosecretory type in the cytoplasm. Immunohistochemically, they show diffuse positive staining for ACTH, GRP, calcitonin, and other substances. These lesions are found in hypoplastic or damaged fibrotic lungs, and they are considered hyperplastic (180). If such a lesion is encountered in an otherwise normal-appearing lung, the possibility of early-stage carcinoid should be considered. Sustentacular

Figure 26.58. Pseudotumor of the lung. A dumbbell-shaped tumor is present beneath the pleura, the cut surface of which is fibromatous.

Figure 26.59. Pseudotumor shown in Figure 26.57. It is made up of bundles of fibroblastic cells admixed with foamy histiocytes.

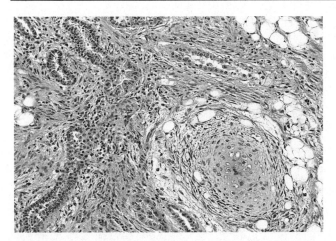

Figure 26.60. Hamartoma. The tumor consists of cartilage, fat, fibrous tissue, and tubular structures lined by cuboidal cells, all of which are normal constituents of the lung.

cells positive for S-100 protein are not found in tumorlets, but they are frequently recognized in carcinoid tumors (144).

When neuroendocrine cell aggregates extend outside the confines of the airway basement membrane (21,165,181), difficulty exists in differential diagnosis of multiple tumorlets, a tumor-like lesion, and diffuse idiopathic pulmonary neuroendocrine hyperplasia with obliterative bronchiolar fibrosis, a preinvasive lesion of peripheral carcinoid tumor; in such instances, tumorlets and carcinoid tumors merge as a pathologic entity.

Hamartoma

Hamartoma is a tumorous lesion consisting of anomalously arranged tissues that are components of the normal lung, such as cartilage, fat, smooth muscle, and tubules lined by bronchial or bronchiolar epithelium, which may be entrapped (Fig. 26.60).

Chondromatous hamartoma (182), which is nodular and well circumscribed, is seen most frequently (Fig. 26.61). The cut

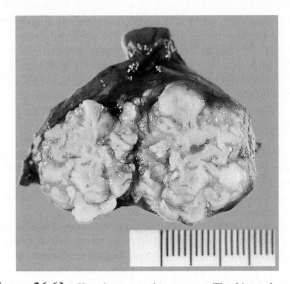

Figure 26.61. Chondromatous hamartoma. The bisected tumor shows a bulging cut surface and an irregularly nodular border. Loose connective tissue is seen among the irregular islands of cartilage.

section reveals irregular lobules of cartilage that may contain calcified areas. Immature myxomatous tissue is seen at the periphery of the cartilage lobules, which lack perichondrium, but this should not be mistaken as a sign of malignancy. Hamartoma without a cartilaginous component does occur, although rarely, and this somewhat resembles adenofibroma of the female genital tract (183) and fibroadenoma of the breast both grossly and histologically. Hamartoma occurs mostly as a solitary nodule, but rarely it appears as a diffuse mass; when adipose tissue is a prominent feature, differential diagnosis from low-grade liposarcoma may be difficult (184).

Most patients with hamartoma are older than 40 years, and the male-to-female ratio is about 1:2. Most patients are asymptomatic, and the lesion is often found on x-ray during a routine checkup. Needle biopsy may disclose fragments of mature cartilage. The lesion may grow very slowly, and recurrence has not been seen even after enucleation. Malignant change does not occur. The multiple nodular leiomyomatous type may be metastatic leiomyosarcoma from other sites (185).

METASTATIC TUMORS OF THE LUNG

The lung is the primary or secondary filter for tumor cells in the bloodstream. Therefore, it is the organ with the highest incidence of hematogenous metastases. Until 1970, surgery for metastasis was rarely performed. However, the indication has been broadened, and metastasis of colorectal cancer, uterine cervical cancer, renal carcinoma, salivary gland tumor, and some types of sarcoma have been surgically treated, particularly for a single metastasis, and the result is an increased number of long-term survivors. However, the results of surgical treatment for metastasis from carcinoma of the lung, stomach, and breast are extremely poor. In general, the longer the interval between the time of resection of the primary tumor and the time of detection of lung metastasis, the better the prognosis and the greater the indication for surgical resection. A single metastasis, as well as metastatic nodules confined within one lobe of the lung, can usually be resected. However, surgery may be performed even when the metastases involve more than two lobes, and bilateral thoracotomy may be carried out for slow-growing tumors.

Making a histologic distinction about whether the tumor is primary or metastatic is easy when the tumor possesses characteristic features, such as those evident in adenocarcinoma of the colon and kidney, as well as those in some sarcomas. Metastatic squamous cell carcinomas of stratified squamous epithelial origin, such as those from the oral cavity, often show extensive cavitation, leaving a thin rim of tumor tissue, and they are somewhat different from squamous cell carcinoma of the lung. However, metastatic squamous cell carcinoma from the uterine cervix may be quite difficult to differentiate from a primary lung tumor. In such instances, the smoking history may be of help because squamous cell carcinoma of the lung among nonsmokers is extremely rare. A histologic finding that may be of help for diagnosing metastasis is the presence of tumor thrombosis in relatively large pulmonary arteries at or near the periphery of the mass. In cases in which the determination of whether a tumor is primary or metastatic cannot be made, it should be resected as a primary tumor in the lung, together with mediastinal node dissection. Conversely, some tumors have been removed under a clinical diagnosis of primary lung carcinoma and then have later been found to be metastatic. Renal cell

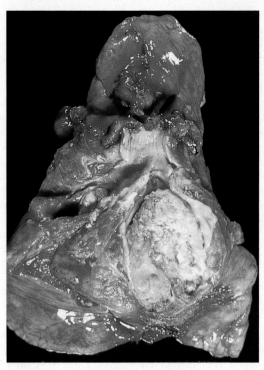

Figure 26.62. Metastatic rectal carcinoma in the lung. A huge tumor grows endobronchially. From: Kameya T. Salivary gland type tumors. In National Cancer Center Hospital. *Cancer of the Lung: Diagnosis and Treatment.* Vol. 1. Tokyo: Kodansha, 1983:179–190 [in Japanese], with permission.

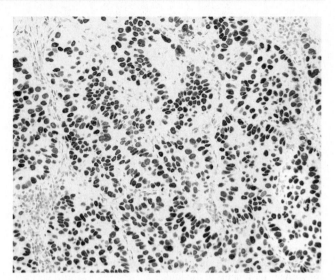

Figure 26.63. Thyroid transcription factor-1 (TTF-1) in acinar adenocarcinoma of bronchial gland cell type with some signet ring–type tumor cells. **(A)** H&E stain. **(B)** TTF-1 immunostaining with positive nuclei is indicative of primary lung cancer.

carcinoma is one such tumor type, the symptoms and signs of which appear late; lung metastasis is not infrequently single. Renal carcinoma and colorectal carcinoma may involve a fairly large bronchus, with occasional polypoid endobronchial growth (Fig. 26.62). This feature mimics primary lung carcinoma.

Squamous cell carcinoma involving both the lung and the anterior mediastinum may present difficulties in the differential diagnosis. However, squamous cell carcinoma possessing vesicular nuclei, prominent nucleoli, and a wide sclerotic stromal zone favors a diagnosis of thymic squamous carcinoma (186). Benign and low-grade malignant tumors of the anterior mediastinum, such as mature teratoma and thymoma, may invade the lung and bronchi and may mislead a clinician to diagnose primary lung cancer (187,188).

To determine whether the tumor is primary or metastatic, a multidisciplinary approach should be adopted; in other words, the clinical course, gross and microscopic appearances, and IHC findings of the tumor should be considered. Adenocarcinoma with immunoreactive surfactant apoprotein can be diagnosed as a primary in the lung, as has been described. IHC for TTF-1 is also useful for the identification of pulmonary adenocarcinoma and nonneuroendocrine large-cell carcinoma because it is present in about 75% of pulmonary adenocarcinomas and in a smaller percentage of large-cell carcinomas (25%) and squamous cell carcinomas (10%), and it is absent in cancer of other sites, excluding the thyroid gland (Fig. 26.63) (95,189).

However, this method should not be used to distinguish primary from metastatic poorly differentiated neuroendocrine carcinoma in extrapulmonary sites (190,191). Pathologists who are well acquainted with the characteristics of each lung tumor can recognize both obvious and minor differences between the primary and metastatic tumors and can arrive at a correct diagnosis in most cases. In the very near future, analysis of some selected genetic abnormalities may become practically feasible for determining whether a tumor is primary or metastatic. For example, gene alterations of *p53* and *EGFR* can be useful in determining whether two histologically similar tumors in a lobe are independent primary tumors by analyzing the site of point mutation for each gene (192).

IMMUNOHISTOCHEMISTRY OF MALIGNANT LUNG TUMORS

Because of the histologic diversity and biologic complexity of lung cancer, IHC must cover many different items, including peptide hormones, specific enzymes, cytoskeleton, altered sugar chains, proliferative properties of the cell, and abnormal gene products. The antigens recognized by polyclonal or monoclonal antibodies used can be divided into differentiation antigens; cancer-associated antigens, including oncofetal antigens; and antigens closely related to cell growth.

AMINE AND PEPTIDE HORMONES

Small-cell carcinoma is known to produce various amine and peptide hormones, such as ACTH and related hormones, antidiuretic hormone, GRP (a human counterpart of bombesin), calcitonin, and serotonin. All of these are substances related to neuroendocrine cells.

Although GRP is present in small amounts in the normal lung and tissue of non–small-cell lung cancers, many small-cell carcinomas do contain larger amounts. In particular, most tumors containing more than 100 ng per g of wet tissue are either small-cell carcinoma or carcinoid tumor, in which the peptide can also often be detected immunohistochemically (56).

The serum level of progastrin-releasing peptide (Pro-GRP)

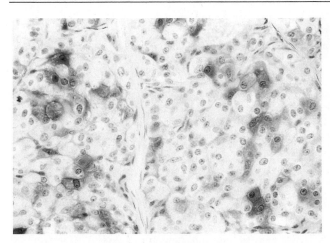

Figure 26.64. Pancreatic polypeptide in carcinoid tumor. Scattered cells possess immunoreactive pancreatic polypeptide, which is not present in small-cell carcinoma (immunostaining).

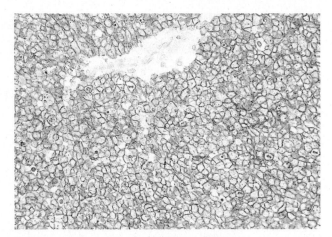

Figure 26.65. Neural cell adhesion molecule (N-CAM) in small-cell carcinoma. Cell membrane of all tumor cells shows staining for N-CAM (immunostaining of AMeX section with NCC-Lu-243).

is a very good marker for the follow-up of patients with small-cell carcinoma of the lung (193). The sensitivity and specificity of Pro-GRP are similar to those of NSE, which is another good serum but not an IHC marker of small-cell carcinoma. Double-staining for calcitonin and cytoplasmic mucus in poorly differentiated adenocarcinoma occasionally shows that some cells produce both mucin and calcitonin (117) and that some non–small-cell lung cancers also produce peptide hormone, although they do so less frequently and in smaller amounts.

The study of small-cell and non–small-cell lung cancers with regard to 17 kinds of peptide hormones has shown that some 80% of small-cell carcinomas produce at least one peptide, whereas only about 10% of non–small-cell cancers do so. Fifty percent of small-cell carcinomas produce more than two kinds of peptides, whereas only 6% of non–small-cell lung cancers simultaneously produce more than two peptide hormones. Small-cell carcinoma is similar to carcinoid tumor with regard to peptide hormone production and enzyme activities. However, pancreatic polypeptide was not produced by any of the small-cell carcinomas examined, but it was produced by some carcinoid tumors (Fig. 26.64) (58).

ENZYMES

NSE, CK-BB, and AADC or l-dopa decarboxylase are rather frequently detected in small-cell carcinoma (194). In our study, NSE was found to be positive in 77% of 47 small-cell carcinomas, and CK-BB stained positively in 91%. AADC can also be stained immunohistochemically; a positive reaction was revealed in (a) Kulchitsky cells of the bronchus, (b) carcinoid tumor, and (c) small-cell carcinoma. A positive reaction was seen in 40% of 47 small-cell carcinomas.

NEUROENDOCRINE MARKERS (CHROMOGRANIN A, NEURAL CELL ADHESION MOLECULE OR CD56, SYNAPTOPHYSIN)

N-CAM (CD56) is one of the best markers of neuroendocrine cells, including small-cell carcinoma, carcinoid tumor, and large-cell neuroendocrine carcinoma and other tumors that show neuroendocrine differentiation. It is superior to chro-

mogranin A and other markers. CD56 antibodies mark almost all small-cell carcinoma cells, some of the small-cell and/or large-cell carcinoma cells, and some tumor cells of a few non–small-cell carcinomas in both histology and cytology specimens (Fig. 26.65 and Table 26.6) (195–197).

Chromogranin A is a structural protein of neuroendocrine granules detected in tumor cells of small-cell carcinoma, carcinoid tumor, and other tumors with neuroendocrine features. It is said to be a good marker for neuroendocrine cells and their neoplastic counterparts, such as carcinoid tumor and small-cell carcinoma (Fig. 26.66) (194), but the percentage of small-cell carcinomas with IHC-positive chromogranin A is not very high.

Synaptophysin is a synaptic vesicle glycoprotein and a unique marker of neuroendocrine cells (Fig. 26.67). The gene encoding the protein is located on the X chromosome. The positivity rate for this protein in neuroendocrine tumors is higher than that of chromogranin A but lower than that of CD56 (198).

BCL-2 protein may be another good marker for neuroendocrine differentiation in small-cell and large-cell carcinomas (128,129).

VIMENTIN

Vimentin is widely believed to be a good marker for mesothelioma, but it is negative in lung cancer. Vimentin is one of the intermediate filaments; it is present in mesenchymal cells, excluding muscle cells, and it is also known to be present in (a) some epithelial cells in culture, and (b) cancer cells in effusion. In 276 cases of surgically resected lung cancer, no squamous cell carcinoma or small-cell carcinoma showed a positive reaction, but 9% of adenocarcinomas and 25% of large-cell carcinomas were proved to contain vimentin immunohistochemically (Fig. 26.68) (93). Coexpression of vimentin and cytokeratin was noted in single cells.

MARKERS OF PERIPHERAL AIRWAY EPITHELIUM (SURFACTANT APOPROTEIN AND THYROID TRANSCRIPTION FACTOR-1)

Surfactant apoprotein, a core protein of surfactant lipoprotein, is expressed mainly in the cytoplasm of type II alveolar epithelial

TABLE 26.6	**Results of Immunocytologic Staining for Neuroendocrine Markers in Various Lung Cancers**					
		Number of Cases with Positive Staining				
Cancer Type	*Number of Cases Studied*	*N-CAM*	*CHG*	*Leu-7*	*GRP*	*NSE*
Small-cell carcinoma	12	12	4	3	1	1
Pure	8	8[a]	2	2	1	1
With large cell	4	4[b]	2	1	0	0
Adenocarcinoma	50	2[c]	4	7	0	16
Squamous cell carcinoma	25	2[c]	0	0	1	6
Large cell carcinoma	6	2[c]	0	0	0	1
Adenosquamous carcinoma	1	1[c]	0	0	0	0
Carcinoid tumor	2	2[a]	2	1	0	0
Malignant lymphoma	1	0	0	0	0	0
Metastatic carcinoma	8	0	0	0	0	0

[a]Almost all tumor cells were positively stained.
[b]Many tumor cells were positive, but a few negative cells were admixed.
[c]A few tumor cells were positively stained. Antibodies against N-CAM are NCC-LU-243 and NCC-LU-246.
CHG, chromogranin A; GRP, gastrin-releasing peptide; Leu-7, antimyelin fiber-associated glycoprotein; N-CAM, neural cell adhesion molecule; NSE, neuron-specific enolase.
From: Tome Y, Hirohashi S, Noguchi M, et al. Immunocytologic diagnosis of small-cell lung cancer in imprint smears. *Acta Cytol* 1991;35:485–490.

cells. It is divided into the following four major subtypes: SPA, SPB, SPC, and SPD. The monoclonal antibody PE-10 is a specific antibody against SPA, and it has been proved useful for the identification of type II alveolar epithelial cells and their neoplastic counterparts (76,199). This antibody is also reactive with nuclear inclusions found in carcinomas of type II alveolar epithelial cell type and Clara cell type. About 50% of all pulmonary adenocarcinomas contain tumor cells reactive with this antibody (Fig. 26.69), not only well-differentiated but also poorly differentiated carcinomas. One study showed no lung cancers of other histologic types or cancers of other organs showed any reaction (Table 26.7) (77). A later investigation disclosed that PE-10 also reacts with lung adenocarcinoma of other cell types, excluding goblet cell–type bronchioloalveolar carcinoma, but not with mesotheliomas or adenocarcinomas of other organs, except for a few thyroid carcinomas (Table 26.7). However, Western blot analysis did not reveal surfactant apoproteins in proteins extracted from positively stained thyroid cancer. This finding indicates that surfactant apoproteins are specific markers for adenocarcinoma of the lung, although the reactivities are noted in only about 50% of cases (94,104).

Conversely, SPC is a specific differentiation marker of type II alveolar epithelial cells. It is detected only in type II alveolar epithelial cells but not in Clara cells or other epithelial cells of the lung. Because SPC is an extremely hydrophobic protein, a monoclonal antibody was produced against pro-SPC protein, which is a useful marker of type II alveolar epithelial cells and which can distinguish type II alveolar epithelial cells from Clara cells (200).

TTF-1 is a transcriptional protein expressed by thyroid and pulmonary epithelia. Therefore, a monoclonal antibody against TTF-1 reacts specifically with thyroid and pulmonary epithelia, and it is an excellent marker for their neoplastic counterpart (Fig. 26.63) (201).

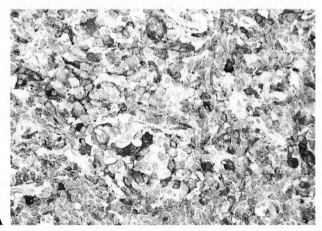
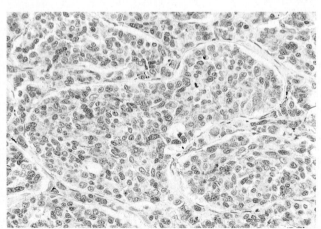

A   B

Figure 26.66. Chromogranin A in neuroendocrine tumors. **(A)** The carcinoid tumor shows marked cytoplasmic staining. **(B)** However, small-cell carcinoma is often weakly stained or unstained (immunostaining).

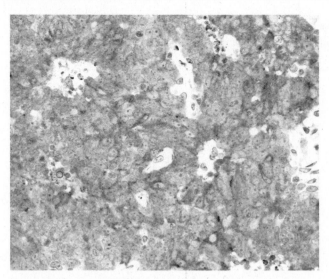

Figure 26.67. Synaptophysin in large cell neuroendocrine carcinoma with frequent rosettes. The tumor is strongly immunoreactive for synaptophysin (immunostaining).

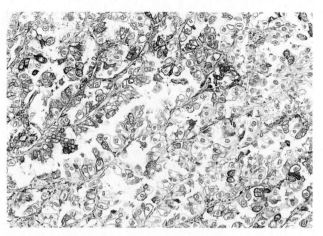

Figure 26.69. Surfactant apoprotein in papillary adenocarcinoma of type II alveolar epithelial cell type. The cytoplasm, which is abundant, vesicular, or clear, shows variable staining for surfactant apoprotein (immunostaining).

MONOCLONAL ANTIBODIES: LEU-7 (CD57)

Leu-7 is known to react with natural killer cells and is considered a marker for amine precursor uptake and decarboxylation (APUD) cells and small-cell carcinoma. Our results indicate that 50% of cases of well to moderately differentiated adenocarcinoma react with Leu-7, although more cases of small-cell carcinoma showed a reaction (57). Cases of squamous cell carcinoma are very rarely reactive to Leu-7.

ALTERED SUGAR CHAINS

The blood group–related antigens include many of the so-called cancer-associated antigens recognized by monoclonal antibodies. Neoplastic mucin has been shown to be positive for I (Ma) antigen, a precursor of H antigen, in every lung cancer

case examined, whereas no such finding has been encountered in nonneoplastic mucin in the lung. Some tumors show deletion of blood group antigens, and, in a few patients with blood group B or O, the tumor cells react positively with anti-A antibody (202). Therefore, in lung cancer, ABH antigens may apparently be lost, the precursor antigen I (Ma) may accumulate, and A-like antigen may be expressed.

CARCINOEMBRYONIC ANTIGEN

Carcinoembryonic antigen (CEA) is a glycoprotein present in the glycocalyx of embryonic entodermal cells. It may be a useful marker in terms of the malignant progression in individual tumors; it is quite often negative in bronchioloalveolar atypical adenomatous hyperplasia, and is frequently positive in pure or focally invasive bronchioloalveolar carcinoma of the Clara cell and/or type II alveolar epithelial cell type. It increases in staining intensity with an increase in atypia and anaplasia of tumors (6).

IDENTIFICATION OF PROLIFERATING OR DNA-SYNTHESIZING CELLS (KI-67 AND PCNA)

DNA-synthesizing cells pick up BrdU, a thymidine analog, which can be stained with the ABC method by using anti-BrdU (203). With this method, the proliferative activity of a solid tumor can be studied. The number of DNA-synthesizing cells in the periphery and central portion of a tumor mass can thus be compared. In most lung tumors, more proliferative activity is seen in the periphery of the tumor than in the central portion, but the reverse is true in most well-differentiated papillary adenocarcinomas with a bronchioloalveolar pattern (6). In addition, more proliferative activity is observed in poorly differentiated tumors than in well-differentiated tumors. Proliferative activity is highest in small-cell carcinoma, followed by squamous cell carcinoma. The proliferative activity of adenocarcinoma cells varies from very low to high according to the case—a finding indicating that some tumors grow very slowly, whereas others grow rapidly (203). Practically, monoclonal antibodies against proliferation-associated nuclear antigen (Ki-67, MIB-1) and PCNA can be used to compare growth properties (Fig. 26.70)

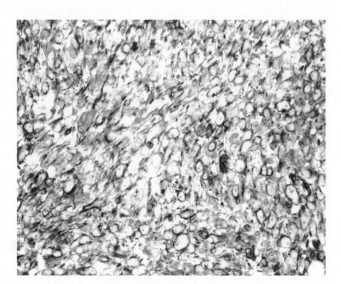

Figure 26.68. Vimentin in large-cell carcinoma. The cytoplasm of many tumor cells is reactive to antivimentin antibody. Endothelial cells serve as a positive internal control (immunostaining).

TABLE 26.7	Immunoreactive Surfactant Apoproteins in Lung Cancer, Adenocarcinomas of Other Organs, and Malignant Mesothelioma		
Cancer Type		*Number of Cases Positive/ Number of Cases Examined*	*Percentage (%)*
Lung cancer			
Adenocarcinoma		36/75	48
Well-differentiated		19/41	46
Moderately differentiated		11/24	46
Poorly differentiated		6/10	60
Squamous cell carcinoma		0/5	0
Large-cell carcinoma		0/8	0
Small-cell carcinoma		0/1	0
Metastases from other organs		0/23	0
Gastric cancer		0/40	0
Pancreatic cancer		0/39	0
Biliary tract cancer		0/27	0
Breast cancer		0/20	0
Thyroid cancer		3/22	14[a]
Malignant mesothelioma (epithelial and biphasic)		0/9	0

[a]Western blot analysis did not reveal surfactant apoproteins.

(204–206). These are usually expressed as the number of positive cells per 1000 tumor cells (MIB-1 index).

CYTOKERATIN

Cytokeratin is useful for identifying sarcomatous transformation in carcinomas (Fig. 26.71). It is subdivided into many subtypes according to their molecular weight. In particular, antibodies against CK7 and CK20 are useful for the differentiation of primary pulmonary adenocarcinoma from metastatic adenocarcinomas originated in the gastrointestinal tract (105–107).

More than 70% of lung adenocarcinomas are positive for anti-CK7 but negative for anti-CK20 (Fig. 26.72). On the contrary, more than 70% of colon carcinomas are positive for anti-CK20 but negative for anti-CK7.

OTHER MARKERS

Secretory component is useful for demonstrating the glandular nature of cancer cells (Fig. 26.73), and lactoferrin is useful for showing differentiation of tumor cells toward bronchial gland cells (Fig. 26.74). Actin and vimentin are helpful for demonstrating neoplastic myoepithelial cells (Fig. 26.75) (207).

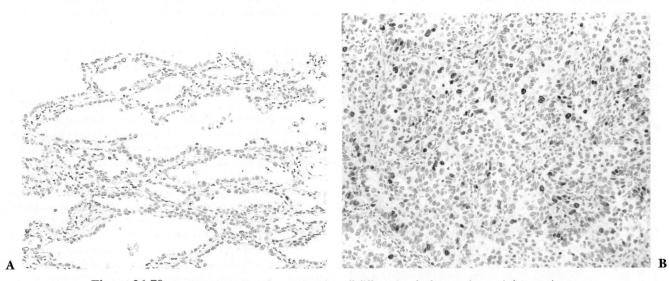

Figure 26.70. Proliferating cell nuclear antigen in well-differentiated adenocarcinoma (adenocarcinoma in atypical adenomatous hyperplasia). **(A)** Nuclear staining is rarely seen in the peripheral portion of the tumor with slight nuclear atypia (atypical adenomatous hyperplasia). **(B)** The central portion of the tumor shows increased nuclear atypia and positive nuclear staining in many tumor cells (well-differentiated adenocarcinoma) (immunostaining). **(A)** and **(B)** are of the same magnification.

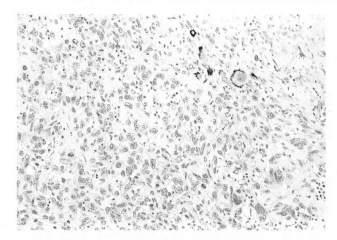

Figure 26.71. Keratin-positive cells in pleomorphic carcinoma (same case as shown in Fig. 26.13). The cytoplasm of a few cells shows immunoreactivity to antikeratin antibody (immunostaining).

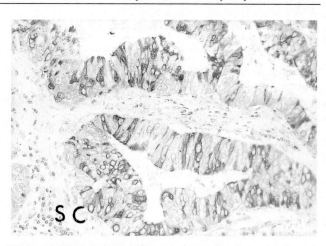

Figure 26.73. Secretory component in adenocarcinoma. Many positively stained tumor cells are present (immunostaining).

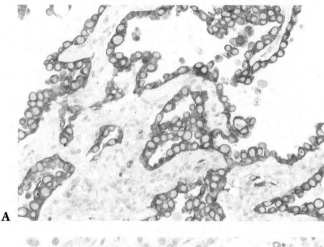

A

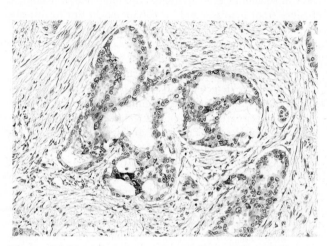

Figure 26.74. Lactoferrin in acinar adenocarcinoma. Immunoreactive lactoferrin is often present in acinar adenocarcinoma of the bronchial gland cell type (immunostaining).

B

Figure 26.72. Cytokeratin immunoreactivity in adenocarcinoma of the lung. **(A)** Positive CK7. **(B)** Negative CK20. **(A)** and **(B)** are the same tumor (immunostaining).

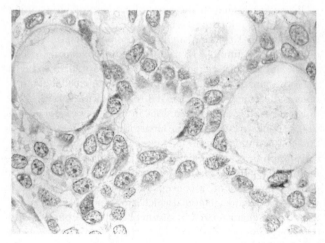

Figure 26.75. Actin in adenoid cystic carcinoma. Crescent-shaped, positively stained cells considered neoplastic myoepithelial cells are facing the cystic lumina (immunostaining).

MOLECULAR PATHOLOGY OF LUNG CARCINOMAS

With advances in molecular biology, particularly in the multiple genetic alterations in neoplasms, the concept of multistep carcinogenesis has been proposed (9,81,208,209). Genetic alterations include chromosomal abnormalities (loss of heterozygosity) and point mutations of dominant oncogenes and tumor suppressor genes. Loss of function of some tumor suppressor genes is mediated by DNA methylation.

Among the four major histologic subtypes of lung carcinoma, small-cell carcinoma shows frequent allelic losses of 3p, and 22q chromosomes and gene amplification of *myc* family oncogenes such as *N-myc*, *L-myc*, and *c-myc* (47,209,210). The abnormal amplifications of *myc* family oncogenes are a prognostic factor in small-cell carcinoma (210). The allelic losses of 3p, 13q, and 17p chromosomes are reported to be involved in the genesis of non–small-cell carcinoma as well, and 2q, 9p, 18q, and 22q play an important role in its progression (211). Especially in squamous cell carcinoma, the sequence of histologic changes from dysplasia and/or carcinoma in situ to invasive carcinoma has been well established, and 3p deletion is detected not only in carcinoma but also in dysplastic and hyperplastic lesions (208).

In adenocarcinoma, deletions at chromosomal loci 5q, 9p, 11q, and 13q are detected in its very early stage, and deletions of 3p, 17p, 18q, and 22q increase significantly during the course of malignant progression (81). The genetic alterations including point mutations of dominant oncogenes such as the *ras* gene and point mutations of tumor suppressor genes such as *p53*, retinoblastoma (*RB*) gene, and *p16* gene have been well characterized (212,213). The point mutation of the *p53* gene is a prognostic factor of adenocarcinoma, and its genetic alterations are useful for the establishment of the diagnosis of multiple primary lung cancers and for distinction of primary pulmonary carcinoma from recurrent or metastatic carcinomas (192,214). Expression of the *p16* gene is considered to be suppressed when there is deletion of one allele and dysfunction of another allele by hypermethylation (215,216). Large-cell neuroendocrine carcinoma not only displays neuroendocrine features but also shows characteristic 3p allelic losses similar to those of small-cell carcinoma.

Recently, targeted chemotherapy for adenocarcinoma using tyrosine kinase inhibitors has been applied for lung carcinomas, especially non–small-cell carcinoma. Among these inhibitors, erlotinib and gefitinib elicit responses in approximately 10% of Caucasian patients and in up to 40% of East Asian patients (217). Systematic resequencing studies have revealed that mutations in the kinase domain of EGFR (deletions in exon 19, insertions in exon 20, and substitutions in exon 21) are correlated with response to EGFR tyrosine kinase inhibitors. Because EGFR that contains mutations in the kinase domain is more sensitive to gefitinib or erlotinib, EGFR inhibitors are beneficial to patients with tumors harboring such mutations (218). Based on detailed observations, a concept of terminal respiratory unit (TRU)-type adenocarcinoma, which shows specific EGFR mutations and is characterized by distinct cellular morphology and the expression of TTF-1 and surfactant apoprotein, has been advocated (219).

Using the microarray technique, several genomewide analyses have been reported. For example, using gene expression profiling, lung carcinomas have been subdivided into several groups, and primary cancers can be discriminated from metastases of extrapulmonary origin. In primary lung carcinomas, gene expression patterns show striking differences between squamous cell carcinoma and small-cell carcinoma (220,221). Neuroendocrine tumors could also be classified into two groups independent of small-cell carcinoma and large-cell neuroendocrine carcinoma (222).

Molecular pathology and IHC based on molecular pathology are useful not only for the study of lung cancer biology but also for routine surgical pathology, including diagnosis of individual tumors, grade of malignancy, metastatic potential, and prediction of therapeutic response. They provide surgical pathologists the objective indications for proper diagnosis.

REFERENCES

1. Woolner LB, David E, Fontana RS, et al. In situ and early invasive bronchogenic carcinoma: report of 28 cases with postoperative survival data. *J Thorac Cardiovasc Surg* 1970;60: 275–290.
2. Melamed MR, Zaman MB, Flehinger BJ, et al. Radiologically occult in situ and incipient invasive epidermoid lung cancer. *Am J Surg Pathol* 1977;1:5–16.
3. Kodama T, Biyajima S, Watanabe S, et al. Morphometric study of adenocarcinomas and hyperplastic epithelial lesions in the peripheral lung. *Am J Clin Pathol* 1986;85:146–151.
4. Nakayama H, Noguchi M, Tsuchiya R, et al. Clonal growth of atypical adenomatous hyperplasia of the lung: cytofluorometric analysis of nuclear DNA content. *Mod Pathol* 1990;3: 314–320.
5. Nomori H, Shimosato Y, Kodama T, et al. Subtypes of small-cell carcinoma of the lung: morphometric, ultrastructural and immunohistochemical analyses. *Hum Pathol* 1986;17: 604–613.
6. Shimosato Y, Noguchi M, Matsuno Y. Adenocarcinoma of the lung: its development and malignant progression. *Lung Cancer* 1993;9:99–108.
7. Noguchi M, Morikawa A, Kawasaki M, et al. Small adenocarcinoma of the lung: histologic characteristics and prognosis. *Cancer* 1995;75:2844–2852.
8. Asamura H, Kameya T, Matsuno Y, et al. Neuroendocrine neoplasms of the lung: a prognostic spectrum. *J Clin Oncol* 2006;24:70–76.
9. Miller RR, Nelems B, Evans KG, et al. Glandular neoplasia of the lung: a proposed analogy to colonic tumors. *Cancer* 1988;61:1009–1014.
10. Miller RR. Bronchioloalveolar cell adenoma. *Am J Surg Pathol* 1990;14:904–912.
11. Shimosato Y, Miller RR. *Biopsy Interpretation of the Lung*. New York: Raven Press, 1994.
12. Kitamura H, Kameda Y, Nakamura N, et al. Atypical adenomatous hyperplasia and bronchioloalveolar lung carcinoma: analysis by morphometry and the expression of p53 and carcinoembryonic antigen. *Am J Surg Pathol* 1996;20:553–562.
13. Yokozaki M, Kodama T, Yokose T, et al. Differentiation of atypical adenomatous hyperplasia and adenocarcinoma of the lung by use of DNA ploidy and morphometric analysis. *Mod Pathol* 1996;9:1156–1164.
14. Kuriyama K, Seto M, Kasugai T, et al. Ground-glass opacity on thin-section CT: value in differentiating subtypes of adenocarcinoma of the lung. *Am J Roentgenol* 1999;173: 465–469.
15. Ikeda S. *Atlas of Flexible Bronchofiberscopy*. Tokyo: Igaku-Shoin, 1974:58–61.
16. Kondo H, Asamura H, Suemasu K, et al. Prognostic significance of pleural lavage cytology immediately after thoracotomy in patients with lung cancer. *J Thorac Cardiovasc Surg* 1993; 106:1092–1097.
17. Tomiyama N, Yasuhara Y, Nakajima Y, et al. CT-guided needle biopsy of lung lesions: a survey of severe complication based on 9783 biopsies in Japan. *Eur J Radiol* 2006;59:60–64.
18. Naruke T, Suemasu K, Ishikawa S. Lymph node mapping and curability at various levels of metastasis in resected lung cancer. *J Thorac Cardiovasc Surg* 1978;76:832–839.
19. Sato Y, Mukai K, Watanabe S, et al. The AMeX method: a simplified technique of tissue processing and paraffin embedding with improved preservation of antigens for immunostaining. *Am J Pathol* 1986;125:431–435.
20. Sato Y, Mukai K, Matsuno Y, et al. The AMeX method: a multipurpose tissue-processing and paraffin-embedding method. II. Extraction of spooled DNA and its application to Southern blot hybridization analysis. *Am J Pathol* 1990;136:267–271.
21. Travis WD, Colby TV, Corrin B, et al. *WHO Histological Typing of Lung and Pleural Tumors*. 3rd edition. Geneva: World Health Organization, 1999.
22. Travis WD, Brambilla EB, Muller-Hermelink HK, et al. *WHO Pathology and Genetics of Tumours of the Lung, Pleura, Thymus and Heart*. Lyon, France: IARC Press, 2004.
23. Shimosato Y, Suemasu K, Suzuki A. Morphology of tumor of probable bronchial gland origin, with particular reference to adenocarcinoma [in Japanese]. *Cancer Clin* 1973;19: 170–177.
24. Kodama T, Shimosato Y, Kameya T. Histology and ultrastructure of bronchogenic and bronchial gland adenocarcinomas (including adenoid cystic and mucoepidermoid carcinomas) in relation to histogenesis. In Shimosato Y, Melamed MR, Nettesheim P, eds. *Morphogenesis of Lung Cancer*. Vol. 1. Boca Raton, FL: CRC Press, 1982:147–166.
25. Shimosato Y, Kodama T, Kameya T. Morphogenesis of peripheral type adenocarcinoma of the lung. In Shimosato Y, Melamed MR, Nettesheim P, eds. *Morphogenesis of Lung Cancer*. Vol. 1. Boca Raton, FL: CRC Press, 1982:65–89.

26. Hammond ME, Sause WT. Large cell neuroendocrine tumors of the lung: clinical significance and histopathologic definition. *Cancer* 1985;56:1624–1629.
27. Kodama T, Shimosato Y, Koide T, et al. Large cell carcinoma of the lung: ultrastructural and immunohistochemical studies. *Jpn J Clin Oncol* 1985;15:431–441.
28. Fechner RE, Bentinck BR. Ultrastructure of bronchial oncocytoma. *Cancer* 1973;31: 1451–1457.
29. England DM, Hochholzer L. Truly benign "bronchial adenoma": report of 10 cases of mucous gland adenoma with immunohistochemical and ultrastructural findings. *Am J Surg Pathol* 1995;19:887–899.
30. Noguchi M, Kodama T, Shimosato Y, et al. Papillary adenoma of type 2 pneumocytes. *Am J Surg Pathol* 1986;10:134–139.
31. Yousem SA, Hochholzer L. Alveolar adenoma. *Hum Pathol* 1986;17:1066–1071.
32. Minami Y, Matsuno Y, Iijima T, et al. Prognostication of small-sized primary pulmonary adenocarcinomas by histopathlogical and karyometric analysis. *Lung Cancer* 2005;48: 339–348.
33. Travis WD, Lubin J, Ries L, et al. United States lung carcinoma incidence trends: declining for most histologic types among males, increasing among females. *Cancer* 1996;77: 2464–2470.
34. Shimosato Y, Amemiya R. Pathology of early stage squamous cell carcinoma of the hilar type [in Japanese]. In Ikeda M, Oho K, Oshibe M, et al., eds. *Atlas of Early Cancer of Major Bronchi.* Tokyo: Igaku-Shoin, 1976:29–37.
35. Asamura H, Nakayama H, Kondo H, et al. Lymph node involvement, recurrence, and prognosis in resected small, peripheral, non-small cell lung carcinomas: are these carcinomas candidate for video-assisted lobectomy? *J Thorac Cardiovasc Surg* 1996;111:1125–1134.
36. Nakanishi K, Kawai T, Suzuki M, et al. Bronchogenic squamous cell carcinomas with invasion along alveolar walls. *Histopathology* 1996;29:363–368.
37. McDowell ME, McLaughlin JS, Merenyl DK, et al. The respiratory epithelium. V. Histogenesis of lung carcinomas in the human. *J Natl Cancer Inst* 1978;61:587–606.
38. Mori K, Kodama T, Shimosato Y. Analysis of cytodifferentiation in squamous cell carcinoma of the lung in relation to the site of origin, sex and smoking history [in Japanese]. *Lung Cancer* 1986;26:117–123.
39. Brambilla E, Moro D, Veale D, et al. Basal cell (basaloid) carcinoma of the lung: a new morphologic and phenotypic entity with separate prognostic significance. *Hum Pathol* 1992;23:993–1003.
40. Moseley JM, Kubota M, Diefenbach-Jagger H, et al. Parathyroid hormone-related protein purified from a human lung cancer cell line. *Proc Natl Acad Sci U S A* 1987;84:5048–5052.
41. Tsuchihashi T, Yamaguchi K, Miyake Y, et al. Parathyroid hormone-related protein in tumor tissues obtained from patients with humoral hypercalcemia of malignancy. *J Natl Cancer Inst* 1990;82:40–44.
42. Matthews MJ, Gazdar AF. Small-cell carcinoma of the lung: its morphology, behavior and nature. In Shimosato Y, Melamed MR, Nettesheim P, eds. *Morphogenesis of Lung Cancer.* Vol. 2. Boca Raton, FL: CRC Press, 1982:1–14.
43. Whang-Peng J, Bunn PA, Jr. Kao-Shan CS, et al. A non-random chromosomal abnormality del 3p (14–23) in human small cell lung cancer (SCLC). *Cancer Genet Cytogenet* 1982;6: 119–134.
44. Kameya T, Kodama T, Shimosato Y. Ultrastructure of small-cell carcinoma of the lung (oat and intermediate types) in relation to histogenesis and carcinoid tumors. In Shimosato Y, Melamed MR, Nettesheim P, eds. *Morphogenesis of Lung Cancer.* Vol. 2. Boca Raton, FL: CRC Press, 1982:15–43.
45. Shimosato Y, Nakajima T, Hirohashi S, et al. Biological, pathological and clinical features of small cell lung cancer. *Cancer Lett* 1986;33:241–258.
46. Minna JD. Genetic events in the pathogenesis of lung cancer. *Chest* 1989;96:17S–23S.
47. Yokota J, Wada M, Shimosato Y, et al. Loss of heterozygosity on chromosomes 3, 13, and 17 in small-cell carcinoma and on chromosome 3 in adenocarcinoma of the lung. *Proc Natl Acad Sci U S A* 1987;84:9252–9256.
48. Barnard WG. The nature of the "oat celled sarcoma" of the mediastinum. *J Pathol Bacteriol* 1926;29:241–244.
49. Azzopardi JG. Oat cell carcinoma of the bronchus. *J Pathol Bacteriol* 1959;78:513–519.
50. Bensch KG, Corrin B, Pariente R, et al. Oat cell carcinoma of the lung: its origin and relationship to bronchial carcinoid. *Cancer* 1968;22:1163–1172.
51. Hattori S, Matsuda M, Tateishi R, et al. Oat cell carcinoma of the lung: clinical and morphological studies in relation to its histogenesis. *Cancer* 1972;30:1014–1024.
52. Pearse AG, Polak JM, Heath CM. Polypeptide hormone production by "carcinoid" APUDomas and their relevant cytochemistry. *Virchows Arch B Cell Pathol* 1974;16:95–109.
53. Gazdar AF, Carney DN, Guccion JG, et al. Small-cell carcinoma of the lung: cellular origin and relationship to other pulmonary tumors. In Greco FA, Oldham RK, Bunn PA Jr, eds. *Small Cell Lung Cancer.* New York: Grune & Stratton, 1981:145–175.
54. National Cancer Center Hospital. *Cancer of the Lung: Diagnosis and Treatment.* Vol. 2. Tokyo: Kodansha, 1983:91–103 [in Japanese].
55. Lee I, Gould VE, Moll R, et al. Synaptophysin expressed in the bronchopulmonary tract: neuroendocrine cells, neuroepithelial bodies, and neuroendocrine neoplasms. *Differentiation* 1987;34:115–125.
56. Abe K, Kameya T, Yamaguchi K, et al. Hormone-producing lung cancers. In Becker KL, Gazdar AF, eds. *Endocrine Lung in Health and Disease.* Philadelphia: WB Saunders, 1984: 549–595.
57. Sato Y, Watanabe S, Kodama T, et al. Stainability of lung cancer cells with Leu-7 and OKT-9 monoclonal antibodies. *Jpn J Clin Oncol* 1985;15:537–544.
58. Yamaguchi K, Abe K, Adachi I, et al. Peptide hormone production in primary lung tumors. *Recent Results Cancer Res* 1985;99:107–116.
59. Simon GR, Turrisi A, American College of Chest Physicians. Management of small cell lung cancer: ACCP evidence-based clinical practice guidelines (2nd edition). *Chest* 2007; 132:324S-339S.
60. Bartter FC, Schwartz WB. The syndrome of inappropriate secretion of antidiuretic hormones. *Am J Med* 1967;42:790–806.
61. Azzopardi JG, Williams ED. Pathology of non-endocrine tumors associated with Cushing's syndrome. *Cancer* 1968;22:274–286.
62. Solva OL, Becker KL, Primack A, et al. Ectopic secretion of calcitonin by oat cell carcinoma. *N Engl J Med* 1974;290:1122–1124.
63. Tsutsumi Y, Osamura Y, Watanabe K, et al. Cytogenesis and pathological alterations of human bronchial neuroendocrine cells: an immunohistochemical study. *Pathol Clin Med* 1983;1:298–319 [in Japanese with English abstract].
64. Cuttitta F, Carney DN, Mulshine J, et al. Bombesin-like peptide can function as autocrine growth factors in human small-cell lung cancer. *Nature* 1985;316:823–826.
65. Valaitis J, Warren S, Gamble D. Increasing incidence of adenocarcinoma of the lung. *Cancer* 1981;47:1042–1046.
66. Travis WD, Travis LB, Devesa SS. Lung cancer. *Cancer* 1995;75:191–202.
67. Kodama T, Watanabe S, Shimosato Y, et al. Endobronchial polypoid adenocarcinoma of the lung: histological and ultrastructural studies of five cases. *Am J Surg Pathol* 1984;8: 845–854.
68. Hirata H, Noguchi M, Shimosato Y, et al. Clinicopathologic and immunohistochemical characteristics of bronchial gland cell type adenocarcinoma of the lung. *Am J Clin Pathol* 1990;93:20–25.
69. Shimosato Y. Bronchial gland type adenocarcinoma. In Corrin B, ed. *Pathology of Lung Tumors.* New York: Churchill Livingstone, 1997:135–147.
70. Shimosato Y, Hashimoto T, Kodama T, et al. Prognostic implications of fibrotic focus (scar) in small peripheral lung cancers. *Am J Surg Pathol* 1980;4:365–373.
71. Tsumuraya M, Kodama T, Shimosato Y, et al. Light and electron microscopic analysis of intranuclear inclusion in papillary adenocarcinoma of the lung. *Acta Cytol* 1981;25: 523–532.
72. Montes M, Binette JP, Chaudhry AP, et al. Clara cell adenocarcinoma: light and electron microscopic studies. *Am J Surg Pathol* 1977;1:93–108.
73. Kimula Y. A histochemical and ultrastructural study of adenocarcinoma of the lung. *Am J Surg Pathol* 1978;2:253–264.
74. Shijubo N, Itoh Y, Yamaguchi T, et al. Clara cell protein-positive epithelial cells are reduced in small airway of asthmatics. *Am J Respir Crit Care Med* 1999;160:930–933.
75. Linnoila RI, Szabo E, DeMayo F, et al. The role of CC10 in pulmonary carcinogenesis: from a marker to tumor suppression. *Ann N Y Acad Sci* 2000;923:249–267.
76. Singh G, Katyal SL, Torikata C. Carcinoma of type II pneumocytes: immunodiagnosis of a subtype of "bronchioloalveolar carcinoma." *Am J Pathol* 1981;102:195–208.
77. Mizutani Y, Nakajima T, Morinaga S, et al. Immunohistochemical localization of pulmonary surfactant apoproteins in various lung tumors, with special reference to lung adenocarcinoma subtypes. *Cancer* 1988;61:532–537.
78. Silver SA, Askin FB. True papillary carcinoma of the lung: a distinct clinicopathologic entity. *Am J Surg Pathol* 1997;21:43–51.
79. Clayton F. The spectrum and significance of bronchioloalveolar carcinomas. *Pathol Annu* 1988;23:361–394.
80. Miyoshi T, Satoh Y, Okumura S, et al. Early-stage lung adenocarcinoma with a micropapillary pattern, a distinct pathologic marker for a significantly poor prognosis. *Am J Surg Pathol* 2003;27:101–109.
81. Aoyagi Y, Yokose T, Minami Y, et al. Accumulation of losses of heterozygosity and multistep carcinogenesis in pulmonary adenocarcinoma. *Cancer Res* 2001;61:7950–7954.
82. Iijima T, Minami Y, Nakamura N, et al. MMP-2 activation and stepwise progression of pulmonary adenocarcinoma: analysis of MMP-2 and MMP-9 with gelatin zymography. *Pathol Int* 2004;54:295–301.
83. Nakamura N, Iijima T, Mase K, et al. Phenotypic differences of proliferating fibroblasts in the stroma of lung adenocarcinoma and normal bronchus tissue. *Cancer Sci* 2004;95: 226–232.
84. Suzuki K, Yokose T, Yoshida J, et al. Prognostic significance of the size of central fibrosis in peripheral adenocarcinoma of the lung. *Ann Thorac Surg* 2000;69:893–897.
85. Yokose T, Suzuki K, Nagai K, et al. Favourable and unfavourable morphological prognostic factors in peripheral adenocarcinoma of the lung 3 cm or less in diameter. *Lung Cancer* 2000;29:179–188.
86. Sakurai H, Maeshima A, Watanabe S, et al. Grade of stromal invasion in small adenocarcinoma of the lung: histological minimal invasion and prognosis. *Am J Surg Pathol* 2004;28: 198–206.
87. Nakatani Y, Kitamura H, Inayama Y, et al. Pulmonary endodermal tumor resembling fetal lung: the optically clear nucleus is rich in biotin. *Am J Surg Pathol* 1994;18:637–642.
88. Bodner SM, Koss MN. Mutations in the p53 gene in pulmonary blastomas: immunohistochemical and molecular studies. *Hum Pathol* 1996;27:1117–1123.
89. Kodama T, Shimosato Y, Watanabe S, et al. Six cases of well differentiated adenocarcinoma simulating fetal lung tubules in pseudoglandular stage. *Am J Surg Pathol* 1984;8:735–744.
90. Nakatani Y, Kitamura H, Inayama Y, et al. Pulmonary adenocarcinoma of the fetal lung type: a clinicopathologic study indicating differences in histology, epidemiology, and natural history of low-grade and high-grade forms. *Am J Surg Pathol* 1998;22:399–411.
91. Warhol MJ, Hickey WF, Corson JM. Malignant mesothelioma: ultrastructural distinction from adenocarcinoma. *Am J Surg Pathol* 1982;6:307–314.
92. Churg A. Immunohistochemical staining for vimentin and keratin in malignant mesothelioma. *Am J Surg Pathol* 1985;9:360–365.
93. Upton M, Hirohashi S, Tome Y, et al. Expression of vimentin in surgically resected adenocarcinoma and large cell carcinomas of lung. *Am J Surg Pathol* 1986;10:560–567.
94. Noguchi M, Nakajima T, Hirohashi S, et al. Immunohistochemical distinction of malignant mesothelioma from pulmonary adenocarcinoma with anti-surfactant apoprotein, anti-Lewis a, and anti-Tn antibodies. *Hum Pathol* 1989;20:53–57.
95. Pecciarini M, Cangi G, Doglioni C. Immunohistochemistry in diagnostic pathology. Identifying the primary site of metastatic carcinoma: the increasing role of immunohistochemistry. *Curr Diagn Pathol* 2001:7:168–175.
96. Yatabe Y, Mitsudomi T, Takahashi T. TTF-1 expression in pulmonary adenocarcinoma. *Am J Surg Pathol* 2002;26:767–773.
97. Sheibani K, Battifora H, Burke JS. Antigenic phenotype of malignant mesotheliomas and

pulmonary adenocarcinoma: an immunohistologic analysis demonstrating the value of Leu M1 antigen. *Am J Pathol* 1986;123:212–219.

98. Warnock ML, Stoloff A, Thor A. Differentiation of adenocarcinoma of the lung from mesothelioma: periodic acid-Schiff, monoclonal antibodies B72.3, and Leu M1. *Am J Pathol* 1988;133:30–38.
99. Attanoos RL, Goddard H, Gibbs AR. Mesothelioma-binding antibodies: thrombomodulin, OV632 and HBME-1 and their use in the diagnosis of malignant mesothelioma. *Histopathology* 1996;29:209–215.
100. Attanoos RL, Webb R, Gibbs AR. CD44H expression in reactive mesothelium, pleural mesothelioma and pulmonary adenocarcinoma. *Histopathology* 1997;30:260–263.
101. Ordoñez NG. The value of antibodies 44-3A6, SM3, HBME-1, and thrombomodulin in differentiating epithelial pleural mesothelioma from lung adenocarcinoma: a comparative study with other commonly used antibodies. *Am J Surg Pathol* 1997;21:1399–1408.
102. Kushitani K, Takeshima Y, Amatya VJ, et al. Immunohistochemical marker panels for distinguishing between epithelioid mesothelioma and lung adenocarcinoma. *Pathol Int* 2007;57:190–199.
103. Ordoñez NG, Mackay B. The roles of immunohistochemistry and electron microscopy in distinguishing epithelial mesothelioma of the pleura from adenocarcinoma. *Adv Anat Pathol* 1996;3:273–293.
104. Nicholson AG, McCormick CJ, Shimosato Y, et al. The value of PE-10, a monoclonal antibody against pulmonary surfactant, in distinguishing primary and metastatic lung tumours. *Histopathology* 1995;27:57–60.
105. Savera AT, Torres FX, Linden MD, et al. Primary versus metastatic pulmonary adenocarcinoma: an immunohistochemical study using villin and cytokeratin 7 and 20. *Appl Immunohistochem* 1996;4:86–94.
106. Chu P, Wu E, Weiss LM. Cytokeratin 7 and cytokeratin 20 expression of epithelial neoplasms: a survey of 435 cases. *Mod Pathol* 2000;13:962–972.
107. Rubin BP, Skarin AT, Pisick E, et al. Use of cytokeratins 7 and 20 in determining the origin of metastatic carcinoma of unknown primary, with special emphasis on lung cancer. *Eur J Cancer Prev* 2001;10:77–82.
108. Takise A, Kodama T, Shimosato Y, et al. Histopathological prognostic factors in adenocarcinomas of the peripheral lung less than 2 cm in diameter. *Cancer* 1988;61:2083–2088.
109. Kitamura H, Kameda Y, Nakamura N, et al. Atypical adenomatous hyperplasia and bronchioloalveolar lung carcinoma. Analysis by morphometry and the expression of p53 and carcinoembryonic antigen. *Am J Surg Pathol* 1996;20:553–562.
110. Niki T, Kohno T, Iba S, et al. Frequent co-localization of Cox-2 and laminin-5 gamma 2 chain at the invasive front of early-stage lung adenocarcinoma. *Am J Pathol* 2002;160:1129–1141.
111. Onn A, Correa AM, Gilcrease M, et al. Synchronous overexpression of epidermal growth factor receptor and HER2-neu protein is a predictor of poor outcome in patients with stage I non-small cell lung cancer. *Clin Cancer Res* 2004;10:136–143.
112. Yatabe Y, Masuda A, Koshikawa T, et al. p27KIP1 in human lung cancers: differential changes in small cell and non-small-cell carcinomas. *Cancer Res* 1998;58:1042–1047.
113. Kawasaki M, Noguchi M, Morikawa A, et al. Nuclear p53 accumulation by small-sized adenocarcinomas of the lung. *Pathol Int* 1996;46:486–490.
114. Saad RS, Liu YL, Han H et al. Prognostic significance of thyroid transcription factor-1 expression in both early-stage conventional adenocarcinoma and bronchioloalveolar carcinoma of the lung. *Hum Pathol* 2004;35:3–7.
115. Gorgoulis VG, Vassiliou LV, Karakaidos P, et al. Activation of the DNA damage checkpoint and genomic instability in human precancerous lesions. *Nature* 2005;434:907–913.
116. Kawasaki M, Noguchi M, Morikawa A, et al. Nuclear p53 accumulation by small-sized adenocarcinomas of the lung. *Pathol Int* 1996;46:486–490.
117. Kameya T, Shimosato Y, Kodama T, et al. Peptide hormone production by adenocarcinomas of the lung: its morphologic basis and histogenetic considerations. *Virchows Arch A Cell Pathol* 1983;400:245–257.
118. Amman RW, Berk JE, Fridhandler L, et al. Hyperamylasemia with carcinoma of the lung. *Ann Intern Med* 1973;78:521–525.
119. Gomi K, Kameya T, Tsumuraya M, et al. Ultrastructural, histochemical and biochemical studies of two cases with amylase, ACTH, and β-MSH producing tumor. *Cancer* 1976;38:1645–1654.
120. Chang YL, Wu CT, Shih JY, et al. New aspects in clinicopathologic and oncogene studies of 23 pulmonary lymphoepithelioma-like carcinoma. *Am J Surg Pathol* 2002;26:715–723.
121. Shimazaki H, Aida S, Sato M, et al. Lung carcinoma with rhabdoid cells: a clinicopathological study and survival analysis of 14 cases. *Histopathology* 2001;38:425–434.
122. Asano S, Urabe A, Okabe T, et al. Demonstration of granulopoietic factor(s) in the plasma of nude mice transplanted with a human lung cancer and in the tumor tissue. *Blood* 1977;49:845–852.
123. Shimosato Y, Kameya T, Hirohashi S. Growth morphology and functions of xenotransplanted human tumors. In Sommers SC, Rosen PP, eds. *Pathology Annual 1979.* Part 2. New York: Appleton-Century-Crofts, 1979:215–257.
124. Fusco FD, Rosen SW. Gonadotropin producing anaplastic large cell carcinoma of the lung. *N Engl J Med* 1966;275:507–515.
125. Gould VE, Chejfec G. Ultrastructural and biochemical analysis of "undifferentiated" pulmonary carcinoma. *Hum Pathol* 1978;9:377–384.
126. Gazdar AF, Linnoila I. The pathology of lung cancer: changing concepts and newer diagnostic techniques. *Semin Oncol* 1988;15:215–225.
127. Travis WD, Linnoila RI, Tsokos MG, et al. Neuroendocrine tumors of the lung with proposed criteria for large-cell neuroendocrine carcinoma: an ultrastructural, immunohistochemical, and flow cytometric study of 35 cases. *Am J Surg Pathol* 1991;15:529–533.
128. Jiang SX, Kameya T, Sato Y, et al. Bcl-2 protein expression in lung cancer and close correlation with neuroendocrine differentiation. *Am J Pathol* 1996;148:837–846.
129. Brambilla E, Negoescu A, Gazzeri S, et al. Apoptosis-related factors p53, Bcl-2 and Bax in neuroendocrine lung tumors. *Am J Pathol* 1996;149:1941–1952.
130. Churg A. The fine structure of large cell undifferentiated carcinoma of the lung: evidence for its relation to squamous cell carcinomas and adenocarcinomas. *Hum Pathol* 1978;9:143–156.
131. Horie A, Ohta M. Ultrastructural features of large cell carcinoma of the lung with reference to the prognosis of patients. *Hum Pathol* 1981;12:423–432.
132. Takamori S, Noguchi M, Morinaga S, et al. Clinicopathologic characteristics of adenosquamous carcinoma of the lung. *Cancer* 1991;67:649–654.
133. Bergmann M, Ackerman LV, Kemler RL. Carcinosarcoma of the lung: review of the literature and report of two cases treated by pneumonectomy. *Cancer* 1951;4:919–929.
134. Koss MN, Hochholzer L, Frommelt RA. Carcinosarcoma of the lung: a clinicopathologic study of 66 patients. *Am J Surg Pathol* 1999;23:1514–1526.
135. Thompson L, Chang B, Barsky SH. Monoclonal origin of malignant mixed tumors (carcinosarcomas): evidence for divergent histogenesis. *Am J Surg Pathol* 1996;20:277–285.
136. Barnard WG. Embryoma of lung. *Thorax* 1952;7:229–301.
137. Spencer H. Pulmonary blastoma. *J Pathol Bacteriol* 1961;82:161–165.
138. Colby TV, Koss MN, Travis WD. Tumors of the lower respiratory tract. In Rosai J, ed. *Atlas of Tumor Pathology.* 3rd series, fascicle 13. Washington, DC: Armed Forces Institute of Pathology, 1995:395–403.
139. Hachitanda Y, Aoyama C, Sato JK, Shimada H. Pleuropulmonary blastoma in childhood: a tumor of divergent differentiation. *Am J Surg Pathol* 1993;17:382–391.
140. Bensch KG, Gordon GB, Miller LR. Electron microscopic and biochemical studies on the bronchial carcinoid tumor. *Cancer* 1965;18:592–602.
141. Bensch KG, Gordon GB, Miller LR. Studies on the bronchial counterpart of the Kultschitzky (argentaffin) cell and innervation of bronchial gland. *J Ultrastruct Res* 1965;12:668–686.
142. Dube VE. Peripheral bronchial carcinoid with spindle-cell pattern. *Arch Pathol* 1970;89:374–377.
143. Patel K, Moore SE, Dickson G, et al. Neural cell adhesion molecule (NCAM) is the antigen recognized by monoclonal antibodies of similar specificity in small-cell lung carcinoma and neuroblastoma. *Int J Cancer* 1989;44:573–578.
144. Barbareschi M, Frigo B, Mosca L, et al. Bronchial carcinoids with S-100 positive sustentacular cells: a comparative study with gastrointestinal carcinoids, pheochromocytomas and paragangliomas. *Pathol Res Pract* 1990;186:212–222.
145. Goodner JT, Berg JW, Watson WL. The non-benign nature of bronchial carcinoids and cylindromas. *Cancer* 1961;14:539–546.
146. Salyer DC, Salyer WR, Eggleston JC. Bronchial carcinoid tumor. *Cancer* 1975;36:1522–1537.
147. Escovitz WE, Reingold IM. Functioning malignant bronchial carcinoid with Cushing's syndrome and recurrent sinus arrest. *Ann Intern Med* 1961;54:1248–1259.
148. Dobek JT. Bronchial carcinoid tumor with acromegaly in two patients. *J Clin Endocrinol Metab* 1974;38:329–333.
149. Arrigoni MG, Woolner LB, Bernatz PE. Atypical carcinoid tumors of the lung. *J Thorac Cardiovasc Surg* 1972;64:413–421.
150. Travis WD, Rush W, Fieder DB, et al. Survival analysis of 200 pulmonary neuroendocrine tumors with clarification of criteria for atypical carcinoid and its separation from typical carcinoid. *Am J Surg Pathol* 1998;22:934–944.
151. Shimosato Y, Kodama T. Low grade malignant and benign tumors. In McDowell EM, ed. *Lung Carcinomas.* Edinburgh: Churchill Livingstone, 1987:310–329.
152. Thurnbull AD, Huvos AG, Goodner JT, Foote FW. Mucoepidermoid tumors of bronchial glands. *Cancer* 1971;28:539–544.
153. Axelsson C, Burcharth F, Johansen A. Mucoepidermoid lung tumors. *J Thorac Cardivasc Surg* 1973;65:902–908.
154. Fechner RE, Bentinck BR, Askew JB. Acinic cell tumor of the lung: a histologic and ultrastructural study. *Cancer* 1972;29:501–508.
155. Wilson RW, Moran CA. Epithelial-myoepithelial carcinoma of the lung: immunohistochemical and ultrastructural observation and review of the literature. *Hum Pathol* 1997;28:631–635.
156. Fulford LG, Kamata Y, Okudera K, et al. Epithelial-myoepithelial carcinomas of the bronchus. *Am J Surg Pathol* 2001;25:1508–1514.
157. Miura K, Harada H, Aiba S, TsuTsui Y. Myoepithelial carcinoma of the lung arising from bronchial submucosa. *Am J Surg Pathol* 2000;24:1300–1304.
158. Kameya T. Salivary gland type tumors. In National Cancer Center Hospital. *Cancer of the Lung: Diagnosis and Treatment.* Vol. 1. Tokyo: Kodansha, 1983:179–190 [in Japanese].
159. Dail DH, Liebow AA. Intravascular bronchioloalveolar tumor [Abstract]. *Am J Pathol* 1975;78:6a.
160. Bhagavan SB, Murthy MS, Dorfman HD, et al. Intravascular bronchiolo-alveolar tumor (IVBAT): a low-grade sclerosing epithelioid angiosarcoma of lung. *Am J Surg Pathol* 1982;6:41–52.
161. Morinaga S, Watanabe H, Genma A, et al. Plasmacytoma of the lung associated with nodular deposits of immunoglobulin: report of a case. *Am J Surg Pathol* 1987;11:989–999.
162. Reid JD, Mehta VT. Melanoma of the lower respiratory tract. *Cancer* 1966;19:627–631.
163. Wilson RW, Moran CA. Primary melanoma of the lung: a clinicopathologic and immunohistochemical study of eight cases. *Am J Surg Pathol* 1997;21:1196–1202.
164. Korn D, Bensch K, Liebow AA, et al. Multiple minute pulmonary tumors resembling chemodectoma. *Am J Pathol* 1960;37:641–672.
165. Corrin B. Unusual tumours and tumour-like conditions of the lung. *Curr Diagn Pathol* 1996;3:1–13.
166. Liebow AA, Castleman B. Benign clear cell tumors of the lung [Abstract]. *Am J Pathol* 1963;43:13a.
167. Hornick JL, Fletcher CD. PEComa: what do we know so far? *Histopathology* 2006;48:75–82.
168. Moran CA, Hochholzer L, Rush W, et al. Primary intrapulmonary meningiomas: a clinicopathologic and immunohistochemical study of ten cases. *Cancer* 1996;78:2328–2333.
169. Haas JE, Yunis EJ, Totter RS. Ultrastructure of a sclerosing hemangioma of the lung. *Cancer* 1972;30:512–518.
170. Hill GS, Eggleston JC. Electron microscopic study of so called "pulmonary sclerosing hemangioma": report of a case suggesting epithelial origin. *Cancer* 1972;30:1092–1106.

171. Katzenstein AA, Fulling K, Weise DL, et al. So-called sclerosing hemangioma of the lung: evidence for mesothelial origin. *Am J Surg Pathol* 1983;7:3–14.

172. Noguchi M, Kodama T, Morinaga S, et al. Multiple "sclerosing hemangioma" of the lung. *Am J Surg Pathol* 1986;10:429–435.

173. Tanaka I, Inoue M, Matsui Y, et al. A case of pneumocytoma (so-called sclerosing hemangioma) with lymph node metastasis. *Jpn J Clin Oncol* 1986;16:77–86.

174. Niho S, Suzuki K, Yokose T, et al. Monoclonality of both pale cells and cuboidal cells of sclerosing hemangioma of the lung. *Am J Pathol* 1998;152:1065–1069.

175. Chan AC, Chan JK. Pulmonary sclerosing hemangioma consistently expresses thyroid transcription factor-1 (TTF-1): a new clue to its histogenesis. *Am J Surg Pathol* 2000;24: 1531–1536.

176. Umiker WO, Iverson L. Postinflammatory "tumors" of the lung: report of four cases simulating xanthoma, fibroma or plasma cell tumor. *J Thorac Surg* 1954;28:55–63.

177. Titus JL, Harrison EG, Clagett OT, et al. Xanthomatous and inflammatory pseudo-tumors of the lung. *Cancer* 1962;15:522–538.

178. Whitwell L. Tumourlets of the lung. *J Pathol Bacteriol* 1955;70:529–541.

179. Bonikos DS, Archibald R, Bensch KG. On the origin of the so called tumorlet of the lung. *Hum Pathol* 1976;7:461–469.

180. Torikata C. Tumorlets of the lung: an ultrastructural study. *Ultrastruct Pathol* 1991;15: 189–195.

181. Miller RR, Muller NL. Neuroendocrine cell hyperplasia and obliterative bronchiolitis in patients with peripheral carcinoid tumors. *Am J Surg Pathol* 1995;19:653–658.

182. McDonald JR, Harrington SW, Clagett OT. Hamartoma (often called chondroma) of the lung. *J Thorac Surg* 1945;14:128–143.

183. Suster S, Moran CA. Pulmonary adenofibroma: report of two cases of an unusual type of hamartomatous lesion of the lung. *Histopathology* 1993;23:547–551.

184. Minami Y, Iijima T, Yamamoto T, et al. Diffuse pulmonary hamartoma: a case report. *Pathol Res Pract* 2005;200:813–816.

185. Wolff M, Silva F, Kaye G. Pulmonary metastases (with admixed epithelial elements) from smooth muscle neoplasms: report of nine cases including three male. *Am J Surg Pathol* 1979;3:325–342.

186. Shimosato Y, Kameya T, Nagai K, et al. Squamous cell carcinoma of the thymus: an analysis of eight cases. *Am J Surg Pathol* 1977;1:109–121.

187. Shimosato Y, Mukai K. Tumors of the mediastinum. In Rosai J, ed. *Atlas of Tumor Pathology.* 3rd series, fascicle 21. Washington, DC: Armed Forces Institute of Pathology, 1997:40–158, 183–207.

188. Asamura H, Morinaga S, Shimosato Y, et al. Thymoma displaying endobronchial polypoid growth. *Chest* 1988;94:647–649.

189. Ordoñez NG. Value of thyroid transcription factor-1, E-cadherin, BG8, WT1, and CD44S immunostaining in distinguishing epithelial pleural mesothelioma from pulmonary and nonpulmonary adenocarcinoma. *Am J Surg Pathol* 2000;24:598–606.

190. Kaufmann O, Dietel M. Expression of thyroid transcription factor-1 in pulmonary and extrapulmonary small-cell carcinomas and other neuroendocrine carcinomas of various primary sites. *Histopathology* 2000;36:415–420.

191. Oliveira AM, Tazelaar HD, Myers JL, et al. Thyroid transcription factor-1 distinguishes metastatic pulmonary from well-differentiated neuroendocrine tumors of other sites. *Am J Surg Pathol* 2001;25:815–819.

192. Noguchi M, Maezawa N, Nakanishi Y, et al. Application of the p53 gene mutation pattern for differential diagnosis of primary versus metastatic lung carcinomas. *Diagn Mol Pathol* 1993;2:29–35.

193. Miyake Y, Kodama T, Yamaguchi K. Pro-gastrin-releasing peptide (31–98) is a specific tumor marker in patients with small cell lung carcinoma. *Cancer Res* 1994;54:2136–2240.

194. Gazdar AF, Helman LJ, Israel MA, et al. Expression of neuroendocrine cell markers l-Dopa decarboxylase, chromogranin A, and dense core granules in human tumors of endocrine and non-endocrine origin. *Cancer Res* 1988;48:4078–4082.

195. Tome Y, Hirohashi S, Noguchi M, et al. Immunocytologic diagnosis of small-cell lung cancer in imprint smears. *Acta Cytol* 1991;35:485–490.

196. Kaufmann O, Georgi T, Dietel M. Utility of 123C3 monoclonal antibody against CD56 (NCAM) for the diagnosis of small-cell carcinomas on paraffin sections. *Hum Pathol* 1997; 28:1373–1378.

197. Lantuejoul S, Moro D, Michalides RJ, et al. Neural cell adhesion molecules (NCAM) and NCAM-PSA expression in neuroendocrine lung tumors. *Am J Surg Pathol* 1998;22: 1267–1276.

198. Ionescu DN, Treaba D, Gilks CB, et al. Nonsmall cell lung carcinoma with neuroendocrine differentiation—an entity of no clinical or prognostic significances. *Am J Surg Pathol* 2007; 31:26–32.

199. Kuroki Y, Dempo K, Akino T. Immunohistochemical study of human pulmonary surfactant apoproteins with monoclonal antibody: pathologic application for hyaline membrane disease. *Am J Pathol* 1986;124:25–33.

200. Yokose T, Ito Y, Ochiai A. High prevalence of atypical adenomatous hyperplasia of the lung in autopsy specimens from elderly patients with malignant neoplasms. *Lung Cancer* 2000;29:125–130.

201. Tanaka H, Yanagisawa K, Shinjo K, et al. Lineage-specific dependency of lung adenocarcinoma on the lung development regulator TTF-1. *Cancer Res* 2007;67:6007–6011.

202. Hirohashi S, Ino Y, Kodama T, et al. Distribution of blood group antigens A, B, H and I(Ma) in mucus-producing adenocarcinoma of human lung. *J Natl Cancer Inst* 1984;72: 1299–1305.

203. Yoshida K, Morinaga S, Shimosato Y, et al. A cell kinetic study of pulmonary adenocarcinoma by an immunoperoxidase procedure after bromodeoxyuridine labeling. *Cancer* 1989;64:2284–2291.

204. Yang WI, Efird JT, Quintanilla-Martinez L, et al. Cell kinetic study of thymic epithelial tumors using PCNA (PC 10) and Ki-67 (MIB 1) antibodies. *Hum Pathol* 1996;27:70–76.

205. Brown DC, Gatter KC. Monoclonal antibody Ki-67: its use in histopathology. *Histopathology* 1990;17:489–503.

206. Murashima A, Takasaki Y, Ohgaki M, et al. Activated peripheral blood mononuclear cells detected by murine monoclonal antibodies to proliferating cell nuclear antigen in active lupus patients. *J Clin Immunol* 1990;10:28–37.

207. Morinaga S, Nakajima T, Shimosato Y. Normal and neoplastic myoepithelial cells in salivary glands: an immunohistochemical study. *Hum Pathol* 1987;18:1218–1226.

208. Wistuba II, Behrens C, Milchgrub S, et al. Sequential molecular abnormalities are involved in the multistage development of squamous cell lung carcinoma. *Oncogene* 1999;18: 643–650.

209. Anami Y, Takeuchi T, Mase K, et al. Amplotyping of microdissected, methanol-fixed lung carcinoma by arbitrarily primed polymerase chain reaction. *Int J Cancer* 2000;89:19–25.

210. Noguchi M, Hirohashi S, Hara F, et al. Heterogeneous amplification of myc family oncogenes in small cell lung carcinoma. *Cancer* 1990;66:2053–2058.

211. Kawanishi M, Kohno T, Otsuka T, et al. Allelotype and replication error phenotype of small cell lung carcinoma. *Carcinogenesis* 1997;18:2057–2062.

212. Westra WH, Baas IO, Hruban RH, et al. K-ras oncogene activation in atypical alveolar hyperplasias of the human lung. *Cancer Res* 1996;56:2224–2228.

213. Kawasaki M, Noguchi M, Morikawa A, et al. Nuclear 53 accumulation by small-sized adenocarcinoma of the lung. *Pathol Int* 1996;46:486–490.

214. Dai Y, Morishita Y, Mase K, et al. Application of the p53 and K-ras gene mutation patterns for cytologic diagnosis of recurrent lung carcinomas. *Cancer* 2000;90:258–263.

215. Hou M, Morishita Y, Iijima T, et al. DNA methylation and expression of p16(INK4A) gene in pulmonary adenocarcinoma and anthracosis in background lung. *Int J Cancer* 1999;84:609–613.

216. Tanaka R, Wang D, Morishita Y, et al. Loss of function of p16 gene and prognosis of pulmonary adenocarcinoma. *Cancer* 2005;103;608–615.

217. Paez JG, Janne PA, Lee JC, et al. EGFR mutations in lung cancer. Correlation with clinical response to gefitinib therapy. *Science* 2004;304:1497–1500.

218. Minami Y, Shimamura T, Shah K, et al. The major lung cancer-derived mutants of ERBB2 are oncogenic and are associated with sensitivity to the irreversible EGFR/ERBB2 inhibitor HKI-272. *Oncogene* 2007;26:5023–5027.

219. Yatabe Y, Kosaka T, Takahashi T, et al. EGFR mutation is specific for terminal respiratory unit type adenocarcinoma. *Am J Surg Pathol* 2005;29:633–639.

220. Garber ME, Troyanskaya OG, Shluens K, et al. Diversity of gene expression in adenocarcinoma of the lung. *Proc Natl Acad Sci U S A* 2001;98:13784–13789.

221. Bhattacharjee A, Richards WG, Staunton J, et al. Classification of human lung carcinomas by mRNA expression profiling reveals distinct adenocarcinoma subclasses. *Proc Natl Acad Sci U S A* 2001;98:13790–13795.

222. Jones MH, Virtanen C, Horioh D, et al. Two prognostically significant subtypes of high-grade lung neuroendocrine tumours independent of small-cell and large-cell neuroendocrine carcinoma identified by gene expression profiles. *Lancet* 2004;363:775–781.

The Pleura

The term *mesothelium* is generally reserved for the monolayer of flattened cells with epithelial features that lines serous cavities. The term derives from a combination of the cells' mesodermal origin and their epithelial phenotype. The major function of mesothelium is to provide a smooth, low-friction surface to facilitate the gliding motion of the lungs in the pleural cavity, the heart in the pericardial sac, and the viscera in the abdominal cavity. This lubrication process is assisted by the presence of myriad bushy surface microvilli coated with hyaluronic acid–rich glycoproteins secreted by the mesothelial cells (1). The mesothelial cells overlie an ill-defined layer of specialized mesenchymal cells involved in the constant repair of the surface mesothelium.

Although neoplasms of mesothelial origin are rare, they have received a disproportionate amount of attention as a result of their relation to occupational and environmental exposure to asbestos. Such neoplasms are a leading cause of lawsuits in developed countries and often present difficult diagnostic problems to the surgical pathologist. This chapter, therefore, focuses primarily on the diagnostic aspects of mesothelioma. However, to better understand some of the various histologic appearances of mesothelium-derived neoplasms, it is helpful to briefly review some features of mesothelial reactions to injury. For a comprehensive review of this subject, see the excellent reviews by Whitaker and colleagues (2,3).

THE REACTIVE MESOTHELIUM

REGENERATION

Following a variety of injuries to the mesothelium, including chemical or mechanical exfoliation, the proximity of an inflammatory or neoplastic process, or its exposure to asbestos fibers, there is an initial loss of the surface cell monolayer followed by the deposition of fibrin, leukocytes, and macrophages (4). Soon—particularly when the irritative stimulus persists—layers of proliferating spindle-shaped cells, indistinguishable from fibroblasts but with a characteristic immunophenotype, appear underneath this layer of fibrin. Evidence suggests that these fibroblast-like cells may play an important role in the restoration of the mesothelial surface layer.

Raftery (5) provided evidence that perivascular cells resembling fibroblasts proliferate under areas of experimentally denuded peritoneum, suggesting that they are the forerunners for a newly formed mesothelial layer. Immunohistochemical studies with antibodies to keratins support this interpretation. Bolen et al. (6) found that normal surface mesothelium expressed both low– and high–molecular-weight keratins, whereas the resting submesothelial cells only expressed vimentin. However, they also found that reactive, proliferating, subserosal fibroblast-like cells coexpressed low–molecular-weight keratins and vimentin. During the process of mesothelial repair, these

specialized fibroblast-like cells gradually acquire more cytoplasm and, as they approach the surface, become rounded and develop epithelial phenotypic and immunophenotypic characteristics, such as expression of high– and low–molecular-weight keratins, and loss or reduction of vimentin expression (Figs. 27.1 and 27.2). This appears to be an exclusive property of the submesothelial mesenchyme.

It is important to emphasize that these subserosal cytokeratin-expressing reactive cells, if not correctly identified, may be a source of diagnostic error, particularly in the distinction between desmoplastic malignant mesothelioma and fibrous pleurisy.

MESOTHELIAL HYPERPLASIA VERSUS MESOTHELIOMA

Unambiguous distinction between malignant epithelial mesothelioma and adenocarcinoma is now relatively easy as a result of recent advances in immunohistochemistry. However, the distinction between mesothelial hyperplasia and mesothelioma continues to be a difficult diagnostic challenge for which immunohistochemistry is still of limited value (7).

EPITHELIAL PROLIFERATIONS

Any chronic irritation may cause hyperplasia of the epithelial-appearing mesothelial cells of the serous mesothelial surface, as well as the submesothelial cytokeratin-expressing spindle cells. Because it may be very difficult to distinguish the epithelial component of such hyperplasias from incipient, well-differen-

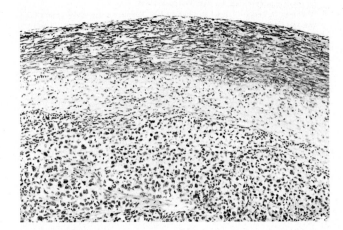

Figure 27.1. Section of small intestine from a case of malignant melanoma with intestinal metastases. Note the bandlike distribution of keratin-positive spindle cells overlying the keratin-negative mesenchymal and neoplastic cells. Stained with a cocktail of monoclonal antibodies to pancytokeratins; hematoxylin counterstained.

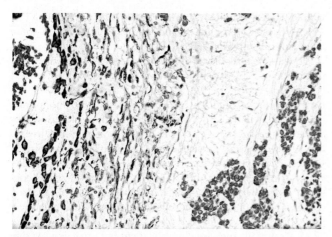

Figure 27.2. Serosal involvement by oat cell carcinoma. Stained with a cocktail of monoclonal antibodies to low–molecular-weight keratins; hematoxylin counterstained. Note a sharply demarcated band of keratin-positive reactive subserosal mesothelial cells. The more superficial cells are plumper and have epithelial features.

tiated epithelial mesothelioma, it is very important to base the diagnosis in such cases on a careful evaluation of the total clinical and radiologic picture (7,8).

True invasion of the underlying tissue, particularly adipose tissue and skeletal muscle of the parietal pleura, remains the most reliable criterion of malignancy in epithelial-appearing mesothelial proliferations. However, it is important not to confuse entrapped mesothelial cells with invasiveness. Entrapped mesothelial cells are usually close to the pleural surface and are well delimited from the underlying adipose tissue, which they do not invade. Reactive fibrosis and inflammatory infiltrates are often present around and near the entrapped mesothelial cells (Fig. 27.3). Clearly, generous and nonfragmented biopsy specimens are essential to avoid error.

The appearance of the pleural surface, particularly at the time of thoracoscopy or thoracotomy, plays an important role in this differential diagnosis. The presence of confluent tumor nodules over large areas of the pleural surface favors malignancy. Absence of such nodules favors a reactive process. Additionally, malignant mesothelioma may be made up of monotonous tumor cells with little or moderate atypia. Additionally, reactive mesothelial cells may show atypical features. Thus, cytologic atypia, unless severe, may not be a reliable criterion for malignancy. The presence of tubular and papillary patterns of growth favors mesothelioma because these patterns are rarely seen in mesothelial hyperplasia.

FIBROUS PROLIFERATIONS

In the distinction between fibrous pleuritis and desmoplastic malignant mesothelioma, particular attention should be placed to the presence of zonation because it strongly favors a reactive process (7). The term *zonation* means a higher cellularity (and at times atypia) of spindle-shaped, cytokeratin-positive mesothelial cells toward the pleural surface, with less cellular and more collagenous layers beneath (see illustrative case 4 presented later in this chapter). Often fibrinous deposits and capillaries growing perpendicular to the surface are noted in reactive processes. However, it is important to emphasize that a reactive and fibrous pleuritis may be caused by the presence of an underlying malignancy, including mesothelioma. Ample and deep sampling, as partial decortication of the parietal pleural lesions, is thus very helpful. It cannot be overemphasized that a diagnosis of desmoplastic malignant mesothelioma must rest on the clear evidence of invasiveness (see illustrative case 5 presented later in this chapter).

ROLE OF IMMUNOHISTOCHEMISTRY IN THE DISTINCTION BETWEEN HYPERPLASIA AND NEOPLASIA

Immunohistochemistry, as will be discussed later in greater detail, helps to identify the mesothelial lineage of the proliferating

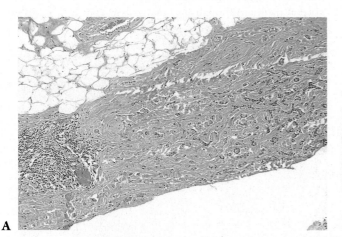

A

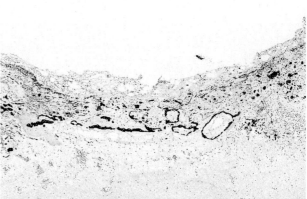

B

Figure 27.3. **(A)** Entrapped reactive mesothelial cells in chronic irritation of serous membrane. Note dense collagen surrounding mesothelial cells, predominance of small glandular spaces, and chronic inflammatory infiltrates. Most important, the reactive cells are sharply demarcated from the underlying adipose tissue (hematoxylin and eosin stained). **(B)** Another example of reactive mesothelium with predominant epithelial maturation. Stained with a cocktail to pancytokeratins. This stain highlights the sharp demarcation from underlying mesenchyme.

cells but is of limited value to distinguish between mesothelial hyperplasia and mesothelioma. However, pancytokeratin stains may be useful to identify invasiveness (see Fig. 27.19).

Although some have reported that p53 protein is frequently overexpressed by mesothelioma and not by reactive mesothelial proliferations (9–11), others have found otherwise (12–14). Moreover, studies using molecular biologic methods have revealed a low rate of p53 mutations in mesothelioma (14). Nonetheless, in an isolated case, strong nuclear immunostaining for p53 by the majority of the mesothelial cells supports mesothelioma over hyperplasia.

Recently, Kato et al. (15) have reported that GLUT-1, a member of the family of glucose transporter isoforms, may be a potential new marker for distinguishing benign reactive mesothelium from malignant epithelial mesothelioma. They reported GLUT-1 expression in 100% of 40 mesotheliomas and in none of 40 cases of reactive mesothelium. If independently validated, this may be a useful marker of mesothelial malignancy.

Chiosea et al. (16) have reported that fluorescence in situ hybridization (FISH) analysis on paraffin-embedded tissue demonstrated the homozygous deletion of the 9p21 locus in 35 (67%) of 52 pleural mesotheliomas and in none of 40 cases of reactive pleural mesothelial proliferations (16). Again, if independently validated, this may be another helpful ancillary test for this differential diagnosis.

PLEURAL FIBROSIS AND PLEURAL PLAQUE

Chronic injury to the pleural surface may result in the formation of dense layers of scarlike tissue involving visceral as well as parietal pleura. Among causes of pleural fibrosis are asbestosis and other pneumoconiosis, inflammatory pleurisy including rheumatoid pleuritis, and, most commonly, bacterial pneumonias. Pleural fibrosis also may result from the intentional introduction of irritants (such as talcum powder) into the pleural cavity to promote therapeutic pleural fusion (pleurodesis).

A frequent area of diagnostic difficulty is the distinction between fibrous pleuritis and desmoplastic malignant mesothelioma, and this is now one of the most common requests to the

United States–Canadian Mesothelioma Reference Panel (7). This difficult differential diagnosis will be discussed in some detail later in this chapter.

These forms of pleural fibrosis should not be confused with pleural plaques, which are, in the vast majority of cases, caused by asbestos exposure (17,18). Pleural plaques arise over the parietal pleura particularly at the lower chest and the diaphragmatic pleura. Usually they develop two to three decades after asbestos exposure. Grossly, they consist of well-delimited, irregularly shaped, raised, grayish-white to ivory plaques ranging in size from tiny specks to several centimeters. They have a cartilaginous consistency and often calcify. Microscopically, they consist of dense strands of virtually acellular, intensely hyalinized collagen fibers that feature a reticulated, meshlike appearance, a pattern that has been referred to as "basket weave" (Fig. 27.4). Pleural plaques are clinically silent but serve as a reliable marker of asbestos exposure. It has been shown that pleural and peritoneal plaques contain asbestos fibers, particularly chrysotile (19–21).

BENIGN TUMORS OF THE PLEURA AND SUBPLEURAL TISSUES

BENIGN LOCALIZED EPITHELIAL MESOTHELIOMA (ADENOMATOID TUMOR)

Benign localized epithelial mesotheliomas of the pleura are exceedingly rare. The few that have been reported were found incidentally at lung resection for other conditions. Histologically, they were similar to the more common pelvic peritoneal adenomatoid tumors (22–24).

LOCALIZED FIBROUS TUMOR

These rare neoplasms, also called solitary fibrous tumors and localized fibrous mesothelioma, usually are discovered as asymptomatic lesions on routine chest radiographs in patients of any age, with no sex predilection and with no evident relation to asbestos exposure. Most of these tumors arise at the level of the visceral pleura. Although they may grossly appear to infiltrate

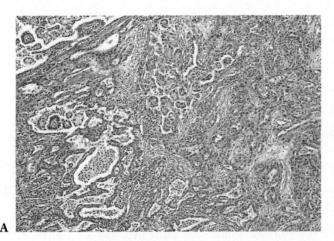

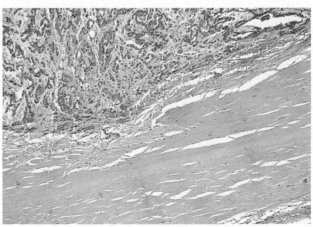

A **B**

Figure 27.4. (A) Malignant epithelial mesothelioma illustrating the typical tubulopapillary pattern of growth. **(B)** Predominantly tubular malignant epithelial mesothelioma overlying typical pleural plaque. Both hematoxylin and eosin stained.

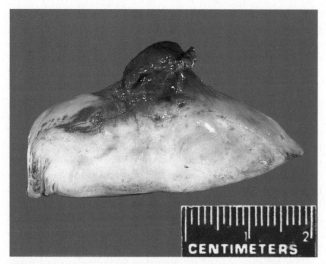

Figure 27.5. Pedunculated localized fibrous tumor of pleura, resected with a small portion of lung, partially transected to show the cut surface. The tumor is predominantly exophytic but mushroom shaped, and the overlying mesothelial surface appears smooth and shiny.

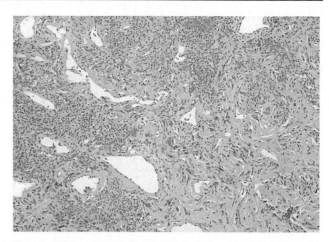

Figure 27.7. Section from another localized fibrous tumor of the pleura showing focal cytologic atypia. However, mitoses are not increased. These changes are not indicative of malignant transformation. Hematoxylin and eosin stained.

the pulmonary parenchyma, they usually have a sharply delimited pushing border and are often pedunculated (Fig. 27.5). They tend to measure several centimeters in diameter and are usually rounded, firm, white, and scarlike in their gross appearance. Histologically, they are composed of a mixture of spindle-shaped fibroblast-like cells lying within a variable amount of collagenous stroma (Fig. 27.6). Although a storiform pattern of growth may be focally present, more commonly, the cells are distributed randomly. Cell atypia and mitoses are uncommon (Fig. 27.7), but foci of degeneration and cystic change may be present, especially in the larger tumors (25). Nuclear pleomorphism and mitoses may be seen in the larger tumors but do not correlate with poor prognosis if the tumor is circumscribed (26,27).

Although most follow a benign course, local recurrence may develop in as many as 16% of the cases, but recurrences can be successfully managed by repeated resection (28,29).

Localized fibrous tumors have a characteristic immunophenotype (CD34 positive, cytokeratin negative) that is useful to distinguish them from fibrous and desmoplastic mesotheliomas, which invariably express cytokeratins and generally are CD34 negative (Figs. 27.8 and 27.9) (30,31).

Although initially thought to be of mesothelial origin, solitary fibrous tumor is now believed to originate in the subpleural nonmesothelial mesenchyme. Indeed, tumors with similar morphologic features and immunophenotype occur at several extrathoracic locations, further supporting a nonmesothelial origin (32–35).

MALIGNANT MESOTHELIOMA

ETIOLOGY, INCIDENCE, AND PATHOGENESIS

Since 1960, after pioneering studies on the incidence of mesothelioma in South African asbestos miners by Wagner et al. (36),

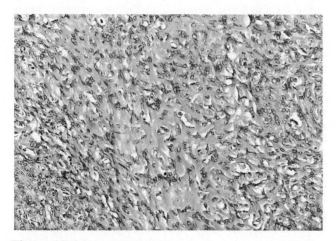

Figure 27.6. Localized fibrous tumor of pleura; typical histologic appearance showing thick hyaline collagen fibers interspersed between bland-appearing spindle cells, singly or in haphazardly distributed short bundles. Hematoxylin and eosin stained.

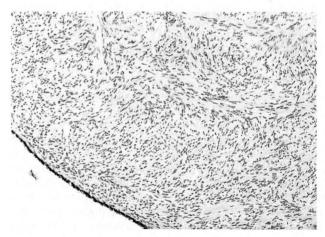

Figure 27.8. Section of the localized fibrous pleural tumor shown in Figure 27.4 immunostained for pancytokeratins. Note the intensely stained, normal-appearing surface mesothelium and absence of staining of the neoplastic cells.

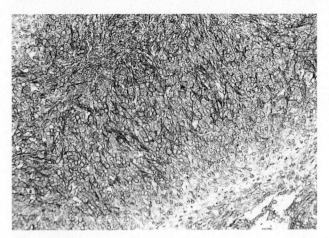

Figure 27.9. Localized fibrous tumor of the pleura immunostained with a monoclonal antibody to CD34. There is strong and uniform staining of the tumor cells, which is a common and diagnostically useful feature of this neoplasm.

the mesothelial carcinogenesis of inhaled asbestos fibers has been firmly established (37–43). Additionally, it is generally accepted that all types of asbestos fibers are capable of causing malignant mesothelioma, usually decades after their inhalation. Moreover, a correlation between the intensity and duration of exposure to asbestos fibers and the risk of developing mesothelioma is well documented (44,45). It also is evident, however, that some mesotheliomas, especially many of those occurring in young people, may not be related to asbestos exposure (46). The incidence of asbestos-related mesothelioma cases has ranged in different series from 10% to 99% (47). Although non–asbestos-related malignant mesotheliomas undoubtedly exist, it is difficult to determine their true incidence for two main reasons: (a) there is no defined threshold of exposure to asbestos fibers in relation to the development of mesothelioma (additionally, the issue of threshold is complicated by the possible effect of individual susceptibility [48]); and (b) there is a decades-long period of latency between the exposure to asbestos and development of the neoplasm (44,49). It was suggested (50) that even a mild exposure, such as that which may occur in the household, may be sufficient to induce mesothelioma. In a review of 668 cases of malignant mesothelioma, McDonald and McDonald (51) found that only 50% of the cases in men and 5% of the cases in women were associated with occupational exposure to asbestos (51). However, Vianna et al. (50) proposed that the wide variation in estimates of asbestos exposure in patients with malignant mesothelioma was a result of inadequate occupational histories.

Experimental and epidemiologic evidence (40,51–55) suggests that other etiologic agents may be associated with mesothelioma as well. Such agents include radiation, minerals such as silica and beryllium, and synthetic fibers, although evidence for the latter is far from conclusive (44). The finding of Simian virus 40–like DNA sequences (SV40) in some cases of human malignant mesothelioma (56,57) suggested that the SV40 virus, which was a contaminant of some polio vaccines, may be implicated as a co-carcinogen or as directly causing mesothelioma. However, more recent studies report a low prevalence of SV40 in mesothelioma patients and suggest that earlier reports were a result of laboratory contamination (58). Of greater signifi-

cance is the fact that several epidemiologic studies have failed to support an etiologic role of SV40 in mesothelioma (59–64).

Malignant mesothelioma is a rare tumor, but its true incidence is difficult to ascertain because it is underreported. McDonald and McDonald (51) estimated the combined United States–Canadian incidence to be 2.8 per million male and 0.7 per million female persons but noted a steady increase in cases in men, which they attributed to occupational exposure to asbestos. A significant increase in the incidence of pleural mesothelioma among white men older than 55 years during the years of 1973 to 1980 was reported by Spirtas et al. (65) after a study of incidence rates based on data from population-based cancer registries in New York State (exclusive of New York City) and Los Angeles County (California) and the Surveillance, Epidemiology and End Results (SEER) Program of the National Cancer Institute. In this study, even after histopathologic review, a notable upward trend remained.

The pathogenesis of malignant mesothelioma remains unclear. The presence of asbestos fibers in the vicinity of the serosal surfaces appears to be a crucial pathogenic factor. In both epidemiologic and experimental studies, differences in the tumorigenicity of asbestos fibers were found, depending of the composition and physical characteristics of the fibers. Contributions of other factors (including heredity and exposure to other carcinogens such as tobacco smoke) to the pathogenesis of mesothelioma are not clear. Nonetheless, there is no compelling evidence that smoking increases the risk for the development of mesothelioma in asbestos workers (66).

CLINICAL FEATURES

Malignant mesothelioma of the pleura is approximately three times more common in men than in women (51,67). Most cases occur in patients between ages 50 and 70 years. Chest pain and shortness of breath are the most frequent initial symptoms; these are followed by weakness, fatigue, and weight loss. Clinical signs of pleural effusion are by far the most common finding at the initial physical examination and, in some cases, may precede the development of clinically detectable mesothelioma by several years (68). Chest roentgenograms or computerized tomography will reveal irregular pleural thickening that is most apparent after evacuation of the pleural fluid. Irregular thickening of the interlobar fissures is another characteristic radiographic feature of pleural mesothelioma. In patients who have had a long or intense exposure to asbestos fibers, the presence of pleural plaque will frequently be discovered by these examinations. The effusions, which often are bloody, tend to recur rapidly after evacuation, but with progressive obliteration of the chest cavity by the growing tumor, they may subside. There may be involvement of pericardium and mediastinum, as well as invasion of the soft tissues of the chest wall, particularly at biopsy sites or at the location of chest tubes after surgery. Metastases are uncommon in the early stages of the disease, but they may be seen in later stages and are a frequent finding at autopsy. Nonetheless, cases of metastatic mesothelioma with initial presentation as lymph node metastases have been reported. However, most of these have been peritoneal mesotheliomas (69).

The average survival time from the onset of symptoms is approximately 15 months, but much longer survivals have been reported (70,71). Patients with pure epithelial mesotheliomas tend to survive longer than those with a sarcomatoid mesothelioma (67,72).

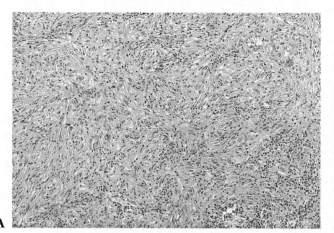
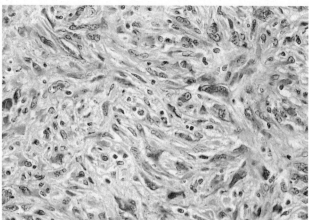

A

B

Figure 27.10. **(A)** Example of sarcomatous mesothelioma. Moderately pleomorphic spindle cells growing in a poorly defined storiform pattern are seen. Hematoxylin and eosin stained. **(B)** Section from same tumor stained for pancytokeratins. Most tumor cells show keratin expression.

The treatment of mesothelioma is generally ineffective. Surgery is of limited benefit for pleural mesothelioma. Radiation therapy and intracavitary instillation of radioactive substances have not been shown to be effective (39,73,74). However, combinations of surgical resection, radiation, and chemotherapy have been found to prolong life in selected cases (75).

PATHOLOGIC FINDINGS

Gross Findings

The gross appearance of mesothelioma depends on its stage at diagnosis. When diagnosed early, it appears as numerous small nodules or plaques extending over the visceral and parietal pleural surfaces. Later, confluence of the nodules results in a rindlike mass encasing and compressing the lungs. Usually, the tumor is thickest in the lower portions of the lung and over the diaphragm. At autopsy, invasion of the chest wall, lung, and mediastinum and distant metastases are common. The tumor may be firm, yellowish, and leathery, particularly in the desmoplastic variant, or it may be soft and gelatinous, especially in

the poorly differentiated epithelial types. In the latter, abundant foci of degeneration and necrosis are commonly seen at autopsy. The gross appearance of mesothelioma may be complicated by its intermingling with asbestos-related fibrous plaque.

CLASSIFICATION

Three major histologic types of diffuse malignant mesothelioma are familiar: epithelial, fibrous (sarcomatous), and mixed (biphasic) (Figs. 27.4, 27.10, and 27.11); in each of these, cellular differentiation varies over a wide range. Diagnostic difficulties are presented by cases at all levels of differentiation. For example, well-differentiated epithelial mesothelioma must be distinguished from reactive mesothelial hyperplasia, poorly differentiated epithelial mesothelioma must be distinguished from metastatic undifferentiated carcinoma and other poorly differentiated neoplasms, and epithelial mesothelioma of intermediate degree of differentiation must be distinguished from pleural involvement by an adenocarcinoma of lung origin or from a distant metastasis from an adenocarcinoma arising elsewhere in the body. The distribution of the various histologic types

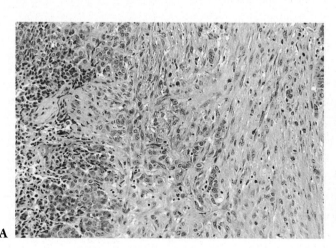
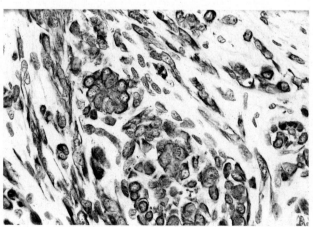

A

B

Figure 27.11. **(A)** Field from a biphasic mesothelioma in which the epithelial and sarcomatous components are well defined. Hematoxylin and eosin stain. **(B)** Another field from the same tumor stained for pancytokeratins. There is generalized distribution of keratin immunostaining in the two components of the neoplasm.

varies from series to series, but usually epithelial mesothelioma predominates. Because virtually all series are composed of consultation cases, they tend to underestimate the percentage of biphasic cases because these are easier to diagnose and less likely to require consultation. I reviewed 100 consecutive malignant pleural mesotheliomas from my consultation files over the years of 2000 and 2001. Of these 100 mesotheliomas, 82 were of the epithelial type, 7 were biphasic, and 11 were sarcomatoid, including 2 cases of the desmoplastic variant.

Unusual Variants of Mesothelioma

Unusual variants include clear-cell mesothelioma, a form of epithelial mesothelioma that resembles metastatic renal cell carcinoma (76,77), and lymphohistiocytoid malignant mesothelioma, which mimics malignant lymphoma or other lymphoproliferative disorders (78,79). In these cases, immunohistochemistry is very helpful because the neoplastic cells express a mesothelial lineage immunophenotype.

Another rare mesothelioma variant is the so-called deciduoid malignant mesothelioma, which is a large-cell type of mesothelioma resembling exuberant ectopic decidual reaction. Although deciduoid mesothelioma is more commonly seen in the peritoneal cavity, cases have also been reported involving the pleura (80,81).

Localized malignant mesothelioma that is histologically and immunophenotypically indistinguishable from diffuse malignant mesothelioma has also been reported. However, these mesotheliomas exhibit a different biologic behavior than their diffuse counterparts, with many patients having a long survival after surgical resection (82,83).

Well-differentiated papillary mesothelioma (WDPM) is more commonly seen in the peritoneal cavity of women. It is characterized by papillary formations lined by bland epithelioid mesothelial cells with no or only superficial invasiveness. Like its peritoneal counterpart, WDPM of the pleura has an indolent clinical course (84,85).

Unusual Mimics of Mesothelioma

Infrequently, epithelioid hemangioendothelioma and epithelioid angiosarcoma involving the pleura may also enter the differential diagnosis with mesothelioma (see illustrative case 6 presented later in this chapter) (86–89).

Thymomas arising from ectopic thymic tissues may rarely present as pleural-based tumors, occasionally with total encasement of the lung and clinically and macroscopically mimicking malignant mesothelioma. Histologically, they are indistinguishable from classical mediastinal thymomas (90,91). However, distinction from mesothelioma, particularly its lymphohistiocytoid variant, may be difficult on morphologic grounds alone, particularly with scant or fragmented biopsies. In these circumstances, immunohistochemistry can be very helpful because the epithelial cells express p63 and the lymphocytes show immunophenotypic features of T lymphocytes and express terminal deoxynucleotidyl transferase (TdT) (92,93).

HISTOLOGIC FEATURES AND DIFFERENTIAL DIAGNOSIS

The epithelial type, if sufficiently differentiated, is characterized by predominantly papillary and tubular patterns of growth (Figs. 27.4 and 27.12). A variable proportion of solid growth, sometimes with a marked discohesiveness of the tumor cells, may be increasingly present in the less differentiated types and is the prevailing histologic pattern in poorly differentiated epithelial mesothelioma (Fig. 27.13A). The tumor cells are usually cuboidal, with a bulging, domelike apical portion, but may be flattened and rarely columnar. A common finding in well-differentiated epithelial mesothelioma is the presence of single or multiple, sharply delimited, clear, round cytoplasmic vacuoles. These resemble those commonly seen in localized benign epithelial mesothelioma (adenomatoid tumor) and, under electron microscopy, are identifiable as intracytoplasmic lumina. Because adenocarcinomas, epithelioid hemangioendotheliomas, and other neoplasms may contain intracytoplasmic lumina, this finding is of limited diagnostic value.

A brush border–like rim—corresponding to the abundant long microvilli seen by electron microscopy—may be seen on the free portions of the cell surfaces in thin sections of well to moderately differentiated epithelial mesothelioma (Fig. 27.14). This is useful in distinguishing epithelial mesothelioma from adenocarcinoma because the latter seldom has thick brush borders. Several immunostains to membrane-based marker mole-

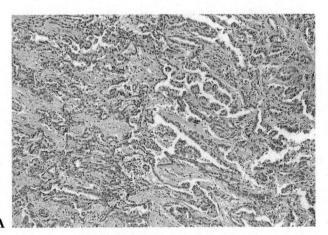

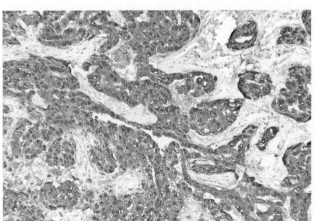

A   **B**

Figure 27.12.   Case 1. **(A)** Hematoxylin and eosin–stained section; typical tubulopapillary pattern of epithelial mesothelioma. **(B)** Section stained with antibody to calretinin. There is strong and generalized nuclear and cytoplasmic staining. All the epithelial markers in this case gave negative results.

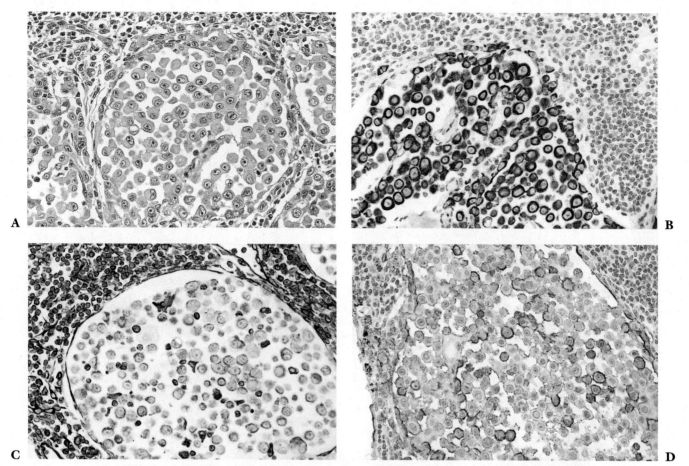

Figure 27.13. Poorly differentiated epithelioid mesothelioma metastatic to a lymph node. **(A)** Hematoxylin and eosin stain. Notice discohesive aggregates of round tumor cells with abundant cytoplasm and fuzzy cell borders. **(B)** Strong and generalized expression of pancytokeratins by the tumor cells. **(C)** The tumor cells express less vimentin than keratin and less than the neighboring stromal and lymphoid cells. **(D)** Stained with antibody HBME-1, which shows the focal presence of thick cell membranes. All epithelial markers were negative in this tumor.

cules help to highlight this feature (Figs. 27.14B, 27.15, 27.16, and 27.17B). Microcalcifications (psammoma bodies) may be seen, particularly in the tubulo-papillary forms of epithelial mesothelioma. They are of no diagnostic value.

Diffuse fibrous mesothelioma (sarcomatoid or sarcomatous mesothelioma) is made up predominantly of malignant-appearing spindle cells growing in short fascicles within a variable amount of fibrous stroma (Fig. 27.10A). A storiform pattern of growth and focal hemangiopericytoma-like patterns are not uncommon (Fig. 27.18B). Although not frequent, multinucleated atypical cells may be present and may give the neoplasm an appearance resembling malignant fibrous histiocytoma. However, sarcomatous mesothelioma may also be well differentiated, with the neoplastic cells having a bland cytologic appearance resembling reactive fibroblasts. Considerable amounts of collagenous stroma may separate the neoplastic cells (Fig. 27.19). Such well-differentiated sarcomatous mesotheliomas closely resemble fibromatoses and are often designated as the desmoplastic variant of malignant fibrous mesothelioma (94,95). They differ from the fibromatoses in that their neoplastic cells consistently express cytokeratins. However, their distinction from reactive pleural fibrosis is often difficult, as will be discussed later (see illustrative cases 4 and 5). Sarcomatoid meso-

thelioma also may imitate hemangiopericytoma, schwannoma, and other sarcomas (96).

The mixed type, also called biphasic malignant mesothelioma, is the most easily diagnosed. As the name implies, it consists of a mixture of epithelial and sarcomatous cellular components (Fig. 27.11). For this reason, it has often been compared with synovial sarcoma, to which, however, it has only a superficial resemblance. Nonetheless, synovial sarcoma may present as a pleural-based lesion and mimic mesothelioma clinically and morphologically (97,98). The epithelial component of synovial sarcoma is often mucicarmine positive. Moreover, several epithelial markers are expressed by synovial sarcoma (99). Additionally the translocation t(X;18) (SYT-SSX) characteristic of synovial sarcoma is not found in sarcomatoid mesothelioma (100). Carcinosarcoma of the lung with pleural involvement, a rare occurrence, may also simulate biphasic mesothelioma. Such cases can be identified by appropriate use of immunohistochemical procedures (101).

Clearly, malignant mesothelioma exhibits a wide range of differential diagnoses, from metastatic carcinoma of various origins to several types of sarcomas, as well as benign reactive processes. Although some cases of mesothelioma are sufficiently typical to permit a relatively firm diagnosis based on routine

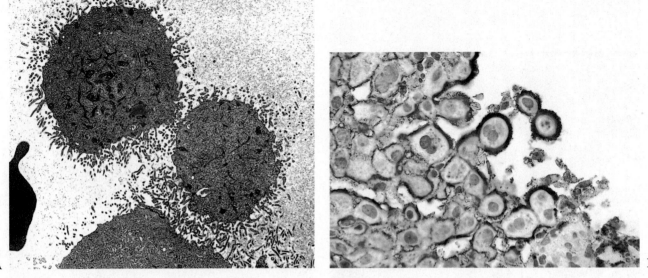

Figure 27.14. Malignant epithelial mesothelioma. **(A)** Electron micrograph showing presence of abundant long and narrow microvilli over much of the free surfaces of the tumor cells. **(B)** Section of same tumor stained with antibody HBME-1 showing a thick, brush border–like staining of the cell surfaces as a result of the presence of microvilli.

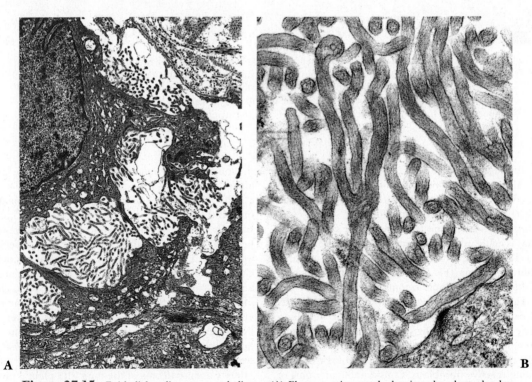

Figure 27.15. Epithelial malignant mesothelioma. **(A)** Electron micrograph showing abundant, slender bushy microvilli, well-developed desmosomes, and bundles of tonofibrils. **(B)** Detail of the microvilli showing tendency to branch.

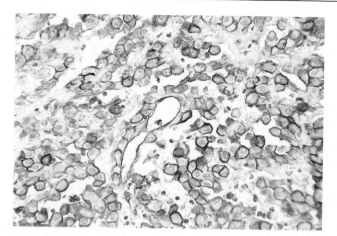

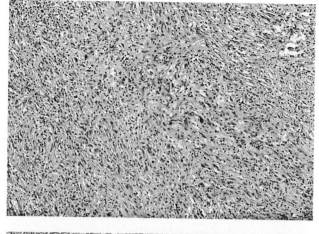

Figure 27.16. Malignant epithelial mesothelioma immunostained for thrombomodulin. There is thick membranous staining of large portions of the cell membranes in many of the tumor cells. Note that endothelial cells are also stained.

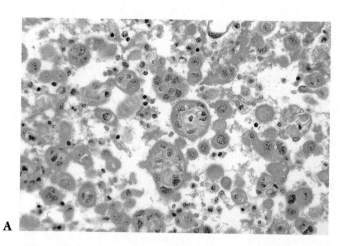

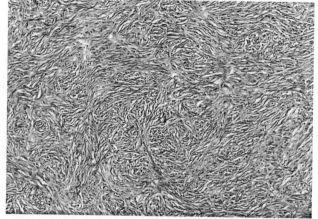

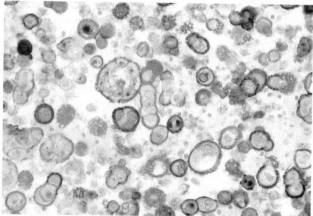

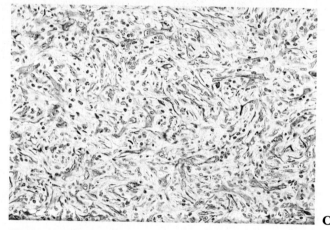

Figure 27.18. Case 3. **(A)** Hematoxylin and eosin–stained section of the pleural biopsy. Neoplastic-appearing spindle cells invade lung parenchyma. **(B)** Masson's trichrome stain is used to demonstrate the storiform pattern of growth that predominates throughout the neoplasm. **(C)** Stained with a cocktail of monoclonal antibodies to pancytokeratins. Virtually all of the neoplastic cells exhibit expression of keratins. Hematoxylin counterstained.

Figure 27.17. **(A)** Pleural fluid cell block (hematoxylin and eosin–stained section). Clusters of cytologically malignant epithelioid mesothelial cells with fuzzy cell borders are seen. **(B)** Parallel section stained with antibody to mesothelin. A thick, brush border–like pattern of membranous staining is typical of this marker.

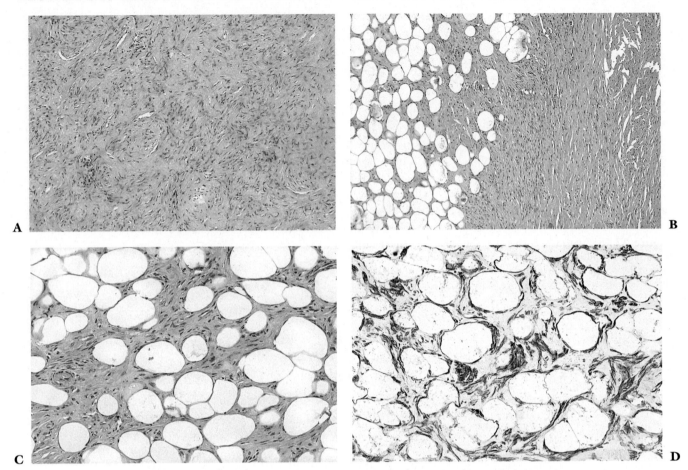

Figure 27.19. Case 5. **(A)** Section of the pleural decortication specimen. A predominantly bland population of spindle cells is seen in a scarlike stroma. **(B)** Low-power view of a portion of the decorticated parietal pleura, showing infiltration of the underlying adipose tissue. **(C)** Higher magnification of the same field to show the invasiveness of the tumor cells; all stained with hematoxylin and eosin. **(D)** Pancytokeratin-stained section of the invaded adipose tissue. All of the tumor cells strongly express keratins.

morphologic examination, in a large proportion of cases, its diagnosis is often imprecise and prone to be controversial. It has been correctly stated that interobserver variability is greater for the diagnosis of malignant mesothelioma than for most other human neoplasms (102). Thus, numerous ancillary procedures, in particular histochemistry, electron microscopy, and immunohistochemistry, have been used in an attempt to improve the accuracy of mesothelioma diagnosis.

ADEQUACY OF BIOPSY MATERIAL

Decades ago, many believed that autopsy was the only way to ascertain a diagnosis of mesothelioma. Currently, with adequate biopsy, a firm diagnosis is nearly always possible. In many instances of differential diagnosis between malignant epithelial mesothelioma versus adenocarcinoma, a needle biopsy, if representative of tumor tissue, may suffice. Indeed, with the help of immunohistochemistry, it is now possible, in many instances, to diagnose malignant epithelial mesothelioma based solely on cytologic preparations of pleural fluid, as will be discussed in further detail later.

However, distinguishing between reactive hyperplasia and epithelial mesothelioma or between fibrous pleuritis and desmoplastic malignant mesothelioma requires more extensive

sampling, preferably using thoracoscopy or thoracotomy. This is so because demonstration of invasiveness is of foremost importance in the differential diagnosis in these cases.

ANCILLARY DIAGNOSTIC PROCEDURES

Because no single test is currently capable of providing an unambiguous confirmation of the histologic diagnosis of mesothelioma, such diagnosis must be based on the accumulation of evidence. Nonetheless, recent advances in immunohistochemistry have markedly improved the accuracy of mesothelioma diagnosis to the point of rendering many older tests obsolete.

Histochemistry

Histochemical stains, such as mucicarmine, periodic acid-Schiff (PAS), and Alcian blue, once considered useful for the distinction between epithelial mesothelioma and adenocarcinoma have been largely superseded by the more specific and sensitive immunohistochemical stains.

Electron Microscopy

Before recent progress in immunohistochemistry, electron microscopy (EM) was often used to distinguish between epithelial mesothelioma and adenocarcinoma. The ultrastructural hallmark of epithelial mesotheliomas consists of the presence of long, thin, branching "bushy" microvilli, devoid of a glycocalyx coating, over much of their free cell surface (Figs. 27.14 and 27.15).

Warhol et al. (103) attempted to establish objective criteria for the ultrastructural diagnosis of mesothelioma and concluded that only the length-to-diameter ratio of the microvilli and the abundance of tonofilaments were of diagnostic value. Adenocarcinomas have fewer and shorter microvilli than do mesotheliomas. Additionally, microvilli in adenocarcinomas are usually present only on the apical portion of the cell surface, whereas in mesothelioma, they tend to involve all free cell surfaces (Fig. 27.14). Burns et al. (104) found a median length-to-diameter ratio of 11.9 in mesothelioma and 5.28 in adenocarcinoma. However, overlapping cases create a relatively wide "gray zone." Dardick et al. (105) emphasized that poorly differentiated epithelial mesothelioma and sarcomatous mesothelioma may show no evidence at all of such long microvilli. Moreover, in my experience, practically all mesotheliomas exhibiting long, sinuous microvilli also have a typical mesothelioma immunophenotype and often reveal thick brush border staining with membrane-based markers (Figs. 27.13C,D, 27.14B, 27.16, and 27.17B).

Distinction of sarcomatous mesothelioma from true sarcomas is also simpler and more accurate by immunohistochemical means than by EM. Thus, EM is no longer needed for the diagnosis of mesothelioma, although it remains an essential tool for the identification and quantification of asbestos fibers in lung and pleural tissue (20,106).

Immunohistochemistry

Immunohistochemistry has evolved into the most important ancillary procedure in the distinction of epithelial malignant mesothelioma from its mimics. However, there is yet no consensus about which is the ideal antibody panel, and there still remain some discrepancies on how best to interpret some of these immunostains.

Not too long ago, we relied chiefly on the use of antibodies binding to molecules expressed predominantly by carcinoma cells such as carcinoembryonic antigen (CEA), B72.3, CD15,

and others. Thus, the diagnosis of mesothelioma was based on negative results, which is an unsatisfactory situation. This has dramatically changed in recent years with the introduction of antibodies of relative specificity for mesothelial cells (Table 27.1). As a result, rarely are cases left undiagnosed when a well-chosen immunohistochemical panel is used. Because none of these new markers is by itself sufficiently specific or sensitive, they need to be used within a diagnostic panel. Clearly, as the number of available markers—particularly those of mesothelial lineage—continues to grow, we need to periodically re-evaluate our antibody panels to keep them reasonably sized with no loss of accuracy.

It is important to remember that specificity in immunohistochemistry is a relative concept because it depends in great part on the differential diagnosis in any particular case. For example, a partially mesothelial-restricted marker, such as Wilms tumor gene product (WT-1), has a very high specificity when the differential diagnosis is between mesothelioma and adenocarcinoma of the lung in a male patient. However, when ovarian carcinoma enters the differential diagnosis, this marker's specificity dramatically decreases because it is expressed by a large proportion of ovarian adenocarcinomas. Thus, awareness of each marker's limitations is fundamental to select the antibody panel most suitable to the differential diagnosis at hand.

Cytokeratins (Keratins)

Keratins comprise a family of at least 20 individually gene-coded filamentous proteins that are the dominant cytoskeletal filament of epithelial cells. Which member(s) of the keratin family is expressed depends on the type of epithelial cell. Neoplasms derived from different epithelia tend to express the same combination of cytokeratins as their cell of origin. Thus, the cytokeratin immunophenotype of tumors is often used as an indicator of cell lineage.

The cytoskeletal phenotype of mesotheliomas closely resembles that of reactive and resting mesothelium. When broad-spectrum antibodies (pancytokeratin antibodies)—recognizing epitopes shared by multiple members of the keratin family—are correctly used, all mesotheliomas and all adenocarcinomas immunostain strongly and diffusely. Therefore, the use of pancytokeratin antibodies is not helpful to distinguish mesothelioma

TABLE 27.1	Antibodies Useful for the Differential Diagnosis between Adenocarcinoma and Epithelial Mesothelioma				
Antibody	*Specificity*	*Clone*	*Source*	*Dilution*	*Pretreatment*
Calretinin	Mesothelial	5A5	Novocastra	1:50	8 minutes pressure cooker citrate buffer pH 6.0
Cytokeratin 5/6	Mesothelial	D5/16B4	Chemicon	1:2000	Steam 20 minutes in citrate + 10 minutes in pronase
D2-40 (podoplanin)	Mesothelial	D2-40	Signet	1:50	Steam 20 minutes in citrate buffer pH 6.0
Mesothelin	Mesothelial	5B2	Novocastra	1:25	8 minutes pressure cooker citrate buffer pH 6.0
WT-1	Mesothelial	Polyclonal	Santa Cruz	1:1000	8 minutes pressure cooker citrate buffer pH 6.0
Thrombomodulin	Mesothelial	1009	Novocastra	1:250	Steam 20 minutes in citrate + 10 minutes in pronase
BG-8	Epithelial	F3	Signet	1:250	Protease XXIV × 5 minutes
MOC-31	Epithelial	MOC-31	DAKO	1:50	Protease XXIV × 5 minutes
Ber-EP4	Epithelial	Ber-EP4	DAKO	1:250	Protease XXIV × 5 minutes
CEA	Epithelial	Polyclonal	DAKO	1:4000	Steam 20 minutes in citrate buffer pH 6.0

Chemicon, Chemicon International Inc., Temecula, CA; DAKO, DAKO Corporation, Carpentaria, CA; Santa Cruz, Santa Cruz Biotechnology, Santa Cruz, CA; Novocastra, Novocastra Laboratories, Newcastle upon Tyne, United Kingdom; Signet, Signet Laboratories, Dedham, MA.

from carcinoma. However, as will be discussed later in more detail, pancytokeratin antibodies are valuable in the diagnosis of sarcomatous mesothelioma and to identify invasiveness, particularly in the desmoplastic type (see illustrative cases 3, 4, and 5).

Many monoclonal antibodies (MoAbs) recognizing epitopes restricted to certain members of the keratin family are currently available. Among these, one binds to an epitope shared by cytokeratins 5 and 6 and is of diagnostic value for epithelial mesothelioma in paraffin-embedded tissues. Although MoAbs to cytokeratins 7 and 20 may help to pinpoint the site of origin of metastatic adenocarcinoma, they are of no value in the differential diagnosis between adenocarcinoma and epithelial mesothelioma.

Vimentin

Vimentin, the chief intermediate filament of mesenchymal cells, is now known to be expressed by a large proportion of epithelium-derived neoplasms (107). Thus, earlier publications claiming usefulness of the demonstration of vimentin for the differential diagnosis between adenocarcinoma and mesothelioma are now less valid. In fact, we found that a majority of epithelial mesotheliomas do not express vimentin or do so minimally (108). However, vimentin, using clone V9 without antigen retrieval, is a useful universal control to detect overfixation and other types of antigen damage (109).

MESOTHELIAL MARKERS (POSITIVE MARKERS)

This group consists of antibodies that bind to epitopes of molecules expressed mainly by normal mesothelial cells and their tumors. These antibodies should thus be regarded as markers of mesothelial lineage, rather than as mesothelioma markers. As already stated, none of these is sufficiently specific or sensitive; thus, they need to be used within a diagnostic panel. Based on the literature and our own studies, the first five markers discussed in the following sections are recommended as the best currently available mesothelial markers.

Calretinin

Calretinin, a calcium-binding protein in the family of S-100 protein, was initially found to be present in central and peripheral neural tissues. Later it was also found in adipocytes, renal tubular cells, Leydig and Sertoli cells, eccrine glands, and mesothelial cells (110,111). As is the case with S-100 protein, it is localized in both cytoplasm and nuclei (Figs. 27.12B and 27.20). Doglioni et al. (110) reported calretinin to be expressed by normal mesothelial cells and mesothelioma and rarely by adenocarcinoma. Several studies have confirmed a high sensitivity of this marker for epithelial mesothelioma, while uncovering its expression by a small fraction of adenocarcinomas (112–114). However, although mesotheliomas usually immunostain strongly and diffusely, in the few positive adenocarcinomas, the staining tends to be weak and focal.

Currently, there are several commercially available antisera and MoAbs to calretinin. It is very important to use the correct one. In an early study, we found calretinin to be of low sensitivity. We had used the only commercially available antibody at that time, a polyclonal antiserum raised against guinea pig calretinin (Chemicon, Temecula, CA) (108). Since then, more sensitive antisera and MoAbs have become available. Using MoAb 5A5

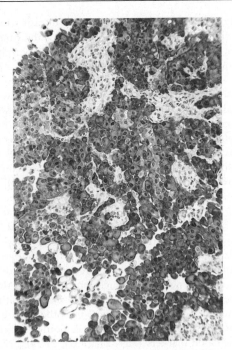

Figure 27.20. Malignant epithelial mesothelioma immunostained for calretinin. Strong cytoplasmic and nuclear staining of virtually every neoplastic cell is typical of well- and moderately differentiated epithelial mesotheliomas.

(Novocastra, Newcastle upon Tyne, United Kingdom) in a recent study comparing a large series of epithelial mesotheliomas with adenocarcinomas of various origins, we found a sensitivity of 96% and a specificity of 83% for this marker (115). Similar results have been reported using polyclonal antisera to human recombinant calretinin (Zymed, San Francisco, CA) (116).

Cytokeratin 5/6

Cytokeratin 5, a member of the cytokeratin family, has a restricted distribution in normal and neoplastic tissues. Normal mesothelial cells, myoepithelium, and squamous and transitional epithelium express cytokeratin 5 (117–120). Most epithelial mesotheliomas and nearly all squamous cell carcinomas also express this cytokeratin (117,119,121). Thus, in the appropriate context of differential diagnosis, it can be a helpful marker for each. However, expression of cytokeratin 5 by adenocarcinoma is infrequent. Thus, for the common differential diagnosis of mesothelioma versus adenocarcinoma, this is a very useful marker.

As expected of intermediate filaments, the pattern of immunostaining for cytokeratin 5 is cytoplasmic and fibrillary. The latter feature is particularly visible if high-resolution chromogen and very thin sections are used (Fig. 27.21). In most cases of mesothelioma and squamous cell carcinoma, the staining affects the majority of the tumor cells.

In a recent study comprising only epithelial mesotheliomas and adenocarcinomas of various origins and excluding squamous cell carcinoma, using an MoAb that binds to an epitope shared by cytokeratins 5 and 6, the sensitivity for epithelial mesothelioma was 76%, and the specificity was 86% (122). Clearly, if squamous cell carcinoma had been included in the series,

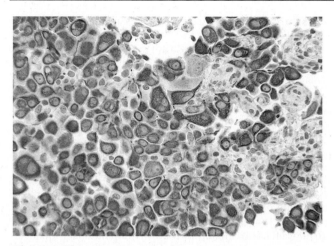

Figure 27.21. Malignant epithelial mesothelioma immunostained for cytokeratins 5/6. There is strong cytoplasmic staining with a fibrillary pattern of most of the tumor cells.

the test specificity would have markedly decreased. However, this is not a serious impediment because squamous cell carcinoma mimicking mesothelioma is rare and is usually easy to diagnose clinically and morphologically. Moreover, with the use of additional immunostains to the panel, such as p63, the correct diagnosis can be readily established in the rare doubtful case (123,124).

Thrombomodulin (CD141)

Thrombomodulin is a transmembrane glycoprotein with anticoagulant properties expressed preferentially by mesothelial and endothelial cells. It has also been reported to be expressed by syncytiotrophoblast, dermal keratinocytes, and urothelial tumors (125–128). Collins et al. (129) reported that all of 31 mesotheliomas and only 4 (8%) of 48 adenocarcinomas stained with this antibody (129). The combined literature concerning this marker reported positive staining in 114 (80%) of 141 mesotheliomas, although up to 17% of adenocarcinomas also stained (129–132). Our recent study with this marker revealed a sensitivity of 64% and a specificity of 92% (122). Thus, although somewhat limited in sensitivity, if it is positive in a case that is otherwise negative to the panel's epithelial markers, the diagnosis strongly favors mesothelioma.

Positive immunostaining with thrombomodulin is predominantly membranous, often exhibiting the thick "brush border" pattern correlating with the presence of long and abundant microvilli (Fig. 27.16). Cytoplasmic staining should not be interpreted as a positive result. Endothelial cell staining is also the rule with this marker, providing a suitable internal control for adequacy of the immunostaining (Fig. 27.16).

Wilms Tumor Gene Product

Wilms tumor gene product (WT-1) is a DNA-binding protein that plays an important role in the morphogenesis of the genitourinary tract and mesothelium. In normal adult tissues, mesangial cells of the kidney, Sertoli cells of the testis, ovarian stromal cells and ovarian surface epithelium, all mesothelial cells, and some stromal cells in the gynecologic tract express WT-1. It is expressed by epithelial mesotheliomas, tumors derived from

the ovarian surface epithelium, desmoplastic small round cell tumors, and Wilms tumors (133–135). Adenocarcinoma of the lung rarely expresses WT-1. Thus, within an appropriate context of differential diagnosis, WT-1 can be a useful marker for mesothelioma (99,136,137).

Positive WT-1 immunostains are localized chiefly in the cell nuclei. In most positive mesotheliomas, the stain involves a large proportion of the tumor cells (Fig. 27.22).

In a recent study, WT-1 had a sensitivity of 81% and a specificity of 61% for mesothelioma. If only adenocarcinomas of lung origin are considered, the specificity of WT-1 increases to 95%. However, as previously stated, this marker is of no value in discerning between epithelioid mesothelioma and serous carcinoma of ovarian or peritoneal origin (116).

Mesothelin

Initially this marker was designated as the CAK1 antigen, identified by the antibody K1 (138). The antigen is a cell surface protein, probably an intercellular adhesion molecule. Now it is identified as mesothelin by "second-generation" MoAbs such as the 5B2 clone. Mesothelin is relatively specific for mesothelial cells and epithelial cells of the ovarian surface. However, a large subset of pancreatic carcinomas and squamous cell carcinomas of various sites of origin have been shown to express this marker (139,140).

In a recent study, we found mesothelin to have a sensitivity of 71% for malignant epithelial mesothelioma and a specificity of 66%. Only immunostains showing discrete membranous distribution should be interpreted as positive. A thick membranous pattern of immunoreactivity is often exhibited by epithelial mesothelioma with this marker (Fig. 27.17B).

D2-40 (Podoplanin)

Recently added to this group, D2-40 antibodies recognize a membrane-based glycoprotein (podoplanin) expressed by lymphatic endothelial cells, type I epithelial cells of pulmonary alveoli, renal glomerular podocytes, and mesothelial cells. Several recent studies have investigated the possible diagnostic role of

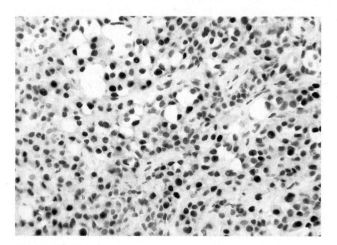

Figure 27.22. Poorly differentiated malignant epithelial mesothelioma immunostained for Wilms tumor gene product (WT-1). Strong to moderate staining of a large proportion of the tumor cell nuclei is present.

this marker in mesothelioma (141–146). The reported range of podoplanin expression by epithelioid mesothelioma is from 86% to 100% (144). D2-40 is often expressed by pulmonary squamous cell carcinoma, serous carcinomas, and angiosarcomas but is not expressed by adenocarcinoma of the lung (144). Thus, in a diagnostic context between epithelioid mesothelioma and lung adenocarcinoma, this is a useful marker. As is the case with mesothelin and thrombomodulin, a membranous pattern of immunostaining is seen in epithelial mesotheliomas stained with antibodies to podoplanin.

h-Caldesmon

An MoAb to the high–molecular-weight isoform of caldesmon (h-caldesmon)—a cytoskeleton-associated protein abundantly present in smooth muscle cells—has been recently reported by Comin et al. (147,148) to immunoreact with the vast majority of epithelioid mesotheliomas but not with adenocarcinoma of the lung and rarely with serous papillary carcinoma of the ovary. Although it is not clear whether this immunoreactivity reflects true expression of this marker, it nonetheless appears to be a promising new marker of mesothelial lineage when applied within the appropriate context of differential diagnosis.

EPITHELIAL MARKERS (NEGATIVE MARKERS)

Under this designation are included several antisera and MoAbs to antigens primarily expressed by carcinoma. Many of these antigens have been characterized as being high–molecular-weight glycoproteins. Until recently, these markers, used as a panel, were the main tools available for distinguishing mesothelioma from adenocarcinoma (108). Best among this group are MoAbs and antisera to CEA, the MoAb designated as Ber-EP4, the MoAb designated as BG-8 (a blood group–related glycoprotein), and the MoAb designated as MOC-31. The MoAbs Leu-M1 (CD15) and B72.3 have also been found to be useful as members of a secondary panel.

Successful application of these antibodies depends, in great part, on their careful titration with a panel of known mesotheliomas and adenocarcinomas to select the titer that stains the lowest number of mesotheliomas. For optimal results, certain rules of interpretation must be observed, as discussed later. It also is important to keep in mind that many early publications using these antibodies antedated the use of heat-induced epitope retrieval (HIER) and are less valid today because the sensitivity of some of these antibodies has been greatly enhanced by HIER, in most instances with no appreciable change in specificity (108).

Carcinoembryonic Antigen

This oncofetal antigen has been found by many investigators to be expressed with variable frequency by adenocarcinoma and rarely by mesothelioma (149–153). The incidence of CEA immunostaining in adenocarcinoma varies from series to series, but in most reports, approximately 70% of the carcinomas are CEA positive. The site of origin of the adenocarcinomas is important in their expression of CEA. Gastrointestinal or lung-derived neoplasms tend to be positive more frequently than adenocarcinomas of other origins. The staining pattern is usually intracytoplasmic. In cases with high expression, some peritu-

moral stromal staining as a result of leaching of CEA is not unusual.

We found CEA to be positive in 175 (83%) of 211 adenocarcinomas of various origins and in none of 57 epithelial mesotheliomas by using the MoAb clone CEJ065 and HIER (108). Results with polyclonal antisera are similar, although a small number of mesotheliomas did stain (122).

MOC-31

MOC-31 is an MoAb binding a glycoprotein of unknown function present in the cell membrane of epithelial cells. In 1994, Ruitenbeek et al. (154) reported that 98% of adenocarcinomas and none of 5 mesotheliomas immunoreacted with MOC-31. Ordóñez (155), in a more extensive study, found that 100% of 40 lung adenocarcinomas and 82% of nonpulmonary adenocarcinomas immunoreacted strongly and diffusely with MOC-31. Only 2 of 38 epithelial mesotheliomas stained, but they stained focally and weakly (116,155).

Our recent re-evaluation of these markers confirms the usefulness of MOC-31 in the differential diagnosis between epithelial mesothelioma and adenocarcinoma (115).

BG-8

The MoAb BG-8 has been found to bind to the blood group antigen Lewis^y. Jordan et al. (156) reported strong, diffuse, and homogeneous staining in 18 primary lung adenocarcinomas with this antibody, whereas mesotheliomas did not stain or did so in less than 10% of the cells. We expanded these studies by including a larger series of adenocarcinomas and mesotheliomas with HIER pretreatment (108). When a 10% cutoff was used, none of 57 epithelial mesotheliomas was considered positive, whereas 114 of 123 pulmonary adenocarcinomas were unambiguously BG-8 positive.

Several points are important to keep in mind in the interpretation of BG-8 immunostains. As already stated, a semiquantitative approach is necessary because, in a small number of mesotheliomas, less than 10% of the tumor cells may stain (usually weakly). However, the staining of adenocarcinomas, particularly those of lung origin, usually involves from 60% to 100% of the tumor cells and is commonly intense. The sensitivity of the antibody is markedly enhanced by the use of HIER (Fig. 27.23). Staining with this antibody is diffusely and homogeneously cytoplasmic, with membrane accentuation. As warned by Jordan et al. (156), for unknown reasons, a coarse granular pattern of staining may occasionally be seen in mesothelioma and should not be misinterpreted as true antigen expression. In our cases, using HIER, such spurious staining was rarely observed (108).

BG-8 is a useful member of the mesothelioma panel and capable (when used together with CEA and Ber-EP4 or MOC-31) of identifying most adenocarcinomas (122).

Ber-EP4

This MoAb recognizes an epitope present in two glycoproteins present in most epithelial cells but not in mesothelial cells. Latza et al. (157) found immunoreactivity with this antibody in 99% of 144 epithelial tumors of various origins, whereas none of 14 mesotheliomas stained. Sheibani et al. (158), a year later, reported Ber-EP4 immunoreactivity in 87 adenocarcinomas of various sites of origin and in only 1 of 115 mesotheliomas. Later, however, Gaffey et al. (159) reported immunoreactivity

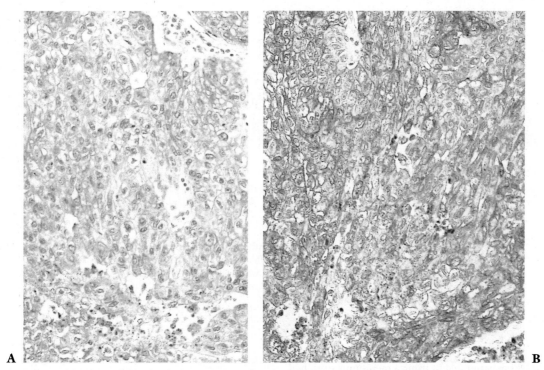

Figure 27.23. Adenocarcinoma stained with antibody BG-8. **(A)** Section stained without heat-induced epitope retrieval (HIER); diffuse but weak immunostaining is noticed. **(B)** Parallel section stained after HIER. There is stronger immunostaining with the typical cytoplasmic pattern with membrane accentuation of this marker.

for this marker in 10 of 48 mesotheliomas. Ordóñez (160) reported up to 26% of 70 mesotheliomas immunostaining for Ber-EP4, albeit focally and affecting only a small proportion of cells, whereas in lung adenocarcinoma, the staining was invariably diffuse and positive in 100% of the cases. Thus, a cutoff level could be reasonably applied to Ber-EP4, as is the case with BG-8.

Moreover, I believe that differences in the interpretation of the immunostains account for much of the discrepancy in the literature about this marker. Latza et al. (157) emphasized the predominant basolateral immunoreactivity when using this MoAb. If predominantly apical membrane staining is found, it should not be interpreted as positive. In my experience, most mesotheliomas show entirely negative stains with Ber-EP4, and those that do stain show a very small percentage of cells staining, usually weakly and without the basolateral accentuation shown by adenocarcinoma (Fig. 27.24). Thus, with a quantitative approach, including careful observation of the pattern of staining, Ber-EP4 is a useful diagnostic marker, particularly to distinguish adenocarcinoma of the lung from mesothelioma.

Thyroid Transcription Factor-1

Thyroid transcription factor-1 (TTF-1) is a tissue-specific nuclear transcription protein important in the morphogenesis of the lung and thyroid gland. Recent immunohistochemical studies have shown that it is often expressed by adenocarcinoma and neuroendocrine carcinoma of the lung. Conversely, TTF-1 is not expressed by mesothelioma, squamous cell and large-cell carcinoma of the lung, or adenocarcinoma of nonlung origin,

with the exception of adenocarcinoma arising in the thyroid gland (135,161–164).

Thus, TTF-1 can be helpful in the distinction between primary adenocarcinoma of the lung and pleural mesothelioma. Only nuclear stains should be interpreted as positive. Usually staining involves a majority of nuclei. Because normal pneumocytes express TTF-1, they provide adequate internal control in biopsies including lung tissue.

Leu-M1 (CD15)

Sheibani et al. (165) reported that the antigen detected by the MoAb Leu-M1, a myelomonocytic marker, was also detectable in a large percentage of nonhematopoietic epithelial neoplasms. Of a group of 179 adenocarcinomas of various origins, 119 (58%) were found to immunoreact with the MoAb Leu-M1, whereas none of 18 mesotheliomas stained. Later the same investigators expanded the study and compared the expression of CD15 in 50 pulmonary adenocarcinomas and in 28 pleural mesotheliomas (166). Focal cytoplasmic staining was found in 47 (94%) of the adenocarcinomas and in none of the mesotheliomas. Subsequent studies showed that addition of HIER did not significantly affect these results (108).

It must be kept in perspective that the expression of CD15 is often focal. Thus, in small biopsies, the number of false-negative results is expected to increase. It also is important to emphasize that areas of necrosis should be avoided in the interpretation of this stain because degenerating leukocytes in and around these foci may lead to false-positive readings.

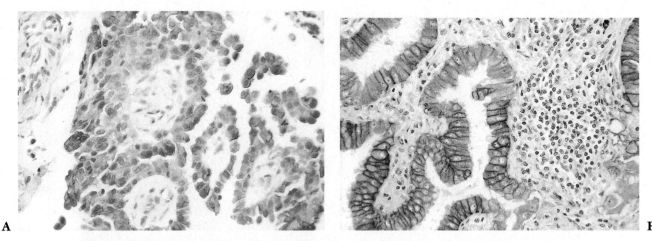

Figure 27.24. **(A)** Epithelial mesothelioma stained with monoclonal antibody Ber-EP4. Faint, predominantly apical immunostaining is present. This was focal, affecting approximately 1% of the neoplastic cells in the sample. **(B)** Adenocarcinoma of the lung also stained with antibody Ber-EP4. There is strong membrane staining involving predominantly the basal and lateral cell membranes. Additionally, the staining was present in nearly all the tumor cells in the sample.

B72.3

The MoAb B72.3 was generated by using a membrane-enriched fraction of a human breast carcinoma (167). It was found to stain a large proportion of adenocarcinomas of nonbreast origin and no mesotheliomas (168). The pattern of staining of adenocarcinomas is membranous and cytoplasmic, often focally distributed. In our post-HIER re-examination of this marker, we found that 80.5% of the adenocarcinomas were positive, whereas only 2 (3.5%) of 57 mesotheliomas stained (169). Omission of HIER greatly decreased the number of B72.3-positive adenocarcinomas without altering its specificity. Although B72.3 may be useful as an epithelial marker in the mesothelioma versus adenocarcinoma panel, CEA, BG-8, MOC-31, and Ber-EP4 have largely superseded it.

Other Epithelial Markers

The tight junction–associated protein claudin-4 (CL-4) has been proposed as a useful marker in the differential diagnosis between epithelial mesothelioma and adenocarcinoma. Data from a recent study by Facchetti et al. (170) suggest a high sensitivity and specificity for this epithelial marker. If supported by further studies by others, this marker could prove to be superior to CD15 and B72.3.

The Mesothelioma Diagnostic Immunohistochemistry Panel

Most cases of differential diagnosis between epithelial mesothelioma and adenocarcinoma can be correctly diagnosed with a six-antibody panel (three mesothelial and three epithelial): calretinin, cytokeratin 5/6, WT-1 (or D2-40), CEA, MOC-31 (or Ber-EP4), and BG-8. It is possible that smaller panels may be sufficient, particularly when dealing with well- or moderately differentiated tumors (115,116). Nonetheless, a practical approach would be to use three mesothelial and three epithelial markers for all cases suspected of being epithelial mesotheliomas. Only a few poorly differentiated tumors will be found to need expansion of this six-antibody panel.

Additionally, the panel should be modified if the differential diagnosis includes carcinoma of ovarian origin or squamous cell carcinoma, as previously discussed. Moreover, if other possibilities beyond adenocarcinoma enter the differential diagnosis, additional markers may become necessary, usually as a secondary panel. For example, markers of vascular lineage such as CD31 and von Willebrand factor should be included if epithelioid hemangioendothelioma is suspected (see illustrative case 6). The *p53*-related gene *p63* should be added if the histologic features suggest squamous cell carcinoma (123).

CYTOLOGIC DIAGNOSIS OF MESOTHELIOMA

It is generally agreed that the cytologic diagnosis of malignant mesothelioma is difficult. Furthermore the distinction between malignant mesothelial cells, adenocarcinoma cells, and atypical irritated mesothelial cells is a common and particularly challenging occurrence in the practice of cytology. Naylor (171), who studied seven cases of malignant mesothelioma, concluded that cytologic examination could only suggest the diagnosis of mesothelioma. According to Naylor, two important criteria need to be met for the cytologic diagnosis of malignant mesothelioma. First, the cells have to exhibit the usual cytologic characteristics of malignancy, and second, they have to display features typical of mesothelial cells. Cytologic features supporting the diagnosis of mesothelioma are the knobby outline of cell clusters (morula formations), cytoplasmic vacuolation, binucleation, and a fuzzy cell surface as a result of the presence of abundant long microvilli (Fig. 27.14A), which are best seen with immunostaining for thrombomodulin, D2-40, mesothelin, or HBME-1 (Fig. 27-17B).

The use of immunohistochemical studies in cell blocks of serous effusions has greatly facilitated the differential diagnosis between epithelial mesothelioma and adenocarcinoma, provided that Naylor's first criterion is met because reactive atypical mesothelial cells will be positive to most of the mesothelial-restricted markers. Thus, if the cytologic features are unquestionably malignant and mesothelial markers are positive and epithelial markers are not, a cytologic diagnosis of malignant mesothelioma is possible. However, even if there is uncertainty about whether suspicious cells are malignant or not, immunohistochemistry may still be useful. If the mesothelial markers are negative and one or more of the epithelial markers are positive in the suspicious cells, then the results would strongly favor adenocarcinoma over atypical mesothelial hyperplasia. A recent study concluded that D2-40 offers the highest specificity and sensitivity for the differential diagnosis between epithelial mesothelioma and adenocarcinoma on cell blocks of effusion fluids (172).

It needs to be emphasized that the criteria mentioned here apply only to epithelial and biphasic forms of mesothelioma. Sarcomatous and desmoplastic mesotheliomas shed infrequently into serous effusions and seldom can be diagnosed by cytologic means.

Flow Cytometry

Determination of DNA aneuploidy on serous effusions may serve as a marker for malignant cells. However, its usefulness to distinguish mesothelioma from carcinoma is controversial. El-Naggar et al. (173) compared the DNA flow cytometric characteristics of 23 epithelial mesotheliomas and 41 pulmonary adenocarcinomas from paraffin-embedded blocks. They reported that 78% of the mesotheliomas were diploid, versus a statistically significant 88% aneuploidy rate for the adenocarcinomas. Additionally, these authors found a significantly higher proliferative rate in adenocarcinoma than in mesothelioma. Similar findings were reported by Esteban and Sheibani (174). Thus, it would appear that the finding of a diploid tumor by flow cytometry favors a diagnosis of mesothelioma over adenocarcinoma. Pyrhönen et al. (175), by using fresh-frozen tumor samples, reported 16 (52%) of 31 mesotheliomas as diploid and found that the ploidy status was of no prognostic value in mesothelioma. Similar lack of prognostic value was reported by Dazzi et al. (176). Frierson et al. (177) studied effusion fluids and compared them with paraffin-embedded samples. They found a 53% rate of aneuploidy in mesothelioma and concluded that aneuploidy in an effusion specimen containing atypical mesothelial cells would strongly support a diagnosis of mesothelioma. Thus, it would appear that, in some circumstances, flow cytometric DNA analysis can be diagnostically useful.

ILLUSTRATIVE CASES

The following consultation cases—most of which were initially misdiagnosed—illustrate common areas of difficult differential diagnosis of pleural-based lesions.

CASE 1: EPITHELIAL MESOTHELIOMA

History

A 73-year-old man developed progressively worsening shortness of breath and nonproductive cough, for which he sought medical attention. A right-sided pleural effusion was evacuated with temporary relief of the symptoms, but it rapidly recurred and required repeated thoracenteses. Chest radiographs revealed marked pleural thickening on the right side and bilateral calcified pleural plaques. He was not a smoker but had been exposed heavily to asbestos dust for two decades, beginning at age 30 years, when his occupation was to grind asbestos to prepare a paste to line boilers. A needle biopsy of the pleura was done at another hospital and was interpreted by the local pathologists as adenocarcinoma. A palliative right parietal pleurodesis with partial pleurectomy was performed to reduce the recurrent effusion.

Discussion

The histologic appearance of the pleurectomy material was similar to that of the initial biopsy. It revealed an epithelial-appearing neoplasm with a tubulopapillary pattern of growth (Fig. 27.12A). The neoplastic cells were predominantly cuboidal and had moderate nuclear pleomorphism and abundant clear to lightly eosinophilic cytoplasm. The cell borders, in many places, had a fuzzy appearance, suggesting the presence of abundant microvilli. EM revealed the presence of abundant long and slender microvilli over the free cell surface of many of the neoplastic cells. The immunohistochemical study was confirmatory of the diagnosis of mesothelioma, as the tumor cells stained strongly and diffusely for the mesothelial-restricted marker calretinin (Fig. 27.12B) and focally for cytokeratin 5/6. Additionally, the epithelial markers CEA, Ber-EP4, and BG-8 gave negative results.

Comment

Although this is a typical example of epithelial mesothelioma, clinically, radiologically, and morphologically, it nevertheless was initially misdiagnosed as adenocarcinoma based only on the examination of the hematoxylin and eosin (H&E) stain.

CASE 2: PSEUDOMESOTHELIOMATOUS ADENOCARCINOMA

History

The patient, a 37-year-old man, worked for approximately 13 years in a brake shop, servicing brakes. He had no respiratory symptoms until shortly before admission, when he developed a nonproductive dry cough. A chest radiograph ordered by his primary care physician revealed opacification of the left lung field. Computerized tomography showed marked pleural thickening throughout the entire left hemithorax that was interpreted as compatible with mesothelioma by the radiologists (Fig. 27.25A). A left thoracotomy was performed, and an open pleural biopsy was obtained.

Discussion

Clusters and sheets of cuboidal cells with moderately abundant eosinophilic cytoplasm within a fibrous, reactive-appearing stroma were seen in the biopsy material (Fig. 27.25B). By conventional light microscopy, this tumor would be difficult to distinguish from mesothelioma. Indeed, this biopsy was initially diagnosed as a mesothelioma after a PAS/diastase PAS (dPAS) stain was found to be negative (undoubtedly the diagnosis was heavily influenced by the radiologic and clinical data) and before it was referred to our laboratory for immunohistochemical study. Strong cytoplasmic immunostaining was noted with the following epithelial markers: Leu-M1, CEA, and B72.3 (Fig. 27.25C,D). None of the mesothelial markers gave positive results. These findings virtually ruled out mesothelioma and spoke

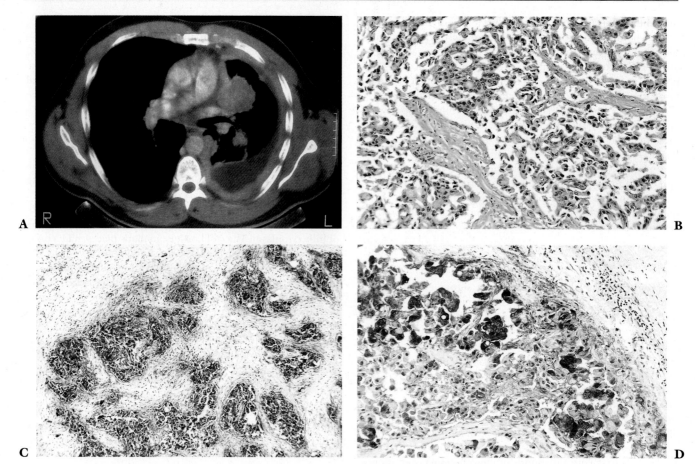

Figure 27.25. Case 2. **(A)** Computed tomography scan of the chest. Note marked thickening of the left pleura, closely simulating a mesothelioma. **(B)** Hematoxylin and eosin–stained section of the pleural biopsy. An epithelial neoplasm, histologically compatible with mesothelioma or adenocarcinoma, is present. **(C)** Section stained with a commercially available monoclonal antibody to carcinoembryonic antigen (CEA). Strong cytoplasmic granular staining is present. **(D)** Section stained for CD15 (Leu-M1). Strong staining is present on a large proportion of the tumor cells.

in favor of adenocarcinoma, probably arising in the lung parenchyma, near the pleura, and with extensive pleural involvement. Such tumors have been reported as examples of pseudomesotheliomatous adenocarcinoma (178,179).

CASE 3: SARCOMATOUS MESOTHELIOMA

History

A 66-year-old man had a clinical history of dry cough of approximately 1 month in duration and no other symptoms. He had worked for more than three decades in a shipyard, where he was repeatedly exposed to asbestos. Chest radiographs showed opacification of the left lung. A thick, leathery pleura was decorticated.

Discussion

In this case, according to the pathologist who referred the case in consultation, a large, firm, white-gray tumor rind covered the lung surface. The clinical history of industrial exposure to asbestos and the gross appearance of the tumor strongly suggested the diagnosis of malignant mesothelioma. However, the neoplasm had a sarcoma-like appearance (Fig. 27.18A), and in many places, a frank storiform pattern was evident (Fig. 27.18B).

Thus, a true sarcoma, possibly a malignant fibrous histiocytoma, involving the pleura secondarily could not be excluded with confidence on morphologic grounds alone. Strong expression of pancytokeratins by the neoplastic cells was readily demonstrable in this case (Fig. 27.18C). This finding, in the context of the narrow differential diagnosis, was sufficient to warrant a firm diagnosis of sarcomatous mesothelioma.

Comment

Although it is unlikely that malignant fibrous histiocytoma would be seen with a clinical and radiologic picture of a pleura-based tumor, in our experience, cases of sarcomatous mesothelioma with extensive involvement of the chest wall would be very difficult to distinguish from true sarcomas without the benefit of the pancytokeratin immunostains.

CASE 4: FIBROUS PLEURITIS

History

The patient, a 51-year-old man, was initially diagnosed with pneumonia. Because of a persistent right pleural effusion, he underwent a pleurocentesis with removal of 700 mL of bloody fluid. He continued a febrile course and developed pain in the right hemithorax. A computed tomography scan revealed marked pleural thickening (Fig. 27.26A). A thoracoscopic biopsy was diagnosed as desmoplastic malignant mesothelioma. He was then treated with a right pneumonectomy and pleurectomy. A firm, thick, white-tan, rindlike pleural thickening covered the entire surface of the resected lung. No gross lesions were found in the lung parenchyma.

Discussion

The histologic appearance on the HE-stained preparations is entirely consistent with desmoplastic malignant mesothelioma.

The bland-appearing spindle cells appear to invade the adipose tissue of the chest wall (Fig. 27.26B). However, immunostains for pancytokeratins reveal a different picture. The cytokeratin-expressing spindle cells are sharply delimited from the underlying adipose tissue (Fig. 27.26C). Sections of the interphase between the fibrous proliferation and the lung show a similar absence of invasiveness and reveal a zonation pattern (Fig. 27.26D,E). Numerous sections from the pleuropneumonectomy were studied, and no invasiveness was detected either in the lung parenchyma or in the thoracic wall. The diagnosis of desmoplastic malignant mesothelioma was changed to fibrous pleuritis, and no further therapy was given to the patient.

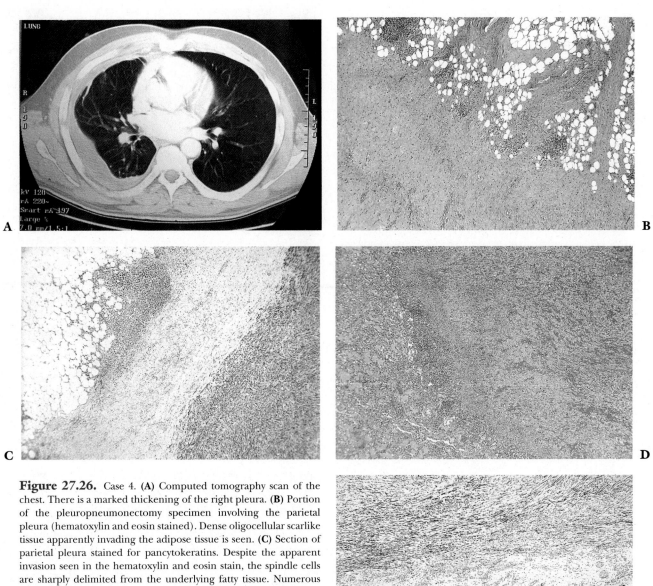

Figure 27.26. Case 4. **(A)** Computed tomography scan of the chest. There is a marked thickening of the right pleura. **(B)** Portion of the pleuropneumonectomy specimen involving the parietal pleura (hematoxylin and eosin stained). Dense oligocellular scarlike tissue apparently invading the adipose tissue is seen. **(C)** Section of parietal pleura stained for pancytokeratins. Despite the apparent invasion seen in the hematoxylin and eosin stain, the spindle cells are sharply delimited from the underlying fatty tissue. Numerous sections similarly stained showed absence of invasiveness. **(D)** Representative section of the lesion near the lung surface (hematoxylin and eosin stained). The lesion at this level is reminiscent of granulation tissue. **(E)** Pancytokeratin-stained section of the lung surface. Note that this stain enhances the layering (zoning) distribution of the lesion. Again, a band of cytokeratin-negative tissue separates the strongly stained lung epithelium and the sharply demarcated reactive cytokeratin-positive spindle cells.

Comment

The patient was alive and well more than 6 years after the pleuropneumonectomy. Given the natural history of desmoplastic malignant mesothelioma, this evolution strongly supports the diagnosis of postpneumonic fibrous pleuritis. Clearly, a diagnosis of desmoplastic malignant mesothelioma should not be made unless invasiveness can be unequivocally identified.

CASE 5: DESMOPLASTIC MESOTHELIOMA

History

The patient, a 71-year-old man, was admitted to a hospital because of mild right chest pain. A chest radiograph revealed a right-sided pleural effusion. He was discharged and treated with antibiotics on an ambulatory basis with no improvement. The chest pain grew worse in the next 2 weeks, and he was readmitted to the hospital. An exploratory thoracotomy revealed a densely fibrotic pleura, and several biopsy samples were taken. There was no history of occupational asbestos exposure.

Discussion

The biopsy material showed scarlike tissue involving visceral and parietal pleura. Within abundant collagenous stroma, a variable number of fibroblast-like cells with bland cytologic features were seen in most of the tissue samples (Fig.

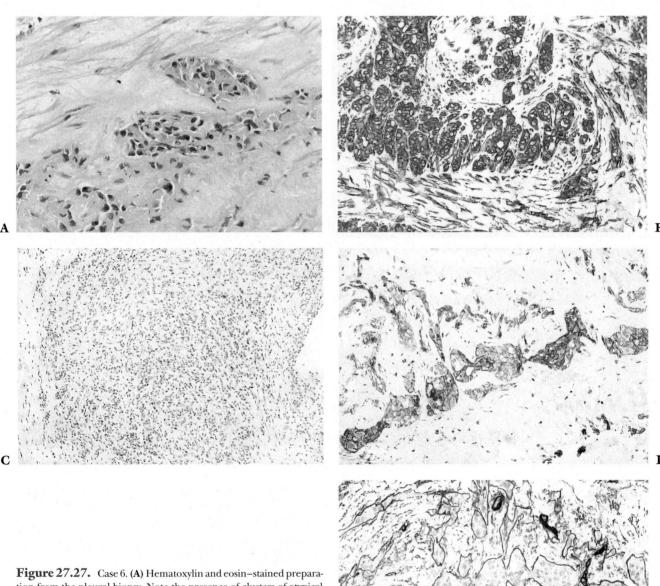

Figure 27.27. Case 6. **(A)** Hematoxylin and eosin–stained preparation from the pleural biopsy. Note the presence of clusters of atypical epithelioid cells within a desmoplastic stroma. **(B)** Vimentin-stained section. The clusters of tumor cells stain intensely. **(C)** Stained with a cocktail of monoclonal antikeratin antibodies. The tumor cells do not express detectable keratins. **(D)** Stained with antibody CD31. There is strong and generalized immunostaining with the typical, predominantly submembranous pattern. Other endothelial markers also were positive. **(E)** Stained with collagen type IV. A basal lamina surrounds the cell clusters.

27.19A,B,C). However, focal areas of cellularity with a moderate degree of pleomorphism were noted. Nevertheless, the pathologists diagnosed the biopsy as fibrous pleurisy without the benefit of immunohistochemistry. The patient's condition deteriorated rapidly, and he died 11 months after the biopsy. At autopsy, there was extensive involvement of the right pleural space with fibrous tumor that completely encased the lung. A focus of metastatic tumor was found in the liver, and another one was found in the body of a lumbar vertebra. Histologically, all of the autopsy tissue, including the metastatic tumor, resembled the original pleural biopsy. Re-examination of the biopsy with immunostains for pancytokeratins revealed intense immunoreactivity by the spindle cells, while at the same time demonstrating their invasiveness of the chest wall (Fig. 27.19D).

Comment

In retrospect, a correct diagnosis of desmoplastic malignant mesothelioma could have been easily made from the ample biopsy material if the pancytokeratin stain had been done at that time.

CASE 6: PSEUDOMESOTHELIOMATOUS HEMANGIOENDOTHELIOMA

History

The patient, a 57-year-old male nonsmoker with a history of exposure to asbestos at a young age, was first seen with a pleura-based tumor and no radiographic evidence of tumor elsewhere. A thoracoscopic pleural biopsy was done.

Discussion

Clusters of pale epithelioid tumor cells surrounded by dense fibrous stroma are seen in the biopsy material (Fig. 27.27A). The architectural and cytologic features of this tumor were considered to be consistent with poorly differentiated epithelial mesothelioma or adenocarcinoma. However, the intermediate filament immunophenotype was unusual because the tumor cells were strongly vimentin positive and negative for keratins (Fig. 27.27B,C). In view of these results, the possibility of an epithelioid endothelial neoplasm was considered. Immunostains for endothelial markers (i.e., von Willebrand factor, CD31, and *Ulex europaeus* lectin) were all positive, confirming the suspected diagnosis (Fig. 27.27D). Additionally, staining for collagen type IV showed a pattern of staining supporting a vascular neoplasm (Fig. 27.27E).

Comment

Although rare, epithelioid hemangioendothelioma and angiosarcoma may be seen as serous membrane neoplasms and closely resemble mesothelioma (180). The diagnostic difficulties may be increased by the history of asbestos exposure, as in this case. This diagnosis should be suspected whenever the tumor cells show stronger staining for vimentin than for keratins.

REFERENCES

1. Wang NS. Anatomy of the pleura. *Clin Chest Med* 1998;19:229–240.
2. Whitaker D, Papadimitriou JM, Walters MN-I. The mesothelium and its reactions: a review. *CRC Crit Rev Toxicol* 1982;10:81–144.
3. Whitaker D, Papadimitriou J. Mesothelial healing: morphological and kinetic investigations. *J Pathol* 1985;145:159–175.
4. Moalli PA, MacDonald JL, Goodglick LA, et al. Acute injury and regeneration of the mesothelium in response to asbestos fibers. *Am J Pathol* 1987;128:426–445.
5. Raftery A. Regeneration of parietal and visceral peritoneum in the immature animal: a light and electron microscopical study. *Br J Surg* 1973;60:969–975.
6. Bolen JW, Hammar SP, McNutt MA. Reactive and neoplastic serosal tissue. A light-microscopic, ultrastructural, and immunocytochemical study. *Am J Surg Pathol* 1986;10:34–47.
7. Churg A, Colby TV, Cagle P, et al. The separation of benign and malignant mesothelial proliferations. *Am J Surg Pathol* 2000;24:1183–1200.
8. Rosai J, Dehner LP. Nodular mesothelial hyperplasia in hernia sacs: a benign reactive condition simulating a neoplastic process. *Cancer* 1975;35:165–175.
9. Kafiri Y, Thomas DM, Shepherd NA, et al. p53 expression is common in malignant mesothelioma. *Histopathology* 1992;21:331–334.
10. Mayall FG, Goddard H, Gibbs AR. p53 immunostaining in the distinction between benign and malignant mesothelial proliferations using formalin-fixed paraffin sections. *J Pathol* 1992;168:377–381.
11. Cagle PT, Brown RW, Lebovitz RM. p53 immunostaining in the differentiation of reactive processes from malignancy in pleural biopsy specimens. *Hum Pathol* 1994;25:443–448.
12. Ramael M, Lemmens G, Eerdekens C, et al. Immunoreactivity for p53 protein in malignant mesothelioma and non-neoplastic mesothelium. *J Pathol* 1992;168:371–375.
13. Metcalf RA, Welsh JA, Bennett WP, et al. p53 and Kirsten-*ras* mutations in human mesothelioma cell lines. *Cancer Res* 1992;52:2610–2615.
14. Mor O, Yaron P, Huszar M, et al. Absence of p53 mutations in malignant mesotheliomas. *Am J Respir Cell Mol Biol* 1997;16:9–13.
15. Kato Y, Tsuta K, Seki K, et al. Immunohistochemical detection of GLUT-1 can discriminate between reactive mesothelium and malignant mesothelioma. *Mod Pathol* 2007;20:215–220.
16. Chiosea S, Krasinkas A, Cagle PT, et al. Diagnostic importance of 9p21 homozygous deletion in malignant mesotheliomas. *Mod Pathol* 2008;21:742–747.
17. Craighead JE. Report of the pneumoconiosis committee of the College of American Pathologists and the National Institute for Occupational Safety and Health. *Arch Pathol Lab Med* 1982;106:544–596.
18. Hillerdal G. The pathogenesis of pleural plaques and pulmonary asbestosis: possibilities and impossibilities. *Eur J Respir Dis* 1980;61:129–138.
19. Suzuki Y, Kohyama N. Translocation of inhaled asbestos fibers from the lung to other tissues. *Am J Ind Med* 1991;19:701–704.
20. Suzuki Y, Yuen SR. Asbestos tissue burden study on human malignant mesothelioma. *Ind Health* 2001;39:150–160.
21. Sebastien P, Janson X, Gaudichet A, et al. Asbestos retention in human respiratory tissues: comparative measurement in lung parenchyma and in parietal pleura. *IARC Sci Publ* 1980;30:237–246.
22. Handra-Luca A, Couvelard A, Abd AI, et al. Adenomatoid tumor of the pleura. Case report. *Ann Pathol* 2000;20:369–372.
23. Kaplan MA, Tazelaar HD, Hayashi T, et al. Adenomatoid tumors of the pleura. *Am J Surg Pathol* 1996;20:1219–1223.
24. Ikuta N, Tano M, Iwata M, et al. A case of adenomatoid mesothelioma of the pleura. *Nihon Kyobu Shikkan Gakkai Zasshi* 1989;27:1540–1544.
25. Dalton WT, Zolliker T, McCaughey WTE, et al. Localized primary tumors of the pleura. An analysis of 40 cases. *Cancer* 1979;44:1465–1475.
26. Briselli M, Mark EJ, Dickersin GR. Solitary fibrous tumors of the pleura: eight new cases and review of 360 cases in the literature. *Cancer* 1981;47:2678–2689.
27. de Perrot M, Fischer S, Brundler MA, et al. Solitary fibrous tumors of the pleura. *Ann Thorac Surg* 2002;74:285–293.
28. Magdeleinat P, Alifano M, Petino A, et al. Solitary fibrous tumors of the pleura: clinical characteristics, surgical treatment and outcome. *Eur J Cardiothorac Surg* 2002;21:1087–1093.
29. Cardillo G, Facciolo F, Cavazzana AO, et al. Localized (solitary) fibrous tumors of the pleura: an analysis of 55 patients. *Ann Thorac Surg* 2000;70:1808–1812.
30. Renshaw AA, Pinkus GS, Corson MC. CD34 and AE1/AE3. Diagnostic discriminants in the distinction of solitary fibrous tumor of the pleura from sarcomatoid mesothelioma. *Appl Immunohistochem* 1994;2:94–102.
31. Flint A, Weiss SW. CD-34 and keratin expression distinguishes solitary fibrous tumor (fibrous mesothelioma) of pleura from desmoplastic mesothelioma. *Hum Pathol* 1995;26:428–431.
32. Mentzel T, Bainbridge TC, Katenkamp D. Solitary fibrous tumour: clinicopathological, immunohistochemical, and ultrastructural analysis of 12 cases arising in soft tissues, nasal cavity and nasopharynx, urinary bladder and prostate. *Virchows Arch Int J Pathol* 1997;430:445–453.
33. Suster S, Nascimento AG, Miettinen M, et al. Solitary fibrous tumors of soft tissue: a clinicopathologic and immunohistochemical study of 12 cases. *Am J Surg Pathol* 1995;19:1257–1266.
34. Westra WH, Gerald WL, Rosai J. Solitary fibrous tumor. Consistent CD34 immunoreactivity and occurrence in the orbit. *Am J Surg Pathol* 1994;18:992–998.
35. Okamura JM, Barr RJ, Battifora H. Solitary fibrous tumor of the skin. *Am J Dermatopathol* 1997;19:515–518.
36. Wagner JC, Sleggs CA, Marchand P. Diffuse pleural mesothelioma and asbestos exposure in the North Western Cape Province. *Br J Ind Med* 1960;17:260–271.
37. Borow M, Conston A, Livornese L, et al. Mesothelioma following exposure to asbestos: a review of 72 cases. *Chest* 1973;64:641–646.

38. Elmes PC, McCaughey WTE, Eade OL. Diffuse mesothelioma of pleura and asbestos. *Br Med J* 1965;1:350–353.

39. Lerner HJ, Schoenfeld DA, Martin A, et al. Malignant mesothelioma. The Eastern Cooperative Oncology Group (ECOG) experience. *Cancer* 1985;52:1981–1985.

40. Newhouse M. Epidemiology of asbestos-related tumors. *Semin Oncol* 1981;8:250–257.

41. O'Donnell W, Mann RH, Grosh JL. Asbestos—an extrinsic factor in the pathogenesis of bronchogenic carcinomas and mesotheliomas. *Cancer* 1966;19:1143–1148.

42. Selikoff IJ, Churg J, Hammond EC. Relation between exposure to asbestos and mesothelioma. *N Engl J Med* 1965;272:560–565.

43. Wanebo HJ, Martini N, Melamed MR, et al. Pleural mesothelioma. *Cancer* 1976;38:2481–2488.

44. McDonald JC. Cancer risks due to asbestos and man-made fibres. *Recent Results Cancer Res* 1990;120:122–131.

45. Rogers AJ, Leigh J, Berry G, et al. Relationship between lung asbestos fiber type and concentration and relative risk of mesothelioma. *Cancer* 1991;67:1912–1920.

46. Grundy GW, Miller R. Malignant mesothelioma in childhood. Report of 13 cases. *Cancer* 1972;30:1216–1218.

47. Peterson JT, Greenberg SD, Buffler P. Non-asbestos-related malignant mesothelioma. A review. *Cancer* 1984;54:951–960.

48. Hammar SP, Bockus D, Remington F, et al. Familial mesothelioma: a report of two families. *Hum Pathol* 1989;20:107–112.

49. Selikoff IJ, Hammond EC, Seidman H. Latency of asbestos disease among insulation workers in the United States and Canada. *Cancer* 1980;46:2736–2740.

50. Vianna NJ, Maslowsky J, Roberts S, et al. Malignant mesothelioma. *NY State J Med* 1981;81:735–738.

51. McDonald AD, McDonald J. Malignant mesothelioma in North America. *Cancer* 1980;46:1650–1656.

52. Davis JMG. The biological effects of mineral fibres. *Ann Occup Hyg* 1981;24:227–234.

53. McDonald AD, Harper A, El Attar OA, et al. Epidemiology of primary malignant mesothelial tumors in Canada. *Cancer* 1970;26:914–919.

54. Oels HC, Harrison EG, Carr DT, et al. Diffuse malignant mesothelioma of the pleura: a review of 37 cases. *Chest* 1971;60:564–570.

55. Roggli VL, McGavran MH, Subach J, et al. Pulmonary asbestos body counts and electron probe analysis of asbestos body cores in patients with mesothelioma: a study of 25 cases. *Cancer* 1982;50:2423–2432.

56. Carbone M, Pass HI, Rizzo P, et al. Simian virus 40-like DNA sequences in human pleural mesothelioma. *Oncogene* 1994;9:1781–1790.

57. Carbone M, Rizzo P, Pass H. Simian virus 40: the link with human malignant mesothelioma is well established. *Anticancer Res* 2000;20:875–877.

58. Ziegler A, Seemayer CA, Hinterberger M, et al. Low prevalence of SV40 in Swiss mesothelioma patients after elimination of false-positive PCR results. *Lung Cancer* 2007;57:282–291.

59. Carbone M, Pass HI. Re: Debate on the link between SV40 and human cancer continues. *J Natl Cancer Inst* 2002;94:229–230.

60. Klein G, Powers A, Croce C. Association of SV40 with human tumors. *Oncogene* 2002;21:1141–1149.

61. Gordon GJ, Chen CJ, Jaklitsch MT, et al. Detection and quantification of SV40 large T-antigen DNA in mesothelioma tissues and cell lines. *Oncol Rep* 2002;9:631–634.

62. Shah KV. SV40 and human cancer: a review of recent data. *Int J Cancer* 2007;120:215–223.

63. Rollison DE. Epidemiologic studies of polyomaviruses and cancer: previous findings, methodologic challenges and future directions. *Adv Exp Med Biol* 2006;577:342–356.

64. Engels EA. Cancer risk associated with receipt of vaccines contaminated with simian virus 40: epidemiologic research. *Expert Rev Vaccines* 2005;4:197–206.

65. Spirtas R, Beebe GW, Connelly RR, et al. Recent trends in mesothelioma incidence in the United States. *Am J Ind Med* 1986;9:397–407.

66. Muscat JE, Wynder EL. Cigarette smoking, asbestos exposure, and malignant mesothelioma. *Cancer Res* 1991;51:2263–2267.

67. Adams VI, Unni KK, Muhm JR, et al. Diffuse malignant mesothelioma of pleura. Diagnosis and survival in 92 cases. *Cancer* 1986;58:1540–1551.

68. Elmes PC, Simpson MJC. The clinical aspects of mesothelioma. *Quart J Med* 1976;45:427–449.

69. Sussman J, Rosai J. Lymph node metastasis as the initial manifestation of malignant mesothelioma: report of six cases. *Am J Surg Pathol* 1990;14:819–828.

70. Fishbein A, Suzuki Y, Selikoff IJ. Unexpected longevity of a patient with malignant pleural mesothelioma. *Cancer* 1978;42:1999–2004.

71. Reichart R, Sherman CD. Prolonged survival in diffuse pleural mesothelioma treated with Au 198. *Cancer* 1959;17:799–805.

72. Johansson L, Lindén CJ. Aspects of histopathologic subtype as a prognostic factor in 85 pleural mesotheliomas. *Chest* 1996;109:109–114.

73. Kucuksu N, Thomas W, Ezdinli EZ. Chemotherapy of malignant diffuse mesothelioma. *Cancer* 1976;37:1265–1274.

74. Ball DL, Cruickshank DG. The treatment of malignant mesothelioma of the pleura: review of a 5-year experience with special reference to radiotherapy. *Am J Clin Oncol* 1990;13:4–9.

75. Bard M, Ruffie P. Malignant pleural mesothelioma. Present data and perspectives for treatment. *Presse Med* 2002;31:412–419.

76. Dessy E, Falleni M, Braidotti P, et al. Unusual clear cell variant of epithelioid mesothelioma. *Arch Pathol Lab Med* 2001;125:1588–1590.

77. Ordóñez NG, Myhre M, Mackay B. Clear cell mesothelioma. *Ultrastruct Pathol* 1996;20:331–336.

78. Henderson DW, Attwood HD, Constance TJ, et al. Lymphohistiocytoid mesothelioma: a rare lymphomatoid variant of predominantly sarcomatoid mesothelioma. *Ultrastruct Pathol* 1988;12:367–384.

79. Khalidi HS, Medeiros LJ, Battifora H. Lymphohistiocytoid mesothelioma. An often misdiagnosed variant of sarcomatoid mesothelioma. *Am J Clin Pathol* 2000;113:649–654.

80. Serio G, Scattone A, Pennella A, et al. Malignant deciduoid mesothelioma of the pleura: report of two cases with long survival. *Histopathology* 2002;40:348–352.

81. Ordóñez NG. Epithelial mesothelioma with deciduoid features: report of four cases. *Am J Surg Pathol* 2000;24:816–823.

82. Crotty TB, Myers JL, Katzenstein AL, et al. Localized malignant mesothelioma. A clinicopathologic and flow cytometric study. *Am J Surg Pathol* 1994;18:357–363.

83. Allen TC, Cagle PT, Churg AM, et al. Localized malignant mesothelioma. *Am J Surg Pathol* 2005;29:866–873.

84. Galateau-Salle F, Vignaud JM, Burke L, et al. Well-differentiated papillary mesothelioma of the pleura: a series of 24 cases. *Am J Surg Pathol* 2004;28:534–540.

85. Butnor KJ, Sporn TA, Hammar SP, et al. Well-differentiated papillary mesothelioma. *Am J Surg Pathol* 2001;25:1304–1309.

86. Attanoos RL, Suvarna SK, Rhead E, et al. Malignant vascular tumours of the pleura in "asbestos" workers and endothelial differentiation in malignant mesothelioma. *Thorax* 2000;55:860–863.

87. Zhang PJ, LiVolsi VA, Brooks JJ. Malignant epithelioid vascular tumors of the pleura: report of a series and literature review. *Hum Pathol* 2000;31:29–34.

88. Lin BT, Colby T, Gown AM, et al. Malignant vascular tumors of the serous membranes mimicking mesothelioma. A report of 14 cases. *Am J Surg Pathol* 1996;20:1431–1439.

89. Yousem SA, Hochholzer L. Unusual thoracic manifestations of epithelioid hemangioendothelioma. *Arch Pathol Lab Med* 1987;111:459–463.

90. Attanoos RL, Galateau-Salle F, Gibbs AR, et al. Primary thymic epithelial tumours of the pleura mimicking malignant mesothelioma. *Histopathology* 2002;41:42–49.

91. Moran CA, Travis WD, Rosado-de-Christenson M, et al. Thymomas presenting as pleural tumors. Report of eight cases. *Am J Surg Pathol* 1992;16:138–144.

92. Pan CC, Chen PC, Chou TY, et al. Expression of calretinin and other mesothelioma-related markers in thymic carcinoma and thymoma. *Hum Pathol* 2003;34:1155–1162.

93. Fukayama M, Maeda Y, Funata N, et al. Pulmonary and pleural thymoma. Diagnostic application of lymphocyte markers to the thymoma of unusual site. *Am J Clin Pathol* 1988;89:617–621.

94. Cantin R, Al-Jabi M, McCaughey WTE. Desmoplastic diffuse mesothelioma. *Am J Surg Pathol* 1982;6:215–222.

95. Kannerstein M, Churg J. Desmoplastic diffuse malignant mesothelioma. In Ferioglio CM, Wolff M, eds. *Progress in Surgical Pathology. Volume II.* New York, NY: Masson Publishing, 1980:19–29.

96. Moran CA, Suster S, Koss MN. The spectrum of histologic growth patterns in benign and malignant fibrous tumors of the pleura. *Semin Diag Pathol* 1992;9:169–180.

97. Cappello F, Barnes L. Synovial sarcoma and malignant mesothelioma of the pleura: review, differential diagnosis and possible role of apoptosis. *Pathology* 2001;33:142–148.

98. Nicholson AG, Goldstraw P, Fisher C. Synovial sarcoma of the pleura and its differentiation from other primary pleural tumours: a clinicopathological and immunohistochemical review of three cases. *Histopathology* 1998;33:508–513.

99. Miettinen M, Limon J, Niezabitowski A, et al. Calretinin and other mesothelioma markers in synovial sarcoma: analysis of antigenic similarities and differences with malignant mesothelioma. *Am J Surg Pathol* 2001;25:610–617.

100. Weinbreck N, Vignaud JM, Begueret H, et al. SYT-SSX fusion is absent in sarcomatoid mesothelioma allowing its distinction from synovial sarcoma of the pleura. *Mod Pathol* 2007;20:617–621.

101. Mayall FG, Gibbs AR. "Pleural" and pulmonary carcinosarcomas. *J Pathol* 1992;167:305–311.

102. Benjamin CJ, Ritchie A. Histological staining for the diagnosis of mesothelioma. *Am J Med Technol* 1982;48:905–908.

103. Warhol MJ, Hickey WF, Corson JM. Malignant mesothelioma. Ultrastructural distinction from adenocarcinoma. *Am J Surg Pathol* 1982;6:307–314.

104. Burns TR, Greenberg D, Mace ML, et al. Ultrastructural diagnosis of epithelial malignant mesothelioma. *Cancer* 1985;56:2036–2040.

105. Dardick I, Jabi M, McCaughey WTE, et al. Diffuse epithelial mesothelioma: a review of the ultrastructural spectrum. *Ultrastruct Pathol* 1987;11:503–533.

106. Roggli VL, Sharma A, Butnor KJ, et al. Malignant mesothelioma and occupational exposure to asbestos: a clinicopathological correlation of 1445 cases. *Ultrastruct Pathol* 2002;26:55–65.

107. Azumi N, Battifora H. The distribution of vimentin and keratin in epithelial and nonepithelial neoplasms. A comprehensive immunohistochemical study on formalin- and alcohol-fixed tumors. *Am J Clin Pathol* 1987;88:286–296.

108. Riera JR, Astengo-Osuna C, Longmate JA, et al. The immunohistochemical diagnostic panel for epithelial mesothelioma. A reevaluation following heat-induced epitope retrieval. *Am J Surg Pathol* 1997;21:1409–1419.

109. Battifora H. Assessment of antigen damage in immunohistochemistry: the vimentin internal control. *Am J Clin Pathol* 1991;96:669–671.

110. Doglioni C, Dei Tos AP, Laurino L, et al. Calretinin: a novel immunocytochemical marker for mesothelioma. *Am J Surg Pathol* 1996;20:1037–1046.

111. Dei Tos AP, Doglioni C. Calretinin: a novel tool for diagnostic immunohistochemistry. *Adv Anat Pathol* 1998;5:61–66.

112. Ordóñez NG. Value of calretinin immunostaining in differentiating epithelial mesothelioma from lung adenocarcinoma. *Mod Pathol* 1998;11:929–933.

113. Comin CE, Novelli L, Boddi V, et al. Calretinin, thrombomodulin, CEA, and CD15: a useful combination of immunohistochemical markers for differentiating pleural epithelial mesothelioma from peripheral pulmonary adenocarcinoma. *Hum Pathol* 2001;32:529–536.

114. Attanoos RL, Webb R, Dojcinov SD, et al. Value of mesothelial and epithelial antibodies in distinguishing diffuse peritoneal mesothelioma in females from serous papillary carcinoma of the ovary and peritoneum. *Histopathology* 2002;40:237–244.

115. Yaziji H, Battifora H, Barry TS, et al. Evaluation of 12 antibodies for distinguishing epithelioid mesothelioma from adenocarcinoma: identification of a three-antibody immunohistochemical panel with maximal sensitivity and specificity. *Mod Pathol* 2006;19:514–523.

116. Ordóñez NG. Immunohistochemical diagnosis of epithelioid mesotheliomas: a critical review of old markers, new markers. *Hum Pathol* 2002;33:953–967.

117. Clover J, Oates J, Edwards C. Anti-cytokeratin 5/6: a positive marker for epithelioid mesothelioma. *Histopathology* 1997;31:140–143.

118. Cury PM, Butcher DN, Fisher C, et al. Value of the mesothelium-associated antibodies thrombomodulin, cytokeratin 5/6, calretinin, and CD44H in distinguishing epithelioid pleural mesothelioma from adenocarcinoma metastatic to the pleura. *Mod Pathol* 2000;13:107–112.

119. Chu PG, Weiss LM. Expression of cytokeratin 5/6 in epithelial neoplasms: an immunohistochemical study of 509 cases. *Mod Pathol* 2002;15:6–10.

120. Nagle RB, Bocker W, Davis JR, et al. Characterization of breast carcinomas by two monoclonal antibodies distinguishing myoepithelial from luminal epithelial cells. *J Histochem Cytochem* 1986;34:869–881.

121. Moll R, Dhouailly D, Sun T-T. Expression of keratin 5 as a distinctive feature of epithelial and biphasic mesotheliomas. An immunohistochemical study using monoclonal antibody AE14. *Virchows Arch B* 1989;58:129–145.

122. Yaziji H, Battifora H, Bachi C, et al. A comprehensive study of immunohistochemical markers in the distinction between pleural mesothelioma and adenocarcinoma: emphasis on specificity and sensitivity of newly defined markers. *Mod Pathol* 2002;15:331A.

123. Kaufmann O, Fietze E, Mengs J, et al. Value of p63 and cytokeratin 5/6 as immunohistochemical markers for the differential diagnosis of poorly differentiated and undifferentiated carcinomas. *Am J Clin Pathol* 2001;116:823–830.

124. Pelosi G, Pasini F, Olsen SC, et al. p63 immunoreactivity in lung cancer: yet another player in the development of squamous cell carcinomas? *J Pathol* 2002;198:100–109.

125. Maruyama I, Bell CE, Majerus PW. Thrombomodulin is found on endothelium of arteries, veins, capillaries, and lymphatics, and on syncytiotrophoblasts of human placenta. *J Cell Biol* 1985;101:363–371.

126. Yonezawa S, Maruyama I, Sakae K, et al. Thrombomodulin as a marker for vascular tumors. Comparative study with factor VIII and *Ulex europaeus* I lectin. *Am J Clin Pathol* 1987;88:405–411.

127. Jackson DE, Mitchell CA, Bird P, et al. Immunohistochemical localization of thrombomodulin in normal human skin and skin tumours. *J Pathol* 1995;175:421–432.

128. Ordóñez NG. Thrombomodulin expression in transitional cell carcinoma. *Am J Clin Pathol* 1998;110:385–390.

129. Collins CL, Ordóñez NG, Schaefer R, et al. Thrombomodulin expression in malignant pleural mesothelioma and pulmonary adenocarcinoma. *Am J Pathol* 1992;141:827–833.

130. Koukoulis GK, Radosevich JA, Warren WH, et al. Immunohistochemical analysis of pulmonary and pleural neoplasms with monoclonal antibodies B72.3 and CSLEX-1. *Virchows Arch B* 1990;58:427–433.

131. Singh G, Whiteside TL, Dekker A. Immunodiagnosis of mesothelioma. *Cancer* 1979;43:2288–2296.

132. Donna A, Betta PG, Bellingeri D, et al. New marker for mesothelioma: an immunoperoxidase study. *J Clin Pathol* 1986;39:961–968.

133. Nagoshi M, Tsuneyoshi M. Expression of proliferating cell nuclear antigen in Wilms' tumors and other pediatric renal tumors: the correlation between histologic classification and proliferative activity. *J Surg Oncol* 1994;55:114–121.

134. Charles AK, Moore IE, Berry PJ. Immunohistochemical detection of the Wilms' tumour gene WT1 in desmoplastic small round cell tumour. *Histopathology* 1997;30:312–314.

135. Ordóñez NG. Value of thyroid transcription factor-1, E-cadherin, Bg8, WT1, and CD44S immunostaining in distinguishing epithelial pleural mesothelioma from pulmonary and nonpulmonary adenocarcinoma. *Am J Surg Pathol* 2000;24:598–606.

136. Hecht JL, Lee BH, Pinkus JL, et al. The value of Wilms tumor susceptibility gene 1 in cytologic preparations as a marker for malignant mesothelioma. *Cancer* 2002;96:105–109.

137. Walker C, Rutten F, Yuan X, et al. Wilms' tumor suppressor gene expression in rat and human mesothelioma. *Cancer Res* 1994;54:3101–3106.

138. Chang K, Pai LH, Batra JK, et al. Characterization of the antigen (CAK1) recognized by monoclonal antibody K1 present on ovarian cancers and normal mesothelium. *Cancer Res* 1992;52:181–186.

139. Argani P, Iacobuzio-Donahue C, Ryu B, et al. Mesothelin is overexpressed in the vast majority of ductal adenocarcinomas of the pancreas: identification of a new pancreatic cancer marker by serial analysis of gene expression (SAGE). *Clin Cancer Res* 2001;7:3862–3868.

140. Chang K, Pastan I, Willingham MC. Frequent expression of the tumor antigen CAK1 in squamous-cell carcinomas. *Int J Cancer* 1992;51:548–554.

141. Kimura N, Kimura I. Podoplanin as a marker for mesothelioma. *Pathol Int* 2005;55:83–86.

142. Ordóñez NG. D2-40 and podoplanin are highly specific and sensitive immunohistochemical markers of epithelioid malignant mesothelioma. *Hum Pathol* 2005;36:372–380.

143. Ordóñez NG. Podoplanin: a novel diagnostic immunohistochemical marker. *Adv Anat Pathol* 2006;13:83–88.

144. Ordóñez NG. What are the current best immunohistochemical markers for the diagnosis of epithelioid mesothelioma? A review and update. *Hum Pathol* 2007;38:1–16.

145. Chu AY, Litzky LA, Pasha TL, et al. Utility of D2-40, a novel mesothelial marker, in the diagnosis of malignant mesothelioma. *Mod Pathol* 2005;18:105–110.

146. Mimura T, Ito A, Sakuma T, et al. Novel marker D2-40, combined with calretinin, CEA, and TTF-1: an optimal set of immunodiagnostic markers for pleural mesothelioma. *Cancer* 2007;109:933–938.

147. Comin CE, Dini S, Novelli L, et al. h-Caldesmon, a useful positive marker in the diagnosis of pleural malignant mesothelioma, epithelioid type. *Am J Surg Pathol* 2006;30:463–469.

148. Comin CE, Saieva C, Messerini L. h-Caldesmon, calretinin, estrogen receptor, and Ber-EP4: a useful combination of immunohistochemical markers for differentiating epithelioid peritoneal mesothelioma from serous papillary carcinoma of the ovary. *Am J Surg Pathol* 2007;31:1139–1148.

149. Dejmek A, Hjerpe A. Carcinoembryonic antigen-like reactivity in malignant mesothelioma: a comparison between different commercially available antibodies. *Cancer* 1994;73:464–469.

150. Wick MR, Loy T, Mills SE, et al. Malignant epithelioid pleural mesothelioma versus peripheral pulmonary adenocarcinoma: a histochemical, ultrastructural, and immunohistologic study of 103 cases. *Hum Pathol* 1990;21:759–766.

151. Whitaker D, Sterret GF, Shilkin K. Detection of tissue CEA-like substance as an aid in the differential diagnosis of malignant mesothelioma. *Pathology* 1982;14:255–258.

152. Otis CN, Carter D, Cole S, et al. Immunohistochemical evaluation of pleural mesothelioma and pulmonary adenocarcinoma. A bi-institutional study of 47 cases. *Am J Surg Pathol* 1987;11:445–456.

153. Battifora H, Kopinski M. Distinction of mesothelioma from adenocarcinoma. An immunohistochemical approach. *Cancer* 1985;55:1679–1685.

154. Ruitenbeek T, Gouw ASH, Poppema S. Immunocytology of body cavity fluids: MOC-31, a monoclonal antibody discriminating between mesothelial and epithelial cells. *Arch Pathol Lab Med* 1994;118:265–269.

155. Ordóñez NG. Value of the MOC-31 monoclonal antibody in differentiating epithelial pleural mesothelioma from lung adenocarcinoma. *Hum Pathol* 1998;29:166–169.

156. Jordan D, Jagirdar J, Kaneko M. Blood group antigens, Lewis* and Lewisy in the diagnostic discrimination of malignant mesothelioma versus adenocarcinoma. *Am J Pathol* 1989;135:931–937.

157. Latza U, Niedobitek G, Schwarting R, et al. Ber-EP4: new monoclonal antibody which distinguishes epithelia from mesothelia. *J Clin Pathol* 1990;43:213–219.

158. Sheibani K, Shin SS, Kezirian J, et al. Ber-EP4 antibody as a discriminant in the differential diagnosis of malignant mesothelioma vs. adenocarcinoma. *Am J Surg Pathol* 1991;15:779–784.

159. Gaffey MJ, Mills SE, Swanson PE, et al. Immunoreactivity for BER-EP4 in adenocarcinomas, adenomatoid tumors, and malignant mesotheliomas. *Am J Surg Pathol* 1992;16:593–599.

160. Ordóñez NG. Value of the Ber-EP4 antibody in differentiating epithelial pleural mesothelioma from adenocarcinoma: the M.D. Anderson experience and a critical review of the literature. *Am J Clin Pathol* 1998;109:85–89.

161. Di Loreto C, Puglisi F, Di Lauro V, et al. TTF-1 protein expression in pleural malignant mesotheliomas and adenocarcinomas of the lung. *Cancer Lett* 1998;124:73–78.

162. Nakamura N, Miyagi E, Murata S, et al. Expression of thyroid transcription factor-1 in normal and neoplastic lung tissues. *Mod Pathol* 2002;15:1058–1067.

163. Folpe AL, Gown AM, Lamps LW, et al. Thyroid transcription factor-1: immunohistochemical evaluation in pulmonary neuroendocrine tumors. *Mod Pathol* 1999;12:5–8.

164. Bejarano PA, Baughman RP, Biddinger PW, et al. Surfactant proteins and thyroid transcription factor-1 in pulmonary and breast carcinomas. *Mod Pathol* 1996;9:445–452.

165. Sheibani K, Battifora H, Burke JS, et al. Leu-M1 antigen in human neoplasms. An immunohistologic study of 400 cases. *Am J Surg Pathol* 1986;10:227–236.

166. Sheibani K, Battifora H, Burke JS. Antigenic phenotype of malignant mesotheliomas and pulmonary adenocarcinomas. An immunohistologic analysis demonstrating the value of Leu M1 antigen. *Am J Pathol* 1986;123:212–219.

167. Szpak CA, Johston WW, Lottich SC, et al. Patterns of reactivity of four novel monoclonal antibodies (B72.3, DF3, B1.1 and B6.2) with cells in human malignant and benign effusions. *Acta Cytol* 1984;28:356–367.

168. Johston WW, Szpak CA, Lottich SC, et al. Use of a monoclonal antibody (B72.3) as a novel immunohistochemical adjunct for the diagnosis of carcinomas in fine needle aspiration biopsy specimens. *Hum Pathol* 1986;17:501–513.

169. Riera JR, Astengo-Osuna C, Longmate JA, et al. The immunohistochemical diagnostic panel for epithelial mesothelioma: a reevaluation after heat-induced epitope retrieval. *Am J Surg Pathol* 1997;21:1409–1419.

170. Facchetti F, Lonardi S, Gentili F, et al. Claudin 4 identifies a wide spectrum of epithelial neoplasms and represents a very useful marker for carcinoma versus mesothelioma diagnosis in pleural and peritoneal biopsies and effusions. *Virchows Arch* 2007;451:669–680.

171. Naylor B. The exfoliative cytology of diffuse malignant mesothelioma. *J Pathol Bacteriol* 1963;86:293–298.

172. Bhalla R, Siddiqui MT, Mandich D, et al. Diagnostic utility of D2-40 and podoplanin in effusion cell blocks. *Diagn Cytopathol* 2007;35:342–347.

173. El-Naggar AK, Ordóñez NG, Garnsey L, et al. Epithelioid pleural mesotheliomas and pulmonary adenocarcinomas: a comparative DNA flow cytometric study. *Hum Pathol* 1991;22:972–978.

174. Esteban JM, Sheibani K. DNA ploidy analysis of pleural mesotheliomas: its usefulness for their distinction from lung adenocarcinomas. *Mod Pathol* 1992;5:626–630.

175. Pyrhönen S, Tiainen M, Rautonen J, et al. Comparison of DNA and karyotype ploidy in malignant mesothelioma. *Cancer Genet Cytogenet* 1992;60:8–13.

176. Dazzi H, Thatcher N, Hasleton PS, et al. DNA analysis by flow cytometry in malignant pleural mesothelioma: relationship to histology and survival. *J Pathol* 1990;162:51–55.

177. Frierson HF, Mills SE, Legier JF. Flow cytometric analysis of ploidy in immunohistochemically confirmed samples of malignant epithelial mesothelioma. *Am J Clin Pathol* 1988;90:240–243.

178. Harwood TR, Gracey DR, Yokoo H. Pseudomesotheliomatous carcinoma of the lung: a variant of peripheral lung cancer. *Am J Clin Pathol* 1976;65:159–167.

179. Koss M, Travis W, Moran C, et al. Pseudomesotheliomatous adenocarcinoma: a reappraisal. *Semin Diag Pathol* 1992;9:117–123.

180. Lin BTY, Colby T, Gown AM, et al. Malignant vascular tumors of the serous membranes mimicking mesothelioma. A report of 14 cases. *Am J Surg Pathol* 1996;20:1431–1439.

The Mediastinum

Although the mediastinum is a relatively small anatomic compartment, the diversity of pathologic processes that may reside in it is impressive. Such lesions are both nonneoplastic and neoplastic, and they include proliferations of somatic epithelial, lymphoid, mesenchymal, and germ cell types. The surgical pathologist's perspective on mediastinal maladies has been one of relatively rapid evolution because operative technique was not advanced enough to allow for direct exploration of this topographic site until the 1940s (1). Since that time, however, a multiplicity of tumors and tumor-like conditions have been well characterized in the mediastinum; moreover, the development of comparatively noninvasive techniques to obtain tissue samples from them (2–6) has presented a new challenge to virtually all histopathologists to be familiar with their salient attributes.

This chapter is devoted to a consideration of differential diagnostic problems that one may encounter in the context just cited. In the course of discussing this topic, most—but not all—of the potential lesions of the mediastinum will be reviewed. A decision was made to present a directed treatment of the subject material and to concentrate on those problems that are most frequent and most difficult for surgical pathologists. For those readers desiring a more encyclopedic exposition on mediastinal diseases, other reference works may be consulted (7–10).

CLINICAL FEATURES OF MEDIASTINAL LESIONS

Relatively few clinical symptoms and signs allow the examining physician to pinpoint the exact location of an intrathoracic lesion in one of the mediastinal subcompartments. Nevertheless, certain observations, when taken together with the knowledge that a mediastinal abnormality is indeed present on chest radiographs, may assist the pathologist in anticipating just which lesion is most likely and, in the process, to narrow the differential diagnosis appreciably.

The mediastinum is a "forgiving" region of the human anatomy, in that space-occupying lesions within it must reach a maximum diameter of several centimeters to produce general symptoms or signs of structural compression and displacement. These include vague anterior or posterior chest pain, dyspnea, dysphagia, cough, and, more rarely, indications of the superior vena caval syndrome or cardiac embarrassment. Save for the last two of these observations (which are usually seen in conjunction with invasive neoplasms), none of them allows for an accurate prediction of whether the lesion at hand is benign or malignant. In fact, the great majority of mediastinal masses, regardless of their biologic attributes, are unaccompanied by any symptoms or signs and are seen incidentally on chest x-rays taken in routine health assessments.

Nevertheless, selected symptoms and signs are of particular diagnostic importance because they are associated with predefined subsets of mediastinal lesions. Systemic complaints, such as weight loss, fever, and night sweats, are predominantly seen with lymphoproliferative diseases (malignant lymphomas [11,12] and Castleman disease [angiofollicular lymphoid hyperplasia] [13]); the same is true of microcytic-hypochromic anemia. Myasthenia gravis is generally a marker of true thymic hyperplasia and thymoma (13–20), as distinguished from thymic carcinoma (discussed later in the chapter); rarely, other mediastinal tumors may be linked to this disorder as well (13,16,21,22). Similarly, acquired hypogammaglobulinemia serves as a potential indicator of thymoma (23,24), as does pure anerythrogenesis (25,26), but both may also occasionally be present in cases of leukemia and malignant lymphoma (27,28).

Additional syndromes that appear to occur excessively in patients with thymoma include aplastic anemia, rheumatoid arthritis, systemic lupus erythematosus, scleroderma, mucocutaneous candidiasis, CD4 lymphopenia, and relapsing polychondritis (14,15,29–32). Isolated examples of cancer-associated retinopathy, myotonic dystrophy, and graft-versus-host disease–like colitis also have been documented in association with thymoma (33–35). On the other hand, Cushing syndrome, syndrome of inappropriate secretion of antidiuretic hormone, Eaton-Lambert (pseudomyasthenic) syndrome, and multiple endocrine neoplasia type 1 (MEN1) serve as clues to the existence of neuroendocrine neoplasms of the mediastinum, both primary and secondary (3,13,36–50). Hypercalcemia and elevations in plasma parathormone (PTH) levels are observed in cases of intrathymic parathyroid neoplasia, examples of primary thymic or metastatic squamous cell carcinoma involving the mediastinum, and rare instances of thymic carcinoid tumor (51–54). Concomitant gynecomastia and impotence in men may potentially be seen in conjunction with intrathymic choriocarcinoma (55). Symptoms and signs simulating those of adrenal pheochromocytomas may be associated with paragangliomas of the anterior or posterior mediastinum (19,56–58), and the syndromes of childhood opsoclonus-myoclonus or hypokalemic diarrhea may identify a posterior mediastinal tumor as neuroblastic in nature (59). The presence of a hematologic dyscrasia (usually represented by acute leukemia showing the marker isochromosome 12p) points to a diagnosis of extragonadal germ cell tumor if a concurrent anterior mediastinal mass is seen, and the stigmata of Klinefelter syndrome (constitutional 47XXY karyotype) have the same contextual association (60,61). Finally, rare cases of primary thymic carcinoma have been allied with pulmonary sarcoidal (noncaseating granulomatous) reactions, which appear to be paraneoplastic in nature (62).

The review of plain film chest roentgenograms, computed thoracic tomograms, and other imaging studies (when necessary) with an experienced radiologist should be considered es-

PERTINENT GROSS FEATURES OF MEDIASTINAL LESIONS

In those cases where the first procedure applied to a mediastinal lesion is an attempt at excision, the pathologist may use selected gross features to begin the process of differential diagnosis. Macroscopic invasion into attached fragments of lung, pericardium, or thoracic blood vessels is generally associated with a potential for aggressive behavior. Not all proliferations with such attributes are overtly malignant cytologically, in that desmoid-type fibromatosis, thymoma, and fibrosing mediastinitis may demonstrate invasive growth. Nevertheless, all of the latter lesions do have the capacity to cause significant morbidity and even mortality.

However, encapsulation is generally a characteristic of biologically indolent processes in the mediastinum; benign cysts of thymic, mesothelial, enteric, and bronchogenic types typically have distinct capsules, as do the majority of thymomas (Fig. 28.2). Conversely, it is uncommon for thymic carcinomas, malignant germ cell tumors, neuroendocrine neoplasms, and sarcomas to be surrounded completely by fibrous tissue at their peripheries, and malignant lymphomas never are encapsulated.

Other macroscopic findings are sometimes useful points of distinction but with a lesser predictive value. For example, thymomas often are subdivided internally (on cut section) by broad fibrous bands that intersect one another at acute angles, whereas sclerosing lymphomas, which may sometimes otherwise simulate thymic epithelial neoplasms, exhibit indistinct fibrous trabeculation or stromal bands that connect with one another obliquely (Fig. 28.3) (7). Also, extensive intralesional hemorrhage and necrosis are worthy of note because they are generally uncommon in lymphomas, as well as in benign tumors of the mediastinum.

HISTOLOGIC FEATURES OF MEDIASTINAL TUMORS, WITH EMPHASIS ON DIFFERENTIAL DIAGNOSTIC CATEGORIES

The microscopic differential diagnosis of mediastinal lesions is facilitated by three rather simple steps. The pathologist must

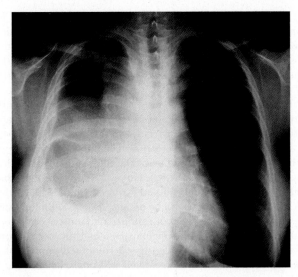

Figure 28.1. Posteroanterior chest radiograph showing a large anterior mediastinal mass with projection into the right superior lung field and accompanying right pleural effusion. This radiologic presentation indicates the presence of a malignant neoplasm.

sential to the diagnostic process (Fig. 28.1) (58–67). This reflects not only the fact that radiologic-pathologic correlation has presently evolved to an advanced state (63,64,68,69), but also the reality that open surgical (incisional) biopsy of mediastinal tumors is being threatened with extinction. Pathologists are infrequently afforded the luxury of a first-hand macroscopic description of such lesions by the surgeon because radiologically assisted needle biopsies (4–5a) now typically represent the first diagnostic procedures used in these cases.

Simple radiographic localization of a mediastinal mass has considerable value in and of itself. Substantial information is available on the relative likelihood of any given lesion in the three anatomically defined regions of the mediastinum. The anterior mediastinal compartment is that which is ventral to the anterior cardiac border and the aortic root; it most commonly harbors thymic epithelial tumors and cysts, germ cell neoplasms, lymphoproliferative lesions, retrosternal thyroid glandular proliferations, parathyroid lesions, aorticopulmonary-type paragangliomas, and nonneurogenic mesenchymal tumors. The "middle" mediastinum is defined on one side by the anterior cardiac silhouette and aortic root and on the other side by the posterior aspect of the tracheal carina; lesions in this region are typically benign cysts, although malignant lymphomas also may be encountered therein. Lastly, the posterior mediastinum is dorsal to the large conducting airways; it principally plays host to neurogenous mesenchymal lesions and enteric cysts.

Radiologic findings that tend to correlate with malignancy in mediastinal lesions also have been well documented. These include obvious infiltration of the mediastinal fat, pulmonary hila, or great vessels (70); "seeding" of the pleural surfaces, lung fields, or pericardium (71); and obvious intratumoral foci of spontaneous necrosis or stippled calcification (72). Conversely, peripheral "eggshell" calcification in an anterior mediastinal mass is used as a relatively reliable marker of benign (mature) teratomas, and the circumscription and attenuation of simple mediastinal cysts are easily recognized diagnostically with computed tomography (73).

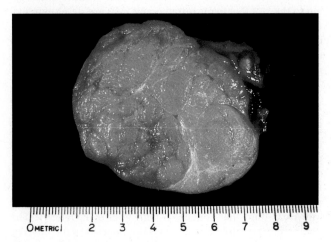

Figure 28.2. Encapsulated thymoma, showing circumscription by fibrous tissue. Internal fibrous septations yield a lobulated macroscopic appearance.

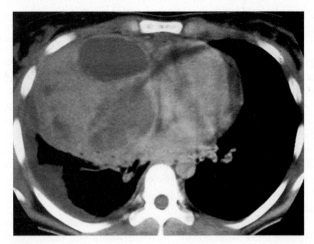

Figure 28.3. A large anterior mediastinal mass is present in this computed tomogram of the thorax. The lesion shows internal bands of fibrous matrix material surrounding rounded masses of tissue. This radiologic appearance is virtually diagnostic of nodular sclerosing Hodgkin disease, correlating well with the macroscopic characteristics of this tumor.

decide first whether the proliferation being studied is cystic and, second, whether it is composed of cytologically bland or cytologically atypical cells. If the lesion is clearly neoplastic and malignant, then it must be placed into one of five generic categories: small cell, large polygonal cell, mixed large cell and small cell, spindle cell/pleomorphic, and myxoid-adipocytic. Accordingly, the following discussion shall present this broad classification system in a workable context, with ancillary information that is of clinical or conceptual interest.

CYSTIC LESIONS OF THE MEDIASTINUM

Even when one includes neoplasms that may undergo cystic degeneration, mediastinal cysts are relatively uncommon and account for only 10% to 15% of radiologically detected masses at this site (74). However, several tissue types can be seen in such lesions, including thymic, pericardial, bronchogenic, enteric, and parathyroid cysts (75,75a). Indeed, selected mediastinal cysts may contain more than one of these constituents, relating to the fact that many intrathoracic cysts are developmental (congenital) rather than acquired and also to the close proximity in which the embryologic foregut anlage, pleuropericardial membranes, and branchial pouches are found during early morphogenesis (76).

Parathyroid and Thymic Cysts

Because the parathyroid glands and the thymus are all derived from the third and fourth pharyngeal pouches, cysts or solid proliferations containing tissue from either source may be located in low cervical or anterosuperior mediastinal positions (77–79). "Pure" parathyroid cysts may be seen at any age; they range from 1 to 10 cm in size, are thin-walled, and are filled with clear fluid that contains a high level of PTH (80). The nonsecretory nature of such lesions is supported by the observation that hypercalcemia is rare in these cases; accordingly, parathyroid cysts typically present themselves as asymptomatic masses that are found radiologically and have an internal density approximating that of serum (80). The lining of these lesions is comprised of attenuated parathyroid epithelium, which may be chief cell, oxyphilic, clear cell, or mixed in character. It is uniform in thickness and nonnodular in contrast to the epithelium of parathyroid adenomas, which undergoes secondary cystic change (76).

Thymic cysts manifest themselves clinically, predominantly between the ages of 20 and 50 years, typically in asymptomatic patients; this observation is germane to the contention offered by some authors that these are all postinflammatory lesions formed by cystic transformation of Hassall corpuscles or medullary epithelial structures (81,82). However, it is now known that both congenital (unilocular) and acquired (multilocular) thymic cysts exist (82,83), as will be discussed later. Radiologically, these cysts assume the form of rounded, circumscribed masses in the anterior mediastinal subcompartment. Unilocular lesions have an internal waterlike density on computed tomography, whereas multilocular cysts are filled with material showing a higher attenuation. Occasionally, plain film x-rays may demonstrate peripheral "rim" calcification. The greatest dimension of thymic cysts may be considerable, extending up to 18 cm (76,84).

As stated previously, macroscopic examination shows two main groups of thymic cysts: unilocular with a thin wall (Fig. 28.4) and multilocular with pericystic fibrous adhesions and a thick wall (82). These may be obviously centered on the thymus or, in some instances, connected to it by a narrow pedicle. Cyst contents have a variable consistency, correlating with other gross findings. Unilocular cysts typically contain only serous fluid, whereas multilocular lesions are filled with turbid, "cheesy," or hemorrhagic material (82,85).

These appearances also correspond to the integrity of the lining as seen microscopically. In unilocular thymic cysts, the epithelial surface of the cyst cavity is only a few layers in thickness—consisting of bland squamoid cells (Fig. 28.5)—and the fibrous wall lacks inflammation, hemorrhage, and cholesterol granulomas. However, the epithelial component of multilocular thymic cysts is often proliferative in nature; multiple layers of squamous cells may be observed alone or in admixture with simple cuboidal, simple columnar, multilayered cuboidal and columnar, or micropapillary glandular epithelium (Fig. 28.6) (82). Rarely, small areas of parathyroid tissue will be seen (76),

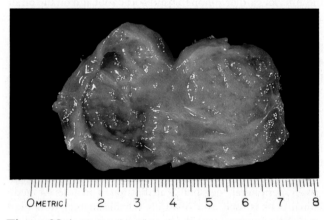

Figure 28.4. Unilocular thymic cyst showing a thin, nearly translucent fibrous wall. The denser mural tissue at the right of the figure represents incorporated thymic remnants.

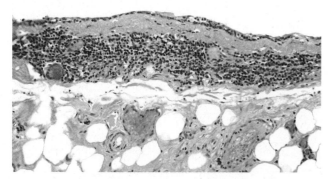

Figure 28.5. A squamoid lining is typical of many thymic cysts.

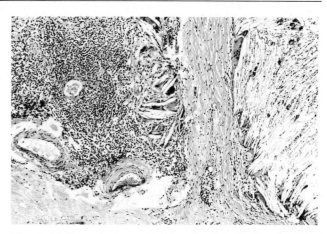

Figure 28.7. A cholesterol granuloma is present in the fibrous wall of this thymic cyst. Such inclusions are seen in virtually all lesions of this type.

and even more uncommonly, salivary glandular epithelium can be observed (85,86). In the latter circumstances, the terms "third pharyngeal pouch cyst" or "mixed multilocular thymic cyst" can be used diagnostically. Abundant lymphocytes, granulation tissue, hemorrhage, and cholesterol granulomas are constant constituents in the fibrous walls and cyst cavities of multilocular thymic cysts (Fig. 28.7) (82,84,85). The cause of the inflammatory process that is putatively the underlying cause of multilocular thymic cysts is presently unknown. Identifiable Hassall corpuscular remnants and identifiable thymic tissue are seen in up to one-half of all cases with careful scrutiny, but specialized mesenchyme, such as cartilage and smooth muscle, is never observed.

A peculiar variant of the multilocular thymic cyst is the "proliferating" subtype (87,88). It has significant histologic similarities to the cutaneous lesions known as "proliferating epidermoid cyst" and "proliferating trichilemmal cyst," in that it exhibits narrow, often interconnecting tongues of squamoid epithelium that extend deeply into the fibrous cyst wall from its luminal aspect (Fig. 28.8). One can rightly consider this change to represent "pseudoepitheliomatous hyperplasia" of the cyst-lining cells. Close inspection shows that they have cytologic attributes like those seen in "hyperplasia with reactive atypia" of mucosal epithelia, rather than truly dysplastic or overtly malignant features (87). Mitoses are indeed present in the proliferating epithelium, but they do not assume pathologic shapes. The importance of the proliferating thymic cyst is not that of an altered prognosis or risk of recurrence. Rather, it

resides in the danger that exists for the pathologist to overinterpret the lesion as a squamous cell carcinoma. It should be remembered that true malignant change in a thymic cyst is a rare phenomenon, with only a few well-documented examples of intracystic cancers in the English-language literature (89–93).

However, Moran et al. (93a) have described three examples of low-grade serous ovarian adenocarcinomas that presented with metastases to the anterior mediastinum, simulating multilocular thymic cysts. This eventuality could be addressed with immunostains for CA-125, a marker that is expected in ovarian epithelial tumors but not in thymic proliferations.

Other potential causes of acquired thymic cysts concern changes that occur in thymuses involved by Hodgkin disease and some that have been "traumatized" surgically. It is now well known that mediastinal Hodgkin lymphoma (HL) may coexist with, or be succeeded by, the appearance of a thymic cyst (94–99). This observation was originally thought to be a reflection of thymic degeneration brought about by thoracic irradiation or systemic chemotherapy (88). Nevertheless, examples have now been reported wherein untreated Hodgkin disease was complicated by thymic cyst formation (97). It is likely that the lymphomatous infiltrate compromises the integrity of thy-

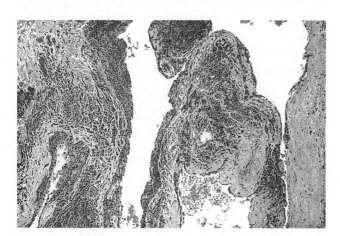

Figure 28.6. This multilocular thymic cyst contains internal septa that focally display papillary excrescences into the luminal spaces.

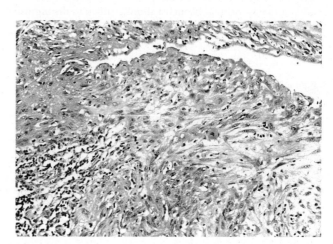

Figure 28.8. Broad but irregular aggregates of squamous cells extend downward into the fibrous wall of this "proliferating" thymic cyst.

mic epithelial nests, potentially leading to acquired cystic transformation. Admittedly, the addition of cytotoxic therapy—with subsequent lysis of intrathymic lymphoid cells—may accentuate this phenomenon through an "ex vacuo" mechanism (76). Curiously, thymic cysts have not been documented to date in association with non-Hodgkin lymphomas of the mediastinum. The other putatively acquired type of thymic cyst is that which is seen after open thoracotomies performed for nonneoplastic diseases. Jaramillo et al. (100) have reported three such cases in which these lesions were detected postoperatively. Those authors speculated that mechanical trauma to the thymus by the surgeon initiated the cystic glandular epithelial transformation, perhaps through microscopic vasodisruption.

Bronchogenic Cysts

Bronchogenic cysts may potentially arise in a broader anatomic distribution than cysts of parathyroid or thymic cysts; the first of these lesions can be seen in the anterior, superior, middle, or posterior mediastinum, and intrapericardial examples have been documented as well (101,102). They are likewise seen over a wide age range, extending from childhood to middle life (75). Whereas intrapulmonary cysts of this type often communicate with large airways and therefore may present with symptoms and signs of superinfection, mediastinal bronchogenic cysts are usually asymptomatic (101,103). The radiographic appearance is that of a round or oval mass that molds itself to contiguous structures; the internal aspect of the lesion is uniformly hypodense, and the wall may contain linear calcification (104). Angiography may demonstrate an independent vascular supply to bronchogenic cysts, in contrast to other mediastinal cysts (103).

Gross examination of excised bronchogenic cysts may show them to be unilocular or multilocular with internal septation. Their contents are variably turbid or viscous (76).

Histologically, the key features of such lesions are the presence of respiratory-type pseudostratified columnar epithelium, which is often ciliated, as well as small islands of predominantly mature cartilage (Figs. 28.9 and 28.10) (75). Smooth muscle also may be observed in small fascicles that are admixed with the chondroid elements, but cholesterol granulomas are uniformly absent. A possible resemblance to mature teratomas (discussed later in the chapter) must be acknowledged, but the overall organization of constituent tissues in bronchogenic cysts (resembling that of normal bronchi) should suffice to distinguish the two lesions.

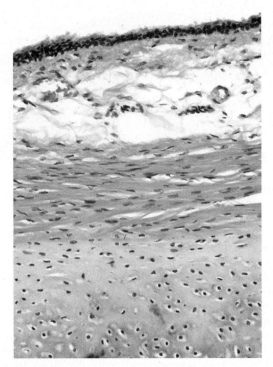

Figure 28.10. Bronchial-type epithelium and cartilage are apparent in this bronchogenic cyst.

Pericardial Cysts

Pericardial cysts of the mediastinum are typically found in the cardiophrenic angle (75,105,106). They may occur in patients of all ages and are generally asymptomatic; nonetheless, rare cases present with dyspnea or substernal chest pain (107). Radiographically, these cysts abut the cardiac contours and are irregularly shaped, with a uniform waterlike internal density (106). Like bronchogenic cysts, they can arise in any of the mediastinal subcompartments (76).

The gross appearance of excised pericardial cysts is banal, being represented by thin fibrous-walled structures that collapse completely when opened. The internal surfaces are uniformly smooth, and the fluid contents are serous in nature (76,107).

Microscopically, this configuration is recapitulated. One observes laminated fibrous tissue that is usually mantled by a single layer of bland mesothelium (Fig. 28.11); uncommonly, the lat-

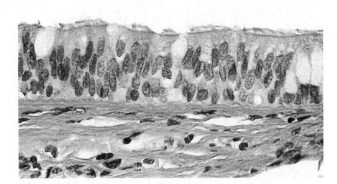

Figure 28.9. A ciliated respiratory epithelial lining is present at least focally in bronchogenic cysts.

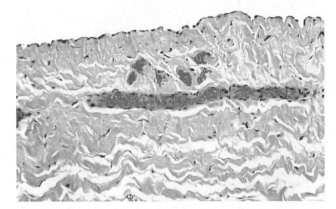

Figure 28.11. Pericardial cysts are typified by an attenuated mesothelial lining and a laminated fibrous wall.

ter tissue may undergo focal papillary hyperplasia (75). Smooth muscle, cartilage, specialized epithelium, and cholesterol granulomas are lacking.

Enteric Cysts

Enteric cysts are almost totally confined to the posterior mediastinum and characteristically occur in children and adolescents (108–116). Those individuals with paraesophageal cysts present with dysphagia or subnormal weight gain (108–110), whereas gastroesophageal cysts are associated with a wider array of symptoms; cough, vomiting, fever, and pneumonia or empyema have all been reported in conjunction with such lesions (111,113, 114,116). Also, it has been shown that enteric mediastinal cysts may be linked to concurrent vertebral anomalies including hemivertebrae and spina bifida (112,115).

Radiographically, enteric cysts range in size from 2 to 10 cm; they are rounded or irregular in shape and may demonstrate obvious loculation on computed tomography. In those cases where leakage of cyst contents has occurred clinically, evidence may be seen of pleural effusions or pulmonary consolidation in the posterior lobe of either lung (113,114).

Macroscopically, one observes a variably thick fibromuscular wall and a smooth mucosal lining. In accord with the previously cited radiologic attributes, multiloculation may be seen (75). Cystic contents are variably mucoid, and an extremely acidic pH is seen in some examples on simple testing with litmus paper.

Histologically, both paraesophageal and gastroesophageal mediastinal cysts are bounded by a double layer of smooth muscle, in recapitulation of that seen in the remainder of the gut (75,76,111,114). The epithelial lining may be squamous, simple columnar, pseudostratified columnar, or mixed, but gastroesophageal lesions typically contain at least some specialized gastric glandular mucosa (potentially with chief and parietal cell differentiation) as well (Fig. 28.12) (75,76). Acid production by the latter tissue accounts for those cases that show spontaneous cystic rupture. Cartilage and cholesterol granulomas are absent.

"Cystic Hygromas" (Lymphangiomas)

Cystic lesions that represent lymphangiomas may be seen in the anterior, middle, and posterior mediastinum as well as the soft tissues of the neck, usually in pediatric patients (117–123). They may become large enough to produce respiratory compromise, cardiac embarrassment, or nerve compression but are just as often found radiographically in asymptomatic individuals (118–120,122–123a). Radiographically, these "cystic hygromas" are often seen to be extensively infiltrating the mediastinal soft tissues. They have a more variegated internal appearance than many other cysts of the thorax because of their potential content of solid tissue (122,124). Discernible septation between cystic spaces may be observed on computed tomography.

Macroscopically, these lesions are edematous-looking, unencapsulated, white-gray masses with variably sized internal cavities and watery contents. The tissue lining the internal spaces is smooth and glistening. Histologically, lymphangiomas are characterized by large, irregularly shaped vascular spaces mantled by bland, flattened endothelial cells, embedded in a fibroblastic and collagenous stroma (117,125). Small collections of lymphocytes are often scattered throughout the lesion; they may be present within the vascular spaces as well, together with flocculent eosinophilic precipitates of proteinaceous lymphatic fluid

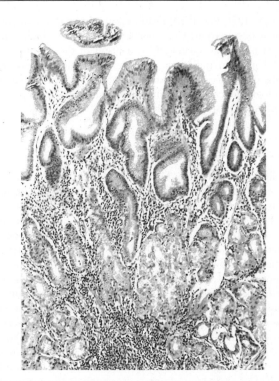

Figure 28.12. Gastric-type epithelium is evident in this gastroenteric paraesophageal cyst of the posterior mediastinum.

(Fig. 28.13) (117). Other specialized mesenchyme and epithelium are uniformly absent, as are cholesterol granulomas.

Cystic Meningoceles

In infants or children, the posterior mediastinum may harbor cystic meningoceles. These are thin-walled paraspinal malformations that demonstrate a communication with the meninges, usually through a defect in the vertebral bodies (126). Meningoceles are filled with clear to amber cerebrospinal fluid, and microscopic examination of such lesions demonstrates a thick fibrous wall lined internally by mature, flattened arachnoidal

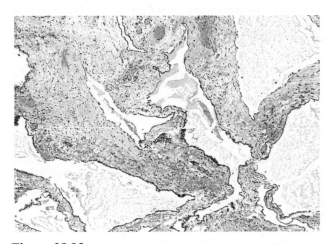

Figure 28.13. This lymphangioma of the anterior mediastinum is composed of large, interanastomosing vascular channels that contain wispy eosinophilic material and an endothelial lining.

cells (105,127). Focal calcification and admixed neural tissue also may be apparent. Meningoceles are typically "incidental" surgical pathology specimens as a result of the sophisticated state of modern radiologic imaging techniques and the fact that the diagnosis is usually suggested clinically by concomitant neurologic deficits. Therefore, these lesions do not represent interpretative histologic problems.

Cystic Teratomas of the Mediastinum

Notwithstanding their highly organized and differentiated nature, most cystic teratomas of the mediastinum are true neoplasms rather than developmental malformations. These lesions have been classically defined by the presence of at least two tissue derivatives of the three germinal cell layers—endoderm, ectoderm, and mesoderm—although "monodermal" teratomas have been recently recognized as well (128).

Teratomatous and germ cell tumors make up 10% to 20% of all mediastinal lesions (126,129), and they are largely, but not exclusively (130), restricted to the anterior subcompartment. These are predominantly neoplasms of children, adolescents, and young adults, with an average age of approximately 20 years at presentation (129). Approximately one-half of the patients with such tumors are asymptomatic, whereas the remainder complain of chest pain, dyspnea, or cough (131). A minority of cases are associated with Klinefelter syndrome (132), but the distribution of cystic teratomas between the sexes is approximately equal (131).

Radiologically, one observes a predominantly cystic or solid and cystic mass with variable attenuation on computed tomography. Internal septation can reliably be considered a radiographic marker of benignancy in teratomas; likewise, calcification is usually an indicator of a biologically innocuous lesion (73,132a).

The gross characteristics of mediastinal teratomas are also important reflections of their behavioral potential. Those tumors that demonstrate dense adherence to contiguous lung, pericardium, or blood vessels are almost certainly malignant, with the exception being those mature teratomas that have spontaneously ruptured and are associated with a fibroinflammatory response in the surrounding tissue (131). Mucoid cyst contents, "cheesy" keratinous debris, or obvious osteocartilaginous foci are most often seen in benign lesions, whereas spontaneous necrosis is a worrisome finding with regard to possible areas of malignancy in a teratoma (128). As Dehner (131) has indicated, one must address the question of adequacy in the sampling of large cystic teratomas; accepted procedure currently dictates that one block be submitted for every centimeter of tumor diameter or for every 10 g of neoplastic tissue. Obviously, the samples should be taken from as broad an area as possible.

The microscopic complexity of teratomas is an immediate clue to their germinal nature, and it virtually eliminates all other differential diagnostic considerations among cystic mediastinal lesions. One commonly observes a mixture of mature squamous epithelium (often with cutaneous appendages), foregut-type columnar epithelium, neuroglial elements, bone, cartilage, fat, and fetal or mature striated muscle tissue (Figs. 28.14 and 28.15). Other potential histologic components include choroid plexus, hepatocytic islands, pancreas, and pigmented neuroepithelium resembling retinal tissue (132–134).

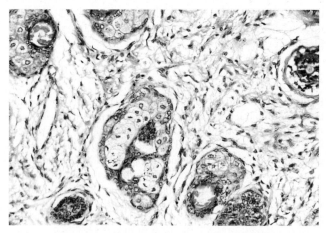

Figure 28.14.   Sebaceous adnexal structures are seen in this mature anterior mediastinal teratoma.

The definition of "immature" teratoma (with that term implying possible recurrence or even metastatic potential) is still somewhat problematic for some observers. In short, it is the author's belief that the presence of immature neuroepithelial tissue is all that is necessary for the diagnosis of this pathologic entity (Fig. 28.16) (134). It would be unwise to broaden the spectrum of immature teratomas to include those lesions containing fetal (but cytologically benign) mesenchyme or somatic epithelium. This opinion stems from the fact that immature neuroepithelium appears to be the sole potentially adverse marker in such tumors from a biologic point of view. In fact, even those neoplasms that do contain this tissue type fail to behave in an aggressive fashion in patients under 15 years of age, as shown by Carter et al. (135). In light of this information, it is likely that broadening the definition of *immaturity* for these neoplasms would only incur needless worry and possible overtreatment.

The foregoing comments notwithstanding, one should also recognize that exceptionally rare examples of otherwise mature mediastinal teratomas exist wherein overtly sarcomatous, gliomatous, or carcinomatous somatic tissue makes up a portion of the lesion. For example, rhabdomyosarcoma, fibrosarcoma,

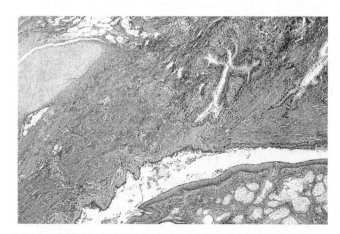

Figure 28.15.   Mature mediastinal teratomas commonly contain a mixture of squamous and glandular somatic epithelium, as well as cartilage or bone.

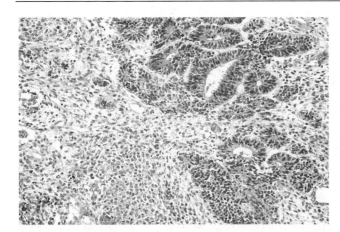

Figure 28.16. This immature mediastinal teratoma is recognizable by its content of primitive neuroepithelial tissue, represented by embryonic tubules (*top right*).

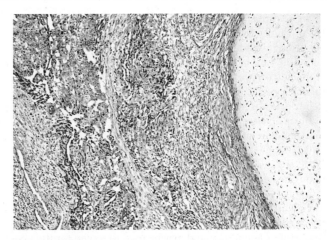

Figure 28.18. Malignant mixed germ cell tumor of the mediastinum. Embryonal carcinoma (*left*) is juxtaposed to mature hyaline cartilage (*right*).

chondrosarcoma, liposarcoma, angiosarcoma, enteric-type adenocarcinoma, carcinoid tumor (neuroendocrine carcinoma), squamous cell carcinoma, and glioblastoma multiforme have all been reported in this setting (Fig. 28.17) (133–139b). The proper diagnostic classification of such tumors is that of "mature teratoma with sarcomatous/carcinomatous transformation." Their prognosis is much more guarded, and specific treatment measures directed at the malignant somatic components are necessary.

Still other teratomatous neoplasms contain obvious foci of seminoma/dysgerminoma, embryonal carcinoma, yolk sac tumor, or choriocarcinoma, as seen in the gonads (Fig. 28.18) (see Chapter 47) (128,131,133,134). The commingling of a mature or immature teratomatous component with the latter elements qualifies the lesion as a "mixed malignant germ cell tumor," the biology of which is largely determined by the non-teratomatous germinal tissues. One should nevertheless clearly inform attending physicians of the presence of mature somatic elements in such cases because the latter tissues may fail to involute after chemotherapy. In this circumstance, treatment converts a mixed malignant germ cell neoplasm into an apparently pure mature teratoma; the latter commonly requires subsequent surgical removal for complete extirpation (140).

Lastly, it should again be mentioned that occasional teratoid tumors of the mediastinum can be associated with antecedent, concomitant, or ensuing hematolymphoid malignancies, with acute myelogenous leukemia predominating (60,141,142). This association is seen even in the absence of potentially mutagenic chemotherapy for the germinal lesion, and common karyotypic abnormalities have been demonstrated in both the teratomatous cells and the aberrant hematopoietic elements (143). Hence, it appears that leukemia in such cases is derived from the germ cell tumors.

Cystic Thymomas and Seminomas

Among all other tumors of the mediastinum, only thymoma (Fig. 28.19) (defined as a cytologically bland proliferation of thymic epithelium) and intrathymic seminoma have any reproducible capacity for cystic change. Indeed, some of these lesions may be so extensively cavitary that numerous microscopic sections are necessary to detect their basically neoplastic nature.

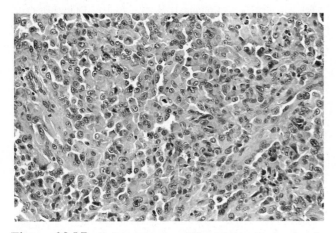

Figure 28.17. Angiosarcomatous differentiation in an otherwise mature teratoma. This finding is rare.

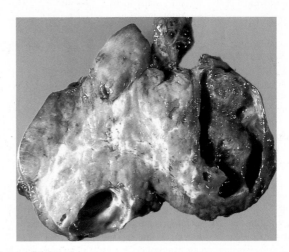

Figure 28.19. This encapsulated thymoma demonstrates multifocal cystification. In occasional cases, degenerative change of this type dominates the mass and may cause confusion with true mediastinal cysts.

In many respects, cystic thymomas (144) may closely resemble thymic cysts microscopically, as described earlier. The two are distinguished from one another histologically in that nodular proliferations of thymic epithelial cells define the former entity but are not "allowed" in the walls of thymic cysts. Parenthetically, cystic thymomas also may exhibit extensive spontaneous necrosis and hemorrhage, neither of which is expected in thymic cysts. Other microscopic characteristics of thymomas in general are presented in the following section titled "Differential Diagnosis of Selected Thymoma Variants." Extensively cystic seminomas—which are presumably formed by spontaneous degenerative change—likewise may contain only small mural nodules of residual viable tumor cells, which are overtly malignant with prominent nucleoli (98,145). The periodic acid-Schiff (PAS) stain is helpful in delineating the glycogen content that typifies seminomas and may be used to screen for the neoplastic cell aggregates in this particular setting.

Additional clues to the identity of cystic thymomas may be gleaned from the clinical history if an appropriate paraneoplastic syndrome is evident; similarly, concomitant hematologic abnormalities or Klinefelter syndrome would be valuable evidence suggesting the existence of a mediastinal germ cell tumor. High-resolution computed tomography and magnetic resonance imaging of the thorax are also valuable. These techniques are capable of delineating the aforementioned mural nodular densities that would not be expected in thymic cysts (63,64,70,146). The most salient facts on cystic mediastinal lesions discussed thus far are summarized in Table 28.1.

DIFFERENTIAL DIAGNOSIS OF SELECTED THYMOMA VARIANTS

General Comments

The microscopic variability of thymomas is considerable, perhaps second only to that of teratomas among all mediastinal

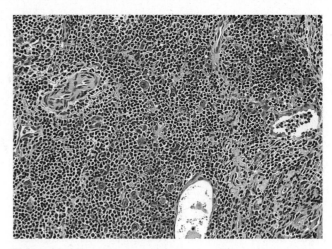

Figure 28.20. Lymphocyte-predominant thymoma showing a preponderance of small stromal lymphocytes. Characteristic perivascular serum "lakes" are seen (right bottom).

neoplasms. There are, however, several nuances in the histologic traits of thymomas that play important roles in differential diagnosis with other lesions. These are outlined in a systematic fashion here, using the simple classification scheme of Bernatz et al. (147). The latter nosologic construct divides thymomas into four discrete categories based on cross-sectional microscopic morphology: lymphocyte predominant (>66% lymphocytes) (Fig. 28.20), epithelial predominant (>66% epithelial cells) (Fig. 28.21), mixed lymphoepithelial (34% to 66% epithelial cells) (Fig. 28.22), and spindle cell (a subtype of epithelial-predominant thymoma featuring a nearly exclusive composition by fusiform tumor cells) (Fig. 28.23). It merits emphasis that thymoma must first be defined as a *cytologically bland epithelial neoplasm* in order for this scheme to have any histopathologic

TABLE 28.1	Differential Diagnosis of Mediastinal Cysts						
Type of Cyst	*Typical Location*	*Contents*	*Chol Gran*	*Cart*	*SM*	*Epith*	*Loculation*
Parathyroid	Anterosuperior	Serous	No	No	No	Cuboidal	Unilocular
Thymic	Anterosuperior	Serous or Turbid	Yes	No	No	Variable[a]	Unilocular or multilocular
Bronchogenic	Middle[b]	Viscous	No	Yes	+/−	Columnar	Unilocular or multilocular
Pericardial	Middle	Serous	No	No	No	Flattened cuboidal	Unilocular
Enteric	Posterior	Mucoid	No	No	Yes[c]	Columnar[d]	Unilocular
Lymphangiomatous	Anterosuperior[b]	Serous	No	No	No	None	Multilocular
Teratoma	Anterosuperior	Turbid or "cheesy"	No	+/−	+/−	Variable[a]	Multilocular
Cystic thymoma	Anterosuperior	Variable	Rare	No	No	Polygonal or spindle cell	Unilocular or multilocular
Cystic seminoma	Anterosuperior	Variable	No	No	No	Polygonal	Unilocular or multilocular

Cart, cartilage in cyst wall; Chol Gran, cholesterol granulomas in cyst wall; Epith, type of epithelium in cyst lining; SM, smooth muscle in cyst wall
[a]Epithelium may be squamous, cuboidal, columnar, or mixed.
[b]May also occur in other mediastinal subcompartments.
[c]Enteric cysts contain an external double layer of smooth muscle.
[d]True goblet cells and specialized gastric glands often present.
+/−, variably present.

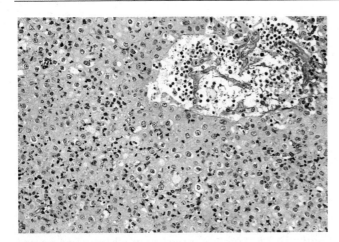

Figure 28.21. Predominantly epithelial thymoma composed of bland polygonal cells in sheets. A perivascular serum lake is again evident within the mass.

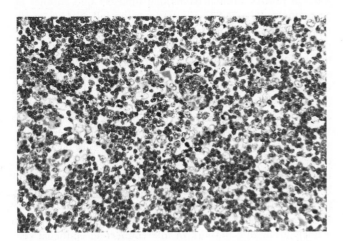

Figure 28.22. Mixed lymphoepithelial thymoma composed of a relatively even admixture of bland thymic epithelial cells and small lymphocytes.

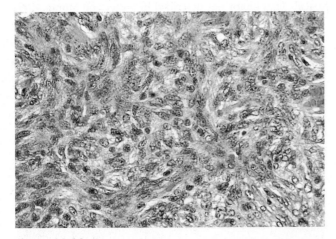

Figure 28.23. Spindle cell thymomas are variants of predominantly epithelial tumors, in which neoplastic elements assume a fusiform shape. These lesions pursue an innocuous course but are sometimes associated with hematologic paraneoplasias.

use (148). Moreover, the author holds to the opinion that, with the exception of spindle cell thymomas, which typically pursue an innocuous course, the Bernatz system does not represent—and was not devised as—a prognostic classification. Rather, its usefulness is in serving as a cue mechanism for well-defined histologic differential diagnostic problems concerning thymomas.

In fact, there is currently no means of microscopically subcategorizing thymomas that correlates perfectly with behavior (149–152), including a scheme proposed by Marino, Muller-Hermelink, and colleagues (149,150). The latter system (usually abbreviated as the MMH classification) is based on the putative resemblance of thymomatous epithelial cells to those of the normal thymic cortex ("cortical" thymomas—usually equating to Bernatz lymphocyte-predominant, mixed lymphoepithelial, and most epithelial-predominant lesions) or medulla ("medullary" thymomas, which are largely synonymous with spindle cell lesions in the Bernatz system) (153–155). It is contended that "medullary" thymomas have a good prognosis, whereas "cortical" lesions (including those with modest cytologic atypia, termed *well-differentiated thymic carcinoma* by Kirchner et al. [156]) have a relatively unfavorable evolution, and "mixed cortical/medullary" tumors manifest an intermediary behavior.

As well summarized by Shimosato and Mukai (13), it would appear that the MMH system is, in actuality, a derivative distillation of information that would already be made available from implementation of the Bernatz classification scheme, albeit using different terminology (157). In light of this, one could question whether the former nosologic strategy can be regarded as "new" or progressive. Moreover, problems with interobserver reproducibility of the classification of thymomas have been reported (150,158), and Moran and Suster (159) have summarized the considerable effects of sampling bias on this process as well. Finally, it must be forthrightly stated that spindle cell ("medullary") thymomas (160) have long been known to have a rather innocuous behavior, regardless of what specific adjectives were used to describe them. In light of that fact, it would seem advisable to re-evaluate the claims of MMH proponents (17,161–169) after pure spindle cell neoplasms have been excluded from formal statistical analyses. In my personal experience with a large number of thymoma cases, the MMH system has failed to equal stage as a significant prognostic factor after this step is taken.

In 1999, Rosai published the second edition of *Histological Typing of Tumors of the Thymus* (170), under the auspices of the World Health Organization (WHO) International Histological Classification of Tumors project. In an effort to reconcile the Bernatz and MMH schemes, a hybrid system was advanced therein. It defines thymomas as:

- *Type A (spindle cell or medullary)*—composed of a population of neoplastic thymic epithelial cells having a spindle or oval shape, lacking nuclear atypia, and accompanied by few or no nonneoplastic lymphocytes.
- *Type AB*—foci having the features of type A thymoma admixed with foci rich in lymphocytes.
- *Type B1*—resembling the normal functional thymus in that it combines large expanses having an appearance practically indistinguishable from normal thymic cortex with areas resembling thymic medulla.
- *Type B2*—the neoplastic epithelial component appears as scattered plump cells with vesicular nuclei and distinct nu-

cleoli among a heavy population of lymphocytes. Perivascular spaces are common and sometimes very prominent. A perivascular arrangement of tumor cells resulting in a palisading effect may be seen.

- *Type B3*—predominantly composed of epithelial cells having a round or polygonal shape and exhibiting no or mild atypia. They are admixed with a minor component of lymphocytes, resulting in a sheetlike growth of the neoplastic cells. This histotype is synonymous with "well-differentiated thymic carcinoma," as cited previously.
- *Type C*—thymomas that are outright thymic carcinomas, with obvious cytologic anaplasia.

Since the introduction of this paradigm, several publications have suggested that the WHO classification is a prognostically oriented system (171–174), even though it was not intended as such (175). The principal goal of the WHO scheme was, in fact, to improve interobserver reproducibility in diagnosis. Another proposal appeared virtually simultaneously with the WHO monograph and was advanced by Suster and Moran. It contends that thymic epithelial neoplasms can be divided into "thymomas" (corresponding to WHO type A, AB, B1, and B2 tumors), "atypical thymomas" (WHO type B3 lesions), and "thymic carcinomas" (WHO type C tumors) (176–177a); this author endorses that practical paradigm.

I continue to believe that the best prognostic observation in thymoma cases is whether the tumor invades its capsule, either macroscopically or microscopically (178–183). Codifications of the degrees of invasion have been published by Masaoka et al. (184) in a formal staging scheme that has been restructured in an attempt to fit the standard tumor-node-metastasis (TNM) protocol advised by the American Joint Committee on Cancer (AJCC) (185). Several publications attest to the value of this process (13,157,186,187). For those conscientious practitioners wishing to use all-inclusive reporting practices in thymoma cases, *both* the Masaoka and AJCC-type stages can be provided to the surgeon (as well as both the Bernatz, Suster-Moran, and MMH classifications of the tumor [188]).

LYMPHOCYTE-PREDOMINANT THYMOMA VERSUS LYMPHOID HYPERPLASIA

Particularly in patients with myasthenia gravis, the pathologist is often asked to distinguish between true thymic hyperplasia (189) and thymoma in surgically resected glands. There are several straightforward histologic guidelines to make this separation.

Thymic lymphoid hyperplasia is defined by the retention of a normal microscopic cortical and medullary glandular distinction, together with the presence of several well-formed intrathymic lymphoid follicles. The latter often contain germinal centers, complete with tingible body macrophages (Fig. 28.24). Small aggregates of proliferating thymic epithelial cells may be seen as well in hyperplastic glands, but they do not alter the normal architecture of the thymus and are not associated with the previously cited lymphoid follicles (190–193).

In contrast, lymphocyte-predominant thymoma (LPT) is characterized by effacement of most or all of the thymic substructure (7,147,148,194). Like all forms of thymoma, this neoplasm often features the presence of a thick fibrous capsule and

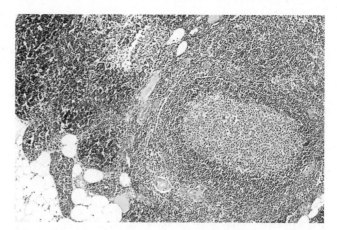

Figure 28.24. Lymphoid hyperplasia in a thymus gland removed in the treatment of myasthenia gravis. A germinal center is apparent (*right*).

internal fibrous stromal bands that intersect one another at acute angles (Fig. 28.25). Close inspection will disclose an admixture of bland thymic epithelial cells with "activated" lymphocytes (Fig. 28.26) that have folded nuclear contours and may be mitotic. The epithelial elements may be relatively inconspicuous, but they exhibit oval nuclei, fine dispersed chromatin, small chromocenters, and a moderate amount of amphophilic cytoplasm. Additional observations that aid in the recognition of LPT are the presence of intratumoral, perivascular serum "lakes" (Fig. 28.27); microcysts; numerous dispersed mast cells as seen with the chloroacetate esterase method; and "medullary differentiation" (multifocal loose aggregates of lymphocytes that simulate thymic medulla on low-power microscopy) (Fig. 28.28) (2,194,195). Medullary differentiation is particularly prominent in lesions that have been termed *organoid thymomas* by Pescarmona et al. (196). Immunostaining for keratin reveals a finely arborizing network of interconnecting epithelial cell processes in LPT, which is not seen in lymphoproliferative lesions (Fig. 28.29) (194,197,198).

A more difficult lesion to distinguish from thymic lymphoid hyperplasias, particularly in small biopsy specimens, is represented by "micronodular thymoma with lymphoid B-cell hyperplasia." That tumor was described by Suster and Moran (199)

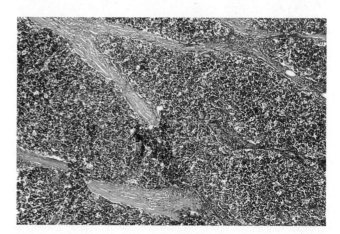

Figure 28.25. Distinct collagenous bands subdivide this lymphocyte-predominant thymoma and intersect one another at acute angles.

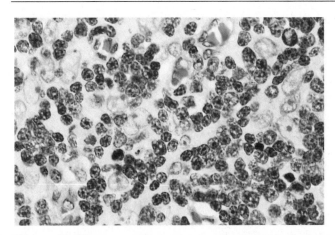

Figure 28.26. "Activated" lymphocytes in lymphocyte-predominant thymomas may demonstrate enlargement, slight nuclear convolution, and mitotic activity.

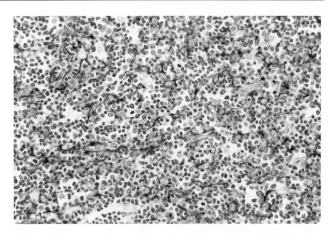

Figure 28.29. An arborizing, delicately interconnecting pattern of keratin immunoreactivity is typical of thymomas.

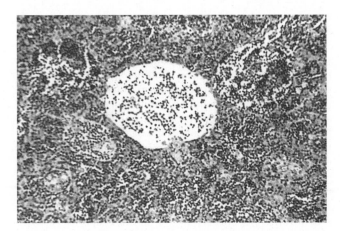

Figure 28.27. Serum "lakes" in thymoma (*center*) are perivascular in location, with suspended erythrocytes and lymphocytes. They are not expected in lymphomas of the mediastinum (also see Figs. 28.20 and 28.21).

and appears to represent a special form of spindle cell ("medullary;" "WHO type A") thymoma in which multiple small nodules of thymic epithelial cells are separated from one another by a prominent lymphoid stroma containing easily seen germinal centers, with a striking resemblance to those of Castleman disease (see next section) (200). Again, immunostains for keratin are helpful in characterizing this tumor type.

LYMPHOCYTE-PREDOMINANT THYMOMA VERSUS CASTLEMAN DISEASE

Castleman disease (also known as angiofollicular lymphoid hyperplasia [AFLH]) is a peculiar hematolymphoid disorder that presents clinically with symptoms of a mass lesion or, alternatively, with systemic findings such as fever, weight loss, and anemia (12,201). AFLH commonly affects the mediastinum and, as such, may be confused with LPT (194). In fact, the seminal paper in the literature on AFLH was focused on this differential diagnostic problem (201).

In contrast to the picture of LPT presented in this chapter, AFLH is rarely centered in the thymus. Instead, it affects mediastinal lymph nodes (Fig. 28.30). These cases demonstrate archi-

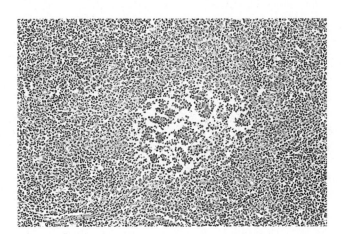

Figure 28.28. "Medullary differentiation" in lymphocyte-predominant thymomas (*center*) is represented by loose aggregates of lymphocytes that passingly resemble thymic medulla.

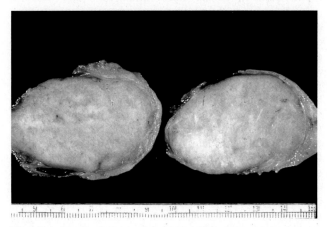

Figure 28.30. Castleman disease (angiofollicular lymphoid hyperplasia) of mediastinal lymph nodes. This process enlarges and distorts the macroscopic appearance of the nodes.

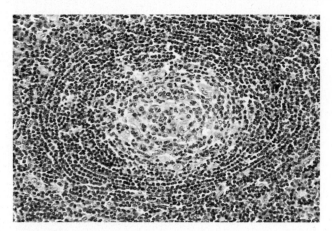

Figure 28.31. "Onion-skinning" of mature lymphoid cells around a sclerotic, hypervascular germinal center in Castleman disease of the mediastinum.

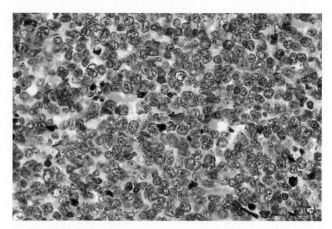

Figure 28.32. Lymphoblastic lymphoma of the mediastinum is characterized by small to intermediate-sized lymphocytes with irregular nuclear contours, delicate chromatin, and numerous mitoses. Compare with Figure 28.26.

tectural distortion by follicular aggregates of small, mature lymphoid cells, with compression of normal nodal sinusoidal channels. The internal aspects of the lymphoid follicles often show an unusual proliferation of small-caliber blood vessels, surrounded by a variable amount of fibrohyaline eosinophilic matrix material. Many of the follicles also are surrounded by "onion skin" arrays of lymphocytes, simulating exaggerated mantles (Fig. 28.31) (11,12,201,202). In one subtype of AFLH—termed the *plasma cellular variant*—interfollicular zones of the affected node are replaced by sheets of mature plasma cells (203). None of these features is seen in thymomas, except for the "micronodular" ("Castlemanoid") variant, as described earlier. Interestingly, Strobel et al. (203a) have reported the coexistence of micronodular thymoma and non-Hodgkin lymphoma in the same patients. I have also seen a singular case in which micronodular thymoma and true Castleman disease were present simultaneously.

LYMPHOCYTE-PREDOMINANT THYMOMA VERSUS LYMPHOMA

A common potential mistake in mediastinal pathology is the confusion of LPT with malignant lymphoma, particularly lymphoblastic lymphoma (LBL). Although the latter lesion is most often seen in the mediastinum in adolescents and young adults (11,204–207), which are patient groups that rather uncommonly develop thymomas (195), there is enough demographic and radiologic overlap between LBL and LPT to make a purely clinical distinction between them extremely difficult (208,209). Even the presence of an elevated peripheral white blood cell count offers no assurance of a diagnosis of LBL because this has been reported in patients with thymoma as well (210). The mimicry of LBL by selected LPT cases is facilitated by the particular attributes of infiltrating lymphocytes in some thymomas; these cells may exhibit "convoluted" nuclear contours, increased nucleocytoplasmic ratios, and many mitotic figures (7,194), as typically seen in LBL (Fig. 28.32). Moreover, the immunophenotypic characteristics of LPT lymphocytes and LBL cells are closely similar. Both populations commonly express the CD1, CD2, CD3, CD99 (MIC-2) (211–213), and bcl-2 (213–215) antigens and terminal deoxynucleotidyl transferase (TdT) (212,213,216–221); consequently, flow cytometric or im-

munohistochemical interpretations obviously must be made with extreme caution.

The most helpful ancillary studies in this differential diagnosis—and ones that the author, through sad experience, has made pro forma—are the immunohistologic detection of reactivity for p63 (an intranuclear transcription factor that is seen preferentially in squamous and transitional epithelium [222]) and keratin. As mentioned earlier, the interconnecting epithelial cells of LPT, which are absent in LBL, demonstrate a distinctive pattern of positivity for keratin, assuming a "lacy" staining configuration. This observation merits special emphasis because LBL and other lymphomas affecting the thymus may entrap scattered residual nonneoplastic thymic epithelial cells that are visible on keratin immunostains (223). p63 is also regularly seen in thymic epithelial cells but not in lymphoid elements (222).

Electron microscopy also plays a role in this differential diagnostic context (224). In contrast to the ultrastructural appearance of LBL, thymoma shows well-formed intercellular junctions between apposed processes of epithelial cells (Fig. 28.33).

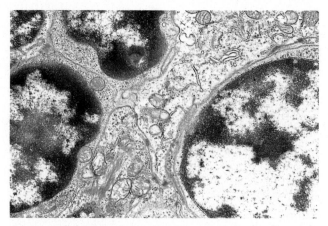

Figure 28.33. Electron micrograph of lymphocyte-predominant thymoma showing desmosomal attachments between apposed epithelial cell processes (*center*).

In addition, the cytoplasm of these elements is usually rich in tonofilaments (7,8,194,195,225,226).

Only one other small-cell, non-Hodgkin lymphoma besides LBL has any reproducible potential to present in the thymic region, thus raising the specified differential diagnosis. Several cases of small noncleaved cell (Burkitt) lymphoma have become manifest with mediastinal masses, in the absence of disease elsewhere (227,228). In the author's experience with such cases, most of the patients have had acquired immunodeficiency syndrome (AIDS), in which Burkitt lymphoma has been reported with some frequency (229). The cells of this tumor have a characteristic coarsely clumped nuclear chromatin pattern, with prominent nucleoli and numerous mitoses (Fig. 28.34) (11,134). Nuclear detail is the most reliable discriminant between the lymphoid cells of Burkitt lymphoma and those of LPT because the "starry sky" pattern of dispersed tingible body macrophages that is often cited as a marker of the former lesion (see Chapter 17) may also be seen in thymomas (7,148,194).

As stated repeatedly heretofore, the isolated presence of still other forms of small-cell lymphoma in the mediastinum is rare, but it has indeed been documented. For instance, several examples of mucosa-associated lymphoid tissue (MALT)–type (mantle cell/low-grade, small-cell lymphoplasmacytoid) lymphoma have been reported to affect the thymus (230,231). The proliferating lymphoid cells in this lesion also may be confused with those of LPT, but the methods of differential diagnosis just described are effective in this specific context as well. Finally, Skinnider et al. (232) have reported the rare but conjoint appearance of thymoma and lymphoma in the same patients, a situation that mandates special studies be performed to distinguish one tumor type from the other.

THYMIC DYSPLASIA VERSUS "MICROSCOPIC" THYMOMA

On purely histologic grounds, the pattern of thymic epithelial growth that one observes in dysplastic glands (233) is somewhat similar to that described as "microscopic thymoma" by Pescarmona et al. (234). Both lesions feature the presence of nodular aggregates of cytologically bland cells that are subdivided by fibrous stromal bands and punctuated by admixed lymphocytes.

However, the congruence ends there. Dysplasia occurs in smaller than normal thymuses. In addition, patients with this condition are children who almost invariably manifest severe clinical immunocompromise, such as the severe combined immunodeficiency syndrome (233). However, all reported cases of "microscopic thymoma" were seen in normally sized or enlarged glands removed in the treatment of myasthenia gravis in adults (234).

"ANCIENT" (SCLEROTIC) THYMOMA VERSUS FIBROSING MEDIASTINITIS

Moran and Suster (234a) have described 10 examples of thymoma in which the tumor mass was dominated by hyalinized collagenous stroma. As such, the lesions microscopically resembled fibrosing mediastinitis (234b), and thorough sampling was required to find diagnostic foci of thymoma.

PREDOMINANTLY EPITHELIAL SPINDLE CELL THYMOMA VERSUS FIBROUS HISTIOCYTOMA AND HEMANGIOPERICYTOMA

Predominantly epithelial thymomas (PETs) that are composed of plump or elongated fusiform cells may be difficult to distinguish from fibrous histiocytomas (FHs) or hemangiopericytomas (HPCs) on purely histologic grounds (7,194). This resemblance is occasioned primarily on the basis of storiform cellular growth (FH-like thymoma) (Fig. 28.35) or the lobulated aggregation of bluntly spindled tumor cells punctuated by "staghorn"-like vascular channels (HPC-like thymoma) (Fig. 28.36). In the absence of biasing clinical information, such as the presence of pure erythroid aplasia or acquired hypogammaglobulinemia, which may be associated with spindle cell thymomas (148,194), one must rely on fine points in the microscopic appearance of each tumor type or on the application of discriminating special studies to make a proper diagnostic interpretation. However, it should be borne in mind that thymomas are far more common than anterior mediastinal mesenchymal tumors, and therefore, the former lesions usually represent the final "answer" in such cases.

Thymic epithelial neoplasms that simulate FH or HPC still retain, in most instances, the microscopic hallmarks of thymomas in general. To reiterate, these include internal fibrous

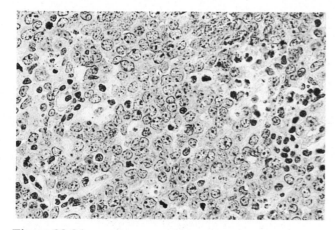

Figure 28.34. Burkitt (small noncleaved cell) lymphoma of the anterior mediastinum is composed of small to intermediate-sized cells with clumped chromatin, multiple distinct nucleoli, and brisk mitotic activity.

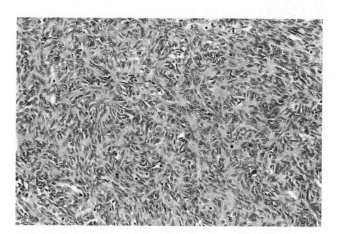

Figure 28.35. Storiform growth in spindle cell thymomas (shown here) may simulate the appearance of a fibrous histiocytoma.

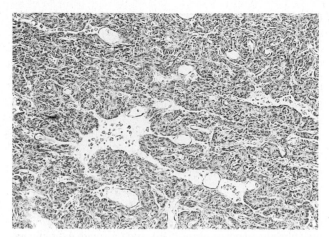

Figure 28.36. Hemangiopericytoma-like growth in a spindle cell thymoma, with irregular "staghorn"-shaped stromal blood vessels.

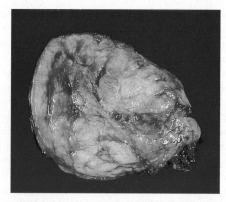

Figure 28.37. This thymolipoma of the anterior mediastinum is dominated by its adipocytic component. Unless an athymic remnant is attached to the mass, distinction from simple mediastinal lipoma is nearly impossible on gross examination.

septa, intralesional microcysts, and perivascular serum lakes. Such findings are not seen in mesenchymal tumors. Reticulin stains are occasionally useful in the differential diagnosis as well because they demonstrate delicate intercellular matrix deposition around individual tumor cells in true HPCs but not thymomas.

Immunohistochemistry and electron microscopy are the surest means of making a final interpretation in cases that are histologically indeterminate, particularly when only small biopsy specimens are available for evaluation. Pseudomesenchymal thymomas uniformly express keratin and lack vimentin (198), whereas FH and HPC show the converse of this immunostaining profile (235). Similarly, the well-developed intercellular junctions and cytoplasmic tonofilaments of thymomas are not shared by the other two lesions (7,125,194,195,235).

DIFFERENTIAL DIAGNOSIS OF BENIGN MESENCHYMAL NEOPLASMS

In general, mesenchymal tumors of the mediastinum are uncommon lesions. Nonetheless, they are potentially distributed among all three anatomic subcompartments and may cause diagnostic consternation in selected cases. The following section considers selected problems that center on benign lesions in this group.

MEDIASTINAL LIPOMA VERSUS THYMOLIPOMA

Lipomas of the thorax may be seen in many sites, including the anterior, middle, and posterior mediastinum; the pericardium; and the deep soft tissues of the chest wall, including the parietal pleura (236,237). They are usually readily recognizable by radiographic means and hence are not excised in many cases. However, those in the anterosuperior mediastinum are similar clinicopathologically to an unusual neoplasm of the thymus known as thymolipoma (discussed later). One microscopic subtype of lipoma that may be unique to the mediastinum is that known as "elastofibrolipoma," as described by DeNictolis et al. (238). This tumor manifests an admixture of ordinary lipoma with areas containing abnormal elastic fibers or dense zones of fibrosis. Verhoeff-van Gieson stains may be necessary to optimally visualize the elastic tissue in elastofibrolipomas.

Thymolipomas are generally asymptomatic tumors that are found radiographically in young to middle-aged adults (7,125, 134,239,240). Only 10% are associated with systemic symptoms, which are like those of thymoma-related paraneoplasias (21,241–243). These tumors may attain a considerable size (up to 20 cm) (244,245) and characteristically show a uniform density on computed tomography that is essentially equivalent to that of adipose tissue (246,247).

Macroscopically, thymolipomas have few if any traits that would dissuade one from a simple diagnosis of lipoma, except for the fact that they are often intimately associated with remnants of unremarkable thymus gland (Fig. 28.37) (248). Their histologic appearance, however, is distinctive. Lobules of unremarkable thymic tissue—complete with cortex, medulla, and Hassall corpuscles—are admixed evenly with mature adipose tissue and bounded by a thin fibrous capsule (Fig. 28.38) (7,125,134). The contention that the lesion is simply an infiltrative lipoma of the thymus is seemingly untenable; careful studies have shown that the absolute mass of thymic tissue in thymolipoma is increased far beyond that seen in normal glands (7). Furthermore, rare examples may demonstrate some degree of thymic epithelial proliferation as well (Fig. 28.39), with elongated cords of polygonal cells amid the fatty component; these

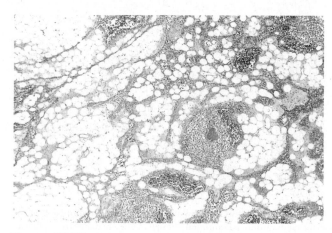

Figure 28.38. Thymolipoma showing an admixture of relatively normal thymic elements and mature adipocytic tissue.

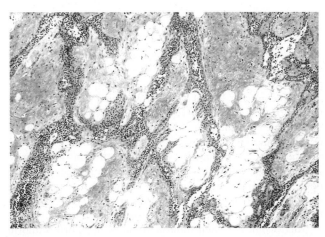

Figure 28.39. Some thymolipomas demonstrate the proliferation of intratumoral thymic epithelium, as shown in this figure by the elongated cords of polygonal cells.

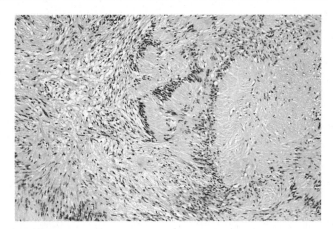

Figure 28.41. "Antoni A" areas of neurilemoma demonstrate a compact cellular architecture, with palisading of tumor cell nuclei.

variants have been termed *proliferating thymolipomas* by Hull et al. (248). Iseki et al. (249) have documented a remarkable thymolipoma in which obvious myoid cells were seen in the medullary areas of the admixed thymic tissue, and Moran et al. (250) have observed two cases in which broad zones of dense fibrosis were present. These last two cases were called "thymofibrolipomas" in recognition of their peculiar morphologic variation. Similarly, Ogino et al. (251) reported a thymolipoma with an extremely prominent vascular stromal component and designated it a "thymohemangiolipoma."

BENIGN PERIPHERAL NERVE SHEATH TUMORS AND GANGLIONEUROMAS

The overwhelming majority of neoplasms encountered in the posterior mediastinum are neurogenic in nature (7–10,13,125). As such, they often show considerable gross and microscopic similarities and may challenge the pathologist to discern one from another. In particular, lesions with Schwann cell differentiation (peripheral nerve sheath tumors [PNST]) require further nosologic separation into neurofibromas and neurilemomas (schwannomas), and they also must be distinguished from ganglioneuromas in this location.

NEURILEMOMA

Neurilemomas are the most common neural tumors of the mediastinum (252–254). They are usually detected radiologically in asymptomatic patients, but occasional cases present with symptoms and signs of esophageal or spinal nerve root compression (254). Most affected individuals are young adults, but these lesions may be observed in all age groups (125,253).

The macroscopic features of neurilemomas are important clues to their distinction from other neural neoplasms. The latter lesion is typically encapsulated and sharply demarcated from adjacent soft tissue. An association with large nerves is common, and the tumor may appear to "hang" from the nerve like a pod on a tree branch (Fig. 28.40) (125). Histologically, one observes a biphasic arrangement of neoplastic fusiform cells; some are densely apposed and may exhibit nuclear palisading (Antoni A areas with Verocay bodies), whereas other foci show only loosely aggregated cells with a myxoid background (Antoni B areas) (Figs. 28.41 and 28.42) (7,125). Intralesional blood vessels are usually prominent with thick walls. Division figures are typically sparse.

Some neurilemomas exhibit specialized differentiation that can cause interpretative consternation. At the same time, this

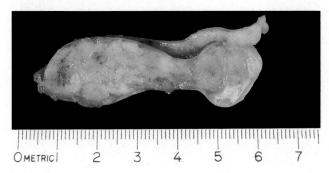

Figure 28.40. Neurilemomas of the posterior mediastinum may "hang" from adjacent nerves, as in this photograph. Note the partially yellow appearance of the fresh cut surface of the neoplasm, which is typical.

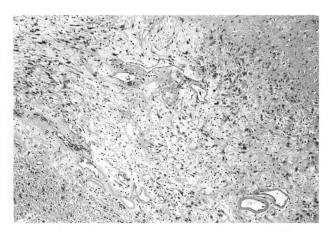

Figure 28.42. "Antoni B" foci of neurilemoma are myxoid and more paucicellular. Typical thick-walled blood vessels are also seen in this illustration.

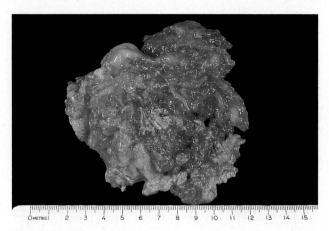

Figure 28.43. Recurrent plexiform neurofibroma of the posterior mediastinum, with a gross appearance like that of a distorted and greatly enlarged neural plexus.

feature is useful in differential diagnosis because neither neurofibromas nor ganglioneuromas demonstrate such complexity. Neurilemomas may show partial pigmentation ("melanotic" schwannoma) (255,256); alarming nuclear pleomorphism and hyperchromasia ("ancient" schwannoma) (125); foci with true epithelial differentiation ("glandular" schwannoma) (257); psammomatous calcification and pigmentation ("psammomatous-melanotic" schwannoma) (258); and dense cellularity with herringbone-like, storiform, or fascicular growth patterns, slight nuclear atypia, and brisk mitotic activity ("cellular" schwannoma) (259–261). In the last of these variations, the tumor may be mistaken for a sarcoma; however, unlike nerve sheath malignancies, cellular schwannomas are encapsulated and lack foci of necrosis or pathologically shaped mitotic figures (261).

Ultrastructurally, neurilemomas also are singular in the degree of neural differentiation that is observed. Elongated overlapping cell processes are present in such tumors; these may be attached to one another by primitive junctions, sometimes yielding structures that simulate embryonic mesaxons. Pericellular basal lamina is usually discernible and may be abundant (259).

NEUROFIBROMA

Mediastinal neurofibroma represents the principal diagnostic alternative to neurilemoma. It has a similar demography and clinical presentation but also possesses the capacity for multiplicity or "plexiform" growth that macroscopically simulates a neural plexus (Fig. 28.43) (252–254). Tumors of this type with the latter characteristics are pathognomonic of von Recklinghausen disease, which is not associated with either mediastinal neurilemoma or ganglioneuroma (262). Also, in contrast to these lesions, neurofibromas often are centered on, or grow within, a large spinal nerve root; in fact, some examples have both intradural and extradural components protruding through neural foramina of the vertebral column with a "dumbbell" configuration (125). They are not encapsulated.

Microscopically, neurofibromas show a more uniform growth pattern than the patterns seen in schwannomas. Bland spindle cells are arranged in fascicles, storiform arrays, or tactoids in neurofibromas. A myxoid stroma is common, but one does not observe biphasic Antoni A/B areas or thick-walled blood vessels as seen in neurilemoma (Fig. 28.44). Mast cells often are numerous in neurofibromas as well (125).

The electron microscopic attributes of neurofibroma are such that evidence of clear-cut schwannian differentiation is often lacking. Often, one observes only fibroblast-like tumor cells with relatively abundant rough endoplasmic reticulum, rudimentary cytoplasmic processes, and sparse formation of pericellular basal lamina (263).

GANGLIONEUROMA

Mediastinal ganglioneuroma is typically a tumor of childhood, but in some cases, it may be detected as late as the third or fourth decade of life (125,264). Patients with this tumor are usually asymptomatic. However, rare individuals present with watery diarrhea because of the ectopic synthesis of vasoactive intestinal polypeptide by the neoplasm (59), and other lesions may cause symptoms relating to spinal nerve root compression (265).

Similar to neurilemoma, ganglioneuroma is an encapsulated tumor that is situated in the paraspinal soft tissue of the posterior mediastinum. Nevertheless, it also may show partially intra-

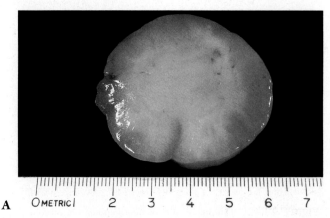

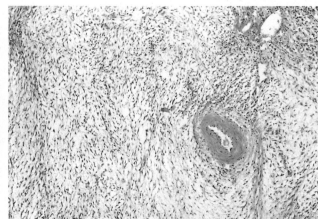

Figure 28.44. **(A)** Myxoid neurofibroma of the posterior mediastinum has a glistening, "slimy" cut surface. **(B)** The lesion is relatively paucicellular; bland fusiform tumor cells are separated by abundant myxoid stroma.

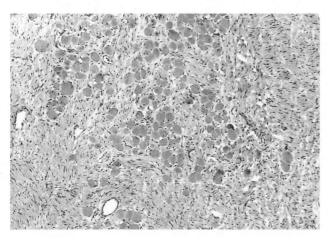

Figure 28.45. Ganglioneuroma of the posterior mediastinum differs from neurofibroma because of the intralesional presence of ganglion cells (*center*). The gross appearance of ganglioneuroma is much like the image shown in Figure 28.44.

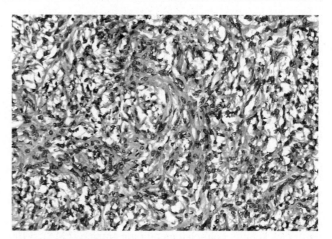

Figure 28.46. Solitary fibrous tumor of the anterior mediastinum showing cytologically bland fusiform cells haphazardly arranged and embedded in a uniformly collagenous stroma.

dural growth and a dumbbell-shaped profile, as seen in some neurofibromas (125).

Attention to the presence or absence of a tumor capsule on gross and microscopic examination is particularly important in the recognition of ganglioneuroma. This is true because the basic pattern of spindle cell proliferation in this tumor is virtually identical to that seen in neurofibroma. The major histologic difference between the two lesions is the presence of well-formed ganglion cells in ganglioneuroma (Fig. 28.45), but these may be observed only regionally and scrutiny of many tissue blocks may be required to document their presence (266). The use of immunostains for synaptophysin—a synaptic vesicle-related protein that is seen in neuronal lesions (267)—can assist in the rapid identification of widely scattered ganglion cells in ganglioneuromas.

FIBROGENIC AND MYOFIBROBLASTIC PROLIFERATIONS

Four cytologically bland spindle cell proliferations of the mediastinum may be histologically mistaken for one another. These are the solitary fibrous tumor, desmoid-type fibromatosis, sclerosing mediastinitis, and inflammatory myofibroblastic tumor (inflammatory pseudotumor).

SOLITARY FIBROUS TUMORS

Solitary fibrous tumors (SFTs) are best known as pleural neoplasms, but they also have been reported as primary lesions of the mediastinum (as well as many other locations) in adults (268–270). All three mediastinal subcompartments appear to be at equal risk. Some lesions are polypoid and protrude into the mediastinum from bases in the medial reflections of the pleura, but others appear to truly take their origin in the soft tissues between the lungs (268). As is true of their counterparts in the serosal investments of the lungs, mediastinal SFTs have no pathogenetic relationship to asbestos exposure (268). These neoplasms are either found incidentally on chest radiographs or they manifest themselves with nonspecific symptoms and signs of structural displacement (268,269).

As just mentioned, a subset of SFT has a circumscribed, polypoid gross configuration and is covered by a smooth layer of mesothelium. The remainder are less well-defined macroscopically, although their demarcation from adjacent soft tissues is usually clear to the surgeon at thoracotomy. On cut section, these lesions are white-gray with a uniformly firm consistency. Occasionally, a whorled, fascicular gross appearance is appreciated, similar to common leiomyomas of the uterus.

The histologic features of SFT include a constituency by cytologically banal spindle cells that are arranged haphazardly in a densely collagenous matrix (Fig. 28.46). The intercellular stroma has a distinctive fibrohyaline character—focally resembling that of keloids—and often circumferentially invests the individual cells in these neoplasms (Fig. 28.47). Tumor vascularity is typically rich, and some supporting blood vessels may assume an irregularly branched appearance like those seen in HPCs (268,269). Mitotic activity is usually limited, but some SFTs do show as many as 10 division figures per 10 high-power (×400) microscopic fields. Spontaneous necrosis is virtually unknown in such tumors, although areas of myxohyaline degeneration are not uncommon (125). Variant microscopic patterns

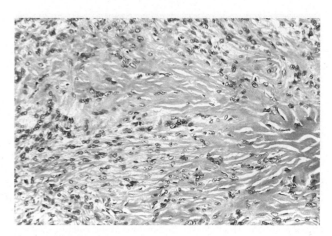

Figure 28.47. Individual tumor cells in solitary fibrous tumor of the mediastinum are often completely encompassed by dense fibrous stroma, as shown here.

include one featuring focal storiform growth, an epithelioid-predominant form (269a), and another wherein considerable nuclear pleomorphism or dense cellularity, or both, are observed focally or regionally (268). The last-cited of these SFT subtypes may be termed "atypical" SFT; however, the "minimal" criteria for a diagnosis of malignant SFT have not yet been codified. With that having been said, it is, perhaps, wise to consider SFT as a "borderline" tumor instead of a completely benign lesion, in light of its potential for recurrence (269b).

Immunohistochemical analysis of SFT has, in the author's experience and that of others (270–272), demonstrated vimentin and CD34 reactivity as consistent findings, similarly to other selected, specialized fibroblastic proliferations. Several authors have also shown that nuclear beta-catenin and cyclin D1 are apparent in SFT (269c,269d). The cells of this tumor consistently lack keratin, epithelial membrane antigen (EMA), S-100 protein, desmin, and actin.

Ultrastructural studies further support the fibroblastic nature of SFT in that they show nondescript spindle cells with notable profiles of rough endoplasmic reticulum and focal intrareticular collagen fibers (272). Features of myofibroblasts or myogenous cells, such as cytoplasmic thin filament skeins and dense bodies, pericellular basal lamina, and subplasmalemmal dense plaques, are generally not observed. Moreover, an absence of intercellular junctions militates against the presence of epithelial differentiation (273).

DESMOID-TYPE FIBROMATOSIS

In contrast to SFT, desmoid-type fibromatosis (DTF) is a poorly demarcated tumefactive proliferation that is centered in the soft tissue. It may affect the anterior or posterior mediastinum and is more often seen in children or young adults (274). These patients may present with the superior vena caval syndrome, a nerve entrapment syndrome, or dysphagia, depending on the location of the lesion.

To the surgeon, the true boundaries of DTF are indistinct; it tends to blend imperceptibly with surrounding fibroadipose soft tissue. Consequently, the pathologist often receives an incompletely excised mass or a "morselized" specimen that reflects the technical difficulty of its resection. Like fibromatoses in general, DTF has a firm, almost gritty cut surface, with a vaguely fascicular white-tan appearance (Fig. 28.48) (275).

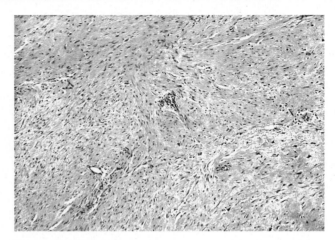

Figure 28.49. Desmoid tumor of the mediastinum showing atypical paucicellular appearance. The lesion is composed of bland fusiform cells in a slightly myxoid and fibrous stroma.

The microscopic features of this lesion include a variably fibromyxoid matrix in which parallel or interweaving fascicles of cytologically bland tumor cells are enmeshed. The latter may have either a stellate or fusiform shape, and their nuclei show dispersed chromatin and inconspicuous nucleoli (Fig. 28.49). The cytoplasm is eosinophilic or amphophilic, and close scrutiny may reveal a slightly fibrillary quality therein (276). One of the most characteristic histologic attributes of DTF is its vascularity; numerous venule-sized supporting vessels with thick walls are interspersed regularly throughout the mass (Fig. 28.50) (277). Despite the obviously fibrogenic nature of the proliferation, the vascular lumina are open and distinct rather than compressed. Nonetheless, staghorn-type blood vessels are not seen in this lesion. Similarly, areas with storiform growth or nuclear pleomorphism are regularly lacking in DTF, and mitotic activity is virtually nonexistent. In fact, the observation of even a few division figures in several high-power microscopic fields should raise the strong diagnostic suspicion of a low-grade fibrosarcoma rather than DTF. Intratumoral inflammation also is not expected in the latter lesion.

Ultrastructural studies of DTF and other fibromatoses have demonstrated that the tumor cells have myofibroblastic proper-

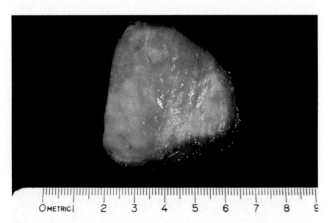

Figure 28.48. Desmoid-type fibromatosis of the anterior mediastinum may have a deceptively circumscribed appearance on gross examination. However, this proliferation extends irregularly into surrounding soft tissue.

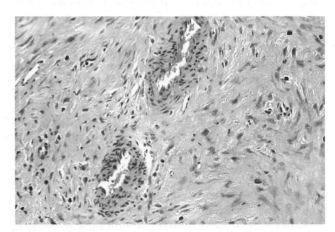

Figure 28.50. Venule-sized supporting blood vessels in desmoid tumor characteristically have thick walls and open lumina.

ties, including intrareticular collagen fibers, thin filament bundles, and cytoplasmic dense bodies (278). Otherwise, they resemble those seen in SFT. This same profile is reflected in the results of immunohistochemical analyses of DTF, which demonstrate reactivity not only for vimentin, but also for actin and desmin (279). Both SFTs and DTFs are potentially reactive for nuclear beta-catenin, unlike most other spindle cell proliferations (269a,279a). However, CD34 is absent in DTF (269d).

SCLEROSING (FIBROSING) MEDIASTINITIS, INFLAMMATORY MYOFIBROBLASTIC TUMOR, AND CALCIFYING FIBROUS TUMOR

DTF is most likely to be confused with sclerosing mediastinitis, which occurs almost exclusively in the anterosuperior mediastinum (280), or with "inflammatory myofibroblastic tumor" (IMT; formerly known as "inflammatory pseudotumor, not further specified" [281]). Sclerosing mediastinitis or IMT may manifest clinically with the superior vena caval syndrome or with symptoms of cardiorespiratory compromise, and both may be observed at any age (280,282–285). All of the cited lesions are characteristically represented by asymmetric widening of the mediastinum on chest films, usually with projection of a mass into an upper lung field (283).

The gross features of sclerosing mediastinitis and IMT are like those of dense but banal fibrosis occurring in other settings. Firm, white tissue is seen on cut section, without any suggestion of fascicular growth, and the junction of the periphery of the process with adjacent adipose tissue is clear cut (281,284).

Microscopically, sclerosing mediastinitis demonstrates the deposition of dense, fibrohyaline, relatively avascular tissue that is extremely paucicellular (280,284). Variably sized collections of mature lymphocytes are entrapped within the fibrotic zones and probably play a pathogenetic role in their formation (Fig. 28.51A) (284). Caseating or noncaseating granulomas are sometimes observed as well, relating to the fact that sclerosing mediastinitis is, in a substantial number of cases, an idiosyncratic response to infection of the mediastinal lymph nodes or lungs.

The most common causative organism in these instances is *Histoplasma capsulatum*, which may be detectable with silver impregnation stains in the granulomatous foci (283). Fungal infection accounts for no more than half of all examples of sclerosing mediastinitis; in addition to histoplasmosis, aspergillosis, cryptococcosis, and mucormycosis have been documented as potentiators of this condition. Other cases have been reported in association with sarcoidosis, nocardiosis, actinomycosis, syphilis, therapy with methysergide (an antimigraine medication), and trauma to the chest (284). The remainder are of indeterminate etiology, but the postulated common pathogenetic thread is that of a delayed cell-mediated hypersensitivity reaction (284). It would appear that a process similar to sclerosing mediastinitis may rarely involve the thymus itself and be relatively limited to it (285,286).

Other examples of mediastinal "pseudotumor" were reported by Brachet et al. (287) and by Coffin et al. (281), but these lesions had the histologic features of IMT rather than those of sclerosing mediastinitis, as noted previously. The former of these two proliferations is currently regarded as a true neoplasm (281), and it is more cellular than the latter lesion. Indeed, IMT is composed of bland fusiform elements that are arranged in variably dense arrays—often being fascicular or randomly configured—admixed with lymphocytes and a scattering of other inflammatory cells. The proliferating spindle cells in most IMTs are immunoreactive for vimentin and α-isoform actin (281), overlapping with the immunophenotypes of DTF and smooth muscle tumors. Approximately 40% of IMTs also are immunoreactive for the ALK-1 protein, in contrast to other diagnostic possibilities (287a).

Nascimento et al. (287b) have documented the presence of calcifying fibrous tumor (CFT) in the mediastinum when examining the possibility that the latter entity was a form of IMT. They instead concluded that the two lesions were distinct from one another. CFTs show a composition by bland spindle cells in a densely hyalinized collagenous stroma, with focal calcification (Fig. 28.51B). Variable immunoreactivity is present in such tumors for CD34 and α-isoform actin, but ALK-1 is absent.

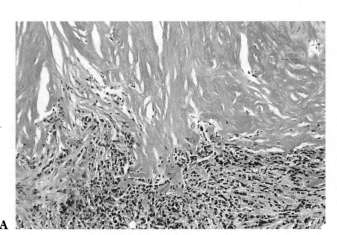
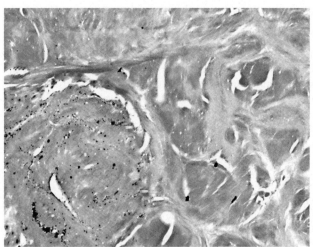

A   B

Figure 28.51. **(A)** Sclerosing mediastinitis is exemplified in this photomicrograph showing dense, acellular hyaline fibrous tissue and a cuff of small lymphocytes. Granulomatous inflammation may be observed focally in this process. **(B)** Calcifying fibrous tumor of the mediastinum, represented by a paucicellular bland spindle cell lesion with a densely collagenized stroma and focal calcification (*lower left*).

An important caveat must be remembered in the evaluation of putative cases of sclerosing mediastinitis. This is the ability of the tumor cells in selected malignant lymphomas (e.g., "obliterative total sclerosis" Hodgkin disease [98,288]), metastatic carcinomas, or malignant desmoplastic mesotheliomas to incite a brisk and obfuscating fibrotic response in the mediastinal soft tissue or lymph node groups. The neoplastic cells in such lesions are rather sparse and may be deceptively bland cytologically. Accordingly, they may be easily overlooked, leading to diagnostic misadventures (285,289,290). Stains for keratin, CD15, CD20, CD30, and CD45 are a prudent part of the workup of such lesions (see "Mediastinal Large-Cell Non-Hodgkin Lymphoma" and "Sarcomatoid Mediastinal Malignant Mesothelioma").

DIFFERENTIAL DIAGNOSIS OF CYTOLOGICALLY ATYPICAL MEDIASTINAL NEOPLASMS

Because of the diversity of cytologically atypical and overtly malignant proliferations that are capable of arising in the mediastinum, differential diagnosis of these lesions can be daunting. However, as mentioned earlier, this process can be simplified significantly by considering generic groupings of tumors that bear reproducible similarities to one another. Accordingly, the following material is organized in that fashion. Each pathologic entity in the respective groups is synopsized briefly from a clinicopathologic perspective, and differential diagnostic summaries are provided thereafter.

SMALL-CELL NEOPLASMS OF THE MEDIASTINUM

The primary considerations among those tumors with a uniform small-cell appearance encompass lesions with epithelial, lymphoid, neuroectodermal, and mesenchymal characteristics. This group includes small-cell neuroendocrine (oat cell) carcinoma (both primary and metastatic), basaloid squamous cell carcinoma, neuroblastoma (and congeners), primitive neuroectodermal tumor, rhabdomyosarcoma, and small-cell malignant lymphomas.

MEDIASTINAL SMALL-CELL NEUROENDOCRINE (OAT CELL) CARCINOMA

The overwhelming majority of small-cell neuroendocrine carcinomas (SCNCs) that present as anterior, middle, or posterior mediastinal masses are metastatic in nature (291), usually from primary sources in the lungs or esophagus. Patients with such lesions will often have symptoms referable to intrabronchial disease (e.g., cough, hemoptysis, dyspnea) or enteric mucosal abnormalities (e.g., dysphagia), but this statement is not absolute. Also, a minority of individuals have evidence of a paraneoplastic endocrinopathy, such as Cushing syndrome or the syndrome of inappropriate secretion of antidiuretic hormone (SIADH) (51). Because it is well known that primary pulmonary SCNC may not be detectable on conventional chest radiographs, computed tomography, or even magnetic resonance scanning, one should not accept negative results from such studies as providing definitive evidence against the existence of these tumors in cases where a mediastinal biopsy shows small-cell carcinoma. Indeed, the diagnosis of primary mediastinal (thymic) SCNC is one to be made with extreme circumspection

in light of the fact that there are less than 100 well-documented cases in the English-language literature (50,90,91,291–298).

The gross characteristics of SCNC are identical, regardless of their anatomic origins. These tumors have a fleshy, white-gray, partially hemorrhagic and necrotic appearance, simulating that of malignant lymphoma in some respects (291,293).

Microscopically, particular attention should be given to whether or not the neoplasm is actually centered in the thymus gland or, instead, represents a nodal metastasis. Even in the former of these circumstances, a secondary lesion still cannot be excluded; however, thymic involvement could provide at least provisional support for the primary nature of such a tumor. The histologic attributes of SCNC are familiar to all surgical pathologists. They include a vaguely clustered or organoid architecture, regional spontaneous necrosis (often in the central areas of tumor cell nests), extremely high nucleocytoplasmic ratios with scanty cytoplasm, dispersed or homogeneously dark nuclear chromatin with inconspicuous nucleoli, "molding" of adjacent nuclei against one another, and numerous mitoses (Fig. 28.52). "Crush" artifact is common in small endoscopic biopsy specimens of SCNC, and one may also observe the "Azzopardi phenomenon," wherein deeply basophilic rings of nuclear material are encrusted on intratumoral blood vessels (Fig. 28.53) (36). Another characteristic of SCNC, be it primary or metastatic in the mediastinum, is its capacity for divergent differentiation. Examples of this tumor showing an admixture of obvious squamous cell carcinoma or adenocarcinoma have been seen in the thymus, lung, gut, and other sites (90,91,294).

A long-standing problem concerning SCNC is its distinction from so-called "atypical carcinoids." The latter tumors have traditionally been defined histologically by a larger cellular size, with more cytoplasm than that of SCNC and a more distinctly organoid growth pattern with potential spindle cell foci (Fig. 28.54) (36). From a practical point of view, the author prefers the term *grade 2 neuroendocrine carcinoma* to *atypical carcinoid* to avoid associating the lesion in clinicians' minds with low-grade tumors ("classic" or "conventional" carcinoids, which are synonymous with grade 1 neuroendocrine carcinomas). More important, the distinction between the small-cell type and other forms of neuroendocrine carcinoma does not appear to be important prognostically in the context under discussion here. All

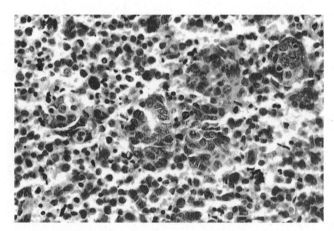

Figure 28.52. Nuclear "molding" and brisk mitotic activity are apparent in this thymic small-cell neuroendocrine carcinoma. These features are shared by both primary and secondary oat cell carcinomas of the thymic region.

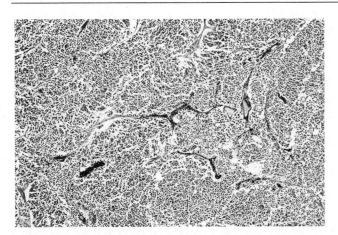

Figure 28.53. Encrustation of free nucleic acid around intratumoral blood vessels is characteristic of small-cell neuroendocrine carcinoma, as shown here.

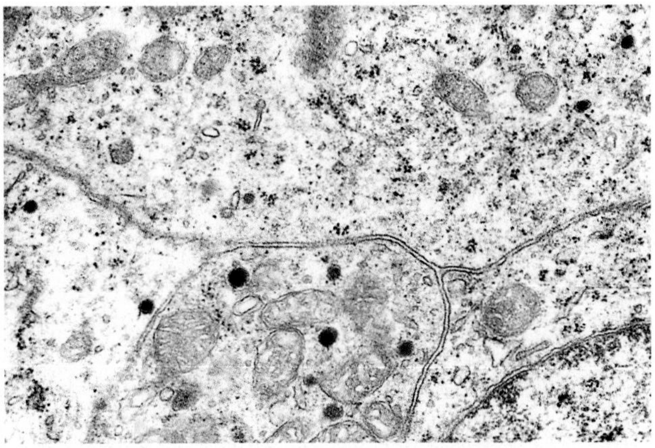

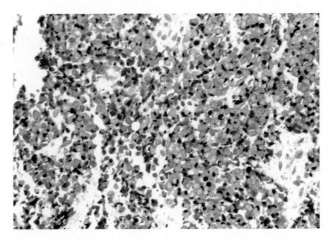

Figure 28.55. Electron microscopy of small-cell neuroendocrine carcinoma of the thymus typically shows a small number of uniformly sized cytoplasmic neurosecretory granules.

of these tumors, whether metastatic or primary, are capable of an aggressive clinical evolution in cases with mediastinal involvement (91).

Ultrastructurally, SCNC is defined by the presence of primitive junctional complexes between apposed tumor cells, as well as the presence of neurosecretory (neuroendocrine) granules in the cytoplasm (36,90,91,292,297). The latter organelles are small (80 to 250 nm) and relatively uniform in appearance (Fig. 28.55). To be assured that they do not represent lysosomes, a clear-cut peripheral "halo" should be seen within each granule around a central, electron-dense core; moreover, clusters of granules are more convincing than isolated inclusions in a minority of cells.

On an immunohistochemical level, SCNC is recognizable either by a distinctive pattern of intermediate filament expression, with perinuclear "globules" of keratin protein (Fig. 28.56) (198), or by its potential reactivity for one of several neuroendocrine markers. These include chromogranin A (a matrix protein of neurosecretory granules), synaptophysin, CD57 antigen, and selected neuropeptides such as adrenocorticotropic hormone (36). Thyroid transcription factor-1 (TTF-1) is present in the

majority of primary pulmonary SCNCs (298a), but to date, insufficient numbers of primary thymic small-cell carcinomas have been studied to make definitive statements on their TTF-1 immunoreactivity.

BASALOID SQUAMOUS CELL CARCINOMA OF THE MEDIASTINUM

Basaloid squamous cell carcinoma (BSCC) shares the same potential as SCNC to involve the mediastinum either primarily as a thymic tumor (90–92) or by metastasis (Fig. 28.57). Potential primary sites in the latter instance include the oropharynx, hypopharynx, larynx, esophagus, lungs, and anorectal region (92). Hence, the same cautions pertain to rushed conclusions that such neoplasms originate in the mediastinum as emphasized previously in connection with mediastinal oat cell carcinoma. Patients with BSCC of the mediastinum are adults who present with generic symptoms and signs of an intrathoracic mass (91,299) and, potentially, other findings that may be referable to the sources of metastatic lesions.

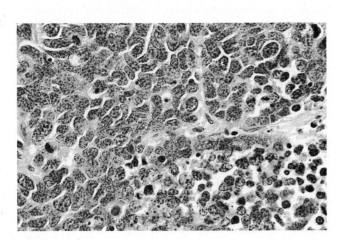

Figure 28.54. "Atypical carcinoid" (moderately differentiated neuroendocrine carcinoma) manifests larger individual tumor cells than those of oat cell carcinoma. Conversely, it has more necrosis and mitotic activity than typical "carcinoid" tumors.

Figure 28.56. Small-cell carcinoma of the thymic region is recognizable as neuroendocrine in nature by its pattern of keratin immunoreactivity. Distinctly globular paranuclear accentuation of staining is seen in this illustration.

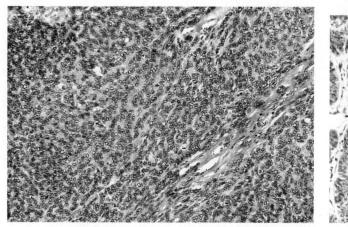
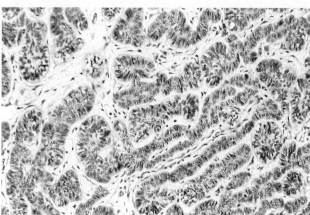

A

B

Figure 28.57. **(A)** Basaloid carcinoma of the thymus is composed of nests, cords, and sheets of compact tumor cells, separated by myxoid or eosinophilic stroma. **(B)** Focally, this tumor may demonstrate peripheral palisading of nuclei within nests of neoplastic cells.

Histologically, BSCC is composed of organoid clusters of small polygonal cells with high nucleocytoplasmic ratios, scanty cytoplasm, uniformly hyperchromatic round nuclei, and abundant mitoses. However, there is no nuclear "molding." In addition, this lesion may show foci of stromal mucin-containing glandlike profiles that may recall the appearance of adenoid cystic carcinomas, globular eosinophilic intercellular deposits of basement membrane material as seen in cylindromas of the skin, and areas of overt squamous differentiation with keratin "pearls" (90,91,194,195). The few cases reported as primary in the thymus have shown a remarkable tendency for association with (and probable origin in) antecedent multilocular thymic cysts (90–92), the remnants of which were obvious in resection specimens.

The electron microscopic attributes of this neoplasm are basically those of a poorly differentiated squamous proliferation (90). Therefore, limited numbers of cytoplasmic tonofilaments are expected, together with well-formed desmosomal-type intercellular junctions (Fig. 28.58). Neurosecretory granules are not observed. In addition, the globular accumulations of basement

membrane seen by optical microscopy are reflected in the presence of focally redundant basal lamina on an ultrastructural level.

Keratin is uniformly detected immunohistochemically in BSCC with a diffuse intracellular distribution, and p63 and EMA reactivity also may be observed (194,299a). However, the author has detected no staining in these lesions for neuroendocrine determinants.

NEUROBLASTOMA OF THE MEDIASTINUM

In its usual form, neuroblastoma is a disease of young children (300). Intrathoracic examples of this tumor are largely (but not totally [37,38,301]) restricted to the posterior mediastinum (302), where they are typically primary and originate in association with nerve roots in a paraspinal location (254). The latter region is only exceptionally involved by metastases of a neuroblastoma arising at another anatomic site.

Symptoms of the mass most often relate to the compression of spinal nerves or interference with esophageal motility. Some children also may have the paraneoplastic neurologic syndrome known as opsoclonus-myoclonus ("dancing feet and dancing eyes") (59). Erosion of contiguous vertebral bones may be seen as well (303). Interestingly, when neuroblastomas involve the thymus and anterior mediastinum, they appear to show an inordinate association with production of SIADH (37,38). Laboratory evaluation of the urine or blood often reveals elevated levels of homovanillic acid and vanillylmandelic acid, representing metabolites of tumoral catecholamine products (293). In accord with information previously mentioned, marked hyponatremia also may be apparent in connection with those tumors synthesizing antidiuretic hormone.

The resectability of neuroblastoma is predicated on its relative circumscription, and in the mediastinum, most cases do demonstrate partial or complete encapsulation (125). Cut surfaces are fleshy and pink-gray, often with foci of necrosis, hemorrhage, and punctate calcification (Fig. 28.59).

Neuroblastoma is potentially one of the prototypical, undifferentiated, small round-cell tumors of childhood (304); in its primitive form, this lesion is composed of sheets of monomorphic elements with uniformly dispersed chromatin, inconspicu-

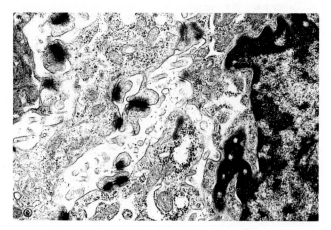

Figure 28.58. Electron micrograph of basaloid squamous cell carcinoma of the thymus showing numerous well-formed desmosomes between adjacent tumor cells. These structures are not expected in the usual case of small-cell neuroendocrine carcinoma.

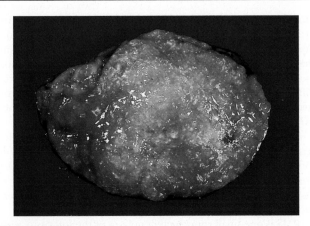

Figure 28.59. Gross photograph of posterior mediastinal neuroblastoma showing a pink-gray cut surface with stippled necrosis and calcification.

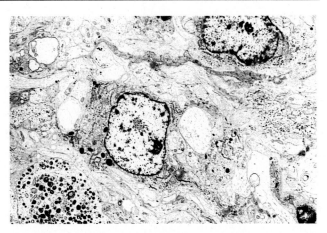

Figure 28.61. Electron photomicrograph of posterior mediastinal neuroblastoma showing elongated cellular processes. Some of these projections (*bottom*) contain neurosecretory granules.

ous nucleoli, and a scant amount of eosinophilic cytoplasm (Fig. 28.60). Mitotic activity and karyorrhexis vary considerably but may be striking. Regional necrosis and superimposed dystrophic calcification also are observed rather frequently, and an arborizing network of delicate stromal blood vessels is a consistent finding (125). Differentiating examples of this entity betray their neuroblastic nature through the formation of a fibrillary eosinophilic intercellular matrix, and even more mature tumors may demonstrate the presence of scattered primitive ganglion cells. If the latter are numerous, the diagnostic term *ganglioneuroblastoma* is more appropriate (305) (see Chapter 14).

Electron microscopy discloses variable neuritic differentiation in the form of complex, long, interdigitating cytoplasmic processes that contain microtubules (Fig. 28.61) (37,301). Some also show synaptic vesicles or scant numbers of neurosecretory granules, but the latter structures are not necessary diagnostically (306). Basal lamina is scarce to absent, intercellular junctions are few in number and primitive, and only a minority of cases exhibit the presence of intracellular glycogen granules (307). Cytoplasmic intermediate filaments are usually not seen; when present, they are inconspicuous and widely separated.

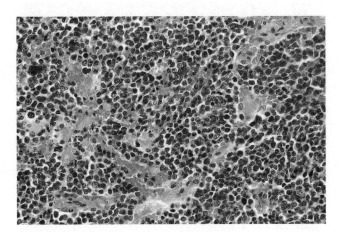

Figure 28.60. Neuroblastoma is typified by sheets of small round cells, traversed by delicate fibrovascular septa. A suggestion of a fibrillary intercellular matrix is also seen in this illustration.

Immunohistochemical assessment of neuroblastoma reveals variable reactivity for vimentin and neurofilament protein; many tumors lack both of these polypeptides altogether (308). Evidence of neural differentiation is manifest by positivity for the CD57 antigen and synaptophysin, both of which are seen in the majority of cases (125). Many neuroblastomas also react with NB84, a monoclonal antibody recognizing a 57-kd tumor-selective moiety (308a,308b). Markers of muscular lesions (desmin, actin), lymphoid tumors (CD45), and epithelial neoplasms (keratin, EMA) are absent (37,271).

MEDIASTINAL PRIMITIVE NEUROECTODERMAL TUMOR

The "primitive neuroectodermal tumor" (PNET) is now an accepted member of the lexicon of diagnostic pathology. In the past, this lesion was considered variously to be synonymous with "peripheral neuroblastoma" or "extraskeletal Ewing sarcoma" and was vaguely defined morphologically (309). However, documentation of the pathologic spectrum of PNET is now well established. This lesion is predominantly a tumor of childhood, but it can indeed be seen throughout life. Patients with PNET complain of a rapidly growing mass, which, when located in the mediastinum (a rare occurrence), may produce symptomatic structural displacement (310). The author has observed single examples in both the anterior and posterior mediastinum, respectively, one of which arose in an adolescent and the other in a young adult. Similar cases have been reported by Glick and Page (311) and Grosfeld et al. (312). For statistical purposes, primary mediastinal PNET should be separated from the Askin tumor (primitive small-cell thoracopulmonary tumor), which has its origin in the soft tissues of the chest wall (313). However, the lineages of these two entities are identical in that both demonstrate unequivocal neuroectodermal differentiation (314).

Mediastinal PNET is a bulky, poorly delimited, necrotic and hemorrhagic, white-gray fleshy mass on macroscopic examination. It may show adherence (or apparent origin) from a spinal nerve root when located in the posterior subcompartment.

The microscopic characteristics of this neoplasm are again those of a primitive round-cell sarcoma in most cases. Nonetheless, some may exhibit a vaguely organoid growth pattern or focal formation of primitive rosettes, suggesting the identity of

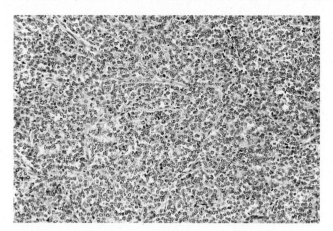

Figure 28.62. Primitive neuroectodermal tumor of the posterior mediastinum composed of vaguely organoid nests of monomorphic small round cells. Focal rosette formation may be seen in this neoplasm.

the lesion as neuroectodermal. The overall histologic appearance is very much like that of "undifferentiated" neuroblastoma, including a prominent network of delicate intratumoral blood vessels, but unlike the latter, PNET does not demonstrate any attempt at cytoplasmic neurofibrillary maturation (Fig. 28.62) (307,309). In other sites, PNETs have been shown to manifest divergent differentiation, with areas resembling rhabdomyosarcoma or even primitive glands (307,309). Although this phenomenon has not yet been reported in mediastinal lesions, it is potentially possible.

The ultrastructural attributes of PNET are somewhat similar to those of neuroblastoma, except that those cytoplasmic processes that are formed are blunt and rudimentary. There are no intracellular microtubules in the tumor cells, and neurosecretory granules or synaptic vesicles are sparse (235,307,314). Intercellular junctions assume a primitive nature. Examples of PNET with divergent differentiation may manifest foci wherein the cells show cytoplasmic thick and thin filaments or form nascent glandular lumina (314,315).

Immunohistochemical characteristics of PNET are again like those of neuroblastoma, but PNET exhibits more uniform reactivity for vimentin, less often shows NB84 positivity (308b), and only exceptionally expresses neurofilament protein (235). Moreover, the CD99 (MIC-2) and MB2 antigens, FLI-1, and β_2-microglobulin are reproducibly present in PNET but not in neuroblastoma (316–319a). Synaptophysin and the CD57 antigen are detectable in many cases, and divergent neoplasms also may show focal reactivity for keratin, desmin, and actin (235,316).

Perhaps the most certain method for securing a firm diagnosis of PNET is the cytogenetic analysis of fresh tumor tissue. A characteristic and distinctive reciprocal chromosomal translocation [t(11;22)(q24;q12)] serves as a definitive marker of PNET among all small-cell tumors of the mediastinum (320). With the benefit of suitable nucleotide primers and polymerase chain reaction, this abnormality can now be identified using paraffin-embedded tissue as well.

RHABDOMYOSARCOMA OF THE MEDIASTINUM

Rhabdomyosarcoma (RMS) of the mediastinum also may arise in either the anterior or posterior subcompartments, and in

pure form, it almost exclusively affects children and adolescents (125,274,310,311,321). The latter demographic point is an important one because another posterior mediastinal neoplasm that can be seen in adults—the so-called malignant triton tumor (see Chapter 5)—may demonstrate partial rhabdomyoblastic differentiation. Childhood RMS produces manifestations of structural displacement but is associated with no other distinctive clinical syndromes (274,310,321).

The macroscopic findings in RMS are also relatively nondescript, being those of a poorly delimited, bulky lesion of the soft tissues with a fleshy, white-gray cut surface and frequent areas of spontaneous hemorrhage or necrosis (274). There is no reproducible association with particular anatomic structures, such as the paraspinal muscles.

RMS is one small round-cell neoplasm of the soft tissue with histologic features that may serve as a clue to the lineage of the lesion on conventional microscopic examination. Although some of these tumors are indeed monomorphic proliferations of primitive cells, more of them demonstrate discernible nuclear and cellular pleomorphism that is not observed in differential diagnostic alternatives. Scattered large cells with multinucleation, eccentric nuclei, fusiform features, or deeply eosinophilic cytoplasm strongly suggest the diagnosis of RMS, as does the presence of focal myxoid stromal change in an otherwise uniform small-cell lesion (Figs. 28.63 and 28.64). Likewise, areas of alveolar growth are distinctive when present (125,307). Begin et al. (322) also have drawn attention to the ability of mediastinal RMS to manifest clear-cell change when the glycogen content of the lesion is high; this variation increases the overall size of the tumor cells, potentially causing confusion with large-cell neoplasms of other lineages (discussed subsequently).

Electron microscopically, RMS is recognized by the tight aggregates of intermediate filaments that are present in the cytoplasm of tumor cells. These may occasionally be organized with thick (myosin) filaments into primitive sarcomeric structures (Fig. 28.65), complete with Z-bands. Glycogen is usually present, together with short segments of pericellular basal lamina. Intercellular junctions, cytoplasmic processes, microtubules, synaptic vesicles, and dense-core granules are lacking (235,319).

Virtually all RMSs are immunoreactive for desmin and muscle-specific actin, together with vimentin. Myoglobin is ob-

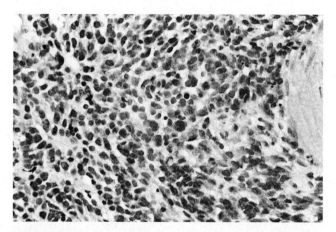

Figure 28.63. This embryonal rhabdomyosarcoma of the anterior mediastinum displays focal nuclear enlargement and pleomorphism (*center*). This feature is not expected in other intrathoracic small round-cell tumors.

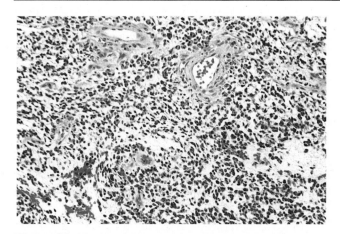

Figure 28.64. Myxoid stroma in mediastinal embryonal rhabdomyosarcoma. This attribute distinguishes this tumor from other small round-cell sarcomas that may occur in the thorax.

served only in large maturing rhabdomyoblasts and is therefore not a particularly useful marker of RMS in its purely small-cell form. Synaptophysin is regularly absent, but some examples of RMS may demonstrate focal positivity for the CD57 antigen (235,271,319). The specificity of desmin and actin for the diagnosis of RMS has been questioned by some because these determinants also are seen in smooth muscle proliferations. Nonetheless, because a small-cell variant of leiomyosarcoma does not exist, that argument seems irrelevant to the author in this context. In any event, other markers that are apparently restricted to striated muscle—particularly MyoD1 and myogenin (323,323a)—can be applied to the differential diagnosis in question. As a final word of caution in this section, it should also be remembered that both RMS of the alveolar subtype and PNET share potential reactivity for CD99 (318,319,323); hence, that determinant should not be used diagnostically in isolation.

SMALL-CELL MALIGNANT LYMPHOMAS OF THE MEDIASTINUM

As alluded to earlier, there are three small-cell non-Hodgkin malignant lymphomas (SCMLs) that may affect the mediasti-

num as primary processes. These are LBL (205,206), small non-cleaved cell (Burkitt/non-Burkitt) lymphoma (SNCL) (227, 228), lymphomas arising in MALT ("MALTomas") (230,231), and primary marginal zone lymphoma of the thymus (324). The first two of these tumors are seen predominantly in children and adolescents, but LBL also has a second incidence peak in the seventh to eighth decades (208), and the author has observed examples of mediastinal SNCL in adults as well. Either LBL or SNCL is capable of peripheralization, with the appearance of acute leukemia (206,207,228). However, this complication is observed at presentation in only a minority of cases with mediastinal masses.

The gross characteristics of all lymphomas are roughly similar and have been described herein. Similarly, the light microscopic attributes of LBL and SNCL have been documented earlier in this discussion. Mediastinal MALTomas, on the other hand, show a constitution by clusters of differentiated, centrocyte-like lymphoid cells that are commingled with mature-appearing lymphocytes as well as lymphoid follicles containing reactive germinal centers. Plasma cells also may be observed. All of these elements must be centered in the thymus, virtually by definition. The centrocyte-like cells diffusely expand the gland and permeate the thymic epithelium in small groups (yielding so-called "lymphoepithelial lesions"); this phenomenon may cause microcystic change as well (230,231). Marginal zone lymphomas demonstrate a composition by small, relatively mature lymphocytes with admixed monocytoid cells and plasma cells (324). With the electron microscope, small-cell non-Hodgkin lymphoma is a diagnosis of exclusion. One should not observe intercellular junctions, cytoplasmic filament bundles, neurosecretory granules, synaptic vesicles, microtubules, basal lamina, cytoplasmic processes, or primitive sarcomeres (325). In addition, most lymphoma cells demonstrate the formation of nuclear "blebs," which are irregular protrusions of the nuclear membranes (Fig. 28.66) (134).

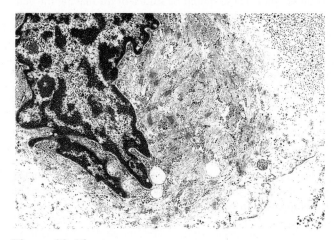

Figure 28.65. Electron micrograph of embryonal rhabdomyosarcoma showing the organization of cytoplasmic thick and thin filaments into primitive sarcomeres. These structures are diagnostic of rhabdomyoblastic differentiation.

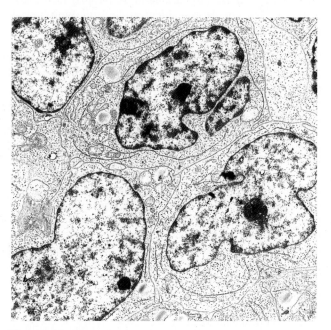

Figure 28.66. Nuclei in this electron micrograph of mediastinal lymphoma are irregular with outward projections or "blebs."

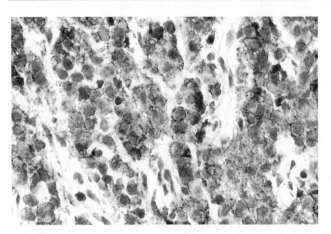

Figure 28.67. Immunoreactivity for CD43 antigen in lymphoblastic lymphoma of the mediastinum. Although characteristic of this lesion, CD43 positivity is also shared by the lymphocytes of lymphocyte-predominant thymoma and should not be interpreted in isolation.

Immunohistochemical analysis is helpful in solidifying the diagnosis of LBL, SNCL, and MALToma of the mediastinum. These lesions express the CD45 (leukocyte common) antigen, as well as show reactivity with other lymphoid-selective monoclonal antibodies. LBL commonly is labeled with CD43 reagents (L60, Leu-22, MT-1) (Fig. 28.67); CD99 antibodies such as O13 or 12E7; and antibodies to CD10, bcl-2 protein, and TdT (213). SNCL is reactive for CD20 and typically lacks all of the other cited determinants, with the possible exception of bcl-2 protein (213). MALTomas are best studied using fresh tissue specimens rather than paraffin sections. With the former preparations, reactivity for monotypic immunoglobulin light chain can be detected by immunohistochemistry or corresponding ribonucleic acid in situ hybridization methods in the centrocyte-like cells (231). Positivity for CD10 (common acute lymphoblastic leukemia antigen) and CD20 is also apparent, but CD43, CD99, bcl-2, and TdT are lacking in MALTomas (326); CD5 is usually—but not always—absent in the latter morphotype. Positivity for keratin, CD57, synaptophysin, desmin, and actin is not observed in any of these three lymphoma morphotypes, but some examples of all of them may exhibit immunoreactivity for vimentin (235). Marginal zone lymphomas are typically immunoreactive for CD20 and usually bcl-2 protein as well (324).

OTHER SMALL-CELL MEDIASTINAL NEOPLASMS

In addition to those small-cell tumors presented in the foregoing sections, others of a metastatic nature also may involve the mediastinum. These include small-cell osteosarcoma and Ewing sarcoma of bone, as well as small-cell malignant melanoma. Except for the last of these possibilities, the primary lesion in such cases is typically obvious, and there is no question of whether the intrathoracic neoplasm might have arisen there. However, it is common knowledge that melanomas have the capability of presenting with distant metastasis in the face of an undetectable primary source, and rare examples are thought to have arisen in the thymus (327,328). Moreover, the potential for melanomas to assume the guise of a small-cell morphology also has been well documented (329).

Ultrastructural analyses may be helpful in these circumstances in demonstrating the presence of cytoplasmic premela-

nosomes in small-cell melanomas (319,325). Also, the immunohistochemical characteristics of such lesions feature reactivity for S-100 protein and the HMB45 antigen (329), neither of which is expected in other small-cell neoplasms of the mediastinum.

SPECIFIC DIFFERENTIAL DIAGNOSTIC CONSIDERATIONS AMONG SMALL-CELL TUMORS OF THE MEDIASTINUM

It should be apparent that the foregoing discussion of mediastinal small-cell neoplasms was structured in part to set the stage for a consideration of particularly vexing differential diagnoses in this group of lesions. These are discussed in the sections immediately following.

Rhabdomyosarcoma Versus Primitive Neuroectodermal Tumor Versus Neuroblastoma

Among all soft tissue tumors, those in the small round-cell category in children are, perhaps, the most challenging for the pathologist. As mentioned earlier, mediastinal RMS, PNET, and neuroblastoma all may assume an "undifferentiated" appearance that is closely similar. Thus, histologic examination alone is unlikely to provide a definitive answer, and other, more specialized techniques must be used to reach a final interpretation. The pathologic features of greatest value in this context are outlined in Table 28.2.

Small-Cell Malignant Lymphoma Versus Small-Cell Carcinomas

Especially in small biopsy specimens of mediastinal tumors, it may be difficult to distinguish SCMLs from small-cell carcinomas. If a distinctly clustered growth pattern is observed, despite obscure nuclear features, the latter of these diagnoses should be favored. Likewise, the presence of the Azzopardi phenomenon suggests the presence of a carcinoma rather than lymphoma. Nonetheless, many cases will require specialized studies to reach a final conclusion. Electron microscopy is not very productive when specimens have been distorted badly during procurement; however, it is fortunate that CD45 and keratin immunostains often can still be performed successfully even on crushed tissue samples. These should be sufficient for making the general diagnostic separation under discussion, but more specific interpretations (e.g., of SCNC) may well require that additional specimens be obtained.

Obtaining additional specimens is important because the ultrastructural and immunohistologic markers separating the types of carcinoma or lymphoma (discussed previously) usually are optimally seen only in well-processed tissue samples. As a practical solution to this problem—mindful of the fact that clinicians are often loath to undertake another surgical procedure without much debate—fine-needle aspiration biopsy of the mediastinal mass is suggested (2,3,5). This technique typically yields sufficiently preserved material to allow for more detailed study of a lesion that is already known to be carcinomatous or lymphomatous in nature.

Small-Cell Neuroendocrine Carcinoma Versus Basaloid Carcinoma

The distinction between carcinoma morphotypes, as just mentioned, is often an important step in the planning of therapy

TABLE 28.2	Differential Diagnosis of Malignant Small Round-Cell Tumors of the Mediastinum												
	Light Microscopy		Electron Microscopy Immunohistochemistry										
Neoplasm	Myxoid Stroma	Pleomorphism	Fibrillar Stroma	PAS	IFS	ECP	NSG	ICJ	LCA	Ker	D/A	NM	S-100
ERMS/ARMS	+/−	Variable	No	+/−	+	0	0	0	0	0	+	0	0
PNET	0	Minimal	No	+/−	0	0	+/−	+[a]	0	+/−	+/−	+[b]	0
NBL	0	Minimal	Variable	0	0	+	+/−	+[a]	0	0	0	+	0
SCNC	0	Minimal	No	+/−	+	0	+	+	0	+	0	+/−	0
SCML	0	Minimal	No	0	0	0	0	0	+	0	0	0	0
BSCC	+/−	Minimal	No	+/−	+	0	0	+	0	+	0	+/−	0
SCMM[c]	0	Minimal	No	+/−	0	0	0[c]	+[a]	0	0	0	0	+

ARMS, alveolar rhabdomyosarcoma; BSCC, basaloid squamous cell carcinoma; D/A, desmin/actin; ECP, elongated cell processes; ERMS, embryonal rhabdomyosarcoma; ICJ, intercellular junctions; IFS, intermediate filament skeins; Ker, keratin; LCA, leukocyte common antigen; NBL, neuroblastoma; NM, neural markers (Leu-7, synaptophysin); NSG, neurosecretory granules; PAS, periodic acid-Schiff stain; PNET, primitive neuroectodermal tumor; S-100, S-100 protein; SCML, small-cell malignant lymphoma; SCMM, small-cell malignant melanoma; SCNC, small-cell neuroendocrine carcinoma.
[a]Rare examples of neuroblastoma may be weakly PAS positive.
[b]PNET is labeled by monoclonal antibodies to CD99.
[c]Rare examples of melanoma may contain NSG.

for a mediastinal tumor. In particular, primary small-cell neuroendocrine thymic carcinoma is usually managed, at least in part, with chemotherapy that would be appropriate for SCNC of the lung. In contrast, primary basaloid thymic carcinomas should be resected surgically (91).

To reiterate selected points made earlier in this chapter, the findings of dispersed nuclear chromatin, inconspicuous nucleoli, and nuclear molding should suggest a diagnosis of SCNC. However, association with remnants of a thymic cyst, cellular nucleolation, and intercellular deposits of eosinophilic basement membrane material (potentially highlighted with a PAS-diastase stain) militate in favor of BSCC. Cases that are histologically indeterminate do exist in this context, but they usually yield themselves to electron microscopy and immunohistochemistry (see earlier sections in this chapter).

Primary Versus Metastatic Carcinoma of the Mediastinum

In cases where a nonmelanocytic lineage of a small-cell malignancy of the mediastinum is observed, the question arises regarding the primary or secondary nature of the proliferation. Although the incidence of certain mesenchymal tumors is skewed in one direction or another in this regard (see previous discussion), the origin of most other neoplasms is questionable.

Unfortunately, there are no reliable pathologic indicators that allow for a definitive resolution of this problem. Accordingly, one must require that the clinician undertake appropriate radiologic or endoscopic procedures to address the potential existence of primary lesions outside of the mediastinum, before assigning a final diagnostic interpretation to the tumor under consideration. This stipulation has more than mere academic significance because, in many cases, it ultimately determines the surgical or nonsurgical management of the lesion.

LARGE POLYGONAL CELL NEOPLASMS OF THE MEDIASTINUM

Malignant large polygonal cell tumors of the mediastinum likewise comprise a heterogeneous group of lesions with respect to

cellular lineage. These include variants of thymic carcinoma, germ cell tumors, carcinoid tumor of the thymus, large-cell lymphoma, granulocytic sarcoma, plasmacytoma, syncytial Hodgkin disease, paraganglioma, parathyroid carcinoma, malignant mesothelioma, and metastatic carcinoma or melanoma.

PRIMARY THYMIC CARCINOMAS

Thymic carcinomas are neoplasms that have been well recognized as distinctive entities only in the recent past (62,90, 176,180,190,297,298,330–343). Before their current characterization, literature on tumors of the thymus often stated that their biologic potential could not be determined by histologic appearance (344–346); this view is only partially correct. It is true that the regional recurrence of conventional thymoma is predicated most on the presence or absence of gross invasion (178), rather than on its cytologic attributes. Moreover, a small number (approximately 7%) of invasive thymomas do show extrathoracic (but idiosyncratic) spread ("metastasizing thymoma"). Thus, these biologic events do not necessarily equate with a diagnostic label of "carcinoma." In this specific context, it is notable that the entity advanced by Kirchner et al. (156) as "well-differentiated thymic carcinoma" (WHO type B3 thymoma) shows a clinicopathologic synonymity with that subset of epithelial-predominant thymomas that manifest modest nuclear atypia, as discussed by Lewis et al. (148).

Outside of the foregoing remarks, there is a distinct subset of thymic epithelial lesions that manifests overt cellular anaplasia and aggressive clinical evolution. These do deserve the designation of carcinoma because of such features.

Thymic carcinomas also differ clinically from thymomas in that they are typically not associated with paraneoplastic syndromes such as myasthenia gravis or pure red-cell aplasia (90,91,297,336,337). The former lesions most often present themselves with symptoms of structural displacement, although a minority are discovered incidentally on screening chest radiographs (296,297). Patients with thymic carcinomas are typically middle-aged or older adults, with a slight predominance in men. Nevertheless, a few cases have been observed in children. Be-

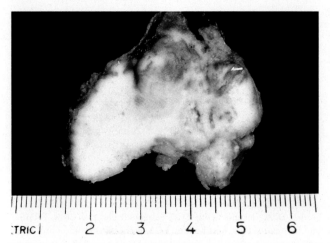

Figure 28.68. In contrast to thymomas, thymic carcinoma (shown here) typically lacks encapsulation and internal fibrous septation and manifests a gritty white-gray cut surface.

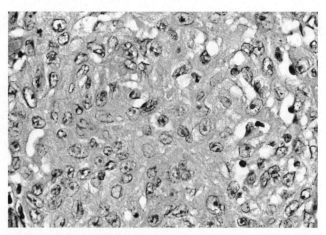

Figure 28.69. Keratinizing squamous cell carcinoma of the thymus is composed of cells with a moderate amount of eosinophilic glassy cytoplasm, as well as vesicular nuclei and prominent nucleoli. Squamous "pearls" also may be evident in this neoplasm.

cause some of these lesions may resemble metastases to the thymic region histologically (discussed subsequently) (347, 348), one must strictly require that clinical attention is given to the possibility of an occult malignancy elsewhere before a definitive diagnosis is made.

Grossly, thymic carcinomas usually lack the encapsulation or internal fibrous septation that is seen in thymomas (Fig. 28.68) (297). They are firm to hard (sometimes gritty) and white-gray on the cut surface, with frequent foci of necrosis and hemorrhage. A particular variant of thymic carcinoma (the basaloid squamous type, discussed earlier) may demonstrate a close association with remnants of a multilocular thymic cyst on macroscopic examination (90,91). Another type, the mucoepidermoid thymic carcinoma, often has a mucoid cut surface and a "slimy" consistency (90).

Several microscopic subtypes of thymic carcinoma are currently recognized (13,90,91,190,291–297,332,349,350). Two of them—basaloid carcinoma and spindle cell (sarcomatoid) carcinoma—are not polygonal cell in nature and are therefore discussed in other sections of this chapter. The remaining variants are presented in the following sections.

Keratinizing Squamous Cell Carcinoma of the Thymus

Keratinizing squamous cell carcinoma (KSCC) of the thymus is identical microscopically to its counterpart in the skin, mouth, pharynx, larynx, lung, and genitourinary tract. It is composed of large polyhedral cells arranged in nests and cords and potentially shows intercellular bridges on high-power examination. The nuclei are vesicular or hyperchromatic, and nucleoli are usually readily apparent (Fig. 28.69). Cytoplasm is eosinophilic, and incipient or well-formed keratin "pearls" are scattered throughout KSCC (91,294,295,298,349). Foci of spontaneous necrosis are frequently seen, as is invasion of intratumoral blood vessels.

A potential point of confusion in cases of thymic KSCC concerns the conjoint presence of a tumor pattern that is diagnostic of conventional thymoma. The two lesional components may be seen in widely separated sections from the same mass or in admixture. Indeed, the author has seen some cases in which a gradual transition between them was evident (194); Shimosato

and Mukai (13) likewise have documented this phenomenon. These observations make it likely that some cases of KSCC (and other thymic carcinoma variants) arise through the "clonal evolution" ("dedifferentiation") of thymomas. Nevertheless, such examples are rare, and the majority of thymic carcinomas probably represent de novo neoplasms.

Nonkeratinizing Squamous Cell Thymic Carcinoma

The nonkeratinizing variant of squamous thymic carcinoma differs from the foregoing description only in that it shows a lesser degree of differentiation (91,297). Intercellular bridges, cytoplasmic eosinophilia, and keratin pearls are absent, yielding a tumor that shows angular cohesive nests of cells with distinct plasmalemmae, set in a desmoplastic fibrous stroma (Fig. 28.70). The latter differs from that of thymoma, however, in lacking a discretely septated configuration. Cytoplasm is more amphophilic than in KSCC. An intralesional inflammatory infiltrate is typically sparse. The author includes tumors labeled by others as "large-cell carcinomas" (13) in the category of

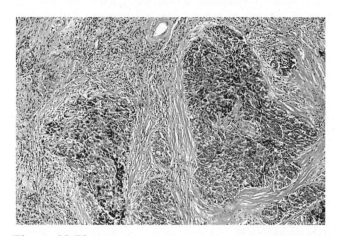

Figure 28.70. This nonkeratinizing squamous cell thymic carcinoma shows irregularly sized nests of polygonal cells embedded in a densely fibrous stroma.

nonkeratinizing squamous carcinoma because of his anecdotal experience with the ultrastructure of such lesions.

Lymphoepithelioma-Like Squamous Thymic Carcinoma

It is now well accepted that "lymphoepitheliomas" of the naso-pharynx, oropharynx, and other anatomic sites actually represent very poorly differentiated and distinctive forms of squamous cell carcinoma, some of which are associated with integration of genomic material from the Epstein-Barr virus (351) (see Chapter 21). Likewise, these same concepts apply in the context of thymic neoplasia (352–354a). Lymphoepithelioma-like thymic carcinoma (LETC) has a distinctive histologic appearance that differs substantially from that of KSCC or non-keratinizing squamous carcinoma. The first of these lesions is composed of syncytial groupings of polyhedral cells with ill-defined boundaries, round to oval and uniformly vesicular nuclei, prominent eosinophilic nucleoli, amphophilic cytoplasm, and an intimate admixture of mature lymphocytes (Fig. 28.71) (13,91,294,295,297). Tumoral stroma varies in density but is usually represented by narrow septa of fibrovascular tissue. Regional necrosis is also a variable finding and may be totally lacking in some examples.

Adenosquamous and Mucoepidermoid Thymic Carcinomas

Rare examples of primary thymic carcinomas have been reported that closely simulate mucoepidermoid carcinoma (MEC) of salivary glands (90,91,332,355) or adenosquamous carcinoma of the lung (13,91,294,295). Both of these lesions show a partially squamous constituency. In MEC, foci that resemble well-differentiated KSCC are admixed with others containing goblet cell–type epithelium arranged around microcysts with mucinous contents (Fig. 28.72). Fibrous stromal partitions were also apparent in one of two examples of primary thymic MEC that the author has seen.

In contrast, adenosquamous carcinoma is a cytologically high-grade tumor that is most like nonkeratinizing squamous cancer histologically. The pertinent difference between these lesions is the presence of small but well-formed glandular lumina that punctuate the neoplastic cellular population ran-

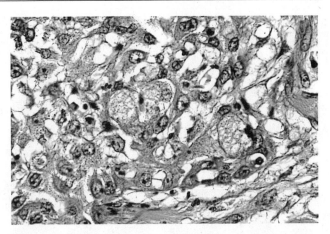

Figure 28.72. Mucoepidermoid thymic carcinoma shows a predominance of keratinizing tumor cells, punctuated by mucin-containing goblet cell–type glandular elements.

domly. The contents of these formations may contain secretions that can be labeled with the mucicarmine or PAS-diastase stains (13,294).

Clear-Cell Carcinoma of the Thymus

Relatively few examples of clear-cell thymic carcinoma have been documented (91,294,330,356,357). This lesion exhibits a uniform composition by polygonal cells with round, vesicular nuclei, nucleoli, and optically lucent cytoplasm (Fig. 28.73) (334). In some cases, cellular clarity was evidently the by-product of abundant cytoplasmic glycogen, as revealed by the PAS stain (91,330,357); in others, hydropic cellular degeneration appeared to explain this histologic feature (356). The tumor has a vaguely organoid growth pattern because of the presence of delicately intersecting fibrovascular stromal septa. Nevertheless, tumoral vascularity is inconspicuous, and there are no "blood lakes" within this neoplasm as seen in some clear-cell carcinomas originating in extrathymic sites (particularly in the kidneys) (348,356).

Primary Adenocarcinoma of the Thymus (Not Further Specified)

Although I have seen only rare cases of non–clear-cell thymic carcinoma in which a purely adenocarcinomatous image was evident (Fig. 28.73A), two such neoplasms have been well documented by Shimosato and Mukai (13). One arose in apparent transition from an epithelial-predominant thymoma and demonstrated micropapillary growth and focal psammomatous calcification. The overtly malignant portion of that lesion was immunoreactive for carcinoembryonic antigen, in likeness to other forms of thymic carcinoma (198). Another lesion described by Shimosato and Mukai was evidently uniform histologically and demonstrated admixed foci of micropapillary and solid growth. A purely mucinous ("colloid") form of thymic adenocarcinoma has also been documented (Fig. 28.73B) (357a), in analogy to tumors of the breast, skin, gastrointestinal tract, and other anatomic sites.

Special Pathologic Features of Thymic Carcinomas

By electron microscopy, there are two "common threads" in the characteristics of most forms of thymic carcinoma just pre-

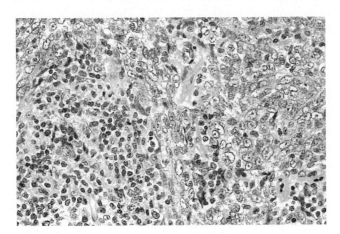

Figure 28.71. Lymphoepithelioma-like carcinoma of the thymus features large anaplastic cells with vesicular nuclei and prominent nucleoli, admixed with small lymphocytes.

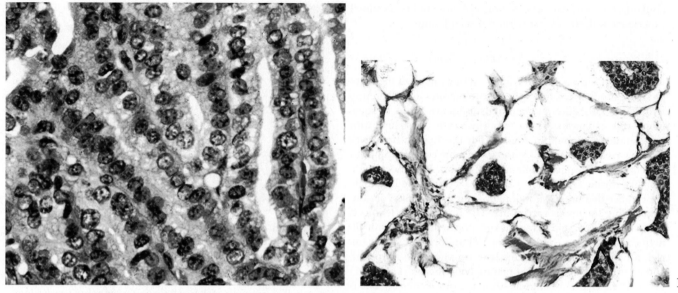

Figure 28.73. Clear-cell carcinoma of the thymus showing relatively uniformly sized, glandlike arrays of polygonal tumor cells, with optically lucent cytoplasm and compact oval nuclei. **(A)** Papillary adenocarcinoma of the thymus, demonstrating a close resemblance to papillary thyroid carcinoma. The thyroid in this case was normal. **(B)** Mucinous ("colloid") thymic adenocarcinoma showing variably sized nests of polygonal cells suspended in a mucomyxoid stroma.

sented. These are the presence of well-formed desmosome-like intercellular junctions and (except in pure adenocarcinomas) the observation of cytoplasmic tonofilaments that may insert into junctional complexes (194). In addition, isolated reports have appeared of divergent neuroendocrine differentiation (at a subcellular level only) as manifested by cytoplasmic neurosecretory granules (Fig. 28.74) (297). Moreover, MEC, adeno-

squamous carcinoma, and some cases of clear-cell thymic cancer have shown the focal presence of cellular microvilli in association with glandular differentiation (295,334,358).

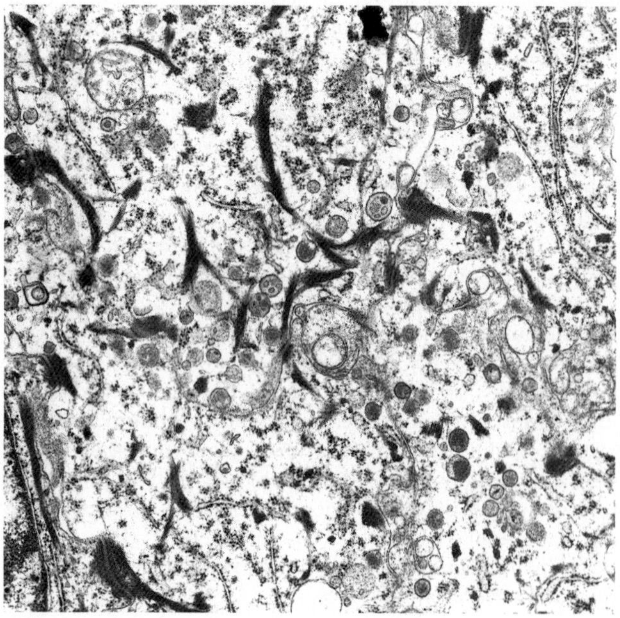

Immunohistochemical analysis of these lesions reveals uniform reactivity for keratin, and many cases also will be labeled by antibodies to EMA. Carcinoembryonic antigen and the TAG-72 antigen may be observed as well, particularly in those tumors that show overt glandular differentiation (358). However, vimentin is typically unexpected in polygonal cell thymic carcinoma variants (398). Finally, TTF-1, an intranuclear marker that is normally present in thymic epithelium and glandular pulmonary epithelial cells, is an effective discriminant between primary thymic carcinoma and metastatic adenocarcinoma of the lung that involves the mediastinum (359).

Several reports have appeared regarding the expression of CD5 by the epithelial cells of thymic carcinoma but not those of conventional thymoma (359–362). This statement must be qualified somewhat, in that *atypical epithelial-predominant thymomas*—that is, those in which there is evidence of cytologic atypia that is insufficient for an outright diagnosis of malignancy (13,148)—also are CD5 positive in 40% of cases (361). Other primary thymic malignancies, such as germ cell tumors and lymphomas, are CD5 negative, as are metastatic mediastinal carcinomas arising in other viscera (360–362). This last piece of information obviously may be useful in the exclusion of secondary malignancies that might histologically simulate thymic carcinomas. Conversely, Chan et al. (211) found that CD99-reactive lymphocytes are lacking in both PTCs and metastatic carcinomas in the thymic region, suggesting that MIC-2 stains have no role in making the distinction between those neoplasms.

CD70 has been described as a similar discriminant between thymic carcinoma and metastatic carcinomas or intrathymic nonepithelial malignancies (363). However, to date, that marker, which is a member of the tumor necrosis factor family,

Figure 28.74. Electron photomicrograph of a thymic carcinoma that exhibits divergent squamous and neuroendocrine differentiation. These elements are represented by cytoplasmic tonofibrils and neurosecretory granules, respectively.

has only been assessed using frozen sections as substrates. As cited earlier, it is known that a proportion of LETC cases exhibit evidence of Epstein-Barr virus integration at a molecular level (364–366). Using in situ hybridization and riboprobes to Epstein-Barr virus early ribonucleic acid-1 (EBER-1), Wu and Kuo (366) found no positivity in 21 encapsulated or invasive thymomas. Nonetheless, they were able to label only one of five LETCs and none of 15 other thymic carcinomas for EBER-1 transcripts, limiting the differential diagnostic use of this assay. Chen et al. (367) obtained comparable results in a methodologic comparison of in situ hybridization and the polymerase chain reaction. Patton et al. (364) have also detected the presence of BZLF1 transactivator in a thymic carcinoma (presumably LETC), which is an indicator of Epstein-Barr virus reactivation. However, those investigators did not compare the tumor in question with other mediastinal neoplasms, and the diagnostic applicability of their findings is therefore uncertain. Evaluations for mutant p53 protein, as undertaken by Tateyama et al. (368), also show a broad range of expression by thymomas and PTC. In light of widespread abnormalities in the *p53* gene in tumors of many other sites (369), it should be obvious that they preclude a meaningful role for that moiety in the differential diagnosis of mediastinal lesions.

PARATHYROID CARCINOMA OF THE MEDIASTINUM

Parathyroid carcinomas (PACs) may arise within the thymus or the perithymic soft tissues of the anterosuperior mediastinum (80,370–376). The diagnosis of these lesions is typically straightforward clinically because patients usually present with extreme hypercalcemia (>14 mg/dL) and marked elevations of plasma parathormone (PTH) levels (377). Nevertheless, this is not always the case; the author has seen one example of PAC in which biochemical hyperparathyroidism was absent (375). In this instance, the tumor manifested itself with symptoms of an intrathoracic space-occupying lesion, and an infiltrative mediastinal mass was apparent on chest radiographs.

Reported examples of mediastinal PAC have shown a gross appearance like that of primary thymic carcinoma, as outlined previously. Obvious invasion of lung, pericardium, and thoracic great vessels is found on surgical exploration (334–377).

Microscopically, this neoplasm may be deceptively bland, but it nonetheless usually exhibits at least a modest degree of nuclear atypia. Sheets, nests, or trabecula of polyhedral cells with round to oval nuclei, occasional nucleoli, nuclear hyperchromasia, and cytoplasmic granularity or clarity are evident (Fig. 28.75) in the absence of a definable peripheral fibrous capsule. Internal collagenous bands may subdivide the tumor (375), although these are not invariably seen. Mitotic activity is characteristically present, but it may be apparent only focally. Small foci of spontaneous tumor necrosis are sometimes observed. The PAS stain frequently reveals abundant intracellular glycogen in PAC (334,375).

In the face of the histologic variation just mentioned, a question arises—as it does in cases of PAC in the neck—regarding the criteria that are necessary for this diagnosis. In the author's opinion, these include a constellation of both clinical and pathologic findings. First, the level of hypercalcemia, when present, should be striking. Second, in the mediastinum, the lesion must at least demonstrate an invasive, unencapsulated pattern of growth. Mitoses, necrosis, cellular anaplasia, and the presence of broad fibrous intratumoral partitions should be factored into the final interpretation, but I do not hold all of these cytoarchitectural elements to be necessary diagnostically. In a general review of this topic, Evans (378) suggested that the major morphologic determinants of adverse biologic potential in parathyroid tumors were mitotic activity of greater than five division figures per ×400 field and a thick lesional fibrous capsule or an obviously infiltrative growth pattern (378).

Electron microscopic analysis shows the presence of primitive intercellular junctional complexes, prominent cytoplasmic glycogen granules, primitive blunt microvilli, and sparse numbers of neurosecretory granules in PAC (334,375,379). Tonofibrils are lacking in this tumor. By immunohistology, one observes the presence of cytoplasmic PTH (380), which may assume a "mosaic" pattern of staining (Fig. 28.76) (375), with or without concomitant reactivity for chromogranin A or synaptophysin.

MALIGNANT MEDIASTINAL GERM CELL TUMORS

Pure or mixed mediastinal germ cell tumors with seminomatous, embryonal carcinomatous, endodermal sinus tumor, and

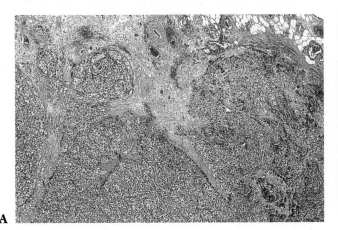
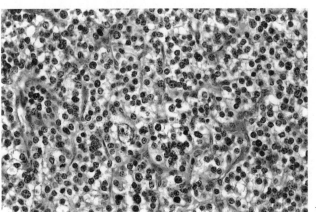

Figure 28.75. **(A)** Parathyroid carcinoma of the mediastinum showing invasive growth of the tumor into surrounding fibroadipose soft tissue. **(B)** Minimal cellular pleomorphism is evident in some parathyroid carcinomas, as shown here.

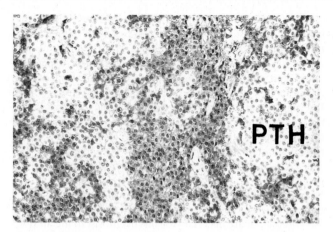

Figure 28.76. "Mosaic" staining for parathormone in a parathyroid carcinoma of the mediastinum.

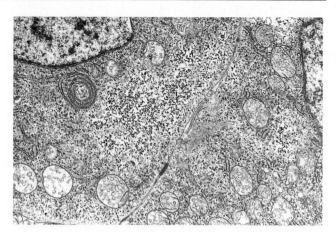

Figure 28.78. Electron micrograph of mediastinal seminoma showing primitive appositional plaque between adjacent tumor cells (*center*), as well as abundant intracytoplasmic glycogen granules. Tonofilaments and neurosecretory granules are absent.

choriocarcinomatous elements are all included in the malignant large polygonal cell category in the context under discussion. These tumors tend to have a marked male predominance and typically appear during young adulthood or early middle age (128,131,145,334,381–382a). Indeed, a cytologically malignant mediastinal epithelial neoplasm in the patient groups just cited should be presumed to represent a germ cell tumor until proven otherwise. Clinical symptoms and signs in such cases are often relatively nonspecific, but elevations in serum levels of α-fetoprotein (AFP), β-human chorionic gonadotropin (β-HCG), human placental lactogen, lactate dehydrogenase, and placental alkaline phosphatase (PLAP) may be important clues to the histologic identity of these lesions in a generic sense (55,131,334,358,383–398).

These lesions typically feature obvious foci of spontaneous necrosis or hemorrhage in a relatively homogeneous, fleshy, unencapsulated mass with indistinct boundaries (Fig. 28.77). Invasion of contiguous mediastinal structures is a frequent finding for the surgeon (131).

The histologic attributes of mediastinal malignant germ cell tumors are identical to those of corresponding lesions in the gonads (131); indeed, recent publications support the notion that thymic lesions of this type may be part of a systemic diathesis involving germ cells, including testicular intratubular germ cell

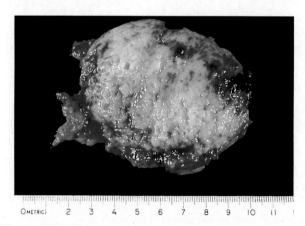

Figure 28.77. Intrathymic seminoma represented by a fleshy, unencapsulated, partially necrotic and hemorrhagic mass.

neoplasia (399). In the interest of brevity, the reader is referred to the excellent expositions on this topic in Chapters 47 and 55.

Ultrastructurally, seminomas exhibit primitive appositional intercellular junctions, prominent and complex nucleoli ("nucleolonemata"), and abundant cytoplasmic glycogen (Fig. 28.78). Embryonal carcinomas show more well-developed junctional complexes between adjacent cells and may also manifest primitive microvillous structures or intracellular lumina. Endodermal sinus tumors (yolk sac carcinomas) feature the presence of redundant basal lamina, as well as globular concretions of moderately dense material (representing AFP) within rough endoplasmic reticulum. These findings are particularly helpful in the differential diagnosis of a peculiar variant of mediastinal endodermal sinus tumor—the "hepatoid" subtype—in which solid sheets of large, somewhat nondescript eosinophilic cells are seen by light microscopy (382). Choriocarcinomas are potentially confused with somatic adenosquamous carcinomas on electron microscopy in that they often show the concurrent presence of cytoplasmic tonofibrils and plasmalemmal microvilli (134).

Immunohistochemistry is helpful in defining the lineage of mediastinal germ cell neoplasms. The typical appearance of seminoma is that of a keratin- and EMA-negative tumor with strong immunoreactivity for PLAP and CD117 (c-kit protein) (Fig. 28.79) (334,358,400,401). Embryonal carcinomas and yolk sac carcinomas differ from the latter profile in their acquisition of positivity for keratin and CD30, a tendency toward CD117 negativity, and the potential expression of AFP (358,400,401). Choriocarcinoma also demonstrates keratin reactivity, but it is additionally defined by the presence of EMA and β-HCG in syncytiotrophoblastic tumor cells (402).

MEDIASTINAL CARCINOID TUMOR/NEUROENDOCRINE CARCINOMA

Aside from oat cell carcinomas of the mediastinum, other neuroendocrine lesions arising in this region belong to the large polygonal cell category. Such neoplasms are overwhelmingly of thymic origin but also may occasionally be seen in the middle or posterior mediastinum. One remarkable case, documented

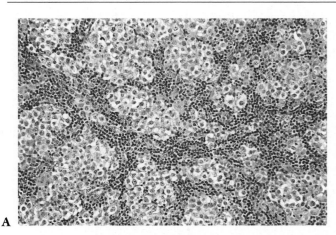
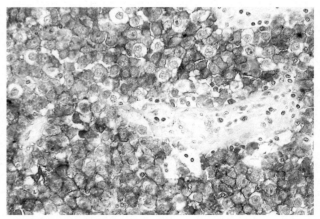

A   B

Figure 28.79. **(A)** Typical microscopic appearance of mediastinal seminoma; clusters of tumor cells with clear cytoplasm and vesicular round nuclei are separated from one another by lymphoid-rich fibrous stroma. **(B)** Strong membrane-based immunoreactivity for placental alkaline phosphatase in thymic seminoma. The latter marker is seen in most germ cell tumors.

by Warren and Yum (139), appeared after chemotherapy for an anterior mediastinal germ cell tumor and probably represented the emergence of a carcinoidal somatic teratomatous constituent that was refractory to the treatment regimen. Other similar examples apparently have arisen spontaneously in mature teratomas or thymic cysts (402a,403); one of them assumed the histologic appearance of "goblet cell carcinoid" as usually seen in the appendix (403). The neoplasms under discussion here are variously known as thymic carcinoid tumors (TCTs) or neuroendocrine carcinomas (3,36,49,50,404–409a), and as stated, they are potentially associated with a distinctive group of paraneoplastic phenomena that are dissimilar from those attending thymomas. The former disorders include Cushing syndrome, SIADH, Eaton-Lambert syndrome, and, very rarely, production of PTH with hypercalcemia (46,47,53,54), one of which is seen in roughly one-third of all cases (410). In this context, TCTs may produce appalling biochemical or neuromuscular abnormalities while they are still very small, being detectable only on high-resolution computed tomography of the chest (72), thoracic magnetic resonance imaging (64), or

radionuclide scanning with labeled octreotide (411). Approximately 20% to 30% of these tumors also are expected to occur in patients with the multiple endocrine neoplasia (MEN) syndromes, either type 1 (with pituitary adenomas, pancreatic endocrine tumors, and parathyroid adenomas) or type 2 (with medullary thyroid carcinoma, pheochromocytoma, parathyroid hyperplasia, and mucosal ganglioneuromatosis) (41,44,45, 412–417). Remaining examples of TCTs manifest themselves as nonspecific intrathoracic space-occupying lesions (42,331, 333,418–420). Despite the diagnosis of "carcinoid," the complete carcinoid syndrome is essentially unknown in association with primary thymic tumors of this type (410).

Grossly, non–small-cell neuroendocrine thymic tumors are unencapsulated, firm, pink-gray masses that may be gritty on cut section (Fig. 28.80). They lack internal fibrous septation and often exhibit foci of necrosis and hemorrhage (418).

The microscopic features of such neoplasms include a strikingly organoid growth pattern, with insulae, ribbons, festoons, and trabeculae of tumor cells, often with the distinct formation of rosettes that simulate glandlike spaces (Figs. 28.81 and

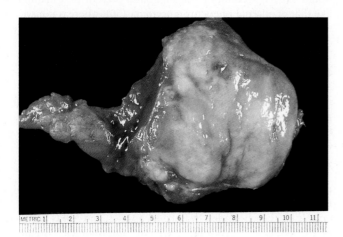

Figure 28.80. Thymic carcinoid is usually unencapsulated, with a firm pink-tan cut surface. Internal fibrous septa are lacking, and small foci of necrosis are evident.

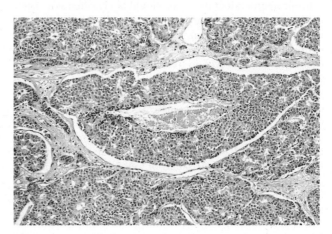

Figure 28.81. Organoid growth of uniform polygonal tumor cells in thymic carcinoid tumor, with typical artifactual detachment of centrally necrotic "balls" of neoplastic cells from surrounding stroma.

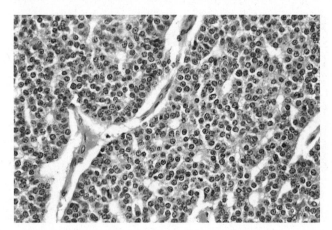

Figure 28.82. Numerous rosettes are seen in this thymic carcinoid.

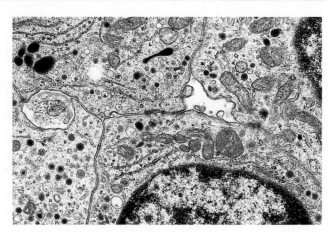

Figure 28.83. Cytoplasmic neurosecretory granules are abundant in this electron micrograph of a thymic carcinoid tumor. In addition, intercellular macular junctions are seen.

28.82). In many cases, cellular nests become artifactually detached from surrounding fibrovascular septa during histologic processing, and foci of central geographic necrosis, which may be dystrophically calcified, are common in these areas. Mitotic activity is reproducibly present (410,412–419). Recognized histologic variants of TCTs include a form with a sheetlike disorganized cellular growth pattern, another showing formation of amyloid-like stroma (with potential foci of spindle cell differentiation), a subtype with extensively sclerotic stroma, a pigmented form in which intracellular melanin or lipofuscin may be observed, a mucinous variant in which mucopolysaccharide-rich matrix is abundant, an oncocytic form, a lipid-rich type, and a "dedifferentiated" form showing an admixture of conventional TCT and sarcomatoid carcinoma (331,333,410, 418,420–423a). Shimosato and Mukai (13), Cho et al. (424), and Mizuno et al. (425) also have described cases in which thymoma and TCT coexisted, either in separate lobes of the thymus or in an intermingled configuration. Nuclei in TCTs are round to oval with stippled chromatin and indistinct nucleoli, and the cytoplasm is eosinophilic or amphophilic and granular (425a). The tumor cells are argyrophilic with the Sevier-Munger or Churukian-Schenk methods, but they do not demonstrate argentinaffinity (410,419).

Similarly to a problem mentioned in connection with mediastinal oat cell carcinomas, it may be vexing to decide whether a thymic neuroendocrine tumor should be classified as a "carcinoid" or as a "neuroendocrine carcinoma" ("atypical" carcinoid). In the mediastinum, most lesions actually best conform to the second of these two choices (408,426); nevertheless, this issue again is not crucial to treatment or prognosis in this context (426–430).

The ultrastructural features of TCTs are very similar to those of mediastinal oat cell carcinomas, except that cytoplasmic neurosecretory granules are much more numerous in the former of these lesions (Fig. 28.83) (418,419,431). Perinuclear whorls of intermediate filaments can be detected in the majority of cases. On occasion, short skeins of tonofilaments also may be observed in the tumor cells as well.

Immunohistochemically, TCTs are regularly reactive for keratin, neuron-specific (γ-dimeric) enolase, synaptophysin, CD56, CD57, and chromogranin A (198). In addition, even those lesions not associated with clinical endocrinopathies may exhibit the synthesis of such neuropeptides as adrenocorticotropic hormone (ACTH), corticotropin-releasing hormone/factor, anti-

diuretic hormone, somatostatin, gastrin, β-endorphin, calcitonin, met-enkephalin, leu-enkephalin, and PTH (40,43,53,54, 429,431,432).

MEDIASTINAL PARAGANGLIOMAS

Intrathoracic paragangliomas are infrequently encountered in the general practice of surgical pathology. This finding is supported by the results of large series on mediastinal tumors, showing an overall incidence of approximately 0.3% (127). These lesions characteristically arise in either the anterior subcompartment, in association with the aorticopulmonary vascular root, or in the posterior mediastinum, in a paravertebral location (57,58,410,433–435).

Aorticopulmonary paragangliomas (APPGs) are seen at an average age of 49 years with a slight predilection for women; in contrast, paravertebral paragangliomas (PVPGs) occur in younger individuals (with a mean age of 29 years), a majority of whom are men (436). The symptoms and signs attending APPG and PVPG are different as well. The former of these tumors synthesizes catecholamines in only 3% of cases, whereas PVPG does so in approximately 50% (56–58,436–437a). As one would expect, secretory paragangliomas present in a manner like that of adrenal pheochromocytoma (56), whereas nonsynthetic tumors produce complaints referable only to structural compression or displacement (437).

Mediastinal paragangliomas share with TCTs the capacity for an association with the familial MEN syndrome, type 2 (410). Also, Carney (438) has described an unusual (seemingly sporadic) syndromic complex featuring the concurrent presence of pulmonary chondromas, multiple gastric stromal tumors, and functioning extra-adrenal paragangliomas. The latter may be observed in the mediastinum in such patients, the great majority of whom are young women.

Macroscopically, all mediastinal paragangliomas are firm, reddish-pink or brown masses, with frequent foci of hemorrhage and necrosis. Most of these lesions are unencapsulated or only partially bounded by fibrous capsules, and APPG particularly tends to infiltrate adjacent intrathoracic organs (436,437).

The microscopic features of paragangliomas are potentially distinctive. A characteristic finding that allows for quick identifi-

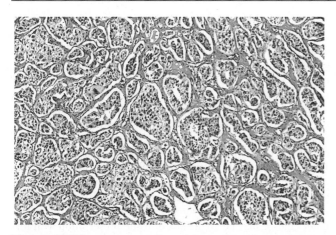

Figure 28.84. Characteristic "zellballen" in mediastinal paraganglioma. These structures are compact nests of tumor cells. They are separated from one another by richly vascular fibrous stroma.

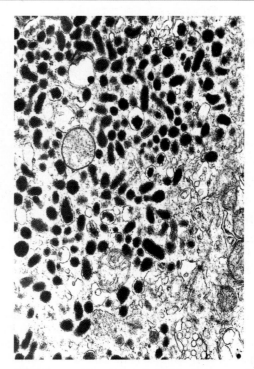

Figure 28.85. Electron micrograph of mediastinal paraganglioma shows pleomorphic cytoplasmic neurosecretory granules, some of which have eccentric "halos."

cation of such lesions on medium-power microscopy is their peculiar tendency to grow in tightly aggregated, roughly equally sized nests of cells, surrounded by a markedly vascular fibrous stroma (Fig. 28.84). These groupings are termed "zellballen" (German for "balls of cells") (433). Tumor cell nuclei vary in shape from round to fusiform to extremely angular and pleomorphic; likewise, the nuclear chromatin may be dispersed, uniformly dense, or vesicular. Nucleoli are variably observed as well. Mitotic figures are usually absent in paragangliomas, but a scant number may be seen in some examples. The cytoplasm is granular and eosinophilic or amphophilic and often contains discrete "hyaline" globules (439).

A report by Plaza et al. (439a) has documented the existence of a peculiar sclerosing variant of paraganglioma. In that lesion, stromal fibrosis is prominent and potentially obscures the basic architecture of the tumor, possibly leading to diagnostic confusion with fibrosing mediastinitis or invasive carcinomas.

Histochemical methods show argyrophilia with the Churukian-Schenk or Grimelius methods, and argentinaffinity is also demonstrable with the del Rio Hortega technique (410,440). Paragangliomas do not contain appreciable cellular glycogen, but the digested PAS stain or the Fontana-Masson method may reveal the presence of ceroid pigment or melanin, respectively, in some cases (433,435). The reticulin stain is a helpful procedure in the assessment of these tumors because it highlights stromal tissue that invests the zellballen (433). In most studies, the presence of spontaneous necrosis, mitotic activity, nuclear atypia and pleomorphism, hemorrhage, and even vascular invasion in paraganglioma cases has correlated poorly with malignant behavior (56,437).

In the author's opinion, with specific regard to mediastinal tumors, the most important and adversely predictive pathologic feature is the extensive invasion of such lesions into contiguous thoracic soft tissues. However, a report by Linnoila et al. (439) has also suggested that the concurrence of confluent tumor necrosis, coarse tumor nodularity, and an absence of globular cytoplasmic inclusions in the tumor cells predicts malignant behavior in more than 70% of extra-adrenal paragangliomas.

The ultrastructural attributes of paragangliomas are variable and parallel their biochemical activity. Those lesions that synthesize norepinephrine tend to contain a large number of pleomorphic neurosecretory granules, with eccentric "halos" (Fig.

28.85). Nonsecretory tumors, on the other hand, often contain more nondescript endocrine granules. Intercellular junctional complexes are relatively unusual in paragangliomas; intermediate filament whorls, tonofibrils, and microvilli are uniformly absent (410,437,441).

Immunohistochemically, the nonepithelial nature of paragangliomas is reflected in their consistent negativity for keratin and EMA. Instead, these neoplasms express neurofilament protein or vimentin (410). The S-100 protein immunostain may be employed to decorate fusiform "sustentacular" cells that surround cellular nests in paragangliomas (442), and the tumor cells themselves often contain one of the enkephalin neuropeptides (443).

Molecular analysis also may play a useful role in the differential diagnosis of paragangliomas and carcinoid tumors. As shown by Komminoth et al. (444), DNA extracted from paraffin sections of such lesions may be evaluated for point mutations in exons 10, 11, 13, 15, and 16 of the *ret* proto-oncogene. Among all sporadic neuroendocrine tumors analyzed in the study just cited, only medullary thyroid carcinomas and paragangliomas showed such aberrations. It must be acknowledged that a low incidence of *ret* mutation in those two neoplasms (44% and 15%, respectively) does limit the practical use of this technique, but its specificity is apparently very high.

MEDIASTINAL LARGE-CELL NON-HODGKIN LYMPHOMA

Except for localized cases of another hematopoietic lesion (Hodgkin disease), large-cell non-Hodgkin lymphoma (LCNHL) is the most common primary malignant neoplasm of the mediastinum (11). This tumor is seen predominantly in

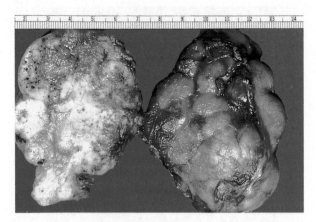

Figure 28.86. Anterior mediastinal, large-cell non-Hodgkin lymphoma is usually a lobulated, fleshy, unencapsulated mass with internal hemorrhage and necrosis.

young women in the third or fourth decade of life; men also may be affected but at a mean of 50 years of age (223). Patients with mediastinal LCNHL present with a bulky intrathoracic mass that is usually centered in the anterior subcompartment. Relatively few of these lesions arise in the middle or posterior mediastinum. Symptoms and signs of the neoplasm include dyspnea, cough, the superior vena caval syndrome, pleural effusions, and hydropericardium (11,223). Most examples of mediastinal LCNHL are confined to the chest at diagnosis; less than 25% of patients are found to have involvement of extrathoracic tissues after completion of staging analyses (223,227,445–450).

Gross characteristics of this neoplasm are those of a fleshy, multilobated, poorly defined, unencapsulated mass that may demonstrate internal foci of necrosis and hemorrhage (Fig. 28.86). Involvement of the lung, pleura, chest wall, great vessels, and pericardium is common, by direct extension of the lesion (134,223,447).

Microscopically, one observes sheets or irregularly shaped groupings of large polyhedral cells with vesicular or hyperchromatic nuclei and variably prominent nucleoli (Fig. 28.87). Some lesions demonstrate overtly immunoblastic cytologic attributes,

and nuclear multilobation, sometimes yielding Reed-Sternberg (RS)–like cells, is a potential finding as well (see Chapter 17) (11,223,450,451). Tsai et al. (451a) also have described a rare variant of mediastinal LCNHL in which rosette formation may cause diagnostic confusion with epithelial or neuroendocrine tumors.

Mediastinal LCNHL is often centered in the thymus, and one may therefore observe entrapped glandular remnants in histologic sections (223). The nuclear contours of the tumor cells are typically irregular, with "blebs" or blunt projections (450,451). Occasionally, marked nuclear pleomorphism may be observed, creating the image of "anaplastic" large-cell lymphoma (452). Cytoplasm is amphophilic in most instances, but it may be optically clear in some neoplasms (334,453–455). The latter change may be an artifact of tissue preservation with formalin, in that it is not often seen with the use of B5 fixative (11). A minor admixture of small lymphocytes, which can either be mature or atypical in cytologic appearance, also may be observed in LCNHL. Mitotic figures are common in the large tumor cells, and widespread apoptosis is a common finding as well. However, broad zones of geographic necrosis are unusual (223,450,451).

A general peculiarity of mediastinal non-Hodgkin lymphomas is their tendency to manifest stromal sclerosis. This may yield a "pseudocompartmentalized" low-power microscopic picture that simulates that of an epithelial tumor (Fig. 28.88) (223); alternatively, the degree of matrix collagen deposition may be so extreme that the diagnosis of fibrosing mediastinitis is considered. As might be expected, sclerosing examples of LCNHL are those that have the greatest clinical association with superior vena caval obstruction (447).

The electron microscopic diagnosis of large-cell lymphoma is tenuous because it is based solely on an exclusionary process. One should not see intercellular junctional complexes, pericellular basal lamina, or tonofibrils in this lesion (134,223). Moreover, potential traps exist for the unwary in this realm of analysis. Some lymphomas (of the "anemone cell" type) manifest elongated filiform projections of their cellular membranes, potentially simulating microvilli (223). In addition, I have seen cases that were misdiagnosed because small lysosomes were erroneously interpreted as neuroendocrine granules.

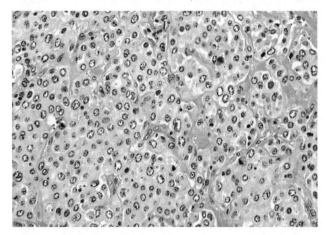

Figure 28.87. Relatively uniform population of large, atypical lymphoid cells with slightly irregular nuclear contours in a mediastinal large-cell lymphoma.

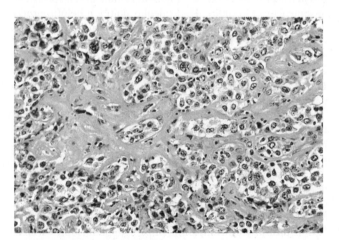

Figure 28.88. Intralesional sclerosis may yield a "pseudocompartmentalized" pattern of growth in mediastinal large-cell lymphoma, leading to potential confusion with an epithelial neoplasm.

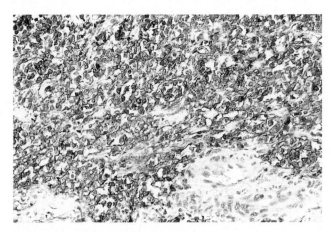

Figure 28.89. Intense immunoreactivity for CD45 antigen in large-cell lymphoma of the anterior mediastinum.

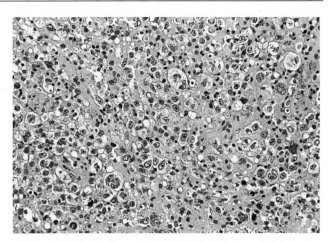

Figure 28.90. Confluent sheets of mononuclear Reed variant cells and classic Reed-Sternberg cells in "syncytial" nodular sclerosing Hodgkin disease. This histologic appearance may be confused with that of large-cell non-Hodgkin lymphoma or carcinoma.

Immunohistochemical studies show distinct cell membranous reactivity for the CD45 antigen in the great majority of mediastinal large-cell lymphomas, securing the diagnosis of a hematopoietic neoplasm (Fig. 28.89) (11,134,450,451,453–455). However, rare examples of "Ki-1" (large-cell anaplastic) lymphoma have been documented at this site (456), some of which have failed to express the leukocyte common antigen. Therefore, it is wise to include antibodies in the CD30 group in the immunohistologic workup of LCNHL; these label the great majority of large-cell anaplastic lesions, and in the context of concomitant keratin negativity, they are specific for a diagnosis of lymphoma (11). The contention that most mediastinal LCNHLs are B-cell lesions is supported by reactivity for CD20 antigens in the majority of cases (457,458), even most of those with anaplastic features (452). Few examples of large-cell lymphomas with T-cell or "true histiocytic" differentiation have been described in this location (11).

"SYNCYTIAL" AND SARCOMATOID MEDIASTINAL HODGKIN DISEASE

As cited, HL is the most frequently encountered, cytologically malignant mediastinal tumor (11). It classically (but not exclusively) affects young women in the third or fourth decade of life, and like LCNHL, it also may involve contiguous intrathoracic structures by direct extension (459–461). Patients have symptoms and signs that are similar to those of LCNHL, except that systemic complaints (e.g., fever, night sweats, weight loss, fatigue) and the incidence of concurrent extrathoracic disease are greater with Hodgkin disease (11,223,462). The propensity for the nodular-sclerosing variant of Hodgkin disease (NSHD) to affect the thymus is reflected in a previous, now antiquated designation for examples of this condition in the anterior mediastinum—namely, "granulomatous thymoma" (27,460).

The macroscopic characteristics of thymic NSHD are such that they partially overlap those of thymoma and sclerosing LCNHL. The first of these conditions may appear to be pseudoencapsulated, and it also may demonstrate internal fibrous bands within the neoplastic mass. Nonetheless, these stromal partitions enclose irregularly rounded islands of tumor tissue rather than angular profiles, as in thymomas. Moreover, they are less well defined than the internal fibrous septa of thymomas

but more distinct than the matrix of sclerosing large-cell lymphomas (134).

These points of dissimilarity notwithstanding, a peculiar histologic subtype of NSHD may further contribute to diagnostic confusion with either an epithelial neoplasm or LCNHL. This pathologic entity has been dubbed "syncytial" Hodgkin disease because it is composed of sheets of highly atypical mononuclear (Reed variant) cells with vesicular chromatin and eosinophilic nucleoli (Fig. 28.90) (463). These cell groups are separated by bands of refractile collagen, which tend to form oblique intersections with one another. An admixture of small lymphocytes often is observed in syncytial NSHD, again similarly to LETC or LCNHL (11,463). However, eosinophilic leukocytes often are interspersed throughout the tumor cell population in syncytial HLs; this observation has a good deal of differential diagnostic importance because tissue eosinophilia is not expected in carcinomas or LCNHLs (134). Likewise, the detection of scattered cells showing artifactual cytoplasmic retraction ("lacunar cells") is strongly in favor of NSHD (463).

Ultrastructural analysis of syncytial NSHD is helpful in eliminating epithelial neoplasms as diagnostic considerations. Nevertheless, it does not allow for a confident exclusion of non-Hodgkin lymphoma because the fine structure of constituent cells in these conditions is closely similar (134).

However, immunohistologic studies typically demonstrate a lack of CD45 antigen in syncytial Hodgkin disease, in contrast to its presence in almost all cases of LCNHL (11,198). Instead, the mononuclear Reed variant (MRV) cells of NSHD coexpress CD15 and CD30 antigens (Fig. 28.91). CD15 is not expected in most anaplastic large-cell non-Hodgkin lymphomas (ALCLs), aiding the distinction between these pathologic entities as well (11); however, it must be acknowledged that a great deal of immunophenotypic similarity is possible between HL and selected examples of ALCL. This makes cytogenetic evaluation—particularly for abnormalities at the 5q35 locus, which typify ALCL (464,465)—a prudent consideration in this context. PAX-5 is an intranuclear transcription factor that also has been observed in RS cells and B-lymphoid elements, but not in ALCL (466). Thus, that determinant may facilitate the latter

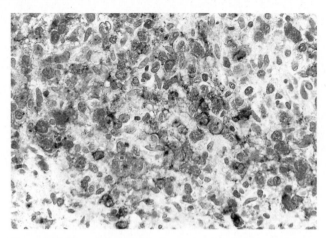

Figure 28.91. Uniform immunoreactivity for CD15 antigen in syn-cytial Hodgkin disease. This marker typically assumes a combined para-nuclear-globular and cell membranous pattern of staining, as shown here.

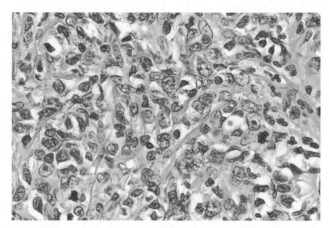

Figure 28.92. Granulocytic sarcoma (extramedullary myelogenous leukemia) of the anterior mediastinum. Tumor cells resemble those of large-cell non-Hodgkin lymphoma or syncytial Hodgkin disease but have slightly more irregular nuclear profiles.

differential diagnosis. Syncytial Hodgkin disease is nonreactive for keratin (139,198), unlike malignant epithelial neoplasms.

Numerous fusiform cells also may be seen in the "reticular" form of lymphocyte-depleted HL, explaining its alternative diag-nostic designation of "sarcomatoid" HL (466a). RS and MRVV cells in the latter tumor subtype are admixed randomly with elements resembling those of IMT or fibrosarcoma. The general immunophenotype of sarcomatoid HL is comparable to that of the syncytial variant, except that CD30 and PAX-5 reactivity is much more focal and CD15 is generally absent, at least in my experience.

OTHER MEDIASTINAL HEMATOPOIETIC TUMORS

Three other hematopoietic neoplasms that may present in the mediastinum (either anteriorly or posteriorly) are worthy of discussion because they may mimic some of the lesions that have been described thus far. These are represented by granulocytic sarcoma (extramedullary myelogenous leukemia), extraosseous plasmacytoma, and dendritic cell sarcoma (DCS).

Mediastinal granulocytic sarcoma may be seen in the setting of antecedent myeloproliferative disease or as a sporadically occurring neoplasm (467–470a). Its clinical presentation is vir-tually identical to that of LCNHL, except that, in some cases, symptoms and signs of evolving acute myelogenous leukemia also are observed (468). Patients with this tumor generally fall into one of two age groups: less than 35 years old or greater than 65 years old. Overt, peripheralized leukemia may coexist with the mediastinal mass in such cases, or it may follow the latter lesion by as much as 24 months (471).

The macroscopic attributes of granulocytic sarcoma are nearly identical to those of large-cell lymphomas. However, the somewhat dated term of "chloroma" has been used to describe tumefactive lesions of extramedullary myeloid leukemia be-cause of their greenish color on cut section, which fades after exposure to ambient air. This feature is distinctive and stems from the presence of a particular enzyme—myeloperoxi-dase—in the neoplastic cells (467).

Histologically, one typically observes sheets of relatively monomorphic, large, polyhedral cells in granulocytic sarcoma,

with irregular nuclear contours, vesicular chromatin, and varia-bly prominent nucleoli (Fig. 28.92) (467,468). Matrix fibrosis may be apparent in admixture with the tumor cell population, much like that seen in sclerosing LCNHL. However, there are some microscopic nuances that enable the astute observer to suspect the true identity of extramedullary leukemic masses. First, eosinophilic leukocytes, some of which may be immature, can often be discerned amid the large tumor cells (467). Sec-ond, attempts to place the proliferation into a nosologically predefined category of "lymphoma" will meet with failure be-cause the leukemic cells do not conform cytologically to a recog-nized lymphoid morphotype. This scenario serves as adequate justification for the routine preparation of touch-imprint prepa-rations from fresh tissue in all cases of mediastinal neoplasia. If a leukemic infiltrate is suspected after initial examination of tissue sections, the imprints can be stained with a Romanowsky method to look for Auer rod inclusions in the malignant cells, and they may also be used for histochemical or immunohisto-chemical confirmation of a myeloid lineage (472).

Electron microscopy is of potential benefit in recognizing granulocytic sarcomas because the myeloid cells may be found to contain distinctive "primary granules" (lysosomal forms) that are not seen in malignant lymphomas. Histochemical analy-ses for myeloperoxidase and chloroacetate esterase can be per-formed on either imprint preparations or paraffin sections; both of these markers are diagnostic of myeloid leukemia, if present in this context (11). Similarly, potential immunoreactiv-ity for CD13, CD15, CD33, CD34, CD68, CD117, and myeloper-oxidase is expected in granulocytic sarcoma but not lymphoma (11,471–473).

Extraosseous plasmacytoma of the mediastinum (EPM) is a potential simulator of neuroendocrine neoplasms, as well as large-cell lymphomas (470a,474–477). Plasmacytomas are typi-cally seen in older individuals, only some of whom will have concurrent multiple myeloma or paraproteinemias at the time of initial diagnosis (474). In the absence of the latter disorders, EPM presents with nonspecific symptoms of a mass-occupying lesion in the anterior or posterior thorax.

The macroscopic characteristics of this tumor are most like those of large-cell lymphomas. Histologically, sheets of poly-gonal cells with round, eccentrically placed nuclei, coarsely stip-

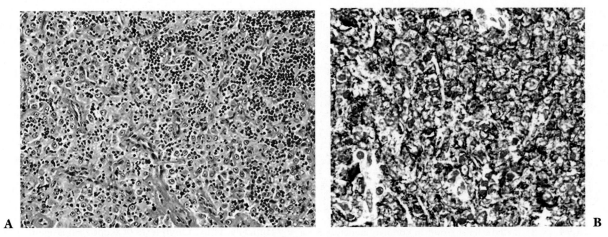

Figure 28.93. **(A)** Follicular dendritic cell sarcoma of the anterior mediastinum, exhibiting a composition by epithelioid and bluntly fusiform cells with admixed lymphocytes. The differential diagnosis includes thymoma, lymphoma, and inflammatory myofibroblastic tumor. **(B)** CD35 immunoreactivity in follicular dendritic cell sarcoma is distinctive and is not expected in differential diagnostic alternatives.

pled chromatin, and homogeneous amphophilic cytoplasm are observed (Fig. 28.93) (474,475). These features may recall those of carcinoids on conventional microscopic examination. However, additional cytologic details may serve as clues to the correct diagnosis of EPM. These include the presence of binucleate cells, zones of perinuclear cytoplasmic clarity ("hofs"), and discohesion of the tumor cells at the peripheral aspects of paraffin tissue sections.

Ultrastructurally, plasma cells are typified by abundant cytoplasmic profiles of rough endoplasmic reticulum; in contrast to endocrine neoplasms, intercellular junctional complexes and neurosecretory granules are absent (478). EPM does not exhibit cellular argyrophilia, and it is immunoreactive for light chain immunoglobulins, CD38, and CD138, rather than for keratin, chromogranin A, or synaptophysin (479). An additional potential diagnostic trap attending this tumor is its potential for EMA reactivity (480), which may further solidify a mistaken interpretation of neuroendocrine neoplasia.

In the past decade, a group of unusual malignant hematopoietic proliferations has been characterized, showing dendritic cell differentiation. Two principal subtypes have been identified—namely, "follicular" and "interdigitating" (480a). These tumors can be encountered in the anterior or posterior mediastinum, and they have been reported mainly in middle-aged or elderly individuals (480b–480f). Such lesions demonstrate a composition by polygonal and bluntly fusiform cells that are arranged in haphazard fascicles or storiform profiles and admixed with mature lymphocytes (Fig. 28.93A). Variable nuclear atypia, necrosis, and mitotic activity are apparent.

In light of these histologic appearances, DCSs may be confused with several other intrathoracic neoplasms, potentially including thymoma, LCNHL, and IMT. A possible likeness to thymoma is particularly troublesome in reference to selected cases of DCS that aberrantly label for keratin (480g).

Nevertheless, additional immunohistologic studies are discriminating. Follicular DCS is reactive for CD21, CD23, and CD35 (Fig. 28.93B) (480a), providing a phenotype that is unlike that of its differential diagnostic alternatives. Similarly, interdigitating DCS labels for S-100 protein, a marker that is comparably exclusionary vis-à-vis thymoma and IMT.

DCSs pursue variably untoward clinical courses. Follicular DCS is generally—but not always—an indolent, "borderline" lesion, whereas interdigitating DCS has greater potential for aggressive behavior.

MALIGNANT EPITHELIOID MESOTHELIOMA OF THE MEDIASTINUM

Although malignant mesotheliomas are usually thought of as lesions of the peripheral pleural surfaces or peritoneum, they also can be seen in the mediastinum. There, such tumors presumably take their origins in the hilar reflections of the pleura and project into the interpulmonary space serendipitously; nonetheless, a clear-cut connection to the serosal surfaces is not always apparent (8). Hence, polygonal cell mesotheliomas of the mediastinum may mimic other epithelial neoplasms.

Patients with mediastinal mesotheliomas are typically middle-aged or older men. As is true with pleuropulmonary neoplasms of this type, a definite history of prolonged exposure to high levels of aerosolized asbestos-containing products is obtained in roughly 50% of cases, with the remainder of cases being etiologically indeterminate (481). Attendant symptoms and signs are those of intrathoracic structural displacement or compression; a pericardial or pleural effusion is seen in a substantial number of cases as well (482).

Histologically, those mesotheliomas that manifest a biphasic or tubulopapillary configuration (see Chapter 27) do not represent diagnostic problems. However, a subset of such tumors is composed of solid sheets or cohesive nests of nondescript but overtly malignant polyhedral cells, which may be similar in appearance to those of metastatic carcinomas (Fig. 28.94) (483).

Electron microscopy and immunohistology are helpful in delineating the cellular lineage of these lesions. Ultrastructurally, epithelioid mesotheliomas exhibit long, branching, "bushy" cellular microvilli, with length-to-diameter ratios that are greater than 10:1 (and usually greater than 15:1) (483,484). Cytoplasmic tonofibrils and elongated intercellular junctional complexes may be seen as well. Immunohistochemically, intense keratin reactivity is present in all of these tumors, and vimentin coexpression also may be documented. Specialized

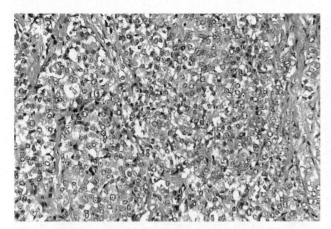

Figure 28.94. Solid, nested cellular growth in a primary mediastinal malignant mesothelioma of the purely epithelioid type. This growth pattern may mimic that of carcinoma.

determinants of adenocarcinoma cells, including carcinoembryonic antigen, CD15, TTF-1, BG8, MOC-31, and the TAG-72 antigen, are absent in mesotheliomas (483,485–487). Conversely, reactivity for calretinin, cytokeratin 5/6, podoplanin, and the intranuclear *WT-1* gene product typifies most epithelioid mesotheliomas, whereas histologically similar carcinomas are negative (486–487a).

Attanoos et al. (488) have described a particular pitfall in reference to the differential diagnosis of those mesotheliomas that may involve the mediastinum and *thymomas* with extensive pleural seeding. Both of those tumor types may express cytokeratin 5/6, and at least in the study just cited, calretinin reactivity was potentially common to both of them as well. *WT-1* lends itself to a solution of this problem because nuclear labeling for that marker is restricted to mesotheliomas (489).

PRIMARY EPITHELIOID LEIOMYOSARCOMA

Moran et al. (490) have drawn attention to the fact that malignant smooth muscle tumors may arise primarily in the soft tissue of the anterior and posterior mediastinum in patients of diverse ages (26 to 71 years). Those with anteriorly situated lesions have nonspecific symptoms and signs of structural displacement, as outlined previously in this chapter. However, posterior mediastinal leiomyosarcomas are typically asymptomatic and are found incidentally.

Grossly, intrathoracic leiomyosarcomas do not differ appreciably from their counterparts in other anatomic locations. They are circumscribed, white-tan, firm masses that commonly exhibit foci of cystic degeneration or myxoid change when cut.

Histologic features of such lesions include the potential for a predominantly or purely epithelioid appearance, accounting for their inclusion with primary epithelioid leiomyosarcomas. In this particular guise, leiomyosarcomas may be confused with carcinomas, mesotheliomas, and other polygonal cell proliferations. Nuclear atypia varies considerably but is invariably present in these tumors, as is mitotic activity.

Ultrastructural findings in epithelioid leiomyosarcoma include plasmalemmal dense patches, pinocytotic activity, and investment by basal lamina. Skeins of thin cytoplasmic filaments and dense bodies also may be evident. Immunophenotypically, the characteristic profile of smooth muscle tumors includes reactivity for desmin, muscle-specific actin, h-caldesmon, calponin, and possibly vimentin, with negative results for epithelial markers, S-100 protein, and the HMB-45 antigen (125,490).

METASTATIC MEDIASTINAL CARCINOMA AND MELANOMA

It cannot be overemphasized that, in the mediastinum, metastatic lesions account for the vast majority of malignant somatic epithelial neoplasms of the polygonal cell type. These tumors usually arise in the trachea, bronchi, peripheral pulmonary parenchyma, or esophagus, although other anatomic sources are implicated in selected cases (330,347,348,491). There may be few, if any, symptoms or signs that are referable to the primary lesion, with those caused by the mediastinal mass predominating clinically. Thus, a high level of skepticism is again appropriate in rendering a diagnosis of primary mediastinal (thymic) carcinoma, and attending physicians should be required to pursue extensive radiographic or endoscopic evaluations of other viscera before such an interpretation is made.

In these circumstances, there are no distinguishing macroscopic features that allow for a definitive separation of primary and metastatic somatic carcinomas of the mediastinum. Moreover, conventional histologic examination is often similarly unfruitful in making such a distinction because a high proportion of the tumors being considered are poorly differentiated.

Immunohistologic analysis may be somewhat more revealing. If determinants are detected that are not synthesized by primary thymic carcinomas, such as thyroglobulin, prostate-specific antigen, S-100 protein, PLAP, CA19-9 (an enteric carcinoma marker), or CA-125 (a serosal and müllerian tract marker) (492), one can conclude that the neoplasm in question is, in all likelihood, a metastasis and attempt a prediction of its primary source. Conversely, the observation of CD5 expression by the tumor cells would, at least tentatively, appear to support a thymic origin for the lesion (362).

Mediastinal metastasis of amelanotic malignant melanoma has, on rare occasions, been documented as the presenting manifestation of this neoplasm (493), despite the absence of discernible cutaneous or mucosal disease. In this setting, melanoma can be confused with primary or metastatic somatic carcinomas, malignant germ cell tumors, or lymphomas. Thus, one should always include the first of these neoplasms in the differential diagnosis of polygonal cell lesions and take appropriate steps to exclude its presence. Electron microscopy may aid in this process because more than half of all amelanotic melanomas still retain a synthesis of premelanosomes at an ultrastructural level (494). Immunohistochemical studies show that melanomas are negative for keratin, EMA, PLAP, and the CD15, CD30, and CD45 antigens. Instead, they react with antibodies to vimentin, S-100 protein, MART-1, tyrosinase, PNL2 protein, and the HMB-45 antigen (492,495).

SPECIFIC DIFFERENTIAL DIAGNOSTIC PROBLEMS CONCERNING MEDIASTINAL POLYGONAL CELL TUMORS

In the foregoing sections, several well-defined differential diagnostic issues have already been considered by way of discussing certain pathologic entities. Nevertheless, either because of their degree of difficulty or their relative frequency, some of these problems merit the special emphasis that is presented here.

Primary Carcinoma Versus Lymphoma Versus Germ Cell Tumor Versus Melanoma Versus Epithelioid Leiomyosarcoma

In situations where an extramediastinal neoplasm has been excluded clinically and one is faced with an undifferentiated large-cell lesion, the chief diagnostic considerations are still multiple. As in other anatomic locations, carcinoma, lymphoma, germ cell tumors (such as seminoma and embryonal carcinoma), metastatic melanoma, and primary epithelioid leiomyosarcoma are all possibilities.

Careful scrutiny of conventional histologic sections may yield some helpful clues in this context. Cohesive cellular growth, regularly round or oval nuclear outlines, eosinophilic nucleoli, and foci of geographic necrosis favor a diagnosis of somatic carcinoma. Nests of clear cells with distinct membranes, complicated nucleolar structures, and admixed lymphocytes suggest an interpretation of seminoma. Eosinophilic intercellular globules or rudimentary lumina may serve as hints for the diagnosis of embryonal carcinoma. Nuclear irregularities, with "blebs" or projections of the nucleolemma, are expected in lymphomas. Small foci of delicate intracellular pigment, intranuclear pseudoinclusions of cytoplasm, and a tendency toward thèque-like growth favor metastatic melanoma. Predominantly epithelioid leiomyosarcomas may contain minute foci of conventional fascicular spindle cell growth.

In most cases of this type, however, the pathologist will want to pursue more detailed avenues of morphologic assessment. Hence, distinguishing features in this class of neoplasms are presented in Table 28.3.

Carcinoid Tumor Versus Paraganglioma Versus Parathyroid Carcinoma Versus Plasmacytoma

Because they are all neuroendocrine neoplasms, carcinoid tumor, paraganglioma, and PAC of the anterior mediastinum may be difficult to distinguish from one another histologically. Among these three lesions, carcinoids are the ones that display

the most notable mitotic activity, and they also commonly exhibit the presence of artifactually detached "balls" of tumor cells that are centrally necrotic. PAC is often composed of tumor cells with cytoplasmic lucency. These are intensely PAS positive but diastase sensitive, in contrast to the neoplastic elements in carcinoids or paragangliomas. Although parathyroid tumors can be labeled with antibodies to PTH (375), this peptide has now been described in rare examples of TCT as well, limiting its differential diagnostic value. Paragangliomas show a much more distinctive "tight" cellular nesting pattern and more nuclear pleomorphism than that seen in carcinoids or PACs; they are also the only lesions in this group that are immunohistologically keratin negative and potentially positive for mutant forms of the *ret* oncogene.

Plasmacytoma has the ability to assume a pseudoepithelial growth pattern, and the "clock face" chromatin pattern of its constituent cells may closely simulate the nuclear features of the aforementioned neuroendocrine neoplasms. However, monotypic immunoreactivity for light chain immunoglobulins and CD38 separates plasma cell tumors from parathyroid tumors, carcinoids, and paragangliomas.

Large-Cell Lymphoma Versus Granulocytic Sarcoma Versus Syncytial Nodular Sclerosing Hodgkin Disease

LCNHL, granulocytic sarcoma, and syncytial Hodgkin disease may be extremely similar to one another microscopically. This differential diagnosis is best resolved through the study of touch preparations stained with Romanowsky methods (discussed previously), together with histochemical techniques and immunohistology. Discriminating observations in this category of tumors are outlined in Table 28.4.

MIXED LARGE- AND SMALL-CELL MALIGNANT MEDIASTINAL TUMORS

Three anterior mediastinal neoplasms are made up of a mixture of cytologically malignant large and small cells: lymphoepitheli-

| TABLE 28.3 | General Differential Diagnosis of Malignant Polygonal Cell Mediastinal Tumors |

	Light Microscopy			Electron Microscopy				Immunohistochemistry						
	Nuclear													
Tumor	Blebs	Geo/Nec	PAS	Comp Nuc	ICJ	Premel	BMV	Ker	EMA	LCA	PLAP	CEA	S-100	MSA
PTC	0	+/−	+/−	0	+	0	0	+	+	0	0	+/−	0	0
LCL	+	0	0	0	0	0	0	0	+/−	+[a]	0	0	+/−	0
Seminoma	0	+/−	+	+	+	0	0	0[b]	0	0	+	0	0	0
Embryonal ca	0	+/−	+	+	+	0	0	+	0	0	+	0	0	0
Melanoma	0	+/−	+/−	0	+/−	+/−[c]	0	0	0	0	0	0	+	0
EMM	0	+/−	+/−	0	+	0	+	+	+	0	0	0	0	0
Met undiff ca	0	+/−	+/−	+/−	+	0	0	+	+	0	+/−	+/−	+/−	0
ELMS	0	+/−	+/−	0	+/−	0	0	0	0	0	0	0	+/−	0

BMV, branching surface microvilli; Ca, carcinomas; CEA, carcinoembryonic antigen; Comp Nuc, complex nucleoli; ELMS, epithelioid leiomyosarcoma; EMA, epithelial membrane antigen; EMM, epithelioid malignant mesothelioma; Geo/Nec, geographic necrosis; ICJ, intercellular junctions; Ker, keratin; LCA, leukocyte common antigen; LCL, large-cell lymphoma; Met undiff Ca, metastatic undifferentiated carcinoma; MSA, muscle-specific actin; PAS, periodic acid-Schiff stain; PLAP, placental alkaline phosphatase; Premel, premelanosomes; PTC, primary thymic carcinoma; S-100, S-100 protein.

[a]Rare large-cell lymphomas may be negative for LCA (and positive for CD30 antigens).

[b]Approximately 10% of seminomas show limited keratin positivity.

[c]Approximately 50% to 60% of metastatic melanomas contain premelanosomes.

TABLE 28.4	Differential Diagnosis of Malignant Large-Cell Hematopoietic Tumors of the Mediastinum								
	Histology and Histochemistry				Immunohistology				
Tumor	Auer Rods on TP	Admixed Eosinophils	Perox	CAE	CD15	CD20	CD30	CD45	CD68
Large-cell NHL	0	Rare	0	0	0	+	+/−	+[a]	0
Granulocytic sarcoma	+/−	Common	+	+	+/−	0	0	+/−	+/−
Syncytial Hodgkin disease	0	Common	0	0	+/−	0	+	0	0

CAE, chloroacetate (von Leder) stain; CD15/20/30/45/68, CD antigen immunostains on paraffin sections or touch-imprint preparations; NHL, non-Hodgkin lymphoma; Perox, peroxidase stain on touch-imprint preparations or with diaminobenzidine on paraffin sections; TP, touch preparations.
[a]Rare cases of CD30-positive large-cell non-Hodgkin lymphoma may lack CD45.

oma-like carcinoma (LELC), mixed large-cell and small-cell non-Hodgkin lymphoma (MNHL), and mixed cellularity Hodgkin disease (MCHD). MNHL is the most frequent of these disorders, followed in relative order by MCHD and LELC. Potential clinical presentations in such cases are virtually identical to those described earlier in the sections on primary large-cell lymphoma, syncytial NSHD, and thymic carcinoma.

Mixed Large-Cell and Small-Cell Non-Hodgkin Lymphoma

Some controversy surrounds the definition of MNHL, as it is distinguished from LCNHL. I use the rather arbitrary criterion that no more than 30% of large cells are "allowed" in the former of these lesions. Both the large-cell and small-cell components typically show nuclear atypia, with hyperchromasia, irregular nuclear contours, and variable nucleolation (Fig. 28.95). Admixed leukocytes of other types (e.g., neutrophils, eosinophils) are not expected in most lesions of this type; nevertheless, those examples of MNHL that manifest T-cell differentiation may indeed contain nonlymphocytic white cells (11). Sclerosis is not a usual feature of MNHLs (134).

The immunohistologic attributes of MNHL are diagnostic. They include reactivity for the CD45 antigen in all lesional cells, as well as similar positivity for CD20 antigen, with or without

PAX-5, in B-cell tumors or CD3, CD43, or CD45R0 determinants in T-cell proliferations (496). Keratin reactivity is never observed.

Mixed Cellularity Hodgkin Disease

MCHD is superficially similar histologically to MNHL; however, the former lesion demonstrates the presence of classic RS cells, defined by their nuclear multilobation, vesicular chromatin, and multiple eosinophilic nucleoli (134). Cells approximating this description are evident only in rare examples of mixed non-Hodgkin lymphomas. Moreover, the small lymphocytes in MCHD are uniformly mature, and the lesion regularly exhibits an admixture of eosinophils, plasma cells, immunoblasts, and MRV cells (Fig. 28.96).

Immunoreactivity for CD45 is not seen in the classic RS cells or MRV elements of Hodgkin disease, regardless of microscopic subtype (6). In addition, these same tumoral components uniformly lack CD3, CD20, CD43, and CD45R0 determinants. Instead, RS and MRV cells can be labeled for CD30, with or without PAX-5 and the CD15 antigen, and with a distinctive staining pattern for CD15 and CD30 (11,462,463,496,497). This features a globular accentuation of positivity in the perinuclear region of the cytoplasm, as well as diffuse reactivity of the cell membranes.

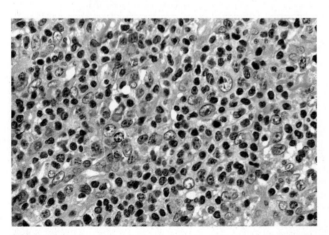

Figure 28.95. Mixed small-cell and large-cell non-Hodgkin lymphoma of the anterior mediastinum. Both neoplastic elements are atypical cytologically.

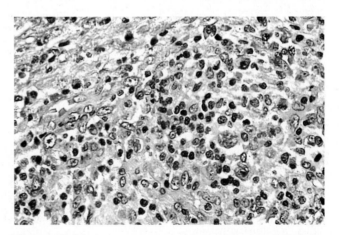

Figure 28.96. Mixed cellularity Hodgkin disease of the mediastinum. Small lymphocytes are mature in this process, and the presence of stromal eosinophils further distinguishes it from mixed non-Hodgkin lymphomas.

EMA may be observed in RS or MRV cells in some cases of HL, but keratin is consistently lacking (134).

Lymphoepithelioma-Like Carcinoma

The histologic and immunohistochemical features of LELC have been described previously, and only pertinent attributes will be recounted here. This neoplasm shows the formation of small syncytia that are made up of large tumor cells with vesicular chromatin. Admixed lymphocytes are mature in appearance, and the presence of background neutrophilia or eosinophilia is uncommon.

All cases of LELC are immunoreactive for keratin and EMA. Conversely, the large tumor cells lack determinants in the CD3, CD15, CD20, CD30, CD43, CD45, and CD45R0 groups (198).

Malignant Spindle Cell/Pleomorphic Mediastinal Neoplasms

The list of malignant spindle cell or pleomorphic tumors that may arise primarily in the mediastinum is considerable. It includes sarcomatoid thymic carcinomas, spindle cell carcinoid tumors, sarcomatoid mesotheliomas, synovial sarcomas, malignant peripheral nerve sheath tumors, leiomyosarcomas, liposarcomas, rhabdomyosarcomas, osteosarcomas, angiosarcomas, malignant fibrous histiocytomas, and fibrosarcomas (125). Of these neoplasms, only the first three types are relatively restricted to the thorax in their topographic distributions. In general, mediastinal sarcomas have few, if any, unique pathologic characteristics that distinguish them from identical tumors elsewhere in the body. In view of this fact and to avoid needless repetition, the reader is referred to Chapter 5 on soft tissue neoplasms to obtain detailed differential diagnostic information on such lesions. However, as a rapid reference, Table 28.5

presents a working outline of discriminating pathologic observations in this category of tumors.

Sarcomatoid Thymic Carcinoma

Few examples of sarcomatoid thymic carcinoma (STC) have been reported (90,91,297,350,498–500). Patients with this tumor are adults who have symptoms and signs of a space-occupying intrathoracic mass (91). In one example seen by the author, irradiation had been given to the mediastinum many years previously for presumably malignant lymphadenopathy, but a biopsy of the latter condition had never been obtained. To date, no cases of STC have been linked to paraneoplastic phenomena of the types that are affiliated with thymomas or thymic neuroendocrine lesions. At the risk of redundancy, it must again be emphasized that metastases to the thymic region must be excluded rigorously before assigning a final diagnosis of STC.

The gross characteristics of STCs are essentially the same as those of poorly differentiated squamous carcinomas affecting this gland (discussed previously). However, probably because of their extremely limited degree of differentiation and conjointly high proliferative rate, the lesions of STC tend to be even larger than other thymic carcinomas. In the author's experience, the mean diameter of such neoplasms has been 15 cm.

Microscopically, STC is characterized by irregularly disposed fascicles of fusiform and pleomorphic tumor cells, with little tendency to assume clustered configurations (Fig. 28.97) (90,91,297). Nuclei are generally densely hyperchromatic, and nucleoli are apparent at least focally in most cases. Mitotic activity is typically brisk, and pathologic division figures may be encountered. The cytoplasm is amphophilic or eosinophilic. Occasional cases have shown small areas wherein cohesive epithelioid cell nests were admixed with the spindle cell elements (90), and it should be reiterated that biphasic STCs with carcinoidal

TABLE 28.5 | **Differential Diagnosis of Malignant Spindle Cell and Pleomorphic Mediastinal Tumors**

Tumor	Histologic Category	Light Microscopy			Electron Microscopy					Immunohistochemistry				
		FECC	FDC	Argyr	ICJ	Myofil	NSG	WPB	ECP	Ker	D/A	EMA	S-100	UELB
Sarc ca	A	+/−	0	0	+	0	0	0	0	+	+/−	+	0	+/−
SCCARND	B	+/−	+	+	+	0	+	0	0	+	0	+/−	0	0
Sarc meso	A	+/−	0	0	+	0	0	0	0	+	0	+/−	0	0
Syn sarc	A	+/−	0	0	+	0	0	0	0	+/−	0	+	0	+/−
MPNST	A	+/−	0	0	+	0	0	0	+	0	0	+/−	+/−	0
LMS	A	+/−	0	0	0	+	0	0	0	0	+	0	0	0
PLPS	C	0	0	0	0	0	0	0	0	0	0	0	+[a]	0
PRMS	C	0	0	0	0	+	0	0	0	0	+[b]	0	0	0
Osteosarc	A	0	0	0	0	0	0	0	0	0	0	0	0	0
Angiosarc	A	+/−	0	0	+/−	0	0	+/−	0	0	0	0	0	0
MFH	C	0	0	0	0	0	0	0	0	0	0	0	0	0
Fibrosarc	B	0	0	0	0	0	0	0	0	0	0	0	0	0

A, may be spindle cell or pleomorphic or both; Angiosarc, angiosarcoma; Argyr, argyrophilic; B, spindle cell growth only; C, pleomorphic growth pattern only; D/A, desmin/actin; ECP, elongated cell processes; EMA, epithelial membrane antigen; FDC, finely dispersed chromatin pattern; FECC, focal epithelioid cell clusters; Fibrosarc, fibrosarcoma; ICJ, intercellular junctional complexes; Ker, keratin; LMS, leiomyosarcoma; MFH, malignant fibrous histiocytoma; MPNST, malignant peripheral nerve sheath tumor; Myofil, myofilaments; NSG, neurosecretory granules; Osteosarc, osteosarcoma; PLPS, pleomorphic liposarcoma; PRMS, pleomorphic rhabdomyosarcoma; S-100, S-100 protein; Sarc ca, sarcomatoid carcinoma; Sarc meso, sarcomatoid mesothelioma; SCCARND, spindle cell carcinoid tumor; Syn sarc, synovial sarcoma; UELB, *Ulex europaeus* I lectin binding; WPB, Weibel-Palade bodies.
[a]S-100 protein in liposarcomas is confined to lipoblastic tumor cells.
[b]Pleomorphic rhabdomyosarcoma is immunoreactive for myoglobin, as well as desmin and actin.

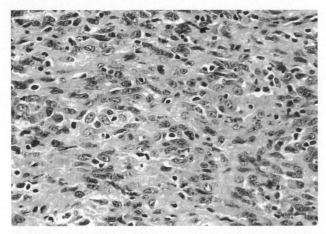

Figure 28.97. Spindle cell (sarcomatoid) carcinoma of the thymus. This tumor may resemble a true sarcoma, as well as sarcomatoid spindle cell malignant mesothelioma.

elements ("dedifferentiated" TCTs) have also been documented (331,333). Snover et al. (90) reported an example of STC with focally well-defined rhabdomyogenic differentiation, complete with cytoplasmic cross-striations. Some observers may choose to label lesions with these attributes as "carcinosarcomas," but it is my belief that all such proliferations are basically epithelial in nature (501).

Electron microscopy often confirms the latter contention by demonstrating at least focal junctional complexes between the spindle cells, possibly with small numbers of cytoplasmic tonofibrils as well (90,501). However, it is also possible that the ultrastructural features of STC will be those of a nondescript spindle cell proliferation of indeterminate lineage.

Immunohistochemically, the fusiform and pleomorphic cells of all sarcomatoid carcinomas are reactive for vimentin. Staining for keratin and EMA is also seen consistently, but it may be focal; the same is true of labeling for p63 (194,498,501). This fact leaves open the possibility that a small biopsy specimen might fail to demonstrate any epithelial markers because of sampling artifact. The latter eventuality should be considered before a final diagnostic report of "mediastinal sarcoma" is issued, and comments should be included that address the problem just cited. Cases showing divergent components, such as cellular foci with myogenic properties, may indeed exhibit immunoreactivity in these areas for desmin, actin, or myogenin (90). Such potential results compound the difficulty in establishing a firm diagnosis of sarcomatoid carcinoma with limited tissue samples.

One particularly vexing differential diagnostic challenge is the distinction between primary mediastinal synovial sarcoma and PTC, inasmuch as their clinical, electron microscopic, and immunophenotypic features are largely similar. The demonstration of consistent t(X;18) chromosomal translocations in synovial sarcoma by fluorescence in situ hybridization has now made that tumor consistently recognizable with diagnostic certainty, even using paraffin-embedded specimens (502).

Spindle Cell Carcinoid Tumor of the Thymus

The existence of a spindle cell variant of thymic carcinoid was first documented in 1976 by Levine and Rosai (503), but it

appears to be a very rare tumor subtype. Relatively few other well-documented examples have appeared in the literature (48,504,505); the author has seen only one representative case among a total of 51 thymic carcinoids. The patient in the seminal report on this lesion showed evidence of inappropriate secretion of antidiuretic hormone, the source of which was thought to be the neoplasm itself. No other paraneoplastic phenomena were present. Other patients have manifested signs of the MEN type 1 syndrome and "ectopic" Cushing syndrome (48,504).

The macroscopic attributes of this lesion are identical to those of other thymic carcinoids. Microscopically, it is composed of interweaving fascicles of plump fusiform cells, and it appears to lack the prototypically organoid appearance of other TCT morphotypes (410,503). A key feature of spindle cell thymic carcinoid is its nuclear chromatin, which, similar to other differentiated neuroendocrine tumors, is dispersed and finely particulate (Fig. 28.98). These details are particularly well seen in touch-imprint preparations or fine-needle aspirates (504). Nucleoli are inconspicuous, but mitoses are easily seen. The cytoplasm is amphophilic and slightly granular; focal positivity is evident with various argyrophilic staining methods (36). Electron microscopic and immunohistologic features of spindle cell TCT are consonant with those seen in other forms of thymic neuroendocrine neoplasia.

Sarcomatoid Mediastinal Malignant Mesothelioma

Aside from its exclusive composition by fusiform and pleomorphic tumor cells, sarcomatoid mediastinal mesothelioma shows only selected clinicopathologic differences from its purely epithelioid, desmoplastic, or biphasic counterparts. The most salient disparity concerns the ultrastructural and immunohistologic features of sarcomatoid mesothelioma. These diverge from those expected in purely epithelioid neoplasms and are largely similar to the specialized pathologic attributes of sarcomatoid carcinoma that were described previously. However, Hinterberger et al. (505a) have suggested that combined immunoreactivity for calretinin and podoplanin favors a diagnosis of mesothelioma. Based only on morphologic information, one often cannot make a distinction between these two neoplasms

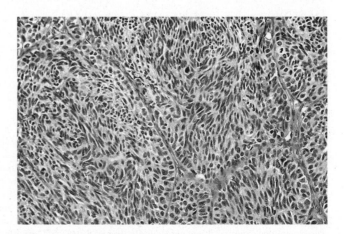

Figure 28.98. Spindle cell variant of thymic carcinoid tumor. Neoplastic cells have dispersed nuclear chromatin, regular oval nuclear contours, and granular cytoplasm, in contrast to other mediastinal tumors that are composed of fusiform cells.

with certainty. The pathologist also must pay careful attention to radiologic findings and consult with the surgeon on exact in situ anatomic relationships between the tumor and adjacent intrathoracic structures to reach a final diagnostic interpretation.

Sarcomatoid Thymic Yolk Sac Tumor

A peculiar variant of primary mediastinal yolk sac tumor (MYST) has been documented by Moran and Suster (506). Despite the fact that it features a predominance of spindle cells and, as such, may be confused with the other neoplastic entities cited in this section, "sarcomatoid" MYST exhibits no other clinicopathologic differences from more conventional forms of endodermal sinus tumor.

The most important microscopic attributes of spindle cell MYST include a tendency for storiform growth, focally myxoid stroma, and the presence of intercellular eosinophilic globules that are labeled with the PAS-diastase method. Other specialized features of an ultrastructural and immunohistologic nature are identical to those of "ordinary" yolk sac tumors of the mediastinum. In particular, Moran and Suster found intense reactivity for keratin and AFP in spindle cell yolk sac tumor. The second of these markers allows for a reproducible separation from STC, which is AFP negative.

Malignant Adipocytic and Myxoid Mediastinal Neoplasms

In addition to thymolipomas and true soft tissue lipomas, other neoplasms that may be seen in the mediastinum demonstrate partial or global adipocytic differentiation. All of the forms of liposarcoma (well differentiated, sclerosing, myxoid, round cell, "dedifferentiated," and pleomorphic) have been documented in this location (125,507–509). Nevertheless, as with the spindle cell sarcomas listed in the previous section, there are no special features of liposarcomas that are dependent on this particular topographic site. Thus, the general discussion of such lesions in Chapter 5 should suffice to enumerate the characteristics of those in the thorax.

Thymoliposarcoma

A malignant counterpart to thymolipoma was originally reported by Havlicek and Rosai (510) and termed *thymoliposarcoma*. Patients with this lesion have been adults, and their tumors tend to have the gross appearance of thymolipomas (507, 510–512b). However, microscopic examination demonstrates malignant mesenchymal components admixed with thymic tissue (Fig. 28.99). The former elements have an appearance ranging from that of well-differentiated liposarcoma to highly pleomorphic and poorly differentiated neoplasms. One reported thymoliposarcoma recurred 32 years after initial diagnosis, with possible metastasis to bone, indicating that prolonged follow-up is necessary in such cases (510).

Epithelioid Hemangioendothelioma and Chordoma

In addition to the myxoid variant of liposarcoma, two other potentially myxoid mesenchymal neoplasms that may arise in the mediastinum warrant comment here. These are epithelioid hemangioendothelioma (EH) and chordoma. EH can be observed in either the anterior or posterior subcompartments (125,513–514a) and often demonstrates a gross association with the adventitia of large blood vessels. It is typically a circumscribed but unencapsulated mass, with a glistening and hemorrhage cut surface (125). Microscopically, EH may be confused with either metastatic carcinoma or liposarcoma because it is composed of markedly vacuolated polygonal cells set in a myxohyaline stroma (Fig. 28.100). The tumor cells may be arranged in cords or in disorganized sheets. Nuclear atypia is variable in severity, as is mitotic activity; however, both of these features are usually not marked (125,514). Electron microscopic studies show numerous Weibel-Palade bodies in the proliferating cells, marking them as endothelial in nature (515). Immunohistochemistry likewise shows uniform reactivity for CD31 and CD34, von Willebrand factor, FLI-1, and thrombomodulin (Fig. 28.101), all of which are potential indicators of endothelial differentiation (125,319a) (see also Chapter 5). Keratin, EMA, and S-100 protein are uniformly absent.

Although it is much more frequently observed at the base of the skull and in the sacrococcygeal region, chordoma also

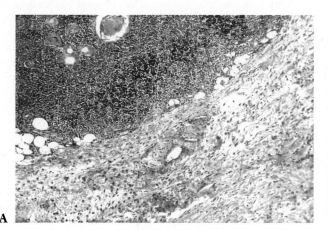
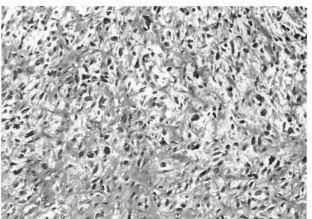

A   **B**

Figure 28.99. **(A)** Thymoliposarcoma showing the junction of normal thymic tissue and an atypical lipomatous component containing spindled and pleomorphic tumor cells. **(B)** Higher power view of sarcomatous element of thymoliposarcoma, assuming an appearance that is most like that of myxoid malignant fibrous histiocytoma. Other foci showed unequivocal lipoblastic differentiation.

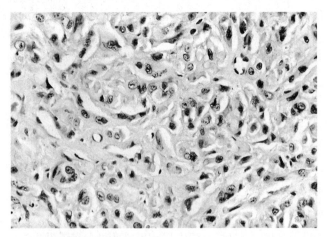

Figure 28.100. Epithelioid hemangioendothelioma of the posterior mediastinum. Tumor cells are arranged in cords and nests, with focal cytoplasmic vacuolization. Background stroma is slightly myxoid.

may present itself as a paramedian posterior mediastinal mass in both children and adults (516). Partial destruction of adjacent vertebral bodies is a common radiographic finding in such cases. Macroscopically, chordomas are circumscribed but not encapsulated, with a mucoid, glistening, white-gray cut surface. They are histologically composed of nests and elongated cords of polygonal cells in a myxochondroid matrix (Fig. 28.102). Nuclear hyperchromasia and nucleolation are variable, but both may be extreme in scope. Mitotic activity is usually apparent. The single most characteristic microscopic feature of chordoma is its content of "physaliphorous" tumor cells, which show multiple small cytoplasmic vacuoles that contain mucopolysaccharide (see Chapter 8).

Ultrastructurally, chordoma exhibits the presence of intercellular junctions, broad skeins of cytoplasmic intermediate filaments, and complexes of rough endoplasmic reticulum and mitochondria. Intrareticular microtubules also may be evident. The immunophenotype of this neoplasm includes reactivity for keratin, EMA, S-100 protein, and CD57 (517).

OTHER NEOPLASMS OF THE MEDIASTINUM

Other mediastinal neoplasms are either extremely rare or present relatively little diagnostic difficulty and thus will merely be

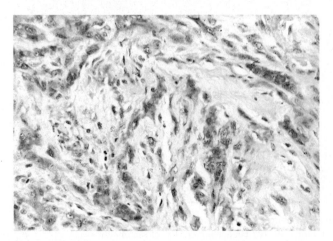

Figure 28.101. Immunoreactivity for CD34 antigen in epithelioid hemangioendothelioma is indicative of its endothelial differentiation.

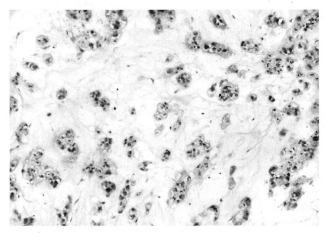

Figure 28.102. Chordoma presenting as a posterior mediastinal mass. Tumor cells are arranged in cords in a myxoid stroma, similar to those in Figure 28.100. However, they are finely vacuolated ("physaliferous") and therefore suggest the correct diagnosis.

mentioned here. These include hemangiomas (both capillary and cavernous types) (125,312,513,518); lymphangiomyomas (125); hyperplasias, adenomas, and carcinomas in ectopic thyroid tissue (76); parathyroid adenomas and lipoadenomas (410); melanotic neuroectodermal tumors of infancy ("melanotic progonomas") (519,520); ependymomas (521,521a); granular cell tumors (522,523); tumefactive extramedullary hematopoiesis (524,525); osteosarcomas (526,527); Langerhans cell histiocytosis (528,529); rhabdomyomas (530) (which must be distinguished from "rhabdomyomatous" thymomas [531]); pleomorphic adenomas (532); oncocytomas (533); chondrosarcomas (534); and malignant rhabdoid tumors (535,536).

Ectopic Lesions with Features of Mediastinal Tumors

Several reports have concerned neoplasms that have the pathologic attributes of mediastinal lesions but are located in other anatomic sites. Thymomas have been documented in the neck (537–539) and pleural surfaces (including interlobar pulmonary septa) (540–544), in the absence of abnormalities in the thymus gland itself. Chan and Rosai (545) introduced the concept that some peculiar tumors of the cervical soft tissue and thyroid—termed "spindle cell epithelial tumors with thymus-like differentiation" (SETTLE) and "carcinomas showing thymus-like differentiation" (CASTLE)—fall into the same category. The latter premise has been generally accepted (365,546–549) and is supported by the observation that ectopic thymic tissue and thymic cysts are frequently found above the clavicles (76,550).

PROGNOSTIC FEATURES OF MEDIASTINAL NEOPLASMS

The surgical pathologist is increasingly asked to provide behavioral information on a variety of neoplasms, including those in the mediastinum. Accordingly, Table 28.6 outlines four groupings of such lesions, two of which represent a miniature spectrum of biologically "borderline" proliferations. In addition, comments are provided on several of these tumors in the following sections.

TABLE 28.6	Prognostic Groups of Mediastinal Neoplasms		
		Borderline	
Benign	Limited Potential for Local Recurrence	High Potential for Local Recurrence; Rare Metastasis	Overtly Malignant
Pericardial cyst	Paravertebral paraganglioma	Aorticopulmonary paraganglioma	Malignant germ cell tumors
Enteric cyst	Solitary fibrous tumor	Desmoid-type fibromatosis/ well-differentiated fibrosarcoma	PNET
Parathyroid cyst	Cellular schwannoma	Epithelioid hemangioendothelioma	Neuroblastoma
Bronchogenic cyst	Encapsulated thymoma	Well-differentiated squamous cell thymic carcinoma	Non-Hodgkin lymphomas
Meningocele	Histiocytosis X	Basaloid squamous thymic carcinoma	Hodgkin disease
Cystic mature teratoma	Melanotic progonoma	Mucoepidermoid thymic carcinoma	Carcinoid tumor
Lymphangioma		Well-differentiated liposarcoma	Neuroendocrine carcinomas
Lipoma		Myxoid liposarcoma	High-grade thymic carcinomas
Thymolipoma		Invasive thymoma	Parathyroid carcinoma
Neurilemoma		Thymoliposarcoma (?)	Malignant mesothelioma
Neurofibroma		Hemangiopericytoma	Rhabdomyosarcomas
Rhabdomyoma		Fibrous histiocytoma	Granulocytic sarcoma
Hemangioma		Carcinoma arising in ectopic thyroid	Multicentric Castleman disease
Ganglioneuroma		Chordoma	Round-cell and pleomorphic liposarcomas
Castleman disease (unifocal)			Leiomyosarcoma
Parathyroid adenoma			Malignant fibrous histiocytoma
Parathyroid lipoadenoma			Synovial sarcoma
Ectopic thyroid adenoma			Metastatic tumors
			Malignant rhabdoid tumor

PNET, primitive neuroectodermal tumor.

THYMOMAS

As stated earlier in this chapter, a great deal of controversy and misunderstanding surrounded the prognostication of thymomas in the past. Some of this unrest continues, concerning the impact—if any—of histologic classification strategies on biologic behavior (148–155,157–167,169–174,178,188,551–553). This issue has already been discussed earlier in this chapter and will not be repeated here. Nonetheless, even with that topic set aside, it is indisputably true that one can predict the probable behavior of these neoplasms with reasonable certainty using other information—namely, the extent of regional invasion demonstrated by the tumors in question. Some might argue that this factual material might not be provided spontaneously by thoracic surgeons, preventing its use by surgical pathologists. I would respond that it is the obligation of the latter practitioners to solicit such an important clinical fact actively, rather than passively dismissing it as unavailable.

Masaoka et al. (184) devised a staging system for thymomas based on the reality that the most important pathologic indicator of the clinical course is the presence or absence of tumor invasion at initial diagnosis. Several studies have endorsed the use of that scheme (154,182,339,554–556). Stage I thymomas are totally encapsulated, both grossly and microscopically. Stage IIA tumors show microscopic invasion of the capsule but have been removed completely by the surgeon. Stage IIB lesions demonstrate transcapsular infiltration of mediastinal soft tissue or pleura. Stage III thymomas invade the pericardium, great vessels, or lungs. Stage IV neoplasms seed the pericardial or pleural surfaces multifocally (substage IVA) or metastasize distantly (substage IVB).

Haniuda et al. (557) have suggested that further modification of the Masaoka system might be useful for stage II cases; those authors proposed appending a "p" designator to describe the precise status of the mediastinal pleura in the specified context. In such a construction, stage II-p0 tumors show no adhesion to the pleura; p1 lesions demonstrate fibrous adhesions between the tumor and pleura without true invasion of the latter structure; and p2 tumors manifest actual pleural infiltration. In their experience, an adverse breakpoint in behavior was seen at the stage II-p1 level (regardless of whether the lesions were stage IIA or IIB), and therefore, they recommended adjuvant treatment with irradiation, chemotherapy, or both at that point. Those interventions also appear, at least in large measure, to ameliorate the poorer prognosis that has attended thymomas that could not be completely resected surgically (187,557–561).

More generally, it can be concluded that the Masaoka scheme definitely has been proven to have clinical validity, with progressive diminution in 5-year postsurgical survival paralleling increasing stage (152,154,157,182,184,186,187,339,554–556,562,563). However, one should keep in mind that even encapsulated thymomas do have some potential for recurrence, which occurs in up to 15% of cases (560,564,565).

As mentioned, there have also been proposals from the same Japanese investigators' attempts to bring the staging of thymoma (and other epithelial neoplasms of the thymus) into line with current American Joint Committee on Cancer staging recommendations (tumor-node-metastasis [TNM]) (185,566). These schemes have claimed to yield predictive values that roughly approximate those of the original Masaoka schema (184). However, in all candor, the author sees no particular benefit in eschewing the Masaoka system for a TNM-based construct. That statement may not apply with specific reference to thymic *carcinomas* (discussed later in the chapter) because an insufficient number of cases of the latter lesions have been analyzed systematically to truly test the merits of TNM coding (567).

Other clinicopathologic observations besides invasion may also have some bearing on the behavior of thymoma. In the Mayo Clinic experience (148), factors with independently adverse statistical significance included the presence of tumor-related symptoms and signs at diagnosis and a tumor diameter greater than 15 cm. Age less than 30 years at diagnosis, a microscopic predominance of epithelial cells, and nuclear atypia were additional interdependent determinants of untoward behavior. Similar results were noted by Cowen et al. (186) and Regnard et al. (167). It is notable that other investigators (148,187,568,569) have shown no statistically significant prognostic effect of myasthenia gravis or any other paraneoplastic syndrome on the biology of thymomas.

In regard to specialized pathologic techniques and the prognosis of thymoma, it can be stated that relatively little appears to be gained by the application of such procedures. Contradictory or noncontributory results have been obtained in reference to flow cytometric determination of DNA content (570); immunohistologic semiquantitation of tumoral proliferative rates with anti–proliferating cell nuclear antigen (PCNA) and Ki-67 (571); and detection of aberrant expression of *bcl-2, fas,* or *p53* gene products by immunostaining or blotting methods (214,215,572). Pich et al. (556,573) have reported that quantitation of silver-stained nucleolar organizing regions (AgNORs) in the tumor cells of thymomas does provide additional predictive information, but that claim appears to be in conflict with data pertaining to PCNA and Ki-67.

LYMPHOPROLIFERATIVE DISEASES

In the category of mediastinal lymphoproliferative diseases, a diversity of behavioral attributes is observed. Castleman disease is curable surgically when it is localized (13), but the 10% of cases in which multifocal disease is present (574) have a relatively poor prognosis. The therapy of limited-stage mediastinal Hodgkin disease has progressed dramatically, so that stage IA through IIB tumors are now curable in more than 90% of cases (575). Nonetheless, HLs that are larger than one-third of the thoracic diameter are treated more aggressively than smaller tumors (576). The histologic subtype (e.g., classic nodular sclerosing, syncytial, mixed cellularity, etc.) does not influence the behavior of this neoplasm appreciably (575). Lymphoblastic and Burkitt lymphomas of the mediastinum are still tumors with a poor overall prognosis, and even with multiagent chemotherapy, the 5-year survival rate is only approximately 50% (11).

Treatment advances for LCNHLs have improved survival to approximately 85% at 5 years (577–577b). Nevertheless, tumors in this category that are larger than 10 cm, lesions with an immunoblastic appearance, and those with extrathoracic involvement at diagnosis have a much more negative outlook (223). Lazzarino et al. (461) also have shown that the presence of a pericardial effusion at diagnosis and poor initial response to multiagent chemotherapy were adverse prognosticators. LCNHLs of B-cell lineage (the majority) appear to behave more adversely than others with T-cell immunophenotypes (11). Granulocytic sarcoma likewise has an ominous prognosis because of its usual

evolution into peripheralized acute myelogenous leukemia (467,470).

GERM CELL TUMORS

The biology of mediastinal germ cell tumors is also heterogeneous. Mature teratomas (that is, with no primitive neuroepithelium or malignant germinal or somatic elements) are entirely benign (73). The age of patients with immature teratomas is the most important predictive factor; patients less than 15 years old have favorable prospects, whereas similar lesions in adults usually behave adversely (135). Teratoid tumors that contain seminomatous or nonseminomatous components must be treated with aggressive chemotherapy and may necessitate resection of residual tumor thereafter. With this approach, Parker et al. (140) reported a high cure rate of such "teratocarcinomas."

In contrast to the current situation with gonadal germ cell tumors, both mediastinal seminomas and nonseminomatous lesions have an extremely guarded prognosis (383). This is probably so because these tumors have attained a large size before the diagnosis is made. It has been suggested that all patients with malignant mediastinal germ cell tumors would benefit from both irradiation and chemotherapy, including those with "pure" seminomas (578,579). Using this regimen, it is expected that 50% to 65% of seminoma patients will achieve 5-year tumor-free survival, but less than 20% of patients with primary embryonal carcinoma, yolk sac tumor, or choriocarcinoma of the thymic region can be cured (383,578).

Favorable prognostic factors in cases of pure mediastinal seminoma include age of 35 years or less at diagnosis (383,580); the absence of the superior vena caval syndrome, mediastinal lymphadenopathy, and fever (383); and (probably) a grossly cystic configuration (98,145). In regard to nonseminomatous tumors of the gonads, it is now recognized that cases showing a rapid decline in serum AFP or β-HCG levels, after tumor excision and administration of multiagent chemotherapy, have a relatively favorable outlook (581), as do those in which vascular invasion is absent and yolk sac or choriocarcinomatous components are lacking histologically (582). Similar factors appear to be equally applicable to mediastinal lesions. For example, Mayordomo et al. (583) found that age less than 22 years, the absence of endodermal sinus tumor components, and AFP levels of less than 1000 ng/mL were favorable predictive elements in that context.

NEUROENDOCRINE TUMORS OF THE MEDIASTINUM

Carcinoid tumors (neuroendocrine carcinomas) of the thymus are biologically capricious, and therefore, all of them must be considered to have the potential for widespread metastasis (410,418). Moreover, an association with the MEN syndromes or with ectopic ACTH production correlates with a particularly adverse prognosis in such cases (413). Results of the author's analyses of tumor size, relative mitotic activity, encapsulation or capsular invasion, and the presence or absence of regional lymph node metastasis at diagnosis have not revealed any prognostic significance for such factors in 38 cases of TCT. Admittedly, this conclusion does contrast with the conclusions of Gal et al. (406) and Yamakawa et al. (566).

In general, recent studies have continued to affirm the contention that thymic carcinoids should be approached by clinicians as "surgical" lesions because radiation treatment and chemotherapy have been rather ineffectual in managing such tumors (36,410,426–430). Recurrence of TCT may be delayed up to almost 10 years after initial diagnosis (418), making evaluation of treatment regimens more difficult.

Primary thymic small-cell neuroendocrine carcinoma is also an aggressive neoplasm. Almost all cases reported thus far have proven to be fatal (13,50,90,91,294–298), and it is logical to suggest that the same therapy should be used for this lesion as would be used for oat cell carcinomas arising in the lungs. The one difference that has been noted between high-grade pulmonary and thymic neuroendocrine carcinomas is the duration of survival after initial diagnosis; this averages 12 to 15 months for cancers arising in the lung but is approximately 36 months for thymic oat cell carcinomas (13,297).

The biology of mediastinal paragangliomas has been partially considered previously. In short, it is more dependent on their location than on any other clinicopathologic feature (57,58,410,434,435). Paragangliomas in the aorticopulmonary region of the anterior mediastinum are all potentially fatal because of their tendency toward extensive local invasion (437). In contrast, paravertebral mediastinal paragangliomas uncommonly cause patient mortality (56).

Too few cases of primary mediastinal PAC have been documented to make any meaningful comment on prognostic variables. Nonetheless, it is logical to expect that the postsurgical recurrence of such lesions would be an ominous event, in light of accrued experience with cervical tumors of this type (583). Accordingly, postoperative irradiation for PAC is often advised on empiric grounds.

PRIMARY NON–SMALL-CELL THYMIC CARCINOMAS

It was originally believed that all primary non–small-cell thymic carcinomas (PTCs), regardless of histotype, were universally fatal. However, several series have addressed the current status of our ability to prognosticate such lesions in more detail (91,294,295,336,337,340). These have concluded that there are, indeed, variants of PTC that may be cured by surgical excision. Well-differentiated squamous cell carcinoma, MEC, and basaloid carcinoma represent this group. Suster and Rosai (91) found no fatalities among patients with the latter tumors in a study of 60 PTC cases. Kuo et al. (294) and Truong et al. (295) also concluded that well-differentiated squamous thymic carcinomas had a favorable outlook, with Hsu et al. (584) being the only authors finding otherwise. Even in regard to other histotypes, several recent series have suggested that aggressive surgical excision and modern adjuvant therapy are capable of effecting cure in low-stage cases (336,337,340). It is still unfortunately true that selected types of PTC (nonkeratinizing squamous carcinoma, LELC, clear-cell carcinoma, sarcomatoid carcinoma, and adenosquamous carcinoma) are associated with high mortality rates (13,91,294–298,330,585–587). Nonetheless, Suster and Rosai (91) found that there was some variation in the length of survival in such cases. This was influenced adversely by the presence of histologically infiltrative tumor margins, mitotic activity greater than 10 division figures per 10 high-power fields, a nonlobular growth pattern, and the nuclear grade of the neoplasms.

PROGNOSTIC FEATURES OF OTHER MEDIASTINAL TUMORS

Biologically predictive pathologic observations associated with various mesenchymal tumor types are covered well in Chapter 5 in regard to lesions of the peripheral soft tissues. There is no reason to believe that mediastinal examples of these proliferations diverge in any way from the portraits presented in Chapter 5. Inasmuch as relatively few thymoliposarcomas have been reported heretofore (507,510–512), only qualified statements can be made regarding their behavior. However, it would appear that those lesions are comparatively indolent biologically, with a good response to irradiation or chemotherapy.

Metastatic carcinomas and melanomas that present as mediastinal masses are universally fatal in a relatively short period of time, usually because of additional spread of these tumors to other anatomic locations (13,347,348). Similarly, malignant mesotheliomas of the mediastinum have a dismal prognosis, regardless of microscopic subtype (289).

REFERENCES

1. Blalock A. Thymectomy in the treatment of myasthenia gravis: report of twenty cases. *J Thorac Cardiovasc Surg* 1944;13:316–339.
2. Sterrett G, Whitaker D, Shilkin KB, et al. The fine needle aspiration cytology of mediastinal lesions. *Cancer* 1983;51:127–135.
3. Gherardi G, Marveggio C, Placidi A. Neuroendocrine carcinoma of the thymus: aspiration biopsy, immunocytochemistry, and clinicopathologic correlates. *Diagn Cytopathol* 1995;35:158–164.
4. Heilo A. Tumors in the mediastinum: ultrasound-guided histologic core-needle biopsy. *Radiology* 1993;189:143–146.
5. Powers CN, Silverman JF, Geisinger KR, et al. Fine needle aspiration biopsy of the mediastinum: a multiinstitutional analysis. *Am J Clin Pathol* 1996;105:168–173.
5a. Assaad MW, Pantanowitz L, Otis CN. Diagnostic accuracy of image-guided percutaneous fine needle aspiration biopsy of the mediastinum. *Diagn Cytopathol* 2007;35:705–709.
6. Yu GH, Salhany KE, Gokaslan ST, et al. Thymic epithelial cells as a diagnostic pitfall in the fine needle aspiration diagnosis of primary mediastinal lymphoma. *Diagn Cytopathol* 1997;16:460–465.
7. Rosai J, Levine GD. Tumors of the thymus. In *Atlas of Tumor Pathology*. Series 2, Fascicle 13. Washington, DC: Armed Forces Institute of Pathology, 1976.
8. Flinner RL, Hammond EH. *Pathology of the Mediastinum*. Chicago, IL: ASCP Press, 1989.
9. Marchevsky AM, Kaneko M. *Surgical Pathology of the Mediastinum*. 2nd edition. New York, NY: Raven Press, 1992.
10. Kornstein MJ. *Pathology of the Thymus and Mediastinum*. Philadelphia, PA: WB Saunders, 1995.
11. Strickler JG, Kurtin PJ. Mediastinal lymphoma. *Semin Diagn Pathol* 1991;8:2–13.
12. Frizzera G. Castleman's disease and related disorders. *Semin Diagn Pathol* 1988;5:346–364.
13. Shimosato Y, Mukai K. Tumors of the mediastinum. In Rosai J, ed. *Atlas of Tumor Pathology*. Series 3, Fascicle 21. Washington, DC: Armed Forces Institute of Pathology, 1997:33–273.
14. Slater G, Papatestas AE, Genkins G, et al. Thymomas in patients with myasthenia gravis. *Ann Surg* 1978;188:171–174.
15. Debono DJ, Loehrer PJ. Thymic neoplasms. *Curr Opin Oncol* 1996;8:112–119.
16. Matsui M, Wada H, Ohta M, et al. Potential role of thymoma and other mediastinal tumors in the pathogenesis of myasthenia gravis. *J Neuroimmunol* 1993;44:171–176.
17. Offner F, Vallaeys J, Roels H, et al. Thymoma: a clinicopathological comparative study of 25 cases. *Eur Respir J* 1991;4:1060–1065.
18. Ohmi M, Ohuchi M. Recurrent thymoma in patients with myasthenia gravis. *Ann Thorac Surg* 1990;50:243–247.
19. Onoda K, Namikawa S, Takao M, et al. Fulminant myasthenia gravis manifested after removal of anterior mediastinal tumor. *Ann Thorac Surg* 1996;62:1534–1536.
20. Wu MH, Low TL. Distribution of thymic hormones in thymic tumors and myasthenic thymus. *Proc Natl Sci Counc Repub China B* 1996;20:1–5.
21. LeMarc'hadour F, Pinel N, Pasquier B, et al. Thymolipoma in association with myasthenia gravis. *Am J Surg Pathol* 1991;15:802–809.
22. Liu KL, Herbrecht R, Tranchant C, et al. Malignant thymic lymphoblastic lymphoma and myasthenia gravis: an exceptional association. *Nouv Rev Fr Hematol* 1992;34:221–223.
23. Gafni J, Michaeli D, Heller H. Idiopathic acquired agammaglobulinemia associated with thymoma: report of two cases and review of the literature. *N Engl J Med* 1960;263:536–541.
24. Rogers BHG, Manaligod JR, Blazek WV. Thymoma associated with pancytopenia and hypogammaglobulinemia: report of a case and review of the literature. *Am J Med* 1968;44:154–164.
25. Hirst E, Robertson TI. The syndrome of thymoma and erythroblastopenic anemia: a review of 56 cases including 3 case reports. *Medicine* 1967;46:225–264.
26. Masuda M, Arai Y, Okamura T, et al. Pure red cell aplasia with thymoma: evidence of a T-cell clonal disorder. *Am J Hematol* 1997;54:324–328.
27. Null JA, LiVolsi VA, Glenn WWL. Hodgkin's disease of the thymus ("granulomatous thymoma") and myasthenia gravis: a unique association. *Am J Clin Pathol* 1977;67:521–525.

28. Nagasawa T, Abe T, Nakagawa T. Pure red cell aplasia and hypogammaglobulinemia associated with T-gamma chronic lymphocytic leukemia. *Blood* 1981;57:1025–1031.

29. Souadjian JV, Enriquez P, Silverstein MN, et al. The spectrum of diseases associated with thymoma: coincidence or syndrome? *Arch Intern Med* 1974;134:374–379.

30. Moysset I, Lloreta J, Miguel A, et al. Thymoma associated with CD4+ lymphopenia, cytomegalovirus infection, and Kaposi's sarcoma. *Hum Pathol* 1997;28:1211–1213.

31. Kuo TT, Shih LY. Histologic types of thymoma associated with pure red cell aplasia: a study of five cases including a composite tumor of organoid thymoma associated with an unusual lipofibroadenoma. *Int J Surg Pathol* 2001;9:29–35.

32. Murakawa T, Nakajima J, Sato H, et al. Thymoma associated with pure red cell aplasia: clinical features and prognosis. *Asian Cardiovasc Thorac Ann* 2002;10:150–154.

33. Katsuta H, Okada M, Nakauchi T, et al. Cancer-associated retinopathy associated with invasive thymoma. *Am J Ophthalmol* 2002;134:383–389.

34. Sader C, Sharma S, Edwards MG. Graft-versus-host disease-type colitis: an unusual association of malignant thymoma. *Ann Thorac Surg* 2002;73:1947–1948.

35. Hirai Y, Yamanaka A, Fujimoto T, et al. Multiple thymomas with myotonic dystrophy. *Jpn J Thorac Cardiovasc Surg* 2001;49:457–460.

36. Wick MR, Rosai J. Neuroendocrine neoplasms of the thymus. *Pathol Res Pract* 1988;183: 188–199.

37. Argani P, Erlandson RA, Rosai J. Thymic neuroblastoma in adults: report of three cases with special emphasis on its association with the syndrome of inappropriate secretion of antidiuretic hormone. *Am J Clin Pathol* 1997;108:537–543.

38. Asada Y, Marutsuka K, Mitsukawa T, et al. Ganglioneuroblastoma of the thymus: an adult case with the syndrome of inappropriate secretion of antidiuretic hormone. *Hum Pathol* 1996;27:506–509.

39. He J, Zhou J, Lu Z. Radiotherapy of ectopic ACTH syndrome due to thoracic carcinoids. *Chin Med J* 1995;108:338–341.

40. Kimura N, Ishikawa T, Sasaki Y, et al. Expression of prohormone convertase, PC2, in adrenocorticotrophin-producing thymic carcinoid with elevated plasma corticotrophin-releasing hormone. *J Clin Endocrinol Metab* 1996;81:390–395.

41. Martinez-Cerezo FJ, Garreta J, Gonzalez T, et al. Thymus carcinoid associated with type I multiple endocrine neoplasia syndrome. *Med Clin (Barc)* 1996;106:21–23.

42. Matejka G, Toubeau M, Bernard A, et al. Thymic carcinoid tumor causing paraneoplastic Cushing's syndrome. *Presse Med* 1996;25:1201–1202.

43. Ozawa Y, Tomoyasu H, Takeshita A, et al. Shift from CRH to ACTH production in a thymic carcinoid with Cushing's syndrome. *Horm Res* 1996;45:264–268.

44. Schaaf L, Nies G, Raue F, et al. Diagnosis, therapy, and screening of multiple endocrine neoplasia type I (MEN-I) in four endocrinologic centers. *Med Klin* 1994;89:1–6.

45. Teh BT, McArdle J, Chan SP, et al. Clinicopathologic studies of thymic carcinoids in multiple endocrine neoplasia, type I. *Medicine (Balt)* 1997;76:21–29.

46. Boix E, Pico A, Pinedo R, et al. Ectopic growth hormone-releasing hormone secretion by thymic carcinoid tumor. *Clin Endocrinol* 2002;57:131–134.

47. Andres R, Mayordomo JI, Ramon-y-Cajal S, et al. Paraneoplastic Cushing's syndrome associated to locally advanced thymic carcinoid tumor. *Tumori* 2002;88:65–67.

48. Kuo TT. Pigmented spindle cell carcinoid tumor of the thymus with ectopic adrenocorticotropic hormone secretion: report of a rare variant and differential diagnosis of mediastinal spindle cell neoplasms. *Histopathology* 2002;40:159–165.

49. de Perrot M, Spiliopoulos A, Fischer S, et al. Neuroendocrine carcinoma (carcinoid) of the thymus associated with Cushing's syndrome. *Ann Thorac Surg* 2002;73:675–681.

50. Hekimgil M, Hamulu F, Cagirici U, et al. Small cell neuroendocrine carcinoma of the thymus complicated by Cushing's syndrome: report of a 58-year-old woman with a 3-year history of hypertension. *Pathol Res Pract* 2001;197:129–133.

51. Faber LP. Lung cancer. In Holleb AI, Fink DJ, Murphy GP, eds. *American Cancer Society Textbook of Clinical Oncology*. New York, NY: American Cancer Society, 1991:194–212.

52. Negron-Soto JM, Cascacde PN. Squamous cell carcinoma of the thymus with paraneoplastic hypercalcemia. *Clin Imaging* 1995;24:122–124.

53. Takayama T, Kameya T, Inagaki K, et al. MEN type I associated with mediastinal carcinoid producing parathyroid hormone, calcitonin, and chorionic gonadotropin. *Pathol Res Pract* 1993;189:1090–1100.

54. Yoshikawa T, Noguichi Y, Matsukawa H, et al. Thymus carcinoid producing parathyroid hormone (PTH)-related protein: report of a case. *Surg Today* 1994;24:544–547.

55. Knapp RH, Fritz SR, Reiman HM. Primary embryonal carcinoma and choriocarcinoma of the mediastinum. *Arch Pathol Lab Med* 1982;106:507–509.

56. Gallivan MVE, Chun B, Rowden G, et al. Intrathoracic paravertebral malignant paraganglioma. *Arch Pathol Lab Med* 1980;104:46–51.

57. Boneschi M, Erba M, Giuffrida GF, et al. Mediastinal functioning paraganglioma: a case report. *Minerva Chir* 1993;48:1455–1458.

58. Neumann DR, Basile KE, Bravo EL, et al. Malignant pheochromocytoma of the anterior mediastinum: PET findings with [18f]FDG and 82Rb. *J Comput Assist Tomogr* 1996;20: 312–316.

59. Rosen EM, Cassady JR, Frantz CN, et al. Neuroblastoma: the Joint Center for Radiation Therapy/Dana Farber Center Institute/Children's Hospital experience. *J Clin Oncol* 1984; 2:719–732.

60. Downie PA, Vogelzang NJ, Moldwin RL, et al. Establishment of a leukemia cell line with i(12p) from a patient with a mediastinal germ cell tumor and acute lymphoblastic leukemia. *Cancer Res* 1994;54:4999–5004.

61. Joos H, Frick J, Wessely K, et al. Mediastinal tumor and Klinefelter's syndrome. *Eur Urol* 1994;26:344–346.

62. Ohmichi M, Hiraga Y, Miyazaki M, et al. Thymic carcinoma associated with pulmonary sarcoidosis. *Nippon Kyobu Shikkan Gakkai Zasshi* 1997;35:571–576.

63. Do YS, Im JG, Lee BH, et al. CT findings in malignant tumors of thymic epithelium. *J Comput Assist Tomogr* 1995;19:192–197.

64. Kushihashi T, Fujisawa H, Munechika H. Magnetic resonance imaging of thymic epithelial tumors. *Crit Rev Diagn Imaging* 1996;37:191–259.

65. Wernecke K, Vassallo P, Rutsch F, et al. Thymic involvement in Hodgkin's disease: CT and sonographic findings. *Radiology* 1991;181:375–383.

66. Sakai S, Murayama S, Soeda H, et al. Differential diagnosis between thymoma and non-thymoma by dynamic MR imaging. *Acta Radiol* 2002;43:262–268.

67. Jung KJ, Lee KS, Han J, et al. Malignant thymic epithelial tumors: CT-pathologic correlation. *Am J Roentgenol* 2001;176:433–439.

68. Kreel L. Computed tomography of the thorax. *Radiol Clin North Am* 1978;16:575–584.

69. Gamsu G, Webb WR, Sheldon P, et al. Nuclear magnetic resonance imaging of the thorax. *Radiology* 1983;147:473–480.

70. Baron RL, Lee JKT, Sagel SS, et al. Computed tomography of the abnormal thymus. *Radiology* 1982;142:127–134.

71. Zerhouni EA, Scott WW, Jr., Baker RR, et al. Invasive thymomas: diagnosis and evaluation by computed tomography. *J Comput Assist Tomogr* 1982;6:92–100.

72. Brown LR, Aughenbaugh GL, Wick MR, et al. Roentgenologic diagnosis of primary corticotrophin-producing carcinoid tumors of the mediastinum. *Radiology* 1982;142:143–148.

73. Lewis BD, Hurt RD, Payne WS, et al. Benign teratomas of the mediastinum. *J Thorac Cardiovasc Surg* 1983;86:727–731.

74. Kirwan WO, Walbaum PR, McCormack RM. Cystic intrathoracic derivatives of the foregut and their complications. *Thorax* 1973;28:424–428.

75. Salyer DC, Salyer WR, Eggleston JC. Benign developmental cysts of the mediastinum. *Arch Pathol Lab Med* 1977;101:136–139.

75a. Wick MR. Cystic lesions of the mediastinum. *Semin Diagn Pathol* 2005;22:241–253.

76. Wick MR. Mediastinal cysts and intrathoracic thyroid tumors. *Semin Diagn Pathol* 1990;7: 285–294.

77. Langman J. *Medical Embryology*. Baltimore, MD: Williams & Wilkins, 1969:183–280.

78. Gilmour JR. The embryology of the parathyroid glands, the thymus, and certain associated rudiments. *J Pathol Bacteriol* 1937;45:507–522.

79. Van Hoeven KH, Brennan MF. Lipothymoadenoma of the parathyroid. *Arch Pathol Lab Med* 1993;117:312–314.

80. Clark OH. Mediastinal parathyroid tumors. *Arch Surg* 1988;123:1096–1100.

81. Krech WG, Storey CF, Umiker WC. Thymic cysts: a review of the literature and report of two cases. *J Thorac Cardiovasc Surg* 1954;27:477–493.

82. Suster S, Rosai J. Multilocular thymic cyst: an acquired reactive process. Study of 18 cases. *Am J Surg Pathol* 1991;15:388–398.

83. Zanca P, Chuang TH, De Avila R, et al. True congenital mediastinal thymic cyst. *Pediatrics* 1965;36:615–619.

84. Bieger RC, McAdams AJ. Thymic cysts. *Arch Pathol* 1966;82:535–541.

85. Leong ASY. Thymic cysts. In Givel JC, ed. *Surgery of the Thymus*. Berlin, Germany: Springer-Verlag, 1990:71–77.

86. Breckler IA, Johnston DG. Choristoma of the thymus. *Am J Dis Child* 1956;92:175–178.

87. Suster S, Barbuto D, Carlson G, et al. Multilocular thymic cysts with pseudoepitheliomatous hyperplasia. *Hum Pathol* 1991;22:455–460.

88. Michal M, Havlicek F. Pseudo-epitheliomatous hyperplasia in thymic cysts. *Histopathology* 1991;19:281–282.

89. Leong ASY, Brown JH. Malignant transformation in a thymic cyst. *Am J Surg Pathol* 1984; 8:471–475.

90. Snover DC, Levine GD, Rosai J. Thymic carcinomas: five distinctive histological variants. *Am J Surg Pathol* 1982;6:451–470.

91. Suster S, Rosai J. Thymic carcinoma: a clinicopathologic study of 60 cases. *Cancer* 1991; 67:1025–1032.

92. Iezzoni JC, Nass LB. Thymic basaloid carcinoma: a case report and review of the literature. *Mod Pathol* 1996;9:21–25.

93. Yamashita S, Yamazaki H, Kato T, et al. Thymic carcinoma which developed in a thymic cyst. *Intern Med* 1996;35:215–218.

93a. Moran CA, Suster S, Silva EG. Low-grade serous carcinoma of the ovary metastatic to the anterior mediastinum simulating multilocular thymic cysts: a clinicopathologic and immunohistochemical study of 3 cases. *Am J Surg Pathol* 2005;29:496–499.

94. Baron RL, Sagel SS, Baglan RJ. Thymic cysts following radiation therapy for Hodgkin's disease. *Radiology* 1981;41:593–597.

95. Murray JA, Parker AC. Mediastinal Hodgkin's disease and thymic cysts. *Acta Haematol* 1984;71:282–284.

96. Lewis CR, Manoharan A. Benign thymic cysts in Hodgkin's disease: report of a case and review of published cases. *Thorax* 1987;42:633–634.

97. Kaesberg PR, Foley DB, Pellett J, et al. Concurrent development of a thymic cyst and mediastinal Hodgkin's disease. *Med Pediatr Oncol* 1988;16:293–294.

98. Suster S, Moran CA. Malignant thymic neoplasms that may mimic benign conditions. *Semin Diagn Pathol* 1995;12:98–104.

99. Katz M, Peikarski JD, Bayle-Weisgerber C, et al. Residual mediastinal mass following radiation therapy for Hodgkin's disease. *Ann Radiol* 1977;20:667–672.

100. Jaramillo P, Perez-Atayde A, Griscom NT. Apparent association between thymic cysts and prior thoracotomy. *Radiology* 1989;172:207–209.

101. Maier HC. Bronchogenic cysts of the mediastinum. *Ann Surg* 1948;127:476–502.

102. Ramenofsky ML, Leape LL, McCauley RGK. Bronchogenic cyst. *J Pediatr Surg* 1979;14: 219–224.

103. Agha FP, Master K, Kaplan S, et al. Multiple bronchogenic cysts in the mediastinum. *Br J Radiol* 1975;48:54–57.

104. Robbins LL. The roentgenologic appearance of "bronchiogenic" cysts. *AJR* 1943;50: 321–333.

105. Abell MR. Mediastinal cysts. *Arch Pathol* 1956;61:360–371.

106. Morrison IM. Tumors and cysts of the mediastinum. *Thorax* 1958;13:294–307.

107. Lillie WI, McDonald JR, Clagett OT. Pericardial celomic cysts and pericardial diverticula: a concept of etiology and report of cases. *J Thorac Surg* 1950;20:494–504.

108. Ladd WE, Scott HW, Jr. Esophageal duplications or mediastinal cysts of enteric origin. *Surgery* 1944;16:815–835.

109. Black RA, Benjamin EL. Enterogenous abnormalities: cysts and diverticula. *Am J Dis Child* 1936;51:1126–1137.

110. Poncher HG, Milles F. Cysts and diverticula of intestinal origin. *Am J Dis Child* 1933;45:1064–1078.

111. Veeneklass GMH. Pathogenesis of intrathoracic gastrogenic cysts. *Am J Dis Child* 1952;83:500–507.

112. Fallon M, Gordon ARG, Lendrum AC. Mediastinal cysts of foregut origin associated with vertebral abnormalities. *Br J Surg* 1954;41:520–533.

113. Sabiston D, Scott HW. Primary neoplasms and cysts of the mediastinum. *Ann Surg* 1961;136:777–797.

114. Chitale AR. Gastric cyst of the mediastinum: a distinctive clinicopathological entity. *J Pediatr* 1969;75:104–110.

115. Crispin RH, Logan WD Jr, Abbott OA. Mediastinal gastroenteric cyst with vertebral anomaly. *Dis Chest* 1965;47:346–347.

116. Spock A, Schneider S, Baylin J. Mediastinal gastric cysts. *Am Rev Respir Dis* 1966;94:97–110.

117. Pachter MR, Lattes R. Mesenchymal tumors of the mediastinum. III. Tumors of lymph vascular origin. *Cancer* 1963;16:108–117.

118. Brown LR, Reiman HM, Rosenow EC III, et al. Intrathoracic lymphangioma. *Mayo Clin Proc* 1986;61:882–892.

119. Feng YF, Masterson JB, Riddell RH. Lymphangioma of the middle mediastinum as an incidental finding on a chest radiograph. *Thorax* 1980;35:955–956.

120. Curley SA, Ablin DS, Kosloske AM. Giant cystic hygroma of the posterior mediastinum. *J Pediatr Surg* 1989;24:398–400.

121. Perkes EA, Haller JO, Kassner EG, et al. Mediastinal cystic hygroma in infants: two cases with no extension into the neck. *Clin Pediatr* 1979;18:168–170.

122. Sumner TE, Volberg FM, Kiser PE, et al. Mediastinal cystic hygroma in children. *Pediatr Radiol* 1981;11:160–162.

123. Scholefield JH, Angwin R. Posterior mediastinal lymphangioma presenting with thoracic inlet compression. *Br J Hosp Med* 1989;41:183–184.

123a. Park JG, Aubry MC, Godfrey JA, et al. Mediastinal lymphangioma: Mayo Clinic experience of 25 cases. *Mayo Clin Proc* 2006;81:197–203.

124. Feutz EP, Yune HY, Mandelbaum I, et al. Intrathoracic cystic hygroma: a report of three cases. *Radiology* 1973;108:61–66.

125. Swanson PE. Soft tissue neoplasms of the mediastinum. *Semin Diagn Pathol* 1991;8:14–34.

126. LeRoux BT, Kallichurum S, Shama DM. Mediastinal cysts and tumors. *Curr Probl Surg* 1984;21:1–77.

127. Wychulis AR, Payne WS, Clagett OT, et al. Surgical treatment of mediastinal tumors: a 40-year experience. *J Thorac Cardiovasc Surg* 1971;62:379–392.

128. Gonzalez-Crussi F. Extragonadal teratomas. In *Atlas of Tumor Pathology*. Series 2, Fascicle 18. Washington, DC: Armed Forces Institute of Pathology, 1982:77–94.

129. Mullen B, Richardson JD. Primary anterior mediastinal tumors in children and adults. *Ann Thorac Surg* 1986;42:338–345.

130. Karl SR, Dunn J. Posterior mediastinal teratomas. *J Pediatr Surg* 1985;20:508–510.

131. Dehner LP. Germ cell tumors of the mediastinum. *Semin Diagn Pathol* 1990;7:266–284.

132. Nichols CR, Heerema NA, Palmer C, et al. Klinefelter's syndrome associated with mediastinal germ cell neoplasms. *J Clin Oncol* 1987;5:266–284.

132a. Wu TT, Wang HC, Chang YC, et al. Mature mediastinal teratoma: sonographic imaging patterns and pathologic correlation. *J Ultrasound Med* 2002;21:759–765.

133. Dehner LP. Gonadal and extragonadal germ cell neoplasms and teratomas in childhood. In Finegold M, ed. *Pathology of Neoplasia in Children and Adolescents*. Philadelphia, PA: WB Saunders, 1986:282–312.

134. Wick MR, Rosai J. Neuroendocrine, germ cell, and nonepithelial tumors. In Givel JC, ed. *Surgery of the Thymus*. Berlin, Germany: Springer-Verlag, 1990:109–150.

135. Carter D, Bibro MC, Touloukian RJ. Benign clinical behavior of immature mediastinal teratoma in infancy and childhood: report of two cases and review of the literature. *Cancer* 1982;49:398–402.

136. Ulbright TM, Clark SA, Einhorn LH. Angiosarcoma associated with germ cell tumors. *Hum Pathol* 1985;16:268–272.

137. Manivel C, Wick MR, Abenoza P, et al. The occurrence of sarcomatous components in primary mediastinal germ cell tumors. *Am J Surg Pathol* 1986;10:711–717.

138. Cushing B, Bhanot PK, Watts FB, Jr., et al. Rhabdomyosarcoma and benign teratoma. *Pediatr Pathol* 1983;1:345–348.

139. Warren JS, Yum MN. Carcinoid tumor arising in a treated primary germ cell tumor of the mediastinum. *South Med J* 1987;80:259–261.

139a. Hsu JS, Kang WY, Chou SH, et al. Mature cystic teratoma in the anterior mediastinum containing a carcinoid. *J Thorac Imaging* 2006;21:60–62.

139b. Malagon HD, Valdez AM, Moran CA, et al. Germ cell tumors with sarcomatous components: a clinicopathologic and immunohistochemical study of 46 cases. *Am J Surg Pathol* 2007;31:1365–1362.

140. Parker D, Holford CP, Begent RHJ, et al. Effective treatment for malignant mediastinal teratoma. *Thorax* 1983;38:897–902.

141. Mihal V, Dusek J, Jarosova M, et al. Mediastinal teratoma and acute megakaryoblastic leukemia. *Neoplasma* 1989;36:739–747.

142. DeMent SH, Eggleston JC, Spivak JL. Association between mediastinal germ cell tumors and hematologic malignancies: report of two cases and review of the literature. *Am J Surg Pathol* 1985;9:23–30.

143. Chaganti RSK, Ladanyi M, Samaniego F, et al. Leukemic differentiation of a mediastinal germ cell tumor. *Genes Chromosomes Cancer* 1989;1:83–87.

144. Moran CA, Suster S. Thymoma with prominent cystic and hemorrhagic changes and areas of necrosis and infarction: a clinicopathologic study of 25 cases. *Am J Surg Pathol* 2001;25:1086–1090.

145. Moran CA, Suster S. Mediastinal seminomas with prominent cystic changes: a clinicopathologic study of 10 cases. *Am J Surg Pathol* 1995;25:1047–1053.

146. Schnyder P, Candardjis G. Computed tomography of thymic abnormalities. *Eur J Radiol* 1987;7:107–113.

147. Bernatz PE, Harrison EG, Jr., Clagett OT. Thymoma: a clinicopathologic study. *J Thorac Cardiovasc Surg* 1961;42:424–444.

148. Lewis JE, Wick MR, Scheithauer BW, et al. Thymoma: a clinicopathologic review. *Cancer* 1987;60:2727–2743.

149. Marino M, Muller-Hermelink HK. Thymoma and thymic carcinoma: relation of thymoma epithelial cells to the cortical and medullary differentiation of thymus. *Virchows Arch A Pathol Anat Histopathol* 1985;407:119–149.

150. Muller-Hermelink HK, Marino M, Palestro G. Pathology of thymic epithelial tumors. *Curr Topics Pathol* 1986;75:207–268.

151. Kornstein MJ. Controversies regarding the pathology of thymomas. *Pathol Annu* 1992;27(Part 2):1–15.

152. Pescarmona E, Rendina EA, Venuta F, et al. Analysis of prognostic factors and clinicopathological staging of thymoma. *Ann Thorac Surg* 1990;50:534–538.

153. Lequaglie C, Giudice G, Brega-Massone PP, et al. Clinical and pathologic predictors of survival in patients with thymic tumors. *J Cardiovasc Surg* 2002;43:269–274.

154. Rios A, Torres J, Galindo PJ, et al. Prognostic factors in thymic epithelial neoplasms. *Eur J Cardiothorac Surg* 2002;21:307–313.

155. Lardinois D, Rechsteiner R, Lang RH, et al. Prognostic relevance of Masaoka and Muller-Hermelink classification in patients with thymic tumors. *Ann Thorac Surg* 2000;69:1550–1555.

156. Kirchner T, Schalke B, Buchwald J, et al. Well-differentiated thymic carcinoma: an organotypical low-grade carcinoma with relationship to cortical thymoma. *Am J Surg Pathol* 1992;16:1153–1169.

157. Koga K, Matsuno Y, Noguchi M, et al. A review of 79 thymomas: modification of staging system and reappraisal of conventional division into invasive and non-invasive thymoma. *Pathol Int* 1994;44:359–367.

158. Dawson A, Ibrahim NB, Gibbs AR. Observer variation in the histopathological classification of thymomas: correlation with prognosis. *J Clin Pathol* 1994;47:519–523.

159. Moran CA, Suster S. On the histologic heterogeneity of thymic epithelial neoplasms: impact of sampling in subtyping and classification of thymomas. *Am J Clin Pathol* 2000;114:760–766.

160. Pan CC, Chen WY, Chiang H. Spindle cell and mixed spindle/lymphocytic thymomas: an integrated clinicopathologic and immunohistochemical study of 81 cases. *Am J Surg Pathol* 2001;25:111–120.

161. Engel P, Pilsgaard B, Francis D. Thymomas and thymic carcinomas: a retrospective investigation with histological reclassification. *APMIS* 1995;103:671–678.

162. Ho FC, Fu KH, Lam SY, et al. Evaluation of a histogenetic classification for thymic epithelial tumours. *Histopathology* 1994;25:21–29.

163. Kuo TT, Lo SK. Thymoma: a study of the pathologic classification of 71 cases with evaluation of the Muller-Hermelink system. *Hum Pathol* 1993;24:766–771.

164. Pescarmona E, Rendina EA, Venuta F, et al. The prognostic implication of thymoma histologic subtyping: a study of 80 consecutive cases. *Am J Clin Pathol* 1990;93:190–195.

165. Quintanilla-Martinez L, Wilkins EW, Jr., Ferry JA, et al. Thymoma—morphologic subclassification correlates with invasiveness and immunohistologic features: a study of 122 cases. *Hum Pathol* 1993;24:958–969.

166. Quintanilla-Martinez L, Wilkins EW, Jr., Choi N, et al. Thymoma: histologic subclassification is an independent prognostic factor. *Cancer* 1994;74:606–617.

167. Regnard JF, Magdeleinat P, Dromer C, et al. Prognostic factors and long-term results after thymoma resection: a series of 307 patients. *J Thorac Cardiovasc Surg* 1996;112:376–384.

168. Schneider PM, Fellbaum C, Fink U, et al. Prognostic importance of histomorphologic subclassification for epithelial thymic tumors. *Ann Surg Oncol* 1997;4:46–56.

169. Tan PH, Sng IT. Thymoma—a study of 60 cases in Singapore. *Histopathology* 1995;26:509–518.

170. Rosai J. *Histological Typing of Tumors of the Thymus [World Health Organization]*. 2nd edition. Berlin, Germany: Springer, 1999:9–15.

171. Chen G, Marx A, Wen-Hu C, et al. New WHO classification predicts prognosis of thymic epithelial tumors: a clinicopathologic study of 200 thymoma cases from China. *Cancer* 2002;95:420–429.

172. Okumura M, Ohta M, Miyoshi S, et al. Oncological significance of WHO histological thymoma classification: a clinical study based on 286 patients. *Jpn J Thorac Cardiovasc Surg* 2002;50:189–194.

173. Okumura M, Ohta M, Tateyama H, et al. The World Health Organization histologic classification system reflects the oncologic behavior of thymoma: a clinical study of 273 patients. *Cancer* 2002;94:624–632.

174. Okumura M, Miyoshi S, Fujii Y, et al. Clinical and functional significance of WHO classification on human thymic epithelial neoplasms: a study of 146 consecutive tumors. *Am J Surg Pathol* 2001;25:103–110.

175. Dadmanesh F, Sekihara T, Rosai J. Histologic typing of thymoma according to the new World Health Organization classification. *Chest Surg Clin N Am* 2001;11:407–420.

176. Suster S, Moran CA. Thymoma, atypical thymoma, and thymic carcinoma: a novel conceptual approach to the classification of thymic epithelial neoplasms. *Am J Clin Pathol* 1999;111:826–833.

177. Suster S, Moran CA. Primary thymic epithelial neoplasms: spectrum of differentiation and histological features. *Semin Diagn Pathol* 1999;16:2–17.

177a. Suster S, Moran CA. Problem areas and inconsistencies in the WHO classification of thymoma. *Semin Diagn Pathol* 2005;22:188–197.

178. Wick MR. Assessing the prognosis of thymomas. *Ann Thorac Surg* 1990;50:521–522.

179. Lara PN, Jr. Malignant thymoma: current status and future directions. *Cancer Treat Rev* 2000;26:127–131.

180. Loehrer PJ, Sr., Wick MR. Thymic malignancies. *Cancer Treat Res* 2001;105:277–302.

181. Moore KH, McKenzie PR, Kennedy CW, et al. Thymoma: trends over time. *Ann Thorac Surg* 2001;72:203–207.

182. Mehran R, Ghosh R, Maziak D, et al. Surgical treatment of thymoma. *Can J Surg* 2002;45:25–30.

183. Matsushima S, Yamamoto H, Egami K, et al. Evaluation of the prognostic factors after thymoma resection. *Int Surg* 2001;86:103–106.

184. Masaoka A, Monden Y, Nakahara K, et al. Follow-up study of thymomas with special reference to their clinical stages. *Cancer* 1981;48:2485–2492.

185. Masaoka A, Yamakawa Y. TNM classification of thymic epithelial tumors. *Gan To Kagaku Ryoho* 1997;24:749–754.

186. Cowen D, Richaud P, Mornex F, et al. Thymoma: results of a multicentric retrospective series of 149 non-metastatic irradiated patients and review of the literature. *Radiother Oncol* 1995;34:9–16.

187. Zhang Z, Ge F, Li S, et al. Factors affecting removal and prognosis of thymic tumors. *Chin Med Sci J* 1995;10:229–231.

188. DeMontpreville VT, Dulmet E. Thymomas and carcinoma of the thymus: which classification should be used? *Ann Pathol (Paris)* 1996;16:159–166.

189. Rice HE, Flake AW, Hori T, et al. Massive thymic hyperplasia: characterization of a rare mediastinal mass. *J Pediatr Surg* 1994;29:1561–1564.

190. Levine GD, Rosai J. Thymic hyperplasia and neoplasia: a review of current concepts. *Hum Pathol* 1978;9:495–515.

191. Grody WW, Jobst S, Keesey J, et al. Pathologic evaluation of thymic hyperplasia and myasthenia gravis and Lambert-Eaton syndrome. *Arch Pathol Lab Med* 1986;110:843–846.

192. Hofmann WJ, Moller P, Otto HF. Thymic hyperplasia. II. Lymphofollicular hyperplasia of the thymus: an immunohistologic study. *Klin Wochenschr* 1987;65:53–60.

193. Hofmann WJ, Moller P, Otto HF. Hyperplasia. In Givel JC, ed. *Surgery of the Thymus*. Berlin, Germany: Springer-Verlag, 1990:59–70.

194. Wick MR, Rosai J. Epithelial tumors. In Givel JC, ed. *Surgery of the Thymus*. Berlin, Germany: Springer-Verlag, 1990:79–107.

195. Walker AN, Mills SE, Fechner RE. Thymomas and thymic carcinomas. *Semin Diagn Pathol* 1990;7:250–265.

196. Pescarmona E, Pisacane A, Rendina EA, et al. "Organoid" thymoma: a well-differentiated variant with distinctive clinicopathological features. *Histopathology* 1991;18:161–164.

197. Battifora H, Sun TT, Bahu RM, et al. The use of antikeratin antiserum as a diagnostic tool: thymoma versus lymphoma. *Hum Pathol* 1980;11:635–641.

198. Wick MR, Simpson RW, Niehans GA, et al. Anterior mediastinal tumors: a clinicopathologic study of 100 cases, with emphasis on immunohistochemical analysis. *Prog Surg Pathol* 1990;11:79–119.

199. Suster S, Moran CA. Micronodular thymoma with lymphoid B-cell hyperplasia: clinicopathologic and immunohistochemical study of eighteen cases of a distinctive morphologic variant of thymic epithelial neoplasm. *Am J Surg Pathol* 1999;23:955–962.

200. Tateyama H, Saito Y, Fujii Y, et al. The spectrum of micronodular thymic epithelial tumors with lymphoid B-cell hyperplasia. *Histopathology* 2001;38:519–527.

201. Tung KSK, McCormack LJ. Angiomatoid lymphoid hamartoma: report of five cases with a review of the literature. *Cancer* 1967;20:525–536.

202. Castleman B, Iverson L, Pardo-Menendez V. Localized mediastinal lymph node hyperplasia resembling thymoma. *Cancer* 1956;9:822–830.

203. Keller AR, Hochholzer L, Castleman B. Hyaline-vascular and plasma-cell types of giant lymph node hyperplasia of the mediastinum and other locations. *Cancer* 1972;29:670–683.

203a. Strobel P, Marino M, Feuchtenberger M, et al. Micronodular thymoma: an epithelial tumor with abnormal chemokine expression setting the stage for lymphoma development. *J Pathol* 2005;207:72–82.

204. Baldit C, Trojani M, Eghbali H, et al. Lymphoblastic lymphoma with convoluted nuclei: a report of 19 cases. *Oncology* 1984;41:252–256.

205. Nathwani BN, Kim H, Rappaport H. Malignant lymphoma, lymphoblastic. *Cancer* 1976; 38:964–983.

206. Nathwani BN, Diamond LW, Winberg CD, et al. Lymphoblastic lymphoma: a clinicopathologic study of 95 patients. *Cancer* 1981;48:2347–2357.

207. Shikano T, Arioka H, Kobayashi R, et al. Acute lymphoblastic leukemia and non-Hodgkin's lymphoma with mediastinal mass—a study of 23 children; different disorders or different stages? *Leuk Lymphoma* 1994;13:161–167.

208. Streuli RA, Kaneko Y, Variakojis D, et al. Lymphoblastic lymphoma in adults. *Cancer* 1981; 47:2510–2516.

209. Coleman CN, Picozzi VJ, Cox RS, et al. Treatment of lymphoblastic lymphoma in adults. *J Clin Oncol* 1986;4:1628–1637.

210. Shachor Y, Radnay J, Bernheim J, et al. Malignant thymoma with peripheral blood lymphocytosis. *Cancer* 1988;61:1222–1227.

211. Chan JKC, Tsang WY, Seneviratne S, et al. The MIC2 antibody O13: practical application for the study of thymic epithelial tumors. *Am J Surg Pathol* 1995;19:1115–1123.

212. Robertson PB, Neiman RS, Worapongpaiboon S, et al. O13 (CD99) positivity in hematologic proliferations correlates with TdT positivity. *Mod Pathol* 1997;10:277–282.

213. Soslow RA, Bhargava V, Warnke RA. MIC2, TdT, bcl-2, and CD34 expression in paraffin-embedded high-grade lymphoma/acute lymphoblastic leukemia distinguishes between distinct clinicopathologic entities. *Hum Pathol* 1997;28:1158–1165.

214. Brocheriou I, Carnot F, Briere J. Immunohistochemical detection of bcl-2 protein in thymoma. *Histopathology* 1995;27:251–255.

215. Chen FF, Yan JJ, Jin YT, et al. Detection of bcl-2 and p53 in thymoma: expression of bcl-2 as a reliable marker of tumor aggressiveness. *Hum Pathol* 1996;27:1089–1092.

216. Chan WC, Zaatari GS, Tabei S, et al. Thymoma: an immunohistochemical study. *Am J Clin Pathol* 1984;82:160–166.

217. Knowles DM II. Lymphoid cell markers: their distribution and usefulness in the immunopathologic analysis of lymphoid neoplasms. *Am J Surg Pathol* 1985;9(Suppl):85–108.

218. Weiss LM, Bindl JM, Picozzi VJ, et al. Lymphoblastic lymphoma: an immunophenotypic study of 26 cases with comparison to T-cell acute lymphoblastic leukemia. *Blood* 1986;67: 474–478.

219. Picker LJ, Weiss LM, Medeiros LJ, et al. Immunophenotypic criteria for the diagnosis of non-Hodgkin's lymphoma. *Am J Pathol* 1987;128:181–201.

220. Berrih-Aknin S, Safar D, Cohen-Kaminsky S. Analysis of lymphocyte phenotype in human thymomas. *Adv Exp Med Biol* 1988;237:369–374.

221. Ito M, Taki T, Mihaye M, et al. Lymphocyte subsets in human thymoma studied with monoclonal antibodies. *Cancer* 1988;61:284–287.

222. DiComo CJ, Urist MJ, Babayan I, et al. p63 expression profiles in human normal and tumor tissues. *Clin Cancer Res* 2002;8:494–501.

223. Perrone T, Frizzera G, Rosai J. Mediastinal diffuse large-cell lymphoma with sclerosis: a clinicopathologic study of 60 cases. *Am J Surg Pathol* 1986;10:176–191.

224. Hammond EH, Flinner RL. The diagnosis of thymoma: a review. *Ultrastruct Pathol* 1991; 15:419–438.

225. Levine GD, Rosai J, Bearman RM, et al. The fine structure of thymoma, with emphasis on its differential diagnosis. *Am J Pathol* 1975;81:49–86.

226. Eimoto T, Teshima K, Shirakusa T, et al. Heterogeneity of epithelial cells and reactive components in thymomas: an ultrastructural and immunohistochemical study. *Ultrastruct Pathol* 1986;10:157–173.

227. Trump DL, Mann RB. Diffuse large cell and undifferentiated lymphomas with prominent mediastinal involvement: a poor prognostic subset of patients with non-Hodgkin's lymphoma. *Cancer* 1982;50:277–282.

228. Majolino I, Marceno R, Magrin S, et al. Burkitt's cell leukemia with mediastinal mass and unusually good prognosis. *Haematologica* 1983;68:287–288.

229. Ziegler J, Beckstead JA, Volberding PA, et al. Outbreak of Burkitt's-like lymphoma in homosexual men. *Lancet* 1982;2:631–633.

230. Isaacson PG, Chan JKC, Tang C, et al. Low-grade B-cell lymphoma of mucosa-associated lymphoid tissue arising in the thymus: a thymic lymphoma mimicking myoepithelial sialadenitis. *Am J Surg Pathol* 1990;14:342–351.

231. Takagi N, Nakamura S, Yamamoto K, et al. Malignant lymphoma of mucosa-associated lymphoid tissue arising in the thymus of a patient with Sjogren's syndrome: a morphologic, phenotypic, and genotypic study. *Cancer* 1992;69:1347–1355.

232. Skinnider LF, Alexander S, Horsman D. Concurrent thymoma and lymphoma: a report of two cases. *Hum Pathol* 1982;13:163–166.

233. Huber J, Zegers BJM, Schuurman HJ. Pathology of congenital immunodeficiencies. *Semin Diagn Pathol* 1992;9:31–62.

234. Pescarmona E, Rosati S, Pisacane A, et al. Microscopic thymoma: histologic evidence of multifocal cortical and medullary origin. *Histopathology* 1992;20:263–266.

234a. Moran CA, Suster S. "Ancient" (sclerosing) thymomas: a clinicopathologic study of 10 cases. *Am J Clin Pathol* 2004;121:867–871.

234b. Kang DW, Canzian M, Beyruti R, et al. Sclerosing mediastinitis in the differential diagnosis of mediastinal tumors. *J Bras Pneumonol* 2006;32:78–83.

235. Wick MR, Swanson PE, Manivel JC. Immunohistochemical analysis of soft tissue sarcomas: comparisons with electron microscopy. *Appl Pathol* 1988;6:169–196.

236. Sarama RF, DiGiacomo WA, Safirstein BH. Primary mediastinal lipoma. *J Med Soc NJ* 1981; 78:901–902.

237. Politis J, Funahasi A, Gehlsen JA, et al. Intrathoracic lipomas: report of three cases and review of the literature, with emphasis on endobronchial lipoma. *J Thorac Cardiovasc Surg* 1979;77:550–556.

238. DeNictolis M, Goteri G, Campanati G, et al. Elastofibrolipoma of the mediastinum: a previously undescribed benign tumor containing abnormal elastic fibers. *Am J Surg Pathol* 1995;19:364–367.

239. Teplick JG, Nedwich A, Haskin ME. Roentgenographic features of thymolipoma. *AJR* 1973;17:873–877.

240. Moran CA, Rosado-de-Christenson M, Suster S. Thymolipoma: clinicopathologic review of 33 cases. *Mod Pathol* 1995;8:741–744.

241. Otto HF, Loning TH, Lachenmayer L, et al. Thymolipoma in association with myasthenia gravis. *Cancer* 1982;50:1623–1628.

242. Reintgen D, Fetter BF, Roses A, et al. Thymolipoma in association with myasthenia gravis. *Arch Pathol Lab Med* 1978;102:463–466.

243. Rios-Zambudio A, Torres-Lanzas J, Roca-Calvo MJ, et al. Thymolipomas in association with myasthenia gravis. *J Thoracic Cardiovasc Surg* 2001;122:825–826.

244. Peake JB, Zeigler MG. Thymolipoma: report of three cases. *Am Surg* 1977;43:477–479.

245. Hirai S, Hamanaka Y, Mitsui N, et al. Gigantic thymolipoma. *Jpn J Thorac Cardiovasc Surg* 2002;50:40–42.

246. Yeh HC, Gordon A, Kirschner PA, et al. Computed tomography and sonography of thymolipoma. *AJR* 1983;140:1131–1133.

247. Rosado-de-Christenson ML, Pugatch RD, Moran CA, et al. Thymolipoma: analysis of 27 cases. *Radiology* 1994;193:121–126.

248. Hull MT, Warfel KA, Kotylo P, et al. Proliferating thymolipoma: ultrastructural, immunohistochemical, and flow-cytometric study. *Ultrastruct Pathol* 1995;19:75–81.

249. Iseki M, Tsuda N, Kishikawa M, et al. Thymolipoma with striated myoid cells: histological, immunohistochemical, and ultrastructural study. *Am J Surg Pathol* 1990;14:395–398.

250. Moran CA, Zeren H, Koss MN. Thymofibrolipoma: a histologic variant of thymolipoma. *Arch Pathol Lab Med* 1994;118:281–282.

251. Ogino S, Franks TJ, Deubner H, et al. Thymohemangiolipoma, a rare histologic variant of thymolipoma: a case report and review of the literature. *Ann Diagn Pathol* 2000;4: 236–239.

252. Chaves-Espinosa JI, Chaves-Fernandez JA, Hoyer OH, et al. Endothoracic neurogenic neoplasms: analysis of 30 cases. *Rev Interamer Radiol* 1980;5:49–54.

253. Gale AW, Jelihovsky T, Grant AF, et al. Neurogenic tumors of the mediastinum. *Ann Thorac Surg* 1974;17:434–443.

254. Davidson KG, Walbaum PR, McCormack RJM. Intrathoracic neural tumors. *Thorax* 1978; 33:359–367.

255. Mandybur TI. Melanotic nerve sheath tumors. *J Neurosurg* 1974;41:187–192.

256. Paris F, Cabanes J, Munoz C, et al. Melanotic spinothoracic schwannoma. *Thorax* 1979; 34:243–246.

257. Woodruff JM. Peripheral nerve tumors showing glandular differentiation (glandular schwannomas). *Cancer* 1976;37:2399–2413.

258. Carney JA. Psammomatous melanotic schwannoma: a distinctive, heritable tumor with

special associations, including cardiac myxoma and the Cushing syndrome. *Am J Surg Pathol* 1990;14:206–222.

259. Woodruff JM, Goodwin TA, Erlandson RA, et al. Cellular schwannoma: a variety of schwannoma sometimes mistaken for a malignant tumor. *Am J Surg Pathol* 1981;5:733–744.

260. Fletcher CDM, Davies SE, McKee PH. Cellular schwannoma: a distinct pseudosarcomatous entity. *Histopathology* 1987;11:21–35.

261. Lodding P, Kindblom LG, Angervall L, et al. Cellular schwannoma: a clinicopathologic study of 29 cases. *Virchows Arch A Pathol Anat Histopathol* 1990;416:237–248.

262. Chalmers AH, Armstrong P. Plexiform mediastinal neurofibromas: a report of two cases. *Br J Radiol* 1977;50:215–217.

263. Lassmann H, Jurecka W, Lassmann G, et al. Different types of benign nerve sheath tumors: light microscopy, electron microscopy, and autoradiography. *Virchows Arch A Pathol Anat Histopathol* 1977;375:197–210.

264. Young DG. Thoracic neuroblastoma/ganglioneuroma. *J Pediatr Surg* 1983;18:37–41.

265. Hamilton JP, Koop CE. Ganglioneuromas in children. *Surg Gynecol Obstet* 1965;121:803–812.

266. Bender BL, Ghatak NR. Light and electron microscopic observations on a ganglioneuroma. *Acta Neuropathol* 1978;42:7–10.

267. Gould VE, Wiedenmann B, Lee I, et al. Synaptophysin expression in neuroendocrine neoplasms as determined by immunocytochemistry. *Am J Pathol* 1987;126:243–257.

268. Witkin GB, Rosai J. Solitary fibrous tumor of the mediastinum: a report of 14 cases. *Am J Surg Pathol* 1989;13:547–557.

269. Balassiano M, Reichert N, Rosenman Y, et al. Localized fibrous mesothelioma of the mediastinum devoid of pleural connections. *Postgrad Med J* 1989;65:788–790.

269a. Marchevsky AM, Varshney D, Fuller C. Mediastinal epithelioid solitary fibrous tumor. *Arch Pathol Lab Med* 2003;127:e212–e215.

269b. Vallat-Decouvelaere AV, Dry SM, Fletcher CDM. Atypical and malignant solitary fibrous tumors in extrathoracic locations: evidence of their comparability to intrathoracic tumors. *Am J Surg Pathol* 1998;22:1501–1511.

269c. Ng TL, Gown AM, Barry TS, et al. Nuclear beta-catenin in mesenchymal tumors. *Mod Pathol* 2005;18:68–74.

269d. Andino L, Cagle PT, Burer B, et al. Pleuropulmonary desmoid tumors: immunohistochemical comparison with solitary fibrous tumors and assessment of beta-catenin and cyclin-D1 expression. *Arch Pathol Lab Med* 2006;130:1503–1509.

270. Hanau CA, Miettinen M. Solitary fibrous tumor: histological and immunohistochemical spectrum of benign and malignant variants presenting at different sites. *Hum Pathol* 1995;26:440–449.

271. Wick MR, Manivel JC, Swanson PE. Contributions of immunohistochemistry to the diagnosis of soft tissue tumors. *Prog Surg Pathol* 1988;8:197–249.

272. England DM, Hochholzer L, McCarthy MJ. Localized benign and malignant fibrous tumors of the pleura: a clinicopathologic review of 223 cases. *Am J Surg Pathol* 1989;13:640–658.

273. Briselli MF, Mark EJ, Dickersin GR. Solitary fibrous tumors of the pleura: eight new cases and review of 360 cases in the literature. *Cancer* 1981;47:2678–2689.

274. Pachter MR, Lattes R. Mesenchymal tumors of the mediastinum. I. Tumors of fibrous tissue, adipose tissue, smooth muscle, and striated muscle. *Cancer* 1963;16:74–94.

275. Coffin CM, Dehner LP. Fibroblastic-myofibroblastic tumors in children and adolescents: a clinicopathologic study of 108 examples in 103 patients. *Pediatr Pathol* 1991;11:559–578.

276. Das Gupta TK, Brasfield RD, O'Hara J. Extra-abdominal desmoids: a clinicopathological study. *Ann Surg* 1969;170:109–117.

277. Yokoyama R, Tsuneyoshi M, Enjoji M, et al. Extra-abdominal desmoid tumors: correlations between histologic features and biologic behavior. *Surg Pathol* 1989;2:29–42.

278. Stiller D, Katenkamp D. Cellular features in desmoid fibromatosis and well-differentiated fibrosarcoma: an electron microscopic study. *Virchows Arch Pathol Anat Histopathol* 1975;369:155–170.

279. Swanson PE, Wick MR. Immunohistochemical diagnosis of soft tissue tumors. In Colvin R, Bhan A, McCluskey R, eds. *Diagnostic Immunopathology*. 2nd edition. New York, NY: Raven Press, 1995:599–632.

279a. Bhattacharya B, Dilworth HP, Iacobuzio-Donahue C, et al. Nuclear beta-catenin expression distinguishes deep fibromatosis from other benign and malignant fibroblastic and myofibroblastic lesions. *Am J Surg Pathol* 2005;29:653–659.

280. Dines DE, Payne WS, Bernatz PE, et al. Mediastinal granulomas and fibrosing mediastinitis. *Chest* 1979;75:320–324.

281. Coffin CM, Watterson J, Priest JR, et al. Extrapulmonary inflammatory myofibroblastic tumor (inflammatory pseudotumor): a clinicopathologic and immunohistochemical study of 84 cases. *Am J Surg Pathol* 1995;19:859–872.

282. Schowengerdt CG, Suyemoto R, Main FB. Granulomatous and fibrous mediastinitis: a review and analysis of 180 cases. *J Thorac Cardiovasc Surg* 1969;57:365–379.

283. Wieder S, Rabinowitz JG. Fibrous mediastinitis: a late manifestation of mediastinal histoplasmosis. *Radiology* 1977;125:305–312.

284. Light AM. Idiopathic fibrosis of the mediastinum: a discussion of three cases and review of the literature. *J Clin Pathol* 1978;31:78–88.

285. Matsubara O, Mark EJ, Ritter JH. Pseudoneoplastic lesions of the lungs, pleural surfaces, and mediastinum. In Wick MR, Humphrey PA, Ritter JH, eds. *Pathology of Pseudoneoplastic Lesions*. Philadelphia, PA: Lippincott-Raven, 1997:97–129.

286. Marchevsky AM. Mediastinal tumor-like conditions and tumors that can simulate thymic neoplasms. In Givel JC, ed. *Surgery of the Thymus*. Berlin, Germany: Springer-Verlag, 1990:151–162.

287. Brachet A, Thevenet F, Gilly FN, et al. Inflammatory pseudotumor of the superior vena cava: rare etiology of mediastinal tumor. *Ann Chir* 1993;47:170–173.

287a. Makimoto Y, Nabeshima K, Iwasaki H, et al. Inflammatory myofibroblastic tumor of the posterior mediastinum: an older adult case with anaplastic lymphoma kinase abnormalities determined using immunohistochemistry and fluorescence in-situ hybridization. *Virchows Arch* 2005;446:451–455.

287b. Nascimento AF, Ruiz R, Hornick JL, et al. Calcifying fibrous "pseudotumor:" clinicopath-

ologic study of 15 cases and analysis of its relationship to inflammatory myofibroblastic tumor. *Int J Surg Pathol* 2002;10:189–196.

288. Lukes RJ, Butler JJ, Hicks EB. Natural history of Hodgkin's disease as related to its pathologic picture. *Cancer* 1966;19:317–344.

289. Crotty TB, Colby TV, Gay PC, et al. Desmoplastic malignant mesothelioma masquerading as sclerosing mediastinitis: a diagnostic dilemma. *Hum Pathol* 1992;23:79–82.

290. Ritter JH, Humphrey PA, Wick MR. Malignant neoplasms capable of simulating inflammatory (myofibroblastic) pseudotumors and tumefactive fibroinflammatory lesions: "pseudopseudotumors." *Semin Diagn Pathol* 1998;15:111–132.

291. Rosai J, Levine GD, Weber WR, et al. Carcinoid tumors and oat cell carcinomas of the thymus. *Pathol Annu* 1976;11:201–226.

292. Wick MR, Scheithauer BW. Oat cell carcinoma of the thymus. *Cancer* 1982;49:1652–1657.

293. Duguid JB, Kennedy AM. Oat cell tumours of mediastinal glands. *J Pathol Bacteriol* 1930;33:93–99.

294. Kuo TT, Chang JP, Lin FJ, et al. Thymic carcinomas: histopathological varieties and immunohistochemical study. *Am J Surg Pathol* 1990;14:24–34.

295. Truong LD, Mody DR, Cagle PT, et al. Thymic carcinoma: a clinicopathologic study of 13 cases. *Am J Surg Pathol* 1990;14:151–166.

296. Ramon-y-Cajal S, Suster S. Primary thymic epithelial neoplasms in children. *Am J Surg Pathol* 1991;15:466–474.

297. Wick MR, Scheithauer BW, Weiland LH, et al. Primary thymic carcinomas. *Am J Surg Pathol* 1982;6:613–630.

298. Shimizu J, Hayashi Y, Morita K, et al. Primary thymic carcinoma: a clinicopathological and immunohistochemical study. *J Surg Oncol* 1994;56:159–164.

298a. Ordonez NG. Value of thyroid transcription factor-1 immunostaining in distinguishing small cell lung carcinoma from other small cell carcinomas. *Am J Surg Pathol* 2000;24:1217–1223.

299. Matsuo T, Hayashida R, Kobayashi K, et al. Thymic basaloid carcinoma with hepatic metastasis. *Ann Thorac Surg* 2002;74:579–582.

299a. Emanuel P, Wang B, Wu M, et al. p64 immunohistochemistry in the distinction of adenoid cystic carcinoma from basaloid squamous cell carcinoma. *Mod Pathol* 2005;18:645–650.

300. DeLorimier AA, Bragg KU, Linden G. Neuroblastoma in childhood. *Am J Dis Child* 1969;118:441–450.

301. Salter JE, Jr., Gibson D, Ordonez NG, et al. Neuroblastoma of the anterior mediastinum in an 80 year old woman. *Ultrastruct Pathol* 1995;19:305–310.

302. Hachitanda Y, Hata J. Stage IVS neuroblastoma: a clinical, histological, and biological analysis of 45 cases. *Hum Pathol* 1996;27:1135–1138.

303. Bar-Ziv J, Nogrady MB. Mediastinal neuroblastoma and ganglioneuroma: the differentiation between primary and secondary involvement on the chest roentgenogram. *AJR* 1975;125:380–390.

304. Carachi R, Campbell PE, Kent M. Thoracic neural crest tumors: a clinical review. *Cancer* 1983;51:949–954.

305. Adam A, Hochholzer L. Ganglioneuroblastoma of the posterior mediastinum: a clinicopathologic review of 80 cases. *Cancer* 1981;47:373–381.

306. Taxy JB. Electron microscopy in the diagnosis of neuroblastoma. *Arch Pathol Lab Med* 1980;104:355–360.

307. Triche TJ, Askin FB, Kissane JM. Neuroblastoma, Ewing's sarcoma, and the differential diagnosis of small-, round-, blue-cell tumors. In Finegold M, ed. *Pathology of Neoplasia in Children and Adolescents*. Philadelphia, PA: WB Saunders, 1986:145–195.

308. Wirnsberger GH, Becker H, Ziervogel K, et al. Diagnostic immunohistochemistry of neuroblastic tumors. *Am J Surg Pathol* 1992;16:49–57.

308a. Thomas JO, Nijjar J, Turley H, et al. NB84: a new monoclonal antibody for the recognition of neuroblastoma in routinely processed material. *J Pathol* 1991;163:69–75.

308b. Miettinen M, Chatten J, Paetau A, et al. Monoclonal antibody NB84 in the differential diagnosis of neuroblastoma and other small round-cell tumors. *Am J Surg Pathol* 1998;22:327–332.

309. Dehner LP. Peripheral and central primitive neuroectodermal tumors: a nosologic concept seeking a consensus. *Arch Pathol Lab Med* 1986;110:997–1005.

310. Crist WM, Raney RB, Newton W, et al. Intrathoracic soft tissue sarcomas in children. *Cancer* 1982;50:598–604.

311. Glick AD, Page DL. Primitive neuroepithelial tumors with vermiform processes (filiform neuroepithelial tumors): immunocytochemical and ultrastructural study of two cases. *Pathol Res Pract* 1992;188:687–691.

312. Grosfeld JL, Skinner MA, Rescorla FJ, et al. Mediastinal tumors in children: experience with 196 cases. *Ann Surg Oncol* 1994;1:121–127.

313. Askin FB, Rosai J, Sibley RK, et al. Malignant small cell tumor of the thoracopulmonary region in childhood. *Cancer* 1979;43:2438–2451.

314. Linnoila RI, Tsokos M, Triche TJ, et al. Evidence for neural origin and PAS-positive variants of the malignant small-cell tumor of thoracopulmonary region ("Askin tumor"). *Am J Surg Pathol* 1986;10:124–133.

315. Pollak A, Friede RL. Fine structure of medulloepithelioma. *J Neuropathol Exp Neurol* 1977;36:712–725.

316. Parham DM, Dias P, Kelly DR, et al. Desmin-positivity in primitive neuroectodermal tumors of childhood. *Am J Surg Pathol* 1992;16:483–492.

317. Fellinger EJ, Garin-Chesa P, Su SL, et al. Biochemical and genetic characterization of the HBA71 Ewing's sarcoma cell surface antigen. *Cancer Res* 1991;51:336–340.

318. Dehner LP. Primitive neuroectodermal tumor and Ewing's sarcoma. *Am J Surg Pathol* 1993;17:1–13.

319. Leong ASY, Wick MR, Swanson PE. *Immunohistology and Electron Microscopy of Anaplastic and Pleomorphic Tumors*. Cambridge, England: Cambridge Press, 1997:109–208.

319a. Rossi S, Orvieto E, Furlanetto A, et al. Utility of the immunohistochemical detection of FLI-1 expression in round cell and vascular neoplasms using a monoclonal antibody. *Mod Pathol* 2004;17:547–552.

320. Whang-Peng J, Triche TJ, Knutsen T, et al. Cytogenetic characterization of selected small round-cell tumors of childhood. *Cancer Genet Cytogenet* 1987;21:185–208.

321. Suster S, Moran CA, Koss MN. Rhabdomyosarcomas of the anterior mediastinum: report of four cases unassociated with germ cell, teratomatous, or thymic carcinomatous components. Hum Pathol 1994;25:349–356.

322. Begin LR, Schurch W, Lacoste J, et al. Glycogen-rich clear-cell rhabdomyosarcoma of the mediastinum: potential diagnostic pitfall. Am J Surg Pathol 1994;18:302–308.

323. Tsokos M. The diagnosis and classification of childhood rhabdomyosarcoma. Semin Diagn Pathol 1994;11:26–38.

323a. Kumar S, Perlman E, Harris CA, et al. Myogenin is a specific marker for rhabdomyosarcoma: an immunohistochemical study in paraffin-embedded tissues. Mod Pathol 2000;13:988–993.

324. Lorsbach RB, Pinkus GS, Shahsafaei A, et al. Primary marginal zone lymphoma of the thymus. Am J Clin Pathol 2000;113:784–791.

325. Mackay B, Osborne BM. The contribution of electron microscopy to the diagnosis of tumors. Pathobiol Annu 1978;8:359–405.

326. Zukerberg LR, Medeiros LJ, Ferry JA, et al. Diffuse low-grade B-cell lymphomas: four clinically distinct subtypes defined by a combination of morphologic and immunophenotypic features. Am J Clin Pathol 1993;100:373–385.

327. Shimizu J, Kawaura Y, Tatsuzawa Y, et al. Malignant melanoma originating in the thymus. Aust N Z J Surg 2000;70:753–755.

328. Fushimi H, Kotoh K, Watanabe D, et al. Malignant melanoma in the thymus. Am J Surg Pathol 2000;24:1305–1308.

329. Nakhleh RE, Wick MR, Rocamora A, et al. Morphologic diversity in malignant melanomas. Am J Clin Pathol 1990;93:731–740.

330. Hasserjian RP, Klimstra DS, Rosai J. Carcinoma of the thymus with clear cell features: report of eight cases and review of the literature. Am J Surg Pathol 1995;19:835–841.

331. Kuo TT. Carcinoid tumor of the thymus with divergent sarcomatoid differentiation: report of a case with histogenetic considerations. Hum Pathol 1994;25:319–323.

332. Moran CA, Suster S. Mucoepidermoid carcinoma of the thymus: a clinicopathologic study of six cases. Am J Surg Pathol 1995;19:826–834.

333. Paties C, Zangrandi A, Vassallo G, et al. Multidirectional carcinoma of the thymus with neuroendocrine and sarcomatoid components and carcinoid syndrome. Pathol Res Pract 1991;187:170–177.

334. Wick MR, Ritter JH, Humphrey PA, et al. Clear cell neoplasms of the endocrine system and thymus. Semin Diagn Pathol 1997;14:183–202.

335. Morgenthaler TI, Brown LR, Colby TV, et al. Thymoma. Mayo Clin Proc 1993;68:1110–1123.

336. Chung DA. Thymic carcinoma—analysis of nineteen clinicopathologic studies. Thorac Cardiovasc Surg 2000;48:114–119.

337. Ogawa K, Toita T, Uno T, et al. Treatment and prognosis of thymic carcinoma: a retrospective analysis of 40 cases. Cancer 2002;94:3115–3119.

338. Liu HC, Hsu WH, Chen YJ, et al. Primary thymic carcinoma. Ann Thorac Surg 2002;73:1076–1081.

339. Hsu HC, Huang EY, Wang CJ, et al. Postoperative radiotherapy in thymic carcinoma: treatment results and prognostic factors. Int J Radiat Oncol Biol Phys 2002;52:801–805.

340. Lucchi M, Mussi A, Ambrogi M, et al. Thymic carcinoma: a report of 13 cases. Eur J Surg Oncol 2001;27:636–640.

341. Zhang Z, Cui Y, Li B, et al. Thymic carcinoma (report of 14 cases). Chin Med Sci J 1997;12:252–255.

342. Kitami A, Suzuki T, Suzuki S, et al. Tiny thymic carcinoma completely surrounded by thymic tissue: the possibility of de novo carcinoma. Jpn J Thorac Cardiovasc Surg 2000;48:670–672.

343. Ritter JH, Wick MR. Primary carcinomas of the thymus gland. Semin Diagn Pathol 1999;16:18–31.

344. Weissberg D, Goldberg M, Pearson FG. Thymoma. Ann Thorac Surg 1973;16:141–147.

345. Gerein AN, Srivastava SP, Burgess J. Thymoma: a ten year review. Am J Surg 1978;136:49–52.

346. Gray GF, Gutowski WT. Thymoma: a clinicopathologic study of 54 cases. Am J Surg Pathol 1979;3:235–249.

347. Hayashi S, Hamanaka Y, Sueda T, et al. Thymic metastasis from prostatic carcinoma: report of a case. Surg Today 1993;23:632–634.

348. Mattana J, Kurtz B, Miah A, et al. Renal cell carcinoma presenting as a solitary anterior superior mediastinal mass. J Med 1996;27:205–210.

349. Shimosato Y, Kameya T, Nagai K, et al. Squamous cell carcinoma of the thymus: an analysis of eight cases. Am J Surg Pathol 1977;1:109–121.

350. Nishimura M, Kodama T, Nishiyama H, et al. A case of sarcomatoid carcinoma of the thymus. Pathol Int 1997;47:260–263.

351. Weiss LM, Gaffey MJ, Shibata D. Lymphoepithelioma-like carcinoma and its relationship to Epstein-Barr virus. Am J Clin Pathol 1991;96:156–158.

352. Leyvraz S, Henle W, Cahinian AP, et al. Association of Epstein-Barr virus with thymic carcinoma. N Engl J Med 1985;312:1296–1299.

353. Dimery IW, Lee JS, Blick M, et al. Association of Epstein-Barr virus with lymphoepithelioma of the thymus. Cancer 1988;61:2475–2480.

354. Weiss LM, Movahed LA, Butler AE, et al. Analysis of lymphoepithelioma and lymphoepithelioma-like carcinomas for Epstein-Barr viral genomes by in situ hybridization. Am J Surg Pathol 1989;13:625–631.

354a. Hsueh C, Kuo TT, Tsang NM, et al. Thymic lymphoepitheliomalike carcinoma in children: clinicopathologic features and molecular analysis. J Pediatr Hematol Oncol 2006;28:785–790.

355. Tanaka M, Shimokawa K, Matsubara O, et al. Mucoepidermoid carcinoma of the thymic region. Acta Pathol Jpn 1982;32:703–712.

356. Wolfe JT III, Wick MR, Scheithauer BW, et al. Clear cell carcinoma of the thymus. Mayo Clin Proc 1983;58:365–370.

357. Stephens M, Khalil J, Gibbs AR. Primary clear cell carcinoma of the thymus gland. Histopathology 1987;11:763–765.

357a. Choi WW, Lui YH, Lau WH, et al. Adenocarcinoma of the thymus: report of two cases, including a previously-undescribed mucinous subtype. Am J Surg Pathol 2003;27:124–130.

358. Nappi O, Mills SE, Swanson PE, et al. Clear cell tumors of unknown nature and origin: a systematic approach to diagnosis. Semin Diagn Pathol 1997;14:164–174.

359. Pomplun S, Wotherspoon AC, Shah G, et al. Immunohistochemical markers in the differentiation of thymic and pulmonary neoplasms. Histopathology 2002;40:152–158.

360. Berezowski K, Grimes MM, Gal A, et al. CD5 immunoreactivity of epithelial cells in thymic carcinoma and CASTLE using paraffin-embedded tissue. Am J Clin Pathol 1996;106:483–486.

361. Hishima T, Fukayama M, Fujisawa M, et al. CD5 expression in thymic carcinoma. Am J Pathol 1994;145:268–275.

362. Kornstein MJ, Rosai J. CD5 labeling of thymic carcinomas and other non-lymphoid neoplasms. Am J Clin Pathol 1998;109:722–726.

363. Hishima T, Fukayama M, Hayashi Y, et al. CD70 expression in thymic carcinoma. Am J Surg Pathol 2000;24:742–746.

364. Patton DF, Ribeiro RC, Jenkins JJ, et al. Thymic carcinoma with a defective Epstein-Barr virus encoding the BZLF1 trans-activator. J Infect Dis 1994;170:7–12.

365. Shek TW, Luk IS, Ng IO, et al. Lymphoepithelioma-like carcinoma of the thyroid gland: lack of evidence of association with Epstein-Barr virus. Hum Pathol 1996;27:851–853.

366. Wu TC, Kuo TT. Study of Epstein-Barr virus early RNA-1 (EBER1) expression by in situ hybridization in thymic epithelial tumors of Chinese patients in Taiwan. Hum Pathol 1993;24:235–238.

367. Chen PC, Pan CC, Yang AH, et al. Detection of Epstein-Barr virus genome within thymic epithelial tumors in Taiwanese patients by nested PCR, PCR in situ hybridization, and RNA in situ hybridization. J Pathol 2002;197:684–688.

368. Tateyama H, Eimoto T, Tada T, et al. p53 protein expression and p53 gene mutation in thymic epithelial tumors: an immunohistochemical and DNA sequencing study. Am J Clin Pathol 1995;104:375–381.

369. Humphrey PA. p53: mutations and immunohistochemical detection, with a focus on alterations in urologic malignancies. Adv Pathol Lab Med 1994;7:579–606.

370. Black BK, Ackerman LV. Tumors of the parathyroids: a review of twenty-three cases. Cancer 1950;3:415–444.

371. Nathaniels EK, Nathaniels AM, Wang CA. Mediastinal parathyroid tumors: a clinical and pathological study of 84 cases. Ann Surg 1970;171:165–170.

372. Van Heerden JA, Beahrs OH, Woolner LB. The pathology and surgical management of primary hyperparathyroidism. Surg Clin North Am 1977;57:557–563.

373. Wang CA, Gaz RD, Moncure AC. Mediastinal parathyroid exploration: a clinical and pathologic study of 47 cases. World J Surg 1986;10:687–695.

374. Russell CF, Edis AJ, Scholz DA. Mediastinal parathyroid tumors: experience with 38 tumors requiring median sternotomy for removal. Ann Surg 1981;193:805–809.

375. Murphy MN, Glennon PG, Diocee MS, et al. Nonsecretory parathyroid carcinoma of the mediastinum. Cancer 1986;58:2468–2476.

376. Pachter MR, Lattes R. Uncommon mediastinal tumors. Dis Chest 1963;43:519–528.

377. Scholz DA, Purnell DC, Woolner LB, et al. Mediastinal hyperfunctioning parathyroid tumors: review of 14 cases. Ann Surg 1973;178:173–178.

378. Evans HL. Pathologic diagnosis of parathyroid carcinoma. Int J Surg Pathol 1993;1:139–142.

379. Altenahr E, Saeger W. Light and electron microscopy of parathyroid carcinoma: report of 3 cases. Virchows Arch A Pathol Pathol Anat 1973;360:107–122.

380. Ordonez NG, Ibanez ML, Samaan NA, et al. Immunoperoxidase study of uncommon parathyroid tumors. Am J Surg Pathol 1983;7:535–542.

381. Moriconi WJ, Taylor S, Hunkatroon M, et al. Primary mediastinal germinomas in females: a case report and review of the literature. J Surg Oncol 1985;29:176–180.

382. Moran CA, Suster S. Hepatoid yolk sac tumors of the mediastinum: a clinicopathologic and immunohistologic study of four cases. Am J Surg Pathol 1997;21:1210–1214.

382a. Dominguez-Malagon H, Perez-Montiel D. Mediastinal germ cell tumors. Semin Diagn Pathol 2005;22:230–240.

383. Knapp RH, Hurt RD, Payne WS, et al. Malignant germ cell tumors of the mediastinum. J Thorac Cardiovasc Surg 1985;89:82–89.

384. Cox JD. Primary malignant germinal tumors of the mediastinum: a study of 24 cases. Cancer 1975;36:1162–1168.

385. Recondo J, Libshitz HT. Mediastinal extragonadal germ cell tumors. Urology 1978;11:369–375.

386. Pachter MR, Lattes R. "Germinal" tumors of mediastinum: a clinicopathologic study of adult teratomas, teratocarcinomas, choriocarcinomas, and seminomas. Dis Chest 1964;45:301–310.

387. Martini N, Golbey RB, Hajdu SI, et al. Primary mediastinal germ cell tumor. Cancer 1974;33:763–769.

388. Hurt RD, Bruckman JE, Farrow GW, et al. Primary anterior mediastinal seminoma. Cancer 1982;49:1658–1663.

389. Bush SE, Martinez A, Bagshaw MA. Primary mediastinal seminoma. Cancer 1981;48:1877–1882.

390. Noronha PA, Noronha R, Rao DS. Primary anterior mediastinal endodermal sinus tumors in childhood. Am J Pediatr Hematol Oncol 1985;7:312–316.

391. Gooneratne S, Keh P, Sreekanth S, et al. Anterior mediastinal endodermal sinus (yolk sac) tumor in a female infant. Cancer 1985;52:1430–1433.

392. Hawkins EP, Finegold MJ, Hawkins HK, et al. Nongerminomatous malignant germ cell tumors in children: a review of 89 cases from the Pediatric Oncology Group, 1971–1984. Cancer 1986;58:2579–2584.

393. Fox MA, Vix VA. Endodermal sinus (yolk sac) tumors of the anterior mediastinum. AJR 1980;135:291–294.

394. DeSmet AA, Silver TM, Hart WR. Endodermal sinus tumor of the anterior mediastinum. South Med J 1977;70:757–758.

395. Kuzur ME, Cobleigh MA, Greco FA, et al. Endodermal sinus tumor of the mediastinum. Cancer 1982;50:766–774.

396. Mukai K, Adams WR. Yolk sac tumor of the anterior mediastinum: case report with light- and electron microscopic examination and immunohistochemical study of alpha-fetoprotein. Am J Surg Pathol 1979;3:77–83.

397. Truong LD, Harris L, Mattioli C, et al. Endodermal sinus tumor of the mediastinum: a report of seven cases and review of the literature. *Cancer* 1986;58:730–739.

398. Sickles EA, Belliveau RE, Wiernik PH. Primary mediastinal choriocarcinoma in the male. *Cancer* 1974;33:1196–1203.

399. Hailemariam S, Engeler DS, Bannwart F, et al. Primary mediastinal germ cell tumor with intratubular germ cell neoplasia of the testis—further support for germ cell origin of these tumors. *Cancer* 1997;79:1031–1036.

400. Leroy X, Augusto D, Leteurtre E, et al. CD30 and CD117 (c-*kit*) used in combination are useful for distinguishing embryonal carcinoma from seminoma. *J Histochem Cytochem* 2002; 50:283–285.

401. Gibson PC, Cooper K. CD117 (KIT): a diverse protein with selective applications in surgical pathology. *Adv Anat Pathol* 2002;9:65–69.

402. Niehans GA, Manivel JC, Copland GT, et al. Immunohistochemistry of germ cell and trophoblastic neoplasms. *Cancer* 1988;62:1113–1123.

402a. Moran CA, Suster S. Cystic well-differentiated neuroendocrine carcinoma (carcinoid tumor): a clinicopathologic and immunohistochemical study of two cases. *Am J Clin Pathol* 2006;126:377–380.

403. Lancaster KJ, Liang CY, Myers JC, et al. Goblet cell carcinoid arising in a mature teratoma of the mediastinum. *Am J Surg Pathol* 1997;21:109–113.

404. DeMontpreville VT, Macchiarini P, Dulmet E. Thymic neuroendocrine carcinoma (carcinoid): a clinicopathologic study of fourteen cases. *J Thorac Cardiovasc Surg* 1996;111: 134–141.

405. Suster S, Moran CA. Neuroendocrine neoplasms of the mediastinum. *Am J Clin Pathol* 2001;115(Suppl):S17–S27.

406. Gal AA, Kornstein MJ, Cohen C, et al. Neuroendocrine tumors of the thymus: a clinicopathological and prognostic study. *Ann Thorac Surg* 2001;72:1179–1182.

407. Goto K, Kodama T, Matsuno Y, et al. Clinicopathologic and DNA cytometric analysis of carcinoid tumors of the thymus. *Mod Pathol* 2001;14:985–994.

408. Fujiwara K, Segawa Y, Takigawa N, et al. Two cases of atypical carcinoid of the thymus. *Intern Med* 2000;39:834–838.

409. Moran CA, Suster S. Neuroendocrine carcinomas (carcinoid tumors) of the thymus: a clinicopathologic analysis of 80 cases. *Am J Clin Pathol* 2000;114:100–110.

409a. Moran CA. Primary neuroendocrine carcinomas of the mediastinum: review of current criteria for histopathologic diagnosis and classification. *Semin Diagn Pathol* 2005;22: 223–229.

410. Wick MR, Rosai J. Neuroendocrine neoplasms of the mediastinum. *Semin Diagn Pathol* 1991;8:35–51.

411. Cadigan DG, Hollett PD, Collingwood PW, et al. Imaging of a mediastinal thymic carcinoid tumor with radiolabeled somatostatin analogue. *Clin Nucl Med* 1996;21:487–488.

412. Rosai J, Higa E, Davie J. Mediastinal endocrine neoplasm in patients with multiple endocrine adenomatosis: a previously unrecognized association. *Cancer* 1972;29:1075–1083.

413. Wick MR, Scott RE, Li CY, et al. Carcinoid tumor of the thymus: a clinicopathologic report of seven cases with a review of the literature. *Mayo Clin Proc* 1980;55:246–254.

414. Marchevsky AM, Dickman SH. Mediastinal carcinoid with an incomplete Sipple's syndrome. *Cancer* 1979;43:2497–2501.

415. Burgess JR, Giles N, Shepherd JJ. Malignant thymic carcinoid is not prevented by transcervical thymectomy in multiple endocrine neoplasia, type I. *Clin Endocrinol* 2001;55:689–693.

416. Hirai S, Hamanaka Y, Mitsui N, et al. Thymic carcinoids in multiple endocrine neoplasia-type I. *Jpn J Thorac Cardiovasc Surg* 2001;49:525–527.

417. Dotzenrath C, Goretzki PE, Cupisti K, et al. Malignant endocrine tumors in patients with MEN1 disease. *Surgery* 2001;129:91–95.

418. Wick MR, Carney JA, Bernatz PE, et al. Primary mediastinal carcinoid tumors. *Am J Surg Pathol* 1982;6:195–205.

419. Rosai J, Higa E. Mediastinal endocrine neoplasm of probable thymic origin, related to carcinoid tumor: clinicopathologic study of eight cases. *Cancer* 1972;29:1061–1074.

420. Suster S, Moran CA. Thymic carcinoid with prominent mucinous stroma: report of a distinctive morphologic variant of thymic neuroendocrine neoplasm. *Am J Surg Pathol* 1995;89:1277–1285.

421. Lagrange W, Dahm HH, Karstens J, et al. Melanocytic neuroendocrine carcinoma of the thymus. *Cancer* 1987;59:484–488.

422. Moran CA, Suster S. Primary neuroendocrine carcinoma (thymic carcinoid) of the thymus with prominent oncocytic features: a clinicopathologic study of 22 cases. *Mod Pathol* 2000; 13:489–494.

423. Smith NL, Finley JL. Lipid-rich carcinoid tumor of the thymus gland: diagnosis by fine-needle aspiration biopsy. *Diagn Cytopathol* 2001;25:130–133.

423a. Gao Z, Kahn L, Bhuiya T. Thymic carcinoid with mucinous stroma: a rare variant of carcinoid with an aggressive clinical course. *Ann Diagn Pathol* 2006;10:114–116.

424. Cho KJ, Ha CW, Koh JS, et al. Thymic carcinoid tumor combined with thymoma—neuroendocrine differentiation in thymoma? *J Korean Med Sci* 1993;13:458–463.

425. Mizuno T, Masaoka A, Hashimoto T, et al. Coexisting thymic carcinoid tumor and thymoma. *Ann Thorac Surg* 1990;50:650–652.

425a. Renshaw AA, Haja JC, Neal MH, et al. Distinguishing carcinoid tumor of the mediastinum from thymoma: correlating cytologic features and performance in the College of American Pathologists Interlaboratory Comparison Program in Nongynecologic Cytopathology. *Arch Pathol Lab Med* 2006;130:1612–1615.

426. Best LA, Westbrook BM, Trastek VF, et al. Surgery in the management of mediastinal carcinoid. *J Cardiovasc Surg (Torino)* 1994;35:133–135.

427. Cupisti K, Dotzenrath C, Simon D, et al. Surgical therapy of neuroendocrine tumors of the thymus. *Chirurg* 1997;68:136–140.

428. Dusmet ME, McKneally MF. Pulmonary and thymic carcinoid tumors. *World J Surg* 1996; 25:189–195.

429. Valli M, Fabris GA, Dewar A, et al. Atypical carcinoid tumor of the thymus: a study of eight cases. *Histopathology* 1994;24:371–375.

430. Wang DY, Chang DB, Kuo SH, et al. Carcinoid tumours of the thymus. *Thorax* 1994;25: 357–360.

431. Wick MR, Scheithauer BW. Thymic carcinoid: a histologic, immunohistochemical, and ultrastructural study of 12 cases. *Cancer* 1984;53:475–484.

432. Herbst WM, Kumner W, Hofmann W, et al. Carcinoid tumors of the thymus: an immunohistochemical study. *Cancer* 1987;60:2465–2470.

433. Glenner GG, Grimley PM. Tumors of the extra-adrenal paraganglion system (including chemoreceptors). In *Atlas of Tumor Pathology.* Series 2, Fascicle 9. Washington, DC: Armed Forces Institute of Pathology, 1974.

434. Assaf HM, Al-Momen AA, Martin JG. Aorticopulmonary paraganglioma: a case report with immunohistochemical studies and literature review. *Arch Pathol Lab Med* 1992;116: 1085–1087.

435. Moran CA, Albores-Saavedra J, Wenig BM, et al. Pigmented extraadrenal paragangliomas: a clinicopathologic and immunohistochemical study of five cases. *Cancer* 1997;79:398–402.

436. Odze R, Begin LR. Malignant paraganglioma of the posterior mediastinum. *Cancer* 1990; 65:564–569.

437. Olson JL, Salyer WR. Mediastinal paraganglioma (aortic body tumor): a report of four cases, and a review of the literature. *Cancer* 1978;41:2405–2412.

437a. Young WF, Jr. Paragangliomas: clinical overview. *Ann NY Acad Sci* 2006;1073:21–29.

438. Carney JA. The triad of gastric epithelioid leiomyosarcoma, pulmonary chondroma, and functioning extra-adrenal paraganglioma: a five-year review. *Medicine* 1983;62:159–169.

439. Linnoila RI, Keiser HR, Steinberg SM, et al. Histopathology of benign versus malignant sympathoadrenal paragangliomas: clinicopathologic study of 120 cases including unusual histologic features. *Hum Pathol* 1990;21:1168–1180.

439a. Plaza JA, Wakely PE, Jr., Moran C, et al. Sclerosing paraganglioma: report of 19 cases of an unusual variant of neuroendocrine tumor that may be mistaken for an aggressive malignant neoplasm. *Am J Surg Pathol* 2006;30:7–12.

440. Rosai J, Mettler EA. Chemodectoma of the mediastinum. *Rev Assoc Med Arg* 1965;79: 242–246.

441. Lack EE, Stillinger R, Colvin R, et al. Aorticopulmonary paraganglioma. *Cancer* 1979;43: 269–278.

442. Schroder HD, Johannsen L. Demonstration of S100 protein in sustentacular cells of phaeochromocytomas and paragangliomas. *Histopathology* 1986;10:1023–1033.

443. DeLellis RA, Tischler AS, Lee AK, et al. Leu-enkephalin-like immunoreactivity in proliferative lesions of the human adrenal medulla and extra-adrenal paraganglia. *Am J Surg Pathol* 1983;7:29–37.

444. Komminoth P, Roth J, Muletta-Feurer S, et al. RET protooncogene point mutations in sporadic neuroendocrine tumors. *J Clin Endocrinol Metab* 1996;81:2041–2046.

445. Levitt LJ, Aisenberg AC, Harris NL, et al. Primary non-Hodgkin's lymphoma of the mediastinum. *Cancer* 1982;50:2486–2492.

446. Lichtenstein AK, Levine A, Taylor CR, et al. Primary mediastinal lymphoma in adults. *Am J Med* 1980;68:509–514.

447. Miller JB, Variakojis D, Bitran JD, et al. Diffuse histiocytic lymphoma with sclerosis: a clinicopathologic entity frequently causing superior vena caval obstruction. *Cancer* 1981; 47:748–756.

448. Bunin NJ, Hvizdala E, Link M, et al. Mediastinal nonlymphoblastic lymphomas in children: a clinicopathologic study. *J Clin Oncol* 1986;4:154–159.

449. Haioun C, Gaulard P, Roudot-Thoraval F, et al. Mediastinal large-cell lymphoma with sclerosis: a condition with a poor prognosis. *Am J Clin Oncol* 1989;12:425–429.

450. Lamarre L, Jacobson JO, Aisenberg AC, et al. Primary large cell lymphoma of the mediastinum: a histologic and immunophenotypic study of 29 cases. *Am J Surg Pathol* 1989;13: 730–739.

451. Yousem SA, Weiss LM, Warnke RA. Primary mediastinal non-Hodgkin's lymphomas: a morphologic and immunologic study of 19 cases. *Am J Clin Pathol* 1985;83:676–680.

451a. Tsai HW, Yen YS, Chang KC. Mediastinal large B-cell lymphoma with rosette formation mimicking thymoma and thymic carcinoid. *Histopathology* 2006;49:93–95.

452. Suster S, Moran CA. Pleomorphic large cell lymphomas of the mediastinum. *Am J Surg Pathol* 1996;20:224–232.

453. Moller P, Lammler B, Eberlein-Gonska M, et al. Primary mediastinal clear-cell lymphoma of B-cell type. *Virchows Arch A Pathol Anat Histopathol* 1986;409:79–92.

454. Moller P, Moldenhauer G, Momburg F, et al. Mediastinal lymphoma of clear cell type is a tumor corresponding to terminal steps of B-cell differentiation. *Blood* 1987;69:1087–1095.

455. Brandter LB, Smith CIE, Hammarstrom L, et al. Clonal immunoglobulin gene rearrangements in primary mediastinal clear cell lymphomas. *Leukemia* 1989;3:122–129.

456. Agnarsson BA, Kadin ME. Ki-1-positive large cell lymphoma: a morphologic and immunologic study of 19 cases. *Am J Surg Pathol* 1988;12:264–274.

457. Addis BJ, Isaacson PG. Large-cell lymphoma of the mediastinum: a B-cell tumor of probable thymic origin. *Histopathology* 1986;10:379–390.

458. Davis RE, Dorfman RF, Warnke RA. Primary large-cell lymphoma of the thymus: a diffuse B-cell neoplasm presenting as primary mediastinal lymphoma. *Hum Pathol* 1990;21: 1262–1268.

459. Fechner RE. Hodgkin's disease of the thymus. *Cancer* 1969;23:16–23.

460. Katz A, Lattes R. Granulomatous thymoma or Hodgkin's disease of thymus? A clinical and histologic study and a re-evaluation. *Cancer* 1969;23:1–15.

461. Lazzarino M, Orlandi E, Paulli M, et al. Treatment outcome and prognostic factors for primary mediastinal (thymic) B-cell lymphoma: a multicenter study of 106 patients. *J Clin Oncol* 1997;15:1646–1653.

462. Grogan TM. Hodgkin's disease. In Jaffe ES, ed. *Surgical Pathology of the Lymph Nodes and Related Organs.* 2nd edition. Philadelphia, PA: WB Saunders, 1995:133–192.

463. Strickler JG, Michie SA, Warnke RA, et al. The "syncytial variant" of nodular sclerosing Hodgkin's disease. *Am J Surg Pathol* 1986;10:470–477.

464. Frizzera G. The distinction of Hodgkin's disease from anaplastic large cell lymphoma. *Semin Diagn Pathol* 1992;9:291–296.

465. Menestrina F, Chilosi M, Scarpa A. Nodular lymphocyte predominant Hodgkin's disease and anaplastic large cell (CD30+) lymphoma: distinct entities or nonspecific patterns? *Semin Diagn Pathol* 1995;12:256–269.

466. Torlakovic E, Torlakovic G, Nguyen PL, et al. The value of anti-Pax5 immunostaining in

routinely fixed and paraffin-embedded sections: a novel pan-pre-B and B-cell marker. *Am J Surg Pathol* 2002;26:1343–1350.

467. Neiman RS, Barcos M, Berard C, et al. Granulocytic sarcoma: a clinicopathologic study of 61 biopsied cases. *Cancer* 1981;48:1426–1437.

468. Banerjee D, Silva E. Mediastinal mass with acute leukemia: myeloblastoma masquerading as lymphoblastic lymphoma. *Arch Pathol Lab Med* 1981;105:126–129.

469. Kubonishi I, Ohtsuki Y, Machida K, et al. Granulocytic sarcoma as a mediastinal mass. *Am J Clin Pathol* 1984;83:730–734.

470. Chubachi A, Miura I, Takahashi N, et al. Acute myelogenous leukemia associated with a mediastinal tumor. *Leuk Lymphoma* 1993;12:143–146.

470a. Nappi O, Boscaino A, Wick MR. Extramedullary hematopoietic proliferations, extraosseous plasmacytomas, and ectopic splenic implants (splenosis). *Semin Diagn Pathol* 2003; 20:338–356.

471. Meis JM, Butler JJ, Osborne BM, et al. Granulocytic sarcoma in nonleukemic patients. *Cancer* 1986;58:2697–2709.

472. Quintanilla-Martinez L, Zukerberg LR, Ferry JA, et al. Extramedullary tumors of lymphoid or myeloid blasts: the role of immunohistology in diagnosis and classification. *Am J Clin Pathol* 1995;104:431–443.

473. Goldstein NS, Ritter JH, Argenyi ZB, et al. Granulocytic sarcoma: potential diagnostic clues from immunostaining patterns seen with "anti-lymphoid" antibodies. *Int J Surg Pathol* 1995;2:199–206.

474. Arbona GL, Lloyd TV, Lucas J. Mediastinal extramedullary plasmacytoma. *South Med J* 1980;73:670–671.

475. Niwa K, Tanaka T, Mori H, et al. Extramedullary plasmacytoma of the mediastinum. *Jpn J Clin Oncol* 1987;17:95–100.

476. Miyazaki T, Kohno S, Sakamoto A, et al. A rare case of extramedullary plasmacytoma in the mediastinum. *Intern Med* 1992;31:1363–1365.

477. Ahmed AR, Marchbank AJ, Nicholson AG, et al. Extramedullary plasmacytoma presenting with myasthenia gravis and mediastinal mass. *Ann Thorac Surg* 2000;70:1390–1392.

478. Fisher ER, Zawadzki Z. Ultrastructural features of plasma cells in patients with paraproteinemias. *Am J Clin Pathol* 1970;54:779–789.

479. Tong AW, Lee JC, Stone MJ. Characterization of a monoclonal antibody having selective reactivity with normal and neoplastic plasma cells. *Blood* 1987;69:238–245.

480. Petruch UR, Horny HP, Kaiserling E. Frequent expression of haematopoietic and non-haematopoietic antigens by neoplastic plasma cells: an immunohistochemical study using formalin-fixed, paraffin-embedded tissue. *Histopathology* 1992;20:35–40.

480a. Jaffe ES, Harris NL, Stein H, et al., eds. *Pathology and Genetics of Tumours of Haematopoietic and Lymphoid Tissues.* Geneva, Switzerland: World Health Organization, 2001:250–300.

480b. Fassina A, Marino F, Poletti A, et al. Follicular dendritic cell tumor of the mediastinum. *Ann Diagn Pathol* 2001;5:361–367.

480c. Krober SM, Marx A, Aebert H, et al. Sarcoma of follicular dendritic cells in the dorsal mediastinum. *Hum Pathol* 2004;35:259–263.

480d. Guettier C, Validire P, Emilie D, et al. Follicular dendritic cell tumor of the mediastinum: expression of fractalkine and SDF-1-alpha as mast cell chemoattractants. *Virchows Arch* 2006;448:218–222.

480e. Jiang L, Admirand JH, Moran CA, et al. Mediastinal follicular dendritic cell sarcoma involving bone marrow: a case report and review of the literature. *Ann Diagn Pathol* 2006; 10:357–362.

480f. Leipsic JA, McAdams HP, Sporn TA. Follicular dendritic cell sarcoma of the mediastinum. *Am J Roentgenol* 2007;188:W554–W556.

480g. Chan AC, Serrano-Olmo J, Erlandson RA, et al. Cytokeratin-positive malignant tumors with reticulum cell morphology: a subtype of fibroblastic-reticulum cell neoplasm? *Am J Surg Pathol* 2000;24:107–116.

481. Peterson JT, Greenberg SD, Buffler PA. Nonasbestos-related malignant mesotheliomas: a review. *Cancer* 1984;54:951–960.

482. Wanebo HJ, Martini N, Melamed MR, et al. Pleural mesothelioma. *Cancer* 1976;38:2481–2488.

483. Wick MR, Loy T, Mills SE, et al. Malignant epithelioid pleural mesothelioma versus peripheral pulmonary adenocarcinoma: a histochemical, ultrastructural, and immunohistologic study of 103 cases. *Hum Pathol* 1990;21:759–766.

484. Warhol MJ, Corson JM. An ultrastructural comparison of mesotheliomas with adenocarcinomas of the lung and breast. *Hum Pathol* 1985;16:50–55.

485. Ordonez NG. The immunohistochemical diagnosis of mesothelioma: differentiation of mesothelioma and lung adenocarcinoma. *Am J Surg Pathol* 1989;13:276–291.

486. Ordonez NG. The immunohistochemical diagnosis of epithelial mesothelioma. *Hum Pathol* 1999;30:313–323.

487. Abutaily AS, Addis BJ, Roche WR. Immunohistochemistry in the distinction between malignant mesothelioma and pulmonary adenocarcinoma: a critical evaluation of new antibodies. *J Clin Pathol* 2002;55:662–668.

487a. Ordonez NG. Podoplanin: a novel diagnostic immunohistochemical marker. *Adv Anat Pathol* 2006;13:83–88.

488. Attanoos RL, Galateau-Salle F, Gibbs AR, et al. Primary thymic epithelial tumors of the pleura mimicking malignant mesothelioma. *Histopathology* 2002;41:42–49.

489. Foster MR, Johnson JE, Olson SJ, et al. Immunohistochemical analysis of nuclear versus cytoplasmic staining of WT1 in malignant mesotheliomas and primary pulmonary adenocarcinomas. *Arch Pathol Lab Med* 2001;125:1316–1320.

490. Moran CA, Suster S, Perino G, et al. Malignant smooth muscle tumors presenting as mediastinal soft tissue masses: a clinicopathologic study of 10 cases. *Cancer* 1994;74:2251–2260.

491. Park Y, Oster MW, Olarte MR. Prostatic cancer with an unusual presentation: polymyositis and mediastinal adenopathy. *Cancer* 1981;48:1262–1264.

492. Wick MR. Immunohistochemistry in the diagnosis of "solid" malignant tumors. In Jennette JC, ed. *Immunohistology in Diagnostic Pathology.* Boca Raton, FL: CRC Press, 1989: 161–191.

493. Feldman L, Kricun ME. Malignant melanoma presenting as a mediastinal mass. *JAMA* 1979;241:396–397.

494. Mackay B, Lichtiger B, Tessmer CF, et al. The pathologic diagnosis of metastatic malignant melanoma. *Cancer Bull* 1971;23:30–45.

495. Wick MR. Immunohistologic features of melanocytic neoplasms. In Dabbs DJ, ed. *Diagnostic Immunohistochemistry.* New York, NY: Churchill-Livingstone, 2002:147–161.

496. Andrade RE, Wick MR, Frizzera G, et al. Immunophenotyping of hematopoietic malignancies in paraffin sections. *Hum Pathol* 1988;19:394–402.

497. Said JW. The immunohistochemistry of Hodgkin's disease. *Semin Diagn Pathol* 1992;9: 265–271.

498. Suster S, Moran CA. Spindle cell thymic carcinoma: clinicopathologic and immunochemical study of a distinctive variant of primary thymic epithelial neoplasm. *Am J Surg Pathol* 1999;23:691–700.

499. Okudela K, Nakamura N, Sano J, et al. Thymic carcinosarcoma consisting of squamous cell carcinomatous and embryonal rhabdomyosarcomatous components: report of a case and review of the literature. *Pathol Res Pract* 2001;197:205–210.

500. Eimoto T, Kitaoka M, Ogawa H, et al. Thymic sarcomatoid carcinoma with skeletal muscle differentiation: report of two cases, one with cytogenetic analysis. *Histopathology* 2002;40: 46–57.

501. Wick MR, Swanson PE. "Carcinosarcomas"—current perspectives and a historical review of nosological concepts. *Semin Diagn Pathol* 1993;10:118–127.

502. DeLeeuw B, Suijkerbuijk RF, Olde-Weghuis D, et al. Distinct Xp11.2 breakpoint regions in synovial sarcoma revealed by metaphase and interphase FISH: relationship to histologic subtypes. *Cancer Genet Cytogenet* 1994;73:89–94.

503. Levine GD, Rosai J. A spindle-cell variant of thymic carcinoid tumor: a clinical, histologic, and fine structural study with emphasis on its distinction from spindle-cell thymoma. *Arch Pathol Lab Med* 1976;100:293–300.

504. Dusenbery D. Spindle cell thymic carcinoid occurring in multiple endocrine neoplasia I: fine needle aspiration findings in a case. *Diagn Cytopathol* 1996;15:439–441.

505. Moran CA, Suster S. Spindle-cell neuroendocrine carcinomas of the thymus (spindle-cell thymic carcinoids): a clinicopathologic and immunohistochemical study of seven cases. *Mod Pathol* 1999;12:587–591.

505a. Hinterberger M, Reineke T, Storz M, et al. D2-40 and calretinin: a tissue microarray analysis of 341 malignant mesotheliomas with emphasis on sarcomatoid differentiation. *Mod Pathol* 2007;20:248–255.

506. Moran CA, Suster S. Yolk sac tumors of the mediastinum with prominent spindle cell features: a clinicopathologic study of three cases. *Am J Surg Pathol* 1997;21:1173–1177.

507. Klimstra DS, Moran CA, Perino G, et al. Liposarcoma of the anterior mediastinum and thymus: a clinicopathologic study of 28 cases. *Am J Surg Pathol* 1995;19:782–791.

508. Mikkilineni RS, Bhat S, Cheng AW, et al. Liposarcoma of the posterior mediastinum in a child. *Chest* 1994;106:1288–1289.

509. Ranz I, Soula R, Ben J, et al. Primary mediastinal myxoid liposarcoma: apropos of a case. *Ann Radiol (Paris)* 1992;35:526–532.

510. Havlicek F, Rosai J. A sarcoma of thymic stroma with features of liposarcoma. *Am J Clin Pathol* 1984;82:217–224.

511. Okumori M, Mabuchi M, Nakagawa M. Malignant thymoma associated with liposarcoma of the mediastinum: a case report. *Jpn J Surg* 1983;13:512–518.

512. Sekine Y, Hamaguchi K, Miyahara Y, et al. Thymus-related liposarcoma: report of a case and review of the literature. *Surg Today* 1996;26:203–207.

512a. Sung MT, Ko SF, Hsieh MJ, et al. Thymoliposarcoma. *Ann Thorac Surg* 2003;76:2082–2085.

512b. Howling SJ, Flint JD, Muller NL. Thymoliposarcoma: CT and pathologic findings. *Clin Radiol* 1999;54:341.

513. Pachter MR, Lattes R. Mesenchymal tumors of the mediastinum. II. Tumors of blood vascular origin. *Cancer* 1963;16:95–107.

514. Mentzel T, Beham A, Calonje E, et al. Epithelioid hemangioendothelioma of skin and soft tissue: clinicopathologic and immunohistochemical study of 30 cases. *Am J Surg Pathol* 1997;21:363–374.

514a. Campos J, Otero E, Dominguez MJ, et al. Epithelioid hemangioendothelioma in the posterior mediastinum. *Eur J Intern Med* 2007;18:331–332.

515. Weiss SW, Ishak KG, Dail DH, et al. Epithelioid hemangioendothelioma and related lesions. *Semin Diagn Pathol* 1986;3:259–287.

516. Castellano GC, Johnston HW. Intrathoracic chordoma presenting as a posterior mediastinal tumor. *South Med J* 1975;68:109–112.

517. Wick MR, Burgess J, Manivel JC. Reassessment of "chordoid sarcomas": immunohistochemical and ultrastructural comparison with chordoma and skeletal myxoid chondrosarcoma. *Mod Pathol* 1988;1:433–443.

518. Parker JR, Knott-Craig C, Min KW, et al. Cellular hemangioma of the posterior mediastinum: unusual presentation of a rare vascular neoplasm. *J Okla State Med Assoc* 1997;90: 7–9.

519. Misugi K, Okajima H, Newton WA, et al. Mediastinal origin of a melanotic progonoma or retinal anlage tumor: ultrastructural evidence for neural crest origin. *Cancer* 1965;18: 477–484.

520. D'Abrera VSE, Burfitt-Williams W. Melanotic neuroectodermal neoplasm of the posterior mediastinum. *J Pathol* 1973;111:165–172.

521. Doglioni C, Bontempini L, Iuzzolino P, et al. Ependymoma of the mediastinum. *Arch Pathol Lab Med* 1988;112:194–196.

521a. Estrozi B, Queiroga E, Bacchi CE, et al. Myxopapillary ependymoma of the posterior mediastinum. *Ann Diagn Pathol* 2006;10:283–287.

522. Harrier KWV, Patchefsky AS. Malignant granular cell myoblastoma of the posterior mediastinum. *Chest* 1972;61:95–96.

523. Robinson JM, Knoll R, Henry DA. Intrathoracic granular cell myoblastoma. *South Med J* 1988;81:1453–1457.

524. Verani R, Olson J, Moake JL. Intrathoracic extramedullary hematopoiesis: report of a case in a patient with sickle cell disease-beta-thalassemia. *Am J Clin Pathol* 1980;73:133–137.

525. Loh CK, Alcorta C, McElhinney AJ. Extramedullary hematopoiesis simulating posterior mediastinal tumors. *Ann Thorac Surg* 1996;61:1003–1005.

526. Valderrama E, Kahn LB, Wind E. Extraskeletal osteosarcoma arising in an ectopic hamartomatous thymus: report of a case and review of the literature. *Cancer* 1983;51:1132–1137.

527. DeNictolis M, Goteri G, Brancorsini D, et al. Extraskeletal osteosarcoma of the mediastinum associated with long-term patient survival. *Anticancer Res* 1995;15:2785–2789.

528. Siegal GP, Dehner LP, Rosai J. Histiocytosis X (Langerhans cell granulomatosis) of the thymus: a clinicopathologic study of four childhood cases. *Am J Surg Pathol* 1985;9:117–124.

529. Nakata H, Suzuki H, Sato Y, et al. Histiocytosis X with an anterior mediastinal mass as its initial manifestation. *Pediatr Radiol* 1982;12:84–85.

530. Miller R, Kurtz SM, Powers JM. Mediastinal rhabdomyoma. *Cancer* 1978;42:1983–1988.

531. Moran CA, Koss MN. Rhabdomyomatous thymoma. *Am J Surg Pathol* 1993;17:633–636.

532. Feigin GA, Robinson B, Marchevsky A. Mixed tumor of the mediastinum. *Arch Pathol Lab Med* 1986;110:80–81.

533. Meijer S, Hoitsma HFW. Malignant intrathoracic oncocytoma. *Cancer* 1982;49:97–100.

534. Chetty R. Extraskeletal mesenchymal chondrosarcoma of the mediastinum. *Histopathology* 1990;17:261–263.

535. Lemos LB, Hamoudi AB. Malignant thymic tumor in an infant (malignant histiocytoma). *Arch Pathol Lab Med* 1978;102:84–89.

536. Lynch HT, Shurin SB, Dahms BB, et al. Paravertebral malignant rhabdoid tumor in infancy. *Cancer* 1983;52:290–296.

537. Martin JME, Randhawa G, Temple WJ. Cervical thymoma. *Arch Pathol Lab Med* 1986;110:354–357.

538. Rosai J, Limas C, Husband EM. Ectopic hamartomatous thymoma: a distinctive benign lesion of the lower neck. *Am J Surg Pathol* 1984;8:501–513.

539. Asa SL, Dardick I, Von Nostrand AWP, et al. Primary thyroid thymoma: a distinct clinicopathologic entity. *Hum Pathol* 1988;19:1463–1467.

540. Yeoh CB, Ford JM, Lattes R, et al. Intrapulmonary thymoma. *J Thorac Cardiovasc Surg* 1966;51:131–136.

541. Honma K, Shimada K. Metastasizing ectopic thymoma arising in the right thoracic cavity and mimicking diffuse pleural mesothelioma: an autopsy study of a case with review of the literature. *Wien Klin Wochenschr* 1986;98:14–20.

542. Green WR, Pressoir R, Roma VG, et al. Intrapulmonary thymoma. *Arch Pathol Lab Med* 1987;111:1074–1076.

543. Moran CA, Travis WD, Rosado-de-Christenson M, et al. Thymomas presenting as pleural tumors: report of eight cases. *Am J Surg Pathol* 1992;16:138–144.

544. Higashiyama M, Doi O, Kodama K, et al. Ectopic primary pleural thymoma: report of a case. *Surg Today* 1996;26:747–750.

545. Chan JKC, Rosai J. Tumors of the neck showing thymic or related branchial pouch differentiation: a unifying concept. *Hum Pathol* 1991;22:349–367.

546. Attaran SY, Omrani GH, Tavangar SM. Lymphoepithelial-like intrathyroidal thymic carcinoma with foci of squamous differentiation. *APMIS* 1996;104:419–423.

547. Mizukami Y, Kurumaya H, Yamada T, et al. Thymic carcinoma involving the thyroid gland: report of two cases. *Hum Pathol* 1995;26:576–579.

548. Nomori H, Morinaga S, Kobayashi R, et al. Cervical thymic cancer infiltrating the trachea and thyroid. *Eur J Cardiothorac Surg* 1994;27:222–224.

549. Su L, Beals T, Bernacki EG, et al. Spindle epithelial tumor with thymus-like differentiation: a case report with cytologic, histologic, immunohistologic, and ultrastructural findings. *Mod Pathol* 1997;10:510–514.

550. Henderson CJ, Gupta L. Ectopic hamartomatous thymoma: a case study and review of the literature. *Pathology* 2000;32:142–146.

551. McCart JA, Gaspar L, Inculet R, et al. Predictors of survival following surgical resection of thymoma. *J Surg Oncol* 1993;54:233–238.

552. Froudarakis ME, Tiffet O, Fournel P, et al. Invasive thymoma: a clinical study of 23 cases. *Respiration* 2001;68:376–381.

553. Johnson SB, Eng TY, Giaccone G, et al. Thymoma: update for the new millennium. *Oncologist* 2001;6:239–246.

554. Sonobe M, Nakagawa M, Ichinose M, et al. Thymoma: analysis of prognostic factors. *Jpn J Thorac Cardiovasc Surg* 2001;49:35–41.

555. Kornstein MJ, Curran WJ Jr, Turrisi AT III, et al. Cortical versus medullary thymomas: a useful morphologic distinction? *Hum Pathol* 1988;14:1139–1147.

556. Pich A, Chiarle R, Chiusa L, et al. Long-term survival of thymoma patients by histologic pattern and proliferative activity. *Am J Surg Pathol* 1995;19:918–926.

557. Haniuda M, Morimoto M, Nishimura H, et al. Adjuvant radiotherapy after complete resection of thymoma. *Ann Thorac Surg* 1992;54:311–315.

558. Ichinose Y, Ohta M, Yano T, et al. Treatment of invasive thymoma with pleural dissemination. *J Surg Oncol* 1993;54:180–183.

559. Mineo TC, Biancari F. Reoperation for recurrent thymoma: experience in seven patients and review of the literature. *Ann Chir Gynaecol* 1996;85:286–291.

560. Nomori H, Horio Y, Iga R, et al. Recurrence of a stage I thymoma after resection. *Nippon Kyobu Shikkan Gakkai Zasshi* 1996;34:833–836.

561. Uematsu M, Yoshida H, Kondo M, et al. Entire hemithorax irradiation following complete resection in patients with stage II-III invasive thymoma. *Int J Radiat Oncol Biol Phys* 1996;35:357–360.

562. Verley JM, Hollmann KH. Thymoma: a comparative study of clinical stages, histologic features, and survival in 200 cases. *Cancer* 1985;55:1074–1086.

563. Park HS, Shin DM, Lee JS, et al. Thymoma: a retrospective study of 87 cases. *Cancer* 1994;73:2491–2498.

564. Fechner RE. Recurrence of noninvasive thymomas: report of 4 cases and review of literature. *Cancer* 1969;23:1423–1427.

565. Ohde Y, Yokose T, Yoshida J, et al. Encapsulated thymoma metastasizing to a pectoralis major muscle. *Jpn J Thorac Cardiovasc Surg* 2002;50:260–262.

566. Yamakawa Y, Masaoka A, Hashimoto T, et al. A tentative tumor-node-metastasis classification of thymoma. *Cancer* 1991;68:1984–1987.

567. Tsuchiya R, Koga K, Matsuno Y, et al. Thymic carcinoma: proposal for pathological TNM and staging. *Pathol Int* 1994;44:505–512.

568. Wilkins EW Jr, Castleman B. Thymoma: a continuing survey at the Massachusetts General Hospital. *Ann Thorac Surg* 1979;28:252–255.

569. Maggi G, Giaccone G, Donadio M, et al. Thymomas: a review of 169 cases, with particular reference to results of surgical treatment. *Cancer* 1986;58:765–776.

570. Kuo TT, Lo SK. DNA flow cytometric study of thymic epithelial tumors with evaluation of its usefulness in the pathologic classification. *Hum Pathol* 1993;24:746–749.

571. Yang WI, Efird JT, Quintanilla-Martinez L, et al. Cell kinetic study of thymic epithelial tumors using PCNA (PC10) and Ki-67 (MIB-1) antibodies. *Hum Pathol* 1996;27:70–76.

572. Tateyama H, Eimoto T, Tada T, et al. Apoptosis, bcl-2 protein, and fas antigen in thymic epithelial tumors. *Mod Pathol* 1997;10:983–991.

573. Pich A, Chiarle R, Chiusa L, et al. Argyrophilic nucleolar organizer region counts predict survival in thymoma. *Cancer* 1994;74:1568–1574.

574. Frizzera G, Peterson BA, Bayrd ED, et al. A systemic lymphoproliferative disorder with morphologic features of Castleman's disease: clinical findings and clinicopathologic correlations in 15 patients. *J Clin Oncol* 1985;3:1202–1216.

575. Leopold KA, Canellos GP, Rosenthal D, et al. Stage IA-IIB Hodgkin's disease: staging and treatment of patients with large mediastinal adenopathy. *J Clin Oncol* 1989;7:1059–1065.

576. Hoppe RT. The management of bulky mediastinal Hodgkin's disease. *Hematol Oncol Clin North Am* 1989;3:265–276.

577. Jacobson JO, Aisenberg AC, Lamarre L, et al. Mediastinal large-cell lymphoma: an uncommon subset of adult lymphoma curable with combined modality therapy. *Cancer* 1988;62:1893–1898.

577a. Boleti E, Johnson PW. Primary mediastinal B-cell lymphoma. *Hematol Oncol* 2007;25:157–163.

577b. Mazzarotto R, Boso C, Viannello F, et al. Primary mediastinal large B-cell lymphoma: results of intensive chemotherapy regimens (MACOP-B/VACOP-B) plus involved field radiotherapy on 53 patients. A single institution experience. *Int J Radiat Oncol Biol Phys* 2007;68:823–829.

578. Boumghar M, Dusmet M. Postoperative evolution and prognosis of thymic tumors. In Givel JC, ed. *Surgery of the Thymus.* Berlin, Germany: Springer-Verlag, 1990:319–331.

579. Nichols CR. Mediastinal germ cell tumors: clinical features and biologic correlates. *Chest* 1991;99:472–479.

580. Harms D, Janig U. Germ cell tumors of childhood: report of 170 cases including 59 pure and partial yolk sac tumours. *Virchows Arch A Pathol Anat Histopathol* 1986;409:223–239.

581. Toner GC, Geller NL, Tan C, et al. Serum tumor marker half-life during chemotherapy allows early prediction of complete response and survival in non-seminomatous germ cell tumors. *Cancer Res* 1990;50:5904–5910.

582. Wishnow KI, Johnson DE, Swanson DA, et al. Identifying patients with low-risk clinical stage I non-seminomatous testicular tumors who should be treated by surveillance. *Urology* 1989;34:339–343.

583. Mayordomo JI, Paz-Ares L, Rivera F, et al. Ovarian and extragonadal malignant germ cell tumors in females: a single institution experience with 43 patients. *Ann Oncol* 1994;5:225–231.

584. Hsu CP, Chen CY, Chen CL, et al. Thymic carcinoma: ten years' experience in twenty patients. *J Thorac Cardiovasc Surg* 1994;107:615–620.

585. Peleg D, Zabari A, Shalev E. Relapsing thymic carcinoma during pregnancy. *Acta Obstet Gynecol Scand* 1992;71:398–400.

586. Seto H, Kageyama M, Shimizu M, et al. Assessment of residual tumor viability in thymic carcinoma by sequential thallium-201 SPECT: comparison with CT and biopsy findings. *J Nucl Med* 1994;35:1659–1661.

587. Yanagawa H, Bando H, Takishita Y, et al. Thymic carcinoma treated with intensive chemotherapy and radiation. *Anticancer Res* 1995;15:1485–1489.

The Heart

Over the past several decades, the management of cardiovascular diseases has advanced in several important areas. Disease prevention, including dietary manipulation, regular resistance exercise, smoking cessation programs, and lipid-modifying drugs, has contributed to a decline in the annual mortality related to cardiovascular disease (1–4). New diagnostic interventions and refinement of existing techniques provide clinicians with remarkable anatomic and functional detail of the heart and peripheral vascular system (5,6). Two- and three-dimensional echocardiography generates detailed spatial information and regional wall function information that is useful in the evaluation of structural abnormalities such as valvulopathies, congenital defects, intracardiac masses, and transient or evolving wall motion abnormalities (7,8). Color flow imaging provides additional information of intracardiac blood flow (9). Intravascular ultrasound (IVUS) generates cross-sectional, three-dimensional images of coronary artery segments. All three layers of the vessel are tomographically outlined, and information about arterial plaque size, length, composition, and luminal diameter can be generated (Fig. 29.1) (10–14). Cardiovascular computed tomography (CT) is used for the evaluation of cardiac function, coronary artery imaging including the identification of calcified plaques, and cardiac morphology (15–18). More recently, the introduction of multidetector CT allows for qualitative and se-

miquantitative assessment of regional and global ventricular function. Cardiac magnetic resonance imaging also provides functional information together with quantitative assessment of ventricular volume and mass (Fig. 29.2) (19). Radionucleotide perfusion scanning is a now a mainstay in the noninvasive assessment of myocardial viability, perfusion, and function (20). In the area of therapeutic intervention, a variety of noninvasive and invasive therapies have emerged. Minimally invasive and beating heart surgical options are available for coronary revascularization and valvular procedures (21,22). Surgery aided by robotic technology is currently being evaluated in adult and pediatric patients. Drug-eluding stents and coated stents, notwithstanding their current controversies, are commonly used in the management of patients with acute coronary syndromes and restenosis lesions (23,24). Other percutaneous interventions include deployment of occlusion devices and coils for the treatment of septal defects and patent ductus arteriosus (25). A fourth area of advancement in cardiovascular disease is the realm of molecular genetics and genomics (26). The current classification of cardiovascular diseases such as the cardiomyopathies has evolved, in large part, from the insights of molecular cardiology. The pathogenesis and treatment of monogenic dis-

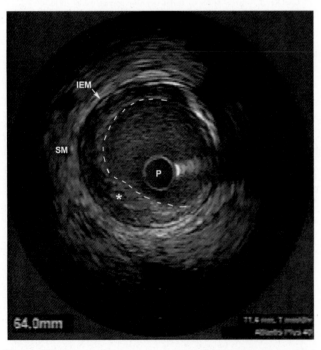

Figure 29.1. Intravascular ultrasound image of cross section of coronary artery. The luminal probe (P) is surrounded by blood. The intimal plaque is outlined by ----. The internal elastic membrane (IEM) separates the smooth muscle (SM) of the medial layer from the plaque*.

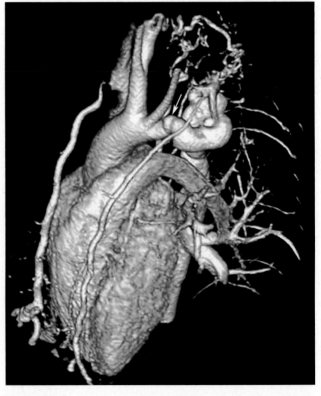

Figure 29.2. Volume rendering of contrast-enhanced magnetic resonance angiography of a corkscrew preductal coarctation of the aorta.

orders, such as hypertrophic cardiomyopathy, and polygenic conditions, such as atherosclerosis and hypertension, are the subject of ongoing investigations influenced by genomic and proteomic studies (27–29). In each of these different areas of cardiovascular advancement (prevention, diagnostics, therapeutics, and molecular), the diagnostic pathologist has assumed an essential role (30,31). As a result, the breadth and complexity of cardiovascular specimens continues to expand in community practice and in academic centers. Herein we will discuss the current classifications, diagnostic criteria, and problematic issues commonly encountered in the surgical pathology laboratory. The discussion of atherosclerotic disease, hypertensive heart disease, and congenital heart disease is beyond the scope of this chapter, and the reader is directed to other excellent resources (32–35). A more detailed discussion of the clinical and imaging findings can be found in many contemporary textbooks of cardiovascular medicine (36–39).

The practicing surgical pathologist is now likely to encounter specimens beyond valve leaflets and pericardiectomy specimens. In centers with active interventional, transplant, and surgical programs, endomyocardial biopsies (EMBs), ventricular core excisions from ventricular assist device (VAD) placement, septal myomectomies, tumor excisions, prosthetic valve and VAD devices, and native hearts are encountered. In each case, careful attention to specimen handling and preparation is essential, and the specific requirements will be addressed in each category.

MYOCARDIAL DISEASES

Over the past 50 years, the terminology, concepts, and classification of myocardial disorders have undergone numerous revisions. The World Health Organization (WHO) originally defined the term *cardiomyopathy* in 1968 as "diseases of different and often unknown etiology in which the dominant feature is cardiomegaly and heart failure" (40). This functional definition was modified in the 1980 WHO classification to "heart diseases of unknown cause" (41). The three types of primary cardiomyopathy consisted of dilated or congestive, hypertrophic (with or without obstruction), and restrictive types. The 1995 classification reflected new knowledge of disease genetics, etiologies, and pathogenesis and expanded the scope to "diseases of the myocardium associated with cardiac dysfunction" (42). Primary cardiomyopathies and specific heart muscle diseases were enumerated. In 2006, a consensus group of the American Heart Association (AHA) defined cardiomyopathies as "a heterogeneous group of diseases of the myocardium associated with mechanical and/or electrical dysfunction that usually (but not invariably) exhibit inappropriate ventricular hypertrophy or dilatation and are a result of a variety of causes that are frequently genetic" (43). In this etiologic/pathogenetic classification, there are primary types that are genetic, nongenetic, or acquired in nature and secondary types that are usually a component of a systemic disease (Table 29.1). In 2007, the European Society of Cardiology proposed a new classification based on the definition of cardiomyopathy as a "myocardial disorder in which the heart muscle is structurally and functionally abnormal, in the absence of coronary artery disease, hypertension, valvular heart disease and congenital heart disease sufficient to cause the observed myocardial abnormality" (44). This clinically oriented classification established familial and nonfamilial

categories for each of the major types of cardiomyopathies and eliminated the primary and secondary types (Table 29.1). Although both of these recent classifications have their individual merits, we prefer a morphologic approach to cardiomyopathy that highlights the key macroscopic and/or histopathologic findings that can be identified in EMBs or larger specimens such as ventricular apical plugs and explanted hearts. In many cases, histochemical and immunohistochemical stains and molecular studies aid in the classification. In some disorders such as dilated cardiomyopathy (DCM), the histopathologic features are nonspecific, and the role of EMB is to exclude treatable causes of ventricular dysfunction (Table 29.2).

THE NORMAL HEART

The macroscopic, histologic, and ultrastructural features of the normal heart have been described in several textbooks and monographs and will only be briefly reviewed here (45,46). The myocardium is composed of bundles of myocytes separated by fibrous bands. Individual myocytes form a syncytium connected by intercalated discs at their terminal ends and occasionally display side-to-side junctions. On average, myocytes measure 15 to 17 μm in diameter and display central round to oval nuclei measuring up to 8 μm in diameter. Lipofuscin granules can be seen in a perinuclear position. The cytoplasm contains actin and myosin filaments, mitochondria, glycogen granules, and Z-bands. The interstitium is composed of collagen and elastic fibers, a proteoglycan- and glycosaminoglycan-rich matrix, basement membrane proteins such as laminin and fibronectin, and a rich capillary vascular network admixed with scattered fibroblasts, leukocytes, and, on occasion, adipocytes and nerve twigs (47).

THE ENDOMYOCARDIAL BIOPSY

In many centers, the evaluation of cardiomyopathic patients includes a detailed history and physical examination, many of the sophisticated techniques described earlier, coronary angiography, and EMB. The indications for EMB have been previously published, including a recent consensus statement (33,48–50). Currently, the major indications include the diagnosis of acute transplantation rejection, the classification of myocarditis, the evaluation of recent-onset heart failure in the absence of coronary artery disease, the grading of anthracycline cardiotoxicity, the evaluation of restrictive heart disease such as amyloidosis, and the diagnosis of storage disorders and cardiac tumors. Complications are uncommon and include hematomas and nerve injury and cardiac problems such as arrhythmias, tricuspid valve apparatus damage, and ventricular perforation.

Proper tissue procurement and handling are essential for optimal diagnostic evaluation. Biopsy specimens should be gently extracted from the bioptome with a needle tip to limit crush artifactual distortion. The clinical indications for the biopsy determine, in large part, the method of tissue handling. For example, for standard light microscopy, the tissue should immediately be placed in a standard fixative such as 10% neutral buffered formalin. To subtype amyloid fibrils in cardiac amyloidosis by immunofluorescence (e.g., AL, AA, or transthyretin) one to two pieces should be submitted in saline or Zeus medium and then snap frozen in a plastic Beem capsule containing an optimal cutting temperature (OCT)–embedding medium. Snap freezing tissue is optimal for preserving tissue for molecu-

TABLE 29.1	Current Classifications of the Cardiomyopathies

AHA Classification (2006)	European Society of Cardiology (2007)
Primary Cardiomyopathies	**Cardiomyopathies**
	(e.g., amyloid, obesity)
	Familial/Genetic
A. Genetic Hypertrophic	**Hypertrophic CMP**
Arrhythmogenic RV CMP/Dysplasia	
LV noncompaction	Non familial
Glycogen storage	(e.g., amyloid, obesity)
Conduction defects	
Mitochondrial disorders	
Ion channelopathies	
	(e.g., familial CMP, mitochondrial CMP)
	Familial/Genetic
B. Mixed Genetic/Acquired Dilated CMP	**Dilated CMP**
Restrictive CMP	
	Non familial
	(e.g., myocarditis, drug-induced CMP)
	(e.g., familial, plakoglobin mutation)
	Familial/Genetic
C. Acquired Inflammatory (myocarditis)	**Arrhythmogenic RV CMP**
Stress-induced (Tako-tsubo)	
Peripartum	Non familial
Tachycardia-induced	
Infants of IDDM mothers	
	(e.g., familial CMP, desminopathy)
	Familial/Genetic
Secondary Cardiomyopathies	**Restrictive CMP**
	Non familial
	(e.g., AL-type amyloidosis, carcinoid)
	(e.g., LV noncompaction, Barth syndrome)
	Familial/Genetic
	Unclassified CMP
	Non familial
	(e.g., Tako-Tsubo/stress-induced CMP)

Modified from References 43 & 44

CMP, cardiomyopathy; IDDM, insulin-dependent diabetes mellitus; LV, left ventricular; RV, right ventricular.

lar analysis such as nested polymerase chain reaction (PCR) and real-time PCR in the evaluation of viral pathogens. The diagnosis of chronic anthracycline cardiotoxicity requires that *all* the biopsy pieces (minimum of three to five pieces) should be fixed for transmission electron microscopy (e.g., 2.5% glutaraldehyde with 2% paraformaldehyde in 0.1 M sodium cacodylate buffer, pH 7.2).

For routine diagnostic evaluation, overnight processing and paraffin embedding are sufficient. For emergent cases, a 90-minute rapid ("ultra") processing cycle is available, and microscopic slides can be prepared within 2 to 3 hours. All of the biopsy pieces should be embedded in the same block. We recommend a minimum of three to six slides prepared at 4- to 5-μm thickness from various depths within the paraffin block. Multiple paraffin ribbons are placed on each slide. We routinely stain with hematoxylin and eosin and use stains such as Masson's trichrome to confirm the presence of myocyte damage or fibrosis, Congo red or sulfated Alcian blue stain for amyloid fibrils, and the Prussian blue stain for iron deposition. Immunohistochemical, immunofluorescence, and molecular studies are used for specific indications. Paraffin section immunohistochemistry is used to evaluate for infectious myocarditis (e.g., cytomegalovirus [CMV] or toxoplasmic myocarditis), posttransplantation lymphoproliferative disorders (PTLD) (e.g., B-cell clonality, Epstein-Barr virus [EBV] latent membrane proteins, anomalous coexpression of B-cell and T-cell antigens), or acute antibody-mediated rejection (intravascular collections of CD68+ histiocytes and deposition of C4d on the microvasculature). In situ hybridization is helpful to demonstrate the presence of EBV or other viral genome or light chain restriction in PTLD.

TABLE 29.2

Morphologic Approach to the Cardiomyopathies

PRIMARY CARDIOMYOPATHY
Dilated cardiomyopathy
Hypertrophic cardiomyopathy
Restrictive cardiomyopathy
RV arrhythmogenic cardiomyopathy/dysplasia
Left ventricular noncompaction
Histiocytoid cardiomyopathy[a]
Unclassified cardiomyopathy
INFLAMMATORY CARDIOMYOPATHY (MYOCARDITIS)
SECONDARY CARDIOMYOPATHY
Infiltrative (amyloidosis, Gaucher disease)
Storage disorders (Fabry disease, glycogen storage, hemochromatosis)
Toxic/Drug/Therapy-related (anthracycline, cyclophosphamide, radiation, heavy metals, recreational drugs, alcohol, chemicals)
Endocrinopathies (pheochromocytoma, acromegaly, hypothyroidism, hyperthyroidism)
Postpartum/Peripartum cardiomyopathy
Neuromuscular Neurologic (Friedreich ataxia, muscular dystrophy, neurofibromatosis)
Autoimmune/Collagen vascular diseases
Nutritional/Electrolyte imbalances

RV, right ventricular.
[a]Discussed in the section titled "Pediatric Tumors and Tumor-Like Lesions."
Modified from Maron et al. (43).

A variety of artifacts in EMB specimens can mimic pathologic lesions. The surgical pathologist must be aware of these patterns to avoid a misdiagnosis that could lead to unnecessary therapeutic interventions. These have been reviewed in detail in a recent publication, and only selected topics will be briefly reviewed (45,50). The most common biopsy artifact is the presence of contraction bands in myocytes that are identical to the linear bands observed in acute ischemic necrosis and catecholamine ("pressor") effect. Another frequent artifact is intussusception or "telescoping" of small arteries that has been confused with luminal occlusion by thrombus and transplantation-related arteriosclerosis. Connective tissue stains such as Masson's trichrome or elastic van Gieson highlight the internal elastic membranes of both vessel segments. Intramyocardial accumulations of mature adipose tissue can simulate epicardial tissue, especially if associated with vessels of relatively large caliber, and both can be found in the right ventricular (RV) apical region. Ventricular perforation is identified by the presence of mesothelial cells. Accumulations of fresh platelet/fibrin-rich thrombus may be identified along the endocardial surface of biopsy fragments. Bioptome-induced tissue distortion or crush artifact can occur, and on occasion, it may not be possible to distinguish the cell types (e.g., lymphocytes, endothelial cells, histiocytes, myocytes). In some instances, additional leveled hematoxylin and eosin–stained sections provide less distorted foci in the deeper aspects of the biopsy sample.

The surgical pathology report should be comprehensive to provide the clinician with as much diagnostic information as possible. The number of pieces of myocardium, the appearance of the myocyte nuclei (hypertrophied, pyknotic, attenuated, or atrophic), the presence of cytoplasmic pigments or other accumulations, the pattern of necrosis (focal vs. diffuse), the composition of the interstitium (e.g., cellularity, fibrosis, edema, amyloid deposits), and the presence of endocardial inflammation should be addressed. It is essential that detailed clinical information be provided to allow clinical-pathologic correlation.

PRIMARY CARDIOMYOPATHIES

Dilated Cardiomyopathy

Dilated or congestive cardiomyopathy is the most common type of idiopathic or primary cardiomyopathy and is one of the most common indications for heart transplantation (44). The estimated prevalence is 1:2500 (43). It is characterized by systolic dysfunction, leading to diminished stroke volumes, elevated left ventricular (LV) end-systolic and end-diastolic volumes, diminished ejection fraction, increased ventricular chamber dimensions and wall tension, and thinning of LV wall (Table 29.3). In most cases, both ventricles are affected, and at the time of transplantation, four-chamber dilatation is common (Fig. 29.3). By definition, significant coronary artery disease, hypertensive heart disease, and valvular causes of contractile dysfunction are absent. The pathogenesis is elusive; approximately 50% of cases are idiopathic, and the remainder is composed of familial cases (25% to 35%), chronic alcohol and heavy metal toxicity, and peripartum causes (51). The genetic determinants are variable and include mutations in genes coding sarcomeric, cytoskeletal, and nuclear proteins and proteins involved in the regulation of calcium metabolism (52). The most common pattern of inheritance is autosomal dominant, but the penetrance is variable; other reported patterns include autosomal recessive, X-linked, and mitochondrial. Of the idiopathic causes, postviral and other infectious events and autoimmune mechanisms are suspected pathogenetic mechanisms. The clinical manifestations of DCM reflect the poor systolic pump function of the heart. Congestive heart failure symptoms are common. Complications include supraventricular and ventricular arrhythmias, thromboembolic events, and sudden death.

The macroscopic and histopathologic findings result from ventricular remodeling. Increased heart weight, globular shape, chamber dilatation of both ventricles and atria, prominent fine reticulation of LV trabecular musculature, mural thrombi in one or more chambers, endocardial fibrous thickening over the

TABLE 29.3

Dilated Cardiomyopathy

KEY GROSS FINDINGS
Globular-shaped heart
Increased heart weight
Biventricular/4-chamber dilatation
Normal or diminished LV thickness
Mural thrombi
Prominent LV endocardial trabeculations
Annular dilatation of AV valves
Endocardial fibrous thickening of Septal portion of LV
KEY MICROSCOPIC FINDINGS
Myocyte hypertrophy (nuclear size/shape)
Interstitial/perivascular fibrosis
Interstitial lymphocytes and macrophages
Attenuated myocytes (myofibrillar loss)

AV, atrioventricular; LV, left ventricular; S, septum.

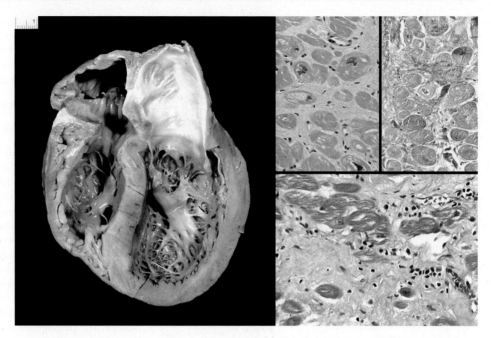

Figure 29.3. Idiopathic dilated cardiomyopathy (DCM). *Left panel*: Four-chamber dilatation with prominent PV trabeculations is noted. *Upper right panel*: Myocyte hypertrophy and interstitial fibrosis are prominent microscopic features. *Lower right panel*: Scattered collections of lymphocytes within fibrous tissue are a common finding in DCM.

septal portion of the LV, annular dilatation of atrial-ventricular valves, and reduced free wall thickness are common macroscopic findings (Fig. 29.3). These features can be best appreciated by a four-chamber view of the heart or by the short axis (bread loafing) method. The microscopic findings are less dramatic and nonspecific. The myocytes appear attenuated usually with increased vacuolization. Myocyte hypertrophy is characterized by enlarged, irregularly shaped, and hyperchromatic nuclei. The interstitium is expanded by collagenous fibrosis that ranges from fine to coarse in composition. Perivascular fibrosis is also conspicuous. Scattered collections of mononuclear inflammatory cells are observed in more than 80% of cases, but myocyte damage is absent (53). At the ultrastructural level, myofibrillar loss, Z-band remnants, and numerous, irregularly shaped mitochondria masses are observed, particularly in the advanced stages of DCM (54).

Several disorders can mimic DCM both clinically and pathologically. The primary role of EMB is to exclude those mimics with specific diagnostic features and therapies such as lymphocytic myocarditis, sarcoidosis, hemochromatosis, anthracycline cardiotoxicity, and so on. A detailed clinical history is required to exclude acquired causes such as collagen vascular disorders, endocrinopathies, nutritional deficiencies, recreational abuse of drugs such as methamphetamines, and tachycardiomyopathy (44). In our experience, the majority of cases of peripartum/postpartum cardiomyopathy that have an EMB as part of the workup show features of DCM. We avoid the term *chronic myocarditis* for cases with scattered lymphocytes embedded in fibrous tissue because we think that these cases fall within the spectrum of DCM. The number of truly idiopathic cases is likely to continue to diminish with the application of newer and more sophisticated molecular studies.

Hypertrophic Cardiomyopathy

Hypertrophic cardiomyopathy (HCM) is the most common genetic disorder of the heart and affects 1 in 500 adults (43). HCM is characterized by myocyte hypertrophy in the absence of abnormal loading disorders such as hypertension and stenotic valvular heart disease or systemic or infiltrative disorders such as amyloidosis or hemochromatosis (55). It has an autosomal dominant pattern of inheritance with variable phenotypic expression depending in large part on age (56). Patients present across a wide age spectrum, including infants, but most manifest symptoms during adolescence. Symptoms include exertional dyspnea and chest pain, palpitations, lightheadedness, syncope, and sudden death; HCM is a common cause of sudden death in young athletes. In some cases, patients are asymptomatic.

In its classic form, HCM is caused by a single gene mutation. In 1990, Geisterfer-Lowrance et al. (57) identified a missense mutation in the beta-myosin heavy chain in a family with HCM. Ten additional mutations that encode sarcomeric proteins have been identified; beta-myosin heavy chain and myosin-binding protein C are the most frequent point mutations. Several metabolic and storage diseases, such as glycogen storage disease, carnitine deficiency, Anderson-Fabry disease, and Danon disease; mitochondrial cytopathies such as Senger syndrome and Friedreich ataxia; and syndromic forms of HCM such as Noonan and LEOPARD syndromes produce cardiomyopathies that resemble the sarcomeric forms (Table 29.4) (55,58).

The original pathologic description of HCM by Teare in 1958 (59) provides many of the key morphologic criteria used today. The macroscopic findings are optimally presented by the short axis method of sectioning or in a long axis cut through the LV outflow; the lines-of-flow approach is best avoided (60). Transverse slices of the myocardium demonstrate the markedly thickened LV, usually with disproportionate enlargement of the septum and normal or reduced LV chamber size. The ratio of septal thickness to LV free wall thickness of more than 1.3 is used by some pathologists to confirm asymmetric hypertrophy (61). In many cases, the musculature of the septum displays a whorled arrangement of the muscle bundles (Fig. 29.4). The RV is also thickened in the majority of cases, particularly in the anterior wall of the RV outflow tract. Most cases of HCM display asymmetric thickening of the interventricular septum, but con-

TABLE 29.4

Hypertrophic Cardiomyopathy

KEY GROSS FINDINGS
Markedly thickened LV (asymmetric/symmetric)
Normal or reduced LV cavity
Endocardial fibrous thickening opposite anterior mitral cusp
Whorled appearance of septal musculature
Increase in RV wall thickness
KEY MICROSCOPIC FINDINGS
Marked myocyte hypertrophy
Myocyte disarray pattern
Interstitial and perivascular fibrosis
Endocardial fibrosis
Fibrous mural changes in intramyocardial arteries

LV, left ventricle; RV, right ventricle.

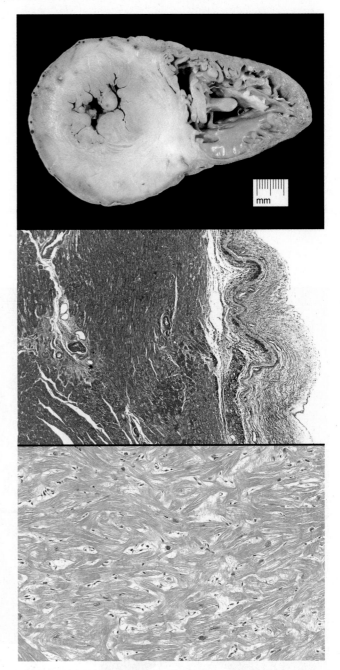

Figure 29.4. Hypertrophic cardiomyopathy (HCM). Upper panel: Marked left ventricular (LV) hypertrophy with diminished LV cavity. The septum is thicker than the LV free wall, indicating the asymmetric form of HCM. Middle panel: Trichrome stain showing endocardial fibrous thickening and perivascular collagenous fibrosis. Lower panel: Myocyte disarray is characterized by irregularly arranged, interwoven myocyte fibers.

centric or symmetric hypertrophy is also reported. For this reason, the diagnosis of HCM requires that hypertensive heart disease and amyloidosis be excluded by clinical and morphologic means, respectively. In patients with outflow tract obstruction, the septum may have a transverse fibrous plaque on the endocardium at the site of repetitive contact with the anterior leaflet of the mitral valve. This repetitive mechanical injury results in thickening of the leaflet. In the late stages of HCM, protracted heart failure may lead to LV dilatation and obscure some of these findings. The disrupted muscular arrangement seen grossly reflects the microscopic disorganization and fibrosis within the more central portions of the septum, particularly toward the base of the heart. Myocytes showing marked hypertrophy with pleomorphic and hyperchromatic nuclear forms alternate with haphazard bands of dense collagenous tissue to create the characteristic interwoven myocyte disarray pattern (Fig. 29.4). The loss of orderly myocyte bundles is often prominent at scanning magnification. The trichrome stain highlights the interstitial fibrosis and the subendocardial plaques. The small intramyocardial arteries show disorganized smooth muscle proliferation with reduced lumens and intramural and perivascular fibrosis (62). Foci of coarse interstitial fibrosis can be found within the central portions of the septum.

Several points must be emphasized about the differential diagnosis of HCM. First, myocyte disarray is observed in cases of HCM as a result of mutations of genes coding for sarcomeric proteins and in the nonsarcomeric forms such as Friedreich ataxia and Noonan syndrome (Fig. 29.5). On occasion, these changes can also be seen in hypertensive heart disease and in some congenital heart diseases, but they are usually patchy (63). Hypertensive heart disease and amyloidosis can mimic some of the macroscopic features of HCM, and careful attention to clinical history and the microscopic findings is essential. Routine amyloid staining of myomectomy specimens of patients more than 65 years old is advocated by many investigators (64). RV EMB is not helpful in establishing the diagnosis of HCM because myocyte disarray is a normal finding in the RV apex and in trabecular muscles. It is, however, useful to exclude other causes such as amyloidosis and hemochromatosis. Distinction of HCM from ''athlete's heart'' is important and at times difficult. Sustained isometric exercise produces a physiologic form of hypertrophy with increased LV muscle mass, LV wall thickening, and normal or reduced chamber dimensions. Importantly, the

septal-to-posterior free wall ratio is not greater than 1.3 and the wall thickness does not exceed 1.6 cm in athlete's heart (65).

Currently, the medical management of HCM is directed at improving myocardial relaxation and increasing diastolic filling. Ventricular septal myotomy-myomectomy removes the portion of the septum beneath the aortic valve and is indicated in patients who fail medical therapy or have severe outflow obstruction (Fig. 29.6) (66). Tazelaar and Billingham (67) found disar-

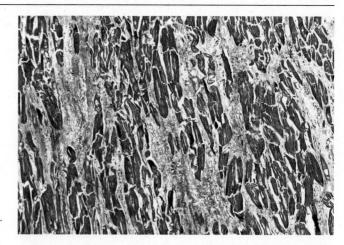

Figure 29.5. Marked hypertrophy and fibrosis in Friedrich ataxia. Myocyte disarray was found elsewhere in the heart.

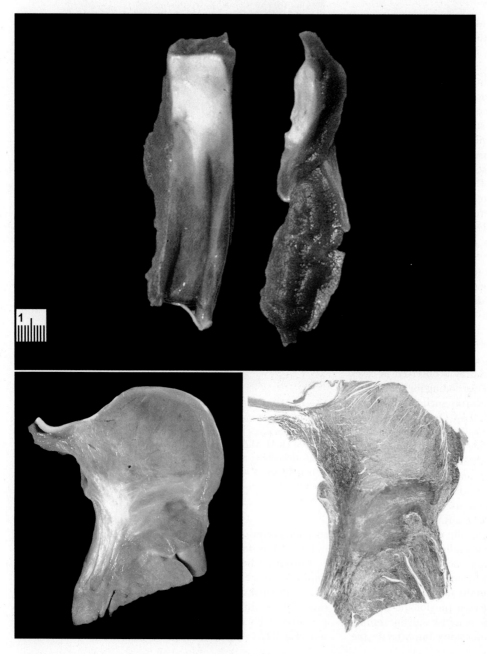

Figure 29.6. Upper panel: Myomectomy specimen from left ventricular (LV) outflow tract in hypertrophic cardiomyopathy (HCM). Note prominent endocardial fibrous thickening. Lower panel: Alcohol ablation of septum showing wedge-shaped fibrous scar. The transeptal scar is highlighted on the trichrome stain.

ray in 58% of myomectomy specimens along with the interstitial and vascular changes described earlier. In a recent series of 204 cases from the Mayo Clinic, the microscopic findings included myocyte hypertrophy (100%), endocardial (96%) and myocardial fibrosis (93%), myocyte disarray (79%), endocardial inflammation (48%), arterial thickening (46%), dilated venules (28%), and arterial dysplasia (16%) (68). In our experience, myocyte disarray is not found in small or superficial myomectomy specimens because it is generally located in the mid region of the septum. Another therapeutic intervention is transcoronary septal ablation with alcohol (69). The septal perforator branch(es) of the left anterior descending artery is infused with 1 to 3 cc of pure alcohol, causing localized infarction and eventually retraction and scarring of the basal portion of the septum (Fig. 29.6). There are very few studies comparing the two techniques, and a controlled randomized study has not yet been reported (70,71).

Restrictive Cardiomyopathy

The disorders comprising the primary restrictive cardiomyopathies are a heterogeneous group characterized by diastolic dysfunction as a result of thickened or "stiff" ventricles. Secondary causes are more common and include several infiltrative disorders, storage diseases, and postradiation disorder. In the setting of restrictive hemodynamics, ventricular compliance is diminished, causing elevated ventricular filling pressure but preservation of systolic function. Other causes of diastolic dysfunction, such as constrictive pericarditis, need to be excluded by clinical and imaging modalities like echocardiography. The EMB is useful for excluding many of the secondary types.

Two forms of the primary disorder have been described (Table 29.5) (72). Primary idiopathic restrictive cardiomyopathy is generally a sporadic disorder that affects children and adults and can be associated with a skeletal myopathy (73–75). Familial forms have also been reported. At transplantation, the heart weight is normal or increased, and the ventricular chamber dimensions and wall thickness and epicardium are normal. Endocardial fibrous plaques are sometimes observed. Biatrial dilatation is present, and thrombi can be found in the appendages. Microscopic sections display variable degrees of myocyte hypertrophy and interstitial fibrosis both in distribution and severity (Fig. 29.7). The second type of restrictive cardiomyopa-

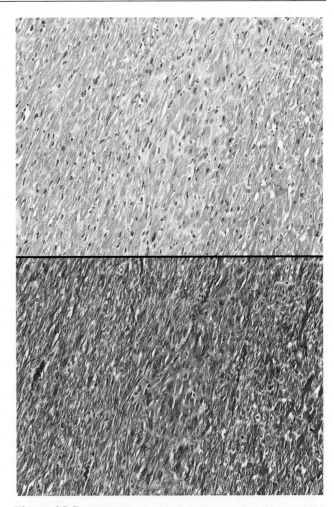

Figure 29.7. Idiopathic restrictive cardiomyopathy in a young child. Fine interstitial fibrosis is noted on routine sections and highlighted by trichrome stain.

TABLE 29.5	Restrictive Cardiomyopathy (RCM)
Primary Idiopathic RCM	*Obliterative CMP*
KEY GROSS FINDINGS	
Normal or increased heart weight	Thrombus in RV and LV inflow tract and apex
Dilatation of both atria	TV and MV dysfunction
Atrial mural thrombi	Diminished ventricular cavities
Endocardial fibrous plaques	
Normal ventricular size and wall thickness	
KEY MICROSCOPIC FINDINGS	
Variable myocyte hypertrophy	Endocardial fibrous thickening
Interstitial and perimyocyte fibrosis	Mural thrombus overlying endocardium
	Eosinophils in thrombus, endocardium, and myocardium
	Interstitial fibrosis
	+/− lymphocytes in endomyocardium

CMP, cardiomyopathy; LV, left ventricle; MV, mitral valve; RV, right ventricle; TV, tricuspid valve.

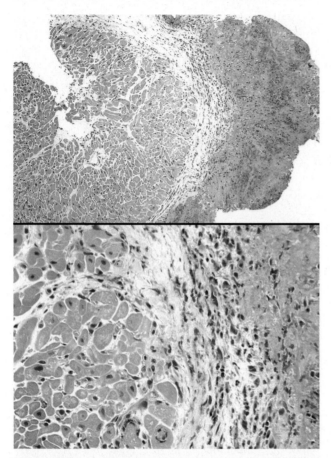

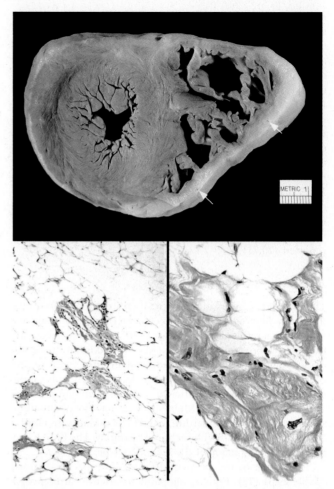

Figure 29.8. Endomyocardial biopsy specimen in obliterative cardiomyopathy. *Upper panel*: The endocardium is thickened and covered by a thrombus. *Lower panel*: Eosinophils and mononuclear inflammatory cells are present in the endocardium and infiltrate into the adjacent myocardium.

Figure 29.9. Arrhythmogenic right ventricular (RV) dysplasia/cardiomyopathy. *Upper panel*: The RV free wall is replaced by fat (*arrows*), and the chamber is dilated. *Lower panel*: Microscopic sections showing marked fatty replacement with scattered islands of myocytes and bands of fibrous tissue.

thy is also called obliterative cardiomyopathy. It is characterized by endomyocardial abnormalities and consists of an acute form (Loffler endocarditis) and a chronic form (endomyocardial fibrosis [EMF]). The endocardium of the inflow tracts and apices are covered by thrombus. The EMB shows thrombus overlying granulation tissue attached to the endocardium as irregular aggregates (Fig. 29.8). Eosinophils are admixed with the thrombus and may extend into the underlying myocardium. In the later stages, the number of eosinophils diminishes, and the endocardial plaques are thick and fibrotic. This resembles the findings in EMF. Inflow tracts and papillary muscles are covered by collagenous fibrosis and calcifications with reduction in the chamber size. Lymphocytic infiltrates and interstitial fibrosis may be found in the myocardium.

Arrhythmogenic Right Ventricular Cardiomyopathy/ Dysplasia

Arrhythmogenic RV cardiomyopathy/dysplasia (ARVC/D) is a recent addition to the primary cardiomyopathy group (42). It is an uncommon disorder affecting adolescents and young adults, with an estimated prevalence of 1:5000, and is more common in parts of Europe than North America. The clinical presentation typically is exercise-induced ventricular arrhythmias and sudden

death. An autosomal dominant pattern of inheritance has been reported, and mutations in six genes encoding desmosomal components like dplakophilin-2 and desmoplakin have been identified (76,77). In its classic form, ARVC/D affects the RV either segmentally or globally with replacement of the myocardium by adipose tissue and fibrous tissue. The RV inflow tract, apex, and outflow tract are involved, and at the time of transplantation or autopsy, the RV is dilated and the free wall is attenuated (Fig. 29.9). In some cases, collections of mononuclear inflammatory cells are found within the adipose tissue. The LV can also be affected but usually in conjunction with RV disease. More recently, left dominant and biventricular forms of the disorder have been reported (78). The role of the EMB in the diagnosis of ARVC/D is limited, and the findings must always be interpreted and reported with the clinical and imaging findings. The RV anterior free wall and apex are sites of fatty infiltration in a variety of conditions including normal hearts and in DCM (79).

Left Ventricular Noncompaction

LV noncompaction (LVNC) is another primary cardiomyopathy that was first included in the 1995 WHO classification. In

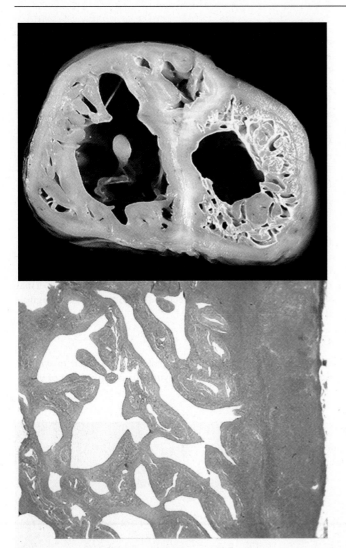

Figure 29.10. Left ventricular (LV) noncompaction. *Upper panel*: The LV exhibits a spongelike appearance caused by deep recesses. Note the presence of a thickened endocardium in the LV. *Lower panel*: Low-power microscopy showing the marked trabeculation deep within the myocardium.

most cases, it is a congenital disorder that features prominent trabeculations of the LV and deep intertrabecular recesses or sinusoids resulting in a "spongy LV" (Fig. 29.10). The sinusoids are in direct communication with the ventricular cavity (80). The lesion is segmental and shows a predilection for the apical region. Microscopic sectioning shows fibroelastotic thickening of the endocardium, anastomosing endocardial trabeculations, and interstitial fibrosis (81). Foci of ischemic necrosis and vacuolization can be found in the subendocardial zone and in the thickened trabeculae. LVNC occurs from arrested embryologic development of the ventricle (43). It may be a solitary abnormality or seen in association with other congenital abnormalities or syndromes. Recently, a gene mutation in the gene *G4.5* was reported (82). Some patients require heart transplantation for intractable heart failure.

Other Types of Primary Cardiomyopathy

In the recent AHA classification of primary cardiomyopathies, several disorders have been included that the pathologist

should be aware of but that do not have specific or recognized histopathologic patterns (43). On occasion, an EMB will be obtained to evaluate an unexplained arrhythmia or conduction defect. In these cases, the pathologist should pay careful attention to the distribution and severity of fibrosis and look for inflammation or granulomas. Molecular studies have identified mutations in several genes responsible for ion channel proteins, and these have been grouped into ion channelopathies. The number of disorders continues to expand and includes long QT syndrome, Brugada syndrome, catecholaminergic polymorphic ventricular tachycardia, short QT syndrome, and idiopathic ventricular fibrillation (83). Frustaci et al. (84) showed a spectrum of histopathologic changes in right and left EMBs in patients with the clinical presentation of Brugada syndrome and normal cardiac structure and function on noninvasive workup. These changes included lymphocytic myocarditis, fibrofatty change, and hypertrophy and fibrosis of DCM. Many investigators now promote the concept of the "molecular autopsy" using genetic testing to further investigate these disorders in patients who experience sudden death (85). We expect that many of the cardiomyopathies that are currently unclassified will be clarified by molecular genetic studies in the future.

SECONDARY CARDIOMYOPATHIES

The term *secondary cardiomyopathy* has been proposed to replace *specific cardiomyopathy* and *specific heart muscle disorder* of previous classifications. As such, it is defined as a disorder that "shows pathological myocardial involvement as part of a large number and variety of generalized systemic (multiorgan) disorders" (43). This group includes infiltrative and storage disorders; drug, radiation, and chemical toxicities; endocrinopathies; neuromuscular disorders; nutritional and electrolyte disturbances; and autoimmune diseases (Table 29.2). The role of the EMB is twofold: (a) to establish the diagnosis in those disorders with characteristic morphologic findings (e.g., amyloidosis, glycogen storage disorder, Fabry disease, anthracycline toxicity, and hemochromatosis) and (b) to identify treatable or reversible causes of myocardial dysfunction (e.g., catecholamine effect, myocarditis, and neoplasia). The more common diseases are discussed herein.

Amyloidosis

In our experience, the majority of patients with cardiac amyloidosis present in one or more of the following manners: (a) restrictive physiology in the absence of constrictive pericarditis; (b) congestive heart failure that remains refractory to maximal medical therapy; (c) low-voltage changes on electrocardiogram in association with marked LV hypertrophy; or (d) myocardial dysfunction in the setting of known plasma cell dyscrasia or connective tissue disorder. With the exception of isolated senile atrial amyloidosis, which is characterized by beaded subendocardial deposits in the left atrial myocardium found incidentally at autopsy, four types of amyloidosis are associated with cardiac or multiorgan symptoms (85–89). The most common type is immunoglobulin-associated amyloidosis (AL type), which occurs in primary amyloidosis, multiple myeloma, and other types of plasma cell dyscrasia and is characterized by deposition of immunoglobulin light chain. This form is associated with a poor prognosis, and therapy is directed at heart failure management and chemotherapy for the underlying malignancy. Familial or hereditary amyloidosis (ATTR type) is an autosomal dominant disease caused by one of 80 different mutations of the transthyretin protein. The mutant TTR protein deposits in the heart and in nerves cause heart failure and peripheral and autonomic neuropathy. The long-term prognosis is better than AL type, and liver transplantation is the definitive treatment. Systemic senile amyloidosis is characterized by deposition of wild-type transthyretin and occurs in middle-aged and older men. Its clinical progression and outcome are much better than AL type; unlike AL type, cardiac transplantation is not a contraindication for advanced cardiac involvement. Cardiac involvement in secondary amyloidosis (AA type) is uncommon, and symptoms are minor. Deposition of the nonimmunoglobulin protein A occurs in the setting of chronic infections and autoimmune disorders such as rheumatoid arthritis.

The macroscopic findings in cardiac amyloidosis range from normal ventricles to dilated ventricles with thinned walls (mimicking DCM) to thickened LV walls with small chambers (mimicking HCM). The cut surface is often described as waxy (Fig. 29.11). Involvement of the endocardium, myocardium, pericardium, valves, and epicardial and intramyocardial vessels is common (90). Microscopically, several different patterns are observed. The most common pattern is interstitial and perimyocyte deposition of pale, finely fibrillar eosinophilic material that envelops individual myocytes in a castlike manner. Attenuated myocytes are frequent and best seen in longitudinally arranged fibers. In

our experience, the Masson's trichrome stain distinguishes the amyloid fibers from collagen by its gray-blue tinctorial appearance (Fig. 29.11). In addition, collagen shows artifactual retraction from the adjacent myocyte whereas amyloid encases the myocytes. Coalescence of interstitial deposits to form nodular aggregates is a common feature. The walls of small intramyocardial arteries and the subendocardial tissues are replaced or expanded by amyloid deposits. Classically, in 10-μm sections stained with Congo red, amyloid shows orangiophilic staining under light microscopy and apple-green birefringence under polarized light microscopy. Other histochemical stains, such as sulfated Alcian blue, stain amyloid deposits green (91). Ultrastructurally, the perimyocytic and intramural vascular deposits are found, and at high magnification, the fibrils are 7 to 10 nm, randomly arranged, beaded, and nonbranching (Fig. 29.12). In most centers, frozen section immunohistochemistry or immunofluorescence is required to subclassify the different types of amyloid. Because this has important therapeutic and prognostic implications, clinicians should routinely submit tissue in Zeus medium or normal saline as part of the biopsy procedure when amyloid is a diagnostic consideration.

Glycogen Storage Disease

Glycogen storage disorder is a group of inherited enzymatic deficiencies responsible for the synthesis or utilization of glyco-

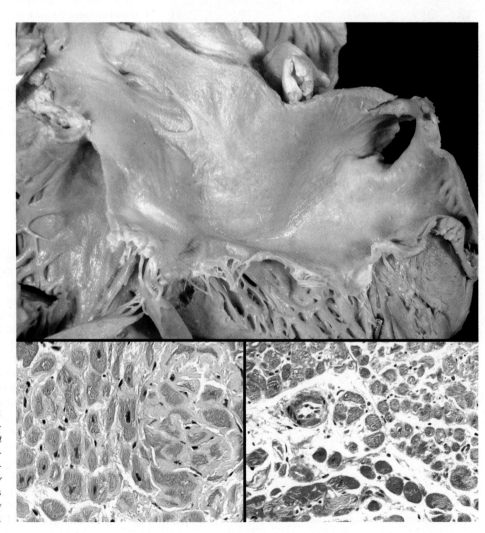

Figure 29.11. Cardiac amyloidosis: *Upper panel*: The dilated left atrium exhibits a waxy glistening appearance. *Left lower panel*: High power showing encasement of individual myocytes by pale eosinophilic amyloid fibers. *Right lower panel*: The trichrome stain highlights the vascular and interstitial deposits by the bluish-purple tinctorial appearance.

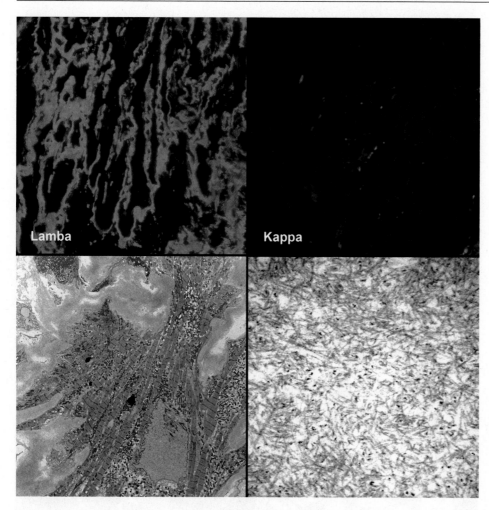

Figure 29.12. Cardiac amyloidosis: *Upper panels*: Immunofluorescent staining of myocardium showing lambda light chain restriction in AL type. *Lower left panel*: Low-power transmission electron microscopy showing amyloid fibers enveloping the attenuated myocyte. *Lower right panel*: High-power image showing randomly arranged and beaded amyloid fibrils.

gen. Of the 12 types currently reported, types II (Pompe), III (Forbe), and IV (Andersen) have cardiac manifestations (92,93). Pompe disease is an autosomal recessive disorder caused by a deficiency of acid maltase (acid alpha-glucosidase). In the infantile form, hepatomegaly, failure to thrive, hypotonia, macroglossia, and massive cardiomegaly occur as a result of accumulations of glycogen within hepatocytes, skeletal muscle, and myocytes. The heart is enlarged and simulates HCM, although DCM and restrictive patterns have also been reported. Endocardial fibroelastosis is observed in up to 20% of cases (92). Histologic sections show enlarged myocytes with vacuolated cytoplasm filled with periodic acid-Schiff (PAS)–positive glycogen (Fig. 29.13). The key feature distinguishing Pompe disease from the vacuolization of normal myocytes is the uniformly massive and diffuse vacuolization of all the myocytes in Pompe disease. Currently, enzyme replacement therapy using recombinant human enzyme is being evaluated in clinical trials (94).

Fabry Disease

Fabry disease is another example of a storage disorder and is caused by a deficiency of the alpha-galactosidase A enzyme. This X-linked disorder results in glycolphospholipid accumulations in the skin, kidneys, liver, pancreas, nervous system, and heart. Cardiac involvement affects endothelial cells, myocytes, valvular

structures, and the conduction system. Marked LV hypertrophy with either concentric or asymmetric patterns mimics HCM both macroscopically and functionally. In EMB sections, the myocytes and endothelial cells are diffusely vacuolated with pinpoint weakly positive predigested PAS granules within these

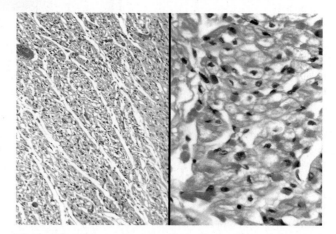

Figure 29.13. Pompe disease. *Left panel*: Scanning power showing marked vacuolization of the myocytes throughout the biopsy. *Right panel*: Uniform clearing of the cytoplasm in every myocyte without inflammation.

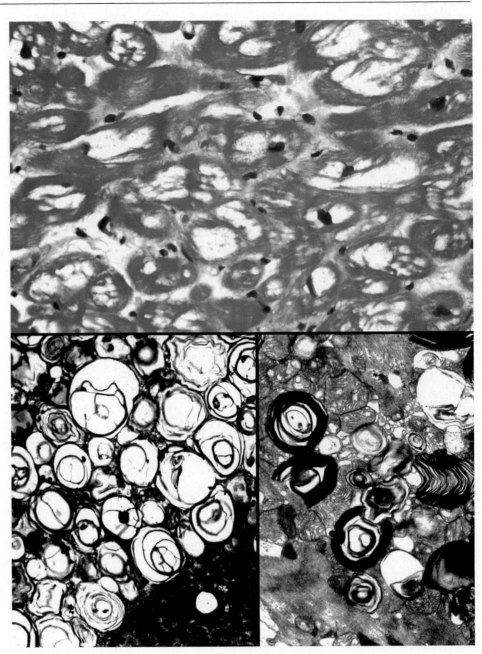

Figure 29.14. Fabry disease. *Upper panel*: The endomyocardial biopsy specimen shows cytoplasmic vacuolization containing fine granularity. *Lower panels*: Transmission electron microscopy showing membrane-bound lamellar myelin bodies.

spaces (Fig. 29.14). The diagnosis is confirmed at the ultrastructural level by the presence of membrane-bound electron-dense lamellar myelin ("zebra") bodies. Valvular deposition can produce stenotic or regurgitant valves, and severe coronary artery disease has been reported (95,96). Recently, enzyme replacement therapy using recombinant human alpha-galactosidase A enzyme has shown tremendous promise for stabilizing and improving symptoms (97).

Chloroquine cardiotoxicity can mimic the clinical and light microscopy features of Fabry disease (98). This potent antimalarial drug is also used in the treatment of sarcoidosis, collagen vascular disorders such as rheumatoid arthritis, and cutaneous discoid lupus. Diffuse myocyte vacuolization is observed. At the ultrastructural level, electron-dense myelin figures and curvilinear bodies are found within myocytes; the latter finding is not seen in Fabry disease.

Hemochromatosis

Hemochromatosis is one of the most common inheritable metabolic disorders, with a reported prevalence of 1:200 to 1:400. It is characterized by increased iron absorption and deposition in the liver, heart, pituitary gland, pancreas, joints, adrenal glands, and skin. The pattern of inheritance is autosomal recessive, but the penetrance is variable, accounting for the difficulty in diagnosis (99). The most common mutations in the *HFE* gene on the short arm of chromosome 6 are C282y, H63D, and S65C. A smaller number of cases are linked to mutations of genes coding SLC11A3 and transferrin receptor 2 (100). The cardiac manifestations reflect the effects of iron deposition in myocytes and include congestive heart failure, conduction defects, and arrhythmias. Systolic pump failure causing a DCM is the most common pattern, although cases presenting with a restrictive

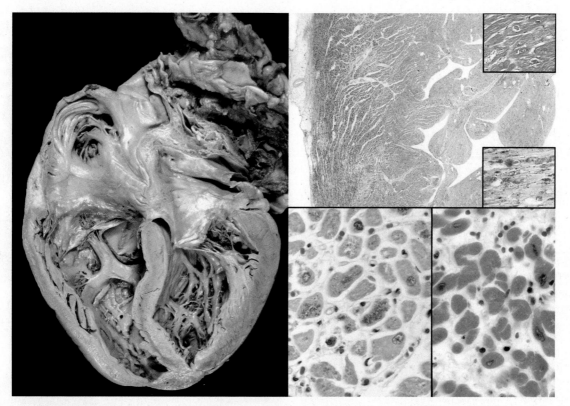

Figure 29.15. Hemochromatosis: *Left panel*: Four-chamber dilatation and hypertrophy mimicking idiopathic dilated cardiomyopathy (DCM). *Right upper panel*: Prussian blue stain showing disproportionate iron accumulations within the outer half of the myocardium. Insets: Hematoxylin and eosin (H&E) and Prussian blue stain of iron deposits within the cytoplasm of the myocytes. *Right lower panels*: The distinction between dark brown iron deposits (*on left*) and golden brown lipofuscin (*on right*) is seen on H&E stains.

physiology are reported (Fig. 29.15). Microscopically, iron is deposited in myocytes throughout the myocardium, although a preferential accentuation in the outer half of the myocardium is often observed. The brown deposits are typically perinuclear and are highlighted by the Prussian blue stain. Lipofuscin pigment is distinguished from iron particles by the small uniform golden yellow appearance and lack of staining on iron stains. In advanced cases, interstitial fibrosis and other features of remodeling are present. After transplantation, repetitive phlebotomy is required to prevent recurrence of the disease (101).

Pheochromocytoma and Other Endocrinopathies

Endocrine disorders may be associated with a variety of cardiomyopathic conditions. Thyroid disorders can produce DCM that is reversible with appropriate interventions (102). Acromegaly produces pronounced LV hypertrophy, interstitial fibrosis, and lymphocytic myocarditis and is influenced by multiple factors such as growth hormone effect, hypertension, longstanding arrhythmias, and vascular changes (103,104). Pheochromocytomas may produce acute or chronic changes in the heart. The release of large amounts of catecholamine produces constriction of small "end vessels" in the myocardium, leading to "microinfarcts" in the myocardium. These lesions are composed of necrotic fibers admixed with scant acute and chronic inflammatory cells (Fig. 29.16) (105). Repetitive and episodic hormone release may lead to arrhythmia- or stress-induced in-

jury that progresses to a DCM. The histopathologic findings are nonspecific, and the diagnosis requires clinical screening (106).

Anthracycline Cardiotoxicity

The most common anthracycline antibiotics used in the treatment of solid tumors and hematolymphoid malignancies are doxorubicin and daunorubicin. Their efficacy is limited by their cardiotoxicity—a complication that has been recognized for more than 30 years. Both acute, early-onset chronic progression and late-onset chronic forms have been described (107). The late-onset chronic form can present many years or decades after treatment and is dose dependent, cumulative, and progressive. Congestive heart failure or arrhythmias are common and may be precipitated by other clinical events such as infection, pregnancy, or surgery (108). As previously discussed, the morphologic assessment of chronic anthracycline toxicity requires special tissue handling. *All* the issue is fixed and processed in a glutaraldehyde solution for transmission electron microscopy. Using the Billingham criteria, a minimum of 10 Epon plastic blocks is required to confidently assess a numeric grade (109). One-micron sections are cut and stained with toluidine blue stain and assessed under light microscopy for distribution and extent of cellular injury. Myocytes with myofibrillar loss appear shrunken with homogeneous pale cytoplasm, and sarcotubular dilatation is depicted by cytoplasmic vacuolization (Fig. 29.17). At the ultrastructural level, myofibrillar loss with partial or complete loss of fibrils and retention of Z-band remnants along the

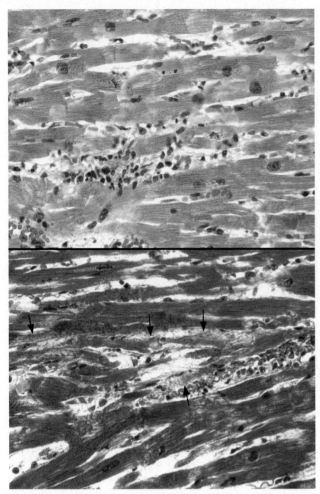

Figure 29.16. Acute myocyte injury in hypertensive crisis of pheochromocytoma. *Upper panel*: High-power magnification showing punctate focus of acute injury with mixed inflammatory cell infiltrate. *Lower panel*: Trichrome stain highlighting attenuated and discolored fibers (*arrows*).

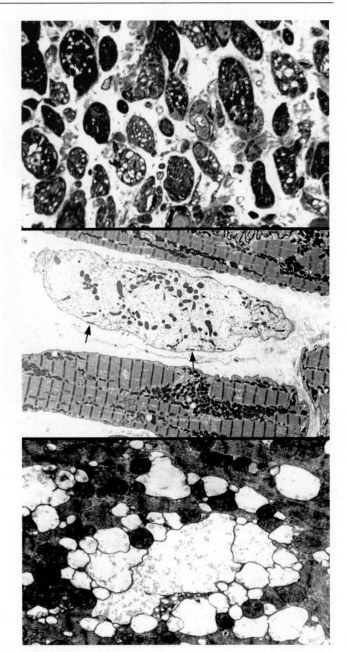

Figure 29.17. Chronic anthracycline cardiotoxicity. *Upper panel*: Toluidine-stained thick section showing vacuolization of numerous attenuated myocytes indicating advanced injury. *Middle panel*: Transmission electron microscopy showing a central damaged myocyte flanked by normal myocytes. Myofibrillar loss and Z-band remnants (*arrows*) are noted. *Lower panel*: Sarcotubular distention is characterized by swollen, dilated sarcotubules.

cytoplasmic membrane is more common than the swelling and coalescence of vacuolar change to form sarcotubular distention. The grading of cardiotoxicity ranges from 0 to 3, and each grade is associated with specific therapeutic recommendations (Table 29.6) (107). Approaches to reducing the incidence of cardiotoxicity include the use of liposomal formulations of the anthracyclines and cardioprotective drugs such as dexrazoxane (110, 111).

An uncommon form of anthracycline toxicity develops after the first dose or within the first week of therapy. Patients present with signs and symptoms of acute pericarditis/myocarditis. The myocardial lesions are typically patchy and are composed of a mixture of neutrophils and lymphocytes in association with myocyte damage (Fig. 29.18) (112).

Cardiotoxicity is reported with other chemotherapeutic drugs (113,114). In many cases, the changes are functional rather than morphologic. Alkylating agents such as busulfan and cyclophosphamide can cause EMF and pericarditis/myocarditis, respectively. DCM is reported in the setting of human immunodeficiency virus (HIV) infection and may be related to the viropathic effects of HIV or the antiviral drugs such as zidovudine (AZT) (115).

INFLAMMATORY CARDIOMYOPATHY (MYOCARDITIS)

In patients with recent onset (<3 months in duration) of unexplained congestive heart failure with normal-sized or dilated heart and/or ventricular arrhythmias, the EMB is used to evaluate for myocarditis (48). This category includes numerous etiologies of myocarditis (Table 29.7) (116). For the purpose of this chapter, we will present the types of myocarditis that may be encountered in surgical pathology and refer the reader to other monographs for more comprehensive discussions (117–120).

TABLE 29.6

Grading of Chronic Anthracycline Cardiotoxicity with Clinical Recommendations

Grade	Morphology/ Clinical Recommendations
0	Normal ultrastructural appearance of myocytes
1.0	Isolated or scattered myocytes showing sarcotubular distention or early/partial myofibrillar loss; damage to <5% of all cells in Epon blocks; therapy is continued
1.5	Changes similar to those in grade 1.0 but involving 6% to 15% of all cells in 10 plastic blocks; therapy is continued
2.0	Clusters of myocytes with myofibrillar loss or sarcotubular distention involving 16% to 25% of all cells; therapy is continued with close hemodynamic/cardiac assessment
2.5	Numerous damaged myocytes (26% to 35%) showing characterized changes; one more dose of anthracycline
3.0	Diffuse or confluent myocyte damage of >35% of cells; necrotic cells may be seen; therapy is discontinued

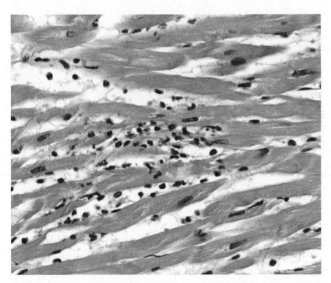

Figure 29.18. Acute doxorubicin toxicity is characterized by an acute toxic myocarditis composed of lymphocytes, neutrophils, and pyknotic debris in association with myocyte damage.

TABLE 29.7

Etiologies of Inflammatory Cardiomyopathy (Myocarditis)

Idiopathic (postviral/lymphocytic) myocarditis
Infectious myocarditis (see Table 29.8)
Drug induced (hypersensitivity amd toxic types)
Myocarditis associated with systemic disease/processes (autoimmune, acute rheumatic disease, Kawasaki disease, peripostpartum, thrombotic thrombocytopenic purpura)
Sarcoidosis
Idiopathic giant-cell myocarditis

In 1984, a consensus definition and classification of myocarditis was proposed (120). Myocarditis was defined as a myocardial process characterized by the presence of *both* an inflammatory infiltrate *and* myocyte damage or necrosis that is not typical of the myocardial damage of ischemic heart disease. In active myocarditis, *both* inflammation and myocyte damage are present. The composition of the cellular infiltrate delineates the specific type of myocarditis (e.g., lymphocytic, eosinophilic, neutrophilic, giant-cell, granulomatous, or mixed cell types). The distribution of inflammatory infiltrate may be focal, confluent, or diffuse, and the severity ranges from mild to severe. The most difficult challenge is the determination of myocyte damage in the biopsy specimen. In our experience, florid myocytolysis and necrosis are not common biopsy patterns. Myocyte damage is characterized by the presence of mononuclear cells that cause encroachment or scalloping of the sarcolemmal membrane of myocytes, fragmentation of myocytes with remnants of cytoplasm or "bare nuclei," architectural displacement or distortion of myocytes by inflammatory cells, or partial replacement of myocytes by inflammatory cells (Fig. 29.19). The liberal use of leveled sections and Masson's trichrome are helpful in difficult cases because damaged myocytes display a basophilic tinctorial quality. Finally, the presence or absence of fibrosis should be noted for reference to changes in subsequent biopsies and the potential development of DCM. Interstitial, perivascular, and endocardial patterns can be seen. Borderline myocarditis is defined by the presence of limited inflammatory cell infiltrates and the absence of definitive myocyte damage. The phrase *no evidence of myocarditis* is used when neither diagnostic feature is present. Deeper sectioning of the paraffin blocks should also be considered before this diagnosis is rendered because the inflammatory process may be patchy in distribution. If myocarditis is absent, attention should be focused on the presence of other myocardial disorders such as myocyte hypertrophy and interstitial fibrosis in the setting of DCM. Connective tissue stains and stains for amyloidosis and hemochromatosis should then be routinely obtained. Follow-up biopsies after therapeutic intervention are less commonly performed

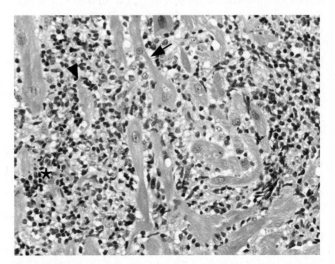

Figure 29.19. The Dallas criteria for myocarditis require both myocyte damage and an inflammatory infiltrate. Myocyte damage is characterized by scalloped myocytes with inflammatory cell encroachment (*arrow*), attenuated fibers (*arrowhead*), or remnants of myocytes ("bare nuclei") (*).

today. Possible diagnostic observations include ongoing or persistent myocarditis, resolving or healing myocarditis, and complete resolution of inflammation and damage. We have observed cases of recurrent myocarditis after rapid tapering of immunosuppressive therapy. Furthermore, the development of myocyte hypertrophy and interstitial fibrosis should be noted in follow-up biopsies and correlated with physiologic and imaging findings because progression to DCM has been observed (121).

Lymphocytic Myocarditis

In developed countries, viral agents are thought to be the primary cause of lymphocytic myocarditis. Historic, clinical, and experimental evidence has identified enteroviruses such as coxsackie B virus, echovirus, and adenovirus as likely causes (116,118). Possible mechanisms include postviral autoimmunity mechanisms; direct viral cytopathic injury; induction of viral-specific immune response through mediators such as interleukin (IL)-1, IL-2, IL-6, tumor necrosis factor (TNF), interferon, and nitrous oxide; and viral-mediated endothelial injury with intimal proliferation and ischemic sequelae. In many clinical cases, however, a direct causative link is not established, and these cases are classified as idiopathic myocarditis. Other terms that have been used include acute myocarditis to reflect the clinical onset of symptoms and absence of fibrosis in the biopsy specimen or rapidly progressive or fulminant myocarditis in cases of multifocal damage and extensive injury.

The incidence and natural history of idiopathic myocarditis remain largely unknown. Discrepancies between clinically suspected cases and EMB findings are well recognized, and the prevalence of myocarditis using the EMB as the gold standard is less than 10% (122).

The macroscopic findings in florid myocarditis typically range from normal cardiac configurations to four-chamber dilatation and cardiac enlargement. The papillary muscles and trabeculae carneae are often flattened, and the myocardium appears pale and flabby. Thrombi within atrial appendages or along ventricular endocardial surfaces are uncommon. The cut surface of the myocardium is usually pale, and foci of hemorrhage or hemorrhagic necrosis are found. Many cases have fibrinous pericarditis and exudative effusions.

The resemblance of this type of myocarditis and acute cellular rejection of the cardiac allograft has been previously noted (123). In many cases, the infiltrates are sparse and are predominantly lymphocytic in nature. In fulminant cases, myocyte damage or necrosis is conspicuous (Fig. 29.20). Architectural patterns include focal, multifocal, or diffuse interstitial infiltrates. Interstitial widening by tissue edema and inflammation is seen. The patterns of confluent myocyte damage and necrosis are similar in biopsies of adult and pediatric patients. The majority of lymphocytes are CD3⁺ T cells with both helper and suppressor subtypes. Macrophages and natural killer cells are also present, but B cells are infrequent or absent.

There are several common histopathologic lesions that can be mistaken for lymphocytic myocarditis, and many are included in Table 29.7. The average number of lymphocytes in normal myocardial tissue is thought to be less than 5.0 per high-power field (124). Tazelaar and Billingham (125) examined EMBs obtained from 86 young disease-free cardiac transplantation donors at the time of transplantation. Foci composed of at least five mononuclear inflammatory cells were found in 9.3%

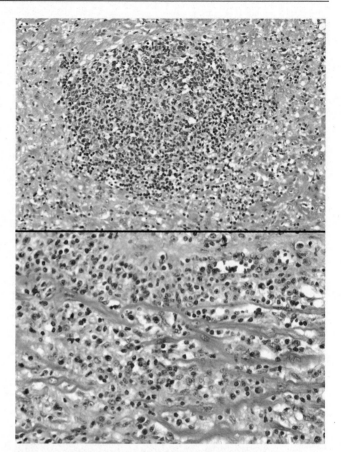

Figure 29.20. Patterns of lymphocytic myocarditis. *Upper panel*: Focal collection of mononuclear cells associated with architectural distortion and myocyte damage. *Lower panel*: Diffuse interstitial inflammation with conspicuous myocyte damage.

of cases. Other types of interstitial cells normally found within the myocardium that can be confused with lymphocytes are endothelial cells, smooth muscle cells, pericytes, fibroblasts, and mast cells. Hill and Swanson (126) reported the presence of extramedullary hematopoietic cells including immature erythroid and myeloid precursors in healing infarcts of ischemic and cardiomyopathic hearts and areas of fibrosis in congenital defects (126). Foci of mononuclear leukocytic cells are found in the interstitial tissues and within fibrosis in most cases of DCM but are not associated with myocyte damage (127). Vasopressor/catecholamine-damaged myocytes appear fragmented and hypereosinophilic and are surrounded by a sparse mixed inflammatory cell infiltrate, which is similar to the lesions seen with pheochromocytomas (15). The distribution of the lesions near or around small intramyocardial arteries and the mixed nature of the infiltrate are important diagnostic clues. The trichrome stain highlights the necrotic myocytes. The damaged myocytes may undergo punctate calcification and mimic infectious myocarditis such as toxoplasmosis. Neoplastic infiltrates are uncommon findings on EMBs. Their atypical cytologic features and the absence of necrosis and fibrosis characterize hematolymphoid malignancies such as leukemia and lymphoma. Immunophenotypic and molecular studies are helpful to confirm the clonality of these processes and to distinguish them from myocarditis.

Infectious Myocarditis

In developed countries, infectious causes of heart muscle inflammation are uncommon in immunocompetent individuals. Patients with acquired immunodeficiency syndrome (AIDS), transplantation-associated immunosuppression to prevent allograft rejection, and advanced stages of malignancy are susceptible to a variety of bacterial, viral, fungal, protozoan, and rickettsial infections. In many developing countries, these remain a significant cause of morbidity and mortality, and cardiac involvement is frequently observed. Careful clinical history, cultures, serologies, and histochemical, immunohistochemical, and molecular studies are usually necessary to establish the diagnosis. More detailed descriptions of these different infections are found in other monographs (Table 29.8) (117).

Drug-Related Myocarditis

Drug-induced myocardial dysfunction remains a significant clinical problem, and the list of implicated drugs continues to expand. Four patterns are recognized: (a) hypersensitivity myocarditis; (b) toxic myocarditis; (c) endocardial fibrosis (e.g., ergotamine tartrate, methysergide, pergolide mesylate, phentermine/fenfluramine); and (d) drug-induced cardiomyopathy (e.g., anthracycline, chloroquine) (128).

HYPERSENSITIVITY MYOCARDITIS. Hypersensitivity myocarditis is the most common form of acute drug-related myocardial injury. More than two dozen drugs have been identified, but the majority of cases are caused by antibiotics, diuretics, and antihypertensive drugs (129). It is also observed in 7% of patients undergoing cardiac transplantation and is likely related to prolonged dobutamine infusion (130–132). Clinical signs can include rash, fever, peripheral eosinophilia, and occasionally arrhythmias, sudden death, and congestive heart failure. It is not dose dependent and may occur at any time during drug administration. The histopathologic features include temporally uniform lesions distributed in the subendocardial, perivascular, and interstitial tissues between bundles of myocytes. The predominant inflammatory cells are eosinophils, but variable numbers of histiocytes and scattered lymphocytes are also found (Fig. 29.21). Myocyte necrosis is usually absent or very focal except in severe cases. Necrotizing vasculitis is not found, but infiltration of vessel walls by eosinophils is common (133,134). Collections of histiocytes centered on degenerated collagen bundles form ill-defined granulomas in up to 25% of cases, but fibrinoid necrosis, well-formed aggregates of epithelioid histiocytes ("hard granulomas"), multinucleated giant cells, interstitial fibrosis, and hemorrhage are absent in our experience. The lymphocytes show a T-cell phenotype and sparse or absent B cells. The absence of diffuse myocardial necrosis and giant cells distinguishes hypersensitivity myocarditis from drug-induced

TABLE 29.8	**Causes of Infectious Myocarditis**	
BACTERIAL, SPIROCHETAL, AND RICKETTSIAL CAUSES OF MYOCARDITIS		
Bacterial	Brucellosis	Mycobacterial
	Diphtheria	Meningococcal
	Gonococcal	*Mycoplasma*
	Streptococcal	Pneumococcal
	Staphylococcal	Tularemia
	Haemophilus	Salmonellosis
	Cholera	Whipple
	Listeriosis	*Campylobacter*
	Actinomycosis	
Spirochetal	Leptospirosis	Relapsing fever
	Lyme disease	Syphilis
Rickettsial	Q fever	Rocky Mountain spotted fever
	Scrub typhus	
VIRAL CAUSES OF MYOCARDITIS		
Adenovirus	Herpes simplex virus	Polio virus
Arbovirus	Herpes zoster	Rabies virus
Arenavirus (Lassa fever)	Human immunodeficiency virus	Respiratory syncytial virus (RSV)
Coxsackie virus	(HIV)	Rubella
Cytomegalovirus	Influenza virus (A and B)	Rubeola
Dengue virus	Junin virus	Vaccinia virus
Echo virus	Lymphocytic choriomeningitis	Varicella virus
Encephalomyocarditis virus	Measles	Variola virus
Epstein-Barr virus	Mumps	Yellow fever virus
Hepatitis virus (HAV, HCV)	Parvovirus	
FUNGAL CAUSES OF MYOCARDITIS		
Candidiasis	Mucormycosis	Histoplasmosis
Aspergillosis	Coccidioidomycosis	
Blastomycosis	Cryptococcosis	
PROTOZOAN/HELMINTHIC CAUSES OF MYOCARDITIS		
Toxoplasmosis	Cysticercosis	Visceral larva migrans
Sarcocystis	Schistosomiasis	Echinococcosis
Trypanosomiasis	Paragonimiasis	Filariasis
Ascariasis	Trichinosis	

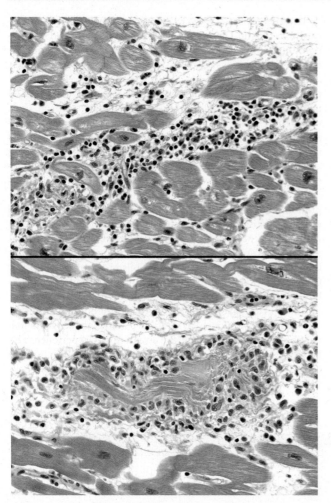

Figure 29.21. Hypersensitivity myocarditis. *Upper panel*: Discrete collections of eosinophils and histiocytes between myocyte bundles. Myocyte damage is inconspicuous or absent. *Lower panel*: Histiocytic cell aggregates around degenerating collagen creating a vague granuloma appearance.

giant-cell myocarditis (135). Acute necrotizing eosinophilic myocarditis differs from classic hypersensitivity myocarditis by the presence of extensive necrosis, dense interstitial inflammatory cell infiltrates, and absence of systemic allergic symptoms (136,137).

TOXIC MYOCARDITIS. Toxic myocarditis is an uncommon form of myocarditis and is characterized by direct myocyte cytotoxicity. Causative agents include antineoplastic agents such as cyclophosphamide and anthracyclines, catecholamines, cocaine, arsenicals, fluorouracil, lithium compounds, and antihypertensives (128). In distinction to hypersensitivity myocarditis, it is usually dose dependent, and the lesions may persist or progress after the cessation of the drug. The pathologic features reflect the cellular response to myocyte damage. The lesions are focal and temporally heterogeneous, reflecting the episodic or cumulative mechanism of injury. Some lesions in the biopsy sample may be acute, whereas others may be in the reparative phases. Fibrosis is not uncommon. The inflammatory infiltrates are polymorphous with lymphocytes, plasma cells, and neutrophils, but eosinophils are rare or absent. A classic example is

the acute form of doxorubicin cardiotoxicity presenting as acute myocarditis (Fig. 29.18).

Myocarditis Associated with Systemic Processes

Myocarditis has been reported in several systemic illnesses and in the peripartum period. Many of these are examples of immune-mediated myocarditis and exhibit lymphocytic myocarditis.

COLLAGEN VASCULAR DISEASES. Myocarditis is reported in connective tissue diseases such as systemic lupus erythematosus (SLE), systemic sclerosis, polyarteritis nodosa, rheumatoid arthritis, polymyositis/dermatomyositis, thrombotic thrombocytopenic purpura, Wegener granulomatosis, and rarely, ankylosing spondylitis and mixed connective tissue disease (138, 139). SLE, rheumatoid arthritis, and polymyositis/dermatomyositis are most commonly associated with myocarditis. The morphologic features on EMB or in postmortem material are lymphocytic myocarditis similar to the idiopathic (postviral) type of myocarditis. This emphasizes the importance of comprehensive clinical information in the evaluation of these cases. In SLE, fibrinoid vasculitis may also be observed in the small intramyocardial arteries in the biopsy. Immunofluorescence studies may demonstrate immunoglobulin, complement, and fibrinogen deposition, indicating an immune complex–mediated form of myocarditis. Immunosuppressive therapy remains the mainstay of treatment. Drug-related toxic myocarditis should be considered in the differential diagnosis, particularly in SLE patients receiving quinidine-based therapy.

ACUTE RHEUMATIC FEVER. Rheumatic fever remains a significant cause of cardiac morbidity and mortality in underdeveloped countries (140). It is a sequel to group A streptococcal pharyngitis and arises as an autoimmune response to extracellular or somatic bacterial antigens that share similar epitopes in human tissues. Cardiac involvement occurs in up to 55% of patients and is characterized by a pancarditis. The diagnosis of rheumatic myocarditis has been made on EMB at the time of transplantation and at autopsy (141,142). The myocardial lesions consist of nonspecific lymphocytic myocarditis and Aschoff nodules. The latter may be found in the valves, endocardium, myocardium, pericardium, and conduction system and are pathognomonic of acute rheumatic fever. They represent oval collections of histiocytes, lymphocytes, plasma cells, and giant cells (Aschoff cells) in the interstitium adjacent to small blood vessels (Fig. 29.22). This "granulomatous stage" of Aschoff nodules arises 1 to 2 months after the onset of clinical symptoms and develops within or near foci of fibrinoid necrosis. They are eventually replaced by collagenous scar tissue.

PERIPARTUM MYOCARDITIS/CARDIOMYOPATHY. Peripartum myocarditis/cardiomyopathy is defined as myocardial dysfunction occurring during the third trimester of pregnancy or in the first 5 or 6 months postpartum (143). Possible etiologies include viral infection, nutritional deficiencies, small vessel coronary disease, and immunologic interactions to fetal and myometrial antigens. Lymphocytic myocarditis is reported in 5% to 30% of cases. DCM has been occasionally found in association with myocarditis. Whether postpartum myocarditis/cardiomyopathy is a distinct entity from idiopathic DCM or idiopathic lymphocytic myocarditis remains unknown.

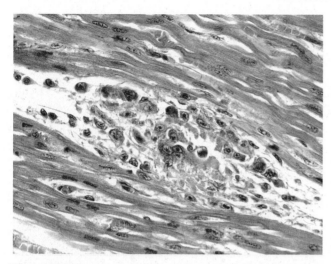

Figure 29.22. An Aschoff nodule composed of multinucleated giant (Aschoff) cells and histiocytes between myocyte bundles.

Sarcoidosis

Cardiac involvement in sarcoidosis occurs in 25% to 60% of patients but remains subclinical in the vast majority of cases. Isolated cardiac involvement in the absence of systemic disease is found in a minority of cases. Cardiac dysfunction manifests as arrhythmias, particularly ventricular types, conduction disturbances with high degrees of atrioventricular (AV) block and complete bundle branch block, sudden death, congestive heart failure, papillary muscle dysfunction, acute myocardial infarction (MI)–like syndrome, ventricular aneurysm, or recurring pericardial effusions. In a recent study of cardiac sarcoidosis, left-sided heart failure and syncope were the most common symptoms at the time of hospital presentation. AV block and ventricular tachycardia accounted for more than 75% of arrhythmias, but sudden death occurred in 2% of cases (144). The sensitivity of RV EMB ranges from 20% to 50% because of the patchy distribution of the granulomatous lesions and the preferential localization in the cephalad portion of the interventricular septum, LV free wall, and papillary muscles (145). A negative biopsy does not exclude the diagnosis, and some have advocated institution of immunosuppressive therapy even in the face of a negative biopsy result (146). Corticosteroid therapy is effective in many cases, and cardiac transplantation remains a therapeutic option for patients who fail medical therapy or progress to DCM. Recurrence in the allograft has been reported but is uncommon; treatment with augmented immunosuppression is efficacious (147).

Several histopathologic patterns can be observed on EMBs in cardiac sarcoidosis. These include the classic noncaseating granulomatous inflammation, lymphocytic myocarditis, DCM, and normal myocardium. Diffuse myocardial involvement progresses to myocyte hypertrophy and interstitial fibrosis resembling DCM; in a minority of cases, a restrictive profile is observed. The classic granulomatous pattern is characterized by firm, white nodules forming discrete masses within the interventricular septum, LV free wall, or papillary muscle (Fig. 29.23). These may be confused for metastatic deposits or fibrous tumors. The histopathologic features are similar to extracardiac lesions and consist of noncaseating, well-formed (so-called "hard") granulomas composed of epithelioid histiocytes and multinucleated giant cells arranged

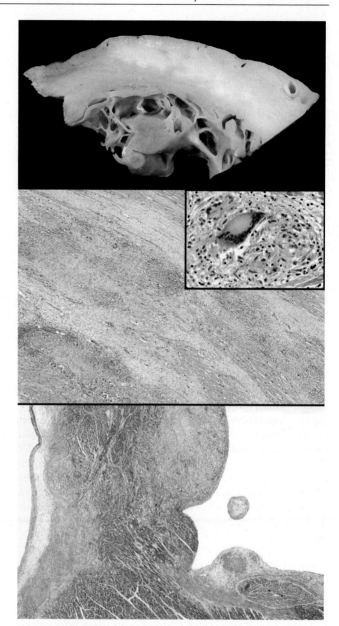

Figure 29.23. Cardiac sarcoidosis. *Upper panel*: Gross appearance of sarcoidosis showing tan-white foci within myocardium. *Middle panel*: Low-power appearance showing coalescence of discrete granulomas embedded in mature fibrous scar tissue. Inset: Classic well-formed granuloma. *Lower panel*: Section of heart near atrioventricular (AV) node showing numerous granulomas.

in round or oval aggregates. These can be found as isolated lesions or may coalesce to form larger zones within the myocardium. Endocardial and pericardial involvement is observed in some cases. Scattered around and within the granulomas are mature lymphocytes, but eosinophils are absent or sparse in number. Mature collagenous fibrosis is present and surrounds the granulomas, but active myocyte necrosis is uncommon. The epithelioid histiocytes express CD68, and the infiltrating lymphocytes are almost exclusively T cells with a predominance of CD4$^+$ cells; B cells are rare (148).

The differential diagnosis includes granulomatous and giant-cell lesions of the heart. Granulomatous infections are uncommon in immunocompetent patients, but we routinely obtain histochemical stains for fungal and mycobacterial microorganisms. In general, infectious lesions demonstrate necrotizing granulomas. Giant-cell myocarditis is characterized by the presence of giant cells, and by definition, granulomas are absent. In hypersensitivity myocarditis, the histiocytic lesions are poorly formed and are centered on collagen fibers. Eosinophils are numerous, but multinucleated giant cells and fibrosis are not found. The granuloma-like lesions of acute rheumatic fever are poorly formed, and the giant cells are generally smaller and do not resemble Langhan type. Foreign body–type giant cells surrounding catheter sheath fragments can be found in biopsies of patients who undergo repeated biopsy procedures. The edge of healing ischemic infarcts can contain giant cells of myogenic origin; lymphocytes and hemosiderin-laden macrophages are seen within the scar tissue. Granulomas are also reported in metabolic disorders such as lipogranulomatosis (Farber disease), oxalosis, and gout; in collagen vascular diseases such as rheumatoid nodules, Wegener granulomatosis, and Churg-Strauss syndrome; and in chronic granulomatous disease of childhood (149).

Idiopathic Giant-Cell Myocarditis

Idiopathic giant-cell myocarditis (IGCM) is a rare but frequently fatal form of myocarditis that occurs in previously healthy young adults. Clinical onset is abrupt and characterized by rapidly progressive heart failure and/or arrhythmias. Death occurs within weeks or months of onset of symptoms unless aggressive immunosuppression and cardiac transplantation are implemented (150). Twenty percent of patients have an associated autoimmune disorder such as ulcerative colitis, cryofibrinogenemia, rheumatoid arthritis, myasthenia gravis, hyperthyroidism, and hypothyroidism. Other associations include drug hypersensitivity, Wegener granulomatosis, thymoma, sarcoidosis, and infections.

Grossly, confluent or multifocal areas of necrosis are easily observed in the heart. The heart weight is normal or slightly increased. The four chambers of the heart are uniformly involved in most cases. In the late or healed stages of the disease, the ventricular wall may appear thin, but this reflects diffuse scarring and not aneurysmal changes as islands of myocytes are found within the collagenous scar tissue (Fig. 29.24). Endocardial and pericardial involvement has been described, but the process is primarily centered on the myocardium. The microscopic features consist of regions of diffuse, serpiginous necrosis containing multinucleated giant cells, lymphocytes, histiocytes, and eosinophils in the absence of sarcoid-like granulomas. The giant cells are distributed throughout the inflammatory infiltrates often in apposition to the sarcolemmal membranes of necrotic myocytes. They measure up to 90×20 μm in size and contain up to 20 nuclei in each cell. The necrotic myocardium is replaced by edematous granulation tissue, and the border between viable and necrotic myocardium is not well delineated. Litovsky et al. (148) have proposed classification of IGCM into acute, healing, and healed phases (148). The acute or active phase is described earlier and is distinguished by the abundant inflammatory response, loose connective tissue stroma, and numerous giant cells of macrophage origin. In the healing or resolving stage, granulation tissue and immature fibrosis replace the myocardium, and the number of giant cells and inflammatory cells is diminished. In the healed or resolved phase, mature

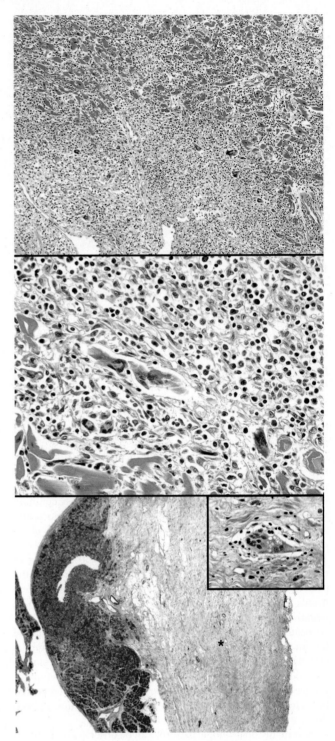

Figure 29.24. Giant-cell myocarditis. *Upper panel*: Low-power appearance showing widespread myocyte damage and replacement by a mixed inflammatory cell infiltrate. *Middle panel*: Collections of multinucleated giant cells, lymphocytes, eosinophils, and histiocytes within the myocardium. *Lower panel*: Trichrome stain showing healed idiopathic giant-cell myocarditis with replacement of the outer half of the myocardium by mature collagen. Inset: Rare multinucleated giant cells are scattered within the scar tissue.

fibrosis is noted with rare or absent giant cells and sparse inflammatory cells (Fig. 29.24). Myocytes are found as islands of single cells or small clusters surrounded by scar tissue. In explanted or postmortem heart specimens, some degree of overlap between the different stages can be seen, suggesting temporal heterogeneity in this disease. This is an important caveat when examining EMB specimens for the purpose of grading the response to immunosuppressive therapy.

Immunohistochemical studies show a macrophage/monocyte origin of the giant cells because they stain with CD68 and not with muscle markers like actin, desmin, and myoglobin (151). CD3$^+$ T cells are the predominant inflammatory cell type; B cells are rare or absent. In the active phase, CD8 cytotoxic/suppressor cells far outnumber CD4 cells. In the healing stages, occasional actin-positive myogenic-type giant cells are found at the edge of inflamed and viable myocytes, suggesting the sequel of inflammatory injury to myocytes.

The differential diagnosis is identical to sarcoidosis. The clinical and morphologic distinction between cardiac sarcoidosis and IGCM can be problematic. In general, however, close attention to the presence or absence of granulomas is the key discriminating feature. In addition, sarcoidosis has significantly more fibrosis and few or no eosinophils in the inflammatory infiltrate. Myocyte necrosis, particularly the broad zonal distribution, is a feature of IGCM, whereas the masslike effect is seen in sarcoidosis (144).

CARDIAC TRANSPLANTATION

More than 3100 adult heart transplantations and 400 pediatric heart transplantations were performed worldwide in 2005 to 2006, and 76,538 registered heart transplantations have been performed through June 2006 (152,153). Current (2002 to 2006) survival rates for the adult recipients are approximately 88% at 1 year, 80% at 3 years, and 75% at 5 years (152). Therefore, many pathologists at many institutions will encounter cardiac allograft specimens. The majority of these will be for the diagnosis of acute rejection.

In the 1980s, the pioneering surgical group at Stanford University dubbed the EMB the "gold standard" for the diagnosis of acute cellular rejection. This designation reflected, in part, their confidence in pathologist Dr. Margaret Billingham based on their collaborations in experimental heart transplantation and in their combined clinical-pathologic correlations for patients on an early immunosuppressive regimen (generally relying on prednisone and azathioprine). The subsequent introduction of cyclosporine and many new immunosuppressive regimens has reduced the incidence of acute rejection, altered the histomorphology of acute cellular rejection, and changed the physiologic correlates for the histopathology. The biopsy, however, remains an important tool in the diagnosis of acute cellular and antibody-mediated rejection and therefore has a critical role in the management of heart transplantation patients.

Early experience and varied grading schemes developed in the 1980s at multiple centers were integrated into a standardized system for the grading of rejection of the International Society for Heart and Lung Transplantation (ISHLT) in 1990 (154). This system facilitated communication between centers and multicenter trials in heart transplantation. In 2004, the ISHLT directed a multidisciplinary review of the grading system to address challenges and inconsistencies in its use and to incor-

TABLE 29.9

ISHLT Endomyocardial Biopsy Grading Schemes for Acute Cellular Rejection (1990 and 2004)

1990 ISHLT Grading Scheme	2004 Revised ISHLT Scheme
No rejection (0)	No rejection (0)
Focal mild rejection (1A): Perivascular +/− interstitial infiltrate without myocyte damage	Mild rejection (1R)
Diffuse mild rejection (1B): Interstitial infiltrate without myocyte damage	
Focal moderate (2): Solitary focus of infiltrate that is associated with myocyte damage	
Multifocal moderate rejection (3A): 2 or more foci of infiltrates that are associated with myocyte damage	Moderate rejection (2R)
Diffuse moderate rejection (3B): "Borderline severe"	Severe rejection (3R)
Diffuse, often polymorphous inflammatory infiltrates in many biopsy pieces with conspicuous myocyte damage	
Severe rejection (4): Findings of 3B rejection + interstitial edema, hemorrhage +/− small vessel vasculitis	

ISHLT, International Society for Heart and Lung Transplantation. Modified from Billingham et al. (154) and Stewart et al. (155).

porate information regarding antibody-mediated rejection (155). In the following description, we incorporate the patterns of both the 1990 scheme and the 2004 revision; the grades designated by the revision have an "R" suffix to distinguish them from the initial grading system (Table 29.9). Most transplantation centers indeed use a "dual reporting" format for reasons noted in the following sections.

GRADING OF ACUTE CARDIAC ALLOGRAFT REJECTION

Inflammatory Infiltrate

The majority of infiltrating cells are lymphocytes and macrophages with occasional eosinophils. The ratio of CD4 to CD8 lymphocytes has not been shown to have any diagnostic or prognostic value. Polymorphonuclear leukocytes may be present in the most severe forms of rejection (which are exceedingly rare); their presence should raise the possibility of ischemic injury, antibody-mediated rejection, or infection. Plasma cells are also not typical of acute cellular rejection but may be prominent in nodular endocardial infiltrates ("Quilty lesions," named for the patient at Stanford in whom they were first recognized), healing ischemic damage related to allograft vasculopathy, or PTLD (reactive plasmacytic hyperplasia or polymorphic PTLD). Interstitial infiltrates of predominantly eosinophils may be seen in hypersensitivity myocarditis or in infectious (parasitic) disease.

1200   *Section VII • Intrathoracic Organs and Blood Vessels*

Myocyte Damage

Identifying definite myocyte injury or damage can be extremely challenging in biopsies. The changes are often modest, with encroachment of inflammatory cells on the edges of myocytes giving them a scalloped appearance; the presence of damage may just be implied, as a dense inflammatory infiltrate occupies space that should contain myocytes.

Contraction bands are a common artifact of the biopsy procedure and therefore cannot be used as definitive proof of myocyte damage. Coagulation necrosis indicates ischemic injury and is not part of acute cellular rejection. Myocytolysis reflects chronic ischemia of myocytes and may be seen in biopsies from hearts with allograft vasculopathy or may be occasionally seen in early posttransplantation biopsies and reflect "preservation" or "reperfusion" injury. It should be noted that the intense immunosuppression in the early posttransplantation period alters the usual course of infarct healing; ischemic damage sustained at the time of transplantation may have less inflammation than expected for the posttransplantation timing of the biopsy.

Grade 0 R (no acute cellular rejection)

There is no mononuclear cell inflammation or myocyte damage (Fig. 29.25).

Grade 1 R

This grade includes the grades 1A, 1B, and 2 of the original working formulation. In the grade 1A histology, there are focal perivascular mononuclear cell infiltrates that do not encroach on myocyte borders (no myocyte damage is seen) and do not distort the normal architecture (Fig. 29.25). In 1B histology, there are diffuse interstitial and/or perivascular mononuclear cell infiltrates also in the absence of myocyte damage. The grade 2 histology includes a single, usually dense, infiltrate of mononuclear cells that distorts the normal architecture and may be associated with myocyte damage.

Grade 2 R

In grade 2 R, there are two or more foci of mononuclear cells (lymphocytes and macrophages) with associated myocyte damage (Fig. 29.25). Eosinophils and interstitial edema may be present. The foci may be in one or more biopsy pieces, and the other biopsy fragments may also include grade 1 R histology. Grade 2 R was grade 3A histology of the 1990 working formulation.

Grade 3 R

A diffuse infiltrate of lymphocytes and macrophages is present in most of the biopsy pieces, and there are multiple foci of myocyte damage (Fig. 29.25). Eosinophils and neutrophils may be present, and interstitial edema is likely to be seen. In the most severe examples, interstitial hemorrhage and vasculitis may be seen.

Reporting of Biopsy Findings

Most transplantation centers report biopsy histology under both the 1990 working formulation and the 2004 revision. Many cen-

ters include some descriptive text in the diagnosis, such as: "Interstitial lymphoid infiltrate in right ventricular biopsy – ISHLT grade 1R / 1B. No histologic features of acute antibody-mediated rejection – ISHLT grade AMR 0." The reason for dual reporting is the belief among many cardiologists that the portent of, and the appropriate response to, grade 1B histology is different from that for grade 1A histology. The more diffuse interstitial infiltrates (grade 1B) may be treated or the patients biopsied more frequently than patients with limited perivascular infiltrates (grade 1A). Although this assessment was largely anecdotal at the time of the 2004 revision of the grading system, subsequent data from the CARGO study (156) indicate potential biologic differences between grades 1A and 1B histology in adults and children (157). Briefly, this eight-center prospective study was initiated in 2001 with 629 patients and 4917 posttransplantation encounters with studies of peripheral blood mononuclear cell gene expression and routine EMBs. The standard for the diagnosis of rejection was histology; biopsies were reviewed by a central panel of three pathologists to standardize diagnoses. The study produced a 20-gene algorithm that reliably distinguishes ISHLT grade 3A rejection from graft quiescence (ISHLT grade 0). Of interest is the observation that the peripheral blood gene expression profiles of patients with ISHLT grades 1A and 2 histology are similar to those of the grade 0 graft quiescence, whereas ISHLT grade 1B biopsies have peripheral blood gene expression profiles similar to those of grade 3A rejection. This confirms the observations that grade 2 histology is not clinically significant and can be grouped with grade 1A and also confirms the suspicion that grades 1A and 1B histology reflect different biologic processes. The clinical significance of these data is yet to be defined.

Technical Considerations

A minimum of three, and ideally more, appropriate samples of myocardium is the standard for grading acute cellular rejection. An appropriate piece of endomyocardium is at least 50% myocardium, excluding healing biopsy site, fat, or blood clot. Fixation in commercially available 10% neutral buffered formalin is adequate for routine histology. Because these are small pieces of tissue, expedited processing in an automated tissue processor is possible. The high quality of the histology makes rapid processing preferable to performing frozen sections for "stat" diagnosis. Hematoxylin and eosin staining of at least three levels though the block is recommended. Special staining (trichrome stain) may help define myocyte damage and fibrosis. Immunohistochemical stains for lymphocyte subsets are not routinely necessary but can be extremely helpful for identifying myocardial extension from nodular endocardial infiltrates, as will be discussed later. Ultrastructural studies are also not routinely necessary. Snap-frozen tissue is necessary if immunofluorescence studies are to be performed in assessing antibody-mediated rejection; most centers have opted for immunoperoxidase staining on formalin-fixed paraffin-embedded tissues for establishing the diagnosis.

Other Pathology in the Allograft Biopsy (Table 29.10)

NODULAR ENDOCARDIAL INFILTRATES (QUILTY EFFECT). Nodular endocardial infiltrates were recognized in posttransplantation biopsies after the introduction of cyclosporine immunosuppression. Some, but not all, cardiac allograft recipi-

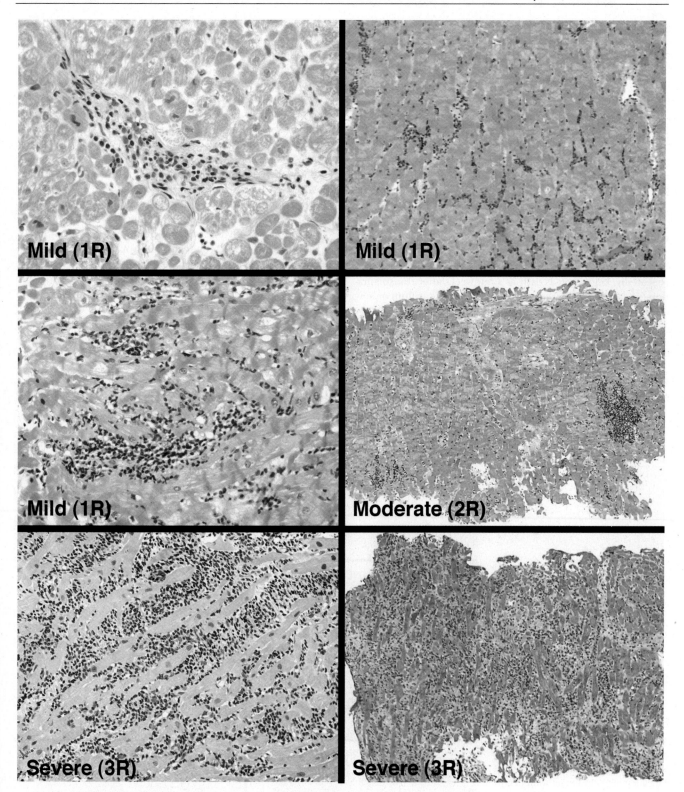

Figure 29.25. Acute cellular rejection. Patterns of acute cellular rejection ranging from mild to severe rejection are seen. See text for detailed description.

TABLE 29.10

Morphologic Mimics of Acute Cellular Rejection

Perioperative ischemic/reperfusion injury
Vasopressor/catecholamine effect
Biopsy site changes
Infectious myocarditis
Quilty effect (nodular endocardial infiltrates)
Posttransplant lymphoproliferative disorder
Recurrence of primary cardiac disease (e.g., sarcoidosis, idiopathic giant-cell myocarditis)
Ischemia related to transplant coronary artery disease

ents form these lesions (74% at Stanford University [158], 58% at Columbia University Medical Center [159], and 39% at Cleveland Clinic [160]). Those who form the lesions tend to do so repeatedly, beginning as early as a few weeks after transplantation. These lesions may be confined to the endocardium or may extend irregularly into the subjacent myocardium (Fig. 29.26). When the lesions extend into the myocardium, a tangential section through the biopsy may not show the connection to the surface endocardium, making differentiation of this dense, space-occupying, inflammatory infiltrate from acute rejection very difficult. The histology, when a single lesion is present, often mimics ISHLT grade 2 histology. Indeed, the vast majority of biopsies called "grade 2 rejection" have been shown to be myocardial extension of Quilty lesions (161). This myocardial extension of nodular endocardial infiltrates is also the cause of significant variability in the diagnosis of ISHLT grades 2, 3A, and 3B rejection (162,163). The distinction of Quilty lesions from rejection may be accomplished with deeper levels demonstrating extension to the endocardium (161). The presence of plasma cells and prominent small vessels also helps identify Quilty lesions. Immunohistochemical staining for T and B lymphocytes may also be useful. The Quilty lesions have central cores of CD20+ B lymphocytes surrounded by a rim of CD3+ T lymphocytes; CD21+ dendritic cells may also be present in the center of the nodule (Fig. 29.26).

The relationship of nodular endocardial infiltrates to acute rejection is not determined. The lesion has generally been considered not to represent acute rejection and is therefore not treated as rejection. Observations of an increased incidence of rejection in association with Quilty lesion formation may reflect

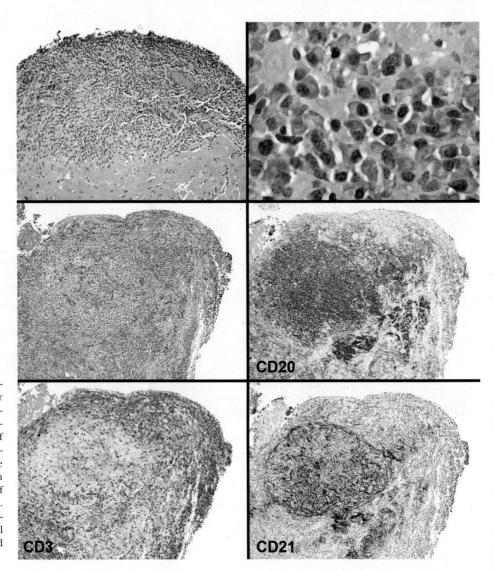

Figure 29.26. Quilty lesions (nodular endocardial infiltrates). Upper panels: Low-power and high-power magnification of Quilty lesions without myocyte encroachment. The presence of plasma cells favors Quilty lesions. Middle panels: Quilty lesion with myocyte encroachment is often associated with myocyte damage. The presence of CD20+ B cells is typical of Quilty lesions. Lower panels: CD3+ T cells ring the B-cell collections. CD21+ dendritic cell networks are seen in Quilty lesions and not cellular rejection.

the challenges noted earlier in the histologic differentiation of the two processes in some biopsies.

PERIOPERATIVE ISCHEMIC DAMAGE. Early ischemic injury is characterized by coagulative necrosis of myocytes; a Masson trichrome stain can be useful if coagulative necrosis is difficult to recognize on the hematoxylin and eosin stain. As noted earlier, contraction bands are commonly seen in EMBs and cannot be reliably used to diagnose reperfusion injury in biopsy material. Healing fat necrosis, involving interstitial fat, may also reflect ischemic injury. Inflammation associated with healing ischemic damage should not be confused with rejection; the presence of a mixed cellular infiltrate including neutrophils helps define ischemic injury, but the time course of healing infarct in these heavily immunosuppressed patients differs from healing of MIs in nonimmunosuppressed persons (Fig. 29.27). "Reperfusion" injury in the peritransplantation period also has histologic features overlapping with antibody-mediated rejection.

ISCHEMIC DAMAGE RELATED TO ALLOGRAFT VASCULO-PATHY. EMBs only very rarely include small vessels that could

show posttransplantation vasculopathy. It is possible in biopsies to see acute MI or myocytolysis, indicating chronic ischemia of subendocardial myocytes. Ischemic myocytes may also accumulate microvesicular fat droplets.

INFECTION AND POSTTRANSPLANTATION LYMPHOPRO-LIFERATIVE DISORDERS. CMV inclusions, *Toxoplasma gondii* tachyzoites in pseudocysts (Fig. 29.27), or amastigotes of *Trypanosoma cruzi* may be seen in the myocardium after transplantation. There may be little or no inflammatory reaction as a result of immunosuppression, or there may be lymphocytic inflammation potentially mistaken for rejection. PTLDs rarely involve the allograft (Fig. 29.27) but have histology similar to that of other extranodal sites.

ANTIBODY-MEDIATED (HUMORAL) REJECTION. Acute antibody-mediated rejection occurs in cardiac allografts, but there is no consensus on the criteria for diagnosis, and there is considerable variation in the apparent incidence at different centers. Recipients may be allosensitized by pregnancy, blood product administration, prior transplantation, or assist device placement. Antibody-mediated rejection does not, compared with

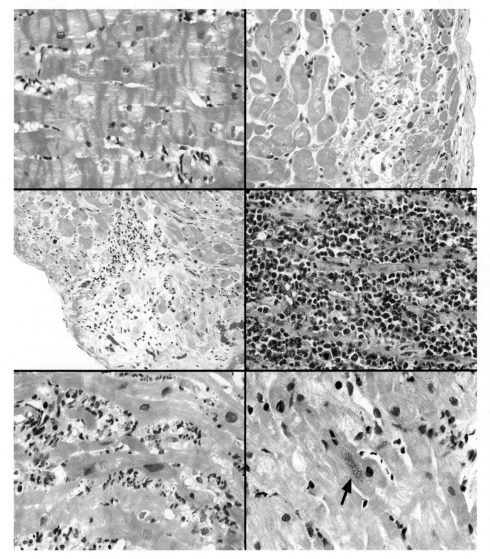

Figure 29.27. Mimics of acute rejection. *Upper left panel*: Contraction bands are the most common biopsy artifact and should not be mistaken for contraction band necrosis. *Upper right panel*: Subendocardial acute ischemic necrosis in which the degree of myocyte necrosis is much greater than the cellular infiltrate is seen in the early posttransplantation period. *Middle left panel*: Healing biopsy site lesion with scattered mononuclear inflammatory cells and variable amounts of organizing fibrin and fibrous tissue. *Middle right panel*: Posttransplantation lymphoproliferative disorder is uncommon in the heart. Cytologic atypia, division figures, and necrosis are helpful clues. *Lower left panel*: Cytomegalovirus myocarditis showing eosinophilic nuclear inclusions and a mixed inflammatory cell infiltrate. *Lower right panel*: Toxoplasmic myocarditis with diagnostic cytoplasmic cyst. The surrounding inflammation may be sparse.

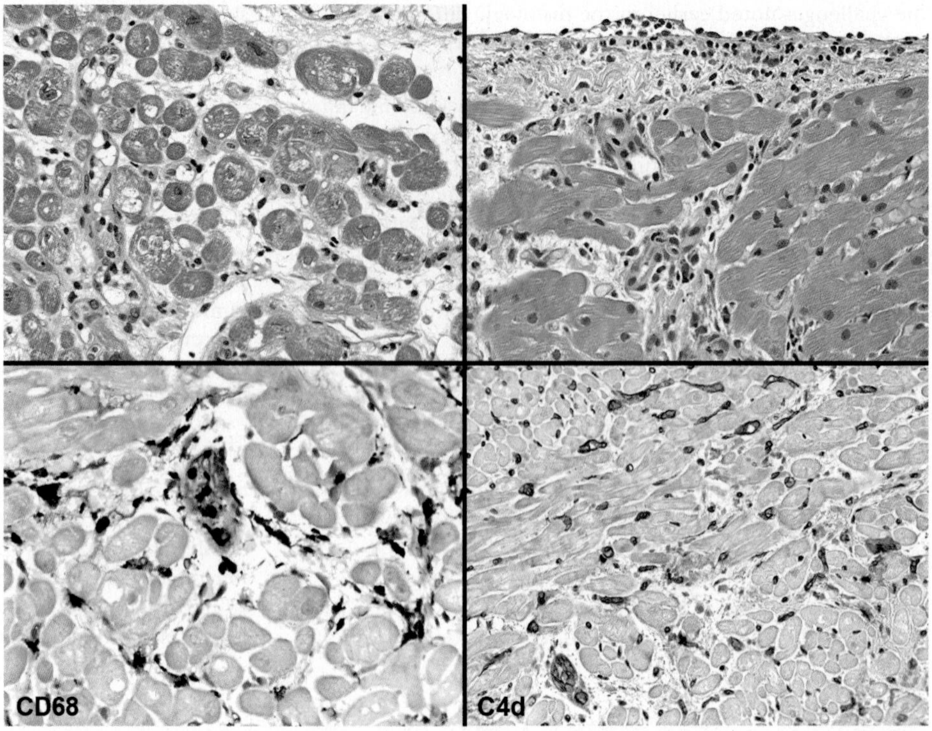

Figure 29.28. Acute antibody-mediated rejection (AMR). *Upper panels:* The range of histologic changes in AMR include interstitial edema and hyperplastic endothelial cells lining the interstitial vessels to neutrophilic endocardial and interstitial infiltrates admixed with the edema and vascular changes. *Lower panels:* CD68$^+$ histiocytes are found within the lumens of the vessels. C4d staining of the small interstitial vessels.

acute cellular rejection, have a distinctive clinical presentation but is associated with a higher rate of graft loss (164–166).

The histopathology of humoral rejection in the heart may be limited to endothelial cell swelling and accumulation of intravascular macrophages or may be pronounced with interstitial edema (Fig. 29.28) and adhesion of neutrophils to capillary endothelium. In extreme instances, interstitial hemorrhage, intravascular thrombi, and myocyte necrosis may be present (165,166). The confirmation of the involvement of antibody in the process requires the demonstration of immunoglobulin and/or complement deposition in the tissues. This may be accomplished with immunofluorescence staining for immunoglobulin (IgG, IgM, and/or IgA) and complement (C3d, C4d, and/or C1q) on frozen sections or immunoperoxidase staining for C4d and/or C3d on formalin-fixed, paraffin-embedded tissue (167). It has been suggested (166) that demonstration of CD68$^+$ macrophages within capillaries (CD31$^+$/CD34$^+$ endothelium-lined capillary channels) by immunohistochemistry can be a surrogate marker for antibody or complement deposition (Fig. 29.28).

For transplantation recipients with hemodynamic compromise and cardiac dysfunction, it has been proposed that immunohistochemical staining be performed. Combined cellular and humoral rejection may occur, so these studies may be requested even if there are significant cellular infiltrates in the biopsy. If there are marked histologic changes with interstitial edema and endothelial swelling and adherent neutrophils, performing the immunohistochemical stains is merely confirmatory. However, when patients have hemodynamic dysfunction and there are minimal cellular infiltrates in the biopsy, performing immunohistochemical studies is warranted even if there is no histologic suggestion of antibody-mediated rejection. The consensus meeting of the ISHLT (155) did not recommend routine screening of all biopsies for antibody-mediated rejection but did recommend that each biopsy be carefully evaluated for the

histologic features noted earlier. If none is found, the biopsy should be designated as negative for antibody-mediated rejection, or "AMR 0." If features suggestive of antibody-mediated rejection are found, then the diagnosis should be confirmed with immunohistochemistry; if these studies are positive, a diagnosis should be made of "AMR 1, Positive for antibody-mediated rejection, Histologic features of AMR and positive for *(listing the immunofluorescence and/or immunoperoxidase studies confirming the diagnosis)*." It was additionally recommended that in the presence of histologic features of rejection, serum should be drawn and tested for donor-specific antibody (155,168,169). If positive, this testing can provide reassuring supporting evidence and, ideally, a surrogate endpoint by which to assess the effects of therapy. However, recipient antibodies may be directed against non–human leukocyte antigen (HLA) antigens not in the test panel, and a negative result does not exclude antibody-mediated rejection. There is, as of the moment, no consensus on a diagnostic algorithm for antibody-mediated rejection in heart transplantations incorporating circulating antibody, histologic findings, immunohistologic findings, and hemodynamic studies of cardiac function (170). In the absence of an accepted definition, there will be considerable variation between centers in diagnostic and therapeutic approaches to antibody-mediated rejection.

Hyperacute rejection is the most fulminant form of antibody-mediated rejection in heart allografts. It is extremely rare (171) in clinical practice. Circulating preformed antibodies (IgG and/or IgM) in the recipient bind to vascular endothelial cells with subsequent complement activation, endothelial damage, neutrophil activation, platelet adhesion, activation of clotting, and fibrinolytic cascades. This results in microvascular thrombosis, hemorrhage, vascular and myocardial necrosis, and rapid graft failure. The heart is swollen and darkly discolored with interstitial hemorrhage and edema (Fig. 29.29).

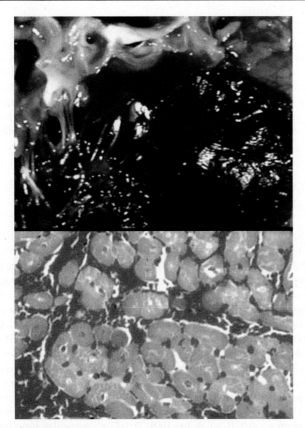

Figure 29.29. Hyperacute rejection (HAR) in an animal model of presensitization. *Upper panel*: The heart is swollen, plum colored, and poorly functioning. *Lower panel*: In early HAR, there is extensive interstitial hemorrhage as a result of endothelial damage by antibody or complement deposition and neutrophils.

Hyperacute rejection may occur with preformed anti-ABO antibodies, preformed anti-HLA antibodies, preformed anti–donor endothelial cell antibodies, and xenotransplantation. Sensitizing events include previous blood transfusions, pregnancy, prior cardiac surgery, and prior transplantation. Successful heart transplantations have, however, been performed across ABO mismatches in neonates who have not yet formed anti-ABO antibodies (172). Naturally forming xenoantibodies are the first immunologic obstacle to successful pig to primate xenotransplantation. The primary antibody response is directed toward the alpha-1,3-galactose antigen (α-Gal), a moiety abundantly present on porcine endothelium but absent from humans and Old World primates (173,174). In experimental conditions when anti-Gal effects are eliminated, grafts are lost in a delayed xenograft rejection (175) with microvascular thrombosis and myocardial necrosis without a cellular infiltrate but with IgG and IgM deposition.

TRANSPLANTATION CORONARY ARTERY DISEASE

Beyond 1 year after transplantation, malignancy and transplantation coronary artery disease (TCAD) become important determinants of graft and patient survival (152). The incidence of TCAD varies substantially between centers and is related to the sensitivity of the method of detection. The most recent summary of angiographic studies shows an incidence of TCAD of 7% at 1 year, 32% at 5 years, and 53% at 10 years after transplantation (152). IVUS is more sensitive than angiography in the detection of the intimal proliferations of TCAD (176).

TCAD (Fig. 29.30) differs morphologically from common atherosclerosis in the following ways: (a) the intimal lesions are concentric rather than eccentric; (b) the intimal lesions are diffuse and extensive rather than discrete and focal; (c) there tends to be more extensive inflammation with lymphocytes; (d) calcification is less common; (e) the lesions more often extend

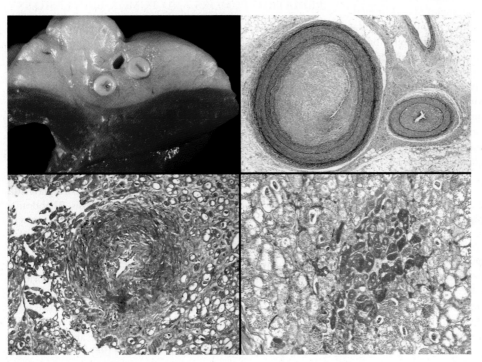

Figure 29.30. Transplantation coronary artery disease (TCAD). *Upper left panel*: Concentric narrowing of bifurcated left anterior descending (LAD) artery with residual slitlike lumen. Note abundant lipid within the lesions. *Upper right panel*: Low-power magnification showing epicardial vessel and its adjacent branch with concentric intimal narrowing and preservation of the internal elastic membrane. *Lower left panel*: TCAD involving intramyocardial vessels is an uncommon finding in the biopsy. The effects of TCAD range from vacuolar degeneration to acute ischemic injury (*lower right panel*).

into small, intramyocardial vessels; and (f) similar but less extensive lesions may be present in cardiac veins.

The relative contributions of intimal thickening and vessel constriction to vessel lumen loss have been detailed with serial IVUS studies. Increase in intimal area is greater in the first year after transplantation than in subsequent years (177). After year 1, lumen narrowing is primarily related to constriction of the vessel wall (with reduction of the area circumscribed by the external elastic lamina, particularly in larger coronary arteries) (178).

Many immunologic and nonimmunologic factors have been implicated in the development of TCAD (179,180). Nonimmunologic factors include warm and cold ischemic time, donor age, pre-existing vessels disease, and the risk factors for nontransplantation atherosclerosis. Generally, TCAD is considered a manifestation of chronic allograft rejection with an immunologic attack directed against the graft's vascular endothelium. The relative roles of prior episodes of acute cellular rejection, T lymphocytes, B lymphocytes, and antibodies in the genesis of endothelial damage and the subsequent intimal proliferations and medial damage have been hotly debated. It is interesting that a discrepancy between acute cellular rejection and vasculopathy is noted in at least one experimental transplantation model (181) and that incremental improvements in immunosuppression and patient care have reduced the incidence of acute cellular rejection but have not significantly reduced the incidence of TCAD as a cause of death (182). Differences in the methods of antigen presentation could account for some of this discrepancy if indirect antigen presentation (donor antigens presented by host antigen-presenting cells) is more important for the development of TCAD and direct presentation (donor antigen presented by donor cells) is more important for acute cellular rejection. The argument would be that different immunosuppressive regimens differ in their effects on direct versus indirect pathways. It is also interesting that circulating recipient stem cells have been described as contributing to TCAD and atherosclerosis (183–185). The many different etiologies (immunologic and/or nonimmunologic) of endothelial/coronary artery damage may each result in homing of circulating stem cells into the area of injury. Subsequent differentiation and proliferation of these cells and cytokine release in response to additional factors may result in the intimal and medial lesions of TCAD with immunosuppression having little effect on the host's stem cells involved in the lesions.

As described earlier, it is uncommon to find the lesions of TCAD in the EMB. The changes of acute ischemia or vacuolar degeneration, however, are occasionally observed, particularly in patients with TCAD involving the small intramyocardial vessels (Fig. 29.30).

Reinnervation of the Heart Allograft

Limited sympathetic reinnervation occurs in the majority (75% to 80%) of heart transplantation recipients studied 1 year or more after transplantation (186). The most frequently reinnervated site is the anterior wall of the LV. Thus, recipients with graft vasculopathy and ischemic damage to the myocardium in the first year after transplantation may not experience chest pain; angina pectoris is reported by some recipients later in the posttransplantation period.

Recurrent Disease in the Allograft

Approximately 25% of patients with giant-cell myocarditis will have recurrence in the allograft (150). Occasional instances of recurrent sarcoid have been reported (187); these generally occur more than 1 year after transplantation when immunosuppression has been diminished. Chagas disease has also been seen to recur in the allograft; the instances we have seen have also recurred in the skin. Amyloidosis may recur if the underlying disease has not been treated.

CARDIAC TUMORS AND TUMOR-LIKE LESIONS

Although primary cardiac tumors in children and adults are rare, improvements in cardiac imaging and interventional techniques including EMB afford clinicians the possibility to diagnose and classify many of these tumors before surgical intervention. In autopsy series, the vast majority of cardiac tumors are metastatic neoplasms (188,189). In large retrospective surgical series of primary tumors, 75% to 80% are benign, with myxomas accounting for 75% to 90% (190,191). The clinical manifestations usually relate to the site of involvement and can produce local symptoms related to valvular obstruction or dysfunction, mural involvement and arrhythmias, fragmentation and embolization, or constitutional symptoms such as fever and weight loss.

Primary cardiac tumors can be classified in several different schemes: (a) left- or right-sided, atrial or ventricular topography; (b) benign versus malignant tumors; (c) pediatric versus adult tumors; (d) localization within the heart layers (e.g., endocardial, myocardial, pericardial); or (e) inflammatory, thrombotic, hamartomatous, or neoplastic. We use a practical approach that incorporates many of these elements for both diagnostic and differential diagnostic considerations (Table 29.11).

PEDIATRIC TUMORS AND TUMOR-LIKE LESIONS

The majority of pediatric masses are hamartomatous in nature and include rhabdomyoma, cardiac fibroma, histiocytoid cardiomyopathy, and hamartoma of adult cardiac myocytes. The nature of inflammatory myofibroblastic tumors is unclear (i.e., inflammatory or neoplastic). Germ cell tumor is an example of a true neoplasm in this age group (192).

Rhabdomyoma

Rhabdomyoma is the most common pediatric tumor arising in the heart. It is closely associated with tuberous sclerosis complex because up to 30% to 80% of patients with this lesion have the clinical or radiologic stigmata of tuberous sclerosis. Rhabdomyoma occurs as a solitary mass or multiple masses in the ventricular wall or chamber (193). Multiple lesions arise almost always in the setting of tuberous sclerosis. The presenting signs and symptoms are related in large part to size, location, and number of masses (e.g., congestive heart failure, conduction abnormalities, and obstruction of flow across a valve). Cases of sudden death have been reported, and intrauterine fetal demise is associated with fetal hydrops. Echocardiography shows homogeneous bright echogenic changes, and the lesions are well delineated from the adjacent cardiac muscle (194). Many of these

TABLE 29.11

Cardiac Tumors and Tumor-Like Lesions

PEDIATRIC
Rhabdomyoma
Fibroma
Histiocytoid cardiomyopathy
Hamartoma of adult cardiac myocytes
Inflammatory myofibroblastic tumor
Teratoma
Vascular masses (e.g., blood cysts, hemangiomas)
Sarcomas (e.g., undifferentiated sarcoma, angiosarcoma, rhabdomyosarcoma, osteosarcoma)
ADULT
Myxoma
Paraganglioma
Lipoma
Sarcomas (e.g., angiosarcoma, undifferentiated sarcoma, leiomyosarcoma, osteosarcoma, synovial sarcoma, rhabdomyosarcoma)
Malignant lymphoma
Metastatic tumors
TUMOR-LIKE LESIONS
Papillary fibroelastoma
Mesothelial/Monocytic incidental cardiac excrescence (MICE)
Mural thrombi including calcified amorphous tumor (CAT)
Cystic tumor of atrioventricular node
Lipomatous hypertrophy interatrial septum

Modified from Burke and Virmani (192) and Miller and Edwards (193).

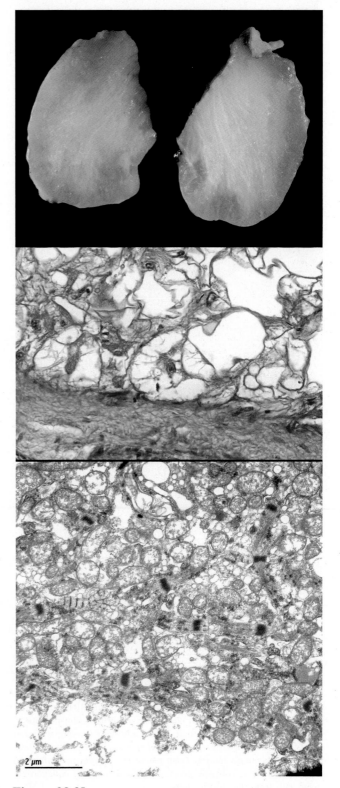

Figure 29.31. Cardiac rhabdomyoma. *Upper panel*: Tan-white circumscribed nodular mass in the myocardium. *Middle panel*: The characteristic spider cells showing strands of cytoplasm across the clear cytoplasm. *Lower panel*: Transmission electron microscopy showing an abundance of mitochondria admixed with scattered fibrils.

lesions regress spontaneously in early childhood, and surgery is reserved for patients with large obstructing lesions or who fail antiarrhythmia therapy.

On cut section, rhabdomyomas are sharply circumscribed, nonencapsulated, pale tan to yellow nodules that range in size from 0.1 to 9.0 cm (Fig. 29.31). They are composed of large vacuolated cells with central round-to-oval nuclei and strands of eosinophilic cytoplasmic bands traversing the cells producing the "spider cells." The cells contain large amounts of glycogen and demonstrate immunoreactivity for desmin, actin, myoglobin, and vimentin. At the ultrastructural level, the spider cells contain abundant glycogen and myofibrils, and mitochondria form the radiating strands (195,196). Z- and A-bands, but not I-bands, are present, and the cells resemble fetal cardiac myoblasts.

Cardiac Fibroma

Cardiac fibromas are the second most common tumor in the pediatric group. These benign hamartomatous proliferations usually present within the first year of life and, unlike rhabdomyomas, rarely spontaneously regress. They are usually solitary lesions within the interventricular septum or free wall of the RV or LV and cause symptoms of congestive heart failure, obstruction, arrhythmias, or sudden death. The majority are sporadic; less than 5% are associated with Gorlin syndrome. Most patients require surgery or transplantation to relieve the cardiac symptoms because the masses can range up to 10 cm or more (197).

The macroscopic appearance resembles the white whorled appearance of uterine leiomyomas (Fig. 29.32). The tumors are sharply delineated from the adjacent myocardium and may

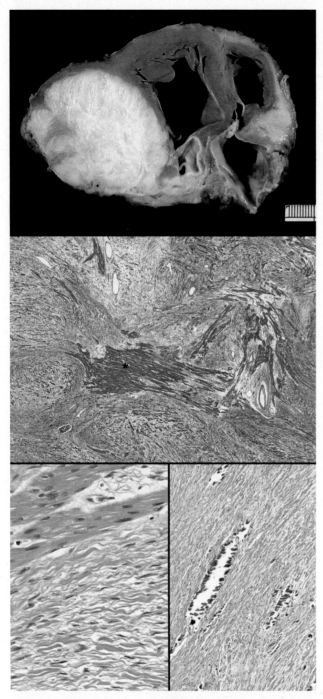

Figure 29.32. Cardiac fibroma. *Upper panel*: Large left ventricular (LV) circumscribed mass with characteristic whorled fibrous appearance on cut section. *Middle panel*: Trichrome stain showing scattered islands of residual myocytes (*) surrounded by a cellular process embedded in a collagenous matrix. *Lower panels*: High-power magnification showing a bland fibroblastic proliferation and bands of collagen admixed with scattered calcifications.

contain central foci of calcifications, but necrosis and hemorrhage are absent. Microscopically, the bland fibroblastic proliferation resembles an extra-abdominal fibromatosis with tumor cells interdigitating into the adjacent myocytes. The cellularity is variable, and the matrix is rich in collagen and elastin fibers (198).

Histiocytoid Cardiomyopathy

Histiocytoid cardiomyopathy is a rare subendocardial lesion that presents in infancy and demonstrates a strong female predominance. It occurs in isolation or with other congenital abnormalities such as ventricular noncompaction, septal defects, and hypoplastic left heart syndrome (81,199). The majority of children present under the age of 2 years with arrhythmias, heart failure, or sudden death. If successfully controlled, many of the lesions spontaneously regress.

Grossly, the lesions appear as solitary or multiple raised, subendocardial-based, tan-yellow nodules (Fig. 29.33). Most measure less than 0.5 cm and are sharply separated from the adjacent tissue. In routine sections, they appear as raised, non-encapsulated nodular collections of cuboidal and polygonal cells with abundant eosinophilic, granular cytoplasm (200). The oncocytic features are confirmed ultrastructurally by the abundance of mitochondria, scattered leptomeric structures, and absence of T-tubules. The myogenic origin is confirmed by weak reactivity for actin, myosin, desmin, and myoglobin and lack of staining for CD68 (193,200). Currently, histiocytoid cardiomyopathy is considered to be a hamartoma of oncocytic cardiac myocytes.

Inflammatory Myofibroblastic Tumor

Inflammatory myofibroblastic tumor of the heart is a rare, endocardial-based proliferation of uncertain etiology that occurs more commonly in children and young adults than in adults (201). These left- or right-sided lesions form an intracavitary polypoid or multilobulated mass with a smooth surface and broad base (Fig. 29.34) (202). Microscopically, inflammatory myofibroblastic tumor is composed of cellular, bland-appearing myofibroblastic cells embedded in a myxoid matrix and admixed with plasma cells and lymphocytes. Cytologic atypia, pleomorphism, and increased mitotic activity are absent, but hyaline necrosis secondary to torsion may be seen. The spindle cells show immunoreactivity for smooth muscle actin but not anti–S-100 protein, cytokeratin, or desmin, and only rare weak staining with ALK-1 has been reported (201). Local recurrence has occurred in some cases, whereas spontaneous regression has also been reported; to date, none has metastasized (203,204).

Neoplasms of the Heart

True neoplasms of the heart are extremely rare in children. Both benign and malignant soft tissue tumors have been reported, including hemangioma, rhabdomyosarcoma, angiosarcoma, undifferentiated sarcomas, and osteosarcoma. They resemble their soft tissue and osseous counterparts.

Germ cell tumors are usually pericardial in location and consist of teratomas and yolk sac tumors. Surgical excision is the primary treatment modality, and patients with malignant germ cell tumors also receive chemotherapy (192).

ADULT TUMORS

Cardiac Myxoma

Cardiac myxoma is defined as a benign neoplasm characterized by an abundant mucopolysaccharide matrix and stellate "myxoma" cells and is also called a benign tumor of pluripotent

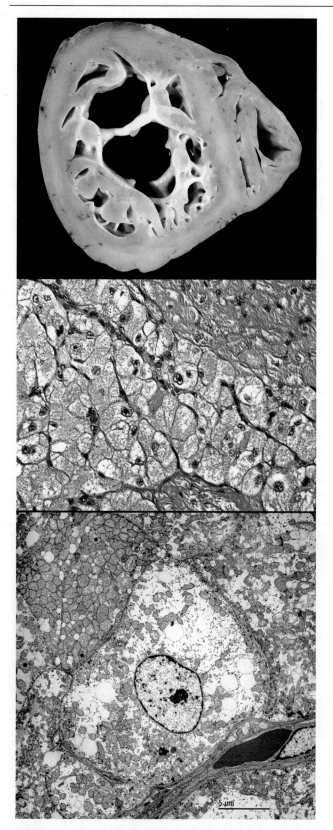

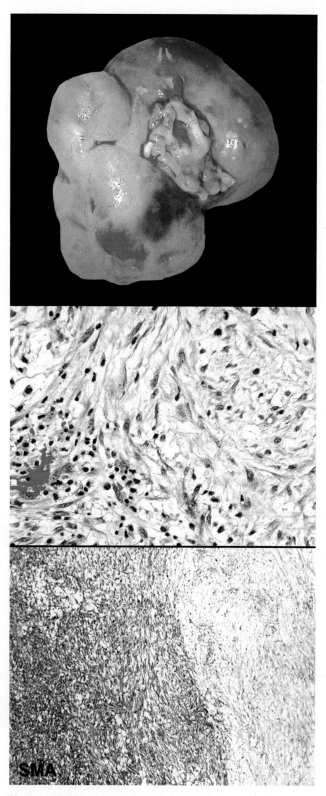

Figure 29.33. Histiocytoid cardiomyopathy. *Upper panel*: Discrete yellow-brown subendocardial nodules are noted throughout the left ventricle (LV). *Middle panel*: Nodular collections of pale eosinophilic cells with granular cytoplasm and central round nuclei with conspicuous nucleoli are separated from the adjacent myocardium. *Lower panel*: Low-power transmission electron microscopy showing abundant mitochondria, glycogen, and absence of T-tubules.

Figure 29.34. Inflammatory myofibroblastic tumor (IMT). *Upper panel*: 2.5-cm endocardial-based bosselated mass in right atrium with narrow stalk. *Middle panel*: High-power magnification showing admixture of inflammatory cells and bland spindled cells. No coagulative tumor cell necrosis, mitotic figures, or pleomorphism is noted. *Lower panel*: The spindled cells stain strongly for smooth muscle actin.

mesenchyme. It is the most common primary neoplasm and constitutes 75% to 80% of tumors in surgical series (205). The majority present as a solitary mass arising on the endocardial surface of the left atrium adjacent to the foramen ovale (75%). The remainder are found in the right atrium (15% to 20%), biatrial (2%), RV (2%), LV (2%), and multifocal locations (3%). Less than 10% of cases occur as part of the Carney complex or as a nonsyndromic familial cardiac myxoma. This group is associated with a higher frequency of multiple lesions at presentation or recurrent tumors (206). Symptoms at presentation depend in large part on location (left vs. right atrium), size, and mobility (e.g., AV valve obstruction, embolization, congestive heart failure).

Grossly, these gelatinous tumors attach by either a broad base or delicate stalk to the endocardium and protrude into the cardiac cavity. They range in size from 1 to 15 cm, but most are 2 to 8 cm. The surface can be either smooth and lobulated or gelatinous and frondlike with a greater likelihood of detachment and embolization (Fig. 29.35). The cut surface may exhibit foci of hemorrhage, calcification, or cystic change, but tumor necrosis is absent. Microscopically, the myxoma or "lepidic" cell is composed of spindled or stellate cells with eosinophilic cytoplasm and uniform, round nuclei with inconspicuous nucleoli. The cellularity can be variable, including foci of increased cellularity, but marked pleomorphism, increased mitotic activity, and abnormal division forms are absent. When present, these features raise the possibility of a malignant myxoid neoplasm such as malignant fibrous histiocytoma and myxoid fibrosarcoma, and thorough tissue sampling is warranted (Fig. 29.36). Toward the surface of the myxoma, the myxoma cells can align around vessels in a more complex ringlike pattern and may be associated with mononuclear inflammatory cells (Fig. 29.35). In 1% to 2% of cases, foci of glandular differ-

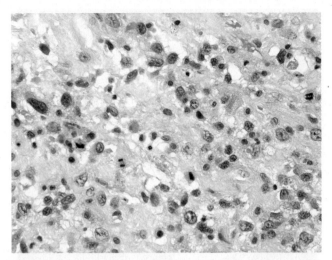

Figure 29.36. The differential diagnosis of atrial myxoma includes high-grade sarcomas with abundant myxoid features. The presence of numerous mitotic figures, cellular pleomorphism, marked cellularity, and tumor cell necrosis (not shown) is seen in cardiac sarcomas but not myxomas.

entiation can be found, particularly toward the base of the tumor. The degree of myxoid stroma is also variable, and collections of pigment-laden macrophages, calcification or ossification, and extramedullary hematopoietic elements have been reported. Organizing thrombotic changes can be found along the surface, and thorough sampling is required to demonstrate the myxoma cells in some cases. Immunohistochemical staining with calretinin is found in myxomas but not thrombi and can be useful in difficult cases (207).

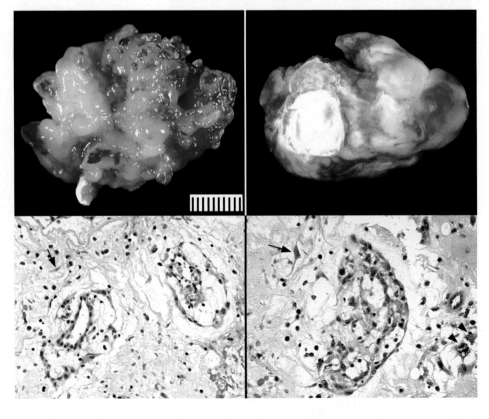

Figure 29.35. Atrial myxoma. *Upper panels*: Gross appearance of atrial myxoma ranges from loose gelatinous friable masses on a narrow stalk (*left*) to a rounded, firmer lesion on broad base. *Lower panels*: Characteristic myxoma cells with stellate, slender nucleus, and eosinophilic cytoplasm embedded in pale edematous myxoid matrix (*arrows*). Alignment of myxoma cells around delicate vessels creates ring forms. Hemosiderin-laden macrophages may be found (*arrowheads*).

The varied histopathologic findings support the primitive pluripotential mesenchymal cell theory currently favored. A recent study demonstrated similar protein and gene expression profiles between myxoma cells and endocardial cushion cells and suggested they may derive from adult developmental remnants (208). Surgical excision is curative, and recurrence of the sporadic type is rare if careful attention is directed to removal of an additional rim of adjacent endocardial tissue. The recurrence rate in the syndromic types is reported to be higher, but this may reflect incomplete excision, multifocal lesions, or intraoperative tumor displacement.

Angiosarcoma

In most published series of surgically excised cardiac tumors, angiosarcoma is the most common type of sarcoma and accounts for one-third of cases (190,191,209). The remainder include high-grade sarcoma not otherwise specified, malignant fibrous histiocytoma, leiomyosarcoma, matrix-producing osteosarcoma and chondrosarcoma, fibrosarcoma, and synovial sarcoma. Angiosarcomas preferentially arise from the right atrium or pericardium; primary left atrial angiosarcoma has been reported but is extremely rare. Clinical symptoms are quite variable and depend on location, extent of intrathoracic spread, and size.

At surgery, angiosarcoma exhibits a multilobulated mass often with frondlike papillae. Infiltration into the atrial chamber and/or extension into or through the pericardium is common (Fig. 29.37). The cut surface is hemorrhagic, and foci of necrosis are visible. The microscopic findings are similar to their soft tissue counterpart and range from well-differentiated sarcomas with anastomosing channels lined by atypical, hyperchromatic endothelial cells with coarse chromatin and mitotic figures to anaplastic or epithelioid tumors (210). Immunohistochemistry is required, particularly in high-grade variants, to demonstrate endothelial origin. A panel of antibodies that in-

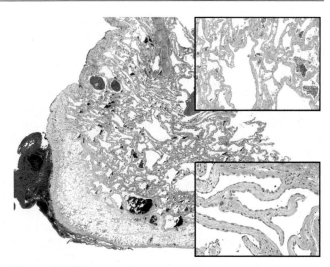

Figure 29.38. Pericardial hemangioma exhibiting an unencapsulated circumscribed mass of dilated vascular spaces. *Upper inset*: Scanning magnification showing variably sized vascular spaces without tissue infiltration. *Lower inset*: The vascular spaces are lined by bland endothelial cells without mitotic figures.

cludes factor VIII–related protein, CD31, and CD34 is helpful. In low-grade angiosarcoma, the distinction from cardiac hemangioma is not usually difficult. Hemangiomas lack complex vascular architecture, mitotic activity, and cytologic atypia (Fig. 29.38). A multimodality treatment approach combing surgery with chemotherapy, irradiation, and immunotherapy has been tried, but overall, the prognosis is poor.

Malignant Lymphoma

Primary malignant lymphoma of the heart is defined by WHO as an intrathoracic malignancy presenting with cardiac symptoms,

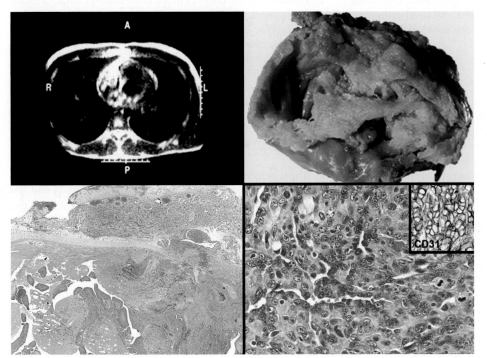

Figure 29.37. Cardiac angiosarcoma. *Upper left panel*: Cardiac magnetic resonance imaging showing large atrial mass with increased uptake. *Upper right panel*: En bloc resection of atrial mass showing infiltration in the wall and protrusion into the right atrial (RA) cavity. *Lower left panel*: Transmural involvement of the neoplasm with extension into the pericardium. *Lower right panel*: High-power magnification showing rudimentary slitlike vascular lumens and large epithelioid tumor cells. *Inset*: Strong staining with CD31.

and the preponderance of the tumor is within the heart or pericardium (211). The right atrium is the most common site of involvement, and clinical findings are often related to obstruction and arrhythmias (212). Widespread involvement of the RV and pericardium is often present. Grossly, multiple tumor masses within the cavity and wall of the right heart are seen (Fig. 29.39). The most common subtype is diffuse large B-cell lymphoma, but Burkitt lymphoma and other subtypes have been reported. Anthracycline-based chemotherapy is used as the primary therapy, but the survival rates are generally poor.

OTHER TUMOR-LIKE LESIONS

Several nonneoplastic proliferations occur in the heart and present as mass lesions that mimic neoplasms. On occasion, they can become large enough to cause obstructive symptoms or embolize.

Papillary Fibroelastoma

This reactive lesion arises on the endocardial surface of valves and cardiac chambers in adults. The aortic and mitral valves are more commonly affected than right-sided valves, with the aortic valve cusps, LV outflow tract, and anterior mitral valve leaflet being the most common sites (213). Papillary fibroelastomas (PFEs) are also reported in patients with chronic rheumatic valvular disease, in patients with prior surgery or irradiation, and along the LV outflow tract in HCM (214). The macroscopic appearance is characteristic, and the resemblance to the sea anemone has been described (Fig. 29.40). The collection of thin delicate fronds attaches by a stalk to the endocardial surface. Most measure less than 1 cm in diameter, but "giant PFEs" of 7 cm in size have been reported. Microscopically, the filiform structures are composed of a collagenous core admixed with elastic fibers, scattered myofibroblasts, and mucopolysaccharide matrix and lined by plump endothelial cells. They are distinguished from Lambl excrescences by their size and location. Lambl excrescences are small frondlike papillae that arise along the ventricular aspect of semilunar valves and involve the free and closing edges of the leaflet or on the atrial surface of AV valves (193).

Mesothelial/Monocytic Incidental Cardiac Excrescences

As the name suggests, these lesions are incidental findings at the time of surgical intervention or EMB (215). They likely represent an iatrogenic or artifactual process and are not neoplastic. The microscopic features consist of an admixture of blood, fibrin, inflammatory cells, and collections of cytokeratin-positive mesothelial cells and CD68[+] macrophages/monocytes (Fig. 29.41).

Thrombotic Lesions Including Calcified Amorphous Tumor

Mural thrombi are common complications of a variety of valvular and myocardial disorders. On occasion, they can become sufficiently large to create a mass effect or embolic episodes. In surgical resection specimens, they can sometimes be confused with cardiac myxomas. Reynolds et al. (216) described 11 cases presenting as endocardial-based masses that protruded into a cardiac cavity. The lesions were found in both right- and left-

sided chambers but more commonly in the ventricles than the atria. Calcified amorphous tumors varied in size from 0.2 to 6.5 cm. Microscopically, they were composed of eosinophilic degenerated fibrin collections and occasional hemosiderin-laden macrophages and erythrocytes. Nodular aggregates of calcium were distributed within the eosinophilic material (Fig. 29.42).

Cystic Tumor of Atrioventricular Node

This rare, nonneoplastic proliferation is now thought to be a proliferating congenital remnant of epithelial cells of endodermal origin and not an AV node mesothelioma (217). It can cause complete heart block or sudden death and is usually diagnosed at autopsy. It ranges in size from 0.2 to 2.0 cm and displays multiple cystic spaces in the large lesions. Flattened cuboidal epithelial cells line the cysts, although foci of transitional or squamous metaplasia can also be present (Fig. 29.43). The cells stain with carcinoembryonic antigen and cytokeratin markers but not mesothelial markers.

Lipomatous Hypertrophy of Interatrial Septum

The normal interatrial septum contains strands of myocytes, adipose tissue, blood vessels, and collagen fibers. In some patients, large accumulations of adipose tissue in the U-shaped limbus of the oval fossa produce a bulging expansion that can mimic a neoplastic or infiltrative disorder such as amyloidosis. By definition, the thickened septum is greater than 2.0 cm in diameter (Fig. 29.44). Varying proportions of brown fat and mature adipose tissue intermixed with hypertrophied myocytes are seen in microscopic sections (218).

METASTATIC TUMORS TO THE HEART

This group of malignant tumors is defined by WHO as cardiac tumors that do not arise either on the pericardium or in the myocardium (219). They are much more common than primary cardiac tumors. They constitute 10% to 15% of surgically resected cardiac tumors. The most common sites of origin are lung, breast, and gastric carcinoma, malignant lymphoma and leukemia, and malignant melanoma. In the absence of clinical history, a panel of immunohistochemical markers can be applied to define the site of origin. The pattern of dissemination to the heart is usually along lymphatic routes.

VALVULAR LESIONS OF THE HEART

A comprehensive approach to the evaluation of an excised valvular specimen requires an understanding of the gross and microscopic features and function of the normal valve (45), a detailed clinical history such as drug history and prior antibiotic therapy, and the operative findings. In many cases, the lesions are part of an isolated process, whereas in other cases, the valvular findings may be part of a systemic process (e.g., carcinoid syndrome, Fabry disease, mucopolysaccharidoses) (220). Moreover, the information provided by clinicians and the macroscopic findings help determine the need for microscopic evaluation and special stains. Careful inspection of specimen and documentation of the number of valve cusps; alterations on atrial and ventricular aspects of the AV valves; the ventricular

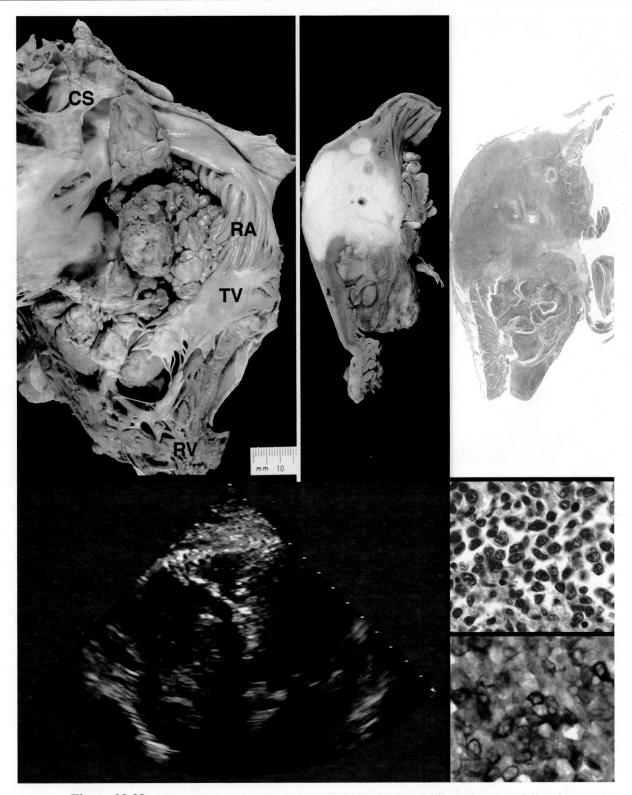

Figure 29.39. Malignant lymphoma. *Upper panels*: Large right atrial mass filling right atrium (RA) and extending across tricuspid valve (TV) into right ventricle (RV). Pale fleshy mass infiltrates the wall of the right-sided chambers and TV apparatus. *Lower left panel*: Echocardiographic image of large mass filling the RA. *Lower right panels*: Large atypical lymphoid cells that strongly stain for CD20.

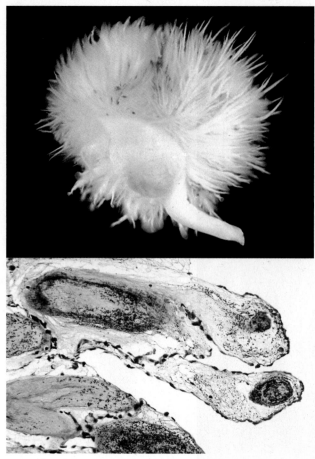

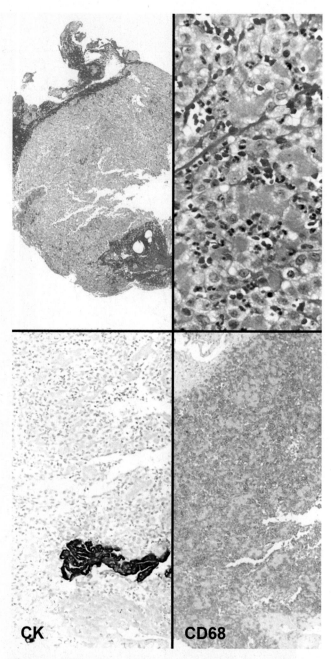

Figure 29.40. Papillary fibroelastoma. *Upper panel*: Delicate thin fronds on a long slender stalk resembling a sea anemone. *Lower panel*: Elastic van Gieson (EVG) staining of fronds showing central core of elastic fibers and edematous stroma lined by plump endothelial cells.

Figure 29.41. Cardiac mesothelial/monocytic incidental excrescences (MICE). *Upper panels*: Low- and high-power magnifications showing aggregates of blood, fibrin, and histiocytic cells found in an endomyocardial biopsy. *Lower panels*: Immunohistochemical stains showing rare collections of cytokeratin-positive mesothelial cells admixed with numerous CD68+ histiocytes.

and arterial surfaces of semilunar valves; severity and distribution of fibrosis, calcifications, tears, perforations, and vegetations; fusion of commissures; annular circumference; and changes in chordae tendineae or papillary muscles are essential (221). The leaflets of semilunar valves can be approximated to their normal positions to evaluate the stenotic and/or regurgitant nature of the lesions. In postrheumatic disease, the mitral valve may be resected intact, but in the setting of mitral valve repair for mitral valve prolapse, only a portion of the valve will be submitted to the surgical pathology lab. Photography of unusual findings can also aid in the clinicopathologic correlation. Microscopic assessment should focus on alterations in the structural layers of the valve from mechanical forces, severity and type of inflammation and postinflammatory changes, changes caused by metabolic disturbances, and degenerative changes. The roles of valve interstitial cells and valve endothelial cells in normal and disease states are currently the focus of investigation (222,223).

Several different classifications of valvulopathies are published, but the most practical paradigm classifies structural lesions based on their functional effect on the patient (i.e., stenotic vs. regurgitant physiology) (224–227). An important point to emphasize is the change in etiology of many of these lesions over the past half century as a result of, in part, antibiotic ther-

apy, increased life expectancy, and expanded patient selection for surgical intervention (228).

AORTIC VALVULAR DISEASE

There are several congenital and acquired lesions of the aortic valve that require surgical replacement. Some produce purely stenotic changes, others produce purely regurgitant alterations, and some lead to a mixed stenotic/regurgitant picture (229).

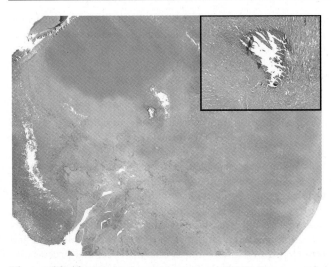

Figure 29.42. Calcified amorphous tumor (CAT). Large organizing thrombus in the atrium that contained variable amounts of calcification. Pockets of organizing cellular thrombus were present. *Inset*: Focus of calcification from center of thrombus.

Aortic valve replacement currently accounts for the majority of valve replacement surgeries.

Aortic Stenosis

The two most common etiologies of aortic stenosis are calcified congenital bicuspid valves and tricuspid calcific or senile/degenerative valvular stenosis. The frequency varies in published series, but these account for more than 85% of all cases (229,230). Other less common causes are postinflammatory/postrheumatic (<10%), congenital valvular/subvalvular stenosis including unicuspid/unicommissural valve, dysplastic valvular formation, and a group of rare metabolic disorders.

BICUSPID AORTIC VALVE. Bicuspid aortic valve (BAV) is the most common cardiovascular malformation and affects 1% to 2% of the population (men more often than women). It can occur in isolation or associated with other abnormalities such as aortic coarctation. There are two cusps instead of three, and one is usually larger than the other with the raphe (a ridge reflecting the incompletely formed commissure) present on the larger cusp (220). Most cases are classified as the anterior-posterior type and develop from fusion of the right and left coronary cusps; the coronary ostia are located behind the anterior cusp. In the right-left variant, the coronary ostia are located behind each cusp, respectively. The classic gross appearance of BAV is profound nodular calcifications in one or both cusps, absence of commissural fusion, and a slitlike orifice (Fig. 29.45). Second-

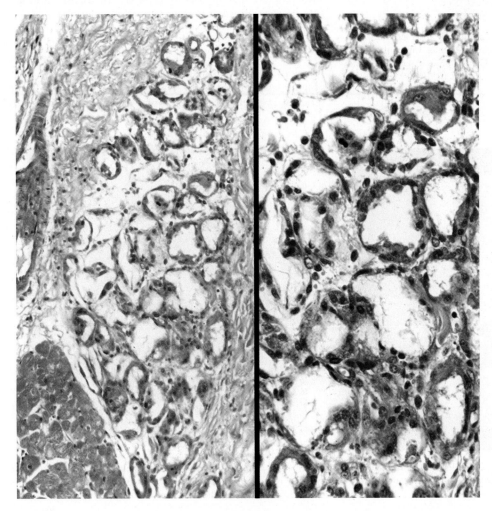

Figure 29.43. Cystic tumor of atrioventricular (AV) node. *Left panel*: Low-power magnification showing circumscribed collection of glandular structures. *Right panel*: Glands are lined by low cuboidal epithelial cells.

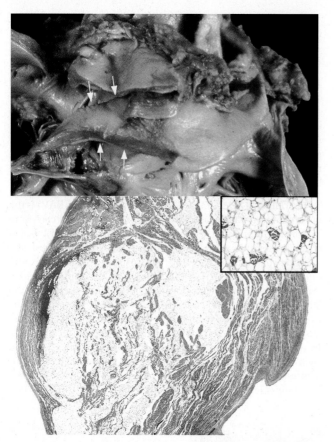

Figure 29.44. Lipomatous hypertrophy of interatrial septum. *Upper panel*: Gross appearance showing bulging pale mass within the atrial septum (*arrows*). *Lower panel* and *inset*: The septum is expanded by mature adipose tissue.

ary infectious endocarditis should be excluded by careful examination. The histopathologic changes reflect the extensive calcific changes that begin in the fibrosa layer and expand into the sinuses (231). Patients with BAV have an increased risk for ascending aortic aneurysm and dissection.

SENILE CALCIFIC TRICUSPID AORTIC STENOSIS. Like BAV, calcification and other fibrodegeneration occur in the valve cusps of an otherwise normal valve. It presents in an older age group than BAV and is not associated with aortic dilatation. Calcifications are arranged as nodular protrusions into the sinuses and are distributed in all three leaflets (Fig. 29.46). The orifice is triangular in shape, and the leaflets are thickened, but the free edge of the leaflet is only minimally thickened. Current molecular insights suggest that this pattern is more complex than simply a "wear and tear" process. The calcification and remodeling of the valve matrix is an active cellular process with interactions of multiple cell signaling pathways (232).

POSTINFLAMMATORY/POSTRHEUMATIC AORTIC STENOSIS. Postrheumatic aortic stenosis is now uncommon in developed countries, but it remains a significant clinical problem worldwide. It is often associated with concurrent mitral valve disease. The characteristic findings are fusion of the commissures and postinflammatory fibrous thickening of the free edge of the leaflets (Fig. 29.47). This progresses to thickened, inflexible leaflets that form a triangular orifice. Calcification is generally less severe than in either BAV or calcific tricuspid disease. Infectious endocarditis is an important complication.

Aortic Insufficiency

Primary valvular abnormalities causing regurgitant valve function are less common today than aortic root dilatation. In the series by Dare et al. (229), 50% of their cases were caused by

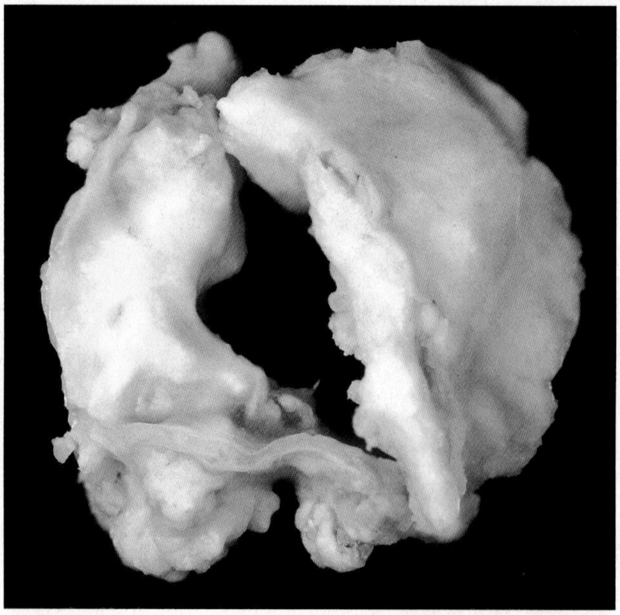

Figure 29.45. Bicuspid aortic valve. Both leaflets are distorted by thick nodular aggregates of fibrocalcific deposits. The leaflet on the left shows a dimpled raphe.

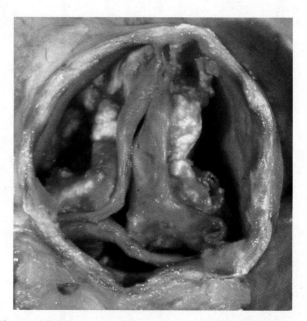

Figure 29.46. Senile calcific tricuspid aortic stenosis (AS). The three leaflets display normal commissures and slight thickening along the valve edge. Large collections of calcific deposits protrude into the sinuses of all three leaflets.

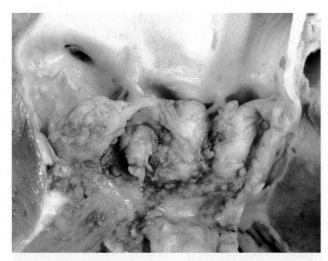

Figure 29.47. Postrheumatic aortic stenosis. The commissures are fused, and the leaflets are thickened and distorted. Acute bacterial endocarditis is also present.

aortic root dilatation either associated with age-related aortic degeneration or coexisting disorders of the aorta in Marfan syndrome or BAV (229). Postrheumatic and prior valvular intervention or septal myomectomy were less frequent causes. Recently, the anorectic drug, fenfluramine-phentermine (fenphen) was reported to cause insufficiency in left- and right-sided valves (233).

The pathologic findings in excised regurgitant valves depend on the underlying etiology (234). In age-related aortic root dilatation, the leaflets show minimal or no degenerative features under the microscope. In root dilatation associated with Marfan syndrome, the leaflets display a range of myxomatous expansion of the spongiosa layer that is highlighted by stains for glycosaminoglycans such as colloidal iron. Aortic insufficiency caused by postrheumatic lesions contains limited amounts of calcific deposits and fibrosis. In other inflammatory causes such as ankylosing spondylitis, both aortic and valvular changes may be seen (220).

The valvular lesion associated with fen-phen shows both macroscopic and microscopic changes (235,236). The cusps are thickened but retain a glistening smooth surface. Nodular thickening in the central portion of the valve can be seen (Fig. 29.48). The microscopic features are plaques composed of myofibroblastic cells embedded in a myxoid stroma that are "plastered" onto the aortic side of the cusps. Inflammation and calcifications are absent or sparse.

Combined Aortic Stenosis and Insufficiency

In the series from the Mayo Clinic of mixed patterns, degenerative/senile calcific changes in a trileaflet valve were the most common cause. Other causes included postinflammatory, BAV, and posttherapeutic (229). This reflects the change in the frequency of postinflammatory causes from earlier studies (237).

MITRAL VALVULAR DISEASE

Disease of the mitral valve can be divided into stenotic and regurgitant lesions. An understanding of the normal anatomy,

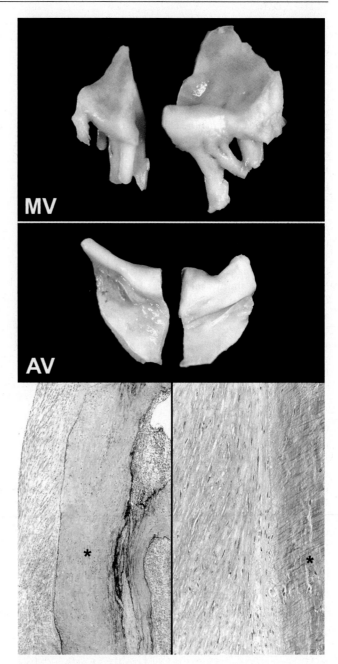

Figure 29.48. Valvular changes associated with fenfluramine-phentermine. *Upper panel*: Mitral valve showing thickened rolled leaflet with shortened and thickened chordae tendineae. *Middle panel*: Aortic valve showing glistening translucent surface and central nodular thickening. *Lower panels*: Elastic van Gieson (EVG) stain showing chordae (*) surrounded by loose edematous myxoid lesion plastered to surface. The trichrome stain shows paucicellular myofibroblastic cells and matrix adherent to valve (*).

function, and histology of the valve and its chordal attachments is important in assessing pathologic states and for correlating with clinical, echocardiographic, and other functional tests (45,220).

Mitral Stenosis

The most common cause of mitral stenosis in both the developed and underdeveloped world remains postrheumatic or postinflammatory disease and accounts for 99% of cases (238–241). In one large series, the autopsy incidence of mitral stenosis remained constant over a 30-year period of observation (238). Rare causes include congenital valvular or supravalvular stenosis, SLE, Whipple endocarditis, and extensive calcification of the mitral annulus (226). Surgical intervention in acute rheumatic valvulitis is not commonly performed, but acute fulminant pancarditis may cause death. The mitral valve leaflets are swollen, and tiny flat vegetations can be seen along the lines of closure (242,243). Microscopically, edema, chronic inflammation, and platelet-fibrin thrombi are present; Aschoff bodies are present in a minority of cases (Fig. 29.49). Progression from the acute stage to the fibrosing phase results in fusion of the commissures and fibrous thickening, retraction, and calcification of the leaflets. The chordae are fused and shortened, and the orifice is reduced to an oval, narrow "fish mouth" opening (Fig. 29.50). Superimposed sterile or infected vegetations, papillary fibroelastomas, and other secondary changes can occur. Microscopically, the typical findings include fibrosis, calcification with or without ossification, neovascularization, and a variable chronic inflammatory cell infiltrate containing lymphocytes, monocytes, and mast cells. At this stage, Aschoff bodies are not found, but 20% of left atrial appendages and 1% to 2% of LV papillary muscles may demonstrate residual Aschoff bodies (244).

Mitral Regurgitation

Currently, the most common cause of pure mitral insufficiency requiring surgical intervention is mitral valve prolapse (MVP). A frequent clinical cause of "functional" mitral insufficiency occurring in the setting of structurally normal valves is annular dilatation caused by papillary muscle dysfunction and marked ventricular dilatation in DCM or ischemic heart disease. Currently, surgical repair, rather than replacement, is initially attempted for cases of MVP, and the surgical pathologist is likely to receive only a small part of the valve and chordae. Careful review of the clinical history and findings in the valve and chordal attachments is necessary in these cases. Uncommon causes of pure insufficiency include postinflammatory disease, infec-

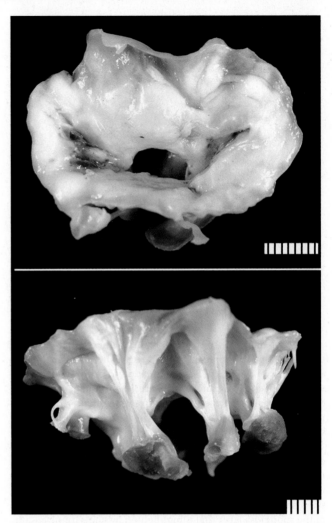

Figure 29.50. Chronic rheumatic mitral valve. *Upper panel*: The fused commissures and thickened, retracted leaflets produce the oval "fish mouth" deformity. *Lower panel*: The chordae are shortened, rigid, and fused.

tive endocarditis, ruptured chordae tendineae, drug induced, and annular calcification (206,245). Drug-induced mitral valve disease is caused by the anorectic drug fen-phen and antimigraine drugs (e.g., ergotamine and methysergide) (233,236, 243). The changes caused by fen-phen include thickening and retraction of the leaflets without fusion of commissures and chordae (Fig. 29.48). Encasement of the chordae and deposition of the myofibroblast-glycosaminoglycan–rich plaques containing collagen and elastin fibers onto the ventricular side of the leaflet are reported and are histologically identical to those described earlier in aortic regurgitant valves (236).

Myxomatous Degeneration of Mitral Valve

Myxomatous valvulopathy or MVP or Barlow disease may be either isolated or a component of Marfan or Ehlers-Danlos syndrome, HCM, ischemic heart disease, or Turner syndrome. Patients with MVP have a range of clinical findings from asymptomatic to congestive heart failure and sudden death. The terms used by Barlow and Popock (246) to describe the intraoperative valvular findings were "billowing, floppy, prolapsed and

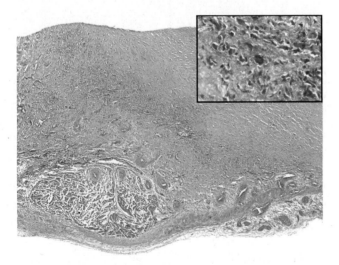

Figure 29.49. Acute rheumatic valvulitis. The mitral valve leaflet shows central necrosis and a mixed inflammatory cell infiltrate containing Aschoff cells (*inset*).

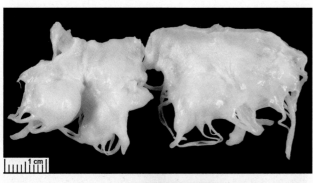

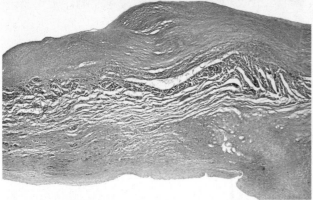

Figure 29.51. Mitral valve prolapse. *Upper panel*: A 7-cm segment of redundant billowing posterior leaflet was removed during mitral valve repair. *Lower panel*: Colloidal iron stain highlights the abundant mucopolysaccharide deposition that expands the spongiosa and fibrosa layers of the valve.

flailed." These descriptively reflect the macroscopic findings that include enlarged, thickened, voluminous, nonfibrotic, redundant portions of the posterior leaflet, particularly the middle scallop (Fig. 29.51). Rupture of the chordae results in flail valves. Microscopically, the spongiosa layer is expanded by acid mucopolysaccharides and focal disruption of the fibrosa layer (247,248).

TRICUSPID AND PULMONIC VALVULAR DISEASE

Stenotic and regurgitant alterations of the tricuspid valve are less common than alterations of the mitral valve. Postinflammatory valvulopathy occurs in association with left-sided lesions. Isolated causes of stenosis include infective endocarditis, congenital tricuspid stenosis, and metabolic abnormalities like Fabry disease and "giant blood cysts" (249). Surgical indications for tricuspid replacement for tricuspid insufficiency include Epstein anomaly, carcinoid heart disease, flail leaflets from chordal disruption after EMB, and occasionally anorectic drug–induced valvulopathy (250–252). In carcinoid heart disease, the right-sided valves are affected if metastatic lesions are present in the heart. On occasion, left-sided valvular lesions develop on account of intracardiac shunts or pulmonary metastasis. The leaflets are thickened, firm, and retracted, and the tips of the papillary muscle insertions appear "pearly white" (Fig. 29.52). The chordae are thickened and fused and can be confused with rheumatic valvulopathy. Microscopically, deposits are found on both surfaces of the leaflets and the chordae

and are composed of the same constituents as fen-phen valvulopathy. Neovascularization, chronic inflammation, and mast cells are also common (251). The pathogenesis involves serotonin receptors, valve interstitial cells, and transforming growth factor-beta activity (253).

Stenotic pulmonic valvular abnormalities are mostly congenital in origin (e.g., tetralogy of Fallot). Annular dilatation associated with pulmonary arterial hypertension is the most common cause of regurgitation. Other causes are infectious endocarditis and carcinoid heart disease (254).

INFECTIVE ENDOCARDITIS

The clinical and morphologic diagnosis of infective endocarditis (IE) is often challenging. IE is defined as a disease caused by microbial infection of the endothelial lining of intracardiac structures, such as valves and chordal attachments, and mural endocardium (255). If unrecognized and untreated, it is a potentially lethal disease. In the case of valvular endocarditis, the majority of patients have an underlying congenital or acquired alteration. Left-sided valves are more commonly affected than right-sided valves (aortic > mitral > tricuspid > pulmonic). In the second half of the twentieth century, the demographics of IE changed as antibiotic therapy became routine and degenerative/senile aortic valve disease increased. Valves with regurgitant alterations are particularly at risk, as are patients with prosthetic valves and pacemaker/intracardiac cardioverter-defibrillator wires, immunosuppressed patients, and intravenous drug abusers.

A variety of Gram-positive and Gram-negative bacterial, fungal, mycobacterial, rickettsial, and chlamydial organisms are responsible for IE. The gross and microscopic changes are a result of, in large part, the virulence of the organisms. The liberal use of Gram stains, fungal stains, and stains for acid-fast organisms is essential, although many patients will have received antibiotic therapy prior to surgical excision of the native or prosthetic valve. Microbiologic culture of excised tissue should be routinely performed. Currently, molecular techniques are being evaluated and will aide in the small percentage of cases where both tissue and microbiologic analysis are unsuccessful (256). Grossly, the lesions can vary in size and shape, and particularly virulent organisms can cause perforations of the leaflets or rupture of the chordae (Fig. 29.53). Extension from the site of initiation at the cusp apposition line (atrial surface of AV valves and ventricular surface of semilunar valves) can proceed to the leaflets, chordae, and annular regions to form abscesses (257). In the untreated, early phase of organization, acute fibrinous exudates with neutrophils and necrotic changes and tissue destruction in the valve are observed (Fig. 29.54). In the healing phases or in the setting of an insidious low-grade infection, neovascularization, chronic inflammation, fibrosis, and calcification replace the damaged tissue.

NONINFECTIVE ENDOCARDITIS

Two patterns of noninfective endocarditis are recognized but rarely require surgical excision. Nonbacterial thrombotic or marantic endocarditis is usually seen at autopsy and is defined as platelet-fibrin vegetations that are devoid of inflammatory cells or bacteria (258). The vegetations are arranged as continuous, linear aggregates along the lines of closure of the left-sided valves (Fig. 29.55). By definition, no inflammatory cell infiltrates or tissue destruction of the underlying valve tissue is present.

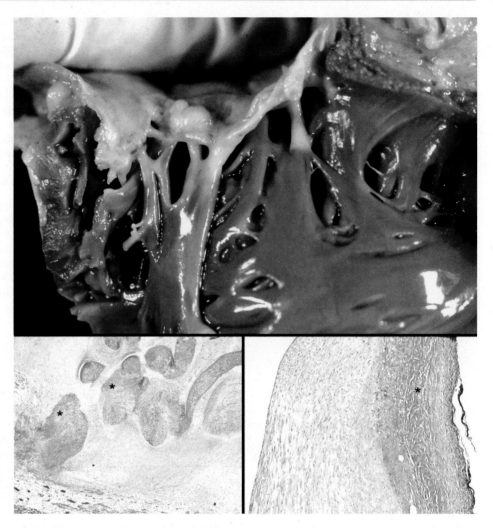

Figure 29.52. Carcinoid valve disease. *Upper panel*: The tricuspid valve shows thickened, retracted leaflets and shortened fused chordae. *Lower panels*: The trichrome stain showing chordae (*) enmeshed by the same myofibroblastic-myxoid material as in fenfluramine-phentermine drug effect. The Elastic van Gieson (EVG) stain on the right shows the leaflet (*) with the same lesion.

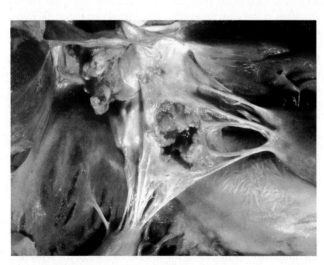

Figure 29.53. Infective endocarditis. Perforation of the mitral leaflet caused by *Streptococcus viridans* infection.

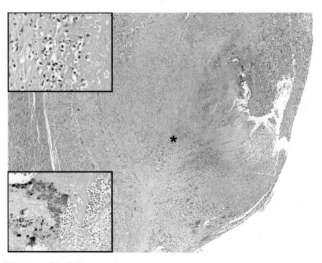

Figure 29.54. Microscopic section of the base of the aortic valve leaflet from Figure 29.47. *Upper inset*: Dense acute inflammatory exudates are present. *Lower inset*: The Gram stain demonstrates numerous colonies of Gram-positive organisms.

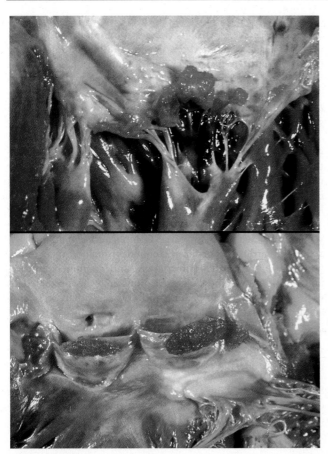

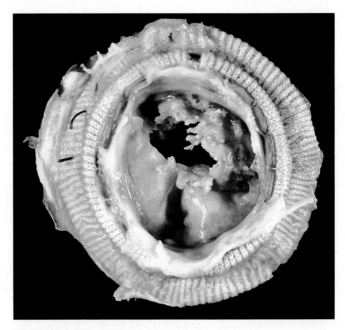

Figure 29.56. Bioprosthetic tissue valve with marked fibrocalcific degeneration and tearing of the leaflets.

Figure 29.55. Marantic endocarditis. *Upper panel*: Linear red fibrinous exudates on the atrial surface along the lines of closure. *Lower panel*: Aortic valve showing fibrinous aggregates on the central nodules. The underlying valves are normal.

thetic valves is also a known complication, and any vegetation should be carefully examined for the presence of infectious organisms. As in the case of IE of native valves, a host of different microbial organisms has been reported.

PERICARDIUM

ACUTE PERICARDITIS

There are many and varied causes of acute inflammation of the pericardium (Table 29.12). The relative proportions of these

In SLE and antiphospholipid syndrome, flat vegetations can develop on the atrial aspect of the posterior mitral valve leaflet and the ventricular aspect of the aortic valve. These may expand to cover both aspects of the valve or extend along the atrial or ventricular endocardium. These Libman-Sacks lesions can mimic IE on account of the presence of fibrin, cores of fibrinous necrosis of the valve, inflammatory cell infiltrates, and hematoxylin bodies.

PROSTHETIC VALVES

Currently, two main types of prosthetic valves are used in clinical medicine: tissue valves and mechanical valves. Tissue-engineered valve replacement is the subject of research and development for future application (221). Tissue valves are composed of either porcine aortic valve or bovine pericardium that has been treated in a dilute aldehyde solution and sewn onto a metallic frame. More than half fail within 10 years because of calcification and/or tissue degeneration leading to tears, perforations, and leakages (Fig. 29.56). Mechanical valves are classified as ball and cage valves, caged disk valves, and tilting disk valves. Fractures of strut components, annular ring abscess formation, and dehiscence and thrombus formation are recognized complications (Fig. 29.57). A specimen photograph is helpful, and in some cases, the specimen should be retained for manufacturer evaluation or medical-legal issues. IE of pros-

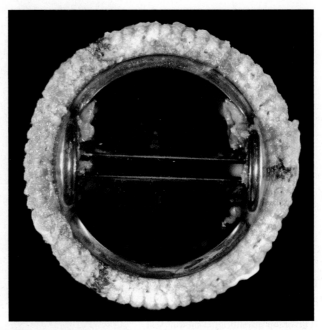

Figure 29.57. Mechanical valve with thrombi on the metal leaflets and at the opening.

TABLE 29.12

Causes of Acute and Chronic Pericarditis

ACUTE PERICARDITIS
Infectious
Bacterial (Gram-positive, Gram-negative bacteria, mycobacteria, spi-
   rochetes)
Fungal
Viral
Parasitic
Idiopathic
Post–myocardial infarction
Iatrogenic (postsurgical, radiation therapy, drug reaction)
Metastatic neoplasm
Systemic disease (autoimmune, renal failure, endocrine)
Traumatic
CHRONIC/CONSTRICTIVE PERICARDITIS
Idiopathic
Following episode of acute pericarditis
Infectious (mycobacteria, fungal)
Postsurgical (including transplantation)
Systemic disease (autoimmune, renal failure)
Radiation therapy
Neoplasms (usually metastatic tumors)

different etiologies will change with the site of practice (259). In general, acute pericarditis is more common in men than in women. Tissue injury and the resultant inflammation may be the result of direct damage by microorganisms or the result of inflammatory mediators released by inflammatory cells. Hypersensitivity and autoimmune mechanisms are most likely causative after MI, surgery, or drug reactions and in association with systemic autoimmune disease (107,260–263).

The pathology of acute pericarditis includes vascular dilation and prominence, exudates of fibrin, and exudates of inflammatory cells (Fig. 29.58). Organisms may be present, and there may be special features reflecting pathogenesis (granulomatous inflammation, vascular endothelial changes after radiation, lupus erythematosus [LE] cells in association with SLE, etc.).

Acute pericarditis after viral infection, MI, or cardiac surgery is generally a self-limited process. Complications of all forms of acute pericarditis (in order of frequency) include recurrence, tamponade, pericardial constriction, and combined effusion and constriction. These complications may be predicted as more likely to occur in patients with fever less than 38°C, subacute course, large effusion or tamponade, or failure to respond to aspirin or nonsteroidal anti-inflammatory therapy (264).

CONSTRICTIVE PERICARDITIS

Some versions of acute pericarditis will organize and heal with dense fibrosis and calcifications resulting in a thickened pericardium that encases the heart and interferes with diastolic filling.

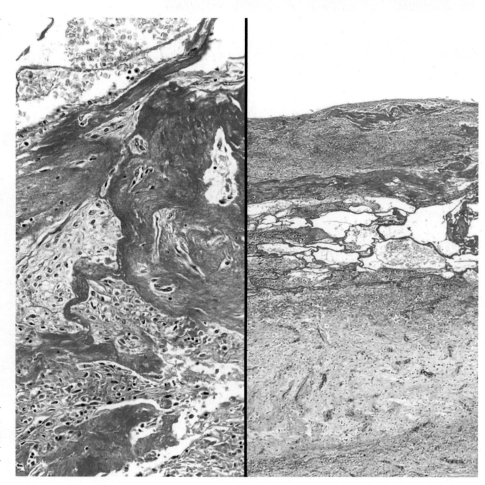

Figure 29.58. Fibrinous pericarditis. *Right panel*: Blood and layered fibrin on the visceral pericardium. *Left panel*: High-power magnification showing scattered inflammatory cells, blood, and fibrin.

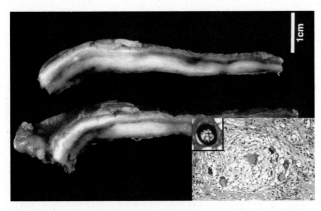

Figure 29.59. Fungal constrictive pericarditis. Pericardiectomy specimen showing a thickening parietal pericardium measuring up to 1 cm in thickness. Inset: Granulomatous pericarditis with *Coccidioides immitis.*

The clinical distinction of constrictive pericarditis from restrictive myocardial disease caused by amyloid or hemochromatosis may be challenging; EMB is often used to exclude infiltrative myocardial disease. In the past, tuberculosis was the most often recognized cause of constrictive pericarditis. Currently, the cause is usually unknown, but multiple sections should be reviewed to exclude tuberculosis and fungal and other known etiologies for pericarditis (Fig. 29.59). Management includes medical therapy to limit volume expansion and anti-inflammatory drugs. For patients who fail conservative therapy, surgical pericardiectomy is usually indicated (265). An uncommon form of constrictive pericarditis is idiopathic cholesterol pericarditis (Fig. 29.60). Originally described in 1919, it can be associated with recurrent pericardial effusions that yield a "scintillating gold paint appearance" on account of the cholesterol crystals in the fluid (266). Other known associations include hypothyroidism, rheumatoid arthritis, and tuberculosis.

PRIMARY PERICARDIAL MASSES

Primary pericardial tumors are much less common than metastatic malignancies. Benign masses include pericardial or meso-

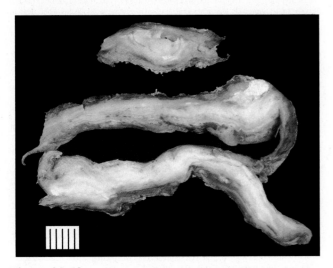

Figure 29.60. Cholesterol pericarditis. Golden yellow collections of cholesterol-rich deposits were found in this pericardial stripping specimen.

thelial cysts. These may be congenital or form after surgical procedures or infarct as the result of trapping of small inclusions of benign mesothelium that continues to function. Pericardial pseudocysts, lacking a mesothelial lining, have walls of collagen and granulation tissue and are the result of trauma or prior pericarditis. Mesothelial papillomas are composed of epithelioid mesothelial cells on papillary connective tissue cores. Like mesothelial/macrophage incidental cardiac excrescence, these rare lesions are likely reactive proliferations (267). Other benign lesions include teratomas in infants, bronchogenic cysts, benign fibrous tumors, lipomas, lymphangiomas, and giant lymph node hyperplasia. Foci of ectopic thyroid or thymic tissue can also be found in the pericardium.

Primary malignant tumors of the pericardium are rare. Most are sarcomas; angiosarcoma is the most commonly seen, but other types including synovial sarcoma and malignant fibrous histiocytoma are reported. Malignant mesotheliomas of the pericardium occur in a similar frequency to sarcoma, although they comprise less than 1% of all malignant mesotheliomas (268). There is an association with asbestos exposure. The tumors may present with symptoms and signs of pericarditis or constriction. Tumor nodules may stud the pericardial surfaces, and at later stages, the pericardial cavity may be filled with tumor causing constriction. The pericardial fluid is usually sanguineous. The histology and diagnostic criteria for pericardial malignant tumors are the same as for the lesions when found in other sites.

FUTURE DIRECTIONS

The impact of new molecular technologies and genomic/proteomic findings in the wide spectrum of cardiac disorders has expanded the role of the diagnostic surgical pathologist. The importance of clinical-pathologic correlation in the evaluation of these insights and the application of new technologies are predicated on accurate and thorough macroscopic and microscopic examinations. Further, emerging infectious diseases and re-emergence of remote diseases require familiarity with uncommon lesions. The EMB remains the "gold" standard for the diagnosis, classification, and monitoring of acute rejection in heart transplantation recipients. It is also an essential diagnostic tool in the distinction of primary and secondary cardiomyopathies. The breadth of cardiovascular pathology continues to expand, and the role of the diagnostic surgical pathologist remains essential.

REFERENCES

1. Williams MA, Kaskell WL, Ades PA, et al. Resistance exercise in individuals with and without cardiovascular disease: 2007 update: a scientific statement from the American Heart Association Council on Clinical Cardiology and Council on Nutrition, Physical Activity and Metabolism. *Circulation* 2007;116:572–584.
2. Fonarow GC. A practical approach to reducing cardiovascular risk factors. *Rev Cardiovasc Med* 2007;8(Suppl 4):S25–S36.
3. Panzer C, Apovian CM. Aggressive diets and lipid responses. *Curr Cardiol Reports* 2004;6: 464–473.
4. Glassberg H, Rader DJ. Management of lipids in the prevention of cardiovascular events. *Ann Rev Med* 2008;59:475–490.
5. Douglas P, Chen J, Gillam L, et al. Achieving quality in cardiovascular imaging: proceedings from the American College of Cardiology-Duke University medical center think tank on quality in cardiovascular imaging. *J Am Coll Cardiol* 2006;48:2141–2151.
6. Berman DS, Hachamovitch R, Shaw LJ, et al. Roles of nuclear cardiology, cardiac computed tomography, and cardiac magnetic resonance: noninvasive risk stratification and a

conceptual framework for the selection of noninvasive imaging tests in patients with known or suspected coronary artery disease. *J Nucl Med* 2006;47:1107–1118.

7. Krishnamoorthy VK, Sengupta PP, Gentile F, et al. History of echocardiography and its future applications in medicine. *Crit Care Med* 2007;35(Suppl):S309–S313.

8. Marx GR, Su X. Three-dimensional echocardiography in congenital heart disease. *Cardiol Clin* 2007;25:357–365.

9. Teske AJ, DeBoeck BW, Melman PR, et al. Echocardiographic quantification of myocardial function using tissue deformation imaging: a guide to image acquisition and analysis using tissue Doppler and speckle tracking. *Cardiovasc Ultrasound* 2007;5:27–45.

10. McKay CR, Shavelle DM. Intravascular ultrasound in the coronary arteries. *Semin Vasc Surg* 2006;19:132–138.

11. Nicholls SJ, Tuzcu EM, Sipahi I, et al. Intravascular ultrasound in cardiovascular medicine. *Circulation* 2006;114:e55–e59.

12. Hamdan A, Assali A, Fuchs S, et al. Imaging of vulnerable coronary artery plaques. *Catheter Cardiovasc Interv* 2007;70:65–74.

13. Mintz GS, Nissen SE, Anderson WD, et al. American College of Cardiology clinical expert consensus document on standards for acquisition, measurement and reporting of intravascular ultrasound studies (IVUS). A report of the American College of Cardiology Task Force on Clinical Expert Consensus Documents. *J Am Coll Cardiol* 2001;37:1478–1492.

14. Yamada R, Okura H, Kume T, et al. Histological characteristics of plaque with ultrasound attenuation: a comparison between intravascular ultrasound and histology. *J Cardiol* 2007; 50:223–228.

15. Beach S, Syed MA. Current and upcoming roles of CT and MRI in clinical cardiac imagery. *Curr Cardiol Rep* 2007;9:420–427.

16. Bogot NR, Durst R, Shaham D, et al. Cardiac CT of the transplanted heart: indications, technique, appearance and complications. *Radiographics* 2007;27:1297–1309.

17. DiCardli MF, Dorbala S. Cardiac PET-CT. *J Thorac Imaging* 2007;22:101–106.

18. Savino G, Zwerner P, Herzog C, et al. CT of cardiac function. *J Thorac Imaging* 2007;22: 86–100.

19. Raman VK, Lederman RJ. Advances in interventional cardiovascular MRI. *Curr Cardiol Rep* 2006;8:70–75.

20. Russell RR, Zaret BL. Nuclear cardiology: present and future. *Curr Probl Cardiol* 2006;31: 557–629.

21. Mack MJ. Beating heart surgery: does it make a difference? *Am Heart Hosp J* 2003;1: 149–157.

22. Soltesz EG, Cohn LH. Minimally invasive valve surgery. *Cardiol Rev* 2007;15:109–115.

23. Kaul S, Shah PK, Diamond GA. As time goes by: current status and future directions in the controversy over stenting. *J Am Coll Cardiol* 2007;50:128–137.

24. Kipshidze NN, Tsapenko MV, Leon MB, et al. Update on drug-eluding coronary stents. *Expert Rev Cardiovasc Ther* 2005;3:953–968.

25. Walsh KP. Interventional paediatric cardiology. *BMJ* 2003;327:385–388.

26. Roberts R, Gollob M. Molecular cardiology and genetics in the 21s century: a primer. *Curr Probl Cardiol* 2006;31:637–701.

27. Scobioala S, Klocke R, Michel G, et al. Proteomics: state of the art and its application in cardiovascular research. *Curr Med Chem* 2004;11:3203–3218.

28. White MY, Van Eyk JE. Cardiovascular proteomics: past, present, and future. *Mol Diag Ther* 2007;11:83–95.

29. Miller DT, Ridker PM, Libby P, et al. Atherosclerosis: the path from genomics to therapeutics. *J Am Coll Cardiol* 2007;49:1589–1599.

30. Thiene G. Evolving role of cardiovascular pathology in clinical and surgical decision making. *J Thorac Cardiovasc Surg* 2005;129:966–969.

31. Thiene G, Basso C, Calbrese F, et al. Twenty years of progress and beckoning frontiers in cardiovascular pathology: cardiomyopathies. *Cardiovasc Pathol* 2005;14:165–169.

32. Davies MJ. *Atlas of Coronary Artery Disease.* Philadelphia, PA: Lippincott-Raven, 1998.

33. Sheppard M, Davies MJ. *Practical Cardiovascular Pathology.* London, United Kingdom: Arnold, 1998.

34. Anderson RH, Becker AE, Robertson WB. *The Cardiovascular System. Part A: General Considerations and Congenital Malformations.* Edinburgh, United Kingdom: Churchill Livingstone, 1993.

35. Yen Ho S, Baker EJ, Rigby ML, et al. *Color Atlas of Congenital Heart Disease: Morphologic and Clinical Correlations.* London, United Kingdom: Mosby-Wolfe, 1995.

36. Gatzoulis MA, Webb GA, Daubeney PEF. *Diagnosis and Management of Adult Congenital Heart Disease.* Edinburgh, United Kingdom: Churchill-Livingstone, 2003.

37. Chang AC, Towbin JA. *Heart Failure in Children and Young Adults: From Molecular Mechanisms to Medical and Surgical Strategies.* Philadelphia, PA: Saunders Elsevier, 2006.

38. Camm AJ, Luscher TF, Serruys PW. *The ESC Textbook of Cardiovascular Medicine.* Oxford, United Kingdom: Blackwell Publishing, 2006.

39. Topol EJ, Califf RM, Prystowsky EN, et al. *Textbook of Cardiovascular Medicine.* Philadelphia, PA: Lippincott Williams & Wilkins, 2007.

40. Fejfar Z. Idiopathic cardiomyopathy. *Bull Wld Hlth Org* 1968;38:979–992.

41. Report of the WHO/ISFC task force on the definition and classification of cardiomyopathies. *Br Heart J* 1980;44:672–673.

42. Richardson P, McKenna W, Bristow M, et al. Report of the 1995 World Health Organization/International Society and Federation of Cardiology Task Force on the definition and classification of cardiomyopathies. *Circulation* 1996;93:841–842.

43. Maron BJ, Towbin JA, Thiene G, et al. Contemporary definitions and classification of the cardiomyopathies: a American Heart Association scientific statement from the Council on Clinical Cardiology, Heart Failure and Transplantation Committee; Quality of Care and Outcomes Research and Functional Genomics and Translational Biology Interdisciplinary Working Groups; and Council on Epidemiology and Prevention. *Circulation* 2006; 113;1807–1816.

44. Elliot P, Andersson B, Arbustini E, et al. Classification of the cardiomyopathies: a position statement from the European Society of Cardiology Working Group on Myocardial and Pericardial Diseases. *Eur Heart J* 2008;29:270–276.

45. Berry GJ, Billingham ME. The normal heart. In Mills SE, ed. *Histology for Pathologists.* 3rd edition. Philadelphia, PA: Lippincott Williams & Wilkins, 2007:527–545.

46. Veinot JP, Ghadially FN, Walley VM. Light microscopy and ultrastructure of the blood vessels and hart. In Silver MD, ed. *Cardiovascular Pathology.* 3rd edition. New York, NY: Churchill Livingstone, 2001:30–53.

47. Spinale FG. Myocardial matrix remodeling and the matrix metalloproteinases: influence on cardiac form and function. *Physiol Rev* 2007;87:1285–1342.

48. Cooper LT, Baughman KL, Feldman AM, et al. The role of endomyocardial biopsy in the management of cardiovascular disease: a scientific statement from the American Heart Association, the American College of Cardiology, and the European Society of Cardiology. *J Am Coll Cardiol* 2007;50:1914–1931.

49. Berry GJ, Billingham ME. The pathology of human cardiac transplantation. In Baumgartner WA, Reitz BA, Kasper E, et al., eds. *Heart and Lung Transplantation.* Philadelphia, PA: WB Saunders Co., 2002:309–330.

50. Hauck AJ, Edwards WD. Histopathologic examination of tissues obtained by endomyocardial biopsy. In Fowles RE, ed. *Cardiac Biopsy.* Mount Kisco, NY: Futura Publishing Inc, 1992:95–153.

51. Kaspar E, Agema W, Hutchins G. The causes of dilated cardiomyopathy: a clinicopathologic review of 673 consecutive patients. *J Am Coll Cardiol* 1994;23:589–590.

52. Karkkainen S, Peuhkurinen K. Genetics of dilated cardiomyopathy. *Ann Med* 2007;39: 91–107.

53. Tazelaar HD, Billingham ME. Leukocytic infiltrates in idiopathic dilated cardiomyopathy: a source of confusion with active myocarditis. *Am J Surg Pathol* 1986;10:405–412.

54. Edwards WD. Cardiomyopathies. In Virmani R, Atkinson JB, Fenoglio J, eds. *Cardiovascular Pathology.* Philadelphia, PA: WB Saunders, 1991:257–309.

55. Elliott P. Investigation and treatment of hypertrophic cardiomyopathy. *Clin Med* 2007;7: 383–387.

56. Charron P, Caier L, Dubourg O, et al. Penetrance of familial hypertrophic cardiomyopathy. *Genet Couns* 1997;8:107–114.

57. Geisterfer-Lowrance AA, Kass S, Tanigawa G, et al. A molecular basis for familial hypertrophic cardiomyopathy: a beta cardiac myosin heavy chain gene missense mutation. *Cell* 1990;62:999–1006.

58. Robbins RC, Bernstein D, Berry GJ, et al. Cardiac transplantation for hypertrophic cardiomyopathy associated with Sengers syndrome. *Ann Thorac Surg* 1995;60:1525–1527.

59. Teare D. Asymmetrical hypertrophy of the heart in young adults. *Br Heart J* 1958;20:1–8.

60. Davies MJ, Mann JM. *The Cardiovascular System. Part B: Acquired Disease of the Heart.* New York, NY: Churchill Livingstone, 1995:119.

61. Rose AG. Evaluation of pathological criteria for diagnosis of hypertrophic cardiomyopathy. *Histopathology* 1984;8:395–406.

62. Maron BJ, Wolfson JK, Epstein SE, et al. Intramural ("small vessel") coronary artery disease in hypertrophic cardiomyopathy. *J Am Col Cardiol* 1986;8:545–557.

63. Hughes SE. The pathology of hypertrophic cardiomyopathy. *Histopathology* 2004;44: 412–427.

64. Allen RD, Edwards WD, Tazelaar HD, et al. Surgical pathology of subaortic septal myomectomy not associated with hypertrophic cardiomyopathy: a study of 98 cases (1996–2000). *Cardiovasc Pathol* 2003;12:207–215.

65. Maron BJ, Pelliccia A. The heart of trained athletes: cardiac remodeling and the risks of sports, including sudden death. *Circulation* 2006;114:1633–1644.

66. Robbins RC, Stinson EB. Long-term results of left ventricular myotomy and myomectomy for obstructive hypertrophic cardiomyopathy. *J Thorac Cardiovasc Surg* 1996;111:586–594.

67. Tazelaar HD, Billingham ME. The surgical pathology of hypertrophic cardiomyopathy. *Arch Pathol Lab Med* 1987;111:257–260.

68. Lamke GT, Allen RD, Edwards WD, et al. Surgical pathology of subaortic septal myectomy associated with hypertrophic cardiomyopathy: a study of 204 cases (1996–2000). *Cardiovasc Pathol* 2003:12:149–158.

69. Alam M, Dokainish H, Lakkis N. Alcohol septal ablation for hypertrophic obstructive cardiomyopathy: a systematic review of published studies. *J Interv Cardiol* 2006;19:319–327.

70. Olivotto I, Ommen SR, Maron MS, et al. Surgical myectomy versus alcohol septal ablation for obstructive hypertrophic cardiomyopathy. *J Am Coll Cardiol* 2007;50:831–834.

71. Heldman AW, Wu KC, Theodore P, et al. Myectomy or alcohol septal ablation: surgery and percutaneous intervention go another round. *J Am Coll Cardiol* 2007;49:358–360.

72. Kushwaha SS, Fallon JT, Fuster V. Restrictive cardiomyopathy. *N Eng J Med* 1997;336: 267–276.

73. Benotti JR, Grossman W. Restrictive cardiomyopathy. *Annu Rev Med* 1984;35:113–125.

74. Katritsis D, Wilmshurst PT, Wendon JA, et al. Primary restrictive cardiomyopathy: clinical and pathologic characteristics. *J Am Coll Cardiol* 1991;18:1230–1235.

75. Angelini A, Calzolari V, Thiene G, et al. Morphologic spectrum of primary restrictive cardiomyopathy. *Am J Cardiol* 1997;80:1046–1050.

76. Vatta M, Marcus F, Towbin JA. Arrhythmogenic right ventricular cardiomyopathy: a 'final common pathway' that defines clinical phenotype. *Eur Heart J* 2007;28:529–530.

77. Thiene G, Corrado D, Basso C. Arrhythmogenic right ventricular cardiomyopathy/dysplasia. *Orphanet J Rare Dis* 2007;2:45–61.

78. Sen-Chowdhry S, Syrris P, Ward D, et al. Clinical and genetic characterization of families with arrhythmogenic right ventricular dysplasia/cardiomyopathy provides novel insights into patterns of disease expression. *Circulation* 2007;115:1710–1720.

79. Burke A, Arbustini E, Dal Bello B, et al. Fat infiltrates in endomyocardial biopsies lack specificity for the diagnosis of right ventricular dysplasia. *Circulation* 1998;31:S68.

80. Engberding R, Yelbuz TM, Breihardt G. Isolated noncompaction of the left ventricle: a review of the literature two decades after the initial case description. *Clin Res Cardiol* 2007; 96:481–488.

81. Burke A, Mont E, Kutys R, et al. Left ventricular noncompaction: a pathological study of 14 cases. *Hum Pathol* 2005;36:403–411.

82. Ichida F, Tsubata S, Bowles KR, et al. Novel gene mutations in patients with left ventricular noncompaction or Barth syndrome. *Circulation* 2003;103:1256–1263.

83. Lehnart SE, Ackerman MJ, Benson DW, et al. Inherited arrhythmias: a National Heart,

Lung and Blood Institute and Office of Rare Diseases workshop consensus report about the diagnosis, phenotyping, molecular mechanisms and therapeutic approaches for primary cardiomyopathies of gene mutations affecting ion channel function. *Circulation* 2007; 116:2325–2345.

84. Frustaci A, Priori SG, Pieroni M, et al. Cardiac histological substrate in patients with clinical phenotype of Brugada syndrome. *Circulation* 2005;112:3680–3687.

85. Tester DJ, Ackerman MJ. The role of molecular autopsy in unexpected sudden cardiac death. *Curr Opin Cardiol* 2006;21:116–172.

86. Steiner I, Hajkova P. Patterns of isolated atrial amyloid: a study of 100 hearts on autopsy. *Cardiovasc Pathol* 2006;15:287–290.

87. Kholova I, Niessen HWM. Amyloid in the cardiovascular system: a review. *J Clin Pathol* 2005;58:125–133.

88. Falk RH. Diagnosis and management of the cardiac amyloidoses. *Circulation* 2005;112: 2047–2060.

89. Shah KB, Inoue Y, Mehra MR. Amyloidosis and the heart: a comprehensive review. *Arch Intern Med* 2006;166:1805–1813.

90. Wittich CM, Neben-Wittich MA, Mueller PS, et al. Deposition of amyloid proteins in the epicardial coronary arteries of 58 patients with primary systemic amyloidosis. *Cardiovasc Pathol* 2007;16:75–78.

91. Pomerance A, Slavin G, McWatt J. Experience with the sodium sulfate-alcian blue stain for amyloid in cardiac pathology. *J Clin Pathol* 1976;29:22–28.

92. Gilbert-Barness E. Metabolic cardiomyopathy and conduction system defects in children. *Ann Clin Lab Sci* 2004;34:15–34.

93. Ozen H. Glycogen storage diseases: new perspectives. *World J Gastroenterol* 2007;13: 2541–2553.

94. Amalfitano A, Bengur AR, Morse RP, et al. Recombinant human acid alpha-glucosidase enzyme therapy for infantile glycogen storage disease type II: results of a phase I/II clinical trial. *Genet Med* 2001;3:132–138.

95. Desnick RJ, Blieden LC, Sharp HL, et al, Cardiac valvular anomalies in Fabry disease: clinical, morphologic and biochemical studies. *Circulation* 1976;54:818–824.

96. Fisher EA, Desnick RJ, Gordon RE, et al. Fabry disease: an unusual cause of severe coronary disease in a young man. *Ann Intern Med* 1992;117:221–223.

97. Desnick RJ, Brady R, Barranger J, et al. Fabry disease, an under-recognized multisystem disorder: expert recommendations for diagnosis, management, and enzyme replacement therapy. *Ann Intern Med* 2003;138:338–346.

98. Roos JM, Aubry MC, Edwards WD. Chloroquine cardiotoxicity: clinicopathologic features in three patients and comparison with three patients with Fabry disease. *Cardiovasc Pathol* 2002;11:277–283.

99. Pietrangelo A. Hereditary hemochromatosis. *Annu Rev Nutr* 2006;26:251–270

100. Bomford A. Genetics of haemochromatosis. *Lancet* 2002;360:1673–1681.

101. Kuppahally SS, Hunt S, Valantine HA, et al. Recurrence of iron deposition in the cardiac allograft in a patient with Non-HFE hemochromatosis. *J Heart Lung Transplant* 2006;25: 144–147.

102. Umpierrez G, Chaallapani S, Pattereson C. Congestive heart failure due to reversible cardiomyopathy in patients with hyperthyroidism. *Am J Med Sci* 1995;310:99–102.

103. Lie JT, Grossman SJ. Pathology of the heart in acromegaly: anatomic findings in 27 autopsied patients. *Am Heart J* 1980;100:41–52.

104. Lombardi G, Galdiero M, Auriemma RS, et al. Acromegaly and the cardiovascular system. *Neuroendocrinology* 2006;83:211–217.

105. Van Vliet PD, Burchell HB, Titus JL. Focal myocarditis associated with pheochromocytoma. *N Engl J Med* 1966;274:1102–1108.

106. Miles CD, Burke M, Radley-Smith R, et al. Pheochromocytoma presenting after cardiac transplantation for dilated cardiomyopathy. *J Heart Lung Transplant* 2001;20:773–775.

107. Berry GJ, Jordan M. Pathology of radiation and anthracycline cardiotoxicity. *Pediatr Blood Cancer* 2005;44:630–637.

108. Pai VB, Nahata MC. Cardiotoxicity of chemotherapeutic agents: incidence, treatment and prevention. *Drug Safety* 2000;22:263–302.

109. Billingham ME, Mason JW, Bristow MR, et al. Anthracycline cardiomyopathy monitored by morphologic changes. *Cancer Treat Rep* 1978;62:865–873.

110. Berry GJ, Billingham ME, Alderman E, et al. The use of cardiac biopsy to demonstrate reduced cardiotoxicity in AIDS Kaposi's sarcoma patients treated with pegylated liposomal doxorubicin. *Ann Oncol* 1998;9:711–716.

111. Lipshultz SE, Alvarez JA, Scully RE. Anthracycline associated cardiotoxicity in survivors of childhood cancer. *Heart* 2008;94:525–533.

112. Bristow MR, Thompson PD, Martin PR, et al. Early anthracycline cardiotoxicity. *Ann Int Med* 1978;65:823–828.

113. Yeh ETH, Tong AT, Lenihan DJ, et al. Cardiovascular complications of cancer therapy: diagnosis, pathogenesis, and management. *Circulation* 2004;109:3122–3131.

114. Floyd JD, Nguyen DT, Lobins RL, et al. Cardiotoxicity of cancer therapy. *J Clin Oncol* 2005; 30:7685–7696.

115. Coplan NS, Bruno MS. Acquired immunodeficiency syndrome and heart disease: the present and the future. *Am Heart J* 1989;117:1175–1180.

116. Magnani JW, Dec GW. Myocarditis: current trends in diagnosis and treatment. *Circulation* 2006;113:876–890.

117. Berry GJ, Atkins KA. Pathology of human myocarditis. In Cooper LT, ed. *Myocarditis: From Bench to Bedside*. Totowa, NJ: Humana Press, 2002:325–370.

118. Esfandiarei M, McManus BM. Molecular biology and pathogenesis of viral myocarditis. *Annu Rev Pathol Mech Dis* 2008;3:125–153.

119. Ellis CR, DiSalvo T. Myocarditis: basic and clinical aspects. *Cardiol Rev* 2007;15:170–177.

120. Aretz HT, Billingham ME, Edwards WD, et al. Myocarditis. A histopathologic definition and classification. *Am J Cardiovasc Pathol* 1986;1:3–14.

121. Spontnitz MD, Lesch M. Idiopathic dilated cardiomyopathy as a late complication of healed viral (Coxsackie B virus) myocarditis: historical analysis, review of the literature, and a postulated unifying hypothesis. *Prog Cardiovasc Dis* 2006;49:42–57.

122. Mason JW, O'Connell JB, Herskowitz A, et al. A clinical trial of immunosuppressive therapy for myocarditis. The Myocarditis Treatment Trial Investigators. *N Engl J Med* 1995;333: 269–275.

123. Billingham ME. Is acute cardiac rejection a model of myocarditis in humans? *Eur Heart J* 1987;8(Suppl J):19–23.

124. Edwards WD, Holmes DR, Jr., Reeder GS. Diagnosis of active lymphocytic myocarditis by endomyocardial biopsy: quantitative criteria for light microscopy. *Mayo Clin Proc* 1982;57: 419–425.

125. Tazelaar HD, Billingham ME. Myocardial lymphocytes. Fact, fancy or myocarditis? *Am J Cardiovasc Pathol* 1987;1:47–50.

126. Hill DA, Swanson PE. Myocardial extramedullary hematopoiesis: a clinicopathologic study. *Mod Pathol* 2000;13:779–787.

127. Tazelaar HD, Billingham ME. Leukocytic infiltrates in idiopathic dilated cardiomyopathy. A source of confusion with active myocarditis. *Am J Surg Pathol* 1986;10:405–412.

128. Billingham M. Pharmacotoxic myocardial disease: an endomyocardial study. In Sekiguchi M, Olsen EGJ, Goodwin JF, eds. *Myocarditis and Related Disorders: Proceedings of the International Symposium on Cardiomyopathy and Myocarditis*. Tokyo, Japan: Springer-Verlag, 1985: 278–282.

129. Gravanis MB, Hertzler GL, Franch RH, et al. Hypersensitivity myocarditis in heart transplant candidates. *J Heart Lung Transplant* 1991;10:688–697.

130. Spear GS. Eosinophilic explant carditis with eosinophils: hypersensitivity to dobutamine infusion. *J Heart Lung Transplant* 1995;14:755–760.

131. Hawkins ET, Levine TB, Goss SJ, et al. Hypersensitivity myocarditis in the explanted hearts of transplant recipients. Reappraisal of pathologic criteria and their clinical implications. *Pathol Annu* 1995;30:287–304.

132. Hawkins ET, Levine TB, Goss SJ, et al. Hypersensitivity myocarditis in the explanted hearts of transplant recipients. Reappraisal of pathologic criteria and their clinical implications. *Pathol Annu* 1995;30:287–304.

133. Takkenberg JJM, Czer LSC, Fishbein MC, et al. Eosinophilic myocarditis in patients awaiting heart transplantation. *Crit Care Med* 2004;32:714–721.

134. Burke AP, Saenger J, Mullick F, et al. Hypersensitivity myocarditis. *Arch Pathol Lab Med* 1991;115:764–769.

135. Daniels PR, Berry GJ, Tazelaar HD, et al. Giant cell myocarditis as a manifestation of drug hypersensitivity. *Cardiovasc Pathol* 2000;9:287–291.

136. Getz MA, Subramanian R, Logemann T, et al. Acute necrotizing eosinophilic myocarditis as a manifestation of severe hypersensitivity myocarditis. Antemortem diagnosis and successful treatments. *Ann Intern Med* 1991;115:201–202.

137. Sabatine MS, Poh KK, Mega JL, et al. Case 36-2007: a 31 year-old woman with rash, fever and hypotension. *N Engl J Med* 2007;357:2167–2178.

138. Ferrans VJ, Rodriguez ER. Cardiovascular lesions in collagen-vascular diseases. *Heart Vessels Suppl* 1985;1:256–261.

139. Clemson BS, Miller WR, Luck JC, et al. Acute myocarditis in fulminant systemic sclerosis. *Chest* 1992;101:872–874.

140. Hutchins SJ. Acute rheumatic fever. *J Infect* 1998;36:249–253.

141. Ursell PC, Albala A, Fenoglio JJ, Jr. Diagnosis of acute rheumatic carditis by endomyocardial biopsy. *Hum Pathol* 1982;13:677–679.

142. Silva LM, Mansur AJ, Bocchi EA et al. Unsuspected rheumatic fever carditis ending in heart transplantation. *Thorac Cardiovasc Surg* 1994;42:191–193.

143. Rizeq MN, Rickenbacher PR, Fowler MB, et al. Incidence of myocarditis in peripartum cardiomyopathy. *Am J Cardiol* 1994;74:474–477.

144. Okura Y, Dec GW, Hare JM et al. A clinical and histopathological comparison of cardiac sarcoidosis and idiopathic giant cell myocarditis. *J Am Coll Cardiol* 2003;41:322–329.

145. Valantine H, McKenna WJ, Nihoyannopoulos P, et al. Sarcoidosis: a pattern of clinical and morphological presentation. *Br Heart J* 1987;57:256–263.

146. Valantine HA, Tazelaar HD, Macoviak J, et al. Cardiac sarcoidosis: response to steroids and transplantation. *J Heart Transplant* 1987;6:244–250.

147. Oni AA, Hershberger RE, Norman DJ, et al. Recurrence of sarcoidosis in a cardiac allograft: control with augmented corticosteroids. *J Heart Lung Transplant* 1992;11:367–369.

148. Litovsky SH, Burke AP, Virmani R. Giant cell myocarditis: an entity distinct from sarcoidosis characterized by multiphasic myocyte destruction by cytotoxic T cells and histiocytic giant cells. *Mod Pathol* 1996;9:1126–1134.

149. Ferrans VJ, Rodriguez ER, McAllister HA, Jr. Granulomatous inflammation of the heart. *Heart Vessels Suppl* 1985;1:262–270.

150. Cooper LT Jr, Berry GJ, Shabetai R. Idiopathic giant-cell myocarditis: natural history and treatment. Multicenter Giant Cell Myocarditis Study Group Investigators. *N Engl J Med* 1997;336:1860–1866.

151. Ariza A, Lopez MD, Mate JL, et al. Giant cell myocarditis: monocytic immunophenotype of giant cells in a case associated with ulcerative colitis. *Hum Pathol* 1995;26:121–123.

152. Taylor DO, Edwards LB, Boucek M, et al. Registry of the International Society for Heart and Lung Transplantation: twenty-fourth official adult heart transplant report–2007. *J Heart Lung Transplant* 2007;26:769–781

153. Boucek MM, Aurora P, Edwards LB, et al. Registry of the International Society for Heart and Lung Transplantation: twenty-fourth official pediatric heart transplant report–2007. *J Heart Lung Transplant* 2007;26:796–807.

154. Billingham ME, Cary NRB, Hammond EH, et al. A working formulation for the standardization of nomenclature in the diagnosis of heart and lung rejection: Heart Rejection Study Group. *J Heart Transplant* 1990;9:587–593.

155. Stewart S, Winters GL, Fishbein MC, et al. Revision of the 1990 working formulation for the standardization of nomenclature in the diagnosis of heart rejection. *J Heart Lung Transplant* 2005;24:1710–1720.

156. Deng M, Eisen H, Mehra M, et al. Noninvasive discrimination of rejection in cardiac allograft recipients using gene expression profiling. *Am J Transplant* 2006;6:150–160.

157. Bernstein D, Williams GE, Eisen H, et al. Gene expression profiling distinguishes a molecular signature for grade 1B mild acute cellular rejection in cardiac allograft recipients. *J Heart Lung Transplant* 2007;26:1270–1280.

158. Joshi A, Masek MA, Brown BW, Jr., et al. Quilty revisited: 1 a 10-year perspective. *Hum Pathol* 1995;26:547–557.
159. Chu KE, Ho EK, de la Torre L, et al. The relationship of nodular endocardial infiltrates (Quilty lesions) to anti-HLA antibodies, coronary artery disease, and survival following heart transplantation. *Cardiovasc Pathol* 2005;14:219–224.
160. Yamani MH, Ratliff NB, Starling RC, et al. Quilty lesions are associated with increased expression of vitronectin receptor (alphavbeta3) and subsequent development of coronary vasculopathy. *J Heart Lung Transplant* 2003;22:687–690.
161. Fishbein MC, Bell G, Lones MA, et al. Grade 2 cellular heart rejection: does it exist? *J Heart Lung Transplant* 1994;13:1051–1057.
162. Winters GL, McManus BM, for the Rapamycin Cardiac Rejection Treatment Trial Pathologists: Consistencies and controversies in the application of the ISHLT working formulation for cardiac transplant biopsy specimens. *J Heart Transplant* 1996;15:728–735.
163. Marboe CC, Billingham ME, Eisen H, et al. Nodular endocardial infiltrates (Quilty lesions) cause significant variability in the diagnosis of ISHLT grades 2 and 3A rejection in cardiac allograft recipients. *J Heart Lung Transplant* 2005;24(7S):S219–S226.
164. Michaels PJ, Espejo ML, Kobashigawa J, et al. Humoral rejection in cardiac transplantation: risk factors, hemodynamic consequences and relationship to transplant coronary artery disease. *J Heart Lung Transplant* 2003;22:58–69.
165. Hammon EH, Yowell RL, Nunoda S, et al. Vascular (humoral) rejection in heart transplantation: pathologic observations and clinical implications. *J Heart Transplant* 1989;8: 430–443.
166. Lones MA, Lawrence SC, Alfredo T, et al. Clinical pathologic features of humoral rejection in cardiac allografts: a study of 81 consecutive patients. *J Heart Lung Transplant* 1995;14: 151–162.
167. Chantranuwat C, Qiao JH, Kobashigawa J, et al. Immunohistochemical staining for C4d on paraffin embedded tissue in cardiac allograft endomyocardial biopsies: comparison to frozen tissue immunofluorescence. *Appl Immunohistochem Mol Morphol* 2004;12:166–171.
168. Vasilescu ER, Ho E, de la Torre L, et al. Anti-HLA antibodies in heart transplantation. *Transplant Immunol* 2004;123:177–183.
169. Taylor DO, Yowell RL, Khoury AG, et al. Allograft coronary artery disease: clinical correlations with circulating anti-HLA antibodies and the immunohistopathologic pattern of vascular rejection. *J Heart Lung Transplant* 2000;19:518–521.
170. Takemoto S, Zeevi A, Fung S, et al. A national conference to assess antibody mediated rejection in solid organ transplantation. *Am J Transplant* 2004;4:1033–1041.
171. Rose AG, Cooper DKC, Human PA, et al. Histopathology of hyperacute rejection of the heart: experimental and clinical observations in allografts and xenografts. *J Heart Lung Transplant* 1991;10:223–232.
172. West L, Phil D, Pollock-Barziv SM, et al. ABO-incompatible heart transplantation in infants. *N Engl J Med* 2001;44:793–800.
173. Galili U, Shohet SB, Kobrin E, et al. Man, apes, and Old World monkeys differ from other mammals in the expression of alpha-galactosyl epitopes on nucleated cells. *J Biol Chem* 1988;263:17755–17759.
174. Cooper DKC, Good AH, Koren E, et al. Identification of alpha-galactosyl and other carbohydrate epitopes that are bound by human anti-pig antibodies: relevance to discordant xenografting in man. *Transplant Immunol* 1993;1:198–204.
175. Bach FH, Winkler H, Ferran C, et al. Delayed xenograft rejection. *Immunol Today* 1996; 17:379–384.
176. Ventura HO, Ramee SR, Jain A. Coronary artery imaging with intravascular ultrasound in patients following cardiac transplantation. *Transplantation* 1992;53:216–219.
177. Pethig K, Klauss V, Heublein B, et al. Progression of cardiac allograft vascular disease as assessed by serial intravascular ultrasound: correlation to immunological and non-immunological factors. *Heart* 2000;84:494–498.
178. Wong C, Ganz P, Miller L, et al. Role of vascular remodeling in the pathogenesis of early transplant coronary artery disease: a multicenter prospective intravascular ultrasound study. *J Heart Lung Transplant* 2001;20:385–392.
179. Mehra MR. Contemporary concepts in prevention and treatment of cardiac allograft vasculopathy. *Am J Transplant* 2006;6:1248–1256.
180. Rahmani M, Cruz RP, Granville DJ, et al. Allograft vasculopathy versus atherosclerosis. *Circ Res* 2006;99:801–815.
181. Hillebrands JL, Rauel HP, Klatter FA, et al. Intrathymic immune modulation prevents acute rejection but not the development of graft atherosclerosis (chronic rejection). *Transplantation* 2001;71:914–924.
182. Mitchell RN, Libby P. Vascular remodeling in transplant vasculopathy. *Circ Res* 2007;100: 967–978.
183. Sata M, Saiura A, Kuknisato A, et al. Hematopoietic stem cells differentiate into vascular cells that participate in the pathogenesis of atherosclerosis. *Nat Med* 2002;8:403–409.
184. Shimizu K, Mitchell RN. Stem cell origins of intimal cells in graft arterial disease. *Curr Atheroscler Rep* 2003;5:230–237.
185. Iwata H, Sata M. Potential contribution of bone marrow-derived precursors to vascular repair and lesion formation: lessons from animal model of vascular diseases. *Front Biosci* 2007;12:4157–4167.
186. Wilson RF, Christensen BV, Olivari MT, et al. Evidence for structural sympathetic reinnervation after orthotopic cardiac transplantation in humans. *Circulation* 1991;83:1210–1220.
187. Yager JE, Hernandez AF, Steenbergen C, et al. Recurrence of cardiac sarcoidosis in a heart transplant recipient. *J Heart Lung Transplant* 2005;24:1988–1990.
188. Lam KY, Dickens P, Chan AC. Tumors of the heart. A 20-year experience with a review of 12,485 consecutive autopsies. *Arch Pathol Lab Med* 1993;117:1027–1031.
189. Butany J, Leong SW, Carmichael K, et al. A 30-year analysis of cardiac neoplasms at autopsy. *Can J Cardiol* 2005;21:675–680.
190. Tazelaar HD, Locke TJ, McGregor CG. Pathology of surgically excised primary cardiac tumors. *Mayo Clin Proc* 1992;67:957–965.
191. Odim j, Reehal V, Laks H, et al. Surgical pathology of cardiac tumors. Two decades at an urban institution. *Cardiovasc Pathol* 2003;12:267–270.
192. Burke A, Virmani R. Pediatric heart tumors. *Cardiovasc Pathol* 2008;17:193–198.
193. Miller DV, Edwards WD. Cardiovascular tumor-like conditions. *Semin Diagn Pathol* 2008; 25:54–64.
194. Liang CD, Ko SH, Huang SC. Echocardiographic evaluation of cardiac rhabdomyoma in infants and children. *J Clin Ultrasound* 2000;28:381–386.
195. Fenoglio JJ, Jr., McAllister HA, Jr., Ferrans VJ. Cardiac rhabdomyoma: a clinicopathologic and electron microscopic study. *Am J Cardiol* 1976;38:241–251.
196. Bruni C, Prioleau PG, Ivey HH, et al. New fine structural features of cardiac rhabdomyoma: report of a case. *Cancer* 1980;46:2068–2073.
197. Cho JM, Danielson GK, Puga FJ, et al. Surgical results of ventricular cardiac fibromas: early and late results. *Ann Thorac Surg* 2003;76:1929–1934.
198. Gotlieb AI. Cardiac fibromas. *Semin Diagn Pathol* 2008;25:17–19.
199. Malhotra V, Ferrans VJ, Virmani R. Infantile histiocytoid cardiomyopathy: three cases and literature review. *Am Heart J* 1994;128:1009–1021.
200. Gelb AB, Van Meter SH, Billingham ME, et al. Infantile histiocytoid cardiomyopathy-myocardial or conduction system hamartoma: what is the cell type involved? *Hum Pathol* 1993;24:1226–1231.
201. Burke A, Li L, Kling E, et al. Cardiac inflammatory myofibroblastic tumor: a "benign" neoplasm that may result in syncope, myocardial infarction, and sudden death. *Am J Surg Pathol* 2007;31:1115–1122.
202. Gandy KL, Burtelow MA, Reddy VM, et al. Myofibroblastic tumor of the heart: a rare intracardiac tumor. *J Thorac Cardiovasc Surg* 2005;130:888–889.
203. Butany J, Dixit V, Leong SW, et al. Inflammatory myofibroblastic tumor with valvular involvement: a case report and review of the literature. *Cardiovasc Pathol* 2007;16:359–364.
204. Pearson PJ, Smithson WA, Driscoll DJ, et al. Inoperable plasma cell granuloma of the heart: spontaneous decrease in size during an 11-month period. *Mayo Clin Proc* 1988;63: 1022–1025.
205. Burke A, Virmani R: Cardiac Myxoma. In *Tumors of the Heart and Great Vessels.* 3rd edition. Bethesda, MD: Armed Forces Institute of Pathology, 1996:21–46.
206. Vaideeswar P, Butany JW. Benign cardiac tumors of the pluripotent mesenchyme. *Semin Diagn Pathol* 2008;25:20–28.
207. Terracciano LM, Mhawech P, Suess K, et al. Calretinin as a marker for cardiac myxomas: diagnostic and histogenetic considerations. *Am J Clin Pathol* 2000;114:754–759.
208. Orlandi Q, Ciucci A, Ferlosio A, et al. Cardiac myxoma cells exhibit embryonic endocardial stem cell features. *J Pathol* 2006;209:231–239.
209. Burke A, Virmani R. Cardiac tumors: an update. *Heart* 2008;94:117–123.
210. Kurian KC, Weisshaar D, Parekh H, et al. Primary cardiac angiosarcoma: case report and review of the literature. *Cardiovasc Pathol* 2006;15:110–112.
211. Rolla G, Calligaris-Cappio, Burke AP. Cardiac lymphomas. In Travis WD, Brambilla E, Muller-Hermelink HK, et al., eds. *Tumours of the Lung, Pleura and Heart.* Lyon, France: IARC Press, 2004:282–283.
212. Nascimento AF, Winters GL, Pinkus GS. Primary cardiac lymphoma: clinical, histologic, immunophenotypic, and genotypic features of 5 cases of a rare disorder. *Am J Surg Pathol* 2007;31:1344–1350.
213. Ngaage DL, Mullany CJ, Daly RC, et al. Surgical treatment of cardiac papillary fibroelastoma: a single center experience with eighty-eight patients. *Ann Thorac Surg* 2005;80: 1712–1718.
214. Kurup AN, Tazelaar HD, Edwards WD, et al. Iatrogenic cardiac papillary fibroelastoma: a study of 12 cases (1990–2000). *Hum Pathol* 2002;33:1165–1169.
215. Veinot JP, Tazelaar HD, Edwards WD, et al. Mesothelial/monocytic incidental cardiac excrescences: cardiac MICE. *Mod Pathol* 1994;7:9–16.
216. Reynolds C, Tazelaar HD, Edwards WD. Calcified amorphous tumor of the heart (cardiac CAT). *Hum Pathol* 1997;28:601–666.
217. Burke AP, Araoz PA. Cystic tumor of atrioventricular node. In Travis WD, Brambilla E, Muller-Hermelink HK, et al., eds. *Tumours of the Lung, Pleura and Heart.* Lyon, France: IARC Press, 2004:272.
218. Xanthos T, Giannakopoulos N, Papadimitrou L. Lipomatous hypertrophy of the interatrial septum: a pathologic and clinical approach. *Int J Cardiol* 2007;121:4–8.
219. Rolla G, Calligaris-Cappio F. Metastatic tumours to the heart. In Travis WD, Brambilla E, Muller-Hermelink HK, et al., eds. *Tumours of the Lung, Pleura and Heart.* Lyon, France: IARC Press, 2004:284.
220. Aretz HT. The heart. In Mills SE, Carter D, Greenson JK, et al., eds. *Sternberg's Diagnostic Surgical Pathology.* Philadelphia, PA: Lippincott Williams & Wilkins, 2004:1323–1367.
221. Schoen FJ. Cardiac valves and valvular pathology: update on function, disease, repair and replacement. *Cardiovasc Pathol* 2005;14:189–194.
222. Liu AC, Joag VR, Gotlieb AI. The emerging role of valve interstitial cell phenotypes in regulating heart valve pathobiology. *Am J Pathol* 2007;171:1407–1418.
223. Waller B, Howard J, Fess S. General concepts in the morphologic assessment of operatively excised cardiac valves—Part I. *Clin Cardiol* 1994;17:41–46.
224. Schoen FJ. Surgical pathology of removed natural and prosthetic heart valves. *Hum Pathol* 1987;18:558–567.
225. Waller B, Howard J, Fess S. General concepts in the morphologic assessment of operatively excised cardiac valves—Part II. *Clin Cardiol* 1994;17:208–214.
226. Rose AG. Etiology of valvular heart disease. *Curr Opin Cardiol* 1996;11:98–113.
227. Bonow RO, Carabello BA, de Leon AC, et al. ACC/AHA 2006 guidelines for the management of patients with valvular heart disease: a report of the American College of Cardiology/American Heart Association task force on practice guidelines (writing committee to revise the 1998 guidelines for the management of patients with valvular heart disease): developed in collaboration with the Society of Cardiovascular Anesthesiologists: endorsed by the Society for Cardiovascular Angiography and Interventions and the Society of Thoracic Surgeons. *Circulation* 2006;114:e84–e231.
228. Passik CS, Ackermann DM, Pluth JR, et al. Temporal changes in the causes of aortic stenosis: a surgical pathologic study of 646 cases. *Mayo Clin Proc* 1987;62:119–123.
229. Dare AJ, Veinot JP, Edwards WD, et al. New observations on the etiology of aortic valve disease: a surgical pathological study of 236 cases from 1990. *Hum Pathol* 1993;24: 1330–1338.

230. Davies MJ, Treasure T, Parker DJ. Demographic characteristics of patients undergoing aortic valve replacement for stenosis: relation to valve morphology. *Heart* 1996;75:174–178.

231. Davies MJ, Mann JM. *The Cardiovascular System. Part B: Acquired Diseases of the Heart.* New York, NY: Churchill Livingstone, 1995:161.

232. Bosse Y, Mathieu P, Pibarot P. Genomics: the next step to elucidate the etiology of calcific aortic valve stenosis. *J Am Coll Cardiol* 2008;51:1327–1336.

233. Connolly HM, Crary JL, McGoon MD, et al. Valvular heart disease associated with fenfluramine-phentermine. *N Engl J Med* 1997;337:581–588.

234. Olson LJ, Subramanian R, Edwards WD. Surgical pathology of pure aortic insufficiency: a study of 225 cases. *Mayo Clin Proc* 1984;59:835–842.

235. Steffee CH, Singh HK, Chitwood WR. Histologic changes in three explanted native cardiac valves following use of fenfluramine. *Cardiovasc Pathol* 1999;8:245–253.

236. Volmar KE, Hutchins GM. Aortic and mitral fenfluramine-phentermine valvulopathy in 64 patients treated with anorectic agents. *Arch Pathol Lab Med* 2001;125:1555–1561.

237. Subramania R, Olson LJ, Edwards WD. Surgical pathology of combined aortic stenosis and insufficiency: a study of 213 cases. *Mayo Clin Proc* 1985;60:247–254.

238. Rose AG. Etiology of acquired valvular heart disease in adults. A survey of 18,132 autopsies and 100 consecutive valve-replacement operations. *Arch Pathol Lab Med* 1986;110:385–388.

239. Olson LJ, Subramanian R, Ackermann DM, et al. Surgical pathology of the mitral valve: a study of 712 cases spanning 21 years. *Mayo Clin Proc* 1987;62:22–34.

240. Dare AJ, Harrity PJ, Tazelaar HD, et al. Evaluation of surgically excised mitral valves: revised recommendations based on changing operative procedures in the 1990s. *Hum Pathol* 1993;24:1286–1293.

241. Waller B, Howard J, Fess S. Pathology of mitral valve stenosis and pure mitral regurgitation. Part 1. *Clin Cardiol* 1994;17:330–336.

242. Josselson A, Bagnall JW, Virmani R. Acute rheumatic carditis causing sudden death. *Am J Forensic Med Pathol* 1984;5:151–154.

243. Davies MJ, Mann JM. *The Cardiovascular System. Part B: Acquired Diseases of the Heart.* New York, NY: Churchill Livingstone, 1995:155.

244. Virmani R, Roberts WC. Aschoff bodies in operatively excised atrial appendages and papillary muscles. Frequency and clinical significance. *Circulation* 1977;55:559–563.

245. Waller BF, Howard J, Fess S. Pathology of mitral valve stenosis and pure mitral regurgitation. Part II. *Clin Cardiol* 1994;17:395–402.

246. Barlow JB, Popock WA. Billing, floppy, prolapsed or flail mitral valve? *Am J Cardiol* 1985;55:501–502.

247. Baker PB, Bansal G, Boudoulas H, et al. Floppy mitral valve chordae tendineae: histopathologic alterations. *Hum Pathol* 1988;19:507–512.

248. Cheunsuchon P, Chuangsuwanich T, Samanthai N, et al. Surgical pathology and etiology of 278 surgically removed mitral valves with pure mitral regurgitation in Thailand. *Cardiovasc Pathol* 2007;16:104–110.

249. Waller BF, Howard J, Fess S. Pathology of tricuspid valve stenosis and pure regurgitation. Part I. *Clin Cardiol* 1995;18:97–102.

250. Waller BF, Howard J, Fess S. Pathology of tricuspid valve stenosis and pure regurgitation. Part II. *Clin Cardiol* 1995;18:167–174.

251. Simula DV, Edwards WD, Tazelaar HD, et al. Surgical pathology of carcinoid heart disease: a study of 139 valves from 75 patients spanning 20 years. *Mayo Clin Proc* 2002,77:139–147.

252. Chan MCY, Giannetti N, Kato T, et al. Severe tricuspid regurgitation after heart transplantation. *J Heart Lung Transplant* 2001;20:709–717.

253. Veinot JP. Pathology of inflammatory native valvular heart disease. *Cardiovasc Pathol* 2006;15:243–251.

254. Waller BF, Howard J, Fess S. Pathology of pulmonic valve stenosis and regurgitation. *Clin Cardiol* 1995;18:45–50.

255. Haldar SM, O'Gara PT. Infective endocarditis. In Fuster V, O'Rouke RA, Walsh RA, et al., eds. *Hurst's The Heart.* 12th edition. New York, NY: McGraw Hill Medical, 2008:1975–2004.

256. Greub G, Lepidi H, Rovery C, et al. Diagnosis of infectious endocarditis in patients undergoing valve surgery. *Am J Med* 2005;118:230–238.

257. Silver MD. Infective endocarditis. In Silver MD, ed. *Cardiovascular Pathology.* 2nd edition. New York, NY: Churchill Livingstone, 1991:895–931.

258. Asopa S, Patel A, Khan OA, et al. Non-bacterial thrombotic endocarditis. *Eur J Cardiothorac Surg* 2007;32:696–701.

259. Soler-Soler J, Permanyer-Miralda G, Sagrista-Sauleda J. A systematic diagnostic approach to primary acute pericardial disease. The Barcelona experience. *Cardiol Clin* 1990;8:609–620.

260. Correale E, Maggioni AP, Romano S, et al. Pericardial involvement in acute myocardial infarction in the post-thrombolytic era: clinical meaning and value. *Clin Cardiol* 1997;20:327–331.

261. Griffiths ID, Kan SP. Sulphaslazine induced lupus syndrome in ulcerative colitis. *BMJ* 1977;ii:1188–1189.

262. Dent MT, Ganapathy S, Holdsworth CD, et al. Mesalazine induced lupus-like syndrome. *BMJ* 1992;305:159.

263. Knockaert DC. Cardiac involvement in systemic inflammatory diseases. *Eur Heart J* 2007;28:1797–1804.

264. Imazio M, Cecchi, Demichelis B, et al. Indicators of poor prognosis of acute pericarditis. *Circulation* 2007;115:2739–2744.

265. Clare GC, Troughton RW. Management of constrictive pericarditis in the 21st century. *Curr Treat Options Cardiovasc Med* 2007;9:436–442.

266. Alexander JAS. A pericardial effusion of "gold paint" appearance due to the presence of cholesterin. *BMJ* 1919;ii:463

267. Hanson RM, Caya JG, Clowry LJ, et al. Benign mesothelial proliferations with effusion: clinicopathologic entity that may mimic malignancy. *Am J Med* 1984;77:887–894.

268. Burke A, Virmani R. Malignant mesothelioma of the pericardium. Tumors of the heart and great vessels. In *Atlas of Tumor Pathology.* 3rd edition. Bethesda, MD: Armed Forces Institute of Pathology, 1996:181–194.

Blood Vessels

HEREDITARY DISEASES OF BLOOD VESSELS

MARFAN SYNDROME

Marfan syndrome is an autosomal dominant condition characterized by skeletal, ocular, and cardiovascular manifestations and is traditionally defined by clinical criteria (1). In most cases, there is a mutation in fibrillin-1 on chromosome 15. Marfan patients with normal fibrillin-1 genotype may have mutations in the transforming growth factor-beta (TGF-β) receptor (2). Cardiovascular manifestations include proximal aortic aneurysms, which may lead to aortic dissections and rupture; aortic incompetence; mitral valve prolapse; and peripheral artery aneurysms. Less than 10% of patients with ascending aortic aneurysms will have extracardiac clinical manifestations of Marfan syndrome, and approximately 3% to 5% of patients with ascending aortic dissections have Marfan syndrome. In a series of 513 patients with aortic root disease necessitating surgical repair, 32 patients had documented Marfan syndrome (3). Most aneurysms in patients with the full-blown syndrome are symptomatic before age 35 years.

The characteristic histologic finding in Marfan syndrome is cystic medial degeneration, with or without features of acute or chronic dissection (Fig. 30.1). Medial degeneration is characterized by the loss of elastic laminae and smooth muscle cells, with replacement by pools of proteoglycan matrix. There is variability in the degree of cystic medial degeneration in patients with inherited aortic root disease; in only 25% of patients is the degree severe, and in approximately 5% of patients, the aortic media is histologically normal (3). Therefore, histologic evaluation is not helpful in assigning a genetic etiology for degenerative aortic root disease. The degree of histologic variability is likely in part a result of sampling, and the changes are patchy.

FAMILIAL NON-MARFAN DISSECTIONS

Familial aortic dissection are about as common in patients without extravascular abnormalities as in patients with Marfan syndrome (3). The genetic basis is not known, although it has been shown that 5% of patients with non-Marfan familial dissection have mutations in the TGF-β receptor (4), as is the case of the recently described Loeys-Dietz syndrome. As with Marfan syndrome, the histologic characteristic is cystic medial degeneration, although the degree is quite variable.

EHLERS-DANLOS SYNDROME

Ehlers-Danlos syndrome type IV, the vascular type, results from mutations in the gene for type III procollagen (COL3A1). Affected patients are at risk for arterial, bowel, and uterine rupture (5). The histologic features of Ehlers-Danlos syndrome are not well characterized; indeed, in many cases, the media is histologically normal, and the pathologic features are that of rupture and pseudoaneurysm formation in an otherwise apparently normal vessel. In the Mayo Clinic series of aortic root resection, primarily for aneurysm, only 2 of 513 patients had evidence of Ehlers-Danlos syndrome, less than 5% of hereditary cases. It is unclear whether cystic medial degeneration is a typical finding of the disease, in contrast to Marfan syndrome and other non-Marfan familial dissections.

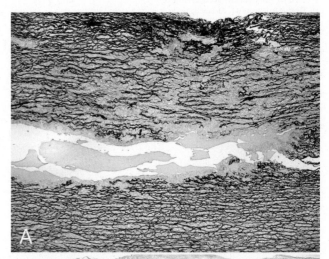

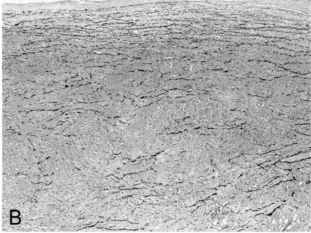

Figure 30.1. Cystic medial degeneration. **(A)** There is a large area in the central media with loss of elastic layers and smooth muscle cells, with a pool of ground substance. **(B)** In this example, there is more diffuse loss and disorganization of elastic laminae, with increased proteoglycan matrix. The degree of cystic medial degeneration varies and does not in an individual patient allow the distinction between inherited forms of the aortic aneurysm without a clear genetic etiology.

AORTIC ROOT DISEASE IN PATIENTS WITH BICUSPID AORTIC VALVE

Bicuspid aortic valve (or congenitally bicommissural valve) has an autosomal dominant inheritance (6). There is a known association with aortic root aneurysm and dissection, with the risk being 5 to 10 times that of the general population (7). In the Mayo Clinic series of surgically resected ascending aorta, more than 10% of patients (67 of 513 patients) had a bicuspid aortic valve; the incidence in the normal population is less than 2%. In this series, the mean age was 53 years, and the degree of cystic medial necrosis was significantly less in patients with congenitally bicuspid aortic valve compared with other inherited connective tissue disease; only 11% of patients had severe cystic medial degeneration (3). However, it should be emphasized that in an individual case, histologic findings of the aortic media cannot distinguish the underlying etiology of medial degeneration. There is genetic evidence that there is a common gene that underlies bicuspid aortic valve and aortic aneurysm and that the most dilated portion of the aorta is distal to the annulus (6). The genetic basis remains unknown, however, and is likely unrelated to fibrillin-1 because patients with Marfan syndrome have trileaflet aortic valves.

PSEUDOXANTHOMA ELASTICUM

Pseudoxanthoma elasticum (PXE) is caused by mutations in the adenosine triphosphate (ATP)–binding cassette transporter C6 (*ABCC6*), also known as multidrug resistance–associated protein 6 (*MRP6*) gene. It is inherited as an autosomal recessive trait and has an incidence of 1 in 25,000 to 100,000. PXE is characterized by progressive calcification and fragmentation of elastic fibers in the skin, the retina, and the cardiovascular system (Fig. 30.2). Patients typically have a normal life span, with the morbidity varying based on the extent of extracutaneous involvement.

PRIMARY HYPEROXALURIA

Type I hyperoxaluria occurs in 1 per 120,000 live births and is transmitted as an autosomal recessive trait. It is caused by a

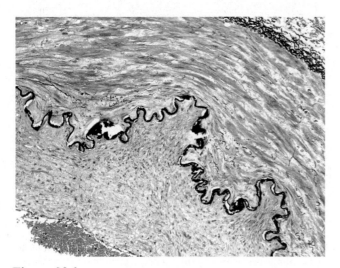

Figure 30.2. Pseudoxanthoma elasticum. The internal elastic lamina of this coronary artery demonstrates duplication of the elastic layer, with focal calcifications. Movat pentachrome.

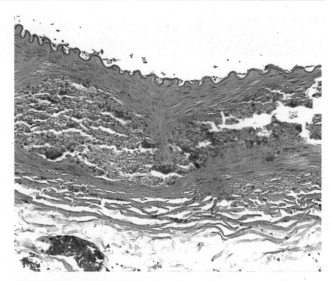

Figure 30.3. Primary hyperoxaluria. Note crystals of oxalate salt within the media of the renal artery.

deficiency of the peroxisomal liver-specific alanine:glyoxylate aminotransferase gene (*AGT*). Most patients develop renal failure in childhood. Occasionally, extensive crystalline deposits within the walls of blood vessels (Fig. 30.3) may result in vasculopathy clinically mimicking systemic vasculitis.

OTHER NONINFLAMMATORY VASCULAR DISEASES

ACQUIRED AORTIC ROOT DILATATION AND DISSECTION

The majority of patients with degenerative aortic medial disease have no family history or evidence of inherited connective tissue disease. Many of the patients, who are on average 10 to 20 years older than patients with inherited diseases and bicuspid aortic valve, have systemic hypertension. In approximately 25% of patients, however, there are no known predisposing factors. It is likely that these patients have a polygenetic predisposition to aortic dissection. The histologic features of idiopathic aortic root aneurysm, with or without dissection, are similar to those of inherited disease, although the degree of cystic medial degeneration is typically mild. Again, the histologic features, per se, do not point to an underlying etiology.

GENERAL APPROACH TO ASCENDING AORTIC ANEURYSM

The surgical pathologist, when evaluating an aortic root aneurysm, should recognize the limitations of histologic assessment in assigning an etiology (Table 30.1). Inflammatory lesions, such as idiopathic aortitis, should be excluded, because there may be foci mimicking cystic medial necrosis in the otherwise inflamed aortic media. In noninflammatory aortic aneurysms, the degree of medial degeneration is quite variable and does not point to a specific etiology. The number of aortic valve leaflets should be noted in cases with concomitant valve replacement, and the presence of acute dissection should be noted. In addition, any areas of healed dissection, characterized by

TABLE 30.1	Histopathologic Differential Diagnosis of Ascending Aorta Aneurysms Seen at Aortic Root Reconstruction with or without Aortic Valve Replacement

Diagnosis	Approximate Relative Frequency	Histologic Features	Associated Histologic Findings	Associated Medical Conditions
Degenerative medial disease	95%	Medial degeneration (cystic medial necrosis): minimal to marked	Acute or healed dissection	Marfan[a] Hypertension[b] Bicuspid aortic valve[c]
Aortitis, necrotizing	<5%	Zonal medial necrosis, with macrophage reaction	Healing lesions mimicking degenerative medial disease or dysplasia; atherosclerosis; intimal and adventitial fibrosis	Takayasu disease[d] Rheumatoid arthritis[e] Giant-cell arteritis[f]
Aortitis, nonnecrotizing	<5%	Medial inflammation, without necrosis	Acute or healed dissection	Giant-cell arteritis
Syphilis[g]	<1%	Transmural inflammation	Adventitial inflammation	

[a]Less than 10% of patients.
[b]Medial degenerative changes are typically minimal in hypertension-related aneurysms and dissections; media can appear nearly normal.
[c]Approximately 15% of patients.
[d]Less than 5% of patients, generally young women with diffuse peripheral extension of disease, resulting in peripheral stenoses and systemic autoimmune symptoms.
[e]Less than 5% of patients; histologically, rheumatoid nodules are not present in aneurysmal disease.
[f]More frequent in nonnecrotizing aortitis; seen in older patients with a female predominance.
[g]Exceptionally rare in Western countries; reported generally as case reports; no reported example in two large series of aortitis in the United States (8,9).

elastic reduplication of the false lumen lining, should be described; these are readily detected by the use of elastic stains. Adequate sampling of the lesions (approximately one section per centimeter of aorta excised) aids in the identification of acute and healed dissections, aortitis, and the extent of cystic medial degeneration.

FIBROMUSCULAR DYSPLASIA

Fibromuscular dysplasia is a generic term for a group of structural abnormalities of one or more layers of medium-sized and large arteries that result in aneurysms and dissections of the media (Fig. 30.4). Imaging studies suggest that the disease may be familial in a significant proportion of patients, with autosomal dominant inheritance (10,11). It occurs most frequently in young to middle-aged white women. Clinical manifestations reflect the arterial bed involved, most commonly hypertension (renal) and stroke (carotid). Dysplasia of the renal arteries and carotid and visceral beds may be localized or part of a systemic process; angiography may be indicated to define the extent of disease in a given patient. The histologic features are not well defined but include disorganization of the media with segmental thinning (classic form of medial dysplasia), diffuse intimal thickening, and primarily adventitial scarring. Mild medial disorganization is characteristic of normal renal arteries, and care should be taken not to overdiagnose fibromuscular dysplasia based on histologic assessment alone.

PERIPHERAL ANEURYSMS AND DISSECTIONS

Aneurysms of the peripheral arteries may be the result of vasculitis (especially polyarteritis nodosa) or septic embolism (infectious aneurysms, especially in patients with infectious endocarditis). More commonly, they are noninflammatory and often of

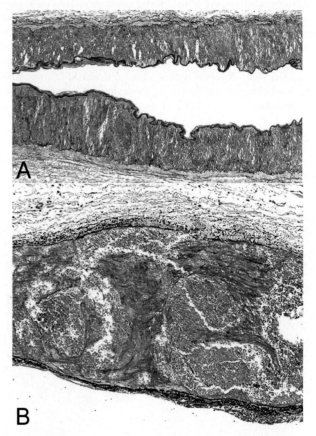

Figure 30.4. Medial dysplasia. **(A)** There is disorganization of the media. Movat pentachrome. **(B)** Higher magnification demonstrates areas of medial smooth muscle cell loss, with hemorrhage within the media (acute dissection). The artery was the mesenteric artery in an elderly man with hemoperitoneum.

uncertain etiology. Noninflammatory aneurysms may be associated with either medial dysplasia or cystic medial degeneration, and hypertension is a frequent clinical finding. Splenic aneurysms, the most common site for visceral aneurysms, are pathologically heterogeneous and may be the result of medial dysplasia or degeneration, vasculitis, adjacent pancreatitis, portal hypertension, or atherosclerosis. The histologic features are typically obscured by secondary changes of calcification and fibrosis, making a specific diagnosis impossible. In addition to medial dysplasia and medial degeneration, potential causes of peripheral aneurysms include atherosclerotic aneurysms (most common in the leg) and cystic adventitial disease of the popliteal artery

Spontaneous dissections may occur in peripheral arteries with or without pre-existing aneurysm (Fig. 30.5). As with aneurysms, predisposing conditions include medial dysplasia and medial degeneration. Spontaneous dissections of the renal arteries often occur in young men without evidence of renal artery dysplasia and may be related to exertion (12).

AMYLOIDOSIS

Amyloidosis may result in bleeding, either secondary to coagulopathy or direct involvement of the arterial wall (13). The protein precursor may be free light chains, prealbumin, or AA protein (14). Microvessels may be involved in amyloidosis secondary to β_2-microglobulin associated with chronic dialysis. Temporal artery biopsy may occasionally disclose amyloid secondary to primary AL amyloidosis (15), mimicking the clinical symptoms of temporal arteritis (Fig. 30.6).

MEDIAL CALCIFICATION: MONCKEBERG AND VASCULAR CALCINOSIS (CALCIPHYLAXIS)

Age-related, modest calcification of the media of small and medium-sized muscular arteries (Monckeberg medial calcifica-

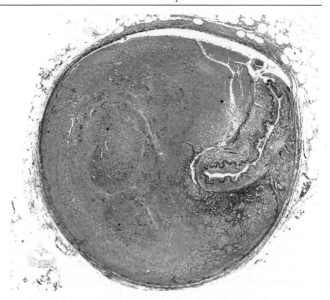

Figure 30.5. Acute arterial dissection. This renal artery demonstrates a large hematoma between the media and adventitia.

tion) is a common finding in the elderly. Calcification involves the media and elastic laminae. Significant luminal narrowing or giant-cell inflammatory reaction occurs uncommonly, typically in the setting of diabetes mellitus and renal failure.

More severe forms of calcification of the media, which result in a marked giant-cell reaction in proximal arteries, extension of calcification into distal vessels, and elevation of acute phase reactants, are termed vascular calcinosis or calciphylaxis. Obstruction of the vessel occurs because of fibrosis of the intima, causing ischemia symptoms or progressive ischemic gangrene. Most patients with severe medial calcification have renal failure with hyperparathyroidism; calciphylaxis affects 1% to 4% of the population with end-stage renal disease. Radiographs demon-

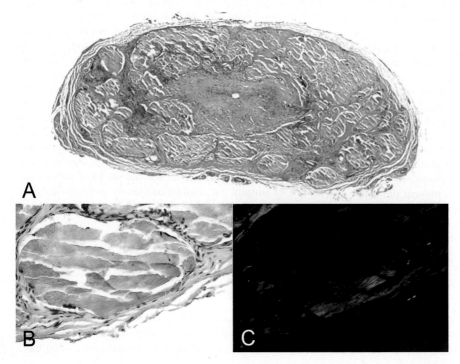

Figure 30.6. Vascular amyloid. The patient had symptoms of temporal arteritis. On biopsy, diffuse amyloid was noted. **(A)** Note replacement of adventitial with nodules of amyloid. **(B)** Higher magnification, Congo red stain. **(C)** Congo red stain viewed with polarized light, focal apple-green birefringence.

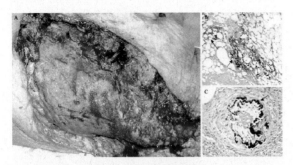

Figure 30.7. Calciphylaxis (from papa).

strate diffuse vascular calcifications of vessels of the extremities, but the diagnosis rests on histologic confirmation of calcification in distal arteries and arterioles (Fig. 30.7). Subcutaneous calcium deposits with panniculitis and fat necrosis may sometimes be found. Vascular microthrombi are frequently evident.

ATHEROSCLEROSIS

AORTIC ANEURYSMS

Atherosclerosis of the aorta progresses from early lesions (fatty streak and fibrous plaque) to late ulcerated plaques. Fatty streaks are lipid rich, grossly yellow, and barely raised. Histologically, there are variable numbers of intimal foam cells, lipid pools without fibroatheroma formation (pathologic intimal thickening), and smooth muscle cells. Fibrous plaques, by contrast, are raised, firm white lesions that generally correspond histologically to fibroatheromas, namely necrotic cores with overlying fibrous caps. Advanced lesions are those with rupture of the fibrous cap and luminal thrombus, grossly identified as ulcerated plaques. Complications of advanced lesions causing clinical symptoms include aneurysm formation, luminal thrombotic obstruction, and atheroembolism. Aortic atherosclerosis is most advanced in the abdominal segment between the renal arteries and iliac bifurcation and is often accompanied by iliac disease. The thoracic aorta, especially the descending portion, may also be involved in aneurysmal disease.

The most common complication of aortic atherosclerosis is atherosclerotic aortic aneurysm, which has been increasing in incidence (16). The reason that only a proportion of patients with severe aortic atherosclerosis develop aneurysms is unknown, leading to doubt that the cause is specifically atherosclerosis. White race, hypertension, and smoking are risk factors, and there are likely genetic factors that contribute to increased elastolysis and collagenolysis within the aortic media.

The surgical pathologist will encounter aortic atherosclerosis most commonly as aortic aneurysm repair. The repair of abdominal aortic aneurysms is performed largely to prevent the complication of rupture, which can lead to hemoperitoneum and sudden death. The wall of the aneurysm is generally left in place, with Dacron conduit interposed between nonaneurysmal areas proximally and distally. Therefore, the pathologist receives only portions of luminal thrombus, atherosclerotic intima, and inflamed media and adventitia.

CAROTID ATHEROSCLEROSIS

Carotid endarterectomy is performed in symptomatic patients as well as in asymptomatic patients with severe stenosis. The

surgeon attempts to remove the specimen in toto. The pathologist should note presence or absence of ruptures or thrombi and section the plaque transversely (after decalcification if necessary) for histologic analysis. As with coronary atherectomy, a proportion of patients will have a history of previous endarterectomy, and the indication for the procedure will be restenosis.

In general, acute thrombi are present in approximately 65% of carotid plaques removed by endarterectomy, ulceration or fissures are present in approximately 75%, and necrotic atheroma is present in approximately 80%. Calcification is common. Morphologic changes associated with ischemic symptoms include plaque ulceration, thrombosis, and intramural hemorrhage, which is often accompanied by neovascularization in the base and shoulder regions of the plaque surrounding the necrotic core (Fig. 30.8) (17). The plaque composition of carotid endarterectomies has been correlated with risk factors. There is an association between hyperfibrinogenemia and hypercholesterolemia and plaque rupture and thrombosis.

AORTIC OCCLUSIVE DISEASE

Some patients with severe aortic atherosclerosis develop primarily occlusive disease (18), with little if any dilatation distal to the renal arteries. These patients are treated with aortobifemoral bypass grafting and often have embolic symptoms and symptoms of severe peripheral vascular disease. There may be a component of coagulopathy contributing to aortoiliac occlusive disease, especially in younger women, and there is an association with atherosclerosis of other arterial beds and chronic renal failure.

INFLAMMATORY AORTIC ANEURYSMS

Approximately 10% of patients with abdominal aortic aneurysm demonstrate an inflammatory variant, defined both grossly and histologically (19,20). Male sex and smoking are even stronger risk factors for this inflammatory variant than they are for atherosclerotic aortic aneurysms. Grossly, there is marked thickening of the aneurysm wall, fibrosis of the adjacent retroperitoneum, and adherence of the adjacent structures to the anterior aneurysm wall. Histologically, there is expansion of the adventitia with fibrosis, lymphocytes, and plasma cells (Fig. 30.9). Inflammatory aortic aneurysm is sometimes considered a manifestation of retroperitoneal fibrosis, and purported etiologies include autoimmune disease, possibly triggered by *Chlamydia pneumoniae*, and immunoglobulin G4 (IgG4)–related sclerosing disease akin to autoimmune sclerosing pancreatitis. Although there is typically superimposed atherosclerosis, inflammatory aortic aneurysm is considered separately from atherosclerotic disease and is treated more as an isolated vasculitis, with a combination of surgery and anti-inflammatory medications (19). However, inflammation of other vessels is not a feature of inflammatory aortic aneurysm.

VASCULITIS

INTRODUCTION

The term vasculitis means different things in different settings. To the clinician, a diagnosis of vasculitis connotes a systemic autoimmune disease, with a variably chronic course, that has a

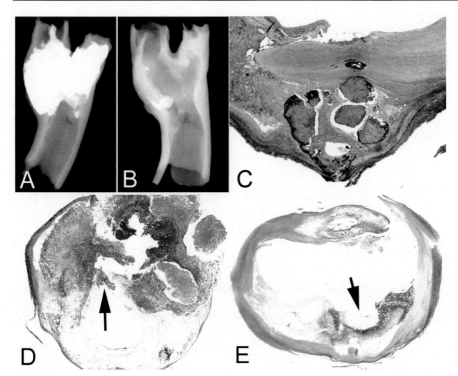

Figure 30.8. Carotid endarterectomy. **(A)** Carotid plaques are often significantly calcified; for adequate histology analysis, decalcification is required. **(B)** The lesions typically occur maximally at the bifurcation of the common carotid artery to the internal and external iliac. **(C)** Nodules of calcification may break up and contribute to plaque instability. **(D)** Intraplaque hemorrhage is common; in this case, there is a small rupture site (*arrow*). **(E)** Typically in carotid plaques, the ruptures ulcerate (*arrow*).

prominent vascular component. To the pathologist, vasculitis generally denotes the presence of primary vascular inflammation, in the absence of infection, infarction, or other secondary cause. Because most of the systemic vasculitis syndromes have isolated variants that are identical to their systemic counterparts, the pathologic definition of vasculitis is, in some sense, more broad than that of the clinical definition. Pathologically, it has been stated that certain histologic features (e.g., fibrinoid necrosis) are a prerequisite for the diagnosis of vasculitis. However, it is well known that the histologic findings in patients with known vasculitis syndromes vary by vessel size and type of vasculitis; for example, necrosis is not a typical feature of giant-cell vasculitis, and vascular inflammation in nerve or muscle

biopsies may not show necrosis in patients with polyarteritis. Therefore, the use of the term vasculitis by the pathologist is generally best qualified by context and explained in a report on what the clinical ramifications may be.

The classification of vasculitis depends on at least three major features: size and type of vessel involved, presence of immune complexes and association with known autoimmune disease, and systemic or localized distribution (21). Two vasculitic syndromes affect elastic arteries: Takayasu disease and giant-cell arteritis (Table 30.2). Two vasculitic syndromes affect muscular arteries in the absence of small vessel involvement: polyarteritis nodosa and Kawasaki disease (Table 30.3). A host of vasculitis syndromes affect small vessels (arterioles, capillaries, and venules). These are generally divided into those that are caused by immune complex deposition (Table 30.4) and pauci-immune (often antineutrophil cytoplasmic antibody [ANCA] related) vasculitis (Table 30.5). The vasculitic syndromes that involve small vessels often affect muscular arteries as well; therefore, histologic features are indistinguishable from polyarteritis if only muscular arteries are sampled histologically.

The pathologist's role in the diagnosis of vasculitis is often limited because clinical and serologic evaluation by a rheumatologist is often necessary for a specific diagnosis. Therefore, if the pathologist initially diagnoses vasculitis, it is recommended that the surgical pathology report indicate that further workup be done to determine if (a) the process is systemic or isolated and (b) there are associated autoimmune syndromes. Of course, if the biopsy is performed specifically to rule in or out vasculitis, specifically in the case of temporal artery, nerve, or muscle biopsy, then the pathologist's role is more straightforward.

TAKAYASU DISEASE

Historically, Takayasu disease was defined as inflammatory peripheral arterial stenoses, first described as ophthalmic artery

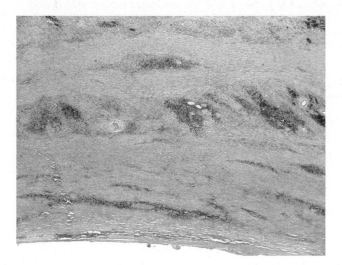

Figure 30.9. Inflammatory abdominal aortic aneurysm. The media of the aorta has been replaced with a fibrous tissue and aggregates of chronic inflammation, which surrounds nerves and adventitial fat.

TABLE 30.2	Classification of Arteritis Involving Elastic Arteries				
Type of Vasculitis	*Vessel Type Involved*	*Typical Distribution*	*Inflammation*	*Necrosis*	*Features*
Giant-cell arteritis	Muscular, elastic	Cranial, aorta, visceral, iliofemoral	Chronic, often with giant cells	Minimal or absent	Elastic lamellar destruction
Takayasu	Elastic, occasionally muscular extension	Aorta, proximal branches	Chronic, usually with giant cells	Zonal medial necrosis with healing	Medial destruction, prominent inflammation of vasa vasorum, intimal and adventitial scarring

TABLE 30.3	Classification of Arteritis Involving Muscular Arteries			
Type of Vasculitis	*Vessel Involved*	*Typical Distribution*	*Inflammation*	*Necrosis*
Kawasaki disease	Muscular	Coronary	Acute in initial phases, chronic	Only in initial stages
Polyarteritis nodosa	Muscular	Visceral, renal, soft tissue, skin (diverse sites)	Acute, chronic	Fibrinoid necrosis typical

TABLE 30.4	Immune-Mediated Small Vessel Vasculitis		
Type of Vasculitis	*Vessel Type Involved*	*Typical Distribution*	*Features*
Henoch-Schönlein purpura	Arterioles, capillaries, venules	Skin, bowel, glomeruli	Leukocytoclastic vasculitis; Glomerulonephritis; Venular thrombosis; IgA specific
Cryoglobulinemia	Arterioles, capillaries, venules	Skin (pan-dermal), glomeruli, lung	Leukocytoclastic vasculitis, Venular thrombosis; Globular endovascular deposits
Mixed connective tissue disease	Arterioles, capillaries, venules	Muscles, small arterioles	Associated with noninflammatory arteriolar thickening
Lupus vasculitis	Pan-vasculitis	Skin (pan-dermal), glomeruli, nervous system	Leukocytoclastic vasculitis; Glomerulonephritis; PAN-like muscular arterial lesions may occur
Rheumatoid vasculitis	Pan-vasculitis, as lupus	Skin (pan-dermal), viscera, nervous system	Leukocytoclastic vasculitis; PAN-like muscular arterial lesions may occur

IgA, immunoglobulin A; PAN, polyarteritis nodosa.

TABLE 30.5	Pauci-immune Small Vessel Vasculitis		
Type of Vasculitis	*Vessels Involved*	*Sites of Predilection*	*Features*
Wegener granulomatosis	Arteries, arterioles, capillaries, venules	Upper airways, lungs, glomeruli, various others	Extravascular necroinflammatory lesions typical, especially in lung; strong association with ANCA, especially C-ANCA
Churg-Strauss angiitis	Arteries, arterioles, capillaries, venules	Lungs, various viscera	Extravascular eosinophilic microabscesses in association with necrotizing arteritis; weaker association with ANCA
Microscopic polyangiitis/ polyarteritis	Arteries, arterioles, capillaries, venules	Glomeruli, lungs, kidney, others	Typically limited to renal capillaries (crescentic GN), lungs (capillaritis), skin; strong association with ANCA, especially P-ANCA

ANCA, antineutrophil cytoplasmic antibody; C-ANCA, cytoplasmic antineutrophil cytoplasmic antibody; GN, glomerulonephritis; P-ANCA, perinuclear antineutrophil cytoplasmic antibody.

occlusion. Subsequently, it was determined in autopsy studies from Japan that the inflammatory process involved the aortic arch as well, and gradually, the concept of Takayasu aortitis with aneurysm and stenosis of arch vessels evolved. Eventually, it has become somewhat accepted to use the term for any noninfectious aortitis, in the absence of other autoimmune disease, in virtually any age group (22). The most common initial finding is aortic root disease with aneurysm in the absence of systemic illness. However, clinical criteria for diagnosis include young age range and specific clinical findings indicating autoimmune syndrome and peripheral stenoses. The use of the term "Takayasu disease" in the medical literature without uniform criteria has resulted in significant confusion in classification of vasculitis of large vessels.

As a unifying concept, Takayasu disease is a necrotizing vasculitis that involves the aorta and branch vessels. In a subset of patients, who are generally women less than age 50 years, there is diffuse involvement, with extension into peripheral arteries, resulting in systemic autoimmune syndrome with peripheral stenoses. Although not accepted, this subset of patients could be termed as having "Takayasu syndrome." In contrast, patients with "Takayasu disease" range in age from 20 to more than 80 years, have no gender predilection, and suffer from aortic root dilatation and valve insufficiency without systemic vasculitis (23,24).

The gross features of aortitis are wrinkling of the intima (so-called tree barking) with variable thickening of the aortic wall (23,24). The histologic features of necrotizing aortitis include zonal medial necrosis rimmed by macrophage giant cells (Fig. 30.10) (25). With healing, there is intimal and adventitial fibrosis. Curiously, healed lesions of the media are relatively devoid of scarring (unlike the fibrosis one sees in the intima and adventitia) (23,24). In old lesions, there is an accumulation of proteoglycans, which impart an appearance of dysplasia. Extensive sampling with elastic stains to demonstrate the zonal necrosis may be necessary to establish a diagnosis.

The surgical pathologist encounters Takayasu disease (necrotizing aortitis) at evaluation of aortic root biopsies in cases of aortic aneurysm repair (Fig. 30.11). Although the majority of these specimens demonstrate nonspecific degenerative medial disease, less than 5% will demonstrate aortitis, which the pathol-

ogist will initially diagnose. In the great majority of these patients, there is no prior clinical history of autoimmune disease or Takayasu syndrome. Although it is unclear what the most appropriate clinical course should be after diagnosis of unsuspected aortitis, the surgical pathologist should recommend rheumatologic evaluation. A small proportion of patients with isolated inflammatory aortic root disease develop subsequent aneurysms (25,26).

ANKYLOSING SPONDYLITIS

HLA-B27–related diseases, including ankylosing spondylitis, may be associated with aortic inflammation that typically extends on to the aortic valve. Unlike Takayasu disease and other types of autoimmune aortitis, aortic dilatation is not a common feature, and the valve disease manifests more often as stenosis

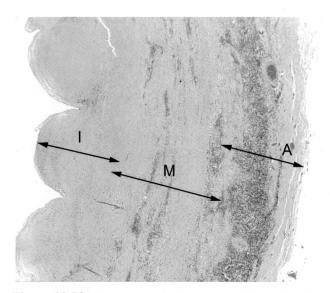

Figure 30.10. Takayasu aortitis. There is marked thickening of the aortic wall, including the intima (I), media (M), and adventitia (A). There is patchy inflammation in the media. There is marked inflammation in the adventitia, centered on vasa vasorum.

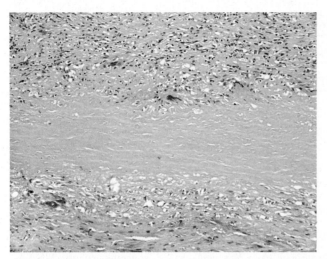

Figure 30.11. Necrotizing aortitis. Often isolated, necrotizing aortitis demonstrates zones of necrosis, surrounded by granulomatous inflammation. The central eosinophilic band is a remnant of necrotic media (so-called laminar necrosis), with ghosts of elastic laminae still intact. Necrotizing aortitis may be associated with Takayasu syndrome and other autoimmune diseases such as rheumatoid arthritis.

compared with regurgitation. The aortic histologic findings are nonspecific, but there is usually adventitial inflammation, and there may be granulomatous inflammation (Fig. 30.12).

GIANT-CELL ARTERITIS

The surgical pathologist encounters giant-cell arteritis primarily in two settings: temporal artery biopsy and aortic root disease. Approximately 10% of patients with giant-cell arteritis demonstrate aortic root dilatation, but there are few reports of histologically documented aortitis in patients with known temporal arteritis (27,28). Nevertheless, it is generally accepted that the two entities represent part of the same spectrum.

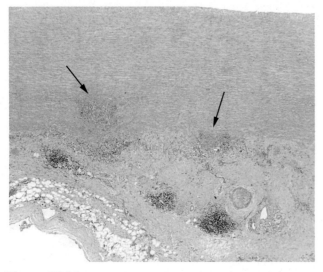

Figure 30.12. Ankylosing spondylitis. This patient demonstrated aortic stenosis, which was repaired with aortic valve replacement and aortic root resection. Aortic histologic findings were adventitial inflammation and granulomas in the outer media and adventitia (arrows).

Giant-cell arteritis of the temporal artery is commonly called "temporal arteritis," but there are rare cases of temporal arteritis caused by other vasculitis syndromes (Table 30.6). Therefore, the use of the nonspecific phrase "temporal arteritis" should be avoided.

The majority of temporal artery biopsies are straightforward. Most are negative, but because of the known spotty nature of the disease, multiple sections should be examined. There are no specific guidelines; however, it is useful in the report to state the number of sections examined. For example, if the artery is cut into eight pieces, placed into a cassette, and 10 levels are taken, then the comment section of the report can state that 80 sections were examined. A negative biopsy does not, of course, exclude the disease; bilateral biopsies are sometimes performed to decrease the rate of false-negative biopsies. The routine use of elastic stains is commonplace, primarily to assess presence and extent of destruction of the elastic laminae as seen in arteritis. CD68 immunohistochemical staining may be of help in cases with minimal inflammation (29).

A positive biopsy consists of medial inflammation, classically with giant cells engulfing fragments of elastic laminae (Fig. 30.13). Chronic inflammation without giant cells occurs in approximately 50% of cases and is still diagnostic for giant-cell arteritis. In most cases with healed arteritis, active inflammation is present (Fig. 30.14). A "borderline" category is the presence of chronic inflammation in branch vessels without temporal artery inflammation (30,31). This finding has been shown to have an intermediate association with clinical features classic for giant-cell arteritis, which include temporal headache, palpable tender temporal artery, high elevations of sedimentation rate, and polymyalgia rheumatica. Not all patients with temporal arteritis have elevated sedimentation rates (32,33), and it is generally accepted that steroid treatment does not affect the rate of positive biopsies for up to 10 days to 2 weeks (34).

Other diagnoses that may be encountered in temporal artery biopsies include Wegener granulomatosis (35) and polyarteritis nodosa (both of which manifest as a necrotizing arteritis), Buerger disease (thromboarteritis obliterans) (36), amyloidosis (15), atherosclerosis, and calcinosis (Table 30.6). These entities are typically straightforward histologically. Traumatic pseudoaneurysms and angiolymphoid hyperplasia may also occur in the temporal artery, and the inflammatory infiltrate should not be mistaken for vasculitis.

Giant-cell aortitis is an uncommon finding in aortic root aneurysm repair. The diagnosis is generally not considered unless the patient is 60 years or older. In patients with previously diagnosed giant-cell arteritis of the temporal artery, the pattern of inflammation in the aorta can be identical to necrotizing aortitis as seen in Takayasu disease. More frequently, however, there is chronic inflammation with destruction of elastic laminae, without zonal necrosis or significant intimal or adventitial scarring (so-called nonnecrotizing aortitis) (Fig. 30.15). The relative lack of scarring in giant-cell aortitis, as opposed to Takayasu disease, accounts for the relatively high rate of dissection in giant-cell aortitis and the low rate of dissection in Takayasu disease. Calcification, dissection, and aortic rupture are potential complications of aortitis regardless of the cause.

Isolated giant-cell arteritis may occur in various organs, especially the visceral arteries, breast, and gynecologic tract (Fig. 30.16) (37). In a small proportion of cases, generalized giant-cell arteritis with temporal artery involvement and autoimmune symptoms such as polymyalgia rheumatica occur (38,39).

TABLE 30.6	Diagnosis of Temporal Artery Biopsies	
Histologic Findings	*Diagnosis*	*Caveats*
RELATIVELY COMMON DIAGNOSES		
Chronic inflammation centered on elastic laminae, with or without giant cells	Giant-cell arteritis	Necrosis is generally minimal; spotty destruction of elastic laminae typical; changes typically persist for 2 weeks after steroid treatment
Chronic inflammation with extensive fibrous destruction of elastic laminae	Healed giant-cell arteritis	Typically, active disease coexists; neovascularity may be present in fibrotic areas; clinical relevance of this subcategory not established
Chronic inflammation of branch vessels, without nvolvement of main artery	Suspicious for giant-cell arteritis, but not diagnostic	See Esteban M-J (31)
Intimal thickening, without destruction of the elastic laminae, sometimes with reduplication of elastic laminae	Age-related changes	Most common finding in temporal artery biopsies; diagnosis should simply state ''negative for arteritis'' with a comment regarding number of levels examined
Medial calcification, centered on elastic laminae	Medial calcification of Monckeberg	Calcification may be present in areas of giant-cell arteritis as well
UNCOMMON AND RARE DIAGNOSES		
Unusual pattern of inflammation (or in patients younger than 55–60 years)	Other types of vasculitis	Wegener may present as temporal arteritis, usually with necrosis; PAN demonstrates fibrinoid necrosis and adventitial inflammation; Buerger demonstrates cellular thrombus with luminal giant cells
Intimal disease with necrotic core, atheroma	Atherosclerosis	Rare in temporal artery; term often misused for age-related intimal thickening
Marked medial calcification with giant-cell reaction and intimal thickening	Calcinosis	Renal failure patients
Amorphous medial deposits	Amyloid	Confirm with Congo red staining, may have giant-cell reaction
Nodular adventitial lymphocytic inflammation with eosinophils, epithelioid capillaries	Epithelioid hemangioma	Also known as angiolymphoid hyperplasia with eosinophilia
Interruption of media with proteoglycan-rich organized thrombus	Traumatic pseudoaneurysm	May have abundant inflammation mimicking epithelioid hemangioma

PAN, polyarteritis nodosa.

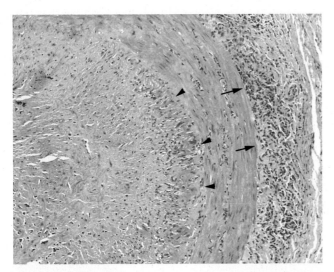

Figure 30.13. Giant-cell arteritis, temporal artery. There is granulomatous inflammation involving the internal elastic lamina (*arrowheads*) and external elastic lamina (*arrows*). The symptoms result from hyperplasia of the intimal smooth muscle cells resulting in luminal obstruction.

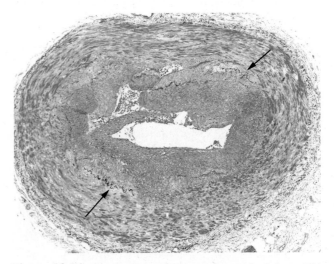

Figure 30.14. Giant-cell arteritis, temporal artery, healed area. This Movat pentachrome stain shows generalized destruction of the internal elastic lamina, with focal residual intact areas (*arrows*). In most cases of healed arteritis, there are active foci present. In this case, an adjacent section shows granulomatous destruction of the elastic laminae.

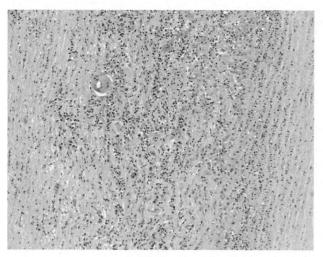

Figure 30.15. Giant-cell aortitis. Although it is unclear whether there are histologic subtypes of aortitis, giant-cell aortitis is characterized by nonnecrotizing inflammation of the media, associated with destruction of the elastic laminae. Many patients have associated temporal arteritis.

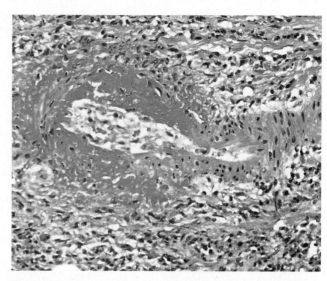

Figure 30.17. Polyarteritis nodosa. There is fibrinoid necrosis with pseudoaneurysm formation. Residual intact media is to the right. Typically, there is extensive periadventitial inflammation. Usually there are uninvolved vessels and scarred vessels in the same section.

POLYARTERITIS NODOSA

Polyarteritis nodosa is a necrotizing arteritis that involves muscular arteries in virtually any organ, with a predilection for the gut and kidneys (40). Fibrinoid necrosis is a defining feature (Fig. 30.17), and there is usually adventitial inflammation, pseudoaneurysm formation, and thrombosis with organization and scarring. Lesions at different stages of development are typical. Capillaries, veins, and venules are not involved. The primary differential diagnosis is nonvasculitic necrosis secondary to infarction or infection. Necrotizing arteritis with fibrinoid necrosis may also occur in Wegener granulomatosis, rheumatoid vasculitis, and Churg-Strauss angiitis. In evaluation of systemic disease, nerve or muscle biopsy may be performed to confirm the diagnosis of vasculitis; in these small biopsies, inflammation in small muscular arteries without fibrinoid necrosis is considered diagnostic.

The pathologist may encounter incidental necrotizing arteritis in the gallbladder, appendix, bowel serosa (41), breast, gynecologic tract, and testis (Fig. 30.18) (37). In most patients, systemic vasculitis does not occur, but because of the small risk of development of systemic symptoms, rheumatologic evaluation should be recommended.

KAWASAKI DISEASE

Also known as mucocutaneous lymph node syndrome, Kawasaki disease is a necrotizing vasculitis occurring in children that in-

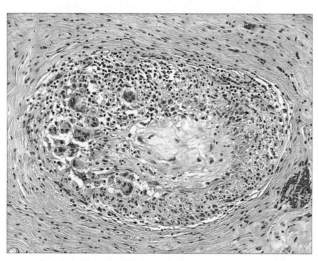

Figure 30.16. Giant-cell arteritis may be seen as an isolated finding in various organs, including the gynecologic tract. This artery demonstrates giant-cell inflammation and was an incidental finding in a hysterectomy with salpingo-oophorectomy. Some patients may develop cranial giant-cell arteritis necessitating steroid therapy, although this patient remained asymptomatic.

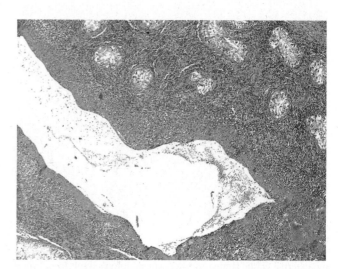

Figure 30.18. Polyarteritis nodosa, isolated, testicular. In this section, the outline of the artery is destroyed, replaced by a layer of fibrin. The artery is dilated. Note surrounding testicular tubules. There is marked periadventitial inflammation. Most cases of testicular arteritis do not develop into systemic disease.

volves muscular arteries, typically coronary, although peripheral aneurysms may occur (40). The diagnosis is generally made clinically. Kawasaki disease is no longer considered a pediatric variant of polyarteritis nodosa because the histologic features are distinct and fibrinoid necrosis is not typical.

BUERGER DISEASE (THROMBOANGIITIS OBLITERANS)

Strongly linked to cigarette smoking, Buerger disease is an inflammatory disease of arteries and veins that results in luminal thrombosis and obstruction (36,42). Because autoimmunity and systemic symptoms are not features, Buerger disease is not typically considered a vasculitis. The distribution is more distal than atherosclerosis, and occlusions of the femoral and popliteal vessels are typical. Other vessels may be involved, including arm vessels and temporal arteries. In most patients, histologic findings are nonspecific and consist of thrombi at different stages of evolution. The surgical pathologist may be asked to make the diagnosis on amputation specimens. In a small proportion of cases, diagnostic findings of intraluminal cellular thrombi with giant cells are seen and considered pathognomonic.

WEGENER GRANULOMATOSIS

Wegener granulomatosis is an ANCA-related vasculitis involving muscular arteries and small vessels (43). In addition, there are extravascular necrotic lesions, most commonly encountered in the lung and upper airways (Figs. 30.19 and 30.20). The triad of organ involvement is the lung, sinonasal area, and kidneys. In some patients, all three histologic manifestations exist, namely necrotizing parenchymal lesions, necrotizing arteritis, and small vessel vasculitis. The necrotizing arteritis of Wegener granulomatosis is indistinguishable from polyarteritis nodosa histologically. If only small vessel involvement exists, then the term microscopic polyangiitis is used. From a surgical pathologist's

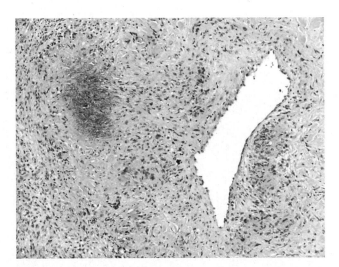

Figure 30.19. Wegener granulomatosis. Histologic manifestations include necrotizing arteritis indistinguishable from polyarteritis nodosa, small vessel vasculitis and capillaritis in the lung, and extravascular necrotizing lesions. This photomicrograph shows a necrotizing lesion at the left and perivenular granulomatous inflammation on the right, with giant cells.

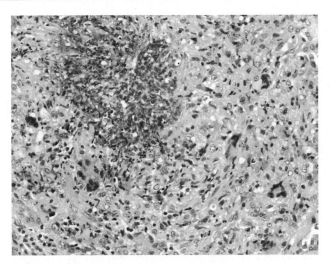

Figure 30.20. Wegener granulomatosis. A higher magnification of the necrotizing lesion shows apoptotic degenerating neutrophils resulting in basophilic necrosis, with surrounding giant cells and chronic inflammation.

standpoint, the diagnosis of necrotizing, cavitary lung lesions with basophilic necrosis should raise the possibility of Wegener granulomatosis. Muscular arteritis and pulmonary capillaritis may or may not accompany parenchymal lesions. In the upper airway, the histologic findings are typically more nonspecific, with necrotizing inflammation or granulation tissue being the sole findings. In these biopsies, it should be stated that the diagnosis of Wegener granulomatosis cannot be excluded because necrotizing arteritis is frequently absent. Wegener granulomatosis can present as soft tissue necroinflammatory lesions in a variety of sites, without specific histologic features. In addition, it may present as necrotizing vasculitis in a variety of arteries.

CHURG-STRAUSS ANGIITIS

Characterized by peripheral eosinophilia and tissue eosinophilic infiltrates, Churg-Strauss syndrome also demonstrates a necrotizing arteritis indistinguishable from polyarteritis nodosa. Similar to Wegener granulomatosis, there are extravascular granulomas, but the histologic features are those of eosinophilic microabscesses with degranulation and palisading necrosis (Figs. 30.21 and 30.22). It is debated whether Churg-Strauss syndrome is ANCA related, but at least a proportion of patients have increased serum levels.

ANTINEUTROPHIL CYTOPLASMIC ANTIBODY SMALL VESSEL VASCULITIS (MICROSCOPIC POLYANGIITIS)

At one end of the spectrum of Wegener granulomatosis is ANCA-related vasculitis limited to small vessels (43). The major sites of involvement are the skin, kidneys, muscles, nerves (resulting in mononeuritis multiplex), and lungs. Small vessel vasculitis limited to the kidneys is occasionally designated pauci-immune necrotizing and crescentic glomerulonephritis. Small vessel vasculitis of the lungs, or capillaritis, can be a histologic manifestation of Wegener and microscopic polyangiitis, as well

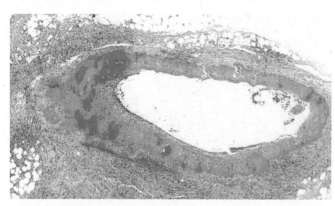

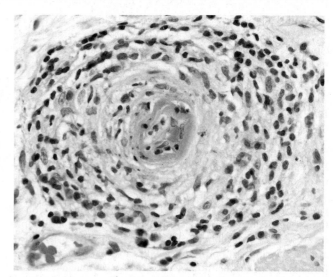

Figure 30.21. Churg-Strauss angiitis. Histologically, Churg-Strauss disease is manifest by necrotizing arteritis, similar to polyarteritis, with eosinophilic inflammation and eosinophilic microabscesses. This figure demonstrates necrotizing arteritis with fibrinoid necrosis.

as immune complex–related vasculitis. North American and European patients with Wegener granulomatosis most frequently exhibit positivity for cytoplasmic ANCA (C-ANCA), which corresponds to antibodies against proteinase 3. In contrast, most patients with microscopic polyangiitis have perinuclear ANCA (P-ANCA), which corresponds to antimyeloperoxidase autoantibodies.

IMMUNE COMPLEX–MEDIATED SMALL VESSEL VASCULITIS

Immune complex vasculitis includes entities that involve exclusively small vessels (arterioles, capillaries, and venules) and autoimmune disorders such as rheumatoid and lupus vasculitis that also involve muscular arteries. In addition to lupus and rheumatoid vasculitis, several diseases result in small vessel vasculitis, generally without larger arterial involvement, typically in the skin (44). There is no histologic difference between immune complex–mediated small vessel vasculitis and pauci-immune small vessel vasculitis, which may affect the skin as microscopic

Figure 30.23. Immune complex small vessel vasculitis, arteriole. The spectrum of immune complex–mediated small vessel vasculitis, similar to pauci-immune polyangiitis, includes involvement of arterioles, capillaries, and venules. In this example, there is fibrinoid necrosis (leukocytoclastic vasculitis) of an arteriole, with surrounding chronic inflammation.

polyangiitis (Figs. 30.23 and 30.24). The distinction between immune complex small vessel vasculitis and microscopic polyangiitis is typically made clinically and serologically, although immunofluorescence for immunoglobulin types and complement may be helpful on frozen sections.

Immune complex small vessel vasculitis includes drug-induced "hypersensitivity" vasculitis (up to 25% of cutaneous leukocytoclastic vasculitis), urticarial vasculitis, immunoglobulin A (IgA)–associated vasculitis (roughly synonymous with Henoch-Schönlein purpura, although the designation is sometimes used only with extracutaneous involvement), pustular vas-

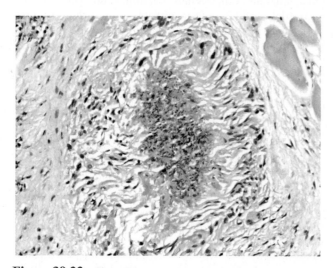

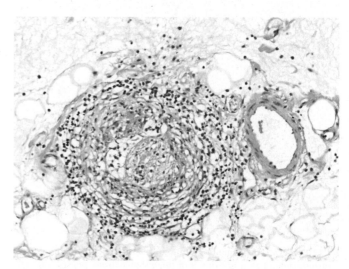

Figure 30.22. Churg-Strauss angiitis. A characteristic features is the eosinophilic granuloma, with apoptotic eosinophils surrounded by palisading macrophages.

Figure 30.24. Immune complex small vessel vasculitis, venule. Note normal arteriole and adjacent venule with vasculitis. The patient had been recently treated with Tegretol, which has been implicated in small vessel vasculitis via an immune complex mechanism.

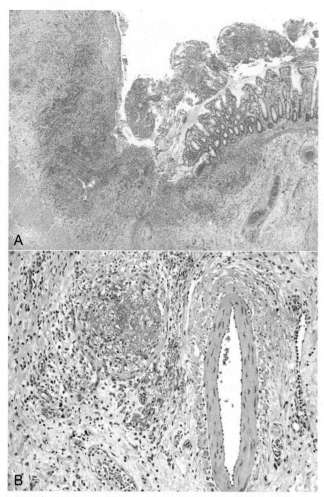

Figure 30.25. Behçet disease. **(A)** There is an aphthous ulcer in the small bowel in a patient with recently diagnosed Behçet disease and small bowel perforation. **(B)** There is a small vessel vasculitis, consisting in this field of a thrombosed inflamed venule (left) with normal accompanying arteriole (right).

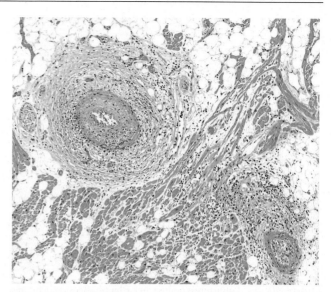

Figure 30.26. Rheumatoid arteritis. Rheumatoid vasculitis may involve muscular arteries and small vessels. The photomicrograph demonstrates epicardial coronary arteries with medial and adventitial inflammation from a patient who died of complications of coronary vasculitis. Fibrinoid necrosis is not prominent in this example.

culitis, Behçet disease (Fig. 30.25), relapsing polychondritis, and Sjögren disease. There are a variety of conditions resulting in thrombosis of small vessels, with variable inflammatory reaction. These do not typically have leukocytoclasia and fibrinoid necrosis and include cryoglobulinemic vasculitis (although a severe form of necrotizing vasculitis may be associated with types II and III cryoglobulinemia), cryofibrinogenemia, and antiphospholipid syndrome (44).

RHEUMATOID VASCULITIS

Vasculitic involvement in patients with rheumatoid arthritis is associated with high titers of rheumatoid factor and febrile illness. All calibers of arteries are involved, with muscular lesions mimicking polyarteritis nodosa and small vessel disease mimicking other types of immune complex vasculitis (Fig. 30.26). Only rarely are rheumatoid nodule–like lesions seen. In the aorta, for example, rheumatoid nodules have been described in the adventitia in autopsies (45), but symptomatic aortitis with aneurysm in patients with rheumatoid arthritis demonstrates no histologic differences from Takayasu aortitis (necrotizing aortitis) (24–26).

LUPUS VASCULITIS

Vasculitis occurs in up to 50% of patients with systemic lupus erythematosus (SLE) (46). The vascular lesions are similar to those of rheumatoid vasculitis, but renal involvement with glomerulopathy is characteristic of lupus, unlike rheumatoid arthritis. Cutaneous lupus vasculitis manifests as palpable purpura and is histologically similar to other causes of immune complex vasculitis.

VASCULITIS IN MUSCLE AND NERVE BIOPSIES

The surgical pathologist encounters systemic vasculitis most frequently in biopsies of the skin and kidney, as well as neuromuscular biopsies. The types of vasculitis most commonly present in nerve and muscular biopsies include polyarteritis nodosa (Fig. 30.27), rheumatoid vasculitis, lupus vasculitis, microscopic polyangiitis (Fig. 30.28), and vasculitis of mixed connective tissue disease (MCTD). They generally cannot be distinguished from one another histologically (47). Polyarteritis nodosa affects primarily epineurial and perineurial vessels, reflecting involvement of muscular arteries with sparing of smaller vessels in the endoneurium (Fig. 30.27). The nerve damage is typically "downstream" and may not be in the same region as the vasculitis; for example, surrounding muscle is often normal. If only muscular artery involvement is present in the absence of small vessel vasculitis, the diagnosis of polyarteritis nodosa can be favored over other forms of vasculitis; however, the muscular arterial lesions are identical to those seen in other causes of vasculitis. MCTD is one of the more common causes of vasculitis in muscle biopsies and consists of capillary, venule, and small arteriolar inflammation with minimal necrosis.

The vascular lesions of dermatomyositis differ in that leukocytoclastic or necrotizing vasculitis is not typical. Dermatomyositis is an autoimmune disorder of children and adults and is associated with the onset of neoplasms. Patients have a characteristic rash appearing as a heliotrope of the eyelids and erythema of the cheeks and trunk. Systemic vasculitis with gastroin-

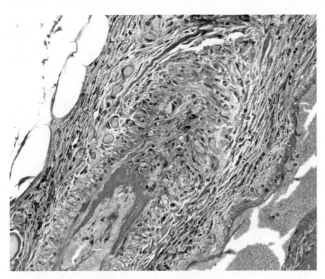

Figure 30.27. Polyarteritis nodosa, nerve biopsy. Because of limited sampling of muscular arteries in nerve and muscle biopsies, any degree of inflammation of a muscular artery is diagnostic of arteritis. In this patient, lack of inflammation of small vessels, with segmental inflammation in the muscular artery in this Masson trichrome stain, was suggestive of polyarteritis nodosa, subsequently corroborated by clinical evaluation.

testinal ulcerations and perforations may occur. Histologic features of muscular biopsies reflect chronic, relapsing immune complex–mediated attack against capillary endothelial cells, manifested by capillary endothelial cell swelling, sparse T-cell infiltrates, tubulovesicular inclusions by electron microscopy, and perifascicular atrophy.

CENTRAL NERVOUS SYSTEM VASCULITIS

Vasculitis involving the brain is most frequently a manifestation of systemic autoimmune disease, especially SLE. Primary angiitis

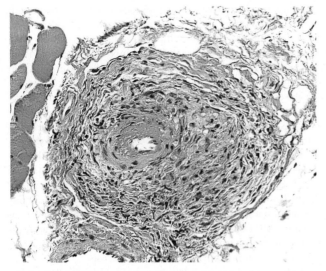

Figure 30.28. Microscopic polyangiitis, muscle biopsy. Microscopic polyangiitis, or pauci-immune small vessel vasculitis, is histologically indistinguishable from immune complex–mediated small vessel vasculitis. Lack of immunoglobulin and complement deposition and the presence of serum antineutrophil cytoplasmic antibody (ANCA) are features of microscopic polyangiitis.

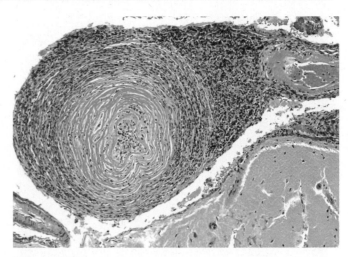

Figure 30.29. Central nervous system (CNS) vasculitis. The histologic features of CNS vasculitis are varied. In this example, there is fibrinoid necrosis of a meningeal artery with prominent layering and adventitial inflammation. Many cases are characterized by prominent giant cells.

of the central nervous system is a rare cause of multifocal neurologic deficits in children and adults. The diagnosis rests on brain biopsy, and the histologic findings are varied, including a giant-cell arteritis and polyarteritis-like necrotizing arteritis (Fig. 30.29). Aggressive treatment with immunosuppressive agents is indicated (48).

VASCULITIS OF THE SPERMATIC CORD

A curious lesion that presents as a testicular mass, isolated spermatic cord vasculitis is typically a giant-cell inflammatory process that involves both arteries and veins. Less commonly, isolated polyarteritis may occur (Fig. 30.30) (49,50). Occasionally, epididymitis may be the initial manifestation of systemic vasculitis, such as Henoch-Schönlein purpura.

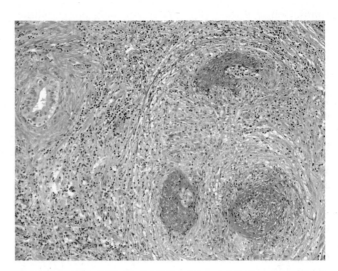

Figure 30.30. Isolated vasculitis of the spermatic cord. There is fibrinoid necrosis of muscular arteries adjacent to an epididymal duct. In many cases of isolated spermatic cord vasculitis, there is a prominent granulomatous component.

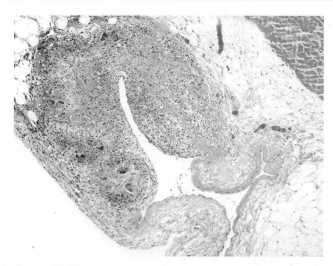

Figure 30.31. Sarcoid venulitis. Typically, sarcoid vasculitis involves veins, as in this example, although arterial granulomas may also occur.

SARCOID VASCULITIS

Although it is unclear whether sarcoid is associated with an increased incidence of systemic vasculitis, vascular involvement with granulomas is not unusual. Veins are involved more frequently than arteries (Fig. 30.31), and sites of predilection for sarcoid vascular involvement include the lung (resulting in secondary veno-occlusive disease) and the central nervous system. Sarcoidal granulomas in veins may be identified in nerve biopsies from patients with sarcoid neuropathy (47,51).

GIANT-CELL PHLEBITIS

Giant-cell phlebitis is an inflammatory process involving veins of the gastrointestinal tract, especially the right colon. There is typically extravascular inflammation and fibrosis resulting in an obstructing mass lesion (Fig. 30.32). The histologic spectrum ranges from granulomas with giant cells to lymphocytic perivenous cuffing. Eosinophils may be prominent. A form of drug reaction has been proposed as an etiology (41).

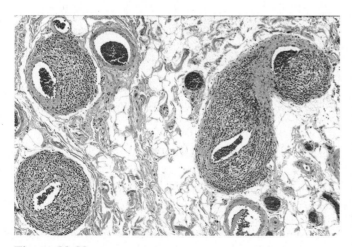

Figure 30.32. Phlebitis, colonic mesentery. Phlebitis of the intestinal mesentery often has a prominent giant-cell component; but in this case, there is marked lymphocytic cuffing of the veins. Note sparing of the accompanying arteries.

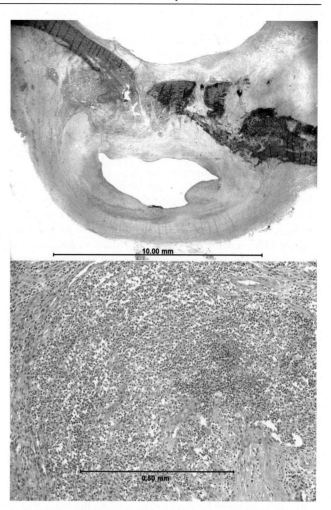

Figure 30.33. Mycotic aneurysm aorta. Infectious (so-called mycotic) aortic pseudoaneurysms usually arise in the setting of bacteremia, especially in patient with endocarditis, or in the setting of congenital aortic disease. **(A)** In this patient with coarctation, there was interruption of the media as seen on this Movat pentachrome stain, with surrounding inflammation and pseudoaneurysm (below). **(B)** A higher magnification of the surrounding inflammation (hematoxylin and eosin) shows purulent inflammation.

SEPTIC VASCULITIS

Infectious vasculitis may involve the wall of the aorta, especially the descending thoracic aorta (Fig. 30.33). Predisposing conditions include underlying vascular abnormalities, especially coarctation, and pre-existing or recent infectious endocarditis. Infectious aortitis typically results in localized pseudoaneurysm. Septic emboli may also result in aneurysms and pseudoaneurysms of visceral and peripheral arteries (52).

TUMORS OF GREAT VESSELS AND MUSCULAR ARTERIES

PULMONARY ARTERY SARCOMAS

Sarcomas of the lung are rare, especially those that arise within the pulmonary arteries. Sarcomas of the pulmonary artery are generally intraluminal tumors that cause symptoms that mimic those of pulmonary embolism. In a center that performs thromboembolectomies for central pulmonary artery embolism and chronic pulmonary hypertension, approximately 3% to 4% of patients with the diagnosis of chronic thromboembolic hypertension had primary sarcomas disclosed at thromboendarterectomy (53). It has been suggested that the true incidence is underestimated because, in many patients, a tissue diagnosis is not rendered until death. The prognosis of pulmonary artery sarcoma is exceptionally poor and significantly worse than that of pulmonary parenchymal sarcomas (54).

The majority of pulmonary artery sarcomas are predominantly intraluminal at early stages of growth, can be readily shelled out of the artery surgically, and appear to arise from the intima histologically. For this reason, the origin is generally considered to be intimal stromal cells. Because of the wide range of differentiation seen in pulmonary artery sarcomas, the term "intimal" as a histologic subtype is not entirely appropriate, and the precursor cell is likely uncommitted or pluripotent. It has been suggested that to classify a pulmonary sarcoma as an arterial intimal sarcoma, there should be predominantly (>50%) intraluminal growth, with at least one cross section of artery demonstrating intact media surrounding the tumor.

The histologic subtypes of pulmonary artery sarcoma are quite varied and include undifferentiated pleomorphic sarcomas (malignant fibrous histiocytomas), leiomyosarcomas, osteosarcoma, and chondrosarcoma (55). Rhabdomyosarcomatous elements are generally combined with other types of sarcoma, such as chondrosarcoma. Pleomorphic sarcomas of the pulmonary artery run a gamut that includes undifferentiated epithelioid neoplasms, typical storiform malignant fibrous histiocytoma (MFH)–like tumors, fibrosarcoma patterns with features of hemangiopericytoma, and myxoid fibrosarcomas (fibromyxosarcoma). These patterns often coexist. Curiously, angiosarcomas are rare. An uncommon finding is that of pleomorphic cells overlying a fibrin-rich surface, which can give a benign appearance and lead to misdiagnosis if adequate sampling is not performed. There is no prognostic significance to histologic subtypes. A recent study has shown that prognosis is dismal, except for a small subset of tumors that resemble inflammatory myofibroblastic tumor, lacking significant mitotic activity and marked atypia with an inflammatory background, "tissue culture" appearance to the tumor cells, and fibrin coating the luminal surface. Intra-arterial pulmonary soft tissue sarcomas that have been reported with benign follow-up have features of inflammatory myofibroblastic tumor as opposed to high-grade sarcoma.

AORTIC SARCOMAS

Aortic sarcomas, similar to those of the pulmonary artery, are predominantly luminal and are therefore also considered of intimal origin (54). Approximately two-thirds are removed because of luminal obstruction, either by embolectomy or aortic repair. The remainder are incidental findings for abdominal aortic aneurysm repair. They occur throughout the aorta, but most commonly occur from the arch to the iliacs. Unlike pulmonary artery sarcomas, osteosarcomas rarely occur (Fig. 30.34), and a relatively high proportion are angiosarcomas, especially epithelioid angiosarcoma. In the authors' consultation files of 35 cases, 11 were epithelioid angiosarcoma, 4 were typical angiosarcoma, 18 were pleomorphic undifferentiated sarcoma, and 2 were chondrosarcoma. The histologic differential diagnosis of

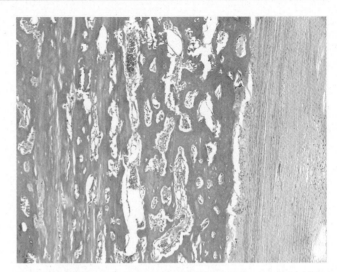

Figure 30.34. Aortic sarcoma, osteosarcoma. The aortic media is on the right, with the intima and luminal surface on the left, replaced by an intimal sarcoma composed of malignant osteoid.

aortic epithelioid angiosarcoma includes metastatic carcinoma. Coexpression of endothelial markers confirms the diagnosis, and carcinoma occurring within the lumen of the aorta is extremely rare.

TUMORS OF THE INFERIOR VENA CAVA

Leiomyosarcomas of the retroperitoneum are sometimes traceable to origin in the wall of the inferior vena cava. These tumors are generally relatively well differentiated, with clear smooth muscle cell differentiation (54). Occasionally, benign leiomyomas occur within the lumen of the inferior vena cava, are generally quite fibrotic, and are extensions of uterine leiomyomas.

TRAUMATIC AND IATROGENIC VASCULAR DISEASES

FOREIGN BODY EMBOLIZATION

The peripheral vessels may receive embolic material from iatrogenic procedures or self-injections, including components of drugs of abuse, hydrophilic gels that coat catheters, and fragments of catheters (Fig. 30.35). Occasionally, there will be vascular symptoms with excision, and the pathologist will be unaware of a prior history of intervention. The presence of foreign material should be excluded in any vascular process with the presence of foreign body giant cells.

TRAUMATIC PSEUDOANEURYSM

Blunt trauma can result in perforation of a superficial artery, especially the temporal artery. Clinically, there will be a pulsatile mass, and when a history of trauma is elicited, the diagnosis is generally suspected. Histologically, the excised lesion demonstrates interruption of the media; organizing thrombus, often with "epithelioid" neovessels within a proteoglycan-rich stroma; and adventitial inflammation and fibrosis (Fig. 30.36). The differential diagnosis may include angiolymphoid hyperplasia with eosinophilia (epithelioid hemangioma).

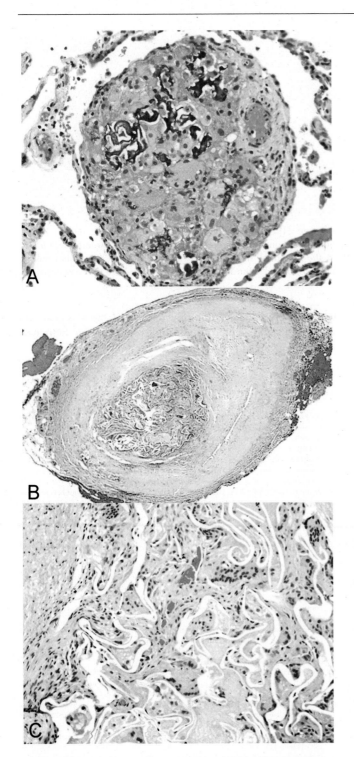

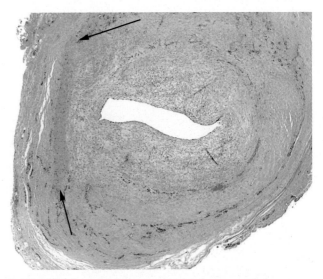

Figure 30.36. Temporal artery pseudoaneurysm. The patient experienced a pulsatile mass and admitted to recent head trauma. The limits of the intact media are delineated by *arrows*. The remainder of the lesion represents organizing thrombus.

Iatrogenic arteriovenous fistulas for dialysis access may develop a pseudoaneurysm or become infected. If removed or revised, the surgical pathologist should note the presence of pseudoaneurysm or purulent inflammation indicative of infection.

VASCULAR THROMBOSIS

GENERAL FEATURES OF THROMBOSIS

Virchow's triad consists of stasis, hypercoagulability, and underlying endothelial dysfunction. In arterial thrombosis, underlying lesions and coagulation defects are paramount, whereas in venous thrombosis, stasis is the most important feature, with underling coagulation defects being an important predisposing factor to thrombosis. The histologic features of thrombosis consist of fibrin platelet layering (lines of Zahn), with organization, progressing from the edges of the thrombus. Organization includes endothelial ingrowth, inflammation with hemosiderin-laden macrophages, fibroblast ingrowth, and eventual recanalization, as a natural mechanism against vascular occlusion. The sequence of events allows for approximate dating of the thrombus, provided that there is adequate sampling.

ETIOLOGY OF VASCULAR THROMBOSIS

Vascular thrombi are more common in the venous circulation, which is more prone to stasis than the arterial circulation. Thrombophlebitis is a descriptive term denoting venous thrombosis, with secondary inflammation. Suppurative venous thrombi arise in infected veins, often after instrumentation or catheterization, and bacterial organisms may be identified. Arterial and venous thrombosis is increased in incidence with a variety of genetic coagulation defects, including factor V Leiden, prothrombin 20210A mutation, and protein C and S deficiency (56), and a host of acquired diseases, including antiphospholipid syndrome, heparin-induced thrombocytopenia (which re-

Figure 30.35. Foreign body embolization. (A) Polyvinylpyrrolidone embolization in the pulmonary artery of a drug addict. (B) Foreign material embolization, temporal artery, in a patient with temporal headaches. (C) Higher magnification demonstrates foreign body embolized material; the patient later elicited a history of multiple angiographic procedures involving the head and central nervous system.

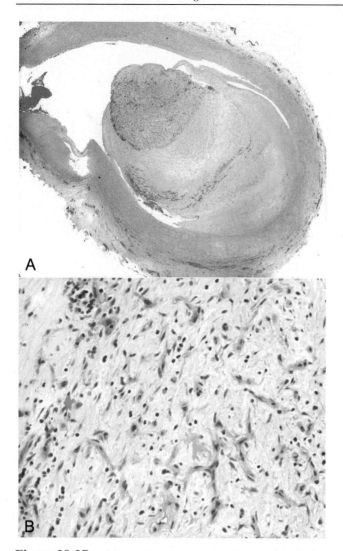

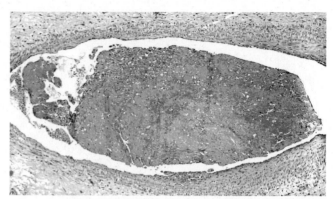

Figure 30.38. Mesenteric thrombosis, mesenteric vein. In this patient with segmental bowel infarction, organizing thrombi were found in the mesentery of the excised necrotic bowel. The patient was on birth control pills but had no other predisposition for coagulopathy.

Figure 30.37. Idiopathic thrombosis, innominate artery. **(A)** A low magnification demonstrates subtotal occlusion in the vessel, which was resected and bypassed in a young woman with right arm ischemia. **(B)** A higher magnification demonstrates typical myxoid features of organizing intraluminal thrombus, with scattered hemosiderin macrophages. The differential diagnosis should include embolic myxoma, but myxoma cells are not identified, and the histologic findings are typical of organizing thrombus.

cent to fibrin platelet thrombi; peripheral blood smear will reveal schistocytes indicative of a microangiopathic hemolytic anemia.

sults in platelet-rich "white" thrombi), and malignancy. Antiphospholipid syndrome is part of the spectrum of thrombotic lupus vasculopathy and may be associated with vascular thromboses involving arteries and veins of all sizes. In a significant proportion of cases of unexplained vascular thrombosis in the absence of underlying vascular disease, no coagulation defect is found (Figs. 30.37 and 30.38) (57,58).

THROMBOSIS IN THE MICROCIRCULATION

Fibrin platelet thrombi in arterioles and capillaries may reflect local inflammation or vasculitis, embolism, and diffuse coagulation syndromes such as disseminated intravascular coagulation. In thrombotic thrombocytopenic purpura and hemolytic uremic syndrome, there is a microangiopathic process characterized histologically by activated, swollen endothelial cells adja-

REFERENCES

1. De Paepe A, Devereux RB, Dietz HC, et al. Revised diagnostic criteria for the Marfan syndrome. *Am J Med Genet* 1996;62:417–426.
2. Disabella E, Grasso M, Marziliano N, et al. Two novel and one known mutation of the TGFBR2 gene in Marfan syndrome not associated with FBN1 gene defects. *Eur J Hum Genet* 2006;14:34–38.
3. Homme JL, Aubry MC, Edwards WD, et al. Surgical pathology of the ascending aorta: a clinicopathologic study of 513 cases. *Am J Surg Pathol* 2006;30:1159–1168.
4. Pannu H, Fadulu VT, Chang J, et al. Mutations in transforming growth factor-beta receptor type II cause familial thoracic aortic aneurysms and dissections. *Circulation* 2005;112:513–520.
5. Pepin M, Schwarze U, Superti-Furga A, et al. Clinical and genetic features of Ehlers-Danlos syndrome type IV, the vascular type. *N Engl J Med* 2000;342:673–680.
6. Loscalzo ML, Goh DL, Loeys B, et al. Familial thoracic aortic dilation and bicommissural aortic valve: a prospective analysis of natural history and inheritance. *Am J Med Genet A* 2007;143:1960–1967.
7. Larson EW, Edwards WD. Risk factors for aortic dissection: a necropsy study of 161 cases. *Am J Cardiol* 1984;53:849–855.
8. Miller DV, Usotalo PA, Weyand CM, et al. Surgical pathology of noninfectious ascending aortitis: a study of 45 cases with emphasis on an isolated variant. *Am J Surg Pathol* 2006;30:1150–1158.
9. Burke AP, Tavora F, Narula N, et al. Aortitis and ascending aortic aneurysm: description of 52 cases and proposal of a histologic classification. *Num Pathol* 2008;39:514–526.
10. Perdu J, Boutouyrie P, Bourgain C, et al. Inheritance of arterial lesions in renal fibromuscular dysplasia. *J Hum Hypertens* 2007;21:393–400.
11. Rushton AR, The genetics of fibromuscular dysplasia. *Arch Intern Med* 1980;140:233–236.
12. Alamir A, Middendorf DF, Baker P, et al. Renal artery dissection causing renal infarction in otherwise healthy men. *Am J Kidney Dis* 1997;30:851–855.
13. Alwitry A, Brackenbury ET, Beggs FD, et al. Vascular amyloidosis causing spontaneous mediastinal haemorrhage with haemothorax. *Eur J Cardiothorac Surg* 2001;20:871–873.
14. Westermark GT, Sletten K, Westermark P. Massive vascular AA-amyloidosis: a histologically and biochemically distinctive subtype of reactive systemic amyloidosis. *Scand J Immunol* 1989;30:605–613.
15. Rodon P, Friocourt P, Blanchet S, et al. Temporal artery involvement revealing AL amyloidosis and IgD monoclonal gammapathy. *J Rheumatol* 1996;23:189–190.
16. Reilly JM, Tilson MD. Incidence and etiology of abdominal aortic aneurysms. *Surg Clin North Am* 1989;69:705–711.
17. Milei J, Parodi JC, Alonso GF, et al. Carotid rupture and intraplaque hemorrhage: immunophenotype and role of cells involved. *Am Heart J* 1998;136:1096–1105.
18. Prager MR, Hoblaj T, Nanobashvili J, et al. Collagen- versus gelatine-coated Dacron versus stretch PTFE bifurcation grafts for aortoiliac occlusive disease: long-term results of a prospective, randomized multicenter trial. *Surgery* 2003;134:80–85.
19. Hellmann DB, Grand DJ, Freischlag JA. Inflammatory abdominal aortic aneurysm. *JAMA* 2007;297:395–400.
20. Yusuf K, Murat B, Unal A, et al. Inflammatory abdominal aortic aneurysm: predictors of long-term outcome in a case-control study. *Surgery* 2007;141:83–89.
21. Jennette JC, Falk RJ. Pathologic classification of vasculitis. *Pathol Case Rev* 2007;12:179–185.
22. Tavora F, Burke A. Review of isolated ascending aortitis: differential diagnosis, including syphilitic, Takayasu's and giant cell aortitis. *Pathology* 2006;38:302–308.
23. Burke AP. Takayasu arteritis and giant cell arteritis. *Pathol Case Rev* 2007;12:186–192.

24. Burke AP, Tavora F, Narula N, et al. Aortitis and ascending aortic aneurysm: description of 52 cases and proposal of a histologic classification. *Hum Pathol* 2008;39:514–526.

25. Miller DV, Isotalo PA, Weyand CM, et al. Surgical pathology of noninfectious ascending aortitis: a study of 45 cases with emphasis on an isolated variant. *Am J Surg Pathol* 2006;30:1150–1158.

26. Rojo-Leyva F, Ratliff NB, Cosgrove DM 3rd, et al. Study of 52 patients with idiopathic aortitis from a cohort of 1,204 surgical cases. *Arthritis Rheum* 2000;43:901–907.

27. Evans JM, O'Fallon WM, Hunder GG. Increased incidence of aortic aneurysm and dissection in giant cell (temporal) arteritis. A population-based study. *Ann Intern Med* 1995;122:502–507.

28. Gonzalez-Gay MA, Garcia-Porrua C, Pineiro A, et al. Aortic aneurysm and dissection in patients with biopsy-proven giant cell arteritis from northwestern Spain: a population-based study. *Medicine (Baltimore)* 2004;83:335–341.

29. Burke AP, Virmani R. Temporal artery biopsy of giant cell arteritis. *Pathol Case Rev* 2001; Volume 6.

30. Disdier P, Pellissier JF, Harle JR, et al. Significance of isolated vasculitis of the vasa vasorum on temporal artery biopsy. *J Rheumatol* 1994;21:258–260.

31. Esteban M-J, Font C, Hernández-Rodríguez J, et al. Small-vessel vasculitis surrounding a spared temporal artery. *Aruhr Rheum* 2001;44:1387–1395.

32. Martinez-Taboada VM, Blanco R, Armona J, et al. Giant cell arteritis with an erythrocyte sedimentation rate lower than 50. *Clin Rheumatol* 2000;19:73–75.

33. Wise C, Agudelo CA, Chmelewski WL, et al. Temporal arteritis with low erythrocyte sedimentation rate: a review of five cases. *Arthritis Rheum* 1991;34:1571–1574.

34. Achkar AA, Lie JT, Hunder GGO, et al. How does previous corticosteroid treatment affect the biopsy findings in giant cell (temporal) arteritis? *Ann Intern Med* 1994;120:987–992.

35. Nishino H, DeRemee RA, Rubino FA, et al. Wegener's granulomatosis associated with vasculitis of the temporal artery: report of five cases. *Mayo Clin Proc* 1993;68:115–121.

36. Lie JT, Michet CJ Jr. Thromboangiitis obliterans with eosinophilia (Buerger's disease) of the temporal arteries. *Hum Pathol* 1988;19:598–602.

37. Burke AP, Virmani R. Localized vasculitis. *Semin Diagn Pathol* 2001;18:59–66.

38. Walsh T, Lyons F, Sinha SK, et al. Giant cell arteritis of the female genital tract. *Ir Med J* 2004;97:23.

39. Bajocchi G, Zamorani G, Cavazza A, et al. Giant-cell arteritis of the female genital tract associated with occult temporal arteritis and FDG-PET evidence of large-vessel vasculitis. *Clin Exp Rheumatol* 2007;25:S36–S39.

40. Takahashi K, Oharaseki T, Yokouchi Y, et al. Kawasaki disease and polyarteritis nodosa. *Pathol Case Rev* 2007;12:193–199.

41. Burke AP, Sobin LH, Virmani R. Localized vasculitis of the gastrointestinal tract. *Am J Surg Pathol* 1995;19:338–349.

42. Lie JT. Thromboangiitis obliterans (Buerger's disease) revisited. *Pathol Annu* 1988;23:257–291.

43. Jennette JC, Falk RJ. ANCA vasculitis: microscopic polyangiitis, Wegener's granulomatosis, and Churg-Strauss syndrome. *Pathol Case Rev* 2007;12.

44. Crowson AN, Magro CM. Small vessel cutaneous vasculitis. *Pathol Case Rev* 2007;12:205–214.

45. Gravallese EM, Corson JM, Coblyn JS, et al. Rheumatoid aortitis: a rarely recognized but clinically significant entity. *Medicine (Baltimore)* 1989;68:95–106.

46. Calamia KT, Balabanova M. Vasculitis in systemic lupus erythematosis. *Clin Dermatol* 2004;22:148–156.

47. Vital C, Vital A, Canron MH, et al. Combined nerve and muscle biopsy in the diagnosis of vasculitic neuropathy. A 16-year retrospective study of 202 cases. *J Peripher Nerv Syst* 2006;11:20–29.

48. Bitter KJ, Epstein LG, Melin-Aldana H, et al. Cyclophosphamide treatment of primary angiitis of the central nervous system in children: report of 2 cases. *J Rheumatol* 2006;33:2078–2080.

49. Kameyama K, Kuramochi S, Kamio N, et al. Isolated periarteritis nodosa of the spermatic cord presenting as a scrotal mass: report of a case. *Heart Vessels* 1998;13:152–154.

50. Halim A, Neild GH, Levine T, et al. Isolated necrotizing granulomatous vasculitis of the epididymis and spermatic cords. *World J Urol* 1994;12:357–358.

51. Said G, Lacroix C, Plante-Bordeneuve V, et al. Nerve granulomas and vasculitis in sarcoid peripheral neuropathy: a clinicopathological study of 11 patients. *Brain* 2002;125:264–275.

52. Javid PJ, Belkin M, Chew DK. Mycotic aneurysm of the superior mesenteric artery: a delayed complication from a neglected septic embolus-a case report. *Vasc Endovascular Surg* 2005;39:113–116.

53. Maruo A, Okita Y, Okada K, et al. Surgical experience for the pulmonary artery sarcoma. *Ann Thorac Surg* 2006;82:2014–2016.

54. Burke AP, Virmani R. Sarcomas of the great vessels. A clinicopathologic study. *Cancer* 1993;71:1761–1773.

55. Yi JE, Tazelaar HD, Burke A, et al. Pulmonary artery sarcoma. In Travis WD, Brambilla E, Muller-Hermelink HK, et al., eds. *Tumours of the Lung, Pleura, Thymus and Heart*. Lyon, France: International Agency for Research on Cancer, 2004:109–110.

56. Esmon CT. The protein C pathway. *Chest* 2003;124:26S–32S.

57. Caprini JA, Glase CJ, Anderson CB, et al. Laboratory markers in the diagnosis of venous thromboembolism. *Circulation* 2004;109:14–18.

58. Tripodi A. Laboratory diagnosis of thrombophilic states: where do we stand? *Pathophysiol Haemost Thromb* 2002;32:245–248.

Index

Page numbers followed by a *t* indicate tables; italicized page numbers indicate figures.

Toxoplasmosis
  in brain, 372, 374, *374*
  cardiac allograft infection with, 1203, *1203*
  in immunocompromised host, 1045, *1045*
  reactive adenopathy of, 692, *692*
  surgery directed toward, 352t
Trabecular carcinoid, of ovary, 2335
Trabecular carcinoma. *See* Polymorphous low-grade adenocarcinoma
Trabecular hepatocellular carcinoma, 1559, *1560*
Tracheobronchial amyloidosis, 1044, *1044*
Tracheopathia osteoplastica, of larynx, 907
Tracking, lymphatic, 1019, *1020*
Traditional serrated adenoma (TSA), 1368, 1373–1374, *1373–1374*
Tragi, accessory, *929*, 929–930
Transbronchial lung biopsy, 995, *996*, 999–1000, 1043–1044
  for diffuse lung disease, 1046–1047, 1046t
Transient acantholytic dermatosis, 16, *16*
Transient migratory osteoporosis, 228
Transient myeloproliferative disorder (TMD), 625
Transient osteoporosis, 228, *228*
Transition zone, of prostate, 1870, *1870*
Transitional cell carcinoma (TCC)
  of nose and paranasal sinuses, 871
  of ovary, *2302*, 2302–2303
Transitional cell papilloma, of nose, paranasal sinuses, and nasopharynx, 867
Transitional cell tumors, of ovary, 2300–2303, *2301–2302*
Transitional meningioma, 357t, 415, *416*
Transitional tumors, hepatocellular, 1569–1570
Translocation-related renal cell carcinoma, 1781
Transmissible spongiform encephalopathies. *See* Prion disease
Transplant recipients
  gastritis in, 1291–1292, *1291–1292*
  lung biopsy in, 1044–1046, *1045–1046*
Transplantation
  of bone marrow, bone cellularity after, 614
  cardiac, 1199–1206, 1199t, *1201–1205*, 1202t
    grading of acute cardiac allograft rejection, 1199–1205, *1201–1205*, 1202t
    transplantation coronary artery disease, *1205*, 1205–1206
  corneal, 967
  liver disease and, 1527–1529, *1527–1529*
  of pancreas, 1436
  renal, pathology of, 1738–1748, *1739–1744*, 1744t, *1746–1747*
  small-bowel, 1354
Transplantation coronary artery disease (TCAD), *1205*, 1205–1206
Transthyretin, 413, *413*, 1188
Transurethral biopsy, cystitis secondary to, 1833, *1833*
Transurethral resection (TUR)
  granuloma after, 1873–1874, *1874*
  of prostate, clinical stages of cancer detected in, 1898–1899
Transverse myelitis, 370
Transverse sectioning, 2
Trastuzumab, 321
Traumatic neuroma, 55
Traumatic pseudoaneurysm, 1244–1245, *1245*
Traumatic vascular diseases, 1244–1245, *1245*
Traumatic-type change, of colon, 1327
Trematode, in brain, 372

T(6;11)(p21;q12) renal cell carcinoma, 1823–1824, *1824*
Trephine biopsy, 611, 611t, 652, 667
Trichilemmal cyst, *42*
Trichoepithelioma, *44*
Trichomonas vaginalis, 2119
Trichophyton mentagrophytes, 14
Tricuspid aortic stenosis, senile calcific, 1216, *1216*
Tricuspid valvular disease, 1219, *1220*
Triphasic Wilms tumor, 1804, *1804*, 1812
Triplication, of gallbladder, 1602
Trisomy 12, 709
Trisomy 21. *See* Down syndrome
TRK-A, 576
Troglitazone, liver toxicity of, 1512
Tropheryma whippelii, 371–372, *372*, 695, 1319
Trophoblast, *2049*, 2049–2051, 2050t
Trophoblastic disease. *See* Gestational trophoblastic disease
Trophoblastic implants, of peritoneum, 2396
Trophoblastic pseudotumor. *See* Placental site trophoblastic tumor
Trophoblastic tumors, 1971–1972, *1971–1972*, 2357
Tropical eosinophilia, 1007–1008
Tropical sprue, 1317, *1317*
TRS. *See* Testicular regression syndrome
True glomerulonephritides. *See* Hypercellular glomerulonephritides
Trypanosoma cruzi, 1203
Tryptase stain, for mast cells, 638, *638*
TSA. *See* Traditional serrated adenoma
TTF-1. *See* Thyroid transcription factor-1
TTP. *See* Thrombotic thrombocytopenic purpura
Tubal carcinoma, 2382–2385, *2383–2385*, 2383t
Tubal pregnancy, 2376, *2376*
Tuberculosis
  adrenal hypofunction with, 550
  arthritis with, 208–209, *209*
  in brain, 371–372
  of fallopian tubes, *2374*, 2374–2375
  in granulomatous gastritis, 1287
  in immunocompromised host, 1045
  in larynx, 907
  nodular vasculitis associated with, 33
  of nose, paranasal sinuses, and nasopharynx, 861
  of ovary, 2358
  of penis, 2009
  pericarditis due to, 1223
  of peritoneum, 2392
  reactive adenopathy of, *693*
  renal, 1730
  of testis, 1933
  of vulva, 2099
Tuberculous cystitis, 1831–1832
Tuberculous prostatitis, of prostate, 1872
Tuberous sclerosis, 600, 1206
  angiofibroma of, 50
  astrocytoma with, 393
  pulmonary lymphangiomyomatosis associated with, 1039–1040
  renal involvement in, 1675, *1675*
Tubers, cortical, 443
Tuboendometrial metaplasia (TEM), of endocervical glands, 2158, *2159*
Tubo-ovarian carcinoma, 2357, 2382
Tubular adenocarcinoma. *See* Acinar adenocarcinoma
Tubular adenoma
  of breast, 333–334, *334*
  intestinal, 1381–1385, *1385*

Tubular adenosis, 301
Tubular atrophy, quantitative criteria for, 1751
Tubular carcinoid tumor. *See* Adenocarcinoid tumor
Tubular carcinoma, 296t, 300, 301t, 324, *324*
Tubular carcinoma NOS, 324
Tubular differentiation, of WT, 1804t, 1805, *1805*
Tubular mixed carcinoma, 324
Tubular sclerosis, infertility associated with, 1926
Tubulitis, quantitative criteria for, 1750
Tubulointerstitial diseases, 1723–1733, *1724–1733*
  acute interstitial nephritis, 1727–1728, *1727–1728*
  acute pyelonephritis, 1725–1727, *1726*
  acute tubular necrosis, 1723–1725, *1724–1725*
  analgesic nephropathy, *1731*, 1731–1732
  chronic interstitial nephritis, 1728–1733, *1729–1733*
  herbal and Balkan nephropathy, 1732, *1732*
  metabolic disorders, 1732–1733, *1732–1733*
Tubulointerstitium, terms relating to, 1752
Tubulolobular infiltrating lobular carcinoma, 322, *323*
Tubulopapillary adenoma, renal, 1769, *1769*
Tubulovillous adenoma, intestinal, 1381–1385
Tufted angioma, 168
Tufting enteropathy, 1322
Tumefactive fibroinflammatory lesions, 145
Tumor budding, of intestinal carcinoma, 1400, *1401*
Tumor necrosis factor (TNF), lymphoma association with, 690
Tumor of probable Wolffian origin, of ovary, *2346*, 2346–2347
Tumor phenotype, 126–127
Tumor stage lesions, 69
Tumor syndromes, inherited, adrenal neoplasia association with, 549t
Tumoral calcinosis, 207, *208*
Tumoral CPPD disease, 943
Tumor-infiltrating lymphocytes, as prognostic factor in malignant melanoma, 94, *94*
Tumorlet
  of lung, 1084–1085
  of pituitary, 467
Tumors of unknown origin, 261–264, *262–264*
  benign, 261–263, *262*
  malignant, 263–264, *263–264*
Tunica albuginea, 2006–2007, *2006–2007*
  tumors of, 1987–1990, *1987–1990*
Tunnel clusters, of cervix, 2154–2155, *2155*
TUR. *See* Transurethral resection
Turcot syndrome, in intestine, 1394–1395
Twin transfusion syndrome, 2092, *2092*
Twins, placenta and, 2091–2092, *2091–2092*
Twists, of umbilical cord, 2080
Tylectomy, of breast, 287
Tympanic cavity, 928
Tympanic paraganglioma, 593, *594*, 600
Tympanosclerosis, in otitis media, 931, *931*
Type 1 fibers, 100, *100*, 100t, 105–106, 105t
Type 2 fibers, 100, *100*, 100t, 105, *105*, 106t
Type grouping, 106, 106t, *107*
Typical carcinoid, of lung, 1081
Tyrosine kinase inhibitors, 1092
Tzanck preparation, 17
T-zone lymphoma, 725–726

UC. *See* Ulcerative colitis
UIP. *See* Usual interstitial pneumonia
Ulcerated carcinoma, of stomach, 1299